GOLDMAN-CECIL MEDICINE

GOLDMAN-CECIL MEDICINE

26TH EDITION

Volume 2

EDITED BY

LEE GOLDMAN, MD

Harold and Margaret Hatch Professor
Chief Executive, Columbia University Irving Medical Center
Dean of the Faculties of Health Sciences and Medicine
Columbia University
New York, New York

ANDREW I. SCHAFER, MD

Professor of Medicine
Director, Richard T. Silver Center for Myeloproliferative Neoplasms
Weill Cornell Medical College
New York, New York

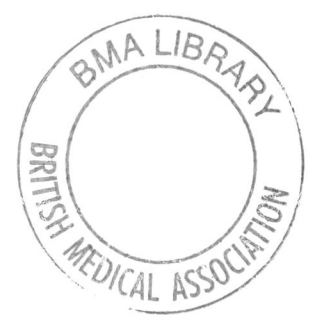

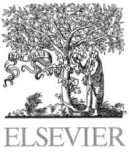

ELSEVIER

Elsevier
1600 John F. Kennedy Blvd.
Ste 1600
Philadelphia, PA 19103-2899

GOLDMAN-CECIL MEDICINE, TWENTY-SIXTH EDITION

ISBN: 978-0-323-53266-2
Volume 1 ISBN: 978-0-323-76018-8
Volume 2 ISBN: 978-0-323-76019-5

INTERNATIONAL EDITION

ISBN: 978-0-323-64033-6
IE Volume 1 ISBN: 978-0-323-75998-4
IE Volume 2 ISBN: 978-0-323-75999-1

Notice

Practitioners and researchers must always rely on their own experience and knowledge in evaluating and using any information, methods, compounds or experiments described herein. Because of rapid advances in the medical sciences, in particular, independent verification of diagnoses and drug dosages should be made. To the fullest extent of the law, no responsibility is assumed by Elsevier, authors, editors or contributors for any injury and/or damage to persons or property as a matter of products liability, negligence or otherwise, or from any use or operation of any methods, products, instructions, or ideas contained in the material herein.

Previous editions copyrighted 2016, 2012, 2008, 2004, 2000, 1996, 1991, 1988, 1982, 1979, 1975, 1971, 1963, 1959, 1955, 1951, 1947, 1943, 1940, 1937, 1933, 1930, 1927 by Saunders, an imprint of Elsevier Inc.
Copyright renewed 1991 by Paul Beeson.
Copyright renewed 1979 by Russell L. Cecil and Robert F. Loeb.
Copyright renewed 1987, 1975, 1971, 1965, 1961, 1958, 1955 by Elsevier Inc.

Library of Congress Control Number: 2019909209

Publishing Director, Medical Reference: Dolores Meloni
Content Development Manager: Laura Schmidt
Publishing Services Manager: Catherine Jackson
Senior Project Manager: Daniel Fitzgerald
Designer: Maggie Reid

Printed in Poland

Last digit is the print number: 9 8 7 6 5 4 3 2

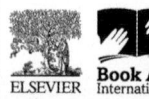
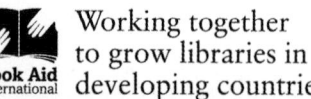

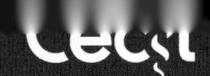

ASSOCIATE EDITORS

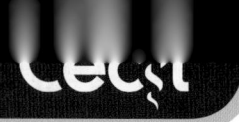

PREFACE

In the more than 90 years since the first edition of the *Cecil Textbook of Medicine* was published, almost everything we know about internal medicine has changed. Progress in medical science is now occurring at an ever-accelerating pace, and it is doing so within the framework of transformational changes in clinical practice and the delivery of health care at individual, social, and global levels. This textbook and its associated electronic products incorporate the latest medical knowledge in multiple formats that should appeal to students and seasoned practitioners regardless of how they prefer to access this rapidly changing information.

Even as *Cecil*'s specific information has changed, however, we have remained true to the tradition of a comprehensive textbook of medicine that carefully explains the *why* (the underlying genetics, genomics, and pathobiology of disease) and the *how* (now expected to be evidence-based from randomized controlled trials and meta-analyses). Descriptions of physiology and pathophysiology include the latest genetic advances in a practical format that strives to be useful to the nonexpert so that care can truly be as precise and personalized as possible.

Medicine has entered an era when the acuity of illness and the limited time available to evaluate a patient have diminished the ability of physicians to satisfy their intellectual curiosity. As a result, the acquisition of information, quite easily achieved in this era, is often confused with knowledge. We have attempted to address this dilemma with a textbook that not only informs but also stimulates new questions and gives a glimpse of the future path to new knowledge. Grade A evidence is specifically highlighted in the text and referenced at the end of each chapter. In addition to the information provided in the textbook, the *Cecil* website supplies expanded content and functionality. In many cases, the full articles referenced in each chapter can be accessed from the *Cecil* website. The website is also continuously updated to incorporate subsequent Grade A information, other evidence, and new discoveries.

The sections for each organ system begin with a chapter that summarizes an approach to patients with key symptoms, signs, or laboratory abnormalities associated with dysfunction of that organ system. As summarized in E-Table 1-1, the text specifically provides clear, concise information regarding how a physician should approach more than 100 common symptoms, signs, and laboratory abnormalities, usually with a flow diagram, a table, or both for easy reference. In this way, *Cecil* remains a comprehensive text to guide diagnosis and therapy, not only for patients with suspected or known diseases but also for patients who may have undiagnosed symptoms or signs that require an initial evaluation.

Just as each edition brings new authors, it also reminds us of our gratitude to past editors and authors. Previous editors of *Cecil* include a short but remarkably distinguished group of leaders of American medicine: Russell Cecil, Paul Beeson, Walsh McDermott, James Wyngaarden, Lloyd H. Smith, Jr., Fred Plum, J. Claude Bennett, and Dennis Ausiello. As we welcome a new associate editor—Nancy Davidson—we also express our appreciation to James Doroshow and other associate editors from the previous editions on whose foundation we have built. Our returning associate editors—Mary K. Crow, Jeffrey M. Drazen, Robert C. Griggs, Donald W. Landry, Wendy Levinson, Anil Rustgi, W. Michael Scheld, and Allen M. Spiegel—continue to make critical contributions to the selection of authors and the review and approval of all manuscripts. The editors, however, are fully responsible for the book as well as the integration among chapters.

The tradition of *Cecil* is that all chapters are written by distinguished experts in each field. Two of those authors, Frank A. Lederle, author of the chapter on "Diseases of the Aorta," and Ronald Victor, author of the chapter on "Arterial Hypertension," passed away after submitting their chapters, and we mourn their passing.

We are also most grateful for the editorial assistance in New York of Timothy Gahr, Maribel Lim, Eva Allen, and Magdalena Fuentes. These individuals and others in our offices have shown extraordinary dedication and equanimity in working with authors and editors to manage the unending flow of manuscripts, figures, and permissions.

This edition of *Goldman-Cecil Medicine* includes many new authors. We would also like to thank outgoing authors, who often provided figures that are included in this edition as well as tables that have been included or modified for this edition. Furthermore, because of the templated format and extensive editing that are characteristic of *Goldman-Cecil Medicine*, some new chapters incorporate principles, concepts, and organizational aspects from those prior chapters, often revised extensively prior to publication. Among prior authors who deserve our appreciation, in the numerical order of their chapters, are Victoria M. Taylor, Steven A. Schroeder, Thomas B. Newman, Charles E. McCulloch, Thomas H. Lee, F. Daniel Duffy, Lawrence S. Neinstein, Steven E. Hyman, Grant W. Cannon, Cem Gabay, Carlo Patrono, Jack Hirsh, Adam Perlman, Sandesh C.S. Nagamani, Paweł Stankiewicz, James R. Lupski, Sekar Kathiresan, David Altshuler, Göran K. Hansson, Anders Hamsten, L. David Hillis, Bruce W. Lytle, William C. Little, Donna Mancini, Yoshifumi Naka, Dennis E. Niewoehner, Frank J. Accurso, Emanuel P. Rivers, Marsha D. Ford, Geoffrey K. Isbister, Itzchak Slotki, Mark L. Zeidel, David H. Kim, Perry J. Pickhardt, Martin J. Blaser, Stephen Crane Hauser, H. Franklin Bunn, Gordon D. Ginder, Martin H. Steinberg, Aśok C. Antony, Ayalew Tefferi, Michael Glogauer, Marc E. Rothenberg, William L. Nichols, Lawrence T. Goodnough, Adrian R. Black, Kenneth H. Cowan, Susan O'Brien, Elias Jabbour, Marshall R. Posner, Charles D. Blanke, Douglas O. Faigel, David Spriggs, John D. Hainsworth, F. Anthony Greco, Clay F. Semenkovich, Stephen G. Kaler, Bruce R. Bacon, Bruce R. Bistrian, Stephen A. McClave, Mark E. Molitch, Matthew Kim, Paul W. Ladenson, Kenneth R. Hande, Robert W. Rebar, Deborah Grady, Elizabeth Barrett-Connor, Samuel A. Wells, Jr., Stephen I. Wasserman, Larry Borish, Suneel S. Apte, Joel A. Block, Carla Scanzello, Robert M. Bennett, Ilseung Cho, S. Ragnar Norrby, Lionel A. Mandell, Donald E. Low, Kenneth L. Gage, Atis Muehlenbachs, Stuart Levin, Kamaljit Singh, Richard L. Guerrant, Dirk M. Elston, Larry J. Anderson, Martin Weisse, Mark Papania, Letha M. Healey, Tamsin A. Knox, Christine Wanke, Kristina Crothers, Alison Morris, Toby A. Maurer, Thomas S. Uldrick, Robert Yarchoan, Robert Colebunders, Ralph F. Józefowicz, Michael Aminoff, Eelco F.M. Wijdicks, Myron Yanoff, Douglas Cameron, David H. Chu, James C. Shaw, Neil J. Korman, and Ronald J. Elin. We also thank Michael G. House, who contributed to the chapter on "Diseases of the Gallbladder and Bile Ducts," and Anna Louise Beavis, who contributed to the chapter on "Gynecologic Cancers." Chapters written by public employees reflect recommendations and conclusions of the authors and do not necessarily reflect the official position of the entity for which they work.

At Elsevier, we are most indebted to Dolores Meloni and Laura Schmidt, and also thank Lucia Gunzel, Dan Fitzgerald, and Maggie Reid, who have been critical to the planning and production.

We have been exposed to remarkable physicians in our lifetimes and would like to acknowledge the mentorship and support of several of those who exemplify this paradigm—Eugene Braunwald, the late Lloyd H. Smith, Jr., Frank Gardner, and William Castle. Finally, we would like to thank the Goldman family—Jill, Jeff, Abigail, Mira, Samuel, Daniel, Morgan, Robyn, Tobin, Dashel, and Alden—and the Schafer family—Pauline, Eric, Melissa, Nathaniel, Caroline, Pam, John, Evan, Samantha, Kate, Sean, Patrick, and Meghan—for their understanding of the time and focus required to edit a book that attempts to sustain the tradition of our predecessors and to meet the needs of today's physician.

LEE GOLDMAN, MD
ANDREW I. SCHAFER, MD

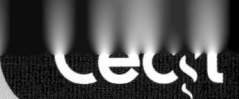

CONTRIBUTORS

Charles S. Abrams, MD
Francis C. Wood Professor of Medicine, University of Pennsylvania
Perelman School of Medicine, Philadelphia, Pennsylvania
Thrombocytopenia

Ronald S. Adler, MD, PhD
Professor of Radiology, New York University School of Medicine; NYU
Langone Health, New York, New York
Imaging Studies in the Rheumatic Diseases

Cem Akin, MD, PhD
Professor of Medicine, Internal Medicine, University of Michigan Medical
School, Ann Arbor, Michigan
Mastocytosis

Allen J. Aksamit, Jr., MD
Professor of Neurology, Mayo Clinic College of Medicine and Science,
Rochester, Minnesota
Acute Viral Encephalitis

Qais Al-Awqati, MB ChB
Robert F. Loeb Professor, Medicine, and Physiology & Cellular Biophysics,
Columbia University Vagelos College of Physicians & Surgeons, New
York, New York
Structure and Function of the Kidneys; Disorders of Sodium and Water

Ban Mishu Allos, MD
Associate Professor of Medicine, Division of Infectious Diseases, Vanderbilt
University School of Medicine, Nashville, Tennessee
Campylobacter Infections

Jeffrey L. Anderson, MD
Professor of Medicine, Division of Cardiovascular Medicine, University of
Utah School of Medicine; Distinguished Clinical and Research
Physician, Intermountain Medical Center Heart Institute, Salt Lake City,
Utah
*ST Elevation Acute Myocardial Infarction and Complications of Myocardial
Infarction*

Derek C. Angus, MD, MPH
Professor and Mitchell P. Fink Endowed Chair, Department of Critical
Care Medicine, University of Pittsburgh School of Medicine, Pittsburgh,
Pennsylvania
Approach to the Patient with Shock

Gerald B. Appel, MD
Professor of Medicine and Director, Glomerular Center, Columbia
University Irving Medical Center, New York, New York
Glomerular Disorders and Nephrotic Syndromes

Frederick R. Appelbaum, MD
Professor of Medicine, University of Washington School of Medicine;
Executive Senior VP and Deputy Director, Clinical Research Division,
Fred Hutchinson Cancer Research Center, Seattle, Washington
The Acute Leukemias

James O. Armitage, MD
Professor of Internal Medicine, University of Nebraska Medical Center
College of Medicine, Omaha, Nebraska
Non-Hodgkin Lymphomas

Deborah K. Armstrong, MD
Professor of Gynecology and Obstetrics, Johns Hopkins University School
of Medicine, Baltimore, Maryland
Gynecologic Cancers

M. Amin Arnaout, MD
Professor of Medicine, Chief Emeritus, Division of Nephrology,
Department of Medicine, Massachusetts General Hospital and Harvard
Medical School, Boston, Massachusetts
Cystic Kidney Diseases

Robert M. Arnold, MD
Distinguished Service Professor, Chief, Section of Palliative Care and
Medical Ethics, University of Pittsburgh School of Medicine; Chief
Medical Officer, UPMC Palliative and Supportive Institute, UPMC
Health Plan, Pittsburgh, Pennsylvania
Palliative Care

David Atkins, MD, MPH
Director, Health Services Research and Development, Office of Research
and Development, Dept. of Veterans Affairs (10P9H), Washington, D.C.
The Periodic Health Examination

John P. Atkinson, MD
Professor of Medicine, Division of Rheumatology, Washington University
School of Medicine in St. Louis, St. Louis, Missouri
Complement System in Disease

John Z. Ayanian, MD, MPP
Alice Hamilton Professor of Medicine; Director, Institute for Healthcare
Policy and Innovation, University of Michigan Medical School, Ann
Arbor, Michigan
Disparities in Health and Health Care

Larry M. Baddour, MD
Professor of Medicine, Mayo Clinic College of Medicine and Science,
Rochester, Minnesota
Infective Endocarditis

Grover C. Bagby, MD
Professor of Medicine, Molecular and Medical Genetics, Oregon Health &
Science University, Portland, Oregon
Aplastic Anemia and Related Bone Marrow Failure States

Barbara J. Bain, MBBS
Professor in Diagnostic Haematology, Haematology, St Mary's Hospital
Campus of Imperial College London, London, United Kingdom
The Peripheral Blood Smear

Dean F. Bajorin, MD
Attending Physician and Member, Memorial Sloan Kettering Cancer
Center; Professor of Medicine, Weill Cornell Medical College, New
York, New York
Tumors of the Kidney, Bladder, Ureters, and Renal Pelvis

Robert W. Baloh, MD
Professor of Neurology, David Geffen School of Medicine at UCLA,
Los Angeles, California
Neuro-Ophthalmology; Smell and Taste; Hearing and Equilibrium

Charles R.M. Bangham, BM BCh
Professor of Medicine, Faculty of Medicine, Imperial College London School of Medicine, London, United Kingdom
Retroviruses Other Than Human Immunodeficiency Virus

Jonathan Barasch, MD, PhD
Samuel W Lambert Professor of Medicine, Professor of Pathology and Cell Biology, Columbia University Vagelos College of Physicians & Surgeons, New York, New York
Structure and Function of the Kidneys

Richard L. Barbano, MD, PhD
Professor of Neurology and Chief of the Movement Disorders Division, University of Rochester School of Medicine & Dentistry, Rochester, New York
Mechanical and Other Lesions of the Spine, Nerve Roots, and Spinal Cord

Bruce Barrett, MD, PhD
Professor, Department of Family Medicine and Community Health, University of Wisconsin School of Medicine and Public Health, Madison, Wisconsin
The Common Cold

John R. Bartholomew, MD
Professor of Medicine and Section Head Vascular Medicine, Cleveland Clinic Lerner College of Medicine, Cleveland, Ohio
Other Peripheral Arterial Diseases

J.D. Bartleson, MD
Professor of Neurology, Mayo Clinic College of Medicine and Science, Rochester, Minnesota
Mechanical and Other Lesions of the Spine, Nerve Roots, and Spinal Cord

Mary Barton, MD, MPP
Vice President, Performance Measurement, National Committee for Quality Assurance, Washington, D.C.
The Periodic Health Examination

Robert C. Basner, MD
Professor of Medicine, Columbia University Vagelos College of Physicians and Surgeons, New York, New York
Sleep Disorders

Anne R. Bass, MD
Professor of Clinical Medicine, Weill Cornell Medical College; Attending Physician, Hospital for Special Surgery, New York, New York
Immunomodulatory Drugs

Stephen G. Baum, MD
Professor of Medicine and of Microbiology and Immunology, Albert Einstein College of Medicine, Bronx, New York
Mycoplasma *Infections*

Julie E. Bauman, MD, MPH
Professor of Medicine, University of Arizona Cancer Center, Tucson, Arizona
Head and Neck Cancer

Daniel G. Bausch, MD, MPH&TM
Director, United Kingdom Public Health Rapid Support Team, Public Health England/London School of Hygiene and Tropical Medicine, London, United Kingdom
Viral Hemorrhagic Fevers

Arnold S. Bayer, MD
Distinguished Professor of Medicine, David Geffen School of Medicine at UCLA; Senior Investigator-LA Biomedical Research Institute At Harbor-UCLA, Los Angeles, California
Infective Endocarditis

Hasan Bazari, MD
Associate Professor of Medicine, Massachusetts General Hospital and Harvard Medical School, Boston, Massachusetts
Approach to the Patient with Renal Disease

Jeffrey J. Bazarian, MD, MPH
Professor of Emergency Medicine, University of Rochester School of Medicine & Dentistry, Rochester, New York
Traumatic Brain Injury and Spinal Cord Injury

John H. Beigel, MD
Associate Director for Clinical Research, Division of Microbiology and Infectious Diseases, National Institute of Allergy and Infectious Diseases, National Institutes of Health, Bethesda, Maryland
Antiviral Therapy (Non-HIV)

Elisabeth H. Bel, MD, PhD
Professor and Head of the Department of Respiratory Medicine, Amsterdam University Medical Center, University of Amsterdam, The Netherlands
Asthma

George A. Beller, MD
Emeritus Professor of Cardiology, Department of Medicine, University of Virginia Health System, Charlottesville, Virginia
Noninvasive Cardiac Imaging

Joseph R. Berger, MD
Professor of Neurology, University of Pennsylvania Perelman School of Medicine, Philadelphia, Pennsylvania
Cytomegalovirus, Epstein-Barr Virus, and Slow Virus Infections of the Central Nervous System; Brain Abscess and Parameningeal Infections

Paul D. Berk, MD
Professor of Medicine, Columbia University Vagelos College of Physicians & Surgeons, New York, New York
Approach to the Patient with Jaundice or Abnormal Liver Tests

Nancy Berliner, MD
H. Franklin Bunn Professor of Medicine; Chief, Division of Hematology, Brigham and Women's Hospital and Harvard Medical School, Boston, Massachusetts
Leukocytosis and Leukopenia; Histiocytoses

James L. Bernat, MD
Professor of Neurology and Medicine, Geisel School of Medicine at Dartmouth, Hanover, New Hampshire and Dartmouth-Hitchcock Medical Center, Lebanon, New Hampshire
Coma, Vegetative State, and Brain Death

Philip J. Bierman, MD
Professor of Internal Medicine, University of Nebraska Medical Center College of Medicine, Omaha, Nebraska
Non-Hodgkin Lymphomas

Leslie G. Biesecker, MD
Chief, Medical Genomics and Metabolic Genetics Branch, National Human Genome Research Institute, National Institutes of Health, Bethesda, Maryland
Clinical Genomics—Genome Structure and Variation

Michael R. Bishop, MD
Professor of Medicine and Director of the Cellular Therapy Program, Section of Hematology and Oncology, University of Chicago Pritzker School of Medicine, Chicago, Illinois
Hematopoietic Stem Cell Transplantation

Joseph J. Biundo, MD
Clinical Professor of Medicine, Tulane Medical Center, New Orleans, Louisiana
Bursitis, Tendinitis, and Other Periarticular Disorders and Sports Medicine

Joel N. Blankson, MD, PhD
Professor of Medicine, Johns Hopkins University School of Medicine, Baltimore, Maryland
Immunopathogenesis of Human Immunodeficiency Virus Infection

William A. Blattner, MD
Chief Executive Officer, Salt Run Global Health and Research, Saint Augustine, Florida
Retroviruses Other Than Human Immunodeficiency Virus

Thomas P. Bleck, MD
Professor of Neurology, Northwestern University Feinberg School of Medicine; Professor Emeritus of Neurological Sciences, Neurosurgery, Medicine, and Anesthesiology, Rush Medical College, Chicago, Illinois
Arboviruses Affecting the Central Nervous System

Karen C. Bloch, MD, MPH
Associate Professor of Medicine (Infectious Diseases) and Health Policy, Vanderbilt University School of Medicine, Nashville, Tennessee
Tularemia and Other Francisella *Infections*

Henk J. Blom, PhD
Professor of Biochemistry of Inherited Metabolic Disease, Department of Clinical Genetics, Center for Lysosomal and Metabolic Diseases, Erasmus MC, Rotterdam, The Netherlands
Homocystinuria and Hyperhomocysteinemia

Olaf A. Bodamer, MD, PhD
Park Gerald Chair of Genetics and Genomics, Department of Medicine, Boston Children's Hospital and Harvard Medical School, Boston, Massachusetts
Approach to Inborn Errors of Metabolism

William E. Boden, MD
Professor of Medicine, Boston University School of Medicine; Lecturer in Medicine, Harvard Medical School; Scientific Director, Clinical Trials Network, Department of Medicine, VA Boston Healthcare System, Boston, Massachusetts
Angina Pectoris and Stable Ischemic Heart Disease

Guy Boivin, MD
Professor of Microbiology, Immunology and Infectiology, CHU de Québec-Laval University, Quebec City, Quebec, Canada
Cytomegalovirus

Jean Bolognia, MD
Professor of Dermatology, Yale University School of Medicine, New Haven, Connecticut
Infections, Hyperpigmentation and Hypopigmentation, Regional Dermatology, and Distinctive Lesions in Black Skin

William Bonnez, MD
Professor Emeritus of Medicine, University of Rochester School of Medicine & Dentistry, Rochester, New York
Papillomavirus

Robert A. Bonomo, MD
Professor of Medicine, Case Western Reserve University School of Medicine; Chief of Medicine, Cleveland VA Hospital, Cleveland, Ohio
Diseases Caused by Acinetobacter *and* Stenotrophomonas *Species*

Sarah L. Booth, PhD
Professor of Nutrition, Tufts University; Director, USDA Human Nutrition Research Center on Aging; Director, Vitamin K Laboratory, USDA Human Nutrition Research Center on Aging, Boston, Massachusetts
Vitamins, Trace Minerals, and Other Micronutrients

Patrick J. Bosque, MD
Associate Professor of Neurology, University of Colorado School of Medicine; Chief, Neurology Division, Department of Medicine, Denver Health Medical Center, Denver, Colorado
Prion Diseases

Lucy Breakwell, PhD, MSc
Epidemiologist, Global Immunization Division, Centers for Disease Control and Prevention, Atlanta, Georgia
Diphtheria and Other Corynebacterium *Infections*

David J. Brenner, PhD, DSc
Higgins Professor of Radiation Biophysics, Center for Radiological Research, Columbia University Irving Medical Center, New York, New York
Radiation Injury

Laurent Brochard, MD
Keenan Chair in Critical Care and Respiratory Medicine and Professor of Medicine and Interdepartmental Division Director for Critical Care, University of Toronto Faculty of Medicine; Division of Critical Care, Saint Michael's Hospital, Toronto, Ontario, Canada
Mechanical Ventilation

Itzhak Brook, MD
Professor of Pediatrics, Georgetown University School of Medicine, Washington, D.C.
Diseases Caused by Non–Spore-Forming Anaerobic Bacteria; Actinomycosis

Enrico Brunetti, MD
Associate Professor, Department of Clinical, Surgical, Diagnostic and Pediatric Sciences and Staff Physician, Department of Infectious and Tropical Diseases, San Matteo Hospital Foundation, University of Pavia, Pavia, Italy
Cestodes

Amy E. Bryant, PhD
Associate Professor of Medicine, University of Washington School of Medicine, Seattle, Washington and Research Career Scientist, Infectious Diseases Section, VA Medical Center, Boise, Idaho
Nonpneumococcal Streptococcal Infections and Rheumatic Fever

David M. Buchner, MD, MPH
Professor Emeritus, Department of Kinesiology & Community Health, University of Illinois Urbana Champaign, Champaign, Illinois
Physical Activity

Pierre A. Buffet, MD, PhD
Professor of Cell Biology, Faculty of Medicine, Paris University and Consultant Physician, Institut Pasteur Medical Center, Paris, France
Leishmaniasis

David A. Bushinsky, MD
John J. Kuiper Distinguished Professor of Medicine and of Pharmacology and Physiology, University of Rochester School of Medicine & Dentistry, Rochester, New York
Nephrolithiasis

Vivian P. Bykerk, MD
Associate Professor of Medicine, Weill Cornell Medical College; Associate Attending Physician, Hospital for Special Surgery, New York, New York
Approach to the Patient with Rheumatic Disease

John C. Byrd, MD
Distinguished University Professor, Ohio State University, Columbus, Ohio
Chronic Lymphocytic Leukemia

Peter A. Calabresi, MD
Professor of Neurology and Neuroscience, Director of the Richard T Johnson Division of Neuroimmunology and Neuroinfectious Diseases; Director of the Multiple Sclerosis Center, Johns Hopkins University School of Medicine, Baltimore, Maryland
Multiple Sclerosis and Demyelinating Conditions of the Central Nervous System

David P. Calfee, MD, MS
Professor of Medicine and of Health Policy & Research, Weill Cornell
  Medical College; Chief Hospital Epidemiologist, NewYork-Presbyterian
  Hospital/Weill Cornell, New York, New York
Prevention and Control of Health Care–Associated Infections

Clara Camaschella, MD
Professor of Medicine, Division of Genetics and Cell Biology, San Raffaele
  Scientific Institute, Milano, Italy
Microcytic and Hypochromic Anemias

Michael Camilleri, MD
Atherton and Winifred W. Bean Professor of Medicine, Pharmacology, and
  Physiology, Mayo Clinic College of Medicine and Science; Consultant,
  Division of Gastroenterology and Hepatology, Department of Medicine,
  Mayo Clinic, Rochester, Minnesota
Disorders of Gastrointestinal Motility

Maria Domenica Cappellini, MD
Professor of Internal Medicine, Department of Clinical Sciences and
  Community Health, University of Milan; and Ca' Granda
  Foundation-Policlinico Hospital, Milan, Italy
The Thalassemias

Blase A. Carabello, MD
Professor of Cardiovascular Sciences and Chief, Division of Cardiology,
  East Carolina University Brody School of Medicine, Greenville, North
  Carolina
Valvular Heart Disease

Edgar M. Carvalho, MD, PhD
Professor of Medicine, Federal University of Bahia, Oswaldo Cruz
  Foundation (Fiocruz), Instituto de Pesquisa Gonçalo Moniz (IGM),
  Salvador-Bahia, Brazil
Trematode Infections

William H. Catherino, MD, PhD
Professor and Chair-Research Division, Department of Obstetrics and
  Gynecology, Uniformed Services University of the Health Sciences,
  Bethesda, Maryland
Ovaries and Pubertal Development; Reproductive Endocrinology and Infertility

Jane A. Cauley, DrPH
Distinguished Professor of Epidemiology, Graduate School of Public
  Health, University of Pittsburgh, Pittsburgh, Pennsylvania
Epidemiology of Aging: Implications of an Aging Society

Naga P. Chalasani, MD
David W. Crabb Professor and Director, Division of Gastroenterology and
  Hepatology, Indiana University School of Medicine, Indianapolis,
  Indiana
Alcoholic and Nonalcoholic Steatohepatitis

Henry F. Chambers, MD
Professor of Medicine and Director, Clinical Research Services, Clinical
  Translational Science Institute, University of California, San Francisco,
  School of Medicine, San Francisco, California
Staphylococcal Infections

Larry W. Chang, MD, MPH
Associate Professor of Medicine, Epidemiology, and International Health,
  Johns Hopkins University School of Medicine and Bloomberg School of
  Public Health, Baltimore, Maryland
*Epidemiology and Diagnosis of Human Immunodeficiency Virus Infection and
  Acquired Immunodeficiency Syndrome*

Lin H. Chen, MD
Associate Professor of Medicine, Harvard Medical School, Boston,
  Massachusetts and Director of the Travel Medicine Center, Division of
  Infectious Diseases and Travel Medicine, Mount Auburn Hospital,
  Cambridge, Massachusetts
Approach to the Patient before and after Travel

Sharon C-A Chen, MB, PhD
Professor of Medicine, University of Sydney and Centre for Infectious
  Diseases and Microbiology, ICPMR and Westmead Hospital, New South
  Wales, Australia
Cryptococcosis

William P. Cheshire, Jr., MD
Professor of Neurology, Mayo Clinic College of Medicine and Science,
  Jacksonville, Florida
Autonomic Disorders and Their Management

Arun Chockalingam, PhD
Professor of Epidemiology, Medicine and Global Health, Dalla Lana School
  of Public Health, University of Toronto, Toronto, Ontario, Canada
Global Health

David C. Christiani, MD
Professor of Medicine, Harvard Medical School; Physician, Pulmonary and
  Critical Care, Massachusetts General Hospital; Elkan Blout Professor of
  Environmental Genetics, Environmental Health, Harvard School of
  Public Health, Boston, Massachusetts
Physical and Chemical Injuries of the Lung

Edward Chu, MD, MMS
Professor and Chief, Division of Hematology-Oncology, Deputy Director,
  UPMC Hillman Cancer Center, University of Pittsburgh School of
  Medicine, Pittsburgh, Pennsylvania
Neoplasms of the Small and Large Intestine

Theodore J. Cieslak, MD, MPH
Associate Professor of Epidemiology, Co-Medical Director, Nebraska
  Biocontainment Unit, College of Public Health, University of Nebraska,
  Omaha, Nebraska
Bioterrorism

George A. Cioffi, MD
Edward S. Harkness Professor and Chair, Jean and Richard Deems
  Professor of Ophthalmology, Columbia University Vagelos College of
  Physicians and Surgeons, New York, New York
Diseases of the Visual System

Carolyn M. Clancy, MD
Clinical Associate Professor of Internal Medicine, George Washington
  University School of Medicine; Assistant Deputy Undersecretary for
  Health, Quality, Safety and Value, Veterans Administration, Washington,
  D.C.
Measuring Health and Health Care

Heather E. Clauss, MD
Associate Professor of Medicine, Section of Infectious Diseases, Lewis Katz
  School of Medicine at Temple University, Philadelphia, Pennsylvania
Listeriosis

Daniel J. Clauw, MD
Professor of Anesthesiology, Medicine (Rheumatology) and Psychiatry,
  Director, Chronic Pain and Fatigue Research Center, University of
  Michigan Medical School, Ann Arbor, Michigan
Fibromyalgia, Chronic Fatigue Syndrome, and Myofascial Pain

David R. Clemmons, MD
Kenan Professor of Medicine, University of North Carolina School of
  Medicine; Attending Physician, Medicine, UNC Hospitals, Chapel Hill,
  North Carolina
Approach to the Patient with Endocrine Disease

David Cohen, MD
Professor of Medicine, Columbia University Vagelos College of Physicians and Surgeons, New York, New York
Treatment of Irreversible Renal Failure

Jeffrey Cohen, MD
Chief, Laboratory of Infectious Diseases, National Institute of Allergy and Infectious Diseases, National Institutes of Health, Bethesda, Maryland
Varicella-Zoster Virus (Chickenpox, Shingles)

Myron S. Cohen, MD
Yeargan-Bates Eminent Professor of Medicine, Microbiology and Epidemiology, Associate Vice Chancellor for Global Health; Director, Institute of Global Health and Infectious Diseases, University of North Carolina School of Medicine, Chapel Hill, North Carolina
Approach to the Patient with a Sexually Transmitted Infection; Prevention of Human Immunodeficiency Virus Infection

Steven P. Cohen, MD
Professor of Anesthesiology & Critical Care Medicine, Neurology and Physical Medicine & Rehabilitation and Chief, Pain Medicine Division, Johns Hopkins School of Medicine; Director of Pain Research and Professor of Anesthesiology and Physical Medicine & Rehabilitation, Walter Reed National Military Medical Center, Uniformed Services University of the Health Sciences, Baltimore, Maryland
Pain

Steven L. Cohn, MD
Professor Emeritus, Department of Medicine, University of Miami Miller School of Medicine, Miami, Florida; Clinical Professor of Medicine Emeritus, SUNY Downstate, Brooklyn, New York
Preoperative Evaluation

Joseph M. Connors, MD
Emeritus Professor, BC Cancer Centre for Lymphoid Cancer and the University of British Columbia, Vancouver, British Columbia, Canada
Hodgkin Lymphoma

Deborah J. Cook, MD, MSc
Professor of Medicine, Clinical Epidemiology & Biostatistics, McMaster University Michael G. DeGroote School of Medicine, Hamilton, Ontario, Canada
Approach to the Patient in a Critical Care Setting

David S. Cooper, MD
Professor of Medicine, Division of Endocrinology and Metabolism, The Johns Hopkins University School of Medicine, Baltimore, Maryland
Thyroid

Joseph Craft, MD
Paul B. Beeson Professor of Medicine and Professor of Immunobiology, Departments of Internal Medicine and Immunobiology, Yale University, New Haven, Connecticut
The Adaptive Immune System

Jill P. Crandall, MD
Professor of Medicine and Chief, Division of Endocrinology, Albert Einstein College of Medicine, Bronx, New York
Diabetes Mellitus

Simon L. Croft, PhD
Professor of Parasitology, Faculty of Infectious and Tropical Diseases, London School of Hygiene & Tropical Medicine, London, United Kingdom
Leishmaniasis

Mary K. Crow, MD
Joseph P. Routh Professor of Rheumatic Diseases in Medicine, Weill Cornell Medical College; Physician-in-Chief and Benjamin M. Rosen Chair in Immunology and Inflammation Research, Hospital for Special Surgery, New York, New York
The Innate Immune System; Approach to the Patient with Rheumatic Disease; Systemic Lupus Erythematosus

John A. Crump, MB ChB, MD, DTM&H
McKinlay Professor of Global Health, Centre for International Health, University of Otago, Dunedin, Otago; Adjunct Professor of Medicine, Pathology, and Global Health, Division of Infectious Diseases and International Health, Duke University Medical Center, Durham, North Carolina
Salmonella *Infections (Including Enteric Fever)*

Merit E. Cudkowicz, MD
Professor of Neurology, Harvard Medical School and Chair of Neurology, Massachusetts General Hospital, Boston, Massachusetts
Amyotrophic Lateral Sclerosis and Other Motor Neuron Diseases

Mark R. Cullen, MD
Professor of Medicine, Stanford University School of Medicine, Stanford, California
Principles of Occupational and Environmental Medicine

Charlotte Cunningham-Rundles, MD, PhD
David S Gottesman Professor of Medicine, Icahn School of Medicine at Mount Sinai, New York, New York
Primary Immunodeficiency Diseases

Inger K. Damon, MD, PhD
Director, Division of High Consequence Pathogens and Pathology, Centers for Disease Control and Prevention, Atlanta, Georgia
Smallpox, Monkeypox, and Other Poxvirus Infections

Troy E. Daniels, DDS, MS
Professor Emeritus of Oral Pathology & Pathology, University of California, San Francisco, School of Medicine, San Francisco, California
Diseases of the Mouth and Salivary Glands

Richard Dart, MD, PhD
Professor of Emergency Medicine, University of Colorado School of Medicine and Director, Rocky Mountain Poison and Drug Center, Denver Health and Hospital Authority, Denver, Colorado
Envenomation, Bites, and Stings

Nancy E. Davidson, MD
Professor of Medicine and Raisbeck Endowed Chair; President, Seattle Cancer Care Alliance; Senior Vice President and Director, Clinical Research Division, Fred Hutchinson Cancer Research Center; Chief, Division of Medical Oncology, University of Washington School of Medicine, Seattle, Washington
Breast Cancer and Benign Breast Disorders

Lisa M. DeAngelis, MD
Lillian Rojtman Chair in Honor of Jerome B Posner, Acting Physician-in-Chief, Memorial Hospital, Chair, Department of Neurology, Memorial Sloan-Kettering Cancer Center, New York, New York
Tumors of the Central Nervous System

Malcolm M. DeCamp, MD
Professor of Surgery and Chair, Division of Cardiothoracic Surgery, K. Craig Kent Chair in Strategic Leadership, University of Wisconsin School of Medicine and Public Health, Madison, Wisconsin
Interventional and Surgical Approaches to Lung Disease

Carlos Del Rio, MD
Hubert Professor and Chair, Hubert Department of Global Health, Rollins School of Public Health of Emory University; Professor, Department of Medicine, Emory University School of Medicine, Atlanta, Georgia
Prevention of Human Immunodeficiency Virus Infection

Gabriele C. DeLuca, MD, DPhil
Associate Professor, Nuffield Department of Clinical Neurosciences, University of Oxford, Oxford, Oxfordshire, United Kingdom
Approach to the Patient with Neurologic Disease

David W. Denning, MBBS
Professor of Infectious Diseases in Global Health and Director of the National Aspergillosis Centre, University of Manchester and Wythenshawe Hospital, Manchester, United Kingdom
Systemic Antifungal Agents

Patricia A. Deuster, PhD, MPH
Professor and Director, Department of Military and Emergency Medicine, Director, Consortium for Health and Military Performance, Uniformed Services University, Bethesda, Maryland
Rhabdomyolysis

Robert B. Diasio, MD
William J and Charles H Mayo Professor of Molecular Pharmacology and Experimental Therapeutics, Mayo Clinic College of Medicine and Science, Rochester, Minnesota
Principles of Drug Therapy

David J. Diemert, MD
Associate Professor, Departments of Medicine and Microbiology, Immunology and Tropical Medicine, George Washington University School of Medicine and Health Sciences, Washington, D.C.
Nematode Infections

Kathleen B. Digre, MD
Professor of Neurology and Ophthalmology, University of Utah School of Medicine, Salt Lake City, Utah
Headaches and Other Head Pain

James. H. Doroshow, MD
Deputy Director for Clinical and Translational Research, Director, Division of Cancer Treatment and Diagnosis, National Cancer Institute, National Institutes of Health, Bethesda, Maryland
Approach to the Patient with Cancer

John M. Douglas, Jr., MD
Executive Director, Tri-County Health Department, Greenwood Village, Colorado
Papillomavirus

Jeffrey M. Drazen, MD
Distinguished Parker B. Francis Professor of Medicine, Harvard Medical School and Senior Physician, Department of Medicine, Brigham and Women's Hospital, Boston, Massachusetts
Asthma

Dimitri Drekonja, MD, MS
Associate Professor of Medicine, University of Minnesota and Chief, Infectious Diseases Section, Minneapolis VA Health Care System, Minneapolis, Minnesota
Approach to the Patient with Urinary Tract Infection

Stephen C. Dreskin, MD, PhD
Professor of Medicine and Immunology, University of Colorado School of Medicine, Aurora, Colorado
Urticaria and Angioedema

W. Lawrence Drew, MD, PhD
Professor Emeritus of Laboratory Medicine and Medicine, University of California, San Francisco, School of Medicine, San Francisco, California
Cytomegalovirus

George L. Drusano, MD
Professor of Medicine and Director, Institute for Therapeutic Innovation, University of Florida College of Medicine, Orlando, Florida
Antibacterial Chemotherapy

Thomas D. DuBose, Jr., MD
Professor Emeritus of Medicine, Wake Forest School of Medicine, Winston-Salem, North Carolina; Visiting Professor of Medicine, University of Virginia School of Medicine, Charlottesville, Virginia
Vascular Disorders of the Kidney

J. Stephen Dumler, MD
Professor and Chairperson, Joint Departments of Pathology, Uniformed Services University, Walter Reed National Military Medical Center, and Joint Pathology Center, Bethesda, Maryland
Zoonoses

Herbert L. DuPont, MD
Professor of Infectious Diseases, University of Texas School of Public Health, Mary W. Kelsey Chair, University of Texas McGovern Medical School, Houston, Texas
Approach to the Patient with Suspected Enteric Infection

Madeleine Duvic, MD
Professor and Deputy Chairman, Department of Dermatology, University Texas MD Anderson Cancer Center, Houston, Texas
Urticaria, Drug Hypersensitivity Rashes, Nodules and Tumors, and Atrophic Diseases

Kathryn M. Edwards, MD
Sarah H. Sell and Cornelius Vanderbilt Chair in Pediatrics, Vanderbilt University School of Medicine, Nashville, Tennessee
Parainfluenza Viral Disease

N. Lawrence Edwards, MD
Professor and Vice Chairman, Department of Medicine, University of Florida College of Medicine; Chief, Section of Rheumatology Medicine, Malcolm Randall Veterans Administration Medical Center, Gainesville, Florida
Crystal Deposition Diseases

Lawrence H. Einhorn, MD
Distinguished Professor of Medicine, Indiana University School of Medicine, Indianapolis, Indiana
Testicular Cancer

George M. Eliopoulos, MD
Professor of Medicine, Harvard Medical School; Physician, Beth Israel Deaconess Medical Center, Boston, Massachusetts
Principles of Anti-Infective Therapy

Perry M. Elliott, MBBS, MD
Professor of Cardiovascular Medicine, Institute of Cardiovascular Science, University College London & St. Bartholomew's Hospital, London, United Kingdom
Diseases of the Myocardium and Endocardium

Jerrold J. Ellner, MD
Professor of Medicine, Rutgers-New Jersey Medical School; Director of Research Innovations, Center for Emerging Pathogens, Newark, New Jersey
Tuberculosis

Ezekiel J. Emanuel, MD, PhD
Vice Provost for Global Initiatives, Office of the Provost; Chair, Department of Medical Ethics and Health Policy, University of Pennsylvania, Philadelphia, Pennsylvania
Bioethics in the Practice of Medicine

Joel D. Ernst, MD
Professor and Chief, Division of Experimental Medicine, University of California, San Francisco, School of Medicine, San Francisco, California
Leprosy (Hansen Disease)

Gregory T. Everson, MD
Professor of Medicine, University of Colorado Denver; Director of Hepatology, Hepatology and Transplant Center, University of Colorado Hospital, Aurora, Colorado
Hepatic Failure and Liver Transplantation

Amelia Evoli, MD
Associate Professor of Neurology, Institute of Neurology, Catholic University, Roma, Italy
Disorders of Neuromuscular Transmission

Matthew E. Falagas, MD, MSc, DSc
Director, Alfa Institute of Biomedical Sciences and Chief, Department of Medicine, Henry Dunant Hospital Center, Athens, Greece; Adjunct Associate Professor of Medicine, Tufts University School of Medicine, Boston, Massachusetts
Pseudomonas and Related Gram-Negative Bacillary Infections

Gary W. Falk, MD, MS
Professor of Medicine, University of Pennsylvania Perelman School of Medicine, Philadelphia, Pennsylvania
Diseases of the Esophagus

James C. Fang, MD
Professor of Medicine, University of Utah School of Medicine; Executive Director, Cardiovascular Service Line, University of Utah Health Sciences, Salt Lake City, Utah
ST Elevation Acute Myocardial Infarction and Complications of Myocardial Infarction

Gene Feder, MBBS, MD
Professor, Centre for Academic Primary Care, Population Health Sciences, Bristol Medical School, University of Bristol; General Practitioner, Helios Medical Centre, Bristol, United Kingdom
Intimate Partner Violence

David J. Feller-Kopman, MD
Professor of Medicine, Anesthesiology, Otolaryngology-Head & Neck Surgery and Director, Bronchoscopy & Interventional Pulmonology, Johns Hopkins University School of Medicine, Baltimore, Maryland
Interventional and Surgical Approaches to Lung Disease

Thomas McDonald File, Jr., MD, MSc
Professor and Chair, Infectious Disease Section, Northeast Ohio Medical University, Rootstown, Ohio; Chair, Infectious Disease Division, Summa Health, Akron, Ohio
Streptococcus Pneumoniae Infections

Gary S. Firestein, MD
Professor of Medicine, Dean, and Associate Vice Chancellor of Clinical and Translational Research, University of California, San Diego, School of Medicine, La Jolla, California
Mechanisms of Inflammation and Tissue Repair

Glenn I. Fishman, MD
William Goldring Professor of Medicine and Director, Leon H. Charney Division of Cardiology, New York University School of Medicine, New York, New York
Principles of Electrophysiology

Lee A. Fleisher, MD
Robert D. Dripps Professor and Chair, Anesthesiology and Critical Care; Professor of Medicine, University of Pennsylvania Perelman School of Medicine, Philadelphia, Pennsylvania
Overview of Anesthesia

Paul W. Flint, MD
Professor and Chair of Otolaryngology-Head & Neck Surgery, Oregon Health & Science University, Portland, Oregon
Throat Disorders

Evan L. Fogel, MD, MSc
Professor of Medicine, Indiana University School of Medicine, Indianapolis, Indiana
Diseases of the Gallbladder and Bile Ducts

Chris E. Forsmark, MD
Professor of Medicine, University of Florida College of Medicine, Gainesville, Florida
Pancreatitis

Pierre-Edouard Fournier, MD, PhD
Professor of Medical Bacteriology-Virology and Hygiene, Faculté de Médecine, Aix-Marseille Université and Institut Hospitalo-Universitaire Méditerranée-Infection, Marseille, France
Rickettsial Infections

Vance G. Fowler, Jr., MD, MHS
Professor of Medicine and of Molecular Genetics and Microbiology, Duke University School of Medicine, Durham, North Carolina
Infective Endocarditis

Manuel A. Franco, MD, PhD
Professor, Instituto de Genética Humana, Facultad de Medicina, Pontificia Universidad Javeriana, Bogotá, Colombia
Rotaviruses, Noroviruses, and Other Gastrointestinal Viruses

David O. Freedman, MD
Professor Emeritus of Infectious Diseases, University of Alabama at Birmingham School of Medicine; Medical Director, Shoreland Travax, Birmingham, Alabama
Approach to the Patient before and after Travel

Martyn A. French, MB ChB, MD
Emeritus Professor in Clinical Immunology, University of Western Australia Medical School and School of Biomedical Sciences, Faculty of Health and Medical Sciences, Perth, Australia
Immune Reconstitution Inflammatory Syndrome in HIV/AIDS

Karen M. Freund, MD, MPH
Professor of Medicine and Vice Chair for Faculty Affairs and Quality Improvement, Tufts University School of Medicine, Boston, Massachusetts
Approach to Women's Health

John N. Galgiani, MD
Professor of Medicine and Director, Valley Fever Center for Excellence, University of Arizona College of Medicine; Chief Medical Officer, Valley Fever Solutions, Tucson, Arizona
Endemic Mycoses

Patrick G. Gallagher, MD
Professor of Pediatrics, Pathology and Genetics, Yale University School of Medicine, New Haven, Connecticut
Hemolytic Anemias: Red Blood Cell Membrane and Metabolic Defects

Leonard Ganz, MD
Director of Cardiac Electrophysiology, Heart and Vascular Center, Heritage Valley Health System, Beaver, Pennsylvania
Electrocardiography

Hasan Garan, MD, MS
Dickinson W. Richards, Jr. Professor of Medicine, Director, Cardiac Electrophysiology, Columbia University Vagelos College of Physicians and Surgeons, New York, New York
Ventricular Arrhythmias

Guadalupe Garcia-Tsao, MD
Professor of Medicine, Yale University School of Medicine, New Haven, Connecticut; Chief of Digestive Diseases, School of Medicine, VA-CT Healthcare System, West Haven, Connecticut
Cirrhosis and Its Sequelae

William M. Geisler, MD, MPH
Professor of Medicine, University of Alabama at Birmingham School of Medicine, Birmingham, Alabama
Diseases Caused by Chlamydiae

Tony P. George, MD
Professor of Psychiatry and Director, Division of Brain and Therapeutics, University of Toronto; Chief, Addictions Division, Centre for Addiction and Mental Health, Toronto, Ontario, Canada
Nicotine and Tobacco

Lior Gepstein, MD, PhD
Sohnis Family Professor in Medicine, Technion - Israel Institute of Technology; Director, Cardiology Department, Rambam Health Care Campus, Haifa, Israel
Regenerative Medicine, Cell, and Gene Therapies

Susan I. Gerber, MD
Chief, Respiratory Viruses Branch, Division of Viral Diseases, National Center for Immunization and Respiratory Diseases, Centers for Disease Control and Prevention, Atlanta, Georgia
Coronaviruses

Dale N. Gerding, MD
Professor (retired) of Medicine, Loyola University Chicago Stritch School of Medicine, Maywood, Illinois; Research Physician, Medicine, Edward Hines Jr. VA Hospital, Hines, Illinois
Clostridial Infections

Morie A. Gertz, MD
Roland Seidler Jr. Professor of the Art of Medicine and Chair Emeritus, Internal Medicine, Mayo Clinic College of Medicine and Science, Rochester, Minnesota
Amyloidosis

Khalil G. Ghanem, MD, PhD
Associate Professor of Medicine, Johns Hopkins University School of Medicine, Baltimore, Maryland
Granuloma Inguinale (Donovanosis); Syphilis; Nonsyphilitic Treponematoses

Christopher J. Gill, MD, MS
Associate Professor of Global Health, Boston University School of Public Health, Boston, Massachusetts
Whooping Cough and Other Bordetella *Infections*

Jeffrey S. Ginsberg, MD
Professor of Medicine, McMaster University Michael G. DeGroote School of Medicine, Hamilton, Ontario, Canada
Venous Thrombosis and Embolism

Geoffrey S. Ginsburg, MD, PhD
Professor of Medicine and Pathology and Director, Duke Center for Applied Genomics & Precision Medicine, Duke University, Durham, North Carolina
Applications of Molecular Technologies to Clinical Medicine

Marshall J. Glesby, MD, PhD
Professor of Medicine, Weill Cornell Medical College, New York, New York
Systemic Manifestations of HIV/AIDS

John W. Gnann, Jr., MD
Professor of Medicine, Medical University of South Carolina, Charleston, South Carolina
Mumps; Herpes Simplex Virus Infections

Matthew R. Golden, MD, MPH
Professor of Medicine, University of Washington School of Medicine; Director, HIV/STD Program, Public Health - Seattle & King County, Seattle, Washington
Neisseria Gonorrhoeae *Infections*

David L. Goldman, MD
Associate Professor of Pediatrics, Microbiology and Immunology, Children's Hospital at Montefiore/Albert Einstein College of Medicine, Bronx, New York
Mycoplasma *Infections*

Lee Goldman, MD
Harold and Margaret Hatch Professor, Chief Executive, Columbia University Irving Medical Center, Dean of the Faculties of Health Sciences and Medicine, Columbia University, New York, New York
Approach to Medicine, the Patient, and the Medical Profession: Medicine as a Learned and Humane Profession; Approach to the Patient with Possible Cardiovascular Disease

Larry B. Goldstein, MD
Ruth L Works Professor and Chairman, Department of Neurology, University of Kentucky College of Medicine; Co-Director, Kentucky Neuroscience Institute, Lexington, Kentucky
Approach to Cerebrovascular Diseases; Ischemic Cerebrovascular Disease

Richard M. Gore, MD
Professor of Radiology, University of Chicago Pritzker School of Medicine; Chief, Section of Gastrointestinal Radiology, NorthShore University HealthSystem, Evanston, Illinois
Diagnostic Imaging Procedures in Gastroenterology

Jason Gotlib, MD, MS
Professor of Medicine, Stanford University School of Medicine, Stanford Cancer Institute, Stanford, California
Polycythemia Vera, Essential Thrombocythemia, and Primary Myelofibrosis

Eduardo Gotuzzo, MD
Professor Emeritus, Alexander von Humboldt Tropical Medicine Institute, Universidad Peruana Cayetano Heredia; Principal Professor of Medicine and Tropical Diseases, National Hospital Cayetano Heredia, Lima, Peru
Cholera and Other Vibrio *Infections; Trematode Infections*

Leslie C. Grammer, MD
Professor of Medicine, Northwestern University Feinberg School of Medicine, Chicago, Illinois
Drug Allergy

Hartmut Grasemann, MD, PhD
Professor of Pediatrics, The Hospital for Sick Children and University of Toronto, Toronto, Ontario, Canada
Cystic Fibrosis

M. Lindsay Grayson, MBBS, MD, MS
Professor of Medicine, University of Melbourne, Director, Infectious Diseases & Microbiology, Austin Health, Melbourne, Victoria, Australia
Principles of Anti-Infective Therapy

Harry B. Greenberg, MD
Professor of Medicine and of Microbiology and Immunology, Stanford University School of Medicine, Stanford, California
Rotaviruses, Noroviruses, and Other Gastrointestinal Viruses

Steven A. Greenberg, MD
Professor of Neurology, Brigham and Women's Hospital and Harvard Medical School, Boston, Massachusetts
Inflammatory Myopathies

David M. Greer, MD, MA
Professor and Chair of Neurology, Boston University School of Medicine, Boston, Massachusetts
Coma, Vegetative State, and Brain Death

Robert C. Griggs, MD
Professor of Neurology, Medicine, Pediatrics, Pathology & Laboratory Medicine, University of Rochester School of Medicine & Dentistry, Rochester, New York
Approach to the Patient with Neurologic Disease

Lev M. Grinberg, MD, PhD
Professor and Chair, Department of Pathology, Ural State Medical University, Ekaterinburg, Russia
Anthrax

Daniel Grossman, MD
Professor of Obstetrics, Gynecology and Reproductive Sciences, University of California, San Francisco, School of Medicine, San Francisco, California
Contraception

Lisa M. Guay-Woodford, MD
Richard L. Hudson Professor of Pediatrics, George Washington University School of Medicine and Health Science and Director, Center for Translational Research, Children's National Medical Center, Washington D.C.
Hereditary Nephropathies and Developmental Abnormalities of the Urinary Tract

Roy M. Gulick, MD, MPH
Professor of Medicine, Weill Cornell Medical School; Attending Physician, NewYork-Presbyterian Hospital, New York, New York
Antiretroviral Therapy for Human Immunodeficiency Virus and Acquired Immunodeficiency Syndrome

Rajesh Gupta, MD, MEd
Associate Professor of Medicine, University of Toronto; General Internist, Medicine, St. Michael's Hospital, Toronto, Ontario, Canada
Medical Consultation in Psychiatry

Colleen Hadigan, MD, MPH
Staff Clinician, National Institutes of Health, Laboratory of Immunoregulation, NIAID, Bethesda, Maryland
Microbial Complications in Patients Infected with Human Immunodeficiency Virus

Melissa M. Hagman, MD
Associate Professor of Medicine, Program Director, Internal Medicine Residency-Boise, University of Washington, Boise, Idaho
Nonpneumococcal Streptococcal Infections and Rheumatic Fever

Klaus D. Hagspiel, MD
Professor of Radiology, Medicine (Cardiology) and Pediatrics; Chief, Division of Noninvasive Cardiovascular Imaging, Department of Radiology and Medical Imaging, University of Virginia School of Medicine, Charlottesville, Virginia
Noninvasive Cardiac Imaging

H. Hunter Handsfield, MD
Professor of Medicine Emeritus, University of Washington School of Medicine, Seattle, Washington
Neisseria Gonorrhoeae Infections

Raymond C. Harris, MD
Anne and Roscoe R. Robinson Chair and Professor of Medicine and Associate Chair, Division of Nephrology, Medicine, Vanderbilt University School of Medicine, Nashville, Tennessee
Diabetes and the Kidney

Frederick G. Hayden, MD
Stuart S. Richardson Professor Emeritus of Clinical Virology and Professor Emeritus of Medicine, Department of Medicine, University of Virginia School of Medicine, Charlottesville, Virginia
Influenza

Frederick M. Hecht, MD
Professor of Medicine, University of California, San Francisco, School of Medicine, San Francisco, California
Complementary, Alternative, and Integrative Medicine

Douglas C. Heimburger, MD, MS
Professor of Medicine, Vanderbilt University School of Medicine; Associate Director for Education & Training, Vanderbilt Institute for Global Health, Vanderbilt University, Nashville, Tennessee
Nutrition's Interface with Health and Disease

Donald D. Hensrud, MD, MPH
Associate Professor of Preventive Medicine and Nutrition, Mayo Clinic College of Medicine and Science, Rochester, Minnesota
Nutrition's Interface with Health and Disease

Erik L. Hewlett, MD
Professor of Medicine, Microbiology, Immunology and Cancer Biology, University of Virginia School of Medicine, Charlottesville, Virginia
Whooping Cough and Other Bordetella Infections

Richard J. Hift, MMed(Med), PhD
Professor of Medicine, University of KwaZulu-Natal, Durban, KwaZulu-Natal, South Africa
The Porphyrias

David R. Hill, MD, DTM&H
Professor of Medical Sciences, Director, Global Public Health, Quinnipiac University Frank H Netter MD School of Medicine, Hamden, Connecticut
Giardiasis

Nicholas S. Hill, MD
Professor of Medicine, Tufts University School of Medicine; Chief, Division of Pulmonary, Critical Care and Sleep Medicine, Tufts Medical Center, Boston, Massachusetts
Respiratory Monitoring in Critical Care

Christopher D. Hillyer, MD
President and Chief Executive Officer, New York Blood Center; Professor of Medicine, Weill Cornell Medical College, New York, New York
Transfusion Medicine

Brian D. Hoit, MD
Professor of Medicine, Physiology and Biophysics, Case Western Reserve University School of Medicine; Director of Echocardiography, Harrington Heart & Vascular Center, University Hospital Cleveland Medical Center, Cleveland, Ohio
Pericardial Diseases

Steven M. Holland, MD
Director, Division of Intramural Research, Chief, Immunopathogenesis Section, National Institute of Allergy and Infectious Diseases, NIH, Bethesda, Maryland
The Nontuberculous Mycobacteria

Steven M. Hollenberg, MD
Professor of Medicine, Cooper Medical School of Rowan University;
Director, Coronary Care Unit, Cooper University Hospital, Camden,
New Jersey
Cardiogenic Shock

Edward W. Hook, III, MD
Professor of Medicine and Director, Division of Infectious Diseases,
University of Alabama at Birmingham School of Medicine, Birmingham,
Alabama
Granuloma Inguinale (Donovanosis); Syphilis; Nonsyphilitic Treponematoses

Jo Howard, MB BChir
Consultant Haematologist and Lead Clinician, Haematology, Guy's and St
Thomas' National Health Service Foundation Trust; Honorary Reader,
King's College London, London, United Kingdom
Sickle Cell Disease and Other Hemoglobinopathies

David J. Hunter, MBBS, MPH, ScD
Richard Doll Professor of Epidemiology and Medicine, Nuffield
Department of Population Health, University of Oxford, Oxford, United
Kingdom
Epidemiology of Cancer

Khalid Hussain, MB ChB, MD, MSc
Professor of Pediatrics, Weill Cornell Medicine-Qatar; Division Chief-
Endocrinology, Vice Chair for Research, Program Director-Research,
Sidra Medicine, OPC, Doha, Qatar
Hypoglycemia and Pancreatic Islet Cell Disorders

Michael C. Iannuzzi, MD, MBA
Professor and Chairman, Department of Internal Medicine,
Northwell-Staten Island University Hospital and Donald and Barbara
Zucker School of Medicine at Hofstra/Northwell, New York
Sarcoidosis

Robert D. Inman, MD
Professor of Medicine and Immunology, University of Toronto and Kremil
Research Institute, University Health Network, Toronto, Ontario,
Canada
The Spondyloarthropathies

Sharon K. Inouye, MD, MPH
Professor of Medicine, Harvard Medical School; Director, Aging Brain
Center, Marcus Institute for Aging Research-Hebrew SeniorLife, Boston,
Massachusetts
Neuropsychiatric Aspects of Aging; Delirium in the Older Patient

Michael G. Ison, MD, MS
Professor of Medicine (Infectious Diseases) and Surgery (Organ
Transplantation), Northwestern University Feinberg School of Medicine,
Chicago, Illinois
Influenza; Adenovirus Diseases

Karen R. Jacobson, MD, MPH
Assistant Professor of Medicine, Medical Director, Boston Tuberculosis
Clinic, Boston University School of Medicine, Boston, Massachusetts
Tuberculosis

Michael R. Jaff, DO
Professor of Medicine, Harvard Medical School, Boston, Massachusetts;
President, Newton-Wellesley Hospital, Newton, Massachusetts
Other Peripheral Arterial Diseases

Joanna C. Jen, MD, PhD
Professor of Neurology, David Geffen School of Medicine at UCLA, Los
Angeles, California
Neuro-Ophthalmology; Smell and Taste; Hearing and Equilibrium

Dennis M. Jensen, MD
Professor of Medicine, David Geffen School of Medicine at UCLA; Staff
Physician, Medicine-GI, VA Greater Los Angeles Healthcare System;
Director, Human Studies Core & GI Hemostasis Research Unit, CURE
Digestive Diseases Research Center, Los Angeles, California
Gastrointestinal Hemorrhage

Michael D. Jensen, MD
Professor of Medicine, Mayo Clinic College of Medicine and Science,
Rochester, Minnesota
Obesity

Robert T. Jensen, MD
Chief, Cell Biology Section, Digestive Diseases Branch, National Institute
of Diabetes and Digestive and Kidney Diseases, National Institutes of
Health, Bethesda, Maryland
Neuroendocrine Tumors

Alain Joffe, MD, MPH
Retired. Most recently, Associate Professor of Pediatrics, Johns Hopkins
University School of Medicine and Director, Student Health and
Wellness Center, Johns Hopkins University, Baltimore, Maryland
Adolescent Medicine

Stuart Johnson, MD
Professor of Medicine/Infectious Disease, Loyola University Chicago
Stritch School of Medicine, Maywood, Illinois; Physician Researcher,
Research Service, Hines VA Hospital, Hines, Illinois
Clostridial Infections

Robin L. Jones, MD, BSc, MB
Consultant Medical Oncologist, Royal Marsden Hospital and Institute of
Cancer Research, London, United Kingdom
Malignant Tumors of Bone, Sarcomas, and Other Soft Tissue Neoplasms

Sian Jones, MD
Associate Professor of Clinical Medicine, Weill Cornell Medical College,
New York, New York
Systemic Manifestations of HIV/AIDS

Jacqueline Jonklaas, MD, PhD
Professor of Medicine, Georgetown University School of Medicine,
Washington, D.C.
Thyroid

Richard C. Jordan, DDS, PhD
Professor of Pathology, Oral Pathology & Radiation Oncology, University
of California, San Francisco, School of Medicine, San Francisco,
California
Diseases of the Mouth and Salivary Glands

Charles J. Kahi, MD, MS
Professor of Clinical Medicine, Indiana University School of Medicine; GI
Section Chief, Richard L. Roudebush VAMC, Indianapolis, Indiana
Vascular Diseases of the Gastrointestinal Tract

Moses R. Kamya, MB ChB, MMed, MPH, PhD
Professor of Medicine, Makerere University School of Medicine, Kampala,
Uganda
Malaria

Louise W. Kao, MD
Associate Professor of Clinical Emergency Medicine and Director, Medical
Toxicology Fellowship Program, Indiana University School of Medicine,
Indianapolis, Indiana
Chronic Poisoning: Trace Metals and Others

Steven A. Kaplan, MD
Professor of Urology, Icahn School of Medicine at Mount Sinai; Director,
Men's Health Program, Mount Sinai Health System, New York, New
York
Benign Prostatic Hyperplasia and Prostatitis

Daniel L. Kastner, MD, PhD
Scientific Director, Division of Intramural Research, National Human Genome Research Institute, National Institutes of Health, Bethesda, Maryland
The Systemic Autoinflammatory Diseases

David A. Katzka, MD
Professor of Medicine, Mayo Clinic College of Medicine and Science, Rochester, Minnesota
Diseases of the Esophagus

Debra K. Katzman, MD
Professor of Pediatrics, The Hospital for Sick Children and University of Toronto; Senior Associate Scientist, Research Institute; Director, Health Science Research, Faculty of Medicine, University of Toronto, Toronto, Ontario, Canada
Adolescent Medicine

Carol A. Kauffman, MD
Professor of Internal Medicine and Chief, Infectious Diseases, Veterans Affairs Ann Arbor Healthcare System, University of Michigan Medical School, Ann Arbor, Michigan
Endemic Mycoses; Cryptococcosis; Candidiasis

Kenneth Kaushansky, MD
Professor of Medicine, Senior Vice President for Health Sciences, and Dean, Stony Brook University School of Medicine, Stony Brook, New York
Hematopoiesis and Hematopoietic Growth Factors

Keith S. Kaye, MD, MPH
Professor of Medicine, University of Michigan Medical School, Ann Arbor, Michigan
Diseases Caused by Acinetobacter *and* Stenotrophomonas *Species*

Armand Keating, MD
Professor of Medicine and Professor, Institute of Biomaterials and Biomedical Engineering, University of Toronto, Toronto, Canada
Hematopoietic Stem Cell Transplantation

Robin K. Kelley, MD
Associate Professor of Clinical Medicine, University of California, San Francisco, School of Medicine, San Francisco, California
Liver and Biliary Tract Cancers

Morton J. Kern, MD
Professor of Medicine and Associate Chief of Cardiology, University of California, Irvine, Orange, California; Chief of Medicine, Long Beach Veterans Health Care System, Long Beach, California
Catheterization and Angiography

Gerald T. Keusch, MD
Professor of Medicine, Boston University School of Medicine, Boston, Massachusetts
Shigellosis

Fadlo R. Khuri, MD
President and Professor of Hematology and Medical Oncology, American University of Beirut; Adjunct Professor of Medicine, Pharmacology and Otolaryngology, Emory University School of Medicine, Atlanta, Georgia
Lung Cancer and Other Pulmonary Neoplasms

Louis V. Kirchhoff, MD, MPH
Professor of Internal Medicine (Infectious Diseases), Psychiatry, and Epidemiology, University of Iowa Carver College of Medicine and College of Public Health, Iowa City, Iowa
Chagas Disease

Ajay J. Kirtane, MD
Associate Professor of Medicine, Columbia University Vagelos College of Physicians and Surgeons; Chief Academic Officer, Center for Interventional Vascular Therapy; Director, Columbia University Irving Medical Center Cardiac Catheterization Laboratories, New York, New York
Catheterization and Angiography

Amy D. Klion, MD
Senior Clinical Investigator, Laboratory of Parasitic Diseases, National Institute of Allergy and Infectious Diseases, National Institutes of Health, Bethesda, Maryland
Eosinophilic Syndromes

David S. Knopman, MD
Professor of Neurology, Mayo Clinic College of Medicine and Science, Rochester, Minnesota
Regional Cerebral Dysfunction: Higher Mental Functions; Cognitive Impairment and Dementia

Christine J. Ko, MD
Professor of Dermatology and Pathology, Yale University School of Medicine, New Haven, Connecticut
Approach to Skin Diseases

Dimitrios P. Kontoyiannis, MD, ScD
Texas 4000 Distinguished Endowed Professor For Cancer Research, Deputy Head, Division of Internal Medicine, University of Texas MD Anderson Cancer Center, Houston, Texas
Mucormycosis; Mycetoma and Dematiaceous Fungal Infections

Barbara S. Koppel, MD
Chief of Neurology, Metropolitan Hospital, New York, New York and Professor of Clinical Neurology, New York Medical College, Valhalla, New York
Nutritional and Alcohol-Related Neurologic Disorders

Kevin M. Korenblat, MD
Professor of Medicine, Washington University School of Medicine in St. Louis, St. Louis, Missouri
Approach to the Patient with Jaundice or Abnormal Liver Tests

Bruce R. Korf, MD, PhD
Professor of Genetics, University of Alabama at Birmingham and Chief Genomics Officer, UAB Medicine, Birmingham, Alabama
Principles of Genetics

Mark G. Kortepeter, MD, MPH
Professor of Epidemiology, College of Public Health, University of Nebraska, Omaha, Nebraska; Adjunct Professor of Preventive Medicine and Medicine, Uniformed Services University of the Health Sciences, Bethesda, Maryland
Bioterrorism

Shyamasundaran Kottilil, MD, PhD
Professor of Medicine and Associate Chief of Infectious Diseases at the Institute of Human Virology, University of Maryland School of Medicine, Baltimore, Maryland
Antiviral Therapy (Non-HIV)

Joseph A. Kovacs, MD
Senior Investigator, Critical Care Medicine Department, National Institutes of Health Clinical Center, Bethesda, Maryland
Pneumocystis Pneumonia

Thomas O. Kovacs, MD
Professor of Medicine, David Geffen School of Medicine at UCLA, Los Angeles, California
Gastrointestinal Hemorrhage

Kris V. Kowdley, MD
Director, Liver Care Network and Organ Care Research, Swedish Medical Center; Clinical Professor of Medicine, Washington State University, Elson S. Floyd College of Medicine, Seattle, Washington
Iron Overload (Hemochromatosis)

Monica Kraft, MD
Robert and Irene Flinn Professor and Chair, Department of Medicine, Deputy Director, Asthma and Airway Disease Research Center, University of Arizona Health Sciences, Tucson, Arizona
Approach to the Patient with Respiratory Disease

Christopher M. Kramer, MD
Ruth C. Heede Professor of Cardiology and Professor of Radiology, University of Virginia School of Medicine, Charlottesville, Virginia
Noninvasive Cardiac Imaging

Donna M. Krasnewich, MD, PhD
Program Director, NIGMS, National Institutes of Health, Bethesda, Maryland
Lysosomal Storage Diseases

Alexander Kratz, MD, PhD, MPH
Professor of Clinical Pathology and Cell Biology, Columbia University Vagelos College of Physicians and Surgeons; Director, Automated Core Laboratory and Point of Care Testing Service, Columbia University Irving Medical Center and NewYork-Presbyterian Hospital, New York, New York
Reference Intervals and Laboratory Values

Virginia Byers Kraus, MD, PhD
Professor of Medicine, Adjunct Professor of Pathology and Orthopaedic Surgery, Duke University School of Medicine, Duke Molecular Physiology Institute, Durham, North Carolina
Osteoarthritis

William E. Kraus, MD
Richard and Pat Johnson Distinguished University Professor, Duke University School of Medicine, Durham, North Carolina
Physical Activity

Peter J. Krause, MD
Senior Research Scientist, Yale University School of Public Health, Yale University School of Medicine, New Haven, Connecticut
Babesiosis and Other Protozoan Diseases

Daniela Kroshinsky, MD, MPH
Associate Professor of Dermatology, Massachusetts General Hospital, Harvard Medical School, Boston, Massachusetts
Macular, Papular, Purpuric, Vesicobullous, and Pustular Diseases

John F. Kuemmerle, MD
Charles M. Caravati Professor of Medicine, Chair, Division of Gastroenterology, Hepatology and Nutrition, Medical College of Virginia, Virginia Commonwealth University, Richmond, Virginia
Inflammatory and Anatomic Diseases of the Intestine, Peritoneum, Mesentery, and Omentum

Ernst J. Kuipers, MD, PhD
Professor of Medicine, Erasmus MC University Medical Center, Rotterdam, Netherlands
Acid Peptic Disease

Daniel Laheru, MD
Ian T. MacMillan Professorship in Clinical Pancreatic Research, Johns Hopkins University School of Medicine, Baltimore, Maryland
Pancreatic Cancer

Donald W. Landry, MD, PhD
Samuel Bard Professor and Chair, Department of Medicine, Columbia University Vagelos College of Physicians and Surgeons and Physician-in-Chief, Columbia University Irving Medical Center, New York, New York
Approach to the Patient with Renal Disease

Anthony E. Lang, MD
Jack Clark Chair in Parkinson's Disease Research and Director, Division of Neurology, University of Toronto; Director, Morton and Gloria Shulman Movement Disorders Clinic and Edmond J Safra Program in Parkinson's Disease, University Health Network, Toronto Western Hospital, Toronto, Ontario, Canada
Parkinsonism; Other Movement Disorders

Richard A. Lange, MD, MBA
Rick and Ginger Francis Endowed Professor and President, Texas Tech University Health Sciences Center, El Paso; Dean, Paul L. Foster School of Medicine, El Paso, Texas
Acute Coronary Syndrome: Unstable Angina and Non–ST Elevation Myocardial Infarction

Frank A. Lederle, MD[†]
Formerly Professor of Medicine, University of Minnesota School of Medicine; Director of the Minneapolis Veterans Administration Center for Epidemiological and Clinical Research, Minneapolis, Minnesota
Diseases of the Aorta

William M. Lee, MD
Meredith Mosle Chair in Liver Disease and Professor of Internal Medicine, University of Texas Southwestern Medical Center at Dallas, Dallas, Texas
Toxin- and Drug-Induced Liver Disease

James E. Leggett, MD
Department of Medical Education, Providence Portland Medical Center; Associate Professor of Medicine Emeritus, Division of Infectious Diseases, Oregon Health & Science University, Portland, Oregon
Approach to Fever or Suspected Infection in the Normal Host

Glenn N. Levine, MD
Professor of Medicine, Baylor College of Medicine; Director, Cardiac Care Unit, Michael E. DeBakey VA Medical Center, Houston, Texas
Antithrombotic and Antiplatelet Therapy

Marc S. Levine, MD
Emeritus Professor of Radiology, University of Pennsylvania Perelman School of Medicine, Philadelphia, Pennsylvania
Diagnostic Imaging Procedures in Gastroenterology

Stephanie M. Levine, MD
Professor of Medicine, University of Texas Health San Antonio, San Antonio, Texas
Alveolar Filling Disorders

Gary R. Lichtenstein, MD
Professor of Medicine, University of Pennsylvania Perelman School of Medicine; Director, Center for Inflammatory Bowel Disease, Department of Medicine, Hospital of the University of Pennsylvania, Philadelphia, Pennsylvania
Inflammatory Bowel Disease

Jeffrey M. Liebmann, MD
Shirlee and Bernard Brown Professor and Vice Chair, Department of Ophthalmology, Columbia University Vagelos College of Physicians and Surgeons, New York, New York
Diseases of the Visual System

[†]Deceased.

Henry W. Lim, MD
Chairman and C.S. Livingood Chair Emeritus of Dermatology, Henry Ford Hospital; Senior Vice President for Academic Affairs, Henry Ford Health System, Detroit, Michigan
Eczemas, Photodermatoses, Papulosquamous (Including Fungal) Diseases, and Figurate Erythemas

Aldo A.M. Lima, MD, PhD
Professor, Institute of Biomedicine, Federal University of Ceara, Fortaleza, Ceará, Brazil
Cryptosporidiosis; Trematode Infections

Geoffrey S.F. Lin, MD, PhD
Professor of Neurology, Johns Hopkins University School of Medicine, Baltimore, Maryland
Traumatic Brain Injury and Spinal Cord Injury

Mark S. Link, MD
Professor of Medicine, University of Texas Southwestern Medical Center, Dallas, Texas
Electrocardiography

Donald M. Lloyd-Jones, MD, ScM
Chair and Eileen M. Foell Professor of Preventive Medicine, Senior Associate Dean for Clinical & Translational Research, Northwestern University Feinberg School of Medicine, Chicago, Illinois
Epidemiology of Cardiovascular Disease

Bennett Lorber, MD, DSc
Thomas M. Durant Professor of Medicine and Professor of Microbiology and Immunology, Lewis Katz School of Medicine at Temple University, Philadelphia, Pennsylvania
Listeriosis

Arnold Louie, MD
Professor of Medicine, Molecular Genetics and Microbiology and Associate Director, Institute for Therapeutic Innovation, University of Florida College of Medicine, Orlando, Florida
Antibacterial Chemotherapy

Daniel R. Lucey, MD, MPH
Adjunct Professor, Department of Medicine/Infectious Diseases, Georgetown University Medical Center, Washington, D.C.
Anthrax

Jeffrey M. Lyness, MD
Professor of Psychiatry & Neurology and Senior Associate Dean for Academic Affairs, University of Rochester School of Medicine & Dentistry, Rochester, New York
Psychiatric Disorders in Medical Practice

C. Ronald MacKenzie, MD
C. Ronald MacKenzie Chair in Ethics and Medicine, Hospital for Special Surgery; Professor of Clinical Medicine and Medical Ethics, Weill Cornell Medical College, New York, New York
Surgical Treatment of Joint Diseases

Harriet L. MacMillan, CM, MD, MSc
Chedoke Health Chair in Child Psychiatry and Professor of Psychiatry & Behavioural Neurosciences and of Pediatrics, Offord Centre for Child Studies, McMaster University Michael G. DeGroote School of Medicine, Hamilton, Ontario, Canada
Intimate Partner Violence

Robert D. Madoff, MD
Professor of Surgery, University of Minnesota, Minneapolis, Minnesota
Diseases of the Rectum and Anus

Frank Maldarelli, MD, PhD
Head, Clinical Retrovirology Section, HIV Dynamics and Replication Program, NCI-Frederick, Frederick, Maryland
Biology of Human Immunodeficiency Viruses

Atul Malhotra, MD
Kenneth M. Moser Professor of Medicine, Chief of Pulmonary and Critical Care Medicine, Director of Sleep Medicine, University of California, San Diego, School of Medicine, La Jolla, California
Disorders of Ventilatory Control

Mark J. Manary, MD
Helene B. Roberson Professor of Pediatrics, Washington University School of Medicine in St. Louis, St. Louis, Missouri; Senior Lecturer, Department of Community Health, University of Malawi College of Medicine, Blantyre, Malawi
Protein-Energy Malnutrition

Peter Manu, MD
Professor of Medicine and Psychiatry, Donald and Barbara Zucker School of Medicine at Hofstra/Northwell, Hempstead, New York; Director of Medical Services, South Oaks Hospital, Amityville, New York
Medical Consultation in Psychiatry

Luis A. Marcos, MD, MPH
Associate Professor of Clinical Medicine, School of Medicine, Stony Brook University, Stony Brook, New York
Trematode Infections

Ariane J. Marelli, MD, MPH
Professor of Medicine and Director, McGill Adult Unit for Congenital Heart Disease, McGill University Health Centre, Montreal, Quebec, Canada
Congenital Heart Disease in Adults

Xavier Mariette, MD, PhD
Professor of Rheumatology, Université Paris-Sud, AP-HP, Le Kremlin Bicêtre, France
Sjögren Syndrome

Andrew R. Marks, MD
Wu Professor and Chair, Department of Physiology and Cellular Biophysics, Director, Helen and Clyde Wu Center for Molecular Cardiology, Columbia University Vagelos College of Physicians & Surgeons, New York, New York
Cardiac and Circulatory Function

Kieren A. Marr, MD
Professor of Medicine and Oncology and Director, Transplant and Oncology Infectious Diseases, John Hopkins University School of Medicine, Baltimore, Maryland
Approach to Fever and Suspected Infection in the Immunocompromised Host

Thomas J. Marrie, MD
Professor of Medicine and Dean Emeritus, Faculty of Medicine, Dalhousie University, Halifax, Nova Scotia, Canada
Legionella Infections

Paul Martin, MD
Professor of Medicine and Chief, Division of Gastroenterology and Hepatology, University of Miami Miller School of Medicine, Miami, Florida
Approach to the Patient with Liver Disease

Fernando J. Martinez, MD, MS
Bruce Webster Professor of Internal Medicine and Chief, Division of Pulmonary and Critical Care Medicine, Weill Cornell Medical College, New York, New York
Interstitial Lung Disease

Joel B. Mason, MD
Professor of Medicine and Nutrition, Tufts University School of Medicine; Director, Vitamins & Carcinogenesis Laboratory, U.S.D.A. Human Nutrition Research Center at Tufts University, Boston, Massachusetts
Vitamins, Trace Minerals, and Other Micronutrients

Henry Masur, MD
Chief, Critical Care Medicine Department, Clinical Center, National
  Institutes of Health, Bethesda, Maryland
  *Microbial Complications in Patients Infected with Human Immunodeficiency
  Virus*

Amy J. Mathers, MD
Associate Professor of Medicine and Pathology, Associate Director of
  Clinical Microbiology, Medical Director Antimicrobial Stewardship,
  University of Virginia School of Medicine, Charlottesville, Virginia
  *Infections Due to Other Members of the Enterobacteriaceae, Including
  Management of Multidrug-Resistant Strains*

Eric L. Matteson, MD, MPH
Professor of Medicine, Mayo Clinic College of Medicine and Science,
  Rochester, Minnesota
  Infections of Bursae, Joints, and Bones

Michael A. Matthay, MD
Professor of Medicine and Anesthesia, University of California, San
  Francisco, San Francisco, California
  Acute Respiratory Failure

Emeran A. Mayer, MD
Professor of Medicine and Psychiatry, Executive Director G. Oppenheimer
  Center for Neurobiology of Stress and Resilience, David Geffen School
  of Medicine at UCLA, Los Angeles, California
  *Functional Gastrointestinal Disorders: Irritable Bowel Syndrome, Dyspepsia,
  Esophageal Chest Pain, and Heartburn*

Stephan A. Mayer, MD
William T. Gossett Endowed Chair of Neurology, Henry Ford Health
  System, Professor of Neurology, Wayne State University School of
  Medicine, Detroit, Michigan
  Hemorrhagic Cerebrovascular Disease

F. Dennis McCool, MD
Professor of Medicine, Warren Alpert Medical School of Brown University,
  Providence, Rhode Island; Memorial Hospital of Rhode Island,
  Pawtucket, Rhode Island
  Diseases of the Diaphragm, Chest Wall, Pleura, and Mediastinum

Iain McInnes, PhD
Professor of Experimental Medicine and Director, Institute of Infection,
  Immunity and Inflammation, University of Glasgow, Glasgow, United
  Kingdom
  Rheumatoid Arthritis

William J. McKenna, MD
Emeritus Professor of Cardiology, Institute of Cardiovascular Science,
  University College London, London, United Kingdom
  Diseases of the Myocardium and Endocardium

Vallerie McLaughlin, MD
Professor of Medicine, University of Michigan Medical School; Director,
  Pulmonary Hypertension Program, Ann Arbor, Michigan
  Pulmonary Hypertension

John J.V. McMurray, BSc, MB ChB, MD
Professor of Medical Cardiology, British Heart Foundation Cardiovascular
  Research Centre, University of Glasgow; Honorary Consultant
  Cardiologist, Queen Elizabeth University Hospital Glasgow, Glasgow,
  Scotland, United Kingdom
  Heart Failure: Management and Prognosis

Kenneth R. McQuaid, MD
Professor of Clinical Medicine and Vice-Chair, Department of Medicine,
  University of California, San Francisco, School of Medicine; Chief of
  Gastroenterology and of the Medical Service, San Francisco Veterans,
  Affairs Medical Center, San Francisco, California
  Approach to the Patient with Gastrointestinal Disease

Paul S. Mead, MD, MPH
Chief, Bacterial Diseases Branch, Division of Vector-Borne Diseases,
  Centers for Disease Control and Prevention, Fort Collins, Colorado
  Plague and Other Yersinia Infections

Robert T. Means, Jr., MD
Professor of Internal Medicine, East Tennessee State University James H.
  Quillen College of Medicine, Johnson City, Tennessee
  Approach to the Anemias

Graeme Meintjes, MB ChB, MPH, PhD
Professor of Medicine, University of Cape Town, Cape Town, South Africa
  Immune Reconstitution Inflammatory Syndrome in HIV/AIDS

Genevieve B. Melton-Meaux, MD, PhD
Professor of Surgery, University of Minnesota Medical School,
  Minneapolis, Minnesota
  Diseases of the Rectum and Anus

Samuel T. Merrick, MD
Professor of Clinical Medicine, Weill Cornell Medical College, New York,
  New York
  Systemic Manifestations of HIV/AIDS

Marc Michel, MD
Professor and Head of the Unit of Internal Medicine, Henri Mondor
  University Hospital, Assistance Publique Hopitaux de Paris, Université
  Paris-Est Créteil, Creteil, France
  Autoimmune and Intravascular Hemolytic Anemias

Jonathan W. Mink, MD, PhD
Professor of Neurology, University of Rochester School of Medicine &
  Dentistry, Rochester, New York
  Congenital, Developmental, and Neurocutaneous Disorders

William E. Mitch, MD
Professor of Medicine, Baylor College of Medicine, Houston, Texas
  Chronic Kidney Disease

Bruce A. Molitoris, MD
Distinguished Professor of Medicine, Indiana University School of
  Medicine, Indianapolis, Indiana
  Acute Kidney Injury

José G. Montoya, MD
Professor of Medicine, Division of Infectious Diseases and Geographic
  Medicine, Stanford University School of Medicine, Stanford, California;
  Director, Palo Alto Medical Foundation Toxoplasma Serology
  Laboratory, National Reference Center for the Study and Diagnosis of
  Toxoplasmosis, Palo Alto, California
  Toxoplasmosis

Ernest Moy, MD, MPH
Executive Director, Office of Health Equity, Veterans Health
  Administration, Washington, D.C.
  Measuring Health and Health Care

Debabrata Mukherjee, MD, MS
Professor and Chairman, Department of Internal Medicine, Chief,
  Cardiovascular Medicine, Texas Tech University Health Sciences Center,
  El Paso, Texas
  *Acute Coronary Syndrome: Unstable Angina and Non–ST Elevation Myocardial
  Infarction*

Andrew H. Murr, MD
Professor and Chairman, Department of Otolaryngology-Head and Neck
  Surgery, University of California, San Francisco, School of Medicine, San
  Francisco, California
  Approach to the Patient with Nose, Sinus, and Ear Disorders

Daniel M. Musher, MD
Distinguished Service Professor of Medicine and Professor of Molecular Virology and Microbiology, Baylor College of Medicine; Staff Physician, Infectious Disease Section, Michael E. DeBakey VA Medical Center, Houston, Texas
Overview of Pneumonia

Robert J. Myerburg, MD
Professor of Medicine and Physiology, Department of Medicine, University of Miami Miller School of Medicine, Miami, Florida
Approach to Cardiac Arrest and Life-Threatening Arrhythmias

Kari C. Nadeau, MD, PhD
Naddisy Family Foundation Professor of Allergy and Director, Sean N. Parker Center for Allergy and Asthma Research at Stanford University, Stanford, California
Approach to the Patient with Allergic or Immunologic Disease

Stanley J. Naides, MD
President, Stanley J. Naides, M.D., P.C., Dana Point, California
Arboviruses Causing Fever and Rash Syndromes

Theodore E. Nash, MD
Principal Investigator, Clinical Parasitology Section, National Institutes of Allergy and Infectious Diseases, National Institutes of Health, Bethesda, Maryland
Giardiasis

Avindra Nath, MD
Chief, Section of Infections of the Nervous System, National Institutes of Neurological Diseases and Stroke, National Institutes of Health, Bethesda, Maryland
Cytomegalovirus, Epstein-Barr Virus, and Slow Virus Infections of the Central Nervous System; Meningitis: Bacterial, Viral, and Other; Brain Abscess and Parameningeal Infections

Genevieve Neal-Perry, MD, PhD
Professor of Obstetrics and Gynecology and Director of the Reproductive Endocrinology and Infertility Center, University of Washington School of Medicine, Seattle, Washington
Menopause

Anne T. Neff, MD
Professor of Medicine, Hematology/Medical Oncology, Cleveland Clinic Lerner College of Medicine; Staff Physician, Cleveland Clinic Foundation, Cleveland, Ohio
Von Willebrand Disease and Hemorrhagic Abnormalities of Platelet and Vascular Function

Eric G. Neilson, MD
Vice President for Medical Affairs and Lewis Landsberg Dean and Professor of Medicine and of Cell and Developmental Biology, Northwestern University Feinberg School of Medicine, Chicago, Illinois
Tubulointerstitial Diseases

Christina A. Nelson, MD, MPH
Medical Officer, Bacterial Diseases Branch, Division of Vector-Borne Diseases, Centers for Disease Control and Prevention, Fort Collins, Colorado
Plague and Other Yersinia Infections

Lewis S. Nelson, MD
Professor and Chair, Department of Emergency Medicine; Director, Division of Medical Toxicology, Rutgers New Jersey Medical School, Newark, New Jersey
Acute Poisoning

Eric J. Nestler, MD, PhD
Nash Family Professor of Neuroscience, Director, Friedman Brain Institute, Icahn School of Medicine at Mount Sinai, New York, New York
Biology of Addiction

Anne B. Newman, MD, MPH
Distinguished Professor and Chair, Department of Epidemiology, Katherine M. Detre Endowed Chair of Population Health Sciences; Director, Center for Aging and Population Health, Professor of Medicine, and Clinical and Translational Science Graduate School of Public Health, University of Pittsburgh; Clinical Director, Aging Institute of UPMC and Pitt, Pittsburgh, Pennsylvania
Epidemiology of Aging: Implications of an Aging Society

Lindsay E. Nicolle, MD
Professor Emeritus, Department of Internal Medicine, University of Manitoba, Winnipeg, Manitoba, Canada
Approach to the Patient with Urinary Tract Infection

Lynnette K. Nieman, MD
Senior Investigator, Diabetes, Endocrinology and Obesity Branch, NIDDK/NIH, Bethesda, Maryland
Approach to the Patient with Endocrine Disease; Adrenal Cortex; Polyglandular Disorders

Gaetane Nocturne, MD, PhD
Associate Professor of Rheumatology, Université Paris-Sud, AP-HP, Le Kremlin Bicêtre, France
Sjögren Syndrome

Christopher M. O'Connor, MD
Adjunct Professor of Medicine, Duke University School of Medicine, Durham, North Carolina; CEO, Inova Heart and Vascular Institute, Fairfax, Virginia
Heart Failure: Pathophysiology and Diagnosis

Francis G. O'Connor, MD, MPH
Professor and Medical Director, Consortium for Health and Military Performance, Uniformed Services University of the Health Sciences, Bethesda, Maryland
Disorders Due to Heat and Cold; Rhabdomyolysis

Patrick G. O'Connor, MD, MPH
Dan Adams and Amanda Adams Professor and Chief, General Internal Medicine, Yale University School of Medicine, New Haven, Connecticut
Alcohol Use Disorders

James R. O'Dell, MD
Bruce Professor and Vice Chair of Internal Medicine, University of Nebraska Medical Center College of Medicine; Chief of Rheumatology, Medicine, Omaha VA, Omaha, Nebraska
Rheumatoid Arthritis

Anne E. O'Donnell, MD
The Nehemiah and Naomi Cohen Chair in Pulmonary Disease Research, Chief, Division of Pulmonary, Critical Care and Sleep Medicine, Georgetown University Medical Center, Washington, D.C.
Bronchiectasis, Atelectasis, Cysts, and Localized Lung Disorders

Jae K. Oh, MD
Professor of Medicine, Mayo Clinic College of Medicine and Science, Rochester, Minnesota; Director, Heart Vascular Stroke Institute, Samsung Medical Center, Seoul, Gangnam, South Korea
Pericardial Diseases

Pablo C. Okhuysen, MD
Professor of Infectious Diseases, Infection Control and Employee Health, University of Texas MD Anderson Cancer Center; Adjunct Professor of Infectious Diseases, Baylor College of Medicine; Adjunct Professor of Epidemiology, Human Genetics and Environmental Health, University of Texas School of Public Health; Adjunct Professor of Infectious Diseases, McGovern Medical School at the University of Texas Health Science Center at Houston, Houston, Texas
Approach to the Patient with Suspected Enteric Infection

Michael S. Okun, MD
Professor and Chair of Neurology, Fixel Institute for Neurological Diseases, University of Florida College of Medicine, Gainesville, Florida
Parkinsonism; Other Movement Disorders

Jeffrey E. Olgin, MD
Gallo-Chatterjee Distinguished Professor and Chief of Cardiology, University of California, San Francisco, School of Medicine, San Francisco, California
Approach to the Patient with Suspected Arrhythmia

Nancy J. Olsen, MD
Professor of Medicine, Penn State Milton S. Hershey Medical Center, Hershey, Pennsylvania
Biologic Agents and Signaling Inhibitors

Walter A. Orenstein, MD, DSc
Professor of Medicine, Pediatrics, Epidemiology & Global Health, Emory University School of Medicine; Associate Director, Emory Vaccine Center, Atlanta, Georgia
Immunization

John J. O'Shea, MD
Scientific Director, National Institute of Arthritis and Musculoskeletal and Skin Diseases, National Institutes of Health, Bethesda, Maryland
Biologic Agents and Signaling Inhibitors

Douglas R. Osmon, MD
Professor of Medicine, Mayo Clinic College of Medicine and Science; Consultant, Division Infectious Disease, Mayo Clinic, Rochester, Minnesota
Infections of Bursae, Joints, and Bones

Catherine M. Otto, MD
J. Ward Kennedy-Hamilton Endowed Chair in Cardiology and Professor of Medicine, University of Washington School of Medicine; Director, Heart Valve Clinic, Associate Director, Echocardiography, University of Washington Medical Center, Seattle, Washington
Echocardiography

Martin G. Ottolini, MD
Professor of Pediatrics and Director, Capstone Student Research Program, Uniformed Services University of the Health Sciences; Consultant, Pediatric Infectious Diseases, Pediatrics, Walter Reed National Military Medical Center, Bethesda, Maryland
Measles

Peter G. Pappas, MD
Professor of Medicine, University of Alabama at Birmingham School of Medicine, Birmingham, Alabama
Candidiasis; Mycetoma and Dematiaceous Fungal Infections

Ben Ho Park, MD, PhD
The Donna S. Hall Professor of Medicine, Vanderbilt University School of Medicine; Co-Leader Breast Cancer Research; Director of Precision Oncology; Associate Director for Translational Research, Vanderbilt-Ingram Cancer Center, Nashville, Tennessee
Cancer Biology and Genetics

Pankaj Jay Pasricha, MD
Professor of Medicine and Neuroscience, Johns Hopkins University School of Medicine, Baltimore, Maryland
Gastrointestinal Endoscopy

Manisha Patel, MD, MS
Measles, Mumps, Rubella, Herpesvirus, and Domestic Polio Epidemiology Team Lead, National Center for Immunization and Respiratory Diseases, Centers for Disease Control and Prevention, Atlanta, Georgia
Mumps

Robin Patel, MD
Elizabeth P. and Robert E. Allen Professor of Individualized Medicine and Professor of Medicine and of Microbiology; Chair, Division of Clinical Microbiology; Consultant, Divisions of Clinical Microbiology and Infectious Diseases; Director, Infectious Diseases Research Laboratory, Mayo Clinic College of Medicine and Science, Rochester, Minnesota
Introduction to Microbial Disease: Pathophysiology and Diagnostics

David L. Paterson, MBBS, PhD
Professor of Medicine and Director, Centre for Clinical Research, University of Queensland, Herston, Queensland; Consultant Infectious Diseases Physician, Department of Infectious Diseases, Royal Brisbane and Women's Hospital, Brisbane, Australia
Infections Due to Other Members of the Enterobacteriaceae, Including Management of Multidrug-Resistant Strains

Jean-Michel Pawlotsky, MD, PhD
Professor, Department of Virology, Henri Mondor University Hospital, Creteil, France
Acute Viral Hepatitis; Chronic Viral and Autoimmune Hepatitis

Thomas H. Payne, MD
Professor of Medicine, University of Washington School of Medicine; Medical Director, Information Technology Services, UW Medicine, Seattle, Washington
Statistical Interpretation of Data and Using Data for Clinical Decisions

Richard D. Pearson, MD
Professor Emeritus of Medicine, University of Virginia School of Medicine, Charlottesville, Virginia
Antiparasitic Therapy

Trish M. Perl, MD, MSc
Jay Sanford Professor of Medicine and Chief of Infectious Diseases and Geographic Medicine, University of Texas Southwestern Medical Center Dallas, Texas
Enterococcal Infections

Michael A. Pesce, PhD
Professor Emeritus of Pathology and Cell Biology, Columbia University Vagelos College of Physicians and Surgeons, New York, New York
Reference Intervals and Laboratory Values

Brett W. Petersen, MD, MPH
Epidemiology Team Lead, Poxvirus and Rabies Branch, Centers for Disease Control and Prevention, Atlanta, Georgia
Smallpox, Monkeypox, and Other Poxvirus Infections

William A. Petri, Jr., MD, PhD
Wade Hampton Frost Professor of Epidemiology and Vice Chair for Research, Department of Medicine, University of Virginia School of Medicine, Charlottesville, Virginia
Relapsing Fever and Other Borrelia Infections; African Sleeping Sickness; Amebiasis

Marc A. Pfeffer, MD, PhD
Dzau Professor of Medicine, Harvard Medical School; Senior Physician, Brigham and Women's Hospital, Boston, Massachusetts
Heart Failure: Management and Prognosis

David S. Pisetsky, MD, PhD
Professor of Medicine and Immunology, Duke University School of Medicine, Chief, Rheumatology, VA Medical Center, Durham, North Carolina
Laboratory Testing in the Rheumatic Diseases

Frank Powell, PhD
Professor of Medicine, University of California, San Diego, School of Medicine, La Jolla, California
Disorders of Ventilatory Control

Reed E. Pyeritz, MD, PhD
Professor of Medicine, University of Pennsylvania Perelman School of Medicine, Philadelphia, Pennsylvania
Inherited Diseases of Connective Tissue

Thomas C. Quinn, MD, MSc
Professor of Medicine and Pathology, Director, Center for Global Health, Johns Hopkins University School of Medicine; Associate Director, National Institute of Allergy and Infectious Diseases, National Institutes of Health, Baltimore, Maryland
Epidemiology and Diagnosis of Human Immunodeficiency Virus Infection and Acquired Immunodeficiency Syndrome

Jai Radhakrishnan, MD, MS
Professor of Medicine, Columbia University Vagelos College of Physicians and Surgeons; Clinical Chief, Division of Nephrology, Columbia University Irving Medical Center, New York, New York
Glomerular Disorders and Nephrotic Syndromes

Jerald Radich, MD
Associate Professor of Medical Oncology, Clinical Research Division, Fred Hutchinson Cancer Research Center and University of Washington School of Medicine, Seattle, Washington
Chronic Myeloid Leukemia

Petros I. Rafailidis, MD, PhD, MSc
Assistant Professor Internal Medicine-Infectious Diseases, Democritus University of Thrace; Beta University Department of Internal Medicine, University General Hospital of Greece, Alexandroupolis, Greece; Senior Researcher, Alfa Institute of Biomedical Sciences, Athens, Greece
Pseudomonas and Related Gram-Negative Bacillary Infections

Ganesh Raghu, MD
Professor of Medicine and Laboratory Medicine (adjunct), University of Washington School of Medicine; Director, Center for Interstitial Lung Diseases, UW Medicine; Co-Director, Scleroderma Clinic, University of Washington Medical Center, Seattle, Washington
Interstitial Lung Disease

Margaret V. Ragni, MD, MPH
Professor of Medicine, and Clinical Translational Science, University of Pittsburgh School of Medicine; Director, Hemophilia Center of Western Pennsylvania, Pittsburgh, Pennsylvania
Hemorrhagic Disorders: Coagulation Factor Deficiencies

Srinivasa N. Raja, MD
Professor of Anesthesiology, Critical Care Medicine, and Neurology; Director of Pain Research, Division of Pain Medicine, Johns Hopkins University School of Medicine, Baltimore, Maryland
Pain

S. Vincent Rajkumar, MD
Edward W. and Betty Knight Scripps Professor of Medicine, Mayo Clinic College of Medicine and Science, Rochester, Minnesota
Plasma Cell Disorders

James D. Ralston, MD, MPH
Senior Investigator, Kaiser Permanente Washington Health Research Institute, Seattle, Washington
Comprehensive Chronic Disease Management

Stuart H. Ralston, MB ChB
Professor of Rheumatology, University of Edinburgh, Edinburgh, United Kingdom
Paget Disease of Bone

Didier Raoult, MD, PhD
Professor, Aix-Marseille Université, Faculté de Médecine, Chief, Institut Hospitalo-Universitaire Méditerranée-Infection, Marseille, France
Bartonella Infections; Rickettsial Infections

Adam J. Ratner, MD, MPH
Associate Professor of Pediatrics and Microbiology and Chief, Division of Pediatric Infectious Diseases, New York University School of Medicine, New York, New York
Haemophilus and Moraxella Infections

Annette C. Reboli, MD
Dean and Professor of Medicine, Cooper Medical School of Rowan University and Cooper University Hospital, Camden, New Jersey
Erysipelothrix Infections

K. Rajender Reddy, MD
Ruimy Family President's Distinguished Professor of Internal Medicine, University of Pennsylvania Perelman School of Medicine, Philadelphia, Pennsylvania
Bacterial, Parasitic, Fungal, and Granulomatous Liver Diseases

Donald A. Redelmeier, MD
Professor of Medicine, University of Toronto; Canada Research Chair, Medical Decision Science; Senior Scientist, Evaluative Clinical Sciences, Sunnybrook Research Institute; Staff Physician, Sunnybrook Health Sciences Centre, Toronto, Ontario, Canada
Postoperative Care and Complications

Susan E. Reef, MD
Medical Epidemiologist, Global Immunization Division, Centers for Disease Control and Prevention, Atlanta, Georgia
Rubella (German Measles)

John Reilly, MD
Richard D. Krugman Endowed Chair and Dean, School of Medicine, and Vice Chancellor for Health Affairs, University of Colorado School of Medicine, Aurora, Colorado
Chronic Obstructive Pulmonary Disease

Megan E. Reller, MD, PhD
Associate Professor of Medicine, Duke University School of Medicine, Durham, North Carolina
Zoonoses

Neil M. Resnick, MD
Thomas Detre Professor of Medicine and Chief, Division of Geriatric Medicine and Gerontology, University of Pittsburgh Medical Center, Pittsburgh, Pennsylvania
Urinary Incontinence

David B. Reuben, MD
Archstone Professor and Chief, Division of Geriatrics, David Geffen School of Medicine at UCLA, Los Angeles, California
Geriatric Assessment

Jennifer G. Robinson, MD, MPH
Professor of Epidemiology and Medicine, Director, Prevention Intervention Center, Department of Epidemiology, University of Iowa Carver College of Medicine, Iowa City, Iowa
Disorders of Lipid Metabolism

Inez Rogatsky, PhD
Professor of Microbiology and Immunology, Weill Cornell Medical College; Senior Scientist, Arthritis and Tissue Degeneration Program, Hospital for Special Surgery, New York, New York
Immunomodulatory Drugs

Joseph G. Rogers, MD
Professor of Medicine, Duke University School of Medicine, Durham, North Carolina
Heart Failure: Pathophysiology and Diagnosis

Jean-Marc Rolain, PharmD, PhD
Professor, Aix-Marseille Université and Institut Hospitalo-Universitaire Méditerranée Infection, Marseille, France
Bartonella Infections

Barrett J. Rollins, MD, PhD
Linde Family Professor of Medicine, Dana-Farber Cancer Institute, Brigham & Women's Hospital and Harvard Medical School, Boston, Massachusetts
Histiocytoses

José R. Romero, MD
Horace C. Cabe Professor of Infectious Diseases, Department of Pediatrics, University of Arkansas for Medical Sciences; Director, Pediatric Infectious Diseases Section, Arkansas Children's Hospital; Director, Clinical Trials Research, Arkansas Children's Research Institute, Little Rock, Arkansas
Enteroviruses

Karen Rosene-Montella, MD
President, Karen Rosene, LLC; Senior Consultant the Levinson Institute; Professor Emerita of Medicine, Warren Alpert Medical School at Brown University, Providence, Rhode Island
Common Medical Problems in Pregnancy

Philip J. Rosenthal, MD
Professor of Medicine, University of California, San Francisco, School of Medicine, San Francisco, California
Malaria

James A. Russell, MD
Professor of Medicine, University of British Columbia, Vancouver, British Columbia
Shock Syndromes Related to Sepsis

Anil K. Rustgi, MD
Irving Professor of Medicine, Director, Herbert Irving Comprehensive Cancer Center; Chief, NewYork-Presbyterian Hospital/Columbia University Irving Medical Center Cancer Service, Columbia University Vagelos College of Physicians and Surgeons, New York, New York
Neoplasms of the Esophagus and Stomach

Daniel E. Rusyniak, MD
Professor of Emergency Medicine, Indiana University School of Medicine, Indianapolis, Indiana
Chronic Poisoning: Trace Metals and Others

George Sakoulas, MD
Associate Adjunct Professor, Division of Host-Microbe Systems & Therapeutics, University of California, San Diego, School of Medicine, La Jolla, California; Infectious Disease Consultant, Sharp Healthcare, San Diego, California
Staphylococcal Infections

Robert A. Salata, MD
STERIS Chair of Excellence in Medicine, Professor and Chairman, Department of Medicine, Case Western Reserve University School of Medicine; Physician-in-Chief, Master Clinician in Infectious Diseases, University Hospitals Cleveland Medical Center, Cleveland, Ohio
Brucellosis

Jane E. Salmon, MD
Collette Kean Research Chair, Hospital for Special Surgery; Professor of Medicine, Weill Cornell Medical College, New York, New York
Mechanisms of Immune-Mediated Tissue Injury

Edsel Maurice T. Salvana, MD, DTM&H
Associate Professor of Medicine and Director, Institute of Molecular Biology and Biotechnology, National Institutes of Health, University of the Philippines College of Medicine, Manila, Philippines
Brucellosis

Nanette Santoro, MD
Professor and E. Stewart Taylor Chair, Department of Obstetrics and Gynecology, University of Colorado School of Medicine, Aurora, Colorado
Menopause

Renato M. Santos, MD
Assistant Professor of Medicine, Emory University School of Medicine, Emory Heart and Vascular Center, John's Creek, Georgia
Vascular Disorders of the Kidney

Peter A. Santucci, MD
Professor of Medicine, Loyola University Medical Center, Maywood, Illinois
Electrophysiologic Interventional Procedures and Surgery

Patrice Savard, MD, MSc
Assistant Professor of Microbiology and Immunology, Université de Montréal; Director, Unité de Prévention, Centre Hospitalier de l'Université de Montréal, Québec, Canada
Enterococcal Infections

Michael N. Sawka, PhD
Professor, School of Biological Sciences, Georgia Institute of Technology, Atlanta, Georgia
Disorders Due to Heat and Cold

Paul D. Scanlon, MD
Professor of Medicine, Mayo Clinic College of Medicine and Science, Rochester, Minnesota
Respiratory Testing and Function

Andrew I. Schafer, MD
Professor of Medicine, Director, Richard T. Silver Center for Myeloproliferative Neoplasms, Weill Cornell Medical College, New York, New York
Approach to Medicine, the Patient, and the Medical Profession: Medicine as a Learned and Humane Profession; Thrombotic Disorders: Hypercoagulable States; Approach to the Patient with Bleeding and Thrombosis; Hemorrhagic Disorders: Disseminated Intravascular Coagulation, Liver Failure, and Vitamin K Deficiency

William Schaffner, MD
Professor of Preventive Medicine, Vanderbilt University School of Medicine, Nashville, Tennessee
Tularemia and Other Francisella Infections

W. Michael Scheld, MD
Bayer-Gerald L. Mandell Professor of Infectious Diseases; Professor of Medicine; Clinical Professor of Neurosurgery; David A. Harrison Distinguished Educator, University of Virginia Health System, Charlottesville, Virginia
Introduction to Microbial Disease: Pathophysiology and Diagnostics

Manuel Schiff, MD, PhD
Associate Professor of Pediatrics and Head of Metabolic Unit, Reference Center for Inborn Errors of Metabolism, Robert Debré University Hospital, Paris, France
Homocystinuria and Hyperhomocysteinemia

Michael L. Schilsky, MD
Professor of Medicine and Surgery, Yale University School of Medicine, New Haven, Connecticut
Wilson Disease

Robert T. Schooley, MD
Professor of Medicine, University of California, San Diego, School of Medicine, San Diego, California
Epstein-Barr Virus Infection

David L. Schriger, MD, MPH
Professor of Emergency Medicine, David Geffen School of Medicine at UCLA, Los Angeles, California
Approach to the Patient with Abnormal Vital Signs

Lynn M. Schuchter, MD
Professor of Medicine, C. Willard Robinson Professor and Chair of the Division of Hematology-Oncology, University of Pennsylvania Perelman School of Medicine, Philadelphia, Pennsylvania
Melanoma and Nonmelanoma Skin Cancers

Sam Schulman, MD, PhD
Professor of Medicine, McMaster University Michael G. DeGroote School of Medicine, Hamilton, Ontario, Canada
Antithrombotic and Antiplatelet Therapy

Lawrence B. Schwartz, MD, PhD
Charles and Evelyn Thomas Professor of Medicine, Medical College of Virginia, Virginia Commonwealth University, Richmond, Virginia
Systemic Anaphylaxis, Food Allergy, and Insect Sting Allergy

Carlos Seas, MD, MSc
Associate Professor of Medicine, Universidad Peruana Cayetano Heredia; Vice Director, Alexander von Humboldt Tropical Medicine Institute, Attending Physician, Infectious and Tropical Medicine, Hospital Nacional Cayetano Heredia, Lima, Peru
Cholera and Other Vibrio *Infections*

Steven A. Seifert, MD
Professor of Emergency Medicine, University of New Mexico School of Medicine; Medical Director, New Mexico Poison and Drug Information Center, Albuquerque, New Mexico
Envenomation, Bites, and Stings

Julian Lawrence Seifter, MD
James G. Haidas Distinguished Chair in Medicine, Brigham and Women's Hospital and Harvard Medical School, Boston, Massachusetts
Potassium Disorders; Acid-Base Disorders

Duygu Selcen, MD
Professor of Neurology and Pediatrics, Mayo Clinic College of Medicine and Science, Rochester, Minnesota
Muscle Diseases

Carol E. Semrad, MD
Professor of Medicine, University of Chicago Pritzker School of Medicine, Chicago, Illinois
Approach to the Patient with Diarrhea and Malabsorption

Harry Shamoon, MD
Professor of Medicine and Senior Associate Dean for Clinical & Translational Research, Albert Einstein College of Medicine; Director, Harold and Muriel Block Institute for Clinical and Translational Research at Einstein and Montefiore, Bronx, New York
Diabetes Mellitus

Pamela J. Shaw, DBE, MBBS, MD
Professor of Neurology, Sheffield Institute for Translational Neuroscience, University of Sheffield, Sheffield, United Kingdom
Amyotrophic Lateral Sclerosis and Other Motor Neuron Diseases

Beth H. Shaz, MD
Chief Medical and Scientific Officer, New York Blood Center; Adjunct Assistant Professor, Department of Pathology and Cell Biology, Columbia University Vagelos College of Physicians and Surgeons, New York, New York
Transfusion Medicine

Robert L. Sheridan, MD
Professor of Surgery, Harvard Medical School and Massachusetts General Hospital, COL (ret), U.S. Army, Boston, Massachusetts
Medical Aspects of Trauma and Burns

Stuart Sherman, MD
Glen A. Lehman Professor of Gastroenterology and Professor of Medicine and Radiology; Clinical Director of Gastroenterology and Hepatology, Indiana University School of Medicine, Indianapolis, Indiana
Diseases of the Gallbladder and Bile Ducts

Wun-Ju Shieh, MD, MPH, PhD
Deputy Chief/Medical Officer, Infectious Diseases Pathology Branch, Centers for Disease Control and Prevention, Atlanta, Georgia
Leptospirosis

Michael E. Shy, MD
Professor of Neurology and Pediatrics, University of Iowa Carver College of Medicine, Iowa City, Iowa
Peripheral Neuropathies

Ellen Sidransky, MD
Chief, Section of Molecular Neurogenetics, Medical Genetics Branch, NHGRI, National Institutes of Health, Bethesda, Maryland
Lysosomal Storage Diseases

Richard M. Siegel, MD, PhD
Clinical Director and Chief, Autoimmunity Branch, National Institute of Arthritis and Musculoskeletal and Skin Diseases, National Institutes of Health, Bethesda, Maryland
The Systemic Autoinflammatory Diseases

Costi D. Sifri, MD
Professor of Medicine and Medical Director, Immunocompromised Infectious Diseases Program, University of Virginia Health System, Charlottesville, Virginia
Approach to Fever and Suspected Infection in the Immunocompromised Host

Robert F. Siliciano, MD, PhD
Professor of Medicine, Johns Hopkins University School of Medicine; Investigator, Howard Hughes Medical Institute, Baltimore, Maryland
Immunopathogenesis of Human Immunodeficiency Virus Infection

Michael S. Simberkoff, MD
Professor of Medicine, New York University School of Medicine and Chief of Staff, VA New York Harbor Healthcare System, New York, New York
Haemophilus and Moraxella Infections

David L. Simel, MD, MHS
Professor of Medicine, Duke University School of Medicine; Chief of Medical Service, Durham Veterans Affairs Medical Center, Durham, North Carolina
Approach to the Patient: History and Physical Examination

Karl Skorecki, MD
Professor and Dean, Azriel Faculty of Medicine, Bar-Ilan University, Ramat Gan, Israel
Regenerative Medicine, Cell, and Gene Therapies

Arthur S. Slutsky, CM, MD
Professor of Medicine, Director, Interdepartmental Division of Critical Care Medicine, University of Toronto; Vice President (Research), St Michael's Hospital; Keenan Research Centre, Li Ka Shing Knowledge Institute, Toronto, Ontario, Canada
Mechanical Ventilation

Eric J. Small, MD
Professor of Medicine, Deputy Director and Chief Scientific Officer, UCSF Helen Diller Family Comprehensive Cancer Center, University of California, San Francisco, School of Medicine, San Francisco, California
Prostate Cancer

Gerald W. Smetana, MD
Professor of Medicine, Harvard Medical School and Physician, Division of General Medicine and Primary Care, Beth Israel Deaconess Medical Center, Boston, Massachusetts
Principles of Medical Consultation

Gordon Smith, MD
Professor and Chair of Neurology, Medical College of Virginia, Virginia Commonwealth University, Richmond, Virginia
Peripheral Neuropathies

Frederick S. Southwick, MD
Professor of Medicine, University of Florida College of Medicine, Gainesville, Florida
Nocardiosis

Allen M. Spiegel, MD
Dean Emeritus and Professor of Medicine, Albert Einstein College of Medicine, Bronx, New York
Principles of Endocrinology; Polyglandular Disorders

Robert Spiera, MD
Professor of Clinical Medicine, Weill Cornell Medical College; Director, Scleroderma, Vasculitis, & Myositis Center, Hospital for Special Surgery, New York, New York
Giant Cell Arteritis and Polymyalgia Rheumatica

Stanley M. Spinola, MD
Professor of Medicine, Microbiology and Immunology, Pathology and Laboratory Medicine and Chair, Microbiology and Immunology, Indiana University School of Medicine, Indianapolis, Indiana
Chancroid

Sally P. Stabler, MD
Professor of Medicine and Cleo Scott & Mitchell Vincent Allen Chair in Hematology Research, University of Colorado School of Medicine, Aurora, Colorado
Megaloblastic Anemias

Stephanie M. Stanford, PhD
Assistant Professor of Medicine, University of California, San Diego, School of Medicine, La Jolla, California
Mechanisms of Inflammation and Tissue Repair

Paul Stark, MD
Professor Emeritus of Radiology, University of California, San Diego, School of Medicine; Chief of Cardiothoracic Radiology, VA San Diego Healthcare System, La Jolla, California
Imaging in Pulmonary Disease

David P. Steensma, MD
Associate Professor of Medicine, Harvard Medical School and Physician, Dana-Farber Cancer Institute, Boston, Massachusetts
Myelodysplastic Syndromes

Theodore S. Steiner, MD
Professor and Associate Head, Division of Infectious Diseases, University of British Columbia, Vancouver, British Columbia, Canada
Escherichia Coli Enteric Infections

David S. Stephens, MD
Stephen W. Schwarzmann Distinguished Professor of Medicine and Chair, Department of Medicine, Emory University School of Medicine, Atlanta, Georgia
Neisseria Meningitidis Infections

David A. Stevens, MD
Professor of Medicine, Stanford University School of Medicine, Stanford, California; President and Principal Investigator, Infectious Diseases Research Laboratory, California Institute for Medical Research, San Jose, California
Systemic Antifungal Agents

Dennis L. Stevens, PhD, MD
Professor of Medicine, University of Washington School of Medicine, Seattle, Washington; Research & Development Service, Veterans Affairs Medical Center, Boise, Idaho
Nonpneumococcal Streptococcal Infections and Rheumatic Fever

James K. Stoller, MD, MS
Professor and Chairman, Education Institute, Jean Wall Bennett Professor of Medicine, Samson Global Leadership Endowed Chair, Cleveland Clinic Lerner College of Medicine, Cleveland Clinic, Cleveland, Ohio
Respiratory Monitoring in Critical Care

John H. Stone, MD, MPH
Professor of Medicine, Harvard Medical School, Director, Clinical Rheumatology, Massachusetts General Hospital, Boston, Massachusetts
The Systemic Vasculitides

Richard M. Stone, MD
Professor of Medicine, Harvard Medical School; Chief of the Medical Staff, Dana-Farber Cancer Institute, Boston, Massachusetts
Myelodysplastic Syndromes

Raymond A. Strikas, MD, MPH
Medical Officer, Immunization Services Division, Centers for Disease Control and Prevention, Atlanta, Georgia
Immunization

Edwin P. Su, MD
Associate Professor of Clinical Orthopaedics, Weill Cornell Medical College; Associate Attending Orthopaedic Surgeon, Hospital for Special Surgery, New York, New York
Surgical Treatment of Joint Diseases

Roland W. Sutter, MD, MPH&TM
Special Adviser to Director, Polio Eradication Department, World Health Organization, Geneva, Switzerland
Diphtheria and Other Corynebacterium Infections

Ronald S. Swerdloff, MD
Professor of Medicine, David Geffen School of Medicine at UCLA, Los Angeles, California; Chief, Division of Endocrinology, Metabolism and Nutrition, Harbor-UCLA Medical Center, Senior Investigator, Los Angeles Biomedical Research Institute, Torrance, California
The Testis and Male Hypogonadism, Infertility, and Sexual Dysfunction

Heidi Swygard, MD, MPH
Professor of Medicine, University of North Carolina at Chapel Hill, Chapel Hill, North Carolina
Approach to the Patient with a Sexually Transmitted Infection

Megan Sykes, MD
Michael J. Friedlander Professor of Medicine, Director, Columbia Center for Translational Immunology, Columbia University Vagelos College of Physicians and Surgeons, New York, New York
Transplantation Immunology

H. Keipp Talbot, MD, MPH
Associate Professor of Medicine, Vanderbilt University School of Medicine, Nashville, Tennessee
Respiratory Syncytial Virus

Marian Tanofsky-Kraff, PhD
Professor of Medical and Clinical Psychology and of Medicine, Uniformed Services University of the Health Sciences, Bethesda, Maryland
Eating Disorders

Susan M. Tarlo, MBBS
Professor of Medicine, University of Toronto; Respiratory Physician, University Health Network, Toronto, Ontario, Canada
Occupational Lung Disease

Paul S. Teirstein, MD
Chief of Cardiology; Director, Interventional Cardiology, Scripps Clinic, La Jolla, California
Interventional and Surgical Treatment of Coronary Artery Disease

Sam R. Telford, III, ScD
Professor of Infectious Disease and Global Health, Tufts University School of Veterinary Medicine, North Grafton, Massachusetts
Babesiosis and Other Protozoan Diseases

Rajesh V. Thakker, MD
May Professor of Medicine, Radcliffe Department of Medicine, University of Oxford, Oxford, United Kingdom
The Parathyroid Glands, Hypercalcemia, and Hypocalcemia

Judith Therrien, MD
Professor of Medicine, Jewish General Hospital, Montreal, Quebec, Canada
Congenital Heart Disease in Adults

George R. Thompson, III, MD
Associate Professor of Clinical Medicine, University of California, Davis School of Medicine, Davis, California
Endemic Mycoses

Antonella Tosti, MD
Fredric Brandt Endowed Professor of Dermatology, Dr. Phillip Frost Department of Dermatology and Cutaneous Surgery, University of Miami Miller School of Medicine, Miami, Florida
Diseases of Hair and Nails

Indi Trehan, MD, MPH, DTM&H
Associate Professor of Pediatrics, Washington University School of Medicine in St. Louis, St. Louis, Missouri; Executive Director and Medical Director, Lao Friends Hospital for Children, Luang Prabang, Lao People's Democratic Republic
Protein-Energy Malnutrition

Ronald B. Turner, MD
Professor of Pediatrics, University of Virginia School of Medicine, Charlottesville, Virginia
The Common Cold

Anthony Michael Valeri, MD
Associate Professor of Medicine, Vagelos College of Physicians and Surgeons; Medical Director, Hemodialysis, Columbia University Irving Medical Center, New York, New York
Treatment of Irreversible Renal Failure

John Varga, MD
John and Nancy Hughes Distinguished Professor of Medicine, Northwestern University Feinberg School of Medicine, Chicago, Illinois
Systemic Sclerosis (Scleroderma)

Bradley V. Vaughn, MD
Professor of Neurology, University of North Carolina, Chapel Hill, North Carolina
Sleep Disorders

Alan P. Venook, MD
Professor of Clinical Medicine, University of California, San Francisco, School of Medicine, San Francisco, California
Liver and Biliary Tract Cancers

Joseph G. Verbalis, MD
Professor of Medicine, Georgetown University; Chief, Endocrinology and Metabolism, Georgetown University Hospital, Washington, D.C.
Posterior Pituitary

Ronald G. Victor, MD[†]
Formerly Burns & Allen Professor of Medicine, Smidt Heart Institute, Cedars-Sinai Medical Center, Los Angeles, California
Arterial Hypertension

Angela Vincent, MBBS, MSc
Emeritus Professor, Nuffield Department of Clinical Neurosciences, University of Oxford, Oxford, United Kingdom
Disorders of Neuromuscular Transmission

Tonia L. Vincent, PhD
Professor of Musculoskeletal Biology, Arthritis Research UK Senior Fellow and Consultant Rheumatologist; Director, Arthritis Research UK Centre for Osteoarthritis Pathogenesis, University of Oxford, Oxford, England
Osteoarthritis

Robert M. Wachter, MD
Holly Smith Professor and Chairman, Department of Medicine, University of California, San Francisco, School of Medicine, San Francisco, California
Quality, Safety, and Value

Edward H. Wagner, MD, MPH
Director Emeritus, MacColl Center for Health Care Innovation, Group Health Research Institute, Seattle, Washington
Comprehensive Chronic Disease Management

Edward E. Walsh, MD
Professor of Medicine, University of Rochester School of Medicine & Dentistry; Unit Chief, Infectious Diseases, Rochester General Hospital, Rochester, New York
Respiratory Syncytial Virus

Thomas J. Walsh, MD
Professor of Medicine, Pediatrics, Microbiology & Immunology and Chief, Infectious Diseases Translational Research Laboratory, Weill Cornell Medical College, New York, New York; Adjunct Professor of Pathology, Johns Hopkins University School of Medicine; Adjunct Professor of Medicine, University of Maryland School of Medicine, Baltimore, Maryland
Aspergillosis

Jeremy D. Walston, MD
Raymond and Anna Lublin Professor of Geriatric Medicine, Johns Hopkins University School of Medicine, Baltimore, Maryland
Common Clinical Sequelae of Aging

[†]Deceased.

Roland B. Walter, MD, PhD, MS
Associate Professor of Medicine, University of Washington School of Medicine and Associate Member, Clinical Research Division, Fred Hutchinson Cancer Research Center, Seattle, Washington
The Acute Leukemias

Christina Wang, MD
Professor of Medicine, David Geffen School of Medicine at UCLA, Los Angeles, California; Clinical and Translational Science Institute, Los Angeles Biomedical Research Institute and Division of Endocrinology, Department of Medicine, Harbor-UCLA Medical Center, Torrance, California
The Testis and Male Hypogonadism, Infertility, and Sexual Dysfunction

Lorraine B. Ware, MD
Professor of Medicine, Pathology, Microbiology, and Immunology, Vanderbilt University School of Medicine, Nashville, Tennessee
Acute Respiratory Failure

Cirle A. Warren, MD
Associate Professor of Medicine, University of Virginia School of Medicine, Charlottesville, Virginia
Cryptosporidiosis

John T. Watson, MD, MSc
Respiratory Viruses Branch, Division of Viral Diseases, Centers for Disease Control and Prevention, Atlanta, Georgia
Coronaviruses

Thomas J. Weber, MD
Associate Professor of Medicine, Duke University School of Medicine, Durham, North Carolina
Approach to the Patient with Metabolic Bone Disease; Osteoporosis

Geoffrey A. Weinberg, MD
Professor of Pediatrics, University of Rochester School of Medicine & Dentistry; Director, Clinical Pediatric Infectious Diseases & Pediatric HIV Program, Golisano Children's Hospital, University of Rochester Medical Center, Rochester, New York
Parainfluenza Viral Disease

David A. Weinstein, MD, MMSc
Professor of Pediatrics, University of Connecticut School of Medicine, Farmington, Connecticut; Director, Glycogen Storage Disease Program, Connecticut Children's Medical Center, Hartford, Connecticut
Glycogen Storage Diseases

Robert S. Weinstein, MD
Professor of Medicine, University of Arkansas for Medical Sciences; Staff Endocrinologist, Central Arkansas Veterans Health Care System, Little Rock, Arkansas
Osteomalacia and Rickets

Roger D. Weiss, MD
Professor of Psychiatry, Harvard Medical School, Boston, Massachusetts; Chief, Division of Alcohol and Drug Abuse, McLean Hospital, Belmont, Massachusetts
Drugs of Abuse

Roy E. Weiss, MD, PhD
Kathleen & Stanley Glaser Distinguished Chair and Chairman, Department of Medicine, University of Miami Miller School of Medicine, Miami, Florida; Esformes Professor Emeritus, Department of Medicine, University of Chicago Pritzker School of Medicine, Chicago, Illinois
Neuroendocrinology and the Neuroendocrine System; Anterior Pituitary

Jeffrey I. Weitz, MD
Professor of Medicine & Biochemistry, McMaster University Michael G. DeGroote School of Medicine; Executive Director, Thrombosis & Atherosclerosis Research Institute, Hamilton, Ontario, Canada
Venous Thrombosis and Embolism

Richard P. Wenzel, MD, MSc
Professor and Former Chairman, Internal Medicine, Medical College of Virginia, Virginia Commonwealth University, Richmond, Virginia
Acute Bronchitis and Tracheitis

Victoria P. Werth, MD
Professor of Dermatology, University of Pennsylvania Perelman School of Medicine; Chief of Dermatology, Corporal Michael J. Crescenz VAMC, Philadelphia, Pennsylvania
Principles of Therapy of Skin Diseases

Sterling G. West, MD
Professor of Medicine, University of Colorado School of Medicine, Aurora, Colorado
Systemic Diseases in Which Arthritis Is a Feature

A. Clinton White, Jr., MD
Professor of Internal Medicine, University of Texas Medical Branch, Galveston, Texas
Cestodes

Christopher J. White, MD
Chairman and Professor of Medicine, Ochsner Clinical School of the University of Queensland, Ochsner Medical Institutions, New Orleans, Louisiana
Atherosclerotic Peripheral Arterial Disease

Julian White, MBBS, MD
Professor and Head, Toxinology Department, Women's & Children's Hospital, North Adelaide, South Australia, Australia
Envenomation, Bites, and Stings

Perrin C. White, MD
Professor of Pediatrics, University of Texas Southwestern Medical Center; Chief of Endocrinology, Children's Medical Center, Dallas, Texas
Sexual Development and Identity

Richard J. Whitley, MD
Distinguished Professor of Pediatrics, Loeb Eminent Scholar Chair in Pediatrics, Professor of Microbiology, Medicine, and Neurosurgery, Pediatrics, University of Alabama at Birmingham School of Medicine, Birmingham, Alabama
Herpes Simplex Virus Infections

Michael P. Whyte, MD
Professor of Medicine, Pediatrics, and Genetics, Washington University School of Medicine in St. Louis; Medical-Scientific Director, Center for Metabolic Bone Disease and Molecular Research, Shriners Hospital for Children, St. Louis, Missouri
Osteonecrosis, Osteosclerosis/Hyperostosis, and Other Disorders of Bone

Samuel Wiebe, MD, MSc
Professor of Clinical Neurosciences, Community Health Sciences and Pediatrics, University of Calgary Cumming School of Medicine, Calgary, Alberta, Canada
The Epilepsies

Jeanine P. Wiener-Kronish, MD
Henry Isaiah Dorr Professor of Research and Teaching in Anaesthesia, Department of Anesthesia, Critical Care and Pain Medicine, Harvard Medical School; Anesthestist-in-Chief, Massachusetts General Hospital, Boston, Massachusetts
Overview of Anesthesia

David J. Wilber, MD
George M Eisenberg Professor of Medicine, Loyola University Chicago Stritch School of Medicine; Director, Division of Cardiology, Loyola University Medical Center, Maywood, Illinois
Electrophysiologic Interventional Procedures and Surgery

Beverly Winikoff, MD, MPH
President, Gynuity Health Projects; Professor of Clinical Population and Family Health, Population and Family Health, Columbia University Mailman School of Public Health, New York, New York
Contraception

Jane N. Winter, MD
Professor of Medicine, Robert H Lurie Comprehensive Cancer Center and the Department of Medicine, Northwestern University Feinberg School of Medicine, Chicago, Illinois
Approach to the Patient with Lymphadenopathy and Splenomegaly

Edward M. Wolin, MD
Professor of Medicine, Albert Einstein College of Medicine; Director, Neuroendocrine Tumor Program, Department of Medical Oncology, Montefiore Einstein Center for Cancer Care, Bronx, New York
Neuroendocrine Tumors

Gary P. Wormser, MD
Professor of Medicine and of Microbiology and Immunology and Pharmacology, New York Medical College; Chief, Division of Infectious Diseases, Valhalla, New York
Lyme Disease

Neal S. Young, MD
Chief, Hematology Branch, NHLBI, National Heart, Lung, and Blood Institute, Bethesda, Maryland
Parvovirus

Vincent B. Young, MD, PhD
William Henry Fitzbutler Professor of Internal Medicine/Infectious Diseases, Professor of Microbiology & Immunology, University of Michigan Medical School, Ann Arbor, Michigan
The Human Microbiome

William F. Young, Jr., MD, MSc
Professor of Medicine, Tyson Family Endocrinology Clinical Professor, Mayo Clinic College of Medicine and Science, Rochester, Minnesota
Adrenal Medulla, Catecholamines, and Pheochromocytoma

Alan S.L. Yu, MB BChir
Harry Statland and Solon Summerfield Professor, University of Kansas Medical Center; Director, The Kidney Institute, University of Kansas Medical Center, Kansas City, Kansas
Disorders of Magnesium and Phosphorus

Anita K. M. Zaidi, MBBS, SM
Director, Enteric and Diarrheal Diseases; and Vaccine Development and Surveillance, Bill and Melinda Gates Foundation, Seattle, Washington
Shigellosis

Sherif Zaki, MD, PhD
Chief, Infectious Diseases Pathology Branch, Centers for Disease Control and Prevention, Atlanta, Georgia
Leptospirosis

Thomas R. Ziegler, MD
Department of Medicine, Division of Endocrinology, Metabolism and Lipids, Emory University School of Medicine, Atlanta, Georgia
Malnutrition: Assessment and Support

Peter Zimetbaum, MD
Richard and Susan Smith Professor of Cardiovascular Medicine, Harvard Medical School; Associate Chief and Director of Clinical Cardiology, Medicine, Beth Israel Deaconess Medical Center, Boston, Massachusetts
Supraventricular Cardiac Arrhythmias

CONTENTS

VOLUME 2

SECTION XXV: HIV AND THE ACQUIRED IMMUNODEFICIENCY SYNDROME

SECTION XXVI: NEUROLOGY

VIDEO CONTENTS

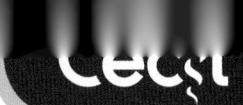

 This icon appears throughout the book to indicate chapters with accompanying video available on Expertconsult.com.

EYE, EAR, NOSE, AND THROAT DISEASES

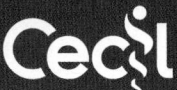

XVII

METABOLIC DISEASES

194

APPROACH TO INBORN ERRORS OF METABOLISM

OLAF A. BODAMER

DEFINITION

The term *metabolism* (Greek: *metabolé*, "change") refers to the network of chemical reactions that sustain the human organism through the digestion, absorption, transport, and utilization of nutrients.

Inborn errors of metabolism (IEM) are genetic disorders that affect the intrinsic metabolic pathways either through deficiencies of enzymes, membrane transporter proteins, signaling peptides, or structural proteins. The resulting clinical phenotype follows a spectrum of different organ manifestations that may be progressive, fluctuating, or stationary in nature and may manifest at any age. Any IEM can principally present during adolescence and/or adulthood, although more severe presentations are typically recognized during infancy and childhood.[1] A growing number of patients with IEM who were diagnosed during infancy or childhood now reach adulthood due to improved management and the advent of novel therapies.

Archibald Garrod pioneered the field of IEM after recognizing alkaptonuria as one of the first metabolic conditions due to homozygosity of mutant alleles in 1902. He had the foresight to recognize the autosomal recessive inheritance of additional IEM, including cystinuria, pentosuria, and albinism, and to speculate about "chemical individuality" as one of the driving forces of selection and evolution. However, it was not until the early 1950s when the deficiency of homogentisate 1,2-dioxygenase (HGD) was recognized as the underlying cause of alkaptonuria, and it took many more years to identify pathogenic mutations in the *HGD* gene.

The advent of novel analytical techniques led to the molecular and biochemical characterization of known IEM and the delineation and recognition of new clinical phenotypes, some of which were previously not presumed to be due to IEM. The completion of the first human genome in 2001 and the following "genomics" revolution laid the foundation for the successive identification of many additional conditions through next-generation sequencing, bringing the total number of cataloged IEM to about 1000.

EPIDEMIOLOGY

Inborn errors of metabolism occur in all populations, although their incidence and prevalence rates may vary considerably due to differences in carrier rates. These variations are readily explained by the presence of founder mutations, for example, in individuals of Ashkenazi Jewish or Amish ancestry, or by an increased rate of parental consanguinity that leads to a relative increase in mutant allele frequency (Table 194-1). Knowledge of the increased carrier frequencies is instrumental for preconception genetic counseling and targeted carrier screening.

PATHOBIOLOGY

The complexity of human metabolism and its spatial relationship with the human proteome, genome, and methylome is poorly understood. Naturally occurring variants in human nucleotide sequences may or may not result in variation of amino acid sequences in peptides and proteins. It is now well established from whole exome and genome sequencing that individuals may carry in excess of 10,000 nucleotide variants, the vast majority of variants being silent, *single nucleotide polymorphic variants*. Up to 4% of variants may be pathogenic in either recessive or dominant genes.[2] These variants in particular will lead to functional changes in proteins that may render the affected individual susceptible to disease, increase the risk of undesired side effects when treated with certain drugs, or increase the risk for genetic conditions in future generations.

Inborn errors of metabolism are monogenic conditions that follow either autosomal recessive or dominant, X-linked recessive/dominant, or mitochondrial inheritance patterns. Of note is the existence of genetic and/or environmental modifiers that contribute to the interindividual and intrafamilial variability of phenotypic expression, although for most inborn errors of metabolism these modifiers remain elusive. In case of mitochondrial inheritance, heteroplasmy (the random distribution and expression of mitochondrial mutations in different organs) may explain by itself the striking variability of clinical symptoms in mitochondrial conditions.

Pathophysiology

The severity of any given IEM depends on the degree of enzyme deficiency and the complex interaction of the underlying pathogenic mutations, genetic modifiers, and environment. Hypomorphic mutations may not lead to overt disease until adulthood, whereas severe mutations in the same gene may lead to infantile-onset disease associated with significant morbidity and mortality. The underlying pathophysiologic mechanisms may contribute individually or in combination to the disease state (Table 194-2). Complete blockage of a catabolic pathway may result in accumulation of toxic substrates, activation of secondary minor pathways, and/or a relative shortage of downstream products. As a consequence, different organs may be affected by the same metabolic defect.

CLINICAL MANIFESTATIONS

Inborn errors of metabolism typically affect multiple organs and, in more than 50% of cases, the central and/or peripheral nervous systems and/or muscles. One or more organ manifestations may dominate the clinical phenotype, although oligosymptomatic cases may occur. The clinical phenotype represents a continuous clinical spectrum ranging from the severe end, presenting during infancy, to the mild end of the spectrum, presenting during adolescence and/or adulthood. Some affected individuals may never come to medical attention due to almost complete absence of symptoms or atypical presentation. Recent data from newborn screening programs suggest much higher incidence rates for some IEM due to the detection of a high rate of mild cases who may never develop disease-related signs or symptoms. Some clinical signs are pathognomonic for IEM, whereas others should raise the suspicion for the presence of an IEM (Table 194-3).

Classification

Inborn errors of metabolism can be classified based on the underlying pathomechanism (see Table 194-2) on the nature and/or localization of the protein involved or on the clinical phenotype (see Table 194-3). A new nosology has been recently proposed for IEM.[3]

● SELECTED INBORN ERRORS OF METABOLISM
Disorders of Protein Metabolism

These conditions are due to cytosolic or mitochondrial enzyme or transport protein deficiencies (Table 194-4 and Table 194-5). Listed next are selected, more frequent inborn errors of protein metabolism, although the list is not exhaustive due to space constraints.

PHENYLKETONURIA

Phenylalanine is an essential amino acid important for growth and production of thyroid hormone, neurotransmitters, and melanin. Phenylketonuria (PKU) is caused by deficiency of tetrahydrobiopterin (BH4)–dependent phenylalanine hydroxylase that catalyzes the conversion of phenylalanine to tyrosine. PKU may also be caused by deficiency of enzymes that are required for BH4 synthesis. PKU is one of the "traditional" IEM and the first to be included in newborn screening programs more than 50 years ago, demonstrating that early diagnosis and continued therapy consistently result in normal intellectual development.[4] The advent of novel therapies, most recently pegylated recombinant phenylalanine ammonia lyase (PEG-PAL), has provided an effective alternative to dietary therapy with the potential of normalization of phenylalanine levels even when individuals with PKU remain on a normal diet.[A1][A2]

Disorders of the Urea Cycle

The role of the urea cycle is to convert ammonium as a byproduct of amino acid metabolism to nontoxic urea that is readily excreted in urine and to synthesize arginine and ornithine.[5] Arginine is an important precursor for the nitric oxide pathway and substrate for creatine/creatine phosphate synthesis. Several mitochondrial and cytosolic enzymes and transporters are required for the function of the urea cycle. Individuals with any of the disorders of the urea cycle are at risk for hyperammonemia during catabolic episodes when there is an increased rate of protein breakdown. All conditions are inherited as an autosomal recessive trait with the exception of ornithine transcarbamylase deficiency (OTCD), which is inherited as an X-linked recessive trait (see Table 194-4). Females with OTCD typically report an aversion to high protein

TABLE 194-1 INCIDENCE OF SELECTED INBORN ERRORS OF METABOLISM

DISORDER	GENE	INCIDENCE*	CARRIER RATE	POPULATION
Familial hypercholesterolemia	*LDLR*	1:500	1:500	United States
Phenylketonuria	*PAH*	1:4000 <1:120,000 1:15,000	1:32 <1:173 1:61	Ireland Finland, Japan United States
Gaucher disease	*GBA*	1:20,000 1:450	1:71 1:11	United States† Ashkenazi Jews
Canavan disease	*ASPA*	Unknown 1:6000	Unknown 1:39	United States Ashkenazi Jews
Glycogen storage disease 1a	*G6PC*	1:100,000 1:1225	1:158 1:18	United States Ashkenazi Jews
Mucolipidosis IV	*MCOLN1*	Unknown 1:3000	Unknown 1:27	United States Ashkenazi Jews
Niemann-Pick disease A	*SMPD1*	<1:250,000 1:40,000	<1:250 1:100	United States Ashkenazi Jews
Tay-Sachs disease	*HEXA*	1:300,000 1:3500	1:274 1:30	United States Ashkenazi Jews

*Per live births.
†Includes Ashkenazi Jews.

TABLE 194-2 PATHOPHYSIOLOGIC MECHANISMS IN INBORN ERRORS OF METABOLISM

MECHANISM	DISORDER
Accumulation of toxic substrates through primary blockage of catabolic pathway	Organic acidopathies (MMA, PA) MSUD, tyrosinemia type 1
Accumulation of nontoxic macromolecules through blockage of catabolic pathway	Lysosomal storage disorders (MPS)
Energy failure through primary blockage of pathway relevant for ATP synthesis	Fatty acid oxidation defects Glycogen storage disorder types I and III Respiratory chain enzyme deficiencies
Impairment of post-translational glycosylation	Congenital disorders of glycosylation
Deficiency of end product through primary blockage of anabolic pathway	Albinism, orotic aciduria, scurvy, disorders of creatine metabolism
Lack of detoxification through primary blockage of catabolic pathway	Urea cycle defects

ATP = adenosine triphosphate; MMA = methylmalonic aciduria; MPS = mucopolysaccharidoses; MSUD = maple syrup urine disease; PA = propionic aciduria.

TABLE 194-3 CHARACTERISTIC SIGNS OF INBORN ERRORS OF METABOLISM

ORGAN	CLINICAL SIGN	DISORDER
Eye (cornea)	Cornea verticillata	Fabry disease
Skeletal system	Ochronosis, black urine	Alkaptonuria
Connective tissue	Carpal tunnel syndrome	MPS I, II, VI, and VII
Central nervous system	Ataxia	Respiratory chain enzyme deficiency
Muscle	Hypotonia	Pompe disease, GSD V Disorders of creatine metabolism
Liver	Hepato(-spleno)megaly Fibrosis/cirrhosis	MPS I, II, VI, and VII GSD I, III GSD IV, IXb/c, LAL deficiency
Kidney	Renal insufficiency	Cystinosis, Fabry disease
Skin	Angiokeratomata	Fabry disease

GSD = glycogen storage disease; LAL = lysosomal acid lipase; MPS = mucopolysaccharidosis.

intake that leads to neurologic symptoms, including migraine headaches. Timely diagnosis and initiation of therapy following careful dietary history and family history to identify additional family members at risk are important determinants for good outcome.[6]

Organic Acidurias

Organic acidurias are disorders due to mitochondrial enzyme deficiencies and accumulation of potentially toxic substrates, activation of alternative pathways, and lack of downstream products. Although the typical clinical presentation is during infancy or childhood, adult cases with mild or atypical symptoms have been reported in the medical literature. Although individuals with organic acidurias are at risk for metabolic decompensation during catabolic episodes, this risk is somewhat lower during adulthood (see Table 194-5).

Lysosomal Storage Disorders

The lysosomal storage disorders comprise a heterogeneous group of more than 50 distinct disorders due to genetic defects in lysosomal enzymes and membrane proteins or transporters, resulting in lysosomal accumulation of specific substrates.[7] The accumulation in tissues and organs is progressive, ultimately causing deterioration of cellular and tissue function. Many lysosomal disorders affect the central nervous system, and most patients have a decreased lifespan and significant morbidity. Lysosomal storage disorders may be categorized based on the type of substrate stored. Disorders of glycosaminoglycan metabolism include the mucopolysaccharidoses (MPSs): MPS I,

Hurler syndrome, Scheie syndrome; MPS II, Hunter syndrome; MPS III a–d, Sanfilippo syndrome A–D; MPS IVa, IVb, Morquio syndrome A and B; MPS VI, Maroteaux-Lamy syndrome; MPS VII, Sly syndrome. Disorders of ganglioside metabolism include Fabry disease, Gaucher disease, Niemann-Pick disease, Tay-Sachs disease, I-cell disease, fucosidosis, mannosidosis, sialidosis, and aspartylglycosaminuria. Danon and Pompe diseases are two lysosomal storage disorders resulting in storage of glycogen in different types of muscle cells.[8]

DIAGNOSIS
Biochemical and Molecular Testing

The path to a diagnosis of an inborn error of metabolism begins with ascertainment of the medical and family history, as well as an in-depth clinical evaluation. The majority of inborn errors of metabolism can be diagnosed through analysis of small molecules (metabolites, peptides, and hormones) in appropriate body fluids (serum, whole blood, urine, and cerebrospinal fluid [CSF]) followed by enzyme testing in tissues (dried whole blood, lymphocytes, leukocytes, fibroblasts, and muscle tissue). Tissue biopsies for histology and histochemistry are still of value in some cases. Selected metabolic tests for diagnosis of IEM include analysis of amino acids in plasma, dried blood spots (DBS), urine, and CSF; analysis of acylcarnitine species in plasma and DBS; analysis of total and free carnitine in plasma and urine; analysis of succinylacetone in DBS and urine; and analysis of orotic acid in plasma and urine.

Molecular confirmation is warranted for prediction of phenotype and as prerequisite for family planning, including preimplantation diagnosis, prenatal

TABLE 194-4 DISORDERS OF PROTEIN METABOLISM

DISORDER	ENZYME DEFECT	METABOLITE(S)	CLINICAL PHENOTYPE
Argininemia	Arginase	Arginine	Hyperammonemia, neurologic disease
Argininosuccinic aciduria	Argininosuccinate lyase	Argininosuccinate*	Hyperammonemia, liver cirrhosis
Citrullinemia	Arginiosuccinate synthetase	Citrulline, orotic acid*	Hyperammonemia, liver cirrhosis
Homocystinuria	Cystathionine β-synthase	Homocysteine, methionine	Marfanoid habitus, intellectual disability, lens dislocation
Maple syrup urine disease	Branched-chain α-keto acid dehydrogenase complex	Alloisoleucine,* leucine, valine, isoleucine	Encephalopathy, ataxia, metabolic decompensation
Ornithine transcarbamylase deficiency	Ornithine transcarbamylase	Orotic acid,* ornithine, arginine	Severe hyperammonemia, X-linked inheritance
Phenylketonuria	Phenylalanine hydroxylase	Phenylalanine	Intellectual disability,† seizures†
Tyrosinemia type I	Fumaryl acetoacetase	Succinylacetone,* tyrosine	Acute liver failure, tubulopathy
Tyrosinemia type II	Tyrosine aminotransferase	Tyrosine, phenylalanine	Corneal lesions, hyperkeratosis of the skin, mild intellectual disability

*Diagnostic compound.
†If untreated.

TABLE 194-5 ORGANIC ACIDURIAS

DISORDER	ENZYME DEFECT	INHERITANCE	URINE METABOLITES
Glutaric aciduria type I	Glutaryl-CoA dehydrogenase	Autosomal recessive	3-Hydroxyglutaric acid, glutaric acid
Holocarboxylase synthetase deficiency	Holocarboylase synthetase	Autosomal recessive	β-Hydroxyisovaleric acid, β-methylcrotonylglycine, β-hydroxypropionic acid, 3-methylcitrate
Isobutyric aciduria	Isobutyryl-CoA dehydrogenase	Autosomal recessive	Isobutyric acid
Isovaleric aciduria	Isovaleryl-CoA dehydrogenase	Autosomal recessive	Isovaleric acid
Methylmalonic aciduria	Methylmalonyl-CoA dehydrogenase	Autosomal recessive	Methylmalonic acid
Mevalonic aciduria	Mevalonate kinase	Autosomal recessive	Mevalonic acid
Propionic aciduria	Propionyl-CoA carboxylase	Autosomal recessive	3-Methylcitrate, propionic acid, 3-hydroxypropionic acid

TABLE 194-6 DIAGNOSTIC TESTS FOR INBORN ERRORS OF METABOLISM

METABOLITE	BIOLOGICAL MATRIX	METHOD	DISORDER
Amino acids	Plasma, urine, CSF	HPLC, MS-MS	Disorders of amino acid metabolism including PKU, MSUD, tyrosinemia, urea cycle defects, lysinuric protein intolerance
Organic acids	Urine, CSF	GC-MS	Organic acidopathies including MMA, PA, IVA Lactic acidosis, mitochondrial disorders including disorders of the Krebs cycle, respiratory chain enzymes, fatty acid oxidation defects
Acylcarnitine species	Plasma, DBS	MS-MS	Fatty acid oxidation defects, organic acidopathies
Total/free carnitine	Plasma, DBS, urine	MS-MS	Carnitine transporter deficiency, CPT-I/II deficiencies (in conjunction with acylcarnitine species), secondary carnitine deficiency
Orotic acid	Plasma, urine	GC-MS, MS-MS	Orotic aciduria, OTC deficiency, citrullinemia type I
Succinylacetone	Plasma, DBS, urine	GC-MS	Tyrosinemia type 1
Glycosaminoglycans	Urine	TLC, MS-MS	Mucopolysaccharidoses

CPT-I/II = carnitine palmitoyl transferase I/II; CSF = cerebrospinal fluid; DBS = dried blood spots; GC-MS = gas chromatography–mass spectrometry; HPLC = high-pressure liquid chromatography; IVA = isovaleric aciduria; MMA = methylmalonic aciduria; MS-MS = tandem mass spectrometry; MSUD = maple syrup urine disease; PKU = phenylketonuria; OTC = ornithine transcarbamylase; PA = propionic aciduria; TLC = thin layer chromatography.

testing, and carrier testing for the partner (Table 194-6). Additionally, next-generation sequencing (NGS) is increasingly used as a first-line test.

Next-Generation Sequencing

NGS enables the rapid and accurate sequencing of whole human genomes and/or exomes that represent the 1 to 2% of the genome that is translated into proteins. The continuous refinement of NGS technologies has led to a rapid decline of sequencing cost, thereby facilitating the sequencing of tens of thousands of individuals in both research and clinical settings. NGS has not been restricted to humans but plays an increasing role in the delineation of other species, including microorganisms, which may help us understand the functionality of the intestinal microbiome and allow the development of new anti-infectious therapies.

Clinical gene panels and whole exome or genome sequencing in accredited laboratories may aid in the diagnosis of rare mendelian disorders, including

IEM, provided all other diagnostic avenues are exhausted. Although sequencing may be relatively straightforward and inexpensive, analytical challenges remain.[9,10]

TREATMENT

The individual treatment strategy follows the general principle of either (1) enhancing enzyme activity through cofactor administration, (2) stabilizing enzyme structure through chaperone therapy, (3) enzyme replacement therapy, (4) reduction of substrate through dietary intervention, (5) substrate inhibition through blockage of the reverse enzyme reaction, (6) replacement of the affected organ (e.g., liver), or (7) stem cell transplantation and/or therapy.[11] Other therapeutic approaches, including "read-through," m-RNA, gene modification (CRISPR), and gene therapies, are either in preclinical development or already in clinical trials (Table 194-7).

The choice of therapy is guided by the underlying diagnosis, but additional factors warrant consideration. A curative approach may be preferred whenever possible, although this may be rarely an option in adults with IEM, as in the case of bone marrow or stem cell transplantation in metachromatic leukodystrophy or X-linked adrenoleukodystrophy. Therapeutic agents that address central nervous system manifestations have to cross the blood-brain barrier to be effective, thereby limiting the use of larger molecules, including enzymes, for treatment of neurologic manifestations.

Individuals with IEM should always be managed by a multidisciplinary team of biochemical geneticists, internists, and genetic counselors at a tertiary center with significant expertise in the management of inborn errors of metabolism. Ideally a biochemical genetics laboratory to facilitate immediate sample testing should be on site.

Genetic Counseling

Genetic counseling through board-certified genetic counselors is an integral part of the evaluation and management of patients with any genetic condition, including complex IEM. A three-generation family history and thorough medical history are the prerequisites for a focused clinical and diagnostic evaluation. Genetic counseling communicates limitations and implications of genetic testing and associated test results to the patient and the family at large.

Enzyme Therapy

The therapeutic goal of enzyme therapy is to increase endogenous enzyme activity. Individuals with cofactor (vitamin)–responsive enzyme deficiencies may benefit from supraphysiologic doses of the respective vitamin. An example is tetrahydrobiopterin (BH4)–responsive PKU due to mutations in the *PAH* gene affecting the binding site of phenylalanine hydroxylase (PAH). In this case 20 mg/kg of BH4 will result in stabilization of the PAH through a chaperone-like effect and as a consequence increase PAH activity. Patients with BH4-responsive PKU will experience improved phenylalanine tolerance and metabolic control when taking BH4 supplementation.

Enzyme replacement therapy has been available for the treatment of Gaucher disease for over 15 years. Initially glucocerebrosidase, the enzyme deficient in Gaucher disease, was purified from human placentas and administered intravenously to affected patients. More recently, glucocerebrosidase has been overexpressed in Chinese hamster ovary cells and produced in large quantities in bioreactors. Recombinant enzyme replacement therapies are now available for Pompe disease (α-glucosidase), Fabry disease (α-galactosidase), mucopolysaccharidosis type I (α-iduronidase), mucopolysaccharidosis type II (α-iduronate sulfatase), mucopolysaccharidosis type IVa (galactosamine-6-sulfatase), and mucopolysaccharidosis type VI (arylsulfatase B). Additional enzyme therapies are currently in different phases of clinical trials (see Table 194-7).

Nutritional Therapy

The therapeutic goal for nutritional therapy is the correction of the metabolic imbalance through reduced substrate accumulation, promoting protein synthesis through anabolism and the prevention of episodes of metabolic decompensation. In addition, supplementation of a reduced product may be needed. An example is the therapy for PKU. The mainstay of its therapy is the reduction of phenylalanine intake through low-protein food and the simultaneous supplementation of phenylalanine-free amino acids for sustained growth and development. This regimen will reduce the phenylalanine levels in plasma and, most important, in the brain to nontoxic, near-normal levels that facilitate age-appropriate intellectual development.[12] Occasionally tyrosine supplementation is needed when tyrosine levels are low. Similar dietary strategies apply to other disorders of amino acid metabolism and organic acidopathies, although natural protein restriction may be more pronounced to reduce the risk for metabolic decompensation during a catabolic episode (intercurrent illness).

Another approach to reduce substrate accumulation is through inhibition of the reverse enzyme reaction that leads to substrate synthesis. This concept has been shown to be effective in reducing glucosylceramide in mild to moderate Gaucher disease type I. Individuals with IEM at risk for metabolic decompensation, such as urea cycle disorders, organic acidopathies, and disorders of fatty acid oxidation, should always carry an "emergency letter" detailing the diagnosis, symptoms of decompensation, emergency treatment, and contact information of the tertiary metabolic center.

Vitamin Therapy

A number of IEM affect transport and/or metabolism of vitamins. These conditions typically benefit from supraphysiologic doses of vitamins. An example is thiamine-responsive megaloblastic anemia, which is due to mutations in the thiamine transporter gene *SLC19A2*. Affected individuals develop sensorineural deafness, vision loss, diabetes mellitus, and megaloblastic anemia. Diabetes and anemia respond to high doses of thiamine. Other examples include disorders of vitamin B_{12} (cobalamin) absorption, transport, and metabolism and disorders of biotin and folic acid metabolism.

Organ, Bone Marrow, and Stem Cell Transplantation

Liver transplantation has been done in patients with tyrosinemia type I, urea cycle defects, methylmalonic aciduria, propionic aciduria, lysosomal lipase deficiency, and glycogen storage diseases affecting the liver. The effect of liver transplantation in these conditions is two-fold. First, metabolic control will be improved in those conditions where the diseased liver is the main contributor to the overall lack of sufficient metabolic control. However, the intrinsic defect will not be corrected elsewhere after liver transplantation, and an affected individual may continue to have significant neurologic disease in methylmalonic aciduria, for example. Second, liver function will be restored in those conditions that lead to chronic liver disease, including liver fibrosis and/or cirrhosis, or where there is a significant risk for malignant transformation. Kidney transplantation may be required in conditions that affect kidney function, as is the case in methylmalonic aciduria or cystinosis.

Bone marrow and/or stem cell transplantation has limited benefits in patients with IEM. Examples include presymptomatic bone marrow and/or stem cell transplantation in severe mucopolysaccharidosis type I, metachromatic leukodystrophy, and X-linked adrenoleukodystrophy. Stem cell therapy is currently under investigation for glycogen storage disease type I.

Grade A References

A1. Thomas J, Levy H, Amato S, et al. Pegvaliase for the treatment of phenylketonuria: results of a long-term phase 3 clinical trial program (PRISM). *Mol Genet Metab*. 2018;124:27-38.
A2. Harding CO, Amato RS, Stuy M, et al. Pegvaliase for the treatment of phenylketonuria: a pivotal, double-blind randomized discontinuation phase 3 clinical trial. *Mol Genet Metab*. 2018;124:20-26.

GENERAL REFERENCES

For the General References and other additional features, please visit Expert Consult at https://expertconsult.inkling.com.

TABLE 194-7 EXAMPLES OF THERAPEUTIC STRATEGIES FOR INBORN ERRORS OF METABOLISM

LEVEL	THERAPEUTIC APPROACH	DISORDER
Gene	Solid organ transplantation	Urea cycle defects, MSUD, tyrosinemia type I
	Stem cell transplantation	Adrenoleukodystrophy, MPS I
	Gene therapy	MPS I and II, Pompe disease (phase I/II trial)
	Read-through therapy	Duchenne muscular dystrophy (phase III), cystic fibrosis (phase III)
Enzyme	Recombinant enzyme infusion	Gaucher, Pompe, Fabry diseases, MPS I, II, IVa, VI
		Phenylketonuria
	Chaperone	Fabry and Pompe diseases
Substrate	Substrate reduction	Phenylketonuria, maple syrup urine disease
	Substrate inhibition	Gaucher disease, Tay-Sachs disease, Niemann-Pick type C

MPS = mucopolysaccharidosis; MSUD = maple syrup urine disease.

195

DISORDERS OF LIPID METABOLISM

JENNIFER G. ROBINSON

Disorders of lipid metabolism are an increasingly common consequence of modern industrial lifestyles.[1] With increasing prosperity, the spread of Western-style diets and sedentary habits is resulting in dramatic rises in obesity in countries around the world. Poor lifestyle habits coupled with genetic predisposition commonly result in dyslipidemia characterized by higher levels of the atherogenic cholesterol- and triglyceride-rich apolipoprotein (apo) B-100 lipoproteins, higher levels of triglyceride-rich apo B-48 lipoproteins, and lower levels of apo A lipoproteins. In the office setting, these apolipoproteins are reflected in levels of low-density lipoprotein cholesterol (LDL-C), triglycerides, high-density lipoprotein cholesterol (HDL-C), and non-HDL-C.

The most common clinical manifestation of lipid disorders is atherosclerotic cardiovascular disease (ASCVD) resulting from elevated levels of apo B-100 lipoproteins.[2,3] The role of apo A lipoproteins in the development of (or protection from) ASCVD is less clear. Severe hypertriglyceridemia is primarily associated with an increased risk of pancreatitis.

LIPID METABOLISM

PATHOBIOLOGY

Cholesterol and Triglycerides

Cholesterol is an essential component of all animal cell membranes and functions as a precursor to fat-soluble vitamins and steroid hormones such as cortisol, estradiol, progestins, and testosterone. Plants utilize sterols rather than cholesterol as structural components of the cell membrane. Triglycerides are composed of 3 fatty acid chains attached to a glycerol molecule. Triglycerides are a source of energy, particularly in the fasting state. Both cholesterol and triglycerides are insoluble in water, requiring transport in lipoprotein particles in plasma (Fig. 195-1). Apolipoproteins are amphipathic molecules located on the surface of the lipoprotein particle that serve as biochemical keys to specific receptors or binding sites that allow delivery, entry, or modification. E-Figure 195-1 provides an overview of cholesterol, triglyceride, and lipoprotein metabolism and sites of lipid-modifying drug action.

Cholesterol and triglycerides are either synthesized or absorbed from the intestine. Adults synthesize about 100 mg of cholesterol per day. The liver synthesizes about 25% of cholesterol; the brain, reproductive organs, adrenal glands and intestines also have higher rates of cholesterol synthesis. Cholesterol is synthesized via multiple steps from acetyl CoA and acetoacetyl-CoA. The rate-limiting step in cholesterol synthesis is the reduction to mevalonate by 3-hydroxy-3-methyl-glutaryl-CoA (HMG CoA) reductase, the target of statins. Downstream metabolites of mevalonate include several bioactive molecules, which have been implicated in some adverse effects of statins.

Diet provides 300 to 500 mg cholesterol per day. Bile acids provide about two thirds of daily cholesterol (800 to 1200 mg) and sloughed intestinal cells about 300 mg. Nonesterified cholesterol is secreted from the liver in bile acids, which are stored in the gallbladder and secreted into the small intestine where they solubilize dietary fats and enhance fatty acid, lipid, and fat-soluble vitamin absorption. Bile acids are largely reabsorbed from the distal ileum and transported back to the liver via the enterohepatic circulation.

Dietary fats and animal products are broken down in the intestine, and the constituents are transported into enterocytes where they are re-esterified into cholesteryl ester and triglycerides. Cholesterol is absorbed from the intestine via the Niemann-Pick C1-Like 1 (NPC1L1) receptor, which can be inhibited with ezetimibe.

Chylomicrons

In the enterocyte, triglycerides and cholesterol are packaged with apo B48 as well as apo CII and CIII and other apolipoproteins for secretion into the blood as triglyceride-rich chylomicrons (Fig. 195-1). Chylomicrons undergo progressive hydrolysis of triglycerides into fatty acids by lipoprotein lipase in the capillary endothelium, which binds apo CII, as well as other apolipoproteins. The fatty acids can be stored in adipose tissue or used as fuel by muscle tissue. Chylomicrons are converted into chylomicron remnants which are relatively enriched in cholesteryl esters. Chylomicrons are the largest lipoproteins and thought unlikely to contribute to atherosclerosis. They are not soluble in plasma, and cause a "tomato soup" appearance to freshly drawn plasma, rising to the top of the serum after overnight refrigeration to cause a "cream" layer. The smaller chylomicron remnants can enter the subendothelial space to be taken up by macrophages, and may be the mechanism through which postprandial hypertriglyceridemia contributes to atherogenesis.

Chylomicrons and chylomicron remnants are also taken up by the liver by the LDL receptor-related protein which interacts with apo E, and to a lesser extent by the LDL receptor and cell surface glycosaminoglycans. The liver breaks down the chylomicron particles, which can be stored as cholesteryl ester and triglycerides, assembled into very low density lipoprotein (VLDL) particles for secretion into the blood, or the cholesteryl esters can be incorporated into bile acids for secretion into the intestine.

VLDL, IDL, LDL

The liver assembles a VLDL particle from one apolipoprotein B100 molecule, cholesteryl esters, triglycerides, and a number of other apolipoproteins and lipids. Triglycerides are the rate limiting step in VLDL synthesis. Microsomal transfer protein (MTP) transfers triglycerides to the growing apo B peptide. Drugs that inhibit MTP can thus cause intrahepatic triglyceride accumulation.

Nascent VLDL is secreted into the blood, where it acquires apo E, apo CII, and apo CIII. Similar to chylomicrons, apo CII activates lipoprotein lipase to hydrolyze triglycerides into fatty acids for transport into tissues. As VLDL continues to deliver cholesterol and triglycerides to tissues, VLDL is transformed into increasingly cholesteryl-rich intermediate density lipoproteins (IDL) and ultimately into low density lipoproteins (LDL) (Fig. 195-1). LDLs comprise the largest fraction of circulating lipoproteins and contain about 60 to 70% of total cholesterol in the circulation.

LDL is removed from the blood predominantly by the LDL receptor. LDL receptor expression is regulated by proprotein convertase subtilisin/kexin type 9 (PCSK9). In response to decreased intracellular cholesterol levels, sterol regulator element-binding proteins (SREBP) 1 and 2 upregulate the hepatic

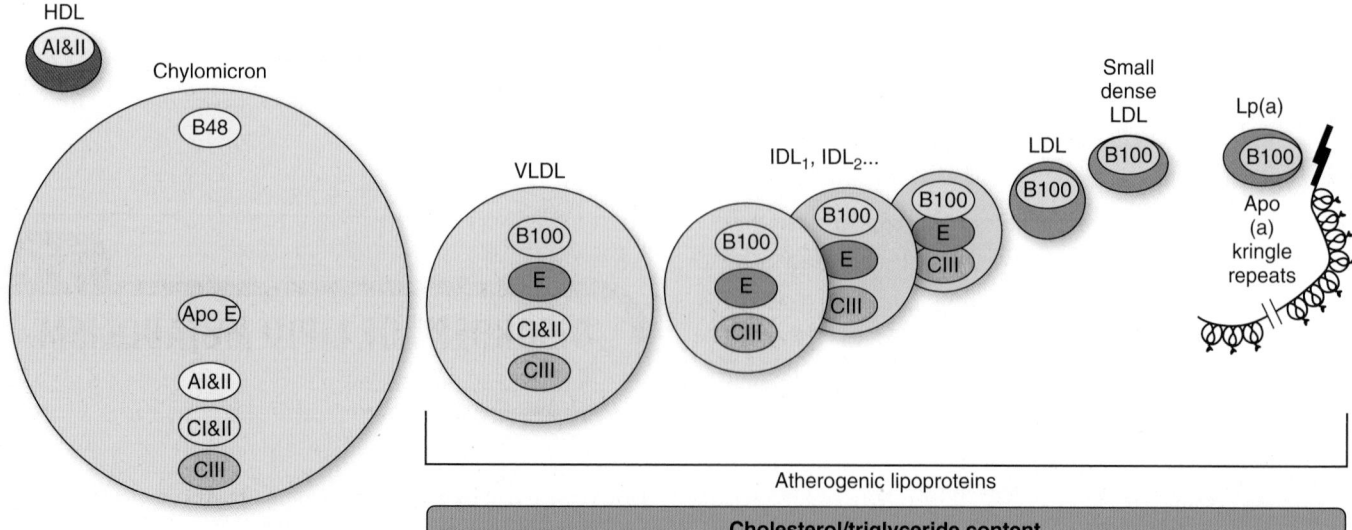

FIGURE 195-1. Relative size (not to scale), triglyceride, and cholesterol composition, major apolipoproteins and atherogenicity of circulation lipoproteins. (Adapted from Robinson J. *Clinical Lipid Management.* 1st ed. West Islip, NY: Professional Communications, Inc; 2016.)

synthesis of both LDL receptors and PCSK9. LDL receptors travel to the cell surface where they bind LDL particles from the blood. The LDL particle–LDL receptor complex is then taken up into vesicles, where the LDL particle undergoes degradation while the LDL receptor remains intact. The LDL receptor is then recirculated intact back to the cell surface to continue to remove LDL particles from the blood.

At the same time that LDL-receptor is traveling to the cell surface, the PCSK9 molecule is secreted into the blood, where it can bind the LDL-LDL receptor complex, tagging both the LDL receptor and the LDL particle for degradation. Inhibition or decreased levels of PCSK9 thus permit greater LDL receptor circulation and enhanced LDL particle removal from the circulation.

The atherogenicity of large VLDL particles is unclear. Smaller VLDL particles, IDL, and LDL are clearly atherogenic.

Lp(a)

The liver assembles lipoprotein(a) (Lp[a]) from an apo(a) moiety connected to the apo B of an LDL-like particle (Fig. 195-1). Apo(a) isoforms are quite variable due to the number of kringle repeats determined by the apo(a) gene. Apo(a) size is inversely related to Lp(a) concentration, and is thought to result from the longer assembly time of an apo(a) isoform with a large number of kringle repeats. The liver removes Lp(a) from the circulation. This process and the function of Lp(a) are not well understood. Lp(a) appears to be atherogenic. It is unknown whether pharmacologically lowering Lp(a) reduces cardiovascular events.

HDL

High density lipoprotein (HDL) is the smallest and densest of the circulating lipoproteins (Fig. 195-1). HDL carries apos AI and AII rather than apo B-100 or apo B-48. HDL is synthesized in the liver from apos AI, AII and phospholipids to form nascent HDL or pre-β HDL (E-Fig. 195-2). As this particle circulates through the body and interacts with peripheral cells, it acquires cholesterol and additional phospholipid by binding to adenosine triphosphate-binding cassette protein (ABC1), through a process called "reverse cholesterol transport."

HDL carries about 30% of blood cholesterol. Inside the HDL particle, unesterified cholesterol is esterified by lecithin-cholesterol acyl transferase (LCAT). Esterified cholesterol can be removed from HDL via the scavenger receptor B1 (SR-B1) in the liver. In the blood, esterified cholesterol can be exchanged for triglycerides from apo B lipoproteins via the cholesteryl ester transfer protein (CETP) in the plasma. Phospholipid transfer protein transfers phospholipids from apo B lipoproteins to HDL. Lipoprotein lipase hydrolyzes triglycerides from VLDL and chylomicrons to HDL. Hepatic lipase removes triglycerides from HDL.

In epidemiologic studies low levels of HDL, HDL-cholesterol (HDL-C), and apo AI are associated with increased cardiovascular risk. It is unclear whether low HDL-C, often accompanied by elevated triglyceride levels, causes cardiovascular disease or is simply a marker of impaired glucose metabolism and insulin resistance. Mendelian randomization studies have failed to find an association between HDL-C-raising genes and cardiovascular risk. In randomized trials, HDL-C-raising drugs have not been shown to decrease cardiovascular risk beyond their effects on LDL-C or non-HDL-C (e.g., niacin and cholesteryl ester transfer protein [CETP] inhibitors). Indeed, there are several genetic polymorphisms that markedly increase HDL-C levels that are associated with increased cardiovascular risk. A number of mechanisms for this increase in risk have been proposed, including conversion of HDL into a more pro-inflammatory state or impairment of reverse cholesterol transport.

The functionality of HDL as measured by in vitro reverse cholesterol assays has been associated with reduced cardiovascular risk, independent of HDL-C levels. An uncommon apo AI mutation, apo AI-Milano, causes low HDL-C levels and is associated with reduced cardiovascular risk that is thought to be mediated by more efficient reverse cholesterol transport. Apo AII is associated with increased cardiovascular risk through unknown mechanisms.

DIAGNOSIS

Lipid Measurement

In the clinical laboratory lipoprotein particles are usually not measured directly, but by density ultracentrifugation, which separates them into bands based on cholesterol and triglyceride content. Hence, the more commonly reported triglyceride, total cholesterol, LDL-cholesterol (LDL-C), and HDL-cholesterol (HDL-C) levels. Patients with high triglyceride levels have elevated numbers of chylomicrons, chylomicron remnants, or VLDL, or have increased triglyceride content in VLDL. It should be understood that triglyceride levels reflect the triglyceride content of the lipoprotein particles and do not exist as independent entities in the blood. (They would be insoluble even if they did.) Patients with high cholesterol levels have increased numbers of LDL, VLDL, IDL, or Lp(a) particles, or increased cholesteryl content in these particles.

On fasting samples (≥8 hours), LDL-cholesterol (LDL-C) is calculated by the Friedewald equation when the triglyceride level is lower than 400 mg/dL:

$$LDL\text{-}C = Total\ cholesterol - HDL\text{-}C - triglycerides/5$$

Calculated LDL-C is not accurate in the presence of Type III hyperlipidemia (see later) or when CETP inhibitors are used.

On nonfasting or fasting samples when triglycerides are greater than 500 mg/dL, non-HDL-C can be calculated:

$$Non\text{-}HDL\text{-}C = Total\ cholesterol - HDL\text{-}C$$

thus, non-HDL-C represents the atherogenic lipid component (see Fig. 195-1). Non-HDL-C is generally about 30 mg/dL higher than LDL-C. A more elaborate method of calculating LDL-C when triglycerides are elevated has been developed but has not been validated in multiple populations.

LDL-C levels can also be measured directly, and are accurate when triglycerides are as high as 1000 mg/dL. Direct LDL-C levels are 5 to 10 mg/dL lower than calculated LDL-C levels, in part because they do not measure lipoprotein (a) (Lp[a]).

Measurement of Lp(a) has been problematic due to inter-individual variation in the number of kringles in the apo(a) moiety. No standardized method exists at this time, and large race-dependent variations support the need to develop race-specific reference ranges.

Advanced lipid testing can measure apo B and apo A directly, but only apo B measurement has been standardized. Other techniques can measure the number of LDL, IDL, and VLDL particles and their size using a variety of methods; none of these methods have been standardized and test-retest variability is often high. The clinical utility of advanced lipid testing is not clearly established. The vast majority of patients can be managed with calculated LDL-C or non-HDL-C levels, which is the least expensive and widely available method. Apo B measurement may be helpful in select patients with hypertriglyceridemia.

Apo B Lipoproteins, Cholesterol, and Atherogenesis

An extensive body of over 50 years of epidemiologic, genetic, and clinical trial evidence has shown a direct and causal relationship between blood cholesterol levels and ASCVD (also see Chapter 46). More recent evidence has shown that it is the accumulation of cholesterol and triglyceride-rich apo B lipoproteins in the arterial subendothelium that is the pathologic initiating factor in the development of an atherosclerotic plaque (Chapter 46 and Fig. 195-2). Apolipoproteins with up to approximately 70 nm diameter (LDL, IDL, smaller VLDL, remnant chylomicron particles, and Lp[a]) more efficiently cross the endothelium. High plasma concentrations increase the probability that these particles will enter the subendothelial space of the artery. This size limitation is likely why very high plasma levels of large apo B-48 chylomicrons in lipoprotein lipase deficiency do not cause atherosclerosis.

Normally, few apo B lipoproteins are retained in the subendothelium and return to the circulation. In the presence of atherosclerotic plaque, the endothelium becomes abnormally permeable to apo B lipoproteins. Treatment of hyperlipidemia results in rapid decreases in permeability and increased fractional degradation of the LDL entering the plaque. However, the key initiating factor of atherogenesis is the subendothelial retention of apo B lipoproteins. Atherosclerosis preferentially develops in specific sites in the arterial tree. Disturbed laminar flow at these sites provokes matrix proliferation in the adjacent arterial wall. In the earliest stages of atherogenesis, negatively charged proteoglycans in the extracellular matrix of the arterial intima trap the positively charged apo B-100 and apo B-48 moieties. Other characteristics of the LDL molecule may affect atherogenicity by influencing apo B binding or proteoglycan interactions, such as surface lipid composition or core lipid composition. Apo E mediates binding to arterial glycosaminoglycans but also facilitates hepatic disposal of apo B lipoproteins. On the other hand, apo CIII increases both the affinity of LDL for arterial wall proteoglycans and decreases hepatic uptake of apo B lipoproteins, thereby promoting retention of the cholesterol and triglyceride-rich apo B lipoproteins.

Following retention in the arterial wall, apo B lipoproteins undergo further enzymatic modifications that promote aggregation and accelerating accumulation. These aggregations release biologically active byproducts that recruit

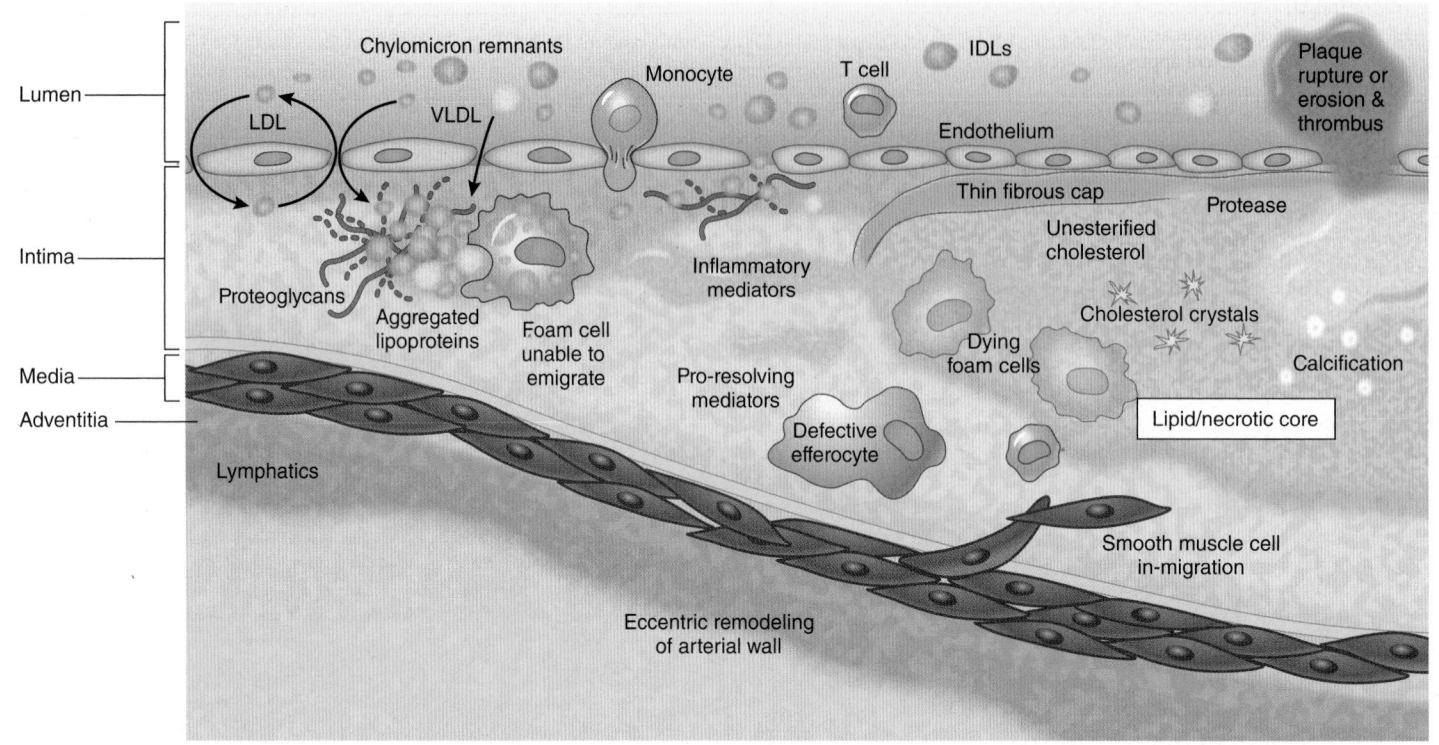

FIGURE 195-2. Apo B lipoprotein response-to-retention model of atherosclerosis initiation and progression. High plasma concentrations of apo B lipoproteins (LDL, IDL, VLDL, chylomicron remnants, Lp[a]) increase entry into intima and retention. Apo B lipoproteins bind to proteoglycans and begin aggregating, a process that accelerates once plaque begins. Retention is influenced by particle composition and diet. Retention leads to a maladaptive cellular response leading to increased inflammation, fibrosis, and necrosis. The lipid/necrotic core forms when normal phagocytotic processes and efferocytosis are overwhelmed by continued retention and accumulation of "toxic" apo B lipoproteins. Plaque rupture or erosion can lead to formation of overlying thrombus, which can precipitate an acute clinical event. Apo = apolipoprotein; IDL = intermediate lipoprotein; LDL = low density lipoprotein; Lp(a) = lipoprotein (a); VLDL = very low density lipoprotein. (From Robinson JG, Williams KJ, Gidding S, et al. Eradicating the burden of atherosclerotic cardiovascular disease by lowering apolipoprotein B lipoproteins earlier in life. *J Am Heart Assoc*. 2018;7:1-12.)

more macrophages and immunoregulatory T cells into the developing lesion. Interestingly, dietary composition can alter LDL aggregability: saturated fats and sucrose increase it, and polyunsaturated fats and fiber decrease it. Aggregated apo B lipoproteins are avidly taken up by vascular smooth muscle cells and macrophages, initiating their transformation into cholesterol-laden foam cells. This results in a maladaptive response that further accelerates atherogenesis. Proatherogenic enzymes and signaling molecules are released, inducing synthesis of more proteoglycans with increased affinity for apo B lipoproteins, other factors that enhance retention, and proteolytic enzymes. Proteases can weaken the overlying fibrous cap, which favors plaque rupture and release of the thrombogenic subendothelial contents. In animal models, injections of HDL, overexpression of apo AI and increased HDL function to inhibit plaque formation and promote plaque stabilization and regression.

Atherogenesis begins in childhood, and may progress to advanced plaque by late adolescence or early adulthood, a process that is accelerated in the presence of other cardiovascular risk factors and genetic predisposition. Most adults have advanced plaque in their 40s and 50s, and begin experiencing clinical ASCVD events such as myocardial infarction and other acute coronary syndromes, stroke, peripheral arterial disease, and death. Apo B lipoproteins, as measured by total, LDL-C and non-HDL-C levels, predict ASCVD risk in all ages, genders, races/ethnicities, and regions. The increase in the relative risk of ASCVD per increment increase in total or LDL-C depends on age and the level and duration of exposure (Fig. 195-3). Elevated cholesterol levels remain a risk factor into old age, although the relative contribution to risk is attenuated.[4] Lp(a) level appears to increase ASCVD risk beyond that expected from the LDL-C level.

Atherosclerosis Regression

Reducing LDL and other apo B lipoproteins levels can regress atheroma. Markedly lowering apo B lipoprotein levels results in reduced subendothelial uptake and retention and decreased monocyte and macrophage recruitment (E-Fig. 195-3). Reducing the inputs allows the normal scavenger and phagocytic clearance mechanisms to clear the apo B lipoprotein overload. Reverse cholesterol transport mechanisms mobilize cholesterol out of the foam cells. Foam cells decrease due to emigration into adventitial lymphatics and transmigration into the lumen. More effective efferocytosis clears apoptotic cells

and necrotic core. Inflammatory cells out-migrate and smooth muscle cells migrate into the subendothelium, collagen synthesis falls, and fibrosis resolves. In animal models, very low LDL-C levels of less than 20 to 40 mg/dL have been shown to completely regress early atheroma and normalize vascular function. In more advanced atheroma, substantial regression can occur but residual stabilized plaque remains.

To date, only lipid-modifying drugs that lower LDL-C or non-HDL-C have been shown to stabilize or regress atherosclerotic plaque and to reduce cardiovascular events. Mendelian randomization studies have consistently found that genetic polymorphisms that increase LDL-C or non-HDL-C increase cardiovascular risk, and that the converse is true for those that cause lower LDL-C or HDL-C levels.[5,6] Polymorphisms causing very elevated Lp(a) levels are also associated with increased cardiovascular risk. Consistent with a causal role for apo B lipoproteins in atherosclerosis, the only hypertriglyceridemic polymorphisms that influence cardiovascular risk are those influencing VLDL levels. In contrast, Mendelian randomization studies have found little association between HDL-C raising polymorphisms and cardiovascular risk, consistent with the findings from randomized trials of pharmacologically raising HDL-C levels.

● CLINICAL DISORDERS OF LIPID METABOLISM
Secondary Causes of Hyperlipidemia

All patients with a first LDL-C of 160 mg/dL or higher or triglycerides of 500 mg/dL or higher should be evaluated for secondary causes of hyperlipidemia (Table 195-1). The most common causes of secondary hypercholesterolemia include obesity, high intake of saturated or *trans*-fats, and glucocorticoids. The most common causes of hypertriglyceridemia are poorly controlled diabetes, obesity, and high refined carbohydrates, alcohol, or fat. Once secondary causes are addressed or stabilized, a repeat fasting lipid panel can be used to guide therapy.

Genetic Lipid Disorders

Blood levels of LDL-C, non-HDL-C, triglycerides and HDL-C are influenced by genetics, lifestyle habits, medications, and medical conditions. Secondary causes of hyperlipidemia should be identified and treated. Severe primary elevations in LDL-C (≥190 mg/dL), non-HDL-C (≥220 mg/dL), or triglycerides (≥1000 mg/dL) almost always occur in the setting of a significant genetic disorder. However, treatment approaches are guided by LDL-C or non-HDL-C as the primary elevation or triglycerides higher than 1000 mg/dL.

In the United States, individuals with LDL-C higher than 190 mg/dL have a five-fold higher lifetime risk of ASCVD, and those with familial hypercholesterolemia (FH) have a 20-fold higher lifetime risk of ASCVD. In the

Netherlands, where nationwide efforts to identify FH patients have resulted in earlier treatment, FH patients who receive statins have an ASCVD risk similar to that of the non-FH population. Therefore, all patients older than 20 years with a primary elevation in LDL-C higher than 190 mg/dL should receive high-intensity statin therapy unless a contraindication is present.

Familial Hypercholesterolemia

EPIDEMIOLOGY

FH is the most common genetic disorder, affecting about 1 in 250 persons in populations around the world. FH may be more common in some populations such as Ashkenazi Jews, some Lebanese groups, and French Canadians. Homozygous FH or compound heterozygous FH is present in about 1 in 500,000 adults.

PATHOBIOLOGY

Heterozygous FH is characterized by LDL-C levels higher than 190 mg/dL and a family history of severe LDL-C elevations or premature cardiovascular disease and/or a genetic FH mutation.[7] Genetic testing is more common in European countries. About 60 to 75% of those with heterozygous FH have a monogenetic autosomal dominant mutation, and the remainder have a polygenic disorder. The most common FH mutations result in loss of function in the LDL receptor. Uncommon are gain-of-function mutations in PCSK9, which results in more rapid LDL receptor degradation, and mutations which alter the apo B LDL receptor binding site.

CLINICAL MANIFESTATIONS

Men and women with heterozygous FH have a 20-fold higher lifetime risk of ASCVD and death due to their genetic disorder. FH is a common cause of premature atherosclerotic coronary heart disease in the 30s and 40s in men and 40s and 50s in women. The first presentation is often sudden death in younger adults, leaving no opportunity for prevention. Clinical ASCVD is markedly accelerated in smokers with FH, with death in the 20s and 30s not uncommon. Homozygous FH manifests with ASCVD events in childhood.

DIAGNOSIS
Screening

Because heterozygous FH is a common and completely reversible genetic disorder if treated early, universal screening with a fasting or nonfasting lipid panel is recommended between the ages of 8 and 11 years. Screening should occur at an even earlier age if there is family history of LDL-C higher than 190 mg/dL or premature onset ASCVD (before age 55 in male first-degree relative or age 65 in a first-degree female relative). All adults should be screened no later than age 20.

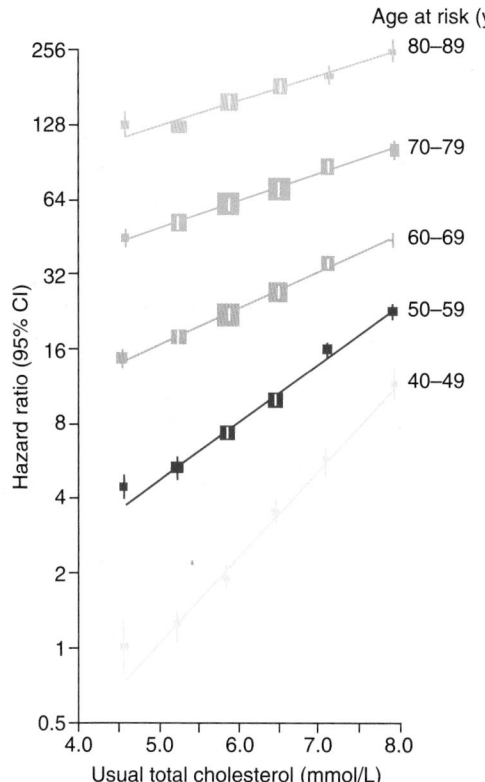

FIGURE 195-3. Age-specific association of atherosclerotic coronary heart disease mortality and total cholesterol level. (From Prospective Studies Collaboration; Lewington S, Whitlock G, Clarke R, et al. Blood cholesterol and vascular mortality by age, sex, and blood pressure: a meta-analysis of individual data from 61 prospective studies with 55,000 vascular deaths. *Lancet.* 2007;370:1829-1839.)

TABLE 195-1 SECONDARY CAUSES OF HYPERLIPIDEMIA

SECONDARY CAUSE	ELEVATED LDL–C OR NON-HDL-C	ELEVATED TRIGLYCERIDES
Diet	<u>**Saturated or *trans* fats**</u>, <u>**large weight gain**</u>, anorexia	<u>**Large weight gain**</u>, high fat intake, <u>**high refined carbohydrate intake**</u>, <u>**excessive alcohol intake**</u>, very-low-fat diets if high in refined carbohydrates
Drugs	**Glucocorticoids**, cyclosporine, anticonvulsants, oral contraceptives, anabolic steroids, diuretics, sirolimus, amiodarone	**Glucocorticoids**, oral estrogens, anabolic steroids, bile acid sequestrants, highly active retroviral therapy, retinoic acid (isotretinoin), sirolimus, tacrolimus, raloxifene, tamoxifen, β-blockers (not carvedilol), thiazides, cyclophosphamide, L-asparaginase, second-generation antipsychotics (clozapine and olanzapine)
Diseases	Biliary obstruction, nephrotic syndrome, monoclonal gammopathy	**Proteinuria**, nephrotic syndrome, chronic renal failure, glomerulonephritis, Cushing syndrome, HIV, lipodystrophies, monoclonal gammopathy, systemic lupus erythematosus, autoimmune chylomicronemia, chronic idiopathic urticaria
Disorders and altered states of metabolism	**Obesity**, hypothyroidism, pregnancy*	<u>**Diabetes (poorly controlled)**</u>, **obesity**, lipodystrophy, hypothyroidism, pregnancy*, polycystic ovarian syndrome

*Cholesterol and triglycerides rise progressively throughout pregnancy
Common causes of secondary hyperlipidemia (most common causes in **bold**; leading causes <u>underlined</u>).
Secondary causes of hyperlipidemia should be evaluated in patients with:
- Newly identified LDL-C ≥160 mg/dL or non-HDL-C ≥190 mg/dL
- Newly identified triglycerides ≥500 mg/dL
- Worsening LDL-C, non-HDL-C, or triglyceride levels despite adherences to lifestyle and drug therapy
Initial laboratory tests should include:
- Fasting glucose or hemoglobin A1C (HbA1C)
- Thyroid-stimulating hormone (TSH)
- Alkaline phosphatase, bilirubin, and alanine aminotransferase (ALT)
- Creatinine/glomerular filtration rate (GFR)
- Urinary albumin
Additional tests include:
- Total protein
- Women of childbearing age—beta human chorionic gonadotropin (βhCG)
Used with permission of author: Robinson JG. *Clinical Lipid Management.* West Islip, NY: Professional Communications Inc; 2015.

FH TREATMENT AND PREVENTION

Cascade Screening

Once an index case of FH is identified, all first-degree relatives should be screened with a fasting lipid panel. As an autosomal dominant genetic disorder, 50% of first-degree relatives will likely have FH and benefit from early treatment.

FH Treatment

Smoking avoidance and risk factor control is imperative for patients with FH. All FH patients should adhere to lifestyle healthy lifestyle habits, but almost all will need statin therapy due to the impaired removal of LDL-C from the blood. Moderate-intensity statin therapy is recommended for children and adolescents with LDL-C over 160 mg/dL after a trial of lifestyle change to healthy habits. High-intensity statin therapy is recommended after age 20 for adults with FH higher than 190 mg/dL. Some individuals will have milder cases of FH with LDL-C levels of 160 to 189 mg/dL. These patients will benefit from earlier statin treatment as well, especially if risk factors are present.

A high-intensity statin on average lowers LDL-C by about 50%. Many patients with FH will achieve LDL-C levels around 100 mg/dL with a high-intensity statin and ezetimibe, in addition to healthy lifestyle habits. For primary prevention of younger patients with FH this level of LDL-C, along with non-HDL-C levels around 130 mg/dL are likely sufficient to prevent significant progression of atherosclerosis. However, patients with more severe FH or those with clinically evident ASCVD may benefit from the addition of a PCKSK9 inhibitor (see later). Bile acid sequestrants and niacin are infrequently used in FH patients due to problems with tolerability and only modest efficacy. LDL apheresis under the direction of a lipid specialist may be an option for statin intolerant or unresponsive FH patients.

Pregnancy and Lactation

Statins, PCSK9 monoclonal antibodies, and niacin are contraindicated during pregnancy and lactation due to potential effects on the fetus and infant. Therefore, early treatment may be helpful for a woman with FH, because she may more comfortably discontinue statin therapy once she contemplates pregnancy and lactation, and then resume statin therapy once childbearing is complete.

Familial Combined Hypercholesterolemia

Familial combined hypercholesterolemia (FCH) is relatively common polygenic cholesterol disorder that often runs in families, although in a less distinct pattern than that of autosomal dominant FH. The genetic predisposition of FCH is expressed with advancing age and increasing adiposity. Most typically, non-HDL-C is elevated to higher than 220 mg/dL and accompanied by elevated triglycerides of 200 to 600 mg/dL. FCH can also be expressed as pure LDL-C or triglyceride elevations. Onset of clinical ASCVD is somewhat later than in FH, with clinical ASCVD presentation in the 50s in men and 60s in women. Screening and treatment is as for FH, with an emphasis on lifestyle, weight control, and statin therapy. If triglycerides remain elevated above 1000 mg/dL after lifestyle and maximal statin therapy, triglycerides should be treated as outlined in the Hypertriglyceridemia section.

Familial Dysbetalipoproteinemia

Familial dysbetalipoproteinemia is an uncommon (1 in 10,000) but extremely high risk genetic disorder for premature coronary heart disease.[8] These patients have two copies of apo E2, which results in impaired clearance of VLDL through the VLDL receptor. However, two copies of apo E2 are insufficient to cause severe hyperlipidemia in the absence of conditions that slow VLDL clearance, such as obesity, diabetes, or hypothyroidism. LDL-C levels are usually over 190 mg/dL and non-HDL-C levels are over 220 mg/dL. Triglycerides of higher than 500 mg/dL are common and are caused by impaired lipolysis of VLDL remnants, in addition to the higher levels of circulating VLDL. Patients with familial dysbetalipoproteinemia respond well to fibrates, but a statin should be added to further reduce ASCVD risk.

Other Rare Monogenetic Lipid Disorders

Low LDL-C

Individuals homozygous for mutations in the gene encoding microsomal triglyceride transfer protein (MTP) can have abetalipoproteinemia, a rare disease characterized by the absence of circulating apo B, VLDL-C, IDL-C, and LDL-C. Fat-soluble vitamins (vitamins A, D, E, K) cannot be transported in the absence of apo B, and patients with abetalipoproteinemia suffer from multiple severe disorders, including severe neurologic dysfunction and retinopathy beginning early in life.

Individuals homozygous for mutations resulting in abnormal or decreased apo B synthesis have hypobetalipoproteinemia with low but not absent levels of circulating apo B, VLDL-C, IDL-C, and LDL-C levels. These individuals appear to be healthy.

Loss-of-function *PCSK-9* mutations result in no breakdown of LDL receptors, and enhanced removal of LDL from the blood. Depending on the degree of loss of function, heterozygotes have lower than average LDL-C levels and reduced risk of cardiovascular disease. Homozygotes have LDL-C levels of 10 to 15 mg/dL and appear to be healthy.

Low HDL-C

HDL-C levels have a U-shaped association with mortality. Recent studies have found that extremely high HDL-C levels (>115 mg/dL in men and >135 mg/dL in women) are associated with increased mortality. The mechanism for this is unclear, but is consistent with the lack of benefit observed in trials of CETP inhibiting drugs.

Sitosterolemia

Beta sitosterolemia results from increased intestinal absorption of plant sterols, which are normally excreted back into the intestine by ABCG5 and ABCG8.

Severe Hypertriglyceridemia

Severe hypertriglyceridemia (>1000 mg/dL) is due to rare monogenetic lipid disorders, typically unmasked in the presence of secondary causes of hypertriglyceridemia (Table 195-1). Treatment of hypertriglyceridemia is outlined in the Hypertriglyceridemia section.

● ASCVD PREVENTION

Despite tremendous advances in acute treatment, and improvements in smoking cessation and risk factor control, ASCVD remains the leading cause of death in almost every country in the world.[9] Lipid-modifying drugs that predominantly lower LDL-C and/or non-HDL-C levels are the first-line approach to reduce the risk of a first or recurrent cardiovascular event.[A1-A5] HDL-C raising has not been shown to reduce cardiovascular events after accounting for the reduction in LDL-C or non-HDL-C levels.[A6] Reduction of elevated triglyceride levels may also be beneficial in selected patients.[10]

Lifestyle is the foundation of all cardiovascular risk reduction efforts. However, most individuals are at increased risk of cardiovascular events during their lifetime, due to genetic predisposition, unhealthy lifestyle habits, or both. Statins are overwhelmingly the first choice for cardiovascular prevention, with more than 25 randomized trials demonstrating cardiovascular risk reduction with an excellent margin of safety in a wide variety of populations around the world. Selected patients remain at high risk after maximizing statin therapy, and may benefit from the addition of a nonstatin cholesterol-lowering therapy to further reduce cardiovascular risk.

The randomized clinical trial evidence that supported the 2018 AHA/ACC Multispecialty Guideline on the Management of Blood Cholesterol[11] provides the basis for the following discussion. Guideline recommendations from other organizations may differ from those of the 2018 AHA/ACC cholesterol guideline. Guidelines from the U.S. Preventive Services Task Force,[12] and National Institutes for Clinical Excellence, among others, have taken an approach similar to that of the 2018 AHA/ACC cholesterol guideline by focusing on statin treatment in patient groups most likely to benefit. Other specialty groups and the European Society of Cardiology guidelines have continued to recommend titrating statin dose aiming for a target LDL-C.

The 2018 AHA/ACC cholesterol guideline recommends periodically monitoring LDL-C levels after initiating statin therapy to evaluate treatment response and adherence. It continues the 2013 ACC/AHA cholesterol guideline move away from treat-to-target approaches for several reasons. There is no clinical trial evidence that titration to a specific cholesterol goal improves outcomes. Nor does titration to goal account for the potential for net benefit from additional therapy, which is a function of both risk reduction benefit as well as the harms from the added therapy. Harms include not only the potential for adverse effects from the drug, but diminished adherence to evidence-based therapy and increased patient costs. Being "at goal" may mean a patient does not receive evidence-based statin therapy, or receives a suboptimal intensity of statin therapy. Treat to goal also means a patient with cholesterol slightly above goal is treated, while the patient with slightly below goal is not, despite identical cardiovascular risk.

The 2018 AHA/ACC guideline uses LDL-C (or non-HDL-C) levels as thresholds for triggering consideration of the potential for net benefit from added therapy. This depends on the absolute ASCVD risk of the patient, the relative risk reduction from the added therapy, and the potential for harm.[13,14]

Lifestyle

Healthy lifestyle habits throughout the lifespan are associated with lower cardiovascular risk, and lifestyle remains the foundation of all cardiovascular risk reduction efforts. Unfortunately, by adulthood, less than 5 to 10% of individuals in industrialized societies remain in a state of ideal cardiovascular health as characterized by healthy diet, regular physical activity, smoking avoidance, and desirable levels of cholesterol, blood pressure, and blood glucose.[15]

Lifestyle modifications can reduce LDL-C levels by about 10 mg/dL (Table 195-2). Referral to a dietician can be helpful for motivated patients seeking to improve their dietary habits. It should be noted that the cholesterol-lowering drug trials were performed in the background of healthy diet advice.

Drug Therapy

Several classes of drugs have been shown to reduce cardiovascular events used as monotherapy. Based on an extensive body of randomized trial evidence, statins are overwhelmingly the first choice for reducing ASCVD events, cardiovascular mortality, and all-cause mortality. More limited data are available from cardiovascular outcomes trials in highly selected populations for other lipid-modifying agents. The LDL-C lowering agents ezetimibe[A7] and PCSK9 monoclonal antibodies[A8,A9] have been shown to further reduce cardiovascular events when added to background statin therapy in very-high-risk patient populations. The relative reduction in ASCVD risk from all of these drugs is proportional to the magnitude of the LDL-C or non-HDL-C lowering.[A10]

STATIN THERAPY

Statins have been shown to reduce nonfatal and fatal cardiovascular events and overall mortality in primary and secondary prevention populations over treatment periods of 2 to 7 years. Those receiving high-intensity statin therapy had greater relative risk reductions than those receiving moderate-intensity statin therapy. In the Cholesterol Treatment Trialists' individual level meta-analysis of 28 statin trials, each 39 mg/dL (1 mmol/L) reduction in LDL-C

was associated with a 22% reduction in cardiovascular events. With the exception of patients with class II to IV heart failure or receiving hemodialysis, all patient subgroups in the clinical trials benefited from statin therapy.[A11]

The 2018 AHA/ACC cholesterol guideline identified four groups of patients for high-intensity statin therapy (unless safety concerns) and at least a 50 percent LDL-C reduction (Fig. 195-4):

1. Clinical ASCVD
2. LDL-C higher than 190 mg/dL
3. Higher risk diabetes (High-risk characteristics or ≥7.5% 10-year ASCVD risk)
4. Primary prevention with at least 20% 10-year ASCVD risk

Based on a high level of clinical trial evidence, two groups of patients were identified for moderate-intensity statin therapy following a clinician-patient discussion:

1. Lower risk diabetes (No risk factors or less than 7.5% 10-year ASCVD risk)
2. Primary prevention with 7.5 to less than 20% 10-year ASCVD risk.

Because the margin of benefit may be less, a clinician patient discussion is recommended to consider the potential for an ASCVD risk reduction benefit, potential for adverse effects, and patient preferences.

There is also moderate evidence from one trial of benefit from statins in primary prevention patients with 5 to less than 7.5% 10-year ASCVD risk.

Based on extensive clinical trial evidence that high-intensity statins reduce cardiovascular events more than moderate-intensity statins, and that the relative reduction in cardiovascular risk is proportional to the magnitude of LDL-C reduction, high-intensity statins are recommended for higher risk patients. Moderate-intensity statins are recommended for lower risk patients, those older than 75 years, or those who have safety concerns such as the potential for drug-drug interactions.[A12] Statins are categorized by intensity in Table 195-3. The primary effect of statins is on LDL-C and non-HDL-C levels.

In patients with heart failure with reduced ejection fraction attributable to ischemic heart disease who have a reasonable life expectancy and are not already on a statin because of ASCVD, clinicians may consider initiation of moderate-intensity statin therapy to reduce the occurrence of ASCVD events. In patients requiring hemodialysis, statin initiation is not recommended but can be continued if already initiated.

Risk Estimation for Primary Prevention Statin Therapy

The ASCVD risk calculator developed as part of the 2018 AHA/ACC guideline process can be used to estimate 10-year ASCVD risk. The ASCVD calculator can be found online or downloaded in an app (http://tools.acc.org/ascvd-risk-estimator-plus/#!/calculate/estimate/). The ASCVD calculator estimates the risk of an incident fatal or nonfatal myocardial infarction or stroke over 10 years. It performs well in the general U.S. population of non-Hispanic white and African American women and men. However, the risk estimate may be adjusted upward or downward based on other characteristics (Table 195-4). Risk estimation in populations outside the United States should use risk calculators developed for that country. For example, in Europe, the SCORE equations are recommended (https://www.escardio.org/Education/Practice-Tools/CVD-prevention-toolbox/SCORE-Risk-Charts), and in the United Kingdom the QRISK equations are recommended (https://www.qrisk.org/).

In patients who remain reluctant to initiate statin therapy for primary prevention after estimating ASCVD risk and considering risk enhancing factors, coronary artery calcification can be measured in selected patients. Coronary artery calcification should not be measured in patients who smoke or have diabetes, a premature family history of ASCVD, or LDL-C levels greater than or equal to 130 mg/dL since these patients are at increased ASCVD risk regardless of the presence of coronary artery calcium. In patients without these characteristics, a calcium score of zero indicates lower ASCVD risk.

Statin Safety

Statins have had an excellent margin of safety in all clinical trial populations, including trials in heart failure and hemodialysis populations, with similar rates of adverse events, including muscle adverse events, in the placebo/control and low-, moderate-, and high-intensity statin arms.[16,A13] Statins are contraindicated during pregnancy and lactation, and women with childbearing potential should be appropriately counseled.

Moderate-intensity statins slightly increase, and high-intensity statins modestly increase, the risk of diabetes in individuals already at risk for diabetes. However, this is not of concern because the diagnosis is only accelerated by about 2 months. Patients receiving statins should be encouraged to adhere to healthy lifestyle habits. Those with diabetes risk factors or glucose intolerance

TABLE 195-2	2013 ACC/AHA LIFESTYLE GUIDELINE RECOMMENDATIONS
	CLASS/LOE
DIET	
Consume a dietary pattern that:	IA
• Emphasizes intake of vegetables, fruits, and whole grains	
• Includes low-fat dairy products, poultry, fish, legumes, nontropical vegetable oils, and nuts	
• Limits intake of sweets, sugar-sweetened beverages, and red meats	
• Adapts to appropriate calorie requirements, personal and cultural food preferences, and nutrition therapy for other medical conditions (including diabetes mellitus)	
• Follows plans such as the DASH dietary pattern, the USDA Food Pattern, or the AHA Diet	
Aim for a dietary pattern that achieves 5 to 6% of calories from saturated fat	IA
Reduce percent calories from saturated fat	IA
Reduce percent calories from trans fat	IA
PHYSICAL ACTIVITY	
In general, advise adults to engage in aerobic physical activity to reduce LDL-C and non-HDL-C	IIaA
• 3 to 4 sessions per week	
• Lasting on average 40 minutes per session	
• Involving moderate to vigorous physical activity	

From Stone NJ, Robinson JG, Lichtenstein AH, et al. 2013 ACC/AHA guideline on the treatment of blood cholesterol to reduce atherosclerotic cardiovascular risk in adults: a report of the American College of Cardiology/American Heart Association Task Force on Practice Guidelines. *J Am Coll Cardiol.* 2014;63(25Pt B):2889-2934.
ADD/AHA = American College of Cardiology/American Heart Association; DASH = Dietary Approaches to Stop Hypertension; HDL-C = high-density lipoprotein cholesterol; LDL-C = low-density lipoprotein cholesterol.

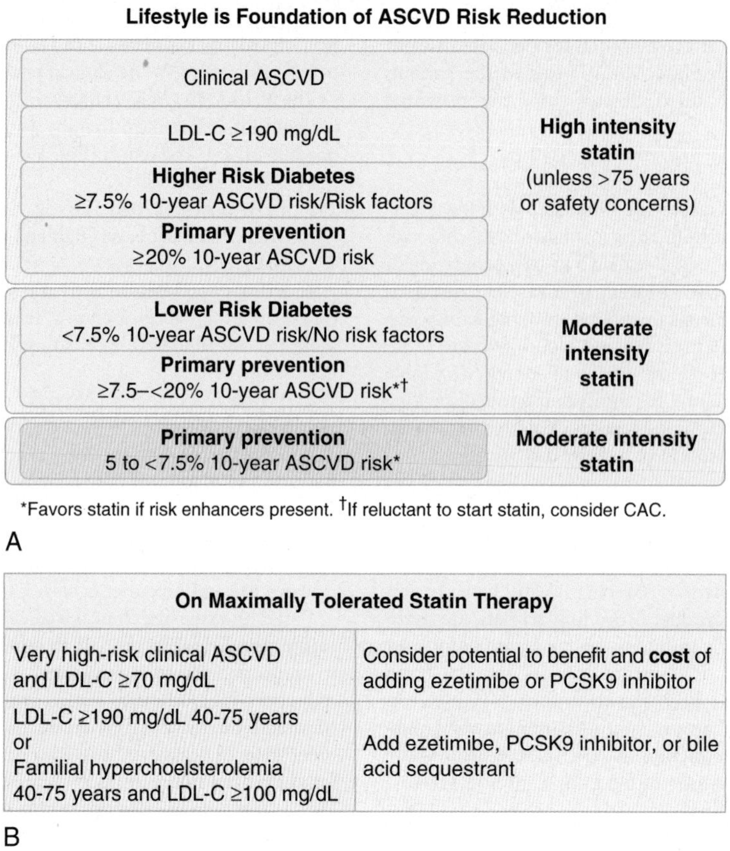

Lifestyle is Foundation of ASCVD Risk Reduction

Clinical ASCVD	High intensity statin (unless >75 years or safety concerns)
LDL-C ≥190 mg/dL	
Higher Risk Diabetes ≥7.5% 10-year ASCVD risk/Risk factors	
Primary prevention ≥20% 10-year ASCVD risk	
Lower Risk Diabetes <7.5% 10-year ASCVD risk/No risk factors	Moderate intensity statin
Primary prevention ≥7.5–<20% 10-year ASCVD risk*†	
Primary prevention 5 to <7.5% 10-year ASCVD risk*	Moderate intensity statin

*Favors statin if risk enhancers present. †If reluctant to start statin, consider CAC.

A

On Maximally Tolerated Statin Therapy	
Very high-risk clinical ASCVD and LDL-C ≥70 mg/dL	Consider potential to benefit and **cost** of adding ezetimibe or PCSK9 inhibitor
LDL-C ≥190 mg/dL 40-75 years or Familial hypercholesterolemia 40-75 years and LDL-C ≥100 mg/dL	Add ezetimibe, PCSK9 inhibitor, or bile acid sequestrant

B

FIGURE 195-4. Summary of 2018 ACC/AHA cholesterol guideline recommendations for statin and nonstatin therapy. Background color denotes Class and level of evidence: Green = Class I (strong) recommendation; yellow = Class IIa (reasonable) recommendation; blue = Grade A (high) level of evidence; orange = Grade B (moderate) level of evidence.

TABLE 195-3 HIGH-, MODERATE-, AND LOW-INTENSITY STATIN THERAPY*

STATIN THERAPY	HIGH INTENSITY† ↓LDL-C ≥50%	MODERATE INTENSITY‡ ↓LDL-C 30-<50%	LOW INTENSITY§ ↓LDL-C <30%
	DAILY DOSE		
Atorvastatin	(40‖)-80 mg	10 (20) mg	
Rosuvastatin	20 (40) mg	(5) 10 mg	
Simvastatin		20-40 mg¶	10 mg
Pravastatin		40 (80) mg	10-20 mg
Lovastatin		40 mg	20 mg
Fluvastatin		80 mg (Fluvastatin XL)	20-40 mg
Fluvastatin		40 mg**	
Pitavastatin		2-4 mg	1 mg

FDA = U.S. Food and Drug Administration; LDL-C = low-density lipoprotein cholesterol; XL = extended-release.

*Individual responses to statin therapy varied in randomized, controlled trials and vary in clinical practice. A less-than-average response may have a biologic basis. Statins and dosages in bold were reduced in major cardiovascular events in randomized, controlled trials. Statins and doses in italics were approved by the FDA but were not tested in randomized, controlled trials.

†Daily dose decreases LDL-C levels by an average of ≥50%.

‡Daily dose decreases LDL-C levels by an average of 30 to <50%.

§Daily dose decreases LDL-C levels by an average of <30%.

‖Evidence from 1 randomized, controlled trial only; down-titration if patient is unable to tolerate atorvastatin, 80 mg.

¶Although simvastatin, 80 mg, was evaluated in randomized, controlled trials, the FDA recommends against initiation of or titration to 80 mg of simvastatin because of increased risk for myopathy and rhabdomyolysis.

**Twice daily.

Reprinted with permission of the authors: Stone NJ, Robinson JG, Lichtenstein AH, et al. 2013 ACC/AHA Guideline on the Treatment of Blood Cholesterol to Reduce Atherosclerotic Cardiovascular Risk in Adults: A Report of the American College of Cardiology/American Heart Association Task Force on Practice Guidelines. *J Am Coll Cardiol.* 2014;63(25, Part B):2889-2934.

TABLE 195-4 RISK ENHANCING FACTORS FAVORING STATIN INITIATION

These characteristics may confer increased ASCVD risk due to genetic or adverse cardiometabolic risk factiors:

Family history of premature ASCVD (males, age < 55 years; females, age < 65 years)

Metabolic syndrome

CKD (eGFR 15-59 mL/min/1.73 m^2 ± albuminuria; no dialysis or transplantation)

Chronic inflammatory conditions (e.g., psoriasis, rheumatoid arthritis, HIV/AIDS)

Premature menopause (before age 40 years)

Pregnancy-associated conditions that increase later ASCVD risk (e.g., preeclampsia)

High-risk race/ethnicities (e.g., South Asian ancestry)

Ankle-brachial index < 0.9

LDL-C 160-189 mg/dL (4.1-4.8 mmol/L)

Non–HDL-C 190-219 mg/dL (4.9-5.6 mmol/L)

Persistently elevated, primary hypertriglyceridemia (≥175 mg/dL)

Lp(a) ≥ 50 mg/dL or ≥125 nmol/L

ApoB ≥ 130 mg/dL

hs-CRP ≥ 2.0 mg/L

2019 AHA/ACC Chol GL.

should be counseled to lose weight and engage in regular physical activity to prevent progression to diabetes.

Statins have no hepatotoxic effects. If baseline hepatic aminotransferase levels are less than two times the upper limit of normal, no further monitoring is needed following statin initiation. Nor is routine monitoring of creatine kinase recommended.

In the Cholesterol Treatment Trialists' meta-analysis of 26 statin trials, rhabdomyolysis, severe myopathy, and hemorrhagic stroke events were rare. The cardiovascular risk reduction benefit from statins far exceeds the risk of these rare events (E-Fig. 195-4).

Muscle or Other Symptoms During Statin Therapy

Many patients have symptoms during statin therapy. The challenge is to determine if the symptoms are caused by the statin. Recent randomized,

TABLE 195-5 APPROACH TO PATIENTS WITH SYMPTOMS DURING STATIN THERAPY

Mild-moderate symptoms	1. Stop statin 2. Wait until symptoms resolve 3. Rechallenge with lower dose of same statin, or another statin, per the patient's preference 4. Increase statin dose/interval as tolerated
Severe muscle pain or weakness	1. Stop statin 2. Check creatine kinase (CK), creatinine/glomerular filtration rate (GFR), urine myoglobin 3. Admit and carefully hydrate if CK >10 × ULN and elevated/worsened creatinine or myoglobinuria 4. Evaluate for predisposing factors and treat 5. If considering restarting statin, refer to lipidologist
Jaundice or persistent hepatic transaminases >5×	1. Stop statin 2. Evaluate for other causes of hepatitis 3. Consider statin reinitiation once condition resolves
Diabetes mellitus	1. Continue statin 2. Encourage weight loss and regular physical activity 3. Treat diabetes

ULN = upper limit of normal

double-blind placebo controlled trials have found that about 75 to 80% of patients reporting intolerance to two or more statins can tolerate atorvastatin 20 mg when received as blinded therapy. Therefore patient expectations of adverse effects, the "nocebo" effect, may play a large role in patients reporting symptoms during statin therapy.

The most straightforward approach in patients with mild to moderate symptoms is to stop the statin, wait until symptoms resolve, and rechallenge with the same statin at a lower dose or another statin at least once a week, depending on the patient's preferences after being informed of statin benefits (heart attack, stroke, and death reduction) (Table 195-5). If symptoms do not resolve within 2 months, the statin is not the cause. Alternative etiologies should be investigated and treated. Once treated, the statin can be reinitiated. After the statin has been tolerated for 3 months, up-titration is desirable. However, even rosuvastatin 10 mg once a week will lower LDL-C by about 25% on average.

Patients with severe muscle pain or weakness or dark urine should be evaluated for the possibility of rhabdomyolysis. Symptomatic creatine kinase elevations more than 10 times the upper limit of normal, elevated creatinine levels, and myoglobinuria are indicative of rhabdomyolysis. The statin should be stopped and the patient should be admitted to the hospital for hydration, close observation, and evaluation for other causes of severe muscle damage. Once any predisposing conditions are addressed, the safety and potential benefits of reinitiating statin therapy need to be carefully considered. Referral to a lipid specialist is advisable.

Statins have no hepatotoxic effects. If transaminases are two to three times the upper limit of normal, then alanine aminotransferase can be retested in 3 months as reassurance of continued statin safety. In patients with transaminases that are more than three times the upper limit of normal, other causes of hepatoxicity or infection should be investigated prior to statin initiation and the potential benefit and safety of statin therapy should be reassessed. If hepatitis symptoms develop during statin therapy, or transaminases more than five times the upper limit of normal persist on retest, the statin should be stopped until the patient's condition has improved.

Cognitive impairment has been reported anecdotally during statin therapy. The statin can be discontinued and rechallenged as outlined above. Persistent cognitive symptoms should be evaluated.

Special Populations

Many groups of patients were excluded from the randomized trials due to concerns regarding safety or the potential to benefit. Little clinical trial evidence is available for primary prevention patients older than 75 years of age. Statin initiation should be individualized in primary prevention patients older than 75 years based on patient preferences and severity of other comorbidities.

Patients with inflammatory or chronic infectious conditions may be at increased cardiovascular risk, and may meaningfully benefit from statin therapy. However, these patients may also be at increased risk of drug-drug interactions due to immunosuppressive or antiviral therapy.

Monitoring Statin Therapy

The 2018 AHA/ACC cholesterol guideline recommends periodically monitoring LDL-C levels after initiating statin therapy to evaluate treatment response and adherence to lifestyle and drug therapy.

NONSTATIN THERAPY

Two PCSK9 monoclonal antibodies, alirocumab and evolocumab, and ezetimibe have been shown to further reduce ASCVD risk when added to background statin therapy in high risk ASCVD patients. Although trials of niacin and fenofibrate reduced cardiovascular events as monotherapy, no benefit, and some evidence of harm, was found when these drugs were added to background therapy. Cholestyramine (a bile acid sequestrant) and gemfibrozil (a fibrate) did reduce cardiovascular events in selected populations of men. No trials have evaluated bile acid sequestrants added to background statin therapy. Gemfibrozil is contraindicated for use with statin therapy due to a greater than 30-fold increased risk of myopathy.

Ezetimibe

Ezetimibe acts in the small intestine to block cholesterol uptake by the Niemann-Pick C1-Like 1 receptor. The resulting lower level of intrahepatic cholesterol stimulates synthesis of LDL-C receptors. Ezetimibe 10 mg daily lowers LDL-C by 15 to 20% as monotherapy and an additional 20 to 25% when added to statin therapy, with similar percent reductions in non-HDL-C.

In IMPROVE-IT (Improved Reduction of Outcomes: Vytorin Efficacy International Trial), ezetimibe further reduced cardiovascular events when added to moderate-intensity statin therapy in patients with acute coronary syndromes and at least one additional high-risk characteristic.[A14] Mean LDL-C levels were 70 mg/dL in the simvastatin 40- to 80-mg group and 54 mg/dL in the ezetimibe-simvastatin 40-mg group. A modest 10% reduction in ASCVD events was observed over the average 6 years of treatment. The greatest reductions in risk occurred in the patients with diabetes, polyvascular ASCVD, or multiple high-risk characteristics.

Ezetimibe has no known significant adverse effects. Ezetimibe should be avoided during pregnancy and lactation.

PCSK9 Monoclonal Antibodies

PCSK9 monoclonal antibodies inactivate PCSK9, which allows the LDL receptor to be recirculated to the cell surface to continue to remove LDL from the blood. Two PCSK9 monoclonal antibodies have been FDA approved, alirocumab and evolocumab. These drugs are injected subcutaneously every 2 to 4 weeks. Alirocumab 75 to 150 mg every 2 weeks or 300 mg every 4 weeks lowers LDL-C by 45 to 65% as monotherapy or added to background statin therapy. Evolocumab 140 mg every 2 weeks or 320 mg every 4 weeks lowers LDL-C by 50 to 70%. Fairly similar reductions in non-HDL-C occur. These drugs also lower Lp(a) by 25 to 30%, the significance of which in unclear.

In the FOURIER (Further Cardiovascular Outcomes Research with PCSK9 Inhibition in Subjects with Elevated Risk) trial, evolocumab further reduced ASCVD risk when added to high- or moderate-intensity statin therapy in more than 27,000 patients with cardiovascular disease and additional high-risk characteristics.[A15] LDL-C levels were 92 mg/dL in the statin-placebo group and 30 mg/dL in the statin-evolocumab group. ASCVD events were reduced by 20% over the average treatment period of 2.2 years. This magnitude of relative risk reduction was somewhat less than expected for the 62 mg/dL (1.6 mmol/L) reduction in LDL-C when compared to the 22% reduction observed per 39 mg/dL (1 mmol/L) reduction in LDL-C observed in the statin trials. The ODYSSEY OUTCOMES trial found that alirocumab further reduced cardiovascular events in patients with acute coronary syndromes treated with high- or moderate-intensity statin therapy.[A16] A reduction in total mortality and the majority of the ASCVD risk reduction occurred in patients with baseline LDL-C levels greater than or equal to 100 mg/dL.

Previous data from evolocumab and alirocumab trials of 11 to 18 months duration found 50% relative risk reductions from approximately 70 mg/dL LDL-C reductions. In contrast to the FOURIER trial population, populations in these trials had mean baseline LDL-C levels of approximately 120 mg/dL, which is similar to the mean level in the Cholesterol Treatment Trialists meta-analysis where each 39 mg/dL reduction in LDL-C was associated with a 22% reduction in cardiovascular events. A subsequent meta-analysis of LDL-C lowering trials found when baseline LDL-C levels were less than 100 mg/dL, no reductions in total or cardiovascular mortality were observed. When baseline LDL-C levels were greater than 100 mg/dL, greater reductions in total and cardiovascular mortality occurred as baseline LDL-C levels increased. These data suggest diminishing returns to further reducing LDL-C levels of less than 100 mg/dL and of achieving very low LDL-C levels.[A17]

PCSK9 monoclonal antibodies have been well tolerated over a period of up to 3 years. The most common adverse effect has been mild, transient injection site reactions occurring in less than 5% of patients. No excess of adverse events was observed in the FOURIER trial or ODYSSEY OUTCOMES trials overall, and adverse event rates were similar across levels of achieved LDL-C levels, including those whose LDL-C remained below 25 mg/dL. PCSK9 monoclonal antibodies are highly selective for PCSK9, and the antibody-antigen complexes are metabolized by the reticuloendothelial system. Evolocumab and alirocumab have no drug interactions. Both antibodies are contraindicated during pregnancy and lactation.

The acquisition price of PCSK9 monoclonal antibodies has limited their use.[17] The 2018 AHA/ACC cholesterol guideline recommended the consideration of PCSK9 monoclonal antibodies only for very high-risk ASCVD patients whose LDL-C remained greater than 70 mg/dL despite maximal statin and ezetimibe therapy. Very high-risk patients include ASCVD patients with heterozygous FH or with several additional high-risk characteristics, including age 65 years or older, previous coronary revascularization, diabetes mellitus, hypertension, renal insufficiency (eGFR 15-59 mg/nL/min/1.73 m^2), current smoking, LDL-C 100 mg/dL or greater despite maximal statin therapy, or a history of congestive heart failure.

Other Nonstatin Therapies
Bile Acid Sequestering Agents
Cholestyramine, colestipol, and colesevelam bind bile acids in the intestinal lumen, interrupting the enterohepatic recirculation of the cholesterol-rich bile acids. Decreased intracellular cholesterol levels upregulate LDL-C receptor synthesis, thereby enhancing removal of LDL from the blood. Bile acid sequestrants are not absorbed and are excreted in the feces. Due to tolerability issues and modest LDL-C lowering effects, bile acid binding agents have limited clinical use.

Colesevelam is an anion-binding resin with greater affinity for the negatively charged bile acids than cholestyramine and colestipol. As a consequence, colesevelam is better tolerated and has fewer drug-drug interactions. At the full recommended doses, the three bile acid sequestering agents have similar efficacy, reducing LDL-C by 15 to 20%, similar to ezetimibe 10 mg used as monotherapy. Cholestyramine reduced cardiovascular events by 19% over a 7-year period in the Lipid Research Clinics trial in hypercholesterolemic men.

Use of bile acid sequestrants is limited by their bulk and significant gastrointestinal adverse effects, including severe constipation. They can also severely exacerbate underlying hypertriglyceridemia, and should be avoided when triglyceride levels are higher than 300 mg/dL. They may cause fat-soluble vitamin deficiencies. Use during pregnancy or lactation requires the potential for benefit to be weighed against the potential for harm.

Niacin
Niacin, or nicotinic acid, has beneficial effects on all lipid parameters, raising HDL-C, lowering LDL-C or non-HDL-C, triglycerides, and Lp(a) in a dose-dependent manner. Niacin's mechanisms of action have not been clearly elucidated. Due to tolerability issues and modest if any cardiovascular benefits, niacin is rarely used in clinical practice.

Niacin was one of the first cholesterol-lowering drugs tested in clinical trials. A trial of niacin in the pre-statin era found a modest benefit for immediate-release niacin 2 grams daily for reducing nonfatal coronary heart disease events in men with coronary heart disease, and a total mortality benefit that emerged on long-term follow-up. However, enthusiasm for niacin waned after the results of the AIM-HIGH[A18][A19] and HPS2-THRIVE[A20] trials, performed in the background of statin therapy, were reported. In AIM-HIGH, where both treatment groups were treated to similar LDL-C levels, the additional increase in HDL-C, reduction in triglycerides, non-HDL-C, and Lp(a) with extended release niacin 1.5 to 2 grams did not reduce cardiovascular events. In HPS2-THRIVE, extended-release niacin 2 grams combined with laropriprant (an antiflushing agent) did not further reduce cardiovascular events. Moreover, the niacin/laropriprant group had more serious adverse events, including disturbances in diabetes control, increased diabetes incidence, and cutaneous, gastrointestinal, bleeding, musculoskeletal, and infectious adverse events.

Mipomersen and Lomitapide
Mipomersen and *lomitapide* are orphan drugs with significant hepatotoxicity that are approved for use only in patients with homozygous familial hypercholesterolemia. They should be used only under the direction of a lipid specialist.

Determining When to Add Nonstatin Therapy
Once statin therapy and lifestyle are optimized, selected high-risk patients may benefit from further LDL-C lowering therapy. As for primary prevention in nondiabetic patients with LDL-C lower than 190 mg/dL, where the margin of benefit may be less and patient preferences are important, a clinician-patient discussion is recommended.

For very high-risk patients with an approximately 30% 10-year ASCVD risk, such as those with cardiovascular disease and familial hypercholesterolemia, diabetes, or polyvascular disease, adding ezetimibe would result in NNTs of more than 50 unless LDL-C levels are above 130 mg/dL (E-Fig. 195-5). Adding a PCSK9 monoclonal antibody is unlikely to be cost-effective unless LDL-C levels are over 100 to 130 mg/dL, dependent upon the level of price discounting.

For high-risk patients with an approximately 20% 10-year ASCVD risk, such as those with cardiovascular disease and well-controlled risk factors, or primary prevention patients with heterozygous familial hypercholesterolemia, adding ezetimibe would result in NNTs of more than 50 unless LDL-C levels are over 190 mg/dL (E-Fig. 195-5). Adding a PCSK9 monoclonal antibody is unlikely to be cost-effective unless LDL-C levels are over 130 to 160 mg/dL, dependent upon the level of price discounting.[17]

HYPERTRIGLYCERIDEMIA
The triglyceride levels reported by the laboratory reflect the triglycerides in the triglyceride-rich lipoproteins and their remnants, predominantly chylomicrons, VLDL, IDLs and to some extent LDL (Fig. 195-1). Since both cholesterol and triglycerides are carried in apolipoprotein B-containing lipoproteins, genetic variants associated with elevated blood triglyceride levels due to elevated triglyceride-rich lipoproteins are associated with increased ASCVD risk. Thus, the increased risk is not due to triglyceride levels per se.[18] However, the increased cardiovascular risk arises from the cholesterol-rich lipoproteins rather than the triglyceride level per se. Therefore, cardiovascular risk reduction efforts should focus primarily on reducing the levels of LDL-C and non-HDL-C. However, pancreatitis risk is increased when triglycerides are in excess of 1000 mg/dL, suggesting that these patients could benefit from therapy targeted specifically at lowering triglycerides.

Mild-moderate hypertriglyceridemia (150 to 499 mg/dL) is common in patients with cardiovascular risk factors, diabetes, or cardiovascular disease.[19] Small effects from a number of common and rare genetic variants contribute to triglyceride levels of 175 to 899 mg/dL. Triglyceride levels over 900 mg/dL usually result from a large-effect monogenetic disorder. Hypertriglyceridemia gene expression is modified by stimuli from the diet, excess adiposity, physical activity, drugs, and other factors. Because hypertriglyceridemia clusters in families due to shared genetic and environmental stimuli, screening and counseling of family members is recommended once severe hypertriglyceridemia (>500 mg/dL) is identified.

TREATMENT   Rx

Patients should be retested after at least a 12-hour fast to confirm fasting hypertriglyceridemia. Reductions in elevated triglyceride levels are likely to benefit selected patients,[20] and the treatment approach is the same for almost all patients with hypertriglyceridemia.

Lifestyle
Successful lifestyle modification often has dramatic effects. All patients with triglycerides higher than 150 mg/dL should be counseled on a healthy diet, with an emphasis on avoiding refined carbohydrates and processed foods as well as saturated, *trans* and overall high fat intake. Increased omega-3 rich fish intake may also be beneficial. Regular physical activity and modest weight loss are also helpful. Alcohol should be avoided. Patients whose triglycerides remain over 1000 mg/dL should also be referred to a dietician for counseling on a very low-fat diet.

Rule Out Secondary Causes
If triglycerides remain elevated above 500 mg/dL, secondary causes should be sought and treated (Table 195-1). The most common secondary cause of hypertriglyceridemia is undiagnosed or inadequately treated diabetes mellitus (Chapter 216). Other common causes include a large weight gain, excessive alcohol or sugar intake, drugs (estrogen, glucocorticoids, protease inhibitors, retinoic acid), pregnancy, and renal disease.

Statins to Reduce ASCVD Risk

Many hypertriglyceridemic patients are at increased cardiovascular risk or may have concomitant elevations in LDL-C or non-HDL-C. Statin therapy to reduce ASCVD risk is recommended for these patients. A direct LDL-C can be obtained when triglyceride levels are over 500 mg/dL.

As monotherapy, gemfibrozil and fenofibrate have been shown to reduce cardiovascular events in selected populations. Subgroup analyses suggest fenofibrate may reduce cardiovascular risk in diabetic patients with both low HDL-C and elevated triglycerides on a moderate-intensity statin. However, the relative reductions in cardiovascular risk observed in these analyses were what would be expected from the reductions in non-HDL-C. Therefore, statins continue to be first-line cardiovascular risk reduction therapy based on the extensive evidence of benefit and safety for statin therapy across all triglyceride and HDL-C subgroups.

Drug Therapy to Lower Triglycerides

Based on observational data, patients with triglyceride levels over 1000 mg/dL or a history of hypertriglyceridemic pancreatitis may benefit from additional drug therapy to lower triglycerides in order to decrease the risk of pancreatitis. The efficacy of various drugs with triglyceride-lowering effects is shown in E-Table 195-1. Low- to moderate-intensity statin therapy should be intensified because high-intensity statins further reduce triglycerides by about 25%.

Fibrates

If additional triglyceride lowering is needed, fenofibrate is the most convenient option and lowers triglycerides 15 to 35%. However, fenofibrate increases the risk of serious myopathy five-fold in patients treated with moderate-intensity statins, with little safety data on use with high-intensity statins. Fenofibrate can also raise LDL-C levels in some patients, which is probably not beneficial. It can also raise creatinine levels without affecting renal function, and needs dose adjustment when the glomerular filtration rate is lower than 60 mL/min/1.73 m^2. Gemfibrozil increases the risk of serious myopathy and rhabdomyolysis 30-fold in statin-treated patients and should be avoided.

Marine Omega-3 Fatty Acids

It is probably safer for patients on high-intensity statin therapy to add omega-3 fatty acids with at least 3.4 mg of docosahexaenoic acid (DHA) or eicosapentanoic acid (EPA). This amount of DHA/EPA can be obtained from 4 capsules containing 850 mg DHA/EPA per 1000 mg marine oil capsule, and can be taken in divided doses. Lower doses (1000 mg daily) can reduce the risk of myocardial infarction but not of all major cardiovascular events.[A21] In the REDUCE-IT trial, icosapent ethyl, a highly purified eicosapentaenoic acid ester (4 grams daily) reduced cardiovascular events in very high-risk ASCVD patients with triglyceride levels 135 to 499 mg/dL. A 25% reduction in the risk of major cardiovascular events occurred over an average of 5 years of treatment.[A22] It is not clear whether this benefit was due to triglyceride-lowering per se or an effect of EPA. Atrial fibrillation, peripheral edema, and adverse bleeding events were more common in the icosapent ethyl group.

Other Lipid Drugs

Niacin has modest triglyceride-lowering effects but may exacerbate hyperglycemia, and along with its other adverse effects has a limited role. Ezetimibe and PCSK9 monoclonal antibodies have no significant triglyceride-lowering effects. Bile acid sequestrants should be avoided when triglycerides are over 300 mg/dL because they have been known to cause hypertriglyceridemic pancreatitis.

Volanesorsen is an orphan drug approved for treatment of patients with familial chylomicronemia syndrome and familial partial lipodystrophy, severe autosomal recessive triglyceride disorders with significant morbidity. Volanesorsen is an antisense olionucleotide that targets the messenger RNA for apo C-III.

In pregnant women, the benefits of fenofibrate and gemfibrozil therapy should be carefully weighed against the risks; fibrates should not be used in nursing mothers.

Grade A References

A1. Fulcher J, O'Connell R, Voysey M, et al. Efficacy and safety of LDL-lowering therapy among men and women: meta-analysis of individual data from 174,000 participants in 27 randomised trials. *Lancet.* 2015;385:1397-1405.

A2. Sabatine MS, Wiviott SD, Im K, et al. Efficacy and safety of further lowering of low-density lipoprotein cholesterol in patients starting with very low levels: a meta-analysis. *JAMA Cardiol.* 2018;3:823-828.

A3. Koskinas KC, Siontis GCM, Piccolo R, et al. Effect of statins and non-statin LDL-lowering medications on cardiovascular outcomes in secondary prevention: a meta-analysis of randomized trials. *Eur Heart J.* 2018;39:1172-1180.

A4. Mills EJ, O'Regan C, Eyawo O, et al. Intensive statin therapy compared with moderate dosing for prevention of cardiovascular events: a meta-analysis of >40 000 patients. *Eur Heart J.* 2011;32:1409-1415.

A5. Chou R, Dana T, Blazina I, et al. Statins for prevention of cardiovascular disease in adults: evidence report and systematic review for the US Preventive Services Task Force. *JAMA.* 2016;316:2008-2024.

A6. Bowman L, Hopewell JC, Chen F, et al. Effects of anacetrapib in patients with atherosclerotic vascular disease. *N Engl J Med.* 2017;377:1217-1227.

A7. Zhan S, Tang M, Liu F, et al. Ezetimibe for the prevention of cardiovascular disease and all-cause mortality events. *Cochrane Database Syst Rev.* 2018;11:CD012502.

A8. Sabatine MS, Giugliano RP, Wiviott SD, et al. Efficacy and safety of evolocumab in reducing lipids and cardiovascular events. *N Engl J Med.* 2015;372:1500-1509.

A9. Schwartz GG, Steg PG, Szarek M, et al. Alirocumab and cardiovascular outcomes after acute coronary syndrome. *N Engl J Med.* 2018;379:2097-2107.

A10. Silverman MG, Ference BA, Im K, et al. Association between lowering LDL-C and cardiovascular risk reduction among different therapeutic interventions: a systematic review and meta-analysis. *JAMA.* 2016;316:1289-1297.

A11. Baigent C, Blackwell L, Emberson J, et al. Efficacy and safety of more intensive lowering of LDL cholesterol: a meta-analysis of data from 170,000 participants in 26 randomised trials. *Lancet.* 2010;376:1670-1681.

A12. Cholesterol Treatment Center Trialists' Collaboration. Efficacy and safety of statin therapy in older people: a meta-analysis of individual participant data from 28 randomised controlled trials. *Lancet.* 2019;393:407-415.

A13. He Y, Li X, Gasevic D, et al. Statins and multiple noncardiovascular outcomes: umbrella review of meta-analyses of observational studies and randomized controlled trials. *Ann Intern Med.* 2018;169:543-553.

A14. Cannon CP, Blazing MA, Giugliano RP, et al. Ezetimibe added to statin therapy after acute coronary syndromes. *N Engl J Med.* 2015;372:2387-2397.

A15. Giugliano RP, Pedersen TR, Park JG, et al. Clinical efficacy and safety of achieving very low LDL-cholesterol concentrations with the PCSK9 inhibitor evolocumab: a prespecified secondary analysis of the FOURIER trial. *Lancet.* 2017;390:1962-1971.

A16. Steg PG, Szarek M, Bhatt DL, et al. Effect of alirocumab on mortality after acute coronary syndromes: an analysis of the ODYSSEY OUTCOMES randomized clinical trial. *Circulation.* 2019. [Epub ahead of print.]

A17. Navarese EP, Robinson JG, Kowalewski M, et al. Association between baseline LDL-C level and total and cardiovascular mortality after LDL-C lowering: a systematic review and meta-analysis. *JAMA.* 2018;319:1566-1579.

A18. Boden WE, Probstfield JL, Anderson T, et al. Niacin in patients with low HDL cholesterol levels receiving intensive statin therapy. *N Engl J Med.* 2011;365:2255-2267.

A19. Probstfield JL, Boden WE, Anderson T, et al. Cardiovascular outcomes during extended follow-up of the AIM-HIGH trial cohort. *J Clin Lipidol.* 2018;12:1413-1419.

A20. HPS2-THRIVE randomized placebo-controlled trial in 25 673 high-risk patients of ER niacin/laropiprant: trial design, pre-specified muscle and liver outcomes, and reasons for stopping study treatment. *Eur Heart J.* 2013;34:1279-1291.

A21. Manson JE, Cook NR, Lee IM, et al. Marine n-3 fatty acids and prevention of cardiovascular disease and cancer. *N Engl J Med.* 2019;380:23-32.

A22. Bhatt DL, Steg PG, Miller M, et al. Cardiovascular risk reduction with icosapent ethyl for hypertriglyceridemia. *N Engl J Med.* 2019;380:11-22.

GENERAL REFERENCES

For the General References and other additional features, please visit Expert Consult at https://expertconsult.inkling.com.

196

GLYCOGEN STORAGE DISEASES

DAVID A. WEINSTEIN

DEFINITION

Glycogen, a highly branched polymer of glucose, is the storage form of glucose in mammals. The major sites of glycogen deposition are skeletal muscle and liver. Several other tissues and organs, including the heart, smooth muscle, kidney, and intestine, are sites of glycogen synthesis that can be impaired in the glycogen storage diseases (GSDs).[1]

EPIDEMIOLOGY

The overall frequency of the GSDs is approximately 1 case per 20,000 to 25,000 births. Sixteen distinct types have been identified, which are referred to either by the deficient enzyme or by a numbering system that reflects the historical sequence of their description. They are all uncommon and some are extremely rare. Six types account for approximately 97% of GSD cases: GSD I (25%), GSD II (15%), GSD III (24%), GSD IV (3%), and GSD VI and IX (30%). It is likely, however, that the mild forms of GSD are underrecognized, and GSD IX may be the most common identifiable cause of recurrent hypoglycemia (Chapter 217) in male patients.

PATHOBIOLOGY

Glucose transporter type 2 (GLUT2) predominates in the liver (and pancreatic beta cells) and has a high K_m ($\approx$15 to 20 mmol/L); consequently, the free glucose concentration in hepatocytes increases in direct proportion to the increase in plasma glucose concentration. Glucose is rapidly phosphorylated by glucokinase to form glucose 6-phosphate, which is converted to glucose 1-phosphate, the starting point for glycogen synthesis (Fig. 196-1). Hepatic glycogen synthase catalyzes the formation of α-1,4 linkages that elongate the chains of glucose molecules. A branching enzyme leads to formation of α-1,6 linkages at branch points along the chain. The concentration of GLUT4 in the plasma membrane of skeletal muscle increases markedly after exposure to insulin and in response to exercise, resulting in increased glucose transport into skeletal muscle, where it is either oxidized to provide energy for contracting muscle or converted to glycogen.

In the intervals between meals and during the overnight fast, a cascade of enzymatic reactions (including adenylate cyclase, phosphorylase *b* kinase, and cyclic adenosine monophosphate–dependent protein kinase) activates hepatic glycogen phosphorylase, the rate-limiting enzyme in glycogenolysis, leading to the formation of glucose 6-phosphate. Glucose-6-phosphatase catalyzes the terminal reaction of both glycogenolysis and gluconeogenesis, the hydrolysis of glucose 6-phosphate, thereby allowing glucose to be released from the liver into the systemic circulation. This process is critically important for the maintenance of glucose homeostasis. Because muscle lacks glucose-6-phosphatase, it cannot release glucose for systemic use. Muscle glycogen is used to meet the energy requirement of contracting muscle and is a source of lactate, pyruvate, and alanine for gluconeogenesis early in starvation. The rate of glycogenolysis in muscle is most rapid during the first 5 to 10 minutes of exercise. As exercise continues and blood flow to muscle increases, blood-borne substrates (glucose and free fatty acids) become increasingly important sources of energy.

The GSDs or glycogenoses comprise several inherited disorders of glycogen synthesis or degradation. All are autosomal recessive with the exception of a subtype of GSD IX that is X-linked. The GSDs are caused by mutations in the genes that code for enzymes involved in the synthesis or degradation of glycogen and may involve the liver, skeletal muscle, and kidney. They are all characterized by an abnormal tissue concentration or structure (or both) of the glycogen molecule.

CLINICAL MANIFESTATIONS AND DIAGNOSIS

Hepatomegaly and hypoglycemia are the principal clinical manifestations of the hepatic glycogenoses; muscle cramps, exercise intolerance, easy fatigability, and progressive weakness are the major manifestations of the muscle glycogenoses. Features of the most common GSDs are shown in Table 196-1. Molecular genetic testing performed on DNA extracted from blood or saliva is used to diagnose all of the common forms of GSD.

TREATMENT   Rx

The goal of treatment of the hepatic forms of GSD is to prevent hypoglycemia and glucose counter-regulation. The specific details of therapy principally depend on whether normal gluconeogenesis can occur. In GSD I, abnormal glucose-6-phosphatase activity impairs both glycogenolysis and gluconeogenesis. In contrast, gluconeogenesis is intact in the other liver forms of GSD, allowing protein to be used as a substrate for endogenous glucose production. Fatty acid oxidation is also intact in all types of GSD except for GSD I, resulting in ketone formation during periods of hypoglycemia.[2]

Treatment of GSD I consists of providing a continuous dietary source of glucose to maintain blood glucose levels at 75 to 90 mg/dL before meals and overnight. Glucose concentrations must be maintained above 70 mg/dL to prevent counter-regulation, which causes shunting of glucose 6-phosphate into alternative pathways, resulting in hyperlactacidemia, hyperuricemia, and hypertriglyceridemia. In infants, continuous glucose can be provided by frequent feeds during the day and continuous intragastric feeds at night through a nasogastric or gastrostomy tube. Beginning at 6 to 12 months of age, uncooked cornstarch (UCS), which is slowly digested and absorbed into the circulation as glucose, can be used as an alternative method of continuously providing

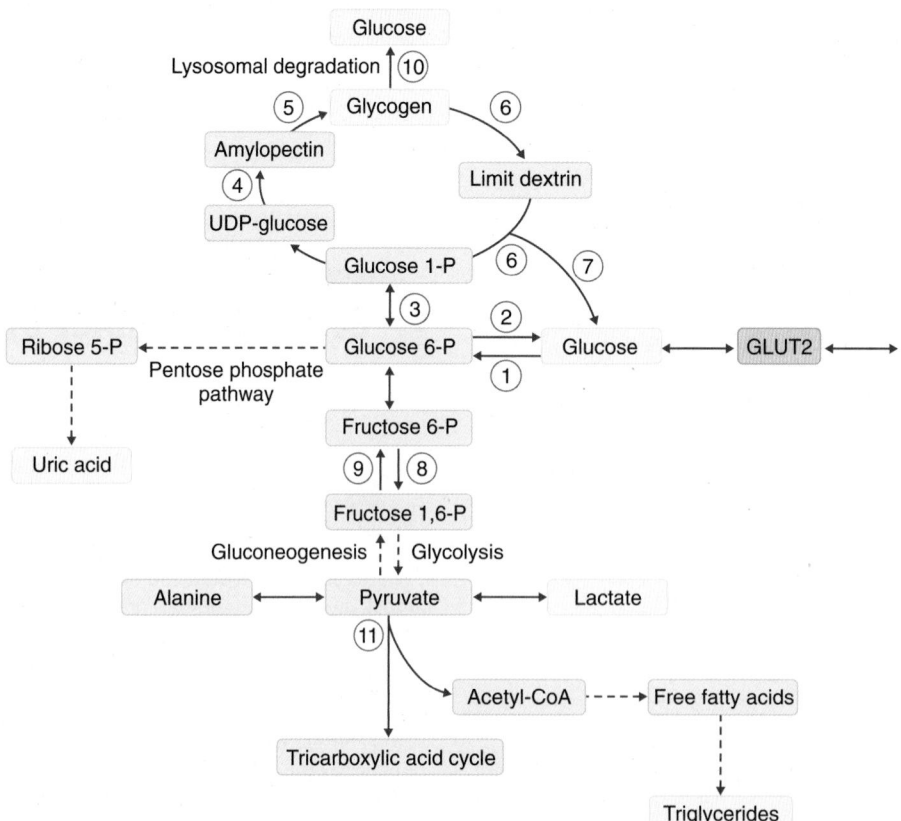

FIGURE 196-1. Simplified scheme of glycogen synthesis and degradation in the liver. Note that in skeletal muscle, glucose transporter type 4 (GLUT4) transports glucose across the cell membrane and glucose-6-phosphatase is absent. CoA = coenzyme A; UDP-glucose = uridine diphosphoglucose; 1, hexokinase/glucokinase; 2, glucose-6-phosphatase; 3, phosphoglucomutase; 4, glycogen synthase; 5, branching enzyme; 6, glycogen phosphorylase; 7, debranching enzyme; 8, phosphofructokinase; 9, fructose-1,6-bisphosphatase; 10, acid maltase; 11, pyruvate dehydrogenase.

TABLE 196-1 PRINCIPAL FEATURES OF THE COMMON GLYCOGEN STORAGE DISEASES

TYPE AND DEFECTIVE ENZYME	CHARACTERISTIC CLINICAL FEATURES	HIGH-RISK POPULATIONS	THERAPY
0 *Hepatic glycogen synthase*	Liver small or normal in size, fasting ketotic hypoglycemia, postprandial hyperglycemia and hyperlactatemia	French Canadians Italians	UCS, especially at bedtime, with high-protein diet
Ia *Glucose-6-phosphatase* *von Gierke disease*	Hepatomegaly, failure to thrive, growth retardation, severe hypoglycemia, lactic acidosis, hyperuricemia, hyperlipidemia	Ashkenazi Jews Mexicans Chinese Japanese	UCS during the day and night or continuous overnight intragastric feeding
Ib *Glucose 6-phosphate transporter*	Same as type Ia; also neutropenia, recurrent bacterial infections, and inflammatory bowel disease	Native Americans Iranian Jews Italians	UCS as for glycogen storage disease Ia; granulocyte colony-stimulating factor, mesalamine
II *Lysosomal acid maltase (α-glucosidase)* *Pompe disease*	Infantile form is characterized by severe generalized hypotonia, muscle weakness, and hypertrophic cardiomyopathy leading to cardiorespiratory failure usually by 1 year of age. Skeletal myopathy with slowly progressing muscle weakness is the primary clinical manifestation of the juvenile- and adult-onset forms. Serum creatine kinase is markedly increased.	None	Intravenous enzyme replacement with recombinant human α-glucosidase
III *Debranching enzyme* *Cori or Forbes disease*	Hepatomegaly, moderate to severe ketotic hypoglycemia, muscle weakness and wasting, hypertrophic cardiomyopathy (IIIa), increased transaminases; without muscle involvement (IIIb)	Faroe Islanders First Nation (Canada) Indian subcontinent	High-protein diet with low-dose UCS supplementation
IV *Glycogen branching enzyme* *Andersen disease*	A clinically heterogeneous disorder The typical presentation is liver disease in early childhood progressing to lethal cirrhosis. The less common neuromuscular presentation is distinguished by age at onset into 4 groups: perinatal, congenital, childhood, and adult.	None	High-protein diet with restriction of carbohydrates Liver transplantation has resulted in decreased glycogen storage in heart and skeletal muscle.
V *Muscle glycogen phosphorylase* *McArdle disease*	Symptoms usually begin in adolescence or early adulthood with exercise intolerance, fatigue, myalgia, muscle cramps, and muscle swelling. Transient myoglobinuria due to rhabdomyolysis may occur after exercise. Severe myoglobinuria may lead to acute renal failure. Later in adult life, persistent and progressive muscle weakness and atrophy with fatty replacement occur. Serum creatine kinase is increased.	None	High-protein diet (50% carbohydrate and 25-30% protein) Oral sucrose before sustained aerobic exercise may be beneficial.
VI *Hepatic glycogen phosphorylase* *Hers disease*	Hepatomegaly; growth retardation; moderate ketotic hypoglycemia; increased serum transaminases, cholesterol, and triglycerides	Mennonites Scottish	UCS dosed to prevent hypoglycemia and ketosis
VII *Muscle phosphofructokinase* *Tarui disease*	Manifested in childhood with fatigue, muscle cramps, exercise intolerance; rhabdomyolysis and myoglobinuria with strenuous exertion; increased serum creatine kinase; may have mild hemolytic anemia and mild hyperbilirubinemia; hyperuricemia	None	No specific treatment; avoid strenuous exercise
IX *Phosphorylase b kinase*	Hepatomegaly, mild ketotic hypoglycemia, growth retardation, increased serum transaminases, hypercholesterolemia, hypertriglyceridemia May be X-linked or autosomal recessive	None	UCS dosed to prevent hypoglycemia and ketosis; high-protein diet to normalize prealbumin

UCS = uncooked cornstarch.

glucose. Initially, UCS is given every 3 hours. As children age and guided by the results of periodic blood glucose and lactate monitoring, the interval between feeds eventually is increased to 4 to 5 hours. An extended-release cornstarch preparation allows many older patients to sleep through the night without awakening, but use is not recommended in children under 5 years of age.[3] Galactose and fructose must be restricted because they cannot be converted to glucose, and consumption of large quantities may exacerbate the biochemical derangements. Optimal care usually ameliorates all biochemical abnormalities; however, if optimal dietary management does not lower serum uric acid and triglycerides to acceptable levels, treatment with allopurinol and gemfibrozil, respectively, is indicated. Neutropenia (Chapter 158) in type Ib responds well to low-dose granulocyte colony-stimulating factor (G-CSF) therapy; however, untoward effects of G-CSF may include splenomegaly and very rare cases of leukemia.[4] The recommended starting dose (2.5 µg/kg/day) is therefore lower than in other conditions, and the lowest possible dose that prevents infections is used. Vitamin E supplementation may improve neutrophil survival and allow lower G-CSF doses.[5] An enterocolitis that resembles Crohn disease (Chapter 132) occurs almost universally in GSD type Ib, and mesalamine (Pentasa) is the first-line therapy because small intestinal disease predominates.

Patients with the other forms of GSD use a high-protein diet (2 or 3 g/kg) supplemented with complex carbohydrates and UCS, which, typically, is administered every 6 to 8 hours to maintain glucose concentrations above 75 mg/dL. Because β-oxidation of fatty acids can occur in these forms of GSD, ketosis can develop rapidly, and UCS doses are titrated to maintain a normal blood ketone concentration (<0.3 mmol/L). Protein dosing is aimed at normalization of total protein and prealbumin concentrations. Strict avoidance of fructose and sucrose is unnecessary; however, intake of simple sugars is still discouraged to avoid excessive storage of glycogen. This is particularly important in GSD III because excessive glycogen storage has been associated with worsening of the associated hypertrophic cardiomyopathy.

Treatment of the muscle glycogenoses is shown in Table 196-1.

Prevention of Complications

Long-term complications previously were common in GSD I and III. There is increasing evidence, however, that complications can be delayed or even prevented with optimal metabolic control.[6] Hepatic adenomas can develop in patients with GSD I during adolescence or early adulthood and may gradually enlarge, undergo malignant transformation, or hemorrhage into the peritoneal cavity. Nephrocalcinosis and nephrolithiasis, caused by hypocitraturia, are also common and can be prevented by oral citrate supplementation. Maintenance of optimal metabolic control can prevent development of hepatic adenomas, renal tubular dysfunction, focal segmental glomerulosclerosis, anemia, gout, and osteoporosis.

In type III GSD, a hypertrophic cardiomyopathy can develop. The cardiac disease appears to be caused by overstorage of glycogen, and restriction of simple sugars and carbohydrates has resulted in normalization of cardiac function. Hepatic adenomas develop in 10% of patients, and hepatocellular cancer is rare. Most patients with type III do not have myopathic symptoms during childhood and early adulthood. Progressive myopathy can develop beginning in the teenage years, and it can become debilitating. A very high protein diet (3 or 4 g/kg) may slow the progression of the muscle disease.[7]

Short stature and osteoporosis are the only common complications in GSD 0, VI, and IX, but these can be prevented by maintenance of optimal metabolic control and avoidance of ketosis. Cirrhosis has been described as a complication in untreated patients with GSD IX, but scarring may be prevented with treatment.

PROGNOSIS

The prognosis for all of the hepatic GSDs is now excellent. Almost all complications can be delayed or prevented with optimal metabolic control. Patients are doing well into adulthood, and pregnancies are now routine. Liver transplantation should be viewed as a treatment of last resort, especially because gene therapy may be available for treatment of these disorders in the future. Gene therapy has been used to successfully treat animal models for GSD I and II, and human gene therapy trials for GSD Ia have recently been started.

The Association for Glycogen Storage Disease website (*http://www.agsdus.org*) provides basic information about the GSDs intended to be of use to people affected by one of the GSDs, their families, and other interested parties. Similar organizations exist in the United Kingdom, France, Spain, the Netherlands, Germany, Italy, Sweden, the Faroe Islands, Russia, Poland, Brazil, and Mexico, as well as an organization for all of South America.

GENERAL REFERENCES

For the General References and other additional features, please visit Expert Consult at https://expertconsult.inkling.com.

197

LYSOSOMAL STORAGE DISEASES

DONNA M. KRASNEWICH AND ELLEN SIDRANSKY

The lysosomal storage diseases encompass a group of more than 50 different inherited disorders, all sharing a defect in lysosomal function. Lysosomes are acidic, membrane-bound organelles located in the cytoplasm that contain enzymes that degrade macromolecules. Lysosomal storage disorders ensue when one or more of the hydrolytic enzymes are deficient or when essential lysosomal transporters, receptors, cofactors, or protective proteins are defective or lacking. Typically, complex macromolecules, including glycolipids, mucopolysaccharides, and glycoproteins, are delivered to the lysosome, where they undergo sequential modification by a series of hydrolases. An enzymatic deficiency becomes clinically important when macromolecules accumulate due to inadequate degradation. Different categories of defects resulting in lysosomal dysfunction are encountered in the lysosomal storage disorders; examples of each type are listed in Table 197-1.

Although most lysosomal storage disorders are rare, as a group their frequency is estimated to be 1 per 7000 to 8000 live births. This is an underestimate because milder or attenuated forms of these disorders are often not identified. Each of the disorders has an autosomal recessive pattern of inheritance, except for Fabry disease and Hunter syndrome (mucopolysaccharidosis II), which are X-linked recessive, and Danon disease, caused by mutations in the lysosome-associated membrane protein 2 (LAMP-2), which is inherited in an X-linked dominant manner. All lysosomal storage disorders are characterized by a broad spectrum of manifestations, sometimes causing them to evade diagnosis. Many were traditionally classified into infantile, juvenile, and adult types, based on the patient's age at the onset of manifestations, but atypical presentations complicate these distinctions. Among the factors contributing to this phenotypic diversity are the amount of residual enzyme activity, the cellular localization of the enzyme, the genotype, and the genetic background of the affected individual, as well as other genetic, environmental, and epigenetic influences.[1]

TABLE 197-1   CLASSIFICATION OF LYSOSOMAL STORAGE DISORDERS BASED ON THE TYPE OF DEFECT*

SPHINGOLIPIDOSES

Fabry disease (α-galactosidase)
Farber disease (ceramidase)
GM$_1$ gangliosidosis/Landing disease (β-galactosidase)
GM$_2$ gangliosidosis/Tay-Sachs disease
Sandhoff disease (α-hexosaminidases A and B)
Gaucher disease (glucocerebrosidase)
Niemann-Pick disease, types A and B (sphingomyelinase)
Metachromatic leukodystrophy (arylsulfatase A)
Krabbe disease (β-galactocerebrosidase)

LIPID STORAGE DISORDERS

Wolman disease (acid lipase)
Ceroid-lipofuscinosis, adult type, Kufs/Parry (CLN4, heterogeneous)

MUCOPOLYSACCHARIDOSES

Type I/Hurler disease (α-L-iduronidase)
Type II/Hunter disease (iduronate-2-sulfatase)
Type III/Sanfilippo disease (four different enzymes in the degradation of heparan sulfate defining types A-D)
Type VI/Maroteaux-Lamy disease (*N*-acetylgalactosamine-4-sulfatase)
Type VII/Sly disease (α-glucuronidase)

OLIGOSACCHARIDOSES

Aspartylglucosaminuria (aspartylglucosaminidase)
Fucosidosis (α-fucosidase)
α-Mannosidosis (α-mannosidase)
Schindler disease (α-*N*-acetylgalactosaminidase)
Sialidosis I (sialidase)
Sialidosis II/mucolipidosis I (sialidase)

MUCOLIPIDOSES

Mucolipidosis II/I-cell disease (*N*-acetylglucosaminylphosphotransferase)
Mucolipidosis III/pseudo-Hurler (*N*-acetylglucosaminylphosphotransferase)
Mucolipidosis IV (*MCOLN1* mutation)

LYSOSOMAL GLYCOGEN STORAGE DISORDERS

Glycogenosis type II/Pompe disease (α-1,4-glucosidase)

LYSOSOMAL TRANSPORT DISORDERS

Sialic acid storage disease/Salla disease (sialin/SLC17A5)
Cystinosis (cystine transporter)
Niemann-Pick disease, type C (intracellular cholesterol transport)

MULTIPLE ENZYME DEFICIENCY DISORDERS

Galactosialidosis (β-galactosidase and sialidase)
Multiple sulfatase deficiency/Austin disease (sulfatases)

*Full chapters describing each of these disorders are available in Valle D, Beaudet AL, Vogelstein B, et al., eds. The Online Metabolic and Molecular Bases of Inherited Disease. http://www.ommbid.com/OMMBID

With the advent of new therapies for some of the lysosomal storage disorders, early establishment of the diagnosis is paramount. Suggestive clinical findings include coarse facial features; organomegaly; specific eye findings, including corneal clouding or a cherry red spot (of the macula); cytopenia; and skeletal abnormalities, notably dysostosis multiplex. Disorders associated with each of these findings are listed in Table 197-2. There should be a greater index of suspicion whenever these features occur in concert, the findings are progressive, there is developmental regression, or the affected individual appears dissimilar to other family members.

The diagnostic work-up includes a careful history, with analysis of the family pedigree and assessment of developmental milestones in childhood and adolescence. A family history of consanguinity, other affected siblings, multiple miscarriages, or early deaths can aid in making the diagnosis. Ethnicity can be a helpful clue because some of the lysosomal disorders occur with increased incidence in specific populations, such as Ashkenazi Jews (Gaucher disease type 1, Tay-Sachs disease, mucolipidosis type IV) and Scandinavians (mannosidosis, aspartylglucosaminuria, Salla disease, Gaucher disease type 3). On physical examination, special attention should be paid to head circumference (micro or macrocephaly), facial appearance (coarse facies), enlargement of the tongue, hepatosplenomegaly, skeletal manifestations including kyphosis, broadening of the long bones, and stiffness of the joints. Skin evaluation may reveal angiokeratoma, especially around the umbilicus and in skin creases.

TABLE 197-2 MANIFESTATIONS ENCOUNTERED IN DIFFERENT LYSOSOMAL STORAGE DISORDERS

FINDING	DISORDERS
Hepatosplenomegaly	GM$_1$ gangliosidosis, Niemann-Pick disease, Gaucher disease, Wolman disease, lysosomal acid lipase deficiency, fucosidosis, Pompe disease, mannosidosis, multiple sulfatase deficiency, sialidosis, galactosialidosis, several mucopolysaccharidoses, cystinosis
Coarse facies	GM$_1$ gangliosidosis, fucosidosis, Pompe disease, mannosidosis, multiple sulfatase deficiency, I-cell disease, several mucopolysaccharidoses, mucolipidosis II, sialic acid storage disease, aspartylglucosaminuria
Skeletal findings	GM$_1$ gangliosidosis, Gaucher disease, fucosidosis, mannosidosis, sialidosis, galactosialidosis, several mucopolysaccharidoses, I-cell disease, mucolipidosis III
Cherry red spot (retina)	Infantile forms of GM$_1$ gangliosidosis, Sandhoff disease, Tay-Sachs disease, Niemann-Pick disease, sialidosis, galactosialidosis, I-cell disease
Corneal clouding	GM$_1$ gangliosidosis, several mucopolysaccharidoses, mannosidosis, I-cell disease, mucolipidosis III and IV, multiple sulfatase deficiency, galactosialidosis
Cognitive impairment	GM$_1$ gangliosidosis, Sandhoff disease, Tay-Sachs disease, Niemann-Pick disease, Gaucher disease type 2, Wolman disease, fucosidosis, mannosidosis, multiple sulfatase deficiency, sialidosis, galactosialidosis, several mucopolysaccharidoses, sialic acid storage disease, aspartylglucosaminuria, I-cell disease, mucolipidosis III and IV, Krabbe disease, metachromatic leukodystrophy, neuronal ceroid lipofuscinosis

Hematologic
  Foam cells
  Granulated or vacuolated white blood cells
	GM$_1$ gangliosidosis, Niemann-Pick disease, Gaucher disease, acid lipase deficiency, fucosidosis
	Several mucopolysaccharidoses, sialidosis, galactosialidosis, neuronal ceroid-lipofuscinosis, Niemann-Pick disease, Wolman disease, fucosidosis, mannosidosis, aspartylglucosaminuria, I-cell disease, mucolipidosis III, multiple sulfatase deficiency

Psychiatric or behavioral manifestations	Several mucopolysaccharidoses (especially Sanfilippo), sialidosis, galactosialidosis, Fabry disease, mannosidosis, neuronal ceroid-lipofuscinosis, metachromatic leukodystrophy, Tay-Sachs disease, Niemann-Pick disease, type C
Newborn presentations	Gaucher disease, type 2; GM$_1$ gangliosidosis; Krabbe disease; Niemann-Pick disease, types A and C; mucopolysaccharidosis I, IVA, VII; Pompe disease; sialidosis, types I and II; mucolipidosis, types I and II; Schindler disease; Wolman disease; infantile sialic acid storage disease; sialuria; Salla disease; galactosialidosis; multiple sulfatase deficiency; prosaposin deficiency

The eye evaluation should include a funduscopic and slit-lamp examination to screen for storage material within the retina (cherry red spots) as well as an assessment for atypical eye movements, which may be pathognomonic for disorders such as neuronopathic Gaucher disease and Niemann-Pick disease type C. Unexplained cardiomyopathy and cryptogenic stroke may be the initial presentation of Fabry disease. A careful neurologic and cognitive evaluation can be fruitful because the later presentations include dementia and psychiatric manifestations in several of these disorders. Regression of developmental milestones can provide an early diagnostic clue. Preliminary clinical diagnostic studies include urine for thin-layer chromatography, blood count with smear for vacuolated white blood cells, skeletal radiography, and ophthalmologic examination.

For the most part, the diagnosis of a specific lysosomal storage disorder is made by assaying enzymatic activity in a blood sample or fibroblast cell line. A lysosomal panel, evaluating the activity of multiple lysosomal enzymes from the same sample, historically has been the first-tier test. If a lysosomal storage disorder is suspected, a tissue biopsy, most often of the bone marrow or liver, might be considered, although this is rarely indicated. Most of the genes encoding the lysosomal enzymes have been identified, and mutation analysis is commonly used when a mutation has already been identified in a family or when specific mutations are known to be common in a given ethnic group. Diagnostic testing based on DNA sequencing of panels of genes implicated in lysosomal storage disease is emerging.

Improved care and new therapeutic modalities have transformed the natural history of several of these disorders. With patients' increased longevity, diseases that were once encountered only by pediatricians have now made their way to the offices of internists. Moreover, many of the classic complications are now avoided by early therapeutic interventions, such as enzyme replacement therapy.[2] However, in some instances, prolonged longevity has unmasked unanticipated clinical manifestations. In addition, the advent of next generation DNA sequencing of affected individuals with unknown diagnoses has led to the identification of lysosomal storage disorders in individuals lacking classic disease manifestations. Physicians' increased awareness of the range of manifestations and presentations of lysosomal disorders may lessen the lengthy delays in diagnosis that patients frequently experience. As the pathogenesis of many of these disorders continues to be investigated, some common themes are emerging, including the involvement of the CLEAR (coordinated lysosomal expression and regulation) network which unites autophagy, lysosomes, and lysosome-like organelles in response to nutrient availability, and downstream inflammatory events. Lysosomal disorders encountered in adult patients are discussed here, with a focus on Gaucher disease and Fabry disease. A brief discussion of specific disorders frequently diagnosed during adulthood, as well as of childhood-onset lysosomal disorders that persist through adulthood is included.

● GAUCHER DISEASE

PATHOBIOLOGY

Gaucher disease, the autosomal recessively inherited deficiency of the lysosomal enzyme glucocerebrosidase, is a disorder primarily of the reticuloendothelial system.[3] Lysosomes within macrophages become engorged with the substrate glucocerebroside, giving rise to the characteristic Gaucher cells, that have a wrinkled-paper appearance resulting from intracytoplasmic substrate deposition. The accumulated glycolipid glucocerebroside is derived from the degradation of senescent leukocytes or erythrocyte membranes.

CLINICAL MANIFESTATIONS

Clinically, Gaucher disease has been divided into three types based on the absence or presence and the rate of progression of neurologic involvement. Type 1, the non-neuronopathic form, is the most common type and can manifest at any age. Type 2, the acute neuronopathic form, manifests before or shortly after birth and has a rapid and progressive course. Type 3 is the subacute neuronopathic form. The spectrum of manifestations encountered in this disorder ranges from asymptomatic octogenarians to infants who succumb in utero. Some patients defy classification into one of the three types. It is a pan-ethnic disorder, although type 1 Gaucher disease is more frequent among Ashkenazi Jews, in whom the carrier frequency is about 1 in 16; in contrast, the approximate carrier frequency in the general population is 1 in 100.

The gene encoding glucocerebrosidase, *GBA1*, is located on chromosome 1q21. More than 300 different mutations have been found in patients, several of which are encountered with increased frequency in type 1 Gaucher disease; for example, among Ashkenazi Jews, mutation N370S is the most common allele. However, the mutations identified do not adequately correlate with the range of manifestations encountered.

In recent years, an association between Gaucher disease and Parkinsonism (Chapter 381) has been reported. Both patients with Gaucher disease and carriers of mutations in *GBA1* have a higher incidence of Parkinson disease and Lewy body disorders. Studies in cohorts of patients with Parkinson disease around the world demonstrate that they have a more than five-fold increased frequency of *GBA1* mutations, rendering this the most common genetic risk factor for Parkinsonism identified to date. However, the majority of affected individuals and carriers do not develop Parkinson disease.

Commonly encountered symptoms in all types of Gaucher disease include easy bruisability, hepatomegaly, splenomegaly, chronic fatigue, and bone pain or pathologic fractures. Laboratory findings include anemia, thrombocytopenia, and elevations of ferritin, acid phosphatase, angiotensin-converting enzyme, and, at times, liver enzymes. Painless splenomegaly is the most common

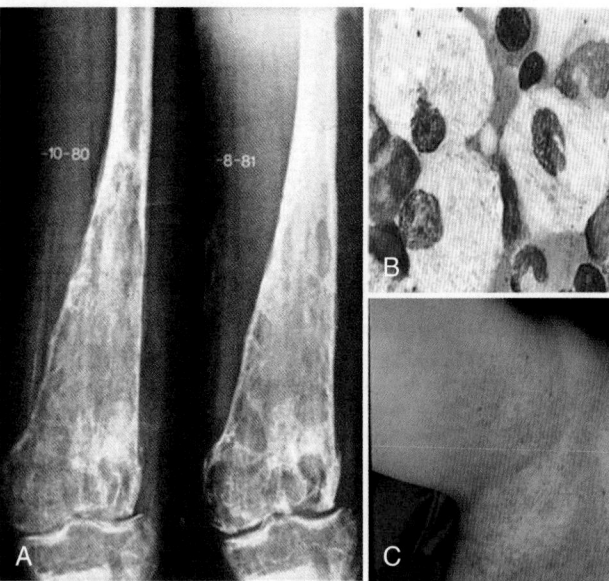

FIGURE 197-1. **A,** Radiographic image showing the Erlenmeyer flask deformity in Gaucher disease. There is cortical thinning and widening of the medullary cavity of the metaphysis and adjacent diaphysis. **B,** Gaucher cells—reticuloendothelial cells storing abnormal amounts of lipid. **C,** Angiokeratomas, the nonblanching punctate skin lesion in Fabry disease.

TABLE 197-3 SUGGESTIVE DIAGNOSTIC FEATURES IN ADULTHOOD FOR GAUCHER DISEASE AND FABRY DISEASE

GAUCHER DISEASE	FABRY DISEASE
Family member with Gaucher disease	Family history of Fabry disease
Hepatomegaly, splenomegaly (sometimes massive)	Cutaneous lesions of capillaries (angiokeratoma)
Frequent epistaxis	Hypohidrosis or heat intolerance
Easy bruising	Intermittent episodes of severe pain in the extremities (acroparesthesias)
Abnormal saccadic eye movements	Left ventricular hypertrophy of unknown etiology in young adulthood
Thrombocytopenia or anemia	
Painful bone crisis	Stroke of unknown etiology in young adulthood
Erlenmeyer flask deformity of the distal femur, aseptic necrosis of the femoral heads	Chronic kidney disease of unknown etiology in young adulthood
Pathologic fractures, unexplained rib fracture	Multiple renal sinus cysts discovered incidentally
Multiple myeloma	Female carriers may have more variable and less severe symptoms with later onset
Parkinsonism	
Elevated serum ferritin, angiotensin-converting enzyme, or tartrate-resistant acid phosphatase	

TABLE 197-4 ENZYME REPLACEMENT THERAPY (ERT) FOR GAUCHER DISEASE AND FABRY DISEASE

GAUCHER DISEASE	FABRY DISEASE
ERT is a costly but effective intravenous therapy generally administered every other week for life.	ERT is costly, and there are not uniform recommendations for its use.
Decreased splenic and hepatic volumes and increases in hemoglobin levels and platelet counts should be expected in the first year of treatment.	On the basis of some current trials, hemizygous males with a low or undetectable level of α-galactosidase A should be treated with ERT, whether or not clinical features are present.
Asymptomatic and mildly symptomatic adults do not always require treatment.	On the basis of current trials, female carriers and atypically affected males with clinical features of Fabry disease (renal, neurologic, cardiovascular) should be treated with ERT.
ERT does not cross the blood-brain barrier and does not correct neurologic features of neuronopathic forms of Gaucher disease.	Other trials suggest that patients with end-stage renal disease due to Fabry disease should be treated with ERT to potentially reduce other organ involvement.
ERT will not prevent the development of Parkinsonism.	

presentation in patients with type 1 Gaucher disease, and the spleen can be massively enlarged. Occasional patients have pulmonary involvement or pulmonary hypertension. Bone involvement is a significant cause of morbidity and can manifest with extreme bone pain or pathologic fractures. Most patients have radiologic evidence of skeletal involvement, including the classic Erlenmeyer flask deformity of the distal end of the femur and osteopenia (Fig. 197-1A). Pathologic fractures (especially of the hip, ribs, or spine), lytic bone lesions, and osteoporosis may occur. Painful bone crises, episodes of bone infarcts, can last for weeks and may require aggressive pain management. Altered macrophage function, complement processing, and an increased risk for multiple myeloma (Chapter 178) have been reported.

Type 2 Gaucher disease, which is rare, is characterized by a rapid neurodegenerative course with extensive visceral involvement and associated with failure to thrive, laryngospasm, strabismus, and seizures. Death usually occurs within the first 3 years of life.

Type 3 disease is clinically variable and is often noted in childhood. In addition to organomegaly and bone involvement, patients have abnormal horizontal eye movements, and some develop myoclonic epilepsy or neurodegeneration. A subgroup of patients have cardiac calcifications, hydrocephalus, and other atypical manifestations. All carry the *GBA1* mutation D409H.

DIAGNOSIS

Gaucher disease should be considered in the differential diagnosis of patients of all ages with unexplained organomegaly, easy bruisability, or bone pain (Table 197-3). The diagnosis can be made by demonstration of deficient glucocerebrosidase activity in leukocytes or cultured cells. In some populations, particularly Ashkenazi Jews, mutation analysis can be diagnostic because mutation N370S accounts for about 70% of mutant alleles. However, the presence of a highly homologous pseudogene sequence nearby can complicate molecular analysis. Bone marrow and liver biopsies show pathologic changes (Fig. 197-1B) but are not indicated for diagnosis. Carrier identification is best achieved by DNA testing when the mutant allele is known. Prenatal diagnosis is possible by determining the enzymatic activity or specific mutations in chorionic villi or cultured amniotic fluid cells.

TREATMENT Rx

Two treatment approaches have been used to lower pathologic glucocerebroside accumulation in Gaucher disease: enzyme replacement therapy and substrate reduction therapy. Enzyme replacement with recombinant glucocerebrosidase is available for the treatment of symptomatic patients with type 1 Gaucher disease (Table 197-4). Studies show that anemia, thrombocytopenia,

and organomegaly are reversed within 12 to 36 months with enzyme doses between 15 and 60 IU/kg given every other week. The treatment is ongoing, administered intravenously, and extremely expensive. Asymptomatic and mildly symptomatic adults do not always require treatment. Several companies are now marketing different forms of recombinantly produced enzyme. The enzyme does not cross the blood-brain barrier and does not alter the neurologic progression of patients with neuronopathic forms of Gaucher disease, but it can still be useful in alleviating visceral manifestations. Enzyme replacement does not prevent the development of Parkinsonism. Efforts are also under way to develop alternative therapies, including substrate reduction therapy, chemical chaperones, and gene therapy. A newer substrate reduction therapy is eliglustat, which is a ceramide analog.[4] It is a potent specific inhibitor of glucosylceramide synthase, which reduces glucosylceramide production to match its impaired rate of degradation. It is administered orally and significantly improves the spleen and liver volume, the hemoglobin level, and the platelet count. However longer-term comparison with standard enzyme replacement therapy is needed.[A1][A2]

Useful supportive therapies include bisphosphonates for osteoporosis, orthopedic surgery for bone fractures, and palliative therapy and hydration for bone crises. Total or partial splenectomy, once commonly performed in patients with Gaucher disease, is now rarely indicated. Hematopoietic stem cell transplantation (Chapter 168) has improved systemic but not neurologic manifestations.

FABRY DISEASE

PATHOBIOLOGY

Fabry disease, an X-linked inherited deficiency of the lysosomal enzyme α-galactosidase A, has intermediate penetrance in females and is considered a systemic vascular disorder. This defect in the hydrolytic cleavage of the terminal molecule of galactose from glycolipids causes lysosomal accumulation of globotriaosylceramide and galabiosylceramide in many cell types. Lysosomal inclusions or lipid deposits can be seen in vascular cells, including both endothelial and smooth muscle cells; cardiac cells, such as endocardial cells, cardiomyocytes, and cardiac valves; kidney epithelial cells, including tubular and glomerular cells and podocytes; and nerve cells, including dorsal root ganglia and some central nervous system neurons.

The gene encoding α-galactosidase A, *GLA*, is located on Xq22.1. More than 400 mutations have been described, including missense/nonsense mutations, small deletions, large deletions, splice defects, and complex rearrangements. Most affected individuals have 2 to 25% of residual enzymatic activity, but the most severe form of Fabry disease has been correlated with complete absence of α-galactosidase A activity.

CLINICAL MANIFESTATIONS

Clinically, angiokeratomas (nonblanching, punctate, blue-black skin lesions), debilitating pain, and corneal opacities can occur in childhood and may lead to the diagnosis. If the diagnosis is missed, the disease can result in progressive renal and cardiac deterioration. Affected adults have a propensity for ischemic stroke, sometimes in their 20s, but more commonly in the fourth and fifth decades of life. As with many metabolic disorders, there is a spectrum of presentations that can mimic more common disorders, and many patients are undiagnosed.

Fabry disease typically manifests in childhood in classically affected males with episodes of extremity pain. Angiokeratomas develop in adolescence, followed by advancing renal disease during adulthood. The progressive cardiac and cerebrovascular involvement accounts for most of the deaths associated with Fabry disease in adulthood. X-linked inactivation and the penetrance of this X-linked disorder are reflected in the fact that approximately 90% of females carrying the mutation have symptoms although they frequently go undiagnosed. However, affected males show more significant clinical manifestations at an earlier age than do heterozygous females.

Although variable, clinical manifestations of Fabry disease occur in a predictable order; acroparesthesia, angiokeratoma, proteinuria, polyuria, polydipsia, heat, cold, exercise intolerance, hypo- or hyperhidrosis, lymphadenopathy, abdominal pain and diarrhea, with increasing risk in adulthood of progressive cardiac and central nervous system involvement.

The majority of patients experience acroparesthesia, or a "Fabry crisis," characterized by excruciating, burning pain that may be either continuous or episodic. This is often the initial clinical manifestation. The pain typically affects the feet first, followed by the hands, and may be triggered by exercise, stress, and extremes in environmental temperatures. Abdominal or flank pain, simulating renal colic, may occur.

Angiokeratomas (Fig. 197-1C) are often an early sign of Fabry disease and may be accompanied by hypohidrosis. These classic skin lesions increase in number and size over time, and are typically most dense between the umbilicus and the knees; however, they may occur anywhere, including the buccal mucosa. Ophthalmologic findings include conjunctival and retinal tortuosity and corneal opacities (cornea verticillata). Characteristic lenticular lesions are observed during slit-lamp examination and are present in affected males and female heterozygotes. Progressive hearing loss may also occur.

Renal involvement is seen in approximately 50% of affected males by age 35 and 20% of affected females, initially manifesting with proteinuria, followed by progressive renal insufficiency, with birefringent "Maltese crosses" sometimes seen in the urinary sediment. Chronic kidney disease is part of the natural history, and end-stage renal disease may develop in the second to fourth decades. Fabry disease should be considered when multiple renal sinus cysts are seen on an imaging study. As affected men and women age, cardiovascular findings may include ventricular hypertrophy, conduction defects, coronary artery disease, aortic and mitral valve insufficiency, and aortic root dilation. Furthermore, atypical Fabry disease can be manifested with concentric left ventricular hypertrophy and no other disease findings. Cerebrovascular involvement, leading to transient ischemic attacks and stroke, occur in approximately 25% of patients, with a mean age at onset of 40 years.

Female carriers of this X-linked disorder tend to have more variable and less severe symptoms, with a later age at onset. Affected women may not have proteinuria, even with pronounced renal impairment, and in almost 40%, stroke is the initial presentation. While angiokeratomas are not typically seen in affected women, half have hypohidrosis and heat intolerance. The onset of cardiomyopathy in affected women is generally 10 years later than the classic presentation in men, and may be the only manifestation of Fabry disease.

DIAGNOSIS

Fabry disease should be considered in individuals with acroparesthesia, angiokeratoma, and corneal lesions as well as in individuals with cryptogenic strokes, idiopathic cardiomyopathy, or renal disease (Table 197-3). Men and women with left ventricular hypertrophy without any other explanation or with a family history of renal, cardiovascular, cerebrovascular, or skin issues should be screened for Fabry disease. Angiokeratoma should be differentiated from Fordyce disease, benign angiokeratomas of the scrotum, and angiokeratoma circumscriptum. Angiokeratomas are also seen in other lysosomal disorders including mannosidosis, fucosidosis, sialidosis, β-galactosidase and β-hexosaminidase deficiency. Corneal abnormalities are like those seen secondary to the use of chloroquine or amiodarone. Exposure to silicone dust can result in similar renal findings.

A presumed diagnosis can be confirmed by low α-galactosidase activity in peripheral white blood cells or cultured skin fibroblasts. Levels below 20% of normal are considered diagnostic, and levels up to 35% of normal should be considered suggestive. *GLA* mutation analysis is available and is critical for confirmation in atypically presenting males and heterozygote females because random X chromosome inactivation may lead to only slightly reduced or normal enzyme activity. An increased awareness of Fabry disease, pilot newborn screening studies, and the implementation of next-generation sequencing strategies in cardiovascular disease have led to the appreciation that Fabry disease is more common than previously recognized. Mutations associated with classic Fabry disease features are present in approximately 1 : 22,000 to 1 : 40,000 males and mutations associated with atypical presentations are present in about 1 : 1000 to 1 : 3000 males and 1 : 6000 to 1 : 40,000 females. As many as 3 to 12 % of adults with hypertrophic cardiomyopathy may have Fabry disease.

TREATMENT

Symptomatic treatment of the clinical manifestations of Fabry disease should follow standard medical care.[5] Antiplatelet agents such as clopidogrel and aspirin or long-acting dipyridamole should be used for the prevention of strokes. Angiotensin-converting enzyme inhibitors and angiotensin receptor blockers are appropriate to manage hypertension and to preserve renal function. Kidney transplantation is effective in individuals with end-stage renal disease. Neuropathic pain can be treated with relatively low doses of antiepileptic medications, antidepressants, topical anesthetics, or pain relievers. Nonsteroidal anti-inflammatory agents should be avoided because of potential renal toxicity.

Enzyme replacement therapy has been available since 2001, and clinical trials suggest a modest benefit in modifying the natural course of the disease.[A3] Although there are no uniform recommendations, it is generally agreed that this therapy is appropriate for classically affected males, symptomatic females, and males with atypical disease (Table 197-4). Recent ongoing studies have revealed potential efficacy of migalastat hydrochloride, an oral pharmacologic chaperone, in affected individuals with specific appropriate mutations in *GLA*.[A4]

OTHER LYSOSOMAL DISORDERS SEEN IN ADULTS

Metachromatic leukodystrophy, the deficiency of arylsulfatase A, results in the accumulation of sulfatides in the central and peripheral nervous systems, leading to demyelination of axons and peripheral nerves. It has a spectrum of manifestations, divided into childhood, juvenile, and adult variants.[6] Peripheral neuropathy is often the presenting feature, with gait disturbance and cognitive regression also seen. The adult form typically presents with dementia and behavioral disturbances, often mistakenly resulting in a diagnosis of psychosis. Metachromatic leukodystrophy is a recognized underlying cause of psychiatric illness in adults, and prominent features include auditory hallucinations, bizarre delusions, behavioral changes, personality changes, disinhibition and disorganization in daily life, and catatonic posturing. The diagnosis can be especially difficult in these individuals. Other neurologic signs, such as dysarthria and spasticity, manifest later as the disease progresses. Metachromatic leukodystrophy should be considered in individuals with the combined findings of reduced nerve conduction velocity and elevated cerebrospinal fluid protein levels. The diagnosis is made by demonstration of low arylsulfatase A activity. However, because there can be a pseudodeficiency, it must be confirmed by molecular diagnosis or the demonstration of the excretion of sulfatides in urine. No specific therapy is currently available. A case series suggests that hematopoietic stem cell gene therapy can potentially prevent the onset of symptoms in presymptomatic children and may slow or even halt progression of the disease.[7]

Tay-Sachs disease, caused by β-hexosaminidase A deficiency, is characterized by an excessive accumulation of the fatty acid derivative ganglioside GM_2 in neurons. There are three clinical variants based on the age at onset: type 1, infantile acute; type 2, subacute (2 to 18 years); and type 3, late onset.[8] The main features of the disease are neurologic and cognitive deterioration as well as blindness, a macular cherry red spot, and deafness. In patients with late-onset GM_2 gangliosidosis, there is typically a history of subtle motor issues. In some patients, psychiatric signs may manifest years before the appearance of significant motor findings. The most common psychiatric signs include acute psychosis, mania, and depression without psychosis. Either recurrent progressive psychosis, consistent with schizophrenia-hebephrenia, or major depression followed by psychotic features may occur. Dysarthria and progressive speech loss are also common. The disorder is diagnosed by measurement of β-hexosaminidase A activity in the serum or white blood cells in the presence of normal or elevated activity of the β-hexosaminidase B isoenzyme. In pregnant women or those taking oral contraceptives, the test should be performed only in leukocytes. Community-based screening efforts in the high-risk Ashkenazi Jewish population have vastly decreased the incidence of this disorder.

Niemann-Pick disease type C results from an error in cellular trafficking of exogenous cholesterol, leading to lysosomal accumulation of unesterified cholesterol, and has been linked to mutations in the *NPC1* (95% of cases) and *NPC2* (5% of cases) genes. Affected individuals present with a spectrum of features ranging from a rapidly progressive, fatal neonatal phenotype to an adult-onset chronic, neurodegenerative course. Glycosphingolipids and cholesterol accumulate in different tissues such as the liver, spleen, bone marrow, and brain. In adults, the presentation may include progressive ataxia, vertical supranuclear ophthalmoplegia, and dystonia. Dementia, depression, bipolar symptoms or schizophrenia may be the presenting features. Hepatosplenomegaly may be present and precede the neurologic deterioration. The diagnosis is made by demonstration of impaired cholesterol esterification in cultured skin fibroblasts, termed the Filipin test. Molecular genetic testing for mutations is available. Miglustat (*N*-butyldeoxynojirimycin) has been shown in clinical trials to stabilize but not to prevent or reverse key neurologic findings. Decisions about starting this therapy typically involve the team of physicians, parents, and caregivers of the affected individual. A trial using intrathecal 2-hydroxypropyl-β-cyclodextrin began in 2017.[9]

Aspartylglucosaminuria, a disorder more common in Finland than elsewhere in the world, is an autosomal recessive defect in glycoprotein degradation with subsequent lysosomal storage of the undegraded compounds. Affected individuals generally have a slow or progressive delay in development. The speech delay and motor defects are often accompanied by repeated upper respiratory infections. Patients typically achieve the developmental competency of a 5- to 6-year-old child at around puberty; subsequently, they may experience progressive deterioration, resulting in the severe cognitive impairment seen in adulthood. The characteristic coarse facial features, thick calvaria, and osteoporosis result from mild connective tissue transformation. About 20% of patients experience seizures during the later stages of the disease, resulting primarily from abnormalities in the differentiation between gray and white matter and delayed myelination. The diagnosis is made by the detection of elevated urine oligosaccharides and deficient aspartylglucosaminidase activity in leukocytes.

The *neuronal ceroid-lipofuscinoses* were historically divided into four major groups—infantile, classic late infantile, juvenile, and adult—reflecting the age at symptom onset and the appearance of autofluorescent ceroid lipopigments in the brain and other tissues. To date, mutations causing neuronal ceroid-lipofuscinoses have been found in thirteen human genes, complicating genetic analysis. Symptoms result from deficiencies in palmitoyl-protein thioesterase 1, cathepsin D, and tripeptidyl-peptidase 1. These diseases, when identified in children and teens, are characterized by visual impairment that leads to blindness, gait abnormalities, seizures, and early death. The two major clinical phenotypes in adults are: (1) progressive myoclonic epilepsy with dementia, ataxia, and late occurring Parkinsonian symptoms or (2) behavior changes and dementia with motor dysfunction, ataxia, extrapyramidal and brain stem involvement. The diagnosis is based on diminished enzyme activity, molecular genetic testing and, in some cases, clinical findings and electron microscopy of biopsied tissues. Distinguishing between the clinical phenotypes can be challenging because of the wide variation in both the age of onset and disease progression. Therefore, molecular testing may be necessary for optimal classification. Intrathecal recombinant human tripeptidyl peptidase 1 replacement therapy may slow the decline in motor and language function.[10]

Lysosomal acid lipase deficiency (LAL-D or Wolman disease in infants) is an autosomal recessive storage disease that is caused by mutations in the *LIPA* gene. Clinical manifestations are due to the lysosomal accumulation of cholesteryl esters and triglycerides, which lead to the reduced generation of free cholesterol, increased production of apolipoprotein B-containing lipoproteins, and reduced formation of high-density lipoprotein cholesterol. In infants, progression of the disease is rapid, typically occurring within 6 months of age. Clinical manifestations of LAL-D are quite diverse.[11,12] The most common manifestations, specifically dyslipidemia, hepatomegaly and liver cell damage, elevated serum transaminases, and progression to fibrosis and cirrhosis, are shared with other, more common cardiovascular, liver, and metabolic diseases. LAL-D is an under-recognized condition, and many affected individuals are not diagnosed or receive the incorrect diagnoses of heterozygous familial hypercholesterolemia, familial combined hyperlipidemia, nonalcoholic steatohepatitis, or nonalcoholic fatty liver disease. Enzyme replacement with sebelipase-alfa therapy is an FDA-approved therapy to reduce hepatic and lipid abnormalities in children and adults with LAD-D.[A5]

Pompe disease is discussed in Chapters 196 and 393.

The *mucopolysaccharidoses* (MPS) are a group of disorders resulting from defective lysosomal degradation and storage of glycosaminoglycans. These chronic, progressive storage disorders show clinical manifestations that vary by type. Findings may include growth impairment, coarse facial features, dysostosis multiplex, organomegaly, and neurologic manifestations with regression. Affected individuals may develop ophthalmologic, cardiovascular, musculoskeletal, neurologic, gastrointestinal, and auditory complications. All types are inherited in an autosomal recessive pattern except for MPS II (Hunter syndrome),[13] which is X-linked. The mucopolysaccharidoses were once typically considered pediatric disorders, but with the advent of enzyme replacement therapy, improved management strategies, and the recognition of milder forms, more patients are being cared for in adult clinics.[14] Clinical features of each type have similarities and distinctions. For example, patients with MPS type IS (Hurler syndrome) may present with normal to short stature, normal intelligence, degenerative joint disease, corneal opacities, and cardiac valve lesions. However, patients with MPS II share the symptoms of MPS I, except that airway involvement may be more significant in individuals with MPS II, and the corneas are clear. Patients with MPS III (Sanfilippo) have primarily central nervous system manifestations, with mild somatic involvement. They develop progressive speech impairment, as well as severe behavioral and sleep disturbances. Later they experience an unrelenting loss of skills and deterioration into a vegetative state, with death in the third decade. Individuals with MPS IV have severe skeletal dysplasia, with normal intelligence in type A and a degenerative course in type B. Medical management is type specific. In general, attention should focus on the need to optimize joint mobility and function by physical therapy and to manage airway involvement resulting from progressive storage in the soft tissue of the upper airway. Patients with MPS I, II, and VI should be monitored for the development of cervical myelopathy due to dural thickening, which may impact endurance before ascending paralysis becomes apparent. Treatment is available in the form of enzyme replacement therapy for MPS IS, MPS II, and MPS IVA and VI, and enzyme therapies for other forms are in development. It is interesting to note that gene therapy directly to the central nervous system appears promising in a mouse model of Hunter syndrome.

Cystinosis is a lysosomal storage disorder with three clinical phenotypes: the most common infantile or nephropathic form, an intermediate or juvenile-onset form, and a benign form typically seen in adults and affecting primarily the eyes. Lysosomal cystine accumulation results from mutations in the gene *CTNS*, which codes for cystinosin, a lysosomal carrier protein. Individuals with the nephropathic form have lysosomal cystine accumulation leading to multiorgan system involvement, including progressive renal disease, corneal crystals, and effects on the thyroid, gonads, pancreas, muscle, and central nervous system. The adult form has only corneal crystals. Treatment is supportive and should include cysteamine, which is an oral medication that decreases cystine accumulation. Cysteamine hydrochloride eyedrops dissolve corneal crystals and relieve photophobia.

Grade A References

A1. Mistry PK, Lukina E, Ben Turkia H, et al. Effect of oral eliglustat on splenomegaly in patients with Gaucher disease type 1: the ENGAGE randomized clinical trial. *JAMA.* 2015;313:695-706.

A2. Mistry PK, Lukina E, Ben Turkia H, et al. Outcomes after 18 months of eliglustat therapy in treatment-naive adults with Gaucher disease type 1: the phase 3 ENGAGE trial. *Am J Hematol.* 2017;92:1170-1176.

A3. El Dib RP, Nascimento P, Pastores GM. Enzyme replacement therapy for Anderson-Fabry disease. *Cochrane Database Syst Rev.* 2013;2:CD006663.

A4. Hughes DA, Nicholls K, Shankar SP, et al. Oral pharmacological chaperone migalastat compared with enzyme replacement therapy in Fabry disease: 18-month results from the randomized phase III ATTRACT study. *J Med Genet.* 2017;54:288-296.

A5. Burton BK, Balwani M, Feillet F, et al. A phase 3 trial of sebelipase alfa in lysosomal acid lipase deficiency. *N Engl J Med.* 2015;373:1010-1020.

GENERAL REFERENCES

For the General References and other additional features, please visit Expert Consult at https://expertconsult.inkling.com.

198

HOMOCYSTINURIA AND HYPERHOMOCYSTEINEMIA

MANUEL SCHIFF AND HENK J. BLOM

DEFINITION

Homocysteine is a nonprotein amino acid and is a key metabolic branch point metabolite between the trans-sulfuration and remethylation pathways of methionine metabolism. The many conditions associated with high homocysteine levels encompass a wide range of clinical manifestations.[1] The normal level of plasma total homocysteine (tHcy) is below 15 µM. However, the threshold of tHcy above which a disorder of homocysteine metabolism should be suspected and a specific therapy should be initiated is around 50 µM. These metabolic conditions mainly include genetic recessively inherited disorders of homocysteine metabolism but also acquired severe nutritional cobalamin (cbl, vitamin B12) or folate deficiencies. Inherited disorders of homocysteine metabolism (Figs. 198-1 and 198-2) comprise *disorders of the transsulfuration pathway* with cystathionine β-synthase (CBS) deficiency (or classical homocystinuria), and *disorders of remethylation* of homocysteine to methionine. The latter include 5,10-methylenetetrahydrofolate reductase [MTHFR] deficiency and inherited disorders of cbl absorption, transport, and intracellular metabolism, as well as the very rare congenital folate malabsorption disorder. Intracellular remethylation defects include disorders which all have defective methionine synthesis in common: MTHFR deficiency impairs 5-methyltetrahydrofolate (5-methylTHF) synthesis, defective lysosomal release of cobalamin (cblF and cblJ), and defects in cytosolic reduction and transport of hydroxocobalamin (cblC and cblD) impair the synthesis of both methyl- and adenosylcobalamin. Isolated deficiencies of methionine synthase (cblE and cblG) are associated with defective methyl cobalamin synthesis as well as the cblD-Hcy variant.

In CBS deficiency, in addition to severe elevations of tHcy, plasma methionine level is also increased. In contrast, in remethylation disorders, the increased tHcy is associated with a low (or low-normal) level of methionine in plasma due to the ineffective conversion (remethylation) of homocysteine to methionine. Among the remethylation disorders, the cblC defect (the most frequent inherited disorder of intracellular cbl metabolism) and MTHFR deficiency are by far the most frequent.

Accordingly, this chapter will focus on CBS deficiency, the cblC defect, and MTHFR deficiency.

EPIDEMIOLOGY

Prevalence and Incidence

The worldwide prevalence of CBS deficiency has been reported at 1 in 344,000. Minimum estimates of the incidence of CBS deficiency by newborn screening programs have ranged from 1 in 60,000 to 1 in 300,000 live births, varying with the population and the screening method. Estimates of its incidence in Europe have been in the area of 1 in 40,000 live births, which corresponds to a carrier (heterozygote) frequency of about 1%, but studies with screening for known mutations suggest that the incidence may be more than twice that rate. Studies from the Saudi Arabian countries have shown incidence rates as high as 1 in 1800 live births. The incidence of severe homocysteine remethylation defects has never been evaluated but may be less than 1 in 500,000 live births.

PATHOBIOLOGY

The homocysteine that accumulates in both CBS deficiency and remethylation defects is a well-known multisystem toxic agent. It exerts its effects either directly or indirectly via conversion to S-adenosylmethionine (AdoHcy) (Fig. 198-1), which potentially inhibits many essential methyltransferases. Direct cellular homocysteine toxicity is found with endothelial damage and neuronal cell death. Homocysteine's effects on vascular endothelium predispose to thrombosis that may occur at any age and involve arteries and/or veins of any size. Specifically in CBS deficiency, accumulation of homocysteine and/or cysteine deficiency induces modification of connective tissue proteins, possibly causing the skeletal and ocular manifestations of the disease. These effects are probably related to fibrillin, which is a component of the matrix of periosteum and perichondrium, the major component of the zonular fibers of the ocular lens, and a protein singularly rich in cysteine. Fibrillin structure can be affected by the linking of homocysteine to cysteine; as a result, some clinical features of homocystinuria overlap with fibrillin mutations (Marfan syndrome; Chapter 244).

Remethylation defects (cblC and MTHFR) not only result in severe elevations of homocysteine, but also in depletion of methionine that is required for protein synthesis and AdoMet synthesis. The latter causes via this route a reduction of cellular methylation capacity in addition to accumulation of AdoHcy, especially in the central nervous system (CNS). The cblC defect is an inborn error of intracellular cobalamin metabolism due to a mutation in *MMACHC*, the gene that encodes methylmalonic aciduria and homocystinuria type C protein. After normal dietary intake, intestinal absorption, blood transport, and cellular uptake, cobalamin is delivered in the cytosol where it becomes bound to MMACHC. This protein has been shown to catalyze dealkylation of alkylcobalamins, such as adenosylcobalamin (Ado-cbl) and methylcobalamin (Me-cbl), and the decyanation of cyanocobalamin. In the absence of normal MMACHC, neither Me-cbl (the cofactor of methionine synthase) nor Ado-cbl (the cofactor of methylmalonyl-CoA mutase) is functional with subsequent secondary defects of the methionine synthase (remethylation defect) and methylmalonyl-CoA mutase (methylmalonic acid [MMA] accumulation), respectively (Fig. 198-2). In MTHFR deficiency, the methyl donor 5-methylTHF cannot be produced, which secondarily reduces methionine synthase function and subsequent remethylation (Fig. 198-2). The pathogenesis of MTHFR deficiency can be ascribed to homocysteine toxicity together with cellular methionine depletion. In addition, 5-methylTHF (the circulating form of folate) formation is hampered, causing in particular cerebral folate deficiency. The pathophysiology of the other remethylation disorder, the cblC defect, remains incompletely understood. One unique mechanism in cblC defect is the trapping of 5-methylTHF due to methionine synthase dysfunction. Because MTHFR activity is irreversible this causes accumulation of 5-methylTHF. Because this form of folate is not available for metabolism in the cblC defect, it results in cellular folate deficiency. Toxic accumulation of MMA in the cblC defect might play an additional role, though it is considered to be minor.

All these disorders are inherited in an autosomal recessive manner (Table 198-1).

CLINICAL MANIFESTATIONS

Cystathionine β-synthase (CBS) Deficiency

Overview of Clinical Presentation

As an autosomal recessive condition, CBS deficiency can clinically affect homozygous or compound heterozygous individuals. Affected individuals are normal at birth after an uneventful pregnancy and delivery. If untreated, they

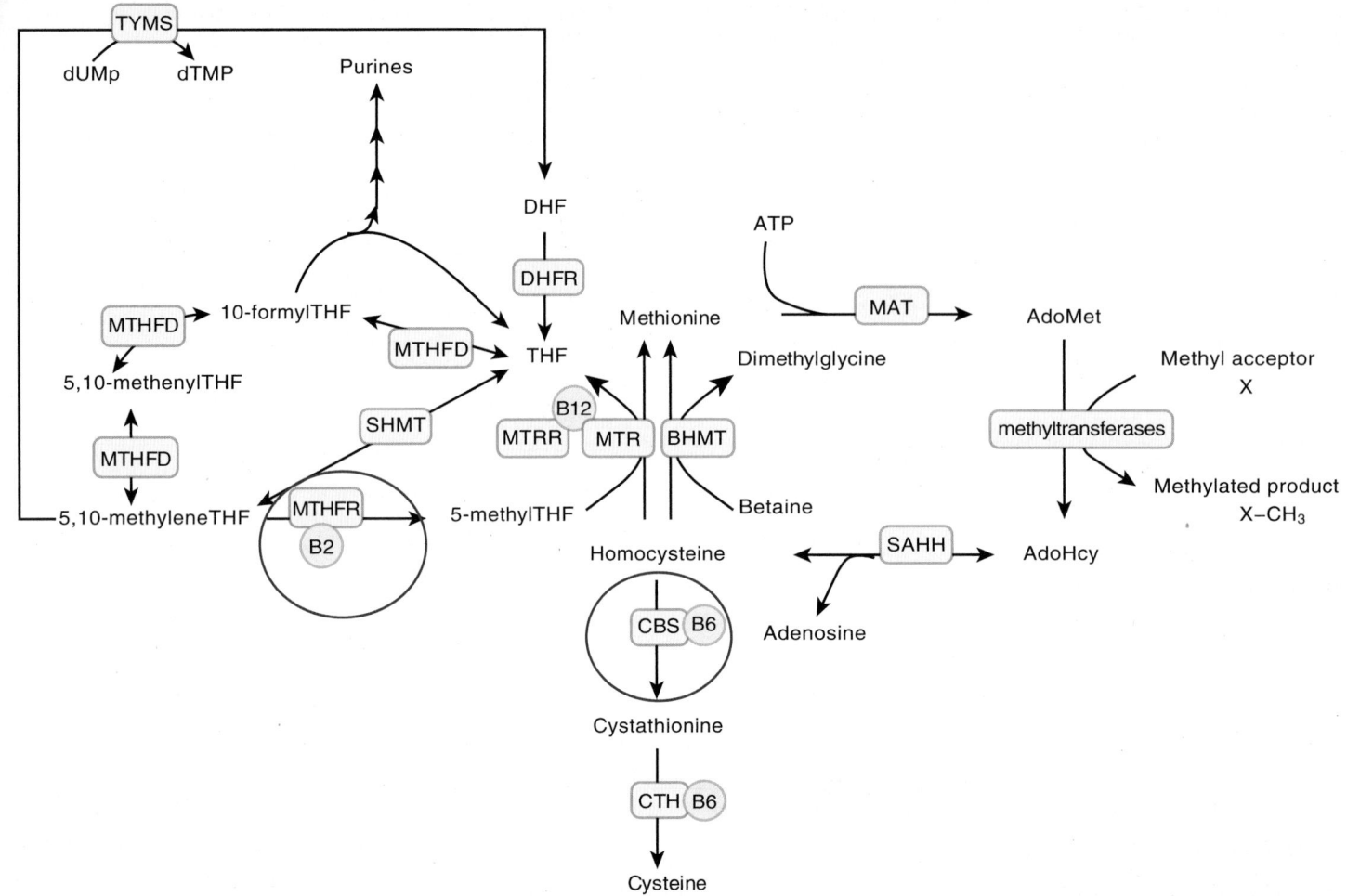

FIGURE 198-1. Homocysteine metabolism and the folate cycle. AdoHcy = S-adenosylhomocysteine, AdoMet = S-adenosylmethionine, AICAR = 5-aminoimidazole-4-carboxamide ribonucleotide, SAHH = S-adenosylhomocysteine hydrolase, ATP = adenosine triphosphate, BHMT = betaine-homocysteine methyltransferase, CBS = cystathionine β-synthase, CTH = cystathionine γ-lyase, DHF = dihydrofolate, DHFR = dihydrofolate reductase, dUMP = deoxyuridine monophosphate, dTMP = deoxythymidine monophosphate, FAICAR = formyl-AICAR, MAT = methionine-adenosyltransferase, MTHFD = methylenetetrahydrofolate dehydrogenase/methenyltetrahydrofolate cyclohydrolase/formyltetrahydrofolate synthetase, MTHFR = methylenetetrahydrofolate reductase, MTR = methionine synthase, MTRR = methionine synthase reductase, SHMT = serine-hydroxymethyltransferase, THF = tetrahydrofolate, TYMS = thymidylate synthase. The two conditions leading to accumulation of homocysteine (CBS and MTHFR) are surrounded by a blue circle.

progressively develop the core clinical symptoms of CBS deficiency,[2,3] which involve four major organ systems.

CENTRAL NERVOUS SYSTEM. Developmental delay and mental retardation affect about 60% of the patients to a variable degree of severity. Seizures, electroencephalogram abnormalities, and psychiatric disturbances have also been reported in approximately half of the cases. Focal neurologic signs may be a consequence of cerebrovascular accidents.

EYE. Dislocation of the ocular lens (ectopia lentis), myopia, and glaucoma are frequent, severe, and characteristic complications. Retinal detachment and degeneration, optical atrophy, and cataracts may eventually appear. Myopia often precedes lens dislocation. Ectopia lentis is detected in most untreated patients from 5 to 10 years of age and in nearly all untreated patients by the end of the fourth decade. In children as well as adults it is often the clue to diagnosis. The dislocation is generally downward, whereas it is usually upward in Marfan syndrome. However, upward lens dislocation may also occur in CBS deficiency. Once ectopia lentis has occurred, a peculiar trembling of the iris (iridodonesis) following eye or head movement may be observed.

SKELETON. Osteoporosis is almost invariably detected, at least after childhood. Frequent consequences are scoliosis and a tendency toward pathologic fractures and vertebral collapse. Homocystinuric patients tend to be tall, with thinning and elongation (dolichostenomelia) of long bones near puberty, enlarged metaphyses and epiphyses, especially at the knees, and arachnodactyly, present in about half of the patients. Other bone deformities include genu valgum, pes cavus, and pectus carinatum or excavatum. Restricted joint mobility, particularly at the extremities, contrasts with the joint laxity observed in Marfan syndrome.

VASCULAR SYSTEM. Thromboembolic complications, occurring in arteries and veins[4] of all parts of the body, constitute the major cause of morbidity

and mortality at any age. Two phenotypic variants are recognized, vitamin B$_6$-responsive homocystinuria and vitamin B$_6$-nonresponsive homocystinuria. B$_6$-responsive homocystinuria is usually milder than the nonresponsive variant.

Adult-Onset Clinical Presentation

Onset of all clinical symptoms is extremely variable and may manifest during childhood, but also during adulthood even up to 60 years of age. Individuals are often tall and slender with a marfanoid habitus and are prone to osteoporosis. The main acute manifestation in adulthood is thromboembolic disease. In all forms of inherited homocystinurias, isolated arterial and venous occlusive disease may present at any age. Thromboembolism is the major cause of early death and morbidity. Adults can also present with isolated quick loss of diopter, which is the most common symptom before diagnosis.

IQ in individuals with untreated homocystinuria ranges widely, from 10 to 138. In B$_6$ (pyridoxine)-responsive untreated individuals the mean IQ is 79 versus 57 for those who are B$_6$-nonresponsive.

The neuropsychiatric symptoms (like schizophrenia or autistic-like features) may remain apparently isolated, but a thorough clinical history and examination will often reveal associated features like marfanoid habitus, skeletal abnormalities, and lens dislocation.

Remethylation Disorders: cblC Defect and MTHFR Deficiency

Clinical signs of remethylation defects are mainly neurologic. Neonatal and early-onset patients exhibit acute neurologic distress. In childhood, patients exhibit nonspecific developmental delay often associated with acquired microcephaly. Without appropriate therapy, remethylation defective patients may develop acute or rapidly progressive neurologic deterioration, sometimes

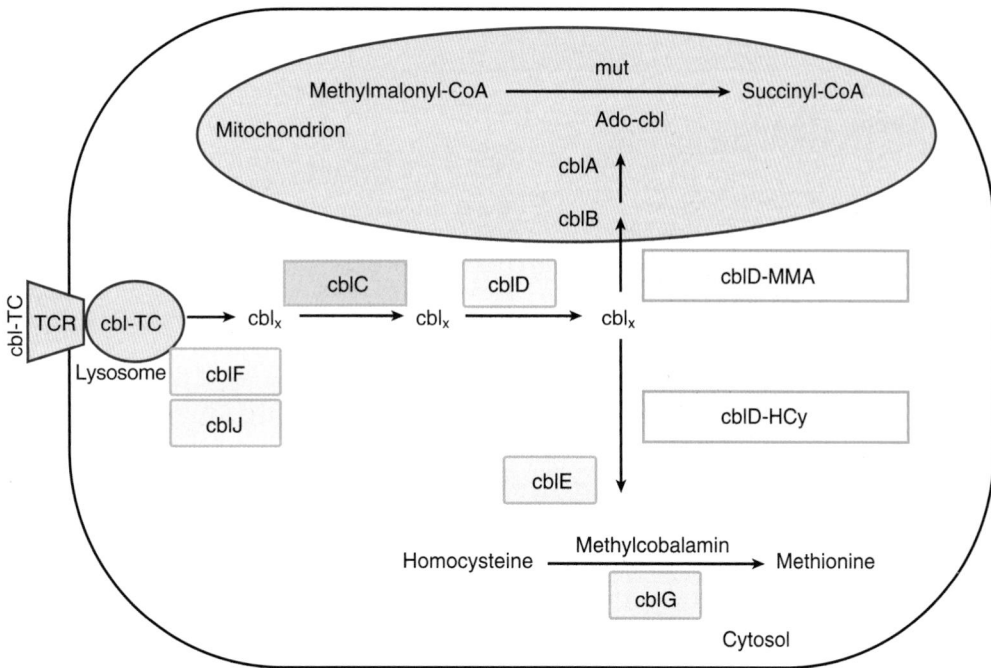

FIGURE 198-2. **Intracellular cobalamin metabolism pathway and its defects.** To date, ten complementation-group defects of the cobalamin pathway have been described. After binding to transcobalamin receptor (TC-R), cobalamin bound to TC enters the cell via lysosome-mediated endocytosis and is released through proteolysis. Export from the lysosome into the cytoplasm is defective in patients with the cblF and recently described cblJ defects. The steps in the cytosol after lysosomal release are defined by the complementation groups cblC and cblD. The exact form of cobalamin at this stage is unclear (as indicated by "cblx"). In the cytosol, cobalamin is reductively methylated by methionine synthase reductase (cblE) to methylcobalamin, the cofactor for methionine synthase (cblG). After its transport into the mitochondrion, cobalamin is converted to adenosylcobalamin, the cofactor for methylmalonyl-coenzyme A (CoA) mutase (mut), by cobalamin adenosyltransferase (cblB). cblD defect can cause isolated methylmalonic aciduria (cblD-MMA complementation group), isolated homocystinuria (cblD-HCy), or both (cblD). In all the above mentioned conditions with defective remethylation (TC and TC-R deficiency, cblF, cblJ, cblC, cblD, cblD-HCy, cblE, and cblG defects), there is homocysteine accumulation due to dysfunction in methionine synthesis.

TABLE 198-1 GENETIC DEFECTS ASSOCIATED WITH HOMOCYSTINURIA

FUNCTIONAL DEFECT	COMMON NAME	ENZYME DEFECT	GENE	CHROMOSOME LOCUS
Trans-sulfuration	"Classical" homocystinuria	Cystathionine β-synthase	*CBS*	21q22.3
Remethylation	Folate-dependent homocystinuria	Methylenetetrahydrofolate reductase	*MTHFR*	1p36.3
	cblE	Methyltransferase reductase	*MTRR*	5p15.2-p15.3
	cblG	Methionine synthase	*MTR*	1q43
Cobalamin transport	TC-II	Transcobalamin	*TCN2*	22q11.2-qter
	cblF	Lysosomal B$_{12}$ translocase	*LMBRD1*	6q13
Cobalamin processing	cblC	Intracellular cobalamin chaperone?	*MMACHC*	1p34.1
	cblD	Cobalamin reductase?	*MMADHC*	2q23.2
	cblJ	Cobalamin processing?	*ABCD4*	14q24.3

leading to death. Adolescents and adults exhibit, after a period of normal development or mild developmental delay, a rapid mental or psychiatric deterioration. These patients may typically have signs of subacute combined degeneration of the spinal cord. In addition, adults can be asymptomatic or present with isolated stroke.

In cblC disease, 5-methylTHF accumulates due to the block at methionine synthase (the 5-methylTHF trap), causing a functional cellular folate deficiency (Fig. 198-1). This explains the hematologic signs (megaloblastic bone marrow leading to macrocytic anemia or pancytopenia) which are not present in MTHFR deficiency. In cblC defect, severe (occasionally fatal) multisystem deterioration may occur. This includes hemolytic uremic syndrome (HUS),[5] cardiomyopathy, and interstitial pneumonia, which all share an identical pathologic hallmark (i.e., thrombotic microangiopathy) (Chapter 163). Pulmonary hypertension has also been reported. In addition, a peculiar and poorly understood retinopathy with nystagmus is often present especially in early onset severe presentations.

Adult-Onset Clinical Presentation
Adult-onset cblC disease is less frequent than childhood-onset and is dominated by neuropsychiatric manifestations such as ataxia, cognitive impairment, and psychosis.[6] HUS (even isolated) can also be present (Chapter 163).

In MTHFR deficiency, the neuropsychiatric presentation is similar and can be subtle. Patients may remain asymptomatic or exhibit isolated stroke.

In both remethylation defects, the neurologic disorder results in many signs similar to the late stage observed in childhood. Previously, most of these patients had either no or mild developmental delay and a striking feature is the rapid mental deterioration occurring in the second decade of life accompanied by bouts of unexplained lethargy and a progressive cerebral, myelopathic, and neuropathic disorder with variable results on neurophysiologic investigations.

In both groups of inherited homocystinurias, isolated arterial and venous occlusive disease may present at any age. Because of the very low incidence of arteriosclerosis and thrombosis in children or adolescents, homocystinurias should therefore be excluded in any case in this age group in the setting of arterial or venous occlusive disease.

DIAGNOSIS
If homocystinuria is suspected clinically, plasma total homocysteine (tHcy) should be determined. If tHcy (normal values 5 to 15 μM) is higher than 50 μM, determination of serum vitamin B$_{12}$ along with folates in serum and in red blood cells, plasma amino acids and urinary organic acids (and/or plasma methylmalonic acid) is warranted. If tHcy is below 50 μM, the

TABLE 198-2 CLINICAL FEATURES OF HOMOCYSTINURIAS

| CLASS | BIOCHEMICAL FEATURES | | | CLINICAL FEATURES | |
	tHcy	METH	MMA	SYSTEM	SIGNS
CBS deficiency	↑	↑	–	Ocular	Ectopia lentis, myopia, glaucoma, optic atrophy, retinal detachment
				Skeletal	Elongated and thinned bones, arachnodactyly, genu valgum, pectus malformation, scoliosis
				Vascular	Thromboembolic events (arterial or venous)
				Neurologic	Mental retardation in untreated cases, cerebrovascular thromboses, seizures
					Psychiatric disorders, personality disorder
MTHFR deficiency	↑	↓	–	Vascular	Thromboses
				Neurologic	Variable: psychiatric to severe neurologic
Transcobalamin	↑	–/↓	+	Hematologic	Early-onset pancytopenia, macrocytosis
cblF, cblJ	↑	–/↓	+	Pansystemic	MMA, macrocytosis, stomatitis, congenital heart defects
cblC, cblD	↑	↓	+	Hematologic	Pancytopenia
				Neuropsychiatric	
				Systemic (cblC)	HUS
cblE, cblG	↑	↓	–	Vascular	Thromboses
				Hematologic	Pancytopenia
				Neurologic	
				Ocular	Retinopathy (macular involvement) in early onset cblC

cbl = cobalamin; HUS = hemolytic uremic syndrome; tHcy = total plasma homocysteine; Meth = plasma methionine; MMA = methylmalonic acid urine or plasma.

probability of a disorder of homocysteine metabolism is very low but not excluded. If methionine is elevated or high-normal with low cysteine, it points to CBS deficiency whereas decreased or low-normal methionine and elevated tHcy points to remethylation defects. In cblC disease, hematologic abnormalities with megaloblastic bone marrow failure are observed along with normal vitamin B_{12} and folate blood levels. Nutritional vitamin B_{12} or folate deficiencies and other genetic causes of cobalamin and folate metabolism should also be considered as other possible causes for remethylation defects. It has to be kept in mind that CBS deficiency can cause secondary vitamin B_{12} and folate deficiency and remethylation defects can cause secondary folate deficiency. In MTHFR, folate levels (red blood cells and/or serum, CSF) are usually low. Blood cell count with blood smear (looking for characteristics of vitamin B_{12}/folate deficiency) (Chapter 155), blood vitamin status, and metabolic biomarkers (tHcy, methionine and MMA) are usually sufficient to differentiate between the different forms of homocystinurias (Table 198-2). Definitive diagnosis can be confirmed at the molecular level by sequence analysis of the putative gene or direct homocystinurias panel sequencing (Table 198-1); if the molecular studies are not conclusive, functional studies can be performed in fibroblasts or lymphocytes.

TREATMENT Rx

In the context of the European network and registry for homocystinurias and methylation defects (E-HOD) consortium (http://www.e-hod.org), published treatment guidelines are now available. None of the treatment options are evidence based due to the rarity of these disorders (grade D).[7]

Therapeutic Goals

The general therapeutic goal is to reduce tHcy accumulation and, for remethylation disorders, to bypass the remethylation defect, thereby maintaining normal methionine and folate concentrations. This should correct the hematologic abnormalities and ensure normal neurologic development or prevent further neurologic deterioration. In both conditions, normalization of plasma tHcy levels would be ideal but in practice is difficult if not impossible to achieve. However, the large experience with CBS defective patients has shown that treatment prevents further thromboembolic events even when the tHcy levels remain clearly above the normal range. Decreasing tHcy to 50 to 70 µM would therefore be a more reasonable goal in many patients with CBS deficiency or remethylation disorders.

Available Treatment Options

To date, all the remethylation disorders are similarly treated with the combined supplementation of vitamin B_{12}, vitamin B_9 (folate), vitamin B_6, betaine, and methionine, although the dosage and route of administration may vary with the type of defect.

With CBS deficiency, therapy is more standardized with a longer experience available. It is based on (1) increasing residual CBS activity with the use of vitamin B_6 (in B_6-responsive patients); (2) decreasing the load on the affected pathway and replacing the deficient products by a low methionine diet, limitation of natural proteins, methionine-free amino acid mixture, special low-protein foods, and supplementation of cystine to increase cysteine; and (3) increasing remethylation to methionine with folate, vitamin B_{12}, and betaine to reduce tHcy accumulation.

Vitamin B_{12}

Vitamin B_{12} is the cofactor of methionine synthase. Its natural form, hydroxocobalamin (OHcbl) is more effective than the synthetic form cyanocobalamin (CNcbl). In CBS deficiency, OHcbl may be given orally (1 mg/day to 1 mg/week) according to the serum B_{12} level to prevent cbl deficiency (Chapter 155).

In remethylation disorders, initial treatment includes daily parenteral administration of OHcbl (1 mg/day). If MTHFR deficiency is confirmed, switching to oral hydroxocobalamin (1 mg/day to 1 mg/week) or even stopping hydroxocobalamin supplementation may deserve discussion. Conversely, in the cblC defect, lifelong high-dose intramuscular hydroxocobalamin injections are needed. The optimal interval between intramuscular injections remains to be determined.

Folate

Folate (or vitamin B_9) is available in three different forms. Folic acid, a stable synthetic form of the vitamin used, for example, in food fortification; folinic acid (5-formyl-THF), the most stable form of the reduced and active vitamin; and 5-methylTHF (CH3-THF), the main natural and circulating form of the vitamin (Chapter 155). A folinic acid formulation for parenteral administration is available for emergency treatment, whereas the other forms are available only for oral use. Whatever the disorder, folinic acid is more appropriate because it is the most stable reduced form, and folic acid may exacerbate cerebral CH3-THF deficiency, especially in MTHFR deficiency. In CBS deficiency, folinic acid should be given orally (1 to 5 mg/day) to avoid folate depletion. Moreover, folate repletion may be necessary to permit a pyridoxine (B_6) response, which means that pyridoxine responsiveness should always be tested after folate depletion correction. In cblC defect, long-term high-dose oral folinic supplementation is added to compensate for the methylfolate trap and to correct the hematologic abnormalities. The daily dose varies from 5 to 30 mg. The same folinic acid doses should be used in MTHFR deficiency.

Vitamin B_6

Vitamin B_6 (or pyridoxine), via its action as the cofactor for CBS, is given orally in pharmacological dose in CBS-deficient patients to detect possible B_6-responsive individuals. There is no consensus on the dose and duration of B_6, which is usually given from 100 to 500 to 1000 mg/day during a period of several weeks, after which tHcy is determined to evaluate whether B_6 has been effective in lowering (or even normalizing) tHcy. As discussed above, B_6 should always be combined with folinic acid. In B_6-responsive patients, long-term therapy with pyridoxine and folate prevents further deterioration. In remethylation disorders, B_6 might theoretically enhance homocysteine removal and may be given at a low dose (50 to 100 mg/day).

For pyridoxine-responsive CBS-deficient patients, pyridoxine should be kept at the lowest dosage able to achieve adequate metabolic control. Due to reported high-dose pyridoxine toxicity on the nervous system, daily dosages of more than 400 to 500 mg/day in children and adults should probably be avoided as long-term treatment. In pyridoxine-nonresponsive patients, a daily dosage of 50 to 100 mg of pyridoxine can be added to the treatment.

Betaine

Betaine is derived from choline and is a substrate for the enzyme betaine-homocysteine methyltransferase and therefore acts as a methyl donor (Fig. 198-1). Oral betaine supplementation decreases homocysteine levels. Despite widespread usage, there is little consensus on betaine dosage and frequency of administration. Case studies and early literature have used doses of 150 to 250 mg/kg/day in children and 5 to 10 g/day in adults, usually given two or three times daily. These early data were further confirmed by pharmacokinetic studies that showed that above 200 mg/kg/day in two to three divided doses, there was no obvious benefit in terms of lowering tHcy (in studies performed in CBS deficient patients).

In CBS deficiency, the use of betaine is usually followed by an increase in plasma methionine, and a fall in plasma tHcy. Methionine levels should be kept below 1000 μM because there is a serious risk for brain edema at levels of methionine greater than 1000 μM. In B_6-nonresponsive early-treated patients, a low-methionine diet alone can be highly successful with very good long-term outcomes provided life-long compliance is good. The clinical benefits of betaine are therefore questionable in compliant patients on a low-methionine diet. However, in some patients (especially when compliance with the diet is poor), betaine has been of benefit and may allow an increase in natural protein intake, thus improving the nutritional status.

In remethylation disorders, betaine increases systemic methionine levels and probably also methionine availability for the CNS, especially in patients with MTHFR deficiency. In cblC defect, there are some data reporting a synergistic action of OHcbl with betaine in terms of lowering tHcy level.

Oral Methionine

Oral methionine may also hold promise as an additional therapeutic measure in remethylation defects for several reasons. Cerebral methionine depletion is a key pathogenic factor. Added methionine might act synergistically with betaine by supplying intracellular methionine, and acute methionine loading does not lead to further homocysteine accumulation (with its attendant risk of thromboembolism). As a whole, whatever the remethylation defect, methionine depletion is rarely corrected by betaine therapy alone, whereas the combination of methionine and betaine usually corrects methionine depletion.

PREVENTION

It is prudent to adopt measures to prevent additional risk of thrombosis, such as using long-term low-dose aspirin or dipyridamole in CBS deficiency and avoiding smoking and oral contraceptives in all homocystinurias. In remethylation disorders, nitrous oxide is contraindicated because it inhibits methionine synthase. In CBS deficiency, surgery poses serious risks and should be avoided if possible, especially when tHcy is above 50 μM. However, it can be performed safely if tHcy is below 50 μM (or has been lowered to such levels after a few days of emergency dietary regimen) as long as attention is paid to the patient's hydration (1.5 times IV maintenance) and coagulation status. Low-molecular-weight heparin can be used.

PROGNOSIS

In CBS deficiency, pyridoxine responsiveness generally correlates with higher residual enzyme activity, and the outcome is significantly better than that for unresponsive cases, with or without treatment. Skeletal, ocular, vascular, and neurologic risks are all reduced with successful treatment. Without the early institution of treatment, the median IQ in a large outcome study was 57 for unresponsive patients and 78 for responsive patients. With early treatment, pyridoxine-unresponsive patients have a nearly normal median IQ. For patients who are responsive and compliant to treatment, the prognosis for intellectual development is very good, especially with diet alone. However, in cases of poor adherence, significant elevations in tHcy generally persist, and some increased risk for vascular complications probably remains.

In the few MTHFR-deficient patients treated in the neonatal period, the outcome is good with respect to the first years of neurologic development despite suboptimal metabolic control. If undiagnosed or untreated or late treated, these patients have a very poor outcome with severe impairments. In spite of some pathogenic similarity (intracellular methionine depletion due to impaired remethylation), early-onset cblC-defective patients have in general a particularly poor long-term outcome with multisystem involvement, thrombotic microangiopathy, and retinopathy.

GENERAL REFERENCES

For the General References and other additional features, please visit Expert Consult at https://expertconsult.inkling.com.

199

THE PORPHYRIAS

RICHARD J. HIFT

DEFINITION

The porphyrias are a group of disorders that arise from disturbances in heme synthesis and are characterized by the accumulation of porphyrins or their precursors, the intermediate metabolites, on the heme biosynthetic pathway. Most porphyrias are genetic and heritable, except for the sporadic form of porphyria cutanea tarda and rare instances of porphyria arising from acquired somatic mutations.

CLASSIFICATION

Approximately 90% of heme biosynthesis occurs within the erythron, leading to the production of heme for incorporation into hemoglobin. The remainder is synthesized in all other nucleated cells of the body, producing heme for incorporation into hemoproteins. The liver is the predominant site of non-erythroid heme synthesis, with much of the product being incorporated into enzymes of the cytochrome P450 (CYP) system.

Thus the porphyrias may be classified into two categories: the erythropoietic and hepatic porphyrias.[1] Disturbances in erythroid heme biosynthesis give rise to congenital erythropoietic porphyria (CEP) and two forms of protoporphyria: erythropoietic protoporphyria (EPP) and X-linked protoporphyria (XLP). A possible third form of protoporphyria, related to mutations in the *CLPX* gene, has recently been described.[2] Disturbances in nonerythroid heme biosynthesis give rise to five forms of hepatic porphyria: acute intermittent porphyria (AIP), variegate porphyria (VP), porphyria cutanea tarda (PCT), hereditary coproporphyria (HCP), and ALA dehydratase porphyria (ALADP).

A clinical classification divides the porphyrias into a further two cross-cutting groups (Table 199-1). The acute hepatic porphyrias (AHP) are those characterized by the potential to develop the potentially fatal acute attack (AIP, VP, HCP, and ALADP), whereas the nonacute porphyrias present with cutaneous manifestations alone (PCT, CEP, EPP, and XLP).

EPIDEMIOLOGY

Each porphyria has a prevalence that varies between populations. Assessment of prevalence is complicated by incomplete penetrance, suboptimal case recognition, and unevenness in the accuracy of biochemical diagnosis performed by different laboratories. The prevalence reported from Europe is 9.2 per million for EPP, 5.9 per million for AIP, and 3.2 per million for VP. The figures for North America are believed to be similar. The prevalence of potentially pathogenic mutations may be higher than these figures suggest, possibly as high as 560 cases per million, but with a low penetrance of approximately 1%.[3] The incidence of PCT in Europe is estimated at 40 to 120 per million. HCP has a lower prevalence whereas CEP and ALADP are very rare, and experience is restricted to small case series and case reports. Founder effects have led to a high prevalence of AIP in northern Sweden of 23 per million, and of VP among the Dutch-descended immigrant population of South Africa of 1.2 per thousand of the white population.

PATHOBIOLOGY

The pathobiology of the porphyrias is easily understood by reference to the heme biosynthetic pathway (Fig. 199-1). There are slight differences in erythroid and nonerythroid heme synthesis. The initial step in the pathway is the synthesis of 5-aminolevulinate (ALA), catalyzed by the enzyme 5-aminolevulinate synthase (ALAS). The nonerythroid enzyme, ALAS1, is strongly expressed in the liver and is encoded by the *ALAS1* gene. The erythroid form, ALAS2, is encoded by the *ALAS2* gene on the X chromosome. The two genes share 73% homogeneity. The remaining genes are common to both systems.

Regulation of Heme Biosynthesis

The synthesis of ALA is under normal circumstances the rate-limiting step in the pathway. ALAS1 and ALAS2 are regulated by different mechanisms as described later. The importance of the regulatory elements and proteins associated with control of heme synthesis is now increasingly recognized.[4] They

TABLE 199-1 SUMMARY OF THE PORPHYRIAS

PORPHYRIA	ENZYME	KEY CLINICAL FEATURES AND LONG-TERM COMPLICATIONS	INHERITANCE
ACUTE PORPHYRIAS			
More Common			
Acute intermittent porphyria (AIP)	Hydroxymethylbilane synthase (HMBS)	Acute attacks Hypertension Chronic kidney disease Hepatocellular carcinoma	Autosomal dominant
Variegate porphyria (VP)	Protoporphyrinogen oxidase (PPOX)	Vesiculo-erosive skin disease Acute attacks Hepatocellular carcinoma	Autosomal dominant
Less Common			
Hereditary coproporphyria (HCP)	Coproporphyrinogen oxidase (CPOX)	Vesiculo-erosive skin disease Acute attacks	Autosomal dominant
Rare			
ALA dehydratase porphyria (ALADP)	Porphobilinogen synthase (PBGS)	Acute attacks Neuropathy	Autosomal recessive
NONACUTE PORPHYRIAS			
More Common			
Porphyria cutanea tarda (PCT)	Uroporphyrinogen decarboxylase (UROD)	Vesiculo-erosive skin disease Associated with iron-loading, alcoholic liver disease, hepatitis C, HIV infection, renal failure, and other disorders	Acquired, sometimes on a background of an inherited mutation
*Erythropoietic protoporphyria (EPP)	Ferrochelatase (FECH)	Immediate photosensitivity Cholelithiasis, liver disease	Autosomal recessive; frequently in association with a common polymorphism in the ferrochelatase gene
*X-linked protoporphyria (XLP)	5-Aminolevulinate synthase (ALAS)	Immediate photosensitivity Cholelithiasis, liver disease	X-linked
Rare			
*Congenital erythropoietic porphyria	Uroporphyrinogen III synthase (UROS)	Vesiculo-erosive skin disease Severe photomutilation	Autosomal recessive

*The three forms of erythropoietic porphyria. The remainder are classified as hepatic porphyrias. Rare instances of phenotypic CEP presenting in association with *GATA1* mutations and of EPP with *CLPX* mutations have recently been described and require further investigation and description.

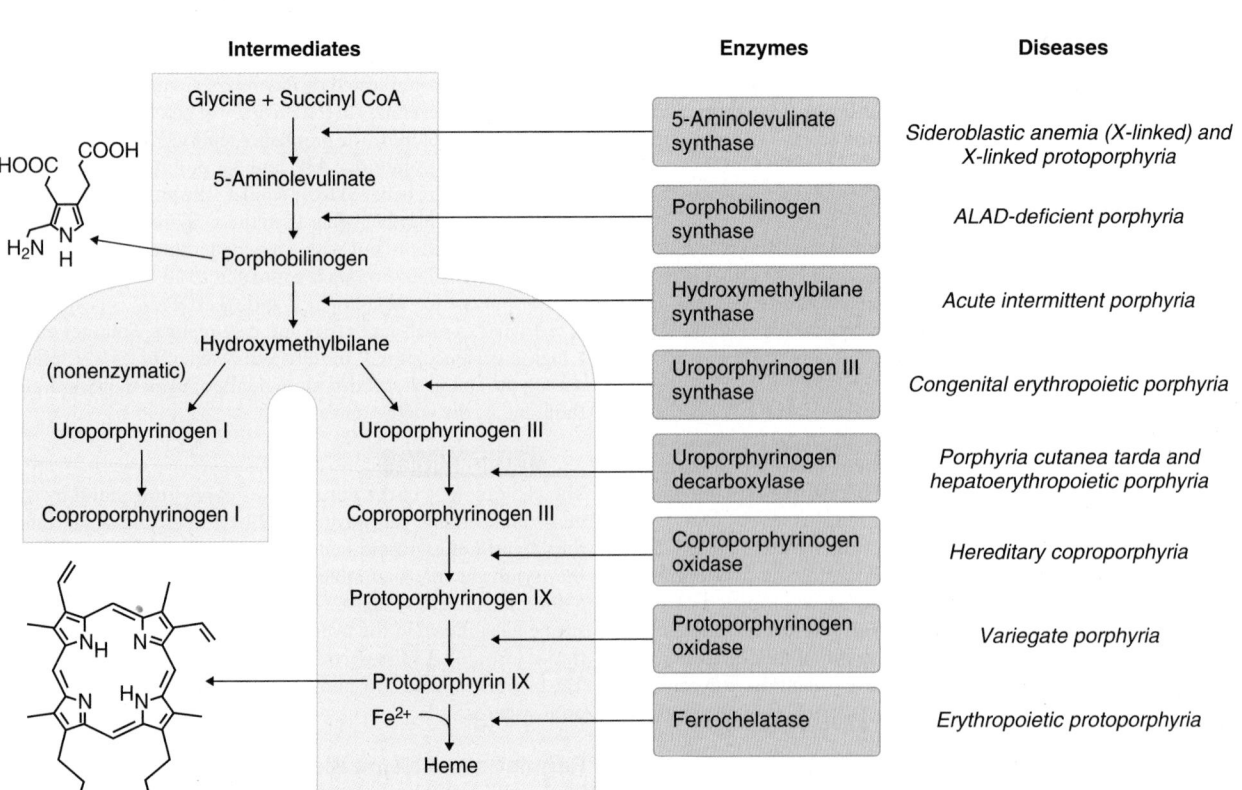

FIGURE 199-1. The heme biosynthetic pathway. Heme is synthesized via a series of porphyrin precursor and porphyrin intermediates, catalyzed by the enzymes listed on the *left* of the figure. The form of porphyria associated with abnormal enzyme function is shown on the *right*.

may be responsible in part for modulating the phenotypic expression of the porphyrias, and in some instances, disturbances may present phenotypically as a porphyria even in the absence of a primary defect within the enzymes of the heme biosynthetic pathway. They constitute potential targets for therapeutic intervention.

Hepatic Heme Biosynthesis
Transcription of *ALAS1* is upregulated in response to a reduction of heme within the hepatocyte and conversely is suppressed by heme replenishment. The mechanisms are less well understood than those for erythroid heme synthesis.

Erythroid Heme Biosynthesis
ALAS2 is not subject to repression by exogenous hemin nor is it induced by factors responsible for induction of hepatic ALAS1. Regulation appears to be exerted at several levels, including ALAS2, HMB synthase, and ferrochelatase. It is primarily regulated by iron availability. When the intracellular iron pool is reduced, iron regulatory proteins IRP1 and IRP2 bind to an iron-responsive element (IRE) in the 5′ region of the *ALAS2* mRNA, preventing translation and hence blocking the synthesis of ALAS2. Erythropoietin has also been shown to directly affect heme synthesis, thus coupling heme production with erythropoiesis.

Heme Biosynthetic Pathway
The structure of the biochemical intermediates of heme biosynthesis, as well as the heme catabolic products biliverdin and bilirubin, are shown in E-Fig. 199-1. After ALAS-mediated synthesis, ALA is converted into porphobilinogen (PBG), which has a monopyrrolic ring structure. Four PBG molecules are then combined to form the linear tetrapyrrole hydroxymethylbilane, which is then enzymatically cyclized by the enzyme uroporphyrinogen-III synthase, resulting in the tetrapyrrolic macrocycle, uroporphyrinogen-III. Sequential modification of the porphyrinogen side chains of uroporphyrinogen-III results in the production of a sequence of porphyrinogens and their oxidized counterparts, the porphyrins. In the final step, iron is incorporated into the tetrapyrrolic macrocycle, resulting in the functional heme molecule. The enzymes ALAS, coproporphyrinogen oxidase, protoporphyrinogen oxidase, and ferrochelatase are all mitochondrial, whereas the remaining enzymes are cytosolic. Heme synthesis therefore begins and ends in the mitochondrion, with intermediate metabolism occurring in the cytoplasm.

Characteristics of the Porphyrins
ALA and PBG are classified as porphyrin precursors, whereas the subsequent tetrapyrrolic structures are known as the porphyrins. The distinction between porphyrin precursors and porphyrins is important in diagnosis and in predicting the clinical presentation of each form of porphyria. The porphyrin precursors and the initial porphyrins in the pathway (ALA, PBG, uroporphyrin, and coproporphyrin) are water soluble, circulate freely in the plasma, and are largely excreted in urine. Protoporphyrin is hydrophobic, may be protein bound in the plasma, and is subject to biliary excretion, eventually being excreted in the stool. Coproporphyrin has intermediate water solubility and is found in both urine and stool. The pattern of accumulation and excretion of precursors and porphyrins is exploited for the biochemical diagnosis of porphyrias and ultimately underlies the varying presentations of the acute and nonacute porphyrias. The acute attack is always associated with elevations in the precursors in urine and plasma, whereas skin disease is characteristic of the disorders in which substantial amounts of porphyrin accumulate in plasma and skin, and variably in urine and feces.

Etiology
Acute Hepatic Porphyrias
AIP, VP, and HCP are inherited as autosomal dominant disorders. ALADP is autosomal recessive and rare. The dominant porphyrias are marked by numerous mutations in different families. The clinical penetrance of each is low; thus the prevalence of asymptomatic carriers exceeds the prevalence of clinically affected patients.[5] Rare cases of homozygous AIP, VP, and HCP have been described. Such patients are severely affected and may have skeletal and neurologic developmental abnormalities.

Nonacute Porphyrias
In approximately 75% of patients with PCT, the *UROD* gene is normal, and symptoms result from the inhibition of UROD enzymatic activity by uroporphomethene, an oxidative product of the normal substrate uroporphyrin. PCT

is associated with hepatic iron overload, alcohol, hepatitis C virus (HCV) infection, HIV infection, estrogen treatment, renal failure, lymphoma, systemic lupus erythematosus, and exposure to toxins such as hexachlorobenzene. In the other 25%, there is an inherited mutation resulting in reduced UROD activity (familial PCT). Since this is insufficient on its own to cause symptoms, clinically expressed patients will be found to have one or more of the associations listed above as well.

Iron loading may be secondary to known causes of iron loading (Chapter 201). Thus the C282Y mutation in the *HFE* gene commonly found in Caucasian patients with hereditary hemochromatosis is overrepresented in PCT. In other cases, the reason for the iron loading is unknown. Alcohol, toxins, and HCV infection may induce PCT via the downregulation of hepcidin and oxidative stress. Rare cases of homozygous PCT had been described. This is known as hepatoerythropoietic porphyria and presents clinically with severe photomutilation resembling that seen in CEP.

EPP is a recessive disorder associated with ferrochelatase mutations. Approximately 5% of cases are homozygous, resulting in sufficiently reduced ferrochelatase activity for the disease to become clinically manifest.[6] The remainder carry a disease-associated mutation on one allele only, but have inherited an *FECH**IVS3-48C polymorphism on the other. This allele is subject to aberrant splicing and decreased stability of the transcript, resulting in low expression. The summative effect of the family-specific mutation and low-expression allele is sufficient to reduce ferrochelatase activities to a level below approximately 35%, at which stage the clinical syndrome may develop. Prevalence of the polymorphism in the population varies from 1% in West African to 12% in European and 47% in Japanese populations. As a result of the high prevalence of the polymorphism, EPP presents clinically more frequently than is expected of a recessive disorder, and its inheritance has been described as "pseudo-dominant."

CEP is an autosomal recessive disorder associated with homozygosity or compound heterozygosity for mutations in the *UROS* gene. Most of the mutations underlying CEP are associated with abnormal folding of the UROS protein and resulting thermodynamic instability. Several patients with CEP have been shown to have normal *UROS* but carry a mutation in the X-linked gene that encodes the GATA1 transcription factor. It is hypothesized that the *GATA1* mutation may impair the *UROS* gene promotor, causing a reduction in gene expression, providing an alternative mechanism for CEP.[7] Several coinherited factors are reported to function as modifier genes, including an *ALAS2* gain-of-function mutation, coinheritance of which in a patient with homozygous *UROS* mutation expressed a markedly severe phenotype.

Somatic Mutations Resulting in Acquired Porphyria
Very rarely, non–germline tissue-specific mutations may result in manifest porphyria. Cases of CEP, EPP, and VP have been described in neoplastic and paraneoplastic settings such as myelodysplasia (Chapter 172), myeloproliferative disorders (Chapter 157), and hepatocellular carcinoma (Chapter 186).

Pathogenesis
Heme Deficiency
Reduced heme production does not appear to result in direct clinical adverse effect in patients with the porphyrias. Though patients with CEP, EPP, and XLP may be mildly anemic, this is in part secondary to hemolysis in CEP and to iron deficiency in XLP. In the acute porphyrias, hemoproteins such as CYP and tryptophan pyrrolase and the cytochromes of the respiratory chain may reveal evidence of heme desaturation without obvious clinical consequences. A possible exception may be the homozygous forms of acute hepatic porphyria, which are accompanied by a range of developmental abnormalities that may possibly be heme dependent. The principal consequence of heme deficiency in the hepatic porphyrias is the induction of *ALAS1*. This upregulates heme biosynthesis with a consequent increase in the flux of porphyrins through the pathway. If this throughput exceeds the capacity of a secondary rate-limiting step downstream (in most cases, a mutant or inhibited enzyme further down the pathway), porphyrins, their precursors, or both will accumulate, potentially precipitating symptoms. This mechanism is the key to understanding the porphyrias.

Photosensitivity
In those porphyrias associated with skin disease, porphyrins are found in high concentrations in plasma, skin, and blister fluid. Porphyrins are fluorescent. Stimulation by light results in an excitation of the porphyrin molecules, the promotion of electrons to a higher energy state, and the production of singlet oxygen. Relaxation to the ground state is accompanied by loss of

energy manifesting as a radiation of red light. In the skin, this energy may be transferred to biologic molecules resulting in oxidation of membrane lipids, polypeptides, and nucleic acids and phototoxic skin damage. The most potent wavelengths for porphyrin excitation lie within the ultraviolet spectrum, in the Soret band between 400 and 410 nm. Four additional absorption bands are present in the range 500 to 700 nm; thus, even visible light, against which most topical sunscreen preparations are ineffective, is harmful to the skin in subjects with a cutaneous porphyria. Pathologic examination will reveal epidermal bullae, duplication of basement membranes, and deposition of hyaline material, which appears to be associated with fibrinogen, immunoglobulins, and complement in and around the blood vessels of the dermis, suggesting that these vessels may be the principal target for light-induced injury.

The Acute Attack

Elevated concentrations of the heme precursors ALA and PBG are always present in patients during the acute attack, and remission is commonly accompanied by a reduction in these concentrations. The development of the acute attack is strongly associated with hyperinduction of *ALAS1*. In patients with AIP, HMBS becomes rate-limiting, resulting in increased ALA and PBG concentrations and acute symptoms. In VP and HCP, the accumulation of coproporphyrinogen and protoporphyrinogen secondarily inhibits HMBS with the same consequences, thus explaining the co-occurrence of acute attacks with skin disease.

Many drugs will induce ALAS1 as part of their metabolism. Such drugs are termed *porphyrogenic,* and exposure to porphyrogenic medication is a common cause of the acute attack. The most powerfully porphyrogenic compounds include multifunctional inducers, which induce multiple hepatic microsomal autosomal enzymes, those which induce the CYP3A and CYP2C9 subclasses, and those which are associated with irreversible mechanism-based inhibition of CYP. Such inhibition results in destruction of the enzyme and the release of heme, which is then catabolized by heme oxygenase, leading to a reduction in the free heme pool, and consequently to *ALAS1* induction. These processes are mediated by nuclear receptors, particularly the constitutively active receptor (CHR) and the pregnane xenobiotic receptor (PXR). Now that these mechanisms are understood, it is possible with high accuracy to predict which drugs are most likely to be porphyrogenic. Patients carrying a gene for an acute porphyria do not respond uniformly or predictably to drug exposure. The reason for this varying susceptibility is not understood. Caloric deprivation is known to induce porphyrin synthesis and potentially the acute attack, whereas glucose administration has a suppressive effect. This is mediated via the transcriptional coactivator, peroxisome proliferator-activated receptor gamma coactivator-1-alpha (PGC-1α), which is upregulated when the liver shifts from the use of glucose as an energy substrate to β-fatty acid oxidation, inducing the transcription of *ALAS1* and increasing heme synthesis.

Women with AIP may show a pattern of regularly recurring attacks associated with the luteal phase of the menstrual cycle. Endogenous hormone production is sufficient to induce ALAS and cause an acute attack. Smoking, stress, and infection have been listed as possible inducers of the acute attack, though the evidence for this is weak. The mechanism may involve induction of the acute-phase protein heme oxygenase 1, which will result in increased catabolism of heme.

Several lines of evidence point to a direct role for ALA in causing the symptoms of the acute attack. ALA is structurally similar to neurotransmitters such as glutamine and γ-aminobutyric acid (GABA). Patients with hereditary tyrosinemia and with lead poisoning, conditions in which ALAD is inhibited and ALA elevated, may experience neurologic symptoms resembling the acute attack of porphyria. Liver transplantation cures AIP and VP; conversely, nonporphyric recipients who received the explanted porphyric liver as part of a domino transplant have developed acute attacks. Studies of the explanted liver have suggested that, although there is elevated *ALAS1* expression and markedly raised hepatic ALA and PBG levels, there is apparently no generalized hepatic heme deficiency. There is, however, evidence to suggest that in the hyperinduced state, there are manifest defects in hepatic mitochondrial nonheme respiratory chain complexes linked to withdrawal of succinyl CoA from the tricarboxylic acid cycle, as well as deficiencies in adrenal steroidogenesis.

Nerve Damage

Nerve damage is characterized by axonal loss, though some degree of segmental demyelination may be present. There may be a reduction in intradermal nerve fiber density on skin biopsy. Skeletal muscle may show neurogenic atrophy.

Nerve conduction studies show a characteristic pattern of axonal necrosis with little evidence of demyelination. Upper limbs may be affected more than the lower limbs. Sensory nerves may be variably affected. Electromyography initially shows a pattern of denervation, with widespread fibrillation, later replaced by a pattern of reinnervation marked by polyphasic motor unit potentials with increased amplitude and duration.

CLINICAL MANIFESTATIONS

Patients with CEP and EPP and patients with the homozygous forms of the acute porphyrias usually present in childhood, though occasional patients with milder expression may present in adult life. The dominant porphyrias usually present clinically after puberty.

The Acute Attack

The cardinal manifestation of the acute hepatic porphyrias is the acute attack. There is often a brief prodrome of mild behavioral disturbance, anxiety, and restlessness followed by a characteristic picture of severe, generalized abdominal pain, felt throughout the abdomen and sometimes in the lower back, buttocks, and thighs. The pain is severe and requires opioids for relief. It is not associated with signs of peritonitis, and typically the abdominal examination is normal. Autonomic overactivity may present as hypertension, tachycardia, and gastrointestinal dysfunction, vomiting, and constipation. Occasionally autonomic overactivity is so severe as to resemble a pheochromocytoma crisis. Hyponatremia is common and may lead to seizures and altered consciousness. Though often ascribed to the syndrome of inappropriate antidiuretic hormone secretion (SIADH), the pattern of electrolyte excretion frequently suggests renal salt-wasting, sometimes associated with marked urinary losses of potassium, calcium, and magnesium. Typically the urine darkens on standing. This is due to the nonenzymatic conversion of PBG to the colored molecules porphobilin and uroporporphyrin-I in the urine.

A severe acute attack may be complicated by a rapid-onset motor neuropathy, usually developing 24 or more hours after the onset of the abdominal pain. Rarely a patient will present with an acute-onset neuropathy with a history of minimal or no abdominal pain. The neuropathy is typically symmetrical and affects proximal muscles predominantly; it may progress to quadriparesis and respiratory paralysis requiring ventilation. Though motor signs predominate, there may be some sensory involvement in a central, "bathing-suit" distribution. Once established, the recovery of motor function is typically slow, but usually near-complete. Cranial nerve or cerebellar involvement is occasionally noted. Patients with severe acute attacks may develop the posterior reversible encephalopathy syndrome (PRES) with radiologic evidence of reversible cerebral ischemia (Chapter 265). Rhabdomyolysis (Chapter 105) complicating the acute attack has been described, as have acute renal failure and potentially fatal cardiac arrhythmias.

Occasionally patients manifest a short-lived psychotic episode, which reverses completely with remission of the attack. There is, however, a widespread misperception that psychiatric manifestations are a prominent part of the symptomatology of the acute porphyrias. Claims that historical figures such as King George III of England and Vincent van Gogh had porphyria are not supported by evidence. A statistical association with chronic anxiety and depression in patients with AIP has been shown but may not differ from that encountered in other chronic disorders. National data in Sweden have suggested a statistical association between porphyria, schizophrenia, and bipolar illness in patients with AIP and their first-degree relatives. This conclusion is provisional; it is now generally accepted by porphyria experts that the link between porphyria and chronic psychotic illness has been greatly overstated.

The acute attack is more common in females than males, is rare before puberty, and becomes uncommon from the sixth decade onward. Acute attacks are more prevalent in patients with AIP and more likely to be associated with hormonal factors than VP. Pregnancy may occasionally precipitate an acute attack. The most characteristic laboratory disturbance is hyponatremia (Chapter 108), which may be present in up to 40% of cases. It may be severe, associated with encephalopathy, seizures, and coma. There may be a slight rise in urea, probably reflecting dehydration and, very occasionally, hypocalcemia and hypomagnesemia in association with hyponatremia reflecting renal tubular dysfunction. Hematologic parameters are usually normal.

Features of the Chronic Phase of Acute Hepatic Porphyrias
Recurrent Attacks

Approximately 3 to 5% of patients, typically young women with AIP, may show a course characterized by recurrent acute attacks.[8] In some of these women there is a clear relationship to the menstrual cycle. In the remainder such an association is not obvious. The worst-affected patients become debilitated and cachectic, show evidence of accumulating neuronal damage, experience a poor quality of life,[9] and may ultimately die.

Chronic Sensory Neuropathy

Patients who have had severe or recurrent attacks may develop a persistent small-fiber neuropathy that presents with generalized dysesthesia and hyperalgesia. This is now increasingly recognized as a problem, particularly as it may be difficult to distinguish a recurrent acute attack from a flare in neuropathic pain centered on the abdomen. Such pain may even appear cyclical. The factors determining the intensity and frequency of such pain are not understood.

Hypertension and Chronic Kidney Disease

At least 40% of patients with AIP will develop chronic hypertension, possibly due in part to chronic activation of the sympathetic nervous system. Many patients with symptomatic AIP will develop chronic kidney disease. It is not a feature of latent disease and is independent of hypertension. It presents as chronic tubulointerstitial nephropathy or focal cortical atrophy. The mechanism is believed to be tubular cell death and tubulointerstitial damage secondary to reabsorption of ALA. The severity of this varies with genetic variation in peptide transporter 2 (PEP2), which mediates the reabsorption of ALA in the proximal tubule.[10] The disease is slowly progressive and may result in end-stage kidney disease requiring dialysis or renal transplantation.

Hepatocellular Carcinoma

A strong association between both AIP and VP and noncirrhotic hepatocellular carcinoma (Chapter 186) has been reported from several countries. Swedish patients with AIP older than age 50 have been shown to be at 86-fold increased risk of hepatocellular carcinoma. The risk is significantly higher in females. There is evidence of an increased risk in VP as well, though surprisingly, such an association has not been seen in South Africa despite the frequency of VP in that population. The mechanism is unknown but may include mutagenesis stimulated by a heightened oxidative state within the hepatocyte in response to chronically elevated ALA levels. Biallelic gene inactivation has been shown in some cases, with a somatic mutation present in tumor tissue in *trans* to the inherited mutation. A population-wide study in Norway has suggested an association between acute hepatic porphyrias, kidney, and endometrial cancers; corroboration is required.

Acute Attacks in Children

The three dominantly inherited acute porphyrias typically present after puberty, most commonly in the third decade. Clinical presentation in prepubertal children is extremely rare. The presentation of affected children is as described for the adult attack, though patients are more likely to be male, tend to have severe attacks, and have complications such as seizures and, occasionally, irreversible neurologic deficits. Prepubertal presentation of VP is less common still.

Vesiculo-erosive Skin Disease

The vesiculo-erosive skin disease of VP, HCP, PCT, and CEP presents as blistering and erosions, typically in response to minor skin trauma, in sun-exposed areas, particularly the dorsal surfaces of the hands and forearms, the face, and the back of the neck. There is no immediate photosensitivity and changes develop insidiously. Therefore patients frequently fail to recognize the association between sun exposure and skin damage. The lesions heal slowly, leaving a residuum of scarring and areas of hypopigmentation or hyperpigmentation (Fig. 199-2). Milia may be present, particularly on the dorsal surfaces of the hands and in the digital clefts. The most severe skin disease is characterized by photomutilation, including loss of skin appendages such as the nose, ears, and lips. This is seen in CEP and HEP. Patients with homozygous VP and HCP may show lesser changes.

PCT usually presents in middle-aged and older subjects who develop characteristic vesiculo-erosive skin lesions in sun-exposed areas.[11] They may develop thickening of the skin of the fingers and hands (so-called pseudosclerodermoid changes), which may lead to a misdiagnosis of scleroderma. Other common features are facial hypertrichosis, skin darkening, and alopecia. There is often evidence of increased iron storage, liver dysfunction, alcohol misuse, or renal dysfunction.

CEP is usually mutilating.[12] Patients typically demonstrate scarring; loss of skin appendages such as ears, nose, and lips; loss of fingernails and

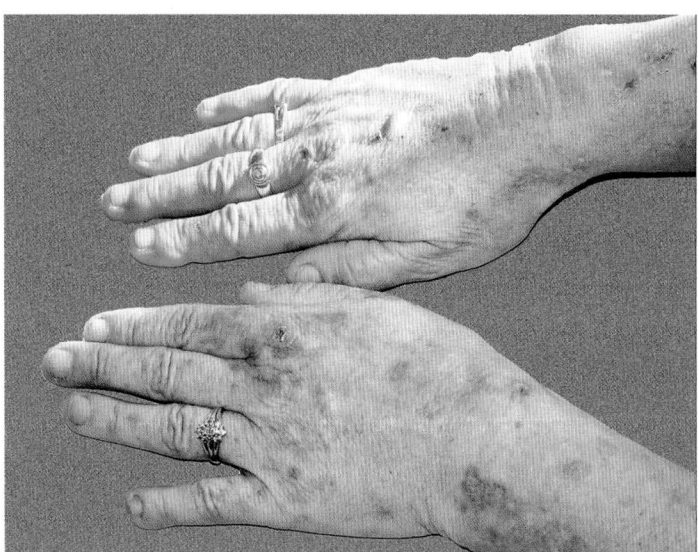

FIGURE 199-2. The hands in variegate porphyria. The characteristic lesions are bullae, shallow erosions that develop scabs and heal slowly, leaving areas of hypopigmentation and hyperpigmentation. The skin disease of porphyria cutanea tarda and hereditary coproporphyria is similar.

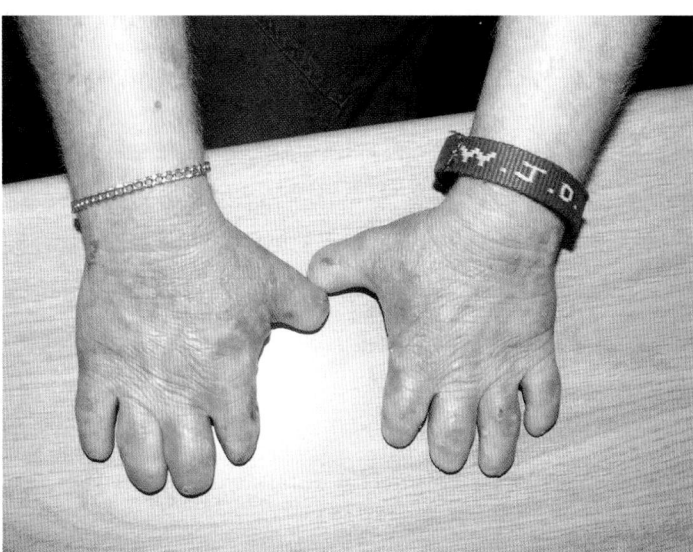

FIGURE 199-3. The hands of a patient with a homozygous form of variegate porphyria. In addition to the characteristic vesiculo-erosive skin lesions, there is marked brachydactyly, representing both photo-osteolysis and a skeletal developmental defect.

digits; ulcerative keratitis; and corneal scarring (Fig. 199-3). Patients may show erythrodontia, osteodystrophy, a hypercellular bone marrow, hemolytic anemia, and splenomegaly. The skin deteriorates progressively with age. Impact on quality of life and psychosocial consequences may be severe. Prenatal cases presenting in utero with severe anemia associated with hydrops fetalis have been described. There is a variable genotype-phenotype correlation, and some patients are less severely affected. Reports have suggested an interaction with modifier genes, including *ALAS2* and *GATA1*, with severity of phenotype being modulated by variants in those genes. The features most predictive of a severe course are early age of onset and the presence of hematologic complications, particularly severe anemia and thrombocytopenia.

Skin Disease Associated with Immediate Photosensitivity
Protoporphyria

Patients with EPP, XLP, and the recently described EPP-like syndrome associated with *CLPX* mutations do not manifest the vesiculo-erosive pattern of skin disease described previously, but develop a characteristic pattern of immediate photosensitivity. Patients report that after a short period of sun exposure, they develop severe discomfort and pain in sun-exposed areas. This may be

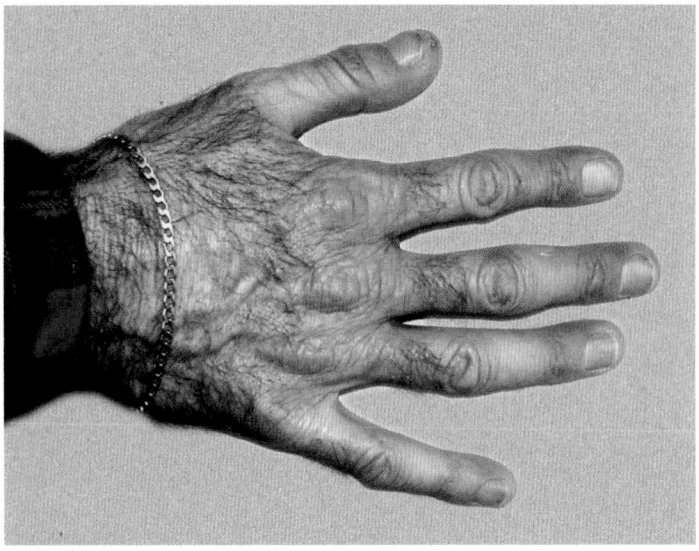

FIGURE 199-4. The hands in erythropoietic protoporphyria. There is thickening and grooving of the skin over the knuckles.

associated with erythema and edema, or there may be no objective visible signs of injury. The discomfort may take 24 to 48 hours to settle after cessation of sun exposure. Photosensitivity is often sufficiently severe to markedly impair quality of life and to restrict the patient's choice of occupation and recreational activity.

The onset of the illness is often in childhood, but typically there is a delay of months or years before the diagnosis is made. Chronic skin changes are minimal and are usually limited to the development of a waxy thickening and grooving of the skin, typically over the bridge of the nose and over the knuckles (Fig. 199-4). Patients who are homozygous or compound heterozygous for ferrochelatase mutations may show seasonal palmar keratoderma. A mild microcytic hypochromic anemia may be present. Cholelithiasis associated with pigment stones in the biliary tract is common. Approximately 1 to 3% of patients with EPP will develop life-threatening liver disease secondary to the massive accumulation of protoporphyrin within hepatocytes.

X-linked Protoporphyria

XLP and EPP cannot for practical purposes be distinguished clinically. XLP is likely to have a higher penetrance as well as a typical X-linked pattern of inheritance. Some patients will report a correlation between iron deficiency and severity of symptoms. Patients with XLP, particularly males, tend to have higher protoporphyrin levels than patients with EPP and appear to be at higher risk of hepatopathy.

Immediate Photosensitivity in Other Settings

A transient immediate acute photosensitivity is occasionally observed in patients with VP as they emerge from an acute attack. This is sometimes associated with acute loss of fingernails. Patients with CEP may manifest immediate photosensitivity in addition to the characteristic vesiculo-erosive skin response. Immediate photosensitivity is observed in patients treated with ALA or synthetic porphyrin analogs as part of photodynamic therapy for cancer.

Homozygous Acute Hepatic Porphyrias

ALA dehydratase deficiency porphyria is an extremely rare recessive disorder, which may present in either childhood or adulthood, depending on the severity of the phenotype, typically with chronic neuropathy, other neurologic symptoms, and acute attacks.

Patients with homozygous AIP present with severe neurodevelopmental abnormalities, including porencephaly, psychomotor and developmental retardation, ataxia, epilepsy, cataracts, and several other neurologic manifestations. It is usually fatal in childhood. Recently a family has been described in which a leukoencephalopathy accompanied by progressive neurologic deficits including slowly progressive spastic paraparesis, cerebellar ataxia, peripheral neuropathy, optic atrophy, nystagmus, and gaze palsies with childhood onset persisted into middle age. Those affected were found to be compound heterozygous for biallelic HMBS mutations previously reported to be associated with symptomatic AIP.[13]

The skin disease of homozygous VP is marked by vesiculo-erosive skin disease, alopecia, skeletal dysmorphism, resorption of digits, nystagmus, seizures, a sensory neuropathy, and cognitive impairment. An association with cerebral demyelination, detectable on magnetic resonance imaging, has been described. Despite the severity of the symptoms, there is no appreciable early mortality, and for reasons yet unknown, acute attacks are not a feature of homozygous VP.

Homozygous HCP takes two forms: the first resembles homozygous VP with small stature, photosensitivity, psychomotor retardation, and neurologic defects; the second presents at birth with hemolytic anemia and severe jaundice. This variant, known as harderoporphyria, is associated with specific mutations in the *CPOX* gene that block an intermediate stage in the oxidation of coproporphyrinogen to protoporphyrinogen, resulting in the accumulation of a tricarboxylic harderoporphyrinogen intermediate.

DIAGNOSIS

Delayed diagnosis may result in unnecessarily impaired quality of life and potentially a fatal acute attack. Conversely it is not unusual for patients to be erroneously labeled as having a porphyria, and an accurate laboratory diagnosis is essential. Physicians need to recognize the acute attack early and should be particularly alerted by the presence of hyponatremia, dark urine, or muscle weakness in the patient with severe abdominal pain.

Biochemical Testing

Biochemical analysis is the first and essential step in the diagnosis and evaluation of the porphyrias. It is highly recommended that diagnostic testing for porphyria be restricted to national reference laboratories that analyze sufficient cases to develop expertise and that cooperate in a quality-enhancement network.[14]

Porphyrin analysis is typically performed with a high-performance liquid chromatographic separation technique with fluorometric detection of the porphyrins. The varying water solubilities of the precursors and porphyrins lead to differential patterns of accumulation in urine, stool, and plasma, whereas the erythropoietic porphyrias are most reliably diagnosed by measuring erythrocyte porphyrin concentrations. Accordingly, urine, stool, and blood samples should be submitted for examination. Examination of urine alone may lead to both misdiagnosis and to misclassification of the porphyria. The series I and III isomers can be distinguished, and the concentration of each individual porphyrin species quantitated by reference to standard specimens. Differentiation of isomers is particularly important in the identification of HCP. Enzyme assays are no longer recommended, given their inaccuracy.

Coproporphyrinuria refers to an elevation of urinary coproporphyrin that is common in patients with liver disease. It results from a diversion of coproporphyrin excretion from bile to urine. It is not related to any disturbance in heme biosynthesis and is essentially irrelevant, yet patients with coproporphyrinuria have frequently been misdiagnosed as having porphyria.

Plasma fluorescence scanning is a useful initial screening test that is suitable for most laboratories. The fluorescence emission maximum varies between different porphyrins and with the extent of their protein binding. When subjected to ultraviolet light, a plasma sample will typically demonstrate an emission peak at approximately 630 nm in EPP, 625 nm in VP, and 619 nm in AIP, HCP, and PCT. The fluorescence emission peak in AIP may be transient, and a negative test does not therefore exclude the diagnosis.

The acute attack is always associated with an elevation of the porphyrin precursors ALA and PBG. It is therefore essential to submit urine with a specific request for measurement of PBG concentration to confirm the presence of an acute attack. Urine porphyrin testing in the acute setting is of little value as it will not confirm the presence of an acute attack. In the appropriate clinical setting, elevated levels are highly confirmatory; conversely, where the PBG concentration is normal, an acute attack is highly unlikely. A quantitative result is recommended. A very dilute sample may produce false-negative results: the PBG concentration should therefore be expressed as a ratio to the urine creatinine concentration, which will correct for concentration or dilution. Since early diagnosis of the acute attack is essential, the specimen should be tested at a laboratory that can return a result within 24 hours. For immediate use in the emergency setting, semiquantitative test kits have been developed that allow the identification of elevated urinary PBG concentrations without the use of specialized equipment. It is recommended that every emergency department have ready access to these.

It may be difficult to confirm the presence of a recurrent acute attack in a patient known to have symptomatic AIP, because the PBG may remain elevated in AIP in remission. It is often a matter of clinical judgment as to whether the patient with known AIP who complains of abdominal pain is experiencing an acute attack or not, as there is no defined diagnostic threshold that reliably distinguishes AIP in the acute phase from AIP in remission.

Genetic Testing

Once a biochemical diagnosis of porphyria has been made, the underlying mutation should be identified. Screening family members for this mutation will then determine carrier status. This is particularly important in the case of the acute hepatic porphyrias, so that as-yet unaffected family members can practice risk avoidance. Where there is a very high prevalence of a single mutation because of a founder effect, screening for that mutation may prove useful in preliminary assessment. This is the case in South Africa, where a single *PPOX* mutation, the R59W mutation, accounts for over 95% of all cases of VP.

Given that the various porphyrias result from mutations in different genes, and that within each porphyria numerous family-specific mutations may give rise to the characteristic phenotype, molecular diagnosis is not well suited to the primary evaluation of a patient. No mutation-specific diagnostic test will exclude any form of porphyria other than the one specifically associated with that gene and that mutation. Conversely, detection of a mutation in the gene for one or more heme-biosynthetic enzymes does not establish the diagnosis as it may represent an incidental polymorphism. Proving that a mutation is indeed associated with clinical disease requires experience and expertise. Genetic testing, unlike biochemical testing, provides no information on the degree of activity of the porphyria at the time of testing.

Differential Diagnosis

Acute Attack

The differential diagnosis of an acute attack includes any cause of severe abdominal pain. About 40% of children with hereditary tyrosinemia type I may develop a syndrome closely resembling the acute attack; this is mediated by the accumulation of succinylacetone, which is a potent inhibitor of ALAD. Lead poisoning may also be accompanied by an acute abdominal crisis, and both these conditions may be distinguished by demonstrating isolated elevation of ALA with a normal PBG concentration. Where patients present with a motor neuropathy or quadriparesis, other causes of acute-onset neuropathy, such as the Guillain-Barré syndrome, should be considered. A careful history may reveal a history of abdominal pain (though very occasionally this is absent), and neurophysiologic testing in acute porphyria will show a pattern of axonal necrosis rather than demyelination. A biochemical analysis for porphyria will confirm the correct diagnosis.

Skin Disease

The differential diagnosis of a typical vesiculo-erosive porphyria is limited. Other chronic bullous diseases require exclusion (Chapter 410). Epidermolysis bullosa is not restricted to sun-exposed areas. Pseudoporphyria is a condition associated with vesiculo-erosive disease resembling porphyria, but there is no underlying enzymatic or genetic defect and plasma porphyrin profiles are normal. Pseudoporphyria is associated with end-stage renal or liver disease, with tanning bed use, or as a class of drug-induced skin reactions, particularly in response to nonsteroidal anti-inflammatory drugs, nalidixic acid or tetracycline, sulfur-containing diuretics, systemic retinoids, cyclosporine, and dapsone. The pathogenetic mechanism is unknown.

TREATMENT

The Acute Attack

Patients should be managed by or in consultation with a physician with experience in porphyria. Pain is severe and requires opioid analgesia in doses sufficient to relieve it. Inexperienced physicians and nurses frequently do not prescribe opioids in the doses and frequency required; they may be misled by the lack of abdominal signs and may incorrectly suspect exaggeration of symptoms or opioid addiction. Morphine and newer opioids should be selected in preference to meperidine, given its addictive potential. It is essential that all porphyrogenic drugs and other potential precipitants are stopped, and no medication should be administered to the patient unless its safety in porphyria has been checked. Patients may require antiemetics. Though β-blockers may assist in slowing the pulse and reducing blood pressure, these are rarely sufficiently elevated to require treatment.

Electrolyte balance requires careful monitoring. Though carbohydrate loading has been shown to have a suppressive effect on porphyrin synthesis,

its effect is minimal in comparison with that of hemin therapy. Enteral glucose administration is more effective and safer than intravenous administration, because infusions of glucose-containing hypotonic fluids may aggravate hyponatremia.

Specific Therapy

Administration of exogenous heme (in the form of hemin, a heme variant in which the iron moiety is in the ferric state, with a coordinating chloride ligand) results in negative feedback inhibition of ALAS1, resulting in a rapid reduction in porphyrin synthesis. This is now the standard of care for the acute attack. It shortens the duration of symptoms, allows earlier discharge, and prevents severe complications such as encephalopathy and motor neuropathy.

Human hemin is marketed in two forms.[1] They are equally efficacious. Lyophilized human hemin (Panhematin, Recordati Rare Diseases Inc., Lebanon, NJ) is licensed for use in the United States. It is presented as a powder that is reconstituted with sterile water for injection and infused intravenously in a dose of 1 to 4 mg per kilogram per day. Heme arginate (Normosang, Orphan Europe, Puteaux, France) is a newer compound in which heme is complexed with arginine. It is not currently licensed for use in the United States but is now widely used in Europe and other areas. It is administered intravenously in a dose of 3 mg/kg daily for 4 days. The manufacturer recommends that the dose be reconstituted in 100 mL of a 0.9 % sodium chloride solution and infused into a large vein over at least 30 minutes. It is common practice, however, to administer heme arginate in human serum albumin as albumin has a buffering effect, which may reduce the incidence of phlebitis at the site of infusion and may facilitate hepatic uptake.

Administration of hemin typically results in clinical improvement within 24 hours. After the third or fourth dose the patient is usually symptom free and may be discharged. It is essential that hemin is administered early as it will prevent neuropathy but not reverse it once established. Treatment of children and pregnant women is safe.

Patients may rarely present with a syndrome of severe, accelerated hypertension, tachycardia, and cerebral complications, which may include coma, seizures, and the posterior reversible encephalopathy syndrome. Administration of intravenous magnesium sulfate in association with combined α- and β-blockade is useful in controlling the autonomic overactivity while the attack is aborted with hemin. Recovery is usually rapid and complete.

Recurrent Attacks

Recurrent acute attacks are an uncommon manifestation of the acute porphyrias, affecting approximately 3 to 5% of all symptomatic patients. Medications should be reviewed and potentially porphyrogenic medication stopped. Smoking and alcohol should be discouraged.

Patients experiencing recurrent attacks need to be under the care of an experienced physician or team. Advance arrangements to ensure that hemin will be readily available when required should be made. It is advisable that patients are admitted directly to a ward where they are known and staff are comfortable with therapy rather than being processed via the emergency department.

Prophylactic Use of Hemin

Some patients with a history of recurrent acute attacks have received prophylactic hemin at scheduled intervals or on demand at the earliest onset of symptoms, reportedly with benefit. Home use has been practiced in the United Kingdom. Frequent administration is associated with high incidence of thrombophlebitis, and a permanent indwelling central venous catheter is often required. Regular administration of prophylactic hemin is not without risk. Frequent administration of hemin may induce heme oxygenase, leading to rapid catabolism of heme, thus initiating a vicious cycle of reduction in hepatocyte free regulatory heme levels, ALAS1 induction, and increased precursor synthesis, promoting the development of a further attack. Hemin contains 9% iron by weight, and patients receiving frequent courses of therapy may become iron overloaded. Ferritin should be measured at regular intervals, and phlebotomy undertaken if necessary. Once-monthly injections of givosiran (an investigational RNA interference therapeutic agent that inhibits hepatic synthesis of delta aminolevulinic acid synthase 1) is an experimental therapy to reduce attack rates in patients with acute intermittent porphyria.[15]

Management of Chronic Pain

The problem of chronic neuropathic pain following recurrent acute attacks is difficult to manage. It may run a relapsing/remitting course, which may make it difficult to distinguish from recurrent acute attacks. It is not responsive to hemin but may respond to drugs used for neuropathic pain, such as anticonvulsants and antidepressants. The advice of a neurologist or pain management specialist should be sought.

Menstrual Attacks

Some patients have had a pattern of menstrual attacks successfully treated with low-dose estrogen-gestagen combinations, whereas others have had attacks precipitated by such treatment. Some patients have responded satisfactorily to prophylactic hemin therapy given just before the luteal phase of the cycle. Oophorectomy is not appropriate. Gonadal suppression using gonadotropin-releasing hormone agonists such as gonadorelin, goserelin, buserelin, leuprorelin, triptorelin, histrelin, or nafarelin may be attempted. This is efficacious in aborting the pattern of recurrent attacks in approximately half the patients treated.[16] Treatment should be initiated within the first 3 days of the cycle as later initiation may precipitate an attack. Therapy results in estrogen deficiency, which is usually symptomatic, and is accompanied by bone demineralization. This may be counteracted by administration of low-dose estrogen, preferably as a cutaneous patch. Adding supplemental gestagen will frequently precipitate an attack.

Orthotopic Liver Transplantation

Orthotopic liver transplantation prevents further acute attacks in both AIP and VP. It should be considered in any patient who develops a pattern of severe repetitive acute attacks, particularly when there is incomplete recovery between attacks, progressive disability, or severely impaired quality of life. Combined liver and kidney transplantation may be necessary when AIP is accompanied by chronic kidney disease.

Skin Disease

There is no specific therapy for vesiculo-erosive skin disease. Sun avoidance is central to its management. This may require behavioral modification as well as careful attention to dress, wearing nontranslucent clothing to reduce the skin's ultraviolet exposure. Trauma to exposed areas should be minimized. Sunscreens must prevent the transmission of ultraviolet (UV) A, UVB, and visible wavelengths. Zinc oxide is more effective than titanium dioxide. Though sunscreens containing micronized zinc oxide or titanium dioxide are translucent and cosmetically more acceptable, they reflect less light and therefore only provide partial protection. Established lesions should be carefully cleaned with nonastringent antiseptics. In our experience, aseptic lancing of bullae may hasten resolution. Where secondary infection is noted, topical or systemic antibiotics are indicated.

Porphyria Cutanea Tarda

PCT will remit once the precipitating factors have been removed. Alcohol use should be severely restricted. Hepatitis C should be treated. Elevated iron stores should be reduced (Chapter 201). A common regimen is to carry out a 500-mL venesection fortnightly until the serum ferritin is in the low-normal range; typically, this requires about 8 to 12 sessions. Iron chelation therapy is effective, though less efficient than phlebotomy. Patients who are anemic, as in those with renal failure, may require concurrent erythropoietin to maintain an adequate hemoglobin concentration and will in addition mobilize hepatic iron.

Oral chloroquine is as effective as venesection in inducing remission in PCT. By disrupting lysosomal structure, it allows the release of porphyrins stored in the liver into the plasma from where they are cleared by the kidneys. Initiation of chloroquine therapy frequently causes an initial, transient increase in plasma porphyrins and severity of skin disease. Chloroquine must be used in low doses, typically 125 mg twice weekly, as larger doses may result in a significant transaminitis.

Specific therapy for HCV infection will induce remission in PCT. Direct-acting antiviral agents are preferable to α-interferon and ribavirin, treatment with which has been reported to induce an initial exacerbation in the severity of the PCT skin disease. Given the deleterious effects of iron overload, however, it would appear prudent to combine treatment with antivirals or chloroquine with iron-lowering therapy where accompanying iron overload is shown. Remission of PCT, once attained, is usually maintained for many years, though occasionally retreatment may be necessary.

Protoporphyrias

Reducing sun exposure requires behavioral change, attention to dress, and use of broad-spectrum sunscreens. Some patients appear to respond positively to the administration of β-carotene in doses sufficiently large to induce carotenodermia, though efficacy has not been convincingly proven. Narrow-band UVB phototherapy has in some cases resulted in increased phototolerance.

Treatment with afamelanotide has been proven effective in controlled trials.[A1] This is a synthetic melanocyte-stimulating hormone analog, administered as a slow-release subcutaneous implant, with a longer duration of action than the natural hormone. It induces the synthesis of both pheomelanin and eumelanin, which together absorb and reflect radiation over a wide light spectrum. Eumelanin synthesis is not dependent on UV exposure. Afamelanotide is now licensed for use in EPP in Europe and is under review in the United States. Treatment is without serious adverse effects, and it may now be recommended as the standard of care.

Anemia and iron deficiency are common in patients with EPP and XLP. It is appropriate to provide iron replacement therapy with careful monitoring of both the clinical response and plasma protoporphyrinogen levels, as some though not all patients have been reported to respond favorably.

Benefit has been claimed for a number of interventions in terms of their utility in reducing the acute pain of EPP, including lotions, steroids, local anesthetics, antihistamines, water immersion, and ice packs. Though individual patients may feel that they were helped by one or the other, no consistent benefit has been shown for any single intervention. A method for dynamically measuring protoporphyrin levels in the skin noninvasively has shown that erythrocyte and skin porphyrin levels are closely correlated with photosensitivity in EPP and offers a potential method for monitoring of such patients to determine photosensitivity and monitor treatment response.

Protoporphyria-associated hepatopathy is not well understood. Certain groups are at elevated risk: those with homozygosity, EPP, XLP, or a family history of liver disease, and those with high erythrocyte protoporphyrinogen levels. Such patients require the care of an experienced hepatologist. The sensitivity of liver chemistry tests in providing early warning of liver involvement has not been established nor are evidence-based recommendations to guide treatment. Administration of oral sorbents such as activated charcoal, cholestyramine, and colestipol, which interrupt hepatic porphyrin recycling, have yielded inconsistent results. Hypertransfusion and administration of hemin may suppress porphyrin synthesis but are not suitable for long-term use. Severely affected patients are candidates for orthotopic liver transplantation. Given that the viscera are porphyrin laden and prone to severe light-induced necrosis, careful preparation of the patient is necessary, and surgery must be carried out using filtered operating lights. Severe motor neuropathy has proven to be an unexpected complication of liver transplantation in patients with protoporphyria. Following transplantation, protoporphyrin will reaccumulate in the liver. Consideration may therefore be given to performing combined bone marrow and liver transplantation.

Congenital Erythropoietic Porphyria

Light avoidance, with protection for both skin and eyes, is essential. Where skin disease is severe—as in CEP—consideration may be given to replacing fluorescent lighting with other forms of illumination with lower short-wavelength light emission and the application of transparent film to windows, spectacles, and windshields to exclude the relevant wavelengths. Afamelanotide has shown benefit in a single case. Some patients require chronic transfusion for anemia and may benefit from splenectomy. Early autologous stem cell transplantation will prevent further disfigurement and inevitable psychosocial consequences in severely affected individuals. There is now consensus that young subjects with severe CEP should be offered stem cell transplantation before mutilating disease becomes established. The phenotype of CEP is extremely variable. It is recommended that bone marrow transplantation be reserved for patients with a mutation known to be associated with a severe phenotype and for those presenting in infancy or with severe hemolytic anemia or thrombocytopenia.

Investigational Therapies for the Porphyrias
Acute Hepatic Porphyrias

Though hemin administration is effective, it is subject to limitations that make the search for better treatments worthwhile. These include a relatively slow onset of action, the frequency of phlebitis requiring administration through a central venous line in patients with recurrent attacks, and tolerance with repeated use.

Intravenous administration of recombinant HMBS protein to patients with AIP has been studied in a small series. Although treatment reduced plasma PBG levels, ALA levels remained high and symptoms were not affected, presumably because of limited access of this preparation to the hepatocyte. Gene replacement for AIP, using a variety of vectors, is under active development and has shown promise in laboratory studies. Administration of a recombinant adenovirus-associated vector expressing HMBS has now been investigated in a small clinical study. Precursor levels did not change in response, though an apparent trend to improvement in clinical course was reported. Further studies are in progress. Hepatocyte transplantation has shown promise experimentally in the treatment of AIP and would have advantages over orthotopic liver transplantation.

Because ALAS1 is central to the pathogenesis of the acute attack, downregulation of ALAS1 is seen as a prime target for therapeutic intervention. Several potential sites have been identified: transcriptional and post-transcriptional regulation, modulation of the rate of import of the precursor enzyme from cytosol into the mitochondrion, enzyme inhibition, and downregulation of LON1P, a protease that controls the turnover of mitochondrial matrix proteins. The effect of exogenous hemin is mediated via at least three of these mechanisms. Gene-silencing directed at ALAS1 mRNA to block ALAS1 induction appears encouraging in the acute hepatic porphyrias. Patients with AIP have higher ALAS1 mRNA levels compared with controls. Use of givoseran, which is an ALAS1 antisense nucleotide (small interfering RNA sequence, siRNA1) complexed with N-acetylgalactosamine to promote hepatocyte uptake has been reported to be safe and effective in reducing ALA and PBG levels and in reducing recurrent attacks in patients with AIP.[17] More studies will be needed to determine its role in clinical care.

Congenital Erythropoietic Protoporphyria

Encouraging results for gene therapy, including reengineered induced pluripotent stem cells, have been shown in animal studies. Where the effect of a mutation is to reduce protein stability, interventions to improve stability may lead to improvement in enzyme concentration and activity. In vitro studies suggest that administration of a proteasome inhibitor may improve UROS function where the enzyme deficiency is due to an unstable protein.

Erythropoietic Protoporphyria

A study has shown that an antisense oligonucleotide directed at the cryptic splice site of FECH coded for by the common low-expression polymorphism increases the use of the wild-type splice site, leading to increased mRNA levels, increased FECH activity, and decreased protoporphyrin accumulation in vitro. This may potentially have therapeutic value.

PREVENTION

Primary Prevention

Given that most of the porphyrias are genetically determined, there is currently no practical way in which these illnesses may be prevented. Genetic counseling and education of patient and family, as well as access to appropriate literature resources for patient support, are important. Diagnosis in utero using molecular methods for the identification of family-specific mutations is possible. Selective abortion is not appropriate given that a very high proportion of carriers will be either unexpressed or will experience symptoms that are easily controlled. The conditions most likely to result in severely impaired quality of life are CEP and the homozygous acute porphyrias. These recessive conditions are extremely rare, and in many instances parents have not previously been recognized as gene carriers, thus preventing prenatal diagnosis. Prenatal testing may, however, be appropriate in cases of known consanguinity, where the possibility of recessive inheritance is increased.

Secondary Prevention
Acute Hepatic Porphyrias

Acute attacks should be prevented. Patients must avoid sudden reductions in caloric intake and must not be exposed to any porphyrogenic medication. All gene carriers, whether the disease is expressed or not, and the health professionals who care for them must understand the importance of consulting a drug safety database before taking or prescribing any medicinal agent. We recommend use of the European web-based database *The Drug Database for Porphyria* (http://www.drugs-porphyria.org) maintained by the Norwegian Porphyria Centre. The recommendations in this database are assigned on the basis of their metabolic fate and predicted porphyrogenicity. Experience has shown that these predictions are reliable and avoid many of the shortcomings of older lists based largely on clinical or animal experience.

Anesthesia is safe in acute hepatic porphyria, provided that nonporphyrogenic anesthetic agents and ancillary drugs are used. Pregnancy is rarely problematic. Occasional patients experience more frequent attacks during pregnancy. Hemin administration is safe in pregnancy. There is a slightly increased risk of fetal loss in patients who have experienced recurrent attacks. Patients should be screened at regular intervals for hypertension, chronic kidney disease, and hepatocellular carcinoma.

Cutaneous Porphyrias

Children at risk for the cutaneous porphyrias, including those known to have inherited a gene for VP or HCP, should be encouraged to develop healthy habits of sun avoidance and sun protection before the onset of symptoms. Patients with established disease need to modify behavior and dress to limit sun exposure. In cases of extreme photosensitivity, filtering of natural and artificial light may be beneficial.

Patients with PCT should be screened for hemochromatosis-associated mutations (Chapter 201). Once in remission, the precipitating factors for PCT described previously should be avoided. Patients should be screened annually for urine porphyrin concentrations and ferritin levels, and a repeat course of phlebotomy commenced if necessary. Some authorities recommend monitoring for diabetes and for hepatocellular carcinoma, particularly in those with hepatitis C or alcoholic cirrhosis.

PROGNOSIS

With few exceptions, the prognosis of the porphyrias is favorable.

Acute Hepatic Porphyrias

Patients may expect a normal lifespan provided that acute attacks are avoided and, if experienced, effectively treated. The prognosis for the individual attack is good if the patient is treated, usually with hemin, before the onset of neuropathy. Even where the patient has developed quadriparesis, the prognosis for ultimate recovery is good provided the patient receives high-quality care, including assisted ventilation if necessary. Typically the patient may be weaned off the ventilator within 4 months and is usually fully ambulant and independent by 8 months. There may be some mild residual footdrop and wristdrop, but recovery is usually near-complete by 12 months. It is important to avoid further acute attacks during the period of convalescence, and if necessary to treat them properly and effectively, to prevent a relapse in neuropathy.

There has been a dramatic decrease in the incidence of acute attacks over the past 5 decades, probably because of increasing awareness, early screening, better education, and changing habits in drug prescription. In expert hands, death is now extremely rare. Yet in countries where historically the acute porphyrias have not previously been recognized, such as India, a proliferation of recent case reports and small series indicate increasing diagnosis of patients experiencing the acute attack, typically made late with a high incidence of serious complications and significant mortality.

The prognosis is less benign in those patients who present with recurrent acute attacks poorly responsive to therapy. The course is frequently one of slow deterioration over several years and may ultimately be fatal. Such patients should be assessed for orthotopic liver transplantation. Patients with homozygous AIP are prone to severe developmental abnormalities and may die in childhood. By contrast, there appears to be no early mortality in patients with homozygous VP, though the photomutilation and neurodevelopmental effects may have psychosocial and educational consequences.

Cutaneous Porphyrias

The skin disease of porphyria is not life threatening. Patients with CEP are subject to severe photomutilation with serious psychosocial consequences and should be assessed for allogeneic stem cell transplantation. PCT is treatable and remission is expected once the precipitating factors, including iron overload, have been corrected. A small proportion of patients with protoporphyria will develop hepatopathy, which may prove fatal. The majority will, however, have a normal lifespan.

Grade A Reference

A1. Langendonk JG, Balwani M, Anderson KE, et al. Afamelanotide for erythropoietic protoporphyria. *N Engl J Med.* 2015;373:48-59.

GENERAL REFERENCES

For the General References and other additional features, please visit Expert Consult at https://expertconsult.inkling.com.

200

WILSON DISEASE

MICHAEL L. SCHILSKY

DEFINITION

Wilson disease is an autosomal recessive disorder of copper transport. Affected individuals accumulate abnormal levels of copper in the liver and later in the brain as a consequence of mutations in both alleles of the Wilson disease gene (*ATP7B*). The gene encodes a copper-transporting ATPase expressed primarily in hepatocytes in the liver, where its major function is excretion of hepatic copper into the biliary tract. The clinical condition of hepatolenticular degeneration with associated cirrhosis was first described in detail in 1912 by S. A. K. Wilson. There are wide differences between patients in the age at onset and the spectrum of symptoms.

EPIDEMIOLOGY

The incidence of Wilson disease, defined as the occurrence of new cases, is approximately 1 in 30,000 to 40,000 live births. For special populations in which consanguinity is common, the incidence is higher. In the general population, the prevalence of heterozygous gene carriers (defined as the ratio of all individuals with one mutant *ATP7B* allele to the population at large) is estimated to be 1 in 90 to 1 in 180. Some consider this incidence an underestimate on the basis of population data of the frequency of *ATP7B* mutation in the United Kingdom.

PATHOBIOLOGY

Individuals normally consume 1 to 3 mg of dietary copper daily, 50% of which is absorbed through the gastrointestinal tract. Most diets contain adequate amounts of copper, and certain foods (e.g., shellfish, liver, mushrooms, chocolate, nuts) contain higher quantities. In normal homeostasis, copper is absorbed from the stomach and duodenum, where absorption at the apical surface of the enterocyte is mediated by a specific copper transporter, hCTR1. *ATP7A*, which encodes a copper transporting ATPase protein with high homology to the one encoded by *ATP7B*, transports copper from intestinal epithelial cells into the blood stream, where it is bound by albumin or amino acids, carried to the liver and other organs and tissues, or excreted by the kidney. Renal copper excretion represents a minor pathway, and adults normally excrete only up to 40 μg of copper per day in the urine.

Within the liver, copper may be (1) incorporated into ceruloplasmin, a multifunctional 132-kD α_2-glycoprotein enzyme containing six or seven copper atoms per molecule; (2) used in the synthesis of other copper-requiring enzymes; (3) bound by metallothionein, a low-molecular-weight, cysteine-rich protein that provides a storage and detoxification depot for copper and other trace metal elements; or (4) excreted into the bile. *ATP7B*, the gene that is mutated in Wilson disease, is expressed primarily in the liver and encodes another copper-transporting protein that facilitates the removal of excess hepatic copper through the bile.[1,2] Biliary copper does not undergo enterohepatic recirculation, and thus fecal loss of copper normally represents a major pathway for copper excretion.

In Wilson disease, copper excretion is impaired due to the abnormal ATPase copper transporter encoded by the mutant *ATP7B* gene, thereby producing massive hepatic copper overload when the condition is unrecognized and untreated.[3] With untreated hepatic copper overload, excess copper enters the circulation and copper subsequently deposits in other tissues, including the brain, which is particularly sensitive to perturbations in trace metal homeostasis. It is because copper first accumulates in the liver before other organs that liver disease tends to precede the onset of copper injury to other organs, most notably the brain.

In Wilson disease, the acquisition of copper by ceruloplasmin is usually reduced, reflecting impaired transport of copper into the trans-Golgi compartment, where glycoprotein processing and the copper incorporation by apoceruloplasmin occur. This results in low circulating levels of holoceruloplasmin (the protein with its full complement of copper) due to the instability of the apoprotein (without copper) in the circulation. Because copper in ceruloplasmin accounts for 90% of circulating copper, total serum copper is low in most Wilson disease patients.

CLINICAL MANIFESTATIONS

Presenting clinical features of Wilson disease include nonspecific liver disease (Fig. 200-1), neurologic abnormalities, psychiatric illness, hemolytic anemia, renal tubular Fanconi syndrome, and various skeletal abnormalities.[4]

There is considerable variation in clinical presentation and phenotype in Wilson disease.[5] Specific presentations differ with age, with liver disease more often presenting at age less than 30 years, sometimes even in the first or second decades of life. By contrast, those presenting with neurologic or psychiatric signs typically do so after age 20, but reports show a range in age from the first to the eighth decade of life. Regardless of clinical presentation, some degree of liver disease is invariably present.[6] In one older series of 400 adult patients with Wilson disease, approximately 50% presented with neurologic and psychiatric symptoms, 20% with neurologic and hepatic symptoms, and 20% with purely hepatic symptoms.

In hepatic presentations, signs and symptoms include fatigue, jaundice, hepatomegaly, edema, and ascites. Secondary endocrine effects of liver disease may include delayed puberty or amenorrhea. Viral hepatitis and autoimmune hepatitis are often initial diagnostic considerations in individuals with Wilson disease. Rare patients have Wilson disease concurrent with another liver disorder, and the diagnosis of Wilson disease is often delayed in these individuals as a consequence.

In patients with neurologic presentations, abnormalities include speech difficulty (dysarthria), dystonia, rigidity, tremor or choreiform movements,

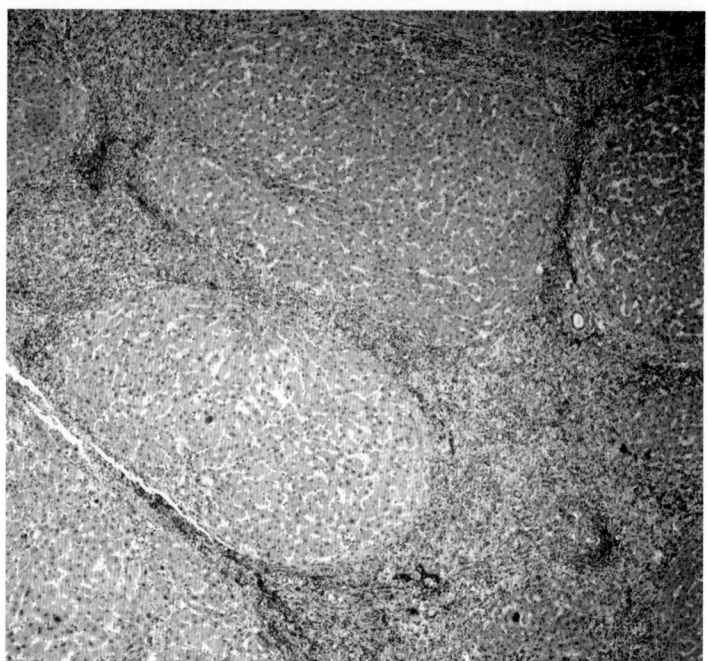

FIGURE 200-1. Hepatic cirrhosis in Wilson disease. (Image courtesy Kisha A. Mitchell, MD.)

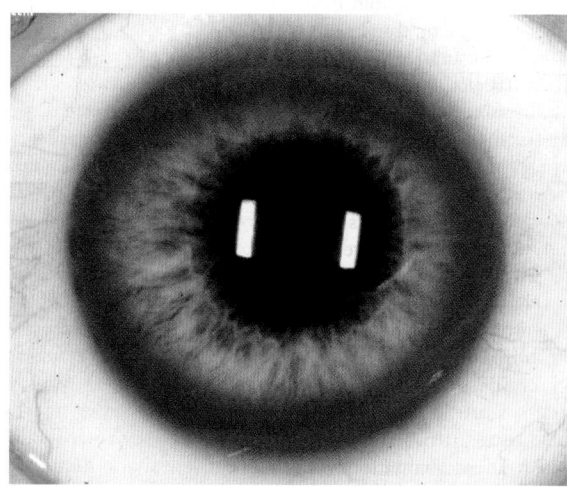

FIGURE 200-2. Kayser-Fleischer ring in a newly diagnosed patient with Wilson disease.

abnormal gait, uncoordinated handwriting, and (rarely) a combined motor and sensory peripheral neuropathy.[7-10] Wilson disease may properly be classified as a movement disorder. The neurologic signs and symptoms reflect a predilection for involvement of the basal ganglia (e.g., caudate, putamen) in the brains of these individuals. Parkinson disease or other movement disorders may be mistakenly diagnosed.

In psychiatric presentations,[11] changes in personality (irritability, anger, poor self-control), depression, and anxiety are common symptoms. Psychosis or bipolar disorder may also occur. Patients presenting with psychiatric symptoms are typically in their late teens or early twenties, a period during which substance abuse and schizophrenia are also prime diagnostic considerations. Wilson disease should be considered and formally excluded in all young adults with new-onset psychiatric symptoms, especially if results of liver function tests are abnormal or a family history of Wilson disease is noted.

In addition to brain and liver, the eye is a site of copper deposition in Wilson disease, producing a benign but characteristic sign, the Kayser-Fleischer ring (Fig. 200-2). The Kayser-Fleischer ring is the annular deposition of copper in the periphery of the cornea. This important diagnostic sign first appears as a golden colored superior crescent, then develops inferiorly and ultimately becomes circumferential. Slit-lamp examinations are required to detect rings in their early stage of formation. Copper can also accumulate in the lens and produce "sunflower" cataracts.

Approximately 95% of patients with neurologic or psychiatric signs have Kayser-Fleischer rings compared with approximately 50 to 65% of those with hepatic presentations. Copper chelation therapy, zinc treatment, and liver transplantation cause fading and disappearance of corneal copper over time.

Hemolytic anemia resulting from the direct toxic effects of copper on red blood cell membranes has been observed in Wilson disease. This is usually associated with the release of massive quantities of hepatic copper into the circulation, a phenomenon that can be sudden and catastrophic due to the development of acute (fulminant) liver failure.[12] On occasion, hemolytic anemia may occur without liver failure.

Renal dysfunction in Wilson disease is tubular in nature and leads to abnormal losses of amino acids, electrolytes, calcium, phosphorus, uric acid, and glucose. This effect is presumably related to direct renal tubular copper toxicity or toxicity of copper complexes with metallothionein. Treatment with copper chelation often improves the renal disturbances.

There can be skeletal involvement in Wilson disease, including osteoporosis and rickets; in part these may be attributable to renal losses of calcium and phosphorus. Osteoarthritis primarily affecting the knees and wrists also occurs in Wilson disease patients and may involve excess copper deposition in the bone and cartilage.

DIAGNOSIS

Wilson disease should be considered in patients with liver disease without a clear etiology; in patients presenting with acute liver failure with associated hemolysis; in patients with neurologic and psychiatric disease, especially if there is concomitant liver disease; and in first-degree relatives of identified patients.[13]

Laboratory findings supporting the diagnosis include low levels of serum copper and serum ceruloplasmin, elevated urine copper excretion (>100 µg/24 hours), elevated hepatic transaminase levels, low serum albumin, elevated prothrombin time (international normalized ratio), aminoaciduria, low uric acid levels, and direct antiglobulin test (Coombs)–negative hemolytic anemia. Analysis of liver biopsy specimens for histologic features and copper content also can assist diagnosis (see later). Clinical signs of the disease include the stigmata of chronic liver disease, neurologic signs and symptoms, and Kayser-Fleischer rings (often requiring slit-lamp examination for detection). A scoring system was developed by experts that uses biochemical, clinical, and molecular genetic data to give a cumulative score that allows establishment of the diagnosis, suggests further evaluation is needed, or provides exclusion of the diagnosis; it has been used in a diagnostic algorithm developed by the European Association for the Study of the Liver.

Molecular diagnostics for *ATP7B* mutations has been extremely helpful, especially for difficult to diagnose cases and for family screening, in which it may be used as first-line testing if the mutations in the proband have been identified.[14] There are over 500 known disease-specific mutations, and most patients have different mutations on each allele.

Incorporation of a stable radioisotope, ^{64}Cu, into serum ceruloplasmin is a highly specific diagnostic test; patients with Wilson disease incorporate very little ^{64}Cu into ceruloplasmin. This test is particularly useful in patients thought to have Wilson disease despite normal ceruloplasmin levels. Clinical availability of this test, however, is limited.

Increased urinary excretion of copper (>100 µg/24 hours) is another diagnostic test for this disorder. Copper-free collection containers should be used. A variation involving serial urine copper measurements is the penicillamine "challenge," in which 500 mg of penicillamine is administered orally once and again after 12 hours during the 24-hour urine collection. A more than 10-fold increase in copper excretion is highly suggestive of Wilson disease, though using a cutoff of basal urine copper excretion of 40 µg/24 hours is equally sensitive for detecting patients.

Percutaneous needle liver biopsy for quantitative measurement of hepatic copper remains a useful test for the diagnosis of Wilson disease. Hepatic copper values higher than 250 µg/g of dry weight (normal, 20 to 50 µg/g dry weight) are characteristic of Wilson disease, although rare patients may have levels as low as 75 µg/g dry weight liver. Copper quantitation by inductively coupled plasma mass spectrometry or by atomic absorption spectrometry on dried and digested specimens is preferred to paraffin-embedded specimens, although paraffin-embedded specimens may be used when the diagnosis is considered retrospectively and adequate tissue was obtained. Histochemical staining of a liver biopsy specimen for copper by rhodanine may suggest Wilson disease but is less reliable.

In summary, in the absence of formal molecular evidence, the diagnosis of Wilson disease should be considered when at least two of the following are present: a positive family history, Kayser-Fleischer rings, Coombs-negative hemolytic anemia, low serum copper and ceruloplasmin levels, elevated hepatic copper content, increased 24-hour urine copper excretion, or a positive penicillamine challenge result. Heterozygous carriers for Wilson disease do not require treatment.

TREATMENT Rx

d-Penicillamine binds copper and greatly enhances its urinary excretion, thereby preventing copper overload and its effects. Faithful compliance with oral penicillamine treatment has enabled the good health of thousands of patients with Wilson disease worldwide during the past 50 years.[15-17] Pyridoxine (vitamin B$_6$) should be prescribed concomitantly to counter the vitamin B$_6$ deficiency that may develop with long-term d-penicillamine administration.

About 20% of patients are intolerant of d-penicillamine. Significant side effects include hypersensitivity; nephrotoxicity; hematologic abnormalities; and a distinctive rash, elastosis perforans serpiginosa, that often involves the neck and axilla. Furthermore, in some patients with neurologic presentations, d-penicillamine treatment induces paradoxical worsening of the neurologic disease.

Even though d-penicillamine is the therapy with the longest experience, other pharmaceutical agents are available and may be considered for use as first-line drugs. For example, zinc acetate and triethylene tetramine dihydrochloride (trientine) are suitable alternative agents with somewhat less significant side-effect profiles.[18]

Oral zinc acetate also has proved highly effective as maintenance therapy in Wilson disease. The mechanism involves decreased copper absorption by the intestine into the blood stream by induction of the copper storage protein metallothionein in intestinal epithelial cells. Zinc monotherapy has particular value in young, presymptomatic patients and in patients who are pregnant, given the possible fetal teratogenic effects of other compounds. Whereas most patients do well with zinc therapy, 10 to 20% experience dyspepsia, and a higher incidence of hepatic decompensation has been observed with long-term zinc therapy compared with chelation therapy. Another drawback to zinc is the relatively long time (4 to 6 months) needed to restore proper copper balance if zinc monotherapy is used as initial treatment.

Tetrathiomolybdate (TTM) remains experimental for the treatment of Wilson disease, and there are ongoing clinical trials of a stabilized form of this compound. TTM forms stable tripartite complexes with albumin and copper and promotes biliary copper excretion. It is fast acting and can restore normal copper balance within several weeks, compared with the several months required with other copper chelators or with zinc. TTM may be especially appropriate for the initial treatment of patients with neurologic presentations on the basis of a completed phase 2 clinical trial.[A1]

Regardless of the specific regimen chosen, treatment of Wilson disease is lifelong. Noncompliance eventually leads to symptomatic disease or liver failure.

Liver transplantation for Wilson disease is curative, but should be considered only for patients with acute liver failure due to Wilson disease or those with end-stage liver disease with irreversible hepatic damage who are unlikely to respond to medical therapy. Long-term outcomes after transplantation for Wilson disease are excellent, and the disease does not recur in the transplanted organ.[19]

Apart from pharmacologic treatment, there are several other important considerations in the treatment of Wilson disease. These include dietary copper restriction, especially of shellfish, liver, and chocolate, which are copper rich.[20] The major sources of patients' drinking water should be tested for copper concentration and avoided if levels approach 1.3 mg/L, which is the current maximum contaminant level goal established by the U.S. Environmental Protection Agency.

In newly diagnosed patients with neurologic manifestations, there is frequently a need for speech therapy and physical or occupational therapy, and for others, psychological and genetic counseling.

PROGNOSIS

The prognosis in Wilson disease is generally favorable. Current therapeutic approaches can prevent, stabilize, or reverse most of the significant clinical signs and symptoms, including Kayser-Fleischer rings. However, if treatment is stopped, recurrence of symptoms and potentially fatal liver damage inevitably occur.

FUTURE DIRECTIONS

Treatment with methanobactin, a peptide that is produced by *Methylosinus trichosporium* OB3b and that has an exceptionally high affinity for copper, can deplete excess copper from hepatocytic mitochondria, as well as prevent subsequent hepatocyte death and liver failure in rats, but it has not been tested in humans.[21] Gene therapy for Wilson disease is also a possibility. Because the Wilson copper transporter is expressed most prominently and functions most critically in the liver, this organ could be specifically targeted by the use of adenoviral or adeno-associated viral vectors (e.g., AAV8). This has been accomplished in an animal model of Wilson disease, and human trials may proceed in the near future. Hepatocyte transplantation, an alternative to gene therapy, may also be applicable to the treatment of liver-specific metabolic disorders through therapeutic liver repopulation.

 Grade A Reference

A1. Weiss KH, Askari FH, Czlonkowska A, et al. Phase 2 study of WTX101 (bis-choline tetrathiomolybdate) in patients with Wilson disease. *Lancet.* 2017;2:869-876.

GENERAL REFERENCES

For the General References and other additional features, please visit Expert Consult at https://expertconsult.inkling.com.

201

IRON OVERLOAD (HEMOCHROMATOSIS)

KRIS V. KOWDLEY

DEFINITION

Iron overload disorders (Table 201-1) represent chronic conditions that result from excess iron accumulation in various tissues and organs, which may result in injury, fibrosis, and organ failure. The most common genetic disorder of iron overload is hereditary hemochromatosis.[1] Of note, hyperabsorption of dietary iron may result from other conditions, including chronic anemias associated with ineffective erythropoiesis (e.g., thalassemia; Chapter 153) or chronic hepatitis (Chapter 140).[2]

EPIDEMIOLOGY

Three common *HFE* mutations have been described, C282Y, H63D, and S65C. The allele carrier frequency of C282Y is greater than 10% among the general Irish population and 5 to 10% in other Northern European countries. Homozygosity for the C282Y mutation in the total U.S. population has been estimated to be 0.26%, whereas compound heterozygosity for C282Y/H63D occurs in approximately 2%. There are significant racial differences in the distribution of the C282Y mutation and therefore the overall prevalence of hereditary hemochromatosis. The prevalence of hereditary hemochromatosis is six times higher in whites than in African Americans. The prevalence of C282Y homozygotes is estimated to be significantly higher in non-Hispanic whites than in other populations such as Native Americans, Hispanics, African Americans, Pacific Islanders, or Asians.

PATHOBIOLOGY

Dietary iron absorption is regulated by body iron needs.[3,4] Under circumstances of iron deficiency, there is increased iron absorption until body iron stores are replete at which time iron absorption decreases to basal levels. Dietary iron is absorbed in the proximal duodenum either as inorganic iron or as heme iron as shown in Figure 201-1. Iron balance in humans is regulated primarily at the level of intestinal absorption, because the body does not have a mechanism for the excretion of iron other than through physiologic loss of desquamated cells or menses. Hepcidin is a 25-amino acid peptide that is synthesized mainly in the liver and secreted into the blood; it is considered to be the master hormone regulator of iron homeostasis.[5] It acts by blocking iron absorption from the intestine and blocking iron release from reticuloendothelial cell storage sites mainly within the liver. Inappropriately low levels of hepcidin are the cause of many iron overload disorders.[6] Primary iron overload disorders are caused by mutations in iron regulatory genes, the net effect

TABLE 201-1	CLASSIFICATION OF IRON OVERLOAD SYNDROMES

HEREDITARY HEMOCHROMATOSIS

HFE **Related**

C282Y/C282Y
C282Y/H63D
C282Y/S65C
Other mutations

Non–*HFE* Related

Hemojuvelin (*HJV*) mutations (autosomal recessive)
Hepcidin (*HAMP*) mutations (autosomal recessive)
Ferroportin (*SLC40A1*) mutations (autosomal dominant)
Transferrin receptor 2 (*TFR2*) mutations (autosomal recessive)
Divalent metal transporter 1 (*SLC11A2*) mutations (rare)
Ferritin regulatory mutations (rare)

Miscellaneous

African iron overload
Neonatal iron overload (rare)

SECONDARY IRON OVERLOAD

Anemia Caused by Ineffective Erythropoiesis

Thalassemia major
Sideroblastic anemias
Congenital dyserythropoietic anemias
Congenital atransferrinemia

Liver Disease

Alcoholic liver disease
Chronic viral hepatitis B and C
Porphyria cutanea tarda
Nonalcoholic steatohepatitis
After portacaval shunt

Miscellaneous

Transfusional iron overload
Excessive parenteral iron administration

From Bruce R. Bacon. Chapter 212. Iron overload (hemochromatosis). *Goldman-Cecil Medicine.* 25th ed. Philadelphia: Elsevier; 2016.

of which is lifelong hyperabsorption of dietary iron. Because the human body does not have a physiologic mechanism to excrete excess iron, progressive iron loading of various organs can eventually cause the characteristic forms of organ damage seen in advanced iron overload states.

Absorption of both forms of iron is increased in hereditary hemochromatosis. Absorption of inorganic iron follows a coordinated process beginning with conversion of iron from ferric to ferrous form by the duodenal cytochrome b–related ferric reductase (dcytb) that is present on the luminal surface of duodenal enterocytes. Ferrous iron then traverses the apical membrane of enterocytes via the divalent metallic transporter 1 (DMT1). The absorbed iron may be utilized for intracellular processes, stored as ferritin in enterocytes, or it can be converted back to ferric iron by hephaestin, thereby allowing it be transferred across the basolateral membrane of enterocytes into circulating plasma via the iron export protein, ferroportin. Iron is bound to transferrin at the transferrin receptor (TfR1) in the circulation. Parenchymal cells in the liver (hepatocytes) take up transferrin-bound iron via the receptors, TfR1, and possibly TfR2, as well as by non–receptor-mediated mechanisms. Hepatocytes may also absorb free iron found in the circulation when transferrin becomes highly saturated. In contrast, reticuloendothelial system (RES) cells (Kupffer cells in the liver) take up iron primarily by phagocytosis of senescent erythrocytes or possibly apoptotic hepatocytes. They can also sequester transferrin-bound iron via TfR1. Hepcidin, a circulating peptide is produced by hepatocytes in response to the status of body iron stores and regulates iron metabolism by reducing iron absorption via binding to ferroportin.[7] Ferroportin is then internalized and degraded, resulting in reduced iron export from enterocytes and reticuloendothelial cells, leading to decreased intestinal iron absorption. Mutations in the *HFE, TfR2,* and *HJV* genes result in markedly depressed hepcidin levels, thereby permitting persistently increased absorption of iron from a normal diet. Mutations in the *HAMP* (hepcidin) gene may likewise lead to inappropriately low levels of hepcidin, thereby resulting in iron overload. Parenchymal iron overload may also be caused by mutations in the ferroportin gene.

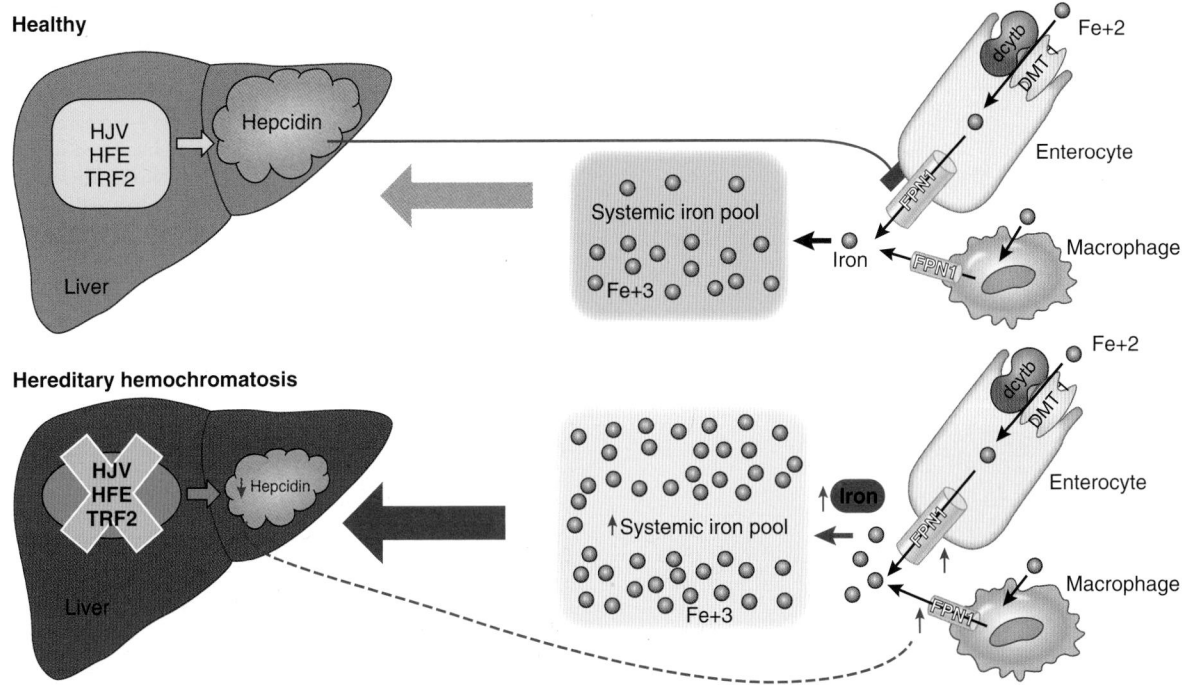

FIGURE 201-1. Regulation of iron homeostasis in healthy individuals and hereditary hemochromatosis individuals. Nonheme iron is reduced from ferric (Fe^{3+}) to ferrous (Fe^{2+}) iron by duodenal cytochrome b (Dcytb) that is present on the apical surface of enterocytes. Fe^{2+} is taken up into the cells via divalent metallic transporter 1 (DMT1). In healthy individuals, plasma transferrin saturation controls the expression of liver hepcidin through an *HFE*, *TFR2*, and *HJV* induced signaling pathway. Hepcidin is secreted into the blood, where it binds to ferroportin (FPN) on the enterocytes in the intestine and macrophages, inducing FPN internalization and degradation, reducing intestinal iron absorption, and recycling by macrophages to maintain plasma transferrin saturation. In individuals with mutations in *HFE*, *HJV* or *TFR2*, hepcidin synthesis is impaired, leading to reduced levels of hepcidin in the blood, in turn leading to increased FPN levels/activity and increased iron release from intestinal cells and macrophages, elevating plasma transferrin saturation and promoting the accumulation of iron in the liver and other tissues.

Approximately 85 to 90% of patients of white descent with phenotypic hemochromatosis are homozygous for the C282Y mutation in the *HFE* gene. In recent years, a greater understanding of iron biology and pathobiology has led to identification of several other genetic forms of hemochromatosis.[8,9] These other forms are rare but may be identified by distinct clinical presentations.

The new Online Mendelian Inheritance in Man (OMIM) classification of hereditary hemochromatosis now defines classical (*HFE* hemochromatosis) as type 1. Other types of hereditary hemochromatosis are now classified as type 2 to 4. Juvenile hemochromatosis, a severe form of hemochromatosis that is associated with severe iron overload presenting in the second to third decade of life, consists of type 2A and type 2B forms. Type 2A is caused by a mutation in the hemojuvelin (*HJV*) gene located on chromosome 1 encoding the hemojuvelin protein. Type 2B is caused by a mutation in the hepatic antimicrobial protein (*HAMP*) gene, which encodes hepcidin. Type 3 is due to a mutation in the transferrin receptor 2 (*TFR2*) gene that is located on the long arm of chromosome 7; *TFR2* is similar to *TFR1* but expressed predominantly in the liver and is now recognized to be involved in iron homeostasis. Type 4 is usually associated with a rare autosomal dominant mutation in the ferroportin (*SLC40A1*) gene encoding ferroportin protein, located on chromosome 2. Type 4 has also been called "ferroportin disease" because the clinical, biochemical, and histologic features are very different from other forms of hereditary hemochromatosis.

CLINICAL MANIFESTATIONS

Our understanding of the clinical features of hereditary hemochromatosis has evolved substantially from the original description of "bronze diabetes." Prior to the identification of the *HFE* gene, the disorder was identified by the phenotype of iron overload and occasionally in siblings of a proband by HLA A and B haplotyping. Subsequently, the C282Y homozygous mutation was found to be present in the majority of white patients expressing the hereditary hemochromatosis phenotype. It is now apparent that many patients carrying *HFE* mutations, whether they are heterozygous or homozygous, do not express the clinical phenotype of iron overload disease (Tables 201-2 and 201-3) or even biochemical evidence of iron overload (increased serum transferrin-iron saturation, ferritin). This finding indicates that the C282Y as well as the H63D mutations of the *HFE* gene have low penetrance.[10] It has been estimated that about 50% of female and 25% of male adults who are homozygous for the

TABLE 201-2 SYMPTOMS IN PATIENTS WITH HEREDITARY HEMOCHROMATOSIS

ASYMPTOMATIC

Abnormalities of serum iron studies on routine screening chemistry panel
Abnormal liver test results
Identified by family screening
Identified by population screening

NONSPECIFIC SYSTEMIC SYMPTOMS

Weakness
Fatigue
Lethargy
Apathy
Weight loss

SPECIFIC ORGAN-RELATED SYMPTOMS

Abdominal pain (hepatomegaly)
Arthralgias (arthritis)
Symptoms of diabetes mellitus (pancreas)
Amenorrhea (cirrhosis)
Loss of libido, impotence (pituitary, cirrhosis)
Congestive heart failure symptoms (heart)
Arrhythmias (heart)

From Bacon BR. Chapter 212. Iron overload (hemochromatosis). *Goldman-Cecil Medicine*. 25th ed. Philadelphia: Elsevier; 2016.

C282Y mutation have normal serum ferritin levels and will never require phlebotomy therapy.[11] Even those homozygotes who have modestly elevated ferritin levels do not necessarily progress to clinical iron overload. Based on these discoveries, hereditary hemochromatosis can be classified into three clinical stages, as shown below:

- Stage 1: genetic predisposition for hereditary hemochromatosis without evidence for increase in iron stores (normal serum iron studies)
- Stage 2: genetic predisposition for hereditary hemochromatosis and some phenotypic characteristics of iron overload in the absence of organ damage
- Stage 3: genetic predisposition for hereditary hemochromatosis accompanied by evidence for iron overload with tissue injury or organ damage

TABLE 201-3	PHYSICAL FINDINGS IN PATIENTS WITH HEREDITARY HEMOCHROMATOSIS

ASYMPTOMATIC

No physical findings
Hepatomegaly

SYMPTOMATIC

Liver

Hepatomegaly
Cutaneous stigmata of chronic liver disease
Splenomegaly
Signs of liver failure: ascites, encephalopathy

Joints

Arthritis
Joint swelling

Heart

Dilated cardiomyopathy
Congestive heart failure

Skin

Increased pigmentation

Endocrine

Testicular atrophy
Hypogonadism
Hypothyroidism

From Bacon BR. Chapter 212. Iron overload (hemochromatosis). *Goldman-Cecil Medicine.* 25th ed. Philadelphia: Elsevier; 2016.

Symptoms and Signs Associated with Hereditary Hemochromatosis

Arthropathy

Arthropathy occurs in 20 to 60% of patients with hereditary hemochromatosis.[12] The second and third metacarpophalangeal joints and knees are most commonly involved but other joints may be affected, causing a mono- or polyarticular arthritis. The axial skeleton can be involved with associated deformities. The mechanism is believed to be deposition of calcium pyrophosphate crystals in joint spaces, leading to inflammation, joint space narrowing, chondrocalcinosis, subchondral cyst formation, and osteopenia. The features of hereditary hemochromatosis-associated arthritis may overlap with those of osteoarthritis and calcium pyrophosphate deposition disease. The classic physical sign is "pain on handshake," reflecting inflammatory changes of the second and third metacarpophalangeal joints. Plain radiography can differentiate hereditary hemochromatosis-associated arthritis from calcium pyrophosphate deposition disease by the finding of specific involvement of the second and third metacarpophalangeal joints and "hook-shaped" osteophytes of the metacarpal heads. Unfortunately, iron depletion by phlebotomy does not reliably improve joint symptoms and patients should be advised as to such.

Fatigue

Fatigue is a nonspecific symptom but may affect up to 60% of hereditary hemochromatosis patients. Hereditary hemochromatosis patients were shown to be significantly more likely to report fatigue compared to coworkers in one study. Fatigue may improve with iron depletion.

Liver Disease

The liver as a major storage site for iron is always involved in patients with significant iron overload in hereditary hemochromatosis, and liver disease is the most common cause of mortality in *HFE*-associated hereditary hemochromatosis.[13] Hepatomegaly is frequently present and may be asymptomatic or be associated with right upper quadrant pain from distension of the liver capsule. Progressive iron accumulation in the liver can lead to hepatic fibrosis and cirrhosis. Advanced fibrosis and even cirrhosis may occur in the absence of inflammation; therefore serum aminotransferase levels are not useful to identify patients with advanced hepatic fibrosis. The presence of coincidental liver disease, particularly steatohepatitis (alcoholic or nonalcoholic) and chronic hepatitis C, may increase the level of hepatic iron overload and the likelihood of cirrhosis in patients with hereditary hemochromatosis. Patients with cirrhosis have a significantly increased risk of hepatocellular carcinoma, especially

in the presence of another coexisting form of liver disease. Hepatocellular carcinoma may develop in hereditary hemochromatosis patients in the absence of cirrhosis, but in the great majority hepatocellular carcinoma develops with underlying cirrhosis. Patients with advanced liver disease from another cause, particularly hepatitis C and alcohol, may have increased serum-transferrin saturation and ferritin levels, in addition to increased hepatic iron content even in the absence of hereditary hemochromatosis. Therefore, *HFE* genotyping is necessary to establish the diagnosis in this setting, although genetic testing will not be helpful in patients with non-HFE hereditary hemochromatosis (types 2 to 4).

Heart Disease

Cardiac manifestations of hereditary hemochromatosis are uncommon but they are the second leading cause of disease-related death. Cardiac iron overload in hereditary hemochromatosis is associated with conduction defects which may lead to arrhythmias or heart block. Patients may initially present with exertional dyspnea due to diastolic dysfunction that creates restrictive hemodynamics and elevated filling pressures. Manifestations of dilated cardiomyopathy and left ventricular systolic dysfunction occur later.[14]

Diabetes Mellitus

The relationship between diabetes mellitus and hereditary hemochromatosis has been best studied in type 1 hereditary hemochromatosis. The prevalence has been estimated at approximately 13 to 23% but reported to be higher in juvenile hereditary hemochromatosis (type 2) and possibly type 4. The putative mechanisms include direct damage to pancreatic beta cells by iron with some component of insulin resistance in the liver due to the organ's iron loading.[15]

Hypogonadism and Thyroid Disease

Hypogonadotropic hypogonadism in hereditary hemochromatosis is due to iron deposition in the anterior pituitary. It is the second most common endocrine complication of hereditary hemochromatosis after diabetes mellitus. It is a predominant feature of juvenile hereditary hemochromatosis (type 2). Clinical manifestations in men include loss of libido, impotence, and early osteoporosis. Amenorrhea, loss of libido, or premature menopause is seen in women. The prevalence of hypothyroidism is 80 times higher in hereditary hemochromatosis than in the general population.

Skin Pigmentation

Hyperpigmentation of the skin in hereditary hemochromatosis is mostly due to primary adrenal insufficiency which leads to increased melanin production that results in the characteristic metallic or slate gray hue commonly referred to as bronzing. It is most pronounced in the face, neck, and extremities. Increased pigmentation of the hard palate and retina has also been reported, as well as epidermal and dermal atrophy.

Infection and Immunity

Iron overload is associated with reduced function in immune cells. It is also associated with altered regulation of CD8 T lymphocytes from both *HFE* patients and *Hfe* null mice. Siderophilic microbes grow rapidly in niches where iron is more available, and these organisms may cause severe infections in patients with iron overload.[16] Possibly as a result, the risk of infections with *Listeria monocytogenes, Yersinia enterocolitica, Aeromonas hydrophila, Cunninghamella bertholletiae,* and *Vibrio vulnificus* is increased in hereditary hemochromatosis.

DIAGNOSIS

The widespread availability of mutation analysis for the common mutations in HFE has revolutionized the diagnosis of hereditary hemochromatosis.[17] Genetic testing for *HFE* mutations has eliminated the need for phenotype-based tests such as liver biopsy to confirm the diagnosis. However, it is important to remember that clinical genetic testing is limited to the C282Y, H63D, and S65C mutations. In addition, because the C282Y mutation is present primarily in white populations, *HFE* gene testing is less likely to be positive in persons of non-white descent. Furthermore, patients who are not C282Y homozygous are more likely to have an additional explanation for hepatic iron overload compared to C282Y homozygotes. One study of 182 U.S. patients with phenotypic hereditary hemochromatosis showed that patients with the C282Y/H63D compound heterozygous mutation and other *HFE* genotypes were more likely to have portal or lobular inflammation and steatosis on liver biopsy than C282Y homozygotes, suggesting that patients with *HFE* genotypes should be evaluated for the presence of concomitant liver disease such as hepatitis or fatty liver disease.

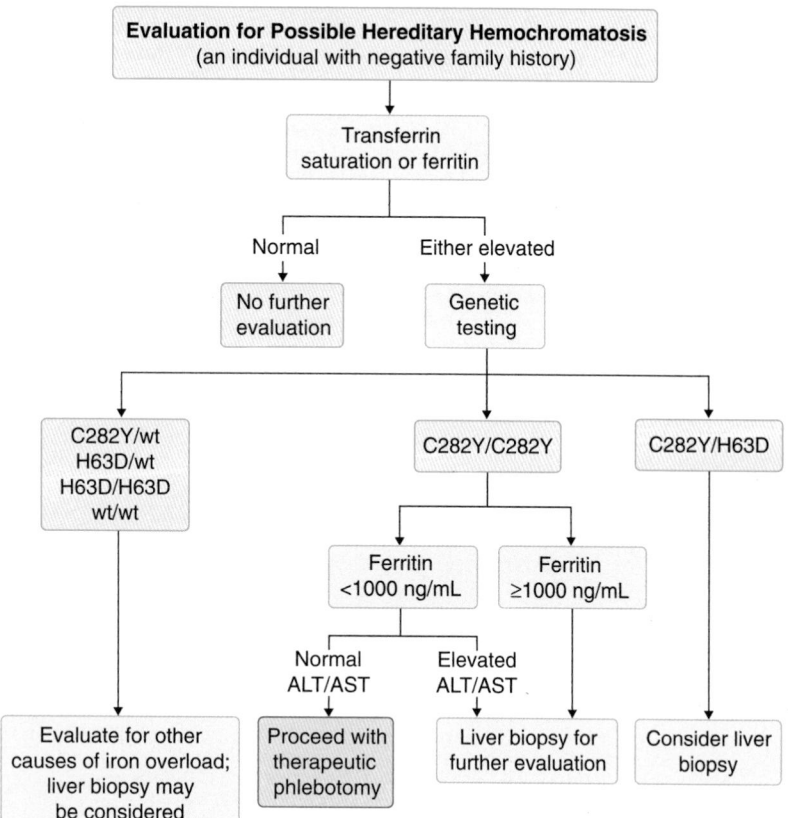

FIGURE 201-2. Proposed algorithm for diagnosis and management of hereditary hemochromatosis. ALT = alanine aminotransferase; AST = aspartate aminotransferase; wt = wild-type (normal).

Screening of first-degree relatives of patients with genotypically confirmed hereditary hemochromatosis is indicated. In addition to *HFE* mutation analysis, measurement of transferrin saturation and ferritin should be part of the basic screening. Relatives of patients with *HFE*-related hereditary hemochromatosis who are negative for *HFE* mutations do not require further testing, whereas those who are positive should be monitored annually for serum ferritin levels, and phlebotomy should be started if and when clinical iron overload appears.

An algorithm for evaluation of patients with suspected iron overload is shown in Figure 201-2. The initial screening test for hereditary hemochromatosis should include serum iron (Fe), total iron binding capacity (TIBC), calculation of transferrin-iron saturation (Fe/TIBC×100), and serum ferritin.[18] A transferrin-iron saturation greater than 45% should prompt further evaluation, which should include *HFE* gene testing and serum ferritin measurement. Patients found to be C282Y homozygous can be confirmed to have hereditary hemochromatosis.

The next step is to assess the degree of hepatic iron overload, the possibility of advanced hepatic fibrosis, and extrahepatic manifestations. Additional measures to evaluate the degree of hepatic fibrosis include serum hyaluronic acid levels, transient elastography or magnetic resonance elastography.[19] Patients with a serum ferritin over 1000 ng/mL have up to a 40% risk of advanced hepatic fibrosis or cirrhosis and should be evaluated for advanced hepatic fibrosis. Magnetic resonance (MR) imaging (T2*-weighted) is the most sensitive and specific imaging modality that is readily available in major medical centers for the diagnosis and quantitation of iron overload in patients with hereditary hemochromatosis. Liver biopsy has been the gold standard for confirming the diagnosis of hereditary hemochromatosis and for the biochemical measurement of hepatic iron concentration (HIC) and calculation of the hepatic iron index (HII), as well as determining the degree of hepatic fibrosis. Liver biopsy can establish the phenotypic diagnosis of hereditary hemochromatosis when *HFE* genotyping is negative. For secondary iron overload (e.g., transfusional iron overload), the pattern of iron distribution within the liver is similar to that observed in type 4 hereditary hemochromatosis, with iron deposition primarily localized in Kupffer RES cells, a scarcity of iron in hepatocytes, and the lack of a periportal to pericentral iron gradient.

Noninvasive methods have gained popularity in recent years to evaluate for advanced hepatic fibrosis and may be considered especially when the diagnosis of hereditary hemochromatosis has been confirmed by *HFE* genotyping. These include serum-based markers as well as transient elastography and MR elastography. Serum-based biomarkers for fibrosis include the European Liver Fibrosis Group score and hyaluronic acid. Vibration-controlled transient elastography is a noninvasive and rapid procedure for detecting hepatic fibrosis by measuring liver stiffness.

In patients with clinical or laboratory evidence of iron overload who do not have a mutation of the *HFE* gene that is associated with classical (type 1) hereditary hemochromatosis, one of the non-*HFE* forms of hereditary hemochromatosis should be considered. Phenotypic analysis of hereditary hemochromatosis caused by one of the 70 different mutations identified to date in the *HJV*, *HAMP*, and *TFR2* genotypes has shown that these patients have an earlier age of onset and a more severe clinical course than *HFE* hereditary hemochromatosis with cardiomyopathy and hypogonadism being particularly prevalent.[20]

TREATMENT   Rx

The cornerstone of therapy of hereditary hemochromatosis has been therapeutic phlebotomy, with removal of one unit of blood at regular intervals, with a goal to reduce serum ferritin to less than 100 ng/mL.[21] Each unit of whole blood (450 to 500 mL) contains about 200 to 250 mg of iron. Most patients tolerate frequent phlebotomies (weekly or biweekly) until they have depleted their total body iron stores. Erythrocytapheresis selectively removes red cells and is more efficient and leads to faster iron depletion than simple phlebotomy, but it requires apheresis equipment and expertise. It is important to monitor serum ferritin levels and hemoglobin levels during treatment because the rate of iron mobilization may vary among patients.[22] Although there is little controversy about the need to institute phlebotomy therapy in patients with hereditary hemochromatosis who have serum ferritin levels greater than 1000 ng/mL, some had advocated "watchful waiting" for those with only modest hyperferritinemia. However, a participant-blinded, randomized controlled trial of erythrocytapheresis versus sham treatment with plasmapheresis in hereditary hemochromatosis patients with moderately elevated serum ferritin levels (300 to 1000 ng/mL) and raised TF saturation found that iron depletion leads to significant improvement in quality of life as measured by (blinded) patient-reported Modified Fatigue Impact Scale scores.[A1]

Hemoglobin levels are routinely checked before each phlebotomy, and phlebotomy is suspended or the schedule is modified if it has dropped to less than 11 g/dL. After reaching the target serum ferritin level of 50 to 100 ng/mL, maintenance phlebotomy is instituted (every 2 to 4 months) because of ongoing hyperabsorption and reaccumulation of iron.[23] Additional therapeutic options include oral or parenteral iron chelators, which may be indicated in patients with iron overload and anemia who are unable to undergo therapeutic phlebotomy.[24] Recent studies suggest that proton pump inhibitors (PPI) may reduce iron absorption and phlebotomy requirements,[A2] although therapeutic administration of PPIs for this purpose is not currently recommended. The future development of hepcidin agonists holds promise.

Liver transplantation has been performed for end-stage liver disease or hepatocellular carcinoma due to hereditary hemochromatosis. There are data to suggest that patients with hereditary hemochromatosis may be at increased risk of infectious or cardiac complications after liver transplantation, and careful attention to degree of cardiac iron overload and attempts at iron depletion prior to liver transplantation should be attempted.

Grade A References

A1. Ong SY, Gurrin LC, Dolling L, et al. Reduction of body iron in HFE-related haemochromatosis and moderate iron overload (Mi-Iron): a multicentre, participant-blinded, randomised controlled trial. *Lancet Haematol.* 2017;4:e607-e614.

A2. Vanclooster A, van Deursen C, Jaspers R, et al. Proton pump inhibitors decrease phlebotomy need in HFE hemochromatosis: double-blind randomized placebo-controlled trial. *Gastroenterology.* 2017;153:678-680.

GENERAL REFERENCES

For the General References and other additional features, please visit Expert Consult at https://expertconsult.inkling.com.

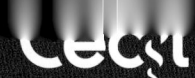

XVIII

NUTRITIONAL DISEASES

202

NUTRITION'S INTERFACE WITH HEALTH AND DISEASE

DONALD D. HENSRUD AND DOUGLAS C. HEIMBURGER

OLD AND NEW PARADIGMS IN THE SCIENCE OF NUTRITION

Nutrition science was characterized by two major phases in the 20th century. During the first phase, nutrition scientists discovered, characterized, and synthesized the essential nutrients and described their deficiency syndromes in detail. The dietary requirements for these nutrients were estimated and periodically updated as recommended dietary allowances (RDAs). The RDAs are the average daily level of intake sufficient to meet the nutrient requirements of nearly all (97 to 98%) healthy people. Beginning in 1997, the RDAs were reformulated in a series of volumes containing dietary reference intakes (DRIs). In addition to the RDAs, the DRIs include adequate intakes (AIs), which are determined when there is inadequate information to determine an RDA, and tolerable upper intake levels (ULs), which are the highest intake levels likely not to pose any adverse health risks.

More fundamentally, the DRIs take into consideration the accumulating evidence on the relationships of diet and nutritional status to chronic diseases, such as coronary heart disease (CHD), cancer, diabetes, and the other leading causes of death.[1] DRIs recommend intake levels that not only prevent deficiencies but also may promote long-term health and disease prevention.

Along with this, diet and nutrition research and dietary guidelines have expanded from focusing on preventing deficiencies through isolated nutrients to chronic disease prevention and dietary patterns that can help accomplish this. The importance of this is underscored by the facts that about one half of all adult Americans have one or more preventable chronic diseases, and two thirds of adults and one third of children are overweight or obese. The 2015-2020 Dietary Guidelines for Americans reflect these changes to prevention of chronic diseases through healthy dietary patterns.

NUTRITION'S INFLUENCE ON MORTALITY AND MORBIDITY

Evidence of Connections Between Diet and Disease

Deficiency conditions of specific nutrients have been well documented. Establishing conclusive relationships between diet and chronic diseases can be much more difficult. In vitro and animal studies may have limited relevance to humans. Epidemiologic studies are susceptible to unrecognized confounding variables and cannot infer causality. Difficulties isolating nutritional variables make randomized controlled trials connecting dietary factors and chronic diseases challenging to perform. Subjecting people to a dietary intervention to prevent a specific cancer, for example, is not feasible because of the time, cost, and behavior change involved.

However, when considering the totality of evidence, relationships have emerged. In some cases, large population studies have reported consistent results that have been further supported through meta-analyses. Randomized controlled trials conducted in at-risk individuals have reported even stronger findings. Although controversies remain in some specific areas, characteristics of dietary patterns that promote optimal health are more apparent now than ever. Further research should continue to build on this body of evidence in an evolutionary manner but will not likely replace it with revolutionary new claims.

Diet should not be considered in isolation because other lifestyle factors also influence the risk of chronic diseases. The greatest nutritional public health problems in the United States and in many other parts of the world are overweight and obesity and their associated comorbidities. Body weight is ultimately determined by the balance between energy intake through diet and energy expenditure through physical activity. Health promotion and disease prevention recommendations must include diet, physical activity, and other lifestyle factors.

Diseases Influenced by Nutrition

Table 202-1 lists the 10 leading causes of death in the United States.[2] Six of the top causes of death are related to diet, four to excess alcohol use, and six to obesity. The table also lists other major medical conditions that are associated with diet and nutrition. Table 202-2 summarizes the 2015-2020 Dietary Guidelines for Americans. It should be noted that the primary audiences for the Dietary Guidelines are policymakers, as well as nutrition and health professionals, not the general public. The Dietary Guidelines are a critical tool for professionals to help Americans make healthy choices. Table 202-3 compares dietary recommendations promulgated by professional societies for risk reduction and/or management of the major chronic diseases. The close agreement among these recommendations enhances their credibility.

Coronary Heart Disease

Nutritional influences on the leading cause of death in the United States, CHD, have been the subject of a great deal of research. Of the seven major risk factors for CHD, four are related to diet: hypercholesterolemia, hypertension, obesity, and diabetes. Elevated plasma low-density lipoprotein (LDL) cholesterol is a strong risk factor for CHD and is raised by increasing consumption of dietary saturated fat and *trans* fat. *Trans* fat also lowers high-density lipoprotein (HDL) cholesterol. Saturated fat is found in meat, full-fat dairy products, and tropical oils. *Trans* fat comes almost entirely from partially hydrogenated oils and has no health benefits, which led the U.S. Food and Drug Administration to require food manufacturers to remove these fats from processed foods by June 2018. Less emphasis is being placed on limiting dietary cholesterol in recent guidelines because dietary cholesterol has a lesser effect on LDL cholesterol than saturated fat and is often found in the same foods. Limiting foods that contain saturated fat also limits dietary cholesterol. LDL cholesterol levels can be lowered by substituting healthier unsaturated fats (polyunsaturated or monounsaturated oils) or carbohydrates (preferably whole grains) for saturated fat. LDL cholesterol can also be lowered modestly by increasing the intake of soluble fiber and phytosterols from legumes, fruits, vegetables, and flax seed, as well as by consuming proteins and isoflavones from soy foods.

In recent decades, it has become clear that diet may influence the risk of CHD through many different mechanisms independent of LDL cholesterol and traditional risk factors, such as inflammation, oxidative stress, endothelial function, insulin sensitivity, and others.[3,4] However, identifying and characterizing the precise mechanisms are not necessary when certain foods and dietary patterns have demonstrated consistent evidence in influencing the risk of CHD. Good evidence from meta-analyses of large cohort studies has shown decreased cardiovascular and total mortality with increasing consumption of fruits and vegetables,[5] whole grains,[6] and nuts and decreased incident CHD and total mortality from fish and olive oil.[7,8] Randomized trials are generally consistent with cohort studies, and a Mediterranean dietary pattern composed of many of these food groups has produced favorable effects on cardiovascular risk factors.[A1] The Prevención con Dieta Mediterránea (PREDIMED) trial conducted in Spain randomized subjects at high risk of heart disease to a control diet versus a Mediterranean diet supplemented with either olive oil or nuts.[A2] Subjects following both of the supplemented diets experienced 30% less cardiovascular disease (CVD) than did those on the control diet. The Optimal Macronutrient Intake Trial for Heart Health (OmniHeart) diet built on the groundwork of the Dietary Approaches to Stop Hypertension (DASH) diet (see Hypertension) and compared three different diets in a randomized trial with a common core built around the DASH diet: higher carbohydrate (similar to DASH), higher unsaturated fat, and higher protein. The higher-carbohydrate diet lowered the risk of CHD in men by 20%, whereas the higher–unsaturated fat and higher-protein diets reduced the risk by 30%. The prognostic nutritional index (PNI), a well-accepted parameter of nutritional status, calculated based on serum albumin level and lymphocyte count, has been found to be an independent prognostic factor for mortality in patients undergoing coronary artery bypass graft (CABG) surgery.[9]

Moderate consumption of alcohol, defined as no more than one drink daily for women and two for men, has been associated with reduced risk of CHD, primarily by raising HDL cholesterol, inhibiting platelet aggregation, and stimulating fibrinolytic activity. Data from the National Health and Nutrition Examination Survey (NHANES) reported that added sugar was associated with increased CVD mortality. In addition, consumption of red and particularly processed meat has been associated with increased CVD and total mortality.[10]

Cancer

It has been consistently estimated that one third of cancers are due to suboptimal habits in diet, physical activity, and weight management. Because cancer consists of many different conditions that share a common feature of uncontrolled abnormal cell division, risk factors, including diet, vary among different types of cancer. Nutrients, non-nutritive dietary constituents, and nutritional status can influence the risk for cancer through many different mechanisms such as free radical scavenging and DNA repair. Supplementation with individual nutrients has had limited success in preventing and treating cancer. Therefore, as with heart disease, a focus on foods and dietary patterns provides the best nutritional approach to preventing cancer. Over the past couple of decades, obesity has emerged as a major risk factor for at least 11 cancers, perhaps by elevating serum levels of insulin and leptin, inducing insulin resistance, and creating a chronic inflammatory state (Chapter 169). Excess alcohol intake also increases the risk for many cancers, including liver, breast, and the entire gastrointestinal tract. The World Cancer Research Fund International has conducted an extensive review of diet and lifestyle risk factors for various cancers and continues to update the literature on an ongoing basis.[11]

Lung Cancer

Although the most important causal factor in the number one cancer killer, lung cancer (Chapter 182), is cigarette smoking, consumption of fruit is inversely associated with lung cancer risk in both smokers and nonsmokers. Two large, randomized trials of supplementation with β-carotene reported increased mortality from lung cancer and all causes, primarily in smokers and former smokers, so β-carotene supplementation should be avoided.

Breast Cancer

The number two cause of cancer deaths in women is breast cancer (Chapter 188). Postmenopausal breast cancer is positively associated with obesity, especially when excess adiposity is located predominantly in the abdomen. Paradoxically, the risk of premenopausal breast cancer is decreased with obesity. Alcohol increases and lactation probably decreases the risk of both types of breast cancer.

Colorectal Cancer

Colorectal cancer (Chapter 184) is the third leading cause of cancer mortality in men and women. The risk for colorectal cancer correlates positively with the intake of red and processed meats, obesity, and alcohol. The World Health Organization has classified processed meat as a carcinogen and red meat as a probable carcinogen based on an International Agency for Research on Cancer monograph on this topic.[12] Foods that contain dietary fiber (as opposed to fiber per se), dairy products, and calcium decrease risk.[13]

Prostate Cancer

Although studies have evaluated different dietary factors on the risk of prostate cancer, the clearest risk factor is obesity.

Liver Cancer

The strongest risk factor for liver cancer is alcohol; obesity also increases risk. Aflatoxins are a strong risk factor, primarily outside the United States where they are more prevalent in the food supply. Coffee is protective against liver cancer.

TABLE 202-1	MAJOR CAUSES OF DEATH (2017) AND MORBIDITY IN THE UNITED STATES RELATED TO DIETARY FACTORS		
CAUSE OF DEATH		**NUMBER**	**%**
1. Heart disease*†		647,000	23
2. Cancer*†‡		599,000	21
3. Accidents†		169,000	6
4. Chronic lower respiratory diseases†		160,000	6
5. Cerebrovascular diseases*†‡		146,000	5
6. Alzheimer*†		121,000	4
7. Diabetes mellitus*†		84,000	3
8. Pneumonia/influenza		56,000	2
9. Kidney disease*		51,000	2
10. Suicide‡		47,000	2
MORBIDITY			
1. Obesity			
2. Chronic liver disease and cirrhosis			
3. Hypertension			
4. Diverticular disease and constipation			
5. Osteoporosis			

*Related to diet.
†Related to obesity.
‡Related to excess alcohol use.

TABLE 202-2	DIETARY GUIDELINES FOR AMERICANS, 2015-2020 AND KEY RECOMMENDATIONS

DIETARY GUIDELINES

1. Follow a healthy eating pattern across the lifespan.
2. Focus on variety, nutrient density, and amount.
3. Limit calories from added sugars and saturated fats and reduce sodium intake.
4. Shift to healthier food and beverage choices.
5. Support healthy eating patterns for all.

KEY RECOMMENDATIONS

Consume a healthy eating pattern that accounts for all foods and beverages within an appropriate calorie level.
A healthy eating pattern includes:
- A variety of vegetables from all the subgroups—dark green, red and orange, legumes (beans and peas), starchy, and other
- Fruits, especially whole fruits
- Grains, at least half of which are whole grains
- Fat-free or low-fat dairy, including milk, yogurt, cheese, and/or fortified soy beverages
- A variety of protein foods, including seafood, lean meats and poultry, eggs, legumes (beans and peas), and nuts, seeds, and soy products
- Oils

A healthy eating pattern limits:
- Saturated fats and *trans* fats, added sugars, and sodium

Key Recommendations that are quantitative are provided for several components of the diet that should be limited. These components are of particular public health concern in the United States, and the specified limits can help individuals achieve healthy eating patterns within calorie limits:
- Consume less than 10% of calories per day from added sugars.
- Consume less than 10% of calories per day from saturated fats.
- Consume less than 2300 mg per day of sodium.
- If alcohol is consumed, it should be consumed in moderation—up to one drink per day for women and up to two drinks per day for men—and only by adults of legal drinking age.

In tandem with the recommendations above, Americans of all ages—children, adolescents, adults, and older adults—should meet the Physical Activity Guidelines for Americans to help promote health and reduce the risk of chronic disease. Americans should aim to achieve and maintain a healthy body weight. The relationship between diet and physical activity contributes to calorie balance and managing body weight. As such, the Dietary Guidelines include a Key Recommendation to:
- Meet the Physical Activity Guidelines for Americans

TABLE 202-3 DIETARY GUIDELINES PROMULGATED BY NATIONAL ORGANIZATIONS*

Indication or Objective	U.S. DEPARTMENT OF AGRICULTURE AND DEPARTMENT OF HEALTH AND HUMAN SERVICES: DIETARY GUIDELINES FOR AMERICANS (2015-2020) *General Health Promotion and Disease Prevention*	AMERICAN HEART ASSOCIATION (2013 AND 2016) *Heart Disease Prevention*	AMERICAN CANCER SOCIETY (2012) *Cancer Prevention*	NATIONAL HIGH BLOOD PRESSURE EDUCATION PROGRAM/ JOINT NATIONAL COMMITTEE: 7 DIETARY APPROACHES TO STOP HYPERTENSION (DASH; 2006) *Prehypertension and Hypertension (2000-calorie level)*	AMERICAN DIABETES ASSOCIATION (2014 AND 2017) *Diabetes Prevention and Treatment*
NUTRIENT/FOOD GROUP					
Total energy	Achieve and maintain a healthy body weight	Achieve and maintain a healthy weight	Achieve and maintain a healthy weight throughout life. Choose foods and beverages in amounts that help achieve and maintain a healthy weight	Reduce energy intake to lose weight if overweight	Modest weight loss achievable by the combination of reduction of calorie intake and lifestyle modification in overweight and obese adults with type 2 diabetes and prediabetes
Fruits and vegetables	Include 2 c fruits, especially whole fruits, and 2½ c of a variety of vegetables from all the subgroups daily	Emphasize vegetables and fruits	Consume a healthy diet, with an emphasis on plant foods. Eat at least 2.5 cups of vegetables and fruits each day	4-5 servings/day of vegetables and 4-5 servings/day of fruit	
Meat	Choose a variety of protein foods, including 5½ oz-equivalents of seafood, lean meat and poultry, eggs, legumes (beans and peas), and nuts, seeds, and soy products	Limit red meat, use lean sources	Limit consumption of processed and red meats	≤6 oz/day lean meat, poultry, or fish	
Dairy	3 c-equivalents daily of fat-free or low-fat dairy including milk, yogurt, cheese, and/or fortified soy beverages	Include fat-free and low-fat dairy products		2-3 servings/day of fat-free or low-fat dairy	
Grains, fiber	Consume 6 oz-equivalents daily with at least half as whole grains.	Emphasize whole grains, 28-30 g/day fiber	Choose whole grains instead of refined grain products	6-8 servings/day of whole grains and whole-grain products, 30 g/day fiber	Achieve U.S. Dietary Guidelines recommendation
Fat	Include 27 g daily of PUFA and MUFA oils Limit saturated fats and *trans* fats		The totality of the evidence does not support a relationship between total fat intake and cancer risk	27% of calories	Individualize the mix of carbohydrate, protein, and fat
Saturated fats	<10% of daily calories, by replacing them with MUFA and PUFA	Limit to 5-6% of calories		6% of calories	Achieve U.S. Dietary Guidelines recommendation
Polyunsaturated fats	Replace solid fats with PUFA	Include nontropical vegetable oils			
Monounsaturated fats	Replace solid fats with MUFA				Emphasize in a Mediterranean style diet
Trans-fats	Keep as low as possible	Avoid			Avoid
Cholesterol				150 mg/day	
Carbohydrates				55% of calories	Replace refined carbohydrates and added sugars with whole grains, legumes, vegetables, and fruits. Individualize the mix of carbohydrate, protein, and fat
Sugar	<10% of calories	Limit added sugars to no more than 100 calories/day for women and 150 calories/day for men	Limit sugar-sweetened beverages and high-sugar foods	≤5 servings/week	Persons with or at risk for type 2 diabetes should avoid sugar-sweetened beverages and minimize added sugars
Protein	Choose a variety of protein foods, which include eggs, beans and peas, soy products, and unsalted nuts and seeds (for more, see Meat)	Include fish, poultry, nuts, and beans		18% of calories from lean meats, poultry, fish, and 4-5 servings/week of nuts, seeds, beans, and peas	Individualize the mix of carbohydrate, protein, and fat. Select lean protein sources

TABLE 202-3 DIETARY GUIDELINES PROMULGATED BY NATIONAL ORGANIZATIONS—cont'd

Indication or Objective	U.S. DEPARTMENT OF AGRICULTURE AND DEPARTMENT OF HEALTH AND HUMAN SERVICES: DIETARY GUIDELINES FOR AMERICANS (2015-2020) *General Health Promotion and Disease Prevention*	AMERICAN HEART ASSOCIATION (2013 AND 2016) *Heart Disease Prevention*	AMERICAN CANCER SOCIETY (2012) *Cancer Prevention*	NATIONAL HIGH BLOOD PRESSURE EDUCATION PROGRAM/ JOINT NATIONAL COMMITTEE: 7 DIETARY APPROACHES TO STOP HYPERTENSION (DASH; 2006) *Prehypertension and Hypertension (2000-calorie level)*	AMERICAN DIABETES ASSOCIATION (2014 AND 2017) *Diabetes Prevention and Treatment*
Alcohol	Up to 2 drinks/day for men and up to 1 drink/day for women; persons in special circumstances (e.g., pregnancy, history of alcoholism) should abstain	If you drink alcohol, do so in moderation. No more than 1 drink/day for women and 2 drinks/day for men	No more than 1 drink/day for women and 2 drinks/day for men	<2 drinks/day for men and <1 drink/day for women	If individuals with type 2 diabetes choose to drink, limit to 2 drinks/day for men and 1 drink/day for women, and take extra precautions to prevent hypoglycemia
Sodium	Reduce daily sodium intake to less than 2300 mg, and further reduce intake to 1500 mg among persons who have prehypertension or hypertension	Consume no more than 2300 mg/day of sodium; further reduction of sodium intake to 1500 mg/day is desirable		1500-2300 mg/day	<2300 mg/day
Potassium				4700 mg/day	

*For further details, see the websites listed in this chapter.
c = cups; LDL = low-density lipoprotein; MUFA = monounsaturated fatty acid; PUFA = polyunsaturated fatty acid.
Adapted from Heimburger DC, Ard JD, eds. *Handbook of Clinical Nutrition*, 4th ed. Philadelphia: Elsevier; 2006.

Pancreas Cancer
Associations exist between pancreas cancer and various dietary factors, but causality is not clear except for obesity, which increases risk.

Summary
Although there are differences among dietary risks for different cancers, the American Cancer Society Guidelines for Cancer Prevention are generally similar to other major dietary guidelines: consuming a plant-based diet, regular physical activity, and maintenance of a healthy body weight. Alcohol intake is the primary difference between guidelines to prevent heart disease, in which moderate consumption is beneficial, and guidelines to prevent cancer, in which consumption even at low levels for some cancers, such as breast, increases risk. Randomized trials with isolated nutrients including carotenoids,[A3] vitamins C and E,[A4] folic acid,[A5] selenium,[A6] and fiber[A7] have not shown benefit on cancer risk. Whole plant foods contain hundreds of different vitamins, nutrients, and other phytochemicals that may collectively reduce the risk of cancer more than specific nutrients.

Hypertension
Elevated blood pressure (Chapter 70) is a major risk factor for stroke, CHD, heart failure, peripheral vascular disease, and renal disease. There are five lifestyle factors that reduce blood pressure: weight loss if overweight or obese, the Dietary Approaches to Stop Hypertension (DASH) diet, increased physical activity, sodium restriction, and alcohol restriction. Obesity, especially abdominal obesity, is associated with hypertension, and weight reduction is the strongest lifestyle change that decreases blood pressure. The DASH diet is a plant-based diet that has been studied extensively, originally for its effect on blood pressure, where it lowered blood pressure as much as drug treatment (11.6/5.3 mm Hg), in people with hypertension.[A8] The DASH-sodium trial found that sodium restriction provided additional benefit when added to the DASH diet.

Diabetes Mellitus
Type 2 diabetes mellitus (Chapter 216) is strongly associated with obesity, especially abdominal obesity, so maintenance of a desirable body weight throughout life is of major importance in both preventing and treating type 2 diabetes. Sugar consumption does not lead to diabetes, except to the extent that it may promote weight gain. However, there is evidence that sugar-sweetened beverages contribute to weight gain and increased

risk of type 2 diabetes. A high–glycemic index (a measure of the amount a food increases blood glucose) diet also increases risk. Red and particularly processed meats increase the risk of type 2 diabetes. Coffee intake decreases the risk of diabetes in a dose-dependent fashion. Similar to the general population, different proportions of macronutrient intakes can be used to treat diabetes, and this allows individualization of dietary practices. A Mediterranean dietary pattern higher in healthy fat has been demonstrated to lead to slightly better glucose control than a high-carbohydrate diet.[A9] However, a higher-carbohydrate diet can still be utilized, as long as calories are controlled and preferably whole grains are included. An overall healthy eating pattern helps reduce risk for CVD, the main killer of persons with diabetes.

Osteoporosis
Adequate intake of calcium, vitamin D, and protein in childhood is important for achieving optimal peak bone mass in adulthood and preventing osteoporosis (Chapter 230) later in life. Dairy products are the primary source of calcium for most children. Adults should try to achieve the RDA for calcium (1000 mg/day until age 50 for women and age 70 for men, then 1200 mg/day), primarily through dietary calcium with supplemental calcium as necessary. The optimum intake and blood level of vitamin D are controversial. Although there are suggestive data of broader health benefits from increased vitamin D status, this depends on interpretation of the data. Therefore, most adults should try to achieve an intake of vitamin D at the level of the RDA (600 IU/day until age 70, then 800 IU/day). Fruit and vegetable intake is associated with increased bone density through various mechanisms. Vitamin K, magnesium, and zinc are involved in bone metabolism, but supplementation has not been demonstrated to be beneficial to bone health. Excessive supplementation with vitamin A increases fracture risk, as does excess alcohol consumption.

Other Conditions
Obesity
The causes and health effects of obesity, the most prevalent nutritional disorder in the United States, are reviewed in Chapter 207. The metabolic syndrome, a constellation that includes obesity with a large waist circumference; increased serum glucose, triglycerides, and blood pressure; and reduced HDL cholesterol, is strikingly prevalent in the United States and is a major risk factor for CHD, cancer, type 2 diabetes, and hypertension (Chapter 70).

Intestinal Diverticular Disease

Low dietary fiber intake causes constipation, and it is thought to be a cause of intestinal diverticular disease.

Dementia

Although physical activity is the strongest lifestyle factor to prevent cognitive decline, dietary factors also play a role. The Mediterranean and DASH diets have some evidence supporting a role in preserving cognitive function. People who followed the Mediterranean-DASH Intervention for Neurodegenerative Delay (MIND) diet experienced less cognitive decline over time compared with either the Mediterranean or DASH diet.[14] This dietary pattern is a hybrid of both diets and emphasizes 10 healthy food groups that have some evidence supporting cognitive protection (e.g., green leafy vegetables, berries, fish, nuts, olive oil) and limiting five less healthy food groups (e.g., red meats, pastries, and sweets).

Congenital Neural Tube Defects

Inadequate maternal folic acid intake has been definitively proven to be a major risk factor for congenital neural tube defects such as spina bifida and myelomeningocele. For this reason, cereal and grain products have been fortified with folic acid in the United States since 1998, and supplementation with folic acid is recommended in all women capable of becoming pregnant.[15]

Dietary Supplements

Relatively few dietary supplements have demonstrated benefit in preventing disease. Meta-analyses of randomized, controlled trials of antioxidants have reported increased total mortality from vitamin A, vitamin E, and β-carotene.[A10] Vitamin D and calcium are necessary for adequate bone health, and vitamin D may have other health benefits, although interpretations of the evidence behind this and the optimal dose of vitamin D are controversial. A recent large randomized trial showed no reduction in cancer, cardiovascular disease, or mortality with vitamin D supplementation in men over age 50 years or women over age 55 years.[A11] Although multivitamins are one of the most widely used dietary supplements, with over one third of Americans taking them, there is little evidence that they prevent CVD or cancer. Fish consumption is associated with decreased CVD, yet randomized trials have found no benefit from omega-3 supplementation.[A12] A condition that has demonstrated benefit from dietary supplements is early macular degeneration. The second Age Related Eye Disease Study (AREDS2) trial demonstrated the most effective combination of supplements to prevent progression of early macular degeneration contained vitamins C and E, zinc, copper, lutein, and zeaxanthin.[A13]

● TRANSLATING EVIDENCE INTO DIETARY CHANGE

The evidence is strong that dietary habits can influence the incidence and severity of many incapacitating or lethal diseases.[16,17] No justification exists for the belief that modification of the "usual" American diet is unnecessary or futile. The following statement from the Scientific Report of the 2015 Dietary Guidelines Advisory Committee concisely outlines the optimal dietary pattern based on current evidence: "The overall body of evidence examined by the 2015 Dietary Guidelines Advisory Committee identifies that a healthy dietary pattern is higher in vegetables, fruits, whole grains, low- or non-fat dairy, seafood, legumes, and nuts; moderate in alcohol (among adults); lower in red and processed meats; and low in sugar-sweetened foods and drinks and refined grains."[18] Various organizations have provided dietary recommendations generally consistent with this statement (see Table 202-3). The U.S. Departments of Agriculture and of Health and Human Services have developed and periodically revised the Dietary Guidelines for Americans (see Table 202-2). The Dietary Guidelines list three patterns of eating that are consistent with the guidelines and people can use as a practical template to follow: the DASH diet, the Mediterranean diet, and the vegetarian diet.[19] A food guidance system, now called MyPlate (Fig. 202-1), is part of a larger communications initiative to help consumers make better food choices. Although the practical applications of nutritional genomics and the microbiome are not yet ready for routine clinical practice, they represent important emerging sciences that may in the future be applied to nutrigenetic testing to provide dietary advice.

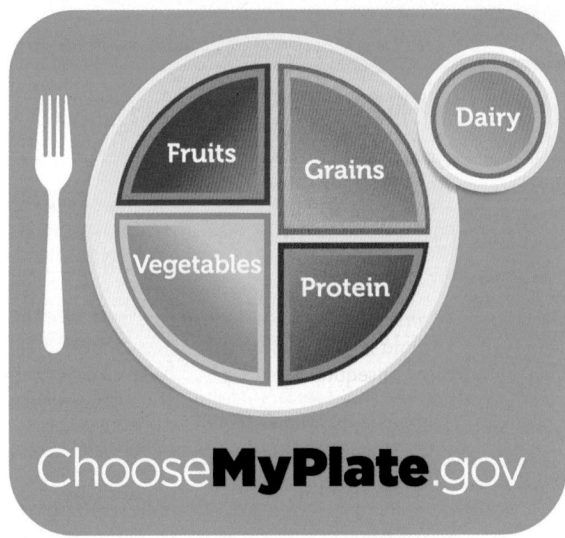

FIGURE 202-1. U.S. Department of Agriculture's MyPlate. MyPlate illustrates that a substantial proportion of dietary intake should be derived from vegetables, fruits, and grains, as contrasted with many Americans' expectation that protein sources should dominate. For more information, see www.ChooseMyPlate.gov.

Physicians can influence their patients' health by encouraging them to optimize their dietary habits and providing them with instructional materials, assistance from dietitians, or behavioral counseling, particularly in patients who are overweight, obese, or have other cardiovascular risk factors. A significant barrier to practical nutritional interventions could be removed if health insurers would expand coverage of dietitians' services.

Grade A References

A1. Rees K, Takeda A, Martin N, et al. Mediterranean-style diet for the primary and secondary prevention of cardiovascular disease. *Cochrane Database Syst Rev.* 2019;3:CD009825.

A2. Druesne-Pecollo N, Latino-Martel P, Norat T, et al. Beta-carotene supplementation and cancer risk: a systematic review and metaanalysis of randomized controlled trials. *Int J Cancer.* 2010;127: 172-184.

A3. Estruch R, Ros E, Salas-Salvadó J, et al. Primary prevention of cardiovascular disease with a Mediterranean diet. *N Engl J Med.* 2018;378:e34.1-e34.14.

A4. Wang L, Sesso HD, Glynn RJ, et al. Vitamin E and C supplementation and risk of cancer in men: posttrial follow-up in the Physicians' Health Study II randomized trial. *Am J Clin Nutr.* 2014;100:915-923.

A5. Vollset SE, Clarke R, Lewington S, et al. Effects of folic acid supplementation on overall and site-specific cancer incidence during the randomised trials: meta-analyses of data on 50,000 individuals. *Lancet.* 2013;381:1029-1036.

A6. Vinceti M, Filippini T, Del Giovane C, et al. Selenium for preventing cancer. *Cochrane Database Syst Rev.* 2018;1:CD005195.

A7. Yao Y, Suo T, Andersson R, et al. Dietary fibre for the prevention of recurrent colorectal adenomas and carcinomas. *Cochrane Database Syst Rev.* 2017;1:CD003430.

A8. Saneei P, Salehi-Abargouei A, Esmaillzadeh A, et al. Influence of dietary approaches to stop hypertension (DASH) diet on blood pressure: a systematic review and meta-analysis on randomized controlled trials. *Nutr Metab Cardiovasc Dis.* 2014;24:1253-1261.

A9. Ajala O, English P, Pinkney J. Systematic review and meta-analysis of different dietary approaches to the management of type 2 diabetes. *Am J Clin Nutr.* 2013;97:505-516.

A10. Bjelakovic G, Nikolova D, Gluud LL, et al. Antioxidant supplements for prevention of mortality in healthy participants and patients with various diseases. *Cochrane Database Syst Rev.* 2012;3:CD007176.

A11. Manson JE, Cook NR, Lee IM, et al. Vitamin D supplements and prevention of cancer and cardiovascular disease. *N Engl J Med.* 2019;380:33-44.

A12. Manson JE, Cook NR, Lee IM, et al. Marine n-3 fatty acids and prevention of cardiovascular disease and cancer. *N Engl J Med.* 2019;380:23-32.

A13. Writing group for the AREDS2 research group. Effect of long-chain ω-3 fatty acids and lutein + zeaxanthin supplements on cardiovascular outcomes: results of the Age-Related Eye Disease Study 2 (AREDS2) randomized clinical trial. *JAMA Intern Med.* 2014;174:763-771.

GENERAL REFERENCES

For the General References and other additional features, please visit Expert Consult at https://expertconsult.inkling.com.

203

PROTEIN-ENERGY MALNUTRITION

MARK J. MANARY AND INDI TREHAN

DEFINITION

The term *protein-energy malnutrition* encompasses at least three distinct clinical syndromes. The first and most common, *stunting*, occurs throughout the developing world. It is a consequence of chronic macronutrient and micronutrient deficiency prenatally and during early childhood and is manifested as low birthweight and irreversible cognitive and physical stunting, including below normal weight and short stature in the first few years of life.[1] A second manifestation takes the form of *acute malnutrition*, a primarily macronutrient deficiency that can also occur in adults. In its most severe forms, it includes kwashiorkor, marasmus (wasting), and marasmic kwashiorkor. The third syndrome is the wasting that occurs secondary to acute or chronic underlying medical or surgical illnesses.

EPIDEMIOLOGY

Global rates of stunting and acute malnutrition are difficult to quantify accurately, given the primarily rural populations where they mostly occur.[2] Nearly 23% of children younger than 5 years are stunted worldwide, and another 8% suffer from wasting.[3] The number with kwashiorkor is unknown and underreported because of minimal high-quality surveillance data; more than half of children with severe acute malnutrition in southern Africa have kwashiorkor. It is estimated that some 15% of the worldwide under-5 mortality is attributable to stunting and another 12% to wasting.

Rates of secondary protein-energy malnutrition among those with medical and surgical illnesses vary widely and are a function of underlying disease processes, comorbidities, nutritional status before illness, and level of financial resources and social support. It is not unusual for malnutrition rates of 25 to 60% among hospitalized patients to be reported in the literature (Chapter 204).

PATHOBIOLOGY

Most stunting in children occurs during the critical "1000 days" window between conception and 2 years of age.[4] Maternal undernutrition contributes to low birthweight, which persists as underweight, short stature, and cognitive stunting. Stunting also places children at elevated risk for acute malnutrition when challenged by food shortages or acute infections. Even children without prenatal stunting are at high risk for stunting and acute malnutrition when raised in impoverished environments.[5] HIV infection and exposure, diarrhea, pneumonia, measles, and malaria lead to anorexia with decreased dietary intake, increased energy expenditure, and poor nutrient absorption, placing the child at risk for stunting and acute malnutrition. The end of exclusive breast-feeding (whether prematurely or at the recommended 6 months of age) and the introduction of complementary feeding also represent a high-risk period as the child ingests a variety of environmental pathogens and often suffers a relative loss of high-quality protein, lipids, and micronutrients.

Aside from chronic food insecurity and repeated gastrointestinal infections, two major pathobiologic factors have been recently appreciated to contribute significantly to the development of protein-energy malnutrition in children. The first is environmental enteric dysfunction (EED), endemic in children and adults throughout the developing world.[6] EED is characterized by blunted and atrophied intestinal villi, hyperplasia of the crypts, and lymphocytic infiltration of the lamina propria, histologically similar in many ways to celiac disease. The net effect of EED is an increase in intestinal permeability with bacterial and toxin translocation due to loss of tight junction integrity, impaired immune functioning, and malabsorption. EED is generally subclinical, predisposing children to growth faltering, and leaves them more susceptible to developing acute malnutrition. A second, related risk factor for the development of acute malnutrition is a disturbed configuration of the intestinal microbiome.[7]

Secondary protein-energy malnutrition that occurs in the context of an underlying illness often results from a triad of decreased energy intake, malabsorption, and catabolic stressors. Virtually any chronic and/or critical illness can precipitate protein-energy malnutrition, but among the most common are cancer,[8] HIV/AIDS, tuberculosis, inflammatory bowel disease, chronic kidney disease, chronic liver disease, and rheumatologic illnesses. The patient is in a state of net negative energy balance manifested by decreased weight and metabolic rate, accompanied to varying degrees by muscle wasting, depletion of fat stores, reduced cardiorespiratory capacity, skin thinning with easy breakdown and ulceration, hypothermia, immunodeficiency with impaired wound healing, and apathy.

The specific pathobiologic etiologies and risk factors for the development of secondary protein-energy malnutrition are numerous. Primary among them is poor dietary intake from nausea, anorexia, depression, poor dentition, and oral-motor weakness accompanying the underlying illness. Even nutrients that are ingested may not be absorbed, for example, because of reduced bile salt secretion leading to steatorrhea, pancreatic insufficiency, and damage to the intestinal mucosa in Crohn disease. Systemic inflammation and oxidative stress are common in critical illness, cirrhosis, patients with HIV/AIDS, tuberculosis, other infections, and hemodialysis patients, contributing to a catabolic state. In patients with chronic renal disease, altered amino acid homeostasis by the kidney, resistance to growth hormone and insulin-like growth factor-1, low testosterone levels, insulin resistance, and altered insulin signaling are all important factors in protein-energy wasting.[9] Patients with chronic liver disease often suffer from protein-energy malnutrition due to a combination of altered gut motility, dyspepsia, cholestasis with poor absorption of fat-soluble vitamins, small intestine bacterial overgrowth, a hypermetabolic state, inadequate hepatic protein synthesis, lack of glycogen reserves, and blood loss from varices and the intestinal lumen.

CLINICAL MANIFESTATIONS

Stunting manifests quite simply as short stature and underweight for age. Brain development, and thus head circumference, may also be small for age, although this is relatively proportional for overall body size.

Acute malnutrition manifests in at least three different forms. Children and adults with wasting are emaciated and weak, having suffered significant weight loss in a relatively short period.[10] The wasting often first manifests in the axilla and groin, progressing to the thighs and buttocks, and eventually becomes visible in the face, taking on an "old man" appearance. Wasting may be mild, moderate, or severe ("marasmus") (Fig. 203-1).

The second form of acute malnutrition, edematous malnutrition or kwashiorkor,[11] was classically described to occur when a child was weaned rapidly from the high-quality protein source that is breast milk,[12] although older children and adults may certainly develop this as well, particularly in the context of extrapulmonary tuberculosis infection. Bilateral peripheral edema begins in the most dependent areas of the body and progresses cephalad as it worsens. Despite what can be a relatively profound edema, they generally do not have ascites, nor is their illness a result of hepatic insufficiency or hypoalbuminemia. The skin may have patchy areas of "flaky paint" depigmentation, commonly with areas of breakdown and resultant infection (Fig. 203-2).

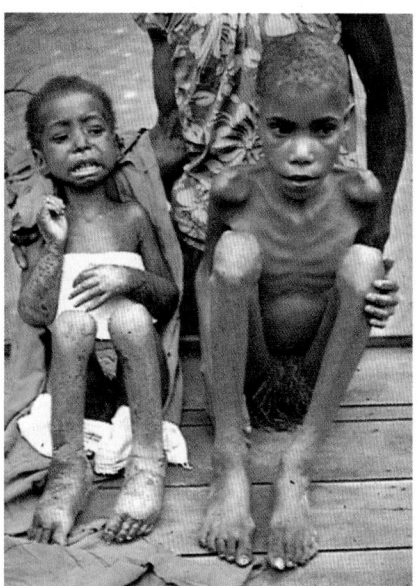

FIGURE 203-1. **Kwashiorkor and marasmus in brothers.** The younger brother, on the left, has kwashiorkor with generalized edema, skin changes, pale reddish yellow hair, and an unhappy expression. The older child, on the right, has marasmus, with generalized wasting, spindly arms and legs, and an apathetic expression. (From Peters W, Pasvol G, eds. *Tropical Medicine and Parasitology*, 5th ed. London: Mosby; 2002, Fig. 986.)

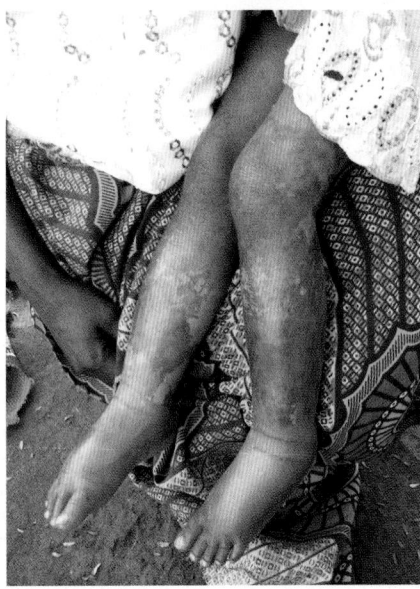

FIGURE 203-2. Edematous malnutrition or kwashiorkor.

Protein-energy malnutrition in patients with severe or chronic underlying disease generally presents as low body-mass index (BMI) or with progressive weight loss.

Virtually every organ system and tissue type is starved of energy in all forms of protein-energy malnutrition, resulting in a homeostatic drive to adapt to the decreased energy available. Fat is increasingly used as the body's primary fuel source within days, having replaced glucose, and ketosis quickly develops. Overall, the marked changes in glucose production and protein breakdown are associated with decreased urea production and urinary fluid losses. The basal metabolic rate declines, accompanied by hypothermia and easy fatigue. As starvation continues, nearly all of the body's fat stores are depleted, and lean muscle tissue may be cut in half. Hypokalemia leads to rapid muscle fatigue. Cardiac muscle is not spared, and the metabolic changes potentially lead to bradycardia, decreased stroke volume, hypotension, and poor tissue perfusion. Intravascular volume may be diminished at the same time that cellular and capillary leakage increases, leading to generalized edema, particularly in kwashiorkor.

Pulmonary capacity is adversely affected by decreased respiratory muscle mass and electrolyte disturbances. The skin and hair often atrophy, depigment, and break down, leaving the patient susceptible to cutaneous infections. Insulin and thyroid hormone levels decrease, and cortisol concentrations increase. A state of immunodeficiency develops as lymphoid tissues atrophy and cell-mediated immunity becomes impaired, placing the malnourished patient at high risk for opportunistic infections. Pancytopenia can occur due to bone marrow suppression, sometimes due to gelatinous transformation of the marrow. Prolonged malnutrition leads to deterioration of all portions of the gastro-intestinal system, including atrophy and blunting of the intestinal villi (thereby complicating therapeutic feeding), impaired exocrine pancreatic function, and decreased gastric and biliary secretions. Hepatomegaly and fatty liver infiltration are seen. Except in cases in which renal pathology is the inciting pathway, kidney function is relatively well preserved until late in the course. Although the brain is preserved longer than other organs, cerebral atrophy is seen in acute malnutrition, and (often permanently) delayed cognitive development is a profound complication with lifelong consequences among survivors.

DIAGNOSIS

Careful anthropometry must be conducted to accurately evaluate any individual for protein-energy malnutrition. In the case of children, it can be particularly challenging to gain their cooperation for anthropometry. Precise measurements of height (to the nearest 0.5 cm or less), weight (to the nearest 100 g or less), mid-upper arm circumference (to the nearest 2 mm or less), and an assessment of peripheral pitting edema should be performed. World Health Organization growth standards should be used for diagnosis and classification.

Children and adults are considered *stunted* when the height-for-age Z-score (HAZ) is 2 or more standard deviations (SD) below the median.[13] Familial short stature, hypothyroidism, growth hormone deficiency, and micronutrient deficiency are all in the differential diagnosis for a stunted child, although

these will be relatively rare compared with stunting in the relevant epidemiologic context.

Wasting may be diagnosed based on a weight-for-height Z-score (WHZ) or BMI-for-age Z-score (BMIZ) more than 2 SD below the median. The mid-upper arm circumference can also be used to diagnose wasting in children under 5, in pregnant women, and in adults. Congenital heart disease, severe diarrhea and dehydration, malabsorption syndromes due to intestinal parasites, malaria, HIV/AIDS, tuberculosis, and malignancy should be considered in the differential diagnosis of a patient presenting with wasting.

The presence of edema in the appropriate epidemiologic context, regardless of other anthropometric parameters, should prompt serious consideration of the diagnosis of kwashiorkor. Edema is most easily detected on the dorsum of the feet and is graded as 1+ if confined to the lower extremities, 2+ if also present on the upper extremities, and 3+ if extending to the face. The usual physiologic causes of edema, including underlying cardiac, hepatic, and renal diseases, should be considered in the differential diagnosis. In rural impoverished populations where kwashiorkor is endemic, routine health care is also generally limited; thus, the possibilities of congenital or rheumatic heart disease, acute proliferative glomerulonephritis (postinfectious or poststreptococcal), profound anemia (from primary iron deficiency, severe malaria, or hookworm, among other causes), and tuberculosis should be considered. Nevertheless, for the majority of children presenting with edema in these populations, kwashiorkor remains the leading diagnosis (E-Fig. 203-1).

Secondary malnutrition due to underlying illness also requires careful anthropometry, with a BMI of less than 18.5 kg/m^2 representing moderate malnutrition and a BMI of less than 15 kg/m^2 representing severe protein-energy malnutrition. Even without a BMI this low, any significant weight loss, especially if associated with lean muscle loss in addition to depletion of fat stores, should prompt consideration of protein-energy malnutrition and necessitates an investigation into an underlying illness if one had not been previously identified. No reliable diagnostic tests are available to identify those with protein-energy malnutrition because serum markers such as albumin, prealbumin, and C-reactive protein are themselves acute phase reactants and nonspecific for this purpose. Diminished grip strength is perhaps the best single clinical measure to assess the degree of malnutrition in this context.

TREATMENT   Rx

Relatively little can be done to reverse stunting because the physical and cognitive growth faltering suffered in the first "1000 days" is due to a confluence of environmental factors not likely amenable to medical therapies. These children remain at high risk for further stunting during childhood, although some degree of catch-up growth is possible in later childhood and adolescence. Attention should be directed to an overall improvement in dietary quality and diversity, particularly with respect to increased complete protein intake. Exclusive breast-feeding until 6 months of age and continued breast-feeding with appropriate supplementary foods until at least 2 years of age should be encouraged whenever possible, with special considerations in the case of an HIV-infected mother.[14] Routine health care, including immunizations, vitamin A supplementation, and periodic deworming, should be ensured. HIV testing and treatment should be sought. Improvements in sanitary living conditions are likely to be the most beneficial.

Children with *uncomplicated* severe acute malnutrition can be treated as outpatients using ready-to-use therapeutic food, most often a fortified peanut paste, if they are able to successfully ingest approximately 30 g of ready-to-use therapeutic food under directly observed therapy (see E-Fig. 203-1). They can then be treated at home with 1 to 2 weeks of 175 kcal/kg/day of ready-to-use therapeutic food, returning for reassessments on a regular basis until they reach anthropometric and therapeutic end points. The inclusion of a week of empiric oral antibiotic therapy decreases mortality and improves nutritional recovery.[A1][A2] Children with *complicated* severe acute malnutrition should be managed as inpatients, with initial attention focused urgently on the infections, hypoglycemia, hypothermia, and dehydration that lead to early mortality. If the child is unable to initially consume ready-to-use therapeutic food, then nutritional rehabilitation can begin with a milk-based formula known as F-75 before transitioning to a more nutrient-dense food (Table 203-1).

Mortality and nutritional recovery outcomes from community-based programs are generally superior to those achieved by inpatient care, making this the current international standard of care and relegating inpatient care only to those children who have anorexia or medical complications or who are in an area where ready-to-use therapeutic food is not available.

Patients with secondary protein-energy malnutrition should, first and foremost, have their underlying illness addressed because this is most likely to lead to long-term recovery of their nutritional status. Concomitantly, nutritional rehabilitation should be undertaken to prevent further energy losses and allow

TABLE 203-1	NUTRITIONAL COMPOSITION OF THERAPEUTIC FOODS FOR SEVERE ACUTE MALNUTRITION		
	F-75 (100 mL)	**F-100 (100 mL)**	**RUTF (100 mg)**
Energy (kcal)	75	100	543
Protein (g)	0.9	2.9	13.6
Lactose (g)	1.3	4.2	
Potassium (mg)	156	246	1111
Sodium (mg)	14	44	189
Magnesium (mg)	10.5	17.7	92
Zinc (mg)	2	2.3	14
Copper (mg)	0.25	0.25	1.78
Osmolarity (mOsm/L)	413	419	
% of total energy from protein	5	12	10-12
% of total energy from fat	36	53	45-60

RUTF = ready-to-use therapeutic food.

for recovery of damaged organic pathways. Fluid, electrolyte, and acid-base status should be corrected cautiously. In general, enteral nutrition (Chapter 204) is preferred over parenteral, assuming the gastrointestinal tract is functioning adequately. Frequent small feedings or slow drip feedings may be necessary. Aggressive tube feeding or parenteral nutrition should be avoided in the early stages of rehabilitation because the refeeding syndrome is a real danger in patients who are malnourished. Hypophosphatemia, hypokalemia, hypomagnesemia, hyperglycemia, fluid overload, muscular weakness, cardiac arrhythmias, and diarrhea are all risks associated with aggressive refeeding. Fluid status, glycemic status, and electrolyte levels should be monitored closely throughout refeeding.[15] Studies are limited with regard to how effective nutritional support is during acute illness,[A3] but much of the benefit is likely to be seen in the longer term, beyond the duration of most clinical studies.

PREVENTION

Prevention of stunting and acute malnutrition remains one of the most challenging and elusive goals in global health, especially given the intergenerational effects of maternal malnutrition. Providing pregnant women with nutritional supplementation, intermittent malaria treatment, timely care for sexually transmitted infections, and comprehensive prenatal care shows some success in improving birthweights and decreasing premature delivery. Adherence to recommendations for exclusive breast-feeding for the first 6 months and continued breast-feeding for at least the first 2 years also shows significant benefits.[16] Early diagnosis and treatment of HIV in mothers and their infants is also beneficial. Nevertheless, impoverished children remain at high risk for stunting and acute malnutrition because of the relative lack of sanitation, high rates of food insecurity, spotty vaccination coverage, and limited access to medical care. Addressing these underlying societal factors and dietary interventions to improve complete protein intake[A4] may provide the most benefit to decreasing childhood protein-energy malnutrition and its adult consequences.

Close attention to the nutritional status of medical and surgical patients, with risk stratification based on BMI and weight trajectory, is necessary to limit the risk for protein-energy malnutrition in these patients as they are treated for their underlying illnesses. Optimizing nutritional status will aid in recovery from their primary conditions, and similarly, recovery from the primary condition will improve benefit to overall nutritional status. Efforts to empirically provide extra protein, calories, and micronutrients during times of particular oxidative stress and catabolism will help limit weight loss and its adverse effects.

PROGNOSIS

The prognosis for stunted children generally remains poor because the physical and cognitive deficits they suffer are mostly carried with them throughout life. Children who recover from an episode of severe acute malnutrition remain more susceptible to further episodes over the next several months than their

peers; those with underlying illnesses such as HIV or tuberculosis remain at significantly elevated risk. The best recovery rates in severe acute malnutrition treatment programs peak at approximately 90%, with about 4 to 5% mortality. Mortality rates are substantially higher, about 35%, in children who require hospitalization.[17] Untreated episodes of severe wasting carry an estimated 10 to 20% mortality risk per month. Although many children will recover spontaneously, most will never return to their baseline nutritional status and fully thrive.

Most relevant for the practicing internist must be the understanding that early childhood protein-energy malnutrition is linked to an increased risk for the metabolic syndrome as adults, contributing to the double epidemic of childhood undernutrition and adult obesity being increasingly observed worldwide.[18] Thus, although the predominant burden of protein-energy malnutrition occurs in young childhood, its intergenerational effects and lifelong consequences make an assessment of nutritional challenges during childhood and adolescence an important consideration when caring for any adult patient with a vulnerable background.

Grade A References

A1. Trehan I, Goldbach HS, LaGrone LN, et al. Antibiotics as part of the management of severe acute malnutrition. *N Engl J Med.* 2013;368:425-435.
A2. Isanaka S, Langendorf C, Berthé F, et al. Routine amoxicillin for uncomplicated severe acute malnutrition in children. *N Engl J Med.* 2016;374:444-453.
A3. Bally MR, Blaser Yildirim PZ, Bounoure L, et al. Nutritional support and outcomes in malnourished medical inpatients: a systematic review and meta-analysis. *JAMA Intern Med.* 2016;176:43-53.
A4. Iannotti LL, Lutter CK, Stewart CP, et al. Eggs in early complementary feeding and child growth: a randomized controlled trial. *Pediatrics.* 2017;140:1-8.

GENERAL REFERENCES

For the General References and other additional features, please visit Expert Consult at https://expertconsult.inkling.com.

204

MALNUTRITION: ASSESSMENT AND SUPPORT

THOMAS R. ZIEGLER

Nutritional assessment is designed to identify and address possible malnutrition or overweight/obesity. Protein-energy malnutrition, which is the focus of this chapter, is present when a patient has unintentionally lost more than 10 pounds or 5% of body weight or developed hypoalbuminemia (not due to fluid overload or inflammation/infection, which are non-nutritional causes of hypoalbuminemia). It is commonly associated with specific dietary deficiencies, which are reviewed in more detail in Chapter 205. Obesity is discussed in Chapter 207.

EPIDEMIOLOGY

Protein-energy malnutrition and depletion of specific micronutrients is common in adult patients with chronic illnesses and in those requiring hospital admission for acute care (Table 204-1), with a typical prevalence of 20 to 40%. Common associated chronic conditions include heart failure, depression, and chronic pulmonary, kidney, or liver disease. Patients with chronic infections, such as HIV, or gastrointestinal conditions (ranging from malabsorption to short bowel syndrome, to intestinal parasites) also become malnourished. Eating disorders (Chapter 206) represent a specific challenge beyond the malnutrition itself. Hospitalization can worsen or even precipitate undernutrition because patients commonly consume or receive inadequate amounts of calories, protein, vitamins, and minerals during their hospital stay.

Patients with acute and chronic illnesses typically have experienced several days to several weeks or months of continuous or intermittent decreased food intake owing to anorexia, gastrointestinal symptoms, depression/anxiety, and other medical factors. They may also have had restricted food intake due to a surgical operation or diagnostic/therapeutic procedure and their subsequent

TABLE 204-1	COMMON CAUSES OF PROTEIN-ENERGY MALNUTRITION AND MICRONUTRIENT DEPLETION IN MEDICAL PATIENTS WITH ACUTE OR CHRONIC ILLNESSES

- Decreased spontaneous food intake due to anorexia from chronic or acute illness, gastrointestinal symptoms (e.g., nausea, vomiting, abdominal pain), depression/anxiety
- Restricted food intake required for surgical operations or diagnostic/therapeutic procedures and gastrointestinal dysfunction that follows these
- Abnormal macronutrient and micronutrient losses from the body due to malabsorption (e.g., celiac sprue, short-gut syndrome, inflammatory bowel disease, cystic fibrosis, diarrhea), maldigestion (e.g., pancreatitis), emesis, polyuria (e.g., in diabetes), wound drainage, or renal replacement therapy
- Periods of increased energy expenditure (calorie needs), protein requirements, and micronutrient needs (e.g., critical illness, increased inflammation)
- Catabolic effects of counter-regulatory hormones (e.g., cortisol, catecholamines, glucagon), release of pro-inflammatory cytokines from stimulated immune cells and endothelial and epithelial cells (interleukins 1, 6, and 8 and tumor necrosis factor-α), and peripheral tissue resistance to the anabolic hormones insulin and insulin-like growth factor-I
- Bedrest, decreased ambulation, and chemical paralysis during mechanical ventilation (skeletal muscle wasting due to impaired protein synthesis)
- Administration of drugs that induce skeletal muscle breakdown, gastrointestinal injury, or electrolyte and water-soluble vitamin losses (e.g., corticosteroids, chemotherapeutic agents, diuretics, and antirejection regimens)
- Socioeconomic deprivation, inadequate caregivers, ambulation difficulties in the home setting
- Inadequate provision of calories, protein, and essential micronutrients (vitamins, minerals, and trace elements) during hospitalization

recovery. Some patients become nutrient-depleted owing to diarrhea, vomiting, polyuria, wound drainage, dialysis, and other causes. Drugs, including corticosteroids, chemotherapeutic agents, anti-rejection drugs, and diuretics are associated with skeletal muscle breakdown, gastrointestinal injury, and losses of electrolytes or water-soluble vitamins.[1] Complete bedrest or limited ambulation are common in outpatient and inpatient settings and are associated with skeletal muscle wasting and impaired muscle anabolic responses.

PATHOBIOLOGY

Catabolic and critical illnesses are associated with concomitantly increased blood concentrations of catabolic hormones (cortisol, catecholamines, glucagon), release of pro-inflammatory cytokines from stimulated immune, endothelial, and epithelial cells (interleukins [e.g., IL-1, IL-6, IL-8] and tumor necrosis factor-α [TNF-α]) and peripheral tissue resistance to anabolic hormones (insulin and insulin-like growth factor-I [IGF-I]). These hormonal and cytokine alterations serve to increase the availability of endogenous metabolic substrates critical for cellular and organ function, wound healing, and host survival (e.g., glucose via glycogenolysis and gluconeogenesis, amino acids via skeletal muscle breakdown, and free fatty acids via lipolysis). This common combination of decreased nutrient intake and increased tissue nutrient losses, coupled with increased energy (calorie), protein, and micronutrient needs owing to inflammation, infection, cytokinemia, and the like is responsible for the wasting and micronutrient depletion common in medical patients with acute and chronic illness.

CLINICAL MANIFESTATIONS AND DIAGNOSIS

Significant erosion of lean body mass or deficiency of specific vitamins and minerals is variously associated with weakness and fatigue, increased rates of infection, impaired wound healing, and delayed convalescence. This relationship is especially apparent in patients with chronic protein-energy malnutrition and body weight loss associated with illness.

Body mass index (BMI; weight in kilograms divided by height in meters squared) can quantify undernutrition. Malnutrition should be suspected in patients (a) with involuntary loss of 5 to 10% or more of their usual body weight in the previous few weeks or months, (b) weighing less than 90% of their ideal body weight, or (c) having a BMI less than 18.5 kg/m^2. Skinfold calipers can be used to measure the skinfold thickness of the triceps as an estimate of body fat; a thickness below the age-adjusted fifth percentile (generally a skinfold thickness of ≤5 mm in men or 12 to 13 in women should raise a suspicion of malnutrition [E-Table 204-1]). Another approach is to measure the circumference of the mid-upper arm muscle: a measurement below 24 cm in men or 19 cm in women suggests malnutrition. In outpatients, tools such

TABLE 204-2	COMPREHENSIVE NUTRITIONAL ASSESSMENT OF MEDICAL PATIENTS

- **Review past medical and surgical history and current illness**
- **Obtain body weight history**
- Determine dietary intake pattern in relation to nutrient needs
- Perform detailed physical examination (consider skeletal muscle wasting, skin, hair, and tongue lesions suggestive of micronutrient deficiency)
- Evaluate gastrointestinal tract function
- Determine ambulatory and mental functional status
- Evaluate standard biochemical tests of organ function indices and obtain blood levels of micronutrients as indicated by clinical status (e.g., zinc, copper, thiamine)
- Consider consultation with multidisciplinary nutrition support team

as the Mini Nutritional Assessment Score (https://www.nestle.com/asset-library/documents/library/events/2010-malnutrition-in-older-people/mna_mini_english.pdf) can identify patients who require formal assessment by a nutritionist.[2,3]

● NUTRITIONAL ASSESSMENT

Accurate assessment of nutritional status is essential for detecting preexisting depletion of body protein, energy reserves, and micronutrients, identifying risk factors for malnutrition, and defining steps to prevent nutrient deficiencies, depletion of lean body mass, and loss of skeletal muscle. Blood concentrations of specific micronutrients (e.g., copper, thiamine, 25-hydroxyvitamin D, vitamin B_{6}, folate, vitamin B_{12}) and electrolytes (e.g., magnesium, potassium, phosphorus) are important to guide needs and repletion responses. Unfortunately, there is not a practical, simple test that can be used as an index of general protein-energy nutritional status. Nutritional assessment involves integration of multiple factors, including medical/surgical history, type and severity of the acute/chronic underlying illness and anticipated medical and surgical course, fluid drainage sites and amounts, physical examination findings, history of body weight change (degree and temporal aspects), dietary intake pattern, use of nutritional supplements, including prior administration of specialized enteral nutrition or parenteral nutrition, evaluation of current organ function and fluid status, and determination of selected vitamin, mineral, and electrolyte concentrations in blood (Table 204-2).[4] In the intensive care unit (ICU) setting, measured body weight typically reflects recent intravenous fluid administration and is generally much higher than their most recent "dry" weight, or preoperative weight, which is the best parameter to use.[5]

In hospitalized patients, especially those in the ICU, circulating concentrations of proteins (e.g., albumin, prealbumin, transferrin) are generally quite low and not useful as protein nutritional status biomarkers given their lack of specificity. Plasma concentrations during active inflammation/infection, critical illness, and the like are markedly affected by non-nutritional factors, including fluid status, capillary leak, iron status (ferritin), impaired hepatic synthetic function, or abnormal protein clearance from blood. Because of the long circulating half-life of albumin (18 to 21 days), levels in blood remain low despite adequate feeding and are slow to respond to nutritional repletion, irrespective of the other confounding factors noted above. Prealbumin has a much shorter circulating half-life than albumin (several days), and serial blood levels can be used as a rough indicator of protein status in clinically stable outpatients.

TREATMENT

Nutritional Requirements

Energy requirements can be estimated using standard methods. These include the Harris-Benedict equation, which incorporates the patient's age, gender, weight, and height to determine basal energy expenditure in kilocalories (kcal) per 24 hours. The Harris-Benedict equation to estimate basal energy expenditure (BEE) for males and females is as follows:

Males (kcal per 24 hours): $= 66 + (13.7 \times$ kg body weight$)$
$\qquad + (5.0 \times$ height in cm$) - (6.8 \times$ age in years$)$

Females (kcal per 24 hours): $= 655 + (9.6 \times$ kg body weight$)$
$\qquad + (1.8 \times$ height in cm$) - (4.7 \times$ age in years$)$

The estimated maintenance energy requirement is approximately 1.3 times the BEE in ambulatory subjects. A simple and relatively accurate method to estimate energy needs is to simply use 20 to 25 kcal/kg/day using actual, dry

TABLE 204-3 ESTIMATED PROTEIN REQUIREMENTS IN ADULT MEDICAL PATIENTS

CLINICAL CONDITION	PROTEIN/AMINO ACID DOSE (G/KG/DAY)
Well-nourished with acute illness	1.2-1.5
Malnourished and/or severe catabolic stress	1.5-2.0
Postoperative	1.2-1.5
Hepatic failure	0.6-1.0 (based on estimated liver function)
Acute encephalopathy	0-0.6
Acute renal failure, not on renal replacement therapy	0.6-1.0 (based on estimated renal function/azotemia)
Renal failure, on renal replacement therapy	1.2-2.0

TABLE 204-4 SOME CLINICAL INDICATIONS FOR SPECIALIZED ORAL/ENTERAL OR PARENTERAL NUTRITION SUPPORT

- Evidence of moderate to severe protein or protein-energy malnutrition or evidence of specific deficiency of one or more essential micronutrients
- Involuntary loss of 5-10% or more of usual body weight
- Dietary food intake likely to be <50% of needs for more than 5 to 10 days
- Severe catabolic stress (e.g., intensive care unit care, serious infection, major operation), prolonged gastrointestinal dysfunction (>5-10 days), or intestinal failure (e.g., short bowel syndrome)
- Chronic obstructive lung disease, chronic infection, and other chronic inflammatory or catabolic disorders with documented poor nutrient intake and recent weight loss

TABLE 204-5 ENTERAL NUTRITION (PROTOCOL FOR NASOGASTRIC FEEDING)

1. Elevate head of bed 30 to 45 degrees at all times.
2. Scrutinize and correct electrolyte abnormalities (esp. K^+, Ca^{2+}, Mg^{2+}, and phosphorus).
3. Place nasal bridle.
   - Place 12-French nasogastric tube into stomach.
   - Secure tube to bridle.
   - Confirm position by abdominal radiograph.
4. Initiate enteral nutrition (EN) feeds with small peptide/medium-chain triglycerides (MCT) oil formula full strength at 10 to 25 mL/hr.
   - Advance by 10 to 25 mL/hr every 8 to 12 hours as tolerated to goal.
   - State goal feeds in kcal/day and the goal infusion rate in mL/hr.
5. Administer chlorhexidine mouthwash with good oral hygiene nursing care twice daily.
6. Check gastric residual volume (GRV) every 4 hours.
   - Return all contents <500 mL to the patient.
7. If GRV >400 mL, initiate the following:
   - Continue EN at the current rate.
   - Turn patient to right lateral decubitus position if possible for 30 minutes.
   - Begin metoclopramide 10 mg IV every 6 hours (if patient is receiving opioid narcotics).
   - Begin naloxone, 8 mg in 10 mL saline per tube every 6 hours.
   - Recheck GRV in 4 hours.
8. Only if second GRV 4 hours later is >400 mL, hold EN.
   - Recheck GRV every 2 hours and restart EN when GRV is <400 mL.
   - If no other signs of intolerance, restart at same rate.
   - If other evidence of intolerance is present, consider reducing rate by 25 mL/hr when GRV <400 mL (or to baseline 25 mL/hr).
9. If tube in small bowel and GRV >50 mL, recheck position of tube by abdominal radiograph. Consider switching to aspirate/feed nasojejunal tube.

or ideal body weight in most patients. This assumes that the body weight used does not reflect intravenous fluid administration or capillary leak syndromes (see above). In ICU patients, even lower caloric doses (equivalent to 15 to 20 kcal/kg dry weight/day) have been advocated by some, based on known complications of overfeeding (see below) and limited clinical outcome data as a function of energy dose. In obese subjects (defined for these calculations as 20 to 25% above ideal body weight), the calculation of energy and protein needs should be based on adjusted body weight as follows:

$$\text{Adjusted body weight} = \text{current weight} - \text{ideal body weight}$$
$$\text{(from standard tables or equations)} \times 0.25 + \text{ideal body weight}$$

Guidelines for protein/amino acid administration are shown in Table 204-3. In most catabolic patients requiring specialized feeding, a generally recommended protein dose is 1.5 g/kg/day in individuals with normal renal function. This is about twice that of the recommended dietary allowance (RDA) for healthy adults, which is 0.8 g/kg/day. The administered protein dose should be adjusted downward as a function of the degree and rate of azotemia (without dialysis) and hyperbilirubinemia.

⬤ NUTRITIONAL SUPPORT

Nutritional support beyond usual oral feeding should be considered when patients have evidence of protein-energy malnutrition or a clinical condition likely to result in malnutrition.[A1] Major indications for specialized oral or enteral nutrition or parenteral nutrition are shown in Table 204-4.

Oral Nutrition Support

Oral nutrition supplementation includes provision of balanced oral diets of usual foods supplemented with complete liquid (or solid) nutrient products, protein supplements (e.g., hydrolyzed whey or casein powder that can be mixed with dietary beverages), high potency multivitamin-mineral supplements, or specific micronutrients required to treat a diagnosed deficiency (e.g., zinc, copper, vitamins B_6, B_{12}, or D). Special supplements designed for patients with chronic renal failure featuring concentrated calories and low amounts of protein and electrolytes are available, as are a variety of formulations designed for other specific disease categories. Several studies show that convalescence is enhanced with the addition of one or two containers per day of complete liquid nutrient supplements to meals following stresses such as total hip replacement. It is prudent to place patients who can tolerate oral medications on a potent oral multivitamin-mineral preparation, at least for several months, particularly for those who either exhibit or are at risk for undernutrition, although this is not specifically evidence supported.

Tube Feeding

Patients with intact gastrointestinal (GI) function may be unable to consume an adequate diet orally due to medical or surgical conditions (e.g., mechanically ventilated patients, those with pancreatitis, dementia, dysphagia, and following trauma or burns). Although parenteral nutrition is commonly administered in these settings, this practice is not evidence based. Current guidelines strongly suggest that oral nutritional supplements or enteral tube feedings should be used if specialized nutrition support is indicated in patients with a functional GI tract.[6] Permissive underfeeding (which provides 80% of caloric requirements)

and trophic feeding (which provides only 25% of caloric requirements) may be as good as full feeding for critically ill adults during the first week or two of hospitalization—with the caveat that, lacking good data, underlying pre-hospitalization protein-energy malnutrition may be the exception with regard to the need to provide more adequate initial nutritional support during this early hospital period.[A2-A4]

Enteral nutrition is associated with improved gut barrier function, decreased infectious complications, less hypermetabolism, and decreased morbidity and mortality, compared to parenteral nutrition.[7] When delivered in recommended amounts, the liquid tube feedings provide complete nutrition for most patients, although some ICU patients and patients with malabsorption may have special needs.

The feedings can be delivered by conventional nasogastric tubes into the stomach, small-bore nasogastric or nasojejunal tubes, percutaneous endoscopic gastrostomy (PEG) or jejunostomy tubes, or percutaneous gastrojejunostomy tubes (in which the gastric port may be used for suction and the jejunal port for feeding).[8] Gastric feedings can be by either continuous or bolus feeds, while small bowel feeds must be via continuous slow administration using an infusion pump to avoid diarrhea (Table 204-5). Tube feedings should be initiated at a slow rate (e.g., 10 to 20 cc/hr) for 8 to 24 hrs and slowly advanced to the goal rate by 8 to 24 hour increments to deliver the calculated caloric and protein needs over the next 24 to 48 hours, depending on clinical tolerance and clinical conditions. Recent guidelines emphasize placing tube-fed patients in the semi-recumbent position (e.g., increase head of bed), advancing feedings cautiously (with serial evaluation for diarrhea, nausea, emesis, abdominal distention, significant gastric residuals), and use of prokinetic agents or postpyloric feedings when gastric feedings are not well tolerated. Recent data suggest that higher volumes of gastric residuals (e.g., >250 mL) are usually well tolerated; lower residual volumes commonly used as a cutoff for temporary discontinuation of feeding (e.g., >100 to 125 mL) may not be necessary if the above safety procedures are maintained.

Most outpatients and hospitalized ICU and non-ICU patients tolerate standard, inexpensive enteral formulas delivered via gastric or intestinal routes that provide between 1.0 and 1.5 kcal/mL. A large variety of enteral tube feeding products are available for clinical use. The specific product chosen should be based both on clinical conditions and underlying organ function, with the assistance of a dietitian or other nutrition support professional.

Diarrhea is common in hospital patients receiving tube feedings but is typically due to factors independent of the feeding, including administration of antibiotics, sorbitol-containing or hypertonic medications (e.g., acetaminophen elixir), and infections. Diarrhea due to tube feeding itself does occur with rapid formula administration, in patients with underlying gut mucosal disease, and those with severe hypoalbuminemia which causes bowel wall edema. Use of a fiber-containing enteral formula is sometimes a useful maneuver to decrease diarrhea. Other complications of tube feeding include aspiration of tube feedings into the lung, mechanical problems with nasally placed feeding tubes including discomfort, sinusitis, pharyngeal or esophageal mucosal erosion due to local tube trauma, and, with percutaneous feeding tubes, entrance site leakage, skin breakdown, cellulitis, and pain. Metabolic complications of tube feeding include fluid imbalances, hyperglycemia, electrolyte abnormalities, azotemia, and occasionally refeeding syndrome. In general, if tube feedings are deemed to be required for more than 4 to 6 weeks, a percutaneous feeding tube should be placed.

In tube-fed patients receiving either subcutaneous or intravenous insulin to control hyperglycemia, significant hypoglycemia due to the continued actions of insulin may occur when tube feedings are discontinued inadvertently or for diagnostic or therapeutic tests. A prudent approach is to have a standing order on the patient's chart to begin dextrose-containing intravenous fluids (e.g., 10% dextrose in one half normal saline at 42 mL/hr) if tube feeds are discontinued for more than 2 hours in patients who are not consuming oral diet.

Hospital patients receiving tube feedings should generally have blood glucose monitored on a daily basis (as frequently as indicated) and blood electrolytes (including magnesium and phosphorus) and renal function monitoring several times weekly (generally daily in the ICU setting). Other blood chemistries should be determined at least weekly. This should be accompanied by close monitoring of intake and output records (including urine, stool, and drainage outputs), gastrointestinal tolerance, vital signs, physical examination changes, and chart review and communication with primary physicians for recent or anticipated changes in the clinical course. When patients are able to consume oral food, tube feeding should be decreased and then discontinued when oral intake is clearly established (e.g., with daily calorie counts by a registered dietitian).

Parenteral Nutrition

Parenteral nutrition support includes administration of standard complete nutrient mixtures, which contain dextrose, L-amino acids, lipid emulsion, electrolytes, vitamins, and minerals (and certain medications as indicated, such as insulin or octreotide) given via either a peripheral or central vein. Parenteral nutrition technically also includes parenteral administration of specific micronutrients or micronutrient combinations to replete a deficiency (e.g., thiamine, copper, electrolytes). Administration of complete parenteral nutrition therapy in patients with GI tract dysfunction has become a standard of care in most hospitals and intensive care units throughout the world, although use in individual institutions varies widely. Parenteral nutrition is lifesaving in patients with intestinal failure (e.g., short bowel syndrome); unfortunately, in patient subgroups with lesser degrees of intestinal failure, few objective data from properly designed, large, randomized, controlled studies are available to determine the true efficacy of and optimal indications for parenteral nutrition.[A5] Enteral nutrition is at least as good as parenteral nutrition in patients who can tolerate the former.[A6][A7] In patients who cannot tolerate enteral nutrition, early parenteral nutrition is no better than delaying for 3 to 4 days.[A8]

As a result, the basic principle in considering parenteral nutrition therapy is that the patient must be unable to achieve adequate nutrient intake via the enteral route.[9] Compared with parenteral nutrition, enteral nutrition is less expensive, probably maintains intestinal mucosal structure and function to a greater extent, is safer in terms of mechanical and metabolic complications (see below), and is associated with reduced rates of nosocomial infections. Thus, the enteral route of feeding should be utilized and advanced whenever possible and the amount of administered parenteral nutrition correspondingly reduced. Generally recognized indications for parenteral nutrition include:

1. Patients with short bowel syndrome or other conditions causing intestinal failure which prohibit adequate intake or absorption of enteral nutrients (e.g., motility disorders, obstruction, severe ileus, severe inflammatory bowel disease), especially in those with preexisting malnutrition;
2. Clinically stable patients in whom adequate enteral feeding (e.g., >50% of needs) is unlikely for 7 to 10 days due to any underlying illness(s);
3. Patients with severe catabolic stress requiring ICU care in whom adequate enteral nutrient intake is unlikely for more than 3 to 5 days.

Generally accepted contraindications for parenteral nutrition include (1) inability to tolerate the extra intravenous fluid that may be required to meet nutrient needs via parenteral nutrition; (2) the presence of severe hyperglycemia or electrolyte abnormalities at the time the start of parenteral nutrition is scheduled; (3) coexistence of uncontrolled bloodstream infection or severe hemodynamic instability; or (4) undue risks posed by the insertion of a new intravenous line just for the purpose of parenteral nutrition.

Parenteral nutrition can be administered either as peripheral vein solutions or as central vein solutions. To minimize the possible development of phlebitis, typical peripheral vein parenteral nutrition solutions provide low concentrations of dextrose (5%; provides 3.4 kcal/g) and amino acids (<3.5 %; provides 4 kcal/g). A major percentage of energy is provided as fat emulsion (50 to 60% of total calories). Because fluid restriction or organ dysfunction often precludes infusion of large fluid volumes for parenteral nutrition, peripheral vein parenteral nutrition is usually avoided in ICU patients or patients with fluid overload or renal, hepatic, or cardiac failure. These solutions are most useful in stable patients who can tolerate the large fluid volumes required to meet amino acid and energy goals (usually 2.5 to 3 L/day) without providing excessive lipid.

Intravenous lipid emulsions (typically added to parenteral nutrition as a 20% soybean oil-based solution) provide both essential linoleic and α-linolenic fatty acids and energy (10 kcal/g); these are generally infused over a 24-hour period in the complete parenteral nutrition administration bag.[10,11] The maximal recommended rate of fat emulsion infusion is approximately 1.0 g/kg/day. Most patients clear triglyceride from intravenous fat emulsion well from plasma. A new intravenous lipid emulsion for use in parenteral nutrition containing a combination of soybean oil, medium-chain triglycerides, fish oil, and olive oil has been approved for clinical use in the United States. Additional intravenous lipid products containing medium-chain triglyceride or olive oil with soybean oil and fish oil are clinically available throughout the world, including recently in the United States. It is important to monitor serum triglyceride levels at the start of intravenous lipid emulsions and then weekly or as frequently as indicated to determine removal of intravenous fat. Triglyceride levels should be kept under 400 to 500 mg/dL to reduce the risk of pancreatitis or impaired pulmonary diffusion capacity in individuals with severe chronic obstructive lung disease.

Central venous administration of parenteral nutrition allows higher concentrations of dextrose and amino acids to be delivered as hypertonic solutions and thus lower amounts of fat emulsion are needed to reach caloric goals. Requirements for potassium, magnesium, and phosphorus are typically higher with central vein parenteral nutrition compared to peripheral vein parenteral nutrition due to the increased dextrose provided (insulin-mediated intracellular electrolyte shift) and needs related to increased glucose metabolism and ATP production. The higher concentrations of dextrose and amino acids possibly allow most patients to attain caloric and amino acid targets with only 1 to 1.5 liters of parenteral nutrition/day. In central vein parenteral nutrition, initial orders typically prescribe 60 to 70% of nonamino acid calories as dextrose and 30 to 40% of nonamino acid calories as fat emulsion. These percentages are adjusted as indicated based on blood glucose and triglyceride levels, respectively. Based on comprehensive data associating hyperglycemia with hospital morbidity and mortality, expert panels now recommend blood glucose in ICU and general ward settings to be maintained between 80 and 180 mg/dL and close blood glucose monitoring. The dextrose amount in central vein parenteral nutrition should be reduced or regular insulin added to the parenteral nutrition bag to maintain blood glucose within the desired range. Separate intravenous insulin infusions may be required in some ICU patients to maintain adequate blood glucose control.

Requirements for intravenous trace elements and vitamins have not been rigorously determined; therefore treatment follows published recommended

TABLE 204-6	COMMON METABOLIC COMPLICATIONS OF PARENTERAL NUTRITION
PARENTERAL NUTRITION PRESCRIPTION PROBLEM	**METABOLIC/CLINICAL CONSEQUENCES**
Excess kcal, CHO, fat	Abnormal liver function tests
Excess kcal, CHO, fat	Hepatic steatosis
Excess CHO	Hypercapnia
Excess fluid, kcal, CHO, fat	Respiratory insufficiency
Excess amino acids	Azotemia
Excess sodium and fluid	Sodium and fluid retention
Excess CHO, inadequate insulin	Hyperglycemia-mediated immune cell dysfunction, infection
Inadequate or excessive electrolytes	Abnormal blood electrolyte levels
Excess fluid, kcal, sodium, CHO, inadequate electrolytes	Cardiac failure, arrhythmias
Excess CHO, inadequate electrolytes, thiamine	Refeeding syndrome

CHO = carbohydrate; kcal = calories.

doses that are aimed at keeping blood levels within normal limits in most stable patients with the use of standardized intravenous preparations.

The most common complication of peripheral vein parenteral nutrition is local phlebitis due to the catheter (a small dose of hydrocortisone and heparin is typically added to such solutions). Alterations in blood electrolytes can be treated with adjustment of concentration in the peripheral parenteral nutrition prescription. Hypertriglyceridemia typically responds well to lowering of the total parenteral nutrition lipid dose. Central vein parenteral nutrition is associated with a much higher rate of mechanical, metabolic, and infectious complications than peripheral vein parenteral nutrition.[12] Mechanical complications include those related to insertion of the central venous catheter (e.g., pneumothorax, hemothorax, malposition of the catheter, and thrombosis). Infectious complications include catheter-related bloodstream infections and noncatheter-related infections by bacteria and fungal species, that may in some cases be due to endogenous bacterial translocation from the gut lumen. The risk for these infections appears to be increased with use of nonsubclavian vein central venous access (e.g., jugular, femoral veins) and multiple-use catheters with nondedicated parenteral nutrition infusion ports used for additional purposes such as blood drawing or medication administration. Poorly controlled blood glucose is not uncommon in patients requiring central vein parenteral nutrition and associated with an increased risk of nosocomial infection. Factors that may contribute to the development of hyperglycemia are (1) poor glucose control at the start of parenteral nutrition; (2) administration of high concentrations of dextrose (>10%) during initiation of parenteral nutrition or an excessively rapid increase in total dextrose load; (3) inadequate exogenous insulin dosing; (4) inadequate monitoring of blood glucose during central vein parenteral nutrition administration; or (5) administration of corticosteroids and pressor agents such as norepinephrine (which stimulate gluconeogenesis and cause insulin resistance).

Overfeeding can induce severe metabolic complications, including carbon dioxide overproduction, azotemia, hyperglycemia, electrolyte alterations, and hepatic steatosis and injury (Table 204-6). Dextrose and lipid doses in parenteral nutrition should be advanced over several days after initiation, and blood glucose, electrolytes, triglycerides, and organ function tests, intake and output measurements, and the clinical course must be closely monitored. Refeeding syndrome[13] with central vein parenteral nutrition administration can occur particularly in patients at risk, including those with preexisting malnutrition, electrolyte depletion, alcoholism, or after prolonged periods of intravenous hydration therapy (e.g., 5% dextrose) without nutrition support, all of which are common in hospital patients. Refeeding syndrome is caused by intravenous infusion of excessive dextrose (>150 to 250 g, such as given in 1 liter of parenteral nutrition with 15 to 25% dextrose). Dextrose

substantially induces the release of insulin, which rapidly reduces blood potassium, magnesium, and especially phosphorus concentrations as a result of intracellular shift and consumption in carbohydrate metabolic pathways. Administration of high doses of carbohydrate also utilizes thiamine, which is required as a cofactor for carbohydrate metabolism and can precipitate symptoms of thiamine deficiency. Hyperinsulinemia can also lead to sodium and fluid retention at the level of the kidney. The combination of fluid and sodium retention, drop in blood levels of electrolytes (which can cause arrhythmias), and hypermetabolism due to excessive calorie provision can lead to heart failure, especially in those with preexisting heart disease and cardiac muscle atrophy due to prolonged protein-energy malnutrition. Prevention of refeeding syndrome requires vigilance to identify patients at special risk, initiation of parenteral nutrition dextrose at relatively low concentrations, and empiric supplementation with higher doses of potassium, magnesium, and phosphorus, based on current blood levels and renal function, and the addition of thiamine (100 mg/day for 3 to 5 days).

For patients in whom home parenteral nutrition is indicated, primary physicians should consult with social service professionals to identify appropriate home care companies and nutrition support professionals to assess intravenous line access, metabolic status, and the home parenteral nutrition order and to arrange for follow-up care and monitoring of parenteral nutrition.[14] It is important not to arrange for rapid hospital discharge in patients newly started on parenteral nutrition; obtaining appropriate venous access and monitoring of fluid and electrolyte status over a 2- to 3-day period is an important aspect of care for most patients started on parenteral nutrition and imperative in those with severe malnutrition and those at risk for refeeding syndrome.

● FUTURE DIRECTIONS

The field of malnutrition, nutritional assessment, and nutritional support should be significantly advanced in the future with developments like those listed below.

- Optimal levels for vitamins and trace elements (e.g., vitamin D, zinc) and other micronutrients will be better defined, thus making clearer the circumstances under which they should be measured and provided.
- Better evidence will be generated on target blood glucose levels that achieve optimal benefit compared with adverse consequences in hospitalized, acutely ill patients with various disorders.
- Better methods to accurately assess underlying nutritional status in hospitalized patients will be developed (e.g., use of metabolomics).

Grade A References

A1. Schuetz P, Fehr R, Baechli V, et al. Individualised nutritional support in medical inpatients at nutritional risk: a randomised clinical trial. *Lancet.* 2019;393:2312-2321.
A2. Arabi YM, Aldawood AS, Al-Dorzi HM, et al. Permissive underfeeding or standard enteral feeding in high- and low-nutritional-risk critically ill adults. Post hoc analysis of the PermiT trial. *Am J Respir Crit Care Med.* 2017;195:652-662.
A3. Arabi YM, Aldawood AS, Haddad SH, et al. Permissive underfeeding or standard enteral feeding in critically ill adults. *N Engl J Med.* 2015;372:2398-2408.
A4. Rice TW, Wheeler AP, Thompson BT, et al. Initial trophic vs full enteral feeding in patients with acute lung injury: the EDEN randomized trial. *JAMA.* 2012;307:795-803.
A5. Bally MR, Blaser Yildirim PZ, Bounoure L, et al. Nutritional support and outcomes in malnourished medical inpatients: a systematic review and meta-analysis. *JAMA Intern Med.* 2016;176:43-53.
A6. Harvey SE, Parrott F, Harrison DA, et al. Trial of the route of early nutritional support in critically ill adults. *N Engl J Med.* 2014;371:1673-1684.
A7. Lewis SR, Schofield-Robinson OJ, Alderson P, et al. Enteral versus parenteral nutrition and enteral versus a combination of enteral and parenteral nutrition for adults in the intensive care unit. *Cochrane Database Syst Rev.* 2018;6:CD012276.
A8. Casaer MP, Mesotten D, Hermans G, et al. Early versus late parenteral nutrition in critically ill adults. *N Engl J Med.* 2011;365:506-517.

GENERAL REFERENCES

For the General References and other additional features, please visit Expert Consult at https://expertconsult.inkling.com.

205

VITAMINS, TRACE MINERALS, AND OTHER MICRONUTRIENTS

JOEL B. MASON AND SARAH L. BOOTH

MICRONUTRIENTS IN NUTRITIONAL SCIENCE

Dietary Requirements

Micronutrients are a diverse array of dietary components necessary to sustain health. The physiologic roles of micronutrients are as varied as their composition. Some micronutrients are used in enzymes as either coenzymes or prosthetic groups, others as biochemical substrates or hormones; in some instances, the functions are not well defined. Under normal circumstances, the average daily dietary intake required to sustain normal physiologic functions for each micronutrient is measured in milligrams or smaller quantities. In this manner, micronutrients are distinguished from macronutrients, which encompass carbohydrates, fats, and proteins as well as macrominerals such as calcium, magnesium, phosphorus, sodium, potassium, and chloride.

Optimal Intake

For orderly homeostasis to proceed, most dietary nutrients must be ingested in quantities that are neither too small nor too great. Disorders may arise, therefore, when intake regularly falls outside of this physiologic window. The size of this physiologic window varies for each micronutrient and should be kept in mind, particularly in this era when the administration of large quantities of certain micronutrients is increasingly explored for possible therapeutic implications. The dietary requirement for a particular micronutrient is determined by many factors, only one of which is the amount needed to sustain those physiologic functions for which it is used (Table 205-1). The U.S. Institute of Medicine of the National Academies Food and Nutrition Board regularly updates dietary guidelines that define the quantity of each micronutrient that is "adequate to meet the known nutrient needs of practically all healthy persons." These *recommended dietary allowances* (RDAs) were most recently revised between 1998 and 2001 (vitamin D and calcium values were updated in 2010), and the values for adults appear in Tables 205-2 and 205-3. Also established for the first time for each micronutrient were *tolerable upper limits* (TULs), which are the "maximal daily levels of oral intake likely to pose no adverse health risks." *Adequate intake,* the amount necessary to prevent a deficiency state, is not necessarily synonymous with *optimal intake.*

TYPES AND FUNCTION OF MICRONUTRIENTS

Vitamins

Vitamins are categorized as either fat soluble (A, D, E, K) or water soluble (all the others), as shown in Table 205-2. This categorization remains physiologically meaningful. Fat-soluble vitamins rarely serve as coenzymes whereas most of the functions of the water-soluble vitamins are as coenzymes. Intestinal absorption of the fat-soluble vitamins is primarily through a micellar phase, and pathophysiologic conditions associated with fat malabsorption frequently are associated with selective deficiencies of the fat-soluble vitamins. In contrast, water-soluble vitamins are not absorbed through the lipophilic phase in the intestine.

Trace Minerals (Alternatively, "Trace Elements")

Fifteen trace minerals have been identified as essential for health: iron, zinc, copper, chromium, selenium, iodine, fluorine, manganese, molybdenum, cobalt, nickel, tin, silicon, vanadium, and arsenic (see Table 205-3), but only for the first 10 of these has compelling evidence indicated that they are essential nutrients in humans. Cobalt appears to be essential solely as a component of vitamin B_{12}, but an isolated deficiency state has never been described. Deficiency syndromes for several of the essential trace elements were not recognized until recently because of their exceedingly small requirements and because of the ubiquitous nature of these elements in foodstuffs. Only under exceptional circumstances, such as long-term reliance on total parenteral nutrition lacking these elements, have some of the deficiency syndromes been observed.

The biochemical functions of trace elements appear to be as components of prosthetic groups or as cofactors for enzymes. Determination of essential trace element status is problematic with the exception of iron. The low concentrations of these elements in body fluids and tissues, the finding that blood levels frequently do not correlate well with levels in the target tissues, and the fact that functional tests cannot be devised until their biochemical functions are better understood preclude an accurate laboratory method of assessing the adequacy of most trace elements.

Additional Compounds with Nutritional Relevance

Evidence indicates that humans also have an absolute requirement for the dietary component choline, which is a necessary precursor for acetylcholine and phospholipids and is needed to sustain normal levels of biologic methylation. To date, the most significant adverse effect of dietary inadequacy has been hepatic inflammation. Deficiency is nevertheless thought to be extremely rare, although pregnancy, and particularly lactation, increases the apparent requirement. Individuals whose long-term nutritional requirements are solely derived from total parenteral nutrition appear to be susceptible to choline deficiency. Both an RDA (425 mg, women; 550 mg, men) and a TUL (3.5 g) have now been established.

L-Carnitine is a dietary component that facilitates the transport of fatty acids into mitochondria, and a deficit therefore limits the fatty acid β-oxidation that occurs in those organelles. Although no evidence exists for a dietary requirement in healthy children or adults, individuals undergoing chronic hemodialysis develop diminished plasma and muscle levels. Controlled clinical trials in hemodialysis patients who suffer from cardiomyopathy, intradialytic hypotension, or anemia refractory to erythropoietin have shown improvements in these parameters with intermittent parenteral supplementation.[A1] Premature infants also have very low stores of skeletal muscle carnitine, although in clinical trials parenteral supplementation has not generally improved clinical end points. Similarly, it has been suggested that individuals on long-term total parenteral nutrition may also be susceptible to the clinical consequences of L-carnitine depletion, but convincing evidence is lacking.

Lutein and zeaxanthin are two carotenoids that are not precursors of vitamin A but appear to play a role in age-related macular degeneration. Low plasma lutein and zeaxanthin concentrations or dietary intake are associated with low macular pigment density and increased risk of macular degeneration. The AREDS2 trial indicated that a combination supplement that included lutein and zeaxanthin (in addition to vitamins C and E, zinc oxide, and cupric oxide) significantly diminished the progression of macular degeneration.[A2]

CONDITIONS THAT INCREASE REQUIRED DIETARY INTAKE

Many physiologic, pathophysiologic, and pharmacologic factors increase the dietary requirements for micronutrients (see Table 205-1), thereby enhancing the risk for development of a deficiency state.

Physiologic Factors

Stages of the life cycle frequently have a significant impact on the requirements of nutrients. Phases of rapid growth and development, such as in utero development, infancy, adolescence, and pregnancy, are associated with increases in the utilization of certain micronutrients on a per-kilogram basis.

Text continued on p. 1413

TABLE 205-1	FACTORS THAT DETERMINE DIETARY REQUIREMENT OF A MICRONUTRIENT

PHYSIOLOGIC FACTORS

Bioavailability: the proportion of an ingested micronutrient that is capable of being assimilated and used for physiologic purposes

Quantity required to fulfill physiologic roles

Extent to which the body can reuse the micronutrient

Distribution of nutrient in the body: storage compartments

Gender

Stage of life cycle: intrauterine development, childhood, adulthood, elder adulthood, pregnancy, lactation

PATHOPHYSIOLOGIC AND PHARMACOLOGIC FACTORS

Inborn errors of metabolism: variously affect assimilation, utilization, or excretion of micronutrients

Acquired disease states that alter the amounts required to sustain homeostasis (e.g., malabsorption, maldigestion, states that increase use)

Lifestyle habits: smoking, ethanol consumption

Drugs: may alter bioavailability or utilization

TABLE 205-2 VITAMINS AND THEIR FUNCTIONS

	BIOCHEMISTRY AND PHYSIOLOGY	DEFICIENCY [RDA*]	TOXICITY [TUL†]	ASSESSMENT OF STATUS
FAT-SOLUBLE VITAMINS				
Vitamin A	A family of retinoid compounds, each member having biologic activity qualitatively similar to retinol. Carotenoids are structurally related to retinoids. Some carotenoids, most notably β-carotene, are metabolized into compounds with vitamin A activity and are therefore considered to be provitamin A compounds. Vitamin A is an integral component of rhodopsin and iodopsins, light-sensitive proteins in rod and cone cells in the retina. *Additional functions:* induction and maintenance of cellular differentiation in certain tissues; signal for appropriate morphogenesis in the developing embryo; maintenance of cell-mediated immunity. 1 μg of retinol = 3.33 IU of vitamin A.	Follicular hyperkeratosis and night blindness are early indicators. Conjunctival xerosis, degeneration of the cornea (keratomalacia), and dedifferentiation of rapidly proliferating epithelia are later indications of deficiency. *Bitot spots* (focal areas of the conjunctiva or cornea with foamy appearance) are an indication of xerosis. Blindness, due to corneal destruction and retinal dysfunction, ensues if left uncorrected. Increased susceptibility to infection is also a consequence. [F: 700 μg; M: 900 μg]	In adults, >150,000 μg may cause *acute* toxicity: fatal intracranial hypertension, skin exfoliation, and hepatocellular necrosis. *Chronic* toxicity may occur with habitual daily intake of >10,000 μg: alopecia, ataxia, bone and muscle pain, dermatitis, cheilitis, conjunctivitis, pseudotumor cerebri, hepatocellular necrosis, hyperlipidemia and hyperostosis are common. Single, large doses of vitamin A (30,000 μg) or habitual intake of >4500 μg/day in early pregnancy can be teratogenic. Excessive intake of carotenoids causes a benign condition characterized by yellowish discoloration of the skin. [3000 μg]	Retinol concentration in the plasma and vitamin A concentrations in the milk and tears are reasonably accurate measures of adequate status. Toxicity is best assessed by elevated levels of retinyl esters in plasma. A quantitative measure of dark adaptation for night vision and electroretinography are useful functional tests.
Vitamin D	A group of sterol compounds whose parent structure is cholecalciferol (vitamin D₃). Cholecalciferol is formed in the skin from 7-dehydrocholesterol (provitamin D₃) by exposure to UVB radiation. A plant sterol, ergocalciferol (provitamin D₂), can be similarly converted into vitamin D₂ and has similar vitamin D activity. The vitamin undergoes sequential hydroxylations in the liver and kidney at the 25 and 1 positions, respectively, producing the most bioactive form of the vitamin, 1,25-dihydroxy vitamin D. Vitamin D maintains intracellular and extracellular concentrations of calcium and phosphate by enhancing intestinal absorption of the two ions and, in conjunction with PTH, promoting their mobilization from bone mineral. It retards proliferation and promotes differentiation in certain epithelia. Purported actions of vitamin D as an anti-diabetes, anti-inflammatory, and cancer preventive agent remain controversial and are under investigation. 1 μg = 40 IU.	Deficiency results in decreased mineralization of newly formed bone called *rickets* in childhood and *osteomalacia* in adults. Deficiency also contributes to osteoporosis and increased fracture risk in later life. Commonly appears following gastric bypass procedures. Expansion of the epiphyseal growth plates and replacement of normal bone with unmineralized bone matrix are the cardinal features of rickets; the latter feature also characterizes osteomalacia. Deformity of bone and pathologic fractures occur. Decreased serum concentrations of calcium and phosphate may occur. [15 μg, ages 19-70 yr; 20 μg, age >70 yr]	Excess amounts result in abnormally high concentrations of calcium and phosphate in the serum; metastatic calcifications, renal damage, and altered mentation may occur. [100 μg for ages ≥9 yr]	The serum concentration of the major circulating metabolite, 25-hydroxyvitamin D, is the best indicator of systemic status except in advanced kidney disease (stages 4 and 5), in which the impairment of renal 1-hydroxylation results in disassociation of the mono- and dihydroxyvitamin concentrations. Measurement of the serum concentration of 1,25-dihydroxyvitamin D is then necessary.
Vitamin E	A group of at least 8 naturally occurring compounds, some of which are tocopherols and some of which are tocotrienols. At present, the only dietary form that is thought to be biologically active in humans is α-tocopherol. Vitamin E acts as an antioxidant and free radical scavenger in lipophilic environments, most notably in cell membranes. It acts in conjunction with other antioxidants, such as selenium.	Deficiency due to dietary inadequacy is rare. It is usually seen in premature infants, individuals with fat malabsorption, and individuals with abetalipoproteinemia. Red blood cell fragility occurs and can produce a hemolytic anemia. Neuronal degeneration produces peripheral neuropathies, ophthalmoplegia, and destruction of posterior columns of spinal cord. Neurologic disease is frequently irreversible if deficiency is not corrected early enough. May contribute to the hemolytic anemia and retrolental fibroplasia seen in premature infants. Reported to suppress cell-mediated immunity. [15 mg]	Depressed levels of vitamin K–dependent procoagulants and potentiation of oral anticoagulants have been reported, as has impaired WBC function. Doses of 800 mg/day have been reported to increase slightly the incidence of hemorrhagic stroke. [1000 mg]	Plasma or serum concentration of α-tocopherol is most commonly used. Additional accuracy is obtained by expressing this value per milligram of total plasma lipid. RBC peroxide hemolysis test is not entirely specific but is a useful functional measure of the antioxidant potential of cell membranes.

TABLE 205-2 VITAMINS AND THEIR FUNCTIONS—cont'd

	BIOCHEMISTRY AND PHYSIOLOGY	DEFICIENCY [RDA*]	TOXICITY [TUL†]	ASSESSMENT OF STATUS
Vitamin K	A family of naphthoquinone compounds with similar biologic activity. Phylloquinone (vitamin K_1) is derived from plants; a variety of menaquinones (vitamin K_2) are derived from bacterial and animal sources. Vitamin K serves as an essential cofactor in the post-translational γ-carboxylation of glutamic acid residues in many proteins. These proteins include several circulating procoagulants and anticoagulants as well as proteins in a variety of tissues.	Deficiency syndrome is uncommon except in breast-fed newborns, in whom it may cause "hemorrhagic disease of the newborn," especially among newborns whose parents refuse prophylactic administration of vitamin K at birth. Also occurs in adults with fat malabsorption or who are taking drugs that interfere with vitamin K metabolism (e.g., coumarin, phenytoin, broad-spectrum antibiotics); and in individuals taking large doses of vitamin E and anticoagulant drugs. Excessive hemorrhage is the usual manifestation. [F: 90 μg; M: 120 μg]	Rapid intravenous infusion of K_1 has been rarely associated with dyspnea, flushing, and cardiovascular collapse; this is likely related to the dispersing agents in the solution. Supplementation may interfere with coumarin-based anticoagulation. Pregnant women taking large amounts of the provitamin menadione may deliver infants with hemolytic anemia, hyperbilirubinemia, and kernicterus. [No TUL established]	Prothrombin time is typically used as a measure of functional K status; it is neither sensitive nor specific for vitamin K deficiency. Determination of fasting plasma vitamin K is an accurate indicator of status. Undercarboxylated plasma prothrombin is also an accurate metric, but only for detecting the deficient state, and is less widely available than plasma vitamin K.
WATER-SOLUBLE VITAMINS				
Thiamin (vitamin B_1)	A water-soluble compound containing substituted pyrimidine and thiazole rings and a hydroxyethyl side chain. The coenzyme form is thiamin pyrophosphate (TPP). Thiamin serves as a coenzyme in many α-ketoacid decarboxylation and transketolation reactions. Inadequate thiamin availability leads to impairments of these reactions, resulting in inadequate adenosine triphosphate synthesis and abnormal carbohydrate metabolism, respectively. It may have an additional role in neuronal conduction independent of the aforementioned actions.	Classic deficiency syndrome (beriberi) remains endemic in Asian populations consuming a polished rice diet. Globally, alcoholism, chronic renal dialysis, and persistent nausea and vomiting after bariatric surgery are also common precipitants. High carbohydrate intake increases need for B_1. *Mild deficiency:* irritability, fatigue, and headaches. *More severe deficiency:* combinations of peripheral neuropathy, cardiovascular dysfunction, and cerebral dysfunction. Cardiovascular involvement (wet beriberi): congestive heart failure and low peripheral vascular resistance. Cerebral disease: nystagmus, ophthalmoplegia, and ataxia (Wernicke encephalopathy); hallucinations, impaired short-term memory, and confabulation (Korsakoff psychosis). Deficiency syndrome responds within 24 hr to parenteral thiamin but is partially or wholly irreversible after a certain stage. [F: 1.1 mg; M: 1.2 mg]	Excess intake is largely excreted in the urine, although parenteral doses of >400 mg/day are reported to cause lethargy, ataxia, and reduced tone of the gastrointestinal tract. [TUL not established]	The most effective measure of B_1 status is the erythrocyte transketolase activity coefficient, which measures enzyme activity before and after addition of exogenous TPP; RBCs from a deficient individual express a substantial increase in enzyme activity with addition of TPP. Thiamin concentrations in blood or urine are also used.
Riboflavin (vitamin B_2)	Consists of a substituted isoalloxazine ring with a ribitol side chain. Riboflavin serves as a coenzyme for a diverse array of biochemical reactions. The primary coenzymatic forms are flavin mononucleotide and flavin adenine dinucleotide. Riboflavin holoenzymes participate in oxidation-reduction reactions in myriad metabolic pathways.	Deficiency is usually seen in conjunction with deficiencies of other B vitamins. Isolated deficiency of riboflavin produces hyperemia and edema of nasopharyngeal mucosa, cheilosis, angular stomatitis, glossitis, seborrheic dermatitis, and a normochromic, normocytic anemia. [F: 1.1; M: 1.3]	Toxicity is not reported in humans. [TUL not established]	The most common method of assessment is to determine the activity coefficient of glutathione reductase in RBCs (the test is invalid for individuals with glucose-6-phosphate dehydrogenase deficiency). Measurements of blood and urine concentrations are less desirable methods.

TABLE 205-2 VITAMINS AND THEIR FUNCTIONS—cont'd

	BIOCHEMISTRY AND PHYSIOLOGY	DEFICIENCY [RDA*]	TOXICITY [TUL†]	ASSESSMENT OF STATUS
Niacin (vitamin B₃)	Refers to nicotinic acid and the corresponding amide, nicotinamide. The active coenzymatic forms are composed of nicotinamide affixed to adenine dinucleotide, forming NAD or NADP. More than 200 apoenzymes use these compounds as electron acceptors or hydrogen donors, either as a coenzyme or as a co-substrate. The essential amino acid tryptophan is a precursor of niacin; 60 mg of dietary tryptophan yields approximately 1 mg of niacin. Dietary requirements thus depend partly on tryptophan intake. Requirement is often determined on basis of calorie intake (i.e., niacin equivalents/1000 kcal). Large doses of nicotinic acid (1.5-3 g/day) effectively lower low-density lipoprotein cholesterol and elevate high-density lipoprotein cholesterol.	*Pellagra* is the classic deficiency syndrome and is often seen in populations in which corn is the major source of energy; it is still endemic in parts of China, Africa, and India. Diarrhea, dementia (or associated symptoms of anxiety or insomnia), and a pigmented dermatitis that develops in sun-exposed areas are typical features. Glossitis, stomatitis, vaginitis, vertigo, and burning dysesthesias are early signs. It is reported occasionally to occur in carcinoid syndrome because tryptophan is diverted to other synthetic pathways. [F: 14 mg; M: 16 mg]	Human toxicity is known largely through studies examining hypolipidemic effects. Includes vasomotor phenomenon (flushing), hyperglycemia, parenchymal liver damage, and hyperuricemia. [35 mg]	Assessment of status is problematic; blood levels of the vitamin are not reliable. Measurement of urinary excretion of the niacin metabolites N-methylnicotinamide and 2-pyridone is thought to be the most effective means of assessment at present.
Vitamin B₆	Refers to several derivatives of pyridine, including pyridoxine, pyridoxal, and pyridoxamine, which are interconvertible in the body. The coenzymatic forms are pyridoxal-5-phosphate (PLP) and pyridoxamine-5-phosphate. As a coenzyme, B₆ is involved in many transamination reactions (and thereby in gluconeogenesis), in the synthesis of niacin from tryptophan, in the synthesis of several neurotransmitters, and in the synthesis of δ-aminolevulinic acid (and therefore in heme synthesis). It also has functions unrelated to coenzymatic activity: pyridoxal and PLP bind to hemoglobin and alter oxygen affinity; PLP also binds to steroid receptors, inhibiting receptor affinity to DNA and thereby modulating steroid activity.	Deficiency is usually seen in conjunction with other water-soluble vitamin deficiencies. Stomatitis, angular cheilosis, glossitis, irritability, depression, and confusion occur in moderate to severe depletion; normochromic, normocytic anemia has been reported in severe deficiency. Abnormalities on electroencephalography and, in infants, convulsions have also been observed. Some sideroblastic anemias respond to B₆ administration. Isoniazid, cycloserine, penicillamine, ethanol, and theophylline can inhibit B₆ metabolism. [Ages 19-50 yr: 1.3 mg; >50 yr: 1.5 mg for women, 1.7 mg for men]	Long-term use with doses exceeding 200 mg/day (in adults) may cause peripheral neuropathies and photosensitivity. [100 mg]	Many useful laboratory methods of assessment exist. The plasma or erythrocyte PLP levels are most common. Urinary excretion of xanthurenic acid after an oral tryptophan load and activity indices of RBC alanine or aspartate transaminase are functional measures of B₆-dependent enzyme activity.
Folate	A group of related pterin compounds. More than 35 forms of the vitamin are found naturally. The fully oxidized form, folic acid, is not found in nature but is the pharmacologic form of the vitamin used in supplements and fortification programs. All folate functions relate to its ability to transfer one-carbon groups. It is essential in the de novo synthesis of nucleotides and in the metabolism of several amino acids; it is an integral component for the regeneration of the "universal" methyl donor, S-adenosylmethionine. Inhibition of bacterial and cancer cell folate metabolism is the basis for the sulfonamide antibiotics and chemotherapeutic agents, such as methotrexate and 5-fluorouracil, respectively.	Women of childbearing age are most likely to be deficient. *Classic deficiency syndrome:* megaloblastic anemia, diarrhea. The hematopoietic cells in bone marrow become enlarged and have immature nuclei, reflecting ineffective DNA synthesis. The peripheral blood smear demonstrates macro-ovalocytes and polymorphonuclear leukocytes with an average of more than 3.5 nuclear lobes. Megaloblastic changes also occur in other epithelia that proliferate rapidly (e.g., oral mucosa and gastrointestinal tract, producing glossitis and diarrhea, respectively). Sulfasalazine and diphenytoin inhibit absorption and predispose to deficiency. [400 μg of dietary folate equivalents (DFE); 1 DFE = 1 μg food folate = 0.6 μg folic acid]	Doses >1000 μg/day may partially correct the anemia of B₁₂ deficiency and may therefore mask (and perhaps exacerbate) the associated neuropathy. Large doses are also reported to lower seizure threshold in individuals prone to seizures. Parenteral administration is rarely reported to cause allergic phenomena, which is probably due to dispersion agents. [1000 μg]	Serum folate measures short-term folate balance, whereas RBC folate is a better reflection of tissue status. Serum homocysteine rises early in deficiency but is nonspecific because B₁₂ or B₆ deficiency, renal insufficiency, and older age may also cause elevations.

TABLE 205-2 VITAMINS AND THEIR FUNCTIONS—cont'd

	BIOCHEMISTRY AND PHYSIOLOGY	DEFICIENCY [RDA*]	TOXICITY [TUL†]	ASSESSMENT OF STATUS
Vitamin C (ascorbic and dehydroascorbic acid)	Ascorbic acid readily oxidizes to dehydroascorbic acid in aqueous solution. Dehydroascorbic acid can be reduced in vivo, so it possesses vitamin C activity. Total vitamin C is therefore the sum of ascorbic and dehydroascorbic acid content. Vitamin C serves primarily as a biologic antioxidant in aqueous environments. Biosyntheses of collagen, carnitine, bile acids, and norepinephrine as well as proper functioning of the hepatic mixed-function oxygenase system depend on this property. Vitamin C in foodstuffs increases the intestinal absorption of nonheme iron.	Overt deficiency is uncommon in developed countries. The classic deficiency syndrome is *scurvy*: fatigue, depression, and widespread abnormalities in connective tissues, such as inflamed gingivae, petechiae, perifollicular hemorrhages, impaired wound healing, coiled hairs, hyperkeratosis, and bleeding into body cavities. In infants, defects in ossification and bone growth may occur. Tobacco smoking lowers plasma and leukocyte vitamin C levels. [F: 75 mg; M: 90 mg; increase requirement for cigarette smokers by 35 mg/day]	≥500 mg/day (in adults) may cause nausea and diarrhea. >1 g/day modestly increases risk for oxalate kidney stones. Supplementation may interfere with laboratory tests based on redox potential (e.g., fecal occult blood testing, serum cholesterol, and glucose). Withdrawal from chronic ingestion of high doses of vitamin C supplements should be done gradually because accommodation appears to occur, raising a concern of "rebound scurvy." [2 g]	Plasma ascorbic acid concentration reflects recent dietary intake, whereas WBC levels more closely reflect tissue stores. Women's plasma levels are approximately 20% higher than men's for any given dietary intake.
Vitamin B_{12}	A group of closely related cobalamin compounds composed of a corrin ring (with a cobalt atom in its center) connected to a ribonucleotide through an aminopropanol bridge. Microorganisms are the ultimate source of all naturally occurring B_{12}. The two active coenzyme forms are deoxyadenosylcobalamin and methylcobalamin. These coenzymes are needed for the synthesis of succinyl CoA, which is essential in lipid and carbohydrate metabolism, and for the synthesis of methionine. The synthesis of methionine is essential for amino acid metabolism, for purine and pyrimidine synthesis, for many methylation reactions, and for the intracellular retention of folates.	Dietary inadequacy is a rare cause of deficiency except in strict vegetarians. Most deficiencies arise from loss of intestinal absorption, which may occur with pernicious anemia, pancreatic insufficiency, atrophic gastritis, small bowel bacterial overgrowth, or ileal disease. Megaloblastic anemia and megaloblastic changes in epithelia (see Folate) are the result of sustained depletion. Demyelination of peripheral nerves, posterior and lateral columns of spinal cord, and nerves within the brain may occur. Altered mentation, depression, and psychoses occur. Hematologic and neurologic complications may occur independently. Folate supplementation, in doses of 1000 μg/day, may partly correct the anemia, thereby masking (or perhaps exacerbating) the neuropathic complication. [2.4 μg]	A few allergic reactions have been reported to crystalline B_{12} preparations and are probably due to impurities, not the vitamin. [TUL not established]	Serum or plasma concentrations are generally accurate. Subtle deficiency with neurologic complications, as described in the Deficiency column, can best be established by concurrently measuring the concentration of plasma B_{12} and serum methylmalonic acid, which is a sensitive indicator of cellular deficiency. This subtle deficiency state has been increasingly recognized among elder populations.
Biotin	A bi-cyclic compound consisting of a ureido ring fused to a substituted tetrahydrothiophene ring. Endogenous synthesis by intestinal flora may contribute significantly to biotin nutriture. Most dietary biotin is linked to lysine, a compound called biotinyl lysine, or biocytin. The lysine must be hydrolyzed by an intestinal enzyme called biotinidase before intestinal absorption occurs. Biotin acts primarily as a coenzyme for several carboxylases; each holoenzyme catalyzes an adenosine triphosphate–dependent carbon dioxide transfer. The carboxylases are critical enzymes in carbohydrate and lipid metabolism.	Isolated deficiency is rare. Deficiency in humans has been produced by prolonged total parenteral nutrition lacking the vitamin and by ingestion of large quantities of raw egg white, which contains avidin, a protein that binds biotin with such high affinity that it renders it biounavailable. Alterations in mental status, myalgias, hyperesthesias, and anorexia occur. Later, a seborrheic dermatitis and alopecia develop. Deficiency is usually accompanied by lactic acidosis and organic aciduria. [30 μg]	Toxicity has not been reported in humans with doses as high as 60 mg/day in children. [TUL not established]	Plasma and urine concentrations of biotin are diminished in the deficient state. Elevated urine concentrations of methyl citrate, 3-methylcrotonylglycine, and 3-hydroxyisovalerate are also observed in deficiency.

TABLE 205-2   VITAMINS AND THEIR FUNCTIONS—cont'd

	BIOCHEMISTRY AND PHYSIOLOGY	DEFICIENCY [RDA*]	TOXICITY [TUL†]	ASSESSMENT OF STATUS
Pantothenic acid	Consists of pantoic acid linked to β-alanine through an amide bond. Pantothenic acid is an essential component of CoA and phosphopantetheine, which are essential for synthesis and β-oxidation of fatty acids as well as for synthesis of cholesterol, steroid hormones, vitamins A and D, and other isoprenoid derivatives. CoA is also involved in the synthesis of several amino acids and δ-aminolevulinic acid, a precursor for the corrin ring of vitamin B_{12}, the porphyrin ring of heme, and of cytochromes. CoA is also necessary for the acetylation and fatty acid acylation of a variety of proteins.	Deficiency is rare; it has been reported only as a result of feeding of semisynthetic diets or consumption of an antagonist such as calcium homopantothenate (which has been used to treat Alzheimer disease). Experimental, isolated deficiency in humans produces fatigue, abdominal pain, vomiting, insomnia, and paresthesias of the extremities. [5 mg]	In doses of 10 g/day, diarrhea is reported to occur. [TUL not established]	Whole blood and urine concentrations of pantothenate are indicators of status; serum levels are not thought to be accurate.

CoA = coenzyme A; NAD = nicotinamide adenine dinucleotide; NADP = nicotinamide adenine dinucleotide phosphate; PTH = parathyroid hormone; RBC = red blood cell; UVB = ultraviolet B; WBC = white blood cell.
*Recommended daily allowance (RDA) established for female (F) and male (M) adults by the U.S. Food and Nutrition Board, 1999-2001 (updated in 2010 for vitamin D and calcium). In some instances, insufficient data exist to establish an RDA, in which case the adequate intake (AI) established by the board is listed.
†Tolerable upper limit (TUL) established for adults by the U.S. Food and Nutrition Board, 1999-2001.

TABLE 205-3   NUTRITIONAL TRACE ELEMENTS AND THEIR CLINICAL IMPLICATIONS

	BIOCHEMISTRY AND PHYSIOLOGY	DEFICIENCY [RDA*]	TOXICITY [TUL†]	ASSESSMENT OF STATUS
Chromium	Dietary chromium consists of both inorganic and organic forms. Its primary function in humans is to potentiate insulin action. It accomplishes this function as a circulating complex called *glucose tolerance factor*, thereby affecting carbohydrate, fat, and protein metabolism.	Deficiency in humans has been described only in long-term total parenteral nutrition (TPN) patients receiving insufficient chromium. Hyperglycemia or impaired glucose tolerance occurs. Elevated plasma free fatty acid concentrations, neuropathy, encephalopathy, and abnormalities in nitrogen metabolism are also reported. Whether supplemental chromium may improve glucose tolerance in glucose-intolerant individuals remains controversial. [F: 25 μg; M: 35 μg]	Toxicity after oral ingestion is uncommon and seems confined to gastric irritation. Airborne exposure may cause contact dermatitis, eczema, skin ulcers, and bronchogenic carcinoma. [no TUL established]	Plasma or serum concentration of chromium is a crude indicator of chromium status; it appears to be meaningful when the value is markedly above or below the normal range.
Copper	Copper is absorbed by a specific intestinal transport mechanism. It is carried to the liver, where it is bound to ceruloplasmin, which circulates systemically and delivers copper to target tissues in the body. Excretion of copper is largely through bile and then into the feces. Absorptive and excretory processes vary with the levels of dietary copper, providing a means of copper homeostasis. Copper serves as a component of many enzymes, including amine oxidases, ferroxidases, cytochrome *c* oxidase, dopamine β-hydroxylase, superoxide dismutase, and tyrosinase.	Dietary deficiency is rare; it has been observed in premature and low-birthweight infants fed exclusively a cow's milk diet and in individuals on long-term TPN lacking copper. It has also been described after gastric bypass surgery and with chronic zinc supplementation. Clinical manifestations include depigmentation of skin and hair, myelopathy and other neurologic lesions, leukopenia, anemia, and skeletal abnormalities. Anemia arises from impaired utilization of iron and therefore often is manifested as a sideroblastic anemia. The peripheral smear and bone marrow may mimic myelodysplasia. A deficiency syndrome is also observed in Menkes disease, a rare inherited condition associated with impaired copper utilization. [900 μg]	Acute copper toxicity has been described after excessive oral intake and with absorption of copper salts applied to burned skin. Milder manifestations include nausea, vomiting, epigastric pain, and diarrhea; coma and hepatic necrosis may ensue in severe cases. Toxicity may be seen with doses as low as 70 μg/kg/day. Chronic toxicity is also described. Wilson disease is a rare, inherited disease associated with abnormally low ceruloplasmin levels and accumulation of copper in the liver and brain, eventually leading to damage to these two organs. [10 mg]	Practical methods to detect marginal deficiency are not available. Marked deficiency is reliably detected by diminished serum copper and ceruloplasmin concentrations as well as by low red blood cell superoxide dismutase activity.

TABLE 205-3 NUTRITIONAL TRACE ELEMENTS AND THEIR CLINICAL IMPLICATIONS—cont'd

	BIOCHEMISTRY AND PHYSIOLOGY	DEFICIENCY [RDA*]	TOXICITY [TUL†]	ASSESSMENT OF STATUS
Fluorine	Known more commonly by its ionic form, fluoride. Fluorine is incorporated into the crystalline structure of bone, thereby altering its physical characteristics. Fluoridation of water has reduced incidence of caries in communities with fluoridation programs.	Intake of <0.1 mg/day in infants and <0.5 mg/day in children is associated with an increased incidence of dental caries. Optimal intake in adults is between 1.5 and 4 mg/day. [F: 3 mg; M: 4 mg]	Acute ingestion of >30 mg/kg body weight is likely to cause death. Excessive chronic intake (0.1 mg/kg/day) leads to mottling of teeth (dental fluorosis), calcification of tendons and ligaments, and exostoses and may increase the brittleness of bones. [10 mg]	Estimates of intake and clinical assessment are used because no good laboratory test exists.
Iodine	Iodine is readily absorbed from the diet, concentrated in the thyroid, and integrated into the thyroid hormones thyroxine and triiodothyronine. These hormones circulate largely bound to thyroxine-binding globulin. They modulate resting energy expenditure and, in the developing human, growth and development.	In the absence of supplementation, populations relying primarily on food from soils with low iodine content have endemic iodine deficiency. Maternal iodine deficiency leads to fetal deficiency, which produces spontaneous abortions, stillbirths, hypothyroidism, cretinism, and dwarfism. Permanent cognitive deficits may result from iodine deficiency during the first 2 years of life. In the adult, compensatory hypertrophy of the thyroid (goiter) occurs along with varying degrees of hypothyroidism. [150 µg]	Large doses (>2 mg/day in adults) may induce hypothyroidism by blocking thyroid hormone synthesis. Supplementation with >100 mg/day to an individual who was formerly deficient occasionally induces hyperthyroidism. [1.1 mg]	Iodine status of a population can be estimated by the prevalence of goiter. Urinary excretion of iodine is an effective laboratory means of assessment. Thyroid-stimulating hormone blood level is an indirect and therefore not entirely specific means of assessment.
Iron	Conveys the capacity to participate in redox reactions to a number of metalloproteins, such as hemoglobin, myoglobin, cytochrome enzymes, and many oxidases and oxygenases. The primary storage form of iron is ferritin and, to a lesser degree, hemosiderin. Intestinal absorption is 15-20% for "heme" iron and 1-8% for iron contained in vegetables. Absorption of the latter form is enhanced by the ascorbic acid in foodstuffs; by poultry, fish, or beef; and by an iron-deficient state. It is decreased by phytate and tannins.	Iron deficiency is the most common micronutrient deficiency in the world. Women of childbearing age are the group at highest risk because of menstrual blood losses, pregnancy, and lactation. The classic deficiency syndrome is hypochromic, microcytic anemia. Glossitis and koilonychia ("spoon" nails) are also observed. Easy fatigability often is an early symptom, before anemia appears. In children, mild deficiency of insufficient severity to cause anemia is associated with behavioral disturbances and poor school performance. [postmenopausal F and M: 8 mg; premenopausal F: 18 mg]	Iron overload typically occurs when habitual dietary intake is extremely high, intestinal absorption is excessive, repeated parenteral administration occurs, or a combination of these factors exists. Excessive iron stores usually accumulate in the reticuloendothelial tissues and cause little damage (hemosiderosis). If overload continues, iron eventually begins to accumulate in tissues such as the hepatic parenchyma, pancreas, heart, and synovium, causing hemochromatosis (Chapter 201). Hereditary hemochromatosis results from homozygosity of a common recessive trait. Excessive intestinal absorption of iron is seen in homozygotes. [45 mg]	Negative iron balance initially leads to depletion of iron stores in the bone marrow; a bone marrow biopsy and the concentration of serum ferritin are accurate indicators of early depletion. As the severity of deficiency proceeds, serum iron (SI) decreases and total iron-binding capacity (TIBC) increases; an iron saturation (SI/TIBC) of <16% suggests iron deficiency. Microcytosis, hypochromia, and anemia ensue. Elevated levels of serum ferritin or an iron saturation of >60% suggests iron overload, although systemic inflammation elevates serum ferritin regardless of iron status.
Manganese	A component of several metalloenzymes. Most manganese is in mitochondria, where it is a component of manganese superoxide dismutase.	Manganese deficiency in the human has not been conclusively demonstrated. It is said to cause hypocholesterolemia, weight loss, hair and nail changes, dermatitis, and impaired synthesis of vitamin K–dependent proteins. [F: 1.8 mg; M: 2.3 mg]	Toxicity by oral ingestion is unknown in humans. Toxic inhalation causes hallucinations, other alterations in mentation, and extrapyramidal movement disorders. [11 mg]	Until the deficiency syndrome is better defined, an appropriate measure of status will be difficult to develop.
Molybdenum	A cofactor in several enzymes, most prominently xanthine oxidase and sulfite oxidase.	A probable case of human deficiency is described as being secondary to parenteral administration of sulfite and resulted in hyperoxypurinemia, hypouricemia, and low sulfate excretion. [45 µg]	Toxicity not well described in humans, although it may interfere with copper metabolism at high doses. [2 mg]	Laboratory means of assessment are not meaningful until the deficiency syndrome is better described.

TABLE 205-3 NUTRITIONAL TRACE ELEMENTS AND THEIR CLINICAL IMPLICATIONS—cont'd

	BIOCHEMISTRY AND PHYSIOLOGY	DEFICIENCY [RDA*]	TOXICITY [TUL†]	ASSESSMENT OF STATUS
Selenium	Most dietary selenium is in the form of an amino acid complex. Nearly complete absorption of such forms occurs. Homeostasis is largely performed by the kidney, which regulates urinary excretion as a function of selenium status. Selenium is a component of several enzymes, most notably glutathione peroxidase and superoxide dismutase. These enzymes protect against oxidative and free radical damage of various cell structures. The antioxidant protection conveyed by selenium apparently operates in conjunction with vitamin E because deficiency of one seems to potentiate damage induced by a deficiency of the other. Selenium also participates in the enzymatic conversion of thyroxine to its more active metabolite, triiodothyronine.	Deficiency is rare in North America but has been observed in individuals on long-term TPN lacking selenium. Such individuals have myalgias or cardiomyopathies. Populations in some regions of the world, most notably some parts of China, have marginal intake of selenium. In these regions *Keshan disease*, a condition characterized by cardiomyopathy, is endemic; it can be prevented (but not treated) by selenium supplementation. [55 µg]	Toxicity is associated with nausea, diarrhea, alterations in mental status, peripheral neuropathy, and loss of hair and nails; such symptoms were observed in adults who inadvertently consumed 27-2400 mg. [400 µg]	Erythrocyte glutathione peroxidase activity and plasma or whole blood selenium concentrations are the most commonly used methods of assessment. They are moderately accurate indicators of status.
Zinc	Intestinal absorption occurs by a specific process that is enhanced by pregnancy and corticosteroids and diminished by coingestion of phytates, phosphates, iron, copper, lead, or calcium. Diminished intake of zinc leads to an increased efficiency of absorption and decreased fecal excretion, providing a means of zinc homeostasis. Zinc is a component of more than 100 enzymes, among which are DNA polymerase, RNA polymerase, and transfer RNA synthetase.	Zinc deficiency has its most profound effect on rapidly proliferating tissues. *Mild deficiency:* growth retardation in children. *More severe deficiency:* growth arrest, teratogenicity, hypogonadism and infertility, dysgeusia, poor wound healing, diarrhea, dermatitis on the extremities and around orifices, glossitis, alopecia, corneal clouding, loss of dark adaptation, and behavioral changes. Impaired cellular immunity is observed. Excessive loss of gastrointestinal secretions through chronic diarrhea and fistulas may precipitate deficiency. *Acrodermatitis enteropathica* is a rare, recessively inherited disease in which intestinal absorption of zinc is impaired. [F: 8 mg; M: 11 mg]	Acute zinc toxicity can usually be induced by ingestion of >200 mg of zinc in a single day (in adults). It is manifested by epigastric pain, nausea, vomiting, and diarrhea. Hyperpnea, diaphoresis, and weakness may follow inhalation of zinc fumes. Copper and zinc compete for intestinal absorption: long-term ingestion of >25 mg/day of zinc may lead to copper deficiency. Long-term ingestion of >150 mg/day has been reported to cause gastric erosions, low high-density lipoprotein cholesterol levels, and impaired cellular immunity. [40 mg]	No accurate indicators of zinc status exist for routine clinical use. Plasma, red blood cell, and hair zinc concentrations are often misleading. Acute illness, in particular, is known to diminish plasma zinc levels, in part by inducing a shift of zinc out of the plasma compartment and into the liver. Functional tests that determine dark adaptation, taste acuity, and rate of wound healing lack specificity.

*Recommended daily allowance (RDA) established for female (F) and male (M) adults by the U.S. Food and Nutrition Board, 1999-2001. In some instances, insufficient data exist to establish an RDA, in which case the adequate intake (AI) established by the board is listed.
†Tolerable upper limit (TUL) established for adults by the U.S. Food and Nutrition Board, 1999-2001.

Pregnancy

Requirements for most micronutrients are increased in pregnancy,[1] but, proportionately, the observed increases in the maternal requirements for iron and folate are particularly great and are related to the rapid proliferation of the placental and fetal tissues. Periods of lactation are similarly associated with remarkable increases in requirements; a lactating woman experiences disproportionately large increases in her requirements for zinc and vitamins A, E, and C to meet the metabolic demands incurred by milk production in addition to the aforementioned needs observed in pregnancy.

Aside from its general role in supporting the rapid proliferation of placental and fetal tissues, folate plays a specific role in the prevention of particular birth defects. A 20 to 85% reduction in births complicated by neural tube defects (NTDs, i.e., spina bifida and anencephaly) has been realized by providing women of childbearing age with a daily supplement of folic acid in the form of supplements or fortified foods. Most women do not receive the recommended daily intake of folate from diet alone. The optimal dose is not well defined, but the U.S. Preventive Services Task Force recently reassessed the balance of the benefits and harms of folate supplementation in women of childbearing age, determined that the net benefit is substantial, and recommended that all women who are planning or capable of pregnancy take a daily supplement of 0.4 to 0.8 mg (400-800 micrograms) of folate.[2] Populations with a high background rate of NTD births attain the largest reductions in NTDs from supplemental folate. However, because the nascent neural tube closes about day 20 after conception, the additional folate must be provided before this time to be effective.

Infancy

Infancy carries particular vulnerabilities to specific micronutrient inadequacies. Healthy infants in the United States are typically supplemented with vitamin K at birth and with iron and vitamin D during the course of the first year because of their particular susceptibility to deficiencies of these nutrients. There has been a recent rise in parental refusal of vitamin K prophylaxis at birth, primarily among couples giving birth in birthing centers who plan to exclusively breast-feed and who refuse vaccinations, enhancing the likelihood of hemorrhagic disease of the newborn.

Women of Childbearing Age

The ability to maintain adequate iron status from menarche through menopause is compromised in women by the additional losses incurred by menstruation, pregnancy, and lactation. Therefore, it is not surprising that the population subset that almost invariably displays the highest rate of iron deficiency is women of childbearing age.

Elderly Persons

Specific dietary recommendations for elderly people have been formally incorporated into the recommended dietary allowances (RDA) because aging has an impact on the need for certain micronutrients.[3] Vitamin B_{12} status declines significantly with aging, in large part because of the high prevalence of atrophic gastritis and its associated impairment in protein-bound vitamin B_{12} absorption.[4] Estimates suggest that 10 to 20% of the elderly population is at risk for clinically significant vitamin B_{12} deficiency. Consequently, elderly persons should consume some of their vitamin B_{12} requirement in the crystalline form rather than solely from the naturally occurring protein-bound forms found in food because absorption of the crystalline form is not impaired by atrophic gastritis. Elderly people also require greater quantities of vitamins B_6 and D to maintain health compared with younger adults, as reflected in the new RDAs (see Table 205-2). The increased need for vitamin D appears to result from less consumption of vitamin D, diminished cutaneous synthesis of the vitamin by senile skin, and from decreased sun exposure, a particularly important factor in elders residing in institutional facilities. The need for crystalline vitamin B_{12} and for a quantity of vitamin D that is difficult to achieve without resorting to a supplement suggests that universal use of a daily supplement pill containing these nutrients would benefit elderly people. Widespread use of a multivitamin that contains a broad spectrum of micronutrients is more controversial, in part because of concerns about subtle toxicity. For example, elders with chronic renal failure appear to have a vulnerability to vitamin A toxicity, suggesting that use of supplements containing this vitamin is contraindicated.

● PATHOPHYSIOLOGIC AND PHARMACOLOGIC FACTORS

Diseases of the Gastrointestinal Tract

Malabsorption and maldigestion predispose to multiple micronutrient deficiencies. Both fat- and water-soluble micronutrients (except vitamin B_{12}) are absorbed predominantly in the proximal small intestine. Therefore, diffuse mucosal diseases affecting the proximal portion of the gastrointestinal tract are likely to result in deficiencies. Even in the absence of mucosal disease of the proximal small intestine, extensive ileal disease, small bowel bacterial overgrowth, and chronic cholestasis can each interfere with the maintenance of adequate intraluminal conjugated bile acid concentrations and thereby impair absorption of fat-soluble vitamins. Maldigestion is usually the result of chronic pancreatitis. Untreated, it frequently causes malabsorption and deficiencies of fat-soluble vitamins. Vitamin B_{12} malabsorption can often be demonstrated in this setting, a result of inadequate R-protein digestion, but clinical vitamin B_{12} deficiency is rarely reported.

Inborn Errors of Metabolism

Myriad rare inborn errors of metabolism have been described for vitamins and minerals that impair an individual's ability to assimilate, to use, or to retain a particular micronutrient (Chapter 194). Such defects are usually partial and can often be overcome, to a certain extent, by administering doses of the nutrient that are several orders of magnitude greater than usually required. Suspicion for such defects should be entertained if a known defect exists in the family, a deficiency syndrome arises at birth or during infancy, or the deficiency syndrome is present despite adequate dietary intake and the absence of any disease that would impair the ability to assimilate the nutrient.

Medications

Long-term administration of many drugs may adversely affect micronutrient status. The manner in which drug-nutrient interactions occur varies; some of the more common mechanisms are outlined in Table 205-4. Some drugs exert their therapeutic effects by specifically inhibiting the actions of a micronutrient. Examples include coumarin, which inhibits γ-carboxylation reactions mediated by vitamin K, and methotrexate, which binds tightly to dihydrofolate reductase, thereby inhibiting folate metabolism.

Toxins

Tobacco smoking alters the metabolism of several vitamins, including folate and vitamins C and E. In large surveys, diminished plasma levels of folate and ascorbic acid have been observed in chronic smokers. Smoking is also associated with diminished levels of folate in cells of the oral mucosa, diminished

TABLE 205-4	DRUG-MEDIATED EFFECTS ON MICRONUTRIENT STATUS: EXAMPLES	
DRUG	**NUTRIENT**	**MECHANISM OF INTERACTION**
Dextroamphetamine, fenfluramine, levodopa	Potentially all micronutrients	Induces anorexia
Cholestyramine	Vitamin D, folate	Adsorbs nutrient, decreases absorption
Omeprazole	Vitamin B_{12}	Modest bacterial overgrowth, decreases gastric acid, impairs absorption
Sulfasalazine	Folate	Impairs absorption and inhibits folate-dependent enzymes
Isoniazid	Pyridoxine	Impairs utilization of B_6
Nonsteroidal anti-inflammatory drugs	Iron	Gastrointestinal blood loss
Penicillamine	Zinc	Increases renal excretion

ascorbic acid levels in leukocytes, and decreased concentrations of vitamin E in the alveolar fluid, indicating that the effect does not simply represent a shift of these micronutrients out of the plasma compartment.

● ADVANCES IN NUTRITIONAL SCIENCE

New Frontiers in Marginal Deficiency States of Micronutrients

Does Optimal Intake of Micronutrients Optimize Health?

Updating the definition of a micronutrient deficiency and establishing recommended daily intakes that are consistent with the most recent evidence have proved difficult for several reasons. In some instances, a novel biochemical or physiologic role for a nutrient has been identified but the question that arises is whether optimization of such functions translates into optimization of health. For example, providing supplemental vitamin E to elderly individuals whose vitamin E status falls within normative standards enhances T-lymphocyte responsiveness; nevertheless, it is unclear whether this translates into diminished infection rates. Another difficulty pertains to the use of micronutrients in supraphysiologic quantities to achieve a pharmacologic effect. The ingestion of gram quantities of niacin to reduce low-density lipoprotein (LDL) cholesterol is an example. Such physiologic effects are not observed at more conventional levels of intake.[5] Thus, the determination of optimal nutrient intake is highly dependent on which physiologic effect is sought. Furthermore, if only a segment of the population will benefit from supraphysiologic quantities of a nutrient, should dietary guidelines for the remainder of the population be established according to this effect?

Defining a desirable level of intake also implies the existence of a means of measuring nutrient status. In seeking an appropriate measure of nutrient status, the diversity of function often makes it difficult to decide which measurement is the most germane. Tobacco smoking, for example, diminishes vitamin E levels in alveolar fluid but not in the serum. Thus, the concepts of localized nutrient deficiencies and tissue-specific requirements add an additional level of complexity to the determination of nutrient status.

Redefining Nutritional Requirements. A Contemporary Example: Folate and B_{12}

Examples of the complexities that have arisen in redefining the criteria for vitamin deficiencies and vitamin requirements are the water-soluble vitamins folate and B_{12}.

In the past, guidelines regarding the necessary intake of folate were straightforward because they were based solely on the prevention of megaloblastic anemia. Measurement of serum and erythrocyte folate concentrations was the most common means of assessing status, and maintaining these levels within accepted normative ranges provided assurance that folate status was adequate to prevent anemia. However, degrees of deficiency that are insufficient to cause anemia may still disturb normal biochemical and physiologic homeostasis and, in some instances, cause clinical disease. Clinical trials have demonstrated that women taking folic acid supplements at the time of conception have a markedly lower chance of delivering a baby with an NTD compared with women who are not folate supplemented but whose folate status falls within a conventionally accepted range (see under "Pregnancy").

Less than optimal intake of folate is also evidenced by an increase in serum homocysteine, an amino acid that is normally metabolized by a folate-dependent pathway. Before the federally mandated fortification of flour, the median intake of folate among adults was half of the present RDA, and a substantial minority of Americans had significantly elevated serum homocysteine levels. Elevated homocysteine (Chapter 198) is associated with the development of occlusive vascular disease and accelerated cognitive decline. In randomized clinical trials, however, supplementation with folate, vitamin B_{12}, and vitamin B_6 has shown no benefit against cardiovascular disease despite its ability to lower homocysteine levels.[A3] Such supplementation also has no clear benefit for cognitive function, except perhaps in patients with low baseline folate levels.

A compelling body of observations in both humans and animals has demonstrated that habitually low consumption of folate substantially increases the risk of colorectal cancer[6] and perhaps cancers of other organs, such as those of the breast and pancreas. This inverse relationship is observed even when dietary folate intake falls within the range of conventionally accepted normative values. This relationship has further complicated the determination of what constitutes an optimal intake of folate because the recent epidemiologic data suggest that about 500 μg constitutes the optimal daily intake for suppressing the risk of colon cancer. The issue is further confounded by observations, albeit controversial, suggesting that exceptionally high doses of supplemental folic acid among those who unknowingly harbor precancerous or cancerous lesions may paradoxically enhance the progression of these neoplasms, thereby underscoring the potential for harm produced by taking a nutrient outside of its physiologic window.

The most recent update of the U.S. RDA for folate raised the value from 200 to 400 μg/day, citing both the prevention of anemia and optimization of serum homocysteine as criteria, and recommended that women capable of becoming pregnant consume an additional 400 μg/day in the form of supplements or fortified food. The issues surrounding the prevention of cardiovascular disease, cancer, and cognitive decline were not incorporated into that 1998 determination because the existing data at the time were inconclusive. However, future revisions of the RDAs may integrate some of this new knowledge. The potential for toxicity, the criterion for which was primarily linked to its ability to mask vitamin B_{12} deficiency, was dealt with by setting the TUL at 1000 μg/day of folic acid obtained from supplements and fortified foods in addition to that obtained from natural food sources (see Table 205-2).

Like folate, the metrics by which we assess vitamin B_{12} status are also evolving. Plasma vitamin B_{12} concentrations were formerly considered to be an accurate indication of vitamin B_{12} status (see Chapter 155 for full discussion of clinical B_{12} and folate deficiency). Values greater than 150 μg/mL were thought to exclude vitamin B_{12} deficiency as a cause of neurologic or psychiatric syndromes.[7] Recent observations now indicate that 7 to 10% of elder individuals who have plasma vitamin B_{12} values between 150 and 400 μg/mL may develop neuropsychiatric complications of vitamin B_{12} deficiency in the absence of any indications of megaloblastic anemia. Such individuals can be identified by the demonstration of an elevated level of methylmalonic acid in the blood that decreases to normal levels with parenteral vitamin B_{12} repletion. An elevation in serum methylmalonic acid is both a sensitive and a specific indication of cellular vitamin B_{12} deficiency. An alternative approach is to administer parenteral injections of vitamin B_{12} to an individual who has an otherwise unexplained neuropsychiatric syndrome and whose plasma vitamin B_{12} level falls in the range of 150 to 400 μg/mL and follow clinical response. Awareness of this phenomenon is particularly important because it has become clear that atrophic gastritis, an asymptomatic condition that affects approximately 30% of the elderly population, frequently produces a modest decrease in vitamin B_{12} status; similarly, long-term use of proton pump inhibitor drugs inhibits absorption and also increases the risk of clinically significant deficiency.[8]

New biochemical functions of vitamins are increasingly being recognized. As the clinical significance of each of these new roles is defined and as quantities of each vitamin needed to optimize such functions are determined, redefinition of the desirable range of vitamin status is likely to occur. Future efforts to refine appropriate dietary goals for each micronutrient will, however, need to take into consideration an important theme that is underscored by the previous discussion: the level of consumption of a particular micronutrient that conveys health benefits to one segment of the population is not necessarily beneficial, or even appropriate, for all segments of society.

Is Routine Multivitamin and Multimineral Supplementation Beneficial?

In a large, nationally representative survey of U.S. adults, use of supplements, including vitamins and minerals, remained stable from 1999 to 2012, with 52% of adults reporting their use in the prior 30 days; trends varied for individual supplements and across age, sex, race/ethnicity, and education.[9] A common query by patients is whether regular use of a multivitamin or

multimineral supplement is safe and efficacious in the maintenance of health. Although there is not a unanimous consensus about the "correct" answer to this question, the weight of available evidence indicates that for the general adult North American population, supplementation offers little or no benefit in regard to the prevention of common chronic degenerative diseases such as vascular disease, cancer, and dementia.[A4][A5] This apparent lack of efficacy has been notably contradicted by two clinical trials conducted in Western industrialized countries in which men taking multivitamins realized modest decreases in the incidence of cancer, but such benefits have not been substantiated by other investigations.

Although daily supplementation at the levels found in most multivitamin preparations probably presents no risk of harm, adverse health effects have been observed in several rigorously performed clinical trials in which long-term supplementation with micronutrients at levels that exceed the RDA (or conventional levels of dietary intake) by several-fold was examined. For example, an increased incidence of prostate cancer was observed in the SELECT trial, in which vitamin E was administered at a dose of 400 IU/day,[A6] and β-carotene supplementation resulted in an increased incidence of lung cancer among heavy smokers in the ATBC and CARET trials at doses of 20 to 30 mg/day.

This is not to say that health benefits cannot be realized from supplementation in select groups of individuals, although some thought needs to be exercised to determine which segments of the population should be targeted and what specific nutrients should be administered. Certainly, health benefits are likely in individuals whose dietary intake is chronically inadequate or in patients whose medical conditions are predictably complicated by micronutrient deficiencies, such as those on chronic renal dialysis or among individuals with marginally controlled intestinal malabsorption. The elderly frequently cannot achieve recommended intakes of vitamin D and calcium to optimize bone health with diet alone, and therefore targeted supplementation with these nutrients is often indicated. Additional extra-skeletal benefits of vitamin D supplementation remain a matter of controversy, and a recent meta-analysis of more than 50,000 patients showed no benefit of vitamin D on musculoskeletal health.[A7] Although a 2014 systematic review of randomized clinical trials in elderly individuals identified a small (7%) but significant decrease in all-cause mortality with vitamin D supplementation, the most definitive vitamin D supplementation trial to date, which post-dated the systematic review, observed no decrease in the incidence of either cancer or cardiovascular events among more than 25,000 enrolled participants.[A8] In addition to elder adults, certain racial and ethnic subgroups and those who are obese may have increased needs for some vitamins. Poorer dietary patterns among those of lower socioeconomic status and among certain race/ethnic groups have also been reported. Before dietary supplements are deemed categorically not beneficial, they need to be studied more extensively in those population subgroups most likely to benefit from them.

Moreover, in many regions of the world, there continues to be a high prevalence of marginal micronutrient status among the general adult population, and in such areas widespread supplementation may be indicated.

Grade A References

A1. Higuchi T, Abe M, Yamazaki T, et al. Levocarnitine improves cardiac function in hemodialysis patients with left ventricular hypertrophy: a randomized controlled trial. *Am J Kidney Dis.* 2016;67:260-270.

A2. Age-Related Eye Disease Study 2 Research Group. Lutein + zeaxanthin and omega-3 fatty acids for age-related macular degeneration: the Age-Related Eye Disease Study 2 (AREDS2) randomized clinical trial. *JAMA.* 2013;309:2005-2015.

A3. Clarke R, Halsey J, Lewington S, et al. Effects of lowering homocysteine levels with B vitamins on cardiovascular disease, cancer, and cause-specific mortality: meta-analysis of 8 randomized trials involving 37,485 individuals. *Arch Intern Med.* 2010;170:1622-1631.

A4. Fortmann S, Burda B, Senger C, et al. Vitamin and mineral supplements in the primary prevention of cardiovascular disease and cancer: an updated systematic evidence review for the U.S. Preventive Services Task Force. *Ann Intern Med.* 2013;159:824-834.

A5. Lamas G, Roineau R, Goertz C, et al. Oral high-dose multivitamins and minerals after myocardial infarction: a randomized trial. *Ann Intern Med.* 2013;159:797-805.

A6. Klein EA, Thompson IM Jr, Tangen CM, et al. Vitamin E and the risk of prostate cancer: the Selenium and Vitamin E Cancer Prevention Trial (SELECT). *JAMA.* 2011;306:1549-1556.

A7. Bolland MJ, Grey A, Avenell A. Effects of vitamin D supplementation on musculoskeletal health: a systematic review, meta-analysis, and trial sequential analysis. *Lancet Diabetes Endocrinol.* 2018;6:847-858.

A8. Manson JE, Cook N, Lee I-M, et al. Vitamin D supplements and prevention of cancer and cardiovascular disease. *New Engl J Med.* 2019;380:33-44.

GENERAL REFERENCES

For the General References and other additional features, please visit Expert Consult at https://expertconsult.inkling.com.

206

EATING DISORDERS

MARIAN TANOFSKY-KRAFF

DEFINITION

Feeding and eating disorders are defined as syndromes "characterized by a persistent disturbance of eating or eating related behavior that results in the altered consumption or absorption of food and that significantly impairs physical health or psychosocial functioning."[1] The *Diagnostic and Statistical Manual of Mental Disorders*, 5th edition (DSM-5), defines anorexia nervosa, bulimia nervosa, and binge eating disorder as primary diagnoses in adolescents and adults. All other diagnoses are identified as Unspecified Feeding or Eating Disorders and represent presentations that do not meet the criteria for the primary eating disorders, but nonetheless cause significant distress and impairment. The severity of each disorder is also specified as mild, moderate, severe, or extreme.

Anorexia Nervosa

Anorexia nervosa (AN) involves a restriction of "energy intake relative to requirements, leading to a significantly low body weight in the context of age, sex, developmental trajectory, and physical health." Individuals with AN experience an intense fear of gaining weight or becoming fat, have an over-concern with weight or shape, and often may not recognize the seriousness of their low body weight. AN has two subtypes, restricting and binge-eating/purging. DSM-5 criteria for AN are listed in Table 206-1.

Bulimia Nervosa

A diagnosis of bulimia nervosa (BN) requires recurrent episodes of binge eating (i.e., the consumption of an unambiguously large amount of food given the context, accompanied by a sense of loss of control over eating). Episodes of binge eating co-occur with behaviors intended to compensate for energy consumed and to prevent weight gain, such as self-induced vomiting and fasting. Binge eating and compensatory behaviors must occur, on average, at least once a week for three months. The self-esteem of individuals with BN is excessively influenced by their body weight and shape. DSM-5 criteria for BN are outlined in Table 206-2.

Binge Eating Disorder

Binge eating disorder (BED)[2] is characterized by recurrent episodes of binge eating in the absence of regular compensatory behaviors that are present in BN. The binge episodes are distinguished by at least three associated characteristics: eating rapidly, eating until feeling uncomfortably full, and feeling disgust and guilt regarding the episodes. Individuals experience marked distress surrounding the binge episodes, and the binge eating episodes must occur, on average, at least once a week for three months. DSM-5 criteria for BED are listed in Table 206-3.

EPIDEMIOLOGY

The lifetime prevalence of AN is approximately 0.6%, with higher rates among women (0.9%) compared to men (0.3%). The lifetime prevalence of BN appears to be about 1%, with higher rates among women (1.5%) than men (0.5%). The lifetime prevalence of BED is estimated at 3.5% for women and 2.0% for men. Among adolescents, lifetime prevalence estimates of AN, BN, and BED have been reported at 0.3%, 0.9%, and 1.6%, respectively. Contrary to the view that eating disorders afflict only non-Hispanic white, affluent females, individuals of all races, ethnicities, and cultures are impacted by these diagnoses.

PATHOBIOLOGY

Several brain regions may be involved in, and potentially interact with, the manifestations of all eating disorders. With regard to *structural neurobiology*, the pathology of ED is associated with general brain atrophy and enlarged ventricles. In terms of *functional neurobiology*, individuals with eating disorders appear to have brain function alterations in emotional/limbic, reward, and cognitive control circuits. Fear circuitry networks involving the amygdala, anterior cingulate cortex, hippocampus, insula, striatum, and prefrontal cortex have demonstrated differential activation among individuals with eating disorders compared with controls. Specifically, there tends to be a hyper-responsiveness in the limbic circuitry in response to potentially threatening cues, such as food, and about body weight/shape.

There also appear to be alterations in reward function in patients with AN, but the direction is unclear. By contrast, individuals with BN and BED consistently demonstrate hyper-responsivity in reward and somatosensory regions upon exposure to food images. Individuals with eating disorders may have dysregulated frontal cortical cognitive neural networks acting in concert with regional reward systems. Individuals with eating disorders have demonstrated impaired cognitive flexibility. Specifically in BN, impulsivity and poor inhibitory control have also been reported.

Individuals with AN appear to have impaired dopaminergic signaling, particularly in striatal circuits, that might contribute to altered reward and affect, decision making, and executive control, as well as compulsivity and decreased food ingestion. Increased dorsal striatal dopaminergic activity is associated with greater anxiety in AN, suggesting that endogenous dopamine release might have an anxiogenic effect that drives restriction of food intake.[3] Increased functional connectivity between the dorsal striatum and the dorsolateral prefrontal cortex (DLPFC) for low- versus high-fat foods and its association with decreased food intake in individuals with AN highlights the role of fronto-striatal circuits in AN pathobiology. Striatal dopamine abnormalities may exist in individuals with BN and BED. Because serotonin 1A and 2A receptors and the serotonin transporter may play a part in eating disorder symptoms such as impulse control and associated mood symptoms, it is likely that interactions between the serotonin and dopaminergic systems contribute to eating disorders. Furthermore, atypical intestinal microbiota may also contribute to altered energy homeostasis and behavior in eating disorders via the brain-gut axis.[4]

TABLE 206-1 DSM-5* DIAGNOSTIC CRITERIA FOR ANOREXIA NERVOSA

A. Restriction of energy intake relative to requirements, leading to a significantly low body weight in the context of age, sex, developmental trajectory, and physical health. *Significantly low weight* is defined as a weight that is less than minimally normal or, for children and adolescents, less than minimally expected.

B. Intense fear of gaining weight or becoming fat, or persistent behaviors that interfere with weight gain, even though at a significantly low weight.

C. Disturbance in the way in which one's body weight or shape is experienced, undue influence of body weight or shape on self-evaluation, or persistent lack of recognition of the seriousness of the current low body weight.

Specify whether:

Restricting type: During the last 3 months, the individual has not engaged in recurrent episodes of binge eating or purging behavior (i.e., self-induced vomiting or the misuse of laxatives, diuretics, or enemas). This subtype describes presentations in which weight loss is accomplished primarily through dieting, fasting, and/or excessive exercise.

Binge-eating/purging type: During the last 3 months, the individual has engaged in recurrent episodes of binge eating or purging behavior (i.e., self-induced vomiting or the misuse of laxatives, diuretics, or enemas).

*Diagnostic and Statistical Manual of Mental Disorders. 5th ed. Washington, DC: American Psychiatric Association; 2013.

TABLE 206-2 DSM-5* DIAGNOSTIC CRITERIA FOR BULIMIA NERVOSA

A. Recurrent episodes of binge eating. An episode of binge eating is characterized by both of the following:
1. Eating, in a discrete period of time (e.g., within any 2-hour period), an amount of food that is definitely larger than most people would eat during a similar period of time and under similar circumstances.
2. A sense of lack of control over eating during the episodes (e.g., a feeling that one cannot stop eating or control what or how much one is eating).

B. Recurrent inappropriate compensatory behavior in order to prevent weight gain, such as self-induced vomiting; misuse of laxatives, diuretics, enemas, or other medications; fasting; or excessive exercise.

C. The binge eating and inappropriate compensatory behaviors both occur, on average, at least once a week for 3 months.

D. Self-evaluation is unduly influenced by body shape and weight.

E. The disturbance does not occur exclusively during episodes of anorexia nervosa.

*Diagnostic and Statistical Manual of Mental Disorders. 5th ed. Washington, DC: American Psychiatric Association; 2013.

TABLE 206-3 DSM-5* DIAGNOSTIC CRITERIA FOR BINGE EATING DISORDER

A. Recurrent episodes of binge eating. An episode of binge eating is characterized by both of the following:
  1. Eating, in a discrete period of time (e.g., within any 2-hour period), an amount of food that is definitely larger than most people would eat during a similar period of time and under similar circumstances.
  2. A sense of lack of control over eating during the episodes (e.g., a feeling that one cannot stop eating or control what or how much one is eating).
B. The binge eating episodes are associated with three (or more) of the following:
  1. Eating much more rapidly than normal.
  2. Eating until feeling uncomfortably full.
  3. Eating large amounts of food when not feeling physically hungry.
  4. Eating alone because of feeling embarrassed by how much one is eating.
  5. Feeling disgusted with oneself, depressed, or very guilty afterward.
C. Marked distress regarding binge eating is present.
D. The binge eating occurs, on average, at least once a week for three months.
E. The binge eating is not associated with the recurrent use of inappropriate compensatory behavior as in bulimia nervosa and does not occur exclusively during the course of bulimia nervosa or anorexia nervosa.

*Diagnostic and Statistical Manual of Mental Disorders. 5th ed. Washington, DC: American Psychiatric Association; 2013.

Risk Factors

Eating disorders develop as a result of multiple biological, psychological, and sociocultural factors. AN, BN, and BED aggregate in families with estimates from twin studies suggesting that 40 to 60% of vulnerability for eating disorders is genetic. Although genetic linkage and association studies have implicated several susceptibility loci for AN, BN, and BED, specific genes that consistently lend vulnerability to eating disorders are less conclusive.

Female sex, age, presence of eating disorders in siblings, and comorbid disorders in family members, pediatric overweight, elevated shape and weight concerns, sexual abuse, trauma, and mood disorders have been identified as risk factors for eating disorders.[5] Personality-related variables, such as impulsivity and perfectionism, appear to be linked to eating disorders. Internalization to the "thin ideal" (a sociocultural emphasis on shape and weight and a marked preference for a thin body type) and resulting weight and shape concerns have been proposed to contribute to eating disorder development, particularly among adolescents who are under strong influence from their peer and family environments. For example, parental over-concern about eating, shape, and weight, as well as weight-related teasing by family members confer risk for eating disorders. Specific to BED, maltreatment, including teasing and bullying, and perceived stress are risk factors for the disorder.

CLINICAL MANIFESTATIONS
Symptoms and Signs

For AN, physical symptoms and signs may include amenorrhea, constipation, cold intolerance, anemia, and lanugo hair. Reduced bone density may predict the onset of premature osteopenia and osteoporosis. Health problems associated with malnutrition impact cardiovascular, gastrointestinal, reproductive, hematologic, and endocrine systems.[6] Many of the medical complications of AN are potentially reversible with refeeding and improved nutrition. Sinus bradycardia caused by heightened vagal tone associated with weight loss is a characteristic finding. However, patients with AN can also develop arrhythmias, prolongation of the QTc interval on electrocardiogram, sudden cardiac death, and structural changes in the heart such as left ventricular atrophy and cardiac fibrosis. Patients with AN can have markedly slowed gastric emptying, manifested by early satiety, nausea, abdominal pain, and bloating. Superior mesenteric artery syndrome, resulting in chronic intermittent or acute duodenal obstruction (that can be complete or partial), can result from the loss of fatty tissue that normally maintains the angle between the superior mesenteric artery and the aorta, leading to extrinsic compression of the duodenum by the superior mesenteric artery. Transient elevations of liver transaminases are common. Hypogonadism, with amenorrhea in females, and transient thyroid function abnormalities are common endocrine manifestations of AN. In advanced AN, pancytopenia can develop as a result of gelatinous transformation of the bone marrow.

Individuals with AN frequently present with comorbid psychiatric disorders, including mood and anxiety disorders (i.e., social phobia, specific phobias, post-traumatic stress disorder), as well as high rates of suicidal ideation and behavior.

Individuals with BN present with signs and symptoms most commonly associated with purging behavior. These include dental enamel erosion secondary to vomiting, gastrointestinal symptoms, including gastric acid reflux leading to dyspepsia and repeated exposure to gastric acid with dysphagia, salivary gland hypertrophy, and electrolyte disturbance. Electrolyte abnormalities and changes in acid-base balance can have dangerous consequences. BN patients are at risk for cardiometabolic conditions (i.e., diabetes, stroke) as well as chronic pain. Metabolic acidosis can also occur in patients who are abusing laxatives as a result of the loss of bicarbonate from the bowel (Chapter 110). The cathartic colon syndrome is caused by permanent damage to the Auerbach plexus in the colon by the chronic laxative abuse. Although the acute therapeutic actions of laxatives stimulate these nerve plexi to promote peristalsis, their chronic use incapacitates the colon's ability to propagate fecal matter and leads to severe constipation.

Noninflammatory swelling of the salivary glands is a common clinical manifestation of BN. The most common psychiatric comorbidities in BN are major depressive disorder, anxiety disorders, substance use disorders, and disruptive behavioral disorders.

Individuals with BED are frequently overweight or obese. However, adults with BED are likely to report the development of diagnoses of metabolic syndrome components (i.e., dyslipidemia, hypertension, type 2 diabetes) after accounting for the contribution of body weight. The presence of BED may impact bariatric surgery (Chapter 207) outcome resulting in less weight loss or more weight regain, but this is not a consistent finding. However, the presence of "loss of control" eating post-surgery consistently predicts less weight loss or greater weight regain. Compared to obese adults without BED, those with the disorder experience significant impairment in a number of domains of psychosocial functioning, including a poorer quality of life and more impaired functioning in their home and social lives. Individuals with BED often have higher levels of disability, health problems, and work productivity impairment compared to obese and healthy controls without binge eating. With regard to comorbid psychiatric diagnoses (Chapter 406), adults with BED experience Axis I psychiatric disorders at a rate comparable to (or higher than) individuals with AN or BN, including major depressive disorder, anxiety disorders, substance use disorders, and disruptive behavioral disorders.

Natural History

AN typically manifests during adolescence, although the disorder can develop prior to puberty. BN frequently develops during later adolescence or early adulthood. BED often manifests in adulthood, but adolescents also present with the disorder. Several retrospective and prospective studies report that binge and "out of control" eating are reported as early as middle childhood.

Data on the natural course of eating disorders in the clear absence of treatment are limited. Eating disorders tend to exhibit a remitting and relapsing natural course across the lifespan, and there appear to be high rates of diagnostic crossover. Treatment outcome data indicate that AN tends to transition to BN or an Unspecified Eating Disorder and those with BN and BED tend to migrate from one to the other.

DIAGNOSIS

A number of structured, well-validated assessments for the diagnosis of eating disorders exist. These include, but are not limited to, the Structured Clinical Interview for the DSM, the Eating Disorder Examination, and the Eating Disorders Assessment for DSM-5 (EDA-5). However, eating disorders are typically diagnosed by review of patient history, symptoms, and behaviors in an interview format. Evaluation of comorbid psychiatric problems, most notably mood, anxiety, substance use disorders, and disruptive behavioral disorders is also required. Information should be gathered on interpersonal relationships, history of sexual and physical abuse, self-harm, and suicidal ideation or behavior. Family involvement is crucial, particularly for pediatric patients. A complete physical examination is recommended for all patients to assess body composition, vital signs, cardiovascular function, hematologic assessment, and blood chemistries.

TREATMENT ℞

Anorexia Nervosa

There is limited evidence on effective treatments for AN, with no FDA-approved medication currently available.[7,8] For severely underweight patients, inpatient medical monitoring and supervised nutrition rehabilitation are required. The optimal setting (inpatient vs. outpatient treatment) remains a subject of debate[9] and the evaluation of treatment costs in AN plays an important role in determining treatment. However, for pediatric patients, family-based psychotherapy, particularly during the early phases of the disorder, has demonstrated effectiveness.[A1] Maudsley's family-based therapy involves both joint family sessions and simultaneous, but independent, patient/family intervention. Antidepressants (e.g., selective serotonin reuptake inhibitors, SSRIs) are associated with high rates of noncompliance and compelling evidence of beneficial effects has not been found. The use of antipsychotic drugs has been explored, but results regarding their effectiveness remain nondefinitive. Furthermore, the treatment potential of neuromodulative techniques such as transcranial direct current stimulation (tDCS), repetitive transcranial magnetic stimulation (rTMS), and deep brain stimulation (DBS) are currently being explored.[10,A2]

Bulimia Nervosa

Cognitive-behavioral therapy (CBT) has been recognized as the treatment of choice for BN.[A3] Interpersonal psychotherapy (IPT) is also effective for the treatment of BN, particularly for those who are nonresponsive to CBT.[11] There is growing support that pharmacotherapy may be helpful for some patients with BN. Antidepressants, especially SSRIs, are modestly effective for reducing binge eating in BN over the short term and long term, with fluoxetine approved by the FDA for treatment of BN.[12] Topiramate has consistently been shown to decrease binge eating in BN, but side effects may limit its usefulness. It is unclear whether combination therapy may be required for optimal outcomes.

Binge Eating Disorder

Psychological treatment for BED aims to reduce binge eating, reduce weight and shape concerns, and prevent excess weight gain and/or induce modest weight loss. The psychotherapies most evaluated in clinical trials include CBT, IPT, behavioral weight loss, and CBT guided self-help approaches (CBTgsh). CBT and IPT are first-line treatments. Given its cost-effectiveness, CBTgsh may be an optimal treatment option when specialist care is not available. Face-to-face CBT leads to quicker and greater reductions in the number of objective binge eating episode days, better abstinence rates, and better eating disorder psychopathologic findings, and may be generally a better initial treatment option than internet-based guided self-help.[A4] With regard to pharmacologic treatment in BED, three medications or classes of medications have been studied in two or more placebo-controlled trials. SSRIs, sibutramine, and topiramate all produce reductions in frequency of binge eating relative to placebo in short-term trials. However, sibutramine was withdrawn from the market and topiramate is frequently associated with problematic cognitive effects, thus limiting its clinical utility. Lisdexamfetamine has been shown to reduce binge eating episodes in RCTs and is currently the only FDA-approved medication for BED in adults.[A5]

PREVENTION

In general, data suggest that media literacy interventions are effective for universal prevention, and cognitive-based approaches are effective for selective prevention of eating disorders.[13] However, most macro-level environmental public health initiatives (i.e., anti-dieting media campaigns and sanctions on advertising practices propagating an ideal of extreme thinness) have not been empirically evaluated. There are more data on individual, micro-level interventions aimed at reducing proximal eating disorder risk factors, as well as current and distal eating pathology. Selected, interactive, multisession programs with adolescent girls may be more effective than universal, didactic, heterogeneous-sampled and single session programs in reducing risk factors for eating disorder symptoms. For example, a dissonance-based program aimed at reducing eating disorder risk factors in adolescent girls has demonstrated effectiveness.[14]

PROGNOSIS

Anorexia Nervosa

Remission rates vary widely for AN. Lower remission rates (29%) have been observed, particularly in studies with the shortest follow-up duration, with relatively higher remission rates (40%) at longer follow-up duration (20 years). However, most individuals with AN (approximately 76%) treated in outpatient settings will remit within 5 years following the initiation of treatment. Most individuals who do not achieve remission from AN during follow-up periods transition to a diagnosis of BN or an Unspecified Eating Disorder, which likely captures partial syndrome AN, though transition to BED or obesity is less likely. Among psychiatric diagnoses, AN consistently has one of the highest mortality rates due to suicide, nutritional deficits, cardiac complications, and substance abuse. The crude cumulative mortality rate is 2.8% with longer

duration of illness prior to receiving treatment and the need for inpatient treatment as negative prognostic indicators for AN. Predictors of relapse include desiring a lower weight at the end of treatment and receiving treatment in a general (versus specialty) clinic, with the highest risk of relapse during the first year after treatment.[15]

Bulimia Nervosa

Similar to AN, most individuals with BN (70% or greater) who receive treatment fully remit when assessed 5 to 20 years later, with remission rates being much lower (27 to 28%) at one-year follow-up. If individuals with BN do not achieve remission within 5 years, however, they are likely to exhibit a chronic course of the illness. Mortality rates for BN range between 0 and 2%. Diagnostic crossover from BN to AN is relatively rare. Yet, there is frequent diagnostic crossover between BN and BED, which may suggest possible common psychological and/or biological maintaining processes. Negative prognostic indicators for BN include endorsement of greater psychiatric comorbidity, multiple impulsive behaviors (e.g., self-harm, substance use disorder), and a family history of alcohol abuse. Individuals who receive inpatient treatment or have a low motivation for engaging in treatment are more likely to relapse.

Binge Eating Disorder

A paucity of data exists on the long-term outcomes for BED patients. There are data to suggest that at 1 year following outpatient treatment, upward of 80% of patients remit. In one clinical trial that examined 4-year outcomes, between 52 and 76% of individuals receiving psychological treatment for BED demonstrated remission from binge eating. These preliminary data suggest that the prognostic trajectory may be similar to BN. Diagnostic crossover from BED to BN is high, whereas crossover to AN is relatively rare. Although examination of prognostic indicators for BED is in its early stages, patients reporting an undue influence of their body shape or weight on self-evaluation are less likely to have remission from binge eating at 12-month follow-up. Rapid remission of binge eating has also been shown to be a positive prognostic indicator for binge remission.

Grade A References

A1. Lock J, Le Grange D, Agras WS, et al. Randomized clinical trial comparing family-based treatment with adolescent-focused individual therapy for adolescents with anorexia nervosa. *Arch Gen Psychiatry.* 2010;67:1025-1032.

A2. Lipsman N, Lam E, Volpini M, et al. Deep brain stimulation of the subcallosal cingulate for treatment-refractory anorexia nervosa: 1 year follow up of an open-label trial. *Lancet Psychiatry.* 2017;4:285-294.

A3. Poulsen S, Lunn S, Daniel SI, et al. A randomized controlled trial of psychoanalytic psychotherapy or cognitive-behavioral therapy for bulimia nervosa. *Am J Psychiatry.* 2014;171:109-116.

A4. de Zwaan M, Herpertz S, Zipfel S, et al. Effect of internet-based guided self-help vs individual face-to-face treatment on full or subsyndromal binge eating disorder in overweight or obese patients: the INTERBED randomized clinical trial. *JAMA Psychiatry.* 2017;74:987-995.

A5. Hudson JI, McElroy SL, Ferreira-Cornwell MC, et al. Efficacy of lisdexamfetamine in adults with moderate to severe binge-eating disorder: a randomized clinical trial. *JAMA Psychiatry.* 2017;74:903-910.

GENERAL REFERENCES

For the General References and other additional features, please visit Expert Consult at https://expertconsult.inkling.com.

207

OBESITY

MICHAEL D. JENSEN

Obesity is the most common nutritional disorder in the United States and directly or indirectly accounts for a significant portion of health-related expenses. The safest treatment approaches (comprehensive lifestyle change with behavior modification) are not commonly employed by physicians and require training and time to implement. The Guideline for the Management of Overweight and Obesity in Adults provides direction for clinicians for the treatment of obesity.

The Guideline for the Management of Overweight and Obesity in Adults produced by the National Institutes of Health and the National Heart, Lung, and Blood Institute (NHLBI) and disseminated by the American College of Cardiology (ACC), the American Heart Association (AHA), and The Obesity Society (TOS) provides evidence-informed, scientifically based recommendations on evaluation and management of overweight and obesity.

Body mass index (BMI) continues to be the recommended approach to categorize weight relative to height for adults. BMI is calculated as weight (in kilograms) divided by height squared (in meters):

$$BMI = \frac{weight\,(kg)}{height^2\,(m^2)}$$

To calculate BMI with pounds and inches, the formula is modified as follows:

$$BMI = \frac{weight\,(lb)}{height^2\,(in^2)} \times 703$$

The guideline did not recommend changes in the weight classifications by BMI, which are summarized in Table 207-1. Individuals who are overweight (BMI of 25.0 to 29.9) are not always overfat—some "overweight" adults have increased muscle mass, which is a straightforward clinical observation. Although, in general, the risk for development of adiposity-related health problems increases continuously as the BMI exceeds 25, the new guideline recommends providers use waist circumference measurements to discriminate among patients who may require more testing. Overweight and class I obese patients with a waist circumference in the high-risk category deserve a discussion of lifestyle issues as they relate to health and weight loss. Some individuals with a BMI of 27 to 29.9 develop serious metabolic complications that improve with weight loss and are candidates for more aggressive treatment, including pharmacotherapy if it is justified. Asian populations, in particular, are at risk for the typical metabolic complications of obesity at lower BMI and waist circumferences than those for whites, Hispanics, blacks, and Polynesians; the guideline for at-risk BMI in Asian populations is 23 to 24.

The prevalence of comorbidities and risk of future morbidities increase considerably at a BMI of more than 30, the cut point for obesity. Obesity is divided into three classes, also depending on BMI (see Table 207-1). Treatment approaches may differ for those who are overweight and for different classes of obesity. Current U.S. Food and Drug Administration (FDA) guidelines indicate that pharmacotherapy can be adjunct treatment for any class of obesity, even if medical complications are not present. Familiarity with the guidelines is important. Supervisory agencies and third-party payers use them to determine who is eligible for treatment benefits. Class III obesity (BMI > 40) is one feature that would prompt consideration of a patient for bariatric surgery when medical treatments have failed. Patients with class II obesity (BMI of 35.0 to 39.9) may be considered for bariatric surgery if medical treatments have failed and if severe, life-threatening complications are present.

Waist circumference measures are recommended as an office assessment tool to help with the treatment decision-making process. The guidelines agree that the waist circumference cut points of more than 102 cm (40 inches) for men and more than 88 cm (35 inches) for women are indicators of increased metabolic risk. The relationships between disease risk and waist circumference are continuous and progressive, with no obvious cut points. The recommendation is to measure waist circumference in overweight and class I obesity adults.

TABLE 207-1	CLASSIFICATION OF OVERWEIGHT AND OBESITY BY BODY MASS INDEX (BMI)	
	OBESITY CLASS	**BMI (kg/m²)**
Underweight		<18.5
Normal		18.5-24.9
Overweight		25.0-29.9
Obesity	I	30.0-34.9
Obesity	II	35.0-39.9
Extreme obesity	III	≥40

From Jensen MD, Ryan DH, Apovian CM, et al. 2013 AHA/ACC/TOS guideline for the management of overweight and obesity in adults: a report of the American College of Cardiology/American Heart Association Task Force on Practice Guidelines and The Obesity Society. *J Am Coll Cardiol.* 2014;63:2985-3023.

Those adults with waist circumferences above the cut points deserve further evaluation to detect other cardiovascular disease risk factors. Adults with class II or class III obesity are at sufficiently high risk that waist circumference information does not add valuable information. These definitions of overweight and obesity and of high-risk waist circumference are generally applicable to those of European and African descent, but lower values are recommended for those of Asian descent. The risks of metabolic abnormalities occur at lower BMI and lower waist circumference in these populations.

Prevalence of Obesity

It has been estimated that a total of 107.7 million children (<20 years of age) and 603.7 million adults were obese worldwide in 2015. Using the Global Burden of Disease study data and methods, excess body weight accounted for about 4 million deaths and 120 million disability adjusted life-years worldwide in 2015.[1] The prevalence of overweight and obese adults in the United States increased dramatically between the 1980s and 2000s, but the increase in the prevalence is now leveling off. The prevalence of obesity was 36.5% (38.3% for women and 34.3% for men) among U.S. adults between 2011 to 2014. Approximately 60% of U.S. men and 51% of U.S. women are overweight or obese. In 2013 to 2016, there were differences in the prevalence of obesity and severe obesity by age, race and Hispanic origin, and household education, and severe obesity was inversely associated with urbanization.[2] There was a significantly greater prevalence of obesity and severe obesity among adults living in nonmetropolitan compared with large metropolitan statistical areas.[3] There are substantial differences in the prevalence of obesity by age, race, and socioeconomic status. The prevalence of obesity in adults tends to rise steadily from the ages of 20 to 60 years, decreasing in later years. It has been estimated that almost 75% of men aged 60 to 69 years in the United States have a BMI of more than 25.

Because young adults will accumulate greater exposure to metabolic and mechanical damage from being overweight or obese throughout their lives, they are at increased risk for chronic health conditions such as coronary heart disease and type 2 diabetes mellitus.[4] By comparison, the increase in mean BMI with age, though deleterious, is not as much of a threat to population health as is a similar increase in the BMI of younger populations. A study involving 62,565 Danish men whose weights and heights had been measured at 7 and 13 years of age and in early adulthood (ages 17 to 26) found that childhood overweight at 7 years of age was associated with increased risk of adult type 2 diabetes only if it continued until puberty or later ages.[5]

The lowest mortality rates for young adults have historically been for a BMI in the normal range (20.0 to 24.9),[6] whereas the BMI associated with the lowest mortality rates is somewhat above 25 kg/m² for those in their 60s and 70s. Data also suggest that the optimal BMI may be evolving as we live longer. For example, a recent large Danish study found a gradual increase in ideal BMI from 23.7 to 27.0 from the late 1970s to the 21st century.[7] Because of this, providers should base their weight recommendations for individual patients on whether adverse health consequences associated with obesity are present.

The differences in overweight and obesity among African Americans, Mexican Americans, and European Americans are not subtle. African American women and Mexican Americans of both sexes have the highest rates of overweight and obesity in the United States. In interpreting these data, however, it is important to keep in mind that there is an inverse relationship between socioeconomic status and obesity, especially among women (Chapter 4). Women in lower socioeconomic classes are much more likely than those in higher socioeconomic classes to be obese. This association reduces but does not eliminate the racial differences in the prevalence of obesity. Whether the remaining racial differences in the prevalence of obesity are due to genetic, constitutional, or social factors is not yet known.

Etiology

Genetic and constitutional susceptibility to obesity are heavily influenced by the environment. Studies of twins adopted into different families indicate that within a given environment, a significant portion of the variation in weight is genetic.[8] That said, the remarkable increase in the prevalence of obesity in the United States during the past 3 decades cannot be explained by changes in the genetic makeup of Americans.

Genetic Aspects of Human Obesity

Although obesity susceptibility is a classic polygenic condition, there are also a number of syndromic and monogenic obesity syndromes. The genetic defects resulting in obesity include Prader-Willi and Laurence-Moon-Biedl syndromes. Rare monogenic forms of human obesity can be due to mutations in the leptin gene, the leptin receptor gene, and the melanocortin signaling system genes.[9] These gene mutations are associated with increased appetite rather than with reduced energy expenditure. Genome-wide association studies have revealed a number of genes associated with higher BMI. Those that appear to predict the greatest amount of variance in BMI include the fat mass and obesity-associated (*FTO*) gene and the melanocortin-4 receptor (*MC4R*) gene. Other genes that have been associated with obesity include *TMEM18*, *KCTD15*, *GNPDA2*, *SH2B1*, *MTCH2*, and *NEGR1*. Together, however, the combined effects of all the identified genetic contributions account for less than 1% of the variance in BMI. This emphasizes both the huge environmental effects and the polygenic nature of susceptibility to obesity.[10]

Constitutional Influences on Obesity

Environmental factors can result in long-term, epigenetic effects that affect body weight regulation and the susceptibility to obesity-related health problems. These epigenetic effects are ascribed to changes in DNA methylation, acetylation, and chromatin remodeling. The effect of the intrauterine environment and the perinatal period on subsequent weight and health is best studied. Undernutrition in the last trimester of pregnancy and in the early postnatal period decreases the risk of adult obesity, although the low birthweight associated with undernutrition (or smoking) in late pregnancy also increases the risk of adulthood hypertension, abnormal glucose tolerance, and cardiovascular disease. In contrast, undernutrition limited to the first two trimesters of pregnancy is associated with an increased probability of adult obesity. The infants of diabetic mothers tend to be fatter than those of nondiabetic mothers, and children of diabetic mothers have a greater prevalence of obesity when they are 5 to 19 years old, independent of whether their mother is obese. Finally, intrauterine exposure to the diabetic environment results in an increased risk of diabetes mellitus and obesity in the offspring. Thus the issue of the genes versus the environment in regard to obesity and metabolic complications of obesity is blurred in the intrauterine and perinatal time intervals. Worrisome aspects of these metabolic effects are the long-term effects on the individual's weight regulation and health and the likelihood that these traits can be passed on to future generations.

Environmental Contributors to Human Obesity

Dramatic changes in the environment of Western countries over the past 50 years include reduced demands for physical activity and alterations in the food supply. These food supply changes appear to have either increased or prevented the expected decrease in energy intake that would be needed to match the reduced energy expenditure from physical activity.

Food

Some of the environmental factors can influence food intake are listed in Table 207-2. Consuming energy-dense foods results in greater energy intake because adults tend to respond to food volume rather than to the energy content. This factor likely accounts for the association between high-fat diets and excess body weight; many high-fat foods are also energy dense. When humans consume diets that are high in fat but low in energy density, energy intake is not greater than would be expected on the basis of the energy density of the foods. There is evidence that consuming sugar-sweetened beverages, such as soft drinks and fruit juices, is not accompanied by a decrease in food

TABLE 207-2	ENVIRONMENTAL FACTORS PROMOTING OBESITY	
DIETARY	**ACTIVITY**
↑ Energy density of foods	↑ Sedentary behavior
↑ Portion size	↓ Activities of daily living
↑ Variety*	↓ Employment-related physical activity
↑ Palatability	
↑ Availability	
↓ Cost	
↑ Caloric beverages (sugar-sweetened beverages)	

*Variety of sweets, snacks, and entrees.

intake to offset the extra energy intake. The implication is that some types of beverages will increase energy intake and promote weight gain. Larger food portion size also increases food intake. The trend to serve larger portions of food and beverages in the United States could contribute to greater obesity risk. Food variety can also affect energy intake. An increased variety of entrees, sweets, snacks, and carbohydrates in the diet is associated with an increase in body fatness and food intake. In contrast, an increase in the variety of vegetables available does not appear to increase energy intake and is not associated with increased body fatness. Other factors that may have broad population effects in the United States include the reduced costs of food, increased availability, and palatability.

Psychological factors such as dietary restraint or disinhibition, as well as the social context in which the food is present, can influence how the food properties affect energy intake.

Physical Activity

Physical activity can be divided into three categories: (1) exercise (fitness- and sports-related activities); (2) work-related physical activity; and (3) nonexercise, nonemployment (spontaneous) activity. Online resources are available that allow one to calculate energy expenditure on the basis of weight, type, and duration of exercise. Only about 20 to 30% of Americans engage in exercise at the recommended frequency, intensity, or duration that could be expected to substantially reduce the chances of developing obesity and related health problems, but this does not seem to have changed in recent decades. The amount of time spent in sedentary activities (e.g., watching television, using the computer) is an independent predictor of metabolic abnormalities associated with obesity over and above the effects of exercise. Thus to the extent that reduced physical activity is contributing to the epidemic of obesity, it is likely that it is reduced employment-related and spontaneous physical activity that is changing.

Although it is becoming easier for individuals to measure the energy expended in nonexercise activity with step counters and electronic motion sensors, there are limited longitudinal, population-based data that quantitates the changes in this activity. Certainly, employment-related physical activity has decreased with the advent of more automated systems in the workplace. Analysis of data from the U.S. Bureau of Labor Statistics indicates that since 1960 employment-related physical activity has decreased enough to reduce mean daily energy expenditure by over 100 calories/day.

The energy Americans expend performing the activities of daily living has probably been reduced by labor-saving conveniences (e.g., drive-through food and banking, escalators, remote controls, e-mail, online shopping). Although there are few hard data to assess how much of a change has actually occurred, a reduction in daily walking trips and an increase in daily automobile trips have been documented.

There is a large amount of information on how differences in sedentary activity (television watching, video games, and computer use) relate to obesity and obesity complications. The evidence indicates that more time spent in sedentary pursuits is associated with an increased risk of overweight and obesity. The striking aspect to these studies is that the adverse effect of sedentary activities is independent of participation in traditional exercise activities.

Providers who are aware of the decreases in work-related physical activity and activities of daily living, as well as the increases in sedentary behavior, can help their patients uncover patterns that may relate to weight gain. Likewise, providers who understand the effects of environmental factors can better help their obese patients identify the environmental factors that are contributing to the problem and thus to help them develop intervention plans. In this regard, patients who regularly use step counters or other types of activity-monitoring devices will be better able to self-identify and modify their behavior to obtain sufficient physical activity.

Regulation of Body Weight and Energy Balance

The regulation of adult body weight is a well-balanced process. The typical U.S. adult will take in and expend approximately 2000 to 3000 kcal/day. Consistent errors of even 1% in excess food consumption can result in body fat gain of 25 to 30 pounds in 10 years, assuming no change in energy expenditure. It follows that many adults regulate their average energy balance with greater than 1% precision. There appears to be regulation of both energy intake and energy expenditure through conscious and unconscious processes.

The excess energy consumed by adults is generally stored as triglycerides in adipocytes. Humans continuously recruit new adipocytes from a large preadipocyte pool to replace dying adipocytes. Although the primary means by which abdominal adipose tissue mass expands is through increased fat cell size (adipocyte hypertrophy), this process can store only a limited amount of fat. Adults who gain leg fat accumulate more rather than larger adipocytes on average, resulting in a net increase in adipocyte number as more new adipocytes are created than needed to replace dying cells. Some adults appear to recruit new adipocytes more readily than others do and if they gain body fat will do so more from adipocyte hyperplasia (increased fat cell number) than from hypertrophy. Those who gain fat with large adipocytes are more likely to be insulin resistant.

Leptin is a hormone that is secreted by adipocytes. As such, leptin is one of the most important of the so-called adipokines.[11] Low leptin, such as is seen with leptin deficiency or extreme loss of body fat, results in extreme hunger, which can be reduced by administering leptin. Leptin also has other hypothalamic-pituitary functions and is proposed to have diverse peripheral physiologic actions. The leptin-deficient animal model of obesity, the *ob/ob* mouse, is severely obese, hyperphagic, hypometabolic, and sexually immature and has low levels of spontaneous activity; leptin administration corrects all of these defects. A few leptin-deficient humans (due to mutations in the leptin gene) have been identified. These severely obese children had very low plasma leptin concentrations, were hyperphagic, and responded to exogenous leptin administration with dramatic weight loss, reduced food intake, and accelerated maturation of the pituitary-gonadal axis. Obese humans are almost never leptin deficient and in fact have high plasma leptin concentrations unless they are in a major negative energy balance circumstance. Screening for leptin deficiency is not warranted except in severe, hyperphagic obesity that begins in early childhood, is accompanied by sexual immaturity, and exists in the absence of other known causes (e.g., Prader-Willi syndrome).

Some animal models of genetic obesity (the *db/db* mouse and *fa/fa* rat) have defective leptin receptors, making them unresponsive to leptin. There are very rare cases of obese humans with defective leptin receptor genes. Clinical screening for leptin receptor mutations is not warranted, given that no treatment exists.

Energy Intake

Much of what has been learned about the biologic regulation of food intake has been from the study of animal models. These signals may affect different aspects of eating behavior. They can affect *hunger,* the compelling need or desire for food; *satiation,* the state of being satisfactorily full and unable to take on more; or *satiety,* the sense of no longer being hungry, a complex set of postprandial events that affect the interval to the next meal or the amount consumed at the next meal. Some of the signals alter just one aspect of eating behavior and others affect multiple aspects. For example, ghrelin, a peptide produced by the stomach, increases hunger but does not appear to affect satiation or satiety. Cholecystokinin causes satiation but has no effect on satiety. Leptin appears to act on multiple pathways; leptin deficiency is associated with increased hunger and reduced satiation and satiety.

Peripheral satiety signals act to inhibit further food intake at some point during meal consumption. Some of the signals reach the brain through the vagus nerve and some through the systemic circulation. Examples of the factors thought to modulate appetite are listed in Table 207-3. The compounds range from gut-derived (ghrelin, cholecystokinin, glucagon-like peptide 1) and pancreas-derived (insulin and amylin) hormones to peptides such as apolipoprotein A-IV, which is secreted with chylomicrons. The signals are thought to be triggered both by mechanical stimuli (e.g., the fullness of the stomach) and by the presence of nutrients in the jejunum and ileum.

The central nervous system regulation of food intake, energy expenditure, and peripheral metabolism (or the so-called gut-brain axis) is becoming better understood.[12] A number of neuropeptides, lipid derivatives, and monoamines have either anabolic (increased food intake with or without decreased energy expenditure) or catabolic (decreased food intake with or without increased energy expenditure) properties. A list of these molecules is provided in Table 207-4. Many of these compounds serve more than one function, such as regulation of hormone secretion (thyrotropin-releasing hormone and corticotropin-releasing hormone), wakefulness (norepinephrine), and behavior-reinforcing systems (endocannabinoids).

Energy Expenditure

There is a wide range of daily energy expenditure in adults, from less than 1400 kcal/day to more than 5000 kcal/day, with larger, more physically active individuals having the greatest energy needs. Typically, daily energy expenditure is divided into resting (or basal) metabolic rate, the thermic effect of food, and physical activity energy expenditure.

Basal Metabolic Rate

The basal metabolic rate (BMR) is the energy expenditure of lying still at rest, awake, in the overnight postabsorptive state. The resting metabolic rate (RMR) is similarly defined but is not necessarily measured before arising from bed. For most sedentary adult Americans, the RMR represents the major portion of energy expended during the day and may range from less than 1200 to more than 3000 kcal/day. Most (~80%) of the variability in BMR can be explained by how much lean and fat tissue an individual has. In addition, BMR is slightly lower in women than men and older than younger adults even after accounting for the amount of lean and fat tissue. There is evidence for heritable or family factors that influence BMR, accounting for as much as 10% of the interindividual differences. There are both obligatory and facultative components to RMR. With an energy-restricted diet, significant reductions in BMR relative to the amount of fat-free mass occur. Reductions in the production of triiodothyronine from thyroxine and the sympathetic nervous system drive are thought to contribute to this phenomenon. Likewise, during brief periods of overfeeding, RMR increases slightly above that which would be expected for the amount of lean tissue present. There are a number of formulas that can be used to estimate BMR. The Harris-Benedict formula (available through numerous online calculators) predicts BMR on the basis of height, weight, age, and sex and is accurate to within 10% in approximately 90% of adults with BMIs of 18.5 to 45 kg/m^2.

In contrast to what is typically thought, muscle accounts for only 25% of RMR, but during exercise muscle can account for 80 to 90% of energy expenditure. Adipose tissue is a minor contributor to daily energy expenditure, consuming only approximately 3 kcal/kg of body fat per day.

Brown fat is adipose tissue that expresses large amounts of uncoupling protein-1, a protein that allows a mitochondrial membrane proton leak,

TABLE 207-3 SUGGESTED BIOLOGIC MODULATORS OF FOOD INTAKE

PERIPHERAL SIGNAL	PROPOSED EFFECT ON FOOD INTAKE
Vagal	−
Cholecystokinin	−
Apolipoprotein A-IV	−
Insulin	−
Amylin	−
Peptide YY$_{3-36}$	−
Glucagon-like peptide 1	−
Oxyntomodulin	−
Leptin	+ when leptin ↓↓
Ghrelin	+
Obestatin	−

TABLE 207-4 CENTRAL NERVOUS SYSTEM MODULATORS OF ENERGY BALANCE

CENTRAL ANABOLIC (↑ INTAKE)	CENTRAL CATABOLIC (↓ INTAKE)
Neuropeptide Y	α-Melanocyte-stimulating hormone
Agouti-related protein	Corticotropin-releasing hormone
Melanin-concentrating hormone	Thyrotropin-releasing hormone
Hypocretins and orexins	Cocaine- and amphetamine-regulated transcript
Galanin	Interleukin-1β
Norepinephrine	Urocortin
Endogenous endocannabinoids (anandamide and 2-arachidonoylglycerol)	Oxytocin
	Neurotensin
	Serotonin

resulting in heat release as opposed to chemical work from adenosine triphosphate—"uncoupling" of substrate oxidation from chemical or mechanical work. This thermogenic tissue was thought to be present only in human infants but does exist in small amounts in adults. Because of the high metabolic activity of brown adipose tissue and its potential role in stimulating energy expenditure (i.e., resting energy expenditure and possibly thermogenesis) it is an attractive target for interventions to reduce adiposity.[13] Methods used to detect brown fat largely rely on ^{18}F-fluorodeoxyglucose positron emission tomography scanning of humans exposed to cold.

Measurement of BMR is sometimes helpful in the evaluation of patients who insist that they are unable to lose weight while following diets containing less than 1000 kcal/day. Almost without fail, if BMR is measured with a reliable instrument, it is substantially greater than the reported food intake. This underscores the fact that most adults are unreliable in assessing their own food intake.

The Thermic Effect of Food

An average of 10% of the energy content of food is expended in the process of digestion, absorption, and metabolism of nutrients. There is a significant interindividual variability in this value, however, ranging from a low of about 3% to a high of about 15% of meal calories that are "wasted" in the postprandial interval.

Secondary Causes of Obesity
Medications

A number of medications cause weight gain in some or most of the patients for whom they are prescribed. Awareness of the medications that have this potential can facilitate weight loss treatment in some patients. Table 207-5 lists a number of medications that are associated with weight gain as well as alternative treatment approaches, if any, for the underlying condition.

Diseases

Less than 1% of obese patients have an underlying disease that can explain the development of their obesity. Endocrinopathies are the most common secondary cause of obesity. These include Cushing syndrome (Chapter 214), hypothalamic damage resulting in overeating (most commonly after pituitary surgery), insulinoma (Chapter 217), and hypothyroidism (Chapter 213). A Cushing syndrome–like fat distribution is common; therefore other physical or laboratory findings are the best clues to whether to test for this condition. These include the classic purple striae, thinning skin, easy bruising, proximal muscle weakness, and electrolyte abnormalities. Correction of Cushing syndrome commonly results in substantial loss of excess body fat. Insulinoma is a rare tumor, and only a small portion of patients with insulinoma develop obesity. The weight gain associated with hypothyroidism is largely due to fluid retention and resolves with thyroid hormone replacement. Unfortunately, successful treatment is not available for hyperphagia due to hypothalamic damage. Adult patients with growth hormone deficiency, most commonly after hypophysectomy, may lose excess body fat with growth hormone replacement therapy.

Psychosocial Aspects of Obesity

Sexual, physical, and emotional abuse, especially in women, can result in long-term adverse consequences, including obesity. The effects of the abuse tend to be most profound if it occurs in childhood and adolescence. These women may be severely obese, suffer from chronic depression, and experience a number of psychosomatic symptoms, particularly chronic gastrointestinal distress. Identifying these issues before initiation of weight loss programs is important because successful weight loss may actually aggravate the distress experienced by these women. In addition, appropriate referral for psychiatric help may be needed before initiation of treatment for obesity.

PATHOPHYSIOLOGY
Metabolic Complications of Obesity

A central or upper body fat distribution is more predictive than total fat mass of the metabolic complications of obesity. Adipose tissue release of free fatty acids (FFAs) and glycerol into the circulation through lipolysis provides 50 to 100% of daily energy needs. Adipose tissue lipolysis is regulated primarily by insulin (inhibition) and catecholamines (stimulation), although growth hormone, cortisol, and atrial natriuretic peptide also stimulate lipolysis. Upper body obesity is associated with several abnormalities of adipose tissue lipolysis, most remarkably with higher postprandial FFA release and concentrations; this abnormality is particularly evident in type 2 diabetes mellitus. Abnormally

TABLE 207-5	PHARMACOLOGIC INFLUENCES IN WEIGHT GAIN AND ALTERNATIVE THERAPIES	
DRUGS THAT MAY PROMOTE WEIGHT GAIN	**ALTERNATIVE TREATMENTS: WEIGHT NEUTRAL OR WEIGHT LOSS**
PSYCHIATRIC AND NEUROLOGIC MEDICATIONS	**ALTERNATIVE PSYCHIATRIC AND NEUROLOGIC MEDICATIONS**
Antipsychotics: olanzapine, clozapine, risperidone, quetiapine, aripiprazole	Ziprasidone
Antidepressants	Nortriptyline, bupropion, nefazodone, fluvoxamine, sertraline, duloxetine
Tricyclics: imipramine, amitriptyline	Topiramate, zonisamide (weight loss), lamotrigine (less weight gain)
Triazolopyridines: trazodone	
Serotonin reuptake inhibitors: paroxetine, fluoxetine, citalopram	
Tetracyclics: mirtazapine	
Monoamine oxidase inhibitors	
Antiepileptic drugs: gabapentin (higher doses), valproic acid, carbamazepine, divalproex	
Mood stabilizers: lithium, carbamazepine, lamotrigine, gabapentin (higher doses)	
STEROID HORMONES	**ALTERNATIVES TO STEROID HORMONES**
Progestational steroids	Barrier methods, intrauterine device
Corticosteroids	Nonsteroidal anti-inflammatory drugs
Hormonal contraceptives	
ANTIDIABETES AGENTS	**ALTERNATIVE ANTIDIABETES AGENTS**
Insulin (most forms)	Metformin
Sulfonylureas	Acarbose, miglitol
Thiazolidinediones	Exenatide
	Dipeptidyl peptidase 4 inhibitors
	Liraglutide
	Sodium-glucose cotransporter 2 inhibitors
ANTIHISTAMINES	**ALTERNATIVES TO ANTIHISTAMINES**
Commonly reported with older agents; also oxatomide, loratadine, and azelastine	Decongestants, mast cell stabilizers, antagonists of endogenous mediators of inflammation
ANTIHYPERTENSIVE AGENTS	**ALTERNATIVE ANTIHYPERTENSIVE AGENTS**
α-Adrenergic and β-adrenergic receptor blockers	Angiotensin-converting enzyme inhibitors
Calcium channel blockers: nisoldipine	Angiotensin receptor blockers
	Calcium channel blockers: most other agents
	Diuretics
HIGHLY ACTIVE ANTIRETROVIRAL THERAPY	

high FFA concentrations can contribute to a number of the metabolic complications of obesity.

Insulin Resistance

The term *insulin resistance* is typically used in referring to the ability of insulin to promote glucose uptake and to inhibit the release of glucose into the circulation. The primary site of insulin-stimulated glucose uptake, oxidation, and storage is skeletal muscle. The principal site of glucose production is the liver. Insulin resistance initially leads to hyperinsulinemia and may eventually lead to the development of type 2 diabetes mellitus if β-cell exhaustion occurs (Chapter 216).

The ability of insulin to promote glucose uptake, oxidation, and storage in muscle and to suppress plasma FFA concentrations is reduced in upper body obesity. High plasma FFA concentrations can induce a state of insulin resistance both in the muscle (glucose uptake) and in the liver (glucose release), independent of obesity. Thus abnormal regulation of adipose tissue FFA export is a significant component of the development of insulin resistance. It is hypothesized that excess FFAs induce muscle insulin resistance by promoting increased synthesis of diacylglycerols and ceramides, both of which can interfere with the normal insulin signaling pathway.

Dysregulated production of a number of adipose-derived hormones, also called adipokines, is hypothesized to contribute to insulin resistance and the metabolic complications of obesity. Adiponectin, an adipocyte-derived hormone that improves insulin action, is secreted at reduced rates in obesity and diabetes. Increased production of resistin, interleukin-6, and tumor necrosis factor by adipose tissue has been linked to insulin resistance in animal models. We currently lack the experimental evidence from human studies to know what role adipokines play in the metabolic complications of obesity.

Islet Cell Failure and Type 2 Diabetes Mellitus

Type 2 diabetes usually results from defects in both insulin secretion and insulin action (Chapter 216). Many obese individuals are insulin resistant, yet only a subset will develop diabetes mellitus. It follows that those who develop type 2 diabetes develop pancreatic β-cell decompensation with subsequent hyperglycemia. Animal (rodent) studies have suggested that a process referred to as lipotoxicity is involved in pancreatic β-cell failure. In this model, increased FFAs are proposed to contribute to the insulin secretory abnormalities seen in obesity and ultimately to lead to β-cell failure. There is some evidence that elevated FFAs have adverse effects on islet β-cell function in humans.

Hypertension

Blood pressure can be increased by a number of mechanisms (Chapter 70). Increased circulating blood volume, abnormal vasoconstriction, decreased vascular relaxation, and increased cardiac output may all contribute to hypertension in obesity. The effect of hyperinsulinemia to increase renal sodium absorption may contribute to hypertension through increased circulating blood volume. Abnormalities of vascular resistance also contribute to the pathophysiologic process of obesity-related hypertension. Under some experimental conditions, elevated FFAs have been found to cause increased vasoconstriction and reduced nitric oxide–mediated vasorelaxation, similar to that seen in the metabolic syndrome. Some obese adults have increased sympathetic nervous system activity, which could contribute to obesity-associated hypertension. Finally, angiotensinogen (also produced by adipocytes) is a precursor of the vasoconstrictor angiotensin II and is proposed to contribute to elevated blood pressure.

Dyslipidemia

Upper body obesity and type 2 diabetes mellitus are associated with increased triglycerides, decreased high-density lipoprotein (HDL) cholesterol, and a high proportion of small, low-density lipoprotein (LDL) particles (Chapter 195). This dyslipidemia contributes to the increased cardiovascular risk observed in the metabolic syndrome. Fasting hypertriglyceridemia is caused by increased hepatic very low density lipoprotein (VLDL) secretion, which may be driven by increased delivery of FFAs to the liver coming from both visceral fat and upper body subcutaneous fat. The reduced HDL cholesterol concentrations and the increased small, dense LDL particle concentrations associated with upper body obesity are likely an indirect consequence of elevated triglyceride-rich VLDL. Increased cholesterol ester transfer protein activity and hepatic lipase activity can theoretically account for the atherogenic shifts in triglycerides and cholesterol between lipoproteins. Genetic influences play a significant role in the expression of these lipid abnormalities. Polymorphisms in the genes for apolipoprotein E, lipoprotein lipase, apolipoprotein B-100, and apolipoprotein A-II are correlated with increased triglycerides and decreased HDL.

Endocrine Manifestations of Obesity

Obesity is associated with abnormalities of the endocrine system, one of the most common being polycystic ovary syndrome. This syndrome (Chapter 223) is characterized by mild hirsutism and irregular menses or amenorrhea with anovulatory cycles. It is most commonly linked with obesity and often improves with weight loss and other treatments that improve insulin resistance.

The insulin resistance associated with obesity may trigger the development of polycystic ovary syndrome in susceptible individuals. Whereas mild to moderate androgen overproduction is a feature of upper body obesity in women, obese men may suffer from mild to severe hypothalamic hypogonadism. This androgen deficiency improves with weight loss, and attempts to treat this condition with testosterone replacement offer little clinical benefit. There has been some concern that testosterone treatment of obese men may increase the risk of obstructive sleep apnea and perhaps even cardiovascular events. Although estrogens are not elevated in obese premenopausal women, they remain somewhat above postmenopausal levels in obese postmenopausal women. Serum growth hormone concentrations are often low in obese adults, but insulin-like growth factor-I concentrations are often normal, and growth hormone concentrations increase with weight loss. Treatment of these patients with growth hormone has been reported to worsen insulin resistance and glucose intolerance and cannot be justified, considering the costs and poor risk-to-benefit ratio.

Mechanical Complications of Obesity

The excess body weight associated with obesity is thought to be responsible for the increased prevalence of lower extremity degenerative joint disease. Extreme obesity can result in premature degenerative joint disease, and this may be especially difficult to treat surgically, given the greater stress on joint replacements. Severely obese individuals may also have problems with venous stasis, which is occasionally aggravated by right-sided heart failure (see later).

Obstructive Sleep Apnea and Sleep Restriction

Sleep apnea (Chapter 377) is common in severely obese patients, tending to be more prevalent in men and in women with an upper body/visceral obesity. Sleep apnea is most likely explained by enlargement of upper airway soft tissue, resulting in collapse of the upper airways with inspiration during sleep. The obstruction leads to apneas, with hypoxemia, hypercarbia, and high catecholamine and endothelin levels. The frequent arousals to restore breathing result in poor sleep quality. Sleep apnea is associated with an increased risk of hypertension, and if sleep apnea is severe, it can lead to right-sided heart failure and sudden death. A history of daytime hypersomnolence, loud snoring, restless sleep, or morning headaches is suggestive of obstructive sleep apnea. Treatment of sleep apnea is important to improve cardiovascular risk, and the failure to recognize and to treat this complication may make weight loss intervention strategies much less successful.

Epidemiologic studies have linked short sleep duration and disruptions of circadian rhythm with increased risk of metabolic syndrome and diabetes. Experimentally induced sleep restriction combined with circadian disruption in humans led to decreased RMR and increased postprandial plasma glucose levels due to inadequate insulin secretion.

Cancer

The risk of breast cancer and endometrial cancer is increased in obese women (Chapter 170). It is thought that this may be due to the increased estrogen levels associated with obesity in the postmenopausal woman. Obese men also have a higher mortality risk from cancers of the prostate and colon. The reasons for this association are unknown. The International Agency for Research on Cancer Working Group identified the following additional cancers for which there is now sufficient evidence that the absence of body fatness lowers cancer risk: esophageal, gastric cardia, colorectal, liver, gallbladder, pancreas, ovary, renal cell, meningioma, thyroid, and multiple myeloma.[14]

Gastrointestinal Disorders

Gastroesophageal reflux disease and gallstones are more prevalent in obese patients. Likewise, fatty liver and nonalcoholic steatohepatitis (Chapter 143) is strongly associated with overweight, obesity, and the metabolic syndrome.[15] Nonalcoholic steatohepatitis can eventually progress to life-threatening hepatic cirrhosis. Weight loss and interventions that improve insulin sensitivity have been shown to improve fatty liver and nonalcoholic steatohepatitis.

DIAGNOSIS

Evaluation of Obesity

In the office practice, obtaining height and weight allows calculation of BMI. For patients with a BMI above 25 and below 35, a second piece of information—the waist circumference—provides an added indicator as to whether the patient is at greater risk for adverse consequences (see earlier). Measurement of blood pressure (which may require a large blood pressure cuff) then provides a third item of health information at almost no cost. The presence or absence of dyslipidemia (HDL cholesterol < 45 mg/dL for women, HDL cholesterol < 35 mg/dL for men, or triglycerides > 150 mg/dL), hypertension, glucose intolerance and diabetes, and hyperuricemia should be documented. A history suggestive of sleep apnea should prompt a referral for overnight oximetry or a sleep disorder evaluation.

A review of the patient's lifestyle, including an assessment of physical activity level and eating habits, may help provide information about why the patient is obese. A family history of obesity, or long-standing obesity, provides evidence against a secondary cause of obesity. A careful medication history, including over-the-counter medications, and social history may help the clinician identify precipitating factors that can be modified. By emphasizing the role of modifiable lifestyle factors that predispose to disease risk, as opposed to focusing solely on the patient's weight, it may be possible to initiate a conversation about weight/disease management in a less threatening manner from the patient's perspective.

Before a patient enters a weight management program, it is helpful to ensure that the patient is interested and ready to make lifestyle changes and has realistic goals and expectations. Patients who expect to lose large amounts of weight in a short time are virtually doomed to disappointment. Medical treatment programs, even if they include pharmacotherapy, struggle to routinely achieve sustained weight loss of more than 10%. Although this amount of weight loss is sufficient to markedly reduce the medical complications of obesity, disappointment with "only" 10% weight loss may cause patients to abandon a medically successful program. Helping the patient to accept that lifestyle changes resulting in achievable (10%) weight loss is a reasonable, initial goal can be challenging for a physician.

It is sometimes necessary to delay entry into any treatment program if a patient is not ready to make lifestyle changes. Every form of treatment currently available requires some degree of lifestyle accommodation, and those uninterested in doing so should be advised to reconsider their goals at a later date. A reasonable strategy is to periodically remind the patient of the health benefits of improved activity and eating habits and reconsider efforts once a willingness to make changes is apparent.

TREATMENT   Rx

Obesity represents an individual's response to the environment based on genetics and learned behavior and is best viewed as a chronic disease. Therefore treatment must be considered a long-term issue, much like diabetes, hypertension, or dyslipidemia. Substantial weight loss can be induced through severe dietary calorie restriction, but without approaches to ensure behavioral changes, body fat is invariably regained. To the extent that environmental factors contribute to a patient's overweight status, and to the extent that the macroenvironment is unlikely to change, patients must learn how to make permanent lifestyle changes (eating and activity behavior) to hope for permanent weight loss. Behavior modification approaches,[16] which can help patients recognize and circumvent environmental cues for sedentary behavior and overeating, can increase the likelihood that patients will accomplish these lifestyle changes.[A1] A randomized study has shown that intensive lifestyle intervention (compared with only support and education) is associated with fewer hospitalizations, fewer medications, and lower health care costs in overweight or obese adults with type 2 diabetes.[A2]

Reducing energy intake is the most efficient and effective means to lose weight.[17] For example, creating a 500 kcal/day deficit by reduced food intake will initially theoretically result in the loss of 1 pound of fat per week. It is more difficult to increase energy expenditure by 500 kcal/day through exercise. Greater amounts of physical activity can prevent weight gain (or weight regain after weight loss). Some patients are able to change eating and activity habits on their own, given the proper information, whereas others require formal or informal behavior modification interventions (see later) to help make these changes. In some instances, pharmacotherapy, endoscopic obesity treatments or bariatric surgery may be needed for treatment of obesity. A flow diagram on how to evaluate and to manage patients with overweight and obesity is presented in Figure 207-1.

Diet

Changes in eating habits must be permanent if weight loss is to be maintained. An experienced registered dietitian can be helpful in the evaluation of a patient's eating habits and will be able to provide the needed education. The diet history may identify eating behaviors that result in excess energy intake. Although it is important to address specific adverse eating behaviors, patients need to understand some general principles regarding diet. Reducing the energy density of food (most commonly accomplished by reducing dietary fat) can allow patients to feel satiated while consuming fewer calories. A consensus recommendation is that providers prescribe 1200 to 1500 kcal/day for women and 1500 to 1800 kcal/day for men.[18] Alternatively, diets that produce an energy deficit of 500 to 750 kcal/day can be recommended. Because there appears to be no clear superiority of one diet over another (e.g., low-carbohydrate compared with low-fat) with regard to weight loss,[A3] it is recommended that providers prescribe one of the evidence-based diets that restricts selected food types (e.g., high-carbohydrate foods, low-fiber foods, or high-fat foods) to create an energy deficit by reduced food intake as well as to address issues such as dyslipidemia, diabetes, and hypertension. Patients should be informed that consuming foods high in water and fiber (fruits, vegetables, legumes, and soups) can provide satiety without excess calories. Patients also should be counseled to reduce the intake of beverages containing substantial calories, most often sugar-sweetened beverages. Finally, a regular pattern of eating should be encouraged.

Commercial weight-loss programs (Weight Watchers, Jenny Craig, Nutrisystem) generally result in 2 to 4% more weight loss than usual education and counseling.[A4] Contrary to expectations, however, the opportunity to choose what diet to follow does not necessarily improve weight loss.

New diets are continually being promoted with the promise of easy weight loss. A common feature of these diets is the claim that special properties of certain foods help people lose weight or are the cause of obesity. If followed, most of these diets result in weight loss because of a reduced energy intake. The reduced intake can often be explained by the monotony of the diet, and no diets have been identified that cause persons to lose weight out of accordance with physiologic principles. Although a number of dietary approaches can be successful in promoting weight loss, if there is no peer-reviewed evidence for safety and success of new diets, a review by a dietitian for nutritional safety is warranted. The NHLBI/AHA/ACC/TOS obesity guideline concluded that many types of diets are able to help patients achieve long-term, medically significant weight loss. Thus it may be less important what specific type of diet (DASH diet, Mediterranean diet, high-carbohydrate/low-fat or high-fat/low-carbohydrate diet) is recommended than for the patient to find dietary adherence to be relatively easy. A comprehensive lifestyle intervention that includes a high-intensity, on-site behavioral intervention provides the best results.

Very low calorie diets (<800 calories per day) are still used to achieve accelerated weight loss. Because the long-term results of these diets are no better and sometimes worse than the results from the standard low-calorie diet combined with behavior modification, these diets are not commonly used. The expensive laboratory monitoring required for very low calorie diets without an improved long-term outcome raises questions about the costs versus benefits of this approach.

Physical Activity

A long-term increase in physical activity, either through the activities of daily living or through regular exercise, is key to preventing weight regain, thereby increasing the amount of successful, long-term weight loss.[A5] Unfortunately, many overweight and obese patients are unfit, being unable to walk even 1 mile continuously. It is not possible for most adults to expend a great deal of energy through exercise. For example, only about 100 kcal are expended by a 70-kg adult walking one mile. Losing weight solely by increasing exercise is impractical for most patients. However, increasing physical activity as a means of maintaining weight loss is an attainable goal for most patients.

Successful maintenance of weight loss usually entails maintaining a daily energy expenditure approximately 80 to 90% above RMR. This is a considerable increase for most patients. For example, someone with an RMR of 1500 kcal/day would need to expend about 1000 kcal/day in physical activity to meet this target. Activities other than exercise are important means to achieve this goal. The most commonly applicable approach is by increasing the amount of walking done throughout the day.

The health benefits from regular physical activity over and above the effects on weight include lower cardiovascular and all-cause mortality as well as improved mood and cognition. The options for increasing physical activity include exercise (sports or fitness pursuits) and use of lifestyle approaches.

Both methods can improve fitness and allow weight stability. In a randomized trial involving 160 obese older adults, a combined aerobic and resistance exercise program with weight management was more effective in improving functional status than either aerobic-only or resistance-only programs combined with weight management.[A6] Persuading obese patients to become more active is not easy. Physicians can begin by asking patients about their current and past activity habits as well as what barriers they see to increasing physical activity. This accomplishes the goal of stimulating patients to think about the

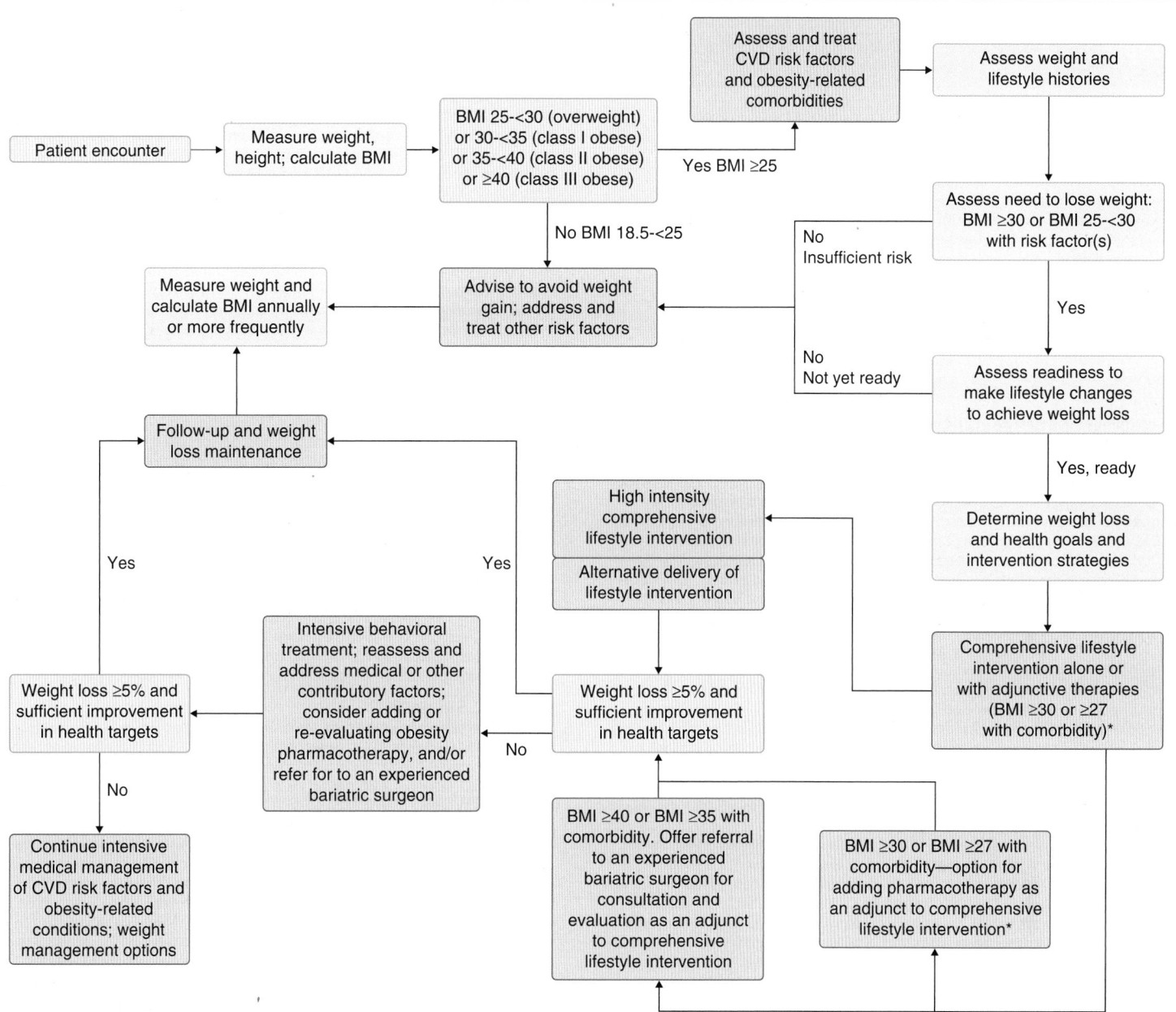

FIGURE 207-1. Flow diagram for the evaluation and management of overweight and obesity. BMI = body mass index; CVD = cardiovascular disease. *BMI cutpoint determined by the U.S. Food and Drug Administration (FDA) and listed on the package inserts of FDA-approved obesity medications. (Modified from Jensen MD, Ryan DH, Apovian CM, et al. 2013 AHA/ACC/TOS guideline for the management of overweight and obesity in adults: a report of the American College of Cardiology/American Heart Association Task Force on Practice Guidelines and The Obesity Society. *J Am Coll Cardiol.* 2014;63:2985-3023.)

issue in a tactful manner. It can help to ask the patient what personal benefits are envisioned as a result of increasing the level of activity. If patients agree to begin an exercise or physical activity program, they will need to set realistic goals for the amount of exercise they are going to achieve and to monitor their activity. The ready availability of step counters and electronic activity monitoring devices built into many "smart phones" offers practical means for patients to track physical activity throughout the day and to assess the effects of changes in lifestyle on their activity level. Patients should be advised to use devices that accurately count steps. Self-monitoring of how many steps are taken each day for 1 to 2 weeks can give patients a good sense of their baseline activity level. Many Americans take as few as 4000 to 5000 steps per day, whereas it may take as many as 15,000 to 17,000 steps per day to help those who have lost significant amounts of weight to maintain that lower weight. Gradually increasing the number of steps regularly taken during the day through a series of changes in habits (e.g., parking farther away, walking during work breaks) is more likely to result in long-term success for most persons than setting aside 2 hours or more for continuous walking.

Behavior Modification

Patients who are unable to make changes in eating activity habits on their own or with informal office counseling may benefit from referral to an interventionist trained in behavior therapy. The goals are to help patients modify their eating, activity, and thinking habits that predispose to obesity and focus on specific pathways to achieve the goals. These pathways may include identifying and removing barriers to development of better eating or activity habits. Small, incremental, and consistent changes in behavior are encouraged. Self-monitoring of food and activity is considered a key feature to success because most obese patients underestimate food intake and overestimate exercise. Cognitive restructuring has been introduced as a way to help overcome the thought processes that can lead to failure of a weight management program. Patients are taught to identify, to challenge, and to correct self-defeating thoughts.

The best weight loss results are provided by in-person, high-intensity (≥14 sessions in 6 months) comprehensive behavioral interventions, which average an 8-kg (5 to 10% of body weight) loss in 6 months. Approaches that provide electronically delivered counseling (telephone or Internet), including some commercial programs, can also achieve weight loss, but generally less than with in-person delivery approaches. Commercial programs that have published their results in peer-reviewed journals are preferred. Physicians who refer patients to programs that offer intensive, comprehensive lifestyle interventions are encouraged to obtain outcomes data from those programs.

Pharmacotherapy

A number of drugs are currently available to help patients with weight loss.[19,20] All of the major studies of obesity medications uses them in concert with a

TABLE 207-6 INDICATIONS FOR PHARMACOLOGIC TREATMENT OF OBESITY

Body mass index > 27 kg/m^2

One or more complications or conditions that are likely to improve with weight loss

Previous failure of conservative treatment with behavioral intervention, diet, and exercise

Agree to 2- to 4-wk trial of making initial changes in diet and exercise before starting pharmacotherapy

Agree to continued treatment with diet, exercise, and behavioral modification while receiving pharmacologic treatment

Agree to periodic follow-up

Premenopausal women (able to have children) must use some form of contraception

Consider a pregnancy test on initiation of treatment if there is any possibility of pregnancy

No contraindications to the specific drug used for pharmacologic treatment

comprehensive lifestyle intervention by knowledgeable providers; prescribing these medications without such support is likely to result in lesser success. Not all overweight or obese patients are candidates for pharmacologic treatment of obesity. Table 207-6 provides criteria that should help select patients for pharmacologic treatment. Because pharmacologic treatment of obesity exposes patients to some risks and expense, it is reasonable to require an objective benefit. A rational argument can be made that prioritization should be given to those with one or more medical complications or conditions that are likely to improve with weight loss. In prescribing antiobesity medications, it is important to set clear goals with respect to both weight loss and health benefits.

Currently Available Medications

The medications currently available for long-term use act through either appetite reduction or inhibition of pancreatic lipase, which results in fat maldigestion. All are better than placebo for achieving weight loss.[A7]

Phentermine is approved only for short-term (3 months) use. Other medications approved by the FDA for chronic treatment of obesity include lorcaserin, a selective serotonin 2C receptor agonist; the combination of topiramate and phentermine (see later); a combination of bupropion with naltrexone; and liraglutide. Because weight that is lost with pharmacotherapy is often regained once the medication is discontinued, agents that are approved for long-term use are better therapeutic choices.

Orlistat at the typical dose of 120 mg three times daily with meals causes about 30% of dietary fat to be malabsorbed. As expected, adverse gastrointestinal side effects, such as oily spotting, abdominal pain, excess flatus, fecal urgency, and fatty or oily stools, are not uncommon. These side effects decrease over time, and the concomitant use of bulk-forming laxatives (e.g., psyllium, methylcellulose) can reduce these symptoms. A daily multivitamin is recommended for those receiving long-term orlistat therapy. It is not necessary to take orlistat if a nonfat meal is being consumed. Orlistat is now available as an over-the-counter medication. Orlistat improves the results of medical treatment programs that include diet, exercise, and behavior modification, resulting in almost twice as many patients achieving goal weight loss (10% of body weight).

The combination of phentermine and topiramate in an extended-release capsule is approved for chronic treatment of obesity. The highest dose (15 mg phentermine/92 mg controlled-release topiramate) resulted in an average of about 10% weight loss at 2 years (8% more than with placebo), with slightly more than half of patients achieving 10% weight loss and 15% of patients achieving 20% weight loss.[A8] As both components of this medication were previously approved (topiramate for seizures and migraine prevention), the side effects are somewhat predictable. The most common side effects are constipation, paresthesia, sinusitis, and dry mouth; the incidence of individual adverse effects diminishes significantly after the first year.

Lorcaserin inhibits the serotonin pathway in a manner similar to fenfluramine, but without the cardiac valvulopathy effects. Patients taking lorcaserin 10 mg/day for 1 year lost an average of 5.8 kg compared with 2.2 kg with placebo. At 1 year, 47% of patients treated with lorcaserin lost 5% or more of their body weight compared with 20% of the placebo group.[A9] Lorcaserin can sustain weight loss without adverse cardiovascular effects, though with a slightly higher risk of hypoglycemia compared with placebo.[A10]

The combination of bupropion and naltrexone was developed to address the issue of dopamine-induced gratification and addictive behavior. The drug results in an average weight loss comparable to other approved drugs, with few side effects and no abuse potential, and probably without an increased risk of major cardiovascular events.[A11]

Liraglutide is FDA approved for the treatment of obesity in patients who have a BMI greater than or equal to 30 or a BMI greater than or equal to 27 in association with dyslipidemia or hypertension. Given as a once-daily subcutaneous injection at a dose of 3 mg, it can reduce weight by an average of about 8% (compared with about 3% for placebo) when used as an adjunct to diet and exercise.[A12]

Success of Medical Therapy

It has been estimated that more than 95% of those embarking on self-diets or fad diets fail to maintain a significant weight loss for a time that would have meaningful health benefits. The published results from two commercial programs have shown better results. These commercial weight loss interventions provided a comprehensive intervention that was delivered in person and resulted in an average weight loss of 4.8 to 6.6 kg at 6 months in trials in which conventional foods were consumed and 6.6 to 10.1 kg at 12 months in trials in which prepared food was provided. Comprehensive weight management programs delivered at academic medical centers that employ behavior modification, dietary instruction, and physical activity can achieve equally or more impressive results. Average 1-year weight losses of about 10% can be achieved and maintained for 1 to 2 years, depending on the intensity of follow-up. Additional evidence that intense lifestyle interventions can provide long-term benefits comes from the control groups of studies comparing bariatric surgery to lifestyle for type 2 diabetes. Even after 5 years (3 of which with virtually no behavioral support), the control groups have maintained 8 to 10% weight loss. The addition of medications, when indicated (see earlier), can produce even greater amounts of weight loss.

Endoscopic Treatment of Obesity

Three different types of gastric balloons have been FDA approved for treatment of obesity, as has one gastric aspiration device. The gastric balloons have been documented to result in significantly greater weight loss than placebo at 6 months (when they need to be removed). Weight regain occurs following removal of the device despite efforts to provide behavioral support. The gastric aspiration device provided significantly greater weight loss than lifestyle alone at 1 year and has been approved for up to 5 years of use by the FDA. Where these devices fit in the growing number of options for treating obesity is not yet clear. An electrical stimulation system that delivers low-level electrical stimuli to the vagus nerve has been approved with the goal of blocking nerve activity between the brain and stomach, thereby reducing food intake. Although this device is placed into the abdomen surgically rather than endoscopically, conceptually this is closer to endoscopic treatments than bariatric surgery. The amount of weight loss obtained from this treatment is modest at best.

Bariatric Surgery

Surgical treatment can provide more weight loss than medications for class II and class III (see Table 207-1) obese patients with medical complications that could be expected to improve with successful weight loss, such as uncontrolled type 2 diabetes,[21] assuming past attempts at medical treatment have failed. Patients with a BMI of 35 to 40 with life-threatening complications can be considered, but more typically patients with a BMI higher than 40 and several complications are candidates for surgery. Because the risks and costs of surgical treatment are greater than for medical treatment, selection of patients who stand to obtain more potential benefit from surgery should optimize the risk-to-benefit ratio. Among patients with severe obesity followed for a median of 6.5 years, bariatric surgery compared with medical treatment was associated with a clinically important increased risk for complication (new-onset depression, treatment with opioids, need for additional surgical procedure) but lower risks of obesity-related comorbidities.[A13] Contraindications to surgery include active substance abuse, defined noncompliance or inability to comply with medical care, and schizophrenia, borderline personality disorder, or uncontrolled depression.

A multidisciplinary team, including a physician, dietitian, psychologist or psychiatrist with expertise in this area, and surgeon experienced in bariatric procedures, is important for optimal outcome. Defining realistic expectations is an important part of the evaluation process. Patients undergoing bariatric surgery are not likely to be reduced to their ideal body weight. Successful weight loss is typically defined as losing an average of 50 to 60% of excess body weight, which is a difficult criterion to explain to patients. An easier explanation is that most successful patients will achieve weight losses of 25 to 35% of body weight. Follow-up to support the necessary changes in long-term behavior is recommended to optimize weight loss outcomes.

A variety of bariatric surgical procedures have been used. Procedures that only modify the capacity of the stomach (laparoscopic gastric banding) are much less effective than Roux-en-Y gastric bypass in terms of long-term weight loss. Procedures that both reduce stomach size and modify other stomach properties (sleeve gastrectomy) are somewhat less effective than the Roux-en-Y gastric bypass in terms of long-term weight loss and outright surgical success. Follow-up at 12 years after Roux-en-Y gastric bypass surgery in a large, prospective trial has confirmed the procedure's durability of weight loss and prevention of type 2 diabetes, hypertension, and dyslipidemia.[A14] Offsetting advantages include the absence of any nutrient malabsorption. The partial pancreaticobiliary bypass, the very long limb Roux-en-Y gastric bypass, and the duodenal switch procedures create malabsorption that results in greater weight loss than with the standard Roux-en-Y gastric bypass. Unfortunately, the incidence of severe, even fatal vitamin and mineral deficiencies (Chapter 205) is much higher with these procedures. Laparoscopic approaches are routinely employed for bariatric surgery because they reduce the hospitalization time and reduce the risk of incisional hernias compared with open procedures. The Swiss Multicenter Bypass or Sleeve Study in patients with morbid obesity reported no significant difference in excess BMI loss between patients randomized between laparoscopic sleeve gastrectomy and laparoscopic Roux-en-Y gastric bypass at 5 years of follow-up.[A15] Also at 5 years of follow-up, the SLEEVEPASS randomized trial reported a statistically insignificant excess weight loss in the gastric bypass group.[A16]

After surgery, almost all of the weight loss that occurs will happen during the first 1 to 2 years. Long-term (>5 year) success rates are outstanding in good programs. Virtually all patients with successful weight loss will have a dramatic improvement in the medical complications of obesity, making bariatric surgery an important treatment for severe, medically complicated obesity.

The results of the Roux-en-Y gastric bypass for treatment of morbid obesity have been favorable. Approximately 70% of patients achieve success as defined previously with this procedure. The mortality and morbidity (e.g., infection, anastomotic leak, wound dehiscence) of this procedure are low in centers with expertise, despite the high-risk population. Laparoscopic gastric banding is less used because of the inferior long-term weight loss results and late complications of band slippage, erosion, and weight regain. After any of the malabsorptive procedures, the patients require permanent follow-up specifically for adverse nutritional consequences.

The long-term follow-up of patients who have undergone gastric bypass surgery is needed to ensure adequate protein, calorie, vitamin, and mineral nutrition. Supplemental vitamin B_{12}, iron, and calcium are routinely added to standard multivitamins. The most common nutritional consequences of malabsorptive procedures are disorders of calcium and vitamin D metabolism, although many severely obese patients have low vitamin D levels even before surgery (Chapter 231). An increase in bone alkaline phosphatase may signal calcium or vitamin D deficiency. Low plasma vitamin D levels and low urinary calcium excretion should prompt aggressive replacement therapy. Iron deficiency, other fat-soluble vitamin deficiencies, and cases of copper deficiency occurring more than 5 to 10 years after surgery have been described. There have also been cases of pancreatogenous hypoglycemia that develop after bariatric surgical procedures. The symptoms are primarily postprandial and can be quite severe. Medical management by specialists in this field is the best approach for these patients.

PREVENTION

The dramatic increase in the prevalence of obesity during the past few decades strongly suggests that preventive strategies are needed. Public health approaches that emphasize education have been almost uniformly unsuccessful at preventing weight gain or producing weight loss. Public health strategies that virtually impose behavior change are more successful in this regard. Unless widespread efforts are made to address the problem of obesity, it is likely that its prevalence and complications will become an ever-increasing health burden.

Grade A References

A1. LeBlanc ES, Patnode CD, Webber EM, et al. Behavioral and pharmacotherapy weight loss interventions to prevent obesity-related morbidity and mortality in adults: updated evidence report and systematic review for the US Preventive Services Task Force. *JAMA.* 2018;320:1172-1191.

A2. Espeland MA, Glick HA, Bertoni A, et al. Impact of an intensive lifestyle intervention on use and cost of medical services among overweight and obese adults with type 2 diabetes: the action for health in diabetes. *Diabetes Care.* 2014;37:2548-2556.

A3. Gardner CD, Trepanowski JF, Del Gobbo LC, et al. Effect of low-fat vs low-carbohydrate diet on 12-month weight loss in overweight adults and the association with genotype pattern or insulin secretion: the DIETFITS Randomized Clinical Trial. *JAMA.* 2018;319:667-679.

A4. Johnston BC, Kanters S, Bandayrel K, et al. Comparison of weight loss among named diet programs in overweight and obese adults: a meta-analysis. *JAMA.* 2014;312:923-933.

A5. Schwingshackl L, Dias S, Hoffmann G. Impact of long-term lifestyle programmes on weight loss and cardiovascular risk factors in overweight/obese participants: a systematic review and network metaanalysis. *Syst Rev.* 2014;3:130.

A6. Villareal DT, Aguirre L, Gurney AB, et al. Aerobic or resistance exercise, or both, in dieting obese older adults. *N Engl J Med.* 2017;376:1943-1955.

A7. Khera R, Murad MH, Chandar AK, et al. Association of pharmacological treatments for obesity with weight loss and adverse events: a systematic review and meta-analysis. *JAMA.* 2016;315:2424-2434.

A8. Garvey WT, Ryan DH, Look M, et al. Two-year sustained weight loss and metabolic benefits with controlled-release phentermine/topiramate in obese and overweight adults (SEQUEL): a randomized, placebo-controlled, phase 3 extension study. *Am J Clin Nutr.* 2012;95:297-308.

A9. Smith SR, Weissman NJ, Anderson CM, et al. Behavioral Modification and Lorcaserin for Overweight and Obesity Management (BLOOM) Study Group. Multicenter, placebo-controlled trial of lorcaserin for weight management. *N Engl J Med.* 2010;363:245-256.

A10. Bohula EA, Wiviott SD, McGuire DK, et al. Cardiovascular safety of lorcaserin in overweight or obese patients. *N Engl J Med.* 2018;379:1107-1117.

A11. Nissen SE, Wolski KE, Prcela L, et al. Effect of naltrexone-bupropion on major adverse cardiovascular events in overweight and obese patients with cardiovascular risk factors: a randomized clinical trial. *JAMA.* 2016;315:990-1004.

A12. Pi-Sunyer X, Astrup A, Fujioka K, et al. A randomized, controlled trial of 3.0 mg of liraglutide in weight management. *N Engl J Med.* 2015;373:11-22.

A13. Jakobsen GS, Smastuen MC, Sandbu R, et al. Association of bariatric surgery vs medical obesity treatment with long-term medical complications and obesity-related comorbidities. *JAMA.* 2018;319:291-301.

A14. Adams TD, Davidson LE, Litwin SE, et al. Weight and metabolic outcomes 12 years after gastric bypass. *N Engl J Med.* 2017;377:1143-1155.

A15. Peterli R, Wölnerhanssen BK, Peters T, et al. Effect of laparoscopic sleeve gastrectomy vs laparoscopic Roux-en-Y gastric bypass on weight loss in patients with morbid obesity: the SM-BOSS randomized clinical trial. *JAMA.* 2018;319:255-265.

A16. Salminen P, Helmiö M, Ovaska J, et al. Effect of laparoscopic sleeve gastrectomy vs laparoscopic Roux-en-Y gastric bypass on weight loss at 5 years among patients with morbid obesity: the SLEEVEPASS randomized clinical trial. *JAMA.* 2018;319:241-254.

GENERAL REFERENCES

For the General References and other additional features, please visit Expert Consult at https://expertconsult.inkling.com.

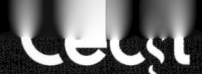

XIX

ENDOCRINE DISEASES

208

APPROACH TO THE PATIENT WITH ENDOCRINE DISEASE

DAVID R. CLEMMONS AND LYNNETTE K. NIEMAN

Most endocrine disorders are due to either an excess or a deficiency of a hormone that is transported in the systemic circulation and therefore result in multiorgan manifestations. Patients rarely present with a single isolated set of symptoms referable to only one organ system. Generalized nonspecific symptoms such as weakness, difficulty concentrating, lack of energy, and change in appetite are common. Often, a constellation of symptoms is required to point to the correct diagnosis, and single symptoms evaluated in isolation are rarely helpful even if one considers an exhaustive differential diagnosis (Table 208-1). As a result, it is critical to obtain a good longitudinal history. The duration of hormone excess or deficiency often dictates the severity of symptoms, and characterizing symptom progression over time can be very helpful in selecting diagnostic tests, and either substantiating the need for treatment or selecting the optimal treatment. Physical examination helps to confirm the likelihood of a diagnosis; for example, the presence of a symmetrically enlarged thyroid gland indicates that Graves disease is the most likely cause of hyperthyroidism. Even if endocrine disorders are diagnosed by biochemical screening in the absence of symptoms or signs of overt disease (e.g., hyperparathyroidism), a thorough history and physical examination are still important; they establish whether the patient is truly in the asymptomatic phase of the disease, and whether therapy or observation is required. A careful temporal history of a symptomatic change may also assist with the differential diagnosis—for example, whether a thyroid mass is due to a hemorrhagic cyst (i.e., occurring suddenly) or is an adenoma that evolved over an extended period. A thorough general history and physical examination may identify diseases associated with endocrinologic abnormalities, such as cancers that ectopically secrete hormones.

As genetic testing to establish the etiology of endocrine syndromes is more available, an accurate family history can indicate a need for genetic testing or familial screening. A thorough evaluation of medication use is also mandatory. Some medications can mask the symptoms of overt endocrine disease, such as β-blockers in hyperthyroidism, and others can exacerbate the findings, such as thiazide diuretic use in hyperparathyroidism. Medications also may confound laboratory evaluation, such as diuretics in patients with hyperaldosteronism or acetaminophen in patients screened for pheochromocytoma. Medication withdrawal may be required before testing. Finally, it may be difficult to obtain an accurate history of certain complaints. For example, in evaluating male sexual dysfunction, a corroborating history from his partner may be needed.

COMMON SYMPTOMS OF ENDOCRINOLOGIC DISEASE

A number of signs and symptoms are common to many endocrine disorders and the general population without endocrine disorders. These include weakness and fatigue, abnormal menstrual function, constipation or diarrhea, generalized hair loss or male pattern balding, recurrent or episodic headaches, altered libido, polyuria and nocturia, weight gain or loss, depression, altered mood, acne, dry skin, and vitiligo. By contrast, pain is not common and usually accompanies an acute endocrine emergency such as diabetic ketoacidosis or adrenal crisis, although chronic bone pain is seen in hyperparathyroidism and osteomalacia. Other signs are not so common in the general population and may more specifically suggest an endocrine disorder. These include striae, plethora, easy bruisability, acanthosis nigricans, and hyperpigmentation.

Any single symptom is unlikely to lead to the correct diagnosis. However, combinations of these symptoms (e.g., weight gain, constipation, cold intolerance, and dry skin in hypothyroidism) are more likely to suggest a diagnosis.

PHYSICAL EXAMINATION

Physical examination can confirm or refute findings ascertained by a medical history (Table 208-2). Thyroid disease is often first suspected based on the physical examination.[1]

Endocrinopathies lead to skin changes that may occur early in the illness and progress over time and may assist in identifying the diagnosis.[2]

By contrast, a number of symptoms are found in multiple endocrine disorders, such as hypertension, hypercalcemia, hyperparathyroidism, acromegaly, Cushing syndrome,[3] diabetes mellitus, pheochromocytoma, obesity, and primary aldosteronism.

The presence of edema may be an early sign of hormone-producing tumors that result in salt retention, including Cushing syndrome and hyperaldosteronism. Measurement of upper to lower segment ratios and arm span is helpful in establishing the timing and onset of puberty in primary gonadal disorders.

Pelvic examination is a major aid to the differential diagnosis of ovarian disorders. Palpation may identify polycystic ovaries and suggest the absence of ovarian tissue. The absence of a uterus is important in the differential diagnosis of pseudohermaphroditism, and the evaluation of external genitalia can be important in establishing the presence of congenital adrenal hyperplasia. Vaginal dryness is a sign of severe estrogen deficiency, as is breast atrophy.

Mental status changes occur frequently with extreme hypercalcemia, Cushing syndrome, and hyperthyroidism. Many primary endocrine disorders are associated with characteristic psychiatric manifestations.[4]

LABORATORY EVALUATION

Endocrine diseases are frequently diagnosed in an asymptomatic state because of radiologic or hormonal testing abnormalities.

The most common radiologic conundrums occur in patients who are noted incidentally to have small pituitary, thyroid, or adrenal masses. Evaluation for a functionally active tumor is usually necessary, even though only a minority will test positive. For pituitary tumors, this includes measurement of a baseline serum prolactin level and, in cases with suggestive symptoms, of 24-hour urine cortisol and growth hormone after glucose suppression. In patients with incidentally found adrenal masses ("incidentalomas"),[5,6] the tumor heterogeneity, size (>4 cm) and density, hypertension or hypokalemia, and symptoms and signs of Cushing syndrome should be evaluated. If any of these are present, evaluation should be done for Cushing syndrome, hyperaldosteronism, and pheochromocytoma.[7]

Measurements of the active hormone in blood, urine, or saliva are generally sufficient. Occasionally, measurement of a metabolite (such as 25-hydroxycholecalciferol, a vitamin D metabolite) is more reliable. Measurement of hormones with a very long plasma half-life (e.g., thyroxine) can be obtained at any time of day. However, other hormones (e.g., growth hormone) are secreted episodically, and therefore a static measurement may or may not be indicative of hormone excess or deficiency. In these cases, suppression or stimulation testing is used to confirm the diagnosis. Usually, an exogenous substance (e.g., adrenocorticotropic hormone [ACTH]) is administered either orally or intravenously, and the production of the hormone (e.g., cortisol) by the gland is either stimulated or suppressed.

Many hormones circulate bound to binding proteins, which can cause problems in interpretation. Medications or concomitant illnesses can result in a major change in the concentration of the binding protein, which in turn alters the total hormone concentration. This problem can be obviated either by measuring the binding protein itself or by direct measurement of the free hormone, such as measurement of free thyroxine.[8]

Static hormone measurements are often used for screening—for example, morning cortisol for hypoadrenalism. Stimulation or suppression testing is then used to confirm the diagnosis. In some cases, plasma measurements are much less reliable than urinary testing (e.g., a single morning cortisol level to identify Cushing syndrome).[9] In these cases, 24-hour urinary measurement of hormone is often required to document overproduction. Urinary assays have the advantage of providing integrative assessment over 24 hours and thus are less likely to be susceptible to errors due to episodic hormonal secretion. Occasionally, measurements of other substances, such as electrolytes or metabolites, are also informative for confirming the diagnosis. For example, measurement of 24-hour urinary calcium can be important in the differential diagnosis of hypercalcemia. Metabolites in the urine may be extremely important in the evaluation of adrenal disorders and in documentation of pheochromocytoma and carcinoid syndrome. Simultaneous measurements of two substances is extremely helpful in the diagnosis of some disorders. Measurement of simultaneous serum calcium and parathyroid hormone (PTH) is important for confirming the presence of hyperparathyroidism. Likewise, simultaneous measurement of blood glucose and insulin are needed to screen for an insulin-producing tumor. Indirect measurement of hormonal status can also be important; for example, insulin-like growth factor (IGF)-I, which is inducible by growth hormone (GH), reflects integrated GH secretion, and

TABLE 208-1 SYMPTOM CONSTELLATIONS SUGGESTING SPECIFIC ENDOCRINE DISORDERS

SYMPTOM CONSTELLATION	DIAGNOSIS
Weakness, fatigue, anorexia, loss of appetite, postural hypotension	Adrenal insufficiency
Cold intolerance, dry skin, constipation, weight gain	Hypothyroidism
Fatigue, easy bruising, striae, proximal muscle weakness, obesity, hypertension, acne	Cushing syndrome
Weight loss, increased appetite, palpitations, tremor, emotional lability, diffuse hair thinning	Hyperthyroidism
Galactorrhea, amenorrhea, headaches	Prolactinoma
Weight loss, anorexia, loss of pubic and axillary hair	Hypopituitarism
Episodic palpitations, tremor, anxiety, headaches, sweating, weight loss	Pheochromocytoma
Episodic flushing, palpitations, abdominal cramping, and diarrhea	Carcinoid syndrome

TABLE 208-2 PHYSICAL SIGNS THAT SUGGEST SPECIFIC ENDOCRINE DISORDERS

Hyperpigmentation of palms, extensor surfaces, and buccal mucosa	Adrenal insufficiency
Facial plethora, moon facies, striae, purpura, proximal muscle weakness	Cushing syndrome
Skin tags, acral enlargement, prognathism, orthodontia, cardiomegaly, increased size of hand/foot/tongue	Acromegaly
Proptosis, lid lag, symmetrically diffuse thyroid enlargement, abnormal extraocular movements	Graves disease
Hyperreflexia, moist skin, thin hair, tachycardia, wide pulse pressure, flow murmur, bruit over thyroid, tremor	Hyperthyroidism
Hyperkeratosis, myxedema, hyporeflexia, coarse hair	Hypothyroidism
Retinal microaneurysms, macular edema, motor nerve defect, inability to detect monofilament or vibratory sensation	Diabetic retinopathy/neuropathy
Short stature, web neck, loss of tears, coarctation of the aorta	Turner syndrome
Shield-like chest, short fourth vertebra	Primary ovarian failure
Bowing of the legs	Hypophosphatemic rickets
Orthostatic blood pressure	Pheochromocytoma
Galactorrhea	Hyperprolactinemia
Purple-hued flushing	Midgut carcinoid

hemoglobin A_{1c} is an integrative measurement of long-term blood sugar control in diabetes.

Imaging studies are commonly used in endocrine diagnosis. Magnetic resonance imaging and computed tomography are helpful in evaluating pituitary and adrenal masses. The ability of the thyroid gland to take up radioactive iodine is used to evaluate its functional status and the etiology of nodules. Bone mineral density testing is used to document osteoporosis and to evaluate established fracture syndromes. Imaging can be combined with hormonal measurements. Specifically, venous sampling can confirm the presence of an aldosteronoma and the location of PTH-secreting tumors. Similarly, intraoperative measurements of hormones that change rapidly, such as intraoperative PTH, can help determine whether surgical removal of the hormone-secreting tumor has been adequate. The primary use of biopsy in endocrinologic diagnosis is ultrasound-guided fine-needle aspiration of the thyroid gland in the outpatient setting. It can determine whether further diagnostic evaluation or therapeutic intervention is necessary.

GENETIC EVALUATION

Genetic testing in endocrinologic diagnosis is commonplace. Polymerase chain reaction amplification of DNA obtained from peripheral blood cells is often used to determine the presence of a specific disorder. This has been extremely useful in differential diagnosis, for determining prognosis, and for deciding whether family screening is required (e.g., in the presence of multiple endocrine neoplasia).

EVALUATION OF THE RESPONSE OF AN ENDOCRINE DISEASE TO TREATMENT

Most hormone excess syndromes are treated surgically by removal of the particular endocrine gland or tumor that is oversecreting the hormone.[10] However, appropriate follow-up of these patients requires that (1) it be established that the disease has truly been cured by the resection, or whether residual disease is present and (2) if the patient has not been cured, one must determine whether a repeat operation is likely to result in remission, or whether some other form of therapy should be undertaken. These decisions generally are made in consultation with surgeons and radiotherapists.

If an endocrine deficiency is present, hormone replacement therapy is most often used to correct the disorder. A combination of return of symptoms and signs to normal, laboratory testing, and indirect tests (e.g., potassium, blood urea nitrogen, and creatinine in the case of adrenal insufficiency) is required to determine the adequacy of replacement therapy. Sometimes the efficacy of substitution therapy can be assessed by laboratory testing, such as measurement of thyroid-stimulating hormone during thyroxine replacement. Understanding the pharmacology of the particular synthetic hormone used is important for proper replacement therapy. For example, synthetic glucocorticoids vary greatly in their half-life, and therefore dosage and timing of administration are important issues for patients receiving these hormones. Some patients, such as those with hypopituitarism, require substitution with multiple hormones, and often these interact and must be coordinated.

Hormones are also used throughout medicine for treatment of other disorders, and sometimes these treatments result in a hormone excess syndrome. The most common example is administration of high-dose glucocorticoid therapy for immune suppression resulting in Cushing syndrome. Similarly, growth hormone may be administered to children with short stature who do not have GH deficiency. A comprehensive knowledge of the actions of these hormones, and understanding of the desired nonphysiologic effect, can intelligently guide the proper use of these agents in treating nonendocrine disorders.

GENERAL REFERENCES

For the General References and other additional features, please visit Expert Consult at https://expertconsult.inkling.com.

209

PRINCIPLES OF ENDOCRINOLOGY

ALLEN M. SPIEGEL

INTRODUCTION

The principal manifestation of most endocrine diseases is over- or undersecretion of one or more hormones, but the causes of endocrine disease are not unique to endocrinology as a subspecialty of medicine. Benign or malignant proliferation of endocrine cells, destruction of endocrine cells by autoimmune, infectious, or other infiltrative processes, mutations in genes expressed by endocrine cells, and alterations in endocrine cell function caused by metabolic abnormalities or drugs are major causes of endocrine disease shared with diseases of other organ systems. If the causes of endocrine disease are not unique, there are nonetheless some general principles of endocrinology that define it as a medical subspecialty. These principles all derive from the study of hormones. Endocrinology was born with the recognition that certain cells secrete specific chemical entities—hormones—directly into the blood stream to act on specific distant targets. This immediately posed a series of questions: how are hormone synthesis and secretion regulated, how are hormones transported and metabolized, and how do hormones exert their actions on specific target tissues? This chapter will provide an overview of the answers to each of these questions and how they inform our current approach to the diagnosis and treatment of endocrine diseases.

WHAT IS A HORMONE?

The initial definition of a hormone was based on physiology rather than chemistry. Action on target cells reached via the blood stream was the operative principle. Secretin, now known to be a peptide hormone secreted by enteroendocrine cells in the gastrointestinal lining and acting on pancreatic exocrine cells, was the first example.[1] In contrast to enteroendocrine cells dispersed in the gut lining with other cell types, discrete collections of hormone-secreting cells, endocrine glands such as the adrenals, gonads, thyroid, and parathyroids, were soon recognized and their hormonal secretions chemically characterized. We now know that peptides, steroids, and many other chemical substances fit the definition of a hormone.

Endocrine action, a hormone secreted into the blood stream acting at a distance, has been contrasted with *paracrine action*, a growth factor or other signaling molecule secreted from one cell and acting on adjacent cells, and *autocrine action*, a cell secreting a signaling molecule that acts on the same cell. The distinction among endocrine, paracrine, and autocrine actions is not sharp. In some cases, a factor such as parathyroid hormone–related peptide (PTHrP) that acts physiologically in paracrine fashion during normal bone development may act as an endocrine factor in the syndrome of humoral hypercalcemia of malignancy. The definition of what constitutes an endocrine gland has also blurred. First came the discovery that specialized neurons could synthesize and secrete hormones directly into the blood stream, so-called neuroendocrine action, exemplified by vasopressin secretion by posterior pituitary cells. This contrasts with the classic neuronal secretion of neurotransmitters into a synaptic cleft. With increasing recognition that many tissues secrete hormones (e.g., erythropoietin by the kidney and leptin and other adipokines by fat cells), the role of endocrine glands as the exclusive purveyors of hormonal secretions has diminished. This blurring of the boundaries between endocrinology and other medical specialties is a general phenomenon in which study of hormones has informed seemingly disparate fields. Radioimmunoassay, the concept of receptors, and other principles of signal transduction first elucidated in studying hormone action are now broadly applied in all fields of medicine.

REGULATION OF HORMONE SYNTHESIS AND SECRETION

There are two broad categories of hormone synthesis: (1) that responsible for the synthesis of peptide hormones and (2) that responsible for the synthesis of steroids, including the active form of vitamin D, thyroid hormones, catecholamines, and other nonpeptide hormones. In the former category, hormone structure is encoded genetically. mRNA translation yields a protein precursor (pre-prohormone) that is generally cleaved through successive steps to yield the mature secreted product. Some protein precursors such as proopiomelanocortin contain within them multiple hormonal products, adrenocorticotropic hormone (ACTH), melanocyte-stimulating hormone (MSH), and endorphins in that example. In certain pathologic conditions, inappropriate immature hormone secretion occurs (e.g., excessive proinsulin secretion by insulinomas). Post-translational modifications occur for some hormones, such as disulfide bond formation for vasopressin and insulin, C-peptide cleavage for insulin, and glycosylation of the pituitary glycoprotein hormones, thyroid-stimulating hormone (TSH), follicle-stimulating hormone (FSH), and luteinizing hormone (LH). Mutations in genes encoding peptide hormones can lead to disruption of normal hormone synthesis or secretion, a rare cause of hormone deficiency. Peptide hormones are typically stored in secretory granules, and they are secreted by exocytosis, a process regulated by calcium (Ca^{2+}) and other factors. For steroids and other nonpeptide hormones, hormone synthesis is accomplished by a series of enzymatic steps acting on precursors (cholesterol for steroid hormones; aromatic amino acids for thyroid hormones, catecholamines, and related compounds). Mutations in genes encoding enzymes responsible for one or more steps in hormone synthesis can lead to hormone deficiency.

Negative feedback regulation is the general principle that governs normal hormone synthesis and secretion. For endocrine glands whose growth and hormone secretion is stimulated by pituitary trophic hormones (gonads, adrenal cortex, thyroid), the hormone secreted by the gland acts directly on cognate pituitary trophic cells (e.g., cortisol acting on ACTH-secreting pituitary corticotrophs) to suppress hormone secretion (Fig. 209-1).[2] Conversely,

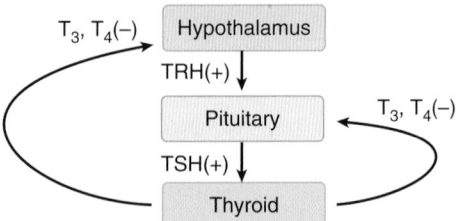

Thyroid Axis

FIGURE 209-1. Hypothalamic-pituitary-thyroid axis illustrating negative feedback regulation. Following thyroid-stimulating hormone (TSH) secretion by the pituitary, the thyroid gland secretes triiodothyronine (T_3) and thyroxine (T_4), which feed back on the hypothalamus and pituitary to suppress further increases in thyrotropin-releasing hormone (TRH) and TSH secretion.

a physiologically meaningful reduction in target gland hormone secretion leads to increased pituitary trophic hormone secretion. In many other cases, negative feedback regulation operates without the pituitary as an intermediate (e.g., PTH secretion from the parathyroid glands regulates extracellular Ca^{2+} homeostasis, and Ca^{2+} feeds back directly on parathyroid cells to regulate PTH secretion). Chronic hormone deficiency with resultant loss of negative feedback can lead to hypersecretion of the cognate trophic hormone and even to neoplastic proliferation of trophic hormone–secreting cells. Examples include Nelson syndrome in which corticotroph tumors form secondary to adrenalectomy, and tertiary hyperparathyroidism in which parathyroid adenomas occur in the setting of chronic hypocalcemia. In some adrenal cortical disorders, hormone deficiency leading to loss of negative feedback of trophic hormone secretion causes pathologic hypersecretion of alternative steroid hormones. The various forms of congenital adrenal hyperplasia are caused by mutations in one of the several enzymes in the cortisol biosynthetic pathway. 21-Hydroxylase deficiency, the most common, can lead to virilization in female infants, with excessive adrenal androgen secretion caused by ACTH stimulation in the face of inability to synthesize cortisol. Inhibition of enzymatic steps in hormone synthesis, such as aromatase inhibitors to decrease estrogen formation in estrogen receptor–positive forms of breast cancer, may be an important therapeutic target.

Hormone hypersecretion syndromes in which excessive hormone secretion occurs in the face of "normal" levels of the factor that ordinarily suppresses the cognate hormone are by definition caused by some intrinsic defect in negative feedback suppression. This may be caused by neoplastic proliferation of hormone-secreting cells, so that "basal" hormone secretion from the increased mass of cells exceeds physiologic levels. This may also be due to alterations in the intrinsic "set-point" for negative feedback suppression of hormone secretion. In practice, it may be impossible to differentiate these two mechanisms, and they are not mutually exclusive.

Hormone secretion is subject to many additional forms of regulation beyond simple negative feedback suppression. These include metabolic, neural, and other internal and environmental inputs. The temporal pattern of hormone secretion is often related to diurnal rhythms, as classically seen for cortisol, and also pulsatility. Changes in gonadotropin secretion during the menstrual cycle and during the course of puberty are striking examples of complex regulation of temporal patterns of hormone secretion.

HORMONE TRANSPORT AND METABOLISM

Most peptide hormones circulate as the free peptide, but insulin-like growth factor-I (IGF-I) uniquely binds to a number of specialized binding proteins. Steroid and thyroid hormones are lipophilic molecules that circulate largely in protein-bound form. Specialized binding proteins for cortisol, androgens, estrogens, and thyroid hormones are selective for their cognate hormone. The free circulating hormone concentration is only a small fraction of the total hormone measured by routine analytic methods. Binding protein abnormalities can occur in liver disease because most are synthesized by the liver. Thus, the determination of free as opposed to total plasma hormone concentration may be critical to accurate diagnosis in certain clinical conditions.

Hormone metabolism is another critical determinant of action for some hormones. For testosterone, thyroxine, and vitamin D, enzymatic conversion to more potent hormones—dihydrotestosterone formation in target tissues such as skin by 5-α reductase, thyroxine conversion to triiodothyronine by deiodinases, and 1,25 dihydroxyvitamin D formation by sequential hydroxylations in the liver and kidney—are all critical to normal hormone action. Defects in these metabolic steps leads to impaired hormone action. Even some peptide hormones such as angiotensin must undergo enzymatic conversion from secreted precursor form to generate the active hormone.

MECHANISM OF HORMONE ACTION

The central question in hormone action is how a hormone circulating in the blood stream in minute concentrations recognizes its specific target cells and regulates physiologic processes within them. Research addressing this question over the past four decades defined receptors, previously a purely theoretical concept, in molecular terms. Receptors are highly selective molecules that bind their cognate hormones with high affinity and specificity. Two broad classes of receptors were identified: (1) cell surface receptors that typically span the plasma membrane one or more times (Fig. 209-2) and (2) so-called nuclear receptors that reside either in the nucleus or in the cytoplasm, with subsequent translocation to the nucleus[3] (Fig. 209-3).

Hormones regulate cellular physiologic processes such as secretion of hormones, enzymes, and other compounds, muscle contraction, growth, and proliferation. *Signal transduction* is the general term for the biochemical steps between hormone binding to receptor and alterations in cell physiology. Most peptide and protein hormones (e.g., insulin, growth hormone, ACTH) bind to cell surface receptors that can be classified according to the mechanism of signal transduction to which they are coupled (e.g., G protein–coupled[4,5] receptor tyrosine or serine kinase, JAK/STAT coupled; see Fig. 209-2). Cell surface receptors may generate "second messengers," which in turn regulate a kinase cascade. Receptor activation may have rapid effects such as exocytosis of secretory granules, but longer-term actions involving gene regulation may also be a consequence of second messenger and kinase cascade activation. Steroid and thyroid hormones and vitamin D bind to members of the nuclear receptor family. The latter act as "ligand-regulated" transcription factors to regulate gene expression (see Fig. 209-3).

Selectivity of hormone binding by receptors is not absolute. "Specificity spillover" is a clinically important phenomenon in which supraphysiologic concentrations of a hormone leads to binding and activation of a noncognate receptor for a closely related hormone. Examples include hypoglycemia seen with nonislet cell tumors secreting IGF-II, which binds to the insulin receptor[6]; skin hyperpigmentation in subjects with Addison disease in whom excessive ACTH secretion activates the melanocortin receptor in melanocytes normally regulated by MSH; and hyperthyroidism in pregnant women with high human chorionic gonadotropin (HCG) concentrations activating the TSH receptor.

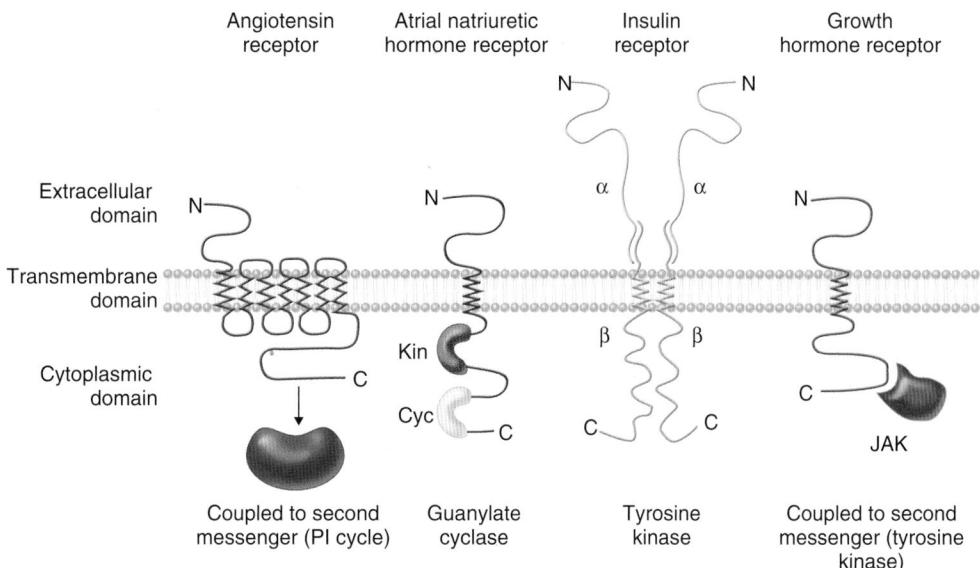

FIGURE 209-2. Structures of different types of peptide hormone receptors. PI = phosphoinositide.

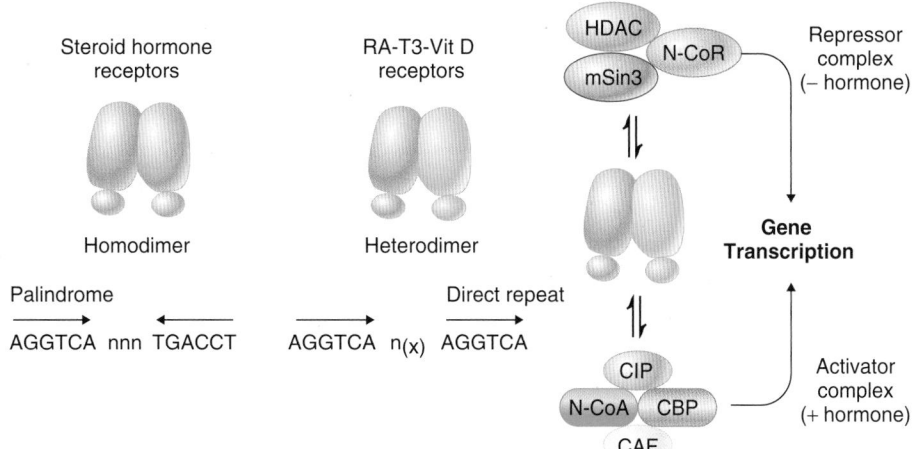

FIGURE 209-3. How steroid hormone receptors function. *Left,* Glucocorticoid receptor family members bind as homodimers to palindromic DNA sites. Thyroid hormone receptor family members bind primarily as heterodimers with retinoid X receptor to direct repeat DNA sites separated by varying numbers of base pairs. *Right,* As a result of hormone binding, repressor complexes dissociate and activator complexes bind to nuclear receptors. Repressor complexes contain histone deacetylase (HDAC), and activator complexes contain histone acetylase (CAF). CBP = CREB Binding Protein (CREB = cAMP response element binding protein); CIP = cyclin-dependent kinase interacting protein; mSin3 = mammalian homologue of the yeast *SIN3* gene; N-CoA = nuclear receptor coactivator protein; N-CoR = nuclear receptor corepressor protein; RA-T3-Vit D = retinoic acid-triiodothyronine-vitamin D.

TABLE 209-1 DISEASES CAUSED BY G PROTEIN–COUPLED RECEPTOR LOSS-OF-FUNCTION MUTATIONS

RECEPTOR	DISEASE	INHERITANCE
V2 vasopressin	Nephrogenic diabetes insipidus	X-linked
ACTH	Familial ACTH resistance	Autosomal recessive
GHRH	Familial GH deficiency	Autosomal recessive
GnRH	Hypogonadotropic hypogonadism	Autosomal recessive
GPR54	Hypogonadotropic hypogonadism	Autosomal recessive
Prokineticin receptor 2	Hypogonadotropic hypogonadism	Autosomal dominant*
FSH	Hypergonadotropic ovarian dysgenesis	Autosomal recessive
LH	Male pseudohermaphroditism	Autosomal recessive
TSH	Familial hypothyroidism	Autosomal recessive
Ca²⁺ sensing	Familial hypocalciuric hypercalcemia, neonatal severe primary hyperparathyroidism	Autosomal dominant Autosomal recessive
Melanocortin 4	Obesity	Autosomal recessive
PTH/PTHrP	Blomstrand chondrodysplasia	Autosomal recessive

*With incomplete penetrance.
ACTH = adrenocorticotropic hormone; Ca²⁺ = calcium; FSH = follicle-stimulating hormone; GH = growth hormone; GHRH = growth hormone–releasing hormone; GnRH = gonadotropin-releasing hormone; LH = luteinizing hormone; PTH = parathyroid hormone; PTHrP = parathyroid hormone–related protein; TSH = thyroid-stimulating hormone.

TABLE 209-2 DISEASES CAUSED BY G PROTEIN–COUPLED RECEPTOR GAIN-OF-FUNCTION MUTATIONS

RECEPTOR	DISEASE	INHERITANCE
LH	Familial male precocious puberty	Autosomal dominant
TSH	Sporadic hyperfunctional thyroid nodules	Noninherited (somatic)
TSH	Familial nonautoimmune hyperthyroidism	Autosomal dominant
Ca²⁺ sensing	Familial hypocalcemic hypercalciuria	Autosomal dominant
PTH/PTHrP	Jansen metaphyseal chondrodysplasia	Autosomal dominant
V2 vasopressin	Nephrogenic inappropriate antidiuresis	Autosomal dominant

Ca²⁺ = calcium; LH = luteinizing hormone; PTH = parathyroid hormone; PTHrP = parathyroid hormone–related protein; TSH = thyroid-stimulating hormone.

Genetic endocrine diseases include those caused by mutations in one component of a signal transduction pathway leading either to hormone "resistance" or hormone-independent activation (Tables 209-1 and 209-2). In the former, subjects present with apparent hormone deficiency, but direct hormone measurement reveals high concentrations of bioactive hormone that fails to act owing to target organ resistance. In the latter, patients present with apparent endocrine hyperfunction, but direct measurement reveals suppressed hormone concentration due to intact negative feedback. Loss-of-function mutations in receptors and in signaling intermediates such as G proteins have been identified in patients with hormone resistance. The converse, mutations that constitutively activate receptors or downstream signaling components,[7] have been identified in endocrine hyperactivity diseases such as familial male precocious puberty and familial nonautoimmune hyperthyroidism. Receptor inactivating mutations that lead to hormone-resistance diseases, such as the androgen receptor mutations responsible for varying degrees of testosterone insensitivity,[8] have been identified for both the cell surface and nuclear classes of receptors. Mutations in genes encoding proteins such as corepressors that form part of the nuclear receptor complex may also cause hormone resistance (e.g., central hypothyroidism caused by TBL1X mutations).[9]

GENERAL REFERENCES

For the General References and other additional features, please visit Expert Consult at https://expertconsult.inkling.com.

210

210
NEUROENDOCRINOLOGY AND THE NEUROENDOCRINE SYSTEM

ROY E. WEISS

NEUROENDOCRINE REGULATION

The interactions between the nervous system and the endocrine system's metabolic and hormonal homeostatic activities is termed neuroendocrinology. One role the nervous system has is to connect the environment with the body. The most important environmental factors are temperature and light, which fluctuate in a predictable way each day. Humans have a circadian clock that makes sure that the physiology and behavior are attuned to the time of day. The nervous system senses temperature and light, and it uses them as clues to guide eating, activity, sleep, and other essential life functions. The neurohypophysial neurons originate from the paraventricular and supraoptic nuclei and traverse the hypothalamic-pituitary stalk to the posterior pituitary, where nerve endings release vasopressin and oxytocin. Hypophysiotropic neurons are localized to specific hypothalamic nuclei, from which they project their axons to the median eminence, where they secrete hormones, which in turn stimulate or inhibit the release of peptides and bioamines into the proximal hypothalamic-pituitary vessels (Fig. 210-1). The blood supply of the median eminence comes from the superior hypophysial artery and its richly arborized capillary beds that extend into the median eminence and then coalesce to form the portal veins that traverse the pituitary stalk and terminate in the pituitary gland. The neuroendocrine system relies on a series of feedback loops, which regulate pituitary hormones as well as the levels of target organ hormones. The target organ hormones regulate both the hypothalamus and the pituitary gland to complete the feedback loop. Perturbations in feedback loops can be altered by factors like circadian rhythms (circadian periodicity), stress, nutritional status, and response to systemic illness.

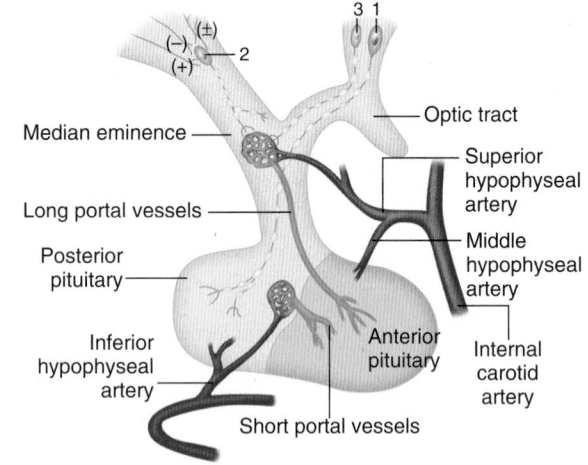

FIGURE 210-1. Neuroendocrine organization of the hypothalamus and pituitary gland. The posterior pituitary is fed by the inferior hypophyseal artery and the hypothalamus by the superior hypophyseal artery, both branches of the internal carotid artery. Most of the blood supply to the anterior pituitary is venous by way of the long portal vessels, which connect the portal capillary beds in the median eminence to the venous sinusoids in the anterior pituitary. Hypophysiotropic neuron 3 in the parvocellular division of the paraventricular nucleus and neuron 2 in the arcuate nucleus are shown to terminate in the median eminence on portal capillaries. These neurons of the tuberoinfundibular system secrete hypothalamic releasing and inhibiting hormones into the portal veins for conveyance to the anterior pituitary gland. Neuron 2 is innervated by monoaminergic neurons. Note that the multiple inputs to such neurons, using neuron 2 as an example, can be stimulatory, inhibitory, or neuromodulatory, in which another neuron may affect neurotransmitter release. Neuron 1 represents a peptidergic neuron originating in the magnocellular division of the paraventricular nucleus or supraoptic nucleus and projecting directly to the posterior pituitary by way of the hypothalamic-neurohypophyseal tract. (From Gay VL. The hypothalamus: physiology and clinical use of releasing factors. *Fertil Steril.* 1972;23:50-63, with permission of the American Society for Reproductive Medicine.)

Hypophysiotropic Hormones

The hypophysiotropic hormones regulate pituitary hormones by releasing various hormones that then affect the secretion of pituitary hormones. Some feedback loops are redundant, and some hypophysiotropic hormones exert effects on more than one pituitary hormone. Furthermore, the hypophysiotrophic hormones themselves are regulated by signals higher in the brain, such as the thalamus and the molecular clocks.

Thyrotropin-Releasing Hormone

The primary neuroendocrine function of thyrotropin-releasing hormone (TRH) is to stimulate the synthesis and release of both thyroid-stimulating hormone (TSH) and prolactin. TRH is synthesized from the precursor prepro-TRH and then processed to biologically active TRH. Tanycytes that line the third ventricle contain an enzyme, pryoglutamyl peptidase II, that degrades TRH to regulate the amount of TRH that is transported to the pars distalis of the anterior pituitary gland. In hypothyroidism, the increased TRH synthesis and binding to the thyrocyte TRH receptors results in increased levels of TSH and prolactin. Correction of the hypothyroidism with thyroid hormone replacement decreases the elevated levels of both TSH and prolactin. Conversely, in primary hyperthyroidism, TSH levels are markedly suppressed owing to a direct effect of thyroid hormone on mRNA expression of TRH in the paraventricular nucleus (Fig. 210-2). While TRH is the major regulator of the synthesis and secretion of TSH, the role of TRH for regulating prolactin-releasing factor is less well understood.

Gonadotropin-Releasing Hormone

Gonadotropin-releasing hormone (GnRH) is a 10–amino acid peptide; its neurons originate outside the central nervous system in the epithelium of the medial part of the olfactory placode. This origin of GnRH-producing neurons from olfactory epithelium is of clinical interest with respect to the entity of Kallmann syndrome (Chapter 220), in which GnRH deficiency is associated with congenital agenesis of the olfactory bulbs. One of its genetic forms is caused by a loss of anosmin, which is a protein that facilitates the embryologic migration of these GnRH-producing neurons.

The primary function of GnRH is to control the reproductive axis. GnRH, which is released in a pulsatile manner into the hypothalamohypophyseal portal circulation, subsequently reaches the anterior pituitary gland where it stimulates the secretion of luteinizing hormone (LH) and follicle-stimulating hormone (FSH). In humans, two different forms of GnRH have been identified: GnRH-1 and GnRH-2. The function of the latter is not well understood, and it does not regulate LH and FSH secretion.

Once the GnRH neuron migrates to the hypothalamus, a GnRH pulse generator is activated. In early postnatal life, GnRH secretion increases, thereby leading to temporary activation of gonadal hormone production, referred to as "minipuberty." During childhood, the gonads respond to exogenous LH and FSH stimulation but remain quiescent because the endogenous pulsatile GnRH release is suppressed until puberty. The processes that cause the infantile and prepubertal quiescent periods are not understood.

GnRH results in the differential secretion of LH and FSH owing to variable sensitivity of the feedback loop for steroid and peptide hormones as well as variable sensitivity to GnRH. The pulsatile secretion of GnRH directly increases its own receptor, whereas continuous administration of GnRH is associated with a decrease. In women, positive and negative regulation of steroid hormone feedback in the hypothalamic-pituitary-gonadal axis occurs at both the hypothalamic and pituitary levels. The hypothalamic effects depend on the amplitude and frequency of the pulsed release of GnRH, whereas the pituitary effects are modulated by the gonadotropin response to GnRH. In males, testosterone decreases pulsatile GnRH secretion, with a resulting decrease in amplitude and frequency of the gonadotropin pulse as well as a decreased gonadotropin response to exogenous GnRH.

In addition to pulsatility and regulation of GnRH receptors, kisspeptin may indirectly stimulate LH and FSH release by stimulating GnRH neurons. Kisspeptin levels rise just before puberty. Mutations in the kisspeptin gene have been associated with hypothalamic hypogonadism and impaired pubertal development, thereby demonstrating its role in the reproductive axis.

The negative feedback effects of inhibin, a peptide produced by testicular Sertoli cells and ovarian granulosa cells, are predominantly on FSH at the pituitary level, where inhibin causes a decrease in the sensitivity of gonadotrophs to GnRH. A related ovarian protein, activin, stimulates the basal and GnRH-stimulated synthesis and release of FSH from the pituitary, but its primary effect is to promote the response of ovarian granulosa cells to FSH. Another gonadal peptide, follistatin, inhibits the GnRH-induced rise in FSH that follows oophorectomy, primarily by binding to activin. These ovarian peptides are also found in the pituitary; therefore they may have additional local effects on gonadotropin secretion.

Pulsatile administration of exogenous GnRH is very successful for restoring normal sexual function and fertility in patients who have hypogonadotropic hypogonadism (Chapter 221) secondary to GnRH deficiency. Long-acting GnRH agonists also are useful to downregulate GnRH receptors and gonadotropin secretion in a variety of conditions, including precocious puberty (Chapter 220), prostate cancer (Chapter 191), breast cancer (Chapter 188), uterine fibroids (Chapter 189), and endometriosis (Chapter 223). Direct GnRH antagonists, which competitively bind to the GnRH receptor, are used for similar conditions.

Somatostatin

Somatostatin (also known as somatotropin release inhibiting factor) inhibits the secretion of growth hormone. The interactions between somatostatin and growth hormone–releasing hormone (GHRH) and their effects on the secretion of growth hormone are complex. Growth hormone secretory episodes are associated with increased secretion of GHRH, often accompanied by low somatostatin levels. By comparison, basal or trough levels of growth hormone are associated with lower levels of GHRH and more elevated levels of somatostatin. Somatostatin also inhibits both the basal and stimulated TSH secretion. However, growth hormone is about 10-fold more sensitive to inhibition by somatostatin than is TSH, thereby suggesting that the physiologic role of somatostatin in inhibiting TSH secretion is limited. Other tissues with somatostatin include the gut mucosa, D cells of the pancreatic islets, and the myenteric neural plexus. By its paracrine and endocrine actions, somatostatin suppresses the secretion of insulin, glucagon, gastrin, secretin, cholecystokinin, vasoactive intestinal polypeptide (VIP), and other gastrointestinal hormones, which in turn regulate functions such as gastric acid secretion, gastric emptying,

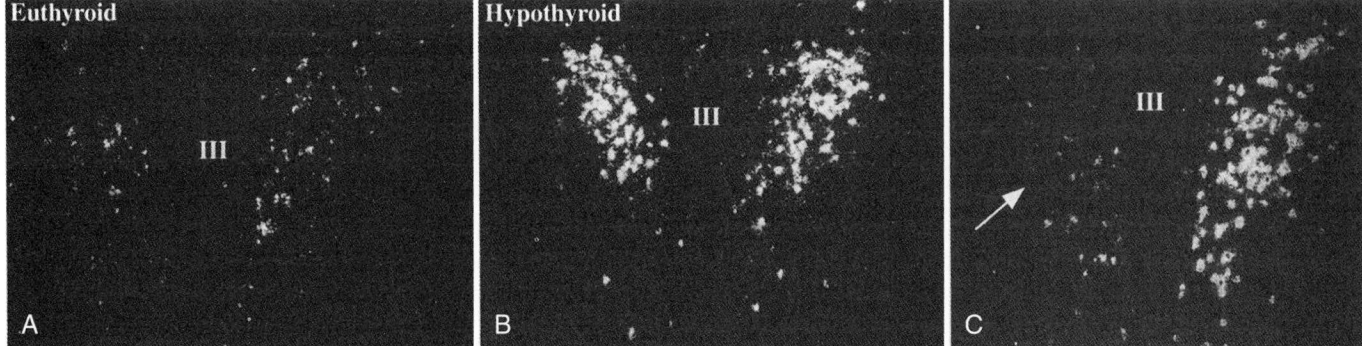

FIGURE 210-2. In situ hybridization autoradiographs of proTRH mRNA in the paraventricular nucleus of (A) euthyroid and (B) hypothyroid rats. Note the marked increase in hydridization signal in (B). C shows the effect of stereotaxic placement of a thyroid hormone implant adjacent to one side of the paraventricular nucleus in a hypothyroid animal. Marked asymmetry of hybridization signal is apparent with diminished signal on the side of the implant (*arrow* III, 3rd ventricle). (From Lechan, RM and Hollenberg A. Thyrotopin releasing hormone [TRH]. In: Henry H, Norman AW. *Encyclopedia of Hormones.* Academic Press: Amsterdam; 2003:519.)

gallbladder contraction, and splanchnic blood flow. Somatostatin analogs are used to treat acromegaly (Chapter 211), carcinoid tumors (Chapter 219), VIP-secreting tumors (Chapter 219), TSH-secreting pituitary tumors (Chapter 211), and islet cell tumors (Chapter 217).

Corticotropin-Releasing Hormone

Corticotropin-releasing hormone (CRH) stimulates the release of equimolar amounts of adrenocorticotropic hormone (ACTH), β-endorphin, β-lipotropin, melanocyte-stimulating hormone (MSH), and other peptides that are generated from proopiomelanocortin. CRH and vasopressin have synergistic effects on the release of ACTH. For example, the release of ACTH in response to stress is mediated 75% via CRH and 25% by vasopressin. However, since the releases of CRH and vasopressin are not always coordinated, stress can selectively activate the vasopressin-containing subset of CRH neurons. In a feedback loop, cortisol decreases ACTH secretion at both the hypothalamic and the pituitary levels. ACTH and β-endorphin also feed back negatively to decrease the release of CRH by the hypothalamus. Central bioamines, opioids, and peptides also influence the secretion of CRH. Inflammatory monokines, including interleukin (IL)-1, IL-6, and tumor necrosis factor (TNF)-α, stimulate the synthesis and release of CRH and vasopressin from the hypothalamus. The resulting increase in cortisol then reduces the intensity of the inflammatory response and the related release of monokines, thereby completing the feedback loop. CRH receptors, which are widely distributed in the brain, are activated by the sympathetic nervous system and suppressed by the parasympathetic nervous system. CRH may also help regulate body weight, because overfeeding increases leptin levels, which stimulate CRH, which in turn inhibits appetite and increases energy expenditure.

Biosynthetic human CRH is helpful for differentiating Cushing disease from ectopic ACTH syndrome, with the finding that patients with Cushing disease respond with a greater than 35% increment, whereas those with ectopic ACTH secretion have a lesser response. If the results are equivocal, CRH testing during bilateral inferior petrosal sinus sampling for ACTH often provides additional discriminatory information.

Growth Hormone–Releasing Hormone

GHRH dose-dependently stimulates growth hormone secretion. Repetitive administration of GHRH can release enough growth hormone in children with GHRH deficiency to increase insulin-like growth factor (IGF)-I levels and accelerate growth. The negative feedback of both IGF-I and growth hormone on the secretion of growth hormone decreases GHRH and increases somatostatin. This feedback effect is clinically relevant, as evidenced by high circulating growth hormone levels in IGF-I–deficient states such as renal insufficiency (Chapter 121) and cirrhosis (Chapter 144). In children in whom mutations in the growth hormone receptor make them unresponsive to growth hormone (also known as Laron-type dwarfism), IGF-I levels are very low and levels of growth hormone are correspondingly elevated.

Prolactin Inhibitory Factor

The inhibitory component of hypothalamic regulation of prolactin secretion predominates over the stimulatory component. Dopamine is the major factor that inhibits prolactin in most physiologic circumstances (e.g., lactation), such as when a rising prolactin level is accompanied by a simultaneous fall in dopamine as well as a rise in prolactin-releasing factors such as VIP. When endogenous dopamine receptors are blocked by drugs, such as the antipsychotic agents, prolactin levels rise. Lesions that interrupt the basal hypothalamic neuronal pathways that carry dopamine to the median eminence or interrupt portal blood flow (e.g., craniopharyngiomas or other large mass lesions) decrease the amount of dopamine that reaches the pituitary and can cause hyperprolactinemia.

Prolactin-Releasing Factor

Hypothalamic peptides other than TRH that have prolactin-releasing factor activity include VIP, which stimulates the synthesis and release of prolactin in hypothalamic-pituitary portal blood. Within the VIP precursor, another similarly sized peptide (peptide histidine methionine) also has prolactin-releasing factor activity.

Endogenous Opioid Peptides

Endogenous opioid peptides, which have a common 5–amino acid sequence at their amino terminals (Tyr-Gly-Gly-Phe-Met [or Leu]), bind to endogenous opioid receptors. The opioid μ-receptor mediates most of the opioid endocrine effects and analgesia (Chapter 27). Its primary peptide ligand is β-endorphin,

which is derived from proopiomelanocortin. For the opioid δ-receptor, which mediates behavioral, analgesic, and endocrine effects, the principal peptide ligands are met- and leu-enkephalins that are derived from proenkephalin A. Naloxone is not as effective for blocking the δ-receptor as for blocking the μ-receptor. The κ-receptor, which mediates sedation and ataxia, binds principally to dynorphin and the neoendorphins. A fourth receptor, which is partly homologous with the δ-receptor, binds to nociception, an endogenous 17–amino acid peptide.

Proopiomelanocortin, which is a 31-kD precursor peptide, contains ACTH, β-lipotropin, and β-endorphin. Its major cleavage products in the anterior pituitary are ACTH and β-lipotropin, and much of the latter is then processed into β-endorphin. In the intermediate lobe of the pituitary, the major products are α-melanocyte stimulating hormone (α-MSH), corticotropin-like intermediate peptide, β-endorphin, and γ-lipotropin. In the brain, however, proopiomelanocortin is processed primarily to β-endorphin, γ-lipotropin, and ACTH, with most of the ACTH then further processed to corticotropin-like intermediate peptide and α-MSH. The pentapeptide enkephalins are derived from the 28-kD precursor proenkephalin A. Neuronal perikarya containing the enkephalins are widely distributed in the brain. Dynorphin is a 17–amino acid peptide that is derived from a 28-kD precursor called proenkephalin B or prodynorphin. This peptide as well as shorter peptides called α-neoendorphin (with 10 amino acids) and β-neoendorphin (with 9 amino acids) react almost exclusively with the κ-receptor. Nociceptin, which is a 17–amino acid peptide that is derived from a κ precursor called pronociceptin, and its receptor, which also is present in the hypothalamus as well as in other areas of the brain, are sources of monoamine neurotransmitters. Nociceptin appears to have an antiopioid or antinociceptive effect. Opioid peptides that influence hormone secretion in the anterior pituitary are produced through modulation of hypothalamic bioamines and hypophysiotropic factors.

The specific functions of the various opioid peptides and their receptors are incompletely understood, although evidence links them to a number of bodily functions, including stress, mental illness, narcotic tolerance and dependence, pregnancy, eating, drinking, gastrointestinal function, learning, memory, reward, cardiovascular responses, respiration, thermoregulation, locomotor activity, seizures, brain electrical activity, and neuroimmune activity. Endogenous opioids inhibit gonadotropin secretion via their action on GnRH secretion. The exogenous administration of analogues of β-endorphin or enkephalin increase serum levels of growth hormone and prolactin, but blocking endogenous opioid pathways with naloxone does not alter basal or stimulated levels of growth hormone or prolactin. Opioids provide negative feedback on the secretion of ACTH and β-endorphin, and naloxone increases basal and stimulated levels of ACTH. Overall, the effects of the endogenous opioids on the normal physiologic regulation of the various pituitary hormones in humans is minimal. However, exogenous opioids in pharmacologic doses can impair the secretion of GnRH and gonadotropin, thereby causing hypogonadism (reduced libido, sexual function, and fertility) and adrenal insufficiency (by impairing the secretion of CRH and ACTH).

Central Nervous System Rhythms and Neuroendocrine Function

Pituitary hormones are secreted in a pulsatile fashion but in the context of underlying rhythms. A pituitary hormone's pulse amplitude reflects the amount of releasing hormone as well as factors that alter the pituitary's sensitivity to that releasing hormone. Thus, the pulse amplitude will be reduced by inhibitory factors (e.g., GHRH versus somatostatin), feedback from target organ hormones, nutritional factors, and prior stimulation that can deplete the releasable hormone pool. Pulse frequency is driven by the frequency at which the hypophysiotropic factor is released, which in turn is regulated by the hypothalamic pulse generator system.

The pituitary has an intrinsic rhythm of small amplitudes at a frequency of every 2 to 10 minutes. The pulsatile release of hypophysiotropic releasing factors is superimposed on this intrinsic rhythm with or without the withdrawal of a corresponding inhibitory factor. Ultradian rhythms are less than 1 day, circadian rhythms have a periodicity of about 24 hours (synchronized by an environmental cue such as the light-dark cycle), and infradian rhythms have a periodicity of more than 24 hours. The suprachiasmatic nucleus functions as a circadian pacemaker and receives light-induced electrical impulses from the retina and then transmits these impulses to the pineal gland, where they are converted to hormonal signals. Infradian rhythms include the gravitational influence of the moon, which guides the menstrual cycle.

Circadian and infradian rhythms are modulated by the sleep-wake cycle. For example, the secretion of growth hormone, prolactin, ACTH, and pubertal LH are linked more to the sleep-wake cycle than to the dark-light cycle

(E-Fig. 210-1). Each of these hormones increases to its maximal level after the onset of sleep. The marked diurnal variation in ACTH and cortisol is often an indication of whether this system is functioning normally (E-Fig. 210-2). Loss of this diurnal rhythm occurs when the regulation of CRH is abnormal, which may occur with depression, excessive alcohol intake, or autonomous secretion of ACTH in Cushing disease (Chapter 214). In fact, a diagnostic test for Cushing syndrome is the diurnal cortisol rhythm.

Interesting changes occur in gonadotropin secretion as a child passes through puberty into adulthood. Early in puberty, the amplitude of the pulses increases during sleep at night, especially for LH, but this nocturnal rise is lost in adulthood. In patients who have anorexia nervosa (Chapter 206), the pattern of gonadotropin secretion often reverts to this pubertal pattern. This phenomenon suggests that body composition may influence the pulsatile secretion of gonadotropins. The percentage of body fat also may influence the timing of the onset of puberty. Recent studies implicate leptin levels as the signal that indicates changes in body composition.

The hypothalamic-pituitary axis also undergoes changes with aging. Whether the cause of abnormal sleep patterns in the elderly is a result of the changes in the circadian rhythm is not known. However, it has been well described that hypothalamic-pituitary axes are blunted with aging (E-Fig. 210-3). Furthermore, changes in the hormonal milieu associated with sleep deprivation and disruption of the axes result in significant metabolic sequelae, such as hypertension and impaired glucose tolerance.

● NEUROENDOCRINE DISEASE
Diseases of the Hypothalamus

Diseases that cause localized hypothalamic changes include generalized central nervous system diseases (e.g., neurosarcoidosis [Chapter 89]) and processes (e.g., hydrocephalus) (Table 210-1). Systemic illnesses also can alter hypothalamic regulation and cause systemic illnesses.

Axons that project to the median eminence contain the various hypophysiotropic factors that are concentrated in the basal portion of the hypothalamus. Thus, lesions located within this final common pathway can decrease secretion of some or all of the pituitary hormones except prolactin, which may increase because its tonic inhibition by dopamine is eliminated. Diabetes insipidus (Chapter 212) may also occur. Symptoms of hypothalamic dysfunction also correlate with the size of the lesion, the area of the hypothalamus involved, and the rapidity at which the lesion grows. Slowly growing lesions typically cause gradual hormone dysregulation rather than sudden symptoms. However, slowly growing but large lesions also can cause acute symptoms if a slight increment in growth eliminates the remaining vestiges of vasopressin or ACTH secretion. The best way to diagnose hypothalamic lesions is magnetic resonance imaging (MRI) with gadolinium enhancement, although computed tomographic (CT) scanning with intravenous contrast is also effective. Visual field testing may detect an impingement on the optic chiasm and nerves by hypothalamic lesions. Detailed hypothalamic-pituitary function testing may reveal functional hypothalamic disruption that is not otherwise clinically evident.

CONGENITAL EMBRYOPATHIC DISORDERS

The most common embryopathic disorders that affect the hypothalamus are the midline cleft syndromes, which cause varying defects of midline structures, especially the optic and olfactory tracts, the septum pellucidum, the corpus callosum, the anterior commissure, the hypothalamus, and the pituitary. The clinical features of midline cleft defects vary from cyclopia to cleft lip and from isolated hypothalamic hormone defects to panhypopituitarism.

Optic nerve hypoplasia is a common but complex congenital disorder of unknown cause. It involves a spectrum of anatomic malformations and clinical manifestations ranging from isolated hypoplasia of one or both optic nerves, with a variable degree of visual impairment, to extensive brain malformations, hypothalamic-pituitary dysfunction, neurocognitive disability, and autism spectrum disorders (Chapter 389). It is the second leading cause of congenital visual impairment, superseded only by cortical visual impairment. More recent, larger studies have demonstrated optic nerve hypoplasia to be an independent risk factor for hypothalamic-pituitary dysfunction. Abnormalities of the septum pellucidum have no independent prognostic value, but the combination of an absent septum pellucidum plus optic nerve hypoplasia (termed septo-optic dysplasia) is associated with abnormalities in the hypothalamus and other diencephalic structures. Some such patients have precocious puberty (Chapter 220), presumably because they lack other inhibitory influences but have intact GnRH-producing structures.[1]

TABLE 210-1 ETIOLOGY OF HYPOTHALAMIC DISEASE

NEONATES

Congenital embryopathic disorders: agenesis of the corpus callosum, cleft palate (*HESX1*)
Congenital disorders: isolated hormone and receptor mutations, combined pituitary hormone deficiency (*PIT1, PROP1*), Laurence-Moon-Bardet-Biedl syndrome, Prader-Labhart-Willi syndrome
Tumors: glioma, hemangioma
Trauma
Hydrocephalus, hydranencephaly, kernicterus

1 MONTH TO 2 YEARS

Tumors: glioma, especially optic glioma, hemangiomas
Infiltrative disease: Langerhans cell histiocytosis, meningitis
Hydrocephalus

2-10 YEARS

Tumors: craniopharyngioma, glioma, dysgerminoma, hamartoma, leukemia, ganglioneuroma, ependymoma, medulloblastoma
Infiltrative disease: Langerhans cell histiocytosis, meningitis, tuberculosis, encephalitis
Irradiation: for nasopharyngeal tumors, intracranial tumors, leukemia
Functional: psychosocial deprivation

10-25 YEARS

Congenital disorders: Kallmann syndrome, gonadotropin-releasing hormone receptor defects
Tumors: craniopharyngioma, pituitary tumors, glioma, hamartoma, dysgerminoma, dermoid, lipoma, neuroblastoma
Trauma: subarachnoid hemorrhage, vascular aneurysm, arteriovenous malformation
Infiltrative diseases: Langerhans cell histiocytosis, sarcoidosis, tuberculosis, meningitis, encephalitis, leukemia
Chronic hydrocephalus or increased intracranial pressure
Functional: hypogonadotropic hypogonadism associated with weight loss, exercise

25-50 YEARS

Tumors: pituitary tumors, meningioma, craniopharyngioma, Rathke cleft cyst, glioma, lymphoma, angioma, colloid cysts, ependymoma
Infiltrative diseases: sarcoidosis, Langerhans cell histiocytosis, tuberculosis, viral encephalitis
Subarachnoid hemorrhage, vascular aneurysms, arteriovenous malformation
Irradiation: for pituitary adenoma, nasopharyngeal tumors, intracranial tumors
Nutritional: Wernicke disease
Functional: hypogonadotropic hypogonadism associated with weight loss, exercise

50 YEARS AND OLDER

Tumors: pituitary tumors, meningioma, craniopharyngioma, sarcoma, glioblastoma, lymphoma, colloid cysts, ependymoma
Vascular: infarct, subarachnoid hemorrhage, pituitary apoplexy, aneurysm
Irradiation: for pituitary adenoma, nasopharyngeal tumors, intracranial tumors
Infiltrative diseases: encephalitis, sarcoidosis, meningitis
Nutritional: Wernicke disease

Modified from Plum F, Van Uitert R. Non-endocrine diseases of the hypothalamus. In: Reichlin S, Baldessarini RJ, Martin JB, eds. *The Hypothalamus.* New York: Raven Press; 1978:415.

Children with very mild midline cleft defects (e.g., cleft lip, cleft palate, or both) are more likely to have deficiencies of growth hormone and other pituitary hormones. Nearly 50% of patients with "idiopathic" growth hormone deficiency will have an absent infundibulum detectable on MRI.

TUMORS

The most common tumors that affect the hypothalamus are pituitary adenomas with significant suprasellar extension. Such tumors typically cause variable degrees of hypopituitarism and hyperprolactinemia, either because they disturb the pituitary stalk and the mediobasal hypothalamus or because the normal pituitary is compressed. A normal or elevated prolactin level indicates the hypothalamus or stalk as the site of the lesion, and normal pituitary function often returns following therapy. Surprisingly, diabetes insipidus (Chapter 212) is rarely caused by pituitary adenomas.

Craniopharyngiomas, which arise from remnants of Rathke pouch, are the next most common tumors affecting the hypothalamus.[2] Microscopically, craniopharyngiomas consist of cysts alternating with stratified squamous epithelium. The cyst's fluid is usually dark and thick, and the lesion is often calcified. A Rathke cleft cyst is a closely related lesion that develops from the space between the anterior and rudimentary intermediate lobes. These cysts are lined with cuboidal (as opposed to squamous) epithelium, and their fluid is usually white and mucoid. Craniopharyngiomas most commonly arise during childhood but can occur in adults and even the elderly.

Tumors cause symptoms because their mass effects precipitate headache, vomiting, visual disturbance, seizures, hypopituitarism, and polyuria. Some patients have galactorrhea, amenorrhea, and hyperprolactinemia suggestive of a prolactinoma. Careful endocrine testing reveals varying degrees of hypopituitarism in 50 to 75% of cases, modest hyperprolactinemia in 25 to 50%, and often diabetes insipidus. Surgical extirpation of craniopharyngiomas commonly worsens pituitary function, often results in complete panhypopituitarism and diabetes insipidus, and may damage the hypothalamic centers that regulate thirst, body temperature, and food intake, thereby resulting in severe obesity. Hypothalamic-sparing surgery may cause less obesity without increasing recurrence rates. It can be difficult to remove craniopharyngiomas completely, but postoperative radiation reduces the risk of recurrence. Rathke cleft cysts are less likely to recur.

Suprasellar dysgerminomas arise from primitive germ cells, which are structurally identical to germ cell tumors and which migrated during fetal development. The tumors occur most commonly in children, in whom they decrease growth because of hypopituitarism, and also cause diabetes insipidus and visual problems. Hyperprolactinemia occurs in more than 50% of affected children, and 10% have precocious puberty because of the production of human chorionic gonadotropin (HCG) by the tumor. The finding of an elevated HCG level in the spinal fluid may be diagnostic. As compared with craniopharyngiomas, these tumors are very radiosensitive, and radiation therapy combined with chemotherapy is the preferred treatment.

A hypothalamic hamartoma is a nodule of hypothalamic neurons, glia, and fiber bundles. It is attached to the hypothalamus by a pedicle between the tuber cinereum and the mammillary bodies, and it extends into the basal cistern.[3] Asymptomatic hamartomas can be identified in up to 20% of routine autopsies. These lesions rarely may enlarge and disrupt hypothalamic function because they compress adjacent tissues. Less commonly, they may cause seizures, especially gelastic seizures. Some hamartomas can be associated with other congenital anomalies and mutations in the transcription factor gene *GLI3*. A choristoma (or gangliocytoma) is a hamartomatous variant composed of similar tissue in the anterior pituitary but not attached to the hypothalamus. These neuronal tumors cause precocious puberty, acromegaly, or Cushing syndrome when they produce GnRH. Surgery can be risky. Treatment with a long-acting GnRH analogue can be used to suppress gonadotropin secretion and may be preferred if the hamartoma does not cause mass effects.

Other tumors and space-occupying lesions in the suprasellar area include arachnoid cysts, meningiomas (Chapter 180), gliomas (Chapter 180), astrocytomas, chordomas, infundibulomas, cholesteatomas (Chapter 400), neurofibromas (Chapter 389), lipomas, and metastatic cancer (especially from the breast and lung). Such lesions can cause varying degrees of hypopituitarism, diabetes insipidus, and hyperprolactinemia. Unfortunately, surgical therapy often worsens the hormonal deficit and may cause other hypothalamic damage.

INFLAMMATORY AND INFILTRATIVE DISORDERS

Sarcoidosis (Chapter 89) involves the central nervous system clinically in 1 to 5% of patients and in up to 16% of patients at autopsy. Isolated central nervous system sarcoidosis, however, is uncommon. When sarcoidosis involves the central nervous system, it affects the hypothalamus in 10% to 20% of cases. Sarcoid granulomas can be seen in the hypothalamus, pituitary, or stalk, either as an infiltrative process or as a mass lesion.[4] The most common endocrinologic sequelae are varying degrees of hypopituitarism, diabetes insipidus, and hyperprolactinemia. Obesity can also result from hypothalamic involvement by sarcoidosis. Examination of cerebrospinal fluid usually shows pleocytosis, elevated protein levels, low glucose levels, and variable elevations of angiotensin-converting enzyme. In a patient who has isolated central nervous system sarcoidosis, the diagnosis may be extremely difficult to establish, and biopsy is often required. Corticosteroid therapy can at least partially reverse the thirst disorders, but deficits in anterior pituitary hormones usually do not improve.

Langerhans cell histiocytosis (Chapter 160) of the hypothalamus can cause diabetes insipidus, varying degrees of hypopituitarism, and hyperprolactinemia.[5] It is the most common cause of diabetes insipidus in children. This infiltration usually thickens the pituitary stalk, but it may cause a mass lesion of the hypothalamus or pituitary (Fig. 210-3). Osteolytic lesions may be seen on radiographs of the jaw or mastoid. Therapy consists of surgery, focal irradiation, or chemotherapy with alkylating agents and high-dose corticosteroids.

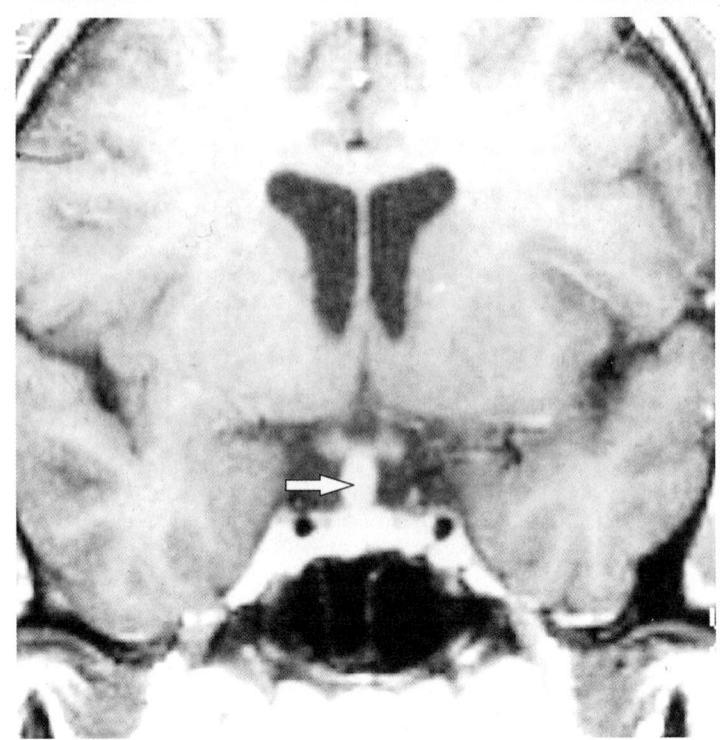

FIGURE 210-3. Thickened pituitary stalk in Langerhans cell histiocytosis. Magnetic resonance image of patient with Langerhans cell histiocytosis who manifested initially with amenorrhea, galactorrhea, and diabetes insipidus. Arrow points to the thickened pituitary stalk. (Reproduced with permission from Purdy LP, Molitch ME. Sudden onset of diabetes insipidus in an adolescent. *Endocr Trends.* 1998;5:1-7.)

Other infiltrative diseases that can cause progressive alteration in the hypothalamic regulation of the secretion of pituitary hormones include tuberculosis (Chapter 308), lymphomas (Chapters 176 and 177), and fungal diseases (E-Fig. 210-4).

VASCULAR DISEASE

An enlarging aneurysm (Chapter 380) may present as a mass lesion in the hypothalamic-pituitary area, where it can cause visual field defects and hypopituitarism. Tumors and aneurysms may also coexist, and careful MRI evaluation is critical. Vascular infarction very rarely causes hypothalamic disease, but almost 50% of cases of subarachnoid hemorrhage (Chapter 380) may be associated with varying degrees of hypopituitarism. Diabetes insipidus is an uncommon complication.

TRAUMA

Traumatic brain injury (Chapter 371) can cause a variety of hormonal perturbations that range from isolated ACTH deficiency to panhypopituitarism with diabetes insipidus. With frontal injuries, the brain travels backward, but the pituitary cannot move; as a result, the pituitary stalk is avulsed, with interruption of the portal vessels. The paraventricular and supraoptic nuclei and median eminence are particularly involved with microhemorrhages, hence the high frequency of panhypopituitarism with diabetes insipidus. Most patients with head injury are hyperprolactinemic, which clinically confirms that the primary site of injury is the hypothalamus or stalk. Blood levels of growth hormone, ACTH, TSH, LH, and prolactin may actually be elevated. These levels subsequently fall, and then pituitary function either may return to normal or hypopituitarism may develop.[6] Overall, about 25% of surviving patients develop hypopituitarism after major traumatic brain injury, but significant hypothalamic, pituitary stalk, or anterior pituitary damage is seen in about 85% of fatal cases. Deficiencies in ACTH (and hence cortisol) may be life-threatening, so cortisol levels should be monitored carefully in the hours and days after major brain trauma.[7] Hypocortisolism must be treated with stress doses of glucocorticoids (Chapter 32). However, hypopituitarism should not be confused with prolonged stress-related endocrine alterations.

IRRADIATION

Whole-brain irradiation frequently causes hypothalamic dysfunction, with resulting endocrine abnormalities and behavioral changes. The loss of pituitary function is so frequent that all patients who have had their pituitary and hypothalamic areas irradiated must be monitored periodically to detect the most common abnormality, which is hyperprolactinemia, as well as hypopituitarism that occurs especially when the radiotherapy is targeted to the hypothalamic area.[8] However, such deficiencies may occur many years later, so annual testing is recommended for up to 20 years. Stereotactic gamma knife irradiation and external beam radiation of pituitary and other parasellar tumors appear to carry a similar risk of subsequent hypopituitarism.

Effects of Hypothalamic Disease on Pituitary Function

Hypothalamic disease can cause both pituitary hyperfunction and hypofunction of varying degrees of severity. Although severe disease can cause absolute deficiencies of the various hormones, milder disease may cause subtle alterations, such as the loss of menstrual cycling and subsequent "hypothalamic" amenorrhea (Chapter 223). Furthermore, these hypothalamic defects may be interrelated. A rather common phenomenon is when hyperprolactinemia owing to hypothalamic dysfunction causes a hypogonadotropic hypogonadism that can be reversed when the elevated prolactin levels are normalized. Oftentimes MRI does not reveal a structural lesion, so a functional defect is presumably related to altered neurotransmitter regulation.

GROWTH HORMONE

Loss of normal secretion of growth hormone is the most common hormonal defect caused by structural hypothalamic disease. About 75% of patients with congenital idiopathic growth hormone deficiency respond normally to exogenous GHRH, thereby implying that the problem is probably disordered hypothalamic regulation. A rare form of growth hormone deficiency is caused by a mutation in the GHRH receptor. Reversible idiopathic growth hormone deficiency, which can be caused by inadequate parental care and affection, is termed the emotional deprivation syndrome or psychosocial dwarfism (e.g., inflammatory bowel disease [Chapter 132]). The disordered regulation of growth hormone is probably caused by psychogenic alterations in the balance of neurotransmitters needed for normal secretion of GHRH and somatostatin. Restoration of proper care promptly normalizes the secretion of growth hormone and subsequent growth. Treatment of systemic illnesses that also may decrease the secretion of growth hormone will correct the growth abnormality. Treatment of children and adults with growth hormone deficiency is discussed in Chapter 211.

GONADOTROPINS

Hypothalamic Hypogonadism

The primary defect in hypothalamic hypogonadism is the diminished secretion of GnRH that impairs the secretion of pituitary gonadotropin and gonadal function.[9] The cause may be congenital or acquired. Depending on the age of onset, these conditions may be manifested as either delayed development or loss of adult gonadal function. Hormonal deficiencies may be isolated to GnRH or involve other hormones as well. Primary growth hormone deficiency is the most common cause; some cases are idiopathic, but mutations in the GnRH receptor may be implicated. Hypothalamic structural damage is the second most common cause, but a substantial portion of these defects are caused by hyperprolactinemia and are reversible if the hyperprolactinemia is corrected.

In children with isolated disorders of GnRH and gonadotropins, growth and development are normal until puberty, when the expected growth spurt does not occur. About 50% of males with GnRH deficiency have undescended testes, probably secondary to the absence of gonadotropins during fetal development. The most common congenital lesion causing prepubertal GnRH deficiency is Kallmann syndrome, which affects 50% of males and 37% of females with isolated gonadotropin deficiency (see earlier). In patients with GnRH deficiency, subcutaneous replacement of GnRH every 2 hours via a portable pump rapidly increases FSH and LH so that testosterone levels rise to normal, and normal spermatogenesis ensues. Similar approaches in women restore the ovulatory cycles in 80% of cases. In men, comparable results can be obtained with a more practical administration of exogenous gonadotropins three times per week. In patients with GnRH receptor mutations, GnRH therapy is not successful. Testosterone replacement alone induces adequate androgenization but does not increase testicular size or generate spermatogenesis.

Acquired loss of previously normal GnRH secretion in adulthood may be caused by structural hypothalamic damage (e.g., a tumor), a functional change without a detectable anatomic lesion, or hyperprolactinemia. A CT or MRI is indicated to evaluate possible structural disease. Most cases of functional hypogonadotropic hypogonadism occur in women, especially related to weight loss, excessive exercise with reduced body fat even if body weight is unchanged, psychogenic stress, or systemic illness, but idiopathic forms also are seen. Pulsatile gonadotropin secretion is usually lost, but the gonadotropin response to injected GnRH is normal. Weight gain and reduced exercise can restore normal gonadal function. Furthermore, leptin administration can also restore the normal pulsatile secretion of gonadotropins and subsequent ovulation, thereby confirming that leptin has a critical mediating influence on reproductive function. Postpuberty hyperprolactinemia can also decrease GnRH as well as the pulsatile secretion of LH and FSH, thereby resulting in anovulation with oligomenorrhea and amenorrhea in women and impotence and infertility in men.

In the idiopathic form, spontaneous resolution does not occur. The treatment of idiopathic functional hypogonadotropic amenorrhea focuses on restoration of a normal estrogen status to promote well-being, to prevent osteoporosis, and to facilitate ovulation.[10] The first two usually can be achieved with cyclic estrogen and progesterone (Chapter 223), whereas the latter may require clomiphene, GnRH, or gonadotropin therapy. In men, similar goals may be achieved with testosterone, GnRH, or gonadotropins.

Hypothalamic Hypergonadism (Precocious Puberty)

Precocious puberty is defined when puberty begins before 8 years of age in girls or 9 years of age in boys. Central (GnRH-dependent) precocious puberty is characterized by hormonal changes similar to what occurs at the time of normal puberty—that is, an increase in the pulsatile release of LH, an increase in the gonadotropin response to GnRH, and an increase in gonadal steroid secretion. Pseudoprecocious puberty results from peripheral (gonadal or adrenal) causes.

The molecular basis for precocious puberty is not well defined. Some patients have activating mutations of *KISS1* and *KISSR1*, and a loss of function mutation in the makorin ring finger protein 3 (MKRN3) can also result in central precocious puberty.[11] GnRH-dependent precocious puberty can be related to premature activation of the GnRH pulse generator by a variety of lesions, or it may also be idiopathic.

Boys represent only about 10% of cases of central precocious puberty, but they often have more serious underlying causes. For example, hypothalamic hamartomas account for about 40% of boys who have central GnRH-dependent precocious puberty, another 30% are caused by central nervous system lesions, familial disease accounts for about 25% of cases, and the remainder are idiopathic. The picture is quite different in girls, in which hypothalamic hamartomas account for only about 15% of cases, other central nervous system lesions for 14%, and the McCune-Albright syndrome (polyostotic fibrous dysplasia [Chapter 218]) for 6%; the remaining 65% are idiopathic.

The treatment of central GnRH-dependent precocious puberty emphasizes surgical removal of the tumor or medical therapy with a long-acting GnRH analogue, either as monthly injections or yearly implants. When therapy is discontinued at the time of normal puberty, sex steroid levels increase, secondary sexual characteristics again develop, growth increases, and regular menses appear spontaneously.

PROLACTIN

Hypothalamic Hyperprolactinemia

Structural or infiltrative hypothalamic lesions can decrease how much dopamine reaches the lactotrophs and thereby cause modest hyperprolactinemia (usually <100 ng/mL).[12] A nonsecreting pituitary adenoma with extensive suprasellar extension can cause elevated prolactin levels that must be distinguished from a prolactin-secreting adenoma, which usually elevates prolactin levels 5 to 50 times higher. In patients with very large tumors, the prolactin level should be measured undiluted and at 1 : 100 dilution to avoid spurious findings. A number of medications, especially antipsychotic agents, can cause hyperprolactinemia, primarily by interfering with central catecholamines.

THYROID-STIMULATING HORMONE

Hypothalamic hypothyroidism (Chapter 213) is due to a central lesion that impairs the secretion of TRH, usually along with the loss of other hormones.[13] It occurs considerably less commonly than hypothalamic deficiencies in growth hormone and gonadotropins. Molecular causes of central hypothyroidism include mutations in the TRH receptor and the TSH beta gene that encodes for the TSH β-glycoprotein. In these patients, TSH is less biologically active than normal, so it binds less well to the TSH receptor.

Prenatal screening with TSH only (as is done in parts of the United States and England) will not detect children sufficiently early to prevent the neuropsychiatric sequelae of hypothyroidism. Screening with both T4 and TSH, as is done in the Netherlands, has the potential to diagnose these children early and perhaps uncover other newborns with life-threatening pituitary deficiencies.

Treatment is with L-thyroxine (Chapter 213), and patients should be monitored with free thyroxine (T_4) levels rather than TSH levels.

ADRENOCORTICOTROPIC HORMONE

Hypothalamic lesions rarely cause ACTH deficiency. ACTH deficiency can be an isolated abnormality or be accompanied by deficiencies in other pituitary hormones. The most common cause is suppression by exogenous or endogenous glucocorticoids, but head trauma or an autoimmune pituitary disorder also can be causative. Glucocorticoid treatment is indicated, but mineralocorticoid treatment is not.

Effects of Hypothalamic Disease on Other Neurometabolic Functions

Other functions that are regulated, at least in part by the hypothalamus, include food intake, carbohydrate metabolism, temperature control, sleep, and behavior.

ALTERATIONS IN FOOD INTAKE
Hypothalamic Obesity

Destruction of the mediobasal hypothalamus can suppress the phenomenon of satiety, thereby resulting in hyperphagia and hypothalamic obesity.[14] Because of the location of the lesions, hypopituitarism and diabetes insipidus often coexist. Whether the obesity seen in rare patients with Prader-Willi (Chapter 220) and Laurence-Moon-Biedl-Bardet (Chapter 220) syndromes is caused by hypothalamic dysfunction is unproven.

Hypothalamic Anorexia

Very rare bilateral lesions of the lateral hypothalamus can destroy nigrostriatal dopaminergic fibers that pass through this area, suppress appetite, increase in peripheral norepinephrine turnover, and raise the metabolic rate. By comparison, the hormonal changes seen in patients with anorexia nervosa (Chapter 206) are as a result of the weight loss, with no evidence that there is a primary preexisting hypothalamic abnormality.

HYPERGLYCEMIA

The hypothalamic response to stress can release growth hormone, ACTH, and prolactin, which then stimulate gluconeogenesis, lipolysis, and insulin resistance, thereby resulting in elevation of blood glucose levels. This hypothalamic response also activates the sympathetic nervous system, which releases catecholamines that inhibit insulin secretion and stimulate glycogenolysis.

TEMPERATURE REGULATION

Although input regarding body temperature comes from a variety of feedback signals, these signals appear to converge on a common set of neurons in the preoptic area of the hypothalamus. The anterior hypothalamus and preoptic area contain temperature-sensitive neurons that respond to internal temperature changes by initiating the thermoregulatory responses that are needed to restore a constant temperature. Measures that dissipate heat include cutaneous vasodilation, sweating, and panting; measures that increase body heat include increasing metabolic heat production, shivering, and cutaneous vasoconstriction.

Rare patients with anterior hypothalamic lesions can develop paroxysmal or sustained hypothermia or hyperthermia because these thermoregulatory activities fail. Some patients respond to anticonvulsant medications, thereby suggesting that the temperature changes are caused by seizure-like discharges.

Poikilothermy results from an inability to dissipate or generate heat to keep the body temperature constant in the face of varying ambient temperatures. This condition results from bilateral lesions in the posterior hypothalamus and rostral mesencephalon, which are the areas responsible for the final integration of thermoregulatory neural efferents. Patients with this condition are not bothered by temperature changes and typically are unaware that they have such a problem. Depending on the ambient temperature, they may experience life-threatening hypothermia or hyperthermia.

GENERAL REFERENCES

For the General References and other additional features, please visit Expert Consult at https://expertconsult.inkling.com.

ANTERIOR PITUITARY

ROY E. WEISS

ANATOMY AND EMBRYOLOGY

The pituitary is located in the sella turcica, which is a part of the sphenoid bone of the skull. It is attached to the base of the brain by a stalk, known as the infundibulum, and is contained in a capsule that is continuous with the dura mater, thus making it technically outside of the blood-brain barrier. The gland itself is composed of two parts, the anterior pituitary (adenohypophysis) and the posterior pituitary (neurohypophysis). The adenohypophysis has three anatomic components: the pars distalis (where the hormone-secreting cells are situated); the pars tuberalis (which hugs the infundibulum); and in children one can appreciate a third structure between the two, known as the pars intermedia, which is essentially absent in adulthood. The infundibulum has direct neural fibers that connect to the neurohypophysis, and, in a network of blood vessels, the infundibulum communicates with the adenohypophysis. The inferior border of the pituitary rests on the floor of the sella turcica, and the superior border is located just under the optic chiasm. Growth of the pituitary inferiorly can lead to erosion of the floor of the sella turcica and invasion into the sphenoid bone and sphenoid sinus, whereas the cavernous sinus and carotids are found laterally. Abnormal superior growth of the pituitary explains the visual problems encountered when the pituitary is enlarged by tumor, bleeding, or infiltration.

An understanding of the vascular supply and drainage of the pituitary is necessary for both diagnosis and treatment of pituitary disease (Fig. 211-1). The superior and inferior hypophyseal arteries provide the main arterial supply to the anterior and posterior pituitary, respectively. These vessels are branches from the internal carotid arteries. The superior hypophyseal artery forms the primary plexus of the hypophyseal portal system at the origin of the infundibulum. Blood from this plexus flows down the portal vessels. The pars distalis receives very little blood from the internal carotid and instead is mainly supplied by the venous system—long portal veins from the plexus and from the neurohypophysis through short portal vessels. This anatomy allows the pars distalis to be exposed to hormones from the hypothalamus, posterior pituitary, and the general blood circulation. Lack of direct arterial supply to the pars distalis makes it vulnerable to ischemia secondary to hypovolemia and hypotension. Venous drainage of the anterior pituitary is by the hypophyseal veins and of the posterior pituitary is via the short portal and hypophyseal veins to the cavernous sinus. The cavernous sinus drains into the inferior petrosal sinuses and then the internal jugular vein. Oftentimes lateralization (left or right sided tumor) of a small secreting tumor of the anterior pituitary can be detected by measuring the concentrations of the hormones in blood from the inferior petrosal sinuses.

IMAGING OF THE PITUITARY

The indication for imaging the pituitary is usually based on the history, physical examination, and laboratory evaluation of the patient. A lesion is suspected in the pituitary when there is evidence of over-secretion or under-secretion of one or more of the pituitary hormones or a visual disturbance consistent with disruption of the optic chiasm. Occasionally, however, there is no prior suspected pituitary or hormonal abnormality, but the imaging study is obtained for a different reason (e.g., a motor vehicle accident, headaches, or a non-pituitary intracerebral mass effect) and a pituitary microadenoma or an empty sella is an incidental finding. These findings are referred to as "incidentalomas" that otherwise would have avoided clinical detection because they are either silent or subclinical.[2]

Magnetic resonance imaging (MRI) is the preferred radiologic method for anatomic definition of the pituitary and its surrounding structures.[3] The normal pituitary is less than 1 cm in height, and a small tumor (microadenoma) can be as small as 1 mm, so high quality imaging is necessary. Sagittal and coronal images are the most useful to obtain (Fig. 211-2). The quality and resolution of an image depends on (1) the thickness of the sections obtained, generally 2 mm; (2) the graininess of the image, which is related to the strength of the magnetic field; and (3) the acquisition time. The longer the acquisition time,

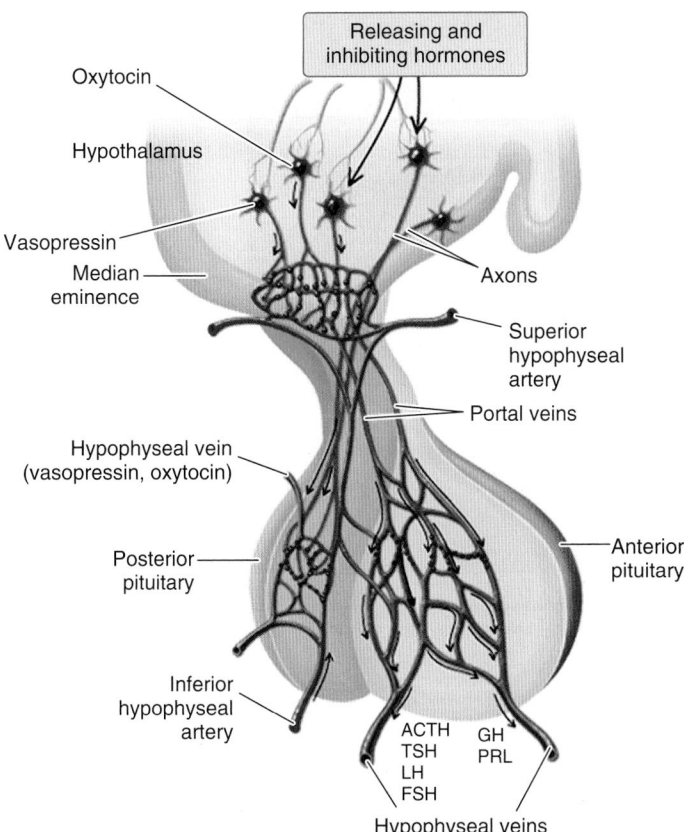

Releasing and
inhibiting hormones

Oxytocin

Hypothalamus

Vasopressin

Median eminence

Axons

Superior hypophyseal artery

Portal veins

Hypophyseal vein (vasopressin, oxytocin)

Posterior pituitary

Anterior pituitary

Inferior hypophyseal artery

ACTH   GH
TSH   PRL
LH
FSH

Hypophyseal veins

FIGURE 211-1. Structural-functional, humoral, endocrine, and neuroendocrine relationships within the hypothalamic-pituitary unit emphasize the unique and intimate interdependence of neural structures and hormone secretion with the circulation. Oxytocin and vasopressin neuron bodies located in the hypothalamus send axons through the pituitary stalk that terminate in the posterior pituitary, where they release oxytocin and vasopressin into blood vessels within the posterior pituitary. Hypothalamic neurons that produce growth hormone–releasing hormone, corticotropin-releasing hormone, thyrotropin-releasing hormone, and gonadotropin-releasing hormone send their axons through the median eminence to terminate and release their hormones into the hypophyseal-portal circulation. This network of blood vessels is located at the median eminence, which surrounds the pituitary stalk and penetrates into the anterior lobe of the pituitary. These hypothalamic neurohormones stimulate responsive anterior pituitary cells to secrete growth hormone (GH), adrenocorticotropic hormone (ACTH), thyroid-stimulating hormone (TSH), luteinizing hormone (LH), and follicle-stimulating hormone (FSH), respectively. Dopamine neurons reaching the median eminence are responsible for tonic inhibition of prolactin (PRL) secretion from the anterior pituitary, whereas somatostatin released from somatostatinergic neurons inhibits GH and TRH release. (From Melmed S. *The Pituitary*. 3rd ed. London: Elsevier; 2011.)

the better the quality but the more likely the image is influenced by movement artifact.

MRI images are usually obtained as either T1 or T2 weighted images. T1 (longitudinal relaxation time) is the time it takes the protons to realign in the tissue when stimulated by disruption of the magnetic field by an external radiofrequency. T2 (traverse relaxation time) is when the protons go out of phase with each other. Different tissues have different properties with T1 or T2. For example, cerebrospinal fluid is black on T1 images and white on T2 images. To enhance the images, intravenous contrast can be used as bolus and directly imaged afterward because normal pituitary generally enhances more than tumors. When the use of a contrast agent is not recommended, the T2 images may be helpful to distinguish normal pituitary from a tumor (Fig. 211-3).

Functional imaging of the pituitary is still in development and not recommended as a routine imaging tool. However, there are several modalities that are most useful when a tumor is actively secreting a hormone. These include positron emission tomography (PET), single photon emission computed tomography (SPECT), and magnetic resonance spectroscopy (MRS). PET is based on the tumor utilizing radiolabelled glucose (^{18}F-fluorodeoxyglucose, FDG) or methionine (^{11}C L-methionine) combined with a simultaneous CT scan to create a three-dimensional image of where the isotopic uptake is relative to the anatomic landmarks. MRS allows spectral analysis coupled with MRI to see changes in peaks of N-acetylaspartate with the use of ^{1}H.

REGULATION OF THE PITUITARY AXIS

Given the multitude of effects that the hormones of the pituitary have on the physiology and metabolism of the entire body, exquisite control of hormone secretion is regulated via multiple feedback loops and other stimuli either from the hypothalamus or higher in the brain or in the environment. The pituitary hormones are regulated and secreted with a highly reproducible diurnal variation and with superimposed episodic secretion throughout the day and night and influenced by sleep and wakefulness (Chapter 210). Therefore, measurement of hormone levels needs to account for the episodic secretion of the hormones, and a single point in time may not reflect the overall activity of the axis. For example, the stress and pain (although minimal) of phlebotomy itself could be sufficient to cause an increase in prolactin and cortisol.

One example of axis regulation is the release of thyroid hormone from the thyroid under the control of TSH from the pituitary thyrotrophs. The more TSH stimulates the TSH receptors on the thyroid cells (thyrocytes), the more thyroid hormone is released. The thyroid hormone then feeds back to the pituitary to downregulate further secretion of TSH, which then turns off thyroid hormone release from the thyrocytes. Superimposed on this process is the hypothalamus, which secretes TRH (thyrotropin releasing hormone) and stimulates the release of TSH. However, thyroid hormone also provides feedback to the hypothalamus and, independent of TSH, turns off TRH secretion. Therefore the pituitary's thyrotrophs need to integrate the positive stimulation

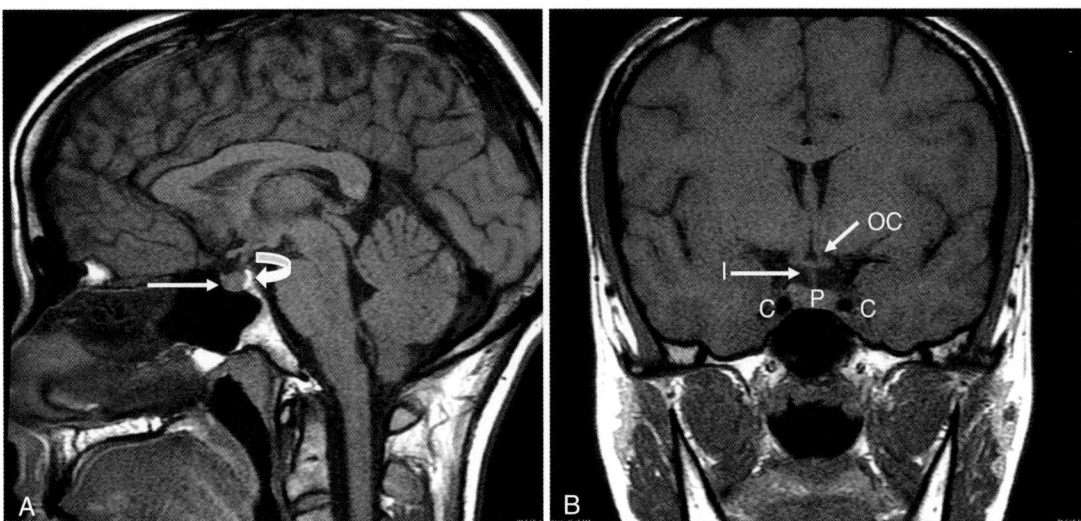

FIGURE 211-2. Magnetic resonance image of normal pituitary. **A,** Sagittal postcontrast. Normal anterior pituitary (*long arrow*), posterior pituitary (*curved arrow*). **B,** Coronal postcontrast image shows homogeneously enhancing gland (P) and stalk (I). Note the carotid arteries (C), easily depicted by their flow voids. Optic chiasm (OC) is the cranial nerves within the cavernous sinuses.

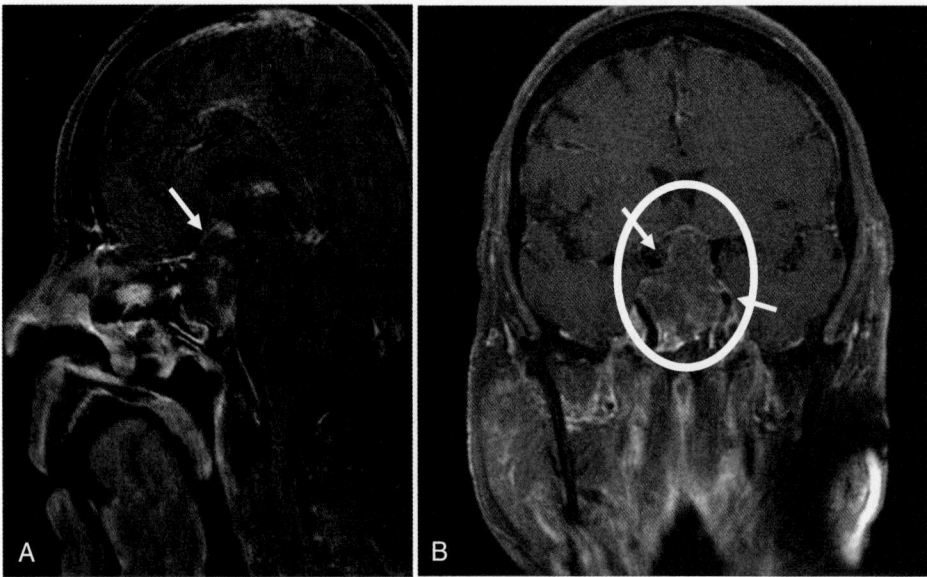

FIGURE 211-3. Magnetic resonance image of a large pituitary macroadenoma. **A,** Sagittal postcontrast. Note the extension of the tumor (*arrow*) below and above the sella. **B,** Coronal postcontrast. Large tumor is encircled with displacement of the carotid arteries (*arrow*), erosion of the floor of the sella turcica, and extension into the sinuses.

of TRH and at the same time the inhibition by the thyroid hormone levels in order to modulate the level of TSH release. The story is still not complete, because dopamine and other neurotransmitters from centers in the brain above the hypothalamus can stimulate and inhibit TRH, thereby providing an additional level of control over thyroid hormone secretion. Similar multilevel feedback control mechanisms can be described for cortisol from the adrenal gland as well as other pituitary hormones such as the gonadotropins, prolactin, and growth hormone. Understanding the basis for hypothalamic-pituitary-target endocrine gland axis regulation is essential for the diagnosis of abnormalities at specific levels of the axis as interpreted from provocative and suppressive tests used clinically to assess the pituitary axes.

HYPOPITUITARISM

PATHOBIOLOGY

Hypopituitarism is a condition in which there is a deficiency of one or more pituitary hormones.[4] The prevalence is between 290 to 455 cases per million, with an incidence of 42 cases per million per year. It is useful to classify hypopituitarism into two main categories: congenital (with known and unknown genetic causes) and acquired (Table 211-1). Although the congenital types may involve deficiency of a single or multiple pituitary hormones, acquired types of hypopituitarism usually simultaneously involve more than one of the pituitary hormones. Panhypopituitarism refers to a defect in all pituitary hormone lines. In addition to congenital and acquired defects, hypopituitarism may result from a hypothalamic disorder. Clinical manifestations of diabetes insipidus and hypopituitarism usually suggest combined hypothalamic and pituitary defects. Furthermore, the presence of hyperprolactinemia suggests interruption of the hypothalamic dopaminergic inhibition of prolactin and can be a result of hypothalamic defects.

Congenital defects are usually noted soon after birth when the consequences of an absent pituitary hormone become evident due to growth retardation or failure to develop. Acquired hypopituitarism usually presents the soonest in women of reproductive age because any perturbation in the hypothalamic pituitary milieu will likely result in an abnormality of the menstrual cycle. Normal menstruation requires orchestration of multiple hormones, which are exquisitely sensitive to changes in the pituitary hormones. Males of all ages and women of post-reproductive age usually have hypopituitarism for several years before the diagnosis is made. In such patients, the symptoms can be nondescript and not appreciated for many years after the onset of hypopituitarism.

A clinical description of each hormone deficiency is found in the following paragraphs. Although growth hormone deficiency can exist in up to 60% of patients with hypopituitarism, such deficiency in an adult is not likely to cause the same remarkable symptoms as the short stature that is seen in children. When multiple hormones are deficient, the manifestations in adulthood may

TABLE 211-1	CONGENITAL AND ACQUIRED CAUSES OF HYPOPITUITARISM

CONGENITAL EMBRYOPATHIC DEFECTS

Anencephaly
Midline cleft defects: septo-optic dysplasia, basal encephalocele, cleft lip and palate
Pituitary aplasia
Kallmann syndrome (GnRH defect with anosmia)

ACQUIRED DEFECTS

Tumors: pituitary adenomas, craniopharyngiomas, dysgerminomas, meningiomas, gliomas, metastatic tumors, hamartomas, Rathke cleft cysts
Irradiation
Trauma: surgery, external blunt trauma
Empty sella syndrome
Vascular
    Pituitary apoplexy
    Sheehan syndrome
    Internal carotid aneurysm
    Vasculitis
    Subarachnoid hemorrhage
Inflammatory and infiltrative diseases
    Sarcoidosis
    Langerhans cell histiocytosis (histiocytosis X, eosinophilic granuloma)
    Tuberculosis, syphilis
    Meningitis
    Lymphocytic hypophysitis, infundibulohypophysitis
Metabolic defects
    Hemochromatosis
    Amyloidosis
    Critical illness
    Malnutrition
    Anorexia nervosa
    Psychosocial deprivation
Idiopathic

GnRH = gonadotropin-releasing hormone.

be as subtle as skin changes, decreased sexual functioning, decreased muscle mass, and increased fat mass.

Genetic defects have been reported at every level of the hypothalamic pituitary axis, including defects in the hypothalamic factors, receptors for the hypothalamic factors, and the genes for the pituitary hormones. These patients present with congenital failure of a specific pituitary function and manifest with early onset growth defects, delayed puberty or hypothyroidism. Defects in the genes coding for the specific hormone almost always result in a low serum concentration of the hormone, and factors such as the *PIT1* and *PROP1* genes may impair pituitary cell differentiation. Furthermore, the pituitary

TABLE 211-2	TESTS OF PITUITARY INSUFFICIENCY

HORMONE	TEST	INTERPRETATION
Growth hormone (GH)	*Insulin tolerance test:* Regular insulin (0.05-0.15 U/kg) is given IV, and blood is drawn at −30, 0, 30, 45, 60, and 90 min for measurement of glucose and GH.	If hypoglycemia occurs (glucose <40 mg/dL), GH should increase to >5 μg/L.*
	Arginine-GHRH test: GHRH 1 μg/kg IV bolus followed by 30-min infusion of L-arginine (0.5 g/kg up to 30 g)	Normal response is GH >4.1 μg/L.
	Glucagon test: 1 mg IM with GH measurements at 0, 60, 90, 120, 150, and 180 min	Normal response is GH >3 μg/L.
	Arginine-L-DOPA test: L-DOPA 500 mg PO at start of Arginine 30 g in 10% solution IV infusion over 30 minutes, blood sampled at 30, 60, 90, 120 min	Normal response is GH > 1.5 μg/L.
Adrenocorticotropic hormone (ACTH)	*Insulin tolerance test:* Regular insulin (0.05-0.15 U/kg) is given IV, and blood is drawn at −30, 0, 30, 45, 60, and 90 min for measurement of glucose and cortisol.	If hypoglycemia occurs (glucose <40 mg/dL), cortisol should increase by >7 μg/dL or to >20 μg/dL.
	CRH test: 1 μg/kg ovine CRH IV at 8 AM, with blood samples drawn at 0, 15, 30, 60, 90, and 120 min for measurement of ACTH and cortisol	In most normal individuals, the basal ACTH increases two- to four-fold and reaches a peak (20-100 pg/mL). ACTH responses may be delayed in cases of hypothalamic dysfunction. Cortisol levels usually reach 20-25 μg/dL.
	ACTH stimulation test: ACTH$_{1-24}$ (cosyntropin), 0.25 mg IM or IV. Cortisol is measured at 0, 30, and 60 min.	A normal response is cortisol >18 μg/dL. In suspected hypothalamic-pituitary deficiency, a low-dose (1-μg) test may be more sensitive.
Thyroid-stimulating hormone (TSH)	*Basal thyroid function tests:* free T$_4$, free T$_3$, TSH	Low free thyroid hormone levels in the setting of TSH levels that are not appropriately increased
Luteinizing hormone (LH), follicle-stimulating hormone (FSH)	*Basal levels of LH, FSH, testosterone, estrogen*	Basal LH and FSH should be increased in postmenopausal women. Low testosterone levels in conjunction with low or low-normal LH and FSH are consistent with gonadotropin deficiency.

*Values are with polyclonal assays.
CRH = corticotropin-releasing hormone; GHRH = growth hormone–releasing hormone; IM = intramuscularly; IV = intravenously; PO = orally; T$_3$ = triiodothyronine; T$_4$ = thyroxine.

TABLE 211-3	HORMONAL REPLACEMENT THERAPY IN HYPOPITUITARISM*

PITUITARY AXIS	HORMONAL REPLACEMENTS
Growth hormone (GH)	In children, GH (0.25 mg/kg) SC daily. In adults, GH (0.3-1.2 mg) SC daily. Titrate dose to achieve IGF-I levels in middle to upper part of normal range. Women receiving oral estrogens require higher doses.
Prolactin	None
Adrenocorticotropic hormone–cortisol	Hydrocortisone (10-15 mg PO q AM; 5-10 mg PO q PM) or prednisone (2.5 mg PO q AM; 2.5 mg PO q PM). Dose adjusted on clinical basis. Stress dosing: 50-75 mg hydrocortisone IV q8h
Thyroid-stimulating hormone–thyroid	L-thyroxine (0.075-0.15 mg) PO daily
Gonadotropins–gonads	FSH and LH (or HCG) can be used to induce ovulation in women. HCG alone or with FSH can be used to induce spermatogenesis in men. In men, testosterone enanthate (100-300 mg) IM q1-3 wk or testosterone cyclopentylpropionate (100-300 mg) IM q1-3 wk. Testosterone transdermal patches can also be used (5 mg daily). Testosterone gel 5-10 g daily In women, conjugated estrogens (0.625-1.25 mg) PO days 1-25 each month, cycled with medroxyprogesterone acetate (5-10 mg) PO days 15-25 each month. Low-dose contraceptive pills may also be used. Estrogen-containing transdermal patches are also available.
Posterior pituitary	Desmopressin, 0.05-0.2 mL (5-20 μg) intranasally once or twice daily, or tablets (0.1-0.4 mg q8-12h) or 0.5 mL (2 μg) SC

*Replacement therapy is dictated by the types of hormone deficiencies and by the clinical circumstances. In each case, the recommended preparations and doses are representative but need to be adjusted for individual patients. Other hormonal preparations are also available.
FSH = follicle-stimulating hormone; GnRH = gonadotropin-releasing hormone; HCG = human chorionic gonadotropin; IGF-I = insulin-like growth factor-I; IM = intramuscularly; LH = luteinizing hormone; PO = orally; SC = subcutaneously.

hormone receptor in the respective glands may be defective, thereby resulting in resistance to the action of the pituitary hormones. Finally, genetic defects in the gene coding for the hormone or the hormone's receptor can result in profound hormone deficiency.

Acquired defects such as a tumor, specifically a macroadenoma in the sella, is the most common cause of hypopituitarism. Tumor enlargement within the confines of the bony sella turcica can compress the normal pituitary cells, resulting in their failure to function. Irradiation of the pituitary, pituitary infarction, surgical intrusion, and infiltrative disease can compromise normal pituitary functioning. In addition to structural damage to the cells, dysfunction can occur in malnutrition, critical illness, and psychiatric disorders.

Diagnosis of hypopituitarism in patients with secreting or non-secreting pituitary masses usually involves a combination of static and stimulatory blood tests (Table 211-2). While there are multiple tests available, each has advantages and disadvantages, and the choice of the test may depend on the age of the patient and the clinical setting. Sometimes multiple tests may be performed if results of one test are equivocal. Treatment is replacement of the deficient hormones (Table 211-3).[5]

Hypophysitis

Inflammation of the pituitary is known as hypophysitis and can be classified clinically as primary hypophysitis when isolated inflammation of the pituitary is not associated with other inflammatory conditions, infections, or medications. Histologically, lymphocytic hypophysitis is the most common form and occurs three times more frequently in women, typically in the fourth decade. It was previously thought that lymphocytic inflammatory hypophysitis was predominately related to the end of pregnancy or the first few months after delivery; however, rare cases have been described in men and children. The other histologic types, granulomatous and xanthomatous hypophysitis, are not associated with pregnancy although they are more common in females. The least common form, plasmacytic or IgG4-related hypophysitis, occurs in males in a 2 : 1 ratio and usually presents in the seventh decade. Furthermore, IgG4-related hypophysitis cases usually have other organ involvement. The etiology of any of the forms of hypophysitis is unknown, and an autoantigen in the pituitary has yet to be clearly identified.[6]

TABLE 211-4	SIGNS AND SYMPTOMS OF PITUITARY APOPLEXY

SYMPTOM	INCIDENCE
Headache	95%
Vomiting	70%
Vision Defects:	
Visual field defect	64%
Decreased visual acuity	52%
Diplopia (CN III, IV, V and VI)	
Hemiplegia	Rare
Meningismus	Rare
Hypotension (cardiovascular collapse)	95%

CN = cranial nerves.

TABLE 211-5	PREDISPOSING CONDITIONS ASSOCIATED WITH PITUITARY APOPLEXY

Pituitary Tumor
   Nonfunctioning pituitary macroadenoma
   Certain functional tumors
Hypertension and/or hypotension
Surgery
   Cardiac surgery (heart lung bypass; coronary artery grafts)
   Major orthopedic procedures
Drugs
   Cabergoline
   Bromocriptine
   Endocrine stimulation tests (thyrotropin-releasing hormone stimulation; insulin tolerance test)
   Anticoagulants
   Estrogen
Head Trauma
Pregnancy and delivery (when significant hemorrhage and hypovolemia occurs, called Sheehan syndrome)
Infections
   Dengue fever
   Hypophysitis
Radiation therapy
Diabetes, poorly controlled
Sickle cell anemia

Patients with hypophysitis usually present with headaches and multiple deficiencies of anterior pituitary hormones. Diabetes insipidus (Chapter 212) is reported in half the patients, and most have associated mild hyperprolactinemia. Diagnosis typically cannot be confirmed by imaging alone. An MRI cannot reliably differentiate hypophysitis from a pituitary adenoma, but hypophysitis usually causes diffuse pituitary enlargement, normal sellar size, and thickening of the midline stalk. Diagnosis can be made based on radiologic and clinical characteristics during or just after pregnancy or if there is a proximal history of use of anti-CTLA-4 agents several months prior to the onset of symptoms (headaches and weakness). Definitive diagnosis, however, is usually made by biopsy. Surgery may be indicated when a biopsy is needed for diagnosis, when the history is unclear or if there is a mass effect. Careful pituitary function testing is mandatory even in patients who do not undergo surgery because they might otherwise die from undiagnosed adrenocortical insufficiency. The prognosis is unclear, but both the structural and functional abnormalities can occasionally resolve spontaneously. Glucocorticoids in physiologic doses may have a direct effect on the lymphocytic invasion in lymphocytic hypophysitis, but there are no prospective treatment trials of this rather rare condition.

Pituitary Apoplexy

Insult to the pituitary can be in the form of hemorrhage, infarction, or both. When abrupt, and sometimes catastrophic hemorrhagic infarction occurs in the pituitary, it is defined as apoplexy. The constellation of headache, vomiting, visual impairment, and altered consciousness with hemodynamic instability is not specific for pituitary apoplexy but raises suspicion for the diagnosis (Table 211-4). Often, this dramatic presentation is the first time the patient is aware of a potential pituitary tumor. Asymptomatic hemorrhage and infarction into a pituitary tumor can occur in 10 to 25% of patients, but true apoplexy occurs in only 2 to 10% of pituitary tumor patients.

The most common presenting complaint, headache, can present variably from retro-orbital to unilateral to bilateral temporal headaches during the acute phase of apoplexy. As the hemorrhagic infarction resolves, the patient often is left with hypopituitarism.

Certain conditions predispose a patient to pituitary apoplexy (Table 211-5). Although all large pituitary tumors are at risk for hemorrhagic infarction, certain functional pituitary tumors, such as those in Cushing disease or acromegaly, may be particularly prone. Nearly 25% of all patients with apoplexy have inadequately treated hypertension.

The main symptoms and consequences of apoplexy are due to the increased pressure present within the bony walls of the sella turcica in which the pituitary resides. A sudden increase in the sellar contents, due to blood and edema, results in increased pressure. This increased pressure and meningeal irritation are responsible for the neurologic symptoms described in Table 211-4, including the increased pressure in the cavernous sinus and the cranial nerve palsies as well as bitemporal hemianopsia. Extravasation of blood into the subarachnoid space causes meningeal irritation.

DIAGNOSIS

Prompt recognition of patients presenting with the triad of headache, vomiting, and visual disturbances is required to prevent death or irreversible neurologic impairment. Clinical evaluation of the patient should begin with a thorough history from the patient, if sufficiently conscious to give one, or from family members. A history of a pituitary tumor should raise the suspicion of apoplexy. More subtle abnormalities associated with pituitary dysfunction

(hypofunctioning of thyroid, adrenal, or gonadal systems) may be helpful. The cornerstone for diagnosis is urgent radiologic assessment. MRI T2-weighted images are the test of choice and should be performed emergently in all patients with visual symptoms. A CT scan can be useful when an MRI is not available or possible. Urgent measurement of blood chemistries, including electrolytes, kidney function, liver function, complete blood count with platelets, and prothrombin time can be useful. Because more than 80% of patients will have endocrine dysfunction, urgent measurement of free T4, TSH, prolactin, and random cortisol can be helpful. Less rapidly available and helpful (and less important in the initial diagnosis and management) are other pituitary hormones such as LH, FSH, estradiol or testosterone, growth hormone, and IGF-I. Examination of cerebrospinal fluid (CSF) is usually not diagnostic and is unnecessary if the diagnosis of apoplexy is certain. However, if there is bleeding into the CSF as a result of the apoplexy, red blood cells as well as an elevated protein level and xanthochromia can be seen.

The differential diagnosis of pituitary apoplexy should include other conditions that result in the symptoms of headache, vomiting, visual disturbances, and hemodynamic instability such as infection (meningitis [Chapter 384]), cavernous sinus thrombosis (Chapter 385), migraine (Chapter 370), Rathke cyst hemorrhage (Chapter 380), and hyperemesis gravidarum (Chapter 226). Each of these conditions is itself a medical emergency that requires specific treatment.

TREATMENT AND PROGNOSIS   Rx

The initial management is stabilization of the hemodynamic status with intravenous 0.9% NaCl boluses to maintain normal tissue perfusion, usually accompanied by high-dose parenteral glucocorticoids (100 mg hydrocortisone every 8 hours intravenously). Although 80% of patients have residual hypopituitarism following apoplexy (with or without surgical decompression), some patients do not display immediate evidence of hypopituitarism. In addition, recurrent apoplexy has been reported to occur. MRI of the pituitary should be obtained at 3- to 6-month intervals until the anatomy is stable and then yearly for 5 years. A month after discharge from the hospital and recovery from the acute event, patients should have repeat endocrine testing to determine if the endocrine defect persists. Repeat testing will confirm whether the patient needs to remain on life-long hormone replacement therapy.

Empty Sella

Empty sella is a radiologic diagnosis that refers to the observation on imaging of the presence of CSF in the sella turcica accompanied by a flattened pituitary gland (Fig. 211-4). It is usually noted as an incidental finding when an MRI or CT scan of the skull is performed because of problems unrelated to the pituitary. It can be primary or acquired when a defect in the diaphragma sella

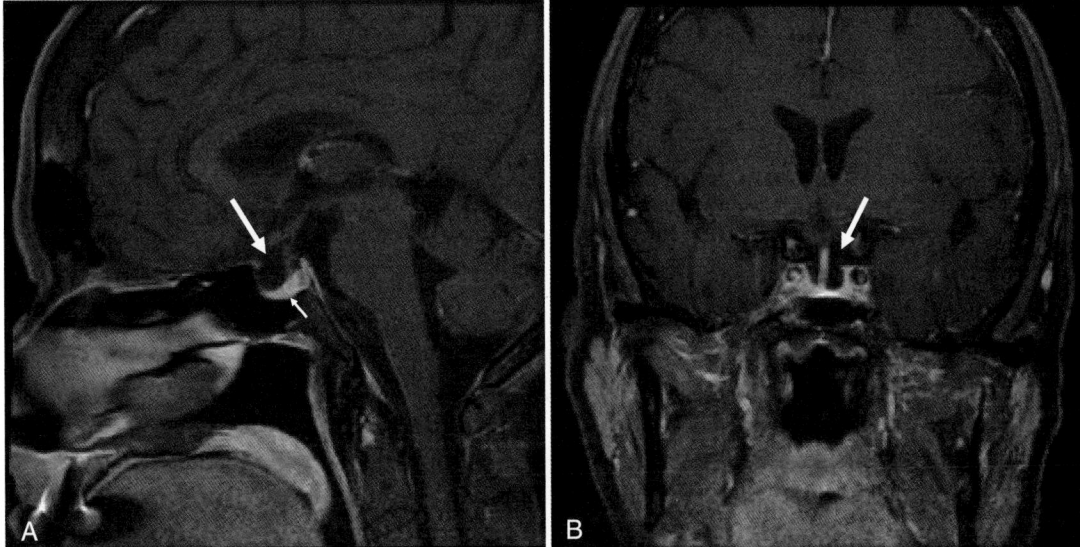

FIGURE 211-4. Magnetic resonance image of an empty sella. **A,** Sagittal postcontrast. Note the void in the sella (*large arrow*) with compression of the normal pituitary against the sella turcica (*small, thin arrow*). **B,** Coronal postcontrast. Sella filled with cerebrospinal fluid and appears as empty.

allows the arachnoid membrane to herniate into the sella. If the herniation has been present for years, the sella enlarges, probably owing to persistent exposure to intracranial pressure. Primary empty sella is more frequent in women and may be accompanied by benign intracranial hypertension (Chapters 180 and 370). Pituitary function is usually normal, but about 10% of patients also have mild hyperprolactinemia, probably owing to stretching of the pituitary stalk. Patients with acquired empty sella may have a prior history of an infarcted pituitary, surgery, or radiation. After the diagnosis of empty sella is made and the patient is asymptomatic, there is no need to measure hormone levels unless there is suspicion of a clinical abnormality related to the pituitary. Because pituitary function is usually normal, no specific treatment is required. However, when there is concern about hypopituitarism, investigation as outlined above should be performed.

Other Causes of Hypopituitarism

Functional causes of defective pituitary function can be seen in severe malnutrition (Chapter 203). Such nutritional deprivation can occur in critically ill patients who are in a state of severe calorie deprivation or in anorexia nervosa (Chapter 206). In both examples, there are likely central (hypothalamic and higher) mechanisms and molecular mediators (e.g., cachexins and tumor necrosis factor) that inhibit the release of pituitary hormone. This form of hypopituitarism is generally reversible when the caloric situation improves. Deposition and infiltration of amyloid protein in amyloidosis (Chapter 179) or iron in hemochromatosis (Chapter 201) can result in hypopituitarism.

⬤ PITUITARY TUMORS

PATHOBIOLOGY

Clonal proliferation of the different cell types in the pituitary result in tumor formation. Although the molecular basis for this clonal proliferation is not well understood, pituitary tumors are classified clinically as "functioning," meaning they produce one or more hormones in excess, or "nonfunctioning," meaning that they do not produce an excess hormone in blood.[7] Because most functional tumors do not have appropriate physiologic feedback due to their oncologic nature, they usually secrete excess hormone(s) that cause a variety of clinical syndromes as described. Not uncommonly, confirmation of the secretory nature of the pituitary tumor is made at the time of removal when the surgical pathologist, based on immunochemistry, demonstrates the immunoreactivity of a hormone(s) in the tumor. However, not all immunohistochemically positive tumors result in excess blood levels of the hormone. The exact reason is unknown but may result when a defect in the intracellular processing of the hormone inhibits release of that hormone. Nevertheless, a functioning pituitary tumor is a diagnosis made clinically and based on provocative testing as discussed below. The five cell types result in different pituitary adenomas. The reported prevalences differ among large surgical series, which represent only patients who undergo surgery rather than being managed medically.

Prolactinomas, which may account for up to 50% of pituitary tumors, are likely caused when proliferation of the lactotroph results in excess prolactin and subsequent galactorrhea and hypogonadism. Somatotrophs producing growth hormone, corticotrophs making ACTH, and gonadotrophs making LH and FSH together account for 10 to 20% of adenomas. Nonfunctioning tumors, which mainly cause a mass effect or hypopituitarism, account for 10 to 25%. The size of the tumor usually is proportional to the amount of hormone it produces when functioning. Depending on the severity of the clinical perturbation caused, certain tumors are usually diagnosed sooner and therefore are usually smaller on diagnosis than others. For example, gonadotropinomas are usually diagnosed as macroadenomas because their symptoms are usually more subtle than in TSH-secreting tumors, where the symptoms present early and the tumors are usually smaller at the time of diagnosis. In addition to functioning and nonfunctioning, tumors are classified by their anatomy based on imaging studies: microadenomas are less than 10 mm in diameter versus macroadenomas which are greater than 10 mm in diameter (and typically with extrasellar extension).

Pituitary adenomas are monoclonal and can be locally invasive, but they are rarely malignant. The somatic mutations causing most pituitary tumors remain unknown, and the hormonal environment may also affect the rate of tumor growth (e.g., the growth of ACTH-secreting tumors following bilateral adrenalectomy as seen in Nelson syndrome).

At least six types of inherited predispositions to pituitary tumors are recognized (Table 211-6). When macroadenomas are found in children or when there is a family history of pituitary adenomas, genetic testing is warranted (Table 211-6) so that appropriate monitoring can occur before the patient is symptomatic.[8]

CLINICAL MANIFESTATIONS

The clinical manifestations of pituitary tumors depend in large part on whether they are functional and whether their size compromises the normal function of the pituitary gland and thereby results in clinical symptoms of hypopituitarism.[9] In general, the diagnosis of a tumor due to excess or diminishing hormone secretion presents the greater clinical challenge. Pituitary tumors have historically been diagnosed more frequently in women of reproductive age because even a slight perturbation in hormonal milieu will disrupt the multiple hormone interactions necessary for a normal menstrual period. In men or postmenopausal women, slight perturbations in hormone levels (either excess or deficiency) are usually not noticed for several years. More recently, the diagnosis of pituitary adenomas is usually an incidental finding on an imaging study obtained for unrelated reasons. Even careful endocrine evaluation of patients with incidental tumors reveals hyper- or hyposecretion of pituitary hormones in only a small percent, and such incidental tumors usually do not increase in size over time.

Other than hormonal effects, reasons for suspicion of a pituitary mass are headaches and visual field abnormalities. A reported 33 to 72% of patients with a pituitary lesion have headaches, a percentage that is greater than the

TABLE 211-6 INHERITED SYNDROMES OF PITUITARY ADENOMAS

SYNDROME	PITUITARY TUMOR	MOLECULAR PATHOGENESIS	MODE OF INHERITANCE	OTHER MANIFESTATIONS
McCune Albright	F/NF	Gsα SU	Somatic mutation	Ovary, bone, thyroid dysfunction
Multiple endocrine neoplasias*	F (30% PRL)/NF	Menin (*MEN1*) and MEN4 (*CDKN1B*)	AD	Parathyroid and pancreas tumors
Familial Isolated Pituitary Adenoma (FIPA) Syndrome*	F/NF	Arylhydrocarbon receptor interacting protein (*AIP*)†	AD with variable penetrance	None
Carney Complex (with or without PPNAD)	1/3 with Cushing	Type 1A regulatory subunit of protein kinase A (*PRKARIA*)	AD	Atrial myxomas, spotty skin pigmentation, schwannomas
Primary Pigmented Nodular Adrenocortical Disease (PPNAD)	Cushing	Succinate dehydrogenase subunit (*SDH*)	AD	Pheochromocytomas, paragangliomas
Early childhood gigantism	GH	*CD40LG, ARHGEF6, RBMX, GPR101*	X-linked	gigantism

*Tumors are generally more aggressive and occur at a younger age.
†About 15% of FIPA and 50% of familial acromegaly
AD = autosomal dominant; F = functioning; GH = growth hormone; NF = nonfunctioning; PPNAD = primary pigmented nodular adrenocortical disease; PRL = prolactin.

TABLE 211-7 SELECTED TESTS OF EXCESS PITUITARY FUNCTION

HORMONE	TEST	INTERPRETATION
Growth hormone (GH)	*Basal IGF-I*	Elevated IGF-I levels are consistent with acromegaly when interpreted in the context of age and nutritional status.
	Oral glucose suppression test: after 75-g glucose load, GH is measured at −30, 0, 30, 60, 90, 120 min.	GH should be suppressed to <1 µg/L in normal persons with polyclonal radioimmunoassays; <0.4 µg/L with two-site monoclonal assays. GH may paradoxically increase in acromegaly.
Prolactin	*Basal prolactin levels*	Elevated prolactin (>200 µg/L) is consistent with a prolactinoma. When prolactin levels are between 20 and 200 µg/L, other causes of hyperprolactinemia should be considered.
Adrenocorticotropic hormone (ACTH)	*Measurement of 24-hr urine free cortisol*	Elevated level is suggestive of Cushing syndrome, but it has several other causes as well.
	Midnight salivary cortisol: special tubes with cotton pledgets available to collect saliva at 11 PM to midnight	In normal persons, the midnight salivary cortisol is very low because of the normal diurnal variation. In patients with Cushing syndrome, the salivary cortisol is elevated.
	Overnight dexamethasone suppression test: dexamethasone (1 mg) PO at midnight, followed by 8 AM plasma cortisol	In normal persons, AM cortisol should be suppressed to <5 µg/dL. Normal test excludes Cushing syndrome. Other disorders can cause failure to suppress normally.
	CRH test: ovine CRH (1 µg/kg) is administered IV, and ACTH and cortisol are drawn at −15, 0, 15, 30, 60, 90, and 120 min.	In Cushing disease, there is usually a 50% increase in ACTH and a 20% increase in cortisol. Adrenal adenoma is associated with suppressed ACTH. Ectopic ACTH is associated with high basal ACTH and cortisol levels that are not affected by CRH.
	Petrosal sinus ACTH sampling: the inferior petrosal sinus is catheterized bilaterally, and plasma ACTH is compared with simultaneous peripheral samples. The sampling can be done in conjunction with CRH stimulation.	In Cushing disease, the ratio of ACTH in the petrosal sinus to the periphery is at least 2 basally and at least 3 after CRH. In ectopic ACTH, the ratio of petrosal sinus to peripheral level is <1.5.
Thyroid-stimulating hormone (TSH)	*Basal thyroid function tests*	An inappropriate normal or elevated TSH in the setting of increased free thyroid hormone levels is consistent with a TSH-producing tumor or other causes of inappropriate TSH secretion.
	Free α-subunit level	Elevated levels associated with inappropriately elevated TSH are suggestive of a TSH-producing tumor.
Follicle-stimulating hormone (FSH), luteinizing hormone (LH)	*Basal FSH, LH, testosterone*	Increased LH and testosterone levels in males are consistent with LH-secreting tumors. Elevated FSH and low-normal testosterone are suggestive of an FSH-producing tumor if primary gonadal failure is not present. In females, assessment of excess hormone secretion is difficult because of changes during the menstrual cycle and at menopause.

CRH = corticotropin-releasing hormone; IGF = insulin-like growth factor; TRH = thyrotropin-releasing hormone.

22% of women and 11% of men in the general population who complain of headaches (Chapter 370). Mass effect of the innervated dura is an explanation for the headache, but discerning which patients have a headache from the pituitary lesion and which ones have an unrelated cause for the headache is challenging. Headaches due to pituitary lesions are more common in females and in patients with Rathke cleft cysts and apoplexy. The mass effect of the tumor is also responsible for the temporal visual field problems associated with macroadenomas that expand into the suprasellar region and abut against the optic chiasm. The superior and temporal visual fields are most affected, and severely impaired visual fields can be revealed on examination by confrontation testing. The degree of visual field loss depends on how the pituitary is fixed to the sella, the mode of expansion, and the degree of growth. If there is any evidence on MRI that the tumor is close to or abuts the chiasm, formal visual field testing should be performed. In general, the sooner treatment is initiated to decompress the chiasm (with surgery, or in the case of a medically responsive prolactinoma, with appropriate medication) the more likely vision will be restored; however, visual improvement has been noted even after months of visual field impairment.

Diagnosis of pituitary adenomas that are actively secreting a hormone is based on provocative testing (Table 211-7).

TREATMENT

Rx

Surgery

The first line of therapy for pituitary tumors that require treatment is surgery (Video 211-1). The major exception is for prolactinomas (even those that are macroadenomas and result in visual field cuts, headaches, and evidence of selected hypopituitarism), for which medical therapy is the first mode of treatment. Indications for surgery include decompression of mass effects, prevention of further tumor expansion, and normalization of hormone levels. The endoscopic transsphenoidal approach is the standard for decompression or extirpation.

Subfrontal craniotomy is reserved for tumors requiring extensive extrasellar exploration. Transsphenoidal surgery is effective, with a less than 5% complication rate and 1% mortality rate in experienced centers, but potential sequelae include sinusitis, hemorrhage, CSF leak, hypopituitarism, and optic nerve injury. About 5% of patients develop transient postoperative diabetes insipidus that rarely persists. About 80 to 90% of microadenomas and only 30 to 60% of macroadenomas are completely cured by transsphenoidal hypophysectomy, but most other patients substantially improve in terms of their hormone levels. Even after apparent surgical cure, about 10 to 20% of tumors recur within several years, as manifested by oversecretion of their hormones, and recurrence is more likely if the tumor extended into the suprasellar space or fragmented upon removal.

Radiation Therapy

Irradiation (typically 45 Gy) can be adjunctive therapy after surgery or used in combination with medical therapy. CyberKnife stereotactic radiotherapy can deliver the same total dose in one treatment as would be provided by traditional external beam radiotherapy over five weeks. CyberKnife therapy spares critical radiosensitive structures, but the response can take months up to several years.[10] Proton beam therapy may be performed for intrasellar lesions but is not widely available. Irradiation provides complete remission, and it is most useful for nonfunctioning macroadenomas and for patients who have some residual postoperative tumor or visible tumor. Complications are generally dose related and include partial or complete hypopituitarism (50 to 70% of patients), second tumors in the radiation field (about 2% of patients over a 20-year period), cognitive dysfunction, damage to the optic nerve, and stroke. Stereotactic radiotherapy appears to cause similar complication rates of hypopituitarism but less stroke compared with conventional external beam therapy.

Medical Therapy

Bromocriptine and cabergoline, which are dopamine agonists, now are the primary treatments for prolactinomas. These agents decrease the tumor's size and induce a rapid decline in prolactin levels. They also can treat acromegaly, but the decline in tumor size and in growth hormone levels is less pronounced than in prolactinomas, and they usually work best if the tumor is also secreting prolactin as well as growth hormone. Somatostatin analogues (octreotide, lanreotide, and pasireotide)—which suppress the secretion of growth hormone, TSH, and ACTH—can treat acromegaly, Cushing disease, and TSH-producing tumors. Other medications (ketoconazole, metyrapone, etomidate, and mitotane) used in Cushing disease inhibit steroid biosynthesis, but these agents have side effects that adversely affect adherence. Furthermore, because most tumors cannot be controlled with these agents, they are used primarily to reduce preoperative cortisol levels or as adjunctive postoperative therapy.

The hormonal effects of functioning pituitary tumors can also be treated with receptor blockers. For example, pegvisomant, which is an analogue of growth hormone, competitively binds the growth hormone receptor and can be used to treat acromegaly. Mifepristone blocks the interaction of cortisol with its receptor and is useful to treat Cushing syndrome, specifically in helping with glucose control. However, these drugs do not affect the size or growth of the tumor, only the biologic effect of its hormone in the peripheral tissues.

GROWTH HORMONE

PATHOBIOLOGY

Growth hormone is the main regulator of the growth of bone and other tissues. The human growth hormone gene along with four other related genes is located at the growth hormone locus on chromosome 17 where, by gene duplication, these genes are interspersed in the same transcriptional orientation. The five genes not only have a high degree of sequence identity but also exist as multiple isoforms based on variable splicing. The variant expressed in the somatotrophs of the pituitary gives rise to two isoforms. Growth can occur in the fetus and early postnatal state independent of growth hormone; but soon after birth, growth hormone controls growth, and its deficiency results in dwarfism.

The metabolic effects of growth hormone are both direct, by interaction with its tissue receptors, as well as mediated by a serum factor secreted by the liver (somatomedin or insulin-like growth factor-I [IGF-I]). IGF-I in turn acts on a variety of tissues to stimulate body growth. IGF-I is also produced in a variety of tissues including smooth muscle, skin, lung, bone, and cartilage. However, in addition to IGF-I production in the various tissues, growth hormone causes hydrolysis of triglycerides in adipose tissue. In skeletal muscle, growth hormone enhances amino acid uptake and nitrogen retention, similar to what would be expected in exercising muscle. Growth hormone also stimulates glycogenolysis and gluconeogenesis.

Growth Hormone Deficiency

PATHOBIOLOGY

Growth hormone deficiency in children may be due to hypothalamic defects in the production, release, or sensing of growth-hormone-releasing hormone (GHRH). Deficiency also can be caused by any congenital disorder of pituitary gland development or from central nervous system defects such as tumors (craniopharyngioma, germinoma, ependymoma, pituitary adenoma, meningioma, medulloblastoma, glioma, Rathke cleft cyst, and arachnoid cyst). Postsurgical disruption of the hypothalamic pituitary axis, trauma, radiation, or infiltration also can cause growth hormone deficiency. Isolated growth hormone deficiency, which is the most common form of nonfamilial deficiency, is responsible for most cases of hypopituitarism in children. Growth hormone deficiency also can occur in combination with other pituitary hormone defects, as discussed above.

CLINICAL MANIFESTATIONS

In children, growth hormone deficiency is primarily manifested by slow growth. The child may present with short stature (>2 standard deviations below normal) or have a height that is crossing the centile on the growth chart. Due to redundancy of other hormones and factors on growth, children usually are not small for gestational age at birth but can manifest hypoglycemia due to the counterregulatory effect of growth hormone. There is an increase in body fat, which may result in an appearance that the child is younger than the stated age, and hypogonadism or small genitalia may variably be present. Children usually are diagnosed when found to be shorter than their peers—at well-baby visits, when they enter school, or at puberty. In the Laron dwarfism syndrome, growth hormone levels are high due to failure of IGF-I stimulation caused by mutations in the growth hormone receptor.

DIAGNOSIS

In children, the diagnosis of isolated growth hormone deficiency is most reliably made by careful growth measurements, a thorough medical history to exclude other causes of growth failure (renal tubular acidosis [Chapter 110], thyroid disease [Chapter 213], Turner syndrome in girls, or other chronic disease) or combined hormone deficiencies. Because growth hormone is secreted episodically, measurements of serum growth hormone, IGF-I, and insulin-like growth factor binding protein-3 (IGFBP-3) are also helpful to confirm the diagnosis.

Provocative tests are usually necessary to diagnose growth hormone deficiency in children (Table 221-2), and similar diagnostic criteria can be applied for adult onset growth hormone deficiency. Children with the diagnosis of idiopathic growth hormone deficiency should be retested as adults if they were inadequately diagnosed or had a mild form that resolved in adulthood. If an adult is deficient in three pituitary hormones and has an IGF-I level below the lower limit of normal, provocative testing is not required.

TREATMENT Rx

The treatment of isolated growth hormone deficiency in childhood is replacement human recombinant growth hormone at 0.3 mg/kg/week divided into 6 or 7 doses. The average growth is 9 to 10 cm in the first year of treatment, and then it begins to slow down to 6 to 7 cm per year for the next two years. At the time of puberty, some pediatric endocrinologists increase the dose to 0.7 mg/kg/week in divided doses while monitoring serum IGF-I and IGFBP-3 levels to be sure they are not greater than 2 standard deviations above the upper limit of normal. If growth slows, thyroid function should be checked because hypothyroidism develops in some children who are treated with growth hormone.

Treatment of adult-onset growth hormone deficiency is with human recombinant growth hormone at 0.2 mg/day in men and 0.3 mg/day in women, but 0.1 mg/day in older individuals. The dose is usually given in the evening to mimic the diurnal variation in growth hormone secretion in the physiologic state. Assessment of fat and muscle mass, as well as objective assessment of quality of life, can be helpful to monitor treatment. Although generally safe, complications of treatment include fluid retention (resulting in lower extremity edema or carpal tunnel syndrome) and mild glucose intolerance. Contraindications for treatment include known malignancy, intracranial hypertension, and proliferative retinopathy.

Growth Hormone Excess: Acromegaly and Gigantism

Acromegaly is a disease of excessive growth and metabolic derangements caused by proliferation of pituitary somatotrophs and excessive secretion of growth hormone. If left untreated, it results in gross acral and facial disfigurement, cardiac disease, cancer, metabolic abnormalities including diabetes, and increased mortality.

PATHOBIOLOGY

There are multiple levels of normal control of growth hormone synthesis and release. The hypothalamic factor, somatotropin release–inhibiting factor, inhibits growth hormone release, whereas growth hormone–releasing hormone stimulates both its synthesis and release. Other growth hormone secretagogues, such as ghrelin in the gastrointestinal tract, directly bind to growth hormone–stimulating receptors in the hypothalamus and induce the release of growth hormone. Furthermore, growth hormone's action is mediated by hepatic IGF-I, which inhibits growth hormone synthesis by stimulating somatotropin release–inhibiting factor in the hypothalamus and pituitary. Acromegaly therefore can be due to pituitary adenomas that produce excessive and uncontrolled amounts of growth hormone, by ectopic production of growth hormone by islet cell tumors (Chapter 217) or lymphomas (Chapters 176 and 177), or by ectopic production of growth hormone–releasing hormone in bronchial carcinoid tumors (Chapter 182), small cell cancers of the lung (Chapter 182), medullary thyroid cancers (Chapter 213), or pheochromocytomas (Chapter 215).

CLINICAL MANIFESTATIONS

When first encountering patients with excess growth hormone, the handshake by a large, enveloping doughy hand and a rough, resonant "Hello Doctor" may be the first hints of acromegaly. Symptoms associated with growth hormone hypersecretion are often not recognized for 10 or more years after their often-subtle onset. The classic coarse facial features are usually not immediately apparent but recognized in retrospect and after looking at past photographs (Fig. 211-5). Because these pituitary tumors are usually diagnosed only years after the onset of symptoms,[11] they are usually macroadenomas by the time of presentation (75%). Headaches are an initial symptom in up to 60% of the patients, and 10% present with the classic temporal hemianopsia. Tall stature may be present depending on when the growth hormone excess began, with younger age of onset correlating with taller stature.

The effects are most apparent in the bones and soft tissue with bony overgrowth, specifically a protruding lower jaw, splayed teeth, malocclusion, mandibular overbite, and macroglossia are frequently noted. Overgrowth of soft tissues of the pharynx may result in sleep apnea. Enlargement of the nose and facial bones results in frontal bossing. Enlargement of bones and soft tissue likewise account for the changes patients may observe in ring, shoe, or hat size. Soft tissue growth, including multiple skin tags, is often associated with premalignant colonic polyps and colon cancer (Chapter 184). Hyperhidrosis at rest is very common. Neuropathy, such as carpal tunnel syndrome (Chapter 392), can be seen secondary to nerve entrapment.

Acromegaly increases mortality rates two- to three-fold, with increased mortality mostly attributable to cardiovascular and cerebrovascular complications. This risk can be explained in part by high frequencies of hypertension (25 to 35%) and diabetes mellitus (10 to 25%). Most patients develop myocardial hypertrophy, which is often ultimately associated with symptomatic ischemic heart disease and heart failure. Sleep apnea (Chapter 377) may contribute to cardiac dysrhythmias. The multiple cosmetic, metabolic, cardiac, and other consequences of acromegaly emphasize why early diagnosis and appropriate therapy is so important.

DIAGNOSIS

Because growth hormone is secreted in a pulsatile manner and at high amplitudes (>50 ng/mL), random measurements are not very useful for diagnosing or excluding acromegaly. Because stress, exercise, and sleep all cause

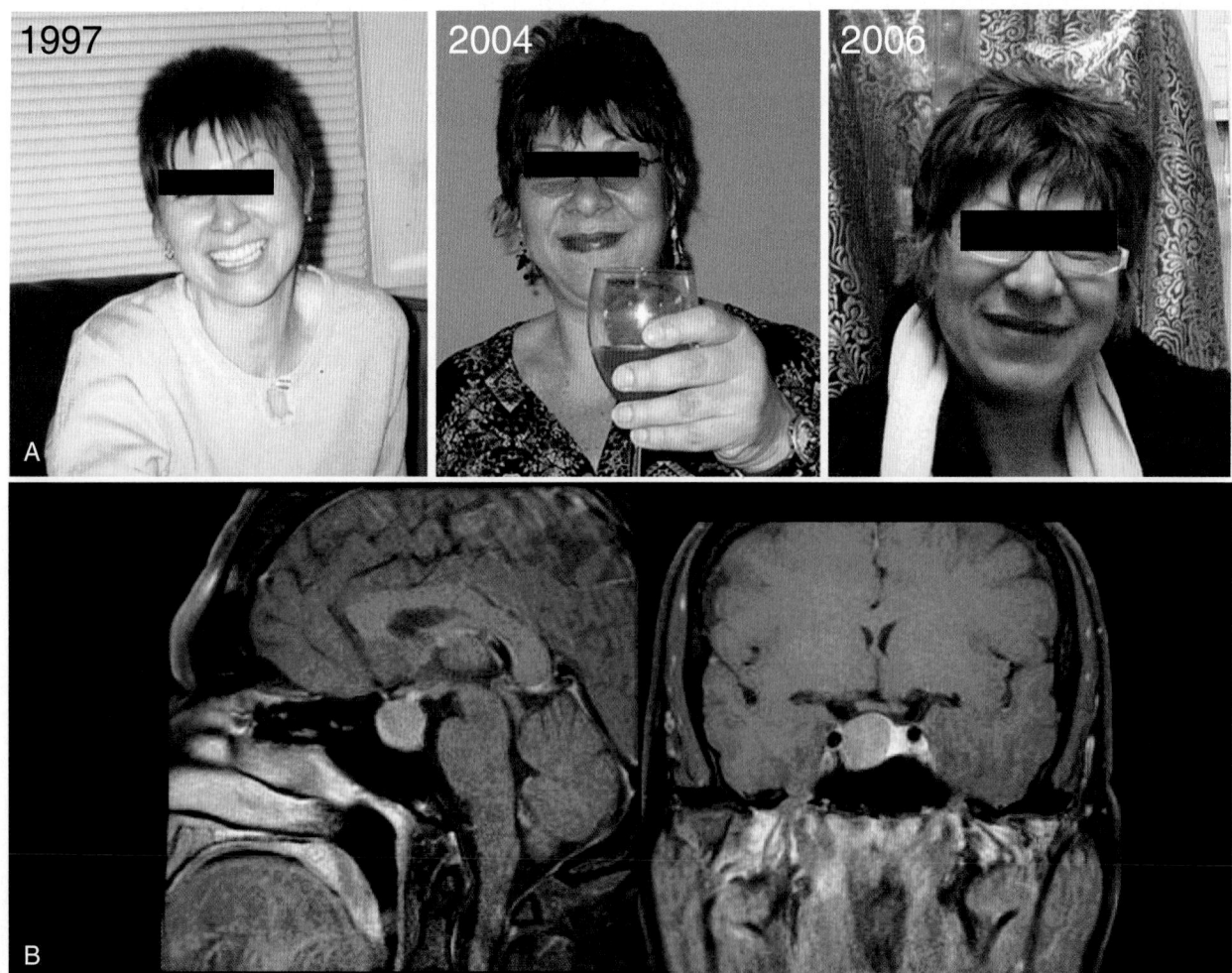

FIGURE 211-5. Clinical features of acromegaly. A, Serial photographs of a woman with acromegaly. Over a 9-year period, there is a progressive coarsening of facial features, including enlargement of the nose and lips and development of prognathism. She also experienced hypertension, arthropathy, and enlargement of the hands. B, MRI of patient's pituitary adenoma at the time of presentation.

physiologic increases in serum growth hormone, a better integrated index of growth hormone production and a more useful way to screen for acromegaly is to measure IGF-I levels (which correlate well with daily secretion of growth hormone and with the activity of the disease) after a 2-hr, 75-g oral glucose tolerance test (Table 211-7). In acromegaly, glucose administration will not suppress growth hormone levels to below 1 ng/mL by a polyclonal antibody immunoassay or below 0.4 ng/mL by a chemiluminescent immunoradiometric assay. The response to a glucose load is also useful to determine the efficacy of therapy because it should normalize quickly after growth hormone levels normalize. Co-secretion of prolactin should be measured, since a significant percentage of tumors co-secrete growth hormone and prolactin, and these findings have implications for medical therapy with dopamine agonists.

After the diagnosis of acromegaly is made based on a full endocrine evaluation, an MRI should be obtained to determine the extent of tumor growth. Although 90% of patients have a visible pituitary adenoma on MRI, 10% of the patients have an empty sella. The rare nonpituitary causes of acromegaly include hypothalamic tumors that make excess growth hormone–releasing hormone or nonendocrine tumors that secrete ectopic growth hormone. Occasionally, selective venous sampling over tumor beds identified radiologically can identify sources of secreted IGF-I or similar compounds.

TREATMENT Rx

The goals of therapy are to shrink the tumor, prevent tumor mass effects, and eliminate the function of the tumor, thereby reducing the long-term morbidity and mortality that result from excess growth hormone production. Treatment is usually successful at reversing many of the soft tissue abnormalities as well as the diabetes and other metabolic derangements. Acral changes, however, are usually arrested, so that physical disfigurement can be prevented rather than corrected. Although any reduction in the growth hormone level can improve symptoms, the goal is to normalize growth hormone and IGF-I levels, to prevent recrudescence of the tumor, and to avoid precipitating hypopituitarism. Cure usually is defined by the normalization of random blood levels as well as levels after provocative testing, such as an oral glucose tolerance test.

Transsphenoidal surgery can reduce growth hormone levels below 2.5 ng/mL in 80 to 90% microadenomas. Macroadenomas have tumor cure rates less than 30%, but the growth hormone level usually is substantially reduced.

Medical therapies for acromegaly include somatostatin analogues (octreotide, lanreotide, and pasireotide), dopamine agonists (e.g., cabergoline), and a growth hormone receptor antagonist (pegvisomant). Somatostatin analogues can be used as adjunctive therapy if surgery or radiation do not cure the tumor or as primary therapy when a surgical cure is not possible, such as when the tumor has invaded the cavernous sinus. Intramuscular octreotide, lanreotide, and especially pasireotide given every 4 weeks almost always reduce growth hormone and IGF-I levels, and they normalize IGF-I levels in about 50 to 60% of cases. Pasireotide LAR (either 40 mg or 60 mg administered once every 28 days for 24 weeks) provides superior efficacy compared with octreotide or lanreotide and is becoming the new standard in patients whose acromegaly is not adequately controlled by a first-generation somatostatin analog. [A1][A2][A3] Tumor size is reduced modestly in about 50% of cases, and about 10 to 20% of patients who achieve normal levels of growth hormone and IGF-I can eventually be successfully withdrawn from treatment after several years. Side effects of somatostatin analogues include diarrhea and cholelithiasis, although cholecystitis and subsequent cholecystectomy are rare. Some patients experience additive benefit when two classes of medications are combined in low doses to avoid adverse effects.

Although cabergoline often can reduce levels of growth hormone and IGF-I, levels return to normal in only about 30% of patients. Pegvisomant, which is a biosynthetic analogue of growth hormone, prevents growth hormone from binding to its receptor. When given by daily subcutaneous injection, it can normalize IGF-I levels in greater than 90% of patients but does not affect the size of the tumor itself. It can be reserved for patients who do not respond to other therapies, be used as initial medical therapy for small tumors, or be combined with somatostatin analogues. The most common adverse effect of pegvisomant is an increase in liver enzyme levels.

Radiation is not an effective primary treatment because it will not reduce growth hormone levels until 5 to 10 years later and carries a high risk of hypopituitarism and other complications. Adjunctive radiation therapy, especially stereotactic radiotherapy, may benefit patients whose macroadenomas persist despite transsphenoidal surgery and medical therapy.

Data show that patients with acromegaly have a mortality similar to the general population if they achieve growth hormone suppression to less than 1 ng/mL during an oral glucose tolerance test and normal IGF-I levels, especially with ongoing use of somatostatin analogs as adjuvant therapy. However, the increased life expectancy has been associated with more deaths due to cancer.

PROLACTIN

Both prolactin and growth hormone have similar amino acid sequences and are present in all vertebrates. During pregnancy, prolactin concentrations increase and, in conjunction with the other hormones of pregnancy, stimulate the breast epithelium to produce milk. Lactotrophs, which are the cells that secrete prolactin, represent 20 to 50% of the anterior pituitary cell population and are the most likely to give rise to pituitary tumors. Prolactin is now implicated in not only lactation, but also inhibition of reproductive function (by suppression of gonadotropins) and support of maternal behavior. The function is less clear when prolactin is expressed outside the pituitary, including in the mammary gland and uterine decidua. A prolactin variant, "big prolactin" or macroprolactin, is a high-molecular-weight variant due to the tendency of prolactin to aggregate and form intermolecular disulfide bridges spontaneously or with IgG. Despite their immunoreactivity, these prolactin variants usually have decreased biologic activity.

Prolactin binds to the prolactin receptor, which is a member of the type 1 cytokine receptor family. Janus kinase-2 is a protein kinase that is associated with the prolactin receptor and mediates prolactin's effect in the target cells in ways that are incompletely understood. The prolactin receptor is also the receptor for placental lactogens, which are hormones synthesized during pregnancy and which are also a result of prolactin or growth hormone gene duplication.

Regulation of prolactin secretion by lactotrophs is primarily under the inhibition of dopamine, which acts through the D_2-type receptors on lactotrophs. Inhibition of the dopamine ("inhibiting the inhibitor") results in a release of prolactin as is seen in nonsecreting pituitary tumors or trauma that disrupts the pituitary stalk, thereby preventing dopamine from inhibiting prolactin release. Estrogen is a potent stimulator of lactotroph proliferation and raises the possibility that exogenous estrogen could increase the growth of prolactinomas, although clinical evidence suggests this phenomenon may be true only for macroprolactinomas. Thyrotropin releasing hormone (TRH) and vasoactive intestinal peptide (VIP) also stimulate the release of prolactin, so when hypothyroidism increases TRH release from the hypothalamus, it causes hyperprolactinemia. In addition to the hypothalamic control, prolactin secretion is induced by sleep, stress, chest wall stimulation, and pregnancy. During pregnancy, high levels of estrogen and progesterone inhibit lactation, and their postpartum decline permits lactation accompanied by the secretion of oxytocin in response to suckling.

Prolactin Deficiency

The normal concentration for prolactin is less than 15 to 20 pg/mL in women and less than 10 to 15 pg/mL in men. The consequences of low prolactin values and the lower limits of normal are not well understood, but the limit of detection of prolactin in most clinical assays is less than 1 pg/mL. Low serum levels of prolactin can be seen in hyperthyroidism because TRH is suppressed. Low prolactin may prevent adequate lactation in nursing mothers and may be a reliable marker for hypopituitarism when seen with another pituitary hormone deficiency. Lactation is not completely absent because nipple stimulation may be sufficient to start milk production. No cases of isolated prolactin deficiency have been reported in men.

Hyperprolactinemia
PATHOBIOLOGY

Among causes of elevated levels of prolactin (Table 211-8) are medications that antagonize dopamine action or increase the activity of endorphins or serotonin. These mechanisms result in mild hyperprolactinemia (<100 pg/mL), but the most common cause of hyperprolactinemia greater than 100 pg/mL is a prolactinoma.

CLINICAL MANIFESTATIONS

In adult premenopausal females, the typical presentation is galactorrhea and oligomenorrhea. Because galactorrhea is enabled by estrogen, postmenopausal women, who are generally deficient in estrogen, do not develop galactorrhea despite elevated prolactin levels. Prolactin can also suppress GnRH, therefore LH and FSH, and in turn estrogen. As a result, symptoms of hyperprolactinemia may also be manifestations of low estrogen levels, such as infertility, decreased libido, and vaginal dryness. Oral contraceptive agents (Chapter 225) can overcome the perturbations in GnRH and induce normal menses even in the presence of elevated prolactin levels. Osteopenia (Chapter 230) may be a direct effect of an elevated prolactin level on the bone as well as its indirect effects on estrogen. If the prolactinoma grows large enough, neurologic symptoms

TABLE 211-8   CAUSES OF HYPERPROLACTINEMIA

DRUG CAUSES	EXAMPLES	MECHANISM	SERUM PRL RANGE PG/ML
Antiemetics	Metoclopramide, domperidone, prochlorperazine	Dopamine receptor blockade	
Antipsychotics	First generation: fluphenazine; halperidol, others; Second generation: paliperidone; risperidone	Dopamine receptor blockade	20-70
Antidepressants, cyclic	Clomipramine	Unknown	20-70
Narcotics	Methadone, morphine, others	Indirect effect of opioid mu receptor activation	20-70
Estrogen	Oral contraceptives	Stimulates PRL at transcription	20-70
NONDRUG CAUSES			
Stress		Hypothalamic	20-70
Pregnancy		Estrogen	20-500
Pituitary adenoma			Macro: 200->10,000 Micro: 20-250
Hypothyroidism		Increase in TRH	Moderate;<100
Chronic renal failure, cirrhosis		Decreased clearance and central effect	Moderate; <100
Chest wall injury, nipple stimulation		Unknown	20-70

PRL = prolactin; TRH = thyrotropin releasing hormone.

(e.g., vision changes and headaches) can appear even before endocrine manifestations.

In adult men, prolactinomas are usually detected late because a large mass is necessary to cause neurologic or endocrine manifestations. However, excess prolactin inhibits GnRH, thereby lowering testosterone and resulting in decreased libido, impotence, reduced muscle mass, and increased fat mass. In rare situations when men have elevated estrogen levels (e.g., cirrhosis), high prolactin levels can include gynecomastia and even galactorrhea. In men with osteopenia (Chapter 230), prolactin should be measured because elevated levels decrease testosterone and osteoblasts.

DIAGNOSIS

The diagnosis of hyperprolactinemia is based on a straightforward measurement of elevated blood prolactin by immunoassay. When an occasional macroprolactinoma causes a prolactin level higher than 1000 pg/mL, falsely low values may be reported because the high level "overwhelms" the antibody and artificially reduces the measured value. Conversely, prolactin can dimerize with itself ("big prolactin") or complex with circulating IgG ("big big prolactin") to form "macroprolactin" complexes that are not biologically active but may result in elevated prolactin values on some immunoassays.

Prolactin values slightly above normal but less than 70 pg/mL are usually due to drug causes. Nondrug causes include chest wall syndrome, pregnancy, lactation, and renal failure as well as prolactin-secreting adenomas. Because dopamine inhibits prolactin, nonprolactin–secreting pituitary or hypothalamic tumors that compress the pituitary stalk can also cause an increase in prolactin by disrupting the flow of dopamine to the lactotrophs. As in most functional adenomas, in which larger tumors generally produce more hormones, macroadenomas can be associated with levels greater than 1000 pg/mL whereas microadenomas may only slightly elevate prolactin levels. In patients who have mildly elevated prolactin levels (<100 pg/mL) but no tumor seen on MRI, the cause may be macroprolactin, a microadenoma too small to be seen on MRI, or "idiopathic" hyperprolactin owing to hypothalamic dysfunction.

TREATMENT   Rx

The goal of therapy is to restore normal gonadal function.[12] An additional goal is to shrink the tumor to alleviate any anatomic or neurologic mass effects. Dopamine agonists, which activate dopamine receptors located on the tumor, are the therapy of choice for patients with prolactinomas. Cabergoline (0.5 mg orally twice weekly) is the most popular drug because it is effective and relatively well tolerated (Fig. 211-6). It is usually preferred over bromocriptine because of fewer side effects and better efficacy for reducing the size of the tumor. Patients should be prescribed the lowest dose that reduces the serum prolactin level to less than 10 pg/mL. In general, patients with macroprolactinomas require higher doses, usually greater than 2.0 mg/week. Between 80 and 90% of patients with macroprolactinomas have a greater than 50% decrease in tumor size, and visual fields can improve within the first week. Patients who cannot tolerate cabergoline due to nausea and dizziness may respond better to bromocriptine, which can be inserted vaginally in women. A patient who appears to be resistant to dopamine agonists may be nonadherent, unable to tolerate the side effects, or have true resistance. Because of the concern that these agents could damage heart valves, it is reasonable to perform yearly echocardiograms in patients who have known valvular heart disease or who require long-term therapy at doses greater than 5 mg/week.

Patients who respond well—with suppression of prolactin levels, disappearance of their tumor, and resolution of symptoms for at least a year—should reduce their dose or stop it completely. Prolactin levels and MRI should be requested at 3 months after stopping the medication, then at 6 months, and then yearly until it is certain there is no recurrence. Macroprolactinomas are more likely to recur than microprolactinomas. If cabergoline is restarted, it should be prescribed at the lowest dose necessary to keep the serum prolactin less than 10 pg/mL.

As a clear second choice, and only in patients in whom pharmacologic intervention is not successful, transsphenoidal tumor resection is recommended. Although cure rates are not as impressive as for medication, prolactin normalizes in 65 to 85% of microadenomas and 30 to 40% of macroadenomas, with recurrent rates of 20% over 10 years. Radiotherapy is rarely used.

● ADRENOCORTICOTROPHIC HORMONE (ACTH)
Introduction

ACTH is a 39–amino acid peptide synthesized as part of a precursor polypeptide, proopiomelanocortin (POMC; 241 amino acids).

In extrapituitary tumors, the processing of POMC is variable, and a number of intermediates are produced. Therefore, tumors that produce ectopic ACTH usually are accompanied by detectable blood levels of other POMC intermediates that are not seen when a pituitary adenoma causes excess ACTH.

Balanced blood ACTH levels, and therefore the cortisol levels, require several layers of control of ACTH secretion by the pituitary gland. The most important stimulator of ACTH secretion is hypothalamic corticotropin-releasing hormone (CRH). Chronic CRH stimulation causes hyperplasia of corticotroph cells, which rarely can be seen in neuroendocrine tumors that secrete CRH. However, other neurotransmitters and brain peptides (including various cytokines that synergize with hypothalamic hormones, leukemia inhibitor factor, and CRH) also traverse the hypothalamic portal axis and stimulate the corticotroph to release ACTH. In addition, hypoglycemia, stress (as from sepsis, surgery, acute illness), and depression can stimulate the peripheral and hypothalamic cytokines that activate the hypothalamic-pituitary-adrenal axis. Cortisol inhibits the release of ACTH, blunts the response of ACTH to CRH, and inhibits the production of CRH. After prolonged administration of exogenous glucocorticoids and the resulting suppression of the hypothalamic-pituitary-adrenal axis, the recovery of endogenous CRH secretion, which appears to be the rate-limiting step for a return to normal function, can take several months.

ACTH is released in an ultradian pulsatile manner, with 10 to 12 pulses each day resulting in plasma levels of less than 10 to 80 pg/mL. The values are highest around 8 AM and spike with meals. The nadir is usually around 1 to 2 AM. Even the stress of a venipuncture can increase plasma ACTH concentrations. Pulse release combined with a short half-life (minutes) explains why random measurement of ACTH is generally unhelpful except when the random level is very high, as can be seen in primary adrenal insufficiency (low cortisol). Nearly undetectable plasma ACTH concentrations in the setting of hypercortisolism suggest a primary adrenal source (an adrenal adenoma making cortisol or congenital adrenal hyperplasia).

Insulin-induced hypoglycemia provides a mechanism for testing the integrity of the hypothalamic-pituitary-adrenal axis (see Table 211-2). Trauma and

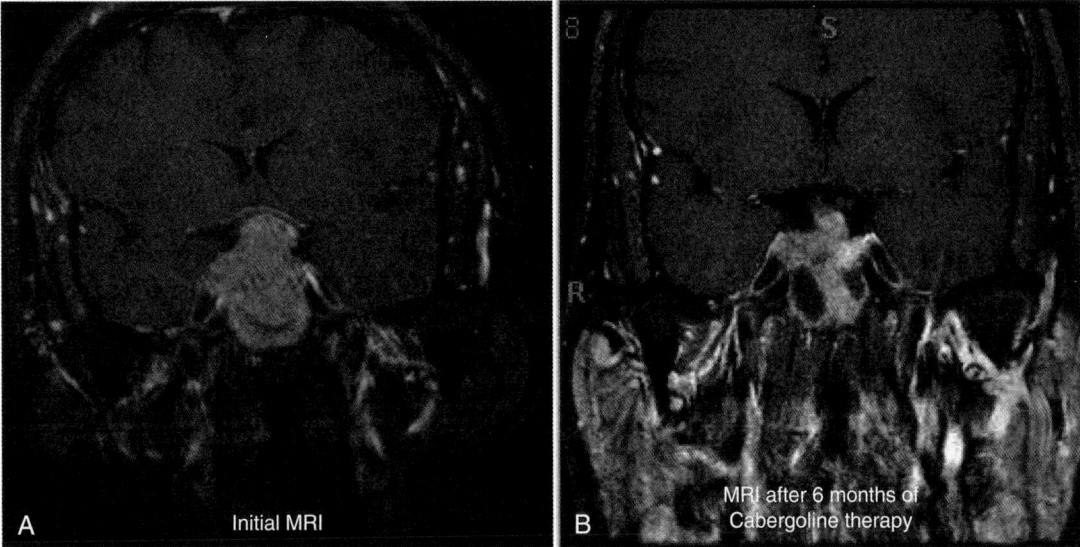

FIGURE 211-6. Magnetic resonance image a macroprolactinoma before (A) and after (B) commencing cabergoline therapy. 43-year-old man presented with headaches for 4 weeks and normal vision. MRI revealed the large mass. Prolactin on presentation was 8000 ng/dL (normal <20). After 2 doses of cabergoline (0.5 mg PO at night) the serum prolactin was 2086; after 6 months of treatment the prolactin was 15 ng/dL, and repeat MRI showed a significant decrease in size of tumor.

infection increase the secretion of CRH, ACTH, and, as a result, cortisol levels. Analogous adjustments in the doses of cortisol replacement therapy are required in seriously ill patients.

Adrenocorticotropic Hormone Deficiency: Secondary Hypocortisolism

Secondary adrenal insufficiency refers to states of low cortisolism due to inappropriately low levels of CRH or ACTH. Any congenital or acquired disease that disrupts normal pituitary function can disrupt the formation and release of ACTH. Symptoms of fever, nausea, vomiting, weakness, and fatigue are typically accompanied by relative or absolute hypotension. Abnormal laboratory test findings can include hypoglycemia, hyponatremia, and eosinophilia. Primary adrenal insufficiency (Chapter 214) usually causes more severe cortisol deficiency and associated mineralocorticoid deficiency, whereas secondary adrenal insufficiency is often not as severe and is not accompanied by mineralocorticoid deficiency, because the mineralocorticoids are controlled primarily through the renin-angiotensin system rather than ACTH-dependent mechanisms. As a result, volume depletion is less pronounced in ACTH deficiency, and hyperkalemia is not a part of the clinical syndrome. Another differentiating feature is that MSH levels are low when ACTH levels are low, so hyperpigmentation is not a feature of primary adrenal insufficiency. In women, a reduction in adrenal androgens can reduce libido and lead to loss of hair in the axillary and pubic areas.

ACTH deficiency is most often caused when exogenous glucocorticoid treatment suppresses the hypothalamic-pituitary-adrenal axis. Because of the lack of ACTH stimulation, the sudden discontinuation of exogenous glucocorticoids or an unmet increased need for them because of intervening severe stress can cause symptoms and signs of glucocorticoid deficiency. When ACTH deficiency otherwise occurs in adults, it is almost always accompanied by deficiencies in other pituitary hormones, especially in women who have lymphocytic hypophysitis. Isolated primary ACTH deficiency is rare,[13] though it can be seen in defects of transcription factors (T-Box19 and pituitary restricted transcription factor), proopiomelanocortin expression, or CRH gene expression.

ACTH reserve is usually assessed by the controlled induction of hypoglycemia with intravenous insulin via an insulin tolerance test that directly tests the hypothalamic-pituitary-adrenal axis by stimulating the brain to release cytokines and CRH, which in turn stimulate ACTH release. The insulin tolerance test is performed following an overnight fast by administering 0.1 U insulin/kg/body weight intravenously (or 0.05 U if there is high suspicion of ACTH deficiency) using 0.9% NaCl to maintain IV access. The blood glucose level is measured every 15 minutes, monitoring for a glucose level less than 40 mg/dL or when symptoms of hypoglycemia appear (whichever is first). Patients with ACTH deficiency may not rebound from the hypoglycemia and may need to receive 50 mL of 50% dextrose solution to normalize their blood sugar. A normal test would be a cortisol level greater than 18 μg/dL at or soon after confirmed hypoglycemia. The insulin tolerance test should be conducted cautiously in patients with seizure disorders because hypoglycemia may lower the seizure threshold.

Another way to determine ACTH reserve when ACTH deficiency is suspected is to administer CRH (1 μg/kg) intravenously at time "zero," with cortisol measurements at 5, 10, 15, and 30 minutes following the injection. This test, which is not as well standardized as the insulin tolerance test, bypasses the hypothalamus. The metapyrone test, which often is poorly tolerated and can be difficult to obtain, is now rarely used.

ACTH deficiency responds to glucocorticoid replacement. In general, isolated ACTH deficiency requires only hydrocortisone, usually 20 mg in the morning and 10 mg in the afternoon, to mimic the physiologic profile of cortisol release. Such doses are usually doubled during mild to moderate stress. Emergency hydrocortisone injection kits are worthwhile in case vomiting prevents oral dosing. Stress doses of steroids (e.g., 50 to 75 mg every 8 hours for severe stress) are required for acute illness. Patients who have been taking long-acting, potent glucocorticoids (e.g., prednisone) for months for chronic inflammatory diseases (e.g., asthma [Chapter 81], systemic lupus erythematosus [Chapter 250], or inflammatory bowel disease [Chapter 132]) can be liberated from chronic glucocorticoid if the hypothalamic-pituitary-adrenal axis is stimulated by switching to shorter-acting glucocorticoids (e.g., hydrocortisone) in gradually diminishing doses, oftentimes slowly titrated over many months. However, if the underlying disease for which the steroids were given is still active, other immunosuppressive drugs must be substituted, or the underlying disease will flare.

Cushing Disease

Cushing syndrome is a clinical syndrome that reflects excessive tissue exposure to glucocorticoids. The diagnosis depends on a suspicion and definitive laboratory testing. The syndrome can be ACTH-dependent and ACTH-independent, but the most common cause is when excess cortisol is produced by the unmitigated release of ACTH from a pituitary adenoma; the term Cushing *disease* is reserved for this specific cause of Cushing *syndrome*. Other causes of ACTH-dependent Cushing syndrome are ectopic ACTH secretion, ectopic CRH secretion, and exogenous administration of ACTH. ACTH-*in*dependent causes of Cushing syndrome are adrenal adenomas, adrenal carcinomas, primary pigmented nodular adrenal disease, ACTH-independent bilateral macronodular hyperplasia (Chapter 214), and the exogenous administration of glucocorticoids.

PATHOBIOLOGY

Approximately 60 to 70% of all cases of Cushing syndrome represent Cushing disease caused by a solitary corticotroph adenoma, although rare cases are caused by corticotroph hyperplasia or even more rarely a corticotroph carcinoma. Cushing disease occurs 8 to 10 times more frequently in women than in men. Although most tumors are small when they are identified because of the profound biologic effects of excess cortisol, 10 to 15% present as macroadenomas. The molecular pathology of most corticotroph adenomas is unknown because the usual oncogenes and tumor suppressor genes do not appear to be commonly involved. In patients with familial endocrine tumor syndromes, corticotroph producing adenomas are more rare than nonsecreting adenomas or adenomas that secrete growth hormone or prolactin.

CLINICAL MANIFESTATIONS

The presence of glucocorticoid receptors on most cells of the body explains why the overproduction of ACTH has multiple manifestations. The symptoms that lead most patients to seek medical care are weight gain, sleep disturbances, emotional lability, and the typical physical changes associated with glucocorticoid excess. Most patients experience depression, and some even have suicidal ideation if left untreated. In menstruating females, the first perturbations can be oligomenorrhea and amenorrhea. Patients may also note proximal muscle weakness when entering or exiting an automobile or even brushing their hair. Occasional patients complain of headaches and vision loss depending on the size of the pituitary adenoma. Women can also present with hirsutism and worsening acne. Because of their immunocompromised state, the initial presentation also can be with life-threatening infections and sepsis. The associated hypercoagulable state can result in deep venous thrombosis or pulmonary embolism (Chapter 74).

Common findings on physical examination include central obesity, owing to muscle wasting. Large, wide, violaceous striae ("stretch marks") are also seen on the abdomen, under the breasts, in the axillae, and in the upper inner thighs. Compared with the stretch marks in pregnancy, Cushing striae are usually wider than a fingerbreadth, purple in color, and can have subcutaneous bleeding that contributes to their pigmentation. Abnormal adipose tissue is usually seen between the scapulae ("buffalo hump") or in the supraclavicular space. In the face, fat deposition causes "moon facies," and the increased hematocrit contributes to facial plethora (ruddy cheeks) (Table 211-9). Hair growth is increased in an androgen-dependent distribution, and male-pattern baldness develops in women (Fig. 211-7). Multiple ecchymoses on the trunk and extremities can be seen due to bruising from capillary fragility.

Patients can have mild glucose intolerance or flagrant diabetes depending on the absolute elevation of the cortisol level as well as its chronicity. Relatively constant high levels of cortisol do not follow the physiologic diurnal variation. An additional finding in ACTH-dependent Cushing disease is hyperpigmentation

TABLE 211-9 CLINICAL FEATURES OF CUSHING DISEASE
GENERAL
Obesity (centripetal distribution)
"Moon facies" and mild proptosis
Increased supraclavicular fat and "buffalo hump"
Hypertension
SKIN
Hyperpigmentation
Facial plethora
Hirsutism
Violaceous striae and thin skin
Capillary fragility and easy bruising
Acne
Edema
Female balding
MUSCULOSKELETAL
Muscle weakness (proximal)
Osteoporosis and back pain
REPRODUCTIVE
Decreased libido
Oligomenorrhea and amenorrhea
NEUROPSYCHIATRIC
Depression
Irritability and emotional lability
Psychosis
Disrupted sleep
METABOLIC
Hypokalemia and alkalosis
Hypercalciuria and renal stones
Glucose intolerance or diabetes mellitus
Impaired wound healing
Impaired resistance to infection
Granulocytosis and lymphopenia
Hypercoagulable state—Pulmonary embolus, deep vein thrombosis
TUMOR MASS EFFECTS
Headache
Visual field loss
Hypopituitarism and mass effect of tumor

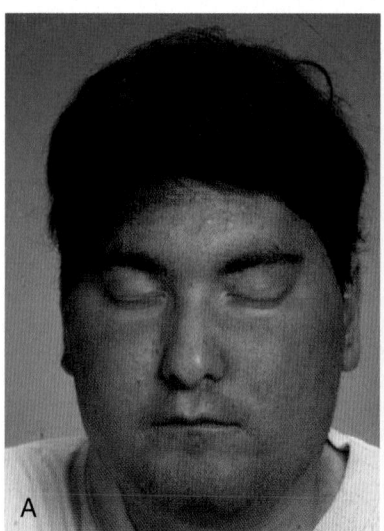
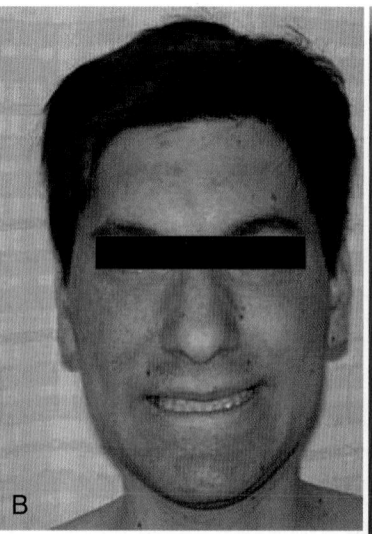
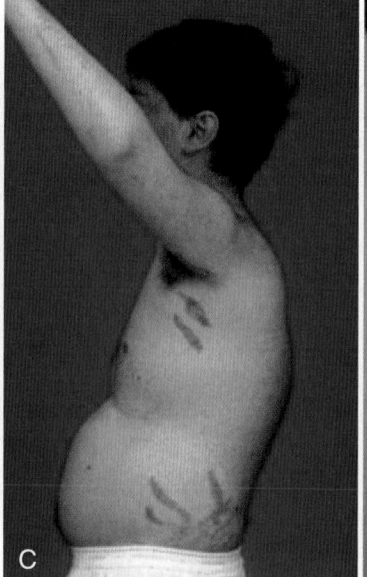
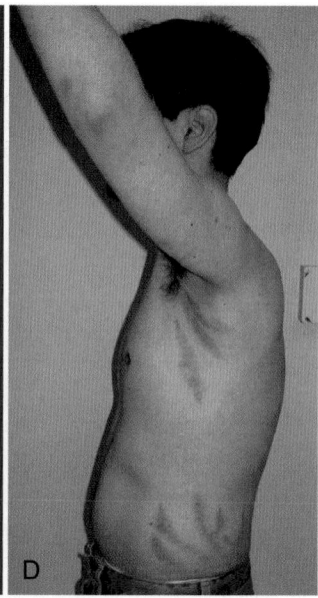

FIGURE 211-7. Clinical features of Cushing disease before (A, C) and after (B, D) transsphenoidal resection of an ACTH-secreting pituitary adenoma. 18-year-male presented with lower back pain secondary to vertebral fractures, depression, and 20-pound weight gain over a 2-year period. Note the "moon facies" and facial plethora (A) and abdominal obesity with thin extremities as well as violaceous striae (C). 1 year after pituitary tumor removal the patient had weight loss and while the striae remained as scar tissue, they were less violaceous. Muscle mass increased and abdominal obesity decreased.

owing to the melanocyte-stimulating hormone (MSH) that is secreted along with ACTH from the adenoma. Although the hyperpigmentation is not as marked as seen in Addison disease (where ACTH levels are usually 10- to 100-fold greater) nor as in ectopic hypercortisolism, it is certainly more than seen in ACTH-independent causes of Cushing syndrome. Hypertension, which is common, is caused by the direct ability of ACTH to stimulate the secretion of mineralocorticoids from the adrenal cortex as well as the excess glucocorticoids. The mineralocorticoid excess also commonly leads to kaliuresis and hypokalemia.

DIAGNOSIS

Most patients with obesity, hypertension, and glucose intolerance or diabetes do not have Cushing syndrome, but the presence of the classic physical findings may suggest the need for further investigation. No single diagnostic test can confirm Cushing disease, but a constellation of test results is usually determinative. The first and often most difficult step is to document hypercortisolism.

Measurement of the Serum Cortisol Level
Hypercortisolism is challenging to confirm by measuring a random serum cortisol level because 80% of serum cortisol is bound to cortisol-binding globulin, 10% is bound to albumin, and only 10% is free. Changes in cortisol-binding globulin (e.g., in pregnancy) and albumin can therefore affect the measurement. Although the liquid chromatography–tandem mass spectrometry (LC-MS/MS) assay provides high analytical sensitivity and specificity, a random serum level is rarely diagnostic because of the episodic secretion of cortisol.

24-Hour Urine Free Cortisol Measurement
A properly collected 24-hour urine specimen that measures urine free cortisol avoids the fluctuations that make serum cortisol levels unreliable and is sufficiently deterministic that an elevated urine free cortisol level in an unstressed patient with normal renal function is usually sufficient to diagnose Cushing syndrome. Conversely, a normal result is strong evidence against that diagnosis. However, biologic variation as well as problems with the over- or under-collection of urine make this test less than ideal for the initial screening of Cushing syndrome.

Late-Night Salivary Cortisol Measurement
Late-night (23:00 to 24:00 hour) salivary cortisol testing is increasingly used as an initial test to evaluate patients with a clinical suspicion of Cushing syndrome. The diagnostic sensitivity of this test is high (80 to 90%), but its specificity is lower (70 to 90%). Nevertheless, its excellent sensitivity make it a good screening test.

Plasma ACTH Measurement
ACTH measurements, although subject to the same circadian variability as cortisol levels, are not subject to the effects of cortisol-binding globulin. ACTH values greater than 100 pg/mL are suggestive of primary adrenal insufficiency, whereas values greater than 500 pg/mL are diagnostic. Low concentrations of plasma ACTH are not diagnostic, except for the undetectable levels observed with cortisol-producing adrenal adenomas. The plasma ACTH concentration is also low in patients taking exogenous steroids.

Dexamethasone Suppression Testing
At least five variations of dexamethasone suppression testing have been described. All versions require patients to self-administer the dexamethasone at inconvenient hours of the day (11 PM) or up to four times a day. Sampling requires either collection of urine for 24 hours or coming to the physician's office or laboratory at 8 AM for multiple blood sampling.

A popular option is a single dose of 1 mg dexamethasone administered at 11 PM, with blood obtained by 8 AM the following morning. A normal response is a serum cortisol concentration of less than 1.8 µg/dL. An alternative cut point, less than 5 µg/dL, is more specific but less sensitive. If the cortisol level is greater than 10 µg/dL, the likelihood of hypercortisolism is high. Patients with corticotroph-secreting macroadenomas or very active tumors may have urine free cortisol levels greater than 1000 µg/dL and will require higher doses of dexamethasone to confirm suppressibility and exclude ectopic ACTH production.

CRH Stimulation Test
The CRH stimulation test is one of the most sensitive to determine if there is an abnormality in the hypothalamic-pituitary-adrenal axis and for diagnosing the etiology of hypercortisolism in ACTH-dependent Cushing syndrome. The mean ACTH concentrations at 15 and 30 minutes after CRH administration should increase by at least 35% above the mean basal value in patients with Cushing disease but not in patients with ectopic ACTH secretion. This measure provides the best sensitivity (93%) and specificity (100%).

MRI
The best next step in the evaluation of patients with documented hypercortisolism (i.e., nonsuppression with low-dose dexamethasone and CRH hyperstimulation) is MRI to confirm the presence of a pituitary mass. Unfortunately, 10% of all normal individuals may have slight MRI abnormalities of their pituitary glands, and many patients with Cushing disease may have tumors that are too small to be seen on MRI. However, subjecting a patient to surgical pituitary exploration in the absence of a demonstrable mass is likely to result in an unsuccessful surgery.

Inferior Petrosal Sinus Sampling
If previous dexamethasone suppression and CRH testing have been equivocal, then inferior petrosal sinus sampling should be performed to confirm the pituitary as the source of the ACTH. Although this test is less reliable in lateralizing the ACTH source (i.e., left vs. right) than it is in confirming that the ACTH is central in origin, it can exclude ectopic ACTH production by a tumor. However, it usually cannot distinguish an ectopic CRH-secreting tumor from true Cushing disease.

TREATMENT

The best chance of curing an ACTH-secreting adenoma is transsphenoidal surgery (Fig. 211-7).[14] Recurrences are seen in 7% of cases when the immediate postoperative plasma cortisol is less than 3 µg/dL compared with 100% when the postoperative plasma cortisol is 3 to 8 µg/dL. In patients with Cushing disease and macroadenomas, only about one third of patients have long-term remission. When initial surgery fails, a second pituitary surgery has a success rate of only about 50%.

Pituitary irradiation or bilateral adrenalectomy may be recommended in patients who have a recurrence, in whom surgery is contraindicated (large tumor with invasion of carotid or cavernous sinus), or when a skilled neurosurgeon is not available. Pituitary radiation can take up to 2 to 5 years to be effective, and panhypopituitarism usually results. If a pituitary tumor cannot be demonstrated with certainty, bilateral laparoscopic adrenalectomies will cure the hypercortisolism, and lifetime postoperative steroid replacement is then required.

Medical therapy to inhibit ACTH release from the corticotroph, to block the synthesis of cortisol by the adrenal glands, or to inhibit the action of cortisol at the tissue level is neither particularly well tolerated nor easy to monitor. Mifepristone, which is a glucocorticoid receptor antagonist, and some newer analogues are effective against hyperglycemia and can improve quality of life, but patients may become severely adrenally insufficient because of the receptor blockade, despite very high cortisol and ACTH levels. In tumors that co-secrete prolactin and ACTH, cabergoline may have some limited effect. The somatostatin analogue pasireotide can normalize cortisol levels in about 20% of patients, but it worsens hyperglycemia in about 75%. Chemical adrenalectomy using ketoconazole, mitotane, metapyrone, or etomidate is poorly tolerated and difficult to titrate to normal adrenal function.

Nelson Syndrome

Nelson syndrome is a rare condition of uncontrolled growth of an ACTH-secreting pituitary adenoma, usually within three years after bilateral adrenalectomy has been performed to treat Cushing disease. The incidence of Nelson syndrome following bilateral adrenalectomy can be as high as 43% in patients with macroadenomas, high plasma concentrations of ACTH, and visible pituitary tumors prior to adrenalectomy. Other risk factors for Nelson syndrome include longer duration of Cushing disease before diagnosis and treatment, younger patients, inadequate glucocorticoid replacement, and tumors with higher mitotic indices.

All patients have high plasma ACTH levels following bilateral adrenalectomy, even those without prior Cushing disease. Such patients should have their hormones measured prior to administration of the AM dose of steroid or 1 hour thereafter. Some experts recommend follow-up MRI every 6 months for several years in patients who have undergone bilateral adrenalectomy after failed transsphenoidal pituitary adenomectomy. Treatment of Nelson syndrome is usually with the same modalities used for ACTH-secreting pituitary adenomas.[15]

GONADOTROPINS (FOLLICLE STIMULATING HORMONE AND LUTEINIZING HORMONE)

PATHOBIOLOGY

The three pituitary glycoprotein hormones—FSH, LH, and TSH—have a common α-subunit and a hormone-specific β-subunit that are combined together to form the hormone. Chorionic gonadotropin (hCG), which is structurally very similar to LH, is made in the placenta. The protein is glycosylated in the Golgi apparatus, and this glycosylation is responsible for the proper synthesis and transport of the molecule from the pituitary into the blood. These peptides interact with their cognate receptors located in the cell membrane of their target cells. These transmembrane receptors classically have an extracellular domain that binds the hormone, an intramembranous domain, and an intracellular domain that transduces the hormone signal to the cell. Mutations in the extracellular or intracellular domain can cause constitutive activation of the receptor even in the absence of the ligand. The result is the appearance of a hormone-rich state in the absence of the hormone (e.g., precocious puberty due to the constitutive activation of the FSH receptor). Similarly, mutations in the receptor can make it insensitive to the ligand, so that even high hormone levels are not recognized by the receptor. Lastly, due to the similarity of the α-subunit among these glycoprotein hormones, there can be some promiscuity of ligand stimulation when ligand levels are high. During pregnancy, for example, the hCG level is very high and can stimulate the TSH receptor as if TSH were present.

Gonadotropins regulate sexual differentiation, the production of sex steroids, and gametogenesis. In males, FSH receptors are located on Sertoli cells and seminiferous tubules, where they stimulate sperm maturation, whereas LH receptors on Leydig cells in the testis stimulate the production of androgen. Together, FSH and LH induce spermatogenesis (Chapter 221). In females, ovarian FSH receptors on granulosa cells induce the biosynthesis of estrogen, whereas LH receptors on ovarian thecal cells stimulate the synthesis of ovarian androgens and steroid precursors that granulosa cells aromatize into estrogens. The secretion of FSH and LH regulate the menstrual cycle (Chapters 222 and 223).

Hypogonadotrophic Hypogonadism

CLINICAL MANIFESTATIONS AND DIAGNOSIS

Hypogonadotrophic hypogonadism or secondary hypogonadism is defined as failure of gonadal function due to pituitary or hypothalamic abnormalities that result in acquired or congenital reductions in LH, FSH, or GnRH.[16] Acquired forms can be due to a tumor that interferes with the normal production of LH or FSH, such as Rathke pouch cysts, craniopharyngiomas, or other brain tumors. Functional gonadotropin deficiency can be transient as seen in chronic illness, starvation, Cushing syndrome, anorexia nervosa (Chapter 206), or alcoholism (Chapter 30). Other causes of acquired hypogonadotrophic hypogonadism include infection (tuberculosis [Chapter 308], HIV [Chapter 366], syphilis [Chapter 303]), trauma, infiltrative diseases (e.g., hemochromatosis [Chapter 201], and sarcoidosis [Chapter 89]), and medications such as opioids and anabolic steroids. Congenital forms of hypogonadotrophic hypogonadism can be due to at least 18 different genes involved in the migration of the GnRH neurons and stimulation of GnRH signaling.

The clinical presentation of hypogonadotrophic hypogonadism depends on the onset (acquired or congenital), the severity of the defect, and any associated conditions. Classically, patients present in the second or third decade of life with poorly or absent sexual characteristics, failure to enter puberty, and primary amenorrhea or infertility. The endocrine diagnosis of hypogonadotrophic hypogonadism is rather straightforward when there are low levels of testosterone in men or estradiol in women in the presence of low or normal levels of gonadotropins. Selective deficiency of LH or FSH can rarely be due to inactivating mutations of the β-subunit.

Occasionally a provocative test is necessary to confirm hypogonadotrophic hypogonadism and to distinguish hypothalamic from pituitary disease. In such instances, leuprolide is administered (10 μg/kg subcutaneously), and then LH and FSH are measured at −10, 0, 30, 60, 90, 180, 240, and 1440 minutes later, with estradiol (or testosterone) also measured at baseline and 1440 minutes.

Replacement of gonadal hormones is usually the best treatment. In females who have not yet started puberty, estrogen should be initiated at low doses to promote breast development. When breakthrough bleeding occurs about 6 months later, cyclical therapy can be started by adding a progestogen and then increasing estrogen doses gradually over a 2- to 3-year period. Vitamin D should also be provided. Chapter 223 provides guidance for inducing ovulation for women who hope to become pregnant.

In men, testosterone can be replaced using intramuscular injections at 2- to 4-week intervals (e.g., testosterone cypionate 200 mg every 2 weeks). Doses and the intervals between injections should be adjusted based on peak and trough testosterone levels (one week after and just before the next dose) and self-reported libido. Oral androgens can cause hepatotoxicity and should be avoided, but transdermal testosterone is effective for maintaining stable levels.

Tumors Producing Follicle-Stimulating Hormone and Luteinizing Hormone

PATHOBIOLOGY

A majority of pituitary tumors are classified clinically as nonsecreting or nonfunctional adenomas. On further investigation, however, the majority (70 to 80% of them) secrete small amounts of either the α-subunit or β-subunit of LH or FSH (which would have no clinical manifestations) or rarely an intact LH or FSH with both alpha and beta subunits. FSH is more common than LH, and free α-subunits are more common than β-subunits. Little is known about the molecular basis of these tumors.

CLINICAL MANIFESTATIONS

Most gonadotrophinomas are clinically silent except when their size results in neurologic findings such as visual field problems or headaches. Patients usually present with hypogonadism because secreted gonadotropins are ineffective for stimulating the gonads. Premenopausal females may have ovarian cysts and menstrual disorders. Men commonly are hypogonadal because of low testosterone levels but also develop testicular enlargement from FSH-secreting tumors. In rare tumors that secrete LH, males have elevated testosterone and hemoglobin levels.

DIAGNOSIS

No clinical syndrome is uniquely associated with these tumors. Some patients may have nonspecific moderate elevations of prolactin, but almost all cases are diagnosed postoperatively when the surgical specimen is analyzed.

Because the major symptoms of the gonadotropin-producing tumors or nonfunctioning adenomas are related to local mass effects and extrasellar extension, the goal of treatment is to reduce the size of the tumor. Transsphenoidal surgery usually can completely or partially reverse any hypopituitarism and visual field impairment but is rarely curative because the tumors are large. Postoperative radiation therapy may benefit patients who have minimal residual tumor. If no tumor is seen on a postoperative MRI, annual monitoring with visual field testing plus CT or MRI is indicated. Tumor markers also can monitor tumor activity. For growing tumors, repeat surgery, radiation therapy, or both are indicated. Medical therapy (e.g., dopamine agonists and somatostatin analogues) usually is not helpful.

THYROID-STIMULATING HORMONE

PATHOBIOLOGY

Thyroid function (Chapter 213) and growth is controlled by the action of TSH. Similar to LH and FSH, TSH is composed of a common α-subunit and a unique β-subunit that is unique to thyrotrophs. Regulation of TSH secretion is by the hypothalamic TRH and by thyroid hormone itself. Feedback by thyroid hormone is dependent on intranuclear thyroid hormone receptors, which bind T3.

TSH is secreted in a pulsatile and diurnal variation; but, unlike other pituitary hormones, random measurements of morning serum TSH are consistent enough so that measurement of TSH is clinically useful in determining the extent of thyroid hormone production. Whereas the range of TSH in the normal population is generally between 0.4 and 4.0 mU/L, each person has an individual "thyroid thermostat" set at a specific level. This variability means that someone who normally has a TSH of 2.0 might feel hyperthyroid when the TSH is 0.5, and conversely someone with a normal TSH of 0.5 might feel relatively hypothyroid when their TSH is 2.0, although both values are within the normal range for the population. In general, screening for thyroid disease is best done by TSH measurement and, if outside the normal range, confers a high likelihood of thyroid dysfunction (see Chapter 213). When thyroid hormone production is low due to a defect in thyroid hormonogenesis, levels of thyroid hormones are low and those of TSH are high, and vice versa. However, when the thyroid hormone levels are low and the TSH is normal or low, secondary or central hypothyroidism exists. Alternatively, when thyroid hormone levels are high and the TSH is not suppressed, secondary hypothyroidism, of which TSH-secreting pituitary adenomas are in the differential diagnosis (see below), is likely.

Central Hypothyroidism

Failure of the pituitary to produce TSH in response to low levels of thyroid hormone is consistent with central or secondary hypothyroidism. An isolated TSH defect is relatively rare and usually related to a genetic factor necessary for thyrotroph differentiation. Pituitary masses that impinge on the thyrotrophs would cause failure to produce sufficient amounts of TSH in the setting of low thyroid hormone levels. Another cause of the constellation of thyroid tests consistent with central hypothyroidism would be in euthyroid sick syndrome (Chapter 213) or nonthyroidal illness. In patients with concurrent critical illness, cytokines inhibit the release of hypothalamic and pituitary hormones. This finding is most noticeable in patients who have low T4, T3, and TSH. Furthermore, euthyroid sick syndrome is characterized by an increase in serum reverse T3, which is formed by 5′ deiodination of T4 and is not biologically active. The conversion to the inactive reverse T3 occurs in the tissues and is thought to preserve metabolic demand during critical illness. The same test results are seen in starvation due to activation of the deiodinase. Other causes of low thyroid hormone levels and inappropriately normal TSH are listed in Table 211-10.

Treatment of secondary hypothyroidism is straightforward once the diagnosis is made. A physiologic replacement dose of T4 (e.g., levothyroxine) is targeted to maintain serum T4 levels at the upper end of normal if not slightly elevated. TSH is not a useful marker as in other forms of hypothyroidism because the thyrotroph is not responsive to the thyroid hormone concentration. Because isolated TSH deficiency is rare, the clinician needs to be certain other hormone replacement is not needed.

Tumors that Secrete Thyroid-Stimulating Hormone

Rarely, pituitary adenomas known as TSHomas or TSH-secreting pituitary adenomas can produce TSH. These tumors account for less than 1% of all cases of hyperthyroidism. In addition to classic findings of hyperthyroidism, clinical findings in TSHoma include a diffuse goiter, visual field defects, headache, and menstrual irregularities in women. Occasionally, patients do not have hyperthyroid symptoms, most likely due to habituation to the mildly elevated hormone concentrations.

A diagnosis of TSHoma should be considered when patients present with high serum levels of total and free thyroxine and triiodothyronine. In some cases, elevated serum levels of the alpha subunit of the TSH molecule and nonsuppressed TSH can be seen. Other causes of elevated T4 and T3 in the presence of nonsuppressed TSH are shown in Table 211-10. The diagnosis is rarely straightforward. A combination of tests (e.g, repeat thyroid tests in another laboratory, α-subunit, other pituitary hormones) can confirm the diagnosis, but no single test is diagnostic. In the absence of any history or testing suggestive of a pituitary adenoma and given the difficulty in distinguishing patients with TSH-secreting tumors from resistance to thyroid hormone, consideration should be given to performing (when available) an analysis for mutations in the thyroid hormone receptor-β gene in patients with elevated free T4 and T3, nonsuppressed TSH, and a normal serum α-subunit.

The goal of treatment is to reduce the size of the tumor. Treatments and outcomes are similar to those for gonadotropin-producing adenomas (see above).

A β-blocker such as propranolol (80 to 160 mg daily) or atenolol (25 to 50 mg daily) can be given to ameliorate some of the symptoms and signs of hyperthyroidism (Chapter 213). Long-term antithyroid drug therapy or thyroid ablation with radioiodine or surgery is not indicated because sustained reductions in thyroid hormone secretion would be expected to increase TSH secretion and stimulate the tumor's growth. However, if euthyroidism cannot be achieved with somatostatin analogs or dopamine agonists, short-term administration of a thionamide is necessary to restore euthyroidism prior to neurosurgery.

● NONFUNCTIONING PITUITARY ADENOMAS

Nonfunctioning pituitary adenomas do not cause hormonal excess,[17] although hyperprolactinemia can occur if the pituitary stalk is sufficiently compressed. As a result, these tumors are usually detected when their size causes neurologic symptoms, especially visual field abnormalities, headaches, and ophthalmoplegias. Elevated prolactin levels from stalk compression are much lower than the levels seen with a macroprolactinoma. Oftentimes a nonfunctioning pituitary adenoma is found incidentally when a pituitary mass is discovered in a patient who has a brain imaging study for an unrelated reason. Evaluation (Table 211-7) reveals no hormone excess. Nonfunctioning pituitary adenomas that cause neurologic symptoms require surgical removal, but asymptomatic nonfunctioning pituitary adenomas can be monitored by hormonal testing, to assure that no abnormal abnormalities develop, and by MRI, to evaluate the tumor's potential growth.

● PITUITARY CARCINOMAS

With few exceptions, pituitary tumors are adenomas that can grow around the sella and invade the carotids and sphenoid sinuses but that do not metastasize. The term *pituitary carcinoma* is restricted to 0.1 to 0.2% of the pituitary tumors that metastasize beyond the immediate vicinity of the sella to the craniospinal region or systemically. The Ki-67 proliferation index of greater than 3% can be useful as a guide to suggest a more aggressive pituitary tumor. Approximately half of these tumors produce either ACTH or prolactin, and the remainder are nonsecreting. Surgical debulking is the standard therapy, but radiotherapy and temozolomide chemotherapy also have been used because pituitary tumors can have multiple recurrences and be resistant to standard treatments. These aggressive tumors generally have a high mortality rate (over 50%), with a median life expectancy of about 10 months after diagnosis (Fig. 211-8).

TABLE 211-10	CAUSES OF DISCORDANT THYROID TESTS

LOW TH AND NORMAL OR LOW TSH

Secondary hypothyroidism
Pituitary dysfunction
TRH mutation
TSH mutation
Low TBG or other binding proteins (free T4 would be normal)
Nonthyroidal illness
Medications

HIGH TH AND NORMAL OR HIGH TSH

TSHoma
Thyroid hormone receptor β resistance to thyroid hormone
Elevated binding proteins (e.g., elevated TBG, familial dysalbuminemic hyperthyroxinemia)
Thyroid hormone habituation
Selenocysteine deficiency syndrome (inability to convert T4 to T3)

TBG = thyroid-binding globulin; TH = thyroid hormone; TRH thyroid-releasing-hormone; TSH = thyroid-stimulating hormone.

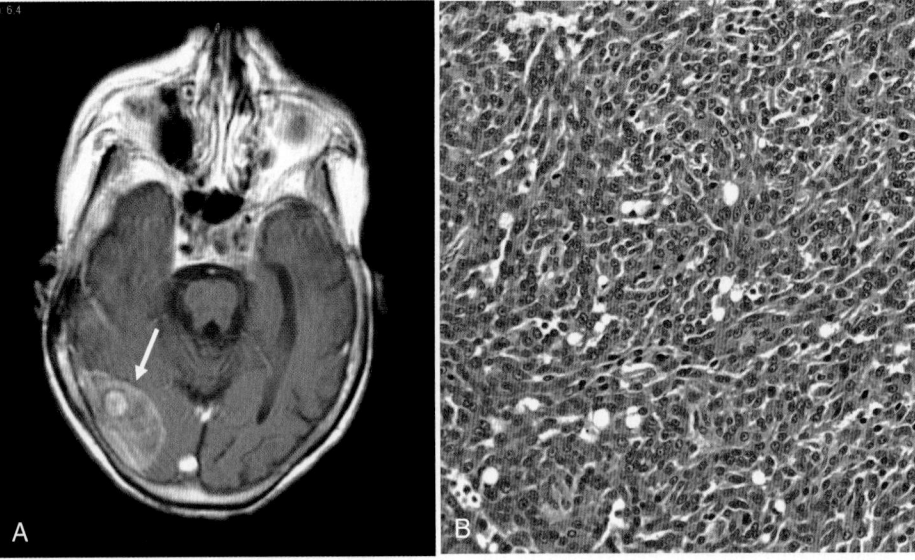

FIGURE 211-8. Pituitary carcinoma. Magnetic resonance image of a cerebral mass in a 43-year-old male patient with an aggressive TSH-secreting adenoma (**A**). Patient presented with seizures. Biopsy of brain lesion revealed sheaths of disorganized pituitary cells (**B**).

Grade A References

A1. Gadelha MR, Bronstein MD, Brue T, et al. Pasireotide versus continued treatment with octreotide or lanreotide in patients with inadequately controlled acromegaly (PAOLA): a randomised, phase 3 trial. *Lancet Diabetes Endocrinol*. 2014;2:875-884.

A2. Sheppard M, Bronstein MD, Freda P, et al. Pasireotide LAR maintains inhibition of GH and IGF-1 in patients with acromegaly for up to 25 months: results from the blinded extension phase of a randomized, double-blind, multicenter, phase III study. *Pituitary*. 2015;18:385-394.

A3. Tahara S, Murakami M, Kaneko T, Shimatsu A. Efficacy and safety of long-acting pasireotide in Japanese patients with acromegaly or pituitary gigantism: results from a multicenter, open-label, randomized, phase 2 study. *Endocr J*. 2017;64:735-747.

GENERAL REFERENCES

For the General References and other additional features, please visit Expert Consult at https://expertconsult.inkling.com.

212

POSTERIOR PITUITARY

JOSEPH G. VERBALIS

ANATOMY AND HORMONE SYNTHESIS

The hormones of the posterior pituitary, vasopressin and oxytocin, are synthesized in specialized neurons in the hypothalamus, the neurohypophyseal neurons. These neurons, notable for their large size, are termed *magnocellular neurons*. In the hypothalamus, the magnocellular neurons are clustered in the paired paraventricular and supraoptic nuclei (Fig. 212-1). Vasopressin and oxytocin are also synthesized in parvocellular (i.e., small cell) neurons of the paraventricular nuclei,[1,2] and vasopressin (but not oxytocin) is also synthesized in the suprachiasmatic nucleus.

Transcription of vasopressin and oxytocin messenger RNA and translation of the vasopressin and oxytocin prohormones occur entirely in the cell bodies of the neurohypophyseal neurons. The prohormones provasopressin and pro-oxytocin are packaged along with processing enzymes into neurosecretory granules that are transported out of the perikaryon of the neurohypophyseal

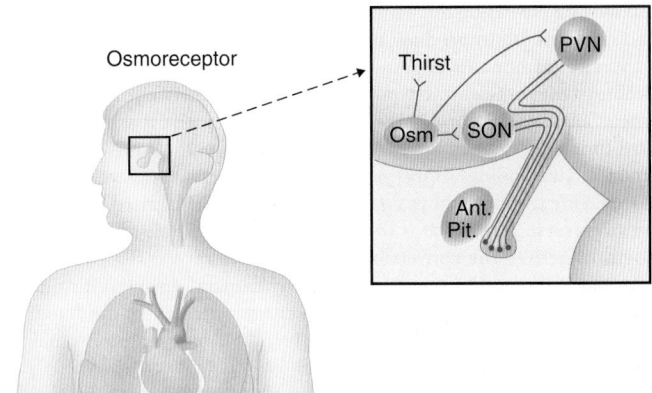

FIGURE 212-1. Sagittal view of the head, demonstrating the position of the neurohypophysis. The magnocellular neurons are clustered in two paraventricular nuclei (PVN) and two supraoptic nuclei (SON). Only one nucleus of each pair is illustrated. The supraoptic nuclei are lateral to the edge of the optic chiasm, whereas the paraventricular nuclei are central along the wall of the third ventricle. The axons of the four nuclei combine to form the supraopticohypophysial tract as they course through the pituitary stalk to their storage terminals in the posterior pituitary. The osmostat (Osm) is in the hypothalamus anterior to the third ventricle; the thirst center (Thirst) is distributed across different brain areas. Ant. Pit. = anterior pituitary. (From Buonocore CM, Robinson AG. Diagnosis and management of diabetes insipidus during medical emergencies. *Endocrinol Metab Clin North Am.* 1993;22:411-423.)

neurons via microtubules and down the long axons that form the supraopticohypophysial tract, which terminates in the posterior pituitary. During transport, the processing enzymes cleave provasopressin into vasopressin (9 amino acids), vasopressin-neurophysin (95 amino acids), and vasopressin glycopeptide, or copeptin (39 amino acids). Pro-oxytocin is similarly cleaved to oxytocin (which differs from vasopressin by only two of nine amino acids) and oxytocin-neurophysin. The neurophysins form neurophysin-hormone complexes that stabilize the hormones. Stimulatory (e.g., glutamatergic, cholinergic, and angiotensin) neurotransmitter terminals and inhibitory (e.g., γ-aminobutyric acid and noradrenergic) neurotransmitter terminals control the release of vasopressin through the activity of synaptic contacts on the neurohypophyseal cell bodies. Physiologic release of vasopressin or oxytocin into the general circulation occurs at the level of the posterior pituitary, where, in response to an action potential, intracellular calcium is increased and causes the neurosecretory granules to fuse with the axon membrane, thereby releasing each hormone into the general circulation. Although each of the other prohormone fragments are released into the circulation, vasopressin and oxytocin are the only known biologically active components of the prohormones. Factors that stimulate the release of neurohypophyseal hormones also stimulate their synthesis. Because synthesis is delayed, maintenance of a large store of hormone in the posterior pituitary is essential to enable the instantaneous release of each hormone that is necessary following acute hemorrhage (vasopressin) or during parturition (oxytocin). In most species, sufficient vasopressin is stored in the posterior pituitary to support maximal antidiuresis for several days and to maintain baseline levels of antidiuresis for weeks.

Vasopressin
Vasopressin and Regulation of Osmolality
The primary physiologic action of vasopressin is its function as a water-retaining hormone. The central sensing system (osmostat) for controlling the release of vasopressin is anatomically discrete, located in a small area of the hypothalamus just anterior to the third ventricle (see Fig. 212-1). The osmostat controls the release of vasopressin to allow water retention and also stimulates thirst to cause water repletion.

Osmotic regulation of vasopressin release and osmotic regulation of thirst are usually tightly coupled, but they can be dissociated under pathologic conditions. The primary extracellular osmolyte to which the osmoreceptor responds is sodium. Under normal physiologic conditions, glucose and urea cross neuron cell membranes and do not stimulate the release of vasopressin. Although basal osmolality in normal subjects ranges between 280 and 295 mOsm/kg H_2O, extracellular fluid osmolality for each individual is maintained within narrow ranges. Increases in plasma osmolality as small as 1 to 2% are sufficient to stimulate vasopressin release. Basal plasma levels of vasopressin are generally 0.5 to 2 pg/mL, which maintains urine osmolality above plasma osmolality and urine volume in the range of 1 to 3 L/day. When vasopressin levels are suppressed below 0.5 pg/mL, maximal urine osmolality decreases to below 100 mOsm/kg H_2O, and a free water diuresis (or "aquaresis") ensues at levels that approach 800 to 1000 mL/hour (18 to 24 L/day). Increases in plasma osmolality cause a linear increase in plasma vasopressin and a corresponding linear increase in urine osmolality. At a plasma osmolality of approximately 295 mOsm/kg H_2O, urine osmolality is maximally concentrated to 1000 to 1200 mOsm/kg H_2O. Thus, the entire physiologic range of urine osmolality is accomplished by relatively small changes in plasma vasopressin levels of 0 to 5 pg/mL (Fig. 212-2).

To maintain fluid balance, water must be not only conserved but also consumed to replace insensible water losses and obligate urine output. Thirst is not stimulated until a somewhat higher plasma osmolality (5 to 10 mOsm/kg H_2O) above the threshold for release of vasopressin. Most humans derive sufficient water from habitual fluid intake and catabolism of food to maintain plasma osmolality below the threshold that activates thirst. Therefore, under normal physiologic conditions, water balance (and hence plasma osmolality) is regulated more by secretion of vasopressin than by thirst. However, with severe degrees of dehydration, thirst is essential to restore body water deficits.

Vasopressin acts on the V_2 subtype of vasopressin receptors in the collecting duct principal cells of the kidney to cause water retention, or antidiuresis. Vasopressin V_2 receptors are G protein–coupled receptors that activate adenylate cyclase, with subsequent increased intracellular cyclic adenosine monophosphate (cAMP) levels upon ligand activation of the receptor. The increased cAMP initiates the movement of aquaporin-2 (AQP2) water channels to the apical (luminal) membrane of the collecting duct cells. These channels allow facilitated rapid transport of water from the collecting duct lumen into the principal cell along osmotic gradients. The water then exits the cell through the basolateral membrane into the kidney medullary circulation through constitutively expressed aquaporin-3 and aquaporin-4 water channels. This entire process is termed *antidiuresis*. In the absence of vasopressin, the AQP2 channels are reinternalized from the apical membrane into subapical vesicles. This prevents active reabsorption of water from the collecting duct lumen, resulting in diuresis. In addition to this rapid "shuttling" of the AQP2 channels to regulate water reabsorption on a minute-to-minute basis, vasopressin also acts through the V_2 receptors to regulate long-term stores of AQP2—that is, increased vasopressin stimulates AQP2 synthesis, and the absence of vasopressin results in decreased AQP2 synthesis. The hypertonic medullary interstitium is the determinant of the maximal concentration of the urine, which is in equilibrium with the osmolality of the inner medulla of the kidney under conditions of maximal antidiuresis (Chapter 107).

Vasopressin and Pressure and Volume Regulation
High-pressure baroreceptors are located in the aorta and carotid sinus, and low-pressure baroreceptors are located in the right and left atria. Decreases

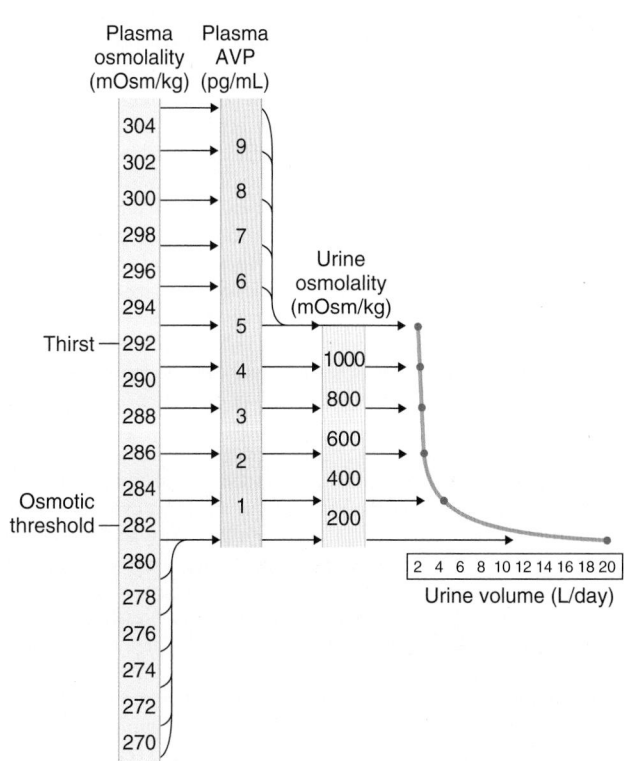

FIGURE 212-2. Idealized schematic of the normal physiologic relationships among plasma osmolality, plasma vasopressin (AVP), urine osmolality, and urine volume. The entire physiologic range of urine osmolality occurs with plasma vasopressin levels from 0 to 5 pg/mL. Increases in plasma osmolality above approximately 290 to 295 mOsm/kg H_2O result in increases in plasma vasopressin but no further concentration of the urine, which is limited by the maximal osmolality in the inner medulla. The relation of volume (calculated on the basis of a constant osmolar load) is inversely exponential to the other parameters. Because of this relationship, urine volume does not change substantially until there is nearly absent vasopressin secretion, after which urine volume increases dramatically. (Calculated from formulas presented in Robertson GL, Shelton RL, Athar S. The osmoregulation of vasopressin. *Kidney Int.* 1976;10:25-37. Figure drawn by J.G. Verbalis, Georgetown University, Washington, DC.)

in blood pressure or intravascular volume stimulate vasopressin release, whereas situations that increase blood volume or left atrial pressure (e.g., negative-pressure breathing) decrease the secretion of vasopressin.[2] The release of vasopressin in response to changes in volume or pressure is much less sensitive than the release in response to osmoreceptors; generally a 10 to 15% reduction in blood volume or pressure is needed to stimulate the release of vasopressin. However, once arterial pressure falls below this threshold, the stimulated response is exponential, resulting in plasma levels of vasopressin that are markedly greater than those resulting from osmotic stimulation.

The pressor effects of vasopressin are mediated through a separate vasopressin receptor subtype, the V_{1a} receptors, located on vascular smooth muscle. The relatively insensitive regulation of vasopressin secretion by changes in volume and pressure and the modest role of vasopressin to regulate blood pressure are consistent with the notion that regulation of sodium homeostasis by the renin-angiotensin-aldosterone system (Chapter 214) is more important for controlling extracellular and blood volume than is the regulation of water homeostasis. However, the pressor effects of vasopressin to increase blood pressure can become prominent when other blood pressure regulatory systems are deficient (e.g., autonomic neuropathy or renin-angiotensin-aldosterone system blockade) or in states of pathologic vasodilation (e.g., liver cirrhosis, septic shock).

Vasopressin and Adrenocorticotropic Hormone
Vasopressin stimulates adrenocorticotropic hormone (ACTH) secretion via stimulation of the vasopressin V_{1b} receptor subtype that is located on anterior pituitary corticotroph cells. Although the major regulator of ACTH secretion is corticotropin-releasing hormone (Chapter 211), vasopressin activates a different signal transduction system in the corticotrophs, so these hormones have synergistic effects on ACTH secretion.

Interaction of Osmotic and Volume Regulation

The vasopressin system has evolved to optimize mammalian water homeostasis. Water is consumed as available in the absence of stimulated thirst, and vasopressin secretion then regulates water excretion to maintain plasma osmolality. Thirst serves as a backup mechanism if dehydration becomes excessive. Because pressure-volume regulation of vasopressin is less sensitive, modest changes in pressure or volume, which are exacerbated by upright posture, do not interfere with the regulation of osmolality. Yet the pressor effect of high vasopressin levels serves to maintain blood pressure if volume depletion or hypotension becomes excessive. Usually, the physiologic regulation of osmolality and pressure-volume are synergistic. Dehydration causes an increase in plasma osmolality and a decrease in blood volume, both of which stimulate the release of vasopressin. Conversely, excess fluid administration causes a decrease in plasma osmolality and an expansion of blood volume, both of which inhibit vasopressin secretion.

Other factors can also modulate osmotic release and action of vasopressin. With volume expansion, natriuretic factors such as atrial natriuretic peptide and brain natriuretic peptide are released from atrial myocytes and act at the kidney to induce a natriuresis. Brain natriuretic peptide is also synthesized in the hypothalamus, where it may act to decrease vasopressin secretion. During pregnancy, there is a decrease of plasma osmolality by approximately 10 mOsm/kg H_2O as a result of a resetting of the osmostat for vasopressin secretion, and the osmostat for thirst is reset downward in parallel. These effects appear to be mediated by the placental hormone relaxin.

Abnormalities in water and electrolyte balance are common in the elderly. This is due in part to age-related changes in body volume (as much as a 50% decrease in total body water occurs in those older than 75 years) and renal function. The elderly also have a decreased sense of thirst. Although there is a normal or even increased ability to secrete vasopressin with age, there is a decreased ability to achieve either maximal urine concentration to retain water or maximal dilution of urine to excrete water. Consequently, the elderly are particularly prone to both hypernatremia and hyponatremia with diseases that affect water balance or from the drugs used to treat various diseases.

Oxytocin

Prolactin is the main hormone necessary for milk production, but oxytocin is essential for milk secretion. Suckling stimulates tactile receptors in the nipple, producing an afferent signal to the hypothalamus that causes a synchronized release of oxytocin from the posterior pituitary. Oxytocin binds to oxytocin receptors in the breast and induces contraction of myoepithelial cells around the alveoli and ductules to eject milk. In addition, upregulation of uterine oxytocin receptors dramatically increases uterine smooth muscle contractions in response to oxytocin secretion at the end of pregnancy. The greatest release of oxytocin occurs with, not before, delivery of the infant, probably secondary to stretching of the vaginal wall. Because transgenic mice lacking either oxytocin or oxytocin receptors have normal parturition, oxytocin release may be more important to induce uterine contraction to inhibit blood loss after delivery than to initiate parturition. No pathologic syndromes of either increased or decreased secretion of oxytocin have yet been defined, but experimental studies have implicated oxytocin in maternal and affiliative behavior as well as bone formation.[3] However, because of the structural similarity between vasopressin and oxytocin, at high plasma levels oxytocin can activate vasopressin receptors, and vasopressin can activate oxytocin receptors, both of which can have pathologic consequences.

⬤ SYNDROME OF INAPPROPRIATE ANTIDIURETIC HORMONE SECRETION

Excess secretion of vasopressin can be caused by abnormally regulated secretion from the posterior pituitary, or by ectopic synthesis and secretion of vasopressin by tumors. Osmotically inappropriate secretion of vasopressin causes renal water retention and volume expansion of body fluids, with consequent dilutional hyponatremia. This disorder is called the syndrome of inappropriate antidiuretic hormone secretion (SIADH) and is discussed in Chapter 108.

⬤ DIABETES INSIPIDUS

❰ DEFINITION ❱

Diabetes insipidus is the excretion of a large volume of hypotonic insipid (tasteless) urine, usually manifested by polyuria (increased urination) and

polydipsia (increased thirst).[4,5] The large urine volume, usually in excess of 50 to 60 mL/kg/day, must be distinguished from an increased frequency of small urine volumes and from large volumes of isotonic or hypertonic urine, both of which have different clinical significance.

❰ PATHOBIOLOGY ❱

Five pathophysiologic mechanisms must be considered in the differential diagnosis of diabetes insipidus.

1. Central diabetes insipidus is caused by the inability of the hypothalamus–posterior pituitary to secrete (and usually to synthesize) vasopressin in response to increased osmolality.[6] No concentration of the dilute glomerular filtrate takes place in the renal collecting duct, and consequently, a large volume of hypotonic (i.e., dilute) urine is excreted. This produces a secondary increase in serum osmolality, with stimulation of thirst and secondary polydipsia. Levels of vasopressin in plasma are unmeasurable or inappropriately low for the plasma osmolality.

2. Nephrogenic diabetes insipidus is caused by the inability of an otherwise normal kidney to respond to vasopressin. As in hypothalamic (central) diabetes insipidus, the dilute glomerular filtrate entering the collecting duct is excreted as a large volume of hypotonic urine. The rise in plasma osmolality that occurs stimulates thirst and produces polydipsia. Unlike central diabetes insipidus, however, measured levels of vasopressin in plasma are high or appropriate for plasma osmolality.

3. Gestational diabetes insipidus[7] is a rare condition produced by elevated levels or activity of placental cysteine aminopeptidase (oxytocinase or vasopressinase) during pregnancy. The rapid destruction of vasopressin produces diabetes insipidus with polyuria and secondary stimulation of thirst with polydipsia. Because of the circulating vasopressinase, plasma vasopressin levels usually cannot be measured.

4. Primary polydipsia is a disorder of excess fluid ingestion rather than of vasopressin secretion or activity. Excessive ingested water produces a mild decrease in plasma osmolality that shuts off the secretion of vasopressin. In the absence of vasopressin action on the kidney, urine does not become concentrated, and a large volume of hypotonic urine is excreted. The amount of vasopressin in plasma is unmeasurable or low but is appropriate for the low plasma osmolality.

5. Osmoreceptor dysfunction is a variant of central diabetes insipidus in which the neurohypophysis is intact, but the osmoreceptive cells in the anterior hypothalamus have been damaged (see Fig. 212-1). Because the osmoreceptor cells are necessary for osmotically stimulated vasopressin secretion, the patient manifests polyuria. However, because the osmoreceptor cells also control thirst, these patients do not have polydipsia. As a result, they are characterized by elevated serum sodium levels and plasma osmolalities. For this reason, this disorder has also been called essential hypernatremia and adipsic diabetes insipidus, in recognition of the profound thirst deficits found in most of the affected patients.[8]

Although the pathophysiologic mechanisms for each of these five disorders are distinct, patients in the first four categories usually manifest polyuria and polydipsia, and the serum sodium level is usually normal because an intact thirst mechanism is sufficiently sensitive to maintain water homeostasis in the first three disorders, and the normal kidney has sufficient capacity to excrete the excess water load in the fourth. The fifth category of osmoreceptor dysfunction is the exception, owing to a defective thirst mechanism leading to hypernatremia.

❰ CLINICAL MANIFESTATIONS ❱
Central Diabetes Insipidus

The sudden appearance of hypotonic polyuria after transcranial surgery in the area of the hypothalamus or after head trauma with basal skull fracture and hypothalamic damage strongly suggests the diagnosis of central diabetes insipidus.[9] In these situations, if the patient is unconscious and unable to recognize thirst, hypernatremia is a common accompaniment. However, even in patients with more insidious progression of a specific disease or in patients with idiopathic central diabetes insipidus, the onset of polyuria is often relatively abrupt and occurs over several days or weeks. Most patients do not notice polyuria until urine volume exceeds 3 to 4 L/day, and as illustrated in Figure 212-2, urine volume does not exceed 4 L/day until the ability to concentrate the urine is severely limited and plasma vasopressin is nearly absent. As few as 10 to 15% of the normal number of vasopressinergic neurons in the hypothalamus is sufficient to maintain an asymptomatic urine volume, but the further loss of just a small number of these neurons produces a rapid increase in urine volume and symptomatic polyuria. Urine volume seldom exceeds the amount of dilute fluid delivered to the collecting duct ($\approx$18 to 24 L in humans); in many cases, urine volume is significantly less because patients voluntarily restrict fluid intake, which causes some mild volume contraction and increased proximal tubular reabsorption of fluid. Patients often express a preference for cold liquids, which are more effective in assuaging thirst. Both thirst and increased urine output persist through the night, impairing sleep. Patients with partial central diabetes insipidus have some ability to secrete vasopressin, but this secretion is markedly attenuated at normal levels of plasma osmolality. Therefore, these patients often have urine volume and symptoms similar to those of patients with complete central diabetes insipidus. Because most patients with central diabetes insipidus have sufficient thirst to drink fluid to match urine output, few laboratory abnormalities are present at the time of initial evaluation. The serum sodium level can be in the high-normal range, whereas the blood urea nitrogen level can be low secondary to the large urine volume. Uric acid is relatively high because of the modest intra-vascular volume contraction and lack of action of vasopressin on V_{1a} receptors in the kidney, which stimulate the clearance of uric acid. Uric acid levels greater than 5 mg/dL can help to differentiate diabetes insipidus from primary polydipsia.

Central diabetes insipidus can be inherited as an autosomal dominant disease that is typically characterized by an asymptomatic infancy and an onset later in childhood. Most genetic defects are either in the signal peptide of the pre-prohormone or in the neurophysin portion of the prohormone.[10] Mutations involving the vasopressin sequence itself are few. Most cases are believed to result from disruption of cleavage from the signal peptide or abnormal folding of the neurophysin, which slows trafficking of the mutant prohormone through the endoplasmic reticulum, leading to neuronal cell dysfunction or death. Because this is a cumulative process, this explains the later onset of central diabetes insipidus with these types of mutations.

Myxedema and adrenal insufficiency both impair the ability to excrete free water by renal mechanisms. The simultaneous occurrence of either of these diseases with central diabetes insipidus (as can occur with a tumor of the hypothalamus or pituitary) can decrease an otherwise large urine output, thereby masking the symptoms of diabetes insipidus. Replacement treatment for the anterior pituitary deficiency, especially glucocorticoids, can then cause a sudden and massive excretion of dilute urine. Similarly, the onset of either hypothyroidism or adrenal insufficiency during the course of diabetes insipidus can decrease the need for vasopressin replacement and in some cases can even cause hyponatremia. Central diabetes insipidus occurs commonly in patients with severe brain ischemia and is often indicative of brain death. Treatment of the diabetes insipidus along with any coexistent anterior pituitary hormone deficiencies can be used to preserve donor organs in such cases.

Osmoreceptor Dysfunction

A variant of central diabetes insipidus is the syndrome of osmoreceptor dysfunction. Physiologic maneuvers demonstrate that when such patients are euvolemic, an increase in plasma osmolality produces neither secretion of vasopressin nor a sensation of thirst. However, vasopressin is still synthesized by the hypothalamus and stored in the posterior pituitary, because stimulation of baroreceptors by hypovolemia or hypotension results in the prompt secretion of vasopressin; the kidney is responsive because vasopressin release by volume receptor stimulation causes urinary concentration. Because patients lack thirst, they are chronically dehydrated, often with markedly increased serum sodium levels (hypovolemic hypernatremia). However, it is the dehydration-induced volume depletion, not the increased osmolality that eventually stimulates the secretion of vasopressin. The volume of urine output depends on the degree of dehydration-induced secretion of vasopressin. If sufficient fluid replacement is given to return extracellular fluid volume to normal, these patients are unable to regulate vasopressin by osmolality and again become polyuric, thereby manifesting their underlying central diabetes insipidus. Lesions that cause osmoreceptor dysfunction are similar to lesions that can cause central diabetes insipidus, but in contrast to central diabetes insipidus these lesions usually occur more rostrally in the hypothalamus, consistent with the anterior hypothalamic location of the primary osmoreceptor cells (see Fig. 212-1). One lesion that is unique to this disorder is an anterior communicating cerebral artery aneurysm, particularly following resection of the aneurysm.

Nephrogenic Diabetes Insipidus

Nephrogenic diabetes insipidus is caused by mutations of the vasopressin V_2 receptor or the vasopressin-induced water channel AQP2, or by impairments in the signal transduction system linking V_2 receptor activation and AQP2

membrane insertion. Familial nephrogenic diabetes insipidus is a rare disease, most cases of which (>90%) are due to mutations of the V_2 receptor.[11] More than 100 different V_2 receptor mutations have been described and can be classified into several different general categories based on differences in transport of the mutant receptor to the cell surface and vasopressin binding or stimulation of adenylate cyclase. Because the gene for the V_2 receptor is located on the X chromosome, this is an X-linked recessive disease. Symptoms are noted only in affected males, who often present with vomiting, constipation, failure to thrive, fever, and polyuria during the first week of life. Hypernatremia with a hypotonic urine is typically present. The phenotype is similar in the less than 10% of patients with mutations of the AQP2 water channel, but because the AQP2 gene is located on chromosome 12, mutations cause autosomal recessive disease; consequently, consanguinity and a family history of the disease in men and women is common, and this disorder should be suspected when the proband is female.

Nephrogenic diabetes insipidus can also be acquired during treatment with certain drugs such as demeclocycline (which can be used to treat inappropriate secretion of vasopressin), lithium carbonate (used to treat bipolar disorders), and fluoride (previously used in fluorocarbon anesthetics), and from electrolyte abnormalities such as severe hypokalemia and hypercalcemia. All causes of acquired nephrogenic diabetes insipidus have in common the decreased synthesis and function of AQP2 due to impaired vasopressin signaling from V_2 receptor binding and activation. Other diseases of the kidney can produce polyuria and inability to concentrate the urine secondary to altered renal medullary blood flow or to other disorders that inhibit maintenance of the hyperosmolar concentrating gradient in the inner medulla. Renal manifestations of such disorders (e.g., sickle cell disease, sarcoidosis, pyelonephritis, multiple myeloma, analgesic nephropathy) are discussed in Chapter 113.

Gestational Diabetes Insipidus

In pregnancy, there is an increased metabolism of vasopressin due to cysteine aminopeptidase (oxytocinase or vasopressinase), an enzyme that degrades oxytocin and prevents premature uterine contractions. Normally, this is compensated for by increased synthesis and secretion of vasopressin. Rarely, women with normal regulation of vasopressin develop diabetes insipidus because of markedly elevated levels of vasopressinase. Some of these patients have accompanying preeclampsia, acute fatty liver, and coagulopathies, but causal relations between diabetes insipidus and these abnormalities have not been identified. In general, diabetes insipidus does not persist after the pregnancy ends and does not recur in subsequent normal pregnancies.

Polyuria can also manifest in patients who have limited vasopressin reserve (partial central diabetes insipidus) or who respond poorly to vasopressin action (compensated nephrogenic diabetes insipidus). Treatment may be required only during the pregnancy, and the patient often returns to her previous baseline function without the need for therapy when the pregnancy ends. Less commonly, central diabetes insipidus of another cause first becomes symptomatic during pregnancy and then persists afterward, following the usual course of diabetes insipidus.

Primary Polydipsia

Excessive fluid intake also causes hypotonic polyuria and, by definition, polydipsia. This disorder must be differentiated from the various causes of diabetes insipidus. Despite normal pituitary and kidney function, patients with this disorder share many characteristics of both central diabetes insipidus (vasopressin secretion is suppressed as a result of decreased plasma osmolality) and nephrogenic diabetes insipidus (kidney AQP2 expression is decreased as a result of suppressed plasma vasopressin levels). Many different names have been used for this excessive fluid intake, but primary polydipsia remains the best descriptor to avoid confusing this order with diabetes insipidus as classically defined.[12]

Primary polydipsia is sometimes due to a severe mental illness such as schizophrenia, mania, or obsessive-compulsive disorder, in which case it is called psychogenic polydipsia. These patients usually deny true thirst and attribute their polydipsia to bizarre motives, such as a need to cleanse the body of poisons. The incidence in psychiatric hospitals can be as high as 40%, and there is no obvious explanation for the polydipsia. Primary polydipsia can also be caused by an abnormality in the osmoregulatory control of thirst, in which case it is called dipsogenic diabetes insipidus. These patients have no overt psychiatric illness and invariably attribute their polydipsia to a nearly constant thirst. Dipsogenic diabetes insipidus is usually idiopathic, but it can also be secondary to organic structural lesions in the hypothalamus identical to those causing central diabetes insipidus, such as neurosarcoidosis of the hypothalamus, tuberculous meningitis, multiple sclerosis, or trauma. Consequently, all polydipsic patients should be evaluated with magnetic resonance imaging (MRI) of the brain before it is concluded that excessive water intake is due to an idiopathic or psychiatric cause. Primary polydipsia can also be produced by diseases or drugs that cause a dry mouth, or by any peripheral disorder causing marked elevations of renin or angiotensin II.

Finally, primary polydipsia is sometimes caused by physicians, nurses, lay practitioners, or health writers who recommend a high fluid intake for valid (e.g., recurrent nephrolithiasis) or unsubstantiated health reasons. These patients lack overt signs of mental illness, but they also deny thirst and usually attribute their polydipsia to habits acquired from years of adherence to a drinking regimen. Laboratory studies in these patients are generally normal, although the serum sodium concentration is sometimes at the low end of the normal range, and the level of uric acid is generally lower than in patients with other forms of diabetes insipidus.

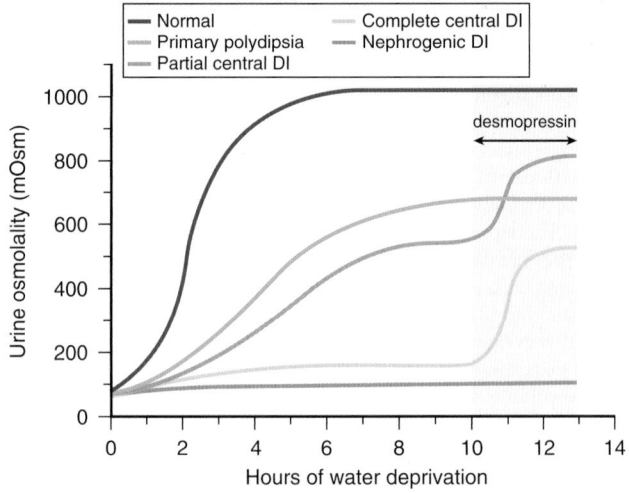

FIGURE 212-3. Responses to the water deprivation test to differentiate various types of diabetes insipidus (DI) and primary polydipsia (as described by Miller M, Dalakos T, Moses AM, et al. Recognition of partial defects in antidiuretic hormone secretion. *Ann Intern Med.* 1970;73:721-729). The response to dehydration reaches a plateau, and the subsequent change in urine osmolality in response to administered desmopressin is illustrated. See the discussion in the text.

DIAGNOSIS

Physiologic Diagnosis

Diabetes insipidus should be considered in all patients presenting with significant polyuria, defined as urine output greater than 50 mL/kg/day. Although osmotic diuresis secondary to hyperglycemia, intravenous contrast agents, or renal injury is a more common clinical cause of polyuria, the medical history, an isotonic urine osmolality, and routine clinical laboratory tests generally distinguish these disorders from diabetes insipidus. A diagnosis of diabetes insipidus can be made when urine osmolality is inappropriately low in the presence of an elevated plasma osmolality as a result of increased serum sodium concentration.[13] These criteria are sometimes met at the initial examination, especially in cases of acute diabetes insipidus occurring after trauma or surgery with inadequate fluid replacement. In such patients with hypernatremia and hypotonic urine osmolality with normal renal function, one need only administer a vasopressin agonist to differentiate central diabetes insipidus, in which a renal response with decreased urine volume and increased urine osmolality occurs, from nephrogenic diabetes insipidus, in which a subnormal renal response is seen. Sometimes in the postoperative state, a water diuresis occurs as a result of water retention during the surgical procedure. Vasopressin is normally secreted in response to surgical stress, causing fluid administered intravenously during the procedure to be retained. During recovery, vasopressin levels fall, and a diuresis of the retained fluid occurs. In this case, the serum sodium level is almost always normal; however, if additional fluid is administered to match the urine output, persistent polyuria can be mistaken for diabetes insipidus. In this situation, the physician should decrease the rate of fluid administered and follow the urine output and serum sodium level. If the urine output decreases and the serum sodium level remains normal, no treatment is necessary; if serum sodium rises above the normal range and the urine remains hypotonic, diabetes insipidus is likely, and the response to a vasopressin agonist can ascertain the type (central versus nephrogenic).

Most outpatients with diabetes insipidus are not hypernatremic, because the polydipsia produced by a normal thirst response is generally sufficient to maintain water homeostasis. Instead, they present with polyuria, polydipsia, and a normal sodium level. In these patients, further testing is necessary to increase serum osmolality and then measure the plasma vasopressin level or the urinary response to an administered vasopressin agonist. The best described test is the water deprivation test (Fig. 212-3), which should be carried out under controlled observation in the hospital or an appropriately equipped outpatient area. The exact timing of the test depends on the patient's symptoms. If the patient has marked polyuria during the night, it is best to begin the test during the day because the patient may become overly dehydrated overnight. However, if the patient has only two or three episodes of nocturia per night, it is best to begin the test in the evening so that the major part of the dehydration takes place when the patient is asleep. In either case, the patient is weighed at the beginning of the test, and all subsequent fluids are withheld. The volume and osmolality of all excreted urine are measured, and the patient is reweighed after each liter of urine output. When three consecutive urine samples have an osmolality differing by no more than 10% and the patient has lost at least 2% of body weight, a blood sample is obtained for the measurement of serum osmolality, sodium, and plasma vasopressin. The patient is then given 2 µg of desmopressin intravenously or subcutaneously and observed for an additional 2 hours.

Adults with normal vasopressin secretion concentrate their urine to greater than 800 mOsm/kg H₂O and have less than a 10% increase in urine osmolality in response to administered desmopressin. Patients with complete central diabetes insipidus have minimal concentration of the urine with dehydration,

and a marked increase in urine osmolality (usually >50%) in response to administered desmopressin. Patients with nephrogenic diabetes insipidus usually have no increase in urine concentration in response to administered desmopressin, although in some cases of acquired nephrogenic diabetes insipidus, some increased urinary concentration (but generally <10%) can occur. Nephrogenic diabetes insipidus is best distinguished from central diabetes insipidus by the measurement of vasopressin in plasma; plasma vasopressin levels are elevated in cases of nephrogenic diabetes insipidus, especially after dehydration.

In patients with partial central diabetes insipidus and patients with primary polydipsia, the urine is often somewhat concentrated in response to dehydration, but not to the maximum of a normal person. The chronically reduced level of vasopressin downregulates the synthesis of AQP2 water channels, and the large urine volume, regardless of cause, washes out the medullary osmotic gradient that is the determinant of maximal urine concentration. When desmopressin is administered, patients with partial central diabetes insipidus have a further increase (usually >10% but <50%) in urine osmolality, whereas most patients with primary polydipsia have no further increase (i.e., <10%). However, the reliability of distinguishing between these two disorders by the water deprivation test is suboptimal. Some patients with primary polydipsia may not become sufficiently dehydrated to secrete maximal vasopressin and hence have an increase in urine osmolality in response to administered desmopressin. Alternatively, some patients with partial central diabetes insipidus can become sufficiently dehydrated that their maximal concentration of urine is reached during the test, and no further concentration is seen with administered desmopressin. Plasma vasopressin levels at the end of dehydration are better at discriminating between these two disorders, but only at high serum sodium concentrations (i.e., >145 mmol/L). Consequently, some investigators recommend a limited infusion of hypertonic (3%) sodium chloride solution to achieve these elevated levels if they are not achieved by the water deprivation itself. Because measurement of vasopressin in plasma is difficult, recent studies have suggested that the C-terminal fragment of the vasopressin prohormone copeptin may be a reliable and more convenient surrogate measure of vasopressin secretion.[14]

Etiologic Diagnosis

If the water deprivation test confirms that inadequate vasopressin secretion is responsible for the polyuria, the underlying cause must be determined. MRI of the hypothalamic-pituitary area is the most important diagnostic tool in these cases. The three areas of interest are the immediate suprasellar region of the hypothalamus, the pituitary stalk, and the posterior pituitary within the sella turcica (see the earlier discussion of anatomy). Most slow-growing tumors confined to the sella do not cause diabetes insipidus. To cause central diabetes insipidus, tumors in the hypothalamic area immediately above the sella must be either sufficiently large to destroy 80 to 90% of the vasopressin cells or located where the paths of the four nuclear groups converge at the origin of the pituitary stalk, just above the diaphragm sella. Primary tumors, especially craniopharyngioma and suprasellar germinoma, metastatic tumors, and infiltrative diseases can also cause diabetes insipidus by involvement of the pituitary stalk, which is then thickened (i.e., >2 mm) on MRI. On T1-weighted MRI, the vasopressin and oxytocin stored in neurosecretory granules in the posterior pituitary are visualized as a bright spot in the sella turcica. Most but not all normal subjects have this bright spot (it is absent more frequently in elderly and dehydrated patients); in most but not all patients with central diabetes insipidus, the bright spot is absent. Thickening of the stalk and absence of the bright spot are therefore especially suggestive of a hypothalamic disease process.[15]

Brain trauma (Chapter 371), especially when severe, can also cause diabetes insipidus. In particular, deceleration injuries can cause a shearing of the pituitary stalk at the level of the diaphragm sella. Patients with basilar skull fractures should always be evaluated for possible accompanying diabetes insipidus.

Tumors that cause central diabetes insipidus are most often benign primary intracranial tumors such as craniopharyngioma, ependymoma (suprasellar germinoma), and pinealoma, which arise in the third ventricle. Primary tumors of the anterior pituitary (Chapter 211) cause diabetes insipidus only when substantial suprasellar extension is present. However, rapidly growing intrasellar lesions, such as metastases from carcinomas of the lung, breast, and melanoma or hemorrhage into pituitary adenomas, can cause diabetes insipidus because there is insufficient time for the vasopressin axons to adapt by releasing vasopressin from the hypothalamus. Metastases to the hypothalamus can also destroy the supraopticohypophysial tract and produce diabetes insipidus.

Granulomatous diseases, such as Langerhans cell histiocytosis, sarcoidosis, tuberculosis, and leukemic infiltrates and lymphomas of the hypothalamus, can cause diabetes insipidus by destroying vasopressin cells. In such patients, the diagnosis is usually suspected on the basis of peripheral manifestations of the respective diseases. Lymphocytic infundibuloneurohypophysitis is an autoimmune disease similar to lymphocytic hypophysitis of the anterior pituitary (Chapter 211) in which lymphocytes infiltrate the neurohypophysis to produce diabetes insipidus. The hallmarks of this process are a thickened pituitary stalk and an absence of the pituitary bright spot in a patient with the abrupt onset of polyuria and polydipsia, particularly a postpartum female. The diagnosis was originally demonstrated by pituitary biopsy, but now is more commonly made by regression of the thickened stalk with continued MRI follow-up. When no specific cause is identified, the diagnosis of exclusion is idiopathic diabetes insipidus; but most such cases are probably caused by an autoimmune disease, and other autoimmune diseases, including anterior pituitary hypophysitis,[16] are often recognized in affected patients. When central nervous system disease is suspected but not diagnosed by MRI or general physical examination, cerebrospinal fluid obtained by lumbar puncture may be helpful in identifying tumor cells or markers of tumors or inflammatory processes (e.g., elevated angiotensin-converting enzyme levels with neurosarcoidosis, elevated β-HCG levels with germinomas).

A family history suggestive of diabetes insipidus should be investigated with genetic testing for inherited mutations in the vasopressin or vasopressin receptor genes depending on the site of the defect.[17]

TREATMENT   Rx

Because excess excretion of water is the primary manifestation of diabetes insipidus, water replacement in adequate quantities avoids the metabolic complications of all forms of this disease. However, oral or intravenous administration of the volume of fluid required to replace the often large urinary losses in diabetes insipidus is difficult and inconvenient. The goal of therapy is therefore to reduce the amount of polyuria and polydipsia to a tolerable level while avoiding overtreatment, which can produce water retention and hyponatremia.

Central Diabetes Insipidus

The best therapeutic agent for the treatment of central diabetes insipidus is the vasopressin agonist desmopressin. Desmopressin is different from vasopressin in that the amino group of the N-terminal cysteine residue has been removed to prolong the duration of action, and D-arginine has been substituted for L-arginine in position 8 to decrease the vasopressor effects. At therapeutic dosages, this agent acts primarily on V_2 or antidiuretic receptors, with minimal activity at V_{1a} or pressor receptors. Desmopressin is available as tablets of 0.1 or 0.2 mg for oral administration and in either a spray bottle that delivers a fixed dose of 10 µg in 100 µL or a bottle with a rhinal catheter that can deliver 50 to 200 µL (5 to 20 µg) for intranasal administration. When therapy is initiated, it is generally best to begin with a low dose (e.g., half of a 0.1-mg tablet, 5 µg by the rhinal tube, or a single 100 µL spray of 10 µg) at bedtime to allow the patient to sleep through the night, and then determine the duration of action

by quantifying the polyuria the next day. The duration of action of a single dose varies from 6 to 24 hours, but in most patients, a good therapeutic response can be achieved on an every-12-hour schedule for the nasal spray or an 8- or 12-hour schedule for the tablets. Desmopressin is also available for parenteral use in 1-mL vials of 4 µg/mL. Parenteral administration is especially useful postoperatively or when a patient is unable to take the nasal preparation. In hospitalized patients, some physicians add vasopressin directly to a crystalloid solution to infuse doses in the range of 0.25 to 2.7 mIU/kg/hour to cause modest but persistent urinary concentration as a treatment of diabetes insipidus. With any form of desmopressin administration, serum sodium levels should be monitored regularly to prevent the development of hyponatremia.[18]

Osmoreceptor Dysfunction

Because the diabetes insipidus of patients with osmoreceptor dysfunction is central, they respond to desmopressin as do patients with central diabetes insipidus. However, because of their thirst defect, this is usually not sufficient to maintain normal plasma osmolality. Consequently, they must be given a "prescription" for amounts of fluids to be consumed each 24 hours in order to maintain normal serum sodium levels and plasma osmolalities. This must be individualized to each patient because overconsumption of fluid coupled with desmopressin administration can produce severe hyponatremia. Body weight using an accurate scale is useful as a guide to preventing under- or overhydration, but frequent monitoring of serum sodium levels is usually necessary as well.

Nephrogenic Diabetes Insipidus

Although most patients with nephrogenic diabetes insipidus do not respond to desmopressin, a small number have a partial response to higher doses (e.g., 10 to 20 µg subcutaneously or intranasally).[19] For the majority of patients who have no response to desmopressin, some orally administered pharmacologic agents are also useful. Chlorothiazide, amiloride, and prostaglandin synthase inhibitors can be used to reduce polyuria in nephrogenic diabetes insipidus. Symptomatic nephrogenic diabetes insipidus is usually treated with a thiazide diuretic, which is enhanced by coadministration of the potassium-sparing diuretic amiloride. Thiazide diuretics cause sodium depletion and volume contraction and decrease urine volume by increasing proximal tubular reabsorption of glomerular filtrate. Prostaglandin synthase inhibitors (e.g., indomethacin) block the action of prostaglandin E to inhibit the action of vasopressin on the kidney. However, none of these agents has been approved by the U.S. Food and Drug Administration for the treatment of diabetes insipidus; therefore, the prescribing physician should be aware of potential toxicities and side effects. When diuretics are used to treat nephrogenic diabetes insipidus, special attention should be paid to the possibility that the induced dehydration may increase the concentration of other drugs. In cases of drug-induced nephrogenic diabetes insipidus, the most direct therapy is discontinuation of the offending agent, if possible. Amiloride can be especially beneficial in cases of nephrogenic diabetes insipidus induced by lithium, because the drug decreases the entrance of lithium into cells in the distal tubule.

Gestational Diabetes Insipidus

During pregnancy, vasopressinase increases the metabolism of vasopressin but not of desmopressin, so desmopressin is the drug of choice for these patients. The vasopressinase activity subsides within a few weeks of delivery, and patients with the onset of partial diabetes insipidus during pregnancy may become asymptomatic after delivery. An additional advantage of desmopressin is that it has little action on the oxytocin receptors of the uterus. During pregnancy, normal serum sodium decreases by approximately 10 mOsm/kg H_2O because of a reset osmostat, so pregnant patients with diabetes insipidus require only enough desmopressin to maintain the plasma osmolality at this lower level.

Correction of Hyperosmolality

Some situations require special attention during therapy. Rarely, if patients with diabetes insipidus are unable to drink or are given a hypertonic solution, severe hypernatremia can develop acutely. Osmotic equilibrium with the intracellular water of neurons and glia produces shrinking of the brain. The brain is in a closed vault (i.e., the skull), and when the brain shrinks, traction on the vasculature of the central nervous system can cause the rupture of blood vessels and subarachnoid or intracerebral hemorrhage. If the hypernatremia persists for a longer time, the neurons accommodate by producing organic osmolytes (previously called idiogenic osmoles), which limit the amount of brain shrinkage. Once this adaptation has occurred, a too-rapid lowering of osmolality in the extracellular fluid will produce a shift of water into the brain and cause cerebral edema. This is especially of concern in children, in whom overly rapid rehydration can produce seizures. In this situation, desmopressin can be administered to produce constant antidiuresis, and the amount of water given can be regulated to decrease osmolality by no more than approximately 12 mEq/L every 24 hours. Postoperatively or after head trauma, diabetes insipidus can be transient (see Prognosis), and the need for long-term maintenance therapy cannot be immediately established.

The prognosis of properly treated diabetes insipidus is excellent. If nephrogenic diabetes insipidus is diagnosed and treated early, intracranial calcification and mental retardation do not occur. When the diabetes insipidus is secondary to a recognized disease process, that disease generally determines the ultimate prognosis. In some specific clinical situations, the course is different and characteristic. The development of diabetes insipidus after surgical or traumatic injury to the neurohypophysis can follow any of several well-defined patterns (Fig. 212-4). In some patients, polyuria develops 1 to 4 days after injury and resolves spontaneously. Less often, the diabetes insipidus is permanent and continues indefinitely. Most interestingly, one can see a "triphasic" response that has been well described after pituitary stalk transection. The first phase of diabetes insipidus is due to axon shock and lack of function of the damaged neurons. This phase lasts several hours to several days and is followed by a second, antidiuretic phase that is due to the uncontrolled release of vasopressin from the disconnected and degenerating posterior pituitary or from the remaining severed neurons. Overly aggressive administration of fluids during this second phase does not suppress the uncontrolled vasopressin release from the damaged neurohypophysis and can lead to hyponatremia. The antidiuresis can last 2 to 14 days, after which diabetes insipidus recurs after depletion of vasopressin from the degenerating posterior pituitary gland (third phase). Transient hyponatremia without preceding or subsequent diabetes insipidus has been reported with surprisingly high frequency after transsphenoidal surgery for pituitary microadenomas, and is a common cause of hospital readmission after pituitary surgery.[20]

Once a deficiency of vasopressin secretion has been present for more than a few weeks, it rarely improves, even if the underlying cause of the neurohypophyseal destruction is eliminated. The major exception to this is postoperative diabetes insipidus, in which spontaneous resolution is the rule. Although recovery from diabetes insipidus that persists more than several weeks postoperatively is less common, and is uncommon after 1 year of continued diabetes insipidus, well-documented cases of recovery as long as 10 years after the initiating event have been reported. Potential return of function is a reason to occasionally withhold therapy transiently (i.e., one dose every 1 to 2 weeks) during long-term treatment. Diabetes insipidus after traumatic brain injury is associated with high mortality, but it usually resolves within a few days to a few weeks. In the minority of cases in which it is permanent, management is similar to nontraumatic central diabetes insipidus.

Diabetes insipidus should not be considered idiopathic until at least 4 years of follow-up. During this interval, annual computed tomography or MRI is indicated to search for a tumor or infiltrative process that may not have been detected at the initial examination.

GENERAL REFERENCES

For the General References and other additional features, please visit Expert Consult at https://expertconsult.inkling.com.

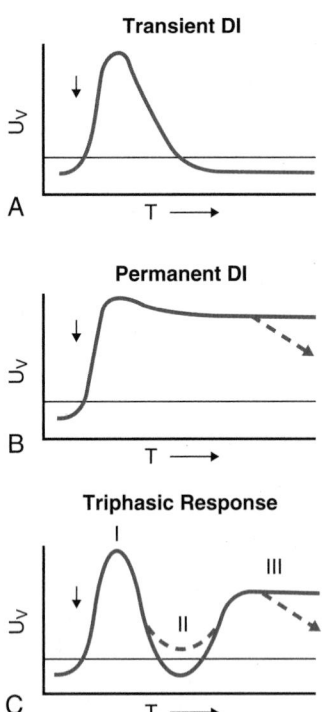

FIGURE 212-4. A to C, **Diagrammatic summary of the major patterns of postoperative and post-traumatic diabetes insipidus (DI).** The abscissa represents time (T) after the initial injury (*arrow*); the ordinate represents urinary volume (Uv) relative to a hypothetical "normal" urine output of 2 to 3 L/24 hours (*solid line*). See the discussion in the text. During the triphasic response (**C**), uncontrolled release of vasopressin from the disconnected or damaged posterior pituitary gland causes an antidiuresis that can lead to water retention and a dilutional hyponatremia. Diabetes insipidus returns as the third phase after the stored hormone in the posterior pituitary has been depleted. (From Verbalis JG, Robinson AG, Moses AM. Postoperative and post-traumatic diabetes insipidus. In: Czernichow AP, Robinson A, eds. *Diabetes Insipidus in Man: Frontiers of Hormone Research.* Basel: S Karger; 1985:247.)

213

THYROID

JACQUELINE JONKLAAS AND DAVID S. COOPER

The function of the thyroid gland is to secrete the thyroid hormones: 3,5,3′,5′-l-tetraiodothyronine (thyroxine, T_4) and a smaller amount of 3,5,3′-l-triiodothyronine (T_3). The main source of circulating T_3 is from the subsequent extrathyroidal deiodination of T_4 in peripheral tissues. In thyroid hormone responsive tissues, T_3 interacts with nuclear T_3 receptors that bind to promoter regions of genes that are positively or negatively regulated by thyroid hormone. Thyroid hormones are critically important for fetal and childhood growth and development; regulate heart rate and contractile function; affect gastrointestinal motility, respiratory function, and renal water clearance; and also modulate the body's energy expenditure, heat generation, weight, and lipid metabolism. In addition, the thyroid contains parafollicular or C cells that produce calcitonin, a 32-amino-acid polypeptide that inhibits bone resorption but has no apparent physiologic role in humans. However, calcitonin is clinically important as a tumor marker produced by medullary thyroid cancers that arise from these cells.

In utero, the thyroid develops at the base of the tongue and descends via the foramen cecum to its normal position along the anterior trachea midway between the thyroid cartilage and the suprasternal notch. The adult thyroid gland is butterfly-shaped, containing two lobes connected by an isthmus. Each lobe is about the size of a teaspoon (5 cc) and measures approximately 4 cm in length, 2 cm in width, and 1 cm in depth. Ectopic thyroid tissue can be present anywhere along the tract of its embryologic descent, starting at the base of the tongue ("lingual thyroid") and moving down toward the mediastinum. Remnants of the tract can form "thyroglossal duct cysts" or can persist as a pyramidal thyroid lobe, which can be palpably enlarged in diffuse thyroid disease (e.g., autoimmune thyroiditis and Graves disease).

When the thyroid enlarges, it can extend laterally, posteriorly, and inferiorly into the superior mediastinum, causing deviation and compression of the trachea, veins at the thoracic outlet, and the esophagus. Important structures around the thyroid also can be compromised during thyroid surgery: the parathyroid glands, which usually are behind the thyroid gland's superior and inferior poles; and the recurrent laryngeal nerves, which course upward through the tracheoesophageal groove and then branch behind each thyroid lobe.

Histologically, thyroid tissue is composed of clustered spherical follicles, each lined by a single layer of epithelial thyrocytes, which in turn surround a colloid-containing lumen. Thyroglobulin, which is the principal component of colloid, is the storage form of thyroid hormones. Calcitonin-producing parafollicular C cells, which are derived from the neural crest, are distributed between follicles.

PHYSIOLOGY

Thyroid Hormone Synthesis and Secretion

Dietary iodine (iodide I^- or iodate IO_3^-) is absorbed and then distributed in extracellular fluid. In the United States, daily iodine intake routinely exceeds the recommended daily need (150 µg) because of the widespread use of iodized salt and iodate preservatives in baked goods. The active transportation of circulating iodine into the thyrocyte is facilitated by a sodium-iodide symporter that is located in its basolateral membrane. After iodide has translocated to the apical membrane, its efflux is mediated by three apical iodide channels. Pendrin, anoctamin-1, and chloride channel-5 have been identified as candidate iodide transporters involved in iodine efflux. An H_2O_2 generation system is present at the apical surface of the thyrocyte in which H_2O_2 is produced by the enzyme dual oxidase 2. Molecules of the enzyme thyroid peroxidase, also present at the apical surface of the thyrocyte, are activated by H_2O_2. Oxidized thyroid peroxidase can then in turn oxidize iodide. The resulting reactive iodinium ion then covalently binds to tyrosyl residues in thyroglobulin, where it generates monoiodotyrosine and diiodotyrosine residues via organification. Thyroid peroxidase also catalyzes the formation of thyroxine (T_4) and triiodothyronine (T_3) by coupling monoiodotyrosine and diiodotyrosine residues.

Thyroglobulin is then pinocytosed at the apical membrane, and T_4 and T_3 are secreted after proteolysis of thyroglobulin. The proteolysis of thyroglobulin also liberates monoiodotyrosine and diiodotyrosine, and these compounds undergo deiodination so that the iodide can be recycled. Release of T_4 and T_3 from the basolateral membrane of the thyrocyte is mediated by thyroid hormone transporters, including monocarboxylate transporter 8 (E-Fig. 213-1). About 100 µg of T_4 and 5 µg of T_3 are normally released daily into the circulation. Thyroglobulin itself can also be measured in the circulation. Pharmacologic amounts of iodine inhibit the trapping and organification of iodide, as well as the release of the thyroid hormones. The release of thyroid hormone can also be blocked by lithium.

Thyroid Hormone Transport and Metabolism

More than 99% of circulating T_4 and T_3 is bound to three classes of plasma proteins. Thyroxine-binding globulin functions as the principal transport protein, whereas thyroxine-binding prealbumin (also known as transthyretin) and albumin make lesser contributions to T_4 and T_3 transport in blood. Pharmacologic doses of estrogens, pregnancy, hepatitis, and some medications (e.g., 5-fluorouracil, tamoxifen, and methadone) increase the serum thyroxine-binding globulin level, and familial excess of thyroxine-binding globulin can also be seen. Conversely, thyroxine-binding globulin levels are decreased with hepatic failure (Chapter 145), severe systemic illness, nephrotic syndrome (Chapter 113), and some medications (e.g., androgens, glucocorticoids, and slow-release nicotinic acid). Although total T_4 and T_3 levels change with changes in thyroxine-binding globulin, the free serum levels of these hormones remain constant. Familial dysalbuminemic hyperthyroxinemia is an autosomal dominant disorder characterized by the production of an albumin molecule that binds T_4 with a higher-than-normal affinity. Affected individuals may present with high total T_4 levels with an apparently inappropriately normal thyroid-stimulating hormone (TSH), and with normal free T_4 when this is measured by equilibrium dialysis.

T_3 is the preferred ligand for the thyroid hormone receptors. More than 80% of the T_3 present in target tissues is derived from T_4 through the action of deiodinase enzymes that remove an outer-ring iodine, converting T_4 to T_3, generating the pool of T_3 in target tissues, and contributing to T_3 in the circulation. The type 2 deiodinase is present in the pituitary gland and brain, whereas type 1 deiodinase predominates in other peripheral tissues such as the liver and kidney. The activity of these deiodinases may be inhibited by iodide-containing compounds (e.g., amiodarone, radiocontrast agents), glucocorticoid therapy, systemic illness, and selenium deficiency. T_4 can also be converted to biologically inactive reverse T_3 (rT_3) when its inner ring is deiodinated by type 1 deiodinase and a type 3 deiodinase that is present in the central nervous system glial cells. Type 3 deiodinase, which is also expressed in placenta, is one of several factors that lead to increased thyroxine dose requirements in pregnant women. Both T_3 and rT_3 can be converted by the action of deiodinases to inactive diiodothyronine (T_2).

Control of Thyroid Function

The hypothalamus and the pituitary gland control the growth of thyroid tissue and its production of thyroid hormones. Thyrotropin-releasing hormone (TRH), which is a tripeptide synthesized in the hypothalamus, is transported to the pituitary gland via the hypothalamic-pituitary portal system (Chapter 211). It binds to receptors on thyrotrophic cells, where it stimulates the synthesis and secretion of TSH (thyrotropin). TSH is a heterodimeric glycoprotein composed of an α-subunit (which is identical to that of follicle-stimulating hormone, luteinizing hormone, and human chorionic

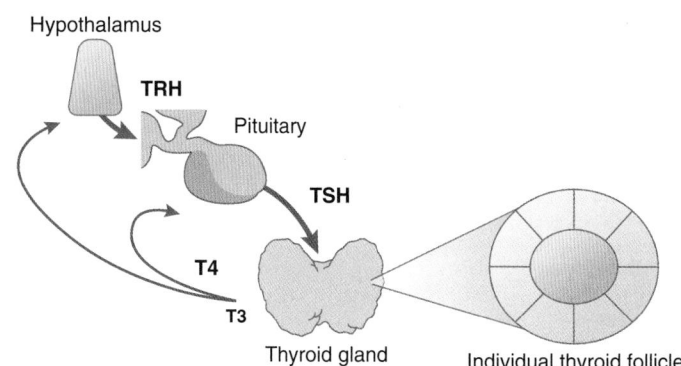

FIGURE 213-1. Schematic of control of thyroid gland. T3 = triiodothyronine; T4 = thyroxine; TRH = thyrotropin-releasing hormone; TSH = thyroid-stimulating hormone.

gonadotropin) coupled to a unique β-subunit. After it is transported by the circulation to the thyroid gland, it binds to the TSH receptor of thyrocytes, where it stimulates growth as well as the synthesis and secretion of thyroid hormone. Circulating T_3 and T_4 exert negative feedback that inhibits the synthesis and secretion of TRH in the hypothalamus and TSH in the pituitary gland (Fig. 213-1).

Thyroid Hormone Action

Although the circulating levels of thyroid hormones are determined by the hypothalamic pituitary axis, the intracellular levels and impact of T_3 are regulated by several distinct factors. These include thyroid hormone transporters, deiodinase enzymes, tissue-specific thyroid hormone receptors, and coregulators.[1] The thyroid hormone receptors that bind T_3 are members of the nuclear receptor superfamily, and there are at least three distinct isoforms, α_1, β_1, and β_2. In the presence of T_3, the various isoforms of the thyroid hormone receptors bind to specific DNA sequences known as thyroid hormone response elements. The regulation of target genes is achieved through the recruitment and release of corepressors and coactivators which interact with the transcriptional machinery.[2] The classic view of thyroid hormone action is positive regulation of gene expression. In the liver, for example, T_3 increases the expression of the low-density lipoprotein (LDL) receptor, thereby accelerating the clearance of LDL cholesterol. In the myocardium, T_3 increases myocyte contractility by promoting expression of alpha myosin heavy chain myocytes and relaxation by promoting sarcoplasmic reticulum adenosine triphosphatase (ATPase). T_3 increases the heart rate by accelerating depolarization and repolarization in the sinoatrial node. Thyroid hormone also increases the basal metabolic rate, thermogenesis,[3] ventilatory drive, gastrointestinal motility, mental alertness, and bone turnover. During fetal development, thyroid hormone is critical for skeletal maturation and brain development. Interestingly, although T_3 up-regulates the expression of many genes, it also down-regulates the expression of other genes, such as those coding for the beta subunit of TSH. Negative regulation takes place in the hypothalamus, pituitary, and liver.

Although T_4 is classically viewed as a prohormone that requires conversion to T_3 to have biologic activity, under certain circumstances T_4 can also bind to the thyroid hormone receptors. The ability of T_4 to bind to the thyroid hormone receptor seems to be determined by alterations in the cellular complement of corepressors and coactivators. Furthermore, the ability of the thyroid hormone receptor to respond to T_4 seems to differ according to the receptor isoform. Thus, T_4 may function directly as a hormone in specific physiologic situations yet to be determined.

DIAGNOSIS

Physical Examination

Examination of the thyroid starts with inspecting the anterior lower portion of the neck to determine whether the gland is diffusely or asymmetrically enlarged, the trachea is deviated, and lymphadenopathy or jugular venous distention is present. Palpation can be performed by an anterior or posterior approach. Anterior palpation uses one thumb to locate the gland's isthmus inferior to the cricoid cartilage. The right thyroid lobe is then palpated by placing the right thumb along the left side of the trachea, thereby displacing the contralateral lobe. Then, by placing the fingertips of the left hand medial to the right sternocleidomastoid muscle at the thyroid isthmus, the fingerpads of the right hand are used to define size, firmness, contour, surface characteristics, and potential tenderness, as well as possible palpable nodules in that thyroid

TABLE 213-1	CAUSES OF EUTHYROID HYPERTHYROXINEMIA (INCREASED TOTAL T$_4$, NORMAL TSH, NORMAL FREE T$_4$)

Increased synthesis of thyroxine-binding globulin
   Pregnancy
   Hepatitis
   Acute intermittent porphyria
   Drugs
      Estrogens
      Tamoxifen
      Raloxifene
      Methadone
      5-Fluorouracil
Increased binding of thyroid hormone to albumin
   Familial dysalbuminemic hyperthyroxinemia
Increased binding of thyroid hormone to transthyretin
   Hereditary variants

T$_4$ = thyroxine; TSH = thyroid-stimulating hormone.

TABLE 213-2	CAUSES OF EUTHYROID HYPOTHYROXINEMIA (DECREASED TOTAL T$_4$, NORMAL TSH, NORMAL FREE T$_4$)

Increased metabolism of thyroid hormone
   Drugs
      Phenytoin
      Phenobarbital
      Carbamazepine
      Rifampin
Decreased synthesis of thyroxine-binding globulin
   Severe liver disease
   Malnutrition
   Drugs
      Androgens
      Danazol
      L-Asparaginase
Increased clearance of thyroxine-binding globulin
   Nephrotic syndrome
   Protein-losing enteropathy
Decreased binding of thyroid hormone to thyroxine-binding globulin
   Drugs
      Salicylates (high dose)
      Phenytoin (high dose)
      Furosemide (intravenous)

T$_4$ = thyroxine; TSH = thyroid-stimulating hormone.

lobe while the patient swallows. The maneuver is reversed to examine the left lobe. The normal thyroid is just barely palpable, and it has a smooth surface and a slightly rubbery consistency. An enlarged thyroid is called a goiter. A goiter can be diffuse or nodular, and thyroid enlargement can be symmetrical or asymmetrical. Other features on physical examination include tracheal deviation from a large thyroid mass, the presence of cervical adenopathy, and a palpable pyramidal lobe. A palpable thrill is often noted over the thyroid in Graves disease due to increased vascularity, which can also be documented as a bruit on auscultation over the gland.

Laboratory Findings
TSH and Thyroid Hormone Levels

The serum level of TSH, which is a sensitive indicator of primary thyroid gland dysfunction, should be measured whenever thyroid dysfunction is suspected,[4] but routine screening of thyroid dysfunction is not of proven value in asymptomatic, nonpregnant adults. Indeed, the exquisitely sensitive inverse relationship between thyroid hormone levels and TSH secretion, which is logarithmic, results in serum TSH levels that are abnormal even when patients' thyroid hormone levels remain within the reference ranges. Subclinical hypothyroidism occurs when the serum free T$_4$ level is normal and the serum TSH is elevated (usually between 5 and 10 mU/L), and subclinical thyrotoxicosis exists when the serum free T$_4$ is normal but the serum TSH is below the reference range. In these circumstances, the serum free T$_4$ is "normal" but has become lower or higher compared with the patient's individual "set point." A single TSH measurement accurately classifies thyroid function, except when TSH deficiency is caused by hypothalamic or pituitary disease, by temporary perturbations in the hypothalamic-pituitary-thyroid axis or analytic problems affecting the TSH immunoassay. Apparently, normal aging is also associated with increased serum TSH levels without any changes in free T$_4$ levels, thereby suggesting that rising TSH levels in many elderly individuals are caused by age-related alterations in the TSH set point or by reduced TSH bioactivity, rather than by actual thyroid disease.

Concurrent measurements of the serum free T$_4$ level can confirm the clinical significance of an abnormal TSH level, define the severity of any thyroid dysfunction, and (together with a serum T$_3$ level in a thyrotoxic patient) suggest an underlying cause. Assays of total T$_4$ and T$_3$ levels are accurate but cannot distinguish the large plasma protein–bound (>99.5%) fractions from the much smaller (<0.5%) free fractions of each hormone. Congenital and acquired derangements of thyroxine-binding globulin (and, less commonly, transthyretin and albumin), which alter the total but not the free T$_4$ and T$_3$ levels, will be misdiagnosed as thyroid dysfunction unless the TSH level is measured (Tables 213-1 and 213-2). Free T$_4$ immunoassays are now widely available and yield reliable results in common conditions that alter plasma protein levels, such as estrogen-induced thyroxine-binding globulin excess. Free T$_4$ measurement after equilibrium dialysis of serum is the most accurate approach, but it is technically demanding and less readily available. Due to the small circulating quantities of free T$_3$, serum free T$_3$ assays are not quite as reliable as free T$_4$ assays, so some experts recommend total T$_3$ assays, recognizing the potential for misinterpretation in pregnancy and when levels of thyroxine-binding globulin are elevated. Serum T$_3$ measurements are useful in patients with various forms of thyrotoxicosis, in whom T$_3$ levels are usually elevated. Because T$_3$ is secreted preferentially in Graves disease and toxic multinodular goiter,

serum T$_3$ levels are often elevated above the T$_3$ reference range to a greater degree than serum T$_4$ or free T$_4$ levels. In contrast, serum T$_4$ and free T$_4$ are elevated to a greater degree than serum T$_3$ in various forms of thyroiditis, because the thyrotoxicosis is due to leakage of thyroid hormonal stores into the circulation, and far more T$_4$ than T$_3$ is stored within the thyroid gland.

Other Laboratory Tests

Thyroid autoantibody titers can aid in the evaluation of thyroid dysfunction. Antithyroid peroxidase and antithyroglobulin antibody titers can confirm the diagnosis of autoimmune thyroiditis. TSH receptor binding and stimulating immunoglobulin levels can be used to confirm the diagnosis of Graves disease. The erythrocyte sedimentation rate (ESR) can be helpful in the diagnosis of subacute thyroiditis. Serum thyroglobulin and calcitonin levels are used as tumor markers when observing patients treated for differentiated and medullary thyroid cancers, respectively.

Imaging
Anatomic Imaging

Ultrasonography can assess the size, texture, vascularity, symmetry, and structural abnormalities of the thyroid, including simple cysts, solid nodules, and cystic nodules.[5] Diffuse ultrasonographic heterogeneity is suggestive of autoimmune thyroiditis. Certain characteristics of nodules—including their number, echogenicity, capsular regularity, vascularity, and patterns of calcification—alter the probability of malignancy but rarely confirm or exclude thyroid cancer with certainty. Imaging of surrounding structures may identify cervical lymphadenopathy not detectable on physical examination.

Computed tomographic (CT) scanning and magnetic resonance imaging (MRI) can detect tracheal narrowing or deviation and determine whether the thyroid extends substernally into the mediastinum. Regional lymphadenopathy can also be detected by cervical CT scanning. Positron emission tomography (PET) can help localize metastatic sites of thyroid cancer.

Nuclear Medicine Imaging

Radioactive iodine-123 (^{123}I) scanning shows the pattern of uptake within the thyroid gland. Scanning can determine whether a nodule is hypofunctional (cold), hyperfunctional (hot), or has apparently equivalent function to the surrounding extranodular thyroid. Radionuclide scanning also can identify ectopic thyroid tissue at the base of the tongue (lingual thyroid), in ovarian teratomas (struma ovarii), or in distant thyroid cancer metastases. However, radionuclide imaging has essentially been replaced by ultrasonography and fine-needle aspiration biopsy (see section on Thyroid Nodules) for the evaluation of thyroid nodules.

The fractional amount of administered radioactive iodine or technetium that the thyroid gland takes up and retains during a defined period is an indicator of the gland's activity. Normal technetium pertechnetate uptake ranges from 0.5 to 3% at 20 minutes, whereas radioiodine uptake ranges from 8 to 28% at 24 hours. Radionuclide uptake is elevated in Graves disease, toxic nodules, and toxic multinodular goiter, but it is low in thyroiditis. Although radioiodine uptake measurements are rarely indicated for making these diagnoses, they remain valuable for calculating the ^{131}I dose needed to treat hyperthyroidism and thyroid cancer.

HYPOTHYROIDISM

DEFINITION

Primary hypothyroidism, which is called *myxedema* when severe, is hormone deficiency caused when intrinsic dysfunction of the thyroid gland reduces the synthesis and secretion of T_4 and T_3 (Table 213-3). In clinically overt primary hypothyroidism, the TSH level is elevated (usually >10 mU/L), in conjunction with a free T_4 level below the lower limit of the reference range. In subclinical hypothyroidism, the TSH level is only modestly elevated; the free T_4 level remains in the low-normal to normal range.

Secondary or central hypothyroidism develops when the pituitary gland does not adequately stimulate the thyroid gland with TSH. The cause can be a congenital or acquired pituitary or hypothalamic disorder, such that TSH is insufficient, either in quantity or functional integrity (Chapter 211).

EPIDEMIOLOGY

The lifetime incidence of primary hypothyroidism is about 5%. As many as 15% of older adults may develop mild hypothyroidism, depending on how subclinical hypothyroidism is defined (see Subclinical and Mild Hypothyroidism below). Hypothyroidism is more common in women, whites, and Latin Americans. More than 99% of all hypothyroidism reflects primary dysfunction of the thyroid gland itself.

PATHOBIOLOGY

Dietary iodine deficiency is a cause of primary hypothyroidism in regions of the world where deficiency of this micronutrient exists and is uncorrected by iodine supplementation. In developed countries, however, primary hypothyroidism

is most commonly an autoimmune disease (Hashimoto thyroiditis) in which altered T-cell-mediated immunity leads to a lymphocytic infiltrate, inflammation, and fibrosis, with linkage studies suggesting a polygenic genetic predisposition. In some patients, autoimmune thyroiditis is accompanied by other endocrine and nonendocrine autoimmune disorders (e.g., the type 2 polyglandular autoimmune syndrome with adrenal insufficiency and type 1 diabetes mellitus or the type 1 autoimmune syndrome with adrenal insufficiency, hypoparathyroidism, and chronic mucocutaneous candidiasis [Chapter 218]). Other associated nonendocrine autoimmune conditions include atrophic gastritis, pernicious anemia (Chapter 155), celiac disease (Chapter 131), Sjögren syndrome (Chapter 252), systemic sclerosis, and vitiligo (Chapter 412). Treatment with interferon-α can also cause transient or permanent autoimmune thyroiditis.

Surgical resection of the thyroid gland predictably leads to hypothyroidism. Radioactive iodine therapy for treatment of hyperthyroidism commonly destroys sufficient thyroid tissue to cause postablative hypothyroidism. External beam radiation therapy for head and neck cancer can also cause thyroid gland failure. Exposure to pharmacologic and radiocontrast agents that contain large amounts of iodine (e.g., amiodarone, radiocontrast dyes, some expectorants, and some topical disinfectants) can disrupt thyroid hormone production, thereby leading to hypothyroidism. Lithium inhibits secretion of T_4 and T_3, leading to hypothyroidism in 10% of treated patients. Other pharmacologic agents reported to cause hypothyroidism include stavudine, thalidomide, lenalidomide, imatinib, sunitinib, sorafenib, motesanib, bexarotene, ipilimumab, and aminoglutethimide. Interestingly, ipilimumab and nivolumab are associated with both primary and secondary hypothyroidism.[6]

Other rare causes of primary hypothyroidism (see Table 213-3) include thyroid agenesis, infiltrative disorders (e.g., hemochromatosis [Chapter 201], amyloidosis [Chapter 179], systemic sclerosis [Chapter 251], and invasive fibrous thyroiditis [Riedel thyroiditis]). Subacute thyroiditis and painless (postpartum) thyroiditis also can result in transient hypothyroidism. Consumptive hypothyroidism can occur with hemangiomas or gastrointestinal stromal tumors that express the type 3 deiodinase, which converts T_4 to biologically inactive reverse T_3.

Central or secondary hypothyroidism can be seen in disorders that impair the normal control of the thyroid gland by the hypothalamus or by the pituitary gland (Chapter 211). Infiltrative hypothalamic disorders include sarcoidosis (Chapter 89), hemochromatosis (Chapter 201), and histiocytosis (Chapter 160). Compression of thyrotrophic cells by pituitary adenomas and other masses can inhibit the synthesis and secretion of TSH, as can radiation therapy or surgery used to treat adenomas. Other disorders that can cause secondary hypothyroidism include lymphocytic hypophysitis, hypophysitis caused by immune checkpoint inhibitors (e.g., ipilimumab, nivolumab), metastatic tumors, pituitary infarction, and traumatic brain injury (Chapter 371).

CLINICAL MANIFESTATIONS

Symptoms of hypothyroidism include lethargy, fatigue, weakness, myalgias, decreased exercise tolerance, cold intolerance, depressed mood, weight gain despite poor appetite, hoarseness, constipation, arthralgias, paresthesias, dry skin, and hair loss.[7] If severe, women can develop amenorrhea, menorrhagia, and galactorrhea. Cognitive changes can range from mild memory lapses to delirium, dementia, seizures, and even myxedema coma. Because these symptoms are nonspecific and because hypothyroidism is often insidious in its onset, it can be under-recognized, especially in older adults.

Physical findings vary by age and the severity. Children may have delayed growth despite weight gain, delayed or precocious puberty, and muscle pseudohypertrophy. Adults can have mild hypothermia, bradycardia, and diastolic hypertension. Heart sounds may be muffled by a pericardial effusion. The skin may be dry, coarse, yellow, and cool to the touch because of peripheral vasoconstriction. Scalp hair thins, sometimes accompanied by thinning of the lateral eyebrows as well. The nails may become brittle. In autoimmune thyroiditis, the gland can be diffusely enlarged, normal in size, or atrophic and difficult to detect on palpation. The gland may be soft and smooth or firm and irregular, and its texture can be lobular or nodular. Diffuse nonpitting edema of the extremities can be a result of the deposition of glycosaminoglycans. The terminal relaxation phase of the deep tendon reflexes can be markedly delayed. Speech and mentation can be impaired in severe hypothyroidism.

Other Routine Test Abnormalities
Typical laboratory abnormalities can include macrocytic anemia (Chapter 155), hyponatremia (Chapter 108), hypoglycemia (Chapter 217), and elevated blood levels of creatine phosphokinase, total and LDL cholesterol, triglyceride,

---

TABLE 213-3 ETIOLOGIES OF HYPOTHYROIDISM

PRIMARY HYPOTHYROIDISM

Insufficient functioning thyroid tissue
  Congenital absence of thyroid tissue
  Autoimmune destruction of thyroid tissue (Hashimoto thyroiditis)
  Surgical removal of thyroid tissue
  Radioablation of thyroid tissue by radioactive iodine or external beam radiation
  Infiltrative destruction of thyroid tissue
    Hemochromatosis
    Scleroderma
    Amyloidosis
Impaired thyroid hormone synthesis
  Iodine deficiency
  Congenital enzymatic defects that disrupt thyroid hormone synthesis
  Drug-mediated inhibition of thyroid hormone production and release
    Thionamides
    Amiodarone
    Lithium
    Bexarotene
    Certain tyrosine kinase inhibitors (e.g., sunitinib)
Altered metabolism of thyroid hormone
  Consumptive hypothyroidism
  Drugs altering thyroid hormone metabolism

SECONDARY HYPOTHYROIDISM

Insufficient secretion of TRH or TSH
  Hypothalamic disorders
    Tumor (lymphoma, germinoma, glioma)
    Irradiation
    Inflammation (sarcoidosis, vasculitis)
  Hypopituitarism
    Mass lesions
    Pituitary surgery
    Pituitary radiation
    Hemorrhagic apoplexy (Sheehan syndrome)
    Infiltration (hemochromatosis, tuberculosis, fungal infection)
    Lymphocytic hypophysitis
Thyroid hormone resistance syndrome

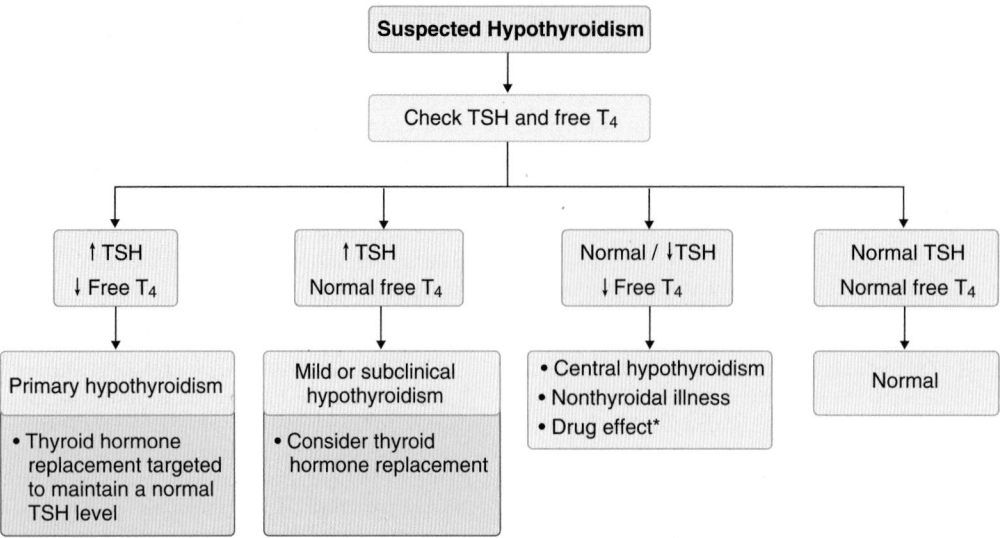

FIGURE 213-2. Laboratory assessment of suspected hypothyroidism. *e.g., suppression of TSH by dopamine, lowering of free T_4 due to increased metabolism by antiseizure medications. TSH = thyroid-stimulating hormone.

homocysteine, and prolactin.[8] On electrocardiography, typical findings are sinus bradycardia and low voltage in the limb leads. Chest radiography may show a widened cardiac silhouette, which echocardiography may confirm as a pericardial effusion.

DIAGNOSIS

Suspected primary hypothyroidism is confirmed by an elevated TSH level (Fig. 213-2). Established reference ranges for TSH levels typically extend from 0.5 to 4.5 mU/L. However, the distribution of values within this range is skewed toward the lower half, such that the mean TSH level in adults is 1.5 mU/L. Measurement of the free T_4 level confirms the diagnosis of primary hypothyroidism and characterizes its severity. A low free T_4 level in conjunction with a persistently elevated TSH level represents overt primary hypothyroidism, whereas a low-normal free T_4 level with an elevated TSH level is termed *mild* or *subclinical primary hypothyroidism*. Other uncommon causes of isolated TSH elevation should be considered in appropriate settings, including recovery from severe systemic illness, renal failure, and adrenal insufficiency. The underlying cause of primary hypothyroidism is usually clinically obvious, and laboratory testing is unnecessary in most cases. When confirmation is helpful (e.g., to enhance patient understanding of the etiology of their condition, or in a female contemplating pregnancy), serum antithyroid antibodies may be assessed. Measurement of thyroid peroxidase antibody is a more sensitive test than thyroglobulin antibody for this purpose. However, 10% of patients with histologically documented autoimmune thyroiditis have no circulating antithyroid antibodies.

If a sellar mass, prior pituitary surgery, or irradiation suggests possible secondary hypothyroidism, the TSH level cannot be relied on to provide an accurate index of thyroid function. However, a low or even low-normal free T_4 level confirms the diagnosis.

TREATMENT   Rx

Levothyroxine sodium (thyroxine T_4) is the preferred replacement hormone and should be dosed to restore normal TSH and thyroid hormone levels. Thyroxine is well absorbed, with a 7-day half-life that permits daily dosing. Although T_3 is the active thyroid hormone at the thyroid hormone receptor, T_4 (which is converted to T_3 by deiodinases present in peripheral tissues) provides steady circulating levels of T_3. By comparison, T_3 is more difficult to use therapeutically because its 1-day half-life is associated with fluctuating T_3 levels.

However, even thyroxine has a relatively narrow therapeutic index, and it requires careful titration in order to avoid iatrogenic thyrotoxicosis. The bioavailability of different preparations may vary by as much as 12%, perhaps because various inert ingredients affect the absorption of the preparation. Consequently, an individual patient should take a single, consistently identifiable thyroxine formulation (i.e., the same generic or brand name formulation).

The optimal thyroxine dose is approximately 1.6 to 1.8 µg/kg, but it is often lower in elderly adults (e.g., 1 µg/kg/day), possibly because of their slower metabolic clearance of the drug. The required dose is often higher in patients

TABLE 213-4   INTERFERENCE WITH THYROXINE REPLACEMENT THERAPY

FACTORS CONTRIBUTING TO UNDERREPLACEMENT

Inadequate prescribed dose
Limited compliance
Decreased absorption due to ingestion of agents that bind thyroxine
    Ferrous sulfate
    Calcium carbonate
    Aluminum hydroxide
    Sucralfate
    Cholestyramine
    Soy protein
Increased metabolism of thyroxine
    Pregnancy
    Drugs
        Phenytoin
        Phenobarbital
        Carbamazepine
        Rifampin
Diminishing residual thyroid function
Changing formulations

FACTORS CONTRIBUTING TO OVERREPLACEMENT

Excessive prescribed dose
Factitious ingestion of additional doses
Decreased metabolism of thyroxine due to aging
Increasing residual thyroid function
Changing formulations

with no residual thyroid function (e.g., postsurgical or postablative hypothyroidism) than in patients with autoimmune thyroiditis, in which the gland may retain some residual function. Malabsorption can interfere with intestinal absorption of thyroxine, as can soy-containing foods and some medications (e.g., oral iron tablets, calcium carbonate, aluminum hydroxide, sucralfate, cholestyramine) (Table 213-4). As a result, thyroxine should be given 4 or more hours before or after such medications.

Thyroxine requirements may increase by as much as 75% in many pregnant women because of the increased production of thyroxine-binding globulin caused by high estrogen levels, their increased clearance of thyroid hormone by placental deiodinase activity, and their increased plasma volume.[9] Patients who have the nephrotic syndrome (Chapter 113) or systemic illnesses, as well as patients being treated with some medications (e.g., phenytoin, carbamazepine, phenobarbital, or rifampin) may require higher daily doses.

Most adults *without* known or suspected heart disease can be started immediately on a full replacement dose, with the TSH level measured 4 to 6 weeks later. The target TSH level typically is the lower half of the normal range (i.e., 0.5 to 2.0 mU/L). Once the dose is appropriate, the TSH level should be checked annually unless substantial weight changes, new potentially interfering medications, symptoms of hyperthyroidism or hypothyroidism, or pregnancy indicate a need for more frequent monitoring. In secondary hypothyroidism, the serum free T_4 level should be checked 2 to 4 weeks after thyroxine is started or adjusted, targeted to a free T_4 level in the upper half of the reference range.

Avoidance of Adverse Effects

Complications of thyroxine therapy are limited to iatrogenic thyrotoxicosis and, rarely, adverse effects of restoring euthyroidism. Typical symptoms and signs of thyrotoxicosis usually accompany significant degrees of overtreatment. However, even a modestly excessive thyroxine dose can induce bone mineral loss, especially in postmenopausal women, and it can increase the risk of atrial fibrillation in older individuals. In patients with underlying coronary artery disease, the positive chronotropic and inotropic effects of thyroxine may exacerbate myocardial ischemia. Consequently, adults with known or suspected ischemic heart disease should be started on a low dose that is titrated upward in small increments once tolerance is ensured (e.g., starting with 25 µg daily, then increasing the dose by 12.5 to 25 µg every 4 to 6 weeks). In some cases, β-blocker therapy may need to be intensified to counter the induction of myocardial ischemia. However, deliberate suboptimal dosing of thyroxine should be avoided. If necessary, coronary revascularization may be required before euthyroidism can be fully restored.[10] Adrenal insufficiency, associated with hypopituitarism or the type 2 polyglandular autoimmune syndrome, may be unmasked when the cortisol clearance is accelerated and cortisol requirement is increased by a return to the euthyroid state. Even a modestly excessive dose of thyroxine can cause loss of bone mineralization, especially in postmenopausal women. Other infrequent adverse effects include transient hair loss and sympathomimetic symptoms.

Approximately 15% of hypothyroid patients continue to report bothersome symptoms despite biochemical evidence of adequate thyroid hormone replacement. Multiple randomized clinical trials have disproven the hypothesis that thyroxine/liothyronine combinations are superior to thyroxine replacement alone. Even combination therapy using desiccated thyroid does not improve performance or cognitive measures, although a patient may prefer desiccated thyroid, in part because it can modestly augment weight loss.[A1]

Subclinical and Mild Hypothyroidism

Individuals with subclinical hypothyroidism (i.e., a free T_4 level within the normal range but an elevated TSH) may benefit from thyroxine therapy if their TSH values are higher than 10 mU/L, are unlikely to benefit if their TSH values are higher than 7 mU/L, but are much less likely to benefit if their TSH values are between 4.5 and 7 mU/L.[11] For example, a randomized trial of thyroxine administration for patients over 65 years of age with a mean TSH value of 6.4 mU/L showed no improvement in hypothyroid symptoms, and thyroid hormone therapy does not improve general quality of life or thyroid-related symptoms in patients with subclinical hypothyroidism.[A2][A3] Another randomized trial found that treatment of subclinical hypothyroidism in pregnant women between 8 and 20 weeks of gestation did not result in significantly better cognitive outcomes in their children through 5 years of age.[A4] In practice, many physicians may try thyroxine therapy in mildly hypothyroid, symptomatic, young or middle-aged patients who have underlying hypercholesterolemia, or have a high likelihood of progressing to overt hypothyroidism. Predictors of progressive thyroid failure include age older than 65 years, TSH level higher than 10 mU/L, and the presence of circulating thyroid autoantibodies, indicating underlying autoimmune thyroiditis.

Myxedema Coma

Myxedema coma is a rare, life-threatening manifestation of severe hypothyroidism. It is characterized by hypotension, bradycardia, hypothermia, altered mental status, and multisystem organ failure. Risk factors for myxedema can include advanced age, poor access to health care, cold weather, and severe underlying diseases. Most patients have long-standing and severe thyroid hormone deficiency, but exposure to iodine-containing contrast agents or other iodine sources can precipitate a severe decline in thyroid hormone release. Treatment is by parenteral thyroxine (1.8 µg/kg/day after a 200- to 400-µg loading dose), but some experts advocate coadministration of liothyronine (5- to 20-µg loading dose followed by 2.5 to 10 µg every 8 hours) to compensate for temporarily impaired peripheral conversion of T_4 to T_3. Intravenous dosing is often recommended because of potential coexisting gastrointestinal dysfunction, but myxedema coma is successfully treated by thyroxine given via a feeding tube in countries where intravenous preparations are not available. Stress doses of glucocorticoids (Chapter 214) are recommended until the result of a cosyntropin stimulation test, performed before treatment to check for concomitant adrenal insufficiency, is available (Chapter 214). Hypothermia should be treated with passive external warming to reduce the risk that peripheral vasodilation will lead to circulatory collapse. Sedative or analgesic agents should be avoided. Older age, need for mechanical ventilation, vasopressors, and unfavorable scores on the Glasgow Coma Scale are associated with higher mortality rates, which can approach 30 to 50%.

Nonthyroidal Illness

Patients with a severe nonthyroidal illness may have thyroid function test results that suggest central hypothyroidism but are consistent with the so-called "sick euthyroid syndrome" (see Fig. 213-2).[12] The T_3 level usually declines and is accompanied by an increase in reverse T_3 (rT_3) concentrations. Reduced activity of type 1 deiodinase and increased activity of type 3 deiodinase are at least partially responsible for these changes. With increasingly severe disease, total T_4 and free T_4 levels progressively decline. TSH levels are usually low-normal or low. During recovery, TSH levels can rise above normal, thereby mimicking primary hypothyroidism. Clinical correlation (e.g., a history of preexisting thyroid or pituitary disease, the presence of a goiter, or features suggesting other elements of hypopituitarism) is essential to determine whether thyroid disease requiring treatment truly exists in severely ill patients. If not, the preferred approach is observation with retesting 6 to 8 weeks after recovery because thyroid hormone replacement is of no benefit for patients with nonthyroidal illness.

● THYROTOXICOSIS

DEFINITION AND EPIDEMIOLOGY

Thyrotoxicosis is a clinical syndrome resulting from tissue exposure to excessive circulating levels of thyroid hormones (Table 213-5).[13] Its prevalence is 1 in 2000 adults, and it affects 2% of women during their lifetime.

PATHOBIOLOGY

Thyrotoxicosis refers to any condition in which thyroid hormone levels are elevated, whether by actual thyroidal secretion or any other means (e.g., exogenous thyroid hormone ingestion). By comparison, hyperthyroidism is the term for thyrotoxicoses that are caused when the thyroid gland itself produces excessive thyroid hormone, either because of a thyrotropic stimulus or because of autonomous hormone secretion (see Table 213-5). Graves disease, which is the most common cause of hyperthyroidism, occurs when the TSH receptor is activated by autoantibodies that bind to it. Excessive TSH causes hyperthyroidism in patients with rare TSH-secreting pituitary adenomas (Chapter 211). Human chorionic gonadotropin (hCG), a glycoprotein with a high degree of TSH homology, can cause transient gestational hyperthyroidism during pregnancy if hCG levels are excessive, as occurs in hyperemesis gravidarum or choriocarcinoma. Alternatively, mutant TSH receptors may bind hCG more avidly, as occurs in a rare syndrome of familial gestational thyrotoxicosis.

Autonomous production of thyroid hormone occurs when thyrocytes function independently of TSH receptor activation. This phenomenon is seen with a benign functioning thyroid adenoma or growth of multiple autonomously functioning nodules in a toxic multinodular goiter. In rare cases, a well-differentiated thyroid cancer can have functioning metastases. In

TABLE 213-5 ETIOLOGIES OF THYROTOXICOSIS

HYPERTHYROIDISM

Antibody-mediated stimulation of thyroid tissue
   Graves disease
Autonomously functioning thyroid tissue
   Toxic multinodular goiter
   Toxic adenoma
   Iodine exposure (in a patient with thyroid nodules)
Autonomously functioning heterotopic thyroid tissue
   Struma ovarii
   Metastatic differentiated thyroid cancer
Excessive secretion of TSH
   TSH-secreting pituitary adenoma

NONHYPERTHYROID THYROTOXICOSIS

Ingestion of exogenous thyroid hormone
   Pharmacologic
      Levothyroxine
      Liothyronine
      Combination preparations
   Nonpharmacologic
      Dietary supplements
      Improperly processed meat products
Inflammation causing release of endogenous thyroid hormone
   Subacute (De Quervain) thyroiditis
   Silent or painless thyroiditis
   Amiodarone-induced thyroiditis

TSH = thyroid-stimulating hormone.

some toxic adenomas, gain of function somatic mutations in the TSH receptor gene and, less commonly, activating mutations in the Gs alpha gene, lead to constitutive activation. In patients whose thyroid glands have the potential for autonomous function, exposure to excessive amounts of iodine in the form of amiodarone or iodinated contrast agents can provoke hyperthyroidism (the so-called "Jod-Basedow phenomenon").

Various forms of transient thyroiditis are the most common cause of thyrotoxicosis without true hyperthyroidism. In these conditions, thyroid inflammation causes the release of an excessive amount of stored thyroid hormone (see section on Thyroiditis below). Examples include subacute thyroiditis (which may be triggered by a viral infection), acute or suppurative thyroiditis (caused by bacterial or fungal infection), radiation-induced thyroiditis, and pharmacologic thyroiditis (as can be caused by amiodarone). Thyroiditis typically occurs after delivery, when it is called "postpartum thyroiditis"; when it occurs in men or nonpostpartum women, it is called silent or painless thyroiditis. Excess thyroid hormone also rarely can be secreted by ectopic thyroid tissue, which can be located anywhere from the mediastinum to the base of the tongue, or by heterotopic thyroid tissue in an ovarian teratoma (a condition known as struma ovarii).

Thyrotoxicosis can also be caused by ingestion of excessive amounts of thyroid hormone. This is most often the result of the prescription of excessive doses of pharmacologic preparations of thyroid hormone, but it can rarely be due to surreptitious or accidental ingestion. An example of the latter is inclusion of thyroid hormones in over-the-counter supplements.

CLINICAL MANIFESTATIONS

Symptoms and Signs

The classic symptoms of thyrotoxicosis include anxiety, irritability, insomnia, weakness, weight loss despite hyperphagia, heat intolerance, tremor, palpitations, and increased frequency of formed bowel movements. Some patients develop chest pain, dyspnea on exertion, and even periodic paralysis (Chapter 393).

Signs of thyrotoxicosis include resting tachycardia, systolic hypertension with a widened pulse pressure, warm moist skin with a velvety texture, onycholysis (separation of the nails from the nailbed), and a staring gaze with lid lag (sclera is visible between the upper eyelid and the superior margin of the iris on downward gaze). A systolic flow murmur is often heard, and the apical impulse may be prominent and accompanied by brisk carotid upstrokes. Neurologic findings may include a restless, impatient demeanor, pressured speech, hand tremor, proximal muscle weakness, and brisk deep-tendon reflexes. Elderly patients may present with "apathetic thyrotoxicosis" typified by weight loss or atrial fibrillation in the absence of adrenergic symptoms and signs.

Several clinical findings are suggestive of a specific underlying cause. In Graves disease, the gland is diffusely enlarged, has a smooth or slightly lobulated contour, and may be associated with a palpable thrill or an audible bruit. Thyroid orbitopathy (ophthalmopathy) and dermopathy are also unique to Graves disease. With a toxic nodular goiter, one or more discrete nodules may be appreciated. By comparison, the gland is extremely tender, firm, and usually modestly enlarged in subacute thyroiditis. A history of recent pregnancy suggests possible painless thyroiditis. Exposure to amiodarone, other iodine-containing compounds, interferon-α, the tyrosine kinase inhibitor sorafenib, or pharmacologic preparations of thyroid hormone suggest thyrotoxicosis precipitated by these agents.

DIAGNOSIS

Laboratory Findings

Occasionally, patients have few symptoms or signs of thyrotoxicosis, and routine laboratory testing provides the first suggestion of thyrotoxicosis. Thyrotoxic patients may have hypercalcemia or hypercalciuria, increased alkaline phosphatase levels, modestly elevated aminotransferase levels, and low or declining levels of total and LDL cholesterol. When they are measured, sex hormone binding globulin, ferritin, and angiotensin-converting enzyme levels are often increased. Electrocardiography typically reveals resting sinus tachycardia or an atrial tachyarrhythmia, especially atrial fibrillation (Chapter 58) at a rapid ventricular rate. In severe thyrotoxicosis, the chest radiograph may show cardiomegaly and high-output heart failure.

The diagnosis is established by an elevated free T_4 level combined with a low TSH level (Fig. 213-3). However, patients with TSH-secreting pituitary tumors or isolated pituitary resistance to thyroid hormone will not have suppressed TSH levels. Free T_4 and T_3 levels define the severity of thyrotoxicosis and may suggest its underlying cause. If only one hormone (the free T_4 or T_3) is elevated, the terms T_4 toxicosis or T_3 toxicosis are used. If the TSH level is suppressed but both free T_4 and T_3 levels are normal, the patient has mild or subclinical thyrotoxicosis.

Specific Causes of Thyrotoxicosis
GRAVES DISEASE

Graves disease is an autoimmune form of hyperthyroidism, associated with ophthalmopathy in about 30% of patients, dermopathy (also called "pretibial myxedema" in 1 to 3% of patients), and acropachy (clubbing of the digits, in about 0.1% of patients).[14] Graves disease is 3- to 4-fold more common in women than men, and as many as 1 in 50 women will develop Graves disease during her lifetime. Graves disease can present at any age, but the onset is most commonly between ages 30 and 60 years.

PATHOBIOLOGY

Graves hyperthyroidism results from production of thyroid-stimulating immunoglobulins that bind to the TSH receptor and activate it, thereby promoting growth of the thyroid gland as well as the synthesis and secretion of thyroid hormone. Stimulating TSH-receptor antibodies are present in over 95% of patients, whereas antithyroid peroxidase antibodies and antithyroglobulin antibodies are found in about 50% of patients. Although the underlying cause is unknown, the higher incidence in monozygotic twins and first-degree relatives indicates a genetic predisposition. Factors potentially implicated in triggering Graves disease include female sex, cigarette smoking, a high dietary intake of

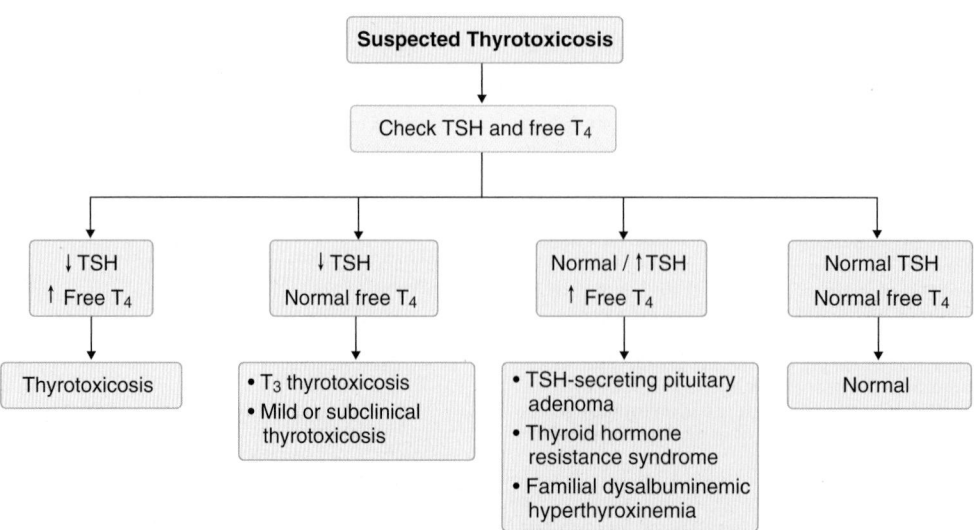

FIGURE 213-3. Laboratory assessment of suspected thyrotoxicosis. TSH = thyroid-stimulating hormone.

iodine, stressful life events, and infection, especially with *Yersinia enterocolitica* (Chapter 296).

CLINICAL MANIFESTATIONS

In addition to thyrotoxicosis, patients typically have a diffusely enlarged, smooth, rubbery gland; a definable pyramidal lobe; and palpable thrill or audible bruit. Thyroid eye disease usually develops within 6 months before or after the diagnosis of hyperthyroidism, but it can develop long before or after the initial presentation. Rare patients may have typical findings of thyroid eye disease without biochemical hyperthyroidism ("euthyroid Graves disease").

Graves Orbitopathy

Graves eye disease is characterized by proptosis (also called exophthalmos; Chapter 395) with inflammation and swelling of orbital fat and extraocular muscles, retraction, periorbital edema, conjunctival swelling, and episcleral vascular injection.[15] Ophthalmopathy is more common when Graves disease has been of longer duration and in patients who smoke. Affected individuals typically note a change in the appearance of their eyes, ocular dryness and irritation, the sensation of a foreign body, and ironically, excessive tearing. More severe disease can cause exposure keratitis with corneal ulceration, diplopia, and blurred vision. On physical examination, patients may have a staring gaze, a scleral rim visible between the upper eyelid and the superior margin of the iris during downward gaze (lid lag), conjunctival inflammation, periorbital edema, and abnormalities of color vision, visual acuity, and even conjugate gaze (Fig. 213-4). Patients can develop diplopia, and, uncommonly, optic nerve compression that may threaten sight and is an ophthalmologic emergency.

The precise degree of proptosis can be measured with an exophthalmometer. Clinical tools such as the "clinical activity score" have been developed to enumerate and quantify the extent and activity of the disease. Orbital CT scanning, MRI, or ultrasonography can confirm the diagnosis and distinguish it from other causes of bilateral and unilateral proptosis, including orbital myositis and tumors, respectively.

Graves Dermopathy and Acropachy

Infiltrative dermopathy or pretibial myxedema, which is typically nonpitting, is an uncommon physical finding caused by the dermal deposition of glycosaminoglycans and associated fibroblast proliferation. Affected individuals, who almost always have concomitant ophthalmopathy, present with a mildly pruritic, orange peel–like thickening that is most prominent along the anterior surfaces of the shins and other areas of repetitive trauma and increased intradermal pressure, including the dorsal aspects of the feet and fingers and

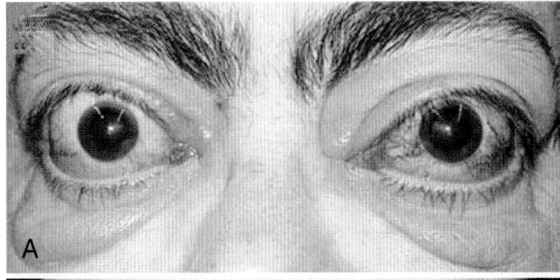
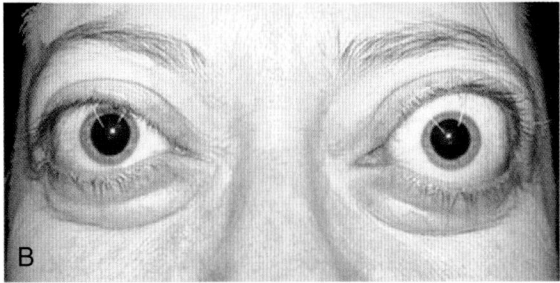

FIGURE 213-4. Graves ophthalmopathy. **A,** A 59-year-old woman with excess proptosis, moderate eyelid edema, and erythema with moderate eyelid retraction affecting all four eyelids. Conjunctival chemosis (edema) and erythema with bilateral edema of the caruncles, with prolapse of the right caruncle, are evident. **B,** A 40-year-old woman with excess proptosis, minimal bilateral injection, and chemosis with slight erythema of the eyelids. On slit lamp examination, she also had evidence of moderate superior limbic keratoconjunctivitis. (From Bahn RS. Graves' ophthalmopathy. *N Engl J Med.* 2010;362:726-738. Copyright 2010, Massachusetts Medical Society. All rights reserved.)

the extensor surface of the elbows. The diagnosis can be confirmed by skin biopsy. Clinically, thyroid acropachy appears similar to the digital clubbing seen in cardiopulmonary disease.

PROGNOSIS

Untreated Graves disease is persistent and progressive, but up to 25% of patients have spontaneous remissions. The likelihood of remission appears to be linked to a decline in the titer of the inciting TSH receptor antibodies.

TOXIC ADENOMA

A toxic adenoma is an almost always benign thyroid neoplasm that autonomously synthesizes and secretes excessive thyroid hormone independent of TSH stimulation. Most adenomas are palpable by the time they produce overt thyrotoxicosis. Some are caused by somatic gene mutations that constitutively activate the TSH receptor. If untreated, the hyperthyroidism persists, except in rare cases of spontaneous hemorrhagic infarction.

TOXIC MULTINODULAR GOITER

A toxic multinodular goiter comprises multiple nodules that autonomously synthesize and secrete excessive thyroid hormone. A goiter typically is felt with multiple palpable thyroid nodules, but the size of the goiter can be difficult to assess because of substernal extension. Toxic multinodular goiters become more common with advanced age. In some euthyroid patients with preexisting multinodular goiters, iodine-containing radiographic contrast material can induce previously quiescent nodules to hyperfunction and cause thyrotoxicosis.

TSH-SECRETING PITUITARY ADENOMA

TSH-secreting pituitary adenomas represent less than 1% of all functioning pituitary tumors (Chapter 211). Patients have the typical clinical manifestations of thyrotoxicosis, but they also usually have symptoms and signs of excess secretion of other anterior pituitary hormones (growth hormone, prolactin, or adrenocorticotropic hormone) or of panhypopituitarism. The key to suspecting the condition is usually recognition of an inappropriately nonsuppressed TSH level in a patient with thyrotoxicosis. The diagnosis can be confirmed by an elevated level of the pituitary glycoprotein α-subunit associated with a sellar mass on pituitary imaging.

DIFFERENTIAL DIAGNOSIS OF THYROTOXICOSIS

The specific cause of thyrotoxicosis guides its treatment.[16] The normal ratio of serum T_3 to free T_4 is elevated in Graves disease and toxic nodular goiter, because of increased relative thyroidal secretion of T_3. In contrast, the T_3 to free T_4 ratio is lower than normal in various forms of thyroiditis, because circulating hormone levels reflect release of thyroid hormonal stores, which contain a higher proportion of T_4 than T_3. Iodine-induced hyperthyroidism is also associated with a lower T_3 to free T_4 ratio.

TSH receptor antibodies are pathognomonic of Graves disease, and their presence excludes other etiologies. Measurement of these antibodies is not necessary in patients with obvious stigmata of Graves disease (i.e., orbitopathy, dermopathy) but can be very helpful when the diagnosis is not clinically apparent.

Thyroid ultrasonography can detect solitary or multiple thyroid nodules. On Doppler imaging, thyroidal blood flow is increased in Graves disease and is normal in thyroiditis. On scintigraphic scanning, uptake of the radiotracer and its distribution can establish a definitive diagnosis (Table 213-6). Chest radiography and CT scanning may help delineate a substernal goiter.

TREATMENT   Rx

Selection of the most effective treatment for thyrotoxicosis requires an understanding of the underlying pathophysiologic process and natural history.[17] For example, toxic multinodular goiter does not remit and usually requires definitive radioiodine treatment or surgery; silent and subacute thyroiditis subsides spontaneously and requires only temporizing symptomatic therapy (see below). For Graves disease, symptomatic therapy provides temporary amelioration while patients undergo primary treatment with antithyroid drugs, radioactive iodine, or surgical total thyroidectomy (Table 213-7).

Symptomatic Therapy: β-Blockers

β-Blockers, which help alleviate the sympathomimetic manifestations of thyrotoxicosis regardless of the underlying cause, often can promptly control tremor, anxiety, and palpitations. However, other clinical features of thyrotoxicosis

TABLE 213-6   RADIOGRAPHIC EVALUATION OF SUSPECTED THYROTOXICOSIS

ETIOLOGY	FRACTIONAL 24-HOUR RADIOIODINE UPTAKE (%)	THYROID SCAN APPEARANCE
Graves disease	35-95	Diffuse increased homogeneous uptake; visible pyramidal lobe extending from isthmus
Toxic adenoma	20-60	Solitary focus of intense uptake; suppression of uptake in remainder of thyroid
Toxic multinodular goiter	20-60	Patchy heterogeneous foci of increased uptake interspersed with regions of diminished uptake
Subacute thyroiditis	0-2	Minimal to absent uptake
Autoimmune thyroiditis	0-2	Minimal to absent uptake; patchy heterogeneous uptake during recovery
Iodine-induced hyperthyroidism	0-2	Minimal to absent uptake
Exogenous thyroid hormone intoxication	0-2	Minimal to absent uptake
Metastatic differentiated thyroid cancer	0-5	Focal uptake in metastases
TSH-secreting pituitary adenoma	30-80	Diffuse increased homogeneous uptake

TSH = thyroid-stimulating hormone.

TABLE 213-7   TREATMENT OF GRAVES DISEASE

TREATMENT	OUTCOME
Antithyroid drugs: methimazole, carbimazole, propylthiouracil	About 50% remission rate; hypothyroidism unusual
Radioactive iodine (^{131}I)	About 75% cure rate (euthyroid or hypothyroid) after one dose; up to 80% risk of hypothyroidism at 1 year
Surgical total thyroidectomy	Definitive cure and universal hypothyroidism, except in very rare cases of ectopic thyroid tissue

(including fatigue, weight loss, and heat intolerance) do not respond to β-blockers. In thyrotoxic patients with marked sinus tachycardia or atrial fibrillation with a rapid ventricular response rate, β-blockers can be used as rate-controlling agents. Propranolol in high doses also partially inhibits the extrathyroidal conversion of T_4 to T_3, so it may particularly benefit patients with severe thyrotoxicosis.

Propranolol can be started as 20 to 40 mg every 8 hours and then titrated to a maximal daily dose of 240 mg as needed to control symptoms. Sustained-release propranolol or longer-acting β-blockers, such as metoprolol and atenolol, can also be used. β-Blockers must be used cautiously in patients with asthma (Chapter 81), chronic obstructive pulmonary disease (Chapter 82), Raynaud phenomenon (Chapter 72), or heart failure (Chapter 53). Esmolol is a short-acting parenteral option if heart rate control is urgent in patients with thyrotoxic heart failure. Calcium channel blockers such as diltiazem can be used to control the heart rate in patients in whom β-blockers are contraindicated.

For transient thyrotoxicosis (subacute thyroiditis, silent thyroiditis, or exogenous thyroid hormone intoxication), a β-blocker may be the only required treatment. In Graves disease and toxic nodular goiter, however, the prompt initial relief provided by β-blockers should be considered a temporary measure until definitive treatment (e.g., antithyroid drugs, radioiodine therapy, or curative surgery) reduces thyroid hormone levels.

Antithyroid Drugs

Methimazole, carbimazole, and propylthiouracil inhibit thyroid hormone biosynthesis by competitively inhibiting iodine organification and iodotyrosine coupling. Propylthiouracil, but not methimazole or carbimazole, inhibits the conversion of T_4 to T_3 in peripheral tissues. These agents are used for the treatment of thyrotoxicosis caused by overproduction of thyroid hormones. Because the thionamides block only new thyroid hormone synthesis, glandular stores of preexisting thyroid hormone must be exhausted before they are fully effective. This may require 3 to 8 weeks in patients with Graves disease or toxic multinodular goiter. Although antithyroid drugs can provide long-term control of hyperthyroidism, they are most appropriately used when there is a possibility that the underlying condition will remit, as in Graves disease, or when thyrotoxicosis must be attenuated before radioiodine treatment or surgery.

Methimazole is the most widely used antithyroid agent. For mild to moderate hyperthyroidism, methimazole is usually started as 5 to 10 mg daily if the free T_4 level is 1 to 1.5 times the upper limit of normal; 10 to 20 mg daily if the free T_4 level is 1.5 to 2 times the upper limit of normal; and 30 to 40 mg daily if the free T_4 level is 2 to 3 times the upper limit of normal. It can be increased to 120 mg daily if needed. Propylthiouracil, which is a second line agent because of its hepatotoxicity, may be used in the first trimester in pregnant women with Graves disease, in thyroid storm because of its ability to block the conversion of T_4 to T_3, or when methimazole is not tolerated.

Chronic medical therapy is generally reserved for patients who are most likely to achieve a remission (defined as maintenance of a euthyroid state for 1 year off methimazole): those with mild biochemical hyperthyroidism, a small thyroid gland, low levels of TSH receptor antibodies, and no active ophthalmopathy.

In patients who are taking antithyroid drugs, thyroid function should be monitored every 3 to 12 weeks while the dose is being titrated. Minor side effects (fever, rash, pruritus, and arthralgias) are common. Agranulocytosis (Chapter 158) develops in approximately 0.2% of patients, typically within the first 90 days. Drug-induced hepatoxicity (1/1000 to 1/10,000 patients) can require liver transplantation. Because these severe adverse reactions are unpredictable and relatively sudden in onset, monitoring of blood counts and liver function usually is not recommended. However, patients should be advised, preferably in writing, to seek medical attention should they experience a high fever, pharyngitis, jaundice, or abdominal pain.

Radioactive Iodine

After oral administration, radioactive iodine (^{131}I) is concentrated in the thyroid gland, where its destruction of thyroid tissue effectively can control thyrotoxicosis, usually within 1 to 2 months. Although the dose can be calculated based on the fractional uptake of radioiodine on imaging and on the size of the thyroid gland, a fixed dose achieves a similar cure rate of about 75%.

The most common adverse effect of radioiodine is a transient exacerbation of thyrotoxicosis, which can occur in the first few weeks after treatment as a result of radiation thyroiditis, and 1 to 3 months after treatment due to worsening Graves disease caused by an increase in TSH receptor antibody levels. Following radioiodine therapy, thyroid function should be assessed every 4 to 8 weeks. Some patients may have transient mild hypothyroidism followed by a return of hyperthyroidism. Postablative hypothyroidism develops in about 50% of patients in the first 6 to 12 months. Lifelong monitoring of thyroid function is required because patients who remain euthyroid or mildly hyperthyroid after the first year subsequently develop postablative hypothyroidism at a rate of approximately 3% per year. The risk of postablative hypothyroidism is much lower in patients with solitary autonomous nodules or toxic nodular goiter, because the paranodular normal tissue does not concentrate the radioiodine because TSH levels are suppressed. An FT$_4$ level below the normal range, accompanied by a persistently low TSH value, also signals the development of hypothyroidism, as recovery of thyrotrophs from prior hyperthyroidism can be delayed. Prompt treatment of hypothyroidism may limit worsening of Graves orbitopathy.

In Graves disease, radioiodine therapy can worsen preexisting thyroid eye disease, so radioiodine is contraindicated in patients who have active moderate to severe eye disease. In patients with milder eye involvement, glucocorticoid therapy (e.g., prednisone 40 mg/day) at the time of therapy and tapered over 2 to 3 months can prevent exacerbations.

Radioiodine-treated patients do not have an increased risk of thyroid cancer, other malignancies, infertility, spontaneous abortion, or children with birth defects. Nevertheless, women should avoid pregnancy until euthyroidism has been confirmed 3 to 6 months after treatment.

Other Drugs

Potassium iodide transiently inhibits the synthesis and release of thyroid hormone from the gland and is rarely used to accelerate recovery after radioactive iodine treatment, to prepare patients for thyroidectomy, and to augment other treatments used to control severe thyrotoxicosis (see later). It can also temporarily control hyperthyroidism if severe allergies preclude the use of other medications.

Surgery

In the United States total thyroidectomy is seldom recommended for hyperthyroid Graves disease, except when radioiodine therapy is contraindicated, when malignancy is suspected in a thyroid nodule, or when concomitant hyperparathyroidism also requires surgical intervention. It may be first-line therapy, however, if a woman with Graves disease wishes to become pregnant and avoid taking antithyroid drugs during pregnancy. Thyroidectomy is the treatment of choice for toxic multinodular goiters that cause cosmetic disfigurement or compressive symptoms. Prior to surgery, patients should be rendered euthyroid with methimazole.

Specific Treatment Scenarios

Treatment of Graves Ophthalmopathy and Dermopathy

Mild thyroid eye disease can be treated with moisturizing ointment or drops, glasses, and even taping the eyelids closed at bedtime. In more severe cases, high-dose systemic glucocorticoid therapy can sufficiently diminish orbital inflammation so that orbital irradiation, which was recommended in the past, does not have added benefit.[A5] Teprotumumab, a humanized monoclonal antibody that inhibits the insulin-like growth factor-I receptor, also reduces proptosis in active ophthalmopathy.[A6] Orbital decompression surgery may occasionally be required for persistent corneal complications, optic nerve compression, or cosmetic reasons. Infiltrative dermopathy may respond to topical glucocorticoids, but intradermal or systemic glucocorticoids, long-acting somatostatin analogues, and surgery have been tried for advanced disease.

Pregnancy

In pregnant patients, Graves disease is almost always the underlying cause of the hyperthyroidism.[18] The diagnosis requires a careful assessment of symptoms, especially heat intolerance, palpitations, and vomiting, which also occur during normal pregnancy. In pregnancy total T_4 levels are elevated because of increased thyroxine-binding globulin, and the TSH level can be suppressed in the first trimester because of hCG-mediated thyroid stimulation. If hyperthyroidism is confirmed, β-blockers should be used only transiently for severe symptoms. Propylthiouracil can cause congenital malformations but is the preferred medication for the first trimester because methimazole has been linked to more severe birth defects. However, methimazole is preferred after the first trimester because of its better side-effect profile. If Graves disease has been well controlled on low-dose methimazole, it can be discontinued with careful monitoring prior to conception with the goal of avoiding its use during pregnancy. Because Graves disease often remits in late pregnancy, the dose of the antithyroid drug often can be reduced. TSH receptor antibody levels can be used to estimate the likelihood that the baby will develop neonatal Graves disease.

Subclinical and Mild Hyperthyroidism

Patients who have mild or subclinical hyperthyroidism (i.e., a suppressed TSH level with normal free T_4 and T_3 levels) may have findings, particularly bone mineral loss (Chapter 230) or atrial fibrillation (Chapter 58), that can justify treatment. It is less clear, however, whether younger asymptomatic patients with modestly suppressed TSH levels (e.g., 0.1 to 0.5 mU/L) require anything more than periodic monitoring.[19]

Thyrotoxic Crisis

Thyrotoxic crisis (thyroid storm) is a rare but potentially life-threatening sequela of sustained and severe thyrotoxicosis.[20] The greatest risk is in patients who have inadequately treated Graves disease, in whom it can be precipitated by the discontinuation of medications, intercurrent illness, trauma, infection, surgery, childbirth, radiocontrast dye, or treatment with radioactive iodine. Clinical findings include fever, atrial tachyarrhythmias, heart failure, nausea, vomiting, diarrhea, and seizures. Agitation, psychosis, delirium, and even coma are seen. Prompt recognition and treatment in a monitored setting are crucial. Treatment should include acetaminophen, external cooling, β-blockers, thionamides, potassium iodide, and glucocorticoids, as well as rapid evaluation and aggressive management of any underlying medical problems. Addition of bile acid sequestrants can lower free T_4 levels faster than antithyroid drugs alone. Salicylates are contraindicated because they can increase serum levels of free T_4 and T_3 by displacing thyroid hormones from thyroid binding proteins. Plasmapheresis has also been used in critically ill patients not responding to traditional pharmacologic therapies.

● THYROIDITIS

Subacute (de Quervain) Thyroiditis

PATHOBIOLOGY

The uncontrolled release of thyroid hormone from an inflamed and damaged thyroid gland can cause transient thyrotoxicosis that resolves spontaneously 2 to 8 weeks later, when the supply of stored hormone has been released. Hypothyroidism then ensues for about one month, after which normal thyroid function returns in most patients.

CLINICAL MANIFESTATIONS

Patients usually have pain that is localized to the thyroid gland, but pain can radiate to the throat, ears, or jaw. Systemic symptoms, including fever, chills, sweats, and malaise, are common and, on occasion, can dominate the clinical picture. Patients typically have symptoms of transient thyrotoxicosis followed by transient hypothyroidism. Many patients report an antecedent upper respiratory infection. On examination, the thyroid gland typically is exquisitely tender, modestly enlarged, and woody or hard on palpation

DIAGNOSIS

Differential Diagnosis

The differential diagnosis includes acute (suppurative) thyroiditis, hemorrhage into an existing thyroid nodule, and rapid growth of anaplastic or infiltrating thyroid cancer or a thyroid lymphoma.

Laboratory Findings

Laboratory testing initially shows evidence of overt thyrotoxicosis, with T_4 levels proportionately higher than T_3 levels. The erythrocyte sedimentation rate is elevated during the acute phase. On scanning, the fractional radioiodine uptake typically is less than 2% at 24 hours (see Table 213-6).

TREATMENT

High-dose aspirin or nonsteroidal anti-inflammatory drugs (NSAIDs) can treat the thyroid pain and systemic inflammatory symptoms, with glucocorticoids reserved for unresponsive patients (and tapered over several weeks to prevent a relapse). Transient symptoms of thyrotoxicosis will respond after 1 to 3 weeks of β-blocker treatment. Subsequent symptomatic hypothyroidism may require short-term thyroxine, but long-term thyroid hormone replacement usually is not required.

Silent Thyroiditis

EPIDEMIOLOGY

Silent thyroiditis (also known as painless or lymphocytic thyroiditis) occurs more commonly in women than men, with a peak age of incidence at ages 30 to 40 years. It appears to be more prevalent in areas of high iodine uptake.

PATHOBIOLOGY

This painless inflammation of the thyroid gland is characterized by diffuse lymphocytic infiltration. Based on this finding and the presence of thyroid peroxidase antibodies in about 50% of patients, this condition is believed to be autoimmune. Silent thyroiditis typically follows the same triphasic course as subacute thyroiditis, with transient thyrotoxicosis followed by transient hypothyroidism and eventual return to euthyroidism. The thyrotoxic phase may be less frequently recognized than the hypothyroid phase. Hypothyroidism may occasionally persist. Each of these phases of thyroid dysfunction can have a variable duration of weeks to months.

CLINICAL MANIFESTATIONS AND DIAGNOSIS

The diagnosis of silent thyroiditis may be suspected when a patient presents with symptoms of hypothyroidism that were preceded by symptoms of hyperthyroidism. The thyroid gland is either normal in size or modestly enlarged and is not tender. The diagnosis of silent thyroiditis can be made by finding a suppressed TSH level during the thyrotoxic phase but an elevated TSH level during the hypothyroid phase. The fractional uptake of radioiodine is very low or absent during the thyrotoxic phase and then returns to normal as the gland recovers (see Table 213-6).

TREATMENT

Silent thyroiditis can often be managed with observation and reassurance. Symptoms of hyperthyroidism can be treated with a course of β-blockers, whereas overt hypothyroidism warrants short-term thyroxine replacement.

PROGNOSIS

Most patients with silent thyroiditis return to a euthyroid state, but 10 to 20% develop persistent hypothyroidism. Recurrences of silent thyroiditis may occur in 5 to 10% of patients.

Postpartum Thyroiditis

EPIDEMIOLOGY

Postpartum thyroiditis is defined as the development of thyroid dysfunction in a previously euthyroid woman within 12 months of pregnancy. It affects 8 to 11% of women within two to 12 months after delivery or miscarriage. Predisposing factors include a history of previous episodes of postpartum thyroiditis, type 1 diabetes mellitus, and circulating antithyroid autoantibodies.

PATHOBIOLOGY

Postpartum thyroiditis, which is an autoimmune condition characterized by lymphocytic infiltration of the thyroid gland, is likely a form of silent thyroiditis specifically related to pregnancy. The inflammation of the thyroid gland is painless but can cause transient thyrotoxicosis followed by transient or persistent hypothyroidism. However, the pattern of thyroid dysfunction can be quite variable, with some patients exhibiting the classic triphasic pattern and others exhibiting only hyperthyroidism or hypothyroidism.

CLINICAL MANIFESTATIONS AND DIAGNOSIS

The diagnosis of postpartum thyroiditis is often overlooked because its nonspecific thyrotoxic symptoms (e.g., weight loss, insomnia, anxiety) or hypothyroid symptoms (e.g., fatigue, depression) are attributed to the postpartum state. Most patients have a small painless goiter. The diagnosis can be confirmed or excluded by a suppressed TSH level during the thyrotoxic phase followed by an elevated TSH level during the hypothyroid phase. The median time of onset of the thyrotoxic and hypothyroid phases are about 13 and 19 weeks postpartum, respectively. Approximately 80% of patients have thyroid peroxidase antibodies, and this condition must be distinguished from postpartum Graves disease, which can occur at about the same time but is associated with TSH-stimulating antibodies. Fractional uptake of radioiodine is either absent or very low in the setting of postpartum thyroiditis, whereas it is increased in active Graves disease (see Table 213-6).

TREATMENT ℞

Postpartum thyroiditis can usually be managed with observation and reassurance. A course of β-blocker therapy can be used for symptomatic thyrotoxicosis. Overt hypothyroidism may require short-term thyroxine replacement. Monitoring of thyroid function after recovery is essential because thyroxine therapy may be required if a subsequent pregnancy is also affected by postpartum thyroiditis or if permanent hypothyroidism ensues.

PROGNOSIS

Although most patients recover from their hypothyroidism, long-term studies show that about 15 to 50% of patients with postpartum thyroiditis eventually develop permanent hypothyroidism. Furthermore, patients have a 70% risk of recurrent postpartum thyroiditis after a subsequent pregnancy.

Acute (Suppurative) Thyroiditis

Infection of the thyroid gland is a rare condition that typically presents with severe thyroid pain, fever, and other systemic manifestations of infection. The bacterial infection can be due to direct spread of bacteria from the skin or piriform sinus, or hematogenous spread (bacteria, mycobacteria, fungi, or parasites, especially *Pneumocystis carinii*) in immunocompromised individuals.

On physical examination, fever is associated with localized erythema and asymmetrical swelling of a tender, warm, and even fluctuant thyroid gland. Thyroid ultrasound may show an abscess, which can be aspirated to identify the pathogen. Prompt antibiotic therapy guided by the Gram stain and culture of the aspirate may need to be accompanied by surgical drainage of any abscesses.

Other Forms of Thyroiditis

Amiodarone can cause painless thyroiditis that may be associated with thyrotoxicosis or lead to iodine-induced thyrotoxicosis. The former should be treated with glucocorticoids, but the latter requires antithyroid drugs.[21] Interferon-α can cause a painless thyroiditis and transient thyrotoxicosis that must be differentiated from interferon-α–induced Graves disease; the former is treated with β-blockers, but the latter requires antithyroid drugs.

Riedel thyroiditis or struma is fibrotic replacement of thyroid tissue. The thyroid becomes substantially enlarged, hardened, and fixed. Adherence and infiltration of adjacent structures can cause local compressive symptoms. Some patients also have mediastinal and retroperitoneal fibrosis (Chapter 259), sclerosing cholangitis (Chapter 146), or orbital pseudotumor as part of the spectrum of IgG4-related diseases that are characterized by lymphoplasmocytic fibro-inflammation (Chapter 259). Diagnosis requires open biopsy. Glucocorticoids are first-line therapy, with tamoxifen and rituximab being second-line agents. Unfortunately, surgical removal is difficult or impossible.

● GOITER

DEFINITION

A goiter can be diffuse or nodular, nontoxic or toxic (i.e., associated with thyroid hormone overproduction), and benign or malignant.[22] It can be the result of the proliferation of thyrocytes stimulated by circulating TSH or thyroid-stimulating autoantibodies, infiltration by inflammatory or malignant cells, or a benign or malignant neoplasm.

EPIDEMIOLOGY

Worldwide, the most common cause of goiter is iodine deficiency. Such goiters are only encountered in the United States among immigrants from iodine-deficient regions. In younger patients, the goiter will shrink if adequate iodine supplementation is provided, whereas iodine supplementation in older individuals with multinodular iodine-deficient goiters will not decrease their size but may provoke thyrotoxicosis.

PATHOBIOLOGY

Mutations in the thyroglobulin, thyroid peroxidase, dual oxidase, and pendrin genes can cause benign multinodular goiters or adenomas. Drugs (e.g., lithium carbonate) that inhibit the synthesis of thyroid hormone can also lead to goiter, but the underlying cause usually is unknown in iodine-replete patients.

Autoimmune thyroiditis can cause a modest goiter because of glandular infiltration with lymphocytes, inflammation, and fibrosis. Hypothyroid autoimmune thyroiditis results in increased TSH levels, which further stimulate enlargement. In Graves disease, diffuse thyroid enlargement is stimulated by thyroid stimulating immunoglobulins. Other forms of thyroiditis and malignant neoplasms also can cause a goiter to develop.

CLINICAL MANIFESTATION AND DIAGNOSIS

Clinical Examination

True thyroid enlargement is confirmed by palpation, but a thyroid ultrasound may help resolve any uncertainty. A childhood history may provide a clue to iodine deficiency. Symptoms of hypothyroidism suggest autoimmune thyroiditis, whereas thyrotoxicosis suggests toxic multinodular goiter or Graves disease. Clinical findings may lead to recognition of one of the various forms of thyroiditis (e.g., pain in subacute thyroiditis or postpartum status in lymphocytic thyroiditis).

On physical examination, the gland should be measured and any evidence of tracheal deviation, cervical lymphadenopathy, or venous distention should be assessed. Diffuse enlargement is consistent with Graves disease, thyroiditis, or a diffusely infiltrating neoplasm. Nodularity suggests a benign multinodular goiter or a malignancy. Subtotal thoracic outlet obstruction may be diagnosed if signs of facial plethora and cervical venous distention are seen when the patient touches his or her hands together above the head (Pemberton maneuver).

Laboratory Findings

A TSH level determines whether there is primary hypothyroidism or thyrotoxicosis. Elevated antithyroid peroxidase antibody titers can confirm suspected autoimmune thyroiditis. Other blood tests (e.g., ESR for subacute thyroiditis or calcitonin for medullary thyroid cancer) may be useful if the clinical examination suggests specific diagnoses.

Imaging

Ultrasonography can accurately determine whether a goiter is diffuse or nodular, impinging on other cervical structures, or associated with lymphadenopathy. Ultrasonography is also essential to guide fine-needle aspiration for cytologic diagnosis. If the goiter extends posteriorly or beneath the sternal notch, CT or MRI may be required for evaluation. Iodine-containing radiocontrast dyes should be avoided because the iodide load may induce hyperthyroidism in patients with nodular goiters. Radionuclide ^{123}I scanning can determine the gland's functional status, the cause of the goiter, and whether any mediastinal mass is truly thyroid tissue. A barium swallow is indicated in patients with swallowing symptoms, and pulmonary function testing (Chapter 79) is indicated if tracheal compression is suspected. Laryngoscopy can evaluate vocal cord function if recurrent laryngeal nerve involvement is suspected.

TREATMENT Rx

If thyroid dysfunction and malignant disease can be excluded, asymptomatic goiters can be observed and monitored with periodic ultrasonography. The suppression of TSH levels with thyroxine therapy shrinks only a minority of goiters and carries the risks of symptomatic thyrotoxicosis, atrial fibrillation, and loss of bone mineralization.

Surgery is often preferred if the goiter causes compressive complications, especially when there is substernal extension of the goiter or an acute worsening of symptoms. If surgery is contraindicated, radioactive iodine therapy can reduce the goiter size by an average of 50% over 12 to 24 months.

THYROID NODULES

Thyroid nodules are detected by palpation in about 6% of women and 2% of men,[23,24] but high-resolution ultrasonography will find a thyroid nodule in up to 75% of all adults, especially women. Although the majority of these represent small, benign adenomatoid nodules or cysts, 5 to 10% of thyroid nodules are malignant. Less commonly, thyroid nodules are clinical problems by virtue of being hyperfunctioning or causing local compressive symptoms or cosmetic dissatisfaction.

DIAGNOSIS

Clinical Manifestations

An otherwise asymptomatic thyroid nodule may be noted by the patient or discovered on a physician's examination, but it also may be detected incidentally on carotid ultrasonography or a cervical spine CT or MRI.[24] Local symptoms of compression or invasion suggest a malignancy. Examples include lower anterior neck pain, cough or dyspnea (owing to tracheal compression), hemoptysis (owing to tracheal invasion), dysphonia (owing to encasement of the recurrent laryngeal nerve), and dysphagia or odynophagia (owing to esophageal compression). A toxic adenoma should be suspected if patients have evidence of thyrotoxicosis, whereas hypothyroid symptoms and signs suggest autoimmune thyroiditis. Symptoms and signs related to metastases of thyroid cancer include chest pain, dyspnea, bone pain, and neurologic findings. Rare thyroid nodules can represent metastatic spread from a primary kidney (Chapter 187), colon (Chapter 184), or breast cancer (Chapter 188).

A history of neck irradiation greatly increases the risk of papillary thyroid cancer. Medullary and papillary thyroid cancers have a strong familial predisposition. Medullary thyroid cancer should be considered if there is a personal or family history of diagnosed or possible multiple endocrine neoplasia type 2 (MEN 2) syndromes, including hyperparathyroidism and pheochromocytoma (Chapter 218). Other genetic syndromes associated with thyroid cancer include Cowden syndrome and familial adenomatous polyposis (Gardner syndrome; Chapter 184).

Physical Examination

The physical examination of a thyroid nodule should define its tenderness, size, consistency, surface texture, and mobility. A hard texture, fixation, ipsilateral adenopathy or vocal cord paresis suggests a malignancy. Multinodularity suggests a benign nodular goiter but is not sufficiently diagnostic to avoid further evaluation. Furthermore, a patient's risk of having thyroid cancer is only marginally lower with multiple nodules compared with a solitary nodule.

Laboratory Findings

A TSH level can identify hyperthyroidism or hypothyroidism. If the TSH level is low or undetectable, radionuclide thyroid scanning can diagnose a benign autonomous toxic adenoma or multiple functioning nodules (see Table 213-6). If the TSH level is elevated, antithyroid peroxidase antibody titers can diagnose autoimmune thyroiditis. If MEN 2 or familial medullary thyroid cancer is a consideration, a calcitonin level should be measured.

Imaging

Thyroid ultrasonography is critical to confirm that a mass is a thyroid nodule and then to define its size, whether it is cystic or solid, and whether more than one nodule is present.[25] Nodules that are more than 50% cystic or have a "spongiform" appearance are rarely malignant. Conversely, hypoechogenicity, microcalcifications, irregular nodule borders, a "taller than wide" orientation, and cervical adenopathy suggest the need for further evaluation with fine-needle aspiration (Fig. 213-5A).

Radionuclide scanning with radioiodine or technetium pertechnetate is helpful only if the TSH level is suppressed. In this situation, scanning can determine whether the nodule is hyperfunctioning, in which case biopsy usually can be avoided.

Invasive Evaluation
Fine-Needle Aspiration Biopsy

Ultrasound-guided fine-needle aspiration is the most accurate way to confirm or exclude malignancy when a nodule is accompanied by a normal TSH level (Fig. 213-5B). The size of the nodule is relevant but less important than its full sonographic features. Nodules less than 1 cm in diameter generally do not require biopsy (see Table 213-8).

An adequate biopsy specimen can be accurately categorized as benign, atypical, suspicious for a follicular neoplasm, suspicious for malignancy, or malignant (Table 213-9). A benign classification is highly accurate, with a false-negative rate of less than 3% in sonographically directed biopsy specimens. Furthermore, the biopsy diagnosis of malignancy typically has a 98% true-positive rate. If a biopsy is judged suspicious for malignancy, approximately 70% will be thyroid cancers when resected.

About 20% of biopsies yield adequate but diagnostically indeterminate cytologic material. Although most indeterminate nodules are benign,

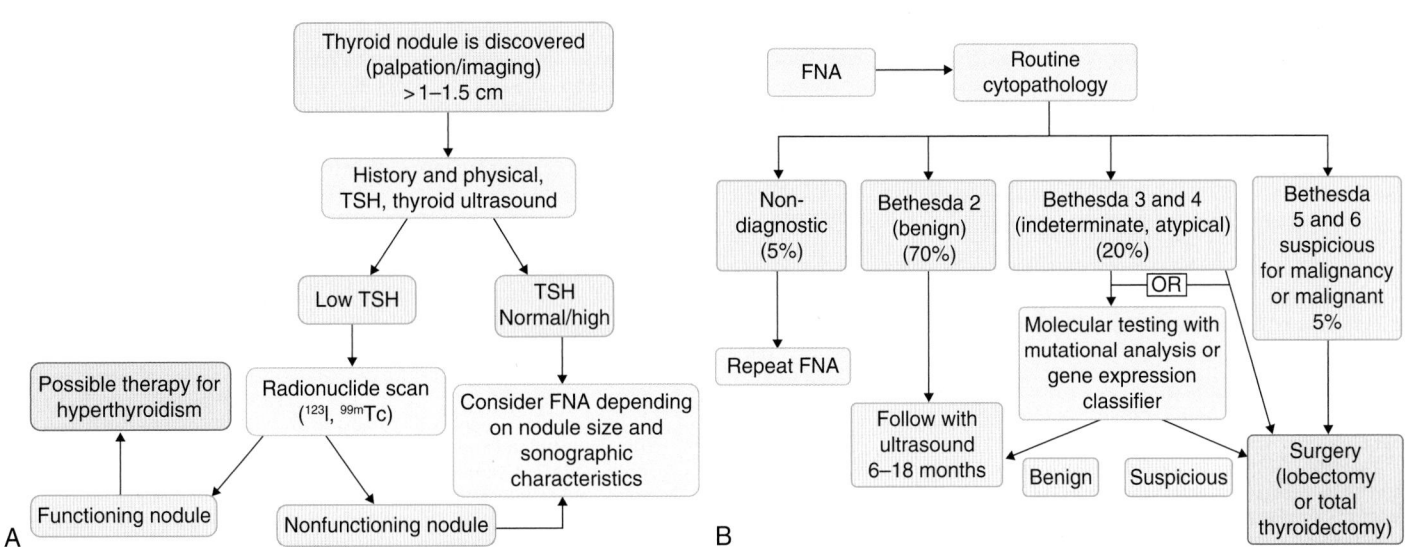

FIGURE 213-5. A, Initial evaluation of a thyroid nodule. TSH = thyroid-stimulating hormone; [123]I = radioactive iodine 123; [99m]Tc = technetium 99m. **B,** Algorithm for evaluation of a thyroid nodule with fine-needle aspiration (FNA). With indeterminate nodules (Bethesda Class 3 and 4), surgery, typically a diagnostic lobectomy, or molecular testing are both potential strategies.

TABLE 213-8 SIZE THRESHOLDS FOR THYROID NODULE FINE-NEEDLE ASPIRATION (FNA) BASED ON SONOGRAPHIC FEATURES

NODULE SONOGRAPHIC FEATURES	RECOMMENDED NODULE THRESHOLD SIZE FOR FNA
High suspicion: Hypoechoic AND microcalcifications, taller than wide configuration, irregular borders	≥1 cm
Intermediate suspicion: Hypoechoic without and other suspicious features	≥1 cm
Low suspicion: Iso- or hyperechoic without any suspicious features	≥1.5 cm
Very low suspicion: Spongiform or partially cystic with no suspicious features	>2 cm or consider not performing an FNA at all
Benign (pure cyst)	Not needed

Data from Haugen BR, Alexander EK, Bible KC, et al. 2015 American Thyroid Association Management Guidelines for Adult Patients with Thyroid Nodules and Differentiated Thyroid Cancer: The American Thyroid Association Guidelines Task Force on Thyroid Nodules and Differentiated Thyroid Cancer. *Thyroid*. 2016;26:1-133.

TABLE 213-9 BETHESDA SYSTEM FOR REPORTING CYTOPATHOLOGY

BETHESDA CLASS	CYTOLOGIC DIAGNOSIS	RISK OF MALIGNANCY*
2	Benign	0-3% (1-10%)
3	Atypia of undetermined significance	14% (6-48%)
4	Suspicious for a follicular neoplasm	25% (14-34%)
5	Suspicious for malignancy	70% (53-97%)
6	Malignant	99% (94-100%)

Diagnostic categories associated with risk of malignancy.
Adapted from Bongiovanni M, Spitale A, Faquin WC, et al. The Bethesda System for Reporting Thyroid Cytopathology: a meta-analysis. *Acta Cytol.* 2012;56:333-339.
*The risk of malignancy is lower than depicted for Class 3,4, and 5 now that the noninvasive encapsulated follicular variant of papillary thyroid cancer is considered to be "nonmalignant" (see text) (Strickland KC, Howitt BE, Marqusee E, et al. The impact of noninvasive follicular variant of papillary thyroid carcinoma on rates of malignancy for fine-needle aspiration diagnostic categories. *Thyroid.* 2015;25:987-92.

approximately 15 to 25% are thyroid carcinomas. Repeat sampling may allow a more specific diagnosis to be made.

For cytologically indeterminate nodules, about 75% of which are histo-pathologically benign,[26] molecular diagnostic testing is helpful.[27] For a typical cytologically indeterminate nodule with a thyroid cancer probability of 20 to 35%, the negative predictive value of oncogenic testing and gene expression profiling is 90 to 95%. For patients with no clinical features of malignancy, particularly middle-aged or older women with multinodular glands in whom the prevalence of malignancy is 5% or less, vigilant observation with serial sonography is an alternative to molecular testing.

TREATMENT AND PROGNOSIS   Rx

Most asymptomatic, sonographically or cytologically benign thyroid nodules do not grow in the subsequent 5 years, and thyroid cancer rarely develops. As a result, conservative observation with periodic sonographic reassessment can be recommended. Further enlargement during observation (i.e., >20% increase in two of three dimensions) should prompt a repeat biopsy. A cytologically benign nodule should be surgically resected only if it causes compressive symptoms or cosmetic disfigurement.

The definitive diagnosis of a suspicious nodule often requires surgical resection for pathological examination. Unilateral lobectomy, which results in fewer surgical complications and a lower risk of postoperative hypothyroidism compared with complete thyroidectomy is typically recommended for definitive diagnosis and treatment of the nodule. Total thyroidectomy is usually needed only when a higher-risk cancer is diagnosed.

● THYROID CANCER

Thyroid gland cancers range from incidental and inconsequential microcarcinomas to aggressive and virtually untreatable anaplastic tumors.[28,29] The U.S. Preventive Services Task Force recommends against screening for thyroid cancer.[30,31] Thyroid cancers usually present as asymptomatic thyroid nodules, although they may present with local symptoms, or with cervical adenopathy. They rarely present with metastatic signs or symptoms, such as a pulmonary mass or bone pain.

Papillary and Follicular (Epithelial or Differentiated) Thyroid Carcinomas

Papillary and follicular thyroid cancers, which arise from follicular epithelium, often retain the characteristics of normal thyrocytes, including responsiveness to TSH, production of thyroglobulin, and concentration of iodide. They are distinguished by their histopathologic appearances and characteristic patterns of progression. Hürthle cell carcinoma is composed of thyrocytes with abundant mitochondria-laden cytoplasm and behaves like a follicular thyroid cancer, although it typically does not have iodine-concentrating ability.

EPIDEMIOLOGY

Approximately 50,000-60,000 new cases of thyroid cancer are diagnosed each year in the United States. Thyroid cancer is three-fold more common in women than men (about 21 vs. 7 per 100,000 population), and the median age at diagnosis is 51 years. The incidence of thyroid cancer has increased in both women and men since 2004, although incidence rates now appear to be stabilizing, with about 52,000 new cases per year. Several factors, including diagnostic aggressiveness, may potentially account for this changing incidence of thyroid cancer (E-Table 213-1). Papillary microcarcinomas also are a common incidental pathologic finding, seen in 10% of thyroid glands excised for other reasons or examined at autopsy. Death rates from thyroid cancer (about 0.5 per 100,000 population) are similar in both sexes, but the percentage of thyroid cancer deaths increases with age and is highest in the 75- to 84-year age group.

PATHOBIOLOGY

Childhood irradiation to the thyroid gland and radioiodine exposure after nuclear incidents are risk factors for thyroid cancer. Gene mutations in *RET/PTC*, *RAS*, and *BRAF* activate the MAP kinase signaling pathway and are implicated in the pathogenesis and progression of papillary thyroid cancer.

CLINICAL MANIFESTATIONS

Papillary thyroid carcinoma, which is the most common form, accounts for 90% of cases. Most papillary thyroid carcinomas are slow growing and either confined to the thyroid gland or spread to local cervical lymph nodes. However, papillary thyroid carcinomas can be more aggressive, with extension into adjacent tissues, extensive nodal involvement, and distant metastatic spread, most commonly to the lungs. Aggressive tumors are more common in older patients and with specific gene mutations, such as combined *BRAF* and *TERT* mutations.

Follicular and Hürthle cell thyroid carcinomas represent 9% of thyroid cancer cases. The noninvasive encapsulated follicular variant of papillary thyroid cancer is now considered a nonmalignant lesion. If these tumors invade only the tumor capsule, they are *minimally invasive* and typically behave like papillary thyroid carcinomas. If, however, follicular and Hürthle cell carcinomas invade the vasculature, they are more likely to metastasize, commonly to the lungs and bones.

TREATMENT   Rx

Treatment of differentiated thyroid cancer entails surgery, selectively followed by radioiodine ablation of remnant thyroid tissue.[32] Total or near-total thyroidectomy with or without selective central compartment lymph node resection is often the appropriate initial surgical procedure. However, lobectomy may be considered for patients with tumors smaller than 4 cm confined to one lobe of the thyroid gland and without other negative prognostic indicators such as cervical node involvement or extrathyroidal extension. Thyroid surgery can be complicated by hypoparathyroidism or recurrent laryngeal nerve injury, which causes hoarseness if it is unilateral and airway obstruction if it is bilateral. Traditionally, the rationale for bilateral surgery is the frequent presence of bilateral disease in papillary thyroid cancer, and the lower risk of recurrence after bilateral gland removal in some but not all studies. In addition, there may be greater accuracy in detecting residual disease after the eradication of all remaining normal thyroid tissue. Recent guidelines have suggested that the selection of initial surgery (thyroidectomy versus lobectomy) can be considered on a case by case basis, considering the suspected extent of disease on the basis of thyroid ultrasonography and preoperative cervical node mapping, and the likelihood that radioactive iodine treatment may be pursued. Use of postoperative cervical ultrasonography and following the trend in thyroglobulin concentration provides sensitive tools for surveillance in those patients who have not had a total thyroidectomy or received radioiodine therapy.

Follow-Up

Once surgery has been performed, adjuvant therapy with radioiodine harnesses the properties that thyroid cancer cells share with normal thyroid tissue, namely the ability to accumulate iodine and responsiveness to TSH stimulation. Postoperatively, ^{131}I administration after TSH stimulation can be employed to ablate the small amount of normal thyroid tissue that usually remains after total thyroidectomy. Thyroglobulin is a more specific tumor marker with essentially a baseline of zero if all remaining normal thyroid tissue has been ablated. Remnant ablation, however, does not improve the mortality rate in low risk disease, which is close to zero, nor does it decrease recurrence rates in individuals with low risk thyroid cancers. Therefore, radioiodine therapy is not recommended for the vast majority of thyroid cancer patients with low risk disease. Although the patient may have detectable circulating thyroglobulin and residual thyroid tissue detectable upon ultrasonography, these measures can be followed for changes in their respective baselines. Similarly, for patients in whom lobectomy alone has been chosen, follow-up relies on assessment of thyroglobulin levels and ultrasound examination of the ipsilateral cervical nodes and the remaining thyroid tissue. Controlled but nonrandomized trials have shown that radioiodine treatment is associated with a lower rate of tumor recurrence in patients with advanced disease (stages 3 and 4) at presentation (see later). Studies of some cohorts also show improved survival. TSH stimulation of residual thyroid tissue, which is essential for effective radioiodine therapy, can be accomplished either by the temporary withdrawal of thyroid hormone therapy to promote endogenous TSH production or, more commonly, by the administration of recombinant human thyrotropin, which avoids the morbidity of hypothyroidism.

Thyroxine therapy is required for all patients who have had a total thyroidectomy. In addition to providing thyroid hormone replacement, thyroxine can be adjusted to suppress the patient's circulating TSH level to the low or low-normal range to reduce the likelihood of tumor recurrence. In determining the extent to which the TSH level should be suppressed, the patient's risk of cancer recurrence must be balanced against potential thyrotoxic complications such as bone mineral loss in postmenopausal women and atrial fibrillation in older patients. In patients who have had a lobectomy, thyroxine replacement may not be required, since many patients will have serum TSH levels that are in the appropriate range (0.5 to 2 mU/L).

Radioiodine imaging is helpful in the early postoperative phase in those patients in whom radioactive iodine therapy is being considered, since it may reveal metastatic disease in cervical nodes or in distant sites. Post-treatment radioiodine imaging is always performed to document areas of radioiodine avidity. Patients who received radioiodine therapy usually have at least one additional diagnostic radioiodine scan 6 to 12 months later to document that previous regions of radioiodine concentration have been ablated. Long-term monitoring of patients entails periodic clinical assessment, measurement of serum thyroglobulin levels, and use of cervical ultrasonography. Clinically, patients should be assessed for local neck symptoms or recurrent cervical masses, as well as for optimization of thyroid hormone therapy. For patients treated with radioactive iodine therapy, who have negative diagnostic scanning and stimulated thyroglobulin values at initial follow-up, and subsequent undetectable thyroglobulin levels on TSH-suppressive thyroid hormone therapy, additional radioiodine imaging is not necessary.

Most differentiated thyroid cancer "recurrences" actually represent persistent disease, typically in cervical nodes or the thyroid bed. Ultrasonography is particularly useful for postoperative monitoring in patients who presented with extensive cervical disease or who have persistently detectable serum thyroglobulin levels. If further follow-up radioiodine imaging is performed to identify disease recurrence, once such imaging is negative, it offers little or no advantage over measurement of thyroglobulin levels or other imaging. Trends in thyroglobulin levels, assessed using thyroglobulin doubling times, are useful for predicting the progression of disease, analogous to the use of calcitonin doubling times for monitoring of medullary thyroid cancer (see later). Unfortunately, thyroglobulin testing is unreliable in the 15 to 20% of patients who have circulating thyroglobulin autoantibodies that interfere with thyroglobulin immunoassays. In such patients, the trend in the thyroglobulin autoantibody titer may be informative. Chest CT scans can detect intrathoracic disease if recurrence outside of the neck is suspected. In patients with substantial detectable thyroglobulin levels (>10 ng/mL) and negative findings on standard imaging studies, FDG-PET scanning can locate residual disease in more than 50% of patients.

Recurrent cervical disease is usually an indication for a comprehensive compartmental neck dissection. Distant and nonresectable metastases that are iodine-avid can be treated with repeated [131]I. External beam radiation can provide symptomatic relief for hilar node and skeletal metastases. Surgery may be useful for isolated metastatic disease sites.

Conventional chemotherapy is of limited use for metastatic differentiated thyroid cancer, but agents that target relevant molecular pathways hold promise.[33] Sorafenib and lenvatinib are FDA-approved for patients with progressive differentiated thyroid cancer that is unresponsive to the usual therapies, including [131]I. Sorafenib (an oral inhibitor of vascular endothelial growth factor receptors, platelet-derived growth factor receptors, RET, and KIT) can double progression-free survival to almost 11 months in patients who have metastatic thyroid cancers.[A7] Lenvatinib (an oral inhibitor of vascular endothelial growth factor receptors, fibroblast growth factor receptors, platelet-derived growth factor receptors, RET, and KIT) at a daily dose of 24 mg per day in 28-day cycles provides at least a partial response in 65% of patients and prolongs median progression-free survival from 3.6 months to 18.3 months.[A8] Multikinase inhibitors have significant adverse effects, including hypertension, diarrhea, anorexia, nausea, weight loss, and fatigue. Because they are only tumoristatic, their discontinuation is associated with resumed tumor growth. Thus, the size and site of metastatic lesions, the possibility of local treatment measures, and the age and comorbidities of the patient must be carefully considered before initiating treatment.

PROGNOSIS

The TNM (tumor, node, metastasis) staging system is commonly used to predict the survival of patients with differentiated thyroid cancer. Tumor size, extra-thyroidal extension, extent of node involvement, presence of distant metastatic disease, and the patient's age are important predictors of outcome (E-Table 213-2, E-Table 213-3). The 10-year survival rates for patients with stage I and stage II disease are now 99% and more than 95%, respectively. However, tumors recur in up to 5% of patients with low-risk thyroid cancer, so all patients must be monitored.

Medullary Thyroid Carcinoma

In contrast to differentiated thyroid cancer, medullary thyroid cancer arises from the parafollicular or C cells, which produce calcitonin. It is a rare malignancy, comprising approximately 2% of all thyroid malignancies. The average age of diagnosis is approximately 50 years. Medullary thyroid cancer can be hereditary or nonhereditary. Hereditary medullary thyroid cancer, which accounts for approximately 25% of cases, is associated with the multiple endocrine neoplasia syndrome 2 (MEN2A and MEN2B; Chapter 218) and with mutations in the RET proto-oncogene. It tends to be bilateral and multifocal. The remaining 75% of medullary thyroid cancers are the results of sporadic mutations, which may be in the RET gene, and are typically associated with a unilateral lesion.

Patients with the familial multiple endocrine neoplasia syndromes (Chapter 218) are often diagnosed by genetic testing in the preclinical phase of their disease. In the more common MEN2A syndrome, medullary thyroid cancer typically occurs in the third decade of life, compared with the first decade of life in patients with the less common MEN2B syndrome. MEN2A may be accompanied by pheochromocytoma (Chapter 215), Hirschsprung disease (Chapter 127), and hyperparathyroidism (Chapter 232), whereas MEN2B is accompanied by pheochromocytoma, mucosal neuromas, intestinal ganglioneuromas, and a marfanoid habitus (Chapter 244). Patients with nonhereditary medullary thyroid cancer typically present with a thyroid nodule and cervical adenopathy. Symptoms of flushing, diarrhea, and pruritus can occur when the circulating calcitonin level is markedly elevated. At presentation, approximately 35% of tumors may have spread to cervical nodes, and 13% may have distant metastases.

After sporadic medullary thyroid cancer has been diagnosed, the treatment is total thyroidectomy and central compartment lymph node dissection. Dissection of lateral neck compartments may be considered depending upon the calcitonin levels. Thyroidectomy is generally recommended before age 5 years in patients with MEN2A and before age 1 in MEN2B, although these recommendations may be modified based on the specific mutation. Serum calcitonin concentrations are used to monitor patients postoperatively, and the serum calcitonin doubling time provides a valuable prognostic indicator of survival. A rising calcitonin level should lead to imaging of the neck, chest, and abdomen. Recurrent or persistent disease is best treated with surgery. However, treatment options for unresectable or advanced disease include radiation and systemic therapy with multikinase inhibitors. Both vandetanib and cabozantinib are approved agents for the treatment of progressive medullary thyroid cancer. Early diagnosis is the key to successful treatment of medullary thyroid cancer:

ten-year survival is 100% for stage I disease, compared with approximately 20% in stage IV.

Anaplastic Thyroid Carcinoma

Anaplastic thyroid carcinoma is a rare, histologically undifferentiated, clinically aggressive malignant neoplasm that typically arises in older patients, about 25% of whom have had a prior differentiated thyroid cancer. This cancer typically presents with a rapidly enlarging anterior or lateral neck mass associated with pain, tenderness, and compressive symptoms, including dysphagia, dysphonia, and stridorous dyspnea. Fine-needle aspiration biopsy of the mass usually yields large, pleomorphic, undifferentiated cells, but open surgical biopsy is sometimes required to confirm the diagnosis.

Most anaplastic thyroid cancers cannot be fully resected because they already have invaded other cervical structures when diagnosed. Surgery targets airway preservation. In the case of esophageal impingement, a percutaneous gastrostomy tube is often required to ensure adequate nutrition. Patients typically relapse within a few months and die within a median of 3 to 7 months.[34] However, overall survival of 22 months has been reported with trimodal therapy including surgery, radiation, and chemotherapy (potentially including targeted therapy and immunotherapy) compared with 6.5 months with just radiation and chemotherapy.

Primary Thyroid Lymphoma

Lymphoma (Chapter 176), which rarely arises in the thyroid gland, nevertheless accounts for 1 to 5% of all thyroid malignancies. It typically presents in older persons, with an average age of diagnosis of 66 years. Hashimoto thyroiditis is the strongest risk factor for primary thyroid lymphoma.

Thyroid lymphoma typically presents as a rapidly enlarging, diffuse goiter with compressive symptoms. Fine-needle aspiration biopsy usually shows abundant lymphocytes, and flow cytometry can identify monoclonal lymphocytes, usually B cells. Surgical biopsy is sometimes required to establish the diagnosis.

Most tumors respond to chemotherapy and external beam radiation therapy (Chapter 176). Surgery is rarely indicated, but tracheal compression occasionally requires elective tracheostomy. Disease-free survival rates vary, but early stage disease localized to the thyroid gland is associated with a 5-year survival rate of over 85%.

Grade A References

A1. Hoang TD, Olsen CH, Mai VQ, et al. Desiccated thyroid extract compared with levothyroxine in the treatment of hypothyroidism: a randomized, double-blind, crossover study. *J Clin Endocrinol Metab.* 2013;98:1982-1990.
A2. Stott DJ, Rodondi N, Kearney PM, et al. Thyroid hormone therapy for older adults with subclinical hypothyroidism. *N Engl J Med.* 2017;376:2534-2544.
A3. Feller M, Snel M, Moutzouri E, et al. Association of thyroid hormone therapy with quality of life and thyroid-related symptoms in patients with subclinical hypothyroidism: a systematic review and meta-analysis. *JAMA.* 2018;320:1349-1359.
A4. Casey BM, Thom EA, Peaceman AM, et al. Treatment of subclinical hypothyroidism or hypothyroxinemia in pregnancy. *N Engl J Med.* 2017;376:815-825.
A5. Rajendram R, Taylor PN, Wilson VJ, et al. Combined immunosuppression and radiotherapy in thyroid eye disease (CIRTED): a multicentre, 2 x 2 factorial, double-blind, randomised controlled trial. *Lancet Diabetes Endocrinol.* 2018;6:299-309.
A6. Smith TJ, Kahaly GJ, Ezra DG, et al. Teprotumumab for thyroid-associated ophthalmopathy. *N Engl J Med.* 2017;376:1748-1761.
A7. Brose MS, Nutting CM, Jarzab B, et al. Sorafenib in radioactive iodine-refractory, locally advanced or metastatic differentiated thyroid cancer: a randomised, double-blind, phase 3 trial. *Lancet.* 2014;384:319-328.
A8. Schlumberger M, Tahara M, Wirth LJ, et al. Lenvatinib versus placebo in radioiodine-refractory thyroid cancer. *N Engl J Med.* 2015;372:621-630.

GENERAL REFERENCES

For the General References and other additional features, please visit Expert Consult at https://expertconsult.inkling.com.

214

ADRENAL CORTEX

LYNNETTE K. NIEMAN

The adrenal glands weigh 6 to 8 g in adults (Fig. 214-1). Each contains a cortex, which makes steroid hormones, and a medulla, which produces catecholamines. Diseases of the adrenal medulla are discussed in Chapter 215. In the adrenal cortex, production of the three major classes of steroids occurs in specific zones: (1) the outermost layer, the glomerulosa, produces mineralocorticoids, primarily aldosterone; (2) the middle layer, the fasciculata, produces glucocorticoids, primarily cortisol; and (3) the innermost layer, the reticularis, produces adrenal "androgens," primarily dehydroepiandrosterone (DHEA) and its sulfated conjugate (DHEA-S) (Fig. 214-2). This division reflects the fact that certain critical enzymes are restricted to specific zones, resulting in the ability or inability to synthesize specific end products.

FUNCTION

The actions and regulation of these steroid classes differ. Mineralocorticoids act through the renal mineralocorticoid receptor[1] to promote the reabsorption of sodium and the secretion of potassium. In addition to this classic action, mineralocorticoids have important action on the vasculature and may exacerbate the metabolic syndrome. Aldosterone secretion is stimulated primarily by hyperkalemia and angiotensin II (which itself is stimulated by hypovolemia and excess renin). These agents increase the production of aldosterone synthase to restore homeostasis through this feedback loop. Aldosterone production is stimulated to a much smaller degree by adrenocorticotropic hormone (ACTH).

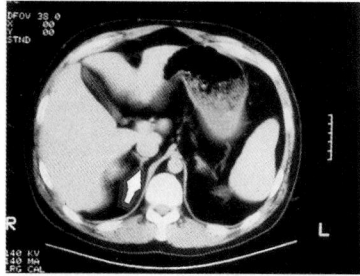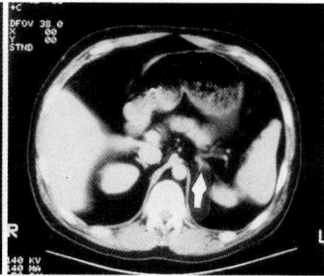

FIGURE 214-1. Magnetic resonance images of the abdomen showing the position and relative size of the normal adrenal glands.

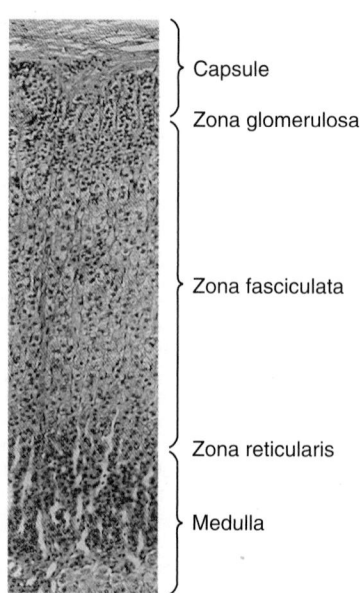

Capsule

Zona glomerulosa

Zona fasciculata

Zona reticularis

Medulla

FIGURE 214-2. Histologic section through a normal adult adrenal gland showing the progression (from outside to inside) of the zona glomerulosa, zona fasciculata, zona reticularis, and medulla.

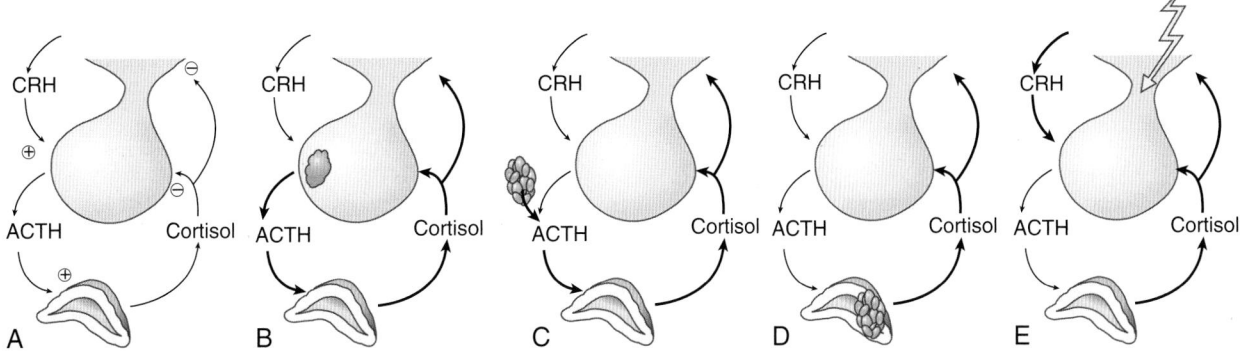

FIGURE 214-3. Physiology of the adrenal axis in health, Cushing syndrome, and pseudo-Cushing states. **A,** In healthy individuals, cortisol production is stimulated by the increased hypothalamic release of corticotropin-releasing hormone (CRH), which then travels down the pituitary stalk to stimulate adrenocorticotropic hormone (ACTH) secretion and release by corticotropes. Circulating ACTH stimulates adrenal gland production and secretion of cortisol. Cortisol then functions in a negative feedback mechanism to inhibit both CRH and ACTH. **B,** In Cushing disease, a pituitary tumor releases excessive amounts of ACTH, which results in increased cortisol secretion by the adrenal glands. **C,** In ectopic ACTH secretion, a nonpituitary ACTH-secreting tumor releases excessive amounts of ACTH, which results in increased cortisol secretion by the adrenal glands. **D,** In ACTH-independent adrenal forms of Cushing syndrome, the adrenal tumor autonomously releases excess amounts of cortisol. In all forms of Cushing syndrome, the negative feedback effects of excessive cortisol inhibit endogenous CRH and ACTH secretion, so that circulating ACTH levels reflect the underlying tumor (levels are normal or increased) or independent cortisol production (levels are suppressed). **E,** In pseudo-Cushing states, central stimulation increases CRH secretion, which in turn increases ACTH and hence cortisol production. In this setting, the negative feedback effects of excessive cortisol inhibit endogenous CRH and ACTH secretion, so that cortisol levels are ultimately constrained, albeit at an increased level.

Cortisol and other glucocorticoids act through the glucocorticoid receptor type 2 and its isoforms. The actions of this class of steroids are much broader, including effects on carbohydrate handling, lipid and calcium metabolism, and the immune and nervous systems. Cortisol production is regulated primarily by ACTH, which is secreted in a circadian rhythm in response to corticotropin-releasing hormone (CRH) so that cortisol levels are highest in the morning and fall to a nadir around midnight. Cortisol coordinates ACTH production through negative feedback at the pituitary (ACTH) and hypothalamus (CRH). Vasopressin secretion also plays a role in stimulating ACTH release.

DHEA and DHEA-S are the most abundant products of the adrenal gland. They exert their estrogenic and androgenic effects as prohormones, being converted to estrogens and testosterone in the peripheral tissues and activating the androgen and estrogen receptors. There is no known regulator of DHEA synthesis, but its production declines with age.

DISORDERS OF ADRENAL FUNCTION

Most disorders of the adrenal cortex reflect overproduction or underproduction of the products of a single synthetic zone—cortisol, aldosterone, or testosterone or estrogen (Fig. 214-3). The congenital adrenal hyperplasias are an exception and are manifested with both overproduction and underproduction. Abnormal secretion is suggested by clinical features of each disorder and is reflected in plasma or urine levels of the relevant hormones or by the consequent increases or decreases in feedback systems, which form the basis of the biochemical diagnostic tests.

Glucocorticoid Excess: Cushing Syndrome

CLINICAL MANIFESTATIONS

Cushing syndrome is a symptom complex that reflects excessive tissue exposure to cortisol. Classic features of Cushing syndrome include weight gain, plethora, hypertension, and striae (Table 214-1). Not all patients have all features; the number and severity of features correlate roughly with the duration and severity of hypercortisolism. Because many of the signs and symptoms are nonspecific, the diagnosis may be confused with psychiatric disorders, polycystic ovary syndrome, the metabolic syndrome, simple obesity, fibromyalgia, or acute illness. However, because worsening hypercortisolism may precipitate hypertension, glucose intolerance, infections, psychiatric disturbances, impaired cognition, and hypercoagulability, it is important to identify this treatable disorder to prevent its associated morbidity and mortality.[2]

Changes in mood and cognition are useful markers of hypercortisolism. These include irritability, crying, and restlessness; depressed mood; decreased libido; insomnia; anxiety; and decreased concentration and impaired memory.

DIAGNOSIS
Clinical Examination
Cushing syndrome screening is most likely to be positive in the presence of signs that are typical of glucocorticoid excess, such as abnormal fat distribution

TABLE 214-1 THE FREQUENCY OF CLINICAL SIGNS AND SYMPTOMS OF CUSHING SYNDROME

SIGN OR SYMPTOM	PERCENTAGE
Decreased libido in men and women	100
Obesity or weight gain	97
Plethora	94
Round face	88
Menstrual changes	84
Hirsutism	81
Hypertension	74
Ecchymoses	62
Lethargy, depression	62
Striae	56
Weakness	56
Electrocardiographic changes or atherosclerosis	55
Dorsal fat pad	54
Edema	50
Abnormal glucose tolerance	50
Osteopenia or fracture	50
Headache	47
Backache	43
Recurrent infections	25
Abdominal pain	21
Acne	21
Female balding	13

in the supraclavicular and temporal fossae, proximal muscle weakness, wide (>1 cm) purple striae, and new irritability, decreased cognition, and decreased short-term memory.[3] Testing is indicated when clinical features have progressed over time and in patients with adrenal masses that are incidentally detected on imaging obtained for unrelated reasons (so-called adrenal incidentalomas).[4] For example, oligomenorrhea is more suggestive of Cushing syndrome if a woman previously had regular menses. Serial seven subtractions and recall of three cities (or objects) are useful bedside strategies to identify deficits in cognition and memory.

Laboratory Findings
Exogenous administration of glucocorticoid should be excluded before screening for endogenous Cushing syndrome. In the absence of pseudo-Cushing states (see later), at least two different screening test results should be abnormal to establish the diagnosis. Tests for the differential diagnosis of Cushing

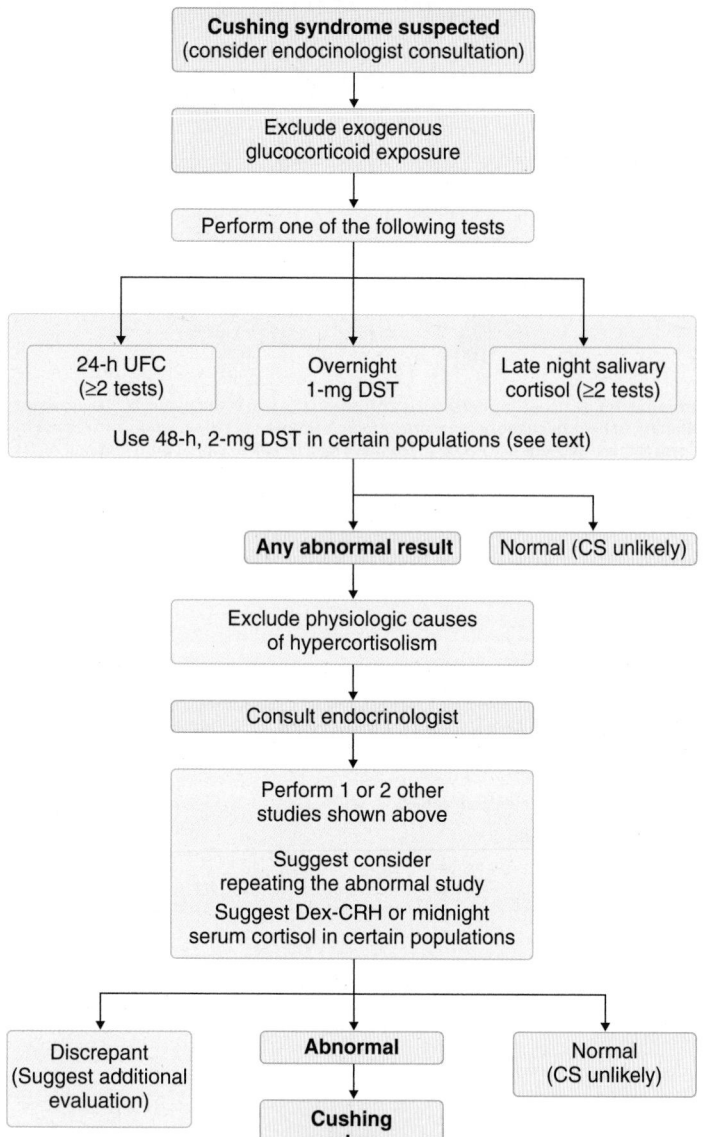

FIGURE 214-4. Algorithm for testing of patients suspected of having Cushing syndrome (CS). All statements are recommendations except for those prefaced by "suggest." Diagnostic criteria that suggest Cushing syndrome are urine free cortisol (UFC) greater than the normal range for the assay, serum cortisol greater than 1.8 μg/dL (50 nmol/liter) after 1 mg dexamethasone (1-mg DST), and late-night salivary cortisol greater than 145 ng/dL (4 nmol/liter). Dex-CRH = dexamethasone–corticotropin-releasing hormone test; DST = dexamethasone suppression test. (Reprinted with permission from Nieman LK, Biller BM, Findling JW, et al. The diagnosis of Cushing syndrome: an Endocrine Society clinical practice guideline. *J Clin Endocrinol Metab.* 2008;93:1526-1540.)

syndrome should not be used to make the diagnosis. Figure 214-4 is the Endocrine Society's recommended algorithm for testing of patients suspected of having Cushing syndrome.

Urine, Saliva, and Serum Cortisol Measurements

Urine free cortisol (UFC) excretion during 24 hours is a good screening test. Specific, structurally based assay techniques, such as high-performance liquid chromatography and tandem mass spectrometry, are the "gold standard." The upper-normal limit of these tests is much lower and more specific than that of antibody-based assays, in which other steroids may cross-react. This cross-reactivity may be an advantage in screening for hypercortisolism.

UFC excretion is elevated in about 20% of adrenal incidentalomas[5] and also may be increased in the so-called *pseudo-Cushing states,* including psychiatric disorders (depression, anxiety disorder, obsessive-compulsive disorder), chronic pain, severe exercise, alcoholism, uncontrolled diabetes, and morbid obesity. Here, it is hypothesized that higher brain pathways stimulate CRH release and activation of the entire hypothalamic-pituitary-adrenal axis (see Fig. 214-3E). Cortisol negative feedback inhibition on CRH and pituitary ACTH release restrains the resulting hypercortisoluria to less than four-fold greater than normal. Thus Cushing syndrome cannot be diagnosed

TABLE 214-2 ETIOLOGY OF CUSHING SYNDROME	
EXOGENOUS	**ENDOGENOUS**
Most common cause of Cushing syndrome: 　Glucocorticoid or ACTH driven 　May be factitious or iatrogenic	ACTH independent—autonomous adrenal activation (20% of all cases) 　Adrenal adenoma (40-50%) 　Adrenal carcinoma (40-50%) 　Primary pigmented nodular adrenal disease 　McCune-Albright syndrome 　　Massive macronodular adrenal disease 　　Gastric inhibitory polypeptide or food induced ACTH dependent—adrenal activation by excessive ACTH (80% of all cases) 　Corticotrope adenoma (80%) 　Ectopic ACTH secretion (20%) 　Ectopic CRH secretion (rare)

ACTH = adrenocorticotropic hormone; CRH = corticotropin-releasing hormone.

with certainty unless values reach this threshold. Conversely, patients with Cushing syndrome may have normal UFC excretion because of mild or intermittent hypercortisolism or altered renal metabolism of cortisol. If UFC is only mildly elevated and clinical features are minimal, it is best to treat any pseudo-Cushing state and to remeasure UFC excretion with the expectation that it will normalize. Alternatively, if UFC values are normal but clinical suspicion is high, repeated measurement might disclose intermittent hypercortisolism.

Measurement of plasma cortisol at midnight distinguishes pseudo-Cushing states from Cushing syndrome with 95% diagnostic accuracy; a level greater than 7.5 μg/dL is required for the diagnosis of Cushing syndrome. Measurement of salivary cortisol at bedtime or at midnight works as well, is more convenient, and may be the best screening test in patients with mild or intermittent hypercortisolism.[6] However, the criteria for its interpretation differ, so each assay must be validated before it is used for this purpose.

Dexamethasone Suppression Tests

The dexamethasone suppression test is a simple screening test that takes advantage of the negative feedback effect of glucocorticoids to reduce ACTH (and hence serum cortisol). Dexamethasone 1 mg is given orally between 11:00 PM and midnight, and plasma cortisol is measured between 8:00 and 9:00 the next morning. The test has an 8% false-negative rate in patients with Cushing disease and a 30% false-positive rate in chronic illness, obesity, psychiatric disorders, and normal individuals. As a result, Cushing syndrome cannot be diagnosed by this test alone unless the result is extremely abnormal.

The 2-day, 2-mg dexamethasone suppression test discriminates patients with a pseudo-Cushing state if plasma cortisol end points of less than 1.4 or 2.2 μg/dL are used. Dexamethasone 500 μg is given orally every 6 hours for eight doses, and plasma cortisol is measured 2 hours after the last dose. The test has excellent sensitivity (90 to 100%) and specificity (97 to 100%) for discriminating Cushing syndrome, but it is costly and requires excellent compliance of the patient. The immediate subsequent administration of CRH (1 mg per kilogram of body weight intravenously) and the measurement of cortisol 15 minutes later increased the sensitivity and specificity to 100% in a small study of patients, with values above 1.4 μg/dL indicating Cushing syndrome. Although this combined dexamethasone-CRH test has high diagnostic accuracy, it has the same disadvantages as the 2-day dexamethasone suppression test and the added cost of CRH testing. Because of these drawbacks, these tests are usually reserved for patients with ambiguous or confusing results on other screening tests. CRH is available commercially (Acthrel), with U.S. Food and Drug Administration–approved labeling for the differential diagnosis of Cushing syndrome. Its use in the dexamethasone-CRH test is an off-label use.

Any dexamethasone test may give false results in patients with abnormal metabolic clearance of the drug. Agents that induce the cytochrome P-450 CYP3A4 enzymes (alcohol, rifampin, phenytoin, phenobarbital) increase dexamethasone clearance, whereas renal or hepatic failure decreases it. Measurement of a dexamethasone level can determine whether its clearance has been altered.

Differential Diagnosis

The causes of endogenous Cushing syndrome can be divided broadly into ACTH-dependent (80%) and ACTH-independent (20%) forms (Table 214-2).

Hypercortisolism from autonomously functioning adrenal tumors suppresses ACTH, whereas in primary disorders of ACTH excess, the adrenal glands respond to tumor-derived ACTH. Plasma ACTH concentration distinguishes between these causes. ACTH is usually less than 10 pg/mL in primary adrenal disorders but is also suppressed by exogenous steroids, whether they are prescribed intentionally (iatrogenic Cushing syndrome) or taken factitiously. Patients in the latter group often have had multiple surgical procedures and do not reveal that they are self-administering steroids. As a result, patients must be queried closely about exogenous steroid administration, recognizing that parenteral, inhaled, and topical steroids can all cause glucocorticoid excess. Patients with endogenous Cushing syndrome and low ACTH concentrations should undergo adrenal imaging to identify the site of adrenal abnormality. Nonautonomous adrenal tissue atrophies when ACTH support is subnormal. Because of this, the common ACTH-independent forms of Cushing syndrome—adrenal adenoma and carcinoma—are manifested as a unilateral adrenal mass, with atrophy of the adjacent and contralateral tissue on magnetic resonance imaging or computed tomography.

Bilateral forms of primary adrenal disease are rare and may be manifested with small or large adrenal nodules. Primary pigmented nodular adrenal disease occurs primarily in children and young adults and is characterized by small to normal-sized adrenal glands containing small (<5 mm) black-brown cortical nodules. About half of these patients have additional features, termed *Carney complex,* which are often inherited in an autosomal dominant fashion.[7] The clinical features of Carney complex include myxomas of the skin, breast, and heart; spotty pigmentation, such as lentigines and blue nevi; and other endocrine overactivity, such as acromegaly and testicular tumors. Some of these patients have mutations leading to a truncated form of protein kinase A regulatory 1α subunit. The resultant increase in protein kinase A activation by cyclic adenosine monophosphate presumably allows tumor formation. Bilateral nodular hyperplasia with Cushing syndrome can occur in the setting of *McCune-Albright syndrome,* mostly in infants or children. Massive macronodular adrenal disease generally is manifested after the age of 40 years with huge adrenal glands and aberrant expression of "illicit" receptors for various ligands (gastric inhibitory polypeptide, β-adrenergic, vasopressin), which presumably mediates autonomous cortisol production.

A normal or elevated plasma ACTH level (>15 pg/mL; 3.3 pmol/L) is consistent with an ACTH-producing tumor. Intermediate ACTH concentrations between 5 and 15 pg/mL (1.1 to 3.3 pmol/L) in a two-site sandwich assay are not diagnostic. In these patients, suboptimal cortisol responses to CRH stimulation may identify the minority of cases of ACTH-independent Cushing syndrome with borderline basal ACTH values. In addition, a suppressed plasma DHEA-S value supports the diagnosis of an ACTH-independent disorder.

Cushing disease,[8] an ACTH-secreting pituitary adenoma, is the most common cause of Cushing syndrome (Chapter 211). It is more common in women than in men (6:1 ratio), with a mean age at onset in the fourth decade. ACTH also may be secreted ectopically by a variety of neuroendocrine tumors, as shown in Table 214-3.

Pituitary magnetic resonance imaging shows a tumor in only about 40 to 50% of patients with Cushing disease, but it is obtained routinely in patients with ACTH-dependent disease to exclude a macroadenoma or abnormal anatomy before petrosal sinus sampling or surgery. A pituitary lesion less than 6 mm is seen in up to 10% of healthy individuals and so does not always indicate Cushing disease. Biochemical tests must be used to distinguish among the ACTH-dependent causes of Cushing syndrome, and they must be performed after a 6- to 8-week period of sustained hypercortisolism sufficient to suppress normal corticotrope function.

Inferior petrosal sinus sampling is the best test to distinguish between a pituitary and an ectopic source of excess ACTH; worldwide, the overall sensitivity and specificity are about 94%. The test involves catheterization of a peripheral vein and also the petrosal sinuses draining the pituitary gland; simultaneous measurement of ACTH levels at each site before and 3, 5, and 10 minutes after administration of CRH; and calculation of the central-to-peripheral ACTH ratio at each time point. Ratios of more than 2 before CRH administration or more than 3 after CRH administration are consistent with Cushing disease.

Although it is accurate in experienced hands, inferior petrosal sinus sampling carries a small risk of stroke, is expensive, and is not widely available. Other tests, such as the CRH test and the 8-mg dexamethasone suppression test, may be useful if both responses indicate Cushing disease. In this setting, the likelihood of ectopic ACTH secretion is low. However, the diagnosis is not clear if both responses are negative or if they are mixed. (Disorders of the anterior pituitary, including Cushing disease, are discussed in detail in Chapter 211.)

If endocrine tests suggest ectopic ACTH secretion, imaging is obtained to localize the tumor. Computed tomography and magnetic resonance imaging of the chest are the best initial screens because these tumors are most often in the thoracic cavity. Octreotide scintigraphy is a useful adjunctive test. Measurement of serum calcitonin and gastrin and measurement of plasma or urine catecholamines may identify medullary carcinoma of the thyroid, gastrinoma, and pheochromocytoma. The process can be repeated every 6 to 12 months; tumors that make ACTH ectopically have a spectrum of malignant potential, and annual screening should continue, regardless of treatment for hypercortisolism.

TABLE 214-3	THE INCIDENCE AND TYPES OF TUMORS CAUSING THE SYNDROME OF ECTOPIC ACTH SECRETION	
TUMOR TYPE		**PERCENTAGE**
Carcinoma of lung (small cell or oat cell)		19-50
Carcinoid of bronchus		2-37
Carcinoid of thymus		8-12
Pancreatic tumors, carcinoid and islet cell		4-12
Pheochromocytoma, neuroblastoma, ganglioma, paraganglioma		5-12
Medullary carcinoma of the thyroid		0-5
Miscellaneous*		<1

*Miscellaneous tumors reported to secrete ACTH in 1-10 cases include carcinoma of the ovary, prostate, breast, thyroid, kidney, salivary glands, testes, gallbladder, esophagus, and appendix; gastric carcinoid and renal carcinoid; acute myeloblastic leukemia; melanoma; and cloacogenic carcinoma of the anal canal.
ACTH = adrenocorticotropic hormone.

TREATMENT Rx

Surgical Therapy

The optimal treatment of Cushing syndrome is surgical resection of the lesion that is producing excessive ACTH or cortisol. In ACTH-dependent Cushing syndrome, if this is unsuccessful or cannot be done, bilateral adrenalectomy is an option.[9]

Transsphenoidal resection of a microadenoma is the optimal therapy for a patient with Cushing disease, with up to a 90% chance of cure in the hands of an experienced neurosurgeon. A successful outcome is less likely if the initial surgery is not curative, in cases of recurrence, and for macroadenomas. Controversy exists about the criteria for remission; although a low postoperative cortisol level is encouraging, it does not preclude later recurrence. If recurrence develops, additional resection or alternative therapy should be considered.

Patients with ectopic ACTH secretion can be cured if the tumor can be removed and is not metastatic. Otherwise, adrenalectomy or medical therapy is chosen (see later). Adrenalectomy is appropriate when the patient cannot tolerate the medical toxicity, cost, or adverse psychological effects of long-term medical therapy and monitoring; when rapid correction of hypercortisolism is needed; or if maximal daily doses of ketoconazole (1600 mg) and metyrapone (2 g) given in combination do not render the patient eucortisolemic.

Nonmalignant primary adrenal causes of Cushing syndrome are cured by resection of the abnormal tissue. Laparoscopy is the preferred approach. Surgery is the mainstay in the treatment of adrenal cancer; multiple operations may be needed to resect primary lesions, local recurrences, and hepatic, thoracic, and intracranial metastases. Adjuvant adrenolytic therapy with mitotane may provide a chemotherapeutic benefit.

Radiation Therapy

Radiation therapy to the pituitary gland, with adjunctive therapy with steroidogenesis inhibitors to normalize cortisol levels, is a good option for patients with Cushing disease who cannot undergo surgery, for those in whom the risk of Nelson syndrome (Chapter 211) is deemed great, and for those with recurrent disease. This is usually delivered in 200-rad daily increments to a total dose of 4500 cGy. The disadvantage of radiation therapy is the length of time needed for a full response—up to 10 years—and the possibility of hypopituitarism. There is less experience with high-energy radiosurgery, such as the gamma knife, which has the advantage of requiring only one or two treatments. Adrenalectomy is preferable if rapid normalization of hypercortisolism is needed, and this option may be chosen by patients who have concerns about radiation-induced hypopituitarism and loss of reproductive function.

Medical Therapy

Medical therapy can also be used for patients with occult ectopic ACTH-secreting tumors or in combination with pituitary irradiation to treat Cushing disease.

Medical therapy with steroidogenesis inhibitors alone is rarely appropriate for Cushing disease because it requires close monitoring and adjustment of dose. Cabergoline or pasireotide may normalize UFC in about 40% of patients.[A1] There are limited data on the long-term efficacy of any medical therapy in Cushing disease.

After complete resection, the recurrence of adrenocortical carcinoma is more common in patients who had a larger tumor size, venous tumor thrombus, and the proliferation tumor marker Ki67.[10] For advanced adrenocortical carcinoma, rates of response and progression-free survival but not overall survival are significantly better with first-line therapy using a combination of etoposide (100 mg/m^2 on days 2 to 4), doxorubicin (40 mg/m^2 on day 1), and cisplatin (40 mg/m^2 on days 3 and 4) plus oral mitotane (to achieve a blood level of 14 to 20 mg/L) than with streptozocin plus mitotane as first-line therapy, with similar rates of toxic events.[A2]

Mineralocorticoid Excess

DIAGNOSIS

Patients with mineralocorticoid excess often have few clinical symptoms apart from fatigue and muscle weakness or cramps related to hypokalemia. Most often the condition is suspected because of hypertension, especially if it occurs at an early age in association with spontaneous hypokalemia or is difficult to control.[11] The prevalence of primary aldosteronism among patients with hypertension is uncertain but is generally felt to be no higher than about 5%.[12] Mineralocorticoid excess can result from primary adrenal disease, in which aldosterone (or another mineralocorticoid) is produced autonomously (and renin levels are low),[13] or it may be due to nonadrenal causes as a result of elevated renin values, which stimulate aldosterone secretion. The latter situations include states of contracted arterial intravascular volume, such as congestive heart failure or cirrhosis with ascites, decreased renal arterial blood flow, and tumor production of renin (Table 214-4).

TABLE 214-4 CAUSES OF MINERALOCORTICOID EXCESS

PRIMARY HYPERALDOSTERONISM: HIGH ALDOSTERONE, LOW RENIN

Aldosterone-producing adenomas (30-50%)
Bilateral zona glomerulosa hyperplasia
Familial hyperaldosteronism
  Type 1: glucocorticoid-remediable hyperaldosteronism—this results from formation of a chimeric gene containing the regulator portion of 11β-hydroxylase (normally regulated by ACTH) and the synthetic region of aldosterone synthase; as a result, ACTH stimulates aldosterone synthase and hence aldosterone production
  Type 2: adrenal adenomas or hyperplasia expressed in a familial pattern
  Type 3: caused by mutant *KCNJ5*, often younger and more severe than type 2
Aldosterone-producing adrenal carcinoma
Ectopic aldosterone secretion (rare): kidney, ovary

SECONDARY HYPERALDOSTERONISM: HIGH ALDOSTERONE, HIGH RENIN

Renovascular hypertension and aortic stenosis
Diuretic use
Renin-secreting tumors
Severe cardiac failure

APPARENT MINERALOCORTICOID EXCESS: LOW ALDOSTERONE, LOW RENIN

Licorice ingestion: licorice (candy or flavored tobacco) containing glycyrrhetinic acid (or similar compounds such as carbenoxolone) inhibits renal 11β-hydroxysteroid dehydrogenase type 2, reducing cortisol conversion to cortisone and enabling cortisol to act as an endogenous mineralocorticoid
Severe hypercortisolism: similar in mechanism to licorice ingestion; very high cortisol levels are thought to overwhelm the ability of 11β-hydroxysteroid dehydrogenase type 2 to convert cortisol to cortisone in the kidney; cortisol itself then acts as a potent mineralocorticoid
Liddle's syndrome: mutation of the gene for the β or γ subunit of the collecting tubule sodium channel leads to a constitutive increase in sodium reabsorption and potassium excretion
11β-Hydroxylase deficiency form of congenital adrenal hyperplasia: 11-deoxycortisol accumulates because of an inability to convert it to cortisol
17-Hydroxylase deficiency form of congenital adrenal hyperplasia: deoxycorticosterone and corticosterone are increased

RENIN-INDEPENDENT MINERALOCORTICOID EXCESS

DIAGNOSIS

Although most of these conditions result from excessive aldosterone production by one or both adrenal glands, excessive production of other mineralocorticoids or constitutive activation of the renal sodium channel must be excluded. In these latter conditions, both aldosterone and renin values are low, resulting in the so-called syndrome of apparent mineralocorticoid excess. In this setting, diagnostic information is obtained by history (licorice ingestion) or measurement of other mineralocorticoids (see Table 214-4).

Primary hyperaldosteronism is diagnosed when there is an increased ratio (>20) of morning aldosterone to plasma renin activity (Fig. 214-5). Except as noted in the figure, one of four tests (usually salt loading) is used to confirm primary hyperaldosteronism by demonstrating a lack of aldosterone suppression.[14]

Differential Diagnosis

Having made the diagnosis of aldosterone-dependent mineralocorticoid excess, one must differentiate between the two most common adrenal causes—hyperplasia and adenoma—after excluding potential rare causes of hyperaldosteronism. Two rare autosomal dominant forms of familial hyperaldosteronism are type 1, a glucocorticoid-suppressible hyperaldosteronism, and type 2. Familial hyperaldosteronism type 1 is caused by a genetic swap of the promoter for *CYP11B1* (11β-hydroxylase) with that of *CYP11B2* (aldosterone synthase), forming a chimeric gene in which ACTH stimulates aldosterone synthase. It should be suspected in the setting of familial disease, particularly if there is a history of early-onset cardiovascular events, and is confirmed by gene testing (see http://www.brighamandwomens.org/Departments_and_Services/medicine/services/endocrine/Services/gra/default.aspx). Analysis of a multiplex family with familial hyperaldosteronism type 2 and 80 additional probands with unsolved early-onset primary aldosteronism revealed that eight had novel heterozygous variants in the *CLCN2* gene that encodes a voltage-gated chloride channel that is expressed in adrenal glomerulosa cells.[15]

For the more common conditions, adrenal computed tomography scans may show nonfunctioning nodules and falsely suggest an adenoma. However, further testing is not recommended in a patient less than 35 years old with marked aldosteronism and an adrenal mass.[14] The responses to physiologic maneuvers, such as upright posture, and salt loading with oral or intravenous sodium tend to be preserved in patients with hyperplasia, but there is significant overlap among groups of patients. The best diagnostic test involves the measurement of cortisol and aldosterone in bilateral adrenal venous effluent and a peripheral vein before and during an ACTH infusion. Cortisol is used to evaluate catheter placement in the adrenal veins, as levels from the two sides should be similar. When an adenoma is present, the aldosterone-to-cortisol ratio on one side is usually at least five-fold greater than the other, which may be similar to the periphery, indicating suppression. Bilateral hyperplasia tends to produce similar values on each side.

TREATMENT   Rx

Treatment of primary hyperaldosteronism includes laparoscopic or robotic resection for adenomas.[16] Afterward, hypokalemia generally resolves, but hypertension persists in up to 65% of patients. A mineralocorticoid antagonist, spironolactone or eplerenone, is used to treat patients unable to undergo surgery or those with hyperplasia. Eplerenone is a more selective mineralocorticoid antagonist (with fewer side effects of sexual dysfunction and gynecomastia compared with spironolactone). A sodium channel blocker (e.g., amiloride) may be helpful, and antihypertensive agents are continued as needed.

Androgen Excess

DEFINITION

Women with excess circulating androgens or increased sensitivity to androgens present with complaints of hirsutism, acne, and anovulation or infertility. When testosterone is secreted in great excess, women may virilize and exhibit a deepened voice, clitorimegaly, masculinized body habitus, and alopecia.

DIAGNOSIS

The adrenal causes of hyperandrogenism—congenital adrenal hyperplasia, Cushing disease, adrenal cancer, and androgen-producing adrenal adenoma—are

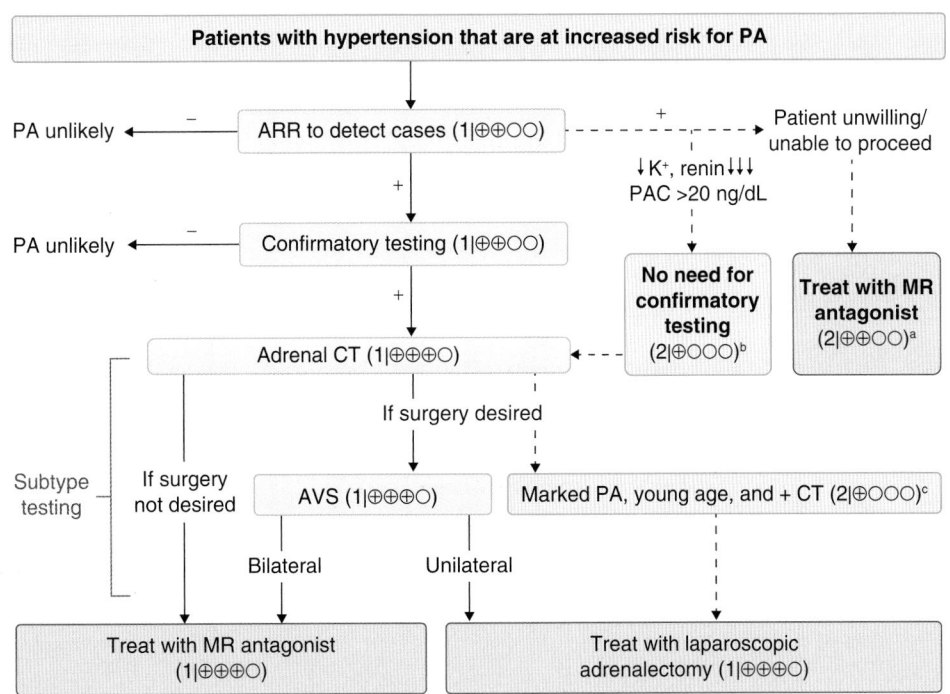

FIGURE 214-5. Algorithm for the diagnosis and treatment of primary aldosteronism (hyperaldosteronism). Cross-filled circles indicate the quality of evidence, such that ⊕○○○ denotes very low quality evidence; ⊕⊕○○, low quality; ⊕⊕⊕○, moderate quality; and ⊕⊕⊕⊕, high quality. ARR = aldosterone-to-renin ratio; AVS = adrenal venous sampling; CT = computed tomography; MR = mineralcorticoid receptor; PA = primary aldosteronism. (Reprinted, with slight modification of text, from Funder JW, Carey RM, Mantero F, et al. The management of primary aldosteronism: case detection, diagnosis, and treatment: an Endocrine Society clinical practice guideline. *J Clin Endocrinol Metab.* 2016;101:1889-916.)

uncommon. Most women have no clear-cut cause (idiopathic hirsutism) or polycystic ovary syndrome. Rarely, androgen-secreting ovarian tumors, hyperprolactinemia, glucocorticoid resistance, or exogenous drugs cause hyperandrogenism. Patients with an adrenal source of hyperandrogenism usually have increased serum levels of DHEA, DHEA-S, or androstenedione, in contrast to the testosterone excess that is more typical of an ovarian source. DHEA and DHEA-S are weak androgens that can be converted locally to testosterone in the hair follicles. Because DHEA and DHEA-S levels decline throughout adult life, these values must be interpreted within age-specific normal ranges. Although a tumor is more likely if DHEA-S is greater than 500 μg/dL or testosterone is greater than 200 ng/mL, it is not excluded at lower levels.

Imaging identifies nearly all adrenal tumors but may miss a small intraovarian one. UFC may be elevated in patients with virilizing adrenal carcinoma or Cushing disease (see earlier) and in those with glucocorticoid resistance. By contrast, androgen-secreting adrenal adenomas do not have glucocorticoid excess. In women suspected of having nonclassic forms of congenital adrenal hyperplasia, precursor and product hormones should be measured before and after ACTH to confirm the diagnosis.

TREATMENT Rx

Treatment of adrenal causes of hyperandrogenism varies according to the disorder. Classic congenital adrenal hyperplasia is treated by glucocorticoids to normalize ACTH and hence androgen levels (typically dexamethasone 0.125 to 0.375 mg at bedtime). The nonclassic forms respond well to oral contraceptive or antiandrogen treatment, with dexamethasone reserved for ovulation induction. Surgery with adjunctive medical treatment may be used in adrenal carcinoma (see earlier).

Mixed Mineralocorticoid and Glucocorticoid Deficiency: Adrenal Insufficiency

PATHOBIOLOGY

Primary Adrenal Insufficiency

Autoimmune Destruction

Autoimmune destruction is the most common cause of primary adrenal insufficiency in industrialized countries and may occur alone or, rarely, in association with autoimmune polyglandular syndromes. These syndromes tend to be manifested either in childhood (type 1), in association with hypoparathyroidism and mucocutaneous candidiasis, or in adulthood (type 2), in association with insulin-dependent diabetes mellitus, autoimmune thyroid disease, alopecia areata, or vitiligo. The glands are small on imaging.

Adrenoleukodystrophy

Adrenoleukodystrophy, a rare (1 in 25,000) X-linked condition, is characterized by a deficiency of peroxisomal membrane adrenoleukodystrophy protein, which transports activated acyl-coenzyme A derivates into the peroxisomes, where they are shortened by β-oxidation. This deficiency results in the accumulation of very long chain fatty acids in the central nervous system and other tissues and increased plasma $C_{26:0}$ fatty acids. Incomplete penetrance of the genetic defect and variable accumulation of very long chain fatty acids in the adrenal gland, brain, testis, and liver account for the clinical phenotypes, which differ by age and presentation.[17]

Replacement of Adrenal Tissue

Infections cause about 15% of primary adrenal insufficiency. Typical infections include tuberculosis and systemic fungal diseases (histoplasmosis, coccidioidomycosis, blastomycosis), in which the adrenal tissue is replaced by caseating granulomas. End-stage AIDS-associated opportunistic infections, such as cytomegalovirus or *Mycobacterium avium-intracellulare,* may reduce adrenal function. Adrenal tissue may be replaced by bilateral metastases (most commonly primary carcinoma of the lung, breast, kidney, or gut) or primary lymphoma, although adrenal insufficiency is uncommon. Intra-adrenal hemorrhage may also lead to insufficient steroidogenesis. Hemorrhage typically occurs in a stressed, hospitalized patient receiving long-term prophylactic anticoagulation and is often accompanied by back pain. The adrenal glands tend to be large on imaging.

Congenital Adrenal Hyperplasias

The congenital adrenal hyperplasias[18] are a disparate group of diseases caused by a genetic deficiency of one of the enzymes needed for adrenal steroidogenesis. Patients with nearly complete deficiency of an enzyme required for cortisol synthesis present in infancy with adrenal insufficiency and salt-wasting crisis. This is most problematic in patients with mutation of the 21-hydroxylase (*CYP21A2*) or 11β-hydroxylase (*CYP11B1*) gene. The increase in ACTH levels caused by cortisol deficiency drives the intact steroidogenic pathways so that there is excessive production of the steroids just proximal to the enzymatic block—17-hydroxyprogesterone and 11-deoxycortisol, respectively,

TABLE 214-5 CAUSES OF ADRENAL INSUFFICIENCY AND ANCILLARY TESTS

SPECIFIC CAUSES	SUGGESTIVE CLINICAL FEATURES	USEFUL ANCILLARY TESTS
Primary adrenal insufficiency	Hyperpigmentation, orthostatic hypotension	Hyperkalemia, elevated ACTH
Idiopathic autoimmune destruction	Most common cause (80%) in developed countries; with or without other endocrinopathies, as below	Antibodies to 21-hydroxylase are present; on imaging, adrenal glands are small
Polyglandular failure type 1	Hypoparathyroidism, mucocutaneous candidiasis, vitiligo; age <20 years	
Polyglandular failure type 2	Insulin-dependent diabetes, autoimmune thyroid disease, alopecia areata, vitiligo; age >40 years	On imaging, adrenal glands are small
Infections: tuberculosis, systemic fungal diseases, AIDS-associated opportunistic infections (e.g., cytomegalovirus)	15% of patients in U.S. series	Adrenal glands tend to be large on CT and may be calcified
Space-occupying adrenal lesions	Metastases from carcinoma of lung, breast, kidney, gut; lymphoma or hemorrhage (heparin use)	Abnormal shape of adrenal glands on CT; evidence of hemorrhage
Bilateral adrenalectomy or treatment with steroidogenesis inhibitors		Ketoconazole, mitotane, aminoglutethimide, trilostane, and metyrapone reduce cortisol levels
Adrenoleukodystrophy	X-linked—screen males; in childhood, cognitive and gait disturbances; in adults, spastic paraparesis	Deficiency of peroxisomal very long chain acyl-coenzyme A synthetase leads to elevated plasma $C_{26:0}$ fatty acid levels
Secondary adrenal insufficiency		
Suppression of the adrenal axis by exogenous or endogenous glucocorticoids	Medication history; history of Cushing syndrome	Adrenal glands are small on imaging
Structural lesions of the hypothalamus or pituitary gland (tumors, destruction by infiltrating disorders, x-irradiation, and lymphocytic hypophysitis)	Other pituitary deficiencies	Adrenal glands are normal or small on imaging; MRI or CT may show pituitary or hypothalamic lesion
Isolated ACTH deficiency		
Head trauma		

ACTH = adrenocorticotropic hormone; AIDS = acquired immunodeficiency syndrome; CT = computed tomography; MRI = magnetic resonance imaging.

in 21-hydroxylase and 11β-hydroxylase deficiency. The increased levels of precursor steroids enable increased adrenal androgen synthesis, so that severely affected girls may be virilized in utero. Girls and women with nonclassic congenital adrenal hyperplasia present later. They have greater enzyme activity, so that cortisol production is adequate, but increased ACTH levels cause hyperandrogenism.

Rare Causes
Other rare causes of primary adrenal insufficiency include ACTH resistance, congenital adrenal hypoplasia, Smith-Lemli-Opitz syndrome, and amyloidosis. Patients with primary adrenal insufficiency should undergo further evaluation to determine its cause (Table 214-5). Detection of antibodies to 21-hydroxylase identifies nearly all patients with idiopathic disease. In a male with negative results, measurement of plasma $C_{26:0}$ fatty acids will detect adrenoleukodystrophy. Taken together, this strategy identifies the cause in nearly all adult patients with idiopathic adrenal insufficiency. Patients with autoimmune disease should be tested for other endocrine deficiencies, and those with adrenoleukodystrophy require neurologic evaluation.

Secondary Adrenal Insufficiency
Suppression of the Pituitary Axis
Suppression of the hypothalamic-pituitary-adrenal axis by exogenous or endogenous glucocorticoids is the most common cause of secondary adrenal insufficiency. This phenomenon depends on the dose, duration, and schedule of glucocorticoid administration. Thus adrenal suppression is unusual with "replacement" doses of glucocorticoid that are roughly equivalent to daily production (e.g., total daily doses of 20 mg hydrocortisone, 5 mg prednisone, or 0.3 to 0.5 mg dexamethasone). At higher doses, adrenal suppression is usually not seen until after 3 weeks of administration, and a single morning administration is less suppressive than are divided doses given during the day. When potentially suppressive doses of glucocorticoids are stopped, symptoms of adrenal insufficiency may occur within 48 hours, and the entire axis may not recover for up to 18 months. During this time, the patient should receive replacement glucocorticoid treatment or supplemental steroids at times of physiologic stress, depending on the degree of impairment (see later). Chronic opiate use may suppress pituitary ACTH secretion, but the frequency of frank adrenal insufficiency appears uncommon.[19]

Lesions of the Hypothalamus or Pituitary
Secondary adrenal insufficiency also may result from structural lesions of the hypothalamus or pituitary gland that interfere with CRH production or transport or with corticotrope function. These causes include tumors, trauma, destruction by infiltrating disorders, x-irradiation, and lymphocytic hypophysitis. In general, these are not reversible conditions. Patients with secondary adrenal insufficiency not ascribed to glucocorticoid use should undergo imaging of the pituitary and hypothalamus to exclude a structural or infiltrating lesion as well as tests of other pituitary function to exclude additional deficiencies.

CLINICAL MANIFESTATIONS
The clinical presentation of adrenal insufficiency reflects the cause and duration of this uncommon condition. Primary adrenal insufficiency eventually destroys the entire adrenal cortex, with loss of both glucocorticoid and mineralocorticoid activity. By contrast, secondary adrenal insufficiency reflects an inability of the hypothalamic-pituitary unit to deliver CRH or ACTH, thus reducing trophic support to otherwise normal glands. As a result, only cortisol production decreases because mineralocorticoid production is not very ACTH dependent (Fig. 214-6).

The characteristic clinical presentation of acute primary adrenal insufficiency includes orthostatic hypotension, agitation, confusion, circulatory collapse, abdominal pain, and fever.[20] These features are most likely to be caused by hemorrhage, metastasis, or acute infection and can lead to death if not treated. In contrast, the typical history and clinical findings of chronic primary adrenal insufficiency include a longer history of malaise, fatigue, anorexia, weight loss, joint and back pain, and darkening of the skin (especially in the creases of the hands, extensor surfaces, recent scars, buccal and vaginal mucosa, and nipples). Patients may crave salt and may develop unusual food preferences, such as drinking the brine from pickles. Associated biochemical features for both acute and chronic presentations include hyponatremia, hypoglycemia, hyperkalemia, unexplained eosinophilia, and mild prerenal azotemia.

Chronic secondary adrenal insufficiency is manifested in a similar way, but without hyperpigmentation or mineralocorticoid abnormalities.

DIAGNOSIS
Biochemical testing confirms the diagnosis of adrenal insufficiency. A morning serum cortisol measurement is an inexpensive but relatively insensitive screening test for adrenal insufficiency in patients who are not acutely ill. The diagnosis is virtually excluded by values greater than 19 µg/dL (524 nmol/L) and is likely if the value is less than 3 µg/dL (83 nmol/L). However, both healthy individuals and patients with adrenal insufficiency may have indeterminate results (3 to 19 µg/dL) that require additional evaluation.

Patients with acute adrenal insufficiency should be evaluated for sepsis, adrenal metastases, and hemorrhage. Imaging of the glands and other testing

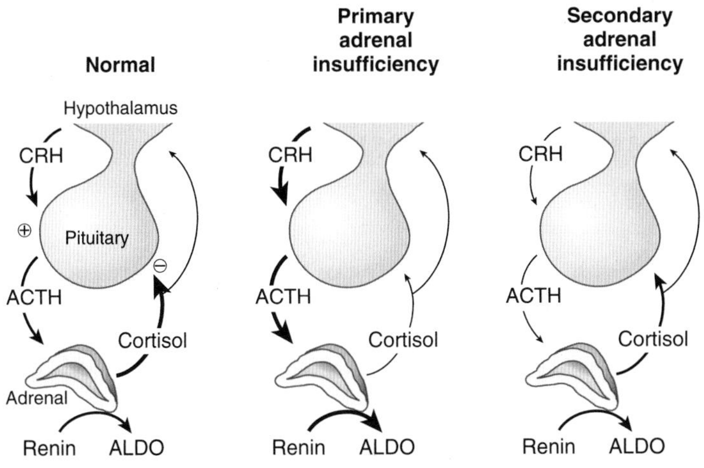

FIGURE 214-6. Physiology of the adrenal axis in health, primary adrenal insufficiency, and secondary adrenal insufficiency. *In healthy individuals* (Normal), cortisol production is stimulated by the increased hypothalamic release of corticotropin-releasing hormone (CRH), which then travels down the pituitary stalk to stimulate adrenocorticotropic hormone (ACTH) secretion and release by corticotropes. Circulating ACTH stimulates adrenal gland production and secretion of cortisol. Cortisol then functions in a negative feedback mechanism to inhibit both CRH and ACTH. *In patients with primary adrenal insufficiency,* destruction or replacement of the entire adrenal cortex results in decreased cortisol, aldosterone, and dehydroepiandrosterone (DHEA, not shown) secretion by the adrenal glands. As a result of decreased cortisol negative feedback, the normal hypothalamus and pituitary gland increase CRH and ACTH secretion. The decreased aldosterone levels lead to an increase in renin levels. *In patients with secondary adrenal insufficiency,* ACTH or CRH secretion is reduced because of destruction or replacement of the hypothalamus or pituitary gland or because of disruption of the pituitary stalk. The decreased ACTH stimulation results in decreased cortisol (and, not shown, DHEA) secretion by the adrenal glands. Aldosterone production is only slightly affected by ACTH stimulation, and levels remain normal. The abnormal hypothalamus and pituitary gland do not increase CRH and ACTH secretion in response to the decreased cortisol negative feedback.

may reveal an infectious cause. In acute adrenal insufficiency, a serum cortisol value is generally inappropriately normal or subnormal in the setting of hypotension, in which cortisol values are usually well above 18 µg/dL.

There is controversy about the best test to diagnose chronic adrenal insufficiency. Many use the cortisol response to exogenous ACTH as a gold standard test of adrenal steroidogenic ability. In the classic test, 250 µg of ACTH (1-24, cosyntropin) is given intravenously at any time of day. This dose of ACTH is a maximal stimulus to the adrenal gland, so that the serum cortisol level measured 30 to 60 minutes later is greater than 18 µg/dL. A 1-µg dose is equally good for establishing the diagnosis, but both doses are unfortunately associated with a substantial risk of a false-negative result.[21] Lower values indicate adrenal insufficiency. Insulin-induced hypoglycemia and metyrapone stimulation have been proposed as better tests for patients with mild or recent secondary adrenal insufficiency, who may respond to pharmacologic doses of ACTH. None of these is ideal. Also, because there is no commercial formulation of ACTH for lower-dose tests, the product must be diluted on site, leading to concerns about the accuracy of the administered dose and the validity of results. Metyrapone has limited availability in the United States.

Cerebral adrenoleukodystrophy, presenting in childhood, is characterized by cognitive and gait disturbances; the adult form, adrenomyeloneuropathy, is characterized by spinal cord and peripheral nerve demyelination. In both forms, the accumulation of very long chain fatty acids in the adrenal cortex alters membrane function and inhibits signal transduction by ACTH. Because a substantial minority of patients in both groups present first with adrenal insufficiency, boys and young men with adrenal insufficiency should be screened for adrenoleukodystrophy.

Differential Diagnosis

Primary and secondary adrenal insufficiency can be distinguished by measurement of plasma ACTH. In primary adrenal insufficiency, ACTH levels are generally above the normal range and may exceed the normal range before the cortisol response to exogenous ACTH stimulation is subnormal. In addition, hyperkalemia and elevated renin values are characteristic of primary but not of secondary adrenal insufficiency, which is identified by a suppressed or inappropriately normal ACTH level.

Acute Adrenal Insufficiency

In suspected acute adrenal insufficiency, hydrocortisone is the treatment of choice because it has both glucocorticoid and mineralocorticoid activity. Treatment with intravenous saline for volume expansion, glucose for hypoglycemia, and intravenous hydrocortisone (100 mg) is started immediately after placement of an intravenous line and withdrawal of blood for documentation of the cortisol value.

Chronic Adrenal Insufficiency

Therapy for chronic adrenal insufficiency[22] aims to provide the physiologic replacement of steroids. Glucocorticoid replacement is achieved by administration of 10 to 12 mg/m² of hydrocortisone daily in one to three oral doses, attempting to mimic the physiologic diurnal variation of cortisol concentrations. Hydrocortisone offers the advantage of multiple-dose tablets, which allows fine adjustment and splitting of the daily dose. Ideally, the morning dose is given as soon after waking as possible; for individuals who feel extremely fatigued in the morning before the agent is absorbed, a strategy of taking the medication 30 minutes before arising may be helpful. Some data suggest that once-daily dosing is preferable in terms of immune function, weight gain, and quality of life.[A3] Although many patients do well with a single dose, others complain of pronounced fatigue in the afternoon and evening. For them, a split-dose regimen, in which about one third of the daily dose is given around 4:00 PM or two afternoon doses are given, may be useful.

Other glucocorticoids may be used for daily replacement therapy. Prednisone, 5 to 7.5 mg daily, has the advantage of a long half-life and may be particularly helpful in patients with afternoon or evening fatigue. Dexamethasone may be used, but because of variable interindividual metabolism, it is difficult to recommend a specific replacement dose; in addition, few options for fixed doses are available, so it is difficult to adjust the dose.

Patients with primary adrenal insufficiency should be encouraged to salt their food and not to limit salt intake. Nearly all patients also require a mineralocorticoid, such as fludrocortisone 50 to 300 µg/day. The dose is adjusted until plasma renin activity is normal. If a mineralocorticoid is not given, the dose of hydrocortisone or other steroid with mineralocorticoid activity is often mistakenly increased to reduce an "unwell" feeling or hyperkalemia or salt craving. However, if a supraphysiologic dose is given, the patient becomes cushingoid.

Patients with primary adrenal insufficiency also have decreased serum DHEA levels. Controversy exists about its replacement. A meta-analysis concluded that there is insufficient evidence to support its routine use in these patients.

Ensuring Proper Dosing
Education of the Patient

All patients receiving chronic glucocorticoid replacement therapy should be instructed that they must take the glucocorticoids as prescribed and that failure to take or to absorb the medication will lead to adrenal crisis and possibly death. They should wear medical information bracelets or necklaces that identify this requirement. It is important to educate patients and their families about glucocorticoid adjustment during physiologic stress conditions, including the emergency administration of intramuscular glucocorticoid by means of a kit containing prefilled syringes with injectable steroid.

Dosing for Stress

The daily oral glucocorticoid dose is usually doubled for "stressful" physiologic conditions, such as fever, nausea, and diarrhea, although there are few data to support this strategy. In addition, this practice may lead to chronic overmedication by the patient because of a liberal interpretation of what constitutes physical stress. Thus education about when and how to change the dose of steroid should be reinforced periodically, preferably with written material, and the dangers of excessive steroid use should be emphasized. If the patient is vomiting, has severe diarrhea, or has collapsed, intramuscular glucocorticoids should be given before transport to a medical facility.

The glucocorticoid dose is increased in proportion to the amount of stress. Thus during maximally stressful situations (e.g., adrenal crisis, major surgery, trauma, labor and delivery), the daily hydrocortisone dose is 100 to 300 mg. Few data support the need for this supraphysiologic dose, but the safety of not following this practice has not been established. The dose may be tapered by 50% per day if the patient is clinically stable. For more moderate stress, such as that of cholecystectomy, 75 to 100 mg of hydrocortisone is given on the day of surgery, and the dose is tapered more rapidly. Patients undergoing minimal stress, such as tooth extraction or short operative orthopedic procedures, may not require any additional supplementation.

Assessment to Ensure Proper Dosing

Clinical assessment is the best way to judge whether the glucocorticoid dose is correct. Symptoms of adrenal insufficiency improve with adequate therapy. The development of cushingoid features or osteopenia suggests frank or subtle overreplacement, respectively, and the presence of adrenal insufficiency symptoms (fatigue, anorexia, weight loss) suggests underreplacement.

In women, DHEA replacement increases testosterone levels, so that hirsutism, acne, or other signs of androgen excess may suggest overreplacement. In primary adrenal insufficiency, adequate hormone replacement results in plasma ACTH levels that decrease but remain elevated, in the range of 100 to 200 pg/mL. Renin values, however, normalize completely and may be used to judge the adequacy of mineralocorticoid replacement. Although hydrocortisone is metabolized to cortisol, plasma cortisol values should not be used to monitor therapy because clearance from the bloodstream is rapid, and circulating values are low for most of the day. UFC does not reflect adequate replacement; the increase in plasma cortisol levels after a single daily dose may exceed corticosteroid-binding globulin capacity, resulting in excessive urine levels and overestimation of integrated cortisol levels.

PROGNOSIS

Even in educated patients with chronic adrenal insufficiency, adrenal crisis develops at a rate of 8.3 crises per 100 patient-years. Common precipitating causes include gastrointestinal infection, fever, and emotional stress (about 20% of cases each), but major pain, surgery, strenuous physical activity, heat, and pregnancy are other precipitants. About 6% of crises are fatal.[23]

Mineralocorticoid Deficiency

Hypoaldosteronism may be classified as a low-normal or a high renin state on the basis of plasma renin activity after 4 hours of upright posture. Renin deficiency is the most common cause of hypoaldosteronism, occurring most often in older patients with mild, nonoliguric renal disease who often have insulin-dependent diabetes and potentially diabetic nephropathy. Indomethacin and other prostaglandin synthesis inhibitors as well as autonomic dysfunction associated with prolonged bed rest can also result in hyporeninemic hypoaldosteronism.

CLINICAL MANIFESTATIONS

There are few clinical features associated with mineralocorticoid deficiency; as a result, it is usually suspected when laboratory results reveal hyperkalemia, hyponatremia, and a mild metabolic alkalosis. If glucocorticoid deficiency is excluded, isolated hypoaldosteronism is established if the circulating level of aldosterone is inappropriately low.

High renin states of hypoaldosteronism include congenital adrenal hyperplasias with mineralocorticoid deficiency and primary adrenal insufficiency when it is treated with pure glucocorticoid replacement.

Treatment of these conditions involves sodium replacement with at least 10 mEq/kg/day, roughly equivalent to the 4 g of sodium chloride found in a typical diet in the United States. For individuals who do not maintain such a diet (often the elderly or the young), fludrocortisone can be given at the same doses used in primary adrenal insufficiency.

Grade A References

A1. Lacroix A, Gu F, Gallardo W, et al. Efficacy and safety of once-monthly pasireotide in Cushing's disease: a 12 month clinical trial. *Lancet Diabetes Endocrinol.* 2018;6:17-26.
A2. Fassnacht M, Terzolo M, Allolio B, et al. Combination chemotherapy in advanced adrenocortical carcinoma. *N Engl J Med.* 2012;366:2189-2197.
A3. Isidori AM, Venneri MA, Graziadio C, et al. Effect of once-daily, modified-release hydrocortisone versus standard glucocorticoid therapy on metabolism and innate immunity in patients with adrenal insufficiency (DREAM): a single-blind, randomised controlled trial. *Lancet Diabetes Endocrinol.* 2018;6:173-185.

GENERAL REFERENCES

For the General References and other additional features, please visit Expert Consult at https://expertconsult.inkling.com.

215

ADRENAL MEDULLA, CATECHOLAMINES, AND PHEOCHROMOCYTOMA

WILLIAM F. YOUNG, JR.

ADRENAL MEDULLA AND CATECHOLAMINES

The adrenal medulla occupies the central portion of the adrenal gland. Adrenomedullary cells are called chromaffin cells (they stain brown with chromium salts). Chromaffin cells differentiate in the center of the adrenal gland in response to cortisol; some chromaffin cells also migrate to form paraganglia. The largest cluster of chromaffin cells outside the adrenal medulla is near the level of the inferior mesenteric artery and is referred to as the organ of Zuckerkandl.

Catecholamines are substances that contain catechol (*o*-dihydroxybenzene) and a side chain with an amino group—the catechol nucleus (Fig. 215-1). Epinephrine is synthesized and stored in the adrenal medulla and released into the systemic circulation. Norepinephrine is synthesized and stored not only in the adrenal medulla but also in the peripheral sympathetic nerves. Dopamine, the precursor of norepinephrine, is found in the adrenal medulla and peripheral sympathetic nerves.

Catecholamines have many cardiovascular and metabolic actions, including increasing the heart rate, blood pressure, myocardial contractility, and cardiac conduction velocity. Three types of specific adrenergic receptors mediate their biologic actions: α, β, and DA. Their receptor subtypes are α_1, α_2, β_1, β_2, β_3, DA_1, and DA_2. The α_1 subtype is a postsynaptic receptor that mediates vascular and smooth muscle contraction; stimulation causes vasoconstriction and increased blood pressure. The α_2-receptors are located on presynaptic sympathetic nerve endings and, when activated, inhibit the release of norepinephrine; stimulation causes suppression in central sympathetic outflow and decreased blood pressure. Stimulation of the β_1-receptor causes positive inotropic and chronotropic effects on the heart, increased renin secretion in the kidney, and lipolysis in adipocytes as well as bronchodilation, vasodilation in skeletal muscle, glycogenolysis, and increased release of norepinephrine from sympathetic nerve terminals. The β_3-receptor regulates energy expenditure and lipolysis. DA_1 receptors are localized to the cerebral, renal, mesenteric, and coronary vasculature; stimulation causes vasodilation in these vascular beds. DA_2 receptors are presynaptic and localized to sympathetic nerve endings, sympathetic ganglia, and brain; their stimulation inhibits the release of norepinephrine, inhibits ganglionic transmission, and inhibits prolactin release.

Catecholamines are synthesized from tyrosine by a process of hydroxylation and decarboxylation (see Fig. 215-1). Tyrosine is derived from the diet or synthesized from phenylalanine in the liver, and it enters neurons and chromaffin cells by active transport. Tyrosine is converted to 3,4-dihydroxyphenylalanine (dopa) by tyrosine hydroxylase, the rate-limiting step in catecholamine synthesis. α-Methyl-*p*-tyrosine (metyrosine) is a tyrosine hydroxylase inhibitor that may be used therapeutically in patients with catecholamine-secreting tumors. Aromatic L-amino acid decarboxylase catalyzes the decarboxylation of dopa to dopamine. Dopamine is actively transported into granulated vesicles to be hydroxylated to norepinephrine by the dopamine β-hydroxylase. These reactions occur in the synaptic vesicle of adrenergic neurons and the chromaffin cells of the adrenal medulla. In the adrenal medulla, norepinephrine is released from the granule into the cytoplasm, where phenylethanolamine N-methyltransferase converts it to epinephrine. Expression of phenylethanolamine N-methyltransferase is positively regulated by glucocorticoids. Thus catecholamine-secreting tumors that secrete primarily epinephrine are localized to the adrenal medulla. In normal adrenal medullary tissue, approximately 80% of the catecholamine released is epinephrine.

The biologic half-life of circulating catecholamines is between 10 and 100 seconds. Thus plasma concentrations of catecholamines fluctuate widely. Catecholamines are removed from the circulation by either reuptake by sympathetic nerve terminals or metabolism through two enzyme pathways (see Fig. 215-1), followed by sulfate conjugation and renal excretion. Almost 90% of catecholamines released at sympathetic synapses are taken up locally by the nerve endings (uptake 1). Uptake 1 can be blocked by cocaine, tricyclic antidepressants, and phenothiazine. Extraneuronal tissues also take up

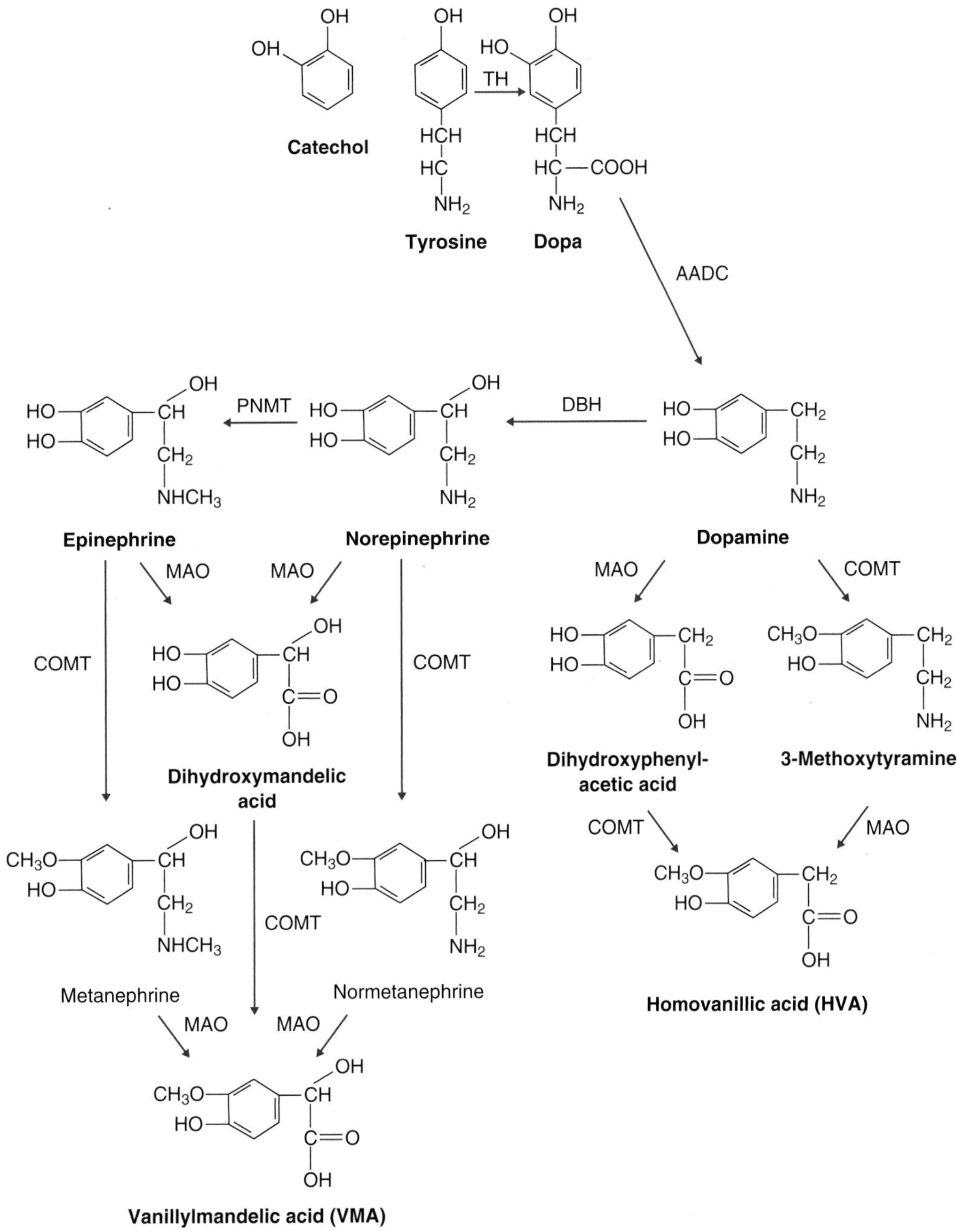

FIGURE 215-1. Biosynthetic and metabolic pathways for catecholamines. The term *catecholamine* comes from the catechol (*o*-dihydroxybenzene) structure and a side chain with an amino group—the catechol nucleus (*top left*). Tyrosine is converted to 3,4-dihydroxyphenylalanine (dopa) in the rate-limiting step by tyrosine hydroxylase (TH). Aromatic L-amino acid decarboxylase (AADC) converts dopa to dopamine. Dopamine is hydroxylated to norepinephrine by dopamine β-hydroxylase (DBH). Norepinephrine is converted to epinephrine by phenylethanolamine *N*-methyltransferase (PNMT); cortisol serves as a cofactor for PNMT, and this is why epinephrine-secreting pheochromocytomas are almost exclusively localized to the adrenal medulla. Metabolism of catecholamines occurs through two enzymatic pathways. Catechol-*O*-methyltransferase (COMT) converts epinephrine to metanephrine and norepinephrine to normetanephrine by meta-*O*-methylation. Metanephrine and normetanephrine are oxidized by monoamine oxidase (MAO) to vanillylmandelic acid by oxidative deamination. Monoamine oxidase also may oxidize epinephrine and norepinephrine to dihydroxymandelic acid, which is then converted by catechol-*O*-methyltransferase to vanillyl-mandelic acid. Dopamine is also metabolized by monoamine oxidase and catechol-*O*-methyltransferase, with the final metabolite homovanillic acid.

catecholamines (uptake 2). Most of these catecholamines are metabolized by catechol-*O*-methyltransferase. Metanephrine and normetanephrine are oxidized by monoamine oxidase to vanillylmandelic acid by oxidative deamination. Monoamine oxidase may also oxidize epinephrine and norepinephrine to 3,4-dihydroxymandelic acid, which is then converted by catechol-*O*-methyl-transferase to vanillylmandelic acid. In the storage vesicle, norepinephrine is protected from metabolism by monoamine oxidase. Monoamine oxidase and catechol-*O*-methyltransferase metabolize dopamine to homovanillic acid (see Fig. 215-1).

PHEOCHROMOCYTOMA AND PARAGANGLIOMA

DEFINITION

Catecholamine-secreting tumors that arise from chromaffin cells of the adrenal medulla and the sympathetic ganglia are referred to as pheochromocytomas

and extra-adrenal catecholamine-secreting paragangliomas, respectively. Because the tumors have similar clinical presentations and are treated with similar approaches, many clinicians use the term *pheochromocytoma* to refer to both entities. However, the distinction between pheochromocytoma and paraganglioma is an important one because there are differences in the risk for associated neoplasms, risk for malignant transformation, and type of genetic testing that should be considered.[1,2]

EPIDEMIOLOGY

Catecholamine-secreting tumors are rare; the annual incidence is 2 to 8 cases per million people. Nevertheless, it is important to suspect, confirm, localize, and resect these tumors. The associated hypertension is curable with surgical removal of the tumor, a risk of lethal paroxysm exists, and at least 10% of the tumors are malignant. Approximately 40% of cases are familial, so detection of this tumor in the proband may result in early diagnosis in other family members.

PATHOBIOLOGY

Genetics

Approximately 40% of patients with catecholamine-secreting tumors have germline mutations (inherited mutations present in all cells of the body) in genes associated with the genetic disease.[3] Hereditary catecholamine-secreting tumors typically are manifested at a younger age than sporadic neoplasms. Sporadic pheochromocytoma is typically diagnosed on the basis of symptoms or incidental discovery on computed imaging, whereas syndromic pheochromocytoma and paraganglioma are frequently diagnosed earlier in the course of disease because of biochemical surveillance or genetic testing.

Multiple Endocrine Neoplasia

Multiple endocrine neoplasia (MEN) type 2A is an autosomal dominant disorder (Chapter 218). The phenotype includes adrenal pheochromocytoma in 50% (usually bilateral and may be asynchronous), medullary carcinoma of the thyroid in 100%, hyperparathyroidism in 20 to 30%, and cutaneous lichen amyloidosis in 5%.[4] Medullary carcinoma of the thyroid is usually detected before pheochromocytoma. Numerous activating mutations in the *RET* proto-oncogene have been documented in persons with MEN type 2A.

MEN type 2B is also an autosomal dominant disorder, and it represents approximately 5% of all MEN type 2 cases. The phenotype includes pheochromocytoma in 50% (usually bilateral), aggressive medullary carcinoma of the thyroid in 100%, mucosal neuromas (typically involving the tongue, lips, and eyelids) in most patients, thickened corneal nerves, intestinal ganglioneuromatosis, and marfanoid body habitus. MEN 2B–associated tumors are caused by mutations in the RET protein's intracellular domain, as described in detail in Chapter 218.

Von Hippel–Lindau Disease

Von Hippel–Lindau (VHL) disease is an autosomal dominant disorder characterized by pheochromocytoma (frequently bilateral), paraganglioma (skull base, mediastinal, abdominal, pelvic), hemangioblastoma (involving the cerebellum, spinal cord, or brain stem), retinal angioma, clear cell renal cell carcinoma, pancreatic neuroendocrine tumor, endolymphatic sac tumor of the middle ear, serous cystadenoma of the pancreas, and papillary cystadenoma of the epididymis and broad ligament.[5] Pheochromocytoma occurs in about 10 to 20% of patients with VHL disease. Nearly 100% of patients have an identifiable gene mutation (VHL tumor suppressor gene).[6] Certain missense mutations appear to be associated with a "pheochromocytoma only" presentation of VHL disease.

Neurofibromatosis

Neurofibromatosis type 1 (NF1) is an autosomal dominant disorder characterized by neurofibromas, multiple café au lait spots, axillary and inguinal freckling, iris hamartomas (Lisch nodules), bone abnormalities, central nervous system gliomas, pheochromocytoma and paraganglioma, macrocephaly, and cognitive deficits. The expression of these features is variable. Approximately 3% of patients with NF1 develop catecholamine-secreting tumors; in these patients, the tumor is usually a solitary benign adrenal pheochromocytoma, occasionally bilateral adrenal pheochromocytomas, and rarely an abdominal paraganglioma.[7] Inactivating *NF1* mutations cause the disorder (*NF1* tumor suppressor gene).

Familial Paraganglioma

Familial paraganglioma is an autosomal dominant disorder characterized by paragangliomas that are located in the skull base and neck, thorax, abdomen, and pelvis. Most cases of familial paraganglioma are caused by mutations in the succinate dehydrogenase (SDH; succinate:ubiquinone oxidoreductase) subunit genes (*SDHB, SDHC, SDHD, SDHAF2, SDHA*), which compose portions of mitochondrial complex II. In patients with *SDHD* mutations, penetrance depends on the mutation's parent of origin. Hence, the disease does not manifest when the mutation is inherited from the mother but is highly penetrant when it is inherited from the father. This phenomenon is known as maternal imprinting. Multiple cofactors are required for normal activity of the SDH complex, including flavin adenine dinucleotide (FAD) in the SDH1 subunit. FAD is covalently attached to Sdh1, and deletion of *SDHAF2* causes a complete loss of FAD cofactor attachment (flavination) of Sdh1. Like families with mutations in *SDHD*, those with mutations in *SDHAF2* also exhibit maternal imprinting and parasympathetic paragangliomas that typically occur in the skull base and neck. Patients with *SDHB* mutations have an increased risk for malignant paraganglioma.

Genetic Testing

Since 1990, 15 different pheochromocytoma and paraganglioma susceptibility genes have been reported: *NF1, RET, VHL, SDHD, SDHC, SDHB, EGLN1/PHD2, KIF1B, SDHAF2, IDH1, TMEM127, SDHA, MAX, HIF2A,* and *FH* gene encoding fumarate hydratase.[8]

Genetic testing should be considered if a patient has one or more of the following: paraganglioma, bilateral adrenal pheochromocytomas, unilateral adrenal pheochromocytoma and a family history of pheochromocytoma or paraganglioma, onset of unilateral adrenal pheochromocytoma at a young age (before 45 years), or other clinical findings suggestive of one of the previously discussed syndromic disorders. Genetic testing can be complex; testing of one family member has implications for related individuals.[9,10] Genetic counseling is recommended to help families understand the implications of genetic test results; to coordinate the testing of at-risk individuals; and to help families work through the psychosocial issues that may arise before, during, or after the testing process. A list of clinically approved molecular genetic diagnostic laboratories is available at www.genetests.org.

CLINICAL MANIFESTATIONS

Catecholamine-secreting tumors occur with equal frequency in men and women, primarily in the third, fourth, and fifth decades of life. These tumors are rare in children; when discovered, they may be multifocal, extra-adrenal, metastatic, and associated with a hereditary syndrome.[11] When symptoms are present, they are due to the pharmacologic effects of excess concentrations of circulating catecholamines (Table 215-1). The resulting hypertension may be

TABLE 215-1 SIGNS AND SYMPTOMS ASSOCIATED WITH CATECHOLAMINE-SECRETING TUMORS

SPELL RELATED

Anxiety and fear of impending death
Diaphoresis
Dyspnea
Epigastric and chest pain
Headache
Hypertension
Nausea and vomiting
Pallor
Palpitation (forceful heartbeat)
Tremor

CHRONIC

Cold hands and feet
Congestive heart failure—dilated or hypertrophic cardiomyopathy
Constipation (megacolon)
Diaphoresis
Dyspnea
Ectopic hormone secretion–dependent symptoms (e.g., CRH/ACTH, GHRH, PTH-RP, VIP)
Epigastric and chest pain
Erythrocytosis
Fatigue
Fever
Grade II to IV retinopathy
Headache
Hyperglycemia
Hypertension
Livedo reticularis
Orthostatic hypotension
Painless hematuria (associated with urinary bladder paraganglioma)
Palpitation (forceful heartbeat)
Raynaud phenomenon
Tremor
Weight loss

NOT TYPICAL OF PHEOCHROMOCYTOMA

Flushing

ACTH = adrenocorticotropic hormone; CRH = corticotropin-releasing hormone; GHRH = growth hormone–releasing hormone; PTH-RP = parathyroid hormone–related peptide; VIP = vasoactive intestinal polypeptide.
Modified from Young WF Jr. Pheochromocytoma: 1926-1993. *Trends Endocrinol Metab.* 1993;4:122-127.

sustained (in approximately half of patients) or paroxysmal (in approximately a third of patients). The remaining patients have normal blood pressure. Episodic symptoms may occur in spells, or paroxysms, that can be extremely variable in presentation but typically include forceful heartbeat, pallor, tremor, headache, and diaphoresis. The spell may start with the sensation of a "rush" in the chest and a sense of shortness of breath, followed by a "pounding" heartbeat in the chest that typically progresses to a throbbing headache. Peripheral vasoconstriction with a spell results in cool or cold hands and feet and facial pallor. Increased sense of body heat and sweating are common symptoms that occur toward the end of the spell. Spells may be spontaneous or precipitated by postural change, anxiety, medications (e.g., metoclopramide, β-adrenergic inhibitors, anesthetic agents, corticosteroids), exercise, or maneuvers that increase intraabdominal pressure (e.g., change in position, lifting, defecation, exercise, colonoscopy, pregnancy, trauma). Although the types of spells experienced by patients are highly variable, spells tend to be stereotypical for each patient. Spells may occur multiple times a day or as infrequently as once a month. The typical duration of a pheochromocytoma spell is 15 to 20 minutes, but it may be much shorter or last several hours. The clinician must recognize that most patients with spells do not have a pheochromocytoma.

Fasting hyperglycemia and diabetes mellitus are caused in part by the α-adrenergic inhibition of insulin release. Some of the cosecreted hormones that may dominate the clinical presentation include corticotropin (Cushing syndrome), parathyroid hormone–related peptide (hypercalcemia), vasopressin (syndrome of inappropriate antidiuretic hormone secretion), vasoactive intestinal peptide (watery diarrhea), and growth hormone–releasing hormone (acromegaly) (see Table 215-1). Cardiomyopathy and congestive heart failure are the symptomatic presentations of pheochromocytoma that are most frequently unrecognized by clinicians. Cardiomyopathy, whether dilated or hypertrophic, may be totally reversible with tumor resection. Some patients with pheochromocytoma may be asymptomatic despite high circulating levels of catecholamines, probably reflecting adrenergic receptor desensitization related to chronic stimulation.

Symptomatic pheochromocytomas are localized to the adrenal glands, with an average diameter of 4.5 cm (Fig. 215-2). Paragangliomas are found where there is chromaffin tissue: along the para-aortic sympathetic chain, within the organs of Zuckerkandl (at the origin of the inferior mesenteric artery), in the wall of the urinary bladder, and along the sympathetic chain in the neck or mediastinum. Paragangliomas in the skull base and neck region (e.g., carotid body tumors, glomus tumors, chemodectomas) usually arise from parasympathetic tissue and typically do not hypersecrete catecholamines and metanephrines, whereas paragangliomas in the mediastinum, abdomen, and pelvis usually arise from sympathetic chromaffin tissue and usually do hypersecrete catecholamines and metanephrines.

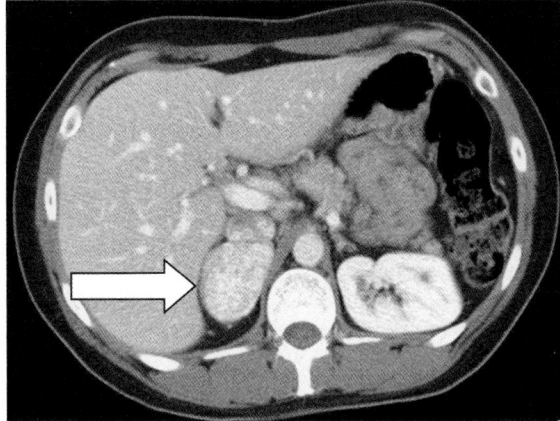

FIGURE 215-2. Contrast-enhanced computed tomography of the abdomen in a 32-year-old second-year medical student with the peripartum discovery of a pheochromocytoma. The plasma fractionated metanephrines were abnormal: metanephrine, 0.19 nmol/L (normal, <0.5 nmol/L); normetanephrine, 28.6 nmol/L (normal, <0.9 nmol/L). The 24-hour urine values were abnormal: norepinephrine, 781 µg (normal, <170 µg); epinephrine, 2.4 µg (normal, <35 µg); dopamine, 197 µg (normal, <700 µg); metanephrine, 117 µg (normal, <400 µg); normetanephrine, 8760 µg (normal, <900 µg). The axial image shows a typical 5-cm heterogeneously enhancing right adrenal mass, consistent with pheochromocytoma (*arrow*). After α- and β-adrenergic blockade, a 5.3 × 5.0 × 2.0–cm, 40-g pheochromocytoma was removed laparoscopically.

DIAGNOSIS
Differential Diagnosis
Numerous disorders can cause signs and symptoms that may lead the clinician to test for pheochromocytoma. These disorders span much of medicine and include endocrine disorders (e.g., primary hypogonadism), cardiovascular disorders (e.g., idiopathic orthostatic hypotension), psychological disorders (e.g., panic disorder), pharmacologic causes (e.g., withdrawal from an adrenergic inhibitor), neurologic disorders (e.g., postural orthostatic tachycardia syndrome), and miscellaneous disorders (e.g., mast cell disease). Indeed, most patients tested for pheochromocytoma do not have it. In addition, fractionated catecholamines and metanephrines may be elevated in several clinical scenarios: withdrawal from medications or drugs (e.g., clonidine, alcohol), any acute illness (e.g., subarachnoid hemorrhage, migraine headache, preeclampsia), and administration of many drugs and medications (e.g., tricyclic antidepressants, levodopa, cocaine, phencyclidine, lysergic acid diethylamide, amphetamines, ephedrine, pseudoephedrine, phenylpropanolamine, isoproterenol) (Table 215-2).

Pheochromocytoma should be suspected in patients who have one or more of the following: hyperadrenergic spells (e.g., self-limited episodes of nonexertional palpitations, diaphoresis, headache, tremor, or pallor); resistant hypertension; a familial syndrome that predisposes to catecholamine-secreting tumors (e.g., MEN type 2, NF1, VHL disease); a family history of pheochromocytoma or a history of a resected pheochromocytoma and a present history of recurrent hypertension or spells; an incidentally discovered adrenal mass with increased precontrast CT attenuation of more than 20 Hounsfield units (HU); hypertension and diabetes; pressor response during anesthesia, surgery, or angiography; onset of hypertension at a young age (before 20 years); and idiopathic dilated cardiomyopathy.

Laboratory Findings
The diagnosis must be confirmed biochemically by increased concentrations of fractionated metanephrines in the plasma or fractionated catecholamines and metanephrines in a 24-hour urine collection (Fig. 215-3). Most laboratories now measure fractionated catecholamines (dopamine, norepinephrine, and epinephrine) and metanephrines (metanephrine and normetanephrine) by high-performance liquid chromatography with electrochemical detection or tandem mass spectroscopy.[12,13] These techniques have overcome the problems with fluorometric analysis (e.g., false-positive results caused by α-methyldopa, labetalol, sotalol, and imaging contrast agents). One of the most reliable methods of identifying catecholamine-secreting tumors is measurement of fractionated metanephrines and catecholamines in a 24-hour urine collection (sensitivity, 98%; specificity, 98%). If clinical suspicion is high, plasma fractionated metanephrines should also be measured. Some groups have advocated the measurement of plasma fractionated metanephrines as a first-line test for pheochromocytoma; the predictive value of a negative test result is extremely high, and the finding of normal plasma fractionated metanephrines excludes pheochromocytoma, except in patients with early preclinical disease and those with strictly dopamine-secreting neoplasms. A plasma test is also attractive because of its simplicity. Although measurement of plasma fractionated metanephrines has a sensitivity of 96 to 100%, the specificity is poor at only 85 to 89%; the specificity falls to 77% in patients older than 60

TABLE 215-2	MEDICATIONS THAT MAY INCREASE MEASURED LEVELS OF CATECHOLAMINES AND METANEPHRINES

Tricyclic antidepressants (including cyclobenzaprine)

Levodopa

Drugs containing adrenergic receptor agonists (e.g., decongestants)

Amphetamines

Buspirone and antipsychotic agents

Monamine oxidase inhibitors (MAO inhibitors)

Prochlorperazine

Reserpine

Serotonin and norepinephrine reuptake inhibitors (SNRIs)

Withdrawal from clonidine and other drugs

Ethanol

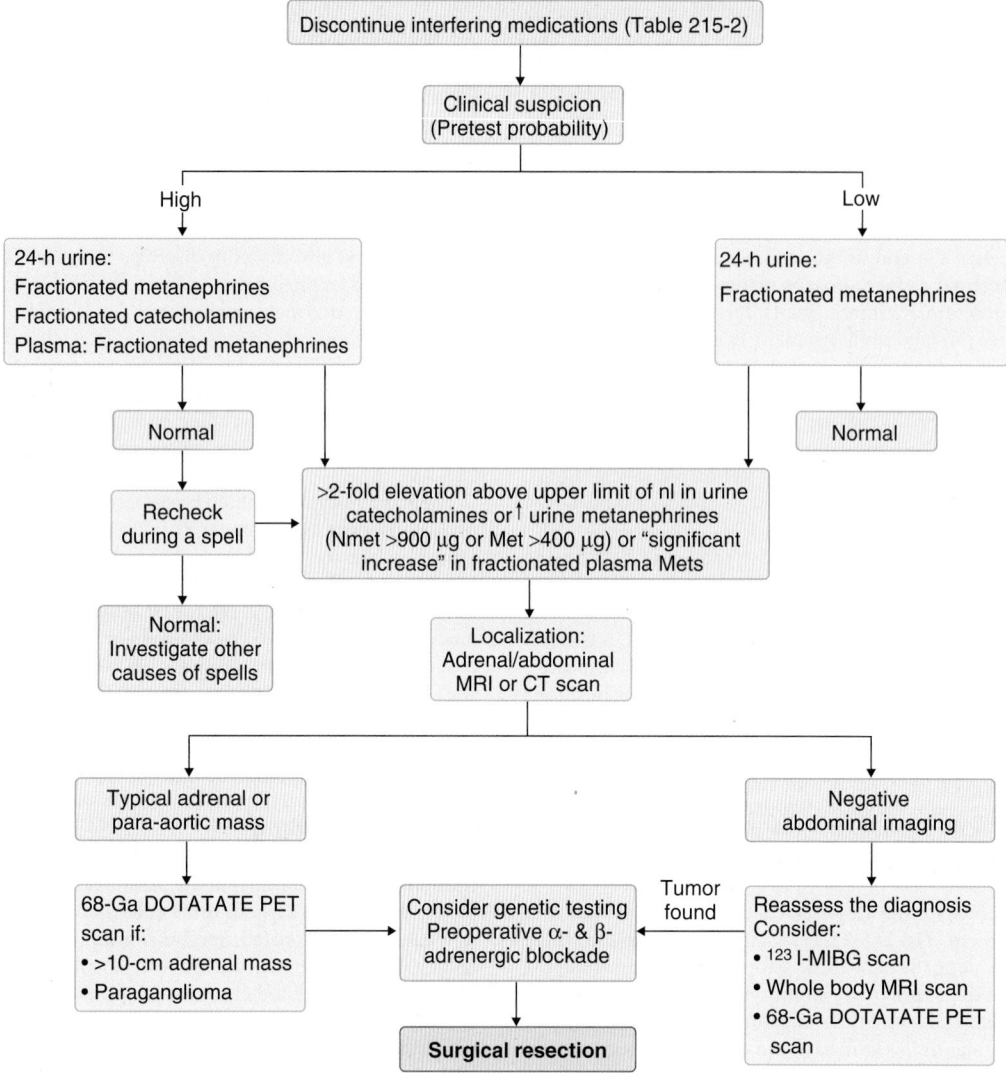

FIGURE 215-3. Evaluation and treatment of catecholamine-secreting tumors. Clinical suspicion is triggered by the following: paroxysmal symptoms (especially hypertension); hypertension that is intermittent, unusually labile, or resistant to treatment; family history of pheochromocytoma or associated conditions; or incidentally discovered adrenal mass. The details are discussed in the text. CT = computed tomography; Ga-68 DOTATATE = gallium 68 1,4,7,10-tetraazacyclododecane-1,4,7,10-tetraacetic acid (DOTA)-octreotate; ^{123}I-MIBG = ^{123}I-metaiodobenzylguanidine; Met = metanephrine; MRI = magnetic resonance imaging; nl = normal; Nmet = normetanephrine; PET = positron emission tomography. (Modified from Young WF Jr. Pheochromocytoma: 1926-1993. *Trends Endocrinol Metab.* 1993;4:122.)

years. It has been estimated that 97% of patients with hypertension seen in a tertiary care clinic who have abnormal plasma fractionated metanephrine measurements do not have pheochromocytoma. This high false-positive rate results in excessive health care expenditures because of subsequent imaging as well as potentially inappropriate surgery. Thus plasma fractionated metanephrines lack the necessary specificity to be recommended as a first-line test; this measurement is reserved for cases in which the index of suspicion is high. However, measurement of plasma fractionated metanephrines is a good first-line test for children, in whom it is difficult to obtain a complete 24-hour urine collection.

The index of suspicion for pheochromocytoma should be high (see Fig. 215-3) in patients with the clinical scenarios described earlier and in those with an incidentally discovered adrenal mass that has imaging characteristics consistent with pheochromocytoma. These include increased precontrast computed tomography (CT) attenuation (e.g., >10 HU), marked enhancement with intravenous contrast medium on CT with slow contrast washout, high signal intensity on T2-weighted magnetic resonance imaging (MRI), cystic and hemorrhagic changes, bilaterality, and large size (>4 cm) (see later).

Although it is preferable for patients not to receive any medications during the diagnostic evaluation, treatment with most medications can be continued. Tricyclic antidepressants interfere most frequently with the interpretation of fractionated catecholamines and metanephrines. For the effective detection of catecholamine-secreting tumors, treatment with tricyclic antidepressants and other psychoactive agents listed in Table 215-2 should be tapered and discontinued at least 2 weeks before any hormonal assessments.

Furthermore, catecholamine secretion may be appropriately increased in situations of physical stress or illness (e.g., stroke, myocardial infarction, congestive heart failure, obstructive sleep apnea). Therefore the clinical circumstances under which catecholamines and metanephrines are measured must be assessed in each case.

Imaging

Localization studies should not be initiated until biochemical studies have confirmed the diagnosis of a catecholamine-secreting tumor (see Fig. 215-3). Computer-assisted imaging of the adrenal glands and abdomen with CT or MRI should be the first localization test (sensitivity, >95%; specificity, >65%). Approximately 85% of these tumors are found in the adrenal glands, and 95% are found in the abdomen. If the results of abdominal imaging are normal, localization with gallium 68 1,4,7,10-tetraazacyclododecane-1,4,7,10-tetraacetic acid (DOTA)-octreotate positron emission tomography (68-Ga DOTATATE PET) is indicated (see Fig. 215-3). Ga-68 DOTATATE PET CT has a lesion-based detection rate of 96-98% and is superior to ^{123}I metaiodobenzyl guanidine (^{123}I-MIBG) scintigraphy.[14–16] If a typical (<10 cm) unilateral adrenal pheochromocytoma is found on CT or MRI, Ga-68 DOTATATE PET CT or MIBG is superfluous. If the adrenal pheochromocytoma is larger than 10 cm in diameter or if a paraganglioma is identified on CT or MRI, Ga-68 DOTATATE PET CT or ^{123}I-MIBG scintigraphy is indicated because the patient has an increased risk of malignant disease and additional paragangliomas. Ga-68 DOTATATE and ^{18}F-fluorodeoxyglucose positron emission tomography are excellent imaging modalities to detect metastatic disease.

Other localizing procedures that can be used but are rarely required include computer-assisted imaging of the chest, skull base, and neck (see Fig. 215-3). Because of marked gradients between the adrenal glands in nonpheochromocytoma patients, adrenal venous sampling for catecholamines is not helpful in the investigation of adrenal pheochromocytoma.

TREATMENT Rx

Medical Therapy

Some form of preoperative pharmacologic preparation is indicated for all patients with catecholamine-secreting neoplasms. However, no randomized controlled trials have compared the different approaches. Combined α- and β-adrenergic blockade is one approach to control blood pressure and to prevent intraoperative hypertensive crises. α-Adrenergic blockade should be started 7 to 10 days preoperatively to normalize blood pressure and to expand the contracted blood volume. A longer duration of preoperative α-adrenergic blockade is indicated in patients with recent myocardial infarction, catecholamine cardiomyopathy, and catecholamine-induced vasculitis. Blood pressure should be monitored with the patient in the seated and standing positions twice daily. Target blood pressure is less than 120/80 mm Hg (seated), with systolic blood pressure greater than 90 mm Hg (standing); both targets should be modified on the basis of the patient's age and comorbid disease. On the second or third day of α-adrenergic blockade, patients are encouraged to start a diet high in sodium content (≥5000 mg daily) because of the catecholamine-induced volume contraction and the orthostasis associated with α-adrenergic blockade. This degree of volume expansion may be contraindicated in patients with congestive heart failure or renal insufficiency. After adequate α-adrenergic blockade has been achieved, β-adrenergic blockade is initiated if the average heart rate is greater than 80 beats per minute.

Phenoxybenzamine is the preferred drug to control blood pressure and arrhythmia preoperatively.[17] It is an irreversible, long-acting, nonspecific α-adrenergic blocking agent. The initial dosage is 10 mg once or twice daily, and the dose is increased by 10 to 20 mg in divided doses every 2 or 3 days as needed to control blood pressure and spells. The final dosage of phenoxybenzamine is typically between 20 and 100 mg daily. By comparison, the more selective α-adrenergic blocking agent doxazosin appears to cause more transient intraoperative hypotension during surgery and a greater need for postoperative blood pressure support.[18]

The β-adrenergic antagonist should be administered only after α-adrenergic blockade is effective; with β-adrenergic blockade alone, hypertension may be more severe from the unopposed α-adrenergic stimulation. Preoperative β-adrenergic blockade is indicated to control the tachycardia associated with both the high concentrations of circulating catecholamines and the α-adrenergic blockade. The clinician should exercise caution if the patient is asthmatic or has heart failure. Chronic catecholamine excess can produce a cardiomyopathy that may become evident with the initiation of β-adrenergic blockade, resulting in acute pulmonary edema.[19] Therefore, the β-adrenergic blocker should be administered cautiously and at a low dose. Other agents that may be used to prepare the patient with pheochromocytoma for surgery include α-methyl-*p*-tyrosine (metyrosine) and calcium-channel blockers. Despite treatment, normotensive patients with pheochromocytomas have roughly comparable perioperative hemodynamic instability to hypertensive pheochromocytoma patients, and both differ markedly from nonpheochromocytoma patients undergoing adrenal surgery.[20] Acute hypertensive crises may occur before or during an operation, and they should be treated with intravenous sodium nitroprusside, phentolamine, or nicardipine.

Surgical Therapy

The treatment of choice for pheochromocytoma is complete surgical resection. Surgical survival rates are 98 to 100% and are highly dependent on the skill of the endocrinologist–endocrine surgeon–anesthesiologist team. Careful preoperative pharmacologic preparation is crucial for successful treatment. Most catecholamine-secreting tumors are benign and can be totally excised. Tumor excision usually cures hypertension.

The laparoscopic approach to the adrenal gland is the procedure of choice for a solitary intra-adrenal pheochromocytoma smaller than 8 cm in diameter. Surgical expertise is key to avoid intraoperative tumor capsule rupture. Laparoscopic adrenalectomy for pheochromocytoma should be converted to open adrenalectomy in cases of difficult dissection, invasion, adhesions, or an inexperienced surgeon. An anterior midline abdominal surgical approach is indicated for abdominal paragangliomas. Paragangliomas of the neck, chest, and urinary bladder require specialized approaches.

Management of Complications

Hypotension may occur during and after surgical resection of the pheochromocytoma, and it should be treated with fluids and colloids and then intravenous pressor agents if necessary. Postoperative hypotension is less frequent in patients who have had adequate preoperative α-adrenergic blockade and volume expansion. If both adrenal glands were manipulated during surgery, adrenocortical insufficiency should be considered a potential cause of postoperative hypotension. Because hypoglycemia can occur in the immediate postoperative period, blood glucose levels should be monitored, and intravenous fluids should contain 5% dextrose.

Approximately 1 to 2 weeks after surgery, fractionated catecholamines and metanephrines should be measured by collection of a 24-hour urine specimen. If the levels are normal, resection of the pheochromocytoma should be considered complete. Increased levels of fractionated catecholamines and metanephrines detected postoperatively are consistent with residual tumor due to either a second primary lesion or occult metastases.

Follow-up

The 24-hour urinary excretion of fractionated catecholamines and metanephrines or plasma fractionated metanephrines should be checked annually for life. Annual biochemical testing assesses for metastatic disease, tumor recurrence in the adrenal bed, or delayed appearance of multiple primary tumors. Follow-up CT or MRI is not needed unless the metanephrine or catecholamine levels become elevated or the original tumor was associated with minimal or no catecholamine or metanephrine excess.

METASTATIC PHEOCHROMOCYTOMA AND PARAGANGLIOMA

Distinguishing between benign and malignant catecholamine-secreting tumors is difficult on the basis of clinical, biochemical, or histopathologic characteristics; thus, malignancy is based on documentation of metastatic disease (e.g., lymph nodes, bone, lung, liver). Metastases develop at a median of 5.5 years (range, 0.3 to 53.4 years) from the initial diagnosis.[21] Median overall and disease-specific survivals are 24.6 and 33.7 years, respectively. However, 13% of patients die within 5 years of diagnosis and shorter survival correlates with male sex, older age at the time of primary tumor detection, synchronous metastases, larger primary tumor size, elevated dopamine, and not undergoing primary tumor resection. The clinician should assess the pace of the malignant disease and base the level of therapy on the aggressiveness of the tumor's behavior. A multimodality, multidisciplinary, individualized approach is indicated to control catecholamine-dependent symptoms, local mass effects, and overall tumor burden.

PHEOCHROMOCYTOMA IN PREGNANCY

Pheochromocytoma in pregnancy can cause the death of both the fetus and the mother. The approach to the biochemical diagnosis is the same as for nonpregnant patients. MRI without gadolinium enhancement is the preferred imaging modality. ^{123}I-MIBG scintigraphy and Ga-68 DOTATATE PET-CT are contraindicated. The treatment of hypertensive crises is the same as for nonpregnant patients, except that nitroprusside should be avoided. Although the most appropriate management is debated, adrenal pheochromocytomas should be removed promptly after α- and β-adrenergic blockade if the diagnosis is made during the first two trimesters of pregnancy.[22] The preoperative preparation is the same as for nonpregnant patients. If the pregnancy is in the third trimester, one operation is recommended for cesarean delivery and removal of the adrenal pheochromocytoma at the same time. Spontaneous labor and delivery should be avoided. The management of catecholamine-secreting paragangliomas in pregnancy may require modification of these guidelines, depending on tumor location.

GENERAL REFERENCES

For the General References and other additional features, please visit Expert Consult at https://expertconsult.inkling.com.

216

DIABETES MELLITUS

JILL P. CRANDALL AND HARRY SHAMOON

Diabetes mellitus is a chronic disorder characterized by abnormal metabolic regulation as well as by the potential for vascular and neuropathic complications. Diabetes comprises a cluster of heterogeneous disorders with elevated blood glucose levels as a common diagnostic feature; however, as genetic and molecular studies have suggested, it is likely that the cluster includes many subcategories, each of which requires tailored prevention, diagnosis, and treatment approaches. Depending on the context in which the patient presents, diabetes can be an acute life-threatening condition, a pregnancy-associated disorder, or a gradually evolving chronic disorder that carries with it secondary complications that may be ultimately more debilitating than hyperglycemia. Other factors make diabetes an unusual clinical challenge, including the need for active participation by patients in their treatment, the varying presentations across the age spectrum, and the unstable and evolving clinical presentation. Because the severity of the underlying metabolic defects does not remain static, diabetes management always requires changes in treatment according to the stage of the disease. These patterns of evolution are superimposed on the phenotypes at presentation and depend on a host of factors, including age, sex, race, societal setting, and others.

It is now established that diabetes-related vascular and neuropathic complications stem from imperfect treatment of the metabolic disturbances, defined principally by hyperglycemia. There is also evidence that genetic factors may predispose or protect individual patients from the deleterious effects of hyperglycemia. Regardless of the specific subtype of diabetes, all have in common some degree of insulin deficiency; insulin deficiency may be absolute, as in type 1 diabetes, or a relative deficit with coexisting insulin resistance, as in type 2 diabetes. Deficient insulin is the primary driver of impaired fuel homeostasis, whereas hyperglycemia plays the dominant role in disease-related complications. Major strides in our understanding of diabetes have been made during the last 40 years, with accompanying additions to the diagnostic and treatment armamentarium.

DEFINITIONS

Despite the heterogeneity of phenotypes, it is possible to generally classify diabetes into two major subgroups, type 1 (previously referred to as juvenile-onset or insulin-dependent diabetes) and type 2 (previously referred to as adult-onset or non–insulin-dependent diabetes). The major clinical features of type 1 and type 2 are shown in Table 216-1 and are described in detail in the corresponding sections later.

In addition to these two large categories, diabetes may occur in association with other disorders, with use of certain medications, or, rarely, as a result of a specific genetic mutation, such as maturity-onset diabetes of youth (MODY).

DIABETES ASSOCIATED WITH OTHER DISORDERS OR SYNDROMES

Diabetes may occur as part of several inherited syndromes, including the Turner, Klinefelter, Prader-Willi, Down, and Wolfram syndromes, among others. The genetic and metabolic defects involved are heterogeneous but usually result in impaired β-cell function. The obesity (and resulting insulin resistance) associated with many of these syndromes also contributes. Diseases of the exocrine pancreas, such as pancreatitis, pancreatic cancer, hemochromatosis, and cystic fibrosis, can be accompanied by impaired pancreatic endocrine function, leading to insulin-deficient diabetes. Several endocrinopathies that are associated with insulin resistance, including acromegaly, Cushing syndrome, and pheochromocytoma, may result in impaired glucose tolerance or frank diabetes in predisposed individuals. Viral infections, such as congenital rubella and cytomegalovirus, may cause diabetes by β-cell destruction. Finally, hyperglycemia may be associated with the use of certain drugs, including those that worsen insulin resistance (e.g., glucocorticoids, nicotinic acid, thiazide diuretics) and those that impair β-cell function (e.g., pentamidine, diazoxide, interferon gamma).

DIAGNOSTIC CRITERIA FOR DIABETES

Diabetes is diagnosed on the basis of one of several criteria, including fasting plasma glucose concentration, plasma glucose concentration after a standard 75-g oral glucose challenge (oral glucose tolerance test), and percentage of glycosylated hemoglobin (HbA_{1c}) (Table 216-2). In most cases, abnormal results require a confirmatory test, but diabetes can be diagnosed in the presence of unequivocal hyperglycemia (casual plasma glucose concentration >200 mg/dL) and typical symptoms of polyuria, polydipsia, and weight loss.

Because plasma glucose levels range on a continuum, the selection of a specific diagnostic threshold is in some respects arbitrary. Current criteria are based on the plasma glucose or HbA_{1c} level above which the risk of diabetes-specific microvascular complications (e.g., retinopathy) is perceptibly increased. In situations of altered red blood cell turnover or certain hemoglobinopathies, HbA_{1c} may not accurately reflect mean plasma glucose levels (see later section on glycosylated hemoglobin), and direct glucose measurement should be used. Separate glucose criteria exist for the diagnosis of gestational diabetes (see section on gestational diabetes under clinical manifestations of type 2 diabetes).

States of impaired glucose regulation, not meeting the criteria for diabetes, have also been defined (fasting glucose concentration of 100 to 125 mg/dL, 2-hour glucose concentration of 140 to 199 mg/dL, or HbA_{1c} level of 5.7 to 6.4%). Individuals in these categories are at increased risk for diabetes, although not all will progress and some may revert to normal glucose regulation. Impaired glucose tolerance (oral glucose tolerance test 2-hour glucose concentration of 140 to 199 mg/dL) has also been associated with increased risk of atherosclerotic cardiovascular disease (CVD), which may be independent of future development of diabetes.

Glycosylated Hemoglobin

Measurements of glycosylated hemoglobin have been in clinical use since the 1980s as a means of assessing glucose control in patients with diabetes and more recently for the diagnosis of diabetes and pre-diabetic states. Hemoglobin A_{1c} (HbA_{1c}) is formed by the nonenzymatic glycosylation of hemoglobin, and its percentage reflects the exposure of the hemoglobin A molecule to glucose during the lifespan of circulating red blood cells (about 120 days). Thus HbA_{1c} has a predictable (but nonlinear) relationship with mean plasma glucose levels during the preceding 3 to 4 months, although more recent glucose exposure

TABLE 216-1 CLASSIFICATION OF DIABETES

	TYPE 1	TYPE 2
Age at onset	Childhood or early adulthood, but can be manifested at any age	Middle age or older, but can be manifested in obese children and adolescents
Family history/genetic factors	Genetic risk defined, but most cases are sporadic	Strong genetic component, polygenic in most cases
Environmental triggers	Largely unknown	Obesity, sedentary lifestyle
Requirement for insulin therapy	Universal	Variable
Frequency among people with diabetes	5-10%	≈90%
Associated disorders	Autoimmunity, especially thyroid, other endocrine disorders	Hypertension, dyslipidemia, metabolic syndrome, polycystic ovary syndrome

TABLE 216-2 DIAGNOSTIC CRITERIA FOR DIABETES

	NORMAL	IMPAIRED (PRE-DIABETES)	DIABETES
Fasting glucose concentration (mg/dL)	<100	100-125	≥126
OGTT 2-hour glucose concentration (mg/dL)	<140	140-199	≥200
HbA_{1c} (%)	<5.7	5.7-6.4	≥6.5

OGTT = oral glucose tolerance test.
Modified from American Diabetes Association Standards of Medical Care in Diabetes—2018. *Diabetes Care* 2018;41(Suppl 1):S13-S27.

(preceding 4 weeks) contributes relatively more to glycosylation. The relationship between HbA$_{1c}$ and mean glucose levels was initially based on data obtained from the Diabetes Control and Complications Trial (DCCT) and recently updated on the basis of data obtained from studies using continuous glucose monitoring in ambulatory individuals, including those with and without diabetes (Table 216-3).

Although several different types of assays (e.g., affinity chromatography, immunoassay) are used to measure HbA$_{1c}$, most methods have been harmonized to a common standard and generally allow results from different laboratories to be used interchangeably. HbA$_{1c}$ results may be influenced by a number of factors, including conditions that alter red cell survival (e.g., hemolytic anemia) or cause interference with a specific assay. In these situations, measurement of fructosamine (a glycosylated serum protein) or glycated albumin, both of which reflect mean glucose levels during the preceding 2 to 3 weeks, may provide more accurate assessment of recent glucose levels. However, these assays have not been as well standardized, and the relationship with mean plasma glucose levels is less well established.

PATHOBIOLOGY OF DIABETES

Figure 216-1 summarizes the effects of insulin deficiency on body fuel metabolism.

Given the dominant role of insulin in carbohydrate metabolism, it is not surprising that its availability and effectiveness play a role in every form of

TABLE 216-3	THE RELATIONSHIP BETWEEN HBA$_{1C}$ AND ESTIMATED AVERAGE GLUCOSE LEVELS DURING THE PRECEDING 3 MONTHS		
	ESTIMATED AVERAGE GLUCOSE LEVEL		
HbA$_{1c}$ (%)	**mg/dL**		**mmol/L**
5	97		5.4
6	126		7.0
7	154		8.6
8	183		10.2
9	212		11.8
10	240		13.4
11	269		14.9
12	298		16.5

From Nathan DM, Kuenen J, Borg R, et al. Translating the A1c assay into estimated average glucose values. *Diabetes Care.* 2008;31:1473-1478.

diabetes. However, because many other diabetogenic factors can be operative and there is interdependence among many of these homeostatic mechanisms, teasing out their individual contributions is virtually impossible in any given patient.

Normal insulin physiology is orchestrated in a complex dynamic involving metabolic fuels, neurotransmitters, and other hormones. Insulin is synthesized as preproinsulin in the ribosomes of the rough endoplasmic reticulum of pancreatic islet β cells and is then converted to proinsulin, which in turn is transported to the Golgi apparatus, where it is packaged into secretory granules. Proinsulin is cleaved into equimolar amounts of insulin and a connecting segment (C-peptide) in the secretory granules. The stimulation of insulin secretion results in release of equimolar quantities of insulin and C-peptide (as well as a small amount of proinsulin) into the hepatic portal vein. Whereas a large proportion of insulin is bound to its hepatic receptor and metabolized in its "first pass" through the liver, C-peptide is much less prone to hepatic metabolism and is a better reflection of insulin secretion, although it is quantitatively of limited usefulness in the clinical diagnosis or treatment of diabetes.

The principal regulator of insulin secretion is glucose. The process of β-cell insulin secretion is shown schematically in Figure 216-2. Glucose is taken up by the β cells through the GLUT2 glucose transporter system and then phosphorylated to glucose 6-phosphate by an islet-specific glucokinase. Thus glucokinase can be considered the "glucose sensor" of the β cell; mutations in this enzyme can lead to a specific diabetes syndrome (MODY2), and there is evidence of its role in common forms of type 2 diabetes. The conversion of glucose to glucose 6-phosphate results in a sequential increase in intracellular adenosine triphosphate (ATP), closing of the ATP-dependent potassium (K_{ATP}) channels in the β-cell membrane, membrane depolarization and influx of calcium, migration of the insulin secretory granules to the cell membrane and their fusion with the membrane, and finally release of insulin into the extracellular fluid. The K_{ATP} channel is made up of the sulfonylurea 1 receptor (SUR1) and an inward potassium channel subunit, Kir6.2. Mutations in either the SUR1 gene or the Kir6.2 gene lead to loss of K_{ATP} activity; as a result, the cell is depolarized, resulting in chronic release of insulin and a syndrome termed *persistent hyperinsulinemic hypoglycemia of infancy*. Mutations in Kir6.2 and SUR1 have also been identified in patients with permanent neonatal diabetes mellitus; treatment with sulfonylurea can normalize insulin secretion in these patients.

The magnitude of the insulin secretory response is determined by the level of blood glucose as well as by the rate and mode of glucose entry. Compared with intravenous administration of glucose, higher insulin levels are produced when glucose is taken orally because of the simultaneous release of gut-derived incretins that include glucagon-like peptide 1 (GLP-1) and glucose-dependent insulinotropic peptide (GIP), both of which augment insulin secretion. In

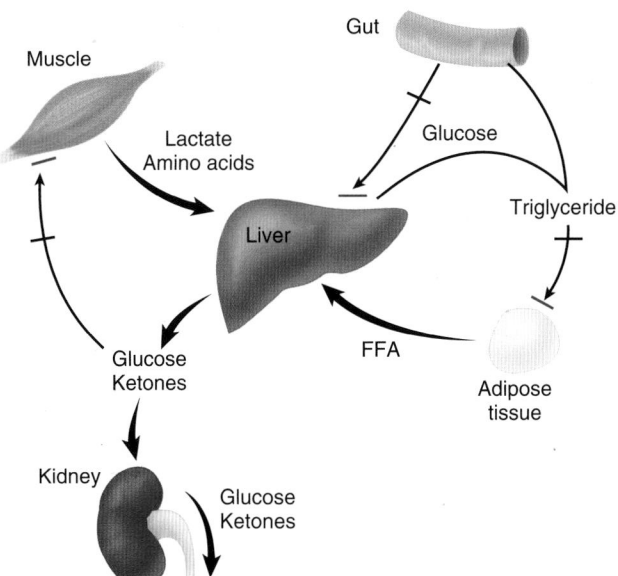

FIGURE 216-1. Effects of insulin deficiency on body fuel metabolism. Lack of insulin leads to mobilization of substrates for gluconeogenesis and ketogenesis from muscle and adipose tissue, accelerated production of glucose and ketones by the liver, and impaired removal of endogenous and exogenous fuels by insulin-responsive tissues. The net results are severe hyperglycemia and hyperketonemia that overwhelm renal removal mechanisms. FFA = free fatty acids.

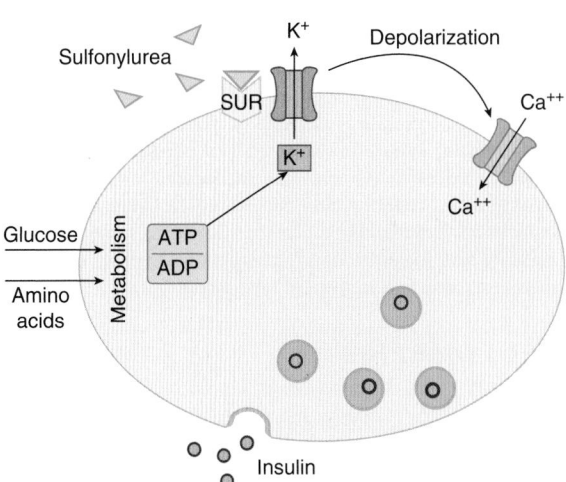

FIGURE 216-2. Nutrient regulation of insulin secretion. Glucose is taken up by the β cell through the GLUT2 glucose transporter and is metabolized (initially through phosphorylation by the glucokinase to glucose 6-phosphate). This leads to an increase in intracellular ATP (and an increase in the cytoplasmic ATP/ADP ratio), which causes closure of the ATP-dependent potassium channel, followed by membrane depolarization and the subsequent opening of voltage-gated calcium channels. The influx of calcium mobilizes the insulin secretory granules to fuse with the cell membrane and to release insulin into the extracellular fluid. The sulfonylurea 1 receptor (SUR1) is a component of the ATP-dependent potassium channel. ADP = adenosine diphosphate; ATP = adenosine triphosphate.

TABLE 216-4	THE METABOLIC EFFECTS OF INSULIN	
METABOLIC EFFECT	**STIMULATED BY INSULIN**	**INHIBITED BY INSULIN**
Carbohydrate metabolism	Glucose transport Glycolysis Glycogen synthesis	Glycogen breakdown Gluconeogenesis
Protein metabolism	Amino acid transport Protein synthesis	Protein breakdown
Lipid metabolism	Triglyceride uptake Lipogenesis	Lipolysis Fatty acid oxidation

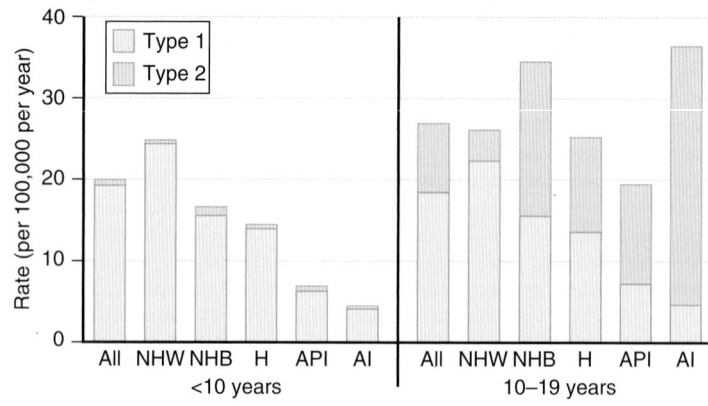

FIGURE 216-3. Rate of new cases of type 1 and type 2 diabetes among people younger than 20 years in the United States, by age and race/ethnicity, 2008–2009. AI = American Indians; API = Asian/Pacific Islander Americans; H = Hispanics/Latinos; NHB = non-Hispanic blacks; NHW = non-Hispanic whites. (From Centers for Disease Control and Prevention. *National Diabetes Statistics Report: Estimates of Diabetes and Its Burden in the United States, 2014.* Atlanta, GA: US Department of Health and Human Services; 2014. Source: SEARCH for Diabetes in Youth Study.)

fact, drugs that mimic or enhance this incretin effect are useful in the treatment of type 2 diabetes.

Rapid increases in blood glucose concentration (e.g., after intravenous administration of glucose) cause a spike of insulin secretion that peaks within a few minutes and declines quickly (so-called first-phase insulin secretion). With more persistent elevations of plasma glucose concentration, insulin secretion is sustained (so-called second-phase insulin secretion). The earliest pathophysiologic indicator of defective β-cell function may be the loss of first-phase secretion of insulin, which precedes by years the decline in insulin secretory reserve sufficient to lead to overt glucose intolerance or diabetes.

Insulin Action

The actions of insulin on its principal target organs (i.e., muscle, fat, liver) have complex and coordinated effects on the metabolism of carbohydrates, proteins, and lipids and are mediated by its interaction with the insulin receptor. Insulin receptor signaling through insulin receptor substrate 1 and phosphatidylinositol 3-kinase is a major pathway in the mediation of insulin-stimulated glucose transport, notably by stimulating the translocation of the glucose transporter GLUT4 to the cell membrane. This pathway is also responsible for the vasodilator effects of insulin (through increased expression of endothelial nitric oxide synthase), which may contribute to glucose utilization by increasing nutrient delivery to tissues. Defects in these intracellular signaling pathways are an important cause of impaired insulin action, or "insulin resistance" (see section on impaired insulin action [insulin resistance] under pathobiology of type 2 diabetes).

The overall actions of insulin tend to promote uptake and storage of nutrients in the fed state and release of nutrients from body stores in the fasting state, as summarized in Table 216-4.

In the *postprandial period*, rising glucose levels simultaneously trigger insulin secretion and suppress glucagon release. The resulting rise in the insulin-to-glucagon ratio increases hepatic glycogen synthesis and inhibits release of glucose from the liver. Insulin stimulates glucose uptake into skeletal muscle and adipose tissue, promoting the synthesis of protein and triglycerides. In the *fasting state*, declining glucose levels inhibit insulin release, thereby increasing glycogenolysis and gluconeogenesis and the resulting delivery of glucose into the circulation. In states of absolute or relative insulin deficiency, inadequate basal insulin levels allow unrestrained hepatic glucose production, which results in fasting hyperglycemia. Inadequate insulin in the fed state impedes peripheral (predominantly skeletal muscle) glucose uptake, thereby contributing to postprandial hyperglycemia. Impaired suppression of hepatic glucose production also contributes to postprandial hyperglycemia in patients with diabetes (see also the section on type 2 diabetes).

● TYPE 1 DIABETES
Epidemiology

Type 1 diabetes may be manifested at any age but most typically appears in childhood, especially around puberty. However, new cases of type 1 diabetes can appear at any time in life, and in the United States approximately 30% of patients are diagnosed after young adulthood.[1]

Worldwide, the incidence of type 1 diabetes varies 50- to 100-fold, with the highest rates occurring in individuals of northern European descent. Both sexes are equally affected in childhood, but men are affected more commonly in early adult life. The incidence of childhood type 1 diabetes is rising rapidly in all populations, especially in the age group younger than 5 years, with a doubling time of less than 20 years in Europe. In the United States, the incidence of type 1 diabetes among youth significantly increased in a linear fashion by 1.8% annually between 2002 and 2012, particularly among youths of minority

racial and ethnic groups.[2] These trends are elaborated below in this section. The increasing incidence of type 1 diabetes suggests a major environmental contribution, but the role of specific pathogenic factors remains largely unsettled. The distinction between type 1 and type 2 diabetes can become blurred in later life, and the true lifetime incidence of the condition is therefore unknown.

In Europe, the highest rates of childhood diabetes are found in Scandinavia, with an incidence for children from birth to 14 years of age ranging from 57 per 100,000 per year in Finland to 4 per 100,000 in Macedonia. In the United States, the overall annual incidence in youths is about 19 per 100,000. Prevalence rates are strikingly different among ethnic groups living in the same geographic region, probably because of genetic differences in susceptibility to the disease. Early-onset diabetes carries a higher familial risk, and affected fathers are more likely to transmit type 1 diabetes to their offspring than affected mothers are, with risks being 6 to 9% and 1 to 3%, respectively.

Given that the United States does not have a systematic health registry and that its population is multiethnic, previous estimates of the prevalence and incidence of type 1 diabetes have been based on extrapolations from limited cohorts. The SEARCH for Diabetes in Youth multicenter study (funded by the U.S. Centers for Disease Control and Prevention and the National Institutes of Health) examined diabetes among children and adolescents in the United States. During 2008–2009, an estimated 18,436 people younger than 20 years in the United States were newly diagnosed with type 1 diabetes and 5089 people younger than 20 years were newly diagnosed with type 2 diabetes. For those younger than 10 years, new cases of type 1 far outweighed type 2 (22.2 per 100,000 per year for type 1 diabetes vs. 0.8 per 100,000 for type 2 diabetes). Among youth aged 10 years or older, the rate of new cases of type 1 was about double that of type 2 (21.9 per 100,000 per year for type 1 diabetes vs. 11.0 per 100,000 for type 2 diabetes). Non-Hispanic white youth had the highest rate of new cases of type 1 diabetes in all age groups. Diabetes incidence rates by age and race/ethnicity are summarized in Figure 216-3.

Higher body mass index (BMI) is associated with younger age at diagnosis of type 1 diabetes, but this appears to be the case only in children with already compromised β-cell function. In addition, low birth weight may be a factor in accelerating the onset of type 1 diabetes, suggesting that the intrauterine environment may be an important determinant of age at onset for type 1 diabetes.

Pathobiology

In type 1 diabetes a complex interplay of genetic, environmental, and autoimmune factors selectively targets insulin-producing pancreatic islet β cells and ultimately destroys the β cells. The role of genetic factors in type 1 diabetes has long been appreciated, emphasized by familial clustering with other autoimmune endocrine disorders[3] and by concordance rates in identical twins of 30 to 40%. Because these concordance rates are not as high as in type 2 diabetes (i.e., >80%), environmental factors must clearly play a major role. Although the presence of an environmental trigger for type 1 diabetes is highly likely, even identical twins do not express identical T-cell receptor and immunoglobulin genes; as a result, total concordance might not be expected. Siblings who are human leukocyte antigen (HLA) identical to the proband have a 12 to 15% risk for development of diabetes by the age of 20 years.

Although many of the genes linked to type 1 diabetes have yet to be identified, about 60 are known.[4] HLA genes, located on the short arm of chromosome 6, contribute about 50% of genetic susceptibility to type 1 diabetes.[5] Two HLA class II haplotypes, DR4-DQ8 and DR3-DQ2, are present in about 90% of children with type 1 diabetes. The genotype containing both haplotypes carries the highest risk of diabetes (about 5%) and is most commonly seen in early-onset disease. In contrast, the DR15-DQ6 haplotype is highly protective, being found in only 1% of children with type 1 diabetes in contrast to 20% in the general population. HLA susceptibility haplotypes are overrepresented in adult-onset type 1, but at lower frequency than in classic type 1 diabetes in youth. Other genes likely contribute to the genetic susceptibility to type 1 diabetes. These include the insulin gene (on chromosome 11) and a number of other loci that are associated with other autoimmune conditions, suggesting the existence of common pathways predisposing to loss of self-tolerance. Another gene, *IFIH1*, located on chromosome 2, encodes a protein involved in innate immunity and plays a role in recognition of the RNA genomes of certain viruses. It is suggested that high IFIH1 levels might provoke exaggerated antiviral immune responses that predispose to autoimmunity. Many other genes have also been implicated, underscoring the polygenic nature of this disease.

Historically, environmental causes of type 1 diabetes focused on viruses because of associations with seasonal pandemics of infections and rarely because of the isolation of a specific pathogen. Epidemics of mumps, rubella, and coxsackievirus infection have been associated with an increased frequency of type 1 diabetes. Moreover, specific and convincing rare examples of virus-induced diabetes have been reported. However, it is believed that virus-mediated β-cell damage is not responsible for the massive destruction of β cells but that it triggers an autoimmune response in genetically predisposed individuals. Thus viruses may contain molecules that resemble a β-cell protein, and viral infection could thus nullify self-tolerance and trigger autoimmune responses.

It has long been recognized that about 80% of patients with new-onset type 1 diabetes have antibodies directed against various islet cell proteins, including insulin, glutamic acid decarboxylase (GAD65 and GAD67), and the secretory granule protein islet cell antigen 512 (IA-2). These antibody biomarkers have been important tools for studying the potential for early identification and prevention of total β-cell destruction in individuals susceptible to type 1 diabetes. β-cell destruction is largely mediated by a variety of cytokines or by direct T-lymphocyte activity that causes apoptosis or cellular destruction, although evidence suggests that islet-directed antibodies may also play a role. Both animal models and human pathologic studies have established that islet-targeted inflammatory cell infiltrates (termed insulitis) that are composed of CD8+ and CD4+ T cells, macrophages, and B cells are linked to the onset of diabetes. Over time, the islets become completely devoid of β cells and inflammatory infiltrates; α, δ, and pancreatic polypeptide cells are left intact, thus illustrating the specificity of the autoimmune attack on β cells.

A critical role for T cells is suggested by studies involving pancreatic transplantation in identical twins. Monozygotic twins with diabetes who received kidney and pancreas grafts from their nondiabetic, genetically identical siblings required little or no therapeutic immunosuppression. However, these patients eventually experienced a resumption of insulitis, with the subsequent recurrence of diabetes. Evidence implicating T cells in diabetes autoimmunity also derives from clinical trials using immunosuppressive drugs. Drugs such as cyclosporine or antibodies directed against a component of the T-cell receptor (anti-CD3) or that alter antigen presentation by B cells (anti-CD20) slow the progression of recent-onset diabetes, but this effect is not sustained if immunosuppression is withdrawn.

Clinical Manifestations

It has been clearly established that type 1 diabetes has a long preclinical phase, best described in Figure 216-4. At the time of clinical diagnosis, about 10 to 20% of the original β-cell mass may still be functional. In most cases, overt hyperglycemia (and ketosis if it is present) may be precipitated by an unrelated medical illness or stress placed on an already-limited islet reserve, thus triggering the diagnostic clinical manifestations. Typically, symptomatic hyperglycemia, manifested by polyuria, polydipsia, weight loss, and fatigue, occurs abruptly in an otherwise healthy child or young adult. For a minority of patients, the initial presentation may be diabetic ketoacidosis (DKA), which can occur if there is a delay in recognizing the symptoms of diabetes. Whereas the disease has an increased incidence in the winter months, classically attributed to respiratory viral infections, this seasonal pattern may be the result of

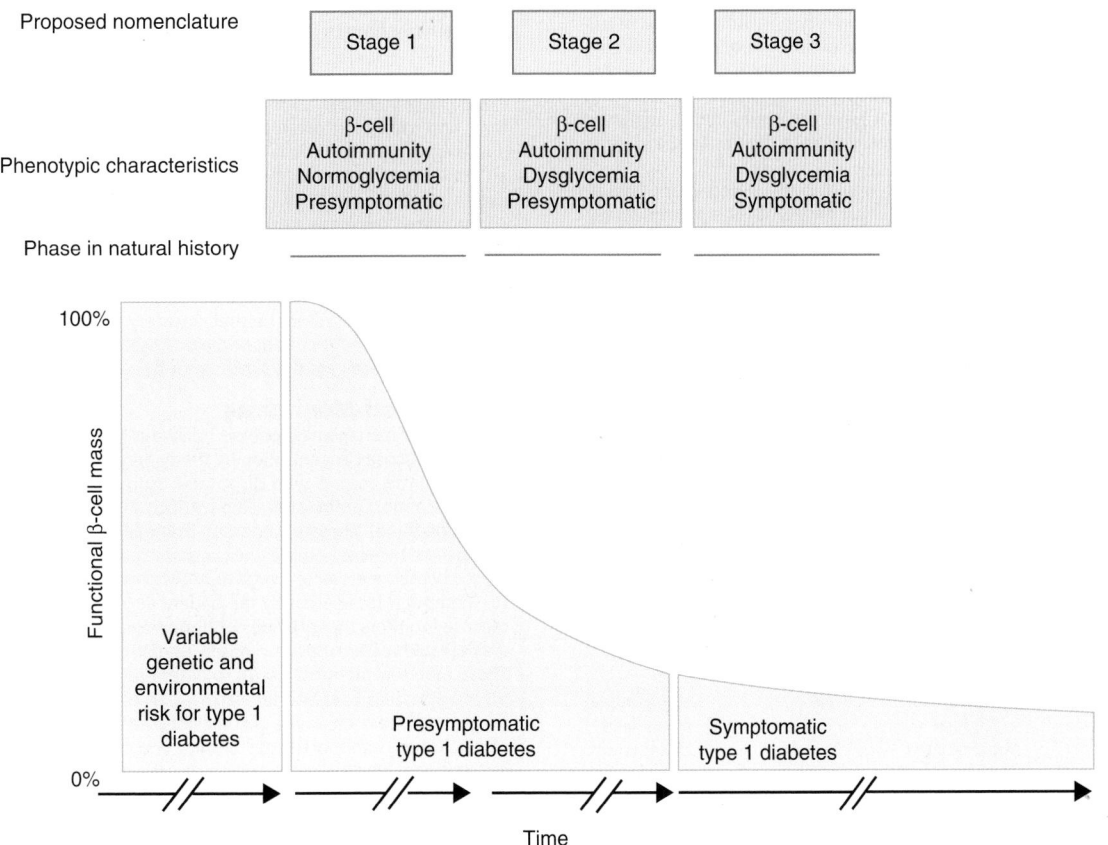

FIGURE 216-4. Summary of the sequence of events that lead to pancreatic β-cell loss and ultimately to the clinical evolution of type 1 diabetes. DKA = diabetic ketoacidosis. (From Insel RA, Dunne J, Atkinson MA, et al. Staging Presymptomatic Type 1 Diabetes: A Scientific Statement of JDRF, the Endocrine Society, and the American Diabetes Association. *Diabetes Care.* Oct 2015;38[10]:1964-1974.)

illness-associated counter-regulatory hormones that drive hyperglycemia in individuals with already compromised β-cell function. Similarly, the coincidence of type 1 diabetes with puberty has been attributed to insulin resistance associated with increases in sex and growth hormone secretion.

The diagnosis of diabetes is made according to symptoms or glucose criteria (see Table 216-2). Rarely, measurement of anti–glutamic acid decarboxylase antibodies is performed, but the determination of type 1 etiology is generally made on clinical grounds. After initiation of insulin therapy and stabilization of plasma glucose levels, the patient may experience a period of weeks to months of relatively easily controlled hyperglycemia. This so-called honeymoon phase of type 1 diabetes results from amelioration of the underlying stress in the face of β-cell function that has not declined further, and reflects the severe but not total β-cell destruction with ongoing (albeit reduced) insulin secretion. Subsequently, the ongoing, progressive, decline in insulin production generally leads to undetectable levels after a few years. However, with highly sensitive C-peptide assays, low levels of insulin production have been detected in some patients with long-standing type 1 diabetes who demonstrate more stable glycemic control. In patients with onset of type 1 diabetes in adulthood, the clinical presentation may follow a more indolent course (termed latent autoimmune diabetes in adults), perhaps because β-cell mass declines at a slower pace. In fact, type 1 diabetes may be misdiagnosed as type 2 in many of these patients until the progression of insulin deficiency reveals the phenotype of permanent and complete insulin dependence.

TREATMENT   Rx

The key to successful treatment of type 1 diabetes is to achieve physiologic insulin replacement, that is, to replicate the normal and tightly regulated relationship between plasma glucose and insulin secretion. Although current technology can only mimic this normal physiology, substantial progress has been made to permit maintenance of relative euglycemia by many patients. Successful glucose management requires substantial commitment by the patient and health care practitioner.[6]

Insulin Therapy

All patients with type 1 diabetes require insulin treatment to maintain life. The approach to insulin replacement in type 1 diabetes requires consideration of both basal insulin requirements (insulin required to maintain homeostasis in the fasting state) and insulin required for the influx of nutrients that occurs with meals. A variety of insulin preparations is available, which differ by patterns of absorption after subcutaneous injection. Most currently used insulin preparations are analogues of human insulin that have been modified (usually by changing one or more amino acids) to alter pharmacokinetics to speed or to delay absorption (Table 216-5).

Patients with type 1 diabetes are treated with both a long-acting "basal" insulin and a shorter-acting "prandial" insulin at mealtime, by a multiple daily insulin injection regimen or a continuous subcutaneous insulin infusion pump. Typically, the daily insulin requirement for patients with type 1 diabetes is between 0.3 and 1.0 unit/kg/day, with half given as basal insulin and the remainder divided into pre-meal boluses. Prandial insulin doses are determined by meal carbohydrate content plus a "correction factor" if glucose is elevated before the meal. For example, a common approach is to use 1 unit for every 10 to

15 g of meal carbohydrate plus a correction factor of 1 unit to lower plasma glucose concentration by 20 to 50 mg/dL. However, insulin requirements are influenced by a number of factors (e.g., age, body size, insulin sensitivity) and vary substantially among patients; therefore these algorithms need to be individualized. A number of mobile phone applications and computer programs are available to assist patients with dose calculation. Critical to the success of physiologic insulin replacement is the need for the patient to monitor blood glucose concentration, generally several times a day (see later).

A continuous subcutaneous insulin infusion pump using a short-acting insulin analogue can be programmed to deliver both a basal infusion and a preprandial bolus. Most insulin pumps contain an insulin reservoir attached by thin flexible tubing to a very small catheter that is inserted subcutaneously by the patient and changed every 2 or 3 days to avoid local inflammation and fibrosis, which can interfere with insulin absorption. The basal insulin delivery rate can be programmed to vary throughout the day and may be especially useful to prevent hyperglycemia associated with the "dawn phenomenon" (rising blood glucose levels in the early morning hours, thought largely to be due to increased growth hormone secretion). Most insulin pumps can be programmed to calculate prandial insulin doses, based on pre-meal glucose level and meal carbohydrate content, which is entered by the patient. However, in the event of pump malfunction, metabolic decompensation, including DKA, can develop within several hours because there is no subcutaneous reservoir of long-acting insulin. Successful use of an insulin pump requires a motivated and educated patient plus the support of a specialized diabetes team, including a certified diabetes educator. Insulin pump therapy can be used successfully in children and adolescents and is associated with reduced rates of acute complications, including severe hypoglycemia and DKA, compared with insulin injection therapy.[7] When used appropriately, continuous subcutaneous insulin infusion provides patients with maximal lifestyle flexibility and the best chance to achieve near-normal blood glucose levels. A1 More recently, hybrid closed-loop insulin delivery systems, in which a control algorithm autonomously and continually increases or decreases the subcutaneous delivery of basal insulin on the basis of real-time glucose levels recorded by a continuous glucose monitor (see below), have become available. These systems can improve glucose control and reduce hypoglycemia, compared with conventional insulin pump use. A2

Some patients who find adherence to a multiple injection or insulin pump regimen difficult can be treated with premixed "biphasic" insulin combinations, for example, a mixture of NPH and regular insulin given twice daily. This approach may be appropriate for patients with recent onset of type 1 diabetes who still maintain some endogenous insulin production. However, for most patients, this regimen is rarely optimal because it lacks flexibility and often increases the risk of hypoglycemia.

Diet and Lifestyle Treatment

In type 1 diabetes, the focus of dietary planning is on accurate estimation of meal carbohydrate content to allow appropriate prandial insulin dosing. This can be approached by promotion of "carbohydrate consistency" from meal to meal and the use of relatively fixed pre-meal insulin dosing. A more flexible approach is for the patient to learn "carbohydrate counting," which specifies an insulin dose per amount of carbohydrate in the meal. With either approach, patients need to monitor the nutrient content of their meals. Avoidance of concentrated sweets and other high-carbohydrate meals, including those with a high "glycemic index," tends to facilitate accurate insulin dosing and to minimize postprandial glycemic excursions. In contrast to type 2 diabetes, most patients with type 1 diabetes are not overweight or obese, and calorie restriction is neither required nor helpful. A variety of eating patterns are considered acceptable, and recommendations for a "heart healthy" diet (low in saturated fat and cholesterol) are the same as for the general population.

Glucose Self-Monitoring

Successful management of type 1 diabetes requires consistent self-monitoring of blood glucose concentration by the patient or caregiver several times a day. Small portable meters with disposable strips are easy to use and reasonably accurate in most ambulatory care settings. Frequent testing (i.e., before meals and at bedtime) allows appropriate prandial insulin dosing and correction of unexpected hyperglycemia as well as detection or confirmation of hypoglycemia. Most current meters store a large number of readings, which can be downloaded to a computer for analysis by the patient and health care team. Subcutaneous glucose monitors that provide continuous reading of interstitial glucose levels are available and are most commonly used in conjunction with an insulin pump. These monitors are most useful to determine glucose patterns and some can be programmed to sound an alarm when the glucose level exceeds a preset range or rate of change. The accuracy of continuous glucose monitoring (CGM) technology has improved substantially and may allow it to be used in place of conventional blood glucose measurement for immediate decision making and use in a closed loop system with an insulin pump. Evidence suggests that use of CGM, compared with usual care, can improve glycemic control for many patients, including those using conventional insulin injection therapy. A3 A4

Patients with type 1 diabetes should be also instructed to test urine ketones (with a reagent strip) in situations in which blood glucose concentration is unexpectedly and persistently elevated, especially if it is accompanied by

TABLE 216-5 INSULIN PREPARATIONS			
TYPE OF INSULIN	**ONSET OF ACTION**	**PEAK EFFECT**	**DURATION OF ACTION**
BASAL INSULIN			
Glargine	Approximately 2 hours	None	Approximately 24 hours
Detemir	Approximately 2 hours	3-9 hours	6-24 hours
Degludec	Approximately 2 hours	None	Approximately 40 hours
NPH/NPL	Approximately 2 hours	6-12 hours	14-24 hours
PRANDIAL INSULIN			
Lispro, aspart, glulisine	5-15 minutes	45-75 minutes	2-4 hours
Regular	Approximately 30 minutes	2-4 hours	5-8 hours

NPH = neutral protamine Hagedorn; NPL = neutral protamine lispro.

symptoms suggestive of DKA (see section on diabetic ketoacidosis under hyperglycemic states in acute metabolic complications of diabetes). Small or trace amounts of urinary ketones are not cause for concern, but moderate or large amounts may indicate the onset of DKA and should prompt the patient to seek urgent medical attention.

Whole Pancreas and Islet Cell Transplantation

The ultimate goal of a "cure" of type 1 diabetes could most likely be achieved by successful transplantation of insulin-producing β cells. Whole pancreas transplantation has been performed for almost three decades, with 5-year graft survival rates of about 70%. However, the surgery is complicated, and lifelong immunosuppression is required, as with any organ transplant. For these reasons, pancreas transplantation is generally reserved for patients who already have or are concurrently receiving a kidney transplant. In the absence of indications for kidney transplantation, pancreas-alone transplantation may be considered for patients who have a history of frequent, acute and severe metabolic complications (especially severe hypoglycemia) or severe and incapacitating psychosocial problems related to insulin therapy. Pancreatic islet cell transplants hold significant potential advantages over whole-gland transplants. However, at this time, islet cell transplantation is an experimental procedure, also requiring systemic immunosuppression, and is performed only within the setting of controlled research studies.

Prevention of Type 1 Diabetes

Given that type 1 diabetes is an immunologically mediated disease, it has long been supposed that immune intervention should alter its natural history and perhaps even prevent it altogether.[8] Furthermore, the significant heritability of type 1 diabetes suggests that treatment could target only susceptible individuals, and the existence of known biomarkers (antibodies that reflect disease activity as well as levels of insulin or C-peptide that reflect islet function) also lends credence to experimental immunologic treatments. Unfortunately, however, the major challenge for most immunologic interventions has been their lack of specificity for immune-mediated insulitis or the risks of spillover immune suppression in otherwise healthy persons. Given the experimental nature of all the tested therapies, we provide only a brief overview here.

Prevention of type 1 diabetes can theoretically be undertaken at three stages: (1) in susceptible individuals before there is evidence of immune attack against islet cells (primary prevention); (2) in nondiabetic people who already have evidence of immune activation (antibodies, insulin defects) to prevent progression to actual diabetes (secondary prevention); and (3) in newly diagnosed patients in whom the goal is to slow the β-cell destructive process (tertiary prevention).

Avoidance of putative environmental triggers of islet autoimmunity (e.g., cow's milk) is one approach, and dietary supplementation with nutrients that may diminish islet autoimmunity (e.g., omega-3 fatty acids or vitamin D) has been attempted. Despite promising results of a pilot study, a large trial of primary prevention by removal of cow's milk from the infant diet failed to reduce incident diabetes over 11 years of follow-up. Secondary prevention trials have also been undertaken with oral, inhaled, or injected insulin and with nicotinamide, but the results have been disappointing.[A5] There are secondary prevention studies with teplizumab (an FcR-nonbinding anti-CD32 monoclonal antibody) and with abatacept (a costimulation modulator) underway. Several tertiary prevention studies (i.e., after the diagnosis of diabetes) have been published. Nonspecific immune interventions, such as cyclosporine, demonstrate that immunotherapy can indeed rescue β cells from ongoing destruction, but it is not an acceptable therapeutic alternative given that it preserves β-cell function only transiently and carries heightened risks of adverse effects, such as nephropathy. Anti-CD3 antibodies currently appear more promising and are being evaluated in clinical trials.

Prognosis

Substantial progress has been made in recent decades in improving the prognosis for patients affected by type 1 diabetes. This is largely due to adoption of more intensive glucose control and more effective nonglycemic treatment of early stages of renal disease and retinopathy. Data from long-term follow-up of the intensively treated DCCT cohort showed that after 30 years' duration of diabetes, rates of serious diabetes complications were substantially lower than in historical controls, and less than 1% became blind, required renal replacement, or had an amputation due to diabetes. In Sweden from 1998 through 2014, mortality and the incidence of cardiovascular complications declined substantially among type 1 diabetic persons.[9,10] In the absence of renal disease, life expectancy for type 1 patients in the United States is comparable to that

of the general population. However, the mortality rate of all type 1 diabetic patients from age 35 onward is about twice as high as in non-diabetics even if the HgbA$_{1c}$ level is 6.9% or lower and becomes progressively higher for HgbA$_{1c}$ levels above 7.9%. Analysis of nationally representative hospitalization and registry data has shown large reductions in the incidence of a broad spectrum of diabetes-related complications between 1985 and 2015 in the U.S. population of adults with diabetes[11]; however, despite the substantial decline in the rates of diabetes-related complications in the past two decades, a large burden of disease persists because of the continued increase in the prevalence of diabetes.

TYPE 2 DIABETES
Epidemiology

Type 2 diabetes is one of the most common chronic diseases, affecting more than 30 million people in the United States and an estimated 366 million worldwide.[12] The prevalence of type 2 diabetes has been increasing in the United States, from approximately 3% of the population in 1995 to more than 9% in 2015.[13,14] This increase is in part due to demographic shifts (i.e., the aging of the population), but incidence rates are also increasing and parallel the rise of overweight and obesity as well as increasingly sedentary lifestyles. A similar pattern is observed globally, with projections of 550 million (approximately half undiagnosed) to be affected by 2030. Although type 2 diabetes is being increasingly recognized in obese adolescents and young adults, older age remains a major risk factor for type 2 diabetes. More than one quarter of adults age 65 years and older have diabetes, and another 50% have glucose or HbA$_{1c}$ levels in the impaired or pre-diabetic range. Type 2 diabetes in the United States is more common among some racial and ethnic groups, with prevalence rates highest among non-Hispanic blacks (18%), Hispanics (16%), and American Indians (16%) and lowest among non-Hispanic whites (9%). Individuals from the Indian subcontinent (i.e., India, Pakistan, Bangladesh) and the Pacific Islands (e.g., Hawaii, Nauru, Samoa) also have high rates of type 2 diabetes. In general, men and women have about equal prevalence of type 2 diabetes.

Pathobiology

Type 2 diabetes is characterized by variable defects in both insulin secretion and insulin action. The underlying metabolic phenotype of type 2 diabetes is distinctly heterogeneous among individuals with the disease; some have a more pronounced defect in insulin secretion, and others have greater resistance to insulin action. The metabolic profile also varies within a given patient over time, as insulin secretion progressively declines with longer duration of disease. Although heterogeneous, type 2 diabetes is characterized in all cases by inadequate insulin secretion for the prevailing glucose level and degree of insulin sensitivity.

IMPAIRED INSULIN SECRETION

The relative insulin deficiency characteristic of type 2 diabetes appears to be a consequence of both functional (i.e., reduced responsiveness to secretagogues) and quantitative (i.e., reduction in β-cell mass) factors. Insulin secretory capacity is difficult to directly measure in humans, but reductions of β-cell mass up to 60% are estimated to occur in type 2 diabetes. However, this alone is insufficient to explain insulin deficiency in type 2 diabetes, as evidenced by the observation that 50% surgical pancreatectomy does not lead to hyperglycemia in otherwise healthy individuals. Classic studies in diabetic patients have demonstrated failure of insulin secretion in response to glucose but a normal response to the amino acid arginine, providing further evidence for the presence of a functional defect specific to glucose sensing. Abnormalities in the usual pulsatile and oscillatory patterns of insulin secretion and inefficient insulin biosynthesis have also been demonstrated in type 2 diabetes. For example, abnormal peptide processing results in increased secretion of intact proinsulin, which serves as a useful biomarker of future diabetes risk. Increased accumulation of amyloid also occurs within diabetic islets and may contribute to impaired secretory function. Ultimately, the β-cell defects in type 2 diabetes appear to be multifactorial, in part genetically determined (see later) but also influenced by environmental exposure, for example, to high levels of circulating glucose (glucotoxicity) and lipids (lipotoxicity). In addition, the β-cell defects are not static but worsen with increasing duration of diabetes.

IMPAIRED INSULIN ACTION (INSULIN RESISTANCE)

Resistance to the metabolic effects of insulin is also a characteristic although variable feature of type 2 diabetes. Hyperinsulinemia, thought to be a compensatory response to impaired insulin action, can be demonstrated in patients with pre-diabetes and in many patients with established type 2 diabetes, particularly early in its course. More precise techniques to measure insulin action (e.g., the euglycemic hyperinsulinemic clamp) have demonstrated resistance to insulin action primarily in peripheral tissues (reduced capacity to stimulate glucose uptake in muscle and fat) but also in the liver (reduced capacity of insulin to suppress hepatic glucose production). Insulin resistance is closely associated with obesity (see later) but also has genetic determinants, reflected by the observation that some obese patients do not have severe insulin resistance. Insulin resistance frequently occurs as part of a constellation of features, termed the *metabolic syndrome*, which include hypertension, abdominal obesity, dyslipidemia, glucose intolerance, and increased cardiovascular risk. Insulin resistance is also a common feature of the polycystic ovary syndrome.

There are multiple molecular mechanisms that can lead to resistance to physiologic insulin action, including pre-receptor defects (e.g., an abnormal insulin molecule) and abnormal insulin receptors (e.g., due to gene mutations). However, common forms of insulin resistance that occur in association with type 2 diabetes are generally due to post-receptor defects, that is, abnormalities in intracellular signaling. In insulin target tissues, signaling through the phosphatidylinositol 3-kinase pathway is responsible for translocation of the glucose transporter GLUT4, which is necessary for uptake of glucose into the cell. Several defects in this pathway have been described in humans with insulin resistance, including abnormalities in insulin receptor substrate 1 and protein kinase B/Akt2. Some specific gene mutations associated with insulin resistance have been identified, but insulin resistance may also be acquired as a consequence of obesity (see later), increases in circulating free fatty acids, certain medications (e.g., glucocorticoids, niacin), and inflammatory states.

Evidence from natural history and genetic association studies (see later) indicates that defects in either insulin action or insulin secretion can remain clinically silent. For example, insulin resistance can induce compensatory hyperinsulinemia, which early in the course of the disease is sufficient to maintain euglycemia. However, in individuals with inherited or acquired defects in β-cell function, this compensation ultimately fails and hyperglycemia ensues. Viewed another way, a subclinical β-cell defect may remain silent in the setting of normal insulin sensitivity but be manifested as hyperglycemia when acquired insulin resistance develops because of weight gain, aging, or some other factor. A unifying theory that explains the coexistence of defects in both insulin action and insulin secretion is appealing but so far elusive.

GENETICS

The evidence for familial aggregation of type 2 diabetes is substantial and supports the presence of an important genetic influence. An individual with one parent with type 2 diabetes has a lifetime risk for development of type 2 diabetes of approximately 40%, with risk increasing to approximately 70% if both parents are affected. Further, the concordance rate among monozygotic twins is as high as 70%. The greater risk of type 2 diabetes among certain racial and ethnic groups also supports an important genetic component. The overall heritability of type 2 diabetes is estimated to be between 25 and 50%, although the specific gene or genes ultimately responsible for common forms of type 2 diabetes have not been established.[15]

Single-Gene Mutations Linked to Type 2 Diabetes Phenotype

A number of syndromes, termed *maturity-onset diabetes of youth* (MODY), characterized by impaired β-cell function have been recognized and linked to specific single-gene mutations. The phenotypes vary with the mutation but generally include early onset of relatively mild hyperglycemia in nonobese children or young adults and an autosomal dominant pattern of inheritance. Although not common (representing 1 to 3% of diabetes cases worldwide), their discovery has provided insight into the role of β-cell function in the more common forms of type 2 diabetes. MODY 2 is associated with a mutation of glucokinase, which acts as a glucose sensor within the β cell. In this case, higher levels of glucose are required to stimulate release of insulin from the β cell. MODY 3 is due to a mutation of the gene for hepatic nuclear factor 1α, which is involved in early pancreatic development and in the regulation of insulin gene expression. Other MODY forms (1, 4, 5, 6) are much less common, having been described in only a few families (Table 216-6).

Other examples of single-gene mutations associated with specific diabetes syndromes include activating mutations of *KCNJ11* (encoding a portion of the β-cell sulfonylurea receptor), which causes severe neonatal diabetes, and *WFS1*, which encodes a protein that is defective in Wolfram syndrome (diabetes insipidus, diabetes mellitus, optic atrophy, and deafness).

TABLE 216-6	SINGLE-GENE MUTATIONS RESPONSIBLE FOR THE MORE COMMON FORMS OF MATURITY-ONSET DIABETES OF YOUTH (MODY)

	MUTATION	METABOLIC DEFECT	CLINICAL PHENOTYPE
MODY 2	Glucokinase	Decreased β-cell sensitivity to glucose	Mild nonprogressive hyperglycemia, may not require pharmacologic treatment; diabetes complications rare
MODY 3	Hepatic nuclear factor 1α	Abnormal regulation of β-cell gene transcription	Mild hyperglycemia, may be progressive; renal glycosuria; increased sensitivity to sulfonylurea drugs; susceptibility to microvascular complications

Polygenic, Common Type 2 Diabetes

Common forms of type 2 diabetes are likely polygenic and multifactorial and represent a complex interaction between genes and environment. In the past several years, more than 100 genetic risk loci for common forms of type 2 diabetes have been identified by genome-wide association studies, but collectively these explain less than 15% of the heritability of the disorder. Outside of rare variants that are unique to specific groups, the gene with the strongest effect size to date (odds ratio for diabetes, 1.4) is *TCF7L2*, which is associated with reduced insulin secretion, as are the majority of other recognized gene variants. Others include a β-cell zinc transporter (ZnT-8; odds ratio, 1.15), the sulfonylurea receptor (*KCNJ11*; odds ratio, 1.1), and melatonin receptor 1B (*MTNR1B*; odds ratio, 1.10). A smaller number of gene variants associated with insulin resistance have been identified and include genes encoding peroxisome proliferator-activated receptor γ (odds ratio, 1.20) and insulin receptor substrate 1 (odds ratio, 1.10). Sequence variants in *SLC16A11*, a gene involved in intracellular lipid metabolism, were discovered to be a relatively common risk allele (odds ratio, 1.29) in Mexican populations. Current knowledge about genetic variants associated with type 2 diabetes risk is not useful for clinical disease prediction, offering no advantage to simple clinical tools based on traditional risk factors.

There is emerging evidence that epigenetic changes may play an important role in development of type 2 diabetes. Epidemiologic studies suggest that "metabolic programming" may occur in utero, with both fetal starvation and fetal overnutrition predisposing to diabetes in adult life. One example comes from experience with the Pima Indians, who have an extremely high prevalence of type 2 diabetes. Children born to mothers who were diabetic during their pregnancy had higher rates of adult diabetes than did children born to the same mothers before they became diabetic, suggesting that intrauterine exposure can have long-lasting metabolic effects. Studies of DNA methylation in animal models support this hypothesis, although human epigenome-wide studies are just now being conducted. Conversely, maternal undernutrition is associated with diabetes in offspring. Low birth weight has been linked to predisposition to cardiovascular disease and diabetes in adulthood. According to the widely cited Barker hypothesis, nutrient deficiency in utero (e.g., due to maternal starvation or placental insufficiency) impairs development of the endocrine pancreas, leading to inadequate insulin production later in life.[16] The available data suggest that maternal nutrition may play an important role in metabolic programming, resulting in increased diabetes susceptibility in adulthood.

OBESITY

The presence of overweight or obesity (Chapter 207) substantially increases the risk for type 2 diabetes and likely accounts for the dramatic increase in diabetes prevalence during the past several decades. In fact, the presence of overweight or obesity is the single most important clinical predictor of type 2 diabetes, particularly for young or middle-aged individuals. The relationship between BMI and type 2 diabetes is linear, and increased risk can be observed even within the BMI range defined as normal (<25 kg/m^2). Related factors, such as sedentary lifestyle and diet (increased consumption of foods with high glycemic load, increased *trans* and saturated fat), may also contribute to diabetes risk, independent of BMI. Distribution of body fat also plays an important role, with visceral adiposity (as assessed by waist circumference or waist-to-hip ratio) being a particularly strong diabetes risk factor in Asian populations, who tend to develop type 2 diabetes at a lower BMI than some other racial or ethnic groups do. Ectopic accumulation of adipose tissue in the liver, often manifested as nonalcoholic fatty liver disease, is also strongly associated with increased diabetes risk.

The increase in adipose tissue mass impairs insulin action by a number of proposed mechanisms, including alterations in fatty acid metabolism, accumulation of triglycerides in the liver, and low-grade systemic inflammation. Adipose tissue macrophages produce proinflammatory cytokines, including tumor necrosis factor–α and interleukin-6, which can interfere with insulin signaling. Obesity is also associated with reduced levels of the fat-derived peptide adiponectin, which exhibits both anti-inflammatory and insulin-sensitizing properties. The increase of circulating free fatty acids that is characteristic of obese states can interfere with insulin action in skeletal muscle and liver, and increased intramyocellular lipid is also associated with insulin resistance. Further, increased lipid accumulation in pancreatic islets may lead to impaired insulin secretion. Interestingly, some obese individuals have apparently normal insulin sensitivity and glucose metabolism, sometimes referred to as the obesity paradox. The mechanisms that may protect someone from the diabetogenic effects of excess adiposity are not known, but intact cardiorespiratory fitness may play a role.

Clinical Manifestations
TYPICAL TYPE 2 DIABETES
The classic hyperglycemic symptoms of polyuria, polydipsia, and weight loss occur when the renal threshold for glucose reabsorption (about 180 mg/dL) is exceeded and glycosuria with osmotic diuresis occurs. Therefore patients may have a plasma glucose concentration that is elevated but below this threshold, for years if not for decades, before specific symptoms appear. In the current era many patients are found to have diabetes during routine screening or in the course of investigation for another disorder (typically CVD). The initial presentation for some patients may be severe decompensated hyperglycemia, with profound dehydration, electrolyte imbalance, and plasma glucose levels of 400 mg/dL or higher, with the most striking examples being hyperosmolar hyperglycemic state (HHS) and DKA (see corresponding sections later).

A key feature of type 2 diabetes is that the metabolic defects are not static but tend to worsen over time. A patient early in the course of type 2 diabetes may maintain acceptable glucose control with simple dietary modification and modest weight loss. For many patients, these measures alone fail over time, and combinations of oral medications and often insulin therapy become necessary to control blood glucose levels.

Although the defining clinical feature of type 2 diabetes is hyperglycemia, it is actually the vascular complications of the disorder that cause the greatest morbidity and mortality. For a minority of patients, the initial clinical presentation of diabetes may be the presence of diabetic microvascular complications (retinopathy, neuropathy, nephropathy), which usually indicates many years of unrecognized hyperglycemia. More typical is the insidious onset of symptomatic microvascular complications after many years of diabetes, especially if it is poorly controlled.

ATYPICAL DIABETES
DKA may be the initial clinical presentation for a minority of patients with type 2 diabetes, who subsequently recover β-cell function and do not require insulin treatment. This entity, referred to as ketosis-prone type 2 or Flatbush diabetes (named for the New York City neighborhood where it was first described), appears to be more common among African Americans and some other ethnic minorities. These patients typically lack markers of β-cell autoimmunity and have a strong family history of type 2 diabetes. Once the initial episode of DKA is treated and glucose levels stabilize, patients may have near-normoglycemic remissions lasting many years. The pathogenesis of this form of diabetes is not clear, but a unique β-cell predisposition to glucose desensitization ("glucose toxicity") has been proposed.

GESTATIONAL DIABETES
Diabetes that appears for the first time during pregnancy and typically regresses after delivery is termed *gestational diabetes* (Chapter 226). Women who develop gestational diabetes usually have risk factors including overweight or obesity, older age (>30 years), and a family history of type 2 diabetes. The majority will develop permanent type 2 diabetes during their lifetime. Hormonal changes (increases in placental lactogen, estrogen, progesterone) induce insulin resistance during pregnancy and may uncover latent β-cell defects in predisposed women. Babies born to mothers with diabetes mellitus are at risk for a number of adverse outcomes, especially macrosomia but also preterm birth, neonatal

hypoglycemia, and hyperbilirubinemia. Routine screening, with an oral glucose tolerance test, of all pregnant women at 24 to 28 weeks of gestation is currently recommended. Because glucose levels tend to be lower than in the nonpregnant state, separate criteria have been developed for the diagnosis of diabetes in pregnancy. These include the presence of any of the following: fasting glucose concentration of 92 mg/dL or higher; glucose concentration of 180 mg/dL or higher at 1 hour or 153 mg/dL or higher at 2 hours after a 75-g oral glucose load. Aggressive glycemic control has been shown to reduce adverse pregnancy outcomes, including macrosomia and traumatic delivery, although its effects on long-term outcomes in offspring have not been established. Medical nutrition therapy is recommended for all women with gestational diabetes, with emphasis on moderate carbohydrate intake and avoidance of excessive weight gain. If diet modification is inadequate to maintain euglycemia, insulin has historically been considered first-line pharmacologic treatment for gestational diabetes. Oral diabetic medications, including glyburide and metformin, are increasingly being used to treat gestational diabetes, although long-term safety has not been established and they are not approved for this indication by the U.S. Food and Drug Administration. A multicenter noninferiority trial in women with gestational diabetes has failed to show that the use of glyburide compared with subcutaneous insulin does not result in a higher frequency of perinatal complications.[A6] After delivery, women with gestational diabetes should continue to be observed for the development of type 2 diabetes.

TREATMENT Rx

Effective treatment of type 2 diabetes is uniquely challenging because it encompasses management of lifestyle factors (including diet, exercise, and weight control), use of multiple oral or injectable medications, self-monitoring of blood glucose concentration, and surveillance and treatment for acute and chronic diabetic complications. The active participation of the patient in this complex program is critical for successful diabetes management, and many patients benefit from participation in a program of diabetes self-management education.

Goals of Therapy Including Glucose Targets
The primary goals of diabetes management are to prevent symptomatic hyperglycemia and hypoglycemia and to prevent the vascular complications associated with diabetes (see later section on chronic vascular complications). Intensive glycemic control (near-normoglycemia) has been shown to reduce microvascular and neuropathic complications of diabetes but not CVD or mortality.[A7][A8] The current consensus view is that lowering of the HbA$_{1c}$ level to 7% or below is an appropriate goal for most patients with diabetes. More stringent glycemic control (HbA$_{1c}$ level close to the normal range) may be appropriate for some individuals (e.g., young patients with short duration of disease) if it can be achieved without excessive hypoglycemia. Conversely, less stringent goals may be suitable for patients with established vasculopathy, significant comorbidities, or reduced life expectancy. Generally accepted targets for fasting and postprandial glucose levels are 80 to 130 mg/dL and less than 180 mg/dL, respectively. Glycemic targets during pregnancy are different, in part because plasma glucose levels normally are lower during pregnancy and because of the risk of adverse fetal outcomes with even modest hyperglycemia (Table 216-7).

Diet and Lifestyle Management
Dietary recommendations for patients with type 2 diabetes have varied over the years and in the past included strict avoidance of sugars and the use of specific diet plans (e.g., "exchange systems") that provided prescribed amounts of carbohydrate, fat, and protein. Current approaches for most patients focus on calorie restriction to achieve and to maintain modest (approximately 5 to

TABLE 216-7 RECOMMENDED GLYCEMIC TARGETS FOR ADULTS WITH DIABETES

	PREPRANDIAL GLUCOSE LEVEL	POSTPRANDIAL GLUCOSE LEVEL	HbA$_{1c}$
Nonpregnant adults	80-130 mg/dL	<180 mg/dL	<7%
Gestational diabetes	≤95 mg/dL	<140 mg/dL (1 hour after meal) or <120 mg/dL (2 hours after meal)	—
Pre–gestational diabetes	<95 mg/dL	<140 mg/dL (1 hour after meal) or <120 mg/dL (2 hours after meal)	6-6.5%

Modified from American Diabetes Association standards of medical care in diabetes—2018. *Diabetes Care.* 2018;41(Suppl 1):S55-S64.

10% of body weight) weight loss, moderate carbohydrate intake, and avoidance of concentrated sweets and foods high in saturated fats and cholesterol. An optimal macronutrient distribution for patients with type 2 diabetes has not been established, and individualization of nutrition plans, depending on such factors as renal function, weight status, and the patient's preference, is recommended. Evidence suggests that a low-fat, low-carbohydrate (Atkins-type) diet and a Mediterranean-type diet can each be effective in promoting weight loss and improving glucose control in patients with diabetes. Moderate alcohol consumption is not prohibited, with the proper consideration of calorie intake (7 kcal/g) and hypoglycemia risk if alcohol is consumed without food, particularly in insulin-treated patients. Referral to a registered dietitian for medical nutrition therapy should be considered for patients newly diagnosed with type 2 diabetes and those who are not achieving glycemic or weight targets.

Regular exercise is an important but often overlooked component of diabetes management. Both aerobic exercise and resistance training can improve blood glucose control, even in the absence of significant weight change. Current recommendations are for a minimum of 150 minutes per week of moderate-intensity physical activity, such as brisk walking, biking, or swimming, and muscle-strengthening exercises two or three times per week. Assessment of cardiovascular status before beginning of an exercise program should be considered for selected patients, but routine screening (e.g., with an exercise stress test) of asymptomatic patients is not recommended. The presence of some diabetic complications may require restriction of certain activities. For example, in patients with proliferative retinopathy, vigorous aerobic or resistance exercise could precipitate retinal hemorrhage or detachment. The presence of significant sensory loss due to peripheral neuropathy can increase the risk of foot injury, including skin ulceration and Charcot joint destruction. Use of proper footwear and careful foot inspection are recommended, and avoidance of weight-bearing exercise may be required for high-risk patients. Finally, exercise-induced hypoglycemia can occur in patients treated with insulin or some secretagogues (i.e., sulfonylureas) and may require adjustment of the medication regimen or added carbohydrate before exercise.

Bariatric Surgery

Weight loss is considered the cornerstone for treatment of patients with type 2 diabetes, the majority of whom are overweight or obese. It has been clearly shown to improve glucose control. As expected, diabetic patients who undergo bariatric (weight reduction) surgery (Chapter 207) also show improvement in glucose control, which in some cases is dramatic. Improvements in glycemia often occur almost immediately after surgery, before significant weight loss has occurred, and appear to be related to changes in gut hormones (including GLP-1 and GIP) or bile acid metabolism. Many patients are able to discontinue diabetes medications, and diabetes remission rates above 50% have been reported. Among obese patients with uncontrolled type 2 diabetes, 3 years of intensive medical therapy plus bariatric surgery was reported to result in glycemic control in significantly more patients than did medical therapy alone; bodyweight, use of glucose-lowering medications, and quality of life also showed more favorable results at 5 years in the surgical groups. [A9][A10]

Pharmacologic Therapy

Although weight control and nutrition form the foundation of effective management, most patients with type 2 diabetes will require use of pharmacologic agents, often multiple, to maintain recommended levels of glycemic control. During the last two decades, several new classes of drugs, targeting different metabolic pathways, have become available for treatment of type 2 diabetes. However, some of the most effective drugs are the oldest, and the long-term safety profile of newer agents remains to be established. Medications can be broadly categorized as those that enhance insulin availability (insulin and insulin secretagogues), those that enhance insulin action, or a miscellaneous group with other targets. Insulin therapy is also covered later and in the section on type 1 diabetes.

Insulin Sensitizers
Metformin

The biguanide drug metformin is the most widely used antidiabetic medication and is considered preferred initial therapy for patients with type 2 diabetes. The pleiotropic effects of metformin are thought to be mediated primarily through inhibition of mitochondrial complex 1 (i.e., effects on mitochondrial oxidative phosphorylation and cellular energy charge) and, in part, through regulation of the activity of 5′-adenosine monophosphate–activated protein kinase and the mammalian target of rapamycin. Metformin lowers glucose levels primarily through suppression of hepatic glucose production, but it also may enhance insulin sensitivity (improved insulin-mediated glucose uptake) and limit intestinal glucose absorption. Modest and sustained weight loss (about 2 to 4 kg) is common with metformin. Metformin is used orally twice a day, and extended-release forms are available for once-daily dosing. Hypoglycemia occurs rarely if at all with metformin monotherapy. The most common adverse effect is gastrointestinal intolerance (dyspepsia, diarrhea), which can be minimized by slow upward dose titration. Vitamin B_{12} malabsorption, leading to clinical B_{12} deficiency, has also been reported. The occurrence of lactic acidosis is the most serious although rare adverse effect, which occurs almost exclusively in patients with renal insufficiency and another precipitating factor, such as sepsis or shock. Renal function should be monitored periodically; metformin must be used with caution in those with an estimated glomerular filtration rate (GFR) of 45 mL/minute or lower and should be discontinued for an estimated GFR of 30 mL/minute or lower. Unique among available antidiabetic therapies, metformin was shown to reduce cardiovascular and all-cause mortality in the U.K. Prospective Diabetes Study (UKPDS), which adds to its appeal as a first-line agent. Metformin has also been used for diabetes prevention and for treatment of polycystic ovary syndrome.

Thiazolidinediones

The thiazolidinediones, which include rosiglitazone and pioglitazone, improve insulin-mediated glucose uptake and reduce hepatic glucose production. They bind to a nuclear receptor, peroxisome proliferator-activated receptor γ, and thus regulate the transcription of a variety of genes involved in carbohydrate and lipid metabolism. Thiazolidinedione therapy has pronounced effects on adipose tissue, reducing lipolysis, increasing fat mass, and causing redistribution of fat away from visceral to subcutaneous depots. Increases in circulating adiponectin, an adipokine with insulin-sensitizing and anti-inflammatory properties, may also play a role in the glucose-lowering effect of these drugs. Thiazolidinediones are given orally in once-a-day dosing. Common adverse effects include weight gain and fluid retention, including precipitation or worsening of congestive heart failure. Also reported have been an increase in fractures in postmenopausal women and increased risk of bladder cancer. The potential cardiovascular toxicity of rosiglitazone remains controversial, and its use has been restricted in many countries; these effects have not been observed for pioglitazone.

Insulin Secretagogues
Sulfonylureas

The sulfonylurea class of insulin secretagogues is among the oldest available oral antidiabetes drugs. Sulfonylureas currently in common use include glipizide, glyburide, and glimepiride; older sulfonylureas (chlorpropamide, tolbutamide) are still sometimes used outside of the United States. Their mechanism of action is to bind to the ATP-sensitive potassium channel in the β-cell membrane (at a site termed the *sulfonylurea receptor*), resulting in membrane depolarization and, ultimately, release of insulin from preformed secretory granules. Therefore the presence of a sufficient mass of intact β cells is required for efficacy of these drugs. They can be used as monotherapy or in combination with other drugs. The major adverse effect of sulfonylureas is their potential to cause hypoglycemia because insulin secretion occurs regardless of ambient plasma glucose. Modest weight gain is also common. Results of a study conducted in the 1970s (University Group Diabetes Program) suggested that sulfonylurea drugs may increase the risk of cardiovascular events and mortality. These findings were not confirmed in other trials, but the issue remains controversial. Despite this, sulfonylureas are among the most widely used antidiabetic medications.

Glinides

Repaglinide and nateglinide are chemically distinct non-sulfonylurea insulin secretagogues that also bind to the ATP-sensitive potassium channel in the β-cell membrane. Their onset and duration of action are much shorter than those of sulfonylureas, and the frequency of fasting hypoglycemia may be less. They are administered orally before each meal, making them somewhat less convenient than medications with a single daily dose but potentially providing an advantage for patients with inconsistent meal timing or content.

Incretin-Based Therapies/GLP-1 Agonists

Exenatide, liraglutide, semaglutide, dulaglutide, and lixisenatide are analogs of the endogenous incretin hormone GLP-1 and stimulate insulin secretion by binding to GLP-1 receptors on β cells. These drugs augment glucose-stimulated insulin secretion and thus have less potential to cause hypoglycemia than sulfonylureas and glinides do. They also suppress hepatic glucose production (by reduction of glucagon secretion), delay gastric emptying, and suppress appetite, resulting in modest weight loss for many patients. GLP-1 agonists are given by injection once or twice a day, and weekly long-acting formulations are also available. Major adverse effects include gastrointestinal intolerance (nausea and vomiting), which can be minimized by initiation with a low dose and gradual titration. In combination with basal insulin treatment, these agents can improve glycemic control without increasing hypoglycemia and often induce significant weight loss. [A11][A12] Liraglutide also reduces all-cause mortality by about 15%, as well as reducing the risk of death from cardiovascular causes, nonfatal myocardial infarction, or nonfatal stroke. [A13] Liraglutide, added to usual care, also resulted in lower rates of the development and progression of diabetic kidney disease than placebo. [A14] Similarly, weekly semaglutide (0.5 or 1.0 mg) significantly reduces the rate of cardiovascular death, nonfatal myocardial infarction, or nonfatal stroke in type 2 diabetes patients who are at high cardiovascular risk. [A15] Improvement in renal outcomes has also been reported for liraglutide and semaglutide. An increased risk of acute pancreatitis has been reported with GLP-1 agonists (and DPP-4 inhibitors; see later), but the magnitude of the risk is uncertain and requires additional research. An increase in C-cell hyperplasia and medullary thyroid cancer was found in laboratory animals, although the relevance of this to humans is unclear.

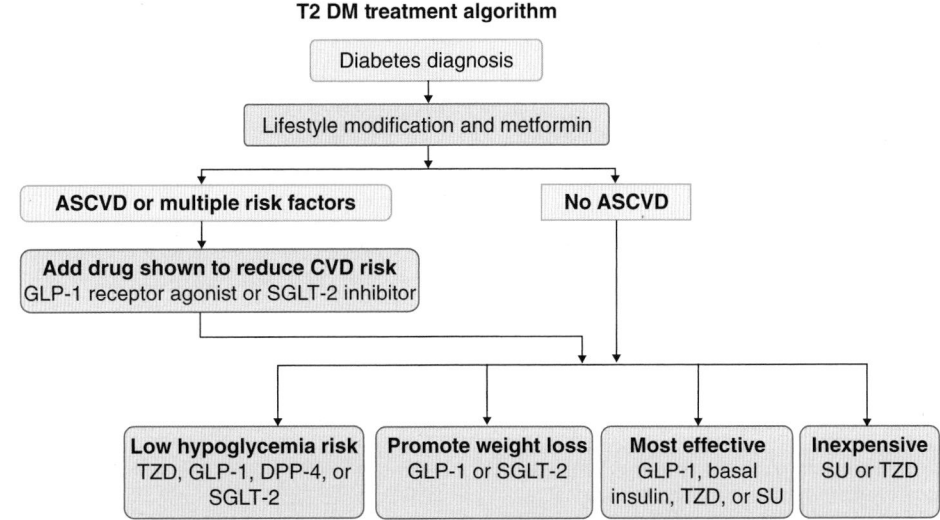

FIGURE 216-5. Algorithm for pharmacologic treatment of type 2 diabetes. ASCVD = Atherosclerotic cardiovascular disease; CVD = cardiovascular disease; DPP-4 = dipeptidyl peptidase 4; DPP-4-i = DPP-4 inhibitor; GLP-1 = glucagon-like peptide 1; HbA$_{1c}$ = glycosylated hemoglobin; SGLT-2 = sodium-glucose cotransporter-2; SU = sulfonylurea; TZD = thiazolidinedione.

Incretin-Based Therapies/DPP-4 Inhibitors

Inhibitors of dipeptidyl peptidase 4 (DPP-4), a ubiquitous serine protease, work by preventing the breakdown of endogenous GLP-1, thus prolonging its effects. DPP-4 inhibitors, including sitagliptin, saxagliptin, and linagliptin, are given orally in a single daily dose. Similar to GLP-1 agonists, they rarely cause hypoglycemia, but they are generally weight neutral and cause fewer gastrointestinal side effects. In a large randomized trial of patients with preexisting CVD, sitagliptin had no effect on future cardiovascular events.[A16] A network meta-analysis has shown that the use of GLP-1 agonists (above) or SGLT2 inhibitors (below) were associated with lower all-cause mortality in patients with type 2 diabetes that DDP-4 inhibitors or placebo or no treatment.[17] Concern about potential risk of pancreatitis and medullary thyroid cancer has also been raised but unconfirmed; however, severe joint pain and skin reactions (bullous pemphigoid) can occur in a small percentage of patients.

Other Pharmacologic Agents

SGLT2 Inhibitors

Canagliflozin, dapagliflozin, and empagliflozin are inhibitors of the sodium glucose cotransporter 2 (SGLT2) in the proximal renal tubule. This inhibition prevents the reabsorption of filtered glucose and results in glycosuria, which is accompanied by mild osmotic diuresis and modest weight loss. The most common adverse effect is an increase in mycotic genital infections; hyperkalemia, urinary tract infections, and reductions in blood pressure have also been reported. Other adverse effects include increased risk of diabetic ketoacidosis, and for canagliflozin, lower extremity amputation. In a large randomized trial of type 2 diabetes patients at high risk for cardiovascular events, empagliflozin reduced cardiovascular and all-cause death by 32% when added to standard care.[A17] Similar cardiovascular benefit has been reported with canagliflozin, but with a greater risk of amputation, primarily at the toe or metatarsal level,[A18] and both drugs appear to prevent decline in renal function. Among patients with evidence of CKD (albuminuria and/or eGFR 30-90 ml/min), canagliflozin can reduce the risk of adverse renal outcomes by 30%.[A19]

Other Drugs

Acarbose and miglitol are inhibitors of α-glucosidase enzymes in the intestinal lumen. They are given with meals to slow the absorption of carbohydrates. Gastrointestinal side effects (e.g. flatulence and bloating) are common and limit their use. Pramlintide, bromocriptine, and colesevelam are also approved for treatment of type 2 diabetes. However, they are used infrequently due to side effects and modest glucose-lowering properties.

Insulin Therapy

Insulin treatment can be considered for patients with type 2 diabetes at any point in the course of the disorder, although typically it is used after "failure" of oral or other noninsulin therapies. Insulin may also be preferred therapy in specific situations, such as during hospitalizations (especially in the perioperative period) or in pregnancy. In contrast to patients with type 1 diabetes, patients with type 2 diabetes may be adequately controlled with basal insulin alone or in combination with other antidiabetic medications. Basal insulin is frequently used in combination with oral medications (e.g., metformin, DPP-4 inhibitors) or GLP-1 agonists (e.g., exenatide, liraglutide). However, reflecting the heterogeneity of type 2 diabetes, some patients may require physiologic insulin replacement similar to that used in type 1 diabetes, and insulin pump therapy is a safe and valuable option in patients who otherwise require multiple daily injections.[A20] Daily insulin requirements tend to be higher for patients with type 2 compared with type 1 diabetes, reflecting the existence of insulin resistance. Use of concentrated insulin preparations (U-200 degludec, U-300 glargine, U-500 regular, U-200 lispro) may be helpful for insulin resistant patients who require insulin doses exceeding 100 units per day. Among patients with type 2 diabetes at high risk for cardiovascular events (CVEs), degludec is noninferior to glargine with respect to the incidence of major CVE and reduces the risk of symptomatic hypoglycemia. Information about available insulin preparations and insulin regimens is provided in the section on insulin therapy under type 1 diabetes (earlier) and in Table 216-5.

Treatment Algorithms

Use of multidrug regimens is common in type 2 diabetes, and algorithms have been developed to guide therapy; however, the current evidence base to support these recommendations is limited. There is general agreement that metformin should be initial therapy for most patients and that subsequent drugs (when needed) are added to but do not replace metformin. The choice of a specific drug combination is driven by a number of factors, including efficacy, cost, side effect profile (e.g., hypoglycemia, weight gain), and preference of the patient (Fig. 216-5). Preferential use of drugs shown to have cardiovascular benefits should be considered for patients with established atherosclerotic heart disease or multiple cardiovascular risk factors.

Metabolic Monitoring

Ongoing assessment of glycemic control is necessary to ensure optimal outcomes in patients with diabetes. Measurement of HbA$_{1c}$, which reflects mean glucose levels during the preceding 2- to 3-month period, should be performed routinely in all patients with diabetes, beginning at diagnosis and periodically thereafter. Quarterly tests should be done for patients whose therapy has been recently changed or who are not meeting glycemic goals. More stable patients can be tested twice a year. Self-monitoring of blood glucose levels is recommended for all patients using insulin and may be useful for any patient trying to achieve target glucose control. Monitoring for the development of vascular complications is addressed in the later section on chronic vascular complications.

Inpatient Management

Management of blood glucose levels during hospitalization is increasingly recognized as an important clinical issue, especially because 40 to 70% of hospitalized patients carry a concomitant diagnosis of diabetes. Frequently, diabetes is not the reason for admission, and attention to glucose management is secondary to other more critical medical problems. However, both hyperglycemia and hypoglycemia are associated with adverse outcomes in hospitalized patients, which has stimulated the development of algorithms and guidelines for inpatient glucose management, although the evidence base to support them is limited. Obviously, all patients with type 1 diabetes require continued insulin use during hospitalization.

Critically Ill Patients

After initial enthusiasm for intensive glucose control (maintenance of near-normoglycemia) for critically ill patients, more recent evidence suggests that it may be harmful, particularly when it is accompanied by hypoglycemia.[A21] Current guidelines recommend intravenous administration of insulin for critically ill patients in intensive care settings, with a goal of maintaining plasma glucose concentration between 140 and 180 mg/dL. Application of standardized infusion protocols, which include frequent glucose monitoring, is recommended.

Non–Critically Ill Patients

The evidence base to support specific treatment guidelines for non–critically ill hospitalized patients is weak because this has not been systematically studied in randomized trials. However, there is agreement that subcutaneous administration of insulin is the preferred therapy to control glucose for most hospitalized (non–critically ill) patients with diabetes. Generally accepted targets are below 140 mg/dL for fasting glucose concentration and below 180 mg/dL for random or postprandial glucose concentration, if this can be achieved with minimal hypoglycemia risk. The patient's status needs to be reassessed frequently and insulin doses adjusted as needed to maintain target glucose levels. Use of basal insulin (see Table 216-5) is sufficient for many type 2 patients, but some may require the addition of prandial or corrective doses of short-acting insulin. However, prolonged dependence on insulin "sliding scales" to manage hyperglycemia should be avoided as this is rarely successful and carries the increased risk of hypoglycemia. For stable patients who are eating consistent meals and those nearing hospital discharge, resumption of their usual oral or noninsulin injectable medications can be considered. Most patients with type 1 diabetes can be managed with their usual insulin injection regimen during hospitalization, but extra attention should be paid to hypoglycemia risk due to missed or delayed meals. Insulin pump therapy can be continued during hospitalization if the patient is able to direct its use and hospital personnel are sufficiently familiar with this form of treatment.

Prevention of Type 2 Diabetes

The substantial burden, both human and societal, that accompanies type 2 diabetes and the difficulty in treating it effectively once it has developed make it an appropriate target for prevention. Further, the existence of a defined state of increased risk, pre-diabetes (i.e., impaired glucose tolerance and impaired fasting glucose), allows identification of patients who are most likely to benefit. Interventions that have been studied to date include lifestyle change (i.e., weight loss and exercise) and several antidiabetic medications.[18]

LIFESTYLE CHANGES

The largest and longest diabetes prevention study to date was the Diabetes Prevention Program, conducted in the United States beginning in the 1990s. Individuals at high risk for type 2 diabetes on the basis of the presence of overweight or obesity and pre-diabetic hyperglycemia (fasting glucose concentration of 95 to 125 mg/dL and 2-hour glucose concentration of 140 to 199 mg/dL) were randomly assigned to an intensive lifestyle program or a medication arm (metformin vs. placebo) and observed for a mean of 3 years. The lifestyle intervention stressed modest weight reduction (minimum 7% of body weight) with a reduced fat, hypocalorie diet and moderate-intensity physical activity for 150 minutes/week. Incident diabetes (determined by oral glucose tolerance test) was reduced by 58% compared with placebo, although the risk reduction was somewhat diminished (34%) with longer-term follow-up of the cohort. Successful weight loss was the major predictor of diabetes prevention, with every kilogram of weight loss reducing diabetes risk by 16%. Primary care–led weight management programs[A22] and locaserin use[A23] can reduce hyperglycemia and lead to remission of type 2 diabetes. Similar findings were reported from other studies, including the Finnish Diabetes Prevention Study. Even among individuals who did not lose weight, achieving the physical activity goal was associated with lower diabetes risk.

MEDICATION

Several classes of antidiabetic drugs have been studied for diabetes prevention, including metformin, which reduced the risk of diabetes by 31% in the Diabetes Prevention Program. In smaller studies, the α-glucosidase inhibitor acarbose showed modest reduction in diabetes risk (approximately 25%). The thiazolidinediones (e.g., troglitazone and rosiglitazone) have also shown diabetes prevention effects but are not widely used for this purpose because of concerns about their long-term safety. Liraglutide used at the dose approved for weight loss (3 mg/day) lowered incident diabetes by 21% in overweight patients with pre-diabetes. None of these drugs is approved by the U.S. Food and Drug Administration for diabetes prevention.

RECOMMENDATIONS

Lifestyle modification and metformin can both be recommended for individuals at high risk of diabetes.[A24] Candidates for prevention include those with defined glucose abnormalities (impaired glucose tolerance, impaired fasting glucose) and those with overweight or obesity plus an additional risk factor, such as family history of diabetes. The curriculum for the lifestyle intervention used in

the Diabetes Prevention Program is available online (http://www.bsc.gwu.edu/dpp/lifestyle/dpp_part.html) and has been widely implemented in community settings, including the YMCA. Both lifestyle modification and metformin have shown positive effects on cardiovascular risk factors, but whether interventions to prevent diabetes will result in lower rates of microvascular or macrovascular complications remains to be determined.

Screening for Type 2 Diabetes

Individuals with risk factors for type 2 diabetes should be considered for screening for diabetes and impaired glucose regulation, even though screening has not been shown to reduce subsequent mortality.[19,20] This is especially important given that hyperglycemia can be present for years without specific symptoms and up to 30% of people with diabetes in the United States are undiagnosed. Screening will also allow identification of people with pre-diabetes, who may benefit from prevention interventions (Table 216-8).

Diabetes screening may be conducted with HbA_{1c} level, fasting glucose concentration, or oral glucose tolerance test, with the choice of test depending on the clinical setting and the preference of the patient. Screening should also be considered for asymptomatic children with BMI above the 85th percentile for age and sex plus any two of the following risk factors: family history of type 2 diabetes, high-risk race/ethnicity, or evidence of insulin resistance or features associated with insulin resistance (acanthosis nigricans, hypertension, dyslipidemia, polycystic ovary syndrome, or small-for-gestational-age birth weight). Pregnant women with risk factors for diabetes should be screened for undiagnosed diabetes at the first prenatal visit. Otherwise, a 75-g oral glucose tolerance test should be performed at 24 to 28 weeks of gestation to detect gestational diabetes.

Prognosis

Type 2 diabetes is a chronic and, in most cases, progressive condition with potentially serious health consequences. However, it is also uniquely sensitive to modification of nutritional and lifestyle factors, which has been shown to be effective for both prevention and treatment of diabetes. Further, several classes of effective antihyperglycemic medications are available. There is substantial evidence that early intervention with a multifactorial approach to achieve and to maintain metabolic control, plus aggressive control of CVD risk factors, will substantially reduce the burden of diabetes complications and improve quality of life.

ACUTE METABOLIC COMPLICATIONS OF DIABETES

Hypoglycemia

Iatrogenic hypoglycemia in people with diabetes is the most frequent cause of low blood glucose concentration. Hypoglycemia (Chapter 217) affects the daily lives of persons with diabetes and can have a dramatic effect on quality of life. It can induce great fear, preclude comfortable engagement in routine activities (e.g., driving, uninterrupted sleep), and lead both patient and clinician to set higher glycemic targets and hence worse metabolic control. Thus hypoglycemia continues to be a major limiting factor in the treatment of diabetes, particularly with the use of insulin.[21]

Whereas insulin-stimulatory drugs (e.g., sulfonylureas) and parenteral insulin are the primary causes of drug-induced iatrogenic hypoglycemia, underlying

TABLE 216-8 CRITERIA FOR DIABETES SCREENING IN ASYMPTOMATIC ADULTS

1. Overweight or obese (BMI >25 kg/m²) with one or more of the following:
   - First-degree relative with type 2 diabetes
   - High-risk race/ethnicity (e.g., African American, Latino, Native American, Asian American, Pacific Islander)
   - History of CVD
   - Hypertension
   - HDL cholesterol level <35 mg/dL or triglyceride level >250 mg/dL
   - Women with polycystic ovary syndrome
   - Physical inactivity
   - Other clinical conditions associated with insulin resistance

   Screening should begin at age 45 and be repeated at least every 3 years.
2. Patients with pre-diabetes (HbA_{1c} ≥5.7%, IGT, or IFG) should be tested annually.
3. Women with history of gestational diabetes should be tested at least every 3 years.

BMI = body mass index; HDL = high-density lipoprotein; IFG = impaired fasting glucose; IGT = impaired glucose tolerance.
Modified from American Diabetes Association. Standards of medical care in diabetes—2018. *Diabetes Care.* 2018;41(Suppl 1):S55-S64.

defects in some parts of the counter-regulatory cascade contribute to the greater frequency and potential morbidity and mortality of hypoglycemia among patients with diabetes. The normal counter-regulatory response to hypoglycemia and the typical adrenergic and neuroglycopenic hypoglycemia symptoms are described in Chapter 217.

The threshold plasma glucose value that results in hypoglycemic symptoms is not constant; it is lower after recent antecedent hypoglycemia and higher in patients with poor glycemic control. However, there is general consensus that a self-monitored glucose level of 70 mg/dL or lower is a value that should alert the patient or caregiver, regardless of the presence of symptoms. A more detailed classification system to describe hypoglycemia has been established and widely adopted in research settings (Table 216-9).

However, these distinctions are not commonly used in clinical practice, and the severity of symptoms is often confused with severity of the actual prevailing physiologic state. Thus a patient may feel intense symptoms at a glucose level of 50 to 60 mg/dL, for which there is no evidence of cognitive impairment or imminent danger, whereas potentially dangerous plasma glucose levels in the range of 20 to 40 mg/dL might go unappreciated owing to lack of classical symptoms. This also has implications for the epidemiology of hypoglycemia; most studies have reliably ascertained only the rates of severe hypoglycemia because other episodes are less likely to be documented. In type 1 diabetes, the DCCT reported 62 severe hypoglycemic episodes per 100 patient-years, although the actual risk may be higher in clinical settings. An episode of severe hypoglycemia can be the immediate cause of death in patients with type 1 diabetes, with recently reported mortality rates ranging from 4 to 10%. There remains uncertainty about the temporal relationship between hypoglycemia and death, and although prolonged episodes of very low circulating glucose (<15 mg/dL) can cause brain death, episodes of fatal hypoglycemia may be due to other mechanisms, such as ventricular arrhythmias. Episodes of severe hypoglycemia are much less common in patients with type 2 diabetes (see later).

In patients with treated diabetes, the initiation of the hypoglycemic event is due to mismatching of prevailing insulin levels to the underlying physiologic state of the individual. Thus even absent overt insulin overdosage, factors such as missed meals, exercise, recent weight loss, alcohol, or insulin-sensitizing drugs create this mismatch and may set the plasma glucose concentration on a downward trajectory. In addition, the counter-regulatory systems that normally would counteract the decline of glucose to dangerous levels may be impaired. In patients with type 1 diabetes, glucagon release during hypoglycemia may become impaired shortly after the onset of diabetes, although glucagon is still secreted in response to other secretagogues, suggesting the presence of a functional defect. Epinephrine release during hypoglycemia also becomes progressively defective in type 1 diabetes; it is not triggered until the plasma glucose level is lower, and the maximal concentration of epinephrine released is significantly reduced. This decrease in epinephrine response during hypoglycemia is accompanied by an attenuated autonomic neural response, which results in the clinical syndrome of *impaired awareness of hypoglycemia*. Without autonomic symptoms, mild hypoglycemia may proceed unnoticed to more advanced and dangerous phases. Patients who have both impaired awareness of hypoglycemia and defective counter-regulation are at the greatest risk for development of severe hypoglycemia.

Hypoglycemia-associated autonomic failure in type 1 diabetes apparently results from antecedent episodes of mild hypoglycemia that further degrade the counter-regulatory response. In experiments in people without diabetes, recurrent or recent episodes of hypoglycemia are associated with reduced autonomic (epinephrine and norepinephrine), symptomatic, and cognitive functional responses to subsequent episodes of hypoglycemia, impairing the endogenous defense mechanisms and the clinical signs required for hypoglycemia detection. Because patients with type 1 diabetes already have a reduced counter-regulatory response, hypoglycemia-associated autonomic failure may play a role in the vicious circle of hypoglycemia begetting hypoglycemia. Meticulous avoidance of hypoglycemia is the only current approach proven to improve the epinephrine response and to reverse impaired awareness of hypoglycemia.

Compared with type 1 diabetes, type 2 diabetes is associated with a much lower risk of hypoglycemia. However, hypoglycemia remains a major clinical problem in this population. Episodes of severe hypoglycemia become progressively more common in patients with longer duration of type 2 diabetes, due in part to progressive β-cell failure and increased dependence on pharmacologic treatments. Use of sulfonylureas accounts for a substantial proportion of cases of drug-induced hypoglycemia, and severe episodes characterized by coma have been reported with all the agents in common use. Other antidiabetic agents, such as metformin, thiazolidinediones, and incretin-based drugs, have been associated with measureable albeit lower risks of hypoglycemia; however, symptomatic hypoglycemia is rare unless these drugs are used in combination with insulin. The elderly are at particularly high risk for iatrogenic hypoglycemia because the intensity of adrenergic symptoms may be reduced and hypoglycemia-induced cognitive impairment greater.

CLINICAL APPROACH TO HYPOGLYCEMIA PREVENTION AND TREATMENT **Rx**

Patients with diabetes need to be well informed about the symptoms of hypoglycemia and the factors that predispose to its occurrence: meal timing and content, exercise, and the expected time course of the drugs in use (especially insulin). Patients should also be made aware that the accuracy of some home glucose meters and continuous glucose monitors may be reduced in the hypoglycemia range and that the typical sympathoadrenal symptoms may wane during years of diabetes. A history of recurrent hypoglycemia should be carefully evaluated and attempts made to determine whether the patient had experienced events that went unrecognized. For example, reports of unexplained night sweats or a clouded mental state on arising in the morning may be due to nocturnal hypoglycemia and should be investigated.

Table 216-10 lists several risk factors for severe hypoglycemia. Patients with these characteristics require greater vigilance, both in selection of treatment regimen and in the recognition and treatment of acute episodes.

Most mild or moderate episodes of hypoglycemia can be self-treated by ingestion of fast-acting carbohydrates such as glucose tablets, glucose gels, or food (juices, soft drinks, or a meal). The suggested amount of carbohydrate to be ingested is about 15 g, which will increase the plasma glucose concentration by about 15 mg/dL. Importantly, foods that are rich in fat delay glucose absorption and are thus less effective. If plasma glucose levels are still below 70 mg/dL and if symptoms have not abated after 15 minutes, the patient should take an additional 15 g of carbohydrate. Because the glycemic response to oral glucose is relatively transient, ingestion of a snack or a meal shortly after correction of hypoglycemia is recommended.

Parenteral treatment of hypoglycemia is recommended if the patient is unwilling or unable to ingest carbohydrates (e.g., due to impaired mental status) or if a patient has sulfonylurea-induced hypoglycemia (which may be prolonged). Intravenous administration of glucose (25 g) is the preferred treatment of hypoglycemia. Parenteral glucagon (1 mg subcutaneously) is an alternative, especially in patients with type 1 diabetes who may have to be treated by

TABLE 216-9 CLASSIFICATION OF IATROGENIC HYPOGLYCEMIA IN TREATED DIABETIC PATIENTS

	CLINICAL FEATURES
Severe hypoglycemia	Episode with neurocognitive impairment that requires another person to administer treatment
Documented symptomatic hypoglycemia	Measured glucose concentration ≤70 mg/dL that coincides with sympathoadrenal or neurologic symptoms. Episode is self-managed.
Asymptomatic hypoglycemia	Measured glucose concentration ≤70 mg/dL, but without concomitant symptoms. Absence of symptoms may be due to hypoglycemia unawareness or hypoglycemia-associated autonomic failure.
Pseudo-hypoglycemia	Typical hypoglycemia symptoms, but with measured glucose concentration >70 mg/dL. Symptoms may be caused by resetting of counter-regulatory system in the setting of chronic poor glucose control.

TABLE 216-10 RISK FACTORS FOR SEVERE HYPOGLYCEMIA IN PATIENTS WITH DIABETES

Youth (children)
Elderly taking sulfonylurea drugs or insulin
Altered consciousness
Ethanol use
Strenuous exercise in the previous 24 hours
Recent antecedent hypoglycemia
Use of pentamidine, quinine, or nonselective β-blocker drugs
Concomitant illnesses, such as sepsis, or hepatic, renal, or cardiac failure
Type 1 diabetes with history of recurrent severe hypoglycemia
Recent rapid improvement in HbA_{1c} into the normal range

family members for severe hypoglycemia. Because glucagon stimulates secretion of insulin in addition to promoting glucose production, it is less effective in patients with type 2 diabetes.

Nocturnal hypoglycemia may be a particular problem for patients with type 1 diabetes. It may be asymptomatic and unsuspected because plasma glucose concentration is rarely measured during the night. Risk factors for nocturnal hypoglycemia include increased physical activity in the last 24 hours, certain insulin regimens (e.g., use of NPH or regular insulin), meal content (e.g., the amount of fat), and alcohol consumption. In addition, sleep is associated with a decrease in the autonomic response to hypoglycemia. Currently, the only practical approaches to detection of nocturnal hypoglycemia are regular nocturnal (3 AM) self-monitoring or the use of continuous glucose monitors with alarm features. Some patients with nocturnal hypoglycemia present with sleep disturbances, morning headache, chronic fatigue, or depression. Children in particular may present with seizures or enuresis. Strategies to prevent nocturnal hypoglycemia include eating "long-acting" bedtime snacks (slowly absorbed carbohydrate, such as uncooked cornstarch) and regular monitoring of blood glucose concentration at bedtime so that corrective action (carbohydrate ingestion) can be taken.

Hyperglycemic States

Diabetic ketoacidosis (DKA) and hyperosmolar hyperglycemic state (HHS) are the most serious acute hyperglycemic complications of diabetes. DKA is typically associated with severe insulin-deficient states (i.e., type 1 diabetes). It may also occur rarely in type 2 diabetes under conditions of extreme stress, such as major infection or trauma or as a presentation of a variant of type 2 diabetes (ketosis-prone or Flatbush diabetes). On the other hand, HHS typically occurs in patients with type 2 diabetes. However, the distinction between the two clinical scenarios is sometimes blurred (e.g., patients with HHS may present with ketosis and acidosis), and these states may be considered as parts of the spectrum of severe metabolic decompensation. Despite aggressive treatment, mortality rates remain high for both conditions, approaching 5% for DKA and 15% for HHS. Mortality is associated not only with the extremes of age (i.e., the very young and the elderly) and comorbidities but also, importantly, with the severity of the precipitating illness or event. Thus in addition to correction of fluid and electrolyte imbalance and administration of insulin, treatment also includes prompt recognition of and therapy for any precipitating illness or event. A list of precipitating conditions commonly associated with DKA and HHS is shown in Table 216-11.

PATHOBIOLOGY

The pathogenesis of DKA and HHS mirrors the underlying respective forms of diabetes. The three fundamental biochemical features of DKA—hyperglycemia, ketosis, and acidosis—result from the combined effects of deficient circulating insulin and counter-regulatory hormone excess. This hormonal milieu promotes the delivery of substrates from muscle (amino acids, lactate, pyruvate) and adipose tissue (free fatty acids, glycerol) to the liver, where they are converted to glucose or to ketone bodies (β-hydroxybutyrate, acetoacetate, acetone). Glucose and ketones are thus released into the circulation at greater rates than their utilization, resulting in severe hyperglycemia (>250 mg/dL), ketoacidosis (arterial pH <7.30), and an osmotic diuresis that

TABLE 216-11	PRECIPITANTS OF DIABETIC KETOACIDOSIS AND HYPEROSMOLAR HYPERGLYCEMIC STATE

MOST COMMON

Inadequate insulin treatment or noncompliance
New-onset diabetes
Infections
Myocardial infarction

OTHER PRECIPITATING FACTORS

Cerebrovascular accident
Acute pulmonary embolism
Acute pancreatitis
Intestinal or mesenteric thrombosis
Alcohol intoxication
Endocrinopathies: Cushing syndrome, thyrotoxicosis, acromegaly
Severe burns, hyperthermia, hypothermia
Drugs: clozapine, olanzapine, cocaine, lithium, sympathomimetics, corticosteroids, thiazide diuretics, SGLT-2 inhibitors

SGLT-2 = sodium-glucose cotransporter-2.

promotes dehydration and electrolyte loss. In HHS, despite comparable elevations of glucagon, the presence of some endogenous insulin modulates the ketosis even though the plasma glucose concentration in HHS typically exceeds 600 mg/dL, whereas in DKA it is usually more than 250 mg/dL.

In both states, fluid depletion plays a major role in causing dramatic elevations in circulating glucose. Indeed, the hyperosmolality accompanying DKA and HHS is best linked to the patient's level of neural and cognitive function, and treatment of both conditions depends on restoration of fluid balance. Finally, other factors have been invoked, including other hormones (such as epinephrine, growth hormone, and cortisol), proinflammatory cytokines (such as tumor necrosis factor–α, interleukin-1β, interleukin-6, and interleukin-8), and lipid peroxidation markers as well as plasminogen activator inhibitor–1 and C-reactive protein. Whether all these factors are simply "stress markers" reflecting the disordered metabolic state or true pathogenetic factors remains uncertain.

Diabetic Ketoacidosis
CLINICAL MANIFESTATIONS
DKA (Chapter 110) may signal the onset of type 1 diabetes, but changes in medical practice in the developed world during the past several decades have enhanced earlier diagnosis of type 1 diabetes, and now the majority of childhood cases are detected and treated before ketoacidosis occurs. Thus DKA is more frequently seen in those with established diabetes, usually in the setting of coexisting illness or poor adherence. For example, a patient may be unable to maintain adequate hydration during an illness, such as a viral gastroenteritis, and may mistakenly omit insulin because of inability to eat. A key component of a diabetes treatment program is education in "sick-day" rules focused on home-based prevention of DKA (e.g., frequent blood glucose monitoring, serum or urine ketone testing, fluid intake, determination of insulin dosing or delivery problems). Behavioral factors may also be involved; some younger patients may omit insulin deliberately to promote weight loss or to call attention to a dysfunctional home situation. This should be suspected in cases of recurrent episodes of DKA.

The clinical history of DKA typically involves deterioration during several hours to days, with progressive polyuria, polydipsia, and other symptoms of hyperglycemia. Other common clinical features are weakness, lethargy, nausea, and anorexia. Nonlocalizing upper abdominal pain in the setting of DKA can mimic an acute abdomen. Reduced motility of the gastrointestinal tract or, in severe cases, paralytic ileus may further contribute to diagnostic confusion. Nausea and vomiting are symptoms that indicate the need for in-hospital treatment because they preclude oral fluid intake. Physical findings in DKA are mainly secondary to dehydration, hyperosmolality, and acidosis; these include dry skin and mucous membranes, reduced jugular venous pressure, tachycardia, orthostatic hypotension, depressed mental function, and deep, rapid respirations (Kussmaul breathing).

DIAGNOSIS
In DKA, glucose levels may vary from modestly elevated to more than 1000 mg/dL, serum bicarbonate concentration drops below 18 mEq/L, and there is an excess anion gap that is generally proportional to the decrease in serum bicarbonate (Table 216-12). Hyperchloremia may be superimposed if the patient maintains an adequate GFR and is able to exchange keto acids for chloride in the kidney. The degree of depression of arterial pH depends largely on respiratory compensation. In mild cases, the pH may range from 7.20 to 7.30; in severe cases, it can fall below 7.00. On occasion, a degree of superimposed metabolic alkalosis (e.g., caused by vomiting or diuretic use) may obscure the true severity of the ketoacidosis. An anion gap out of proportion to the fall of bicarbonate should suggest this possibility. Other laboratory abnormalities commonly seen in DKA include a reduced measured serum sodium concentration (due to hyperosmolarity and the resulting osmotic shift of intracellular water into the intravascular space), prerenal azotemia, and elevated serum amylase. The last is usually of nonpancreatic origin and can lead to an erroneous diagnosis of pancreatitis. Normal, elevated, or reduced concentrations of potassium, phosphate, and magnesium may exist when DKA is diagnosed; however, large deficits of these electrolytes invariably accompany the osmotic diuresis and become readily apparent during the course of treatment. The serum triglyceride concentration is frequently elevated, a reflection of deranged lipid metabolism in the setting of insulin deficiency. The white blood cell count is typically elevated; the hemoglobin and hematocrit may be elevated, reflecting intravascular volume contraction (hemoconcentration).

Special care should be taken in interpreting serum or urine ketone results. Because quantitative measurements of β-hydroxybutyrate and acetoacetate

TABLE 216-12	DIAGNOSTIC CRITERIA FOR DIABETIC KETOACIDOSIS (DKA) AND HYPEROSMOLAR HYPERGLYCEMIC STATE (HHS)			
CRITERION	MILD DKA	MODERATE DKA	SEVERE DKA	HHS
Plasma glucose concentration (mg/dL)	≥250	≥250	≥250	≥600
Effective serum osmolality (mOsm/kg)	Variable	Variable	Variable	≥320
Urine or serum ketones (nitroprusside reaction)	Positive	Positive	Positive	Negative to small
Arterial pH	7.25-7.30	7.00-7.24	<7.00	>7.30
Serum bicarbonate (mEq/L)	15-18	10-15	<10	>15
Anion gap (mEq/L)	>10	>12	>12	Variable, usually <12
Typical mental status	Alert	Drowsy	Stupor or coma	Stupor or coma

are not readily available, rapid diagnosis usually requires qualitative assessment of serum ketones by the use of serum dilutions and reagent strips (e.g., Ketostix) or tablets (e.g., Acetest), which depend on a nitroprusside reaction with acetoacetate. However, acetone reacts weakly with nitroprusside, and β-hydroxybutyrate does not react at all; thus the results of qualitative testing for ketones can be misleadingly low. Furthermore, because of the presence of intracellular acidosis, β-hydroxybutyrate levels are often much higher than acetoacetate levels, which may further conceal the true degree of ketoacidosis. Conversely, after insulin therapy is begun, the nitroprusside reaction may give the "false" impression of sustained ketoacidosis for hours or even days. This occurs because nonacidic acetone is slowly cleared from the circulation and also because, as acidosis improves, β-hydroxybutyrate is converted to acetoacetate, giving the false impression that ketosis is worsening.

TREATMENT ℞

An overview of the treatment of DKA and HHS is shown in Figure 216-6.

In the early hours of treatment, the primary considerations are to restore intravascular volume, to correct tissue hypoperfusion, and to restore insulin sensitivity. With DKA, large total body deficits of water (5 to 10 L), sodium (5 to 10 mEq/kg), and other electrolytes may exist (Chapter 110). These losses are even more profound in HHS, which typically develops during a longer time. Although water loss usually exceeds the loss of sodium, it is almost always preferable to begin fluid replacement with isotonic normal saline (0.9% NaCl solution) for efficient intravascular volume restoration. Fluid replacement regimens vary, but it is common to administer 1 L of normal saline within the first hour, followed by a continuous infusion with either 0.45% NaCl or 0.9% NaCl, depending on the corrected serum sodium concentration, the patient's hemodynamic status, and the clinical assessment of tissue perfusion. Likewise, the rate of infusion (commonly 250 to 500 mL/hour) should be adjusted according to both biochemical responses and the age and clinical status of the patient (e.g., oliguria or underlying CVD). In children, isotonic solutions are generally preferred because they are less likely than hypotonic solutions to accelerate water shifts into the intracellular space and contribute to cerebral edema. As the blood glucose concentration falls below 250 mg/dL, dextrose should be added to intravenous fluids to avoid later insulin-induced hypoglycemia because continued insulin delivery may be required to correct the persistent acidemia.

Although insulin resistance is present in both DKA and HHS, supraphysiologic doses of insulin are unnecessary and are more likely to provoke hypokalemia, hypophosphatemia, and delayed hypoglycemia. A typical insulin replacement regimen uses an intravenous 0.1 U/kg bolus of rapid-acting (e.g., regular) insulin, followed by 0.1 U/kg/hour thereafter. Intravenous administration is the most predictable way to deliver insulin to target tissues, particularly in severely hypovolemic patients with reduced peripheral blood flow. If intravenous administration is not possible, intramuscular or subcutaneous routes of administration can be used. It is ideal if blood glucose levels fall at a steady and predictable rate (50 to 75 mg/dL/hour), so it is important to monitor blood glucose levels hourly during insulin therapy to ensure an appropriate rate of decline. Blood glucose levels should not fall too rapidly, especially in young children, in whom accelerated correction of plasma glucose concentrations has been associated with cerebral edema.

After a stable blood glucose level of 150 to 250 mg/dL is achieved, with resolution of the anion gap acidosis, subcutaneous administration of insulin can be started and the intravenous insulin infusion discontinued. With DKA, it is important to overlap the intravenous and subcutaneous routes by at least 1 to 2 hours to avoid the rebound ketoacidosis if insulin levels drop precipitously. After stabilization, and with resumption of oral food intake, long-term medical management should be initiated (or resumed), with both long-acting and short-acting insulins, to approximate the desired outpatient regimen. A temporary "regular insulin sliding scale" should be avoided because such therapy is reactive to hyperglycemia and the swings in glycemia will not allow safe discharge of the patient. The eventual dosage and frequency of insulin depend on multiple factors, including body weight, comorbidity, insulin sensitivity, and effectiveness of prior therapeutic regimens.

Potassium replacement is usually required in DKA. Overt hypokalemia can result in muscle weakness, cramps, and nausea; both hyperkalemia and hypokalemia are associated with cardiac arrhythmias. Even absent severe hypokalemia, patients have a significant total body potassium deficit (about 3 to 7 mEq/kg), and measured serum potassium levels may be normal or high as acidosis and renal failure can mask the potassium deficiency. As insulin is infused, potassium will move into the intracellular space, further lowering serum potassium to levels that may trigger life-threatening arrhythmias. In addition, fluid replacement causes extracellular dilution of potassium, leading to improved renal perfusion and increased urinary potassium excretion. Thus potassium replacement should be initiated as soon as it is established that the patient is not in renal failure. A low potassium level (<3.5 mEq/L) requires prompt treatment with up to 40 mEq/hour, whereas "normal" serum levels (3.5 to 5.0 mEq/L) call for less aggressive repletion of potassium (20 to 30 mEq/hour), assuming adequate urine output. In patients who may have lost potassium for additional reasons, such as diuretic use or gastrointestinal loss, there will be need for greater potassium supplementation.

In the majority of patients with mild to moderate DKA, keto acids clear spontaneously with standard therapeutic measures, and correction of the pH with alkali (as bicarbonate) is unnecessary. Suppression of lipolysis by insulin reduces free fatty acid flux to the liver and blocks ketogenesis, and circulating keto acids are then cleared or oxidized, with subsequent regeneration of bicarbonate and restoration of arterial pH. However, in cases of severe acidosis (pH <6.9 to 7.0), bicarbonate administration may be indicated if the clinical picture dictates (e.g., hypotension that is unresponsive to fluids, cardiac dysfunction, respiratory exhaustion).[22] Bicarbonate therapy should be used with caution and only at the minimal doses required to stabilize the patient because it can further provoke hypokalemia. In addition, by causing a sudden left shift of the dissociation curve for oxyhemoglobin, bicarbonate may impair oxygen delivery to the tissues. Therefore if alkali therapy is given, small amounts should be administered slowly: 50 mEq of $NaHCO_3$ during 1 hour for arterial pH 6.9 to 7.0, and 100 mEq during 2 hours for pH below 6.9. After bicarbonate administration, arterial pH (and serum potassium levels) should be rechecked every 2 hours, and alkaline therapy should be discontinued when the pH rises above 7.0.

In the setting of DKA, phosphate losses average 3 to 7 mmol/kg; magnesium losses reach 1 to 2 mEq/kg. Phosphate is shifted extracellularly during hyperosmolar states, so initial serum levels may be falsely elevated and may drop rapidly during therapy. Complications of hypophosphatemia generally occur at serum levels below 1.0 mg/dL and include respiratory and skeletal muscle weakness, impaired cardiac systolic performance, and hemolytic anemia. Phosphate repletion should be used in patients with serum phosphate levels below 1.0 mg/dL and in patients with evidence of cardiac or respiratory compromise, hypoxia, or hemolytic anemia. An effective means of replacing phosphate is to replace one third to one half of the potassium losses (discussed previously) as potassium phosphate. In severe hypophosphatemia, cautious intravenous administration of additional small amounts of potassium phosphate may be necessary. Because of calcium binding, hypocalcemic tetany may complicate phosphate therapy unless magnesium supplements are also provided; for this reason, serum calcium, phosphate, and magnesium levels should be monitored during any phosphate infusion.

Hyperosmolar Hyperglycemic Syndrome
CLINICAL MANIFESTATIONS

The metabolic state formerly known as the hyperglycemic hyperosmolar nonketotic state or coma has been renamed the *hyperosmolar hyperglycemic syndrome* (HHS) to highlight two important points: (1) ketosis (and acidosis) may in fact be present to varying degrees in HHS, and (2) alterations in sensorium most commonly occur in the absence of coma. In fact, only 10% of HHS patients present with frank coma, and an equal percentage show no signs whatsoever of mental status change. Major risk factors for HHS include older

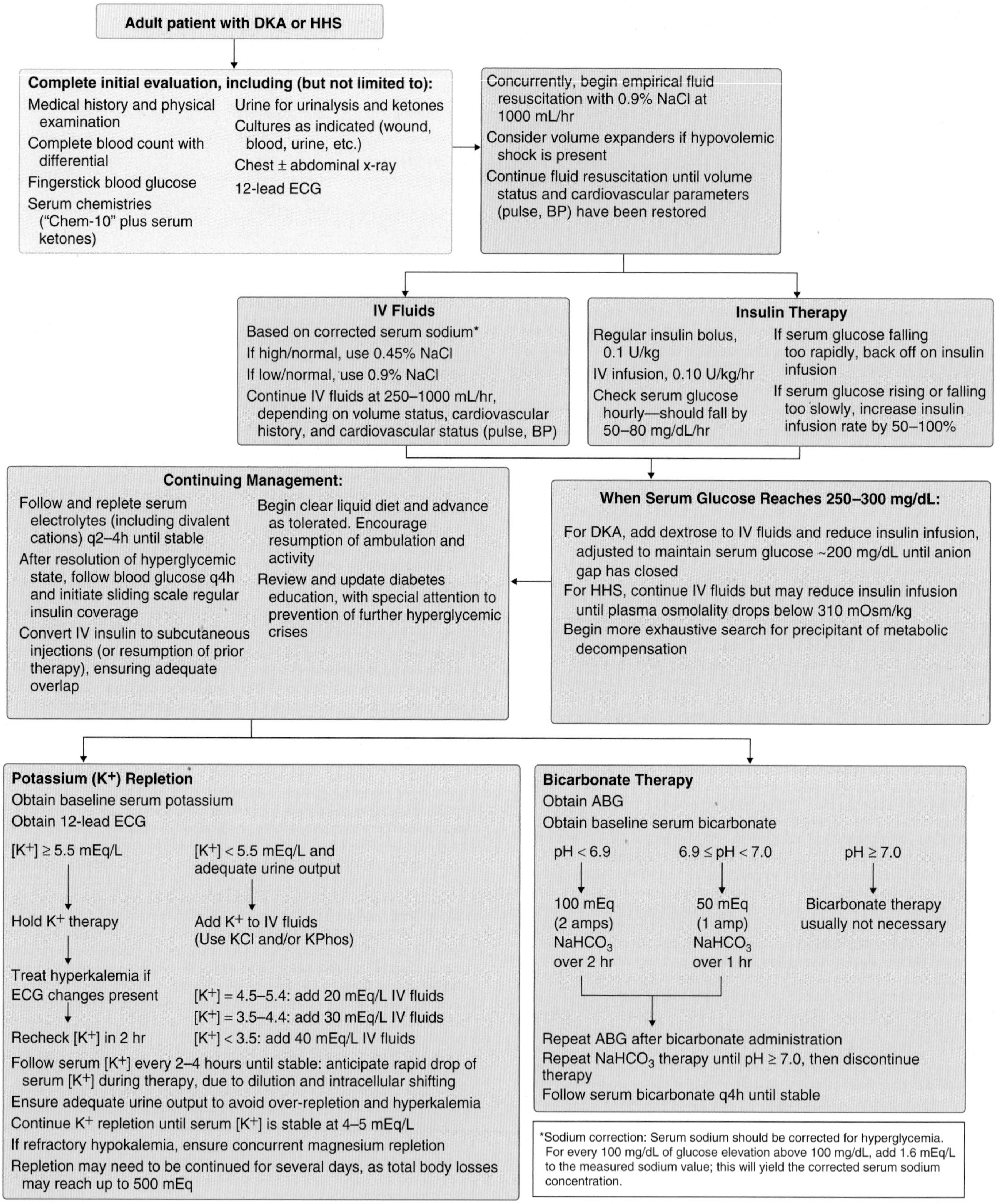

Adult patient with DKA or HHS

Complete initial evaluation, including (but not limited to):

Medical history and physical examination

Complete blood count with differential

Fingerstick blood glucose

Serum chemistries ("Chem-10" plus serum ketones)

Urine for urinalysis and ketones

Cultures as indicated (wound, blood, urine, etc.)

Chest ± abdominal x-ray

12-lead ECG

Concurrently, begin empirical fluid resuscitation with 0.9% NaCl at 1000 mL/hr

Consider volume expanders if hypovolemic shock is present

Continue fluid resuscitation until volume status and cardiovascular parameters (pulse, BP) have been restored

IV Fluids

Based on corrected serum sodium*

If high/normal, use 0.45% NaCl

If low/normal, use 0.9% NaCl

Continue IV fluids at 250–1000 mL/hr, depending on volume status, cardiovascular history, and cardiovascular status (pulse, BP)

Insulin Therapy

Regular insulin bolus, 0.1 U/kg

IV infusion, 0.10 U/kg/hr

Check serum glucose hourly—should fall by 50–80 mg/dL/hr

If serum glucose falling too rapidly, back off on insulin infusion

If serum glucose rising or falling too slowly, increase insulin infusion rate by 50–100%

Continuing Management:

Follow and replete serum electrolytes (including divalent cations) q2–4h until stable

After resolution of hyperglycemic state, follow blood glucose q4h and initiate sliding scale regular insulin coverage

Convert IV insulin to subcutaneous injections (or resumption of prior therapy), ensuring adequate overlap

Begin clear liquid diet and advance as tolerated. Encourage resumption of ambulation and activity

Review and update diabetes education, with special attention to prevention of further hyperglycemic crises

When Serum Glucose Reaches 250–300 mg/dL:

For DKA, add dextrose to IV fluids and reduce insulin infusion, adjusted to maintain serum glucose ~200 mg/dL until anion gap has closed

For HHS, continue IV fluids but may reduce insulin infusion until plasma osmolality drops below 310 mOsm/kg

Begin more exhaustive search for precipitant of metabolic decompensation

Potassium (K⁺) Repletion

Obtain baseline serum potassium

Obtain 12-lead ECG

[K⁺] ≥ 5.5 mEq/L

[K⁺] < 5.5 mEq/L and adequate urine output

Hold K⁺ therapy

Add K⁺ to IV fluids (Use KCl and/or KPhos)

Treat hyperkalemia if ECG changes present

[K⁺] = 4.5–5.4: add 20 mEq/L IV fluids

[K⁺] = 3.5–4.4: add 30 mEq/L IV fluids

Recheck [K⁺] in 2 hr

[K⁺] < 3.5: add 40 mEq/L IV fluids

Follow serum [K⁺] every 2–4 hours until stable: anticipate rapid drop of serum [K⁺] during therapy, due to dilution and intracellular shifting

Ensure adequate urine output to avoid over-repletion and hyperkalemia

Continue K⁺ repletion until serum [K⁺] is stable at 4–5 mEq/L

If refractory hypokalemia, ensure concurrent magnesium repletion

Repletion may need to be continued for several days, as total body losses may reach up to 500 mEq

Bicarbonate Therapy

Obtain ABG

Obtain baseline serum bicarbonate

pH < 6.9

6.9 ≤ pH < 7.0

pH ≥ 7.0

100 mEq (2 amps) NaHCO₃ over 2 hr

50 mEq (1 amp) NaHCO₃ over 1 hr

Bicarbonate therapy usually not necessary

Repeat ABG after bicarbonate administration

Repeat NaHCO₃ therapy until pH ≥ 7.0, then discontinue therapy

Follow serum bicarbonate q4h until stable

*Sodium correction: Serum sodium should be corrected for hyperglycemia. For every 100 mg/dL of glucose elevation above 100 mg/dL, add 1.6 mEq/L to the measured sodium value; this will yield the corrected serum sodium concentration.

FIGURE 216-6. Management of diabetic ketoacidosis (DKA) and hyperosmolar hyperglycemic syndrome (HHS). ABG = arterial blood gas; BP = blood pressure; ECG = electrocardiogram; IV = intravenous.

age (most cases occur in patients aged 65 years and older) and impaired cognition (i.e., impaired ability to recognize thirst or to obtain access to water).

As shown in Table 216-12, the hallmarks of the HHS are severe hyperosmolarity (>320 mOsm/L) and hyperglycemia (>600 mg/dL). Severe hyperglycemia occurs because patients cannot consume enough liquid to keep pace with a vigorous osmotic diuresis. The resulting impairment in renal function eventually further reduces glucose excretion through the kidney, leading to remarkable blood glucose elevations, sometimes exceeding 1000 mg/dL. In contrast to DKA, even though glucose concentrations are generally higher, severe acidosis and ketosis are usually absent in the HHS. This is probably explained by the presence of some residual insulin secretory capacity that is sufficient to suppress lipolysis and to avoid significant keto acid production. Some type 2 patients with depressed endogenous insulin secretion may be unable to suppress ketone production fully in the face of elevated counterregulatory hormones produced by physical illness. However, because HHS patients have higher portal vein insulin concentrations than do patients with

DKA, keto acid production by the liver is quantitatively less, yielding only mild acidosis. In the HHS, in the absence of concurrent acid-base disturbances, arterial pH rarely drops below 7.30, and serum bicarbonate levels typically do not fall below 18 mEq/L.

In the HHS, clinical severity and levels of consciousness generally correlate with the severity and duration of hyperosmolarity. Clinical signs indicate profound dehydration; gastrointestinal symptoms are seen less frequently than in DKA. A variety of often reversible neurologic abnormalities may exist, including grand mal or focal seizures, extensor plantar reflexes, aphasia, hemisensory or motor deficits, and worsening of a preexisting organic mental syndrome. The laboratory picture is dominated by the effects of uncontrolled diabetes and dehydration; renal function is impaired, hemoglobin and hematocrit are elevated, and liver function test results may be abnormal because of baseline hepatic steatosis. Although severe hyperglycemia would be expected to lower measured serum sodium concentration, it is not uncommon to see normal or even elevated sodium levels because of the severity of dehydration. The serum osmolarity can be measured directly or estimated.

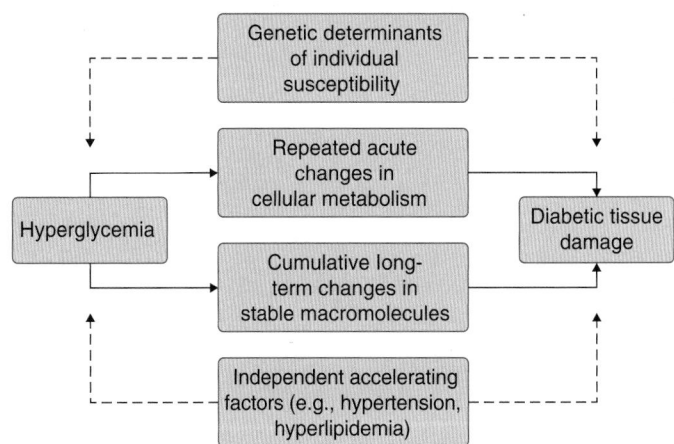

FIGURE 216-7. Factors related to the pathogenesis of diabetes complications. (From Brownlee M. The pathobiology of diabetic complications: a unifying mechanism. *Diabetes.* 2005;54:1615-1625.)

TREATMENT   Rx

The approach to treatment of HHS is similar to that of DKA and requires aggressive management of fluids and electrolytes (see Fig. 216-6).[23] Importantly, patients with HHS tend to have more dramatic volume contraction, and by definition, acidosis is not present or is minimal in degree. It is important to volume resuscitate the patient adequately before insulin is administered because intracellular fluid shifts that occur as glucose levels are reduced may worsen systemic tissue perfusion. In fact, glucose levels usually drop substantially with hydration alone, in part because of improved renal perfusion, thus promoting glycosuria. Coadministration of dextrose along with insulin, as is recommended in patients with DKA to allow ketones to clear and the acidosis to resolve, is rarely required. Further, because recurrent acidosis is less of a concern, patients may be transitioned directly from insulin infusion to subcutaneous injections. Because altered mental status (and, in some cases, coma) is a frequent feature of HHS, attention should be paid to respiratory status and appropriate airway protection. A diligent search for underlying precipitating illness should be made, keeping in mind that the typical HHS patient is elderly and may well have overt or subclinical CVD. The presence of impaired cardiac function, also more common among the elderly, needs to be considered in the management of intravenous fluid resuscitation.

After resolution of the HHS episode, some patients may ultimately be able to be managed with oral agents alone. However, the development of HHS signifies a significant degree of insulin deficiency. As a consequence, it is always best to prescribe insulin injections before the patient is discharged and to reserve judgment about the appropriateness of using non-insulin therapies until the patient's progress can be monitored and reassessed in the outpatient setting.

CHRONIC VASCULAR COMPLICATIONS
Epidemiology

The major clinical burden associated with long-standing diabetes is the development of vascular disease, which includes characteristic microvascular complications (retinopathy, nephropathy, neuropathy) and accelerated medium- and large-vessel atherosclerosis. Diabetes is the leading cause of kidney failure, nontraumatic lower limb amputations, and new cases of blindness among adults in the United States. Diabetes is also a major cause of coronary heart disease, heart failure, and stroke and is the seventh leading cause of death in the United States. The microvascular complications are directly linked to hyperglycemia, with both the duration of diabetes and the degree of glucose elevation constituting the major risk factors. Other factors, including genetic susceptibility, smoking, and concomitant conditions like hypertension, also contribute to the risk of complications (Fig. 216-7). Diabetic microvascular complications occur in both type 1 and type 2 diabetes; given that most patients with type 1 diabetes develop it when younger, they may face greater lifetime risk of complications.

The central role for hyperglycemia in the development of diabetic complications was long suspected and ultimately confirmed by the landmark DCCT, which was reported in 1993. In this study, 1441 adolescents and younger adults with type 1 diabetes were randomly assigned to conventional treatment designed to avoid symptomatic hypoglycemia or hyperglycemia (standard therapy at the time) or to an experimental treatment group designed to achieve near-normoglycemia. The experimental group received intensive management with multiple daily insulin injections or use of a continuous subcutaneous

insulin pump; frequent self-monitored blood glucose determinations; and adoption of detailed algorithms to guide the patient in determining insulin dosing in response to meals, glucose, and exercise. During the course of the study, mean HbA$_{1c}$ levels were 7.2% in the intensive group compared with 9% for the conventional treatment group. The unequivocal DCCT results showed substantially lower rates of retinopathy, nephropathy, and neuropathy in the intensively treated group and led to major changes in the approach to diabetes treatment in the United States and worldwide. Results of the UKPDS, conducted in a cohort of recently diagnosed patients with type 2 diabetes, later confirmed the benefits of more intensive glucose control in the prevention of microvascular complications. These and other studies have provided convincing evidence that hyperglycemia is the driving force behind diabetic microvascular disease. Indeed, the long-term follow-up studies of the DCCT cohort showed that the benefits seen in the intensively treated group persisted for at least a decade after the study ended, even after HbA$_{1c}$ levels between the two treatment groups converged, suggesting that the mechanisms underlying microvascular complications are conditioned by the prevailing metabolic milieu.

Pathobiology

The cellular and molecular mechanisms that mediate hyperglycemic tissue damage are complex and still being elucidated. We now know that multiple interrelated pathways are involved, including four that have received the most attention as key mediators of vasculopathy (Fig. 216-8).

ADVANCED GLYCATION END PRODUCTS
Advanced glycation end products (AGEs) are a heterogeneous group of compounds that form by the nonenzymatic interaction of glucose with amino groups on proteins. This process occurs continuously in vivo but is markedly accelerated in the presence of hyperglycemia. Indeed, the HbA$_{1c}$ test to monitor the chronic level of glycemia was the result of observations of the glycosylation of subfractions of adult hemoglobin. Levels of AGEs in serum and tissues (e.g., skin collagen) correlate with diabetic vascular complications and mean glucose levels over time. AGEs can alter the properties and function of long-lived proteins, such as collagen and elastin, leading to vascular stiffness and increases in basement membrane thickness. AGE binding to specific cell surface receptors (e.g., receptors for AGE, RAGE), particularly on macrophages and endothelial cells, stimulates activation of signaling cascades that promote inflammation and oxidative stress. For example, AGE-RAGE interaction activates the transcription factor NF-κB, leading to multiple pathologic changes in gene expression. Further, AGEs formed intracellularly alter the function of many important cellular proteins. Studies in animal models provide strong evidence that AGE formation is a key process mediating hyperglycemic damage. However, to date, studies of anti-AGE compounds (e.g., aminoguanidine) have failed to demonstrate efficacy in preventing or ameliorating diabetic complications in humans.

INCREASED POLYOL PATHWAY FLUX
Metabolism of glucose through the aldose reductase pathway is generally minor because this enzyme has a low affinity for glucose. However, in the setting of intracellular hyperglycemia (most likely to occur in tissues that cannot

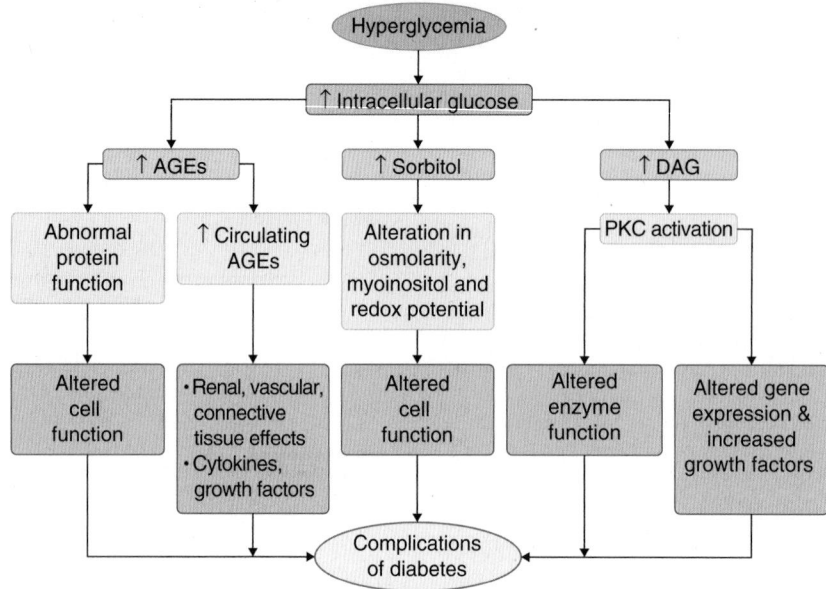

FIGURE 216-8. Proposed mechanisms of hyperglycemia-induced vascular complications. See text for discussion. AGEs = advanced glycation end products; DAG = diacylglycerol; PKC = protein kinase C.

downregulate glucose uptake, such as neurons and endothelial cells), there is increased flux through this pathway, leading to an accumulation of osmotically active sorbitol within the cell. Increased cellular osmolarity occurs, along with an increase in redox stress due to depletion of the reduced form of nicotinamide adenine dinucleotide phosphate and reduced glutathione. Inhibitors of aldose reductase have been proposed as a therapeutic strategy to reduce diabetic complications. Current evidence from clinical trials does not support their use, but this remains an active area of research.

ACTIVATION OF PROTEIN KINASE C

Intracellular hyperglycemia leads to increased de novo synthesis of diacylglycerol, which is a major activator of the protein kinase C family of enzymes. Activation of protein kinase C initiates a complex network of intracellular signaling that alters gene expression and results in enhanced angiogenesis, vasoconstriction, vascular permeability (by increases in vascular endothelial growth factor), cytokine activation, and extracellular matrix expansion. These alterations in cellular function have been linked to the development of microvascular complications (especially retinopathy) and atherosclerosis. Inhibitors of specific protein kinase C isoforms are being studied in clinical trials as agents specific for diabetic retinopathy and macular edema.

INCREASED HEXOSAMINE PATHWAY FLUX

In the setting of hyperglycemia and excess fatty acid oxidation, there is also increased flux of glucose through the hexosamine pathway, leading to increases in glucosamine 6-phosphate and ultimately post-translational modification of certain cytoplasmic and nuclear proteins. Associated with this are increases in expression of key genes, including those for transforming growth factor (α and β_1) and plasminogen activator inhibitor–1, and inhibition of endothelial nitric oxide synthase activity. Whereas the pathway has been linked to defective insulin action, its role in specific complications remains unclear.

These multiple and complex pathways are not mutually exclusive but are interconnected and may have a common antecedent process, which is overproduction of superoxide by the mitochondrial electron transport chain. Superoxide generates the production of other reactive oxygen species that can lead to cellular damage in a variety of ways. Data from animal models support the possibility that correction of diabetes-induced superoxide overproduction will have positive downstream effects on the various pathways leading to hyperglycemic tissue damage, but this remains to be confirmed in human studies.

Microvascular Complications

DIABETIC RETINOPATHY

Diabetic retinopathy (Chapter 395) is a highly prevalent, pathognomonic, microvascular complication, eventually affecting more than 50% of patients with long-term diabetes, although it causes vision impairment less frequently. The occurrence of vision loss due to diabetic retinopathy has declined during the past few decades as glucose and blood pressure control have improved in the population with diabetes. Nonetheless, it remains an important cause of preventable blindness, especially among patients with poor metabolic control. Both vascular and neural tissues in the retina are affected by chronic hyperglycemia. Early changes include the loss of retinal supporting cells (pericytes), basement membrane thickening, and retinal blood flow changes. Damaged retinal capillaries leak protein, red blood cells, and lipids, leading to retinal edema. Chronic retinal hypoxia (due to capillary occlusion) promotes neovascularization; these new vessels are abnormal and prone to rupture. Retinal hemorrhage, inflammation, and scarring can ultimately lead to traction retinal detachment and permanent vision loss (Table 216-13).

Diabetic retinopathy can be detected by dilated funduscopy, with early signs being the presence of microaneurysms, exudates, and intraretinal hemorrhages. Additional tests, including fluorescein angiography and ocular coherence tomography, are helpful to detect abnormal vessel permeability and macular edema, which can threaten vision. Regular screening by an eye care specialist (an ophthalmologist or optometrist) is recommended for all patients with diabetes because significant and potentially vision-threatening retinopathy can be present in the absence of any symptoms.[24] Screening should begin at diabetes diagnosis for patients with type 2 diabetes because hyperglycemia has typically been present for years before it is recognized clinically. For patients with type 1 diabetes, screening can begin at 5 years after diagnosis or after puberty for childhood onset. Because retinopathy can progress rapidly during pregnancy, screening and follow-up should be more aggressive during this time (Table 216-14).

As with other diabetic complications, intensive glycemic control can prevent diabetic retinopathy, delay its progression, and reduce the long-term need for

TABLE 216-13	CLASSIFICATION OF DIABETIC RETINOPATHY
	CLINICAL FEATURES
Mild NPDR	At least one microaneurysm
Moderate NPDR	Microaneurysms, intraretinal (blot) hemorrhage, soft exudates, venous beading, intraretinal microvascular abnormalities
Severe NPDR	More extensive intraretinal hemorrhages (>20 in each of four quadrants) *or* venous beading in at least two quadrants *or* prominent intraretinal microvascular abnormalities
PDR	Neovascularization and/or vitreous or pre-retinal hemorrhage; traction retinal detachment
Clinically significant macular edema	Retinal thickening or hard exudates approaching or involving the center of the macula

NPDR = nonproliferative diabetic retinopathy; PDR = proliferative diabetic retinopathy.

TABLE 216-14	RECOMMENDED INTERVALS FOR DIABETIC RETINOPATHY SCREENING	
DIABETES TYPE	**FIRST EXAMINATION**	**FOLLOW-UP**
Type 1	5 years after diagnosis	Annual
Type 2	At time of diagnosis	Annual
Established diabetes during pregnancy	Before or soon after conception	At least every 3 months

ocular surgery.[A25] However, it has limited effects on advanced retinal disease. Blood pressure control is also important to prevent worsening of retinopathy; there is some evidence that renin-angiotensin system (RAS) blockers may be especially beneficial.

Treatment of diabetic retinopathy (Chapter 395) includes laser photocoagulation, which can ablate abnormal vessels (thus reducing the risk of hemorrhage) and treat macular edema. Laser photocoagulation can be focal (to treat clinically significant macular edema or nonproliferative diabetic retinopathy) or panretinal (to treat severe nonproliferative diabetic retinopathy or proliferative diabetic retinopathy). Vitrectomy is a surgical procedure to remove hemorrhage and scar tissue that is obscuring vision. Nonsurgical therapies include intravitreal injection of glucocorticoids or anti–vascular endothelial growth factor monoclonal antibodies (e.g., ranibizumab) to treat macular edema.[A26] The established efficacy of retinopathy treatment, particularly photocoagulation, in preventing vision loss provides strong justification for routine retinopathy screening. There is evidence that treatment with fenofibrate reduces the progression of retinopathy, although the medication has not been approved for this indication in the United States. In addition to its well-known effects on lipid metabolism, fenofibrate appears to have significant anti-inflammatory, antiangiogenic, and antioxidant properties that are relevant to retinal disease. The presence of retinopathy is not considered a contraindication to the use of aspirin for CVD prevention.

Other eye conditions also affect patients with diabetes. Transient osmotically induced refractive error is common, especially at the time of diabetes diagnosis, but resolves with glucose control. Age-related eye conditions, such as cataracts and glaucoma, tend to occur at younger ages among diabetic patients. Diplopia and other gaze disorders due to acute mononeuropathy involving the cranial nerves (typically III or VI) are also more common in diabetes.

DIABETIC NEPHROPATHY

Diabetic nephropathy (Chapter 116) remains the most common single cause of end-stage renal failure, accounting for up to 50% of the cases in Western societies. Further, despite advances in the management of glucose and hypertension, the prevalence of chronic kidney disease among patients with diabetes has declined little, if at all, in the past several decades. Overall, 20 to 30% of type 1 and type 2 diabetic patients develop evidence of nephropathy, although fewer type 2 patients progress to end-stage renal disease (ESRD). This may be because of competing mortality from CVD, with fewer surviving to ESRD. However, because of their much greater frequency in the population, the majority of diabetes patients presenting for treatment of ESRD (dialysis or transplantation) have type 2 diabetes.[25] The major risk factor for the development of diabetic nephropathy is the duration and severity of hyperglycemia, but there is evidence for variation in genetic susceptibility. For example, African Americans and individuals with a family history of diabetic or nondiabetic renal disease are at higher risk for diabetic nephropathy. An insertion/deletion polymorphism in the gene encoding angiotensin-converting enzyme (ACE) has been widely reported to be associated with increased risk of diabetic nephropathy, but variants in genes involved in the polyol pathway, lipid metabolism, inflammatory cytokines, angiogenesis, and oxidative stress have also been identified.

Diabetic nephropathy develops during many years to decades, with a prolonged "silent" period before clinical detection, followed by more rapid progression to overt renal disease (Chapter 116). In the classic view, the hallmark of diabetic nephropathy is the development of proteinuria, which is due to alteration in glomerular basement membrane permeability and increases in intraglomerular pressure. The first clinical evidence of incipient nephropathy is the development of albuminuria, which is quantitatively minor at first (microalbuminuria, urine albumin-to-creatinine ratio of 30 to 300 mg/g) and then progresses to overt proteinuria, sometimes in the nephrotic range (>2 g/day). During the microalbuminuria phase, GFR is preserved but begins to

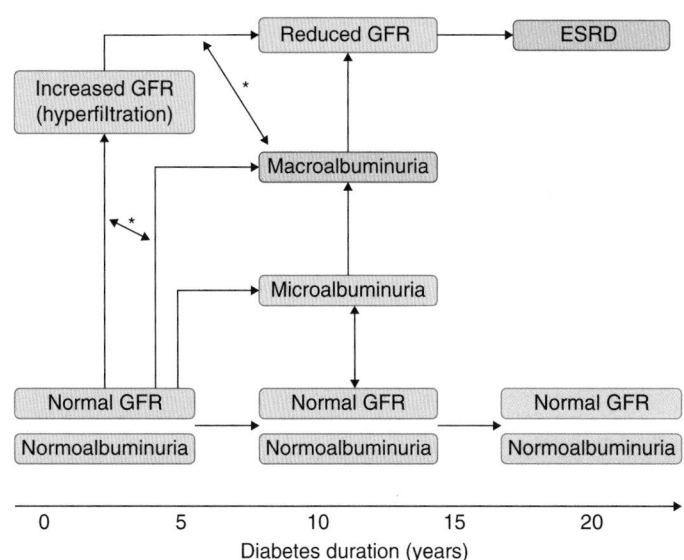

FIGURE 216-9. Development of diabetic nephropathy. See text for discussion. GFR = glomerular filtration rate; ESRD = end-stage renal disease. *GFR and albuminuria may progress independently of each other, that is, patients may have microalbuminuria or macroalbuminuria even though their GFR is normal or even slightly elevated. However, macroalbuminuria is usually associated with reduced GFR and is a strong risk for progressive ESRD. (From Boger CA, Sedor JR. GWAS of diabetic nephropathy: is the GENIE out of the bottle? *PLoS Genet.* 2012;8:e1002.)

decline in parallel with increasing proteinuria, leading to ESRD 5 to 15 years after the first detection of abnormal albumin excretion. However, recent evidence suggests that chronic kidney disease in diabetes is more heterogeneous than previously thought, with some patients progressing to advanced stages of chronic kidney disease in the absence of albuminuria (Fig. 216-9). Nonalbuminuric diabetic kidney disease appears more likely to occur in older patients with type 2 diabetes and may reflect, in part, the concurrence of multiple renal risk factors, including hypertension, obesity, and dyslipidemia. Further, microalbuminuria does not inevitably progress, with some patients regressing to normal or maintaining small but stable amounts of albuminuria. However, persistent and increasing albuminuria is a marker of high risk for progression to clinical nephropathy. Pathologic changes that are typical of diabetic nephropathy include an increase in glomerular basement membrane thickness and increased accumulation of extracellular matrix leading to mesangial expansion and the classic Kimmelstiel-Wilson nodular lesion.

Patients with diabetes should be screened annually for renal involvement (Chapter 116) by measurement of albumin on a spot urine sample with a sensitive immunoassay to detect microalbuminuria and by measurement of serum creatinine for calculation of estimated GFR. The finding of moderately increased urine albumin-to-creatinine ratio (30 to 300 mg albumin per gram of creatinine) should be confirmed on two of three repeated tests because transient increases are not uncommon but may not be clinically important. Data from the DCCT and other studies provide strong evidence that aggressive glycemic control can prevent the development of diabetic nephropathy and can retard the progression of microalbuminuria. However, there is little evidence that glycemic control can modulate the course once clinical albuminuria (>300 mg/day) and declining GFR occur. Central to the treatment of patients with albuminuria (micro or clinical) is intensive blood pressure control, preferentially by blockade of the RAS. Both ACE inhibitors and angiotensin receptor blockers have been shown to delay the progression of diabetic nephropathy and are recommended for patients with albuminuria even in the absence of hypertension. Despite initial enthusiasm, combined ACE inhibitor and angiotensin receptor blocker therapy is not recommended because of high rates of hyperkalemia and acute renal injury. In hypertensive patients, other drugs, such as calcium-channel blockers, diuretics, and β-blockers, can be used as additional therapy if needed to achieve adequate blood pressure control.[A27] There is little evidence to support use of RAS blockade in diabetic patients who are normotensive and normoalbuminuric, although there may be a therapeutic rationale for use of these agents in patients who cannot achieve adequate glycemic control. Dietary protein restriction has been recommended in the past for patients with nephropathy, but recent trials have been unable to demonstrate an effect of a low-protein diet on the rate of deterioration of GFR.

DIABETIC NEUROPATHY

Diabetic neuropathy (Chapter 392) is a common complication of diabetes, with an estimated lifetime prevalence of about 50%. Diabetic neuropathy can be manifested in a variety of syndromes, including radiculoplexopathy and autonomic neuropathy, but the most common form is a characteristic distal symmetrical polyneuropathy (DSP).[26] Despite its high prevalence, there is no distinct neuropathic symptom or lesion that is specific to diabetes, and separation of diabetic neuropathy from other causes can be problematic. As for other microvascular complications, the etiology of DSP is attributed to hyperglycemia, as demonstrated by the dramatic 60% reduction in neuropathy in the intensive treatment group in the DCCT study. However, the possibility that the pathogenesis of DSP may differ in type 2 diabetes, with dyslipidemia and insulin resistance also contributing, has recently emerged. Support for this view comes from largely negative neuropathy results of clinical trials of intensive glucose control in type 2 diabetes (e.g., Action to Control Cardio-vascular Risk in Diabetes [ACCORD] trial, VA Cooperative study) and the observation that the prevalence of DSP is already increased in the setting of pre-diabetes and the metabolic syndrome.

The clinical manifestations of DSP include symptoms of pain, paresthesias, and numbness that typically begin in the feet and progress more proximally in a "stocking and glove" distribution (Chapter 392). Loss of sensation, which may not be noticed by the patient, constitutes an important risk factor for falls due to gait instability. Ulceration, uncontrolled infection, and amputation can also occur from altered foot mechanics and inability to perceive repetitive trauma or other foot injury. For some patients, neuropathic pain can be severe and disabling, resulting in a major reduction in quality of life. DSP can be diagnosed by the presence of classic symptoms and by loss of ability to perceive pressure from a nylon (Semmes-Weinstein) monofilament, impaired vibration sense or loss of pinprick sensation. Additional tests, such as nerve conduction studies or electromyography, are occasionally indicated to distinguish DSP from radiculopathy. Current treatment options are mostly limited to control of metabolic risk factors (i.e., glucose, lipids) and symptoms. The chronic pain of DSP can be difficult to manage. Available therapies include tricyclic anti-depressants, serotonin-norepinephrine reuptake inhibitors, and anticonvulsants (such as gabapentin and pregabalin); opioids are not specifically useful and their use has major addiction potential.

Other forms of diabetic nerve damage (Chapter 392) include small-fiber predominant neuropathy, radiculoplexopathy (diabetic amyotrophy), non-compressive radiculopathy, and mononeuritis multiplex. Autonomic neuropathy can be manifested as gastroparesis, urinary retention, erectile dysfunction, sudomotor dysfunction (typically anhidrosis of the extremities with or without hyperhidrosis of the trunk), cardiac arrhythmias, and disturbance of gut motility (diabetic diarrhea or constipation). Cardiac autonomic neuropathy is an especially ominous form of diabetic autonomic neuropathy. Typical clinical manifestations of cardiac autonomic neuropathy include resting tachycardia, diminished heart rate variability, and orthostatic blood pressure changes. Patients with cardiac autonomic neuropathy are at high risk for myocardial infarction, congestive heart failure, and sudden cardiac death.

DIABETIC FOOT

The combination of sensory impairment due to peripheral neuropathy and reduced tissue perfusion due to large-vessel atherosclerosis (peripheral arterial disease) or microvascular dysfunction can result in ulceration, infection, and ultimately lower extremity amputation. A typical case involves development of an ulceration (often surrounded by callus formation) on the plantar surface of the foot, often underneath the metatarsal heads.[27] Ulceration can be slow to heal because of repetitive trauma from walking and impaired blood flow; hyperglycemia may also impair wound healing by effects on white blood cell migration and function. In the absence of protective sensation, an infection may fester for weeks and eventually invade the bone, leading to osteomyelitis. Altered foot mechanics can also lead to repeated (and usually undetected) fractures that destroy normal foot architecture and result in the classic Charcot foot deformity.

For many patients, foot amputation is the most feared diabetic complication; fortunately, it can be prevented in most cases but requires vigilance on the part of the patient and health care team. Routine foot examination, especially for patients who have evidence of sensory loss, should be performed at every medical visit, and patients should be instructed to inspect their feet daily for cracks, fissures, ulcers, or inflammation. Patients should avoid walking barefoot (even at home) and should wear protective covering (avoid sandals) outside. Thermal injuries can be prevented by avoiding use of heating pads or hot-water bottles on the feet. Referral to a foot care specialist should be considered for patients with sensory loss, foot deformity, extensive callus formation, and nonhealing ulcers. Ulcers are treated with aggressive débride-ment of necrotic tissue and systemic antibiotics (guided by culture of infected tissue) if infection is present. Pressure "off-loading" by use of special shoes, orthotics, or application of total contact casts may be necessary to allow healing. Additional treatments include use of topical platelet-derived growth factor, bioengineered skin substitutes, hyperbaric oxygen, and negative-pressure wound therapy, although none of these has shown conclusive evidence of effectiveness in promoting wound healing.

Other Associated Conditions

Patients with diabetes can develop a number of electrolyte and acid-base abnormalities,[28] even in the absence of ketoacidosis or hyperosmolarity. In type 4 renal tubular acidosis (Chapter 110), for example, hyperkalemia can require dietary and medical interventions.

Although not traditionally recognized as diabetic complications, there are a number of disorders that are increased in frequency or severity in patients with diabetes and that have a plausible or established relationship with hyper-glycemia. These include periodontal disease, Alzheimer dementia, and mus-culoskeletal disorders, such as limited joint mobility, adhesive capsulitis, Dupuytren contracture, and trigger finger (flexor tenosynovitis). Patients with poorly controlled diabetes are widely thought to have increased susceptibility to infection, particularly with fungal pathogens. Defects in immune function (impaired neutrophil chemotaxis) have been described in diabetes, but whether this occurs in reasonably controlled diabetes or contributes to clinical infec-tion is unclear. The incidence of osteoporotic fractures appears to be increased in women with diabetes, despite the presence of normal or even increased bone density. There is also emerging evidence that the frequency of some cancers (e.g., pancreatic, endometrial, colorectal, breast) is increased among people with diabetes.

● CARDIOVASCULAR DISEASE IN DIABETES

Atherosclerotic CVD is the major cause of morbidity and mortality for patients with diabetes and contributes substantially to its economic costs. The clinical and pathologic features of CVD in diabetes are generally not distinguishable from those occurring in nondiabetic individuals, but they are manifested at an earlier age, are more aggressive, and are associated with mortality rates that are two to four times higher in patients with diabetes (Chapter 46). This increased CVD risk is true for both type 1 and type 2 diabetes, with CVD in type 1 diabetes being strongly associated with concurrent presence of renal disease. Diabetes is also an important risk factor for peripheral vascular disease and stroke, which carries greater mortality risk than in nondiabetic patients.

Pathobiology of Cardiovascular Disease in Diabetes

The pathogenesis of atherosclerotic CVD in diabetes is complex and multi-factorial, with several mechanisms playing key roles. *Metabolic factors*, including hyperglycemia, insulin resistance, dyslipidemia, and increases in circulating free fatty acids, contribute to atherosclerotic plaque formation. Increases in *oxidation and glycoxidation* of lipoproteins increase their atherogenicity and enhance foam cell formation. *Endothelial dysfunction*, an early event in the development of atherosclerosis, has been described in association with several metabolic syndrome components, including hyperglycemia, insulin resistance, hypertension, and dyslipidemia. Systemic *inflammation*, which contributes to accelerated plaque formation, is increased in diabetes and obesity as a conse-quence of increased cytokine production by adipose tissue. Finally, diabetes is characterized by a *prothrombotic* state due to enhanced platelet reactivity and alterations in coagulation factors, including increased circulating levels of fibrinogen and plasminogen activator inhibitor–1.

Diabetic Cardiomyopathy and Heart Failure

Diabetic cardiomyopathy is defined as alterations in cardiac structure and function that are not directly attributable to coronary artery disease or hyper-tension (Chapters 52 and 53). Characteristic features include cardiac hyper-trophy, left ventricular dysfunction (diastolic may precede systolic), and altered myocardial metabolism. Diabetes is a recognized risk factor for the development of heart failure, even in the absence of atherosclerotic heart disease. For example, in the Framingham Heart Study, the frequency of heart failure was twice in diabetic men and five times in diabetic women compared with age-matched controls and persisted despite correction for hypertension, obesity, dyslipid-emia, and coronary artery disease. Increased activation of the renin-angiotensin-aldosterone system and formation of AGEs are thought to contribute to myocardial fibrosis and stiffness, and altered substrate utilization (preferential use of free fatty acids) can promote myocyte dysfunction by enhanced production of reactive oxygen species and other mechanisms. Characteristic changes in myocardial function and structure were reported in type 1 diabetes in the DCCT and Epidemiology of Diabetes Interventions and Complications (EDIC) study and were related to long-term glycemic control.

Prevention of Cardiovascular Disease in Diabetes

Aggressive control of CVD risk factors is recommended for most patients with diabetes, keeping in mind that the presence of diabetes is considered the risk equivalent of a prior myocardial infarction by most risk assessment algorithms (e.g., Framingham risk score, Adult Treatment Panel III Report of the National Cholesterol Education Program). Assessment of blood pressure, lipid profile, and smoking status should be included as part of routine diabetes care. Determination of the optimal targets for risk factor control has been the subject of several large randomized trials, which have informed consensus guidelines.

GLUCOSE CONTROL

Hyperglycemia is a major risk for atherosclerotic CVD. In population-based studies including diabetic and nondiabetic cohorts, HbA$_{1c}$ has been reported as an independent predictor of all-cause and CVD mortality, and among individuals with diabetes, every 1% rise in HbA$_{1c}$ is associated with a 30% increase in all-cause mortality and a 40% increase in CVD mortality. Compelling evidence for the benefit of intensive glucose control in patients with type 1 diabetes was shown in the DCCT/EDIC study, in which CVD events were reduced by 58%. However, in type 2 diabetes, hyperglycemia occurs in the setting of multiple other CVD risk factors, including hypertension, dyslipidemia, and obesity, which also contribute to risk, so the contribution of glucose control is less clear. Several large clinical trials in patients with type 2 diabetes have failed to show that aggressive control of hyperglycemia has important effects on CVD outcomes (see later), highlighting the complex pathogenesis of vascular disease in diabetes. Similarly, an intensive lifestyle program designed to achieve weight loss and exercise goals also failed to demonstrate significant effects on CVD outcomes in type 2 diabetes patients.[A28]

The strongest evidence in favor of intensive glucose control comes from the long-term follow-up of the UKPDS, which demonstrated 15% reduction in myocardial infarction and 13% reduction in all-cause mortality in the intensive versus conventional treatment group. More recently, in the ACCORD trial, an intensive treatment arm, designed to maintain HbA$_{1c}$ below 6%, was compared with conventional treatment with HbA$_{1c}$ goal of 7.5% in a cohort of type 2 diabetes patients at high risk for CVD. This trial was stopped early because of unexpected increased mortality, largely CVD related, in the intensive treatment group. The reasons for increased mortality with intensive treatment are not known for certain, but increased frequency and severity of hypoglycemia or the toxicity of specific drugs or combinations has been proposed. Secondary analysis of ACCORD data showed a reduction in nonfatal myocardial infarction in the intensive treatment group, leading to speculation that some patients might still benefit. Other studies designed to address this, including the VA Cooperative Study and ADVANCE, also failed to show CVD benefit for intensive glucose control.[A29] These trials differed somewhat in patient characteristics, HbA$_{1c}$ goal, and specific treatment regimens, and the largely negative results stimulated controversy. However, some consensus views have emerged[29]: (1) in the current era of effective treatment of other CVD risk factors (i.e., with statins, RAS blockers, antiplatelet therapy), the additional benefits of intensive glycemic control are modest at best; (2) patients with long-standing diabetes or established CVD are least likely to benefit from intensive glucose lowering; (3) the benefits of glucose lowering in the prevention of microvascular complications provide an independent rationale for strict glucose control for many patients; and (4) specific glycemic targets should be individualized according to the patient's characteristics (e.g., comorbidities, life expectancy, hypoglycemia risk) and preferences.

HYPERTENSION

Hypertension (Chapter 70) is a common comorbidity in diabetes, affecting the majority of patients with type 2 diabetes, and constitutes an important modifiable CVD risk factor. Further, in even the earliest stages of diabetic nephropathy (i.e., microalbuminuria), hypertension is further accelerated. In type 1 diabetes, hypertension is generally the result of concurrent renal disease, with both contributing to CVD risk. The importance of blood pressure control in reducing CVD events as well as microvascular outcomes in patients with diabetes was established by several major trials, including the

UKPDS, Systolic Hypertension in the Elderly Program (SHEP), Hypertension Optimal Treatment (HOT) study, and others.[A30] However, analysis of these and other trials failed to show evidence of improved outcomes (i.e., in myocardial infarction or mortality) with systolic blood pressure targets of 130 mm Hg or lower.[A31] An even more aggressive target systolic blood pressure of less than 120 mm Hg was shown to be of no additional benefit in reducing CVD events in the ACCORD trial. Current guidelines from the American Heart Association and the American College of Cardiology recommend a blood pressure goal of less than 130/80 for most patients, including those with diabetes. Other guidelines, including those from the American Diabetes Association (ADA), suggest a blood pressure target of less than 140/90 mm Hg for patients with diabetes but with the further recommendation that a lower target may be considered for selected patients if it can be achieved without excessive treatment burden. However, many of these recommendations are based on expert opinion rather than on evidence from randomized trials, and some uncertainty remains.

The choice of antihypertensive agent has also received considerable study, which is complicated by the fact that many patients will require treatment with two or more drugs to achieve target blood pressure. ACE inhibitors and angiotensin receptor blockers are generally considered first-line therapy for patients with diabetes, in part on the basis of their demonstrated renoprotective benefits. In addition, results from several randomized trials, including the Heart Outcomes Protection Study (HOPE), Fosinopril versus Amlodipine Cardiovascular Events Trial (FACET), and Appropriate Blood Pressure Control in Diabetes (ABCD), indicated improved cardiovascular outcomes with ACE inhibitors compared with other antihypertensive drugs, although this was not the case for the UKPDS, in which β-blockers were equally effective. Calcium-channel blockers and low-dose diuretics are also recommended as add-on therapy if needed to achieve blood pressure targets. Use of β-blockers should be considered in the setting of established CVD because of their proven benefits in patients with prior myocardial infarction and congestive heart failure. However, β-blockers should be used with caution in patients at high risk for hypoglycemia because they may blunt the autonomic warning symptoms associated with low glucose concentration. Both β-blockers and thiazide diuretics have been reported to increase the risk for development of diabetes, although there is little evidence for significant deterioration of glycemic control in patients with diabetes.

DYSLIPIDEMIA

The characteristic dyslipidemia of type 2 diabetes and insulin-resistant states, which includes low levels of high-density lipoprotein (HDL) cholesterol, elevated triglycerides, and small dense low-density lipoprotein (LDL) particles, is highly atherogenic (Chapter 195). LDLs also are prone to oxidative modification in the setting of hyperglycemia, which enhances their atherogenicity. There is substantial clinical trial evidence to support lowering of LDL cholesterol levels with statin drugs in the majority of patients with diabetes older than 40 years. These findings come from trials limited to diabetes (Collaborative Atorvastatin Diabetes Study [CARDS]) and to diabetes subset analysis of larger trials (Heart Protection Study), all of which report similar CVD benefits of statin therapy among diabetics and nondiabetics. ADA recommendations are for target LDL levels of less than 100 mg/dL for most adult patients with diabetes and less than 70 mg/dL for diabetic patients with established CVD or multiple risk factors. Recent guidelines from the American Heart Association (AHA) and American College of Cardiology (ACC) have focused on CVD risk stratification to determine the need for and intensity of statin therapy. With this approach, virtually all patients with diabetes (aged 40 to 75 years) would be candidates for statin therapy, regardless of baseline level of LDL cholesterol. Diabetic patients with established atherosclerotic CVD or estimated 10-year CVD risk of more than 7.5% would receive high-intensity statin treatment (regimens sufficient to lower LDL cholesterol >50% from untreated baseline); all others would be considered for moderate-intensity treatment (lowering of LDL cholesterol 30 to <50%). The evidence base to support these new recommendations is considered relatively strong. Although the ADA and the AHA/ACC guidelines differ in structure, ultimately the recommendations for most patients with diabetes will be similar with either approach.

Recent observations from several trials (e.g., JUPITER) and observational cohort studies of an increase in incident diabetes with statin therapy have generated concern, although the risk appears to be small in magnitude (hazard ratio, ≈1.2) and is outweighed by the substantial benefits of CVD protection.[30] Clinically relevant effects of statins on glucose control among established diabetics have not been reported. In patients intolerant of statins, nicotinic acid (niacin) can be used, although CVD outcome trials have been disappointing despite substantial improvement in lipid parameters, including lowering of LDL cholesterol and increasing of HDL cholesterol levels. Further, nicotinic acid may worsen insulin resistance and glycemic control in some patients. Bile acid sequestrants, such as colesevelam or cholestyramine, can also be used but may exacerbate the hypertriglyceridemia characteristic of diabetic dyslipidemia.

In contrast to the definitive benefits of LDL lowering, there is less evidence that pharmacologic treatment of hypertriglyceridemia or of low HDL cholesterol levels reduces CVD risk. This may be in part due to the lesser efficacy of available drugs to alter these lipid subfractions. Trials with fibrate derivatives (gemfibrozil and fenofibrate) have yielded mixed results, and the addition of fenofibrate to a statin did not reduce the rate of major CVD events compared with statin alone in the ACCORD trial. Because most statins have some triglyceride-lowering effect, maximizing statin dose should be considered for patients with high triglyceride levels. Lifestyle factors are also effective, including weight loss and dietary modification (reduced fat diet, avoidance of alcohol). Omega-3 fatty acid supplementation can lower triglyceride levels but is not effective for the routine primary prevention of cardiovascular events in diabetic patients.[A32] Pharmacologic treatment (i.e., with fibrates or fish oil supplements) of severe hypertriglyceridemia (triglyceride level >1000 mg/dL) is indicated to prevent acute pancreatitis.

ANTIPLATELET THERAPY

Prophylactic low-dose aspirin therapy is widely used for prevention of cardiovascular events in high-risk patients (i.e., those with prior myocardial infarction or stroke), with reported risk reductions of about 12%. In patients with diabetes, aspirin is not effective for the primary prevention of cardiovascular disease and increases bleeding events.[A33] Current guidelines recommend aspirin therapy for diabetic patients with a prior CVD event (secondary prevention), but it is uncertain whether primary prevention is beneficial even in higher risk patients, because the potential adverse effects from bleeding may outweigh the potential benefits. The optimal dose (balancing thrombosis prevention with the risk of bleeding) of aspirin has not been established and may differ according to patient characteristics, but 75 to 162 mg/day is commonly recommended. For high-risk patients who are unable to tolerate aspirin, clopidogrel is an effective alternative.

TREATMENT OF ESTABLISHED CARDIOVASCULAR DISEASE IN DIABETES   Rx

In general, treatment of clinically established CVD, including acute coronary syndromes and stable angina, is similar in diabetic and nondiabetic patients. There is some evidence that ischemic symptoms may be less intense, atypical, or absent in diabetic patients, leading to higher rates of "silent" myocardial infarction. However, a strategy of screening for ischemic heart disease, by exercise stress testing, in asymptomatic patients did not result in lower event rates or improved outcomes. Therefore current recommendations are for coronary artery disease screening in patients with symptoms suggestive of ischemia.

The role of intravenous insulin (with or without potassium and glucose infusion) in the setting of acute myocardial infarction has been considered in a few studies. In the Diabetes and Insulin-Glucose Infusion in Acute Myocardial Infarction (DIGAMI) study, acute myocardial infarction patients with diabetes were treated with standard therapy or with insulin infusion during the first 48 hours, followed by continued insulin use after hospital discharge. Mortality after 1 year was reduced by 30% in the insulin-treated group. However, the implications of these results have been debated because factors other than insulin treatment differed between the two groups (i.e., sulfonylureas were routinely used in the standard therapy group but withdrawn from the insulin group). These findings subsequently were not confirmed in a follow-up study, and this approach has largely been abandoned.

Several studies have addressed the roles of medical therapy and revascularization in diabetic patients with coronary artery disease. Among them, the Bypass Angioplasty Revascularization Investigation 2 Diabetes (BARI 2D) study demonstrated that a policy of medical management (including aggressive risk factor modification) was as effective as early revascularization in diabetic patients with stable angina. In the Future Revascularization Evaluation in Patients with Diabetes Mellitus: Optimal Management of Multivessel Disease (FREEDOM) trial, diabetic patients with multivessel coronary disease had better outcome (reduced rates of death from any cause or nonfatal myocardial infarction) with coronary bypass surgery compared with percutaneous intervention with drug-eluting stents, although strokes were more frequent in the surgical group.

Grade **A** References

A1. Misso ML, Egberts KJ, Page M, et al. Continuous subcutaneous insulin infusion (CSII) versus multiple insulin injections for type 1 diabetes mellitus. *Cochrane Database Syst Rev.* 2010;1:CD005103.

A2. Tauschmann M, Thabit H, Bally L, et al. Closed-loop insulin delivery in suboptimally controlled type 1 diabetes: a multicentre, 12-week randomised trial. *Lancet.* 2018;392:1321-1329.

A3. Beck RW, Riddlesworth T, Ruedy K, et al. Effect of continuous glucose monitoring on glycemic control in adults with type 1 diabetes using insulin injections. The DIAMOND randomized clinical trial. *JAMA.* 2017;317:371-378.

A4. Lind M, Polonsky W, Hirsch IB, et al. Continuous glucose monitoring vs conventional therapy for glycemic control in adults with type 1 diabetes treated with multiple daily insulin injections: the GOLD randomized clinical trial. *JAMA.* 2017;317:379-387.

A5. The Type 1 Diabetes TrialNet Oral Insulin Study Group. Effect of oral insulin on prevention of diabetes in relatives of patients with type 1 diabetes. A randomized clinical trial. *JAMA.* 2017;318:1891-1902.

A6. Senat MV, Affres H, Letourneau A, et al. Effect of glyburide vs subcutaneous insulin on perinatal complications among women with gestational diabetes: a randomized clinical trial. *JAMA.* 2018;319:1773-1780.

A7. Hemmingsen B, Lunc S, Gluud C, et al. Targeting intensive glycaemic control versus targeting conventional glycaemic control for type 2 diabetes mellitus. *Cochrane Database Syst Rev.* 2013;11:CD008143.

A8. Hayward RA, Reaven PD, Wiitala WL, et al. Follow-up of glycemic control and cardiovascular outcomes in type 2 diabetes. *N Engl J Med.* 2015;372:2197-2206.

A9. Schauer PR, Bhatt DL, Kirwan JP, et al. Bariatric surgery versus intensive medical therapy for diabetes—5-year outcomes. *N Engl J Med.* 2017;376:641-651.

A10. Mingrone G, Panunzi S, De Gaetano A, et al. Bariatric-metabolic surgery versus conventional medical treatment in obese patients with type 2 diabetes: 5 year follow-up of an open-label, single-centre, randomised controlled trial. *Lancet.* 2015;386:964-973.

A11. Eng C, Kramer CK, Zinman B, et al. Glucagon-like peptide-1 receptor agonist and basal insulin combination treatment for the management of type 2 diabetes: a systematic review and meta-analysis. *Lancet.* 2014;384:2228-2234.

A12. Davies MJ, Bergenstal R, Bode B, et al. Efficacy of liraglutide for weight loss among patients with type 2 diabetes: the SCALE diabetes randomized clinical trial. *JAMA.* 2015;314:687-699.

A13. Marso SP, Daniels GH, Brown-Frandsen K, et al. Liraglutide and cardiovascular outcomes in type 2 diabetes. *N Engl J Med.* 2016;375:311-322.

A14. Mann JFE, Ørsted DD, Brown-Frandsen K, et al. Liraglutide and renal outcomes in type 2 diabetes. *N Engl J Med.* 2017;377:839-848.

A15. Marso SP, Bain SC, Consoli A, et al. Semaglutide and cardiovascular outcomes in patients with type 2 diabetes. *N Engl J Med.* 2016;375:1834-1844.

A16. Green JB, Bethel MA, Armstrong PW, et al. Effect of sitagliptin on cardiovascular outcomes in type 2 diabetes. *N Engl J Med.* 2015;373:232-242.

A17. Zinman B, Wanner C, Lachin JM, et al. Empagliflozin, cardiovascular outcomes, and mortality in type 2 diabetes. *N Engl J Med.* 2015;373:2117-2128.

A18. Neal B, Perkovic V, Mahaffey KW, et al. Canagliflozin and cardiovascular and renal events in type 2 diabetes. *N Engl J Med.* 2017;377:644-657.

A19. Perkovic V, Jardine MJ, Neal B, et al. Canagliflozin and renal outcomes in type 2 diabetes and nephropathy. *N Engl J Med.* 2019;380:2295-2306.

A20. Reznik Y, Cohen O, Aronson R, et al. Insulin pump treatment compared with multiple daily injections for treatment of type 2 diabetes (OpT2mise): a randomised open-label controlled trial. *Lancet.* 2014;384:1265-1272.

A21. Finfer S, Liu B, Chittock DR, et al. The NICE-SUGAR Study Investigators. Hypoglycemia and risk of death in critically ill patients. *N Engl J Med.* 2012;367:1108-1118.

A22. Lean ME, Leslie WS, Barnes AC, et al. Primary care-led weight management for remission of type 2 diabetes (DiRECT): an open-label, cluster-randomised trial. *Lancet.* 2018;391:541-551.

A23. Bohula EA, Scirica BM, Inzucchi SE, et al. Effect of lorcaserin on prevention and remission of type 2 diabetes in overweight and obese patients (CAMELLIA-TIMI 61): a randomised, placebo-controlled trial. *Lancet.* 2018;392:2269-2279.

A24. Diabetes Prevention Program Research Group. Long-term effects of lifestyle intervention or metformin on diabetes development and microvascular complications over 15-year follow-up: the Diabetes Prevention Program Outcomes Study. *Lancet Diabetes Endocrinol.* 2015;3:866-875.

A25. Aiello LP, Sun W, Das A, et al. Intensive diabetes therapy and ocular surgery in type 1 diabetes. *N Engl J Med.* 2015;372:1722-1733.

A26. Nguyen Q, Brown D, Marcus D, et al. Ranibizumab for diabetic macular edema: results from 2 phase III randomized trials: RISE and RIDE. *Ophthalmology.* 2012;119:789-801.

A27. Fried L, Emanuele N, Zhang J, et al. Combined angiotensin inhibition for the treatment of diabetic nephropathy. *N Engl J Med.* 2013;369:1892-1903.

A28. Wing RR, Bolin P, Brancati FL, et al. Cardiovascular effects of intensive lifestyle intervention in type 2 diabetes. *N Engl J Med.* 2013;369:145-154.

A29. Zoungas S, Chalmers J, Neal B, et al. Follow-up of blood-pressure lowering and glucose control in type 2 diabetes. *N Engl J Med.* 2014;371:1392-1406.

A30. Emdin CA, Rahimi K, Neal B, et al. Blood pressure lowering in type 2 diabetes: a systematic review and meta-analysis. *JAMA.* 2015;313:603-615.

A31. Brunström M, Carlberg B. Effect of antihypertensive treatment at different blood pressure levels in patients with diabetes mellitus: systematic review and meta-analyses. *BMJ.* 2016;352:1-10.

A32. Bowman L, Mafham M, Wallendszus K, et al. Effects of n-3 fatty acid supplements in diabetes mellitus. *N Engl J Med.* 2018;379:1540-1550.

A33. Bowman L, Mafham M, Wallendszus K, et al. Effects of aspirin for primary prevention in persons with diabetes mellitus. *N Engl J Med.* 2018;379:1529-1539.

GENERAL REFERENCES

For the General References and other additional features, please visit Expert Consult at https://expertconsult.inkling.com.

217

HYPOGLYCEMIA AND PANCREATIC ISLET CELL DISORDERS

KHALID HUSSAIN

DEFINITIONS

Hypoglycemia is a common biochemical abnormality observed in clinical practice. Hypoglycemic disorders are more frequent in neonates, infants, and children as compared to adults. Inappropriately treated hypoglycemia can have severe consequences, including seizures, permanent brain injury, or death. This is especially the case in neonates with persistent forms of hypoglycemia, who are at high risk of brain injury from delays in diagnosis and effective therapy.

Hypoglycemic disorders in neonates, infants, and children differ from adults in important aspects. First, they are most often due to congenital or genetic disorders, such as disorders of insulin secretion, as well as a range of metabolic and endocrine diseases. Second, during a transitional period of 1 to 3 days after birth, low plasma glucose concentrations are common in normal neonates, thus making it difficult to identify the minority that might have a persistent genetic disorder associated with hypoglycemia. The importance of early recognition and treatment of such persistent hypoglycemia disorders in neonates is emphasized by reports that developmental handicap, which might have been avoidable by early recognition and treatment, occurs in 25 to 50% of cases with congenital hyperinsulinism.[1]

The current adult recommendations define clinical hypoglycemia as a plasma (or serum) glucose concentration low enough to cause symptoms or signs, including impairment of brain function. Because its clinical manifestations and symptoms of hypoglycemia are nonspecific, it is not possible to state a single plasma glucose concentration that categorically defines hypoglycemia. The measured plasma or serum glucose concentration may be low owing to an artifact (e.g., when the blood sample is collected in a tube that does not contain an inhibitor of glycolysis and when separation of the plasma or serum from the formed elements is delayed).

For these reasons, guidelines in adults emphasize the value of the Whipple triad for confirming hypoglycemia: (1) symptoms and/or signs compatible with hypoglycemia, (2) a low measured plasma glucose concentration, and (3) resolution of symptoms and signs when glucose concentrations are raised. Because circulating fuels such as ketone bodies can be used by the brain, lower plasma glucose concentrations can occur in healthy individuals, particularly in women and children, without symptoms or signs during extended fasting. The Pediatric Endocrine Society (PES) recently recommended guidelines for the evaluation and management of persistent hypoglycemia in neonates, infants, and children.[2]

The aim of this chapter is to outline the physiologic and biochemical changes associated with maintenance of a normal blood glucose level, describe the role of the counter-regulatory hormones, review the different hypoglycemia disorders observed in adults and children, and then finally discuss the various management strategies.

PATHOBIOLOGY

Physiologic and Biochemical Changes During Fasting and Feeding

Overview

Plasma glucose concentration is regulated by a balance between glucose production and utilization. Glucose is derived from three sources: (1) intestinal absorption that follows digestion of dietary carbohydrates; (2) glycogenolysis, the breakdown of glycogen, which is the polymerized storage form of glucose; and (3) gluconeogenesis, the formation of glucose from precursors (lactate, pyruvate, alanine, glutamine, and glycerol). Normally the, rate of endogenous glucose influx into the circulation and glucose efflux out of the circulation into insulin-dependent tissues (skeletal muscle, adipose tissue, and liver) is regulated so that despite periods of feeding and fasting, the plasma glucose concentration is maintained in a relatively narrow range between 70 and 110 mg/dL (3.8 to 6 mmol/L). Figure 217-1 shows an outline of glucose physiology.

Glucose is an obligate metabolic fuel for the brain under physiologic conditions. Unlike other body tissues, the brain cannot oxidize fatty acids, and neither can it synthesize/store glucose for later use. It is dependent on a continuous supply of glucose from the circulation. Given the vital importance of brain function and the above circumstances, it is not surprising that physiologic mechanisms have evolved for the maintenance of normal plasma glucose concentrations.

Changes During Fasting

During fasting, the basal rate of glucose output by the liver (2.2 mg/kg/minute in healthy adults after an overnight fast) is precisely matched to glucose uptake by various body tissues. In infants, these rates are much higher ($\approx$6 mg/kg/minute) because of their greater brain mass relative to their body weight. The brain is responsible for nearly two thirds of basal glucose utilization. The remaining one third is used by red blood cells, renal medulla, and to some extent muscle and fat.

Hepatic glucose production results from a combination of glycogenolysis and gluconeogenesis. Endogenous glucose production is also contributed by gluconeogenesis in the kidneys. Breakdown of stored hepatic glycogen is a readily available source of free glucose. However, in an average adult, this process can only provide less than an 8-hour supply of free glucose. (In infants, this may provide only 4 hours of free glucose.) Considering this limited capacity of glycogenolysis, gluconeogenesis is very important in supporting hepatic glycogen stores during an overnight fast.

The key enzymes involved in gluconeogenesis are pyruvate carboxylase, phosphoenolpyruvate carboxykinase (PEPCK), and fructose-1,6-bisphosphatase. Muscle and adipose tissue, which utilize glucose in the fed state, respond to prolonged fasting by reducing their glucose uptake and satisfying their energy requirements by the β-oxidation of fatty acids. Additionally, through the process of proteolysis, muscle tissue provides amino acids to the liver to serve as gluconeogenic precursors for net glucose formation. Changes in the hormonal milieu during fasting (suppressed insulin and elevated counter-regulatory hormones) stimulate ketogenesis. Ketones become a major source of fuel for the brain when glucose utilization by the brain declines. This leads to a decrease in the rate of gluconeogenesis required to maintain plasma glucose concentration and hence in diminished protein wasting.

Changes During Feeding

After a meal, plasma glucose concentrations increase, which stimulates secretion of insulin from the pancreatic β cells and suppresses secretion of glucagon from the pancreatic α cells. This change in the hormonal milieu switches off endogenous hepatic glucose production and accelerates glucose utilization by liver, muscle, and adipose tissue. Glucose concentration then returns gradually to the postabsorptive level, at which endogenous glucose production is equal to the glucose uptake by peripheral tissues.

Counter-Regulatory Hormonal Responses to Hypoglycemia

Counter-regulatory hormones play a key role in the maintenance of normal plasma glucose concentration. During the counter-regulatory hormonal response a reduction in the plasma glucose concentration will result in a decrease in insulin secretion and an increase in glucagon, epinephrine, norepinephrine, cortisol, and growth hormone (GH) secretion. Glucagon secretion increases rapidly in response to decreasing plasma glucose level, and studies have shown that the glucagon response is the primary essential defense mechanism against acute hypoglycemia. GH and cortisol have numerous effects on glucose metabolism, including increasing the rate of gluconeogenesis and antagonizing the effects of insulin. In adults, the glycemic thresholds for the activation of glucose counter-regulatory hormones such as GH and cortisol lie within or just below the physiologic plasma glucose concentration and slightly higher than the threshold for symptoms. This suggests that GH and cortisol secretion increase in response to plasma glucose concentrations within the normoglycemic range, and these increases are inversely proportional to the nadir in plasma glucose. Figure 217-2 outlines the role of the counter-regulatory hormones.

Insulin secretion from β cells of the pancreas in healthy individuals is inhibited as plasma glucose concentration falls below 72 mg/dL (4.0 mmol/L). As insulin secretion is reduced, the repressive effect of insulin on pancreatic α-cell function is removed, thereby rapidly increasing glucagon secretion. Glucagon acts on the liver to increase hepatic glycogenolysis and gluconeogenesis. When the plasma glucose concentration falls further ($\approx$68 mg/dL [3.8 mmol/L]), epinephrine and norepinephrine are released both from the adrenals and directly into interstitial fluid from nerve terminals, further

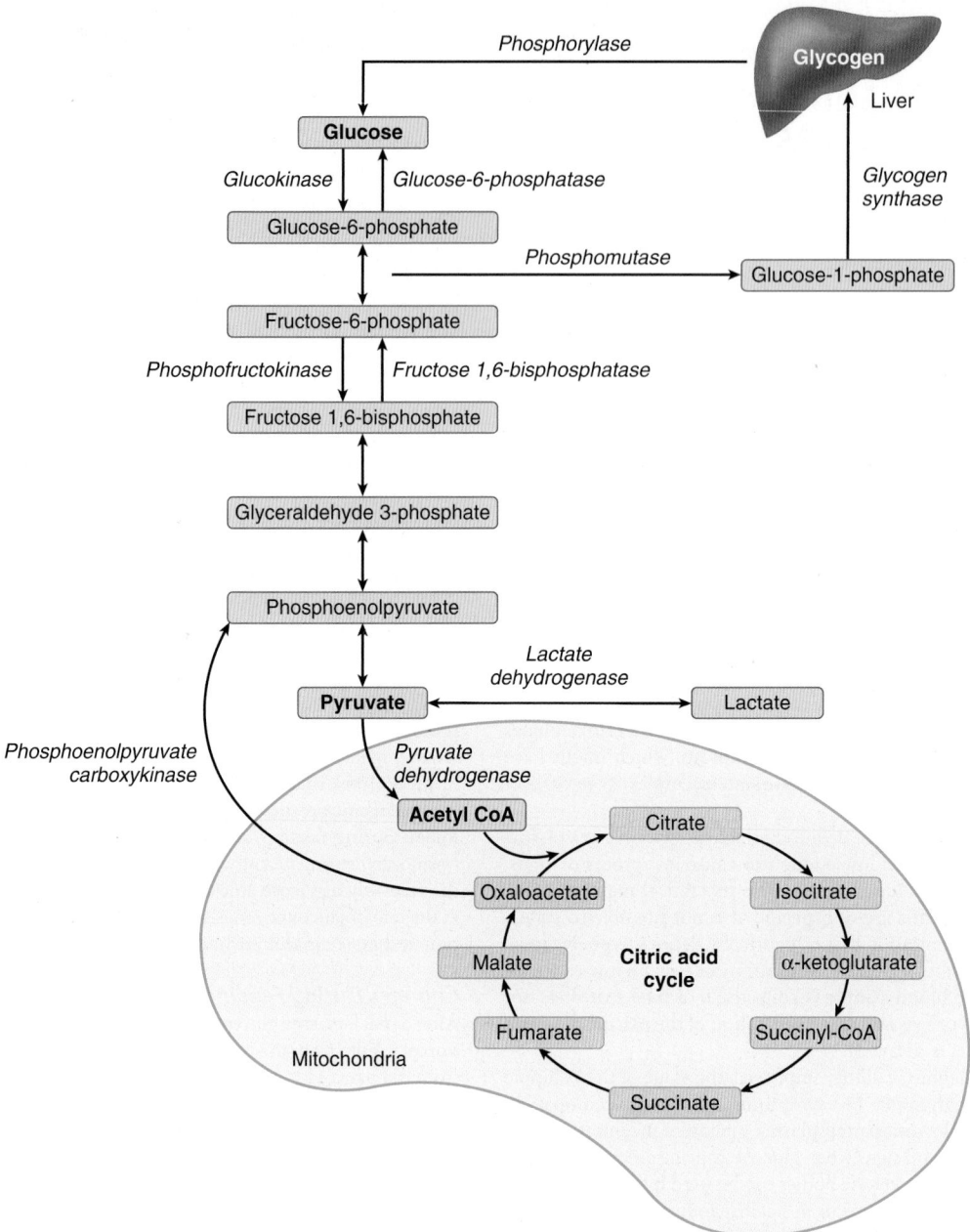

FIGURE 217-1. Outline of the biochemical pathways involved in glucose physiology.

suppressing insulin secretion, increasing glucagon secretion, and decreasing peripheral glucose utilization in the muscle and increasing lipolysis in the adipose tissues.

Additional responses include GH and cortisol secretion, which occur below a plasma glucose concentration of around 66 mg/dL ($\approx$3.7 mmol/L) and are initiators of the adaptive response to hypoglycemia (e.g., during prolonged starvation); glucose-raising actions are much slower in onset (several hours). These hormone responses stimulate lipolysis, ketogenesis, and gluconeogenesis. Permissive amounts of cortisol and GH are required for a normal hepatic response to glucagon and epinephrine. In healthy individuals, this system ensures that hypoglycemia is rarely experienced and would only occur during starvation or ultra-endurance sports. Drugs or diseases that inhibit counter-regulatory secretion or action predispose patients to hypoglycemia.

CLINICAL MANIFESTATIONS
Symptoms of Hypoglycemia
The symptoms of hypoglycemia reflect the responses of the brain to a decrease in the blood glucose level; such symptoms may be nonspecific and vague, especially in the childhood period. Children and those with impaired consciousness may not be able to communicate their hypoglycemic symptoms. The symptoms of hypoglycemia may be categorized into two main groups:

(1) those that arise as a result of the central nervous system being deprived of glucose (neuroglycopenic) and (2) symptoms arising from the perception of physiologic changes caused by the central nervous system–mediated sympatho-adrenal discharge triggered by hypoglycemia (neurogenic or autonomic). The neurogenic symptoms of hypoglycemia are largely the result of sympathetic neural, rather than adrenomedullary, activation.

Neuroglycopenic symptoms (e.g., dizziness, confusion, tiredness, difficulty with speaking, headache, inability to concentrate, coma, and seizures) arise from the failure of brain function itself and are caused by deficient supply of glucose to the brain. Neurogenic symptoms include both adrenergic responses (catecholamine-mediated symptoms such as palpitations, tremor, and anxiety) and cholinergic responses (acetylcholine-mediated symptoms such as sweating, hunger, paresthesias). Awareness of hypoglycemia chiefly depends on perception of the central and peripheral effects of neurogenic (as opposed to neuroglycopenic) responses to hypoglycemia.

In nondiabetic adults during acute insulin-induced hypoglycemia, autonomic symptoms become apparent at a threshold of approximately 60 mg/dL (3.3 mmol/L), and impairment of brain function manifested by neuroglycopenic symptoms occurs at a threshold of approximately 50 mg/dL (2.8 mmol/L) in arterialized venous blood (venous levels would be $\approx$3 mg/dL [0.16 mmol/L] less). However, in patients with recurrent hypoglycemia, the glycemic

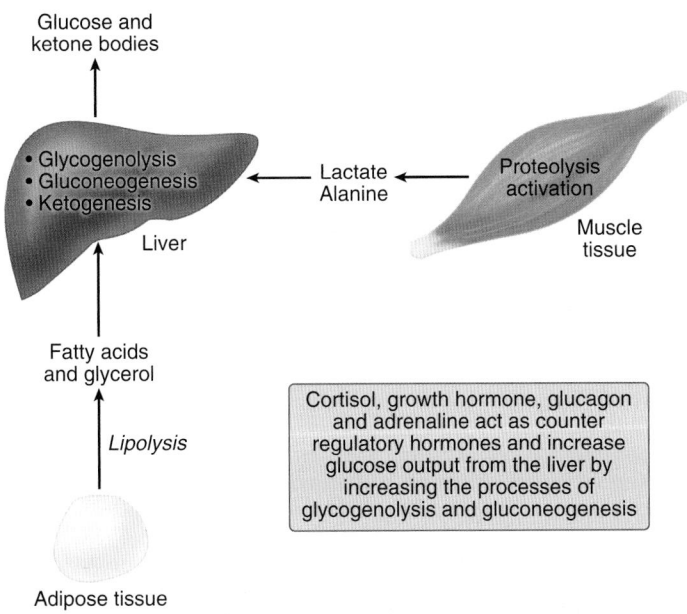

FIGURE 217-2. The role of the counter-regulatory hormones, glycogenolysis, gluconeogenesis, and lipolysis in glucose physiology.

thresholds for responses to hypoglycemia are reset at a lower plasma glucose concentration. The glucose thresholds for the activation of neuroglycopenic and autonomic symptoms in children are not as clearly defined as in adults. The symptoms and signs of hypoglycemia are not influenced by the rate of blood glucose decline in nondiabetic individuals.

Clinical Approach to the Patient with Hypoglycemia

A careful clinical history, description of symptoms, physical examination, and a systematic step-by-step approach is the cornerstone of establishing a diagnosis. The symptoms of hypoglycemia may be very nonspecific, hence any symptomatic child or adult must have the blood glucose level measured and documented.

The relationship of a hypoglycemic episode to the most recent meal can be important diagnostically. Hypoglycemia occurring after a short fast (2 to 3 hours) may be suggestive of hyperinsulinism or glycogen storage disease. Hypoglycemia occurring after a long fast (12 to 14 hours) may suggest a disorder of gluconeogenesis. Postprandial hypoglycemia may indicate galactosemia, hereditary fructose intolerance, dumping syndrome, insulinoma, insulin autoimmune syndrome, and noninsulinoma pancreatogenous hypoglycemia syndrome. In both children and adults, a clear documentation of the medication history is important.

DIAGNOSIS

After the clinical history has been taken and the examination completed, a diagnostic cascade of appropriate tests is necessary. These may be guided in the context of the most common causes of hypoglycemia as listed in Table 217-1.

The current adult recommendations state that evaluation and management of hypoglycemia should only be undertaken in patients in whom Whipple triad—symptoms, signs, or both consistent with hypoglycemia, a low plasma glucose concentration, and resolution of those symptoms or signs after the plasma glucose concentration is raised—is documented. However, this does not apply to children for the reasons discussed earlier.

Causes of Hypoglycemia

Hypoglycemia is more common in the childhood period than in adults and can be due to a large number of causes. Table 217-1 summarizes the differential diagnosis of hypoglycemia.

Hypoglycemia Due to Excess Production of Hormones

Inappropriate and excess production of certain hormones can lead to hypoglycemia. The two most common conditions associated with excess production of a hormone are hyperinsulinemic hypoglycemia and non–islet cell tumor hypoglycemia or IGF-2-oma (insulin-like growth factor–secreting tumor).

TABLE 217-1 DIFFERENTIAL DIAGNOSIS OF HYPOGLYCEMIA*
HYPERINSULINEMIC HYPOGLYCEMIA (INCLUDING POSTPRANDIAL)
Transient: infant of diabetic mother, perinatal asphyxia, Rhesus disease, intrauterine growth retardation, Beckwith-Wiedemann syndrome
Congenital: *ABCC8, KCNJ11,* **GCK***, GDH, HADH, HNF4A, HNF1A,* **SLC16A1, UCP2, HK-1, PGM-1**
Dumping syndrome
Insulin receptor mutations and antibodies
Hypoketotic hypoinsulinemic hypoglycemia with overgrowth
Activating mutations in *AKT2, AKT3* and *PIK3CA*
Insulinoma
Noninsulinoma pancreatogenous hypoglycemia (adults)
Gastric bypass surgery for morbid obesity
Non–islet cell tumor hypoglycemia or IGF-2-oma
Insulin autoimmune syndrome
Insulin factitious hypoglycemia
HORMONAL DEFICIENCY/RESISTANCE
Adrenocorticotropic hormone
Cortisol
Growth hormone
Glucagon[†]
Adrenaline[†]
DEFECTS IN HEPATIC GLYCOGEN RELEASE/STORAGE
Glycogen storage diseases: **glucose-6-phosphatase deficiency, amylo-1,6-glucosidase deficiency,** liver phosphorylase deficiency, glycogen storage disease type 0
DEFECTS IN GLUCONEOGENESIS
Fructose-1,6-bisphosphatase deficiency, phosphoenolpyruvate carboxykinase deficiency, pyruvate carboxylase deficiency
CARNITINE METABOLISM
Carnitine deficiency (primary and secondary)
Carnitine palmitoyltransferase deficiency (CPT 1 and 2)
Carnitine transporter defects
FATTY ACID OXIDATION
Medium-chain acyl-CoA dehydrogenase (MCAD) deficiency
Very long-chain acyl-CoA dehydrogenase (VLCAD) deficiency
Short-chain acyl-CoA dehydrogenase (SCAD) deficiency
Long/short-chain L-3-hydroxyacyl-CoA (L/SCHAD) deficiency
DEFECTS IN KETONE BODY SYNTHESIS/UTILIZATION
HMG-CoA synthase deficiency, HMG-CoA lyase deficiency
Succinyl-CoA: 3-oxoacid-CoA transferase (SCOT) deficiency
METABOLIC CONDITIONS (COMMON ONES)
Organic acidemias (propionic, methylmalonic)
Maple syrup urine disease, galactosemia, fructosemia, tyrosinemia
Hereditary fructose intolerance
Mitochondrial respiratory chain complex deficiencies
Congenital disorders of glycosylation (CDG)
DRUG INDUCED
Oral hypoglycemic agents
Insulin
β-Blockers
Salicylates
Alcohol
Quinine
Haloperidol
Pentamidine
Levofloxacin
Methadone
Disopyramide
Indomethacin
Cibenzoline
Gatifloxacin
TOXIN INDUCED
Lychee fruit
MISCELLANEOUS CAUSES (MECHANISM[S] NOT CLEAR)
Idiopathic ketotic hypoglycemia (diagnosis of exclusion)
Infections (sepsis, malaria), congenital heart disease

*Boldface indicates more common in adults.
[†]No human case yet reported with glucagon or adrenaline deficiency.
HMG = 3-hydroxy-3-methylglutaryl; IGF = insulin-like growth factor.

Inappropriate production of insulin can lead to either fasting hypoglycemia or postprandial hypoglycemia.

Hyperinsulinemic Hypoglycemia

Hyperinsulinemic hypoglycemia is a heterogeneous group of disorders characterized by unregulated insulin secretion from pancreatic β cells. In the face of hypoglycemia, patients have inappropriately detectable serum insulin levels, low ketone bodies, and low fatty acids and show a glycemic response to glucagon.

Congenital Forms of Hyperinsulinemic Hypoglycemia

In patients with congenital forms of hyperinsulinemic hypoglycemia, mutations in the key genes (ABCC8, KCNJ11, GLUD1, GCK, HADH, SLC16A1, HNF4A, HNF1A, HK-1, PGM-1 and UCP2) regulating insulin secretion have been identified.[3] Children with inactivating mutations in the genes ABCC8 and KCNJ11 present with the most severe forms of congenital hyperinsulinemic hypoglycemia, typically in the newborn period. Hyperinsulinism-hyperammonemia syndrome due to activating mutations in the GLUD1 gene and activating mutations in the GCK gene, leading to hyperinsulinemic hypoglycemia, have both been described in adults as well as children. Exercise-induced hyperinsulinemic hypoglycemia due to activating mutations in the SLC16A1 gene has also been recognized in adults.

Hypoketotic Hypoinsulinemic Hypoglycemia with Overgrowth

Activating mutations in the genes encoding AKT2, AKT3 and PIK3CA lead to autonomous activation of the insulin signaling pathway but no detectable insulin in the blood. These conditions are associated with various overgrowth manifestations and biochemically with hypoketotic hypoglycemia.[4]

Insulinoma

An insulinoma is the commonest cause of endogenous hyperinsulinemic hypoglycemia in adults. Insulinomas have the highest incidence in the fifth and sixth decades.[5] Insulinomas are insulin-secreting tumors of pancreatic origin, with an incidence of 1 to 4 per million. The majority (90%) of them are benign, solitary, intrapancreatic, and less than 2 cm in diameter. Classically, symptoms become evident in the fasting state or following exercise. However, it is now known that insulinoma can also present with postprandial symptoms. Diagnosis is based on findings of abnormal serum levels of insulin and C-peptide (also proinsulin) at the time of fasting hypoglycemia. An insulinoma can occur either in isolation or in association with multiple endocrine neoplasia type 1 (MEN 1), with a lifetime prevalence of 10% among adults carrying mutations in MEN1 (Chapter 218). Around 6% of insulinomas occur in patients with MEN 1, and most insulinomas are benign, but 5 to 10% are malignant. Recurrent somatic mutations in the YY1 gene occur in some sporadic insulinomas, and some insulinomas show increased expression of hexokinase-1.

Postprandial Hyperinsulinemic Hypoglycemia

Postprandial hyperinsulinemic hypoglycemia refers to hypoglycemia within a few hours of meal ingestion, secondary to inappropriate insulin secretion in response to a meal. If postprandial hyperinsulinemic hypoglycemia is clinically suspected, then an oral glucose tolerance test (OGTT) or a mixed-meal provocation test is performed. (See later in section "Investigations for Hypoglycemia.") A physiologic dip in the blood glucose level seen in OGTT might lead to misdiagnosis. However, corresponding biochemical evidence of endogenous hyperinsulinemic hypoglycemia and symptoms of neuroglycopenia during a hypoglycemic episode would help distinguish between pathologic postprandial hyperinsulinemic hypoglycemia and reactive hypoglycemia. A decrease of more than 108 mg/dL (6 mmol/L) between peak and nadir blood glucose during OGTT has been used as a diagnostic criterion for dumping syndrome in adults.

DUMPING SYNDROME. Dumping syndrome seen in infants after Nissen fundoplication is a classic example of postprandial hyperinsulinemic hypoglycemia. Precipitous emptying of hyperosmolar carbohydrate-containing solutions into the small bowel results in rapid glucose absorption, hyperglycemia, and reactive hypoglycemia. These children also tend to have abnormally exaggerated secretion of glucagon-like peptide-1 (GLP-1), which may contribute to the exaggerated insulin surge and resultant hypoglycemia.

INSULIN AUTOIMMUNE SYNDROME. Insulin autoimmune syndrome, or Hirata disease, is a rare condition characterized by hyperinsulinemic hypoglycemia associated with high titers of antibodies to endogenous insulin in the absence of prior exposure to exogenous insulin.[6] The disease is extremely uncommon in Western countries. Insulin autoimmune syndrome affects men and women equally and is seen more frequently in patients older than 40 years. The binding kinetics of endogenous insulin by the antibodies are thought to lead to physiologically inappropriate levels of bioavailable insulin, causing either hyper- or hypoglycemia.

In this syndrome, the insulin levels are markedly elevated, usually above 100 mU/L. After a meal or glucose load, these patients often demonstrate initial hyperglycemia, followed by hypoglycemia a few hours later. The hyperglycemia is caused by the anti-insulin antibodies that bind the insulin secreted in response to rising blood glucose levels after a meal. This binding reduces the bioavailability of the secreted insulin to the receptors in the liver and peripheral tissues, resulting in hyperglycemia and further insulin secretion. As blood glucose concentrations begin to decrease and insulin secretion declines, the insulin bound to the antibodies is released, resulting in inappropriately high free insulin concentrations for the blood glucose, causing hypoglycemia.

POSTPRANDIAL HYPERINSULINEMIC HYPOGLYCEMIA IN PATIENTS WITH INSULIN-RECEPTOR MUTATIONS. Postprandial hyperinsulinemic hypoglycemia has been described in patients who carried a heterozygote mutation (Arg1174Gln) in the insulin-receptor gene. Hyperinsulinism seems to be associated with decreased degradation rather than increased secretion of insulin, as evidenced by increased fasting levels of serum insulin despite normal levels of serum C-peptide and reduced clearance of exogenous insulin during clamp studies.

POSTPRANDIAL HYPERINSULINEMIC HYPOGLYCEMIA AFTER GASTRIC BYPASS SURGERY. The increasing use of Roux-en-Y gastric bypass for extreme obesity (Chapter 207) has led to reports of postprandial hyperinsulinemic hypoglycemia.[7] This is independently associated with lower age, greater weight loss, as well as higher β-cell function and insulin sensitivity but not with β-cell mass. In a review of the Swedish Bariatric Surgery registry, the incidence of hospitalization for hypoglycemia in post–gastric bypass patients was reported as less than 1%.

A number of different explanations have been suggested to explain hypoglycemia following gastric bypass surgery. Pancreatic nesidioblastosis (islet cell enlargement, β cells budding from ductal epithelium, and islets in apposition to ducts) has been proposed as the underlying mechanism for this disorder, but this remains controversial. The hypoglycemia may be due to an effect on the enteroinsular axis induced by the diversion of nutrients into the small intestine.

The enhanced postprandial insulin secretion involves increased secretion of glucagon like peptide 1 (GLP-1), and glucose-dependent insulinotropic polypeptide (GIP) GLP-1 levels are increased two- to five-fold after gastric bypass. The elevations of incretins tend to be seen early, even as early as 2 days after gastric bypass, and levels may decline as substantial weight loss and normalization of insulin sensitivity occurs. In patients with postprandial hyperinsulinemic hypoglycemia, elevated levels of GIP and GLP-1 persist for years after surgery.

Increased postprandial insulin secretion by incretins is mediated by islet cell hypertrophy and hyperplasia. Both GIP and GLP-1 have been implicated in increasing pancreatic β-cell mass in rodent models. GLP-1 regulates islet growth by inducing the expression of the transcription factor pancreatic-duodenum homeobox-1 (PDX-1).

Overexpression of IGF-2 and IGF-1 receptor alpha (IGF1Rα) have been found in pancreatic tissue removed from patients with persistent postprandial hyperinsulinemic hypoglycemia after gastric bypass surgery as compared to controls. These findings are suggestive of the role of growth factors in islet hyperfunction seen in post–gastric bypass patients.

NONINSULINOMA PANCREATOGENOUS HYPOGLYCEMIA SYNDROME. Noninsulinoma pancreatogenous hypoglycemia syndrome (NIPHS) is characterized by postprandial neuroglycopenia in the presence of negative prolonged fasting tests and negative perioperative localization studies for insulinoma.[8] However, in some patients the selective arterial calcium stimulation test is positive, with the histology of the resected pancreas showing nesidioblastosis. The underlying genetic basis of NIPHS is not known.

These patients are negative for ABCC8/KCNJ11 mutations and show islet hypertrophy histologically (as observed in diffuse congenital hyperinsulinemic hypoglycemia).

Immunohistologic studies of the resected pancreatic tissue have failed to show an increased rate of proliferation of β cells or abnormal synthesis or processing of either proinsulin or amylin. Neither has there been any evidence of overexpression of pancreatic differentiation factors, PDX-1, and Nkx-6.1, nor the calcium-sensing receptor (CaSR).

Insulin Factitious Hypoglycemia

Hypoglycemia can also be induced pharmacologically, either intentionally as a diagnostic tool, accidentally as a complication of the treatment of diabetes mellitus, or as a consequence of poisoning either with insulin itself or with drugs (e.g., sulfonylureas) that stimulate insulin release. Whenever severe hypoglycemia occurs with documented hyperinsulinism, the possibility of Munchausen syndrome by proxy should be considered in children. The possibility of malicious administration of insulin or an oral sulfonylurea should always be suspected in cases of sudden onset of hypoglycemia in a previously healthy individual. In the case of insulin administration, the clue in the biochemistry will be a raised insulin level accompanied by normal C-peptide.

Non–Islet Cell Tumor Hypoglycemia, or IGF-2-oma

Non–islet cell tumor hypoglycemia, or IGF-2-oma, denotes the syndrome of hypoglycemia produced by or associated with any neoplasm other than an insulinoma. These are usually tumors of mesenchymal and epithelial origin (including hepatomas, fibromas, and fibrosarcomas). The underlying mechanism of hypoglycemia in nearly all patients with this syndrome is overproduction of IGF-2 by the tumor, which includes mature IGF-2 and incompletely processed forms of IGF-2, referred to collectively as "big" IGF-2.[9] The elevated IGF-2–related peptides mimic the fasting hypoglycemia characteristic of patients with insulin-producing islet cell tumors. Rarely, markedly elevated IGF-2 levels produce somatic changes suggestive of acromegaly. Typically, the elevated IGF-2 levels are associated with suppressed plasma levels of insulin, IGF-1, and GH. Hypoglycemia can also occur due to paraneoplastic secretion of insulin-like growth factor-I (IGF-1).

Hypoglycemia Due to Hormone Deficiency

Glucagon and adrenaline deficiency must be extremely rare as, to date, no true human, genetically proven defects in glucagon and adrenaline deficiency have been described. Hormonal deficiency might be either in isolation (e.g., isolated GH, adrenocorticotropic hormone [ACTH], or cortisol deficiency) or in combination with other hormones, such as in patients with hypopituitarism. GH and cortisol deficiency lead to hypoglycemia by reducing gluconeogenic substrate availability (decreased mobilization of fats and proteins) and increasing glucose utilization due to increased insulin sensitivity of tissues in the absence of these two hormones.

Acquired hypopituitarism may result from tumors (most commonly craniopharyngioma), radiation, infection, hydrocephalus, vascular anomalies, and trauma. Addison disease (AD) results from adrenal cortex hypofunction/dysfunction, with deficient production of glucocorticoids, mineralocorticoids, and androgens, and with high levels of both ACTH and plasma renin activity (Chapter 214). Autoimmune AD is the most frequent etiologic form in adult patients, accounting for about 80% of cases, followed by post-tuberculosis AD in 10 to 15%; the remaining 5% of cases are due to vascular, neoplastic, or rare genetic forms.

The markers of autoimmune AD are adrenal cortex (ACA) or 21-hydroxylase autoantibodies (21-OHAbs), and they are present at diagnosis in more than 90% of cases. In autoimmune AD, the adrenal cortex is infiltrated by lymphocytes and plasma cells, and the glands are sclerotic and reduced in volume. Autoimmune AD occurs mainly in middle-aged women, alone or associated with other (clinical, subclinical, or potential) autoimmune diseases, giving rise to various forms of autoimmune polyglandular syndrome. Replacement therapy with gluco- and mineralocorticoids is life-saving for patients with chronic adrenal insufficiency.

Hypoglycemia Due to Defects in Hepatic Glycogen Release/Storage

Glucose-6-phosphatase deficiency (glycogen storage disease [GSD] type I, Von Gierke disease) is the commonest of the glycogen storage diseases causing hypoglycemia (Chapter 196). Deficiency of this enzyme results in the inability to release free glucose from glucose-6-phosphate, with resultant hepatomegaly due to stored glycogen. These children and adults present with recurrent hypoglycemia associated with lactic acidosis, hyperuricemia, and hyperlipidemia. The two other glycogen storage diseases causing hypoglycemia are due to deficiencies of the enzymes amylo-1,6-glucosidase (GSD type III) and liver phosphorylase (GSD type VI). The clinical and biochemical features of GSD-III subjects are quite heterogeneous.

Hypoglycemia Due to Defects in Gluconeogenesis

Gluconeogenesis, or the formation of glucose from mainly lactate/pyruvate, glycerol, glutamine, and alanine, plays an essential role in the maintenance of normoglycemia during fasting. Inborn deficiencies are known in each of the four enzymes of the glycolytic-gluconeogenic pathway that ensure a unidirectional flux from pyruvate to glucose: pyruvate carboxylase, phosphoenolpyruvate carboxykinase (PEPCK), fructose-1,6-bisphosphatase, and glucose-6-phosphatase. Gluconeogenesis can essentially be viewed as a reversal of glycolysis but with a few important differences. Patients with defects in gluconeogenesis present with fasting hypoglycemia and lactic acidosis. Pyruvate carboxylase deficiency may lead to a more widespread clinical presentation, with lactic acidosis, severe mental and developmental retardation, and proximal renal tubular acidosis.

Hypoglycemia Due to Disorders of Carnitine Metabolism and Defects of Fatty Acid Oxidation

Serious clinical consequences may occur if fatty acid oxidation (FAO) is impaired, including hypoglycemic seizures, muscle damage, cardiomyopathy, metabolic acidosis, and liver dysfunction. Fatty acids are taken up by hepatocytes and muscle, where they are subsequently activated to their coenzyme A (CoA) esters. FAO disorders are individually rare, but they are collectively common because of the number of different enzymes affected. When defects occur in fatty acid degradation, excess acylcarnitine intermediates accumulate in the tissues, including heart, liver, and skeletal muscle, which can lead to organ dysfunction. The diversion of acyl-CoA intermediates into β-oxidation results in accumulation of toxic dicarboxylic acids. Acylcarnitines that spill into the blood provide a marker for diagnosis.

Primary carnitine deficiency is an autosomal recessive disorder of fatty acid oxidation that can present at different ages with hypoketotic hypoglycemia and cardiomyopathy or skeletal myopathy (Chapter 194). This disease is suspected based on reduced levels of carnitine in plasma and confirmed by measurement of carnitine transport in the patient's fibroblasts. Carnitine transport is markedly reduced (usually <5% of normal) in fibroblasts from patients with primary carnitine deficiency. Patients with the hepatic isoform of carnitine palmityltransferase (CPT)-1 deficiency present with hypoketotic hypoglycemia in the neonatal period.

The commonest disorder of fatty acid β-oxidation is medium-chain acyl-CoA dehydrogenase (MCAD) deficiency, an autosomal recessive disease presenting in children who are typically asymptomatic except during times of fasting and metabolic stress, usually associated with a viral illness, when they present with fasting nonketotic hypoglycemia; if undiagnosed, 20 to 25% of affected patients will die during the first episode.

Metabolic Diseases

Hypoglycemia can also be due to a number of metabolic conditions (Chapter 194), including galactosemia, fructosemia, tyrosinemia, organic acidemias, maple syrup urine disease, glutaric aciduria type II, and in mitochondrial respiratory chain defects. Hereditary fructose intolerance, caused by catalytic deficiency of aldolase B (fructose-1,6-phosphate aldolase), is a recessively inherited condition in which affected homozygotes develop hypoglycemia and severe abdominal symptoms after taking foods containing fructose and cognate sugars. Continued ingestion of noxious sugars leads to hepatic and renal injury and growth retardation.

Noninsulinoma Islet Cell Tumors

Islet cell tumors present an important challenge to the clinician because of their protean manifestations and potential lethality. These tumors can be clinically silent or active (functioning). Early diagnosis is essential and depends on recognition of the classic and variant clinical syndromes followed by confirmation of elevated peptide levels by radioimmunoassay.[10] Glucagonoma, gastrinoma, VIPoma (VIP = vasoactive intestinal peptide), somatostatinoma, and ACTHoma are functioning tumors that may occur in isolation but can also be part of MEN 1 syndrome (Chapter 218) and von Hippel-Lindau disease (Chapter 389).

Tumor marker measurement gives useful information for the follow-up and management of patients with noninsulinoma islet cell tumors (neuroendocrine tumors). The currently used tumor markers are neuron-specific enolase (NSE) and chromogranin A (CgA). The clinical accuracy of these biomarkers depends on histotype and disease extent. CgA is thought to be the optimal marker for most neuroendocrine tumors, because it is independent of the biologic characteristics of the tumor.

Glucagonoma

Glucagonomas are α-cell tumors that, when they are active, produce a syndrome characterized by necrolytic migratory erythema, diabetes mellitus, weight loss, anemia, glossitis, thromboembolism, neuropsychiatric disturbances, and hyperglucagonemia. Tumor characterization is made by computed tomography (CT) and/or pancreatic endoscopic ultrasonic and indium-labeled octreoscan. The diagnosis is established by documenting the presence of hyperglucagonemia, with diagnostic levels being generally above 500 pg/mL (normal, <120). It is important to remember that other diseases can also cause hyperglucagonemia, including cirrhosis, pancreatitis, diabetes mellitus, prolonged fasting, sepsis, burns, renal failure, acromegaly, and familial hyperglucagonemia. Surgery is the main component of treatment, in some cases in association with chemotherapy.

Gastrinoma

Gastrinomas are uncommon tumors of the endocrine system, occurring within the pancreas and duodenum. Overproduction of the hormone gastrin by these tumors produces a sustained increase in gastric acid secretion, leading to complications of peptic ulceration known as the Zollinger-Ellison syndrome (ZES). Gastrinomas can occur sporadically or in a familial pattern as a component of the MEN 1 syndrome. Gastrinomas have the potential to metastasize to regional lymph nodes, the liver, and other distant sites.

VIPoma

VIPoma is very rare, with 80% of these tumors originating from the pancreas, mostly in the tail. The majority of cases are sporadic. About 50 to 60% of cases have metastasized by the time the diagnosis is made. Most patients have secretory watery diarrhea, resulting in electrolyte disturbances, such as hypokalemia, hypophosphatemia, hypomagnesemia, and metabolic acidosis (Verner-Morrison syndrome, pancreatic cholera, WDHA syndrome). Hypochlorhydria or achlorhydria occurs in 75% of cases, owing to the inhibition of gastric acid production by VIP. Hyperchloremic acidosis can also occur as a result of low bicarbonate levels from severe intestinal loss. Occasionally, hypercalcemia, glucose intolerance, and hypotension may be present. The VIP level is elevated in almost all cases, but it can also be normal between episodes of diarrhea.

Somatostatinoma

Somatostatinomas are rare neuroendocrine tumors with an incidence of 1 in 40 million. These unusual tumors arise predominantly in the pancreas and peripancreatic duodenum, and patients often present with nonspecific symptoms. Rarely, patients present with somatostatinoma syndrome (diabetes, gallstones, and steatorrhea) when the tumor is secretory.

Drug and Toxin-Induced Hypoglycemia

A number of drugs have been linked to hypoglycemia (see Table 217-1). Mechanisms vary, and, except for insulin and oral hypoglycemic agents, the risks in any individual are very low.

The white-fleshed lychee berry has been implicated as the cause of large-scale, severe hypoglycemia in the Bihar state of India. The likely cause is a lychee toxin that is known to cause hypoglycemia in rats. Similar illnesses have been reported in lychee-growing regions of Bangladesh and Vietnam.[11]

Investigations for Hypoglycemia

From the clinical history, description of symptoms, and physical examination, there might be important clues to the underlying cause of hypoglycemia, and the investigations can then be tailored to the particular cause. However, in some cases the clinical history and physical examination may not provide any clues, and in these cases the patient will need to be investigated more extensively.

Reagent strips in combination with a reflectance meter are the most common method of measuring bedside blood glucose levels. However, it is important to remember that these should be used only as a guide (they can be inaccurate), and the blood glucose concentration should always be checked in the laboratory. Whole-blood glucose is approximately 15% lower than serum glucose levels because of the lower glucose content and intracellular water content of the red cells. Glucose concentrations in venous blood are 10% lower than arterial blood. The blood sample for glucose measurement should be collected in a fluoride container to inhibit glycolysis. It should also be analyzed immediately because, even in the presence of fluoride, the blood glucose concentration will decrease over time.

In an ideal situation, the blood glucose level should be measured at the time of a spontaneous episode of hypoglycemia, and samples for plasma glucose, insulin, C-peptide, proinsulin, and β-hydroxybutyrate concentrations and toxicology screen for oral hypoglycemic agents taken. The blood glucose must be considered in the context of the whole fuel economy and in the light of concurrent hormone concentrations. However, this is not always possible, and patients may require further tests (e.g., fasting, mixed-meal, or provocation testing) to unravel the cause of the hypoglycemia. The various tests used for eliciting hypoglycemia in adults and children are described next. Table 217-2 shows the routine baseline investigations that should be performed in children and adults presenting with hypoglycemia.

Fasting Tests

Controlled fasting tests are important procedures for eliciting the cause of hypoglycemia in both children and adults. In adults it is recommended that a prolonged supervised (72-hour) fast be conducted in a standardized fashion (Table 217-3). During the fast, if patients have any signs or symptoms of hypoglycemia, with a documented low blood glucose level, the fast should be terminated. It is currently recommended that the fast not be prolonged beyond 72 hours if patients do not have any symptoms or signs of hypoglycemia and no documentation of low blood glucose. Monitoring for symptoms or signs of hypoglycemia during the fast is essential because patients may experience some symptoms but have serum glucose levels higher than the hypoglycemic range. In some healthy women (thin and lean) and men, blood glucose levels may drop to 40 mg/dL (2.2 mmol/L) during prolonged fasting. Some patients have lower glycemic thresholds without symptoms or signs of hypoglycemia.

In an adult patient where Whipple triad has been demonstrated, the 72-hour fast may be terminated if the plasma glucose concentration is 55 mg/dL (3 mmol/L) or less. The interpretation of serum insulin, C-peptide, and proinsulin during the 72-hour fast will depend on the concurrent plasma glucose concentration. Pancreatic β-cell insulin secretion becomes undetectable in healthy persons when the plasma glucose concentration is down to 55 mg/dL (3 mmol/L). Most patients with an insulinoma become hypoglycemic before 72 hours. However, continuation of the fast to 72 hours is necessary to rule out the likelihood of organic hypoglycemia.

Hyperinsulinemic hypoglycemia in adults is characterized by plasma insulin concentrations of 3 μU/mL or greater (C-peptide of 200 pmol/L or more

---

TABLE 217-2 ROUTINE BASELINE INVESTIGATIONS IN PATIENTS WITH SUSPECTED HYPOGLYCEMIA

BLOOD	URINE
Glucose	Ketones
Insulin	Reducing substances
Cortisol	Organic acids
Lactate	
Growth hormone	
Nonesterified fatty acids	
3β-Hydroxybutyrate	
Carnitine (free and total)	
Blood spot acylcarnitine	
Ammonia	

TABLE 217-3 PROTOCOL FOR 72-HOUR FAST IN ADULTS

1. Start the fast from the last ingestion of a meal. Stop all medications that might interfere with test.
2. The patient can drink water during the test.
3. The patient must be active during waking hours.
4. Measure plasma glucose, insulin, C-peptide, and β-hydroxybutyrate (on the same venipuncture specimen) every 6 hours until plasma glucose reaches 60 mg/dL (3.3 mM). Then measure every 1 to 2 hours.
5. End the fast when the plasma glucose is 45 mg/dL (2.5 mM) and the patient has symptoms or signs of hypoglycemia, or plasma glucose is 55 mg/dL if Whipple triad had been demonstrated previously.
6. At the end of the fast, measure plasma glucose, insulin, C-peptide, β-hydroxybutyrate, and sulfonylurea (on the same venipuncture specimen). Then inject glucagon, 1 mg intravenously, and measure plasma glucose every 10 minutes three times. Once the fast is completed, allow the patient to eat normally.

Adapted from Cryer PE, Axelrod L, Grossman AB, et al. Evaluation and management of adult hypoglycemic disorders: an Endocrine Society clinical practice guideline. *J Clin Endocrinol Metab.* 2009;94:709-728.

and proinsulin 5 pmol/L or more). Insulinoma patients have plasma insulin concentrations that rarely exceed 100 μU/mL, and plasma insulin levels greater than 1000 μU/mL suggest exogenous insulin administration or the presence of insulin antibodies. In the childhood period, any detectable plasma insulin in the presence of hypoglycemia is inappropriate and is highly suggestive of hyperinsulinemic hypoglycemia.

Measurement of the plasma β-hydroxybutyrate concentration is used as a surrogate marker of insulin action at the end of the 72-hour fast in healthy adult individuals and when Whipple triad is fulfilled in patients during a diagnostic fast. In patients with hyperinsulinemic hypoglycemia, because of the suppressive action of insulin on ketogenesis, plasma concentrations of β-hydroxybutyrate are typically less than 2.7 mmol/L. This is in contrast to healthy individuals, who will show a progressive rise in the concentration of β-hydroxybutyrate during the 72-hour test. If a value above 2.7 mmol/L is documented at any time point in the fast, the test can be terminated. In the childhood period, there is no clear-cut plasma level of β-hydroxybutyrate that can be used to confirm hyperinsulinemic hypoglycemia.

Another useful marker of insulin action in both adults and children is the glycemic increment in response to an intravenous/intramuscular injection of glucagon (1-mg dose in adults). Patients with hyperinsulinemic hypoglycemia will have increased glycogen stores, and giving glucagon will result in glycogenolysis. A positive response is defined as a maximal increment at least 25 mg/dL (1.3 mmol/L) greater than the terminal fasting serum glucose.

During the 72-hour prolonged fast, blood should also be collected for measurement of plasma sulfonylureas and meglitinides if the patient develops hypoglycemia. Sulfonylureas stimulate pancreatic β-cell insulin and C-peptide secretion, and the biochemical pattern is similar to that of an insulinoma.

Mixed-Meal Test

A mixed-meal test is performed in patients in whom there is a history suggestive of neuroglycopenic symptoms for up to 5 hours after food ingestion (Table 217-4). A positive test is defined as the onset of neuroglycopenic symptoms in association with a documented low blood glucose level (e.g., ≤50 mg/dL). In postprandial hyperinsulinemic hypoglycemia, plasma insulin and C-peptide levels might be inappropriately elevated. Neuroglycopenic symptoms after a meal are reported in patients with insulinoma, patients with NIPHS, and patients who have undergone surgery for obesity.

The combination of a positive mixed-meal test and a negative 72-hour fast may occur in a patient with insulinoma or with NIPHS. The 5-hour oral glucose tolerance test should not be used as a sole diagnostic test for hypoglycemia, because a substantial percentage of healthy persons may have a serum glucose concentration of 50 mg/dL (2.7 mmol/L) or less.

Insulin Antibodies

In patients with insulin autoimmune hypoglycemia the insulin antibodies may be monoclonal or polyclonal and are present in very high titers, in contrast to the much lower titers in insulin-treated diabetes. It is important to test for the presence of insulin antibodies, because even low titers—which may have no diagnostic significance—may cause spurious results of the assay for insulin.

TABLE 217-4 SUGGESTED PROTOCOL FOR A MIXED-MEAL DIAGNOSTIC TEST IN ADULTS

1. Fast patient overnight. Stop all medications that might interfere with test.
2. Use a mixed meal similar to one that causes patient to experience symptoms.
3. Collect samples for plasma glucose, insulin, C-peptide, and proinsulin before ingestion and every 30 minutes through 300 minutes after meal ingestion.
4. Observe the patient for symptoms and/or signs of hypoglycemia, and ask the patient to keep a written log of all symptoms, timed from the start of meal ingestion.
5. The mixed-meal test should be interpreted on the basis of laboratory measured plasma glucose concentrations, not those estimated with a point-of-care glucose monitor. If it is judged necessary to treat before 300 minutes because of severe symptoms, obtain samples for all the following *before* administering carbohydrates: plasma insulin, C-peptide, and proinsulin (sent for analysis only in those samples in which plasma glucose is <60 mg/dL [3.3 mmol/L]), and a measurement of oral hypoglycemic agents. If Whipple triad is demonstrated, antibodies to insulin should also be measured.

Adapted from Cryer PE, Axelrod L, Grossman AB, et al. Evaluation and management of adult hypoglycemic disorders: an Endocrine Society clinical practice guideline. *J Clin Endocrinol Metab.* 2009;94:709-728.

Hypoglycemia due to IAS typically occurs in the fasting period but can occur postprandially as well.

Radiologic Investigations

Noninvasive imaging procedures such as CT and magnetic resonance imaging (MRI) are used when a diagnosis of insulinoma has been made to localize the source of pathologic insulin secretion. Invasive modalities, such as endoscopic ultrasonography (EUS) and arterial stimulation venous sampling (ASVS), are highly accurate in the preoperative localization of insulinomas and have frequently been shown to be superior to noninvasive localization techniques. Intraoperative manual palpation of the pancreas by an experienced surgeon and intraoperative ultrasonography are both sensitive methods with which to finalize the location of insulinomas.

The sensitivity of transabdominal ultrasonography in the localization of insulinomas is poor (ranging from 9% to 64%). However, insulinomas demonstrate characteristic features when imaged with both CT and MRI, and the sensitivity of these techniques is 33 to 64% and 40 to 90%, respectively. The sensitivity and specificity of MRI is generally superior to that of CT, as is the detection of extrapancreatic extensions. Insulinomas generally demonstrate low signal intensity on T1-weighted images and high signal intensity on T2-weighted images.

Invasive modalities such as EUS and ASVS have been shown to be highly accurate in the preoperative localization of insulinomas and have frequently been shown to be superior to noninvasive localization techniques. EUS is currently the test of choice in most Western centers, with reported detection rates of 86.6 to 92.3%.

ASVS has greatly facilitated the precise regionalization of insulinomas smaller than 2 cm, which noninvasive techniques like ultrasonography, CT, and MRI often fail to localize. This test requires access to intra-abdominal vessels, including the right hepatic vein, splenic artery, gastroduodenal artery, and superior mesenteric artery. A two- to three-fold increase in insulin concentration in the right hepatic vein in response to calcium injection into one or more of the arteries supplying the pancreas suggests that the region served by that artery may harbor abnormally functioning β cells, whether from insulinoma or islet hypertrophy or nesidioblastosis. Calcium injection will stimulate a brisk response of insulin, C-peptide, and proinsulin simultaneously, and the magnitude of increase of both insulin and C-peptide appears to be correlated well with the degree of differentiation of the tumor cells.

Insulinomas have been shown to express GLP-1R in high density, and GLP-1R imaging has been used in some patients for insulinoma localization.[12] Fluorine-18-L-dihydroxyphenylalanine (18F-DOPA) positron emission tomography (PET) has also been used in localizing neuroendocrine tumors. In children with congenital hyperinsulinemic hypoglycemia, 18F-DOPA PET/CT is the gold standard for localizing focal lesions prior to surgery. 18F-DOPA PET has been found to be useful in some patients with insulinoma who had negative CT, MRI, and ultrasound results.

The positive responses to selective arterial calcium stimulation in some patients with NIPHS, despite negative radiologic localizing studies, establish that this technique should be performed in all adults with hyperinsulinemic hypoglycemia of unknown etiology.

Protein/Leucine Sensitivity Testing

Protein sensitivity is observed in some patients with congenital hyperinsulinemic hypoglycemia due to mutations in the genes *ABCC8/KCNJ11*, *GDH*, and *HADH* that lead to protein-induced hypoglycemia. These patients will demonstrate severe hypoglycemia in response to a protein or leucine load.

Exercise Test

In some patients, exercise can trigger unregulated insulin secretion. This is referred to as exercise-induced hyperinsulinism. Promoter-activating mutations induce expression of the *SLC16A1* gene in β cells, where this gene is not usually transcribed, permitting pyruvate uptake and pyruvate-stimulated insulin release despite ensuing hypoglycemia. A physical exercise test will identify this group of patients.

Genetic Studies

Genetic testing should be undertaken in children who have been diagnosed with congenital hyperinsulinemic hypoglycemia and other causes of hypoglycemia that might have a genetic basis. Mutation in the genes *ABCC8/KCNJ11* is the commonest cause of medically unresponsive congenital hyperinsulinemic hypoglycemia. All patients with insulinoma and noninsulinoma islet cell tumors should be tested for mutations in the *MEN1/YY1* genes.

The correct management of hypoglycemia will depend on the underlying cause. Therefore, establishing the correct diagnosis is fundamentally important.

Emergency Management

Acute management of hypoglycemia[13] involves giving a bolus of intravenous glucose (in adults a bolus of 50% dextrose) to correct the blood glucose level. In children a 2 mL/kg bolus of 10% dextrose is used. This will then need to be followed by an infusion of 10% dextrose to maintain normoglycemia. Glucagon can be used in the emergency management of hypoglycemia (in emergency, give 1 mg stat intramuscularly). Glucagon can cause rebound hypoglycemia, so the patient will need blood glucose monitoring after the administration of glucagon.

Management of Specific Causes of Hypoglycemia

The long-term management of hypoglycemia depends on the underlying cause. Below is a summary of the management of the different types of hypoglycemia.

Hyperinsulinemic Hypoglycemia

Diazoxide (5 to 20 mg/kg/day given orally three times daily) is the first-line medical therapy in children and adults with hyperinsulinemic hypoglycemia. Fluid retention is a major side effect. Diazoxide may be combined with a diuretic to reduce the side effect of fluid retention. Second-line therapies include the use of octreotide (5 to 35 µg/kg/day as an infusion or injection 3 or 4 times daily) and glucagon (1 to 10 µg/kg/hour given as a subcutaneous or intravenous infusion). mTOR inhibitors have been tried in some patients.

For adult patients with insulinoma, pancreatectomy is the treatment of choice. However, there are reports of insulinoma in adults responding to therapy with diazoxide and octreotide (including long-acting octreotide). The mTOR inhibitor everolimus has been reported to be effective in controlling hypoglycemia in patients with malignant insulinomas or those who cannot undergo surgical resection. Adult patients with postprandial hyperinsulinemic hypoglycemia after gastric bypass surgery can be treated with diazoxide and octreotide, but some will require pancreatectomy. The insulin autoimmune syndrome will respond to therapy with glucocorticoids, but some patients have responded to diazoxide and octreotide. Non–islet cell tumor hypoglycemia or IGF-2-oma patients will require resection of the primary tumor.

Hypoglycemia Due to Hormonal Deficiencies

Adult patients and children with GH and cortisol deficiency will require replacement therapy with recombinant GH and hydrocortisone (prednisolone), respectively. Replacement therapy with gluco- and mineralocorticoids can be life-saving in patients with adrenal insufficiency.

Hypoglycemia Due to Glycogen Storage Diseases

Patients with hypoglycemia due to disorders of hepatic glycogen storage and release need to avoid prolonged periods of fasting. Children will require overnight continuous feeding. Raw, uncooked cornstarch is commonly used as a slow-release source of glucose and helps with prolonging the period of fasting.

Hypoglycemia Due to Defects in Fatty Acid Oxidation, Disorders of Gluconeogenesis, and Disorders of Ketone Body Metabolism

Principles similar to those already discussed also apply to these patients. However, patients with fatty acid oxidation disorders should have carnitine supplementation.

GENERAL REFERENCES

For the General References and other additional features, please visit Expert Consult at https://expertconsult.inkling.com.

218

POLYGLANDULAR DISORDERS

LYNNETTE K. NIEMAN AND ALLEN M. SPIEGEL

DEFINITION AND CLINICAL SIGNIFICANCE

Polyglandular syndromes are disorders in which there is dysfunction and pathology of more than one endocrine gland. These disorders can be classified into (a) neoplastic syndromes in which there is abnormal endocrine cell proliferation and often, but not invariably, hormone hypersecretion, and (b) autoimmune syndromes in which there is evidence of immune destruction of endocrine cells, often resulting in hypofunction and reduced hormone secretion. Both the neoplastic and autoimmune polyglandular syndromes often have nonendocrine manifestations that are relatively syndrome specific.

With few exceptions, the polyglandular syndromes are due to germline mutations of key growth regulatory genes (neoplastic syndromes) or immune regulatory genes (autoimmune syndromes).[1] It is important to recognize these disorders and differentiate them from sporadic single–endocrine gland diseases for several reasons. First, recognition of a specific polyglandular syndrome should alert the clinician to look for other endocrine and extra-endocrine manifestations of the syndrome. Although some patients will present with multiple endocrine gland manifestations, some will initially present with only a single endocrine gland affected. Careful family history and screening for other endocrine and characteristic extra-endocrine manifestations is needed in such cases. Second, treatment of polyglandular disease may differ from treatment of individual gland disease. Third, because of the genetic basis of most of these syndromes, taking a careful family history and, in some cases, screening other family members to allow disease prevention in affected individuals is indicated.

This chapter discusses the best-characterized polyglandular disorders. Other chapters on the anterior pituitary (Chapter 211), thyroid (Chapter 213), adrenal cortex (Chapter 214), adrenal medulla (Chapter 215), pancreatic islets (Chapters 217 and 219), and parathyroids (Chapter 232) should be consulted for more detailed discussion of the diseases of individual glands.

NEOPLASTIC SYNDROMES

Six distinct neoplastic syndromes involve more than one endocrine gland. These include multiple endocrine neoplasia type 1 (MEN 1), multiple endocrine neoplasia types 2A (MEN 2) and 2B (sometimes referred to as MEN 3), multiple endocrine neoplasia type 4 (MEN 4), Carney complex,[2] von Hippel-Lindau disease (VHL), and McCune-Albright syndrome (MAS) (Table 218-1).[3] All but the latter are caused by heterozygous germline mutations and are inherited in autosomal dominant fashion. The genes responsible for MEN 1[4] and 4, Carney complex, and von Hippel-Lindau disease act as tumor suppressor genes. Germline loss-of-function mutations in one allele are followed by somatic mutations inactivating the second normal allele, leading to tumorigenesis. The basis for the tissue-specific expression of both the endocrine and extra-endocrine manifestations of these syndromes is not well understood, but the germline nature of the mutation and the expression of the affected gene in more than one endocrine gland explains the polyglandular aspect of the disorder. MEN 2A and 2B, in contrast, are caused by germline activating mutations of an oncogene, *RET*. The pattern of expression of this gene, involving chromaffin cells, helps explain the specific clinical manifestations. McCune-Albright syndrome is caused by a somatic rather than germline mutation that constitutively activates the ubiquitously expressed *GNAS* gene. This mutation, which may occur early in embryogenesis, leads to unregulated cyclic adenosine monophosphate (cAMP) formation in affected cells. The resultant mosaic distribution of the mutant gene helps explain the pleiotropic manifestations of the disease.

Patients with polyglandular neoplastic syndromes typically present with their respective endocrine tumors at a younger age than patients with single-gland sporadic endocrine tumors. Treatment of the polyglandular neoplastic syndromes, both in terms of the neoplastic component and the hormone hypersecretion, poses greater challenges than treatment of individual endocrine tumors.[5] For disorders with high risk of fatal cancer, such as medullary thyroid cancer in MEN 2, early genetic diagnosis and prophylactic surgical removal of the thyroid is indicated.[6] In other disorders such as MEN 1 and Carney complex, less aggressive approaches such as selective tumor resection and

TABLE 218-1 POLYGLANDULAR NEOPLASIA SYNDROMES

SYNDROME	GENETIC BASIS*	ENDOCRINE TUMORS	NONENDOCRINE FEATURES
MEN 1	*MEN1*	Parathyroid Anterior pituitary Pancreatic islet	Subcutaneous lipomas Skin collagenomas
MEN 2 (A and B)	*RET*	Medullary thyroid cancer Pheochromocytoma Parathyroid (2A)	Mucosal neuromas (2B) Megacolon (2B)
MEN 4	*CDNK1B*	Anterior pituitary Parathyroid	Renal tumors
Carney complex	*PKAR1A*	Adrenal cortex Anterior pituitary Thyroid	Atrial myxomas Skin lentigines Blue nevi
von Hippel-Lindau disease	*VHL*	Pheochromocytoma Pancreatic islet	Renal cell cancer CNS hemangioblastoma
McCune-Albright syndrome	*GNAS* (mosaic)	Thyroid Anterior pituitary Adrenal cortex Gonads	Fibrous dysplasia Café au lait skin lesions

*With the exception of McCune-Albright, all syndromes are caused by heterozygous germline mutations of the gene listed and show autosomal dominant inheritance.
CNS = central nervous system.

TABLE 218-2 CLINICAL FEATURES OF AUTOIMMUNE POLYGLANDULAR SYNDROMES

FEATURE	TYPE 1	TYPE 2
Mucocutaneous candidiasis	Very common	Not seen
Hypoparathyroidism	Common	Rare
Addison disease	Common	Common
Primary hypogonadism	Common	Occurs
Autoimmune thyroid disease	Rare	Common
Autoimmune diabetes	Occurs	Common
Hypophysitis	Occurs	Occurs
Autoimmune hepatitis	Occurs	Not seen
Pernicious anemia	Occurs	Occurs
Vitiligo	Occurs	Occurs
Malabsorption syndrome	Occurs	Occurs as celiac disease
Alopecia	Common	Occurs
Myasthenia gravis	Not seen	Occurs
Keratopathy	Common	Not seen
Tympanic membrane calcification	Common	Not seen
Inheritance	Autosomal recessive	HLA association
Age at onset	Usually childhood	Usually adulthood

HLA = human leukocyte antigen.

pharmacologic treatment to reduce hormone hypersecretion may be more appropriate. More detailed discussion of the clinical features, diagnosis, and treatment of these neoplastic syndromes may be found in other chapters (MEN 1 in Chapter 232; MEN 2 and 3 in Chapter 219; McCune-Albright syndrome in Chapters 220 and 222).

● AUTOIMMUNE SYNDROMES

Organ-specific autoimmune disease, characterized by lymphocytic infiltration and organ-specific autoantibodies, commonly results in endocrine hypofunction. Not uncommonly, however, disorders of more than one endocrine gland appear in families or individual patients. Characteristic patterns of disease presentation and genetic inheritance allow the definition of two syndromes with overlapping manifestations (Table 218-2).[7]

Autoimmune Polyglandular Syndrome Type 1

DEFINITION

Autoimmune polyglandular syndrome (APS) type 1 is a rare disease that is also known as autoimmune polyendocrinopathy, candidiasis, and ectodermal dystrophy syndrome. It typically manifests in early childhood.

PATHOGENESIS

APS type 1 is an autosomal recessive disorder caused by a variety of inactivating mutations in the gene encoding autoimmune regulator-1 (AIRE-1),[8] which controls the expression of autoantigens by medullary epithelial cells of the thymus. These antigens are also expressed in peripheral tissues. Their expression in the thymus is important for negative selection (elimination) of autoreactive T cells, which underlies the development of (self-) tolerance. These autoreactive T cells escape to the periphery in the absence of AIRE, and if activated, induce autoimmune destruction of the specific tissue. The appearance of organ-specific autoantibodies precedes disease presentation and predicts the development of specific end-organ damage. The role of these antibodies is unknown, however.

CLINICAL MANIFESTATIONS

Mucocutaneous candidiasis (Chapter 318) occurs in virtually all patients and is usually the first manifestation of disease.[9] Hypoparathyroidism and Addison disease are the most common endocrine manifestations; each of these diseases occurs in 70 to 80% of patients. Hypoparathyroidism usually precedes Addison disease; both diseases typically manifest before age 15 years. Premature ovarian failure (in 60% of affected women) usually presents as secondary amenorrhea; testicular failure occurs less frequently. Insulin-dependent diabetes mellitus occurs in 12% of patients, usually in adulthood; hypothyroidism is uncommon.

Nonendocrine components of this syndrome, in addition to the mucocutaneous candidiasis, include alopecia, vitiligo, ocular complications (including keratitis, blepharitis, retinitis, corneal opacities, and ptosis), cerebellar ataxia, autoimmune hepatitis, enamel hypoplasia of teeth, tympanic membrane calcification, obstructive respiratory disease, nail dystrophy that correlates only loosely with obvious candidiasis, parietal cell atrophy and vitamin B_{12} malabsorption, and more general intestinal malabsorption with steatorrhea. Asplenism, with Howell-Jolly bodies on peripheral blood smears (Chapter 148), has been noted in several patients. Each of the disease components should be sought when any patient presents with hypoparathyroidism, primary adrenal insufficiency, or mucocutaneous candidiasis.

TREATMENT ℞

The hypoparathyroidism is treated, like the sporadic disease, with oral calcium and 1,25-dihydroxyvitamin D, although variable intestinal malabsorption can present a particular therapeutic challenge. Synthetic parathyroid hormone (PTH) 1-34 or 1-84 is a new treatment option.[10] The candidiasis can be satisfactorily controlled with ketoconazole. Primary adrenal insufficiency is treated with glucocorticoid and mineralocorticoid replacement.

PROGNOSIS

The prognosis of the variably expressed hormonal disorders is similar to that of their sporadic counterparts. When the diagnosis of APS type 1 is made, surveys for other components of the syndrome can allow earlier treatment than would otherwise occur.

Autoimmune Polyglandular Syndrome Types 2, 3, and 4

PATHOGENESIS

APS types 2 and 3 are usually inherited in families with characteristic (normal) variants of genes that regulate the presentation of antigens to T cells and subsequent T-cell function. The most common genetic locus associated with this syndrome is the human leukocyte antigen (HLA) locus, particularly the B8, DR3, and DR4 alleles. The HLA associations do not predict disease absolutely, even in identical twins, so environmental or other genetic factors must influence disease presentation. Variants of the genes encoding cytotoxic T-lymphocyte antigen-4 (CTLA-4), the MHC class I chain-related gene A (MICA) allele 5.1, signal transducer and activator of transcription 4 (STAT4), and GATA binding protein 3 (GATA) can also predispose to Addison disease (APS type 2). The protein tyrosine phosphatase nonreceptor type 22 gene that encodes the lymphoid tyrosine phosphatase opposes signaling from the activated T-cell receptor. A variant of this gene is enriched in families with both type 1 diabetes mellitus and autoimmune thyroid disease. Genome-wide association studies have identified a large number of genes associated with type 1 diabetes that influence immune responsiveness. It seems likely that some of these genes will prove relevant to APS types 2 and 3, but this remains to be evaluated. Genotyping is not widely available for clinical testing.

CLINICAL MANIFESTATIONS

APS types 2 and 3 are considerably more common than type 1 and typically manifest in the fourth decade of life.[11] Insulin-dependent diabetes mellitus and thyroid dysfunction, either autoimmune hypothyroidism or Graves disease, are the most frequent manifestations.[12] Addison disease (Chapter 214) is the third major endocrine component of this disorder; when present, the disorder may be referred to as APS type 3. Although most patients who present with autoimmune diabetes or thyroid disease have clinical involvement of only one gland, many patients with autoimmune Addison disease develop clinically evident disease in other endocrine glands. Less common components of type 2 or 3 APS include primary hypogonadism and hypophysitis. Pernicious anemia, vitiligo, celiac disease, alopecia, and myasthenia gravis are also associated with this syndrome.

APS type 4 is a combination of endocrine and autoimmune diseases, including insulin-dependent diabetes, pernicious anemia, alopecia, vitiligo, or neuromuscular junction disorder, but without Addison disease, thyroid disease, or hypoparathyroidism. A substantial proportion of these patients may also have positive autoantibodies against glutamic acid decarboxylase (GAD).

Organ-specific antibodies appear before clinical disease and predict subsequent disease. The role of these antibodies in organ hypofunction has not been established, however.

PROGNOSIS

The prognosis of the individual components of APS types 2 and 3 is the same as for the sporadic versions of each component.

TREATMENT   Rx

The treatment of each component of this syndrome is identical to the treatment of each disorder in isolation, although possible clustering of diseases must be kept in mind during the evaluation and follow-up of all patients with each individual component disorder. Thyroid hormone therapy can precipitate symptoms of adrenal insufficiency in patients with both disorders. Consequently, a careful history (including family history), physical examination, and a low threshold for specific laboratory testing for adrenal insufficiency should be part of the evaluation of every patient with autoimmune hypothyroidism. Further, combinations of hypothyroidism, adrenal insufficiency, and hypogonadism can mimic hypopituitarism, although specific hormonal testing (Chapter 211) can easily distinguish these disorders. Because multiple components of the syndrome can appear asynchronously, periodic evaluation for the early appearance of additional disease components is indicated.

GENERAL REFERENCES

For the General References and other additional features, please visit Expert Consult at https://expertconsult.inkling.com.

219

NEUROENDOCRINE TUMORS

EDWARD M. WOLIN AND ROBERT T. JENSEN

GENERAL ASPECTS

DEFINITION

Neuroendocrine tumors (NETs) include pancreatic neuroendocrine tumors (pNETs) and NETs in other locations, which in the past were generally called carcinoid tumors.[1] These two groups of NETs have many similarities, which will be discussed together, and several important differences, which are considered separately.

EPIDEMIOLOGY

The incidence of NETs in the United States increased 6.4-fold from 1973 (1.09 per 100,000) to 2012 (6.98 per 100,000), with the highest rates in the lung (1.5 per 100,000); 50% occur in the gastrointestinal (GI) tract, 21% in the lung, and 12% with an unknown primary.[2] pNETS account for 1 to 10% of all pancreatic tumors, with a prevalence of 1 per 100,000 and an annual incidence of 1 to 4 per million, which is also increasing. However, pNETs occur in 0.5 to 1.5% of autopsies. In recent studies, nonfunctional pNETs (NF-pNETs) have accounted for 60 to 80% of all pNETs (Table 219-1). For the functional pNETs (F-pNETs) associated with clinical syndromes, insulinomas and gastrinomas are the most common, with annual incidences of 0.5 to 3 per million (see Table 219-1). In general, insulinomas and gastrinomas are 8-fold more frequent than VIPomas, 17-fold more than glucagonomas, and greater than 20-fold more than the others.

PATHOBIOLOGY

Pathology/Classification

NETs originate from the diffuse neuroendocrine system, which is present throughout the body. All NETs share cytologic features and were once called APUDomas (for *a*mine *p*recursor *u*ptake and *d*ecarboxylation tumors). Although originally proposed to be of neural crest origin, current studies support more of an endodermal origin. Ultrastructurally they have electron-dense granules containing multiple peptides/amines, neuron-specific enolase, synaptophysin, and chromogranins. Histologically, they characteristically show small cells with uniform nuclei and low rates of mitotic figures. Chromogranin immunoreactivity in the tumor is now widely used to identify them as NETs. Malignancy can be reliably determined only by demonstrating the presence of metastatic disease; light microscopic or ultrastructural findings cannot clearly establish malignant behavior.

Recently several classification systems for staging/grading NETs have been developed (WHO [World Health Organization], ENETs [European Neuroendocrine Tumor Society], AJCC/UICC [Union for International Cancer Control and the American Joint Committee on Cancer]) and are becoming essential to manage NET patients because they have prognostic significance and are coupled to different therapeutic approaches in some cases. These classification systems use differentiation (good vs. poor), tumor size, invasion, and extent. The NETs are divided into three grades depending on proliferative indices, including mitotic rate and Ki-67 expression.

Molecular Pathogenesis

The molecular pathogenesis of NETs is still largely unknown and differs from nonendocrine tumors in rarely having mutations of common oncogenes (*ras, fos, myc,* etc.) and common tumor suppressor genes (*p53,rb*).[3] Numerous studies using comparative-genomic hybridization, sequencing, and microarrays show that pNETs, GI-NETs, and lung NETs all have a different molecular pathogenesis.

pNETs most commonly have allelic losses at chromosomal loci 1p, 1q, 3p, 11p, and 22p, whereas GI-NETs have losses at 18q, 18p, 9p, and 16q.[4] Sequencing studies of pNETs have shown that 44% have inactivating mutations of the multiple endocrine neoplasia type 1 gene (*MEN1*); 43% have mutations in genes encoding either of two subunits of a transcription/chromatin remodeling complex composed of DAXX (death-domain associated protein) and ATRX (α thalassemia/mental retardation syndrome X-linked chromatin remodeler)

TABLE 219-1 PANCREATIC NEUROENDOCRINE TUMORS (PNETS)

NAME OF TUMOR	NAME OF SYNDROME	MAIN SIGNS OR SYMPTOMS	LOCATION (%)	MALIGNANCY (%)	HORMONE CAUSING SYNDROME
I. FUNCTIONAL pNET					
Gastrinoma	Zollinger-Ellison syndrome	Abdominal pain, diarrhea, esophageal symptoms	Pancreas—10-30 Duodenum—70-90 Other—0-10	60-90	Gastrin
Insulinoma	Insulinoma	Hypoglycemic symptoms	Pancreas—100	5-15	Insulin
Glucagonoma	Glucagonoma	Dermatitis, diabetes/ glucose intolerance, weight loss	Pancreas—100	60	Glucagon
VIPoma	Verner-Morrison, Pancreatic cholera, WDHA	Severe watery diarrhea, hypokalemia	Pancreas—90 Other—10 (neural, adrenal, periganglionic tissue)	80	Vasoactive intestinal peptide (VIP)
Somatostatinoma	Somatostatinoma	Diabetes mellitus, cholelithiasis, diarrhea	Pancreas—56 Duod/jejunum—44	60	Somatostatin
GRFoma	GRFoma	Acromegaly	Pancreas—30 Lung—54 Jejunum—7 Other—13 (adrenal, foregut, retroperitoneum)	30	Growth hormone–releasing factor (GRF)
ACTHoma	ACTHoma	Cushing syndrome	Pancreas—4-16% of all ectopic Cushing syndrome cases	>95	Adrenocorticotropic hormone (ACTH)
pNET causing carcinoid syndrome	pNET causing carcinoid syndrome	Diarrhea, flushing	Pancreas—<1% of all carcinoids	60-90	Serotonin, tachykinins
pNET causing hypercalcemia	pNET causing hypercalcemia	Signs/symptoms of hypercalcemia	Pancreas (rare cause of hypercalcemia)	>85	PTHrP, other unknown
pNET secreting erythropoietin	pNET secreting erythropoietin	Polycythemia	Pancreas	Unknown	Erythropoietin
pNET secreting renin	pNET secreting renin	Hypertension	Pancreas	Unknown	Renin
pNET secreting Luteinizing hormone syndrome	pNET secreting luteinizing hormone	Masculinization, loss of libido	Pancreas	Unknown	Luteinizing hormone
CCKoma	CCKoma	Diarrhea, peptic ulcer, gallstone	Pancreas	Unknown	Cholecystokinin
pNET secreting enteroglucagon	pNET secreting enteroglucagon	Small intestinal hypertrophy	Pancreas, renal, duodenal	Unknown	Enteroglucagon
pNET secreting IGF-2 or GLP-1	pNET secreting IGF-2 or GLP-1	Hypoglycemic symptoms	Pancreas	Unknown	IGF-2/GLP-1
II. NF-pNET					
NONFUNCTIONAL/PPoma	NONFUNCTIONAL/PPoma	Weight loss, abdominal mass, hepatomegaly	Pancreas—100%	60-90	None: pancreatic polypeptide, chromogranin released but no known symptoms due to hypersecretion

CCKoma = cholecystokinin-secreting NET; Duod = duodenum; GLP-1 = glucagon-like peptide 1; IGF-2 = insulin-like growth factor 2; pNET = pancreatic neuroendocrine tumor; PP = pancreatic polypeptide; PPoma = pancreatic polypeptide secreting NET; PTHrP = parathormone-related peptide; WDHA = watery diarrhea, hypokalemia, and achlorhydria.

and 14% have mutations in the mTOR pathway. Somatic mutations in pNETs are commonly found in four main pathways, including genes involved in chromatin remodeling, DNA repair, mTOR signaling, and telomere maintenance. In contrast, in small intestinal carcinoids sequencing studies demonstrate a low mutation rate with recurrent somatic mutations and deletions in 8% in *CDKN1B*, the cyclin-dependent kinase inhibitor gene that encodes p27. Recent studies suggest that epigenetic dysregulation may play an important role in the pathogenesis of NETs.

Four autosomal dominant inherited disorders are associated with the occurrence of pNETs: (a) MEN1 (80 to 100% develop pNETs), (b) von Hippel–Lindau disease (VHL; 10 to 17% have pNETs), (c) von Recklinghausen disease (neurofibromatosis-1 [NF-1]; 12% develop duodenal somatostatinomas), and (d) tuberous sclerosis (<1% develop pNETs). Familial syndromes associated with GI/pulmonary NETs (carcinoids) are uncommon.[5]

Tumor Localization

To assess the primary location and extent of an NET, the initial tumor localization study is generally a cross-sectional imaging examination, such as triphasic computed tomography (CT) or magnetic resonance imaging (MRI) with contrast, because of their widespread availability. Greater than 90% of well-differentiated NETs overexpress one of the five subtypes of somatostatin receptors (sst1-5), with sst2 the most frequently overexpressed (>80%). Somatostatin receptor imaging (SRI) using radiolabeled somatostatin analogs

with high affinity for sst2 is now the most sensitive NET imaging modality.[6] Most frequently used for SRI is single-photon emission CT (SPECT) after injection of indium-111–[diethylenediamine penta-acetic acid-d-phenylalanine-1] octreotide or ^{68}Ga-DOTA (1,4,7,10-tetraazacyclododecane-1,4,7,10-tetraacetic acid)–labeled somatostatin analogs with positron-emission-tomography combined with CT (PET/CT) or MRI (PET/MRI). More recently, SRI with ^{68}Ga-labeled somatostatin analogs has been approved in the United States, with numerous studies showing that it has greater sensitivity than SRI with ^{111}In-somatostatin analogs and greater sensitivity than cross-sectional imaging. Endoscopic studies are particularly important for localizing duodenal, gastric, and rectal NETs. Endoscopic ultrasound is widely used to localize pancreatic pNETs and to assess the depth of penetration of gastric and rectal NETs.

● SPECIFIC NEUROENDOCRINE TUMORS
Pancreatic Neuroendocrine Tumors (pNETS)

DEFINITION

pNETs are also called islet-cell tumors, but because the cell of origin of most of these tumors is unknown, the general term *pNET* is preferred. This term is also a misnomer, however, because pNETs can occur outside the pancreas. The established pNET syndromes are listed in Table 219-1 and comprise 16 functional pNETs that cause specific clinical syndromes and nonfunctional pNETs. Nonfunctional pNET is also a misnomer in that these tumors secrete multiple peptides (chromogranin, pancreatic polypeptide [PP], etc.), but these do not cause a specific clinical syndrome. Several of the functional pNET syndromes are very uncommon (fewer than 5 cases reported), including pNETs that secrete renin, erythropoietin, enteroglucagon, luteinizing hormone, and cholecystokinin (CCKoma) (see Table 219-1), as well as pNETs secreting GLP1 and IGF-2 that cause hypoglycemia (2 cases). In addition, pNETs synthesizing neurotensin, calcitonin, and ghrelin have been reported, but no distinct syndromes related to them have been generally established.

PATHOBIOLOGY AND TREATMENT

Except for insulinomas, pNETs are frequently malignant (>50%). Therefore patients with functional pNETs have two treatment problems: both the hormone-excess state needs to be controlled and treatment needs to be directed against the tumor itself because of its malignant nature. Surgical resection would solve both problems, but unfortunately in many cases patients present with advanced, unresectable disease.

Functional Pancreatic Neuroendocrine Tumor Syndromes (F-PNETs)
Zollinger-Ellison Syndrome (Gastrinomas)
DEFINITION

Zollinger-Ellison syndrome (ZES) is a clinical syndrome caused by a gastrin-secreting neuroendocrine tumor usually located in the pancreas or duodenum and characterized by clinical symptoms/signs resulting from gastric acid hypersecretion (peptic ulcer disease, diarrhea, esophageal reflux disease).[7,8]

PATHOBIOLOGY

Currently, gastrinomas are found in the duodenum (80 to 100%) more frequently than in the pancreas (0 to 20%). Duodenal gastrinomas are generally small (<1 cm), whereas pancreatic gastrinomas are generally larger. Occasionally ZES results from a gastrinoma in the splenic hilum, mesentery, or stomach, or only in a lymph node or an ovary. Extrapancreatic gastrinomas producing ZES have been reported in the heart and with small cell lung cancer.

Gastrin stimulates parietal cells to secrete acid and has a growth effect on the gastric mucosa. Chronic hypergastrinemia thus leads to increased gastric mucosal thickness, prominent gastric folds, and increased numbers of parietal cells and gastric enterochromaffin-like cells. Patients with gastrinomas have increased basal and maximal acid outputs from the stomach. *Helicobacter pylori* appears not to be important in the pathogenesis of the ulcer disease in ZES, in contrast to that of common peptic ulcers (Chapter 130). Diarrhea is common because the large-volume gastric acid output leads to structural damage to the small intestine (inflammation, blunted villi, edema), interference with fat transport, inactivation of pancreatic lipase, and precipitation of bile acids. These same mechanisms, if prolonged, can lead to steatorrhea. If acid hypersecretion is controlled, the diarrhea will stop.

From 20 to 25% of ZES patients have MEN1 (MEN1/ZES) (Chapter 130). These patients have hyperplasia or tumors of multiple endocrine glands (parathyroid hyperplasia [>90%], pituitary tumors [60%]). In MEN1/ZES patients, 80 to 95% of the gastrinomas are in the duodenum. They are frequently small (<0.5 cm), almost always multiple, and in 40 to 60% of cases associated with lymph node metastases.

CLINICAL MANIFESTATIONS

ZES is diagnosed most frequently between ages 35 and 65 years, but has been reported in both children and the elderly. Abdominal pain resulting from a peptic ulcer is the most common symptom (>80%). Most ulcers occur in the duodenum (>85%), but they occasionally occur in the postbulbar area, jejunum, or stomach, or in multiple locations. Initially, the pain is usually like that of patients with typical peptic ulcer disease (Chapter 130). With time, however, the symptoms become persistent and generally respond poorly to treatments aimed at eliminating *H. pylori* and to conventional doses of histamine-2 receptor antagonists, as well as to the now rarely used surgical treatments for ulcer disease. By comparison, conventional doses of proton pump inhibitors (PPIs) (e.g., omeprazole, lansoprazole, pantoprazole, esomeprazole, rabeprazole) frequently control the symptoms of most patients with ZES.

Heartburn is also common (20%). Diarrhea (60 to 70%) occurs frequently and may be the first symptom (10 to 20%). In MEN1, ZES is the most common functional pNET syndrome (54%), although patients typically first develop renal stones related to hypercalcemia from the associated hyperparathyroidism or have elevated prolactin levels resulting from pituitary tumors that only later develop. However, studies show that 20 to 40% of patients with MEN1/ZES initially present with ZES symptoms.

Almost all the initial symptoms of ZES result from the effects of acid hypersecretion, but late in the disease patients can have tumor-related symptoms. Approximately one third of patients have metastatic liver disease at presentation, but less than 20% of other patients develop metastatic disease to the liver during a 10-year follow-up period.

Up to 5% of patients with ZES develop ectopic Cushing syndrome (Chapter 214) because of adrenocorticotropic hormone (ACTH) secretion by the gastrinoma. These patients usually have a metastatic gastrinoma in the liver, have ZES without MEN1, and have a poor prognosis.

DIAGNOSIS

ZES should be suspected in any patient whose peptic ulcer disease (PUD) is accompanied by diarrhea, is recurrent, does not heal with treatment, is not associated with *H. pylori* infection, is associated with a complication (bleeding, obstruction, esophageal stricture), is multiple or occurs in unusual locations, or is associated with a pancreatic tumor. ZES should also be suspected in patients with chronic secretory diarrhea (Chapter 131), as well as when PUD is associated with large gastric folds, a family/personal history of nephrolithiases/endocrinopathies, or the finding of hypercalcemia, hypergastrinemia, or acid hypersecretion.

When suspected, the initial test is a fasting serum gastrin level, which is elevated in 99 to 100% of ZES patients. After this, the further steps to establish the diagnosis have become controversial. Recent studies report that up to 60% of commercial gastrin assays are unreliable (overestimate/underestimate of true value), so a reliable assay should be used.[9] Besides ZES, other causes of fasting hypergastrinemia include those also associated with hyperchlorhydria (retained antrum, antral hyperfunction/hyperplasia, renal failure, *H. pylori* infections) and those associated with hypochlorhydria/achlorhydria (physiologic hypergastrinemia) because of pernicious anemia, atrophic gastritis, or the use of proton pump inhibitors (PPIs). All guidelines recommend that if the serum gastrin level is elevated, fasting gastric pH should be determined. If the serum gastrin is greater than 1000 pg/mL (normal <100) and the gastric pH less than 2.0, the patient almost certainly has ZES; approximately 40% of patients have this combination. If the gastrin is increased less than 10-fold and the gastric pH is less than 2.0, basal acid output (BAO), a secretin test should be performed. BAO is increased in patients with ZES with greater than 95% having a BAO greater than 15 mEq/hr if no previous gastric acid–reducing surgery has been performed and 94% having a positive secretin test (stimulating a >120 pg/mL increase in serum gastrin). Because most patients when initially seen are already being treated with PPIs, which have a long duration of action, PPIs should be stopped for up to 1 week, if possible, to ensure that the cause of the hypergastrinemia is not the drug itself. Stopping a PPI in an undiagnosed ZES patient can lead to PUD complications, so this approach is controversial and not performed by many physicians. If it is performed, it needs to be done with care, and it is best to consult a group well versed in making the diagnosis.

Differential Diagnosis

A positive secretin test excludes other causes of hypergastrinemia and hyperchlorhydria that may mimic ZES. No false-positive results are reported except in patients with achlorhydria, and thus it is not reliable if the patient is taking PPIs. In all patients with ZES, evaluation must exclude MEN1 syndrome by searching for other endocrinopathies and assessing family history.

TREATMENT   Rx

Medical Therapy

Patients need medical therapy directed at controlling the gastric acid hypersecretion and, if possible, surgical therapy to remove the gastrinoma. PPIs are now the drugs of choice. Because of their long duration of action, acid hypersecretion can be controlled in almost every patient with once- or twice-daily doses. The recommended starting dose for omeprazole is 60 mg once a day. In 30% of patients, higher doses are needed, particularly in patients with complicated disease (MEN1), previous gastric surgery, or a history of severe esophageal reflux. With time the omeprazole dose can be reduced in most patients with uncomplicated disease to 20 to 40 mg/day. Patients must be treated indefinitely unless surgically cured. Long-term therapy is generally safe, and patients have been treated for up to 20 years with omeprazole without loss of efficacy, although reduced vitamin B12 levels may occur. Histamine-2 receptor antagonists are also effective, but frequent (every 4 to 6 hours) and high doses are needed. Long-acting somatostatin analogs can also control the acid hypersecretion but are uncommonly used because parental administration is needed, whereas PPIs are effective with oral dosing.[10] Total gastrectomy, the historical treatment, is now performed only for patients who cannot or will not take oral antisecretory medications. Selective vagotomy reduces acid secretion, but many patients continue to require a low dose of drug, and it is now rarely performed. Parathyroidectomy should be performed in MEN1 patients with hyperparathyroidism and ZES because the procedure reduces acid secretion and increases the sensitivity to antisecretory drugs.

Surgical Therapy

Surgical exploration for cure is recommended in all patients without unresectable liver metastases, MEN1, or complicating medical conditions that limit life expectancy. Tumors are found by experienced endocrine surgeons in 95% of patients at surgery. Surgical resection decreases the metastatic rate, increases survival, and results in a 5-year cure rate of 30 to 40%. At exploration, a duodenotomy to locate small duodenal gastrinomas is essential, as is the use of operative ultrasound to find and stage small pancreatic tumors. Patients with metastatic gastrinoma in the liver have a poor prognosis, with a 5-year survival rate of 30%. Surgical treatment of MEN1/ZES patients is controversial, because 80 to 90% have multiple small duodenal tumors with 50 to 60% having metastatic lymph nodes, and thus cannot be cured without extensive resections (usually a Whipple procedure). MEN1/ZES patients with an imaged tumor that is less than 2 to 2.5 cm have an excellent prognosis without surgery. Therefore most guidelines recommend surgery only in these cases.[11]

Treatment of Metastatic Disease in ZES

If the metastatic disease can be resected, surgery should be considered (5 to 15% of cases). Additional treatment of metastatic disease is considered later.

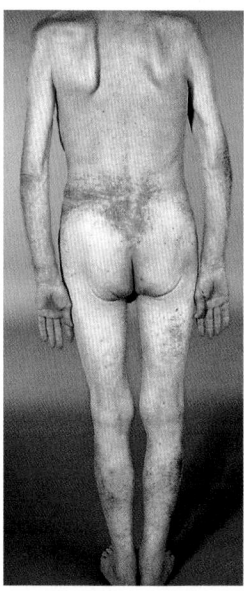

FIGURE 219-1. A patient with a glucagonoma with the characteristic rash (necrolytic migratory erythema). The rash is usually at intertriginous areas or periorificial sites and shows various stages of erythema and crusting. (From Forbes CD, Jackson WF. *Color Atlas and Text of Clinical Medicine.* 3rd ed. London. Mosby; 2003.)

PROGNOSIS

Approximately 25% of gastrinomas show aggressive growth. The most important prognostic predictor is the development of liver metastases. The presence of advanced gastrinoma grade or stage, large primary tumor, a pancreatic tumor, bone metastases, development of ectopic Cushing syndrome, or a high fasting gastrin level is associated with aggressive growth.

Glucagonomas

DEFINITION

Glucagonomas are neuroendocrine tumors of the pancreas that ectopically secrete glucagon, causing a specific syndrome.

PATHOBIOLOGY

Glucagon hypersecretion explains the glucose intolerance. The exact origin of the rash (necrolytic migratory erythema; see later) is unclear; some studies report that prolonged glucagon infusions can cause the characteristic skin lesions. A role for possible zinc deficiency has been proposed because of the similarity of the rash to that seen with zinc deficiency (acrodermatitis enteropathica) and because the rash improves in some patients who are given zinc. The hypoaminoacidemia is thought to be secondary to the effect of glucagon on amino acid metabolism by altering gluconeogenesis. The wasting and weight loss are intrinsic parts of the glucagonoma syndrome, and recent studies suggest that a novel anorectic substance distinct from glucagon may be responsible.

CLINICAL MANIFESTATIONS

The cardinal clinical features are a distinct dermatitis (necrolytic migratory erythema [NME], seen in 70 to 90%) (Fig. 219-1), diabetes mellitus and glucose intolerance (40 to 90%), weight loss (70 to 96%), anemia (30 to 85%), hypoaminoacidemia (80 to 90%) with deficiencies of essential fatty acids, thromboembolism (10 to 25%), diarrhea (15 to 30%), and psychiatric disturbances (0 to 20%).[12] NME is usually found at intertriginous and periorificial sites, especially in the groin and buttocks. It is initially erythematous, becomes raised, and develops central bullae whose tops detach, with the eroded areas becoming crusty. Healing occurs with hyperpigmentation.

DIAGNOSIS/DIFFERENTIAL DIAGNOSIS

The diagnosis is established by demonstrating elevated plasma glucagon levels with accompanying symptoms/signs. Normal levels are 150 to 200 pg/mL; in patients with glucagonomas, levels usually (>90%) are greater than 1000 pg/mL. However, in some recent studies, up to 40% of patients have lower plasma glucagon values. Increased plasma glucagon levels also occur in renal insufficiency, acute pancreatitis, hypercorticism, hepatic diseases, celiac disease, severe stress, and prolonged fasting; in patients treated with danazol; and in familial hyperglucagonemia. In these conditions, the level is usually less than

500 pg/mL except in patients with hepatic diseases or in those with familial hyperglucagonemia. NME is not specific for glucagonomas, and is also seen in short bowel syndrome, myelodysplastic syndromes, malnutrition, hepatitis B infections, cirrhosis, celiac disease, other malignancies, inflammatory bowel disease, and nutritional deficiencies. Two new glucagonoma-related syndromes have been described: (1) Mahvash disease (characterized by mutations in the glucagon receptor gene, glucagon cell hyperplasia, hyperglucagonemia, but no symptoms of the glucagonoma syndrome) and (2) glucagon cell adenomatosis (characterized by glucagon cell hyperplasia and occasional symptoms mimicking the glucagonoma syndrome).

Glucagonomas are generally large when discovered (mean, 5 to 10 cm), and they most frequently occur in the pancreatic tail (>50%). Liver metastases are commonly present at the time of diagnosis (45 to 80%).

TREATMENT Rx

Subcutaneous administration (monthly) of a synthetic long-acting somatostatin analog, octreotide (octreotide [LAR]/lanreotide [Autogel]), controls the rash in 80% of patients and improves weight loss, diarrhea, and hypoaminoacidemia, but it usually does not improve the diabetes mellitus. Zinc supplementation and infusions of amino acids or fatty acids, or both, can diminish the severity of the rash. After tumor localization, surgical resection is preferred; even debulking of metastatic tumor may be of benefit. For advanced disease, treatment is similar to that outlined for other advanced, nonresectable pNETs outlined later.

PROGNOSIS

The prognosis is now largely determined by the growth of the tumor per se, because the symptoms of glucagon excess can be largely controlled by somatostatin analogs. This is particularly true with glucagonomas. In many series, more than 50 to 80% are metastatic at presentation, and patients usually present late with large primary tumors. The mean 5-year survival rate is 50%; however, extended survivals (>15 years) are reported in some patients with treatment with somatostatin analogs and other tumor-directed therapies.

VIPomas

DEFINITION

The VIPoma syndrome, also called the Verner-Morrison syndrome, pancreatic cholera, and the WDHA syndrome (for watery diarrhea, hypokalemia, and achlorhydria), results from a neuroendocrine tumor, usually in the pancreas, that ectopically secretes vasoactive intestinal polypeptide (VIP).[13]

EPIDEMIOLOGY AND PATHOBIOLOGY

VIPomas in adults are found in the pancreas in 80 to 90% of cases; rare cases result from intestinal carcinoids, ganglioneuromas, ganglioneuroblastomas, and pheochromocytomas. In children less than 10 years and rarely in adults, the VIPoma syndrome is caused by ganglioneuromas or ganglioneuroblastomas at extrapancreatic sites. VIPomas are usually large and solitary; 50 to 75% occur in the pancreatic tail, and 40 to 70% have metastasized at the time of diagnosis. VIPomas frequently secrete both VIP and peptide histidine methionine, but VIP is responsible for the symptoms. VIP is a potent stimulant of secretion in the small and large intestine, which causes the cardinal clinical features. VIP also causes relaxation of GI smooth muscle, and this may contribute to the dilated loops of bowel that are common in this syndrome, as well as a dilated atonic gallbladder. Hypochlorhydria is thought to result from the inhibitory effect of VIP on gastric acid secretion, the flushing is related to the vasodilatory effects of VIP, and the hyperglycemia is caused by the glycogenolytic effect of VIP. The mechanism of the hypercalcemia remains unclear.

CLINICAL MANIFESTATIONS

The cardinal clinical feature is severe, large-volume, watery diarrhea (>1 L/day) in all cases, which is secretory and occurs during fasting. Hypokalemia (67 to 100%) and dehydration (83%) commonly occur because of the volume of the diarrhea. Achlorhydria is only occasionally noted, but hypochlorhydria is usually found (34 to 72% of cases). Flushing occurs in 20% of patients, hyperglycemia in 25 to 50%, and hypercalcemia in 41 to 50%. Steatorrhea is uncommon (16%) despite the volume of diarrhea.

DIAGNOSIS/DIFFERENTIAL DIAGNOSIS

The diarrhea of VIPomas characteristically persists during fasting and is large in volume (>3 L/day in 70 to 80%); the diagnosis is excluded when fasting stool volume is less than 700 mL/day. To differentiate VIPomas from other causes of large-volume fasting diarrhea, fasting plasma VIP levels should be determined. The normal value in most laboratories is less than 190 pg/mL, and elevated levels are present in 90 to 100% of patients. The differential diagnosis of large-volume fasting diarrhea (>700 mL/day) includes ZES, diffuse islet-cell hyperplasia, surreptitious use of laxatives, the pseudopancreatic cholera syndrome, and, rarely, HIV infection (Chapter 366). Serum gastrin levels identify patients with ZES, and plasma VIP levels are normal in most patients who abuse laxatives, in 82% of patients with pancreatic islet cell hyperplasia, and in patients with HIV-induced secretory diarrhea.

TREATMENT   Rx

The symptoms caused by the VIP are controlled initially in greater than 85% of patients by daily doses of octreotide (50 to 400 µg 1 to 3 times/daily) or by monthly injections of a depot form (octreotide [LAR]/lanreotide [Autogel]), but increased doses may be needed over time. Before the availability of octreotide, small numbers of patients were reported to respond to a variety of agents, including high-dose prednisone (60 to 100 mg/day; 40 to 50%), clonidine, lithium carbonate, indomethacin, loperamide, metoclopramide, and phenothiazines. After tumor localization studies, surgical resection should be attempted if it is possible to remove all visible tumor; however, greater than 50% of patients have generalized liver metastases at diagnosis, so complete resection may not be possible. For patients with unresectable advanced disease, treatment is similar to that for other advanced nonresectable pNETs (outlined later).

PROGNOSIS

The prognosis is now largely determined by the growth of the tumor per se, because the symptoms of VIP excess can be largely controlled by somatostatin analogs. The mean 5-year survival rate is 50 to 70%.

Somatostatinomas

DEFINITION AND PATHOBIOLOGY

Somatostatinomas are neuroendocrine tumors that occur primarily in the pancreas or upper small intestine and ectopically secrete somatostatin. In the GI tract, somatostatin inhibits basal and stimulated gastric acid secretion, pancreatic secretion, intestinal absorption of amino acids, gallbladder contractility, and release of numerous hormones, including cholecystokinin and gastrin. Pancreatic somatostatinomas occur in the pancreatic head in 60 to 80% of cases; 70 to 92% will have metastasized at the time of diagnosis, and they are usually large (mean, 5 cm) and solitary. In contrast, duodenal somatostatinomas are smaller (mean, 2.4 cm), frequently associated with psammoma bodies on histologic examination (11%), and less frequently have metastases at diagnosis (30 to 40%).

CLINICAL MANIFESTATIONS

Most reported somatostatinomas are diagnosed histologically as a neuroendocrine tumor containing somatostatin-like immunoreactivity and are not associated with a distinct clinical syndrome (the somatostatinoma syndrome). The somatostatinoma syndrome includes diabetes mellitus, gallbladder disease, diarrhea, steatorrhea, and weight loss. Sixty percent of somatostatinomas occur in the pancreas, and 40% are found in the duodenum or jejunum.

The somatostatinoma syndrome occurs much more commonly in patients with pancreatic than duodenal or intestinal somatostatinomas. Duodenal somatostatinomas occur in up to 10% of patients with von Recklinghausen disease and are usually asymptomatic.

DIAGNOSIS/DIFFERENTIAL DIAGNOSIS

Somatostatinomas are usually found incidentally, particularly during exploratory laparotomy or cholecystectomy, during endoscopy, or on imaging studies. The presence of psammoma bodies on histologic examination of a duodenal neuroendocrine tumor or any duodenal lesions in patients with von Recklinghausen disease should raise the suspicion of a duodenal somatostatinoma. The diagnosis of the somatostatinoma syndrome requires the demonstration of increased concentrations of somatostatin-like immunoreactivity in the plasma and the resected tumor. However, other tumors outside the pancreas or intestine, such as small cell lung cancer, medullary thyroid carcinoma, pheochromocytomas, and paragangliomas, may also have elevated concentrations of somatostatin-like immunoreactivity. Somatostatinomas can be imaged using somatostatin receptor scintigraphy or, if needed, other conventional imaging studies to assess the tumor's location.

TREATMENT   Rx

Treatment with octreotide or lanreotide can improve symptoms. Surgery, if possible, should be performed. For patients with unresectable advanced disease, treatment is similar to that for other advanced nonresectable pNETs (outlined later).

PROGNOSIS

Patients with intestinal somatostatinomas, which uncommonly cause the somatostatinoma syndrome, and are less malignant, have an excellent prognosis (5-year survival rate >80%), whereas those with pancreatic somatostatinomas, which frequently cause the somatostatinoma syndrome and present with metastatic disease (>70%), have a much reduced 5-year survival rate (<50%).

GRFomas

DEFINITION

GRFomas are neuroendocrine tumors that can originate in the pancreas, but also occur in other extrapancreatic locations and ectopically release growth hormone–releasing factor (GRF). The GRF causes acromegaly that is clinically indistinguishable from that caused by a pituitary adenoma.

PATHOBIOLOGY

GRFomas most commonly occur in the lung (54%). Most of the remainder occur in the GI tract, including 30% in the pancreas. Pancreatic GRFomas are usually large (mean, 6 cm), 39% are metastatic at diagnosis, 40% occur in combination with ZES, and 33% are in patients with MEN1.

DIAGNOSIS/DIFFERENTIAL DIAGNOSIS

GRFomas are an uncommon cause of acromegaly. They occurred in none of 177 unselected patients with acromegaly in one study. However, any patient with acromegaly and abdominal complaints, with acromegaly but no pituitary tumor (Chapter 211), or with acromegaly and hyperprolactinemia (which occurs in 70% of GRFomas) should be suspected of having a GRFoma. The intra-abdominal features of GRFomas result from its metastases. The diagnosis is confirmed by performing a plasma assay for GRF and growth hormone.

The effects of the GRF can be controlled with octreotide or lanreotide in more than 90% of patients. Treatment should be directed at the GRFoma per se, as described for the other more common pNETs. For patients with unresectable advanced disease, treatment is similar to that for other advanced nonresectable pNETs (outlined later).

Nonfunctional Pancreatic Neuroendocrine Tumors

DEFINITION

Nonfunctional pancreatic neuroendocrine tumors (NF-pNETs) are neuroendocrine tumors that originate in the pancreas and either secrete no peptides or secrete products that do not cause clinical symptoms.[14]

PATHOBIOLOGY

NF-pNETs frequently secrete nonfunctional peptides, including chromogranin A (100%), pancreatic polypeptide (60%), and the α-subunit (40%) and β-subunit of human chorionic gonadotropin. Immunocytochemically, even higher percentages contain these peptides, as well as insulin (50%), glucagon (30%), and somatostatin (13%).

CLINICAL MANIFESTATIONS

In older series NF-pNETs were frequently diagnosed only in late disease stages after the patient presented with symptoms or signs of metastatic disease and a liver biopsy revealed metastatic pNET. In more recent series, an increasing percentage of NF-pNETs are found incidentally during investigation of unrelated symptoms or on screening. Any symptoms or signs in these patients result from the tumor per se and include abdominal pain (36 to 56%), abdominal mass or hepatosplenomegaly (8 to 40%), weight loss or cachexia (8 to 46%), and jaundice (27 to 40%).

DIAGNOSIS/DIFFERENTIAL DIAGNOSIS

Any patients with a long survival (>5 years) after a diagnosis of metastatic pancreatic adenocarcinoma should be suspected of having an NF-pNET. In older series of symptomatic patients, primary tumors were large (70% were >5 cm) and liver metastases were frequent (38 to 62%) at presentation, whereas in recent series of asymptomatic patients, the NF-pNETs detected incidentally have been frequently less than 2 cm, without metastases. An elevated plasma chromogranin A or pancreatic polypeptide level or a positive somatostatin receptor scintigraphic scan is strong evidence that a pancreatic mass is a pNET. Malignancy correlates with vascular/perineural invasion, a proliferative index of greater than 2%, a mitotic rate of greater than 2, a size of at least 4 cm, capsular penetration, nuclear atypia, lack of progesterone receptors, and the presence of calcitonin immunoreactivity in the tumor.

Survival is better in patients with smaller tumors, patients who are asymptomatic at presentation, patients with no metastases, and patients in whom surgical resection can be performed.

Surgical resection should be performed, whenever possible, in patients with NF-pNETs greater than 2 to 3 cm, if duct compression is found, or if a higher grade tumor is present. The role of surgery in NF-pNETs that are less than 2 to 2.5 cm is controversial, with some recommending observation with reevaluation and others surgery.[15] For patients with unresectable advanced disease, treatment is similar to that outlined later for other advanced nonresectable pNETs.

PROGNOSIS

The overall 5-year survival rate varies in different series from 30% to greater than 90%, but it is heavily dependent on the extent of the disease at diagnosis, with survival rates of 96% in patients without metastases at presentation, decreasing to 30 to 50% with metastatic disease.

ACTHomas and Other Uncommon Tumors

pNETs that ectopically secrete ACTH cause 4 to 16% of the cases of ectopic Cushing syndrome.[16] Cushing syndrome (Chapter 214) occurs in 5% of all cases of ZES, but in patients with sporadic ZES it is a late feature, occurring

with metastatic liver disease. Its development is associated with a poor prognosis, and the response to chemotherapy is generally poor; however, some patients benefit from the use of long-acting somatostatin analogs (octreotide, lanreotide).

Paraneoplastic hypercalcemia (Chapter 169) can result from a pNET that releases parathormone-related peptide or an unknown hypercalcemic substance. Tumors are generally large, with metastatic liver disease at diagnosis. Somatostatin analogs may help control the hypercalcemia, but surgery, chemotherapy, hepatic embolization, and chemoembolization are the mainstays of treatment.

pNETs causing the carcinoid syndrome (see later) are usually large, and 68 to 88% are malignant. Octreotide may control the symptoms and the newly released tryptophan hydrolase 1 inhibitor, telotristat, may be helpful to control the diarrhea. Surgery, chemotherapy, hepatic embolization, chemoembolization, or molecular targeted therapy (everolimus, sunitinib) may be helpful.

A single case of a pNET that secreted renin manifested with severe hypertension; the tumor was localized with somatostatin receptor scintigraphy, and the patient's symptoms improved significantly after tumor resection. A single case of an erythropoietin-secreting pNET resulting in polycythemia and a single case of a pNET secreting IGF-II or GLP-1 causing hypoglycemia have been described. Two symptomatic cases of pNETs that secreted luteinizing hormone have been described; virilization occurred in the female patient, whereas the male patient had increased acne and a rash. In both cases, the tumors were resectable, and symptoms improved postoperatively. A single case of a pNET secreting cholecystokinin (CCKoma) has been described, with the patient demonstrating PUD, gallbladder disease, diarrhea, and weight loss. A case of a pNET secreting enteroglucagon causing small intestinal hypertrophy has also been described.

Neuroendocrine Tumors of the Gastrointestinal Tract and Thorax (Carcinoids, non-pNETs)

These well-differentiated NETs, also called carcinoid, occur most often in the GI tract (about 25% in the small intestine, 15% in the rectum, 10% in the appendix, and 5% in the stomach) and the lung (30%), but they also can occur in many other organs.[17]

Stomach Neuroendocrine Tumors

Gastric NETs occur in several subtypes with differing pathophysiology, natural history, and treatment.[18,19] Type 1 gastric NET (carcinoid) arises in the body and fundus of the stomach in the setting of autoimmune atrophic gastritis. This is the most common type, comprising 80% of cases.

In type 1 lesions gastrin is markedly elevated due to the absence of negative feedback from gastric acid, not because the tumors are secreting gastrin. The high gastrin stimulates proliferation of gastric enterochromaffin-like (ECL) neuroendocrine cells in the body and fundus of the stomach, resulting in neuroendocrine cell hyperplasia and small multifocal neuroendocrine lesions, which occasionally progress to type 1 gastric carcinoids. These NETs are generally of low grade and have a low metastatic potential when less than 2 cm in size and are usually removed endoscopically. Multifocal NETs with multiple recurrences can be treated with laparoscopic antrectomy to normalize gastrin level, and cause regression of the NET and neuroendocrine hyperplasia.

Type 2 NETs, which are associated with Zollinger-Ellison syndrome with MEN1, comprise only about 5% of gastric NETs, thereby making them the least common type. These tumors are almost invariably multifocal. Unlike type 1, which is also associated with elevated gastrin, the gastric mucosa is hypertrophic rather than atrophic. The type 2 lesions are usually small and of low to intermediate aggressiveness, best treated with endoscopic excision.

Type 3 NET is sporadic gastric NET. In comparison to types 1 and 2 NET, type 3 NETs are not associated with hypergastrinemia and are usually of higher stage/grade, giving a worse prognosis. They can produce an atypical carcinoid syndrome. In most cases, patients require a partial gastrectomy, as in adenocarcinoma of the stomach.

Small Bowel and Cecum Neuroendocrine Tumors

Patients with small bowel and cecal NET may present with symptoms that are related to the tumor mass or with symptoms caused by biologically active peptides that are released into the circulatory system (e.g., carcinoid syndrome).[20,21] Abdominal primary tumors or metastases can cause abdominal pain and even intestinal or bowel obstruction owing to growing tumor and associated desmoplasia. A primary tumor may infrequently cause GI bleeding. Massive liver metastases can cause palpable hepatomegaly. 5-HIAA, serotonin, chromogranin A, pancreastatin, and neurokinin A are frequently measured biomarkers.

Most small bowel NETs arise within 60 cm of the ileocecal valve, approximately 25% having multiple primary small bowel foci. Localized tumors should be treated with right hemicolectomy or resection of the involved segment of small bowel depending on location. Metastatic potential increases with size, from less than 5% in tumors less than 1 cm to approximately 50% in tumors greater than 2 cm. When metastatic, 5-year overall survival ranges from 40 to 85% and 10-year survival ranges from 40 to 60%.

Duodenal carcinoids can produce several types of hormonal syndromes. Duodenal gastrinomas can be sporadic or can occur in a background of MEN-1, where they are often associated with ZES. In MEN-1–associated cases, hyperplasia of background G cells can be observed. Duodenal somatostatinomas may be associated with psammoma bodies and type-1 neurofibromatosis. The nonfunctional duodenal NET can still produce calcitonin and serotonin. Ampullary NETs have metastatic potential even when small, and are also associated with neurofibromatosis. These tumors are treated with endoscopic resection when possible, although larger, more aggressive tumors, particularly those of the ampulla, may require a modified Whipple resection.

Appendix Neuroendocrine Tumors

Appendix NETs are frequently found incidentally at the time of simple appendectomy. If less than 2 cm in diameter and there are no unfavorable pathologic features, prognosis is outstanding and no additional surgery is needed. However, if these tumors are greater than 2 cm, a right hemicolectomy should be done. Goblet cell carcinoid (GCC) contains both carcinoid elements and adenocarcinoma elements. These tumors arise most commonly in the appendix and because of their aggressive nature should be treated with a right hemicolectomy, even when less than 2 cm in diameter. These tumors can present as solid masses of GCC, as mucinous tumors, which can lead to peudomyxoma peritoneii, or as an adenocarcinoma, which overgrows the GCC. GCCs should be distinguished from "tubular carcinoids," which often have focal mucin present but have an excellent prognosis and are treated as usual appendiceal NETs rather than as GCCs.

Rectum Neuroendocrine Tumors

Hindgut NETs arise in the distal colon and rectum and are almost never associated with functional syndromes.[22] These are frequently detected at screening colonoscopy and if less than 2 cm can be treated with endoscopic mucosal resection or transrectal excision with low risk of recurrence. However, if greater than 2 cm or of higher histologic grade, a low anterior resection of the rectum or anterior posterior resection of the rectum is necessary, and metastatic risk is greater than 50%. Mixed adeno-neuroendocrine carcinomas may also rarely occur in the colon, containing high-grade neuroendocrine and adenocarcinoma elements, which should be differentiated from high-grade adenocarcinoma of the rectum with neuroendocrine differentiation (latter not a neuroendocrine tumor).

Lung Neuroendocrine Tumors

Lung NETs (bronchial carcinoids) comprise 1 to 2% of lung malignancies (Chapter 182) in adults and 20 to 30% NET cases.[23] The annual incidence is 1.35 per 100,000 population/year. There is no definite relationship to cigarette smoking. Among the lung NETs, 90% are sporadic, 5% are associated with MEN-1, and occasional cases arise from diffuse idiopathic pulmonary neuroendocrine cell hyperplasia (DIPNECH). There is a 5:1 female preponderance. Typical carcinoid (low-grade NE) has a mitotic count less than 2 per 10 high-powered fields and no necrosis. Atypical carcinoid (intermediate grade) has a mitotic count of 2 to 20 per 10 high-powered fields and/or focal necrosis. Staging is exactly the same as lung cancer (Chapter 182). Carcinoid syndrome (see later) with serotonin production occurs in less than 10% of cases, but can be severe even in the absence of metastatic disease. Histamine-mediated atypical flushing, which can last over 30 minutes, is bright red and can involve limbs and upper trunk, and is associated with sweating, tearing, wheezing, and burning, and sometimes rosacea. Cushing syndrome from ACTH or CRH secretion occurs in less than 5% of patients with lung carcinoid tumors. This can be cured by resection of a localized tumor. Laparoscopic bilateral adrenalectomy is the treatment of choice, if caused by unresectable or metastatic NET, because medical management is usually inadequate. Acromegaly from ectopic production of GHRH can occur with bronchial NET, and often responds to somatostatin analogs or surgical debulking.

DIPNECH is characterized by infiltration of lung parenchyma with neuroendocrine cells and tumorlets (<0.5 mm) and can lead to the development of multifocal bilateral lung NET. Over many years, it can lead to bronchiectasis, interstitial fibrosis, and bronchiolitis obliterans. CT of the chest, which typically shows numerous subcentimeter pulmonary nodules, should be repeated every 6 months along with pulmonary function tests, including diffusing capacity. The temptation for radical surgery should be avoided to preserve as much lung parenchyma as possible. If the patient becomes symptomatic from progressive disease, somatostatin analog therapy might be considered.

Surgery is the treatment of choice for localized disease. Endoscopic laser debulking may be helpful to allow for recovery from distal obstructive pneumonia and to allow for a more conservative resection. In the absence of locally advanced disease, sleeve resection can often be performed with minimal loss of functional lung tissue. A video-assisted thoracoscopic surgery (VATS) lobectomy and lymphadenectomy for accurate staging and maximizing the chance of cure is usually needed. Ten-year survival rates for typical carcinoid are 82 to 87%.

Thymus Neuroendocrine Tumors

Thymus NET is a rare neoplasm, with an annual incidence of 0.02 per 100,000 per year, and accounting for 2% of all mediastinal tumors and 5% of thymic lesions. Most cases are sporadic, but 25% are associated with MEN-1. Functional syndromes, including Cushing syndrome and acromegaly, may occur, as in lung NETs. Criteria for pathologic grade are the same as in lung NET. There is no accepted staging system, but thymus NETs are usually divided into 3 groups: encapsulated, invasive, and metastatic. Late presentation with invasion of vital structures is common, but complete resection is the only possible curative procedure. Careful preoperative staging is important. Definitive surgery, which typically requires median sternotomy and mediastinal node dissection and may require cardiopulmonary bypass with cardioplegic arrest, should not be done if significant extrathoracic metastasis is present or if the patient is not a good surgical candidate.

⬤ CARCINOID SYNDROME

The *carcinoid syndrome* develops when neuroendocrine mediators released by NETs, most commonly metastatic NETs arising from the small intestine, cause systemic symptoms and signs.[24,25] Symptoms include episodic flushing, diarrhea, wheezing, tachycardia, and blood pressure fluctuations. There can be eventual development of intraperitoneal and retroperitoneal fibrosis, as well as endomyocardial fibrosis leading to valvular heart disease. Approximately 8 to 35% of all NETs develop carcinoid syndrome, most commonly NETs of small bowel origin with liver metastasis. Foregut NETs (e.g., bronchus, stomach, pancreas, and thymus) as well as hindgut NETs rarely cause carcinoid syndrome. Carcinoid syndrome results from NET cell production of biologically active substances including serotonin, tachykinins, histamine, and prostaglandins. Foregut carcinoids frequently produce an atypical carcinoid syndrome due to the release of 5-hydroxytryptophan rather than serotonin.

Diarrhea of secretory type is a major feature of the carcinoid syndrome. Stool volume is typically greater than 1 L/day and persists with fasting (when on intravenous fluids). No "osmotic gap" is present when stool osmolality is measured. Flushing from carcinoid syndrome involves attacks of skin redness without sweating, which may be associated with burning, warmth, and redness of face and neck, sometimes extending to the trunk and abdomen. It is caused by tumor-produced vasodilators increasing blood flow to the skin. Psychiatric manifestations of tryptophan deficiency occur when a large percentage of dietary tryptophan is shunted to produce serotonin, thereby leaving less tryptophan to form nicotinic acid and protein. Pellagra (nicotinic acid deficiency) can be seen when the urinary excretion of 5-HIAA is greater than 100 mg/day as a result of this shunting.

Carcinoid heart disease is endomyocardial fibrosis caused by serotonin.[26] The serotonin level is typically greater than 1000 pg/mL and urinary 5-HIAA greater than 57 mg/24 hours. Cardiac fibrotic manifestations commonly include tricuspid valve regurgitation (65%), pulmonary valve regurgitation (20%), and right ventricular myocardial restrictive disease, but about 10% of patients may develop left-sided cardiac involvement. Symptoms of right-sided heart failure include swelling in legs and abdomen, shortness of breath, and fatigue. Diagnosis often is easily made by echocardiography. Diuretics help, but more than 80% of patients die in 4 to 5 years without valve replacement. With replacement of the damaged tricuspid and pulmonic valves, 4-year survival is 50%. Bioprosthetic valves can develop carcinoid fibrosis, but mechanical valves require lifetime anticoagulation, so the choice of therapy must be individualized. Best results for valve replacement occur when the serotonin level is not massively elevated, age is less than 60 years old, and heart muscle function is still good (Chapter 66).

Intraperitoneal and retroperitoneal fibrosis also results from the high level of serotonin in carcinoid syndrome. This development causes intense fibrosis in the peritoneal cavity leading to bowel obstructions in about 50% of patients, as well as mesenteric vessel occlusion and bowel ischemia. Retroperitoneal fibrosis can cause ureteral obstruction.

Carcinoid crisis is an attack of severe and sustained flushing with life-threatening hemodynamic compromise and bronchoconstriction, precipitated by anesthesia, surgery, tumor necrosis, or catecholamine infusion. Other manifestations include generalized fatigue, bronchoconstriction, tachycardia, rosacea, and proximal myopathy.

Diagnosis of carcinoid syndrome should be considered if at least one clinical manifestation is present in patients with biopsy-proven NET. The diagnostic hallmark is increased excretion of urinary 5-HIAA. Normally, urinary excretion of 5-HIAA does not exceed 6 to 10 mg/day when patients have been placed on a low-serotonin diet and have avoided medications known to falsely elevate 5-HIAA before urine collection. Under these circumstances, urinary excretion of greater than or equal to 25 mg/day of 5-HIAA usually establishes the diagnosis of the carcinoid syndrome. Levels of 9 to 25 mg/day can also be found in patients with vomiting, acute intestinal obstruction, or nontropical sprue. Measurement of fasting plasma 5-HIAA without requiring a low-serotonin diet or a 24-hour urine collection is now becoming available. Plasma chromogranin A and multiple other biomarkers are frequently elevated in NET and in some nonmalignant conditions, but none are diagnostic of carcinoid syndrome.

Treatment of carcinoid syndrome is initiated with a somatostatin analog.[A1] Octreotide causes a reduction of 50% in 5-HIAA excretion and can dramatically reduce the frequency and intensity of diarrhea and flushing. It is recommended that octreotide therapy be initiated subcutaneously every 8 hours, with the dose increased as rapidly as can be tolerated by the patient from 50 to 300 μg three times per day. At that point, octreotide (LAR), 20 to 30 mg intramuscularly every 4 weeks (or lanreotide [Autogel], 40 to 60 mg/month) can be started. To maintain a steady-state therapeutic blood level, patients should continue the subcutaneous dosing until 2 weeks after the long-acting somatostatin analog therapy has been initiated. Telotristat ethyl is a potent inhibitor of tryptophan hydroxylase, the rate-limiting enzyme in serotonin biosynthesis from tryptophan. It does not lower serotonin production in the brain, and toxicity is low. Telotristat ethyl 250 mg orally twice daily[A2] reduces 5-HIAA by 40%, resulting in marked reduction of carcinoid syndrome diarrhea (in combination with continued somatostatin analog therapy), if diarrhea is inadequately controlled by somatostatin analog therapy alone. Reducing the bulk of hormone-producing tumor cells by surgery, embolization, or ablation of liver metastasis is also an important component of long-term control of carcinoid syndrome. Systemic therapy with biologic agents such as everolimus, peptide receptor radiotherapy, or interferon may also improve the symptoms of carcinoid syndrome.

CONTROL OF TUMOR GROWTH IN METASTATIC NEUROENDOCRINE TUMORS
Primary Debulking Surgery/Regional Therapy/Liver Transplantation

If it is possible to surgically remove at least 90% of metastases, survival as well as symptoms of hormone secretion can be improved. Cholecystectomy at the time of abdominal surgery prevents cholelithiasis from somatostatin analog therapy and makes subsequent liver embolization safer. The primary tumor should be removed with carcinoid syndrome that is caused by ileal-jejunal NETs to prevent or treat bowel obstruction, bleeding, and other local complications. Liver metastasis can be treated with radiofrequency or microwave ablation of lesions less than 4 cm diameter, with a probe inserted into metastasis at surgery or under CT guidance, and tumor obliteration using localized heat. Irreversible electroporation (Nanoknife), stereotactic radiosurgery, alcohol injection, and other locally destructive techniques can also help to reduce the volume of liver metastasis. Excellent destruction of liver metastases can be achieved by embolization, because their blood supply is from the hepatic artery. When liver metastasis is too extensive for these techniques, transcatheter hepatic artery embolization can be used to control liver metastasis. Hepatic artery embolization should be bland embolization or chemoembolization, not radioembolization in treating NET, because radioembolization appears to increase the risk of radiation-induced liver disease when peptide receptor radiotherapy is subsequently used. Liver transplantation is occasionally used for patients with refractory symptoms with metastatic disease restricted to the liver.

Somatostatin Analog Therapy

Somatostatin is a peptide hormone that mediates its inhibitory effects on hormone secretion and tumor growth through binding to specific cell-surface G-protein–coupled somatostatin receptors.[27] The somatostatin analogs, octreotide and lanreotide, have a longer half-life than somatostatin and bind preferentially to receptor subtype 2, the receptor most responsible for controlling cell proliferation and secretion, and are effective treatments for pancreatic and gastrointestinal neuroendocrine tumors.[A3] In one trial, 85 patients with locally inoperable or metastatic small bowel NET were randomized to receive either octreotide (LAR) 30 mg monthly or placebo. The median time to tumor progression was significantly longer with octreotide compared with placebo (14.3 vs. 6 months), whether or not carcinoid syndrome was present. The much larger randomized phase 3 trial,[A4] of lanreotide (Autogel) versus placebo, known as the CLARINET trial, has established lanreotide as an effective first-line therapy in patients with metastatic NET who expressed somatostatin receptors. In the CLARINET study, 204 patients with grade 1 or 2 nonfunctioning NET of GI or pancreatic origin were randomly assigned to either 120 mg of lanreotide (Autogel) ($n = 101$) or placebo ($n = 103$) every 4 weeks for 96 weeks. Progression-free survival (PFS) was greater than 96 weeks for lanreotide versus 18 months for placebo when data were published at 2 years. Longer follow-up on the lanreotide open-label extension trial demonstrated the actual real-time PFS to be 38.5 months. Prolongation of PFS was significant, whether NET was grade 1 or grade 2, whether metastatic or locally advanced, and whether high or low liver tumor burden was present. Lanreotide reduced risk of tumor progression or death by 53%.

Peptide Receptor Radionuclide Therapy

Peptide receptor radionuclide therapy (PRRT) utilizes the binding of a radio-labeled somatostatin analog to the somatostatin receptor to selectively irradiate sites of metastasis with minimal injury to the surrounding normal tissues. The phase 3 NETTER-1 clinical trial[A5] randomized patients with advanced midgut carcinoid tumors who had become resistant to treatment with maximum approved doses of a somatostatin analog to receive either PRRT with ^{177}Lu-Dotatate 200 mCi every 8 weeks ×4 plus octreotide 30 mg intramuscularly every 28 days or only octreotide 60 mg intramuscularly every 28 days. Progression-free survival (PFS) was increased from 8.4 months in the non-PRRT arm to a median PFS not yet reached in the PRRT arm, although estimated to be at least 40 months ($P < 0.0001$). An interim analysis suggested an increase in overall survival from 3 to 18%. ^{177}Lu-Dotatate PRRT, as used in this trial with nephron-protective amino acids, demonstrated a favorable safety profile, with no grade 3 to 4 nephrotoxicity, and grade 3 to 4 myelotoxicity of 1%. In multiple phase 2 trials, PRRT has demonstrated similar efficacy on tumor control of NETs arising in the GI tract, pancreas, and lung. It is anticipated that in individuals with NETs progressing on somatostatin analog therapy who have high-affinity, high-specificity binding of somatostatin analog to tumor, as demonstrated by somatostatin receptor imaging (e.g., ^{68}Ga-Dotatate PET), PRRT will play an important role in management.

Therapy Targeting PI3K/Akt/mTOR

Several observations point to inhibition of mTOR to be a logical approach to treatment of pancreatic NET.[A6] Pancreatic NET frequently occurs when there are defects in the *TSC2* gene (whose protein product inhibits mTOR activation) and if there is loss of the *NF1* gene (which regulates mTOR activity). Sporadic pNETs coexpress IGF-1 and the IGF-1 receptor (IGF-1R), activating the PI3K-mTOR pathway. Pancreatic NETs demonstrate downregulation of *TSC2* and *PTEN* genes (negative regulators of the PI3K/Akt/mTOR pathway). This led to the 410-patient phase 3 trial (RADIANT-3)[A7] randomizing patients with advanced, progressive pancreatic NETs to the mTOR inhibitor, everolimus 10 mg orally daily, versus placebo. Everolimus increased PFS from 5.4 months to 11.4 months ($P < 0.0001$). The RADIANT-4 trial[A8] showed a similar improvement in PFS (3.9 to 11 months) in NETs arising from the GI tract and lung, leading to U.S. Food and Drug Administration (FDA) approval for all of these indications.

Antiangiogenics

Neuroendocrine tumors are highly vascular and can be controlled with antiangiogenic agents. Sunitinib is an oral tyrosine kinase inhibitor that inhibits VEGFR, PDGFR, KIT, FLT3, and RET.[28] A phase 3 trial[A9] of 159 patients with progressive pancreatic NET randomized patients to sunitinib 37.5 mg/day versus placebo. PFS was 11.4 months for sunitinib versus 5.5 months for placebo, leading to FDA approval for pancreatic NET. Significant toxicities (all less than 10%) included neutropenia, hypertension, abdominal pain, diarrhea, hypoglycemia, and hand-foot syndrome. Cabozantinib, another TKI targeting VEGF receptors, MET, AXL, and RET, shows promise in pancreatic NET, and pazopanib in carcinoid tumors. Bevacizumab plus everolimus versus everolimus has been studied in pancreatic NET and bevacizumab plus octreotide (LAR) versus interferon-alfa plus octreotide in carcinoid.[A10] In both cases bevacizumab improved the response rate, but not the PFS, and for that reason it is currently not recommended therapy.

Chemotherapy

Cytotoxic chemotherapy has a low response rate in NETs arising outside the pancreas.[29] However, pancreatic NETs treated with streptozotocin combinations (with doxorubicin, cyclophosphamide, or 5-fluorouracil [5-FU]) have had response rates reported as high as 70%. The combination of two oral cytotoxic drugs, temozolomide plus capecitabine, appears to have similar activity in pancreatic NET, and results of a recently completed phase 3 trial of temozolomide with or without capecitabine are pending. For grade G3 poorly differentiated NETs, chemotherapy with etoposide and cisplatin analogs has a response rate of 30 to 70%, but it is usually short lasting.

Immune Therapy

In patients with advanced refractory NET randomized to octreotide (LAR) plus either interferon alfa-2 or bevacizumab there was no difference in PFS between the 2 groups, indicating similar antitumor activity. Because immune checkpoint inhibitors targeting PD-1 have demonstrated effectiveness in controlling poorly differentiated small cell carcinoma of the lung, several studies are now underway to evaluate such agents in NET.

Summary of Clinical Approach to Therapy

Somatostatin analogs (octreotide, lanreotide), everolimus, interferon-alfa, PRRT, observation, telotristat for carcinoid syndrome, and participation in a clinical trials are all options for intestinal carcinoids.[30,31] Somatostatin analogs (octreotide, lanreotide), everolimus, sunitinib, temozolomide plus capecitabine, streptozotocin plus 5-FU, PRRT, observation, and clinical trials are all options for pancreatic NETs. Treatment should be initiated urgently if there is a heavy tumor burden with mass-related symptoms, an uncontrolled functional tumor, compromised liver function, poorly differentiated or high-grade tumor, or rapid growth on imaging. Treatment has little urgency, on the other hand, if tumors have small volume, are low grade, and are asymptomatic. Surgery is always an option when either locoregional or metastatic NET is potentially resectable. Liver-dominant metastasis can potentially be treated with hepatic artery embolization, ablation, or metastasectomy. Metastatic NET progressing on a somatostatin analog and positive somatostatin receptor imaging can be treated with PRRT. The systemic biologic agents and chemotherapy have a role in selected cases as listed in the beginning of this section.

Grade A References

A1. Vinik AI, Wolin EM, Liyanage N, et al. Evaluation of lanreotide depot/autogel efficacy and safety as a carcinoid syndrome treatment(ELECT): a randomized, double-blind, placebo-controlled trial. *Endocr Pract.* 2016;22:1068-1080.

A2. Kulke MH, Horsch D, Caplin ME, et al. Telotristat ethyl, a tryptophan hydroxylase inhibitor for the treatment of carcinoid syndrome. *J Clin Oncol.* 2017;35:14-23.

A3. Kaderli RM, Spanjol M, Kollár A, et al. Therapeutic options for neuroendocrine tumors: a systematic review and network meta-analysis. *JAMA Oncol.* 2019;5:480-489.

A4. Caplin ME, Pavel M, Cwikla JB, et al. Lanreotide in metastatic enteropancreatic neuroendocrine tumors. *N Engl J Med.* 2014;371:224-233.

A5. Strosberg J, El-Haddad G, Wolin E, et al. Phase 3 trial of 177Lu-Dotatate for midgut neuroendocrine tumors. *N Engl J Med.* 2017;376:125-135.

A6. Pavel ME, Hainsworth JD, Baudin E, et al. Everolimus plus octreotide long-acting repeatable for the treatment of advanced neuroendocrine tumours associated with carcinoid syndrome(RADIANT-2): a randomised, placebo-controlled, phase 3 study. *Lancet.* 2011;378:2005-2012.

A7. Yao JC, Shah MH, Ito T, et al. Everolimus for advanced pancreatic neuroendocrine tumors. *N Engl J Med.* 2011;364:514-523.

A8. Yao JC, Fazio N, Singh S, et al. Everolimus for the treatment of advanced, non-functional neuroendocrine tumours of the lung or gastrointestinal tract (RADIANT-4): a randomised, placebo-controlled, phase 3 study. *Lancet.* 2016;387:968-977.

A9. Raymond E, Dahan L, Raoul JL, et al. Sunitinib malate for the treatment of pancreatic neuroendocrine tumors. *N Engl J Med.* 2011;364:501-513.

A10. Yao JC, Guthrie KA, Moran C, et al. Phase III prospective randomized comparison trial of depot octreotide plus interferon Alfa-2b versus depot octreotide plus bevacizumab in patients with advanced carcinoid tumors: SWOG S0518. *J Clin Oncol.* 2017;35:1695-1703.

GENERAL REFERENCES

For the General References and other additional features, please visit Expert Consult at https://expertconsult.inkling.com.

SEXUAL DEVELOPMENT AND IDENTITY

PERRIN C. WHITE

DEFINITION

This chapter reviews the concepts underlying the initial evaluation and management of patients with disorders of sexual development. By definition, such an individual has lack of concordance of various aspects of gender. These include chromosomal sex (46,XX, 46,XY, or other), gonadal or reproductive sex (ovaries, fallopian tubes, and uterus vs. testes, seminal vesicles, prostate gland, and ejaculatory ducts), genital sex (vagina and clitoris vs. scrotum and penis), and gender-specific behavior.[1] Depending on chromosomal sex, most patients can be classified as incompletely masculinized 46,XY males, virilized 46,XX females, and patients with abnormalities of sex chromosomes, such as those with mixed gonadal dysgenesis. (In the past, 46,XY and 46,XX patients with disorders of sexual development were referred to as male and female pseudohermaphrodites, respectively, but these terms are no longer preferred.) Many conditions can cause disorders of sexual development (Table 220-1).

Normal Sexual Differentiation
Gonadal Differentiation

At 4 to 5 weeks' gestation, the gonadal primordia (gonadal ridges) develop from the coelomic epithelium overlying the medial surface of the mesonephros (primitive kidneys; Fig. 220-1). These primitive gonads are identical in both sexes. Germ cells form at 3 to 4 weeks' gestation and migrate through the gut mesentery into the gonads at this early bipotential stage. Whether germ cells are directed toward male or female gametogenesis depends largely on the environment generated by surrounding somatic cells rather than on factors intrinsic to the germ cells.

During the seventh week, XY male gonads begin to differentiate under the influence of testis-determining genes.[2] The first to be expressed is *SRY*, the key gene on the Y chromosome controlling male differentiation, which initiates the development of Sertoli cells by increasing expression of the SOX9 transcription factor. Sertoli cells surround germ cells to form testis cords, which nourish primordial germ cells and direct them into the pathway for male gametogenesis. Recruitment of endothelial cells leads to development of a testis-specific vasculature that is required for normal organization of the testis.

Steroidogenic cells develop from the mesonephros and migrate into the developing adrenal cortex and testis at 8 weeks. In the testis, they become Leydig cells, which secrete the testosterone required for subsequent male reproductive development. In the first trimester, testosterone secretion is mainly under the control of human chorionic gonadotropin (HCG); it subsequently requires luteinizing hormone (LH) secreted by the fetal anterior pituitary.

Ovaries are recognizable at approximately 10 weeks. The signaling molecules WNT4 and RSPO1 play an active role in ovarian development, stabilizing intracellular expression of β-catenin and repressing expression of testis-specific genes and vascular development. The FOXL2 transcription factor is also required for ovarian development.[3] Germ cells in the ovary continue into the first meiotic prophase beginning at 12 weeks' gestation and continuing until 7 months' gestation.

Development of Male and Female Internal Reproductive Tracts

The reproductive tracts are derived from intermediate mesoderm. The male reproductive tract develops from the mesonephric (wolffian) ducts, and the female reproductive tract develops from the paramesonephric (müllerian) ducts (Fig. 220-2). Both sets of ducts are present in normal embryos.

Development of wolffian or müllerian structures depends on the presence or absence of normally functioning testes, respectively. The Sertoli cells secrete antimüllerian hormone (also termed müllerian inhibiting substance) starting when the testes differentiate.[4] Expression of antimüllerian hormone is controlled by several transcription factors, including SOX9. SF1 and WT1 (Wilms tumor locus) synergize to promote transcription, whereas DAX1 antagonizes it. The overall effect of antimüllerian hormone is to induce regression of müllerian structures between 8 and 12 weeks' gestation. In its absence,

TABLE 220-1 DISORDERS OF SEXUAL DEVELOPMENT*

VIRILIZATION OR SEX REVERSAL IN XX FEMALES	MICROPENIS
Virilizing forms of congenital adrenal hyperplasia 21-Hydroxylase deficiency (1:16,000 births) [CYP21A2]: salt-wasting or simple virilizing forms 11β-Hydroxylase deficiency [CYP11B1] 3β-Hydroxysteroid dehydrogenase deficiency [HSD3B2] Cytochrome P-450 oxidoreductase deficiency (also has a maternal effect) [POR] **Maternal or exogenous androgens** Drugs (danazol, progestins) Luteoma Aromatase deficiency [CYP19A1] Transcription factor mutations **Mutations in genes affecting gonadal differentiation** SRY (translocation to X) SOX9 (duplication) SOX3 (duplication) SOX10 (duplication) WT1 (Denys-Drash syndrome) NR5A1(the Arg92Trp mutation causes ovotesticular DSD) FOXL2 (ovarian failure associated with blepharophimosis, ptosis, and epicanthus inversus; BPES) RSPO1 WNT4 Structural/idiopathic	Panhypopituitarism (combined pituitary hormone deficiency) [PROP1, FGF8, PROKR2, WDR1] Septo-optic dysplasia [HESX1, FGFR1] Isolated hypogonadotropic hypogonadism [GNRH1, GNRHR, KISS1, KISS1R, TAC3, TACR3] Other syndromes, including hypogonadotropic hypogonadism Kallmann syndrome [KAL1, AXL, FEZF1, HS6TS1, NSMF, OL14RD, PROK2, SEMA3A, SEMA7A] Prader-Willi syndrome [paternal chromosome 15q11deletion] Adrenal hypoplasia congenita [NR0B1(DAX1)] CHARGE complex (colobomata, heart defects, choanal atresia, growth retardation, genital anomalies, ear defects or deafness) [CHD7] Dandy-Walker syndrome (hypoplasia of the cerebellar vermis and cystic dilation of the fourth ventricle) [FGF17] Leptin and leptin receptor deficiency (severe obesity) [LEP, LEPR] Proprotein convertase 1/3 deficiency (obesity and endocrinopathy due to impaired processing of prohormones) PCSK1 Polyendocrine deficiencies and polyneuropathy [DMXL2] Gordon-Holmes syndrome (cerebellar ataxia and adult onset neurodegeneration) [RNF216, OTUD4, PNPLA6] Waardenburg syndrome (pigmentary abnormalities of the hair, skin, and eyes; congenital sensorineural hearing loss) [SOX10] Vanishing testes (may also cause ambiguous genitalia)
UNDERVIRILIZATION OR SEX REVERSAL IN XY MALES	**OTHER SYNDROMES AFFECTING REPRODUCTIVE SYSTEMS**
Biosynthetic defects Lipoid adrenal hyperplasia [STAR] 17α-Hydroxylase/17,20 lyase [CYP17A1] 3β-Hydroxysteroid dehydrogenase [HSD3B2] 17-Ketosteroid reductase [HSD17B3] 5α-Reductase [SRD5A2] Cytochrome P-450 oxidoreductase deficiency [POR] Smith-Lemli-Opitz syndrome (1:20,000) [DHCR7] Androgen insensitivity (1:20,000) [AR]: complete or partial Luteinizing hormone insensitivity [LHR] **Mutations in genes affecting gonadal differentiation** SRY SOX9 (campomelic dysplasia) NR5A1 (steroidogenic factor-1; sometimes associated with adrenal hypoplasia) WT1 (WAGR and Denys-Drash syndromes) NR0B1 (DAX1) or WNT4 duplications DHH (associated with peripheral neuropathy) ATRX (X-linked α-thalassemia and mental retardation) GATA4 ZFPM2(FOG2) MAP3K1 HHAT DMRT1 Exposure to 5α-reductase inhibitors, other endocrine disruptors	Chromosomal aneuploidy Turner syndrome (1:2500): 45,X; 45,X/46,XX mosaics; 46,XXr; 46,XXq– Klinefelter syndrome (1:1000): 47,XXY Mixed gonadal dysgenesis (1:20,000): 45,X/46,XY; 45,X/47,XXY Other: trisomy 13, trisomy 18, triploidy, 4p–, 13q– Persistent müllerian duct syndrome in XY males Type 1 [AMH] Type 2 [AMHR2] Mayer-Rokitansky-Küster-Hauser syndrome (vaginal atresia) (1:6000)

*Frequencies of relatively common (at least 1:20,000) diseases are noted in parentheses. When causative genetic mutations have been identified, the affected locus is noted in square brackets.
WAGR = Wilms tumor, aniridia, genitourinary abnormalities or gonadoblastoma, and mental retardation.

development of the müllerian ducts proceeds, and the female internal structures (fallopian tubes, uterus, cervix, and upper vagina) are formed.

Development of the structures derived from the wolffian ducts, including the epididymis, ductus deferens, ejaculatory ducts, and seminiferous tubules, requires high local concentrations of testosterone secreted from Leydig cells of the testis beginning at approximately 7 weeks' gestation. In the absence of testosterone, wolffian ducts regress. Levels of testosterone in the circulation are insufficient to develop wolffian structures. Thus in conditions in which the gonads develop asymmetrically (e.g., ovotesticular disorders of sexual development or mixed gonadal dysgenesis; see later), wolffian structures develop asymmetrically as well. Development of wolffian structures requires an intact androgen receptor.

Development of the External Genitalia

External genital structures are also bipotential in early gestation and consist of the genital tubercle, genital folds (later, urethral-labial folds), and genital swelling (later, labioscrotal folds) (see Fig. 220-2). Differentiation to male genitalia occurs from approximately 8 to 14 weeks' gestation under the influence of dihydrotestosterone, which must interact with an intact androgen receptor. The genital tubercle becomes the glans penis; the genital folds fuse to become the shaft of the penis and penile urethra, and the labioscrotal folds

(derived from the genital swelling) fuse to become the scrotum. Without androgens, these structures become the clitoris, labia minora, and labia majora, respectively.

Normal Gonadal and Adrenal Steroidogenesis

Many forms of genital ambiguity result from defects in steroid biosynthesis in the testes or adrenal cortex or from defective steroid metabolism in the placenta or in target tissues (Fig. 220-3 and E-Fig. 220-1).

Steroid biosynthesis in the testes and adrenals begins with the importation of cholesterol into mitochondria, a highly regulated process controlled largely by the steroidogenic acute regulatory (StAR) protein. Levels of StAR are controlled within the adrenals by adrenocorticotropic hormone (ACTH) and within the testis by HCG during the first trimester and by LH later in pregnancy.

Within mitochondria, the side chain of cholesterol is cleaved between carbons 20 and 22 by the cholesterol side-chain cleavage enzyme (cholesterol desmolase, CYP11A), a cytochrome P-450 enzyme. The product is pregnenolone, which is transported to the endoplasmic reticulum. Some pregnenolone is converted by 17α-hydroxylase (CYP17) to 17-hydroxypregnenolone. Both 17-hydroxypregnenolone and the remaining pregnenolone are converted by 3β-hydroxysteroid dehydrogenase (HSD3B2) to 17-hydroxyprogesterone and

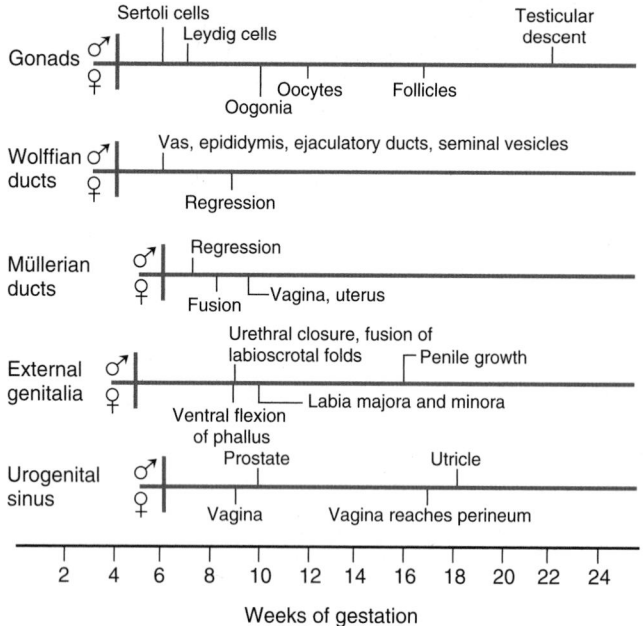

FIGURE 220-1. Time course of prenatal sexual differentiation in male and female fetuses. (Modified from Barthold JS, Gonzalez R. Intersex states. In: Gonzales ET, Bauer SB, eds. *Pediatric Urology Practice.* Philadelphia: Lippincott Williams & Wilkins; 1999.)

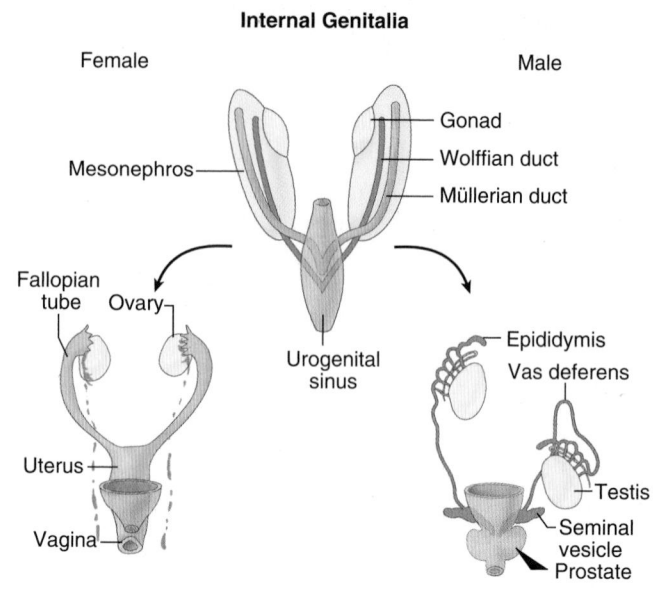

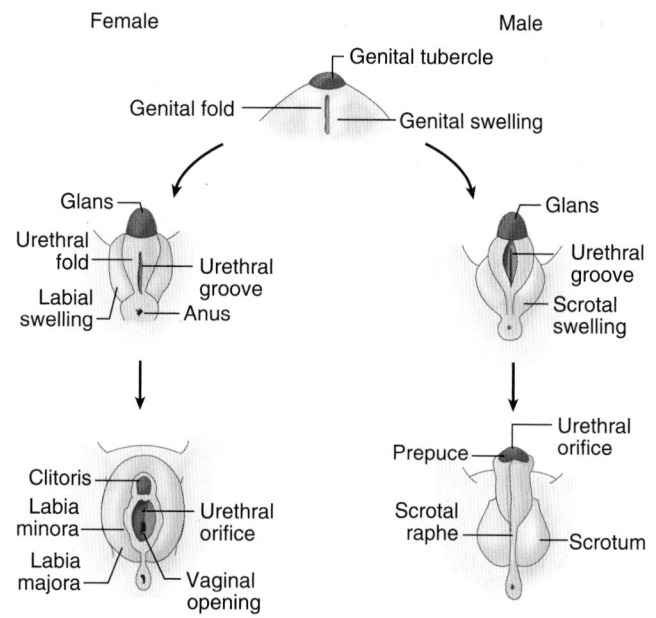

FIGURE 220-2. Differentiation of the internal and external genitalia of the human fetus. (Modified from Griffen JE, Ojeda SR, eds. *Textbook of Endocrine Physiology.* New York: Oxford University Press; 1996.)

progesterone, respectively. The side chain of 17-hydroxypregnenolone is cleaved by the 17,20-lyase activity of CYP17 to dehydroepiandrosterone (DHEA). DHEA may also be converted to androstenedione by HSD3B2.

All the preceding steps can occur in the adrenal cortex, in Leydig cells of the testis, and (after puberty) in theca cells of ovarian follicles. Subsequent biosynthetic steps are specific to different glands. In the adrenal cortex, 17-hydroxyprogesterone is converted by 21-hydroxylase (CYP21, also termed CYP21A2, a microsomal P-450) to 11-deoxycortisol, which is then converted in mitochondria to cortisol by 11β-hydroxylase (CYP11B1). Additionally, progesterone is converted to deoxycorticosterone by CYP21, which is then converted to aldosterone by aldosterone synthase (CYP11B2).

In Leydig cells of the testis, androstenedione is converted to testosterone by 17-ketosteroid reductase (17β-hydroxysteroid dehydrogenase type 3 [HSD17B3]); the same reaction occurs in theca cells of the ovary, catalyzed by 17β-hydroxysteroid dehydrogenase type 1 (HSD17B1). In granulosa cells of the ovary (after puberty), androstenedione and testosterone are converted by aromatase (CYP19) to estrone and estradiol, respectively. In skin of the developing male external genitalia, steroid 5α-reductase (SRD5A2) converts testosterone to a more potent androgen, dihydrotestosterone.

The placenta is a steroid-synthesizing and steroid-metabolizing tissue as well; it has high steroid sulfatase activity that converts DHEA sulfate from the fetal adrenal gland back to DHEA. This is then successively converted by 3β-hydroxysteroid dehydrogenase type 1 (HSD3B1) and aromatase (CYP19) to androstenedione and estrone, respectively, which are then converted to estradiol by HSD17B1.

● DEFECTS OF SEX DIFFERENTIATION
Defects of Steroidogenesis

PATHOBIOLOGY

Genital ambiguity in genetic females is usually the result of exposure to excessive levels of androgens. Virilizing congenital adrenal hyperplasia, the most common cause of genital ambiguity in female infants, occurs in 1 in 16,000 births.

Conversely, severe deficiencies of androgens, if present early in gestation, cause ambiguous or female-appearing external genitalia in male infants. Usually, müllerian structures such as the uterus, cervix, and upper vagina are not present because the testes are able to secrete müllerian inhibitory substance. Thus individuals with these conditions have a short vagina ending in a blind pouch.

CONGENITAL ADRENAL HYPERPLASIA
The fundamental defect among patients with any form of congenital adrenal hyperplasia is inadequate synthesis of cortisol (see Fig. 220-3 and E-Fig. 220-1).[5]

Inefficient cortisol synthesis signals the hypothalamus and pituitary to increase corticotropin-releasing hormone and ACTH, respectively (Chapter 210). Consequently, the adrenal glands become hyperplastic, and steroid precursors accumulate proximal to the block in biosynthesis. In some conditions, these precursors can be converted to androgens.

Lipoid Hyperplasia
Lipoid hyperplasia results from mutations in the *STAR* gene. Cholesterol is not imported efficiently into mitochondria and thus accumulates in cells. Steroid biosynthesis is drastically reduced because of the lack of substrate, and the lipid accumulation quickly kills steroid-synthesizing cells in both the adrenals and the testes. Thus affected male patients are born as phenotypically female because they cannot synthesize testosterone. Affected female patients may undergo transient spontaneous puberty because human ovarian granulosa cells do not synthesize steroid hormones (and thus do not accumulate cholesterol) until puberty. Both sexes have adrenal insufficiency and are unable to synthesize either cortisol or aldosterone.

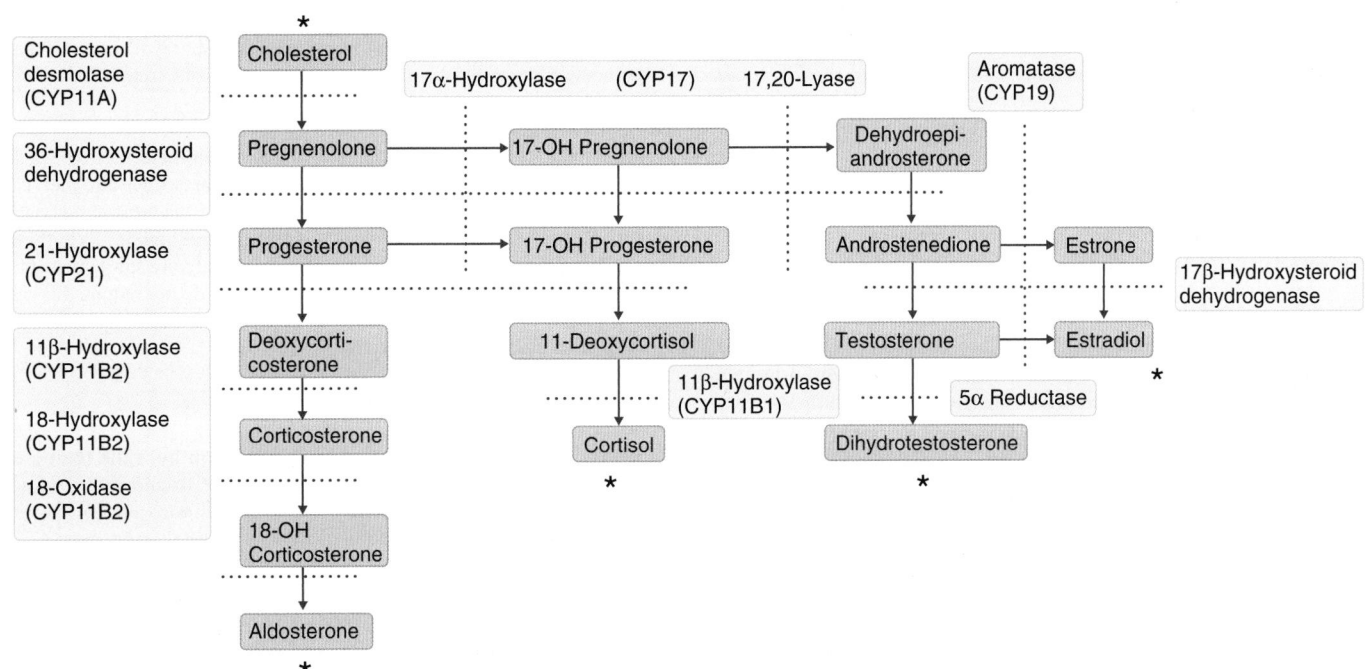

FIGURE 220-3. **Steroidogenesis.** Pathways for the synthesis of progesterone and mineralocorticoids (aldosterone), glucocorticoids (cortisol), androgens (testosterone and dihydrotestosterone), and estrogens (estradiol) are arranged from left to right. The enzymatic activities catalyzing each bioconversion are written in boxes. For those activities mediated by specific cytochrome P-450 subsets, the systematic name of the enzyme (CYP followed by a number) is listed in parentheses. CYP11B2 and CYP17 have multiple activities. (For an expanded version of this image, including planar structures for cholesterol and the end products of each pathway, see E-Fig. 220-1.)

17α-Hydroxylase/17,20 Lyase Deficiency

Severe mutations in the *CYP17* gene prevent the synthesis of any sex hormones.[6] Affected male patients have female-appearing external genitalia but have no müllerian structures because the testes synthesize antimüllerian hormone. Affected female patients remain sexually infantile without hormone replacement. Milder mutations result in ambiguous genitalia in male patients. Although cortisol synthesis is also abolished, even severely affected individuals are able to synthesize corticosterone, an active glucocorticoid, as well as aldosterone. Thus they do not develop adrenal insufficiency. On the contrary, they secrete excessive amounts of deoxycorticosterone, which has mineralocorticoid activity, and are therefore prone to develop hypertension.

Whereas most *CYP17* mutations affect both the hydroxylase and lyase activities, rare mutations can affect the lyase activity alone. Additionally, mutations in genes other than *CYP17* can have the same phenotype as 17,20, lyase deficiency (i.e., deficient androgen synthesis with normal cortisol synthesis). These include an accessory electron transfer protein, cytochrome b5, and mutations in the genes for two aldo-keto reductases, AKR1C2 and AKR1C4. These AKR1C isozymes normally catalyze 3α-hydroxysteroid dehydrogenase activity, which allows synthesis of the potent androgen, dihydrotestosterone, through an alternative "backdoor" biosynthetic pathway that does not include testosterone as an intermediate.

3β-Hydroxysteroid Dehydrogenase Deficiency

Severe mutations in the *HSD3B2* gene prevent the synthesis of aldosterone, cortisol, testosterone, and estrogens. Because DHEA, a weak androgen, is synthesized and secreted at high levels, some degree of phallic growth is present. Thus affected male patients have severely ambiguous genitalia, but affected female patients may have clitorimegaly. Both sexes develop adrenal insufficiency if they are untreated.

Because many children with premature adrenarche (early development of axillary and pubic hair), as well as many women with polycystic ovary syndrome, have elevated levels of DHEA, it was once thought that such individuals could have a mild form of HSD3B2 deficiency. However, mutations in *HSD3B2* are rarely if ever found in such individuals, who instead have an imbalance in the relative levels of HSD3B2 and CYP17 activity within the adrenal cortex.

21-Hydroxylase Deficiency

More than 90% of cases of congenital adrenal hyperplasia are caused by 21-hydroxylase deficiency resulting from mutations in the *CYP21* (or *CYP21A2*)

gene.[7] *CYP21* and a highly homologous pseudogene, *CYP21P* (or *CYP21A1P*), are located within the major histocompatibility complex on chromosome 6p21.3, a genomic region noteworthy for a high rate of recombination. More than 90% of all mutations are the result of intergenic recombination between *CYP21* and *CYP21P*. Most are transfers of deleterious mutations from *CYP21P* to *CYP21*, whereas 20% are net deletions of *CYP21* resulting from unequal meiotic crossover.

In patients with 21-hydroxylase deficiency, the adrenals produce excess 17-hydroxyprogesterone, 17-hydroxypregnenolone, and progesterone, which are further metabolized to DHEA and androstenedione. Once secreted, these substances are further metabolized to active androgens (testosterone and dihydrotestosterone) and, to a lesser extent, to estrogens (estrone and estradiol).

Adrenal secretion of excess androgen precursors does not significantly affect male sexual differentiation. In affected female patients, the urogenital sinus is in the process of septation when the fetal adrenal begins to produce excess androgens, which function to prevent the formation of separate vaginal and urethral canals. Further adrenal-derived androgens interact with androgen receptors in genital skin and induce clitoral enlargement, promote fusion of the labial folds, and cause rostral migration of the urethral/vaginal perineal orifice. However, internal wolffian structures such as the prostate gland and spermatic ducts are usually not virilized, presumably because development of the wolffian ducts requires markedly higher local concentrations of testosterone than the external genitalia. Nevertheless, severely affected female patients occasionally have some development of typically male internal genital structures.

Thus the typical result in severely affected girls is ambiguous or male-appearing external genitalia with perineal hypospadias and chordee, but without palpable testes (Fig. 220-4). The severity of virilization is often quantitated using a five-point scale developed by Prader (Fig. 220-5). The degree of genital ambiguity in female patients with classic congenital adrenal hyperplasia is correlated with the severity of enzymatic compromise conferred by each patient's mutations.

Most patients (75%) cannot synthesize sufficient aldosterone to maintain sodium balance and are termed *salt wasters*. These patients are predisposed to episodic and potentially life-threatening hyponatremic dehydration. Patients with sufficient aldosterone production to prevent salt wasting and who have signs of prenatal virilization and/or markedly increased production of hormonal substrates of 21-hydroxylase (e.g., 17-hydroxyprogesterone) are termed *simple virilizers*.

11β-Hydroxylase Deficiency

Patients with 11β-hydroxylase deficiency have mutations in the *CYP11B1* gene. They have elevated levels of deoxycorticosterone and 11-deoxycortisol, as well as earlier cortisol precursors such as 17-hydroxyprogesterone. These patients secrete excess adrenal androgens, with consequences similar to those seen in 21-hydroxylase deficiency. However, patients with 11β-hydroxylase deficiency synthesize aldosterone normally and do not have problems with salt wasting. Instead, they are likely to become hypertensive as a result of elevated levels of deoxycorticosterone and its metabolites.

DEFECTS OF ANDROGEN BIOSYNTHESIS

Lipoid hyperplasia, 17-hydroxylase/17,20 lyase deficiency, and HSD3B2 deficiency affect the biosynthesis of both corticosteroids and sex hormones. In contrast, two enzymatic defects affect only androgen biosynthesis. They have similar phenotypes. Affected male patients are born with ambiguous genitalia, but they virilize at puberty and often reassign themselves to a male gender if they were raised as females. They have absent müllerian structures as a result of the secretion of antimüllerian hormone by the testes.

17-Ketosteroid Reductase (17-Hydroxysteroid Dehydrogenase 3) Deficiency

This disorder is caused by mutations in the *HSD17B3* gene.[8] Although testosterone is not synthesized well, androstenedione, an active androgen, is

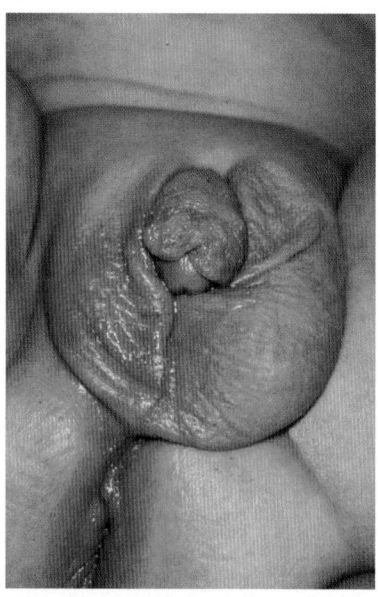

FIGURE 220-4. Virilized external genitalia in a female infant with congenital adrenal hyperplasia caused by 21-hydroxylase deficiency. No gonads are present in the scrotum.

synthesized. Because several other isozymes have 17-ketosteroid reductase activity in other tissues, some testosterone is invariably synthesized, especially at puberty, when circulating levels of androstenedione increase.

5α-Reductase Deficiency

Patients with 5α-reductase deficiency resulting from mutations in the *SRD5A2* gene synthesize entirely normal amounts of testosterone, but they cannot synthesize adequate amounts of dihydrotestosterone, the most potent naturally occurring androgen.[9] This enzyme is not expressed at high levels in the testes (circulating levels of dihydrotestosterone are relatively low); instead, it is expressed in genital skin. Internal wolffian structures do not require this enzyme and are intact; high testosterone levels at puberty induce significant phallic growth without 5α-reductase activity.

OTHER DEFECTS OF STEROIDOGENESIS

Aromatase Deficiency

Mutations in *CYP19* cause aromatase deficiency in both the fetus and the placenta. The placenta can convert DHEA sulfate to androstenedione and testosterone normally, but it cannot convert these androgens to estrone and estradiol. These androgens accumulate in both the fetal and maternal circulations and virilize both the mother and the affected fetus if it is female. Affected male infants are phenotypically normal. Affected female patients virilize further at puberty if they are untreated. The lack of aromatase activity within bone leads to tall stature in both sexes (because estrogens are required to close the growth plates) and later to osteoporosis.

Cytochrome P-450 Oxidoreductase Deficiency

This deficiency is one form of Antley-Bixler syndrome, which is characterized by skeletal anomalies and craniosynostosis; most patients also have ambiguous genitalia associated with mutations in the *POR* gene.[10] Antley-Bixler syndrome without genital abnormalities is caused by mutations in the FGF receptor (*FGFR2*) gene.

Because this disorder affects the activity of all microsomal cytochrome P-450 subsets, complete deficiency of cytochrome P-450 oxidoreductase (POR) is lethal, and identified mutations in humans yield POR with partial activity. *POR* mutations may cause skeletal anomalies by interfering with cholesterol synthesis. Genital ambiguity is caused by several mechanisms. Decreased activity of 17α-hydroxylase/17,20 lyase (CYP17) affects androgen synthesis and leads to undervirilization in males. Conversely, decreased activity of 21-hydroxylase (CYP21) can virilize affected females. These two deficiencies also can cause adrenal insufficiency. Finally, decreased activity of placental aromatase (CYP19) virilizes both the mother and the affected fetus (if female).

Smith-Lemli-Opitz Syndrome

This relatively frequent (1 in 20,000 northern Europeans) disorder of the final step of cholesterol biosynthesis (conversion from 7-dehydrocholesterol) is caused by mutations in the *DHCR7* gene encoding 7-dehydrocholesterol

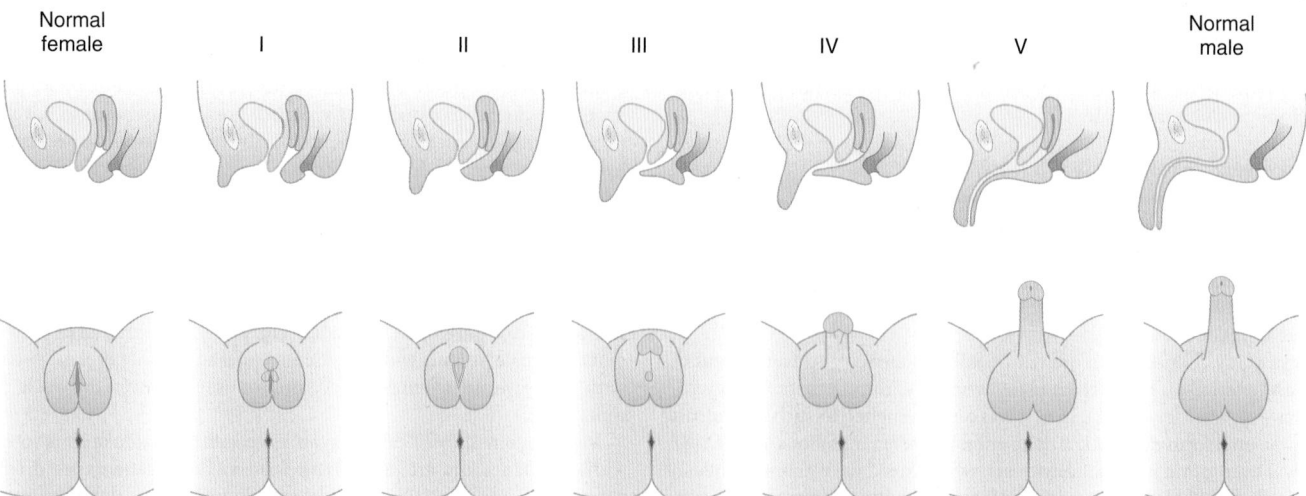

FIGURE 220-5. Abnormal differentiation of the urogenital sinus and external genitalia. Schematic representations of normal female and male anatomy flank a series of schematics illustrating different degrees of virilization of females, graded using the scale developed by Prader. The uterus (*shaded*) persists in virilized females even when the external genitalia have a completely masculine appearance (Prader grade V). (Modified from Prader A. Der Genitalbefund beim Pseudohermaphroditismus femininus der kengenitalen adrenogenitalen Syndroms. *Helv Paediatr Acta.* 1954;9:231-248.)

reductase. The syndrome is characterized by multiple congenital anomalies, including being small for gestational age, short stature, microcephaly, mental retardation, aggressive behavior, seizures, hypotonia, polydactyly, cleft palate, cardiac defects, lung hypoplasia, and renal anomalies. Male patients have ambiguous genitalia. The range of clinical severity is wide and depends on the nature of the mutations. Pathogenetic mechanisms for the ambiguous genitalia may include insufficient provision of cholesterol for steroid hormone biosynthesis or toxic effects of the precursor, 7-dehydrocholesterol, on steroidogenic cells.

⬤ MATERNAL CONDITIONS AFFECTING THE FETUS
LUTEOMA OF PREGNANCY

Luteomas are the most common causes of maternal virilization during pregnancy. They often occur bilaterally. Although many luteomas are discovered incidentally during cesarean sections or postpartum tubal ligations, one fourth of mothers virilize during the latter half of pregnancy, and half of female infants born to these mothers also exhibit signs of virilization, most typically clitorimegaly and labial fusion. Spontaneous regression of the luteoma generally begins within days after delivery.

DRUG EXPOSURE

Depending on the agent, maternal drug exposure may affect either male or female fetuses. Females may be virilized by androgens such as 19-nor-testosterone or progestins administered to prevent spontaneous abortion. Undervirilized males can be born to women exposed to 5α-reductase inhibitors such as finasteride. The antifungal agent fluconazole can inhibit many cytochrome P-450 enzymes and can lead to a condition closely resembling Antley-Bixler syndrome.

The synthetic estrogen diethylstilbestrol was used several decades ago to prevent spontaneous abortion (it was actually ineffective for this purpose). Males exposed to this agent in utero were born with testicular hypoplasia, cryptorchidism, hypospadias, and/or microphallus. Females had uterine, cervical, and vaginal abnormalities and an increased risk for clear cell adenocarcinoma of the vagina. Considering that many cases of genital ambiguity are idiopathic, it is likely that additional endocrine disruptors in the environment have not yet been identified.

⬤ HORMONE INSENSITIVITY SYNDROMES AND OTHER HORMONE DEFICIENCIES
ANDROGEN INSENSITIVITY

Males normally carry a single copy of the X-linked androgen receptor (AR) gene.[11] Thus a single mutation can completely inactivate the receptor in males and lead to complete androgen insensitivity (formerly termed *testicular feminization syndrome*).[12] This is one of the most frequent forms of 46,XY disorders of sexual development, occurring in approximately 1 in 20,000 male births.

Patients with the complete form of androgen insensitivity have normal female external genitalia. Unless suspicion is raised by prior knowledge of the infant's karyotype, the condition is rarely discovered before puberty unless the testes are palpated in the groin or labia on routine examination. Because the testes secrete antimüllerian hormone, müllerian structures are absent, including the uterus, fallopian tubes, and cervix. Thus the vagina is usually shallow and ends blindly. Wolffian structures are also absent. The testes may be located in the abdomen or in the labia majora and do not undergo spermatogenesis. Antimüllerian hormone levels are elevated during the first year and (if the testes have not been removed) after puberty. Testosterone and LH levels in infancy and at puberty are elevated as a result of defective feedback regulation caused by androgen resistance at the level of the hypothalamus.

At puberty, pubic and axillary hair is scant or absent. Testosterone can be aromatized to estradiol by CYP19 in breast fat, and estrogen receptors are unaffected in this condition. Thus breast development is that of a normal female.

Partial androgen insensitivity (Reifenstein syndrome) is characterized by a variable degree of genital ambiguity, and both virilization and breast development occur at puberty. Mild androgen insensitivity also can occur with a male phenotype, with gynecomastia and infertility as the sole manifestations. Mutations in the androgen receptor are not detected in many mild cases, which may result from defects in other transcription factors affecting actions of the receptor.

LEYDIG CELL AGENESIS

Leydig cell agenesis or hypoplasia is a rare autosomal recessive syndrome caused by mutations in the *LHGCR* gene encoding the LH receptor. Without stimulation by LH (or by HCG early in gestation), Leydig cells do not differentiate normally and do not secrete testosterone. Thus affected male infants are born with female-appearing or ambiguous external genitalia. Müllerian structures are absent because of unaffected secretion of antimüllerian hormone by Sertoli cells. LH levels are high in infancy and at puberty, and they respond normally to gonadotropin-releasing hormone, whereas testosterone levels are low and do not respond to stimulation by HCG. Affected females are phenotypically normal but may have oligomenorrhea resulting from primary ovarian dysfunction.

PERSISTENT MÜLLERIAN DUCT SYNDROME

Persistent müllerian duct syndrome (PMDS) is a rare autosomal recessive condition that results from mutations in the genes for either antimüllerian hormone (PMDS type I) or the antimüllerian hormone receptor (*AMHR2* gene, PMDS type II).[13] The two are distinguished clinically by low or absent antimüllerian hormone levels in patients with antimüllerian hormone mutations and by antimüllerian hormone levels in the high-normal range in those with antimüllerian hormone receptor mutations.

Affected male patients have unimpaired testosterone secretion and thus have normal external genitalia and wolffian structures. However, the lack of antimüllerian hormone action prevents regression of müllerian structures, so these patients also retain a uterus and fallopian tubes. These structures are often closely approximated to the vas deferens. The müllerian structures are usually dragged into the inguinal canal by the descending testes. However, these structures typically prevent the testes from descending into the scrotum and thus cause bilateral inguinal hernias (with the uterus on one side) and bilateral or occasionally unilateral cryptorchidism. The condition is usually discovered only at surgery. Fertility in affected patients may be normal or impaired, with an increased risk for malignant disease in undescended testes left in the abdomen.

HYPOGONADOTROPIC HYPOGONADISM

Milder or later appearing deficiencies of androgen biosynthesis (after 13 to 14 weeks) may allow complete fusion of the labioscrotal folds and normal positioning of the urethral meatus, but subsequent growth of the phallus is suboptimal. Such individuals have a micropenis. The most common cause is lack of gonadotropin (specifically, LH) secretion; even when LH is lacking, early male development is normal because testosterone secretion is controlled mostly by HCG during the first trimester.

Defective LH and follicle-stimulating hormone secretion can result when the neurons that normally secrete gonadotropin-releasing hormone fail to migrate into the hypothalamus. This condition, *Kallmann syndrome*,[14] is often X-linked, resulting from mutations in the *KAL1* gene, but many other genes have been implicated (see Table 220-1). It is often associated with hyposmia or anosmia. Other conditions that affect hypothalamic development and cause hypogonadotropic hypogonadism include *Prader-Willi syndrome*, which is a result of paternal deletions, methylation defects, and maternal uniparental disomy of imprinted loci on chromosome 15q12.[15] Children with this syndrome have a characteristic appearance consisting of a narrow bitemporal diameter, almond-shaped eyes with an antimongoloid slant, and small hands and feet. They typically have marked hypotonia as infants, with subsequent moderate developmental delay and slow somatic growth. Hypothalamic obesity develops during childhood. Patients with adrenal hypoplasia congenita resulting from mutations in the DAX1 transcription factor have defective development of the ventromedial hypothalamus and consequent hypogonadotropic hypogonadism associated with adrenal insufficiency that typically manifests with aldosterone deficiency and salt wasting. Steroidogenic factor-1 (SF-1), encoded by the *NR5A1* gene, is an orphan nuclear receptor that is critical for the development and function of the adrenal glands, gonads, pituitary gonadotropes, ventromedial nucleus of the hypothalamus, and male sexual differentiation. Heterozygous null mutations or homozygous milder mutations have been identified mainly among undervirilized 46,XY individuals and 46,XX women with premature ovarian failure. Only a minority have adrenal insufficiency.

Hypogonadotropic hypogonadism often results from failure of the entire anterior pituitary gland, or particular cellular populations therein, to develop.[16] Pituitary gland abnormalities can be associated with other midline defects, including hypoplasia of the optic nerves and the septum pellucidum, a condition termed *septo-optic dysplasia*. Associated pituitary hormone deficiencies may include growth hormone, ACTH, and thyroid-stimulating hormone. These deficiencies may manifest in the neonatal period as hypoglycemia or hypothyroidism (detected by newborn screening programs). Optic nerve dysfunction is difficult to detect by routine examination in the neonatal period, but it causes a characteristic wandering nystagmus after a few months of age.

Although panhypopituitarism is most often sporadic, mutations in transcription factors controlling pituitary development have been documented (Chapter 211), particularly PROP1, and septo-optic dysplasia has been associated with mutations in the *HESX* gene. Rarely, mutations in the gene encoding the β-subunit of LH may yield a phenotype similar to hypogonadotropic hypogonadism.

⬤ OTHER GENETIC CONDITIONS
ANEUPLOIDY OF SEX CHROMOSOMES
Turner Syndrome
Patients with Turner syndrome have normal female external genitalia and a normal uterus and fallopian tubes, but they have dysgenetic streak ovaries.[17,18] Most fetuses with Turner syndrome spontaneously abort, but the incidence in live births is approximately 1 in 2500. Classically, the karyotype is 45,X, but many patients retain an abnormal second X chromosome or even a fragment of a Y chromosome lacking *SRY*. Other patients are mosaic for 46,XX and 45,X cells and may have relatively mild phenotypes.

Untreated patients are short. Many have typical dysmorphic features, including lymphedema of the neck at birth, webbed neck, low posterior hairline, increased carrying angle of the arms, shield chest with widely spaced nipples, low-set ears, and micrognathia. Patients typically have primary amenorrhea and are infertile, but they occasionally have menarche followed by premature ovarian failure. Estrogen therapy can significantly improve bone density, but it is unclear whether it reduces fractures or improves long-term outcome.[19,20][A1]

Klinefelter Syndrome
In this condition, male patients have normal development of the penis and scrotum, but the testes are small and firm. Patients tend to be tall. At adolescence, gynecomastia is frequent. Signs of testosterone deficiency occur in most affected adults, and most have azoospermia. The usual karyotype is 47,XXY. Hormonal findings include elevated gonadotropin levels and a decreased serum testosterone concentration. Klinefelter syndrome is a common disorder that occurs in 1 in 500 to 1000 men.[21]

Mixed Gonadal Dysgenesis
Mixed gonadal dysgenesis, a frequent cause of sexual ambiguity, occurs in approximately 1 in 20,000 births.[22] The karyotype is usually mosaic 45,X/46,XY. Gonadal pathologic features can vary from fibrous streaks indistinguishable from those in Turner syndrome to normally developed testes and a normal male phenotype. Typically, patients have a testis on one side and a fibrous streak on the other. Some patients may have a Turner-like phenotype. A fallopian tube is usually present on the side of the streak gonad. Leydig cell function, evaluated by testosterone response to HCG, and Sertoli cell function, evaluated by serum antimüllerian hormone levels, vary from poor to normal.

XX MALE SYNDROME
Males with a 46,XX karyotype have normal external and internal male genitalia; however, they resemble patients with Klinefelter syndrome in that they have small testes, azoospermia, and infertility. Translocation of the *SRY* gene to the X chromosome is detected in 75 to 90% of sporadic cases; this can occur because the gene is located very near the pseudoautosomal region, where the short arms of the X and Y chromosomes are homologous and meiotic recombination is possible. Duplication of the SOX9 transcription factor may be responsible for some familial cases of XX sex reversal.

XY FEMALE SYNDROMES
Patients with pure XY gonadal dysgenesis (Swyer syndrome) have a normal female phenotype, including a uterus and fallopian tubes, but they have streak gonads. These patients are free of Turner-like malformations and attain normal height. Mutations of the *SRY* gene have been identified in 15% of cases. Unlike 45,X patients with Turner syndrome, these patients have an increased risk for gonadoblastoma.

Similar phenotypes result from duplication of the region of the X chromosome containing the *DAX1* gene, from duplication of the *WNT4* gene, or from

haploinsufficiency of the SF1 transcription factor (see earlier). XY sex reversal also can result from mutations in the SOX9 transcription factor associated with campomelic dysplasia, a form of dwarfism. Mutations of *DHH* cause XY gonadal dysgenesis, associated with peripheral neuropathy.

Some 46,XY patients with absent gonads have various degrees of sexual ambiguity and no müllerian derivatives. The implication that some testicular tissue was functional at least up to 10 weeks' gestation and subsequently regressed led to the name *fetal testicular regression syndrome*. Testicular regression may occur in late pregnancy or even postnatally; these fully virilized male patients have isolated anorchia.

VAGINAL ATRESIA
Mayer-Rokitansky-Küster-Hauser syndrome refers to aplasia of the uterus and upper vagina, occurring in approximately 1 in 5000 women. In approximately one third of cases, it occurs along with other abnormalities including unilateral renal aplasia and cervicothoracic somite dysplasia (MURCS association). The genetic basis is unknown in most cases. Rare affected individuals have heterozygous mutations of *WNT4*; such patients usually have clinical and biochemical signs of androgen excess.

OVOTESTICULAR DISORDER OF SEXUAL DEVELOPMENT (TRUE HERMAPHRODITISM)
Ovotesticular disorder of sexual development (true hermaphrotidism), a rare and usually sporadic disorder, is defined as the coexistence of seminiferous tubules and ovarian follicles. Most patients have an ovotestis with either an ovary or a testis on the opposite side; a gonad in the scrotum is usually a testis but may be an ovotestis.

The genitalia are usually ambiguous, but they may appear completely masculine or feminine. The anatomy of the internal reproductive tract depends on the nature of the gonads, particularly whether they secrete antimüllerian hormone. A uterus or uterine horn is present in 90% of cases. Testosterone response to HCG is variable, and antimüllerian hormone levels are usually low. Most patients experience breast development, ovulation, and even menstruation at puberty; pregnancy and successful childbirth are possible if selective removal of testicular tissue is feasible. Unless sex of rearing has already been chosen, male gender assignment should be restricted to patients with no uterus and descended testicular tissue because the latter is usually dysgenetic and prone to malignant degeneration. Most patients with ovotesticular disorder of sexual development have a 46,XX karyotype. Despite the presence of testicular tissue, they usually lack *SRY*. Some patients in different ethnic groups and locales carry a specific mutation in NR5A1, Arg92Trp.

⬤ MANAGEMENT OF INDIVIDUALS WITH DISORDERS OF SEXUAL DEVELOPMENT: GENDER ROLE AND IDENTITY
The influence of prenatal sex steroid exposure on personality is controversial.[23] In considering this question, it is important to distinguish among gender role, sexual orientation, and gender identity.

Gender Role
Gender role refers to gender-stereotyped behaviors, such as the choice of toys by young children. For example, parents of young girls with congenital adrenal hyperplasia often report that their daughters prefer to play with trucks rather than dolls and tend to be tomboyish later in childhood. Decreased interest in maternal behavior, beginning with infrequent doll play in early childhood and extending to lack of interest in child rearing in older girls and women, occurs frequently.[24]

Sexual Orientation
Sexual orientation refers to homosexual versus heterosexual preferences. In many studies, a significant minority of women with congenital adrenal hyperplasia have been actively homosexual or bisexual or have had an increased tendency toward homoerotic fantasies. These characteristics occur more frequently in women with the salt-wasting form of 21-hydroxylase deficiency, suggesting that they are a consequence of prenatal exposure of the brain to androgens. However, the vast majority of both male and female homosexuals have no identifiable endocrinologic abnormality.

Gender Identity
Gender identity refers to self-identification as male or female. Gender self-reassignment back to male has been reported in cases of male patients with

penile trauma or exstrophy of the bladder who were raised as girls. This may also occur in 46,XY patients with disorders of sexual development raised as girls, especially in cases of 5α-reductase or 17-ketosteroid reductase deficiencies, in which the fetal brain may be exposed to high circulating levels of androgens. Self-reassignment to the male gender is unusual in women with congenital adrenal hyperplasia. When it occurs, it may be related to delays in gender assignment or genital surgery or to inadequate suppression of adrenal androgens with glucocorticoid therapy.

Transgender individuals rarely have identifiable hormonal abnormalities; nonhormonal mechanisms governing gender identity are poorly understood. Gender identity disorders are much more likely to occur in both identical twins than in fraternal twins, suggesting a high degree of heritability. Neuroanatomic studies suggest that the bed nucleus of the stria terminalis is larger in males and trans males (female-to-male transsexuals) and smaller in females and trans females (male-to-female transsexuals). Similar findings involving other sexually dimorphic brain regions have been identified by MRI. Thus gender identity disorder may be considered a brain-limited disorder of sexual development.

DIAGNOSIS

Management of a child born with ambiguous genitalia presents a difficult challenge to medical personnel.[25] It is important to refrain from assigning sex until diagnostic information can be gathered. Usually, test results can be obtained within 24 to 48 hours and parents can be advised about the child's chromosomal and gonadal sex and the anatomy of internal sexual structures.

In addition, the physician must keep in mind that disorders of sexual development may be associated with life-threatening biochemical or anatomic abnormalities. In particular, the most common cause of severely masculinized external genitalia in females, the salt-wasting form of congenital adrenal hyperplasia resulting from steroid 21-hydroxylase deficiency, may cause hyponatremia, hyperkalemia, hypovolemia, and shock. In contrast, male patients with ambiguous genitalia may have lipoid adrenal hyperplasia or a salt-wasting form of 3/3-hydroxysteroid dehydrogenase (HSD3B2) deficiency. Males with micropenis may have panhypopituitarism; in this case they are at risk for significant hypoglycemia and hyponatremia resulting from low cortisol (because of low ACTH) and low growth hormone levels, or they may have adrenal hypoplasia congenita, in which case they could have adrenal insufficiency. Finally, patients with ambiguous genitalia are at increased risk for renal anomalies, or they may have chromosomal syndromes with other associated anomalies.

History

The gestational history should concentrate on potential exposure to agents that could interfere with normal sexual differentiation. For a female infant with virilized genitalia, these include progestational agents, whereas the mother of a male with incompletely masculinized genitalia may have been exposed to a 5α-reductase inhibitor through her husband's use of such an agent for male pattern baldness or prostate enlargement. It should be determined whether amniocentesis and karyotyping have been performed. A family history should elicit similar cases of genital ambiguity or cases of sudden death, which could raise suspicion of undiagnosed salt-wasting congenital adrenal hyperplasia or adrenal hypoplasia congenita.

Physical Examination

The physical examination should document the size of the phallus (clitoris or penis), the degree of chordee (ventral bowing of the phallus), and the extent of fusion of the labioscrotal folds. The urethral meatus should be identified, and there must be careful palpation for gonads in the inguinal canals and labia or scrotum. Bilateral cryptorchidism, even if an isolated finding in a phenotypic male patient, should always lead to evaluation for a possible disorder of sexual development.

Biochemical Evaluation of the Virilized Female

The minimal diagnostic tests should include measurement of basal serum 17-hydroxyprogesterone, androstenedione, and testosterone. Preferably, a complete profile of adrenocortical hormones is obtained before and 1 hour after stimulation of the adrenal cortex with 125 to 250 μg of cosyntropin (ACTH$_{1-24}$). These assays should be deferred until after the first 24 hours of life. They will identify potential defects in adrenal steroidogenesis (i.e., congenital adrenal hyperplasia); 21-hydroxylase deficiency is identified by elevations in 17-hydroxyprogesterone, whereas 11-deoxycortisol and 11-deoxycorticosterone are high in 11β-hydroxylase deficiency.

Biochemical Evaluation of the Undervirilized Male

In 46,XY patients with disorders of sexual development, it is necessary to test adrenal and gonadal function as well as extragonadal androgen metabolism. With regard to adrenal defects, 11-deoxycorticosterone and the ratio of pregnenolone to 17-hydroxypregnenolone are high in 17α-hydroxylase deficiency, 17-hydroxypregnenolone and DHEA are high in HSD3B2 deficiency, and all steroids are low in lipoid hyperplasia.

Defects in gonadal steroidogenesis are best evaluated after stimulation with HCG (1500 IU intramuscularly on days 1, 3, and 5, with blood drawn on day 6). However, 17-hydroxylase and HSD3B2 deficiencies affect both the gonads and the adrenal cortex and thus are often diagnosed by cosyntropin stimulation testing. Low levels of all androgen precursors suggest lipoid hyperplasia, 17α-hydroxylase/17,20 lyase deficiency, or a generalized defect in testicular function, such as the vanishing testes syndrome (testicular regression-syndrome) or gonadotropin insensitivity. A high ratio of androstenedione to testosterone is indicative of 17-ketosteroid reductase (HSD17B3) deficiency, and a high ratio of testosterone to dihydrotestosterone is diagnostic of 5α-reductase deficiency. The diagnosis of androgen insensitivity syndrome is suspected when a 46,XY patient has ambiguous or female-appearing external genitalia despite normal or high circulating levels of testosterone and dihydrotestosterone.

Gonadal Biopsies

Patients with mixed gonadal dysgenesis, ovotesticular disorders of sexual development, or unclear diagnoses should undergo bilateral gonadal biopsies (histology of the two gonads is often not identical). Dysgenetic gonads have a high potential for malignant transformation and usually need to be removed in childhood.

TREATMENT ℞

Initial Medical Management

Patients with congenital adrenal hyperplasia resulting from 21-hydroxylase or HSD3B2 deficiencies or those with lipoid hyperplasia or adrenal hypoplasia congenita require replacement of both glucocorticoids and mineralocorticoids, usually with hydrocortisone (15 to 20 mg/m^2/day in divided doses) and fludrocortisone (usually 0.1 mg/day, but as much as 0.4 mg/day in neonates with salt-wasting crises). Neonates with severe salt losses may require sodium chloride supplementation (≤8 mEq/kg/day). Patients with 11β-hydroxylase or 17α-hydroxylase deficiencies have normal aldosterone biosynthesis and usually require only glucocorticoids. Patients with panhypopituitarism usually require treatment with hydrocortisone, thyroxine, and growth hormone.

All male infants with ambiguous genitalia or micropenis in whom rearing as a boy is contemplated should have a 3- or 4-month therapeutic trial of monthly depot testosterone injections (25 mg) to attempt to increase the size of the phallus during infancy. This treatment may improve social acceptability of the genitalia later in childhood and adolescence and may make reconstructive surgery easier. In cases of suspected partial androgen insensitivity, this treatment also documents the degree to which the patient is androgen responsive and thus may provide useful information about whether rearing as a boy is feasible. Higher doses of testosterone (75 mg every 4 weeks) may be used under these circumstances.

Considerations Related to Sex Assignment

In large medical centers, a multidisciplinary team consisting of a neonatologist, a pediatric endocrinologist, a urologist, and preferably an experienced social worker and/or child psychiatrist or psychologist should promptly review the early diagnostic data and make a recommendation to the family as to the sex of rearing and any medical or surgical treatments. These recommendations should be based on both current knowledge of psychosexual development in individuals with disorders of sexual development and the feasibility of surgical treatment (see later).

In general, the recommended sex assignment should be that of the genetic/gonadal sex, if for no other reason than to retain the possibility of reproductive function. This is especially true for female infants with congenital adrenal hyperplasia who have normal internal genital structures and the potential for childbearing. An exception may be considered in a genetically female infant with completely male-appearing genitalia, especially if the child has been raised as a boy for more than a few months. Such children need to be castrated at puberty to avoid feminization.

Conversely, genetic male infants with completely female-appearing external genitalia (usually resulting from complete androgen insensitivity syndrome, but also seen with severe testosterone biosynthetic defects) should be raised as female because the potential for reconstruction of male genitalia is poor. However, male infants with 17-ketosteroid reductase or 5α-reductase deficiency should usually be reared as boys because they have normal levels of androstenedione or testosterone, respectively, and often virilize significantly at puberty. Indeed, many of these patients reassign themselves to the male gender when they are made aware of the diagnosis. The same considerations pertain to male patients with normal testosterone biosynthesis who have penile trauma or anatomic abnormalities such as bladder exstrophy.

Recommendations for sex assignment are to some extent culture specific. In cultures that value boys over girls, parents may strongly resist rearing a female infant with ambiguous genitalia as a girl, and many girls with severely virilized external genitalia will be raised as boys.

Surgical Management
Surgery for Ambiguous Genitalia

Whether, how, and when to intervene surgically in the treatment of genital anomalies are the subject of continuing debate.[26,27] Some adult patients with disorders of sexual development are unhappy with their gender assignments or surgical outcomes. Some physicians advocate postponing cosmetic genital surgery until the affected individual is able to provide informed consent, thus keeping all the options open if the adult patient wishes to function sexually with abnormal genitalia that nevertheless have sensation undiminished by surgery, or if the patient chooses to reassign his or her gender. Declining or postponing surgery should not be confused with raising the child with an indeterminate gender, a concept currently outside the mainstream. The option of deferring surgery should always be presented as part of the informed consent process.

The greatest change in practice over the past few decades probably pertains to male infants with ambiguous (but not completely female) external genitalia. Physicians are far less likely to recommend that such patients be reared as female because it is now recognized that many of these patients reassign themselves as male at puberty. Thus the ambiguous genitalia in such patients should rarely be "corrected" to female. On the contrary, surgical techniques for hypospadias repair have advanced significantly, and reconstruction of male genitalia is attempted more often, particularly if the infant responds to a course of testosterone with significant phallic growth.

Surgery for female infants with ambiguous genitalia may need to address an enlarged clitoris, the lack of a vaginal introitus, and the presence of a urogenital sinus. The clitoris is normally prominent in many infant girls. Even when enlarged in a girl with virilizing congenital adrenal hyperplasia, the clitoris can be prevented from growing larger with adequate suppression of adrenal androgens by glucocorticoids, and it will become less prominent as the patient grows. Thus mild-to-moderate clitorimegaly is often best managed without surgery. When clitoroplasty is attempted, one must keep in mind the important role of clitoral sensation in the female sexual response. Such surgery must be performed only by experienced operators with scrupulous attention to the preservation of clitoral innervation.

Consensus is lacking regarding the best age for vaginoplasty. Although many surgeons advocate a first procedure in infancy, it is difficult to maintain a functionally adequate introitus in the absence of estrogen exposure and mechanical dilation (with dilators or through sexual intercourse), and many patients require reoperation as young adults. Conversely, many women with atresia of the upper vagina (owing to complete androgen insensitivity or Mayer-Rokitansky-Küster-Hauser syndromes) can use dilators to lengthen the vagina without the need for surgery.

There is a dearth of large longitudinal studies comparing outcomes in patients who have had early genital surgery versus those who have had no surgery or surgery in adolescence. According to self-assessment surveys among sexually active women with congenital adrenal hyperplasia who have had genital surgery, most are able to have satisfactory sexual intercourse. As surgical and medical treatment regimens have improved in recent years, more women with congenital adrenal hyperplasia have successfully conceived spontaneously, completed pregnancies, and given birth.

Hypospadias repair is usually begun in the first year of life, after testosterone treatment (if necessary to increase phallic size). Depending on the degree of hypospadias, more than one surgical procedure may be required.

Removal of Intra-abdominal Testes in 46,XY Patients with Disorders of Sexual Development

Intra-abdominal testes are at increasing risk for malignant transformation over time. In a boy with cryptorchidism who is being reared as male, orchiopexy should be performed as quickly as possible; this also maximizes the possibility of fertility when the underlying condition does not preclude it. Dysgenetic gonads that cannot be brought into the scrotum should be removed soon after diagnosis because the risk for malignant transformation in childhood is relatively high.

There is a lack of consensus regarding nondysgenetic testes in severely undervirilized genetic male infants in whom rearing as female is planned. In patients with complete androgen insensitivity or complete defects in testosterone biosynthesis, no possibility of fertility exists, and so there seems to be no reason to retain the testes. Conversely, the risk for malignant transformation in such gonads is low before puberty, and patients with complete androgen insensitivity can undergo spontaneous breast development at puberty. At that

time, patients themselves can assent or consent to gonadectomy, which can usually be accomplished laparoscopically. This is of particular importance in genetic male patients with partial androgen insensitivity or incomplete defects of testosterone biosynthesis, because such patients may eventually desire a male gender role.

Patients with persistent müllerian duct syndrome have a reduced but still appreciable potential for fertility, and virilization is unaffected. Thus the testes should be removed only if they cannot be brought into the scrotum. Because the müllerian and wolffian structures are closely approximated in these patients, surgical excision of the uterus and fallopian tubes may result in ischemic and/or traumatic damage to the vas deferens and testes; thus salpingectomy and hysterectomy are indicated only in patients whose müllerian structures limit intrascrotal placement of the testes.

Space does not permit extensive discussion of surgical management of transgender adults; options for male-to-female transsexuals include genitoplasty and, for those who did not have hormonal management during adolescence (see the next section), breast augmentation, body contouring, and facial and/or laryngeal surgery to produce a more feminine appearance. Female-to-male transsexuals often desire breast reduction surgery or complete mastectomies.

Treatment of Transgender Individuals
Children and Adolescents

Transgender individuals should be treated by multidisciplinary teams that can provide psychosocial evaluation and support.[28-30] Prepubertal children do not require medical management. The majority of such children do not persist in their identification with the opposite sex, although many will be homosexual as adults. Persistently transgender children may develop significant gender dysphoria (distress at functioning in their natal gender) when puberty commences and are at increased risk for self-injury and suicide as adolescence progresses. If at all possible, such children should be allowed to function in the desired gender role. The current standard of care in many centers for children who have lived in a transgender role for at least 6 months is to delay pubertal progression until midadolescence (around 16 years old), with use of gonadotropin-releasing hormone (GnRH) agonists such as leuprolide depot injections or histrelin implants. This will prevent the development of secondary sexual characteristics that may be distressing to the patient and may present cosmetic barriers to functioning in the desired, non-natal gender. These include breast enlargement, widened hips, and gynecoid adipose distribution in natal females or penile enlargement, facial and body hair, laryngeal enlargement and deep voice, and prominent jaw in natal males.

Increasing evidence suggests that social and medical gender transition reduces the distress that accompanies the incongruence between one's natal sex and identified gender. When the patient is confirmed in the desired gender role (e.g., by living completely in that role for at least 1 year), treatment may begin with the appropriate sex hormones. In high doses, such treatment will itself suppress gonadotropin secretion, and the GnRH agonist may be discontinued. Female-to-male transsexuals can be treated with depot testosterone, and male-to-female transsexuals can be treated with parenteral forms of estradiol. Oral estrogen preparations should be avoided because they tend to increase production of clotting factors by the liver and may thus increase the risk for thromboembolism.

Adults

The medical treatment of transgender adults follows the same principles as for adolescents, except that because secondary sexual characteristics have already developed, prolonged treatment with GnRH agonists is unnecessary. However, continuing such treatment in male-to-female transsexuals permits use of much lower estradiol doses with a concomitant reduction in the risks associated with high-dose estrogen treatment. Nevertheless, cost represents a barrier to the long-term use of GnRH agonists.

Psychosocial Support

Families of patients with disorders of sexual development should be assessed for emotional health, initially by the pediatrician and/or pediatric endocrinologist.[31,32] Parents should be offered psychological counseling soon after the diagnosis is made. Intermittent assessment of family functioning may be a useful tool in predicting future problems. As children mature, they should repeatedly be informed about their condition by parents and physicians in a sensitive and age-appropriate manner. When psychotherapy is undertaken, medical and psychiatric caregivers should communicate with each other so both are aware of the patient's and family's status. Unfortunately, many locales lack mental health professionals with experience in counseling patients with disorders of sexual development and their families.

Although the psychosexual development of individuals with disorders of sexual development cannot be predicted with confidence, patients' families should receive anticipatory counseling. For example, counseling of parents of girls affected with congenital adrenal hyperplasia should address the high likelihood that such girls will exhibit tomboyish behavior and masculine play preferences. The endocrinologist and/or mental health professional (depending on inclination and experience) caring for adolescents with disorders of sexual development should address sexual orientation, both fantasized and actual.

For example, some women with congenital adrenal hyperplasia are most comfortable as homosexuals; such individuals should receive appropriate psychosocial support. Adult patients also should be made aware of relevant patient advocacy groups.

Grade A Reference

A1. Cintron D, Rodriguez-Gutierrez R, Serrano V, et al. Effect of estrogen replacement therapy on bone and cardiovascular outcomes in women with Turner syndrome: a systematic review and meta-analysis. *Endocrine.* 2017;55:366-375.

GENERAL REFERENCES

For the General References and other additional features, please visit Expert Consult at https://expertconsult.inkling.com.

221

THE TESTIS AND MALE HYPOGONADISM, INFERTILITY, AND SEXUAL DYSFUNCTION

RONALD S. SWERDLOFF AND CHRISTINA WANG

PHYSIOLOGY

The testis is a bifunctional organ serving as the site of sex steroid (i.e., testosterone) synthesis and sperm production in the male. Androgens and their metabolites (including estrogens) also act on nonreproductive organs and serve essential roles in muscles, adipose tissues, bones, metabolism, and brain functions.

The male reproductive axis consists of six main components: (1) extrahypothalamic central nervous system (CNS), (2) hypothalamus, (3) pituitary, (4) testes, (5) sex steroid–sensitive end organs, and (6) sites of androgen transport and metabolism (Fig. 221-1). The components of this system function in an integrated fashion to control the concentrations of circulating gonadal steroids required for normal male sexual development and function and for androgen- and estrogen-mediated effects on critical end organs. The reproductive axis is also responsible for normal germ cell development and maturation. Accessory sexual organs, including the epididymides, seminal vesicles, and prostate gland, are important for sperm maturation (epididymis) and seminal fluid production. An anatomically functional sperm transport and ejaculatory system are necessary to ensure male fertility.

Hypothalamic-Pituitary Function

The hypothalamus is responsible for the normal pulsatile secretion of gonadotropin-releasing hormone (GnRH) (Chapter 211). The pulsatile release of GnRH provides the signals for the timing of the release of luteinizing hormone (LH) and follicle-stimulating hormone (FSH), which occurs every 60 to 90 minutes in men. The secretion of GnRH is regulated mainly by Kisspeptin/neurokinin B/dynorphin (KNDy) neurons in the hypothalamus and by circulating levels of sex steroids and peptide hormones such as prolactin and leptin (Chapter 210). Testosterone or its metabolic products (i.e., estradiol and dihydrotestosterone [DHT]) inhibit the secretion and release of GnRH, LH, and FSH. Prolactin is also a potent inhibitor of GnRH secretion.

Testosterone

The testis is a complex organ consisting of (1) seminiferous tubules containing Sertoli cells and germ cells and (2) the interstitium, which contains the steroid-secreting (Leydig) cells. Leydig cells synthesize steroid hormones under the regulation of LH. The LH receptors on the cell surface of the Leydig cells lead to G protein–, adenyl cyclase–, and cyclic adenosine monophosphate–mediated activation of steroid biosynthesis.

Testosterone is the principal male hormone secreted by the testes; approximately 5 to 10 mg/day is produced in adult men. Testosterone synthesis occurs in the human testes through either the Δ^4 or the predominant Δ^5 pathway. The enzymatic rate-limiting steps in the process are the LH-inducible steroid acute regulatory (StAR) protein and translocator protein that converts cholesterol to pregnenolone by the cholesterol side-chain cleavage enzyme P450SCC (Fig. 221-2).

Testosterone circulates mainly bound to two plasma proteins: sex hormone–binding globulin (SHBG) and albumin. In young adult men, approximately 54% of testosterone is bound to albumin, 44% is bound to SHBG, and 2 to 3% is unbound. Bioavailable testosterone refers to the sum of albumin-bound and free testosterone and is measured by separating SHBG-bound testosterone from total testosterone. Serum SHBG levels are increased in hyperestrogenic states, hyperthyroidism, aging, phenytoin treatment, anorexia nervosa, and prolonged stress. SHBG levels are lowered in hyperandrogenic states

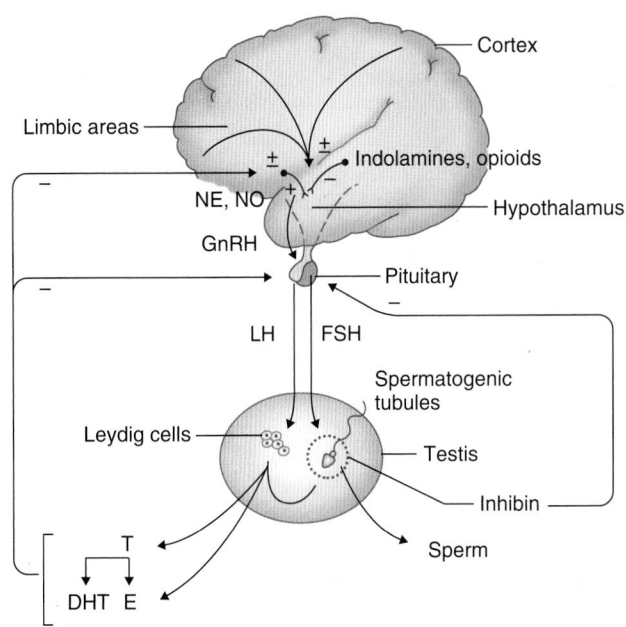

FIGURE 221-1. The hypothalamic-pituitary-gonadal axis in the male. DHT = dihydrotestosterone; E = estrogen; FSH = follicle-stimulating hormone; GnRH = gonadotropin-releasing hormone; LH = luteinizing hormone; NE = norepinephrine; NO = nitric oxide; T = testosterone.

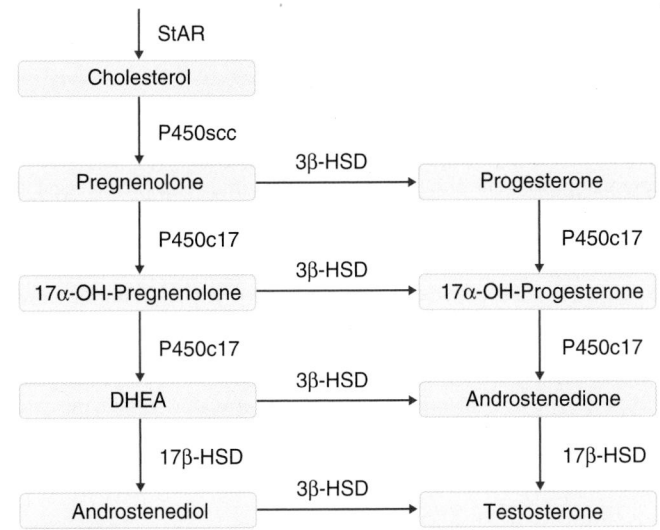

FIGURE 221-2. The steroid acute regulatory (*StAR*) protein mobilizes cholesterol from cellular stores to the mitochondria. Intratesticular steroidogenic pathways for the synthesis of testosterone. Although both the Δ^5 (*left*) and Δ^4 (*right*) pathways exist, the Δ^5 pathway predominates in the testis. DHEA = dehydroepiandrosterone; HSD = hydroxysteroid dehydrogenase.

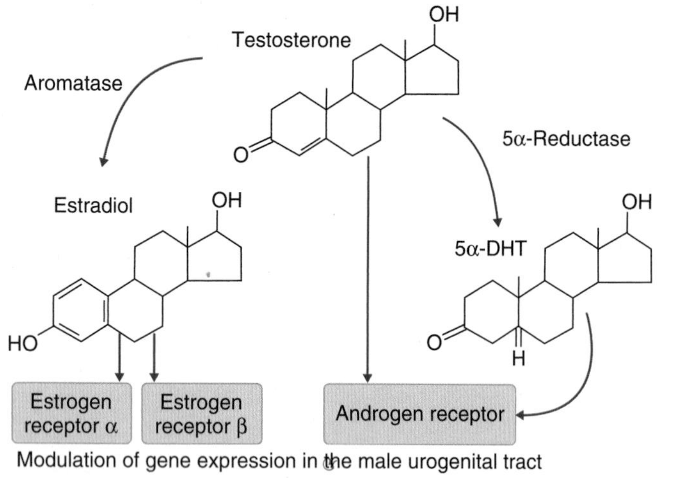

FIGURE 221-3. Testosterone action is mediated directly (androgen receptor), after conversion to estradiol (estrogen receptor α or β), or after conversion to dihydrotestosterone (DHT; androgen receptor). (From Kuiper GCJM, Carlquist M, Gustafsson JA. Estrogen is a male and female hormone. *Sci Med.* 1998;5:36-45.)

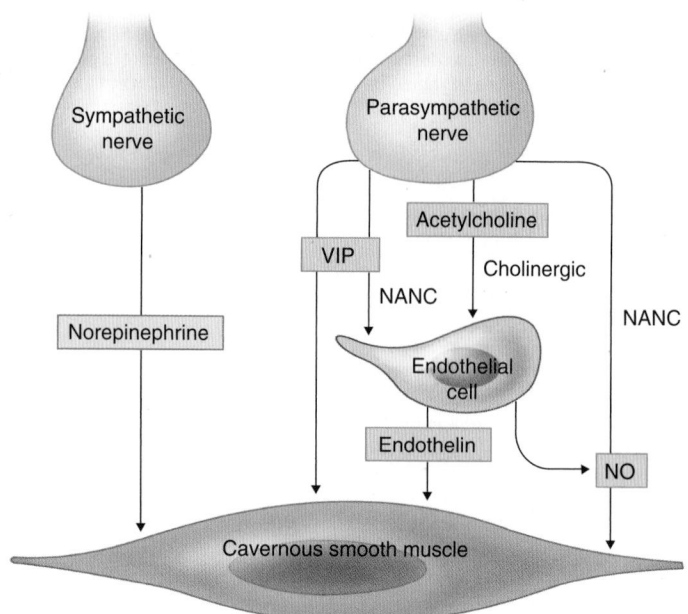

FIGURE 221-4. The interaction among cholinergic, adrenergic, and nonadrenergic, noncholinergic (*NANC*) neuronal pathways and their contribution to penile smooth muscle contraction and dilation (*arrows*). NO = nitric oxide; VIP = vasoactive intestinal polypeptide. (From Lue TF. Physiology of penile erection and pathophysiology of erectile dysfunction and priapism. In: Walsh P, Retick A, Vaughn E, Wein A, eds. *Campbell's Urology,* 7th ed. Philadelphia: WB Saunders; 1998:1164.)

(endogenous and exogenous as in androgen treatment), obesity, acromegaly, and hypothyroidism. In most instances, measurement of serum total testosterone provides biochemical support for the diagnosis of testosterone deficiency. In conditions with abnormal SHBG levels, however, the total testosterone measurement may be misleading, and measurement of non–SHBG-bound testosterone may allow better interpretation of the active testosterone levels. This can be done by direct measurement of free testosterone by the equilibrium dialysis method, measurement of bioavailable testosterone, or calculation of the free testosterone by formulae requiring the serum testosterone and SHBG concentrations. Most guidelines recommend against measurement of free testosterone by a "direct" or analogue displacement method because of lack of accuracy traceable to a standard.[1]

Testosterone exerts its effects either through direct action or after conversion to DHT by two separate 5α-reductase isozymes (1 and 2) or to estradiol by the aromatase enzyme (Fig. 221-3). Both testosterone and DHT bind efficiently to the androgen receptor. Different tissues have coactivators or coinhibitors that modify the action of the androgen-receptor complex, providing tissue selectivity and amplification. Testosterone also can serve as a precursor for estradiol, notably in bone and adipose tissues. After conversion, estrogen binds the estrogen receptors (α or β) to induce its effects. Various end organs differ in their 5α-reductase isoenzyme and aromatase concentrations or activity. Congenital and acquired defects in these two enzymes, as well as in the estrogen and androgen receptors, result in distinct syndromes with characteristic phenotypes that are experiments in nature and provide understanding of the actions of specific receptors and enzyme activities (Chapter 220).

Spermatogenesis

The spermatogenic compartment of the testis consists of the Sertoli and germ cells that are intimately interactive with the interstitial compartment. The Sertoli cells bridge the entire space between the basement membrane and the lumen of the tubules. They are the target of androgenic and FSH stimulation of spermatogenesis and also the source of a multitude of paracrine regulators of spermatogenesis (e.g., inhibin, activin, growth factors, cytokines).

Germ cell development and maturation depend on the proper hormonal (FSH) and paracrine (testosterone) milieu. Both testosterone and FSH stimulate progression of spermatogonia to mature spermatozoa, limit the amount of germ cell death (apoptosis), and regulate sperm release from the germinal epithelium.

After spermatogenesis is completed, mature spermatozoa are released into the excretory system and travel through the rete testes and epididymis, where they become functionally mature and acquire fertilizing capacity before traversing the vas deferens. The seminal fluid gains constituents from the seminal vesicles, prostate, and bulbourethral glands before ejaculation.

Sexual Function and Erectile Physiology

Sexual function in men requires normal sexual desire (libido) and erectile, ejaculatory, and orgasmic capacity. The process is complex, involving cognitive, sensory, hormonal, autonomic neuronal, and penile vascular integrative actions for normal function. Defects can occur at multiple levels.

The brain is the integrative center of the sexual response system. It processes sensory input and hormonal signals to create the hypothalamic neuronal message that traverses the spinal cord to the T9-12 sympathetic and sacral parasympathetic outflow tracts. The nonadrenergic, noncholinergic autonomic plexus nerves initiate vasodilation of the cavernosal arterial and corpora cavernosal sinusoids of the penis through the release of local vasodilators (e.g., nitric oxide and vasoactive intestinal peptide) from the vascular endothelium and the sinusoidal smooth muscle cells of the sinusoids (Fig. 221-4). Nitric oxide produces smooth muscle dilation by the generation of cyclic guanosine monophosphate (cGMP) and the modification of calcium flux. The neurogenic mechanisms leading to vasodilation of the cavernosal arterioles and sinusoids lead to a rapid increase in penile blood flow and expansion of the vascular channels; this, in turn, inhibits venous return through compression of the venous channels against the tunica albuginea and limits venous drainage.

Testosterone's primary effect on erectile function is to enhance libido. Testosterone also increases penile nitric oxide synthase activity and enhances smooth muscle cell growth. Sexual desire and fantasy are highly sensitive to testosterone, explaining the preservation of erectile capacity in many men with partial androgen deficiency.

Physiology in Development and Aging
Reproductive Axis Development during Childhood and Puberty
Adrenarche and Puberty

Adrenarche occurs at approximately 7 or 8 years of age when the zona reticularis of the adrenal gland undergoes maturation and secretes adrenal androgens including androstenedione, dehydroepiandrosterone (DHEA), and DHEA sulfate (DHEA-S). The process is under the control of adrenocorticotropic hormone, not LH or FSH. Androstenedione and DHEA are androgenic prehormones, and the prepubertal growth spurt and development of pubic and axillary hair, are mediated by the conversion of these precursors to testosterone and DHT in peripheral tissues.

Initiation of puberty is determined by an increase in the pulsatile pattern of hypothalamic GnRH secretion. The secretory pulses of GnRH are synchronized by increased kisspeptin and neurokinin B/dynorphin (KNDy) secretion from the hypothalamic neurons. This is marked by nocturnal bursts of LH secretion. As puberty progresses, feedback sensitivity of the hypothalamus and pituitary to circulating steroids lessens, thus increasing the secretion of gonadotropins. The increasing concentrations of intratesticular testosterone and circulating FSH stimulate the Sertoli cell to produce factors leading to the maturation of spermatogenesis. As spermatogenesis advances, the first

TABLE 221-1 PUBERTAL STAGES IN BOYS		
STAGE/AGE (YEARS)	**PUBIC HAIR**	**GENITAL**
I	Absence of pubic hair	Childlike penis, testes, and scrotum (testis 5.0 ± 3.6 cm³)
II 11.7 ± 1.3	Sparse, lightly pigmented hair mainly at base of penis	Scrotum enlarged with early rugation and pigmentation; testes begin to enlarge (6.7 ± 3.5 cm³)
III 13.2 ± 0.8	Hair becomes coarse, darker, more curled, and more extensive	Penis has grown in length and diameter; testes now 14.7±6.3 cm³; scrotum more rugated
IV 14.7 ± 1.1	Hair adult in quality, but distribution does not include medial aspect of thighs	Penis further enlarged, with development of glans; scrotum and testes (20.1 ± 6.2 cm³) further enlarged
V 15.5 ± 0.7	Hair is adult and extends to thighs	Penis and scrotum fully adult; testes 29.3 ± 9.1 cm³

Modified from Marshall WA, Tanner JM. Variation in pattern of pubertal changes in boys. *Arch Dis Child.* 1970;45:13-23. Daniel WA Jr, Feinstein RA. Howard-Peebles P et al. Testicular volumes of adolescents. *J Pediatrics.* 1982: 101:1010-2

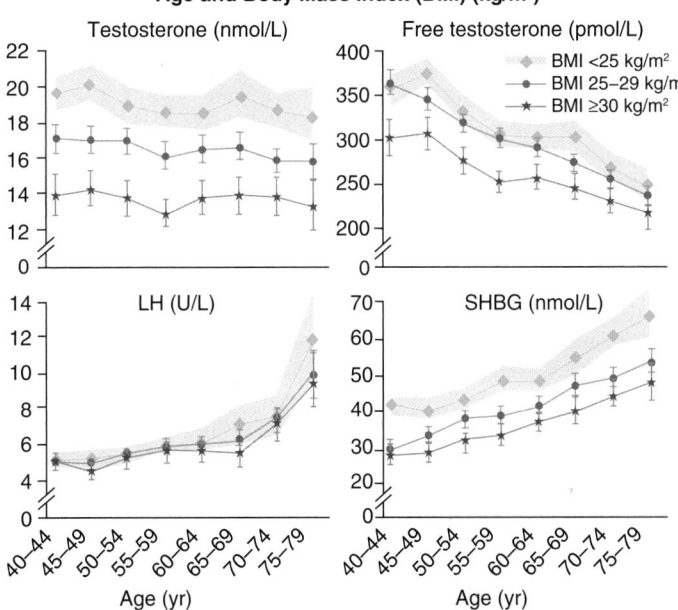

FIGURE 221-5. Relationship between age, BMI, and hormones. The cohort was stratified according to BMI into three groups: nonobese (BMI < 25 kg/m²), overweight (BMI 25 to 30 kg/m²), and obese (BMI > 30 kg/m²). Mean (95% CI in shaded area and vertical lines) total and free T and SHBG were significantly lower in the overweight and obese at all ages, compared with nonobese. The total T and SHBG age trends in the three BMI categories were similar (indicating no interaction between BMI and age); the free T age trend in the obese group was less steep than in the other two groups (indicating an interaction between BMI and age). Mean LH was not significantly different among the three groups at the median age of 60 years. LH was higher in the older than 70 years nonobese, compared with the overweight and obese groups, due to a negative BMI-age interaction. (Wu FC, Tajar A, Pye SR, et al. Hypothalamic-pituitary-testicular axis disruptions in older men are differentially linked to age and modifiable risk factors: the European Male Aging Study. *J Clin Endocrinol Metab.* 2008;93:2737-2745).

sign of puberty is marked by testes increasing in size from 3 to 5 mL at the outset of puberty to 15 to 35 mL in adulthood. The majority of the extratesticular end-organ events of puberty are secondary to the increased testosterone and its metabolic products (DHT and estradiol) (Table 221-1). The penis and scrotum grow and become pigmented. There is a progressive increase in facial, axillary, chest, abdominal, thigh, and pubic hair; frontal scalp hair regresses, and the voice deepens. Genital and sexual hair development and temporal scalp hair regression require DHT. The increased levels of sex steroids result in closure of the epiphysis and achievement of adult height.

Aberrations of Timing of Puberty

Delayed puberty, more common in boys than in girls, is usually assigned to boys when sexual development has not begun by age 14 years. The majority of boys with delayed development have a functional hypothalamic-pituitary disorder and family history of delayed puberty; eventually they attain full sexual maturation. Once initiated, puberty is normally completed within 4.5 years. There are many other causes of delayed puberty including genetics, drugs, chronic illnesses, and diseases of the hypothalamus and pituitary. Careful documentation of changing physical findings and measurement of serum LH, FSH, and testosterone concentrations may provide valuable clues to the beginning of puberty. An increase in testicular size to more than 3 mL usually heralds other signs of pubertal onset. Inquiring and testing for hyposmia or anosmia and other midline defects may indicate a common variant of congenital hypogonadotropic hypogonadism (Kallmann syndrome). The decision to institute early treatment depends on the perceived degree of psychological stress associated with the maturational delay. The major concern is early fusion of the epiphyses induced by treatment with testosterone, which compromises optimal height; however, with judicious dosing and monitoring of bone age, this is unusual. In adolescent boys with delayed puberty and low levels of gonadotropins, periodic withdrawal of treatment is used to determine whether spontaneous puberty has occurred. Many adult men diagnosed with and treated as adolescents for a presumed diagnosis of hypogonadotropic hypogonadism achieve normal reproductive function when they discontinue therapy.

Precocious puberty in boys is defined as the onset of pubertal (secondary sexual characteristics) development before 9 years of age. Sexual precocity can be subcategorized as central or true isosexual precocious puberty and pseudo–precocious (peripheral) puberty. Central or true precocious puberty is associated with increases in GnRH-stimulated LH and FSH secretion (hypothalamic-pituitary origin), whereas pseudo–precocious puberty is independent of GnRH stimulation of LH and FSH secretion. Central precocious puberty in boys is often associated with CNS disease (two thirds of boys), including hypothalamic tumors, cysts, inflammatory conditions, and seizure disorders. Diagnostic findings include sexual precocity, inappropriately elevated serum LH levels, and associated elevations of testosterone. Magnetic resonance imaging can localize most lesions. Another cause of central precocious puberty is human chorionic gonadotropin secretory germinomas (testicular,

hepatic, hypothalamic, or pineal tumors). Pseudo–precocious puberty is characterized by increased testosterone with suppressed LH. Causes of pseudo–precocious puberty include congenital virilizing adrenal hyperplasia, testicular testosterone-secreting neoplasms, and constitutively active LH receptor mutations; the latter condition results in uncontrolled testosterone secretion (testotoxicosis). Treatment of true precocious puberty is removal or correction (with surgery or radiation therapy) of the CNS lesion, if possible, and treatment with GnRH analogues to temporarily suppress LH and FSH secretion. Treatment of pseudo–precocious puberty depends on the cause but includes glucocorticoids for congenital virilizing adrenal hyperplasia and ketoconazole (to suppress steroidogenesis), with or without antiandrogens (e.g., spironolactone, flutamide).

Male Senescence: Decreased Testosterone and Other Anabolic Hormones

Testosterone Deficiency in the Elderly

Blood concentrations of testosterone and androgen prehormones (e.g., DHEA, DHEA-S) are significantly lower in older men than in young adult men.[2] Both total and free serum testosterone levels progressively decrease with aging (Fig. 221-5). The percentage decline in serum testosterone has been estimated as high as 1 to 2% per year although more recent assessments in the European Male Aging Study show a more gradual slope.[3] Serum SHBG levels also rise with age in men, resulting in a higher percentage of circulating testosterone that is tightly bound and thus a more steep decline of free testosterone with aging. Obesity lowers serum testosterone and SHBG and affects the decline of testosterone and free testosterone with age (Fig. 221-5). In men between 40 and 70 years of age the crude prevalence rate of symptomatic testosterone deficiency has been estimated to be approximately 2 to 6%. Low testosterone levels are associated with comorbidities such as obesity, metabolic syndrome, chronic drug use (e.g., opioids), and the commonest symptoms associated with low total or free testosterone in older men are sexual.

Many of the effects of low testosterone levels in aging men are similar to those observed in younger hypogonadal men. These include decreases in libido, erectile function, muscle mass, muscle strength, bone mass, and impaired

TABLE 221-2   CAUSES OF PRIMARY TESTICULAR FAILURE AND END-ORGAN RESISTANCE

Congenital disorders
   Chromosome disorders
   Klinefelter and related syndromes (e.g., XXY, XXY/XY, XYY, XX males)
   Testosterone biosynthetic enzyme defects
   Myotonic dystrophy
Developmental disorders
   Prenatal diethylstilbestrol syndrome
   Cryptorchidism
Acquired defects
   Orchitis
   Mumps and other viruses
   Granulomatous disease (e.g., tuberculosis, leprosy)
   Human immunodeficiency virus infection
   Infiltrative disease (e.g., hemochromatosis, amyloidosis)
   Surgical, traumatic injuries, torsion of testis
   Irradiation
Toxins (e.g., alcohol, fungicides, insecticides, heavy metals, cottonseed oil, DDT, other environmental "endocrine disruptors")
Drugs
   Cytotoxic agents
   Inhibitors of testosterone synthesis and antiandrogens (e.g., ketoconazole, cimetidine, flutamide, cyproterone, spironolactone)
   Ethanol, opioids, other recreational drugs
Autoimmune testicular failure
   Isolated
   Associated with other organ-specific disorders (e.g., Addison disease, Hashimoto thyroiditis, insulin-dependent diabetes)
Androgen resistance syndromes
5α-Reductase deficiency
Systemic diseases* (e.g., cirrhosis, chronic renal failure, sickle cell disease, acquired immunodeficiency syndrome, amyloidosis)
Aging*

*Systemic diseases and aging produce a mixed pattern of testicular and hypothalamic-pituitary dysfunction.

TABLE 221-3   CAUSES OF HYPOGONADOTROPIC HYPOGONADISM

IDIOPATHIC OR CONGENITAL

Isolated deficiency of gonadotropin-releasing hormone
   With anosmia (Kallmann syndrome)
   With other abnormalities (Prader-Willi syndrome, Laurence-Moon-Biedl syndrome, basal encephalocele)
Partial deficiency of gonadotropin-releasing hormone (fertile eunuch syndrome)
Multiple hypothalamic and pituitary hormone deficiency
Pituitary hypoplasia or aplasia

ACQUIRED

Traumatic brain injury, after surgery or irradiation
Neoplastic
Pituitary adenoma (prolactinoma, other functional and nonfunctional tumors)
Craniopharyngioma, germinoma, glioma, leukemia, lymphoma
Pituitary infarction, carotid aneurysm
Infiltrative and infectious diseases of hypothalamus and pituitary (sarcoidosis, tuberculosis, coccidioidomycosis, histoplasmosis, syphilis, abscess, histiocytosis X, hemochromatosis)
Autoimmune hypophysitis
Aging and systemic diseases*
Obesity
Malnutrition
Anorexia nervosa, starvation, renal failure, liver failure
Exogenous hormones and drugs
   Antiandrogens, estrogens and antiestrogens, progestogens, glucocorticoids, cimetidine, spironolactone, digoxin, drug-induced hyperprolactinemia (metoclopramide, tranquilizers, antihypertensives)

*Aging and systemic diseases produce a mixed pattern of central and testicular dysfunction.

---

mood and sense of well-being. Older men have increased body fat, particularly visceral fat. There is considerable controversy as to whether age-associated hypogonadism is a pathological or physiological condition.

Deficiency of Adrenal Androgen in Older Men

A marked decline in the circulating levels of adrenal androgens, especially DHEA and DHEA-S, has been recognized in elderly men and women. Serum levels of DHEA and DHEA-S peak at approximately the third decade of life and then decline at about 2% per year, resulting in levels 10 to 20% of baseline by 80 years of age. DHEA is a precursor to androgens such as testosterone and DHT.

MALE HYPOGONADISM

DEFINITION

Hypogonadism (androgen deficiency) is diagnosed in men with consistent symptoms and signs and unequivocally low circulating levels of testosterone. Most men with more severe androgen deficiency have very low intratesticular testosterone concentrations and are infertile. Primary hypogonadism indicates that the abnormality originates in the testis; it is characterized by increased serum LH and FSH levels. Secondary hypogonadism indicates a defect at the hypothalamus or pituitary, resulting in decreased gonadotropins (LH, FSH, or both).[4] Combined primary and secondary hypogonadism occurs in aging and in a number of systemic diseases, such as alcoholism, liver disease, metabolic syndrome, type 2 diabetes mellitus, human immunodeficiency virus (HIV) infection, hemochromatosis, and sickle cell disease. Obesity leads to low total and free testosterone levels. Greater decreases are seen in the total testosterone level because obesity not only decreases testosterone secretion but also lowers SHBG levels. Decreased androgen action with normal or elevated testosterone levels, mimicking androgen deficiency, may occur in patients with androgen receptor defects (androgen resistance), post-receptor signaling abnormalities, and inability to convert testosterone to the active metabolite DHT (5α-reductase abnormalities).

Many of the causes of primary and secondary hypogonadism are listed in Tables 221-2 and 221-3 (see also Chapter 220).

Primary Testicular Hypogonadism

Primary hypogonadism refers to a condition of androgen deficiency with or without infertility in which the pathologic process lies at the testis level. A list of common causes is given in Table 221-2.

CONGENITAL DEFECTS

The commonest congenital defect is due to chromosomal abnormalities (Klinefelter syndrome), and other causes are listed in Table 221-2 and described in Chapter 220.

ACQUIRED DEFECTS

Mumps, Orchitis, Leprosy, Human Immunodeficiency Virus Infection, and Hemochromatosis

After puberty, mumps (Chapter 345) is associated with clinical orchitis in 25% of cases, and 60% of those affected become infertile. During acute orchitis, the testes are inflamed, painful, and swollen. This is followed by a gradual decrease in size. The testes may return to normal size and function, or they may atrophy. Spermatogenic defects occur more often and earlier than Leydig cell dysfunction. Thus, patients with post-orchitic infertility may have normal testosterone and LH levels with increased serum FSH levels. Over time, elevations in LH and lower serum testosterone levels may appear. Leprosy (Chapter 310) also may cause orchitis and gonadal insufficiency. HIV infection is often associated with hypogonadism, which can be either hypogonadotropic or hypergonadotropic. Hemochromatosis (Chapter 201) may affect the hypothalamus-pituitary, as well as act directly on the testis.

Trauma

The exposed position of the testes in the scrotum makes them particularly susceptible to injury. Surgical injury during scrotal surgery for hernia, varicocele, and vasectomy can result in permanent testicular damage.

Irradiation

Exposure of the testes to irradiation in the treatment of malignant diseases produces testicular germ cell, and less commonly, Leydig cell damage.

DRUGS AND TOXINS

Chemotherapy, in particular alkylating agents, such as cyclophosphamide and busulfan, frequently leads to irreversible germ cell damage. Heavy metals (lead, cadmium) and cottonseed oil (gossypol) cause damage to the germ cells. Leydig cells are relatively less susceptible to most chemotherapeutic drugs than are Sertoli and germ cells. Some medications may interfere with testosterone biosynthesis (e.g., ketoconazole, spironolactone) or action (e.g., cyproterone, flutamide). Ethanol, independent of its role in causing liver disease, inhibits testosterone biosynthesis. Marijuana, heroin, methadone, medroxyprogesterone acetate, other progestins, and estrogens lower testosterone, mainly by decreasing LH. Medical treatment with androgens such as testosterone, DHT, and synthetic anabolic steroids or their illicit use (e.g., in athletes, bodybuilders) lowers serum LH and FSH and sperm counts. Serum testosterone levels are low after the use of DHT and synthetic anabolic agents. Environmental toxins such as fungicides and insecticides (e.g., DBCP, metabolites of DDT, vinclozolin) and byproducts of the plastics industry (e.g., phthalates, bisphenol A) are called "endocrine disruptors" because these chemicals may have either weak estrogenic or antiandrogenic effects and have been shown to cause testicular dysgenesis in male offspring when administered in large doses to pregnant female rodents. Data linking "endocrine disruptors" to male reproductive dysfunction in humans are principally associations studies and do not prove causality.[5]

AUTOIMMUNE TESTICULAR FAILURE
Antibodies against the microsomal fraction of the Leydig cells may occur either as an isolated disorder or as part of a multiglandular disorder (Chapter 218) involving, to variable degrees, the thyroid, pituitary, adrenals, pancreas, and other organs.

ANDROGEN RESISTANCE (ANDROGEN-SENSITIVE END-ORGAN DEFICIENCY)
Certain conditions have clinical phenotypes mimicking testosterone deficiency in the absence of lowered testosterone levels. These androgen-resistant states may be drug-induced (antiandrogens) or genetic defects in the androgen receptor, congenital or acquired post–androgen receptor signaling defects, or 5α-reductase deficiency (Chapter 220).

Hypogonadism Associated with Systemic Diseases

Abnormalities of the hypothalamic-pituitary-testicular axis occur in a number of systemic diseases, including liver failure, renal failure, severe malnutrition, sickle cell anemia, advanced malignant disease, severe obesity, metabolic syndrome, type 2 diabetes, cystic fibrosis, and amyloidosis, as well as in those on chronic hemodialysis. The effects of cirrhosis of the liver on testicular function are complex and may be either independent of or associated with the direct toxic effects of the continued use of alcohol. Gynecomastia, testicular atrophy, and impotence are concomitant signs of cirrhosis. Decreased spermatogenesis with peritubular fibrosis occurs in 50% of cases. Estradiol levels are usually elevated. This results in an increased ratio of serum estradiol to testosterone, often associated with gynecomastia. In sickle cell anemia and thalassemia major, boys may have impaired sexual maturation, and men are often infertile. Diabetes and obesity are two major factors in hypogonadism.[6] Emerging data show that type 2 diabetes is associated with low blood testosterone levels mainly as a result of hypothalamic-pituitary dysfunction; the decrease in serum testosterone correlates with the degree of hyperglycemia.

Secondary Gonadal Insufficiency (Hypogonadotropic Hypogonadism)
CONGENITAL HYPOGONADOTROPIC HYPOGONADISM
Hypogonadotropic hypogonadism represents a deficiency in the secretion of gonadotropins (LH and FSH) because of an intrinsic or functional abnormality in the hypothalamus or pituitary glands (see earlier and Chapter 220). Abnormalities of kisspeptin/neurokinin B/dynorphin (KNDy) release by hypothalamic neurons and receptor deficiencies has emerged as a major cause of GnRH deficiency. Such disorders result in secondary Leydig cell dysfunction (see Table 221-3). The clinical manifestations depend on the age of the patient at the onset of the disorder.

ACQUIRED HYPOGONADOTROPIC DISORDERS AND FUNCTIONAL DISORDERS
Anorexia Nervosa and Weight Loss
Anorexia nervosa (Chapter 206) and weight loss are examples of functional defects resulting in low serum testosterone levels. Men and women with anorexia nervosa present with manifestations of hypogonadotropic hypogonadism. Starvation also may reduce gonadotropic secretion. Strenuous exercise has minimal effects on testicular function in men.

Stress and Illness
Severe stress (e.g., surgery, trauma) and systemic illness also lower gonadotropin and testosterone levels. Organic hypothalamic-pituitary disorders include neoplastic, granulomatous, infiltrative, and post-traumatic lesions in the region of the hypothalamus and pituitary.

Pituitary Tumors
Prolactinomas manifest differently in men than in women (Chapter 211). In men, these tumors are usually large (>1 cm in diameter; macroadenomas) by the time they are detected. Male patients with prolactin-secreting macroadenomas usually present with hypogonadism, erectile dysfunction, and visual manifestations from suprasellar extension. In small tumors, hypogonadotropic hypogonadism may be due to suppressive effects on GnRH described earlier, but in large tumors, it also may be due to a mass effect damaging the non-neoplastic gonadotrophs.

Large non–prolactin-secreting pituitary tumors (growth hormone, adrenocorticotropic hormone, glycopeptide, and null cell) also may produce gonadotropin insufficiency from damage to the adjacent normal pituitary gland (Chapter 211), resulting in decreased serum LH and testosterone levels.

CLINICAL MANIFESTATIONS AND DIAGNOSIS OF HYPOGONADISM
The diagnosis is based on clinical symptoms and signs and a reduced serum testosterone level. The reference range of serum total testosterone in a young adult male population varies across different laboratories and populations. The harmonized normal range in a healthy nonobese population of European and American men from 4 large cohort studies, 19 to 39 years, is 264 to 916 ng/dL.

History
The medical history should focus on testicular descent, pubertal development, shaving frequency, changes in body hair, and present and past systemic illnesses. A complete sexual history includes changes in libido, erectile and ejaculatory functions, frequency of masturbation, coital activity, and fertility (including that of present and previous partners). Information should be obtained on previous orchitis, sinopulmonary complaints, sexually transmitted diseases, human immunodeficiency virus (HIV) status, genitourinary infections, and previous surgical procedures that might affect the reproductive tract (e.g., vasectomy, hernia repair, prostatectomy, varicocele ligation). Social history includes tobacco and alcohol intake. Medication and self-prescribed drug history includes recreational drugs; opioids; anabolic steroids; glucocorticoid use; 5α-reductase inhibitors; and psychiatric, antihypertensive, antiandrogenic, cytotoxic, and alternative medicine therapies; environmental toxins; and exposure to heat (including saunas and Jacuzzis) and irradiation.

Physical Examination
The general physical examination is supplemented by height and span measurements; characterization of facial, pubic, and body hair distribution; presence of acne and facial wrinkling; breast examination for gynecomastia; assessment of muscle mass and adiposity; measurement of penile length and urethral meatus localization; digital rectal prostate examination; and visual field assessment if secondary hypogonadism is suspected. The scrotal examination should include an assessment of midline fusion (e.g., bifid scrotum, hypospadias); testicular size and consistency; presence of intratesticular masses; abnormalities of the epididymis; bilateral presence of vas deferens; and varicoceles, hydroceles, or hernias. Normal testicular size ranges from 3.6 to 5.5 cm in length, 2.1 to 3.2 cm in width, and 15 to 35 mL in volume in white and black men. Asian men have a slightly smaller mean testicular size. A decrease in testicular volume usually implies decreased spermatogenic cells because the seminiferous tubules account for more than 80% of testicular volume.

Laboratory Studies
Because there is a strong diurnal rhythm in testosterone secretion in young men (highest in the morning), testosterone, LH, and FSH are routinely determined from morning blood samples. There is a broad range of reference values of these hormones due partly to measurement variability but also influenced by the selection criteria for the reference population. Most hospital laboratories have used immunoassay methods to measure serum testosterone, which may lack precision at low serum testosterone levels. Recent studies suggest that methods using liquid or gas chromatography and mass spectrometry give more accurate results even at very low serum testosterone levels. The U.S.

Centers for Disease Control (CDC) has developed an external system to harmonize laboratory measurements to a validated standard method.

Total testosterone measurements may be misleading indicators of Leydig cell secretory status in conditions in which SHBG levels are abnormal (see earlier section). In these circumstances, a measurement of free testosterone (by an equilibrium dialysis method), bioavailable testosterone (consisting of free plus albumin bound), or calculated free testosterone (by total testosterone and SHBG measurements) may be useful.

Elevated LH and FSH levels distinguish primary from secondary hypogonadism (both have low serum testosterone levels), but many older men with low serum testosterone levels may have a normal LH concentration. Serum prolactin levels should be measured in all low testosterone, low LH cases (hypogonadotropic hypogonadism) and in men with known pituitary mass lesions, or galactorrhea. DHT is measured in cases of abnormal differentiation of the genitalia and when 5α-reductase deficiency is suspected. Serum estradiol should be measured in cases of gynecomastia. Assessment of other testosterone precursors and products may be required in special circumstances, including suspected congenital enzyme defects. The semen analysis is the "cornerstone" of the laboratory examination for male infertility.

The following rules on measurement of serum testosterone apply to most young and middle-aged men thought to have hypogonadism. If a morning serum total testosterone level is repeatedly below 230 ng/dL (8 nmol/L), and he has symptoms or signs compatible with low testosterone state, the patient is probably hypogonadal, and testosterone replacement is indicated. If the serum testosterone level is between 230 and 320 ng/dL with normal serum LH levels, the patient may or may not be clinically hypogonadal and androgen replacement may not improve the symptoms (e.g., sexual dysfunction). Thus, when serum total testosterone is borderline and LH is not increased, one of the measurements of bioactive testosterone is indicated (e.g., free testosterone). The guidelines for men older than 60 years are less certain. Because SHBG levels are often increased, total testosterone levels may overestimate the biologically active forms. A serum total testosterone level above 350 to 400 ng/dL indicates that hypogonadism is very unlikely to be the cause of the symptoms, and the clinician should look for other etiologies for the symptoms.

TREATMENT   Rx

Indications

The main medical indication for androgen replacement therapy is male hypogonadism (Table 221-4). In approximately 10% of men with idiopathic hypogonadism reversed by testosterone therapy, the reversal is sustained after therapy is stopped. This suggests that some patients with low serum testosterone may have a transient cause of the deficiency.

Beneficial effects of testosterone replacement have been demonstrated in elderly men with relatively low serum testosterone levels. Testosterone replacement therapy (up to 3 years) decreases fat mass, increases lean body mass, improves strength, and increases bone mineral density in older men.[A1] Treatment with testosterone gel sufficient to raise serum testosterone to the mid-normal young male range improves sexual activity libido, erectile function, and mood,[A2][A3] corrects unexplained anemia,[A4] and increases bone mineral density and strength.[A5] The effect on physical activity is modest at best, and no improvement is seen in cognition.[A6] Testosterone-treated men have significantly increased noncalcified plaque volume by coronary computed tomographic angiography,[A7] but cardiovascular adverse events were not increased over the less than 3 year or so duration of the various randomized trials.[A8] In cohort studies with longer-duration follow-up, however, the data on cardiovascular risk are less clear.[7-9] Testosterone replacement therapy does not appear to affect lower urinary tract symptoms.[A9]

At present, testosterone treatment is not recommended for older men with or suspected of having prostate cancer, moderate-to-severe heart failure, severe uncorrected sleep apnea, or high red blood cell mass.[10-12] A digital rectal examination should be performed, prostate-specific antigen level determined, and symptoms of severe urinary tract obstruction evaluated before testosterone treatment is instituted.

In older men with DHEA deficiency, oral administration of DHEA raises serum DHEA and DHEA-S concentrations to the levels found in young men. However, serum testosterone levels do not change, and patients have not reported beneficial effects on quality of life, sexual function, mood, body composition, or exercise capacity.[A10]

Absolute contraindications to androgen replacement therapy include carcinoma of the prostate and the male breast. Androgens should be used with caution in older men with an enlarged prostate and urinary symptoms, elevated hematocrit, and sleep-related breathing disorders.

Testosterone Delivery Systems

The various methods of delivering testosterone treatment are shown in Table 221-5.

Testosterone esters, such as testosterone enanthate (or cypionate) injections, are widely used in the United States and throughout the world. The recommended dose is 150 to 200 mg administered intramuscularly once every 2 to 3 weeks. More recent studies showed that these medium long–acting testosterone esters can be administered by subcutaneous (SC) injections weekly, producing more stable testosterone levels compared to intramuscular injections. Testosterone undecanoate injections, 750 mg administered every 10 weeks or 1000 mg every 12 weeks, are the preferred testosterone replacement therapy in many parts of the world but not in the United States because of the regulatory requirement of an observation period for about 30 minutes after injection for cough episodes.

Modified 17α-alkylated androgens (methyl testosterone and many anabolic steroids), which are available in oral preparations, are not recommended as androgen replacement. These agents may lead to abnormalities in liver function, marked decreases in high-density lipoprotein cholesterol, and increases in total cholesterol levels compared with the testosterone esters. Oral testosterone undecanoate capsules have recently been approved in the United States. The capsules, containing from 158 to 396 mg testosterone undecanoate in a self-emulsifying drug delivery system, have to be taken twice a day with food. Transbuccal delivery of testosterone by mucoadhesive tablets (30 mg applied twice daily) results in physiologic-range testosterone levels through direct absorption into the systemic circulation, thus avoiding first-pass effects on the liver. The tablets may be dislodged from the buccal mucous membrane.

Implants (pellets) of crystalline testosterone are available for chronic treatment of hypogonadism. Serum testosterone levels are maintained in the physiologic range for 4 to 6 months depending on the number of pellets that are inserted SC. Implants are not usually used but are gaining some popularity with urologists in the United States; they are widely used in Australia and the United Kingdom.

TABLE 221-4   INDICATIONS FOR ANDROGEN THERAPY

Androgen deficiency (hypogonadism) (symptoms, signs and low testosterone level)
Microphallus (neonatal)
Delayed puberty in boys
Angioneurotic edema
Other possible uses or under investigation
 Hormonal male contraception
 Sarcopenia associated with cancer, human immunodeficiency virus infection, chronic infection, frailty in older men and women
 Hypoactive sexual disorder in postmenopausal women

TABLE 221-5   ANDROGEN PREPARATIONS

ROUTE	PREPARATION	DOSE AND FREQUENCY OF ADMINISTRATION
Oral*	Testosterone undecanoate	158 to 396 mg PO two or three times daily with food
Buccal	Transbuccal testosterone, mucoadhesive tablets	30 mg two times daily
Injection	Testosterone enanthate and cypionate	100 mg/wk IM or 150-200 mg IM every 2 wk; 50 to 100 mg/week SC
	Testosterone undecanoate	750-1000 mg IM every 10-12 wk
Implant	Testosterone implants	75-mg pellets (in United States), 6-10 inserted once every 4-6 months
Transdermal	Nonscrotal patch Androderm	Two patches, each delivering testosterone 2.5 mg/day; or one patch delivering testosterone 5 mg/day
	Testoderm TTS	One patch delivering testosterone 5 mg/day
Transdermal gels	AndroGel or Testogel; Testim; Axiron; Fortesta	1 to 2% gel applied once daily delivering 50-100 mg testosterone on skin and 5 to 10 mg to body

*Oral modified 17α-alkylated androgens such as methyltestosterone, fluoxymesterone, oxymetholone, stanozolol, and oxandrolone are not recommended for the treatment of androgen-deficient states because of potential hepatotoxicity and adverse effects on serum lipids.
IM = intramuscularly; PO = orally; SC = subcutaneously.

TABLE 221-6 ANDROGEN THERAPY: RISKS VERSUS BENEFITS

BENEFITS	RISKS
Development or maintenance of secondary sex characteristics	Fluid retention
Improved libido and sexual function	Gynecomastia
Increased muscle mass and strength	Acne, oily skin
Increased bone mineral density	Increased hematocrit, erythrocytosis
Improves anemia	Decreased high-density lipoprotein cholesterol (oral agents produce more effect)
Decreased body and visceral fat	Sleep apnea
Improved mood	Aggressive behavior (?)
Effect on cognition (?)	Prostate disease
Effect on vitality and quality of life (?)	Benign prostatic hyperplasia (?)
Decreased cardiovascular disease risk (epidemiologic studies); clinical study no benefits/risk	Carcinoma of prostate (aggravate existing cancer)
	Increased cardiovascular adverse events in one study in frail elderly men with multiple comorbid conditions

TABLE 221-7 MALE INFERTILITY: BASIC LABORATORY TESTS

SEMEN ANALYSES	HORMONE ANALYSES (IN PATIENTS WITH ABNORMAL SEMEN ANALYSES)
Volume, pH	Serum luteinizing hormone and follicle-stimulating hormone
Microscopy: Agglutination, debris	Serum testosterone
Sperm: Concentration, motility, morphology, vitality	If luteinizing hormone and testosterone levels are low, serum prolactin
Leukocytes	
Immature germ cells	
Sperm autoantibodies (sperm and semen biochemistry, sperm function tests)	

TABLE 221-8 SEMEN ANALYSIS: REFERENCE RANGE FROM FERTILE MEN*

PARAMETER	REFERENCE RANGE
Semen volume	>1.5 mL
Sperm	
Concentration	>15 million/mL
Total count	>39 million/ejaculate
Motility	>40% motile
	>32% progressively motile
Morphology	>4% normal†
Vitality (live)	>58%
Leukocytes	<1 million/mL

*Men whose partners had a time-to-pregnancy of ≤12 months were chosen to provide reference distributions for semen parameters.
†This value is based on the strict criteria for assessing sperm morphology in studies using in vitro fertilization as an end point.

Transdermal testosterone delivery through skin patches and gels have been available in the United States for over 15 years. The nonscrotal patches deliver 5 mg/day of testosterone, which is the physiologic production rate. These patches deliver levels of testosterone within the normal range but have a high incidence of skin irritability (redness, swelling, and blisters). Hydroalcoholic and nonalcoholic testosterone gels/lotion have been developed for transdermal application and have become the most widely used testosterone formulations in the United States. The usual dosage is 50 to 100 mg of 1, 1.62, and 2% testosterone gel applied daily to the skin, delivering 5 to 10 mg of testosterone to the body. Transdermal delivery results in a more consistent serum concentration and causes little skin irritation. Transfer from the user to other people is possible during routine use and may be a concern if there is close skin contact with women and children. Protective clothing or a shower is necessary to avoid transferring testosterone through skin-to-skin contact.

Table 221-6 shows the benefits and potential side effects of androgen treatment. In hypogonadal men, androgen replacement leads to the development and maintenance of secondary sexual characteristics. Testosterone has important anabolic effects on muscle and bone and improves libido and sexual dysfunction. It has less effect on erectile dysfunction. It has no major short-term effects on the prostate gland but increases prostatic volume by an average of about 4.5 mL after 12 months of testosterone gel treatment.[13]

MALE INFERTILITY

DEFINITION

Infertility is defined as the failure of a couple to achieve pregnancy after at least 1 year of frequent unprotected intercourse. If a pregnancy has not occurred after 3 years, infertility will most likely persist without medical treatment.

EPIDEMIOLOGY

Studies in the United States and Europe showed a 1-year prevalence of infertility in 15% of couples. The prevalence in developing countries is likely to be higher because of the higher prevalence of genital tract infection. Of subfertility cases, 30 to 35% can be attributed to predominantly female factors, 25 to 30% to male factors, and 25 to 30% to problems in both partners.

PATHOBIOLOGY

Hypothalamic-pituitary disorders are infrequent causes of male infertility and are discussed in the section on hypogonadism and androgen deficiency. Testicular disorders are the most frequent identifiable cause of infertility (see Table 221-2). Y chromosome microdeletions are increasingly recognized as a genetic cause of azoospermia and severe oligozoospermia. Up to 25% of infertile men have microdeletions in the long arm of the Y chromosome, many of which map to the Yq11 region of the chromosome, which is called the azoospermic factor (AZF). Mutations in the AZFa and b regions are associated with azoospermia, whereas mutations of AFZc region may be associated with oligozoospermia. The gr/gr deletion removes a large segment of the AFZc gene and represents a significant risk factor for oligozoospermia in some but not all populations. Mutations in the testis-expressed 11 gene (*TEX11*) and other genes such as NR5A1, DMRT1, have been described and are a common

cause of meiotic arrest and azoospermia in infertile men.[14,15] Y chromosome defects are transmissible to male offspring if cases are successfully treated by ART. Thus, genetic testing and counseling should be done before technologies such as intracytoplasmic sperm injection (ICSI) are considered.

DIAGNOSIS

The approach to the diagnosis of an infertile couple includes management of both the male and the female partner (Figs. 221-6 and 221-7).

Examination of the ejaculate is the cornerstone for the investigation of an infertile man (Table 221-7). Semen samples are collected at the physician's office or at home, preferably after 2 to 7 days of abstinence from ejaculatory activity. The generally accepted reference values for a semen analysis are given in Table 221-8. A normal sperm concentration is greater than 15 million/mL, with a total sperm number greater than 39 million per ejaculate; however, men with lower sperm counts can be fertile. More than 40% of the spermatozoa should be motile, and more than 32% should demonstrate a progressive motility pattern. Using strict criteria to assess sperm morphology, the percentage of morphologically normal forms should be above 4%. There is considerable overlap in the semen quality of fertile and subfertile men. Low sperm concentration or poor sperm morphology is associated with lower chances of natural conception in the female partner. In patients with abnormal semen analyses, measurements of serum FSH, LH, and testosterone are indicated (see Fig. 221-6). Elevated FSH levels usually indicate severe germinal epithelium damage. A decreased serum inhibin B level also reflects poor Sertoli cell function and may indicate spermatogenic dysfunction. Elevated serum LH and FSH concentrations together with a low serum testosterone level indicate pantesticular failure leading to hypogonadism and infertility. Low serum FSH, LH, and testosterone concentrations suggest hypothalamic-pituitary dysfunction; serum prolactin should be measured, and additional investigations may be required. A low sperm concentration and suppressed LH level with an increased, normal, or low serum testosterone level (without clinical manifestations of androgen deficiency) may suggest exogenous androgen use. The hormonal pattern in androgen insensitivity (an uncommon cause of male infertility) is elevated LH, normal FSH, and high-normal to increased serum testosterone levels. Normal hormonal parameters in azoospermic (no sperm in the ejaculate) men with normal-sized testes may suggest congenital or acquired obstruction in the epididymis or vas deferens.

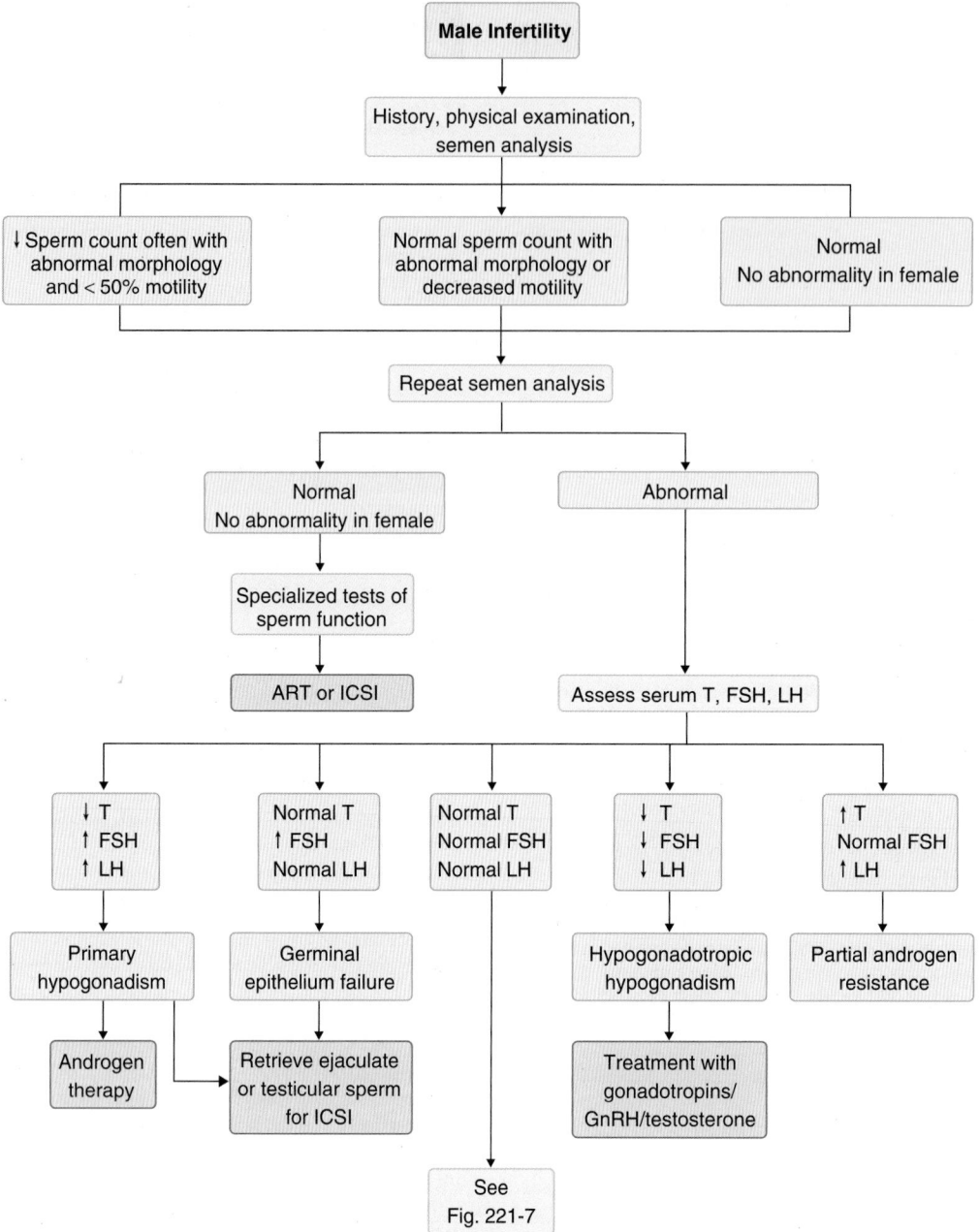

FIGURE 221-6. **Algorithmic approach to the diagnosis and treatment of male infertility.** ART = assisted reproductive technology; FSH = follicle-stimulating hormone; GnRH = gonadotropin-releasing hormone; ICSI = intracytoplasmic sperm injection; LH = serum luteinizing hormone; T = serum testosterone.

TREATMENT Rx

An algorithmic approach to the treatment of male infertility is illustrated in Figures 221-6 and 221-7. The principles of managing male infertility can be summarized as follows. (1) Men with mild-to-moderate oligozoospermia, with or without decreased sperm motility and some impairment of motility, are subfertile rather than infertile. Spontaneous pregnancies can occur in this group. (2) Reliable pharmaceutical treatment is limited to the 1 to 2% of infertile men with gonadotropin insufficiency. (3) Assisted reproductive technologies, including in vitro fertilization and intracytoplasmic sperm injection, have dramatically improved pregnancy rates. (4) In male factor infertility azoospermia (absence of sperm in the ejaculate) may occur with obstruction of the ejaculatory system. In these patients, in vitro fertilization and intracytoplasmic sperm injection after either percutaneous epididymal sperm extraction or microsurgical epididymal sperm extraction are highly successful. (5) Azoospermia resulting from impaired spermatogenesis may not be a sterile state, because sperm may be present within the testes. Microsurgical testicular extraction of sperm from the testis followed by intracytoplasmic sperm injection can be performed with good success, even in patients with Klinefelter syndrome.

● SEXUAL DYSFUNCTION

Sexual dysfunction can be divided into four main categories: (1) loss of desire (libido), (2) erectile dysfunction, (3) ejaculatory insufficiency, and (4) anorgasmic states.

Decreased Libido

Loss of libido refers to a reduction in sexual interest, initiative, and frequency and intensity of responses to internal or external erotic stimuli. Causal factors include psychogenic factors, CNS disease, androgen deficiency and resistance, and side effects from medications (e.g., antihypertensives, psychotropics, alcohol, narcotics, dopamine blockers, antiandrogens, and possibly 5α-reductase inhibitors). Total and free testosterone are consistently but not very strongly associated with sexual desire, erectile function, and sexual activity in symptomatic older men,[16,17] and treatment with testosterone improves sexual desire in symptomatic older men with testosterone deficiency.

Treatment is directed toward the causal mechanism.

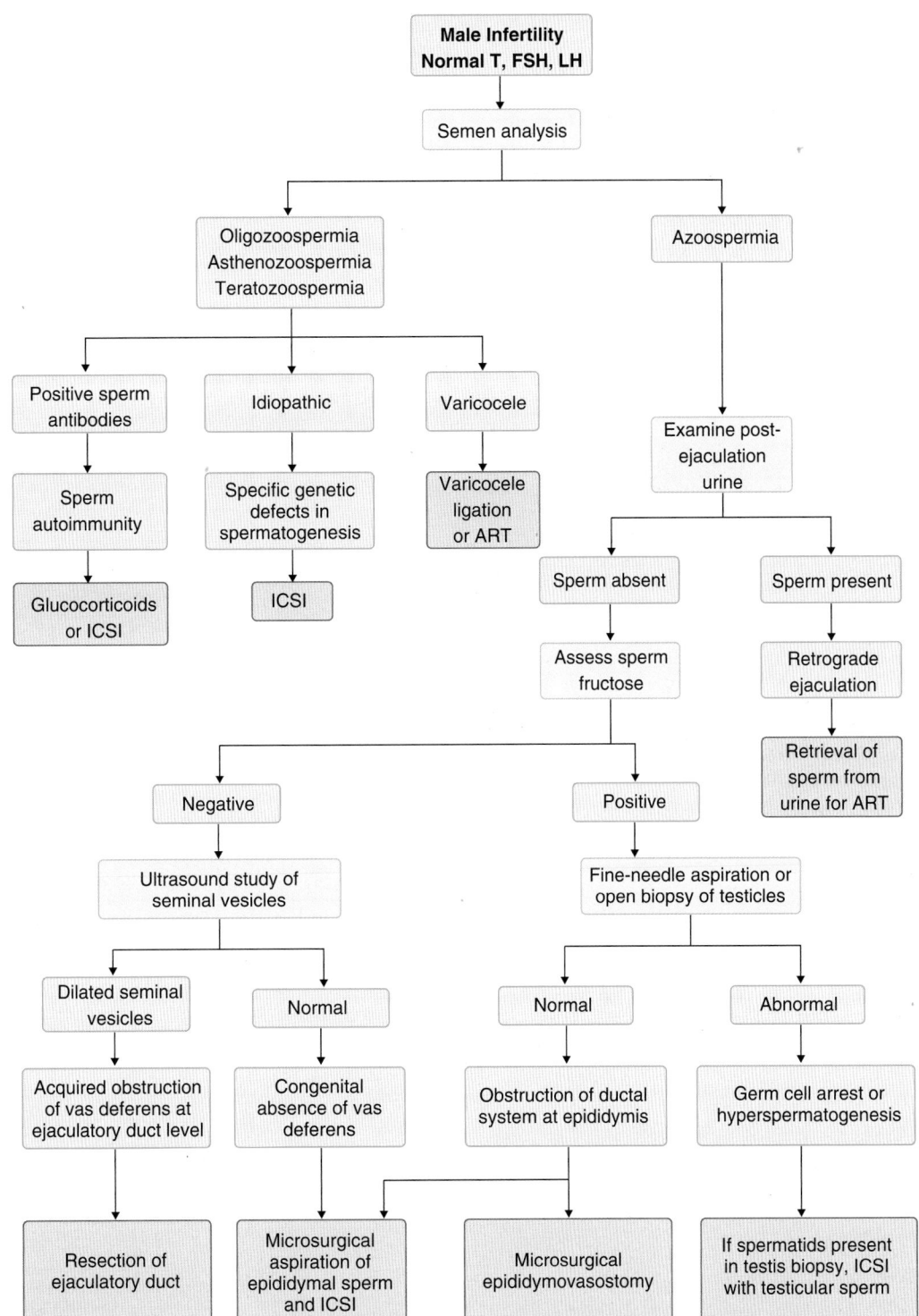

FIGURE 221-7. Algorithmic approach to the diagnosis and treatment of male infertility in patients with normal serum hormone concentrations. ART = assisted reproductive technology; FSH = follicle-stimulating hormone; ICSI = intracytoplasmic sperm injection; LH = serum luteinizing hormone; T = serum testosterone.

Ejaculatory Failure and Impaired Orgasm

Ejaculatory insufficiency refers to absent or reduced seminal emission or impaired ejaculatory contraction. It is usually associated with neurologic conditions and medication therapy. An anorgasmic state is a distressing but relatively uncommon condition in men in which the normal process of erection and ejaculation occurs in the absence of the subjective sensation of pleasure initiated at the time of emission and ejaculation. Premature ejaculation is the most common form of male sexual dysfunction. Estimates of prevalence vary, but 25 to 30% seems to be a reasonable estimate. The *Diagnostic and Statistical Manual of Mental Disorders-5* (2013) defines premature ejaculation as ejaculation occurring within approximately 1 minute of vaginal penetration before the person wishes it on 75% of occasions for at least 6 months and causing personal distress. The pathobiology of premature ejaculation is unknown. It may be associated with marked distress or interpersonal difficulty and is not a direct effect of substance abuse such as opiate withdrawal. The diagnosis is based mainly on sexual history and includes assessment of intravaginal ejaculatory latency time, perceived control, distress, and interpersonal difficulty. The first-line treatment is with selective serotonin reuptake inhibitors (SSRI) or a serotonin transporter inhibitor (e.g., dapoxetine 60 mg or clomipramine 15 mg as on-demand therapy)[A11] together with behavioral therapy and relationship counseling. Meta-analysis of addition of a phosphodiesterase 5 (PDE5) inhibitor to a SSRI has better effect on than a SSRI alone in prolonging the latency time before ejaculation.[18] Topical anesthetic creams can be used as alternatives.[19]

Erectile Dysfunction

DEFINITION

Erectile dysfunction can be defined as a man's inability to obtain rigidity sufficient to permit coitus of adequate duration to satisfy himself and his partner.

EPIDEMIOLOGY

Current estimates suggest that 10 to 15% of all American men suffer from erectile dysfunction, with the incidence progressively increased as men become older. Data from the Massachusetts Aging Study report that 52% of men 40 to 70 years of age experience some degree of erectile dysfunction. The prevalence of erectile dysfunction is even higher in men with type 2 diabetes mellitus and after radical prostatectomy for prostate cancer. Epidemiologic studies in the United States and Europe in men between 50 to 80 years indicate that erectile dysfunction is associated with lower urinary tract obstructive symptoms/benign prostatic hyperplasia.

PATHOBIOLOGY

The causes of erectile dysfunction are many, but they can generally be categorized as follows: vasculogenic, psychological, endocrine, neurologic, iatrogenic (post-radical prostatectomy), drug related, systemic illness, and aging. Erectile dysfunction is common in older men, despite normal serum testosterone levels; this effect appears to be the result of impaired penile vasodilatory capacity as a result of endothelial dysfunction. Decreased nonadrenergic, noncholinergic nerve activity, and reduced production of nitric oxide by endothelial cells result in decreased cavernous smooth muscle relaxation, decreased filling of the cavernous sinusoids, and reduced compression of the venous plexus against the tunica, leading to failure of erection. Men presenting with erectile dysfunction share common risk factors with cardiovascular disease (smoking, obesity, metabolic syndrome, hyperlipidemia, and type 2 diabetes mellitus). Evidence indicates that men presenting with mild erectile dysfunction should be assessed for cardiovascular disease, particularly when other risk factors are present. A retrospective pharmacoepidemiologic study showed that prescription of PDE5 inhibitors did not trigger cardiovascular risks assessment and that this may be a missed opportunity for early intervention to prevent cardiovascular disease.[20]

DIAGNOSIS

The diagnosis of erectile dysfunction is based mainly on a detailed medical and sexual history of the patient and his partner when available. The history may reveal the underlying cause, such as medication use (Table 221-9), or other common disorders associated with erectile dysfunction. Physical examination should focus on genitourinary, cardiovascular, endocrine, and neurologic systems. Prostate examination is important because erectile dysfunction is commonly associated with symptomatic benign prostatic hyperplasia. Laboratory tests should include a morning serum testosterone, and, if indicated, prostate-specific antigen, fasting glucose (or hemoglobin A_{1C}), and cholesterol. Specific diagnostic tests are rarely required.

TREATMENT   Rx

The treatment of erectile dysfunction is to find the cause and treat the cause if found.[21] Symptoms can be effectively treated by the oral administration of penile-selective phosphodiesterase-5 inhibitors (sildenafil, vardenafil, tadalafil) which have similar efficacy.[22] A treatment algorithm for erectile dysfunction is given in Figure 221-8. Lifestyle interventions reduce obesity and improve erectile function. For patients after radical prostatectomy, early penile rehabilitation with PDE5 inhibitors contributes to recovery of erectile dysfunction.[A12] In patients with androgen deficiency (a serum testosterone concentration of less than 275 ng/dL and symptoms suggesting testosterone deficiency), sexual function responds moderately well to testosterone gel which also may have some benefit for improving mood and depressive symptoms but not vitality or walking

TABLE 221-9	DRUGS COMMONLY ASSOCIATED WITH ERECTILE DYSFUNCTION

ANTIDEPRESSANTS

Selective serotonin reuptake inhibitors
Tricyclic antidepressants
Monoamine oxidase inhibitors

ANTIHYPERTENSIVES

β-blockers
Verapamil
Clonidine

CARDIAC DRUGS

Amiodarone
Digoxin

DIURETICS

Thiazides
Spironolactone

HISTAMINE RECEPTOR 2 ANTAGONISTS

Cimetidine
Ranitidine

HORMONAL AGENTS

Corticosteroids
Antiandrogens (flutamide, cyproterone acetate)
Luteinizing hormone releasing hormone agonists (leuprorelin, goserelin)
5α reductase inhibitors

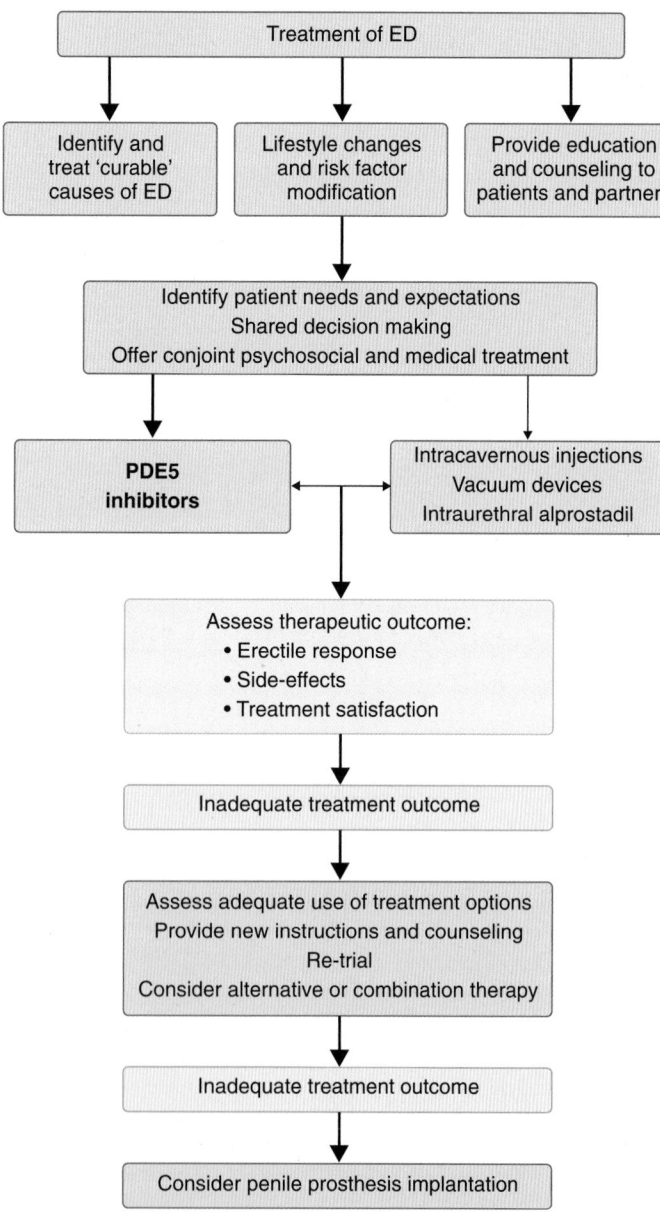

FIGURE 221-8. Treatment algorithm for erectile dysfunction (**ED**). PDE₅ = cyclic GMP phosphodiesterase-5. (Reprinted with permission from Hatzimouratidis K, Amar E, Eardley I, et al. Guidelines on male sexual dysfunction: erectile dysfunction and premature ejaculation. *Eur Urol.* 2010;57:804-814. 2015 update: http://uroweb.org/guideline/male-sexual-dysfunction/. Accessed March 26, 2015.)

distance. Combined androgen deficiency with decreased libido and decreased penile responsiveness resulting from impaired nitric oxide synthase activity may be common in elderly men. With the availability of effective penile vasodilatory medications to ensure erectile capacity, complaints of diminished libido can be effectively treated with androgen supplementation.

Medical Therapy
Oral Medications

Oral and selective inhibitors of cGMP phosphodiesterase-5 (the primary phosphodiesterase in the penile cavernosal tissue) are effective for at least 60% of men. Inhibition of phosphodiesterase-5 causes persistence of normally (sexually) stimulated cGMP in the corpora cavernosa, resulting in protracted cavernosal tumescence and rigidity. Patients with diabetes mellitus, spinal cord injuries, prostatic surgery, and pelvic irradiation also benefit, but with a somewhat lower response rate. The usual starting dose of sildenafil is 50 mg, increasing in 25-mg increments up to 100 mg. Because of its mechanism of action, sildenafil is used on demand with recommended administration 20 to 60 minutes before intercourse. Two other potent phosphodiesterase-5 inhibitors (vardenafil and tadalafil) are widely used for the treatment of erectile dysfunction and appear to be equally effective. Vardenafil (5, 10, and 20 mg) has a relatively longer duration of action (4 to 6 hours), and tadalafil (10 or 20 mg) has an even longer duration of action (up to 36 hours). Randomized controlled trials showed that daily administration of tadalafil (5 mg) improved erectile function compared to on-demand treatment. Daily dosing of tadalafil is well tolerated and effective. Thus, daily dosing starting with 2.5 mg of tadalafil may be an alternative to on-demand administration if intercourse is expected to be more frequent—for example, more than twice per week. Hypogonadal men with erectile dysfunction and low libido may benefit from combined treatment with testosterone and phosphodiesterase-5 inhibitors (PDE-5). However, the addition of testosterone to sildenafil does not further improve erectile dysfunction. PDE-5 inhibitors should not be administered with nitrates because the accumulation of cGMP may result in lowering of blood pressure and hypotension. PDE-5 inhibitors also may interact with antihypertensive agents, including α-blockers, resulting in orthostatic hypotension.

Intracavernosal Injection

Second-line treatment of erectile dysfunction involves intracavernosal injection with vasodilators such as prostaglandin E_1 (Alprostadil) alone or with other vasodilators (papaverine, phentolamine). These medications are injected into the cavernosal space with a 27- to 30-gauge needle and may be useful in men who are refractory to oral agents. The main side effects of penile injections are pain and cavernosal fibrosis which usually resolves after discontinuation of injections. Presence of tunica fibrosis may suggest early Peyronie disease, and injections should be stopped. The intraurethral prostaglandin E_1 suppository alprostadil is believed to work locally on the corpora cavernosa as a vasodilatory agent. The suppository is apparently successful in improving erectile function in 30 to 66% of cases.

Penile Prostheses

Surgical implantation of penile prostheses that include inflatable and malleable devices are the third line of treatment for men who prefer a permanent solution of their problem or for those who do not respond to other therapies. (Adapted from Muneer A, Kalsi J, Nazareth I, et al. Erectile dysfunction. *BMJ.* 2014;348:g129.)

Grade A References

A1. Basaria S, Harman SM, Travison TG, et al. Effects of testosterone administration for 3 years on subclinical atherosclerosis progression in older men with low or low-normal testosterone levels: a randomized clinical trial. *JAMA.* 2015;314:570-581.

A2. Snyder PJ, Bhasin S, Cunningham GR, et al. Effects of testosterone treatment in older men. *N Engl J Med.* 2016;374:611-624.

A3. Cunningham GR, Stephens-Shields AJ, Rosen RC, et al. Testosterone treatment and sexual function in older men with low testosterone levels. *J Clin Endocrinol Metab.* 2016;101:3096-3104.

A4. Roy CN, Snyder PJ, Stephens-Shields AJ, et al. Association of testosterone levels with anemia in older men: a controlled clinical trial. *JAMA Intern Med.* 2017;177:480-490.

A5. Snyder PJ, Kopperdahl DL, Stephens-Shields AJ, et al. Effect of testosterone treatment on volumetric bone density and strength in older men with low testosterone: a controlled clinical trial. *JAMA Intern Med.* 2017;177:471-479.

A6. Resnick SM, Matsumoto AM, Stephens-Shields AJ, et al. Testosterone treatment and cognitive function in older men with low testosterone and age-associated memory impairment. *JAMA.* 2017;317:717-727.

A7. Budoff MJ, Ellenberg SS, Lewis CE, et al. Testosterone treatment and coronary artery plaque volume in older men with low testosterone. *JAMA.* 2017;317:708-716.

A8. Rastrelli G, Dicuio M, Reismann Y, et al. Cardiovascular impact of testosterone therapy for hypogonadism. *Expert Rev Cardiovasc Ther.* 2018;16:617-625.

A9. Ponce OJ, Spencer-Bonilla G, Alvarez-Villalobos N, et al. The efficacy and adverse events of testosterone replacement therapy in hypogonadal men: a systematic review and meta-analysis of randomized, placebo-controlled trials. *J Clin Endocrinol Metab.* 2018;103:1745-1754.

A10. Corona G, Rastrelli G, Giagulli VA, et al. Dehydroepiandrosterone supplementation in elderly men: a meta-analysis study of placebo-controlled trials. *J Clin Endocrinol Metab.* 2013;98:3615-3626.

A11. Kim SW, Choi JB, Kim SJ, et al. Tolerability and adequate therapeutic dosage of oral clomipramine for the treatment of premature ejaculation: a randomized, double-blind, placebo-controlled, fixed-dose, parallel-grouped clinical study. *Int J Impot Res.* 2018;30:65-70.

A12. Jo JK, Jeong SJ, Oh JJ, et al. Effect of starting penile rehabilitation with sildenafil immediately after robot-assisted laparoscopic radical prostatectomy on erectile function recovery: a prospective randomized trial. *J Urol.* 2018;199:1600-1606.

GENERAL REFERENCES

For the General References and other additional features, please visit Expert Consult at https://expertconsult.inkling.com.

222

OVARIES AND PUBERTAL DEVELOPMENT

WILLIAM H. CATHERINO

DEFINITION

The ovaries or female gonads episodically release female gametes (oocytes or eggs) and secrete sex steroid hormones, principally androstenedione, estradiol, and progesterone. Oocytes are released only during the adult reproductive years, when sex steroid secretion is also greatest, but the ovaries are physiologically active throughout life.

Sex steroids affect the growth, differentiation, and function of a variety of tissues and organs throughout the body; therefore abnormalities of the ovaries and of sex steroid secretion should be recognized by all physicians. A rational approach to the diagnosis and treatment of reproductive disorders in women requires an understanding of the functions of the ovaries and of their most important unit, the follicle, throughout life.

Ovarian Function in Childhood and Puberty
Physical Changes at Puberty

Puberty extends from the earliest signs of sexual maturation until the attainment of physical, mental, and emotional maturity. Pubertal changes in girls result directly or indirectly from maturation of the hypothalamic-pituitary-ovarian (HPO) unit.[1] Human puberty is characterized hormonally by a resetting of the negative gonadal steroid feedback loop, the establishment of new circadian and ultradian (frequent) gonadotropin rhythms, and the acquisition in the female of a positive estrogen feedback loop controlling the menstrual cycle as interdependent expressions of the gonadotropins and ovarian steroids. In girls, pubertal development generally occurs between 7 and 14 years of age. The age at onset and the rate of progress through puberty are variable and depend on genetic, socioeconomic, nutritional, physical, and psychological factors. It appears that there are racial differences in the onset of pubertal development. In the United States development begins earlier in African American than in white girls.

Physical changes occur in an orderly sequence during a definite time frame in puberty (Fig. 222-1). Breast budding in girls is usually the first pubertal change, followed shortly by the appearance of pubic hair, with menarche occurring late in pubertal development. The time from breast budding (mean age of 10.0 years in white girls and 8.9 years in African Americans) to menarche is 2 years. Breast development results from increasing ovarian estrogen production, and pubic and axillary hair results from increasing androgen production. Estrogens are required for the growth of pubic hair as well.

The ovarian sex steroids join with growth hormone and adrenal androgens to produce the adolescent growth spurt.[2] Peak growth velocity is achieved relatively early, with little growth observed after menarche. It has been estimated that more than 50 genes play roles in determining final adult height. It is now clear that estrogen, and not testosterone, is the primary hormone mediating pubertal bone growth in both males and females. Lean body mass, skeletal mass, and body fat are equal in prepubertal boys and girls, but by maturity, women have twice as much body fat as men and less lean body mass and skeletal mass as a result of differences in sex steroid secretion. Estrogens are necessary for the normal formation, mineralization, and maturation of

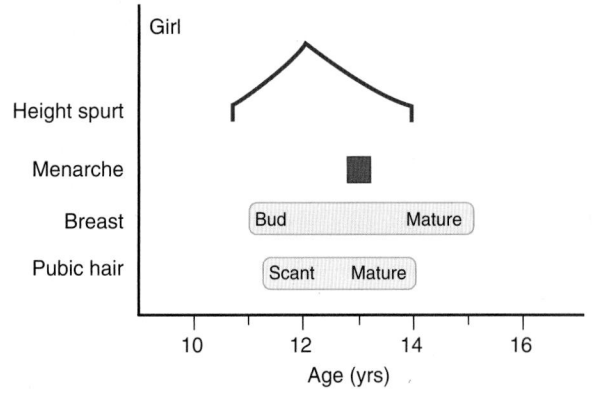

FIGURE 222-1. Temporal sequence of events for the "average" girl during puberty. (From Rebar RW. Practical evaluation of hormonal status. In: Yen SSC, Jaffe RB, Barbieri RL, eds. *Reproductive Endocrinology: Physiology, Pathophysiology, and Clinical Management,* 4th ed. Philadelphia: WB Saunders; 1999:710.)

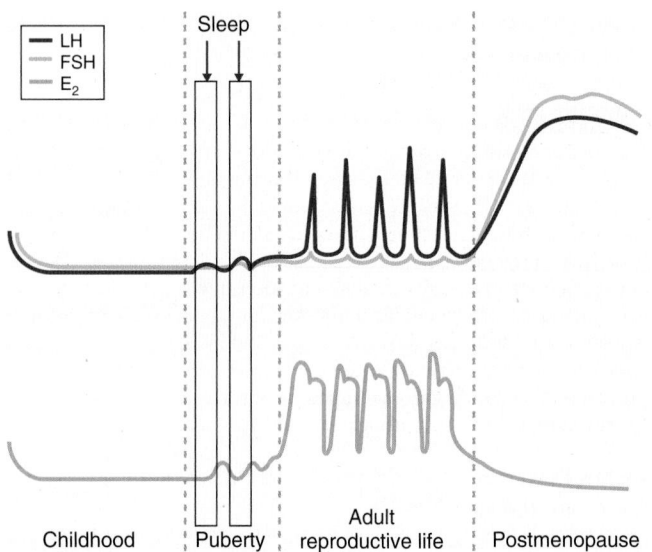

FIGURE 222-2. The changing patterns of luteinizing hormone (LH), follicle-stimulating hormone (FSH), and estradiol (E$_2$) concentrations in peripheral blood throughout the life of a woman. Not shown is the fact that both LH and FSH are secreted in a pulsatile fashion. The pubertal period has been expanded to illustrate the sleep-associated increases in LH and FSH followed by morning increases in E$_2$ that are observed during puberty. (Reprinted with permission from Endocrine and Metabolism Continuing Education Quality Control Program, 1982. Copyright American Association for Clinical Chemistry Inc.)

bones. Well-established standards exist for determining whether bone age is appropriate for chronologic age, typically by examining radiographs of the bones of the wrist. Estrogen deficiencies retard, and excesses advance, bone age in relation to chronologic age.[3]

Hormonal Changes

The ovaries function even in early childhood. Low levels of luteinizing hormone (LH) and follicle-stimulating hormone (FSH) are normally present, and these levels increase if the ovaries are removed before puberty, just as they do later in life, indicating the exquisite sensitivity of the hypothalamic-pituitary unit to extremely low circulating sex steroid levels. As puberty nears, there is a progressive decrease in sensitivity of the hypothalamic-pituitary unit to sex steroids, leading to the increased secretion of pituitary gonadotropins, stimulation of sex steroid output, and development of secondary sex characteristics. Increased secretion of both LH and FSH initially occurs at night with sleep and is associated with increased estradiol secretion the next morning (Fig. 222-2). As is true for most hormones, LH and FSH are secreted in an episodic or pulsatile rather than a continuous fashion. Later in puberty, secretion of LH and FSH is increased throughout the 24-hour period, except during the early follicular phase, when nighttime increases still occur. Basal levels of estradiol, the major estrogen secreted by the ovaries, increase throughout

puberty. A "critical body mass" may be required for positive estrogen feedback and ovulation. During the first 2 years after menarche, up to 90% of menstrual cycles may be anovulatory because of a delay in synchronization of the HPO axis.

Ovarian Cysts and Adnexal Masses

Follicular growth, resulting in an ovarian cyst, is an expected finding during the reproductive years. However, palpable masses before or after the reproductive years require thorough investigation to rule out various cancers. A pelvic mass during the reproductive years could represent an ovarian cyst, but could also represent an endometrioma, ovarian fibroma, intrauterine pregnancy, ectopic pregnancy, uterine fibroid, tubo-ovarian abscess, peritubal cyst, or less likely ovarian or tubal cancer.[4] History, physical examination, pregnancy test, and pelvic ultrasound would assist in focusing the differential diagnosis. CA-125 during the reproductive years is nonspecific and should not be used to rule out ovarian cancer. Incidentally detected adnexal lesions are found in approximately 4 to 5% of women undergoing computed tomography (CT) scan and in 9 to 10% undergoing ultrasound. The overwhelming majority of these masses are benign, and magnetic resonance imaging (MRI) allows for decreased rates of resection or oophorectomy for benign lesions.[5]

● ABERRATIONS IN PUBERTAL DEVELOPMENT

Abnormalities of pubertal development[6] can be divided into four major categories (Table 222-1):
1. *Precocious puberty* represents any pubertal changes before age 9 years in white girls and before age 8 years in African American girls. This remains controversial. Some clinicians believe evaluation is warranted only if pubertal development begins before age 7 years in white girls and 6 years in African American girls. A compromise may involve careful screening by history and physical examination of girls with early-onset puberty, looking for central nervous system (CNS) symptoms, behavioral concerns, and any other abnormal findings that might warrant further evaluation. The nearer pubertal development begins to the mean age of puberty onset, the less likely it is to have a pathologic basis. Precocious development is isosexual when it is common to the phenotypic sex of the individual and heterosexual when the development is characteristic of the opposite sex. True or central precocious puberty is due to premature maturation of the hypothalamic-pituitary axis. In the absence of increased hypothalamic-pituitary activity, precocious pseudopuberty exists.
2. *Delayed (or interrupted) puberty* is defined as the absence of any secondary sex characteristics by age 13 years, the absence of menarche by age 16 years, or the passage of 5 years or more from breast budding to menarche.
3. *Asynchronous pubertal development* occurs when there is deviation from the normal pattern of pubertal development.
4. *Heterosexual pubertal development* occurs at the appropriate time but has some features characteristic of the opposite sex.

Precocious Puberty

DIAGNOSIS

The overall incidence of precocious puberty has been estimated at 1 in 5000 to 10,000 children.[7] About 10 times as many girls as boys are affected.

Differential Diagnosis

The temporal sequence in which the signs and symptoms of sex steroid hormone excess appear is most important. *Incomplete isosexual precocious puberty* indicates premature development of only a single pubertal feature. If breast budding occurs before age 8 years in the absence of any other development, the diagnosis may be *premature thelarche*. Premature thelarche is believed to be due to transient increases in estrogen secretion or increased breast sensitivity to the small quantities of circulating estrogens present before puberty. Simple ovarian cysts may be present in some girls with this disorder and may be due in some cases to the same genetic abnormality found in girls with McCune-Albright syndrome (Chapters 211 and 234). If pubic or axillary hair develops alone and persists, *premature pubarche* and *adrenarche* must be considered. These abnormalities are associated with slight increases in adrenal androgen secretion but not with clitorimegaly or other signs of virilization. These syndromes require no treatment, and affected girls typically begin true puberty at the usual age. Careful follow-up is required to distinguish these disorders from true precocious puberty.

When precocious development is isosexual, the purpose of the evaluation is to determine whether the cause is central (true precocious puberty) or

TABLE 222-1 ABERRATIONS OF PUBERTAL DEVELOPMENT

PRECOCIOUS DEVELOPMENT	Hypogonadotropic or normogonadotropic hypogonadism (LH and FSH <10 mIU/mL, or LH and FSH 6-25 mIU/mL with at least one being >10 mIU/mL)

PRECOCIOUS DEVELOPMENT

Isosexual precocity
  Incomplete sexual precocity
    Premature thelarche
    Premature pubarche
    Premature adrenarche
  True (central) precocious puberty
    Idiopathic (constitutional)
    Due to central nervous system lesions
    Primary hypothyroidism
    Silver-Russell syndrome
  Precocious pseudopuberty (of peripheral origin)
    Ovarian neoplasms
    Adrenal neoplasms
    Iatrogenic (estrogen-containing preparations)
    Human chorionic gonadotropin–secreting neoplasms distinct from central nervous system and ovarian tumors
    McCune-Albright syndrome
Heterosexual precocity
  Ovarian neoplasms
  Adrenal neoplasms
  Congenital adrenal hyperplasia
  Other rare disorders of sexual differentiation

DELAYED PUBERTAL DEVELOPMENT*

Anatomic abnormalities
  Müllerian agenesis or dysgenesis (Rokitansky-Küster-Hauser syndrome)
  Distal genital tract obstruction
    Transverse vaginal septum
    Imperforate hymen
    Vaginal agenesis
Hypergonadotropic hypogonadism (FSH >30-40 mIU/mL)
  Gonadal dysgenesis
    With stigmata of Turner syndrome
    Pure (46,XX or 46,XY)
    Mixed
  Ovarian failure with normal ovarian development
    Genetic disorders
    Autoimmune disorders
    Gonadotropin receptor or postreceptor defects (resistant ovary or Savage syndrome?)
    Enzymatic defects (17α-hydroxylase deficiency, galactosemia)
    Physical causes: irradiation, chemotherapeutic agents, viral agents
    Idiopathic

Hypogonadotropic or normogonadotropic hypogonadism (LH and FSH <10 mIU/mL, or LH and FSH 6-25 mIU/mL with at least one being >10 mIU/mL)
  Isolated gonadotropin deficiency
    In association with midline defects (Kallmann syndrome)
    Independent of associated disorders
  Neoplasms of the hypothalamic-pituitary axis
    Craniopharyngiomas
    Pituitary tumors
    Others
  Infiltrative processes (Langerhans-type histiocytosis)
  Idiopathic hypopituitarism
  "Hypothalamic" forms of amenorrhea
    Psychogenic
    Exercise associated
    Associated with malnutrition
    Anorexia nervosa
  Miscellaneous disorders
    Prader-Labhart-Willi syndrome
    Laurence-Moon-Bardet-Biedl syndrome
    Primary hypothyroidism
Constitutional delayed puberty

ASYNCHRONOUS PUBERTAL DEVELOPMENT

Incomplete forms of androgen insensitivity
Complete forms of androgen insensitivity

HETEROSEXUAL PUBERTAL DEVELOPMENT

Polycystic ovary syndrome
Congenital adrenal hyperplasia (female pseudohermaphroditism)
  21-Hydroxylase deficiency
  11β-Hydroxylase deficiency
  3β-ol-Hydroxysteroid dehydrogenase deficiency
Male pseudohermaphroditism due to 5α-reductase deficiency
Male pseudohermaphroditism due to partial androgen insensitivity
Mixed gonadal dysgenesis
Androgen-producing neoplasms
  Ovarian
  Adrenal
Cushing syndrome

*No development by age 13 yr, absence of menarche by age 15 yr, or passage of ≥5 yr from breast budding without menarche.
FSH = follicle-stimulating hormone; LH = luteinizing hormone.

peripheral, in which case it is considered gonadotropin-releasing hormone (GnRH)–independent precocious puberty or precocious pseudopuberty. Careful questioning of the patient and her parents may indicate the inadvertent ingestion or absorption of sex steroids (iatrogenic or factitious). As many as 20% of individuals with true precocious puberty have one of several organic brain diseases, including any of several neoplasms, tuberous sclerosis, neurofibromatosis, encephalitis, meningitis, vascular malformations, and hydrocephalus. Because of the seriousness of intracranial lesions, girls with precocious puberty must have radiographic evaluation of the CNS, most effectively by MRI. In at least 75% of girls with true precocious puberty, however, no cause is identified (idiopathic or constitutional).

The physical examination may also provide critical information about the cause of the precocious development. Cutaneous café au lait spots, facial asymmetry, polyostotic fibrous dysplasia and other skeletal abnormalities, cranial nerve deficits, and multiple ovarian follicular cysts suggest McCune-Albright syndrome (Chapters 211 and 234) in a girl with precocious development. It is now known that various clones of cells in the endocrine glands of girls with this disorder function autonomously with respect to cyclic adenosine monophosphate production as a consequence of a mutation within exon 8 of the G protein α–subunit. This same mutation probably accounts for the bone lesions and café au lait hyperpigmentation. Other endocrine cells may be similarly affected and lead to pituitary adenomas (usually secreting growth hormone), hyperthyroidism, and, rarely, adrenal hyperplasia.

Studies on the etiologic causes for precocious puberty are in their infancy, but one molecule, kisspeptin, is known to be involved in pubertal development. Kisspeptin and its receptor GPR54 are essential regulators of GnRH-induced gonadotropin secretion and pubertal onset. Activation results in stimulation of the HPO axis, and elevated kisspeptin levels are associated with precocious puberty. Additionally, kisspeptin loss-of-function mutations result in normosmic idiopathic hypogonadotropic hypogonadism.

Abdominal and rectal examination may reveal a mass, suggesting an adrenal or ovarian tumor. Because palpable ovarian cysts may rarely develop before ovulation in true precocious puberty, the presence of a mass does not confirm the diagnosis of precocious pseudopuberty.

When vaginal bleeding is the only sign of development, the diagnosis of sexual precocity should be suspect. Common causes of bleeding in this age group include irritation from a vaginal infection or foreign body, sexual assault, prolapse of the urethral meatus, and ingestion of estrogen-containing medications (most commonly, oral contraceptive preparations). A vaginal or cervical neoplasm is also a rare possibility. Thus vaginal bleeding requires a vaginal examination, which is often best performed with the patient under anesthesia, before further evaluation is undertaken.

Heterosexual precocity in an apparent prepubertal female is almost always due to congenital adrenal hyperplasia or to an androgen-secreting adrenal or ovarian neoplasm. Only rarely must another disorder of sexual differentiation be considered (Chapter 220). It is important to examine the external genitalia carefully, because congenital adrenal hyperplasia is usually associated with some degree of sexual ambiguity.

Excessive androgens produced endogenously by abnormal fetal adrenal glands in utero or diffusing across the placenta to the fetus from the mother can virilize the external genitalia and result in female pseudohermaphroditism. The extent of virilization varies from only an enlarged clitoris to sexual ambiguity sufficient to make gender assignment difficult.

Excessive maternal androgen secretion, typically from an ovarian or adrenal neoplasm, can lead to virilization of a female fetus. This occurs very rarely because of the great capacity of the placenta to aromatize naturally occurring androgens to estrogens. Virilization of a female fetus is much more likely to occur if a pregnant woman has ingested a synthetic steroid preparation with androgenic properties, because synthetic compounds generally cannot be aromatized.

Excessive androgen secretion beginning in utero is usually associated with defective cortisol synthesis. As a consequence, pituitary corticotropin secretion is increased, resulting in congenital adrenal hyperplasia and excessive androgen secretion. The three different enzyme defects in the steroidogenic pathway that can lead to virilization of the female fetus are described in Chapter 220. The most common form of congenital adrenal hyperplasia is 21-hydroxylase deficiency, accounting for the disorder in more than 90% of affected individuals. The defect may vary from partial to complete deficiency of the enzyme.

Diagnostic Tests
Measurement of Peptide and Steroid Hormones
Increased levels of immunoreactive human chorionic gonadotropin (HCG) may suggest an HCG-secreting neoplasm, most commonly an ovarian teratoma or dysgerminoma.[8] In such cases, the HCG, which is antigenically and biologically similar to LH, stimulates ovarian steroid secretion and pseudopubertal development. Because even specific LH immunoassays show some cross-reactivity with HCG, values for serum LH may be elevated in individuals with HCG-secreting tumors. Immunoreactive HCG is always elevated in the presence of such tumors. Levels and ratios of FSH and LH typical of pubertal as opposed to prepubertal girls help in the diagnosis of true precocious puberty. Timed urine collections rather than blood samples can be used to measure gonadotropin secretion if necessary. The use of exogenous GnRH to stimulate endogenous LH and FSH secretion can help differentiate gonadotropin-dependent from gonadotropin-independent precocious puberty and is regarded as the "gold standard" in the diagnosis of central precocious puberty. If GnRH is not available, a GnRH analog can be substituted. Excessively high circulating levels of estrogen (>100 pg estradiol) suggest an estrogen-producing neoplasm or a functioning ovarian cyst. High levels of serum testosterone suggest an ovarian source of excess androgen in girls with heterosexual development, whereas increased levels of dehydroepiandrosterone or its sulfate (the principal precursors of 17-ketosteroids) suggest an adrenal source. High levels of serum l7-hydroxyprogesterone imply congenital adrenal hyperplasia secondary to 21-hydroxylase deficiency, whereas high levels of serum 11-deoxycortisol imply an 11β-hydroxylase deficiency (Chapter 220). In congenital adrenal hyperplasia, these hormone levels should decrease promptly after the oral administration of suppressive doses of dexamethasone. Suppression in response to exogenous corticoids occurs much less consistently in individuals with adrenal cortical adenomas and carcinomas (Chapter 214) and rarely in those with ovarian androgen-secreting neoplasms.

Additional Studies
Imaging of the CNS is the most important test if true precocious puberty is present or if there are any neurologic deficits. Ultrasonography of the adrenals and ovaries or computed tomography (CT) of the adrenals may be indicated to confirm clinical suspicions. In girls with ovarian or adrenal neoplasms, the tumor can almost always be localized radiographically. Catheterization of the ovarian and adrenal veins and measurements of the effluent steroids from each gland should be pursued only when CT, ultrasonography, or MRI fails to identify a suspected neoplasm. Radiographic estimation of bone age is also indicated and serves as a useful tool to follow the results of treatment.

TREATMENT

Treatment of precocious puberty should be initiated promptly so that the patient's ultimate height is not compromised as a result of sex steroid–induced premature epiphyseal closure and to prevent or attenuate emotional disturbances in the patient and her parents.[9-11]

GnRH analogs are now the preferred therapy for suppressing gonadotropin secretion, and they also may prevent early bone maturation. No randomized trials have been conducted, but there is universal acknowledgment that GnRH

analogs increase ultimate adult height in girls presenting before 6 years of age. Two unresolved issues are whether to initiate treatment with GnRH analogs in girls between 6 and 8 years of age and at what age to stop treatment. In addition, some data suggest that oral contraceptive pills or metformin may improve hirsutism and oligomenorrhea in the teenage years.[12] The analogs are not effective in children with McCune-Albright syndrome, and ketoconazole and testolactone have been only marginally successful. Aqueous depot medroxyprogesterone acetate (100 to 200 mg intramuscularly every 2 to 4 weeks) also may be used to suppress gonadotropin secretion; however, it does not always prevent premature epiphyseal closure and the resultant short stature.

Individuals with CNS or steroid-secreting neoplasms must undergo therapy appropriate for the particular lesion. Girls with congenital adrenal hyperplasia are appropriately managed with glucocorticoids (plus mineralocorticoids when indicated), as outlined in Chapter 220.

Delayed Puberty

Girls who have no evidence of thelarche by age 13 or who fail to undergo menarche by age 15 have delayed puberty and should be evaluated.[13] Ovarian failure, congenital absence of the uterus and vagina, and constitutional delay constitute about two thirds of cases in large series. Because of the anxiety generated by delayed puberty, some evaluation is always indicated regardless of the age of the patient.

When pubertal development progresses normally but menstruation does not begin, an abnormality in the genital tract should be considered. Congenital malformations of the müllerian ducts are uncommon, occurring in 0.02% of all women. Most do not cause amenorrhea, and many do not impair reproduction. The anomalies associated with amenorrhea vary in severity from an imperforate hymen to complete aplasia of all müllerian duct derivatives, with vaginal atresia. Although aplasia generally involves all the müllerian duct derivatives, defects may involve only a single part of the distal genital tract. Family aggregates of the most common disorders of müllerian differentiation in females—müllerian aplasia and incomplete müllerian fusion—do occur and are best explained by polygenic or multifactorial inheritance. The HOX genes, a family of regulatory genes that encode transcription factors, are essential for proper development of the müllerian tract.

A müllerian duct anomaly is suggested by (1) normal levels of serum gonadotropins and steroids, (2) an abnormal outflow tract, (3) a history of cyclic abdominal pain with or without a palpable mass, and (4) normal development of secondary sex characteristics. Normal ovarian function still induces endometrial growth and shedding after menarche if the uterus is normal. In the absence of a normal outflow tract, however, the menstrual effluent is retained and may or may not escape into the abdominal cavity. Free in the abdominal cavity, the effluent may cause endometriosis. Constrained to the uterine cavity, the effluent causes hematometra and a large abdominal mass. In the absence of a mass or cyclic pain, karyotyping is indicated in girls with evidence of an abnormal genital tract to rule out disorders of sexual differentiation (Chapter 220). Such disorders, however, almost never occur together with completely normal pubertal development. In girls with a normal karyotype and a genital tract anomaly, examination under anesthesia and diagnostic laparoscopy should be undertaken to delineate the extent of the defect. When the abnormality consists of an imperforate hymen or transverse vaginal septum only, surgical restoration can be accomplished relatively simply. Attempts to provide an outflow tract for the uterus should not be undertaken if there is no cervix because of the high risk of recurrent pelvic infection. Even with a functional cervix, the construction of an outflow tract that permits successful pregnancy is unlikely. A functional vagina can be constructed surgically or by the daily use of ever-larger dilators. To prevent shrinkage and scarring, surgery should be deferred until the patient is willing to use dilators on a daily basis or she is about to become sexually active.

Other causes of delayed puberty and primary amenorrhea are the same as those that cause amenorrhea in older women (Chapter 223).[14] When no apparent cause of delayed development is found, constitutional delayed puberty must be entertained as a diagnosis of exclusion.[15] A strong family history of delayed maturation supports this presumption. Small doses of estrogen can be administered to induce some pubertal development, but this may obscure a pathologic cause of the delay and may compromise linear growth and ultimate height.

Asynchronous Pubertal Development

Asynchronous pubertal development is characteristic of male pseudohermaphroditism due to androgen insensitivity, especially complete testicular feminization. This syndrome of androgen insensitivity is inherited as either an X-linked recessive trait or a sex-limited autosomal dominant trait. Despite the presence of intra-abdominal or inguinal testes, there is complete failure of virilization. Affected individuals develop breasts (but only to Tanner stage 3) and a typical female habitus with unambiguous female external genitalia, but with the absence of internal female structures and generally only a foreshortened, blind-ending vagina. Little or no pubic and axillary hair develops. The karyotype is 46,XY in these individuals. Circulating testosterone levels are equivalent to or higher than those found in normal men, LH levels are elevated, and FSH levels are normal compared with those in menstruating women. For a more detailed description, see Chapter 220.

Heterosexual Pubertal Development
POLYCYSTIC OVARY SYNDROME
Polycystic ovary syndrome (PCOS), by far the most common cause of heterosexual pubertal development, is associated with the development of some secondary sex features characteristic of males at the normal age of puberty.[16] Feminization occurs in affected girls, and they develop normal breasts and a typical female habitus, but masculinization also occurs (in contrast, girls with congenital adrenal hyperplasia generally show little if any female development at puberty). A heterogeneous syndrome, PCOS typically begins at or near puberty with hirsutism and irregular menses from the time of menarche. Many girls who develop PCOS are overweight in childhood, and obesity is clearly a risk factor. It now appears that many girls who develop PCOS have alterations in insulin signaling.[17] Menarche may be delayed in a few cases, so young women may present with primary amenorrhea. Basal LH levels tend to be somewhat elevated in perhaps two thirds of cases, and circulating levels of all androgens are moderately elevated. Some degree of insulin resistance is commonly present as well, and hypercholesterolemia may predispose to cardiovascular disease later in life. This is discussed more completely in Chapter 223.

CONGENITAL ADRENAL HYPERPLASIA
Congenital adrenal hyperplasia is generally diagnosed before puberty, and heterosexual precocious pseudopuberty is typical.[18] However, if the defect is mild and changes to the external genitalia are minimal, masculinization may occur at the expected age of puberty. This attenuated or nonclassic form of 21-hydroxylase deficiency seems to occur in families with a strong history of hirsutism. Affected girls generally have some defeminization, with flattening of the breasts, severe hirsutism, relatively short stature, and obesity. For a more detailed description, see Chapter 220.

MIXED GONADAL DYSGENESIS
Mixed gonadal dysgenesis designates asymmetrical gonadal development, with a germ cell tumor or a testis on one side and an undifferentiated streak, rudimentary gonad, or no gonad on the other.[19] The extent of genital virilization before puberty is variable in this rare disorder. Most individuals are reared as girls, in whom virilization occurs at puberty; some may note breast development as well. Affected individuals generally have a mosaic karyotype, with 45,X/46,XY being most common. Short stature and other stigmata associated with a 45,X karyotype in Turner syndrome are less common in patients with tumors than in patients with testes. Gonadectomy is indicated in all individuals with a Y chromosome to eliminate the increased neoplastic potential of such dysgenetic gonads and in all patients in whom virilization occurs at puberty to remove the source of androgen. Estrogen replacement therapy is warranted after gonadectomy. Other causes of male pseudohermaphroditism associated with heterosexual pubertal development are described in Chapter 220.

OTHER CAUSES
An androgen-producing adrenal neoplasm or Cushing syndrome may occur rarely during the pubertal years and lead to heterosexual development (Chapter 214).

GENERAL REFERENCES

For the General References and other additional features, please visit Expert Consult at https://expertconsult.inkling.com.

223

REPRODUCTIVE ENDOCRINOLOGY AND INFERTILITY

WILLIAM H. CATHERINO

THE NORMAL MENSTRUAL CYCLE
Endometrium
The endometrium undergoes histologic and cytologic changes that culminate with menstrual bleeding when the corpus luteum ceases to secrete progesterone (Fig. 223-1). The basal layer of the endometrium then regenerates the superficial layer of compact epithelial cells lining the uterine cavity and an intermediate layer of spongiosa. Both superficial layers are shed at menstruation. Endometrial glands proliferate under the influence of estrogen, and the mucosa thickens. In the luteal phase, the glands become coiled and secretory, with increased vascularity and edema of the stroma. When estradiol and progesterone decline, the stroma becomes edematous, endometrial and blood vessel necrosis occurs, and bleeding ensues. Local release of prostaglandins may initiate vasospasm with ischemic necrosis and uterine contractions that accompany menstrual flow. Prostaglandin synthetase inhibitors can relieve menstrual cramping. The histologic changes are characteristic; therefore endometrial biopsies can be used to characterize the stage of the cycle and to assess the tissue response to gonadal steroids.

Cervix and Cervical Mucus
During the follicular phase, cervical vascularity, congestion, and edema increase as a result of estrogen. Cervical mucus increases in quantity (10- to 30-fold)

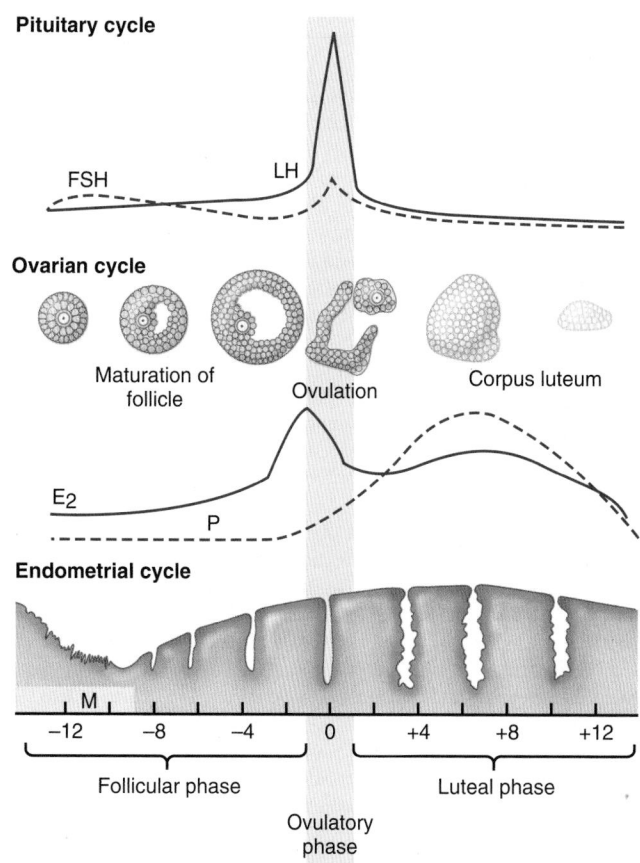

FIGURE 223-1. The idealized cyclic changes observed in gonadotropins, estradiol (E_2), progesterone (P), and uterine endometrium during the normal menstrual cycle. The data are centered on the day of the luteinizing hormone (LH) surge (day 0). Days of menstrual bleeding are indicated by M. FSH = follicle-stimulating hormone; LH = luteinizing hormone. (From Endocrine and Metabolism Continuing Education Quality Control Program, 1982. Copyright American Association for Clinical Chemistry, Inc.)

and in elasticity. So-called ferning becomes prominent. Progesterone stimulates cervical mucus thickening and loss of elasticity and ability to fern. These characteristics are useful in evaluating the stage of the cycle and the amount of estrogen present.

Vagina

Low estrogen is associated with pale, thin vaginal epithelium. As estrogens rise, the number of cornified epithelial cells increases. Subsequently, progesterone decreases the percentage of cornified cells and increases the number of precornified intermediate cells. There is also increased cellular debris and clumping of shed desquamated cells. Histologic changes in the vaginal epithelium are sensitive indicators of estrogen status.

Ovary

The ovaries produce a single dominant graafian follicle that grows and develops to the preovulatory stage during the follicular phase. This process is brought about by combined action of follicle-stimulating hormone (FSH) and luteinizing hormone (LH) on the follicle wall to increase estradiol biosynthesis. The LH surge acts on the preovulatory follicle to cause the secretion of the mature fertilizable oocyte. After ovulation, the follicle wall transforms into the corpus luteum, which produces progesterone and estradiol. If implantation does not occur, the corpus luteum undergoes luteolysis and stops hormone production. In the late luteal phase, another dominant follicle develops, and a new menstrual cycle begins.

Chronology of Folliculogenesis

The preovulatory follicle begins its development when a primordial follicle is recruited into the pool of growing follicles. There are two major phases of folliculogenesis: the preantral (gonadotropin-independent) and the antral (gonadotropin-dependent) periods (see Fig. 223-1). The first phase is characterized by growth of the oocyte and granulosa proliferation. Preantral folliculogenesis proceeds slowly, requiring at least 300 days. During the second phase, granulosa and theca cells proliferate, and the antrum enlarges. The graafian follicle increases relatively rapidly as it develops. The mature graafian follicle that will ovulate requires 40 to 50 days to complete the antral phase.

Selection

The dominant follicle is selected from a cohort at the end of the luteal phase of the previous menstrual cycle. The selected follicle requires 20 days to develop to the ovulatory stage.

Shortly after the midluteal phase of the cycle, the granulosa cells show a sharp increase in the rate of mitosis. The first indication of selection is that the granulosa cells continue dividing at a high rate. As a consequence of the high sustained mitotic rate and the progressive accumulation of follicular fluid, the dominant follicle undergoes remarkable growth. The increase in plasma FSH levels that begins at the end of luteal phase and continues through the early follicular phase evokes follicle selection. The concentration of FSH in the follicular fluid of the healthy (dominant) follicle increases but does not increase in the nondominant atretic follicles. The manner in which this selective increase in FSH is controlled is unknown. More than 99.9% of all follicles are not selected and undergo atresia.

Ovulation

At midpoint in the menstrual cycle, the preovulatory surges of LH and FSH act on the preovulatory follicle to initiate the events leading to ovulation (see Fig. 223-1). The LH surge induces meiotic maturation, a process that converts the oocyte into a fertilizable egg arrested at the second meiotic metaphase. During meiotic maturation, the granulosa cells next to the oocyte are stimulated by FSH to undergo cumulus expansion (Fig. 223-2). This is a prerequisite for the oocyte's pickup and transport by the oviduct. The LH surge also stimulates production of proteolytic enzymes in the vicinity of the presumptive stigma. This process requires the LH stimulation of progesterone and prostaglandins, which are obligatory for stigma formation. After 36 hours, the fertilizable egg and surrounding cumulus cells are secreted through the stigma (see Fig. 223-1). A serum progesterone level higher than 3 ng/mL 1 week before menses is probably diagnostic of ovulation.[1]

Luteogenesis

Ovulation leads to changes in the granulosa and theca cells of the ovulated follicle that result in increased production of progesterone and estradiol during the first week of the luteal phase. This event, termed *luteinization,* is important for the formation and development of a secretory endometrium. Three major

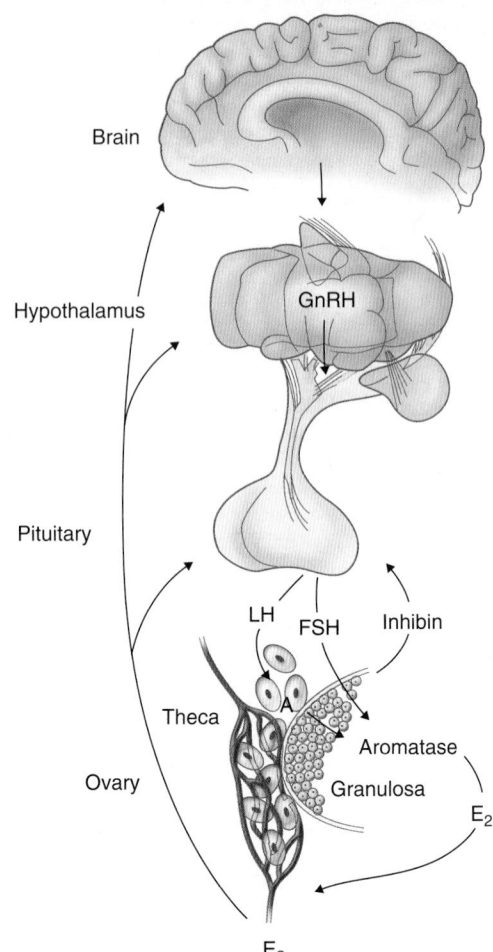

FIGURE 223-2. The hypothalamic-pituitary-ovarian axis in the regulation of follicular maturation and steroidogenesis. A = androgens; E_2 = estradiol; FSH = follicle-stimulating hormone; GnRH = gonadotropin-releasing hormone; LH = luteinizing hormone. (Modified from Endocrine and Metabolism Continuing Education Quality Control Program, 1982. Copyright American Association for Clinical Chemistry, Inc.)

physiologic mechanisms are responsible for luteinization: removal of luteinization inhibitors, secretion of LH by the pituitary, and delivery of high levels of cholesterol. The induction of steroidogenic acute regulatory protein StAR, P450c22, and 3β-hydroxysteroid dehydrogenase in the granulosa lutein cells leads to progesterone production by the corpus luteum. The two-cell, two-gonadotropin mechanism is responsible for estradiol production. If implantation does not occur, the corpus luteum initiates luteolysis, leading to decreases in progesterone, estradiol, and apoptosis. When luteolysis occurs, another dominant follicle is selected, and a new menstrual cycle begins.

ABNORMALITIES OF THE REPRODUCTIVE YEARS

Dysmenorrhea and Endometriosis

DEFINITION

Dysmenorrhea, defined as painful menstruation, affects about 50% of postpubertal women and can be classified as primary or secondary. *Endometriosis,* which may result in dysmenorrhea, infertility, and dyspareunia (i.e., painful intercourse), is the ectopic occurrence of endometrial tissue, most commonly within the abdominal cavity but sometimes in surgical scars, on the vulva, in the umbilicus, and elsewhere.

PATHOBIOLOGY

Primary dysmenorrhea occurs only in ovulatory cycles. Prostaglandins produce dysmenorrhea by initiating painful, exaggerated uterine contractions and myometrial ischemia. Associated systemic symptoms include nausea, diarrhea, headache, and emotional changes. In secondary dysmenorrhea, there is a pathologic cause, with endometriosis being the most common. Other causes include pelvic inflammatory disease; congenital abnormalities, such as atresia of a portion of the distal genital tract and cystic duplication of the paramesonephric ducts; and cervical stenosis. Studies have suggested the possibility that the pain of endometriosis is caused by the presence of nerve fibers within ectopic endometrium.

TREATMENT Rx

Prostaglandin synthetase inhibitors, such as naproxen, ibuprofen, mefenamic acid, and indomethacin, are used to treat primary dysmenorrhea.[A1] If the dysmenorrhea persists, addition of an oral contraceptive to inhibit ovulation and limit prostaglandin release is generally effective. In cases in which the pelvic pain remains intractable, additional evaluation is warranted.[2] If thorough evaluation of the gastrointestinal and urinary tracts fails to reveal a definitive cause, examination under anesthesia and diagnostic laparoscopy may be indicated.

If endometriosis is diagnosed at laparoscopy, treatment varies according to the severity of the disease and the goals of the patient regarding fertility.[3] It may be possible to fulgurate implants or to lyse adhesions. Available data do not demonstrate a benefit of excision over ablation at the time of initial diagnosis as the preferred approach to controlling symptoms. From this point onward, efforts should be directed toward treating endometriosis medically, with additional surgery deferred until infertility (if present) becomes manifest. Medical therapy can consist of continuous suppression with oral contraceptives,[A2] progestins (oral, injectable, or implantable),[A3] or gonadotropin-releasing hormone (GnRH) analogs or danazol for 3 to 6 months. GnRH analogs[A4,A5] are currently the most frequently used form of medical suppressive therapy.[4] After a course of treatment, use of oral contraceptive agents should probably be continued until fertility is desired. Conservative surgical resection of endometriotic tissue should almost always be deferred until it is established as the cause of infertility. Surgery may be required, however, for continuing severe pain, severe endometriosis, or large ovarian cysts containing endometriosis (endometriomas). If symptoms continue despite adequate treatment or if psychological overlay is suspected, psychiatric evaluation may be indicated. Medical causes of dysmenorrhea, however, should be eliminated first.

Premenstrual Syndrome

DEFINITION

Premenstrual syndrome (PMS), also known as *premenstrual tension*, is a complex of physical and emotional symptoms that occur repetitively in a cyclic fashion before menstruation and that diminish or disappear with menstruation.[5]

DIAGNOSIS

The cyclic symptoms typically are sufficiently severe to interfere with some aspects of life. More than 150 different symptoms are now thought to vary with the menstrual cycle (Table 223-1). Estimates of the prevalence of PMS range from 25 to 100%. The *Diagnostic and Statistical Manual of Mental Disorders* classifies severe PMS as premenstrual dysphoric disorder (PMDD). For most women, PMS is merely annoying; severe PMS (or PMDD) causes serious

difficulties for 3 to 5% of women of reproductive age. The diagnosis of both PMS and PMDD is best established by requiring affected individuals to keep prospective daily records of symptoms during a 2- to 3-month period. Less than 50% of women complaining of PMS are found to have the syndrome when such records are examined.

Most women seek help for PMS in their 30s after 10 or more years of symptoms. Many report that their symptoms began at menarche; approximately half state that symptoms followed childbirth. Severity and duration of symptoms are often reported to increase after each successive pregnancy and to become more severe with advancing age. Women with severe long-standing PMS almost always describe associated psychological reactions, including social difficulties, such as marital discord, difficulty relating to their children, difficulty maintaining friendships, and withdrawal from social activities.

TREATMENT Rx

General Measures

The cause of PMS is unknown, and patients should be informed that no one therapy has been effective in all women. Women with mild premenstrual symptoms often benefit from simple changes in lifestyle, including daily mild aerobic exercise; reduction in intake of caffeine-containing beverages, salt, and refined sugar, particularly in the luteal phase; stress reduction; and adequate rest.

Medical Therapy

Women with more severe PMS may benefit from symptomatic treatment.[6] Continuous oral contraceptives have inconsistent but generally positive therapeutic benefit,[7] although intermittent drospirenone/ethinyl estradiol dosed on a 21-7 schedule has been found to have comparable efficacy to the continuous combined oral contraceptive.[A6] Bromocriptine (generally 2.5 mg twice a day) or danazol (100 to 400 mg/day in two divided doses) may be given continuously for relief of mastalgia (breast pain), although this use is not listed in the manufacturer's directive or approved by the U.S. Food and Drug Administration (FDA) and efficacy has not been documented by rigorous randomized trials. Prostaglandin synthetase inhibitors may help reduce dysmenorrhea and may alleviate headaches. Mild sedatives and tranquilizers may help reduce insomnia and anxiety. Low doses of fluoxetine (10 to 20 mg) and other selective serotonin reuptake inhibitors, administered either daily or for the last 2 weeks of each menstrual cycle, are highly effective in reducing the emotional symptoms associated with PMS.[A7] Mild diuretics (especially spironolactone at doses up to 100 mg each morning) may benefit cyclic edema.

Natural progesterone, given in the form of vaginal suppositories, has been used, but results of double-blind placebo-controlled trials show no efficacy.[8] Likewise, the value of large quantities of multiple vitamins or of oil of evening primrose, containing the essential fatty acid γ-linolenic acid, a precursor of prostaglandins, is unsubstantiated.

Surgical Therapy

Because PMS requires the occurrence of cyclic ovulation, oophorectomy is occasionally considered for patients with particularly intractable symptoms. However, oophorectomy may create new problems related to estrogen deficiency for women with PMS treated in this permanent fashion. Several trials employing a GnRH agonist together with exogenous steroids have been described as reducing PMS. Whether such therapy can be used in the long term remains to be determined.

Abnormal Uterine Bleeding

DIAGNOSIS

Differential Diagnosis

Because there is considerable confusion about terminology of abnormal uterine bleeding, it is important to determine just what is being included in any term used other than *abnormal uterine bleeding*.[9] Postmenarchal bleeding in adolescents secondary to immaturity of the hypothalamic-pituitary-ovarian axis (resulting in anovulation) accounts for about 20% of cases, and perimenopausal bleeding consequent to incipient ovarian failure constitutes more than half.

The causes of abnormal uterine bleeding in the reproductive years include complications from the use of oral contraceptives; complications of pregnancy, especially threatened, incomplete, or missed miscarriages and ectopic pregnancy; coagulation disorders, most commonly idiopathic thrombocytopenic purpura and von Willebrand disease; and pelvic disease, such as intrauterine polyps, leiomyomas, and tumors of the vagina and cervix. Clear cell adenocarcinoma of the vagina or cervix may occur in women exposed to diethylstilbestrol during fetal life. Affected women may also have congenital abnormalities of the upper vagina, cervix, and uterus. Women with a history

TABLE 223-1	COMMON SYMPTOMS OF CYCLIC PREMENSTRUAL SYNDROME
SOMATIC SYMPTOMS	
Abdominal bloating	Constipation or diarrhea
Acne	Headache
Alcohol intolerance	Peripheral edema
Breast engorgement and tenderness	Weight gain
Clumsiness	
EMOTIONAL AND MENTAL SYMPTOMS	
Anxiety	Insomnia
Change in libido	Irritability
Depression	Lethargy
Fatigue	Mood swings
Food cravings (especially salt and sugar)	Panic attacks
Hostility	Paranoia
Inability to concentrate	Violence toward self and others
Increased appetite	Withdrawal from others

of diethylstilbestrol exposure should be reassured that the incidence of malignant change is extremely low. Trauma (coital or otherwise), foreign bodies, systemic illnesses including various endocrinopathies (such as diabetes mellitus, hypothyroidism and hyperthyroidism, Cushing syndrome, and Addison disease), leukemia, and renal disease may also be associated with abnormal bleeding as the presenting manifestation.

Abnormal uterine bleeding with no demonstrable organic genital or extragenital cause (75% of cases) is most frequently associated with anovulation and is appropriately termed *anovulatory* (sometimes termed *dysfunctional*) *bleeding*. Most anovulatory bleeding is due to either estrogen withdrawal or estrogen breakthrough bleeding. In anovulatory women, estrogen stimulates the endometrium unopposed by progesterone. The endometrium proliferates, becomes thicker, and may shed irregularly. Anovulatory bleeding tends to occur at less frequent intervals, and organic lesions tend to cause bleeding more frequently than cyclic menses.

Clinical Evaluation

All cases of abnormal bleeding should be evaluated, beginning with a thorough history emphasizing the amount and duration of blood loss. Prospective charting of the days on which bleeding occurs may be required to evaluate the bleeding pattern. Complications of pregnancy or a bleeding diathesis must always be ruled out.

The findings on physical examination (including the Papanicolaou smear) are normal in anovulatory bleeding except for signs of anemia in the more severe cases. Laboratory tests should include a complete blood count, platelet count, coagulation studies, including von Willebrand disease screening, thyroid function tests, and fasting blood glucose concentration. Anovulatory bleeding must be a diagnosis of exclusion, with management depending on the age of the patient and the extent of the bleeding. A sample of the endometrium should be obtained by biopsy or by dilation and curettage from all women older than 35 years and from those at increased risk for endometrial carcinoma because of prolonged anovulatory bleeding.

TREATMENT   Rx

Even profuse bleeding in hemodynamically stable anovulatory women can almost always be successfully treated by the administration of one combination oral contraceptive pill every 6 hours for 5 to 7 days, although this use is not listed in the manufacturer's directive or approved by the FDA. Bleeding should cease within 24 hours, but patients should be warned to expect heavy bleeding 2 to 4 days after therapy is stopped. If anemia is profound, blood transfusion may be necessary. If the bleeding continues despite therapy, curettage can be carried out. Recurrence can be prevented by giving the patient combination oral contraceptive agents cyclically if pregnancy is not desired. If pregnancy is desired, ovulation can be induced.

Acute episodes of anovulatory bleeding can also be treated with conjugated estrogens administered intravenously (25 mg every 4 hours for up to three doses) until bleeding ceases, although this use is not listed in the manufacturer's directive or approved by the FDA. Progestin therapy (medroxyprogesterone acetate, 5 to 10 mg orally for 10 days) should be started simultaneously. Withdrawal bleeding occurs after cessation of therapy, and the patient can then be treated with oral contraceptive agents for at least three cycles.

For individuals with anovulatory bleeding without an episode of profuse bleeding, treatment with cyclic oral contraceptive agents or progestin can be provided unless pregnancy is desired, in which case ovulation must be induced.

Endometrial ablation by any of several methods is being used increasingly to treat persistent bleeding. However, ablation is not 100% effective, and medical management remains the first line of therapy for most women. Hysterectomy may be an appropriate choice for a small number of women.

Amenorrhea

DEFINITION

Amenorrhea is the absence of menstruation for 3 months or more in women with past menses (secondary amenorrhea) or the absence of menarche by the age of 15 years regardless of the absence or presence of secondary sex characteristics (primary amenorrhea).

PATHOBIOLOGY

If an intact genital outflow tract exists and there is no primary disease of the uterus, amenorrhea is a sign of failure of the hypothalamic-pituitary-ovarian axis to produce cyclically the hormones necessary for menses. Amenorrhea is physiologic in the prepubertal girl, during pregnancy and early in lactation, and after menopause. At any other time, it is pathologic and demands evaluation. Use of the term *postpill amenorrhea* to refer to failure to resume menses within 3 months of discontinuation of oral contraceptives is inappropriate. Women so affected should be evaluated in the same manner as any woman with amenorrhea. Similarly, individuals with menses occurring at infrequent intervals of more than 40 days or having fewer than nine menses per year, termed *oligomenorrhea*, should be evaluated identically to women with amenorrhea.

DIAGNOSIS

Clinical Evaluation

In patients with amenorrhea, even subtle hormonal abnormalities may lead to signs and symptoms. Breast development indicates exposure to estrogens, and the presence of pubic and axillary hair indicates androgenic stimulation.

Patients should be questioned especially closely for evidence of psychological disturbances, dietary and exercise habits,[10] lifestyle, environmental stresses,[11] family history of genetic anomalies, abnormal growth and development, and signs of hyperandrogenism, including hirsutism, temporal balding, deepening of the voice, increased muscle mass, clitorimegaly, and increased libido, and signs of defeminization, including decreasing breast size and vaginal atrophy. Any history of galactorrhea should be determined. A history of symptoms related to thyroid and adrenal dysfunction should also be sought (Chapters 213, 214, and 215).

The physical examination should focus on the evaluation of body dimensions and habitus, extent and distribution of body hair, breast development and secretions, and genitalia. In normal adult women, the arm span is similar to the height; in hypogonadal women, the span is generally more than 5 cm greater than the height. The distribution and quantity of body hair should be considered in view of the family history. The extent of any hirsutism should be recorded, preferably by photographs. Other signs of virilization should be sought carefully. Breast development should be graded according to the method of Tanner (Table 223-2).[12] Breast secretion should be sought by applying pressure to the breasts while the patient is seated. Any secretion should be examined microscopically for the presence of perfectly round fat globules of

TABLE 223-2	CRITERIA FOR DISTINGUISHING TANNER STAGES 1–5 DURING PUBERTAL MATURATION	
TANNER STAGE	**BREAST**	**PUBIC HAIR**
1 (Prepubertal)	No palpable glandular tissue or pigmentation of areola; elevation of areola only	No pubic hair; short, fine vellus hair only
2	Glandular tissue palpable with elevation of breast and areola together as a small mound; areolar diameter increased	Sparse, long, pigmented terminal hair chiefly along the labia majora
3	Further enlargement without separation of breast and areola; although more darkly pigmented, areola still pale and immature; nipple generally at or above midplane of breast tissue when individual is seated upright	Dark, coarse, curly hair, extending sparsely over mons
4	Secondary mound of areola and papilla above breast	Adult-type hair, abundant but limited to mons and labia
5 (Adult)	Recession of areola to contour of breast; development of the Montgomery glands and ducts on areola; further pigmentation of areola; nipple generally below midplane of breast tissue when individual is seated upright; maturation independent of breast size	Adult-type hair in quantity and distribution; spread to inner aspects of the thighs in most racial groups

Data from Ross GT. Disorders of the ovary and female reproductive tract. In: Wilson JD, Foster DW, eds. *Textbook of Endocrinology*, 7th ed. Philadelphia: WB Saunders; 1985:206; Speroff L, Glass RH, Kase N. *Clinical Gynecologic Endocrinology and Infertility*, 3rd ed. Baltimore: Williams & Wilkins; 1983:377; and Kustin J, Rebar RW. Menstrual disorders in the adolescent age group. *Primary Care*. 1987;14:139-166.

TABLE 223-3	CAUSES OF AMENORRHEA

ANATOMIC CAUSES

Pregnancy
Various disorders of sexual differentiation
    Distal genital tract obstruction (müllerian agenesis or dysgenesis)
    Gonadal dysgenesis*
    Ambiguity of external genitalia (male and female pseudohermaphroditism)
Intrauterine adhesions (Asherman syndrome)
Gestational trophoblastic disease

CHRONIC ANOVULATION

Due to CNS-hypothalamic-pituitary dysfunction
With inappropriate steroid feedback (e.g., polycystic ovary syndrome)
Due to thyroid or adrenal disorders

OVARIAN "FAILURE"

Menopause
Genetic abnormalities
Physical and environmental causes (e.g., chemotherapeutic agents, irradiation)
Autoimmune disorders
Idiopathic

*Gonadal dysgenesis may be viewed as both a disorder of sexual differentiation and a form of gonadal "failure."
CNS = central nervous system.

varying size, which indicate galactorrhea. Finally, the female genitalia should be examined carefully because they are such sensitive indicators of the hormonal milieu. The Tanner stage of pubic hair development should be noted (see Table 223-2).

Because the sensitivity of the genitalia to androgens decreases onward from early in fetal development, the extent of any virilization is important. Fusion of the labia and enlargement of the clitoris with or without formation of a penile urethra are observed in women exposed to androgens during the first 3 months of fetal development (Chapter 220). Significant clitorimegaly in the absence of other signs of sexual ambiguity and in the presence of other signs of virilization requires marked androgenic stimulation and strongly implicates an androgen-secreting neoplasm. The development of the labia minora in postpubertal women indicates the influence of estrogens. Overt anomalies of the distal genital tract and any evidence of obstruction to the escape of menstrual blood should be sought. Under the influence of estrogen, the vaginal mucosa changes during sexual maturation from a tissue with a shiny, bright red appearance with sparse, thin secretions to a dull, gray-pink rugated surface with copious, thick secretions.

The history and physical examination quickly differentiate among several causes of amenorrhea (Table 223-3). The various disorders of sexual differentiation and other anatomic causes are often apparent on inspection. Distal genital tract obstruction should be identified at the time of pelvic examination even if the specific abnormality is not obvious. The physical stigmata of Turner syndrome, discussed subsequently, generally make the diagnosis simple. Any sexual ambiguity indicates the need for chromosomal analysis and the measurement of 17α-hydroxyprogesterone to rule out congenital adrenal hyperplasia. Pregnancy and gestational trophoblastic disease may be diagnosed by measurement of human chorionic gonadotropin (hCG). The possibility of intrauterine synechiae or adhesions (Asherman syndrome) must be considered in individuals in whom amenorrhea develops after curettage or endometritis. Tuberculous endometritis, especially in younger women, may also lead to this disorder. Without hormonal measurements, it may be impossible to distinguish between individuals with chronic anovulation, in whom hypothalamic-pituitary-ovarian function is insufficiently coordinated to produce cyclic ovulation, and those with ovarian failure. However, it is generally possible to form a clinical impression about the cause of the amenorrhea. It can be noted whether the patient has absence of, incomplete, or complete development of secondary sex characteristics. The presence of excess body hair or galactorrhea may provide clinical evidence of the pathogenesis of the amenorrhea. Signs and symptoms of adrenal or thyroid dysfunction may be important as well. Administration of a progestin (typically medroxyprogesterone acetate, 5 to 10 given orally for 5 to 10 days, or progesterone in oil, 100 mg given intramuscularly) has been advocated to assess the level of endogenous estrogen. This test is of limited value, however, because almost half the young women with premature ovarian failure experience withdrawal bleeding in response to progestin.

To ascertain whether the outflow tract is intact, an orally active estrogen, such as 2.5 mg of conjugated estrogen daily for 21 days, with 5 to 10 mg of oral medroxyprogesterone acetate for the last 5 to 10 days, is administered. Withdrawal bleeding should occur if the endometrium is normal. Still, hysterosalpingography and hysteroscopy may be required for the diagnosis of Asherman syndrome because some patients with a normal endometrium may not have a withdrawal bleed due to obstruction of the cervical os by scar tissue.

Laboratory Findings

Basal levels of FSH, prolactin, and thyroid-stimulating hormone (TSH) should be measured in all amenorrheic and oligomenorrheic women to confirm the clinical impression (Fig. 223-3).

Increased TSH levels with or without increased levels of prolactin imply primary hypothyroidism, and further evaluation for this disorder is indicated (Chapter 213). Although hypothyroidism commonly results in anovulation, amenorrhea occurs in only some hypothyroid women. Menorrhagia and oligomenorrhea may occur as well. The sensitive immunoassays for TSH permit identification of women with hyperthyroidism as well because TSH levels are suppressed in those individuals.

If the prolactin concentration is minimally increased and the TSH level is normal, measurement of the prolactin concentration should be repeated before more extensive evaluation is undertaken because prolactin levels are increased by nonspecific stressful stimuli, sleep, and food ingestion. Prolactin levels may be elevated in as many as one third of women with amenorrhea.

Increased FSH levels (generally above 30 mIU/mL) imply ovarian failure and require further evaluation. Incipient ovarian failure should be considered in any woman with basal FSH levels of 15 mIU/mL or higher other than during the midcycle LH surge. Many clinicians believe that chromosomal evaluation is indicated in all individuals with elevated FSH levels before age 40 years, and it is certainly indicated if hypergonadotropic amenorrhea begins before age 30 years.

If FSH levels are low or normal, the measurement of total testosterone levels may be helpful whether or not there is any evidence of hirsutism or virilization. Hyperandrogenic women need not be hirsute because some have relative insensitivity of the hair follicles to androgens. Mildly increased levels of testosterone (and perhaps dehydroepiandrosterone sulfate as well) suggest polycystic ovary syndrome (PCOS). However, total circulating androgen levels need not be elevated because of the alterations in metabolic clearance rate and sex hormone–binding globulin that are present in PCOS. Consequently, some clinicians prefer to measure circulating free testosterone levels.

Circulating levels of LH and FSH may aid in differentiation of PCOS from hypothalamic-pituitary dysfunction. LH levels are often elevated in PCOS so that the ratio of LH to FSH is increased; however, LH levels may be identical to those observed in normal women in the follicular phase. In contrast, levels of LH and FSH are normal or slightly reduced in hypothalamic-pituitary dysfunction. There is some overlap between women with "polycystic ovarian-like" disorders and those with hypothalamic-pituitary dysfunction. Radiographic assessment of the sella turcica is indicated in all amenorrheic women in whom both LH and FSH levels are consistently low (both below 10 mIU/mL) to exclude a pituitary or parapituitary neoplasm (Chapter 211). Other pituitary functions should be evaluated in any individual with significantly impaired LH and FSH secretion. Both total testosterone and dehydroepiandrosterone sulfate levels should be measured in hirsute or virilized women. Testosterone levels greater than 200 ng/dL should lead to investigation for an androgen-producing neoplasm, most likely of ovarian origin. Dehydroepiandrosterone sulfate levels greater than 7.0 μg/mL should lead to evaluation for an adrenal neoplasm, and levels between 5.0 and 7.0 μg/mL should lead to evaluation for adult-onset congenital adrenal hyperplasia (Chapter 220).

Hypergonadotropic Amenorrhea (Presumptive Ovarian Failure, Primary Hypogonadism, Primary Ovarian Insufficiency)

(DIAGNOSIS)

Differential Diagnosis

Gonadal failure may begin at any time during embryonic or postnatal development and may result from many causes. Normally, the ovaries fail at menopause, when virtually no functioning follicles remain. However, premature loss of oocytes before the age of 40 years may occur and lead to premature ovarian failure. Circulating gonadotropin levels increase whenever

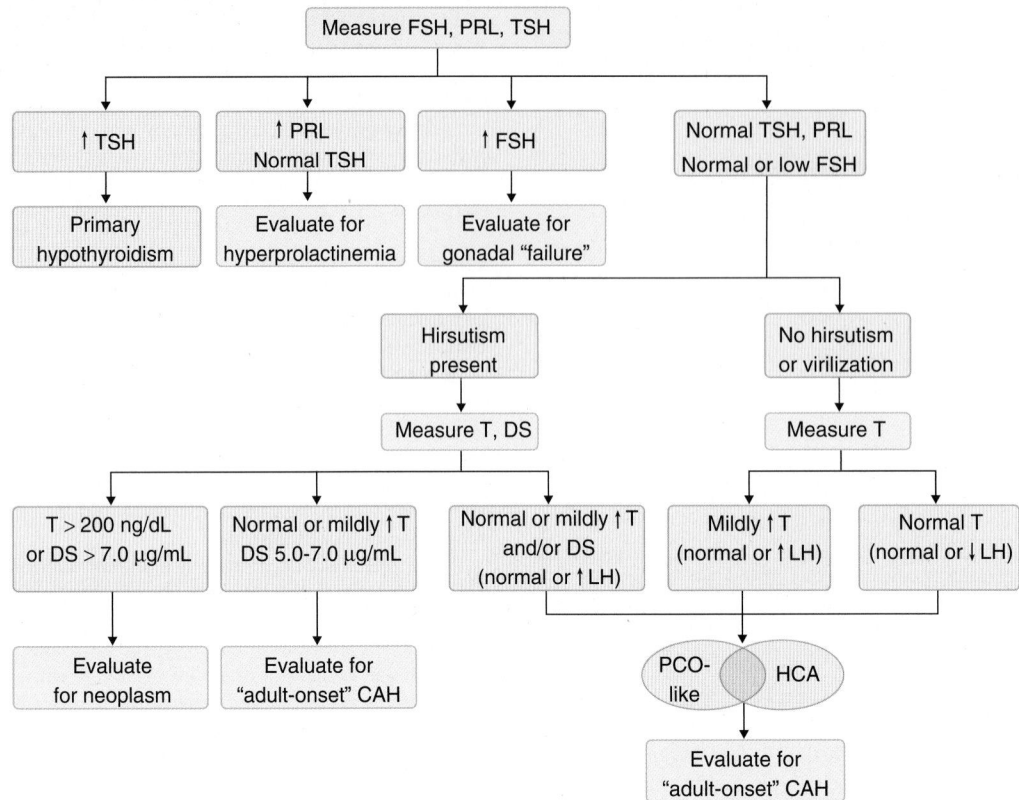

FIGURE 223-3. Biochemical evaluation of amenorrhea. This schema must be considered an adjunct to the clinical evaluation of the patient. See text for details. CAH = congenital adrenal hyperplasia; DS = dehydroepiandrosterone sulfate; FSH = follicle-stimulating hormone; HCA = hypothalamic chronic anovulation; LH = luteinizing hormone; PCO-like = polycystic ovarian syndrome–like; PRL = prolactin; T = testosterone; TSH = thyroid-stimulating hormone.

ovarian failure occurs because of decreased negative estrogen feedback to the hypothalamic-pituitary unit.

PATHOBIOLOGY

There are several causes for premature ovarian failure, including genetic causes (a growing list that includes karyotypic abnormalities, single gene mutations, and complex multifactorial polygenic inheritance), physical and environmental causes, and autoimmune disturbances. In addition, there may be families in which menopause begins earlier than the expected age without any further pathologic cause.

Genetic Abnormalities

Several pathologic conditions with dysgenetic gonads involve elevated gonadotropin levels and amenorrhea as well as abnormalities of the X chromosome. The term *gonadal dysgenesis* refers to individuals with undifferentiated streak gonads without any association with either extragonadal stigmata or sex chromosome aberrations. Because individuals with gonadal dysgenesis have the normal complement of oocytes at 20 weeks of fetal age but virtually none by birth, this disorder is a form of premature ovarian failure.

Turner Syndrome

Turner syndrome (also see Chapter 220) describes patients with streak gonads composed of fibrous stroma and four cardinal features: a female phenotype; sexual infantilism; short stature; and several physical abnormalities, sometimes including webbed neck, low-set ears, multiple pigmented nevi, double eyelashes, micrognathia, epicanthal folds, shieldlike chest with microthelia, short fourth metacarpals, increased carrying angle of the arms, and certain renal and cardiovascular defects (most commonly coarctation of the aorta and aortic stenosis). The diagnosis can sometimes be made at birth because of unexplained lymphedema of the hands and feet. The syndrome is associated with an abnormality of sex chromosome number, morphology, or both. Most commonly, the second sex chromosome is absent (45,X). Turner syndrome is the single most common chromosome disorder in humans, but more than 95% of such fetuses are aborted, and the incidence in newborns is approximately 1 in 3000 to 5000. Chromosome breakage and mosaicism occur as well. In mosaic individuals with a normal 46,XX cell line, sufficient follicles may persist postnatally

to initiate pubertal changes and to cause ovulation so that pregnancy is possible. Deletions of the X-chromosome-linked *SHOX* gene explain many of the dysmorphic skeletal features that are present, including the short stature. It is believed that the number of phenotypic findings may be related to the percentage of cells that are 45,X. There also may be an effect of imprinting with the variation in phenotype partly explained by the parental origin of the one remaining X chromosome.

Pure Gonadal Dysgenesis

Pure gonadal dysgenesis is the term given to phenotypically female individuals with streak gonads who are of normal stature and have none of the physical stigmata associated with Turner syndrome. Such individuals have either a 46,XX or 46,XY karyotype. The 46,XX defect may be inherited as an autosomal recessive, with 10% having associated nerve deafness. The 46,XY defect may be inherited as an X-linked recessive, with clitorimegaly occurring in 10 to 15% and gonadal tumors developing in 25% if the gonads are not removed.

Mutations in the X Chromosome Associated with Premature Ovarian Failure

Several regions of the X chromosome are now recognized to contain mutations in genes that may result in premature ovarian failure. Of particular note is the fragile X mental retardation (*FMR1*) gene. More than 5% of women with 46,XX spontaneous premature ovarian failure have mutations of the *FMR1* gene. This risk is increased if there is a family history of premature ovarian failure. A family history of fragile X syndrome, unexplained mental retardation, dementia, developmental delay of a child, or tremor-ataxia syndrome is reason for genetic counseling. Mutations in the *FMR1* gene are known to be associated with a neurodegenerative disorder. Women with mutations in the *FMR1* gene are at risk of having a child with mental retardation, should they be one of the 6 to 8% of women with premature ovarian failure who conceive spontaneously. For *FMR1*, a CGG repeat sequence occurs, with up to 60 repeats being normal. Expansion to more than 200 repeats leads to the fragile X syndrome, with the high level of repeats causing hypermethylation of the gene promoter and silencing of the gene. Female carriers of the permutation have an unstable intermediate number of repeats (i.e., 60 to 199) and the predisposition for premature ovarian failure.

Trisomy X

Trisomy X (46,XXX karyotype) is also associated with premature menopause, although many such individuals have normal reproductive lives. Premature menopause can also occur in mosaic individuals with cell lines with excess X chromosomes. When gonadal abnormalities occur in women with excess X chromosomes, they seem to occur after ovarian differentiation so that some ovarian function is possible. Only later in life do such women develop secondary amenorrhea and premature ovarian failure.

Known Genetic Alterations of Specific Genes

In girls with the rare syndrome of 17α-hydroxylase deficiency involving *p450c17* who survive until the expected age of puberty, sexual infantilism and primary amenorrhea occur together with elevated levels of gonadotropins (also see Chapter 220). Defects in the 20,22-lyase (*p450scc*) or aromatase (*p450arom*) enzymes may also lead to ovarian failure. Women with galactosemia also experience ovarian failure early in life, even when a galactose-restricted diet is introduced early in infancy.

Mutations of several autosomal genes result in premature ovarian failure. Included in this growing list are mutations involving *FSHR* (the FSH receptor gene), *FOXL2* (a forkhead transcription factor associated with the blepharophimosis-ptosis-epicanthus inversus syndrome), *INHA* (the inhibin-α gene), *E1F2B* (a family of genes associated with central nervous system leukodystrophy and ovarian failure), *PMM2* (the gene for phosphomannomutase), *GALT* (the gene for galactose-1-phosphate uridyltransferase), and *AIRE* (leading to the autoimmune polyendocrinopathy-candidiasis-ectodermal dystrophy syndrome). Myotonic dystrophy (Chapter 393) is caused by an autosomal triple repeat mutation, like the fragile X syndrome, that is similarly associated with premature loss of germ cells from the ovary. The list of mutations associated with early ovarian failure continues to increase as the function of more genes is determined.

Mutations Involving Reproductive Hormones, Their Receptors, and Action

The resistant ovary (Savage) syndrome occurs in young amenorrheic women who have elevated peripheral gonadotropin concentrations, normal (although immature) follicles present on ovarian biopsy, 46,XX karyotype with no evidence of mosaicism, fully developed secondary sex characteristics, and ovarian resistance to stimulation with human menopausal or pituitary gonadotropins. At least some of these women have mutations in the FSH receptor. It is probably inappropriate to use the term "resistant ovary syndrome" because it is likely that this is a heterogeneous disorder due to various genetic mutations.

Other Causes
Physical and Environmental

Irradiation and chemotherapeutic agents used to treat various malignant diseases may also cause premature ovarian failure. Ovulation and cyclic menses return in some of these patients even after prolonged intervals of hypergonadotropic amenorrhea associated with signs and symptoms of profound hypoestrogenism. In general, the younger the individual at the time of treatment, the less likely is she to have permanent ovarian failure after the completion of therapy. Rarely, mumps affects the ovaries and causes ovarian failure.

Autoimmune Disorders

Premature ovarian failure may occur in conjunction with a variety of autoimmune disorders. The most well known syndrome (autoimmune polyglandular syndrome type 1) involves hypoadrenalism, hypoparathyroidism, and mucocutaneous candidiasis together with ovarian failure (Chapter 218). Testing for adrenal antibodies by indirect immunofluorescence will identify the 4% of women with spontaneous premature ovarian failure who have steroidogenic cell autoimmunity and are at risk for adrenal insufficiency. Thyroiditis is the most commonly associated abnormality. Antibodies to the FSH receptor have been identified in a few cases. These associations make it mandatory to rule out other potentially life-threatening endocrinopathies in young women with hypergonadotropic amenorrhea.

TREATMENT Rx

Women with hypergonadotropic amenorrhea and ovarian failure should be treated identically whether or not they have signs of hypoestrogenism or desire pregnancy. Counseling and psychological support are indicated in women in

---

whom the diagnosis of premature ovarian failure is made. Ovarian biopsy is not indicated to document the existence of follicles because only a small portion of each ovary can be sampled and because pregnancies have resulted in patients who had biopsy samples devoid of follicles. Estrogen replacement is warranted to prevent the accelerated bone loss known to occur in affected women (Chapter 230). The estrogen should be given sequentially with a progestin to prevent endometrial hyperplasia. Young women with ovarian failure may require twice as much estrogen as postmenopausal women for relief of signs and symptoms of hypoestrogenism. Inexplicably, women with premature ovarian failure may conceive while taking exogenous estrogen, even in the form of oral contraceptive agents, at the same rate as those not taking estrogen, so barrier contraception should be discussed if pregnancy is not desired.

Women with hypergonadotropic amenorrhea are rarely able to become pregnant. It is not clear why pregnancy may rarely occur in such women, but the pregnancy and delivery rate is 6 to 8%. Infertility treatment of young women with hypergonadotropic amenorrhea involves hormone replacement to mimic the normal menstrual cycle and embryo transfer by use of donor oocytes. Whether women with gonadal dysgenesis should be offered pregnancy by use of donor oocytes is now the subject of debate because a markedly increased incidence of aortic rupture during pregnancy secondary to medial necrosis has been documented. Women with Turner syndrome contemplating pregnancy should be counseled regarding the risks.

● CHRONIC ANOVULATION

Chronic anovulation, the most frequent form of amenorrhea encountered in women of reproductive age, implies that functional ovarian follicles remain and that cyclic ovulation can be induced with appropriate therapy (Table 223-4). The cause of the anovulation should be determined. The pathophysiologic

---

TABLE 223-4 CAUSES OF CHRONIC ANOVULATION

Chronic anovulation of hypothalamic-pituitary origin
  Hypothalamic chronic anovulation
    Psychogenic
    Exercise associated
    Associated with diet, weight loss, or malnutrition
    Anorexia nervosa and bulimia
    Pseudocyesis
  Forms of isolated (idiopathic) hypogonadotropic hypogonadism (including Kallmann syndrome)
  Due to hypothalamic-pituitary damage
    Pituitary and parapituitary tumors
    Empty sella syndrome
    Following surgery
    Following irradiation
    Following trauma
    Following infection
    Following infarction
  Idiopathic hypopituitarism
  Hypothalamic-pituitary dysfunction or failure with hyperprolactinemia (multiple causes)
  Due to systemic diseases
Chronic anovulation due to inappropriate feedback (i.e., polycystic ovary syndrome)
  Excessive extraglandular estrogen production (i.e., obesity)
  Abnormal buffering involving sex hormone–binding globulin (including liver disease)
  Functional androgen excess (adrenal or ovarian)
  Neoplasms producing androgens or estrogens
  Neoplasms producing chorionic gonadotropin
Chronic anovulation due to other endocrine and metabolic disorders
  Adrenal hyperfunction
    Cushing syndrome
    Congenital adrenal hyperplasia (female pseudohermaphroditism)
  Thyroid dysfunction
    Hyperthyroidism
    Hypothyroidism
  Prolactin or growth hormone excess
    Hypothalamic dysfunction
    Pituitary dysfunction (microadenomas and macroadenomas)
    Drug induced
  Malnutrition

bases for several forms of anovulation are unknown, but the anovulation can be interrupted transiently by nonspecific induction of ovulation in most affected women. Anovulation can result in either amenorrhea or irregular (generally less frequent) menses.

Hypothalamic Chronic Anovulation

DEFINITION

Hypothalamic chronic anovulation (HCA) represents a heterogeneous group of disorders with similar manifestations. Emotional and physical stress, excessive exercise, nutritional deficiencies, weight loss, reduced body fat, and other unrecognized factors may contribute in varying proportions to the anovulation. Women with HCA have normal neuroanatomic findings.

ANOREXIA NERVOSA

Individuals with amenorrhea and significant weight loss should be examined for the possibility of anorexia nervosa (Chapter 206).

ISOLATED HYPOGONADOTROPIC HYPOGONADISM

Affected individuals have absence of spontaneous pubertal development. Most have functional GnRH deficiency, but some have abnormalities of gonadotropin deficiency localized to the pituitary gland.

Kallmann syndrome is a familial disorder consisting of gonadotropin deficiency, anosmia or hyposmia, and color blindness in men or, more rarely, in women (Chapter 210). Partial or complete agenesis of the olfactory bulb is present on autopsy, accounting for use of the term *olfactogenital dysplasia*. Isolated gonadotropin deficiency in the absence of anosmia occurs as well. Sexual infantilism with a eunuchoid habitus is the clinical hallmark of this disorder, but moderate breast development may occur. Circulating LH and FSH levels are low but almost always detectable. Ovulation induction requires use of exogenous gonadotropins and hCG or pulsatile GnRH. Estrogen replacement therapy is indicated in these women until pregnancy is desired. It may not be possible to distinguish between partial isolated gonadotropin deficiency and functional HCA in all cases.

HYPOPITUITARISM

Hypopituitarism may be obvious on cursory inspection or sufficiently subtle to require endocrine testing (Chapter 211). The clinical presentation depends on the age at onset, the cause, and the nutritional status of the individual. Failure of development of secondary sex characteristics must always raise the question of hypopituitarism. Ovulation can be induced successfully with exogenous gonadotropins when pregnancy is desired and after the hypopituitarism is treated appropriately. Replacement therapy with estrogen is indicated.

HYPERPROLACTINEMIA

Galactorrhea associated with hyperprolactinemia, whatever the cause, almost always occurs together with amenorrhea caused by hypothalamic-pituitary dysfunction or failure. Many conditions can cause excess prolactin secretion (Chapter 211). A prolactinoma must be excluded. Hirsutism may be observed occasionally in association with amenorrhea-galactorrhea and hyperprolactinemia. Elevated levels of the adrenal androgens dehydroepiandrosterone and dehydroepiandrosterone sulfate may be observed and may account for the polycystic-type ovaries present in some hyperprolactinemic women.

FAILURE OF THE HYPOTHALAMIC-PITUITARY UNIT

The hypothalamic-pituitary unit may also fail to function normally in a number of stressful, debilitating, systemic illnesses that interfere with somatic growth and development. Chronic renal failure, liver disease, and diabetes mellitus are the most prominent examples.

DIAGNOSIS

Abrupt cessation of menses in women younger than 30 years who have no anatomic abnormalities of the hypothalamic-pituitary-ovarian axis and no other endocrine disturbances suggests a diagnosis of HCA. Affected individuals tend to be bright, educated, and engaged in intellectual occupations and may well give a history of psychosexual problems and socioenvironmental trauma. HCA is characterized by low to normal levels of gonadotropins and relative hypoestrogenism. Rarely, however, do affected women present with signs and symptoms of estrogen deficiency. It is important to rule out a central lesion as the cause of the hypogonadotropic hypogonadism in women who appear to have HCA.

TREATMENT Rx

Psychological counseling or a change in lifestyle, especially for women engaged in strenuous exercise programs, may be effective in inducing cyclic ovulation and menses in women with functional HCA. Cognitive-behavioral therapy is effective in a proportion of women with functional HCA. For women desiring pregnancy, ovulation can also be induced with clomiphene citrate (50 to 100 mg/day for 5 days beginning on the third to fifth day of withdrawal bleeding). Treatment with exogenous gonadotropins to induce follicular maturation followed by hCG to induce follicular rupture may be effective in women who do not ovulate in response to clomiphene. Because women with HCA have low circulating levels of leptin, investigators have given recombinant leptin and documented that ovulation may resume in some affected women. Given the heterogeneous nature of the disorder, it is not surprising that exogenous leptin is not effective in all women.

Most physicians advocate the use of exogenous gonadal steroids to prevent osteoporosis. A regimen can consist of daily oral conjugated or esterified estrogens (0.625 to 1.25 mg), ethinyl estradiol (20 μg), or micronized estradiol-17β (1 to 2 mg) or transdermal estradiol-17β (0.05 to 0.10 mg) daily, with oral medroxyprogesterone acetate (5 to 10 mg) added for the first 12 to 14 days of each month. Sexually active women can be given oral contraceptive agents as an alternative. If steroid therapy is administered, patients must be informed that the amenorrhea will probably be present when therapy is discontinued. Other physicians believe that only periodic observation is indicated, with barrier methods of contraception recommended for fertility control. Adequate ingestion of calcium should be ensured regardless of therapy. Contraception is needed for sexually active women with HCA because the functional defect is mild in these disorders and may resolve spontaneously at any time, with ovulation occurring before any episode of menstruation.

Chronic Anovulation Related to Inappropriate Feedback

POLYCYSTIC OVARY SYNDROME

DEFINITION

Polycystic ovary syndrome (PCOS) is a heterogeneous disorder in which there is considerable clinical and biochemical variability among affected individuals.[13] PCOS is currently considered to exist in women with any two of the following: (1) oligo-ovulation or anovulation, (2) hyperandrogenism, or (3) polycystic ovaries on ultrasound, and in whom other etiologies have been eliminated. PCOS is the classic disorder in which the amenorrhea or oligomenorrhea results from inappropriate feedback of gonadal steroids from the ovaries.[14]

PATHOBIOLOGY

Current evidence suggests that the hypothalamic-pituitary unit is intact and that a functional derangement, perhaps involving insulin-like growth factors such as IGF-I within the ovary, results in abnormal gonadotropin secretion. PCOS is characterized by insulin resistance and compensatory hyperinsulinemia. The insulin resistance has been found in affected women of many racial and ethnic groups, implying that it is a universal characteristic and that a common defect may be present. There is increasing evidence of specific genetic abnormalities in some women with PCOS.

CLINICAL MANIFESTATIONS

Although patients usually present with amenorrhea, hirsutism, and obesity, affected women may instead complain of irregular and profuse uterine bleeding, may not have hirsutism, and may be of normal weight. Excess androgen from any source or increased extraglandular conversion of androgens to estrogens can lead to the typical findings of PCOS. Included are such diverse disorders as Cushing syndrome, mild congenital adrenal hyperplasia, virilizing tumors of adrenal or ovarian origin, hyperthyroidism and hypothyroidism, obesity, and primary PCOS with no other recognizable cause.

In the primary syndrome, the irregular menses, mild obesity, and hirsutism begin during puberty and typically become more severe with time, although there is increasing evidence of improvement in the years just before menopause. Obesity alone can lead to a polycystic ovarian-like syndrome, with the degree of obesity required to cause anovulation varying widely. The increase in the prevalence of obesity is leading to an increased prevalence of PCOS. All such patients are well estrogenized regardless of whether they present with primary or secondary amenorrhea or dysfunctional bleeding. LH concentrations tend to be elevated, with relatively low and constant FSH levels, but both may be in the normal range for the follicular phase of the menstrual cycle. Levels of most circulating androgens, especially testosterone, tend to be mildly elevated.

DIAGNOSIS

A consensus conference in Rotterdam in 2003 concluded that after exclusion of other etiologies, two of the following three are required for diagnosis of PCOS: (1) hyperandrogenism (clinical or biochemical), (2) oligo-ovulation or anovulation, (3) polycystic ovaries on ultrasound examination or at surgery.

This definition is confusing to clinicians because it implies that hirsute women with polycystic ovaries on ultrasound examination who ovulate regularly should be considered to have PCOS. Moreover, it is clear that polycystic ovaries may be identified on ultrasound examination in normal women. In any case, the aim of the diagnostic evaluation is to rule out any causes (such as neoplasms) that require definitive therapy. Hirsutism should be evaluated as detailed in Chapter 413.

A particularly severely affected subset of women present with marked obesity, anovulation, mild glucose intolerance with high levels of circulating insulin, acanthosis nigricans, hyperuricemia, severe hirsutism, and elevated circulating androgen levels. These women have hyperthecosis of the ovaries, in which the androgen-producing cells in the stromal, hilar, and thecal regions are increased greatly in number. Hyperthecosis should probably be viewed as a part of the spectrum of disorders constituting PCOS.

TREATMENT

Rx

Patients generally require therapy for hirsutism, for induction of ovulation if pregnancy is desired, and for prevention of estrogen-induced endometrial hyperplasia and cancer. No ideal therapy exists; the therapeutic approach must be individualized. The risks for metabolic syndrome, cardiovascular disease, and diabetes mellitus are increased in women with PCOS, at least in part because of the increased androgens and insulin resistance. Moreover, many women have elevated cholesterol levels.

Medical Therapy

In the anovulatory woman not desiring pregnancy who is not hirsute, therapy with intermittent progestin administration (such as medroxyprogesterone acetate, 5 to 10 mg orally for 10 to 14 days each month) or oral contraceptives can be provided to reduce the increased risk for endometrial carcinoma that is present in such a woman with unopposed estrogen. All women using intermittent progestin administration should be cautioned about the need for effective contraception if they are sexually active because these agents do not inhibit ovulation when they are administered intermittently.

Improvements in insulin sensitivity in women with polycystic ovaries, either through lifestyle changes (e.g., exercise and diet) or through pharmacologic intervention, consistently result in improvements in the reproductive and metabolic abnormalities. Resumption of ovulation may occur in up to 60 to 70% of affected women.[15]

The longest and largest published experiences with any agent that improves insulin sensitivity in PCOS is with metformin, a biguanide that functions primarily by suppressing hepatic gluconeogenesis and also improves insulin sensitivity. Its use in PCOS leads to reductions in insulin and androgen levels and resumption of menses in some women. Divided doses of 1500 to 2000 mg/day have proved effective.

Some clinicians advocate giving metformin to all women with polycystic ovaries, whereas others would administer such an agent only to those with documented insulin resistance. Some clinicians also advocate giving metformin first to women who desire pregnancy and then adding an agent to induce ovulation if the metformin proves ineffective. These agents are not approved for use in pregnant women or for the induction of ovulation.

Treatment Considering Pregnancy

Oral contraceptive agents are the first line of therapy for hirsute anovulatory woman not desiring pregnancy and offer protection from endometrial hyperplasia. In women with PCOS desiring pregnancy, clomiphene citrate or letrozole can be used to induce ovulation.[A8][A9] Letrozole is not approved for this use by the FDA, but a large multicenter randomized trial has demonstrated its superiority to clomiphene in obese women with PCOS. About 75 to 80% conceive with such therapy. In addition to insulin-sensitizing agents, other possible methods of inducing ovulation include use of exogenous gonadotropins and hCG, and laparoscopic ovarian surgery with multiple punctures of the ovary by diathermy or laser. A large clinical trial documented that clomiphene citrate is more effective than metformin in inducing ovulation and resulting in

pregnancy; there was no further improvement when the two agents were used concurrently.[16]

Surgical Treatment

Laparoscopic ovarian surgery can achieve unifollicular ovulation or make it easier for medical ovulation induction, but increases the risk for development of ovarian adhesions (themselves leading to infertility). It may be successful in a small subset of women with PCOS who are geographically removed from good medical care.

Chronic Anovulation Related to Other Endocrine and Metabolic Disorders

Adrenal hyperfunction appears to cause chronic anovulation by inducing a polycystic ovarian-like syndrome secondary to increased adrenal androgen secretion. Both hyperthyroidism and hypothyroidism are associated with a variety of menstrual disturbances, including dysfunctional uterine bleeding and amenorrhea as a result of alterations in the metabolism of androgens and estrogens. These metabolic changes in turn result in inappropriate steroid feedback and chronic anovulation.

INFERTILITY

DEFINITION

The World Health Organization (WHO) has defined *infertility* as "a disease of the reproductive system defined by the failure to achieve a clinical pregnancy after 12 months or more of regular unprotected sexual intercourse." *Sterility* is total inability to reproduce. More than 10% of couples in the United States seek medical assistance for infertility.

The requirements for pregnancy to occur are several:
- The male must produce adequate numbers of normal, motile spermatozoa.
- The male must be capable of ejaculating the sperm through a patent ductal system.
- The sperm must be able to traverse an unobstructed female reproductive tract.
- The female must ovulate and release an ovum.
- The sperm must be able to fertilize the ovum.
- The fertilized ovum must be capable of developing and implanting in appropriately prepared endometrium.

In approximately 40% of cases, infertility is caused by the male (Table 223-5). In one third of couples, more than one cause contributes to the infertility.

Peak age for fertility in the female is 25 years. For nulliparous women of this age, the average time during which unprotected intercourse occurs until conception is 5.3 months. For parous women, the average duration of intercourse until conception is 2.7 months. The reproductive performance of couples is influenced by the ages of the female and male partners, the frequency of intercourse, and the length of time the couple has been attempting to conceive. There is a decline in both female and male reproductive performance after the age of 25 years.

DIAGNOSIS

Couples who complain of infertility merit evaluation regardless of the length of infertility. Evaluation is warranted in all women after 12 months and in women 35 years of age or older after 6 months of regular unprotected intercourse.

The evaluation begins with a detailed history obtained from both partners and physical examinations of both individuals. If possible, the couple should be seen together. Each couple should be questioned together and separately because separate interviews may uncover information that would not be imparted in the presence of the partner.

Initial evaluation for infertility includes assessment of semen; documentation of ovulation by basal body temperature, serum progesterone determination 6 to 8 days before menses, serum thyroid hormone, or (rarely) endometrial biopsy less than 3 days before onset of menses; and evaluation of the female genital tract by hysterosalpingography or sonohysterography. Diagnostic laparoscopy with tubal dye instillation may be performed if results of all previous tests are normal because 30 to 50% of women are found to have endometriosis or tubal disease on surgical evaluation; alternatively, patients with initial normal findings may be merely treated as having idiopathic infertility.

TABLE 223-5   CAUSES OF INFERTILITY AND THEIR APPROXIMATE INCIDENCE

Male factors (40%)
    Decreased production of spermatozoa
        Varicocele
        Testicular failure
        Endocrine disorders
        Cryptorchidism
        Stress, smoking, caffeine, nicotine, recreational drugs
    Ductal obstruction
        Epididymal (after infection)
        Congenital absence of vas deferens
        Ejaculatory duct (after infection)
        After vasectomy
    Inability to deliver sperm into vagina
        Ejaculatory disturbances
        Hypospadias
        Sexual problems (i.e., impotence), medical or psychological
    Abnormal semen
        Infection
        Abnormal volume
        Abnormal viscosity
    Immunologic factors
        Sperm-immobilizing antibodies
        Sperm-agglutinating antibodies

Female factors
    Fallopian tube disease (20-30%)
        Pelvic inflammatory disease or puerperal infection
        Congenital anomalies
        Endometriosis
        Secondary to past peritonitis of nongenital origin
    Amenorrhea and anovulation (15%)
    Minor ovulatory disturbances (<5%?)
    Cervical and uterine factors (10%)
        Leiomyomas and polyps
        Uterine anomalies
        Intrauterine synechiae (Asherman syndrome)
        Destroyed endocervical glands (after surgery or after infection)
    Vaginal factors (<5%)
        Congenital absence of vagina
        Imperforate hymen
        Vaginismus
        Vaginitis
    Immunologic factors (<5%)
        Sperm-immobilizing antibodies
        Sperm-agglutinating antibodies
    Nutritional and metabolic factors (5%)
        Thyroid disorders
        Diabetes mellitus
        Severe nutritional disturbances

Idiopathic or unexplained (<10%)

TREATMENT Rx

Treatment must be predicated on the findings of the infertility evaluation. Abnormalities of sperm are difficult disorders to treat. Low sperm count or poor motility is best treated either by donor insemination or in vitro fertilization with intracytoplasmic injection of a single viable sperm into each oocyte. Obstruction of the fallopian tubes may be amenable to surgical intervention, but success rates are often greater with in vitro fertilization. Endometriosis causing infertility may be treated by surgery or various suppressive drugs as indicated; however, here, too, in vitro fertilization may be indicated.

Induction of ovulation is one of the most successful therapies when used in anovulatory women. Induction of ovulation should never be attempted until serious disorders precluding pregnancy are ruled out or treated. Furthermore, ovulation induction should not be used in women with ovarian failure because they are unresponsive to any form of ovulation induction.

Clomiphene citrate is the agent that usually induces ovulation most easily. Clomiphene should be used in individuals without hyperprolactinemia who have the ability to release LH and FSH. A typical course of clomiphene therapy is begun on the third to fifth days after either spontaneous or induced uterine bleeding. The initial dosage is 50 mg daily for 5 days. Clomiphene appears to act as an antiestrogen and stimulates gonadotropin secretion by the pituitary gland to initiate follicular development. If ovulation is not achieved in the first cycle of treatment, the daily dosage is increased to 100 mg. If ovulation is still not achieved, dosage is increased in a stepwise fashion in 50-mg increments to a maximum of 200 to 250 mg daily for 5 days. The highest dose should be continued for 3 to 6 months before the patient is regarded as unresponsive to clomiphene. The quantity of drug and the length of time that it can be used, as suggested here, are greater than those recommended by the manufacturers and the FDA but conform to published series. Despite absence of FDA approval, letrozole is being used increasingly in place of clomiphene. In one randomized trial, ovarian stimulation with letrozole was equivalent to clomiphene but resulted in a slightly lower frequency of multiple gestation and also a lower frequency of live birth compared with gonadotropin treatment.[A10][A11]

The ovulatory surge of LH may occur 5 to 12 days (average, 7 days) after the completion of the last day of clomiphene treatment. Couples are advised to have intercourse every other day during this interval. Ovulation can be documented by monitoring changes in basal body temperature or preferably by measuring serum progesterone 14 days after the last clomiphene dose. Menses should occur after 3 weeks. Withdrawal bleeding with progestin can be induced if the patient fails to bleed within 4 weeks of therapy and if a serum hCG level documents that the patient is not pregnant. Testing the urine for an LH surge may also be useful in timing ovulation.

Some clinicians give 5000 to 10,000 IU of hCG intramuscularly 7 days after the last day of clomiphene therapy to trigger ovulation, but this approach has not been established to increase effectiveness. The administration of hCG, however, does serve to time ovulation and may be helpful in selected couples. Ovulation can be expected to occur approximately 36 hours after hCG administration.

Of appropriately selected patients, 75 to 80% ovulate, and 40 to 50% can be expected to become pregnant. About 15% of pregnancies can be expected with each ovulatory cycle. The multiple pregnancy rate is about 8%, with almost all being twins. The incidence of congenital anomalies is not increased.

Side effects of clomiphene are uncommon and rarely serious. The most serious ones include vasomotor flushes (10%), abdominal discomfort (5%), breast tenderness (2%), nausea and vomiting (2%), visual symptoms (1.5%), and headache (1%). Ovarian enlargement may occur but is rare (5%). Concern has been raised about the potential for clomiphene to increase the risk for epithelial ovarian cancer. The bulk of the evidence now indicates that clomiphene does not increase this risk.

The addition of dexamethasone, 0.5 mg orally at bedtime, to blunt the nighttime secretion of adrenocorticotropic hormone may be useful in hyperandrogenic women who fail to ovulate in response to clomiphene. Other individuals who do not respond to clomiphene typically require exogenous gonadotropins and hCG or perhaps pulsatile GnRH to induce ovulation.

Both bromocriptine and cabergoline are effective in inducing ovulation in hyperprolactinemic women. The drug should be stopped when pregnancy is confirmed. Ovulatory menses and pregnancy are achieved in about 80% of patients with galactorrhea and hyperprolactinemia. Most women with prolactin-secreting pituitary tumors remain asymptomatic during pregnancy. It is rare for a patient with either a microadenoma or a macroadenoma to develop a problem related to the tumor that affects either the mother or the fetus during pregnancy. Monitoring during pregnancy need consist only of questioning the patient about the development of visual symptoms and headaches. Formal assessment of visual fields and computed tomography or magnetic resonance imaging should be carried out in any patient experiencing suggestive symptoms. Symptoms generally abate with institution of therapy with a dopamine agonist. No adverse effects of dopamine agonists on fetuses or pregnancies have been reported. Concerns have been raised that ergot-derived dopamine agonists, in the large doses used in the treatment of Parkinson disease, may increase the risk for cardiac valve regurgitation. Although there is no evidence of risk in women treated with much lower doses for hyperprolactinemia, they should be counseled about this potential side effect.

Several preparations of purified and synthetic biochemically engineered gonadotropins for use for induction of ovulation now exist. Synthetic preparations consist entirely of FSH, whereas most purified preparations contain some LH as well. Each vial typically contains 75 IU of gonadotropin. Individuals with gonadotropin deficiency require a preparation containing some LH. Exogenous gonadotropins are typically administered at doses of two to four vials (intramuscularly or subcutaneously, depending on the preparation) for 5 to 12 days to achieve follicular development as monitored by ultrasonography and serum or urinary estradiol concentrations; hCG, 5000 to 10,000 IU, is administered as a single intramuscular dose when follicular maturation is apparent. The hCG should be withheld if more than three follicles mature together. GnRH analogs are now being used to suppress endogenous follicular activity before initiation of therapy with exogenous gonadotropins and continued until hCG is given in older women and those with poor responses to exogenous gonadotropins. Use of the analogs necessitates administration of larger doses of exogenous gonadotropins. Success rates, however, appear to be somewhat improved with this combined therapy. Because of the expense and the complication rate, thorough evaluation should be carried out to exclude other causes of infertility before exogenous gonadotropins and hCG are used. Ovulation can be induced in almost 100% of patients, but pregnancy occurs in only 50 to 70%. There is no increased risk for congenital anomalies with exogenous gonadotropins and hCG. The rate of multiple pregnancies with exogenous gonadotropins and hCG may approach 30%, with 5% being triplets or more.

Ovarian hyperstimulation (*ovarian hyperstimulation syndrome,* or OHSS) is the major side effect and may be life-threatening. The ovaries enlarge remarkably, and multiple follicle cysts, stromal edema, and multiple corpora lutea are present. There is a shift of fluid from the intravascular space into the abdominal cavity with resultant hypovolemia and hemoconcentration. The cause of the ascites is unknown. The most serious complications of OHSS may include thromboembolism, renal failure, adult respiratory distress syndrome, and hemorrhage from ovarian rupture. Treatment is conservative, with monitoring of fluid and electrolyte status. Pelvic examinations should not be performed for fear of rupturing the ovaries. The hyperstimulation generally resolves slowly during about 7 days but lasts longer if the cycle results in pregnancy.

Clomiphene citrate or exogenous gonadotropins together with intrauterine insemination of spermatozoa may be used in women with unexplained infertility as so-called controlled ovarian hyperstimulation (COH). The intent is to stimulate several oocytes to be ovulated, but multiple (sometimes high-order) gestations are a significant risk. A randomized trial has noted that the risk for multiple gestation and the costs are reduced if COH with gonadotropins is not used and patients are advanced immediately to treatment by in vitro fertilization.

Assisted Reproductive Technologies

The assisted reproductive technologies, in which by definition both eggs and sperm are handled outside of the body, are being used commonly to treat infertile couples with tubal disease, endometriosis, oligospermia and azoospermia, sperm antibodies, and unexplained infertility. The procedure consists of in vitro fertilization and several variants. In vitro fertilization involves ovarian hyperstimulation, oocyte retrieval, fertilization, embryo culture, and embryo transfer. Ovarian hyperstimulation with clomiphene citrate and exogenous gonadotropins, gonadotropins alone, or a GnRH agonist or antagonist plus gonadotropins typically causes 1 to 20 oocytes to mature, depending on the patient's age and ovarian "reserve." After follicular growth is judged sufficient by ultrasound examination, hCG is given to induce final follicular maturation. About 34 hours after hCG administration, the oocytes are retrieved by direct needle puncture of each follicle, usually transvaginally with ultrasound guidance. The oocytes are then inseminated in vitro with washed sperm, or a single sperm is injected directly into a single egg (so-called intracytoplasmic sperm injection). The embryos are cultured for about 40 to 120 hours, after which one or more embryos are transferred to the uterine cavity. Embryos may be cultured to the blastocyst stage (at 120 hours) before transfer. Additional embryos can be frozen in liquid nitrogen for transfer in a subsequent natural cycle. The success rate is most dependent on the age of the woman. In the United States the percentage of cycles resulting in live births ranges from 40.1% in women younger than 35 years to 12.2% in women age 41 to 42 years. Approximately 30% are twins and 1% are triplets or higher-order multiples. Women with unexplained infertility can be offered intrauterine insemination with ovarian stimulation as an alternative to in vitro fertilization. Intrauterine insemination with ovarian stimulation is a safe and effective treatment for women with unexplained infertility and an unfavorable prognosis for natural conception.[A12]

It is now possible to test the early embryo for genetic abnormalities by trophectoderm biopsy from an embryo in vitro and testing it by next generation sequencing to identify aneuploidy or mutations causing known familial diseases.[17] Identification of normal and abnormal embryos allows only normal embryos to be transferred in families with recognized and testable genetic abnormalities. In addition, concerned future parents can undergo preconception screening to identify diseases for which each is an autosomal recessive carrier for hundreds of syndromes. Preimplantation genetic diagnosis for such diseases can then be performed to select unaffected embryos.[18]

● SEXUAL FUNCTION AND DYSFUNCTION
Sexual Function

DEFINITION

Sexual responses historically have been divided into four phases: excitement, plateau, orgasm, and resolution. With sexual arousal and excitement, vasocongestion and muscle tension increase progressively, primarily in the genital region, manifested by vaginal lubrication in the female. The lubrication is due to formation of a transudate in the vagina. Sexual excitement is initiated by any of a variety of psychogenic or somatogenic sexual stimuli and must be reinforced to result in orgasm. With continued stimulation, the excitement phase increases in intensity into a plateau phase during which a high state of sexual interest is maintained. The plateau phase may be short or long, and it is from this phase that an individual can shift to orgasm. The orgasmic phase tends to be brief and is characterized by rapid release from the developed vasocongestion and muscle tension. The orgasmic release is also known as

the climax because peak psychological and physical intensity is achieved, and there is an attendant feeling of satisfaction. Copious secretions and transudate may flow during orgasm in women. Characteristic genital and extragenital responses occur during these phases. Estrogens magnify the sexual responses, but responses may occur in estrogen-deficient women. For women, these changes occur in the breasts and in the pudendal region and are variable from one response cycle to another. For some women, excitement proceeds quickly through plateau to orgasm, and orgasm is explosive and accompanied by vocalization and involuntary contractions of the pelvic skeletal muscles. For other women, the responses are slow in building, controlled in amplitude, and long lasting. For a few women, orgasm never occurs; for many, it is intermittently absent.

The somatic sensate focus enabling orgasmic release is variable and may include stimulation of the breasts, vagina, or clitoris. The psychological aspect of coitus may involve concentration on the current partner or act or fantasies about other times and persons. Although orgasms may vary in physiologic intensity, what is important is psychological satisfaction. Satisfaction for both men and women may be had without orgasm.

Many clinicians have noted several limitations of this traditional human sex response cycle. Many clinicians and researchers see the cycle as circular with stimuli of different types leading to arousal. Clinicians in this field now have extended this theory to include desire and arousal. Women seek sexual experiences for intimacy as well as for sexual gratification. Women may be receptive to or seek out sexual stimuli to enhance intimacy. Biologic and psychological factors contribute to the processing of these stimuli and can enhance arousal and desire simultaneously.

Sexual Dysfunction

Women may seek consultation because of disturbances in normal sexual arousal or orgasm.[19,20] Such sexual dysfunction may be due to either organic or functional disturbances.

A variety of diseases affecting neurologic function, including diabetes mellitus and multiple sclerosis, may prevent sexual arousal. So, too, may local pelvic disorders, such as endometriosis and vaginitis, which cause dyspareunia and lead to sexual avoidance. Estrogen deficiency causing vaginal atrophy and dyspareunia is a relatively common cause of sexual dysfunction. Debilitating systemic diseases such as malignant disease may also affect sexual function indirectly.

In many cases, the cause of sexual dysfunction is psychological, and psychological interventions can be successful.[A13] For instance, vaginismus involves involuntary contractions of the muscles surrounding the introitus and leads to dyspareunia. It is a conditioned response engendered by a previous real or imagined traumatic sexual experience. Feelings of guilt (caused by incest or rape, as examples), of inadequacy (caused by hysterectomy or mastectomy), or of depression or anxiety may lead to failure to be aroused. Failure to achieve orgasm may be viewed as a dysfunction if the woman is frustrated or dissatisfied.

TREATMENT

Treatment of sexual dysfunction should eliminate functional causes and provide the patient, often together with her partner, with appropriate psychological counseling.[21] Behavioral modification is effective in treating many women with psychological sexual dysfunction. In one randomized trial, self-reported sexual satisfaction was increased in women treated with testosterone. However, dosing guidelines are not clear, and the therapy cannot be considered standard care based on current evidence.

Grade A References

A1. Marjoribanks J, Ayeleke RO, Farquhar C, et al. Nonsteroidal anti-inflammatory drugs for dysmenorrhoea. *Cochrane Database Syst Rev.* 2015;7:CD001751.

A2. Brown J, Crawford TJ, Datta S, et al. Oral contraceptives for pain associated with endometriosis. *Cochrane Database Syst Rev.* 2018;5:CD001019.

A3. Andres Mde P, Lopes LA, Baracat EC, et al. Dienogest in the treatment of endometriosis: systematic review. *Arch Gynecol Obstet.* 2015;292:523-529.

A4. Brown J, Farquhar C. Endometriosis: an overview of Cochrane Reviews. *Cochrane Database Syst Rev.* 2014;10:CD009590.

A5. Taylor HS, Giudice LC, Lessey BA, et al. Treatment of endometriosis-associated pain with elagolix, an oral GnRH antagonist. *N Engl J Med.* 2017;377:28-40.

A6. Eisenlohr-Moul TA, Girdler SS, Johnson JL, et al. Treatment of premenstrual dysphoria with continuous versus intermittent dosing of oral contraceptives: results of a three-arm randomized controlled trial. *Depress Anxiety.* 2017;34:908-914.

A7. Marjoribanks J, Brown J, O'Brien PM, et al. Selective serotonin reuptake inhibitors for premenstrual syndrome. *Cochrane Database Syst Rev.* 2013;6:CD001396.

A8. Liu C, Feng C, Huang W, et al. Comparison of clomiphene citrate and letrozole for ovulation induction in women with polycystic ovary syndrome: a prospective randomized trial. *Gynecol Endocrinol.* 2017;33:872-876.

A9. Wang R, Kim BV, van Wely M, et al. Treatment strategies for women with WHO group II anovulation: systemic review network meta-analysis. *BMJ.* 2017;356:1-11.

A10. Diamond MP, Legro RS, Coutifaris C, et al. Letrozole, gonadotropin, or clomiphene for unexplained fertility. *N Engl J Med.* 2015;373:1230-1240.

A11. Eskew AM, Bedrick BS, Hardi A, et al. Letrozole compared with clomiphene citrate for unexplained infertility: a systematic review and meta-analysis. *Obstet Gynecol.* 2019;133:437-444.

A12. Farquhar CM, Liu E, Armstrong S, et al. Intrauterine insemination with ovarian stimulation versus expectant management for unexplained infertility (TUI): a pragmatic, open-label, randomised, controlled, two-centre trial. *Lancet.* 2018;391:441-450.

A13. Frühauf S, Gerger H, Schmidt HM, Munder T, et al. Efficacy of psychological interventions for sexual dysfunction: a systematic review and meta-analysis. *Arch Sex Behav.* 2013;42:915-33.

GENERAL REFERENCES

For the General References and other additional features, please visit Expert Consult at https://expertconsult.inkling.com.

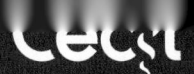

XX

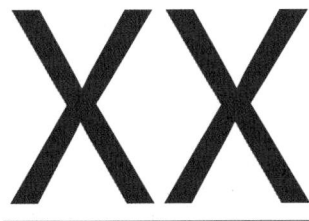

WOMEN'S HEALTH

224

APPROACH TO WOMEN'S HEALTH

KAREN M. FREUND

An approach to the care of women must go beyond an understanding of differences in the incidence of disease between men and women. Providers need to consider the impact of sex differences (those based on genetic and hormonal differences) and gender differences (those attributable to the roles men and women are ascribed in society). Therapeutic decisions should take into account both genetic and environmental differences in the presentation of disease and the effectiveness of therapeutic options, the patient's reproductive life stage, comorbidities, and social and cultural contexts of care. Empirical evidence about care for women has expanded since 1994, when the National Institutes of Health required the inclusion of women as research subjects. The increased number of women participating in clinical research, coupled with initiatives through the Office on Research and Women's Health, has led to a broad expansion of knowledge; however, there is a continued need for gender-specific analyses of data to evaluate the impact of any therapeutic intervention. The NIH requirement that both basic and clinical research address sex as a biologic variable will expand our knowledge base.[1]

LIFESPAN GROUPS

Many important women's health issues are linked to the social, psychological, and biologic context at certain ages and stages of life. When considering both preventive care and common causes of mortality and morbidity, these lifespan stages provide a context for organizing care (Table 224-1).

For most women, young adulthood (15 to 44 years) is marked by social transitions in family structure, such as forming one's own family and parenting, and entering the work force. Mortality rates are low, and health visits can focus on behavioral decisions that will influence the risk for future disease, such as those pertaining to sexual behavior, smoking, alcohol and drug use, diet, and exercise. Major sources of morbidity include intentional and unintentional injury, including interpersonal violence (Chapter 228) and motor vehicle crashes. HIV is a leading cause of morbidity and mortality in this age group. Depression and anxiety are common in this and all life stages. Reproductive issues are considered in most therapeutic decisions.

The middle years (ages 45 to 65 years) continue to be influenced by behavioral decisions, especially diet, exercise, and alcohol and substance use. The social context includes role changes as children reach adulthood; caregiving responsibilities are now for dependent children and possibly grandchildren, as well as aging parents. The menopausal transition may be accompanied by new symptomatic concerns. Common causes of morbidity, including diabetes and obesity, now reflect earlier behavioral decisions. Cancer is the leading cause of mortality.

Health issues in older women (65+ years) may occur in the context of loss of function and independence, and because women commonly survive their male partners, they are more likely at this stage of life to be single and possibly more isolated. Cardiovascular disease is the major cause of mortality, followed by cancer, cerebrovascular disease, chronic obstructive lung disease, and pneumonia. Loss of independence is related to cognitive decline, osteoarthritis, osteoporotic fractures, and incontinence.

HEALTH DISPARITIES AMONG WOMEN

It is critical to consider the racial and ethnic differences in outcomes for most common causes of mortality and morbidity when addressing the health status of women. American women with a minority racial or ethnic affiliation, including those of African descent (whether born in the United States or abroad), women from many Asian and Pacific Island nations, Native Americans, and women of Latino background, share poorer outcomes for a wide variety of conditions. This broad finding of poorer outcomes across many diverse ethnic and racial groups points away from specific genetic differences in these populations and toward social determinants of health. Data are accumulating on the benefits of screening for social determinants of health (income, education, violence, housing, and food insecurity, among others). Minority racial and ethnic affiliation is correlated with lower educational attainment, lower income, residence in neighborhoods with higher crime and more environmental health hazards, less access to comprehensive health insurance, and less access to care

even when insured. Common recommendations for health promotion, including a diet low in animal fats and processed sugars but high in whole grains, fruits, nuts, and vegetables, along with regular exercise, such as walking, may be difficult to follow in high-crime neighborhoods or in those without markets offering a variety of affordable, nutritious food options. Barriers to health care access and poor adherence to medical therapy are more common in low-income women. For instance, they may have difficulty scheduling appointments that do not interfere with their work schedules or unpaid time off from clerical or service jobs. The need to care for dependent children or elders may interfere with women's ability to address their own health care needs. Low health literacy and cultural barriers can add to health care access issues (Chapter 4).

COMMON CAUSES OF MORTALITY IN WOMEN

Cardiovascular Disease

Cardiovascular disease (CVD; Chapter 46) is the overall leading cause of death in women. However, because CVD-related death occurs most often in women older than 65 years, its impact is often under-recognized or underestimated. Racial ethnicity plays a large role in the risk for CVD; African American women have much higher rates of CVD and death from CVD than any other racial or ethnic group, and Latinas and Asian women also have higher rates of CVD and CVD death than white populations.

The incidence rate of CVD in women lags 10 years behind that of men from ages 40 through 70 years; that is, a 65-year-old woman has a similar risk to a 55-year-old man. There is no abrupt increase in CVD risk at menopause in women, suggesting that menopausal changes in estrogen or progesterone do not account for this sex difference. Furthermore, randomized clinical trials have confirmed that hormone therapy in women does not prevent CVD and is not indicated for CVD prevention. Re-analysis of the Women's Health Initiative confirmed the increased risk for CVD *with* hormone therapy, even when treatment is initiated within 10 years of menopause. However, estrogen or estrogen plus progestin therapy has complex systemic effects, and their net rates of adverse outcomes when used for chronic disease prevention may vary according to an individual woman's risk factor profile. Therefore, an individualized risk stratification approach has been advocated in women who are otherwise potential candidates for hormone therapy because of other indications.[1] There has been some controversy about the impact of calcium supplementation for bone health on increased risk for myocardial infarction, but not CVD deaths. However, most observational studies do not find an association in women, and calcium and vitamin D supplementation are still recommended for women regardless of CVD risk (Chapter 230). Other risk factors for CVD in women are the same as those in men: elevated lipids, lack of physical activity, obesity, smoking, hypertension, and diabetes. Women with diabetes have the same risk for CVD as men of the same age with diabetes.

However, there are notable disparities in the burden of coronary heart disease among some groups of women, especially women who are disadvantaged because of race, ethnicity, income level, and educational attainment. For example, because smoking rates in current cohorts of young women continue to increase, cigarette smoking continues to be an important behavioral risk factor for CVD, especially in younger women, American Indian women, and women with low incomes and low educational attainment. The incidence of many known risk factors, including obesity, hypertension, and hypercholesterolemia, is greater in African American women than in white women. Furthermore, data suggest that women are less likely to receive risk factor reduction therapy, reflecting an inertia caused by misperception by clinicians and patients of heart disease risk.

The presentation of coronary artery disease in women differs from that in men. Although chest pain is the most common presentation in women, atypical and noncardiac pain is a more frequent presentation in women than in men, and fewer women have typical chest tightness or pressure as their presenting complaint.[2] For this and other reasons, there are delays in seeking and provision of emergency care at all steps from home to arrival to hospital for women compared with men, which can limit some therapeutic options and increase the severity of disease complications, including congestive heart failure.

The current guidelines for the management of lipid disorders (Chapter 195) are based on 10-year risk of CVD as well as absolute lipid levels alone.[3] Although these guidelines are not gender specific, they do note that the focus on overall risk avoids overtreatment of younger women with low risk, and avoids undertreatment of those with the lower low-density lipoprotein (LDL)-C level but much higher CVD risk. High-intensity statin therapy is recommended for women with clinical vascular disease under age 75 years, and for primary prevention for women with a 10-year calculated risk of atherosclerotic cardiovascular disease greater than 7.5%.

TABLE 224-1 IMPORTANT HEALTH ISSUES FOR WOMEN THROUGH THE LIFESPAN

ISSUE	AGES		
	15-44 yr	45-65 yr	65+ yr
Behavioral issues	Risk behaviors Sexual behavior Smoking Alcohol and drug use Exercise Diet	Risk behaviors Smoking Alcohol and drug use Exercise Diet	Risk behaviors Smoking Exercise
Social roles	Entering work force Relationship transitions Parenting	Caregiving to several generations Transitions in family and work environments	Losses and social isolation
Reproductive issues	Reproductive health issues	Menopause transition	
Injury	Intentional and unintentional interpersonal violence Motor vehicle crashes		Falls
Common causes of mortality and morbidity	Depression Anxiety HIV/AIDS	Cancer Obesity Diabetes Depression Anxiety	Cardiovascular disease Cancer Cognitive decline Osteoporosis Osteoarthritis Incontinence Depression Anxiety

Medical management is similar for men and women with acute coronary syndromes, including unstable angina and acute myocardial infarction (Chapter 63).[4,5] The use of aspirin, β-blockers, angiotensin-converting enzyme (ACE) inhibitors, heparin, and thrombolytic therapy and recommendations for non-invasive testing are the same for women and men. Randomized controlled trial data show that low-risk women with unstable angina or non–ST segment elevation myocardial infarction do not benefit from early revascularization and that medical management is indicated.

Type 2 Diabetes

The rates of type 2 diabetes (Chapter 216) continue to rise, with a greater risk in women who are overweight or obese and physically inactive. Rates are higher in many racial and ethnic groups than among white women, including African Americans, Asians, Native Americans, and Latinas. No randomized clinical trials to date on low- to moderate-risk populations have shown a mortality benefit of screening, and most guidelines do not currently recommend universal screening. Screening women for known risk factors (e.g., hypertension [blood pressure >130/85 mm Hg], obesity, family history) is recommended by some. Asian populations have higher rates of diabetes at a lower body mass index (BMI) than other groups, prompting the American Diabetes Association to recommend screening for DM with a BMI greater than 23. For women who develop gestational diabetes (Chapter 226), the risk of developing type 2 diabetes later in life increases five-fold; therefore, screening with hemoglobin A_{1C} 6 to 12 weeks postpartum and every 3 years thereafter is recommended by some.

The incidence of diabetes is rising in women at younger ages, with significant perinatal implications. Ongoing discussion of fertility control and family planning is critical in diabetic women with childbearing potential. Tight glycemic control before conception and through the first trimester is critical to reduce the risk for birth anomalies, and it is important later in pregnancy to reduce the risk for adverse fetal events, including macrosomia (large for gestational age) and preterm birth (Chapter 226). Ideally, women planning a pregnancy should switch from oral agents to insulin, with home glucose monitoring for tight control (Table 224-2).

Cancer

Cancer is the leading cause of death in women 40 through 65 years, and it is the leading cause of years of life lost in women younger than 65. Breast cancer (Chapter 188) is the most common type of cancer and the second leading cause of cancer death in women, although most women who develop breast cancer do survive. Studies indicate that many women significantly overestimate their personal risk for the disease. The lack of understanding of the cause of most breast cancers and the limitations of the imaging modalities used as screening tests have hampered efforts at breast cancer control. Recent data suggesting overdiagnosis of breast cancer, especially in women 40 to 50 years of age, has prompted growing interest in shared decision making regarding screening in this age group.[6] After decades of an increasing incidence of breast cancer in the United States, incidence rates have fallen in the past decade. The cause of this decline is not understood; reduced use of postmenopausal hormone therapy and recent declines in screening rates have both been implicated. In women who are known carriers of the BRCA1 and BRCA2 mutations, estimates now can be made for age-specific risks of breast, ovarian, and contralateral breast cancer.[7]

Lung cancer (Chapter 182) is now the leading cause of cancer death in women, and rates continue to rise, commensurate with the number of women who took up smoking in the 1940s and 1950s and the lower rates of smoking cessation in women compared with men. Most lung cancers are smoking related, although women are more likely than men to have lung cancers that are not tobacco related. Low-dose chest tomography has been shown to reduce death from lung cancer in those with greater than a 30 pack-year smoking history who are current smokers or quit within the previous 15 years; the harms are false-positive scans and potential overdiagnosis.[A2] The National Lung Screening Trial found a borderline significant greater benefit of screening in women than men. Because of the harms of screening, smoking cessation efforts continue to be recommended as the most effective strategy to prevent lung cancer.

Colorectal cancer (Chapter 184) has a similar incidence in both women and men. Screening for occult blood in the stool using a fecal immunochemical test with or without sigmoidoscopy or colonoscopy is effective at detecting precancerous lesions and thereby reducing rates of both new cancers and later stage disease. Rates of screening in women lag behind men, but neither reach Healthy People 2020 goals for this effective preventive screening.

Ovarian cancer (Chapter 189) is relatively rare, with 21,500 cases in the United States annually, but mortality is high owing to its presentation at late stages in most cases. Lower abdominal or pelvic pain, urinary symptoms, and changes in bowel habits are nonspecific and common in many women, limiting the ability to detect this cancer at an early stage. There is no effective screening test for women at average risk, and screening pelvic examination is no longer recommended in asymptomatic women.[8] CA-125 has both low sensitivity and low specificity. The original and long-term follow-up of the ovarian cancer screening arm of the PLCO trial, with now a median of 14.7 years follow-up, did not show a mortality benefit of screening.[A3] The UK Collaborative Trial of Ovarian Cancer Screening (UKCTOCS) randomized 202,638 women and found a nonsignificant 15% mortality reduction from multimodal screening with ultrasound and CA-125, with a significant 20% mortality reduction after an average of 11 years when removing prevalent cases.[A4] Given these nondefinitive results, we await longer follow-up from the trials before recommending screening.

The greatest recent advance in cancer prevention is the development of vaccines against the most carcinogenic subtypes of human papillomavirus (HPV) associated with cervical cancer (Chapters 189 and 349)[A5] and anal cancer. The vaccine has the potential to reduce significant morbidity caused by the management of premalignant lesions, including the risk for cervical incompetence and preterm labor. Vaccine rates in the United States remain low, especially in minority communities. Despite this, there is evidence of reduced HPV prevalence since the vaccine became available. Although concern of tacit approval resulting in increased sexual activity among young adolescents has been cited by parents as a reason to delaying vaccination, evidence does not demonstrate this concern to be founded. Guidelines now suggest delaying Pap test screening in women until age 21 years and increasing the screening interval to every 2 years in women aged 20 to 29 years and to every 3 to 5 years in women aged 30 years and older if previous screening has demonstrated no high-risk subtypes of the HPV and negative HPV serology.[9] Pap tests are not recommended for women after hysterectomy for nonmalignant indications, or for women older than 65 years with adequate recent screening and no high-risk factors.

Osteoporosis

Hip fracture due to osteoporosis (Chapter 230) is one of the major causes of disability, loss of independence, and mortality in older women. Osteoporosis

TABLE 224-2 PREFERRED MEDICATIONS FOR WOMEN OF REPRODUCTIVE POTENTIAL

COMMON CONDITIONS IN WOMEN OF REPRODUCTIVE POTENTIAL	ISSUES TO BE AWARE OF	PREFERRED MEDICATIONS OR GROUPS OF MEDICATIONS
Depression	Must consider effects of untreated depression on mother and infant	Avoid newer medications when older drugs with more information are available SSRIs are generally considered safe; fluoxetine has most safety data
Anxiety	Commonly associated with depression in women	Benzodiazepines generally considered safe
GERD	No data on harmful effects of either H$_2$-blockers or PPIs Misoprostol is contraindicated; can cause miscarriage, fetal death, congenital anomalies	Calcium-containing antacids are first-line therapy H$_2$-blockers preferred over PPIs
Acne	Oral isotretinoin and topical tazarotene are contraindicated owing to congenital defects	Most other topical agents are considered classes B and C
Asthma	Extensive data on safety of common drug categories: benefit ratios far exceed risk in treating women	Cortisone inhalers Systemic prednisone for flares Short- and long-acting bronchodilators
Seizure disorders	Difficult to separate effects of medication from effects of seizure on fetal development All agents associated with some increased risk for fetal abnormality (4-8%, compared with 1-2% in general population). Valproate and phenobarbital with highest risks	Monotherapy at lowest doses recommended Avoid medication changes in first trimester Folate supplementation in preconception period
Hypertension (not preeclampsia)	ACE inhibitors and ARBs are contraindicated in pregnancy; possibly associated with cardiovascular and neurologic anomalies in first trimester; may cause abnormalities in renal hemodynamics in third trimester Most data suggest thiazide diuretics are safe if stable use before pregnancy	β-blockers, especially labetalol, and methyldopa are first-line choices Calcium-channel blockers are also considered safe
Lipid disorders	Circulating lipid levels are elevated with pregnancy and breast-feeding	No medications during pregnancy; ideally, stop statins before conception
Analgesics for fever and pain management	Controversy about whether NSAIDs slightly increase risk for miscarriage in first trimester	Acetaminophen preferred; aspirin also considered safe
Headache	Controversy about whether NSAIDs slightly increase risk for miscarriage in first trimester	Acetaminophen preferred; aspirin also considered safe
Diabetes	First-generation sulfonylureas contraindicated in pregnancy; may cause fetal hyperinsulinemia and birth defects	Conversion to insulin during planned preconception period Insulin, metformin, and glyburide preferred in women of childbearing potential
Autoimmune conditions	Must weigh benefits of immunosuppressive use against potential risks to both mother and infant Methotrexate is contraindicated in pregnancy because it induces miscarriage Limited data on TNF-alpha and IL-17 inhibitors; available data indicate minimal transfer of IgG across placenta and no known birth defects or premature birth	Prednisone generally considered safe in pregnancy Azathioprine, sulfasalazine, cyclosporine, and hydroxychloroquine generally preferred if required
Tobacco control	Cigarette smoking has known harmful effects on fetus In one small randomized controlled trial, nicotine replacement was associated with reduced levels of nicotine and improved birth outcomes Bupropion is linked with reports of some fetal anomalies	Try nonpharmacologic approaches to cessation first Short course of nicotine replacement likely better for fetus than smoking
Polycystic ovarian disease	Metformin can restore ovulatory cycles; use with contraception	
Bacterial infections	Tetracyclines accumulate in fetal bone and teeth Sulfa drugs may increase risk for neural tube defects with use in first trimester and kernicterus with use in third trimester Trimethoprim interferes with folic acid metabolism Streptomycin and kanamycin associated with bilateral deafness	Penicillins, cephalosporins, erythromycin, azithromycin considered safe

ACE = angiotensin-converting enzyme; ARB = angiotensin receptor blocker; GERD = gastroesophageal reflux disease; IL-17 = interleukin-1; NSAID = nonsteroidal anti-inflammatory drug; PPI = proton pump inhibitor; SSRI = selective serotonin re-uptake inhibitor; TNF = tumor necrosis factor.

prevention through calcium and vitamin D intake and weight-bearing exercise begins at puberty and extends throughout adulthood. Women require a calcium intake of 1000 mg/day, increasing to 1300 mg in puberty and breast-feeding and 1200 mg after menopause, in order to maintain the structural strength of bone. Vitamin D is a necessary element for the absorption of calcium (Chapter 205), and it is available through direct sun exposure or vitamin D supplementation of milk (not most other dairy products) and some juices. Epidemiologic data suggest widespread vitamin D deficiency in women in the United States. This is attributed to low levels of dietary replacement, decreased sun exposure with the use of sunscreens, and lack of vitamin D production in the skin (even with sun exposure) in northern climates during the winter months. Screening for a single baseline serum 25-hydroxyvitamin D level can provide women with useful information about the adequacy of their diets, with levels above

20 ng/mL considered sufficient or ideal. Daily replacement of vitamin D of 600 IU is recommended for women, with 800 IU recommended after age 70 years.

Although no long-term outcome data exist on the benefits of dual-energy x-ray absorptiometry (DXA) screening (DEXA bone densitometry), most guidelines recommend DXA screening at age 65 years in women, and in women ages 50 to 65 years who have one risk factor (smoking, family history, body mass index < 22, or alcohol use). An algorithm to assess risk for bone fracture based on DXA and individual risk factors is available through the World Health Organization and can guide decision making on preventive therapy.[10] Long-term estrogen therapy is not recommended for osteoporosis prevention. Complications from bisphosphonate therapy include gastroesophageal erosions, preventable in most women with weekly doses on an empty stomach while sitting upright for 30 minutes. Rare but debilitating jaw osteonecrosis (Chapter 234) has been seen in women with and without risk factors, such as dental disease. Raloxifene, a selective estrogen receptor modulator, has the benefits of preventing osteoporosis while reducing breast cancer risk without increasing the risk for CVD; it has been underused as a preventive agent. Parathyroid hormone is the only agent associated with increased bone density, and preliminary data suggest it may have greater benefit in those who have not used bisphosphonates; antiabsorptive agents including bisphosphonates are recommended after completion of 2 years of treatment to maintain bone strength gained.

COMMON CAUSES OF MORBIDITY IN WOMEN

Obesity

Obesity rates continue to rise, and the prevalence of obesity is higher in women than men, especially among minority and low-income women (Chapter 207). The rates of increase in obesity in women have doubled from 1976-80, when it was at 17%, to the rate of 36.5% in 2011-14. Dietary reduction in calories and increased caloric output with aerobic exercise are the short- and long-term strategies for care. Studies suggest that no single diet is superior to others, and many common diet strategies can reduce weight. Increasing activity during the course of one's daily routine is as effective as shorter intervals of more strenuous activity. The most effective programs include a combination of behavioral therapy, either individually or in groups, to address behavioral patterns in food intake, and with diet and exercise. Weight loss targets of 1 to 2 lb/week and a total loss of up to 5 to 10% of body weight are realistic goals. Even modest changes in weight and modest increases in physical activity reduce morbidity and mortality on a population basis.

Exercise and diet changes are difficult for many people to achieve for a wide variety of reasons. The physical environment may not be conducive to physical activity owing to the sedentary nature of most workplaces, the lack of safe areas to exercise, and architectural design features, such as the lack of easy access to stairs instead of elevators. The use of prepared foods and the consumption of fast foods, high in calories and low in nutritional content, increase the risk for obesity.

There are currently no evidence-based interventions to support weight reduction in the setting of a brief office visit. Most guidelines focus on assessing BMI in all women and recommending weight reduction with diet restriction and behavioral therapy to support these behavioral changes. Excessive postpartum weight retention (≥4.5 kg over prepregnancy weight at 6 to 12 months after delivery) also occurs disproportionately in minority and low-income women and is associated with similarly increased risk of complications such as diabetes and cardiovascular disease. In contrast to current general obesity treatment guidelines that emphasize intensive, in-person interventions to affect lifestyle modification, it was shown that management of specifically postpartum weight retention is more effective using remote internet-based methods. [AG]

Orlistat and sibutramine are U.S. Food and Drug Administration (FDA)-approved medications with moderate weight reduction efficacy that should be used in conjunction with an exercise and diet program, and not as sole therapy. For obese women with a BMI greater than 40, or those with a BMI greater than 35 and major comorbidities such as diabetes, sleep apnea, or osteoarthritis, bariatric surgery (Chapter 207) is indicated after other weight loss methods have failed. Bariatric surgery leads to short- and long-term benefits in multiple comorbidities and reduced mortality because of improvements in comorbidities. Critical to the success of this intervention is a team approach, with psychological assessment and diet and exercise programs beginning before and continuing after surgery. Management of obesity in general is discussed in detail in Chapter 207.

Depression

Major depression and other related disorders, including dysthymia, predominate in women (Chapter 406). Multiple short screening tools have been developed to identify depression. Women with depression are highly likely to come to the attention of the health care system. Depression is a significant comorbidity in many chronic medical conditions and is also a disabling but treatable complication of the postpartum period.[11] Somatic complaints are a common presentation of depressive disorders. All specialties are likely to see patients with unexplained symptoms, such as chest pain, headache, abdominal pain, and other complaints. It is critical to consider depression as either a primary or a secondary diagnosis and to treat depression as part of the overall management plan.

Anxiety Disorders

Anxiety disorders also predominate in women. They commonly coexist with depressive disorders. Anxiety disorders, including post-traumatic stress disorder, may be a consequence of violence against women, which often remains unidentified (Chapter 228). Benzodiazepines have been demonstrated to be safe and effective in trials for short-term use. Selective serotonin re-uptake inhibitors (SSRIs) and cognitive behavioral therapies are effective for the long-term management of anxiety disorders.

Osteoarthritis

Osteoarthritis (Chapter 246) is one of the most common causes of morbidity and functional status limitation, especially as women age. Assessment of pain and functional status is at the core of management. Physical and occupational therapy to restore functional status is a critical component of care. Joint replacement (Chapter 260) should be considered and recommended when functional status interferes with activities of daily living and supportive care and other symptom management strategies are ineffective.

Smoking

Tobacco use, most commonly cigarette smoking, continues to be one of the major preventable causes of morbidity and mortality in women (Chapter 29). Although there has been much progress in smoking cessation efforts, lower-income women and younger women continue to start smoking and fail to quit smoking at high rates. Health care providers can achieve 1 to 2% smoking cessation rates by asking all patients about their smoking status and making a simple statement encouraging smokers to quit. Further gains in smoking cessation are possible with targeted counseling, which involves assessing the patient's stage of readiness to change and providing counseling relevant to that stage.

Nicotine replacement is equally effective in women and men. Smokers with a physiologic addiction to nicotine (those who smoke more than one pack daily or smoke within 20 minutes of awakening) benefit the most from nicotine replacement. Many women report weight gain as a major barrier to smoking cessation. Chapter 29 describes approaches to smoking cessation in detail.

Alcohol Use and Substance Use

Alcohol dependence is estimated in 5% of women; however, this is underrecognized in clinical practice (Chapter 30). It is well established that lower amounts of alcohol cause alcohol-related liver and other disease in women compared with men and increase the risk for breast cancer. Also worrisome is the frequency of binge drinking (defined as four drinks or more at a sitting) by women, with reports that one in eight women drink with this pattern, with risk for poor judgment in personal safety.

Women in general have lower rates of most substance abuse than men, and women account for about half as many opioid-related deaths as men.[12] They have similar rates of nonmedical use of narcotic medications (about 2% of population), a problem that has more than doubled in the past decade, and narcotic overdose deaths have increased five-fold in women in the same time frame. Current recommendations include specific training for all prescribing physicians; in addition, all nononcology patients who are prescribed more than 30 days of narcotics should be part of a narcotics program, with signed consent on risks and benefits, agreement to obtain medications from a single practice source, and agreement to monitoring, including random pill counts and drug testing, for the presence of the prescribed medication and the absence of other medications.

Alcohol abuse and dependence and drug abuse and dependence are described and discussed in detail in Chapters 30 and 31, respectively.

Incontinence

Urinary incontinence (Chapter 23) is a frequently overlooked cause of major functional status limitations in middle-aged and older women. As many as half of affected women underreport this problem to their physicians and alter their lifestyles to adapt to the problem, including reducing fluid intake, avoiding activities that exacerbate the problem, and restricting travel where access to facilities is uncertain. There are two broad categories of incontinence—stress incontinence and urge incontinence—although women commonly have aspects of both types. Stress incontinence is defined as leaking with increases in intra-abdominal pressure, such as occurs with sneezing or coughing as well as running or walking. The most common reasons are pelvic floor laxity, often from childbirth. Kegel exercises are frequently recommended but are of limited value. A number of surgical procedures are available to address this condition.

Less invasive procedures may be tried first, including the fitting of a vaginal pessary or periurethral injections with biodegradable materials such as collagen or with nonbiodegradable materials. Urge incontinence, described as detrusor muscle instability, results in the urge to void with low volumes. Anticholinergic medications and bladder training are both effective. Urodynamic evaluation should be considered if the history does not clearly identify a cause. The problem of incontinence is discussed in more detail in Chapter 23.

HIV Infection

The risk factors for HIV infection in women are heterosexual contact in 80% of new cases and injection drug use in 20%. HIV continues to affect minority women disproportionately, with 61% of incident cases affecting African American women. Incidence rates remain lower in women than in men, with only 27% of incident cases affecting women; in large part, this is due to the fact that male-to-male sexual contact continues to account for 72% of new cases in men. However, the absolute number of new infections from heterosexual contact is twice as high in women as it is in men. Women with HIV/AIDS continue to have poorer survival than men, despite the availability of antiretroviral therapies. There are no data of differential effectiveness of therapy by gender, and there are no gender-specific recommendations regarding timing and type of antiretroviral therapy. Some data suggest that women are less likely than men to adhere to an antiretroviral therapy regimen. The gender difference in therapy adherence was associated with caring for dependent children in one study, suggesting that women's caregiving roles may be a barrier to their own care. Cervical and anal dysplasia and cancer are more common among women with HIV than those without. Therefore, annual Pap tests are recommended for all women with HIV infection, even in the absence of positive HPV test results. There is insufficient evidence to support anal screening for dysplasia, but providers should be aware of the increased risk and perform an external examination for evidence of lesions.

Prophylaxis and management of complications of HIV/AIDS are discussed in detail in Chapter 365, and other aspects of HIV/AIDS are covered in individual chapters in Section XXV.

⬤ REPRODUCTIVE HEALTH ISSUES

All providers caring for women with reproductive potential should consider the reproductive implications of preventive and therapeutic decisions. With half of all pregnancies in the United States unplanned, providers should routinely inquire about contraceptive practices and consider these in their care plans.

All primary care providers should be comfortable counseling patients about contraceptive choices and prescribing oral contraceptives. The absolute contraindications to oral contraceptives are a personal history of CVD, thromboembolic disease, migraine headache with aura, and gynecologic or breast cancer. A family history of cancer is not considered a contraindication; in fact, data suggest that the use of oral contraceptives decreases the risk for both endometrial and ovarian cancer. Smoking while using oral contraceptives increases the risk for thromboembolic events in all women, but especially in those older than 30 years. Oral contraceptive use is considered safe in nonsmoking women until menopause. Although factor V Leiden and other thrombophilias (Chapter 73) have been associated with an increased risk for deep vein thrombosis in those taking oral contraceptives, the absolute risk to any woman is still very low; therefore, routine screening for this and other genetic thrombophilias is not indicated. Preexisting hypertension is a relative contraindication to oral contraceptive use. Some women develop elevated blood pressures on oral contraceptives; therefore, blood pressure should be monitored at 3 months after starting the drug and then at least annually.

Medical abortion was initially provided by clinicians able to conduct a curettage procedure for prolonged bleeding and incomplete abortion. However, with increased experience and with a new evidence-based regimen, medical abortion is safe for primary care providers to implement with appropriate backup. The evidence-based regimen is approved for use up to 63 days of gestation, using mifepristone 200 mg orally for a single dose, followed by 800 μg of misoprostol buccally 24 to 72 hours later. Recent studies have demonstrated its safety even as telemedicine with counseling but without observed administration. Success rates range from 94 to 98%; rates of complications are similar to surgical abortion and include bleeding requiring blood transfusion in 0.05% of cases, and rare infections, usually with non–evidence-based methods. Women should be counseled on side effects, including nausea and abdominal pain, with bleeding and expulsion of conception products usually following misoprostol. Providers should review local regulations: providers must register with the company to prescribe mifepristone. Some locales require

that the original protocol be used and have additional regulations regarding counseling.

Providers should consider the reproductive implications of all chronic medications in women of reproductive potential (Chapter 226). Given that the teratogenic effects of medications may occur during the first trimester and before an initial obstetric assessment, the principle when choosing chronic medications for women during their reproductive years is to select those with the greatest safety profile during the first trimester of pregnancy. Table 224-2 outlines common drug categories and recommendations for use in pregnancy.

Antidepressant medications deserve particular attention because of the conflicting data regarding their use in pregnancy.[13] Some initial reports suggested that antidepressants, especially paroxetine, were associated with congenital defects and preterm birth. However, in studies that are able to assess whether prescriptions were filled or not and account for severity of depression and other risk factors of birth defects, specifically smoking, the risks from antidepressants are no greater than in the overall population. There may be an increased risk of postpartum hemorrhage with the use of SSRIs. For women who wish to take no medication during pregnancy, the recommendation is to gradually reduce the dosage over the course of several weeks and not to abruptly stop taking the medication. The risk for untreated depression during pregnancy and the risk for postpartum depression to the woman and her infant are substantial. Therefore, screening for depression is worthwhile.[14] Treatment goals should be to provide adequate and even increased dosing to prevent the worsening of depression during this period and to provide close surveillance of women, whether or not they stop antidepressant medications.

Ⓐ Grade A References

A1. Marjoribanks J, Farquhar C, Roberts H, et al. Long-term hormone therapy for perimenopausal and postmenopausal women. *Cochrane Database Syst Rev.* 2017;1:CD004143.
A2. Kovalchik SA, Tammemagi M, Berg CD, et al. Targeting of low-dose CT screening according to the risk of lung-cancer death. *N Engl J Med.* 2013;369:245-254.
A3. Pinsky PF, Yu K, Kramer BS, et al. Extended mortality results for ovarian cancer screening in the PLCO trial with median 15 years follow-up. *Gynecol Oncol.* 2016;143:270-275.
A4. Jacobs IJ, Menon U, Ryan A, et al. Ovarian cancer screening and mortality in the UK Collaborative Trial of Ovarian Cancer Screening (UKCTOCS): a randomised controlled trial. *Lancet.* 2016;387:945-956.
A5. Arbyn M, Xu L, Simoens C, et al. Prophylactic vaccination against human papillomaviruses to prevent cervical cancer and its precursors. *Cochrane Database Syst Rev.* 2018;5:CD009069.
A6. Phelan S, Hagobian T, Brannen A, et al. Effect of an internet-based program on weight loss for low-income postpartum women: a randomized clinical trial. *JAMA.* 2017;317:2381-2391.

GENERAL REFERENCES

For the General References and other additional features, please visit Expert Consult at https://expertconsult.inkling.com.

225

CONTRACEPTION

BEVERLY WINIKOFF AND DANIEL GROSSMAN

⬤ CONTRACEPTIVE USE

Contraception enables women and men to avoid unwanted fertility by preventing pregnancy. Methods can be classified in many different ways. Some classification schemes distinguish among mechanisms (e.g., barriers to the encounter of sperm and ovum versus methods that prevent ovulation); other categories emphasize the timing of use (at the time of intercourse versus ongoing); still other classifications focus on the permanence of the method (sterilization, which is intended as a permanent method; long-acting methods that last for years; and short-term methods that depend on the behavior of the user periodically, every day, or at every exposure to pregnancy). There are advantages and disadvantages of each contraceptive method.[1,2] These advantages and disadvantages should be thoroughly explained so that the individual or couple will choose the most acceptable method that suits their lifestyles and will be used most effectively. Because medical contraindications to individual methods are uncommon among young women, in most cases the choice of contraceptive method depends most on the user's preferences.

In the United States, about 61 million women are in the reproductive age group (15 to 44 years), and about 38 million (62%) are using a method of contraception. Of the remainder, most were either noncontraceptively sterile (about 3%), pregnant or trying to conceive (9.5%), or never sexually active or had no recent sexual activity (19%). About 8% of women were sexually active in the prior 3 months but were not using a method of contraception. About 45% of U.S. pregnancies are unintended, meaning that they are mistimed or unwanted,[3] and more than half of such pregnancies occur in women who are not practicing contraception.[4]

In the United States in 2011 to 2013, the most common methods of pregnancy prevention were oral contraceptives (OCs) and female sterilization, used by 16.0% and 15.5% of women aged 15 to 44 years, respectively.[5] Use of long-acting reversible contraception has increased rapidly in recent years, with 6.4% reporting use of the intrauterine device (IUD) and 0.8% using the implant. Other methods reported include male condoms (9.4%), male sterilization (5.1%), the injectable progestin (2.8%), and the contraceptive ring or patch (1.6%). Use of withdrawal was reported by 3.0% in 2011 to 2013. Between 1982 and 2013, there was a marked decrease in diaphragm use and an increase in condom use.

Unintended Pregnancy and Contraceptive Use

After years of stagnation, recent data indicate a significant reduction in unintended pregnancy, likely due to improved use of contraception. Of the 6.1 million pregnancies that occurred in the United States in 2011 (the most recent data available), 45% were unintended; in 2008, 51% were unintended. Data indicate that 95% of unintended pregnancies occur among women who do not use contraception (54%) or use it inconsistently (41%). In recent years, teen pregnancy rates have declined, and women aged 18 to 24 years have the highest unintended pregnancy rates. Poor women and those who are unmarried and living with a partner have significantly higher rates of unintended pregnancy compared with women with higher incomes and those who are married or not living with a partner. Research has identified a variety of factors associated with nonuse of contraception or gaps in use, including side effects (both experienced and feared), not liking a method, personal or religious reasons, and barriers to access, including difficulty obtaining a prescription or with the method itself, and high cost of a method.

Although there is certainly a need to develop new contraceptive methods with fewer side effects, as well as methods for men, much more could be done to improve access to the full range of existing methods at low or no cost. Women have different preferences regarding contraceptive methods, and matching those preferences with the most appropriate method is a critical role of the practicing physician.

Perfect Use versus Typical Use

"Perfect use" and "typical use" are different approaches to characterizing the effectiveness of the various contraceptive methods. *Perfect use* refers to use of the method as intended and covering all acts of exposure to pregnancy. So, for user-dependent methods such as oral pills or condoms, for example, this measure can be applied only to situations in which the user reliably uses the method every day or at every act of intercourse. Perfect use is a measure of the maximum possible efficacy of the method. *Typical use,* on the other hand, is a measure of how effective methods are when used as a group of people under study actually use them. These rates may be considerably lower than perfect use rates, especially if there is the possibility of not using the method at every intercourse or in other ways not using the method as intended. Methods used at the time of coitus have higher failure rates than OCs, implants, injections, IUDs, and sterilization. IUDs, implants, and sterilization have lower failure rates than pills, patches, and injections because they act over a long period of time, and there is nothing a user needs to do to keep using them. Table 225-1 illustrates the differences in failure rates among the contraception methods under conditions of perfect and typical use.

Cumulative failure rates for use of long-acting methods are low. The effectiveness of long-acting reversible contraception is superior to that of contraceptive pills, patch, or ring and is not altered in adolescents and young women. The cumulative failure rates of all types of tubal sterilization are 1.31% during the first 5 years after the procedure and 1.85% after 10 years; rates are higher for tubal fulguration and lower for segmental resection. The cumulative pregnancy rate for 5 years' use of the levonorgestrel (LNG)-releasing IUD is 0.5%, and for 10 years' use of the copper T380 IUD, it is 1.7%.

The World Health Organization (WHO) has developed a chart that nicely represents the actual use (typical) failure rates of most contraceptives, dividing them into three main classes of effectiveness (Fig. 225-1).

Contraindications, Risks, and Benefits

Most contraceptives can be used safely by most people, but some conditions or concomitant medications are considered contraindications to use. The U.S. Centers for Disease Control and Prevention has developed evidence-based Medical Eligibility Criteria (MEC) for contraceptive use, based on a similar document developed by the WHO.[6,7] The MEC categorizes conditions or medications into four groups for each contraceptive method: 1—no restriction on use; 2—advantages of use generally outweigh theoretical or proven risks; 3—theoretical or proven risks generally outweigh advantages of using the method; and 4—the condition represents an unacceptable health risk if the method is used. For conditions that represent relative contraindications (MEC category 3), it is important to recognize that pregnancy may also be risky, and if the method is the best choice to avoid an unintended pregnancy, it may be worth the risk.

Aside from prevention of unintended pregnancy, many contraceptive methods have additional benefits. Some of the most significant noncontraceptive benefits include the reduced risk for transmission of human immunodeficiency virus (HIV) and other sexually transmitted infections associated with the use of male and female condoms, as well as the reduction in dysmenorrhea and menorrhagia associated with the use of combined hormonal contraception.

TYPES OF CONTRACEPTIVES

Natural Methods

Methods that rely on the natural infertility of different times in the menstrual or life cycle are often called "natural" methods. These methods are not really more natural than other methods because they involve disruptions in the "natural" desire for sexual intimacy; however, they do not rely on any specific external technologies to create a state of low fertility potential. Because male sperm can live only 5 days in the female genital tract and female ova have a lifespan of only about 24 hours, the window for fertilization is only 5 to 6 days each month. In theory, if couples avoid unprotected intercourse on those 5 to 6 days, the potential for pregnancy is markedly reduced. The calendar method counts the days of the cycle to predict fertile and infertile days, and the symptothermal method relies on the calendar plus the biologic signals of impending ovulation (changes in vaginal mucus) and of ovulation itself (rise in basal body temperature) to enhance prediction of "safe" days for intercourse. Breast-feeding in the postpartum period also lowers fertility and is considered another natural method of contraception. Exclusive breast-feeding during the first 6 months after a birth provides a good level of protection against pregnancy. However, once a baby is older than 6 months or if foods other than breast milk become part of the infant's diet, then a woman is at much higher risk for ovulation and possible pregnancy.

Withdrawal, or coitus interruptus, when the penis is removed from the vagina before ejaculation, is a commonly used method, with up to 60% of women reporting ever using it. Although the method can be effective with perfect use, with a pregnancy rate of only 4% in the first year of use, failure is much more common in typical use. One study reported that among U.S. women aged 15 to 24 years using withdrawal as their primary method, 21% experienced an unintended pregnancy, which was a significantly higher pregnancy rate than that among users of other contraceptive methods.

Barriers

Barrier methods are so called because their mechanism of action is to impose a chemical or physical barrier between ovum and sperm so that fertilization is not possible. Barrier methods include spermicides, diaphragm, and male and female condoms, among others.

Spermicides

All spermicidal agents contain a surfactant (in U.S. products this chemical is nonoxynol-9) that immobilizes or kills sperm on contact. The spermicidal products are available in foams, creams, and vaginal suppositories that need to be placed into the vagina before each coital act—and reapplied even if coital acts follow immediately after each other. The typical-use effectiveness of spermicides as a sole contraceptive is among the lowest of modern methods (about 28% of women using the method report an unintended pregnancy during 1 year of use.) There is no increased risk for birth defects in the offspring of women who conceive while using spermicides.

TABLE 225-1 PERCENTAGE OF WOMEN EXPERIENCING AN UNINTENDED PREGNANCY DURING THE FIRST YEAR OF TYPICAL USE AND THE FIRST YEAR OF PERFECT USE OF CONTRACEPTION AND THE PERCENTAGE CONTINUING USE AT THE END OF THE FIRST YEAR—UNITED STATES

METHOD	WOMEN EXPERIENCING AN UNINTENDED PREGNANCY WITHIN THE FIRST YEAR OF USE (%)		WOMEN CONTINUING USE AT 1 YEAR (%)[‡]
	TYPICAL USE*	PERFECT USE[†]	
No method[§]	85	85	—
Spermicides[‖]	28	18	42
Fertility awareness–based methods[¶]	24	—	47
Standard-days method	—	5	—
2-day method	—	4	—
Ovulation method	—	3	—
Symptothermal method	—	0.4	—
Withdrawal	22	4	46
Sponge			
Parous women	24	20	36
Nulliparous women	12	9	—
Condom**			
Female	21	5	41
Male	18	2	43
Diaphragm[††]	12	6	57
Combined pill and progestin-only pill	9	0.3	67
Evra patch	9	0.3	67
NuvaRing	9	0.3	67
Depo-Provera	6	0.2	56
Intrauterine devices			
Paragard (copper containing)	0.8	0.6	78
Mirena (levonorgestrel releasing)	0.2	0.2	80
Implanon	0.05	0.05	84
Female sterilization	0.5	0.5	100
Male sterilization	0.15	0.10	100
Lactational amenorrhea method[‡‡]	—	—	—

*Among typical couples who initiate use of a method (not necessarily for the first time), the percentage who experience an accidental pregnancy during the first year if they do not stop use for any other reason. Estimates of the probability of pregnancy during the first year of typical use for spermicides and the diaphragm are taken from the 1995 National Survey Growth (NSFG) and corrected for underreporting of abortion; estimates for fertility awareness-based methods, withdrawal, the male condom, the pill, and Depo-Provera are taken from the 1995-2002 NSFG corrected for underreporting of abortion.

[†]Among couples who initiate use of a method (not necessarily for the first time) and who use it perfectly (both consistently and correctly), the percentage who experience an accidental pregnancy during the first year if they do not stop use for any other reason.

[‡]Among couples attempting to avoid pregnancy, the percentage who continue to use a method for 1 year.

[§]The percentages who become pregnant in the second and third columns are based on data from populations in which contraception is not used and from women who cease using contraception to become pregnant. Among such populations, approximately 89% become pregnant within 1 year. This estimate was lowered slightly (to 85%) to represent the percentage who would become pregnant within 1 year among women not relying on reversible methods of contraception if they abandoned contraception altogether.

[‖]Foams, creams, gels, vaginal suppositories, and vaginal film.

[¶]The ovulation and 2-day methods are based on evaluation of cervical mucus. The standard-days method avoids intercourse on cycle days 8 to 19. The symptothermal method is a double-check method based on evaluation of cervical mucus to determine the first fertile day and evaluation of cervical mucus and temperature to determine the last fertile day.

**Without spermicides.

[††]With spermicidal cream or jelly.

[‡‡]This is a highly effective, temporary method of contraception. However, to maintain effective protection against pregnancy, another method of contraception must be used as soon as menstruation resumes, the frequency of duration of breast-feeds is reduced, bottle-feeds are introduced, or the baby reaches age 6 months.

Adapted from Trussell J. Contraceptive failure in the United States. *Contraception.* 2011;83:397-404.

Diaphragm

A diaphragm is a dome-shaped latex or silicone device with a flexible rim that seals off the upper genital tract from contact with deposited semen. It is usually used with a spermicide applied inside and around the rim. Traditional diaphragms must be fitted by a health care provider using the largest size that does not cause discomfort or undue pressure on the vagina. A new silicone diaphragm called Caya was recently approved by the U.S. Food and Drug Administration (FDA) that is available in a single size that fits women who are sized between 65 mm and 80 mm, which is the majority of women. The woman will need to insert the diaphragm before every act of intercourse. It should be left in place for 6 hours after intercourse, but should not be left in place for more than 24 hours because it may cause ulceration of the vaginal epithelium. In actual use, the diaphragm is more effective than other barrier methods (12% unintended pregnancy rate in first year of use) and provides contraceptive protection almost as well as hormonal pills in actual use. Diaphragm size for any one woman may change after a birth, miscarriage or abortion after 14 weeks, abdominal or pelvic surgery, or a substantial change in weight. The diaphragm may provide some protection against gonorrhea and *Chlamydia* infection, but not against HIV and herpes. A condom is recommended if infection is a concern. Diaphragm users have an increased risk for urinary tract infection.

Male Condom

The male condom, also called an external condom, is one of the oldest contraceptives known. It is safe, easy to use, and widely available. The modern version is a stretchy latex or plastic sheath that fits over the erect penis and captures the man's ejaculate during intercourse. It is the most effective way to prevent transmission of infections (including HIV) during sex and can be used during vaginal, oral, or anal intercourse. However, natural membrane condoms (made from sheep intestine) do not prevent sexually transmitted infections. Condoms can be used for protection against infection even if another method is used for protection against pregnancy. If the condom is used alone for contraception, in typical use about 18% of women will experience an unintended pregnancy in 1 year. For optimum protection, the condom must be used at every sex act and requires the active participation of the man. Lubricants containing oil-based products may weaken latex condoms and

Effectiveness of Family Planning Methods

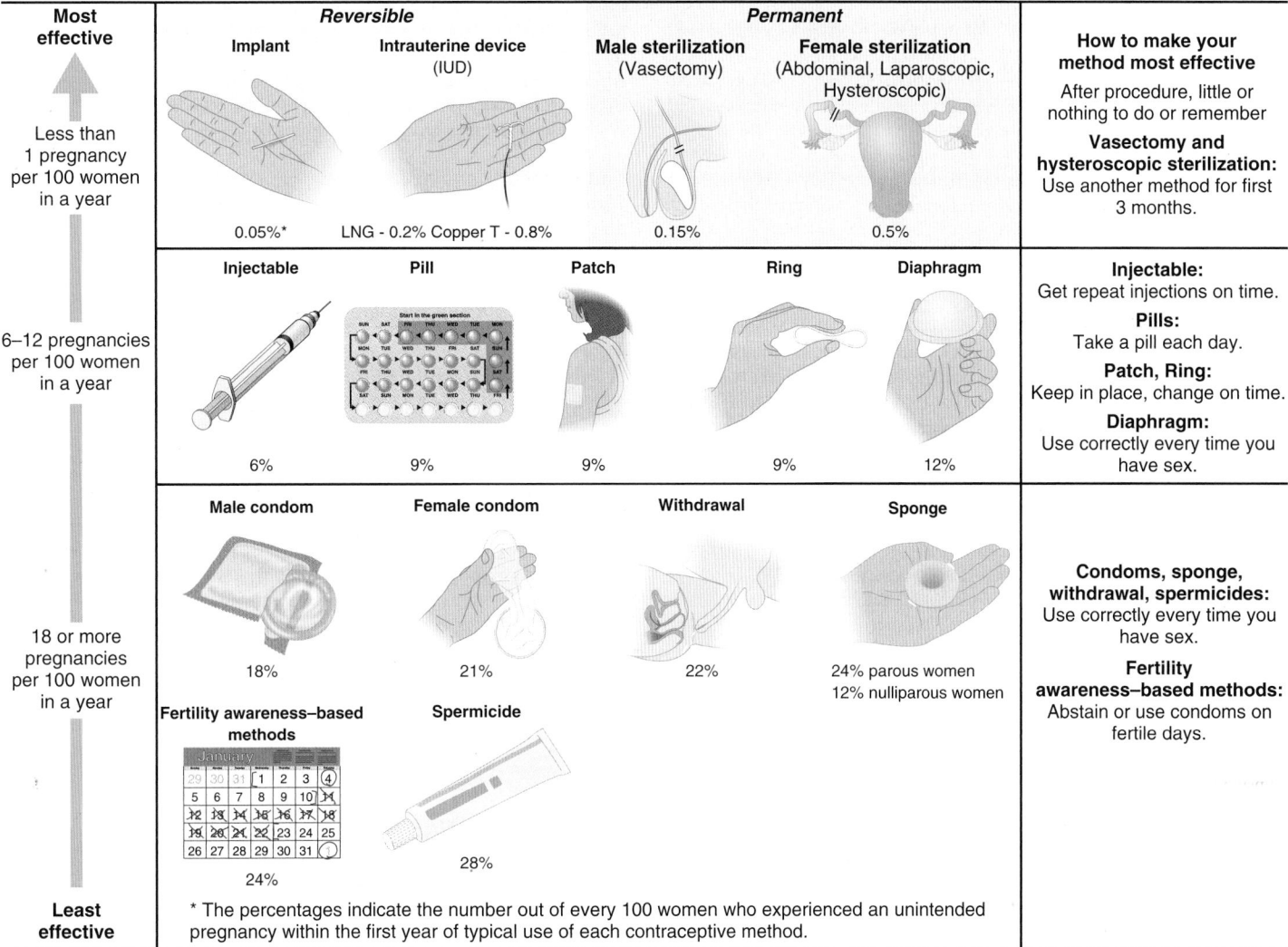

FIGURE 225-1. Detailed chart of the effectiveness of family planning methods with instructions for subjects. LNG = levonorgestrel. (Adapted from World Health Organization [WHO] Department of Reproductive Health and Research, Johns Hopkins Bloomberg School of Public Health/Center for Communication Programs [CCP], Knowledge for Health Project. *Family Planning: A Global Handbook for Providers.* 2011 updates. Baltimore, Geneva: CCP and WHO; 2011, and Trussell J. Contraceptive failure in the United States. *Contraception.* 2011;83:397-404.)

should not be used with them; water-based lubricants (K-Y jelly is one) are safe to use. The male condom causes no side effects except possible irritation or allergy.

Female Condom

The female condom, also called an internal condom, is a soft, loose-fitting prelubricated pouch with two flexible polyurethane rings, one at each end. The smaller ring at the closed end is inserted well into the vagina, creating a barrier to sperm. The larger ring remains outside the vagina, covering the vulva and providing additional protection. The female condom can be inserted before beginning sexual activity and left in place for a longer time than the male condom after ejaculation occurs. Because polyurethane is stronger than the latex used in most male condoms, the female condom is less likely to rupture. Both polyurethane and latex prevent virus transmission and should reduce the risk for acquiring HIV infection.

Hormonal (Steroidal) Contraception

Contraception using steroid hormones has been available since the 1960s. The use of hormones (or derivatives/analogues of hormones) that occur naturally in the female reproductive cycle can alter the reproductive system so that ovulation does not occur or so that physical factors (such as mucus production,

tubal motility, and endometrial thickness) that enhance the probability of fertilization or implantation are altered. All modern hormonal formulations are made from synthetic steroids. The hormones are either a combination of an estrogen and a progestin or, in some formulations, a progestin alone. There are two major types of synthetic progestins: derivatives of 19-nortestosterone (which are used in OCs) and derivatives of 17α-acetoxyprogesterone (pregnanes). Pregnanes are structurally related to progesterone and are used in injectable contraceptives, but are not used in pills.

After the discontinuation of hormonal contraceptives, the rate of return of fertility is slightly lower for users of OCs than for users of barrier methods—but faster than for users of Depo-Provera. OCs do not cause permanent infertility or adversely affect pregnancies that occur after their discontinuation. OCs are not teratogenic if they are accidentally ingested during pregnancy.

From the user's point of view, the main differences are route of administration, length of action, how much attention the user needs to pay to the administration of the drug, and side effects. All these methods are very effective, and if used consistently they have very low pregnancy rates. Even with typical use, they are among the more effective methods, although, with the exception of the implants, they are less effective than sterilization or the IUD. The most commonly used of these methods is the OC ("the pill"), which was also the first hormonal contraceptive and the one most widely used globally.

Oral Contraceptives

There are three major types of OC formulations: fixed-dose combination, combination phasic, and daily progestin. The combination formulations are the most widely used and are most widely prescribed. They consist of tablets containing both an estrogen and a progestin, usually given continuously for 3 weeks. Generally, no steroids are given for the fourth week. Three types of pills provide active tablets for 24 days, with 4 days of inactive tablets. Other types provide active tablets for 84 days followed by 7 days without active tablets or with a low dose of estrogen to allow withdrawal bleeding. The endometrium usually begins to slough 1 to 3 days after steroid ingestion is stopped, causing withdrawal bleeding, which usually lasts 3 to 4 days (and which users interpret as menstrual bleeding). The uterine blood loss with OC use averages about 25 mL per cycle, less than the 35 mL average for ovulatory cycles.

Three estrogens (ethinyl estradiol and its 3-methyl ether, mestranol, as well as one formulation with estradiol valerate) are used in combined OCs. They are combined with one of two major types of 19-nortestosterone progestins—estranes and gonanes—both of which have androgenic activity. The estranes currently used in several OCs are norethindrone and its acetates, norethindrone acetate and ethynodiol diacetate. Gonanes have greater progestational activity per unit weight than estranes, and thus a smaller amount of these progestins is used in OC formulations. One other progestin that is structurally related to spironolactone has been formulated in an OC. This progestin is called drospirenone and has antimineralocorticoid and antiandrogenic actions as well as progestational activity without androgenic activity. There are also daily progestin-only formulations that include norethindrone, norgestrel, LNG, or desogestrel.

Combined OCs, which contain both estrogen and progestin, consistently inhibit the midcycle gonadotropin surge and thus prevent ovulation. The progestin-only formulation has a lower dose of progestin than the combined agents and does not consistently inhibit ovulation, even though it is ingested every day. Progestin-only pills containing desogestrel appear to more consistently inhibit ovulation than other progestin-only formulations. Both combined OCs and progestin-only formulations also act on the cervical mucus and tubal motility to interfere with sperm transport. Progestins also alter the endometrium so that if fertilization occurs, implantation may be prevented. For contraceptive effectiveness to be maintained with the combination formulations, it is important that the pill-free interval be limited to no more than 7 days. This is made easier to remember by inclusion of placebo pills in the packet for the hormone-free days. Continuous or extended cycle combined OCs are an equally safe option for women who prefer them.[A1]

Side Effects

The synthetic steroids in OC formulations have many metabolic effects in addition to their contraceptive actions. These effects can cause the more common, less serious side effects as well as the rare, serious complications. The magnitude of these effects is directly related to the dosage and potency of the steroids in the formulations.

The most frequent symptoms produced by the estrogen component include nausea, breast tenderness, and fluid retention (bloating). The progestins can produce certain androgenic effects, such as weight gain, acne, and depression. But because estrogens decrease sebum production, women who have acne may experience improvement in their symptoms. Insufficient estrogen, too much progestin, or a combination of both may result in unscheduled (breakthrough) bleeding. This problem is more common with formulations containing 20 μg of estrogen than with those containing 30 to 35 μg and is increased in women who also smoke cigarettes. Shortening the pill-free interval to 3 or 4 days may decrease the incidence of unscheduled bleeding with low-estrogen formulations.

The synthetic estrogens used in OCs cause an increase in the hepatic production of several proteins. Some of the proteins that are increased by ethinyl estradiol, such as factors V, VIII, and X and fibrinogen, have the potential to enhance thrombosis (see later), and an increase in angiotensinogen levels may elevate blood pressure in some users. The incidence of both venous and arterial thrombosis is higher with 50-μg estrogen formulations than with those with 20 to 35 μg of estrogen. Blood pressure should be followed in all users of combined OCs and the drug discontinued if there is a clinically significant increase. The progestins do not affect protein synthesis except to reduce levels of sex hormone–binding globulin.

High-progestin formulations have an adverse effect on the lipid profile. However, estrogen has a beneficial effect on the arterial wall and on serum lipids, so users of these agents do not have an increased risk for cardiovascular disease. The newer combination formulations with less androgenic progestins have a more favorable effect on the lipid profile. The effect of OCs on glucose metabolism is directly related to the dose, potency, and type of progestin. Although high-progestin formulations caused peripheral insulin resistance, the low-progestin formulations in current use do not significantly alter levels of glucose, insulin, or glucagon after a glucose load.

Complications and Risk Factors
Thrombosis

The background rate of venous thrombosis and embolism in women of reproductive age is about 3 per 10,000 woman-years. Women of reproductive age who are not pregnant or using OCs experience thrombosis at a rate of 1.9 to 3.7 per 10,000 woman-years. Evidence-based guidelines for the risk of venous thromboembolism with combined hormonal contraception were published in 2017 by the American Society for Reproductive Medicine.[8] Among users of OCs, the relative risk is 3.5 (95% confidence interval, 2.9 to 4.3) compared with nonusers, but less than the rate of 5 to 20 per 10,000 woman-years that occurs in association with pregnancy.[A2] The risk for venous thrombosis and embolism is higher for women using OCs with 50 μg of ethinyl estradiol than for those using 30 to 35 μg. In the presence of an inherited hypercoagulable state (Chapter 73), the risk for venous thrombosis is increased several-fold. Screening for coagulation deficiencies before women are started on OCs is not recommended unless the individual has a personal or significant family history of thrombotic events. Women with known inherited or acquired thrombogenic conditions should not use estrogen-containing steroid contraceptives in pills, rings, or patches because each of these agents has thrombogenic effects. Some epidemiologic studies have found that the risk for venous thromboembolism is greater in individuals ingesting OCs with the newer, less androgenic progestins than those containing LNG with the same amount of estrogen. However, other studies have reported that the risk is similar with formulations[9] containing these two types of progestins. These studies are all observational and thus subject to bias.

Myocardial Infarction and Stroke

Myocardial infarction is rare among women of reproductive age, with a rate of 10.1 per 100,000 person-years in a recent Danish cohort. Although the absolute risks for myocardial infarction and thrombotic stroke associated with the use of hormonal contraception were found to be low, the risk was increased by a factor of 0.9 to 1.7 with OCs that included ethinyl estradiol at a dose of 20 μg and by a factor of 1.3 to 2.3 with those that included ethinyl estradiol at a dose of 30 to 40 μg, with relatively small differences in risk according to progestin type. The use of high-dose OCs by women who smoke cigarettes increases the risk for myocardial infarction by about 10-fold. Therefore, combination OCs should not be prescribed to women older than 35 years who smoke cigarettes or use alternate forms of nicotine. Epidemiologic studies indicate that use of low-dose OCs by nonsmoking women without hypertension is not associated with a significantly increased incidence of either myocardial infarction or either hemorrhagic or thrombotic stroke.

Cancers of the Reproductive System

An analysis of worldwide epidemiologic data in 1988 showed that the risk for breast cancer diagnosis was increased by about 25% in young women who were currently using OCs, but this increased risk was no longer present 10 years or more after they stopped using OCs. A very large cohort study in Great Britain of OC users and aged-matched nonusers was initiated in 1968. Data accumulated until 2004 showed a similar incidence of breast cancer in both groups. More recently, a much larger, nationwide prospective cohort study involving all women in Denmark between 15 and 49 years of age (1.8 million women) followed on average for 10.9 years similarly to the worldwide epidemiologic data observed a 20% higher risk of breast cancer among those who were currently using or had recently used hormonal contraceptives than those who had never used them, in this case using contemporary rather than older, often higher-dose formulations.[10,11] The risk increased with a longer duration of use. However, absolute increases in risk were small.

Several studies have reported that use of OCs by women with a family history of breast cancer does not increase their risk for developing breast cancer.

The epidemiologic data are conflicting regarding OC use and the risk for invasive cervical cancer or cervical intraepithelial neoplasia.[12] Most well-controlled studies indicate that there is no change in risk for cervical intraepithelial neoplasia with OC use. Studies that do indicate an increased risk are often confounded by a lack of information on condom use. Regardless, these studies indicate that the risk declines with interval since last use.

Several studies have shown that the use of OCs has a protective effect against endometrial cancer. Moreover, the decrease in risk persists for many years after OCs are stopped. This protective effect is related to duration of use, increasing from a 20% reduction with 1 year of use to a 60% reduction with 4 years of use. The level of protection declines with time after use is stopped.

In addition, OCs reduce the risk for development of epithelial ovarian cancer, as well as cancers with low malignant potential. The magnitude of the decrease in risk is directly related to the duration of OC use, increasing from about a 40% reduction with 4 years of use to a 60% reduction with 12 years of use. The protective effect continues for at least 20 years after the use of OCs ends. As with endometrial cancer, the protective effect occurs only in women of low parity (fewer than four), who are at greatest risk for this type of cancer.

Studies have reported that OCs significantly reduce the risk for development of colorectal cancer by about 20%, as well as the risk of hematologic malignancies.

Benign Hepatocellular Adenoma

The development of a benign hepatocellular adenoma was a rare occurrence in long-term users of high-dose OCs containing mestranol, but it is not increased by use of ethinyl estradiol OCs. There is no increased risk for liver cancer associated with OC use.

Contraindications

OCs can be prescribed for most women of reproductive age.[13] According to the U.S. MEC for contraceptive use, adapted from the WHO criteria, several conditions are considered absolute contraindications to use of combined hormonal contraceptives (category 4), including smoking 15 cigarettes or more per day, at age 35 or older, and severe hypertension, among others. There is no evidence that individuals with asymptomatic mitral valve prolapse should avoid using OCs. The presence of migraine headaches without aura is also not a contraindication to OC use, but if aura is present, combination OCs should not be prescribed because of a possible increased risk for stroke. OC use does not increase the risk for development of malignant melanoma or prolactin-secreting pituitary adenomas.

Management of OC Therapy

If a healthy woman has no contraindications to OC use, it is unnecessary to perform any laboratory tests, including cervical cytology, before she uses them. A pelvic examination is not required. Starting pills on the day of the visit is associated with better long-term use of the method. There is no reason to discontinue OC use unless pregnancy is desired. Intermittent discontinuation is unnecessary and puts women at risk for an unwanted pregnancy.

Although synthetic sex steroids can retard the biotransformation of certain drugs (e.g., phenazone and meperidine) as a result of substrate competition, such interference is usually not important clinically. However, some drugs can interfere clinically with the action of OCs by inducing liver enzymes that convert the steroids to more polar and less biologically active metabolites. These drugs include barbiturates, sulfonamides, cyclophosphamide, griseofulvin, and rifampin. There is a high incidence of OC failure in women ingesting rifampin as well as systemic griseofulvin, and neither should be given concurrently with OCs. Products containing St. John's wort reduce contraceptive effectiveness and cause breakthrough bleeding. Women taking certain medications for epilepsy should be treated with 50-μg estrogen formulations because many antiepileptic medications lower ethinyl estradiol levels and cause breakthrough bleeding, which may cause premature discontinuation of use.

Because of their many health benefits, including reduction in risk for endometrial and ovarian cancer and induction of regular cyclic uterine bleeding, OC use can be continued until menopause in normotensive, nonsmoking women without contraindications.

A common clinical question is what to do if a pill is missed. The standard advice for combined OCs is to take the first missed pill as soon as possible and take the remaining pills at the usual time, even if it means taking two pills in one day (discarding any additional missed pills). If two or more pills are missed, take the most recent missed pill as soon as possible, continue taking the remaining pills at the usual time, even if it means taking two or more pills on the same day, and use back up contraception (e.g., condoms) or avoid sexual intercourse until pills have been taken for at least 7 consecutive days. If pills were missed in the last week of hormonal pills (third week of cycle), omit the hormone-free interval and start a new pack the next day. Emergency

contraception should be considered. Vomiting and diarrhea for up to 48 hours should be considered as one missed pill; vomiting and diarrhea for more than 48 hours should be treated as two or more missed pills. For norethindrone-containing progestin-only pills, a pill is considered "missed" if it is more than 3 hours late.

Emergency Contraception

There is now a way that women can avoid pregnancy even after unprotected sex acts. The method is termed *emergency contraception* because it should be used as early as possible after the unprotected sex.[14] A formulation of 1500 μg (1.5 mg) LNG in a single tablet prevents about 85% of expected pregnancies, if used within 72 hours after coitus.[15] Another approved agent for emergency contraception is the selective progesterone receptor modulator ulipristal acetate given as a single 30-mg dose. This agent is more effective than LNG and is effective for 5 days after intercourse.[A2][A3] Another option is the immediate insertion of a copper intrauterine device (see later), which virtually eliminates the risk of pregnancy.

Transdermal and Intravaginal Steroid Contraceptives
Transdermal Patch

In the United States, there is one transdermal contraceptive patch that contains both estrogen and progestin (Xulane). The patch has an area of 20 cm² and delivers 150 μg of the progestin norelgestromin, the active metabolite of norgestimate, and 35 μg of ethinyl estradiol daily. It may be applied to the buttocks, lower abdomen, upper arm, or upper torso (but not the breasts). The patch should be removed after 7 days and a new patch applied to a different area of skin. A woman using this method uses three patches sequentially, each for 7 days. After the third patch is removed, she waits 7 days before starting her next patch, thus mimicking the 28-day combined OC cycle (21 hormone days, followed by 7 hormone-free days, during which withdrawal bleeding occurs). Because the patch does not require daily attention, adherence with the patch is somewhat higher than with OCs. Contraceptive efficacy, bleeding patterns, and side effects are similar to those associated with OCs, and the contraindications are similar. Although the effectiveness of the patch may be decreased among women weighing more than 90 kg, there does not appear to be an association between pregnancy risk and body mass index (BMI). For all combined hormonal contraceptives, a BMI of 30 kg/m² or greater is considered category 2 (benefits of use outweigh potential risks) by the MEC.

Intravaginal Ring

Another option for nonoral hormonal contraception is the vaginal ring (NuvaRing in the United States). This soft, flexible ring measures 58 mm in diameter and is 4 mm thick. The ring is composed of ethinyl vinyl acetate and contains the progestin etonogestrel, a major metabolite of desogestrel, and ethinyl estradiol. The ring is inserted and removed by the woman herself. There is no "wrong" position or placement of the ring as long as it is inside the vagina. Each ring is left in place for 3 weeks, after which time it is removed for 1 week to allow withdrawal bleeding. Each day, 120 μg of etonogestrel and 15 μg of ethinyl estradiol are released from the ring, and bleeding with the ring in place is uncommon. Contraceptive efficacy and side effects are similar to those of combined OCs, as are contraindications. Women may keep the ring in place during intercourse, or it can be safely removed for up to 3 hours and then reinserted. Tampons may also be used concurrently with the ring without affecting efficacy.

Injectable Steroid Contraceptives
Constituents and Use

Although several types of injectable steroid formulations are in use for contraception throughout the world, currently the only injectable available in the United States is depot medroxyprogesterone acetate (DMPA). The initial formulation of this contraceptive was administered as an intramuscular injection of 1 mL of an aqueous suspension containing 150 mg of crystalline medroxyprogesterone acetate once every 3 months. There is also a formulation that is administered subcutaneously (DMPA-SC) that contains 104 mg of DMPA in 0.65 mL of solution. This lower-dose formulation has a lower peak medroxyprogesterone acetate concentration than DMPA and a long duration of action that suppresses ovulation for at least 13 weeks and is not affected by body mass. The formulation for subcutaneous administration allows the possibility for women to self-inject the medication. Other injectable contraceptives include norethindrone enanthate, given in a dose of 200 mg every 2 months, and several once-a-month injections of combinations of different progestins and estrogens.

DMPA has a low failure rate, 0.1% at 1 year and 0.4% at 2 years. The major contraceptive action of DMPA is inhibition of ovulation, and it also impedes sperm transport by thickening cervical mucus. With DMPA and DMPA-SC, serum medroxyprogesterone levels rapidly increase to contraceptively effective blood levels (>0.5 ng/mL) within 24 hours after the injection. With DMPA, medroxyprogesterone levels plateau for about 3 months, after which there is a gradual decline until levels become undetectable 7 to 9 months after the injection. With DMPA-SC, medroxyprogesterone levels steadily decline after the initial peak and reach 0.2 ng/mL 3 to 4 months after the injection.

Side Effects

With both formulations, mean endogenous estradiol levels remain above the postmenopausal range (40 to 60 pg/mL), and symptoms of estrogen deficiency do not occur. Although DMPA may decrease bone mineral density during use, it is unnecessary to measure bone mineral density or to administer bone antiresorptive agents in DMPA users because the bone loss is temporary and reversible after stopping DMPA.

Because of the lag time it takes to clear DMPA from the circulation, resumption of ovulation is delayed for a variable time after the last injection. It may take as long as 1 year for ovulatory cycles to return. After this initial delay, fecundity resumes at a rate similar to that found after discontinuation of a barrier contraceptive.

The major side effect of DMPA is complete disruption of the menstrual cycle. Because this formulation contains only a progestin, without an estrogen, endometrial integrity is not maintained, and usually light uterine bleeding occurs at irregular and unpredictable intervals. As duration of therapy increases, the incidence of frequent bleeding steadily declines and the incidence of amenorrhea steadily increases so that at the end of 2 years, about 70% of users are amenorrheic. Because the major reason for discontinuance of all progestin-injectable contraceptives is menstrual irregularity, several combined progestin-estrogen injectables that are given once monthly and produce regular withdrawal bleeding have been developed, but these are not available in the United States.

Most DMPA users gain between 1.5 and 4 kg in their first year of use and continue to gain weight thereafter. Because there is no estrogen in DMPA, its use does not cause hypertension or thromboembolism. DMPA use is associated with a reduction in seizures among women with epilepsy, as well as a reduction in painful crises among women with sickle cell disease.

Subdermal Implants
Constituents and Use

The only subdermal implant[16] currently available in the United States is a single 4-cm by 2-mm ethylene vinyl acetate rod containing 68 μg of etonogestrel, the active metabolite of desogestrel (Implanon or Nexplanon, which is radiopaque). It provides effective contraception for 3 years. The rod is packaged in a disposable metal trocar inserter and does not require a skin incision for insertion, only for removal. Ovulation is inhibited by the circulating etonogestrel levels, and no pregnancies were reported in three large clinical trials. As with other progestin-only implants, irregular bleeding is the most common clinical complaint. Because implants are not user dependent, the typical-use and perfect-use failure rates are identical and very low, making this method essentially as effective as IUDs and sterilization. Another subdermal implant, Jadelle, consists of two 4.3-cm rods each containing 75 mg of LNG and is approved for 5 years of contraception; it is not yet available in the United States.

Intrauterine Devices

Two options for intrauterine contraception are available in the United States: the copper-containing IUD and the LNG intrauterine system (LNG-IUS). Both methods are exceedingly effective with perfect- and typical-use failure rates of less than 1%.

The copper T380A IUD is approved for use in the United States for 10 years and maintains its high levels of effectiveness for at least 12 years. The LNG-IUS is approved for 5 years of use, and it releases a dose of 20 μg of LNG from the device into the endometrial cavity each day. This causes atrophy of the endometrial lining, which markedly reduces the amount of uterine bleeding, and it is approved to treat menorrhagia. A newer LNG-containing IUD is smaller and designed for use by nulliparous women; it releases up to 14 μg of LNG and is approved for 3 years of use.

The main mechanism of action for the copper IUD is spermicidal. This effect is caused by a local sterile leukocytic response produced by the copper as well as the plastic IUD. The LNG-releasing IUD acts mainly by preventing transport of spermatozoa through the cervical mucus and thus preventing fertilization of the ovum. In addition, some women do not ovulate because of the systemic absorption of LNG. After removal of each type of IUD, the inflammatory reaction rapidly disappears, and resumption of fertility is prompt.

The main difference between the two IUDs is the menstrual bleeding pattern. With the copper IUD, women generally continue to have a regular menstrual period, which may be associated with more pain and heavier bleeding. With the LNG-IUS, irregular bleeding is common in the first 4 to 6 months of use, but after that time, most women develop amenorrhea.

Both IUDs can be easily inserted by any clinician who has been trained. No special tests are needed routinely before insertion, and if it is reasonably certain that the woman is not pregnant, the IUD may be inserted on the same day she presents requesting it. It is not necessary to wait for the next menstrual period. Almost all women, including nulliparous and young women, are considered good candidates for the IUD. Uterine perforation is a rare complication of IUD insertion, occurring in less than 0.1% of cases. Spontaneous expulsion of the IUD after insertion is also rare and happens in less than 5% of users. An IUD may be safely inserted immediately after a delivery or abortion, although the expulsion rate may be slightly higher.[Ad]

Development of acute salpingitis more than 1 month after insertion of the IUD is due to infection with a sexually transmitted pathogen and is unrelated to the presence of the device. All IUD-related upper genital tract infections occur only during the insertion process. If there is clinical suspicion that cervicitis is present, an endocervical test for chlamydia and gonorrhea should be performed and the insertion delayed until negative results are obtained. It is not recommended to administer antibiotics routinely with IUD insertion.

Sterilization

Considering both tubal ligations for women and vasectomy for men, sterilization is the most common contraceptive method used by couples in the United States. Female sterilization may be performed transabdominally, such as at the time of cesarean delivery; through a minilaparotomy incision immediately postpartum; laparoscopically; or hysteroscopically. Both laparoscopic tubal ligation and hysteroscopic sterilization may be performed as outpatient procedures. Hysteroscopic tubal occlusion using the Essure device requires evaluation with a hysterosalpingogram 3 months after the procedure to confirm tubal occlusion. As of December 2018, the Essure device is no longer sold in the United States.

Vasectomy is a simple outpatient procedure that can be performed using local anesthesia. Although many men are concerned about the possibility, sexual function is not affected by vasectomy. There are often programs that support contraceptive services for low-income women, but it is often more difficult for low-income men to access vasectomy.

Medical Abortion

Mifepristone was the first medication designed for early termination of pregnancy without a hands-on procedure. Mifepristone for pregnancy termination has now been registered in more than 60 countries and is used for the majority of all terminations in several countries in Europe.[17] In the United States, mifepristone (Mifeprex), an antiprogestin, was licensed for sale in the year 2000 and labeled to be used with misoprostol, a synthetic prostaglandin E₁ analogue, for termination of early first trimester pregnancies. The use of this combination therapy has been increasing every year since. By 2014, mifepristone followed by misoprostol was used in 45% of all pregnancy terminations before 9 weeks' gestation.

This therapy can be provided as a completely outpatient service and hence is used by many types of providers, including family medicine and internal medicine physicians, midwives, physician assistants, and nurse practitioners. The standards of service provision have evolved with experience to allow a much more woman-centered treatment, where the user can decide where to be when she takes the medication and with whom.

Based on a revised and updated label approved by the FDA in March 2016, several aspects of the medical abortion experience have been officially changed to conform to the best researched medical practices. The current recommended regimen, according to the FDA, is one 200 mg tablet of mifepristone followed 24 to 48 hours later by four 200-μg tablets of misoprostol (800 μg total) administered buccally (between the gum and the cheek). The therapy is recommended for pregnancy termination through 70 days after last menstrual period (LMP). Women can take the medications at home or take the first pill in the clinic.

Treatment with this medical abortion regimen is highly successful, with approximately 97% efficacy (defined as not undergoing vacuum aspiration). Efficacy is slightly higher if used at the earlier gestational ages. The main side effects are uterine cramping and bleeding (which are in fact main effects of the treatment), as well as less frequently reported instances of nausea, vomiting, and diarrhea. Serious adverse events are quite rare and mainly fall into two categories: consequences of excessive bleeding (e.g., blood transfusion and/or surgical completion of the abortion) or infection, which is even rarer. Major complications occur in approximately 0.3% of cases. The risk of death among users of this method is 0.00063%, 14 times lower than the risk associated with live birth.

In the United States, access to mifepristone is possible only directly from providers. The medication cannot be prescribed and obtained in pharmacies like most drugs. Instead, providers need to order the pills from the distributor and dispense them to women wanting to use this treatment. Other countries, such as Canada, have made access more consistent with the procurement of other prescribed medications.

Grade A References

A1. Edelman A, Micks E, Gallo MF, et al. Continuous or extended cycle vs. cyclic use of combined hormonal contraceptives for contraception. *Cochrane Database Syst Rev.* 2014;7:CD004695.

A2. Piaggio G, Kapp N, von Hertzen H. Effect on pregnancy rates of the delay in the administration of levonorgestrel for emergency contraception: a combined analysis of four WHO trials. *Contraception.* 2011;84:35-39.

A3. Shen J, Che Y, Showell E, et al. Interventions for emergency contraception. *Cochrane Database Syst Rev.* 2019;1:CD001324.

A4. Hohmann HL, Reeves MF, Chen BA, et al. Immediate versus delayed insertion of the levonorgestrel-releasing intrauterine device following dilation and evacuation: a randomized controlled trial. *Contraception.* 2012;85:240-245.

GENERAL REFERENCES

For the General References and other additional features, please visit Expert Consult at https://expertconsult.inkling.com.

226

COMMON MEDICAL PROBLEMS IN PREGNANCY

KAREN ROSENE-MONTELLA

There are 62 million women of childbearing age in the United States, 85% of whom will give birth by the age of 44 years. The majority of these women will not have obtained preventive health services in any given year, and more than half the pregnancies will be unplanned or unintended. At least 25% will enter pregnancy with a chronic medical illness, and more than half will be overweight or obese, making the role of the internist paramount in maternal health. In the most recent Confidential Enquiry into maternal mortality in the United Kingdom, more than half of all women who died of direct or indirect causes were overweight or obese, and more than 15% of all deaths were in morbidly obese women. Sixteen percent of pregnant women have depression in the perinatal period, and depression rates are even higher in those with chronic illnesses, such as diabetes and asthma.

By the time pregnant patients are seen by their obstetricians, most major teratogenic abnormalities have already occurred (Fig. 226-1), and the window of opportunity to enter pregnancy in a quiescent disease state, on the safest possible medication profile, may have passed. For this reason, internists caring for women of childbearing age have a unique responsibility to provide preconception care at a time when interventions will be of maximum benefit to both the fetus and the mother. Table 226-1 describes preconception interventions for women with chronic medical illnesses.

The basic principles involved in the care of pregnant patients with medical disorders are reviewed here, followed by a more detailed discussion of certain medical conditions, selected because of their contribution to maternal mortality or because of the frequency with which they occur.

TABLE 226-1	PRECONCEPTION INTERVENTIONS FOR WOMEN WITH MEDICAL ILLNESSES

TYPE 1 AND TYPE 2 DIABETES

Discuss importance of a normal hemoglobin A_{1c} before conception and importance of using contraception until that is achieved
Evaluate for microvascular complications
　Obtain remission for proliferative retinopathy
　Emphasize need to discontinue ACE inhibitor after first missed period
Discontinue thiazolidinediones and statins
Consider change to insulin therapy for type 2 diabetic patients on oral agents unless using metformin for ovulation induction in PCOS
Discuss probable need to reduce insulin dose in first trimester

THYROID DISEASE

Screen for hypothyroidism in women at risk
Normalize TSH and free T_4 before pregnancy
Counsel women taking levothyroxine on need to increase dose soon after conception
Diagnose cause of hyperthyroidism and consider ablative therapy for women with Graves disease requiring high doses of PTU

CHRONIC HYPERTENSION/RENAL DISEASE

Rule out secondary causes of hypertension if appropriate
Evaluate extent of end-organ disease
Quantify GFR and proteinuria
Discuss drugs of choice for hypertension and replace ACE inhibitor
Discuss risk for superimposed preeclampsia and use of low-dose aspirin for women at significant risk for preeclampsia

THROMBOEMBOLIC DISEASE

Consider evaluation for congenital or acquired thrombophilias in women with previous VTE, previous poor obstetric outcome, or family history
Discuss risks of warfarin in pregnancy, need to discontinue warfarin by 4 to 6 weeks' gestation, and conversion to unfractionated or low-molecular-weight heparin
Discuss options to combined oral contraceptives

EPILEPSY

Determine whether patient is a candidate for withdrawal of antiepileptic drugs
Consider monotherapy with most effective agent at lowest dose possible
Prescribe folate at 1 to 4 mg/day
Discuss possible ineffectiveness of low-dose contraceptives with phenobarbital, phenytoin, and carbamazepine
Consider discontinuing valproate

CARDIAC DISEASE

Obtain baseline echocardiography if congenital disease, stenotic lesion, or pulmonary hypertension suspected
Evaluate for coronary artery disease in women with multiple risk factors

ASTHMA

Verify patient's asthma action plan and peak flowmeter use
Discuss relative safety of all asthma medications except leukotriene modifiers

SYSTEMIC LUPUS ERYTHEMATOSUS AND AUTOIMMUNE DISEASE

Evaluate for renal and cardiopulmonary disease and antiphospholipid, anti-Ro, anti-La antibodies
Avoid pregnancy if disease is active
Discuss relative safety of most immunosuppressants

ACE = angiotensin-converting enzyme; GFR = glomerular filtration rate; PCOS = polycystic ovary syndrome; PTU = propylthiouracil; T_4 = thyroxine; TSH = thyroid-stimulating hormone; VTE = venous thromboembolism.
From Rosene-Montella K, Keely EJ, Lee RV, Barbour LA, eds. *Medical Care of the Pregnant Patient.* 2nd ed. Philadelphia: ACP Press/American College of Physicians; 2008.

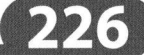 BASIC PRINCIPLES

Pregnancy is associated with significant but normal physiologic changes that have an impact on the diagnosis and management of disease states and the pharmacokinetics of most drugs (Table 226-2). The physiologic changes required during pregnancy may stress the woman's ability to adapt, particularly in the presence of an underlying disease. The mother's response to pregnancy often unmasks diseases or predicts future risk, so pregnancy is an opportunity to identify women at risk for other non–pregnancy-related illnesses. For example, gestational diabetes is predictive of an increased risk for type 2 diabetes; preeclampsia is predictive of increased risk for ischemic heart disease and stroke; and thrombosis, late fetal loss, or preeclampsia may unmask an underlying thrombophilia.

Fetal well-being depends on maternal well-being. Although there is often thought to be a dichotomy between maternal and fetal needs, they are usually

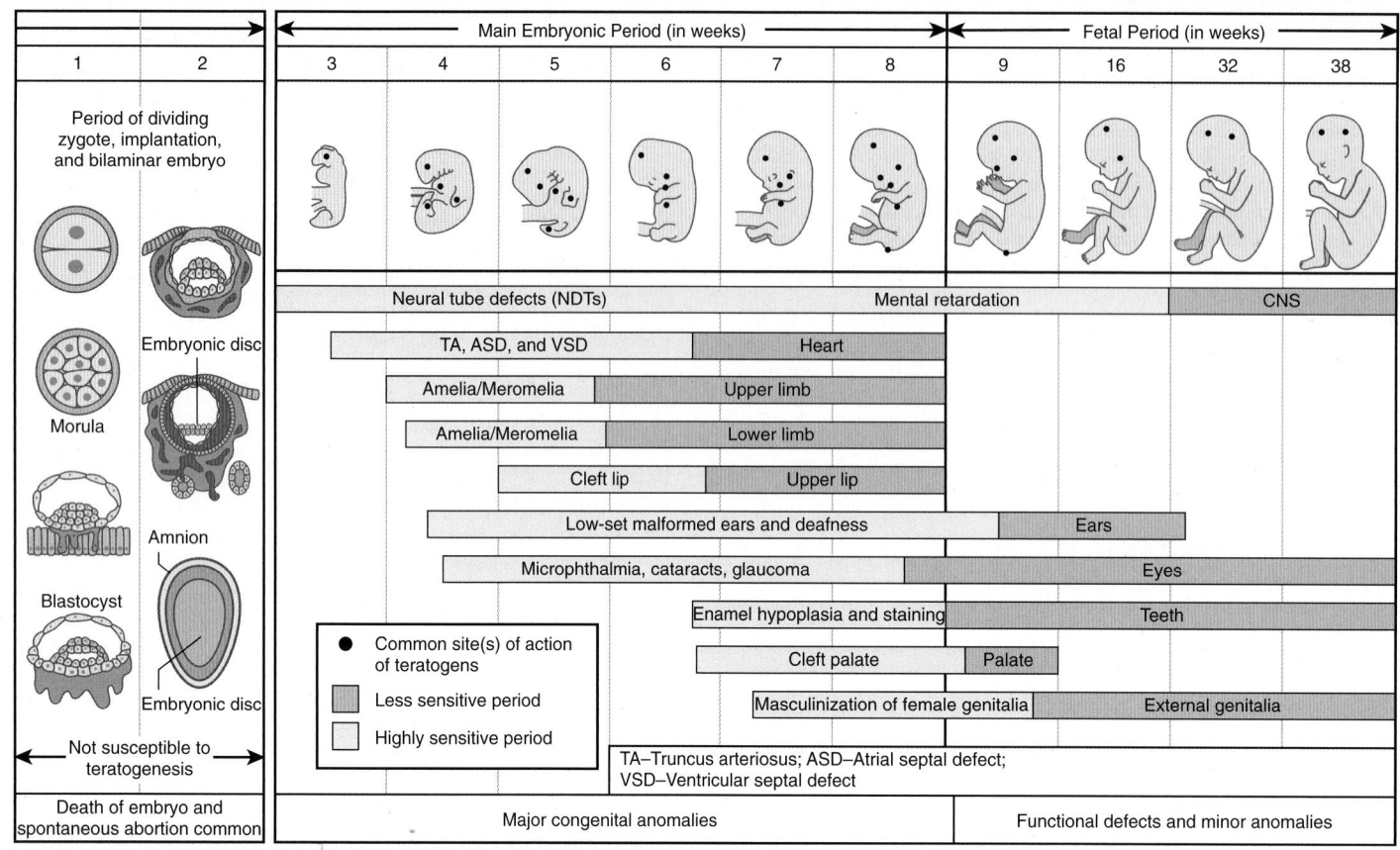

FIGURE 226-1. The developing fetus. CNS = central nervous system. (From Moore K. *The Developing Human: Clinically Oriented Embryology.* Philadelphia: WB Saunders; 1982, with permission from Annals of Internal Medicine.)

TABLE 226-2 NORMAL PHYSIOLOGIC CHANGES IN PREGNANCY

CARDIAC

Cardiac output increased 40%
Blood volume increased 30-50%
Heart rate increased 10-20 beats/min
Blood pressure decreased 10-15 mm Hg
ECG changes related to widened thorax, dextrorotation of heart, elevation of diaphragm

PULMONARY

Upper airway hyperemia and glandular hyperactivity leading to increased edema and friability
Nasal congestion, gestational rhinitis, snoring
Difficult airway management and failed intubation
Minute ventilation increased (owing to an increase in tidal volume, *not* respiratory rate, which remains unchanged), which leads to relative respiratory alkalosis (pH 7.4-7.45)
  Normal Pao_2 100-105 mm Hg
  Normal $Paco_2$ 28-32 mm Hg

RENAL

Increased GFR to 150-180 mL/min/1.73 m^2
Normal serum creatinine concentration <0.8 mg/dL
Increased renal excretion of bicarbonate, limiting buffering capacity in patients who become acidotic
Decreased oncotic pressure

ALTERED PHARMACOKINETICS

Increased renal and hepatic clearance of drugs
Altered absorption
Altered protein binding
Increased volume of distribution

ECG = electrocardiogram; GFR = glomerular filtration rate.
These physiologic changes generally progress throughout gestation.

TABLE 226-3 NATIONAL COMMISSION ON RADIATION PROTECTION (NCRP) RECOMMENDED PREGNANCY EXPOSURES

TOTAL EXPOSURE DURING PREGNANCY (rad)	NCRP RECOMMENDATIONS
≤5	Acceptable; low likelihood of problems
5-10	Low risk for problems
10-15 (at ≤8 wk gestation)	Higher risk; consideration of termination
>15	Termination of pregnancy recommended

From Rosene-Montella K, Keely EJ, Lee RV, Barbour LA, eds. *Medical Care of the Pregnant Patient.* 2nd ed. Philadelphia: ACP Press/American College of Physicians; 2008.

one and the same. The fetus is dependent on maternal perfusion, oxygenation, and nutrition. Thus, more harm may be done by withholding necessary treatments and investigations from pregnant women than by providing them. Uninvestigated symptoms lead to the progression of untreated disease, and untreated maternal disease compromises fetal safety, growth, and development. The major cause of asthma exacerbations and seizures during pregnancy is abrupt discontinuation of medications, exposing the fetus to hypoxemia and acidosis in an effort to save the fetus from drug exposure. A population analysis of prescriptions for asthma medications in The Netherlands showed that prescriptions for controller medications decreased by 30% during the first months of pregnancy. In the U.K. Confidential Enquiry, in more than half the cases of maternal death from pulmonary embolism, failure to make the diagnosis was due to the unfounded fear that diagnostic testing would be harmful to the fetus. Most diagnostic imaging can be used safely in pregnancy. The effects of radiation in utero depend on both the gestational age at exposure and the level of exposure. Recommendations on fetal exposure from the National Commission on Radiation Protection are summarized in Table 226-3. Radiation exposure from specific diagnostic tests is provided in Table 226-4.

The effect of contrast agents is related to the bioavailability of iodine, and there is concern about the impact on the fetal thyroid. Iodine availability is

TABLE 226-4 RADIATION EXPOSURE

STUDY	RADIATION EXPOSURE (rad)
Chest radiography	<0.001
Lung scan	0.01-0.02 ventilation 0.01-0.03 perfusion
Pulmonary angiography	<0.050 by brachial route 0.2-0.3 by femoral route
CT angiography	0.2-0.3
Ultrasound	None
MRI, MRA, MRV	None
Upper gastrointestinal series	0.1
Lumbar spine series	0.9
Barium enema	1
Complete IVP	0.5
Head CT	<0.01
CT of abdomen	2.0-3.0

CT = computed tomography; IVP = intravenous pyelography; MRA = magnetic resonance angiography; MRI = magnetic resonance imaging; MRV = magnetic resonance venography.

extremely low, and single-dose exposures, even if they are high, are unlikely to be harmful. Therefore, contrast agents may be used when necessary. There are limited data on gadolinium, so the current recommendation is to avoid gadolinium exposure if possible.

The use of medications to treat pregnant women requires a rational risk-benefit analysis and a good understanding of the maternal indications. It is helpful to view treatment as justifiable or not justifiable rather than as safe or not safe. It is important to consider whether the condition is self-limited or harmless, what the maternal and fetal consequences of discontinuing a medication will be, and the safety data for the drug. U.S. Food and Drug Administration (FDA) categories may be misleading and often do not include adequate data for a proper risk-benefit analysis.

Recently the FDA has eliminated the categories in favor of descriptive language for this reason. Resources such as the Teratology Information Service, found at http://depts.washington.edu/terisweb/teris, offer more complete information.

The list of known human teratogens is small and includes warfarin, cyclophosphamide, diethylstilbestrol, lithium, thalidomide, penicillamine, isotretinoin, methotrexate, acetazolamide, and the antiepileptic drugs phenytoin, carbamazepine, phenobarbital, and valproic acid. Of the antiepileptic drugs, valproate has the most significant data, and it is the only antiepileptic drug for which discontinuation during pregnancy is recommended if there is an effective alternative. Angiotensin-converting enzyme (ACE) inhibitors and angiotensin II receptor blockers (ARBs) should be added to this list on the basis of data confirming that first-trimester exposure is associated with fetal renal agenesis and renal failure. Tetracyclines should be avoided because of later effects on fetal teeth and bone.

HYPERTENSIVE DISORDERS OF PREGNANCY

DEFINITION

Hypertension in pregnancy is defined as a blood pressure (BP) of 140/90 mm Hg or higher. It is defined as chronic hypertension when it predates pregnancy, is diagnosed before 20 weeks' gestation, or persists postpartum. Transient late or gestational hypertension occurs toward term and resolves postpartum in the absence of any other signs or symptoms of preeclampsia.[1]

EPIDEMIOLOGY

Chronic hypertension is the most common medical condition encountered in women of childbearing age. The incidence is increasing parallel to the increase in obesity, insulin resistance, and pregnancies in women older than 30 years. Hypertension complicates 5 to 8% of pregnancies and is associated with a 20% risk for the development of preeclampsia.

PATHOBIOLOGY

Systemic arterial BP decreases by 10 to 15 mm Hg during normal pregnancy, with a greater fall in diastolic than in systolic pressures, probably because of the decreased sensitivity to angiotensin II that has been demonstrated in pregnant women. BP begins to fall in the first trimester, reaching a nadir toward the end of the second trimester and returning toward baseline at term. This decrease may be exaggerated in women with chronic hypertension, making the diagnosis of chronic hypertension difficult during pregnancy and affecting both diagnostic and therapeutic considerations.

DIAGNOSIS

The diagnosis of hypertension relies simply on a BP measurement, in the sitting position at the level of the heart, of 140/90 mm Hg or higher on two occasions 6 hours apart. Later in pregnancy, inferior vena cava compression by the gravid uterus may lower BP substantially in the supine position, so it is critical to measure maternal BP in the sitting position. The initial evaluation should document target organ damage (such as left ventricular hypertrophy), renal disease (creatinine concentration, urinalysis, and potassium concentration), and retinopathy so that a baseline is established. Consideration of secondary causes is necessary in this young population (Chapter 70), but the diagnosis of secondary causes of hypertension is complicated by normal pregnancy-related changes. The diagnosis of Cushing syndrome is complicated by increased levels of cortisol and the placental production of adrenocorticotropic hormone and corticotropin-releasing hormone, so the best test is a 24-hour urine free cortisol measurement with higher pregnancy-specific reference ranges. Primary hyperaldosteronism (Chapter 214) may also be difficult to diagnose in the face of normal pregnancy-related elevations in plasma renin activity and aldosterone and because progesterone ameliorates both the hypertensive and the kaliuretic effects of aldosterone. Primary hyperaldosteronism should be strongly considered in any patient with chronic hypertension in whom there is a marked increase in BP toward term or postpartum. Pheochromocytoma (Chapter 215) is associated with a high maternal and fetal mortality rate, in large part owing to a delay in diagnosis. Both magnetic resonance imaging and magnetic resonance angiography (which do not require gadolinium) can be used safely in pregnancy to evaluate the adrenal glands and renal arteries.

TREATMENT Rx

Patients previously receiving drug therapy can often discontinue antihypertensives and restart them when BP gradually rises to prepregnant values toward term. It is difficult to determine whether rising BP represents a normal physiologic return to earlier pressure or the development of preeclampsia. Baseline preeclampsia laboratory tests (see later), very close follow-up, and comanagement with the patient's obstetrician are required. Patients with good BP control may prefer to continue safe medications or switch to another regimen. The drugs for which there is grade A evidence of efficacy and safety are methyldopa and labetalol (Table 226-5). Nifedipine, hydralazine, and other β-blockers, especially those with intrinsic sympathomimetic activity, have also been studied and are acceptable second- and third-line agents.

Dosing should take into consideration the increase in renal and hepatic clearance and the increased volume of distribution, which may require higher doses or narrowed dosing intervals during pregnancy. ACE inhibitors and ARBs should be discontinued at the diagnosis of pregnancy because of their teratogenicity and their association with fetal and neonatal renal agenesis and renal failure even when they are used later in gestation.

The goal of antihypertensive therapy in pregnancy is not clear. In a randomized trial, there was no significant difference in the risk for pregnancy loss, high-level neonatal care, or overall maternal complications with tight blood pressure control (target diastolic blood pressure, 85 mm Hg) compared with less-tight control (target diastolic blood pressure, 100 mm Hg), although less-tight control was associated with a significantly higher risk for severe maternal hypertension.[A1] Most current consensus recommendations, which address fetal concerns and short-term maternal safety only, recommend keeping BP below 160/100 mm Hg. Given the long-term maternal data, most centers prefer to keep maternal BP, particularly in patients with diabetes or renal disease, below 140/90 mm Hg. Consensus recommendations agree that maintaining BP above 120/80 mm Hg is necessary to preserve placental perfusion. There is no evidence that salt restriction or dietary changes improve BP control in pregnancy, and weight loss is not recommended. Likewise, there is no evidence that BP control decreases the risk for preeclampsia. It is important to obtain baseline preeclampsia laboratory tests (complete blood count, platelet count, creatinine concentration, uric acid level, aspartate transaminase level, urinalysis) in all patients with hypertension, given the 20% risk for preeclampsia, and low-dose aspirin and calcium supplementation should be considered to prevent preeclampsia (see later). Fetal monitoring with serial ultrasound for growth and amniotic fluid volume, nonstress testing (fetal heart rate acceleration in response

TABLE 226-5 ODDS RATIOS FOR FETAL AND MATERNAL COMPLICATIONS: 1995-2008

VARIABLE	PREGESTATIONAL DIABETES		CHRONIC RENAL DISEASE		COLLAGEN VASCULAR DISEASE		THYROID DISORDERS	
	WITH CHRONIC HYPERTENSION	WITHOUT CHRONIC HYPERTENSION	WITH CHRONIC HYPERTENSION	WITHOUT CHRONIC HYPERTENSION	WITH CHRONIC HYPERTENSION	WITHOUT CHRONIC HYPERTENSION	WITH CHRONIC HYPERTENSION	WITHOUT CHRONIC HYPERTENSION
FETAL OUTCOMES								
Stillbirth*	4.30 (3.81-4.85)	3.05 (2.88-3.23)	7.29 (5.59-9.52)	1.74 (1.51-2.02)	7.42 (5.37-10.25)	2.74 (2.35-3.20)	1.86 (1.48-2.33)	0.98 (0.92-1.05)
Poor fetal growth*	2.66 (2.40-2.94)	1.20 (1.14-1.27)	7.94 (6.67-9.44)	2.29 (2.12-2.49)	7.99 (6.44-9.91)	3.87 (3.55-4.22)	3.59 (3.20-4.02)	1.29 (1.25-1.34)
Spontaneous delivery <37 wk gestation*	4.88 (4.63-5.15)	2.90 (2.83-2.98)	8.60 (7.64-9.67)	2.25 (2.15-2.35)	7.19 (6.22-8.30)	3.15 (2.98-3.33)	3.24 (3.02-3.48)	1.24 (1.21-1.27)
MATERNAL OUTCOMES								
Preeclampsia*	13.96 (13.29-14.66)	3.80 (3.69-3.91)	27.87 (24.85-31.25)	3.28 (3.10-3.47)	17.41 (15.09-20.09)	2.96 (2.76-3.18)	9.74 (9.15-10.35)	1.38 (1.35-1.42)
Stroke/cerebrovascular complications*	7.14 (4.90-10.40)	1.85 (1.41-2.44)	13.73 (6.63-28.44)	3.52 (2.34-5.31)	23.00 (11.47-46.14)	7.60 (5.26-10.97)	3.87 (2.07-7.23)	1.58 (1.29-1.94)
Acute renal failure*	35.41 (28.39-44.16)	4.43 (3.57-5.48)	253.4 (199.5-321.9)	62.40 (54.37-71.63)	191.5 (141.4-259.4)	12.60 (8.88-17.88)	14.17 (9.65-20.82)	1.27 (0.97-1.65)
Pulmonary edema*	11.97 (7.86-18.24)	4.01 (3.07-5.25)	23.29 (10.32-52.56)	9.06 (5.84-14.06)	15.52 (4.92-48.95)	6.08 (3.46-10.69)	9.85 (5.64-17.19)	1.54 (1.16-2.05)
Ventilation*	11.87 (9.22-15.26)	3.34 (2.80-4.00)	19.29 (11.36-32.76)	8.25 (6.43-10.60)	26.20 (15.04-45.63)	11.09 (8.46-14.52)	5.71 (3.69-8.86)	1.84 (1.55-2.18)
Cesarean delivery†	5.75 (5.46-6.05)	3.33 (3.26-3.41)	5.73 (5.03-6.53)	1.74 (1.68-1.81)	4.38 (3.74-5.12)	1.89 (1.80-1.98)	3.16 (2.97-3.36)	1.27 (1.25-1.29)
Length of stay >6 days‡	14.74 (13.68-15.89)	5.34 (5.09-5.60)	42.16 (36.78-48.32)	6.52 (6.12-6.95)	30.29 (25.45-36.04)	6.18 (5.69-6.71)	8.40 (7.60-9.28)	1.77 (1.71-1.84)
In-hospital mortality*	6.02 (2.71-13.40)	2.58 (1.59-4.17)	27.02 (8.72-83.73)	6.88 (3.56-13.29)	88.81 (41.90-188.2)	23.81 (14.67-38.66)	1.74 (0.24-12.40)	1.72 (1.06-2.77)

For each analysis, reference group was delivery admissions without chronic hypertension and without comorbidity of interest. Admissions with chronic hypertension but without comorbidity of interest were included as a group in each analysis. Because of similarity of estimates of association in these groups to those obtained when analyzing effect of overall chronic hypertension, results are not shown.

*Adjusted for multiple birth, year of study, insurance status, region, and age.

†Adjusted for previous cesarean delivery, multiple birth, year of study, insurance status, region, and age.

‡Adjusted for disposition status, admission status, multiple birth, year of study, insurance status, region, and age.

From Bateman BT, Bansil P, Hernandez-Diaz S, et al. Prevalence, trends, and outcomes of chronic hypertension: a nationwide sample of delivery admissions. *Am J Obstet Gynecol* 2012;206:134.e1-134.e8, 2012.

to movement) once or twice a week after 32 weeks, and consideration of Doppler flow velocimetry are recommended.

Most antihypertensives are safe for breast-feeding, which should be encouraged. Hydrochlorothiazide, α-methyldopa, nifedipine, acebutolol, and metoprolol are all approved by the American Academy of Pediatricians. There is no evidence that hydrochlorothiazides affect milk volume. There is evidence that propranolol and atenolol are concentrated in breast milk, so they should be avoided. Enalapril and captopril are the preferred ACE inhibitors in breast-feeding women, but it may be prudent to delay ACE inhibitors for the first few weeks of the baby's life and for mothers of premature babies, given the adverse pregnancy data.

PROGNOSIS

Hypertension may increase the risk for placental abruption, intrauterine growth restriction (IUGR), and low-birthweight babies. The major risk, however, is its contribution to the risk for preeclampsia and the associated increase in perinatal morbidity and mortality. In addition, chronic hypertension in patients with other comorbidities, including diabetes, renal disease, collagen vascular disease, and thyroid disorders, significantly increases the risk for maternal and fetal complications (see Table 226-5).

Women who develop hypertension during pregnancy are at increased lifetime risk for the development of chronic hypertension, even if the BP normalizes postpartum.

⬤ PREECLAMPSIA

DEFINITION

Preeclampsia is a multisystem disorder, previously defined as hypertension and proteinuria. Based on the observation that preeclampsia often presented in the absence of proteinuria, the definition was revised in 2013. It is now defined as BP of 140/90 mm Hg or higher, accompanied by the abnormalities listed in the section on "Diagnosis" later. When it is diagnosed in a patient with preexisting chronic hypertension, it is referred to as chronic hypertension with superimposed preeclampsia.

A urine protein-creatinine ratio of at least 0.3 may be used instead of a 24-hour urine, which was previously required to demonstrate proteinuria. Edema and hyperreflexia are no longer considered diagnostic criteria, and the 30-mm Hg increase in systolic pressure or 15-mm Hg increase in diastolic pressure has been dropped from the criteria for hypertension. Severe preeclampsia is defined as the presence of one of the following symptoms or signs with preeclampsia: systolic BP of 160 mm Hg or higher, or diastolic BP of 110 mm Hg or higher; pulmonary edema; oliguria (<400 mL in 24 hours); persistent headaches; epigastric pain or impaired liver function; thrombocytopenia; or intrauterine growth restriction (IUGR).

EPIDEMIOLOGY

Preeclampsia complicates 6 to 8% of pregnancies worldwide. Preeclampsia/eclampsia is a leading cause of maternal mortality in the developing world and continues to contribute to maternal mortality in the United States despite the availability of antihypertensives and antiseizure medications. In the United States, preeclampsia is believed to be responsible for 15% of premature deliveries and 17.6% of maternal deaths. Worldwide, preeclampsia and eclampsia are estimated to be responsible for approximately 14% of maternal deaths per year (50,000 to 75,000).

Primigravida and multigravida women with new partners are at increased risk, suggesting a role for paternal antigens. Additional risk factors include prior history of preeclampsia, black race, diabetes or insulin resistance, obesity, systemic lupus erythematosus (SLE), especially in the presence of antiphospholipid antibodies, renal disease, hypertension, thrombophilia, obesity, molar pregnancy, multiple gestation, and extremes of age (younger than 20 years or older than 40 years). Gestational hypertension or preeclampsia is also more likely in kidney donors than in matched nondonors.[2]

PATHOBIOLOGY

Preeclampsia is a disorder of abnormal placentation that begins early in gestation, well before its manifestations are clinically apparent. Some data suggest an association with the fetal apoprotein L1 level.[3] In normal pregnancy, uterine spiral arteries undergo remodeling when they are invaded by fetal cytotrophoblastic cells, resulting in an adhesion receptor switch from cells with characteristics of epithelial cells to cells with the phenotype of endothelial cells.

This leads to the transformation of previously narrow, high-resistance maternal uterine blood vessels into dilated, high-capacitance blood vessels. The proximal portions of the spiral arteries are further dilated by the hormonal effects of estrogen and progesterone, resulting in an overall increase in uterine blood flow from 45 mL/minute during menstruation to 750 mL/minute at term. In preeclampsia, this cell switching does not occur, and the fetal cells' only superficial invasion into maternal vasculature results in limited placental perfusion. As the pregnancy progresses, abnormal placentation produces relative hypoxia and ischemia because this compromised uterine blood flow cannot keep up with the growing demands of the fetus and the placenta. The result is diffuse endothelial dysfunction that is manifested as the clinical syndrome of preeclampsia (Fig. 226-2). With severe preeclampsia, both right and left ventricular dysfunction may occur.[4]

DIAGNOSIS

The diagnosis of preeclampsia depends on a BP of 140/90 mm Hg or higher, accompanied by proteinuria of more than 300 mg/24 hours, platelet count of <100,000, creatinine >1.1 or doubling of baseline, liver function test abnormality more than two times the upper limit of normal, pulmonary edema, or new-onset cerebral or visual disturbance after the 20th week of gestation in a previously normotensive patient. Eclampsia is diagnosed when a patient with preeclampsia has a seizure. The HELLP syndrome (hemolysis, elevated liver enzymes, and low platelets) (Chapter 163) is likely to be a more severe form of preeclampsia. The diagnosis of severe preeclampsia depends on the criteria previously listed.

Diagnostic evaluation should include a careful history, asking about headache, visual complaints, epigastric pain, weight gain, and edema and reviewing the presence of risk factors. The physical examination should include a careful neurologic examination, looking for funduscopic changes (retinal vasospasm, edema, or hemorrhage) or hyperreflexia, and examination for any focal findings suggestive of mass effect, hepatic tenderness, and edema. Laboratory testing for preeclampsia includes a complete blood count, platelet count, urine protein-creatinine ratio or 24-hour urine protein, liver function tests, creatinine concentration, and uric acid level. Additional evaluation includes fetal testing and close maternal monitoring for life-threatening consequences, such as severe hypertension, seizures, pulmonary edema, cerebral hemorrhage, hepatic infarction or rupture, disseminated intravascular coagulation, and renal failure.

Currently, diagnosis depends on development of the full clinical syndrome, but earlier diagnosis may be possible on the basis of biomarkers. It is likely that a combined model that looks at soluble endoglin, soluble filmlike tyrosine kinase 1, pregnancy-associated plasma protein A, ADAM12, and placental growth factor concentrations will be a better prediction instrument before 20 weeks' gestation than any individual marker. A ratio of 38 or lower for soluble FMS-like tyrosine kinase 1 to placental growth factor accurately predicts the short-term absence of preeclampsia in women in whom the syndrome is suspected clinically.[5]

The differential diagnosis of each individual manifestation of preeclampsia is broad, so the diagnosis centers on the constellation of signs and symptoms that suggest preeclampsia. The clinical conditions that can mimic preeclampsia include SLE with nephritis (Chapter 250), thrombotic thrombocytopenic purpura, and hemolytic-uremic syndrome (Chapter 163). Differentiation of preeclampsia from a flare of SLE with nephritis (Chapter 250) is difficult because both can cause hypertension, proteinuria, thrombocytopenia, and rises in serum creatinine concentration. The differential diagnostic features that favor SLE include falling serum complement levels, rising anti-DNA antibodies, and extrarenal manifestations of SLE such as rash and arthralgias. The proteinuria and hypertension in preeclampsia are more likely to be of sudden onset.

TREATMENT   Rx

The only known treatment of preeclampsia is delivery as soon as it is obstetrically feasible. Outcomes are better with immediate delivery after 36 weeks of gestation, but expectant care may be preferred between 24 to 36 weeks of gestation.[A2] Nevertheless, preeclampsia can be manifested postpartum, and both preeclampsia and eclampsia have been reported up to 21 days after delivery. Management of preeclampsia includes treatment of hypertension, seizure prophylaxis, and limitation of fluids because of the risk for pulmonary

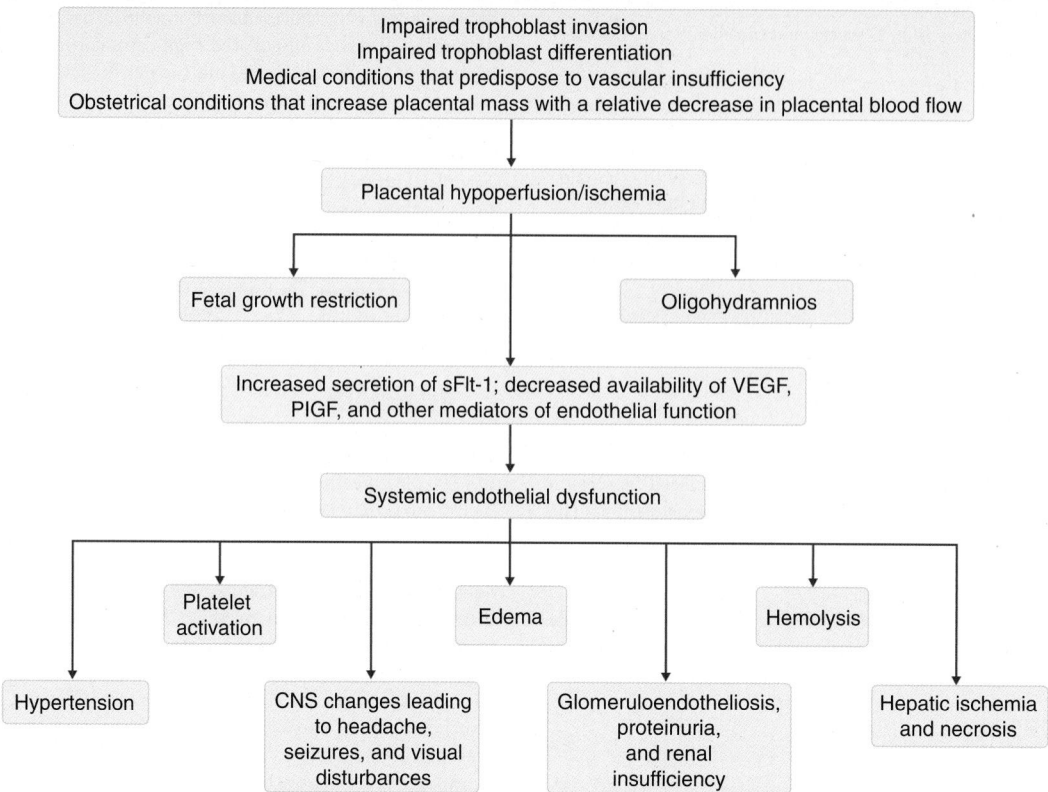

FIGURE 226-2. Model for the pathogenesis of preeclampsia. CNS = central nervous system; PIGF = placental growth factor; sFlt-1= soluble film-like tyrosine kinase; VEGF = vascular endothelial growth factor. (From Rosene-Montella K, Keely EJ, Lee RV, Barbour LA, eds. *Medical Care of the Pregnant Patient.* 2nd ed. Philadelphia: ACP Press/American College of Physicians; 2008.)

edema.[6] Treatment of severe hypertension in preeclampsia is reviewed in Table 226-6. Magnesium sulfate is recommended as first-line treatment of eclampsia as well as for prophylaxis against eclampsia in women with severe and nonsevere preeclampsia.[A3] Phenytoin and benzodiazepines should not be used for eclampsia prophylaxis or treatment unless there is a contraindication to magnesium sulfate or it is ineffective. There is evidence from two randomized controlled trials that magnesium is superior to phenytoin for the prevention of both primary seizures and recurrent seizures in eclampsia.

Treatment of acute seizures in eclampsia includes airway protection, fetal monitoring, magnesium, BP control, and benzodiazepines as needed to stop seizures acutely. Treatment of severe hypertension is as outlined in Table 226-6.

Severe maternal manifestations of preeclampsia that may warrant early delivery include seizure, renal failure, severe hypertension, severe thrombocytopenia or hemolysis, aspartate transaminase or alanine transaminase elevation of more than two to three times normal, pulmonary edema, retinal hemorrhage, and other symptoms suggestive of end-organ damage (headache, visual disturbance, epigastric or right upper quadrant pain). Fetal indications for delivery may include significant IUGR, oligohydramnios, and nonreassuring fetal testing. Women with preeclampsia before 34 weeks' gestation should receive a corticosteroid that crosses the placenta, such as betamethasone or dexamethasone, to accelerate fetal lung maturation.

PREVENTION

Multiple trials of antihypertensives, antioxidant supplementation with vitamins C and E, magnesium, protein or salt restriction, fish oil, and other dietary changes have failed to prevent preeclampsia. Low-dose aspirin in high-risk populations is the only intervention with data to support a positive effect. Low-dose aspirin (<100 mg/day) decreases both the risk for preeclampsia and fetal and neonatal deaths[A4][A5] and is preferred in all patients with risk factors for preeclampsia. Trials of calcium supplementation have shown conflicting results, but given the inverse relationship between dietary calcium intake and BP in the general population, calcium supplementation of at least 1 g/day is recommended for women with a low dietary intake of calcium (<600 mg/day). An alternative to supplementation may be to increase dietary calcium by eating three or four servings per day of dairy products (assuming 250 to 300 mg of calcium per serving).

TABLE 226-6   TREATMENT OF SEVERE HYPERTENSION IN PREECLAMPTIC PATIENTS

MEDICATION	ONSET AND DURATION OF ACTION	ACUTE DOSING FOR SEVERE HYPERTENSION	MAINTENANCE DOSE
Labetalol	Begins to work in 5-10 min Lasts 3-6 hr	Given as a series of boluses until BP reaches the desired level: 10 mg IV push; then in 10 min, 20 mg IV push; then in 10 min, 40 mg IV push; then in 10 min, 80 mg IV push; then in 10 min, 80 mg IV push, up to a total dose of no more than 300 mg Follow with PO labetalol or labetalol drip	100-200 mg PO bid-tid (100-600 mg bid-tid; maximum 2400 mg/day) IV infusion 0.5-2.0 mg/min (labetalol comes in vials of 100 mg/20 mL) Put 5 vials (100 mL) labetalol into 150 mL IV fluid (D₅W, LR, or NS) to get a solution of 2 mg/mL; start at 15 mL/hr (0.5 mg/min); titrate up to as high as 60 mL/hr (2 mg/min)
Nifedipine	Begins to work in <30 min Lasts 4-5 hr	10-20 mg PO q30min to a maximum of 50 mg	10-20 mg PO tid of short-acting nifedipine or 30-120 mg once daily of long-acting formulation
Hydralazine	Begins to work in 10-20 min Lasts for 3-6 hr	2.5-10 mg IV q30min	Start at 10 mg PO qid; can be gradually increased to 50 mg PO qid

BP = blood pressure; D₅W= dextrose 5% in water (solution); LR = lactated Ringer (solution); NS = normal saline.
From Rosene-Montella K, Keely EJ, Lee RV, Barbour LA, eds. *Medical Care of the Pregnant Patient.* 2nd ed. Philadelphia: ACP Press/American College of Physicians; 2008.

PROGNOSIS

Women who have had preeclampsia are at increased risk for heart disease, stroke, and cardiovascular death. Preeclampsia is also a marker for increased risk for end-stage renal disease. One year after delivery, preeclampsia patients observed longitudinally have been shown to have evidence of increased insulin resistance, BP, cholesterol, and triglycerides, which may be the first manifestations of the metabolic syndrome. In one study, the 10-year, 30-year, and lifetime risks for development of cardiovascular disease compared with women who did not have preeclampsia were 18.2% versus 1.7%, 31.3% versus 5.1%, and 41.4% versus 17.8% in matched controls, respectively. It is unclear whether there is a shared pathogenesis, an unmasking of already established disease, or a contribution to the development of disease. It is possible that preexisting abnormal endothelial function predisposes to renal and vascular disease later in life and is, in fact, the same abnormality that disturbs implantation, resulting in preeclampsia and fetal loss. It is also possible that preeclampsia itself contributes to the later development of disease.

Continuing care beyond 6 weeks postpartum is strongly recommended. Women with a history of severe preeclampsia should be screened for preexisting hypertension, underlying renal disease, thrombophilia, and possibly secondary causes of hypertension. They should also be informed of the risk for preeclampsia in subsequent pregnancies, particularly if the birth interval is less than 2 years or more than 10 years. Women who are overweight should be advised to normalize their body mass index before another pregnancy and to reduce long-term risk. Both women with preexisting hypertension and those whose BP normalizes are likely to benefit from an overall assessment of cardiovascular risk that includes a lipid profile, smoking cessation, and early interventions to reduce risk.

● DEEP VENOUS THROMBOSIS, PULMONARY EMBOLISM, AND THROMBOPHILIA

Pulmonary embolism (PE) is one of the leading medical cause of maternal mortality in the developed world. It was responsible for 30% of direct maternal deaths in the most recent U.K. Confidential Enquiry. Despite our best efforts, mortality rates from PE in pregnancy have not changed in more than two decades, and the incidence of PE in the United States is rising, likely owing to the increase in obesity and cesarean deliveries. Current strategies to reduce risk from PE must address the widespread use of appropriate prophylaxis, early detection of venous thromboembolism (VTE), and prompt, safe, and effective therapy (Chapters 73 and 74).

EPIDEMIOLOGY

More than half of the VTE events in women younger than 40 years occur in association with pregnancy. VTE is 10 times more common in pregnant than in nonpregnant women of comparable age. It occurs in 5 to 12 of 10,000 pregnancies antepartum and in 3 to 7 of 10,000 postpartum. The risk for VTE with pregnancy is increased by the presence of additional risk factors, including prolonged bedrest, cesarean section, preeclampsia, three or more children, smoking, obesity, previous superficial thrombophlebitis, previous VTE, thrombophilia, and family history of VTE.

PATHOBIOLOGY

Pregnancy is a hypercoagulable state (Chapter 73) characterized by venous stasis, maternal prothrombotic imbalance in which activation of the coagulation system exceeds the fibrinolytic response progressively through the course of pregnancy, and endothelial disruption. Venous stasis occurs as a result of progesterone-induced venodilation early in pregnancy and is later increased by the compressive effects of the gravid uterus. Compression of the left common iliac vein by the right common iliac artery (May-Thurner syndrome, a congenital anomaly that has been noted in 20% of the general adult population)[7] further increases venous stasis on the left, which may explain the finding that more than 90% of cases of deep vein thrombosis (DVT) in pregnancy occur in the left leg. Endothelial damage occurs with preeclampsia and with both vaginal and operative delivery, further contributing to VTE risk.

Genetic and Acquired Thrombophilias

A positive family history for VTE (possibly a marker for thrombophilia) or a known thrombophilia significantly increases the risk for VTE in pregnancy (Chapter 73). The best-described genetic thrombophilias include deficiencies in protein C, protein S, and antithrombin III, all of which appear to have autosomal dominant inheritance with variable penetrance, and the presence of the single-gene mutations factor V Leiden and prothrombin G202010. Of these, antithrombin-deficient homozygotes (rare) and compound heterozygotes have the highest risk for VTE in pregnancy. The thrombophilias have also been associated with obstetric complications in some studies, including IUGR, abruption, both early and late pregnancy loss, and preeclampsia (early, severe, or recurrent). The antiphospholipid antibody syndrome is the major acquired thrombophilia for which there are compelling pregnancy data supporting a link with both thrombosis risk and obstetric complications. The most recent American College of Obstetricians and Gynecologists technical bulletin and the American College of Chest Physicians guidelines recommend against prophylaxis for prevention of adverse pregnancy outcome in patients with thrombophilias other than the antiphospholipid antibody syndrome.

DIAGNOSIS

The diagnosis of VTE during pregnancy is complicated by both normal pregnancy-related physiologic changes and the reluctance to use diagnostic imaging in pregnancy.[8] Clinical signs are unreliable, and leg swelling and complaints of dyspnea are common during pregnancy, making it difficult to decide when to investigate for VTE. The finding that 90% of DVT occurs in the left leg led to the observation that the combination of symptoms in the left leg, calf circumference difference of 2 cm or more, and first-trimester presentation (when leg swelling is less likely) is highly predictive of DVT. Most DVTs occur antepartum, and events are evenly distributed throughout gestation. The majority of fatal PEs in most studies occurred in the postpartum period, so vigilance is required for a prolonged period after delivery. Diagnosis of DVT requires compression ultrasonography that includes the iliac veins and the inferior vena cava at the level of the liver (Chapter 74). It also requires repeated compression ultrasonography if study findings are normal but there is high pretest probability and continuing symptoms. In patients with suspected iliac or pelvic vein thrombosis and normal findings on ultrasound studies, magnetic resonance imaging or magnetic resonance venography is recommended.

The diagnosis of PE is even more of a problem, given the frequency of dyspnea, the likelihood of normal oxygenation in young patients with no underlying cardiopulmonary disease, and the more invasive nature of diagnostic testing. Arterial blood gas analysis is not helpful; the A-a gradient was normal in 60% of pregnant patients with documented PE in a retrospective review done at two centers.

The radiation exposure from imaging required for the diagnosis of PE is well below that allowed by the National Commission on Radiation Protection (see Table 226-3), so testing should never be withheld out of concern for fetal exposure. Ventilation-perfusion (V/Q) scanning is still the diagnostic test of choice in most centers outside the United States. It is better validated in pregnancy, involves no administration of contrast material, and has good negative predictive value in normal scans and in low-probability scans when it is paired with leg studies. If V/Q is used, it must be understood that there is still a significant risk for PE in patients with scans interpreted to be "intermediate" and "indeterminate," so additional testing is required in those cases. Computed tomography angiography has replaced V/Q scanning in most U.S. centers on the basis of its use in the nonpregnant population. The technique is dependent on cardiac output and plasma volume, both of which are increased during pregnancy. This may lead to poor opacification of the vessels, causing artifacts to be read as filling defects or the failure to visualize clots, so the technique must be adjusted for pregnancy. It is a sensitive, cost-effective test that offers an alternative diagnosis in 25 to 40% of cases, and it is preferred if there is an abnormality on the chest radiograph. It is well tolerated and has a shorter breath-holding time than V/Q scans, so it is also preferred in unstable patients, especially if an alternative diagnosis is suspected. Computed tomography angiography exposes the maternal breast to 2 to 3.5 rad, and exposure of the breast to 1 rad increases the lifetime risk of breast cancer by 13%. The use of breast shields decreases this exposure by about 50% without compromising the integrity of the test, so breast shields are strongly recommended.

The role of D-dimer testing in pregnancy has not yet been elucidated because D-dimer is elevated during normal pregnancy. It may have some use for its negative predictive value, but studies are inadequate to recommend its use at this time.

TREATMENT ℞

The safety of unfractionated heparin (UFH) and low-molecular-weight heparin (LMWH) (Chapter 76) for the fetus is well established, however LMWH is now the drug of choice for both the treatment and the prevention of VTE.[9] Warfarin is a teratogen that crosses the placenta and has been associated with fetal bleeding and central nervous system abnormalities later in gestation, so it is not used for this indication in pregnancy. Initial treatment of VTE in the pregnant patient is either intravenous UFH, followed by subcutaneous UFH or LMWH, or an initial adjusted dose of LMWH that is then continued; both are acceptable.

LMWH causes a much lower incidence of heparin-induced thrombocytopenia than UFH (Chapter 163) and also less osteoporosis, so, given the prolonged exposure during pregnancy, it is the preferred agent. The 2012 American College of Chest Physicians consensus guidelines recommend LMWH as the preferred agent in pregnancy. The same consensus conference suggests limiting the use of fondaparinux and parenteral direct thrombin inhibitors to patients with severe allergic reactions to heparin (e.g., heparin-induced thrombocytopenia) who cannot receive danaparoid. The use of direct oral anticoagulants (against factor Xa or thrombin) is not recommended (Table 226-7). LMWH has increased bioavailability, but the ease of administration in pregnancy is mitigated by the need for twice-daily dosing and frequent monitoring. Dosing requirements increase with increasing gestation, so it is necessary to follow anti-Xa levels. Because LMWH has limited reversibility with protamine and because it has been associated with epidural hematomas in nonpregnant patients given spinal or epidural anesthesia, some centers recommend a switch to UFH by 34 to 36 weeks, although recent guidelines do not support this change. This allows patients the option of epidural anesthesia for delivery, and in the event of an emergent delivery before holding of anticoagulation, UFH can be reversed with protamine. Specific treatment recommendations are outlined in Table 226-8.

PREVENTION

The overall recurrence risk for VTE during pregnancy ranges from 5 to 20%, depending in part on the circumstances of the index clot. The highest risk patients for recurrence include patients with a previous idiopathic VTE (while not pregnant) or a secondary VTE that occurred during a previous pregnancy or while taking oral contraceptives and patients with a positive history of thrombophilia or a family history of thrombophilia. The thrombophilias with the highest recurrence risk are the antiphospholipid antibody syndrome and homozygosity or compound heterozygosity with more than one mutation and antithrombin deficiency.

Unfortunately, randomized trials of *antepartum* prophylaxis with LMWH have found no reduction in VTE, pregnancy loss, or placenta-mediated pregnancy complications in women with thrombophilia and at high risk for these complications[A6]; furthermore, it was associated with an increased risk for minor bleeding.[A7] However, patients with the antiphospholipid syndrome and a prior pregnancy loss have not been well studied and still are recommended for antepartum prophylaxis.

The American College of Chest Physicians consensus guidelines (see Table 226-8) suggest surveillance with postpartum thromboprophylaxis in patients without a family history of thrombophilia in whom the previous VTE occurred in association with a transient risk factor other than pregnancy or oral contraceptive use. Antepartum prophylaxis is recommended by most U.S. centers in patients with prior idiopathic or estrogen-related DVT and patients with high-risk thrombophilias. When prophylaxis is instituted, it should be continued for at least 6 to 8 weeks postpartum, when the hemostatic changes of pregnancy return to prepregnant values. Additional groups that should be considered for thromboprophylaxis are patients who have undergone cesarean section, particularly if they have an additional risk factor for VTE, and patients on prolonged bedrest. Patients receiving continued prophylactic or treatment doses postpartum have the option of switching to warfarin, which is also safe in breast-feeding women.

PROGNOSIS

VTE during pregnancy may be the first manifestation of a hypercoagulable state because pregnancy acts as a "stress test" for thrombophilia. Fifty percent of initial episodes of VTE in women younger than 40 years are manifested in association with pregnancy. A thrombophilia evaluation is indicated in all patients who present with VTE during pregnancy to assess long-term maternal and family risk and to guide future secondary prophylaxis recommendations. Patients with an identified thrombophilia and an adverse pregnancy outcome may be at risk for a similar outcome in a subsequent pregnancy and should be counseled about this risk and considered for thromboprophylaxis. Patients who have had DVT during pregnancy have a high risk for post-phlebitic syndrome and venous insufficiency. Two randomized controlled

trials demonstrated a 50% risk reduction in symptoms of postthrombotic syndrome when compression stockings were used within 1 month of diagnosis and continued for a minimum of 1 year after diagnosis.

ASTHMA

Maintaining adequate control of asthma during pregnancy is important for both maternal and fetal outcome. Asthma may be associated with increased perinatal mortality, preterm birth, IUGR, gestational diabetes, and preeclampsia. Well-controlled asthma reduces the likelihood of these adverse outcomes to baseline, so it is safer for both mother and fetus to treat maternal asthma than to allow exacerbations to occur (Chapter 81).

EPIDEMIOLOGY

Asthma is the most common respiratory disease in pregnancy. It affects 3.7 to 8.4% of pregnancies in the United States and 12 to 13% of pregnancies in Australia and the United Kingdom. Approximately 10% of U.S. women of reproductive age have asthma, and the rates of asthma reported during labor and delivery have doubled during the past decade.

Effect of Pregnancy on Asthma

The course of asthma in pregnancy is unpredictable, and most studies have found that one third of patients improve, one third worsen, and one third stay the same. The most likely predictor in any individual patient is her course during a previous pregnancy. In most studies, the majority of exacerbations occurred between 17 and 32 weeks, with some improvement reported by 36 weeks' gestation. Patients with mild asthma do well during labor and delivery, but almost 50% of patients with severe asthma worsen during labor and delivery. Risk factors for exacerbations include severe asthma, poor compliance with medications (especially inhaled corticosteroids), obesity, viral infections, rhinitis, gastroesophageal reflux, and poor prenatal care. The highest morbidity and mortality rates are reported in African American patients.

Effect of Asthma on Pregnancy

Pregnancy and perinatal outcome are improved when asthma is well controlled. Poorly controlled asthma increases the risk for spontaneous abortion, low birthweight, IUGR, and cesarean section. Preterm delivery, gestational diabetes, and preeclampsia have also been associated with poorly controlled asthma, but it is unclear how systemic steroids contribute to these complications. Systemic steroids have been associated with an increased risk for premature rupture of membranes, preeclampsia, prematurity and low birthweight, and gestational diabetes. A retrospective study suggested that some complications may increase even in patients with mild asthma or asthma in good control.

PATHOBIOLOGY

The normal physiologic changes of pregnancy may contribute to variations in asthma severity. Factors contributing to the worsening of asthma include gastroesophageal reflux disease and rhinitis or sinusitis, triggers for asthma that are common during pregnancy. Gastroesophageal reflux may be manifested initially during pregnancy or worsen in patients with preexisting reflux owing to both hormonal and mechanical effects. Progesterone acts as a smooth muscle dilator that reduces lower esophageal sphincter pressure and contributes to delayed gastric emptying. Later in gestation, uterine enlargement further contributes to gastric displacement and increased reflux. Rhinitis and sinusitis clearly contribute to asthma exacerbations in nonpregnant patients. Gestational rhinitis related to hormonal effects is present in most pregnant women, and its behavior seems to parallel that of asthma. Bacterial sinusitis is five to six times more common in pregnancy and should be treated aggressively.

Hormonal effects on the airway may also contribute to asthma status. There is a progressive increase in serum cortisol and estradiol, which affects the quality of mucus production, and in progesterone, which decreases smooth muscle contractility and thereby causes airway dilation and improves minute ventilation. Immunologic factors during normal pregnancy may also contribute to the course of asthma. There is a suppression of cell-mediated immunity, with a predominant T_H2 environment and high interleukin-5 and tumor necrosis factor messenger RNA. In pregnant women with asthma (not receiving inhaled corticosteroid therapy), the T_H2/T_H1 ratio is even higher, possibly contributing to exacerbations.

The mechanism by which asthma exacerbations affect perinatal outcome is probably related to chronic maternal hypoxia, with consequent placental

TABLE 226-7 SAFETY AND PHARMACOKINETICS OF ANTICOAGULANTS IN PREGNANCY

	UFH	LMWH	SEMISYNTHETIC HEPARINOIDS (DANAPAROID)	SYNTHETIC HEPARINS AND FACTOR Xa INHIBITOR (FONDAPARINUX, RIVAROXABAN)	THROMBIN INHIBITORS (RECOMBINANT HIRUDINS)	THROMBIN INHIBITORS (ARGATROBAN, DABIGATRAN)	WARFARIN (COUMADIN)
Monitoring	aPTT	Anti-Xa level	Anti-Xa level	Anti-Xa level	aPTT	aPTT	INR
Half-life	1.5 hr	Enoxaparin: 4.5-7 hr; Tinzaparin: 3-4 hr; Dalteparin: 3-5 hr; All prolonged in renal impairment	24 hr; Prolonged in severe renal impairment	17-21 hr; Prolonged in severe renal impairment	Lepirudin: 1.3 hr; Bivalirudin: 25 min; Desirudin: 2 hr; All prolonged in renal impairment	Argatroban: 39-51 min; Dabigatran: 12-17 hr	20-60 hr
Clearance	Liver, reticuloendothelial system	Liver 40% urine excretion	Plasma; Urine excretion	Metabolism unknown; Urine excretion	Lepirudin: metabolism unknown; 48% urine excretion; Bivalirudin: plasma (80%); urine (20%) excretion; Desirudin: kidney	Argatroban: liver; urine and fecal excretion; Dabigatran: liver; urine excretion	Liver 92% urine excretion
Safety	Does not cross the placenta; No known risk for teratogenicity	Enoxaparin, tinzaparin, and dalteparin: do not appear to cross the placenta and are not believed to increase risk for birth defects on the basis of animal studies and some human studies outcomes.	No longer available in the United States. Many case reports of use of danaparoid in pregnancy in various doses and duration have shown successful pregnancy outcomes.	Fondaparinux: on the basis of experimental animal studies, use of fondaparinux in pregnancy is not expected to increase the risk for malformations. Small amounts cross the placenta, but clinical significance of such is unknown. Recommended only if severe allergic reaction to LMWH in patients who cannot receive danaparoid. Rivaroxaban: postimplantation pregnancy loss, increased fetal toxicity, and maternal hemorrhagic complications have been observed in animal studies. There are no adequate and well-controlled human studies.	Lepirudin: on the basis of experimental animal studies, it is not expected to increase the risk for congenital malformations, although it is known to cross rat placenta. Case reports of its use during various times of pregnancy did not show adverse events in exposed neonates. Bivalirudin: no epidemiologic studies of congenital anomalies among infants born to women treated with bivalirudin during pregnancy have been reported. Desirudin: teratogenic effects were observed in some animal reproductive studies.	Argatroban: did not produce malformations in rats and rabbits, but dosing was low compared with human therapeutic dose levels. Few case reports describing its use during pregnancy with no adverse newborn outcomes. Not recommended for use in pregnancy. Dabigatran: adverse events were observed in some animal reproductive studies. There are no adequate and well-controlled studies in pregnant women. Not recommended for use in pregnancy.	Warfarin crosses the placental barrier. Risk for birth defect with early exposure; potential for fatal hemorrhage to the fetus in utero. Not recommended for use in pregnancy.
Lactation	Safe	Enoxaparin: excretions in milk unknown; Tinzaparin, dalteparin: no data available	Little or no danaparoid appears in breast milk and would likely be inactivated in infant's stomach	Fondaparinux: appears in rat milk. Possible adverse effects of exposure through milk have not been described. Rivaroxaban: no data available	Lepirudin: in one case report, it was used during lactation without adverse events. It was not detectable in milk. Bivalirudin and desirudin: no data available	Argatroban, dabigatran: no data available	Safe
Administration	SC and IV	SC and IV	SC and IV	Fondaparinux: IV; Rivaroxaban: PO	IV	Argatroban: IV; Dabigatran PO	PO

aPTT = activated partial thromboplastin time; INR = international normalized ratio; LMWH = low-molecular-weight heparin; UFH = unfractionated heparin.
From Mazer J, Zouein J, Bourjeily G. Treatment of pulmonary embolism in pregnancy. *US Respir Dis.* 2012;8:30-35.

TABLE 226-8 TREATMENT OF VENOUS THROMBOEMBOLISM IN PREGNANCY: ANTEPARTUM ANTICOAGULATION

| DRUG | PROPHYLAXIS | | AGGRESSIVE PROPHYLAXIS | | FULL TREATMENT |
	First 20 Weeks	20-37 Weeks	First 20 Weeks	20 Weeks to Term	
Dalteparin	5000 U/day	5000 U q12h	100 U/kg/day	100 U/kg/day	100 U/kg q12h or 200 U/kg q24h with anti-Xa monitoring
Enoxaparin	40 mg/day	30-40 mg q12h	1 mg/kg/day	1 mg/kg/day	1 mg/kg q12h with anti-Xa monitoring
Tinzaparin	3500-4500 U/day	3500-4500 U q12h	88 U/kg/day	88 U/kg/day	88 U/kg q12h or 175 IU per kg q24h with anti-Xa monitoring
Heparin	Alternative if LMWH unaffordable: 750 U bid first 20 wk; 10,000 U bid wk 20-37		Alternative if LMWH unaffordable: 10,000 U bid to achieve anti-Xa level of 0.1-0.3 U/mL		Adjusted to mid-interval anti-Xa of 0.35-0.67 with q12h SC injections

LMWH = low-molecular-weight heparin.
Modified from Bourjeily G, Rosene-Montella K, eds. Venous thromboembolism in pregnancy. In: *Pulmonary Problems in Pregnancy, Respiratory Medicine*. New York: Humana Press; 2009.

dysfunction and decreased uteroplacental flow, which contributes to decreased fetal growth. Poorly controlled asthma increases low birthweight 2.5-fold. Relative placental ischemia in asthma, particularly in disease that was poorly controlled before conception, is likely the link to an increased risk for preeclampsia. Placentas from women with asthma show a change in response to vasodilators and constrictors in vitro, similar to that seen in preeclampsia.

DIAGNOSIS

The diagnosis of asthma during pregnancy is the same as in the nonpregnant state (Chapter 81): normal forced expiratory volume in 1 second (FEV_1)/forced vital capacity on baseline pulmonary function tests with an obstructive physiology during exacerbations that is reversible either spontaneously or with medications. Airway hyperresponsiveness, as demonstrated by a methacholine challenge causing a 20% drop in FEV_1 from baseline, is also useful for diagnosis in pregnancy. Asthma severity in pregnancy is classified the same as in nonpregnant patients by the new classification of asthma severity that incorporates short-acting β-agonist use. The new classification includes both the level of impairment (daytime and nighttime frequency, quality of life and interference with normal activities, lung function) and the risk for exacerbations based on frequency and severity of prior exacerbations.

Differential Diagnosis

Dyspnea of pregnancy is a benign condition that often occurs later in pregnancy and is characterized by an increased awareness of the work of breathing that is disturbing for many patients. It is not likely to be acute, occurs less with rest, and should not interfere with normal daily activities. Dyspnea of pregnancy should not be accompanied by an increase in respiratory rate, wheezing, or hypoxia. It is important to consider pulmonary edema in any pregnant patient complaining of shortness of breath (Chapter 53). Pregnancy-related causes of pulmonary edema and acute respiratory distress syndrome include tocolytics (drugs that slow contractions), preeclampsia, gastric aspiration, amniotic fluid embolism, sepsis (related to pyelonephritis, chorioamnionitis, endometritis, septic abortion), abruption, and obstetric hemorrhage. Cardiac causes should be suspected when pulmonary edema is manifested at the peak of blood volume (28 to 32 weeks), when occult valvular disease (Chapter 66) is most likely to be unmasked. Additional cardiac considerations are peripartum cardiomyopathy, preeclampsia, and ischemic heart disease, which in pregnancy may also be caused by coronary dissection.

TREATMENT Rx

Management of asthma during pregnancy does not differ greatly from that of the nonpregnant patient (Chapter 81).[10] However, normal arterial carbon dioxide pressure ($PaCO_2$) in pregnancy is 28 to 32 mm Hg, so a tachypneic pregnant patient with a $PaCO_2$ above this range may be in impending respiratory failure. Minute ventilation in pregnancy increases by an increase in tidal volume, but respiratory rate is unchanged by pregnancy, so tachypnea is always an abnormal finding.

The goal of asthma therapy during pregnancy is to maintain adequate control to ensure maternal and fetal health. It is always safer for pregnant women with asthma to be treated with asthma medications than to experience symptoms and exacerbations.[A8] Careful monitoring during all prenatal visits, preferably with spirometry, and stepped-up therapy are required both for maternal asthma control and to ensure appropriate oxygenation of the fetus. Maternal arterial oxygen saturation should be maintained at 95% or more, or the arterial oxygen pressure (PaO_2) should be maintained at 80 mm Hg or more, to maintain fetal oxygenation. E-Figure 226-1 outlines the classification of asthma and care for pregnant patients with asthma. More detailed recommendations for the home management of exacerbations and for hospitalization and emergency care for pregnant patients can be found in the *National Asthma Education and Prevention Program Working Group Report for Managing Asthma During Pregnancy*.

Albuterol is the preferred short-acting β-agonist because it has an excellent safety profile and the most data related to safety during human pregnancy. Inhaled corticosteroids are the preferred medication for long-term control. Budesonide is the preferred inhaled corticosteroid solely because of the amount of reassuring data on its use in pregnant patients. There are, however, no adverse data on the other inhaled corticosteroids. Data on the effectiveness and safety of long-acting β-agonists during pregnancy are limited, although it is reasonable to assume that they have a safety profile similar to that of albuterol. Salmeterol is the preferred agent, based only on its longer availability and lack of reports of adverse outcomes in exposed pregnancies. Cromolyn has an excellent safety profile but has limited effectiveness compared with inhaled corticosteroids.

Minimal published reports are available on the use of leukotriene receptor antagonists during pregnancy; however, animal safety data are reassuring. Current guidelines do not recommend leukotriene receptor antagonists because of the limited data, unless a patient's asthma was well controlled with this type of drug before pregnancy.

Intranasal corticosteroids are recommended for the treatment of allergic rhinitis, given the limited systemic effect. The current nonsedating antihistamines of choice are loratadine and cetirizine.

Patients at risk for fatal asthma are those with a large bronchodilator response, overreliance on short-acting bronchodilators, marked circadian variation in lung function, history of hospitalization or intubation, and frequent systemic steroid use. There are specific considerations based on pregnancy physiology in pregnant patients who may require airway intubation. Pregnant patients have a low functional residual capacity and oxygen reserve, a more profound response to sedatives, airway edema, and larger airways. Intubation failure is much higher in pregnant women, so intubation should be performed by the most experienced professional available.

Breast-feeding should be encouraged in all patients with asthma because there is some evidence that it decreases atopy in offspring. Data are conflicting regarding the development of asthma in offspring.

● DIABETES

Diabetes affects 1.85 million women of reproductive age, and it is estimated that preconception management could reduce the risk for 113,000 births per year (Chapter 216). All women of reproductive age with diabetes should be counseled about the relationship between glucose control and congenital anomalies. Hyperglycemia is a teratogen, and the incidence of congenital anomalies is directly related to the hemoglobin A_{1c} level at conception (Fig. 226-3). The anomaly rate was as high as 11% in women without preconception care, including cardiac anomalies, neural tube defects, and sacral agenesis. The single most important contribution an internist can make to the prevention of congenital anomalies is to address pregnancy risk with all women of childbearing age with diabetes. The responsibility to normalize hemoglobin A_{1c} before conception falls to the medical care provider; after pregnancy is diagnosed and the patient is seen by her obstetrician, the teratogenic effects of glucose have already occurred.

DEFINITION

Gestational diabetes mellitus (GDM) is defined as glucose intolerance that first occurs or is first identified during pregnancy. Either type 1 or type 2

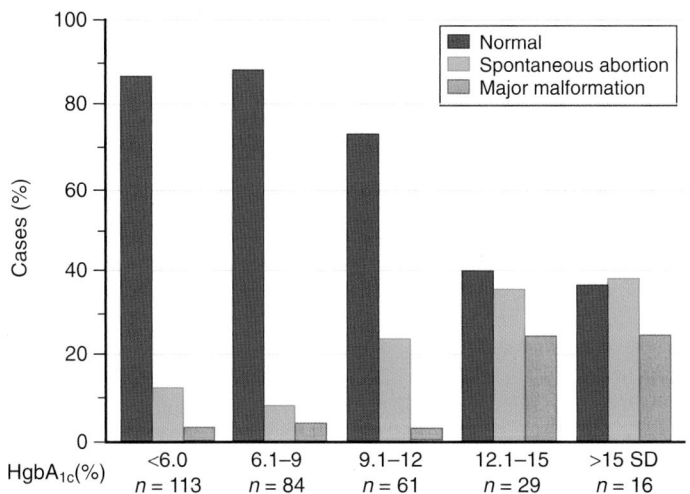

FIGURE 226-3. Relationship of hemoglobin A$_{1c}$ (HgbA$_{1c}$), congenital anomalies, and spontaneous abortion.

diabetes in a pregnant patient is referred to as preexisting or pregestational diabetes.

EPIDEMIOLOGY

The frequency of GDM is rising in the United States; it now occurs in 4 to 14% of all pregnancies, depending on the patient's characteristics. The epidemic of type 2 diabetes has resulted in a higher prevalence at a younger age; in the United States, there has been a 70% increase in the prevalence of diabetes in the 30- to 39-year-old group versus 33% overall. The proportion of women with type 2 versus type 1 pregestational diabetes has also increased, from 26% in 1980 to 65% in 2000, and it is still increasing. The perinatal morbidity and mortality associated with type 2 diabetes is at least as great as that associated with type 1 during pregnancy.

PATHOBIOLOGY

Type 1 diabetes is caused by autoimmune destruction of pancreatic beta cells, resulting in an absolute insulin deficiency. Ninety percent of cases are diagnosed before the age of 25 years and are often associated with other autoimmune illnesses or a family history of autoimmune illness, including thyroid disorders, Addison disease, and celiac disease. Type 2 diabetes is part of the metabolic syndrome, which includes insulin resistance, hyperinsulinemia, dyslipidemia, abdominal obesity, and hypertension with premature atherosclerosis; it probably has a genetic component. GDM may also be a manifestation of the metabolic syndrome, unmasked by the insulin-resistant state of pregnancy. Patients with GDM have a 50% chance for development of type 2 diabetes in the ensuing 5 to 10 years and a long-term risk of approximately 70%.

Pregnancy is a state of accelerated starvation and marked insulin resistance. Lower fasting glucose levels are seen early in the first trimester, and nocturnal hypoglycemia is common. There is blunted hypoglycemic awareness due to decreased epinephrine and norepinephrine release, with falls in blood glucose concentration and increased ketogenesis, resulting in an increased risk for diabetic ketoacidosis. Insulin requirements may decrease 20% in weeks 7 to 12 but then gradually rise later in gestation, such that insulin doses need to be increased by 16 weeks' gestation. Marked insulin resistance is related to the presence of elevated levels of cortisol, prolactin, human placental lactogen, and human placental growth hormone. Insulin sensitivity is decreased by about 50% in the third trimester, resulting in increased serum insulin and postprandial glucose levels, explaining the timing of the onset of GDM.

DIAGNOSIS

The diagnosis of pregestational diabetes is based on the finding of a fasting blood glucose level of more than 125 mg/dL or a 2-hour or random blood glucose level of 200 mg/dL or more. The American Diabetes Association recently added a hemoglobin A$_{1c}$ level of 6.5% or higher as an acceptable alternative diagnostic criterion. GDM is based on the results of a blood glucose screen after a 50-g glucose challenge test (≥140 mg/dL), followed by a 3-hour confirmatory 100-g oral glucose tolerance test. Positive results are any two of the following: fasting, 95 mg/dL or more; 1 hour, 180 mg/dL; 2 hours, 155 mg/dL; and 3 hours, 140 mg/dL. It may be difficult to distinguish between GDM

and type 2 diabetes that was not diagnosed before pregnancy. Elevated fasting glucose levels before 24 weeks' gestation and elevated hemoglobin A$_{1c}$ are both suggestive of type 2 diabetes. Any diabetes diagnosed during pregnancy is referred to as GDM; if it persists postpartum, it is reclassified as type 2.

TREATMENT

Dietary recommendations are for 30 kcal/kg, with 40 to 50% carbohydrates, divided into three meals and three snacks. Aerobic exercise may decrease insulin resistance and reduce maternal glucose levels and may be an effective adjunct to diet in patients with GDM. Adjustment of medications should include the discontinuation of ACE inhibitors, ARBs, and statins and the institution of folate and prenatal vitamins. An assessment of baseline disease status in all patients with diabetes should include hemoglobin A$_{1c}$, ophthalmologic examination, electrocardiogram, assessment of urine protein excretion, serum creatinine concentration, and thyroid-stimulating hormone level. Baseline preeclampsia laboratory studies are also recommended.

The fetal assessment plan includes ultrasound to confirm dates and viability; this is done by the patient's obstetric care provider. There will also be a quad screen (second-trimester prenatal screening), looking for serum markers that suggest neural tube defects or Down syndrome; an ultrasound nuchal translucency and a level 2 ultrasound to assess for congenital anomalies; and a fetal echocardiogram.

Control of Blood Glucose

The goal of treatment for pregestational diabetes is the best hemoglobin A$_{1c}$ level possible, without excessive hypoglycemia.[11] This is achieved by frequent insulin adjustments and self-monitoring of blood glucose level at least four times a day. The specific goals for both GDM and pregestational diabetes are fasting glucose concentration of 65 to 95 mg/dL, 1-hour postprandial glucose concentration of less than 140 mg/dL, and 2-hour glucose concentration of less than 120 mg/dL. This is best achieved by continuous glucose monitoring,[A9] whether by an insulin pump or by using multiple doses of insulin, including basal, intermediate, and long-acting insulin, with preprandial bolus rapid-acting insulin to cover the anticipated carbohydrate load. This regimen requires self-monitoring of blood glucose levels six or seven times a day, so it may be difficult to comply with. Further, the risk for serious hypoglycemia may limit these glycemic targets, particularly in women with type 1 diabetes. Extreme vigilance is required to avoid serious hypoglycemia, particularly in weeks 7 to 12, when insulin requirements are the lowest during pregnancy. In patients with decreased glycemic awareness, the risk for nighttime hypoglycemia is significant, and patients' partners should be counseled about this risk.

Insulin analogues are being used with increasing frequency. Of the rapid-acting analogues, there are data that lispro does not cross the placenta; there are no data yet on aspart. Although long-acting glargine is being used in pregnancy, its placental transfer is unknown, and there are theoretical concerns about its binding to the insulin-like growth factor receptor and its mitogenic potential.

Of the oral agents for which there are data, glyburide is safe and efficacious in women with GDM, and it is more efficacious than metformin in this setting.[A10] Oral agents are less useful with significant insulin resistance and type 2 diabetes, so insulin continues to be the "gold standard" in this group. Metformin does not appear to increase the risk for congenital anomalies or spontaneous abortion, but it does cross the placenta. Women with polycystic ovary syndrome treated with metformin may regain their fertility and should be advised to use contraception. Recent trials support the safety of metformin in the second and third trimesters. In the United States, metformin is not yet recommended for the treatment of type 2 diabetes in pregnancy or for GDM. There are inadequate pregnancy data for the meglitinides and glitazones.

Maternal and Fetal Monitoring

During pregnancy, increased vigilance and continual assessment for the development of complications, including hypertension, preeclampsia, worsening nephropathy, and retinopathy, are required. The incidences of retinopathy in pregnant women with type 1 and type 2 diabetes are 34 to 50% and 3 to 5%, respectively. Nephropathy is found in 4% of diabetic pregnancies and is associated with increased maternal and perinatal morbidity. Most studies agree that pregnancy may accelerate the progression of nephropathy, but the reversibility of this complication is unclear. Most studies show a worsening of retinopathy in pregnant patients similar to that occurring during the same period in nonpregnant patients. The level of severity of retinopathy before pregnancy is most predictive of worsening during pregnancy, and treatment is recommended before conception.

Labor and Delivery

During labor and delivery, tight glucose control is necessary to avoid neonatal hypoglycemia due to hyperinsulinemia at birth. The goal is to maintain serum glucose levels of 72 to 144 mg/dL. The use of an insulin drip with dextrose infusion in active labor is recommended. Immediately after delivery, insulin requirements decrease to prepregnancy levels. Insulin needs should be one half to two thirds prepregnancy requirements, with a further decreased need found in breast-feeding patients.

Postpartum Considerations

Fifteen percent to 25% of pregnant patients with type 1 diabetes develop postpartum thyroiditis, so all patients require postpartum measurements of thyroid-stimulating hormone and follow-up for 6 months. Other postpartum recommendations are to restart ACE inhibitors and to monitor closely for infection. It is important to discuss diabetes prevention in the offspring and to address contraception. It is most important to recommend an effective contraceptive method that is acceptable to the patient. Oral estrogens can increase triglycerides, and both oral and injectable progesterone-only contraceptives may increase insulin resistance. Low-dose combined oral contraceptives and the progesterone-releasing intrauterine device appear to have little effect on glucose.

Insulin is acceptable in breast-feeding women, and limited data suggest that glyburide and metformin are safe as well. One small study found that glyburide is not excreted in breast milk and that metformin is excreted in a small amount that is probably not clinically significant.

PROGNOSIS AND COMPLICATIONS

The maternal complications of diabetes may be affected by pregnancy and may affect the course of the pregnancy. Patients with nephropathy experience an increase in proteinuria and a risk for progression of renal disease, especially if the serum creatinine concentration is more than 1.4 mg/dL. There is an increased risk for hypertension, which is seen in 30% of patients during the first trimester and 75% of patients by the third trimester. Autonomic neuropathy may worsen, as manifested by increasing gastroparesis, orthostatic hypotension, and decreased hypoglycemic awareness. Patients with long-standing diabetes may need to be evaluated for ischemic heart disease, which may impair the heart's ability to meet the cardiovascular demands of pregnancy. Pregnant patients are also at risk for hyperlipidemia and for preeclampsia. Diabetes increases the risk for operative delivery and for infections, the most common of which are wound, urinary tract, and respiratory.

Diabetic ketoacidosis may be precipitated by steroid use for fetal lung maturity, hyperemesis, infection, and noncompliance with insulin regimens. Acidosis may occur more quickly and at lower glucose levels in pregnant than in nonpregnant patients. There is a high fetal mortality associated with diabetic ketoacidosis (9 to 10%), and patients should be monitored in an intensive care setting.

Fetal and Neonatal Effects

There is an increased risk for spontaneous abortion, fetal loss, congenital anomalies, preeclampsia, and preterm delivery in patients with diabetes (Fig. 226-4). Poor glycemic control during pregnancy, especially in type 2 diabetes and GDM, is also associated with macrosomia (baby weighing >4000 g) and fetal intraventricular septal hypertrophy. Poor control is also associated with the effects of maternal vascular and renal disease and ketoacidosis, which include fetal loss, preeclampsia, and low birthweight. A study looking at differences in causes of pregnancy loss in type 1 and type 2 diabetic mothers compared the placental histology of patients with type 1 and type 2 diabetes and found an increase in histologic infarcts in type 2, suggesting a vascular rather than a glycemic cause of pregnancy complications and signs of abnormal development of placentas from patients with type 1 disease.

Neonatal complications include respiratory distress syndrome, hypoglycemia, hypocalcemia, cardiac hypertrophy, hyperbilirubinemia, and polycythemia. The risk for hypoglycemia may be ameliorated by careful control of maternal glucose concentration during labor and delivery. Normalization of maternal glucose concentration prevents hyperinsulinemia in the fetus and mitigates the risk for neonatal hypoglycemia.

Maternal Effects

GDM is a marker for type 2 diabetes; 50% of patients will develop type 2 diabetes within 7 to 10 years, and overall, 70% will develop the disease. Patients who have had GDM need directed testing at their 6-week postpartum visit, annual screening, and recommendations for lifestyle modification and cardiovascular risk reduction. Offspring of patients with GDM and type 2 diabetes are at increased risk for obesity and glucose intolerance.

⬤ LIVER DISEASE IN PREGNANCY

Liver disease found during pregnancy may be unique to pregnancy, represent underlying liver disease unmasked during pregnancy, or develop during pregnancy.[12] Most liver function test results are unchanged by pregnancy with the exception of an increase in alkaline phosphatase (which is produced by the placenta), an increase in fibrinogen, and a decrease in serum albumin.

Table 226-9 outlines pregnancy-related liver disease. This discussion focuses on diseases unique to pregnancy and those diseases for which there are specific management considerations during pregnancy.

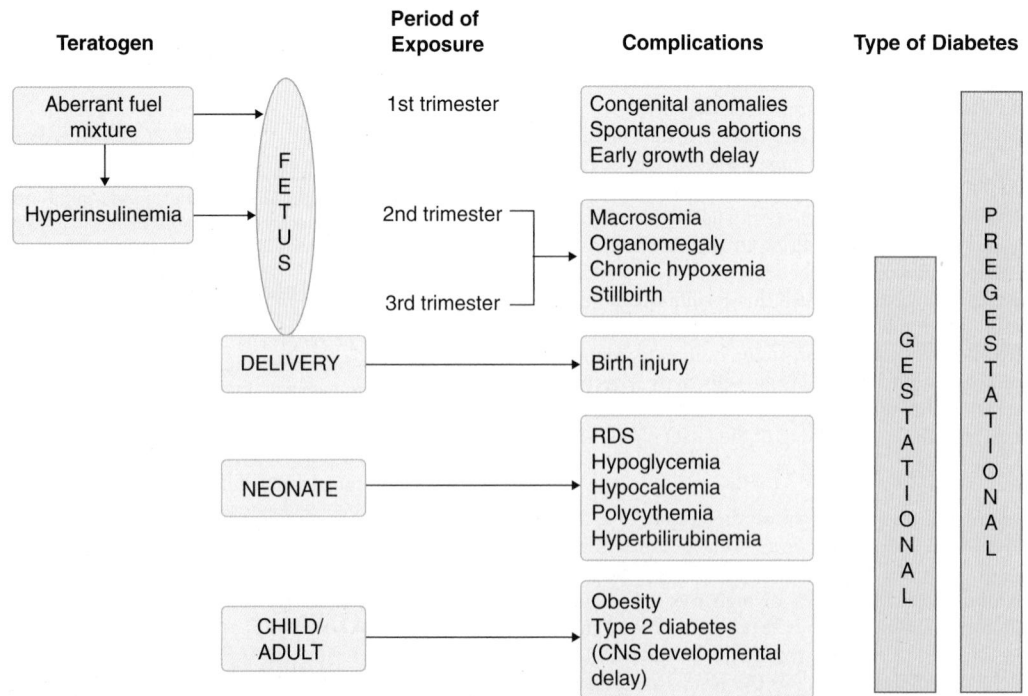

FIGURE 226-4. Fetal, neonatal, and childhood effects of exposure to hyperglycemia. CNS = central nervous system; RDS = respiratory distress syndrome.

TABLE 226-9 LIVER DISEASE AND PREGNANCY

UNIQUE TO PREGNANCY

Acute fatty liver of pregnancy
HELLP syndrome (hemolysis, elevated liver enzymes, and low platelets)
Hyperemesis gravidarum
Intrahepatic cholestasis of pregnancy
Preeclampsia and eclampsia

INCREASED INCIDENCE DURING PREGNANCY

Budd-Chiari syndrome
Drug-induced hepatotoxicity
Gallstones
Liver transplantation
Sepsis
Viral hepatitis

UNDERLYING CONDITION THAT MAY BE REVEALED

Autoimmune hepatitis
Cirrhosis
Hepatitis B and C
Primary biliary cirrhosis
Primary sclerosing cholangitis
Wilson disease

Modified from Mufti AR, Reau N. Liver disease in pregnancy. *Clin Liver Dis.* 2012;16:247-269.

Liver Diseases Unique to Pregnancy

INTRAHEPATIC CHOLESTASIS OF PREGNANCY (OBSTETRIC CHOLESTASIS)

DIAGNOSIS

Intrahepatic cholestasis of pregnancy (ICP) or obstetric cholestasis affects 0.5 to 2% of pregnant women, although in Bolivia and Chile, rates of 4 to 28% have been observed. ICP is manifested most commonly in the late second or third trimester with intense pruritus accompanied by an increase in serum bile acids and often transaminases and prothrombin time. ICP is likely to be a metabolic disease of multifactorial etiology characterized in most cases by a genetic variation in the biliary transporters and receptors that govern bile acid homeostasis. It is more common in patients with underlying hepatitis C, so it is important to screen all patients with hepatitis C serology. ICP is associated with preterm labor, meconium staining, fetal hypoxia, and sudden fetal demise.

TREATMENT Rx

Because no antenatal testing has been able to predict those patients at risk for fetal demise, consensus guidelines recommend delivery at 37 to 38 weeks of gestation in patients with a significant elevation in serum bile acids (≥40 μmol/L). The treatment of choice is ursodeoxycholic acid at 10 to 15 mg/kg, which leads to both symptomatic and biochemical improvement. There are no studies demonstrating a beneficial effect on pregnancy outcome.

PREECLAMPSIA AND ECLAMPSIA

As discussed previously, preeclampsia can be associated with liver abnormalities, including liver edema and infarction, subcapsular hematoma, liver laceration, and HELLP syndrome (hemolysis, elevated liver enzymes, and low platelets).

HYPEREMESIS GRAVIDARUM

Hyperemesis gravidarum, defined as severe persistent nausea and vomiting of pregnancy with weight loss, ketosis, or dehydration, can be associated with transaminase elevations in 50 to 60% of cases.

TREATMENT Rx

Treatment is supportive with rehydration, antiemetics, and vitamin replacement, often requiring hospitalization. Oral fluid repletion can often be accomplished because indwelling intravenous catheters have been associated with a significant risk for thrombosis and infections. Hyperemesis gravidarum is usually a reversible condition with no permanent liver damage.

TABLE 226-10 SWANSEA DIAGNOSTIC CRITERIA FOR ACUTE FATTY LIVER OF PREGNANCY

Six or more of the following features in the absence of another explanation:

- Vomiting
- Abdominal pain
- Polydipsia/polyuria
- Encephalopathy
- Elevated bilirubin
- Hypoglycemia
- Elevated urate
- Leukocytosis
- Ascites or bright liver on ultrasound scan
- Elevated transaminases
- Elevated ammonia
- Renal impairment
- Coagulopathy
- Microvesicular steatosis on liver biopsy

From Ch'ng CL, Morgan M, Hainsworth I, et al. Prospective study of liver dysfunction in pregnancy in Southwest Wales. *Gut.* 2002;51:876-880.

ACUTE FATTY LIVER OF PREGNANCY

DIAGNOSIS

Acute fatty liver of pregnancy is a rare condition that is estimated to occur in 5 per 100,000 pregnancies. It most commonly is manifested in the third trimester and postpartum; in its most severe form, it can be associated with fulminant liver failure and the need for liver transplantation. Maternal mortality rates were earlier thought to be as high as 20%, but a more recent U.K. study found a 2% maternal and 11% perinatal mortality rate. The Swansea criteria have recently been validated as a diagnostic tool for the diagnosis of acute fatty liver of pregnancy (Table 226-10).

PROGNOSIS

The maternal mortality rate has been estimated at 18%. Acute fatty liver of pregnancy is associated with an inherited defect in mitochondrial fatty acid B oxidation. The defect results in accumulation of toxic metabolites produced by the fetus and placenta that, after entering the maternal circulation, are deposited in maternal liver. Diagnosis is clinical, based on the constellations of findings described in Table 226-10. Liver function abnormalities can be severe, and hypoglycemia is a poor prognostic sign. Anyone with evidence of liver failure should be seen at a transplant center as early in the course as possible.

Preexisting or New-Onset Liver Disease during Pregnancy

The major importance of recognition of underlying liver disease in pregnancy is both for maternal health and for those diseases in which lack of treatment results in a high rate of vertical transmission to the fetus or neonate.

VIRAL HEPATITIS

Hepatitis C virus (HCV) infection (Chapter 139) has become an increasingly important and prevalent issue in pregnancy; maternal-to-child HCV vertical transmission rates are 5 to 10% and as high as 22% with HIV coinfection. New screening guidelines will lead to more universal screening in this age group. The mode of delivery does not have an impact on vertical transmission rates. The higher the viral load and the longer the duration of ruptured membranes, the higher the risk for transmission. Infection with hepatitis E virus and herpes simplex virus is much more likely to be severe in pregnant women. Particularly in the third trimester, it can be associated with fulminant disease and high maternal and perinatal mortality. All pregnant patients with new-onset hepatitis should also be screened for cytomegalovirus and Epstein-Barr virus.

TREATMENT Rx

All pregnant women in the United States are screened for hepatitis B virus (HBV) with hepatitis B surface antigen (Chapter 139). All neonates born to positive mothers are treated with hepatitis B immune globulin within 12 hours of birth and given their first dose of HBV vaccine at birth. This regimen is less effective in mothers with a high viral load or in the presence of hepatitis B e antigen positivity.

Fetal risks involved in the use of interferon during pregnancy outweigh its benefits. All current oral anti-HBV drugs (including lamivudine, entecavir, and adefovir) are categorized as FDA pregnancy category C, except telbivudine and tenofovir, which are pregnancy category B drugs. Vertical transmission of HCV occurs, but data supporting recommendations for prevention are limited. Both ribavirin and interferon are contraindicated during pregnancy.

CHRONIC LIVER DISEASE

Chronic liver disease may be associated with anovulation, amenorrhea, and infertility. Thus, it is unusual to see pregnant patients with significant liver decompensation and cirrhosis. Patients with portal hypertension, autoimmune hepatitis, Wilson disease, hepatic masses, and successful liver transplantation will be seen during pregnancy.

TREATMENT   Rx

The management of these patients requires an understanding of their course in pregnancy and a recognition of the importance of continuing prepregnant treatment.

Portal hypertension (Chapter 144) of any cause will be affected by the increase in blood volume during pregnancy, requiring careful follow-up and management of esophageal varices and splenic artery aneurysm. β-Blockers should be continued, and baseline endoscopy should be done early to consider banding of larger varices.

Autoimmune hepatitis (Chapter 140) improves dramatically with immunosuppression, so many women regain fertility with treatment. Immunosuppression with steroids and azathioprine should be continued to avoid relapse and progression of disease. The cholestasis associated with primary biliary cirrhosis can be treated with ursodeoxycholic acid as outlined for ICP.

Similar to women with autoimmune hepatitis, patients with treated Wilson disease (Chapter 200) regain fertility. Chelation therapy should be continued because discontinuation is associated with marked rises in copper levels and can lead to fulminant liver failure.

Hepatic masses are most commonly benign adenomas, focal nodular hyperplasia, or hemangiomas in women of childbearing age. Careful follow-up of these estrogen-sensitive masses is important because enlargement and hemorrhage may be complications of pregnancy.

SUMMARY

Women of childbearing age with chronic medical conditions benefit greatly from preconception counseling and interventions that address control of their disease and safety of their medications. Pregnant patients with acute or chronic medical illnesses require a multidisciplinary team that understands the maternal and fetal risks related to both the underlying illness and untreated disease. Pregnancy is a window of opportunity to address maternal health, and the maternal response to pregnancy may be predictive of future risk. The 6-week postpartum visit, rather than being the end of pregnancy care, should represent the beginning of a woman's long-term health care.

Grade A References

A1. Magee LA, von Dadelszen P, Rey E, et al. Less-tight versus tight control of hypertension in pregnancy. *N Engl J Med.* 2015;372:407-417.
A2. Churchill D, Duley L, Thornton JG, et al. Interventionist versus expectant care for severe preeclampsia between 24 and 34 weeks' gestation. *Cochrane Database Syst Rev.* 2018;10:CD003106.
A3. Roberts JM, Myatt L, Spong CY, et al. Vitamins C and E to prevent complications of pregnancy-associated hypertension. *N Engl J Med.* 2010;362:1282-1291.
A4. Rolnik DL, Wright D, Poon LC, et al. Aspirin versus placebo in pregnancies at high risk for preterm preeclampsia. *N Engl J Med.* 2017;377:613-622.
A5. Henderson JT, Whitlock EP, O'Connor E, et al. Low-dose aspirin for prevention of morbidity and mortality from preeclampsia: a systematic evidence review for the U.S. Preventive Services Task Force. *Ann Intern Med.* 2014;160:695-703.
A6. Skeith L, Carrier M, Kaaja R, et al. A meta-analysis of low-molecular-weight heparin to prevent pregnancy loss in women with inherited thrombophilia. *Blood.* 2016;127:1650-1655.
A7. Rodger MA, Hague WM, Kingdom J, et al. Antepartum dalteparin versus no antepartum dalteparin for the prevention of pregnancy complications in pregnant women with thrombophilia (TIPPS): a multinational open-label randomised trial. *Lancet.* 2014;384:1673-1683.
A8. Bain E, Pierides KL, Clifton VL, et al. Interventions for managing asthma in pregnancy. *Cochrane Database Syst Rev.* 2014;10:CD010660.
A9. Feig DS, Donovan LE, Corcoy R, et al. Continuous glucose monitoring in pregnant women with type 1 diabetes (CONCEPTT): a multicentre international randomised controlled trial. *Lancet.* 2017;390:2347-2359.
A10. Moore LE, Clokey D, Rappaport VJ, et al. Metformin compared with glyburide in gestational diabetes: a randomized controlled trial. *Obstet Gynecol.* 2010;115:55-59.

GENERAL REFERENCES

For the General References and other additional features, please visit Expert Consult at https://expertconsult.inkling.com.

227

MENOPAUSE

NANETTE SANTORO AND GENEVIEVE NEAL-PERRY

DEFINITION AND EPIDEMIOLOGY

Menopause is defined as the permanent cessation of menses and is the culmination of a process of reproductive aging that typically occurs in the fifth to sixth decades of life, with a median age of 52.5 years. Menopause is typically defined by a duration of amenorrhea of a minimum of 12 months. However, this definition relies on a woman having menstrual cycles of some degree of regularity. Women who are age 45 or older have a 90% probability of never having another menstrual period once they attain the milestone of 12 months' amenorrhea. In contrast, younger women have a substantially greater probability of experiencing subsequent menses. The final menstrual period (FMP) is most often preceded by several years of instability in menstrual cyclicity and hormone secretion; this process is called the menopausal transition and usually lasts for 4 years, with wide variation about this median.[1] Women who enter the transition at a younger age tend to have more symptoms and a longer duration, whereas those who enter it later in life are more likely to have a more rapid transit to the FMP.

A host of factors influence the timing of the FMP for any given woman. Genetic and familial factors play a large role. Knowing one's mother's age at FMP is a strong predictor of when a woman is likely to have her own. The known genetic, environmental, racial/ethnic, and gynecologic factors associated with the timing of the FMP are summarized in Table 227-1.

The menopausal transition refers to the processes of reproductive aging that involve menstrual cycle change, irregularity, and a breakdown of the normal reproductive hormonal patterns and feedback mechanisms that characterize the fertile cycles of midreproductive-age women.[2] Patterns of reproductive

TABLE 227-1	SOME KNOWN FACTORS THAT INFLUENCE THE AGE AT MENOPAUSE	
FACTOR	**DIRECTION**	**DEGREE**
GENETIC/FAMILIAL		
CYP3A4 and *CYP1B1*	Earlier menopause	Interaction with smoking
MSH6	Earlier menopause	DNA mismatch repair
MCM8	Earlier menopause	
PvuII ER polymorphism	Earlier menopause, hysterectomy	6 mo
Mosaic Turner syndrome	Earlier menopause	Variable
Fragile X	Earlier menopause	Variable
ENVIRONMENTAL		
EDCs	Earlier menopause	1.8-3.8 yrs
High altitude	Earlier menopause	1-1.5 yrs
LIFESTYLE		
Smoking	Earlier menopause	1-2 yrs
Low socioeconomic status	Earlier menopause	1-2 yrs
Oral contraceptive use	Later menopause	6 mo
RACIAL/ETHNIC		
African American race	Earlier menopause*	2 yrs
Hispanic ethnicity	Earlier menopause	2 yrs
Asian ethnicity	Later menopause	1-2 yrs
MENSTRUAL CHARACTERISTICS		
Shorter cycles (<26 days)	Earlier menopause	1.4 yrs
Higher parity	Later menopause	

*Relative to Caucasian women.
EDCs = endocrine-disrupting chemicals; ER = estrogen receptor.

TABLE 227-2 STAGING REPRODUCTIVE AGING

STAGE	REPRODUCTIVE (−5 to −3)	MENOPAUSAL TRANSITION (−2 to −1)		POSTMENOPAUSE (+1 to +2)
Subdivisions	Early, peak, late	Early (−2)	Late (−1)	Early, late
Age ranges (approximate)	13-47	47-49	49-52	50+
Menses	Mostly regular	Minor irregularity	≥60-364 days amenorrhea	Amenorrhea
Hormonal hallmarks	FSH—low (rises sporadically at stage −3) AMH—high	FSH sporadically elevated AMH—normal to low	FSH more consistently elevated AMH—low	FSH consistently elevated (>25 IU/L) AMH—undetectable

The diagram distills the evidence from the STRAW paradigm (Harlow SD, Gass M, Hall JE, et al. *J Clin Endocrinol Metab.* 2012;97:1159-1168) into a brief referable item to help "place" a woman along the menopause transition. Stage 0 is the Final Menstrual Period (FMP). Clinically helpful milestones are mostly related to menstrual regularity. FSH can be used as a confirmatory test when clinical context is unclear. Newer, highly sensitive AMH assays may allow distinction between Stages −1 and +1.
AMH = antimüllerian hormone; FSH = follicle-stimulating hormone.

hormone production are altered such that cycles become shorter and more sporadic and display less progesterone production. Follicle-stimulating hormone (FSH) increases sporadically as remaining ovarian follicular pool (ovarian reserve) requires more and more stimulation to produce a preovulatory follicle. Eventually, FSH cannot sustain folliculogenesis, and menses begin to skip. Because ovarian reserve waxes and wanes over the course of the transition, cycles do not stop abruptly. Instead, ovulatory and anovulatory cycles generally alternate in a random fashion. This results in hormonal fluctuations that can be debilitating for many women. Therefore symptoms of menopause do not simply appear with the FMP, they are usually present throughout the transition, although they can intensify with progress through the transition. For many, symptom onset begins in the early menopausal transition and worsens by the late transition through the early postmenopausal period. The stages of reproductive aging are shown in Table 227-2.

Determining a woman's proximity to her FMP has implications that are important for her health in several ways. A woman who has an early FMP will spend a greater proportion of her lifetime in a state of relative estrogen deficiency, which will have consequences on her bone health and may have consequences for her cardiovascular health. Women with later FMPs are more prone to estrogen-related diseases such as breast and endometrial cancer. Women who have not yet undergone 12 months of amenorrhea may wish to know when they can safely discontinue the use of contraception. Finally, many women who are symptomatic may want to be able to predict how long their symptoms are likely to last.

Unfortunately, a definitive diagnostic test that can predict the FMP in a foolproof fashion does not exist. Nonetheless, serum level of antimüllerian hormone (AMH), a transforming growth factor beta family peptide synthesized by granulosa cells, is a reliable proxy of ovarian reserve. If AMH is low, it can be used to help approximate the timing of the FMP. Other measures, such as FSH or the inhibins, are generally not recommended for this purpose, in part because—unlike AMH—they fluctuate throughout the menstrual cycle.

Current guidelines for menopausal management concur that symptomatic treatment only is indicated for this normal life transition. The remainder of this chapter will therefore focus on the common symptoms of menopause, the effectiveness of hormonal and nonhormonal treatments, and the balancing of risks and benefits of treatment that facilitate shared decision making with patients.

BIOLOGIC CONSEQUENCES OF MENOPAUSE AND THE MENOPAUSE TRANSITION

The brain is enriched with estrogen receptors (ERs), and ER signaling is hypothesized to mediate multiple key processes in the central nervous system (CNS), including but not limited to neurotrophic effects and neuroprotection.[3] Menopause and advancing age both impose adverse effects on CNS function.

Human as well as nonhuman studies demonstrate sex differences in the structure and function of the hippocampus and the temporal lobe that are thought to be related to differences in the activational and organizational effects of estradiol on memory performance. Estrogen-mediated structural differences in the hypothalamus are hypothesized to translate into higher executive functioning in women. Consequently, anxiety and mood changes are more common in perimenopausal and recently menopausal women, especially in women who have a history of mood dysfunction.[4,5] The hypogonadism of menopause may provide a reason for why perimenopausal and early postmenopausal women frequently complain of memory loss and the inability to

focus. However, studies in menopausal women report conflicting results regarding the benefit of hormone therapy on attention and executive functions such as nonspatial and spatial working memory, as well as verbal memory.[6] Moreover, many of these executive functions spontaneously recover within a few years of the menopause. Last, age-related changes in brain-derived steroids are hypothesized to account for the increased incidence of dementia.

Bone health is significantly affected by gonadal steroids.[7] Over the menopausal transition, serum estradiol and estrone concentrations decrease by as much as 90%. This decline closely parallels a period of accelerated and progressive bone loss. Reduced estrogen signaling in the menopause disrupts the balance of receptor activator nuclear factor-κβ ligand (increased) and osteoprotegerin (decreased) concentrations, with the end effect being increased osteoclast activity, accelerated bone reabsorption, and attenuated rates of bone remodeling. Consequently, markers of bone reabsorption and formation are significantly increased in the serum and urine of menopausal women. Bone mineral density changes begin slowly during the early perimenopause. With the advent of the early postmenopause bone mineral density loss accelerates, with annual rates of loss approximately 1.8 to 2.3% in the spine and 1.0 to 1.4% in the hip and as much as 30% loss of trabecular and 10% loss of cortical bone over the 6 to 10 years spanning the perimenopausal and early menopausal period. Altered bone physiology results in increased risk for osteoporosis and anywhere from 50 to 100% higher fracture rates. Estrogen attenuates bone loss in a dose-dependent manner.

Increased weight gain and altered fat distribution is a common complaint in perimenopausal and menopausal women that transcends race and socioeconomic status. Midlife women tend to gain approximately 1.5 pounds. Of particular note, adipose tissue, an endocrine organ, expresses estrogen receptors and estrogen is hypothesized to increase adipocyte lipolysis. Thus it is reasonable to hypothesize that menopause may drive adipose tissue pathophysiology.

Increased central adiposity,[8] a physiologic state that is characterized by chronic low-grade inflammation, is also a common complaint of midlife women. Central/metabolic adiposity is associated with metabolic syndrome and a higher overall mortality risk with more than a four-fold increased risk in cardiovascular death. Additionally, obese perimenopausal and early menopausal women experience more frequent and severe hot flashes as well as sexual dysfunction. Alterations in fat distribution may in part contribute to increased risk of cardiovascular events in menopausal women.

MENOPAUSAL SYMPTOMS

Although there are many symptoms that women report as they traverse the menopause, it is challenging to disentangle those related to aging from those related to menopause per se. There are four cardinal symptoms that are considered to be directly related to menopause, based on their association with the transition and their ability to be treated with hormones. These include vasomotor symptoms/hot flashes, vaginal dryness, sleep disturbances, and mood/cognition problems.

Vasomotor symptoms (VMS) are one of the cardinal symptoms of menopause and are experienced by up to 80% of women. In a multiethnic, longitudinal cohort study of the menopausal transition, VMS were observed to have a median duration of 7.4 years, with a mean post-FMP persistence of 4.5 years.[9] However, further clinical history can help predict the duration of VMS with more precision. Knowing a woman's onset of VMS and its timing in relation to her transition is important because women with an earlier age of onset who are earlier in their transition at onset will have a longer duration of symptoms, with some women having total durations of more than a decade. About 50%

of women with onset of VMS preceding entry into the menopausal transition will have persistence of VMS 10 years or longer after their FMP. African American women are also more likely to have persistent VMS compared with other racial/ethnic groups; approximately 40% will report post-FMP persistence of 10 years or longer. Additional factors that may result in a longer duration of VMS include lower educational level, greater perceived stress, symptom sensitivity, higher depressive symptoms, and the existence of anxiety at the time of the first report of VMS. Last, whereas a higher body mass index (BMI) at the time of the early menopause is associated with greater VMS, a greater BMI at the time of the late menopause is associated with fewer VMS. Shared decision making about treatment type and duration can be facilitated by taking these additional factors into account.[10]

Vaginal dryness, dyspareunia, and urogenital symptoms are less common than VMS but still widely prevalent. Depending on the study sample and how they are queried, between 25 and 57% of menopausal women report symptoms of urogenital atrophy. There is evidence that these symptoms are inadequately treated. Newer terminology includes symptoms of vaginal dryness apart from intercourse, dyspareunia, and associated urinary symptoms under the term *genitourinary syndrome of menopause* (GSM). Women may report dryness, chronic irritation, or burning of both the vagina and vulva; among those who are sexually active, lack of lubrication with attempted intercourse, pain during intercourse, or bleeding after intercourse may be present. Urinary frequency, urethritis, and frequent urinary tract infections may also occur. All of these symptoms are believed to reflect hypogonadism and the absence of estrogen exposure to the vaginal and urinary tract epithelium. Unlike VMS, symptoms of GSM do not spontaneously resolve over time. Treatment is therefore best considered long term.

Sleep disturbances are more common in women but also worsen with age. It is therefore challenging to differentiate between changes related to aging compared with menopause. Whereas some epidemiologic studies indicate that the menopausal transition worsens preexisting sleep problems and is associated with worse sleep, others have seen little independent effect of ovarian failure on sleep, except for a small, vulnerable subset of women with relatively poor sleep at baseline. Studies of premenopausal women given a gonadotropin-releasing hormone (GnRH) agonist to produce abrupt estrogen withdrawal indicate significant alterations in sleep, largely related to subjective, and less so to objective, measurement of nighttime hot flashes. VMS appear to mediate sleep disruption in women in the menopausal transition, in part by prompting nighttime awakenings. Studies of sleep architecture in menopausal women demonstrate greater sleep disturbances in the second half of the night, in association with compromise of rapid eye movement (REM) sleep.

An additional complexity in attributing sleep disturbances to menopause is the possibility that concomitant acquired sleep disorders are present. These include sleep apnea and restless legs syndrome (RLS). Sleep apnea is diagnosed by an overnight sleep assessment. Typically, questionnaire testing is performed beforehand to identify women with a history of snoring, daytime sleepiness, and less perceived restfulness of sleep. Diagnostic criteria for RLS include (1) irresistible urges to move one's legs; (2) symptoms present at rest; (3) urge relieved by movement; and (4) peak symptoms at night or in the evening. Insomnia may appear at the time of the menopausal transition, but it may also be longstanding in duration. Women age 35 or over with insomnia have the highest rates of persistence of the problem. Table 227-3 provides brief diagnostic assessment criteria for common sleep problems.

Adverse mood is associated with traversal of the menopause in a complex manner. Abrupt estrogen withdrawal using a GnRH agonist in premenopausal women

results in a deterioration of mood.[11] Depressive symptoms are associated with nighttime hot flashes and sleep disruption, indicating the intimate relationship between sleep and mood. Multiple cohort studies have identified the late transition as a period of vulnerability for depression in midlife women. Women are two- to four-fold more likely to experience new onset of major depression during the menopausal transition than they are before they become perimenopausal or after their FMP. Concomitant anxiety and hot flashes are predictors of major depression during this time of life. Although absolute levels of hormones are not clearly associated with major depression or depressive symptoms, greater variability in FSH, luteinizing hormone, and estradiol have been linked to depressive symptoms.

● TREATMENT OF MENOPAUSAL SYMPTOMS

Hormonal options should be reserved for women with bothersome VMS. Hormonal therapies include estradiol, estrogens, and, when women have a uterus, progestin. Risks and side effects of hormonal therapy are modulated by the route of administration, hormonal formulation, age, time since the FMP, and the presence or absence of a uterus, as well as coexisting morbidities such as cardiovascular disease, dementia, and diabetes.[12,13]

Uterine neoplasia is increased under conditions of chronic unopposed estrogen exposure in a woman with an intact uterus. Thus the primary indication of progestin therapy during the menopause is to prevent estradiol-induced endometrial hyperplasia and cancer. Commonly used progestins include medroxyprogesterone acetate (MPA), norethindrone acetate, and micronized progestin (native progesterone). Progestin administered continuously or sequentially provides adequate endometrial protection. However, controversy exits as to whether micronized progestin protects the uterus as effectively as synthetic progestin.

Breast cancer risk and menopausal hormone therapy are reported in both randomized control trial and observational studies. Different types of menopausal hormone formulations, the duration of therapy, and the time in which menopausal hormone therapy is initiated may modify and increase the risk for breast cancer.

- *Combined estrogen and progestin menopausal therapy:* Several epidemiologic studies have reported that the addition of progestin to estrogen increases the risk of breast cancer compared with estrogen alone.
  - The Women's Health Initiative (WHI) study reported an increased risk for invasive breast cancer in the combined equine estrogen (CEE) and MPA group compared with the placebo and CEE alone group. A nonsignificant increase was first noted after 3 years, became significant after 5+ years, and remained elevated at 13 years in the postintervention study.[A1] The risk for breast cancer translated into 1 additional case per 1000 users or 9 additional breast cancer cases per 10,000 person-years. Breast cancer clustered in women who used menopausal therapy before randomization. These data suggest a link between the duration of treatment and progestin with an increased risk for breast cancer.
  - The French E3N cohort study, which investigated the association of menopausal hormone formulation with risk for breast cancer in 80,377 postmenopausal women, found that breast cancer risk was significantly increased in women who used a progestin other than progesterone or dydrogesterone and in women who reported greater than 5 years of menopausal hormone use.
- *Estrogen-only menopausal therapy:* Estrogen-only menopausal hormone therapy has revealed mixed outcomes with regard to the risk for breast cancer.
  - In the WHI study, compared with women assigned to the placebo group, there was no increased risk for invasive breast cancer in women assigned to the CEE alone. Instead, compared with women who were previously exposed to hormone therapy, women assigned to the CEE arm exhibited a significantly decreased risk for invasive breast cancer. This finding is consistent with the Estrogen for the Prevention of Re-Infarction Trial, a randomized clinical control study designed to determine the effect of unopposed estradiol on all-cause death and cancer incidence.[A2] These findings are in contrast with a large retrospective Finnish study designed to determine whether the risk of estrogen-only therapy on breast cancer varied by dose, constituent, and route of administration. The Finnish study found that oral as well as transdermal estradiol for 6 months to less than 5 years was not associated with breast cancer. However, the risk changed with more than 5 years of therapy and was equivalent with transdermal and oral estradiol formulations. The investigators also reported that neither estriol nor vaginal estradiol was associated with breast cancer.

TABLE 227-3   DIAGNOSTIC CRITERIA FOR SLEEP PROBLEMS

RESTLESS LEGS SYNDROME	SLEEP APNEA	INSOMNIA
Irresistible urge to move one's legs	Overnight sleep assessment generally required	Difficulty falling asleep/staying asleep at least 3 nights/wk
Symptoms prevalent at rest	Snoring, apneic episodes	Insomnia Severity Index
Urge relieved by leg movement	Epworth Sleepiness Scale	Pittsburgh Sleep Quality Index
Peak symptoms at night or in the evening		Use of sleep-promoting medication

Criteria for restless legs syndrome are described and can be obtained by history. For sleep apnea, an overnight test is usually necessary to initiate treatment; for sleep apnea and insomnia, suggested supportive survey instruments can be helpful in establishing the diagnosis.

Menopausal Hormone Therapy and Age Affect Risk of Cardiovascular Disease

Premenopausal women are at reduced risk for cardiovascular events compared with age-matched men and postmenopausal women, suggesting that estradiol may mediate the cardioprotection observed in premenopausal women. However, observational studies and clinical trials did not uniformly support the hypothesis that hormone therapy was cardioprotective.

In 1985 the Nurses' Health Study, a large prospective observational study, published results after 4 years of study suggesting that hormone therapy was cardioprotective in postmenopausal women. In contrast, the Framingham study reported adverse effects of hormone therapy on cardiovascular disease. However, the 10-year follow-up study by the Nurses' Health Study in 1991 reaffirmed its original finding that hormone therapy was cardioprotective. Subsequent to the Nurses' Health Study, the Heart and Estrogen/progestin Replacement Study (HERS), a clinical trial designed to investigate the cardioprotective benefits of hormone therapy, failed to generate data supportive of the hypothesis that estrogens are cardioprotective.

The Women's Health Initiative (WHI) study, the largest randomized controlled double-blinded study, was designed to test the hypothesis that hormone therapy was cardioprotective in postmenopausal women. The hormone therapy arm of WHI was stopped prematurely after 5.2 years because the study found increased hazard ratios for coronary heart disease (1.29), breast cancer (1.26), stroke (1.41), and pulmonary embolism (2.13). Additionally, women enrolled in the hormone therapy arm had increased risk for cognitive dysfunction, decreased bone disease, and gastroenterological cancer.[A3] However, long-term follow-up showed no differences in overall mortality at 18 years.[A4] Although WHI changed the entire landscape of menopausal medicine, many investigators raised concerns about the applicability of the findings because the mean age of the women was greater than 60, and many of the study participants were more than 10 years postmenopause. Moreover, this age group of women does not represent the primary patient population who use or request hormone therapy, perimenopausal women. Consequently, a secondary analysis of WHI data comparing placebo with estrogen alone was done, and the study suggested 19 fewer cardiovascular events per 10,000 person-years in women 50 to 59 compared with 51 more cardiovascular events per 10,000 person-years in women 70 to 79. These observations led to two studies designed to determine whether the time since menopause affected ability of hormone therapy to attenuate the risk for cardiovascular events, a hypothesis known as the timing hypothesis.

- *Kronos Early Estrogen Prevention Study (KEEPS):* KEEPS was a randomized clinical trial composed of 728 women ages 42 to 58 years and 6 to 36 months postmenopausal. KEEPS was designed to determine whether a critical window of time exists before which cardiovascular risk is increased or decreased by hormone therapy. Patients were treated with CEE, transdermal estradiol, or placebo with sequential micronized progestin or placebo for 4 years. Initial results suggest appropriate management of vasomotor symptoms without an increased incidence for venous thromboembolism, cardiovascular events, or breast or endometrial cancer. The investigators also did not find accelerated progression of carotid intima-media thickness (CIMT) or coronary artery calcium (CAC). Future follow-up studies of this cohort will provide more information about the importance of the timing of hormone therapy.
- *Early vs. Late Intervention Trial with Estradiol (ELITE):* ELITE was a 5-year randomized, double-blinded study of 643 postmenopausal women designed to determine whether cardiovascular outcome after hormone therapy reflects the time (less than 6 or more than 10 years postmenopause) after menopause when treatment is commenced.[A5] The median age for the two groups of participants was 55.4 and 63.6 years. Similar to KEEPS, the primary and secondary outcomes were change of CIMT and CAC over time of treatment. Participants were treated with estradiol 1 mg plus sequential vaginal progesterone (45 mg) or placebo. Compared with placebo, menopausal hormone therapy was associated with decreased progression of subclinical atherosclerosis (CIMT) when therapy was initiated within 6 years of the menopause. In contrast, when hormone therapy was initiated more than 10 years after menopause there was no benefit.[A6] These studies are provocative in their suggestion that hormone therapy may provide a cardioprotective benefit. However, additional studies are needed to confirm the suggested outcomes.

VENOUS THROMBOEMBOLIC EVENTS

Increased risk for venous thromboembolism (VTE) with the use of oral estrogen is well documented. Moreover, the risk for VTE is increased in women who use combined estrogen and progestin or estrogen-only hormone therapy. The risk for thromboembolism increases with advancing age and is related to the route of administration and the estradiol dose. When taken orally, estrogen enters the enterohepatic circulation and increases the production of liver proteins involved in coagulation and associated with inflammation. First-pass effects of estrogen in the liver most likely explain why meta-analysis of observational studies strongly suggests increased risk for VTE with oral compared with transdermal estrogen. VTE events tend to occur within the first year of hormone therapy, and the risk is magnified if a preexisting risk factor such as obesity or thrombophilia is present. Equally relevant, progestin also modulates VTE risk; VTE risk is not significantly affected by micronized progesterone, medroxyprogesterone acetate, or norethindrone but increased by norpregnane derivatives.

Ischemic stroke risk is also increased with the use of hormone therapy. The risk for stroke is greatest with oral estrogen use and in women who have thrombophilia.

COGNITIVE DYSFUNCTION

Observational studies investigating the effect of hormone therapy on cognition suggested that hormone therapy was beneficial to cognitive function. In contrast, the WHI Memory Study reported an increased incidence of dementia in women over 65 initiating hormone therapy. Similarly, a risk for reduced global cognitive function was not observed when women 50 to 55 initiated hormone therapy. However, clinical trials such as KEEPS[7] and ELITE[A2] suggest that hormone therapy taken by younger women in the early menopause does not adversely affect cognitive function.

VAGINAL SYMPTOMS AND TOPICAL THERAPY

Topical treatments involving estrogen alone, or two U.S. Food and Drug Administration (FDA)–approved nonestrogenic treatments, are now available.[14] Unlike hot flashes, symptoms of vaginal atrophy, including urinary tract irritation, vaginal itching and burning, and dyspareunia (collectively referred to as genitourinary syndrome of menopause [GSM]), do not subside over time.[A7][A8] Therefore long-term treatment may be required to preserve quality of life. Table 227-4 lists common forms of local estrogen treatment. Ospemifene, a selective estrogen receptor modulator that has estrogen receptor beta stimulation properties, is available as a nonestrogenic treatment; however, it is administered systemically. Dehydroepiandrosterone (DHEA) has also recently been FDA approved for vaginal use to treat dyspareunia. Recent uncontrolled studies have raised the possibility that laser treatment of the vagina may provide relief from GSM symptoms[15]; there is insufficient information to recommend this approach at this time.

	TABLE 227-4	NONHORMONAL PHARMACOLOGIC THERAPY FOR HOT FLASHES	
MEDICATION	**USUAL DAILY DOSES**	**RELATIVE EFFICACY[†]**	**SIDE EFFECTS**
Citalopram	20-40 mg	50%	Nausea, somnolence or insomnia, dry mouth, dyspepsia
Clonidine	Transdermal: 0.1-0.2 mg Oral: 0.1-0.3 mg	30%	Dry mouth, orthostatic hypotension, dizziness
Desvenlafaxine	100-150 mg	60%	Nausea, dry mouth, insomnia/somnolence, constipation, high blood pressure, sexual dysfunction
Escitalopram	10-20 mg	50%	Nausea, insomnia, headache, sexual dysfunction
Fluoxetine	10-20 mg	50%	Nausea, insomnia, headache, sexual dysfunction
Gabapentin	100-900 mg	60%	Drowsiness, dizziness, weight gain
Paroxetine mesylate*	7.5 mg	30%	Nausea, insomnia, headache, sexual dysfunction
Venlafaxine	37.5-150 mg	60%	Nausea/vomiting, anorexia, dry mouth, sexual dysfunction, high blood pressure

*Food and Drug Administration approved.
†Relative efficacy: estimated effectiveness compared with estrogen.

Extended Hormone Therapy Use

Women who use combined estrogen and progestin hormone therapy for more than 5.6 years demonstrated an increased risk of invasive breast cancer in the WHI cohort. Women who continue use beyond 4 to 5 years should be monitored carefully. However, for many healthy women, hormones need not be discontinued as long as they continue to serve a purpose. This is especially true for women who are approaching 5 to 10 years on hormone therapy and continue to have severe symptoms. Such women may be tried on nonhormonal options (reviewed later); if they cannot be weaned, extended hormone therapy may be needed to preserve quality of life.

Discontinuing Hormone Therapy

Many women choose to discontinue hormones after the worst of their menopausal symptoms have subsided. Symptoms appear to be subjectively worst in the year before the FMP and up to 2 years afterward. For the majority of women, hormone doses may be reduced, or they may attempt to discontinue either by weaning slowly off of hormones or by stopping "cold turkey." There is limited evidence to suggest that a weaning strategy is less disruptive, but it does not necessarily lead to a greater proportion of women who successfully discontinue hormone therapy. However, a small proportion of women, estimated at 3 to 15%, will have persistence of severe symptoms and will require continued hormones or nonhormonal alternatives.

Nonhormonal management of menopausal symptoms can include behavioral, nonpharmacologic, and pharmacologic methods. For mild to moderate symptoms, behavioral and nonpharmacologic approaches may be preferred. However, for more severe symptoms, it is likely that pharmacologic management will be required

Behavioral and Nonpharmacologic Approaches for Hot Flashes

1. Cognitive-behavioral therapy (CBT) has demonstrated efficacy in the treatment of hot flashes in women with breast cancer.[A9][A10] An approximately 50% reduction in subjective hot flash "problem rating" was observed in the intervention group compared with baseline, and versus an approximately 15% reduction in the comparison group (women who received usual care without a six-session CBT instruction). Given its negligible potential for harm, it can be readily recommended. This intervention is limited to programs that have a CBT-trained therapist.
2. Women may experience hot flash "triggers" from caffeine or alcohol and may modify consumption accordingly. Reducing the ambient room temperature and layering clothing to accommodate sudden changes in heat perception may also be helpful, but these recommendations are not based on medical evidence.[16]
3. Acupuncture has some evidence for efficacy, but not all trials have demonstrated benefit.[A11]
4. Weight loss has shown some efficacy in pilot and observational studies.
5. Yoga, exercise, and consumption of black cohosh and omega-3 fatty acids have been demonstrated to be ineffective in several randomized trials.

There are a number of nonhormonal prescription medications that can be used to treat hot flashes for women who cannot or do not wish to use hormones. Although many of these treatments are supported by well-conducted randomized, clinical trials, only paroxetine mesylate is FDA approved as of this writing. Table 227-4 summarizes the known nonhormonal treatments for hot flashes with the available supporting evidence, along with current FDA approval status.

For vaginal symptoms or GSM, there are fewer options. Nonhormonal treatments that are recommended include vaginal moisturizers (which must be used regularly to achieve effectiveness) and vaginal lubricants, which are specifically helpful during intercourse. Little attention has been paid to the exact composition of these products, which are available over the counter. A recent review has recommended that women choose products that are pH balanced (i.e., relatively acidic) with a physiologic osmolality.[17]

Nonhormonal treatment of adverse mood includes psychotherapy and antidepressants, with or without antianxiety medication as needed. For moderate to severe mood disturbances, hormonal therapy should not be used as a first-line treatment.

Difficulty sleeping can be addressed behaviorally. A recent trial of telephone-based CBT intervention in menopausal women indicated that 84% of women with moderate insomnia at screening improved into the no-insomnia range after treatment.[A12] A self-help smartphone app is available to enable patients to readily implement treatment (https://mobile.va.gov/app/cbt-i-coach). For

patients who wish to use over-the-counter treatments, low-dose diphenhydramine or hydroxyzine may facilitate sleep onset. Low-dose melatonin may be effective in reducing sleep-onset latency, although high-quality clinical trials are lacking in a menopausal population. A wide variety of hypnotics and melatonin receptor agonists are available for treatment of sleep difficulties; a comprehensive review is beyond the scope of this chapter. Judicious, short-term use of these agents may be beneficial for women traversing the menopause.

Mood and sleep issues are often intertwined, and treatment that addresses one of these conditions is likely to affect the other.[14] To make matters more complex, hot flashes or night sweats that interrupt sleep can be a contributing factor to deteriorations of both mood and sleep. A recent small clinical trial comparing venlafaxine and citalopram observed a relatively greater effect of citalopram on reducing hot flashes, but a relatively greater effect of venlafaxine in improving depression.[A13] It can be difficult to disentangle these overlapping contributory factors to adverse mood in a clinical setting. When symptoms are compound or overlapping, rather than using multiple agents specific for mood, sleep, and hot flashes, if possible, a brief trial of hormone therapy may be the most effective way to determine which symptoms are due to the menopausal transition and which are independent of it.

SUMMARY

Menopause is a universal phenomenon among women, and its lived experience varies by individual. The advent of menopause and the coincident loss of gonadal steroids significantly affect multiple organ systems in affected women, resulting in an increased risk for morbidities such as osteoporosis, dementia, and heart disease. Observational and randomized clinical trials suggest that the risk for morbidity is increased with advanced age and time since the onset of the menopause. Additionally, the risks and benefits of hormone therapy vary by organ system, the hormone therapy formulation, and the time since the FMP. Observational as well as randomized clinical trials also suggest that hormone therapy, when administered within the first 5 years of the final menopause, attenuates some but not all of the adverse effects of menopause-related hypogonadism.

Symptoms most commonly associated with menopause include hot flashes, sleep dysfunction, mood, and genitourinary syndrome of menopause and are readily improved with hormone therapy. Nonetheless, fear of hormones has led to widespread undertreatment of symptoms and a proliferation of non-rigorously tested but popular treatments such as custom-compounded hormones, pellets, and a large variety of herbal preparations. Clinicians should assess the patient's symptoms and offer evidence-based treatment, with periodic reevaluation of the necessity of treatment. Whereas the need for treatment of hot flashes, sleep problems, and mood problems will very likely no longer be present over time, a minority of women will continue to have significant symptoms and require long-term treatment, either with extended hormonal therapy or nonhormonal alternatives. Genitourinary syndrome of menopause symptoms are long lasting, and therefore long-term treatment may be necessary.

Grade A References

A1. Chlebowski RT, Rohan TE, Manson JE, et al. Breast cancer after use of estrogen plus progestin and estrogen alone: analyses of data from 2 Women's Health Initiative randomized clinical trials. *JAMA Oncol.* 2015;1:296-305.

A2. Cherry N, McNamee R, Heagerty A, et al. Long-term safety of unopposed estrogen used by women surviving myocardial infarction: 14-year follow-up of the ESPRIT randomised controlled trial. *BJOG.* 2014;121:700-705.

A3. Gartlehner G, Patel SV, Feltner C, et al. Hormone therapy for the primary prevention of chronic conditions in postmenopausal women: evidence report and systematic review for the US Preventive Services Task Force. *JAMA.* 2017;318:2234-2249.

A4. Manson JE, Aragaki AK, Rossouw JE, et al. Menopausal hormone therapy and long-term all-cause and cause-specific mortality: the Women's Health Initiative randomized trials. *JAMA.* 2017;318:927-938.

A5. Harman SM, Black DM, Naftolin F, et al. Arterial imaging outcomes and cardiovascular risk factors in recently menopausal women: a randomized trial. *Ann Intern Med.* 2014;161:249-260.

A6. Hodis HN, Mack WJ, Henderson VW, et al. Vascular effects of early versus late postmenopausal treatment with estradiol. *N Engl J Med.* 2016;374:1221-1231.

A7. Archer DF, Kimble TD, Lin FDY, et al. A randomized, multicenter, double-blind, study to evaluate the safety and efficacy of estradiol vaginal cream 0.003% in postmenopausal women with vaginal dryness as the most bothersome symptom. *J Womens Health (Larchmt).* 2018;27:231-237.

A8. Kroll R, Archer DF, Lin Y, et al. A randomized, multicenter, double-blind study to evaluate the safety and efficacy of estradiol vaginal cream 0.003% in postmenopausal women with dyspareunia as the most bothersome symptom. *Menopause.* 2018;25:133-138.

A9. Ayers B, Smith M, Hellier J, et al. Effectiveness of group and self-help cognitive behavior therapy in reducing problematic menopausal hot flushes and night sweats (MENOS 2): a randomized controlled trial. *Menopause.* 2012;19:749-759.

A10. Mann E, Smith MJ, Hellier J, et al. Cognitive behavioural treatment for women who have menopausal symptoms after breast cancer treatment (MENOS 1): a randomised controlled trial. *Lancet Oncol.* 2012;13:309-318.

A11. Ee C, Xue C, Chondros P, et al. Acupuncture for menopausal hot flashes: a randomized trial. *Ann Intern Med.* 2016;164:146-154.

A12. McCurry SM, Guthrie KA, Morin CM, et al. Telephone-based cognitive behavioral therapy for insomnia in perimenopausal and postmenopausal women with vasomotor symptoms: a MsFLASH randomized clinical trial. *JAMA Intern Med.* 2016;176:913-920.

A13. Davari-Tanha F, Soleymani-Farsani M, Asadi M, et al. Comparison of citalopram and venlafaxine's role in treating sleep disturbances in menopausal women, a randomized, double-blind, placebo-controlled trial. *Arch Gynecol Obstet.* 2016;293:1007-1013.

GENERAL REFERENCES

For the General References and other additional features, please visit Expert Consult at https://expertconsult.inkling.com.

228

INTIMATE PARTNER VIOLENCE

GENE FEDER AND HARRIET L. MACMILLAN

DEFINITION

Intimate partner violence (IPV) is defined as any behavior within an intimate relationship or ex-relationship that causes physical, psychological, or sexual harm.[1] This includes physical aggression, such as hitting, kicking, and beating; psychological violence, such as intimidation or constant humiliation; various controlling behaviors, such as isolation from family and friends, monitoring movements, financial control, and restricting access to services; and sexual violence, including forced intercourse and other sexual coercion. Lifetime prevalence of isolated violent acts within relationships is comparable for men and women, but repeated coercive, sexual, or severe physical violence is perpetrated largely against women by men. IPV also occurs in same-sex relationships[2,3]; although research evidence on the health consequences of IPV and the care of survivors is largely confined to women in heterosexual relationships, there is increasing evidence of similar types of impairment.

Historically, there has been the stereotype of a male batterer as one who uses severe, repeated, and unilateral violence against a nonviolent female victim. It is now recognized that *bilateral violence* is a common form of IPV, even though the overwhelming burden of morbidity and mortality related to IPV is experienced by women. Bilateral violence, sometimes referred to as *common couple violence*, is considered less severe than the pattern of abuse known as *battering* or *intimate terrorism*—a severe and escalating form of IPV characterized by threats, terrorization, multiple forms of abuse, and controlling behavior on the part of the abuser. Current research suggests that women rarely subject men to battering.

IPV is a risk factor for a wide range of medical and psychiatric conditions that requires a clinical and public health response. Yet violence perpetrated by an intimate partner or ex-partner is essentially a violation of human rights and a preventable psychosocial problem that needs to be addressed through social and educational policies.

EPIDEMIOLOGY

The prevalence of IPV against women varies internationally but is universally high, comparable to chronic conditions like diabetes and asthma. A synthesis of 151 surveys in 81 countries worldwide reported that almost one third (30%) of all women who have been in a relationship have experienced physical and/or sexual violence by their intimate partner. In some regions, 38% of women have experienced intimate partner violence. A more recent systematic review highlights the increased risk of IPV among indigenous women.[4] Another systematic review, which included data from 66 countries, concluded that one in seven homicides globally are committed by an intimate partner. This figure is six times higher for female homicides compared with male homicides.[5]

Causation

Several theories about the causes of IPV have been proposed over the years. Social learning theory suggests that IPV is a learned behavior. The fact that male perpetrators and female victims are more likely to report histories of exposure to violence in childhood supports this theory. However, most individuals exposed to violence in childhood do not go on to commit violence as adults, and not all abusers have violent upbringings. Furthermore, the link between poor parenting generally, including neglect, and subsequent IPV in adulthood suggests that the effect is not simply one of modeling abusive behavior. Exposure to rejecting or neglectful parenting is associated with adverse effects on intrapersonal (e.g., poor self-worth) and interpersonal development, which are associated with IPV.

A feminist perspective understands IPV against women as a form of coercive control rooted in society's patriarchal structure, reflecting the persistent inequality in economic and social relationships between men and women. Lending support to this perspective is the finding that IPV appears to be less common in more democratic and less economically polarized societies. Although IPV occurs more often in contexts in which there is support for male authority in the family and women have less access to economic security, it is not clear why some individuals are more likely to be violent under such conditions than others.

With regard to psychological theory, there are conflicting views about the association between IPV and psychopathology. Some researchers argue that abusive males have deficits in one or more coping mechanisms, anger control, and communication skills, whereas others suggest that IPV results from dysfunctional interactional patterns between partners. Because types of IPV are not the same for all couples, there are likely multiple causes for its occurrence. Most of the research has focused on factors associated with increased risk of men abusing women (Table 228-1); however, we do not know to what extent these factors are causal from cross-sectional studies.

An explanatory framework that can guide etiologic and intervention research on IPV (and other public health problems) is the ecologic model. It attempts to integrate evidence on individual (genetic and life course), family, community, and socioeconomic structural factors. The ecologic model has recently been further developed to incorporate the impact of globalization on violence against women.[6]

CLINICAL MANIFESTATIONS

Most of the research examining clinical manifestations associated with IPV exposure has focused on women. However, recent studies of male victims suggest that they also experience increased risk of poor health as well as chronic physical and emotional health problems and injuries.[7,8]

Patients seldom present with a chief complaint of IPV. Injuries are the most obvious manifestation; a clinician should have increased suspicion for IPV if there are multiple injuries, the presenting history of injuries is not consistent with the physical examination, and there is a delay in seeking medical care for injuries. Patients exposed to physical violence may present with injuries that vary from minor abrasions to life-threatening trauma. Although there can be overlap between injuries resulting from IPV and injuries from other causes, the former typically involve trauma to the head, face, and neck, whereas the latter are more typically injuries of the extremities. Multiple facial injuries are suggestive of IPV rather than from other causes, and those that are more specific for IPV include zygomatic complex fractures, orbital blow-out fractures,

TABLE 228-1	FACTORS ASSOCIATED WITH A MAN'S RISK FOR ABUSING HIS PARTNER		
INDIVIDUAL	**RELATIONSHIP**	**COMMUNITY**	**SOCIETAL**
Young age	Poor family functioning	Weak community sanctions against intimate partner violence	Traditional gender norms
Heavy drinking	Marital instability		Social norms supportive of violence
Depression	Marital conflict	Poverty	
Personality disorders	Male dominance	Economic inequality	
Low academic achievement	Economic stress	Low social capital	
Low income			
Exposure to violence in childhood			

Adapted from WHO. *World Report on Violence and Health.* Geneva: WHO; 2002.

and perforated tympanic membrane. Although facial injuries are the most common injuries associated with IPV, they have low specificity. Musculoskeletal injuries are considered the second most common type of injuries, including sprains, fractures, and dislocations. Blunt-force trauma to the forearms should raise suspicion of IPV because these can occur when trying to block being struck.

Victims of IPV often experience multiple mechanisms of injury; being struck by a hand is the most common, followed by use of a household object. Injuries from weapons such as knives and guns are far less common (<1%) but are associated with higher risk of mortality. Strangulation also occurs frequently, but less is known about the types of clinical manifestations that result from this form of IPV. Other injuries that raise suspicion of IPV include fractures of the spine or trunk, bites, hair pulling, and open wounds. Those exposed to sexual abuse may show signs of trauma to the genital area, but sexual assault is associated with signs of injury in less than one third of cases.

Most victims of IPV presenting in health care settings do not have signs of obvious trauma, but rather a constellation of overlapping physical and mental health problems. A patient presenting with vague signs and symptoms or chronic somatic complaints, including pain, suggests the possibility of IPV. Other behaviors that suggest IPV include delay in seeking medical care or multiple cancellations of medical appointments or a partner always being present in the consultation.

There are no systematic reviews of studies on the overall physical health consequences of IPV, but an overview of studies reported increased rates of chronic physical conditions, particularly gynecologic, gastrointestinal, and nervous system disorders, although most of the studies were small and poorly adjusted for other risk factors. Systematic reviews and meta-analyses have uncovered an association between violence against women and their cancer diagnosis[9] and cardiovascular risk,[10] the latter including significant relationships to development of hypertension and self-reported cardiac disease. A cause-and-effect relationship between IPV and these medical conditions has not been established, however. It has also been found that women with a history of abuse, particularly physical or sexual violence, were more likely to experience chronic pain and nonspecific symptoms, although an association between abuse and number of physical symptoms is also found in women who experience emotional abuse without any physical abuse. A World Health Organization (WHO) study of 24,097 women in 10 countries reported significant associations between women's lifetime experiences of partner violence and self-reported poor health and specific health problems in the previous 4 weeks, such as difficulty walking, difficulty with daily activities, pain, memory loss, dizziness, and vaginal discharge. Other physical conditions that should raise suspicion of IPV include chronic gynecologic or gastrointestinal symptoms, such as chronic pelvic pain or irritable bowel syndrome. It should not be assumed, however, that there is a specific association between functional disorders such as irritable bowel syndrome or fibromyalgia over and above the greater reporting of physical syndromes in general. IPV exposure is associated with an increased risk for sexually transmitted infections, including human papillomavirus.

Exposure to any type of IPV can be associated with a wide range of emotional and behavioral symptoms; depression and post-traumatic stress disorder (PTSD) are the two most commonly associated emotional conditions, but anxiety disorders and substance abuse are also associated with IPV exposure. In the WHO study, women who reported IPV at least once in their life reported three to four times more emotional distress, suicidal thoughts, and suicide attempts than nonabused women. There is strong evidence of increased risk for depression, anxiety, substance abuse, and PTSD. A meta-analysis examining the association between IPV against adult women and depressive conditions found a 2- to 3-fold increase in risk of major depressive disorder and 1.5- to 2-fold increased risk of postpartum depression and elevated depressive symptoms. The cross-sectional design of most studies measuring associated impairment precludes definite conclusions about the causal role of IPV in these conditions, but the few published longitudinal studies show the onset or worsening of depression, PTSD, and substance abuse *after* exposure to IPV, with some evidence for increased vulnerability to IPV of women with preexisting mental health conditions.

Pregnant women deserve special mention because IPV can threaten the health of both mother and fetus. Injury patterns during pregnancy are more likely to be central, including blunt trauma to the head, torso, abdomen, breasts, and genitalia.[11] Abuse directed to the abdomen may lead to poor pregnancy outcomes and perinatal death. A systematic review of 50 observational studies found an association between IPV in pregnancy and both preterm birth and low birthweight; there is no clear evidence for an increased risk of intrauterine growth retardation.[12]

Additionally, there is increasing recognition that children's exposure to IPV shows a significant association with children's internalizing and externalizing problems, including trauma symptoms, developmental delay, educational problems, and long-term mental health conditions.

Although intimate partner violence against women has tended to be studied separately from violence against children and other forms of interpersonal violence, an important study has now demonstrated significant intersections between them that should have implications for health programs, policies, and research in the future.[13] The United Nations Multi-Country Study on Men and Violence in Asia and the Pacific has uncovered a cycle of abuse, with child abuse leading to increased violence against women and additional child maltreatment, which in turn increases the risk of adult violence.[14]

Identification

Despite some guidelines recommending universal screening for IPV,[15] a systematic review has confirmed the findings from earlier studies concluding that although such screening increases the identification of women with IPV, it has not been shown to improve women's health outcomes or reduce the occurrence of IPV. **A1** However, it is important to be alert to the signs and symptoms associated with IPV, including those associated with the broad range of physical and mental health conditions referred to previously, and for clinicians to have a low threshold for asking about abuse. Indicators that suggest a higher likelihood of IPV include symptoms of depression, somatization, and PTSD in the female patient and a history of alcohol or drug abuse and unemployment in the male partner (or ex-partner). It is important, when asking about exposure to IPV, to do so privately, with no one else present, including a child (beyond infancy) or partner. If the inquiry or response is overheard, it could put the patient at risk for further IPV. A meta-analysis of qualitative studies of women's expectations and experiences reported that when the topic of IPV is raised, patients want questioning that is nonjudgmental, compassionate, and caring. Women want to be asked about IPV with confidentiality assured, but do not want to be pressured to disclose. In some jurisdictions, however, disclosure of IPV when a patient has children in the home can lead to mandatory reporting to child protection services. It is important that patients be advised about the limits of confidentiality before being asked about IPV exposure.

Possible questions to ask if IPV is suspected include the following: (1) Sometimes partners or ex-partners use physical force. Has this ever happened to you? (2) Have you felt humiliated or emotionally harmed by your partner or ex-partner? (3) Are you now or have you ever been afraid of your partner or ex-partner? (4) Have you ever been physically threatened or hurt by your partner or ex-partner? (5) Have you been forced to have any kind of sexual activity by your partner or ex-partner? (6) Has your partner or ex-partner ever tried to control your behavior, for example, control where you go or whom you see?

The initial clinical response when IPV is identified should include validation of the experience (e.g., everyone deserves to feel safe at home), affirmation that violence is unacceptable, and expression of support. The clinician needs to acknowledge the complexity of IPV and respect the patient's individual concerns and decisions. The assessment should include an evaluation of safety; the patient should be asked if it is safe for her (or him or any children) to return home. The following are examples of safety considerations: (1) Has the frequency or severity of the violence increased? (2) Is the partner or ex-partner obsessed with the patient? (3) How safe does she (he) feel? (4) Does the partner or ex-partner have a weapon or access to one? (5) Has she (he) been threatened with a weapon? Although a general discussion of gun violence is beyond the scope of this section, having firearms in the home is associated with an increased risk for homicide associated with IPV. Another predictor of domestic homicide is threats of deadly violence.

It has also been noted that primary care physicians often interact with male patients who perpetrate IPV and are therefore in a role potentially to intervene.[16] If a male patient discloses IPV perpetration, physicians should asses for lethality, readiness to change, and comorbid medical conditions that could affect treatment, such as substance abuse and mental illness. Referrals to a qualified therapist or batterer intervention program should be offered, but requirement to disclose IPV is dependent on local jurisdictions.

TREATMENT Rx

The initial response of clinicians to the disclosure of IPV by female patients, whether the disclosure is spontaneous or in response to inquiry from the clinician, is crucial in gaining trust and is the basis of further management. IPV is a highly stigmatized condition, akin to sexually transmitted infection or substance abuse, with the added dimension of risk for further harm from breach of confidentiality. A meta-analysis of 25 qualitative studies of women's expectations and experiences (847 informants) reported consistent messages about how clinicians can respond appropriately to disclosure. *Before questioning,* they should understand the problem, including knowing about the available community services and appropriate referral systems; ensure that the clinical environment is supportive, welcoming, and nonthreatening; place brochures and posters in the clinical setting; try to ensure continuity of care; inform abused women about matters of privacy, safety, and confidentiality; be alert to the signs of abuse and raise the matter when indicated; use verbal and nonverbal communication skills to develop trust; and be compassionate, supportive, and respectful toward abused women. *When the topic of IPV is raised,* they should be nonjudgmental, compassionate, and caring when questioning about abuse; be confident and comfortable asking about domestic violence; not pressure women to disclose abuse because simply raising the topic may be helpful to women; ask about abuse over the course of several interviews because a woman may disclose abuse at a later date; ensure that the environment is private and confidential; and provide time. *Immediate response to disclosure* should be nonjudgmental, with compassion, support, and convey belief of experiences; acknowledge the complexity of the problem and respect the woman's unique concerns and decisions; prioritize the needs identified by the woman and help to ensure that social and psychological needs are met; take time to listen, provide information, and offer referrals to specialist help; validate her experiences, challenge assumptions, and provide encouragement; and respond to any concerns about safety. *Response in later interactions* should be patient and supportive, allowing her to progress at her own therapeutic pace; understand the chronicity of the problem and provide follow-up and continued support; respect the woman's wishes and not pressure her into making any decisions; be nonjudgmental if a woman does not follow up with referrals immediately; and give abused women an opportunity to disclose abuse at a later date.

Beyond their initial response and managing the medical sequelae of abuse, most generalists have neither the expertise nor the capacity to meet the specific needs of women experiencing IPV, which include legal, financial, housing, and safety needs. A key step, particularly in the context of current or recent violence, is an offer of referral to some sort of specialist support. Two main types of services have been evaluated: advocacy programs and psychological interventions (individual or group based). Generally, advocates engage with individual clients who are being abused, aiming to empower them and linking them to community services. Core activities of advocacy include provision of legal, housing, and financial advice; facilitating access to and use of community resources, such as refuges (shelters, safe houses) and emergency housing; and provision of safety planning advice. Advocates can also provide ongoing support and informal counseling. A Cochrane review of 13 randomized controlled trials (2141 participants) of domestic violence advocacy concluded that there were some physical and psychosocial benefits from advocacy, but uncertainty about the magnitude of benefit, the impact of abuse severity, and the applicability to women receiving advocacy in or referred from health care settings.[A2] Only two of the studies had participants referred from health care settings. Clinicians should be able to refer patients to specialist IPV advocacy and are more likely to ask about abuse if they have the support of these services. If such services are not immediately available, shelters and refuges often provide these kinds of services for women both in residences and on an outreach basis.

A wide range of individual psychological interventions have demonstrated improvements in psychological outcomes, including depression, PTSD, and self-esteem. Trials of individual cognitive therapy–based interventions for women with PTSD who were no longer experiencing violence provided reasonable evidence for this intervention, but this cannot be extrapolated to women still in an abusive relationship.[A3][A4] All the studies of group psychological interventions showed improvement in one or more psychological or mental health outcomes, but with the exception of one study, they were poorly conducted. Consequently, the effectiveness of this type of intervention remains uncertain, particularly for women who are still experiencing IPV, although trauma-focused treatments hold at least some promise for reducing symptoms.

Although the assessment and treatment of the abuser should be carried out by professionals with expertise in this area, it can be helpful for general clinicians to have some awareness of the effects of treatment, as noted previously. The evidence for batterer treatment is mixed, with randomized controlled trials generally indicating little or no benefit or potential harm (i.e., increased recidivism),[A5] whereas other study designs with longer follow-up suggest that cognitive-behavioral interventions with an emphasis on gender relations may be effective in reducing violence. To date there is insufficient evidence to recommend specific treatment for those committing IPV. There is little trial evidence for couples therapy and uncertainty about its appropriateness or safety when IPV is present in a relationship. One trial in a military population showed some reduction in further violence, but it excluded couples in which the man had been violent in the past 6 months.[A6] Most authors caution that these couple therapy programs are not safe for many abused women, particularly those experiencing "intimate terrorism." Furthermore, when abusers are enrolled in treatment programs, it is important that women are provided with concurrent advocacy and support. There is some evidence to suggest that permanent, but not temporary, civil protection orders may be effective in reducing future violence.

With IPV now clearly identified as a health problem, there is increasing recognition of the need for education of all health care providers who encounter patients exposed to IPV. Two systematic reviews—one focused on physicians[A7] and a second on allied health care practitioners[A8]—found some improvements in knowledge and attitudes and, to a lesser extent, skills and behaviors, but there is no evidence to date for the effect of such training on patient outcomes.

PREVENTION

From a public health perspective, primary prevention of IPV is a priority, although most of the available research focuses on the health care response to the survivors of IPV, both while a woman is still exposed to abuse (secondary prevention) and when she is experiencing the long-term health problems associated with IPV (tertiary prevention).

Efforts aimed at primary prevention of IPV through educational programs have generally focused on changes in attitude, knowledge, skills, or self-reports of dating (relationship) violence. No studies to date have measured physical or emotional health outcomes. A meta-analysis assessing the efficacy of interventions aimed at preventing dating or relationship violence in adolescence and young adults (such violence is often considered a precursor to IPV in adulthood) concluded that there was no evidence that the interventions were effective in improving attitudes, behaviors, or skills related to relationship violence or reducing episodes of relationship violence.[A9]

There is no clinical trial evidence for the effectiveness of interventions provided in general medical settings with the aim of secondary prevention. A systematic review concluded that there is insufficient evidence to determine the effectiveness of interventions in preventing IPV against pregnant women.[A10] However, an advocacy and empowerment program in antenatal clinics reduced psychological and minor physical violence, and a program for pregnant African American women based on individual counseling sessions reduced violence and improved pregnancy outcomes.[A11] Within an Australian family medicine setting, there was equivocal benefit in terms of mental health and safety of a brief counseling intervention delivered by doctors.[A12] Outside of health care settings, intensive advocacy (12 hours or more duration) may reduce physical abuse among women leaving shelters or refuges after 12 to 24 months of follow-up, but not for shorter or longer follow-up. There is evidence that a training and support program for primary care clinicians improves identification of women experiencing abuse and referral to advocacy services.[A13] The WHO has published guidelines for the health care response to IPV with recommendations linked to the current evidence base.[17] Table 228-2 outlines the key recommendations related to prevention of IPV and treatment of conditions associated with exposure to IPV. Particularly noteworthy are the recommendation on training for clinicians in first-line support to women who have disclosed IPV and the recommendations against screening and mandatory reporting.

PROGNOSIS

The prognosis of IPV with and without intervention is uncertain. Trials of interventions have small samples and short follow-up, and most have substantial attrition of participants. As far as the "natural history" of the condition is concerned, cohort studies are rare, and cross-sectional studies are potentially misleading. In a 3-year follow-up of participants who received an advocacy intervention after leaving a shelter, 36% had been assaulted by their original partner or a new partner in the 6 months before the interview. The difference in re-victimization at 2 years between intervention and control arms did not persist, but there was still a significant difference in quality of life and social support among women receiving advocacy. In a U.S. cohort study, 37% of participants were still being abused after 3½ years.

TABLE 228-2   SUMMARY OF SELECTED INTIMATE PARTNER VIOLENCE RECOMMENDATIONS FROM THE WORLD HEALTH ORGANIZATION

CATEGORY	RECOMMENDATION	QUALITY OF EVIDENCE	STRENGTH OF RECOMMENDATION
Woman-centered care	Women who disclose any form of violence by an intimate partner (or other family member) should be offered immediate support by clinicians, at a minimum. If clinicians are unable to provide this first-line support, they should ensure that someone else (within their health care setting or another that is easily accessible) is immediately available to do so.	Indirect	Strong
Identification of survivors	Universal screening is not recommended.	Low-moderate	Conditional
	Ask about exposure to IPV when assessing conditions that may be caused or complicated by abuse.	Indirect	Strong
	Written information about IPV should be available in all health care settings.	No relevant evidence	Conditional
Care for survivors	Women with preexisting diagnosed or IPV-related mental disorders should receive mental health care delivered by health care professionals with a good understanding of violence against women.	Indirect	Strong
	Cognitive-behavioral therapy or eye movement desensitization and reprocessing interventions, delivered by health care professionals with a good understanding of violence against women, should be offered to women with post-traumatic stress disorder who are no longer experiencing violence.	Low-moderate	Strong
	Women who have spent at least 1 night in a shelter, refuge, or safe house should be offered a structured program of advocacy, support, and/or empowerment.	Low	Conditional
	Pregnant women should be offered brief- to medium-duration empowerment counseling (by counselors with specific training about IPV) and IPV advocacy/support, including a safety component.	Low	Conditional
	For children exposed to IPV at home, a psychotherapeutic intervention should be offered.	Moderate	Conditional
Training of clinicians	Training at prequalification level in first-line support for women who have experienced IPV should be given to clinicians (in particular physicians, nurses, and midwives).	Very low	Strong
	Clinicians offering care to women should receive in-service training integrated with training on managing sexual assault.	Low-moderate	Strong
Health care policy	Care for women experiencing IPV should be integrated into existing health services rather than as a stand-alone service.	Very low	Strong
Mandatory reporting	Mandatory reporting to the police by clinicians is not recommended; clinicians should offer to report the incident to the appropriate authorities (including the police) if the woman wants this and is aware of her rights.	Very low	Strong

IPV = intimate partner violence.
Reproduced from Feder G, Wathen CN, MacMillan HL. An evidence-based response to intimate partner violence: WHO guidelines. *JAMA* 2013;310:479-480.

Grade A References

A1. Feltner C, Wallace I, Berkman N, et al. Screening for intimate partner violence, elder abuse, and abuse of vulnerable adults: evidence report and systematic review for the US Preventive Services Task Force. *JAMA*. 2018;320:1688-1701.

A2. Rivas C, Ramsay J, Sadowski L, et al. Advocacy interventions to reduce or eliminate violence and promote the physical and psychosocial well-being of women who experience intimate partner abuse. *Cochrane Database Syst Rev*. 2015;12:CD005043.

A3. Tirado-Muñoz J, Gilchrist G, Farre M, et al. The efficacy of cognitive behavioural therapy and advocacy interventions for women who have experienced intimate partner violence: a systematic review and meta-analysis. *Ann Med*. 2014;46:567-586.

A4. Arroyo K, Lundahl B, Butters R, et al. Short-term interventions for survivors of intimate partner violence: a systematic review and meta-analysis. *Trauma Violence Abuse*. 2017;18:155-171.

A5. Nesset MB, Lara-Cabrera ML, Dalsbo TK, et al. Cognitive behavioural group therapy for male perpetrators of intimate partner violence: a systematic review. *BMC Psychiatry*. 2019;19:1-13.

A6. Taft CT, Creech SK, Gallagher MW, et al. Strength at Home couples program to prevent military partner violence: a randomized controlled trial. *J Consult Clin Psychol*. 2016;84:935-945.

A7. Zaher E, Keogh K, Ratnapalan S. Effect of domestic violence training: systematic review of randomized controlled trials. *Can Fam Physician*. 2014;60:618-624.

A8. Sawyer S, Coles J, Williams A, et al. A systematic review of intimate partner violence educational interventions delivered to allied health care practitioners. *Med Educ*. 2016;50:1107-1121.

A9. Fellmeth GL, Heffernan C, Nurse J, et al. Educational and skills-based interventions for preventing relationship and dating violence in adolescents and young adults. *Cochrane Database Syst Rev*. 2013;6:CD004534.

A10. Jahanfar S, Janssen PA, Howard LM, et al. Interventions for preventing or reducing domestic violence against pregnant women. *Cochrane Database Syst Rev*. 2013;2:CD009414.

A11. Kiely M, El-Mohandes AA, El-Khorazaty MN, et al. An integrated intervention to reduce intimate partner violence in pregnancy: a randomized controlled trial. *Obstet Gynecol*. 2010;115:273-283.

A12. Hegarty K, O'Doherty L, Taft A, et al. Screening and counselling in the primary care setting for women who have experienced intimate partner violence (WEAVE): a cluster randomised controlled trial. *Lancet*. 2013;382:249-258.

A13. Feder G, Davies RA, Baird K, et al. Identification and Referral to Improve Safety (IRIS) of women experiencing domestic violence with a primary care training and support programme: a cluster randomised controlled trial. *Lancet*. 2011;378:1788-1795.

GENERAL REFERENCES

For the General References and other additional features, please visit Expert Consult at https://expertconsult.inkling.com.

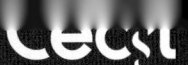

XXI

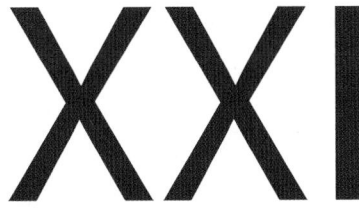

DISEASES OF BONE AND MINERAL METABOLISM

229

APPROACH TO THE PATIENT WITH METABOLIC BONE DISEASE

THOMAS J. WEBER

DIAGNOSIS

History

Patients with metabolic bone disease may present to the clinician in a number of ways, ranging from no symptoms to disabling musculoskeletal pain, depending on the nature of the underlying disorder. The most common conditions, osteoporosis and primary hyperparathyroidism, encompass a clinical spectrum that ranges from asymptomatic (diagnosed by low bone density and an elevated serum calcium, respectively) to severe disease (fractures and bone pain).[1,2] Less common conditions, such as osteomalacia, have more predictable presentations. In osteoporosis, fractures of the long bones (humerus, distal forearm, femur, and tibia) are clearly evident, whereas fractures at other sites (vertebrae, ribs, pelvis) may not be clinically apparent (see later and Chapter 230). Patients with osteomalacia may complain of deep bone pain or aches, although often it is difficult for them to distinguish such pain from muscular pain. They may also report proximal muscle weakness that impairs their ability to ascend stairs. Vitamin D deficiency, the most common cause of osteomalacia, may confer similar bone and muscle complaints as well. In hyperparathyroidism, either self-reported or elicited fatigue may be a common complaint, along with mildly impaired cognition and memory. A history of recurrent nephrolithiasis is a hallmark of symptomatic primary hyperparathyroidism. Patients with hypophosphatasia typically present with musculoskeletal pain and history of fractures.[3]

Physical Examination

Patients may exhibit physical clues to their skeletal condition. Height loss of more than 2 inches from a self-reported maximum, measured accurately with a calibrated stadiometer, may suggest the presence of vertebral compression fractures, which are clinically silent in up to three fourths of patients. Corresponding thoracic kyphosis may be present, and tenderness to palpation or percussion over the spinous process may suggest a recent vertebral fracture. Thoracic kyphosis will also impart quantifiable physical characteristics, including decreased and increased rib to pelvis and wall to occiput distances, respectively, which may be followed clinically in patients and significantly predict the presence of vertebral fractures. The method for the rib to pelvis distance measurement is illustrated in Figure 229-1. The wall to occiput distance is the space between the wall and the occiput of the head when a patient stands straight with the heel, buttocks, and back against the wall: it reflects the degree of kyphosis. Patients may also exhibit signs of secondary causes of osteoporosis (e.g., blue sclerae with osteogenesis imperfecta, goiter and proptosis with hyperthyroidism, facial plethora and purple striae with Cushing syndrome). Patients with Paget disease may have a skeletal deformity and warmth over the affected sites. Patients with osteomalacia often have tenderness to palpation over the tibia or other long bones due to expansion of the subperiosteal space by undermineralized osteoid with resultant periosteal nerve irritation. These patients may also have a wide-based, "waddling" gait due to pain. Hyperparathyroid patients may have flank tenderness if active nephrolithiasis is present and can rarely have corneal calcification if hypercalcemia is severe and long-standing. Such patients rarely have a palpable parathyroid adenoma. If present, however, a diagnosis of parathyroid carcinoma should be entertained.

Laboratory and Radiologic Investigations

Laboratory studies are a useful adjunct in the evaluation of metabolic bone disease, although their specificity depends somewhat on the disease in question. In particular, studies performed in the work-up of osteoporosis are generally not solely diagnostic but rather are supportive of secondary etiologies that may contribute to bone loss. Examples include thyroid-stimulating hormone, 25(OH)D, and testosterone levels (Table 229-1). In addition to a cursory work-up as detailed, additional investigations may also be required as clinically indicated and in individuals with a greater dual-energy x-ray absorptiometry (DXA) bone density deficit than expected for age (see later and Chapter 230).[4] In contrast, the diagnosis of other conditions is more securely based on abnormal biochemical studies, such as alkaline phosphatase (elevated in Paget disease and depressed in hypophosphatasia), serum phosphorus (abnormal in disorders of fibroblast growth factor 23 metabolism[5]), and parathyroid hormone (elevated in hyperparathyroidism). More sophisticated studies that target a specific diagnosis should be based on the history and examination (e.g., genetic testing for hypophosphatasia or osteogenesis imperfecta). Bone turnover markers, which are cellular products of bone formation and resorption that can be measured in the blood and urine of patients, may provide noninvasive information on skeletal turnover (i.e., high or low) but cannot be used for diagnosis. They also have unacceptable biologic and measurement variability that precludes their clinical usefulness at this time.

Radiologic studies are critical to the diagnosis and management of these patients. Because the most common clinical event is fracture, plain radiographs of the involved skeletal sites are often indicated. It is important to note that radiographs are relatively insensitive in identifying stress fractures and may also lag behind a frank fracture by hours or days. As such, additional, more sensitive modalities may be employed, including computed tomography and magnetic resonance imaging, to confirm a fracture. These studies also reveal characteristic patterns of skeletal involvement in certain conditions (e.g., Paget disease). Whole body bone scintigraphy with the radioisotope techneticum-99m is the most sensitive tool to identify an active skeletal process but is nonspecific as to the nature of the underlying process (e.g., fracture, infection, malignancy). Perhaps most widely used and critical to management of osteoporosis is bone mineral density (BMD) testing, generally by DXA. As detailed in Chapter 230, DXA is a low-radiation, noninvasive examination of the spine, proximal femur, and distal forearm that may be used to make serial assessments of the likelihood of future fracture[6] and to identify and subsequently follow the treatment response to pharmacologic or conservative therapies. Finally, although rarely needed, tetracycline-labeled, transcortical bone biopsy of the iliac crest, with subsequent histomorphometric analysis, may be useful in the

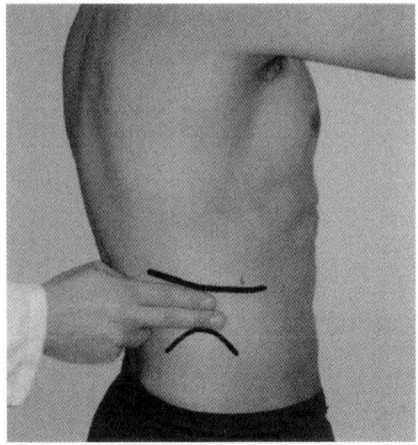

FIGURE 229-1. **Method of assessing rib-pelvis distance.** While standing behind the subject, the examiner holds his or her hands vertically and places them into the space between the inferior margin of the ribs and the superior surface of the pelvis in the mid-axillary line. The vertical distance is then measured in fingerbreadths.

TABLE 229-1 LABORATORY WORK-UP OF OSTEOPOROSIS

ALL OSTEOPOROSIS/OSTEOPENIA PATIENTS	AS CLINICALLY INDICATED
Serum creatinine, calcium, total protein, albumin, phosphorus, alkaline phosphatase, liver function tests	Serum and urine protein electrophoresis (SPEP and UPEP) (if total protein-to-albumin ratio is >2.0)
Complete blood count	Intact parathyroid hormone
Thyroid-stimulating hormone	24-Hour urine cortisol
24-Hour urine calcium and creatinine	Celiac panel (antigliadin/antiendomysial antibodies)
Serum 25(OH)D	Fasting morning testosterone (men)

management of patients. Bone biopsy, which is generally performed by an orthopedic surgeon under conscious sedation, may be indicated to guide management in patients with excessive bone fragility that cannot be adequately characterized by noninvasive means (e.g., patients with renal osteodystrophy, suspected osteomalacia, fractures with normal BMD by DXA).

TREATMENT   Rx

Management of patients with metabolic bone disease is generally directed by the disease process, although there are some unifying aspects of treatment. Adequate intake of calcium and vitamin D, usually through a combination of diet and supplements, is recommended for patients with osteoporosis. High-dose vitamin D is indicated for low-vitamin D–related osteomalacia. Phosphorus in combination with vitamin D analogues (i.e., calcitriol) is necessary to heal osteomalacia and facilitate normal longitudinal growth in children and adolescents and to promote mineralization and heal stress fractures in adults with certain osteomalacic conditions (e.g., X-linked hypophosphatemic rickets and tumor-induced osteomalacia). Weight bearing and resistive exercise are also advisable for osteoporotic patients, although physical therapy consultation may be indicated in patients at high risk for fracture (previous fractures, frequent falls). Pharmacotherapy with oral and parenteral bisphosphonates is frontline therapy for patients with both osteoporosis and Paget disease because of the anticatabolic effect on excessive osteoclastic bone resorption that underlies these diseases. In addition, other antiresorptive drugs, such as raloxifene and denosumab, are approved for the treatment of osteoporosis. Parenteral bisphosphonates and denosumab also are effective in combating malignancy-related bone disease (e.g., metastatic breast cancer, multiple myeloma). Finally, the anabolic bone agents teriparatide and abaloparatide, which are recombinant parathyroid hormone and parathyroid hormone–related peptide analogues respectively, are useful in "building" bone density and reducing fracture risk in patients with severe osteoporosis, defined as very low BMD, high fracture risk, and/or multiple fractures. Newer drugs in development that target more recently identified aspects of bone physiology (e.g., the Wnt pathway in bone formation), as well as specific derangements in less common diseases (e.g., FGF-23 antibody in X-linked hypophosphatemia), will undoubtedly further improve the management of patients with metabolic bone disease.

GENERAL REFERENCES

For the General References and other additional features, please visit Expert Consult at https://expertconsult.inkling.com.

230

OSTEOPOROSIS

THOMAS J. WEBER

DEFINITION

Osteoporosis is defined as a skeletal disorder characterized by compromised bone strength predisposing to an increased risk for fracture. The pertinent clinical outcomes of this disease include fractures, bone pain, height loss, and physical deformity. This definition was developed by the National Institutes of Health in 2000 to help clinicians better diagnose and treat patients with the disease. The concept of bone strength is central to understanding the disorder because patients who suffer an osteoporotic or fragility fracture may or may not have osteoporosis by bone mineral density (BMD) criteria. The World Health Organization defines *osteoporosis* as a BMD that is equal to or greater than 2 standard deviations below that of an average individual at peak bone mass (generally aged 20 to 30 years, depending on the measured skeletal site). However, it is well established that most fragility fractures, which are defined as fractures occurring from the energy imparted from a fall from a standing height or less, occur in individuals who have low (*osteopenia*) or even normal BMD. (Osteopenia, or low bone density, is defined as a BMD between −1.0 and −2.5 standard deviations below young average normal.) This

observation is consistent with the lack of a specific BMD threshold for fracture. Given these observations, it is clear that other factors must also significantly influence fracture risk. Certainly, falls and traumatic injuries are a significant, independent risk factor for fractures. Excluding falls and trauma, however, studies to date have also identified qualitative factors that are integral to bone strength, including skeletal microarchitecture, bone turnover, damage accumulation (e.g., microfractures), and pattern or degree of mineralization. Newer technologies are currently in development to improve our understanding of how these qualitative changes in bone compromise skeletal strength, including high-resolution peripheral quantitative computed tomography and high-resolution magnetic resonance imaging (MRI) (Fig. 230-1).[1] Although promising, these newer techniques are not widely available. More important, they have not enhanced fracture prediction to date over known risk factors and BMD. Indeed, the availability and widespread application of Internet-based fracture prediction tools such as FRAX, which incorporate independent, additive clinical risk factors for fracture with or without femoral neck BMD, are currently used to identify individuals at risk for and most likely to benefit from treatment to prevent fragility fractures.

EPIDEMIOLOGY

Approximately half of white women will develop an osteoporosis-related fracture in their lifetime,[2] which is greater than their risk for breast cancer, heart attack, and stroke combined. In addition, one in five men will also fracture. More than 2 million fractures occur annually in the United States, at an estimated total direct cost of $17 billion. Nearly three fourths of them occur in women, with most occurring in white women. Nonetheless, there are no ethnic exclusions to developing the disorder. The most common site of osteoporotic fracture is the spine, accounting for more than 750,000 fractures annually. Fractures of the proximal femur, which disproportionately confer a greater cost than other osteoporotic fractures, account for 14% of incident fractures but nearly three fourths of costs. Additional sites of fracture include the distal forearm, proximal humerus, and pelvis, with the latter two more commonly occurring in elderly people. The risk for fracture increases markedly with age, although the pattern of fracture risk does differ by skeletal site. The risk for Colles fractures increases until the mid-60s and then plateaus, whereas the risk for hip fractures increases exponentially in woman after the age of 65 years. Vertebral fracture risk rises earlier than that of hip, although many spine fractures are not clinically apparent and are only identified through radiographic assessment. Although clinically silent, such fractures do confer a significant independent risk for future fractures, particularly if they are of recent occurrence. Men also ascribe to an age-independent increase in fracture risk, although the increase in incidence generally lags at least 5 to 10 years behind that of women (Fig 230-2). The reason for the gender-based difference in fracture incidence is likely related to anatomic differences. Specifically, although men and woman have similar volumetric bone density at a given skeletal site, bone size is larger in men than in women and confers an independent mechanical protection against fracture. Nonetheless, the independent contribution of age to fracture risk necessarily predicts a higher morbidity and cost related to osteoporosis in older men as well as women, with an increase in the United States alone by the year 2025 to greater than 3 million fractures with an associated annual cost of $25.3 billion. Despite these ominous predictions, recent data suggest that less than one third of women who incur a low-trauma hip fracture undergo bone mass measurement or initiate pharmacologic antifracture

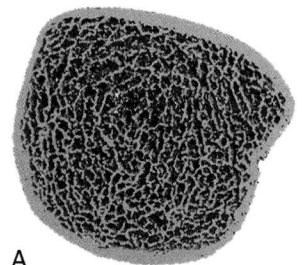 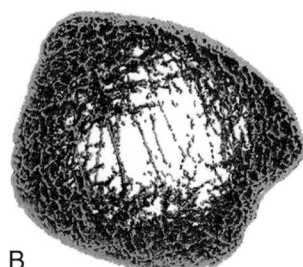

A   B

FIGURE 230-1. High-resolution peripheral computed tomography (Xtreme CT) of distal tibia in subject with normal bone mineral density (A) and severe osteoporosis (B). The deterioration in trabecular architecture with reduced trabecular number, trabecular thinning, increased trabecular spacing, generalized cortical thinning, and increased cortical porosity is readily appreciable in the osteoporotic subject. (From Griffith JF, Genant HK. New advances in imaging osteoporosis and its complications. *Endocrine.* 2012;42: 39-51.)

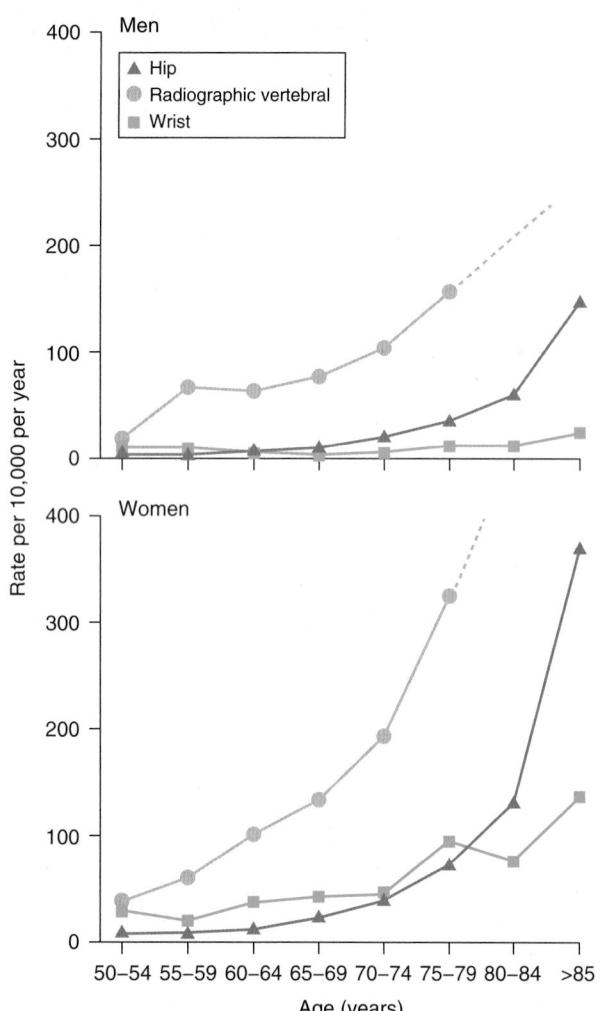

FIGURE 230-2. Age-specific and sex-specific incidence of radiographic vertebral, hip, and distal forearm fractures. (Data derived from European Prospective Osteoporosis Study and General Practice Research Database; from Sambrook P, Cooper C. Osteoporosis. *Lancet.* 2006;367:2010-2018.)

therapy, underscoring the need for significant improvement in the delivery of osteoporosis care.[3]

There are also significant ethnic and geographic differences in the rate of osteoporotic fractures. African Americans have a lower lifetime risk for osteoporotic fracture, approximately half that of whites. Differences in bone size, bone microarchitecture (thicker trabeculae in blacks), body composition, calcium absorption in youth, and life expectancy are potential reasons for this observation. Asian Americans and Hispanics have a fracture risk that is intermediate between that of whites and blacks, despite the fact that the former have a BMD that generally approximates that of whites. Indeed, the risk for hip fracture in U.S. Asian men and women is actually equal to or lower than that of U.S. blacks. The U.S. data are consistent with the global experience as well because hip fracture rates in China are lower than those observed in the United States, despite similar bone density at the hip. Differences in hip geometry, physical activity, and diet have been proposed as possible explanations. Despite this, rates of hip fracture have actually been increasing in the Far East, while declining in the United States for unclear reasons. Changing patterns of nutrition and physical activity could be responsible for the former, although the latter observation remains heretofore unexplained. Based on the most recent data, however, there is evidence that the observed decline in hip fracture rates in the United States has plateaued, perhaps in part because of concomitant declines in femoral neck BMD.[4]

PATHOBIOLOGY
Normal Bone Biology

BMD in adults is determined by the magnitude of bone acquisition during adolescence and young adulthood and the rate of bone loss that ensues thereafter. These processes are generally referred to as bone modeling and

remodeling, respectively. Heritable factors, including gender and ethnicity, account for 60 to 80% of the variability in skeletal development, including peak bone mass, bone size, and bone geometry, although nutrition, lifestyle, and other factors also have a significant impact. Peak bone mass is achieved in most individuals by the early to late 20s and differs in timing by skeletal site (ages 18 to 20 years for proximal femur, 25 to 30 years for spine). Modeling of the skeleton occurs during this time and represents a true increase in bone mass and bone size through endochondral ossification of the axial skeleton and periosteal apposition of the appendicular skeleton.

To best understand the underlying pathophysiology of osteoporosis, one must first appreciate the concept of bone remodeling. Skeletal remodeling is a finely orchestrated process of bone resorption and subsequent formation. It is a necessary physiologic function that results in repair of damaged bone and redistribution of the skeleton to adapt to changes in mechanical stress and to provide calcium to the systemic circulation for critical cellular processes. Recent evidence suggests that the osteocyte, which accounts for 90 to 95% of all bone cells, is the critical cell that regulates both resorption and formation. Osteocytes are derived from osteoblasts that are embedded within the bone matrix. During this maturation phase, this "osteoid-osteocyte" cell actively secretes and calcifies bone matrix material. In addition, mature osteocytes within bone contain dendritic processes that may directly regulate osteoblast recruitment and bone formation. Recent studies also suggest that mature osteocytes may form new bone within their lacunae. In addition, osteocytes produce proteins that regulate mineralization, including positive (PHEX, DMP-1) and negative (FGF-23) factors.

Osteocytes also regulate bone resorption, both directly through apoptosis proximate to skeletal microcracks or fatigue damage in need of repair and indirectly through enhancement of pre-osteoblast or mesenchymal stromal cell development. (Mesenchymal stromal cells may also develop into adipocytes, chondrocytes, and muscle cells, depending on developmental stimuli.) These events result in the production, expression, and release of cytokines critical to osteoclast recruitment and development, including interleukin-1 (IL-1), IL-6, osteoprotegerin (OPG), and receptor activator of nuclear factor-κB ligand (RANKL). The cognate receptor for RANKL, RANK, is expressed on the surface of the developing and mature osteoclast, which itself is a derivative of cells of the monocyte-macrophage lineage. RANKL is a critical determinant of osteoclast recruitment, development, and survival, such that disruption of RANKL signaling results in high bone density fragility disorders (e.g., osteopetrosis). OPG, which is also produced by pre-osteoblasts, is a decoy receptor for RANK that binds to RANKL, preventing RANKL binding to RANK and thereby serving as an endogenous suppresser of osteoclast function. In essence, RANKL/OPG represent a "yin/yang" paradigm in which osteoclast biology and bone resorption are intricately regulated and controlled (E-Fig. 230-1).

Factors Affecting Peak Bone Mass and Remodeling

As mentioned, peak bone mass is achieved by the third decade. Longitudinal studies in children and adolescents suggest that hormonal, physical activity, nutritional, and genetic factors are all important in this process. Hereditary influence is the most important determinant and to date the least well understood. Growth hormone and sex hormones play critical roles in growth of the appendicular (long bones) and axial (vertebrae) skeleton, with the former maturing earlier than the latter (end of puberty vs. young adulthood). Males have larger bones as a result of greater periosteal (outer surface of bone) expansion of bone than occurs in females. Current evidence supports a positive effect of exercise and loading on bone size and mineral density, although a subsequent potential antifracture benefit later in adult life is not proved. Poor nutrition and concomitant disease may also affect bone accrual, primarily through delayed pubertal onset and progression, although studies do support a potential for "catch-up" growth, which depends on the degree of insult and timing of resolution.

Although these factors are all important, genetic factors appear to account for 60 to 80% of the variance in peak BMD. Genome-wide association studies have identified 62 distinct loci that are significantly associated with BMD. Additionally, it has become clear that genetic determination of BMD is relatively skeletal site-specific (E-Fig. 230-2).[5] Three known obligatory pathways of bone metabolism were identified by genome-wide association studies, namely Wnt, RANK-RANKL-OPG, and endochondral ossification. The RANK pathway was discussed previously. The Wnt signaling pathway is obligatory for bone formation, owing to its role in osteoblast proliferation and differentiation. Endochondral ossification, a process that involves the cartilage growth plate and subsequent ossification of the cartilaginous skeleton, is dependent on transcription factors (SOX6, RUNX2) and proteins (parathyroid hormone–related peptide, bone sialoprotein 2, and osteopontin) that are necessary for the development of the cartilage growth plate, bone matrix mineralization, and osteoblast differentiation. All three pathways are now the target of existing and developing therapies for osteoporosis.

In adults, bone remodeling is a physiologic process through which skeletal repair and adaption to changes in biomechanical stress occur. The bone remodeling cycle occurs in the basic multicellular unit, which itself is composed of bone-resorbing osteoclasts, bone-forming osteoblasts, bone lining cells, and embedded osteocytes and is the apparatus that facilitates remodeling (E-Fig. 230-3). After the age of 30 years, this process is reasonably matched, resulting in rates of bone loss of only 0.3 to 0.5% per year from the third through fifth decades of life. As individuals age, mismatches in bone remodeling, either due to reduced formation, increased resorption, or a combination of both, result in greater rates of bone loss. Biologic changes, such as menopause and aging, systemic disease, personal vices, and medications (most notably glucocorticoids), may contribute to this imbalance. In addition, there is evidence that genetic factors influence rates of bone loss and fracture,[6] even if current information is not adequate for true genetic profiling.[7]

Mechanisms of Bone Loss
"Natural" and Aging-Related Bone Loss
The rate of net bone loss accelerates during the latter decades because of a number of factors. Perhaps most important for women, rates of bone loss increase substantially in the perimenopausal and early postmenopausal years, amounting to losses of 1 to 5% per year. Unfortunately, there are currently no biologic markers that help determine which women a priori are "rapid losers." Bone loss is slower in obese women, likely because of higher estrogen levels afforded by production through aromatization in adipose tissue. A decline in circulating estrogen is primarily responsible for bone loss following both natural and surgical menopause, which is mediated primarily through upregulation of cytokines (most notably RANKL) and a resultant increase in the number, activity, and depth of osteoclast-mediated bone resorption sites. In addition, OPG production is diminished, further amplifying bone resorption, although estrogen replacement can restore OPG production while reducing RANKL expression and thereby help mitigate bone loss during this period. Although bone resorption and formation do occur sequentially during this period, resorption outpaces formation because of potentiation of the former aided by the release of soluble cytokines, resulting in a significant uncoupling of bone remodeling and accelerated bone loss. Fortunately, this phase of rapid bone loss is typically limited to 5 to 7 years in most women. Finally, there is emerging evidence for regulation of coupling between bone formation and resorption by other factors in the bone microenvironment (e.g., transforming growth factor-β1, sphingosine 1-phosphate) that could be therapeutically exploited for skeletal benefit in the future.

Secondary Causes and Clinical Impact of Bone Loss
Bone loss also occurs as a result of secondary processes, such as diseases and medications. In fact, such processes are identifiable in more than one fourth of individuals with osteoporosis and may be more likely with greater degrees of skeletal deficit. A list of secondary causes of osteoporosis, using a systems-based approach, is detailed in Table 230-1. As expected, endocrine disorders, including hypogonadism and Cushing syndrome, predominate. Nonetheless, bone loss in several conditions is mediated indirectly through attendant effects on vitamin D metabolism (e.g., malabsorption, chronic liver disease) and is the case with certain medications as well (antiepileptic drugs phenytoin and phenobarbital). In the case of vitamin D deficiency, undermineralization of bone may confound the clinical picture of bone loss (Chapter 231) and should be considered first before initiation of bone active medications (see later). Rarely, malignancies can be the principal cause of osteoporosis, with the best example being multiple myeloma (Chapter 178). Myeloma causes bone loss through uncoupling of bone resorption and formation. Medications also cause bone loss through both osteoclastic activation and osteoblastic inhibition. Reduced bone formation is the mechanism by which glucocorticoids cause bone loss, through both exogenous administration and endogenous overproduction.[8] Previous work has confirmed reduced osteoblast and osteocyte function and survival as the principal mechanism of glucocorticoid-induced osteoporosis. Anorexia nervosa likely interferes with the anabolic effect of insulin-like growth factor-I on bone. Alcohol excess appears to suppress osteoblast function, perhaps both directly and indirectly through associated malnutrition, but it may also possibly cause bone loss through hypogonadism,

TABLE 230-1 SECONDARY CAUSES OF OSTEOPOROSIS
ENDOCRINE DISORDERS
Hypogonadism: female and male
Hypercortisolism: endogenous and exogenous
Hyperthyroidism
Hyperparathyroidism
Idiopathic hypercalciuria
Diabetes mellitus: type 1 and type 2
NUTRITIONAL AND GASTROINTESTINAL DISORDERS
Malabsorption: celiac disease, gastrointestinal bypass
Vitamin D deficiency
Cirrhosis (including primary biliary cirrhosis)
Pancreatic insufficiency
Inflammatory bowel disease
Cystic fibrosis
Anorexia nervosa, bulimia
HEMATOLOGIC AND ONCOLOGIC DISORDERS
Multiple myeloma
Hemolytic anemia
Hemoglobinopathies: thalassemia, sickle cell
Myeloproliferative neoplasms
Skeletal metastases
Pompe disease
Mastocytosis
CONNECTIVE TISSUE AND METABOLIC DISORDERS
Osteogenesis imperfecta
Ehlers-Danlos syndrome
Marfan syndrome
Homocystinuria
Gaucher disease
Pompe disease
MEDICATIONS
Glucocorticoids
Aromatase inhibitors
Thyroxine (excessive)
Antiepileptics
Heparin
Gonadotropin-releasing hormone agonists
Depo-Provera
Immunosuppressants: tacrolimus, cyclosporine
Chemotherapy
Selective serotonin reuptake inhibitors*
Proton pump inhibitors*
Thiazolidinediones*
Sodium glucose cotransporter 2 inhibitors*
Alcohol
MISCELLANEOUS
Rheumatoid arthritis
Immobilization
Juvenile osteoporosis
Pregnancy-associated osteoporosis

*Association based.

which results in accelerated bone turnover. Finally, relatively rare connective tissue disorders, such as osteogenesis imperfecta and Marfan syndrome, increase skeletal fragility by means of disturbances in the skeletal matrix and mechanical integrity rather than altered bone remodeling.

The resulting clinical impact of bone loss and the persistence of effect depend on a number of factors, both potentially modifiable and nonmodifiable. The age at which bone loss occurs (e.g., young adult vs. 80-year-old) affects the ability to recover BMD with resolution or treatment of the condition (younger people have more robust recovery than elderly people) and also appears to hold for conditions of accelerated bone resorption (e.g., immobilization) or reduced bone formation (e.g., glucocorticoids). Predicated on and paralleling this observation, BMD response to treatment is generally more pronounced in individuals with higher rates of bone turnover, likely reflecting to some extent a "filling in" of bone remodeling space. Menopausal stage in women also influences rate of bone loss as described previously, with greater rates of decline occurring within the first 5 to 7 years of cessation of menses (Chapter 227). Concomitant vitamin D deficiency and resulting secondary hyperparathyroidism also potentiate rates of BMD loss, particularly in elderly people;

this is thought to be a major contributing factor to the increase in hip fracture incidence in this group. Tobacco and alcohol overuse may also accelerate bone loss, owing to global effects that include reduced sex hormones, altered calcium metabolism, and weight loss and frailty, resulting in uncoupled bone remodeling. Therefore, a distinct appreciation of the clinical context is critical to defining an appropriate diagnostic and treatment approach to patients with osteoporosis.

CLINICAL MANIFESTATIONS

Historically, osteoporosis was diagnosed in an individual presenting with a low trauma or fragility fracture, typically of the vertebrae or hips. Classic representations of women with the so-called dowager's hump or kyphotic deformity were common depictions of the disease. Currently, however, the disease is appreciated both for its clinical and subclinical manifestations, because of both the advent of bone density testing and the appreciation that many vertebral fractures are clinically silent. This approach is akin to paradigms that identify a surrogate marker for both diagnosis and risk stratification, such as hypertension for stroke and hyperlipidemia for myocardial infarction.

A history of fragility fracture is strongly suggestive of osteoporosis, although there is evidence that a history of high-trauma fractures also identifies persons with low BMD and those at higher risk for low-trauma fractures. The National Osteoporosis Foundation considers fractures of the spine, proximal femur, distal forearm, and proximal humerus "major" osteoporotic fractures, although other skeletal sites are also prone to fragility fractures. These include the pelvis, ribs, and proximal tibia, although there is controversy about whether ankle fractures should be considered as such. Fractures of the spine are generally from the midthoracic region through the lower lumbar region, with the greatest frequency at T11 through L2.[9] Patients often present after a fall or a spinal flexion-loading event in which they may hear a "pop" and complain of sharp midline back pain that may radiate to the flanks. Patients may also present with complaints of back "tiredness," which is improved with sitting or lying down. This symptom is likely related to paraspinal weakness or spasm from abnormal spinal curvature that occurs with chronic vertebral compression. Back pain may commonly be related to other pathology, such as degenerative disc and spine disease that is concomitantly present. This is important to note because low bone mass in and of itself does not cause pain, unless it is due to osteomalacia (see later). Vertebral fractures may occur without acute symptoms as well, as noted later. In contrast, nonvertebral fracture events are always clinically evident. Hip fractures generally occur with falls, although they may rarely occur with limited force such as twisting.

Physical examination may also indicate the presence of osteoporosis and associated fractures, as well as potentially identifying underlying secondary processes contributing to the disease. Measured height loss, best confirmed using a calibrated device such as a stadiometer, of greater than 4 cm since young adult maximum height is suggestive of prior vertebral fractures. Height loss also occurs with scoliosis and aging (approximately ⅓ inch of height is lost per decade after age 50 years). A kyphotic deformity of the upper thoracic spine may be present, although it is important to distinguish it from accentuated cervical lordosis with associated prominence of T1. Spinal tenderness to palpation and percussion can occur with an acute vertebral compression fracture. Palpable tenderness of the long bones may suggest underlying osteomalacia instead, due to periosteal expansion and nerve irritation. Reduced rib-pelvis and increased wall-occiput distances are correlated with vertebral fractures as well.

In addition to the history and physical examination, radiologic findings may identify the presence of osteoporosis, sometimes somewhat surreptitiously. Plain films can detect bone loss by means of accentuation of vertical striations on spine radiographs that represent loss of horizontal trabeculae, although this generally indicates BMD loss of at least 25% or more. Kyphosis and compression fractures may be present, and patients often are unaware of the deformities because nearly three fourths of such fractures occur without acute pain. Furthermore, radiologic reporting of these fractures is inconsistent, suggesting that, if possible, the clinician should review available digitized lateral chest radiographs and even lateral scout films often available from computed tomography (CT) to identify such fractures (Fig. 230-3). This is critical for optimal management, given the aforementioned risk conferred by previous fractures on future fracture events. The degree of compression fracture is also important because more severe fractures (>25% vertebral height loss) appear to predict future fractures better, as do nonvertebral fractures. When recent fractures are suspected, CT and MRI may be used, given that plain radiographs have a lower sensitivity acutely and with stress fractures. MRI also can be used to define a vertebral fracture with persistent swelling and edema based

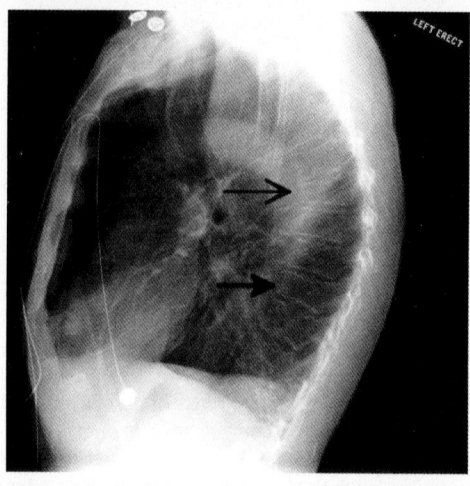

FIGURE 230-3. Incidental vertebral compression fractures on chest radiograph. Lateral radiograph of the chest of a 74-year-old man studied for cough. No relevant pulmonary abnormality was noted on the frontal radiograph (not shown). Examination of the thoracic spine shows the presence of a mild anterior wedge compression fracture of T9 (*thick arrow*) and moderate anterior wedge fracture of T6 (*thin arrow*). Neither fracture was reported on the radiographic report.

on T2 characteristics, potentially identifying patients who could benefit from vertebroplasty or kyphoplasty (see later). Finally, whole body bone scintigraphy is the most sensitive test for fracture but can be falsely positive because of inflammation, infection, or tumor and usually is positive for 6 to 12 months after a fracture event.

DIAGNOSIS

Although a recent fragility fracture is a reasonable basis for diagnosis of osteoporosis, other skeletal conditions should also be entertained, including inherited and acquired osteomalacias and pathologic fracture due to malignancy. These disorders can often be distinguished by history and physical examination, although additional investigations may be required. This distinction is critical because therapies may differ greatly between disorders. Most patients with osteoporosis are diagnosed on the basis of BMD measurement, generally by dual-energy x-ray absorptiometry.[10] Dual-energy x-ray absorptiometry is a low-radiation-based radiologic measurement of the areal bone density (g/cm^2) of the lumbar spine, proximal femur, and distal radius. Osteoporosis can be diagnosed if the BMD of a postmenopausal woman or man older than 50 years is more than 2.5 standard deviations below young average normal individuals (T score ≤−2.5). A T score between −1.0 and −2.5 is considered low bone density or osteopenia, and a Z score (age-matched BMD) in premenopausal women and men younger than 50 years that is more than 2 standard deviations below that of an average age-matched individual is considered low bone density for age. BMD is an independent predictor of fracture risk, such that the relative risk for fracture increases by 1.5- to 2-fold for each 1 standard deviation decrease in T score. In addition, fracture risk increases exponentially below a T score of −2.5. Furthermore, BMD of the femoral neck may be used in fracture prediction models such as FRAX to define better an individual's risk for subsequent fracture (see later). In addition to dual-energy x-ray absorptiometry, other modalities are also used to diagnose osteoporosis, including quantitative CT of the spine (quantitative CT) and wrist and tibia (peripheral quantitative CT), finger dual-energy x-ray absorptiometry, and ultrasound of the calcaneus or wrist. Measurement of BMD by all of these techniques has been shown to predict fractures globally, akin to dual-energy x-ray absorptiometry. Quantitative CT and peripheral quantitative CT provide additional information on cortical and trabecular bone compartments but are accompanied by higher radiation exposure and poorer reproducibility compared with dual-energy x-ray absorptiometry. Ultrasound is radiation free and easy to operate but is less sensitive in diagnosing osteoporosis and does not measure change in a reliable fashion in response to age or treatment, making it useful as a screening modality but not for longitudinal care. Finally, continued development of additional imaging tools (HRpQCT and mMRI) may well further refine the risk for fragility fractures.

Although dual-energy x-ray absorptiometry is an effective diagnostic tool, several potential limitations and caveats need to be considered by the clinician. First, dual-energy x-ray absorptiometry cannot distinguish between low bone density and undermineralized bone matrix, the latter of which occurs in osteomalacia (Chapter 231). BMD may also be quite disparate between regions, perhaps in more than one third of individuals. This inconsistency results from a number of factors, including differences in bone composition (predominantly trabecular bone in the spine and cortical bone in the one-third radius), with resultant variations in rates of bone loss due to aging and disease (vertebral bone loss with menopause and glucocorticoid use vs. cortical bone loss in hyperparathyroidism). Degenerative changes due to aging, such as facet osteoarthritis and aortic calcification, may artifactually raise spine BMD value. Given these considerations, the lowest skeletal site should be used for diagnosis. Finally, BMD should be measured longitudinally on the same dual-energy x-ray absorptiometry machine if possible, because of intermachine and inter-manufacturer differences that may confound the ability to measure change over time validly. Despite these caveats, dual-energy x-ray absorptiometry remains the best method to diagnose and manage osteoporosis by bone density testing.

Despite its utility, bone density has been limited historically in optimally predicting fracture risk in individual patients.[11] In addition, BMD does not take into account clinical factors that independently predict fracture. Under this premise, fracture prediction models have been developed that combine BMD and risk factors to stratify fracture risk better. The best known and most widely used of these prediction models is FRAX. FRAX was developed by the World Health Organization in collaboration with national and international osteoporosis foundations as an Internet-based computer algorithm that defines a person's 10-year risk for hip and major osteoporotic fracture (hip, clinical spine, forearm, and proximal humerus all combined). The model uses country-specific data on clinical risk factors and femoral neck BMD to calculate fracture probability and is available as a Web-based tool that can be used by clinicians with their patients to assist in making informed decisions on osteoporosis management (http://www.shef.ac.uk/FRAX/). A modified FRAX tool is also available to define better the risk for major osteoporotic fracture in individuals with disparately lower lumbar spine than proximal femur BMD. FRAX can be also be used to define country-specific recommended diagnostic and treatment thresholds. An example of this is the National Osteoporosis Foundation guidance that 10-year risks equal to or exceeding 3 and 20% for hip and major fracture risk, respectively, warrant consideration of pharmacologic treatment, which is based on cost-effective analyses in the United States. Furthermore, the number needed to treat (NNT) can be determined to inform patients of their expected risks and benefits of treatment (e.g., bisphosphonate use roughly reduces hip fracture risk by half, or from 10 to 5%, with NNT of 1/0.05, or 20 patients treated to prevent one hip fracture). Despite its utility and ease of use, FRAX does have limitations. These include inability to use patients who are not treatment naïve, absence of fall history/fall risk in the model, and use of fixed clinical risk factors. The 2018 updated Recommendation Statement on osteoporosis screening[12,13] revised its 2011 endorsement of FRAX to identify candidates for screening women aged 50 to 64 years (young postmenopausal) in view of studies published in the interval that found FRAX to be inferior to other tools in screening this group. The 2018 U.S. Preventive Services Task Force now recommends that screening women younger than 65 years for osteoporosis should use a number of formal clinical risk assessment tools, including FRAX, the Simple Calculated Osteoporosis Risk Estimation (SCORE), and the Osteoporosis Self-Assessment Tool (OST). Modifications have been suggested for the latest guidelines, including adjusting FRAX score up or down based on glucocorticoid dose. In addition, although fracture risk calculators that incorporate fall risk are available (e.g., from the Garvan Institute), they do not include the competing risk for mortality as FRAX does. As such, FRAX should be viewed as a complementary tool to BMD in best defining a person's risk for fracture and candidacy for pharmacologic intervention.[14] Finally, recent evidence suggests that the use of a Trabecular Bone Score with FRAX, which is a textural index surrogate measure of bone architecture that can be performed at the same time as dual-energy x-ray absorptiometry, can better predict the risk for FRAX-calculated hip and major osteoporotic fractures (Fig. 230-4).[15]

Finally, all patients presenting with osteoporosis require an assessment for secondary causes of bone loss, given that 20 to 25% of women and perhaps an even greater portion of men will have identifiable additional etiologies that may contribute to bone loss (see Table 230-1). Most patients will have had routine chemistry, hematology, and thyroid studies as part of their annual examination. The 25(OH)D level should be measured in all patients for multiple reasons, as previously discussed. Additional investigations may also be considered, as directed by the clinical history and physical examination. In addition, a greater degree of BMD deficit (i.e., lower Z score) indicates a need for more extensive testing, given the greater likelihood of secondary causes being present. Bone turnover markers are serum and urinary products of bone formation or resorption that can also be used to assist in management. Available tests include bone-specific alkaline phosphatase, osteocalcin, type I procollagen amino-terminal propeptide, and type I procollagen carboxy-terminal propeptide as formation markers, and serum and urine C- and N-terminal peptides of type I collagen as resorption markers, among others.[16] Their use is predicated on studies showing that high bone turnover increases fracture risk independent of BMD. In addition, fracture risk reduction correlates well with reduction in bone turnover based on clinical trials with anticatabolic agents. Nonetheless, their clinical utility has been tempered to date by several issues. First, there is significant biologic variability due to nonmodifiable (e.g., age, gender, underlying comorbid disease, medications) and modifiable (e.g., time of day, food intake, presence of fracture) factors that limit the ability to detect meaningful change over time in an individual patient. Second, optimal specimen processing is required for valid results and interpretation. Finally, and perhaps in part secondary to these issues and others, evidence to date

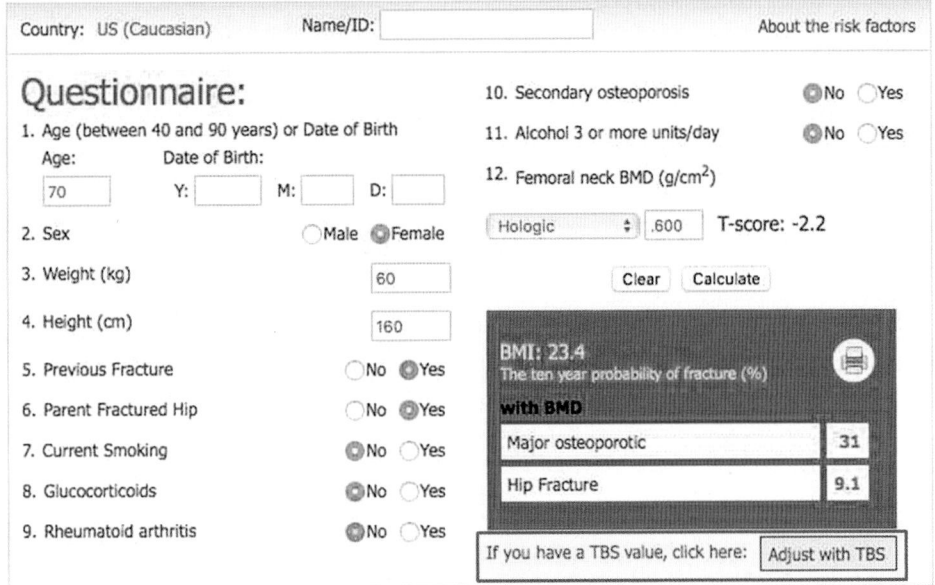

FIGURE 230-4. The FRAX® tool (http://www.shef.ac.uk/FRAX) is an online fracture risk estimation application that can be used to determine an individual patient's 10-year risk for hip fracture and major osteoporotic fracture (hip, clinical spine, distal forearm, and proximal humerus). It can also be used with a patient's Trabecular Bone Score (TBS iNsight) to analyze the quantity and quality of bone matrix and significantly add to the FRAX estimation of fracture risk.

does not demonstrate significant benefit of bone turnover markers in individual patients in securely predicting bone density increase, fracture risk reduction, or cost-effectiveness through patient feedback and improved adherence. Therefore, at present, bone turnover markers should not be used in routine clinical practice, although they could help inform management in more complicated cases of metabolic bone disease.

PREVENTION AND TREATMENT   Rx

Calcium

Adequate intake of calcium is critical to the optimal accumulation and maintenance of BMD. Calcium supplementation has meaningful impact on BMD (modestly improved by 1 to 2%), but evidence of a definitive reduction in hip and nonvertebral fracture risk when given without vitamin D is lacking at present.[A1] Given the established increase in rate of nephrolithiasis and a possible, albeit unproved, potential increase in nonfatal cardiac events with higher dose calcium supplementation, it would seem prudent to recommend that adults with osteoporosis obtain 1200 to 1500 mg of calcium from a combination of supplements and dietary sources. In support of this approach, a recent meta-analysis and resultant guidelines have not supported the restricted use of calcium supplements on the basis of cardiovascular concerns.[17]

Vitamin D

Appropriate circulating levels of 25(OH)D are necessary for optimal intestinal absorption of calcium and skeletal accrual and maintenance. Despite this, a significant proportion of children and adults have vitamin D levels that would be deemed insufficient (i.e., 25[OH]D <20 ng/mL). Data in adults with osteopenia and osteoporosis confirm a benefit of vitamin D supplementation for fracture risk reduction,[A2] although the effect is dependent on the patient population and the amount of supplementation. Doses of 400 to 800 IU of vitamin D combined with 1000 mg of calcium reduce the risk for hip fracture in postmenopausal women and men aged 65 years and older, although the benefit is less certain for community-dwelling individuals than for those in assisted living centers.[A3] Although some data suggest that a 25(OH)D level of at least 30 ng/mL is needed to reduce the risk for hip fracture, there is considerable controversy as to whether a vitamin D level above 30 ng/mL reduces the overall risk for fracture.[A4]

By comparison, routine vitamin D (with or without calcium supplementation) does not appear to prevent falls or fractures in community-dwelling adults without osteoporosis, vitamin D deficiency, or prior fractures.[A5][A6] Although activated vitamin D analogues such as calcitriol and α-calcidiol have been shown to reduce fracture risk, they are generally not indicated based on unacceptable risk for hypercalcemia. The exception to use of vitamin D analogues is possibly patients with stages 3 and 4 chronic kidney disease, wherein treatment of secondary hyperparathyroidism could provide skeletal benefit.

Exercise and Lifestyle

Physical activity is also a critical element of osteoporosis management, which can be indirectly inferred based on the known profound effects of decreased gravitational force (i.e., immobilization, paraplegia, weightlessness in space) on inducing bone loss.[A7] Physical activity likely also confers additional benefits through enhanced muscle strength, improved cardiovascular status, and reduction in fall risk. Meta-analysis confirmed a modest benefit of exercise on lumbar spine (mean difference = 0.85%) and trochanteric BMD (mean difference = 1.03%) in postmenopausal women compared with placebo, although it did not show significant changes in femoral neck or total hip BMD.[A8] However, studies to date have not confirmed an improvement in bone strength with exercise in this patient group. Studies concerning middle-aged and older men are much more limited in number and quality, although preliminary evidence suggests that resistance training with or without impact-loading activities has the greatest BMD benefit. Importantly, although none of the aforementioned studies have demonstrated a clear antifracture benefit from exercise, there are abundant data that multiple targeted exercise interventions do reduce either the risk for falling (Tai Chi) or both the rate and risk for falling (group and home-based exercise programs), which is the most likely inciting event in older patients incurring an osteoporotic fracture (Chapter 22). Finally, modification of aberrant lifestyles is also indicated in patients with osteoporosis, especially tobacco cessation and moderation of caffeine, carbonated beverage, and alcohol intake. Data are lacking, however, on whether these reduce overall fracture risk.

Medications

There is robust evidence that pharmacologic therapy significantly reduces the risk for osteoporotic fracture in a clinically meaningful and cost-effective manner.[18] Medications approved for osteoporosis can be classified based on their mechanism of action: anticatabolic (i.e., antiresorptive) and anabolic (i.e., bone building).

Anticatabolic Agents

Anticatabolic (or antiresorptive) medications inhibit osteoclast recruitment, function, and/or survival, resulting in reductions in skeletal turnover and bone loss. These agents, depending on the potency and persistence of bone effect, reduce the number of new activation sites (basic multicellular units) and the bone remodeling space, thereby improving BMD while strengthening the skeletal microstructure and reducing fracture risk.

Bisphosphonates

Bisphosphonates are the most widely prescribed and used medications for the treatment of osteoporosis, owing in large part to good tolerability and an ability to dose them infrequently (from once weekly to once yearly, depending on the drug). Bisphosphonates are chemically engineered analogues of the naturally occurring molecule pyrophosphate in which a carbon is substituted for an oxygen. As a result, bisphosphonates have an extremely high affinity for hydroxyapatite crystals within bone. After incorporation into bone, bisphosphonates are taken up by osteoclasts and thereafter inhibit cellular attachment, function, and survival. The carbon side-chain molecules largely determine skeletal affinity and potency of bisphosphonate effect. The first-generation bisphosphonate etidronate, which is not approved in the United States for treatment of osteoporosis, is the least potent agent of the class. It must also be given in an interrupted fashion for 2 weeks every 3 months owing to the potential to cause focal osteomalacia, and it may cause lower gastrointestinal symptoms (i.e., abdominal pain and diarrhea). Nonetheless, it is has been shown to reduce the risk for vertebral but not nonvertebral nor hip fractures.

Three oral bisphosphonates are approved by the U.S. Food and Drug Administration (FDA) and currently available in the United States: alendronate, risedronate, and ibandronate, in order of time since initial FDA approval. All three drugs are also available as generic preparations, although some differences do exist between the brand name and generic drugs in regard to the inactive excipients. The oral bisphosphonates may be administered once weekly (alendronate and risedronate) or once monthly (risedronate and ibandronate), fasting in the morning with water only, and the patient must remain fasting in a sitting or standing position for 30 to 60 minutes after the dose. Recently, a delayed-release formulation of risedronate (Atelvia) was approved that may be taken immediately after breakfast. The most common side effect is precipitation or aggravation of gastroesophageal reflux, although most patients tolerate the drugs without difficulty. In light of this side effect and a potential risk for esophageal irritation and ulceration, these drugs are contraindicated in patients with functional or anatomic disorders of esophageal transit (i.e., esophageal stricture, achalasia). All three drugs significantly reduce the risk for vertebral fractures, although high-strength evidence for hip and nonvertebral fracture risk reduction exists for alendronate and risedronate but not ibandronate (Table 230-2).[A9] Finally, and perhaps most important, studies confirm a persistent BMD response and likely antifracture benefit after 5 years of therapy.

Parenteral bisphosphonates are also approved and available for osteoporosis treatment, although they should be considered second line to oral bisphosphonates based on overall risk-benefit assessment in most osteoporotic patients. They may be considered for use in patients with contraindications to oral

TABLE 230-2   STRENGTH OF EVIDENCE FOR THE REDUCTION OF RISK FOR FRACTURE TYPES WITH PHARMACOTHERAPY IN WOMEN WITH POSTMENOPAUSAL OSTEOPOROSIS

	FRACTURE SKELETAL SITES			
	VERTEBRAL	**NONVERTEBRAL**	**HIP**	**WRIST**
Alendronate	• • •	• • •	• • •	•
Ibandronate	• • •	• •	•	I
Risedronate	• • •	• • •	• • •	I
Zoledronate	• • •	• • •	• • •	I
Denosumab	• • •	• • •	• • •	I
Teriparatide	• • •	• •	•	I
Raloxifene	• • •	I	I	I
Bazedoxifene*	• • •	I	I	I
Abaloparatide*	• • •	• •	I	I

*Based on author's review of clinical trial data.
Strength of evidence symbol legend: I = insufficient strength of evidence; • = low strength of evidence; • • = moderate strength of evidence; • • • = high strength of evidence.
Adapted with permission from Levis S, Theodore G. Summary of AHRQ's comparative effectiveness review of treatment to prevent fractures in men and women with low bone density or osteoporosis: update of the 2007 report. *J Manag Care Pharm.* 2012;18(4 Suppl B):S1-S15, discussion S13.

bisphosphonates (e.g., esophageal disease, inability to sit upright and/or fast after dose), documented or expected poor adherence to oral bisphosphonates, or failure to respond to oral bisphosphonates or other FDA-approved therapies (with recurrent fractures and declining BMD). Zoledronic acid, 5 mg once yearly, and ibandronate, 3 mg quarterly, may be given, although high-strength evidence would favor the use of zoledronic acid, given its unequivocal effect on spine, hip, and nonvertebral fracture risk reduction in women and men.[A10] Zoledronic acid has also been shown to reduce mortality in women and men following a low-trauma hip fracture, although the mechanism of the mortality benefit is unknown. BMD remains stable and the antifracture effect likely persists for 3 years after three to six annual doses of zoledronic acid.[A11][A12] Furthermore, zoledronate significantly reduces the risk for vertebral and nonvertebral fragility fractures in older women with osteopenia who do not meet criteria for osteoporosis.[A13]

Both intravenous bisphosphonates are associated with an approximately 15 to 20% likelihood of a flulike reaction, typically consisting of fever, arthralgias, and myalgias, usually limited to the first infusion and generally lasting 24 to 48 hours, although symptoms lasting weeks to months have rarely been reported to the FDA. Both drugs confer a higher risk as well for delayed healing of exposed bone in the oral cavity compared with oral bisphosphonates (see later).

Rare, considerably more serious adverse effects have been associated with both oral and intravenous bisphosphonates. Osteonecrosis of the jaw, which is defined as exposed bone within the oral cavity for more than 8 weeks following an invasive dental procedure (e.g., tooth extraction, dental implant) or spontaneous tooth loss, occurs in roughly 1 in 10,000 to 100,000 patients treated with oral bisphosphonates, although it likely occurs in 1 in 1000 to 10,000 in intravenous bisphosphonate–treated patients with osteoporosis. Current evidence suggests that microbial biofilm formation on an acellular bone surface, perhaps facilitated by bisphosphonates and the nonbisphosphonate drug denosumab (see later), may be operative in the development of this disorder. As such, patients on intravenous bisphosphonates should maintain optimal oral hygiene and consider a bisphosphonate holiday or delay in dose if invasive oral procedures are planned. Atypical femoral fractures have also been recently described in patients on long-term bisphosphonate therapy, generally after 5 years or more of treatment. Patients will typically have prodromal thigh or groin pain, which can refer to a stress fracture of a thickened lateral femoral cortex, inferior to the greater trochanter. These fractures can be bilateral in nature and may be identified radiographically with plain films, MRI, or CT. New dual-energy x-ray absorptiometry software allows for identification of characteristic changes in the femur (cortical thickening, periosteal reaction, medial spike) that may help better identify patients at risk for these fractures. These patients are at risk for low-trauma, severe, oblique, "chalk-stick" fractures, which often represent orthopedic repair and healing challenges. Fortunately, the estimated prevalence of atypical femoral fractures is low (~1 in 5000 to 10,000). Nonetheless, the severe manifestations of osteonecrosis of the jaw and atypical femoral fractures make it prudent for clinicians to consider a bisphosphonate drug holiday, particularly given strong evidence of continued benefit on discontinuation after 3 to 5 years of continuous therapy (3 years for intravenous and 5 years for oral).[19]

Selective Estrogen Receptor Modulators

Selective estrogen receptor modulators are compounds that bind to the estrogen receptor and thereby influence bone and reproductive biology. As with estrogen (see later), selective estrogen receptor modulators are anticatabolic agents in bone, acting through a reduction in cytokines (RANKL, tumor necrosis factor-α) that engender osteoclast activation and function. Raloxifene was the first FDA-approved drug for prevention and treatment of osteoporosis in menopausal women, although the breast cancer drug tamoxifen likely has skeletal benefits as well. Both drugs have antiestrogenic effects in the breast and are FDA approved for the prevention of breast cancer in high-risk patients. Raloxifene does reduce the risk for vertebral fractures by approximately 30 to 50% but does not reduce the risk for hip and nonvertebral fractures. This antifracture profile positions it as an alternative to bisphosphonates in postmenopausal women with osteopenia and a relatively low risk for hip and other nonspine fractures. The most common side effects include hot flushes and leg cramps in about 10 to 15% and about 5% of patients, respectively. Selective estrogen receptor modulators also increase the risk for deep vein thrombosis, with an absolute risk of roughly 1 in 400, akin to that seen with oral estrogen hormone replacement therapy. Raloxifene has also been associated with an increased risk for fatal stroke in women at higher baseline risk for stroke, likely precluding its general consideration in women older than 65 years. More recently, a second selective estrogen receptor modulator (bazedoxifene) was shown to reduce vertebral fracture risk by 42 % and is available in combination with conjugated estrogens 0.45 mg for osteoporosis prophylaxis.[A14]

Estrogen

Estrogen replacement therapy, either alone or in combination with a progestin in women with an intact uterus, had historically been a frontline agent in the management of osteoporosis in postmenopausal women (Chapter 227). Estrogen replacement therapy prevents bone loss if administered to women at menopause and significantly increases BMD by approximately 3 to 5% in woman who are well into their menopausal years. Although lower doses of estrogen may have skeletal benefits, more standard doses of estrogen (0.625 mg of conjugated equine estrogen and 1.0 mg of ethinyl estradiol) have been proved efficacious. Long-term estrogen therapy reduces the risk for all clinical fractures by about 27%, based on the available moderate-quality evidence.[A15] Estrogen replacement therapy is also the most efficacious agent available for treatment of vasomotor symptoms. These data notwithstanding, estrogen replacement therapy is associated with an increased risk for stroke (34% increase), and the use of continuous combined hormone replacement therapy confers an unacceptable greater global risk than benefit in women initiating hormone replacement therapy, based on the results of the Woman's Health Initiative. These results, however, may not be applicable to the younger postmenopausal population, based on differences in cardiovascular risk, although data confirming this are currently lacking. Both estrogen replacement therapy and hormone replacement therapy are also associated with a two- to three-fold increase in the risk for venous thromboembolic disease. Therefore, estrogen replacement therapy/hormone replacement therapy is generally recommended only for postmenopausal women at significant risk for fracture for whom other antifracture therapies are unsuitable.

Denosumab

As detailed previously, increased osteoclast activation through the RANKL pathway is a key mechanism through which bone loss occurs in menopause and other osteoporotic conditions. Intuitively, a therapy that targets this process directly would be desirable. Denosumab is a fully human monoclonal antibody to RANKL that is approved by the FDA for the treatment of osteoporosis in postmenopausal women and in men, as well as for individuals with breast and prostate cancer, to reduce bone loss associated with hormonal deprivation therapy. It is administered twice yearly as a subcutaneous injection in the clinic and clearly reduces the risk for spine, hip, and nonvertebral fractures in women and men.[A16] Denosumab does not undergo hepatic or renal metabolism and thus can potentially be used in patients with more advanced renal dysfunction, unlike bisphosphonates. In contrast to bisphosphonates, it is reversible, such that robust bone loss ensues after the medication is stopped. Indeed, there is emerging evidence that "rebound" fractures may occur in some individuals if denosumab is discontinued without a switch to an alternative antifracture therapy.[20] Recent studies also strongly suggest that teriparatide (see information on drug later) should not be used after denosumab therapy, based on suboptimal BMD response. Denosumab is well tolerated in clinical studies, although a higher incidence of skin conditions (eczema and erysipelas) and infections, including serious infections that required hospitalization, were observed in drug- versus placebo-treated subjects. Therefore, the drug is likely not suitable for patients on immunosuppressant therapy who are at higher baseline risk for infection.

Anabolic Agents

Although anticatabolic drugs are effective at retarding bone loss and reducing fracture risk, anabolic or "bone-building" drugs would be preferred. Teriparatide is a recombinant human parathyroid hormone analogue that encompasses amino acids 1 to 34 and was approved by the FDA in 2002. Given as a self-administered once-daily subcutaneous injection, teriparatide is truly anabolic based on robust increases in bone density (~10% over 2 years in the lumbar spine) and bone formation as determined by bone biopsies and other sophisticated imaging studies. More important, teriparatide significantly reduces the risk for vertebral and nonvertebral fractures by approximately two thirds and one half, respectively. Because bone resorption increases along with bone formation, bone loss generally ensues on cessation of therapy, necessitating the initiation of an anticatabolic bone drug to preserve the increase in BMD facilitated by teriparatide. Finally, although it is plausible to consider that a combination of teriparatide and an anticatabolic drug is more beneficial than either drug alone, evidence from randomized controlled trials to date has failed to confirm this. Recent studies, however, suggest that the combination of teriparatide and denosumab may have a truly synergistic effect on BMD.

Teriparatide is more expensive than other treatments for osteoporosis, although it is generally covered by insurance in patients who have severe osteoporosis (based on BMD and/or fracture risk) and who cannot tolerate or have contraindications to other antifracture agents. The drug is generally well tolerated, with the most common adverse effects being dizziness and leg cramps. Teriparatide has a black box warning, based on the fact that toxicology studies in rats revealed an increase in risk for osteosarcoma in animals treated with supra-pharmacologic doses of the drug, particularly in growing animals. Given this, the drug is contraindicated for patients who are at a higher baseline risk for osteosarcoma, including patients with Paget disease and previous therapeutic radiotherapy as well as younger individuals with open epiphyses. Fortunately, the observed rate of osteosarcoma in patients treated with teriparatide has been significantly lower than that expected in the general population since the drug was approved in 2002.

Other Therapies and Treatment Considerations
Currently Available and Emerging Therapies

Newly approved in 2017, abaloparatide (a selective activator of the parathyroid hormone type 1 receptor; administered as 80 μg subcutaneously daily), was shown to be as effective as teriparatide for reducing fracture risk in postmenopausal women with osteoporosis, with less treatment associated hypercalcemia.[A17] Similar to teriparatide, it is potentially linked to a higher risk for osteosarcoma based on rat toxicology data. Nasal calcitonin is FDA approved and available at the time of this writing for treatment of postmenopausal osteoporosis, although it is widely considered the weakest antifracture agent based on marginal vertebral fracture benefit. In addition, recent human studies have suggested a possible link to cancer, potentially further limiting its clinical utility and future availability in the United States. Strontium ranelate is approved in Europe for the treatment of osteoporosis and may have a dual proformation-anticatabolic effect on bone. It has been shown to reduce the risk for vertebral and nonvertebral fractures as well as clinical osteoporotic fractures.[A18] It is not available for use in the United States, and alternative forms of strontium salts cannot be assumed to be effective as well. In addition, BMD by dual-energy x-ray absorptiometry cannot be followed in patients on strontium because of artifactual increases in BMD related to the incorporation into bone of the strontium salt.

Emerging therapies on the horizon will likely provide additional tools to treat this debilitating disease, including new anabolic therapies (e.g., sclerostin antibody). Sclerostin is a naturally occurring inhibitor of the Wnt pathway and bone formation, and clinical studies confirm a significant increase in BMD and a 75% reduction in the risk for osteoporotic vertebral fractures with romosozumab (a monoclonal antibody that binds sclerostin at a dose of 210 mg subcutaneously monthly for 1 year).[A19][A20] Unlike teriparatide, inhibition of sclerostin does not appear to stimulate bone resorption, potentially affording greater and more persistent gains in BMD.

Glucocorticoid-Induced and Male Osteoporosis

As detailed previously, glucocorticoids are a major cause of and the most common etiology of medication-related secondary osteoporosis. Glucocorticoids are prescribed for a number of common inflammatory conditions, often in a chronic, long-term manner. They are potent suppressors of bone formation and at higher doses likely increase bone resorption, principally through central suppression of sex steroid production. This resultant "uncoupling" of bone turnover can result in dramatic declines in BMD within the first 6 months of starting therapy. In addition to bone loss, there is good evidence to support that individuals on glucocorticoids may fracture at a higher level on BMD compared with non-glucocorticoid-treated patients. Fracture rates are increased as well with doses of prednisone as low as 2.5 mg per day, although the increase in risk appears to attenuate with glucocorticoid discontinuation. The treatment approach to glucocorticoid-induced osteoporosis is similar to osteoporosis in general, with the exception that attempts should be made to reduce the steroid dose to as low as the underlying treated disease will permit.[21] Calcium and vitamin D are important adjuncts but are insufficient to prevent bone loss or fractures. Although not clearly evidence-based, replacement of deficient sex steroids is a reasonable strategy in younger individuals who are at lower risk for fracture. The bisphosphonates alendronate, risedronate, and zoledronic acid are FDA approved for glucocorticoid-induced osteoporosis in women and men.[A21] In a randomized, double-blind, noninferiority study, 60 mg subcutaneous denosumab every 6 months was both noninferior and superior to 5 mg oral risedronate daily at 12 months for effect on BMD in patients with glucocorticoid-induced osteoporosis.[A22] A more logical and indeed superior treatment of glucocorticoid-induced osteoporosis is teriparatide, which as an anabolic drug more directly addresses the primary mechanism of bone loss in glucocorticoid-induced osteoporosis: osteoblast inhibition. Teriparatide is FDA approved for treatment of glucocorticoid-induced osteoporosis in women and men and is superior to alendronate in improving BMD and vertebral fracture risk reduction.[A23] Although the drug was used for 36 months in this head-to-head trial, treatment is advised for no more than 24 months based on previously mentioned safety considerations.

Male osteoporosis historically has been underrecognized and underappreciated by primary care clinicians and patients alike, although the current data support a significantly more prevalent and clinically significant disorder. More than 2 million men in the United States have osteoporosis, and one in four men older than 50 years will suffer a fragility fracture in their remaining lifetime. Roughly 30% of vertebral and hip fractures combined occur in men, and these are the more common fractures in older men. In addition, men have a substantially higher mortality after hip fracture compared with women. As in women, aging, low body weight, and prior fragility fractures are independent predictors of fracture. In some contradistinction to women, however, osteoporosis in men is more commonly multifactorial in etiology, with the most common secondary causes being excess glucocorticoids, hypogonadism, and alcohol overuse. Despite these associations and others (current smoking, history of falls), there is not at present sufficient evidence to warrant use of a specific testing or screening strategy to identify men at higher risk for fracture. The laboratory work-up of male osteoporosis is similar to that for women, with

the exception of a morning fasting testosterone level. Idiopathic osteoporosis may also occur, particularly in younger men with no discernable cause. Genetic factors may well be important in these men, with studies suggesting an association with lower production and circulating levels of estrogen. As in women, primary treatment of male osteoporosis is targeted at lifestyle changes, adequate nutrition (calcium and vitamin D), and exercise. Bisphosphonates (oral and intravenous), denosumab, and teriparatide are all effective at improving BMD in men, although a recent meta-analysis confirmed antifracture efficacy for vertebral and possibly for nonvertebral fractures with bisphosphonates alone, whereas the antifracture efficacy of nonbisphosphonates in men remains unconfirmed.[A24] Although more limited in scope, antifracture efficacy appears evident for denosumab in men with prostate cancer on androgen deprivation therapy. True antifracture efficacy for the other agents and clinical scenarios is either less convincing or absent, based on the paucity of randomized controlled trial data, although this should not be construed as a reason not to treat. Testosterone replacement in men with significant biochemical hypogonadism (total T score <200 ng/dL) does improve bone density, although data on fracture risk reduction are lacking. In older men (>50 years) at a substantial risk for fracture based on history and risk factors, androgen replacement should be considered second line behind the aforementioned other therapies, based on overall risk-benefit and lack-of-fracture data.

Vertebroplasty and Kyphoplasty and Low-Intensity Vibration

Although often clinically silent, vertebral fractures may cause acute and severe back pain. In addition, up to one third of vertebral fractures remain chronically painful, perhaps related to incomplete healing or instability of the fracture. Over the past two decades, vertebroplasty and kyphoplasty have been developed and advanced to reduce the morbidity associated with acute spine fractures. These invasive procedures introduce, through the spinal pedicles, a cement-like substance (polymethylmethacrylate) to the compressed vertebral body, with (kyphoplasty) or without (vertebroplasty) use of saline-infused balloon tamps that permit a few millimeters of elevation of the vertebral end plates. Initial randomized trials suggested a benefit of vertebroplasty over conservative management in patients with acute vertebral fractures, although a recent meta-analysis of patient-level data from two randomized controlled trials did not confirm this finding,[A25] and sham-controlled trials show conflicting results even if the procedure is performed soon after the acute fracture.[A26][A27]

Low-intensity vibration is also under active investigation as an anticatabolic and possibly anabolic intervention for osteoporosis. Animal studies using low-intensity vibration appear to show enhanced osteoblast and hindered osteoclast development, thereby "coupling" bone remodeling. Clinical studies suggest a modest but significant BMD benefit in postmenopausal women and other groups (children with cerebral palsy, adults on prolonged bed rest), although a more recent randomized, placebo-controlled trial did not show an effect on BMD or bone turnover markers in older individuals.[A28] Further studies are clearly needed to confirm a true clinical and ideally an antifracture benefit of this intervention.

PROGNOSIS

The osteoporotic burden incurred by individual patients and society as a whole can be significantly lessened through a combination of diagnostic, preventive, and therapeutic interventions. Although there is no true "cure" for osteoporosis, current pharmacotherapies reduce the risk for fracture roughly by half. This reduction is critical because there is robust evidence to suggest an independent increase in mortality after an osteoporotic fracture, including fractures of the spine, humerus, tibia, and pelvis as well as the proximal femur. Moreover, available data, primarily from randomized controlled trials with bisphosphonates, confirm a statistically significant reduction in death with pharmacologic treatment of osteoporosis, although the mechanism of this effect is not known. Data also indicate that treatment-related increases in BMD are associated with reduced risk for subsequent fractures.[22] These data further underscore the importance of identifying and treating patients with osteoporosis.

Grade A References

A1. Zhao JG, Zeng XT, Wang J, et al. Association between calcium or vitamin D supplementation and fracture incidence in community-dwelling older adults: a systematic review and meta-analysis. *JAMA.* 2017;318:2466-2482.

A2. Cesareo R, Iozzino M, D'Onofrio L, et al. Effectiveness and safety of calcium and vitamin D treatment for postmenopausal osteoporosis. *Minerva Endocrinol.* 2015;40:231-237.

A3. Avenell A, Mak JC, O'Connell D. Vitamin D and vitamin D analogues for preventing fractures in post-menopausal women and older men. *Cochrane Database Syst Rev.* 2014;4:CD000227.

A4. Hansen KE, Johnson RE, Chambers KR, et al. Treatment of vitamin D insufficiency in postmenopausal women: a randomized clinical trial. *JAMA Intern Med.* 2015;175:1612-1621.

A5. Kahwati LC, Weber RP, Pan H, et al. Vitamin D, calcium, or combined supplementation for the primary prevention of fractures in community-dwelling adults: evidence report and systematic review for the US Preventive Services Task Force. *JAMA.* 2018;319:1600-1612.

A6. Bolland MJ, Grey A, Avenell A. Effects of vitamin D supplementation on musculoskeletal health: a systematic review, meta-analysis, and trial sequential analysis. *Lancet Diabetes Endocrinol.* 2018;6:847-858.

A7. Xu J, Lombardi G, Jiao W, et al. Effects of exercise on bone status in female subjects, from young girls to postmenopausal women: an overview of systematic reviews and meta-analyses. *Sports Med.* 2016;46:1165-1182.

A8. Howe TE, Shea B, Dawson LJ, et al. Exercise for preventing and treating osteoporosis in postmenopausal women. *Cochrane Database Syst Rev.* 2011;7:CD000333.

A9. Sanderson J, Martyn-St James M, Stevens J, et al. Clinical effectiveness of bisphosphonates for the prevention of fragility fractures: a systematic review and network meta-analysis. *Bone.* 2016;89:52-58.

A10. Chen L, Wang G, Zheng F, et al. Efficacy of bisphosphonates against osteoporosis in adult men: a meta-analysis of randomized controlled trials. *Osteoporos Int.* 2015;26:2355-2363.

A11. Black DM, Reid IR, Boonen S, et al. The effect of 3 versus 6 years of zoledronic acid treatment of osteoporosis: a randomized extension to the HORIZON-Pivotal Fracture Trial (PFT). *J Bone Miner Res.* 2012;27:243-254.

A12. Black DM, Reid IR, Cauley JA, et al. The effect of 6 versus 9 years of zoledronic acid treatment in osteoporosis: a randomized second extension to the HORIZON-Pivotal Fracture Trial (PFT). *J Bone Miner Res.* 2015;30:934-944.

A13. Reid IR, Horne AM, Mihov B, et al. Fracture prevention with zoledronate in older women with osteopenia. *N Engl J Med.* 2018;379:2407-2416.

A14. Palacios S, Silverman SL, de Villiers TJ, et al. A 7-year randomized, placebo-controlled trial assessing the long-term efficacy and safety of bazedoxifene in postmenopausal women with osteoporosis: effects on bone density and fracture. *Menopause.* 2015;22:806-813.

A15. Marjoribanks J, Farquhar C, Roberts H, et al. Long-term hormone therapy for perimenopausal and postmenopausal women. *Cochrane Database Syst Rev.* 2017;1:CD004143.

A16. Langdahl BL, Teglbjaerg CS, Ho PR, et al. A 24-month study evaluating the efficacy and safety of denosumab for the treatment of men with low bone mineral density: results from the ADAMO trial. *J Clin Endocrinol Metab.* 2015;100:1335-1342.

A17. Miller PD, Hattersley G, Riis BJ, et al. Effect of abaloparatide vs placebo on new vertebral fractures in postmenopausal women with osteoporosis: a randomized clinical trial. *JAMA.* 2016;316:722-733.

A18. Kanis JA, Johansson H, Oden A, et al. A meta-analysis of the effect of strontium ranelate on the risk of vertebral and non-vertebral fracture in postmenopausal osteoporosis and the interaction with FRAX. *Osteoporos Int.* 2011;22:2347-2355.

A19. Saag KG, Petersen J, Brandi ML, et al. Romosozumab or alendronate for fracture prevention in women with osteoporosis. *N Engl J Med.* 2017;377:1417-1427.

A20. Cosman F, Crittenden DB, Adachi JD, et al. Romosozumab treatment in postmenopausal women with osteoporosis. *N Engl J Med.* 2016;375:1532-1543.

A21. Allen CS, Yeung JH, Vandermeer B, et al. Bisphosphonates for steroid-induced osteoporosis. *Cochrane Database Syst Rev.* 2016;10:CD001347.

A22. Saag KG, Wagman RB, Geusens P, et al. Denosumab versus risedronate in glucocorticoid-induced osteoporosis: a multicentre, randomised, double-blind, active-controlled, double-dummy, non-inferiority study. *Lancet Diabetes Endocrinol.* 2018;6:445-454.

A23. Saag KG, Agnusdei D, Hans D, et al. Trabecular bone score in patients with chronic glucocorticoid therapy-induced osteoporosis treated with alendronate or teriparatide. *Arthritis Rheumatol.* 2016;68:2122-2128.

A24. Nayak S, Greenspan SL. Osteoporosis treatment efficacy for men: a systematic review and meta-analysis. *J Am Geriatr Soc.* 2017;65:490-495.

A25. Staples MP, Kallmes DF, Comstock BA, et al. Effectiveness of vertebroplasty using individual patient data from two randomised placebo controlled trials: meta-analysis. *BMJ.* 2011;343:1-11.

A26. Clark W, Bird P, Gonski P, et al. Safety and efficacy of vertebroplasty for acute painful osteoporotic fractures (VAPOUR): a multicentre, randomised, double-blind, placebo-controlled trial. *Lancet.* 2016;388:1408-1416.

A27. Firanescu CE, de Vries J, Lodder P, et al. Vertebroplasty versus sham procedure for painful acute osteoporotic vertebral compression fractures (VERTOS IV): randomised sham controlled clinical trial. *BMJ.* 2018;361:1-9.

A28. Kiel DP, Hannan MT, Barton BA, et al. Low-magnitude mechanical stimulation to improve bone density in persons of advanced age: a randomized, placebo-controlled trial. *J Bone Miner Res.* 2015;30:1319-1328.

GENERAL REFERENCES

For the General References and other additional features, please visit Expert Consult at https://expertconsult.inkling.com.

231

OSTEOMALACIA AND RICKETS

ROBERT S. WEINSTEIN

DEFINITION

Rickets can no longer be considered a historical disorder limited to third world countries or poor people. The recent increased migration to Europe and the United States has been accompanied by a resurgence of deficiency diseases, and vitamin D deficiency is particularly prevalent.[1] The primary function of vitamin D is to provide adequate levels of calcium and phosphorus[2] by increasing their intestinal absorption, thus making them available for normal mineralization of bone and epiphyseal cartilage. Rickets occurs in growing children, and both the cartilaginous growth plate and bone are affected, causing characteristic deformities. Osteomalacia occurs after growth has ceased, and the manifestations are more subtle and frequently overlooked. Normal mineralization requires the availability of sufficient calcium and phosphorus, the presence of normal bone collagen, the absence of inhibitors of mineralization, and an adequate amount of bone alkaline phosphatase activity. Defects in these requirements are the cause of most forms of osteomalacia. Deficiency of vitamin D in isolation has traditionally been incriminated as the cause of the osteomalacia, but today, considerable evidence indicates that the abnormal mineralization associated with vitamin D deficiency is due to inadequate calcium and phosphorus rather than the absence of a direct effect of vitamin D on bone cells. Optimal therapy requires precise identification of the etiology of the abnormal mineralization (Table 231-1). However, after a correct diagnosis is made, therapy is often gratifying.

EPIDEMIOLOGY

Nutritional rickets continues to be an evolving and multifactorial problem worldwide.[3,4] About 25% of women in the United States have 25-hydroxyvitamin D levels below 20 ng/mL (adequate values are greater than 30 ng/mL), and 8% have levels below 12 ng/mL, indicating that at the least, impaired bone mineralization could be a confounding factor in the treatment of their osteoporosis and, at worst, osteomalacia is the correct diagnosis (defective mineralization) rather than osteoporosis (reduced amount of normally mineralized bone). Osteomalacia and vitamin D deficiency must be excluded before administration of the antiresorptive drugs used for postmenopausal osteoporosis. This is particularly important before the use of zoledronate or denosumab. Vitamin D deficiency is more common in nonaffluent elderly people, especially during the winter at more polar latitudes. Osteomalacia may occur with self-imposed diets avoiding dairy products and fish or in vegans. Vitamin D

TABLE 231-1 CAUSES OF OSTEOMALACIA

VITAMIN D DEFICIENCY

Dietary deprivation and lack of solar exposure

VITAMIN D MALABSORPTION

Postgastrectomy
Gastric bypass for obesity
Gluten enteropathy
Inflammatory bowel disease
Pancreatic insufficiency
Cholestyramine therapy
Laxative abuse
Phytates in some cereals and flatbreads

IMPAIRED 1-HYDROXYLATION OF 25-HYDROXYVITAMIN D

Chronic kidney disease
X-linked hypophosphatemia
Tumor-induced osteomalacia
Vitamin D–dependent rickets type I

IMPAIRED TARGET-ORGAN RESPONSE TO 1,25-DIHYDROXYVITAMIN D

Vitamin D–dependent rickets type II

HYPOPHOSPHATEMIA

X-linked hypophosphatemia
Autosomal dominant hypophosphatemic rickets
Tumor-induced osteomalacia
Antacid-induced osteomalacia
Chronic metabolic acidosis
Fanconi syndrome
Paraproteinemia
Saccharated ferric oxide
Tenofovir or adefovir
Cadmium

INHIBITORS OF MINERALIZATION

Etidronate
Fluoride
Aluminum
Iron
Hypophosphatasia

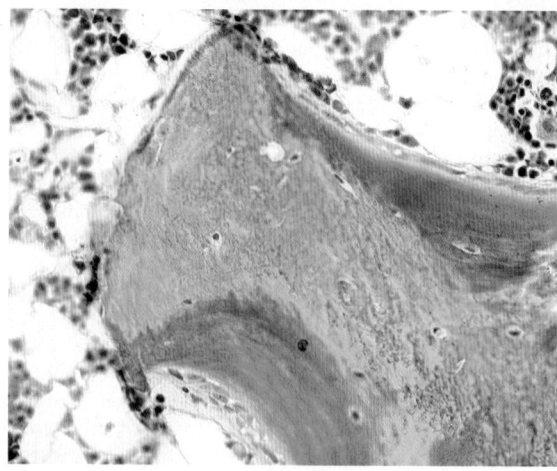

FIGURE 231-1. An undecalcified bone biopsy specimen shows the characteristic abundant osteoid and flattened osteoblasts of osteomalacia. (Normally, mineralized bone appears blue and osteoid is carmine.)

deficiency is also commonly found in medical inpatients and in postmenopausal women with an acute hip fracture. Immigrants from tropical regions are at particularly high risk because of darker skin, movement to more temperate climates, full-body clothing and cosmetics that block sunlight, indoor living, and dietary choices (high phytate cereal or flour that binds calcium [such as that used in chapatti flat bread] and avoidance of dairy products). The prevalence of osteomalacia due to vitamin D deficiency varies with the referral source. The disorder is far more frequent when patients are referred from geriatricians, gastroenterologists (osteomalacia may be found in up to 30% of patients with gastric surgery or bypass for obesity), nursing homes, or orthopedists concerned about symmetrical lesions or nonhealing fractures.

PATHOBIOLOGY

The abnormal mineralization characteristic of osteomalacia is due to slowed or terminated mineral deposition in the organic matrix of bone (osteoid) because of one or more of the defects mentioned earlier. However, osteoblasts continue to make osteoid, which then accumulates in excessive amounts. Histologically, the osteoid width may become dramatically augmented (Fig. 231-1). Depending on the extent of the mineralization delay, overt osteomalacia may take many years to develop. After normalization of the serum calcium and phosphorous levels, bone healing may take at least 6 to 18 months.

CLINICAL MANIFESTATIONS

The clinical presentation of osteomalacia depends on three overlapping manifestations: those due to the underlying disorder such as gastrointestinal disease or surgery (especially troublesome are gastric resection, or bypass for obesity, celiac disease, and intestinal malabsorption); those due to hypocalcemia or hypophosphatemia; and those directly due to the bone disease. The most common symptoms and signs are pelvis and leg pain, muscle weakness, and bone tenderness. When the knees are involved and magnetic resonance imaging (MRI) reveals an increased T2 signal, the osteomalacia can be mistaken for spontaneous osteonecrosis of the knee. A check of the serum 25-hydroxyvitamin D and alkaline phosphatase activity levels will reveal the correct diagnosis. Bone pain is usually nonspecific and poorly localized. Because of the paucity of findings, the pains are often attributed to rheumatism or neurosis. They may be worse at night and after sudden movements, such as turning in bed or the change from sitting to standing. The pain is worse on weight bearing, resulting in a characteristic flat-footed, springless, waddling gait made worse by proximal muscle weakness. The gait has been referred to as "mother penguin's walk." Patients may complain that they can only climb stairs by pulling themselves up with the hand rail or rise from a chair or the toilet by using their hands to push off. The decrease in strength is usually far greater than the degree of muscle wasting. Fasciculations are absent, and both reflexes and sensation remain normal. The bulbar, facial, and ocular muscles are always spared. However, muscle weakness is conspicuously mild or absent when the osteomalacia is due to X-linked hypophosphatemia (XLH, the most common inherited form of hypophosphatemic osteomalacia [the prevalence is 1:20,000]) but is profound, often requiring a wheelchair, in autosomal dominant hypophosphatemic rickets (ADHR) and tumor-induced osteomalacia (TIO). Nevertheless, all three disorders are due to increased (or inappropriate for

the low serum phosphate) fibroblast growth factor 23 (FGF-23) causing excessive phosphaturia and inhibition of 25-hydroxyvitamin D-1α-hydroxylase. The hypophosphatemia is intensified by the inappropriately low levels of 1,25-dihydroxyvitamin D. In XLH, the family history is positive, and the typical presentation is short stature with lower leg deformity. ADHR is characterized by a positive family history, spontaneous remissions, rather abrupt fatigue and weakness, fractures, bone pain, and recurrent dental abscesses. This disorder may be triggered by iron deficiency. TIO is a rare form of acquired, paraneoplastic, hypophosphatemic osteomalacia due to a small and often hard-to-find benign mesenchymal tumor.[5] TIO merits consideration in adults who present with hypophosphatemia, little or no deformities, and no family history of skeletal disease. However, if the family history is vague or absent, ADHR can masquerade as TIO, but serum FGF-23 levels are generally much higher in TIO than in ADHR. Included in the differential diagnosis is Fanconi syndrome, but in this disease, the hypophosphatemia is accompanied by hypokalemia, glycosuria, and hyperchloremic acidosis.

In osteomalacia, bone tenderness often can be elicited by rib cage compression or pressing on the tibiae, wrists, pubic rami, or iliac crests. Hypocalcemia is usually mild to moderate but rarely can be severe enough to present with fingertip paresthesias, muscle cramps, a positive Chvostek or Trousseau sign, or seizures. If the osteomalacia is mistaken for osteoporosis and treatment is started with a bisphosphonate or denosumab, the patient may experience new-onset paresthesias, muscle cramps, and palpitations. This not uncommon scenario occurs because the antiresorptive treatment interferes with the mobilization of calcium from bone by parathyroid hormone (PTH), thereby aggravating the hypocalcemia. The secondary hyperparathyroidism will also worsen the hypophosphatemia by the effect of PTH on renal excretion at the same time that intestinal absorption is impaired and mobilization from bone is blocked.

DIAGNOSIS

Biochemical changes depend on the stage of the disease and its etiology. In vitamin D deficiency, hypophosphatemia precedes and is more severe than the hypocalcemia because of the secondary hyperparathyroidism (Chapter 232) that usually accompanies the disorder by the time that osteomalacia has occurred. However, it remains unclear why some patients do not demonstrate increased PTH levels when severely vitamin D deficient. In malabsorption, hypomagnesemia may contribute to the hypocalcemia by impairing PTH secretion, and hypoalbuminemia may lead to a spurious diagnosis of hypocalcemia. Increased serum alkaline phosphatase activity is classically associated with osteomalacia due to vitamin D deficiency but usually is not an early clue. The serum 25-hydroxyvitamin D levels are often less than 10 to 15 ng/mL. In contrast, serum 1,25-dihydroxyvitamin D levels are usually elevated owing to the concomitant secondary hyperparathyroidism and usually do not contribute to the diagnosis of osteomalacia. However, in the rare autosomal recessive condition of a defective vitamin D receptor (vitamin D–dependent rickets type II), serum 1,25-dihydroxyvitamin D and PTH levels may be extraordinarily high (see Table 231-1). This condition is characterized by consanguinity, alopecia, and early-onset hypocalcemia. In another rare autosomal recessive disorder with defective 1α-hydroxylation of 25-hydroxyvitamin D (vitamin D–dependent rickets type I), serum 1,25-dihydroxyvitamin D levels may be undetectable. This disorder also is characterized by consanguinity and early-onset hypocalcemia. Quite a different pattern occurs with the inherited disease hypophosphatasia: serum 25-hydroxyvitamin D and calcium are normal, phosphorus is high-normal or slightly elevated, and alkaline phosphatase activity is below the normal age-matched range.[6] This disease is caused by a deficiency of the tissue-nonspecific (liver, bone, and kidney) isoenzyme of alkaline phosphatase, which normally prevents extracellular accumulation of inorganic pyrophosphate. If alkaline phosphatase activity is deficient and inorganic pyrophosphate collects adjacent to bone, mineralization is inhibited. The adult form of the disease may present with mild or severe osteomalacia. Calcium pyrophosphate dihydrate (CPPD) crystal deposition disease (chondrocalcinosis) is often associated.

In any form of osteomalacia, radiographic findings may be subtle or absent, and only blurred margins of the cancellous bone with thin cortices may be noted. The presence of bilaterally symmetrical, thin (2 to 3 mm) radiolucent bands known as pseudofractures (Fig. 231-2) found perpendicular to the periosteal surface in ribs, pubic and ischial rami, neck of the femur, metatarsals, and below the glenoid fossa on the outer border of the scapulae is generally considered to be pathognomonic of osteomalacia. However, this radiographic finding may be seen in disorders lacking excessive osteoid. Distinguishing features of pseudofractures in osteomalacia are the lack of callus or adjacent sclerosis and absence of an inciting event. Usually, there are at least two or three of these

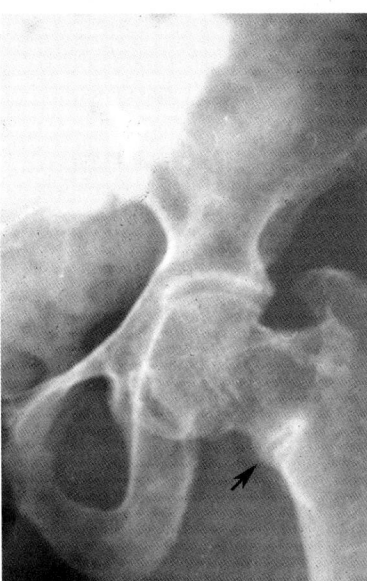

FIGURE 231-2. Radiographic evidence of a pseudofracture of the femoral neck is suspicious for osteomalacia (*arrow*).

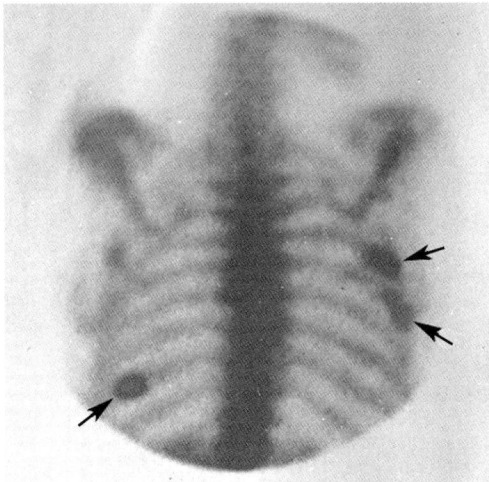

FIGURE 231-3. In osteomalacia, focal increased uptake of radionuclide on a bone scan may erroneously suggest metastatic disease (*arrows*).

fractures with at least one in the rib, pubic rami, or femora, and biochemical clues (hypocalcemia and hypophosphatemia) are present. If what appears to be a pseudofracture is accompanied by normal serum calcium, phosphorus, and alkaline phosphatase activity, osteomalacia is unlikely. Pseudofractures show increased uptake on bone scans (Fig. 231-3) and may lead to an inappropriate search for a malignancy. Pseudofractures are typically located in the medial cortex of long bones and must be distinguished from atypical femoral fractures, which are located in the lateral cortex with cortical thickening and a cortical beak. Both may occur in patients receiving treatment with bisphosphonates. Subtrochanteric femoral pseudofractures also may occur in the lateral cortex in hypophosphatasia. In Paget disease, cortical stress or fissure fractures may resemble pseudofractures but have a predilection for the anterior aspects of a bowed femur or tibia. In contrast to osteomalacia, the surrounding bone has a distinctly abnormal radiographic appearance. In osteomalacia, bone mineral density T-scores are often −3 or −4, with the radial diaphyseal density T-scores lower than those of the lumbar spine and total proximal femur.

Although characteristic clinical, radiographic, and biochemical findings may suggest osteomalacia, the absence of these findings cannot exclude the diagnosis. Bone biopsy is needed to establish the unequivocal presence of osteomalacia (see Fig. 231-1). However, this is rarely necessary unless the patient has unusually painful disease or progressive loss of bone density and the results of the physical examination, radiographs, and biochemical findings are ambiguous. When biopsy is necessary, the best solution is to refer the patient to a bone histomorphometry center. This ensures satisfactory communication

among the clinician, operator, and pathologist and is the best insurance against incomplete, broken, fragmented, or accidentally decalcified specimens.

Several presumed causes of osteomalacia (anticonvulsant drugs, metabolic acidosis without hypophosphatemia, pseudohypoparathyroidism, and chronic renal failure) have not demonstrated accumulation of osteoid due to delayed mineralization and primarily represent secondary hyperparathyroidism. Patients with the nephrotic syndrome lose albumin and vitamin D metabolites in the urine, but their serum ionized calcium and PTH levels are normal and metabolic bone disease in adults with the nephrotic syndrome is absent. Unexplained elevations of the serum alkaline phosphatase activity are usually due to drugs (e.g., anticonvulsants, anabolic steroids, phenothiazines, or antibiotics) or Paget disease of bone (Chapter 233). These possibilities may be distinguished by measurement of the serum bone alkaline phosphatase by immunoassay, although there is up to 15 to 20% cross-reactivity with hepatic alkaline phosphatase. Isoenzyme determination by heat fractionation is not helpful. The bone contribution can also be estimated from the serum procollagen type I amino-terminal propeptide concentration. However, increased serum alkaline phosphatase activity is rarely the only biochemical clue to osteomalacia in a patient with skeletal discomfort.

TREATMENT   Rx

Understanding the treatment of osteomalacia is facilitated by dividing the disease into three subgroups. The first subgroup is osteomalacia due to disorders of vitamin D absorption or metabolism; the second is osteomalacia due to chronic hypophosphatemia. Cadmium, tenofovir, or adefovir may induce Fanconi syndrome and cause osteomalacia due to the resultant hypophosphatemia. Most patients with osteomalacia will be in these first two subgroups. Recently, an anti-FGF-23 antibody (burosumab) has become available for children[7] and adults with X-linked hypophosphatemia.[A1] The third subgroup includes osteomalacia caused by inhibitors of mineralization such as etidronate (the first oral bisphosphonate, now rarely used in North America), high doses of fluoride (in gallons of bulk tea), accumulation of a skeletal burden of aluminum from water used for dialysis or as a contaminant in solutions used for parenteral nutrition (now rarely seen), iron overload as in thalassemia, and hypophosphatasia. In hypophosphatasia, bone-targeted enzyme replacement therapy (asfotase alfa) has been shown to be effective in adults.[8] General measures remain important and include routine nutritional advice and avoidance of further bone loss due to postmenopausal osteoporosis or vitamin D deficiency. High-dose vitamin D therapy in hypophosphatasia has caused nephrocalcinosis, nephrolithiasis, and renal insufficiency and should be avoided.

Osteomalacia Due to Vitamin D Disorders

Iron deficiency anemia, hypocalcemia, weight loss, glossitis or rash, and bone discomfort in a patient with low bone mineral density point to celiac disease (Chapter 131), even without gastrointestinal symptoms. These patients may also have persistently low serum 25-hydroxyvitamin D levels despite high-dose vitamin D supplementation. This scenario suggests the need to test for anti-endomysial immunoglobulin A and tissue transglutaminase antibodies. Advice on nutrition and sun exposure, discontinuation of offending drugs, adherence to a gluten-free diet, and pancreatic enzyme replacement may cure the mineralization defect in some patients with mild disease without the need for additional treatment. Cholestyramine therapy for cholestasis or laxative abuse may also cause malabsorption and resistance to vitamin D supplements.

Patients with severe disease require vitamin D[9] and calcium supplementation. A loading dose accelerates recovery and depends on the serum 25-hydroxyvitamin D level, as shown in Table 231-2. Although vitamin D_3 supplementation may be somewhat more potent than with D_2, the differences are not clinically important with the doses recommended for osteomalacia. Because pharmacologic doses of any vitamin D preparation carry the risk for vitamin D intoxication, increases in the dose must be made carefully. The interval between increments in dosage should be at least the time required to reach maximal effects plus about 50%. However, experience with the doses given in Table 231-2 indicates that serum 25-hydroxyvitamin D levels rarely reach 80 to 100 ng/mL. Vitamin D intoxication is unlikely even with levels of 150 ng/mL. The goal is to raise the serum 25-hydroxyvitamin D level well above 30 ng/mL and reduce the elevated PTH concentration to normal without hypercalcemia or hypercalciuria. Urinary calcium excretion should be monitored after treatment has normalized the serum calcium level. The urinary calcium-to-creatinine ratio (mg/mg) should be kept below 0.22. Approximately 1 to 1.5 g per day of oral elemental calcium is a reasonable initial dose depending on the degree of malabsorption (Table 231-3). Frequent small doses (three times a day) are more effective and tolerable than fewer larger ones, and the absorbability of calcium supplements is enhanced with meals.

In patients with malabsorption, vitamin D requirements may rise during periods of increased diarrhea, and calcitriol may be easier for these patients

TABLE 231-2 VITAMIN D PREPARATIONS FOR TREATMENT OF OSTEOMALACIA

	VITAMIN D$_2$ (ERGOCALCIFEROL)	VITAMIN D$_3$ (CHOLECALCIFEROL)	CALCITRIOL[†] [1,25(OH)$_2$D$_3$]
Trade name	Drisdol and others*	Bio-Tech D3-50	Rocaltrol
Dosage form	Caps: 50,000 U = 1.25 mg	Caps: 50,000 U = 1.25 mg	Caps: 0.25 and 0.50 µg
Loading dosage:			
If 25(OH)D = 20-30 ng/mL	50,000 U once/wk for 10 wks[‡] and once/mo thereafter (or 2000 units/day)	50,000 U once/wk for 10 wks[‡] and once/mo thereafter (or 2000 units/day)	
If 25(OH)D = 10-20 ng/mL	50,000 U twice/wk for 10 wks[‡] and twice/mo thereafter	50,000 U twice/wk for 10 wks[‡] and twice/mo thereafter	
If 25(OH)D = <10 ng/mL	50,000 U three times/wk for 10 wks[‡] and three times/mo thereafter	50,000 U three times/wk for 10 wks[‡] and three times/mo thereafter	
Dosage in resistant cases	Up to 50,000 units/day	Up to 50,000 units/day	2-8 µg/day
Time to reach maximal effects	4-10 wks	4-10 wks	3-7 days
Persistence of effects after cessation	6-30 wks	6-30 wks	3-4 days
Cost	$203/100 gel caps	$20.70/100 capsules	$120.95/100 generic calcitriol capsules of 0.25 µg $91.86/100 Rocaltrol capsules of 0.25 µg $193.38/100 generic calcitriol capsules of 0.5 µg $294.00/100 Rocaltrol capsules of 0.5 µg $179/15 mL (1 µg/mL) generic calcitriol oral solution $235.20/15 mL (1 µg/mL) Rocaltrol oral solution

*Gel caps are best because hard capsules may be indigestible and unreliable.
[†]Calcitriol is reserved for patients with persistent elevation of parathyroid hormone despite normalization of the serum 25-hydroxyvitamin D level. Hypercalcemia and hypercalciuria must be avoided.
[‡]If not >30 ng/mL after 10 weeks, exclude malabsorption, celiac disease, and noncompliance. Weekly tanning bed treatments may be used if oral vitamin therapy fails, or a switch to the more costly calcitriol may be necessary.

TABLE 231-3 CALCIUM PREPARATIONS FOR TREATMENT OF OSTEOMALACIA

PREPARATION	PERCENT ELEMENTAL CALCIUM	AMOUNT OF ELEMENTAL CALCIUM IN THE SUGGESTED DOSE	COST PER MONTH OF THERAPY
Calcium carbonate 600 mg tablets	40	4 tabs = 960 mg	$5
TUMS Ultra 1000 mg (chewable)	40	2 tabs = 800 mg	$5
Citracal Slow Release 1200 mg (85% calcium carbonate and 15% calcium citrate) plus 1000 units vitamin D		4 tabs = 892 mg	$7

to absorb. Its rapid onset of action and disappearance after cessation add to the safety of treatment, albeit at greater cost (see Table 231-2). Use of calcitriol requires great care to avoid hypercalcemia and hypercalciuria. Calcium, phosphorus, potassium, magnesium, and multivitamins may also be beneficial in patients with malabsorption (Table 231-4; see Table 231-3). Rare patients do not tolerate any form of oral vitamin D, and the parenteral calciferol preparations available in North America are ineffective. These patients can be improved, although not restored to normal, by the use of weekly tanning bed treatments to areas of their bodies not normally exposed to the sun, with an attempt to minimize risk for solar-induced skin cancer (Chapter 193). Calcitriol is the drug of choice in patients with vitamin D–dependent rickets type I. In patients with vitamin D–dependent rickets type II and diminished receptor sensitivity to 1,25-dihydroxyvitamin D, extraordinarily high doses of calcitriol may partially overcome the defect. If oral treatment fails, nocturnal infusions of calcium and phosphorus have been successful, providing additional evidence that the osteomalacia is due to inadequate calcium and phosphorus rather than from the defect in vitamin D metabolism.

An increase in the serum alkaline phosphatase activity (the healing "flare") and a small increase in the serum and urine calcium levels are the earliest signs of effective treatment. Thereafter, the serum alkaline phosphatase activity level falls progressively as healing occurs. At the start of therapy, serum calcium levels should be measured every 2 to 3 weeks. If hypoalbuminemia is present, serum ionized calcium determinations or albumin-adjusted calcium values are useful. When therapy appears stabilized, repeat determinations at 6- to 8-week intervals are usually sufficient, but even with long-term therapy, measurements should be at least three times a year. In some patients with severe osteomalacia, bone pain and paresthesias may increase and the serum calcium levels decrease during the first few weeks of therapy. This is due to the increased skeletal avidity for mineral during healing and indicates the need for additional calcium supplementation.

Osteomalacia Due to Hypophosphatemia

Therapy of chronic hypophosphatemia is aimed at maintaining normal concentrations of serum phosphorus without inducing secondary hyperparathyroidism or nephrocalcinosis.[10] This considerably difficult task requires divided doses of phosphorus supplements and calcitriol to increase the absorption of phosphorus and calcium and to prevent the resultant increase in PTH. Regrettably, this regimen is often poorly tolerated, causing diarrhea, secondary or tertiary hyperparathyroidism, nephrocalcinosis, or nephrolithiasis. Therefore, starting therapy should be with no more than 250 mg of elemental phosphorus four times daily and 0.25 to 0.5 µg of calcitriol twice daily, advanced slowly. Lab review should be within 3 to 4 weeks in order to trend the values. If the serum phosphorus has not changed or decreased and the PTH level has increased, advance the calcitriol rather than the phosphorus. Otherwise, the phosphorus-induced secondary hyperparathyroidism will result in rapid excretion of the phosphorus and also cause the additional bone disease of hyperparathyroidism (Chapter 232). Baseline and yearly renal ultrasound examinations are necessary to recognize early nephrocalcinosis or nephrolithiasis.

TIO is also treated with phosphorus supplementation and calcitriol until the offending tumor can be located and resected. Complete resection of these tumors results in cure of the osteomalacia, but they are notoriously hard to find. Encouraging recent information suggests that as many as 60% of these elusive tumors can be localized using scintigraphy with technetium-99m octreotide or gallium-68 conjugated to somatostatin peptide analogues or with fluoro-dexoxyglucose-18 positron emission tomography/computed tomography.[11] If the tumor remains evasive and treatment with phosphorus and calcitriol is not tolerated, the anti-FGF-23 antibody (burosumab) may be useful when it becomes available. The calcium-sensing receptor agonist, cinacalcet (30 mg/day), has been added to the phosphorus and calcitriol used in the management of TIO when the doses of the phosphorus supplements are intolerable. This causes medically induced hypoparathyroidism and an increase in the serum phosphorus level despite the elevated FGF-23, thereby permitting a reduction in the phosphorus supplementation. Hypercalciuria may occur with the fall in PTH combined with the calcitriol treatment, requiring the addition of a small dose of hydrochlorothiazide. Urinary calcium excretion and serum creatinine must be monitored.

TABLE 231-4 PHOSPHATE PREPARATIONS FOR TREATMENT OF OSTEOMALACIA					
PREPARATION	**PHOSPORUS CONTENT (mg/cap or tab)**	**SODIUM CONTENT (mEq/cap or tab)**	**POTASSIUM CONTENT (mEq/cap or tab)**	**AMOUNT THAT CONTAINS 1 G OF ELEMENTAL PHOSPHORUS**	**COST**
Neutra-Phos	250	7	7	4 unit dose caps*	
Phos-NaK	250	7	7	4 packets*	$39/100 packets
Neutra-Phos-K	250	0	14	4 unit dose caps*	
K-Phos Neutral	250	13	1.1	4 tabs	$72/100 tablets
K-Phos Original	114	0	3.7	9 tabs	$52/100 tablets
Phospha 250 Neutral	250	13	1.1	4 tabs	$91/100 tablets
K-Phos No 2	250	5.8	2.3	4 tabs	$99/100 tablets

*Each unit dose cap is reconstituted with at least 75 mL of water, fruit juice, or cola. The unit dose cap or packet contains the powder concentrate and is not to be swallowed undiluted. The powder preparations are cost savers.

PREVENTION

Nutritional rickets and osteomalacia are common in dark-skinned and migrant populations, and their global incidence is rising because of changing population demographics, failing prevention policies, and inadequate implementation strategies. High-risk populations require lifelong supplementation and food fortification with vitamin D or calcium. Advice about vitamin D supplementation should help to prevent osteomalacia caused by vitamin D deficiency, but this has proved to be difficult because routine over-the-counter supplements may be insufficient and compliance with nutritional supplements is poor. The optimal vitamin D supplementation dosage is not clear, but most bone and mineral problems are avoided by 50,000 units of cholecalciferol given once monthly (or, 1600 to 2000 units per day). Notable exceptions occur in patients with celiac disease, gastric surgery, or bypass for obesity, who often require much larger amounts (see Table 231-2). In patients with osteomalacia due to hypophosphatemia, the need for phosphorus supplementation may be lifelong (see Table 231-4).

PROGNOSIS

The response to appropriate treatment in most forms of osteomalacia is usually excellent. Improvements in bone pain and muscle weakness usually occur within 2 or 3 months and healing of skeletal lesions within 6 to 18 months. Depending on the quantity of excess osteoid, repeat bone mineral density determinations may show as much as 20% gains at the lumbar spine and total proximal femur. However, bone density at the radial diaphysis may not improve owing to the irreversible loss of cortical bone resulting from prolonged secondary hyperparathyroidism. Furthermore, if decreased bone volume is present in addition to excess osteoid, skeletal recovery may be incomplete, resulting in residual osteoporosis. However, great caution must be exercised before adding an antiresorptive agent. Addition of drugs for osteoporosis should wait for normalization of the serum calcium, phosphorus, and alkaline phosphatase activity. Bone density improvement from treatment of the osteomalacia may continue for up to a year.

 Grade A Reference

A1. Insogna KL, Briot K, Imel EA, et al. A randomized, double-blind, placebo-controlled, phase 3 trial evaluating the efficacy of burosumab, an anti-GFG23 antibody in adults with X-linked hypophosphatemia: week 24 primary analysis. *J Bone Miner Res.* 2018;33:1383-1393.

GENERAL REFERENCES

For the General References and other additional features, please visit Expert Consult at https://expertconsult.inkling.com.

THE PARATHYROID GLANDS, HYPERCALCEMIA, AND HYPOCALCEMIA

RAJESH V. THAKKER

CALCIUM METABOLISM

A healthy adult body has a total of 1 kg of calcium; about 99% of this is present within the crystal structure of bone mineral, and less than 1% is in soluble form in the extracellular and intracellular fluid compartments. In the extracellular fluid compartment (ECF), about half of the total calcium is ionized, and the rest is principally bound to albumin or complexed with counter-ions. Ionized calcium in the ECF plays an important role in many physiologic pathways, including muscle contraction, secretion of neurotransmitters and hormones, and coagulation pathways. Ionized serum calcium concentrations range from 4.65 to 5.25 mg/dL (1.16 to 1.31 mmol/L), and the total serum calcium concentration ranges from 8.5 to 10.5 mg/dL (2.12 to 2.62 mmol/L).[1] However, the usual 2 : 1 ratio of total to ionized calcium may be disturbed by disorders such as metabolic acidosis, which reduces calcium binding by proteins, or by changes in protein concentration, caused by cirrhosis, dehydration, venous stasis, or multiple myeloma. In view of this, total serum calcium concentrations are adjusted, or "corrected," to a reference albumin concentration: the actual total serum calcium value is adjusted by adding or subtracting 0.8 mg/dL (0.016 mmol/L) for every 1 g/dL (1 g/L) of albumin below or above a reference albumin concentration of 4 g/dL (40 g/L), respectively.

The control of body calcium involves a balance between the amounts that are absorbed from the gut, deposited into bone and into cells, and excreted from the kidney (Fig. 232-1). This fine balance, involving three organs, is chiefly under the control of parathyroid hormone (PTH), which is synthesized and secreted by the parathyroid glands. Hypocalcemia leads to an increased secretion of PTH, whereas hypercalcemia results in diminished PTH secretion. Regulation of extracellular calcium takes place through complex interactions (Fig. 232-2) at the target organs of the major calcium-regulating hormone, PTH, and vitamin D and its active metabolites, 1,25-dihydroxyvitamin D $(1,25[OH]_2D)$.

PARATHYROID GLANDS, PARATHYROID HORMONE, *PTH* GENE, AND PARATHYROID HORMONE ACTIONS

Parathyroid Glands

There are usually four parathyroid glands, which are located in close proximity to the superior and inferior poles of the lobes of the thyroid gland. The superior parathyroids are derived from the endoderm of the embryonic fourth

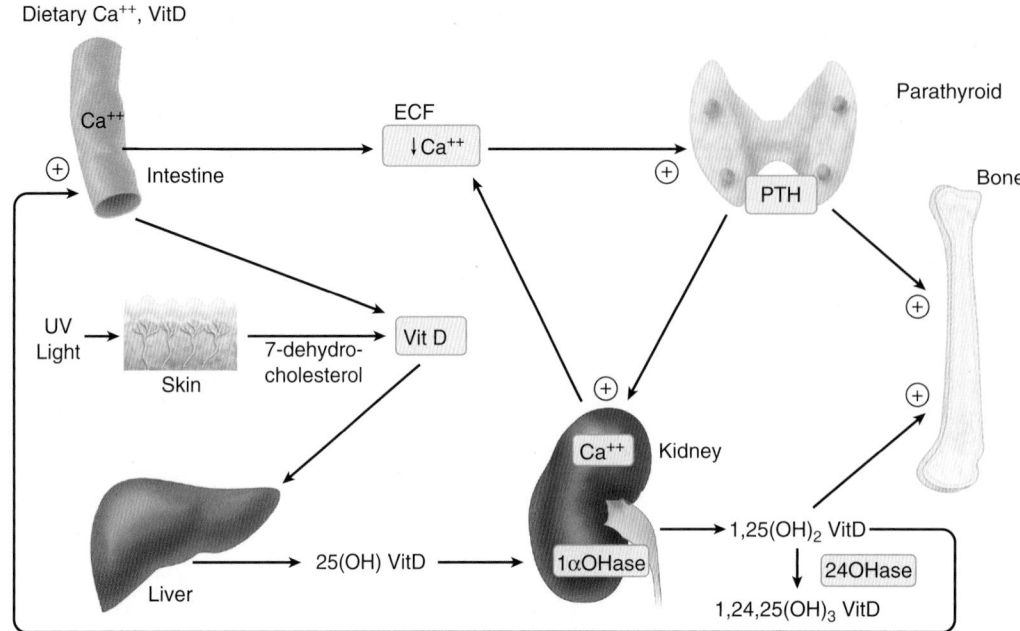

FIGURE 232-1. Regulation of extracellular fluid (ECF) calcium (Ca²⁺) by parathyroid hormone (PTH) action on kidney, bone, and intestine. A decrease in ECF Ca²⁺ is sensed by the calcium-sensing receptor (see Fig. 232-2), and this leads to an increase in PTH secretion and a reduction in PTH degradation. The increased circulating PTH predominantly acts directly on kidney and bone that possess the PTH receptor (PTHR, Fig. 232-2). The skeletal effects of PTH are to increase (+) osteoclastic bone reabsorption. However, because osteoclasts do not have PTHRs, this action is mediated by the osteoblasts, which do have PTHRs and in response release cytokines and factors in turn that activate osteoclasts. In the kidney, PTH stimulates (+) the 1α-hydroxylase (1αOHase) to increase the conversion of 25-hydroxyvitamin D [25(OH)VitD] to the active metabolite 1,25-dihydroxyvitamin D [1,25(OH)₂VitD]. In addition, PTH increases (+) the reabsorption of Ca²⁺ from the renal distal tubule and inhibits the reabsorption of phosphate from the proximal tubule, thereby leading to hypercalcemia and hypophosphatemia. PTH also inhibits Na⁺, H⁺ antiporter activity and bicarbonate reabsorption, thereby causing a mild hyperchloremic acidosis. The elevated 1,25(OH)₂VitD acts on the intestine to increase (+) absorption of dietary calcium and phosphate. It is important to note that PTH does not appear to have a direct action on the gut. Thus, in response to hypocalcemia and the increase in PTH secretion, all of these direct and indirect actions of PTH on the kidney, bone, and intestine will help to increase ECF Ca²⁺, which in turn will act through the calcium-sensing receptor to decrease PTH secretion. (From Thakker RV, Bringhurst FR, Jüppner HH. Regulation of calcium homeostasis and genetic disorders that affect calcium metabolism. In: Jameson JL, De Groot LJ, Giudice LC, et al., eds. *Endocrinology: Adult & Pediatric.* 7th ed. Philadelphia: Saunders; 2016.)

pharyngeal pouches, and the inferior parathyroids are derived with the thymus from the endoderm of the third pharyngeal pouches. Extra parathyroid glands are commonly found in aberrant locations along this migrating path and also within the thymus and thyroid. Parathyroid cells express a G protein–coupled receptor (GPCR), referred to as the *calcium-sensing receptor* (CaSR), that detects changes in extracellular calcium and leads to alterations in PTH secretions.[2,3] For example, activation of the CaSR, which is also expressed in renal tubular cells as a result of elevated extracellular calcium concentrations, causes G protein–dependent stimulation of phospholipase C activity through Gαq and Gα11, which leads to accumulation of inositol 1,4,5-trisphosphate and an increase in intracellular calcium concentrations. These changes, in turn, lead to reduced circulating PTH concentrations and increased urinary calcium excretion. Disorders of the parathyroid glands may cause hypercalcemia or hypocalcemia, and these can be classified according to whether they arise from an excess of PTH, its deficiency, or insensitivity to its effects (Table 232-1; see Fig. 232-2).

Parathyroid Hormone and *PTH* Gene
PTH is an 84–amino acid peptide encoded by the *PTH* gene, which is located on chromosome 11p15. The mature PTH peptide is secreted from the parathyroid chief cells as an 84–amino acid peptide; however, when the *PTH* mRNA is first translated, it is as pre-proPTH peptide. The "pre" sequence consists of a 25–amino acid signal peptide (leader sequence) that is responsible for directing the nascent peptide into the endoplasmic reticulum to be packaged for secretion from the cell. The "pro" sequence is 6 amino acids in length and, although its function is less well defined than that of the "pre" sequence, is also essential for correct PTH processing and secretion. After the 84–amino acid mature PTH peptide is secreted from the parathyroid cell, it is cleared from the circulation with a short half-life of about 2 minutes, by nonsaturable hepatic uptake and renal excretion.

Parathyroid Hormone Actions
PTH shares a receptor with PTH-related peptide (PTHrP); this PTH/PTHrP receptor (see Fig. 232-2) is a member of a subgroup of the G protein–coupled receptor family. PTH/PTHrP receptors are expressed in kidney and bone,

where PTH is its predominant agonist, and thus PTH acts directly on kidney and bone cells and indirectly on intestinal cells (see Fig. 232-1) to enhance renal calcium reabsorption, release stored calcium in bones into the ECF, and increase gut calcium absorption, respectively. Expression of the PTH/ PTHrP receptor also occurs in the brain, heart, skin, lung, liver, and testis, where it mediates the actions of PTHrP. Mutations involving the genes that encode these proteins and receptors in this calcium-regulating pathway (see Fig. 232-2) are associated with hypercalcemic and hypocalcemic disorders (see Table 232-1).

Renal Actions
Calcium is absorbed by the kidneys at multiple sites and by different mechanisms, which include passive paracellular or active transcellular transport, along the renal tubule. The renal actions of PTH are to (1) stimulate activity of the proximal tubular cell 1α-hydroxylase; (2) increase reabsorption of calcium by the cells of the distal tubule, connecting tubules and the thick ascending loop of Henle (TAL); and (3) inhibit phosphate reabsorption by proximal tubular cells (see Fig. 232-1). PTH increases the formation of biologically active 1,25(OH)₂D from its precursor 25-OH-D by stimulating the activity of the renal 1α-hydroxylase and inhibiting the 24-hydroxylase, which metabolizes 1,25(OH)₂D to the inactive 24,25(OH)₂D form (see Fig. 232-1). PTH regulates calcium reabsorption by distal tubular cells by upregulating expression of the transient receptor potential vanilloid 5 (TRPV5), thereby promoting calcium entry into the cell and increasing calbindin-D28K expression to enhance transcellular calcium reabsorption by increased buffering of subapical Ca²⁺ ions. In the TAL, PTH may increase active transcellular transport of calcium, as well as paracellular calcium transport, by augmenting the transepithelial voltage gradient. Phosphate transport in proximal tubular cells is mediated by the luminal membrane sodium-phosphate cotransporters 2a and 2c (NPT2a and NPT2c), and PTH actions lead to internalization and degradation of NPT2a and NPT2c, thereby resulting in decreased reabsorption of phosphate.

Skeletal Actions
PTH acts directly on osteoblasts and indirectly on osteoclasts to increase their numbers and activity, thereby enhancing bone turnover and release of stored

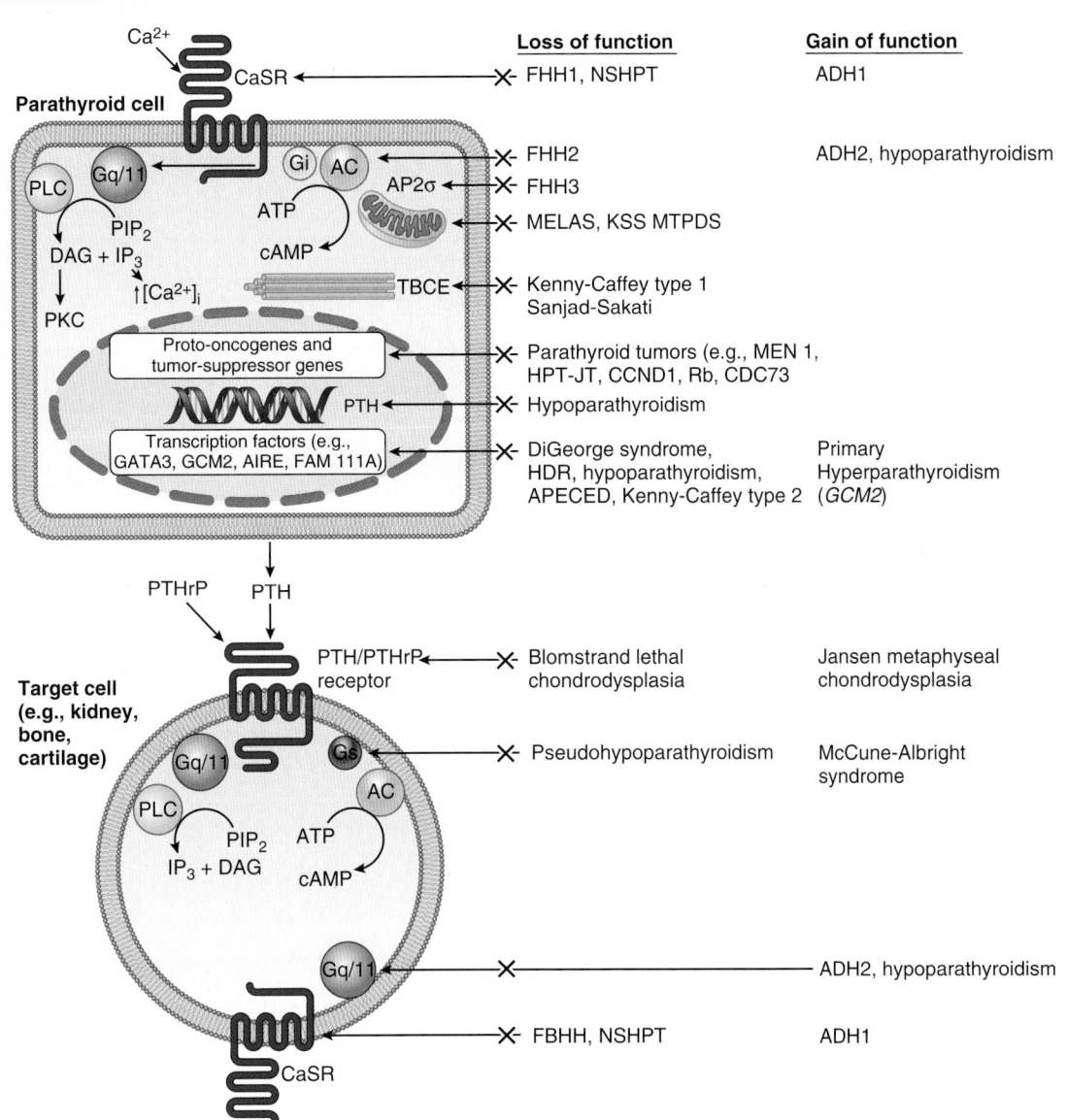

FIGURE 232-2. Schematic representation of some of the components involved in calcium homeostasis. Alterations in extracellular calcium are detected by the calcium-sensing receptor (CaSR), which is a 1078–amino acid G protein–coupled receptor. The PTH/PTHrP receptor, which mediates the actions of PTH and PTHrP, is also a G protein–coupled receptor. Thus, Ca^{2+}, PTH, and PTHrP involve G protein–coupled signaling pathways, and interaction with their specific receptors can lead to activation of Gs, Gi, and Gq/α11, respectively. Gs stimulates adenylcyclase (AC), which catalyzes the formation of cyclic adenosine monophosphate (cAMP) from adenosine triphosphate (ATP). Gi inhibits AC activity. cAMP stimulates protein kinase A (PKA), which phosphorylates cell-specific substrates. Activation of Gq/α11 stimulates phospholipase C (PLC), which catalyzes the hydrolysis of the phosphoinositide (PIP₂) to inositol triphosphate (IP₃), which then increases intracellular calcium, and diacylglycerol (DAG), activating protein kinase C (PKC). These proximal signals modulate downstream pathways, which result in specific physiologic effects. Loss- and gain-of-function mutations in several genes, shown with their respective sites of action on the right, have been identified in specific disorders of calcium homeostasis (also see Table 232-1). (From Thakker RV, Bringhurst FR, Jüppner H. Regulation of calcium homeostasis and genetic disorders that affect calcium metabolism. In: Jameson JL, De Groot LJ, Giudice LC, et al., eds. *Endocrinology: Adult & Pediatric*. 7th ed. Philadelphia: Saunders; 2016.)

calcium. Thus, PTH increases the size of the osteoblast precursor pool, increases the bone-forming activity of mature osteoblasts, and stimulates osteoblasts to release cytokines such as colony-stimulating factor 1 and receptor activator of nuclear factor-κB (NF-κB) ligand (RANKL), which stimulate the formation of new osteoclasts and activate mature osteoclasts. PTH also inhibits osteoblast production of osteoprotegerin (OPG), which is a soluble decoy receptor for RANKL that inhibits osteoclast development. Calcium transport involves TRPV4 and TRPV5 in bone cells; TRPV4 regulates intracellular calcium concentrations in osteoblasts and osteoclasts, whereas TRPV5, expressed in osteoclasts, participates to remove the mineral bone matrix. The net result of persistent elevations of PTH is linked to an increase in osteoclast activity more than osteoblast activity, hence liberating the stores of calcium to the ECF (see Fig. 232-1).

Intestinal Actions
Calcium is absorbed throughout the intestine by passive paracellular routes and active transcellular routes, which involve TRPV6 and calbindin D9K. PTH exerts indirect actions on intestinal calcium absorption by increasing the circulating 1,25(OH)₂D concentrations (see Fig. 232-1). The increased

1,25(OH)₂D concentrations increase TRPV6 expression, which facilitates enhanced calcium entry into the cell from the lumen, and cytosolic calbindin D9K expression, thereby facilitating transcellular transport of calcium.

HYPERCALCEMIA

DEFINITION
Hypercalcemia is defined as a serum calcium concentration greater than 2 standard deviations above the normal mean, and this is usually a total serum calcium above 10.5 mg/dL (2.62 mmol/L) and an ionized serum calcium of above 5.25 mg/dL (1.31 mmol/L). There is no formal grading system for defining the severity of hypercalcemia, but mild, moderate, and severe hypercalcemia is generally considered for total serum calcium concentrations less than 12 mg/dL (3 mmol/L), between 12 and 14 mg/dL (3 to 3.5 mmol/L), and greater than 14 mg/dL (3.50 mmol/L), respectively.

PATHOBIOLOGY
Hypercalcemia may arise through one of three mechanisms: increased bone resorption, increased gastrointestinal absorption of calcium, and decreased

TABLE 232-1 PARATHYROID DISEASES AND THEIR CHROMOSOMAL LOCATIONS

METABOLIC ABNORMALITY	DISEASE	INHERITANCE	GENE/GENE PRODUCT	CHROMOSOMAL LOCATION
HYPERCALCEMIA				
	Multiple endocrine neoplasia type 1	Autosomal dominant	Menin	11q13
	Multiple endocrine neoplasia types 2 and 3	Autosomal dominant	*RET*	10q11.2
	Multiple endocrine neoplasia type 4	Autosomal dominant	*CDNK1B*	12p13.1
	Hereditary hyperparathyroidism and jaw tumors (HPT-JT)	Autosomal dominant	CDC73 Parafibromin	1q31.2
	Familial isolated hyperparathyroidism	Autosomal dominant	Menin, *CDC73, CaSR* *GCMB*	11q13, 1q31.2, 3q21.1, 6p24.2
	Sporadic hyperparathyroidism	Sporadic	*PRAD1/CCND1, PTH* Retinoblastoma Unknown	11q13, 11p15 13q14 1p32-pter
	Parathyroid carcinoma	Autosomal dominant or sporadic	Parafibromin Retinoblastoma	1q31.2 13q14
	Familial benign hypercalcemia (FBH)			
	FBH1	Autosomal dominant	*CaSR*	3q 21.1
	FBH2	Autosomal dominant	Gα11	19p13
	FBH3	Autosomal dominant	*AP2S1*	19q13
	Neonatal severe hyperparathyroidism (NSHPT)	Autosomal recessive or autosomal dominant	*CaSR*	3q21.1
	Jansen disease	Autosomal dominant	PTHR/PTHrP receptor	3p21.3
	Williams syndrome	Autosomal dominant	*Elastin, LIMK* (and other genes)	7q11.23
	Infantile hypercalcemia	Autosomal recessive	CYP24A	20q13.2-q13.3
	McCune-Albright syndrome	Mutations during early embryonic development?	Gsα	20q13.3
HYPOCALCEMIA				
	Isolated hypoparathyroidism	Autosomal dominant	*PTH, GCMB*	11p15*
		Autosomal recessive	*PTH, GCMB*	11p15*, 6p24.2
		X-linked recessive	SOX3	Xq26–27
	Autosomal dominant hypocalcemia type 1 (ADH1)	Autosomal dominant	*CaSR*	3q21.1
	Autosomal dominant hypocalcemia type 2 (ADH2)	Autosomal dominant	Gα11	19p13
	Hypoparathyroidism associated with polyglandular autoimmune syndrome (APECED)	Autosomal recessive	*AIRE-1*	21q22.3
	Hypoparathyroidism associated with Kearns-Sayre and MELAS	Maternal	Mitochondrial genome	
	Hypoparathyroidism associated with complex congenital syndromes			
	DiGeorge syndrome type 1	Autosomal dominant	*TBX1*	22q11.2
	DiGeorge syndrome type 2	Autosomal dominant	*NEBL*	10p14.p13
	HDR syndrome	Autosomal dominant	*GATA3*	10p15
	Blomstrand lethal chondrodysplasia	Autosomal recessive	PTHR/PTHrP receptor	3p21.3
	Kenney-Caffey syndrome type 1, Sanjad-Sakati syndrome	Autosomal dominant	*TBCE*	1q42.3
	Kenney-Caffey syndrome type 2	Autosomal recessive	*FAM111A*	11q12.1
	Barakat syndrome	Autosomal recessive†	Unknown	?
	Lymphedema	Autosomal recessive	Unknown	?
	Nephropathy, nerve deafness	Autosomal dominant†	Unknown	?
	Nerve deafness without renal dysplasia	Autosomal dominant	Unknown?	?
	Pseudohypoparathyroidism (type 1a)	Autosomal dominant parentally imprinted	*GNAS exons 1-3*	20q13.3
	Pseudohypoparathyroidism (type 1b)	Autosomal dominant parentally imprinted	*GNAS* Upstream deletion	20q13.3

HDR = hypoparathyroidism, deafness, and renal dysplasia; MELAS = mitochondrial encephalopathy, stroke-like episodes, and lactic acidosis; ? = location not known.
*Mutations of PTH gene are identified only in some families.
†Most likely inheritance.

renal calcium excretion (see Fig. 232-1). For example, lytic bone metastases cause increased bone resorption; thiazide diuretics lead to a decrease in calcium excretion; and excessive PTH will either directly or indirectly increase $1,25(OH)_2D$ production, stimulate bone resorption and calcium absorption from the gut and renal tubules. The causes of hypercalcemia may be classified according to whether serum PTH concentrations are elevated (i.e., primary or tertiary hyperparathyroidism due to parathyroid tumors) or reduced (i.e., not due to parathyroid tumors but instead to an excessive production of PTHrP by a cancer; a defect in the PTH receptor, for example, the PTH/PTHrP receptor; an excess production of downstream mediators, for example, $1,25(OH)_2D$; or an altered set point in the calcium-sensing receptor) (Table 232-2; Fig. 232-2). Primary hyperparathyroidism and malignancy are the most common causes and account for more than 90% of patients with hypercalcemia. Detailed clinical history and examination will usually help to differentiate between these two diagnoses. In primary hyperparathyroidism, the hypercalcemia is often less than 12 mg/dL (3 mmol/L), asymptomatic, and may have been present for months or years. If symptoms, such as nephrolithiasis, are noted, then they have usually been present for several months. However, in malignancy, the patients are usually acutely ill, often with neurologic symptoms; the hypercalcemia is more than 12 mg/dL (3 mmol/L); and the cancer (e.g., lung, breast, or myeloma) is often readily apparent. Hypercalcemia from causes other than primary hyperparathyroidism or malignancy may also occur (see Table 232-2), and a careful history (e.g., for vitamin D ingestion, drugs, renal disease) and examination (e.g., for thyrotoxicosis, adrenal disease, granulomatous diseases), together with appropriate investigations (Table 232-3; Fig. 232-3),[4] are essential for establishing the diagnosis.

CLINICAL MANIFESTATIONS AND DIAGNOSIS

The clinical presentation of hypercalcemia varies from a mild, asymptomatic, biochemical abnormality detected during routine screening to a life-threatening

TABLE 232-2 CAUSES OF HYPERCALCEMIA

HIGH PARATHYROID HORMONE LEVELS

Primary hyperparathyroidism* (adenoma, hyperplasia, or carcinoma): nonfamilial or familial, e.g., MEN 1, MEN 2, HPT-JT, FIHP

Tertiary hyperparathyroidism (hyperplasia or adenoma in chronic renal failure)

LOW PARATHYROID HORMONE LEVELS

Malignancy*
  Primary
    • Parathyroid hormone–related peptide (PTHrP): carcinoma of lung, esophagus, renal cell, ovary, and bladder
    • Excess production of 1,25(OH)$_2$D (lymphoma)
  Secondary
    • Lytic bone metastases* (multiple myeloma* and breast carcinoma*)
    • Other location, ectopic factors (e.g., cytokines)

Excess vitamin D
  Exogenous vitamin D toxicity by parent D compound, 25(OH) vitamin D$_3$, or 1,25(OH)$_2$ vitamin D$_3$ in vitamin preparations, cod liver oil, herbal medicines
  Endogenous production of 25(OH) vitamin D$_3$—Williams syndrome
  Endogenous production of 1,25(OH)$_2$ vitamin D$_3$, e.g., granulomatous disorders (sarcoidosis, HIV, TB, histoplasmosis, coccidioidomycosis, leprosy), lymphoma, and infantile hypercalcemia

Drugs
  Thiazide diuretics
  Lithium
  Total parenteral nutrition
  Estrogens/antiestrogens, testosterone
  Milk-alkali syndrome
  Vitamin A toxicity
  Aluminum intoxication (in chronic renal failure)
  Aminophylline

Nonparathyroid endocrine disorders
  Thyrotoxicosis
  Pheochromocytoma
  Acute adrenal insufficiency
  Vasoactive intestinal polypeptide hormone producing tumor (VIPoma)
  Immobilization

INAPPROPRIATE PARATHYROID HORMONE LEVELS DUE TO ALTERED SET POINT

Familial benign hypocalciuric hypercalcemia (FBH or FHH) types 1-3

*Most common causes.
FIHP = familial isolated hyperparathyroidism; HIV = human immunodeficiency virus; HPT-JT = hyperparathyroidism with jaw tumors; MEN = multiple endocrine neoplasia; TB = tuberculosis.

TABLE 232-3 PRELIMINARY INVESTIGATIONS FOR HYPERCALCEMIA

BLOOD

× 2-3 estimations of serum calcium, phosphate, albumin, urea and electrolytes, creatinine, alkaline phosphatase, liver function tests
Parathyroid hormone
Complete blood count
Electrophoretic protein strip, serum protein electrophoresis, or immunofixation
25-OH-D$_3$ (and if indicated, 1,25[OH]$_2$D$_3$)
Thyroid function tests
Magnesium
Parathyroid hormone–related peptide (if malignancy suspected)

URINE

× 2-3 estimations of 24-hr urinary calcium and creatinine clearance, and clearance ratios
Imaging
  Chest radiograph
  Radiograph of hands
  Ultrasound of kidneys

TABLE 232-4 CLINICAL FEATURES OF HYPERCALCEMIA

Renal
  Stones (nephrolithiasis) and nephrocalcinosis, polyuria, polydipsia
Musculoskeletal
  Bone pain, osteopenia, fractures, muscular weakness, especially proximal myopathy
Gastrointestinal
  Nausea, vomiting, lack of appetite, constipation, peptic ulcers, and pancreatitis
Neurologic
  Tiredness, lethargy, inability to concentrate, increased sleepiness, depression, confusion, coma
Cardiac
  Bradycardia, first-degree atrioventricular block, arrhythmias, shortened QT interval

TABLE 232-5 SUMMARY OF GUIDELINES FOR PARATHYROID SURGERY IN PRIMARY HYPERPARATHYROIDISM PATIENTS

Surgery* recommended if patient meets any one of the following criteria:
• Serum calcium >1 mg/dL (0.25 mmol/L) above upper limit of normal
• Any complication of primary hyperparathyroidism (e.g., nephrolithiasis, nephrocalcinosis or bone erosions of osteitis fibrosa cystica)
• An episode of acute primary hyperparathyroidism with life-threatening hypercalcemia
• Marked hypercalciuria (>10 mmol/L per 24 hr or >400 mg/24 hr), and increased stone risk by biochemical stone risk analysis
• Significant reduction in creatinine clearance (i.e., <60 mL/min)
• Reduction in bone mineral density (i.e., T score <–2.5, at lumbar spine, total hip, femoral neck or distal 1/3 of radius and/or previous vertebral fracture)
• Age <50 years

*Surgery is also indicated in patients for whom medical surveillance is neither desired nor possible.
Adapted from Bilezikian JP, Brandi ML, Eastell R et al. Guidelines for the management of asymptomatic primary hyperparathyroidism: summary statement from the fourth international workshop. *J Clin Endocrinol Metab.* 2014;99:3561-3569.

are similar, regardless of etiology. Indeed, the clinical manifestations of hypercalcemia involve several organ systems that include the renal, musculoskeletal, gastrointestinal, neurologic, and cardiac systems (Table 232-4), and many of these have been referred to as "moans, groans, pains, and stones." Investigations should be directed at confirming the presence of hypercalcemia and establishing the cause (Table 232-3; see Table 232-5).

TREATMENT

The treatment of hypercalcemia depends on the severity of the hypercalcemia and the presence of symptoms.[5] Thus, asymptomatic patients with mild hypercalcemia do not usually need urgent treatment, whereas patients with severe hypercalcemia would require treatment regardless of symptoms, and patients with moderate hypercalcemia would require urgent treatment if symptomatic. Before instituting treatment, it is always important to consider the underlying causes (see Table 232-2) and to initiate investigations (see Table 232-3). In addition, drugs such as thiazides and vitamin D compounds, which cause hypercalcemia, should be discontinued and, if appropriate, dietary calcium restricted.

The acute management of hypercalcemia involves general measures to enhance hydration and diuresis and specific measures using drugs to lower serum calcium. Dehydration due to hypercalcemic symptoms, such as anorexia, nausea, vomiting, and polyuria because of defective urinary concentration, is very common, and patients may require 5 to 10 liters of 0.9% sodium chloride over a 24- to 48-hour period. This vigorous hydration with normal saline may lower serum calcium by 1 to 3 mg/dL (0.25 to 0.75 mmol/L); saline enhances urinary calcium excretion by increasing glomerular filtration and reducing proximal and distal renal tubular reabsorption of calcium and sodium. This saline diuresis may need adjuvant therapy with a loop diuretic (e.g., furosemide, 10 to 20 mg) as necessary to control complications due to volume overload, especially in elderly patients and those with impaired cardiovascular and renal function. Note that excessive use of furosemide before intravascular volume has been restored with intravenous normal saline may worsen the hypercalcemia by exacerbating volume depletion. Saline diuresis may lead to hypokalemia, hypomagnesemia, and electrolyte imbalance, which will need correction.

If saline diuresis is not successful, particularly if the hypercalcemia is very severe, then more specific measures, such as dialysis or drugs, will be required.

medical emergency. In general, the presence or absence of symptoms correlates with the severity and rapidity of onset of the hypercalcemia. Thus, symptoms do not usually develop when serum calcium is below 12 mg/dL (3 mmol/L) and are invariably present when the hypercalcemia exceeds 14 mg/dL (3.5 mmol/L). However, there is considerable variability, and some patients may be symptomatic with mild hypercalcemia. Although there are many causes of hypercalcemia (see Table 232-2), the signs and symptoms of hypercalcemia

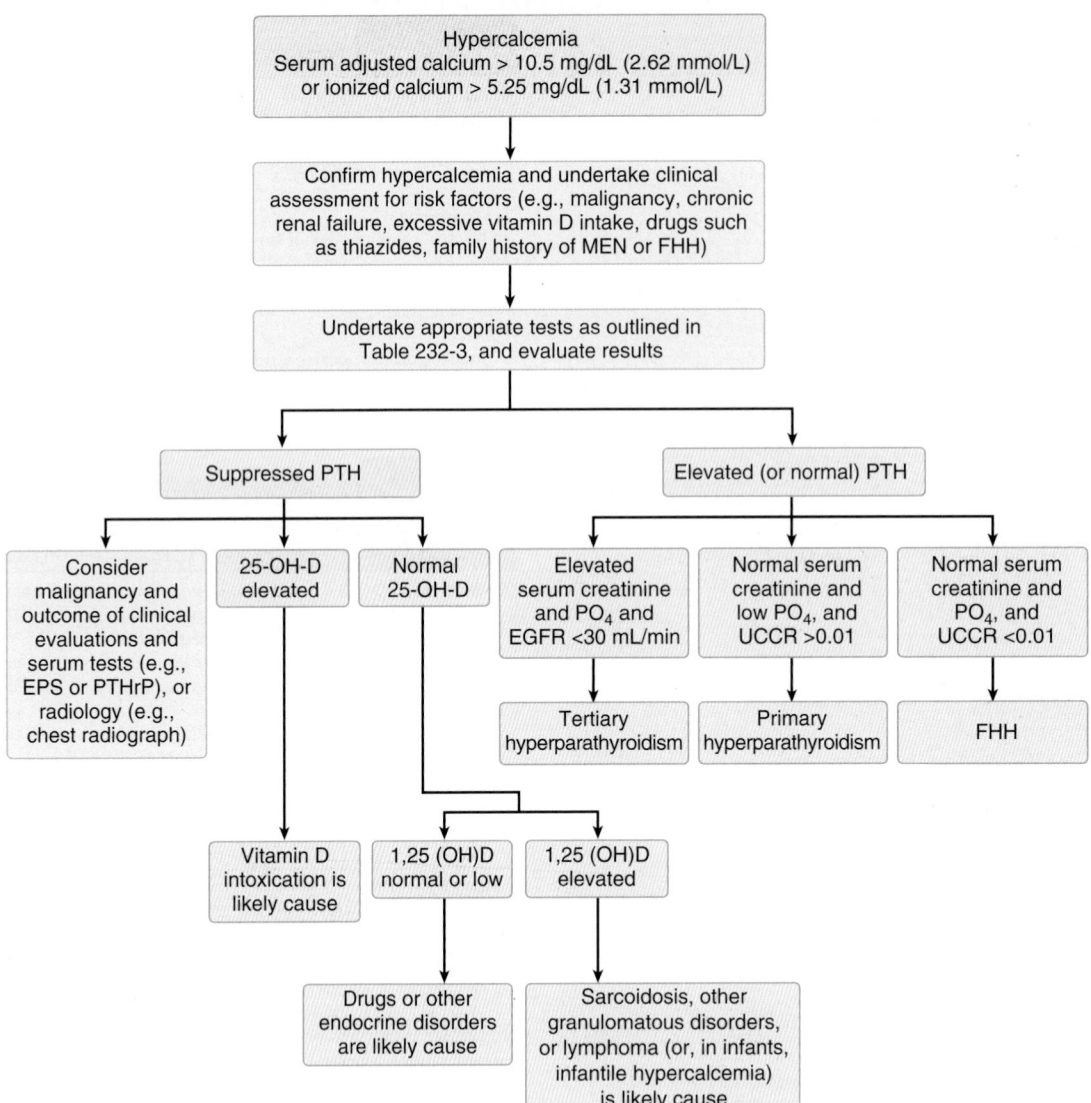

FIGURE 232-3. Clinical approach to the investigation of causes of hypercalcemia. $1,25(OH)_2D = 1,25$-dihyroxyvitamin D; 25-OH-D = 25-hydroxyvitamin D; EGFR = estimated glomerular filtration rate; EPS = electrophoretic strip (serum protein electrophoresis); FHH = familial hypocalciuric hypercalcemia; MEN = multiple endocrine neoplasia; PTH = parathyroid hormone; PTHrP = parathyroid hormone–related peptide; UCCR = 24-hour urinary calcium clearance-to-creatinine clearance ratio.

The drugs of choice are pamidronate and zoledronic acid, which are potent bisphosphonates, but these should not be used if the hypercalcemia is due to primary or tertiary hyperparathyroidism. Recommended treatments are to administer pamidronate (15 to 60 mg, depending on serum calcium concentration, in a single IV infusion or in divided doses, depending upon renal function and responses, over 2 to 4 days; maximum of 90 mg per treatment course) or zoledronic acid (4 mg as a single IV infusion). Other bisphosphonates (e.g., etidronate and clodronate) and other agents, such as mithramycin, calcitonin, and gallium nitrate, have also been used in the past. Glucocorticoid therapy (e.g., hydrocortisone, 120 mg/day in three divided doses, in adults) is particularly effective when the hypercalcemia is mediated by the actions of $1,25(OH)_2D$, for example in granulomatous disease, lymphoma, or myeloma. Dialysis using a low or zero calcium dialysate should be considered if these treatments are not effective or if the patient has renal failure. When the acute management of hypercalcemia has been completed, appropriate treatment for the underlying cause needs to be undertaken.

HYPERPARATHYROIDISM

DEFINITION

Hyperparathyroidism is characterized by high concentrations of serum immunoreactive PTH, and three types, referred to as primary, secondary, and tertiary, are recognized. Primary and tertiary hyperparathyroidism are associated with hypercalcemia (see Table 232-2), whereas secondary hyperparathyroidism is associated with hypocalcemia (see later). Primary hyperparathyroidism usually occurs as an isolated nonsyndromic endocrinopathy and less commonly as part of complex syndromic disorders such as multiple endocrine neoplasia (MEN) and hyperparathyroidism with jaw tumors (HPT-JT). Syndromic and nonsyndromic forms of primary hyperparathyroidism may also occur as hereditary (i.e., familial), usually autosomal dominant disorders, or they may occur as nonfamilial (i.e., sporadic) diseases. Tertiary hyperparathyroidism usually arises in association with chronic renal failure.

Primary Hyperparathyroidism

EPIDEMIOLOGY

Primary hyperparathyroidism, which affects 3 in 1000 adults, is one of the two most common causes of hypercalcemia and is due to an excessive secretion of PTH from one or more parathyroid tumors. Studies have estimated that the global prevalence of parathyroid tumors is 4 million. Primary hyperparathyroidism usually occurs as a nonsyndromic isolated endocrinopathy, between the ages of 40 and 65 years, and is three times more common in females than males.

PATHOBIOLOGY

Eighty percent of patients with primary hyperparathyroidism will have a solitary parathyroid adenoma, and 15 to 20% of patients will have hyperplasia involving all four parathyroid glands. Parathyroid carcinoma occurs in less than 0.5% of patients with primary hyperparathyroidism. The underlying causes of primary hyperparathyroidism are largely unknown. However, more than 10% of patients with clinically nonfamilial primary hyperparathyroidism occurring before 45 years of age have a germline mutation in 1 of 12 genes, including those of MEN 1 (*MEN1*), cell division cycle 73 (*CDC73*), and *CaSR*. In addition, studies of nonfamilial sporadic parathyroid adenomas have shown that 35 to 50% have somatic mutation of the *MEN1* gene; 15% have overexpression of cyclin D1; and more than 85% have an abnormality of the Wnt/β-catenin pathway.[6,7]

CLINICAL MANIFESTATIONS

Many patients with primary hyperparathyroidism are asymptomatic, and the hypercalcemia, which is usually mild, is detected by chance at the time of biochemical screening for other reasons.[8] However, it is important to note that nearly half the patients have subtle neuromuscular symptoms such as fatigue and weakness, and this becomes apparent only in retrospect after a successful parathyroidectomy.

Symptomatic hypercalcemia (see Table 232-4) predominantly affects the skeletal, renal, and gastrointestinal systems; peptic ulcers and pancreatitis may develop. The skeletal changes of osteitis fibrosa cystica due to subperiosteal resorption of the distal phalanges, tapering of the distal clavicles, a salt-and-pepper appearance of the skull, bone cysts, and brown tumors of the long bones are now identified in less than 5% of patients. However, osteopenia, as assessed by bone mineral density, occurs in 25% of patients. Renal stone disease (nephrolithiasis and nephrocalcinosis) occurs in 20% of patients, and hypercalciuria occurs in 30% of patients; renal impairment may complicate this disease.

DIAGNOSIS

In the presence of hypercalcemia, the finding of elevated circulating PTH concentrations establishes the diagnosis because PTH is elevated in approximately 90% of patients with primary hyperparathyroidism, who invariably have hypercalcemia (see Fig. 232-3). However, it is important to make sure that the immunoradiometric (IRMA) and immunochemiluminometric (ICMA) assays for PTH are being used to measure the intact molecule, rather than the older radioimmunoassays, which were not as reliable. The only other hypercalcemic disorders in which PTH may occasionally be elevated are those related to familial benign hypocalciuric hypercalcemia (FBH or FHH), immobilization, or lithium or thiazide use (see Table 232-2). A careful history and cessation of drug use help to exclude the latter possibilities.[9] The hypercalcemia of primary hyperparathyroidism, unlike that of malignancy or granulomatous disease, is usually not suppressible by a 10-day course of oral hydrocortisone (120 mg/day given in three divided doses). This test, referred to as the *steroid suppression test,* was previously used to differentiate primary hyperparathyroidism from other causes of hypercalcemia; however, with the advent of more reliable PTH assays, this test is rarely used now. About one third of patients with primary hyperparathyroidism have a low serum phosphate level (see Fig. 232-3), and in the others, it is in the lower range of normal. In addition, some patients have a small increase in serum chloride concentration and a concomitant decrease in bicarbonate concentration. Serum alkaline phosphatase activity may be elevated in some patients, and urinary calcium excretion is increased in 30% of patients. The circulating $1,25(OH)_2D$ concentration is elevated in some patients with primary hyperparathyroidism, although it is not of diagnostic value because it is also elevated in other hypercalcemic disorders such as sarcoidosis and lymphomas (see Fig. 232-3). The serum 25-OH-D concentration is within the normal range. Densitometric scanning is of use in detecting early skeletal changes. Patients with primary hyperparathyroidism develop reduced bone mineral densities (osteopenia) primarily of the cortical bone (e.g., distal third of forearm) rather than the cancellous bone (e.g., lumbar spine). The hip bones, which are an equal mixture of cortical and cancellous bone, show intermediate reductions in bone mineral density. Overall, the risk for bone fractures in patients with mild primary hyperparathyroidism is similar to those in matched, normal controls. However, successful parathyroidectomy does lead to an increase in bone mineral density over a 6- to 12-month period, and this continues for up to 10 years. Indeed, bone mineral density measurements are used in the evaluation of patients with primary hyperparathyroidism and in deciding on conservative as opposed to surgical management (see Table 232-5).

Preoperative localization to define the sites of the parathyroid tumors may be undertaken.[10] The noninvasive tests consist of ultrasonography, computed tomography (CT), magnetic resonance imaging (MRI), and scintigraphy with technetium-99m sestamibi. Sestamibi scintigraphy has now become established as the best and most convenient localization test; this can be performed with CT techniques (e.g., single-photon emission computed tomography [SPECT]) to give a three-dimensional image with greater anatomic resolution. It is important to note that there is an appreciable incidence of false-positive rates with all

the noninvasive localization procedures, so a confirmation using two methods is preferable. Invasive localization tests consist of arteriography and selective venous sampling for PTH in the veins draining the thyroidal region. These tests are time consuming, expensive, difficult, and dependent on the skill of the radiologist. It is generally accepted that these preoperative localization tests are indicated in those patients who have had previous neck surgery. However, their role in patients who have not had prior surgery remains to be established, and at present, the preferences and expertise of the local medical, radiology, and surgery teams usually determine the use of venous sampling procedures.

TREATMENT   Rx

Parathyroidectomy, which is the definitive cure, is a generally successful and safe procedure if undertaken by an experienced surgeon. There have also been major advances in surgery that have facilitated a surgical approach to be undertaken under local, as opposed to general, anesthesia. An example of this is the use of minimally invasive parathyroidectomy (MIP) in the patient with single gland disease that has been successfully localized by the combined use of sestamibi scintigraphy and ultrasonography. Surgery is recommended for symptomatic patients and for those who have skeletal and renal complications (see Table 232-5). Complications of parathyroid surgery include damage to the recurrent laryngeal nerve and permanent hypoparathyroidism. The decision to recommend surgery may be difficult in asymptomatic patients, who may constitute more than 50% of patients with primary hyperparathyroidism. The natural history of primary hyperparathyroidism in most patients is to progress slowly or not at all. For example, among asymptomatic patients, only 25% have progressive disease, which is usually manifested as a decrease in bone mineral density during a 10-year period. This has led to a controversy regarding the indications for surgery, and guidelines have been provided by the Fourth International Workshop (2013) on the Management of Asymptomatic Primary Hyperparathyroidism (see Table 232-5), and the American Association of Endocrine Surgeons.[11] However, these guidelines may not exclusively influence the decision for or against surgery, and a careful evaluation and assessment of the risks and benefits is considered by most medical and surgical teams in conjunction with the patient.

Patients who do not undergo parathyroidectomy (e.g., those with asymptomatic primary hyperparathyroidism) should be evaluated clinically and also monitored for serum calcium, creatinine, and estimated glomerular filtration rate (eGFR) at 12-month intervals; bone mineral density at 3 sites, at 1- to 3-year intervals with X-ray, or vertebral fracture assessment of the spine if there has been height loss or back pain, and if nephrolithiasis is suspected then appropriate assessments of 24-hour urine collections and renal imaging.[5] In addition, the following medical guidelines are recommended for patients with primary hyperparathyroidism.[12] First, they should avoid dehydration and remain ambulant. Second, vitamin D deficiency should be corrected, and the serum 25-hydroxy vitamin D should be maintained above 50 nmol/L. Third, the dietary intake of calcium should be normal; limiting dietary intake is not recommended. Fourth, thiazide diuretics and herbal and tonic remedies that may contain vitamin D or vitamin A should be avoided. Drugs that have been used for the treatment of primary hyperparathyroidism include oral phosphate, estrogens, or selective estrogen receptor modulators (SERMs) in postmenopausal women; bisphosphonates; and the calcimimetic, cinacalcet. Phosphate is not used because of concerns that it may promote soft tissue ectopic calcification. Estrogens and SERMs (e.g., raloxifene) do increase bone density in postmenopausal women with primary hyperparathyroidism, but they have only small effects on the serum calcium and PTH concentrations. The bisphosphonates (e.g., alendronate) inhibit bone resorption and improve BMD at the lumbar spine, without altering serum calcium and PTH concentrations. Daily high-dose (70 mg or 2800 U) cholecalciferol also can decrease PTH and improve bone density when used for 6 months before and after parathyroidectomy.[A1] However, these effects are not sustained. In a randomized, double-blind, placebo-controlled clinical trial, cinacalcet was effective in lowering serum calcium concentrations to normal values with modest reductions in PTH levels in patients with primary hyperparathyroidism.[A2] These effects were maintained with long-term treatment without major adverse effects. However, bone mineral density in the treated patients remained unchanged, although there was a reduction in biochemical markers for bone resorption and formation. The use of cinacalcet is approved for adult (i.e., over age of 18 years) patients, who have severe hypercalcemia due to primary hyperparathyroidism and are unable to undergo parathyroidectomy, or have hypercalcemia due to inoperable parathyroid carcinoma, or are on dialysis with uncontrolled secondary hyperparathyroidism. The use of these drugs should be dictated by the aims of the treatment. For example, bisphosphonate therapy should be chosen if the aim is to increase BMD, and cinacalcet should be chosen if the aim is to reduce serum calcium concentrations. Combined use of cinacalcet and alendronate has been reported, by one study, to normalize hypercalcemia and improve BMD in patients with primary hyperparathyroidism.

FAMILIAL PRIMARY HYPERPARATHYROIDISM

Primary hyperparathyroidism is most frequently encountered as a nonfamilial (sporadic) disorder. However, approximately 10% of patients with primary hyperparathyroidism have a hereditary form that may either be part of the multiple endocrine neoplasia (MEN) 1, MEN 2, MEN 3, and MEN 4 syndromes or part of the HPT-JT syndrome (see below). In addition, hereditary primary hyperparathyroidism may develop as a solitary endocrinopathy, and this has also been referred to as familial isolated hyperparathyroidism (FIHP). Patients with these familial forms of primary hyperparathyroidism, including the MEN syndromes, have important differences from those developing nonfamilial forms; these include an earlier age of onset (20 to 25 years versus 55 years) and an equal male-to-female ratio (1:1 versus 1:3). In addition, MEN syndromes are associated with the occurrence of multiple parathyroid tumors, rather than the solitary parathyroid adenomas typically found in the sporadic form, and HPT-JT is associated with the occurrence of parathyroid carcinoma in 15% of patients. This has implications for the treatment of parathyroid tumors in patients with these disorders. Thus, minimally invasive parathyroidectomy is an unsuitable approach in MEN patients because of multigland disease, and patients with HPT-JT are likely to require earlier surgery because of the higher risk for parathyroid carcinoma. Investigations of the hereditary and sporadic forms of primary HPT have helped to identify some of the genes and chromosomal regions that are involved in the etiology of parathyroid tumors (see Table 232-1 and Fig. 232-2). FIHP has been reported in several kindreds, and some have been shown to harbor mutations of the *MEN1*, *CDC73*, *GCM2* or *CaSR* genes.[13] The familial syndromes associated with MEN 1, MEN 2, MEN 3, and MEN 4 are reviewed in detail in Chapter 218.

HYPERPARATHYROIDISM–JAW TUMOR SYNDROME

The HPT-JT syndrome is an autosomal dominant disorder characterized by the occurrence of parathyroid tumors, which may be carcinomas in approximately 15% of patients, and ossifying fibromas that usually affect the maxilla or mandible. In addition, some patients may also develop Wilms tumors, renal cysts, renal hamartomas, renal cortical adenomas, papillary renal cell carcinomas, uterine tumors that may be malignant, pancreatic adenocarcinomas, testicular mixed germ cell tumors with a major seminoma component, and Hurthle cell thyroid adenomas. Mutations of the *CDC73* gene, which is located on chromosome 1q31.2 and encodes a 531–amino acid protein, parafibromin, cause HPT-JT.[14] Parafibromin is associated with the human homologue of the Paf1 protein complex, which interacts with RNA polymerase II. As part of this protein complex, parafibromin may regulate post-transcriptional events and histone modification. Patients with nonfamilial parathyroid carcinomas frequently harbor germline *CDC73* mutations.

UREMIC HYPERPARATHYROIDISM

PATHOBIOLOGY

Serum PTH levels rise in response to hypocalcemia, and this secondary hyperparathyroidism usually resolves with treatment of the underlying cause of hypocalcemia (Table 232-6). However, in chronic renal failure (Chapter 121), the secondary hyperparathyroidism may persist for a longer time, and eventually the parathyroid cells gain an autonomous function, secreting excessive PTH despite hypercalcemia; this state is referred to as tertiary hyperparathyroidism (see Table 232-2). The cause of progression from the early, presumably polyclonal, secondary hyperplasia of the parathyroids to the later, presumably monoclonal, tumors is not understood and appears to involve genes other than those involved in the etiologies of the sporadic and familial forms of primary hyperparathyroidism (see Table 232-2).

TABLE 232-6 CAUSES OF HYPOCALCEMIA

LOW PARATHYROID HORMONE LEVELS (HYPOPARATHYROIDISM)

Parathyroid agenesis
  Isolated or part of complex developmental anomaly (e.g., DiGeorge syndrome)
Parathyroid destruction
  Surgery*
  Radiation
  Infiltration by metastases or systemic disease (e.g., hemochromatosis, amyloidosis, sarcoidosis, Wilson disease, thalassemia)
Autoimmune
  Isolated
  Polyglandular (type 1)
Reduced parathyroid function (i.e., parathyroid hormone secretion)
  Parathyroid hormone gene defects
  Hypomagnesemia*
  Neonatal hypocalcemia (may be associated with maternal hypercalcemia)
  Hungry bone disease (postparathyroidectomy)
  Calcium-sensing receptor or Gα11 mutations

HIGH PARATHYROID HORMONE LEVELS (SECONDARY HYPERPARATHYROIDISM)

Vitamin D deficiency*
  As a result of nutritional lack,* malabsorption,* liver disease, or vitamin D receptor defects
  Inadequate production of active vitamin D (1,25[OH]$_2$D) as a result of chronic renal failure*
Vitamin D resistance (rickets)
  As a result of renal tubular dysfunction (Fanconi syndrome) or vitamin D receptor defects
Parathyroid hormone resistance
  (e.g., pseudohypoparathyroidism, hypomagnesemia)
Drugs
  Calcium chelators (e.g., citrated blood transfusions, phosphate—cow's milk is rich in phosphate)
  Inhibitors of bone resorption (e.g., bisphosphonates, calcitonin, plicamycin)
  Altered vitamin D metabolism (e.g., phenytoin, ketoconazole)
  Foscarnet
Miscellaneous
  Acute pancreatitis
  Acute rhabdomyolysis
  Massive tumor lysis
  Osteoblastic metastases (e.g., from prostate or breast carcinoma)
  Toxic shock syndrome
  Hyperventilation

*Most common causes.

---

phosphate in the intestines, and with calcitriol (1,25[OH]$_2$D). The use of the most appropriate phosphate binder is not well established, but it is clear that aluminum-containing compounds are to be avoided. Aluminum in these preparations and as a contaminant of dialysis solutions contributed in the recent past to the osteomalacic osseous disease and other aspects of metal toxicity in patients with renal failure (e.g., hypochromic anemia and encephalopathy). Early treatment of the metabolic disturbance will prevent or delay the onset of severe secondary hyperparathyroidism and tertiary hyperparathyroidism, which requires parathyroidectomy. For patients who have end-stage renal failure and are on dialysis, cinacalcet, the allosteric activator of the CaSR, can be used to treat the severe secondary hyperparathyroidism. Cinacalcet will reduce the PTH concentrations and may also have an antiproliferative effect,[15] but subtotal parathyroidectomy is better than cinacalcet for controlling hypercalcemia in kidney allograft recipients.[A3]

CLINICAL MANIFESTATIONS AND TREATMENT ℞

In chronic renal failure (Chapter 121), the ensuing phosphate retention and decreased production of 1,25(OH)$_2$D result in hypocalcemia and secondary hyperparathyroidism. This combination of biochemical abnormalities results in a severe bone disease that shows combined features of hyperparathyroidism and vitamin D deficiency (i.e., osteomalacia). Thus, in renal osteodystrophy, bone erosions and osteomalacia are simultaneously observed. Treatment is based on correcting the hypocalcemia, for example, with oral administration of calcium salts, which also ameliorates the hyperphosphatemia by chelating

---

● DISORDERS AND SYNDROMES ASSOCIATED WITH HYPERCALCEMIA

Endocrine Causes of Hypercalcemia Other than Hyperparathyroidism

Several nonparathyroid disorders (see Table 232-2) are associated with hypercalcemia, and these include thyrotoxicosis, pheochromocytoma, Addison disease, vasoactive intestinal polypeptide hormone producing tumor (VIPomas), familial benign hypocalciuric hypercalcemia, Jansen disease, and Williams syndrome.

THYROTOXICOSIS

Mild hypercalcemia (<12 mg/dL, or 3 mmol/L) frequently accompanies thyrotoxicosis, which leads to increased bone turnover and resorption. The hypercalcemia may respond to treatment with β-adrenergic blockers.

FAMILIAL BENIGN HYPOCALCIURIC HYPERCALCEMIA

Familial benign hypercalcemia (FBH), which is also referred to as familial hypocalciuric hypercalcemia (FHH), is an autosomal dominant disorder characterized by lifelong asymptomatic hypercalcemia in association with an inappropriately low urinary calcium excretion (i.e., calcium clearance-to-creatinine clearance ratio [CCR] <0.01), and normal circulating PTH concentrations in 80% of patients. Hypermagnesemia is also typically present. Although most patients with FBH are asymptomatic, chondrocalcinosis and acute pancreatitis have occasionally been observed. Patients with FHH have been misdiagnosed as having primary hyperparathyroidism because 20% of FHH patients may have elevated plasma PTH concentrations. In addition, 20% of FHH patients may have a CCR greater than 0.01 and therefore be indistinguishable from patients with primary hyperparathyroidism. Moreover, low CCRs are observed in patients with primary hyperparathyroidism who have vitamin D deficiency or renal insufficiency or are of African American origin. It is important to distinguish FHH patients from those with primary hyperparathyroidism because the hypercalcemia in FHH is generally benign and does not result in sequelae (see Table 232-4). Moreover, parathyroidectomy does not correct the hypercalcemia in FHH. Mutational analysis may help in identifying FHH patients from those with primary hyperparathyroidism.

AUTOIMMUNE HYPOCALCIURIC HYPERCALCEMIA

Some patients, who have the clinical features of FHH1 but not CaSR mutations, may have autoimmune hypocalciuric hypercalcemia (AHH).[16] Such patients may have multiple clinical autoimmune manifestations, including antithyroid, antigliadin, or antiendomyseal antibodies. These patients were shown to have circulating antibodies to the extracellular domain of the CaSR. The CaSR-bound autoantibodies stimulate PTH release from dispersed human parathyroid cells in vitro, probably by inhibiting the activation of the CaSR by extracellular calcium. The effects of treatment with glucocorticoids have been variable, with the hypercalcemia responding in one patient but not in another. Thus, AHH is a disorder of extracellular calcium sensing that should be considered in FHH1 patients who do not have CaSR mutations.

NEONATAL SEVERE PRIMARY HYPERPARATHYROIDISM

Neonatal severe primary hyperparathyroidism (NSHPT) is defined as symptomatic hypercalcemia with skeletal manifestations of hyperparathyroidism in the first 6 months of life. NSHPT children often present in the first few days or weeks of life with failure to thrive, dehydration, hypotonia, constipation, rib cage deformities, and multiple fractures due to bony undermineralization. They often have life-threatening hypercalcemia and require urgent parathyroidectomy, which corrects the PTH-dependent hypercalcemia and bone demineralization. Cinacalcet has been reported to be effective in reducing the hypercalcemia of some children with NSHPT. FBH or FHH is due to heterozygous inactivating mutations of the CaSR, and NSHPT is often associated with inactivating homozygous CaSR mutations when the children are from consanguineous parents with FHH1 (see Fig. 232-2). However, NSHPT has also been observed in children for whom one parent had clinically apparent FBH, and many other NSHPT patients appear to be sporadic; that is, both parents have normal serum calcium concentrations. In such NSHPT patients with heterozygous CaSR mutations, the mutant CaSR may exert a dominant negative action on the normal CaSR.

WILLIAMS SYNDROME

Williams syndrome is an autosomal dominant disorder characterized by supravalvular aortic stenosis, elfin-like facies, psychomotor retardation, and infantile hypercalcemia. The underlying abnormality causing hypercalcemia, which affects 5 to 50% of patients, remains unknown, but abnormal $1,25(OH)_2D_3$ metabolism and decreased calcitonin production have been implicated, although no abnormality has been consistently demonstrated. Hemizygosity for a microdeletion of chromosome 7q11.23 involving the ELASTIN and LIM-KINASE genes, which may explain the respective cardiovascular and neurologic features, have been reported in Williams syndrome patients. However, the calcitonin receptor gene, located on chromosome 7q21 and close to the region deleted

in Williams syndrome, was not involved in the deletion found in four patients with Williams syndrome, indicating that it is unlikely to be implicated in the hypercalcemia of such children. Another, as yet uncharacterized gene that is within this contiguously deleted region is likely to be involved to explain the abnormalities of calcium metabolism.

INFANTILE HYPERCALCEMIA

Infantile hypercalcemia is associated with failure to thrive and is characterized by severe hypercalcemia, hypercalciuria, and nephrocalcinosis and elevated circulating $1,25(OH)_2D$ concentrations. Some infants with this disorder have homozygous or compound heterozygous mutations of the gene encoding the 24-hydroxylase (CYP24A1) enzyme, which metabolizes the active $1,25(OH)_2D$ to the inactive $1,24,25(OH)_3D$ form (see Fig. 232-1).

Malignancy

Hypercalcemia may occur in 20 to 30% of patients with a malignancy, and this is usually due to increased bone resorption, which may either be directly due to skeletal metastases or indirectly due to tumor production of a humoral factor that stimulates osteoclastic bone resorption.[17] The cancers that typically metastasize to produce lytic bone lesions are from the breast, lymphomas, or multiple myeloma (see Table 232-2). The associated osteolysis, mediated by recruitment and activation of osteoclasts, involves cytokines. Denosumab, a humanized neutralizing monoclonal antibody to RANKL, may be used to prevent the recruitment and activation of osteoclasts and the resulting hypercalcemia. The cancers that are typically associated with the humoral hypercalcemia of malignancy (HHM) are squamous carcinomas of the lung, esophagus, cervix, vulva, skin, head, or neck, but other types from the kidney, bladder, ovary, and breast may also occur. HHM accounts for up to 80% of patients with malignancy-associated hypercalcemia. The most common factor causing HHM is PTHrP, which can be measured in the serum by immunoassay. However, these assays are relatively insensitive, and the failure to detect serum PTHrP does not exclude the diagnosis of HHM. Patients with HHM generally have hypercalcemia associated with lower or undetectable serum PTH levels, marked hypercalcemia, and a reduced plasma $1,25(OH)_2D$ level. Therapy of HHM is aimed at (1) reducing the tumor load by surgery, radiotherapy, or chemotherapy; (2) reducing osteoclastic bone resorption by use of denosumab, A6|A5 bisphosphonates (e.g., zoledronate), or calcitonin; and (3) increasing renal calcium clearance by a saline diuresis.

Granulomatous Disorders

Several granulomatous disorders are associated with hypercalcemia (see Table 232-2), and this is invariably associated with elevated circulating concentrations of $1,25(OH)_2D$, which is due to extrarenal synthesis. Sarcoidosis is the most frequently encountered granulomatous disorder associated with hypercalcemia; 10% of patients with sarcoidosis have hypercalcemia, and about half become hypercalciuric. The finding of raised serum angiotensin-converting enzyme (ACE) activity may help confirm the diagnosis. Glucocorticoids (e.g., 40 to 60 mg of prednisolone daily) decrease $1,25(OH)_2D$ production and restore the calcium concentration to normal. Failure to achieve normal serum calcium concentrations within 10 days of glucocorticoid therapy (e.g., hydrocortisone, 40 mg three times per day), the steroid suppression test, should suggest the coexistence of another cause for the hypercalcemia, such as primary hyperparathyroidism or malignancy.

Drugs

Several drugs (see Table 232-2) can cause hypercalcemia by different mechanisms. Compounds containing vitamins D and A are common and frequently associated with hypercalcemia. The use of thiazide diuretics is often associated with hypercalcemia. The hypercalcemia appears to be largely renal in origin because thiazides enhance distal renal tubular calcium reabsorption. Hypercalcemia reverses rapidly with discontinuation of the drug.

The milk-alkali syndrome was first described in the 1930s, generally in the context of ulcer treatment with large quantities of milk together with sodium bicarbonate. Today, the responsible agent is usually calcium carbonate, although consumption of large quantities of dairy products (milk, cheese, and yogurt) may still contribute. Classic features include moderate to severe hypercalcemia with alkalosis and renal impairment. The amount of calcium ingested by patients with this syndrome is usually 5 to 15 g/day. Treatment consists of (1) discontinuing the ingestion of the calcium-containing compounds and antacids, (2) rehydration, and (3) saline diuresis.

HYPOCALCEMIA

DEFINITION

Hypocalcemia is defined as a serum calcium concentration below the lower limit of normal range, and this is usually an ionized serum calcium below 4.65 mg/dL (1.16 mmol/L) and a total serum calcium below 8.5 mg/dL (2.12 mmol/L). Mild hypocalcemia is defined as a total serum calcium of 8 to 8.5 mg/dL (2 to 2.12 mmol/L) and severe hypocalcemia as a total serum calcium below 7.6 mg/dL (1.9 mmol/L).

PATHOBIOLOGY

Hypocalcemia (see Table 232-6) can be classified by cause, according to whether serum PTH concentrations are low (i.e., hypoparathyroid disorders) or high (i.e., disorders associated with secondary hyperparathyroidism). Hypocalcemia is most commonly caused by hypoparathyroidism, a deficiency or abnormal metabolism of vitamin D, acute or chronic renal failure, or hypomagnesemia. Hypocalcemic diseases (see Table 232-6) may arise because of a destruction of the parathyroid glands, failure of parathyroid gland development, or reduced PTH secretion or PTH-mediated actions in target tissues. Thus, these diseases may be classified as being due to a deficiency of PTH, a defect in the PTH receptor (i.e., the PTH/PTHrP receptor), or insensitivity to PTH caused by defects downstream of the PTH/PTHrP receptor (see Fig. 232-2). The diseases may also be classified as being part of the hypoparathyroid disorders, of the CaSR abnormalities, or of the pseudohypoparathyroid disorders.[18]

CLINICAL MANIFESTATIONS AND DIAGNOSIS

The clinical presentation of hypocalcemia ranges from an asymptomatic biochemical abnormality to a severe, life-threatening condition.[19] In mild hypocalcemia, patients may be asymptomatic. Those with more severe and long-term hypocalcemia may develop acute symptoms of neuromuscular irritability (Table 232-7), ectopic calcification (e.g., in the basal ganglia, which may be associated with extrapyramidal neurologic symptoms), subcapsular cataracts, papilledema, and abnormal dentition. Investigations should be directed at confirming the presence of hypocalcemia and establishing the cause (Fig. 232-4).

In hypoparathyroidism, serum calcium is low, phosphate is high, and PTH is undetectable; renal function and concentrations of the 25-hydroxy and 1,25-dihydroxy metabolites of vitamin D are usually normal (see Fig. 232-4). The features of pseudohypoparathyroidism are similar to those of hypoparathyroidism except for PTH, which is markedly increased. In chronic renal failure, which is the most common cause of hypocalcemia, phosphate is high, and alkaline phosphatase, creatinine, and PTH are elevated; 25-OH-D_3 is normal, and $1,25(\text{OH})_2\text{D}_3$ is low (see Fig. 232-1). In vitamin D deficiency osteomalacia, serum calcium and phosphate are low, alkaline phosphatase and PTH are elevated, renal function is normal, and 25-OH-D_3 is low (see Fig. 232-4). The most frequent artifactual cause of hypocalcemia is hypoalbuminemia, such as occurs in liver disease or the nephrotic syndrome.

TREATMENT Rx

Acute Hypocalcemia

The management of acute hypocalcemia depends on the severity of the hypocalcemia, the rapidity with which it developed, and the degree of neuromuscular irritability (see Table 232-7). Treatment should be given to symptomatic patients (e.g., with seizures or tetany) and asymptomatic patients with a serum calcium of less than 7.6 mg/dL (1.90 mmol/L) who are at high risk for developing complications. The preferred treatment for acute symptomatic hypocalcemia

TABLE 232-7 HYPOCALCEMIC CLINICAL FEATURES OF NEUROMUSCULAR IRRITABILITY

Paresthesia, usually of fingers, toes, and circumoral regions
Tetany, carpopedal spasm, muscle cramps
Chvostek sign*
Trousseau sign†
Seizures of all types (i.e., focal or petit mal, grand mal, or syncope)
Prolonged QT interval on electrocardiogram
Laryngospasm
Bronchospasm

*Chvostek sign is twitching of the circumoral muscles in response to gentle tapping of the facial nerve just anterior to the ear; it may be present in 10% of normal individuals.
†Trousseau sign is carpal spasm elicited by inflation of a blood pressure cuff to 20 mm Hg above the patient's systolic blood pressure for 3 minutes.

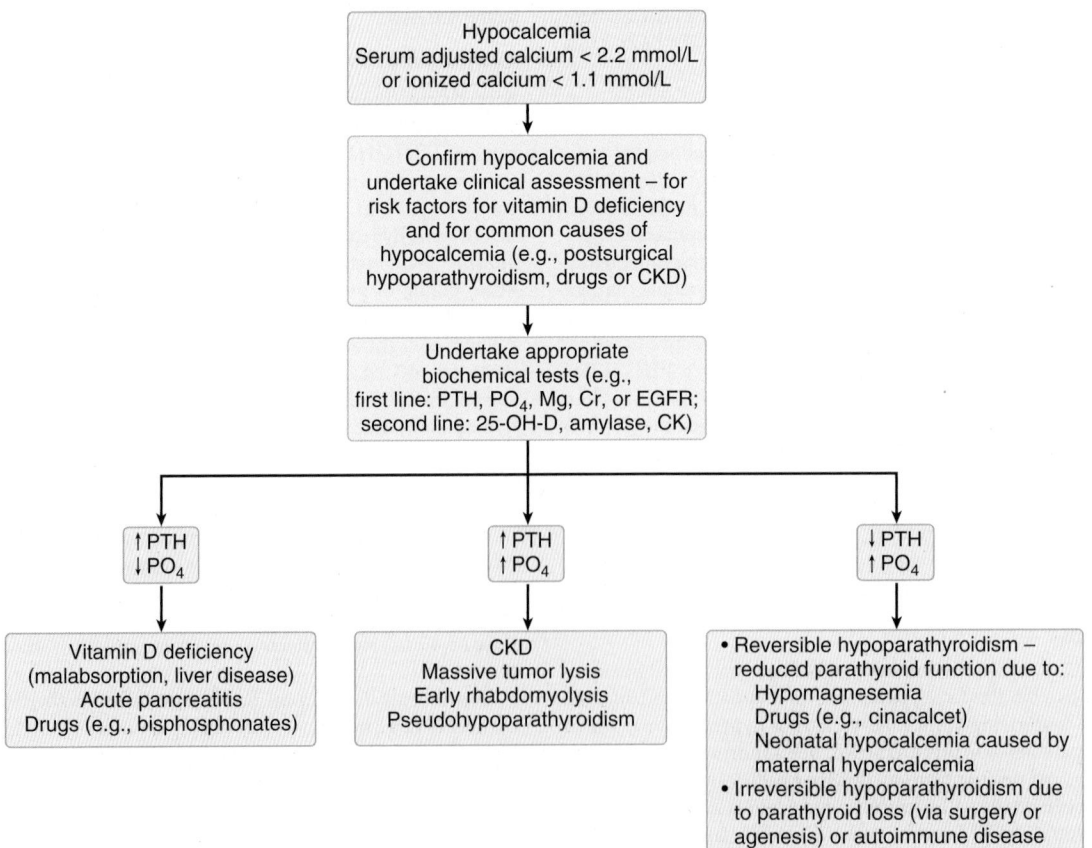

FIGURE 232-4. Clinical approach to investigation of causes of hypocalcemia. 25-OH-D = 25-hydroxyvitamin D; CK = creatinine kinase; CKD = chronic kidney disease; Cr = creatinine; EGFR = estimated glomerular filtration rate; PTH = parathyroid hormone.

is calcium gluconate, 10 mL 10% w/v (2.20 mmol of calcium) intravenous, diluted in 50 mL of 5% dextrose or 0.9% sodium chloride and given by slow injection (>5 minutes); this can be repeated as required to control symptoms. Serum calcium concentrations should be assessed regularly. Persistent hypocalcemia may be managed acutely by administration of a calcium gluconate infusion; for example, dilute 10 ampules of calcium gluconate, 10 mL 10% w/v (22 mmol of calcium), in 1 liter of 5% dextrose or 0.9% sodium chloride, start infusion at 50 mL/hour, and titrate to maintain serum calcium concentrations in the normal range. Generally, 1.2 to 1.6 mg/kg (0.3 to 0.4 mmol/kg) of elemental calcium infused over 4 to 6 hours increases serum calcium by 2 to 3 mg/dL (0.5 to 0.75 mmol/L). If hypocalcemia is likely to persist, oral vitamin D therapy (see later) should also be administered. In hypocalcemic patients who are also hypomagnesemic, the hypomagnesemia must be corrected before the hypocalcemia will resolve. This may occur in the postparathyroidectomy period or in patients with severe malabsorption, for example, those with established celiac disease (Chapter 131).

Chronic Hypocalcemia

The two main agents available for the treatment of chronic (long-term) hypocalcemia are supplemental calcium, about 10 to 20 mmol calcium every 6 to 12 hours, and vitamin D preparations. Patients with hypothyroidism seldom require calcium supplements after the early stages of stabilization with vitamin D. A variety of vitamin D preparations have been used. These include vitamin D_3 (cholecalciferol) or vitamin D_2 (ergocalciferol), 10,000 to 50,000 units (0.25 to 1.25 mg/day); dihydrotachysterol (now seldom used), 0.25 to 1.25 mg/day; alfacalcidol (1α-hydroxycholecalciferol), 0.25 to 1 µg/day; and calcitriol (1,25-dihydroxy cholecalciferol), 0.25 to 2 µg/day. In children, these preparations are prescribed in doses based on body weight. Cholecalciferol and ergocalciferol are the least expensive preparations but have the longest durations of action and may result in prolonged toxicity; however, they are the preparations of choice for treating hypocalcemia associated with vitamin D deficiency (see Table 232-6). The other preparations, which do not require renal 1α-hydroxylation, have the advantage of shorter half-lives and thereby minimize the risk for prolonged toxicity. For treatment of hypocalcemia due to hypoparathyroidism or chronic renal failure, calcitriol is the drug of choice because it is the active metabolite and, unlike alfacalcidol, does not require hepatic 25-hydroxylation. Close monitoring (at about 1- to 2-week intervals) of the patient's serum and urine calcium concentrations are required initially, and follow-up at 3- to 6-month intervals is appropriate once stabilization is achieved. The aim is to avoid hypercalcemia, hypercalciuria, nephrolithiasis, and renal failure. It should be noted that hypercalciuria may occur in the absence of hypercalcemia. The use of PTH (1-84) in hypoparathyroid patients has been reported to be associated with improvement in the biochemical and skeletal indices, as well as in mental and physical health.[20,21]

● HYPOPARATHYROIDISM

Hypoparathyroidism is characterized by hypocalcemia and hyperphosphatemia, which are the result of a deficiency in PTH secretion or action.[22,23] The incidence of hypoparathyroidism is approximately 0.8 per 100,000 person-years, with a prevalence estimated to be 22 to 37 per 100,000 person-years.

▬ PATHOBIOLOGY

The most common cause of hypoparathyroidism is postsurgical hypoparathyroidism. Hypoparathyroidism also may result from agenesis (e.g., DiGeorge syndrome) or destruction of the parathyroid glands (e.g., autoimmune diseases), from reduced secretion of PTH (e.g., neonatal hypocalcemia or hypomagnesemia), or from resistance to PTH (which may occur as a primary disorder (e.g., pseudohypoparathyroidism or secondary to hypomagnesemia) (see Table 232-6). In addition, hypoparathyroidism may occur as an inherited syndromic disorder (see Table 232-1) that may either be part of a complex congenital defect (e.g., DiGeorge syndrome) or part of a polyglandular autoimmune disorder (see Table 232-6 and Fig. 232-2). Hypoparathyroidism may also occur as a nonsyndromic solitary endocrinopathy, which has been referred to as isolated or idiopathic hypoparathyroidism. Familial occurrences of isolated hypoparathyroidism with autosomal dominant, autosomal recessive, and X-linked recessive inheritances have been established.[24]

▬ CLINICAL MANIFESTATIONS AND DIAGNOSIS

Patients with hypoparathyroidism may present with symptoms and signs of acute or chronic hypocalcemia, as described above. The diagnosis requires accurate measurement of PTH. Serum concentrations of immunoreactive PTH are low or undetectable despite the presence of hypocalcemia.

Concentrations of $1,25(OH)_2D_3$ are usually in the low-normal to low range, but alkaline phosphatase activity is normal (see Fig. 232-4). The daily urinary excretion of calcium may be reduced, although the fractional excretion of calcium is invariably increased.

TREATMENT **Rx**

The main treatments for the hypocalcemia due to hypoparathyroidism are vitamin D preparations and supplemental calcium, as described above. Recombinant human PTH (1-84), rhPTH, has been approved by the U.S. FDA for the treatment of patients whose hypocalcemia is refractory to treatment with vitamin D preparations and calcium supplements. Treatment with rhPTH at a dose of 50 µg once daily can provide a specific approach to management with reduced doses of calcium and vitamin D.[25] Doses should be titrated every 4 weeks, with the goal to reduce oral calcium supplements to as low as 500 mg/day and to discontinue vitamin D supplements while keeping serum calcium within the low-normal range. After a stable dose is achieved, serum calcium and phosphate levels should be monitored every 3 to 6 months and urinary calcium excretion at least yearly.

Specific Causes of Hypoparathyroidism
ISOLATED HYPOPARATHYROIDISM
Isolated hypoparathyroidism may either be inherited or acquired by damage to the parathyroids at surgery, by infiltrating metastases, or by systemic disease (see Table 232-6).

Acquired Forms of Hypoparathyroidism
Hypoparathyroidism may occur after neck surgery, after irradiation, or because of infiltration by metastases or systemic disease, for example, hemochromatosis, amyloidosis, sarcoidosis, Wilson disease, or thalassemia (see Table 232-6). Surgical damage to the parathyroids occurs most commonly after a radical neck dissection, such as for laryngeal or esophageal carcinoma treatment, after a total thyroid resection, or after repeated parathyroidectomies for polyglandular disease (e.g., in MEN 1 or MEN 2, discussed previously). Hypocalcemic symptoms begin 12 to 24 hours after surgery and may need treatment with oral or intravenous calcium. Parathyroid function often returns, but persistent hypocalcemia requires treatment with vitamin D preparations.

Neonatal hypoparathyroidism resulting in hypocalcemia may occur in the infant of a mother with hypercalcemia caused by primary hyperparathyroidism (see Table 232-6). Maternal hypercalcemia results in increased calcium delivery to the fetus, and this fetal hypercalcemia suppresses fetal PTH secretion. Postpartum, the infant's suppressed parathyroids are unable to maintain normocalcemia. The disorder is usually self-limited, but occasionally therapy may be required. In addition, the feeding of cow's milk, which has a high phosphate content, to infants may result in hypocalcemia in some children.

Functional hypoparathyroidism may result from severe hypomagnesemia (<0.4 mmol/L), which may be due to a severe intestinal malabsorption disorder (e.g., Crohn disease) or a renal tubular disorder (see Table 232-6). It is associated with hypoparathyroidism because magnesium is required for the release of PTH from the parathyroid gland and also for PTH action through adenyl cyclase. Magnesium chloride, 35 to 50 mmol intravenously in 1 liter of 5% glucose or other isotonic solution given over 12 to 24 hours, may be repeatedly required to restore normomagnesemia.

Inherited Hypoparathyroidism
Patients with inherited forms of hypoparathyroidism may develop hypocalcemic seizures in the neonatal or infantile periods and require lifelong treatment with oral vitamin D preparations, such as calcitriol. Autosomal dominant, autosomal recessive, and X-linked recessive inheritances for hypoparathyroidism have been observed (see Table 232-1). Some of the autosomal forms are due to mutations of the *PTH* gene, the *CaSR* (see later), the *Gα11* subunit (see later), and the transcriptional factor *GCMB* (glial cells missing B). The X-linked forms likely alter regulation of SOX3 (see Fig. 232-4).

Autosomal Dominant Hypocalcemia Type 1 and Type 2
Autosomal dominant hypocalcemia type 1 (ADH1) is characterized by lifelong mild or severe hypocalcemia in association with normal serum PTH concentrations in about 40% of patients or low serum PTH concentrations in about 60% of patients. Serum phosphate and magnesium concentrations may be

elevated or low, respectively. Approximately 50% of ADH1 patients have asymptomatic hypocalcemia, and the remaining 50% may experience paresthesia, muscle cramps, carpopedal spasms, and seizures, which may be associated with a febrile illness. In addition, about 10% of ADH1 patients may have absolute hypercalciuria, which may be associated with nephrocalcinosis and kidney stones in 35% of patients. Vitamin D preparations and calcium supplementation to correct the hypocalcemia may worsen the hypercalciuria and lead to renal impairment. Basal ganglia or ectopic calcification may be found in more than 35% of patients. About 20% of ADH1 patients do not have a previously reported family history because they have de novo mutations. ADH1 is due to gain-of-function mutations of the *CaSR* (see Table 232-1 and Fig. 232-2). ADH2 is due to gain-of-function mutations of the *Gα11* subunit, and ADH2 patients appear to have clinical features that are similar to those in ADH1 patients.

COMPLEX SYNDROMES ASSOCIATED WITH HYPOPARATHYROIDISM

Hypoparathyroidism may occur as part of a complex syndrome that may be associated with either a congenital developmental anomaly or an autoimmune syndrome. The congenital developmental anomalies associated with hypoparathyroidism, which occurs in 1 in 4000 live births, include DiGeorge syndrome, hypoparathyroidism, deafness, and renal anomalies (HDR) syndrome, Kenney-Caffey and Barakat syndromes, and also syndromes associated with either lymphedema or dysmorphic features and growth failure (see Table 232-1 and Fig. 232-2).

Polyglandular Autoimmune Hypoparathyroidism

Polyglandular autoimmune hypoparathyroidism comprises hypoparathyroidism, Addison disease, candidiasis, and two or three of the following: type 1 diabetes mellitus, primary hypogonadism, autoimmune thyroid disease, pernicious anemia, chronic active hepatitis, steatorrhea (malabsorption), alopecia (totalis or areata), and vitiligo. The disorder has also been referred to as either the autoimmune polyendocrinopathy candidiasis ectodermal dystrophy (APECED) syndrome or the polyglandular autoimmune type 1 syndrome (see Table 232-1). Antibodies directed against the adrenal, thyroid, and parathyroid glands are detected in the sera of some patients. The polyglandular autoimmune type 2 syndrome is characterized by adrenal insufficiency, type 1 diabetes mellitus, and thyroid disease and does not involve hypoparathyroidism. APECED, which has an autosomal recessive inheritance, has a high incidence in Finland and among Iranian Jews. The *APECED* gene, which has been located to chromosome 21q22.3, encodes a 545–amino acid protein that contains motifs associated with a transcriptional factor and includes two zinc-finger motifs, a proline-rich region, and three LXXLL motifs. The gene is referred to as *AIRE* (autoimmune regulator) (see Fig. 232-2). Four *AIRE* mutations are commonly found in APECED families, and these likely abolish the E3 ubiquitin ligase activity of the AIRE1 protein. AIRE1 has been shown to regulate the elimination of organ-specific T cells in the thymus, and APECED is likely to be caused by a failure of this specialized mechanism for deleting forbidden T cells and establishing immunologic tolerance.

Autoimmune Acquired Hypoparathyroidism

Twenty percent of patients who have acquired hypoparathyroidism (AH) in association with autoimmune hypothyroidism have autoantibodies to the extracellular domain of the CaSR (see Table 232-1 and Fig. 232-2). The CaSR autoantibodies do not persist for long; 72% of patients who had AH for less than 5 years had detectable CaSR autoantibodies, whereas only 14% of patients with AH for more than 5 years had such autoantibodies. The majority of the patients who have CaSR autoantibodies were female, a finding that is similar to that found in other autoantibody-mediated diseases. Indeed, a few acquired hypoparathyroidism patients also have features of autoimmune polyglandular syndrome type 1. The epitopes for the anti-CaSR antibodies are localized to the N terminal of the extracellular domain of the receptor. These findings establish that the CaSR is an autoantigen in acquired hypoparathyroidism.

DiGeorge Syndrome

Patients with the DiGeorge syndrome suffer from neonatal hypoparathyroidism, T-cell immunodeficiency, congenital heart defects, and deformities of the ear, nose, and mouth (e.g., cleft lip and/or palate). Children with DiGeorge syndrome often die from infections related to the immunodeficiency. The disorder arises from a congenital failure in the development of the derivatives of the third and fourth pharyngeal pouches with resulting absence or hypoplasia of the parathyroids and thymus. Most cases are sporadic, but an autosomal dominant inheritance of DiGeorge syndrome has been observed, and an association between the syndrome and an unbalanced translocation and deletions involving chromosome 22q11.2 has also been reported (see Table 232-1). In some patients, deletions of another locus on chromosome 10p13-p14 have been observed in association with DiGeorge syndrome, and this is referred to as DGS2, whereas patients with the 22q11.2 deletions are referred to as having DGS1. Studies of the DGS1 deleted region on chromosome 22q11.2 have revealed four genes (*RNEX40*, *NEX2.2-NEX3*, *UDFIL*, and *TBX1*) to be involved. However, point mutations in DGS1 patients have been detected only in the *TBX1* gene, and *TBX1* is now considered to be the gene causing DGS1 (see Table 232-1 and Fig. 232-2). *TBX1* encodes a DNA-binding transcriptional factor of the T-BOX family that is known to have an important role in organogenesis and pattern formation. The *TBX1* gene is deleted in approximately 96% of all DGS1 patients, and some of those without deletions have mutations of *TBX1*.

PSEUDOHYPOPARATHYROIDISM

Patients with pseudohypoparathyroidism (PHP), which may be inherited as an autosomal dominant disorder, are characterized by hypocalcemia and hyperphosphatemia due to PTH resistance rather than PTH deficiency (see Table 232-6).[26] Five variants, which form part of a group of inactivating PTH/PTHrP signalling disorders (iPPSDs),[27] are recognized on the basis of biochemical and somatic features (Table 232-8), and three of these—PHP type 1a (PHP 1a), PHP type 1b (PHP 1b), and pseudopseudohypoparathyroidism (PPHP)—will be reviewed in further detail. Patients with PHP 1a exhibit

---

TABLE 232-8 CLINICAL, BIOCHEMICAL, AND GENETIC FEATURES OF HYPOPARATHYROID AND PSEUDOHYPOPARATHYROID DISORDERS

	HYPOPARATHYROIDISM	PSEUDOHYPOPARATHYROIDISM				
		PHP 1a	PPHP	PHP 1b	PHP 1c	PHP 2
AHO manifestations	No	Yes	Yes	No	Yes	No
Serum calcium	↓	↓	N	↓	↓	↓
Serum PO$_4$	↑	↑	N	↑	↑	↑
Serum PTH	↓	↑	N	↑	↑	↑
Response to PTH:						
Urinary cAMP* (Chase-Aurbach test)	↑	↓	↑	↓	↓	↑
Urinary PO$_4$ (Ellsworth-Howard test)	↑	↓	↑	↓	↓	↓
Gsα activity	N	↓	↓	N	N	N
Inheritance	AD, AR, X	AD	AD	AD	AD	Sporadic
Molecular defect	PTH, CaSR, GATA3, Gcm2, others	*GNAS1*	*GNAS1*	*GNAS1*†	?Adenyl cyclase	?cAMP targets
Other hormonal resistance	No	Yes	No	No	Yes	No

↓ = decreased; ↑ = increased; ? = presumed, but not proved; AD = autosomal dominant; AHO = Albright hereditary osteodystrophy; AR = autosomal recessive; N = normal; PHP = pseudoparathyroidism; PPHP = pseudopseudoparathyroidism; PTH = parathyroid hormone; X = X-linked.
*Plasma cyclic adenosine monophosphate (cAMP) responses are similar to those of urinary cAMP.
†Involves deletions that are located upstream of GNAS1.

PTH resistance (hypocalcemia, hyperphosphatemia, elevated serum PTH, and an absence of an increase in serum and urinary cAMP and urinary phosphate following intravenous human PTH infusion), together with the features of Albright hereditary osteodystrophy (AHO), which includes short stature, obesity, subcutaneous calcification, mental retardation, round facies, dental hypoplasia, and brachydactyly (i.e., shortening of the metacarpals, particularly the third, fourth, and fifth). In addition to brachydactyly, other skeletal abnormalities of the long bones and shortening of the metatarsals may occur. Patients with PHP 1b exhibit PTH resistance only and do not have the somatic features of AHO, whereas patients with PPHP exhibit the somatic features of AHO in the absence of PTH resistance. The absence of a normal rise in urinary excretion of cAMP after an infusion of PTH in PHP 1a indicates a defect at some site of the PTH receptor–adenyl cyclase system (see Fig. 232-2). This receptor system is regulated by at least two G proteins, one of which stimulates (Gsα) and another of which inhibits (Giα) the activity of the membrane-bound enzyme that catalyses the formation of the intracellular second messenger cAMP. Patients with PHP 1a may also show resistance to other hormones, such as thyroid-stimulating hormone, follicle-stimulating hormone, and luteinizing hormone, that act through GPCRs. Inactivating mutations of the Gsα gene (referred to as *GNAS1*), which is located on chromosome 20q13.2, have been identified in PHP 1a and PPHP patients (see Table 232-1 and Fig. 232-2). However, *GNAS1* mutations do not fully explain the PHP 1a or PPHP phenotypes, and studies of PHP 1a and PPHP that occurred within the same kindred revealed that the hormonal resistance is parentally imprinted. Thus, PHP 1a occurs in a child only when the mutation is inherited from a mother affected with either PHP 1a or PPHP; and PPHP occurs in a child only when the mutation is inherited from a father affected with either PHP 1a or PPHP. PHP 1b is due to deletions that are located upstream of the *GNAS1* gene. Moreover, in affected individuals, the deletion involves the maternal allele, whereas its occurrence on the paternal allele results in unaffected healthy carriers. This is consistent with parental imprinting of the *GNAS1* abnormality causing PHP 1b.

Grade A References

A1. Rolighed L, Rejnmark L, Sikjaer T, et al. Vitamin D treatment in primary hyperparathyroidism: a randomized placebo controlled trial. *J Clin Endocrinol Metab.* 2014;99:1072-1080.

A2. Peacock M, Bilezikian JP, Bolognese MA, et al. Cinacalcet HCl reduces hypercalcemia in primary hyperparathyroidism across a wide spectrum of disease severity. *J Clin Endocrinol Metab.* 2011;96:E9-E18.

A3. Cruzado JM, Moreno P, Torregrosa JV, et al. A randomized study comparing parathyroidectomy with cinacalcet for treating hypercalcemia in kidney allograft recipients with hyperparathyroidism. *J Am Soc Nephrol.* 2016;27:2487-2494.

A4. Henry D, Vadhan-Raj S, Hirsh V, et al. Delaying skeletal-related events in a randomized phase 3 study of denosumab versus zoledronic acid in patients with advanced cancer: an analysis of data from patients with solid tumors. *Support Care Cancer.* 2014;22:679-687.

A5. Diel IJ, Body JJ, Stopeck AT, et al. The role of denosumab in the prevention of hypercalcaemia of malignancy in cancer patients with metastatic bone disease. *Eur J Cancer.* 2015;51:1467-1475.

GENERAL REFERENCES

For the General References and other additional features, please visit Expert Consult at https://expertconsult.inkling.com.

233

PAGET DISEASE OF BONE

STUART H. RALSTON

DEFINITION

Paget disease of bone is a focal disorder of the skeleton characterized by increased and disorganized bone remodeling. Affected bones enlarge, become deformed, and are at increased risk for pathologic fractures.

EPIDEMIOLOGY

The prevalence of Paget disease is about 1% in the United Kingdom. It is also common in Western Europe and in people of European descent who have migrated to other parts of the world. Paget disease is rare in Scandinavians, Africans, and Asians. These differences are thought to have a genetic basis occurring as the result of founder mutations in North West Europe many centuries ago, with subsequent spread to the rest of the world through emigration. The incidence of Paget disease increases with age; in the United Kingdom, the incidence is 0.3 to 0.5 per 10,000 person years in those aged 55 to 59 years but doubles in frequency each decade thereafter to reach an incidence of 5.4 per 10,000 person years in women and 7.6 per 10,000 person years in men in those 85 years and older. The prevalence and severity of Paget disease have diminished in many countries over the past 25 years.[1] The mechanisms are unclear, but suggested explanations include influx of migrants from low prevalence areas in some populations, improved nutrition, a more sedentary lifestyle with a reduction in skeletal injuries, and reduced exposure to infections.

PATHOBIOLOGY

Susceptibility to Paget disease is strongly influenced by genetic factors, but environmental factors are also important.[2] The importance of genetics is emphasized by the fact that between 15 and 40% of patients have a positive family history and that the risk for developing Paget disease in a first-degree relative of a patient is about seven-fold higher than in the general population. In many families, the disease is transmitted in an autosomal dominant manner, although penetrance is incomplete. The most important susceptibility gene for classical Paget disease is *SQSTM1*. Mutations of *SQSTM1* are present in up to 40% of patients with a family history and 5 to 10% of people without a family history. The *SQSTM1* gene encodes a protein called p62 that is involved in regulating signal transduction downstream of the receptor activator of nuclear factor κB (RANK), which plays a critical role in regulating osteoclastogenesis when activated by RANK ligand (RANKL) (Fig. 233-1). The disease-causing mutations cluster in the ubiquitin-associated domain and have the effect of upregulating nuclear factor κB (NFκB) signaling and stimulating osteoclastogenesis by complex mechanisms that are reviewed in detail elsewhere. Genome-wide association studies have identified seven other loci that predispose to Paget disease, which individually increase the risk between 1.4- and 1.7-fold.[3] These loci have additive effects such that individuals who carry several predisposing alleles have a substantially increased risk for developing Paget disease. Many lie close to genes that play key roles in osteoclast function, including *CSF1*, which encodes macrophage colony-stimulating factor (M-CSF); *TNFRSF11A*, which encodes RANK; *TM7SF4*, which encodes DC-STAMP; *OPTN*, which encodes optineurin, and *RIN3*, which encodes a guanine exchange factor that is expressed in osteoclasts (see Fig. 233-1). Several rare inherited diseases with clinical features overlapping with those of Paget disease have also been described.[4] They include familial expansile osteolysis and related syndromes caused by mutations affecting the signal peptide of RANK; juvenile Paget disease caused by loss of function mutations affecting osteoprotegerin; multisystem proteinopathies caused by mutations in *VCP*, *hnRNPA2B1*, and *hnRNPA1*, in which Paget disease may be accompanied by dementia, myopathy, or amyotrophic lateral sclerosis; and a syndrome wherein Paget disease is accompanied by giant cell tumors and that is caused by mutations in *ZNF687*, which encodes a zinc finger protein whose function is as yet incompletely understood.

Bone is normally renewed and repaired in an orderly and tightly regulated fashion through the process of bone remodeling. Bone remodeling is highly abnormal in Paget disease. Osteoclasts are increased in number and size and are hypernucleated. Some contain nuclear inclusion bodies. These were originally thought to be paramyxovirus nucleocapsids, but more recent studies suggest that they may be aggregates of un-degraded proteins caused by defects in the autophagy pathway. Bone formation is markedly increased, and the amount of new bone that is formed exceeds that which has been removed by osteoclast activity, leading to enlargement and deformity of affected bones (Fig. 233-2). The newly formed bone is laid down in a disorganized fashion (woven bone) and has impaired mechanical strength. Other features include increased vascularity and marrow fibrosis. The focal nature of Paget disease remains a puzzle. Suggested explanations include the occurrence of somatic mutations in affected bones, which locally increase osteoclast activity, or excessive mechanical loading or skeletal injuries early in life, which by causing microdamage act as a focus for localized increases in bone remodeling.

CLINICAL MANIFESTATIONS

It has been estimated that between 7 and 16% of patients with Paget disease come to medical attention, but the mode of presentation in those that do is highly variable. About 20% have no symptoms, and, in these subjects, Paget disease is detected as the result of a raised serum alkaline phosphatase (ALP) or an abnormal radiograph in people who are being investigated for another

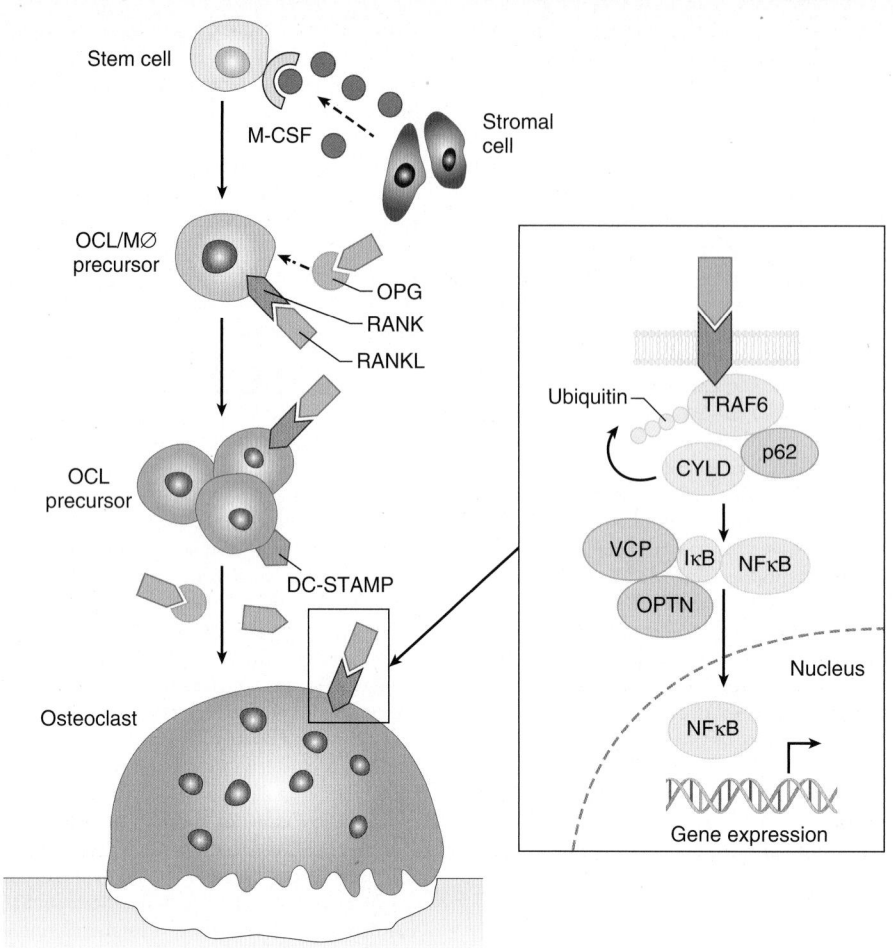

FIGURE 233-1. Regulators of osteoclast dysfunction in Paget disease. Some of the key molecules that have been implicated in the pathogenesis of Paget disease are illustrated. Macrophage colony-stimulating factor (M-CSF) encoded by *CSF1* is required for differentiation of stem cells to the osteoclast/macrophage (OCL/MØ) lineage. Osteoclast differentiation and activity are enhanced when RANK (encoded by *TNFRSF11A*) is activated by RANKL but inhibited by OPG (encoded by *TNFRSF11B*). Fusion of osteoclast precursors to form mature osteoclasts requires DC-STAMP (encoded by *TM7SF4*). Within the cell (*inset*), p62 (encoded by *SQSTM1*) is required for signal transduction downstream of the RANK receptor and is also involved in regulating autophagy. Both VCP (encoded by *VCP*) and OPTN (encoded by *OPTN*) also play a role in regulating NFκB signaling and autophagy.

reason. In the remainder, symptoms attributable to Paget disease are observed. The most common is pain, which can be due to either increased bone turnover or a complication such as osteoarthritis, spinal stenosis, pseudofractures, enlarged skull, bowing of long bones, or nerve compression syndromes. Deafness may occur in patients with skull involvement, but this is usually conductive rather than due to auditory nerve compression. Osteosarcoma occurs in less than 0.5% of cases but should be suspected in patients who experience a sudden increase in bone pain or swelling of an affected site. Other, rare complications include obstructive hydrocephalus, high-output cardiac failure, and hypercalcemia in patients who are immobilized. The risk for cardiovascular disease is increased in patients with Paget disease compared with age- and gender-matched controls, probably owing to an increased prevalence of vascular calcification. Most patients have no clinical signs, but some present with bone deformity (see Fig. 233-2) or warmth of the skin overlying an affected bone.

DIAGNOSIS

The diagnosis can usually be made by radiograph, which shows the typical features of focal osteolysis with coarsening of the trabecular pattern, bone expansion, and cortical thickening (see Fig. 233-2). Occasionally, the disease may be predominantly lytic in nature (see Fig. 233-2). The most sensitive way of defining the extent of Paget disease is a radionuclide bone scan in which tracer uptake is intensely increased at affected sites (see Fig. 233-2).[5] Imaging with magnetic resonance imaging and computed tomography is not usually required unless complications such as spinal stenosis or osteosarcoma are suspected. Laboratory testing should include assessment of renal function, calcium, albumin, ALP, and 25(OH)D levels; liver function should be assessed to rule out the possibility that elevations in ALP are of hepatic origin. Typically, Paget disease presents with an elevation in ALP with otherwise

normal biochemistries, but normal levels of ALP do not exclude the diagnosis. Vitamin D deficiency is a common finding but most likely reflects the fact that Paget disease predominantly affects older people in whom vitamin D deficiency is prevalent. Specialized markers such as bone-specific ALP or procollagen type 1 N-terminal propeptide can be useful in patients with coexisting liver disease but otherwise offer no advantage over total ALP in diagnosis and assessing treatment response. Analysis of genetic markers is being explored in the prediction of people at risk for developing Paget disease,[6] but genetic testing for susceptibility is not generally performed in routine clinical practice.

The differential diagnosis includes hyperostosis frontalis interna (a benign condition characterized by osteosclerosis of the frontal bones of the skull), fibrous dysplasia, pustulotic arthro-osteitis (which can present with mixed osteosclerotic and osteolytic lesions of the clavicle and ribs), and osteosclerotic metastases, particularly from carcinoma of the prostate. Usually, Paget disease can be distinguished from these conditions biochemically and through imaging, but occasionally, biopsy of an affected site may be required.

TREATMENT   Rx

The most common indication for medical treatment of Paget disease is bone pain localized to an affected site.[7,8] Bone pain may be caused by increased metabolic activity, but other causes may be operative, such as nerve compression syndromes, pseudofractures, secondary osteoarthritis, and other musculoskeletal conditions. Careful assessment of the patient is therefore necessary to decide on the most appropriate treatment.[7] Bone pain caused by increased metabolic activity is localized to the affected site and is usually accompanied

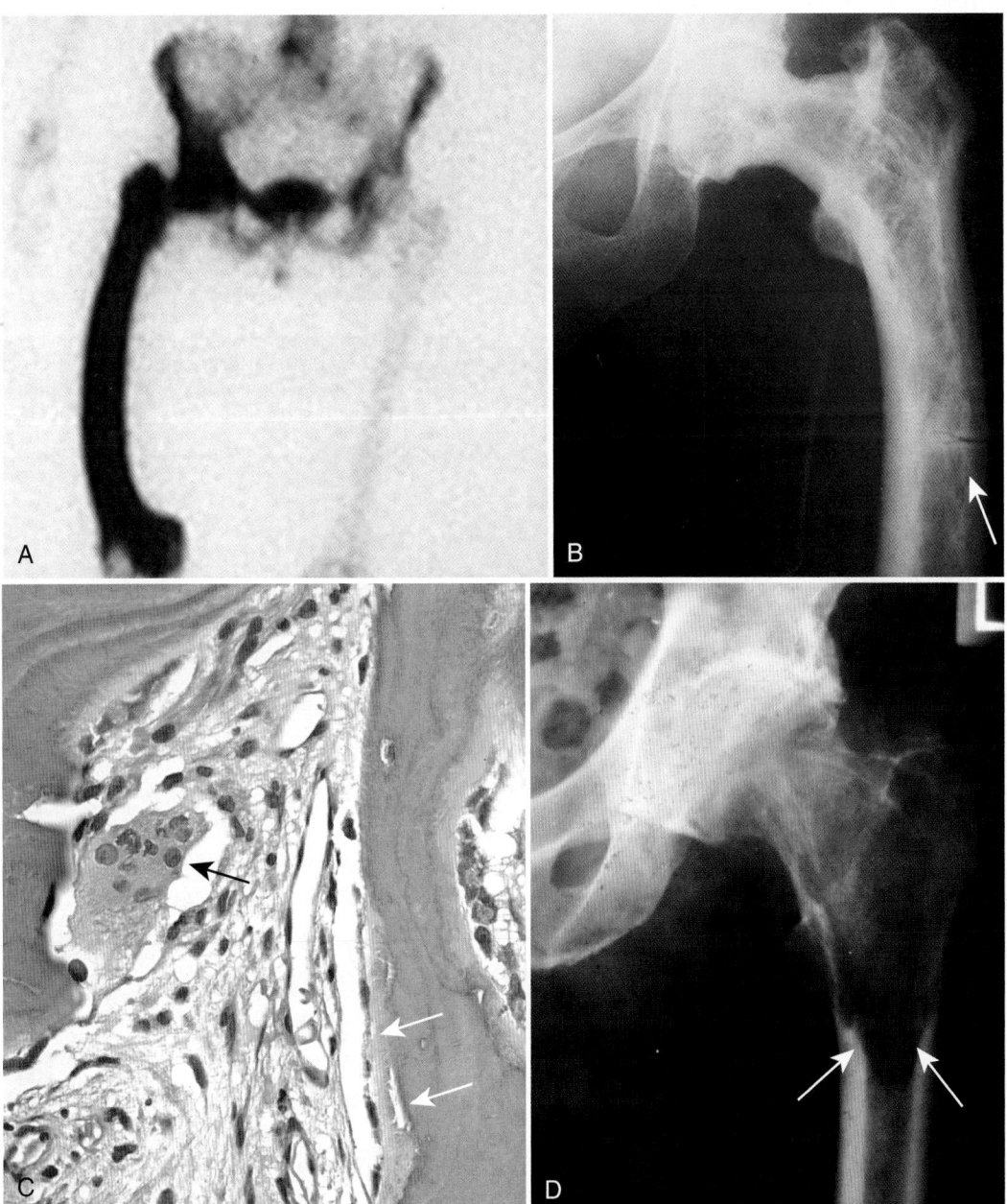

FIGURE 233-2. Radiographic and histologic features of Paget disease. A, Radionuclide bone scan image showing intense tracer uptake, typical of Paget disease of bone affecting in the right femur. B, Radiograph of an affected left femur showing bone expansion with mixed osteolytic/osteosclerotic areas and loss of normal trabecular pattern. A pseudofracture is visible in the lateral cortex (*arrow*). C, Histologic features from a hematoxylin and eosin stained section. A large osteoclast is visible (*black arrow*) close to an area of new bone formation (*white arrows*). There is extensive marrow fibrosis. Irregular cement lines typical of woven bone are apparent to the right of section. D, Predominantly lytic Paget disease of the left femur. The lytic area involves the intertrochanteric region and extends down the femoral shaft (*white arrows*).

by a raised ALP level. It is common to encounter patients in whom pain occurs in the presence of coexisting osteoarthritis, bone deformity, or other musculoskeletal conditions. In such cases, it can be difficult to be sure about the origin of the pain, and many clinicians give a therapeutic trial of bisphosphonates to aid diagnosis. If the pain responds, it is assumed to be due to increased metabolic activity; if it does not, further evaluation should be undertaken to identify the cause and treat the patient appropriately. Pseudofractures represent a distinct management problem. These are areas of focal osteolysis that traverse the lateral cortex of weight-bearing bones of the lower limbs. Some remain stable for prolonged periods without causing symptoms; others regress spontaneously; and others progress to pathologic fracture, often in association with a localized increase in pain at the affected site.

Bisphosphonates

Bisphosphonates are the drugs of first choice for the treatment of pain that is thought to be due to increased metabolic activity, and there is strong evidence that they are more effective than placebo at improving bone pain in Paget disease. Several bisphosphonates are licensed for treatment of Paget disease (Table 233-1), but nitrogen-containing bisphosphonates (aminobisphosphonates)

are now used almost exclusively in preference to older bisphosphonates because of their greater potency in suppressing ALP levels.

There are limited data comparing different aminobisphosphonates, but zoledronic acid has been found to be superior to pamidronate and risedronate at lowering ALP. Randomized trials also suggest that pain relief with zoledronic acid is superior to pamidronate and risedronate.[A1] A comparative trial of a single infusion of 5 mg zoledronic acid with oral risedronate 30 mg daily for 2 months showed that those randomized to zoledronic acid had greater improvement in some domains of health-related quality of life, but the differences between the groups were small (1 to 2 points) and below the 5-point threshold that is considered clinically significant.[A2] A long-term follow-up of this study showed that the suppressive effect of zoledronic acid on ALP lasted in some cases up to 6.5 years, significantly longer than with risedronate.

Another randomized trial with an average follow-up of 3 years compared the effects of giving repeated courses of bisphosphonates with the aim of normalizing ALP (intensive treatment), with therapy primarily aimed at controlling symptoms (symptomatic therapy) in Paget disease. This showed no difference in response of pain, quality of life, or complications between the groups.

TABLE 233-1	BISPHOSPHONATES USED IN THE TREATMENT OF PAGET DISEASE	
DRUG	**DOSE**	**COMMON ADVERSE EFFECTS**
ORAL		
Risedronate	30 mg/day orally for 2 mo	Dyspepsia, esophagitis
Alendronic acid[†]	40 mg/day orally for 6 mo	Dyspepsia, esophagitis
INTRAVENOUS		
Pamidronate	180 mg IV in divided doses, typically 60 mg on 3 consecutive days	Acute phase response, hypocalcemia
Zoledronic acid	5 mg IV	Acute phase response, hypocalcemia

[†]Not licensed in the United Kingdom or Europe for Paget disease. Pamidronate and risedronate should be avoided if estimated glomerular filtration rate (eGFR) <30; zoledronic acid and alendronic acid should be avoided if eGFR <35.

In a 3-year extension of this study,[A3][A4] in which zoledronic acid was the treatment of choice in the intensive treatment group, there was similarly no clinical benefit of intensive bisphosphonate therapy and a nonsignificant trend for an increased risk for fractures and orthopedic procedures with intensive treatment. This indicates that trying to restore ALP to normal with potent bisphosphonates confers no clinical benefit over symptom-directed treatment in patients with established Paget disease.

After initiation of bisphosphonate therapy, levels of ALP start to fall within about 10 days and reach a nadir between 3 and 6 months. Levels of ALP can remain suppressed for many months or years thereafter, particularly with zoledronic acid. Symptoms can improve while ALP levels are still falling, and good clinical responses are observed in patients whose ALP levels are not restored to normal. Conversely, symptoms may recur before ALP values have become elevated again.

Intravenous bisphosphonates can cause transient bone pain, myalgia, headache, nausea, pyrexia, and fatigue within 1 to 3 days of the infusion in about 25% of cases (acute phase response). These symptoms can be ameliorated by acetaminophen given before and for a few days after the infusion, but they almost always subside within 7 days even without treatment. The acute phase response is much less common after second and subsequent infusions. Hypocalcemia may occur, particularly in patients with substantial elevations in bone turnover and vitamin D deficiency. The risk can be minimized by correcting vitamin D deficiency before treatment and providing calcium and vitamin D supplements for the first 1 or 2 weeks after the infusion.

Patients taking oral bisphosphonates must fast before dosing and for at least 30 minutes afterward to achieve adequate absorption. The most common adverse effect is dyspepsia. Other rare side effects of bisphosphonates include uveitis, skin rashes, atrial fibrillation, and osteonecrosis of the jaw, as well as atypical subtrochanteric fractures. Bisphosphonates can cause kidney injury and are contraindicated in patients with significant renal impairment.

Other Drug Treatments

Analgesics, anti-inflammatory drugs, and antineuropathic agents are often required in patients with Paget disease, particularly when there is coexisting osteoarthritis or a nerve compression syndrome. Calcitonin can improve bone pain due to metabolic activity in Paget disease but is seldom used except in patients for whom bisphosphonates are contraindicated. Adverse effects such as nausea and flushing can be problematic, and resistance may develop owing to the formation of neutralizing antibodies. Anecdotal reports suggest that the osteoclast inhibitor denosumab may also be effective at reducing ALP levels in Paget disease of bone,[9] but it is not licensed nor recommended for this indication.

Nonpharmacologic Treatments

Nonpharmacologic approaches (acupuncture, physiotherapy, hydrotherapy, and transcutaneous electrical nerve stimulation) are often used to control pain, but their effectiveness has not been specifically investigated in controlled trials. Clinical experience suggests that specific problems such as limb shortening and deformity can be helped by aids and devices such as walking sticks and shoe raises.

Monitoring Disease Activity and the Effects of Treatment

Metabolic activity and the response to treatment are typically assessed by measuring ALP, but levels can be normal in patients with localized disease that is metabolically active. Further courses of treatment should be considered in patients with recurrent or persistent pain in whom ALP levels remain or become elevated.

Surgery

Orthopedic surgery may be required for the management of coexisting osteoarthritis, pseudofractures, fractures, bone deformity, and spinal stenosis. Osteotomy is performed infrequently, but analyses of small cases series have reported good results. Surgery is much more frequently required to repair fractures and to replace joints that are affected by osteoarthritis. Surgical treatment of Paget disease can be technically challenging because of deformity, osteosclerosis, and increased vascularity, but evidence from case series indicate that fractures through pagetic bone heal normally except when they affect the proximal femur and that joint replacement surgery has a good outcome. It has been suggested that a bisphosphonate should be given before orthopedic and spinal surgery with the aim of reducing operative blood loss, but there is no robust evidence to suggest that this is effective.[8] There is a theoretical concern that previous bisphosphonate therapy might impair fracture union and bone repair, but there is little evidence to suggest that this is a problem in clinical practice. Orthopedic surgery may also be required in patients who develop osteosarcoma, but the prognosis is poor even with aggressive operative treatment.

PROGNOSIS

The prognosis of Paget disease is highly variable. Some patients remain completely symptom free throughout life, but those who present clinically frequently have complications and have a significant reduction in quality of life. Although modern bisphosphonates are highly effective at suppressing bone turnover in Paget disease, they have not as yet been shown to alter the natural history of the disease or prevent complications.[8] Disease severity and extent can be predicted by genotyping for *SQSTM1* mutations and other risk alleles, and studies are currently in progress to determine whether genetic testing can be combined with prophylactic bisphosphonate therapy to prevent or delay the onset of disease.

Grade A References

A1. Corral-Gudino L, Tan A, del Pino Montes J, et al. Bisphosphonates for Paget's disease of bone in adults. *Cochrane Database Syst Rev.* 2017;12:CD004956.
A2. Reid IR, Lyles K, Su G, et al. A single infusion of zoledronic acid produces sustained remissions in Paget disease: data to 6.5 years. *J Bone Miner Res.* 2011;26:2261-2270.
A3. Langston AL, Campbell MK, Fraser WD, et al. Randomised trial of intensive bisphosphonate treatment versus symptomatic management in Paget disease of bone. *J Bone Miner Res.* 2010;25:20-31.
A4. Tan A, Goodman K, Walker A, et al. Long-term randomized trial of intensive versus symptomatic management in paget's disease of bone: the PRISM-EZ study. *J Bone Miner Res.* 2017;32:1165-1173.

GENERAL REFERENCES

For the General References and other additional features, please visit Expert Consult at https://expertconsult.inkling.com.

234

OSTEONECROSIS, OSTEOSCLEROSIS/HYPEROSTOSIS, AND OTHER DISORDERS OF BONE

MICHAEL P. WHYTE

OSTEONECROSIS

DEFINITION

Osteonecrosis (aseptic, avascular, or ischemic necrosis of bone) refers to skeletal infarction. Bone infarcts may be asymptomatic, cause self-limited discomfort, or engender painful collapse of subarticular bone that leads to joint destruction.

EPIDEMIOLOGY AND PATHOBIOLOGY

Many conditions are associated with osteonecrosis (Table 234-1). In adults, the most common causes are prior hip fracture, osteomyelitis, renal dialysis, ethanol abuse, and long-term glucocorticoid therapy.[1]

Skeletal infarction can result from blood vessel destruction (e.g., joint dislocation, fracture), obstruction (e.g., thromboemboli, sickle cell disease, fat emboli, caisson disease), or, hypothetically, compression from local expansion of fatty tissue (e.g., ethanol abuse, glucocorticoid treatment, diabetes mellitus). However, symptoms may not occur unless, weeks later, resorption of dead bone during skeletal repair leads to pathologic fracture. Certain skeletal sites (often subarticular) are predisposed to osteonecrosis, but the locations differ for traumatic and nontraumatic processes and for children and adults. *Osteochondrosis* refers to necrosis of ossification centers; more than 50 eponymic types have been recorded. The susceptibility of children to osteochondrosis and its pathogenesis are poorly understood. At all ages, however, the femoral head is especially prone to infarction. Nontraumatic osteonecrosis commonly affects the humeral head, femoral condyles, distal end of the tibia, and talus. Although the pathogenesis is uncertain, administration of potent bone antiresorptive agents, especially to patients with malignant disease, has been associated with osteonecrosis of the jaw (Fig. 234-1).[2]

TABLE 234-1 CAUSES OF ISCHEMIC NECROSIS OF CARTILAGE AND BONE

Endocrine/metabolic
    Ethanol abuse
    Glucocorticoid therapy
    Cushing disease
    Diabetes mellitus
    Hyperuricemia
    Osteomalacia
    Hyperlipidemia
    Bone antiresorptive therapy (osteonecrosis of the jaw)
Storage diseases (e.g., Gaucher disease)
Hemoglobinopathies (e.g., sickle cell disease)
Trauma (e.g., dislocation, fracture)
Human immunodeficiency virus (HIV) infection
Dysbaric conditions (e.g., caisson disease)
Collagen vascular disorders
Irradiation
Pancreatitis
Organ transplantation
Hemodialysis
Burns
Intravascular coagulation
Idiopathic, familial
Pregnancy

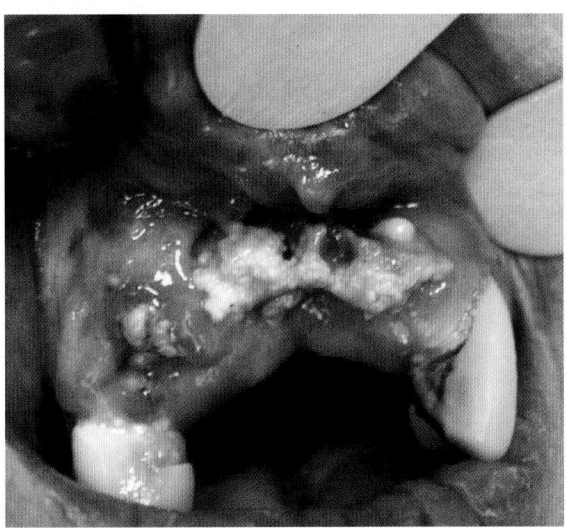

FIGURE 234-1. Exposed dead bone characterizes osteonecrosis of the jaw.

CLINICAL MANIFESTATIONS

Pain occurs acutely if there is skeletal collapse. Chronic arthralgia results from desquamated necrotic tissue and articular destruction.

DIAGNOSIS

Magnetic resonance imaging that demonstrates bone marrow edema is especially sensitive for detection of early osteonecrosis. Bone scintigraphy discloses skeletal reconstitution with or without fracture. Relatively late in the pathologic process, radiographs first show patchy areas of osteopenia and osteosclerosis that reflect skeletal repair. A linear subchondral radiolucency (crescent sign) indicates bone collapse.

TREATMENT   Rx

Nonweight bearing is advisable for the affected limb. Decompression by trephine insertion is used at some sites. Arthrotomy to remove debris, transpositional osteotomy, arthroplasty, or joint replacement may be necessary. Medical treatments for osteonecrosis of the jaw have been disappointing,[A1][3] but surgical resection can be beneficial.[4]

● OSTEOSCLEROSIS/HYPEROSTOSIS

Many conditions are associated with radiographic evidence of increased bone density. Skeletal dysplasias, metabolic disturbances, and various other disorders can cause generalized or focal increases in bone mass (Table 234-2). Aberrations in skeletal growth, modeling (shaping), or remodeling (turnover) may be at fault. *Osteosclerosis* refers to thickening of trabecular (spongy, cancellous) bone.[5] *Hyperostosis* describes widening of cortical (compact) bone. Increases in trabecular bone, cortical bone, or both may augment skeletal density. Most of the dysplasias can be diagnosed by gene mutation analysis.

Osteosclerosis

Neoplastic, hematologic, and metabolic disorders may preferentially sclerose trabecular bone because it houses marrow and remodels more rapidly than cortical bone.

FIBROGENESIS IMPERFECTA OSSIUM
DEFINITION

This rare, usually sporadic condition features generalized osteopenia, but coarsening of the remaining trabeculae places it among the disorders that manifest osteosclerosis.

PATHOBIOLOGY

The cause is unknown, but it is possibly genetic. Subperiosteal bone formation and collagen synthesis in nonosseous tissues seem to be normal.

CLINICAL MANIFESTATIONS

Intractable skeletal pain typically begins gradually during middle age or later and then rapidly increases with a debilitating course and eventual immobility. Spontaneous fractures are a prominent complication. Physical examination reveals marked bone tenderness.

DIAGNOSIS

On radiography, only the skull is spared. Initially, osteopenia and a slightly abnormal appearance of trabecular bone are noted. Subsequently, the changes suggest osteomalacia. Corticomedullary junctions become indistinct as compact bone is replaced by an abnormal cancellous pattern. Generalized osteopenia causes the remaining spongy bone to appear coarse and dense in a fishnet pattern of mixed lytic and sclerotic areas. Alkaline phosphatase activity in serum is increased.

The skeletal lesion is a localized form of osteomalacia that varies considerably in severity from area to area.

Hyperostosis
PROGRESSIVE DIAPHYSEAL DYSPLASIA (CAMURATI-ENGELMANN DISEASE)
PATHOBIOLOGY

Progressive diaphyseal dysplasia affects all races and is inherited as an autosomal dominant trait with variable expressivity. New bone formation gradually

TABLE 234-2 DISORDERS THAT CAUSE DENSE BONES

DYSPLASIAS

Central osteosclerosis with ectodermal dysplasia
Craniodiaphyseal dysplasia
Craniometaphyseal dysplasia
Dysosteosclerosis
Endosteal hyperostosis
   van Buchem disease
   Sclerosteosis (types 1 and 2)
   Worth type (LRP5 and LRP6 activation)
Frontometaphyseal dysplasia
Infantile cortical hyperostosis (Caffey disease)
Juvenile Paget disease
Lenz-Majewski syndrome
Melorheostosis
Metaphyseal dysplasia (Pyle disease)
Mixed sclerosing bone dystrophy
Oculodento-osseous dysplasia
Osteodysplasia of Melnick and Needles
Osteopathia striata
Osteopetrosis (multiple types)
Osteopoikilosis
Progressive diaphyseal dysplasia (Engelmann disease)
Pyknodysostosis
Trichodentosseous dysplasia

METABOLIC CONDITIONS

Carbonic anhydrase II deficiency
Fluorosis
Heavy metal poisoning
Hepatitis C–associated osteosclerosis
Hyperparathyroidism, hypoparathyroidism, pseudohypoparathyroidism
Hypervitaminosis A, D
Hypophosphatemic rickets or osteomalacia (several types)
Milk-alkali syndrome
Renal osteodystrophy

OTHER DISORDERS

Axial osteomalacia
Erdheim-Chester disease
Fibrogenesis imperfecta ossium
Ionizing radiation
Lymphoma
Mastocytosis
Multiple myeloma
Myelofibrosis
Osteomyelitis
Osteonecrosis
Paget bone disease
Sarcoidosis
Skeletal metastases
Tuberous sclerosis

envelops both the periosteal and endosteal surfaces of long bone diaphyses. In patients with severe disease, osteosclerosis also affects the axial skeleton.

Mutations alter the gene that encodes transforming growth factor-β1. Osteoblast differentiation may be deranged.

CLINICAL MANIFESTATIONS

During childhood, limping or a broad-based, waddling gait is noted. Muscular dystrophy can be diagnosed erroneously. Severely affected individuals may have a characteristic body habitus featuring an enlarged head with a prominent forehead, proptosis, and thin limbs with little subcutaneous fat or muscle mass and tender, thickened bones. Cranial nerve palsies and raised intracranial pressure can occur. Some patients have hepatosplenomegaly and Raynaud phenomenon. Symptoms may remit after puberty.

DIAGNOSIS

Irregular hyperostosis of the diaphyses of the major long bones slowly develops as a result of periosteal and endosteal new bone formation. The femur and tibia are most commonly affected. Metaphyses may be involved. The age at onset, rate of progression, and severity are variable. Clinical, radiographic, and bone scan findings are generally concordant. Serum alkaline phosphatase activity, biochemical markers of skeletal turnover, and erythrocyte sedimentation rate

may be elevated. Histopathologic study reveals newly formed woven bone that matures and becomes incorporated into cortical bone. Electron microscopy of muscle may show myopathic changes and vascular abnormalities.

TREATMENT   Rx

Glucocorticoid therapy (typically a low dose of prednisone on alternate days) can relieve bone pain and may normalize skeletal histology. Bisphosphonates or losartan sometimes seem useful.

ENDOSTEAL HYPEROSTOSIS
PATHOBIOLOGY

Sclerosteosis, types 1 and 2, and van Buchem disease are the most severe forms of endosteal hyperostosis. Sclerosteosis is caused by deactivating mutations in the genes called *SOST* and *LRP4*. Van Buchem disease involves a deletion downstream of *SOST*. Enhanced osteoblast activity from impaired sclerostin action, with failure of osteoclasts to compensate for the increased bone formation, leads to the skeletal changes.

CLINICAL MANIFESTATIONS

Sclerosteosis (generalized hyperostosis with syndactyly) affects primarily people of Dutch ancestry. The gender distribution appears equal. Patients are tall and heavy beginning in childhood; have a prominent, square mandible; and are deaf and experience facial nerve palsy from cranial nerve entrapment. Raised intracranial pressure and headache may reflect a small cranial cavity that can shorten life expectancy. Van Buchem disease causes progressive asymmetrical enlargement of the jaw during puberty. Patients may be symptom free, or, beginning as early as infancy, they may have recurrent facial nerve palsy, deafness, and optic atrophy from narrowing of cranial foramina. Long bones may hurt with applied pressure but are strong.

DIAGNOSIS

In sclerosteosis, the skeleton is radiographically normal in early childhood. Congenital syndactyly involves soft tissues and bone in type 1 versus 2, respectively. Progressive bone thickening widens the skull and causes prognathism. Osteosclerosis also involves the skull base, facial bones, vertebrae, pelvis, and ribs. Endosteal thickening homogeneously widens diaphyseal cortices and narrows medullary canals. Computed tomography has shown fusion of ossicles and narrowing of the internal auditory canals and cochlear aqueducts. Serum alkaline phosphatase activity can be increased from enhanced bone formation.

TREATMENT   Rx

Surgical decompression of narrowed foramina may alleviate cranial nerve palsies. Craniectomy may become necessary.

PACHYDERMOPERIOSTOSIS
PATHOBIOLOGY

Pachydermoperiostosis (hypertrophic osteoarthropathy, primary or idiopathic) features clubbing of the digits, hyperhidrosis with thickening of the skin (especially of the face), and periosteal new bone formation, most prominently in the distal ends of the limbs. Not all patients manifest all three principal features. Loss-of-function mutations are found in the gene that encodes 15-hydroxyprostaglandin dehydrogenase in the autosomal recessive form. Autosomal dominant inheritance is also recognized.

CLINICAL MANIFESTATIONS

Men seem more severely affected than women, and blacks more commonly than whites. Symptoms typically begin during adolescence, intensify during the next decade, but then become quiescent. Arthralgia and fatigue are common. Stiffness and limited mobility occur in both the appendicular and the axial skeleton. Clubbing, with slowly progressive enlargement of the hands and feet, results in a pawlike appearance. Cutaneous changes include thickening, furrowing, pitting, and oiliness, especially of the scalp and face.

DIAGNOSIS

Periostitis thickens the distal portions of the tibia, fibula, radius, and ulna. Clubbing is obvious, and acro-osteolysis can occur. Periosteal proliferation is exuberant, with an irregular texture, and it often involves the epiphyses, whereas secondary hypertrophic osteoarthropathy (pulmonary or otherwise) typically causes a smooth and undulating periosteal reaction. Ankylosis of the joints, especially in the hands and feet, may trouble older patients. Bone scanning reveals symmetrical regular uptake along the cortical margins of long bones, especially in the legs—the double stripe sign.

TREATMENT Rx

Patients with painful synovial effusions may respond to nonsteroidal anti-inflammatory drugs. Contractures or neurovascular compression by osteosclerotic lesions may require surgical intervention.

Osteosclerosis with Hyperostosis
OSTEOPETROSIS
DEFINITION

Osteopetrosis (marble bone disease) is a group of rare disorders featuring elevated bone mass due to lack of osteoclast formation or action during growth.[6] There are two major clinical categories: the autosomal recessive or "malignant" type, which often results in death by early childhood if untreated; and the autosomal dominant or "benign" type (Albers-Schönberg disease), which causes lesser complications. Autosomal recessive types can also feature intermediate severity, neuronal storage disease, or renal tubular acidosis with cerebral calcification due to carbonic anhydrase II deficiency. Bisphosphonate-induced osteopetrosis has been reported.

PATHOGENESIS

The defective gene causing autosomal dominant osteopetrosis encodes a chloride channel important for osteoclasts to release hydrochloric acid. Bi-allelic mutations in this gene, or ones that encode components of a vacuolar hydrogen (H^+) pump, result in malignant osteopetrosis. Carbonic anhydrase II deficiency is caused by deactivating mutations in the gene that encodes this isoenzyme. Especially rare autosomal recessive cases involve deficient osteoclastogenesis from loss-of-function mutations within the genes for either receptor activator of nuclear factor κB (RANK) or its ligand (RANKL).

Histopathologic studies show that all true forms of osteopetrosis feature profound deficiency of osteoclast action. Bone-embedded primary spongiosa (calcified cartilage deposited during endochondral bone formation) persists away from growth plates and constitutes the pathognomonic finding. Defective endosteal bone resorption impairs the formation of marrow space. Quiescent skeletal remodeling leads to bone fragility from diminished interconnection of osteons, delayed conversion of immature (woven) bone to mature (compact) bone, and failure of microcracks to heal. Neuronal storage disease (ceroid-lipofuscin) may reflect a lysosomal defect. Deficient superoxide production (necessary for bone resorption) has been considered a pathogenetic factor.

CLINICAL MANIFESTATIONS

Malignant osteopetrosis can present during infancy as nasal "stuffiness" from underdeveloped mastoid and paranasal sinuses. Small cranial foramina may cause optic, oculomotor, or facial nerve palsy. Failure to thrive, delayed dentition, and fractures are common. Hypersplenism and recurrent infection, bruising, and bleeding reflect myelophthisis. Short stature, large head, frontal bossing, nystagmus, hepatosplenomegaly, and genu valgum are characteristic physical findings. Untreated children usually die during the first decade of life of hemorrhage, pneumonia, severe anemia, or sepsis. Benign osteopetrosis can cause fracture, facial palsy, deafness, mandibular osteomyelitis, bone marrow failure, impaired vision, psychomotor delay, carpal tunnel syndrome, or osteoarthritis. Carbonic anhydrase II deficiency can lead to failure to thrive, fracture, developmental delay, mental subnormality, and short stature. Cerebral calcification develops during childhood, but defective skeletal modeling and osteosclerosis may resolve. Both proximal and distal renal tubular acidosis have been described.

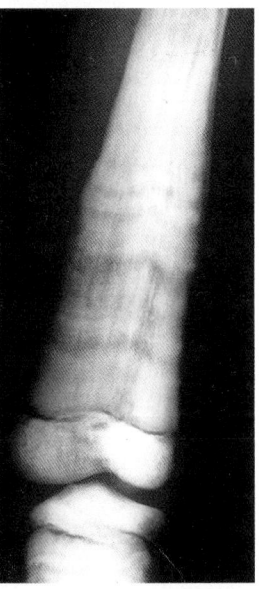

FIGURE 234-2. Osteopetrosis. Anteroposterior radiograph of the distal end of the femur shows a widened metadiaphyseal region, with characteristic alternating dense and lucent bands. (From Whyte MP, Murphy WA. Osteopetrosis and other sclerosing bone disorders. In: Avioli LV, Krane SM, eds. *Metabolic Bone Disease.* 2nd ed. Philadelphia: WB Saunders; 1990.)

DIAGNOSIS

A generalized increase in apparent bone density is the radiographic hallmark of osteopetrosis. In severe disease, modeling defects in long bones produce an "Erlenmeyer flask" deformity (Fig. 234-2). Alternating dense and lucent bands commonly occur in the metaphyses and pelvis. The cranium is usually thickened and dense, especially at the base, and the paranasal and mastoid sinuses are underpneumatized. Vertebrae may show, on a lateral view, a "bone-in-bone" (endobone) configuration or end-plate sclerosis causing a "rugger jersey" appearance. Skeletal scintigraphy can disclose fractures and osteomyelitis. Magnetic resonance imaging helps monitor the response to bone marrow transplantation.

Serum levels of acid phosphatase and creatine kinase (brain isoenzyme) are often increased. In malignant osteopetrosis, hypocalcemia with secondary hyperparathyroidism and elevated serum concentrations of calcitriol can accompany radiographic changes that resemble rickets. In benign osteopetrosis, biochemical indices of mineral homeostasis are typically unremarkable, although serum parathyroid hormone and lactate dehydrogenase isoenzyme levels may be elevated.

TREATMENT Rx

Because the molecular pathogenesis, prognosis, and treatment of the more than 10 types of osteopetrosis can differ, precise diagnosis is crucial.[7] Commercially available mutation analysis can delineate most patients. For the malignant form, prompt use of human leukocyte antigen–identical bone marrow transplantation to supply functional osteoclasts has remarkably benefited only some children. Calcium-deficient diets have been tried but may be limited by hypocalcemia and rickets and have uncertain efficacy. Pharmacologic doses of calcitriol (1,25-dihydroxyvitamin D_3) administered orally, together with dietary calcium restriction (to prevent hypercalciuria and hypercalcemia) were hoped to stimulate osteoclast activity. Prednisone alone or with a low-calcium, high-phosphate diet can sometimes be effective. Glucocorticoid therapy or human interferon-γ, believed to enhance superoxide production, stabilizes pancytopenia and hepatosplenomegaly. Hyperbaric oxygenation helps treat osteomyelitis. Surgical decompression of optic and facial nerves can be beneficial.

DIFFUSE IDIOPATHIC SKELETAL HYPEROSTOSIS
This condition is discussed in Chapter 257.

PYKNODYSOSTOSIS
EPIDEMIOLOGY

Pyknodysostosis is believed to have affected French impressionist painter Henri de Toulouse-Lautrec (1864-1901). Most descriptions have come from

Europe and the United States, but the disorder seems to be especially common in Japan.

PATHOBIOLOGY

This autosomal recessive condition is caused by loss-of-function mutations in *CTSK*, the gene that encodes cathepsin K. Consequently, bone collagen degradation and skeletal turnover are diminished. In chondrocytes and osteoblasts, inclusions have been described.

CLINICAL MANIFESTATIONS

Characteristic features seen during infancy or early childhood include a relatively large cranium, fronto-occipital prominence, proptosis, bluish sclerae, beaked and pointed nose, small facies and chin, obtuse mandibular angle, high-arched palate, dental malocclusion with retention of primary teeth, and disproportionate short stature. Cranial sutures remain open. Fingers are short and clubbed from acro-osteolysis or aplasia of the terminal phalanges, and the hands are small and square. Repeated fractures cause a knock-knee deformity. Mental retardation occurs in approximately 10% of patients. Adult height ranges from 4 feet 3 inches to 4 feet 11 inches. Life expectancy can be shortened by recurrent respiratory infections and right-sided heart failure from chronic upper airway obstruction secondary to micrognathia.

DIAGNOSIS

Osteosclerosis is uniform, first becoming apparent in childhood and increasing with age. Skeletal modeling defects do not distort the shaping of long bones, but they appear to have thick cortices because of narrow medullary canals. Clavicles are gracile and hypoplastic at their lateral segments. The calvarium and skull base are sclerotic, orbital ridges are dense, and wormian bones are present.

TREATMENT Rx

No medical therapy is available. Fractures of the long bones usually mend satisfactorily. Internal fixation of long bones is formidable because of their narrow medullary space and hardness. Tooth extraction is difficult. Osteomyelitis of the mandible may require antibiotic, surgical, or hyperbaric therapy.

HEPATITIS C–ASSOCIATED OSTEOSCLEROSIS

Rarely, achy and tender limbs develop in individuals infected with hepatitis C virus. Radiographic studies reveal a marked generalized increase in bone mass from osteosclerosis and hyperostosis. Disturbances in the insulin-like growth factor system may explain the enhanced bone formation. Calcitonin or bisphosphonate therapy to slow bone turnover or antiviral treatment has benefited some patients.

Focal Osteosclerosis/Hyperostosis

OSTEOPOIKILOSIS

Osteopoikilosis ("spotted bones"), transmitted as a highly penetrant autosomal dominant trait, is generally a radiographic curiosity due to a deactivating mutation of the *LEMD3* gene. The bone lesions are usually asymptomatic. However, incorrect diagnosis may lead to confusion with serious conditions, including metastatic disease.[8] Some patients have connective tissue nevi called *dermatofibrosis lenticularis disseminata* (or Buschke-Ollendorff syndrome). On radiologic examination, numerous small, round or oval foci of bone sclerosis appear in cancellous bone in the metaepiphyseal regions of tubular, tarsal, carpal, and pelvic bones.

OSTEOPATHIA STRIATA

This is usually an autosomal dominant curiosity of asymptomatic linear striations in the metaphyseal regions of long bones and in the ilium. However, two clinically important X-linked dominant disorders with osteopathia striata affect predominantly females: osteopathia striata with cranial sclerosis due to mutation of the *WTX* gene and osteopathia striata with widespread linear areas of dermal hypoplasia and various bone defects in the limbs due to mutation of the *PORCN* gene (Goltz syndrome).

MELORHEOSTOSIS
DEFINITION

Melorheostosis is a sporadic disorder that features bone changes often with the appearance of wax that has dripped down a candle. No mendelian basis

has been established. The anatomic distribution suggests a postzygotic segmental defect, with evidence now of *KRAS* or *MAP2K1* mutation in some patients.[9,10]

CLINICAL MANIFESTATIONS

Involvement of a single limb is usual; bilateral disease is generally asymmetrical. Cutaneous changes over affected bones are common (e.g., linear scleroderma-like areas and hypertrichosis) and often appear before the hyperostosis. Symptoms typically begin during childhood, with pain and stiffness as the major complaints. Joints may become contracted and deformed from ectopic bone. Leg length inequality results from soft tissue contractures and premature fusion of epiphyses. Skeletal changes seem to progress most rapidly throughout childhood. During adult life, melorheostosis may or may not gradually spread, but pain is especially common.

DIAGNOSIS

As seen radiographically, irregular, dense, eccentric periosteal and endosteal hyperostosis affects a single bone or several adjacent bones. The lower limbs are most commonly involved. Endosteal thickening predominates during infancy and childhood, and periosteal new bone formation is prominent during adulthood. Ectopic bone formation may occur, particularly near joints.

TREATMENT Rx

Surgical correction of contractures may worsen ectopic mineralization. Recurrent deformity is common.

MIXED SCLEROSING BONE DYSTROPHY

This typically sporadic disorder features enigmatic combinations of osteopoikilosis, osteopathia striata, melorheostosis, cranial sclerosis, and other skeletal aberrations in one individual. Complications derive from the specific types of osteosclerosis or hyperostosis, such as nerve palsy with cranial sclerosis and bone pain with melorheostosis.

● OTHER DISORDERS OF BONE
FIBROUS DYSPLASIA

This sporadic developmental disorder features one or more expansile fibrous lesions within bone. Polyostotic disease is typically seen before the age of 10 years; monostotic disease begins in adolescence or early adulthood. *McCune-Albright syndrome* refers to polyostotic fibrous dysplasia, café au lait spots (Fig. 234-3), and endocrine hyperfunction.[11]

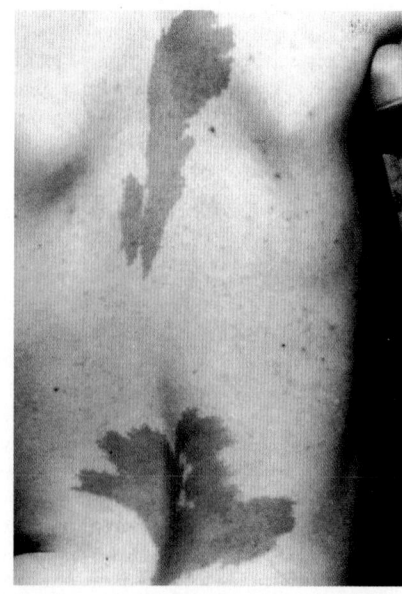

FIGURE 234-3. McCune-Albright syndrome. Typical rough-border ("coast of Maine"), pigmented café au lait spots. (From Whyte MP. Metabolic and dysplastic disorders. In: Coe FL, Favus MJ, eds. *Disorders of Bone and Mineral Metabolism.* New York: Raven Press; 1992.)

PATHOBIOLOGY

Fibrous dysplasia and McCune-Albright syndrome (also see Chapters 211 and 218) are caused by postzygotic mosaicism of an activating mutation in the gene that encodes the α subunit of the receptor subunit/adenylate cyclase–coupling G protein, *GNAS*. Imperfect bone forms because mesenchymal cells do not fully differentiate to osteoblasts.

CLINICAL MANIFESTATIONS

Monostotic fibrous dysplasia is more common than polyostotic disease. The skull and long bones are affected most often. The skeletal lesions can deform bones, cause fractures, and occasionally entrap nerves. Sarcomatous degeneration is rare (<1%) but typically occurs within the facial bones or femur and is more frequent with polyostotic disease. Pregnancy may reactivate quiescent lesions. McCune-Albright syndrome usually causes pseudo-precocious puberty in girls. Less commonly, one sees pseudo-precocious puberty in boys. There can also be thyrotoxicosis, Cushing disease, acromegaly, hyperprolactinemia, or hyperparathyroidism. In some patients, acquired renal phosphate wasting causes hypophosphatemic rickets or osteomalacia (see Chapters 211 and 232).

DIAGNOSIS

The skeletal lesions have a characteristic radiographic appearance early on. In the long bones, they are found in either the metaphysis or diaphysis, typically are well defined with thin cortices, and have a ground-glass appearance (Fig. 234-4). With aging, the defects can become lobulated, with trabeculated areas of radiolucency.

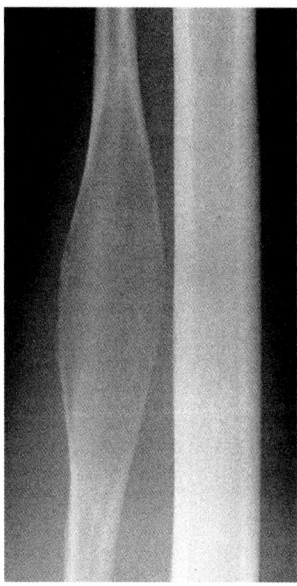

FIGURE 234-4. Fibrous dysplasia. A characteristic expansile lesion with a ground-glass appearance has caused thinning of the cortex in the mid-diaphysis of the fibula. (From Whyte MP. Fibrous dysplasia. In: Favus MJ, ed. *Primer on the Metabolic Bone Diseases and Disorders of Mineral Metabolism*. 3rd ed. Philadelphia: Lippincott-Raven; 1996.)

TREATMENT Rx

In mild disease, bone lesions may not expand. In severe cases, defects can progress and new ones may appear during childhood. Spontaneous healing does not occur, but pathologic fractures generally mend well. Stress fractures, however, can be difficult to detect and to treat. When the skull is involved, nerve compression may require surgical intervention. In McCune-Albright syndrome, search for and pharmacologic control of associated endocrinopathies are important. Bone antiresorptive treatment has helped some patients.

HEREDITARY MULTIPLE EXOSTOSES

This relatively common, highly penetrant, autosomal dominant disorder features irregular bone excrescences that protrude from expanded metaphyses.[12] Mutations have been identified in the *EXT1* and *EXT2* genes. Osteocartilaginous exostoses arise from growth plates and increase in size until linear growth ceases. Lesions may become detached from the parent bone. Their structure is relatively unremarkable, with an outer cortex and an inner spongiosa. Disability results primarily from limb length discrepancies when linear bone growth suffers at the expense of transverse expansion. Compression of nerves, the spinal cord, or the vascular system occurs occasionally. Sarcomatous degeneration (0.5 to 2% of patients) should be suspected when an exostosis enlarges rapidly, especially in an adult.

ENCHONDROMATOSIS (DYSCHONDROPLASIA, OLLIER DISEASE)

This sporadic disorder features cartilaginous masses within the trabecular bone that arise from growth plates.[13] It begins in childhood with localized swelling and interferes with linear bone growth. After puberty, expansion of cartilage masses ceases, and these lesions can be replaced by mature bone. Enchondromas appear radiographically as lucent defects in flat bones or in metaphyses of tubular bones, often with central calcific stippling. When enchondromatosis occurs together with multiple hemangiomas (Maffucci syndrome), the enchondromas or hemangiomas undergo malignant transformation in 15% of cases.

Ollier disease and Maffucci syndrome are caused by somatic mosaic mutations in the *IDH1* and *IDH2* genes.

ACHONDROPLASIA

Chondrodystrophies are disorders of cartilage growth that result in disproportionate short stature. Achondroplasia is the most common.[14] A defect occurs in the gene that encodes fibroblast growth factor receptor type 3; 80% of cases represent new autosomal dominant mutations, which are more prevalent with increasing paternal age. Short tubular bones form because of abnormal endochondral ossification in the limbs. In the chondrocranium, membranous ossification is undisturbed; hence the skull vault is normal. However, the cranial base and foramen magnum are small. The head is large, with frontal bossing and midface hypoplasia. Lumbar lordosis is greatly exaggerated, and the spinal canal narrows from the upper to lower segments of the vertebral column. This disturbance is revealed radiographically by a decreasing interpediculate distance. Trunk length is relatively normal, but the limbs show rhizomelic shortening, and the hands have a trident configuration. The long bones appear massive because of their disproportionately normal width. Growth plates are not grossly disorganized, and chondrocytes appear normal. Complications can include hydrocephalus and compression of the brain stem, spinal cord, or nerve roots. Minimal impingement by a disc or osteophyte on the small spinal canal can cause neurologic disturbances. Despite these problems, achondroplasia is compatible with good health and a normal lifespan.

  Grade A Reference

A1. Rollason V, Laverriere A, MacDonald LC, et al. Interventions for treating bisphosphonate-related osteonecrosis of the jaw (BRONJ). *Cochrane Database Syst Rev.* 2016;2:CD008455.

GENERAL REFERENCES

For the General References and other additional features, please visit Expert Consult at https://expertconsult.inkling.com.

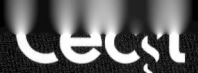

XXII

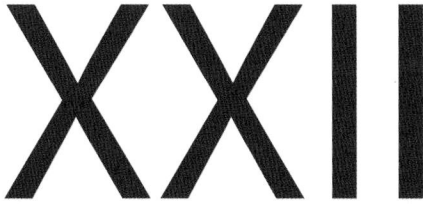

DISEASES OF ALLERGY AND CLINICAL IMMUNOLOGY

235

APPROACH TO THE PATIENT WITH ALLERGIC OR IMMUNOLOGIC DISEASE

KARI C. NADEAU

Allergic diseases and disorders of the immune system affect multiple organ systems. This chapter addresses approaches to common allergic disorders and primary immune deficiencies. Specific disorders are discussed in detail in the chapters to follow.

● ALLERGIC DISEASE

DEFINITION

Diseases characterized by hypersensitivity of the immune system and inappropriate reactions to common environmental, food, and drug substances are termed *allergic diseases*. In the sensitized individual, common foods (e.g., peanut, milk, eggs), airborne particles (e.g., grass pollen, cat dander), drugs (e.g., aspirin, penicillin), insect stings (e.g., bees, wasps), or others (e.g., latex, dyes) can trigger an allergic reaction. Reactions can range from mild to severe to life-threatening, and disease symptoms can occur in one or many organs by skin contact, inhalation, ingestion of allergens, stings, or injections. The prevalence of allergic diseases has increased in recent decades. Although genetics plays a role in their etiology, current hypotheses implicate improvements in hygiene, increased exposure to environmental pollutants, and alterations in diet and lifestyle for the observed increases.

Allergic diseases can be classified based on organs affected, causal allergen type, time taken for symptoms to appear on exposure to allergens, and underlying effector mechanisms. Allergic reactions may be immediate (minutes to 1 to 2 hours) or delayed (hours or days). Based on effector mechanisms, allergies are often classified as immunoglobulin E (IgE)-mediated, mixed IgE- and cell-mediated, and non-IgE-mediated allergic diseases. Although this classification oversimplifies the complexities associated with allergic diseases, at the current time, it plays an essential role in diagnosis and treatment.[1] IgE-mediated diseases are best characterized, and allergic diseases with high IgE levels are termed *atopic diseases*. Table 235-1 details the major IgE-mediated, mixed IgE- and cell-mediated, and non-IgE-mediated allergic diseases, along with their prevalence, major symptoms, and examples of causal allergens.

PATHOBIOLOGY

The mechanisms underlying IgE-mediated allergies are the best understood. Patients with IgE-mediated allergic reactions undergo an initial sensitization phase during which IgE antibodies recognizing a specific allergen are produced and are bound to high-affinity FcεRI receptors on mast cells or basophils. Further exposure to allergens can lead to cross-linkage of IgE antibodies with subsequent degranulation of mast cells or basophils.[2] The initial sensitization phase occurs as epithelial cytokines interleukin-25 (IL-25), IL-33, and thymic stromal lymphopoietin are produced in response to increased allergen permeability caused by loss of epithelial barrier integrity. These cytokines enable differentiation of naïve T cells to T_H2 cells and upregulation of cytokines IL-4, IL-5, and IL-13 and IgE class-switching by B cells. Degranulation of mast cells and basophils lead to the release of histamine and other inflammatory chemical mediators (cytokines, interleukins, leukotrienes, and prostaglandins) into the surrounding tissue causing several systemic effects, such as vasodilation, mucous secretion, tissue eosinophilic infiltration, and smooth muscle contraction (Fig. 235-1). Non-IgE-mediated reactions are poorly defined and are generally T-cell mediated.

Endotypes and Phenotypes

Differences in treatment responses in those with similar clinical characteristics (phenotype) reinforce the heterogeneity of allergic diseases and the need for further classification based on common mechanistic characteristics. These subtypes are termed *endotypes* and are characterized by a distinct pathophysiologic mechanism. Recent advances in high-throughput methods (e.g., genome-wide association studies, RNA-Seq, cytometry by time of flight, 16S rRNA sequencing), big data analytics, and bioinformatics have enabled a better understanding of the molecular changes occurring with allergen sensitization and have spurred research into better diagnostic and prognostic markers and treatments. These technologies are paving the way for better classification of patients based on phenotypes and endotypes, precision medicine, and personalized care.[3]

EPIDEMIOLOGY

Food Allergy

Food allergy is an immune reaction triggered by common food substances.[4] Exposure to very small amounts of allergenic foods can trigger clinical symptoms in one or many organs ranging in severity from mild to life-threatening. The prevalence of food allergies is rising, and current standard of care consists of food allergen avoidance and treatment of severe systemic reactions with adrenaline. Immunotherapy has shown promise in clinical trials, but safety concerns and recurrence of allergen sensitivity after a period of treatment discontinuation have to be addressed before it can become mainstream therapy. In general, allergic reactions occur within minutes to 2 hours after ingestion of the causal allergen. Oral allergy syndrome is a food allergy that requires prior sensitization to a cross-reacting inhalant allergen. Common symptoms include pruritus of the lips, tongue, and mouth. Eosinophilic esophagitis (Chapter 129), food protein–induced enterocolitis syndrome, food protein–induced allergic procolitis, and food protein enteropathy are among the disorders in which food allergy may play a role.

Drug Allergy

Allergic reactions to drugs are a serious public health concern. Drug reactions mediated by immunologic reactions (antibodies or specific T lymphocytes) may occur immediately after exposure to the drug or may be delayed, may affect single or multiple organs, and may be mild, severe, or life-threatening. A careful history of exposure, timing of reactions, and clinical symptoms can help narrow the causal drug allergy because there is no definitive diagnostic test for confirmation of drug allergy. Risk factors for developing a drug allergy include age (young and middle-aged adults), gender (women), genetic polymorphisms (e.g., human leukocyte antigen), and certain viral infections (e.g., HIV, Epstein-Barr virus). Other factors include increased frequency of exposure and prolonged high doses, intravenous or intramuscular route of administration, high molecular weight of drug, and drugs that haptenate tissue or blood proteins.

Environmental Allergy

Outdoor and indoor environmental allergens can sensitize or exacerbate allergic disease (allergic rhinitis, allergic conjunctivitis, and allergic asthma) through IgE-mediated mechanisms. Major indoor aeroallergens are derived from dust mites, cockroaches, cigarette smoking, animal dander (e.g., dog, cat, mice), and mold. Pollutants generated from diesel exhaust, gas-burning stoves, fireplaces, or heaters can also exacerbate allergies and asthma. Children living in close proximity to major highways are more likely to be affected.[5]

Occupational Allergy

A number of substances used in different occupations can cause the development of allergic disease affecting the respiratory tract and skin. Examples include compounds with both low (dyes, isocyanates, metals) and high (latex, flour) molecular weight. Recurring high levels of exposure are the most important determinant in sensitizing individuals to occupational allergens.

CLINICAL SYNDROMES

Allergic diseases affect different organs, such as the nose, lungs, eyes, gastrointestinal tract, or skin. Symptoms may be limited to one or more organs or, as in the case of anaphylaxis, may be systemic. Further, the same allergic sensitization may manifest in different ways at different times in an individual. The concept of the atopic march has been put forth to describe the temporal relationship in the natural and commonly observed progression of atopic disorders from atopic dermatitis in infants to allergic rhinitis, food allergy, and allergic asthma in children and adults.

Skin

Allergic disorders involving the skin include angioedema, urticaria (acute and chronic), and dermatitis (atopic and contact). Symptoms of urticaria and angioedema include pruritus and transient, raised, erythematous cutaneous lesions that range in size from a few millimeters to several centimeters. Acute urticaria is defined as the recurrence of lesions for a period of up to 6 weeks, and chronic urticaria is defined as recurrence of lesions over more than 6 weeks. Acute urticaria may be triggered by aeroallergens, foods, infections,

TABLE 235-1 COMMON IgE-MEDIATED, MIXED (IgE-MEDIATED AND CELL-MEDIATED), AND NON-IgE-MEDIATED ALLERGIES

DISEASE	PREVALENCE	KEY SYMPTOMS	EXAMPLES OF CAUSAL ALLERGENS
IgE-MEDIATED ALLERGIES			
Oral allergy syndrome (pollen-food syndrome)	1-12.2% (children)	Rapid-onset, tingling and pruritus of the lips, mouth, and oropharynx. Pharyngeal swelling in severe cases	Fresh fruits and vegetables, commonly seen in those with birch, ragweed, or grass pollen allergy
Food allergy	8% (children), 5% (adults)	Rapid-onset, abdominal pain, vomiting, hives, wheezing, shortness of breath. Anaphylaxis in severe cases	Food allergens (e.g., egg, peanut, milk)
Anaphylaxis	0.3-5.1%	Rapid-onset, progressive, multiorgan. Rapid progression to cardiovascular and/or respiratory collapse in severe cases	Foods (e.g., peanuts, shellfish), drugs, insect stings
Atopic dermatitis	12.98% (children), 7.2-10.2% (adults)	Pruritus, *Staphylococcus aureus* infection, lichenification, xerosis, excoriations	Foods, aeroallergens, exogenous irritants (e.g., wool, soaps)
Acute, seasonal, and perennial allergic conjunctivitis	10-30%	Conjunctivitis, eyelid edema, watery discharge, ocular itching, conjunctival hyperemia	Aeroallergens
Allergic asthma	7.3%	Chest tightness, shortness of breath, wheezing	Animal dander, mold, house dust mites
Allergic rhinitis	10-40% (children), 10-20% (adults)	Sneezing, rhinorrhea, lacrimation	House dust mites, grass pollen, tree pollen, animal dander
MIXED IgE-MEDIATED AND NON-IgE-MEDIATED ALLERGIES			
Eosinophilic GI disorders (eosinophilic esophagitis, eosinophilic colitis; eosinophilic gastritis; eosinophilic gastroenteritis)	Eosinophilic esophagitis: 5-10/100,000 Eosinophilic colitis: 2.1 per 100,000 Eosinophilic gastroenteritis: 5.1/100,000	Symptoms dependent on region and nature of eosinophilic infiltration (mucosal, muscular, or serosal) and may include nausea, dysphagia, vomiting, failure to thrive, epigastric pain, food impaction, inflammation of some or all regions of the GI tract	Milk, egg, wheat, soy, peanuts
Urticaria (acute and chronic) and angioedema	Acute urticaria: 20% of the general population Chronic urticaria: 5 to 40% of patients with urticaria have angioedema	Pruritus and raised erythematous cutaneous lesions	Aeroallergens, foods, infections, insect stings, or drugs. Many cases are idiopathic
AKC and VKC	VKC: 3.2/10,000 of the population AKC: 20-40% of patients with AD	Clinical symptoms in AKC and VKC can include photophobia and tearing in addition to commonly noted itching and grittiness as observed in ocular allergy. Ropy mucous, giant papillae, and Trantas dots are also often present. AKC patients have concurrent AD	Environmental allergens
NON-IgE-MEDIATED ALLERGIES			
Food protein–induced enterocolitis syndrome (FPIES)	0.34% (CM mediated)	Vomiting, diarrhea, and failure to thrive	Milk, soy
Food protein–induced allergic proctocolitis (FPIAP)	0.16-64% of infants with isolated rectal bleeding	Rectal bleeding	Cow's milk
Food protein–induced enteropathy (FPE)	Prevalence unknown	Steatorrhea from malabsorption, diarrhea, and failure to thrive	Cow's milk proteins and soy proteins
Contact dermatitis	Significant variations with causal allergen	Inflammation, skin rash, and blisters	Poison oak, nickel

AD = atopic dermatitis; AKC = atopic keratoconjunctivitis; CM = cow's milk; GI = gastrointestinal; VKC = vernal keratoconjunctivitis.

insect stings, or drugs. Idiopathic cases of chronic urticaria account for 80 to 90% of cases.[6] Co-occurrence of angioedema with urticaria is common and is found mainly on the face, lips, mouth, upper airways, and genitalia. Symptoms of acute urticaria or angioedema occur rapidly (often within minutes); however, even without treatment, individual urticarial lesions typically resolve within 1 to 24 hours. The use of angiotensin-converting enzyme inhibitors has become the leading cause of acquired angioedema, with those of African American heritage being at higher risk. Urticaria is caused by both IgE- and non-IgE-mediated mechanisms. Additionally, antibodies to IgE and the high-affinity IgE receptor have been detected in some patients, indicating an autoimmune component; however, the clinical significance of these autoantibodies is not clear. Hashimoto thyroiditis has been associated with chronic urticaria, and in 10 to 30% of these patients, antithyroid antibodies have been detected.[7]

Atopic dermatitis is an IgE-mediated disease and is common in infants and children. Increased risk for the disease has been linked to a mutation in the filaggrin gene, a gene essential for skin barrier function. Loss-of-function mutations of filaggrin have been observed in up to 30% of patients with atopic dermatitis. Increased colonization of *Staphylococcus aureus* has been seen in more than 90% of patients with atopic dermatitis and may lead to secondary infections. In individuals, it often precedes the development of other atopic diseases. Further, the severity of atopic dermatitis is correlated with increased risk for asthma and other atopic diseases. Although 20% of children with mild atopic dermatitis develop asthma, more than 60% with severe atopic dermatitis develop asthma.[8]

Allergic contact dermatitis is a common skin disease. It can be caused by direct contact, airborne particles, vapors, or light. The allergens that mediate allergic contact dermatitis are generally low-molecular-weight substances that combine with skin proteins to form complete allergens. Examples include metals (e.g., nickel), plants (e.g., poison oak), or drugs (e.g., neomycin). It is a delayed-type, T-cell-mediated, non-IgE reaction to common substances. Relapse is common, even with prolonged allergen avoidance. Patch testing is the "gold standard" for diagnosis.

Eyes
Ocular allergic conjunctivitis includes seasonal allergic conjunctivitis, perennial allergic conjunctivitis, vernal keratoconjunctivitis, and atopic keratoconjunctivitis (Chapter 395). Seasonal allergic conjunctivitis and perennial allergic conjunctivitis are IgE-mediated leading to an immediate or early response (within minutes). Further activation of chemokines leads to late-phase-mediated reactions. Vernal keratoconjunctivitis and atopic keratoconjunctivitis, however, appear to be mediated by both IgE and non-IgE cellular pathways.

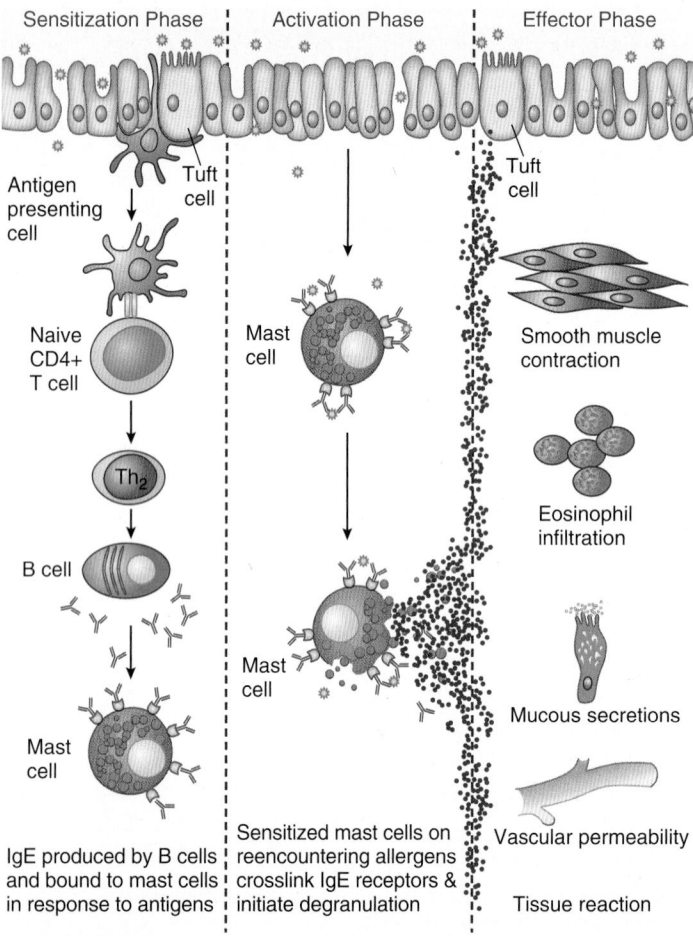

Sensitization Phase	Activation Phase	Effector Phase

Antigen presenting cell

Tuft cell

Tuft cell

Naive CD4+ T cell

Mast cell

Smooth muscle contraction

Th₂

B cell

Eosinophil infiltration

Mast cell

Mucous secretions

Mast cell

Vascular permeability

IgE produced by B cells and bound to mast cells in response to antigens

Sensitized mast cells on reencountering allergens crosslink IgE receptors & initiate degranulation

Tissue reaction

FIGURE 235-1. Mechanism of immunoglobulin E–mediated allergic disease. The right column illustrates the various systemic effects of IgE-mediated allergic reactions, including smooth muscle contraction, tissue eosinophilic infiltration, mucous secretion, and vasodilation with vascular permeability.

Ocular allergies can be caused by numerous factors, such as exposure to air pollutants, insects (cockroaches and house dust mites), pet dander, or pollen. Seasonal allergic conjunctivitis and perennial allergic conjunctivitis primarily affect the conjunctiva and possibly the eyelids. In vernal keratoconjunctivitis and atopic keratoconjunctivitis, the cornea is also affected and has the potential for vision impairment. In seasonal allergic conjunctivitis and perennial allergic conjunctivitis, itching, redness, and swelling of the conjunctiva, along with tearing and discharge of white mucus, is common. One of the main characteristics of vernal keratoconjunctivitis is the presence of giant papillae (several millimeters in diameter) on the upper tarsal conjunctiva, which can be seen easily on the underside of the upper eyelid. Other symptoms include ropy mucous discharge, Trantas dots (aggregation of epithelial cells and eosinophils that appear as gelatinous, mucoid nodules at the superior limbus of the conjunctiva), creasing of the lower eyelids, and pseudomembrane formation on the upper lid. A punctate keratitis may also appear in the central cornea, leading to the formation of a grayish plaque, corneal scarring, and vision impairment. In atopic keratoconjunctivitis, giant papillae and Trantas dots, similar to those found in vernal keratoconjunctivitis, may also be present. However, patients with atopic keratoconjunctivitis are generally older (30 to 50 years) than patients with vernal keratoconjunctivitis (10 years and younger) and often have concurrent atopic dermatitis or a positive family history of atopy. Atopic keratoconjunctivitis and vernal keratoconjunctivitis are two to three times more likely in males than females.

Upper Airway
Allergic rhinitis affects the upper airways and may be either seasonal or perennial. Symptoms include sneezing, nasal pruritus, nasal airflow obstruction, and nasal discharge. In seasonal allergic rhinitis, symptoms usually occur in either spring, summer, or fall and are generally associated with pollen from trees, grass, and weeds. Pollen count and type vary with geographic regions. Even within a specific region, changes in weather patterns can cause yearly

variations in pollen count and overall prevalence and severity of allergic rhinitis. In perennial allergic rhinitis, exposure to indoor and outdoor air pollutants, pet dander, cockroaches, house dust mites, molds, and others should be taken into consideration. In some individuals, seasonal allergies may overlap, leading to perennial symptoms. Forty percent of individuals with allergic rhinitis eventually develop asthma.[9] Because asthma and allergic rhinitis frequently occur in the same patient, one hypothesis is that both are different manifestations of the same disease.

Lower Airway
The most common asthma phenotype is allergic asthma, a chronic inflammatory disease of the airways. It is characterized by contraction of airway smooth muscles, wheezing, cough, and dyspnea on exposure to causal allergens. Both genetic susceptibility and allergen exposure are thought to play a role in the pathogenesis of the disease. Examples of allergens include air pollutants, respiratory viruses, tobacco smoke, drugs, endotoxins, pollen, animal dander, cockroaches, house dust mites, and foods. IgE plays a central role in allergic asthma pathophysiology and has been implicated in both the early (wheezing, shortness of breath, chest tightness, and cough) and late (inflammatory infiltration, bronchoconstriction, and tissue remodeling) phases. The success of anti-IgE therapies in reducing asthma exacerbations has further emphasized the key role of IgE in allergic asthma.[10]

Diseases associated with allergic asthma include eosinophilic granulomatosis with polyangiitis (Chapter 161), formerly known as Churg-Strauss syndrome, and allergic bronchopulmonary aspergillosis (Chapter 319). Eosinophilic granulomatosis with polyangiitis is a rare allergic disease that also affects the lower airways. Asthma is found in 95 to 100% of patients with eosinophilic granulomatosis with polyangiitis and generally precedes it by many years.[11] It is generally characterized by an allergic phase with asthma and rhinosinusitis, an eosinophilic phase with hypereosinophilia in the lungs and other organs, and a vasculitic eosinophilic granulomatosis with a polyangiitis phase leading to impaired blood flow and damage to tissues and organs. It is thought to be mediated by non-IgE mechanisms. A number of studies have shown it to develop after anti-IgE treatment in patients with severe asthma, in whom in may be unmasked when corticosteroids are weaned. The diagnostic criteria for allergic bronchopulmonary aspergillosis include the presence of asthma or cystic fibrosis with deterioration of lung function, positive skin test for *Aspergillus* sp, total serum IgE level of at least 416 IU/mL, increased specific IgE and IgG antibodies for *Aspergillus* sp, and chest radiographic infiltrates.

Gastrointestinal Tract
Allergic inflammatory diseases that affect the gastrointestinal tract include eosinophilic gastrointestinal diseases, food protein–induced enterocolitis syndrome, food protein–induced allergic procolitis, and food protein enteropathy. All three conditions are non-IgE-mediated gastrointestinal food allergic disorders. All three are typically present in infancy and are triggered most commonly by cow's milk protein. Symptoms of food protein–induced enterocolitis syndrome include vomiting, lethargy, and dehydration. Patients with food protein–induced allergic procolitis present with bloody and mucous stools. Diarrhea, malabsorption, and failure to thrive are observed with food protein enteropathy. These diseases have a favorable prognosis, and most resolve by 3 to 5 years of age. Eosinophilic gastrointestinal diseases are inflammatory gastrointestinal disorders in which eosinophils infiltrate the gut. Pathophysiology indicates mixed IgE and non-IgE mechanisms.

Eosinophilic esophagitis (Chapter 129) is the most common and well characterized of the eosinophilic gastrointestinal diseases. It is an inflammatory disorder of the esophagus. Symptoms include nausea, dysphagia, vomiting, failure to thrive, epigastric pain, food impaction, and inflammation of the esophagus. Patients with eosinophilic esophagitis often have comorbid atopic diseases such as allergic rhinitis, asthma, food allergy, and atopic dermatitis. Diagnosis is confirmed if an esophageal biopsy shows at least 15 eosinophils per high-power field.[12] Eosinophilic esophagitis is a food allergy, and elimination diets excluding causal allergens from the diet are effective in reducing and eliminating symptoms.

Eosinophilic gastritis (Chapter 161), eosinophilic colitis (Chapter 161), and eosinophilic gastroenteritis (Chapter 161) are rare and often found in patients with a history of atopy.[13] All three disorders show increased numbers of eosinophils in gastrointestinal biopsies. Symptoms vary based on region of the gastrointestinal tract affected and extent of eosinophilic infiltration (mucosal, muscular, or serosal). In rare cases, eosinophilic ascites is observed with eosinophilic infiltration into the serosal layer.

Vascular

Anaphylaxis is a serious systemic reaction to allergens and is rapid in onset (seconds to minutes) and, in severe cases, can quickly progress to cardiovascular and/or respiratory collapse within minutes of inception. It is associated with skin (flushing, urticaria, and angioedema), pulmonary (asthma, laryngeal edema), cardiac (arrhythmia), vascular (hypotension, extravascular fluid loss), gastrointestinal (abdominal pain, nausea, vomiting, diarrhea), and nonspecific symptoms (metallic taste, sense of impending doom). Common triggers include insect stings, drugs, and food allergens. In addition to IgE mechanisms, non-IgE mechanisms such as IgG immune complexes, complement, neuropeptides, opiates, and radiocontrast also play a role.[14] Patients who have elevated basal levels of serum tryptase are at increased risk for anaphylaxis, especially after an insect sting. All patients should have their baseline tryptase determined as a follow-up to an anaphylactic episode and, if elevated, should be further evaluated for occult mast cell disorders.

Hereditary angioedema is a rare, genetic disease characterized by spontaneous episodes of subcutaneous and submucosal swelling of the face, lips, oral cavity, larynx, and gastrointestinal tract. It is potentially life-threatening, and affected individuals are at risk for laryngeal angioedema and asphyxiation. It is caused by decreases in C1 inhibitor protein level or function and overproduction of bradykinin. The typical duration of episodes is 3 days.[15]

DIAGNOSIS

Allergy is a systemic immune disease and a multifocal approach should be employed when examining a patient with suspected allergies. Because many of the diseases comprise distinct heterogeneous subtypes, a precision medicine approach to personalized diagnosis and treatment should be undertaken. A final diagnosis of allergy should be based on correlations between patient history, clinical symptoms, and laboratory test results.

Patient History

Obtaining an accurate patient history is a crucial first step in diagnosing allergic disease. A family history of atopic disease increases risk for allergic disease. Patient history should include the nature of the patient's symptoms (frequency and severity) and potential allergen exposures, such as seasonal (e.g., pollen from trees or grasses), perennial (e.g., dust mites, cockroaches), food (e.g., peanuts, tree nuts, egg, raw fruits), environmental (e.g., pets, pollutants, cockroaches, molds, fungi), drug (e.g., penicillin), and occupational (e.g., flour, latex, paints) allergen exposures. Table 235-2 details common symptoms and approaches to treatment.

Physical Examination

Skin should be examined for possible urticaria (see Fig. 411-1 in Chapter 411), angioedema, or atopic dermatitis (see Table 411-4 in Chapter 411). Urticarial lesions typically consist of small, pink, raised, irregular wheals and may be associated with angioedema. Angioedematous lesions are most often found on the face and acral areas. Atopic dermatitis is prominent over the trunk and face during infancy, and a typical flexural distribution is observed in childhood. Signs of atopic dermatitis include flexular papulae, thickening of skin due to hyperkeratinization, excoriations, and lichenification. Patients with urticaria should be tested for dermatographism.

The eyes should be examined for signs of excessive tear production, injection and swelling of the palpebral conjunctivae, and swollen or darkened periorbital tissues. "Cobblestone papillae" may be present.

Internal inspection of the nasal mucosa should be focused on deviations or perforations of the nasal septum, nasal patency, presence of polyps or foreign bodies, mucosal appearance, and presence and nature of secretions. Decreases in nasal patency caused by swelling of the lower turbinates are often observed. In allergic patients, the nasal mucosa typically appears pale, watery, edematous, and bluish, and secretions are clear and watery to mucoid in nature.

In patients with acute asthma, clinical examination can help detect wheezing, prolonged expiration, tachypnea, and shortness of breath. Extremities should be checked for cyanosis. Chronic hyperinflation (increased diameter or barrel chest) can be seen in chronic asthma. Wheezing, if unilateral, may suggest a foreign body or tumor. Wheezing may only be present during expiration (mild or moderate asthma) or during both inspiration and expiration (severe asthma), or it may be absent (when airflow is severely limited or when it predominantly affects the small airways).

Anaphylaxis is a systemic event and affects many organs. Signs of anaphylaxis generally include flushing and presence of urticaria and angioedema. Hoarseness caused by upper airway obstruction from angioedema of the tongue, oropharynx, or larynx, or wheezing secondary to asthma, may be observed. Other symptoms may include pruritus, chest tightness, cough, wheezing, rhinitis, sneezing, congestion, rhinorrhea, abdominal pain, uterine cramping, urinary and fecal urgency or incontinence, nausea, vomiting, and diarrhea. Patients may become hypoxic, and anaphylaxis with hypotension may signal shock (Chapter 98) and cardiovascular collapse.

Laboratory Evaluation

Allergen-specific IgE (sIgE) measurements are the most common diagnostic tool for allergy. Total IgE measurements have limited utility for diagnoses of patients with allergic disease. Normal values of total IgE do not exclude the presence of allergic disease, and elevated concentrations can be found in smokers and in a number of other diseases besides allergy. In some cases, however, such as allergic bronchopulmonary aspergillosis, serum IgE levels may measure the severity of disease or risk for an exacerbation.

sIgE can be measured either by in vitro blood tests or in vivo tests (skin prick tests and intradermal testing). The specific allergens tested in sIgE should be based on patient history and environmental exposures. During skin prick tests, a small break in the epidermis (usually forearm or upper back) is made using a lancet or needle to allow penetration of the allergen. In intradermal skin testing, a small amount of the suspected allergen is injected under the surface of the skin. Although studies indicate that intradermal testing is more sensitive and reproducible, it is less common than skin prick tests because of concerns about patient safety and comfort. After about 15 to 30 minutes of allergen introduction, the maximal diameter of both the wheal and the flare is obtained, and results are compared with positive (histamine) and negative (saline) controls. Contraindications include individuals at high risk for anaphylaxis, certain skin conditions such as dermographism, urticaria, cutaneous mastocytosis, and skin affected by atopic dermatitis. Medications that may affect skin prick test results when taken concurrently include antihistamines (including topical forms), tricyclic antidepressants, omalizumab, and topical steroids in the test area.[16] Angiotensin-converting enzyme inhibitors and β-blockers do not interfere with skin prick test results but may be problematic if anaphylaxis occurs and requires treatment.

Several new innovative high-throughput in vitro tests for measuring sIgE have recently been commercialized, such as the ImmunoCAP Immunosorbent Allergen Chip, Immuno Solid Phase Allergen Chip (VBC Genomics-Phadia), and AdvanSure AlloScreen assay, and these tests can be used in conjunction with in vivo sIgE tests for further confirmation of a diagnosis of allergy. Both in vitro and in vivo measurements of sIgE, however, are associated with high rates of false-positive results and only indicate allergen sensitization rather than clinically significant allergy. For some types of allergy, such as IgE-mediated food allergy, food challenges (particularly a double-blind, placebo-controlled food challenge) can provide a definitive diagnosis. The test should be conducted only in carefully supervised settings because of the risk for severe reactions.

Non-IgE tests include inhalation tests and patch tests. Inhalation testing of specific allergens or chemicals may help diagnose occupational allergy or asthma (Chapter 87). Patch tests are used to diagnose contact dermatitis. Patches containing potentially allergenic substances (e.g., dyes, latex, metals)

TABLE 235-2	ALLERGIC DISEASES: SYMPTOMS AND APPROACHES TO TREATMENT
SYMPTOMS	**APPROACH TO TREATMENT**
Cutaneous: pruritus, rash	H_1-antihistamine
Ocular: gritty sensation, pruritus	Topical H_1-antihistamine or mast cell–stabilizing agent
Upper respiratory: palatal pruritus, clear rhinorrhea, sneeze, nasal obstruction	Topical corticosteroid, oral H_1-antihistamine, leukotriene receptor antagonist, topical nasal H_1-antihistamine
Lower respiratory: wheezing, cough, dyspnea	β_2-Agonist, inhaled corticosteroid, inhaled β_2-agonist, leukotriene receptor antagonist, oral methylxanthine, parenteral corticosteroid, parenteral anti–immunoglobulin E
Gastrointestinal: nausea, vomiting, cramping pain	Epinephrine (if caused by anaphylaxis), oral corticosteroid, oral cromolyn

TABLE 235-3 CLINICAL FINDINGS TYPICALLY ASSOCIATED WITH COMMON TYPES OF PRIMARY IMMUNE DEFICIENCY DISEASES

ANTIBODY DEFICIENCY DISORDERS	CELLULAR IMMUNE DEFECTS	COMPLEMENT DEFICIENCIES	NEUTROPHIL DYSFUNCTION
Onset after 6 months of age	Onset before 6 months of age	Recurrent bacterial infection	Late separation of umbilical cord
Recurrent respiratory infection	Recurrent viral, fungal, or parasitic (opportunistic) infection	Recurrent *Neisseria* infection (deficiency of late components)	Persistent neutrophilic leukocytosis
Infection with bacteria, especially encapsulated organisms	Defective delayed hypersensitivity skin responses	Associated rheumatic disorder (especially systemic lupus erythematosus)	Recurrent or persistent gingivitis or periodontitis
Absence of isohemagglutinins	Malabsorption or diarrhea		Recurrent bacterial infection with granuloma formation

are placed on the back for about 48 hours, and a reading is obtained after 72 to 96 hours.

Other Laboratory Aids in Allergic Disease

Chest radiographs can be useful for determining the presence of a tumor, hyperinflation, or bronchiectasis (indicating possible allergic bronchopulmonary aspergillosis). In patients with asthma, both airflow and volumes can determine disease severity and response to treatment. Bronchial response to β_2-adrenergic agonist medication or a short-acting anticholinergic agent should be assessed in those with bronchoconstriction to determine reversibility of bronchoconstriction. A failure to develop bronchoconstriction using methacholine or histamine as triggers argues against a diagnosis of asthma. Another test for airway inflammation that is currently being used is exhaled nitric oxide measurement.

Serum tryptase, a mast cell–specific protease, is currently the best biologic marker of anaphylaxis. However, because it has a short serum half-life of 2 hours, tryptase levels should be measured close to the onset of anaphylaxis.

Two new tests are currently used primarily in research settings. Component-resolved diagnosis measures sIgE using purified or recombinant components of allergens, such as Ara h2 from peanuts. The basophil activation test measures levels of surface proteins (CD63 and CD203c) that are expressed on stimulation with allergenic proteins.

⬤ IMMUNOLOGIC DISEASE

Primary immune deficiency diseases (Chapter 236) are rare genetic disorders with defects in one or more components of the immune system. Primary immune deficiency diseases are characterized by increased incidence of infections and autoimmune diseases. More than 250 primary immunodeficiency diseases have been discovered[17]; however, most of them are rare. The International Union of Immunological Societies Expert Committee for Primary Immunodeficiency 2015 classified primary immune deficiency diseases into (1) immunodeficiencies affecting cellular and humoral immunity; (2) combined immunodeficiencies with associated or syndromic features; (3) predominantly antibody deficiencies; (4) diseases of immune dysregulation; (5) congenital defects of phagocyte number, function, or both; (6) defects in intrinsic and innate immunity; (7) autoinflammatory disorders; (8) complement deficiencies; and (9) phenocopies of primary immune deficiency disease.[18]

The prevalence of primary immune deficiency in the United States has been estimated to be about 1 in 1200 persons. Antibody disorders, which are the most common, constitute one half or two thirds of all primary immune deficiency diseases. Of these diseases, IgA deficiency disorders are the most common (about 30%). Combined B-cell and T-cell disorders, phagocytic defects (abnormalities in neutrophils or monocytes), and complement disorders account for 9 to 10.5%, 8.5 to 12.5%, and 2 to 3% of all primary immune deficiency disease disorders, respectively.

DIAGNOSIS

The presentation of primary immune deficiency (Chapter 236) is highly variable (Table 235-3). Patients with recurrent, persistent, severe, or unusual infections should be suspected for primary immune deficiency disease. Severity is usually correlated with younger age of onset.

History and Physical Examination

Patient history can assist with raising suspicion and recognition of the need for further specialized testing. Clinical symptoms are those often seen in routine care and may go unrecognized in primary care settings. Many primary immunodeficiency diseases are hereditary. Patient history should include details of infections (age of onset of infections, number, site, and type), including family

history of frequent infections and the presence of other abnormalities, because these many provide clues to the underlying disorder.

Laboratory Evaluation

Laboratory tests are essential for the diagnosis of primary immune disorders. Blood counts, including enumeration of total eosinophil, neutrophil, and lymphocyte (T-cell, B-cell, natural killer [NK]-cell) counts, cytokines produced by activated lymphocytes, and determination of serum immunoglobulin levels (IgA, IgE, IgG, IgM) can assist with diagnosis of a suspected immunodeficiency disorder. A significant lymphopenia often can be the first indication of T-cell immunodeficiency. Reduced antibody levels may be indicative of B-cell and antibody immunodeficiency disorders. However, additional tests measuring specific antibody titers in response to defined stimuli (e.g., vaccinations, tetanus toxoid, or pneumococcus) may be useful in patients who have frequent infections and borderline immunoglobulin levels.

When defects in neutrophils are suspected, a nitroblue tetrazolium test or dihydrorhodamine response test can assist with diagnosis. The standard screening test for deficiencies in the complement system is the total hemolytic complement assay or CH50. The AH50 can also be used for screening complement abnormalities in the alternative pathway.

Chest radiographs can detect thymic shadows and cupping and flaring of the costochondral junction, which can assist with the diagnosis of certain T-cell disorders. An abdominal ultrasound can determine abnormalities of spleen size.

GENERAL REFERENCES

For the General References and other additional features, please visit Expert Consult at https://expertconsult.inkling.com.

236

PRIMARY IMMUNODEFICIENCY DISEASES

CHARLOTTE CUNNINGHAM-RUNDLES

Since the descriptions of the first genetic immune defects, severe combined immunodeficiency (SCID) and X-linked agammaglobulinemia (XLA), in the 1940s, the number of known primary immune defects (now over 330) has expanded exponentially. To keep pace, every 2 years the International Union of Immunological Societies has compiled the known defects into general categories[1] (Table 236-1). Auto-inflammatory syndromes are covered in Chapter 245. Complement and phagocyte disorders are discussed in more detail in Chapters 44 and 160, respectively. In this chapter, our current understanding of primary immune defects is considered, with emphasis on primary immune defects found in adults.

⬤ AN APPROACH TO EVALUATION OF THE IMMUNE SYSTEM

Because of the numbers and types of immune deficiencies, recognition of the clinical phenotypes can be difficult,[2] leading in some cases to a delayed diagnosis. In general, the spectrum of immune defects varies with the age of the patient. Defects of both T and B cells, phagocytes, immune dysregulation, and innate immunity are more commonly recognized in early childhood, whereas defects of complement and antibody production and auto-inflammatory diseases are more characteristic of teens and adults. However, there are many exceptions to this generalization. In addition, even if an immune defect has been diagnosed in childhood, adequate treatment has allowed these patients to increasingly present to internists and adult specialists.[3]

For most patients, the first symptom of an immune defect is a series of relatively common infections, particularly involving the respiratory tract. These usually include chronic sinusitis, otitis, and bacterial pneumonia. For adults with immune defects, infections are likely to last longer, may require additional courses of antibiotics, and tend to recur. Infections may also lead to additional complications or procedures, such as empyema after bacterial pneumonia or the need for myringotomy tubes in an adult with chronic otitis. For infants and children, chronic infections lead to poor appetite and growth failure; for adults, some weight loss may occur, but it is less apparent. Because of lack of immunity, shingles (Chapter 351) is relatively common in patients with T-cell defects or antibody deficiencies. Other common clinical presentations include acute gastrointestinal infections with characteristic organisms such as *Giardia* (Chapter 330) and chronic intestinal inflammatory diseases leading to malabsorption and weight loss mimicking Crohn disease (Chapters 131 and 132). In this chapter, primary immune defects are divided into topics, as listed in Table 236-1. General guidelines to approach the laboratory evaluation of the main immune defects, based on clinical presentations, are provided in Table 236-2. A general flow chart of the workup of immune defects presenting with infection is provided in Figure 236-1, but more detailed flow charts, based on extended clinical phenotypes, have been published.[4] (An update of this is available on a smart phone application available at https://play.google.com/store/apps/details?id=com.horiyasoft.pidclassification and https://itunes.apple.com/us/app/pid-phenotypical-diagnosis/id1160729399?mt=8.)

Although susceptibility to infection is a common manifestation of immune defects, the recognition of the molecular defects leading to immune dysregulation syndromes, including auto-inflammatory disorders and interferonopathies, has enhanced our understanding of normal immune functions, leading to therapeutic advances applicable to other immune-based diseases. Another major advance has been the observation that certain mutations in the innate immune system create susceptibility to selected pathogens only, permitting wide-scale screening of populations, based on infection phenotype. Although selected gene panels allow assignment of genetic causes, high-throughput genomic sequencing has become economically practical. These methods can identify a likely molecular diagnosis in up to 40% of unrelated probands with selected characteristic phenotypes, influencing management in nearly 25% of families.[5] With the advent of genetic testing and its use in clinical medicine, autosomal dominant genes with variable penetrance are increasingly being identified. In addition, it is also clear that defects in the same gene can lead to either loss or gain of function.

SEVERE T- AND B-CELL COMBINED DEFECTS

DEFINITION

Combined immune defects are diseases in which both the T- and B-cell compartments are greatly impaired. With the early onset and severe nature of these defects, this group contains all forms of severe combined immunodeficiency (SCID) and other syndromes in which both T- and B-cell limbs of the immune system are markedly abnormal. Increasing recognition of a number of less severe syndromes that affect both T and B limbs as well as natural killer cells, and cells of the myeloid linage, has recently greatly expanded this group of defects. These disorders often include additional inflammatory features such as autoimmunity and loss of T-cell regulatory function.

EPIDEMIOLOGY

Because of newborn screening for SCID, which began in 2009 and, as of December 2018, is performed in all newborns in the United States, the incidence of SCID has undergone a downward revision from the estimated 1 : 100,000 a few years ago, to about 1 : 54,000.[6] Some of these severe forms are listed in E-Table 236-1.

PATHOBIOLOGY AND GENETICS

The hallmark of combined defects is that they eliminate or greatly impair T-cell development, in most cases leading to profound lymphopenia. Infants with disorders that affect the formation of T- and B-cell receptors, such as defects of the recombinase activating genes *RAG1* and *RAG2*, which impair VDJ recombination, have few if any T and B cells. Similarly, other defects of DNA recombination or repair genes (ARTEMIS, the product of *DCLREIC*, and DNA-PKcs) will have a similar phenotype. When T-cell immunity is absent, B cells may be present, but they will have no function. This is the case for one of the more common forms of SCID (X-linked) due to mutations in the cytokine γ chain, an essential signaling component of six cytokine receptors: interleukin (IL)–2, IL-4, IL-7, IL-9, IL-15, and IL-21. Defects of the *JAK3* gene, downstream from the cytokine γ chain, or of the IL-7 receptor itself lead to a similar immune profile.

TABLE 236-1 CATEGORIES OF PRIMARY IMMUNODEFICIENCY DISEASES

T- and B-cell combined deficiencies
Combined defined defects with syndromic features
Antibody deficiencies
Complement disorders
Phagocyte defects
Immune dysregulation syndromes
Auto-inflammatory defects
Defects of intrinsic and innate immunity

TABLE 236-2 CLINICAL PRESENTATION AND EVALUATION OF THE IMMUNE SYSTEM

CLINICAL PRESENTATION	DEFECTS	IMMUNE DEFECTS	CONDITIONS	LABORATORY TESTING
Recurrent or chronic bacterial, viral, or fungal infections Opportunistic infections	Cell-mediated immunity	Impaired killing of intracellular organisms Impaired viral immunity Hypogammaglobulinemia	SCID and other combined syndromes	Absolute lymphocyte count Enumeration of T cells and T-cell subsets Proliferative tests for T-cell function
Bacterial infections Viral infections Autoimmunity Inflammatory diseases Enteropathy Giardiasis	B cells	Hypogammaglobulinemia Impaired bacterial killing Impaired clearance of virus or toxins Autoimmunity	Hypogammaglobulinemia Agammaglobulinemia IgA deficiency CVID IgG subclass defects Antibody deficiency	Enumeration of B cells Serum IgG, IgA, and IgM Antibody testing (e.g., tetanus, diphtheria) Vaccine challenge and antibody testing (pneumococcal vaccine)
Bacterial infections Susceptibility to meningococcal disease Autoimmunity Angioedema	Complement	Impaired opsonization Impaired bacterial killing Lack of clearance of immune complexes	Complement C2 deficiency Other complement defects HAE	CH50 AH50 Measuring individual components C1 inhibitor protein and function
Bacterial infections Poor skin healing Fungal infections Stomatitis Periodontal disease	Phagocytic cells	Impaired neutrophil mobilization Impaired opsonization Impaired bacterial killing	Chronic neutropenia Cyclic neutropenia Autoimmune neutropenia LAD CGD	Absolute neutrophil counts Neutrophil oxidative burst examined by dihydrorhodamine test by flow cytometry Examination of the blood smear Antineutrophil antibodies

CGD = chronic granulomatous disease; CVID = combined variable immunodeficiency; HAE = hereditary angioedema; LAD = leukocyte adhesion deficiency; SCID = severe combined immunodeficiency.

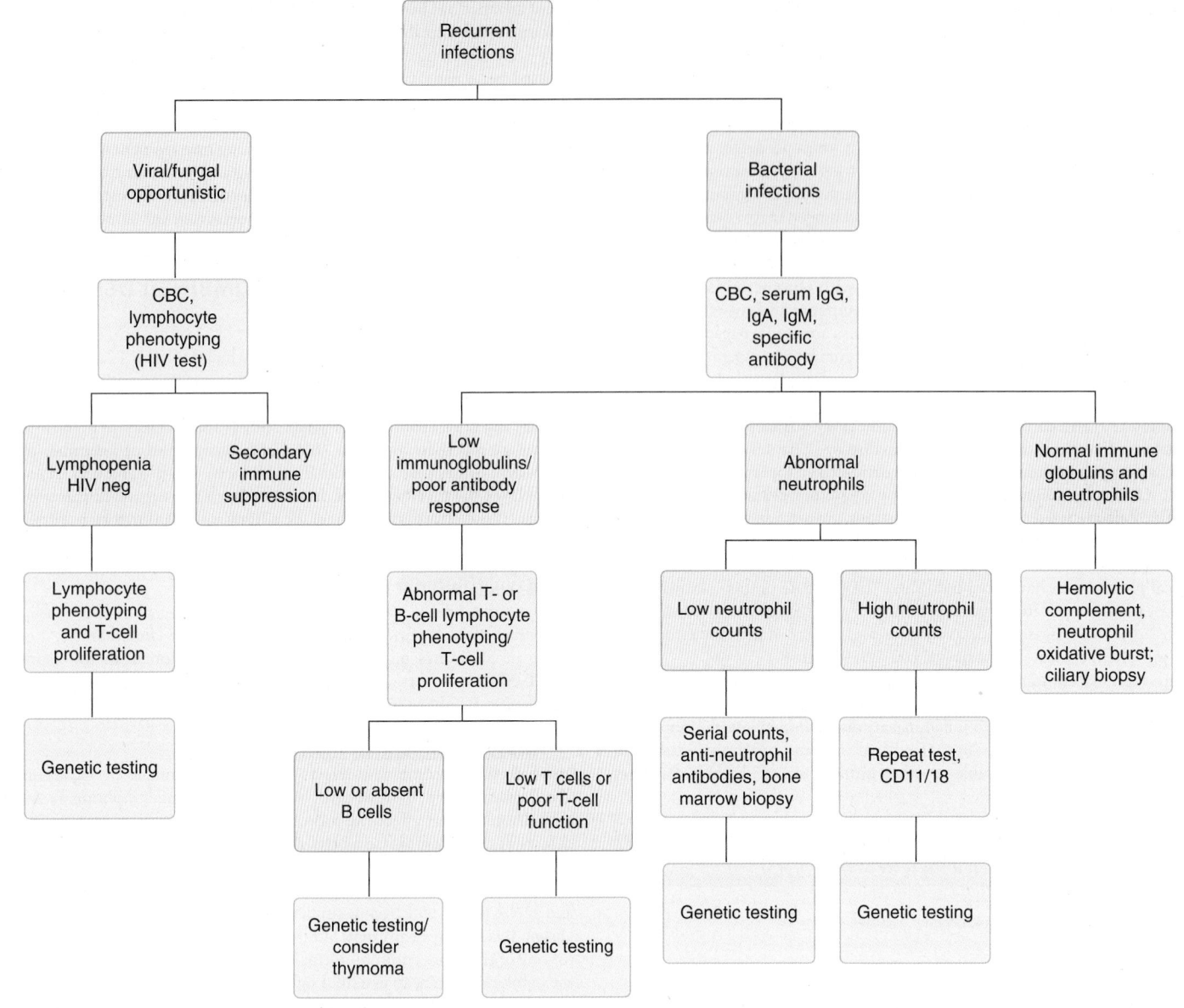

FIGURE 236-1. Evaluation of immune defects presenting with recurrent infections.

CLINICAL MANIFESTATIONS

With loss of both essential limbs of the adaptive immune system, infants with combined immune defects have severe and recurrent infections due to bacteria, viruses, and fungi. Other common features include diarrhea, dermatitis, and failure to thrive. Clinically, most patients present before the age of 3 months, but a significant number of infants may present later, although still usually in the first year of life. Without intervention, SCID commonly results in severe infections and death by the age of 2 years. In some cases, the immune defect is such that a few T cells can develop, but these are often self-reactive; such cases are often termed "leaky" SCID. When the presentation of these cases includes rashes and evidence of autoimmunity, infants are said to have Omenn syndrome.

DIAGNOSIS

The majority of states now perform a sensitive and specific DNA-based newborn screening for SCID, based on standard blood spot (Guthrie) cards to determine if the signature for normal numbers of T cells emigrating from the infant thymus (T-cell excision circles or TRECS) can be detected, leading to rapid clinical recognition and proper treatment. Whereas newborns normally have a mean absolute lymphocyte count of 4000/μL or higher, most infants with SCID have significant lymphopenia. The first step after a newborn screen has indicated low or absent TREC numbers is a flow cytometer panel that is used to enumerate T, B, and natural killer (NK) cells. This will also suggest genes that may be responsible. Further genetic testing is commonly done, but stem cell transplant approaches must also be launched. Note that the less severe forms of combined immune deficiency (E-Table 236-2) are not identified by newborn screening due to the development of some T cells.

Without immune reconstitution, infants with the severe forms of combined immunodeficiency will die, and prompt recognition is essential. Early reconstitution with stem cells from human leukocyte antigen (HLA)–matched bone marrow or mobilized peripheral blood is mandatory. When the diagnosis is made early and no severe infections have occurred, hematopoietic stem cell transplantation (HSCT; Chapter 168) is likely to be curative in 90% of selected cases.[7] For other cases, gene therapy has been developed as a method to correct a patient's own stem cells, which has been used for several primary immunodeficiencies, including forms of SCID and Wiskott-Aldrich syndrome.[8] More recently, new methods for gene editing, allowing the endogenous gene to be repaired and expressed under normal regulatory controls, may offer another option in time.[9]

LESS SEVERE T- AND B-CELL COMBINED DEFECTS

In addition to the severe forms of SCID, a number of other genetic defects also impair both T- and B-cell limbs, but newborn screening will not identify these infants as T-cell numbers are not sufficiently affected. In these forms, in addition to infections, the phenotype is extended to include atopy, severe viral infections, autoimmunity, and, in some, cancer (see E-Table 236-2).

DEFINITION

Examples of these defects include syndromes in which major histocompatibility complex (MHC) class I or class II is not expressed (sometimes called bare lymphocyte syndromes), additional defects of T-cell signaling (such as Zap-70), and syndromes resulting from defects of the actin cytoskeleton that prevent T-cell activation, including the dedicator of cytokinesis proteins, DOCK2 and DOCK8.[10]

DIAGNOSIS AND CLINICAL MANIFESTATIONS

Like the more severe combined immunodeficiency states, these syndromes lead to defects of both T- and B-cell compartments, and infants present with severe and recurrent bacterial, viral, or fungal infections, diarrhea, dermatitis, and usually failure to thrive. Some of these syndromes have unique clinical features as shown in E-Table 236-2. One notable example, with atopic disease and high immunoglobulin E (IgE), is DOCK8 deficiency, which was first recognized in subjects with autosomal recessive hyper-IgE syndrome.

TREATMENT AND PROGNOSIS

More complex is the management of the other combined defects, but hematopoietic transplant is the only curative measure at present.

COMBINED DEFECTS WITH SYNDROMIC FEATURES

Another group of combined primary immune defects are those that have distinctive systemic characteristics, aside from the obvious abnormities in the immune system (Table 236-3). The best known of these are the Wiskott-Aldrich syndrome, ataxia-telangiectasia, DiGeorge syndrome, hyperimmunoglobulin E (Buckley-Job) syndrome, cartilage-hair hypoplasia, ectodermal dysplasia with immune deficiency, and purine nucleoside phosphorylase (PNP) deficiency. These are distinct from each other and are discussed separately.

Wiskott-Aldrich Syndrome
DEFINITION AND EPIDEMIOLOGY

Wiskott-Aldrich syndrome (WAS) is an X-linked recessive disease characterized by eczema, thrombocytopenia, and immune deficiency. WAS is rare, estimated at 1 to 10 cases per million males. Ethnic differences are not known.

PATHOBIOLOGY AND CLINICAL MANIFESTATIONS

WAS is inherited as an X-linked disease, and the main manifestations in early childhood include eczema, chronic thrombocytopenia sometimes leading to bloody diarrhea, and immune deficiency with recurrent infections. Not uncommonly, autoimmunity or inflammatory disease including autoimmune hemolytic anemia, splenomegaly, arthritis, inflammatory bowel disease, and vasculitis appear. There is a clear increase in the incidence of lymphoma in WAS. The syndrome is caused by mutations in the *WAS* gene, which codes for the protein called WASP, an intracellular cytoplasmic scaffold protein important for the activation and mobility of all blood cells. WASP is involved in actin polymerization and in establishing an interface between immune cells (the immune synapse). Partly depending on the location of the mutation in the *WAS* gene, milder versions are known, leading to X-linked thrombocytopenia in some cohorts. Another, much rarer version leads to X-linked neutropenia.

DIAGNOSIS

The diagnosis is commonly made in the first few years of life in males with the characteristic symptoms of eczema with thrombocytopenia leading to petechiae. Typically, IgM levels are low, whereas IgA (and sometimes IgE) levels are increased. Platelet sizes are smaller than normal, and clot retraction is poor. Family history may include male relatives with WAS or thrombocytopenia. The diagnosis can be suggested by lack of the WAS protein as detected by flow cytometry in reference laboratories, but definitive diagnosis requires gene testing.

TABLE 236-3	EXAMPLES OF COMBINED DEFECTS OF IMMUNITY WITH SYNDROMIC FEATURES					
TYPE	**GENES**	**INHERITANCE**	**LABORATORY FEATURES**	**ALTERED FUNCTIONS**	**DISEASE AND COMPLICATIONS**
Wiskott-Aldrich syndrome	*WAS*	XL	Thrombocytopenia, small platelets	Impaired cell activation, mobility	Eczema; lymphoma; autoimmune disease; bacterial and viral infections
Ataxia-telangiectasia	*ATM*	AR	Some have IgA deficiency; IgG defects, lymphopenia in some	Impaired DNA double-stranded break repair	Ataxia; telangiectasia; pulmonary infections; lymphoreticular and other malignant neoplasms; increased α-fetoprotein; x-ray sensitivity
DiGeorge/velocardiofacial syndrome/ chromosome 22q11.2 deletion syndrome	22q11.2 deletion; rarely a deletion in 10p	De novo (majority) or AD	Lymphopenia; low T-cell numbers; large deletion in chromosome 22 on fluorescence in situ hybridization	Impaired T-cell immunity	Cardiac abnormalities; hypoparathyroidism, abnormal facies
Hyper-IgE syndrome (Buckley-Job syndrome)	*STAT3*	AD	Eosinophilia, high IgE	Loss of normal cytokine activation, defective IL-17	Bacterial infections; eczema, distinctive facial features, osteoporosis, fractures, scoliosis, delay of shedding primary teeth, hyperextensible joints, candidiasis
Cartilage-hair hypoplasia	*RMRP*	AR	Lymphopenia, low T-cell numbers	Impaired processing of mitochondrial RNA	Short-limbed dwarfism, sparse hair, celiac disease, Hirschsprung disease, bone marrow failure, autoimmunity, susceptibility to lymphoma
Ectodermal dysplasia with immunodeficiency (EDA-ID)	*IKBKG* (NEMO)	XL	Decreased IgG and IgA, elevated IgM, poor specific antibody responses, absent antibody to polysaccharide antigens	Normal B cell numbers, impaired BCR activation, low memory and isotype switched B cells	Anhidrotic ectodermal dysplasia (in some), various infections (bacteria, mycobacteria, viruses and fungi), colitis, conical teeth, variable defects of skin, hair and teeth, monocyte dysfunction
Purine nucleoside phosphorylase (PNP) deficiency	*PNP*	AR	Progressive T-cell loss Immune globulins normal or low	Impaired T cell functions	Autoimmune hemolytic anemia, neurologic impairment

AD = autosomal dominant; AR = autosomal recessive; ATM = ataxia telangiectasia mutated; BCR = B-cell receptor; IL = interleukin; NEMO = NF-κB essential modulator; PNP = purine nucleoside phosphorylase; RMRP = RNA component of mitochondrial RNA processing endoribonuclease; STAT3 = signal transducer and activator of transcription 3; WASP= Wiskott-Aldrich protein; XL = X-linked.

TREATMENT AND PROGNOSIS

Treatment strategies in WAS are diverse and usually considered on a case-by-case basis. Conservative management includes prophylactic antibiotics, immunization with conjugated polysaccharide vaccines, and intravenous or subcutaneous immune goblin for subjects with repeated infections. For eczema, standard measures are used (Chapter 409). For significant thrombocytopenia (Chapter 163), splenectomy has been performed but is discouraged as lifelong post-splenectomy sepsis poses a significant risk. For these subjects, lifelong antibiotic prophylaxis is mandatory. More recently eltrombopag, a thrombopoietic agent, has been used with benefit.[11] Platelet transfusions should be reserved for active bleeding that cannot be managed with usual methods (e.g., aminocaproic acid) and avoided for subjects for whom transplantation is considered. Autoimmunity can be difficult to control, and immune suppression should be used with caution. Treatment of lymphomas is by standard regimens (Chapter 176).

The prognosis in WAS is highly variable. Some have mild thrombocytopenia leading to occasional nose bleeds, whereas other subjects have inflammatory disease or other complications that require additional, sometimes intensive medical management. HSCT (Chapter 168) offers a cure, but this is best done early and requires careful matching and standard protocols. Trials with gene therapy are also ongoing.

Ataxia-Telangiectasia
DEFINITION AND EPIDEMIOLOGY

Ataxia-telangiectasia (AT) is a rare neurodegenerative disease that leads to cerebellar atrophy, skin telangiectasia, and immune defects. AT is estimated to occur in 1 in 40,000 to 100,000 but is more common in selected isolated populations. Sexes are affected equally.

PATHOBIOLOGY AND CLINICAL MANIFESTATIONS

AT is due to recessive mutations in the gene that encodes the ATM protein, important in both cell division and DNA repair. With the loss of the ATM protein, DNA breakage cannot be repaired, leading to cell death. The clinical manifestations include progressive difficulty in walking, with ataxia beginning around the age of 5 years. Skin telangiectasias develop on the bulbar conjunctiva and behind the ears. The immune defects include IgA deficiency, IgG subclass defects, and cellular defects leading to recurring pulmonary infections and lung damage in some. Subjects with AT have radiosensitivity, and the development of lymphomas is common with increasing age.

DIAGNOSIS

The diagnosis can usually be made by the characteristic clinical phenotype, coupled with an increase in α-fetoprotein in the blood. Radiosensitivity can be assessed in vitro in fibroblast cell lines. Definitive diagnosis is by *ATM* gene sequencing.

TREATMENT AND PROGNOSIS

Treatment for AT includes a medical team providing supportive measures and physical therapy as needed.[12] The life expectancy for subjects with AT varies greatly, but most live into early adulthood.

DiGeorge Syndrome
DEFINITION AND EPIDEMIOLOGY

DiGeorge syndrome is an autosomal dominant defect and one of the members of the 22q11.2 deletion syndrome that includes velocardiofacial syndrome, conotruncal anomaly face syndrome, congenital thymic aplasia, and thymic hypoplasia.[13] DiGeorge syndrome is one of the most common of the immune defects, estimated at 1:4000. Sexes are affected equally.

PATHOBIOLOGY AND CLINICAL MANIFESTATIONS

Although it is classified as an immune defect because of thymic hypoplasia or aplasia, patients with DiGeorge syndrome are likely also to have congenital heart disease, cleft palate or pharyngeal closure defects, characteristic facies, hypocalcemia due to parathyroid insufficiency, and learning disability. The more common cardiac defects include tetralogy of Fallot, interrupted aortic arch, ventricular septal defects, vascular rings, and anomalous return of brachial arteries. The mnemonic CATCH-22 has been applied: cardiac issues, abnormal facies, thymic aplasia, cleft palate, and hypocalcemia. With loss of thymic tissue, cellular immunity is mildly to moderately impaired, leading to recurrent infections. Hypogammaglobulinemia is not uncommon and may be associated with autoimmune cytopenias, especially thrombocytopenia.

DIAGNOSIS

The diagnosis of DiGeorge syndrome for most patients is based on genetic testing with fluorescence in situ hybridization, which detects the loss of the 22q11.2 gene segment or, more rarely, a loss of 10p14-p13. However, about 10% do not have a gene defect but have the syndrome due to maternal diabetes, fetal alcohol syndrome, or prenatal exposure to isotretinoin (Accutane).

TREATMENT AND PROGNOSIS

Treatment of DiGeorge syndrome is based on individual need and may require cardiac surgery, cleft palate repair, and calcium and vitamin D supplementation if hypocalcemia is found. Some subjects are hypothyroid, requiring thyroid supplementation. The immune defect in DiGeorge syndrome varies widely, from complete loss of thymic development with no circulating T cells to normal T-cell numbers. For most, the thymus is hypoplastic, and whereas the level of T cells may be subnormal for age, sufficient T-cell function remains and no specific treatment is needed. Withholding of live viral vaccines may not be necessary as reports of ill effects are rare and the protection afforded is likely to outweigh any risk. For complete loss of the thymus, thymic transplantation[14] can supply sufficient reconstitution. For most subjects, the prognosis depends on the concomitant medical issues, such as results of cardiac surgery, surgical repair of cleft palate, management of swallowing difficulties, and resources to enhance muscle strength and to overcome speech impediments and learning disabilities. For most, the T-cell defect is a minor component and a normal lifespan is likely; but with age, autoimmunity may become more prominent.

Hyperimmunoglobulin E Syndrome
DEFINITION

Hyperimmunoglobulin E syndrome (HIES), also called Buckley-Job syndrome, is an immune deficiency syndrome characterized by eczema, skin and lung abscesses, hyperextensible joints and recurrent bone fractures, distinctive coarse facies, eosinophilia, and high levels of serum IgE.

PATHOBIOLOGY AND CLINICAL MANIFESTATIONS

HIES is an autosomal dominant defect resulting from mutations in the gene *STAT3* encoding a transcription factor, signal transducer, and activator of transcription 3. After activation by selected cytokines and growth factors, STAT3 protein is phosphorylated and translocated to the cell nucleus. Whereas loss of STAT3 signaling affects many cellular processes, the syndrome itself is often clinically recognizable from the characteristic clinical findings of eczema, recurrent skin boils, unusual facies with tubular nose, cyst-forming pneumonias often due to *S. aureus*, and increased serum IgE. Other common manifestations include a rash in the newborn period; mucocutaneous candidiasis; and skeletal abnormalities, such as scoliosis, osteoporosis, fractures with minimal trauma, and delayed shedding of primary teeth. Features of the HIES syndrome have been found in a few patients with rare autosomal recessive defects in genes encoding tyrosine kinase 2 (Tyk2) and dedicator of cytokinesis 8 (DOCK8), but in both of these, viral infections are also prominent.

DIAGNOSIS

The diagnosis can be strongly suspected on clinical grounds, but a useful scoring system composed of a composite of laboratory and clinical characteristics has been shown to aid in the dissection of hyperimmunoglobulin E subjects from other subjects with high serum IgE levels, for example, severely atopic subjects. IgE levels may range from 1000 to 40,000 IU or more; some references note that IgE levels may normalize in older subjects. Eosinophilia is common. However, a definitive diagnosis is best confirmed by identifying a *STAT3* mutation.

TREATMENT AND PROGNOSIS

There is no definitive treatment for HIES syndrome. Because of the propensity for staphylococcal infections, prophylaxis with appropriate antibiotics (trimethoprim-sulfamethoxazole, 5 mg/kg/day trimethoprim divided twice daily) is commonly used, along with oral antifungals such as itraconazole (100 mg daily for patients <13 years old or weighing <50 kg; 200 mg daily for those >13 years old or weighing >50 kg). Surgical drainage of abscesses is also important, but wound healing may be poor. Skin care for eczema may include bleach baths to reduce bacterial burden and antihistamines to control pruritus. Optimization of calcium and vitamin D levels may be useful to strengthen bones. HIES is a lifelong disease, and infections or other complications require individual care. With increasing age, worsening respiratory dysfunction is likely. Recent reports note vascular, especially arterial, abnormalities, which are important to define.

Cartilage-Hair Hypoplasia

DEFINITION AND EPIDEMIOLOGY

Cartilage-hair hypoplasia (CHH) is a rare autosomal recessive form of short-limbed dwarfism associated with a variable cellular immune deficiency. In the Old Order Amish population, CHH affects 1 in 1300 newborns; for those of Finnish descent, the incidence is about 1 in 20,000. A common point mutation in the gene is prevalent in the particularly affected populations.

PATHOBIOLOGY AND CLINICAL MANIFESTATIONS

The genetic defect in CHH is in the *RMRP* gene, which encodes the RNA in a mitochondrial RNA-processing endoribonuclease that helps copy mitochondrial DNA and process ribosomal RNA. In CHH, the encoded RNA is unstable, leading to skeletal dysplasia, sparse hair, and the predominantly T-cell deficiency disease. For unclear reasons, the cellular defect is varied, ranging from mildly impaired immunity to severe defects requiring HSCT (Chapter 168). Other clinical features of CHH include short stature, anemia, autoimmunity, celiac disease, Hirschsprung disease, and several cancers, including lymphoma.[15]

DIAGNOSIS

The diagnosis can be suspected by inheritance patterns and clinical phenotype, but definitive diagnosis is made by genetic sequencing of the *RMRP* gene.

TREATMENT AND PROGNOSIS

For patients with severe T-cell defects and infections (essentially SCID phenotype) suggesting a significantly impaired immune system, HSCT is required (Chapter 168). Aside from the cellular defect, treatment is directed at the other presenting clinical issues. The prognosis of CHH is varied, and the prognosis depends on the extent of the cellular defect, the therapies required, and the associated clinical complications. As the defect is so variable, normal lifespans may be achieved.

● ANTIBODY DEFECTS

DEFINITION

The antibody defects are due to loss of B-cell development, loss of production of one or more of the immunoglobulin (Ig) isotypes, or loss of functional antibody production.

EPIDEMIOLOGY

As a group, antibody defects are the most prevalent immune defects and are found in patients of all ages. Selective IgA deficiency is most common in patients of white background, but the incidence varies with the population studied from 1 : 400 to more than 1 : 10,000. IgA deficiency is found in 1 : 400 in Finland but much less commonly in African Americans or Asians (1 : 14,000 or fewer). Common variable immune deficiency (CVID) has an estimated incidence of 1 in 50,000; IgG subclass or selective antibody defects are also common, but the incidence is unknown.

PATHOBIOLOGY AND CLINICAL MANIFESTATIONS

Whereas the genetic causes have been elucidated for many of the combined forms of immune deficiency, the genes are not yet known for many of the more common B-cell defects (Table 236-4). Antibody defects can be considered

in three main forms: B cells are absent; B cells are present but one or more immunoglobulin isotypes are not made; and B cells and immunoglobulin levels are normal but the produced immunoglobulins have no function.

Lack of B Cells Leading to Agammaglobulinemia
Genetic Defects of the B-Cell Receptor or Signaling Pathways
The first described severe antibody defect was the X-linked form of agammaglobulinemia (XLA). The gene affected, a tyrosine kinase (BTK) located on the X chromosome, is essential for downstream signaling from the B-cell receptor. Without these signals, B cells do not survive, leading to profound hypogammaglobulinemia. The incidence of this disease is approximately 1 in 100,000. The main clinical manifestations appear in the first year of life, but males may come to clinical attention later, in some cases not until the second decade. Whereas X-linked inheritance is a central feature, the family history may or may not be positive because of de novo mutations. Infections are usually bacterial, generally with encapsulated organisms such as *Streptococcus pneumoniae, Haemophilus influenzae, Staphylococcus aureus,* and *Pseudomonas* species. A particular propensity for *Mycoplasma* infections in XLA has been long noted; these may occur in joints or the urinary tract and can be difficult to diagnose as appropriate culture techniques are not widely available.

In addition to XLA, there are other genetic forms of agammaglobulinemia. These are gene defects of the B-cell receptor itself, such as the μ heavy chain, the surrogate light chain λ5, Igα, and Igβ. Similarly, mutations in signaling proteins immediately downstream from the B-cell receptor lead to the same outcome, with loss of all B cells. As these genes are not on the X chromosome, these defects, although rare, are found in both sexes.

Good Syndrome
A special case of agammaglobulinemia with loss of B cells in adults is a poorly understood immune defect associated with thymomas (Good syndrome). This appears to be a secondary immune defect, but it is important to include it here as the loss of B cells, with either agammaglobulinemia or hypogammaglobulinemia, leads to many of the same infectious manifestations as with the other profound antibody defects. Quite rare, Good syndrome occurs in adults, most often after 40 years of age. There is an increased incidence of opportunistic infections, such as *Pneumocystis jiroveci, Candida* infections with nail or other cutaneous involvement, viral infections, autoimmunity, and inflammatory complications such as lichen planus. The connection between thymoma, loss of B-cell function, and the unusual infections remains unclear.

Hypogammaglobulinemia with B Cells Present
Common Variable Immune Deficiency
Patients with CVID have varying degrees of hypogammaglobulinemia ranging from almost total loss of immunoglobulins to more modest reductions of IgG and IgA or IgM.[16] From the clinical point of view, CVID is a noteworthy disorder as it is relatively common (1 : 25,000 to 1 : 50,000), has a later onset than other immune defects (generally between 20 and 40 years of age), and has a highly heterogeneous clinical presentation. Delays in diagnosis are common. Before diagnosis, about 80% of subjects with CVID will have had one or more episodes of pneumonia, sometimes leading to empyema. Over time, bronchiectasis may develop. The bacterial species most commonly found include *S. pneumoniae, H. influenzae, S. aureus,* and *Mycoplasma* species. The gastrointestinal tract is not uncommonly involved; this may be infectious (e.g., *Giardia, Campylobacter,* norovirus) or inflammatory, including lymphoid hyperplasia and forms of inflammatory bowel disease leading to malabsorption. However, a biopsy will show loss of plasma cells in the gastrointestinal mucosa. About one quarter of subjects with CVID have autoimmune conditions such as thrombocytopenia, hemolytic anemia, achlorhydria, pernicious anemia, and granulomatous disease in lymphoid organs, lungs, brain, or skin, suggesting sarcoidosis. Clinically, lymphadenopathy is common, and splenomegaly is noted in 28%. Malignant disease is also increased, usually B-cell lymphomas, but other cancers also appear more commonly in CVID. An increasing number of genes leading to loss of B-cell function and the CVID phenotype have been identified. This is especially true for the roughly 30% of CVID subjects with inflammatory or autoimmune complications; causative genes are found in up to 32%[17] (see Table 236-4). However, the majority of subjects with hypogammaglobulinemia do not have a known gene defect.

Hyperimmunoglobulin M Syndromes
The hyperimmunoglobulin M (hyper-IgM) syndromes are defects in which there is a loss of isotype switch; that is, whereas B cells do produce IgM, they

TABLE 236-4	EXAMPLES OF ANTIBODY DEFECTS			
TYPE	**GENES**	**INHERITANCE**	**LABORATORY FEATURES**	**DISEASE AND COMPLICATIONS**
ABSENT B CELLS: SEVERE REDUCTIONS IN IgG, IgA, and IgM				
X-linked agammaglobulinemia	*BTK*	XL	IgG, IgA, and IgM are very low or absent	Severe bacterial infections
Autosomal forms of agammaglobulinemia	Defects of the B-cell receptor or its signaling pathways; λ5, Igα, Igβ	AR	IgG, IgA, and IgM are very low or absent	Severe bacterial infections
Good syndrome	Unknown	Unknown	Few or absent B cells; variable hypogammaglobulinemia	Associated with thymoma; may have opportunistic infections
B CELLS PRESENT: BUT LOW SERUM IgG, IgA, and/or IgM				
Common variable immune deficiency	Unknown	Unknown	Low IgG, IgA and/or IgM	Bacterial infections, autoimmunity, other inflammatory complications
Defects of B-cell receptors	CD19, CD81, CD20, CD21 TACI, BAFFr, TWEAK	AR, AD and sporadic	Low IgG, IgA and/or IgM	Recurrent infections
Defects of signaling, activation and/or regulation	ICOS, NFKb1, NFKb2; PI3KCD; CTLA4, IKAROS, LRBA, STAT3, etc.	AR, AD with variable penetrance; sporadic	Variably low IgG, IgA and/or IgM; antibody defects. Increased IgM in PI3KCD	Recurrent infections and autoimmunity; variable clinical expression
B CELLS PRESENT: SEVERE REDUCTION IN SERUM IgG AND IgA BUT NORMAL OR ELEVATED IgM				
X-linked hyper-IgM syndrome	*CD40L*	XL	IgG and IgA decreased; IgM may be normal or increased; B-cell numbers may be normal or increased	Bacterial and opportunistic infections, neutropenia, autoimmune disease
CD40 deficiency	*CD40*	AR	Low IgG and IgA; normal or increased IgM	Bacterial and opportunistic infections, neutropenia, autoimmune disease
Defects of DNA recombination	*AID and UNG*	AR	IgG and IgA decreased; IgM increased	Bacterial infections; enlarged lymph nodes and germinal centers
B CELLS PRESENT: ISOTYPE DEFICIENCIES				
Selective IgA deficiency	Unknown	Unknown	IgA absent	Usually asymptomatic; allergies and autoimmunity may be more common
IgA with IgG subclass deficiency	Unknown	Unknown	Reduced IgA with decrease in one or more IgG subclass (usually IgG2/4)	Infections in some with loss of antibody
IgG subclass deficiency	Unknown	Unknown	Reduction in one or more IgG subclass	Asymptomatic in many; infections in some with loss of antibody
B CELLS PRESENT: NORMAL IgG, IgA, AND IgM				
Antibody deficiency	Unknown	Unknown	Normal serum immunoglobulins but no vaccine responses to protein and carbohydrate antigens or vaccines	May lead to recurrent infections

AD = autosomal dominant; AR = autosomal recessive; BAFF-R = B-cell activating factor receptor; *Btk* = Bruton tyrosine kinase; CTLA4 = cytotoxic T-lymphocyte–associated protein 4; ICOS = inducible T-cell costimulator; LRBA = LPS responsive beige-like anchor protein; *PI3KCD* = phosphatidylinositol-4,5-bisphosphate 3-kinase catalytic subunit delta; STAT3 = signal transducer and activator of transcription 3; TACI = transmembrane activator and CAML interactor; TWEAK = tumor necrosis factor ligand superfamily member 12; XL = X-linked.

do not secrete IgG or IgA. The prototypic form is the X-linked version in which an essential T-cell activation receptor, the CD40 ligand encoded on the X chromosome, is missing or nonfunctional. Mutations in the gene for its receptor partner, the CD40 on B cells, lead to a similar defect. Several other genetic disorders lead to a similar immunologic phenotype, including defects of the gene for enzyme activation-induced cytidine deaminase (*AICDA*) and uracil-DNA glycosylase, both important for DNA recombination. The complications of the hyper-IgM syndromes include bacterial infections, autoimmunity, and enteropathy similar to CVID but also *P. jiroveci* pneumonia, neutropenia, and unusual cancers.[18] A predilection to infections with *Cryptosporidium* has been noted in the X-linked hyper-IgM syndrome, which unfortunately can lead to irreversible liver disease. Two other gene defects may present with increased serum IgM: *PI3KCD* and, as noted also in Table 236-3, NEMO (*IKBKG*).

Selective IgA Deficiency

Selective IgA deficiency (IgA <7 mg/dL with other isotypes normal) is the most common of the primary immunodeficiency disorders, but most subjects are asymptomatic. Lack of infections in most subjects is generally ascribed to the overlapping and compensatory role of other immune functions, but this is not clearly understood. However, allergies, autoimmunity, increased serum IgE, asthma, rheumatoid arthritis, gluten intolerance, and inflammatory bowel disease are found more commonly in selective IgA-deficient subjects than in other populations. Presumably owing to the loss of secretory IgA, *Giardia* infections may occur (Chapter 330). The treatments used in subjects with IgA deficiency are based on the clinical conditions observed. Some subjects with IgA deficiency are IgG2 and IgG4 deficient, with loss of

antibacterial antibody leading to severe infections and, in some cases, chronic lung disease.[19]

IgG Subclass Defects

Another variable immune deficiency is represented by the IgG subclass defects. The incidence of these is difficult to determine, partly because laboratory normal ranges vary. The clinical consequences depend on how much antibody function is lost. Whereas there are structural differences in IgG isotypes, their functional roles have considerable overlap; thus the importance of isotype defects can be controversial, especially if loss of antibody is not demonstrable. In adults, IgG3 deficiency appears to be the most common but is likely to have no significance. However, low IgG2 or IgG4, most often found in subjects with selective IgA deficiency, may lead to a profound deficiency of antibody production, especially to carbohydrate antigens such as contained in the pneumococcal vaccine.

Antibody Deficiency with Normal Immunoglobulins

More complex and heterogeneous is the loosely described defect termed *antibody deficiency with normal serum immunoglobulins*, also termed *specific antibody deficiency*.[20] The incidence is unknown; all ages are affected, but in general, children younger than 5 years are not included to allow transient forms of physiologic immune deficiency to resolve. Although B cells are present and there are normal levels of IgG, IgA, and IgM, these subjects do not form protective levels of serum antibodies after having an infection exposure or vaccination with protein and/or carbohydrate vaccines. In the most severe cases, even strong immunogens such as herpes zoster or tetanus vaccines are ineffective; in milder cases, the pneumococcal vaccine does not result in titers of antibody considered sufficient for protection.

DIAGNOSIS

The diagnosis of antibody defects is based on the laboratory tests of numbers of B cells, the serum immunoglobulin levels (IgG, IgA, and IgM), and an evaluation of a panel of vaccine responses to determine the levels of functional antibody. If B cells are absent and the levels of immunoglobulins are very low, further antibody testing is not required. For a young male with a family history of males with immune deficiency, the diagnosis of XLA or hyper-IgM can be investigated by flow cytometry (to determine numbers of B cells for XLA) or by genetic tests (hyper-IgM). For older subjects (generally older than 45 years), a thymoma may be sought by chest computed tomography, which may show a mass in the mediastinum. Most subjects with hypogammaglobulinemia will be found to have B cells in peripheral blood and some amount of serum IgG, IgA, or IgM. In these cases, the loss of functional antibody should be tested by commercial laboratories to determine if protective titers of antibody to common vaccine antigens (i.e., tetanus, diphtheria, *H. influenzae*, and pneumococci) can be detected. In some cases, revaccination may be needed to determine if a response occurs (tested again in 4 to 6 weeks). Most authorities use the laboratory-stipulated protective ranges for protein vaccines and for pneumococcal vaccination, usually 1.3 μg/mL for individual serotypes. When high levels of B cells are found in adults, the possibility of a clonal B-cell expansion should be considered (e.g., chronic lymphocytic leukemia). For subjects with IgG subclass defects or normal immunoglobulins levels, the use of a panel of antibody titers is also recommended to have a clear understanding of immune competence or immune defect. Genetic testing to define causative genes is often used when genetic counseling is important, or to guide therapeutic decisions when autoimmune or inflammatory complications are present.

TREATMENT   Rx

The essential treatment of significant IgG antibody defects is intravenous or subcutaneous immune globulin, usually given in doses of 400 to 600 mg/kg body weight per month. The intravenous forms are usually given every 3 or 4 weeks, the subcutaneous forms weekly, biweekly, or monthly, depending on product and body weight. Indwelling ports are not required and are discouraged. Most patients also require occasional courses of antibiotics, chosen on the basis of culture results, at intervals dictated by clinical events. As many subjects with antibody defects have experienced one or more bouts of pneumonia, lung functions may be abnormal and intermittent or prophylactic antibiotics required, but there is no consensus on the medications, dose, or intervals to use. Referring to Table 236-4, the defects that require IgG replacement are those in which B cells are absent (XLA, other agammaglobulinemias, the hyper-IgM syndromes, IgG subclass defects with demonstrable loss of antibody function, and some cases of loss of antibody with normal immunoglobulins). Subjects

with IgA deficiency do not require immune globulin replacement unless there is clear loss of functional antibody. For unclear reasons, some of the antibody defects have an increased incidence of autoimmune or inflammatory complications. These require treatments commonly prescribed for immunocompetent subjects but with a view to minimizing courses of immune suppressants. Immune cytopenias may be treated with rituximab with some success; splenectomy is to be avoided.

PROGNOSIS

The prognosis for subjects with antibody defects is variable and depends on the degree of the defect, the response to treatment, whether organ damage has occurred, and whether other complications develop. Subjects with loss of B cells have a pure B-cell defect; when they are diagnosed and treated early with sufficient immune globulin, the prognosis appears excellent. Subjects with selective IgA deficiency can be indistinguishable from age-matched healthy peers. CVID subjects with varying degrees of hypogammaglobulinemia ranging from almost total loss of immunoglobulins to more modest reductions of IgG and IgA or IgM often have additional complications, in some cases because the diagnosis has been delayed and pulmonary or other damage has occurred. Autoimmune cytopenias can be treated with rituximab, but chronic interstitial lung disease, lymphoid hyperplasia, and gastrointestinal enteropathy may be difficult to treat, leading to increased morbidity. Improved survival relative to prior years is likely overall in CVID, but the inflammatory complications still present additional challenges. For subjects with IgG subclass defects or antibody deficiency, with immune reconstitution if required, no increased morbidity or mortality is expected.

COMPLEMENT DISORDERS

DEFINITION

The complement system is a network of proteins that both amplify and control many actions of the immune system. It is generally considered to have three main branches, the classical, alternative, and lectin pathways; deficiencies of individual components lead to increased susceptibility to infections, autoimmunity, and inflammatory diseases (Table 236-5). For further details of these disorders, see Chapter 44.

EPIDEMIOLOGY

Complement C2 deficiency is found in 1 : 10,000 white subjects and usually in those with a conserved major histocompatibility complex haplotype due to a founder defect; more than 95% of C2-deficient individuals are homozygous for the same *C2* mutation. The other complement component defects are rare but found in unequal distribution in selected populations; C6 deficiency is more common in persons of African descent and C9 deficiency in Asians, with an estimated incidence of 0.036 to 0.095%. Disorders of components of these pathways are discussed here; deficiency of C1 inhibitor is discussed separately.

TABLE 236-5 EXAMPLES OF COMPLEMENT DEFECTS

TYPE	GENES	INHERITANCE	LABORATORY FEATURES	ALTERED FUNCTIONS	DISEASE AND COMPLICATIONS
C1q, C1r, C1s deficiency	*C1qA, C1qB, C1qC; C1r, C1s*	AR	Absent CH50 hemolytic activity	Loss of early complement activation; impaired dissolution of immune complexes; impaired clearance of apoptotic cells	Bacterial infections; SLE-like syndrome, rheumatoid disease, multiple autoimmune diseases, infections
C4 deficiency	*C4A and C4B*	AR	Absent CH50 hemolytic activity	Loss of early complement activation	Bacterial infections
C2 deficiency	*C2*	AR	Absent CH50 hemolytic activity	Loss of early complement activation	Bacterial infections; SLE-like syndrome, vasculitis, early atherosclerosis, polymyositis, glomerulonephritis
C3 deficiency	*C3*	AR	Absent CH50 hemolytic activity	Loss of classical and alternative pathways of complement activation	Life-threatening pyogenic infections; SLE-like disease; glomerulonephritis; atypical hemolytic-uremic syndrome
C5, C6, C7, C8 deficiency	*C5*	AR	Absent CH50 hemolytic activity	Loss of complement activation	Neisserial infections, SLE
C9 deficiency	*C9*	AR	Reduced CH50 and AP50 hemolytic activity	Partial loss of complement activation	Some *Neisseria* infections
C1 inhibitor deficiency	*C1 inhibitor*	AD	Activation of complement; low levels of C4 and C2	Loss of regulation of activities of complement C1	Angioedema

AD = autosomal dominant; AR = autosomal recessive; SLE = systemic lupus erythematosus.

PATHOBIOLOGY

The classical pathway is triggered by interaction of the Fc portion of an IgG1, IgG2, IgG3, or IgM antibody with C1q, which subsequently engages C1r, C1s, C2, and C3, leading to activation of C4, C5, C6, C7, C8, and C9, resulting in lysis of bacteria (discussed in Chapter 44). As opsonization of bacteria is essential for antibody function, patients with these defects have infections similar to those of subjects with loss of immunoglobulin. The alternative pathway is activated in an antibody-independent manner and involves opsonization of bacteria with subsequent involvement of C3 and the alternative pathway. The lectin pathway includes other serum binding proteins that coat bacteria or fungi, leading to downstream complement activation and the assembly of the membrane attack complex, the C7, C8, C9 components responsible for microbial lysis. The genes of the complement system are located on many chromosomes, and in general the defects are autosomal recessive in inheritance, with the exception of defects of X-linked properdin. In addition to the three pathways of activation, the complement system also includes an even larger number of control proteins that, when genetically defective, also lead to severe infections, hemolytic-uremic syndrome, severe eclampsia, glomerulonephritis, thrombosis, and macular degeneration, which are outside the scope of this chapter.

CLINICAL MANIFESTATIONS

With genetic loss of the classical and alternative pathways, severe bacterial infections are likely; this is particularly true of subjects with defects of C3, which lies at the convergence of the three pathways. For unclear reasons, with loss of C6, C7, C8, and C9 or properdin, *Neisseria gonorrhoeae* or *Neisseria meningitidis* infections are more common. More complex but equally potent is the role that the complement proteins play in immune regulation. With loss of the early components of the classical system, C1q, C1r, C1s, C2, and C4, autoimmunity, especially systemic lupus erythematosus, is common; this complication is estimated at 93% for subjects with defects of C1q and 75% for defects of C4. Complement is important for clearing immune complexes and possibly apoptotic cells, potentially explaining this observation.

DIAGNOSIS

Deficiencies of complement are diagnosed by testing total serum hemolytic complement (CH_{50}) and the alternative hemolytic complement (AP_{50}). The CH_{50} tests for deficiencies in the classical pathway by determining whether the patient's serum can lyse antibody-coated sheep erythrocytes; this will be zero if the proteins of the classical pathway are defective. The AP_{50} tests for alternative pathway activity. Further testing usually includes measurement and function of individual serum complement proteins to determine the most applicable diagnosis. (Note that the most common reason for low levels in CH_{50} and AP_{50} is improper blood handling.)

TREATMENT   Rx

There are no treatments for complement deficiencies. Whereas loss of these classical components may lead to severe clinical consequences, for C2 in particular but also for C4 and C5–C9, there may be no history of illness. Prompt antibiotic therapy for acute infections and control of autoimmunity are the important therapeutics. However, periodic immunizations with pneumococcal, *H. influenzae*, and meningococcal vaccines may be helpful to boost antibody titers to enhance bacterial clearance.

PROGNOSIS

The prognosis of complement defects is highly variable because of the clinical complications; also, most of these defects have been found in healthy subjects. However, for defects of the classical pathway, prompt recognition and treatment of bacterial infections and possibly preemptive vaccination with appropriate vaccines would be important. The prognosis for subjects with autoimmunity will depend on disease manifestation and response to treatment. Whereas C2 deficiency is commonly viewed as usually asymptomatic, some data suggest a higher incidence of premature arteriosclerotic heart disease.

● C1 INHIBITOR DEFICIENCY

The pathobiology, clinical manifestations, diagnosis, and treatment of C1 inhibitor (C1 INH) deficiency are discussed in detail in Chapter 237. A diagnosis of C1 INH deficiency is suggested by a history of recurrent attacks of angioedema or in some cases (25%) episodes of recurrent abdominal pain due to edema.

● PHAGOCYTE DEFECTS

DEFINITION

Abnormalities of the phagocytic system are presented in detail in Chapters 158 and 160. They are categorized as neutropenia, abnormal neutrophil morphology, defective cell adhesion and migration, or defective microbial killing (E-Table 236-3). Examples of major phagocyte defects are presented in E-Table 236-3.

EPIDEMIOLOGY

Genetic defects impairing neutrophil development, adhesion, locomotion, or intracellular killing are rare. The most common genetic abnormality is chronic granulomatous disease (CGD), with an estimated incidence of 1 : 100,000 to 1 : 200,000.

PATHOBIOLOGY AND GENETICS

Circulating neutrophils are attracted to sites of inflammation by complement components C5a, chemokines, and bacterial byproducts, but traveling to these sites requires migration through capillaries and into tissues. The best known diseases in which neutrophil adhesion is impaired are the leukocyte adhesion defects (LAD types 1, 2, and 3). Other defects of neutrophil motility include juvenile periodontitis, Shwachman-Diamond syndrome, and Chédiak-Higashi syndrome.

About two thirds of patients with CGD are males as they have defects in an X-linked gene encoding gp91^{phox}. Autosomal defects in p47^{phox} are the next most common form, occurring in 20% of patients and often due to the same deletion. Other autosomal forms are due to defects in the gene encoding the p22^{phox} or p67^{phox} subunits (about 5% each).

CLINICAL MANIFESTATIONS

The genetic neutrophil disorders have specific clinical associations: delayed separation of the umbilical cord and poor wound healing in LAD-1; growth delay, mental retardation, and Bombay blood group in LAD-2; peripheral nerve conduction defects, pigmentary dilution with partial oculocutaneous albinism, easy bruising, and risk of hemophagocytic disease in Chédiak-Higashi syndrome; and pancreatic insufficiency (fat malabsorption), growth failure, and skeletal abnormalities in Shwachman-Diamond syndrome. For both Shwachman-Diamond syndrome and the severe congenital neutropenias, there is a risk for development of myelodysplastic disease and leukemia.

The clinical manifestations of CGD usually include bacterial or fungal infections. Males with the X-linked form will generally present in the first decade of life, whereas subjects with autosomal forms may have a later onset of symptoms (into the second decade). Regardless of the genetic cause, most patients with CGD have one or more episodes of pneumonia; the most common causes of infection are *Staphylococcus*, *Burkholderia cepacia*, *Klebsiella*, *Aspergillus*, *Serratia*, and *Nocardia* species. Common clinical manifestations include acute or chronic lymphadenitis, colitis leading to recurrent diarrhea, *Staphylococcus* liver abscess, osteomyelitis, and rectal abscess. Patients with CGD are also prone to infections with unusual organisms, for example, *Chromobacterium violaceum*, *Trichosporon inkin*, *Francisella philomiragia*, and *Granulibacter bethesdensis*. For this reason, exposure to contaminated water or decaying plant material (compost, mulch) presents significant risk to subjects with CGD.

DIAGNOSIS

The differential diagnosis of neutropenia is presented in Table 158-4; the genetic diagnosis of congenital neutropenia syndromes, in Table 158-5; and a diagnostic approach to suspected phagocyte defects, in Table 160-4.

TREATMENT   Rx

The management of patients with neutropenia is discussed in Chapter 158.

● IMMUNE DYSREGULATION SYNDROMES

These mostly monogenic diseases have in common lymphoid proliferation, immune activation, and inflammatory or autoimmune complications. These

TABLE 236-6 EXAMPLES OF DISEASES OF IMMUNE DYSREGULATION

TYPE	GENES	INHERITANCE	LABORATORY FEATURES	ALTERED FUNCTION	DISEASE AND COMPLICATIONS
Familial hemophagocytic lymphohistiocytosis syndromes	PRF1, UNC13D, STX11, STXBP2, FAAP24	AR, AD	Anemia, neutropenia, thrombocytopenia, abnormal liver functions, high ferritin and serum IL-2 receptor, hemophagocytosis in bone marrow and liver	Decreased to absent NK cells and cytotoxic activities	Fever, hepatosplenomegaly, cytopenias, hemophagocytic lymphohistiocytosis, neurologic disease in some
Chédiak-Higashi syndrome	LYST	AR	Neutrophils with giant inclusions; hair: pigment clumps	Impaired chemotaxis	Partial albinism, recurrent infections, late-onset primary encephalopathy, increased lymphoma risk
Lymphoproliferative syndromes (susceptibility to EBV)	SAP, XIAP, ITK, CD27, CTPS1, CD70, RASGRP1, MAGT1	XL, AR	Epstein-Barr virus infection; decreased NK cells and CD8+ CTL activation; deficient NK-T cells; anemia; hypogammaglobulinemia in some	Loss of function of NK-T cells leading to impaired viral control	Clinical and immunologic features triggered by Epstein-Barr virus infection; lymphoproliferation, lymphoma
Autoimmune polyendocrinopathy–candidiasis ectodermal dystrophy (APECED)	AIRE	AR	Endocrine dysfunction; hepatitis	Loss of thymic self-tolerance	Autoimmunity leading to hypoparathyroidism, hypothyroidism, diabetes, and adrenal and gonadal dysfunction; cutaneous candidiasis; hepatitis
Autoimmune lymphoproliferative syndrome (ALPS)	FAS, FAS ligand; Caspase 10; Caspase 8, KRAS; NRAS	AD	Increased double-negative T cells (CD4−/CD8−), increased serum B_{12}	Defects in lymphocyte apoptosis	Splenomegaly, lymphadenopathy, autoimmune cytopenias; increased risk of lymphoma
Genetic defects of T-regulatory cells	FOXP3, CD25, CTLA4, LRBA, STAT3 (GOF) BACH2, STAT5B and STAT1; STAT5b	XL, AR	Autoimmunity, diabetes, anemia, eosinophilia, high serum IgE in some	Lack of (or impaired function of) CD4+, CD25+, FOXP3+ regulatory T cells (Tregs)	Enteropathy, dermatitis, eczema, early-onset diabetes, thyroiditis, hemolytic anemia, thrombocytopenia, elevated IgE and IgA
Immune dysregulation leading to colitis	IL-10, IL-10Ra, IL-10Rb, NFAT5	AR, AD	Normal lymphocyte panels	Defects of immune responses to resident microbes	Severe IBD, recurrent sinopulmonary infections

AD = autosomal dominant; AIRE = autoimmune regulator; AR = autosomal recessive; BACH2 = BTB domain and CNC homolog 2; CTL = cytotoxic T lymphocyte; CTLA4 = cytotoxic T-lymphocyte-associated protein 4; CTPS1 = CTP synthase 1; FAAP24 = Fanconi anemia core complex associated protein 24; FAS = Fas cell surface death receptor; FOXP3 = Forkhead box P3; IBD = inflammatory bowel disease; IL = interleukin; ITK = IL2 inducible T-cell kinase; KRAS = KRAS proto-oncogene; LRBA = LPS responsive beige-like anchor protein; LYST = lysosomal trafficking regulator; MAGT1 = magnesium transporter 1; NFAT5= nuclear factor of activated T cells 5; NRAS = NRAS proto-oncogene; PRF1 = perforin; RASGRP1 = RAS guanyl releasing protein 1; SAP = SLAM-associated protein; STAT1 = signal transducer and activator of transcription 1; STAT3 (gain of function) = signal transducer and activator of transcription 3; STAT5B = signal transducer and activator of transcription 5B; STX11 = Syntaxin 11; STXBP2 = Syntaxin binding protein 2; UNC13D = Unc-13 homolog D; XIAP = X-linked inhibitor of apoptosis; XL = X-linked.

include the hemophagocytic lymphohistiocytosis (HLH) diseases (Chapter 160), the lymphoproliferative syndromes linked to Epstein-Barr virus (EBV) infection, autoimmune polyendocrinopathy–candidiasis–ectodermal dystrophy (APECED), autoimmune lymphoproliferative syndromes (ALPS), defects of T-regulatory cells, and immune defects that lead to severe early-onset inflammatory bowel disease (Table 236-6).

EPIDEMIOLOGY

The estimated incidence of the genetic HLH syndromes is 1 : 50,000; the incidence of X-linked lymphoproliferative disease is 1 to 3 in 1,000,000; and the incidence of APECED is high in Finland (1 in 25,000) and in Sardinians and Iranian Jews (1 in 9000) but otherwise much rarer. The incidence of ALPS and defects of T-regulatory cells is unknown.

PATHOBIOLOGY AND CLINICAL MANIFESTATIONS

HLH is a form of extreme and potentially life-threatening immune activation. It is further discussed under the section Hemophagocytic Lymphohistiocytosis and Macrophage Activation Syndrome in Chapter 160. There are two forms: genetic, due to mutations in genes that control cellular cytotoxicity; and secondary, due to acute viral illnesses, autoimmune activation, or underlying malignant disease. The familial form is a heterogeneous autosomal recessive disorder due to mutations in one of five genes essential for control of T-cell cytotoxicity. Immune activation leads to expansion of poorly controlled cytotoxic T cells and macrophages, leading to the release of interferon-γ (IFN-γ), IL-1, IL-6, and IL-10. Patients have high fevers, cytopenias, liver dysfunction, coagulopathy, and sometimes neurologic symptoms. HLH may be fatal unless it is treated with aggressive measures and may require HSCT (Chapter 168). Life-threatening accelerated immune activation syndromes are also characteristic of other genetic defects that impair cytotoxicity, such as the Chédiak-Higashi syndrome.

Monogenic defects leading to impaired immunity to EBV produce another group of immune dysregulation syndromes.[21] The first described (and the most common, 70 to 80%) is the X-linked proliferative disorder (XLP) due to mutations of the X-linked gene SH2D1A, which encodes the gene SAP, a signaling lymphocytic activation molecule (SLAM)–associated protein. Other genetic causes for loss of control of EBV are due to mutations in XIAP (20 to 30%) or, rarely, ITK CD27, MAGT1, or CD70. XLP, XIAP, and MAGT1 are on the X chromosome; the other defects are inherited as autosomal recessive traits. In each case, infection with EBV leads to an acute illness with lymphoproliferation, progressive but variable hypogammaglobulinemia, and lymphoma in XLP, ITP, and CD27 defects. A unifying theme of these syndromes is loss of function of NK-T cells, a subset of T cells important in viral immunity.

A unique member of the genetic immune dysregulation diseases is APECED or autoimmune polyglandular syndrome type 1 (Chapter 218). Whereas the clinical presentation is usually due to endocrine disease (hypoparathyroidism, Addison disease, hypogonadism, and secondary amenorrhea), the disease is caused by loss of thymic recognition of self-antigens due to mutations in the autoimmune regulator gene (AIRE). Chronic mucocutaneous candidiasis is common, probably due to circulating anticytokine antibodies (interferon and IL-17). The transcription factor encoded by the AIRE gene, found in thymic epithelial cells, is involved in the early negative selection of cells with autoimmune potential. Clinically, cutaneous candidiasis or the endocrine defect may be the first sign of the syndrome; for unclear reasons, chronic diarrhea with malabsorption is also common. Other autoimmune complications may include hepatitis, alopecia, vitiligo, diabetes mellitus, anemia, and pernicious anemia.

Defects in lymphocyte apoptosis lead to another form of immune dysregulation; in these subjects, because of impaired death of lymphocytes, lymph nodes and spleen enlarge, and autoimmunities, especially autoimmune thrombocytopenia and hemolytic anemia, occur. Together, these are commonly referred to as autoimmune lymphoproliferative syndrome (ALPS). The most common of these defects are due to autosomal dominant mutations in the *FAS* gene, which encodes the important FAS death receptor, and less commonly in FAS ligand.[22] Both are dominant but have variable penetrance. Much less common forms of autoimmune lymphoproliferation are due to mutations in caspase 8 or 10 or even more rarely the oncogenes *KRAS* and *NRAS* or protein kinase Cδ. In addition, mutations in somatic genes may mimic the clinical presentation of the congenital forms.

The defects of T-regulatory cells are the final member of this set of genetic defects leading to loss of regulation. The first to be described was the immune dysregulation, polyendocrinopathy, enteropathy, X-linked (IPEX) syndrome, a generally lethal disease in males, characterized by early-onset insulin-dependent diabetes mellitus, enteropathy with severe diarrhea, and eczema-like dermatitis.[23] Other manifestations include anemia, thrombocytopenia, and neutropenia, as well as liver or kidney autoimmune disease. The defect is generally due to mutations of the X chromosome forkhead box protein 3 (*FOXP3*) gene, a gene essential for the development of regulatory T cells. However, other genetic defects may lead to a similar clinical syndrome.

DIAGNOSIS

The diagnosis of these syndromes may be suspected from the clinical manifestations, family history, and laboratory grounds, but genetic validation is required for definitive diagnosis.

TREATMENT   Rx

For the HLH diseases and related syndromes, prompt immune suppression by established protocols and intense supportive care are necessary (see Chapter 160). For the genetic forms, HSCT (Chapter 168) is often required. The lymphoproliferative syndromes associated with EBV are similar in that prompt supportive care is required and transplantation is potentially curative. Rituximab has been used in these defects to reduce B-cell numbers and EBV burden if infection occurs. Treatment of the cytopenias in ALPS includes corticosteroids, rapamycin, mycophenylate, and other agents. For unclear reasons, rituximab may lead to permanent hypogammaglobulinemia in ALPS, and splenectomy is to be avoided. Patients with APECED usually require endocrine and possibly nutritional management as well as treatment for cutaneous candidiasis. For the defects of T-regulatory cells due to mutations in IPEX, HSCT is the only curative measure.

PROGNOSIS

The diseases of immune dysregulation have a varied prognosis. For the genetic HLH syndromes, EBV-related lymphoproliferative diseases, and IPEX, immune reconstitution is required. Because of the broad spectrum of manifestations for ALPS and APECED, management of the clinical issues may be sufficient.

DEFECTS OF INNATE IMMUNITY LEADING TO SELECTED INFECTIONS

DEFINITION

As opposed to the adaptive immune system (in which a previous exposure is required to form immune memory; Chapter 40), many components of the immune system function quickly with no pre-exposure. These components of the innate immune system (Chapter 39) include, for example, complement, phagocytic cells, and natural killer cells. Screening of large populations for selected microbial diseases has revealed a number of novel defects of innate immunity. Some of these defects are discussed here (Table 236-7).

PATHOBIOLOGY AND CLINICAL MANIFESTATIONS

Innate immunity defects causing selected infections appear to be rare and the incidence is not known. Anhidrotic ectodermal dysplasia with immunodeficiency, a syndrome due to mutations in the *IKBKG* gene that encodes nuclear factor κB (NF-κB) essential modulator (NEMO), is an X-linked disease and was initially assigned to the category of hyper-IgM syndromes. However, the

TABLE 236-7   EXAMPLES OF DISEASES OF INNATE IMMUNITY

DISEASE	GENES	INHERITANCE	LABORATORY FEATURES	ALTERED FUNCTION	ASSOCIATED FEATURES
Anhidrotic ectodermal dysplasia with immunodeficiency	*IKBKG*, (NEMO), *IKBA*	XL, AD	Variable hypogammaglobulinemia with increased IgM in some; lack of antibody response to polysaccharides	Defective NF-κB signaling pathway	Bacterial and mycobacterial infections, ectodermal dysplasia, hair loss, heat intolerance due to loss of sweat glands, tooth abnormalities
IRAK4, MYD88	*IRAK4, MYD88, IRAK1, TIRAP*	AR, XL	Impaired cytokine responses to toll receptor activators	Defective TIR-IRAK signaling pathway	Bacterial infections, especially *Staphylococcus* and *S. pneumoniae*
Herpes simplex encephalitis	*TLR3* *UNC93B1* *TRAF3, TRIF, (TICAM1), TBK1, IRF3*	AD AR	Impaired cytokine responses to TLR3 activators	Defective IFN-α, IFN-β, and IFN-γ induction	Herpes simplex virus 1 encephalitis
Predisposition to fungal diseases	*CARD9*	AR	Fungal cultures positive	Defective CARD9 signaling pathway	Invasive candidiasis and other fungal diseases
Chronic mucocutaneous candidiasis	*IL17RA* *IL17F* *STAT1* *AIRE* *ACT1*	AR, AD	Fungal cultures positive	Defective IL-17R signaling pathways	Mucocutaneous candidiasis
IL-12, IL-23 receptor deficiency	*IL12RB* *IL12* *IL23*	AR	Mycobacterial cultures positive	Defective cytokine receptor binding and signaling	Mycobacterial and salmonella infections
IFN-γ receptors 1 and 2 deficiency	*IFNGR1* *IFNGR2*	AR	Mycobacterial cultures positive	Defective IFN-γ binding and signaling	Mycobacterial and salmonella infections
GATA2 deficiency	*GATA2*	AR, AD	Multilineage cytopenias; very low monocyte numbers		Infections with mycobacteria, papillomaviruses, histoplasmosis, alveolar proteinosis, but also myelodysplasia and leukemias

AD = autosomal dominant; *AIRE* = autoimmune regulator; AR = autosomal recessive; *GATA2* = a member of the GATA family of zinc-finger transcription factors; IFN = interferon; *IFNGR1* = ligand-binding chain (alpha) of the gamma interferon receptor; *IFNGR2* = ligand-binding chain (beta) of the gamma interferon receptor; *IKBA* = NF-kappa-B inhibitor alpha; IL = interleukin; *IL12* = interleukin 12; *IL12RB* = interleukin 12 receptor B; *IL17* = interleukin 17; IL-17R = interleukin-17 receptor; *IL17RA* = interleukin 17 receptor A; *IRAK1* = interleukin 1 receptor associated kinase 1; *IRAK4* = interleukin 1 receptor associated kinase 4; *IRF3* = interferon regulatory factor 3; *MYD88* = myeloid differentiation primary response protein; NEMO (*IKBKG*) = NF-kappa-B essential modulator; NF-κB = nuclear factor-κB; *STAT1* = signal transducer and activator of transcription 1; *TBK1* = TANK binding kinase 1; TIR = intracytoplasmic toll and IL-1 receptor; *TIRAP* = TIR domain containing adaptor protein; TLR = toll-like receptor; *TLR3* = toll receptor 3; *TRAF3* = TNF-receptor associated factor 3; *TRIF (TICAM1)* = TIR-domain-containing adapter-inducing interferon-β; *UNC93B1* = Unc-93 homolog B1; XL = X-linked.

actual phenotype is broad due to impairment of NEMO, which is essential for both cytokine and toll-like receptor signaling pathways. Impairment in this gene leads to severe bacterial infections and mycobacterial disease as well as to the characteristics of ectodermal dysplasia: sparse hair, abnormal tooth development, and lack of sweat glands. A series of other genetic defects in toll-like receptors and their signaling pathways have been recognized, for example, autosomal recessive defects in *IRAK4* and *MyD88*, both of which lead to severe pneumococcal and staphylococcal infections. In contrast, defects of the TLR3 pathway lead to early herpes simplex encephalitis. Much more clinically heterogeneous are the genetic disorders that lead to chronic muco-cutaneous candidiasis. These defects may be autosomal dominant or recessive and lead to simple onychomycosis in some to invasive fungal infections in others. Patients of any age may have defects in these pathways. The pathogenesis of some of these includes genes that disrupt the dectin-1 pathway. Dectin-1 is a surface lectin receptor that recognizes the β1-3 glucan of fungi; downstream mutations in *CARD9* impair the secretion of IL-17A, IL-17F, and IL-22, cytokines that are essential in fungal clearance.

A separate and unique category of innate defects are the cytokine/receptor mutations that impair the functions of cytokines IL-12, IL-23, and IFN-γ, which are needed for control of mycobacterial and other intracellular infections, such as salmonella. Chronic mycobacterial infections may also occur in patients with autosomal recessive mutations in the gene for signal transducer and activator of transcription 1 (*STAT1*),[24] a gene downstream of both IFN-γ and IFN-α receptors. However, as the functions of both cytokines are impaired, these patients may also have severe viral or fungal infections. Dominant (activating) mutations in *STAT1* may lead to simple cutaneous candidiasis in some or more complex clinical outcomes in others. More complex is the syndrome of GATA2 deficiency,[25] in which mycobacterial disease may also develop, but other organisms (papillomaviruses, fungi) and serious complications (cytopenias, myelodysplasia, pulmonary alveolar proteinosis, peripheral edema) may be foremost. Whereas *GATA2* defects are dominantly inherited, members of the same family with the same mutations may have very different clinical manifestations.

DIAGNOSIS

The diagnosis of innate defects is first based on exclusion of other causes and then confirmed by genetic testing. The family history may be helpful, but for patients with mutations in *STAT1* or *GATA2*, although dominant inheritance is likely, the extreme range of clinical phenotypes may obscure easy recognition.

TREATMENT AND PROGNOSIS   Rx

The treatment of innate defects includes antimicrobial therapy to clear active infections and, probably, relevant prophylactic therapy on an ongoing basis. For the more severe defects, HSCT (Chapter 168) is required.

GENERAL REFERENCES

For the General References and other additional features, please visit Expert Consult at https://expertconsult.inkling.com.

237

URTICARIA AND ANGIOEDEMA

STEPHEN C. DRESKIN

URTICARIA

Urticaria (hives) consists of pruritic, edematous, erythematous, blanching papules that are round or oval; have pale, raised centers (wheals); are several millimeters to a few centimeters in size; and are transient, lasting minutes to days (Fig. 237-1).[1] Angioedema appears as a brawny nonpitting edema,

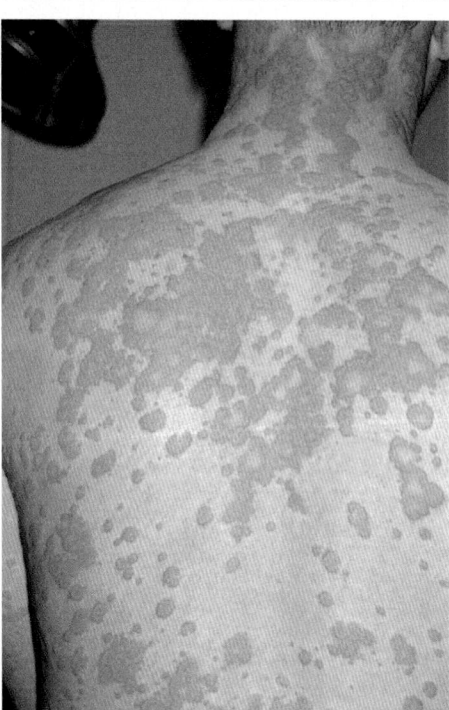

FIGURE 237-1. Extensive urticaria. Many presentations are more subtle. (From Roitt I, Brostoff J, Male D, eds. *Immunology.* 6th ed. London: Mosby; 2001.)

typically without well-defined margins and without erythema. Angioedema can be accompanied by a sense of burning, pressure, or aching but not pruritus; it is distinguished from other edematous states by its frequent involvement of the lips, tongue, eyelids, hands, feet, or genitalia and its rare occurrence in dependent areas of the body. Episodes (daily or almost daily symptoms) of recurrent hives or angioedema during a period of less than 6 weeks are considered acute, and those lasting longer are said to be chronic. Patients typically present with urticaria alone or urticaria with angioedema. Rarely, patients present with angioedema alone, and this becomes a diagnostic dilemma because angioedema as an isolated finding may be due to activation of mast cells (called idiopathic, spontaneous, or histaminergic angioedema) or may be due to activation of the kinin system (see later). The terms *urticaria* and *urticaria/angioedema* are used interchangeably here to refer to illnesses characterized by urticaria or angioedema in which mast cells are activated.

EPIDEMIOLOGY

Urticaria/angioedema occurs in 15 to 25% of individuals at some time during their lives and can affect both genders and all races. Acute urticaria is more common in young adults and children. Chronic urticaria is more common in adults, affecting women (75% of cases) more often than men, and has severe adverse consequences on quality of life.[2,3]

PATHOBIOLOGY

Mast cells, the primary effector cells in urticaria/angioedema, are found in high numbers throughout the body, particularly within the subcutaneous tissue. After activation of mast cells, there is a rapid (<10 minutes) release of histamine, leukotriene C$_4$, and prostaglandin D$_2$, leading to vasodilation, subcutaneous and intradermal leakage of plasma from postcapillary venules, and pruritus. In addition, there is the delayed (4 to 8 hours) production and secretion of inflammatory cytokines such as tumor necrosis factor–α, interleukin-4, and interleukin-5, leading to an inflammatory infiltrate and perpetuation of longer-lived lesions. Angioedema is formed by a similar extravasation of fluid, not superficially in the skin but in deeper dermal and subdermal sites.

Most episodes of acute urticaria/angioedema are caused by immediate hypersensitivity reactions to drugs or foods or result from inflammatory processes initiated by viral illnesses. The most common drugs that cause acute urticaria/angioedema are penicillins, sulfonamides, muscle relaxants, diuretics, and nonsteroidal anti-inflammatory drugs (NSAIDs), although any drug acting as a hapten can generate an allergic response (Chapter 239). The predominant allergenic foods are milk, eggs, and peanuts for children and peanuts, tree nuts, fish, and shellfish for adults, although sensitization can occur to many other foods as well. These allergens cross-link immunoglobulin (Ig) E bound to the high-affinity receptor for IgE (FcεRI), leading to activation of mast cells. Some drugs (e.g., opioids, vancomycin, NSAIDs) and radiocontrast dye can activate mast cells by an IgE-independent (pseudoallergic) mechanism. Ingestion of fish contaminated with bacteria that produce histamine leads to hives as part of a toxic reaction to the histamine (scombroid food poisoning).

The largest subgroup of chronic urticaria/angioedema is idiopathic urticaria, accounting for approximately 70 to 80% of cases. Recently an effort has been made to replace the term *chronic idiopathic urticaria* with the more descriptive term *chronic spontaneous urticaria*. These patients have symptoms in the absence of a specific physical trigger, allergen exposure, or coexistent disease. Half the patients with spontaneous urticaria have evidence of autoimmunity based on the presence of IgG antibodies that can cross-link FcεRI or antithyroid antibodies. Some experts consider these patients to have a separate entity called autoimmune urticaria, whereas others consider these patients to have idiopathic urticaria with evidence of autoimmunity.[4]

Physical stimuli activate mast cells by unknown mechanisms and account for about 20 to 30% of cases of chronic urticaria. The most common of the physical urticarias is dermographism (also called dermatographism), in which wheals can be "written on the skin" by simple stroking or scratching. Cholinergic urticaria is a physical urticaria in which the trigger leading to mast cell activation is related to cholinergic stimuli occurring after exposure to heat or after exercise. Other physical stimuli can cause urticaria, including cold, solar radiation, pressure, vibration, and water. Cold-induced urticaria needs to be distinguished from the cryopyrin-associated periodic fever syndromes (see later and Chapter 245).

In approximately 1 to 2% of patients with chronic urticaria/angioedema, symptoms appear to be caused by ingestants (e.g., foods, medications, dietary supplements), contactants (e.g., soaps, detergents, cosmetics, hair or nail products, latex), concomitant infections, hormonal changes, or systemic illnesses. A food must be consumed regularly to cause chronic urticaria. Multicellular parasites (e.g., those causing strongyloidiasis or filariasis) elicit strong IgE responses and are important causes of chronic urticaria in endemic areas. Chronic urticaria/angioedema can be associated with flares of rheumatic conditions, other autoimmune conditions (including Hashimoto thyroiditis), or neoplastic conditions. Occult neoplasia is exceedingly unlikely to be the cause of chronic urticaria.

CLINICAL MANIFESTATIONS

Patients often report that the first sensation of urticaria is poorly localized pruritus that quickly develops into the typical lesions of urticaria. Groups of hives often appear together during a short period, and episodes of hives can come in waves starting several times a day. Patients with cholinergic urticaria usually have a distinctive clinical presentation of diffuse, pinpoint, intensely pruritic, urticarial lesions following exertion sufficient to cause sweating. A self-rated quality-of-life survey of patients with chronic urticaria revealed dramatic impairment in terms of loss of sleep, fatigue, and emotional discomfort. Angioedema can originate near a wheal or independently in other parts of the body. Symptoms vary from minor discomfort to an intense sense of pressure and may lead to other symptoms, such as severe shortness of breath if there is compromise of the upper airway. Rarely, patients report angioedema beginning 4 to 6 hours after application of local pressure, and this is called delayed pressure urticaria, a debilitating condition that is often difficult to treat.

DIAGNOSIS

The first episode of acute urticaria/angioedema may occur in the absence of an identifiable stimulus. If hives occur 5 to 30 minutes after ingestion of a drug or a food, the patient often can identify the association. If a physician is consulted, the best approach is to take a careful history, with attention to ingestants, contactants, and intercurrent illnesses. Unnecessary drugs and food supplements should be discontinued, and any recently added medication should be changed to a structurally different agent. In the majority of cases, no causative agent is identified, and the hives are treated symptomatically (see the later discussion) for days or weeks before they resolve spontaneously. Most guidelines recommend nothing more than a complete blood count and differential, erythrocyte sedimentation rate (ESR), and C-reactive protein (CRP) as initial laboratory testing in the evaluation of a patient with chronic urticaria.[5]

Differential Diagnosis

The differential diagnosis of chronic urticaria/angioedema includes the subgroups of urticaria discussed earlier: idiopathic, autoimmune, physical, ingestant mediated, and associated with a variety of systemic illnesses.[6] Other conditions that can be confused with chronic urticaria/angioedema include diffuse pruritus complicated by dermographism, flushing disorders, urticarial

TABLE 237-1 CLASSIFICATION OF URTICARIA AND ANGIOEDEMA

I. Acute urticaria/angioedema
  A. Hypersensitivity reactions
    1. Drug allergy
    2. Food allergy
    3. Insect allergy
  B. Idiopathic
  C. Pseudoallergic reactions
    1. Drugs
    2. Radiocontrast dye
  D. Toxic reactions
  E. Immune complex
    1. Serum sickness
    2. Transfusion related
    3. Postviral
II. Chronic urticaria/angioedema
  A. Idiopathic
    1. Autoantibody associated
      a. Anti-IgE receptor (FcεRI)
      b. Anti-IgE
      c. Antithyroid
      d. Other
    2. Not associated with autoantibodies
  B. Physical
    1. Dermographism
    2. Cholinergic
    3. Delayed pressure
    4. Solar
    5. Cold
    6. Vibratory
    7. Aquagenic
  C. Immune complex
    1. Urticarial vasculitis
    2. Collagen vascular disease associated
III. Urticaria pigmentosa and systemic mastocytosis
IV. Complement-related and kinin-mediated angioedema
  A. Hereditary angioedema
  B. Acquired angioedema
  C. Angiotensin-converting enzyme inhibitor–induced angioedema
  D. Renin inhibitor–induced angioedema

IgE = immunoglobulin E.

vasculitis, urticaria pigmentosa, systemic mastocytosis, exercise-induced anaphylaxis, exercise-induced food-associated anaphylaxis, idiopathic anaphylaxis, hereditary angioedema, acquired angioedema, angioedema associated with angiotensin-converting enzyme (ACE) inhibitors, hypereosinophilic syndrome, systemic lupus erythematosus, autoinflammatory disease, and polymorphous eruption of pregnancy; these conditions are considered to be mimics of urticaria[7] (Table 237-1).

Approximately 95% of patients with urticaria/angioedema are not reacting to an ingestant and do not have another illness that is causing their hives. However, it is sometimes difficult for patients (and some physicians) to accept this fact, prompting an extensive, invasive, expensive, and unnecessary investigation. The best "test" to identify patients with a specific underlying cause (i.e., physical trigger, autoimmune condition, allergen, or systemic disease) is a careful and detailed history and physical examination by a specialist knowledgeable in urticarial disease.

A good place to begin is by excluding possible physical triggers. Specific tests are available to establish the diagnosis of most physical urticarias, including scratching the skin and exposing the skin to heat, ice, vibration, pressure, ultraviolet radiation, or water. Cold urticaria must be distinguished from cryopyrin-associated periodic fever syndromes that are characterized by a cold-induced papular rash (not urticaria) and are now classified in the family of hereditary periodic fever syndromes. Solar urticaria must be distinguished from other types of light sensitivity, including metabolic abnormalities (e.g., erythrogenic porphyria) and photosensitivity due to drugs.

Even though foods and drugs are infrequent causes of chronic urticaria, many patients focus on ingestants and are not satisfied until these causes are ruled out. As in the evaluation of acute urticaria, the patient should discontinue all food supplements and medications that are not absolutely necessary and, if possible, change essential medications to structurally unrelated compounds. The patient then keeps a food diary to identify suspect foods that can be eliminated. Some allergists use skin tests with foods to identify "suspects" (Chapter 238), but this approach is unproven. Antihistamines and other medications used to control the urticaria must be discontinued. If the urticaria resolves, it is critical to reintroduce foods in a controlled fashion to identify the specific food causing the urticaria and to reinstate a healthy diet.

Chronic infections, including sinus infection, dental abscess, *Helicobacter pylori* gastric infection, cholecystitis, onychomycosis, and tinea pedis, have been associated with urticaria. Case reports indicate the resolution of urticaria after treatment of these infections, although rigorous proof of an association is lacking.

Laboratory evaluation in a patient with typical urticaria should always include a complete blood count with differential, basic metabolic panel, liver enzymes, and urinalysis. Specialists are not in full agreement about the necessity of additional laboratory testing. Levels of thyroid-stimulating hormone and antithyroid antibodies may be measured in otherwise euthyroid-appearing patients to screen for subclinical Hashimoto thyroiditis. Skin tests for immediate hypersensitivity to foods may be ordered for patients with a suggestive history. Some specialists order no screening tests at all. As in vitro tests for anti-FcεRI autoantibodies have become more widely available, some specialists will perform this test. A positive test response for anti-FcεRI autoantibodies is useful because this reassures the patient that the urticaria is being driven by an internal process and is not caused by an ingestant or occult illness. Other tests should be ordered only as a result of positive findings in the history and physical examination.[8]

Although it is not routinely indicated, a skin biopsy can provide useful information. The most common indication for this procedure is to rule out urticarial vasculitis when the hives are more painful than pruritic, last longer than 24 hours, or leave discolored skin. The presence of vascular destruction, fibrinoid necrosis, and immune complex deposition on microscopic examination (including immunofluorescence) should lead to a consideration of the specific causes of urticarial vasculitis (e.g., systemic lupus erythematosus) and the rapid initiation of more aggressive treatment.

Primary mast cell disorders (Chapter 240) rarely manifest as chronic urticaria. Systemic mastocytosis is a very rare condition characterized by increased numbers of atypical mast cells in the bone marrow, skin, and other organs. Hereditary angioedema, acquired angioedema, and angioedema associated with ACE inhibitors are discussed later in this chapter. Briefly, these syndromes are characterized by episodic swelling without urticaria and are best identified by a careful history, physical examination, and focused laboratory evaluation. An approach to the evaluation and treatment of patients with urticaria or angioedema is summarized in Fig. 237-2.

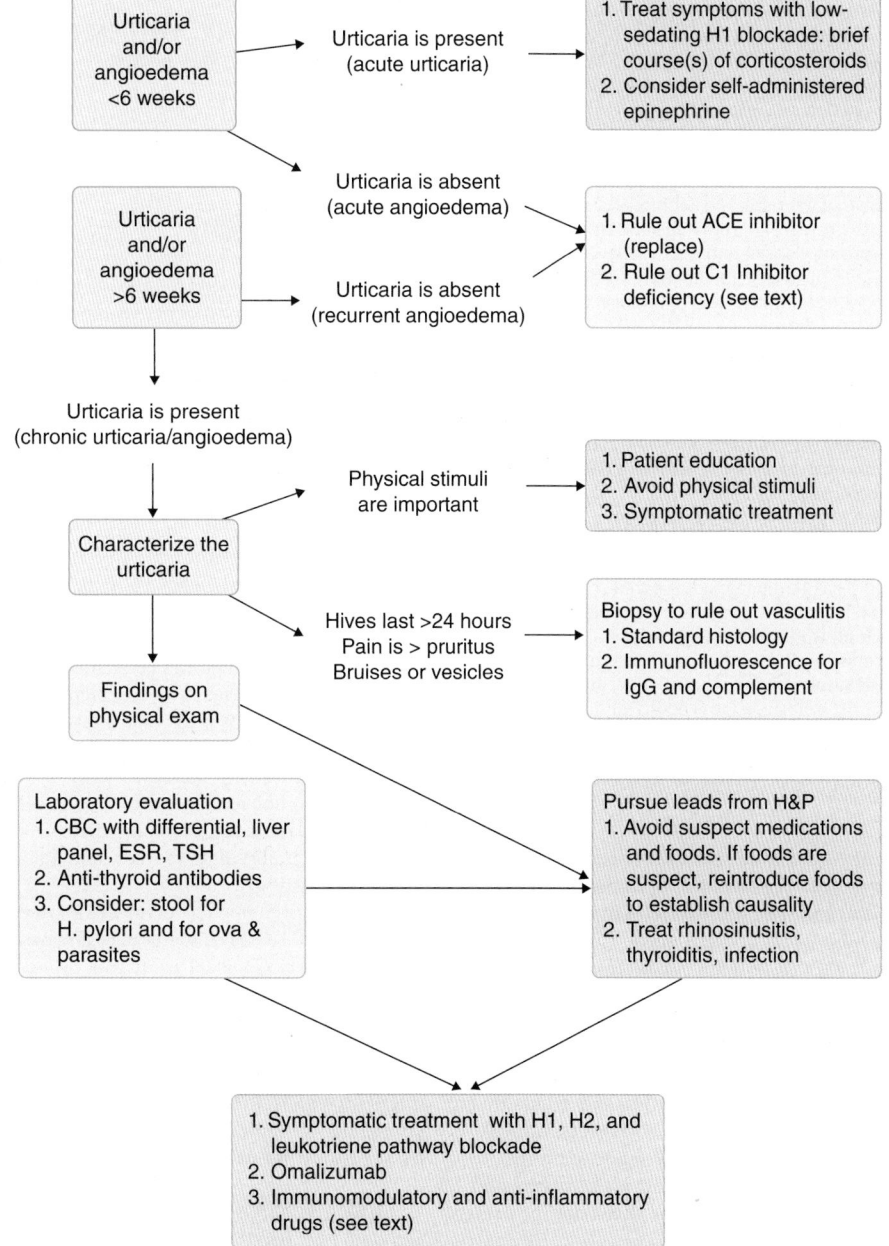

FIGURE 237-2. Evaluation and treatment of urticaria/angioedema. Treatment of urticaria with or without angioedema (AE) can be similar. However, treatment of AE without urticaria depends on the cause. If the AE is caused by an angiotensin-converting enzyme (ACE) inhibitor, discontinuation of the medication is required. Treatment of AE caused by a deficiency or dysfunction of C1 inhibitor (C1 INH) is discussed in the text. Idiopathic AE often responds to treatments described for urticaria/angioedema. CBC = complete blood count; ESR = erythrocyte sedimentation rate; FcεR1 = high-affinity receptor for IgE; H & P = history and physical examination; H₁ = histamine₁-receptor antagonist; H₂ = histamine₂-receptor antagonist; IgE = immunoglobulin E; IgG = immunoglobulin G; TSH = thyroid-stimulating hormone.

TREATMENT

Acute urticaria is usually self-limited and responds well to histamine$_1$ (H$_1$)–type antihistamines. Antihistamines work better if they are taken prophylactically rather than after histamine has been released and is bound to the receptor. Patients often self-medicate with or are prescribed diphenhydramine (25 to 50 mg every 6 hours) or hydroxyzine (25 to 50 mg every 6 hours), but they may experience significant sedation. Second-generation antihistamines such as cetirizine (10 mg nightly at bedtime), fexofenadine (180 mg/day), and loratadine (10 mg/day) cause minimal sedation, are much better tolerated, and can be effective. On occasion, a brief course of corticosteroids is warranted to control severe symptoms. Epinephrine (0.3 mL of 1 : 1000 intramuscularly) quickly (but transiently) reverses the signs and symptoms of urticaria and angioedema. Patients who have experienced potentially life-threatening angioedema or anaphylaxis should have ready access to self-injectable epinephrine and be knowledgeable about its indications, administration, and brief duration of action. β-Blockers not only can aggravate urticaria but also can interfere with the action of epinephrine. NSAIDs and codeine can lead to IgE-independent mast cell activation. These medications should be discontinued if it is clinically safe to do so.

For chronic urticaria/angioedema, multiple randomized, placebo-controlled studies have shown the efficacy of both sedating and low-sedating antihistamines.[A1] Second-generation antihistamines are commonly used at up to four times the standard dose.[A2] If sedating antihistamines must be used, doxepin (10 to 100 mg nightly at bedtime) is more effective than diphenhydramine, but its use can be limited by significant sedation and its tendency to stimulate the appetite, leading to significant weight gain.

Approximately 15% of histamine receptors in the skin are of the H$_2$ subtype. H$_2$-receptor antagonists alone are ineffective, but a meta-analysis of four studies with a total of 144 subjects demonstrated that they are effective when combined with H$_1$-receptor antagonists.[A3] Therefore the addition of an H$_2$ antihistamine, such as ranitidine (150 mg twice daily) or famotidine (20 mg twice daily), is a logical adjunct to H$_1$ antihistamine therapy, providing additional clinical benefit.

Symptoms often persist despite the use of maximal or supramaximal doses of antihistamines.[9] This is not surprising, considering the number of vasoactive and pruritogenic mediators released by mast cells, of which histamine is only one. Antileukotriene medications, such as montelukast (10 mg/day) or zafirlukast (20 mg twice daily), can be added to antihistamines, with some success. Especially severe symptoms may require systemic corticosteroids (prednisone 10 to 60 mg/day) to achieve symptomatic control, but strong concerns about side effects limit their usefulness. Omalizumab (a humanized monoclonal antibody that binds and inactivates IgE[10]; 300 mg subcutaneously every 4 weeks) has been shown to be effective in patients with chronic spontaneous urticaria who have failed standard and even maximal doses of low-sedating antihistamines in a large randomized placebo-controlled trial.[A4][A5]

Refractory symptoms have been treated with a wide variety of other medications. Some of these medications (adrenergic agents, calcium-channel blockers) are thought to decrease the ability of mast cells to release mediators. Other drugs are anti-inflammatory (hydroxychloroquine, sulfasalazine, dapsone, colchicine), immunomodulatory (cyclosporine, tacrolimus, mycophenolate), or antimetabolic (azathioprine, cyclophosphamide, methotrexate). Cyclosporine (4 mg/kg/day) was shown to be effective in a randomized, placebo-controlled, parallel study of 30 patients with autoimmune urticaria. Other treatments of refractory autoimmune chronic urticaria include intravenous immune globulin and plasmapheresis.

PREVENTION

It is essential to encourage patients with chronic urticaria to accept the chronicity of their illness and to focus on achieving reasonable symptomatic control with effective treatments that cause the fewest side effects. Many patients with physical urticaria can learn to avoid or to minimize triggers. The few patients for whom chronic urticaria is a feature of systemic illness may find relief if the underlying condition is appropriately treated. An excellent example is that chronic urticaria in patients with clinically apparent thyroid disease often resolves once the thyroid disease is treated. For many patients, other factors that exacerbate their specific symptoms can be identified, including stress or anxiety, hormonal fluctuations, aspirin and other NSAIDs, and agents that cause cutaneous vasodilation (e.g., alcohol, hot baths or showers, exercise, heated waterbeds). Psychosocial stress is a commonly reported trigger of worsening symptoms. A plausible biochemical mechanism is likely increased release of cutaneous neuropeptides known to lower the threshold for mast cell degranulation.

PROGNOSIS

The prognosis for most patients with chronic urticaria/angioedema is excellent. Spontaneous resolution occurs within 12 months in 50% of patients and within 5 years in an additional 20%. However, 10 to 20% of patients, particularly those with physical or autoimmune urticaria, continue to have symptoms for as long as 20 years. Patients who had one episode of chronic urticaria that lasted for months or years and then resolved may experience one or more similar recurrences later in life.

FUTURE DIRECTIONS

The current trend in the treatment of urticaria/angioedema is to begin with low-sedating antihistamines and anti-leukotriene drugs to block the actions of the mediators produced by mast cells. If these fail, patients are treated with omalizumab. Those who fail omalizumab are treated with anti-inflammatory and immunomodulatory drugs. Some agents under development for asthma and rhinitis may be useful for the treatment of urticaria/angioedema, including 5-lipoxygenase inhibitors, prostaglandin D$_2$-receptor antagonists, and more potent nonsedating antihistamines. Agents that decrease the sensitivity of mast cells to degranulation, such as phosphodiesterase 4 inhibitors and tyrosine kinase inhibitors, may also find a role in the treatment of this condition. In spite of the fact that chronic urticaria/angioedema is not thought to be an IgE-mediated disease, as mentioned before, omalizumab (anti-IgE) has been shown to be very effective. This may be due to unexpected effects of IgE on mast cell activation. This finding could have a significant impact on future therapies.

HEREDITARY ANGIOEDEMA AND RELATED DISEASES

DEFINITION

Hereditary angioedema and related illnesses are characterized by recurrent attacks of angioedema mediated by vasoactive peptides such as bradykinin.[11]

EPIDEMIOLOGY

Hereditary angioedema affects approximately 1 in 50,000 people. It is an autosomal dominant disease and therefore affects 50% of offspring of both genders. Frequently, a history of several generations with this disease is obtained, but new mutations do occur, and a negative family history is not uncommon. Acquired angioedema is rarer, affecting older persons who often have a monoclonal gammopathy or a malignant disease such as lymphoma. Angioedema associated with ACE inhibitors occurs in less than 1% of treated patients and can be fatal.[12]

PATHOBIOLOGY

Hereditary angioedema and acquired angioedema are caused by either low levels or abnormal function of a regulatory protein in the plasma, C1 inhibitor (C1 INH deficiency), which exerts control of the complement, fibrinolytic, and kinin-generating pathways.[13] Because there is one normal gene, levels of C1 INH are detectable but, because of the abnormal gene, are not sufficient to control the generation of kinins. The C1 esterase enzyme, when activated, cleaves two complement products, C4 and C2. Without proper inhibition, this leads to low levels of circulating C4 and C2. C1 INH is also a critical modulator of the bradykinin pathway, and decreased C1 INH function leads to increased levels of bradykinin. Increased generation of bradykinin, not mediators from mast cells or activation of complement, leads to capillary leakage and angioedema. Changes in levels of C4 and C2, although not important in the pathophysiologic mechanism of the disease, are useful diagnostically.

In hereditary angioedema type I (85% of patients), the abnormal gene does not produce C1 INH. In hereditary angioedema type II (15%), an antigenically detectable C1 INH protein is produced, but it is not functional. In hereditary angioedema type III (very rare), C1 INH is present and functional, but there is a yet-to-be-defined abnormality in the generation of vasoactive compounds. In acquired angioedema, unknown factors activate C1 and deplete the C1 INH activity in plasma, or there is an autoantibody to C1 INH that interferes with its function.[14] ACE inhibitor–associated angioedema is due to unintended inhibition of the enzyme that inactivates bradykinin; the complement pathway is unaffected.

CLINICAL MANIFESTATIONS

Children with hereditary angioedema can have attacks shortly after birth, but these tend to be mild. For most patients, the severity of the attacks worsens at puberty, with episodes of swelling that can affect any external body surface, including the genitalia. Mucosal surfaces are also affected, and patients can have life-threatening swelling of the uvula and posterior pharynx, leading to asphyxiation. Swelling of the submucosa of the gastrointestinal tract can cause symptoms of an "acute abdomen," leading to unnecessary exploratory laparotomy. About half of patients report that trauma, particularly trauma associated with local pressure, precipitates an attack, and about half note an increased frequency of attacks during times of emotional stress. Attacks in patients with acquired angioedema are clinically similar to those in patients with hereditary angioedema. In patients taking ACE inhibitors, angioedema may be manifested as severe swelling or simply as a chronic cough beginning days to months after ACE inhibitor therapy is initiated.

DIAGNOSIS

The best tests to support the diagnosis of hereditary angioedema or acquired angioedema are measurements of C1 INH levels, C1 INH function, and C4 levels, particularly during an attack. The distinguishing features of acquired angioedema are onset later in life and the presence of a malignant disease or paraproteinemia. However, in addition to having low levels of C2 and C4, patients with acquired angioedema can have profound depressions in the level of C1, a protein that is commonly normal in hereditary angioedema. Patients with ACE inhibitor–associated angioedema can present within hours after initiation of therapy or after many months and even years. The angioedema seen in urticaria/angioedema is distinctive in that it is usually associated with a pruritic urticarial rash, laboratory evaluation is normal, there is no history of treatment with an ACE inhibitor, and it responds to antihistamines, steroids, and epinephrine.

TREATMENT Rx

Current therapy for hereditary angioedema in the United States includes both prophylactic treatment and on-demand, patient-centered treatment of attacks.

Acute Attacks of Hereditary Angioedema

C1 INH concentrate purified from human plasma (Berinert; 20 units/kg intravenously), a human recombinant C1 esterase inhibitor purified from the milk of transgenic (genetically modified) rabbits (Ruconest; 50 U/kg, IV),[A6] icatibant,[A7][A8] a bradykinin receptor 2 antagonist (Firazyr; 30 mg subcutaneously), and ecallantide,[A9] a kallikrein inhibitor (Kalbitor; 30 mg subcutaneously),[A10] are all FDA approved for on-demand treatment of acute attacks of hereditary angioedema.

If these agents are not available, treatment of angioedema of the airway should include racemic epinephrine (1:1000) delivered in the airway by nebulization and by intramuscular injections (0.2 to 0.3 mL of 1:1000 at intervals of 20 to 30 minutes). The addition of antihistamine for sedation may be helpful. Treating physicians must be prepared to perform nasotracheal intubation, preferably in the operating room under conditions in which tracheostomy can be performed if needed. Acute attacks can be terminated by administration of 2 units of fresh-frozen plasma (FFP) to supply the missing C1 INH; but in rare instances, patients may become more edematous, presumably reflecting the increased availability of substrates for the generation of kinins. Therefore although FFP can be useful for treatment of non–life-threatening acute attacks, it is not recommended for life-threatening laryngeal edema.

Long-term Treatment of Hereditary Angioedema

C1 INH concentrate (Cinryze; 1000 units IV every 3 to 4 days) is approved for long-term treatment. Many patients with relatively mild disease or infrequent attacks are treated with "on-demand" therapy with either C1 INH, icatibant, or ecallantide (see above).[15] Attenuated androgens, such as danazol (50 to 200 mg up to twice daily), increase the production of C1 INH and lead to a marked amelioration of symptoms in patients with hereditary angioedema. Masculinizing side effects are usually mild but can be problematic. Prophylactic administration of androgens, C1 INH concentrate,[A11] or a C1 esterase inhibitor[A12] have been shown in a double-blind, placebo-controlled trial to significantly reduce the number of acute attacks. Androgens are absolutely contraindicated in pregnancy.

Prophylaxis

Patients should be treated prophylactically before dental work or other procedures that involve trauma to tissue. Those treated with attenuated androgens, antifibrinolytic agents, FFP (2 units intravenously), or C1 INH concentrate (500 units subcutaneously) have fewer attacks.

Plasma kallikrein inhibitors offer promise of efficacy for prophylaxis in hereditary angioedema. In a small, double-blind, placebo-controlled trial, lanadelumab, a monoclonal inhibitor of plasma kallikrein, was administered to patients with hereditary angioedema in two subcutaneous injections 14 days apart at total doses 30 mg, 100 mg, 300 mg, or 400 mg, and compared with placebo injections. Lanadelumab at the 300 mg and 400 mg doses reduced cleavage of high-molecular-weight kininogen in plasma and also reduced the frequency

of attacks.[A13] An oral plasma kallikrein inhibitor was administered once daily to patients with hereditary angioedema in escalating doses or as placebo; at a dose of 125 mg or higher, it reduced the attacks of angioedema over a 28-day period.[A14] Likewise, C1 inhibitor replacement with a subcutaneous preparation has shown promise as a prophylactic agent in hereditary angioedema. In a prospective, double-blind, placebo-controlled trial, a nanofiltered C1 inhibitor preparation or placebo was self-administered subcutaneously twice weekly in a crossover design involving two 16-week treatment periods. In patients the prophylactic use of the C1 inhibitor significantly reduced the frequency of acute attacks.[A15]

Acquired Angioedema

Treatment of acquired angioedema is similar to that of hereditary angioedema, but definitive treatment requires amelioration of the underlying disease.

ACE Inhibitor–Associated Angioedema

Treatment of angioedema associated with the use of an ACE inhibitor includes antihistamines, epinephrine, or both, as appropriate, and discontinuation of the ACEI. In a randomized trial of icatibant, a subcutaneously administered selective bradykinin B2 receptor antagonist, edema in patients with ACEI-induced angioedema resolved more rapidly than with combination therapy with a glucocorticoid and an antihistamine.[A16]

The direct renin inhibitor aliskiren is also associated with a significant risk of angioedema. Rarely, patients continue to have episodic angioedema when changed from an ACEI to an angiotension receptor blocker. These patients are more likely to have idiopathic angioedema or persistence of angioedema from the ACEI rather than angioedema due to the angiotension receptor blocker.

PROGNOSIS

The long-term outlook for patients with hereditary angioedema is largely dependent on the phenotype of the illness (frequency of laryngeal attacks), the ability of the patient to tolerate attenuated androgens, and the patient's access to C1 INH concentrate, icatibant, or ecallantide. Repeated use of these medications for recurrent acute episodes appears to be safe and effective.[16] For most patients, life expectancy should be normal. Acquired angioedema usually resolves with treatment of the underlying condition, but the ultimate prognosis depends on the nature of that illness. Angioedema associated with the use of an ACE inhibitor can be fatal but usually resolves after the medication is removed.

FUTURE DIRECTIONS

In the past several years, there has been dramatic progress in the availability of medication for hereditary angioedema. In the near future, the focus will be on tailoring therapy to individual patients and controlling costs.

Grade A References

A1. Sharma M, Bennett C, Carter B, et al. H1-antihistamines for chronic spontaneous urticaria: an abridged Cochrane Systematic review. *J Am Acad Dermatol.* 2015;73:710-716.

A2. Guillén-Aguinaga S, Jáuregui Presa I, Aguinaga-Ontoso E, et al. Updosing nonsedating antihistamines in patients with chronic spontaneous urticaria: a systematic review and meta-analysis. *Br J Dermatol.* 2016;175:1153-1165.

A3. Fedorowicz Z, van Zuren EJ, Hu N. Histamine H$_2$-receptor antagonists for urticaria. *Cochrane Database Syst Rev.* 2012;3:CD008596.

A4. Maurer M, Rosen K, Hsieh HJ, et al. Omalizumab for the treatment of chronic idiopathic or spontaneous urticaria. *N Engl J Med.* 2013;368:924-935.

A5. Dressler C, Werner RN, Eisert L, et al. Chronic inducible urticaria: a systematic review of treatment options. *J Allergy Clin Immunol.* 2018;141:1726-1734.

A6. Riedl MA, Bernstein JA, Li H, et al. Recombinant human C1-esterase inhibitor relieves symptoms of hereditary angioedema attacks: phase 3, randomized, placebo-controlled trial. *Ann Allergy Asthma Immunol.* 2014;112:163-169.

A7. Cicardi M, Banerji A, Bracho F, et al. Icatibant, a new bradykinin-receptor antagonist, in hereditary angioedema. *N Engl J Med.* 2010;363:532-541.

A8. Lumry WR, Li HH, Levy RJ, et al. Randomized placebo-controlled trial of the bradykinin B2 receptor antagonist icatibant for the treatment of acute attacks of hereditary angioedema: the FAST-3 trial. *Ann Allergy Asthma Immunol.* 2011;107:529-537.

A9. Cicardi M, Levy RJ, McNeil DL, et al. Ecallantide for the treatment of acute attacks in hereditary angioedema. *N Engl J Med.* 2010;363:523-531.

A10. Lewis LM, Graffeo C, Crosley P, et al. Ecallantide for the acute treatment of angiotensin-converting enzyme inhibitor-induced angioedema: a multicenter, randomized, controlled trial. *Ann Emerg Med.* 2014;65:204-213.

A11. Zuraw BL, Busse PJ, White M, et al. Nanofiltered C1 inhibitor concentrate for treatment of hereditary angioedema. *N Engl J Med.* 2010;363:513-522.

A12. Riedl MA, Grivcheva-Panovska V, Moldovan D, et al. Recombinant human C1 esterase inhibitor for prophylaxis of hereditary angio-oedema: a phase 2, multicentre, randomised, double-blind, placebo-controlled crossover trial. *Lancet.* 2017;390:1595-1602.

A13. Banerji A, Busse P, Shennak M, et al. Inhibiting plasma kallikrein for hereditary angioedema prophylaxis. *N Engl J Med.* 2017;376:717-728.

A14. Aygören-Pürsün E, Bygum A, Grivcheva-Panovska V, et al. Oral plasma kallikrein inhibitor for prophylaxis in hereditary angioedema. *N Engl J Med.* 2018;379:352-362.

A15. Longhurst H, Cicardi M, Craig T, et al. Prevention of hereditary angioedema attacks with a subcutaneous C1 inhibitor. *N Engl J Med.* 2017;376:1131-1140.

A16. Baş M, Greve J, Stelter K, et al. A randomized trial of icatibant in ACE-inhibitor-induced angioedema. *N Engl J Med.* 2015;372:418-425.

GENERAL REFERENCES

For the General References and other additional features, please visit Expert Consult at https://expertconsult.inkling.com.

238

SYSTEMIC ANAPHYLAXIS, FOOD ALLERGY, AND INSECT STING ALLERGY

LAWRENCE B. SCHWARTZ

DEFINITION

Systemic anaphylaxis arises when mast cells and possibly basophils secrete mediators with potent vasoactive and smooth muscle contractile activities, eliciting a systemic response.[1] Although mast cells in any organ system may be involved, dictated by the distribution of the instigating stimulus, the principal targets are the cardiovascular, cutaneous, respiratory, and gastrointestinal systems, sites where mast cells are most abundant. Systemic anaphylaxis occurs when these cells are activated to secrete mediators such as histamine by multivalent allergens that bind to and aggregate immunoglobulin E (IgE) and high-affinity IgE receptors (FcεRI) on the surfaces of these cells, causing mediator secretion and a classical immediate hypersensitivity reaction.

EPIDEMIOLOGY

Assessments of the annual incidence of systemic anaphylaxis and the prevalence of those at risk for systemic anaphylaxis are compromised by imprecise diagnostic measures. Approximately 1500 to 2000 deaths in the United States per year are attributed to systemic anaphylaxis. The lifetime incidence of systemic anaphylaxis in adults is estimated at 2 to 8% based on a random nonbiased public telephone survey of adults conducted in 2011, and 82% or more of physicians practicing allergy/immunology, emergency medicine, general medicine, or pediatrics report having witnessed systemic anaphylaxis.[2] In children, for whom food allergy is more common, the incidence of anaphylaxis is likely to be higher. Respiratory or cutaneous symptoms occur in more than 50% of cases, whereas cardiovascular, neurologic, or gastrointestinal symptoms are recognized in less than 50%. Medications are the most common trigger, followed by insect stings, foods, environmental allergens, and latex, but in some cases the cause is unknown (Table 238-1). About half of the reactions occur at home, 14% at a medical facility, and 6 to 7% at another person's home, at work, or at a restaurant. Antibiotics and radiocontrast media are the most common triggers in hospitals. In the perioperative setting, systemic anaphylactic reactions occur with a frequency of about 1 in 2000 to 10,000, muscle relaxants or antibiotics being the most common, but latex, induction drugs, chlorhexidine, and other drugs can also be the culprit.[3]

TABLE 238-1 CAUSES OF SYSTEMIC ANAPHYLAXIS

IgE-MEDIATED	NON–IgE-MEDIATED
Insect stings	Aspirin
Foods (with or without exercise)	Radiocontrast media
Drugs	Exercise, cold, heat, vibration, pressure
Latex	Narcotics (except fentanyl)
Allergen extracts	Vancomycin
	Autoimmune
	Complement anaphylatoxins
	Neuropeptides
	Idiopathic

IgE = immunoglobulin E.

Anaphylaxis to foods and insect stings each account for about 100 deaths per year. Most fatal anaphylactic reactions to injected venom proteins begin within 30 minutes after the sting.[4] Most fatal food and insect sting reactions and many drug reactions are preceded by a mild immediate hypersensitivity reaction to the same allergen. Recognition of these earlier events as an important risk factor for future fatal anaphylaxis should lead to implementation of an action plan to prevent and deal with such reactions. Advanced age and concomitant mastocytosis are also important predictors for an increased risk of severe anaphylaxis.[5]

Some type of food allergy is self-reported in 19% of adults and likely is present in as many as 11%. However, only about half of these allergies are classified as serious.[6] Most children lose their allergic sensitivities to cow's milk, egg, wheat, or soy by 5 years of age, whereas sensitivities to peanut, tree nuts, or seafood are typically long-lasting. About 20% of children lose peanut sensitivity by school age, but a small portion of these regain peanut sensitivity later in life, particularly if they continue to avoid this food.

Latex provokes anaphylaxis in a small but significant group of individuals, particularly patients who have undergone multiple surgical procedures early in life such as those with spina bifida or congenital urinary tract disorders, and those with frequent exposure later in life, such as medical personnel.[7] Estimates of the prevalence of latex hypersensitivity range from 1 to 6% in the general population and about 10% among regularly exposed health care workers. Over a 5-year period, the Food and Drug Administration (FDA) collected approximately 1100 reports of latex-induced anaphylaxis, including 15 deaths. Elimination of latex powdered gloves and availability of nonlatex nitrile or polyvinyl gloves have diminished the prevalence of this problem among medical personnel. Contact hypersensitivity is diagnosed by patch testing, and immediate hypersensitivity by latex-specific IgE tests performed in vitro.

PATHOBIOLOGY

Etiology

The mediators produced by activated mast cells and basophils initiate many of the signs and symptoms of anaphylaxis. These cells constitutively express the high affinity receptor for IgE, FcεRI, on their cell surfaces, enabling them always to be armed by antigen-specific IgE and triggered by antigens that aggregate IgE:FcεRI complexes. Therapeutic interventions aim to prevent the activation of these cells or to block the production or actions of their mediators. Cells other than mast cells and basophils also likely participate in systemic anaphylaxis, particularly those expressing inducible FcεRI such as eosinophils, monocytes, antigen-presenting cells, and epithelial cells, thereby affecting the intensity, duration, or character of anaphylactic reactions.

Most IgE-dependent mast cell activation events occur at local sites and result in local disease, such as allergic conjunctivitis, rhinitis, or asthma when allergens land on the corresponding mucosal surface of a sensitive individual and diffuse into the tissue where mast cells reside. Systemic anaphylaxis presumably requires the allergen (or nonallergen agonist) to distribute systemically to activate mast cells at remote sites. However, activation of the contact system by mast cell products such as heparin or tryptase, resulting in bradykinin production, may also enhance anaphylactic severity. Impaired metabolism of the mast cell mediator, platelet-activating factor, also may enhance severity. Activation of mast cells in perivascular locations should have the greatest effect on vascular responses. Additionally, the responsiveness of various organ systems to mast cell mediators may vary.

Allergens

Most allergens are proteins or glycoproteins that serve as complete antigens, having at least two epitopes recognized by different IgE antibodies, and thereby capable of aggregating IgE in a sensitized subject. The protease activity of some allergens (e.g., house dust mite Der p1) may facilitate their penetration and allergenicity at mucosal sites. Others have lipid binding domains (e.g., Der p2) that increase their antigenic potency. Anaphylactic reactions to a humanized IgG monoclonal antibody, cetuximab, can occur on first exposure, due to host IgE against a nonhuman carbohydrate moiety, galactose-alpha-1,3-galactose (alpha-gal), which was made by the animal hybridoma cell and conjugated to the IgG antibody during its expression. IgE anti–alpha-gal sensitization is elicited by Lone Star tick bites, most common in the U.S. southeast. Such sensitized subjects also present with delayed anaphylactic reactions, 3 to 7 hours after ingestion of alpha-gal–containing red meats, perhaps due to transformation during digestion of monovalent to polyvalent alpha-gal allergens. In contrast to complete antigens, most drugs act as haptens. They become covalently linked to self-proteins in the circulation, in tissues or on cells, emerging as multivalent allergens able to bind and aggregate IgE:FcεRI to activate mast cells.

An allergen exposure must lead to sensitization before an immediate hypersensitivity reaction can occur. This process, which takes at least 1 week, involves antigen processing by antigen-presenting cells, which then present peptide antigens to T$_H$2 cells (T helper lymphocytes), which in turn instruct allergen-specific B cells to switch from production of allergen-specific IgM or IgG to IgE. Production of IL-4 or IL-13 by T$_H$2 cells and binding of T$_H$2 CD40 ligand to B cell CD40 are essential for this antibody class switch. Consequently, anaphylaxis does not occur on first exposure to an allergen (sensitization phase), because the antigen is likely gone by the time antigen-specific IgE is made, but can occur with subsequent exposures.

Food

Most cases of food-induced anaphylaxis in children occur in response to egg, peanut, cow's milk, wheat, or soy, whereas peanuts, tree nuts, and seafood account for most reactions in adults.[8] Reactions to seeds such as sesame seem to be growing in importance, and a variety of different foods have proved to be important allergens in specific individuals. Some patients have the oral allergy syndrome, which typically occurs in subjects sensitive to pollen allergens, whose IgE against ragweed pollen cross-reacts with melon, or IgE against birch pollen with peach or apple. Such food allergen epitopes are typically conformational (rather than linear), and more easily destroyed by heat (cooking), by acid in the stomach, or by proteases in the intestines, and thus rarely progress to systemic reactions.

Food allergy–associated exercise-induced anaphylaxis occurs when a sensitive subject exercises within several hours after eating the food to which he or she is sensitive, but not when eating the food without exercise. Shrimp and wheat are most commonly implicated.[9] Exercise appears to increase intestinal permeability to food antigens, which enter into the systemic circulation. Aspirin, nonsteroidal anti-inflammatory drugs, and alcohol also act to increase intestinal permeability and may help trigger food-induced anaphylaxis. Avoiding the implicated food for 4 to 6 hours before exercise is recommended.

Insect Sting Venom

Hymenoptera families primarily responsible for sting venom-triggered anaphylactic reactions include the Apidae (honey bees and bumble bees), Vespidae (hornets, yellow jackets, and paper wasps), and Formicidae (fire ants). Major allergens of honey bees include phospholipase A$_2$ (Api m 1), hyaluronidase (Api m 2), and melitin (Api m 4). Bumble bee venom proteins exhibit immunologic cross-reactivity with those of the honey bee, but lack melitin. Vespid venoms cross-react among themselves and include phospholipase and hyaluronidase, the latter allergen cross-reacting with bee hyaluronidase. Fire ant venom contains various alkaloids that are not allergenic, but produce sterile pustules, and various allergenic proteins that cross-react with vespid allergens such as phospholipase and scorpion venom allergens. A person may exhibit an anaphylactic reaction on first exposure to one insect's sting if previously sensitized to cross-reactive venom from a different insect. Allergens from biting insects of the Diptera order (mosquitoes, gnats, midges, true flies) are salivary in origin and do not cross-react with Hymenoptera venom allergens. Anaphylaxis to these salivary proteins appears to be uncommon, but precise epidemiologic data are problematic because people are often unaware of a mosquito bite, and commercial diagnostic reagents of high quality are not yet available.

Latex

Latex allergenic proteins are derived from the rubber tree, *Hevea brasiliensis*. Irritant dermatitis is the most frequent contact reaction and does not involve acquired immunity. Contact hypersensitivity, which results from cell-mediated immunity to haptenic chemicals used to process latex, produces a poison ivy–like local reaction that may begin the day after a sensitive subject is exposed. In contrast, IgE-dependent immediate hypersensitivity occurs against latex proteins, seen with cutaneous (elastic materials), mucosal or intravascular (catheters), oral (balloon), and inhaled (powdered latex gloves) routes of exposure, eliciting signs and symptoms within minutes. IgE-mediated cross-reactions occur between IgE anti–latex allergens and those in certain fresh foods such as banana, chestnut, avocado, kiwi, peach, bell pepper, and tomato and may necessitate avoidance of these foods.

Vaccines

Systemic anaphylaxis to vaccines is rare, occurring in about 1.31 per million recipients.[10] Anaphylaxis to influenza vaccine, occurring in about 1.3 to 1.9 per million recipients, seems unrelated to a history of egg allergy. Instead, vaccine-triggered anaphylaxis may relate to sensitivities to a variety of vaccine components.

Non–IgE-Dependent Agonists

Many non–IgE-dependent activators of mast cells do not require processing and can elicit a response on first exposure. These include radiocontrast dyes, most narcotics except for fentanyl, and vancomycin. The dose and rate of administration and individual variations in reactivity are determinants of severity. For radiocontrast dyes, those of low ionic strength and iso-osmolarity are less likely than those of high ionic strength and hyper-osmolarity to elicit a systemic reaction. Vancomycin produces a non–IgE-dependent mast cell activation event known as "red man syndrome," typically involving pruritic flushing, but without cardiovascular compromise unless infused too rapidly. These reactions usually are avoided by reducing the rate of administration of the antibiotic, thereby reducing peak levels.

Endogenous mast cell activators include neuropeptides such as substance P, neurokinin A, and calcitonin gene-related peptide, defensins, and the complement anaphylatoxins C3a and C5a. Although C3a and C5a have their own receptors on mast cells, neurokinins, vancomycin, and narcotics activate a G protein–coupled receptor selectively expressed on mast cells, called Mas-related G protein–coupled receptor X2 (MRGPCR-X2), causing histamine secretion.

Aspirin and Nonsteroidal Anti-inflammatory Drugs

Aspirin hypersensitivity typically manifests as either a respiratory reaction with bronchospasm, nasal congestion, and rhinorrhea or a cardiovascular reaction with hypotension and urticaria, although sometimes overlap occurs, including gastrointestinal signs and symptoms. In most cases, such reactions appear to be pharmacologically (not IgE) mediated, and in sensitive subjects they can occur in response to any of the cyclooxygenase 1 (COX1) inhibitors. Although COX1 inhibitors may shunt arachidonic acid metabolism to the lipoxygenase pathway, a mechanism to explain mast cell activation has not yet emerged. COX2-selective inhibitors appear to be safe in aspirin-intolerant asthmatics, but not always in the cardiovascular group. Less commonly, sensitivity occurs to only one of the drugs within this class, a clue that IgE against a unique chemical moiety on that particular drug is involved.

Physical Stimuli

Physical stimuli may precipitate urticaria or systemic anaphylaxis in certain individuals. Episodes can occur in response to exercise, heat, solar radiation, vibration, pressure, or cold. Exercise-dependent anaphylaxis is sometimes associated with ingestion of any food, regardless of whether sensitivity to the food can be documented, occurring within several hours of ingestion and might be avoided by delaying exercise until several hours after eating. In some cases of familial cold- or vibration-triggered urticaria, genetic defects have been found.[11,12]

Autoimmunity, Activating Kit Mutations, and Hereditary Alpha Tryptasemia

Some patients experience spontaneous bouts of anaphylaxis without an obvious exogenous stimulus. Those with systemic mastocytosis (Chapter 240) or hereditary alpha tryptasemia are particularly prone to systemic anaphylaxis, perhaps because they have too many mast cells and because the mast cells they do have harbor either a somatically acquired activating mutation of Kit tyrosine kinase that primes their activation status or a copy number increase in *TPSAB1* when that gene encodes alpha-tryptase, respectively. A corollary of this is that systemic anaphylaxis to a Hymenoptera insect sting may be a presenting manifestation of these conditions, particularly if a baseline serum tryptase level is elevated.[13-15] A related disorder, mast cell activation syndrome, includes patients with clonal mast cell disease, reflected by these same Kit mutations or hereditary alpha tryptasemia, who have recurrent bouts of anaphylaxis but do not meet diagnostic criteria for systemic mastocytosis. Hereditary alpha tryptasemia, an autosomal dominant disorder, presents with an elevated serum tryptase level (8-100 ng/mL) and multiple-organ signs and symptoms, including cutaneous flushing, pruritus and vibratory urticaria, dysautonomia with irritable bowel syndrome, hyperextensible joints, anaphylaxis, and/or retained primary dentition. Another autosomal dominant syndrome of urticaria caused by vibration or rubbing results from an activating mutation in adhesion G protein–coupled receptor E2.

Some cases of chronic urticaria are known to be associated with IgG and IgM antibodies against FcεRI or IgE. Perhaps complement activation synergizes with FcεRI aggregation to preferentially activate mast cells in the skin or in blood vessel walls, where they express C5a and C3a receptors, as opposed to most mast cells in the lung that lack such receptors. Autoimmune progesterone-mediated anaphylaxis, catamenial anaphylaxis, tends to occur just before menses, and may respond to medical or surgical interventions that prevent menses. Human mast cells also express the low-affinity IgG receptor, FcγRIIa, which, when aggregated by IgG immune complexes, is capable of activating mast cells, and may contribute to some episodes of anaphylaxis.[16]

Pathophysiology

Mast cells participate in both acquired and innate forms of immunity. They arise from bone marrow progenitors and complete their development in peripheral tissues, primarily under the influence of stem cell factor, the ligand for the tyrosine kinase receptor called Kit. Armed with allergen-specific IgE, mast cells are activated by multivalent allergens that bind IgE and aggregate FcεRI on their cell surface. This may be important in the defense against certain microbes such as helminths that elicit a strong IgE response or to protein toxins that are destroyed by mast cell proteases.[17] Mast cells exposed to interferon-gamma become capable of antigen processing and presentation to T cells.[18] Whether human mast cells have a critical, nonredundant role in these biologic and immunologic processes remains controversial. However, their central role in immediate hypersensitivity is clear.

DIAGNOSIS

Systemic anaphylaxis can be diagnosed clinically in real time by consensus criteria outlined in Figure 238-1.[19] Acute concurrent onset of cutaneous signs of immediate hypersensitivity along with either hypotension or respiratory compromise in the apparent absence of allergen exposure; rapid onset of hypersensitivity signs involving at least two organs from among cutaneous, gastrointestinal, respiratory, and cardiovascular systems after exposure to a likely allergen; or rapid onset of hypotension after exposure to a known allergen can be used to diagnose systemic anaphylaxis. Antigen-specific IgE, indicating sensitization, is precisely measured by either laboratory or skin tests. Such tests should be delayed for at least 2 weeks after an anaphylactic event to prevent false-negative results. IgE sensitization is necessary but not sufficient to diagnose allergic disease, because many subjects sensitized to an aeroallergen, particularly at a low antigen-specific IgE level, do not have symptoms when exposed. When food allergy is suspected but not confirmed by IgE testing, oral food challenges can be performed, using protocols to minimize the risk for severe systemic anaphylaxis. Food-allergic reactions involving IgE should be distinguished from a variety of other types of adverse reactions, including lactose intolerance (due to lactase deficiency), food-induced enterocolitis (T-cell responses to cow's milk, soy, or grains), and celiac disease (T-cell response to gluten in wheat and other grains).

An increased level of tryptase in acute (over baseline) serum, which peaks 30 to 90 minutes after the onset of signs or symptoms of anaphylaxis and then declines with a half-life of about 2 hours, indicates that mast cell activation has occurred. An increase in the acute serum tryptase level (collected 30 min to 4 hours after clinical onset) of at least $2 + 1.2 \times$ baseline serum tryptase level (collected either before onset or at least 24 hours after all clinical signs and symptoms have resolved) is considered clinically significant. The elevation magnitude correlates with clinical severity, i.e., hypotension, in experimental insect sting–mediated anaphylaxis. Although an increased serum total tryptase level is quite specific for anaphylaxis, the sensitivity is low for detecting anaphylaxis triggered by food ingestion, or, in general, if anaphylactic severity is either modest (no hypotension) or local (laryngeal edema), or if the acute sample was collected outside of the optimal times. Whether there are anaphylactic IgE-dependent pathways not involving mast cell activation, but instead involving basophil activation, is unknown, but has been considered for anaphylaxis triggered by food allergen ingestion. Baseline tryptase levels in serum are stable in healthy subjects, reflecting genetic rather than environmental factors, and range from 1 to 11 ng/mL. Baseline levels above 20 ng/mL occur in most patients with systemic mastocytosis (Chapter 240), representing a minor criterion for that diagnosis, and greater than 8 ng/mL in all patients diagnosed to date with hereditary alpha tryptasemia. Elevated baseline tryptase levels also appear to increase the risk for severe insect sting–triggered systemic anaphylaxis, likely due to the higher prevalence of a clonal mast cell disorder with an activating c-kit mutation or to increased copies of the gene encoding alpha-tryptase.[13,14]

Plasma histamine, because it is rapidly metabolized, is not as practical as serum or plasma tryptase for detecting anaphylaxis. However, urinary N-methylhistamine levels also may reflect overall levels of released histamine, accumulating in urine during anaphylaxis and stored in the bladder until micturition. However, levels are affected by ingested histamine-containing foods, histamine-producing mucosal bacteria, and variability in histamine metabolism. Prostaglandin D_2 (PGD_2) and leukotriene C_4 (LTC_4), arachidonic acid–derived mediators that are made by several cell types, including activated mast cells, are rapidly metabolized to $PGF2\alpha$ and LTE_4, respectively, and urinary or serum levels of these metabolites may be elevated in urine formed during anaphylaxis.

Low serum levels of platelet-activating factor (PAF) acetyl hydrolase, which metabolizes PAF, and of angiotensin-converting enzyme (ACE), which metabolizes bradykinin, have been associated with more severe food-induced systemic anaphylaxis. Whether slow metabolism of PAF and bradykinin might allow these mediators to play a role in such reactions and whether mediator-specific therapies would be clinically useful in such reactions remain to be determined.

Differential Diagnosis

Anaphylaxis should be distinguished from a variety of disorders with overlapping presentations. Vasovagal syncope causes diaphoresis, nausea, hypotension, and bradycardia, but without urticaria and tachycardia. Flushing disorders may be benign and unrelated to anaphylaxis, or they could be a manifestation

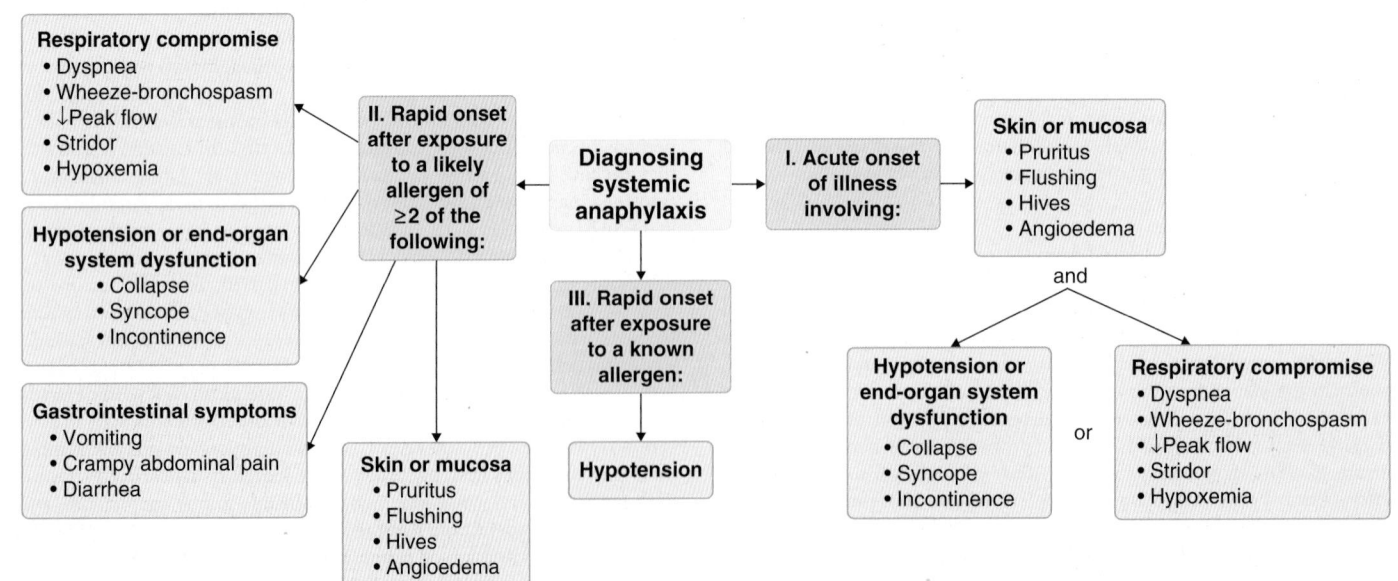

FIGURE 238-1. Diagnosing systemic anaphylaxis in a clinical setting. Acute onset of systemic anaphylaxis in the apparent absence of allergen exposure means that the signs and symptoms, once they begin, develop over minutes to an hour, whereas rapid onset after exposure to a likely or known allergen means that these signs and symptoms begin to occur within minutes to several hours after that exposure. (From Sampson HA, Muñoz-Furlong A, Campbell RL, et al. Second symposium on the definition and management of anaphylaxis: summary report—second National Institute of Allergy and Infectious Disease/Food Allergy and Anaphylaxis Network symposium. *J Allergy Clin Immunol.* 2006;117:391-397.)

of pathologic conditions such as the carcinoid syndrome, with which urticaria and profound hypotension are not typically associated; pheochromocytoma, which causes episodic hypertension; or VIPomas, which cause facial flushing and voluminous diarrhea with hypokalemia but not episodic hypotension or urticaria. Panic attacks and vocal cord dysfunction can be a challenge to distinguish from anaphylaxis, especially by history alone, but nevertheless must be considered. Acute attacks of angioedema caused by C1 esterase inhibitor deficiency are not associated with pruritus or urticaria and evolve slower and persist longer than attacks of anaphylaxis. Shock due to complement activation, generating complement anaphylatoxins, or to activation of the contact system leading to the production of bradykinin, can occur without involving mast cell activation. Scombroidosis occurs 5 to 60 minutes after ingestion of histamine, typically in poorly stored fish, and manifests with flushing, palpitations, headache, and gastrointestinal symptoms. The condition lasts several hours, both duration and severity depending on the amount of histamine ingested, and usually responds to H_1-receptor and H_2-receptor antihistamines, but occasionally requires epinephrine and intravenous fluids. Acute serum sickness, various cell activation syndromes, endotoxin-mediated septic shock, and superantigen-mediated toxic shock syndromes manifest with fever, which is not characteristic of anaphylaxis by itself. Also, hypoglycemia, seizure, and primary pulmonary or cardiac events should be considered. In some cases, systemic anaphylaxis may provoke another disorder (e.g., myocardial infarction, with acute serum levels of both tryptase and troponin being elevated).

Systemic mastocytosis (Chapter 240) and hereditary alpha tryptasemia are important conditions to consider in the setting of anaphylaxis.[20] In adults with mastocytosis, a somatic activating mutation in the gene for Kit in mast cell progenitors results in the accumulation of mast cells, particularly in bone marrow and skin, and increases the risk for anaphylaxis. Hereditary alpha tryptasemia is an autosomal dominant disorder associated with increased copy numbers of *TPSAB1* when that gene encodes alpha-tryptase. Both disorders can be precisely diagnosed by specific genetic tests and can present with systemic anaphylaxis particularly when spontaneous or elicited by an insect sting. Diagnostic tests for systemic mastocytosis are discussed in detail in Chapter 240.

TREATMENT   Rx

Acute

Fatal outcomes in anaphylaxis are principally the result of either airway constriction or hypotension. Accordingly, the acute treatment of systemic anaphylaxis requires that airway patency, blood pressure, and cardiac status be addressed (Fig. 238-2). Intubation, tracheostomy, volume expanders, and vasopressors may be needed. Patients exhibiting any signs or symptoms of hypotension

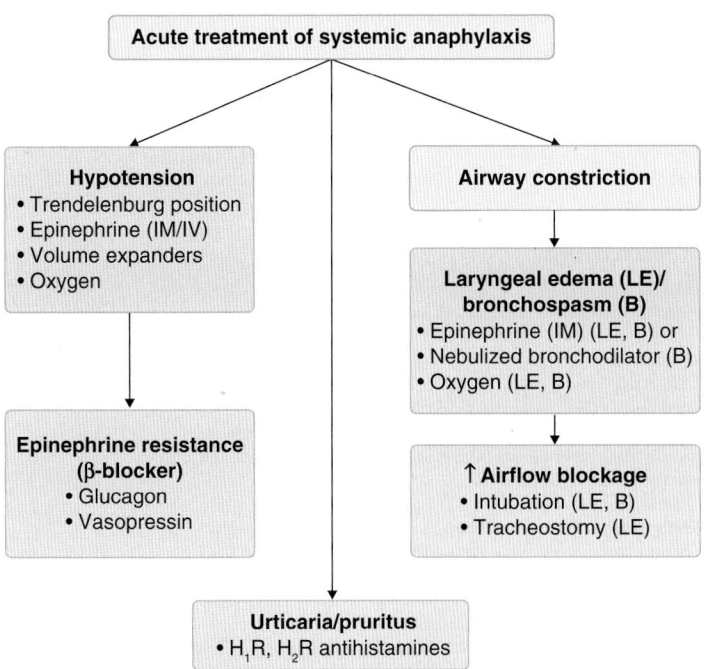

FIGURE 238-2. Acute treatment of systemic anaphylaxis. B = bronchospasm; H_1R = H_1 histamine receptor; H_2R = H_2 histamine receptor; IM = intramuscular; LE = laryngeal edema.

should immediately assume a supine position with lower extremities slightly elevated, which may prevent progression to anaphylactic shock or what has been called in postmortem examinations the *empty ventricle syndrome*—because almost all hypotensive anaphylactic deaths are preceded by syncope occurring in a sitting or upright posture. Epinephrine injected intramuscularly into the thigh (0.2 to 0.5 mg for adults, 0.01 mg/kg up to 0.3 mg for children, repeated every 5 to 30 minutes as indicated) is the most effective drug to administer, the earlier during the course of an anaphylactic event the better. Alternatively, calibrated intravenous administration of a solution of epinephrine (1 mg/100 mL solution starting at 30 to 100 mL/hour) and titrated to the lowest effective rate of infusion can be considered. Epinephrine relaxes bronchial smooth muscle and improves vascular tone and permeability, thereby counteracting bronchospasm, hypotension, and tissue edema. Although there is no absolute contraindication to its use for treating systemic anaphylaxis, the benefits of epinephrine need to be weighed against its disadvantages in elderly subjects and in those with cerebrovascular or coronary artery disease, hypertension, diabetes, hyperthyroidism, cardiomyopathy, or narrow-angle glaucoma, in whom adverse events such as myocardial infarction, stroke, or pulmonary edema can be precipitated. Also, patients taking a β-blocker, particularly if nonselective, may be resistant to epinephrine; in such a case, glucagon (1 mg intravenously [IV], or 1 to 5 mg/hour IV) or vasopressin (5 to 40 IU IV) may be used. Oxygen should be administered by nasal cannula. Inhaled bronchodilators can relieve bronchospasm. Parenteral administration of H_1-receptor (diphenhydramine, 1 to 2 mg/kg up to 50 mg) and H_2-receptor (ranitidine, 300 mg IV over 5 minutes) antihistamines may prevent progression of urticaria and pruritus but is not likely to reverse hypotension or tissue edema. Evidence to support use of glucocorticosteroids to treat anaphylaxis is lacking and in an emergency department setting does not appear to affect relapse rate.[A1]

PREVENTION

Patients who have experienced an anaphylactic reaction are at greatest risk for another episode. Such individuals should wear a Medic-Alert bracelet, carry an epinephrine autoinjector (e.g., EpiPen or AuviQ), and be instructed in its use. Avoidance of nonspecific β-blockers and ACE inhibitors is recommended, because either may worsen the severity of an anaphylactic episode, and β-blockers might interfere with epinephrine treatment. In subjects with recurrent anaphylaxis, prophylactic use of H_1- and H_2-receptor antihistamines is beneficial. A leukotriene antagonist and cyclooxygenase inhibitor theoretically would provide additional prophylactic benefit. Cyclosporine A (≤5 mg/kg/day) might be considered in difficult cases of recurrent anaphylaxis because of its ability to inhibit mast cell activation (e.g., in chronic urticaria).[21] Omalizumab, which neutralizes free IgE, has been reported to be helpful in controlling urticaria, anaphylaxis, and immunotherapy reactions in mastocytosis patients, but it currently is approved by the FDA only for poorly controlled cases of asthma or chronic urticaria. Glucocorticosteroids do not inhibit mast cell activation in vitro or immediate skin test wheal/flare responses to allergens in vivo; whether of benefit in selected patients with recurrent anaphylaxis is anecdotal.

Specific anaphylactic syndromes have unique considerations. Anti-IgE therapy in peanut-allergic subjects can increase the threshold of sensitivity, on average, from the equivalent of half a peanut to almost nine peanuts,[A2] thereby providing protection against accidental exposures. Experimental oral[A3] or epicutaneous[A4] biologic immunotherapies have also shown promising results. Insect venom allergy can be treated by venom immunotherapy, dramatically decreasing the risk of anaphylaxis to future stings.[A5] Reactions to radiocontrast media can be prevented or attenuated by prior administration of H_1- and H_2-receptor antihistamines. Patients who are hypersensitive to penicillin should avoid β-lactam antibiotics in general, but can be desensitized if an antibiotic in this class is critically needed (e.g., penicillin for neurosyphilis). However, desensitization is temporary; once the drug has cleared, sensitivity is likely to return. However, most people with a history of penicillin or amoxicillin allergy lose their sensitivity, which can be determined by allergy skin testing and oral challenge. Catamenial anaphylaxis may respond to the luteinizing hormone–releasing hormone analog Lupron, to oophorectomy, or to conjugated estrogens. Patients with systemic mastocytosis, in addition to prophylactic pharmacologic measures, should avoid using direct mast cell agonists such as vancomycin and most narcotics with the exception of fentanyl. Aspirin-intolerant asthmatics with sinus polyps can be desensitized to aspirin and placed on a daily dose to maintain desensitization status, resulting in better control of asthma, shrinkage of polyps, and reduction of hyposmia. Food- and latex-allergic subjects must practice avoidance of the provocative agent, though data for food allergy support anti-IgE neutralization therapy or oral immunotherapy to protect against inadvertent food allergen exposures; feeding peanuts to children at risk for developing peanut allergic disease may prevent the majority of them from becoming allergic.[A5] Future research should yield more effective therapeutic interventions to achieve longer-lasting clinical tolerance.

FUTURE DIRECTIONS

Ongoing research will provide more precise diagnostic tools for delineating different pathways of systemic anaphylaxis, indicating which cell types and biochemical pathways are involved, thereby revealing the most appropriate treatments. Predictors for anaphylactic risk will be better understood. Consequently, interventions that reduce this risk (including better desensitization regimens) and that more effectively reverse the signs and symptoms of this potentially fatal disorder will be developed.

 Grade A References

A1. Grunau BE, Wiens MO, Rowe BH, et al. Emergency department corticosteroid use for allergy or anaphylaxis is not associated with decreased relapses. *Ann Emerg Med.* 2015;66:381-389.
A2. Vickery BP, Vereda A, Casale TB, et al. AR101 Oral immunotherapy for peanut allergy. *N Engl J Med.* 2018;379:1991-2001.
A3. Wang J, Sampson HA. Safety and efficacy of epicutaneous immunotherapy for food allergy. *Pediatr Allergy Immunol.* 2018;29:341-349.
A4. Boyle RJ, Elremeli M, Hockenhull J, et al. Venom immunotherapy for preventing allergic reactions to insect stings. *Cochrane Database Syst Rev.* 2012;10:CD008838.
A5. Du Toit G, Sayre PH, Roberts G, et al. Effect of avoidance on peanut allergy after early peanut consumption. *N Engl J Med.* 2016;374:1435-1443.

GENERAL REFERENCES

For the General References and other additional features, please visit Expert Consult at https://expertconsult.inkling.com.

239

DRUG ALLERGY

LESLIE C. GRAMMER

DEFINITION

Adverse drug reactions (ADRs) are recognized as an important public health problem because they result in both morbidity and mortality. An ADR is defined by the World Health Organization as an unintended, noxious response to a drug that occurs at a dose usually prescribed for human patients. The classic pharmacologic definition of ADRs by Rawlins and Thompson separates these into two major types: type A reactions, which are predictable and dose dependent; and type B reactions, which are unpredictable and not dose dependent. Type B reactions account for 10 to 25% of all ADRs and include drug allergy. The World Health Organization Nomenclature Review Committee defines *drug allergy* as a hypersensitivity reaction for which a definite immunologic mechanism, either a B-cell-mediated (antibody) or a T-cell-mediated process, is documented. Most published epidemiologic studies refer to ADRs in general and not to drug allergy specifically because the demonstration of drug-specific B-cell-mediated or T-cell-mediated mechanisms is often difficult, and the immunologic culprit may be a drug metabolite.

EPIDEMIOLOGY

Drug allergy is responsible for significant mortality, morbidity, and socioeconomic costs that are probably underestimated. Current data must be evaluated carefully because they involve different populations, different definitions of ADRs and drug allergy, and different methodologies, especially in terms of data analysis. The Boston Collaborative Drug Surveillance Program collected information on all ADRs in 4031 hospitalized patients during a period of 6 months. An incidence of 6.1% was reported, of which 42% were severe; 1% of the severe reactions resulted in the patient's death. Using an automatic detection system in a Salt Lake City hospital, 731 ADRs were identified among 36,653 hospitalized patients. Of note, only 12.3% of these were reported by physicians in the hospital. A meta-analysis of 33 U.S. prospective studies from 1966 to 1996 reported that 15% of hospitalized patients experienced ADRs and that the frequency of drug-related hospital admissions varied from 3 to

6%. Most other subsequent studies reported similar data. Epidemiologic information on drug allergy in nonhospitalized people and in the general population is even more limited and is confined mainly to studies of antibiotics.

Primary care physicians are often the first point of contact for a nonhospitalized patient with a suspected adverse drug reaction. They therefore have a key role in deciding whether to dismiss the diagnosis or refer the patient for further investigation. Having a structured diagnostic approach to distinguishing between hypersensitivity and nonhypersensitivity reactions can avoid life-threatening reactions and at the same time reduce the frequent overdiagnosis of drug hypersensitivity.[1]

Risk Factors

Some risk factors have been identified for the development of drug allergy. Certain drugs more commonly cause adverse reactions, and some drugs lead to more severe reactions (Table 239-1). The dosage and route of administration of a drug can also be risk factors; intermittent, repeated administrations of a drug can be more sensitizing than uninterrupted therapy. Medications that are most likely to cause intraoperative anaphylaxis are neuromuscular blocking agents, antibiotics (especially β-lactams), latex, and opioids.[2] Drug allergy is more commonly reported in women and in patients with HIV infection or reactivation of some herpesviruses. Some ethnic groups appear to be more prone to certain ADRs. For example, white Americans are at a higher risk than other ethnic groups for hypersensitivity reactions to abacavir, a reverse transcriptase inhibitor. For drug allergy caused by angiotensin-converting enzyme inhibitors, the more vulnerable population is African American. There are individuals who have multiple drug hypersensitivity (MDH), which is a syndrome that occurs as a consequence of excessive T-cell stimulation and is characterized by prolonged drug hypersensitivity reactions to several drugs.[3] Mechanistically, it should be noted that T-cell activation characterized by $PD1^+/CD38^+$ expression on $CD4^+$ T cells can be found in the circulation of MDH patients for many years.

In the United States, approximately 10% of individuals who seek health care have a history of penicillin allergy.[4] However, if tested with an appropriate panel of skin tests, less than 10% of those individuals would be deemed to have a hypersensitivity to penicillin. The overreporting of penicillin allergy is a significant obstacle to antimicrobial stewardship with important implications, including more antimicrobial resistance, increased cost of care, and increased length of stay.[5] Individuals with a positive history and negative skin test results tolerate penicillin-type antibiotics at the same rate as the general population with a negative history; in addition, there is a very low rate of resensitization.

PATHOBIOLOGY

Hypersensitivity reactions to drugs can be classified according to the type of immunologic reaction. An immunologic response to any antigen may be diverse and the resulting reaction complex; drugs are no exception. Drugs that are more frequent perpetrators of significant allergy are listed in Table 239-1.

Most pharmacologic agents are simple structures with a molecular mass of less than 1000 D. Alone, they are unable to induce hypersensitivity-type immunologic responses. However, most of these drugs have the ability to covalently bind to proteins and form hapten-carrier complexes, with the

TABLE 239-1	DRUGS FREQUENTLY IMPLICATED IN ALLERGIC DRUG REACTIONS

Allopurinol
Amiodarone
Antiarrhythmic drugs (procainamide, quinidine)
Antibiotics (β-lactams, sulfas, nitrofurans)
Anticonvulsants (hydantoin, phenobarbital, carbamazepine)
Antihypertensive agents (angiotensin-converting enzyme inhibitors)
Antipsychotic tranquilizers
Antisera (antitoxins, antivirals)
Antituberculous drugs (isoniazid, rifampicin)
Aspirin and nonsteroidal anti-inflammatory drugs
Biologics (monoclonal antibodies such as anti–tumor necrosis factor and other recombinant DNA protein products)
Chemotherapy agents (platins, doxorubicin, taxanes)
Enzymes (L-asparaginase, streptokinase, chymopapain)
Muscle relaxants (rocuronium, succinylcholine)
Opioids
Radiocontrast media
Vaccines (egg protein, gelatin)

low-molecular-weight agent acting as the hapten and the protein being the carrier. Hapten-carrier complexes can induce immunologic responses, with most responses being directed at the hapten. In addition to low-molecular-weight drugs acting as haptens, there is evidence that they may activate immune receptors by binding to them directly.[6]

A well-known example of a low-molecular-weight agent is penicillin. Benzylpenicillin has a molecular mass of approximately 300 D and is metabolized into a penicilloyl hapten moiety. The penicilloyl moiety, which constitutes about 95% of all penicillin metabolites, is referred to as the major determinant because it is the major metabolite in terms of quantity. It has been conjugated to poly-D-lysine to form penicilloyl-polylysine, which is now commercially available as Pre-Pen (ALK-Abelló, Round Rock, TX) for skin testing. The other 5% of penicillin metabolites are referred to as the minor determinants. Although they are minor in quantity, these determinants actually cause most of the immediate-type anaphylactic reactions, whereas the major determinant is associated with later and less severe reactions. Minor determinant reagents have never been commercially available in the United States. Penicillin skin testing is not widely used by U.S. physicians; annually, only 40,000 doses of the major determinant are sold.

In contrast to simple low-molecular-weight drugs, therapeutic agents that are proteins with a molecular mass exceeding 5000 D can be recognized by the human immune system and can result in sensitization and hypersensitivity reactions on subsequent exposure. Because these proteins are complete antigens, they can be used as skin testing reagents or as antigens or allergens in in vitro assays. Included among therapeutic protein reagents that reportedly cause hypersensitivity are antithymocyte globulin (rabbit or equine), streptokinase, latex, and vaccines such as tetanus toxoid. Biologics, including monoclonal antibodies, are increasingly recognized causes of drug hypersensitivity. As anticipated, murine antibodies are most immunogenic, followed by chimeric and then humanized monoclonals. Unexpectedly, a variety of human recombinant proteins, including insulin and fully human monoclonal antibodies, can cause hypersensitivity reactions. In addition to hypersensitivity reactions, biologics such as monoclonal antibodies can cause other immunologic reactions (Chapter 33). One such reaction is the *cytokine release syndrome*, in which high cytokine levels result in systemic symptoms, including fever, arthralgia, and capillary leak; interleukin-2 is the original biologic agent in which this was described. Immune imbalance is another immunologic reaction, exemplified by anti–tumor necrosis factor therapy that results in immune dysregulation consisting of increased susceptibility to infection or autoimmunity.

CLINICAL MANIFESTATIONS

The clinical manifestations of drug allergy often include a dermatologic component (Chapter 411). It is estimated that 80 to 90% of drug allergies result in one of the following cutaneous manifestations: exanthematous or morbilliform eruption; urticaria, angioedema, or both; contact dermatitis; fixed drug eruption; erythema multiforme–like eruption; or photosensitivity.[7] Severe cutaneous adverse reactions[8,9] are generally induced by drugs and encompass the conditions of Stevens-Johnson syndrome and toxic epidermal necrolysis[10]; drug-induced eosinophilia and systemic syndrome, also known as drug-induced hypersensitivity syndrome; and acute generalized exanthematous pustulosis. Drug reaction with eosinophilia and systemic symptoms (DRESS), also called drug-induced hypersensitivity syndrome, typically presents with a maculopapular exanthema (Chapter 411), fever, and an elevated alanine aminotransferase level, with about 75% of cases related to anticonvulsant medications.[11] These conditions, although rare, cause significant morbidity and even mortality, which is why it is important for the treating physician to promptly recognize severe cutaneous adverse reactions and to discontinue implicated drugs. Some features of severe cutaneous adverse reactions that distinguish them from nonserious cutaneous reactions include involvement of other organs (e.g., liver, kidneys); fever; eosinophilia; mucosal involvement; and lesions that are painful, blistering, or pustular.[12]

DIAGNOSIS

The diagnosis of drug allergy may be simple if a patient has recently started therapy with a single agent known to cause hypersensitivity, such as a β-lactam antibiotic. In contrast, in a hospitalized patient in whom multiple drugs have been started and stopped, identifying the offending drug may be difficult, requiring a complete and exhaustive history along with a physical examination. It also requires compatible clinical manifestations and temporal relationships. In vitro tests are rarely useful clinically. In vivo testing, such as cutaneous tests and provocative test dosing, may be indicated in some situations.

TABLE 239-2	ORGAN-SPECIFIC REACTIONS AND IMPLICATED DRUGS
REACTION	**IMPLICATED DRUG**
PULMONARY MANIFESTATIONS	
Pulmonary infiltrates with eosinophilia	Minocycline, nitrofurantoin
Pneumonitis and fibrosis	Bleomycin, amiodarone
Noncardiogenic pulmonary edema	Hydrochlorothiazide, cocaine, heroin, methadone
AUTOIMMUNE MANIFESTATIONS	
Drug-induced lupus	Hydralazine, procainamide
DRUG-INDUCED IMMUNE CYTOPENIAS	
Thrombocytopenia	Quinidine, gold salts, sulfonamides, heparin
Hemolytic anemia	Penicillin, methyldopa
Agranulocytosis	Sulfonamides, propylthiouracil, quinidine, procainamide, phenytoin
HEPATIC MANIFESTATIONS	
Cholestasis	Aminosalicylic acid, dapsone
Hepatocellular damage	Phenothiazines, erythromycin
Mixed pattern	Halothane, isoniazid, diclofenac
	Phenytoin, sulfonamides
RENAL MANIFESTATIONS	
Nephrotic syndrome	Gold salts, captopril, NSAIDs, penicillamine
Acute interstitial nephritis	β-Lactam antibiotics, NSAIDs, sulfonamides
LYMPHOID SYSTEM MANIFESTATIONS	
Pseudolymphoma	Phenytoin, lamotrigine
Infectious mononucleosis–like syndrome	Aminosalicylic acid, dapsone
CARDIAC MANIFESTATIONS	Sulfonamides, β-lactam antibiotics
NEUROLOGIC MANIFESTATIONS	
Peripheral neuritis	Colchicine, nitrofurantoin, sulfonamides

NSAIDs = nonsteroidal anti-inflammatory drugs.

Differential Diagnosis

To distinguish drug allergy from other ADRs, several criteria are helpful. Allergic reactions occur in a tiny fraction of individuals who receive the drug, and they cannot be predicted. The observed clinical effects do not resemble known pharmacologic actions of the drug. In the absence of prior exposure to the drug, allergic or hypersensitivity symptoms rarely appear before 1 week of continuous therapy. In general, drugs used consistently for several months or longer are rarely responsible.

Drug allergy often resembles other allergic or hypersensitivity reactions, such as anaphylaxis, urticaria, and serum sickness–like illness. Although most drug reactions include cutaneous manifestations, some involve only other organ systems, for example, pulmonary infiltrates with eosinophilia, hepatitis, and acute interstitial nephritis. A list of drugs that cause organ-specific reactions is provided in Table 239-2. Drug-specific antibodies or T-cell receptors have been identified that react with the suspected drugs or relevant drug metabolites. As with ADRs in general, the reaction often subsides after the drug is discontinued. However, a hypersensitivity reaction may persist or even intensify because of the formation of drug metabolites, which act as haptens and bind to carrier proteins such as human serum albumin.

TREATMENT Rx

Evidence-Based Treatments

There is a paucity of evidence-based information regarding drug allergy, a disease that is generally iatrogenic.[13] One study evaluated HIV patients who previously had an adverse reaction to cotrimoxazole; it was concluded that desensitization resulted in fewer adverse reactions and fewer treatment discontinuations in patients with a previous history of mild or moderate hypersensitivity. A second study, evaluating treatment for toxic epidermal necrolysis, concluded that there are no randomized controlled trials of the most commonly used therapies (i.e., systemic steroids, cyclosporine, intravenous immune globulins).

There are published clinical guidelines for the management of infusion-related hypersensitivity reactions caused by the administration of chemotherapeutic or biologic therapy. These guidelines were developed as part of a performance improvement initiative and resulted in a standardized approach to the management and reporting of ADRs.

PREVENTION

Although the outcome of ADRs is generally favorable, prevention is the obvious goal. The physician should prescribe medications only if they are clinically appropriate and, if possible, should avoid drugs that are known to produce significant hypersensitivity reactions (see Table 239-1). Before starting a medication, the patient should be asked about prior ADRs to the medication or to other pharmacologically related medications. If appropriate, oral administration is probably preferable to parenteral administration; anaphylaxis is less likely, as is sensitization. Protocols for skin testing to foreign antisera and for management of medication hypersensitivity reactions (e.g., premedication, test dosing, desensitization) are available.[14] A general algorithm is provided in Figure 239-1.

The risk for an anaphylactic reaction to a drug such as penicillin is a function of the history of onset, severity, and proximity (Table 239-3). If an individual

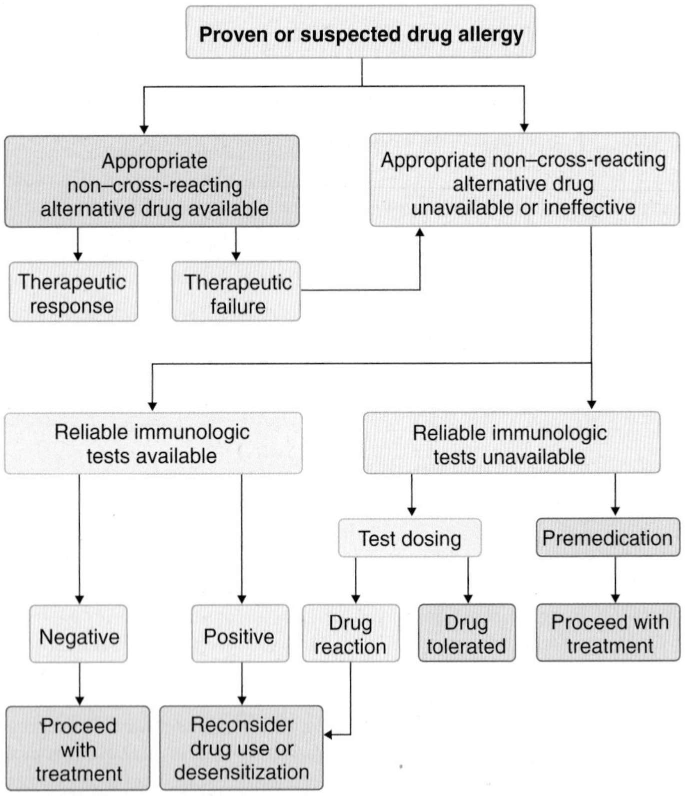

FIGURE 239-1. Guidelines for the treatment of patients with a history of drug allergy. In patients with a suspected or known drug allergy, the first choice is to use an appropriate non–cross-reacting drug. If such a drug is not available, or if the patient does not respond to it, further evaluation is based on the availability of a reliable immunologic test to detect drug hypersensitivity.

TABLE 239-3	RISK FOR ANAPHYLACTIC REACTION TO PENICILLIN OR OTHER PHARMACOTHERAPEUTIC AGENTS	
FACTOR	LOW RISK	HIGH RISK
Onset of previous reaction	>24 hr	<30 min
Signs and symptoms of previous reaction	Morbilliform eruption Urticaria alone	Life-threatening symptoms: hypotension, upper airway angioedema, bronchospasm
Time elapsed since previous reaction	>20 yr	<1 yr

experienced an immediate-type reaction that was rapid in onset, involved life-threatening symptoms or signs, and occurred relatively recently, that individual is at high risk for a severe anaphylactic reaction on subsequent exposure.

Even with a negative Pre-Pen skin test result, a patient could have reactivity against minor determinants; therefore, the approach to a patient who needs a β-lactam antibiotic depends on the risk as listed in Table 239-3. Risks and benefits should be thoroughly discussed and documented. In a high-risk individual, cautious test dosing can be performed. If a reaction occurs, desensitization can be considered if the clinical risks and benefits so warrant.

PROGNOSIS

Most drug allergies involve cutaneous eruptions that are self-limited and resolve shortly after the offending agent has been discontinued. However, severe, life-threatening reactions occur in approximately 1 in every 1000 hospitalized patients. Severe cutaneous adverse reactions are especially likely to cause morbidity and mortality. In 1998 the death rate for hospitalized Medicare patients was 20% higher in those who experienced an ADR. The proportion of ADRs that were allergic reactions was not determined in this study, but it can be estimated at about one fifth.

Most drug reactions resolve, but relapses may occur days to several weeks after discontinuation of the offending drug, especially with carbamazepine, phenytoin, valproic acid, sulfasalazine, allopurinol, and antivirals. In such cases, corticosteroids may be beneficial.[15]

One of the most severe reactions associated with drug allergy is anaphylactic shock (Chapter 238).[16] It is usually immunoglobulin E (IgE) mediated, but it may occur with non-IgE-mediated reactions to drugs such as nonsteroidal anti-inflammatory drugs or radiocontrast media. It is estimated that approximately 1500 people die annually in the United States owing to anaphylaxis from medications. In the United Kingdom, drugs are the leading cause of anaphylactic fatalities.

FUTURE DIRECTIONS

Pharmacogenomics will be an important method of identifying individuals at risk for a significant allergic reaction to a given drug.[17] Human leukocyte antigen (HLA) genotyping can reportedly identify individuals who are at increased risk for drug hypersensitivity. For example, individuals with HLA-B*5701 are at greater risk for a drug hypersensitivity reaction to abacavir, an HIV transcriptase inhibitor. Severe cutaneous adverse reactions to allopurinol are highly associated with the genetic marker HLA-B*5801. In patients of Asian ancestry, HLA-B*1508 is highly associated with development of Stevens-Johnson syndrome if carbamazepine is prescribed. Why this genetic variant is not a risk factor in patients of African or European ancestry is unclear. Other avenues by which susceptible individuals may be identified include polymorphisms in genes for immune recognition molecules, drug-metabolizing enzymes, and macromolecular adduct repair systems.

GENERAL REFERENCES

For the General References and other additional features, please visit Expert Consult at https://expertconsult.inkling.com.

240

MASTOCYTOSIS

CEM AKIN

DEFINITION

Mastocytosis is a heterogeneous group of disorders characterized by pathologic accumulation of mast cells in tissues such as skin and bone marrow. According to the classification of the World Health Organization (WHO), based on clinical presentation and pathologic findings, there are seven distinct categories of mastocytosis (Table 240-1).[1] The term *cutaneous mastocytosis* describes skin disease alone without any evidence of internal organ involvement, whereas the term *systemic mastocytosis* describes the disorder when it involves internal organs (most commonly the bone marrow) with or without skin disease.

TABLE 240-1	WORLD HEALTH ORGANIZATION CLASSIFICATION OF MASTOCYTOSIS

Cutaneous mastocytosis
Indolent systemic mastocytosis
Systemic smoldering mastocytosis
Systemic mastocytosis with associated hematological neoplasm (AHN)
Aggressive systemic mastocytosis
Mast cell leukemia
Mast cell sarcoma

From Horny HP, Akin C, Arber, DA et al. Mastocytosis. In: Swerdlow SH, Campo E, Harris NL, et al, eds. *WHO Classification of Tumours of Haematopoietic and Lymphoid Tissues.* Lyon, France: IARC Press; 2017:60-69.

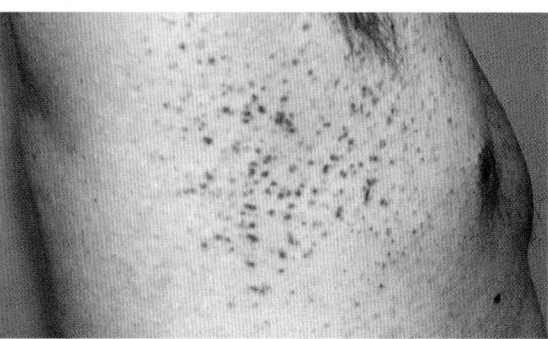

FIGURE 240-1. Urticaria pigmentosa.

EPIDEMIOLOGY

Mastocytosis can be diagnosed at any age.[2] Pediatric-onset and adult-onset forms are distinguished on the basis of the age of the patient at initial diagnosis. These forms display differences in their clinical course, molecular pathology, and prognosis. The most common clinical scenario leading to diagnosis in the pediatric population is a child presenting with skin lesions of cutaneous mastocytosis within the first year of life. Patients with a later onset of skin lesions are more likely to have systemic mastocytosis, as are most patients with adult-onset mastocytosis. The disease has been diagnosed in all ethnic populations. Estimates of the prevalence of patients with cutaneous mastocytosis range from 1 in 500 to 1 in 8000 patients presenting in dermatology clinics. The prevalence of systemic mastocytosis is more difficult to estimate because the diagnosis requires biopsy of an involved tissue and a high degree of clinical suspicion, especially if skin lesions are absent. Systemic mastocytosis is likely to be underdiagnosed, considering the fact that there are neither physical examination findings nor routine hematologic or chemistry laboratory abnormalities specifically associated with the disease. Consequently, it is not unusual to encounter several years' delay after the onset of symptoms in many patients before a diagnosis of mastocytosis is reached. The disease is sporadic, although rare cases of familial occurrence have been described.

PATHOBIOLOGY

Pathogenesis

The pathogenesis of mastocytosis involves the accumulation of mast cells in tissues, with mediators released by activated mast cells. The primary reason for the increased mast cell numbers in tissues appears to be defective apoptosis rather than uncontrolled proliferation. It is unusual to see increased mitotic activity in biopsy specimens from patients with mastocytosis, and, in most patients, the disease follows an indolent course. Tissue microenvironment and altered chemotaxis may also contribute to the final level of tissue mast cell burden.

Genetics

Mast cells are derived from hematopoietic progenitors (Chapter 147). Systemic mastocytosis is associated with somatic gain-of-function point mutations in the *KIT* (formerly *c-kit*) gene of the mast cell progenitor, leading to a clonal neoplastic expansion of mast cells. *KIT* encodes a transmembrane receptor (Kit) whose intracellular portion functions as a tyrosine kinase enzyme. The extracellular portion of Kit binds the cytokine stem cell factor (SCF or Kit ligand). The interaction between SCF and Kit provides the single most important growth and differentiation stimulus for mast cells from their progenitors. Under physiologic conditions, homodimeric SCF binds and cross-links two Kit receptor molecules, which leads to autophosphorylation of the tyrosine amino acids of the intracellular portion of the Kit molecule. Phosphorylated tyrosine residues in turn act as docking sites for downstream adaptor and signal transduction molecules that regulate the differentiation, proliferation, chemotaxis, and functional activation of mast cells.

The most common mutation reported in mastocytosis[3,4] involves codon 816 in *KIT* (located in exon 17), resulting in the replacement of an aspartic acid by a valine residue (D816V) in the Kit protein, leading to ligand-independent autophosphorylation. The D816V mutation has been shown in lesional mast cells from the skin or bone marrow tissue of more than 90% of adults and approximately 40% of pediatric patients with mastocytosis. Another 40% of pediatric patients carry *KIT* mutations in other exons, most commonly in exons 8 and 9. *KIT* mutations can be demonstrated in non–mast cell hematopoietic lineages in advanced variants of systemic mastocytosis, similar to the multilineage involvement observed in myeloproliferative neoplasms (Chapter 157). The sensitivity of detecting the mutation is much higher when a lesional tissue such as bone marrow or skin is analyzed compared with peripheral blood. Other pathogenetic factors, some yet to be determined, appear to be responsible for the final disease phenotype because the presence of the D816V *KIT* mutation alone does not explain the remarkable heterogeneity in the clinical presentation and prognosis of the disease. Molecular aberrations in *TET2, SRSF2, ASXL1, CBL, RUNX1,* and *DNMT3A* have been the other most frequently identified mutations in advanced forms of systemic mastocytosis. In advanced systemic mastocytosis, most patients carry three or more mutations.

CLINICAL MANIFESTATIONS

Symptoms

The symptoms of mastocytosis are primarily related to the release of mast cell mediators and rarely by the destructive infiltration of mast cells into tissues or consequences of an associated hematologic neoplasm. Mast cell activation[5] results in the release of various preformed mediators stored in mast cell granules, *de novo* synthesis of sulfidopeptide leukotrienes such as LTC_4 and prostaglandins (mostly PGD_2) from membrane lipids, and cytokine synthesis. Preformed mediators stored in mast cell granules include histamine; proteases such as tryptase, chymase, and carboxypeptidase A; and proteoglycans such as heparin and chondroitin sulfate. Vasoactive mediators such as histamine, LTC_4, and PGD_2 at local or distant tissues cause vasodilation, which may lead to flushing, tachycardia, hypotension, presyncope, and syncope. Histamine also causes pruritus and stimulates gastric acid hypersecretion from parietal cells. Mast cells are rich sources of cytokines. Elevated serum levels of tumor necrosis factor-α and interleukin-6 have been found in patients with mastocytosis and may contribute to the pathophysiologic process of fatigue and accelerated osteoporosis observed in some patients. Rare aggressive categories of mastocytosis may be associated with an extensive destructive infiltration of mast cells into tissues such as the gastrointestinal tract, which may result in malabsorption, and the liver, which may cause portal fibrosis with associated portal hypertension.

Mast cell activation and mediator release may occur after triggers, such as temperature changes (e.g., hot showers), exercise, ingestion of alcohol or spicy foods, emotional stress, insect stings, and exposure to certain drugs (such as opioid analgesics, nonsteroidal anti-inflammatory drugs, or muscle relaxants), and sometimes spontaneously without an obvious trigger. The prevalence of atopic disease in patients with mastocytosis is similar to that in the general population, and the serum immunoglobulin E (IgE) level is often found to be low. However, patients with anaphylactic sensitivity to hymenoptera venoms appear to have a disproportionately high incidence of mastocytosis.

Mastocytosis is a disease with protean clinical manifestations.[6] Although in some patients the only complaint is the cosmetic appearance of urticaria pigmentosa lesions (Fig. 240-1), others suffer from frequent episodes of vascular instability or have life-threatening hematologic disease. In general, patients with mastocytosis belong to one of two broad categories, according to the site of tissue involvement: those with cutaneous disease alone, or those with systemic disease with or without skin involvement. Cutaneous mastocytosis (i.e., disease limited to the skin in the absence of internal organ involvement) is commonly diagnosed in children within the first year of life, whereas systemic mastocytosis is mostly diagnosed in adults by a bone marrow biopsy and aspirate.

Cutaneous Manifestations

Maculopapular skin lesions of urticaria pigmentosa (known as maculopapular cutaneous mastocytosis) are the most common presentation of cutaneous mastocytosis (Fig. 240-1). They are also present in 50 to 90% of patients with systemic mastocytosis, depending on the disease category. Remarkably different in appearance from urticaria or hives, lesions of urticaria pigmentosa are fixed, tan- to salmon-colored lesions varying in size from a few millimeters to a few centimeters. They are most prominently observed on the trunk and extremities and tend to spare the face and the sun-exposed areas of the skin, although facial and scalp involvement may be seen in children. Blistering of the lesions may occur in children mostly in the first 3 years of life. The lesions are generally not pruritic at rest but may urticate after exposure to a number of triggers (see Pathobiology). Many patients note that the skin lesions become more prominent after exposure to heat or after physical irritation such as rubbing. The lesions may be found concentrated in skin areas that are prone to irritation, such as the axillae and groin.

Uncommon presentations of cutaneous mastocytosis include mastocytomas, and diffuse cutaneous mastocytosis. Mastocytomas are benign and generally solitary mast cell tumors, although they have been known to precede urticaria pigmentosa lesions in some cases. They occur almost exclusively in children, and physical irritation of the lesion may result in generalized flushing and other symptoms of mast cell mediator release. Diffuse cutaneous mastocytosis is another form of skin involvement seen exclusively in children. It is characterized by diffuse thickening of the skin and appendages with a peau d'orange appearance without individual urticaria pigmentosa lesions. Telangiectasia macularis eruptive perstans (TMEP) is a rare form of cutaneous mastocytosis characterized by the presence of diffuse telangiectatic macules. Because TMEP lesions are generally seen in the presence of urticaria pigmentosa, there is debate about whether TMEP represents a distinct form of cutaneous mastocytosis.

Patients with cutaneous mastocytosis may manifest other symptoms such as abdominal pain, diarrhea, and flushing.

Systemic Manifestations

Symptoms caused by mast cell degranulation may be experienced as brief, recurrent, and self-limited episodes with multiorgan manifestations or as chronic complaints during a prolonged time course. A typical mast cell degranulation episode may variably involve flushing, conjunctival hyperemia, nausea, vomiting, abdominal cramping, diarrhea, tachycardia, and lightheadedness. Symptoms of mast cell activation (or "mast cell activation syndromes") may occur in conditions other than mastocytosis (see Chapter 238) where the activation of mast cells is a reactive process secondary to stimuli generated by another pathologic process. Hypotension may develop, and the episode may progress to full loss of consciousness in some patients. Therefore, mastocytosis should be considered in all patients with recurrent anaphylaxis before a diagnosis of idiopathic anaphylaxis can be made. Tryptase, a protease stored in mast cell granules, may be elevated above the patient's baseline level in the serum or plasma if it is measured within 4 hours after the onset of the episode in patients with suspected mast cell degranulation or anaphylaxis, regardless of the cause. Angioedema, hives, and wheezing are uncommon in mastocytosis. Flushing usually involves the face and upper chest area. A consistent trigger can be identified in only a small number of patients (see Pathobiology). The episodes usually last 30 minutes to a few hours. Hypotensive episodes can be life-threatening, particularly in the presence of comorbidities, such as cardiac or pulmonary disease. Systemic mastocytosis should be suspected in all patients with systemic reactions to hymenoptera stings, especially those involving hypotensive syncope or near-syncope.

Gastrointestinal Symptoms

Gastrointestinal symptoms are observed in more than 50% of patients with mastocytosis. Epigastric pain, lower abdominal cramping, nausea, vomiting, or diarrhea can occur episodically in the context of an acute mast cell degranulation episode or on a chronic basis. Gastric acid hypersecretion induced by mast cell–derived histamine may lead to esophagitis, gastritis, and peptic ulcer disease, although measurements of basal acid output have shown great variability in different studies, ranging from hypersecretion in the range of Zollinger-Ellison syndrome to achlorhydria. Mucosal edema, thickened gastric or duodenal mucosal folds, or nodular lesions may be observed in radiographic or endoscopic evaluations. Diarrhea alternating with constipation may be seen. Severe persistent diarrhea may be complicated by clinically significant malabsorption in patients with aggressive systemic mastocytosis. Hematochezia, hematemesis, and melena are uncommon symptoms and should prompt endoscopic evaluation to rule out coexisting disease. Mast cells are constituents of the normal lamina propria in gastrointestinal mucosa, and their numbers may be increased in inflammatory states affecting the gastrointestinal tract. However, quantitation of mast cell numbers in gastrointestinal biopsy

specimens is generally not helpful, and diagnosis of mast cell disease by a gastrointestinal biopsy, solely based on increased mast cell numbers without evidence for other WHO criteria, should be avoided. Mild to moderate hepatomegaly with or without abnormalities in serum transaminases may be observed, although portal hypertension and ascites are rare and indicate the presence of advanced categories of mastocytosis. Jaundice and findings on cholangiography resembling those of primary sclerosing cholangitis have been reported in some patients.

Musculoskeletal Symptoms

Musculoskeletal pain is common in patients with mastocytosis and is mostly caused by soft tissue pain resembling fibromyalgia. Accelerated osteoporosis may be seen in a subgroup of patients, particularly those with other risk factors, such as postmenopausal women, and those receiving glucocorticoid therapy. Pathologic compression fractures and other fragility fractures due to bone involvement may be the initial finding in some patients.[7] A bone densitometry measurement should be recommended as part of the standard evaluation of women with mastocytosis and of any patient with a history of pathologic fractures. Radiographic abnormalities have been reported in up to 75% of patients with mastocytosis. In addition to generalized osteoporosis, bone surveys may show a mixture of sclerotic or lytic lesions, and skeletal scintigraphy may reveal focal or diffuse radiotracer uptake.

Hematologic Manifestations

Peripheral blood abnormalities have been noted in up to 50% of patients with systemic mastocytosis. Mild normochromic normocytic anemia is the most common abnormality, followed by thrombocytopenia, eosinophilia, monocytosis, and leukopenia. Eosinophilia in mastocytosis rarely causes organ damage, as is observed in chronic eosinophilic leukemia or idiopathic hypereosinophilic syndrome (Chapter 161). It is important to differentiate a primary eosinophilic disorder from mastocytosis with eosinophilia. Some cases of chronic eosinophilic leukemia are associated with the FIP1L1-PDGFRA fusion gene and respond to the drug imatinib, whereas systemic mastocytosis is associated with codon 816 point mutations of the KIT gene, which confers resistance to this drug.

Approximately 20% of patients with systemic mastocytosis have been reported to display evidence of another clonal non–mast cell hematologic disease. Non–mast cell clonal hematologic neoplasms associated with mastocytosis are commonly myeloid in nature (myeloproliferative neoplasms, myelodysplastic syndromes, or myeloid leukemias) but may also involve lymphoproliferative disorders, such as lymphomas, myelomas, and lymphocytic leukemias.

DIAGNOSIS

The diagnosis and classification of mastocytosis are carried out according to the guidelines published by the WHO. A suggested algorithm for the diagnosis of mastocytosis is shown in Figure 240-2.

Cutaneous Mastocytosis

Diagnosis of cutaneous mastocytosis is made by observing the typical hyperpigmented maculopapular lesions of urticaria pigmentosa and is confirmed by skin biopsy, which shows infiltration of mast cells in the upper dermis, particularly in perivascular locations. Mild increases in mast cell numbers can be observed in inflammatory and neoplastic skin diseases, and establishing a diagnosis of cutaneous mastocytosis by a blind skin biopsy or biopsy of a lesion that does not have the typical appearance of urticaria pigmentosa should be avoided. A localized wheal-and-flare reaction limited to the lesional skin within a few minutes after rubbing or scratching of the skin is known as the Darier sign. Diagnosis of urticaria pigmentosa in adults should always prompt investigation of possible systemic mastocytosis.

Systemic Mastocytosis
Biopsy

The recommended diagnostic procedure to evaluate the presence of WHO diagnostic criteria for systemic disease (discussed later) is a bone marrow biopsy and aspiration. This procedure is recommended for all patients with adult-onset urticaria pigmentosa, patients with recurrent symptoms suggestive of mast cell degranulation (such as flushing and hypotension accompanied by abdominal complaints), patients with unexplained osteoporosis, and patients with suspected hematologic disease (see Clinical Manifestations). Children with an onset of lesions within the first year of life usually do not require a bone marrow biopsy unless they have abnormal blood counts, lymphadenopathy,

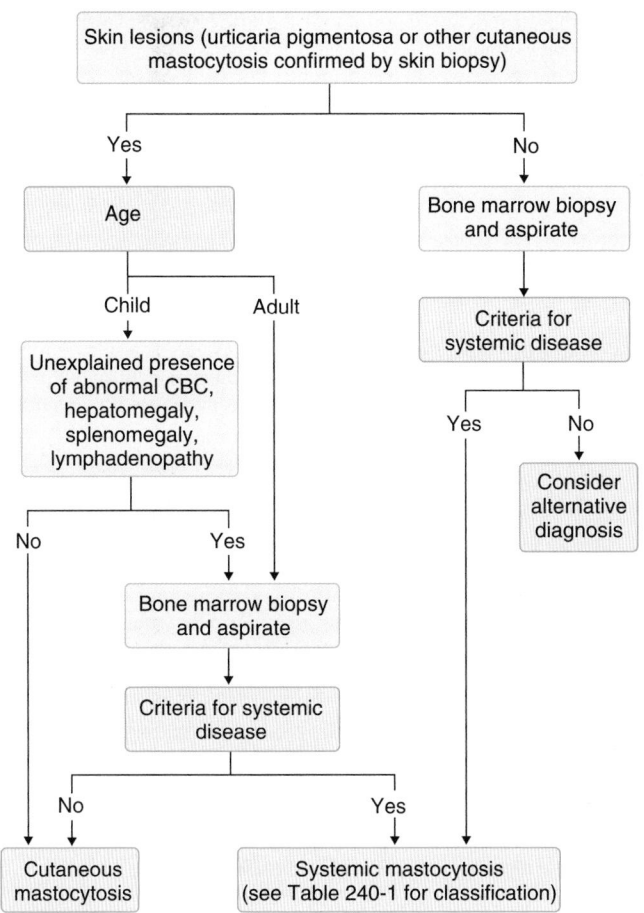

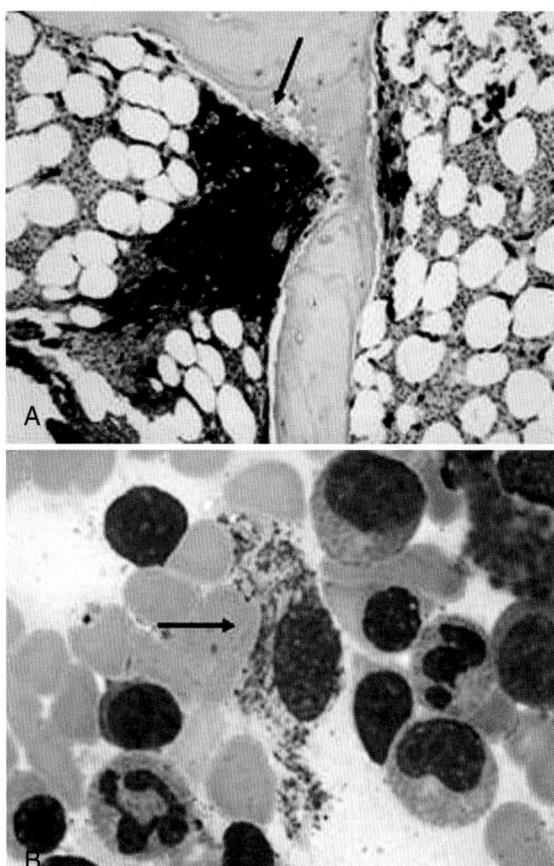

FIGURE 240-3. Diagnostic findings in the bone marrow biopsy specimen and aspirate smear. **A,** Characteristic mast cell aggregates on tryptase staining (major criterion) in biopsy section (*arrow*). **B,** Mast cells with atypical spindle shapes in aspirate smear (*arrow*).

TABLE 240-2	WORLD HEALTH ORGANIZATION DIAGNOSTIC CRITERIA FOR SYSTEMIC MASTOCYTOSIS

MAJOR

Multifocal, dense infiltrates of mast cells consisting of 15 or more mast cells in aggregates detected in sections of bone marrow and/or other extracutaneous organs, confirmed by tryptase immunohistochemistry or other special stains

MINOR

a. More than 25% of mast cells in the infiltrate in biopsy sections or bone marrow aspirate smears showing spindle shape or atypical morphology

b. Detection of a *KIT* codon 816 point mutation in bone marrow, blood, or other extracutaneous organs

c. Expression of CD25 with or without CD2 by mast cells in bone marrow, blood, or extracutaneous organs

d. Persistent elevation of serum total tryptase >20 ng/mL*

*Criterion not valid if there is an associated clonal myeloid disorder.
Diagnosis requires at least 1 major plus 1 minor *or* 3 minor criteria.
From Valent P, Akin C, Metcalfe DD. Mastocytosis: 2016 updated WHO classification and novel emerging treatment concepts. *Blood.* 2017;129:1420-1427.

hepatomegaly, or splenomegaly. Children with late-onset skin lesions, (especially those with uniform morphology as opposed to polymorphic lesions of various sizes) and those who experience persistence of maculopapular cutaneous mastocytosis into adulthood should be considered for diagnostic evaluation for systemic disease.

World Health Organization Diagnostic Criteria

WHO guidelines for diagnosis of systemic mastocytosis consist of one major and four minor criteria (Table 240-2). Presence of the major criterion with at least one minor criterion, or demonstration of three minor criteria in the absence of the major criterion, is needed to establish a diagnosis of systemic mastocytosis and to distinguish it from reactive mast cell hyperplasia. The major diagnostic criterion is the presence of multifocal, dense aggregates of

15 or more mast cells in bone marrow or other extracutaneous tissue biopsy sections (Fig. 240-3A). Such clusters are frequently observed around blood vessels and next to bone trabeculae in bone marrow biopsy sections. Immunohistochemical staining for tryptase and CD117 is the recommended method for visualization of mast cells. Routine hematoxylin and eosin or metachromatic stains such as toluidine blue are not sufficiently sensitive to demonstrate subtle mast cell infiltrates or abnormal morphologic features of mast cells within the infiltrates in decalcified bone marrow biopsy sections.

Mast cell morphology in bone marrow provides important clues to the diagnosis of systemic mastocytosis. Bone marrow mast cells in systemic mastocytosis often display atypical morphology, such as an elongated (spindle) shape, hypogranularity, and an eccentric or lobulated nucleus (Fig. 240-3B). These atypical mast cells are usually observed in close association with bone marrow spicules in the aspirate smear. Mast cells in mast cell leukemia may be very sparsely granulated.

Flow cytometric analysis of the mast cells in a bone marrow aspirate, when it is performed appropriately, is a sensitive diagnostic aid. The mean percentage of mast cells in a healthy bone marrow aspirate is approximately 0.02%, and it does not exceed 1% in most patients with mastocytosis. Therefore, to visualize the mast cell population correctly, the total cell numbers analyzed by flow cytometry should be significantly higher than those in other, more routine evaluations (e.g., leukemia phenotyping). The characteristic flow cytometric finding of systemic mastocytosis is the aberrant expression of CD25 with or without CD2 on CD117+ mast cells. CD25 is more sensitive than CD2 as CD2 may be absent or weakly expressed in some cases of advanced mastocytosis. Aberrant CD25 expression can also be demonstrated by immunohistochemical staining of bone marrow biopsy specimens.[8] Serum tryptase level may be elevated in patients with mastocytosis.[9] Currently available commercial tryptase immunoassays measure levels of total tryptase, the sum of mature tryptase, and tryptase precursors. Mature tryptase enzyme is a serine protease stored in mast cell granules and is transiently elevated in serum or plasma after mast cell degranulation episodes, such as anaphylaxis. In contrast, tryptase precursor proenzymes (α and β protryptases) are constitutively secreted outside the cell, and their serum levels at baseline correlate with mast cell burden. The median serum tryptase level in a healthy population is approximately 5 ng/mL. A serum tryptase level higher than 20 ng/mL raises suspicion for systemic mastocytosis in the appropriate clinical setting. A normal tryptase level does not rule out a diagnosis of mastocytosis, and increased tryptase levels can be seen in other conditions, such as hereditary alpha-tryptasemia, myelodysplastic syndromes, acute myeloid leukemias, chronic eosinophilic leukemia, and chronic renal insufficiency. Metabolites of histamine, such as N-methylhistamine, and prostaglandin D_2 can be elevated in a 24-hour urine specimen but are neither more sensitive nor more specific than the baseline serum tryptase measurement in mastocytosis.

Demonstration of a codon 816 *KIT* mutation (D816V) may be necessary to fulfill the diagnostic criteria in patients lacking the major criterion (see Pathobiology).[10] Examination of lesional tissues, such as skin and bone marrow, affords the highest sensitivity. Codon 816 *KIT* mutations have been detected in a variety of other neoplastic diseases, such as core binding factor acute myeloid leukemias, sinonasal lymphomas, and seminomas, in addition to mastocytosis.

A rare histologic variant with clustering of mature round mast cells without CD25 expression termed well-differentiated systemic mastocytosis has been described. These patients generally have a history of childhood-onset mastocytosis without the D816V *KIT* mutation and therefore may respond to imatinib as opposed to those with typical systemic mastocytosis carrying the D816V mutation (see Treatment).

World Health Organization Disease Categories

Each patient diagnosed with mastocytosis should be assigned a category of disease according to the WHO classification (see Table 240-1).[11] *Cutaneous mastocytosis* in the absence of bone marrow and internal organ involvement is the most common category in patients with pediatric-onset disease.

Systemic mastocytosis is divided into the categories of indolent systemic mastocytosis, smoldering systemic mastocytosis, systemic mastocytosis with an associated hematologic neoplasm (SM-AHN), aggressive systemic mastocytosis, and mast cell leukemia. An algorithm for classification of systemic mastocytosis is presented in Figure 240-4. *Indolent systemic mastocytosis* is the most common category in adults. Patients in this category usually have a normal life expectancy compared with age-matched general populations,

although they experience symptoms related to the release of mast cell mediators. Indolent systemic mastocytosis follows a persistent course, and progression to a more advanced category is unusual (<5% of cases). *SM-AHN* is the second most common category in adults, and a non–mast cell hematologic disease is usually diagnosed at the time that the diagnosis of mastocytosis is made. Therefore, bone marrow biopsy and aspirate specimens should be carefully evaluated for the presence of other hematologic disease in every patient with newly diagnosed systemic mastocytosis. *Aggressive systemic mastocytosis* is a rare category characterized by the presence of organ dysfunction resulting from destructive mast cell infiltration. Aggressive systemic mastocytosis may involve the hematopoietic, gastrointestinal, and skeletal systems in the form of cytopenias, hypersplenism, malabsorption with weight loss, hepatomegaly with portal hypertension and ascites, and large osteolytic lesions with pathologic fractures; these constitute so-called C-findings as defined by the WHO criteria. *Smoldering systemic mastocytosis* denotes patients with high mast cell burden as evidenced by 2 or more B-findings (more than 30% infiltration by mast cells in bone marrow biopsy or tryptase >200 ng/ml; signs of dysplasia or myeloproliferation without meeting the criteria for an AHN; hepatomegaly or splenomegaly without liver dysfunction or hypersplenism) in the absence of C-findings or mast cell leukemia. *Mast cell leukemia* is characterized by 10% or more mast cells in the peripheral circulation or 20% or more mast cells in bone marrow aspirate smears, or both. To diagnose mast cell leukemia, the mast cell percentage in bone marrow aspirate smears should be assessed in an area of the slide that is sufficiently distant from the spicules. *Mast cell sarcoma* is a rare diagnosis characterized by malignant and invasive solid mast cell tumor.

There is a subset of patients with recurrent idiopathic or hymenoptera venom–induced anaphylaxis who have evidence of clonal mast cells carrying the D816V *KIT* mutation or aberrantly expressing surface CD25, without fully meeting the WHO diagnostic criteria and without displaying urticaria pigmentosa skin lesions. Such patients are provisionally referred to as having a monoclonal mast cell activation syndrome.

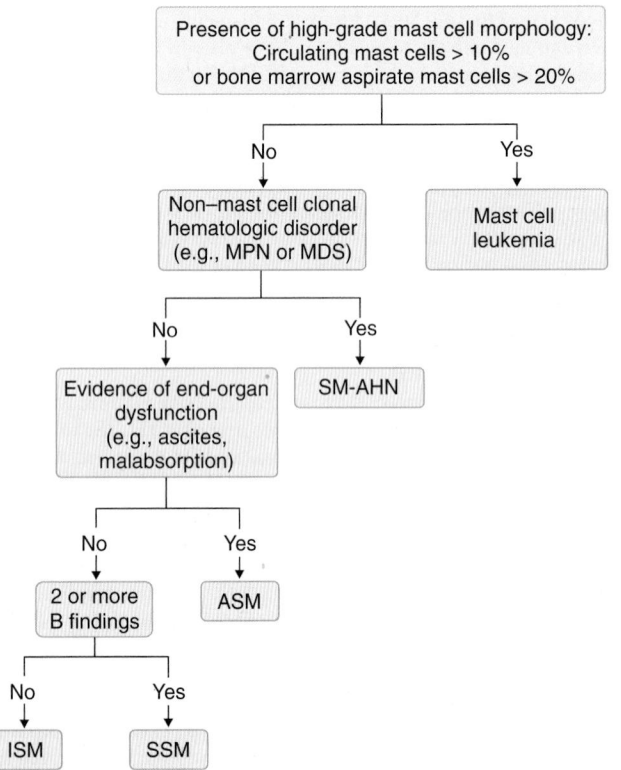

FIGURE 240-4. **An algorithm for classification of systemic mastocytosis.** ASM = aggressive systemic mastocytosis; ISM = indolent systemic mastocytosis; MDS = myelodysplastic syndromes; MPN = myeloproliferative neoplasms; SM-AHN = systemic mastocytosis with associated clonal hematologic non–mast cell lineage disease; SSM = systemic smoldering mastyocytosis.

TREATMENT   Rx

The major goal of treatment for all categories of mastocytosis is symptom control. A reduction in mast cell numbers is considered only in disease categories with a poor prognosis (i.e., SM-AHNMD, aggressive systemic mastocytosis, mast cell leukemia, and mast cell sarcoma).[12] Current treatment modalities have not been shown to change the natural course of the disease.

Medical Therapy

Adults with cutaneous and indolent systemic mastocytosis are treated symptomatically. Pruritus in mastocytosis usually responds to scheduled doses of histamine₁-receptor blocker antihistamines, such as loratadine (10 mg daily), fexofenadine (180 mg with water daily), or cetirizine (5 to 10 mg daily).[13] These doses may be doubled to twice daily if needed in symptomatic patients. Sedating antihistamines, such as hydroxyzine (25 mg three times daily) or diphenhydramine, may be used before bedtime. Photochemotherapy (oral psoralen plus ultraviolet A) or phototherapy may be helpful in patients with refractory pruritus; it results in symptomatic improvement and temporary fading of the pigmented skin lesions in up to 50% of patients. The side effects of phototherapy, including increased risk of skin cancer, should be taken into account when this treatment is considered.

Histamine₂-receptor blocker antihistamines, such as ranitidine (150 mg twice daily) or famotidine (20 mg once or twice daily), are usually prescribed as a first-line treatment for patients with gastrointestinal complaints, such as heartburn, nausea, and abdominal pain. The dual H₁- and serotonin-receptor antagonist cyproheptadine (4 mg three times daily) may be used for diarrhea, flushing, or headaches. Proton pump inhibitors may be added in patients whose abdominal symptoms are refractory to histamine₂-receptor blockers. Oral cromolyn sodium (adult dose, 200 mg four times daily) has been effective in reducing abdominal pain, diarrhea, nausea, vomiting, and pruritus in various studies, although the beneficial effects are variable among patients. Finally, low to moderate doses of systemic glucocorticoids can be beneficial in unusual cases of aggressive mastocytosis presenting with recalcitrant diarrhea associated with malabsorption or hepatomegaly with ascites.

Cysteinyl leukotrienes, such as LTC₄, that are produced after mast cell activation are thought to contribute to symptoms in mastocytosis. Therefore, drugs targeting the synthesis or receptor binding of leukotrienes are usually added to the treatment regimens of patients who derive suboptimal relief of itching and abdominal pain from histamine receptor–blocking therapy. For example, montelukast (10 mg daily) or zileuton may be useful when used in conjunction with H₁- and H₂-receptor antagonists. Patients should be warned about psychiatric side effects.

Self-administered epinephrine should be considered for all patients even if they do not have any history of hypotensive or anaphylactic episodes resulting in presyncope or syncope from acute mast cell degranulation. These episodes should be treated like systemic anaphylaxis (Chapter 238).

Masitinib, a KIT and LYN kinase inhibitor, has been shown in a randomized trial to be an effective and well-tolerated agent for the treatment of severely symptomatic indolent or smoldering systemic mastocytosis. However, the response rate, in terms of 75% improvement from baseline, is less than 20%. Omalizumab (a humanized anti-IgE monoclonal antibody) has been shown to be beneficial in reducing recurrent anaphylactic or mast cell activation symptoms in case reports.

Cytoreductive Therapies

Cytoreductive therapy is generally considered in aggressive disease variants associated with poor prognosis. Some patients with recurrent life-threatening episodes of mast cell mediator release unresponsive to conventional therapy may also be candidates for cytoreductive therapy after careful consideration of risks and benefits. Approaches to cytoreductive treatment of mastocytosis have included tyrosine kinase inhibitors,[14] interferon alfa-2b, and the nucleoside analogue cladribine. No cytoreductive therapy has been shown to result in complete remission.

Most patients with mastocytosis have the D816V *KIT* mutation, which confers resistance to imatinib, and therefore are not appropriate candidates for this therapy. Midostaurin (100 mg twice daily), which inhibits the common KIT D816V driver mutation, provided a 60% response rate in patients with advanced systemic mastocytosis, including mast-cell leukemia.[15] Due to its favorable toxicity profile, midostaurin is emerging as a first-line therapy in patients needing cytoreduction. Otherwise, mast cell leukemia usually is treated with polychemotherapy as acute myeloid leukemia (Chapter 173), although successful treatment regimens have not yet been identified. Imatinib, a tyrosine kinase inhibitor with activity against wild-type *KIT*, *PDGFR*, and *abl*, has been effective in a small number of patients without D816V *KIT* mutation or with the *FIP1L1-PDGFRA* fusion gene, who present with chronic eosinophilic leukemia (Chapter 161) with a modest increase in bone marrow mast cells.

Interferon alfa-2b (0.5 to 5 million units, three to five times per week), alone or with prednisone, has been reported to partially improve clinical and laboratory abnormalities in approximately 50% of patients with aggressive systemic mastocytosis, patients with osteoporosis and pathologic fractures, and patients with recalcitrant recurrent anaphylaxis, although complete histopathologic and molecular remissions appear to be rare. Interferon alfa is difficult to tolerate because of its many side effects, including influenza-like symptoms, bone pain, and depression.

Cladribine is a synthetic purine analog (0.14 mg/kg in infusion or subcutaneously, days 1-5; repeated at 4 to 12 weeks until 1 to 9 courses). In one series, it was effective for indolent and aggressive mastocytosis, with an overall 22% response rate. However, it is associated with a high risk for lymphopenia, neutropenia, and opportunistic infections.[16]

Ancillary and Other Therapies

Avoidance of the triggers of mast cell degranulation is an important adjunct to the pharmacologic treatment of symptoms. These show remarkable individual variation among systemic mastocytosis patients (see Pathobiology), and the individual medical history can be helpful in identifying such triggers. General anesthesia and surgery impose an additional risk to patients with mastocytosis because several agents that are used perioperatively, such as muscle relaxants, opioid analgesics, and nonsteroidal anti-inflammatory drugs, can induce acute mast cell degranulation. Prior surgical and anesthesia records should be obtained if available, and an appropriate strategy for the anesthetic management of the patient should be determined, with close communication involving the patient, anesthesiologist, surgeon, and an allergist.

Non–mast cell clonal hematologic disorders associated with mastocytosis should be treated according to the standard-of-care guidelines for those disorders, regardless of the presence of mastocytosis. Hematopoietic stem cell transplantation (Chapter 168) has yielded variable results for the treatment of mast cell disease, and occasional cases resulting in complete remission have been reported.

Venom immunotherapy is recommended for those with a history of systemic reactions to hymenoptera who have evidence of IgE-mediated sensitization (by blood or skin allergy testing). Most experts recommend the duration of the therapy to be indefinite as fatalities have been reported after discontinuation of immunotherapy.

Because of the high prevalence of osteoporosis and pathologic bone fractures in mastocytosis, bone densitometry should be considered a standard diagnostic procedure in adult patients with mastocytosis. If osteoporosis is detected, it should be treated per standard recommendations (Chapter 230).

PROGNOSIS

The prognosis for mastocytosis varies by the category of disease. At least 50% of patients with pediatric-onset cutaneous mastocytosis have complete resolution of the disease by adolescence, and the great majority of the rest of those patients experience improvement or fading of the skin lesions. Indolent systemic mastocytosis is a persistent disease but has a good prognosis without a decrease in life expectancy, and progression to a more aggressive disease category is rare. Factors associated with poorer prognosis have been reported as the absence of urticaria pigmentosa, older age at onset of symptoms, elevated serum lactate dehydrogenase or alkaline phosphatase, thrombocytopenia, anemia, peripheral blood smear abnormalities, and detectability of the D816V *KIT* mutation in peripheral blood.[17] The prognosis for SM-AHN is determined by the prognosis for the associated hematologic disorder. Aggressive systemic mastocytosis and mast cell leukemia have poor prognoses, with median survival times of less than 3 years and less than 1 year, respectively.

Grade A Reference

A1. Lortholary O, Chandesris MO, Bulai Livideanu C, et al. Masitinib for treatment of severely symptomatic indolent systemic mastocytosis: a randomised, placebo-controlled, phase 3 study. *Lancet.* 2017;389:612-620.

GENERAL REFERENCES

For the General References and other additional features, please visit Expert Consult at https://expertconsult.inkling.com.

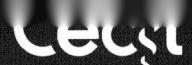

XXIII

RHEUMATIC DISEASES

241

APPROACH TO THE PATIENT WITH RHEUMATIC DISEASE

VIVIAN P. BYKERK AND MARY K. CROW

Rheumatic diseases are common, and they are an important cause of reduced quality of life, increased comorbidity, and reduced life expectancy. They incur a significant socioeconomic burden and warrant expertise on the part of all physicians who treat patients. This chapter provides a framework to approach the evaluation of patients who present with signs and symptoms suggesting a rheumatic disease. An algorithmic approach is provided that allows the physician to integrate presenting features, patient characteristics, and anatomic structures, along with diagnostic tests, to develop a diagnosis and treatment plan.

DEFINITION AND CATEGORIZATION

Rheumatic diseases are disorders of connective tissue in which general or localized inflammation frequently manifests as pain attributable to peripheral joints, the spine, or muscles and related soft tissues. Systemic features such as stiffness, fever, or weight loss and a multitude of extramusculoskeletal features, ranging from skin rashes to renal dysfunction, often accompany rheumatic diseases. In most cases, the basic underlying pathology is understood, although this is less true of pain disorders appearing alone or accompanying a rheumatic disease (Chapter 27). For most rheumatic disorders, underlying molecular processes thought to be triggered by environmental factors in genetically susceptible individuals drive specific patterns of connective tissue disease, making up the clinical phenotype of a particular rheumatic disease. Research is ongoing to define more precisely the molecular pathophysiology unique to these diseases.[1-3] Rheumatic diseases can be broadly considered as those that are primarily degenerative, with inflammation occurring secondarily, and those in which inflammation is the primary pathway leading to the disease characteristics. In the latter, the pathogenesis can be mediated through aberrant immune responses or as a result of metabolic abnormalities.

Histopathology

Rheumatic diseases are often also termed *connective tissue diseases* because connective tissue is most often the target of inflammatory and/or autoimmune processes. Connective tissue is the most abundant tissue in the body, supporting and connecting other tissues and organs, and the cells and mediators of the immune system are widely distributed. Together, these features explain the frequent systemic nature of rheumatic diseases. Loose and dense connective tissues include cellular components and extracellular matrix. Loose connective tissue fills spaces between muscle sheaths, encases blood and lymphatic vessels, and holds fibroblasts that synthesize collagen fibers. It includes reticular fibers that provide the skeleton of muscle cells, nerves, and capillaries. Dense connective tissue supports the body's soft tissues and includes more collagen fibers and fewer cells. It is found in the dermis, joint capsules, cartilage, bone, and fascia of muscles, and it forms tendons, ligaments, and points of connection where these insert into bone (aponeurosis). Cells included in connective tissue may be migratory, such as mast cells or macrophages, or resident cells, such as fibroblasts, fibrocytes, and reticular cells. Fibroblasts are responsible for synthesizing collagen, elastic reticular fibers, and ground substance of extracellular matrix, including tissue fluids and collagen fibers. Importantly, connective tissue is integrated with cells associated with the body's defense system: lymphocytes, plasma cells, macrophages, dendritic cells, and eosinophils. The close proximity of connective tissue to blood vessels and cells of the immune system provides the setting for a group of disorders that are mediated by impaired immune system regulation and disruptions of the vascular system.

Classification of Rheumatic Diseases

More than 100 types of rheumatic diseases have been described. Although these can be considered to be based primarily on one of two (degenerative or inflammatory) overarching processes, one can further subdivide rheumatic diseases as follows (and also outlined in Table 241-1): (1) those associated with degeneration of connective tissues (Chapter 246) attributable to (a) trauma, (b) structural/mechanical imbalances, or (c) inherent early demise of cellular components; (2) those associated with systemic autoimmunity, often linked with measurable autoantibodies that can manifest primarily with (a) synovitis, (b) widespread organ involvement, (c) inflamed blood vessels (vasculitis), or (d) inflammation of muscle (myositis); (3) other inflammatory connective tissue diseases involving more dense tissues, not associated with the formation of autoantibodies and hence termed *seronegative rheumatic diseases* or *spondyloarthropathies* (Chapter 249); (4) diseases in which inflammation of the vasculature (vasculitis), particularly small, medium, or large arteries, is the predominant feature (Chapter 254); (5) autoinflammatory diseases (Chapter 245) that can be associated with crystal deposition or genetic mutations involving cytokine pathways; and (6) pain syndromes that must often be considered in the context of these diseases, in which some appear to be comorbid and closely linked to the underlying rheumatic disease, such as diffuse pain associated with Sjögren syndrome, hypermobility of connective tissue, or those regional pain syndromes that are anatomically linked to mechanical disruption. Patients presenting with generalized pain syndromes (Chapter 27) require investigation to exclude a connective tissue disease. Increasingly, genotypes have been identified that are associated with diseases that fall into each of these categories, and in some cases specific immunologic pathways have allowed grouping of a set of rheumatic diseases previously considered more distinct.

Mimics of rheumatic diseases exist, and clinicians need to be mindful of considering these when evaluating a patient for a rheumatic disease. For instance, arthropathies and syndromes resembling a rheumatic disease can occur in the settings of both infection and malignancy (Chapter 259). Autoimmune phenomena are increasingly being recognized in the setting of malignancy[4] or as a consequence of treatment of malignancy with immune checkpoint

TABLE 241-1	COMMON RHEUMATIC DISEASES BROADLY CLASSIFIED ACCORDING TO PATHOGENESIS				
DEGENERATIVE DISEASES OF BONES AND JOINTS	**SYSTEMIC AUTOIMMUNE DISEASES**	**SERONEGATIVE SPONDYLOARTHROPATHIES**	**VASCULAR RHEUMATIC DISEASES**	**AUTOINFLAMMATORY DISEASES**	**PAIN DISORDERS**
Osteoarthritis	Rheumatoid arthritis	Ankylosing spondylitis	ANCA-associated vasculitis	Adult-onset Still disease	Regional myofascial pain syndromes
DISH	Systemic lupus erythematosus	Psoriatic arthritis	Temporal artery vasculitis	Crystal diseases	Tendonitis/bursitis
Degenerative disc disease	Sjögren syndrome	Reactive arthritis	Polymyalgia rheumatica	Pediatric periodic fever syndromes	Adhesive capsulitis
Spinal stenosis	Inflammatory myopathies (polymyositis, dermatomyositis)	Enteropathic arthritis	Behçet disease		Complex regional pain syndrome type 1 (reflex sympathetic dystrophy)
Osteoporosis	Systemic sclerosis				Pain with hypermobility syndromes
					Fibromyalgia*

*The only pain disorder that has not been associated primarily with inflammation.
ANCA = antineutrophil cytoplasmic antibody; DISH = diffuse idiopathic sclerosing hyperostosis (also linked to metabolic factors, including elevated growth hormone).

TABLE 241-2 WORLDWIDE PREVALENCE* AND INCIDENCE OF RHEUMATIC DISEASES ASSOCIATED WITH AUTOIMMUNITY

DISEASE	NORTH AMERICA	CENTRAL AMERICA	SOUTH AMERICA	EUROPE	MIDDLE EAST	ASIA	SUB-SAHARAN AFRICA	AUSTRALIA
Rheumatoid arthritis	600-1000 (40)	400-2000	100-500	200-900 (2-7)	200-1500	100-800 (40-90)	Rare - 900	2000
Systemic lupus erythematosus	20-60 (2-7)	50-60 (5)	N/A	20-70 (2-7)	N/A	20-70 (3)	Rare	20-80 (11)
Systemic sclerosis	13-28	N/A	N/A	<10-15 (<2)	N/A	<10	N/A	23 (2)
Spondyloarthropathy (primarily ankylosing spondylitis)	50-130 (7)	N/A	N/A	100-850 (2-9)	500	10-240	Rare	N/A
Sjögren syndrome	320 (4)	N/A	N/A	200-600 (4-5)	N/A	330-700 (China)	N/A	N/A

*Prevalence (annual incidence) per 100,000 by world regions.
Data from Shapira Y, Agmon-Levin N, Shoenfeld Y. Geoepidemiology of autoimmune rheumatic diseases. *Nat Rev Rheumatol.* 2010;6(8):468-476; and Chaaya M, Slim ZN, Habib RR, et al. High burden of rheumatic diseases in Lebanon: a COPCORD study. *Int J Rheum Dis.* 2012;15(2):136-143.

inhibitors.[5,6] Red flags for each need to be considered in the assessment of a patient for possible rheumatic disease.

No classification of rheumatic disease can completely explain its genesis. However, considering these in a classification schema can aid in the approach to a patient in whom these disorders are being considered (see Table 241-1).

EPIDEMIOLOGY

Although connective tissue diseases can generally be categorized as noted in Table 241-1, in adults there are six prototypical rheumatic diseases that are most often assessed and managed by rheumatologists: rheumatoid arthritis, systemic lupus erythematosus (SLE), systemic sclerosis, spondyloarthropathies (primarily ankylosing spondylitis), Sjögren syndrome, and vasculitis. These diseases are ubiquitous and for the most part have a similar incidence and prevalence throughout the world (Table 241-2). Each is associated with characteristic immune aberrations and mechanisms of inflammatory damage, although the cause and reasons for chronicity still remain unknown. Autoimmune rheumatic diseases are also among the leading causes of death and morbidity in the industrial world, in part related to associated comorbid diseases, particularly cardiovascular disease. They represent a significant socioeconomic burden. Increasing evidence points to risks for their genesis relating to environmental factors, socioeconomic factors, and exposure to infectious agents, ultraviolet radiation, and pollutants. Smoking, in particular, has been associated with an increased risk for SLE and rheumatoid arthritis in genetically susceptible individuals in Western cultures. Effects of migration elucidate some of these risks. For instance, Africans who migrate far away from their native environmental and cultural origins appear to have an increased susceptibility to SLE. Also, reports have linked occupational exposures, such as silica dust, mercury, pesticides, solvents, and metals, to an increased risk for SLE and rheumatoid arthritis.

In some cases, geographic clusters of a rare autoimmune disease indicate specific genetic determinants. For example, with systemic sclerosis, higher incidence, prevalence, and mortality rates have been reported in African American populations compared with white populations, and the prevalence has been reported as higher in southern Europe, particularly Italy (prevalence of 7 to 33 per 100,000). Additionally, social and demographic factors may contribute to the epidemiology of rheumatic diseases. For example, the prevalence of SLE is reported as very high in Georgia, United States, whereas the prevalence of ankylosing spondylitis is rare in malaria endemic regions where HLA-B27 genotypes are rare. Inflammatory arthropathies, including rheumatoid arthritis and ankylosing spondylitis, have a higher prevalence in North American Native populations.

CLINICAL MANIFESTATIONS

Primary care and hospital-based health care providers are often the first to evaluate a patient with an evolving rheumatic disease, and they need to be attuned to the presenting features to make a timely diagnosis. In many cases, the presentation could signal a life- or organ-threatening condition. Evaluation of constitutional, systemic, and joint symptoms should always include rheumatic disease in the differential diagnosis.

Joint Symptoms as a Common Presenting Feature

Almost all rheumatic diseases can manifest with joint-related symptoms as a significant and frequently presenting feature. This can include symptoms of pain, stiffness, swelling, and erythema, or all of these symptoms, as in the case

of autoinflammatory diseases such as gout or pseudogout. The pattern of joint involvement, particularly duration and timing of maximal symptoms, can help the health care provider diagnose patients who present with spondyloarthropathy or any inflammatory arthritis, regardless of pathogenetic classification. For instance, joint pain that is worse in the morning, is associated with prolonged stiffness, and improves with activity is a classic presentation of inflammatory pain. In contrast, pain that is worse with activity, better with rest, and associated with a very short period of stiffness signals that it most likely has a degenerative etiology. Location provides a clue to broad classification. Patients describing "pain all over" may have a primary pain syndrome. However, pain with an inflammatory pattern localized to the spine or an enthesis (site of ligament insertion) is more likely to indicate a seronegative spondyloarthropathy. A patient presenting with an inflammatory pattern of symptoms predominantly involving the small joints of the hands and feet suggests the presence of one of the autoimmune rheumatic diseases associated with either a positive antinuclear antibody (ANA), rheumatoid factor (RF), or anticitrullinated peptide antibody (ACPA). Thus, the pattern of joint involvement is central to the evaluation and diagnosis of any rheumatic disease.

Nonspecific Clinical Presentations

All of the rheumatic diseases can be associated with joint involvement. However, joint symptoms are not always present in many of these diseases. Thus, a working knowledge of nonarticular patterns of disease presentation is important. Fever or cutaneous manifestations, including rashes, are common in vasculitis and in the presentation of SLE. Sicca symptoms are characteristic of Sjögren syndrome. Both Sjögren syndrome and inflammation of blood vessels can occur concurrently in patients with SLE. Systemic features such as myalgias or fatigue are common to almost all rheumatic diseases regardless of their classification, whereas true weakness may be the only presenting complaint of an inflammatory myopathy. Renal involvement is common to seropositive systemic autoimmune diseases and vasculitis and can present with anasarca if proteinuria is severe or prolonged. Consequently, specific and nonspecific features associated with various connective tissue diseases must be identified to develop correctly a differential diagnosis that fits within the classification described in Table 241-1. Features may evolve sequentially over time; thus, rheumatic diseases from more than one category must often be considered in a patient whose disease has not yet fully manifested before diagnosis, leaving the patient with a label of a nonspecific or undifferentiated connective tissue disease. Most rheumatic diseases have specific classification criteria. When these are not yet met, features are considered in the context of the broad classifications, and terms such as *undifferentiated inflammatory polyarthritis* or *undifferentiated spondyloarthropathy* may be used in the interim to aid in diagnosis and management. When a patient's disease is not yet diagnosed, testing and monitoring over time, as indicated in Figure 241-1, can help to identify an emerging rheumatic disease.

Cutaneous Manifestations

Although cutaneous manifestations are frequent in patients with seropositive autoimmune diseases, particularly SLE, they can be important findings in all autoimmune diseases. A nonblanching purpuric rash can indicate a vasculitis, and rashes involving specific extensor regions are common to dermatomyositis. In cases of SLE or dermatomyositis, rashes are triggered or worsened by exposure to ultraviolet light and tend to occur in a light-exposed distribution. Rashes of vasculitic origin can indicate either the presence of an autoimmune

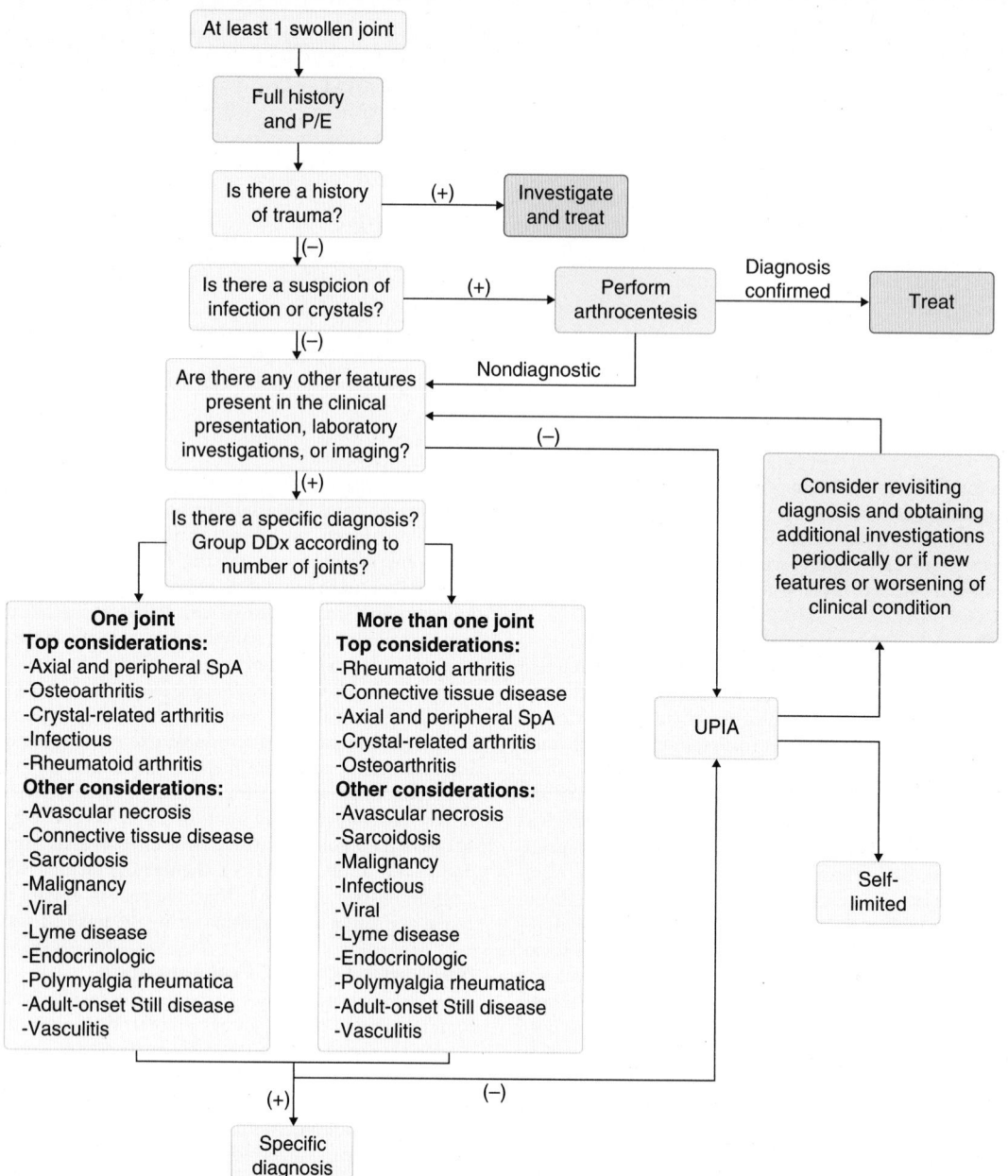

FIGURE 241-1. Algorithm for identification of undifferentiated peripheral inflammatory arthritis. Recommended minimum investigations in all patients: rheumatoid factor and/or anti–citrullinated peptide antibodies, erythrocyte sedimentation rate and/or C-reactive protein, complete blood count, and radiographs of affected joints. DDx = differential diagnosis; P/E = physical examination; SpA = spondyloarthritis; UPIA = undifferentiated peripheral inflammatory arthritis. (From Hazlewood G, Alethaha D, Carmona L, et al. Algorithm for identification of undifferentiated peripheral inflammatory arthritis: a multinational collaboration through the 3e initiative. *J Rheumatol Suppl.* 2011;87:54-58.)

disease such as SLE or an inflammatory vascular disease such as antineutrophil cytoplasmic antibody (ANCA)-associated vasculitis. These tend to be present for days and are often palpable, and a tissue biopsy of the lesions is very helpful in diagnosis. Rashes can be transient. In adult-onset Still disease (an adult form of systemic inflammatory arthritis classified as an autoinflammatory disease), patients present with daily spiking fevers, peaking late in the day, associated with a salmon-colored evanescent blanching rash lasting only 1 to 2 hours. The specific location of a rash aids in diagnosis. A facial rash that spares the nasolabial folds is classic for lupus. A rash that does not spare the nasolabial folds suggests rosacea. Psoriasis is almost always present in psoriatic arthritis (a spondyloarthropathy variant). Although psoriasis is often widespread, involving extensor surfaces, it can be missed if there are very few lesions or if it is located in areas that are not easily seen (intertriginous regions, such as in the ear, umbilicus, buttock creases, or scalp) or if it only involves the nails. The rash of psoriasis can be seen in any of the variants of the spondyloarthropathies. Occasionally rheumatoid arthritis manifests with nodules over the extensor surfaces or rashes in the same areas, but this is increasingly rare. However, the presence of nodules over extensor surfaces may also indicate gouty tophi. In systemic sclerosis, distal tightening of the skin, presence of telangiectasias, and digital ulcers can be seen. These should also be sought in

the context of Raynaud syndrome, characterized by vascular spasm in the hands.

Pattern of Onset of Rheumatic Diseases by Category

Most rheumatic diseases appear spontaneously and often insidiously or with a subacute onset. Not all will manifest with all typical features at the time of presentation, and a diagnosis can take time to make as defining features present themselves. Almost all rheumatic diseases have had classification criteria published that account for the typical and specific features of the disease. (These are detailed in other chapters.) Although classification criteria are generally published to ensure homogenous recruitment of participants in research studies, they can also aid in diagnosis. However, in an individual patient a diagnosis can be made without meeting all classification criteria because some features of a rheumatic disease are highly specific and are not associated with other diseases. For example, SLE is the only disease that presents with a classic malar rash and a particular autoantibody, anti-Sm, in the serum.

The natural history of each rheumatic disease is related to the severity of presentation, the specific additional organs that become involved, and the development of comorbidities. Rheumatoid arthritis may present with one or two swollen joints or pain in the forefoot. However, when the patient has a high titer of anti-cyclic citrullinated peptide antibody (ACPA), an autoantibody associated with development of erosive joint disease, the diagnosis can be made quickly and treatment initiated early. Autoimmune and vascular rheumatic diseases are associated with high morbidity and mortality when left untreated, and efforts to investigate for all manifestations early on are warranted.

Degenerative Rheumatic Diseases

These refer to rheumatic diseases commonly associated with advancing age. Degenerative joint disease is usually thought to include osteoarthritis and degenerative disc disease. Degenerative joint disease is heralded by breakdown of articular collagenous structures (cartilage or intervertebral discs) and development of bony hypertrophy. Controversy remains as to which occurs first. As collagenous structures degrade, associated inflammation commonly occurs. Resultant pain from varying causes contributes to immobility, secondary comorbidities, and disability. Degenerative joint disease represents, by far, the most common of the rheumatic diseases and is described in detail in Chapter 246. In general, these diseases are not associated with rashes or non-specific constitutional symptoms.

Autoimmune Rheumatic Diseases

These diseases include SLE, rheumatoid arthritis, systemic sclerosis, primary Sjögren syndrome, idiopathic inflammatory myositis, and the systemic vasculitides. They involve multiple organ systems and are therefore heterogeneous in clinical manifestations. Each symptom presentation is associated with specific signs and should be further characterized by additional investigations (Table 241-3), including measurement of characteristic autoantibodies in serum. Defined autoantibody specificities can discern subtypes of rheumatic diseases (Chapter 242; see Table 241-3). Many of these diseases affect females more than males. This is most striking in SLE (Chapter 250), which affects 8 to 10 women for every 1 man and typically has its onset in the childbearing years. As noted, cutaneous manifestations, sicca symptoms (of dry eyes or mouth), mucosal ulceration, fevers, alopecia, and Raynaud syndrome are common and often described by patients. These occur alone or in addition to symptoms affecting the joints and muscles. Rheumatoid arthritis (Chapter 248) has a female-to-male ratio of approximately 3 : 1 and typically has its onset in the later adult decades, with symmetrical small-medium joint synovitis as the classic presenting feature. Skin tightness is the hallmark of systemic sclerosis (Chapter 251), often referred to as scleroderma, which most often involves the extremities. Skin manifestations initially present with swelling of the digits,

followed by tightness of the hands and ultimately tightness of the skin. Raynaud phenomenon, although not specific to systemic sclerosis, frequently precedes its onset, often by many years. Skin tightness can go on to involve the face, arms, and, in the case of diffuse systemic sclerosis, the trunk, back, and legs. When features of rheumatic diseases present as the classical phenotype, making the diagnosis is straightforward. Diagnosis is more challenging when presenting features overlap between diseases. For instance, sicca symptoms, which are the prototype of primary Sjögren syndrome (Chapter 252) and are associated with Sjögren-specific autoantibody patterns, can occur concurrently in SLE and rheumatoid arthritis. Autoimmune vasculitides and SLE can share similar organ system manifestations, including those involving the lungs, kidneys, skin, and nervous systems. One or more of certain features, including constitutional disturbances such as fatigue, fever, weight loss, arthralgia, arthritis, and myalgias, are commonly seen in almost all rheumatic diseases. Overlap of symptoms expands the differential diagnosis, and a clear distinction is often not readily apparent, even after serologic testing. Tissue biopsy may help to provide a definitive answer.

Spondyloarthropathies

Ankylosing spondylitis (Chapter 249) manifesting with lower spine disease and earlier spinal fusion is more common in males than females. Disease in females may present more atypically with cervical or thoracolumbar symptoms in the primary presentation. Sacroiliitis is the hallmark of this disease. Localization of symptoms to the neck and thoracolumbar spine, sacroiliac joints, and large upper and lower extremity "root" joints can be used to differentiate ankylosing spondylitis from rheumatoid arthritis. The typical presence of psoriatic skin lesions in patients with psoriatic arthritis can be a distinguishing feature from rheumatoid arthritis. Spinal inflammation can also be associated with inflammatory bowel disease, not infrequently in the mid or upper spine as opposed to the sacroiliac joints.

Forms of Vasculitis

There are many vasculitis syndromes, and these are generally grouped based on vessel size (Chapter 254). Some are classified as such, although not always proved to be of vascular origin. Polymyalgia rheumatica (Chapter 255) is a common inflammatory rheumatic disease of the elderly and shares many pathogenetic and epidemiologic features with giant cell arteritis, a form of older-onset vasculitis.[7] Patients complain of aching around the neck and bilateral involvement of the shoulder and hip girdles, along with significant stiffness that is most problematic in the morning. Symptom onset can be abrupt or

---

TABLE 241-3 CLINICAL FEATURES AND CLUES TO FACILITATE DIAGNOSIS FOR EACH CATEGORY OF RHEUMATIC DISEASE

DEGENERATIVE DISEASES OF BONES AND JOINTS	SYSTEMIC AUTOIMMUNE DISEASES	SERONEGATIVE SPONDYLO-ARTHROPATHIES	VASCULAR RHEUMATIC DISEASES	AUTO-INFLAMMATORY DISEASES	PAIN DISORDERS
Investigate if persistent symptoms of pain >6 wk or failure of conservative measures (physical therapy, acetaminophen, NSAIDs). If at risk for bone loss and possible fragility fracture, consider osteoporosis.	Frequently associated with inflammatory joint pain and/or swelling with or without constitutional symptoms and other organ involvement. Perform ANA, RF, ESR, CRP.	Consider if psoriasis is present, or if back pain has inflammatory features; consider when known associated nonarticular features are present (e.g., uveitis, inflammatory bowel disease, urethritis, enthesitis, dactylitis).	Consider whenever infarction of tissue has occurred or if vasculitic rashes, pulmonary hemorrhage, or acute or subacute renal syndromes are present.	All can present with fever. In children, these are usually genetically determined syndromes mediated through interleukin-1 or TNF-α. In adults, consider crystal diseases.	Consider in situations where pain is in excess of findings, or if history of resolved trauma or repetitive strain, referred pain symptoms, diffuse pain, or colorful descriptions of pain.
INITIAL INVESTIGATIVE APPROACH TO CONFIRM SUSPECTED RHEUMATIC DISEASE IN EACH CATEGORY					
Image specific region associated with persistent pain (consider additional imaging in areas that may be referring pain). If osteoporosis is a concern, perform BMD and investigate using laboratory tests including calcium, 25(OH)D, and/or PTH to begin evaluation for metabolic bone diseases.	Investigations should specifically target suspected diseases. Specific testing should include CPK if weakness or myalgia; anti-CCP (ACPA) and RF if synovitis is present; ANA in screening rheumatic disease, and dsDNA, C3, C4, ENA if SLE or sicca symptoms present.	Imaging of sacroiliac (SI) joints (radiographs if long-standing symptoms, MRI if more recent onset). HLA-B27 testing if inflammatory back pain or SI pain most predominant, clinical suspicion high for inflammatory back pain, but imaging is negative.	Laboratory testing should include ANCA Anti-PR3 Anti-MPO Acute phase reactants (ESR, CRP) Tissue sampling of involved organs to facilitate pathophysiologic classification.	For suspected crystal disease, perform aspiration of synovial fluid or tophus and examine under polarized light microscopy.	Usually a diagnosis of exclusion, based on physical exam. In complex regional pain syndrome, tendonitis, or enthesitis, specific physical findings and imaging can facilitate diagnosis.

ACPA = anti–citrullinated peptide antibodies; ANA = antinuclear antibodies; ANCA = antinuclear cytoplasmic antibodies; anti-CCP = anti–cyclic citrullinated peptide; anti-MPO = anti-myeloperoxidase; anti-PR3 = antiproteinase-3; BMD = bone mineral density scan; CPK = creatinine phosphokinase; CRP = C-reactive protein; dsDNA = anti-double-stranded DNA; ENA = antibodies to extractable nuclear antigens (e.g., Ro, La, Sm, RNP, Scl70, Jo-1); ESR = erythrocyte sedimentation rate; MRI = magnetic resonance imaging; NSAIDs = nonsteroidal anti-inflammatory drugs; RF = rheumatoid factor; SLE = systemic lupus erythematosus; TNF-α = tumor necrosis factor-α; 25(OH)D = 25-hydroxyvitamin D; PTH = parathormone.

insidious over weeks to months. The diagnosis of polymyalgia rheumatica is primarily clinical. Recent diagnostic classification criteria are based on the typical clinical presentation and laboratory evidence of acute phase reactants. Mimics of polymyalgia rheumatica can include elderly onset rheumatoid arthritis; thus, tests to exclude this may be indicated. When considering polymyalgia rheumatica, it is important to include giant cell arteritis in the differential diagnosis, particularly when acute phase reactants are very high or there are nonmusculoskeletal symptoms or manifestations. These often involve inflammation of the temporal arteries. A high index of suspicion for temporal artery inflammation or large vessel disease involving the aorta is needed because clinical consequences of associated vascular inflammation in giant cell arteritis can be damaging, sometimes leading to blindness or stroke, or to more severe vascular destruction and organ ischemia, which can be life-threatening.

Autoinflammatory Diseases

Rare autoinflammatory diseases are based on mutations in genes involved in inflammatory pathways. They are more typically diagnosed in children and are covered in detail in Chapter 245. Gout (Chapter 257) is the most common and prototypical autoinflammatory disease, occurring more often in middle-aged and older men, and is increasing in prevalence. Exquisitely painful joint and periarticular erythema and swelling are presenting features. Tophi that might be confused with rheumatoid nodules can be seen. High serum uric acid is associated with gout, although levels may lower during acute attacks.

Pain and Pain Syndromes

Pain (also see Chapter 27) is a common and nonspecific, but very important, symptom central to nearly all rheumatic diseases. Pain is the key presenting feature of joint disease reported by patients. Location, distribution, and patterns should be elicited along with temporal features, triggers, migratory or alleviating features, and prior history of physical or psychological trauma. In regional pain syndromes, the distribution of pain is the key clue to the diagnosis. Diffuse pain without evidence of underlying pathology associated with inordinate levels of fatigue, difficulty coping, and intricately detailed descriptions of pain using colorful analogies herald fibromyalgia (Chapter 258). Fibromyalgia is defined as widespread pain involving the right and left sides and upper and lower extremities, as well as the neck and back. Most pain syndromes are regional pain syndromes. For instance, a regional pain syndrome relating to a mechanical neck and shoulder syndrome will result in the patient having pain in the involved neck and shoulder but also the trapezius, upper chest, axilla, and upper and/or lower arm and hand. A large proportion of patients presenting with musculoskeletal pain will have regional pain relating to muscular imbalances, postural factors with or without underlying degenerative arthritis, tendinopathy, or enthesopathy. As an example, pain syndromes in the trapezial region, referring down the arm to the deltoid and even forearm, can be multifactorial and associated with a combination of muscular spasm, underlying degenerative arthritis in the cervical spine, or rotator cuff impingement, not infrequently relating to repetitive activities. Pain in a distal extremity after trauma or surgery associated with a cold, shiny extremity is suggestive of complex regional pain syndrome. The etiology of these will become apparent with taking a careful history of pain features along with a medical history, physical examination, and exclusion of "red flags" or factors that indicate an underlying pathology specific to a related organ from which pain can be referred. Pain in the setting of a history of malignancy should suggest the possibility of metastases. A tick bite may indicate prior Lyme disease. Dermatomal distributions are seen with disc herniations or shingles. Most pain syndromes warrant a full medical evaluation before making a definitive diagnosis.

DIFFERENTIAL DIAGNOSIS AND DIAGNOSTIC EVALUATION

A comprehensive history is needed to complete an evaluation of a patient with a rheumatic disease. In addition to considering age and gender, a patient's personal history, including marital status, occupation, and psychosocial factors, helps to elucidate a patient's diagnosis, prognosis, and treatment options. Clues helpful in making a diagnosis of one of the rheumatic diseases are summarized in Table 241-3.

Assessing clinical signs and symptoms is the cornerstone of diagnosis. Most rheumatic disorders will present with symptoms that involve, or seem to involve, joints. This can be limited to pain involving a specific joint or group of joints or periarticular structures. Querying the patient to determine the pattern of symptoms—whether pain, swelling, or stiffness associated with joints—is key to narrowing the differential diagnosis of a rheumatic disease. Joint symptoms should be assessed for inflammatory features such as prolonged stiffness, pain at rest, or noninflammatory and mechanical features, such as instability or giving way, locking, or increased symptoms with use. Patterns of joint

involvement—whether primarily small joints of the hands, wrist, and feet; large joints of the elbows, knees, ankles, or "root" (shoulders or hips); or spinal involvement—will further point to a specific diagnosis. Moreover, questions regarding recent illnesses, travel, exposure to possible infectious pathogens, and presence or absence of systemic features such as fever, fatigue, or weight loss will provide important clues. Appreciation of signs and symptoms indicating extra-articular features, particularly cutaneous, pulmonary, renal, neurologic, or vascular manifestations, will guide the differential diagnosis, and further investigations will help to determine the definitive diagnosis as well as the prognosis and required intensity of therapy.

The presence of one rheumatic disease can be associated with comorbid manifestations unrelated to connective tissue. For example, myocardial infarction is more common in many patients with rheumatic diseases. Immobility or treatment-related factors leading to obesity can increase risks for diabetes and lower joint degeneration.

Factors in the Medical History that Contribute to Diagnosis and Prognosis

Age and Gender

Certain rheumatic diseases typically manifest in childhood. These include genetically based disorders, such as hemophilia associated with arthritis, and a number of autoinflammatory conditions that are by definition childhood diseases. Juvenile idiopathic arthritis refers to forms of arthritis in which the onset occurs before the age of 16 years. Autoimmune rheumatic diseases, and inflammatory rheumatic diseases such as spondyloarthropathies, rheumatoid arthritis, and SLE, can begin in young adulthood, whereas degenerative conditions such as osteoarthritis rarely do and more often begin to manifest in the middle and late middle years. The peak onset of rheumatoid arthritis occurs in the late middle years, although onset can occur at almost any time in life. Elderly people are more prone to osteoarthritis and polymyalgia rheumatica, but the latter has a wide differential diagnosis and should be considered at all ages. Autoimmune diseases are more common in women, whereas spondyloarthropathies can be equally common in men and women. Gouty arthritis is more common in men and rarely attacks women before menopause.

Occupation and Recreation

Occupation and recreational activities may give rise to physical and psychological stresses. The demands of a patient's occupation need to be understood, particularly when repetitive activities may contribute to the development of degenerative joint disease or to regional pain syndromes. Similarly, trauma from sports, including prior injuries, can be a significant contributor to degenerative joint disease.

Family History

It is important to obtain a complete family history because autoimmune diseases, spondyloarthropathies, and gout occur with an increased incidence in families. It is common to see family pedigrees in which different forms of autoimmunity occur throughout a family. This does not mean that any one autoimmune disease has specific heritability. Also, generalized osteoarthritis that involves the hands and other joints commonly runs in families.

Concomitant Medication Use

Concomitant medications may contribute to the genesis of a rheumatic disease. For example, diuretics can increase hyperuricemia and risk for gouty arthritis. Minocycline can be associated with lupus-like presentations. Antibiotics in the fluoroquinolone class have been associated with enthesopathies. A full medication history needs to be considered in the assessment of patients with rheumatic diseases.

Habits and Social Circumstances

Smoking has increasingly been associated with rheumatoid arthritis and SLE. Also, poor socioeconomic circumstances and psychosocial or physical stress may contribute to the severity of symptoms and should be considered in planning management strategies. Similarly, patients of different ethnic and cultural origins may have differences in their ability to describe symptoms and in preferences around treatment choices.

Onset and Evolution of Symptoms

Knowledge of the pattern of onset, location, and evolution of symptoms is essential to make an accurate diagnosis of a rheumatic disease. Symptoms that develop over hours to days typically suggest an inflammatory, or possibly an infectious or traumatic, process. When they persist for more than 6 weeks, symptom onset is considered subacute, and the disease chronic. Early in the presentation of some rheumatic diseases, the symptoms can be intermittent or palindromic before becoming constant. Sudden onset of joint pain and swelling, particularly involving one or a few joints, should be considered to be due to an infectious or crystalline etiology during the course of investigation.

Pain and Stiffness

Pain assessment should include a description of its onset, constancy/chronicity, severity, quality, factors that trigger or improve it, and location and radiation of the pain. Stiffness, often described as tightness or linked to difficulty with movement or function, should be determined in terms of location (e.g., is it in a particular joint or more diffuse) and timing and duration (e.g., occurring after a period of rest). Stiffness that resolves in 10 to 15 minutes is more characteristic of osteoarthritis. In inflammatory disease, stiffness typically lasts longer, often at least 1 hour and even all day.

Joint Involvement

The distribution of joint involvement is key to making a diagnosis of a rheumatic disease. Monoarthritis describes symptoms in a single joint; oligoarthritis (or pauciarthritis) refers to symptoms in two to four joints; and polyarthritis indicates involvement of at least five joints. Peripheral arthritis involves an extremity, whereas spinal involvement is termed *axial disease*. Symmetrical as opposed to asymmetrical peripheral joint disease is more commonly associated with autoimmune rheumatic disorders, whereas asymmetrical arthritis can be associated with spondyloarthropathies or osteoarthritis. Similarly, predominant small joint involvement is more typical in rheumatoid arthritis or SLE, whereas large joint involvement is classic for spondyloarthropathies. In addition, the presence of associated enthesitis and axial symptoms herald spondyloarthropathy. Joint or spine symptoms associated with inflammatory causes often include predominance of symptoms in the morning, associated with stiffness for more than 60 minutes, worsening with rest, and improvement over the day and with activity. Joint or spine symptoms associated with degenerative joint disease typically worsen with activity, are often worse later in the day, are associated with stiffness, and typically resolve quickly over 15 to 30 minutes. Joint pain is usually felt at the joints (exceptions include shoulder pain, felt over the deltoid, and hip pain, felt in the groin). Joint pain from degenerative or inflammatory causes can vary in severity. Most patients will describe joint pain as aching and rarely rate the pain higher than 8/10 on an ascending severity scale. Pain relating to localized myofascial pain syndromes, including tendinopathies and enthesopathies, may be described as being close to joints, and being worse with specific movements. In people suffering from generalized pain syndromes, pain is often rated very highly (10/10) and is poorly localized, involving upper and lower body regions, with descriptions including qualifiers to impress the severity of the pain ("like a truck ran over me").

It is also important to distinguish between arthralgia (subjective joint pain without objective signs) and arthritis, where pain and tenderness are associated with objective signs of joint swelling and warmth (synovitis), deformity, or limitation of movement. Objective findings on physical examination must be identified for a diagnosis of arthritis to be made.

Function

Function is commonly compromised in patients with rheumatic disease. Although this can be related to fatigue or muscular weakness, in the case of rheumatic disorders in which there is no articular involvement, most commonly functional impairment is related to joint involvement. Function should be assessed in terms of a patient's ability to perform activities of daily living, work, and participation. Validated questionnaires of function are available to identify functional limitations.

Physical Examination
Essential Concepts

There is an increased understanding of the ontogenic and cellular and molecular basis of specific patterns of joint involvement and affected organ systems, which tend to associate with each class of rheumatic disease.[8] Once familiar with these, physical examination readily augments the diagnostic process. A complete examination by a physician is required to identify and classify a rheumatic disease. This should include an assessment of constitutional symptoms such as temperature, body mass index, affect, pain behaviors, gait, and posture as well as organ-specific examination of the scalp, skin, eyes, lymphatic system, cardiovascular system, lungs, abdomen, joints, spine, and skeletal muscles. A systematic joint examination is key to the rheumatic disease examination and should include all regions, with comparisons of right and left sides. The pattern of joint involvement, including symmetry and axial versus peripheral

involvement, should be recorded. Use of a joint diagram (homunculus) helps to track joint involvement. The joint examination should include documentation of the presence or absence of tenderness, periarticular wasting, erythema, swelling, limitation in range of motion (ROM), sites of prior surgery and trauma, and joint deformity, allowing for comparison over time and between different examiners. Using a four-step systematic approach to joint examination facilitates a thorough examination. This should include (1) inspection (looking for asymmetry, erythema, swelling, and deformity), (2) palpation (feeling for tenderness, specifically joint line tenderness, warmth, synovial thickening and effusion, bony hypertrophy, and crepitus), (3) ROM (both active and passive for each joint), and (4) special tests specific to each joint or region. A complete examination should also consider relevant extra-articular manifestations.

Examples of Musculoskeletal Findings that Help to Classify a Rheumatic Disease

When considering the joint examination, a finding of redness (erythema) can indicate more acute and/or severe inflammation. The presence of erythema is more typically seen in the case of infection or crystalline (autoinflammatory) arthritis. Joint warmth also signifies underlying inflammation. Joint swelling, a definitive sign of joint inflammation or arthritis, may indicate the presence of a joint effusion (excess synovial fluid) or synovial thickening indicating an active inflammatory process involving increased vascularization, cellular recruitment, and transudate and edema in the synovial membrane (synovitis). All rheumatic diseases short of specific neurologically mediated pain syndromes can present with synovitis. Palpable bony thickening around a joint, particularly distal or proximal phalangeal joints or first metacarpal joints, is due to bone reaction and proliferation or osteophytes, characteristic of osteoarthritis. Examiners should palpate for crepitus, which feels like a grinding sensation under the examiner's hand during active or passive joint motion. Fine or velvety crepitus may indicate chronic proliferative synovitis, whereas coarse crepitus may indicate either roughening of the cartilage surface or complete loss of hyaline cartilage with bone moving on bone. The end result of any chronic arthritic process will lead to primary or secondary joint degeneration and will manifest as loss of cartilage or bony hypertrophy. In some diseases such as rheumatoid arthritis, psoriatic arthritis, or Jaccoud arthropathy (a form of SLE-related deforming arthropathy), deformity occurs as a result of joint subluxation or contracture related to nature's forces on weakened, lax, distended joint capsules and lax ligaments and tendons as a consequence of chronic swelling from synovitis. Typically, muscle atrophy occurs around arthritic joints and contributes to feelings of weakness or instability. Interarticular cartilage becomes more prone to rupture.

Assessing Range of Motion

Both active and passive ROM should be assessed to appreciate joint function. Generally, active ROM is assessed first by asking patients to demonstrate full ROM of a joint; active ROM requires intact strength, innervation, muscle and tendon function, and joint mobility. Passive ROM is assessed by the examiner and for the most part assesses joint mobility or in some cases ligament or tendon impingement. First assessing active ROM enables the examiner to appreciate potential areas of pain and where to examine carefully. If mobility is full on passive ROM, other causes can be considered for loss of mobility.

Establishing a Diagnosis

The findings from a thorough history and physical examination, along with an appropriate set of investigations, can be used to guide diagnosis. Table 241-3 and Figure 241-1 inform the clinical phenotype typical of a rheumatic disease, with diagnosis based on the broad classifications in Table 241-1. By using this algorithm and patterns and findings denoted in Table 241-3, clinicians can hone-in on a differential diagnosis and then use investigations to confirm the suspected diagnosis.

Laboratory and Imaging in Rheumatic Diseases

Identifying the presence of specific laboratory (Chapter 242) or imaging features can support a diagnosis and aid in specific classification of a rheumatic disease.[9] For example, a positive antinuclear antibody test is nonspecific,[10,11] but testing ANCAs or imaging the vascular tree of an involved area can be key to establishing a diagnosis in patients with vasculitis.[12] Similarly, in seronegative spondyloarthropathies, imaging of the sacroiliac joints using radiographs when symptoms are sustained, or magnetic resonance imaging (MRI) if the disease is of more recent onset, is key. Radiographs and MRIs of specific joint areas in degenerative joint disease not only help establish diagnosis but also aid in staging the disease. In the case of rheumatoid arthritis, testing of rheumatoid factor and ACPA is critical. When considering other prototypical seropositive systemic rheumatic diseases, the list of potential autoantibodies is much longer, and depending on the degree of difficulty in making the diagnosis, or appreciating the extent of disease and associated organ involvement, many of these can be considered for testing. It should be noted that no test alone should be used to diagnose a rheumatic disease, but rather the tests should support the diagnosis.

TREATMENT   Rx

The treatment approaches to each rheumatic disease are highlighted in detail in the following chapters. Therapeutic approaches to degenerative rheumatic diseases focus on control of symptoms of pain with either nonsteroidal anti-inflammatory drugs or analgesics. Physical modalities, strengthening, and encouraging activity are a key part of managing degenerative arthritis; at times, injections of glucocorticoids or other agents can manage symptoms. When conservative approaches fail, orthopedic surgery is warranted. However, the approach to systemic and inflammatory rheumatic diseases usually requires more intense or immunomodulatory therapies. Glucocorticoids are a major component of treatment regimens, particularly when organs are at risk for damage, when other agents take time to become fully effective, and in situations in which there are no alternative options for therapy. However, glucocorticoids are not without risk, and these should be discussed with each patient. Depending on the disease, glucocorticoid-sparing therapies are usually initiated early, with potency tailored to the severity and risk for the illness itself, while considering patients' other comorbid conditions and other medications being used. For example, SLE patients presenting with only a rash or synovitis may require a relatively weak agent, hydroxychloroquine, whereas patients with renal disease may need mycophenolate mofetil, cyclophosphamide, or other parenteral immunomodulatory therapies to treat effectively that disease manifestation. Similarly, in rheumatoid arthritis, patients presenting with high-titer ACPA levels and a high swollen joint count, with erosions having been observed on baseline radiographs of the hands and feet, are candidates for rapidly escalating doses of methotrexate with or without other disease-modifying antirheumatic drugs and earlier use of biologic or targeted synthetic drugs as outlined in Chapter 33. More detail regarding specific approaches and use of glucocorticoid-sparing therapies is presented in chapters addressing each rheumatic disease. Current thinking is to use glucocorticoids as transitional therapy with a plan to taper these as soon as possible and to use them again only for disease exacerbations.

SUMMARY

A broad-based set of rheumatic disease classifications can provide an overall construct for consideration of a multitude of possible rheumatic diseases. When the classifications are based on pathogenic mechanisms as well as clinical features, this facilitates identification of specific symptoms and signs and guides a further line of investigation. Although all rheumatic diseases will not fit within this classification, a systematic and directed analysis will accelerate achieving the correct diagnosis of the patient.

GENERAL REFERENCES

For the General References and other additional features, please visit Expert Consult at https://expertconsult.inkling.com.

242

LABORATORY TESTING IN THE RHEUMATIC DISEASES

DAVID S. PISETSKY

The rheumatic diseases are a heterogeneous group of conditions that involve inflammation and damage of the musculoskeletal system as well as other organs. These conditions range from mild, diffuse joint and muscle pain to severe life-threatening kidney failure and stroke. Although the rheumatic diseases have diverse origins, immune disturbances are frequently the etiology. The diagnostic approach therefore entails laboratory tests to assess functional disturbances of individual organs and their relationship to inflammation and autoimmunity.

Laboratory testing in patients suspected of having a rheumatic disease involves determination of biomarkers of the following kinds: antecedent (risk for disease), screening (subclinical disease), diagnostic (overt disease), staging (disease severity or activity), and prognostic (disease course, response to therapy, monitoring therapy). Of these tests, some are useful in all contexts. Because of the increasing efficacy of treatment for diseases such as rheumatoid arthritis (RA), laboratory screening may be important to improve outcomes by identifying individuals who have symptoms (e.g., arthralgias) that could represent the first manifestations of disease (preclinical autoimmunity); serologic screening could also be useful in identifying individuals at risk for disease (e.g., siblings or first-degree relatives). In many diseases, prognosis can reflect ongoing disease activity as well as damage from past disease activity and effects of treatment, with laboratory testing needed to assess these various processes.

MARKERS OF INFLAMMATION

For many patients, the initial goal of evaluation is to determine the presence of inflammation. Inflammation is the body's response to injury and is characterized by a cascade of cellular and molecular events that arise irrespective of stimulus or locale (Chapter 42). The immediate response to inflammatory stimuli is termed the *acute phase response* and includes a set of proteins produced primarily in the liver in response to cytokines such as interleukin-6 (IL-6), tumor necrosis factor-α (TNF-α), and IL-1. These cytokines are expressed by macrophages and dendritic cells after stimulation of pattern recognition receptors (PRRs) that include both toll-like receptors (TLRs) and other non-TLR sensing systems that trigger a system called the *inflammasome*; PRRs recognize intracellular as well as extracellular bacterial and viral products as well as large and small (e.g., adenosine triphosphate, uric acid) molecules released from damaged cells. The result is stimulation of innate immunity (Chapters 40 and 42). Of acute phase proteins, C-reactive protein (CRP) has received the most attention as a marker of inflammation. CRP is a member of the pentraxin family; although its function is not fully known, its ability to bind to phosphocholine suggests a scavenger function to eliminate bacterial products or damaged cells and thereby attenuate the consequences of infection or tissue injury. Other molecules, such as serum amyloid protein (SAP), fibrinogen, and complement, also show marked elevations in levels during the acute phase response, signifying a broad-based effort at host defense.

The CRP level provides a nonspecific but very useful measure of inflammation and can convey information for categorization of a clinical process (e.g., inflammatory versus noninflammatory arthritis) as well as assessment of disease activity or prognosis (e.g., activity of RA or likelihood of joint erosion). The advantage of measuring CRP in the blood, rather than cytokines, is that the protein levels are much higher. Furthermore, CRP levels remain elevated for a longer period (days) than do cytokines; the latter may appear only transiently in the blood. Although CRP testing is commonly performed to assess the risk for atherosclerosis (presumably because of the intimate pathophysiological relationship between inflammation and atherogenesis), the application of this screening in a patient with an inflammatory condition must take into account the various determinants of this marker.[1]

Another simple laboratory test reflecting the acute phase response is the erythrocyte sedimentation rate (ESR). In this test, commonly called the *sed rate*, anticoagulated blood is drawn into a long, thin tube and allowed to settle under the influence of gravity for 1 hour. The distance the blood falls depends on a number of factors, including the concentration of serum proteins such as immunoglobulins and fibrinogen as acute phase reactants. The sedimentation rate is nonspecific with respect to disease association and also depends on the age and gender of the person. Other simple laboratory tests (e.g., complete blood count) can reflect ongoing inflammation. For example, patients with inflammation frequently exhibit a leukocytosis or thrombocytosis, most likely reflecting the action of cytokines and other mediators, including glucocorticoids, during this process. With chronic inflammation, anemia of chronic disease can also occur. In this regard, in systemic lupus erythematosus (SLE), lymphopenia, thrombocytopenia, and low CRP values often characterize active disease, with the discordance between laboratory and clinical findings a clue to diagnosis.

LABORATORY EVALUATION OF MUSCULOSKELETAL DISEASE

The most common presentation of musculoskeletal disease is pain in and around the joints in association with functional impairment. Collectively, diseases causing joint symptoms are called arthritis, implying inflammation. The extent of inflammation in these diseases varies markedly, however, with some forms such as osteoarthritis (Chapter 246) showing only limited evidence of inflammation either locally or systemically.

Arthritis can be characterized by the number and size of joints affected, symmetry, and involvement of the axial as well as peripheral joints. For each pattern (e.g., chronic polyarthritis), a key issue in diagnosis concerns its place in the spectrum of inflammatory versus noninflammatory arthritis. Furthermore, although many diseases can cause arthritis, their prevalence varies enormously, with osteoarthritis or degenerative joint disease being the most common form of noninflammatory arthritis and RA the most common form of inflammatory arthritis.

The differential diagnosis of arthritis is based on a comprehensive history and physical examination to assess symptoms suggesting inflammation (e.g., morning stiffness and fatigue), the presence of synovitis, and results of laboratory tests indicative of inflammation. Of these tests, the ESR and CRP are nonspecific indicators of inflammation. Depending on the stage of disease and prior therapy of the patient, however, both the CRP and ESR may not be elevated at the time of an initial evaluation because many treatments, especially those directed against cytokines, can reduce the acute phase response. Two autoantibody tests, rheumatoid factor (RF) and antibodies to citrullinated proteins, provide more specific diagnostic information. Given the demographics of inflammatory arthritis, testing for antinuclear antibodies (ANAs) is often part of this evaluation as well.

Rheumatoid Factor

RF comprises a family of antibody specificities that bind to the immunoglobulin G (IgG) molecule, reacting with antigenic determinants that are most likely conformational in origin in the Fc portion. IgM RFs are the most abundant of these antibodies and are the easiest to measure, using agglutination assays with red blood cells or latex beads coated with IgG. More recently, enzyme-linked immunosorbent assays (ELISA) and nephelometry have been used to detect RFs.

RFs occur in approximately 60 to 80% of patients with RA (Chapter 248) and represent one criterion for the classification or diagnosis of this disease.[2] Furthermore, high levels of RFs are often associated with a worse prognosis, the occurrence of joint erosion as measured by radiographs, and deformity. Despite these associations, RFs occur in the sera of patients with a wide range of autoimmune and inflammatory diseases as well as in normal individuals, especially with age (Table 242-1). As a result, the 94% specificity of the test for RA results in a positive predictive value (the proportion of people with a positive test who have RA) of only about 20 to 35%.[3] The frequent occurrence of RFs may reflect their etiology and role in innate immune responses to promote the binding of IgG to antigen by Fc cross-linking.

Antibodies to Citrullinated Proteins

Antibodies to citrullinated proteins are other autoantibody specificities important in the diagnosis of RA (Chapter 248). Citrulline is a post-translational modification of the amino acid arginine that results from deamidation. This chemical reaction is catalyzed by the enzyme peptidylarginine deiminase (PAD) and may occur in the setting of inflammation; the function of this modification is unknown. Citrullination can affect many different proteins, creating antigenic sites on proteins that include vimentin, enolase, and filaggrin.[4]

Although antibodies are directed to citrullinated residues on intact proteins, they can be measured using synthetic peptides containing citrulline. Among these synthetic antigens, a citrulline-containing peptide with a cyclic structure provides sensitive and specific assays in an ELISA format. Antibodies directed to this type of antigen are known as anti-CCP (cyclic citrullinated peptide) and can be formally distinguished from antibodies to the citrullinated proteins themselves (ACPA, or anti–citrullinated protein antibodies). The term anti-CCP is commonly used for these specificities, although it is not formally synonymous with ACPA. ACPA can be assessed by a variety of analytic techniques using as antigens both modified proteins as well as arrays of peptides. For detection of anti-CCP antibodies, the formulation of peptides has changed over the years as designated by assay generation. Furthermore, among commercially available assays, results can vary, making it important to know the performance characteristics of assays in interpreting the results of testing.

Anti-CCP antibodies are highly associated with RA and represent a criterion in the classification of patients with this disease.[5] Depending on the assay, these antibodies occur in 60 to 70% of patients with RA and uncommonly in those with other forms of inflammatory arthritis. Significantly, anti-CCP antibodies can occur before the onset of other signs and symptoms of RA,

TABLE 242-1 RHEUMATIC DISEASES AND NONRHEUMATIC CONDITIONS ASSOCIATED WITH A POSITIVE RHEUMATOID FACTOR

DISEASES	FREQUENCY
Rheumatoid arthritis	50-90%
Systemic lupus erythematosus	15-35%
Sjögren syndrome	75-95%
Systemic sclerosis	20-30%
Polymyositis/dermatomyositis	5-10%
Cryoglobulinemia	40-100%
Mixed connective tissue disease	50-60%
Aging (>70 yr)	10-25%
Infection	
Bacterial endocarditis	25-50%
Liver disease	15-40%
Tuberculosis	8%
Syphilis	Up to 13%
Parasitic diseases	20-90%
Leprosy	5-58%
Viral infection	15-65%
Pulmonary disease	
Sarcoidosis	3-33%
Interstitial pulmonary fibrosis	10-50%
Silicosis	30-50%
Asbestosis	30%
Miscellaneous diseases	
Primary biliary cirrhosis	45-70%
Malignancy	5-25%

Modified from Shmerling RH, Delbanco TL. The rheumatoid factor: an analysis of clinical utility. *Am J Med.* 1991;91:530.

suggesting utility for screening of at-risk patients. In addition, in patients with arthralgias without evidence of synovitis by examination, the presence of anti-CCP may predict the development of subsequent arthritis. Thus, because of the specificity of anti-CCP for RA, the presence of these antibodies in patients with early signs and symptoms of disease may indicate the diagnosis of RA and allow initiation of therapy before disease is fully manifest. In this regard, although RA can occur in the absence of anti-CCP antibodies, the presence of these antibodies may define disease subsets that differ in etiology, clinical course, and response to therapy.

Joint Fluid Analysis

Analysis of joint fluid can provide decisive data in the evaluation of arthritis and, in some instances, a definitive diagnosis. This analysis is essential in the setting of acute monoarthritis to investigate the possibility of infection; for chronic forms of arthritis, joint fluid should be analyzed if there is uncertainty about the diagnosis and involvement of one joint out of proportion to others. Joint aspiration is a sterile procedure performed with a local anesthetic. Although fluid can be analyzed by tests to assess viscosity and mucin content, the cell count, examination of crystals, and stains and cultures to evaluate infection are the most informative.

On the basis of cell counts, joint fluids can be categorized into four main types: noninflammatory, inflammatory, septic, and hemorrhagic. A noninflammatory fluid has fewer than 2000 cells/μL with mononuclear cell predominance. An inflammatory fluid has more than 2000 cells/μL, with 50,000 cells/μL frequently used as the upper limit for this type of fluid. In an inflammatory fluid, polymorphonuclear cells predominate. A septic fluid is an inflammatory fluid in which culture or staining for microorganisms demonstrates infection. Suspicion of infection is especially high for fluids with cell counts greater than 50,000/μL. However, crystal-induced arthritis can produce cell counts of this magnitude, and an infected fluid can have counts below this level. Hemorrhagic fluids have red cell predominance that can approximate that of blood.

In the setting of an acute monoarthritis, crystal-induced disease is much more common than infection, with the presence of crystals demonstrated by polarization microscopy. With this technique, monosodium urate crystals in gout appear needle shaped and are negatively birefringent. On careful microscopic analysis, urate and calcium pyrophosphate crystals coexist in a single joint in about 2.5% of cases of crystal arthritis.[6] In contrast, calcium pyrophosphate dihydrate crystals in pseudogout are rhomboidal in shape and are weakly positively birefringent. Infection can coexist with crystal-induced disease, necessitating microbiologic evaluation even when crystals are found. Hemorrhagic fluids can also result from infection, although their presence suggests malignancy or trauma. Figure 242-1 provides an algorithm for the analysis of joint fluid.

Depending on the clinical findings and the results of initial laboratory testing, other studies may be performed to investigate less common diagnostic possibilities such as metabolic disease or malignancy. The laboratory evaluation of inflammatory arthritis may also include serologic tests for infections such as Lyme disease, human immunodeficiency virus (HIV) infection, or hepatitis.

LABORATORY EVALUATION OF SYSTEMIC INFLAMMATORY DISEASE

Among rheumatic diseases, some cause organ-threatening and life-threatening manifestations. These diseases can have arthritis as a component and presenting complaint, although the prominence of extra-articular manifestations, especially

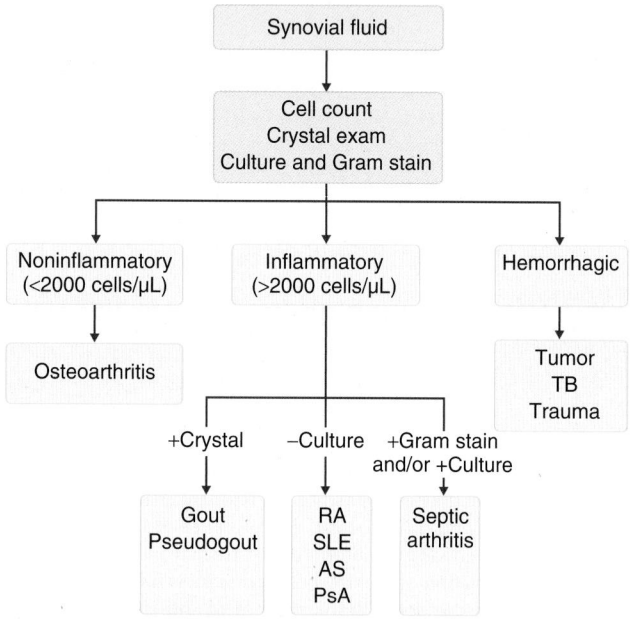

FIGURE 242-1. Algorithm for analysis of joint fluid. Examples of inflammatory arthritis are indicated, although many conditions can produce these findings. AS = ankylosing spondylitis; PsA = psoriatic arthritis; RA = rheumatoid arthritis; SLE = systemic lupus erythematosus; TB = tuberculosis.

as they develop over time and involve organs such as the kidney, points to their systemic nature. These diseases can be categorized on the basis of clinical, serologic, and pathologic findings, with the presence of vasculitis, irrespective of blood vessel size, providing a unifying feature in disease classification.

The terms *connective tissue disease* (CTD) and *collagen vascular disease* are both used to denote a group of diseases that includes RA, SLE, Sjögren syndrome, polymyositis, dermatomyositis, and progressive systemic sclerosis. Diseases in this group can have common clinical features, especially early in their course, when their presentations may be similar. In this stage of disease, the condition may be called *undifferentiated CTD*, with serologic markers sometimes predictive of the eventual diagnosis.

Antinuclear Antibodies

The expression of antibodies to components of the cell nucleus (antinuclear antibodies, or ANAs) is characteristic of CTD and is essentially invariable in patients with SLE (Chapter 250).[7] ANA positivity is also seen in 90 to 95% of patients with systemic sclerosis (Chapter 251).[8] These antibodies target a host of nuclear macromolecules, including DNA, RNA, and proteins as well as complexes of proteins with nucleic acid. These antigens are ubiquitously expressed in cells and subserve critical processes related to chromosomal structure, cell division, transcription, and translation. The basis for the antigenicity of these molecules is unknown, although DNA and RNA both have intrinsic immunologic activity and can stimulate cytokine production through their action on both TLR and non-TLR PRRs, especially when in the form of immune complexes. Furthermore, these antigens may undergo post-translation modification as well as enzymatic cleavage reactions during cell death, perhaps increasing their immunogenicity.

ANAs are commonly measured by immunofluorescence (IF) assays in which sera are incubated with tissue culture cells (e.g., HEp2 cells) fixed to a glass slide. Antibody binding is revealed by fluorescence microscopy after incubation of the slide with a fluoresceinated anti-immunoglobulin reagent. Results are reported in terms of the pattern of fluorescence as well as the end-point titer of sera at which fluorescence can be observed. The patterns of binding differ depending on the location of the macromolecular target, although a few patterns predominate. These patterns include homogeneous, rim, nucleolar, and speckled; in addition, ANA tests can detect antibodies to cytoplasmic antigens. Table 242-2 presents a list of major ANAs with their pattern and disease associations.

A major limitation of ANA assays concerns the frequency of positive reactivity in the sera of otherwise healthy individuals who lack evidence of a CTD. Depending on the titer for screening, the sera of as many as 20% of normal individuals express reactivity in the IF ANA test.[9] The basis of this reactivity, which occurs more commonly in women than men, is not well understood, although it may reflect a predisposition to autoimmunity that occurs in the absence of other immunopathologic disturbances for the complete development of a CTD. Because ANA testing is often performed to evaluate nonspecific

DISEASE PATTERN	ANTIBODY	ANTIGEN	ASSOCIATION
Homogeneous	Antihistone	Histones H1, H2A, H2B, H3, H4	Drug-induced lupus (>95%)
Rim	Anti–double-stranded DNA	Double-stranded DNA	SLE (50%)
Speckled	Anti-Sm	snRNP proteins	SLE (30%)
	Anti–U1-RNP	U1 snRNP proteins	SLE (30%); MCTD (>95%)
	Anti-Ro (SS-A)	Protein complexed to small RNAs Y1-Y5	SLE (30%); Sjögren syndrome (70-80%)
	Anti-La (SS-B)	Single protein plus RNA polymerase III transcript	SLE (15%); Sjögren syndrome (50-70%)
	Anti-Ku	DNA binding protein	SLE (10%)
	Anti–SCL-70	DNA topoisomerase I	PSS (40-70%); CREST (10-20%)
Nucleolar	Anti–PM-Scl	Nucleolar protein complex	PSS (3%); PM (8%)
	Anti–Mi-2	Nuclear protein complex	DM (15-20%)
	Anti-RNA polymerase	Subunits of RNA polymerase I	PSS (4%)
Dividing cell	Anticentromere	Centromere/kinetochore protein	CREST (80%); PSS (30%)
	Antiproliferating cell nuclear antigen	Auxiliary protein of DNA polymerase δ	SLE (3%)
Cytoplasmic	Anti–Jo-1	Histidyl tRNA synthetase	ILD in PM/DM (18-25%)
	Anti–PL-7	Threonyl tRNA synthetase	PM/DM (3%)
	Anti–PL-12	Alanyl tRNA synthetase	PM (4%)
	Anti–SRP	Signal recognition particle	PM/DM (3%)
	Anti–ribosomal P	Large ribosomal subunit	SLE (10%)

TABLE 242-2   SELECTED ANTINUCLEAR ANTIBODIES AND RHEUMATIC DISEASES

CREST = calcinosis, Raynaud phenomenon, esophageal dysmotility, sclerodactyly, and telangiectasia; DM = dermatomyositis; ILD = interstitial lung disease; MCTD = mixed connective tissue disease; PM = polymyositis; PSS = progressive systemic sclerosis (diffuse scleroderma); SLE = systemic lupus erythematosus; snRNP = small nuclear ribonucleoprotein; tRNA = transfer RNA.

complaints such as arthralgias, fatigue, and fever, a positive test must be interpreted with caution and not used as proof of a CTD in the absence of correlative clinical or laboratory findings.

Because the molecular target of many ANAs is now known, testing of individual antibodies can now be performed by ELISA or LINE-based approaches. Furthermore, multiplex assays provide simultaneous assessment of antibodies to a limited number of specificities and therefore may fail to detect certain ANAs. Although multiplex assays are operationally easier than conventional ANA testing by immunofluorescent staining, in clinical situations, the IF assay remains an important laboratory test for patient evaluation and can be used to verify results from a multiplex assay

Among many ANA specificities now identified, only a few are performed routinely because of their value for diagnosis and prognosis. For certain CTDs, diagnosis can be readily determined from clinical findings or other laboratory tests. In these instances, the ANA determination provides confirmatory information as well as clues to the occurrence of certain clinical manifestations.

Antibodies to DNA

Antibodies to DNA (anti-DNA) are serologic markers of SLE and represent a criterion in the classification of patients with this disease (Chapter 250).[10] These antibodies bind sites on both single-stranded (ss) and double-stranded (ds) DNA, although anti-dsDNA antibodies are more specific for SLE and therefore routinely measured. Although these antibodies can bind free DNA, DNA in the cell occurs in association with histones to form a structure called the *nucleosome*, with DNA wrapped around a histone core. Anti-DNA may therefore be considered a subset of antibodies to nucleosomes, with nucleosomes probably serving as the driving antigen for this response.

Anti-DNA determinations, in addition to their value in diagnosis, can serve as an index of disease activity. The association with disease activity appears strongest with glomerulonephritis, most likely because of the role of DNA–anti-DNA immune complexes in immunopathogenesis. The association of anti-DNA antibodies with other disease manifestations is less certain, limiting the use of this marker as a measure of overall disease activity. The presence of anti-DNA may nevertheless be important in assessing likelihood of response to therapies such as belimumab (anti-BLyS or anti-BAFF), an agent indicated for treatment of patients with active disease as evidenced by the presence of either anti-DNA antibodies or a positive test for ANA.[11]

Several immunochemical approaches can be used to detect anti-DNA antibodies. The assays vary with regard to the spectrum of anti-DNA antibodies detected, and results between assays may not correlate. Nevertheless, for each assay, the dynamic range for testing is large. With treatment and disease quiescence, anti-DNA antibodies may essentially disappear; with flare, levels may increase dramatically. This property distinguishes anti-DNA antibodies from other ANAs in SLE, levels of which tend to be more consistent over time.

As is the case for other ANAs, the appearance of anti-DNA antibodies in the serum may precede other manifestations of SLE, suggesting vigilance if these antibodies are present in patients who have symptoms that suggest a CTD but lack other evidence to establish a firm diagnosis.

Other Antinuclear Antibodies

Anti-Sm and anti-RNP antibodies are related specificities that commonly occur together in the sera of patients with SLE, a phenomenon called *linkage*. These antibodies bind proteins on subcellular particles called *snRNPs* (small nuclear ribonucleoproteins) that are composed of a set of proteins and uridine-rich RNAs. Anti-Sm and anti-RNP antibodies differ in protein specificity and in the ability to cause immunoprecipitation of the bound RNA molecules. Anti-Sm antibodies occur only in patients with SLE and represent a serologic marker for disease classification. In contrast, anti-RNP antibodies can appear in the sera of patients with other clinical presentations and, in the absence of anti-Sm, may characterize patients with overlapping CTD features, so-called mixed CTD or MCTD. In SLE, the frequencies of anti-Sm and anti-RNP antibodies vary among racial and ethnic groups, although a clear association with particular clinical manifestations has not been established.

Anti-Ro and anti-La antibodies (or anti–SS-A and anti–SS-B), another set of linked ANAs, are directed to protein-RNA complexes that are involved in cellular metabolism of RNA. Two forms of Ro exist. Ro60 is an RNA-protein complex, whereas Ro52 is a protein known as TRIM22. Anti-Ro and anti-La antibodies are expressed more widely in patients with CTD and appear in the sera of patients with SLE, RA, and Sjögren syndrome, among others. Assessment of these antibodies is important because of their association with the neonatal lupus syndrome, which results from the transplacental passage of antibodies

and causes congenital heart block as well as rash in the neonate. Although both Sm/RNP and Ro/La are complexes of proteins and RNA, these antibodies appear to be expressed by different patient subsets, suggesting distinct mechanisms of induction and clinical associations. Although ANAs are directed to ubiquitous antigens, they nevertheless are expressed in disease-specific patterns and may show association with particular organ-specific manifestations. These associations include anti–ribosomal P antibodies with central nervous systemic involvement in SLE, antibodies to DNA topoisomerase 1 (anti–SCL-70) with progressive systemic sclerosis (diffuse scleroderma), antibodies to centromeres with CREST syndrome (calcinosis, Raynaud phenomenon, esophageal dysmotility, sclerodactyly, and telangiectasia), and antibodies to histidyl transfer RNA synthetase (anti–Jo-1) with interstitial lung disease in scleroderma (Chapter 251). In inflammatory myopathies, the presence of certain autoantibodies may be associated with particular patterns of disease, with antibodies to the enzyme 3-hydroxy-3-methylglutaryl-coenzyme A (HMG-CoA) reductase present in a syndrome of necrotizing myositis; the syndrome can occur in patients treated with statins, which can inhibit the enzyme.[12]

In addition to their association with specific disease manifestations, antibodies to both DNA- and RNA-binding proteins such as Sm and RNP may contribute to overall immune dysregulation in patients with autoimmune disease because of their formation of immune complexes containing DNA or RNA. These complexes can stimulate the production of type 1 interferon by triggering both TLR and non-TLR nucleic acid sensors as well as other cellular receptors (e.g., Fc receptors). Because immunoassays of interferon with patients' sera are limited, the presence of interferon is observed more clearly in the pattern of gene expression known as the interferon signature in peripheral blood cells. This signature can be assessed by both microarray assays and measurement of more limited sets of messenger RNA molecules. Because antibodies to RNA-binding proteins in particular may promote this pattern, the serologic assay of these ANAs may allow assessment of the likelihood of both nonspecific and specific immunologic disturbances.

Antibodies to Phospholipids

Originally defined by their effects on in vitro clotting tests, antibodies to phospholipids (APLs) are associated with in vivo thrombosis and have been termed *lupus anticoagulants* (LACs).[13] Patients with these antibodies display a clinical condition, termed the *antiphospholipid antibody syndrome*,[14] which is characterized by arterial or venous thrombosis, thrombocytopenia, and first trimester spontaneous abortions (Chapter 73). This syndrome may occur by itself or in the context of SLE, where it may contribute to the acceleration of atherosclerosis, premature stroke, and myocardial infarction. The laboratory evaluation of this condition involves specific assays of antibodies to phospholipids and related proteins as well as functional assays of clotting. Because expression of these antibodies may vary over time, testing must be performed on more than one occasion at least 6 weeks apart. Furthermore, the results of immunochemical and functional assays may not be congruent, likely related to the heterogeneity of antibodies.

The serology of APLs is complicated because it is related to the nature of the antigenic targets as well as heterogeneity among patients. These antigens include phospholipids such as cardiolipin. Cardiolipin, however, can bind to the protein β_2-glycoprotein 1, which is also a target for antibodies in this condition. Serologic evaluation thus involves assays with a complex of cardiolipin and β_2-glycoprotein 1 as well as β_2-glycoprotein in an ELISA format using reagents to measure IgG, IgA, and IgM, although the association of antibodies with thrombosis appears strongest with IgG antibodies. In interpreting these assays, it is important to know the cutoff values used to define positivity.

Functional assays for LACs involve tests directed at inhibition of in vitro clotting (e.g., activated partial thromboplastin time, dilute Russell viper venom time), recognizing the discordance between in vivo thrombosis and in vitro anticoagulation. Functional assays to detect LACs involve a mixing step in which patient plasma is mixed with normal plasma to determine the presence of an inhibitor (i.e., an antibody) as opposed to a deficiency state. The mechanisms by which antibodies to phospholipids and related proteins may cause thrombosis in vivo are unknown, although these antibodies may interact with the surface of cells (e.g., endothelium) to promote a prothrombotic state. Assessing the likelihood of the syndrome is best accomplished by considering assay results in the context of the individual patient.

Complement

Assessment of the complement system can provide valuable information on the activity of diseases in which immune complex deposition may promote inflammation and tissue injury (Chapter 44).[15] This system involves a large number of proteins that function in enzyme cascades to generate degradation products that amplify immunologic reactions and promote the destruction or removal of foreign organisms as well as damaged cells. In the setting of SLE and in certain forms of vasculitis and glomerulonephritis, immune complexes activate complement, which can be measured in terms of the total complement level, levels of C3 and C4, and levels of complement fragments bound to red blood cells. Proteins of the complement system are acute phase reactants and can increase with inflammation, including active disease. Correspondingly, low levels may reflect inherited complement deficiency or copy number variations rather than consumption; genetic deficiency of C1q, for example, is highly associated with SLE.

Antineutrophil Cytoplasmic Antibodies

Antineutrophil cytoplasmic antibodies (ANCAs)[16,17] are autoantibodies that react to determinants in the neutrophil and occur prominently in patients with certain forms of necrotizing vasculitis or rapidly progressive glomerulonephritis. Reflecting the serology, conditions have been called ANCA-associated vasculitis (AAV). Two main forms of ANCA have been distinguished on the basis of the target antigens and pattern of immunofluorescence staining of fixed neutrophils: PR3-ANCA (C-ANCA), which reacts with proteinase-3 (PR3), and MPO-ANCA (P-ANCA), which reacts with myeloperoxidase (MPO). By immunofluorescence, PR3-ANCA shows staining in the cytoplasm; staining by MPO-ANCA localizes in the perinuclear area. ANCAs can occur in other conditions including an immune syndrome resulting from the drug levamisole, which is used as an adulterant in cocaine.

In the evaluation of severe, multisystem inflammatory disease, ANCA testing is important to evaluate diagnostic possibilities. ANCAs occur in association with varying clinical manifestations in patients with AAV and help define patterns of clinical involvement in terms of organ system involvement as well as histopathology (e.g., presence of granulomatous inflammation).[18,19] PR3-ANCA occurs commonly in patients with granulomatosis with polyangiitis (GPA, formerly called Wegener granulomatosis) as well eosinophilic granulomatosis with polyangiitis (EGPA, formerly called Churg-Strauss disease); MPO-ANCA marks the course of vasculitis caused by microscopic polyangiitis. Although there is overlap between serology and clinical features, PR3-ANCA occurs commonly in patients with upper airway disease, whereas MPO-ANA occurs commonly patients with patients with rapidly progressive renal disease (Chapter 254).

In patients with ANCA-associated glomerulonephritis, the kidney lacks evidence of immune deposits, as indicated by the lack of staining for immunoglobulins or complement. Kidney disease of this kind is termed *pauci-immune glomerulonephritis*. Although ANCA testing is useful in initial diagnosis, its role for assessing disease activity is less certain. Occasionally, in patients who are desperately ill and cannot tolerate a lung or kidney biopsy, the presence of an ANCA can be used as preliminary evidence for diagnosis to allow the initiation of immunosuppressive therapy. ANCA testing is also useful for assessing the likelihood for relapse because patients who express PR3-ANCA appear at risk for recurrent disease.

Cryoglobulins

Cryoglobulins are serum immunoglobulins that precipitate in the cold and can mediate disease through tissue deposition.[20] The presence of a cryoglobulin is detected by allowing blood, collected warm, to remain cool at 2° to 4° C for 1 or more days. After centrifugation, the amount of cryoprecipitate is measured and expressed as a cryocrit. In the preanalytical phase, it is important that the blood remain at a temperature of 37° C during all steps.[21]

Subsequent analysis of the cryoprecipitate by immunochemical assays allows determination of its components. Cryoglobulins can be classified into three main types on the basis of their composition: (1) single, or type I; (2) mixed, type II; and (3) mixed, type III. A type I cryoglobulin consists of only a monoclonal immunoglobulin that precipitates in the cold. A mixed-type cryoglobulin contains RFs bound to polyclonal IgG to form an immune complex. In type II cryoglobulins, the IgM RF is monoclonal, and in type III, the IgM RF is polyclonal.

Type I cryoglobulins occur in patients with lymphoproliferative disorders such as Waldenström macroglobulinemia, multiple myeloma, or chronic lymphocytic lymphoma (Chapters 174 and 178). In contrast, patients with mixed cryoglobulins can present with a wide range of signs and symptoms resulting from vasculitis. These manifestations include purpura (a sign of leukocytoclastic vasculitis), weakness, arthritis, and neuropathy, representing a syndrome known as *essential mixed cryoglobulinemia*. Most patients with this condition have infection with hepatitis C virus, with viral components present in the complexes. These patients have serologic evidence of this infection as well as manifestations attributable to the underlying liver disease. As in the case of other CTDs and systemic inflammatory diseases, the evaluation of patients with essential mixed cryoglobulinemia demands attention to the entire patient and the impact of disease on multiple organs.

GENERAL REFERENCES

For the General References and other additional features, please visit Expert Consult at https://expertconsult.inkling.com.

243

IMAGING STUDIES IN THE RHEUMATIC DISEASES

RONALD S. ADLER

Historically, rheumatic disorders have been well characterized by conventional imaging. In as much as these disorders often manifest in characteristic distributions and present with specific alterations in the appendicular and/or axial skeleton and adjacent soft tissues, radiographic evaluation has been sufficient to characterize the abnormalities as well as provide a relatively small number of differential possibilities as to the specific disease. The most well-studied example is rheumatoid arthritis (RA), in which symmetric involvement of the metacarpophalangeal joints, uniform joint space narrowing, periarticular osteopenia, and juxta-articular erosions along the "bare areas" are pathognomonic.

The development of new therapeutic alternatives for the inflammatory arthritides, so-called disease-modifying antirheumatic drugs (DMARDs), and chondroprotective strategies in the case of osteoarthrosis, require methods to diagnose these diseases at an earlier stage, characterize the degree of inflammation, and provide a useful metric to assess therapeutic response (Chapters 32 and 33). Indeed, it has become necessary to assess for possible joint and soft tissue abnormalities before irreversible tissue damage when the radiographic findings are not yet abnormal. Fortunately, the requirement to achieve earlier diagnosis has paralleled advances in imaging. Ultrasonography and magnetic resonance imaging (MRI) have largely supplanted conventional radiographic evaluation in the imaging work-up of patients with suspected rheumatologic disorders and negative radiographs. The term *molecular imaging* has been applied, particularly in the case of MRI and positron emission tomography (PET), in as much as these modalities reflect local tissue environment or metabolic activity.[1,2]

RADIOGRAPHIC EVALUATION

Radiographic evaluation is among the first studies ordered in patients with a suspected rheumatologic disorder. In the current digital era, conventional analog-based radiographs have been largely replaced by computed radiography. Images are usually displayed on workstations with high-resolution monitors within the context of a picture archiving system (PACS). Digital radiographs are of high spatial resolution but relatively poor soft tissue contrast. These images are amenable to a variety of image processing schemes, resulting in enhanced definition of the cortical surfaces and cancellous bone, which may be of value in displaying subtle erosions.

It is important to recognize that radiographs are projection images. To detect an abnormality, it may be necessary to view a joint or other structure at a specific angle. For instance, subtle erosions may be apparent only when viewed tangentially, as opposed to en face. It is therefore necessary to have specific image protocols to optimally display the joint, cortical surface, or soft tissue structure. Most radiographic evaluations contain at least two orthogonal projections. The addition of an oblique view or other specialized projection may be necessary to address a specific clinical question.

The nature and distribution of joint space narrowing, presence of osteopenia, new bone formation, soft tissue swelling, soft tissue calcification, chondrocalcinosis, presence and nature of erosions, and assessment for joint malalignment may allow a specific diagnosis, as well as help determine the severity of disease (Fig. 243-1). For instance, the presence of a juxta-articular erosion

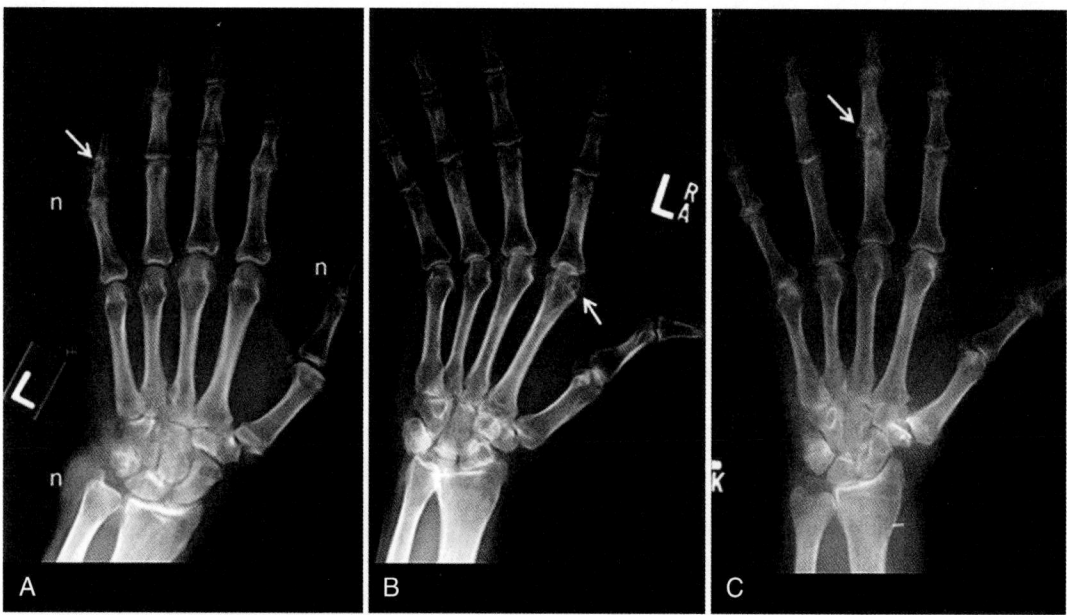

FIGURE 243-1. **Three hands with different diagnoses. A, Gout.** Radiograph of the left hand showing multiple dense soft tissue nodules (n) with multiple small erosions affecting the ulnar styloid, triquetrum, and fifth ray. A large erosion (*arrow*) at the fifth distal interphalangeal (DIP) joint demonstrates bone formation extending circumferentially about the adjacent tophaceous deposit typical of an overhanging edge. Bone mineralization and joint spaces are preserved. **B, Rheumatoid arthritis (RA).** There is ulnar deviation of the second through fifth metacarpophalangeal (MCP) joints with uniform joint space loss involving the MCP joints and the carpus. There is mild ulnar translation of the carpus. The DIP joints are spared. Periarticular demineralization is present with small erosions along the radiovolar aspect of the second (*arrow*) MCP joint. L = left. **C, Osteoarthrosis.** Soft tissue swelling affecting the third digit with joint space narrowing and bone production affecting the DIP joints, third and fifth proximal interphalangeal (PIP) joints, basal joint of the thumb, and scaphotrapezio-trapezoid joint. There are subchondral cystic changes at the third PIP joint having an erosive character (*arrow*). Mineralization is preserved, and radiocarpal as well as MCP joint spaces are preserved.

TABLE 243-1 DISTINGUISHING RADIOGRAPHIC FEATURES OF SEVERAL COMMON RHEUMATIC DISEASES

CONDITION	COMMON SITES	DISTRIBUTION	RADIOGRAPHIC FEATURES
Rheumatoid arthritis	Hands: MCP, PIP; wrists: intercarpal, DRUJ, ulnar styloid; feet: fifth MTP; cervical spine (atlantoaxial, apophyseal)	Bilateral, symmetric, polyarticular	Juxta-articular osteopenia, periarticular swelling, subluxations (e.g., ulnar, volar), uniform joint space loss, erosions (bare areas)
Osteoarthritis (primary)	Hands (DIP), wrists (basal joint, STT), feet (first MTP), hips (superolateral), knees (medial), spine (discs, facet, or apophyseal, uncovertebral)	Symmetric, weight-bearing joints	Normal or increased density, nonuniform joint space loss, subchondral sclerosis, cysts, bone formation (osteophytes) Spine: disc space narrowing, end plate sclerosis, and bone formation
Psoriatic arthritis	Hands (DIP, terminal tufts), feet (IP joints), entheses (calcaneus-plantar, posterior), spine, SI joints	Asymmetric (single ray), polyarticular, segmental (intervertebral, apophyseal)	Normal or increased density, periosteal bone formation, soft tissue swelling, ankylosis (SI joints), thick hyperostosis spine (nonmarginal syndesmophytes), juxta-articular and periarticular erosions
Ankylosing spondylitis	Spine, SI joints, fibrous joints (pubic symphysis), entheses (adductor origin), rhizomelic joints (hips, shoulders)	Symmetric, continuous (may affect entire spine: bamboo spine)	Normal or increased density, erosions (spine: squaring, shining corner) with superimposed bone formation (ankylosis: SI, thin [marginal] syndesmophytes)
Gout	Feet (first MTP), other damaged joints, elbow, knee, hindfoot	Asymmetric, extensor surfaces (elbow), abnormal joints (e.g., osteoarthritic joints)	Normal joint space, normal or increased density, dense soft tissue nodules (tophi), para-articular and subchondral erosions with bone formation along tophi (overhanging edge)
CPPD	Hands (second, third MCP), wrists (radiocarpal, TFC), knees (lateral compartment and patella-femoral, menisci)	Symmetric, fibrocartilaginous joints	Normal or increased density, hypertrophic bone formation, subchondral or periarticular cysts, chondrocalcinosis (hyaline, fibrocartilage), periarticular, peritendinous, periligamentous calcification
Infection	Any joint (pyogenic, TB)	Monoarticular (mostly), any joint	Pyogenic: osteopenia (days), joint space widened (early), joint space loss (rapid development), soft tissue swelling, erosions—both sides of joint, sequestra, periostitis TB: joint space and mineralization may be preserved, juxta-articular erosions Spine: disc space loss and end plate erosion

CPPD = calcium pyrophosphate deposition disease; DIP = distal interphalangeal; DRUJ = distal radial ulnar joint; IP = interphalangeal; MCP = metacarpophalangeal; MTP = metatarsophalangeal; PIP = proximal interphalangeal; SI = sacroiliac; STT = scaphotrapeziotrapezoid; TB = tuberculosis; TFC = triangular fibrocartilage.

extending over an adjacent area of slightly hyperdense soft tissue swelling in the setting of normal bone mineralization with maintenance of the adjacent joint space is diagnostic of gout, in contrast to RA noted earlier. The seronegative arthritides, such as psoriatic arthritis, have a characteristic appearance in the small joints of the hand and feet, with a predilection for distal joints, asymmetry, and appositional new bone formation.

Table 243-1 summarizes some of the features of several of the more common diseases that may be encountered in clinical practice.

Finally, radiographs provide a direct means for needle localization during percutaneous procedures, predominantly joint injections, aspirations, and some biopsies. These are generally performed while imaging in real time (fluoroscopy) using short bursts of low-intensity x-rays enhanced through an image intensifier. Injection of joints under fluoroscopic guidance provides a convenient means to ensure intra-articular deposition of the therapeutic agent or for diagnostic aspiration. Intra-articular location is verified by injection of a small amount of a standard iodinated contrast material. Arthrography using fluoroscopic guidance can be used as a primary diagnostic tool, but this application has largely been replaced by intra-articular injection of contrast followed by computed tomography (CT) or MRI.

For some procedures, CT may be preferable, depending on the location of the abnormality. The principal disadvantages of fluoroscopy relate to the use of ionizing radiation and poor soft tissue contrast. The latter becomes important with needle placement near neurovascular structures that may be potentially compromised by poor needle position. CT allows greater control over needle placement at the cost of greater levels of radiation exposure. Ultrasonography has replaced fluoroscopy and CT for a large number of percutaneous procedures. MRI provides another method to perform a variety of procedures without the necessity of ionizing radiation. These options will be discussed in greater detail below.

COMPUTED TOMOGRAPHY

CT provides a two-dimensional map of tissue attenuation obtained from external x-ray source(s) located on a rotating gantry, whose radiation is detected by a series of detectors opposite the source. The current generation of CT scanners employs multiple detectors (16, 32, 64, and so on), allowing rapid image acquisition that can be displayed in a single plane in real time (CT-fluoroscopy) or as extremely thin section contiguous or overlapping acquisitions in the axial plane. The acquired images can be reconstructed in multiple planes with equivalent (isotropic) resolution elements (voxels) or as a three-dimensional rendering. Image data are generally obtained with the scanner operating in a helical mode (as the subject is advanced continuously while data are obtained), enabling rapid acquisitions. Image reconstruction has traditionally been performed using a technique known as filtered back-projection. Newer techniques involve iterative reconstruction, which is promising as a method to achieve significant decrease in image reconstruction times, as well as radiation dose reduction. Some scanners use dual energy sources, taking advantage of differences in the attenuation characteristics of various tissues at different energies. This has received greatest attention in the setting of gout, enabling a definitive diagnosis with greater sensitivity in depicting tophaceous deposits even in anatomic locations not conducive to radiographs or ultrasound.[3]

CT allows the best assessment of trabecular and cortical bone, providing an excellent means to assess fractures and erosions, the presence of new bone formation (e.g., fracture callus), and degenerative or inflammatory arthritis. Soft tissue mineralization can likewise be well characterized, providing important information as to its etiology. Joints that are difficult to assess on radiographs, including the sacroiliac, temporomandibular, wrist, and sternoclavicular joints, are well seen on CT (Fig. 243-2).

CT generally has poor soft tissue contrast. Nevertheless, it is still very useful in performing a number of guided procedures because of its tomographic nature and rapid image acquisition capability. Improved soft tissue contrast can be obtained with use of iodinated contrast material. A number of soft tissue tumors, inflammatory synovitis, and infectious processes display pathologic enhancement after contrast administration. CT can likewise be used to produce angiographic displays (CTA) when used in combination with contrast, providing exquisite detail of central and peripheral vascular disease, including in patients with suspected vasculitis. These agents are typically administered intravenously following well-defined enhancement characteristics. CTA has become the method of choice in evaluating patients with suspected pulmonary embolism. Likewise, contrast agents may be used to improve intra-articular contrast (CT arthrography), currently the method of choice in assessing internal derangement in the postoperative shoulder, knee, and so on and in patients who are unable to undergo MRI (e.g., those with claustrophobia, aneurysm clips, or cardiac pacemakers). Imaging of cartilage and soft tissue abnormalities usually depends on pathologic inhibition of contrast material, indicative of degeneration or tearing. A limitation of this approach resides in the fact that some abnormalities may remain occult. An example is the inability to detect a bursal-sided rotator cuff tear after shoulder CT arthrography.

The radiation dose from CT can be high, especially when using the newer scanners. This is most significant when one is looking to minimize exposure, such as in children, requiring protocols specifically designed for the pediatric population. Newer iterative image reconstruction techniques as well as sparse sampling (compressed sensing) may allow for compensatory dose reduction. Intravenous (IV) use of iodinated contrast agents is contraindicated in patients with impaired renal function or a history of allergic reaction. Nonionic agents can diminish the associated risks but still should be used with caution.

ULTRASONOGRAPHY

Ultrasound imaging takes advantage of the near uniform speed of sound and predictable attenuation characteristics of sound propagation in soft tissue. Diagnostic frequencies used in musculoskeletal ultrasound range from approximately 5 to 20 megahertz (MHz). Images are formed using a pulse-echo technique, whereby a transducer produces a short duration series of pulses (lasting on the order of microseconds) and then goes into a receive mode from which image information is acquired and processed. In general, anatomic images derive from specular surfaces whose dimensions exceed the ultrasound wavelength; inherent noise (speckle) within the image derives from small scatterers, smaller than the resolution element of the transducer. Modern ultrasound equipment contains various methods to reduce speckle in the image, resulting in a more anatomic rendition of the soft tissues. Rapid image acquisition and processing enables ultrasound to be performed in real time (approximately 30 frames per second). Ultrasonography is also conducive to evaluation of blood flow from which estimates of flow velocity can

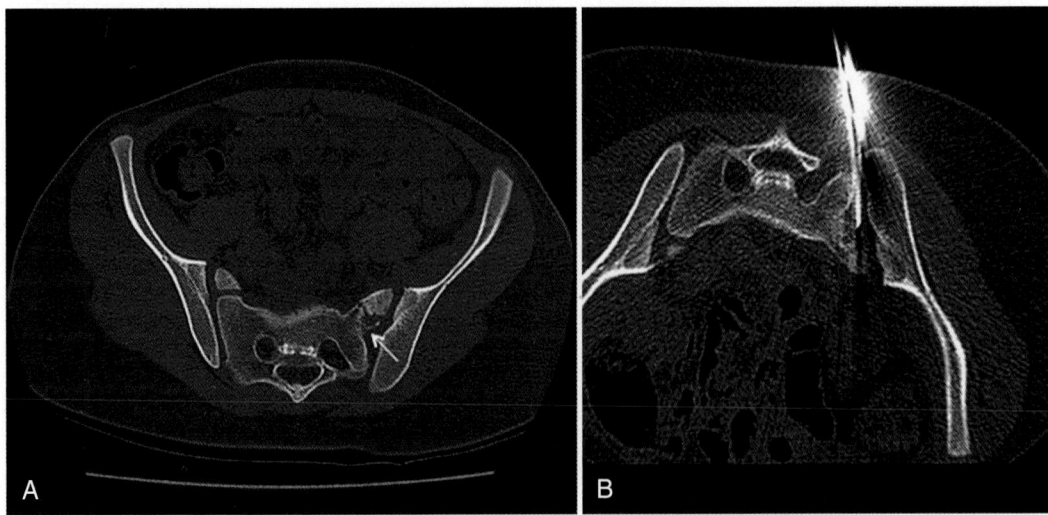

FIGURE 243-2. Infectious sacroiliitis in a 12-year-old boy with a 2-week history of back and left hip pain. A, Axial computed tomography (CT) image of the pelvis at the level of the sacroiliac (SI) joints photographed using window settings optimized for bone detail. There is clear asymmetry in the two SI joints, with the left appearing more irregular. The cortical margins of the left sacral ala are less distinct, and there is an isolated bone fragment (*arrow*) surrounded by soft tissue suspicious for a sequestrum. B, CT-guided aspiration of the left SI joint confirmed an infectious origin.

be obtained through the Doppler equation. Doppler information is typically reported by either continuously estimating velocity at a specific depth (spectral Doppler) or through a color encoded two-dimensional map (color or power Doppler).

There is great appeal for using ultrasonography in patients with rheumatic disorders. There is no ionizing radiation, and it is real-time, inexpensive, relatively portable, and well tolerated. Historically, however, ultrasonography has played only a limited role in the diagnostic assessment and treatment of patients with suspected musculoskeletal abnormalities, being used to differentiate fluid-filled from solid masses. The detection of a Baker cyst in the knee or the presence of a joint effusion constituted two major applications. There has also been limited application of ultrasonography to perform image-guided aspirations and biopsies. Within the United States in particular, the development of MRI further limited the musculoskeletal applications of ultrasonography.

With the development of linear high-frequency small parts transducers, new imaging capabilities of ultrasound scanners, and the evolution of a new class of compact and portable (laptop) ultrasound units that have excellent image quality, the role of ultrasonography has dramatically changed in recent years.[4,5] These new applications have paralleled the development of new classes of DMARDs for which diagnosis of inflammatory synovitis prior to joint destruction is a prerequisite.

The current generation of ultrasound scanners enables examination of the small joints of the hands and feet, allowing early detection of synovitis (Fig. 243-3). Typically, a 10-MHz or higher-frequency linear transducer is used. The displacement of the joint capsule by hypoechoic (dark) soft tissue that displays vascularity on Doppler imaging or is incompressible with direct pressure by the transducer is characteristic, allowing differentiation of synovitis from an effusion. In addition to the detection of synovitis, ultrasonography has been shown to be more sensitive than conventional radiographs in the detection of erosions. Erosions appear as discrete irregular discontinuities in the normally smooth hyperechoic (bright), reflecting cortical surfaces, often seen in continuity with adjacent inflammatory soft tissue. There is some variation in the appearance of synovitis among various arthritides. The distribution, presence, or lack of symmetry and other concomitant findings may be necessary to obtain a specific diagnosis.

The level of vascularity on color flow imaging can reflect active inflammation, correlating with clinical and biochemical parameters. A parametric image encoding either mean Doppler shift (color Doppler) or amplitude (power Doppler) is typically used as a standard Doppler map. Both maps can be used to detect abnormal levels of vascularity. Whereas power Doppler provides an indirect measure of the number of moving scatterers within the region being scanned, color Doppler provides a velocity map and therefore is more subject to artifact (angle dependence and sampling errors). When combined with color flow imaging, the activity of the synovitis can be estimated. Ultrasound contrast agents can depict capillary flow, resulting in significantly improved detection sensitivity of synovial inflammation and are used extensively in Europe. They constitute microbubble agents encased in a lipid or polysaccharide shell that can be instilled as either bolus or constant infusion, with the shell being metabolized in the liver and the gas exhaled in the lungs. These agents have biologic half-lives on the order of minutes and are best suited to examining target joints. Contrast agents have received U.S. Food and Drug Administration

approval for only cardiovascular and abdominal applications at this time and therefore can be used only off label for the assessment of synovitis.

Articular cartilage and fibrocartilage have characteristic appearances on ultrasonography. Whereas the former appears as a thin hypoechoic band paralleling the articular surface, fibrocartilage appears hyperechoic. Chondrocalcinosis appears as discrete hyperechoic foci within the substance of the cartilage, in which case its presence is suggestive of calcium pyrophosphate deposition disease. Calcification along the margin of the articular cartilage gives rise to the double-line sign seen in gout.

Tendons and muscles have characteristic appearances on ultrasonography. The presence of tendinosis, tendon tears, muscle edema or inflammation, atrophy, and tears can be diagnosed. Ultrasonography is very sensitive, although not specific, for the detection of small amounts of calcification or ossification. It is an excellent method to assess for calcific peritendinitis or periarthritis and to provide guidance for treatment. Abnormal fluid distention of synovial lined structures can be assessed and treated under ultrasound guidance. Ultrasonography is an excellent modality to provide image guidance for therapeutic aspiration and injection of small and large joints, tendon sheaths, and cysts (e.g., bursae, ganglion, paralabral cysts, hematomas, abscesses) (Fig. 243-4). The real-time capability of ultrasonography is useful to demonstrate the presence of subluxations, to evaluate painful snapping, to document the distribution of injected material, and to assess adhesions. Ultrasonography is considered the method of choice to detect foreign bodies. Newer ultrasound techniques provide a map of soft tissue mechanical properties, also known as ultrasound elastography (USE). These techniques fall into two categories, compression-based or shear wave elastography. The former employs speckle tracking to estimate local tissue strain following minimal external compression of the tissue being examined, thereby producing a color-encoded strain map or map of tissue hardness. The latter method employs a shear-wave produced either by an external source or by the transducer itself, the speed of the shear wave being an indirect measure of local Young modulus; a color-encoded map or quantitative estimate of local shear wave speed or elastic modulus can be derived. Both techniques provide information regarding alterations of mechanical properties of tendons and muscles in a variety of degenerative, traumatic, and reparative states. For example, fatty infiltration resulting from chronic myopathic disorders produces measurable alterations in local muscle elastic modulus.

Nerves also have a characteristic appearance on ultrasonography. In cross-section, a nerve often has a "cluster of grapes" or "honeycomb" appearance, with nerve fascicles appearing hypoechoic and surrounded by hyperechoic internal and external epineural fat. In long axis, nerves display a characteristic "tram-track" appearance. Ultrasonography has been shown to be useful in the diagnosis and treatment of carpal tunnel syndrome and cubital tunnel syndrome. It is an excellent modality to assess for the presence of post-traumatic or post-surgical and interdigital neuromas and to provide image guidance for treatment, including therapeutic injections, nerve blocks, and ablative therapy.

Although ultrasonography is well suited to the evaluation of superficial structures, it is less well suited to assess deep structures. Frequency and penetration are reciprocally related: the higher the frequency, the better the axial resolution but poorer the degree of penetration. A 15-MHz linear transducer

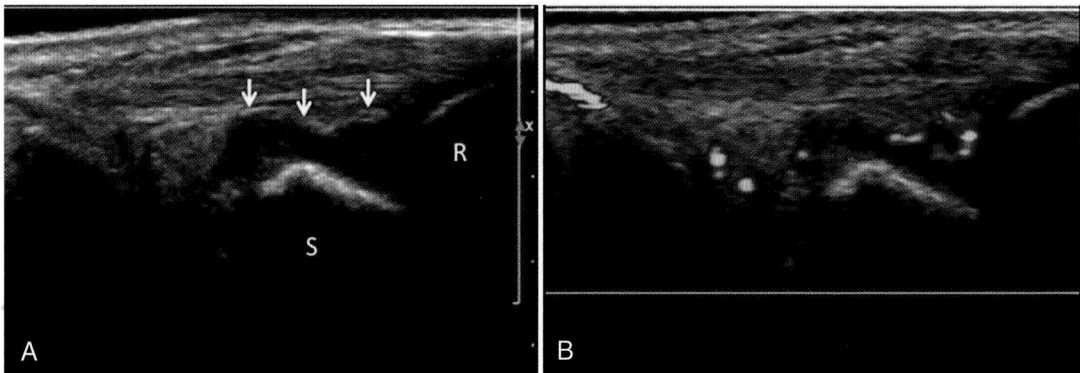

FIGURE 243-3. Synovitis on ultrasound in a female patient with normal hand radiographs. **A,** Gray scale ultrasound image obtained along the dorsal aspect of the radioscaphoid joint shows hypoechoic soft tissue (*arrows*) distending the dorsal recess. The cortical margins of the scaphoid (S) and radius (R) appear as bright reflectors on ultrasound. **B,** Power Doppler image depicts the marked vascularity (red hues) of the soft tissue illustrating the level of disease activity.

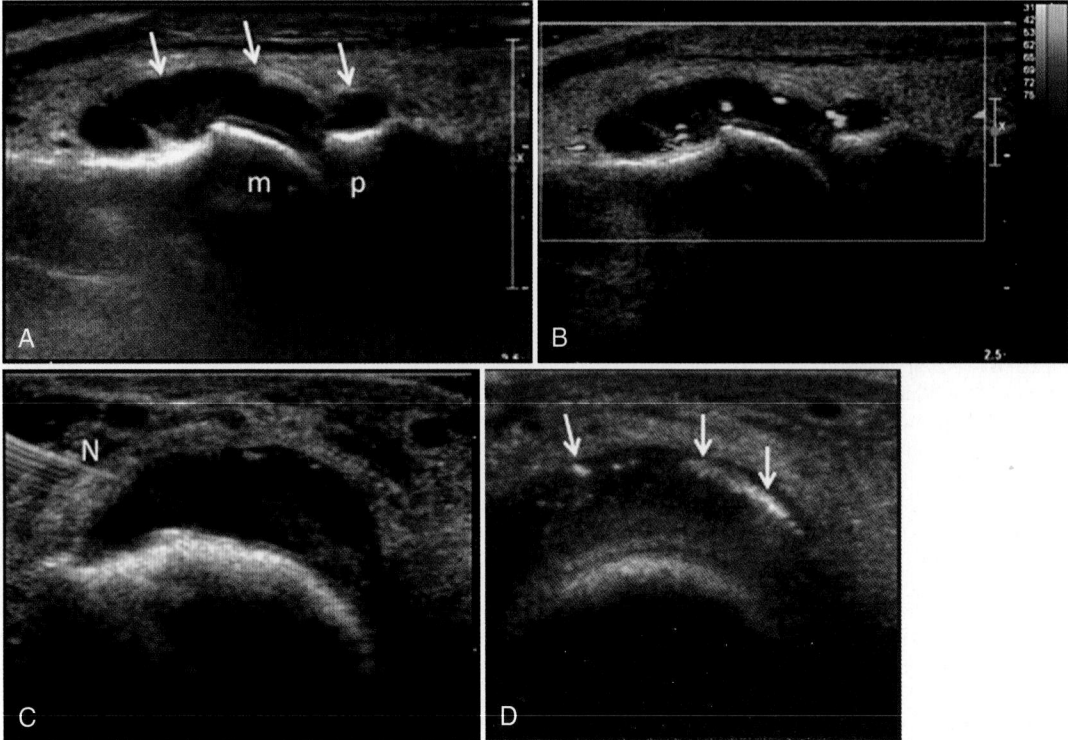

FIGURE 243-4. Ultrasound-guided therapy in the first metatarsophalangeal (MTP) joint of a female patient with pain and swelling. **A,** Longitudinal gray scale image of the dorsal recess of the first MTP joint. Fluid and soft tissue distend the joint capsule (*arrows*). The metatarsal (m) and proximal phalanx (p) are labeled. Note that a thin hypoechoic (dark) band parallels the surface of the metatarsal head, corresponding to the overlying articular cartilage. **B,** Increased vascularity (red hues) demonstrated on power Doppler imaging within the dorsal recess reflects the level of disease activity. **C,** Transverse gray scale ultrasound image shows a needle (N) within the distended dorsal recess from which several drops of synovial fluid were aspirated, followed by therapeutic injection. **D,** Postinjection transverse sonogram depicts low-level echoes (small echogenic foci within dorsal recess) and microbubbles (*arrows*) within the distended joint capsule from injected material. Microbubbles will aggregate along the nondependent portion of the distended joint capsule, whereas injected material tends to settle to the deep potion of the joint.

would work well in the hand but not in the hip. Examination of a hip might require a 5-MHz transducer and curved transducer geometry with reduced image quality. Excessive abdominal fat can further limit acoustic penetration and distort the ultrasound beam, limiting image quality. Diagnostic ultrasonography does not penetrate bone, resulting in limited acoustic access to joint structures. In some instances, soft tissue contrast can be poor. An inexperienced scanner may find ligaments and tendinous insertions difficult to differentiate from adjacent fibrofatty structures.

MAGNETIC RESONANCE IMAGING

The natural abundance of hydrogen in biologic systems and an inherent property of hydrogen, called *spin*, form the basis of conventional MRI. When placed in a strong magnetic field, protons tend to align themselves along the direction of the field. Magnetic field strengths are specified as Tesla and can be variable between clinical scanners. The majority of scanners in clinical usage vary between 1 and 3 Tesla. Application of a radiofrequency (RF) pulse to a system of protons induces the spins to rotate away from the direction of the field, during which time they precess about the direction of the magnetic field at a characteristic frequency, called the Larmor frequency. When the RF pulse is turned off, the spins relax toward their initial state determined by two tissue-dependent relaxation times, T1 and T2, which vary with field strength. T1 (also known as the spin-lattice relaxation) and T2 (or the transverse relaxation time) along with proton density are the principal determinants of signal intensity. The image can emphasize either the T1 or T2 characteristics of the tissue, impacting tissue contrast. By applying a system of gradient coils, one can effectively spatially encode the distribution of Larmor frequencies. Different tissues have varying appearance often based on levels of fat and water content, reflected by their inherent T1 and T2 relaxation times. Tissue morphology is often characterized by their appearance on T1-weighted or proton density images: tendon, muscle, fat, marrow, cortical bone, articular, and fibrocartilage have characteristic appearances. Many pathologic states, alternatively, are characterized by increased mobile water or effective T2 lengthening. Examples include soft tissue edema, inflammatory infiltrates, and neoplasm (Fig. 243-5). Images that emphasize T2 contrast are therefore helpful to display most pathologic states. Selective maps of T2 have been used to characterize the state of articular cartilage in early degenerative disease. Other cartilage-specific

properties that relate to water content, glycosaminoglycan (GAG) content, and integrity of collagen architecture can be assessed using T2 and other parametric maps that can be derived from the MR data (Fig. 243-6).

Measures and parametric images of apparent diffusion coefficient (ADC) provide a method to quantify soft tissue edema present in inflammatory states and may help to differentiate tissue inflammation from other potential sources of increased T2 contrast.[6] The loss of restrictive diffusion has likewise been employed as a quantitative metric and imaging tool to assess collagen breakdown in articular cartilage that occurs in early osteoarthritis.[7] The latter utilizes a technique known as diffusion tensor imaging (DTI) to estimate the loss asymmetry in the axial versus radial diffusion coefficients present following cartilage injury and has been shown to correlate with both alterations in proteoglycan content and altered collagen architecture.

The widely used contrast for MRI studies is a neutral hydrophilic salt of the gadolinium chelate, gadolinium diethylenetriamine-penta-acetic acid (Gd-DTPA). Gadolinium can be injected intravenously or directly into the joint. IV injection (indirect magnetic resonance arthrography) carries the contrast in the vascular system to areas of hyperemia and inflammation (Fig. 243-7). It can be used for assessment of synovial activity in inflammatory joint diseases. Gadolinium is taken up in inflamed synovium and is able to demonstrate thickened pannus. The slope of the early time-signal intensity curve provides a measure of tissue perfusion and can quantify inflammatory activity. Contrast material excreted into the synovial fluid provides excellent depiction of intra-articular structures and can be used in lieu of arthrographic direct techniques. In GAG-depleted cartilage, there can be delayed uptake of contrast into the cartilage, which would normally be inhibited by the negatively charged GAG molecules.

Patients with renal disease who receive IV injection of gadolinium can develop nephrogenic systemic fibrosis (NSF) (see Chapter 251). When the kidney cannot sufficiently clear out the gadolinium, it produces fibrosis of many tissues, including the skin, muscle, heart, nerves, and pleura. To date, NSF has been seen only in patients who have been given IV gadolinium with acute or chronic renal insufficiency. The changes in the skin with NSF are usually bilateral and symmetric, primarily involving the extremities and the trunk. These changes can mimic systemic sclerosis but, unlike that disease, the face is usually spared. If renal function improves, the skin lesions may

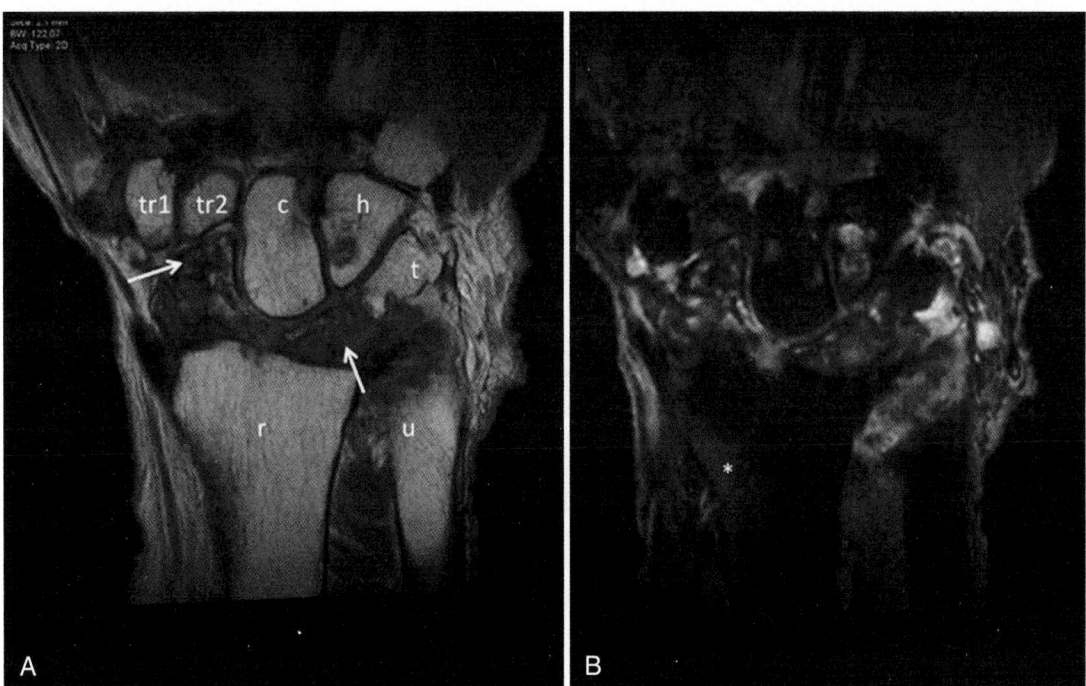

FIGURE 243-5. **Magnetic resonance imaging of the right wrist in a female patient with advanced rheumatoid arthritis. A,** Proton density coronal image shows loss of normally bright marrow signal within the scaphoid and lunate bones (*arrows*). The proximal scaphoid is eroded, and the lunate appears deformed and translocated and volarly tilted (not shown), giving rise to its triangular appearance. The distal ulna (u) is poorly visualized due to a large erosion. Intermediate-intensity material (appears dark gray) within the carpus and distal radioulnar joint is difficult to separate from the distal ulna, lunate, and scaphoid. The triquetrum (t), hamate (h), trapezium (tr1) and trapezoid (tr2), capitate (c), and radius (r) are labeled. **B,** Fluid-sensitive coronal image emphasizing T2 relaxation demonstrates increased signal intensity (bright) within the inflammatory pannus, compatible with increase in mobile water associated with inflammation. Increased signal intensity is evident within the lunate, scaphoid, and distal ulna, including focal areas within the distal row of carpal bones, corresponding to small erosions. Diffuse increased signal within the distal radius likely reflects reactive marrow edema (*asterisk*).

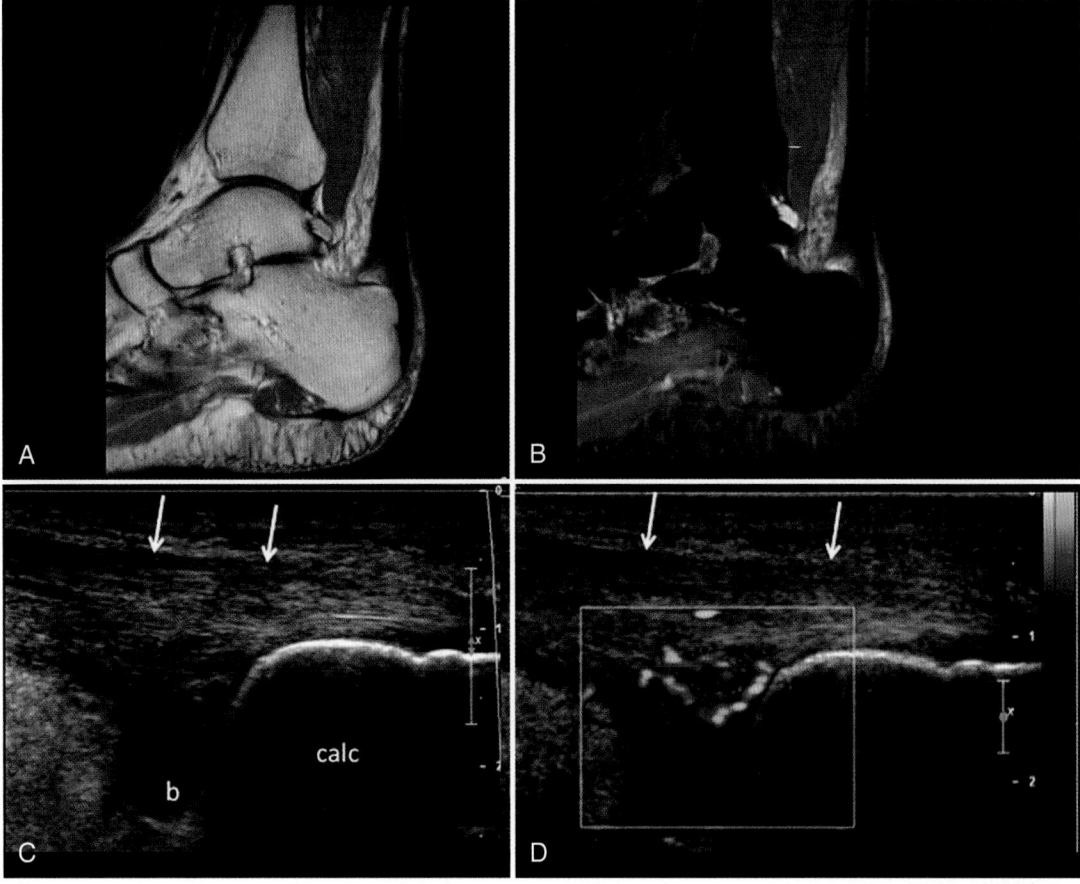

FIGURE 243-6. **Imaging of the soft tissues in a patient with retrocalcaneal pain demonstrating complementary nature of magnetic resonance imaging and ultrasound. A,** Proton density sagittal image emphasizes anatomic detail, whereas **(B)** fluid-sensitive image depicts thickening and increased signal intensity within the distal Achilles tendon reflecting tendinosis, retrocalcaneal bursitis, or tear of the deep surface of the tendon. Surrounding increased signal intensity (bright areas) within the adjacent soft tissue reflects adjacent soft tissue edema. **C,** Long axis gray scale and **(D)** power Doppler images of the same patient obtained when the patient presented for ultrasound-guided therapeutic injection. The tendon (*arrows*) is inhomogeneous. A prominent hypoechoic collection deep to the tendon is compatible with retrocalcaneal bursitis (b). There is prominent increased vascularity on power Doppler imaging at the margin of the bursa and tendon. The calcaneus (calc) is labeled.

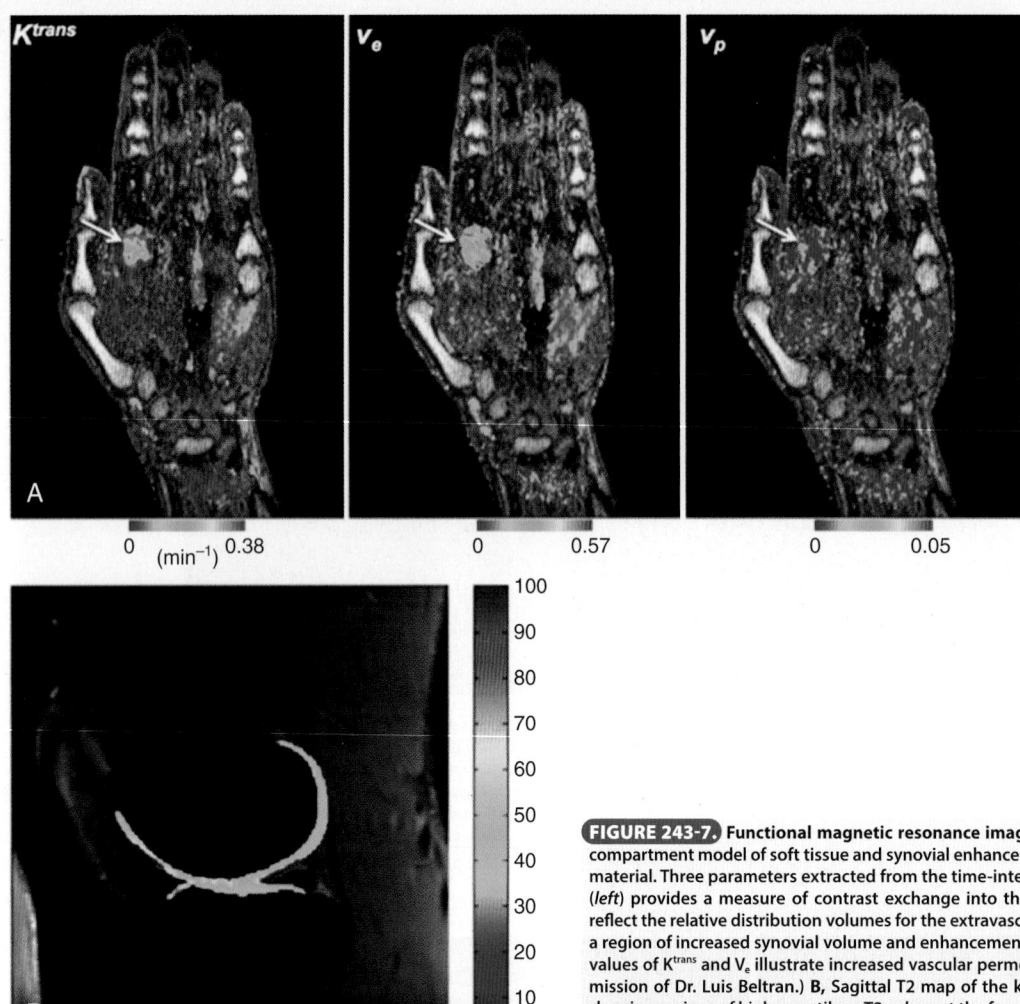

FIGURE 243-7. Functional magnetic resonance imaging. **A,** Parametric image derived from fitting a two-compartment model of soft tissue and synovial enhancement following intravenous administration of contrast material. Three parameters extracted from the time-intensity curves are displayed as parametric images: K^{trans} (*left*) provides a measure of contrast exchange into the extravascular soft tissues; V_e (*center*) and V_p (*right*) reflect the relative distribution volumes for the extravascular space and plasma, respectively. The *arrows* depict a region of increased synovial volume and enhancement at the second metacarpophalangeal joint. Increased values of K^{trans} and V_e illustrate increased vascular permeability at the site of inflammation. (Printed with permission of Dr. Luis Beltran.) **B,** Sagittal T2 map of the knee in which relative T2 relaxation is color encoded, showing regions of higher cartilage T2 values at the femoral condyle and tibial plateau. This reflects alterations in cartilage collagen architecture and water content and possibly early osteoarthritis. (Printed with permission of Dr. Gregory Chang.)

stabilize or get better, although in some patients, the process progresses, affecting mobility and causing severe pain.

Injection of dilute gadolinium into the joint (direct MR arthrography) is helpful for outlining structures to determine whether there is morphologic damage. Injection is usually performed either under fluoroscopic or ultrasound guidance. This technique is particularly effective for visualization of small structures such as the labrum of the hip or shoulder if there is no joint effusion. It is also helpful for demonstrating breakdown of soft tissue structures that normally prevent communication between joint compartments such as the rotator cuff, triangular fibrocartilage of the wrist, and ligaments in the various joints. Newer techniques that enable image acquisition in near real time as well as the development of MR-compatible needles now permit a variety of percutaneous procedures to be performed directly under MR guidance.

● SCINTIGRAPHY

Scintigraphy by its nature represents physiologic imaging because it derives from labeling physiologically occurring substances with a gamma-emitting radionuclide and uses detectors in the form of gamma cameras arranged in a planar or circumferential configuration to determine the distribution of radionuclide within the tissue. Scintigraphy can provide a global assessment of abnormal tracer uptake or can be performed using a targeted approach (Fig. 243-8). Images often provide high tissue contrast but are of relatively poor spatial resolution. Commonly employed agents vary from tagged red blood cells to assess blood flow; agents that reflect bone metabolism (technetium-99m methylene diphosphate [Tc-MDP]); agents that reflect glucose metabolism (18-fluorine deoxyglucose [18-FDG]), in the case of PET; and agents that concentrate at sites of inflammation, such as autologous white blood cells labeled with ^{111}In (indium) and ^{67}Ga-citrate (gallium). Clinical applications

include detection of a variety of malignancies, osteomyelitis, vascular graft infection, multifocal infectious disease, inflammatory diseases such as RA, vasculitis, inflammatory bowel disease, sarcoidosis, fever of unknown origin, and infection of joint prostheses.

Traditional nuclear medicine involves use of single gamma photon emissions as a product of nuclear decay. The information can be displayed using planar imaging through a single (or multiple) pinhole camera or displayed tomographically in a manner similar to CT (single-photon emission CT [SPECT]). Bone scintigraphy employs Tc-MDP as the radioactive tracer. The isotope goes to areas of high bone turnover and vascular flow as well as areas of calcium or bone deposition. Three-phase bone scans are obtained at different intervals after injection, reflecting the early vascular phase, the intermediate blood pool phase, and the late phase. Each phase allows for further characterization of the disease process. Abnormal tracer uptake is seen in areas of inflammation, infection, neoplasm, osteonecrosis, and fracture. The scan is most useful to identify the location of lesions within the skeleton but is nonspecific.

PET scans use the appearance of two simultaneously produced 511-KEV gamma rays following annihilation of a positron and electron pair to localize the distribution of radionuclide. The near-simultaneous detection of the photons (coincidence counting) provides an estimate of source tracer concentration. Newer PET scanners are often used in combination with either CT or MRI in order to achieve improved spatial registration, allow accurate estimates of soft tissue attenuation, provide high-quality anatomic images, and quantify metabolic activity.[8] Combined PET-CT or PET-MRI provides high-resolution images of abnormal metabolic activity and may ultimately provide the most definitive maps of inflammatory activity in patients with rheumatic disease. Early results to date have been promising and are expected to provide sensitive evaluation of the response to DMARDs in patients with inflammatory arthritis.

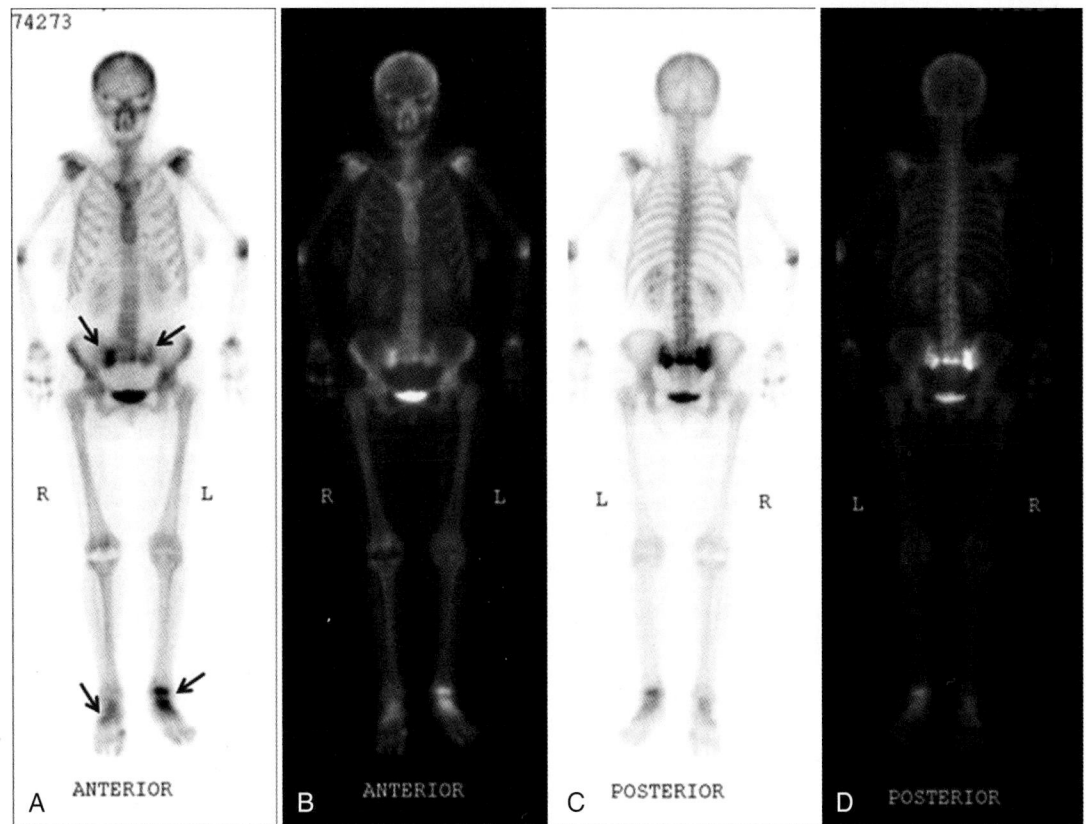

FIGURE 243-8. Rectilinear bone scan in a patient with back pain. **A, B,** Anterior and **(C, D)** posterior delayed images of the axial and appendicular skeleton demonstrate increased tracer uptake in the region of the sacral ala, left ankle, and right midfoot (*arrows*). Follow-up radiographs confirmed the presence of bilateral sacral ala fractures. Note that the central pooling of tracer in the expected location of the urinary bladder is normal. Bone scans provide a sensitive but nonspecific method to evaluate the appendicular and axial skeletal. Increased uptake in the feet in this patient was attributed to degenerative change. L = left; R = right.

GENERAL REFERENCES

For the General References and other additional features, please visit Expert Consult at https://expertconsult.inkling.com.

244

INHERITED DISEASES OF CONNECTIVE TISSUE

REED E. PYERITZ

MUCOPOLYSACCHARIDOSES

DEFINITION

Proteoglycans are ubiquitous components of the extracellular matrix and the surfaces of cells, and they are among the largest and most complex of human molecules. Proteoglycans consist of a protein core to which are covalently bound glycosaminoglycans (GAGs; formerly called mucopolysaccharides) of several types: dermatan sulfate, heparan sulfate, keratan sulfate, and chondroitin sulfate. During normal degradation, these four polymeric molecules are cleaved from their protein core in lysosomes; then they, plus hyaluronan (a GAG lacking a protein core), are catabolized further in lysosomes in a stepwise fashion by more than a dozen enzymes. Genetic defects in any one of these enzymes lead to the accumulation of GAG metabolites in lysosomes, with profound disruption of cellular physiology. The phenotypes resulting from deficiencies of these catabolic enzymes are termed *mucopolysaccharidoses* and are classified into seven types (Table 244-1).[1] Several additional storage disorders, termed *mucolipidoses,* are caused by a genetic defect in post-translational modification of lysosomal enzymes and share features with the mucopolysaccharidoses.

EPIDEMIOLOGY

All mucopolysaccharidosis disorders are rare, each with an incidence of one or fewer cases per 100,000 births, and are without ethnic predilection.

PATHOBIOLOGY

With the exception of mucopolysaccharidosis II (Hunter syndrome), which is X-linked, each of these disorders is autosomal recessive. All mucopolysaccharidoses are caused by deficiency of a single lysosomal enzyme responsible for a specific step in GAG metabolism. Catabolism of GAG proceeds normally until the step requiring the defective enzyme, when further normal metabolism halts. Although a minor degree of nonspecific breakdown occurs, resulting in urinary excretion of cleaved GAG that can be useful diagnostically, the accumulation of GAG within lysosomes of cells of mesenchymal origin, endothelium, and, in most cases, neurons causes widespread, progressive cellular dysfunction and clinical effects. Lysosomal enzymes are targeted to lysosomes by post-translational addition of mannose 6-phosphate. Deficiency of the phosphotransferase that catalyzes the first step in this reaction results in an inability to catabolize any GAG molecules. The catabolic enzymes, which normally would be transported into lysosomes, instead are secreted from the cell and are found in unusually high concentrations in plasma, providing one diagnostic test for mucolipidoses.

Pathology

All pathologic manifestations of mucopolysaccharidosis and mucolipidosis disorders worsen with age, and some are present from early developmental stages. Gross anatomic hallmarks are hepatosplenomegaly, marked skeletal alterations (termed *dysostosis multiplex*)[2] that result in short stature and thoracic cage deformity, thickening and narrowing of airways and arteries, and coarsening of facial features. Although mental retardation is a prominent feature of some of these conditions, the brain may show only ventriculomegaly

TABLE 244-1 MUCOPOLYSACCHARIDOSES AND MUCOLIPIDOSES

TYPE	EPONYM OR COMMON NAME	CLINICAL FEATURES	INHERITANCE	OMIM*	ENZYMATIC DEFECT
MPS IH	Hurler syndrome	DM and short stature; MR; corneal clouding; HS; heart disease; death in childhood	AR	252800	α-L-iduronidase
MPS IS	Scheie syndrome	Coarse facies; stiff joints, corneal clouding; aortic valve disease; normal intelligence and life span	AR	252800	α-L-iduronidase
MPS II	Hunter syndrome	Severe form: coarse facies, DM and short stature, HS; MR; no corneal clouding; death by late adolescence. Mild form: coarse facies, short stature; normal intelligence; survival to adulthood	XL	309900	Iduronate sulfatase
MPS IIIA	Sanfilippo A	Severe MR and hyperactivity; mild somatic changes	AR	252900	Heparan N-sulfatase
MPS IIIB	Sanfilippo B	Same as MPS IIIA	AR	252920	α-N-acetylglucosaminidase
MPS IIIC	Sanfilippo C	Same as MPS IIIA	AR	252930	Acetyl-coenzyme A: α-glucosaminide acetyltransferase
MPS IIID	Sanfilippo D	Same as MPS IIIA	AR	252940	N-acetylglucosamine 6-sulfatase
MPS IVA	Morquio A	Short stature and distinct skeletal dysplasia with odontoid hypoplasia and myelopathy; corneal clouding; normal intelligence; valvular heart disease	AR	253000	Galactose 6-sulfatase
MPS IVB	Morquio B	Same as MPS IVA	AR	253010	β-Galactosidase
MPS VI	Maroteaux-Lamy	DM and short stature; corneal clouding; normal intelligence; aortic stenosis; leukocyte inclusions; hydrocephalus in severe form	AR	253200	N-acetylgalactosamine
MPS VII	Sly syndrome	DM; HS; widely variable, including MR	AR	253220	β-Glucuronidase
MPS IX	—	Short stature; periarticular soft tissue masses	AR	601492	Hyaluronidase
ML II	I-cell disease	Similar to but more severe than MPS IH but with cellular inclusions; no mucopolysacchariduria	AR	252500	UDP-N-acetylglucosamine: lysosomal enzyme N-acetylglucosaminyl-1-phosphotransferase
ML III	Pseudo-Hurler polydystrophy	Short stature and mild DM; stiff joints, mild MR; survival to adulthood	AR	252500	Same as ML II arthropathy, coarse facies; variable but milder

*Entries in Online Mendelian Inheritance in Man, OMIM. McKusick-Nathans Institute of Genetic Medicine. Baltimore: Johns Hopkins University. http://omim.org.
AR = autosomal recessive; DM = dysostosis multiplex; HS = hepatosplenomegaly; MR= mental retardation; UDP = uridine diphosphate; XL = X-linked.

secondary to communicating hydrocephalus. On microscopy, mesenchymal cells show a cytoplasm full of apparently empty vacuoles; these are lysosomes from which GAG has been removed by fixation. Cells cultured from patients show greatly enlarged lysosomes filled with granular material. In the severe form of mucolipidosis, dense inclusions are present, which gave rise to the common name, *I-cell disease*.

CLINICAL MANIFESTATIONS

Each of the disorders in Table 244-1 shows a wide spectrum of clinical severity. This wide spectrum has led to a classification that gives the impression of separate disorders within some of the mucopolysaccharidosis and mucolipidosis types, but these represent the apparent ends of the continuum. Some of the disorders without treatment result in death by adolescence (Hurler syndrome, severe Hunter syndrome, mucolipidosis II), but others are commonly compatible with survival to adulthood. The latter group of disorders is emphasized here.

The milder end of the mucopolysaccharidosis I spectrum, Scheie syndrome, may not be diagnosed until adulthood; patients present with stiffened joints, corneal clouding and glaucoma, carpal tunnel syndrome, and aortic valvular disease. Stature and intelligence are not affected. The main health risks are cardiac valvular involvement, thickening of meninges that can produce a myelopathy, and thickening of the upper airways that can produce obstructive symptoms and sleep apnea.

The milder form of mucopolysaccharidosis II, Hunter syndrome, is distinctive because it is X-linked (affecting males almost exclusively), and the cornea shows little overt clouding. Cervical myelopathy, obstructive airway disease, and cor pulmonale are important concerns. A combined conductive and neurosensory hearing loss is common.

Neither mucopolysaccharidosis IV (Morquio syndrome) nor mucopolysaccharidosis VI (Maroteaux-Lamy syndrome) affects intelligence. Both syndromes often are associated with severe skeletal changes, which are distinct radiographically but produce similar problems of kyphoscoliosis, pectus carinatum, restrictive lung disease, severe short stature, and joint degeneration. Cervical myelopathy resulting from a thickened dura is common to both disorders and is accentuated by odontoid hypoplasia in mucopolysaccharidosis IV.

Thickening of the aortic and mitral valves may produce severe dysfunction necessitating their replacement. General anesthesia is especially hazardous because of the narrow upper and middle airways and cervical instability.

Patients with mucolipidosis III (pseudo-Hurler polydystrophy) resemble patients with mucopolysaccharidosis VI but often have mild to moderate mental retardation. Aortic regurgitation is common.

DIAGNOSIS
Differential Diagnosis

Diagnosis of these conditions is difficult in young children, before most of the clinical features have progressed, but should be considered in any person with hepatosplenomegaly and coarsening of the facial features. Evaluation requires a pedigree analysis, ophthalmologic examination, skeletal radiographic survey, echocardiography, and analysis of the urine for excretion of GAGs. Often the specific mucopolysaccharidosis is evident from radiographs, the presence or absence of corneal clouding, and the pattern of mucopolysacchariduria. Enzymatic analysis of leukocytes confirms the diagnosis. Patients with mucolipidoses do not show mucopolysacchariduria but have marked elevation of all the GAG catabolic lysosomal enzymes in plasma.

TREATMENT   Rx

Ventriculoperitoneal shunting is necessary if intracranial pressure is elevated. Close attention to hearing and visual problems is essential throughout life. Many adults with mucopolysaccharidosis or mucolipidosis require surgery for carpal tunnel syndrome. Cardiovascular surgery for valvular or coronary disease may be necessary. All use of anesthesia is high risk because of the narrow airways and, in the case of mucopolysaccharidosis IV, atlantoaxial instability. For patients who remain ambulatory, selective joint replacement can be beneficial. Because of the morbidity associated with thoracic cage deformity, consideration should be given to stabilizing the spinal deformity before it becomes severe.

Replacement of the deficient enzyme by intravenous infusion is being studied for most of the mucopolysaccharidosis disorders.[3] Laronidase (Aldurazyme) has been approved in the United States for treatment of mucopolysaccharidosis I. An infusion every 2 weeks for 1 year in adolescent and adult patients resulted in substantial reduction in hepatosplenomegaly and modest improvement in pulmonary function, sleep apnea, and joint mobility. Whether early institution of therapy in young children modulates mental retardation in the Hurler variant of mucopolysaccharidosis I is uncertain. Galsulfase (Naglazyme) has been approved for the treatment of mucopolysaccharidosis VI, in which somatic rather than neurologic problems predominate. Bone marrow transplantation has been attempted in many of the mucopolysaccharidosis disorders,[4] with mixed success. The earlier transplantation occurs, the better the outcome in terms of somatic problems, but prevention of mental retardation has not occurred. Current recommendations based on consensus in Europe calls for hematopoietic stem cell transplantation for patients with Hurler syndrome before the age of 2.5 years. Enzyme replacement should be started in all patients when diagnosed. Gene therapy has been successful in a mouse model of Hunter syndrome, thereby providing proof of concept for the treatment of Hunter syndrome patients with cognitive impairment.[5]

MARFAN SYNDROME

DEFINITION

Marfan syndrome is an autosomal dominant, pleiotropic disorder caused by defects in the principal component of the extracellular microfibril, the large glycoprotein fibrillin-1.[6] The disease manifestations occur in multiple systems, especially the eye, skeleton, heart, aorta, lung, and integument. Notable features include dislocation of the ocular lens, tall stature with particularly long limbs and digits, deformity of the thoracic cage by pectus carinatum or excavatum with abnormal curvature of the spine, mitral and tricuspid valve prolapse, dilation of the sinuses of Valsalva and predisposition to aortic dissection, spontaneous pneumothorax, abnormal skin stretch marks, hernias, and dural ectasia. If untreated, patients often die before 30 or 40 years of age from aortic dissection or congestive heart failure.

EPIDEMIOLOGY

Marfan syndrome is a common mendelian disorder, with an estimated incidence of about 1 per 5000 births. Marfan syndrome is found throughout the world, without ethnic or geographic predilection.

PATHOBIOLOGY

Pathogenesis

Mutations in *FBN1*, which maps to human chromosome 15q21.1 and encodes fibrillin-1, cause Marfan syndrome and related connective tissue disorders. More than 1500 distinct mutations have been found, and few occur in more than one family. Patients are heterozygous for mutations in *FBN1*, leading to autosomal dominant inheritance. Extracellular microfibrils are polymers of many fibrillin-1 molecules and are ubiquitous in the extracellular matrix of most tissues. Latent transforming growth factor-β (TGF-β) binding protein, which keeps the cytokine inactive, bears striking homology to regions of fibrillin. Abnormalities of either the quality or the quantity of microfibrils disrupt normal signaling by TGF-β, especially during embryonic development and postnatal growth. Studies in mice engineered to harbor human mutations in *FBN1* showed that excessive TGF-β signaling causes abnormal lung septation (the precursor to pneumothorax), bone overgrowth, mitral valve prolapse, muscular hypoplasia, and aortic dilation. This fundamental shift in understanding of the pathogenesis of Marfan syndrome has suggested novel therapies, such as with small molecules that affect the activity of TGF-β or its downstream signaling.

The features of Marfan syndrome are highly variable, even among relatives who share the same mutation in *FBN1*. This variability persists after accounting for the effects of age. Men tend to be affected more severely, for unclear reasons.

Pathology

The features of Marfan syndrome are age dependent. Some severely affected infants have flagrant features and often die of mitral regurgitation and heart failure despite aggressive management. At the other end of the clinical spectrum, Marfan syndrome merges with several related disorders, and patients may not come to medical attention, let alone receive a definitive diagnosis, until adulthood.

None of the gross or microscopic pathologic changes is specific for Marfan syndrome. The medial degeneration of the aortic wall, characterized by disarray and fragmentation of the elastic fibers and increased proteoglycan (often inappropriately termed *cystic medial necrosis*), also can be seen in other disorders and in older people with hypertension. Aortic dissection (Chapter 69) usually begins just superior to the aortic valve (type A) and often progresses to the bifurcation. Death usually results from retrograde dissection and hemopericardium. About 10% of dissections begin in the descending thoracic aorta (type B).

CLINICAL MANIFESTATIONS

The lens tends to be displaced superiorly, and usually the zonules remain intact. The retina is at increased risk for detachment, especially in patients who are highly myopic. Tubular bones overgrow, accounting for the disproportionate tall stature (dolichostenomelia), long digits (arachnodactyly), and sternal deformity. Ligaments may be lax, causing scoliosis and joint hypermobility. Alternatively, congenital contractures are common, especially of the elbows. The palate typically is highly arched, and the dentition can be crowded and maloccluded. Mitral valve prolapse occurs in about 80% of cases, and the valve leaflets become progressively thickened (myxomatous on histopathology). The mitral annulus may dilate and calcify. Aortic root dilation begins in the sinuses of Valsalva and progresses with age, albeit at highly variable rates (Chapters 61 and 69).[7,8] Most males with Marfan syndrome have an aortic root dimension above the upper limit of normal for their body surface area by adolescence. Some females show a slower progression and may have a root diameter near the upper limit of normal well into adulthood. The dilation usually does not involve the distal ascending aorta. Spontaneous pneumothorax, resulting from rupture of apical blebs, occurs in about 5% of patients. Stretch marks (striae atrophicae) occur over areas of flexural stress, such as the shoulders, breasts, and lower back. The neural canal in the lumbosacral region is enlarged in most people with Marfan syndrome; this may be visible on plain radiographs, especially if the neuroforamina are widened. Imaging by computed tomography or magnetic resonance imaging is diagnostic and should be used in patients with back pain and radicular symptoms. Dural ectasia progresses with age; large anterior meningoceles in the pelvis are a severe manifestation. Simple cysts in the liver and kidneys are common, increase with age, and seldom cause clinical problems. Sleep apnea is of increased frequency in adults.[9]

DIAGNOSIS

Differential Diagnosis

The conditions that overlap clinically and genetically with Marfan syndrome include familial aortic aneurysm, familial ectopia lentis, mitral valve prolapse, mild aortic dilation, striae, skeleton (MASS) phenotype (which includes many families with mitral valve prolapse syndrome), and Loeys-Dietz syndrome. Most of these conditions are diagnosed clinically, so differentiating among them is arbitrary. A careful family history is essential to this process. Molecular genetic testing has a limited role. However, if the mutation in *FBN1* is known in a family, analysis of DNA can be used effectively for presymptomatic or prenatal diagnosis. Loeys-Dietz syndrome, which is associated with generalized arterial tortuosity and susceptibility to dissection, is caused by mutation in either of two receptors for TGF-β, *TGFBR1* and *TGFBR2*, and molecular analysis is clinically available. Most mutations in *TGFBR1* and *TGFBR2* do not cause Loeys-Dietz syndrome but do predispose to familial thoracic aneurysm and dissection.

A question of Marfan syndrome arises most commonly in tall, lanky adolescents who have several minor skeletal features, nearsightedness, and athletic desires. A detailed ophthalmologic examination with full pupillary dilation and a transthoracic echocardiogram are essential components in the evaluation. If these test results are negative and no one in the family has a history of Marfan syndrome or aortic dissection, the patient probably can be reassured.[10]

TREATMENT   Rx

All patients should be seen at least annually by a physician who manages the overall care. Most patients require annual ophthalmologic and cardiologic consultation and orthopedic consultation as required by specific problems. Lens subluxation often requires surgical correction.[11] A number of studies, but only one randomized clinical trial, support the prophylactic use of β-adrenergic blockade from an early age to slow the rate of aortic root dilation and protect against aortic dissection. Based on studies of the Marfan mouse, therapies that interfere with excess signaling through pathways mediated by TGF-β are being studied in human clinical trials. One large European trial suggested a benefit of the angiotensin receptor blocker losartan on aortic root dilation rate,[A1] but three trials found no benefit of losartan compared with atenolol.[A2-A4] Prophylactic surgical repair of the aortic root has had the greatest beneficial impact. The composite graft, involving a prosthetic valve in a Dacron tube and implantation of the coronary ostia into the graft, was the first approach to produce markedly improved survival in these patients. More recently, replacement of the aneurysm and preservation of the native aortic valve have shown promise and should be considered first.[12] For adults, aortic root surgery should be strongly considered when the maximal aortic diameter reaches 45 mm, and a family history of aortic dissection should prompt earlier repair (Chapter 61).

PROGNOSIS

Life expectancy for people with Marfan syndrome has improved markedly, to the point that many patients can expect survival to advanced years. Some data suggest that aortic dissection and cardiovascular death are more likely in patients with *FBN1* haploinsufficiency with expression of the nonmutated allele than in patients with dominant-negative mutations in which abnormal fibrillin 1 coded by the mutated allele interacts with normal fibrillin 1 coded by the normal allele.[13]

EHLERS-DANLOS SYNDROMES

DEFINITION

The Ehlers-Danlos syndromes are clinically variable and genetically heterogeneous. Diagnoses still are based largely on the bedside examination. The unifying themes among these disorders are fragility of tissues, joint hypermobility, and skin hyperextensibility.[14]

EPIDEMIOLOGY

No accurate data exist, but an incidence of about 1 in 5000 births is a reasonable estimate of how many individuals qualify for one of the Ehlers-Danlos syndrome diagnoses. Each type represents something of a clinical spectrum, with the mild end merging with what might be considered normal variation. Just as the diagnostic criteria are arbitrary, so would be any determination of prevalence based on phenotypic criteria. The extent to which normal variation in joint hypermobility, skin elasticity, and tissue fragility represents genetic variation at loci that encode collagen or other extracellular matrix genes requires considerable research.

PATHOBIOLOGY

Pathogenesis

Defects in collagen and other proteins in the extracellular matrix of various tissues underlie all forms of Ehlers-Danlos syndrome that have been elucidated so far. The specific mutations occur in a variety of genes, with the effect of altering the structure, synthesis, post-translational modifications, or stability of the collagens involved. The known molecular defects are listed in Table 244-2.

Pathology

Few findings in the routine pathologic evaluation distinguish among the various types of Ehlers-Danlos syndrome or even distinguish individual types from normal. Thickness of the dermis is decreased in some forms, especially the vascular type, and the walls of arteries are reduced in thickness in this type. By electron microscopy, the classic, hypermobile, and kyphoscoliotic types have abnormal collagen fibers, especially when viewed in cross section (variable and often increased fiber diameter with an irregular outline). In the vascular type, some patients have dilated endoplasmic reticulum consistent with aberrant secretion of type III collagen molecules.

CLINICAL MANIFESTATIONS

The major and minor features of each Ehlers-Danlos syndrome are detailed in Table 244-2. Infants with classic Ehlers-Danlos syndrome often are born prematurely by 4 to 8 weeks because of rupture of fetal membranes. Diagnosis of the vascular and kyphoscoliotic types is important because of their cardiovascular features. The vascular type, previously termed *Ehlers-Danlos syndrome IV*, is characterized by spontaneous rupture of large arteries and hollow organs, especially the colon and uterus, and pneumothorax. Because these events carry considerable morbidity, life expectancy is reduced, on average, by more than half. During pregnancy, women with this form of Ehlers-Danlos syndrome are especially vulnerable to rupture of major arteries and the uterus. In the kyphoscoliotic type, aortic root dilation and aortic regurgitation can develop. Patients with most forms of Ehlers-Danlos syndrome are prone to develop mitral valve prolapse, and progression to mitral regurgitation (Chapter 66) occurs more often than in the common form of mitral valve prolapse.

DIAGNOSIS

Differential Diagnosis

By careful adherence to the clinical features shown in Table 244-2 and judicious use of laboratory tests, the various defined types of Ehlers-Danlos syndrome can be differentiated. Many other specific syndromes need to be excluded.

TABLE 244-2 EHLERS-DANLOS SYNDROMES

TYPE	FORMER NAME	CLINICAL FEATURES*	INHERITANCE	OMIM†	MOLECULAR DEFECT
Classic	EDS I and II	Joint hypermobility; skin hyperextensibility; atrophic scars; smooth, velvety skin; subcutaneous spheroids	AD	130000 130010	Structure of type V collagen caused by mutations in COL5A1 or COL5A2
Hypermobility	EDS III	Joint hypermobility; some skin hyperextensibility, with or without a smooth, velvety texture	AD AR	130020 225320	? Tenascin-X (TNX)
Vascular	EDS IV	Thin skin; easy bruising; pinched nose; acrogeria; rupture of large- and medium-caliber arteries, uterus, and large bowel	AD	130050 (225350) (225360)	Deficient type III collagen (COL3A1)
Kyphoscoliotic	EDS VI	Joint hypermobility; congenital, progressive rupture; scoliosis; scleral fragility with globe rupture; tissue fragility, aortic dilation, MVP	AR	225400	Deficiency of lysyl hydroxylase
Arthrochalasis	EDS VII A	Joint hypermobility, severe, with subluxations, congenital hip dislocation; and skin hyperextensibility; tissue fragility	AD	130060	No cleavage of amino terminus of type I procollagen caused by mutations in COL1A1 or COL1A2
Dermatosparaxis	EDS VII C	Severe skin fragility; decreased skin elasticity, easy bruising; hernias; premature rupture of fetal membranes	AR	225410	No cleavage of amino terminus of type I procollagen caused by deficiency of peptidase
Unclassified types	EDS V	Classic features	XL	305200	?
	EDS VIII	Classic features and periodontal disease	AD	130080	?
	EDS X	Mild classic features, MVP	?	225310	?
	EDS XI	Joint instability	AD	147900	?
	EDS IX	Classic features; occipital horns	XL	309400	Allelic to Menkes syndrome
	EDS, progeroid form	Classic features and premature aging	AR	130700	Deficiency of galactosyltransferase I

*Listed in order of diagnostic importance.
†Entries in Online Mendelian Inheritance in Man, OMIM. McKusick-Nathans Institute of Genetic Medicine. Baltimore: Johns Hopkins University. http://omim.org.
AD = autosomal dominant; AR = autosomal recessive; EDS = Ehlers-Danlos syndrome; MVP = mitral valve prolapse; XL = X-linked.

The kyphoscoliotic type of Ehlers-Danlos syndrome in infants shares some features with severe Marfan syndrome. Patients with Larsen syndrome may resemble patients with the arthrochalaxis type of Ehlers-Danlos syndrome. The skin redundancy and loss of elasticity of the dermatosparaxis type of Ehlers-Danlos syndrome is reminiscent of autosomal dominant cutis laxa, which is not associated with easy bruising or tissue fragility.

The most difficult decision is whether any diagnosis of Ehlers-Danlos syndrome is warranted.[15] Patients who have only joint hypermobility without skin changes should not be labeled with Ehlers-Danlos syndrome; a diagnosis of familial joint hypermobility might be more appropriate. Familial joint instability involves a predisposition to dislocations of major joints that is rare in most types of Ehlers-Danlos syndrome except for arthrochalaxis.

TREATMENT Rx

Management of most skin and joint problems should be conservative and preventive. Sutures need to be placed with careful attention to approximating the margins and avoiding tension; removable sutures should be left in place for twice the usual time. Most instances of joint hypermobility and pain in Ehlers-Danlos syndrome do not require surgical treatment. Benefit often is derived from physical therapy designed to strengthen the muscles that provide support for the loose ligaments. All patients should receive genetic counseling about the mode of inheritance and their risk for having children affected with Ehlers-Danlos syndrome. The possibility of prenatal diagnosis exists for all of the Ehlers-Danlos syndrome types with defined molecular or biochemical defects.

The vascular type of Ehlers-Danlos syndrome requires particular surgical care; the ruptured arteries are difficult to repair because of the pronounced vascular fragility. Experienced vascular surgeons are having some success with prophylactic repair of vessels deemed to be at risk for dissection or rupture. One clinical trial suggested improved outcomes with prophylactic β-adrenergic blockade.[A5] Rupture of the bowel is a surgical emergency. Because the risk for uterine and vascular rupture is especially high during pregnancy in women with the vascular form, affected women should be advised that there is a substantial risk for death related to pregnancy and delivery. Patients should be advised to avoid contact sports and to treat blood pressure elevations aggressively. Arteriography and arterial lines should be avoided if possible. Biochemical and genetic screening holds the potential for reassuring relatives at risk that they do not have a defect in type III collagen.

The kyphoscoliotic type of Ehlers-Danlos syndrome may improve with large doses of vitamin C (1 to 4 g/day) because ascorbate is a cofactor for the enzyme that is deficient. No other metabolic or genetic therapy is effective in other forms of Ehlers-Danlos syndrome.

OSTEOGENESIS IMPERFECTA SYNDROMES

DEFINITION

The heterogeneous group of disorders called *osteogenesis imperfecta* includes, at one end of the severity spectrum, a type that is lethal prenatally or in the neonatal period and, at the other, such mild features that make distinguishing affected individuals from the general population is difficult.[16,17] The unifying feature is hereditary osteopenia (insufficient bone), with primary defects in the protein matrix in bone and other tissues. The clinical syndromes all involve osteoporosis with liability to fracture (Chapter 230).

EPIDEMIOLOGY

No careful epidemiologic study has been performed, and the milder forms of type I osteogenesis imperfecta merge with the phenotypes of familial osteoporosis, fracture susceptibility, and joint hypermobility found in the general population. A crude estimate of the overall prevalence of osteogenesis imperfecta is 1 to 2 per 20,000 births. The neonatal lethal form (type II), which is almost always caused by a new mutation in a parental gamete, has an incidence of about 1 in 50,000 births.

PATHOBIOLOGY
Pathogenesis
Most patients in whom mutations have been found usually have defects in the two genes that encode the procollagen chains of type I collagen, *COL1A1* and *COL1A2*. Type I collagen is composed of two $\alpha1(I)$ and one $\alpha2(I)$ procollagen chains; the mature fiber requires considerable post-translational modification, which occurs appropriately only if the three procollagen chains have intertwined to form a triple helix that is perfect and completed at the right speed. A mutation that affects formation of the triple helix, such as substitution of one of the mandatory glycine residues that occurs at every third position, also has adverse effects on the modifications that render the molecule capable of forming effective mature fibers. As a result, a single nucleotide change resulting in a missense mutation can have profound effects on the extracellular matrix and produce a severe condition. Alternatively, and at first glance paradoxically, a mutation that eliminates an entire allele, or at least production of any product capable of intertwining with normal procollagen chains, has a much milder effect on the extracellular matrix and on the severity of osteogenesis imperfecta. Examples of the most common classes of mutations are shown in Table 244-3. Hundreds of mutations have been described. Patients with mutations in *COL1A1* or *COL1A2* are heterozygous, and thus the most common forms of osteogenesis imperfecta are inherited as autosomal

TABLE 244-3	OSTEOGENESIS IMPERFECTA			
TYPE	**CLINICAL FEATURES**	**INHERITANCE**	**OMIM***	**BASIC DEFECTS**
I	Fractures variable in number; little deformity; stature normal or nearly so; blue sclerae; hearing loss common but not always present; DI uncommon	AD	166200	Typically, one nonfunctional *COL1A1* allele
II	Lethal in utero or shortly after birth; many fractures at birth typically involving ribs (may appear "beaded") and other long bones; little calvaria; pulmonary hypertension	AD	166210	*COL1A1* or *COL1A2*: substitution of glycyl residues; occasionally deletions of a portion of the triple-helical domain
		AR	259400	Deletion in *COL1A2* plus a nonfunctional allele
III	Fractures common, but long bones progressively deform starting in utero; stature markedly reduced; sclerae often blue but become lighter with age; DI and hearing loss common	AD	259420	One single amino acid substitution
		AR (rare)	259440	Two mutations in *COL1A1* and/or *COL1A2* (rarely)
IV	Fractures common; stature usually reduced; bone deformity common but rarely severe; scleral hue normal to grayish; hearing loss variable; DI common	AD	166220 166240	Point mutations in *COL1A1* or *COL1A2* Exon skipping mutations in *COL1A2*
V	Similar to type IV without DI or blue sclerae; fractures develop hyperplastic callus; calcification of the interosseous membrane between the radius and ulna	AD	610967	?
VI	Similar to type IV without DI, blue sclerae or wormian bones; excess osteoid present in bone	?	610968	?
VII	Similar to types II or III with fractures at birth, blue sclerae, no DI; presence of rhizomelic limb shortening and coxa vara	AR	610682	Mutations in *CRTAP*
VIII	Similar to types II or III with fractures at birth	AR	610915	Mutations in *LEPRE1*
IX	Similar to types II or III with fractures at birth	AR	259440	Mutations in *PPIB*

*Entries in Online Mendelian Inheritance in Man, OMIM. McKusick-Nathans Institute of Genetic Medicine. Baltimore: Johns Hopkins University. http://omim.org.
AD = autosomal dominant; AR = autosomal recessive; DI = dentinogenesis imperfecta.

dominant traits. Several autosomal recessive forms of osteogenesis imperfecta occur because of mutations in genes that encode enzymes that process type I collagen into mature fibrils.

Pathology

Other than the gross pathology associated with the clinical manifestations, the most characteristic pathology is a primary reduction in bone matrix with secondary undermineralization.

CLINICAL MANIFESTATIONS

The major phenotypic features of osteogenesis imperfecta are shown in Table 244-3. Among the most common forms, the most severe type is type II, followed in decreasing order by types III, IV, and I. In type II, infants either are stillborn or die soon after birth of pulmonary failure secondary to the small thorax, which usually is compromised further by myriad rib fractures. A few infants have survived for at least a few years but require enormous attention to their medical needs.

Type III osteogenesis imperfecta may be confused with type II at birth, but survival alone helps make the distinction. Bony deformity is pronounced and not necessarily caused by fractures. Mobility is impaired, and most patients require a wheelchair at an early age. Stature may be severely compromised. Because of progressive vertebral column deformity and rib fractures, restrictive lung disease is a common problem as patients age; many die of pulmonary complications. Basilar impression causing compression of the brain stem and the craniocervical junction can produce central sleep apnea, headache, and upper motor neuron signs.

Patients with type IV osteogenesis imperfecta generally have reduced stature, some bony deformity, and abnormal teeth that are opalescent and wear easily (dentinogenesis imperfecta). As in type I osteogenesis imperfecta, the tendency to fracture is highest in childhood and lessens with adolescence. A distinguishing characteristic of type IV osteogenesis imperfecta is a normal scleral hue.

Type I osteogenesis imperfecta is probably the most common form and is associated with a bluish or blue-gray scleral hue. People with type I osteogenesis imperfecta who also have dentinogenesis imperfecta tend to have more severe skeletal problems. The risk for fracture diminishes during adulthood but reemerges as a major concern for women after menopause. Hearing impairment in all forms of osteogenesis imperfecta is common and age related, being rare before adolescence. The deficits are of either a mixed or a predominantly conductive form.

The recessive forms of osteogenesis imperfecta (types VI to IX) range in severity from type IV to type II and may have distinctive radiologic or histopathologic findings.

DIAGNOSIS

Differential Diagnosis

The range of diagnostic possibilities in a person with multiple fractures largely depends on age. In infancy, the genetic conditions hypophosphatasia, severe osteochondrodysplasias (e.g., achondrogenesis and forms of spondyloepiphyseal dysplasia), and Menkes syndrome need to be excluded when a diagnosis of type II or type III osteogenesis imperfecta is considered. The radiographic features eventually become entirely diagnostic, but often the neonatologist has to arrive at a definitive answer in short order. Analysis of serum alkaline phosphatase and copper can be helpful. In childhood, the most common situation leading to consideration of a mild form of osteogenesis imperfecta is child abuse. In this situation, the pattern of fracture is usually distinct, and bone mineralization should be normal if the child is the object of nonaccidental or repeated accidental trauma. Abnormal scleral hue, dentinogenesis imperfecta, and wormian bones (microfractures along the cranial sutures) all support the diagnosis of osteogenesis imperfecta. The legal and child-protective systems often request exclusion of osteogenesis imperfecta by analysis of collagen production from cultured skin fibroblasts or analysis of DNA for a mutation.

In older children, the disorder idiopathic juvenile osteoporosis should be considered in any patient seen initially with repeated fractures. Many osteochondrodysplasias are associated with short stature, skeletal deformity, and a tendency to fracture. Pyknodysostosis and osteopetrosis are associated with sclerotic bones rather than osteoporotic ones. In adulthood, early-onset osteoporosis may be confused with osteogenesis imperfecta (Chapter 230). Mutations in type I collagen also cause familial osteoporosis, and the skeletal phenotypes merge; patients with true osteogenesis imperfecta may have scleral, hearing, or dental abnormalities and a positive family history.

Analysis of the specific enzymes defective in the recessive forms of osteogenesis imperfecta is useful for establishing the diagnosis and enabling reproductive counseling and prenatal diagnosis if desired.

TREATMENT   Rx

Management of the skeletal complications largely depends on orthopedic, physical, and occupational therapy approaches. Risedronate (2.5 or 5 mg daily) increases bone mineral density and reduces both first and recurrent fractures in children with osteogenesis imperfecta.[A6][A7] The long-term goals are for the patient to maintain function and independence as an individual. These goals can be advanced in some patients by judicious use of intramedullary rods in the long bones of the legs; if mobility and especially ambulation can be maintained, the demineralization associated with inactivity can be avoided.

Unaffected parents of a child with osteogenesis imperfecta and all affected individuals should have genetic counseling. For the parents of a child with type II osteogenesis imperfecta, the possibility of germinal mosaicism (which has been well documented in this condition) should not be overlooked. If one parent has a "new" mutation in one of the type I procollagen genes and multiple gonadal cells carry this mutation, the risk for recurrence in future children is not negligible. If the mutation in the affected child can be defined, the risk for recurrence can be quantified (through molecular analysis of sperm) if the mutation arose in the father.

PSEUDOXANTHOMA ELASTICUM

DEFINITION

Pseudoxanthoma elasticum is a heritable disorder of connective tissue with pleiotropic manifestations wherever elastic fibers are found but primarily in the skin, eye, and vasculature.[18] Life expectancy is reduced, on average, because of a predisposition to myocardial infarction and gastrointestinal hemorrhage.

EPIDEMIOLOGY

The exact frequency of pseudoxanthoma elasticum is unknown, but it is probably underdiagnosed. Rough approximations suggest a prevalence of 1 in 25,000 to 100,000 births. Males and females are equally affected, although women are more likely to seek medical attention out of concern for the skin changes.

PATHOBIOLOGY

Pathogenesis

In most families, pseudoxanthoma elasticum occurs as an autosomal recessive trait, which means, given relatively small sibships, that many patients will have no affected relatives. Apparent autosomal dominant inheritance may reflect expression in occasional heterozygotes. The gene for pseudoxanthoma elasticum maps to human chromosome 16 and encodes one of the adenosine triphosphate (ATP)-binding cassette transporters (*ABCC6*). Because of the prominent histopathologic feature of calcification of elastic tissue, this gene may be important in calcium homeostasis. It is unclear, however, whether calcification is a primary or a secondary phenomenon in pseudoxanthoma elasticum.

Pathology

The hallmark of pseudoxanthoma elasticum, and an important diagnostic clue, is the histopathologic finding of hyperproliferated elastic fibers in the middermis; these fibers become fragmented, clumped, and calcified. An arteriolar sclerosis develops in the media of muscular arteries and arterioles; the lumen may become progressively and concentrically narrowed. Alternatively, microaneurysms can form. Thickening of the endocardium, especially in the atria, develops in some patients. In the eye, Bruch membrane becomes calcified and fragmented.

CLINICAL MANIFESTATIONS

Because of the pleiotropic nature of pseudoxanthoma elasticum, the diagnosis initially may be suspected by any of a variety of clinicians, especially dermatologists, ophthalmologists, cardiologists, and gastroenterologists. The condition gains its name from the dermatologic feature of yellowish papules that appear at areas of flexural stress, especially the neck, groin, and popliteal and cubital fossae; in periumbilical regions; and on the buccal mucosa. The appearance of affected skin has been likened to that of a "plucked chicken." Over time, affected areas coalesce and become thickened.

Changes in the eye begin as a generalized, subtle, mottled pattern in the retina (peau d'orange) and progress to the characteristic angioid streaks.[19] The latter changes are not specific for pseudoxanthoma elasticum and can be seen in diabetes mellitus, sickle cell disease, and a variety of other conditions. Streaks represent breaks in Bruch membrane, an elastic lamina that lies between the retinal vasculature and the choroid. Spontaneous hemorrhages, especially those involving the macula, lead to progressive visual loss.

Involvement of arteries of various calibers produces problems because of occlusion and hemorrhage.[20] The lifetime risk for serious gastrointestinal hemorrhage from any site, but especially the stomach, is about 10%. Hypertension is relatively common, in part because of involvement of the renal vasculature. Progressive occlusion of peripheral arteries leads to absence of pulses; acral ischemia is rare because of the development of collaterals. The risk for stroke, myocardial infarction, abdominal angina, and intermittent claudication is increased independent of other risk factors. Impaired left ventricular function is common in adults.

DIAGNOSIS
Differential Diagnosis
Whole exome sequencing is an efficient and sensitive way to make the diagnosis.[21] An acquired form of pseudoxanthoma elasticum has been reported and is also of unclear etiology. This form is difficult to differentiate from a sporadic case in a family because of heterozygosity in the parents, but it tends to affect only the skin. As suggested by the name, the cutaneous features of pseudoxanthoma elasticum need to be differentiated from those of true xanthoma, which results from a disorder of lipid metabolism (Chapter 195). The dermatologic manifestations need to be differentiated from those of Miescher elastoma, elastic tissue nevi (Buschke-Ollendorff syndrome), and solar elastosis.

TREATMENT Rx

No cure for or means of preventing pseudoxanthoma elasticum is known. In many instances, careful attention to the ocular features by a retinal specialist experienced in pseudoxanthoma elasticum can delay but not prevent loss of vision. The risk for gastrointestinal hemorrhage suggests that patients should avoid gastric irritants such as aspirin, nonsteroidal anti-inflammatory drugs, and excessive alcohol. Stool should be checked regularly for occult blood, and angiography may be necessary to detect the source of bleeding. All standard risk factors for atherosclerosis should be managed aggressively. Complaints of chest pain should prompt a rigorous investigation for coronary artery disease. Angioplasty has not been reported to be effective, and the coronary lesions tend to be diffuse. Coronary artery bypass graft surgery has been performed, but long-term results have not been reported. It may be theoretically advantageous to use vein grafts rather than the internal mammary artery for bypass. The excessive wrinkling and pseudoxanthoma in exposed areas can be ameliorated by plastic surgery.

FUTURE DIRECTIONS
Each of these disorders poses special considerations in clinical diagnosis, utility of molecular testing, genetic counseling, and management. For the storage disorders, the clinical utility of enzyme replacement therapy is actively being pursued by several pharmaceutical companies. For several of the other conditions, somatic stem cell therapy offers some promise but is years away from routine clinical use. In Marfan syndrome, clinical trials of drugs that modulate activity of TGF-β are underway. Additionally, close medical management for individuals detected as being at heightened risk for cardiovascular, skeletal, and ocular complications will remain a mainstay.

Grade A References

A1. Groenink M, den Hartog AW, Franken R, et al. Losartan reduces aortic dilatation rate in adults with Marfan syndrome: a randomized controlled trial. *Eur Heart J.* 2013;34:3491-3500.
A2. Lacro RV, Dietz HC, Sleeper LA, et al. Atenolol versus losartan in children and young adults with Marfan's syndrome. *N Engl J Med.* 2014;371:2061-2071.
A3. Milleron O, Arnoult F, Ropers J, et al. Marfan Sartan: a randomized, double-blind, placebo-controlled trial. *Eur Heart J.* 2015;36:2160-2166.
A4. Teixido-Tura G, Forteza A, Rodríguez-Palomares J, et al. Losartan versus atenolol for prevention of aortic dilation in patients with Marfan syndrome. *J Am Coll Cardiol.* 2018;72:1613-1618.
A5. Ong KT, Perdu J, De Backer J, et al. Effect of celiprolol on prevention of cardiovascular events in vascular Ehlers-Danlos syndrome: a prospective, randomized, open, blinded-endpoints trial. *Lancet.* 2010;376:1476-1484.
A6. Bishop N, Adami S, Ahmed SF, et al. Risedronate in children with osteogenesis imperfecta: a randomised, double-blind, placebo-controlled trial. *Lancet.* 2013;382:1424-1432.
A7. Dwan K, Phillipi CA, Steiner RD, et al. Bisphosphonate therapy for osteogenesis imperfecta. *Cochrane Database Syst Rev.* 2014;7:CD005088.

GENERAL REFERENCES

For the General References and other additional features, please visit Expert Consult at https://expertconsult.inkling.com.

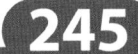

THE SYSTEMIC AUTOINFLAMMATORY DISEASES

RICHARD M. SIEGEL AND DANIEL L. KASTNER

DEFINITION
The systemic autoinflammatory diseases (Table 245-1) are a group of disorders characterized by seemingly unprovoked inflammation, without evidence of high-titer pathogenic autoantibodies or antigen-specific T cells, thus distinguishing them from the more classic autoimmune diseases.[1] The first conditions recognized as autoinflammatory were the hereditary recurrent fevers, a group of mendelian disorders characterized by episodic or fluctuating degrees of fever and localized inflammation. The scope of autoinflammatory disease has been broadened to include other heritable illnesses, including disorders in which purulent or granulomatous inflammation predominates, as well as inherited disorders of the complement system (Chapter 44).[2,3] In addition, in numerous autoinflammatory conditions, some of which manifest in childhood and others that occur later in life, there is a complex interaction of genetic susceptibilities and environmental factors. These illnesses include systemic-onset juvenile idiopathic arthritis (Still disease), Behçet disease, and even the crystalline arthritides. Recent advances in the genetics and pathophysiology of the inherited autoinflammatory diseases suggest that these conditions are inborn errors of innate immunity, the phylogenetically more primitive part of the immune system that uses germline membrane and intracellular receptors expressed in granulocytes and macrophages to mount the body's first line of defense against pathogens (Chapters 39 and 42). Autoinflammatory syndromes can be grouped by key pathogenic cytokines and inflammatory pathways that are dysregulated and may be targets for effective therapies. Here we group diseases into those driven by interleukin-1 (IL-1), type I interferons, and activation of the NF-κB inflammatory signaling pathway. For other diseases, such as the newly described deficiency of adenosine deaminase 2 (DADA2), therapies have been found to be effective empirically, even before the pathogenic signaling pathways have been worked out.

INTERLEUKIN-1–RELATED PERIODIC FEVER SYNDROMES
The IL-1–associated autoinflammatory diseases are linked by markedly increased expression of or cellular responsiveness to this cytokine, and resolution of symptoms with IL-1 blockade. Interleukin-1α and interleukin-1β (IL-1α and IL-1β) are structurally related cytokines released from cells triggered by a number of inflammatory stimuli, such as lipopolysaccharide. They mediate inflammatory responses by binding to a common receptor that is present on the surface of a wide variety of cell types and signals to activate inflammatory genes through the nuclear factor kappa B (NF-κB) transcription factor complex. IL-1 is part of a larger family of cytokines including IL-18, IL-33, and IL-36, which bind to related receptors and share the property of not having a characteristic signal peptide that normally targets cytokines to secretory vesicles. Because of this, IL-1 family cytokines may be secreted only by dead or dying cells, functioning as molecular markers of cellular stress, which can trigger beneficial inflammatory responses to infection and injury. IL-1β and IL-18 are unique in that they are not biologically active until cleaved by the protease caspase-1, which also cleaves intracellular gasdermin D to induce an inflammatory form of cell death known as pyroptosis. Caspase-1 is itself activated

TABLE 245-1 SYSTEMIC AUTOINFLAMMATORY DISEASES: A PARTIAL LISTING

INHERITED AUTOINFLAMMATORY DISEASES	INHERITANCE	GENES OR RISK FACTORS	OMIM*
INTERLEUKIN-1-BETA–RELATED DISORDERS			
Familial Mediterranean fever (FMF)	Autosomal recessive	*MEFV*†	249100
Tumor necrosis factor receptor–associated periodic syndrome (TRAPS)	Autosomal dominant	*TNFRSF1A*†	142680
Hyperimmunoglobulinemia D with periodic fever syndrome (HIDS)	Autosomal recessive	*MVK*†	260920
Neonatal-onset multisystem inflammatory disease (NOMID)/Muckle-Wells syndrome (MWS)/familial cold autoinflammatory syndrome (FCAS)	Autosomal dominant/de novo	*NLRP3* (formerly *CIAS1*)†	607115 191900 120100
Schnitzler syndrome	Sporadic	*NLRP3* mosaic mutations (some)	
Multiple self-healing palmoplantar carcinoma	Autosomal dominant	*NLRP1*	606636
Familial keratosis lichenoides chronica			
Autoinflammation with arthritis and dyskeratosis			
Deficiency of interleukin-1 receptor antagonist (DIRA)	Autosomal recessive	*IL1RN*†	612852
Deficiency of the IL-36R antagonist (DITRA)	Autosomal recessive	*IL36RN*†	605507
INTERFERON-RELATED AUTOINFLAMMATORY SYNDROMES (INTERFERONOPATHIES)			
Aicardi-Goutières syndrome	Autosomal recessive or Autosomal dominant	*TREX1, RNASEH2A, 2B, 2C SAMHD1 ADAR (DRADA) IFIH1 (MDA5)*	225750
STING-associated vasculopathy with onset in infancy (SAVI)	Autosomal recessive	*TMEM173*	612374
Chronic atypical neutrophilic dermatosis with lipodystrophy and elevated temperature (CANDLE), Nakajo-Nishimura syndrome, JMP syndrome	Autosomal recessive	*PSMB8*, genes encoding other proteasome subunits†	256040
NF-KAPPA-B–RELATED AUTOINFLAMMATORY SYNDROMES			
Haploinsufficiency of A20 (HA20) syndrome	Autosomal dominant	*TNFAIP3*†	191163
OTULIN deficiency	Autosomal recessive	*FAM105B (OTULIN)*†	615712
Immunodeficiency and autoinflammatory disease associated with C-terminal NEMO mutations	X-linked	*IKBKG*	300248
Immunodeficiency, autoinflammation, and amylopectinosis	Autosomal recessive	*HOIL1/RBCK1, HOIP/RNF31*	610924 612487
Pediatric-onset inflammatory polyarthritis	Autosomal dominant (de novo)	*Myd88*	602170
GRANULOMATOUS DISORDERS			
Early-onset sarcoidosis/Blau syndrome	Sporadic, autosomal dominant	*NOD2/CARD15*†	186580, 605956
Crohn disease	Complex inheritance	*NOD2/CARD15*†	266600
COMPLEMENT DISORDERS			
Hereditary angioedema	Autosomal dominant	*C1NH*	106100
Early-onset protein-losing enteropathy, and thrombosis, intestinal lymphangiectasia, and intestinal inflammation	Autosomal recessive	*CD55*	125240
Hemolytic-uremic syndrome	Autosomal dominant, sporadic	*CFH* (complement factor H)	235400
Age-related macular degeneration	Complex inheritance	*CFH* (complement factor H)	603075
OTHER AUTOINFLAMMATORY SYNDROMES			
Deficiency of ADA2 (DADA2)	Autosomal recessive	*ADA2*†	607575
Syndrome of periodic fever with aphthous stomatitis, pharyngitis, and cervical adenopathy (PFAPA)	Idiopathic	—	—
Autoinflammatory disease associated with *NLRC4* mutations	Autosomal dominant	NLRC4	606831
Systemic-onset juvenile idiopathic arthritis (SOJIA)/adult-onset Still disease	Complex inheritance	*HLA-DRB1*11, LACC1, IL6, MIF* polymorphisms	604302
Behçet disease	Complex inheritance	*HLA-B*51*, polymorphisms in *IL10, IL23R, CCR1, STAT4, KLRC4, ERAP1, MEFV, TLR4, IL1A-IL1B, IRF8, CEPB-PTPN1, ADO-EGR2, RIPK2, LACC1, FUT2*	109650
Syndrome of pyogenic arthritis with pyoderma gangrenosum and acne (PAPA)	Autosomal dominant	*PSTPIP1*†	604416
Chronic recurrent multifocal osteomyelitis (CRMO)	Sporadic, autosomal recessive	*LPIN2*,† when associated with congenital dyserythropoietic anemia (Majeed syndrome)	259680
Synovitis acne pustulosis hyperostosis osteitis syndrome (SAPHO)	Idiopathic		—
Crystalline arthropathies	Complex inheritance	*SLC2A9/GLUT9, ABCG2*	—

*Online Mendelian Inheritance in Man, an online catalogue of genetic disorders, available at http://www.ncbi.nlm.nih.gov/entrez/query.fcgi?db=OMIM. Accessed September 29, 2014.
†An updated list of disease-associated mutations is available online at http://fmf.igh.cnrs.fr/infevers. Accessed January 7, 2018.
AGS https://www.nature.com/articles/nri3850
HOIP http://mirror.omim.org/entry/612487?search=HOIP&highlight=hoip#1
HOIL-1 https://www.ncbi.nlm.nih.gov/pubmed/23104095
OTULIN https://www.ncbi.nlm.nih.gov/pubmed/27523608
https://www.ncbi.nlm.nih.gov/pubmed/27559085
ADA2 = adenosine deaminase 2; A20 = TNF-γ–induced protein 3; JMP = joint contractures, muscle atrophy, microcytic anemia, panniculitits-induced lipodystrophy; NEMO = NF-κB essential modulator.

in cytoplasmic protein complexes containing various sensor proteins such as NLRP3 and the adapter protein ASC. These complexes are referred to as inflammasomes because of their ability to trigger IL-1–mediated inflammation. Autoinflammatory diseases described below are caused by mutations in genes encoding proteins that process or sense IL-1 or affect this process indirectly.

Familial Mediterranean Fever
DEFINITION

Familial Mediterranean fever (FMF) is a recessively inherited disease that typically manifests with 12- to 72-hour episodes of fever and localized serosal, synovial, or cutaneous inflammation. Between attacks, patients usually feel completely well, although biochemical evidence of inflammation may remain, and some patients eventually develop systemic amyloidosis. Before the identification of the causative gene, FMF was defined purely clinically; clinical features remain an important part of the diagnosis, because some patients with typical disease have only one, or sometimes no, demonstrable mutation in *MEFV*, the only known causative gene.

EPIDEMIOLOGY

FMF is most common in individuals of Jewish, Arab, Armenian, Turkish, and Italian ancestry. The frequency of asymptomatic carriers of a single *MEFV* mutation in these populations is as high as 1 in 5, a finding that suggests a selective advantage for heterozygotes. With genetic testing, FMF is now frequently recognized in both Ashkenazi (eastern European) and non-Ashkenazi Jewish populations, as well as in Mediterranean populations previously thought not to be at risk. Mutation-positive individuals with typical symptoms have been documented worldwide. FMF usually manifests in childhood, sometimes even in infancy, although approximately 10% of patients experience their first attack as adults; infrequently, FMF first occurs in persons older than 40 years.

PATHOBIOLOGY

MEFV, the gene for FMF, was identified by positional cloning in 1997. It encodes a 781–amino acid protein denoted pyrin (or marenostrin) that is expressed in granulocytes, monocytes, and dendritic cells, as well as in peritoneal, synovial, and dermal fibroblasts. The N-terminal 92 amino acids of pyrin are the prototype for a motif, the PYRIN domain, that is involved in protein-protein interactions; this domain defines a family of more than 20 human proteins, including pyrin itself, involved in the regulation of cytokine production (particularly the IL-1 family), NF-κB activation, and cell death. Most of the pathogenic FMF-associated mutations in pyrin reside in the C-terminal domain encoded by exon 10 of *MEFV*. An even larger number of variants of unknown significance have been described in individual patients with a spectrum of inflammatory phenotypes, and some patients with clinical presentations similar to FMF have been found to have pyrin mutations on only one allele. The assembly of pyrin-containing inflammasomes is activated by bacterial toxins that inactivate the GTPase RhoA, including toxins derived from *Clostridia, Yersinia,* and *Vibrio* species.[4] RhoA inactivates pyrin by inducing phosphorylation of pyrin on N-terminal serine residues, which leads to sequestration of pyrin by 14-3-3 proteins and inhibition of pyrin's ability to promote processing of the cytokine IL-1β. These discoveries identified a physiological role for pyrin in host defense against bacteria, and as FMF-associated mutations in *MEFV* render pyrin resistant to RhoA-mediated inactivation, provided a mechanism for the heightened secretion of IL-1β by cells harboring FMF-associated pyrin mutations.[5] These findings also suggest that heightened resistance to pandemic bacterial infections, such as *Yersinia pestis* (the agent of plague in humans), may explain the extraordinarily high FMF carrier frequencies in certain populations. Additional evidence for the importance of pyrin phosphorylation in the regulation of IL-1β production came from the identification of mutations in one of the phosphorylation sites of pyrin associated with a severe early-onset syndrome of autoinflammation and neutrophilic dermatosis (PAAND).[6,7]

CLINICAL MANIFESTATIONS

Episodes of FMF are more properly termed *recurrent* than *periodic,* and some patients associate attacks with psychological stress or physical exertion. Women of childbearing age sometimes experience their attacks with menses, with remissions during pregnancy. Some patients are unaware of fever during the attacks, but it is almost always observed when sought. Serosal involvement in FMF is usually peritoneal or pleural. Abdominal attacks are the most frequent, and they may vary from mild discomfort to frank peritonitis, with boardlike rigidity, direct and rebound tenderness, and air-fluid levels on upright films of the abdomen. Regardless of the severity of the abdominal attack, constipation is much more common than diarrhea. If a laparotomy or laparoscopy is performed during an attack, a small amount of sterile exudate rich in polymorphonuclear leukocytes may be found. Except for serosal inflammation, the appendix is normal. Repeated abdominal attacks may cause peritoneal adhesions, but ascites is rare. Pleurisy, usually unilateral, may accompany abdominal pain, or it may occur independently. Physical findings, if present, may include diminished breath sounds and a pleural friction rub, whereas chest radiograms may show a small effusion or atelectasis. With multiple attacks, pleural thickening may develop. Symptomatic nonuremic pericardial involvement in FMF has been reported but is unusual.

In adults, the arthritis of FMF typically manifests as monoarticular involvement of the knee, hip, or ankle, and attacks of arthritis may persist for up to

1 week at a time. In children, oligoarticular or polyarticular joint involvement may occur. Large joint effusions are sometimes present, and the synovial fluid may have as many as 100,000 leukocytes/mL. In approximately 5% of patients who are not treated with prophylactic colchicine, chronic arthritis (usually of the hip or knee) may develop, often necessitating joint replacement surgery. Regardless of colchicine treatment or a particular human leukocyte antigen (HLA-B27) status, some patients with FMF develop sacroiliitis. Arthralgia without frank arthritis is common in FMF.

Cutaneous manifestations of FMF tend to be less common than serosal or synovial involvement. The characteristic skin lesion of FMF is erysipeloid erythema, a painful, demarcated erythematous area most often seen on the lower leg, ankle, or dorsum of the foot. This rash may occur independently, or it may accompany an episode of arthritis. Histologically, a mixed perivascular cellular infiltrate is seen. Other acute manifestations of FMF include unilateral scrotal inflammation (the tunica vaginalis is an embryologic remnant of the peritoneal membrane) and myalgia, either with fever or, especially in children, without fever and induced by vigorous exercise. Various forms of vasculitis also have been associated with FMF; Henoch-Schönlein purpura may occur in children with FMF; less frequently, polyarteritis nodosa is seen.

COMPLICATIONS

Before the widespread use of colchicine prophylaxis, systemic AA amyloidosis (Chapter 179) was a frequent complication of FMF, caused by the ectopic deposition of a misfolded fragment of serum amyloid A (SAA), an acute phase reactant, in the gastrointestinal tract, kidneys, spleen, lung, testes, and adrenals. Malabsorption and nephrotic proteinuria leading to renal failure are the most common manifestations of AA amyloidosis. Cardiomyopathy is less common, and neuropathy and arthropathy are rare. Several risk factors for amyloidosis development in FMF have been identified, including late diagnosis of FMF, colchicine noncompliance, male gender, and specific genotypes of the *MEFV* and *SAA* genes. Amyloidosis in FMF is less common in the United States than in the Middle East. Abdominal fat aspirates are much less sensitive than rectal or renal biopsy in detecting the amyloidosis of FMF. The latter procedure may be preferred, because of the increasing recognition of nonamyloid glomerular disease in FMF. With early diagnosis, aggressive suppression of the acute phase response with colchicine or adjunctive agents may lead to improvement, but for patients with renal failure, early renal transplantation is preferred.

DIAGNOSIS

Based on a simple recessive model of inheritance, two mutations in *MEFV*, in *trans,* should be identified to establish the genetic diagnosis of FMF. Nevertheless, the interpretation of genetic testing is complicated by complex alleles consisting of various combinations of mutations in *cis,* as well as by the observations that as many as one third of patients with clinically typical FMF have only one demonstrable mutation in *MEFV,* and a few patients with typical disease have no identifiable *MEFV* mutations. These latter two findings suggest that, under some circumstances, one *MEFV* mutation may be sufficient for symptoms or that additional genes for FMF exist.

For these reasons, clinical data remain an essential part of the diagnosis of FMF, and genetic testing plays an adjunctive role in settings in which clinical experience is limited.[8] Clinical criteria emphasize attack duration (12 to 72 hours); recurrence of symptoms (three or more episodes); documented fever (rectal temperature >38° C); painful manifestations in the abdomen, chest, joints, or skin; and the absence of other causative factors. The differential diagnosis includes the other hereditary recurrent fever syndromes (Table 245-2), as well as other conditions specific to the clinical setting. For patients with recurrent abdominal pain, considerations include gynecologic disorders, porphyria (Chapter 199; which can be distinguished by hypertension during attacks, dominant inheritance, and urine porphyrins), and hereditary angioedema (Chapter 237; which usually does not cause fever). The syndrome of periodic fever with aphthous stomatitis, pharyngitis, and cervical adenopathy is probably the most common cause of unexplained recurrent fever in children and is also included in the differential diagnosis. In patients presenting primarily with recurrent monoarthritis, joint aspiration for cultures and crystals may aid in excluding bacterial and crystalline arthritis. Still disease in children (systemic-onset juvenile idiopathic arthritis) and adults (adult-onset Still disease) is also considered in the differential diagnosis. Adult-onset Still disease[9] (see Table 245-1) is an uncommon autoinflammatory condition of unknown cause that is not considered to be hereditary. It is characterized by spiking fever, an evanescent salmon-pink maculopapular rash, arthritis, and neutrophilic leukocytosis. It can be clinically distinguished from FMF by the pattern of fever (intermittent quotidian in Still disease vs. discrete episodes in FMF),

TABLE 245-2 CLINICAL CHARACTERISTICS OF SELECTED AUTOINFLAMMATORY DISEASES

CLINICAL FEATURE	FMF	TRAPS	HIDS	FCAS/MWS/NOMID	DADA2
Typical ethnicity	Arab, Armenian, Italian, Jewish, Turkish	Any ethnicity	Dutch, other North European	European	Georgian Jewish origin for PAN-like disease
Age of onset	Childhood or adult	Childhood or adult	Childhood, especially tied to immunizations	Childhood or adult (FCAS) Childhood (MWS) Infancy (NOMID)	Usually childhood
Attack duration	12-72 hr	Days to weeks	3-7 days	12-24 hr (FCAS) 1-2 days (MWS) Continuous, with flares (NOMID)	Occasional fevers Can have long asymptomatic periods
Abdominal involvement	Sterile peritonitis, constipation > diarrhea	Severe pain, vomiting, peritonitis	Sterile peritonitis, diarrhea, rarely constipation	Nausea (FCAS) Abdominal pain (MWS) Uncommon (NOMID)	Can be seen associated with abdominal vasculitis and infarctions, portal hypertension
Pleural attacks	Common	Common	Rare	Rare (MWS, NOMID)	Rare
Joint/bone involvement	Monoarthritis, rarely protracted arthritis in knee or hip	Arthritis in large joints, arthralgia	Arthralgia, symmetrical polyarthritis	Polyarthralgia (FCAS, MWS) Oligoarthritis (MWS) Clubbing (MWS, NOMID) Epiphyseal overgrowth, contractures, intermittent or chronic arthritis (NOMID)	Uncommon
Skin rash	Erysipeloid erythema on lower leg, ankle, foot	Migratory rash, underlying myalgia	Diffuse maculopapular rash, urticaria	Urticaria-like rash (cold-induced in FCAS)	Livedo reticularis, cutaneous vasculitis, scarring lesions, and necrosis can occur
Hematologic	Splenomegaly, occasional lymphadenopathy	Splenomegaly, occasional lymphadenopathy	Cervical adenopathy in children	Hepatosplenomegaly, adenopathy (NOMID, rare in MWS)	Cytopenias including pure red-cell aplasia, hypo-Ig, hepatosplenomegaly
Neurologic involvement	Aseptic meningitis?	Controversial	Headache	Headache (FCAS) Sensorineural deafness (MWS, NOMID) Chronic aseptic meningitis, intellectual disability (NOMID)	Recurrent ischemic strokes
Ophthalmologic involvement	Rare	Conjunctivitis, periorbital edema, rarely uveitis	Uncommon	Conjunctivitis (all) Uveitis (MWS, NOMID) Progressive vision loss (NOMID)	Retinal artery occlusion
Vasculitis	Henoch-Schönlein purpura (HSP), polyarteritis nodosa	HSP, lymphocytic vasculitis	Cutaneous vasculitis common, rarely HSP	Not seen Occasional in NOMID	Small and medium vessels, can present as polyarteritis nodosa
Systemic amyloidosis	Risk depends on *MEFV* and *SAA* genotypes; more common in Middle East	Occurs in ≈10%; risk increased with cysteine mutations	Rare	Rare (FCAS) 2-5%(MWS) May develop in adulthood (NOMID)	Can occasionally develop
Autoantibodies	Not usually seen	Not usually seen	Not usually seen	Not usually seen	ANCA usually negative
Effective treatments	Colchicine, IL-1 blockade	IL-1 blockade Etanercept	IL-1 blockade	IL-1 blockade	TNF blockade

the pattern of arthritis (chronic polyarthritis vs. intermittent monoarthritis), the characteristic skin involvement (evanescent rash vs. erysipeloid erythema), and the presence of lymphadenopathy (more common in Still disease).

TREATMENT ℞

The mainstay of therapy for FMF is daily oral colchicine, which can prevent both acute attacks of FMF and the development of systemic amyloidosis.[A1] Although colchicine has been used as an anti-inflammatory medication since ancient times, and its particular efficacy in FMF was discovered empirically, new insights into pyrin's negative regulation by the RhoA GTPase may explain its mechanism of action in FMF. As a consequence of its ability to depolymerize microtubules, colchicine activates RhoA, probably through the release of the RhoA guanine-nucleotide-exchange factor GEF-H1 from microtubules. Activated RhoA leads to increased phosphorylation of pyrin, inactivating its pro-inflammatory function, even in cells harboring FMF-associated pyrin mutations.

In adults, the therapeutic dose is 1.2 to 1.8 mg/day, and nearly 90% of patients note significant improvement at this dose. The major side effects are gastrointestinal, and they can usually be minimized by gradually increasing the dosage and avoiding milk products in patients who develop lactose intolerance. Most experts continue to prescribe colchicine to patients during pregnancy, with the recommendation that amniocentesis be performed to exclude trisomy 21,

for which there may be a slightly increased risk. Use of colchicine in lactating women is considered safe. Intravenous colchicine should be used with extreme caution, if at all, in FMF, because fatal toxicity has been reported in patients already receiving oral colchicine who are given the drug intravenously.

IL-1 inhibitors are usually effective in patients who are poorly responsive to colchicine or who cannot tolerate therapeutic doses.[A2] Canakinumab, a recombinant human anti–human-IL-1β antibody, was recently approved by the Food and Drug Administration (FDA) for the treatment of FMF in adults and children. In a randomized, placebo-controlled trial in patients with genetically confirmed colchicine-resistant FMF, mevalonate kinase deficiency, or TRAPS at the time of a flare, canakinumab, 150 mg subcutaneously, with the option for an add-on injection at the same dose, was found to be effective in controlling and preventing flares.[A3]

Hyperimmunoglobulinemia D with Periodic Fever Syndrome (Mevalonate Kinase Deficiency)

Hyperimmunoglobulinemia D with periodic fever syndrome (HIDS) was first described in 1984 as an FMF-like illness seen in six patients of Dutch ancestry. Besides the difference in ethnicity, a key distinction was the observation of extremely high levels of immunoglobulin D (IgD) in the serum of these patients, thus prompting the HIDS nomenclature. HIDS is now recognized in a broader ethnic distribution, although northern Europeans still predominate. Overall, HIDS is still quite rare. Family studies documented autosomal recessive inheritance. The elevated IgD levels seen in HIDS appear to be an epiphenomenon and do not correlate with disease severity either among patients or in a given patient over time, although IgD may contribute to the release of pro-inflammatory cytokines in vitro. In 1999, patients with HIDS were found to have mutations in *MVK*, which encodes the mevalonate kinase enzyme involved in the biosynthesis of cholesterol and nonsterol isoprenes.[10,11] Enzyme activity in patients is markedly reduced but not absent. Recent data link the isoprenoid deficiency resulting from *MVK* mutations to the manifestations of HIDS and make an interesting connection with FMF and other IL-1–related autoinflammatory diseases. Reduced prenylation inactivates the GTPase RhoA, abrogating its negative regulation of the pyrin inflammasome, resulting in increased IL-1β production. IL-1β and increased body temperature can further decrease mevalonate kinase enzymatic activity, thereby creating a vicious circle in which infection or immunization can precipitate HIDS attacks. One of the well-recognized clinical characteristics of HIDS is the provocation of attacks by immunizations. Other distinguishing clinical features include a very early age of onset (average age, 6 months), a duration of attacks intermediate between FMF and TRAPS (3 to 7 days), prominent cervical lymphadenopathy during attacks, polyarticular joint involvement, a diffuse maculopapular rash, the predominance of diarrhea over constipation with abdominal attacks, and the infrequency of pleuritic attacks or systemic amyloidosis.

The diagnosis of HIDS can be established in a patient with recurrent episodes of fever and typical associated findings by documenting either two mutations in *MVK* or elevated levels of mevalonic acid, the substrate for mevalonate kinase, in the urine during attacks. Approximately 10% of patients with otherwise typical disease have only a single identifiable *MVK* mutation. As modestly increased IgD levels can be seen in other inflammatory conditions, and up to 20% of patients (particularly young children) with typical recurrent fevers and *MVK* mutations can have normal serum IgD levels, IgD levels alone are an unreliable diagnostic tool. Consequently, some experts prefer the term *mevalonate kinase deficiency* (MKD) to denote this illness. Nonsteroidal anti-inflammatory drugs (NSAIDs) or corticosteroids are sometimes useful in the treatment of the arthritic manifestations of HIDS. Colchicine is generally not effective. IL-1 inhibitors are generally effective in HIDS, and recently the FDA approved canakinumab for the treatment of this disorder. Patients with HIDS have a normal lifespan, and attacks may become somewhat less frequent in adulthood.

Tumor Necrosis Factor Receptor–Associated Periodic Syndrome

DEFINITION

Worldwide, the tumor necrosis factor (TNF) receptor–associated periodic syndrome (TRAPS) is the second most frequently diagnosed hereditary recurrent fever syndrome, behind FMF. TRAPS is defined by recurrent episodes of fever and localized inflammation, in many ways resembling FMF, but differing in key details (noted later) and caused by mutations in *TNFRSF1A*, encoding the 55-kD receptor for TNF (TNFR1, p55, CD120a). Whereas a positive genetic test is not necessary to diagnose FMF, the diagnosis of TRAPS requires the identification of a TNF receptor mutation. One of the first well-characterized families with what was later defined as TRAPS was of Irish ancestry, and the condition was termed familial Hibernian fever to emphasize the ethnic background and clinical differences from FMF. However, with the discovery of TNF receptor mutations in families of other ancestries, the ethnically neutral TRAPS nomenclature was proposed.

PATHOBIOLOGY

The p55 TNF receptor comprises four cysteine-rich extracellular domains, a transmembrane region, and an intracellular death domain. To date, nearly all of the coding mutations described are in the extracellular domains and approximately one third are missense substitutions of cysteine residues that abolish highly conserved disulfide bonds. The initial description of TRAPS documented a defect in activation-induced ectodomain cleavage of the p55 receptor in patients with the C52F *TNFRSF1A* mutation, possibly leading to a defect in homeostasis by impaired downregulation of membrane receptors and diminished shedding of potentially antagonistic soluble receptor molecules. However, not all TRAPS-associated *TNFR1* mutations exhibit this shedding defect, and recent studies indicate a more complex pathogenetic picture, with the extracellular mutations causing defective trafficking and intracellular accumulation of mutant TNFR1 protein. Spontaneous signaling and possibly activation of the unfolded protein response leads to production of mitochondrial reactive

oxygen species, constitutive activation of mitogen-activated protein (MAP) kinases, and increased production of pro-inflammatory cytokines by myeloid cells harboring the mutant receptor.[12,13]

DIAGNOSIS

Although genetic testing is necessary for the diagnosis of TRAPS, certain clinical clues can help distinguish TRAPS from FMF. These include ethnicity (FMF is seen predominantly in Mediterranean and Middle Eastern populations, whereas TRAPS has a more widespread distribution), mode of inheritance (autosomal recessive in FMF, dominant in TRAPS), and duration of attacks, which tends to be longer in TRAPS and sometimes approaches continuous symptoms. The rash of FMF is typically erysipeloid erythema on the lower extremity, whereas patients with TRAPS often have a distinctive erythematous rash, often with underlying myalgia, which may migrate on the trunk or centrifugally on the extremities. Ocular involvement, with periorbital edema, conjunctivitis, and occasionally even uveitis, is observed in TRAPS but not in FMF. Finally, whereas colchicine is much more effective than corticosteroids in FMF, the opposite is true in TRAPS. Nevertheless, aside from the difference in duration and susceptibility to pharmacologic intervention, the abdominal, pleural, synovial, and even scrotal manifestations of the two diseases are rather similar. The usual age of onset for TRAPS is also in childhood, and systemic AA amyloidosis is seen in approximately 10% of untreated patients with TRAPS. As in FMF, life expectancy in TRAPS is normal in patients whose disease is not complicated by amyloidosis.

As noted earlier, the diagnosis of TRAPS is established by the identification of *TNFRSF1A* mutations in the appropriate clinical setting. One variant, the substitution of glutamine for arginine at residue 92 (R92Q), is present in more than 1% of individuals with European ancestry and may be associated with a broader spectrum of symptoms than is typically seen in TRAPS, including early inflammatory arthritis or, in some cases, no symptoms at all. The substitution of lysine for proline at residue 46 (P46L) has been described in African American patients with TRAPS and is associated with a receptor shedding defect, but it is also seen among healthy West African controls. These findings establish a "gray zone" for the diagnosis of TRAPS and emphasize the potential role of polymorphisms in the recurrent fever genes in other more common inflammatory phenotypes.

TREATMENT   Rx

The treatment of TRAPS depends on the frequency and severity of attacks.[14] Patients with relatively infrequent, mild episodes may respond to NSAIDs. Patients with more severe attacks that occur infrequently may be treated with corticosteroids, although increasing doses may be required as the episodes become more frequent and toxicities may become limiting. For patients with severe attacks occurring once a month or more frequently, treatment with etanercept, the soluble p75 TNF receptor:Fc fusion protein, may be warranted. This may be a unique effect of etanercept, because there is anecdotal evidence that monoclonal antibodies against TNF may actually exacerbate TRAPS. Consistent with a model implicating upregulation of components of the NLRP3 inflammasome by the aberrant inflammatory signaling in TRAPS, IL-1 inhibitors have also been found to be highly effective in TRAPS, and canakinumab recently gained regulatory approval for this indication following a randomized trial that demonstrated efficacy in controlling flares (see Treatment section under FMF).

Cryopyrin-Associated Periodic Syndromes: The Cryopyrinopathies

Three rare, recurrent febrile disorders usually beginning early in life have been associated with mutations in *NLRP3* (formerly *CIAS1*), the gene encoding a protein variously named cryopyrin, NLRP3, NALP3, PYPAF1, or CATERPILLER 1.1, a key component of the NLRP3 inflammasome that activates caspase-1. These disorders are referred to as cryopyrinopathies or cryopyrin-associated periodic syndromes (CAPS). The least severe clinical phenotype is familial cold autoinflammatory syndrome (FCAS; formerly called familial cold urticaria), which is dominantly inherited and is notable for day-long attacks of chills, fever, headache, diffuse urticarial skin rash, arthralgia, and conjunctivitis, precipitated by generalized cold exposure. Amyloidosis is rare in FCAS. Of intermediate severity is Muckle-Wells syndrome (MWS), also dominantly inherited, in which 1- to 2-day episodes of chills, fever, urticarial rash, limb pain, and arthritis occur independently of cold exposure. Sensorineural hearing loss is common in MWS, and systemic amyloidosis may occur. The most severe *NLRP3*-associated phenotype is neonatal-onset multisystem inflammatory disease (NOMID), known in Europe as chronic infantile neurologic cutaneous and articular (CINCA) syndrome. It is usually sporadic owing to the reduced reproductive fitness of most affected individuals. Fever and constitutional symptoms occur almost daily, often from birth, with generalized urticarial skin rash, a peculiar arthropathy characterized by epiphyseal overgrowth of the long bones, and central nervous system (CNS) involvement that includes chronic aseptic meningitis, uveitis, and cochlear inflammation, which may lead to intellectual disability, blindness, and deafness. In all three cryopyrinopathies, the rash is not true urticaria because there is a neutrophilic rather than a mast cell infiltrate and serum histamine levels are normal.

Because there are patients with FCAS, MWS, and NOMID/CINCA without demonstrable germline *NLRP3* mutations, these diagnoses remain clinical, although genetic testing serves as a valuable adjunct and has greatly increased the recognition of all three conditions. Deep sequencing has identified somatic *NLRP3* mutations in some patients with symptoms consistent with CAPS who are negative for mutations by standard genetic testing. In addition, overlap syndromes that are intermediate between FCAS and MWS and NOMID/CINCA have been reported. NLRP3 is only one of a number of inflammasomes nucleated by other members of the NLR gene family, and gain-of-function mutations in *NLRP1*, encoding an NLR family member prominently expressed in the skin, underlie a spectrum of diseases characterized by keratotic skin lesions, arthritis, systemic inflammation and self-healing palmoplantar carcinomas.[15] Gain-of-function mutations in *NLRC4*, another intracellular NLR family member, have been reported in patients with a spectrum of symptoms ranging from FCAS-like disease to severe inflammatory disease with infantile-onset enterocolitis and macrophage activation syndrome. IL-18, a cytokine related to IL-1 which is also intracellularly processed by NLR inflammasomes, is particularly elevated in patients with *NLRC4* mutations, and blockade of IL-18 has been successful in ameliorating symptoms in one severely affected individual resistant to other therapies.[16]

TREATMENT   Rx

Blockade with anakinra, a recombinant IL-1 receptor antagonist, is effective in controlling fever and acute phase reactants in all three cryopyrinopathies, and longitudinal analysis of a large series of patients at the U.S. National Institutes of Health showed that long-term treatment with anakinra markedly decreased CNS inflammation and end-organ damage in NOMID/CINCA, which led to the regulatory approval of anakinra for the treatment of this condition in the United States and Europe. More recent studies have also documented the efficacy of rilonacept, another soluble IL-1 blocker, and canakinumab in FCAS and MWS. The latter two agents may be less effective against NOMID/CINCA because of reduced penetration into the CNS.

Deficiencies of IL-1 and IL-36 Receptor Antagonists

Deficiency of the IL-1 receptor antagonist (DIRA) is characterized by the neonatal onset of a pustular skin rash, multifocal osteomyelitis, periostitis, and, rarely, vasculitis. Fever is not a prominent finding, although acute phase reactants are markedly elevated. DIRA is caused by recessively inherited loss-of-function mutations in *IL1RN*, which encodes the IL-1 receptor antagonist (IL-1Ra). Patients usually present within the first 2 weeks of life with skin lesions ranging from discrete crops of pustules to generalized severe pustulosis or ichthyosiform lesions. Histologic examination demonstrates extensive neutrophilic infiltrates in the dermis and epidermis. Typical radiographic findings include multifocal osteolytic lesions, periosteal elevation of the long bones, heterotopic ossification of the proximal femurs, and widening of the anterior rib ends. Bone biopsies demonstrate sterile purulent osteomyelitis, fibrosis, and sclerosis. In DIRA, the lack of IL-1Ra leads to unopposed IL-1β and IL-1α signaling, whereas in the cryopyrinopathies, *NLRP3* mutations lead to inflammasome activation and increased IL-1β production. DIRA patients respond dramatically to anakinra, a recombinant form of the protein they lack.

Loss-of-function mutations in IL36RN, coding for a protein that serves a similar function as IL1RA in blocking the activity of the IL-1 family member IL-36, are associated with autosomal recessive inheritance of a syndrome termed *DITRA* (for deficiency of the IL-36 receptor antagonist) characterized by generalized pustular psoriasis, periodic fevers, and elevation of systemic inflammatory markers.

THE INTERFERONOPATHIES: TYPE-I-INTERFERON ASSOCIATED AUTOINFLAMMATORY DISEASES

A group of hereditary syndromes marked by systemic inflammation has emerged that share induced gene expression of type I interferon target genes and cytokines and have been termed *interferonopathies*.[17] Although a wide variety of genetic lesions can cause these diseases, the common induction of this cytokine signaling pathway has raised hopes that blocking type I interferons or interferon signaling may be beneficial for these patients. These diseases mimic some aspects of the antiviral state and congenital infection syndromes without a role for a known pathogen and also make an interesting counterpoint to systemic lupus erythematosus (SLE) and Sjögren syndrome, polygenic autoimmune diseases where type I interferon–induced gene expression is also seen in peripheral blood. Unlike most other autoinflammatory syndromes, autoantibodies can be found in some type I interferonopathies, placing them on the spectrum between autoinflammatory and autoimmune disease.

Aicardi-Goutières Syndrome and Associated Diseases

A neonatal syndrome characterized by severe neurologic dysfunction and CSF pleocytosis, Aicardi-Goutières syndrome (AGS) was first associated with mutations in the *TREX1* gene encoding a 3′–5′ DNA exonuclease. The definition of this syndrome has expanded to encompass mutations in a number of other genes associated with DNA or RNA modification or sensing; delayed onset past 1 year of age in some patients, particularly those with *IFIH1* or *ADAR* mutations; and extracerebral features such as glaucoma, hypothyroidism, and inflammatory bowel disease. Certain features, such as "chilblains," cold-induced vascular-based inflammatory lesions in the hands and feet, overlap with those seen in pediatric lupus, and a small number of AGS patients meet clinical criteria for SLE.

Proteasome Associated Autoinflammatory Syndromes

A constellation of diseases have been described linked to recessive loss-of-function mutations in *PSMB8*, which encodes the β5i subunit of the proteasome, also known as LMP7. An autosomal recessive syndrome in adults characterized by recurrent fevers, progressive lipodystrophy, joint contractures, and cardiac manifestations has been linked to homozygous missense mutations in *PSMB8*.[18] Patients with a syndrome termed *CANDLE* (chronic atypical neutrophilic dermatosis with lipodystrophy and elevated temperature) were found to have homozygous missense and nonsense mutations in *PSMB8*, with some patients having only one known *PSMB8* mutation, or compound mutations with other proteasome subunits.[19] It is not yet clear whether these syndromes represent identical diseases related to loss of function of β5i. The β5i proteasome subunit is one of the subunits that are induced in immune cells through immune stimuli such as interferons, altering the proteasome so that it more efficiently processes peptides for antigen presentation to T cells. However, there is no indication of a T-cell component to this disease, and studies have shown that the β5i proteasome subunit can be expressed in nonimmune cells such as adipocytes. A striking interferon transcriptional signature, similar to that seen in SLE, has been observed in circulating blood cells from patients with CANDLE. Defective degradation of proteins in cells lacking β5i may result in buildup of ubiquitinated proteins, which somehow triggers interferon production, or PSMB8 deficiency may enhance interferon signaling by stabilizing components of the interferon signal transduction machinery that are negatively regulated by ubiquitin-proteasome degradation. Whichever the mechanism, the link to interferon hyperactivity suggests that blocking interferons with antibodies or inhibitors of interferon signal transduction may be effective in the therapy of CANDLE and possibly other proteasome-associated autoinflammatory syndromes (PRAAS).

AUTOINFLAMMATORY DISEASES ASSOCIATED WITH ACTIVATION OF NF-κB

Although the NF-κB family of transcription factors was one of the first to be described that transduces extracellular signals into induction of inflammatory gene expression, until recently, no mutations in this pathway were known to cause human autoinflammatory disease. Loss-of-function mutations in *IKBKG*, encoding NEMO (NF-kappa-B essential modulator), a structural component of the I-κB kinase (IKK) complex, cause an X-linked immunodeficiency syndrome, and inherited mutations in *TNFRSF13B*, encoding TACI, a member of the TNF-family cytokine receptor gene family, cause some cases of common variable immunodeficiency. More recently, a number of kindreds have been described with heterozygous loss-of-function mutations in *TNFAIP3*, encoding the A20 protein, which negatively regulates induction of NF-κB through promoting K48 linked ubiquitination and degradation of intracellular components of TNF-family receptor signaling complexes such as RIP1.[20] In these kindreds, individuals with these mutations develop symptoms with some features of Behçet disease, such as oral and genital ulcers, uveitis, and skin abscesses. Biochemical hyperinduction of NF-κB and inflammatory cytokine production by stimuli such as LPS and TNF could be seen in peripheral blood myeloid cells from these patients. Mutations in *IKBKG* that lead to truncations in NEMO that are unable to bind A20 have also been found to lead to inflammatory disease in addition to the immunodeficiency resulting from defects in other functions of NEMO. Recently, a patient with a de novo gain-of-function mutation in the *MYD88* gene coding for the signal transduction protein Myd88 was described with pediatric-onset severe destructive polyarthritis.[21] This mutation is similar to those seen in somatic activating mutations associated with lymphoma. Myd88 activates NF-κB downstream of TLR and IL-1 receptors, and cells from this patient exhibit increased NF-κB activation and enhanced production of pro-inflammatory cytokines. These findings and other syndromes listed in Table 245-1 have validated the role of NF-κB and A20 in regulating clinically relevant inflammatory responses and point to the need for better therapeutic agents which can effectively regulate NF-κB activation in genetic and acquired diseases where this pathway is hyperactive.

● OTHER INHERITED SYSTEMIC AUTOINFLAMMATORY DISEASES

Syndrome of Pyogenic Arthritis with Pyoderma Gangrenosum and Acne

The syndrome of pyogenic arthritis with pyoderma gangrenosum and acne (PAPA) is a rare, dominantly inherited autoinflammatory disease characterized by intermittent episodes of sterile pyogenic arthritis, pyoderma gangrenosum, and severe cystic acne. It is caused by mutations in the gene encoding proline-serine-threonine phosphatase–interacting protein 1 (PSTPIP1), also known as CD2BP1. PSTPIP1 is a cytoskeletal protein that interacts with certain other proteins involved in the immune response, including CD2; the Wiskott-Aldrich syndrome protein (WASP); a phosphatase denoted PTP-PEST; and pyrin, the FMF protein. PAPA mutations abrogate the binding of PSTPIP1 to PTP-PEST, leading to hyperphosphorylation of PSTPIP1 and increased binding to pyrin. Both in patients and in cell lines, this finding is associated with markedly increased IL-1β production. Early in life, PAPA tends to present with monoarticular or pauciarticular pyogenic arthritis, sometimes induced by trauma. In the absence of treatment, arthritis may progress to severe joint damage and ankylosis. As patients reach puberty, skin manifestations begin to predominate, including disfiguring cystic acne. Pathergy also may develop, and extensive pyoderma gangrenosum may require opiates for pain control. The diagnosis of PAPA syndrome is made by documenting *PSTPIP1* mutations in the appropriate clinical setting. High doses of corticosteroids have been used in PAPA, with varying success, and patients with arthritis sometimes require aspiration, intra-articular corticosteroids, or open drainage. Newer investigational approaches for PAPA syndrome focus on the use of targeted cytokine inhibitors. Anecdotal evidence supports the use of anakinra or canakinumab for the arthritis and monoclonal anti-TNF antibodies for the pyoderma gangrenosum of PAPA.

Granulomatous Inflammatory Arthritis, Dermatitis, and Uveitis (Blau Syndrome)

Blau syndrome is a rare, dominantly inherited illness characterized by the following features: early-onset granulomatous synovitis often complicated by cyst formation and camptodactyly (flexion contractures of the fingers and toes); granulomatous anterior and posterior uveitis, sometimes causing retinal detachment, glaucoma, cataracts, and blindness; and an intermittent papular rash with noncaseating granulomas. Lung or other visceral involvement is generally not present. However, visceral involvement of the liver and spleen is observed in early-onset sarcoidosis (Chapter 89), which is phenotypically quite similar to Blau syndrome. Both Blau syndrome and some cases of early-onset sarcoidosis are caused by mutations in *NOD2/CARD15*. Distinct variants of *NOD2/CARD15* have been associated with susceptibility to Crohn disease, which manifests as granulomatous inflammation of the gastrointestinal tract (Chapter 132). The protein encoded by this gene is thought to be an intracellular sensor of bacterial products. Crohn disease–associated mutations in the ligand-binding, leucine-rich repeat region of the protein may alter responses to bacterial products in the gastrointestinal tract to cause inflammation, whereas Blau syndrome mutations in the nucleotide binding domain may lead to constitutive extraintestinal inflammation. Topical and systemic corticosteroids are currently the mainstay of treatment of Blau syndrome. There are case reports of the efficacy of TNF and IL-1 inhibitors in this disease.

Deficiency of ADA2 (DADA2)

A syndrome characterized by fevers, early-onset strokes, and vasculopathy or frank vasculitis mimicking polyarteritis nodosa has been found to be caused by autosomal recessive mutations in *ADA2* (formerly *CECR1*), encoding adenosine deaminase 2 (ADA2).[22] Although sharing enzymatic activity with intracellular adenosine deaminase encoded by the ADA gene, ADA2 is not necessary for lymphocyte development and DADA2 patients do not initially present with severe combined immunodeficiency (SCID), as is the case for ADA deficiency. ADA2 is a secreted extracellular protein, and functional studies have found that ADA2 plays a role in vascular development and regulation of macrophage differentiation. Although this disease is generally diagnosed in childhood, it should be considered in the differential diagnosis of young adults with unexplained lacunar strokes and/or vasculitic skin lesions. As ADA2 is expressed by myeloid cells, bone marrow transplantation may be therapeutic, and TNF inhibition has also shown efficacy in preventing recurrent strokes, though the underlying mechanisms are not yet clear.[23]

● NEW AUTOINFLAMMATORY SYNDROMES AND THE PROMISE OF WHOLE-EXOME SEQUENCING

Recent years have seen a dramatic acceleration in the pace of discovery of new mendelian inflammatory diseases as a result of the availability of whole-exome sequencing, which allows unbiased identification of disease-causing mutations in protein coding sequences, although it should be noted that accurate clinical description of these syndromes is as important as the genetic tools for identification of new syndromes. These discoveries have confirmed the role of gene products in human inflammation that were identified in animal model systems and identified new genes and proteins not previously thought to be involved in the regulation of inflammation. More sensitive deep sequencing techniques have also allowed discovery of subgenomic mosaic mutations in *NLRP3* and *TNFRSF1A*, causing similar or related syndromes to those associated with de novo or inherited mutations in these genes. For example, mosaic mutations in *NLRP3* account for some cases of cryopyrinopathies that were found to be "negative" for these mutations by standard whole-exome sequencing analysis, and low-percentage *NLRP3* mutations have been found in Schnitzler syndrome, which is characterized by monoclonal gammopathy, neutrophilic skin lesions resembling those in cryopyrinopathies, and systemic inflammation.[24] Early-onset, apparently sporadic, cases of inflammatory syndromes have often turned out to be due to de novo mutations in a child when screened against parental DNA. For example, inherited gain-of-function mutations in *CARD14*, encoding an adapter protein in innate immune sensing, cause dominantly inherited familial psoriasis, and a more severe gain-of-function de novo mutation in the same gene causes infantile-onset severe pustular psoriasis. Recessive mutations in *HOIL1/RBCK1* that impair the addition of linear ubiquitin chains to receptor signaling complexes cause a complex syndrome marked by autoinflammation and immunodeficiency and intramuscular glycogen deposition. Gain-of-function mutations in *PLCG2*, encoding phospholipase Cγ2, an enzyme with essential functions in B-cell receptor and Fc receptor signaling, cause a dominantly inherited autoinflammatory syndrome characterized by blistering skin lesions, bronchiolitis, arthralgia, ocular inflammation, and enterocolitis in the absence of autoantibodies.

 Grade A References

A1. Ozen S, Demirkaya E, Erer B, et al. EULAR recommendations for the management of familial Mediterranean fever. *Ann Rheum Dis*. 2016;75:644-651.

A2. Hashkes PJ, Spalding SJ, Giannini EH, et al. Rilonacept for colchicine-resistant or -intolerant familial Mediterranean fever: a randomized trial. *Ann Intern Med*. 2012;157:533-541.

A3. De Benedetti F, Gattorno M, Anton J, et al. Canakinumab for the treatment of autoinflammatory recurrent fever syndromes. *N Engl J Med*. 2018;378:1908-1919.

GENERAL REFERENCES

For the General References and other additional features, please visit Expert Consult at https://expertconsult.inkling.com.

246

OSTEOARTHRITIS

VIRGINIA BYERS KRAUS AND TONIA L. VINCENT

DEFINITION

Osteoarthritis (OA) presents in many phenotypic forms and can involve any joint in the body. Although it is the most prevalent form of arthritis, it has been likened to a collection of orphan diseases because of the heterogeneity of presentations.[1] Characteristic patterns of joint involvement are recognizable and can often provide clues to specific etiologies of disease (Table 246-1). For instance, there is clear evidence for a polyarticular subset of hand OA in women. There are three major determinants of the pattern of polyarticular involvement: symmetry, clustering by row, and clustering by ray. There are also indications that subtle morphometric abnormalities of the hip, such as acetabular depth and shape and femoral head morphometry, can increase the risk for hip OA.[2] It is estimated that at least half of the susceptibility to the various major forms of OA (spine, hands, knees, hip) in the population is explained by genetic factors. In contrast, any joint can develop OA as a consequence of a severe injury or repetitive overuse. Although the characteristic radiographic features (joint space narrowing and osteophytes) have long been accepted as the *sine qua non* of OA, a long preradiographic stage is now recognized. This has prompted a new focus on the disease process, relating to underlying endotypes and distinct pathobiologic mechanisms. Despite different patterns of joint involvement, the end stage of OA represents a common pathology.

Despite its prevalence, OA has attracted relatively modest research attention over recent decades compared with the autoimmune arthritides, and this has contributed to the perpetuation of a number of unhelpful paradigms such as, "OA is due to wearing down of joint surfaces," "OA is an inevitable consequence of aging," "non–weight-bearing joints do not get true OA," and "damaged joints do not have the ability to repair themselves." In recent years, much progress has been made in understanding the pathophysiology of disease. In efforts to further the understanding of the pathophysiology of the disease, to facilitate communication across the field, and to help advance research and drug development for OA, the Osteoarthritis Research Society International (OARSI) supported an initiative to create a pathobiologic definition of OA. The current definition is as follows: "Osteoarthritis is a disorder involving movable joints characterized by cell stress and extracellular matrix degradation initiated by micro and macro injury that activates maladaptive repair responses including pro-inflammatory pathways of innate immunity. The disease manifests first as a molecular derangement (abnormal joint tissue metabolism) followed by anatomic, and/or physiologic derangements (characterized by cartilage degradation, bone remodeling, osteophyte formation, joint inflammation and loss of normal joint function), that can culminate in illness."[3] The proposed definition was not intended to distinguish an OA patient uniquely from patients with other forms of arthritis, but rather to spur scientific advances and serve as the building blocks for defining OA phenotypes and molecular endotypes.

TABLE 246-1	RECOGNIZED DISTINCT PATTERNS OF OSTEOARTHRITIS	
JOINT SITE	**COMMON PRESENTATION**	**INFORMATIVE VARIATIONS**
Knee	Medial dominant: idiopathic or injury related	Lateral dominant: injury related
Hip	Central (medial, concentric) cartilage loss in women, commonly bilateral, associated with hand OA, with less tendency to progress	Superolateral pole in men, unilateral and progressive
Hand	Nodal generalized OA—"arthritis of menopause" involving multiple finger joints and predominating in women	Predisposition to OA of knee, hip, and spine; erosive subset*
Ankle	Injury related	Increased ankle OA risk contralateral to knee OA
Spine	Lumbar and cervical spine associated with hand OA	

*Erosion is often present in hand osteoarthritis (OA) if the detection method is sensitive, e.g., magnetic resonance imaging.
Information in part taken from Doherty M, ed. *Color Atlas and Text of Osteoarthritis*. Barcelona: Wolfe Publishing; 1994.

EPIDEMIOLOGY

Prevalence and Societal Burden

Among the approximately 100 different arthritic conditions, OA is the most prevalent. It affects more than 320 million individuals globally, including an estimated 30.8 million adults in the United States (13.4% of the civilian adult U.S. population).[4] Because the global burden estimates only consider hip and knee OA, and not OA at other sites, it is highly likely that the real burden of OA has been underestimated. Estimates may also be conservative because they do not account for the current trend of increased obesity, which contributes to OA, and the "graying" (aging) of society, a leading contributor to the increasing prevalence of OA. Recent estimates suggest that arthritis prevalence in the United States has also been substantially underestimated, especially among adults younger than 65 years of age, owing to the low sensitivity of the single screening question on the National Health Interview Survey for physician-diagnosed arthritis.[5] Given that OA is by far the most prevalent of all arthritides, these findings underscore the major underestimated societal impact of OA in the U.S. population and, by analogy, worldwide.

Osteoarthritis as a Serious Disease

OA has all the hallmarks of a serious condition. Lower extremity OA is the leading cause of mobility impairment in older adults in the United States. Disability and loss of function associated with OA are higher in women, those with lower education levels, the socially disadvantaged, and those reliant on manual labor, weight bearing, or positions that involve walking or knee bending for their livelihood. Pain from arthritis is one of the key barriers to maintaining physical activity. The more severe the walking disability, the higher the risk for death, largely due to cardiovascular disease. Overall, knee OA is associated with a 1.55-fold increased risk for all-cause mortality compared with the general population.

PATHOBIOLOGY

OA is the oldest known disease, affecting ancient hominids millions of years ago through modern-day humans. Some joints are commonly affected, whereas others are rarely involved. An evolutionary perspective attributes the pattern of joint involvement in generalized OA to the fact that some joints have undergone recent rapid evolutionary change and are underdesigned to cope with the new mechanical stresses placed on them.

Mechanical Factors

Mechanical factors are the most important etiological agents in OA development. The epidemiology is compelling: mechanical joint injury or overuse, joint malalignment, and dysplasia are strong independent risk factors for developing disease, even in young individuals. Chondrocytes have several mechanosensing mechanisms and can perceive loads above a defined threshold as injurious. As we age, our ability to reduce the impact of joint loading during normal activities is reduced by loss of muscle mass (e.g., quadriceps strength across the knee), loss of gait reflexes, and poor response times. In vitro, threshold strains above 10% at 0.5 Hz for 12 hours of loading leads to a predominance of cartilage catabolism. In essence, OA will occur when abnormal loads traverse a normal joint or when normal loads are experienced by a joint that has lost its mechanoprotective mechanisms (Table 246-2), pointing to a "Goldilocks principle" with respect to loading that is context specific (Fig. 246-1). This understanding of the prime role of mechanosensing by chondrocytes in the etiology of OA fits well with the traditional adage that OA is an "inside-out" disease, in contrast to rheumatoid arthritis, which is an "outside-in" disease (having its origin in synovitis).

Conversely, joints that are immobilized do not develop disease. This is evident in individuals who have sustained a stroke (Fig. 246-2) or previous polio as well as in animal studies where casting of limbs after induction of disease halts development. Importantly, the most significant load comes from

TABLE 246-2	MECHANICAL ETIOLOGIES OF OSTEOARTHRITIS	
ABNORMAL LOAD ON NORMAL JOINT	**NORMAL LOAD ON AN UNPROTECTED JOINT**	
Direct articular trauma	Aging by loss of muscle support and gait reflexes	
Obesity	Chondrodysplasia through maladapted joint shape and weakened joint tissues	
Repetitive occupational load, e.g., "coal miner's back," "cotton-picker's thumb"	Joint destabilization, e.g., ruptured anterior cruciate ligament, meniscal tear	
Joint malalignment, e.g., valgus and varus deformities	Cartilage weakened by previous arthritis, e.g., gout, rheumatoid arthritis, sepsis (in the past referred to as *secondary osteoarthritis*)	

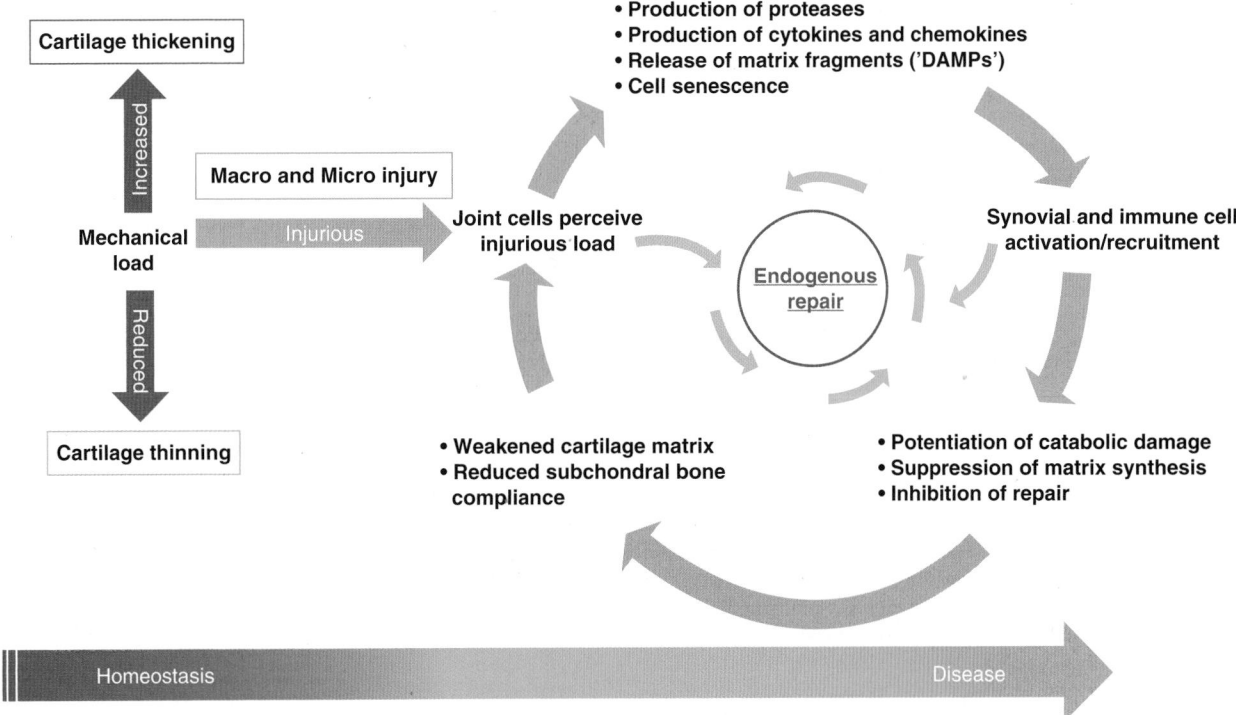

FIGURE 246-1. Vicious cycle of mechanically induced sterile inflammation in osteoarthritis.

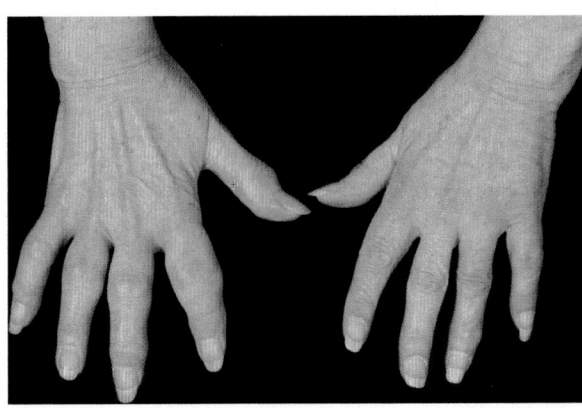

FIGURE 246-2. Asymmetrical osteoarthritis (OA) in a patient with left-sided hemiparesis. This demonstrates that joints that are immobilized do not develop OA.

the action of muscle across the joint rather than from weight, and this explains why OA affects upper limb joints such as the fingers and why these are also protected by immobility (see Fig. 246-2). Thresholds of perceived load can be observed in exercise dosage studies in rodents; increasing exercise in a modest way increases the thickness of cartilage, consistent with a hypertrophic tissue response, but forced treadmill exercise leads to cartilage degradation and disease.[6]

Aging

Age is a very strong risk factor for disease. The contribution of age to disease occurs at a number of levels. Probably the most important impact comes from loss of mechanoprotective muscle support across joints with aging (mentioned previously). It is also the case that the tissues of the joint become stiffer because of increased cross-linking of the matrix, and this changes how cells of the joint are able to respond both to physiologic and injurious mechanical load. Cellular aging also changes the metabolic phenotype of the cell, making it more susceptible to free radical–induced damage and driving cell death or cellular senescence. These features likely contribute to a reduction in regeneration potential with age.

Genetic Factors

Genetic factors play an important role in risk because OA is highly heritable. Although rare monogenic forms of OA exist (often associated with chondrodysplasia—abnormal joint formation), its most common forms are complex, that is, polygenic involving multiple genes, each contributing a low risk of disease.[7] Although *genetic etiologies* are thought to account for as much as 60% of hip OA, 39% to 65% of hand and knee OA, and 70% of spine OA, it is estimated that only 22.5% of the heritable causes of OA have been discovered to date in a genome-wide association study for OA of 77,052 cases and 378,169 controls.[8] Genome-wide association studies in large-joint OA have identified over 60 candidates that reach genome-wide significance, although the clinical relevance of each of these is yet to be determined; some of these may turn out to be genes that determine developmental joint shape rather than pathways that might be modifiable, nonetheless, certain strong pathways are emerging (e.g., members of the TGF-beta family TGFβ-signaling-pathway). In general, genetic factors involved in risk for OA often act by modulating gene regulation and may be characterized by polymorphisms that lead to transcriptional differences—termed *allelic expression imbalance*—whereby one allele produces fewer transcripts than the other allele.[9]

Metabolic Factors

Metabolic factors play a role in OA risk. The jury is still out on whether "metabolic OA" exists as a discrete entity. This terminology is variously applied to features associated with the metabolic syndrome (obesity, dyslipidemia, diabetes, and hypertension). Epidemiology appears to show that body mass index (BMI) alone accounts for the increased risk in this group, although hypertension may also be an independent risk factor.[10] *Obesity* contributes to disease risk through mechanical overload as well as poor joint muscle support as a result of sedentary behavior. Despite low BMI, elderly subjects in Beijing, China had an equal (men) or higher (women) prevalence of radiographic and symptomatic knee OA compared with individuals in the Framingham, Massachusetts, cohort, pointing to genetic and environmental factors (such as squatting or heavy physical activity) that underlie these differences. Adiposity is also associated with increased systemic inflammation driven in part by inflammatory cytokines, so-called adipokines, that are made by adipocytes.[11] This systemic inflammatory component of obesity appears to be tied to the microbiome and the ability of very pro-inflammatory microbiome-related factors, such as lipopolysaccharide, to evade clearance by a fatty liver. Thus, the presence of nonalcoholic fatty liver disease may be a superior indicator of adverse inflammatory effects of obesity compared with BMI alone.

Gender

Gender influences both radiographic and symptomatic OA incidence that is more common in women after menopause. This association is largely absent before menopause, indicating that female sex hormones protect joints from OA. Hand OA in particular has a peak incidence around the time of menopause in women.

Molecular Pathophysiology: From Bench to Bedside
The Role of Proteases in Osteoarthritis

The finding of specific fragments of aggrecan in OA synovial fluid was the first indication that proteases were important in the pathophysiology of OA. Although several matrix metalloproteinases (MMPs) were, by then, characterized, the fragments in the joint did not appear to resemble those generated by known MMPs, and the term *aggrecanase* was coined. In 1999, the first aggrecanase, a disintegrin and metalloproteinase with thrombospondin motif 5 (ADAMTS5), was identified. The subsequent demonstration that mice deficient in ADAMTS5 were protected from surgically induced OA provided definitive evidence that OA was a potentially targetable disease. Aggecanase inhibitors were shelved, but there has been recent renewed interest in this enzyme as a therapeutic target for OA. Unwanted side effects were partly to blame, as was the challenge of taking these types of drugs into clinical trial in the absence of good disease biomarkers.

Mechanobiology in Osteoarthritis

The discovery of proteases as targets in disease appeared, at first, to be at odds with the strong mechanical etiology. However, the observation that cells of cartilage and synovium could induce proteases in response to mechanical injury provided a mechanism to explain how abnormal mechanical load could provoke disease. This may also explain how the elimination of surface chondrocytes also blocks OA development after injury. In mice, joint immobilization after induction of OA not only protects joints from cartilage loss but also abrogates the up-regulation of catabolic genes.[12] A number of intracellular pathways are activated in response to mechanical injury, driving both reparative and degradative responses. Mechanisms include release of growth factors from the cartilage matrix in response to tissue injury and activation of mechanosensitive receptors on the cell surface (see E-Fig. 246-1). Once the cartilage matrix is weakened by proteolytic activity, even noninjurious load may then be perceived as injurious by the chondrocyte, setting up a cycle of chronic, mechanically induced matrix degradation (Fig. 246-1).

Inflammatory Cytokines in Osteoarthritis

Inflammation is recognized as a hallmark of OA, although whether it is a cause or consequence of disease is still debated. Sensitive imaging (by ultrasound, magnetic resonance imaging (MRI), and etarfolatide that identifies sites of activated macrophages) demonstrates inflammation (effusions and synovial thickening) in the majority (~75%) of knees with radiographic OA. MRI effusion synovitis and Hoffa synovitis (inflammation of the intra-articular fat pad) predict about a three-fold increased risk for incident radiographic OA with a year. Unlike rheumatoid arthritis, OA, like many other chronic diseases, involves the innate immune system. All the previously discussed factors suggest a robust whole joint model of a failed wound healing response that integrates the key role of mechanics as an inciting factor and innate immune wound healing response and inflammation as a perpetuating process (see E-Fig. 246-1). A normal wound healing response entails an initial autodébridement phase followed by a cellular proliferation and fibrotic wound remodeling phase. A joint with active OA appears to be in a perpetual state of autodébridement, with macrophages taking on dual roles of both pro- and anti-inflammatory (M1 and M2) phenotypes simultaneously. Mouse strains with less susceptibility to OA after injury have an attenuated inflammatory response. Despite the fact that inflammatory cytokines such as interleukin-1 (IL-1) and tumor necrosis factor-α (TNF-α) are potent inducers of proteolytic activity in chondrocytes and are capable of driving proteoglycan and type II collagen degradation in cartilage explants in vitro, to date there is little evidence from knockout mice or clinical trials that IL-1β, IL-1α, or TNF-α are drivers of cartilage breakdown in vivo.

Senescence in Osteoarthritis

Cellular senescence is a collection of cellular phenotypes that often coexist in a stressed cellular environment.[12] Senescence, a well-established hallmark of aging, is a biological state in which cells have lost the ability to divide but remain metabolically active; they produce senescence-associated secretory proteins (SASPs) with pro-inflammatory and cytotoxic functions. In addition to replicative senescence (from telomere shortening), the concept of cellular senescence has now been expanded to include premature senescence (from cell stress). Senolytics are currently being explored as antiarthritics; preliminary evidence suggests that clearing senescence cells and alleviating a cell checkpoint control (through elimination of p21) are promising strategies based on decreased susceptibility to post-traumatic OA and ability to turn a nonhealer mouse strain to a healer for ear wound regeneration, respectively.

Regeneration of Articular Cartilage in Osteoarthritis

OA incidence and progression are due to the net effects of joint breakdown and repair in response to adverse mechanics and micro and macro injury events. Although it was long believed that cartilage had no innate repair capacity, cartilage regeneration is seen in OA patients undergoing procedures in which the abnormal mechanical stress in the joint is corrected or temporarily removed. Examples of this include high tibial osteotomy and joint distraction, a procedure in which the OA joint is held rigid and under tension by an external metal frame secured into the bone above and below the joint. Both procedures demonstrate regrowth of articular cartilage on MRI and sustained clinical improvement. Injury can also trigger a tissue repair response due to release of growth factors from the matrix and recruitment of intra- and extra-articular progenitor cells. The ability to repair is affected by genetics, joint site, depth of cartilage lesion, age, and inflammation (both positively and negatively according to inflammatory phenotype).

Just like humans, mouse strains differ in their susceptibility to OA after joint injury. Repair of focal cartilage lesions in the mouse demonstrates both genetic and age dependence. Analyses of a range of selected healer and nonhealer mouse strains demonstrate a range of regeneration phenotypes and correlation of wound healing capacities of ear and knee cartilages; genes representing DNA repair and Wnt signaling pathways are related to regenerative phenotype suggesting the existence of underlying mechanisms for regeneration that significantly affect susceptibility to OA. Direct evidence for an innate cartilage repair capacity is also provided by analyses of the cartilage content of post-translationally modified proteins (indicative of "older" protein forms with long residence time in vivo) relative to their native nonmodified forms (indicative of "younger," more recently synthesized protein forms in vivo); compared with healthy cartilage, OA ratio of is characterized by a site-specific (ankle > knee > hip) regenerative capacity with a lower older/younger protein forms.[13] The clinical importance of endogenous repair in the pathogenesis of OA is also supported by the knowledge that polymorphic variants in GDF5, TGFβ1 (as well as other family members), and FGF18 (and its receptor FGFR3) have all emerged from the recent genome-wide association study described earlier and loss of stress defense mechanisms, such as autophagy, are associated with increased risk for OA.[14] This points to the possibility that disease is a failure of repair and regeneration rather than increased degradation. In addition, the mechanisms that drive cartilage repair likely involve injury-induced release of matrix-bound growth factors that contribute to the recruitment and differentiation of local mesenchymal progenitor cells. Delivery of intra-articular fibroblast growth factor 18 (FGF18) to promote cartilage regeneration in OA is in clinical trial and shows early success.

Mechanical load has both mechanoadaptive (homeostatic) and pathogenic consequences in the joint. A reduction in load will lead to reversible cartilage thinning or atrophy. Increased load on an otherwise healthy joint will cause an increase in the cartilage volume. By contrast, micro or macro injury (mechanical load that exceeds a defined injury threshold) triggers a cascade of events driven by the cells of the joint (chondrocytes, synoviocytes, osteocytes) to incite an inflammatory sterile tissue injury response, including production and activation of matrix degrading enzymes. Subsequent tissue remodeling leads to weakened cartilage and reduced bone compliance, and this loss of protection means that even physiologic load is perceived as injurious. When the catabolic process overwhelms the endogenous repair response (that differs by joint site), the cycle continues (E-Fig. 246-1).

CLINICAL MANIFESTATIONS
Clinical Course

OA has traditionally been identified by two major characteristic radiographic alterations of joints; these are joint space narrowing, representing cartilage erosion due to extracellular matrix catabolism, and osteophyte formation, representing an anabolic cartilage response (chondrophyte) that ossifies (Fig. 246-3). These two major radiographic characteristics are often scored using the 1957 Kellgren and Lawrence criteria (see Fig. 246-3 legend) or generally some variation of it. However, as with many other chronic diseases, such as osteoporosis, OA also has a long "silent" phase during which the aneural articular cartilage transitions from a healthy joint tissue to a disease state involving the whole joint organ (see Fig. 246-3) and that is recognizable as abnormalities on a radiograph. Rates of progression vary by joint site. It is therefore probable that progression from subclinical to clinically manifest OA is influenced by mechanical, biologic, developmental, and genetic factors. The reclassification of disease—to one that is no longer a purely radiographic entity, but a disease process that includes molecular, preradiographic, and radiographic stages provides a scenario amenable to the development of primary

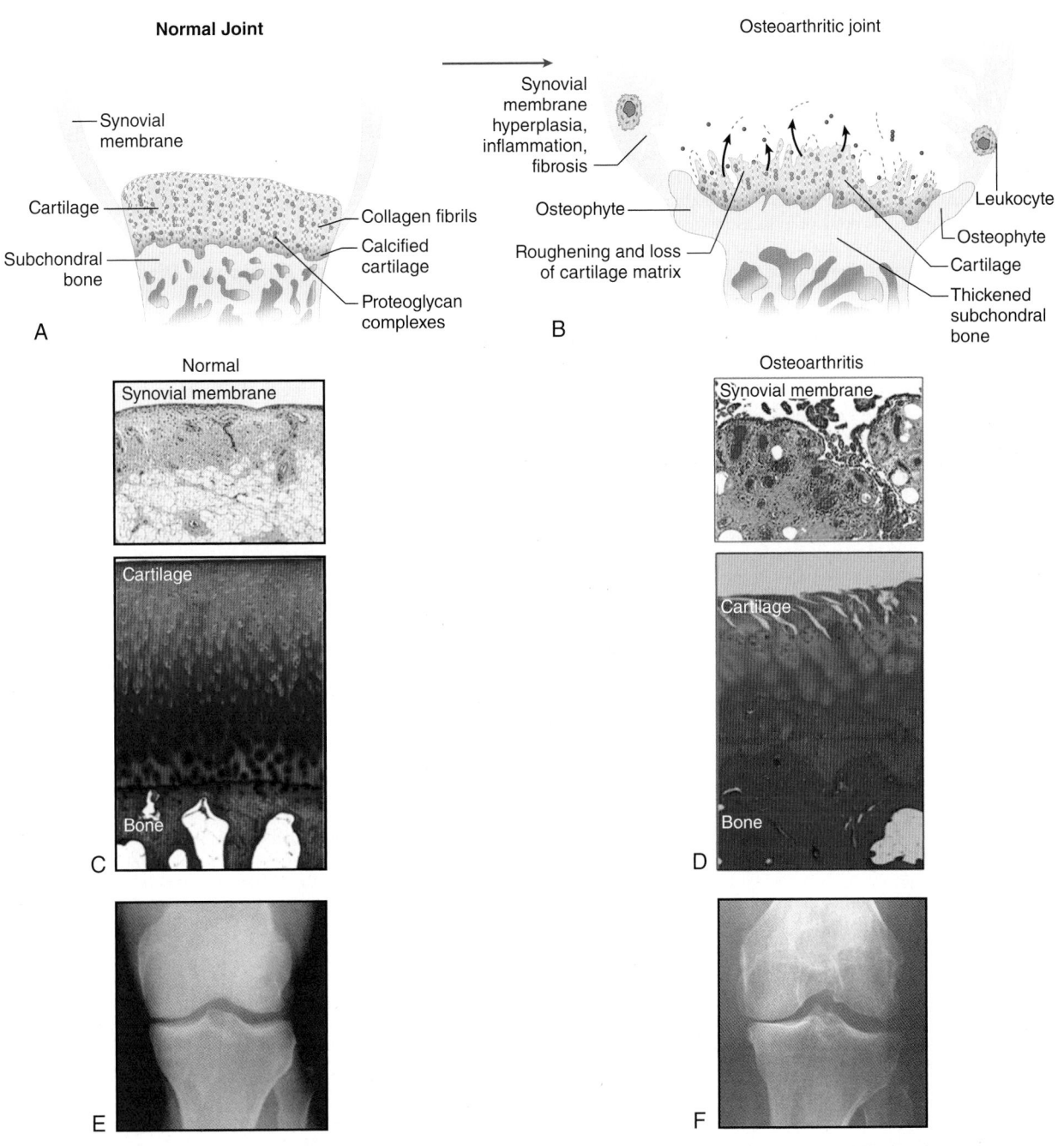

FIGURE 246-3. Pathologic features of osteoarthritic joint tissues. **A,** Features of a normal adult synovial joint. Healthy adult articular cartilage is characterized by a smooth surface and extracellular matrix (ECM) composed of a collagen type II fibrillar network and large proteoglycan complexes. The ECM is produced and maintained by the cellular components of cartilage, chondrocytes. The subchondral bone consists of a thin cortical layer and underlying trabecular bone. The synovial membrane lines the joint capsule and attaches at the cartilage-bone interface. In the normal state, it consists of a lining layer one or two cells thick, with underlying vascularized loose connective tissue. **B,** Typical changes to tissues seen in osteo-arthritis (OA). Enzymatic activities (ADAMTS4,5 and MMP-13 in particular) cleave proteoglycan and collagen components of the ECM, leading to loss of these molecules from the matrix. As the process advances, the articular cartilage thins and fibrillates, and eventually fissures down to the underlying bone are seen. Simultaneously, a remodeling response in the bone is observed. Thickening of the cortical subchondral bone layer occurs, and new bone growth at the margins appears as osteophytes. The synovial membrane changes observed in OA patients include lining layer hyperplasia, inflammation in the form of leukocyte infiltration, and fibrosis, which can be seen to varying degrees. Photomicrographs of human joint tissues showing these features are depicted in **C** (normal tissues) and **D** (OA tissues). (**C** and **D,** Courtesy Edward F. DiCarlo, MD, Hospital for Special Surgery, New York, NY.) **E, F,** Radiographic features of osteoarthritic joint. Patient baseline (**E**) vs. 3 years later (**F**) showing typical features of OA progression including the development of medial joint space narrowing and osteophyte (spur outgrowth) at joint margins. The classical Kellgren & Lawrence grading system scores radiographs by 5 categories (scores 0-4) as follows: 0 = no osteoarthritis; 1 = small osteophyte of doubtful significance; 2 = definite osteophyte(s), possible joint space narrowing; 3 = multiple osteophytes, definite joint space narrowing, some subchondral sclerosis and possible deformity of bony ends; 4 = large osteophytes, marked narrowing of joint space, severe sclerosis of subchondral bone and definite deformity of bone ends.

(for pre-illness), secondary (for early disease), and tertiary (for late disease) prevention strategies.

Clinical Symptoms (Illness)

Illness symptoms of OA are protean and include joint pain and/or aching at rest or on use or motion, loss of normal joint motion and function, short duration (<30 minutes) morning stiffness and stiffness after joint disuse such as sitting ("gel" phenomenon), and intermittent, usually localized disease flares. In contrast to rheumatoid arthritis, profound fatigue, fever, and generalized weakness are rare in OA. Pain is a complex feature of illness that has biologic,

psychological, and social components. General guiding principles regarding pain (Chapter 27) suggest an association of pain on use with a mechanical or enthesopathic etiology, pain at rest with inflammation, and pain at night with intraosseous hypertension due to bone edema and overload in the context of loss of normal cartilage "cushioning" or mechanical function in OA. Stiffness is convincingly explained by accumulation of hyaluronan (HA) fragments, generated by reactive oxygen species in an inflamed joint, in the deep layers of arthritic synovium, excluding water within the synovial tissue and decreasing tissue compliance. Joint movement mobilizes HA fragments from the tissue to the joint cavity and blood with attendant hydration of synovial tissue and improvement in joint stiffness. In OA, HA fragments are mobilized fairly readily with joint movement typically resulting in resolution of stiffness within 30 minutes, in contrast to a severely inflamed rheumatoid arthritic joint, wherein stiffness may last for several hours.

Clinical Signs (Illness)

On physical examination of the joint, a number of disease features can be noted, including bony enlargement secondary to chondrophyte and/or osteophyte formation, joint tenderness to palpation, limited range of motion, crepitus (the grating sensation from the joint felt under the examining hand), joint malalignment and/or instability, atrophy of muscle adjacent to an involved joint due to self-splinting and/or disuse due to pain, synovitis characterized by varying degrees of warmth, effusion (joint swelling), and synovial thickening.

In considering OA clinical manifestations, it is very important to realize that disease worsening and illness exacerbations are phasic. Several studies have demonstrated that molecular abnormalities (for instance, type II collagen N-telopeptide or CTXII and cartilage oligomeric matrix protein) indicative of elevated cartilage catabolism predict radiographic OA worsening.[15] Based on a synthesis of 34 studies, an annual risk for radiographic progression (by at least one Kellgren-Lawrence grade) is estimated to be 5.6 ± 4.9%. Nodal hand OA provides an interesting example of the phasic nature of the OA disease and illness process. Affected hand joints are warmer than normal at the onset of radiographic OA; as the severity of OA worsens, joint surface temperatures decline. These data support the concept that digital OA progresses in phases with dynamic variation of an inflammatory process. The role of use in clinical manifestations of disease is illustrated in the reverse; that is, asymmetrical hand OA in a patient with a stroke with OA absence on the stroke-affected side (see Fig. 246-2).

Molecular Biomarkers (Disease)

The strongest evidence for the existence of a purely molecular disease stage of OA is provided by the sequence of biomarker changes and pathologic joint changes observed after a major joint injury. Immediately after major joint trauma, such as anterior cruciate ligament rupture, cartilage constituents are released into synovial fluid in high amounts. By 6 weeks after the acute injury, the profile of synovial fluid biomarkers predicts the 50% of individuals on an OA trajectory defined by MRI proteoglycan and collagen loss.[16] Progressive anatomic abnormalities, detectable by MRI (T2 mapping and T1 rho imaging) are evident beginning 6 months after injury and worsen over the course of the subsequent 2½ years. In contrast, once the initial pain and swelling subside, and despite ongoing cartilage degradation by MRI, there is typically a "honeymoon" period during which individuals experience little in the way of illness and often return to sports.[17] However, 2 years after joint injury, some individuals no longer maintain a patient acceptable symptom state (PASS). The inability to maintain a satisfactory PASS 2 years after injury is predicted by an early (6 weeks after injury) pro-inflammatory synovial fluid biomarker profile (characterized by higher concentrations of IL-1α); these observations provide a rationale for studying early molecular markers as potential stage indicators for clinical outcome after injury and may identify targets to prevent anatomic (structural) and illness (symptomatic) manifestations of OA.

Prolonged observation of injury cohorts demonstrates sometimes decades of subclinical and preradiographic molecular changes before development of anatomic (radiographic) abnormalities of OA. Of note, these serologic abnormalities reflect joint tissue degradation and turnover (aggrecan fragments, collagen fragments, high bone turnover) as opposed to the laboratory findings typically associated with autoimmune arthritides such as high erythrocyte sedimentation rate, rheumatoid factor, or antinuclear antibody titer.

DIAGNOSIS

The cell count in OA synovial fluid generally varies from 50 to 2000 white blood cells/μL. Higher synovial fluid white blood cell counts correlate with more severe OA and synovitis by MRI and identify a joint with likelihood for greater reduction in knee pain following an intra-articular steroid injection.[18] Synovial fluid white blood cell counts as high as 65,000 to 100,000/μL can occur in the absence of infection in association with calcium pyrophosphate dihydrate crystal disease (pseudogout) that can accompany OA; however, high synovial fluid white counts in OA should trigger prompt investigation for infection. Because the molecular constituents of cartilage differ by joint site and cartilage depth, the synovial fluid and possibly serum biomarker measures of specific cartilage matrix components, released as a result of OA-related processes, could hold promise as diagnostic and prognostic indicators of OA stage for specific joints.

Imaging Joint Pathology (Disease)

It is now possible to evaluate joint physiology. In contrast to purely anatomic measures (a "snapshot in time") provided by classical joint ultrasound and MRI, various functional imaging modalities yield information on joint physiology; these include sodium-23 MRI, diffusion imaging, and positron emission tomography (PET) scanning,[19,20] MRI stress tests with imaging before and after dynamic loading of the joint, PET-MRI,[21] etarfolatide imaging of activated macrophages whose presence in OA is characteristic of symptomatic and actively progressing joints,[22] and bone scintigraphy reflecting sites of high bone turnover and specifically new bone formation in OA characteristic of actively progressing joints.

Correlation Between Illness and Disease

The relationship of illness to disease features is highly variable. The correlation of illness with anatomic disease by radiograph is relatively poor, although controlling for interpatient variation improves the correlation between pain and joint space narrowing; in so doing, there is a dose-response relationship between severity of radiographic knee OA and knee pain that is stronger for joint space narrowing than for osteophytes.[23] Lack of correlation in other studies is partly due to the heterogeneous etiologies of illness in OA (e.g., biologic and psychosocial components are all involved with pain perception), the insensitive detection of disease features provided by radiographs and misclassification due to the intermittent nature of OA symptoms. Radiographs can only indirectly visualize articular and meniscal cartilage pathology as a loss of joint space. In contrast, MRI directly visualizes articular and meniscal cartilage. Because osteophytes are formed from chondrophytes (invisible on radiographs), this important anatomic feature of OA is identified by MRI before it is visible by radiograph. Although the threshold of disease that is associated with illness is unknown, there is a consistent and strong association of OA pain and joint pathology including synovitis, bone marrow edema, and cartilage loss identified by multiple means.[24] This shows that disease is a clinically important determinant of illness of OA.

TREATMENT   Rx

The mainstay or core nonsurgical treatments for OA are nonpharmacologic, including land- and water-based exercise, strength training, weight management, assistive devices to help patients perform activities of daily living, thermal modalities, and joint splints and braces.[25] Based on the 2018 scientific report on physical activity and health to the U.S. Secretary of Health and Human Services (updated each decade), for individuals with lower extremity OA, physical activity provides pain relief, improves physical function, and improves quality of life without concern of worsening the condition for exposures less than 10,000 steps per day. Measurable benefits of physical activity seem to persist for periods of up to 6 months following cessation of a defined program. Exercise raises high-density lipoprotein that helps clear lipopolysaccharide and, by dynamic fluid pressurization, provides nutrition to cartilage, which is avascular.

Consensus recommendations conditionally endorse additional treatments on the basis of the risk-to-benefit ratio and comorbidities of the patient; this group of treatments includes analgesics such as acetaminophen, oral and topical nonsteroidal anti-inflammatory drugs (NSAIDs),[26] opioids (such as tramadol), and intra-articular agents such as steroids and hyaluronates, although the benefit of these various treatments is limited.[A1] For example, a randomized clinical trial of the effectiveness of opioid versus nonopioid drugs (acetaminophen, NSAIDs) for chronic back, hip, or knee pain in patients with OA found that treatment with opioids was not superior to treatment with nonopioid medications for improving pain-related function over 12 months.[A2] The presence of comorbidities, such as renal, cardiovascular, and/or gastrointestinal ulcer history limit the use of existing OA therapies such as oral NSAIDs. Older age is also a contraindication to opioid use.

In the light of concerns about increased risk for cardiovascular events with the use of selective cyclooxygenase 2 (COX2) inhibitors, a randomized trial compared the relative risks for cardiovascular as well as gastrointestinal and renal adverse events during long-term treatment with celecoxib (COX2 inhibitor) compared with the nonspecific COX1/COX2 NSAIDs ibuprofen and naproxen in patients with OA and rheumatoid arthritis. At approved dosages, celecoxib conferred a similar or lower risk for cardiovascular, gastrointestinal, and renal adverse events compared with treatment with ibuprofen or naproxen in both groups of patients.[A3] In a trial to test the effectiveness of intra-articular steroids in OA, 2 years of intra-articular triamcinolone, compared with intra-articular saline for knee OA, resulted in significantly greater cartilage volume loss and no significant difference in knee pain.[A4] However, a 24-week, placebo-controlled, multinational study of intra-articular injection of a microsphere-based, extended-release triamcinolone acetonide formulation, compared with saline solution placebo, in knee OA patients showed significant, clinically meaningful pain reduction at week 12 (the primary end point).[A5] Intra-articular injection of anakinra, a modified human IL-1 receptor antagonist, has been found to be well tolerated as a single 50 mg or 150 mg dose but was not associated with improvements in OA symptoms compared with placebo.

Although early diagnosis and intervention in OA would improve the likelihood of disease modification and thereby reduce medical costs, morbidity, and disability, there are presently no drugs approved that can prevent, stop, or restrain progression of OA. In a randomized clinical trial, hydroxychloroquine was found to be no more effective than placebo for pain relief in patients with moderate to severe hand pain and radiographic OA.[A6] The ultimate treatment option currently available is surgical, including joint distraction (emerging therapy), osteotomy, and joint replacement (Chapter 260).[27,28] Unfortunately, undergoing a joint replacement does not equate with remission or reversal of disability, but rather is associated with a lessening of disease severity in the replaced joint; up to 30% of individuals continue to experience pain and disability after total joint replacement, and one in five require joint replacement in another joint within 2 years. In a randomized clinical trial, patients with knee OA who were eligible for unilateral knee replacement, treatment with knee replacement was associated with a higher number of serious adverse events than was nonsurgical treatment, and most patients who were assigned to receive nonsurgical treatment alone did not undergo total knee replacement during the 12-month follow-up period.[A7] The operation has also reflected racial disparities, with African American patients being less likely to undergo total knee replacement than white patients, despite worse baseline knee pain and function in the former. The efficacy of arthroscopic surgery is limited, with some improvement commonly seen at 3 months but little improvement at 2 years.[A8]

Future Targeted Approaches

Given that established OA is a chronic disease, intermittent administration of long-acting agents or chronic administration of short-acting agents is likely required. In further support of this concept, intra-articular IL-1 receptor antagonist for knee OA provided brief (up to 4 days) pain relief but not beyond in keeping with its known brief (4 hours) intra-articular half-life. Drug and molecule entry into the joint cavity from the systemic circulation is size dependent (through arterioles and venules in synovium) and increased with synovial inflammation due to increased vascular permeability. However, drug and molecule exit from the joint cavity is size independent and rapid through lymphatics in synovium as well as through capillaries (in the case of small molecules); increased rates of exit occur with synovial inflammation due to increased lymphatic flow. Intra-articular half-lives of substances within joints range from 1 to 4 hours for NSAIDs and soluble steroids to 26.3 hours for non–cross-linked hyaluronic acid (molecular weight 3×10^6 D). This problem of rapid clearance of drugs from the joint has been the motivation for developing strategies to improve intra-articular drug efficacy based on increasing residence time of drugs in joints; current strategies for prolonging treatment effects include, to name a few examples, using nanoparticles (steroids), molecular cross-linking (hyaluronans), cell-based delivery (TGF-β1), and targeting gene expression and chondrogenic differentiation (Wnt signaling inhibition) (E-Table 246-1).[29]

The identification of patients with an inflammatory phenotype will likely be necessary to adequately determine the feasibility of anticytokine therapies for OA. Recent experience with an anti-IL-1α/β dual variable domain immunoglobulin (ABT-981), administered systemically to humans, showed that the subset of patients with large osteophyte burden had a lower placebo response rate and greater treatment-to-placebo response ratio. This suggests that identification of the right subset of individuals for a particular class of agents may improve the overall outcome. A strategy of "tunable" or on-demand cytokine inhibition has also been in development; this strategy relies on inflammatory cytokine–driven promoters to activate inhibitors appropriate to the particular inflammatory stimulus, thereby yielding a dynamic anti-inflammatory response modulated by the varying conditions of the inflammatory milieu. The jury is still out for cytokines of the IL-6 family; results of in vivo preclinical studies in IL-6 knockout mice are conflicting. A current clinical trial is evaluating the effects of an IL-6 receptor antagonist (tocilizumab) in patients with refractory hand OA. Other therapeutic approaches under investigation include neutralization of granulocyte-macrophage colony-stimulating factor.

Cellular senescence and autophagy is a state of proliferation arrest in response to cellular stress. It is characterized by changes in cell morphology and secretion of SASPs such as IL-6, IL-8, and vascular endothelial growth factor. Although chondrocytes are not highly proliferative cells, senescence is likely to contribute to the age-related reduction in tissue repair and may be responsible in part for driving tissue catabolism. Strategies that target and remove senescent cells, so-called senolytics, have shown promise in murine models of OA.[30] Increased senescence with age is often associated with a reduction in autophagy—the process by which dysfunctional cellular organelles are destroyed. Promoting autophagy to keep the cell healthy may also be amenable to therapeutic targeting.

Nerve Growth Factor (NGF) Neutralization

The drivers of pain in OA have remained surprisingly difficult to elucidate. Pain correlates have been described for most pathologies in the OA joint, including synovitis, bone edema, and cartilage loss. The most convincing molecular target to date is *nerve growth factor* (NGF), a neurotrophic factor that sensitizes pain fibers. Both human and in vivo murine studies demonstrate the analgesic power of *NGF neutralization*. NGF is regulated by inflammatory processes, by TGF-β as well as by direct cartilage mechanical injury, so could be expressed by several tissues of the joint. This class of inhibitors is associated with rapidly progressive OA in 1 to 2% of treated patients. These adverse events are both dose related and associated with concomitant administration of NSAIDs, suggesting these adverse events may represent a Charcot joint (analgesic arthropathy) phenomenon. This has led to a slow and cautious approach to trial conduct with regular signal and nonsignal joint health monitoring by MRI.

Although disease-modifying OA drugs are not yet available, the greater understanding of the etiopathogenesis of OA in general and advances in drug development tools for OA (imaging and soluble biomarkers) are now providing a strong impetus for renewed interest in development of therapeutics for this highly prevalent and disabling condition.

Grade A References

A1. Gregori D, Giacovelli G, Minto C, et al. Association of pharmacological treatments with long-term pain control in patients with knee osteoarthritis: a systematic review and meta-analysis. *JAMA.* 2018;320:2564-2579.

A2. Krebs EE, Gravely A, Nugent S, et al. Effect of opioid vs nonopioid medications on pain-related function in patients with chronic back pain or hip or knee osteoarthritis pain: the SPACE randomized clinical trial. *JAMA.* 2018;319:872-882.

A3. Solomon DH, Husni ME, Wolski KE, et al. Differences in safety of nonsteroidal antiinflammatory drugs in patients with osteoarthritis and patients with rheumatoid arthritis: a randomized clinical trial. *Arthritis Rheumatol.* 2018;70:537-546.

A4. McAlindon TE, LaValley MP, Harvey WF, et al. Effect of intra-articular triamcinolone vs saline on knee cartilage volume and pain in patients with knee osteoarthritis: a randomized clinical trial. *JAMA.* 2017;317:1967-1975.

A5. Conaghan PG, Hunter DJ, Cohen SB, et al. Effects of a single intra-articular injection of a microsphere formulation of triamcinolone acetonide on knee osteoarthritis pain: a double-blinded, randomized, placebo-controlled, multinational study. *J Bone Joint Surg Am.* 2018;100:666-677.

A6. Kingsbury SR, Tharmanathan P, Keding A, et al. Hydroxychloroquine effectiveness in reducing symptoms of hand osteoarthritis: a randomized trial. *Ann Intern Med.* 2018;168:385-395.

A7. Skou ST, Roos EM, Laursen MB, et al. A randomized, controlled trial of total knee replacement. *N Engl J Med.* 2015;373:1597-1606.

A8. Brignardello-Petersen R, Guyatt GH, Buchbinder R, et al. Knee arthroscopy versus conservative management in patients with degenerative knee disease: a systematic review. *BMJ Open.* 2017;7:1-12.

GENERAL REFERENCES

For the General References and other additional features, please visit Expert Consult at https://expertconsult.inkling.com.

247

BURSITIS, TENDINITIS, AND OTHER PERIARTICULAR DISORDERS AND SPORTS MEDICINE

JOSEPH J. BIUNDO

DEFINITION

An array of painful and sometimes disabling musculoskeletal syndromes exist that are not articular in origin but arise from tendons and bursae. These conditions are referred to by various names, in addition to *tendinitis* and *bursitis*, including the terms *nonarticular rheumatism, soft tissue diseases, regional rheumatic pain syndromes, overuse syndromes,* and *repetitive use syndromes* (Tables 247-1 and 247-2). These entities are often ignored, misdiagnosed as arthritis, or attributed to the aging process; awareness of the existence of these conditions and knowledge of basic musculoskeletal anatomy (Figs. 247-1 and 247-2) are the fundamental requirements for diagnosis.[1] This knowledge is coupled with brief but specific physical diagnosis techniques. The accurate diagnosis and successful treatment of these conditions is gratifying to the clinician because many people can be relieved of their chronic painful syndromes.

Various terms regarding tendon injuries are used and may be confusing. The main term used is *tendinitis*. *Tendinosis* has been proposed as the correct terminology because there are degenerative changes in the tendon but very few inflammatory cells. In addition, fatty mucoid degeneration and hyaline features occur in these tendon syndromes. These tendon conditions are described by some as a *tendinopathy* because use of this term avoids the need to decide whether inflammation is a factor. Also, tendons may *rupture* or *tear*, partially or completely. The term *tendon insufficiency* is used when the tendon is stretched or is partially or even completely torn. The terms *tenosynovitis* and *peritendinitis* refer to an inflammatory response of the tenosynovium or peritendon, respectively. Tendinitis may occur when the tendon repeatedly bears more load than it can withstand. This may result from excessively high loads across normal tendons or from normal loads across degenerated tendons. In addition to load and repetitiveness, tendon changes resulting from immobility and from aging may play a role, as may the use of certain medications such as fluoroquinolones and corticosteroids.[2]

Bursae are closed sacs lined by a synovial membrane and serve as a cushion. They are located between tendon and bone, tendon and tendon, or bone and skin and allow smooth gliding between these structures. A bursa, which normally has a small amount of bursal fluid, can become inflamed from trauma or overuse, or become infected, producing a bursitis. When this occurs, some swelling and pain of the bursa may be present.

EPIDEMIOLOGY

The incidence of the nonarticular syndromes of bursitis and tendinitis is high. They are more common than both rheumatoid arthritis (RA) and systemic lupus erythematosus (SLE). For example, the incidence of shoulder pain, largely a result of rotator cuff tendinitis and rotator cuff tear, was approximately 20% in a population older than 70 years of age.

DIAGNOSIS

A precise history is needed to identify the conditions present, and more than one syndrome can occur concomitantly. A working knowledge of regional anatomy and an approach that uses a regional differential diagnosis will help in obtaining a specific diagnosis. A complete neuromusculoskeletal examination should be performed, emphasizing careful palpation, passive range of motion (ROM), and active ROM alone or sometimes with resistance. Systemic and infectious causes must be considered. Diagnostic ultrasonography is becoming increasingly useful in confirming a musculoskeletal diagnosis.[3] Magnetic resonance imaging (MRI) is also sometimes useful in confirming a diagnosis.

TABLE 247-1 MUSCULOSKELETAL CONDITIONS BY ETIOLOGY

TENDINITIS	TENDON RUPTURE	BURSITIS
Rotator cuff	Rotator cuff	Subacromial
Bicipital	Bicipital	Olecranon
Volar flexor	Quadriceps	Trochanteric
de Quervain	Patellar	Ischial
Patellar	Posterior tibialis	Iliopsoas
Posterior tibialis	Achilles	Pes anserine
Achilles		Prepatellar
Epicondylitis		Retrocalcaneal

TABLE 247-2 TENDINITIS AND BURSITIS CONDITIONS BY REGION

SHOULDER

Rotator cuff tendinitis
Rotator cuff tear
Bicipital tendinitis
Subacromial bursitis
Adhesive capsulitis

ELBOW

Olecranon bursitis
Medial epicondylitis
Lateral epicondylitis

WRIST AND HAND

de Quervain tenosynovitis
Volar flexor tenosynovitis
Ganglion

HIP

Trochanteric bursitis
Iliopsoas bursitis
Ischial bursitis
Coccydynia

KNEE

Prepatellar bursitis
Pes anserine bursitis
Popliteal cyst (Baker cyst)
Patellar tendinitis
Patellar/quadriceps tendon tear

ANKLE AND FOOT

Achilles tendinitis
Achilles tendon tear
Posterior tibial tendinitis
Posterior tibial tendon tear
Retrocalcaneal bursitis
Plantar fasciitis

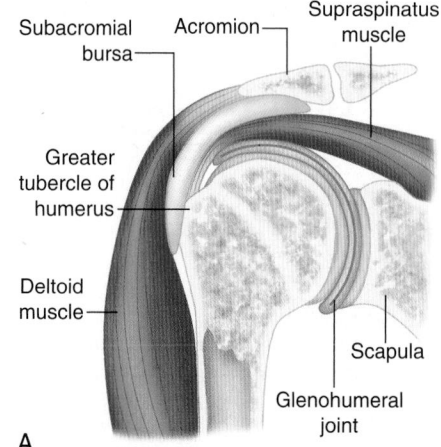
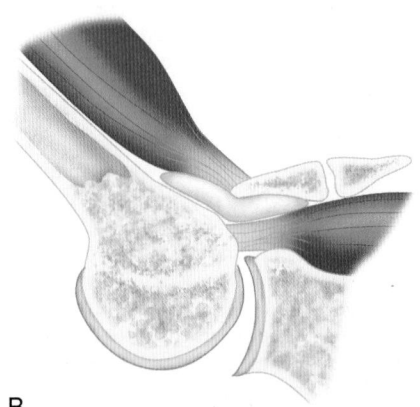

FIGURE 247-1. Relationship of subacromial bursa (shown in *blue*) to supraspinatus muscle and acromion process. **A,** In the position of adduction of the humerus, to show this bursa more clearly, it is in *blue*. The synovial membrane of the glenohumeral joint is not shown. **B,** In the position of abduction of the humerus, the acromion impinges on the subacromial bursa and the insertion of the supraspinatus tendon. (From Polley HF, Hunder GG, eds. *Rheumatologic Interviewing and Physical Examination of the Joints,* 2nd ed. Philadelphia: WB Saunders; 1978:65.)

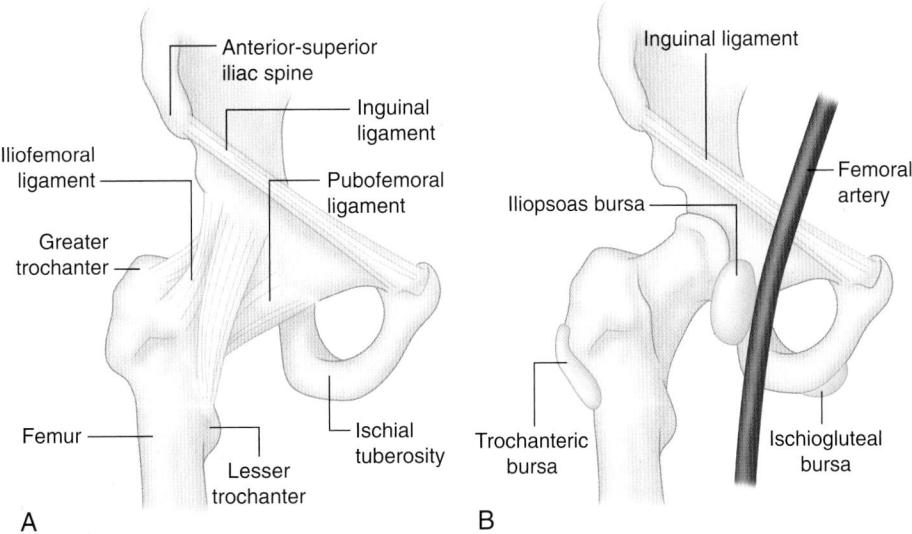

FIGURE 247-2. Musculoskeletal anatomy of the hip. **A,** Anterior aspect of the hip joint and bony structures. **B,** Relationship of the distended iliopsoas, trochanteric, and ischiogluteal bursae (shown in *blue*) to the hip joint and adjacent structures. (From Polley HF, Hunder GG, eds. *Rheumatologic Interviewing and Physical Examination of the Joints,* 2nd ed. Philadelphia: WB Saunders; 1978:183.)

TREATMENT Rx

Treatment of tendinitis and bursitis includes use of nonsteroidal anti-inflammatory drugs (NSAIDs), relative rest of the injured site, stretching and strengthening exercises, friction massage, use of modalities (heat, ice, and ultrasound), splinting, corticosteroid injections,[A1] and surgery. A comprehensive management of these regional syndromes should be undertaken, rather than relying on oral medications alone. The causative aspects should be evaluated, and activity modification should be advised as needed. The goals of therapeutic exercise are to increase flexibility by stretching, increase muscle strength by resistive exercises, and improve muscle endurance by some repetitive regimen. Caution should be exerted in performing corticosteroid injections; the injections should not be placed into the tendon proper, but rather into the peritendinous sheath. The injected solution should be placed beneath the subcutaneous tissue, to avoid skin and subcutaneous fat atrophy, and injections should not be given too frequently, to avoid the possibility of weakening and rupture of the tendon. The accuracy of injections may be improved with concomitant use of diagnostic ultrasonography to assist with determining the correct needle site. Also, fluoroscopically guided injections can be used to increase accuracy.

SPORTS MEDICINE INJURIES

An overlap exists between commonly occurring conditions of tendinitis and bursitis and those attributed to sports injuries (Table 247-3). For example, lateral epicondylitis, frequently referred to as *tennis elbow,* occurs more commonly secondary to non–sports-related causes. In contradistinction, iliotibial band syndrome is usually related to sports. Other entities that occur more often in relation to sports include ligamentous knee injuries, patellar tendinitis, ankle sprains, turf toe, and acromioclavicular separations. It is important in both categories to know the anatomy and biomechanics of the condition to better diagnose and treat the problem. Sports-related injuries are helped with the classic RICE treatment, consisting of *r*est, *i*ce, *c*ompression, and *e*levation. Often, anti-inflammatory and analgesic drugs are used. However, there is less use of corticosteroid injections in athletic injuries than in routine cases of tendinitis and bursitis.

DISORDERS OF THE SHOULDER REGION

Shoulder pain is one of the most common musculoskeletal complaints in people older than 40 years of age. In younger people, athletic injuries are a frequent source of such pain.[4]

Rotator cuff tendinitis, or impingement syndrome, is the most common cause of shoulder pain.[5] Tendinitis (and not bursitis) is the primary cause of pain, but secondary involvement of the subacromial bursa occurs in some cases. The condition may be acute or chronic and may or may not be associated with calcific deposits within the tendon. The key finding is pain in the rotator cuff on active abduction, especially between 60 and 120 degrees, and

TABLE 247-3	ADDITIONAL SPORTS-RELATED CONDITIONS
SHOULDER	
Acromioclavicular separation	
Glenoid labial tear (SLAP lesion)	
Glenohumeral instability with dislocation	
ELBOW	
Triceps tendinopathy	
Little League elbow (apophysitis)	
Distal biceps tendinitis	
WRIST AND HAND	
Gamekeeper's thumb (skier's thumb)	
Mallet finger (baseball finger)	
Extensor carpi ulnaris tendinitis	
Rupture of flexor digitorum profundus tendon	
Injury to triangular fibrocartilage	
HIP	
Adductor strain (groin pull)	
Hip pointer	
Hamstring strain	
KNEE	
Anterior cruciate tear	
Posterior cruciate tear	
Medial collateral ligament tear/strain	
Lateral collateral ligament tear/strain	
Popliteal tendinitis	
Medial and lateral meniscal tears	
Patellar tendinitis	
Iliotibial band syndrome	
ANKLE AND FOOT	
Ankle sprain	
Turf toe	
Stress fracture	

sometimes when lowering the arm. In more severe cases, pain may begin on initial abduction and continue throughout the ROM. Typically, chronic rotator cuff tendinitis manifests as an ache in the shoulder, usually over the lateral deltoid, and occurs with various movements, especially abduction and internal rotation. Other symptoms include difficulty in dressing oneself and night pain because of difficulty in positioning the shoulders. The physical findings include pain and loss of active abduction and internal rotation, less pain on passive motion, tenderness of the area of supraspinatus insertion, and a positive impingement sign (Fig. 247-3), Neer sign, which is pain occurring in forced flexion. The causes of rotator cuff tendinitis are multifactorial, but relative

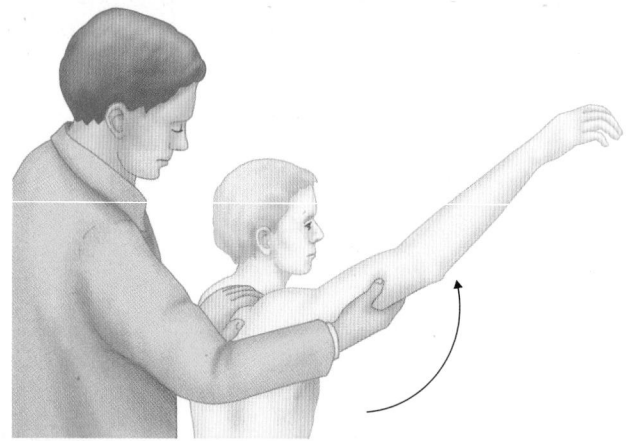

FIGURE 247-3. The impingement sign is elicited by forced forward elevation of the arm. Pain results as the greater tuberosity impinges on the acromion. The examiner's hand prevents scapular rotation. This maneuver may be positive in other periarticular disorders. (From Neer CS II. Impingement lesions. *Clin Orthop.* 1983;173:70-77.)

overuse, especially from overhead activity causing impingement of the rotator cuff, is commonly implicated. Treatment consists of rest and modalities such as hot packs, ultrasound, or cold applications, with specific ROM exercises as soon as tolerated.[6] NSAIDs are often beneficial, but the most frequent treatment is injection of a depot corticosteroid[A2] into the subacromial bursa, the floor of which is contiguous with the rotator cuff. Disodium ethylenediaminetetraacetic acid (EDTA) administered by phonophoresis and mesotherapy to patients with calcific tendinitis of the shoulder has been found to be effective in pain reduction, improvement in shoulder function, and disappearance of calcifications. Extracorporeal shock wave therapy can also be beneficial for chronic calcific tendinitis.[A3][A4]

In a rotator cuff tear, an acute tear after trauma is usually easily recognized. The trauma may be superimposed on an already degenerative and possibly even partially torn cuff. In cases of trauma resulting in a ruptured cuff, fracture of the humeral head and dislocation of the joint also should be considered. However, most patients with a tear recall no trauma. In these cases, degeneration of the rotator cuff occurs gradually, resulting ultimately in a complete tear. Rotator cuff tears are classified as small (≤1 cm), medium (1 to 3 cm), large (3 to 5 cm), or massive (>5 cm). Shoulder pain, weakness on abduction, and loss of motion occur in varying degrees, ranging from severe pain and mild weakness to no pain and marked weakness. A positive drop-arm sign with inability to maintain actively 90 degrees of passive shoulder abduction may be present in patients with large or massive tears. Small complete tears and incomplete tears of the rotator cuff are treated conservatively with rest, physical therapy, and NSAIDs. Although its role has not yet been established by careful studies, a subacromial injection of a corticosteroid may relieve pain. Surgical repair may be indicated in younger patients.

Bicipital tendinitis is manifested by pain, most often in the anterior region of the shoulder and occasionally more diffusely. The pain may be acute but is usually chronic and is related to impingement of the biceps tendon by the acromion. Tenosynovitis of the long head of the biceps is present, and the tendon may be frayed and fibrotic. Palpation over the bicipital groove reveals localized tenderness. The patient's response should be compared with the response to palpation of the opposite side (i.e., tendon with normal tenderness). Pain may be reproduced over the bicipital tendon in some cases by supination of the forearm against resistance (Yergason sign), shoulder flexion against resistance (Speed test), or extension of the shoulder. Treatment of bicipital tendinitis consists of rest, hot packs, ultrasound, and, as pain subsides, passive and then active ROM exercises. NSAIDs may be helpful, and occasionally a small amount of corticosteroid carefully injected into the tendon sheath may be of benefit. Rupture of the biceps tendon can occur at the superior edge of the bicipital groove, producing a characteristic bulbous enlargement of the lateral half of the muscle belly.

Adhesive capsulitis (frozen shoulder) is associated with generalized pain and tenderness and severe loss of active and passive motion in all planes. It is rare before 40 years of age but may occur secondary to any type of shoulder problem. However, not every stiff and painful shoulder is necessarily adhesive capsulitis. Inflammatory arthritis and diabetes can cause adhesive capsulitis. Additional factors such as immobility, low pain threshold, depression, and

neglect or improper initial treatment also favor the development of a frozen shoulder. Many cases, however, are idiopathic. The joint capsule adheres to the anatomic neck, and the axillary fold binds to itself, causing restricted motion. The capsule becomes thickened and contracted. Arthrography can help confirm this diagnosis by showing a decrease in volume of the shoulder joint capsule. Oral steroids improve pain and range of motion in the short term, but a frozen shoulder is probably best treated with a comprehensive program involving NSAIDs and corticosteroid injections into the glenohumeral joint and the subacromial bursa. Physical therapy consists of ice packs, ultrasound, transcutaneous electrical nerve stimulation, and gentle ROM exercises, beginning with pendulum exercises and wall climbing with the fingers and progressing to active ROM and strengthening exercises. The duration of a frozen shoulder may last up to 9 to 12 months. In prolonged duration, manipulation of the shoulder under anesthesia can be considered.

DISORDERS OF THE ELBOW REGION

Olecranon bursitis occurs frequently and involves the subcutaneous olecranon bursa, either secondary to trauma or as an idiopathic condition. The bursa is characteristically swollen and tender on pressure, but pain may be minimal and usually no motion is lost. Aspiration may yield clear or blood-tinged fluid with a low viscosity or grossly hemorrhagic fluid. Inflammatory olecranon bursitis may be caused by gout, RA, or calcium pyrophosphate deposition disease, and infection can also cause a bursitis. Aspiration alone and protection from trauma are usually sufficient to resolve the condition. A small dose of corticosteroid may be injected into the bursa. With septic olecranon bursitis, localized erythema is the major clue. Heat, pain, and a positive culture are also frequently present.

Lateral epicondylitis, or tennis elbow, is a common condition in those who overuse their arms.[7,8] Localized tenderness directly over or slightly anterior to the lateral epicondyle is the hallmark of this disorder. Pain may occur during handshakes, while lifting a briefcase, or with other similar activities. Probably less than 10% of patients actually acquire lateral epicondylitis through playing tennis. Job and recreational activities, including gardening and athletics, are the usual causes. Pathologically, the condition consists of degeneration of the common extensor tendon, particularly of the extensor carpi radialis brevis tendon. Treatment is aimed at altering activities and preventing overuse of the forearm musculature. Ice packs, heat, and NSAIDs are of some benefit. A forearm brace also can be used. A local corticosteroid injection with a 25-gauge needle over the lateral epicondyle often produces satisfactory initial relief. Isometric strengthening is important as the initial part of a rehabilitation program.

Medial epicondylitis, or golfer's elbow, which mainly involves the flexor carpi radialis, is less common and less disabling than lateral epicondylitis. Local pain and tenderness over the medial epicondyle are present, and resistance to wrist flexion exacerbates the pain.

DISORDERS OF THE WRIST AND HAND

A ganglion is a cystic swelling that arises from a joint or tendon sheath and occurs most commonly over the dorsum of the wrist. It is synovial lined and contains thick, jelly-like fluid. Ganglia apparently develop secondary to trauma or prolonged wrist extension. Usually, the only symptom is swelling, but occasionally a large ganglion produces discomfort on wrist extension.

De Quervain tenosynovitis may result from repetitive activity that involves pinching with the thumb while moving the wrist. The symptoms are pain, tenderness, and occasionally swelling over the radial styloid. Pathologic findings include inflammation and narrowing of the tendon sheath around the abductor pollicis longus and extensor pollicis brevis. A positive Finkelstein test result is usually seen; pain increases when the thumb is folded across the palm and the fingers are flexed over the thumb as the examiner passively deviates the wrist toward the ulnar side. However, this test also may be positive in patients with osteoarthritis (OA) of the first carpometacarpal joint and must be differentiated from this common condition. Treatment involves splinting, local corticosteroid injection (Fig. 247-4), and NSAIDs as indicated. Rarely, surgical removal of the inflamed tenosynovium is needed.

Volar flexor tenosynovitis consists of inflammation of the tendon sheaths of the flexor digitorum superficialis and flexor digitorum profundus tendons in the palm. It is extremely common but often unrecognized. Pain in the palm is felt on finger flexion, but in some cases the pain radiates to the proximal interphalangeal (PIP) and metacarpophalangeal (MCP) joints on the dorsal side, misleading the examiner. The diagnosis is made by palpation and identification of localized tenderness and swelling of the volar tendon sheaths. The middle and index fingers are most commonly involved, but the ring and little fingers also can be affected. Often a nodule composed of fibrous tissue

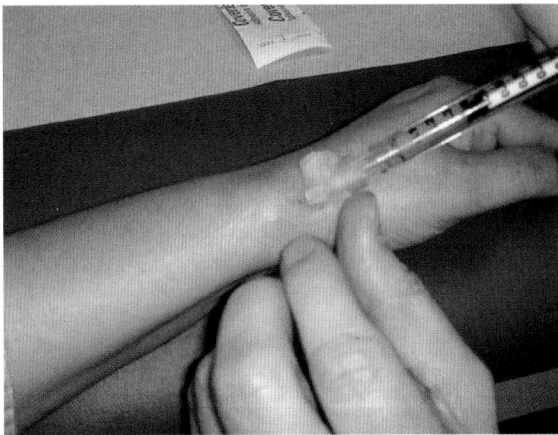

FIGURE 247-4. Injection of de Quervain tenosynovitis.

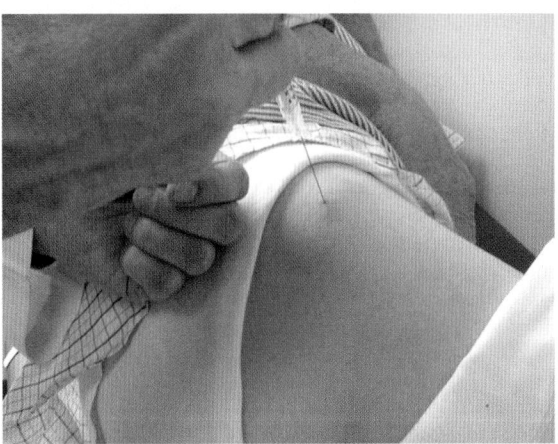

FIGURE 247-5. Injection of trochanteric bursitis.

can be palpated in the palm just proximal to the MCP joint on the volar side. The nodule interferes with the normal tendon gliding and can cause a triggering or locking, which may be intermittent and may produce an uncomfortable sensation. Similar involvement can occur at the flexor tendon of the thumb. The most common cause is overuse trauma of the hands from gripping with increased pull on the flexor tendons. It may be part of inflammatory conditions, such as RA, psoriatic arthritis, or apatite crystal deposition disease. It is seen frequently in conjunction with OA of the hands. Injection of a long-acting steroid into the tendon sheath usually relieves the problem, although surgery on the tendon sheath may be needed in unremitting cases.

Gamekeeper's thumb (skier's thumb) is caused by trauma to the thumb resulting in instability of the first MCP joint. This instability is due to laxity or rupture of the ulnar collateral ligament. It is treated by immobilization, but surgical repair may be necessary.

Avulsion of flexor digitorum profundus (jersey finger) may result from trauma, usually in football, when a player grabs onto a jersey. The distal phalanx, usually the fourth, is hyperextended while the digitorum profundus is contracting maximally. The avulsion of the tendon results in an inability to flex the distal phalanx of that digit. Surgery is required to correct the problem.

DISORDERS OF THE HIP REGION

Although trochanteric bursitis is common, it frequently goes undiagnosed. It occurs predominantly in middle-aged to elderly people, and somewhat more often in women. The main symptom is aching over the trochanteric area and lateral thigh. Walking, various hip movements, and lying on the involved hip may intensify the pain. Onset may be acute, but more often it is gradual, with symptoms lasting for months. In chronic cases, the patient may fail to locate or describe the pain adequately, or the physician may fail to note the symptoms or interpret them correctly. Occasionally, the pain has a pseudoradiculopathic quality, radiating down the lateral aspect of the thigh.[9] In a few cases, the pain is so severe that the patient cannot walk and complains of diffuse pain of the entire thigh. The best way to diagnose trochanteric bursitis is to palpate over the trochanteric area and elicit point tenderness. In addition to specific pain on deep pressure over the trochanter, other tender points may be noted throughout the lateral aspect of the thigh muscle. Pain may be worse with external rotation and abduction against resistance. Although bursitis has historically been described as the principal problem, the condition may actually arise at the insertions of the gluteus medius and gluteus minimus tendons. Local trauma and degeneration play a role in the pathogenesis, leading to tendinosis and/or tendon tears. Conditions that may contribute to trochanteric bursitis, apparently by adding stress to the area, include OA of the lumbar spine or of the hip, leg-length discrepancy, and scoliosis. Treatment consists of local injection of depot corticosteroid using a 22-gauge, 3.5-inch needle to ensure that the bursal area is reached (Fig. 247-5). NSAIDs, weight loss, and strengthening and stretching of the gluteus medius muscle and iliotibial band help in management.

Coccydynia is manifested by pain in the coccyx area when pressure is applied to the area. This most notably occurs on sitting. The patient squirms from buttock to buttock to relieve the pressure and consequent pain and often chooses to sit on a cushion. The symptoms may be chronic and severe. The condition may relate to a fall on the coccyx, dropping to a hard chair when sitting, or some related trauma to the coccyx. However, at times no obvious cause can be detected. Women are much more frequently affected, perhaps because the lordosis that often occurs in women exposes the coccyx to more trauma. The diagnosis is confirmed by finding localized tenderness over the coccyx on palpation. A plain x-ray film can be obtained to exclude a fracture or dislocation of the coccyx. Treatment with a local injection of 1 mL of a long-acting corticosteroid and 2 mL of a 2% lidocaine solution is usually very effective. The exact nature of the pathology of coccydynia has not been studied, but it is presumed to be a bone bruise.

In iliopsoas bursitis, groin and anterior thigh pain are present and worsen on passive hip hyperextension and sometimes on flexion, especially with resistance. Tenderness is palpable over an involved bursa. The patient may hold the hip in flexion and external rotation to eliminate pain and may limp to prevent hyperextension of the hip. The iliopsoas bursa lies behind the iliopsoas muscle, anterior to the hip joint and lateral to the femoral vessels. It communicates with the hip in 15% of cases. The diagnosis is more apparent if a cystic mass is seen (approximately 30% of cases); however, other causes of cystic swelling in the femoral area must first be excluded. A bursal mass can cause femoral venous obstruction or femoral nerve compression. As with most cases of bursitis, acute or recurrent trauma and inflammatory conditions such as RA may lead to iliopsoas bursitis (also called *iliopectineal bursitis*). Iliopsoas tendinitis may overlap with the bursitis or occur independently in a similar clinical picture. The diagnosis is confirmed by plain x-ray with injection of a contrast medium into the bursa, or by ultrasonography, computed tomography, or MRI. Iliopsoas bursitis/tendinitis usually responds to conservative treatment including physical therapy and corticosteroid injections. With recurrent involvement, excision of the bursa may be necessary.

Ischial or ischiogluteal bursitis is caused by trauma or by prolonged sitting on hard surfaces, as evidenced by the name *weaver's bottom*. Pain is often exquisite when sitting or lying down. The hamstring muscles originate from the ischial tuberosity, and the ischiogluteal bursa is superficial to the tuberosity. Because the bursa is superficial to the tuberosity, separating the gluteus maximus from the tuberosity, the pain may radiate down the back of the thigh. Point tenderness over the ischial tuberosity is present. Use of cushions, hamstring stretching, and local injection of a corticosteroid are helpful.

DISORDERS OF THE KNEE REGION

Anserine bursitis is seen predominantly in overweight, middle-aged to elderly women with large legs and OA of the knees. The symptoms are pain and tenderness over the medial aspect of the knee approximately 2 inches below the joint margin, with the pain worsened by climbing stairs. The pes anserinus (Latin for "goose foot") is composed of the conjoined tendons of the sartorius, gracilis, and semitendinosus muscles. The bursa extends between the above tendons and the tibial collateral ligament. Tendinitis of these tendons, rather than bursitis, is the predominant cause of the syndrome. The diagnosis is made by eliciting exquisite tenderness over the bursal area. Anserine bursitis is often overlooked because it frequently occurs concomitantly with OA of the knee, which, when present, is the assumed cause of pain; however, in some cases of dual involvement, anserine bursitis is the principal source of pain.

The treatment is rest, stretching of the adductor and quadriceps muscles, and a corticosteroid injection into the bursa and tendon insertion site.

Prepatellar bursitis manifests as a swelling superficial to the kneecap and results from trauma such as frequent kneeling, leading to the name *housemaid's knee*. The prepatellar bursa lies anterior to the lower half of the patella and the upper half of the patellar ligament. The pain is generally slight unless pressure is applied directly over the bursa. The infrapatellar bursa, which lies between the patellar ligament and the tibia, is also subject to trauma and swelling. Chronic prepatellar bursitis can be treated by protecting the knee from the irritating trauma.

Patellar tendinitis (jumper's knee) is seen predominantly in athletes engaging in activities such as repetitive running, jumping, or kicking. Pain and tenderness are present over the patellar tendon.

Iliotibial band syndrome manifests by lateral knee pain caused by friction between the iliotibial band and the lateral femoral condyle. It is an overuse injury and is seen in runners, cyclists, and other athletes performing repetitive knee flexion activities.

Popliteal cysts, also known as Baker cysts, are not uncommon, and the clinician should be well aware of the possibility of their dissection or rupture. A cystic swelling behind the knee with mild or no discomfort can be the only initial finding. With further distention of the cyst, however, a greater awareness and discomfort are experienced, particularly on full flexion or extension. The cyst is best seen when the patient is standing and examined from behind. Any knee disease having a synovial effusion can develop into a popliteal cyst. Popliteal cysts are most common secondary to RA, OA, or internal derangements of the knee. There are a few reported cases secondary to gout and reactive arthritis. A syndrome of pseudothrombophlebitis may occur as a result of cyst dissection into the calf or actual rupture of the cyst. Findings include diffuse swelling of the calf, pain, and sometimes erythema and edema of the ankle. An ultrasound or arthrogram of the knee confirms both the cyst and the possible dissection or rupture.[10] A cyst related to an inflammatory arthritis is treated by injection of a depot corticosteroid into the knee joint, and possibly into the cyst itself, which usually resolves the problem. If the cyst results from OA or an internal derangement of the knee, surgical repair of the underlying joint lesion is usually necessary to prevent a recurrence of the cyst.

In the knee area, tendon ruptures may occur, and quadriceps tendon rupture is involved approximately 50% of the time; otherwise, patellar tendon rupture occurs. Quadriceps tendon rupture is generally caused by sudden violent contractions of the quadriceps muscle when the knee is flexed. A hemarthrosis of the knee joint may follow. Patients with chronic renal failure, RA, hyperparathyroidism, or gout and patients with SLE taking steroids have been reported to have spontaneous ruptures of the quadriceps tendon. The patient experiences a sudden sharp pain and cannot extend the leg. X-ray studies may show a high-riding patella. The tendon is usually found to be degenerated, and surgical repair is often indicated. Rupture of the patellar tendon has been associated with a specific episode of trauma, repetitive trauma from sporting activities, and systemic diseases.

Meniscal tears are common causes of knee "locking" and pain. Physical examination may show pain, with or without clicking, when the hip and knee are bent to 90 degrees. MRI is the diagnostic test of choice. Physical therapy is often as effective as surgery,[A5-A7] even for patients who complain of knee catching or occasional locking.[A8] Intra-articular injection of mesenchymal stem cells is of limited if any benefit.[A9]

● DISORDERS OF THE ANKLE AND FOOT REGION

Achilles tendinitis usually results from trauma, athletic overactivity, or improperly fitting shoes with a stiff heel counter, but it also can be caused by inflammatory conditions such as ankylosing spondylitis, reactive arthritis, gout, RA, and calcium pyrophosphate dihydrate crystal deposition disease.[11] Pain, swelling, and tenderness occur over the Achilles tendon at its attachment and in the area proximal to the attachment. Crepitus on motion and pain on dorsiflexion may be present. Management includes NSAIDs, rest, shoe corrections, heel lift, gentle stretching, and sometimes a splint with slight plantar flexion. Local injection of platelet-rich plasma (PRP) has become an increasingly used treatment for releasing growth factors into degenerative tendons[12]; however, more recent randomized, placebo-controlled trials for treatment of chronic Achilles and other tendinopathies have found PRP injections to be ineffective in improving pain and activity.[A10] The Achilles tendon is vulnerable to rupture when involved with tendinitis, and treatment with a corticosteroid injection could increase this possibility.

Achilles tendon rupture is well known and occurs with a sudden onset of pain during forced dorsiflexion. An audible snap may be heard, followed by difficulty in walking and standing on toes. Swelling and edema over the area usually develop. Diagnosis can be made with the Thompson test, in which the patient kneels on a chair with the feet extending over the edge and the examiner squeezes the calf and pushes toward the knee. Normally this produces plantar flexion, but in a ruptured tendon, no plantar flexion occurs. Achilles tendon rupture usually occurs during athletic events or with trauma from jumps or falls. The tendon is more prone to tear in people with preexisting Achilles tendon disease and in those taking corticosteroids. Orthopedic consultation should be obtained, and immobilization or surgery may be selected, depending on the situation.

For acute, severe ankle sprain, a below-knee cast or Aircast produces a faster recovery than a tubular compression bandage, but there is no difference in outcomes at 9 months. Plantar fasciitis, which is seen primarily in persons between 40 and 60 years of age, is characterized by pain in the plantar area of the heel. The onset may be gradual, or it may occur with trauma or overuse from some activity, such as athletics, prolonged walking, using improper shoes, or striking the heel with some force. Plantar fasciitis may be idiopathic; it also is likely to be present in younger patients with spondyloarthritis (Chapter 249). The pain characteristically occurs in the morning on arising and is most severe for the first few steps. After an initial improvement, the pain may worsen later in the day, especially after prolonged standing or walking. The pain is burning, aching, and occasionally lancinating. Palpation typically reveals tenderness anteromedially on the medial calcaneal tubercle at the origin of the plantar fascia. Treatment includes relative rest with a reduction in stressful activities, NSAIDs, use of heel pad or heel cup orthosis, arch support, and stretching of the heel cord and plantar fascia. A local corticosteroid injection, using a 25-gauge needle, is often of help.

In posterior tibial tendinitis, pain and tenderness occur just posterior to the medial malleolus; it can be caused by trauma, excessive pronation, RA, or spondyloarthropathy. Extension and flexion may be normal, but pain is present on resisted inversion or passive eversion. The discomfort is usually worse after athletic activity, and swelling and localized tenderness may be present. Treatment usually includes rest, NSAIDs, and possibly a local injection of corticosteroid. Immobilization with a splint is sometimes needed.

Posterior tibialis tendon rupture, which is not commonly recognized, is a cause of progressive flat foot. It can result from trauma, chronic tendon degeneration, or RA. An insidious onset of pain and tenderness may be noted along the course of the tendon just distal to the medial malleolus, along with swelling medial to the hind foot. The unilateral deformity of hind foot valgus and forefoot abduction is an important finding. The forefoot abduction can best be seen from behind; more toes are seen from this position than would be seen normally. The result of the single heel rise test is positive when the patient is unable to rise onto the ball of the affected foot while the contralateral foot is off the floor. Treatment usually includes rest, NSAIDs, and possibly an orthosis. Surgical repair of the tendon is sometimes indicated. Manifestations of retrocalcaneal bursitis include pain at the back of the heel, tenderness of the area anterior to the Achilles tendon, and pain on dorsiflexion. Local swelling is present, with bulging on the medial and lateral aspects of the tendon. Retrocalcaneal bursitis, also called sub-Achilles bursitis, may coexist with Achilles tendinitis, and distinguishing the two is sometimes difficult. This condition may be secondary to RA, spondylitis, a reactive arthritis, gout, or trauma.

Turf toe is an injury of the big toe originally described during play on artificial turf. It results from hyperextension of the first metatarsophalangeal (MTP) joint when a fixed, dorsiflexed foot is forced into the ground. The plantar capsular ligament may be sprained or torn.

Stress fracture is also known as march fracture or fatigue fracture because it was first associated with spontaneous fracture after long marches in army recruits. Pain, swelling, tenderness, and occasionally erythema develop over the metatarsal area, usually without any clear history of trauma. On questioning, however, the episode of spontaneous pain related to onset of the fracture can be identified in some cases. The neck of the second metatarsal bone is most frequently involved, but the third metatarsal is also a site of fracture and less commonly seen in the fourth and fifth metatarsals. Aside from prolonged marching, other athletic events with overactivity, including jogging, are common causes. Stress fractures may be seen in patients with RA and in elderly people. The difficulty in diagnosing stress fractures is that the initial x-ray films usually show no abnormalities or, at most, only a faint fracture line. A repeat x-ray examination several weeks later shows healing with callus formation. Bone scans aid the early diagnosis of stress fractures by showing an increase in uptake over the fracture site. Usually these fractures heal spontaneously, and rest and strapping of the foot are helpful. Occasionally, a cast is needed.

Grade A References

A1. Coombes BK, Bisset L, Vicenzino B. Efficacy and safety of corticosteroid injections and other injections for management of tendinopathy: a systematic review of randomised controlled trials. *Lancet*. 2010;376:1751-1767.

A2. Rhon DI, Boyles RB, Cleland JA. One-year outcome of subacromial corticosteroid injection compared with manual physical therapy for the management of the unilateral shoulder impingement syndrome: a pragmatic randomized trial. *Ann Intern Med*. 2014;161:161-169.

A3. Wu YC, Tsai WC, Tu YK, et al. Comparative effectiveness of nonoperative treatments for chronic calcific tendinitis of the shoulder: a systematic review and network meta-analysis of randomized controlled trials. *Arch Phys Med Rehabil*. 2017;98:1678-1692.

A4. Bannuru RR, Flavin NE, Vaysbrot E, et al. High-energy extracorporeal shock-wave therapy for treating chronic calcific tendinitis of the shoulder: a systematic review. *Ann Intern Med*. 2014;160:542-549.

A5. Katz JN, Brophy RH, Chaisson CE, et al. Surgery versus physical therapy for a meniscal tear and osteoarthritis. *N Engl J Med*. 2013;368:1675-1684.

A6. Sihvonen R, Paavola M, Malmivaara A, et al. Arthroscopic partial meniscectomy versus sham surgery for a degenerative meniscal tear. *N Engl J Med*. 2013;369:2515-2524.

A7. Kise NJ, Risberg MA, Stensrud S, et al. Exercise therapy versus arthroscopic partial meniscectomy for degenerative meniscal tear in middle aged patients: randomised controlled trial with two year follow-up. *BMJ*. 2016;354:i3740.

A8. Sihvonen R, Englund M, Turkiewicz A, et al. Mechanical symptoms and arthroscopic partial meniscectomy in patients with degenerative meniscus tear: a secondary analysis of a randomized trial. *Ann Intern Med*. 2016;164:449-455.

A9. Kim SH, Ha CW, Park YB, et al. Intra-articular injection of mesenchymal stem cells for clinical outcomes and cartilage repair in osteoarthritis of the knee: a meta-analysis of randomized controlled trials. *Arch Orthop Trauma Surg*. 2019;139:971-980.

A10. Moraes VY, Lenza M, Tamaoki MJ, et al. Platelet-rich therapies for musculoskeletal soft tissue injuries. *Cochrane Database Syst Rev*. 2014;4:CD010071.

GENERAL REFERENCES

For the General References and other additional features, please visit Expert Consult at https://expertconsult.inkling.com.

248

RHEUMATOID ARTHRITIS

IAIN MCINNES AND JAMES R. O'DELL

DEFINITION

Rheumatoid arthritis is a chronic systemic inflammatory disease of unknown etiology that primarily targets synovial tissues. It is relatively common, with a prevalence of slightly less than 1% in adults all over the world. Rheumatoid arthritis shortens survival and significantly affects quality of life in many patients.[1] Essentially all patients exhibit some systemic features such as fatigue, low-grade fevers, anemia, and elevations of acute phase reactants (erythrocyte sedimentation rate [ESR] or C-reactive protein [CRP]). This systemic inflammation is believed to be responsible for a variety of coexistent comorbid conditions including cardiovascular disease, osteoporosis, cognitive dysfunction and psychiatric disease, and cancer.[2] However, the primary target of rheumatoid arthritis is the joint. Synovial tissues proliferate in an uncontrolled fashion, resulting in excess fluid production, destruction of cartilage, erosion of marginal bone, and mechanical disruption of the tendons and ligaments. Such damage predicates long-term disability and increased mortality.

In the past two decades, the treatment of rheumatoid arthritis has changed dramatically. Current therapeutic strategies should result in over 50% of patients achieving clinical remissions with treatment with appropriate disease-modifying antirheumatic drugs (DMARD), biologic DMARDs, and targeted synthetic DMARDs used either as monotherapy or in combination and according to rigorous treat-to-target principles.

EPIDEMIOLOGY

Rheumatoid arthritis is a global disease with a variable geographic prevalence of 0.5 to 1% of adults. For reasons that are still unclear, the prevalence in women is around three times greater than that in men prior to the menopause. Rheumatoid arthritis can occur at any age. Overall, the annualized incidence of rheumatoid arthritis is approximately 40 per 100,000 for women and about half that for men. Because rheumatoid arthritis is a lifelong disease and its incidence increases or is stable with age, the prevalence of rheumatoid arthritis increases with each decade. The incidence of rheumatoid arthritis may be decreasing though the reasons for this are unclear. Geographic variations in prevalence and phenotype can be remarkable. Most notably, cohorts have been described in rural Nigeria in which no individuals are affected with rheumatoid arthritis (though case ascertainment bias needs to be excluded); in contrast, a prevalence of 5% has been found in some studies of Chippewa, Yakima, and Inuit Native American tribes. Such extreme phenotypes are as yet poorly understood but likely will reflect the impact of genetics, the gastrointestinal or respiratory microbiome, or other environmental influences. Detailed study of such populations is now generating significant insight into pathogenesis.

PATHOBIOLOGY

Genetics

A combination of candidate association, twin, and genome-wide association studies (GWAS) has established a strong genetic component to the risk for developing rheumatoid arthritis and the severity of the disease.[3] Twin studies reveal a concordance rate of approximately 12 to 15% for monozygotic twins and 2 to 5% for dizygotic twins. Heritability is reported to be around 60%, with lower values for patients who are seronegative.

GWAS in European, North American, and recently Asian populations, combined with subsequent meta-genome analyses, demonstrate that rheumatoid arthritis is a polygenic disorder. The majority of more than 100 thus far identified informative single nucleotide polymorphisms (SNPs) implicate immune genes, indicative of a primary immunologic etiology of disease a priori. Around 40% of genetic risk accrues in the HLA region. Certain HLA-DR alleles (e.g., DRB*0401, DRB*0404, DRB*0101, DRB*1402) associate with an increased risk for developing rheumatoid arthritis and thereafter progressing to more severe disease. Hypervariable regions on DR molecules are particularly important for antigen recognition by binding to antigenic peptides and presenting them to the T-cell receptor (TCR). The amino acid sequence of disease associated DRβ1 chains share a common structural motif, called the *shared epitope* (E-Table 248-1).

Peptides derived from post-translationally modified proteins (e.g., via citrullination, acetylation, carbamylation) may bind with altered avidity to the shared epitope, providing a potential mechanism whereby this genetic factor can mediate disease risk at the molecular level. Thus, altered binding of such peptides to the HLA molecule (expressed on dendritic cells or B cells) may alter the dynamics of HLA-TCR interactions and thereby confer loss of self-tolerance upon (self-reactive) T cells inappropriately activated by this abnormal receptor engagement.

Many other immune related genes are now implicated and add considerable depth to our understanding of pathogenetic pathways. Although individual SNPs usually exhibit modest risk contribution (odds ratios ≈1.05 to 1.2-fold) they nevertheless could confer significant functional impact. Risk genes can be usefully defined on the basis of their contribution to functional immune system compartments. **Adaptive immunity** associated SNPs include a functional polymorphism in protein tyrosine phosphatase nonreceptor 22 (*PTPN22*) that has been reproducibly associated with rheumatoid arthritis and a number of other autoimmune diseases, including type 1 diabetes, systemic lupus erythematosus, Graves disease, and Hashimoto thyroiditis. The co-stimulation receptors, CTLA, CD28, CD40, and signal protein kinase TYK2 have similarly been associated with disease. These could alter the maintenance of central thymic or peripheral tolerance mechanisms, or could confer altered quantitative and functional outcomes from interactions between T cells, B cells, and other antigen presenting cells with increased potential for autoimmunity to emerge. Recently, an association with peptidyl arginase deiminase has been recognized. Because this enzyme converts arginine to citrulline, this raises the possibility of a genetically predisposed risk conferred via increased generation of a major rheumatoid arthritis autoantigen. Pathways that regulate **innate immune** pathways are also identified (e.g., *TRAF1-C5*, *STAT4*, TNF-AIP3, IRAK1) together with pathways concerned with cell migration (*ELMO1*) and fetal development (*LBH*). Several SNPs identify cytokine or cytokine receptor coding loci, including TNF, IL-6R.

Finally, there is increased interest in the role of epigenetics in disease risk and especially propagation. Thus, altered DNA methylation, histone modification (e.g., via acetylation), and microRNA expression patterns have emerged that associate with increased or perpetuation of inflammation. These have been best defined in fibroblast-like synoviocytes (e.g., differential methylation and thus gene expression has been found particularly for pathways related to cell growth and differentiation). Recently the presence of differentially expressed microRNAs has also attracted attention in myeloid lineage cells, T cells, and

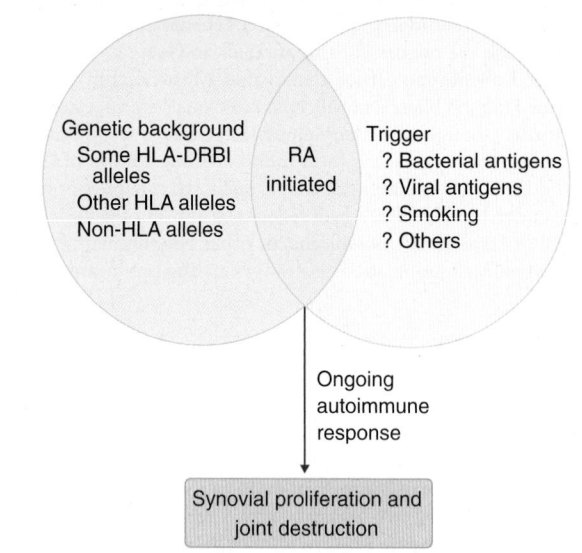

FIGURE 248-1. Initiation of rheumatoid arthritis (RA). HLA = human leukocyte antigen.

fibroblast-like synoviocytes. For example, dysregulation of miR146 and miR155 promotes cytokine and inflammatory pathways in macrophages.

Etiology

Increasing evidence supports a substantial role for environmental factors including smoking, other pulmonary exposures (e.g., silica), obesity, vitamin D deficiency, and lower educational attainment as enhancing factors for rheumatoid arthritis risk. Low levels of alcohol intake may be protective (Fig. 248-1). Smoking in particular has long been associated with a significant increase in the risk for developing rheumatoid arthritis, but this is true only for anticitrullinated peptide antibody (ACPA)-positive disease, especially those who have the shared epitope. Induction of epigenetic changes by smoking provides the most likely explanation for this etiologic link. Infectious triggers are also implicated, such as *Mycobacteria, Streptococcus, Mycoplasma, Escherichia coli, Helicobacter pylori*, and viruses (rubella, Epstein-Barr, parvovirus). The mechanisms whereby infections drive disease are poorly understood. Rheumatic fever (Chapter 274) and reactive arthritis (Chapter 249) are prime examples. Reactive arthritis in particular may occur following one of a myriad of different but specific infectious triggers presented to a specific location in the body (e.g., the gastrointestinal or genitourinary tract) on a predisposed genetic background, in most cases HLA-B27. In this syndrome, age and gender and hence immune system maturity may be critical in the development of clinical disease, which occurs primarily between the ages of 15 and 40 years in males. More recently, Lyme arthritis (Chapter 305) is an example of an arthritic syndrome for which an infectious trigger has clearly been demonstrated. Many other examples exist in animal models of arthritis, including arthritis induced by mycobacteria and streptococci. Currently most interest resides in the role of the microbiome in induction of rheumatoid arthritis. Studies of the gastrointestinal and oral microbiome (the latter particularly in periodontal disease) have identified dysbiosis associated with early rheumatoid arthritis. Specific microbes (e.g., *P. gingivalis, P. coprie, A. actinomycetemcomitans*) have all been implicated. Whether this operates via molecular mimicry, altered immune homeostasis (the GI tract is a vital area for maintenance of peripheral immunologic tolerance) or direct stimulation of immune function (e.g., via enhanced citrullination) remains under investigation.

Finally, the use of oral contraceptives has been associated with a decrease in the incidence of rheumatoid arthritis. Because the effect appears to be strongest for oral contraceptives that have high estrogen content, it is postulated that estrogen is responsible for this protective effect. Studies that have tried to address the question of postmenopausal estrogen use and its effect on rheumatoid arthritis have yielded conflicting results.

Pathogenesis and Tissue Pathology

The overarching pathogenesis of rheumatoid arthritis remains unknown. Taking the foregoing together, the best current model is as follows. The earliest signs of inflammation often occur in the lung: abnormal high-resolution CT scans of pre-RA patients have been reported. Pulmonary mucosal citrullination is increased, perhaps reflecting smoking or other pulmonary irritants. Increased

local inflammation is observed, supporting initial B-cell and then T-cell activation, with consequent "breach of tolerance" to post-translationally modified self proteins. Similar events in the oral mucosa, in periodontal disease, or conceivably in the gastrointestinal tract may also contribute in some patient subgroups. The physico-chemical properties of these self-protein derived peptides that confer increased immune activation presumably arise within the genetic architecture described above and especially the structure of the shared epitope. A prearticular clinical phase ("Pre-RA") ensues that may last up to several years, during which rheumatoid factor and autoantibodies against post-translationally modified proteins (AMPA), particularly anti-citrullinated peptide antibodies (ACPA), rise in titre and with increasingly broad specificity (epitope spreading). ACPAs, for example, can recognize citrullinated residues on a variety of self-proteins (e.g., type II collagen, vimentin, α-enolase, fibronectin, fibrinogen, and histones). The abnormalities thus appear to represent a broad failure to regulate immune homeostasis, rather than one individual (auto)antigen driving disease overall. One autoantigen may, however, serve as a trigger. In parallel, elevated levels of serum cytokines and chemokines are detected, indicative of generalized increased levels of systemic inflammation, along with lipid dysmetabolism. Biopsies of synovial tissue during this pre-RA phase are essentially normal, consistent with its systemic nature.

Thereafter, a transitional event occurs that heralds the onset of clinically detectable arthritis. Systemic disease becomes localized to the joint. This process is ill-defined.[4] ACPA specifics are broadest (they expand during pre-RA), and cytokine concentrations are highest immediately prior to disease onset (imminent RA). Early changes in synovial vascularization, deposition of immune complexes, altered neurologic supply, local infection, and microtrauma have all been postulated as articular localizing mechanisms. An elegant recent notion has ACPA specific for citrullinated vimentin binding to and activating osteoclasts, in turn leading to local bone erosion and pain and the release of chemokines, particularly IL-8. The latter may initiate synovial cellular recruitment.

Established rheumatoid arthritis is associated with development of a dense synovial cellular infiltrate that has some degree of organization (Fig. 248-2). A lining layer forms of 4 to 8 cells in depth including macrophages and fibroblast-like synoviocytes (FLS). The interstitial area contains large numbers of T cells, B cells, plasma cells, mast cells, and FLS. In some patients, lymphocytic aggregates form (ectopic germinal centers) that confer a poorer clinical prognosis. These likely serve as a source of autoantibody production. Intriguing prospective biopsy studies have identified discrete synovial appearances across patient subgroups; myeloid, lymphocytic, and fibroblastic pathotypes have been described at the transcriptional and histologic level. These pathotypes may represent clinically discrete endotypes that in the future could define useful biomarkers to determine optimal choices of immune targeted therapies.

The synovial T-cell response is primarily of T_H1 and T_H17 type. T cells are activated via antigen presented in a CD28/CD80/86 dependent manner by macrophages, B cells, or FLS, by the local cytokine milieu (e.g., IL-7, IL-15, TNF, IL-6), or by cognate cellular activation through cell contact with macrophages. Abatacept that blocks costimulation mediates its effects via interference with some of these pathways. The T cells secrete cytokines (e.g., IL-17 and GM-CSF) that drive further synovial proliferation. The predominant source of synovial cytokines is, however, macrophages, mast cells, and FLS. Macrophage-derived cytokines, particularly interleukin-1 (IL-1), IL-6, and tumor necrosis factor-α (TNF-α), play central roles in this ongoing inflammatory process. TNF and IL-6 in particular appear to have hierarchical functional dominance, reflected in successful therapeutic targeting (e.g., TNF inhibitors, tocilizumab, and JAK inhibitors) and commensurate with their functional profiles that include leukocyte activation, endothelial activation, angiogenesis, or osteoclast activation.

The humoral immune system also plays a role, reflected in the success of rituximab therapy. Rheumatoid factor (RF) and ACPA presence correlate with more severe disease, including erosions of bone, and with the presence of extra-articular features. RF and ACPAs likely have a pathologic role. Via immune complex formation, or perhaps functioning in isolation, they increase complement activation, promote macrophage activation to release lysosomal enzymes, kinins, prostanoids, and oxygen/nitrogen free radicals via Fc receptor (FcR) binding and may activate osteoclasts. ACPAs also activate macrophages via TLR/FcR cross-talk mediated via citrullinated fibronectin.

Articular damage is driven primarily by FLS and osteoclasts. FLS are partially transformed cells, with a distinct epigenetic profile, that exhibit anchorage independence, loss of contact inhibition, low-grade proliferation, and TLR expression, rendering them immunologically competent to sense tissue damage. They release prostanoids, cytokines, chemokines, and matrix metalloproteinases

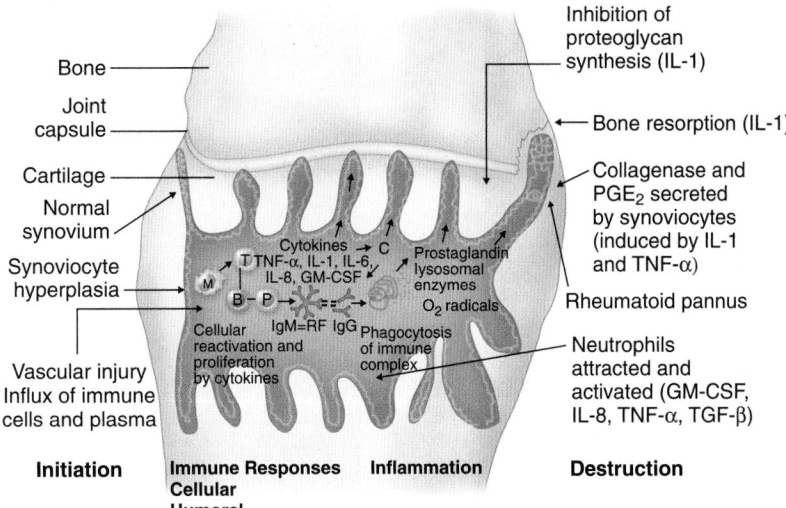

FIGURE 248-2. Events involved in the pathogenesis of rheumatoid synovitis (progressing from *left* to *right*). B = B lymphocyte; C = complement; GM-CSF = granulocyte-macrophage colony-stimulating factor; IgG, IgM = immunoglobulin G, M; IL = interleukin; M = macrophage; P = plasma cell; PGE₂ = prostaglandin E₂; RF = rheumatoid factor; T = T lymphocyte; TGF-β = transforming growth factor-β; TNF-α = tumor necrosis factor-α.

(MMPs) such as MMP1, MMP3, and MMP13, in disproportion to the release of tissue inhibitors of MMPs (TIMPs). In consequence, FLS promote cartilage damage; this local tissue damage area is known as the *cartilage-pannus junction*. Macrophages and mast cells are also likely to contribute to this local process. Bone damage requires cells with capacity to acidify the local milieu—osteoclast maturation and activation is a localized feature of rheumatoid arthritis synovium, arising as a consequence of RANKL, IL-1, TNF, and IL-17 activity. Thus activated osteoclasts localize in periarticular bone and in the adjacent bone marrow, leading to the characteristic erosions detected on plain radiography. The inflammatory process underlying erosion is detected as "bone edema" on MRI. Synovitis thus results in the destruction of cartilage in marginal bone and in the stretching or rupture of the joint capsule or tendons and ligaments. Damage is directly related to disability.

Finally, generalized inflammation promotes systemic comorbidities. Circulating cytokines and immune complexes are proposed to activate endothelium and accelerate atherosclerosis, may provoke systemic osteoporosis, and can drive cognitive impairment, fatigue, and frank psychiatric presentations (e.g., depression). Inhibition of such processes should reduce comorbidities in the clinic.

CLINICAL MANIFESTATIONS
Articular Manifestations
Rheumatoid arthritis can affect any of the synovial (diarthrodial) joints (Fig. 248-3). Most commonly, clinically apparent disease starts in the metacarpophalangeal (MCP), proximal interphalangeal (PIP), and metatarsophalangeal (MTP) joints, followed by the wrists, knees, elbows, ankles, hips, and shoulders, in roughly that order. Early treatment limits the joints involved. Less commonly, and usually later, rheumatoid arthritis may involve the temporomandibular, cricoarytenoid, and sternoclavicular joints. Rheumatoid arthritis may involve the upper part of the cervical spine, particularly the C1-C2 articulation (E-Fig. 248-1), but, unlike the spondyloarthropathies (Chapter 249), it rarely involves the rest of the spine. Patients are also at an increased risk for osteoporosis (Chapter 230), and this risk should be considered and dealt with early.

Hands
The hands are a major site of involvement; a significant proportion of the disability caused by rheumatoid arthritis is due to damage and dysfunction of the hands. Typically disease starts with swelling of the PIPs and MCPs. The distal interphalangeal (DIP) joints are almost never involved; significant involvement of the DIP joints should suggest the possibility of a different diagnosis (i.e., osteoarthritis or psoriatic arthritis). Figure 248-4 illustrates the classic ulnar deviation of the MCP joints and swan-neck deformities (hyperextension of the PIP joints) that are commonly seen in late disease. Boutonnière (or buttonhole) deformities also occur as a result of hyperflexion of the PIP joints. If the clinical disease remains active, hand function deteriorates. Sudden loss of function of individual fingers may occur as a result of tendon rupture, which requires the expertise of a hand surgeon to repair.

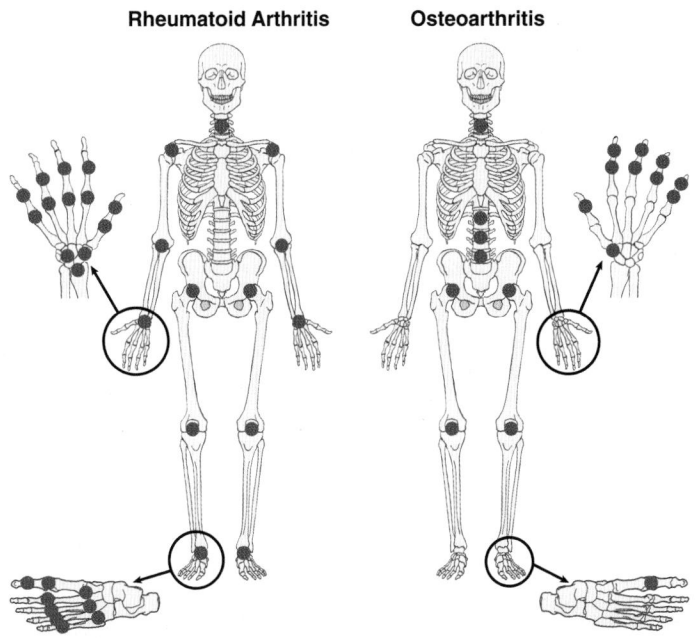

FIGURE 248-3. Distribution of involved joints in the two most common forms of arthritis: rheumatoid arthritis and osteoarthritis. *Black circles* are shown over the involved joint areas.

Feet
Feet, particularly the MTP joints, are involved early in most patients. Radiographic erosions occur at least as early in the feet as in the hands. Subluxation of the toes is common and leads to the dual problem of breakdown of the skin and ulcers on the top of the toes and malalignment of the MTP heads. Painful ambulation develops owing to dislocation of the cushioning pads that usually protect the heads of the MTP joints.

Wrists
The wrist joints are involved in most patients with rheumatoid arthritis. Radial deviation is the rule, and patients with severe involvement may progress to volar subluxation. Even early in the course of the disease, synovial proliferation in and around the wrists may compress the median nerve, causing carpal tunnel syndrome (Fig. 248-5). Later, this synovial proliferation may invade tendons and lead to rupture, most commonly of extensor tendons.

Large Joints
Involvement of knees, ankles, elbows, hips, and shoulders is common. Characteristically, the whole joint surface is involved in a symmetrical fashion.

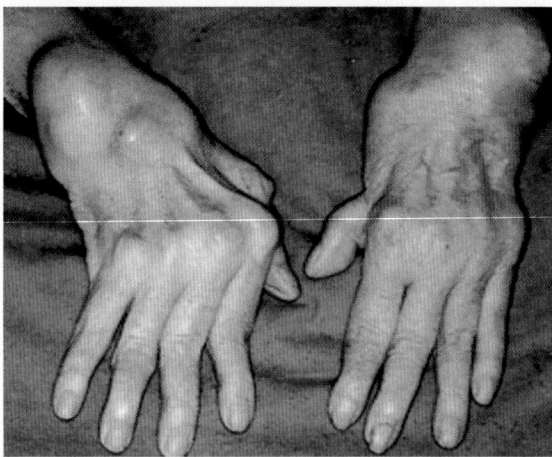

FIGURE 248-4. Severe advanced rheumatoid arthritis of the hands. There is massive tendon swelling over the dorsal surface of both wrists, severe muscle wasting, ulnar deviation of the metacarpophalangeal joints, and swan-neck deformity of the fingers. (From Forbes CD, Jackson WF. *Color Atlas and Text of Clinical Medicine,* 3rd ed. London: Mosby; 2003.)

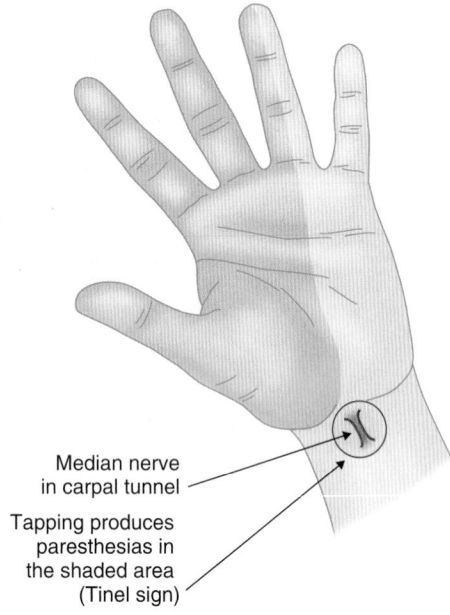

Median nerve in carpal tunnel

Tapping produces paresthesias in the shaded area (Tinel sign)

FIGURE 248-5. Carpal tunnel syndrome. Distribution of pain and/or paresthesias *(shaded area)* when the median nerve is compressed by swelling in the wrist (carpal tunnel).

Rheumatoid arthritis is symmetrical not only from one side of the body to the other but also within the individual joint. In the case of the knee (Fig. 248-6A), the medial and lateral compartments are both severely narrowed. In contrast, in patients with osteoarthritis (Fig. 248-6B) variably only one compartment of the knee may be involved.

Synovial cysts may occur around any of the joints (large or small), and they occasionally manifest as soft, fluctuant masses that present diagnostic challenges. When the knee produces excess synovial fluid, it may accumulate in the popliteal fossa (popliteal or Baker cyst) (E-Fig. 248-2). These cysts can compress the popliteal nerve, artery, or veins. Baker cysts may dissect into the tissues of the calf (usually posteriorly), or they may rupture. Dissection may produce only minor symptoms, such as a feeling of fullness; rupture of the cyst with extravasation of its inflammatory content produces significant pain and swelling and may be confused with thrombophlebitis, the so-called pseudothrombophlebitis syndrome. Ultrasonography of the popliteal fossa and calf is useful to establish the correct diagnosis and rule out thrombophlebitis, which may be precipitated by popliteal cysts. Treatment of popliteal or any other cyst should be directed at interrupting the inflammatory process initially with an intra-articular injection of corticosteroid into the associated joint.

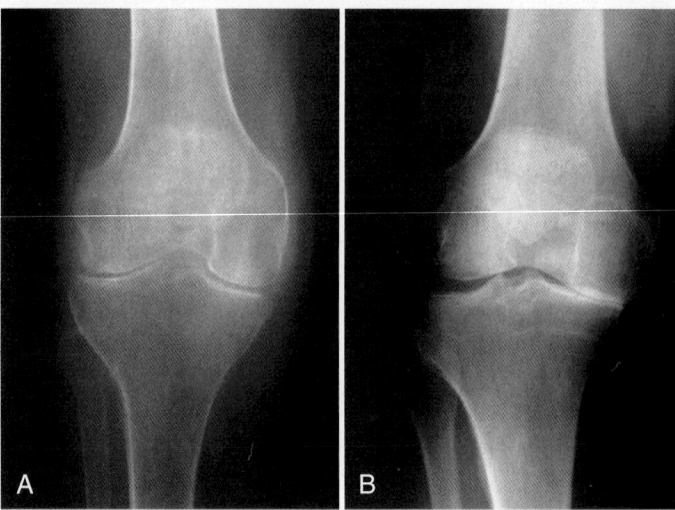

FIGURE 248-6. Radiographs of the knees in the two most common forms of arthritis: rheumatoid arthritis and osteoarthritis. A, Severe involvement in rheumatoid arthritis, with almost complete symmetrical loss of joint space in both the medial and the lateral compartments, but with little subchondral sclerosis or osteophyte formation. B, Typical osteoarthritis, with severe, near-total loss of joint space of one compartment and a normal or actually increased joint space of the other compartment. Note also the significant subchondral sclerosis in the involved area, typical of osteoarthritis.

Neck

Although most of the axial skeleton is spared in rheumatoid arthritis, the cervical spine is commonly involved, particularly the C1-C2 articulation. Bony erosions and ligament damage can occur in this area and may lead to subluxation (see E-Fig. 248-1). Most often, subluxation at C1-C2 is minor and without accompanying symptoms; patients and caregivers need only be cautious and avoid actively forcing the neck into positions of flexion. Occasionally, subluxation at C1-C2 is severe and leads to compromise of the cervical cord with neurologic symptoms and in some cases death. If surgery is planned for a patient with long-standing rheumatoid arthritis, preoperative flexion and extension films of the cervical spine should be obtained looking for significant subluxation.

Other Joints

Wherever synovial tissue exists, rheumatoid arthritis can cause problems. The temporomandibular, cricoarytenoid, and sternoclavicular joints are examples of other joints that may be involved. The cricoarytenoid joint is responsible for abduction and adduction of the vocal cords. Involvement of this joint may lead to a feeling of fullness in the throat, to hoarseness, and, rarely, when the cords are essentially fused in a closed position, to a syndrome of acute respiratory distress with or without stridor. In this latter situation, emergent tracheotomy may be life-saving.

Extra-Articular Manifestations

Systemic features of rheumatoid arthritis such as fatigue, weight loss, and low-grade fevers occur frequently. As with all the other extra-articular features, they are more common in those patients who are positive for rheumatoid factor (RF) or ACPA antibodies or both (Table 248-1) and respond to treatment.

Skin

Subcutaneous nodules are seen in approximately 20% of patients with rheumatoid arthritis, almost exclusively in those who are RF or ACPA positive. Patients with nodules who are seronegative should be carefully scrutinized for a different diagnosis, such as chronic tophaceous gout. Nodules may occur almost anywhere (e.g., lungs, heart, eye), but most commonly develop subcutaneously on extensor surfaces (particularly the forearms) (Fig. 248-7), over joints, or over pressure points. Rheumatoid nodules are firm on examination, usually are not tender, have a characteristic histologic picture, and are thought to be initiated by small vessel vasculitis. A syndrome of increased nodulosis, despite good control of the joint disease, has been described with methotrexate therapy (Fig. 248-8).

Small vessel vasculitis,[5] manifested as digital infarcts or leukocytoclastic vasculitis, may occur in rheumatoid arthritis (Fig. 248-9) and should prompt more aggressive DMARD treatment. A vasculitis of small and medium arteries

TABLE 248-1	EXTRA-ARTICULAR MANIFESTATIONS OF RHEUMATOID ARTHRITIS
Skin	Nodules, fragility, vasculitis, pyoderma gangrenosum
Heart	Pericarditis, premature atherosclerosis, vasculitis, valve disease, and valve ring nodules
Lung	Pleural effusions, interstitial lung disease, bronchiolitis obliterans, rheumatoid nodules, vasculitis
Eye	Keratoconjunctivitis sicca, episcleritis, scleritis, scleromalacia perforans, peripheral ulcerative keratopathy
Neurologic	Entrapment neuropathy, cervical myelopathy, mononeuritis multiplex (vasculitis), peripheral neuropathy
Hematopoietic	Anemia, thrombocytosis, lymphadenopathy, Felty syndrome, large granular lymphocyte syndrome
Kidney	Amyloidosis, vasculitis
Bone	Osteopenia

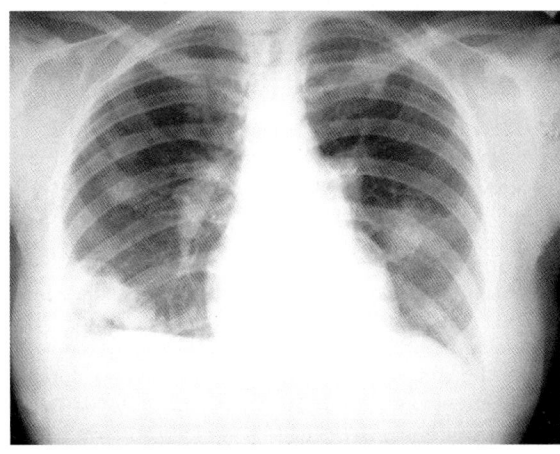

FIGURE 248-10. Rheumatoid nodules in the lung. Chest radiograph demonstrates discrete rheumatoid nodules in both right and left lower lobes. (Courtesy Dr. Martin Lidsky, Houston, TX.)

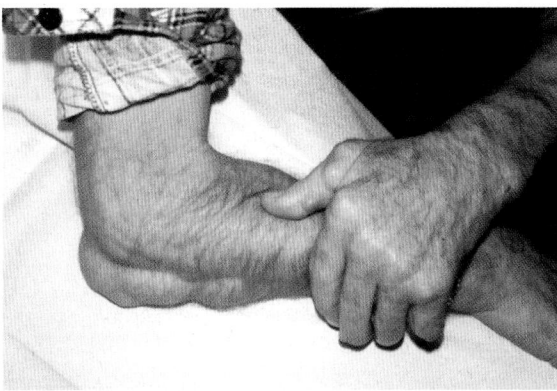

FIGURE 248-7. Rheumatoid nodules. Large rheumatoid nodules are seen in a classic location along the extensor surface of the forearm and in the olecranon bursa.

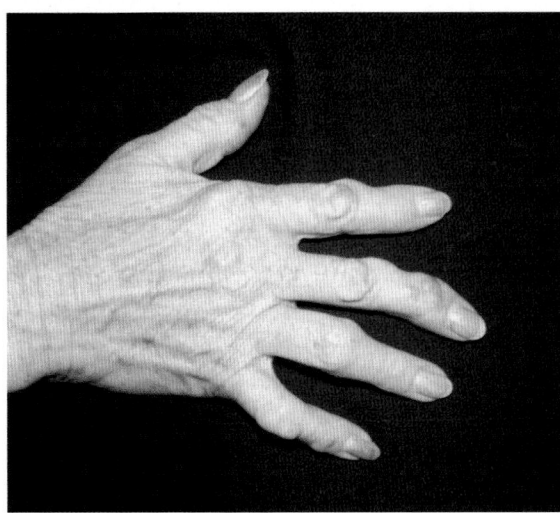

FIGURE 248-8. Rheumatoid nodulosis. In this patient, multiple rheumatoid nodules are present over joints. In some cases, nodules may dominate the clinical picture. Rarely, this may be seen as a side effect of methotrexate therapy.

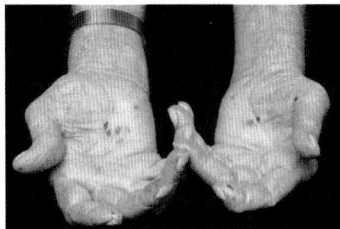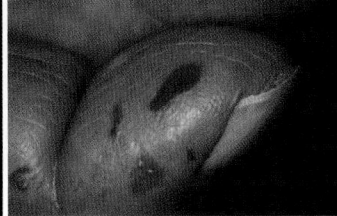

FIGURE 248-9. Small vessel vasculitis. A and B, Rheumatoid vasculitis with small brown infarcts of palms and fingers in chronic rheumatoid arthritis. (Courtesy Dr. Martin Lidsky, Houston, TX.)

that is indistinguishable from polyarteritis nodosa also can be seen and requires aggressive systemic therapy. Finally, pyoderma gangrenosum occurs with increased frequency in association with rheumatoid arthritis.

Cardiovascular Involvement

Cardiac involvement directly related to rheumatoid arthritis is uncommon; however, patients with rheumatoid arthritis have significantly increased morbidity and mortality from coronary artery disease and heart failure. A meta-analysis of observational studies has shown that the risk for incident cardiovascular disease is increased by 48% in patients with rheumatoid arthritis compared with that in the general population. The reasons are not clear, but chronic inflammation appears to be the major cause, superimposed upon the prevalence of conventional risk factors (e.g., smoking, obesity). Some of the medications used to treat rheumatoid arthritis like glucocorticoids and a sedentary lifestyle may be additional risk factors for the development of coronary artery disease. Pericardial effusions are common (50% by echocardiography) but usually are asymptomatic. Rarely, long-standing pericardial disease may result in a fibrinous pericarditis, and patients may present clinically with constrictive pericarditis (Chapter 68). A population-based inception cohort of rheumatoid arthritis patients in Olmstead County, Minnesota, has shown an increased incidence of venous thromboembolism compared with controls.

Pulmonary Manifestations

Pulmonary manifestations include pleural effusions, rheumatoid nodules, and parenchymal lung disease. Pleural effusions occur more commonly in men and are usually small and asymptomatic. Of interest, pleural fluid in rheumatoid arthritis is characterized by low levels of glucose and low pH and, therefore, may at times be confused with empyema. Rheumatoid nodules may occur in the lung, especially in men (Fig. 248-10); these are usually solid but may calcify, cavitate, or become infected. Rarely, pulmonary nodules rupture and produce a pneumothorax. If patients with rheumatoid arthritis are exposed to coal or silica dust, diffuse nodular densities may occur (Caplan syndrome). Differentiating rheumatoid nodules from lung cancer can be problematic, particularly if the lesion is solitary. Therefore, the presence of pulmonary nodules in a patient with rheumatoid arthritis should precipitate an aggressive diagnostic evaluation.

Diffuse interstitial fibrosis occurs in rheumatoid arthritis and rarely may occur prior to joint manifestations. It may progress to a honeycomb appearance on radiography with increasing dyspnea. Rarely, bronchiolitis obliterans can be seen, with or without organizing pneumonia.

Ophthalmologic Manifestations

The most common eye manifestation of rheumatoid arthritis is keratoconjunctivitis sicca (dry eyes) from secondary Sjögren syndrome (Chapter 252). Patients may have associated xerostomia (dry mouth), parotid gland swelling, or, occasionally, lymphadenopathy. Scleritis also can occur and may be painful, with progression to thinning of the sclera, with deep pigment showing through on physical examination, and may progress to perforation (scleromalacia perforans). Rarely, tendonitis of the superior oblique muscles can result in double vision (Brown syndrome).

Neurologic Manifestations

Peripheral nerve entrapment syndromes, including carpal tunnel syndrome (median nerve at the wrist), and tarsal tunnel syndrome (anterior tibial nerve at the ankle), are common in rheumatoid arthritis. Vasculitis can lead to a stocking and glove neuropathy or mononeuritis multiplex, both of which may require aggressive therapy. Subluxations at C1-C2 may produce myelopathy (see E-Fig. 248-1). Rheumatoid nodules in the central nervous system have been described but are rare and usually asymptomatic.

Felty Syndrome

Felty syndrome is the triad of rheumatoid arthritis, splenomegaly, and neutropenia. This complication is seen in patients with severe RF/ACPA-positive disease and may be accompanied by hepatomegaly, thrombocytopenia, lymphadenopathy, and fevers. Most patients with Felty syndrome do not require special therapy; instead, treatment should be directed toward their severe rheumatoid arthritis and when this is done white blood counts improve. If severe neutropenia (Chapter 158) exists (<500 cells/μL) and is accompanied by recurrent bacterial infections or chronic, nonhealing leg ulcers, splenectomy may very rarely be indicated.

Some patients who were previously thought to have Felty syndrome have peripheral white blood cell counts dominated by large granular lymphocytes with almost complete absence of neutrophils. This condition is known as the *large granular lymphocyte (LGL) syndrome* and is thought to be a low-grade lymphoproliferative disorder characterized by the clonal proliferation of large granular lymphocytes. In the setting of rheumatoid arthritis or Sjögren this syndrome has a good prognosis, with the neutropenia often responding dramatically to therapies, particularly methotrexate.

Clinical Course

Although the presentation is variable, most patients with rheumatoid arthritis have the insidious onset of pain, stiffness, or swelling in multiple small joints over the course of weeks to months. Systemic features such as fatigue, low-grade fevers, and weight loss also may be present. Less commonly, the onset can be fulminant, occurring almost overnight, or patients may exhibit persistent monoarthritis or oligoarthritis for prolonged periods before manifesting the more typical pattern of joint involvement. Rarely, particularly men develop extra-articular features of rheumatoid arthritis, especially lung disease, before the joint problems appear.

The distribution of involved joints is a critical clue to the underlying diagnosis. The joints that are involved at presentation are variable; typically, the symptoms start in the small joints of the hands (PIP and MCP joints) and in the toes (MTP joints). Importantly, rheumatoid arthritis usually spares the DIP joints and the small joints of the toes (see Fig. 248-3). Later, it moves, or some would say "metastasizes," to larger joints: wrists, knees, elbows, ankles, hips, and shoulders (roughly in that order). Although the patient's history of joint symptoms (arthralgia) is important, the diagnosis of rheumatoid arthritis requires the presence of inflammation (swelling, warmth, or both) on examination of the joints.

Morning stiffness is a hallmark of inflammatory arthritis and is a prominent feature of rheumatoid arthritis. Patients are characteristically at their worst in the morning or after prolonged periods of rest. This stiffness in and around joints often lasts for hours, and quantifying it is one way to measure improvement. Stiffness is relieved by warmth and activity, and reducing or eliminating joint stiffness is a clear goal of therapy.

DIAGNOSIS

All current treatment paradigms for rheumatoid arthritis stress the early and aggressive use of disease-modifying antirheumatic drugs (DMARDs). Therefore, the importance of accurate early diagnosis cannot be overemphasized. There is no one single pathognomonic finding on physical examination or laboratory testing. Instead, the diagnosis of rheumatoid arthritis requires a collection of historical and physical features, as well as an alert and informed clinician.

Classification

There are currently two classification systems for rheumatoid arthritis: one designed for clinical use and one designed for studies (Table 248-2). Although designed for classification, these criteria are also widely used as diagnostic aids. In the older clinical classification the first five criteria are all clinical; in other words, they are established by physical examination or by talking with the patient. Only the last two criteria require laboratory tests or radiographs. The first four criteria must be present for at least 6 weeks before a diagnosis of

---

TABLE 248-2 CLASSIFICATION CRITERIA FOR RHEUMATOID ARTHRITIS*

Morning stiffness (≥1 hr)
Swelling (soft tissue) of three or more joints
Swelling (soft tissue) of hand joints (PIP, MCP, or wrist)
Symmetrical swelling (soft tissue)
Subcutaneous nodules
Serum rheumatoid factor
Erosions and/or periarticular osteopenia in hand or wrist joints seen on radiograph

*Criteria 1 through 4 must have been continuously present for 6 wk or longer, and criteria 2 through 5 must be observed by a physician. A classification of rheumatoid arthritis requires that 4 of the 7 criteria be fulfilled.
MCP = metacarpophalangeal; PIP = proximal interphalangeal.

TABLE 248-3 DIFFERENTIAL DIAGNOSIS OF RHEUMATOID ARTHRITIS

DISORDER	SUBCUTANEOUS NODULES	RHEUMATOID FACTOR
Viral arthritis (hepatitis B and C, parvovirus, rubella, others)	−	±
Bacterial endocarditis	±	+
Rheumatic fever	+	−
Sarcoidosis	+	+
Reactive arthritis	−	−
Psoriatic arthritis	−	−
Systemic lupus erythematosus	±	+
Primary Sjögren syndrome	−	+
Chronic tophus gout	+	−
Calcium pyrophosphate disease	−	−
Polymyalgia rheumatica	−	−
Osteoarthritis (erosive)	−	−

− = Not present; + = frequently present; ± = occasionally present.

---

rheumatoid arthritis should be made. This caveat is important, because a host of conditions, including many virus-related syndromes, can cause self-limited polyarthritis that looks identical to rheumatoid arthritis, including at times the presence of RF. Such conditions usually last only 2 to 3 weeks. American College of Rheumatology/European League Against Rheumatism criteria for rheumatoid arthritis do not require 6 weeks of disease and give significant weight to the presence of high-titer RF or ACPA positivity.[6] The presence of ACPA antibodies, even in the first few weeks of an inflammatory arthritis, is strongly suggestive of ongoing aggressive rheumatoid arthritis.[7] The 2010 American College of Rheumatology/European League Against Rheumatism collaborative initiative classification criteria are shown in E-Figure 248-3.

Laboratory Findings

Historically, the most characteristic laboratory abnormality is the presence of rheumatoid factor (RF), which is found in approximately 75% of patients. RF is an antibody that recognizes the Fc portion of immunoglobulin G as its antigen. The presence of RF is strongly associated with more severe articular disease, as well as with essentially all the extra-articular features previously discussed. Importantly, RF is seen in association with many diseases other than rheumatoid arthritis, particularly in disease processes that induce chronic stimulation of the immune system (Table 248-3). ACPA (the most commonly detected of the anti-modified protein antibodies [AMPAs]), found in approximately 70% of patients with rheumatoid arthritis, have a high specificity (93 to 98%), and may be present years before clinical disease is diagnosed. They are associated with aggressive erosive disease. Approximately 15% of rheumatoid arthritis patients are negative for both RF and ACPA (seronegative). Rheumatoid arthritis is associated with many other autoantibodies beyond AMPAs, including antinuclear antibodies (≈30%) and antineutrophil cytoplasmic antibodies, particularly of the perinuclear type (≈30%) (Chapter 242).

Most patients with rheumatoid arthritis have an anemia of chronic disease (or anemia of chronic inflammation), and the degree is proportional to the activity of the disease (Chapter 149). Therapy that controls the disease will normalize the hemoglobin levels. Other causes of anemia should also be considered in rheumatoid arthritis, particularly iron deficiency anemia from gastrointestinal blood loss. Thrombocytosis is common, with platelet counts returning to normal as the inflammation is controlled. Acute phase reactants such as ESR and CRP levels parallel the activity of the disease, and their persistent elevation portends a poor prognosis in terms of both joint destruction and mortality. White blood cell counts may be elevated, normal, or, in the case of Felty syndrome, depressed. Eosinophilia is present in some patients with rheumatoid arthritis.

Synovial fluid in rheumatoid arthritis is characterized by white blood cell counts in the range of 5000 to 100,000/μL, with approximately two thirds of the cells being polymorphonuclear leukocytes. There are no synovial fluid findings that are pathognomonic of rheumatoid arthritis.

Differential Diagnosis

The accurate diagnosis of rheumatoid arthritis early in its course, although challenging, is critical if patients are to benefit maximally from therapeutic intervention. Once disease has been present and active for years and the characteristic deformities and radiographic changes have occurred, the diagnosis is all too obvious. Once rheumatoid arthritis has progressed to that point, deformities may no longer be amenable to medical therapy.

Many diseases can mimic rheumatoid arthritis (see Table 248-3). Early in the course of disease, self-limited viral syndromes need to be considered, especially hepatitis B and C, parvovirus, rubella (infection or vaccination), and Epstein-Barr virus. At any time, systemic lupus erythematosus, psoriatic arthritis, and reactive arthritis may present differential diagnostic challenges. In the case of these three mimics, a targeted history and examination to elucidate their associated clinical features, such as rashes, oral ulcers, nail changes, dactylitis, urethritis, and renal, pulmonary, gastrointestinal, or ophthalmologic involvement, is critical. Especially in elderly patients with fulminant-onset rheumatoid arthritis, remitting RF-negative symmetrical synovitis with pitting edema (the so-called RS3PE syndrome) and paraneoplastic syndromes should be considered. Chronic tophaceous gout also may mimic severe nodular rheumatoid arthritis. Hypothyroidism not only causes many rheumatic manifestations but also occurs commonly in conjunction with rheumatoid arthritis and, therefore, should be considered.

TREATMENT ® (Rx)

General Measures

Rheumatoid arthritis is a lifelong disease process that has no known cure; the diagnosis is made based on clinical criteria, and many different options exist for treatment. These factors magnify the importance of the patient-physician relationship and place a premium on the art as well as the science of medicine. Optimal patient care requires effective ongoing interactions between primary care physicians and rheumatologists, and, in some cases, physical therapists, occupational therapists, and orthopedic surgeons.[A1] Because of the serious nature of the disease, the rapid introduction of new treatments, and the need for expertise in monitoring these therapies, all patients with rheumatoid arthritis should be evaluated early and followed closely by a rheumatologist.

The goal of therapy, which is disease remission (Table 248-4) or very low disease activity, should always be kept in mind.[8] When rheumatoid arthritis is treated early, remission is possible in over 50% of patients and low disease activity in at least another 35%. However, continued response requires the ongoing use of DMARDs. Essentially all rheumatoid arthritis patients should be treated with DMARDs.[9] In many patients, combinations of different DMARDs (conventional and biologic) are necessary for optimal control.[A2] Therapy should be escalated rapidly to ensure maximal suppression of disease while minimizing toxicity and expense. Patients with rheumatoid arthritis should be educated about their disease and its treatment. Patients should have an opportunity to spend time with physical therapists and occupational therapists to learn about range-of-motion exercises, joint protection, and assistive devices.

Medical Therapy

Three types of medical therapies are used for rheumatoid arthritis: NSAIDs, glucocorticoids, and DMARDs (both conventional and biologic)[10] (Table 248-5). Initial therapy should always include a DMARD.

Nonsteroidal Anti-inflammatory Drugs

NSAIDs are important for the symptomatic relief they provide; however, they play only a minor role in altering the underlying disease process. Therefore, NSAIDs should rarely, if ever, be used to treat rheumatoid arthritis without the concomitant use of DMARDs. Many clinicians waste valuable time switching from one NSAID to another before starting DMARD therapy.

TABLE 248-4 KEYS TO OPTIMIZE OUTCOME OF TREATMENT OF RHEUMATOID ARTHRITIS

Early, accurate diagnosis
Early DMARD therapy
Strive for remission in all patients
Monitor carefully for treatment toxicities
Consider and treat comorbid conditions*

*Important comorbid conditions include cardiovascular disease, increased susceptibility to infections, and osteoporosis.
DMARD = disease-modifying antirheumatic drug.

TABLE 248-5 TREATMENT OPTIONS FOR RHEUMATOID ARTHRITIS

MEDICATION	DOSE
NONSTEROIDAL ANTI-INFLAMMATORY DRUGS*	
Celecoxib	100 mg PO twice daily or 200 mg PO daily
Diclofenac/misoprostol	50 mg/200 mg PO 2 to 4 times daily
Etodolac	300 mg PO 2 or 3 times daily; or 400 or 500 mg PO twice daily
Ibuprofen	800 mg PO three times daily
Ketoprofen	75 mg PO three times daily; or 50 mg PO four times daily
Naproxen	500 mg PO twice daily
Naproxen/esomeprazole	375 mg/20 mg or 500 mg/20 mg PO twice daily
Tolmetin	400 mg PO three times daily
GLUCOCORTICOIDS*	
Prednisone	5-10 mg PO once daily
DISEASE-MODIFYING ANTIRHEUMATIC DRUGS (DMARDs)	
Conventional DMARDs	
Hydroxychloroquine	200-400 mg PO daily (5 mg/kg)
Leflunomide	10-20 mg PO once daily
Methotrexate	7.5-25 mg PO[†] once weekly (orally or subcutaneously)
Sulfasalazine	500 mg PO once or twice daily for first two weeks; then 2 g daily in two evenly divided doses
Tofacitinib	5 mg PO twice daily
Azathioprine	1 mg/kg (50-100 mg) PO as a single dose or twice daily; may be increased up to 2.5 mg/kg
Minocycline	100 mg PO twice daily
Biologic DMARDs	
Abatacept	500-1000[‡] mg IV at 0, 2, and 4 weeks, then every 4 weeks[§]
Adalimumab	40 mg SC every other week
Certolizumab	400 mg SC at weeks 2 and 4, followed by 200 mg every other week
Etanercept	50 mg SC once weekly
Golimumab	50 mg SC once a month[§]
Infliximab	In conjunction with methotrexate, 3-5 mg/kg at 0, 2, and 6 weeks, then every 4-8 weeks
Rituximab	In combination with methotrexate, two 1000-mg intravenous infusions separated by 2 weeks (one course) every 16-24 weeks
Tocilizumab	4 mg/kg IV every 4 weeks followed by 8 mg/kg every 4 weeks**

*Initial treatment should always include a DMARD; see text.
[†]May be administered SC to reduce side effects and when higher doses are needed
[‡]500 mg if <60 kg; 750 mg if 600-100 kg; 1000 mg if >100 kg
[§]May be administered SC once weekly with or without an intravenous loading dose
[¶]May be administered IV at a dose of 2 mg/kg at weeks 0 and 4, then every 8 weeks
**May be administered SC at a starting dose of 162 mg every other week if <100 kg, or 162 mg every week if >100 kg
DMARD = disease-modifying antirheumatic drug; PO = orally; IV = intravenously; SC = subcutaneously.

TABLE 248-6 GUIDELINES FOR USE OF GLUCOCORTICOIDS

Avoid use of glucocorticoids without DMARDs
Prednisone, >10 mg/day, is rarely indicated for articular disease
Taper to the lowest effective dose
Use as "bridge therapy" until DMARD therapy is effective
Remember prophylaxis against osteoporosis

DMARD = disease-modifying antirheumatic drug.

TABLE 248-7 CAVEATS FOR MONITORING DISEASE-MODIFYING ANTIRHEUMATIC DRUG THERAPIES*

MEDICATION	CAVEATS
Prednisone	Use as bridge to effective DMARD therapy. Prophylaxis for osteoporosis? (see Table 248-6)
Hydroxychloroquine	Keep dosage lower than 5.0 mg/kg/day. Yearly eye checkup by ophthalmologist after 5 years of therapy
Sulfasalazine	CBC for neutropenia, initially every month, then every 6 mo
Methotrexate	CBC and SGOT/SGPT every 8-12 wk when dose is stable. Many toxicities respond to folic acid or small dose reduction. If pneumonitis, stop and do not restart. Decreasing renal function may precipitate toxicities. Absolute contraindication in pregnancy
Leflunomide	CBC and SGOT/SGPT every 4-8 wk; long half-life may require cholestyramine washout; absolute contraindication in pregnancy
TNF inhibitors	If fevers or infectious symptoms of any kind, stop until symptoms resolve; aggressively work up and treat possible infections. May precipitate congestive heart failure, demyelinating syndromes, or lupus-like syndromes

*Patients receiving DMARDs, both conventional and biologic, should be monitored by a rheumatologist.
CBC = compete blood count; DMARD = disease-modifying antirheumatic drug; SGOT = serum glutamate oxaloacetate transaminase (aspartate aminotransferase); SGPT = serum glutamate pyruvate transaminase (alanine aminotransferase); TNF = tumor necrosis factor.

Much has been written about the gastrointestinal toxicity of NSAIDs, and these concerns are particularly relevant to patients with rheumatoid arthritis, who often have significant risk factors, including age and concomitant steroid use. Therefore, cyclooxygenase-2 (COX2)-selective agents have been a popular choice for rheumatoid arthritis patients. The evidence linking these agents to increased cardiovascular toxicity is, however, particularly troubling for patients with rheumatoid arthritis, who are already at high risk for myocardial infarction. In a randomized clinical trial, a cyclooxygenase-2 (COX-2) selective NSAID, celecoxib, was compared to two nonselective NSAIDs, naproxen or ibuprofen, in patients with rheumatoid arthritis and osteoarthritis, and celecoxib was found to be noninferior with regard to cardiovascular outcomes.[A5] If COX2-selective agents are used, they should be kept at a low dose. Consideration should be given to low-dose aspirin prophylaxis, but this therapy may increase the gastrointestinal toxicity of NSAIDs. The use of concomitant misoprostol or proton pump inhibitors should be considered in all patients with rheumatoid arthritis who are taking NSAIDs. Additionally, the potential for NSAIDs to decrease renal blood flow and to increase blood pressure should be kept in mind.

Glucocorticoids

Glucocorticoids have had a significant role in the treatment of rheumatoid arthritis for more than half a century (Chapter 32). Indeed, it was chosen as the first disease to be treated with this new therapy. As was the case with the first patient treated in 1948, glucocorticoids are dramatically and rapidly effective in patients with rheumatoid arthritis. Not only are glucocorticoids useful for symptomatic improvement but they also significantly decrease the radiographic progression of rheumatoid arthritis. However, the toxicities of long-term therapy are extensive and potentially devastating. Therefore, the optimal use of these drugs requires an understanding of several principles (Table 248-6).

Glucocorticoids remain among the most potent anti-inflammatory treatments available; for this reason, and because of their rapid onset of action, they are ideally suited to help control the inflammation in rheumatoid arthritis while the much slower-acting DMARDs are starting to work. Prednisone, the most commonly used glucocorticoid, should rarely be used in doses higher than 10 mg/day to treat the articular manifestations of rheumatoid arthritis. At this dose at the start of methotrexate-based treatment, the addition of prednisone reduces erosive joint damage, disease activity, physical disability, and the use of biologic treatment at 2 years. The dose should be slowly tapered to the lowest effective dose, and the concomitant DMARD therapy should be adjusted to make this possible. Glucocorticoids should rarely, if ever, be used without concomitant DMARD therapy. The paradigm is to shut off inflammation rapidly with glucocorticoids and then to taper them as the DMARD is taking effect ("bridge therapy"). The clear goal is to have all patients off or on very low doses of glucocorticoids with their disease controlled by DMARDs. In all patients receiving glucocorticoids, strong measures should be taken to prevent osteoporosis. Bisphosphonates have been shown to be particularly effective in this regard but are contraindicated in women of childbearing age. Higher doses of glucocorticoids may be necessary to treat extra-articular manifestations, especially vasculitis and scleritis.

Disease-Modifying Antirheumatic Drugs

DMARDs are a group of medications that have the ability to halt the disease process in the synovium and to modify or change the disabling potential of rheumatoid arthritis.[11] These drugs also can halt or slow radiographic progression of the disease.

Conventional Disease-Modifying Antirheumatic Drugs

Included in this group of medications are methotrexate, sulfasalazine (Azulfidine), gold, antimalarials (hydroxychloroquine [Plaquenil] and others), leflunomide (Arava), azathioprine (Imuran), minocycline, and the recently approved tofacitinib (Xeljanz). It is critically important that clinicians and patients understand that conventional DMARDs take 2 to 6 months to exert their maximal effect, and all require some monitoring (Table 248-7). Monitoring of serum drug levels of biologic agents may be especially useful in patients in remission, because higher blood levels predict a longer relapse-free period.[12] Other measures, such as glucocorticoid therapy, may be needed to control the disease while DMARDs are starting to work.

These DMARDs have been shown to be effective in treating both early and more advanced rheumatoid arthritis. Until additional research elucidates factors that allow selection of the best initial therapy for each patient, the choice will depend on patient and physician concerns about toxicity and monitoring issues,

as well as the activity of disease and presence of comorbid conditions. The critical issue is not which DMARD to start first but rather getting the DMARD therapy started early in the disease process.

Methotrexate

Methotrexate should be the initial DMARD for most patients; it is economical, serious toxicities are rare, and when used in combination it makes essentially all other DMARDs work better.[A4] Methotrexate is contraindicated in pregnancy and in patients with significant renal impairment. Methotrexate is dramatically effective in slowing radiographic progression and is usually given orally in doses ranging from 5 to 30 mg as a single weekly dose. This once-per-week administration is worthy of emphasis; prior experience with daily therapy in psoriasis has demonstrated the importance of allowing the liver time to recover between doses. Oral absorption of methotrexate is variable; subcutaneous injections of methotrexate are often effective when oral treatment is not and should be strongly considered before giving up on methotrexate. Side effects of methotrexate include oral ulcers, nausea, hepatotoxicity, bone marrow suppression, and pneumonitis. With the exception of pneumonitis, these toxicities respond to dose adjustments. Monitoring of blood counts and liver blood tests (albumin and aspartate aminotransaminase [AST] or alanine aminotransferase [ALT]) should be done every 3 months, with adjustments in the dose of methotrexate as needed. Renal function is critical for clearance of methotrexate; previously stable patients may experience severe toxicities if renal function deteriorates. Pneumonitis, although rare, is less predictable and can be fatal, particularly if the methotrexate is not stopped or is restarted. Folic acid, 1 to 4 mg/day, can significantly decrease most methotrexate toxicities without interfering with efficacy. If methotrexate alone does not sufficiently control disease, it is combined with other DMARDs.[A5] Methotrexate in combination with virtually any of the other DMARDs (conventional or biologic) has been shown to be more effective than either drug alone.

Leflunomide

Leflunomide, a pyrimidine antagonist, has a very long half-life and is most commonly started at 10 to 20 mg/day orally. Diarrhea is the most common toxicity and responds to dose reduction. Doses of leflunomide of 10 to 20 mg three to five times per week are frequently used. Also, because of the long half-life and teratogenic potential of leflunomide, women wishing to become pregnant who have previously received leflunomide, even if therapy was stopped years ago, should have blood levels drawn. If toxicity occurs or if pregnancy is being considered, leflunomide can be rapidly eliminated from the body by treatment with cholestyramine. Laboratory monitoring for hematologic and hepatic toxicity should be done during treatment with leflunomide, as recommended for methotrexate.

Antimalarial Drugs

The antimalarial drugs hydroxychloroquine (Plaquenil) and chloroquine are frequently used to treat rheumatoid arthritis. They have the least toxicity of any of the DMARDs and do not require monitoring of blood tests. Yearly monitoring by an ophthalmologist after 5 years of therapy is recommended to detect any signs of retinal toxicity (rare). Hydroxychloroquine is the most commonly used preparation and is given orally at 200 to 400 mg/day (5 mg/kg). These drugs are frequently used in combination with other DMARDs, particularly methotrexate. Hydroxychloroquine decreases cholesterol levels, improves HDL function, and recently has been shown to decrease the incidence of diabetes in patients with rheumatoid arthritis.

Sulfasalazine

Sulfasalazine is an effective treatment when given in doses of 1 to 3 g/day. Monitoring of blood counts, particularly white blood cell counts, in the first 6 months is recommended. Sulfasalazine and hydroxychloroquine are often combined with methotrexate, a regimen referred to as triple therapy, which has been shown to have equal efficacy to the combination of a TNF inhibitor and methotrexate and is much more economical.

Minocycline

Minocycline 100 mg twice daily is an effective treatment for rheumatoid arthritis, particularly when used in early RF-positive disease. Chronic therapy (>2 years) with minocycline may lead to cutaneous hyperpigmentation which reverses when the drug is stopped. Minocycline has also been associated with drug-induced lupus.

Tofacitinib

Tofacitinib (Xeljanz) was the first JAK kinase inhibitor to be approved for rheumatoid arthritis. It is given orally at a dose of 5 mg twice daily, and complete blood count and liver function tests should be monitored. Additional toxicity concerns include infections, including tuberculosis, malignancies, and reactivation of herpes zoster. Tofacitinib has been shown to be effective as initial DMARD therapy,[A6] when combined with methotrexate in patients who have incomplete responses to methotrexate, and in patients who have failed TNF inhibitors.

Another JAK inhibitor is baricitinib. In initial reports in patients whose rheumatoid arthritis had not responded to a DMARD, it has shown a consistent beneficial effect compared with placebo.[A7] Furthermore, baricitinib is better than placebo or adalimumab for patients who had inadequate response to methotrexate.[A8] Emerging drugs target distinct members of the JAK family (namely JAK1, JAK2, JAK3, and TYK2). For example, upadacitinib (15 or 30 mg weekly) is effective either as monotherapy or when added to other DMARDs.[A9][A10]

Biologic Disease-Modifying Antirheumatic Drugs

Cytokines, most notably TNF-α, IL-1, and IL-6, play a central role in the pathophysiology of rheumatoid arthritis (Chapter 42). This understanding led to the development and clinical use of biologic agents directed against TNF-α (etanercept [Enbrel], infliximab [Remicade], adalimumab [Humira], golimumab [Simponi], and certolizumab [Cimzia]), IL-1 (anakinra [Kineret]), and IL-6 (tocilizumab [Actemra] and sarilumab [Kevzara]). Additionally, monoclonal antibodies that deplete B cells (anti-CD20, rituximab [Rituxan])[A11] and that block the second signal for T-cell activation (abatacept [Orencia]) are effective treatments for rheumatoid arthritis. All patients with rheumatoid arthritis receiving biologic therapies should be monitored by a rheumatologist, and their physicians should be aware of the risk for infections that are often atypical.[13] All the biologics, when combined with methotrexate, have been shown to decrease disease activity and slow radiographic progression in patients with active disease despite methotrexate.[A12] Early treatment with tocilizumab plus methotrexate was shown to result in greater sustainable clinical, functional, and radiographic benefits than methotrexate alone, with acceptable safety and tolerability, in early erosive rheumatoid arthritis. Sirukumab, which is another anti-IL-6 agent, also may become a useful agent in patients who are refractory in anti-TNF therapy.[A13]

However, standard-dose and high-dose biological drugs (with or without traditional DMARDs) are associated with an increase in serious infections.[A14] Biologic agents also should not be used in combination with each other because they significantly increase the risk of infections (see Chapter 33).

The Order of Therapy in Rheumatoid Arthritis

Several randomized double-blind trials have elucidated the order of therapy in rheumatoid arthritis. The Treatment of Early Aggressive Rheumatoid Arthritis (TEAR) trial nicely showed that initial therapy with methotrexate in patients with poor-prognosis rheumatoid arthritis was not inferior at 2 years to initial combinations of either conventional DMARDs or the combination of methotrexate and etanercept.[A15] The Rheumatoid Arthritis: Comparison of Active Therapies (RACAT) trial has also shown that in those patients who are not controlled on methotrexate alone, the strategy of initially adding sulfasalazine and hydroxychloroquine to methotrexate (triple therapy) was not inferior to the addition of etanercept to methotrexate.[A16] Patients who have not been controlled by methotrexate and other standard treatments can achieve equivalent benefits, with no demonstrable difference in the prevention of joint damage, with combined conventional disease-modifying drugs as with biologics.[A17] Therefore, because of the huge economic advantages, the typical rheumatoid arthritis patient should be started on methotrexate monotherapy, and, if not controlled after 3 to 6 months on maximum methotrexate, the

patient should be advanced to triple therapy. If the patient does not achieve adequate control after 3 to 6 months on triple therapy, either a TNF inhibitor or another biologic should be added to methotrexate.[14] Among patients whose rheumatoid arthritis was previously treated with anti-TNF drugs but who had an inadequate primary response, a non-TNF biologic agent is more effective in achieving a good or moderate response than is a second anti-TNF medication.[A18]

Treatment of Underlying Conditions

Optimal care of patients with rheumatoid arthritis requires recognition of the associated comorbid conditions, including an increased risk for cardiovascular death, osteoporosis, infections (especially pneumonia), and certain cancers such as lymphomas and lung cancers.

Cardiovascular Disease

Cardiovascular disease is being recognized as the cause of much of the excess mortality in rheumatoid arthritis. Various factors contribute to this mortality, including sedentary lifestyle and glucocorticoid therapy. However, a strong association between chronic inflammation and cardiovascular disease has been identified, and it is likely that this is the most significant factor. Therapies that control rheumatoid arthritis earlier and better can be expected to decrease cardiovascular morbidity and mortality. Both methotrexate and TNF inhibitors have been shown to significantly decrease cardiovascular mortality. Clinicians should consider rheumatoid arthritis a risk factor for cardiovascular disease and should aggressively address other cardiovascular risk factors (Chapter 45).

Other Associated Diseases

Osteoporosis is common in patients with rheumatoid arthritis, and early treatment results in long-term dividends. Patients with rheumatoid arthritis are at an increased risk for infections, and some forms of treatment further increase this risk. Patients should be cautioned to seek early medical attention for even minor symptoms suggestive of infection, especially if receiving biologic therapy. All patients with rheumatoid arthritis should receive a pneumococcal vaccine, yearly influenza vaccinations (Chapter 15), and one of the zoster vaccinations. Finally, patients with rheumatoid arthritis have an increased risk for lymphoma. Occasionally, B-cell lymphomas are associated with immunosuppression and regress after immunosuppression is discontinued. Patients with rheumatoid arthritis have significantly decreased risk of developing colon cancer, probably because of chronic inhibition of COX by NSAIDs.

PROGNOSIS

Rheumatoid arthritis is not a benign disease and is not limited to the joints. Once established, it is a lifelong progressive disease that produces significant morbidity in most patients and premature mortality in many. However, all-cause mortality in patients with rheumatoid arthritis is now similar to the general population.[15]

Older studies found that 50% of patients have had to stop working after 10 years ($\approx$10 times the average rate). By comparison, a recent cohort study has shown that the aggressive use of disease-modifying agents and biologic agents, if needed, is associated with substantial reductions in disability. Therefore, early DMARD therapy is critical. Although limited long-term data are available, the current information strongly suggests that patients have the opportunity to benefit greatly if the newer principles of therapy are practiced.

Patients who are RF or ACPA positive and those who are positive for the shared epitope have a worse prognosis, with more erosions and more extra-articular disease (see E-Table 248-1). The HLA-DRB1 locus, which is associated with disease susceptibility, may also be associated with radiologic severity, mortality, and treatment response.[16] Once deformities are found on examination or erosions on radiography, the damage is largely irreversible. Erosions usually occur in the first 1 to 2 years, and the rate of radiographic damage can be reduced by early therapy.

FUTURE DIRECTIONS

Significant advances in the effective treatment of rheumatoid arthritis have come from an understanding of the cytokine imbalance that accompanies this disease. Much research is focused on the further development of biologic products to modulate this balance. There remains a critical need for a cytokine thermostat that titrates the desired cytokine balance to control disease without altering critical immune functions.

Even with existing therapies, many different effective options are available for rheumatoid arthritis. The challenge for the clinician is to pick the right option for each patient. Few data are currently available to aid in this choice, and the establishment of parameters, genetic or otherwise, that would allow selection of the best initial option for each patient would be a major breakthrough. In this respect the option to adopt precision medicine principles is most enticing. Finally, elucidation of the trigger or triggers for rheumatoid arthritis may allow the development of strategies to prevent the onset of clinical disease.

Grade A References

A1. Lamb SE, Williamson EM, Heine PJ, et al. Exercises to improve function of the rheumatoid hand (SARAH): a randomised controlled trial. *Lancet.* 2015;385:421-429.

A2. Nam JL, Takase-Minegishi K, Ramiro S, et al. Efficacy of biological disease-modifying antirheumatic drugs: a systematic literature review informing the 2016 update of the EULAR recommendations for the management of rheumatoid arthritis. *Ann Rheum Dis.* 2017;76:1113-1136.

A3. Nissen SE, Yeomans ND, Solomon DH, et al. Cardiovascular safety of celecoxib, naproxen, or ibuprofen for arthritis. *N Engl J Med.* 2016;375:2519-2529.

A4. Lopez-Olivo MA, Siddhanamatha HR, Shea B, et al. Methotrexate for treating rheumatoid arthritis. *Cochrane Database Syst Rev.* 2014;6:CD000957.

A5. Moreland LW, O'Dell JR, Paulus HE, et al. A randomized comparative effectiveness study of oral triple therapy versus etanercept plus methotrexate in early aggressive rheumatoid arthritis: the treatment of Early Aggressive Rheumatoid Arthritis Trial. *Arthritis Rheum.* 2012;64:2824-2835.

A6. Lee EB, Fleischmann R, Hall S, et al. Tofacitinib versus methotrexate in rheumatoid arthritis. *N Engl J Med.* 2014;370:2377-2386.

A7. Genovese MC, Kremer JM, Kartman CE, et al. Response to baricitinib based on prior biologic use in patients with refractory rheumatoid arthritis. *Rheumatology (Oxford).* 2018;57:900-908.

A8. Taylor PC, Keystone EC, van der Heijde D, et al. Baricitinib versus placebo or adalimumab in rheumatoid arthritis. *N Engl J Med.* 2017;376:652-662.

A9. Genovese MC, Fleischmann R, Combe B, et al. Safety and efficacy of upadacitinib in patients with active rheumatoid arthritis refractory to biologic disease-modifying anti-rheumatic drugs (SELECT-BEYOND): a double-blind, randomised controlled phase 3 trial. *Lancet.* 2018;391:2513-2524.

A10. Burmester GR, Kremer JM, Van den Bosch F, et al. Safety and efficacy of upadacitinib in patients with rheumatoid arthritis and inadequate response to conventional synthetic disease-modifying anti-rheumatic drugs (SELECT-NEXT): a randomised, double-blind, placebo-controlled phase 3 trial. *Lancet.* 2018;391:2503-2512.

A11. Porter D, van Melckebeke J, Dale J, et al. Tumour necrosis factor inhibition versus rituximab for patients with rheumatoid arthritis who require biological treatment (ORBIT): an open-label, randomised controlled, non-inferiority, trial. *Lancet.* 2016;388:239-247.

A12. Nam JL, Ramiro S, Gaujoux-Viala C, et al. Efficacy of biological disease-modifying antirheumatic drugs: a systematic literature review informing the 2013 update of the EULAR recommendations for the management of rheumatoid arthritis. *Ann Rheum Dis.* 2014;73:516-528.

A13. Aletaha D, Bingham CO 3rd, Tanaka Y, et al. Efficacy and safety of sirukumab in patients with active rheumatoid arthritis refractory to anti-TNF therapy (SIRROUND-T): a randomised, double-blind, placebo-controlled, parallel-group, multinational, phase 3 study. *Lancet.* 2017;389:1206-1217.

A14. Genovese MC, Kremer J, Zamani O, et al. Baricitinib in patients with refractory rheumatoid arthritis. *N Engl J Med.* 2016;374:1243-1252.

A15. O'Dell JR, Curtis JR, Mikuls TR, et al. Validation of the methotrexate-first strategy in patients with early, poor-prognosis rheumatoid arthritis: results from a two-year randomized, double-blind trial. *Arthritis Rheum.* 2013;65:1985-1994.

A16. O'Dell JR, Mikuls TR, Taylor TH, et al. Therapies for active rheumatoid arthritis after methotrexate failure. *N Engl J Med.* 2013;369:307-318.

A17. Scott DL, Ibrahim F, Farewell V, et al. Tumour necrosis factor inhibitors versus combination intensive therapy with conventional disease modifying anti-rheumatic drugs in established rheumatoid arthritis: TACIT non-inferiority randomised controlled trial. *BMJ.* 2015;350:1-9.

A18. Gottenberg JE, Brocq O, Perdriger A, et al. Non-TNF-targeted biologic vs a second anti-TNF drug to treat rheumatoid arthritis in patients with insufficient response to a first anti-TNF drug: a randomized clinical trial. *JAMA.* 2016;316:1172-1180.

GENERAL REFERENCES

For the General References and other additional features, please visit Expert Consult at https://expertconsult.inkling.com.

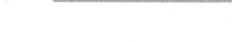

249

THE SPONDYLOARTHROPATHIES

ROBERT D. INMAN

COMMON FEATURES OF SPONDYLOARTHRITIS

DEFINITION

Spondyloarthritis encompasses a group of clinical syndromes that are linked in terms of disease manifestations and genetic susceptibility. The clinical subsets most commonly recognized are ankylosing spondylitis, reactive arthritis, psoriatic arthritis, and enteropathic arthritis (Fig. 249-1). In addition, a sizable

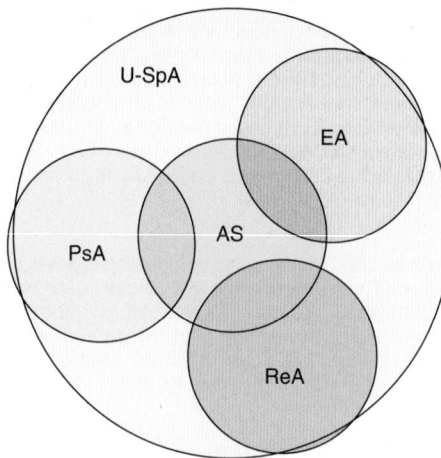

FIGURE 249-1. Schematic relationships among the different spondyloarthritis (SpA) subsets. Ankylosing spondylitis (AS), considered the classic SpA, encompasses the essential features of this family of diseases. AS may overlap with psoriatic arthritis (PsA), enteropathic arthritis (EA), or reactive arthritis (ReA). Many patients have clinical features of SpA that do not meet the diagnostic criteria for any of the four defined subsets. Such cases are termed *undifferentiated SpA* (U-SpA).

number of patients do not fit into one of these distinct diagnostic categories but share some of the common clinical features described in this chapter. This syndrome is termed *undifferentiated spondyloarthritis*; it may evolve over time into a classic pattern such as ankylosing spondylitis, or it may retain an undifferentiated pattern in long-term follow-up studies.

PATHOBIOLOGY

Family studies involving multiple individuals with spondyloarthritis have emphasized some of the common features among the four distinct subsets. The impression from such studies is that there is a shared common path of immunogenetic susceptibility, with further genetic and environmental influences that lead to characteristic clinical subsets. Thus, enteropathic arthritis may occur in one such family, but in another family the disease may be psoriatic arthritis. In this sense, the subsets of spondyloarthritis seem to "breed true." It should be recognized, however, that some distinct clinical features can be very similar in their manifestations (e.g., guttate psoriasis and keratoderma blennorrhagicum), making simple discrimination difficult.

Genetic Susceptibility

Recent genome-wide association studies in ankylosing spondylitis have identified additional genetic markers of susceptibility for ankylosing spondylitis. Polymorphisms in the *IL-23R* gene are associated with ankylosing spondylitis, and these particular variants are the same as those seen in inflammatory bowel disease and psoriasis.[1] Thus the clinical convergence of these different diseases, well known to clinicians, now appears to have a common genetic element. Polymorphisms in the endoplasmic reticulum aminopeptidase (*ERAP*) gene constitute the strongest genetic risk factor for ankylosing spondylitis after HLA-B27, and the association with ankylosing spondylitis is restricted to HLA-B27+ ankylosing spondylitis patients, suggesting a gene-gene interaction. ERAP plays a key role in trimming peptides in the endoplasmic reticulum before loading these peptide complexes onto a nascent class I MHC molecule. This finding continues to attribute a central role to MHC class I peptide presentation in the pathogenesis of ankylosing spondylitis. With larger numbers studied, the list of candidate genes conferring susceptibility to ankylosing spondylitis has now extended to more than 20, but the odds ratio for any one gene is modest, with the notable exception of HLA-B27.

It is believed that the prevalence of ankylosing spondylitis in various parts of the world closely parallels the prevalence of B27 in that population, and in general, this pattern is valid. What introduces complexity into this concept is the recognition that there are more than 30 subtypes of B27. HLA-B2705 is regarded as the primordial subtype, with variability developing over time on the basis of alterations in genomic DNA. Some subtypes, notably B2706 and B2709, do not seem to confer increased susceptibility to the development of ankylosing spondylitis. This observation has led to a search for "arthritogenic peptides" that are presented by the disease-associated subtypes such as B2705 and B2704, but not by the non–disease-associated subtypes. To date, no simple peptide-susceptibility relationship has been demonstrated, but this is an important clue to the pathogenic role of B27, and studies are ongoing to explore this relationship. Recent studies have suggested that certain B27 subtypes have specific interactions with ERAP, which might fundamentally alter MHC structure and function.

Genome-wide screening studies of multiplex families with spondyloarthritis, particularly ankylosing spondylitis, are ongoing in several countries to identify other genes involved in the predisposition to these diseases. The strongest association of spondyloarthritis to date remains with the HLA complex, so at least in familial ankylosing spondylitis, B27 may to a certain extent be necessary (but not sufficient) to confer disease susceptibility. MRI studies in asymptomatic B27-positive individuals indicate that there is a much higher prevalence of sacroiliitis than previously recognized, and studies are continuing to define that prevalence and indeed the prevalence of spondyloarthritis in the general population. Some investigators have concluded that spondyloarthritis is as common as rheumatoid arthritis.

CLINICAL MANIFESTATIONS

There are several common features in the clinical subsets of spondyloarthritis that serve to both link them with and distinguish them from the other major contributor to chronic polyarthritis—rheumatoid arthritis (Chapter 248).[2] Spondyloarthritis has a strong predilection for the spine, in particular the sacroiliac joints. There is a shared tendency for new bone formation at sites of chronic inflammation, with joint ankylosis as a consequence. When peripheral arthritis occurs, it is commonly in the lower extremity and asymmetrical. There is a predilection for involvement at sites of tendon insertion into bone (entheses), so enthesitis is one of the most specific clinical manifestations of spondyloarthritis. Theories postulating the basis for this target organ involvement have invoked biomechanical factors, innervation, local vascularity, and bone marrow–derived inflammatory mediators, but the precise mechanism remains incompletely defined. Whatever the reason, inflammation in the enthesis and contiguous subchondral bone is a characteristic feature of this form of arthritis, and the appearance of this inflammation on magnetic resonance imaging (MRI) is distinct enough to be increasingly used for diagnostic purposes, particularly when the x-rays are not diagnostic. A predilection for ocular inflammation, particularly acute anterior uveitis, is a common feature of spondyloarthritis. Indeed, some investigators consider anterior uveitis to be a feature of spondyloarthritis in its own right because it may occur in the same susceptible population of patients even in the absence of joint involvement, and it may have a unique genetic predisposition. Finally, all spondyloarthritis subsets have an association with the class I HLA allele B27, with the strength of the association varying somewhat among them. Newer genetic risk associations such as *IL23R*, which are shared between spondyloarthritis, psoriatic arthritis, and inflammatory bowel disease, further link the clinical subsets of spondyloarthritis.

DIAGNOSIS

Diagnostic criteria (Table 249-1 [Assessment in Spondyloarthritis International Society criteria]) emphasize the common clinical features—namely, inflammatory spinal pain or asymmetrical lower extremity synovitis. Several distinct features differentiate spondyloarthritis from rheumatoid arthritis, the other main contributor to the differential diagnosis of chronic polyarthritis (Table 249-2). Imaging is often critical for making a diagnosis of axial spondyloarthritis or peripheral spondyloarthritis, monitoring inflammation and damage, predicting outcome, determining response to treatment, and detecting spinal

fractures and osteoporosis.[3] These features include sex predilection, HLA association, pattern of joint involvement, and presence of rheumatoid factor, which becomes the serologic distinction between seropositive disease (rheumatoid arthritis) and seronegative disease (spondyloarthritis).[4]

At the level of joint histopathology, sites of chronic inflammation in rheumatoid arthritis are associated with erosions, but in spondyloarthritis such sites are associated with new bone formation. This distinction suggests a fundamental difference in the cytokine profile in the microenvironment of the joint, but this issue has not been resolved, and the mediators of neo-ossification await identification. Dysregulation of the wnt/β-catenin pathway may play a key role in the ankylosing process. Synovial histopathology in spondyloarthritis is characterized by abundant neutrophils, macrophages, and hypervascularity, whereas in rheumatoid arthritis the prominent features are lymphoid aggregates, dendritic cells, lining cell hyperplasia, and citrullinated proteins. These differences suggest that spondyloarthritis reflects a fundamental alteration in innate immunity, whereas rheumatoid arthritis reflects dysregulation of adaptive immunity.

CLINICAL SUBSETS OF THE SPONDYLOARTHROPATHIES
Ankylosing Spondylitis
EPIDEMIOLOGY

Ankylosing spondylitis is the most common inflammatory disorder of the axial skeleton. The following is a useful rule of thumb: ankylosing spondylitis occurs in 0.2% of the general population, in 2% of the B27-positive population, and in 20% of B27-positive individuals with an affected family member.[5] There is a male preponderance in the disease, with the male-to-female ratio ranging from 2.5 : 1 to 5 : 1; however, recent epidemiologic studies have found more female involvement than these earlier estimates indicate. The basis for the gender bias has not been resolved. It is held, however, that ankylosing spondylitis is underrecognized in women, perhaps because of milder axial

TABLE 249-1	ASAS CLASSIFICATION CRITERIA FOR AXIAL SPONDYLOARTHRITIS	
Sacroiliitis* *Plus* ≥1 SpA feature†	OR	HLA-B27 *Plus* ≥2 other SpA features†
*Sacroiliitis (x-rays or MRI)		†SpA features:
• Definite radiographic sacroiliitis according to modified New York criteria (see Table 249-3) *Or* • Active (acute) inflammation on MRI highly suggestive of sacroiliitis associated with SpA		• IBP • Arthritis • Enthesitis (heel) • Dactylitis • Psoriasis • Crohn disease/ulcerative colitis • Good response to NSAIDs • Family history of SpA • Elevated CRP • HLA-827

ASAS = Assessment in Spondyloarthritis International Society; CRP = C-reactive protein; IBP = inflammatory back pain; MRI = magnetic resonance imaging; NSAIDs = nonsteroidal anti-inflammatory drugs; SpA = spondyloarthritis.

TABLE 249-2	DIFFERENTIAL DIAGNOSIS OF CHRONIC POLYARTHRITIS				
FEATURE	**RHEUMATOID ARTHRITIS**	**ANKYLOSING SPONDYLITIS**	**ENTEROPATHIC ARTHRITIS**	**PSORIATIC ARTHRITIS**	**REACTIVE ARTHRITIS**
Male-female ratio	1 : 3	3 : 1	1 : 1	1 : 1	10 : 1
HLA association	DR4	B27	B27 (axial)	B27 (axial)	B27
Joint pattern	Symmetrical, peripheral	Axial	Axial and peripheral	Axial and asymmetrical, peripheral	Axial and asymmetrical, peripheral
Sacroiliac	0	Symmetrical	Symmetrical	Asymmetrical	Asymmetrical
Syndesmophyte	0	Smooth, marginal	Smooth, marginal	Coarse, nonmarginal	Coarse, nonmarginal
Eye	Scleritis	Iritis	+/−	0	Iritis and conjunctivitis
Skin	Vasculitis	0	0	Psoriasis	Keratoderma
Rheumatoid factor	>80%	0	0	0	0

HLA = human leukocyte antigen.

disease and a more delayed disease onset, but alternative diagnoses of pelvic and low back pain in women may hinder clinician awareness of the disease in female patients.

CLINICAL MANIFESTATIONS

Ankylosing spondylitis typically begins in young adulthood, but symptoms may arise in adolescence or earlier. Up to 15% of children with juvenile idiopathic arthritis are classified as having juvenile ankylosing spondylitis. Such children may have a pauciarticular pattern, with a predilection for the tarsal joints and frequently minimal spinal complaints. During the adolescent years there is an increasing prevalence of radiographic sacroiliitis, with a significant proportion of patients manifesting this feature by the end of the teenage years. At the other end of the age spectrum, a small number of patients with late-onset ankylosing spondylitis may have sacroiliitis and oligoarthritis. The axial involvement and asymmetrical lower extremity involvement may serve to differentiate such patients from those with late-onset rheumatoid arthritis, although there may be overlapping clinical features. Recent studies indicate that the rate of radiographic progression may be less in juvenile-onset ankylosing spondylitis than in adult-onset ankylosing spondylitis.

The classic manifestation of ankylosing spondylitis is the onset of low back pain that persists for more than 3 months, is accompanied by early-morning stiffness, and is typically improved by exercise but not by rest (Table 249-3). Some studies would include a response to NSAID therapy as an additional feature differentiating ankylosing spondylitis from mechanical low back pain. Back pain that awakens the patient from sleep is often a clue to inflammatory back pain that may have been misdiagnosed as the pain of degenerative disc disease, the latter being a much more common cause of low back pain in the population at large. The pain typically occurs in the region of the sacroiliac joints, with or without slight radiation to the buttock area. Midthoracic pain and cervical pain, particularly at night, are less common but strongly suggest inflammatory back pain when they occur. Fatigue is also a suggestive symptom and is often a major concern for the typical young male patient who has a high functional target in terms of sports and recreation. If the inflammation is inadequately controlled, there is increasing stiffness that may persist most of the day, as well as progressive loss of mobility and flexibility.

Peripheral oligoarthritis is seen in up to 30% of patients with ankylosing spondylitis. Typically, it is an asymmetrical oligoarthritis with a predilection for the lower extremities. It is important to ask about concurrent or previous tendinitis (e.g., Achilles tendinitis) or heel pain (e.g., plantar fasciitis), because either may reflect an enthesitis that is part of the clinical picture. Involvement of the hip can occur at any point in the course of ankylosing spondylitis and can follow a course to joint destruction. A hip flexion contracture on this basis may contribute to increasing stoop on standing and walking, which may otherwise be attributed to spinal involvement in the disease.

Extra-articular features most commonly involve the eye. Ocular involvement may occur in up to 40% of ankylosing spondylitis patients, most typically acute anterior uveitis (iritis). The uveitis often manifests as a slight impairment in visual acuity, with accompanying photophobia and eye pain. Typically, it is unilateral and recurrent. Inflammatory bowel disease and psoriasis occur in approximately 10% of ankylosing spondylitis cohorts. Less common manifestations include aortic insufficiency, cardiac conduction defects, and pulmonary fibrosis.

DIAGNOSIS
Physical Examination

Physical examination of the spine characteristically indicates restricted movement, which in the early stages may reflect paraspinal muscle spasm in part; late in the course it reflects ankylosis of the zygapophyseal joints and syndesmophyte bridging of the vertebral bodies. Forward flexion is restricted and can be monitored by the Schober test. This test is used to measure mobility in the lower part of the back: with the patient standing upright, a 10-cm span is marked from the fifth lumbar vertebra upward. On maximal forward flexion, the distance between the marks is remeasured. With normal spinal mobility, the flexed distance should register as 15 cm or an increment of 5 cm. Thoracic involvement is measured in chest expansion, with the chest circumference at maximal inspiration being more than 5 cm greater than the circumference at maximal expiration. Changes in cervical mobility can be measured as the occiput-to-wall distance, with the patient's heels against the wall as the patient attempts to touch the back of the head to the wall. Restricted spinal mobility early in the course of the disease may best be detected by lateral spinal flexion, measured as the difference in the finger-to-floor distance when standing erect compared with maximal bending to the side. Inflammation in the sacroiliac joint may be reflected by joint line tenderness to direct pressure or by the FABERE test (for Flexion, ABduction, External Rotation, and Extension) or Gaenslen maneuver. In the former, the patient lies supine while the examiner flexes and externally rotates the hip. In the latter, the examiner extends the hip by letting the leg dangle off the side of the examining table. In both cases, stress is placed on the sacroiliac joint and may reproduce the back pain if it derives from this site.

Laboratory Findings

Laboratory tests in the evaluation of inflammatory back pain are relatively nonspecific. The ESR and CRP are typically elevated, but normal levels do not exclude inflammatory back pain, and the degree of elevation is typically less than would be seen in acute rheumatoid arthritis. Anemia of chronic disease may be observed if the condition is long-standing. HLA-B27 is rarely the definitive factor for diagnosis, and the false-positive and false-negative rates have already been discussed; however, in the setting of characteristic back symptoms, the test has reasonably high sensitivity and specificity.

Imaging

Radiographic assessment is important for confirmation of disease, but early in the course there may be no radiographic changes in the sacroiliac joints. If the clinician has a high index of suspicion in such cases, MRI may improve the sensitivity of the plain radiograph because inflammatory changes on MRI predate radiographic changes. When ordering x-rays, specific views of the sacroiliac joints can be requested. A routine anteroposterior pelvic radiograph is generally the standard diagnostic x-ray. The classic findings are bilateral changes in the sacroiliac joints (Fig. 249-2). Abnormalities include erosions in the joint line, pseudowidening, subchondral sclerosis, and, finally, ankylosis, reflecting complete bony replacement of the sacroiliac joints.

TABLE 249-3	MODIFIED NEW YORK CRITERIA FOR ANKYLOSING SPONDYLITIS (1984)

CLINICAL CRITERIA

Low back pain and stiffness for >3 mo that improve with exercise but are not relieved by rest
Limitation of motion of the lumbar spine in both sagittal and frontal planes
Limitation of chest expansion

RADIOLOGIC CRITERIA

Sacroiliitis: grade ≥2 bilateral or grade 3 or 4 unilateral

GRADING

Definite AS if the radiologic criterion is associated with at least one clinical variable
Probable AS if:
  The three clinical criteria are present
  The radiologic criterion is present without the clinical criteria

AS = ankylosing spondylitis.

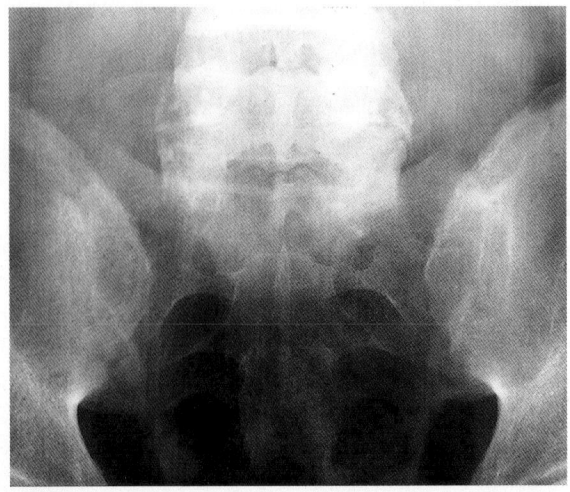

FIGURE 249-2. Bilaterally symmetrical sacroiliitis in ankylosing spondylitis.

Radiographs of the spine may reveal squaring of the vertebral bodies (loss of the normal anterior concavity of the lumbar vertebra) and "shiny corners" (subchondral sclerosis at the upper edge of the vertebral body), both of which are manifestations of enthesitis. Syndesmophytes, which represent marginal bridging of the vertebrae (Figs. 249-3 and 249-4), eventually develop and make the diagnosis clear. Because ankylosis of the apophyseal joints may occur without syndesmophyte formation, it is important to assess the posterior joints on the lateral lumbosacral spine views, as well as the anterior margin of the vertebrae. Eventually, the changes may result in a "bamboo spine," so called because the bridging syndesmophytes can mimic the appearance of bamboo. It is now appreciated that osteoporosis (Chapter 230) is a significant feature of ankylosing spondylitis, probably reflecting both the local chronic inflammation and the abnormal biomechanical loading of the vertebrae as the disease progresses.

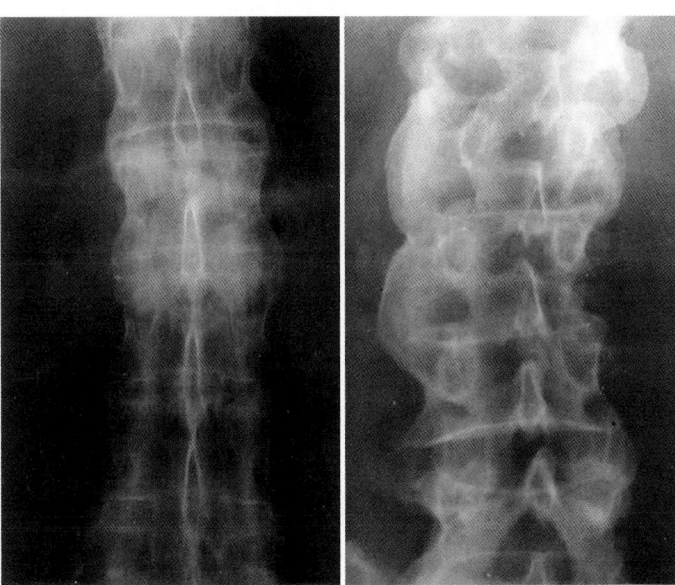

FIGURE 249-3. *Left,* Lumbar spondylitis in ankylosing spondylitis, with symmetrical marginal bridging syndesmophytes and calcification of the spinal ligament. *Right,* The bulky, nonmarginal, asymmetrical syndesmophytes of reactive arthritis with lumbar spondylitis.

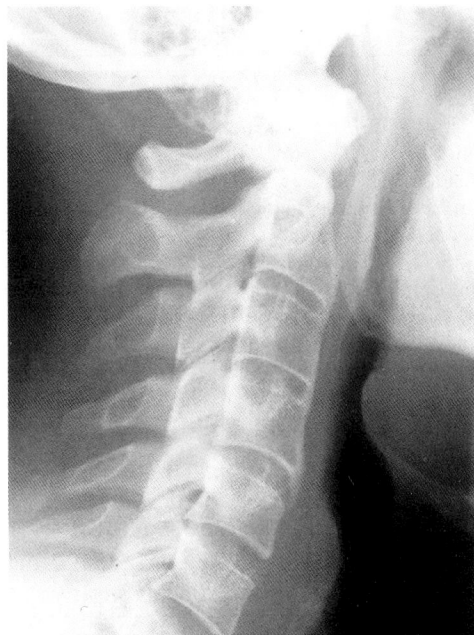

FIGURE 249-4. A 34-year-old man who has had ankylosing spondylitis for 9 years and neck pain. Radiographs demonstrate narrowing of the C2-C3 apophyseal joints posteriorly and anterior bridging marginal syndesmophytes extending from C2 to C5.

Differential Diagnosis

The differential diagnosis of ankylosing spondylitis includes the following: osteitis condensans ilii; diffuse idiopathic skeletal hyperostosis (DISH; Chapter 243); the syndrome of synovitis, acne, pustulosis, hyperostosis, and osteomyelitis (SAPHO); and some induced hyperostotic states (vitamin A intoxication, fluorosis). New bone formation occurs in degenerative disc disease, but the bulky horizontal appearance of osteophytes is usually easily distinguished from that of syndesmophytes, and narrowing of the disc space is not a feature of ankylosing spondylitis. Osteoarthritis of the sacroiliac joint has recently been recognized as having a higher prevalence than previously appreciated.

The clinical course and severity of ankylosing spondylitis are highly variable. Inflammatory back pain and stiffness dominate the picture in the early stages, whereas chronic pain and deformity may develop over time. In both early and late phases of the disease, there may be a significant impact on work disability and quality of life. In only a minority of patients does the full-blown picture of a bamboo spine eventually develop, but there are few variables that can reliably aid in prognosticating the course. At present, the strongest predictor of new syndesmophyte formation is the presence of syndesmophytes at baseline. In ankylosing spondylitis patients in whom new, refractory spinal pain develops, an intervertebral fracture should be considered, which can occur after only minimal trauma.

Additional late complications may include cauda equina syndrome, osteoporotic compression fractures, spondylodiscitis, and restrictive lung disease.

Reactive Arthritis
DEFINITION

Reactive arthritis is an aseptic arthritis that occurs subsequent to an extra-articular infection, most typically of the GI or GU tract.[6] In the GI tract, the key pathogens are *Salmonella typhimurium, Yersinia enterocolitica, Shigella flexneri,* and *Campylobacter jejuni.* In the GU tract, *Chlamydia trachomatis* is the most common offender.

EPIDEMIOLOGY

The true incidence and prevalence of ReA are not well defined. In epidemics involving *Salmonella* (Chapter 292) or *Yersinia* (Chapter 296), it is estimated that reactive arthritis develops in 2 to 7% of infected individuals but in as many as 20% of B27-positive infected individuals. In such epidemic studies, B27 confers risk not only for the onset of arthritis but also for axial involvement and chronicity. Genetic variants in toll-like receptor 2 (TLR-2) are associated with acute reactive arthritis, thus implicating host innate immunity as central in reactive arthritis. The variability in the rate of reactive arthritis is determined by the heterogeneity of the cohorts reported, which introduces confounding variables of different genetic backgrounds in the population and different species of pathogens. Even in the setting of an epidemic point source outbreak, the inoculum varies widely among the exposed individuals, and the genetic makeup of the population at risk (e.g., the prevalence of B27) may differ greatly among different studies. Case ascertainment and relative risk are even more difficult to determine for post-*Chlamydia* reactive arthritis. Young adults in the United States have a high prevalence of asymptomatic *Chlamydia* carriage in the GU tract, and establishing a causal link between *Chlamydia* and synovitis can be difficult. Nevertheless, it is with *Chlamydia* that reactive arthritis has been most intensively studied.

PATHOBIOLOGY

Although immunofluorescence studies have identified bacterial antigens in the joints of patients with reactive arthritis after both GI and GU infections, it is primarily in post-*Chlamydia* reactive arthritis that results of polymerase chain reaction studies on synovial tissues have most consistently been positive, suggesting that viable *Chlamydia* may persist in the joints of such patients, albeit in a metabolically altered state.

Typically, the onset of arthritis occurs 1 to 3 weeks after the GI or GU infection, but the temporal details are often difficult to define precisely.

Although the definition of aseptic arthritis after an extra-articular infection may include a broader range of pathogens (e.g., *Chlamydia pneumoniae*), sites of infection (e.g., streptococcal pharyngitis), and types of infections (e.g., *Giardia* infections of the GI tract), these clinical scenarios have not generally been included in the category of reactive arthritis. They lack the other associated clinical features of the spondyloarthritis group of diseases, and they lack an association with B27.

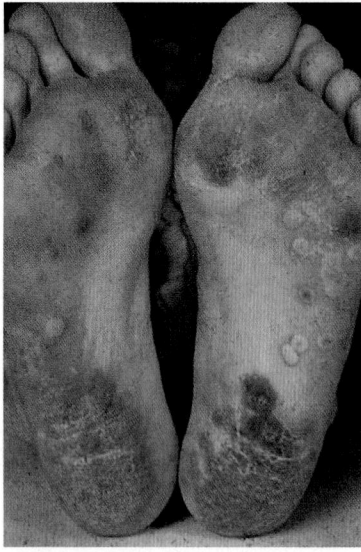

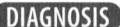

FIGURE 249-5. Keratoderma blennorrhagicum of the feet in reactive arthritis.

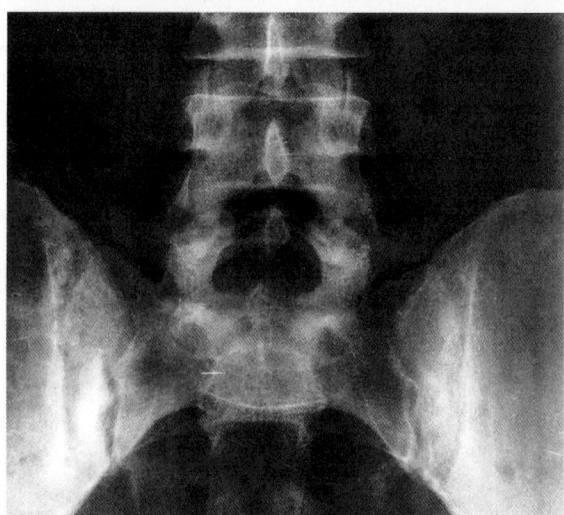

FIGURE 249-6. Bilaterally asymmetrical sacroiliitis in reactive arthritis. Erosions, pseudowidening, and ileal sclerosis are present.

DIAGNOSIS

The pattern of joint involvement in reactive arthritis is one of asymmetrical oligoarthritis with a predilection for the lower extremity, a pattern shared by most spondyloarthritis syndromes. Enthesitis may present as Achilles tendinitis or plantar fasciitis. Dactylitis, appearing as a sausage digit, may also be seen. Dactylitis is the net result of inflammatory changes affecting the joint capsule, entheses, periarticular structures, and periosteal bone. Sacroiliitis may be seen in the acute phase, but radiographic changes are seen largely in patients with a more chronic course.

When reactive arthritis is accompanied by certain extra-articular features such as urethritis, conjunctivitis, or mucocutaneous lesions, the term *Reiter syndrome* has been applied historically, but it is no longer in common use. The urethritis may manifest as dysuria or discharge, and the rash as circinate balanitis, which appears as vesicles or shallow ulcerations on the glans penis. Painless lingual or oral ulcerations may also be seen. The fact that the cervicitis may be less symptomatic could partially account for the underdiagnosis in women. The classic skin manifestation of reactive arthritis is keratoderma blennorrhagicum, a painless papulosquamous eruption on the palms or soles (Fig. 249-5). Occasionally, nail dystrophy with pitting and onycholysis or subungual keratosis can be seen. The conjunctivitis can be bilateral and painful; in contrast, the acute anterior uveitis that can also be seen in this setting tends to be less painful and unilateral.

Radiographic changes of reactive arthritis can be seen in the involved peripheral joints, with early findings consisting of soft tissue swelling and juxta-articular osteopenia. Areas of periostitis and new bone formation may develop in peripheral joints. When changes in the sacroiliac joints are seen, they are typically asymmetrical (Fig. 249-6), in contrast to the symmetrical pattern seen in ankylosing spondylitis. In the chronic phase, syndesmophytes may develop, but they are described as bulky, nonmarginal, often asymmetrical formations that differ from the classic syndesmophytes of ankylosing spondylitis. The frequency with which reactive arthritis evolves into bona fide ankylosing spondylitis has not been determined definitively.

Differential Diagnosis

The most important differential diagnosis for such reactive arthropathies is septic arthritis. Both *Yersinia* and *Salmonella* can cause septic arthritis, so an appropriate culture of synovial fluid should precede the diagnosis of reactive arthritis whenever possible. The course of reactive arthritis is variable, and few prognostic markers are available for the clinician to predict the course in an individual case. The majority of patients have an initial episode lasting 2 to 3 months, but synovitis may persist for a year or longer. In one 5-year follow-up of a point source cohort of post-*Salmonella* reactive arthritis, 20% of patients had ongoing inflammatory joint disease, and some degree of functional disability was observed in 30% of patients 5 years after the onset of disease.

REACTIVE ARTHRITIS AND HUMAN IMMUNODEFICIENCY VIRUS

An aggressive form of spondyloarthritis may be seen in patients who are concomitantly infected with HIV. There is no increased frequency of reactive

TABLE 249-4   ENTEROPATHIC ARTHRITIS

FEATURE	PERIPHERAL ARTHRITIS	SACROILIITIS, SPONDYLITIS
CROHN DISEASE		
Frequency in Crohn disease	10-20%	2-7%
HLA-B27 associated	No	Yes
Pattern	Transient, symmetrical	Chronic
Course	Related to activity of Crohn disease	Unrelated to activity of Crohn disease
Effect of surgery	Remission of arthritis uncommon	No effect
Effect of anti-TNF therapy	Effective	Effective
ULCERATIVE COLITIS		
Frequency in ulcerative colitis	5-10%	2-7%
HLA-B27 associated	No	Yes
Pattern	Transient	Chronic
Course	More common in pancolitis than proctitis; related to activity of ulcerative colitis	Unrelated
Effect of surgery	Remission of arthritis	No effect

HLA = human leukocyte antigen; TNF = tumor necrosis factor.

arthritis in patients with HIV, but HIV may alter the course of these arthropathies, with a tendency for a more aggressive and more refractory joint disease. Aggressive skin and joint disease may be seen in patients in whom psoriatic arthritis develops in the setting of HIV infection. Most North American patients with the HIV-reactive arthritis constellation are B27 positive, but studies of comparable patients in Africa have found a sizable B27-negative component in such patients. The arthritis in these patients falls into two clinical patterns: (1) an additive, asymmetrical polyarthritis or (2) an intermittent oligoarthritis that most commonly affects the lower extremities. Enthesitis, fasciitis, conjunctivitis, and urethritis can all be seen in such patients. Sacroiliitis can occur, although extensive spinal syndesmophyte formation is not common.

Enteropathic Arthritis
DEFINITION

Enteropathic arthritis refers to the arthritis associated with Crohn disease or ulcerative colitis (Chapter 132; Table 249-4).

PATHOBIOLOGY

The association of bowel inflammation and arthritis is supported by ileocolonoscopic studies in which subclinical inflammation of the bowel has been demonstrated in diseases covering the entire spectrum of spondyloarthritis.

Histologic evaluation demonstrates that changes of acute ileitis are seen in postdysenteric reactive arthritis, whereas chronic inflammatory changes are more likely to be seen in patients with ankylosing spondylitis. Altered bowel permeability, with enhanced bacteremia or antigenemia, may provide the link in both cases.

CLINICAL MANIFESTATIONS

All extraenteric manifestations, including arthritis, occur more commonly in Crohn disease than in ulcerative colitis. Peripheral arthritis occurs in 10 to 20% of Crohn disease patients and in 2 to 7% of ulcerative colitis patients. This pattern of arthritis occurs more commonly in patients with other extraenteric features (e.g., erythema nodosum, iritis). It is typically an inflammatory nonerosive polyarthritis, predominantly of large joints. In general, the clinical activity of the peripheral arthritis parallels the activity of the gut inflammation, and measures that control the GI disease usually control the joint disease as well. The peripheral arthritis of enteropathic arthritis is not associated with B27.

In contrast, the sacroiliitis or spondylitis of enteropathic arthritis follows a pattern in which the joint inflammation waxes and wanes independently of the bowel inflammation. Axial disease occurs in 2 to 7% of both Crohn disease and ulcerative colitis patients. HLA-B27 is found in 50% of patients with axial arthritis. The course tends to be chronic, as opposed to the transient course of peripheral arthritis.

DIAGNOSIS

It is important to recognize that the musculoskeletal features of enteropathic arthritis may precede any GI symptoms or signs. Conversely, the diarrhea preceding the onset of peripheral or axial arthritis in a young patient could just as likely represent a food-borne pathogen (e.g., *Salmonella, Yersinia*), with secondary reactive arthritis as inflammatory bowel disease and accompanying enteropathic arthritis. In the initial assessment of such a patient, it is important to carry out careful and complete stool cultures. If the GI symptoms persist, diagnostic colonoscopy is often required to resolve the issue.

Psoriatic Arthritis
EPIDEMIOLOGY

One in five patients with psoriasis also have psoriatic arthritis.[7] Although most cases arise in patients with established cutaneous disease, some patients (particularly children) have arthritis that antedates the appearance of the skin lesions. Although the extent of psoriatic skin disease correlates poorly with the development of arthritis, the risk for psoriatic arthritis increases with a family history of spondyloarthritis. The age at onset can range from 30 to 55 years, with an equal predilection for psoriatic arthritis in women and men. Psoriatic spondylitis has a slight male preponderance. Large prospective studies also suggest that obesity is a significant risk factor for psoriatic arthritis.

PATHOBIOLOGY

The genetic associations with psoriatic arthritis are complex. Psoriasis itself is associated with several HLA loci; some B alleles have been reported, but the dominant element is HLA-Cw6. HLA-B39 and HLA-B27 have been associated with sacroiliitis and axial involvement. No etiologic agent has been proved in psoriatic arthritis, although some investigators have proposed that the disease process represents reactive arthritis in response to cutaneous bacteria. The histopathology of the synovitis of psoriatic arthritis is comparable to that of the other forms of spondyloarthritis, with the absence of the local production of immunoglobulin and rheumatoid factor differentiating this disease from rheumatoid arthritis.[8] There is the potential for aggressive osteolysis, fibrous ankylosis, and heterotopic new bone formation to occur in psoriatic arthritis. As mentioned earlier, the coexistence of HIV and psoriatic arthritis seems to set the stage for an aggressive course of joint destruction in some patients. Patients with psoriatic arthritis can experience substantial physical impairment.[9]

DIAGNOSIS

Psoriatic arthritis has a variable manifestation and disease course, but several clinical patterns have been identified in prospectively monitored cohorts of patients.[10] The clinical subsets are not mutually exclusive, nor are they static over time. The most common form, which affects 30 to 50% of patients, is an asymmetrical oligoarthritis that may involve both large and small joints. Dactylitis, arising as sausage digits, can be seen in fingers and toes and actually represents an enthesitis. In the second subset there is selective targeting of the distal interphalangeal joints, seen in 10 to 15% of patients. These changes

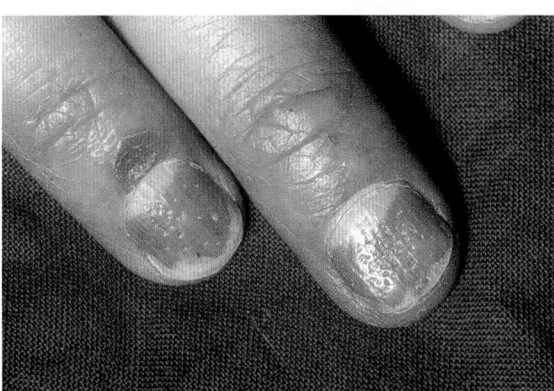

FIGURE 249-7. Nail pitting in psoriasis. The pits are more discrete and regular compared with pits affecting the nail plate in dermatitis.

are strongly associated with nail dystrophy, of which the features are onycholysis, subungual keratosis, pitting, and oil drop–like staining (Fig. 249-7). The third subset (15 to 30% of patients) has a symmetrical polyarthritis that mimics rheumatoid arthritis in many ways, except for the absence of rheumatoid nodules and rheumatoid factor. The fourth clinical variant is psoriatic spondylitis, which occurs in 20% of patients; 50% of such patients are B27 positive. Finally, arthritis mutilans (5% of patients) is a destructive, erosive arthritis that affects large and small joints and can be associated with marked deformities and significant disability.

Radiographic changes in psoriatic arthritis involve soft tissue swelling (particularly in the case of dactylitis), erosions, and periostitis. Axial involvement may lead to the appearance of asymmetrical sacroiliitis with syndesmophytes that are bulky, asymmetrical, and nonmarginal. The classic "pencil-in-cup" deformity may be seen in patients with distal interphalangeal joint disease or arthritis mutilans. Acro-osteolysis is noted in a minority of patients and reflects an aggressive erosive process.

Differential Diagnosis

The diagnosis of psoriatic arthritis depends on finding the typical skin or nail changes in association with one of the articular variants described previously. The differential diagnosis for the skin lesions can include seborrheic dermatitis, dyshidrotic eczema, fungal infection, keratoderma blennorrhagicum, and palmoplantar pustulosis.

Undifferentiated Spondyloarthritis

Despite careful clinical and radiographic assessment, there are still a substantial number of patients who do not fall into one of the classic diagnostic subsets of spondyloarthritis outlined previously. These patients are often defined as having undifferentiated spondyloarthritis with peripheral enthesitis, asymmetrical arthritis or sacroiliitis, or iritis in the absence of identifiable antecedent infection or concurrent inflammatory bowel disease or psoriasis. The natural history of undifferentiated spondyloarthritis has not been well defined, and case heterogeneity and diagnostic dilemmas plague a systematic or multicenter approach to the problem. When the clinical course is examined, a number of patients may finally meet the diagnostic criteria for ankylosing spondylitis, but many retain a distinct undifferentiated spondyloarthritis pattern for prolonged periods.

TREATMENT   Rx

General Measures

Spondyloarthritis necessitates a global approach to management in which education of patients is the cornerstone.[11] Because the typical onset is during young adulthood, these patients may experience significant frustration or depression if their acute arthritis evolves into a chronic disease that significantly impairs their functional capabilities and quality of life. A clinician managing patients with spondyloarthritis should be aware that these psychosocial aspects are an important part of the burden of illness. Similarly, there may be important implications for the workplace, particularly if a job demands significant bending or twisting. It is important to include the mechanical demands of the workplace in the global assessment of patients with spondyloarthritis.

Exercise is an important part of the treatment plan for patients with ankylosing spondylitis.[12] Generally, high-impact sports should be avoided, whereas swimming is an ideal exercise. Stretching to maintain mobility and maintenance of posture should be emphasized, and an experienced physiotherapist can greatly assist in instructing patients in daily exercises. Long car trips and air travel should include periodic stretching. Sleep position should emphasize a straight back position rather than one curled on the side. Deep breathing exercises and avoidance of smoking should be stressed.

One key area of concern for patients is prognosis, because spondyloarthritis, particularly reactive arthritis, often occurs in young, active individuals for whom athletic activity is a priority. There is general recognition that reactive arthritis has a greater propensity for chronicity than was previously appreciated, and this should temper an overly optimistic projection of the disease's natural history. At the 5-year follow-up of a cohort of patients with *Salmonella*-induced reactive arthritis, two thirds continued to have subjective complaints, and one third demonstrated objective changes in their joints. The variability in prognosis for the large group of patients falling into the undifferentiated spondyloarthritis group is perplexing. At present, there is a lack of reliable predictors of progression in patients with this heterogeneous cluster of articular and extra-articular features.

Medical Therapies

Nonsteroidal Anti-inflammatory Drugs

In general, joint inflammation in spondyloarthritis improves significantly after the introduction of nonsteroidal anti-inflammatory drugs (NSAIDs). Indomethacin and diclofenac (up to 150 mg/day in divided doses) or naproxen (up to 1000 mg/day in divided doses) are generally well tolerated in this population.[A1] These agents have to be used with caution in enteropathic arthritis because of concern about exacerbating possible underlying inflammatory bowel disease. In the case of ankylosing spondylitis, the goal with anti-inflammatory treatment is to achieve sufficient relief of pain and stiffness to allow an active, sustained program of exercise and physical activity that maintains posture and improves quality of life. Some studies have suggested that NSAIDs have disease-modifying capability, but this effect appears to be restricted to those patients with elevated C-reactive protein (CRP) or erythrocyte sedimentation rate (ESR).

Biologic Therapies

The pathogenic role of immunomodulatory cytokines in the pathogenesis of spondyloarthritis has remained unresolved, but the advent of biologic agents has changed the landscape for spondyloarthritis. Biologic agents such as monoclonal antibodies to TNF-α (infliximab, adalimumab, golimumab, and certolizumab) or the soluble TNF receptor (etanercept) have been used in the treatment of spondyloarthritis. So far, these five anti-TNF agents have been comparably effective in trials of ankylosing spondylitis and psoriatic arthritis.[A2] These studies have generally reported a prompt response in clinical outcome measures and in laboratory indicators of inflammation, and MRI evaluations have shown improvement in local inflammation in the sacroiliac joints and spine. The anti-TNF treatments have been well tolerated, with no significant incidence of serious adverse events, but patients appear to relapse when treatment is discontinued. In patients whose active nonradiographic axial spondyloarthritis went into sustained remission with adalimumab, continued therapy reduces subsequent flares compared with withdrawing treatment.[A3] Experience with longer-term treatment with anti-TNF agents has been encouraging with regard to the persistence of the therapeutic effect and the infrequency of late adverse events.[A4] These biologic agents also have been shown to retard radiographic progression.[13] Other potential FDA-approved alternatives for ankylosing spondylitis include the interleukin-17A inhibitors secukinumab (given intravenously 10 mg/kg at weeks 0, 2, and 4, followed by 150 mg or 75 mg subcutaneously every 4 weeks starting at week 8) and ixekizumab (80 mg subcutaneously every 2 or 4 weeks), each of which significantly reduces the signs of ankylosing spondylitis.[A5][A6] Filgotinib (an oral Janus kinase inhibitor, given as 200 mg daily for 12 weeks) is a promising potential option.[A7]

Corticosteroids

The response to the intra-articular injection of steroids in the peripheral joints of patients with spondyloarthritis is often neither as dramatic nor as sustained as in those with rheumatoid arthritis. Corticosteroid injection into the sacroiliac joints is usually performed under imaging guidance (fluoroscopy or computed tomography [CT]). One study found that such injections resulted in a good response in 79% of patients and that the improvement could persist for many months. Systemic corticosteroids (either orally or via an intravenous bolus protocol) are not generally recommended but have been used for severe symptomatic flares, despite few controlled trials to validate their effectiveness. The goal should be prompt tapering of the dose when symptomatic control is achieved. The recognition that osteoporosis (Chapter 230) is a significant problem in ankylosing spondylitis provides further impetus to use corticosteroids sparingly. Topical steroids are usually effective for the treatment of the mucous membrane and skin manifestations of reactive arthritis. For uveitis, topical corticosteroid eye drops are an integral component of management, and treatment should be monitored jointly with an ophthalmologist.[14]

Drugs

Sulfasalazine

Randomized placebo-controlled trials have provided some support for the use of sulfasalazine, mostly in psoriatic arthritis. Three 36-week randomized double-blind multicenter studies of patients with ankylosing spondylitis, psoriatic arthritis, and reactive arthritis, respectively, were undertaken to compare sulfasalazine (2 g/day) with placebo in each case. An analysis of these studies stratified the patients into those having axial disease and those having peripheral disease. In patients with only axial disease, response criteria were met equally in the sulfasalazine group and the placebo group. In patients with peripheral arthritis, significantly superior responses were seen with sulfasalazine: 59% of the sulfasalazine group and 43% of the placebo group responded ($P < .0005$).[A8] These findings are useful in guiding the selection of patients for sulfasalazine treatment. A recent study comparing sulfasalazine with etanercept in ankylosing spondylitis demonstrated the superiority of tumor necrosis factor (TNF) inhibitor therapy with respect to symptomatic improvement as well as MRI evidence of inflammation.

Methotrexate

Concurrent with the widespread use of methotrexate in patients with rheumatoid arthritis, there has been increasing use of methotrexate in patients with spondyloarthritis, but responses have been good only for peripheral joint disease. There is no evidence that methotrexate is effective for the spinal inflammation characteristic of ankylosing spondylitis, nor is there evidence that methotrexate changes the course of axial involvement in ankylosing spondylitis. Experience with long-term methotrexate therapy in patients with psoriatic arthritis has increased, although there has been little in the way of randomized controlled trials. Long-term follow-up may be required to resolve whether methotrexate has a joint-sparing effect in psoriatic arthritis.

Antibiotic Therapy

The current concept of the pathogenesis of reactive arthritis postulates that a bacterial infection, usually gastrointestinal (GI) or genitourinary (GU), is the triggering event in an immunogenetically susceptible host. For the other subsets of spondyloarthritis, there is less compelling evidence that infection plays a causal role. It is sound clinical practice to treat any culture-proven chlamydial urethritis in conjunction with treatment of the sexual partner. For this indication, a single 1-g dose of azithromycin is as effective as doxycycline 100 mg twice a day for 7 days. The role of antibiotics in the management of reactive arthritis has been controversial in reactive arthritis,[A9] but rifampin/azithromycin or rifampin/doxycycline therapy may be useful for *Chlamydia*-induced reactive arthritis.[A10]

● APPROACH TO SPECIFIC SPONDYLOARTHROPATHIES

Ankylosing Spondylitis

Consensus guidelines from the American College of Rheumatology/Spondylitis Association of America/Spondyloarthritis Research and Treatment Network can help guide medical therapy (Table 249-5).[15]

Psoriatic Arthritis

Patients typically receive aggressive treatment for psoriasis (Chapter 409), and tight control of inflammation significantly improves outcomes.[A11] The advent of biologic agents has had a major impact on the treatment of psoriatic arthritis. The anti-TNF agents have been studied most extensively, indicating the efficacy of infliximab, etanercept, adalimumab, and golimumab.[16] For example, treatment of psoriatic arthritis with subcutaneous golimumab (50 mg to 100 mg every 4 weeks) inhibits the progression of structural damage, with continued clinical efficacy and safety through 1 year.[A12]

Other FDA-approved biologic agents can also be efficacious. Ustekinumab (a monoclonal antibody against interleukin-12/23) is safe, well tolerated, and reduces the extent and severity of psoriasis, as is guselkumab (a monoclonal antibody against the P19 subunit of interleukin-23, given as 100 mg subcutaneously at weeks 0 and 4, 12, 20, and 28, and then every 8 weeks).[A13] Brodalumab, a human monoclonal antibody against interleukin-17 receptor A (IL17RA), significantly improves response rates among patients with psoriatic arthritis.[A14] Secukinumab (10 mg/kg intravenously at weeks 0, 2, and 4, followed by either 150 mg or 75 mg subcutaneously every 4 weeks)[A15] is another alternative. In patients whose psoriatic arthritis has responded inadequately to TNF inhibitors, tofacitinib (an oral Janus kinase inhibitor at 5 mg or 10 mg twice daily) is more effective than placebo over 3 months for reducing disease activity.[A16] Filgotinib (a Janus kinase inhibitor at 200 mg orally daily for 16 weeks) is a potential future option.[A17]

TABLE 249-5 TREATMENT RECOMMENDATIONS FOR THE SPONDYLOARTHROPATHIES

Nonsteroidal anti-inflammatory drugs (NSAIDs) on demand (and chronically only if needed)

If inadequate response to trials of two different NSAIDs, add a tumor necrosis factor (TNF)-α inhibitor and try to discontinue NSAIDs if the response is good; options are:
etancercept (50 mg subcutaneously once weekly)
infliximab* (5 mg/kg intravenously at 0, 2, and 6 weeks, then every 6 or 8 weeks[†])
adalimumab* (40 mg subcutaneously every other week)
golimumab* (50 mg subcutaneously once a month)
certolizumab (400 mg subcutaneously initially and at 2 and 4 weeks, followed by 200 mg every other week or 400 mg every 4 weeks)

If no response to trials of two different TNF-α inhibitors or contraindication to using them, add a slow-acting anti-rheumatic drug
sulfasalazine (2 to 3 g orally daily in evenly divided doses with dosage intervals not exceeding 8 hours) or
methotrexate (10 to 25 mg once weekly) for psoriatic arthritis and enteropathic arthritis

Short-term treatment with locally injected corticosteroids is useful, but systemic corticosteroids are not recommended

*Preferred over etanercept in patients with inflammatory bowel disease.
[†]6 weeks for ankylosing spondylitis; 8 weeks for psoriatic arthritis.
Adapted from Ward MM, Deodhar A, Akl EA, et al. American College of Rheumatology/Spondylitis Association of America/Spondyloarthritis Research and Treatment Network 2015 recommendations for the treatment of ankylosing spondylitis and nonradiographic axial spondyloarthritis. *Arthritis Rheumatol*. 2016;68:282-298.

As a general approach, nonsteroidal anti-inflammatory drugs are recommended to relieve musculoskeletal signs and symptoms. Treatment with disease-modifying drugs—such as methotrexate, sulfasalazine, or leflunomide—is recommended in patients with swollen joints, structural damage in the presence of inflammation, or clinically relevant extra-articular manifestations. Anti-TNF agents are recommended in patients with active enthesitis or dactylitis and insufficient response to other medications. Patients should be switched to another anti-TNF agent if the first is not successful. Interleukin-17 receptor antibodies and other newer agents currently are usually reserved for otherwise poorly responsive patients.

Reactive Arthritis

The treatment of reactive arthritis begins with therapy of the triggering infection. For example, in patients who are PCR-positive either in blood or joint fluid for *C. trachomatis* or *C. pneumonia*, a 6-month course of combination therapy with rifampicin (300 mg/day) plus either doxycycline (200 mg/day) or azithromycin (500 mg/day followed by 5 days of 2 to 500 mg once a week) yields a response in 63% of patients (versus 22% with placebo), and complete remission is observed in 20% (versus 0% with placebo). For spondyloarthritis, NSAIDs and glucocorticoid injections are effective. In more severe cases, sulfasalazine is often effective if started in the first three months. Biologic therapies are often used in chronic HLA-B27 positive spondyloarthritis, although their efficacy is unproven, especially since about 50% of patients recover within about six months.

Enteropathic Arthritis

For enteropathic arthritis, sulfasalazine is more helpful in ulcerative colitis than in Crohn disease (Chapter 132), whereas the opposite is generally true for methotrexate. TNF-α inhibitors (see Table 249-5) are effective in spondyloarthritis related to both ulcerative colitis and Crohn disease.[17] A multidisciplinary approach has been shown to improve the management of rheumatic disease in patients with inflammatory bowel disease, allowing more comprehensive care.[18]

Grade A References

A1. Kroon FP, van der Burg LR, Ramiro S, et al. Non-steroidal anti-inflammatory drugs (NSAIDs) for axial spondyloarthritis (ankylosing spondylitis and non-radiographic axial spondyloarthritis). *Cochrane Database Syst Rev*. 2015;7:CD010952.
A2. Maxwell LJ, Zochling J, Boonen A, et al. TNF-alpha inhibitors for ankylosing spondylitis. *Cochrane Database Syst Rev*. 2015;4:CD005468.
A3. Landewé R, Sieper J, Mease P, et al. Efficacy and safety of continuing versus withdrawing adalimumab therapy in maintaining remission in patients with non-radiographic axial spondyloarthritis (ABILITY-3): a multicentre, randomised, double-blind study. *Lancet*. 2018;392:134-144.
A4. Song IH, Hermann KG, Haibel H, et al. Consistently good clinical response in patients with early axial spondyloarthritis after 3 years of continuous treatment with etanercept: longterm data of the ESTHER trial. *J Rheumatol*. 2014;41:2034-2040.
A5. Baeten D, Sieper J, Braun J, et al. Secukinumab, an interleukin-17A inhibitor, in ankylosing spondylitis. *N Engl J Med*. 2015;373:2534-2548.
A6. van der Heijde D, Cheng-Chung Wei J, Dougados M, et al. Ixekizumab, an interleukin-17A antagonist in the treatment of ankylosing spondylitis or radiographic axial spondyloarthritis in patients previously untreated with biological disease-modifying anti-rheumatic drugs (COAST-V): 16 week results of a phase 3 randomised, double-blind, active-controlled and placebo-controlled trial. *Lancet*. 2018;392:2441-2451.
A7. van der Heijde D, Baraliakos X, Gensler LS, et al. Efficacy and safety of filgotinib, a selective Janus kinase 1 inhibitor, in patients with active ankylosing spondylitis (TORTUGA): results from a randomised, placebo-controlled, phase 2 trial. *Lancet*. 2018;392:2378-2387.
A8. Braun J, van der Horst-Bruinsma IE, Huang F, et al. Clinical efficacy and safety of etanercept versus sulfasalazine in patients with ankylosing spondylitis: a randomized, double-blind trial. *Arthritis Rheum*. 2011;63:1543-1551.
A9. Barber CE, Kim J, Inman RD, et al. Antibiotics for treatment of reactive arthritis: a systematic review and metaanalysis. *J Rheumatol*. 2013;40:916-928.
A10. Carter JD, Espinoza LR, Inman RD, et al. Combination antibiotics as a treatment for chronic *Chlamydia*-induced reactive arthritis: a double-blind, placebo-controlled, prospective trial. *Arthritis Rheum*. 2010;62:1298-1307.
A11. Coates LC, Moverley AR, McParland L, et al. Effect of tight control of inflammation in early psoriatic arthritis (TICOPA): a UK multicentre, open-label, randomised controlled trial. *Lancet*. 2015;386:2489-2498.
A12. Kavanaugh A, van der Heijde D, McInnes IB, et al. Golimumab in psoriatic arthritis: one-year clinical efficacy, radiographic, and safety results from a phase III, randomized, placebo-controlled trial. *Arthritis Rheum*. 2012;64:2504-2517.
A13. Deodhar A, Gottlieb AB, Boehncke WH, et al. Efficacy and safety of guselkumab in patients with active psoriatic arthritis: a randomised, double-blind, placebo-controlled, phase 2 study. *Lancet*. 2018;391:2213-2224.
A14. Mease PJ, Genovese MC, Greenwald MW, et al. Brodalumab, an anti-IL17RA monoclonal antibody, in psoriatic arthritis. *N Engl J Med*. 2014;370:2295-2306.
A15. Mease PJ, McInnes IB, Kirkham B, et al. Secukinumab inhibition of interleukin-17A in patients with psoriatic arthritis. *N Engl J Med*. 2015;373:1329-1339.
A16. Gladman D, Rigby W, Azevedo VF, et al. Tofacitinib for psoriatic arthritis in patients with an inadequate response to TNF inhibitors. *N Engl J Med*. 2017;377:1525-1536.
A17. Mease P, Coates LC, Helliwell PS, et al. Efficacy and safety of filgotinib, a selective janus kinase 1 inhibitor, in patients with active psoriatic arthritis (EQUATOR): results from a randomised, placebo-controlled, phase 2 trial. *Lancet*. 2018;392:2367-2377.

GENERAL REFERENCES

For the General References and other additional features, please visit Expert Consult at https://expertconsult.inkling.com.

250

SYSTEMIC LUPUS ERYTHEMATOSUS

MARY K. CROW

DEFINITION

Systemic lupus erythematosus (SLE) is a multisystem autoimmune disease that results from immune system–mediated tissue damage. Manifestations of SLE can involve the skin, joints, kidney, central nervous system (CNS), cardiovascular system, serosal membranes, and hematologic and immune systems. The disease is highly heterogeneous, with individual patients manifesting variable combinations of clinical features. In most patients with SLE, the disease is characterized by a waxing and waning clinical course, although some demonstrate a pattern of chronic activity. The molecular triggers of the disease are not known, but the pathogenesis involves the production of autoantibodies specific for nucleic acids and nucleic acid–binding proteins. Immune complexes, along with immune system cells and soluble mediators, generate inflammation and tissue damage. Therapeutic approaches generally involve immunosuppression, although promising biologic agents targeting specific molecular mechanisms are in development.

EPIDEMIOLOGY

A notable feature of SLE is that it occurs much more frequently in females than in males. Like Hashimoto thyroiditis and Sjögren syndrome, the female-to-male ratio is approximately 8 : 1 to 10 : 1 in adults, and most cases are diagnosed between the ages of 15 and 44 years. In children and women older than

55 years, the ratio is closer to 2 : 1. The prevalence of SLE in the United States is estimated to be approximately 62.2 to 84.8 per 100,000, and the incidence of new cases is 4.6 to 5.6 per 100,000 per year.[1,2] The prevalence, severity, and characteristics of disease differ in different ethnic groups, with SLE being three- to four-fold more prevalent in African American and American Indian women than in white women.[3] The severity of disease is also greater in Hispanic individuals than in whites, although data for Hispanic populations are less abundant.[4] Asians may also have a higher prevalence of disease than whites. Studies of lupus in minority populations indicate that socioeconomic factors are major contributors to the increased prevalence and severity of disease in African Americans and Hispanic Americans.

PATHOBIOLOGY

Current understanding of lupus pathogenesis incorporates roles for genetic susceptibility based on a cumulative hit model involving multiple genes[5]; environmental triggers, including microbial infection, sunlight, and certain drugs; and altered immune system function. Recent advances in immunology have focused attention on the mechanisms that account for innate immune system activation.[6] At least some of the genetic and environmental contributions to lupus are likely to promote innate immune system activation and subsequent autoimmunity. Others may contribute to inflammation and tissue damage. Induction of cellular stress responses, including oxidative modification of cell proteins, is of current interest as a mechanism that links environmental triggers to altered immune function.

Murine models have proved useful in identifying genes that could contribute to lupus susceptibility or define patterns of disease. Production of autoantibodies characteristic of SLE and development of nephritis and accelerated death have been demonstrated in numerous murine strains in which immune system genes have been modified. In most cases, no alterations have been noted in the homologous human genes. The ease of induction of lupus-like disease in murine models suggests that there are numerous possible pathogenic paths that might lead to the clinical manifestations of the disease. One prominent immune mechanism involves components of the immune response to viral infection, particularly the type I interferon response, that are associated with lupus in both murine and human systems and are likely to be important in disease pathogenesis.[7]

Genetics

An important role for a genetic contribution to lupus susceptibility is suggested by the high concordance of disease in monozygotic twins (24%). Rare mutations in genes encoding components of the complement pathway, including C1q, C2, and C4A, contribute to increased lupus susceptibility or severity. Impaired production of these early complement components may decrease the clearance of apoptotic cells, thereby augmenting the pool of available autoantigens, or decrease the solubility of immune complexes. Association of SLE with the major histocompatibility complex (MHC) class II alleles human leukocyte antigen (HLA)-DR3 (DRB1*03:01-DQA1*05:01-DQB1*02:01) and HLA-DR15 (DRB1*15:01/03-DQA1*01:02-DQB1*06:01) shows the strongest risk, and these class II alleles are associated with the production of particular autoantibodies. A large transancestral genome-wide association study (GWAS) of subjects of European, African, and Hispanic Amerindian ancestry has identified 80 non-HLA single-nucleotide polymorphisms associated with SLE at a false discovery rate P value < .001 in a meta-analysis. Some associations at a high level of significance were related to ancestry (E-Table 250-1).[8,9] Polymorphic variants in components of the toll-like receptor (TLR) pathways that regulate type I interferon production, including interferon regulatory factor 5 (IRF5) and IRF7, are associated with a diagnosis of SLE and increased plasma interferon activity in some populations. Polymorphisms in the Fc receptor genes FCGR2A and FCGR3A have been associated with SLE nephritis, possibly based on altered clearance of immune complexes. Variants of the PTPN22 gene, which encodes a phosphatase that regulates T-cell activation, are also associated with SLE. GWASs have identified variations in regulators of innate immune system activation (e.g., TNFAIP3, ITGAM, IFIH1) and signaling molecules important in lymphocyte activation (e.g., STAT4, BANK1, and BLK). Rare mutations in genes encoding proteins that regulate nucleic acid integrity and degradation, including TREX1, encoding a DNase; SAMHD1, a triphosphohydrolase; RNASEH2A, B and C; and ADAR, an RNA-specific adenosine deaminase, have been documented in some patients with a lupus-like disorder called Aicardi-Goutieres syndrome, characterized by skin lesions, CNS disease, autoantibodies, and high levels of interferon.[10] Mutations in these genes have also been documented in rare patients with SLE and have provided new insights into the likely contribution of endogenous

nucleic acids to innate immune system activation and lupus pathogenesis.[11] The available data suggest a common theme: the genes associated with lupus confer either increased activation or impaired regulation of innate or adaptive immune responses, with increased type I interferon often observed in association with the risk genotype.

Environmental Triggers

Several classes of potential environmental triggers for lupus have been studied.[12] Although the female preponderance of SLE implies a role for hormonal factors in the disease, recent concepts describe a contribution of epigenetic modification or dosage effects of the X chromosome as accounting for at least some of the sex skewing. A role for microbial triggers—particularly virus infection—has been postulated, consistent with the constitutional symptoms that often characterize the earliest stage of the disease. Epstein-Barr virus has garnered particular interest among investigators because the frequency of previous infection in SLE patients is significantly higher than in the general population (99 vs. 94%). Evidence of exposure to other viruses, including cytomegalovirus, is equivalent between SLE patients and healthy control subjects. Recent data implicate orthologs of human Ro60, a common target of lupus autoantibodies, in commensal bacteria and demonstrate cross-reactivity of human Ro-specific T-cell clones with bacteria-derived Ro60.[13] Ultraviolet light exposure is a well-described trigger of lupus flares. Possible mechanisms include DNA damage, induction of cellular stress responses, and induction of apoptosis of skin cells, which result in concentration of nucleic acids and associated proteins in cell membrane blebs that can be processed by antigen-presenting cells. Data also support an association between current tobacco use and anti-double-stranded DNA antibodies and lupus disease activity. Certain drugs, including procainamide and hydralazine, can induce a lupus-like syndrome, but the symptoms usually abate after discontinuing use of the drug. These agents may promote demethylation of DNA, thereby altering gene expression and potentially increasing the availability of immunostimulatory DNA. Sulfa antibiotics have been reported to induce lupus flare in some patients. Administration of recombinant interferon-α to patients with hematologic malignancies or hepatitis C infection has been associated with induction of a lupus-like syndrome. In addition, anti–tumor necrosis factor agents have induced lupus autoantibodies and occasionally clinical lupus in patients with rheumatoid arthritis.

Immunologic Triggers

Genetic and environmental factors that increase the probability of development of SLE are likely to act on the immune system to induce autoimmunity and consequent tissue inflammation and damage.[14] In addition to mechanisms that increase the availability of self-antigens (such as ultraviolet light), altered expression of gene products that mediate or regulate apoptosis, or impaired clearance of apoptotic debris, results in generalized activation of the immune system and contributes to autoimmunity in lupus. In parallel with the events that account for effective immune responses directed at exogenous microbes, the autoimmunity that occurs in SLE patients is likely to require activation of both innate and adaptive immune responses. The innate immune system (Chapter 39) recognizes common molecular patterns expressed on the microbe and augments antigen-presenting cell capacity and successful generation of an antigen-specific adaptive immune response. The characterization of the TLR family of pattern recognition receptors has provided new understanding of the mechanisms through which the innate immune system is activated by exogenous and endogenous stimuli, including nucleic acid–containing immune complexes, and promotes induction of a self-directed adaptive immune response (Chapter 40).

Type I Interferon

Studies of gene expression in peripheral blood mononuclear cells of SLE patients using microarray and RNA sequencing technology have demonstrated a sustained and broad "signature" of type I interferon–induced gene transcripts that reflect innate immune system activation. Interferon-α (IFN-α), along with other type I IFNs (e.g., IFN-β, IFN-ω) may be responsible for many of the immunologic alterations observed in SLE and is identified as a promising therapeutic target. Immune complexes containing DNA or RNA are postulated to induce the production of type I interferon in SLE. Demethylated CpG-rich DNA or RNA associated with nucleic acid–binding proteins can activate plasmacytoid dendritic cells and other immune system cells through TLRs and thereby result in the production of type I interferon (IFN-α or IFN-β) and other proinflammatory cytokines (E-Fig. 250-1). Sensing of intracellular RNA or DNA by cytosolic nucleic acid sensors represents another potential molecular pathway leading to type I interferon production. Diverse effects of type I interferon on immune system function are consistent with the altered immune responses observed in SLE patients, including maturation of dendritic cells, increased immunoglobulin class switching to mature immunoglobulin isotypes (immunoglobulin G [IgG] and IgA), induction of soluble mediators that increase B-cell differentiation and inflammatory responses, such as B-lymphocyte stimulator (BLyS) and IFN-γ, and modulation of effector T-cell programs. Induction of an immunostimulatory microenvironment by IFN-α may support the development of a humoral immune response directed at self-antigens, particularly intracellular particles that contain nucleic acids and nucleic acid–binding proteins. It is not known why some individuals initiate immune system activation directed at self-antigens and others do not. In addition to its effects on immune system function, type I interferon has been associated with altered endothelial cell function and microglial function in the brain and may contribute to the development of atherosclerotic vascular pathology and CNS disease in patients with lupus.[15,16]

Autoantibodies

The most characteristic lupus autoantibodies target intracellular particles containing both nucleic acid and nucleic acid–binding proteins. Understanding the significance of induction of these particular autoantibody specificities may provide clues to the etiology of SLE. An analysis of the spectrum of autoantibodies present in the sera of individuals in whom SLE is later diagnosed has suggested that autoantibodies reactive with certain RNA-binding proteins, including the Ro protein, occur early in the preclinical stage of the disease, along with a positive antinuclear antibody (ANA) test. These are often followed by anti-double-stranded DNA antibodies and, finally, by the development of antibodies specific for the spliceosomal proteins Smith (Sm) and ribonucleoprotein (RNP) at approximately the time of diagnosis (Fig. 250-1). These observations suggest that individuals who demonstrate progression from antibodies targeting RNA to those targeting DNA and spliceosomal proteins are those in whom sufficient autoimmunity develops to manifest clinical symptoms. Approximately one third of SLE patients have autoantibodies reactive with phospholipids or the proteins associated with them, particularly β$_2$-glycoprotein I. These autoantibody specificities can also be present independently of SLE in primary antiphospholipid antibody syndrome (Chapter 162).

Immune Complexes and Complement

Tissue and organ damage in SLE is mediated by the deposition or in situ formation of immune complexes and subsequent complement activation and inflammation. The complement system (Chapter 44), composed of more than 30 proteins that act in concert to protect the host against invading organisms, initiates inflammation and tissue injury. Complement activation promotes chemotaxis of inflammatory cells and generates proteolytic fragments that enhance phagocytosis by neutrophils and monocytes. The classical complement pathway is activated when antibodies bind to antigen and generate potent effectors. Alternative pathway activation mechanisms differ in that they are initiated by the binding of spontaneously activated complement components to the surfaces of pathogens or self-tissues. C3a, an anaphylatoxin that binds to receptors on leukocytes and other cells, causes activation and release of inflammatory mediators. C5a is a potent soluble inflammatory, anaphylatoxic, and chemotactic molecule that promotes recruitment and activation of neutrophils and monocytes and mediates endothelial cell activation through its receptor. The release of reactive oxygen and nitrogen intermediates is an additional mechanism that contributes to tissue damage.

Tissues targeted by immune system activity in lupus include the skin, where immune complexes and complement are deposited in a linear pattern (as demonstrated in the lupus band test, in which deposited antibodies are identified by a fluorescent tag), the glomeruli, and heart valves. Antibodies reactive with hippocampal neurons in the brain can mediate excitotoxic death. Immune and inflammatory mechanisms responsible for the vasculopathy of lupus are multifactorial and not clearly defined. Microvascular damage is observed in splenic arteries and is characterized by the typical onion-skin pattern of concentric connective tissue deposition. In addition to vascular damage mediated by inflammation, thrombosis, including microthrombi, contributes to ischemia and cell necrosis in the brain and other organs.

CLINICAL MANIFESTATIONS

Symptoms and Signs

Constitutional Symptoms

SLE is a disease that involves virtually all components of the immune system and can be accompanied by constitutional symptoms similar to those seen in the setting of microbial infection. Fatigue, headaches, weight loss, and fevers are common, along with generalized arthralgias, myalgias, and lymphadenopathy. The level of activity of lupus typically follows a pattern of flares and remissions, although some patients sustain active disease for prolonged periods. Careful monitoring for the development of major organ system disease is important to ensure timely adjustments in medical therapy.

Cutaneous and Mucous Membranes

The skin and mucous membranes are affected in most lupus patients (Table 250-1). The erythematous facial rash with a butterfly distribution across the malar and nasal prominences and sparing of the nasolabial folds is the classic rash of SLE and is seen in 30 to 60% of patients (Fig. 250-2). The butterfly rash is often triggered by sun exposure, but photosensitivity can also be demonstrated diffusely in other areas of the body.

The discoid skin lesions are erythematous plaques with central scarring and may be covered with scale. These lesions are seen in about 25% of patients,

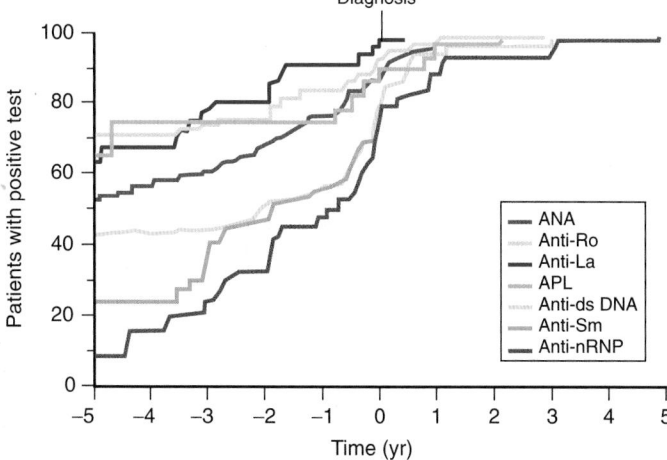

FIGURE 250-1. Proportion of patients with positive antibody tests relative to the time of diagnosis or appearance of the first clinical manifestation of systemic lupus erythematosus (SLE). For each autoantibody, the proportion of patients testing positive relative to the time of diagnosis or to the time of appearance of the first clinical criterion was assessed. In analyses of the time from antibody development to the diagnosis of SLE, antinuclear antibodies (ANAs) appeared significantly earlier than anti-Sm antibodies and antinuclear ribonucleoprotein (anti-nRNP) antibodies, but not significantly earlier than anti-Ro, anti-La, antiphospholipid (APL), or anti-double-stranded DNA antibodies (anti-ds DNA). (From Arbuckle MR, McClain MT, Rubertone MV, et al. Development of autoantibodies before the clinical onset of systemic lupus erythematosus. *N Engl J Med.* 2003;349:16.)

TABLE 250-1	CLINICAL MANIFESTATIONS OF SYSTEMIC LUPUS ERYTHEMATOSUS
MANIFESTATION	**APPROXIMATE FREQUENCY (%)**
Cutaneous	88
Arthritis/arthralgias	76
Neuropsychiatric	66
Pleurisy/pericarditis	63
Anemia	57
Raynaud phenomenon	44
Vasculitis	43
Atherosclerosis	37
Nephritis	31
Thrombocytopenia	30
Sensorimotor neuropathy	28
Cardiac valvar disease	18
Pulmonary alveolar hemorrhage	12
Pancreatitis	10
Myositis	5
Myocarditis	5

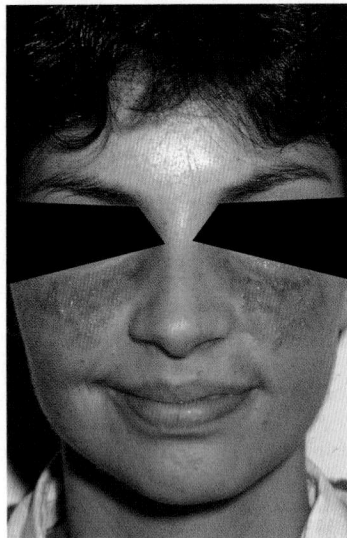

FIGURE 250-2. Malar rash in a patient with systemic lupus erythematosus. Note that the rash does not cross the nasolabial fold. (From Gladman DD, Urowitz MB. Systemic lupus erythematosus: clinical features. In: Klippel JH, Dieppe PA, eds. *Rheumatology*. 2nd ed. London: Mosby; 1998.)

involve the scalp or the face and ears, and may be associated with alopecia. Discoid lesions can be present in the absence of systemic manifestations of SLE (discoid lupus). In addition to the scarring alopecia of discoid lupus, more transient alopecia may be a clinical sign of increased disease activity and is associated with apoptosis of cells in the hair follicle.

Inflammation of the deep dermis and subcutaneous fat can result in lupus panniculitis, with firm painful nodules that sometimes adhere to the epidermis, causing irregularities in the superficial skin. Subacute cutaneous lupus erythematosus is seen in sun-exposed areas and can involve erythematous plaques or psoriasiform lesions. It is associated with autoantibodies to the Ro (SSA) RNA-binding protein. Mucosal ulcerations, especially of the buccal mucosa and upper palate, result from mucositis and are typical of SLE. Manifestations of vasculopathy are also common in SLE, including arteriolar spasm or infarcts in the nail folds, a diffuse lacey pattern over the skin described as livedo reticularis, and petechial-purpuric or urticarial lesions on the extremities. Vasculopathy in SLE is often associated with the presence of antiphospholipid antibodies.

Musculoskeletal System

Arthralgias and nonerosive arthritis are among the most common clinical features of SLE and are experienced by more than 85% of patients. The proximal interphalangeal and metacarpophalangeal joints of the hand are most commonly symptomatic, along with the knees and wrists. In some patients ($\approx$10%), deformities resulting from damage to periarticular tissue can occur, a condition termed *Jaccoud arthropathy*. The heavy use of corticosteroids in many lupus patients can be accompanied by the development of osteoporosis, including osteoporotic fractures or osteonecrosis, most commonly of the hips, although the underlying vasculopathy can also contribute to joint damage.

Inflammation of the muscles with elevated creatine phosphokinase can occur rarely in SLE, and myopathy may be observed as a consequence of corticosteroid therapy. Fibromyalgia, characterized by painful trigger points at characteristic locations, commonly accompanies SLE and can contribute to fatigue and depression.

Renal System

Kidney involvement in SLE (Chapter 113) is common, with 74% of patients being affected at some time in the course of disease, and is a poor prognostic indicator. Renal pathology is generally attributed to the deposition of circulating immune complexes or in situ formation of these complexes in glomeruli and results in the activation of complement and subsequent recruitment of inflammatory cells. In addition to glomerular inflammation, necrosis, and scarring, renal pathology is characterized by vascular lesions, including thrombotic microangiopathy and extraglomerular vasculitis. Tubulointerstitial disease, including infiltration of the interstitium with mononuclear cells, tubular atrophy, and interstitial fibrosis, is increasingly recognized as associated with a poor prognosis for persistent nephritis and renal survival.[17] Hypertension may be a consequence of significant renal involvement.

Most cases of lupus nephritis present a complex immunopathologic picture, but in general, the pattern of renal disease reflects the site of deposition of immunoglobulins and the quality of the effector mechanisms they induce. Mesangial deposition of immunoglobulin induces mesangial cell proliferation and is associated with microscopic hematuria and mild proteinuria (Fig. 250-3). Subendothelial deposition of immune complexes results in proliferative and exudative inflammation, together with hematuria, mild to moderate proteinuria, and reduced glomerular filtration rate. Subepithelial deposition of immune complexes adjacent to podocytes and along the glomerular basement membrane can result in membranous nephritis with nephrotic-range proteinuria. In addition, antiphospholipid antibodies may support the development of thrombotic or inflammatory vascular lesions within or external to glomeruli.

A World Health Organization classification of lupus nephritis lesions was first published in 1975, with subsequent revisions. These classifications were reviewed and rigorously reexamined in the revised International Society of Nephrology and Renal Pathology Society classification criteria for lupus glomerulonephritis (GN) published in 2004, with additional review in 2018.[18] (Table 113-7 in Chapter 113, and also E-Table 250-2). Class I and II GN involves mesangial deposition of immune complexes (class I without and class II with mesangial hypercellularity); class III describes focal GN involving less than 50% of total glomeruli; class IV includes diffuse GN involving 50% or more of glomeruli; class V designates membranous lupus nephritis; and class VI is characterized by advanced sclerotic lesions. Classes III and IV have subdivisions for active and sclerotic lesions, and class IV currently also has subdivisions for segmental and global involvement. Recent recommendations from these societies include elimination of the IV-S and IV-G subdivisions and replacement of the active and chronic designations for class III/IV lesions with application of activity and chronicity indices for all classes. They also suggest eliminating the term "endocapillary proliferation" and are considering a more appropriate definition of endocapillary hypercellularity. Validation of candidate revised classification criteria is planned by these groups. Pathologic diagnosis should include descriptions of tubulointerstitial and vascular disease as well as glomerular involvement. Several renal pathologic lesions seen in SLE patients that are not encompassed in the classification scheme for lupus GN include lupus podocytopathy, collapsing glomerulopathy, and thrombotic microangiopathy, the latter often associated with antiphospholipid syndrome.

The prognosis of class I and class II disease is usually good, whereas class IV, the most common form of lupus nephritis, has the worst prognosis, particularly when the serum creatinine level is elevated at the time of diagnosis. Class V nephritis occurs in 10 to 20% of patients, and the implication for long-term outcome depends on the degree of proteinuria, with mild proteinuria having a good prognosis and nephrotic syndrome with chronic edema having a more negative prognosis. It should be noted that renal veins can occasionally become involved with thrombosis, which then also contributes to nephrotic syndrome. This complication can be evaluated by renal ultrasound (Chapter 113).

Cardiovascular System

Pericarditis and valve nodules were among the first clinical manifestations described in SLE. It is now recognized that premature atherosclerotic disease represents a significant contributor to morbidity and mortality in SLE patients. Pericarditis (Chapter 68) is the most common cardiac manifestation, but it is sometimes recognized only on imaging studies or at autopsy. It is a component of the generalized serositis that is often a feature of SLE and is associated with local autoantibodies and immune complexes. Pericarditis is usually manifested as substernal chest pain that is improved by bending forward and can be exacerbated by inspiration or coughing. The symptoms and effusions associated with pericarditis are quite responsive to moderate-dose (20 to 30 mg/day of prednisone) corticosteroid treatment.

Structural valve abnormalities in SLE range from sterile nodules (originally described by Libman and Sacks) to nonspecific valve thickening (Chapter 66). The nodules are immobile and usually located on the atrial side of the mitral valve and sometimes on the arterial side of the aortic valve. Right-sided lesions are rare. These structural changes may in some cases result in valvular regurgitation. Although valve nodules are detected in most patients with SLE at autopsy, clinically significant valvular heart disease is much less common (1 to 18%). The verrucous valvular lesions of Libman and Sacks are most likely inflammatory in nature and may be associated with the presence of antiphospholipid antibodies.

Premature and accelerated atherosclerosis is prevalent in lupus patients, and preclinical atherosclerotic carotid plaque has been documented in 37% of SLE patients as opposed to 15% of age- and sex-matched controls. Traditional

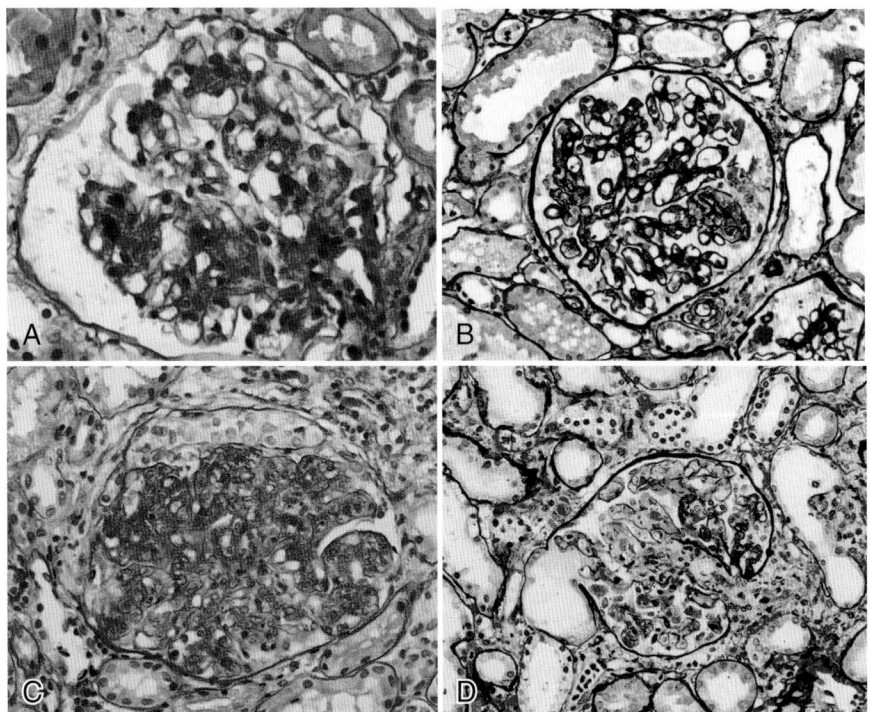

FIGURE 250-3. **Histopathology of lupus nephritis. A,** Lupus nephritis class II. A light micrograph of a glomerulus shows mild mesangial hypercellularity (periodic acid–Schiff). **B,** Lupus nephritis class III (A). Light micrograph showing a glomerulus with segmental endocapillary hypercellularity, mesangial hypercellularity, capillary wall thickening, and early segmental capillary necrosis (methenamine silver). **C,** Lupus nephritis class IV-G (A/C). A glomerulus manifests global endocapillary proliferation, leukocyte influx and apoptotic bodies, double contours, crescent formation with tubular transformation, early sclerosis, and disruption of Bowman capsule (periodic acid–Schiff). **D,** Thrombotic microangiopathy in a patient with systemic lupus erythematosus and circulating lupus anticoagulant. A glomerulus shows severe capillary and arteriolar thrombosis, endothelial cell swelling and necrosis, neutrophil influx, and stasis of erythrocytes. No signs of immune deposits were found (methenamine silver). (From Wenning JJ, D'Agati VD, Schwartz MM, et al. The classification of glomerulonephritis in systemic lupus erythematosus revisited. *J Am Soc Nephrol.* 2004;15:241.)

cardiovascular risk factors apply, but the diagnosis of SLE is itself a significant risk factor for premature atherosclerosis (Chapter 62). Among the lupus-related mechanisms that confer additional risk for atherosclerosis, IFN-α and oxidative modification of lipid-associated proteins contribute to the accumulation of vascular damage.[19] Mortality from atherosclerosis may be up to 10 times greater in patients with SLE than in age- and sex-matched controls.

Although not specific to SLE, Raynaud phenomenon (Chapter 72), characterized by episodic vasospasm and occlusion of the digital arteries in response to cold and emotional stress, is a feature in up to 60% of SLE patients and contributes to pain and sometimes necrosis of the distal ends of extremities. The character of the digits classically changes from pallor to cyanosis and then to rubor as vascular perfusion becomes impaired and then reperfusion ensues. In addition, small arteries, arterioles, and capillaries can be affected by vasculitis and fibrinoid necrosis, with clinical manifestations that include periungual telangiectases, abdominal pain, and neuropsychiatric symptoms.

Pulmonary System
Pleuritis is the most frequent manifestation of pulmonary involvement in SLE and occurs in about 30% of patients at some point in their disease course. Pleuritis is characterized by pain on respiration and exudative effusions (Chapter 92). Parenchymal disease is less common but may be based on several distinct mechanisms, including pneumonitis in the absence of documented infection and sometimes involving alveolar hemorrhage (in up to 12% of patients), pulmonary embolism secondary to deep vein thrombosis, or pulmonary hypertension with increased pulmonary resistance and impaired diffusing capacity.

Neuropsychiatric Involvement
Clinical features of SLE that involve the nervous system include both neurologic and psychiatric manifestations.[20] The central and peripheral nervous systems can be affected by the disease. The American College of Rheumatology has identified 19 neuropsychiatric syndromes that can be associated with SLE, and validation of these neuropsychiatric findings has been substantiated in several independent studies. The most common manifestations that are probably attributable to SLE cerebritis include cognitive dysfunction, present in 17 to 66% of SLE patients; psychosis or mood disorder, the former reported

in up to 8% of patients; cerebrovascular disease in 5 to 18% of patients; and seizures, present in 6 to 51% of patients. Headaches are also common. Although none of these CNS manifestations is found exclusively in SLE, global SLE disease activity is associated with concurrent neuropsychiatric manifestations attributable to SLE.

Evaluation of neuropsychiatric lupus depends on a careful clinical history and physical and laboratory examinations and, in some cases, imaging studies and analysis of cerebrospinal fluid to rule out infection. Magnetic resonance imaging is useful for detecting intracranial abnormalities, which are seen in 19 to 70% of patients and include white matter lesions, cerebral infarction, venous sinus thrombosis, and sometimes atrophy. Magnetic resonance angiography and magnetic resonance spectroscopy can be used to assess cerebral blood flow or neuronal metabolism.

Cranial nerve and ocular involvement, most likely based on vasculopathy and focal ischemia, can sometimes affect vision. Ocular examination of the retina can reveal cotton-wool spots as a result of retinal ischemia or necrosis. Although rare, transverse myelopathy, frequently associated with antiphospholipid antibodies, can have devastating consequences, including paraplegia. Sensorimotor neuropathies, often asymmetrical, are more common (up to 28%) and are based on damage to small nerve fibers with vasculopathy in the small arteries that supply the nerve fibers.

As is the case with lupus nephritis, the pathophysiologic mechanisms that account for the neuropsychiatric manifestations of SLE are diverse and complex. Recent data suggest that autoantibodies cross-reactive with neuronal cell surface glutamate receptors and DNA may mediate excitotoxic death of neurons and are proposed to contribute to cognitive dysfunction. Antibodies directed against ribosomal P protein have also been associated with neuropsychiatric lupus, and antiphospholipid antibodies can contribute to a procoagulant state, vascular thrombosis, and cerebral ischemia. Cerebral vasculopathy has been clearly demonstrated by angiographic and pathologic studies. Noninflammatory small vessel vasculopathy is the most common lesion and can be associated with microinfarcts. Inflammatory mediators, including the cytokines interleukin-6 (IL-6) and IFN-α, and matrix metalloproteinases may also contribute to the neuropsychiatric manifestations of SLE. Recent data from studies of murine lupus indicate that IFN-α mediates microglial activation and excessive synaptic pruning, a possible mechanism of cognitive dysfunction in patients with SLE.

Gastrointestinal System

Although uncommon, vasculitis of the gastrointestinal tract or mesentery can result in pain and bowel necrosis. Less common than pleuritis and pericarditis, peritonitis can manifest as peritoneal effusion and abdominal pain. Pancreatitis occurs in less than 10% of patients but may also be due to vascular pathology. Lupoid hepatitis, a syndrome that was named for the presence of positive ANAs in patients with chronic active hepatitis, is a misnomer because elevated transaminases are only rarely seen in lupus patients.

Lymphadenopathy

About one third of SLE patients demonstrate diffuse lymphadenopathy at some time during the course of their disease. The nodes are often nontender, and lymphoma is sometimes considered in the differential diagnosis. Biopsy usually reveals follicular hyperplasia, although some histopathologic findings appear similar to the histiocytic necrotizing lymphadenitis that is a feature of Kikuchi disease, a self-limited syndrome characterized by fever and lymphadenopathy. Recent multicenter studies have determined the frequency of malignancies in patients with SLE and have found a significant increase in hematologic malignancies, particularly non-Hodgkin lymphoma. Splenomegaly is sometimes seen in SLE, and spleen pathology is characterized by a classic onion-skin histology that appears as concentric circles of collagen matrix surrounding splenic arteries and arterioles.

Hematologic System

In addition to autoantibody specificities that are fairly specific for SLE (anti-DNA, anti-Sm), antibodies that target each of the cellular blood elements are also common. Anemia is present in about 50% of patients and is multifactorial. It can be associated with a positive Coombs test or microangiopathic hemolysis (Chapter 151) or reflect chronic disease (normochromic, normocytic) (Chapter 149). Leukopenia, particularly lymphopenia, is observed, with the lymphocyte count decreasing in the setting of increased disease activity. Antibodies that bind to lymphocytes and neutrophils have been described, and an increased tendency for lymphocytes to undergo spontaneous apoptosis may contribute to lymphopenia. Idiopathic thrombocytopenic purpura (Chapter 163) can be an early manifestation of SLE, and thrombocytopenia induced by antiplatelet autoantibodies can sometimes lead to a life-threatening risk for hemorrhage. Autoantibodies to clotting factors can also occur and contribute to impaired clot formation and hemorrhage.

Lupus Pregnancy and Neonatal Lupus

Whether pregnancy increases the likelihood of lupus exacerbation has been debated, with differences on this point presented by different investigators. However, abundant data indicate that patients with SLE have worse fetal outcomes than healthy individuals.[21] Gestational hypertension, fetal growth restriction, and fetal distress are increased in patients with SLE and may lead to fetal loss or premature delivery. Preeclampsia can contribute to a poor outcome in both the mother and fetus and can be difficult to distinguish from a lupus flare associated with lupus nephritis.

Neonatal lupus is a distinct entity that can occur in infants of mothers with or without a diagnosis of SLE.[22] The syndrome is characterized by cutaneous lesions and congenital heart block in the infant and the presence of antibodies to the Ro (SSA) or La (SSB) RNA-binding proteins (or both) in the mother. The mortality rate in babies with a congenital heart block is 15 to 31%. Deposition of anti-Ro IgG in the fetal heart, indicative of transplacental transfer of maternal autoantibody, and dense connective tissue encompassing the conduction system have been demonstrated in autopsy specimens. Prenatal testing of lupus mothers for the presence of anti-Ro and anti-La antibodies is appropriate, and careful monitoring with fetal echocardiography starting at week 16 of pregnancy can detect conduction defects. Fluorinated corticosteroids such as dexamethasone have been effective in reversing heart block in some cases. The role of hydroxychloroquine in prevention of neonatal lupus manifestations is under investigation.

Antiphospholipid Antibody Syndrome

Antiphospholipid antibodies represent a distinct class of autoantibodies that are seen in about one third of SLE patients but can also be present in individuals who do not carry a diagnosis of SLE (Chapter 162). Although these antibodies were initially thought to be specific for phospholipids exposed in cell membranes, particularly after "flipping" of the membranes of apoptotic cells, extensive data support their primary reactivity with phospholipid-binding proteins, particularly β_2-glycoprotein I. Whether in primary antiphospholipid syndrome or in SLE, antiphospholipid antibodies have been associated with venous and arterial thromboses.[23] In addition to vascular thromboses, clinical manifestations of antiphospholipid syndrome include thrombotic microangiopathic glomerular disease, cardiac valve lesions, livedo reticularis, thrombocytopenia, hemolytic anemia, and CNS disease. Recent data indicate that these autoantibodies can contribute to fetal loss and growth restriction by binding to the placenta, activating the complement system, and inducing inflammation. Catastrophic antiphospholipid syndrome, triggered by the acute onset of multisystemic (three or more organs) thrombosis, is resistant to anticoagulation treatment and is fatal in approximately 50% of cases.[24]

DIAGNOSIS

Classification

Criteria for the classification of patients with SLE for the purpose of clinical studies were developed by the American College of Rheumatology, with the most recent full revision published in 1982 and an update published in 1997 (Table 250-2). The criteria include 11 features that encompass manifestations of skin and mucosal involvement, arthritis, serositis, renal disorder, neurologic disorder, hematologic disorder, immunologic disorder, and an abnormal titer in the ANA test, with at least four criteria required for classification as SLE. ANA has low specificity but strengthens the sensitivity of the criteria because it is positive in virtually all lupus patients. These criteria are not intended for use as diagnostic criteria because more than 50% of patients with SLE do not meet four criteria at any point in time, although all do meet these criteria at some point during the course of the disease.[25] Classification criteria for SLE are currently under review through a project co-sponsored by the American College of Rheumatology and the European League Against Rheumatism. The criteria are useful in reminding the clinician of the most characteristic features of SLE, but a careful history with detailed review of systems and triggering factors, as well as a family history, is essential in raising suspicion for a diagnosis of SLE. Because drugs can trigger a lupus-like syndrome, a careful drug history should be taken. Procainamide and hydralazine present the greatest risk for development of lupus, with quinidine, isoniazid, minocycline, and recombinant IFN-α presenting a lower risk. At the onset of clinical symptoms, the diagnosis of SLE can be uncertain because many of the systemic manifestations of lupus can mimic other conditions, particularly viral infections or malignancy, and only some of the typical clinical symptoms may be expressed at any one point in time. Important features of SLE are its multisystemic nature and characteristic serology. The differential diagnosis of SLE includes other rheumatic disorders, such as rheumatoid arthritis and vasculitis; infections, including gonococcal arthritis, parvovirus B19, and mononucleosis; inflammatory bowel disease; thrombotic thrombocytopenic purpura; drug reactions; and malignancies, particularly lymphoma.[26] It should be recognized that the clinical manifestations of lupus can demonstrate overlap with those of other autoimmune rheumatic diseases and can evolve over time. Many genetic, environmental, and immunologic factors associated with lupus are also associated with other systemic autoimmune diseases, often contributing to a complex clinical picture.

Laboratory Findings

Laboratory tests can be very helpful in supporting the diagnosis of SLE. All cellular elements of blood can be affected in lupus, so the complete blood count is an essential test that aids in diagnosis and management. A prolonged activated partial thromboplastin time (aPTT) can indicate the presence of pathogenic antiphospholipid antibodies (Chapter 162). These antibodies are also associated with a false-positive result in the serologic test for syphilis, an observation that is mainly of historical interest.

Evaluation of renal disease in SLE includes urinalysis with microscopic analysis of urine sediment, serum blood urea nitrogen and creatinine, and 24-hour urine collection (or alternatively, spot urine protein-to-creatinine ratio) for estimation of protein and creatinine clearance. Low serum albumin would be consistent with persistent proteinuria and membranous GN, whereas red and white blood cell casts in the urinary sediment suggest proliferative GN. Although a renal biopsy is usually performed only when the result may influence therapeutic decisions, pathologic classification of the features of renal disease can provide prognostic information.

The erythrocyte sedimentation rate (ESR), although a very nonspecific indicator of systemic inflammation, is often monitored and in many patients can provide an indication of disease activity. Interestingly, C-reactive protein, an acute phase reactant, is relatively uninformative in SLE because it is often low in comparison to an ESR performed on the same occasion.

Assaying and monitoring characteristic lupus serologic tests can strongly support the diagnosis of SLE and, in some cases, can assist in the assessment

TABLE 250-2 UPDATE OF THE 1982 REVISED CRITERIA FOR CLASSIFICATION OF SYSTEMIC LUPUS ERYTHEMATOSUS

CRITERION*	DEFINITION
1. Malar rash	Fixed erythema, flat or raised, over the malar eminences that tends to spare the nasolabial folds
2. Discoid rash	Erythematous raised patches with adherent keratotic scaling and follicular plugging; atrophic scarring may occur in older lesions
3. Photosensitivity	Rash as a result of unusual reaction to sunlight, by history or physician observation
4. Oral ulcers	Oral or nasopharyngeal ulceration, usually painless, observed by a physician
5. Nonerosive arthritis	Involving 2 or more peripheral joints and characterized by tenderness, swelling, or effusion
6. Pleuritis or pericarditis	A. Pleuritis—convincing history of pleuritic pain or rubbing heard by a physician or evidence of pleural effusion *or* B. Pericarditis—documented by electrocardiography, a rub, or evidence of pericardial effusion
7. Renal disorder	A. Persistent proteinuria >0.5 g/day or >3+ if quantitation is not performed *or* B. Cellular casts—may be red cell, hemoglobin, granular, tubular, or mixed
8. Neurologic disorder	A. Seizures—in the absence of offending drugs or known metabolic derangements (e.g., uremia, ketoacidosis, electrolyte imbalance) *or* B. Psychosis—in the absence of offending drugs or known metabolic derangements (e.g., uremia, ketoacidosis, electrolyte imbalance)
9. Hematologic disorder	A. Hemolytic anemia—with reticulocytosis *or* B. Leukopenia—<4000/μL total on ≥2 occasions *or* C. Lymphopenia—<1500/μL on ≥2 occasions *or* D. Thrombocytopenia—<100,000/μL in the absence of offending drugs
10. Immunologic disorder	A. Anti-DNA: antibody to native DNA in abnormal titer *or* B. Anti-Sm: presence of antibody to Sm nuclear antigen *or* C. Positive finding of antiphospholipid antibodies on: (1) an abnormal serum level of IgG or IgM anticardiolipin antibodies; (2) a positive test for lupus anticoagulant using a standard method; or (3) a false-positive test result for syphilis known to be positive for at least 6 months confirmed by *Treponema pallidum* immobilization or fluorescent treponemal antibody absorption test
11. Positive antinuclear antibody	An abnormal titer of antinuclear antibody by immunofluorescence or an equivalent assay at any point in time and in the absence of drugs

*The proposed classification is based on 11 criteria. For the purpose of identifying patients in clinical studies, a person shall be said to have systemic lupus erythematosus if any 4 or more of the 11 criteria are present, serially or simultaneously, during any interval of observation.

Modified from Tan EM, Cohen AS, Fries JF, et al. The 1982 revised criteria for the classification of systemic lupus erythematosus. *Arthritis Rheum*. 1982;25:1271. Modifications described in Hochberg MC. Updating the American College of Rheumatology revised criteria for the classification of systemic lupus erythematosus. *Arthritis Rheum*. 1997;40:1725.

TABLE 250-3 AUTOANTIBODIES ASSOCIATED WITH SYSTEMIC LUPUS ERYTHEMATOSUS

TARGET ANTIGEN	APPROXIMATE FREQUENCY
Nuclear antigens	99
Double-stranded DNA	70
Sm nuclear antigen	38
RNP (U1-RNP)	33
Ro (SSA)	49
La (SSB)	35
Phospholipids	21
Ribosomal P	10

of disease activity. The ANA test is positive in virtually all patients and does not need to be repeated after it has been documented to be positive (Table 250-3). Anti-double-stranded DNA antibodies are common in SLE, and some studies have found that monitoring their titer can be useful in assessing the activity of lupus nephritis. Autoantibodies specific for proteins that associate with nucleic acids in intracellular particles are present in many patients and can provide support for a diagnosis of SLE. Anti-Sm antibodies are highly specific for SLE and, along with anti-RNP antibodies, react with the spliceosome particle. Anti-Ro (SSA) and anti-La (SSB) antibodies are specific for proteins in an RNA-containing particle and are common in patients with Sjögren syndrome and in mothers of babies with neonatal lupus, as well as being a feature of SLE. It is useful to document the presence of anti-Sm, anti-RNP, anti-Ro, and anti-La antibodies when the diagnosis of SLE is being made, but the titers of these autoantibodies are not helpful in monitoring disease activity.

Proteins of the complement system are activated by immune complexes, such as those that form in patients with SLE. The activation products that result from enzymatic cleavage of the complement components promote inflammation directly by binding to cell surface receptors on mononuclear phagocytes, and indirectly by acting as chemotactic agents to recruit inflammatory cells. Decreased levels of two of the more stable complement components, C3 and C4, are typically measured in serum, and decreased C3 and C4 levels are often indicators of enhanced consumption and increased disease

activity. Some laboratories also use a functional measure of total hemolytic complement activity (CH_{50}).

It is the global picture provided by a careful history, physical examination, and blood, urine, and serologic data that supports a diagnosis of SLE. It should be recognized that there is considerable heterogeneity among patients and that different combinations of clinical features will characterize any one individual. As is the case with many systemic diseases, infection and some malignancies may have a similar picture and should be included in the differential until the diagnosis of SLE is secure.

TREATMENT

Although current knowledge of genetic risk factors for SLE is not sufficient to predict those in whom the disease will develop, after the diagnosis has been made, regular counseling and education are fundamental to the treatment of SLE patients. Patients should be advised to avoid known triggers of disease exacerbation, such as ultraviolet light, and should be instructed regarding the need for adequate rest. Pregnancy should be undertaken with caution and with careful monitoring. Lupus patients can be informed that data indicate that oral contraceptive agents do not contribute to disease exacerbations.[A1]

Conventional Medical Therapy

Clinical manifestations of lupus that do not involve major organ systems can often be managed with nonsteroidal anti-inflammatory drugs, low-dose corticosteroids, and antimalarials. Corticosteroids (Chapter 32) are immunosuppressive agents that modulate many functions of lymphocytes and monocytes, including the production of pro-inflammatory cytokines. Oral prednisone in doses ranging from 5 to 30 mg daily is effective in treating constitutional symptoms, arthralgias, pericarditis and pleuritis, and skin disease. Topical corticosteroids are sometimes applied to cutaneous lesions. Although effective, corticosteroids also have toxicities that add to the morbidity associated with lupus. The broad immunosuppression mediated by these drugs contributes to the susceptibility to infection that is an inherent feature of SLE. Osteonecrosis, osteoporotic fractures, posterior subcapsular cataracts, diabetes, myopathy, hypertension, hypoadrenalism, and emotional disturbance are additional deleterious effects of corticosteroids.

Antimalarial agents, most commonly hydroxychloroquine administered at 200 to 400 mg/day, have long been used to control skin involvement and arthralgias and are now routinely used in most lupus patients. An important Canadian study demonstrating an increased frequency of disease flares in patients who discontinued hydroxychloroquine contributed to its recent use in lupus for a broader range of clinical manifestations. Hydroxychloroquine has been associated with a decreased incidence of thrombosis, a mechanism that could affect vasculopathy and end-organ damage. An additional potential mechanism of action implicates the TLR pathway, which is responsible for activation of the innate immune response. The effects of antimalarial agents on acidification of the intracellular vesicles where TLRs associate with their ligands may inhibit immune cell activation mediated by stimulatory nucleic acids. Antimalarials are well tolerated. Because they can rarely cause eye toxicity, ophthalmologic examinations should precede initiation of therapy and take place every 6 to 12 months thereafter.

Management of Serious Organ-System Disease

For more serious disease, particularly active nephritis, CNS disease, or systemic vasculitis, prednisone at 60 mg daily or 1 g of intravenous methylprednisolone administered daily for 3 days can sometimes gain control of disease activity. In many situations, additional immunosuppressive, cytotoxic, or biologic therapies are required. Because lupus nephritis is the most common severe clinical organ-system manifestation of SLE, an algorithm describing guidelines for medical management of lupus nephritis developed by a Task Force Panel assembled by the American College of Rheumatology is useful (Fig. 250-4). A similar approach can be applied to other serious clinical disease flares. Lupus flares involving rapid decompensation of renal function, CNS disease (including seizures, strokes, or psychosis), or widespread vasculitis or vasculopathy can be life-threatening and must be recognized and treated early and aggressively. Careful attention to monitoring for concurrent or superimposed infection is an important priority during management of a severe lupus flare, and distinguishing sepsis from active lupus or catastrophic antiphospholipid syndrome can be a particular challenge. In general, cyclophosphamide can be added to high-dose corticosteroid therapy in the setting of severe flare,[A2] although mycophenolate mofetil has gained increased use in situations in which the physician or patient wishes to avoid the potential toxicities associated with cyclophosphamide.[A3] For example, multitarget therapy consisting of tacrolimus (4 mg per day), mycophenolate mofetil (1 gram per day), and oral prednisone provides superior efficacy compared with intravenous cyclophosphamide as induction therapy for lupus nephritis.[A4] Randomized controlled studies have investigated options for maintaining improvement in those patients who respond to induction therapy in the setting of lupus nephritis flare, with current data favoring mycophenolate mofetil over azathioprine.[A5] One biologic agent, belimumab, a monoclonal antibody reactive with BLyS, has been approved by the U.S. Food and Drug Administration (FDA) for treatment of active autoantibody-positive SLE in conjunction with standard therapies,[A6] but belimumab has not yet been documented to be effective in patients with lupus nephritis or other severe manifestations of lupus. Testing of additional candidate therapeutic agents holds promise, including positive phase II clinical trials for a monoclonal antibody against the type I interferon receptor,[A7] a monoclonal antibody that inhibits IL-12 and IL-23, and a Janus-associated kinase inhibitor. Additional therapeutic agents have initiated clinical testing. Agents used in management of lupus are reviewed below.

Immunosuppressive Agents
Alkylating Agents

Approximately 33% of lupus patients receive cytotoxic therapy during the course of their disease. Cyclophosphamide is a cytotoxic agent that has been one of the more reliable and studied treatments for severe organ system manifestations of lupus, particularly lupus nephritis and CNS involvement. Studies performed at the National Institutes of Health in the 1980s led to recommendations of a standard regimen of cyclophosphamide, 0.5 to 1 g/m² body surface area administered intravenously monthly for 6 months, followed by quarterly doses through 2 years. Cyclophosphamide is usually given with oral prednisone in tapering doses or sometimes with pulse methylprednisolone. Although this regimen is often effective in controlling GN, overall patient survival has not been demonstrated to be increased, and high-dose cyclophosphamide is associated with significant toxicity, including cytopenia, infection, and gonadal failure. A modified therapeutic regimen for administration of cyclophosphamide,

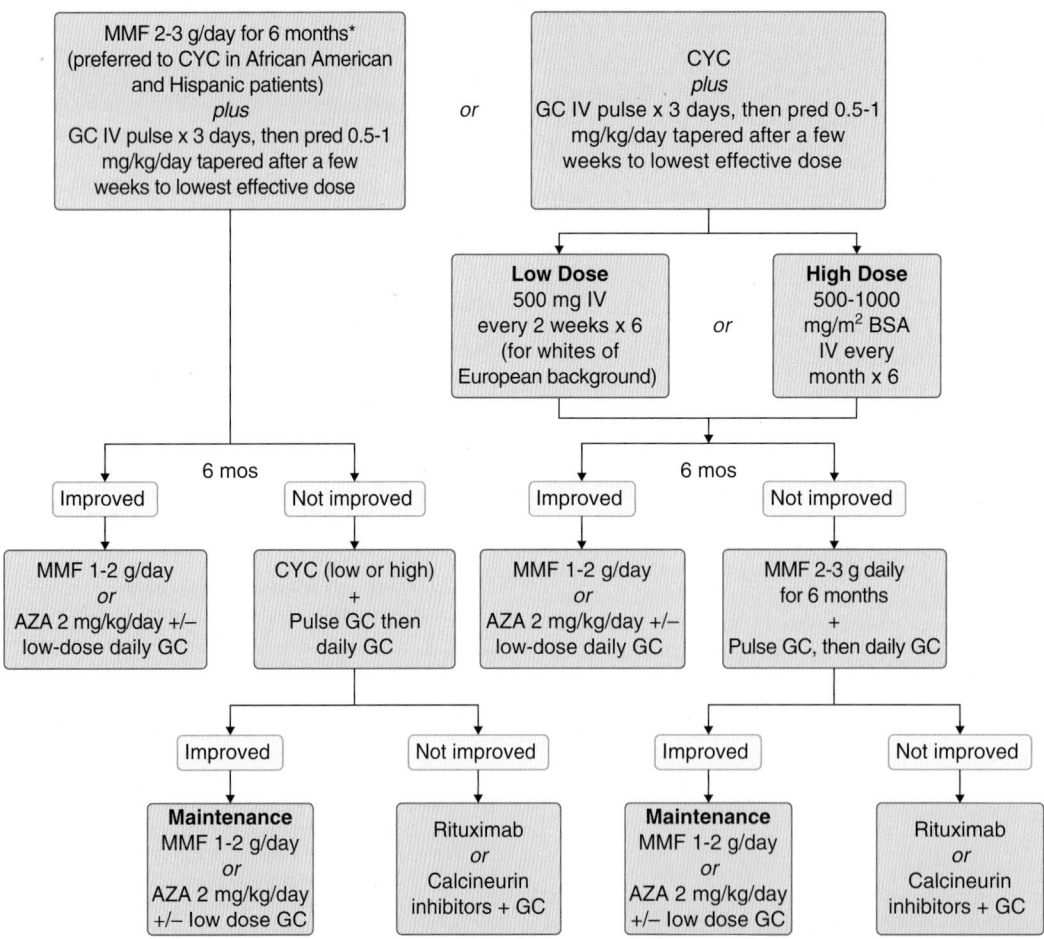

Induction Therapy: Class III/IV

FIGURE 250-4. Algorithm for induction therapy for lupus nephritis. Guidelines developed by the Task Force Panel of the American College of Rheumatology for management of class III/IV lupus nephritis. Refer to reference 29 for guidelines for management of class III/IV lupus nephritis with crescents and class V membranous lupus nephritis without proliferative changes and nephrotic range proteinuria. *The Task Force Panel preferred MMF over CYC in patients who desire to preserve fertility. AZA = azathioprine; BSA = body surface area; CYC = cyclophosphamide; GC = glucocorticoid; IV = intravenous; MMF = mycophenolate mofetil; pred = prednisone. (From Hahn BH, McMahon MA, Wilkinson A, et al. American College of Rheumatology guidelines for screening, treatment, and management of lupus nephritis. *Arthritis Care Res [Hoboken].* 2012;64:797-808.)

termed the "Euro-Lupus regimen," involves 500 mg administered intravenously every 2 weeks for 6 doses, followed by azathioprine. This approach provides long-term efficacy comparable to the high-dose cyclophosphamide regimen and is superior in maintaining ovarian reserve.[27] A recent meta-analysis of randomized clinical trials of therapies for lupus nephritis was overall inconclusive but suggested that mycophenolate mofetil (MMF), calcineurin inhibitors, or the combination were effective in inducing remission compared with intravenous cyclophosphamide, and that MMF is the most effective maintenance therapy.[A8] Cyclophosphamide is relatively contraindicated in pregnant women.

Purine Synthesis Inhibitors

Azathioprine has been used for the treatment of lupus nephritis and as a steroid-sparing agent in SLE for many years. Azathioprine inhibits DNA synthesis and inhibits key signaling pathways in T lymphocytes. Azathioprine is commonly dosed at 2 to 3 mg/kg/day administered as a tablet. Toxicities of azathioprine target the bone marrow (and result in cytopenias) as well as the liver, occasionally resulting in transaminitis. Its use is rarely associated with non-Hodgkin lymphoma (Chapter 176). It has been used safely in pregnant women.

MMF is an inhibitor that binds to the isoform of inosine monophosphate dehydrogenase that mediates purine synthesis in activated lymphocytes. It has a good track record of utility in inhibiting allograft rejection. Recent clinical trials have compared MMF with low-dose intravenous cyclophosphamide for induction therapy in lupus nephritis; the results demonstrated equivalence of MMF and cyclophosphamide in patients with lupus nephritis, although some patients with active acute disease were excluded.[A9] In a randomized trial, MMF (1 g twice daily) was more effective than azathioprine for the maintenance treatment of lupus nephritis, with treatment failure rates reduced from 32 to 16%.[A10] Like cyclophosphamide, MMF should not be used in pregnancy.

Methotrexate

Methotrexate is a folate antagonist that is commonly used in rheumatoid arthritis. A double-blind randomized placebo-controlled trial of oral methotrexate (15 to 25 mg/week for 6 months) in SLE controlled disease and allowed tapering of prednisone. The most responsive clinical manifestations were cutaneous and articular.

Ancillary and Other Therapies
Intravenous Gamma Globulin

Although positive data from controlled trials of intravenous gamma globulin are not available, case reports and clinical experience indicate that administration of pooled IgG fractions can sometimes be efficacious in gaining control of lupus disease activity that is refractory to other therapies. A common regimen is 2 g/kg in divided doses over a 3- to 5-day period. Several mechanisms have been proposed for this therapy, including blockade of Fc receptors, modulation of lymphocyte function through Fc receptors, increased catabolism of pathogenic immunoglobulin, and actions of the anti-idiotype antibody that is a component of the administered IgG.

Plasmapheresis

Removal of pathogenic antibodies and immune complexes is the goal of plasmapheresis, but there are scant data supporting the utility of this therapy. Nonetheless, plasmapheresis has been occasionally useful in lupus patients with life-threatening complications in which the clinical manifestations can be clearly attributed to pathogenic autoantibodies. In particular, plasmapheresis has been effective in cases of thrombotic thrombocytopenic purpura associated with SLE (Chapter 163).

Biologic Therapies

Biologic therapies (Chapter 33) are being actively investigated in clinical trials, but only one agent has been successful as yet in phase III studies. Belimumab, a monoclonal antibody, blocks a B-cell survival and differentiation signal. At a dose of 1 mg/kg or 10 mg/kg intravenously on days 1 and 28 and then every 28 days for 48 weeks, belimumab reduced disease activity by both validated measures and physician global assessment and decreased autoantibody levels. In a second study, belimumab at a dose of 10 mg/kg administered intravenously on days 0, 14, and 28 and then every 28 days, the currently recommended regimen, for 72 weeks, added to standard therapy, significantly improved response rate, disease activity, and severe flares and was generally well tolerated in SLE.[A11] The clinical settings that are most appropriate for the use of belimumab, which was approved by the FDA, will be determined by future clinical trials and clinical experience. Additional agents under investigation target B cells, T-cell activation, and cytokines.[28]

Rituximab, a monoclonal antibody specific for the cell surface B-cell molecule CD20, is approved for use in B-cell lymphomas and has been used in some patients with SLE who are poorly responsive to other therapies. Rituximab depletes B cells, often for many months, and may limit T-cell activation by eliminating activated B cells that can serve as antigen-presenting cells. However, controlled clinical trials of rituximab in lupus have not shown efficacy. In a randomized double-blind placebo-controlled phase III trial in patients with active proliferative lupus nephritis, rituximab therapy led to more responders and greater reductions in anti-double-stranded DNA and C3/C4 levels, but did not improve clinical outcomes after 1 year of treatment.[A12] Nonetheless,

rituximab is increasingly used in patients with lupus nephritis or cytopenias refractory to more conventional therapies.[29]

Other agents that block B-cell survival and differentiation factors or target B-cell surface molecules are under study. T-cell targets include CD28 and CD40 ligand (CD154), a T-cell surface molecule involved in supporting B-cell differentiation. Blockade of T-cell activation by CTLA4-Ig, a soluble inhibitor of CD28 ligation, or inhibition of CD40-CD40 ligand interaction might inhibit B-cell differentiation in the germinal center. Monoclonal antibodies specific for the type I IFN receptor or for subtypes of type I IFN are under study. Small molecule inhibitors of signaling molecules are in development, and inhibitors of mammalian target of rapamycin may prove useful in controlling lupus disease activity.[30]

Adjunctive Therapies

In addition to controlling autoimmunity and inflammation in SLE, it is essential to control hypertension adequately when it occurs. In those with lupus nephritis, treatment with an angiotensin inhibitor or an angiotensin receptor blocker reduces intraglomerular pressure, thus reducing proteinuria. In patients with a history of thrombosis, who will usually have antiphospholipid antibodies, long-term warfarin is recommended. The potential use of statins in lupus is of interest because those agents have anti-inflammatory as well as lipid-lowering effects, but statins have not yet been shown efficacious in controlling lupus disease activity in controlled trials. The value of supplementation with vitamin D and omega-3 fatty acids, such as krill oil, in lupus is under study.

Future Directions

Recent advances in basic immunology, together with detailed molecular and clinical characterization of cohorts of SLE patients, have directed attention to the role adjuvant-like factors play in activating the innate immune response through TLRs. The primary triggers of that response are not known, but abundant data support production of type I interferon as an important consequence of immune activation that has an impact on many aspects of lymphocyte function, probably including induction of self-antigen–specific immune responses. In addition to the biologic therapies currently under study that target T and B lymphocytes, future therapies may be designed that can inhibit TLR activation, signaling components downstream from TLRs, cytoplasmic sensors of stimulatory nucleic acids, or type I interferon itself. Recognition that the complement system is an essential contributor to inflammation triggered by antiphospholipid antibodies, as well as by immune complexes, provides additional targets that might be inhibited therapeutically and limit tissue damage. Continued investigation of the genetic and environmental factors that contribute to disease susceptibility may permit identification of individuals at risk for the development of SLE and may elucidate the primary stimuli that lead to autoimmunity. Identification of informative biomarkers that reflect or even predict disease flares would improve medical management of lupus patients.

PROGNOSIS

Although survival of patients with a diagnosis of SLE is good, lupus remains a disease that is potentially fatal. SLE demonstrates a bimodal pattern of death, with deaths within the first year attributable to active lupus and infection and late deaths attributable to atherosclerotic cardiovascular disease. Recent cohort studies have estimated 5-year survival rates greater than 90%, with improvement in medical management probably contributing to improved outcomes, as opposed to earlier studies, and 85% survival rates at 10 years. However, after a diagnosis of SLE has been made, prolonged remission is rare. Of 702 patients registered in a lupus clinic in Canada, 6.5% achieved complete remission (score of 0 on the SLE Disease Activity Index), and only 1.7% maintained remission for at least 5 years with no treatment. The presence of any permanent organ damage within the first year after a diagnosis of SLE is associated with poorer survival at 10 years (compared with a 75 vs. 95% rate in those without permanent organ damage). Regarding renal outcome, an elevated level of serum creatinine at the time of diagnosis has been correlated with an adverse outcome.

Recent studies of minority populations in the United States have indicated that predictors of high lupus disease activity include Hispanic Texan and African American ethnicities, lack of health insurance, and poor social support. African admixture and anti-double-stranded DNA antibodies also predicted high levels of disease activity, as did previous disease activity.

Data from a multicenter study of nearly 10,000 patients has supported an increased risk for hematologic malignancies in SLE patients, particularly non-Hodgkin lymphoma. Prognostic factors for an adverse fetal outcome in pregnant lupus mothers are maternal renal disease and hypertension.

Grade A References

A1. Rojas-Villarraga A, Torres-Gonzalez JV, Ruiz-Sternberg AM. Safety of hormonal replacement therapy and oral contraceptives in systemic lupus erythematosus: a systematic review and meta-analysis. *PLoS ONE.* 2014;9:1-11.

A2. Houssiau FA, Vasconcelos C, D'Crus D, et al. The 10-year follow-up data of the Euro-Lupus Nephritis Trial comparing low-dose and high-dose intravenous cyclophosphamide. *Ann Rheum Dis.* 2010;69:61-64.

A3. Houssiau FA, D'Cruz D, Sangle S, et al. MAINTAIN Nephritis Trial Group. Azathioprine versus mycophenolate mofetil for long-term immunosuppression in lupus nephritis: results from the MAINTAIN Nephritis Trial. *Ann Rheum Dis.* 2010;69:2083-2089.

A4. Liu Z, Zhang H, Liu Z, et al. Multitarget therapy for induction treatment of lupus nephritis: a randomized trial. *Ann Intern Med.* 2015;162:18-26.

A5. Ordi-Ros J, Saez-Comet L, Perez-Conesa M, et al. Enteric-coated mycophenolate sodium versus azathioprine in patients with active systemic lupus erythematosus: a randomised clinical trial. *Ann Rheum Dis.* 2017;76:1575-1582.

A6. Navarra SV, Guzmán RM, Gallacher AE, et al. Efficacy and safety of belimumab in patients with active systemic lupus erythematosus: a randomised, placebo-controlled, phase 3 trial. *Lancet.* 2011;377:721-731.

A7. Furie R, Khamashta M, Merrill JT, et al. Anifrolumab, an anti-interferon-α receptor monoclonal antibody, in moderate-to-severe systemic lupus erythematosus. *Arthritis Rheumatol.* 2017;69:376-386.

A8. Palmer SC, Tunnicliffe DJ, Singh-Grewal D, et al. Induction and maintenance immunosuppression treatment of proliferative lupus nephritis: a network meta-analysis of randomized trials. *Am J Kidney Dis.* 2017;70:324-336.

A9. Rathi M, Goyal A, Jaryal A, et al. Comparison of low-dose intravenous cyclophosphamide with oral mycophenolate mofetil in the treatment of lupus nephritis. *Kidney Int.* 2016;89:235-242.

A10. Dooley MA, Jayne D, Ginzler EM, et al. Mycophenolate versus azathioprine as maintenance therapy for lupus nephritis. *N Engl J Med.* 2011;365:1886-1895.

A11. Furie R, Petri M, Zamani O, et al. A phase III, randomized, placebo-controlled study of belimumab, a monoclonal antibody that inhibits B lymphocyte stimulator, in patients with systemic lupus erythematosus. *Arthritis Rheum.* 2011;63:3918-3930.

A12. Rovin BH, Furie R, Latinis K, et al. Efficacy and safety of rituximab in patients with active proliferative lupus nephritis. *Arthritis Rheum.* 2012;64:1215-1226.

GENERAL REFERENCES

For the General References and other additional features, please visit Expert Consult at https://expertconsult.inkling.com.

251

SYSTEMIC SCLEROSIS (SCLERODERMA)

JOHN VARGA

TABLE 251-1 CONDITIONS THAT MAY BE ASSOCIATED WITH SCLERODERMA-LIKE SKIN INDURATION

Systemic sclerosis (SSc)
  Limited cutaneous SSc
  Diffuse cutaneous SSc
Localized scleroderma
  Morphea (plaque, guttate, generalized)
  Linear scleroderma, "coup de sabre"
Pansclerotic morphea
Paraneoplastic syndromes
Scleredema and diabetic scleredema
Scleromyxedema (papular mucinosis)
Nephrogenic fibrosing syndrome (nephrogenic systemic fibrosis)
Chronic graft-versus-host disease
Diffuse fasciitis with eosinophilia (Shulman disease, eosinophilic fasciitis)
Eosinophilia-myalgia syndrome
Chemical exposure-associated scleroderma-like conditions
- Vinyl chloride–induced disease, other solvents
- Pentazocine-induced skin fibrosis
- Other drug associations

TABLE 251-2 CLASSIFICATION OF SYSTEMIC SCLEROSIS

CHARACTERISTIC FEATURES	LIMITED CUTANEOUS SYSTEMIC SCLEROSIS	DIFFUSE CUTANEOUS SYSTEMIC SCLEROSIS
Skin induration	Limited to fingers, distal to elbows, face; progression slow	Diffuse: fingers, extremities, face, trunk; progression rapid; tendon friction rubs
Raynaud phenomenon	Precedes skin involvement; often severe; associated with critical ischemia	Onset occurs coincident with or subsequent to skin involvement
Pulmonary fibrosis	Occasional, rarely severe	Frequent, early, can be progressive and severe
Pulmonary arterial hypertension	Frequent, late, may be isolated	Occasional, commonly in association with pulmonary fibrosis
Scleroderma renal crisis	Very rare	Occurs in up to 15%; early
Calcinosis cutis	Frequent, prominent	Infrequent
Characteristic autoantibodies	Anticentromerase	Antitopoisomerase I (Scl-70), anti-RNA polymerase III

DEFINITION

Systemic sclerosis, originally termed *scleroderma,* is a chronic autoimmune disease of unknown cause associated with considerable morbidity and mortality. The disease shows marked clinical heterogeneity, has protean clinical manifestations, and may follow a stable, indolent, or rapidly progressive course.[1] The hallmark of systemic sclerosis is thickening and hardening of the skin (scleroderma), but the lungs, gastrointestinal tract, kidneys, and heart are also affected. In the earliest stages of the disease, evidence of inflammation, autoimmunity, and altered microvascular function are prominent. Over time, progressive and irreversible structural alterations in small blood vessels and fibrosis in multiple organs ensue. There is no cure or approved disease-modifying therapy for systemic sclerosis. Nonetheless, current treatment strategies are frequently effective in controlling symptoms, slowing disease progression, improving quality of life, and prolonging survival. The presence of scleroderma (hard skin) distinguishes systemic sclerosis from other autoimmune and rheumatic diseases, but skin induration also features prominently in localized forms of scleroderma, as well as scleroderma-like conditions, paraneoplastic syndromes, and diverse unrelated disorders (Table 251-1).

Classification
Systemic Sclerosis
A widely used classification for systemic sclerosis divides patients into two subsets: diffuse cutaneous systemic sclerosis and limited cutaneous systemic sclerosis. These two subsets are defined by the pattern of skin involvement, associated clinical and laboratory manifestations, and natural history (Table 251-2). In limited cutaneous systemic sclerosis, skin involvement is restricted to the distal extremities and face. Diffuse cutaneous systemic sclerosis is characterized by skin involvement proximal to the elbows and knees, including the trunk. In patients with limited cutaneous systemic sclerosis, Raynaud phenomenon commonly precedes other disease manifestations, and skin involvement is indolent and limited. In contrast to limited cutaneous systemic sclerosis, diffuse cutaneous systemic sclerosis is generally rapidly progressive and may be complicated by early pulmonary fibrosis, accelerated hypertension, and acute renal failure. The constellation of calcinosis cutis, Raynaud phenomenon, esophageal dysmotility, sclerodactyly (scleroderma of the fingers), and telangiectasia in a subset of patients with limited cutaneous systemic sclerosis is termed *CREST syndrome.* Raynaud phenomenon and other clinical and laboratory findings characteristic of systemic sclerosis in the absence of obvious skin thickening is the hallmark of systemic sclerosis sine scleroderma.

Mixed Connective Tissue Disorder
Mixed connective tissue disorder (MCTD) is an overlap syndrome that is characterized by features of systemic lupus erythematosus, systemic sclerosis, and myositis, all occurring in the same patient. In the early phase, most patients have Raynaud phenomenon in association with edema of the hands and evidence of inflammatory muscle disease. Over time, these patients sequentially manifest other features of connective tissue diseases, including pericarditis, esophageal dysmotility, sclerodactyly, neuropathy, and pulmonary arterial hypertension. Erosive arthritis does not occur. On the other hand, some patients develop acute renal involvement similar to scleroderma renal crisis. In the early stage of this disorder, it can be difficult to predict whether the patient will progress to develop a distinct connective tissue disease such as systemic sclerosis or systemic lupus erythematosus. A diagnostic hallmark of MCTD

is the presence of autoantibody specificity against U1-ribonuclear protein (U1-RNP), often at very high titer. Overall, patients with MCTD generally have a better prognosis than those with systemic sclerosis.

Localized Scleroderma

Localized scleroderma refers to a family of relatively benign skin conditions characterized by discreet areas of skin induration in the absence of Raynaud phenomenon or systemic involvement.[2] Lesional skin is discolored and indurated and histologically may be indistinguishable from systemic sclerosis. Localized scleroderma has multiple distinct forms. When it occurs as single or multiple solitary patches of induration, it is called morphea. When these patches coalesce, the condition is called generalized morphea. The lesions are generally asymmetrical in distribution and spare the digits. Induration may follow in a linear distribution, most commonly on the lower extremities (linear scleroderma). In children, linear scleroderma can be complicated by growth retardation and joint contractures. A rare but severe variant with extensive, disabling, and treatment-resistant skin induration, but lacking significant internal organ involvement, is called pansclerotic morphea.

EPIDEMIOLOGY

Systemic sclerosis is a sporadic disease with a worldwide distribution. It is considered an orphan disease in the United States, with an incidence of 9 to 19 cases per million per year. Like other connective tissue diseases, systemic sclerosis shows a marked female predominance, particularly in the childbearing years. The peak age of onset is 40 to 60 years for both the limited and diffuse cutaneous forms. African Americans have a higher incidence and an earlier age of disease onset compared with whites, and they are more likely to have the diffuse cutaneous form of systemic sclerosis associated with interstitial lung involvement and a worse prognosis.

Etiology and Environmental and Occupational Exposures

Although the cause of systemic sclerosis is unknown, it is commonly ascribed to an interplay between environmental factors and genetic susceptibility. Suspected environmental triggers include occupational, dietary, medical, and lifestyle exposures.

Occupational exposures tentatively linked with systemic sclerosis include silica (in miners), polyvinyl chloride, epoxy resins, and aromatic hydrocarbons including toluene and trichloroethylene. Certain drugs, including bleomycin, pentazocine, hormone replacement therapy, cocaine, and appetite suppressants, have been anecdotally linked with systemic sclerosis or pulmonary arterial hypertension. Although earlier studies implied a possible association of systemic sclerosis with silicone breast implants, large-scale epidemiologic investigations failed to establish an increased risk.

Genetic Factors

A genetic contribution to systemic sclerosis susceptibility is indicated by the fact that 1.6% of patients have a first-degree relative with systemic sclerosis, a prevalence rate substantially higher than in the general population (0.026). Indeed, a family history is the strongest identified risk factor for systemic sclerosis. Moreover, patients with systemic sclerosis are more likely to have first-degree relatives with Raynaud phenomenon and interstitial lung disease, as well as other autoimmune diseases including multiple sclerosis, rheumatoid arthritis, and thyroiditis. Genomewide association and candidate-gene studies have identified significant systemic sclerosis association with multiple human leukocyte antigen (HLA) loci. Associated non-HLA loci include *STAT4*, *IRF4*, *PTPN22*, *TNFAIP3*, *TNIP-1*, *IRAK1*, *CD247*, and *BANK1*, each of which encodes genes involved immune regulation or autoimmunity. Remarkably, most of these risk alleles are not unique for systemic sclerosis, and are also linked with other autoimmune diseases, especially systemic lupus erythematosus.

PATHOBIOLOGY

The protean clinical and pathologic manifestations of systemic sclerosis reflect a complex underlying biology encompassing three interrelated cardinal pathomechanistic processes: autoimmunity and inflammation, vascular injury and obliteration, and fibrosis and excessive matrix accumulation in multiple tissues and organs (Fig. 251-1).

Pathology

The distinguishing pathologic hallmark of systemic sclerosis is the constellation of capillary loss (rarefaction) and obliterative vasculopathy coexisting with fibrosis in most organs. In early-stage disease, perivascular inflammation can be seen even before the appearance of fibrosis. The vascular lesion is characterized by intimal proliferation in the small and medium-sized arteries, resulting in luminal narrowing and obliteration,[3] and is commonly complicated by platelet activation and hypercoagulability. In later-stage systemic sclerosis, fibrosis is prominent in the skin, lungs, gastrointestinal tract, heart, tendon sheath, perifascicular tissue surrounding skeletal muscle, and some endocrine organs such as the thyroid gland. Accumulation of connective tissue rich in fibrillar collagens, fibronectin, cartilage oligomeric matrix protein, and proteoglycans disrupts normal architecture, resulting in functional impairment of affected organs.

In the skin, dermal collagen deposition causes obliteration of the hair follicles, sweat glands, and other adnexae. Fibrosis invades the subjacent adipose layer with entrapment of fat cells (adipocytes) and disappearance of the fat layer. The epidermis is atrophic, and the rete pegs are effaced. In late-stage disease, there is a paucity of vascular and lymphatic endothelium. In the lungs, the interstitium and alveolar spaces are infiltrated with inflammatory cells in early disease. With progression, interstitial fibrosis and vascular damage, often coexisting within the same lesions, dominate the pathologic picture. The most common histologic pattern in systemic sclerosis-associated lung disease is nonspecific interstitial pneumonitis. Progressive thickening of the alveolar septae results in obliteration of the air spaces, honeycombing, and loss of pulmonary blood vessels.

Intimal thickening of small pulmonary arteries (Fig. 251.2), best seen with elastin stain, underlies pulmonary arterial hypertension (Chapter 75). These vascular lesions resemble those of, but are distinct from, idiopathic pulmonary arterial hypertension, but the hallmark plexiform lesions are uncommon in systemic sclerosis.[4] In the gastrointestinal tract, pathologic changes can be found at any level from the mouth to the rectum.[5,6] Fibrosis of the lamina propria and submucosa with atrophy of the muscular layers are prominent in the lower esophagus, whereas striated muscle in the upper third of the esophagus is generally spared (Chapter 129). Replacement of the normal gut architecture leads to disordered peristaltic activity with gastroesophageal reflux and dysmotility, gastroparesis, and small bowel obstruction. Chronic reflux can be complicated by esophageal inflammation, ulcerations, stricture formation, and Barrett metaplasia.

Pathologic changes in the heart are common in systemic sclerosis, with involvement of the myocardium and pericardium.[7] Characteristic microvascular lesions include concentric intimal hypertrophy and luminal narrowing. Contraction band necrosis reflecting ischemia-reperfusion injury is prominent and may be accompanied by patchy myocardial fibrosis. In the kidneys, noninflammatory lesions occur in the interlobular arteries. Scleroderma renal crisis[8] (Chapter 116) is associated with striking changes in small renal arteries, with reduplication of elastic lamina, marked intimal proliferation, and concentric narrowing of the lumen (onion-skin), frequently accompanied by thrombosis and microangiopathic hemolysis.

Tripartite Pathophysiology: Vasculopathy, Immune Dysregulation, and Fibrosis

Vasculopathy

Early vascular injury affects primarily the small and medium-sized arteries and arterioles in multiple vascular beds. The initial vascular endothelial injury might be caused by viruses or other infectious agents, oxygen radicals, circulating cytotoxic factors, complement activation, or autoantibodies. Endothelial cell injury and apoptosis result in altered balance of endothelium-derived vasodilatory (nitric oxide and prostacyclin) and vasoconstricting (endothelin-1) molecules, vascular permeability, and upregulation of adhesion molecules with transendothelial leukocyte diapedesis. Increased reactivity of platelets, activation of intravascular coagulation, defective fibrinolysis, and the resulting thrombosis further compromise vascular function. Small blood vessels show intimal hyperplasia with thickening and reduplication of the basement membrane. In the vascular media, myointimal cells proliferate, whereas the adventitial layers develop fibrosis; the net result is obliteration of capillaries, arterioles, and even large vessels, impaired blood flow and widespread tissue ischemia. Recurrent ischemia-reperfusion is associated with the generation of reactive oxygen species that further damage the endothelium.

Raynaud Phenomenon

The earliest and most common vascular complication of systemic sclerosis is Raynaud phenomenon.[9,10] Raynaud phenomenon (also see Chapter 72) reflects abnormal thermal regulation of blood flow and can precede other disease manifestations by years. Raynaud phenomenon in systemic sclerosis is characterized by autonomic and peripheral nervous system changes leading to impaired production of calcitonin gene–related peptide from sensory afferent

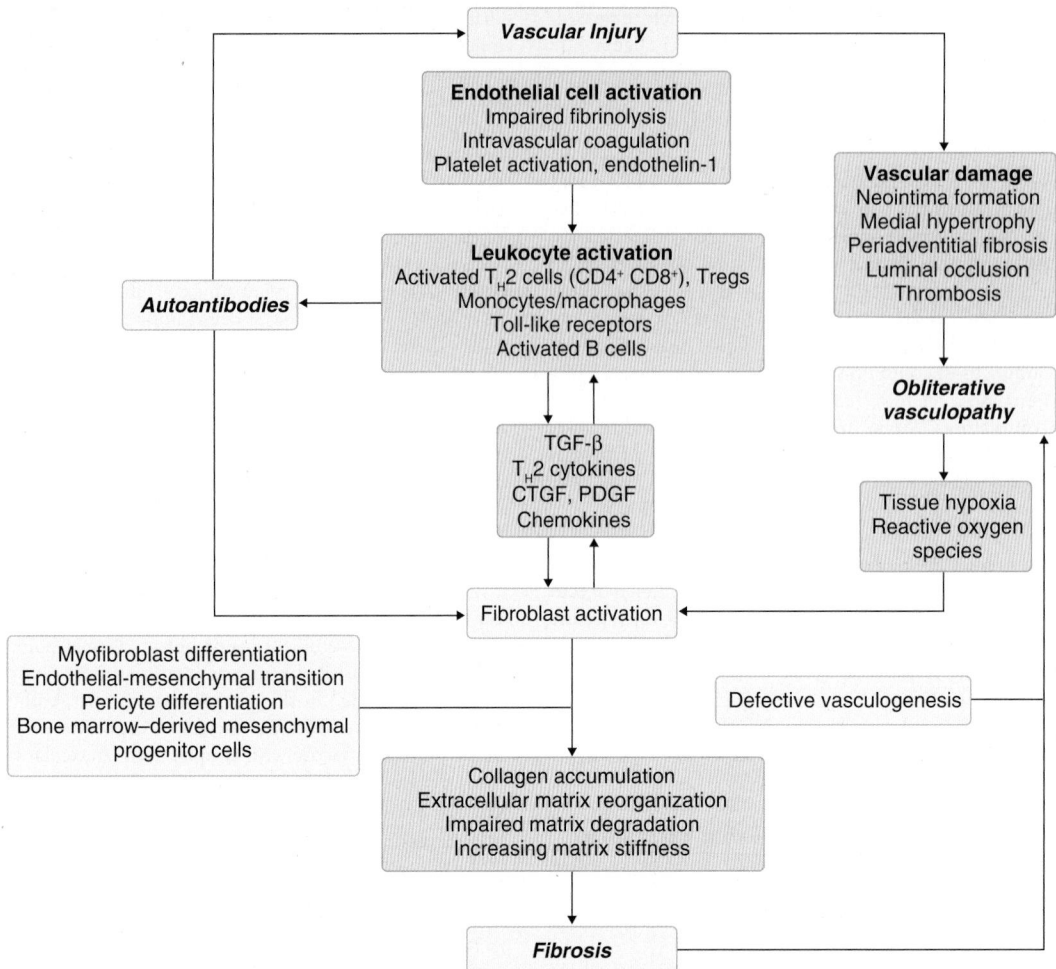

FIGURE 251-1. The tripartite pathogenesis of systemic sclerosis: vasculopathy, autoimmunity, fibrosis. Initial endothelial injury in a genetically susceptible individual is potentially the primary event of disease pathogenesis. Injury leads to vascular damage, inflammation, and autoimmunity. The inflammatory and immune responses generate cytokines and growth factors that initiate fibroblast activation, resulting in matrix remodeling and intractable fibrosis. Vasculopathy, loss of microvasculature, and reduced blood flow result in ischemia and generation of reactive oxygen species that contribute to and further aggravate vascular damage, tissue fibrosis, and atrophy. CTGF = connective tissue growth factor; PDGF = platelet-derived growth factor; TGF-β = transforming growth factor–β.

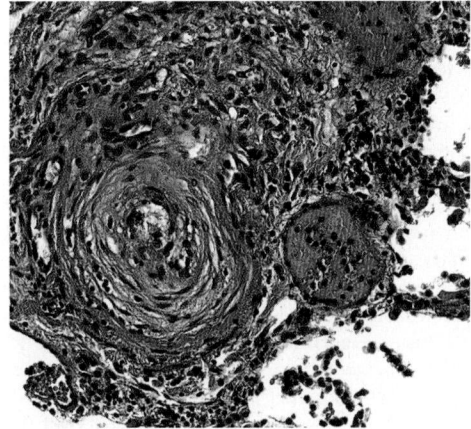

FIGURE 251-2. Pulmonary artery obliterative vasculopathy. Striking intimal hyperplasia and narrowing of the lumen of a small pulmonary artery, coexisting with interstitial pulmonary fibrosis, in a patient with diffuse cutaneous systemic sclerosis.

nerves and heightened sensitivity of α_2-adrenergic receptors on vascular smooth muscle cells. In contrast to *primary* Raynaud phenomenon (called Raynaud disease), which is a common and relatively benign condition, *secondary* Raynaud phenomenon is generally progressive and frequently complicated by vascular remodeling with irreversible structural changes that result in tissue damage.

Inflammation and Autoimmunity
Cellular Immunity
Immune dysregulation is a hallmark systemic sclerosis shares with other autoimmune diseases. In early disease, activated T cells, B cells, dendritic cells and monocyte-macrophages accumulate in lesional tissues.

Infiltrating CD4+ T cells in lesional tissues display restricted TcR receptor signatures indicative of their oligoclonal expansion in response to unknown antigens. T cells show T_H2 polarization with secretion of interleukin (IL)–4, IL-13, and IL-21, and low levels of interferon (IFN)–γ. T_H2 cytokines induce TGF-β and promote the synthesis of collagen and other extracellular matrix molecules.[11] Increased levels of IL-17 detected in the serum suggest a role for T_H17 cells in systemic sclerosis. While the frequency of FOXP3-positive regulatory T cells (Tregs) is elevated, their immunosuppressive function appears to be defective. Myeloid dendritic cells show abnormally high secretion of inflammatory cytokines and chemokines such as CXCL. Macrophages can be prominent in the lesional skin and lungs in early disease and show evidence of alternative activation. Aberrant innate immune responses in dendritic cells and stromal fibroblasts might be triggered and perpetuated by damage-associated nucleic acids and matrix macromolecules via toll-like receptors. Elevated expression of type I interferon-regulated genes (IFN signature) in systemic sclerosis is consistent with innate immune activation and may contribute to vascular injury.

Autoantibodies and B Cells
In addition to antinuclear antibodies that are detected in virtually all patients with systemic sclerosis, a number of highly disease-specific and mutually exclusive autoantibodies occur in systemic sclerosis and have well-established clinical utility in systemic sclerosis as diagnostic and prognostic markers

(Table 251-3). Systemic sclerosis–specific autoantibodies are commonly directed against intracellular proteins, such as topoisomerase-I, centromere, and RNA polymerases I and III. Autoantibodies have been identified in systemic sclerosis that are directed against endothelial cells or recognize cell surface receptors (platelet-derived growth factor receptor [PDGFR], angiotensin II receptor, and endothelin-1 receptor) and might directly contribute to vascular injury or tissue fibrosis. B cells are implicated in mediating both the autoimmune and fibrotic components of systemic sclerosis. In addition to antibody production, B cells also present antigen, produce IL-6 and other profibrotic cytokines, and modulate the function of T cells and dendritic cells.

Fibrosis

Fibrosis of the skin and multiple internal organs distinguishes systemic sclerosis from other rheumatic diseases. Fibrosis is characterized by the accumulation of a collagen-rich and rigid extracellular matrix elaborated by resident fibroblasts and myofibroblasts, and the replacement of normal tissue architecture.

Effector Cells in Fibrosis

Myofibroblasts are smooth muscle cell–like mesenchymal cells with both contractile and biosynthetic properties that normally transiently appear in wounds to promote healing through production of collagen and TGF-β and contraction of the surrounding extracellular matrix. In systemic sclerosis, activated myofibroblasts accumulate in lesional tissue because of one of three pathways: (1) in situ activation of quiescent resident fibroblasts, (2) through transdifferentiation from injured epithelial cells, endothelial cells pericytes, or (3) by migration and terminal differentiation of bone marrow–derived monocytic progenitor cells.

TABLE 251-3 CHARACTERISTIC AUTOANTIBODIES IN SYSTEMIC SCLEROSIS

AUTOANTIBODY (FREQUENCY IN SSc)	SSc SUBSET	CLINICAL ASSOCIATION
Topoisomerase-I (10-40%)	Diffuse cutaneous (less commonly limited)	Tendon friction rubs, ILD, cardiac involvement, scleroderma renal crisis; isolated PAH rare
Centromere (15-40%)	Limited cutaneous	Digital ischemia, calcinosis cutis, isolated PAH, PBC; severe ILD and scleroderma renal crisis rare
RNA polymerase III (4-25%)	Diffuse cutaneous	Extensive skin involvement; tendon friction rubs, scleroderma renal crisis, increased cancer risk
U3-RNP/fibrillarin (1-5%)	Diffuse cutaneous	PAH, ILD, myositis
Th/To (1-7%)	Limited cutaneous	ILD, isolated PAH
PM/Scl (0-6%)	Limited cutaneous	Calcinosis, myositis, arthritis
U1-RNP (5-35%)	MCTD	Severe PAH, myositis

ILD = interstitial lung disease; MCTD = mixed connective tissue disease; PAH = pulmonary arterial hypertension; PBC = primary biliary cirrhosis; SSc = systemic sclerosis.

CLINICAL MANIFESTATIONS

Overview

Multiple organs can be affected in patients with systemic sclerosis, but the relative frequency, tempo, and severity shows considerable patient-to-patient variability. Patients with diffuse cutaneous systemic sclerosis characteristically develop extensive skin induration and joint stiffness associated with early internal organ involvement. In contrast, patients with limited cutaneous systemic sclerosis commonly present with long-standing Raynaud phenomenon, limited skin changes, and insidious progression of internal organ disease. However, many patients defy easy subclassification or show overlap of typical systemic sclerosis features coexisting with clinical and laboratory evidence of another autoimmune disease such as polymyositis, Sjögren syndrome, inflammatory polyarthritis, or systemic lupus erythematosus.[12]

Initial Clinical Presentation
Diffuse Cutaneous Systemic Sclerosis

Patients with diffuse cutaneous systemic sclerosis typically present with soft tissue swelling and puffy fingers, erythema, and pruritus, often accompanied by fatigue, stiffness, muscle weakness, and carpal tunnel syndrome. Raynaud phenomenon may not be present until later in the course of the disease. In the ensuing weeks to months, the inflammatory edematous phase evolves into a chronic "fibrotic" phase with skin induration accompanied by hyperpigmentation, loss of body hair, dry skin, and impaired sweating. Advancing skin changes commonly herald onset of internal organ involvement that is most rapidly progressive during the initial 4 years from disease onset. Thereafter, the risk for new organ involvement subsides.

Limited Cutaneous Systemic Sclerosis

In the case of limited cutaneous systemic sclerosis, the diagnosis is generally made at a later stage of the disease. These patients give a history of long-standing Raynaud phenomenon, sometimes complicated by ischemic ulcerations at the fingertips. Disease course is indolent, with insidious progression of gastroesophageal reflux, mucocutaneous telangiectasia, or calcinosis. Vascular manifestations tend to be more pronounced in limited cutaneous systemic sclerosis compared with diffuse cutaneous systemic sclerosis, whereas scleroderma renal crisis is uncommon.

Organ Involvement
Skin

Skin thickening typically starts in the fingers and is generally preceded by puffy fingers and hands.[13] Skin involvement typically advances in a centripetal pattern from distal extremities. The skin may become hyperpigmented, but dark-skinned individuals may develop vitiligo-like "salt-and-pepper" changes, most prominently on the scalp, upper back, and chest. Obliteration of eccrine and sebaceous glands decreases sweating and oil secretion, causing dry and itchy skin. Facial changes include a beaklike nose, thinning and retraction of the lips, fine wrinkles (radial furrowing) around the mouth, and occasionally a masklike facies due to reduced mobility of the eyelids, cheeks, and mouth (Fig. 251-3). Decreased oral aperture (microstomia) is common and can interfere with eating and oral hygiene.

In long-standing systemic sclerosis, the skin is atrophic and tethered to the subcutaneous tissue. Telangiectasias due to dilation of postcapillary venules in the upper dermis are prominent on the face, hands, lips, and oral mucosa.

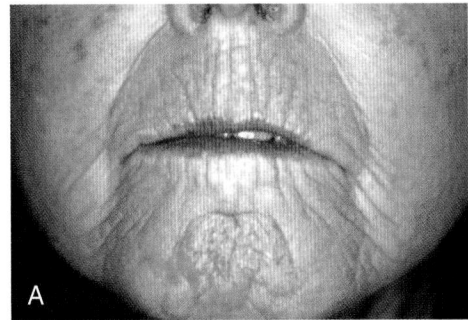
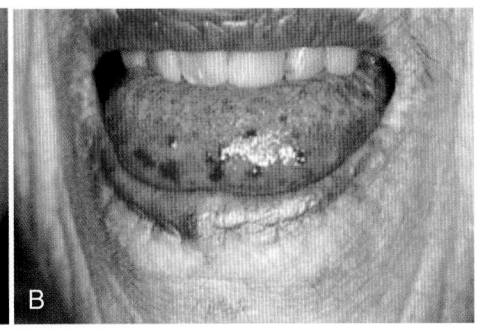

FIGURE 251-3. Facial features in systemic sclerosis. **A,** Perioral furrowing. Note vertical lines around the mouth in a patient with diffuse cutaneous systemic sclerosis. **B,** Telangiectasia on the lips and tongue in a patient with long-standing limited cutaneous systemic sclerosis.

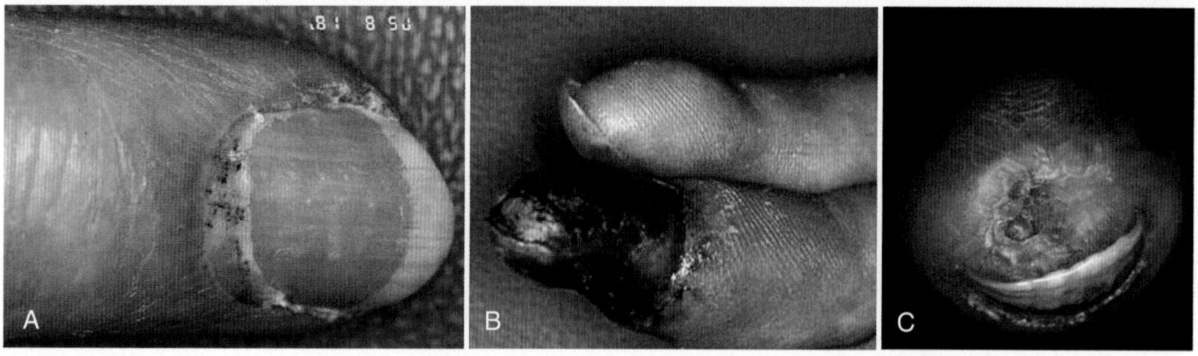

FIGURE 251-4. Vascular complications of systemic sclerosis in the fingers. **A,** Nailfold microvascular changes. **B,** Digital infarction. Sharply demarcated necrosis of the fingertip in a patient with limited cutaneous systemic sclerosis associated with severe Raynaud phenomenon. **C,** Digital tip ulceration and pitting.

Breakdown of atrophic skin leads to painful and nonhealing ulcerations at the extensor surfaces of the interphalangeal joints, fingertips, and bony prominences such as the elbows and malleoli. Ischemic fingertip ulcerations heal slowly, become secondarily infected and give rise to pathognomonic digital tip "pits." Ischemic soft tissue loss at the fingertips is associated with bony resorption of the terminal phalanges (acro-osteolysis) (Fig. 251-4).

Calcinosis of the skin and soft tissues is common. Concrete deposits composed of calcium hydroxyapatite crystals vary in size from tiny punctate lesions to large conglomerate masses. They can be readily visualized on plain radiographs and precisely localized and measured with dual-energy CT imaging (Fig. 251-5).

Frequent locations for calcinosis cutis include the hands (finger pads), extensor surfaces of the forearms, and olecranon and prepatellar bursae. Calcific deposits can ulcerate through the overlying skin, producing drainage of chalky white material, pain, and local inflammation, and may become secondarily infected.

Raynaud Phenomenon

Raynaud phenomenon (Chapter 72) is an episodic vasospastic event in virtually all patients with systemic sclerosis.[14] Typical attacks start with pallor (vasoconstriction) followed by cyanosis (ischemia) and erythema (reperfusion), commonly triggered by exposure to cold or emotional stress. Primary Raynaud phenomenon (called Raynaud disease) is a benign condition representing an exaggerated physiologic response to cold. It occurs in 3 to 5% of the population and is more frequent in women. Secondary Raynaud phenomenon occurs in systemic sclerosis but can also complicate other connective tissue diseases, as well as hematologic and endocrine conditions, and occupational disorders. Raynaud phenomenon also occurs with the use of β-blockers and anticancer drugs such as cisplatin and bleomycin.

Distinguishing primary from secondary Raynaud can present a challenge. Secondary Raynaud typically develops at an older age (>30 years) and tends to be more severe. Nailfold capillaroscopy is a noninvasive bedside method for visualizing cutaneous capillaries using an ophthalmoscope. Patients with primary Raynaud phenomenon have nailfold capillaries that appear as regularly spaced parallel vascular loops, whereas in systemic sclerosis, capillaries are distorted with widened and irregular loops, dilated lumen, areas of vascular "dropout," and microhemorrhages (Fig. 251-4A).

Gastrointestinal Involvement

Gastrointestinal tract involvement is very common in both limited cutaneous systemic sclerosis and diffuse cutaneous systemic sclerosis. A pathologic picture of smooth muscle atrophy and obliterative small vessel vasculopathy with or without fibrosis is seen throughout the length of the gastrointestinal tract, contributing to altered peristaltic activity and consequent complications. Severe intestinal involvement can be associated with malnutrition and has a high mortality.

Upper Gastrointestinal Tract

Oropharyngeal manifestations of systemic sclerosis include xerostomia, reduced oral aperture, periodontal disease, and resorption of the mandibular condyles. The frenulum of the tongue may be shortened. Gastroesophageal reflux is associated with heartburn, regurgitation, and dysphagia; however, in some patients with systemic sclerosis it can also be asymptomatic (Chapter 129). Reduced lower esophageal sphincter pressure frequently coexists with impaired

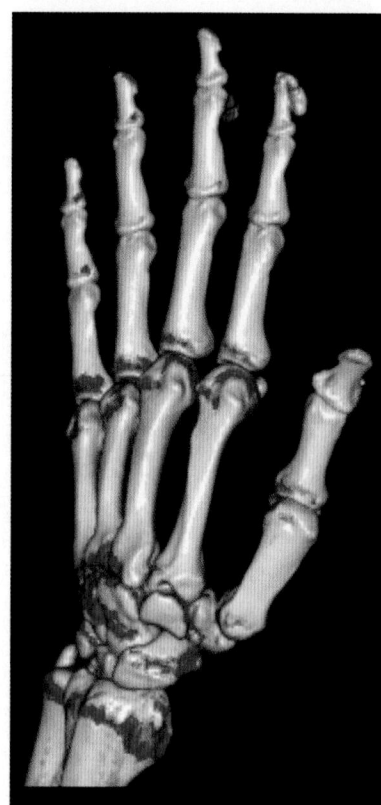

FIGURE 251-5. Calcinosis cutis in systemic sclerosis. Dual-energy CT image of the hand of a 56-year-old woman with long-standing limited cutaneous systemic sclerosis. Note calcification along the distal pulp of the index finger extending focally to the skin. Another calcific deposit along the palmar surface of the long finger middle phalangeal head. (Courtesy of Imran Omar MD.)

esophageal clearance of refluxed gastric contents due to diminished motility in the distal esophagus. Delayed gastric emptying further aggravates the problem. On high-resolution computed tomography (HRCT) of the chest, the esophagus is dilated and shows intraluminal air. Endoscopy may show severe erosive esophagitis in patients with minimal reflux symptoms. Esophageal strictures and Barrett esophagus (Chapter 129) can complicate long-standing reflux. Hoarseness and chronic cough or throat clearing are common and may be extraesophageal manifestations of gastroesophageal reflux disease. Recurrent microaspiration of gastric contents may aggravate underlying interstitial lung disease. A distinct interstitial lung disease called centrilobular fibrosis, associated with esophageal dilation and chronic gastroesophageal reflux, is occasionally seen in systemic sclerosis.

Stomach

Gastroparesis and delayed gastric emptying manifest as early satiety, abdominal distention, and aggravated reflux symptoms. Gastric vascular ectasia or "watermelon stomach" develops in 5% of patients and is more common in those with an anti-RNA Polymerase III antibody. On endoscopy, parallel longitudinal mucosal folds resembling the stripes of a watermelon are seen in the gastric antrum. The histologic features of dilated thrombosed mucosal capillaries and fibromuscular dysplasia of the lamina propria represent the characteristic microangiopathy of systemic sclerosis. Patients with gastric vascular ectasia may have recurrent gastrointestinal bleeding and present with unexplained iron deficiency anemia.

Lower Gastrointestinal Tract

Impaired small bowel motility in systemic sclerosis can cause chronic diarrhea due to bacterial overgrowth. Ensuing fat and protein malabsorption, vitamin B_{12} and D deficiency, and malnutrition are associated with high mortality. Malabsorption is diagnosed by hydrogen breath test or 14C-D-xylose test, and serum prealbumin (transthyretin) is useful for monitoring malnutrition (Chapter 131). Disturbed intestinal motor function can also cause recurrent intestinal pseudo-obstruction with acute abdominal pain, nausea, and vomiting. Differentiating pseudo-obstruction, which responds to supportive care and intravenous supplementation, from mechanical bowel obstruction is a diagnostic challenge. Colonic and anorectal involvement cause constipation, rectal prolapse, and fecal incontinence and is the source of much distress. In late-stage disease wide-mouth colonic sacculations can cause perforation and bleeding. An occasional radiologic finding is pneumatosis cystoides intestinalis due to air trapping in the bowel wall. Rupture of these lesions can cause pneumoperitoneum. Although the liver is rarely affected in systemic sclerosis, primary biliary cirrhosis associated with antimitochondrial antibodies can complicate limited cutaneous systemic sclerosis.

Lung Involvement

There are two major forms of lung involvement in systemic sclerosis: interstitial lung disease and pulmonary arterial hypertension, with many patients developing both. Less frequent pulmonary manifestations include aspiration pneumonitis complicating gastroesophageal reflux, pulmonary hemorrhage, obliterative bronchiolitis, pleural reactions, restrictive ventilatory disease due to chest wall fibrosis, spontaneous pneumothorax, and drug-induced lung toxicity. The incidence of lung cancer, particularly bronchoalveolar carcinoma, is increased.

Interstitial Lung Disease

Interstitial lung disease (Chapter 86) in systemic sclerosis can remain asymptomatic until it is quite advanced.[15] The most frequent presenting symptoms are exertional dyspnea, fatigue, and reduced exercise tolerance. A chronic dry cough may be present. Physical examination may reveal "Velcro" crackles at the lung bases. Pulmonary function testing (Chapter 79) is a commonly used method for detecting early interstitial lung disease but appears to be less sensitive than radiologic imaging using HRCT. The most common pulmonary function abnormalities are reductions in forced vital capacity (FVC) or single breath diffusing capacity (DLCO). However, a reduction in DLCO that is significantly out of proportion to the reduction in FVC (FVC/DLCO ratio >1.6) suggests pulmonary vascular disease.

Evidence of interstitial lung disease can be found in almost all patients with systemic sclerosis and is clinically significant in up to 50%. Risk factors include male sex, African American race, diffuse skin involvement, severe gastroesophageal reflux, and the presence of topoisomerase-I autoantibodies. The most rapid progression in interstitial lung disease occurs within the first 3 years of the onset of the disease.

Plain chest radiography is relatively insensitive for detection of early interstitial lung disease. In contrast, HRCT is highly sensitive (Chapter 78). Prominent HRCT findings in systemic sclerosis include reticular interstitial opacities, predominantly in the lower lobe periphery, in isolation or in combination with ground-glass opacification. Additional findings include mediastinal lymphadenopathy and, rarely, honeycombing. The extent of lung disease on initial HRCT correlates with progression and prognosis of interstitial lung disease and may provide useful information regarding the need for initiating therapy. Bronchoalveolar lavage (Chapter 79) is sometimes indicated for ruling out infection, while lung biopsy is generally indicated only if lung cancer is suspected.

Pulmonary Arterial Hypertension

Approximately 15% of systemic sclerosis patients develop pulmonary hypertension, defined as a mean resting pulmonary arterial pressure of 25 mm Hg or greater, with a pulmonary capillary wedge pressure of 15 mm Hg or less (Chapter 75). In the setting of systemic sclerosis, pulmonary hypertension can be an isolated abnormality (World Health Organization [WHO] group I), or it can coexist with interstitial lung disease (WHO group III). Although the natural history of systemic sclerosis-associated pulmonary hypertension is variable, patients follow a progressive course, with development of right heart failure and increased mortality. Risk factors include limited cutaneous disease, older age of disease onset, severe Raynaud phenomenon, numerous cutaneous telangiectasias, and positivity for anticentromere, U1-RNP, U3-RNP (fibrillarin), Th/To, B23, or β_2-glycoprotein I autoantibodies.

The initial symptoms of pulmonary hypertension are exertional dyspnea and reduced exercise capacity, but early-stage disease is often clinically silent. With progression, angina, syncope, and symptoms and signs of right-sided heart failure develop. Physical examination shows tachypnea, a prominent pulmonic S_2 heart sound, palpable right ventricular heave, elevated jugular venous pressure, and dependent edema. Pulmonary arterial systolic pressures above 40 mm Hg (determined by screening Doppler echocardiography) suggest the presence of pulmonary hypertension, as does an isolated reduction in DLCO or a FVC/DLCO ratio over 1.6. Right heart catheterization is virtually always required for confirming the diagnosis of pulmonary hypertension, assessing its severity, and evaluating ventricular function. The serum levels of N-terminal brain natriuretic peptide (NT-pro-BNP) are elevated in pulmonary hypertension and correlate with severity and survival.

Kidney Involvement

Scleroderma renal crisis is an uncommon but life-threatening acute complication of systemic sclerosis, but chronic and indolent kidney disease also occurs.

Scleroderma Renal Crisis

Scleroderma renal crisis, the most dreaded complication of systemic sclerosis, occurs in 10 to 15% of patients. It almost invariably occurs within 4 years of disease onset.[16] Before the advent of angiotensin-converting enzyme (ACE)–inhibiting drugs in the 1980s, scleroderma renal crisis was invariably fatal, often within weeks. It is thought that vascular injury triggers obliterative vasculopathy and luminal narrowing in the renal arcuate arteries. Progressive reduction in renal blood flow, aggravated by vasospasm, leads to juxtaglomerular hyperplasia and increased renin secretion, with further renal vasoconstriction resulting in a vicious cycle that culminates in accelerated hypertension and oliguric renal failure (Chapters 70 and 116).

Scleroderma renal crisis is a medical emergency. Although patients typically present with abrupt onset of hypertension and progressive renal insufficiency, in some cases the blood pressure remains normal or only modestly elevated. Normotensive renal crisis is associated with a poor outcome. Hypertensive encephalopathy and retinopathy, pericarditis, and arrhythmias may complicate scleroderma renal crisis. Urinalysis shows mild proteinuria, granular casts, and microscopic hematuria. Thrombocytopenia and microangiopathic hemolysis with fragmented red blood cells can sometimes erroneously lead to the diagnosis of thrombotic thrombocytopenic purpura or hemolytic-uremic syndrome (Chapter 163). In many patients, oliguric renal failure develops over a period of weeks. Kidney biopsy can be useful for diagnosis and prognosis, but the characteristic lesions of intimal and medial proliferation and luminal narrowing are indistinguishable from the changes of accelerated hypertension.

In addition to early-stage disease, risk factors for scleroderma renal crisis include rapidly progressive or extensive skin involvement and the presence of tendon friction rubs, African American race, male sex, and positivity for anti-RNA polymerases I and III antibodies. In contrast, the presence of anticentromere antibodies signals a low risk for scleroderma renal crisis. Pericardial effusion, new-onset anemia, and thrombocytopenia may be harbingers of impending scleroderma renal crisis, and a history of recent corticosteroid use is associated with a more than 10-fold increased risk. Accordingly, systemic sclerosis patients with early and progressive cutaneous disease and other risk factors should be counseled to self-monitor their blood pressure daily. In these patients, corticosteroids should be used only when absolutely required and at low doses.

Once scleroderma renal crisis sets in, hospitalization and prompt initiation of short-acting ACE inhibitors is essential. The goal is to achieve adequate blood pressure control before the onset of renal failure. Despite timely intervention, more than half of patients with scleroderma renal crisis require hemodialysis, although some ultimately recover sufficient renal function to be able to discontinue hemodialysis. Oliguria or a serum creatinine level higher than 3 mg/dL at presentation predicts poor outcome. The "prophylactic" use of ACE inhibitors in systemic sclerosis has not been shown to either prevent or improve outcomes in future renal crisis, and therefore its use for this indication is not recommended.

Chronic Kidney Disease

Kidney biopsies in patients with systemic sclerosis commonly show chronic changes including reduplication of elastic fibers, sclerosed glomeruli, tubular atrophy, and interstitial fibrosis. In one study, abnormal renal function or proteinuria was detected in more than one third of patients, none of whom progressed to end-stage renal disease. Rarely, glomerulonephritis associated with lupus serologies or antineutrophil cytoplasmic antibody–positive renal vasculitis occurs.

Cardiac Involvement

Although frequently detected using sensitive diagnostic tools, cardiac involvement in systemic sclerosis is commonly clinically silent.[17] Clinical cardiac involvement is more frequently seen in patients with diffuse cutaneous systemic sclerosis; it generally develops early in the course of the disease and is a poor prognostic factor. The endocardium, myocardium, and pericardium may be affected in isolation or in combination. Clinical manifestations include tachyarrhythmias, conduction abnormalities, valvular regurgitation, diastolic heart failure, and pericardial effusion. Systemic and pulmonary arterial hypertension, as well as lung and renal involvement, also affect the heart. Conventional echocardiography has a low sensitivity for detecting systemic sclerosis-associated heart involvement. In contrast, tissue Doppler echocardiography, single-photon emission computed tomography, and especially cardiac magnetic resonance imaging (cMRI) reveal a high prevalence of myocardial abnormalities in systemic sclerosis. Common findings include abnormal ventricular relaxation and reversible perfusion defects. An elevated level of serum NT-pro-BNP in systemic sclerosis is a sensitive marker for increased pulmonary artery pressure but may also indicate primary cardiac involvement. Myocarditis can develop in association with muscle inflammation. Pericardial effusion develops in more than 15% of patients but is not always clinically significant.

Musculoskeletal Complications

Carpal tunnel syndrome (Chapter 392) may be a presenting manifestation of systemic sclerosis. Joint mobility is progressively impaired, especially in the hands. Large joint contractures can be accompanied by audible or palpable tendon friction rubs that are caused by fibrosis and adhesion of the tendon sheaths and fascial planes at the affected joint. The presence of tendon friction rubs often signals aggressive disease. Frank joint inflammation is uncommon in systemic sclerosis; however, erosive polyarthritis in the hands can occur. Muscle weakness may be a sign of deconditioning, disuse atrophy, and malnutrition. Inflammatory myositis indistinguishable from idiopathic polymyositis (Chapter 253) may be seen, generally in early disease. A noninflammatory myopathy characterized by atrophy and fibrosis in the absence of elevated muscle enzyme levels is common in late disease. Bone resorption affects the distal tufts of terminal phalanges (acro-osteolysis), mandibular condyles, ribs, and distal clavicles.

Other Clinical Manifestations

In addition to microangiopathy, involvement of larger blood vessels (>100 μm) can occur in systemic sclerosis. Manifestations include occlusion of the digital and ulnar arteries, leading to ischemic ulcerations and even loss of digits or limbs. Epidemiologic studies indicate increased risk of coronary artery disease in patients with systemic sclerosis. Dry eyes and dry mouth are common in systemic sclerosis, but in contrast to Sjögren syndrome (Chapter 252), salivary gland biopsy in such cases shows fibrosis rather than focal lymphocytic infiltration. Hypothyroidism due to thyroid fibrosis is common and may be associated with antithyroid autoantibodies. Although the central nervous system is generally spared in systemic sclerosis, autonomic neuropathy, as well as a primarily sensory neuropathy of the trigeminal nerve due to fibrosis or vasculopathy, can occur. Pregnancy in women with active systemic sclerosis has been associated with an increased rate of adverse fetal outcomes. Furthermore, cardiopulmonary involvement might worsen during pregnancy, and scleroderma renal crisis can occur. Inability to attain or maintain penile erection due to vascular insufficiency and fibrosis is frequent and may be the presenting disease manifestation in males with systemic sclerosis.

Systemic Sclerosis and Cancer

Patients with systemic sclerosis have an increased risk of cancer.[18] In these patients, lung cancer and esophageal adenocarcinoma typically occur in the setting of long-standing interstitial lung disease or gastroesophageal reflux disease, and chronic inflammation and tissue damage may be contributing factors. In contrast, breast, lung, and ovarian carcinoma and lymphoma in systemic sclerosis tend to occur in close temporal association with the onset

of systemic sclerosis and are often associated with anti-RNA polymerase III antibodies. In these cases, systemic sclerosis might represent a paraneoplastic syndrome that is triggered by the antitumor immune response.

DIAGNOSIS

Skin induration in the fingers or proximally (associated with Raynaud phenomenon) and characteristic visceral organ manifestations are usually sufficient to establish the diagnosis of systemic sclerosis, although these features may be absent in patients with early disease. Standardized criteria for the diagnosis of systemic sclerosis have been developed and validated and show high degree of specificity and sensitivity. Rarely, diagnostic full-thickness skin biopsy is required for ruling out scleroderma mimics such as scleredema, scleromyxedema, or pansclerotic morphea (see Table 251-1). Primary Raynaud (disease) is differentiated from systemic sclerosis by normal-appearing nailfold capillaries and absence of autoantibodies. Diagnosing systemic sclerosis can be difficult in the early stages of the disease because initial symptoms and findings are often nonspecific and can be mistaken for rheumatoid arthritis, systemic lupus erythematosus, myositis, or undifferentiated connective tissue disease. Occasional patients with systemic sclerosis present with accelerated hypertension or gastrointestinal bleeding caused by watermelon stomach as the initial disease manifestation, which poses diagnostic challenges.

Laboratory Features

Anemia is commonly seen in patients with systemic sclerosis; it may reflect chronic inflammation, gastrointestinal bleeding from gastric vascular ectasia, erosive gastritis or chronic esophagitis, or folate and vitamin B_{12} deficiency due to small bowel bacterial overgrowth and malabsorption. Microangiopathic hemolytic anemia (Chapter 151) caused by mechanical trauma and red blood cell fragmentation in the damaged microvasculature is a laboratory hallmark of scleroderma renal crisis. In contrast to other connective tissue diseases, the erythrocyte sedimentation rate and C-reactive protein generally show only modest elevation. Monitoring serum levels of prealbumin and vitamin K is useful in patients with small bowel bacterial overgrowth and malabsorption.

Antinuclear autoantibodies are present in virtually all patients with systemic sclerosis and can be detected at, or even before, disease onset. Autoantibodies specific for systemic sclerosis are described in Table 251-3. Anticentromere antibodies are associated with pulmonary hypertension, whereas significant cardiac involvement, pulmonary fibrosis, or scleroderma renal crisis occurs only rarely in these patients. Topoisomerase-I antibody positivity is associated with pulmonary fibrosis and reduced survival, whereas anticentromere antibody–positive patients have improved survival compared with those without this antibody. Antibodies to RNA polymerase III are associated with increased risk for scleroderma renal crisis. Antibodies to β_2-glycoprotein I are not specific but in systemic sclerosis identify increased risk for critical ischemia.

TREATMENT AND PREVENTION   Rx

With the exception of ACE inhibitors used for scleroderma renal crisis, no therapy to date has been shown to significantly alter the natural history of systemic sclerosis, and none have been approved specifically for this indication. In contrast, organ-based treatments are commonly effective in alleviating symptoms and slowing progression of the cumulative organ damage. Treatment must be tailored to each patient's unique needs.[19] Because of the marked variability in clinical presentation, a thorough and individualized baseline evaluation is paramount. Optimal management should be guided by the following principles: prompt diagnosis, accurate classification and risk stratification, early recognition and assessment of organ-based complications, and long-term monitoring of progression, disease activity, and response to therapy. Management of disease complications should be proactive, with regular screening and initiation of appropriate intervention at the earliest possible opportunity. Given the multisystemic nature of systemic sclerosis, an integrated team-based management approach, typically at specialized medical centers, is most desirable. The team should incorporate appropriate medical specialists and facilitate coordinated holistic care of the patient.

Disease-Modifying Therapy
Immunosuppressive Agents

Immunosuppressive agents, often highly effective in other connective tissue diseases, have generally shown modest or no benefit in systemic sclerosis. Corticosteroids alleviate stiffness, fatigue, and aching in early-stage disease, but do not slow disease progression and are associated with an increased risk for scleroderma renal crisis. Therefore corticosteroids should be avoided if possible; when absolutely necessary, they should be given at the lowest dose possible and for brief periods only.

Cyclophosphamide was shown to reduce the progression of symptomatic interstitial lung disease in early systemic sclerosis.[A1] Compared with placebo, patients treated with oral cyclophosphamide showed stabilization and, rarely, modest improvement in respiratory symptoms, pulmonary function, and abnormalities on chest HRCT after 1 year of treatment, but these benefits were short-lived. The use of cyclophosphamide in systemic sclerosis needs to be balanced against its potential for side effects, including bone marrow suppression, opportunistic infections, hemorrhagic cystitis, bladder cancer, and premature ovarian failure. Rituximab is an equally effective and safe alternative.[A2]

In small clinical trials, methotrexate was associated with a modest improvement in skin involvement. Mycophenolate mofetil was shown to improve skin involvement and stabilize lung disease as well as cyclophosphamide, and it was well tolerated in a randomized controlled clinical trial.[A3] There is some support in the literature for the use of immunomodulatory agents including, tocilizumab, intravenous immunoglobulin, and extracorporeal photopheresis for the treatment of systemic sclerosis. Recent reports suggest that rituximab might be effective in ameliorating skin and lung involvement.

In patients with severe systemic sclerosis who fail to respond to other treatments (Chapter 168), autologous hematopoietic stem cell transplantation improves long-term, event-free survival despite an increased treatment-related mortality in the first year.[A4] More recently, adults with severe systemic sclerosis were randomized to undergo myeloablative autologous hematopoietic stem cell transplantation (36 patients) or to receive cyclophosphamide immunosuppression by means of 12 monthly infusions (39 patients). The rate of event-free survival at 54 months was 79% in the transplantation group and 50% in the cyclophosphamide group (P = 0.02); at 72 months it was 74% versus 47% (P = 0.03). Overall survival at 72 months also favored transplantation (86% vs. 51%, P = 0.02). Treatment-related mortality in the transplantation group was 3% at 54 months and 6% at 72 months, compared with 0% in the cyclophosphamide group.[A5] Because of potential morbidity and mortality and its substantial cost, hematopoietic stem cell transplantation is presently considered only for carefully selected systemic sclerosis patients with aggressive or treatment-unresponsive disease.

Antifibrotic Therapy

Because tissue fibrosis causes progressive and irreversible organ damage, drugs that block or slow the fibrotic process represent a rational approach to therapy. To date, however, no antifibrotic drug has been shown to be effective in modifying disease course in SSc. D-Penicillamine has been extensively used as an antifibrotic agent. However, in a randomized controlled clinical trial, there was no difference in the extent of skin involvement between patients treated with standard-dose (750 mg/day) or very low-dose (125 mg every other day) D-penicillamine. Minocycline, bosentan, relaxin, interferon-γ, and inhibitors of tumor necrosis factor are putative antifibrotic agents that have failed to show meaningful benefit in systemic sclerosis clinical trials. Small-molecule tyrosine kinase inhibitors used in malignancies (e.g., imatinib, nilotinib, and dasatinib) block signaling by TGF-β and PDGF and thereby prevent fibrotic responses in vitro and in vivo.[17] Antifibrotic drugs that had been recently approved for the treatment of idiopathic pulmonary fibrosis (nintedanib and pirfenidone) may have a role in the treatment of systemic sclerosis-associated interstitial lung disease. These two drugs are currently in clinical trials for this indication.

Treatment of Organ-Specific Complications

Gastrointestinal Complications

Because significant gastroesophageal reflux may be asymptomatic, all patients with systemic sclerosis should be treated for this complication. Proton pump inhibitors may need to be given in relatively high doses and for prolonged periods, and patients should be instructed to elevate the head of the bed and eat frequent small meals. Recurrent gastrointestinal bleeding due to gastric vascular ectasia can be treated with laser or argon plasma photocoagulation. Bacterial overgrowth due to small bowel hypomotility causes bloating and diarrhea and may lead to malabsorption, weight loss, and malnutrition. Treatment with short courses of rotating broad-spectrum antibiotics such as metronidazole, erythromycin, and tetracycline can sometimes eradicate bacterial overgrowth. However, many patients relapse when antibiotics are stopped. In patients with malnutrition but intact small bowel function, enteral nutrition via a jejunostomy can be effective. In others, total parenteral nutrition may be indicated. Refractory hypomotility of the small bowel may respond to subcutaneous octreotide injections. Anorectal complications may respond to sacral neuromodulation.

Vascular Therapy and Raynaud Phenomenon

The goal of vascular therapy in systemic sclerosis is to reduce the frequency and duration of vasospastic episodes, prevent ischemic complications, and enhance their healing, and slow the progression of obliterative vasculopathy. Patients should dress warmly, minimize cold exposure, and avoid drugs that could precipitate or exacerbate vasospastic episodes. Calcium-channel blockers such as nifedipine and diltiazem are used commonly for Raynaud phenomenon but show only moderate benefit, and their use is often limited by side effects (palpitations, dependent edema, lightheadedness). Angiotensin II receptor blockers such as losartan are effective and generally well tolerated. Patients with severe Raynaud phenomenon require α_1-adrenergic receptor blockers (e.g., prazosin), 5-phosphodiesterase inhibitors (e.g., sildenafil), topical nitroglycerine, intradigital botulin toxin injections, or intravenous prostaglandins. Low-dose aspirin and dipyridamole prevent platelet activation and may have a role as adjunctive agents but must be used with caution in light of the risk of bleeding from gastric vascular ectasia lesions.

The endothelin-1 receptor antagonist bosentan reduces development of new ischemic ulcers,[A6] and sildenafil may promote ulcer healing.[A7] Patients with ischemic digital ulcerations may require surgical débridement, especially if necrotic tissue is present. Empirical long-term therapy with statins and antioxidants may slow the progression of vascular damage.

Pulmonary Arterial Hypertension

All patients with systemic sclerosis should be screened for pulmonary hypertension at initial evaluation, and those at high risk on a yearly basis. Treatment for symptomatic pulmonary hypertension should be started with an endothelin-1 receptor antagonist or a 5-phosphodiesterase inhibitor. Diuretics, oral anticoagulation, and digoxin, and supplemental oxygen, may be used when appropriate. If clinical response is inadequate, 5-phosphodiesterase inhibitors may be used in combination with endothelin-1 receptor antagonists. Prostacyclin analogs can be administered intravenously, by continuous subcutaneous infusion, or by frequent inhalations. Lung transplantation remains an option for selected patients with systemic sclerosis–associated pulmonary hypertension or interstitial lung disease who fail medical therapy.

Treatment and Prevention of Scleroderma Renal Crisis

Prompt recognition of impending or early scleroderma renal crisis is essential. Because patients with early-stage systemic sclerosis and progressive skin involvement are at highest risk, they should be instructed to monitor their blood pressure daily and report significant alterations immediately. Corticosteroids should be used only when absolutely necessary and at the lowest possible doses. When scleroderma renal crisis occurs, patients should be hospitalized and treatment with short-acting ACE inhibitors started immediately to achieve prompt blood pressure normalization. There is no evidence that "prophylactic" use of ACE inhibitors can prevent the development of scleroderma renal crisis or ameliorate its severity. Although up to two thirds of patients who develop renal crisis require dialysis, delayed recovery of renal function can occur. Kidney transplantation is appropriate for patients unable to discontinue dialysis after 2 years. Survival with renal transplantation in systemic sclerosis is comparable to that in other connective tissue diseases, and recurrence of scleroderma renal crisis in the kidney graft is rare.

Skin Care

Skin involvement in early systemic sclerosis is inflammatory and may respond to systemic antihistamines or short-term low-dose corticosteroids. Because of the increased risk for scleroderma renal crisis, blood pressure should be carefully monitored. Cyclophosphamide, methotrexate, D-penicillamine, and mycophenolate have been associated with modest improvement in skin induration in early-stage systemic sclerosis.[20] Skin dryness can be managed with the use of hydrophilic ointments and emollient bath oils. Fingertip ulcerations should be protected by occlusive dressing to promote healing and prevent infection. Infected skin ulcers are treated with topical or oral antibiotics and may necessitate surgical débridement. No medical therapy has been shown to be effective in preventing soft tissue calcification or in promoting its dissolution, and surgical therapy and lithotripsy are only occasionally effective.

PROGNOSIS AND NATURAL HISTORY

Patients with diffuse cutaneous systemic sclerosis have a more rapidly progressive disease course, greater internal organ involvement, and generally worse prognosis compared with those with limited cutaneous systemic sclerosis. However, the outcome of the disease is difficult to predict.

Early inflammatory symptoms of diffuse cutaneous systemic sclerosis such as fatigue, edema, arthralgia, and pruritus commonly subside after 2 to 4 years. Skin thickening typically reaches a plateau, followed by slow regression, which characteristically occurs in an order that is the reverse of initial involvement, with softening on the trunk followed by proximal and finally the distal extremities. Sclerodactyly and finger contractures generally fail to resolve. Relapse or recurrence of skin thickening may occur. Visceral organ involvement develops and progresses most rapidly during the initial 2 to 4 years of the disease. New organ involvement rarely occurs once the skin involvement has reached a plateau. Similarly, scleroderma renal crisis almost invariably occurs within the first 4 years of disease. In patients with limited cutaneous systemic sclerosis, Raynaud phenomenon may precede other disease manifestations by years or even decades, and visceral organ complications such as pulmonary hypertension and primary biliary cirrhosis generally occur late in the course of the disease.

Age- and gender-adjusted standardized mortality ratios (SMRs) in patients with systemic sclerosis have ranged from 1.05 to 5.40 across studies, but an overall SMR of 2.72 higher than in the general population has been determined.[21] The 10-year survival rate is 55% for patients with diffuse cutaneous systemic sclerosis and 75% for patients with limited cutaneous systemic sclerosis. Survival correlates with the extent of skin involvement, which represents a surrogate for visceral organ involvement. The leading causes of death are pulmonary fibrosis, pulmonary hypertension, renal and severe gastrointestinal involvement, and cardiac disease. Markers of poor prognosis include male sex, African American race, older age of disease onset, low body mass index, extensive skin thickening with truncal involvement, and evidence of significant or progressive visceral organ involvement. Autoantibodies to topoisomerase-I or absence of anticentromere antibodies are markers of poor prognosis. In one study, systemic sclerosis patients who had extensive skin involvement, vital capacity less than 55% of predicted, significant gastrointestinal involvement, and clinically evident cardiac involvement or scleroderma renal crisis had a less than 40% 10-year survival. The severity of pulmonary hypertension is correlated with mortality, and systemic sclerosis patients with a mean pulmonary arterial pressure of 45 mm Hg or higher had a 33% 3-year survival rate. In scleroderma renal crisis, therapy with ACE inhibitors has had a dramatic effect on survival, increasing from less than 10% at 1 year in the pre-ACE inhibitor era to better than 70% 3-year survival at the present time.

The topic of immunoglobulin (Ig)G4–related disease is discussed in Chapter 259.

Grade A References

A1. Barnes H, Holland AE, Westall GP, et al. Cyclophosphamide for connective tissue disease-associated interstitial lung disease. *Cochrane Database Syst Rev.* 2018;1:CD010908.

A2. Sircar G, Goswami RP, Sircar D, et al. Intravenous cyclophosphamide vs rituximab for the treatment of early diffuse scleroderma lung disease: open label, randomized, controlled trial. *Rheumatology (Oxford).* 2018;57:2106-2113.

A3. Tashkin DP, Roth MD, Clements PJ, et al. Mycophenolate mofetil versus oral cyclophosphamide in scleroderma-related interstitial lung disease (SLS II): a randomised controlled, double-blind, parallel group trial. *Lancet Respir Med.* 2016;4:708-719.

A4. van Laar JM, Farge D, Sont JK, et al. Autologous hematopoietic stem cell transplantation vs intravenous pulse cyclophosphamide in diffuse cutaneous systemic sclerosis: a randomized clinical trial. *JAMA.* 2014;311:2490-2498.

A5. Sullivan KM, Goldmuntz EA, Keyes-Elstein L, et al. SCOT study investigators. Myeloablative autologous stem-cell transplantation in severe scleroderma. *N Engl J Med.* 2018;378:35-47.

A6. Matucci-Cerinic M, Denton CP, Furst DE, et al. Bosentan treatment of digital ulcers related to systemic sclerosis: results from the RAPIDS-2 randomised, double-blind, placebo-controlled trial. *Ann Rheum Dis.* 2011;70:32-38.

A7. Hachulla E, Hatron PY, Carpentier P, et al. Efficacy of sildenafil on ischaemic digital ulcer healing in systemic sclerosis: the placebo-controlled SEDUCE study. *Ann Rheum Dis.* 2016;75:1009-1015.

GENERAL REFERENCES

For the General References and other additional features, please visit Expert Consult at https://expertconsult.inkling.com.

252

SJÖGREN SYNDROME

XAVIER MARIETTE AND GAETANE NOCTURNE

DEFINITION

Sjögren syndrome is a systemic autoimmune disease characterized by lymphocytic infiltrates of salivary and tear glands, leading to oral and ocular dryness, and by autoantibody secretion. It can be encountered either alone (primary Sjögren syndrome) or in the presence of other systemic autoimmune diseases (secondary Sjögren syndrome) like rheumatoid arthritis, systemic lupus erythematosus, inflammatory myositis, and systemic sclerosis.[1] Sjögren syndrome in the setting of rheumatoid arthritis usually follows the diagnosis of rheumatoid arthritis by many years and is mainly manifested by keratoconjunctivitis sicca, with systemic features being rather uncommon. Associated with other systemic autoimmune disease, the presentation of secondary Sjögren syndrome closely resembles that of primary Sjögren syndrome.

EPIDEMIOLOGY

Primary Sjögren syndrome is a common disease that affects 0.1 to 0.6% of the general adult female population.[2,3] A higher prevalence of the disease has been reported (0.5 to 2%), but this must be considered with caution because the reported prevalence of Sjögren syndrome depends on the classification criteria used in the various studies, and the prevalence of sicca symptoms in the general population is high. Conversely, in recent studies with strict criteria, a lower prevalence has been found: 1.02 per 10,000 adults.[4] Primary Sjögren syndrome has a female preponderance (female-to-male ratio at least 9 : 1). The age peak of the disease occurs after menopause in the mid-50s.

PATHOPHYSIOLOGY

Recent years have witnessed major advances in the pathophysiologic mechanisms of the disease. Several studies have confirmed the role of innate immunity, genetics, and B-cell activation and the relation between abnormalities in them.

The presence of an interferon (IFN) signature (the expression of type 1 IFN–inducible genes) has been shown both in salivary glands and blood. Plasmacytoid dendritic cells, the professional cells secreting type 1 IFN, are present within the glands. Type 2 IFN–dependent genes can be overexpressed in salivary glands. Natural killer (NK) cells, another actor of innate immunity able to secrete type 2 IFN, are present in salivary glands of patients and play a role in the disease.

In line with this IFN signature, multiple viral agents have been incriminated as etiologic factors for either the development or the modulation of Sjögren syndrome; these include Epstein-Barr virus, retroviruses, and coxsackieviruses, but in all cases the data remain controversial.

The genetics of primary Sjögren syndrome[5] are now better understood with the reports of two genome-wide association studies (GWASs). Like in other systemic autoimmune diseases, human leukocyte antigen (HLA) is the most important region associated with the disease, especially HLA-DR3-DQ1 in patients with autoantibodies.

Other genes associated with the disease are involved in the IFN response. These include IFN regulatory factor 5 (*IRF5*), a pivotal transcription factor in the type 1 IFN pathway; signal transducer and activator of transcription 4 (*STAT4*); and *IL12A*, involved in the type 2 IFN pathway. Other genes found to be associated with the disease are *TNIP1*, playing a role in control of nuclear factor (NF)-κB activation, and *CXCR5*, involved in germinal center formation.

The presence of ectopic salivary gland germinal centers demonstrates the importance of B-cell activation in primary Sjögren syndrome. Different cytokines may explain this B-cell activation. Several studies have focused on the role of BAFF (B-cell activating factor of the tumor necrosis factor [TNF] family), a cytokine that promotes B-cell maturation, proliferation, and survival. It has been shown that BAFF is enhanced in sera and in salivary glands from primary Sjögren syndrome patients. Interestingly, BAFF can be secreted by salivary gland epithelial cells, the target of autoimmunity, after stimulation by the innate immune system (type 1 or type 2 IFN, or viral infections). Thus, this cytokine is likely to be a link between innate immunity and autoimmunity.

The current hypothetical scenario for the development of primary Sjögren syndrome is based on the successive activation of innate and adaptive immune systems (Fig. 252-1). Environmental factors such as viral infections or hormonal imbalance may act at the initial stage of the disease by activating epithelial cells. This epithelial cell activation is promoted in patients who carry susceptibility factors in the genes for IFN pathway proteins. These patients experience a greater degree of IFN pathway activation, which leads to BAFF overproduction, B- and T-cell activation,[6] and secretion of autoantibodies, especially in predisposed patients. These autoantibodies constitute immune complexes that participate in the maintenance of IFN-α production. Altogether, these steps promote a vicious cycle of immune system activation leading to tissue damage.

CLINICAL MANIFESTATIONS
Glandular

Decreased salivary secretion results in mouth dryness and increased incidence of oral infections, mucosal friability, and dental caries due to loss of the lubricating, buffering, and antimicrobial capacities of saliva.[7,8] Fungal infections (primarily candidiasis) are also common. Parotid salivary gland or other major salivary gland enlargement can also occur. Persistent enlargement should be carefully followed, however, to exclude bacterial superinfection and, more important, the development of lymphoma.

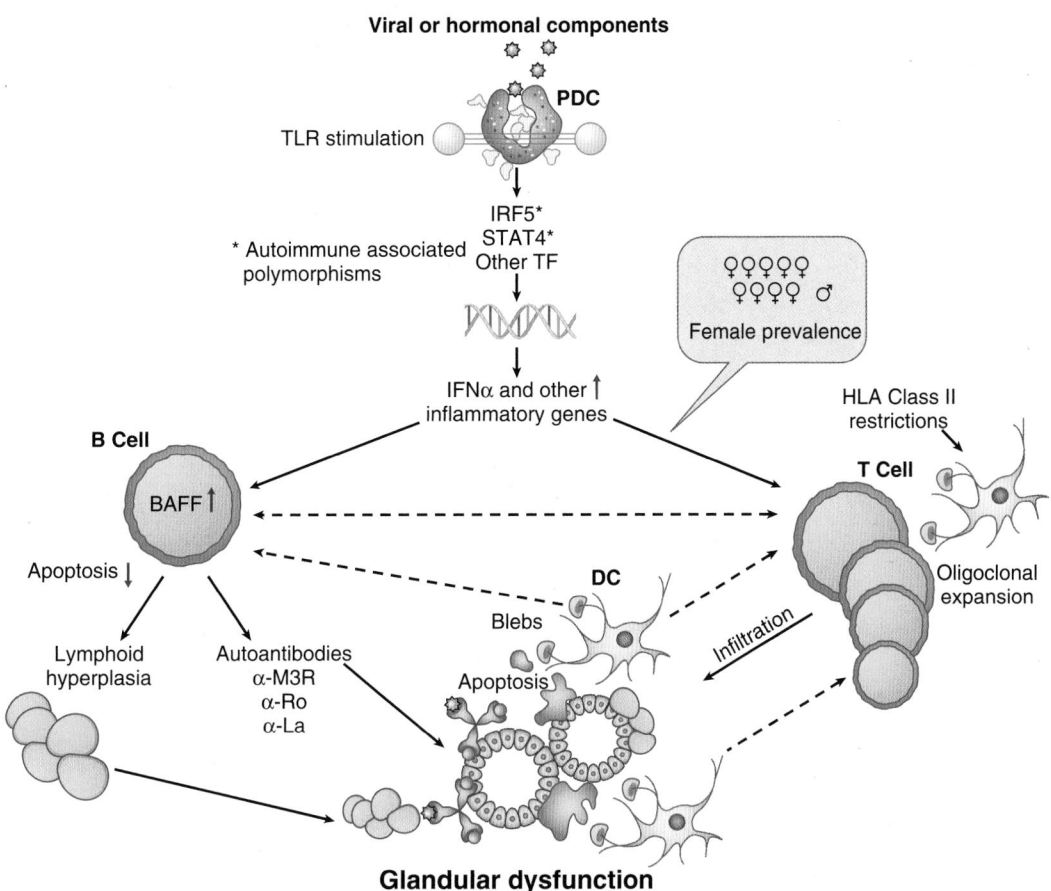

FIGURE 252-1. Hypothetical scenario for development of primary Sjögren syndrome. An environmental factor (e.g., virus) causes epithelial cell and dendritic cell (DC) activation. Plasmacytoid DCs are also activated by immune complexes, promoting interferon (IFN) pathway activation, which leads to BAFF overproduction and to B- and T-cell activation. B-cell activation leads to autoantibody production within germinal center–like structures. Interleukin-12 secreted by myeloid DCs leads to natural killer cell and helper T-cell type 1 activation, which promotes tissue damage and IFN-γ production. IFN-α and IFN-γ enhance BAFF secretion. Epithelial cells release autoantigens that participate in immune complex formation and perpetuate the vicious cycle of immune system overactivation. BAFF = B-cell activating factor of the tumor necrosis factor family; IRF5 = interferon regulatory factor 5; PDC = plasmacytoid dendritic cell; STAT4 = signal transducer and activator of transcription 4; TF = transcription factors; TLR = toll-like receptors.

Decreased lacrimal flow and impaired lacrimal composition lead to damage of the corneal and conjunctival epithelia, a condition known as keratoconjunctivitis sicca. As a result of keratoconjunctivitis sicca, Sjögren syndrome patients might experience foreign-body sensation, grittiness, irritation, photosensitivity, and thick rope-like secretions at the inner canthus, all leading to increased discomfort and possibly visual impairment, with considerable functional disability. Furthermore, ocular complications include corneal ulceration and scarring, bacterial keratitis, and eyelid infections that require continuous ophthalmologic care and treatment.

Systemic

In addition to the sicca features, systemic manifestations occur in approximately 20 to 30% of primary Sjögren syndrome patients.[9,10] Of note, it has been increasingly appreciated that the extraglandular manifestations in Sjögren syndrome can be divided into two major types according to the underlying pathophysiologic mechanism. Thus, lymphocytic infiltration of the epithelia of organs beyond the exocrine glands (e.g., renal, liver, and bronchial epithelial cells) results in interstitial nephritis, autoimmune cholangitis, and obstructive bronchiolitis, respectively. These clinical features appear early and usually have a benign course. On the other hand, immune complex deposition as a result of the ongoing B-cell hyperreactivity can give rise to the extraepithelial manifestations—palpable purpura, glomerulonephritis, interstitial pneumonitis, and peripheral neuropathy—that are linked to increased morbidity and risk for lymphoma development. The main systemic manifestations are listed in Table 252-1. Peripheral neuropathy may occur through various mechanisms. Vasculitis may be present with cryoglobulinemia, leading to both sensory and motor symptoms. More frequently, pure sensory neuropathy is present, sometimes purely ataxic and sometimes in the form of small-fiber neuropathy. This latter entity is difficult to diagnose because clinical and electromyographic examinations are normal. The diagnosis may be made by skin biopsy showing rarefaction of sensory small fibers.

Sjögren Syndrome and Non-Hodgkin Lymphomas

Chronic polyclonal B-cell activation is commonly present in primary Sjögren syndrome, which may explain why this autoimmune disease has the strongest association with the development of B-cell lymphoma (relative risk, 15 to 20). More recent studies have estimated this risk at a lower level: 6 in Denmark and Sweden, 7 in Taiwan, and 9 in Norway.

Lymphomas complicating primary Sjögren syndrome have specific features (Chapter 176).[11,12] They are mostly B-cell non-Hodgkin lymphomas with a predominance of low-grade, marginal-zone histologic type. Mucosal localization is predominant, notably as mucosa-associated lymphoid tissue (MALT) lymphomas. Interestingly, lymphomas often develop in organs where primary Sjögren syndrome is active, such as salivary glands.

In the setting of Sjögren syndrome, chronic autoimmune B-cell activation plays the major role in the lymphomagenesis process, and the identified predictors of lymphoma development in primary Sjögren syndrome are in line with this phenomenon. The main clinical predictors are permanent swelling of salivary glands, splenomegaly, lymphadenopathy, and palpable purpura. The main biologic predictors are positivity of rheumatoid factor (RF), cryoglobulinemia, lymphopenia (especially CD4 lymphopenia), low complement levels, and a monoclonal component in serum or urine. Three novel predictive factors for lymphoma development have been recently described: (1) the presence of ectopic germinal centers associated with the occurrence of lymphoma in primary Sjögren syndrome patients; (2) demonstration that BAFF levels are increased in primary Sjögren syndrome patients with current or previous lymphoma compared with patients without lymphoma; and (3) abnormalities of the gene *TNFAIP3* coding for the A20 protein that regulates NF-κB activation, found in up to 77% of MALT lymphomas complicating primary Sjögren syndrome. In half of the cases, *TNFAIP3* mutations or deletions occur within lymphoma cells; in the other 50%, they involve germline *TNFAIP3* mutations with functional consequences.

TABLE 252-1 EXTRAGLANDULAR MANIFESTATIONS OF PRIMARY SJÖGREN SYNDROME

CONSTITUTIONAL SYMPTOMS

Fatigue
Low-grade fever

SKIN AND VASCULAR

Small vessel vasculitis
Palpable purpura
Raynaud phenomenon
Photosensitivity reactions similar to subacute cutaneous systemic lupus
    erythematosus
Xerosis

UPPER AND LOWER AIRWAYS

Pyogenic sialoadenitis or parotitis
Interstitial pneumonitis or fibrosis
Chronic bronchitis
Bronchiectasis
Bronchiolitis obliterans with organizing pneumonia
Chronic obstructive pulmonary disease

MUSCULOSKELETAL

Polyarthralgia, polyarthritis
Myopathy, polymyositis

RENAL

Type I renal tubular acidosis
Tubular interstitial nephritis
Cryoglobulinemia-associated glomerulonephritis

NEUROLOGIC

Peripheral motor sensory neuropathy
Pure sensory neuropathy (including pure ataxic neuropathy)
Small-fiber sensitive neuropathy
Multiple sclerosis–like focal lesions
Spinal cord dysfunction, including transverse myelitis

HEPATOBILIARY

Autoimmune primary biliary cholangitis

NEOPLASIA

Lymphadenopathy, MALT (mucosa-associated lymphoid tissue) lymphoma

TABLE 252-2 DRUGS AND TOXINS THAT MIGHT DECREASE LACRIMAL AND SALIVARY SECRETION

STRONG EFFECT	MODERATE EFFECT
Atropine, atropinic antiparkinsonian drugs, anticholinergic antihistaminic drugs	β-Adrenergic blockers
	α-Adrenergic blockers
Antidepressants: imipramine (amitriptyline) and inhibitors of monoamine oxidase	Calcium-channel blockers
	Benzodiazepines
Neuroleptics	Inhibitors of serotonin reuptake (very slight effect)
Morphine, codeine, tramadol	
A-type botulinum toxin	Histamine-1 antihistaminic drugs
Class IA antiarrhythmic (disopyramide)	Diuretics
Isotretinoin	Some antiretroviral drugs
Toxins and psychotropic drugs: tobacco, ecstasy, cannabis, cocaine	

TABLE 252-3 THE DIFFERENT CAUSES OF SICCA SYMPTOMS

Drugs, particularly psychotropic drugs (see Table 252-2)
Aging, postmenopausal estrogen deficiency
Prolonged use of contact lenses
Fibromyalgia and chronic fatigue syndrome
Anxiodepressive syndromes
Head and neck radiotherapy
Diabetes (uncontrolled)
Severe hyperlipidemia
Amyloidosis
Sarcoidosis
Lymphoma
Graft-versus-host disease
Some viral infections (HIV, HCV, HTVL-1)
IgG4-related sialoadenitis
Sjögren syndrome

HCV = hepatitis C virus; HIV = human immunodeficiency virus; HTVL-1 = human T-lymphocytic virus-1; IgG4 = immunoglobulin G4.

Laboratory Findings

The most common serologic finding in primary Sjögren syndrome is hypergammaglobulinemia. The elevated γ-globulins contain several autoantibodies directed against non-organ-specific antigens,[13] such as RF and antinuclear antibody (ANA).[14] Specific ANA, anti-SSA/Ro, and anti-SSB/La antibodies are present in 60 to 80% and 30 to 40% of patients, respectively, and anti-SSB/La is never present without anti-SSA/Ro. Of note, the presence of anti-SSA/Ro, possibly with anti-SSB/La, may mediate complete heart block of newborns owing to cross-mimicry between specific fetal myocardial antigens and epitopes of the SSA/Ro-SSB/La complex.

Anemia of chronic inflammation and high erythrocyte sedimentation rates (due to hypergammaglobulinemia) are frequently encountered, whereas C-reactive protein levels are usually within normal limits. Cytopenias (most frequently lymphopenia and neutropenia) can also occur. In the setting of interstitial nephritis, the presence of hypokalemic, hyperchloremic acidosis might reveal distal renal tubular acidosis.

A monoclonal immunoglobulin can be detected in 10 to 15% of patients with Sjögren syndrome, depending on the technique used. Approximately 20% of patients with Sjögren syndrome have cryoglobulins in their sera. Complement levels may be decreased, especially C4. This low C4 level may be either genetically determined or secondary to consumption (in immune complexes or cryoglobulinemia).

DIAGNOSIS

Differential Diagnosis

The definition of primary Sjögren syndrome had suffered for a long time from the absence of accurate and consensus-driven diagnostic criteria. This is important because the patients' main symptoms (dryness, fatigue, and pain) are frequent in the general population. They can be caused by numerous drugs (Table 252-2), anxiety and/or depression, other comorbidities, or aging (Table 252-3). Sarcoidosis can mimic the clinical picture of Sjögren syndrome.

However, in sarcoidosis, minor salivary gland biopsy reveals noncaseating granulomas, and autoantibodies are typically absent. Other Sjögren syndrome mimickers include chronic graft-versus-host disease, amyloidosis, infection with viruses such as HIV, human T-lymphotropic virus 1 (HTLV-1), hepatitis C virus, and immunoglobulin G4 (IgG4)-related disease (Chapter 259). The latter disease is important in the differential diagnosis of Sjögren syndrome. It more often involves men with salivary or lacrimal gland enlargement (previously called Mikulicz syndrome) with previous organ-specific autoimmune disease (like autoimmune pancreatitis) without anti-SSA/SSB antibodies. Sicca symptoms without salivary lymphoid infiltrate and without anti-SSA/SSB antibodies may be part of the fibromyalgia syndrome (Chapter 258), and several acronyms have been proposed for designating these patients: sicca asthenia polyalgia syndrome or dry eyes and mouth syndrome. The arthralgias and arthritis can also sometimes mimic rheumatoid arthritis (Chapter 248).[15]

Diagnostic Criteria

International agreement has established a definition of Sjögren syndrome based on the American-European Consensus Group (AECG) criteria, which require the presence of either focal lymphocytic infiltrates in minor salivary glands with a focus score of 1 or more, or anti-SSA/SSB autoantibodies (Table 252-4). A new set of preliminary criteria for Sjögren syndrome classification was proposed by an expert consensus panel (American College of Rheumatology [ACR]-Sjögren International Collaborative Clinical Alliance [SICCA]).[16] According to these criteria, classification of an individual as a patient with primary Sjögren syndrome requires the presence of two out of three of the following objective items: (1) a positive serum test for anti-Ro/SSA and/or anti-La/SSB antibodies, or positive RF and ANA (titer >1: 320); (2) presence of keratoconjunctivitis sicca, defined by an ocular staining score higher than 3; and (3) presence of focal lymphocytic sialoadenitis, defined by a focus score of 1 focus/4 mm^2 or higher in a labial salivary gland biopsy.

Assessment of Activity of the Disease

An international expert group recently set up a Sjögren syndrome activity score under the umbrella of the European League Against Rheumatism (EULAR). Two indices have been developed: (1) a patient-administered questionnaire to assess subjective features, the EULAR Sjögren Syndrome

TABLE 252-4	2016 ACR/EULAR SS CLASSIFICATION CRITERIA OF PRIMARY SJÖGREN SYNDROME*	
INCLUSION CRITERIA	**ITEM**	**SCORE**
• At least one symptom of ocular or oral dryness (based on AECG questions), *or* • Suspicion of SS from ESSDAI questionnaire (at least one domain with positive item)	Focus Score ≥ 1	3
	Anti-SSA Ab+	3
	Ocular Staining Score ≥ 5	1
	Schirmer test ≤ 5 mm/5 min	1
	Unstimulated Salivary Flow ≤ 0.1 mL/min	1
	Total	**9.0**
SS CLASSIFICATION CRITERIA		
pSS case defined by a score ≥ 4		
Based on 98% consensus among clinician experts		

Note:
- Exclusion criteria similar to AECG and ACR criteria except past lymphoma and cured HCV infection
- Patients taking anticholinergic drugs should be evaluated for OSS, Schirmer, and UWS flow after a sufficient interval off these medications

*2016 American College of Rheumatology/European League Against Rheumatism Sjögren's Syndrome Classification Criteria for Primary Sjögren's Syndrome
AECG = American-European Consensus Group; Anti-SSA = anti-Ro antibody; ESSDAI = EULAR Sjögren's Syndrome (SS) Disease Activity Index; HCV = hepatic C virus; UWS = unstimulated whole saliva.
Shiboski CH, Shiboski SC, Seror R, et al; International Sjögren's Syndrome Criteria Working Group. 2016 American College of Rheumatology/European League Against Rheumatism classification criteria for primary Sjögren's syndrome: a consensus and data-driven methodology involving three international patient cohorts. *Ann Rheum Dis.* 2017;76:9-16.

Patient Reported Index, based on three different visual analogue scores: dryness, fatigue, and limb pain; and (2) a systemic activity index to assess systemic complications, the EULAR Sjögren Syndrome Disease Activity Index. The latter index comprises 12 domains with three or four levels of activity for each domain. Determination of the threshold of moderate activity as well as the minimal clinically important improvement is in progress, with the objective to base inclusion criteria and primary end points of future clinical studies on EULAR Sjögren Syndrome Disease Activity Index levels.

Ultrasound findings in major salivary glands correlate with subjective and objective oral and ocular dryness and with systemic autoimmune features in patients with primary Sjögren syndrome. Ultrasound also can be useful for follow-up assessments.[17]

TREATMENT   Rx

Symptomatic Treatment

Muscarinic agonists (pilocarpine hydrochloride and more recently cevimeline hydrochloride) are effective for treating sicca features (oral dryness and, to a lesser extent, ocular dryness).[A1][A2] Topical cyclosporine collyrium (0.05%) also was effective for moderate or severe ocular dryness and inflammation in a randomized controlled trial versus placebo, as were 0.1% clobetasone butyrate eye-drops.[A3] Environmental measures (avoidance of hot air heating systems or excessive air conditioning, use of a humidifier, appropriate glasses to protect the eye from evaporating air flow) and "little means" (sugar-free chewing gums, regular water drinking, salivary substitutes) might be useful. Regular dental examinations and oral hygiene are crucial for reducing subsequent oral health issues (i.e., caries and periodontal disease associated with xerostomia). To treat pain, simple analgesics should be used first, particularly acetaminophen/paracetamol, which does not cause dryness.

Immunomodulatory Drugs

To date, no immunomodulatory drug has proved efficacious in primary Sjögren syndrome.[18] Severe organ manifestations of primary Sjögren syndrome have to be treated in accordance with treatment modalities used in systemic lupus erythematosus or other connective tissue diseases. Randomized trials have assessed hydroxychloroquine in primary Sjögren syndrome and failed to demonstrate any clinical efficacy.[A4] Despite these negative results on clinical outcomes, hydroxychloroquine is frequently used in primary Sjögren syndrome, especially to treat arthralgia with or without synovitis or purpura. Controlled studies are needed to assess the use of methotrexate, leflunomide, mycophenolate sodium, azathioprine, and cyclosporine. Intravenous immunoglobulin (IVIG) has been used in the treatment of Sjögren syndrome–associated sensorimotor neuropathies or nonataxic sensory neuropathy without any necrotizing vasculitis.

Biologics

Randomized trials of infliximab and etanercept did not show any efficacy of TNF-blocker agents in primary Sjögren syndrome on a composite primary outcome including limb pain, fatigue, and dryness visual analogue scales. B-cell targeting appears to be a promising strategy in primary Sjögren syndrome.[19] Although cohort registries and several randomized controlled trials have reported at least some short-term efficacy using rituximab (a monoclonal anti-CD20 antibody),[A5][A6] other trials and a meta-analysis have shown no benefit.[A7][A8] Rituximab may be useful in cases of persistent parotid swelling or systemic complications, especially in cryoglobulinemia-induced vasculitis. Data are also inconclusive for belimumab (an anti-BAFF monoclonal antibody).

FUTURE DIRECTIONS

Sjögren syndrome is a model of autoimmune disease because it can be primary or associated with other autoimmune diseases; it represents autoimmunity where the risk for lymphoma is most important and where increased risk for cardiovascular and cerebrovascular disease has been found in a systematic review and meta-analysis. Sjögren syndrome is the autoimmune disease for which the target tissue of autoimmunity is the most easily available, with the lip biopsy being necessary for diagnosis. Recent progress in pathophysiology has emphasized a number of similarities with systemic lupus erythematosus that support consideration of Sjögren syndrome as a form of lupus of the mucosa. Even if the pathogenetic mechanisms of the disease remain largely unknown, improved knowledge of the effector mechanisms will allow identification of new targets for future therapy. Moreover, with the validated composite activity scores of EULAR Sjögren Syndrome Patient Reported Index and EULAR Sjögren Syndrome Disease Activity Index,[20] the tools are now available to begin new clinical trials with novel drugs for this disease that will improve the poor quality of life currently associated with it.

Grade A References

A1. Hamad A, Lodi G, Porter S, et al. Interventions for dry mouth and hyposalivation in Sjögren's syndrome: a systematic review and meta-analysis. *Oral Dis.* 2019;25:1027-1047.
A2. Shih KC, Lun CN, Jhanji V, et al. Systematic review of randomized controlled trials in the treatment of dry eye disease in Sjögren syndrome. *J Inflamm (Lond).* 2017;14:1-11.
A3. Aragona P, Spinella R, Rania L, et al. Safety and efficacy of 0.1% clobetasone butyrate eyedrops in the treatment of dry eye in Sjögren syndrome. *Eur J Ophthalmol.* 2013;23:368-376.
A4. Wang SQ, Zhang LW, Wei P, et al. Is hydroxychloroquine effective in treating primary Sjögren's syndrome? A systematic review and meta-analysis. *BMC Musculoskelet Disord.* 2017;18:1-13.
A5. Meijer JM, Meiners PM, Vissink A, et al. Effectiveness of rituximab treatment in primary Sjögren's syndrome: a randomized, double-blind, placebo-controlled trial. *Arthritis Rheum.* 2010;62:960-968.
A6. Devauchelle-Pensec V, Mariette X, Jousse-Joulin S, et al. Treatment of primary Sjögren syndrome with rituximab: a randomized trial. *Ann Intern Med.* 2014;160:233-242.
A7. Bowman SJ, Everett CC, O'Dwyer JL, et al. Randomized controlled trial of rituximab and cost-effectiveness analysis in treating fatigue and oral dryness in primary Sjögren's syndrome. *Arthritis Rheumatol.* 2017;69:1440-1450.
A8. Letaief H, Lukas C, Barnetche T, et al. Efficacy and safety of biological DMARDs modulating B cells in primary Sjögren's syndrome: systematic review and meta-analysis. *Joint Bone Spine.* 2018;85:15-22.

GENERAL REFERENCES

For the General References and other additional features, please visit Expert Consult at https://expertconsult.inkling.com.

253

INFLAMMATORY MYOPATHIES

STEVEN A. GREENBERG

OVERVIEW

The inflammatory myopathies are a heterogeneous group of acquired disorders in which the immune system is thought to play a major pathogenic role.[1] Though some genetic disorders affecting muscle also have significant involvement of the immune system and are treated with immunosuppressive therapy as standard of care (e.g., treatment of Duchenne muscular dystrophy with

TABLE 253-1 CLASSIFICATION OF INFLAMMATORY MYOPATHIES

DISORDER	AGE RANGE	CLINICAL FEATURES	MUSCLE PATHOLOGY
Dermatomyositis	Juvenile and adult forms	Proximal weakness plus skin	Perimysial and perivascular inflammation, perifascicular atrophy
Polymyositis	Adult (rare in childhood)	Proximal weakness	Endomysial inflammation with invasion of non-necrotic muscle fibers
Immune-mediated necrotizing myopathy	Adult	Proximal weakness	Multifocal necrotic muscle fibers
Inclusion body myositis	Adult >40 years old	Prominent quadriceps and finger flexor weakness; treatment refractory	Endomysial inflammation with invasion of non-necrotic muscle fibers plus rimmed vacuoles
Overlap syndromes	Adult	Myositis plus defined connective tissue disease	Nonspecific inflammation
Other (granulomatous myositis, eosinophilic myositis)	All ages	Proximal or distal weakness	Specific to type (e.g., granulomas present with granulomatous myositis)

corticosteroids), these genetic disorders are not classified as inflammatory myopathies. The four major subtypes of inflammatory myopathy are dermatomyositis, polymyositis, immune-mediated necrotizing myopathy, and inclusion body myositis (also called sporadic inclusion body myositis). These disorders have distinct clinical and pathologic features and pathophysiologies (Table 253-1). Whereas dermatomyositis and polymyositis have been described in the medical literature for over 100 years, immune-mediated necrotizing myopathy and inclusion body myositis have only become defined as syndromes distinct from polymyositis within the last few decades.

The original classification of inflammatory myopathies (collectively also referred to as "myositis"[2]) was developed in 1975 (the Bohan and Peter classification). Since then much progress has been made with the discovery of myositis-*specific* and myositis-*associated* autoantibodies, improvements in defining their morphologic features and histopathology, and refining the phenotypic distinctions between the different inflammatory myopathies. These developments necessitated the new 2017 European League Against Rheumatism/American College of Rheumatology diagnostic criteria and classification for adult and juvenile inflammatory myopathies and their major subgroups.[3-5]

EPIDEMIOLOGY

The prevalence of dermatomyositis has been estimated at 100 to 210 per million. The estimated prevalence of polymyositis is confounded by frequent misdiagnosis of inclusion body myositis and muscular dystrophies as polymyositis. Traditionally, polymyositis has been considered more prevalent (70 per million), but comparative studies with attention to inclusion body myositis have found a prevalence of polymyositis of 35 per million, approximately half the prevalence of inclusion body myositis of 70 per million. Inclusion body myositis is the most common acquired muscle disease after age 50.[6] The prevalence of immune-mediated necrotizing myopathy is unknown.[7]

Dermatomyositis has biphasic peaks in prevalence in childhood (7 to 15 years) and in midlife (30 to 50 years), whereas polymyositis peaks in prevalence in midlife. Inclusion body myositis is rarely diagnosed before the age of 40 and is most common after the age of 50. Dermatomyositis and polymyositis have female predominance; inclusion body myositis has male predominance. Ethnicity and worldwide distribution influence the development of various inflammatory myopathies.

PATHOBIOLOGY

The pathophysiologies of various forms of inflammatory myopathy are poorly understood. These disorders do share in common injury to muscle by the immune system. Much of the theory of pathophysiology of these disorders comes from microscopic examination of muscle biopsies and the distinct pathologies of these disorders (Fig. 253-1).

The muscle pathology of dermatomyositis involves loss of blood vessels and injury to myofibers at the edges of muscle fascicles (i.e., perifascicular atrophy; see Fig. 253-1). The relationship of these two features to each other is uncertain but has been postulated to be due to a primary injury to muscle capillaries, followed by ischemic injury to myofibers. An alternative view is that a common factor injures both myofibers and capillaries. Skin pathology shows features analogous to that of muscle, with an interface dermatitis consisting of injury to the basal layer of keratinocytes.

Much evidence points toward dermatomyositis as mediated by the type 1 interferon cytokine family, consisting mainly of interferon (IFN)-α and IFN-β.

Studies of dermatomyositis skin and muscle samples show marked upregulation of type 1 IFN-inducible transcripts and proteins uniquely in dermatomyositis among muscle diseases and similarly to systemic lupus erythematosus among skin diseases. The presence of autoantibodies in some patients with dermatomyositis, such as antibodies to the type 1 IFN-inducible protein MDA5, is of uncertain significance but seems likely due to an immune reaction to proteins that are not normally expressed at high levels or exposed to the immune system.[8] The paraneoplastic associations of dermatomyositis suggest that in such patients an immune reaction against an underlying malignancy results in bystander injury to muscle and skin.

Because polymyositis is a diverse group of disorders, the mechanisms involved are likely to be varied. Pathologically, there is an appearance of invasion of muscle fibers by adaptive immune system cells (T cells) that appears to be antigen driven, so that cytotoxic T cell–mediated autoimmunity directed against an unknown target has been a favored hypothesis. The antigens targeted by this process and the fundamental cause are unknown.

Immune-mediated necrotizing myopathy is also a poorly understood disorder.[9] It can also be paraneoplastic, suggesting cross-reactions by the immune system with the underlying malignancy and with muscle antigens. More commonly, immune-mediated necrotizing myopathy occurs in association with treatment with statin drugs. The identification of autoantibodies against the target of statins, 3-hydroxy-3-methylglutaryl-coenzyme A reductase (HMGCR), in the majority of patients who develop immune-mediated necrotizing myopathy in association with statin use suggests that the upregulation of HMGCR in muscle is directly toxic to muscle and triggers an immune reaction against it. Anti–signal recognition particle (SRP) autoantibodies have also been identified in some patients with immune-mediated necrotizing myopathy. Anti-SRP myopathy, anti-HMGCR myopathy, and autoantibody-negative myopathy have been considered to be three distinct subtypes of immune-mediated necrotizing myopathy.[10]

The pathogenesis of inclusion body myositis is complex. Two dual pathologies have been noted: degeneration of myofibers and of myonuclei in particular, evident as formation of rimmed vacuoles (see Fig. 253-1A and B) and involvement of the immune system.[11] The accumulation of more than 75 different proteins into sarcoplasmic aggregates in a small percentage of inclusion body myositis myofibers has been reported and has given rise to a number of molecular toxicity hypotheses in which certain specific protein aggregates are theorized as injurious to myofibers.

The immune system involvement in inclusion body myositis is notable in that whereas most other forms of inflammatory myopathy are generally responsive to immunomodulatory treatments, inclusion body myositis is refractory to treatment. This is particularly remarkable in that inclusion body myositis has the greatest evidence of all the inflammatory myopathies of a highly refined antigen-driven adaptive immune system involvement. Pathology shows very chronic and often marked but variable inflammatory infiltrates of T cells, myeloid dendritic cells, and plasma cells in muscle. Studies of the T-cell receptors have strongly suggested that T-cell autoimmunity is driven by one or more specific antigens, though the identity of any of these antigens is unknown.

Studies of a B-cell pathway in inclusion body myositis have led to identification of an autoantibody that is highly specific to inclusion body myositis among muscle diseases. Circulating autoantibodies against a 43-kD muscle protein have been identified as cytoplasmic 5′ nucleotidase 1A (cN1A; NT5C1A). cN1A is a nucleotidase that is most abundant in skeletal muscle and involved

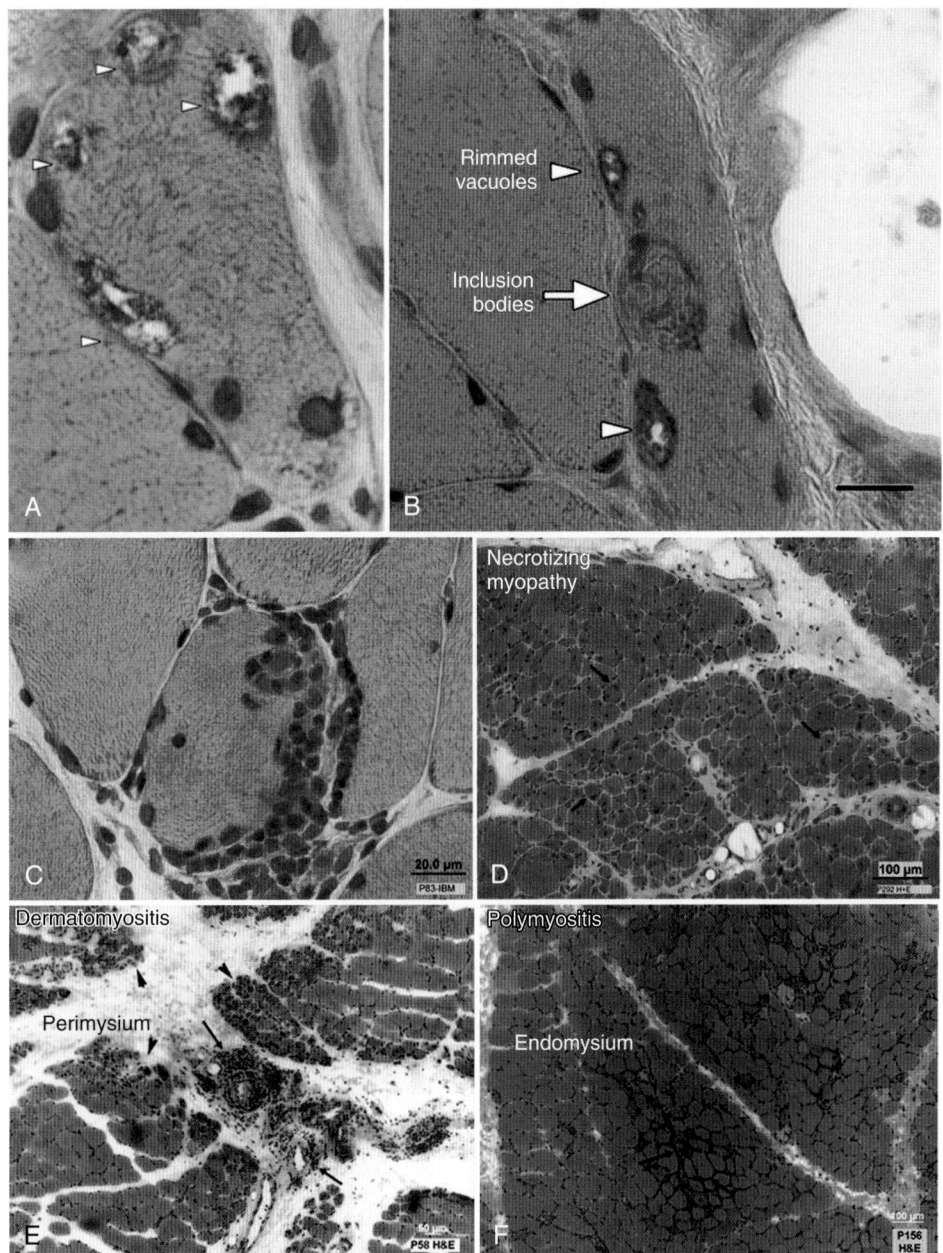

FIGURE 253-1. Pathologies of inflammatory myopathies. **A and B,** Rimmed vacuoles (*arrowheads*) of inclusion body myositis (IBM). **C,** Invasion of non-necrotic muscle fiber in IBM. **D,** Scattered necrotic and regenerating myofibers in immune-mediated necrotizing myopathy. **E,** Perivascular and perimysial inflammation (*arrows*), with perifascicular atrophy (*arrowheads*), in dermatomyositis. **F,** Endomysial inflammation in polymyositis. (With permission from the Inclusion Body Myositis Foundation, Inc.)

in the metabolism of nucleic acids. Serum anti-cN1A autoantibodies are present in 50 to 70% of patients with inclusion body myositis, depending on which assays and what cutoffs are used, and they are highly specific to inclusion body myositis (>90 to 95%) among muscle diseases. The role of blood testing for anti-cN1A autoantibodies in the diagnosis and management of patients with suspected inclusion body myositis is currently being defined, potentially shortening the time to diagnosis, reducing the misdiagnosis rate, and avoiding more invasive muscle biopsy in some patients.

A genetic basis of inclusion body myositis has been suggested by its significant association with the class II MHC allele HLA-DRB1*03:01.[12]

CLINICAL MANIFESTATIONS AND DIAGNOSIS

A diagnosis of inflammatory myopathy is considered when a patient presents with proximal or distal weakness without sensory symptoms or in patients with the characteristic skin lesions of dermatomyositis. Less frequently, asymptomatic elevated creatine kinase (CK) levels lead to a diagnosis of inflammatory myopathy.[13] Most patients with dermatomyositis, polymyositis, or immune-mediated necrotizing myopathy present with subacute proximal weakness of the arms and legs progressing over months, though these diseases may present acutely. Patients with inclusion body myositis present later in

life, usually symptomatic from slowly progressive weakness of knee extensors and finger flexors. More specific diagnostic features of these disorders are considered individually (Table 253-2). Most patients undergo muscle biopsy, or skin biopsy in the case of suspected dermatomyositis, as part of the diagnostic evaluation.

Dermatomyositis

Patients with dermatomyositis typically present with characteristic skin lesions or muscle weakness.[14,15] Virtually pathognomonic skin features are a heliotrope rash, a violaceous periorbital macular erythema, sometimes with edema, and Gottron papules, violaceous papules over dorsal metacarpophalangeal and interphalangeal joints of the hands (Fig. 253-2). Periungual telangiectasias and thrombosed capillaries, poikiloderma over photoexposed areas such as the upper back ("shawl sign"), nonscarring alopecia, and subcutaneous calcification are other suggestive signs. Prominent pruritus is also a common feature of dermatomyositis. Muscle weakness in dermatomyositis is less specific, occurring in a pattern indistinguishable from many other muscle diseases.

Useful laboratory studies for the evaluation of suspected dermatomyositis include serum CK (though CK can be normal or even below typical laboratory lower limits of normal in patients with highly active disease) and

TABLE 253-2 CLINICAL DIAGNOSTIC CRITERIA FOR INFLAMMATORY MYOPATHIES

DISORDER	DIAGNOSIS
Dermatomyositis	1. Diagnostic skin involvement (heliotrope rash, Gottron papules) _OR_ diagnostic muscle biopsy finding of perifascicular atrophy _OR_ 2. All of the following: • Suggestive skin involvement • Subacute or chronic proximal or distal weakness • Muscle biopsy showing perimysial or perivascular inflammation without features suggesting another disorder (e.g., endomysial inflammation, rimmed vacuoles) _OR_ skin biopsy showing interface dermatitis along with clinical exclusion of systemic lupus erythematosus
Polymyositis	All of the following: 1. Subacute or chronic proximal weakness 2. Elevated serum creatine kinase (CK) 3. Muscle biopsy showing invasion of endomysial inflammation 4. Response to immunotherapy _OR_ appropriate consideration and exclusion of limb-girdle muscular dystrophies and inclusion body myositis
Immune-mediated necrotizing myopathy	Both of the following: 1. Subacute or chronic proximal weakness 2. Muscle biopsy showing necrotizing myopathy, with scattered necrotic or regenerating myofibers and a lack of inflammation other than macrophage invasion of necrotic muscle fiber
Inclusion body myositis	All of the following: 1. Adult >40 years old 2. Finger flexion or quadriceps weakness 3. Muscle biopsy showing endomysial inflammation _OR_ the presence of serum anti-cN1A autoantibodies 4. Muscle biopsy showing rimmed vacuoles _OR_ invasion of non-necrotic muscle fibers _OR_ the presence of serum anti-cN1A autoantibodies

cNIA = cytoplasmic 5′ nucleotidase 1A.

dermatomyositis-associated autoantibody studies (e.g., anti-Jo-1, anti-Mi2, and anti-MDA5). Occasional patients have abnormal serum aldolase but normal serum CK. Skin biopsy showing a cell-poor interface dermatitis supports the diagnosis of dermatomyositis. Muscle biopsy showing perimysial and perivascular inflammation also supports a diagnosis of dermatomyositis, whereas the presence of perifascicular atrophy in a muscle biopsy is pathognomonic for dermatomyositis. Because dermatomyositis is associated with malignancy, appropriate laboratory and radiologic studies should be performed to search for underlying malignancy in all newly diagnosed patients. The most common dermatomyositis-associated malignancies tend to reflect the overall age and gender cancer rates within the individual patient's population (i.e., breast, lung, and colorectal cancer in Western countries; nasopharyngeal cancer in Asian populations). This observation supports the notion of dermatomyositis as a paraneoplastic process that can develop in virtually any kind of cancer.

Clinical diagnostic criteria are outlined in Table 253-2. The clinical features of muscle weakness in dermatomyositis are entirely nonspecific, with no particular pattern indicative of dermatomyositis compared with other muscle diseases. In practice, certain dermatologic clinical findings (heliotrope rash, Gottron papules) or muscle biopsy findings (perifascicular atrophy) are considered nearly pathognomonic for dermatomyositis.

Polymyositis

The diagnosis of polymyositis is often problematic, with historically many patients with genetically defined limb-girdle muscular dystrophies and inclusion body myositis being misdiagnosed as polymyositis. The 1975 criteria for polymyositis that are frequently cited allow for a diagnosis of "definite" polymyositis without a muscle biopsy. In clinical practice today, the core criteria for the diagnosis of polymyositis are subacute proximal weakness, elevated serum CK, and muscle biopsy showing endomysial inflammation without features suggestive of another diagnosis such as inclusion body myositis (see Table 253-2). Patients with defined connective tissue disorders such as Sjögren syndrome or mixed connective tissue disease have "overlap syndromes," often also classified as polymyositis.[16] Patients with immune-mediated necrotizing myopathy have historically been classified as polymyositis but are increasingly classified separately. Patients with inclusion body myositis are frequently misdiagnosed as polymyositis because of a lack of appreciation of the characteristic inclusion body myositis finger flexor weakness and because muscle biopsies

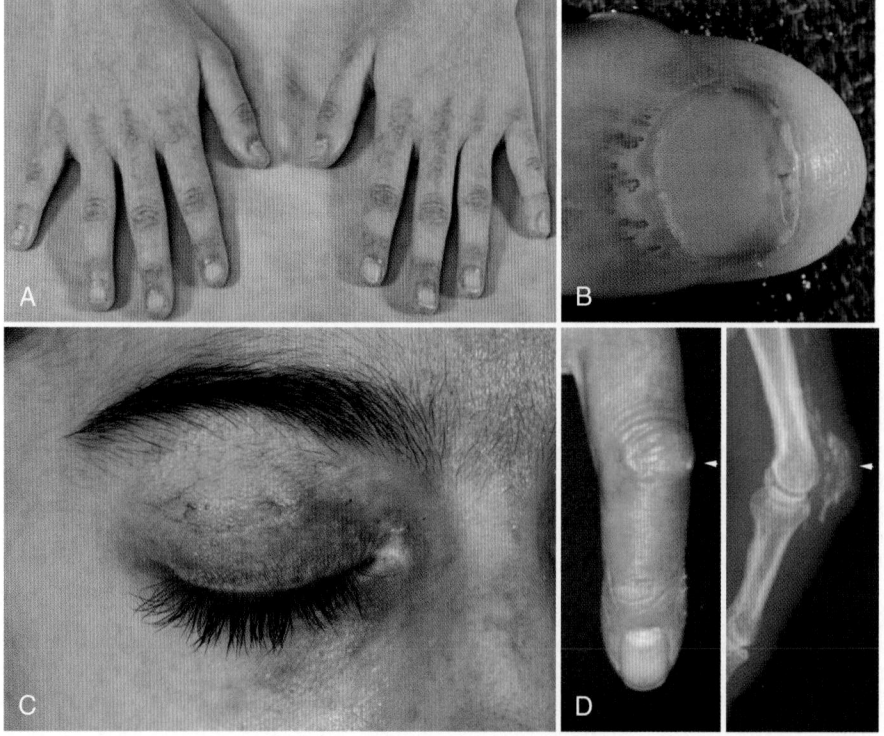

FIGURE 253-2. Clinical findings in dermatomyositis. **A,** Erythematous to violaceous raised papules overlying the metacarpal and interphalangeal joints, known as Gottron papules. These are considered the hallmark finding in dermatomyositis. **B,** Cuticular overgrowth and periungual capillary changes, which include dilated and tortuous blood vessels with areas of atrophy, telangiectasia, vessel dropout, and bushy loop formation along the fingernail bed. **C,** Erythema and minimal edema involving the upper eyelids, with occasional telangiectasia, known as the heliotrope rash. **D,** Subcutaneous calcification erupting through skin (_arrowhead_), seen clinically and by x-ray.

show endomysial inflammation. The presence of autoantibodies such as anti-Jo-1 argue more for polymyositis than inclusion body myositis, though these may be seen in dermatomyositis as well.

Immune-Mediated Necrotizing Myopathy

Immune-mediated necrotizing myopathy has increasingly been separated from the polymyositis category. Acute or subacute proximal weakness indistinguishable from that of polymyositis or dermatomyositis and an elevated CK are nonspecific, but muscle biopsy showing scattered necrotic or regenerating myofibers without inflammation other than macrophages invading these necrotic myofibers is typical of immune-mediated necrotizing myopathy. The presence of anti-HMGCR (3-hydroxy-3-methylglutaryl-coenzyme A reductase) or anti-SRP (signal recognition particle) antibodies both suggest immune-mediated necrotizing myopathy. Immune-mediated necrotizing myopathy, particularly when associated with anti-SRP antibodies, may be paraneoplastic, and laboratory and radiologic evaluation for malignancy should be considered.

Inclusion Body Myositis

Inclusion body myositis has a clinical presentation distinct from other inflammatory myopathies.[17] Inclusion body myositis weakness is always slowly progressive rather than the acute or subacute weakness more typically seen in other forms of inflammatory myopathies. Clinical diagnostic criteria are shown in Table 253-2. Inclusion body myositis has a high misdiagnosis rate, estimated at approximately 50% of patients. Symptoms of inclusion body myositis rarely are present before the age of 40 years and most commonly occur after the age of 50. The distribution of weakness is usually in finger flexors or quadriceps rather than proximal arms (shoulder abduction) or proximal legs (hip flexion), more typical of polymyositis or dermatomyositis. Inclusion body myositis is a highly atrophying muscle disease,[18] and loss of bulk in medial and lateral anterior thighs and ventral forearms is characteristic. Patients present with difficulty walking, buckling of knees, or weakness of grip. The diagnosis of inclusion body myositis can be highly suspected in such patients of appropriate age and findings on examination of quadriceps atrophy and weakness of finger flexors, especially flexor digitorum profundi, responsible for flexion of distal fingertips. Examination of the strength in these distal fingertips, which needs to be done one finger at a time, is often the single most helpful approach to the diagnosis of inclusion body myositis.

Serum CK is either normal or modestly elevated (typically less than five times the upper limit of normal). A serum autoantibody, anti-cN1A (also called anti-NT5C1A), appears highly specific to inclusion body myositis among muscle diseases and may be of diagnostic value. Most patients undergo muscle biopsy, with characteristic features being the presence of rimmed vacuoles seen on hematoxylin and eosin (H&E) and Gomori trichrome staining, along with endomysial inflammation or invasion of non-necrotic muscle fibers. Immunohistochemical stains detecting p62 or TDP-43 are of additional highly specific diagnostic value.

TREATMENT

Generally, most patients with dermatomyositis, polymyositis, and immune-mediated necrotizing myopathy respond to immunomodulatory therapies, whereas patients with inclusion body myositis are almost universally refractory. A general approach to treatment is shown in Fig. 253-3.

Treatment of Dermatomyositis and Polymyositis

Most patients with muscle involvement from dermatomyositis and polymyositis are treated with and respond to corticosteroids.[19,20] Dosing is typically prednisone at 1 mg/kg/day orally until significant improvement occurs (typically 1-3 months), followed by gradual taper of 10 mg/day/month. Second-line agents include methotrexate, azathioprine, cyclosporine, and intravenous immunoglobulin. Second-line agents are used for two reasons: they may have a better side-effect profile than chronic higher doses of corticosteroids, and they may be necessary for patients whose responses are insufficient to corticosteroids alone. An important decision is whether to start second-line agents concurrently with initial corticosteroid treatment or wait and see how low a dose of corticosteroids offers satisfactory control and then add agents only if the corticosteroid dose cannot be lowered sufficiently. Thus in the former approach, prednisone 60 mg/day and methotrexate 7.5 mg PO weekly might be started concurrently, and the methotrexate dose increased weekly to 15 to 20 mg PO weekly. Once improvement is substantial, the dose of prednisone may be tapered over 3 to 6 months. Stability on methotrexate alone would then be followed by gradual reduction in its dose. For patients with severe initial presentations, the combination of corticosteroids and periodic intravenous immunoglobulin (1 g/kg every 2 weeks) may offer a better chance for more rapid improvement.

A number of randomized placebo-controlled trials have shown no benefit for treating dermatomyositis or polymyositis.[A1][A2] These studies have almost always used the Bohan and Peter criteria for the diagnosis, which may result in inclusion of patients with limb-girdle muscular dystrophies and inclusion body myositis misdiagnosed as having polymyositis. In the single largest trial, which used rituximab, all subjects received active drug, but the comparison

---

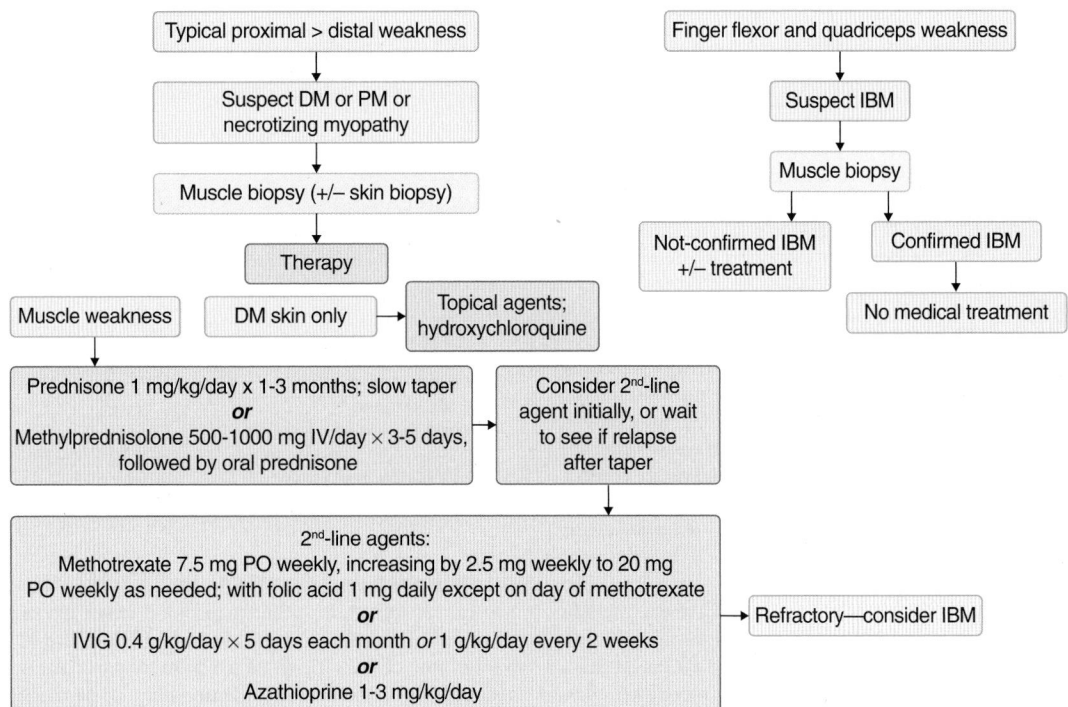

Suspected Inflammatory Myopathy

FIGURE 253-3. Approach to treatment of suspected inflammatory myopathy. DM = dermatomyositis; IBM = inclusion body myositis; IVIG = intravenous immunoglobulin; PM = polymyositis. (With permission from the Inclusion Body Myositis Foundation, Inc.)

was treated "early" or "late" (8 weeks later), and no significant differences were found.[A3]

Treatment of Inclusion Body Myositis

No therapies have demonstrated efficacy for inclusion body myositis, with negative results for prednisone, intravenous immunoglobulin, methotrexate, antithymocyte globulin, etanercept, interferon-β, and alemtuzumab. Current management of patients with inclusion body myositis is supportive, involving avoidance of falls and the use of ankle supports and gait assistive devices. Tendon transfer to improve hand function has been used.

PROGNOSIS

Most patients with adult dermatomyositis, polymyositis, and statin-associated immune-mediated necrotizing myopathy have a good prognosis but require long-standing immunomodulatory therapy. Many patients with juvenile dermatomyositis may go into long-standing remission or cure with aggressive initial treatment. Patients with anti-SRP–associated immune-mediated necrotizing myopathy may have severe and difficult-to-treat disease. Patients with inclusion body myositis generally have a slowly progressive course, with one series showing a mean time to loss of ambulation of 12 years.

Grade A References

A1. Gordon PA, Winer JB, Hoogendijk JE, et al. Immunosuppressant and immunomodulatory treatment for dermatomyositis and polymyositis. *Cochrane Database Syst Rev*. 2012;8:CD003643.
A2. Vermaak E, Tansley SL, McHugh NJ. The evidence for immunotherapy in dermatomyositis and polymyositis: a systematic review. *Clin Rheumatol*. 2015;34:2809-2095.
A3. Oddis CV, Reed AM, Aggarwal R, et al. Rituximab in the treatment of refractory adult and juvenile dermatomyositis and adult polymyositis: a randomized, placebo-phase trial. *Arthritis Rheum*. 2013;65:314-324.

GENERAL REFERENCES

For the General References and other additional features, please visit Expert Consult at https://expertconsult.inkling.com.

254

THE SYSTEMIC VASCULITIDES

JOHN H. STONE

DEFINITION

The vasculitides are a heterogeneous group of disorders linked by the common finding of destructive inflammation within blood vessel walls. The most current nomenclature scheme identifies at least 27 different forms of primary vasculitis (Table 254-1). The major forms of vasculitis are discussed in this chapter.

CLASSIFICATION

Classification by Vessel Size

The etiology of most forms of vasculitis remains unknown, and major gaps exist in our understanding of the pathophysiologic processes. The most valid basis for classification of the vasculitides is the size of the predominant blood vessels involved. The vasculitides are categorized initially by whether the vessels affected are primarily large, medium, or small (Table 254-2). Large vessels are considered the aorta, its primary branches, and any vessel that is not located within an organ such as a muscle, kidney, nerve, or the skin. Medium-sized vessels, in contrast, consist of the main visceral arteries and their branches. (Thus, the renal artery is considered a large vessel, but its intrarenal branches—the interlobar and arcuate arteries—are medium-sized vessels). Finally, small vessels include smaller intraparenchymal arteries as well as arterioles, capillaries, and venules.

Medium-vessel vasculitis and even large-vessel vasculitis can also affect small arteries. However, large-vessel vasculitis affects large arteries more often than medium- or small-vessel vasculitis, medium-vessel vasculitis affects predominantly medium arteries, and small-vessel vasculitis affects predominantly arterioles, capillaries, and venules.

TABLE 254-1 NAMES FOR VASCULITIDES ADOPTED BY THE 2012 INTERNATIONAL CHAPEL HILL CONSENSUS CONFERENCE ON THE NOMENCLATURE OF VASCULITIDES

LARGE-VESSEL VASCULITIS

Takayasu arteritis
Giant cell arteritis

MEDIUM-VESSEL VASCULITIS

Polyarteritis nodosa
Kawasaki disease
Buerger disease*

SMALL-VESSEL VASCULITIS

Antineutrophil cytoplasmic antibody (ANCA)-associated vasculitis
  Microscopic polyangiitis
  Granulomatosis with polyangiitis (formerly Wegener granulomatosis)
  Eosinophilic granulomatosis with polyangiitis (formerly Churg-Strauss syndrome)
Immune complex small-vessel vasculitis
  Antiglomerular basement membrane disease
  Cryoglobulinemic vasculitis
  Immunoglobulin (Ig)A vasculitis (Henoch-Schönlein purpura)
  Hypocomplementemic urticarial vasculitis

VARIABLE-VESSEL VASCULITIS

Behçet syndrome
Cogan syndrome

SINGLE-ORGAN VASCULITIS

Cutaneous leukocytoclastic angiitis
Cutaneous arteritis
Primary central nervous system vasculitis
Isolated aortitis

VASCULITIS ASSOCIATED WITH SYSTEMIC DISEASE

Lupus vasculitis
Rheumatoid vasculitis
Sarcoid vasculitis
Others (e.g., IgG4-related aortitis)

VASCULITIS ASSOCIATED WITH PROBABLE ETIOLOGY

Hepatitis C virus–associated cryoglobulinemic vasculitis
Hepatitis B virus–associated vasculitis
Syphilis-associated aortitis
Drug-associated immune complex vasculitis
Drug-associated ANCA-associated vasculitis
Cancer-associated vasculitis
Others

*Buerger disease (thromboangiitis obliterans) is not always considered to be a primary form of vasculitis and was not included in this consensus statement on nomenclature.
From Jennette JC, Falk RJ, Bacon PA, et al. 2012 Revised International Chapel Hill Consensus Conference Nomenclature of Vasculitides. *Arthritis Rheum*. 2013;65:1-11.

TABLE 254-2 CONSIDERATIONS IN THE CLASSIFICATION OF SYSTEMIC VASCULITIS

Size of predominant blood vessels affected
Epidemiologic features:
  Age
  Sex
  Ethnic background
Pattern of organ involvement
Pathologic features:
  Granulomatous inflammation
  Immune complex deposition vs. "pauci-immune" histopathology
Presence of ANCA in serum

ANCA = antineutrophil cytoplasmic antibody.

Additional Considerations in Classification

Several considerations other than blood vessel size are relevant to the classification of vasculitis (see Table 254-2). These are (1) age, sex, and ethnic background of the patient; (2) tropism for particular organs; (3) presence or absence of granulomatous inflammation; (4) participation of immune complexes in the pathophysiologic process; and (5) detection of characteristic autoantibodies in the patients' serum, such as antineutrophil cytoplasmic antibodies (ANCAs).

Age, sex differences, and ethnic variation are discussed later in the section on Epidemiology. The organ tropisms of these disorders are illustrated by the following examples. Whereas immunoglobulin (Ig)A vasculitis (IgAV, also known as Henoch-Schönlein purpura) typically affects the skin, joints, kidneys, and gastrointestinal (GI) tract, granulomatosis with polyangiitis (GPA; formerly Wegener granulomatosis) classically involves the upper airways, lungs, and kidneys. In contrast to both IgAV and GPA, Cogan syndrome involves the eyes, the audiovestibular apparatus of the inner ear, and (in 10 to 15% of cases) the large arteries.

The presence or absence of granulomatous inflammation is a crucial element of vasculitis diagnosis and classification. Granulomatous inflammation implicates a small number of vasculitides that bear this hallmark, including GPA, giant cell arteritis, Takayasu arteritis, and eosinophilic granulomatosis with polyangiitis (EGPA; Churg-Strauss syndrome).

Immune complexes are essential to the pathophysiologic mechanism of some forms of small- and medium-vessel vasculitis. Complexes of IgA1, for example, are found in IgAV. Immune complexes consisting of IgG, IgM, complement components, and the hepatitis C virion characterize most cases of mixed cryoglobulinemia. In contrast, "pauci-immune" types of small- and medium-vessel vasculitis, such as GPA and microscopic polyangiitis, have little immunoglobulin or complement deposition within diseased tissues. Many but not all patients with pauci-immune forms of vasculitis are ANCA positive.

EPIDEMIOLOGY

The epidemiologic features of individual forms of systemic vasculitis vary tremendously by geography (Table 254-3). This may reflect genetic influences, variation in environmental exposures, and other unknown disease risk factors. For example, whereas Behçet syndrome is rare in North Americans, affecting only 1 person in approximately 300,000, this condition is several hundred times more common among inhabitants of countries bordering the ancient Silk Route. Similarly, although Takayasu arteritis is rare in the United States—on the order of 3 new cases per million people per year—this disease is reportedly the most common cause of renal artery stenosis in India, where the incidence may be as high as 200 to 300 per million per year.

Age is an important consideration in the epidemiology of vasculitis. Eighty percent of patients with Kawasaki disease are younger than 5 years. In contrast, giant cell arteritis virtually never occurs in patients younger than 50 years, and the mean age of patients with this disease is 72. Age may also have an impact on disease severity and outcome. In IgAV, the overwhelming majority of cases in children (who represent 90% of all cases) have self-limited courses, resolving within several weeks. In adults, however, IgAV has a higher likelihood of chronicity and a poor renal outcome.

The distribution of sex varies across many forms of vasculitis. Buerger disease is the only form of vasculitis with a striking male predominance. The greater prevalence of smoking among males in most societies probably explains this predilection. In contrast, Takayasu arteritis has an overwhelming tendency to occur in females (a 9 : 1 female-to-male ratio). The pauci-immune forms of vasculitis, such as GPA, EGPA, and microscopic polyangiitis, occur in males and females with approximately equal frequencies, but the phenotypic expression of these conditions may be affected by both age and sex.

The strongest link between any single gene and vasculitis is the association of HLA-B51 with Behçet syndrome. In Behçet syndrome, 80% of Asian patients have the HLA-B51 gene. The prevalence of HLA-B51 is significantly higher among patients with Behçet syndrome in Japan than among nondisease control subjects (55% versus <15%). Among the sporadic cases of Behçet syndrome involving whites in the United States, however, HLA-B51 occurs in fewer than 15% of cases.

With the exception of Buerger disease and smoking, no definitive associations have been confirmed between disease and environmental or occupational exposures. Associations have been reported but not confirmed between exposures to silica and some types of pauci-immune vasculitis. Studies of potential associations between exposures of any type and vasculitis, however, are complicated frequently by difficulties in obtaining reliable measurements of the levels of the relevant exposure, the likelihood of recall bias among patients who are diagnosed with vasculitis, and the choice of appropriate control groups.

PATHOBIOLOGY

Table 254-4 illustrates the pathologic characteristics of selected forms of vasculitis. Specific pathologic features are discussed in the subsections on each disease. The type of inflammatory cell infiltrate in vasculitis is independent of the size of blood vessels involved. Mixed cell infiltrates in vasculitis are the rule rather than the exception, and histopathologic patterns of vasculitis may

---

TABLE 254-3 EPIDEMIOLOGY OF SELECTED VASCULITIDES

DISEASE	UNITED STATES	ELSEWHERE	AGE, SEX, AND ETHNIC PREDISPOSITIONS
Giant cell arteritis	Incidence: 240/million (Olmsted County, MN)	220-270/million (Scandinavian countries)	Age >50 yr, mean age 72 yr; females 3 : 1; northern European ancestry
Takayasu arteritis	Incidence: 3/million	200-300/million (India)	Age <40 yr; females 9 : 1; Asian
Behçet syndrome	Prevalence: 3/million	3000/million (Turkey)	Silk Route countries
Polyarteritis nodosa	Incidence: 7/million	7/million (Spain)	Slight male predominance
Kawasaki disease	Incidence: 100/million*	900/million (Japan)	Children of Asian ancestry
Wegener granulomatosis†	Incidence: 4/million	8.5/million (United Kingdom)	Whites ≫ blacks

*Among children younger than 5 years.
†Now named granulomatosis with polyangiitis.
From Gonzalez-Gay MA, Garica-Porrua C. Epidemiology of the vasculitides. *Rheum Clin North Am.* 2001;27:729-749.

TABLE 254-4 PATHOLOGIC CHARACTERISTICS OF SELECTED FORMS OF VASCULITIS

	TAKAYASU ARTERITIS	POLYARTERITIS NODOSA	GRANULOMATOSIS WITH POLYANGIITIS (WEGENER GRANULOMATOSIS)	EOSINOPHILIC GRANULOMATOSIS WITH POLYANGIITIS*	HENOCH-SCHÖNLEIN PURPURA	CUTANEOUS LEUKOCYTOCLASTIC ANGIITIS
Vessels involved	Elastic (large) or muscle (medium-sized) arteries	Medium-sized and small muscle arteries	Small arteries and veins; sometimes medium-sized vessels	Small arteries and veins; sometimes medium-sized vessels	Capillaries, venules, and arterioles	Capillaries, venules, and arterioles
Organ involvement	Aorta, aortic arch and major branches, and pulmonary arteries	Skin, peripheral nerves, gastrointestinal tract, and other viscera	Upper respiratory tract, lungs, kidneys, skin, eyes	Upper respiratory tract, lungs, heart, peripheral nerves	Skin, joints, gastrointestinal tract, kidneys	Skin, joints
Type of vasculitis and inflammatory cells	Granulomatous with some giant cells; fibrosis in chronic stages	Necrotizing, with mixed cellular infiltrate	Necrotizing or granulomatous (or both); mixed cellular infiltrate plus occasional eosinophils	Necrotizing or granulomatous (or both); prominent eosinophils and other mixed infiltrate	Leukocytoclastic, with some lymphocytes and variable eosinophils; IgA deposits in affected tissues	Leukocytoclastic, with occasional eosinophils

*Formerly named Churg-Strauss syndrome.

include leukocytoclasis (degranulation and destruction of neutrophils within blood vessel walls), granulomatous findings (with or without giant cells), lymphoplasmacytic infiltrates, varying degrees of eosinophilic infiltration, necrosis, and combinations of all these findings.

PATHOPHYSIOLOGY

Some pathophysiologic mechanisms are common to many different forms of vasculitis, regardless of the size of the predominant blood vessels involved. Immune complex deposition, for example, is present in several types of vasculitis that involve both medium-sized and small blood vessels. In this section, the general concepts related to the pathogenesis of large-vessel vasculitides are discussed separately from those of medium- and small-vessel vasculitides.

Large-Vessel Vasculitides

The pathologic process in large-vessel vasculitis appears to begin in the adventitia. In both Takayasu arteritis and giant cell arteritis, abundant numbers of activated T lymphocytes are found within inflamed arterial walls, centering on the adventitia. In Takayasu arteritis, most of these T cells appear to be of the CD8+ subtype. Current evidence suggests that the cytotoxic functions of these cells, mediated by perforin and granzyme B, contribute to smooth muscle cell damage in this disease. CD4+ T-cell responses in Takayasu arteritis have not been well defined.

In giant cell arteritis (Chapter 255), much evidence now suggests an antigen-driven disease, with the site of immunologic recognition events being the adventitia. CD4+ T cells that secrete interferon (IFN)-γ appear to be recruited to the adventitia by a specific antigen(s), the identity of which remains unknown. Both the T cells that orchestrate the transmural inflammation and the inciting antigens are theorized to reach the adventitia through the vasa vasorum. Subsequently, T-cell signals from the adventitia stimulate macrophages and multinucleated giant cells to elaborate an array of downstream mediators, including metalloproteinases and platelet-derived growth factor. Interleukin (IL)-6, known to be a crucial cytokine in giant cell arteritis and probably Takayasu arteritis as well, is produced by macrophages residing in the blood vessel wall. The results of this inflammatory cascade are granulomatous inflammation, destruction of the internal elastic lamina, arterial wall hyperplasia, smooth muscle cell proliferation, intimal thickening, vascular occlusion, and in some cases, weakening of the vessel wall, leading to dilation and aneurysm formation. Matrix metalloproteinases appear to play important roles in destruction of the internal elastic lamina, damage to other vascular tissues, and weakening of the arterial wall.

Medium- and Small-Vessel Vasculitides

Several different pathophysiologic mechanisms are operative among the medium- and small-vessel vasculitides. In many cases, the mechanisms outlined in the following sections overlap.

Immune Complex–Mediated Vascular Injury

Immune complex–mediated tissue injury does not produce a single clinical syndrome but rather applies to many forms of vasculitis and overlaps with injuries caused by other immune mechanisms. Numerous variables influence immune complex–mediated injury, including the physical properties of the immune complexes (e.g., their size), the ability of the immune complexes to activate complement, the antigen-to-antibody ratio, and the hemodynamic features of specific vascular beds. Immune complexes participate in the pathophysiologic process of some forms of both medium- and small-vessel vasculitis, including polyarteritis nodosa, cryoglobulinemia, IgAV, cutaneous leukocytoclastic angiitis, and rheumatoid vasculitis.

Role of Antineutrophil Cytoplasmic Antibodies

ANCAs are directed against antigens that reside within the primary granules of neutrophils and monocytes. Two types of ANCA are relevant to vasculitis: (1) those directed against proteinase 3 (PR3), known as PR3-ANCA; and (2) those directed against myeloperoxidase (MPO), termed MPO-ANCA. ANCA interact with cytokines, neutrophils, monocytes, and other elements of the immune system to amplify ongoing inflammation in certain forms of vasculitis. A striking and still unexplained feature of ANCA-associated vasculitis (AAV) is that patients with primary forms of these conditions virtually never have antibodies to both PR3 and MPO. Despite the specificity of these antibodies, however, evidence for a primary role of ANCA in the etiology of human disease is still tenuous.

In GPA, abnormal cytokine regulation interacts with the production of ANCA to fuel the inflammatory response. T_H1 cytokines such as interferon

(IFN)-γ, interleukin (IL)-12, and tumor necrosis factor (TNF) appear to play important roles. Under the direction of IL-12, CD4+ T cells from patients with GPA produce elevated levels of TNF, and peripheral blood mononuclear cells secrete increased amounts of IFN-γ. Serum levels of soluble receptors for TNF are elevated in patients with active GPA and normalize with the induction of remission. In vitro priming of activated neutrophils with TNF markedly enhances the ability of ANCA to stimulate neutrophil degranulation. Despite the strong rationale for anti-TNF strategies in GPA, however, a randomized trial of etanercept showed no efficacy in the maintenance of disease remissions.

B-cell depletion is a more effective approach to the treatment of AAV. The efficacy of this treatment strategy probably relates to the removal of several B-cell functions beyond their evolution into plasma cells and the production of ANCA. Such other functions include cytokine production, antigen presentation, and B cell–T cell crosstalk.

Superantigen Model

The degree of immune activation in Kawasaki disease and the acute but generally self-limited nature of this illness imply a potential role for superantigens. Superantigens are proteins produced by microbial pathogens (e.g., *Staphylococcus aureus* or *Streptococcus* species) that are capable of stimulating large populations of T cells in a manner unrestricted by the class II major histocompatibility complex (MHC). Superantigens bind directly to conserved amino acid residues outside the antigen-binding groove on class II MHC molecules, thereby selectively stimulating T cells that express particular β-chain variable gene segments. Through the binding of this MHC-superantigen complex to its cognate T-cell receptors, as many as 20% of circulating lymphocytes may become activated, leading to a potentially enormous outpouring of cytokines. With regard to the etiology of Kawasaki disease, substantial attention has focused on toxic shock syndrome toxin 1, an exotoxin produced by *S. aureus*. Superantigens have also been postulated to play roles in the susceptibility to disease flares in GPA. Nasal carriage of *S. aureus* and superantigens associated with these organisms has been linked to a greater likelihood of disease flares in some studies.

Anti–Endothelial Cell Antibodies

Anti–endothelial cell antibodies can induce endothelial cell injury and lysis through either complement-mediated cytotoxicity or antibody-dependent cellular cytotoxicity. Both of these mechanisms have been demonstrated to cause endothelial injury in in vitro assays employing sera from patients with systemic vasculitis. The ability of these antibodies to damage endothelial cells is an appealing argument for their potential role in forms of vasculitis in which the endothelium is the focus of the inflammation (as opposed to the more external vessel wall layers). However, the true relevance of anti–endothelial cell antibodies to human disease and their importance within the larger context of other disease mechanisms remain unclear.

CLINICAL MANIFESTATIONS

Large-Vessel Vasculitides

Takayasu Arteritis

Takayasu arteritis (Chapter 69) affects the aorta and its major branches. In contrast to atherosclerosis, which is characterized by focal irregular lesions, the lesions of Takayasu arteritis are long, smooth, tapered stenoses (E-Fig. 254-1). The most commonly involved arteries are the subclavian and innominate arteries. Takayasu arteritis has been termed "pulseless disease" because of its ability to obliterate peripheral pulses (particularly in the upper extremities). Exuberant collateral circulation develops over time in response to the gradual narrowing of major arteries, making the loss of digits or limbs from ischemia extremely rare. The extensive development of collateral circulation usually renders unnecessary any attempts to revascularize stenoses of primary aortic branches, such as the subclavian artery. The pulmonary circulation is involved in approximately 50% of cases of Takayasu arteritis.

Patients with severe narrowing of the aortic arch vessels supplying the head may develop Takayasu retinopathy, the hypotensive retinopathy leading to neovascularization originally described by Takayasu. In contrast, patients with prolonged hypertension associated with renal artery stenosis demonstrate the classic ocular features of hypertension: "copper wiring" and multiple retinal infarctions. This complication is particularly difficult to diagnose[1] and dangerous because vascular narrowings of large arteries to the arms and legs often lead to underestimations of the true central aortic pressure. Takayasu arteritis involvement of the ascending aorta may lead to aortic dilation, aortic regurgitation, aneurysm formation, and aortic rupture.

(Chapter 255)

TREATMENT   Rx

For patients with marked symptoms and signs of an inflammatory phase, glucocorticoids (prednisone 1 mg/kg/day) are usually effective in controlling the disease. The toxicity of high doses of glucocorticoids in young women, however, urges the early consideration of alternative agents.[2] IL-6 inhibition, shown to be highly effective in giant cell arteritis,[A1] also appears to be effective in Takayasu arteritis.[A2] Patients can be treated with tocilizumab, administered either intravenously (8 mg/kg each month) or subcutaneously (162 mg each week). Once tocilizumab has been initiated, prednisone should be tapered to low doses (10 mg daily or less) within 3 months and ultimately discontinued altogether, if possible. The optimal duration of tocilizumab in Takayasu arteritis is uncertain. Consideration may be given to tapering (to either 4 mg/kg intravenously each month or 162 mg subcutaneously every other week) after one year. Large-vessel imaging may be useful in guiding decisions regarding the duration of therapy. About 50% of patients will relapse within 10 years,[3] so some Takayasu arteritis patients may require chronic treatment with tocilizumab plus (possibly) low-dose glucocorticoids.

Giant Cell Arteritis

Giant cell arteritis is the other primary form of vasculitis that involves arteries far larger than vasculitides of any other category.[4] This disease is discussed in detail elsewhere (Chapter 255).

Medium-Vessel Vasculitides
Polyarteritis Nodosa

Polyarteritis nodosa has a striking predilection for certain organs, particularly the skin, peripheral nerves, GI tract, and kidneys.[5] This disease usually begins with nonspecific symptoms such as malaise, fatigue, fever, myalgias, and arthralgias. Overt signs of vasculitis may not occur until weeks or months after onset of the first symptoms. Skin lesions of polyarteritis nodosa include livedo reticularis, subcutaneous nodules, ulcers, and digital gangrene. A majority of patients with polyarteritis nodosa (>80% in some series) have vasculitic neuropathy, typically in the pattern of a mononeuritis multiplex.

The classic GI manifestation of polyarteritis nodosa is "intestinal angina," the occurrence of postprandial abdominal pain. Polyarteritis nodosa can also affect individual GI tract organs such as the gallbladder or appendix, presenting as cholecystitis or appendicitis, respectively. The typical renal manifestation of polyarteritis nodosa is vasculitic involvement of the medium-sized intrarenal arteries, leading to renin-mediated hypertension and renal infarctions. Cardiac lesions, which usually remain subclinical, may lead to myocardial infarction or congestive heart failure. Polyarteritis nodosa usually spares the lungs.

The diagnosis of polyarteritis nodosa requires either a tissue biopsy or an angiogram that demonstrates microaneurysms (Fig. 254-1).[6] Simultaneous nerve and muscle biopsies (e.g., sural nerve and gastrocnemius muscle) are of high yield if there is a clinical suspicion of vasculitic neuropathy. Symptoms suggestive of a neuropathy can be confirmed by electrodiagnostic studies that demonstrate a sensorimotor axonal neuropathy, often in a mononeuritis multiplex pattern. The pathologic changes in polyarteritis nodosa are limited to the arterial circulation, and the lesions are segmental, favoring the branch points of arteries. In gross pathologic specimens, aneurysmal bulges of the arterial wall may be visible. Histologic sections reveal infiltration and destruction of the blood vessel wall by inflammatory cells, accompanied by fibrinoid necrosis. Granulomatous inflammation is absent.

TREATMENT   Rx

Therapeutic regimens involving entecavir or tenofovir combined with plasma exchange and short-term (two-week) courses of glucocorticoids have substantially improved the treatment of hepatitis B virus (HBV)-associated polyarteritis nodosa. Because of increasing use of the HBV vaccine, however, fewer than 10% of polyarteritis nodosa cases now are associated with HBV infections. Patients with idiopathic polyarteritis nodosa and multiorgan involvement require high-dose glucocorticoid treatment initially. Approximately half of patients with idiopathic polyarteritis nodosa achieve remissions or cures with high doses of glucocorticoids alone. Severe cases of multiorgan disease, particularly vasculitic neuropathy, should be treated with cyclophosphamide (2 mg/kg/day, adjusted for renal dysfunction). For patients with idiopathic polyarteritis nodosa limited to the skin, tumor necrosis factor inhibitors may be effective glucocorticoid-sparing agents. Most patients with either HBV-associated or idiopathic polyarteritis nodosa ultimately achieve cures of their disease.

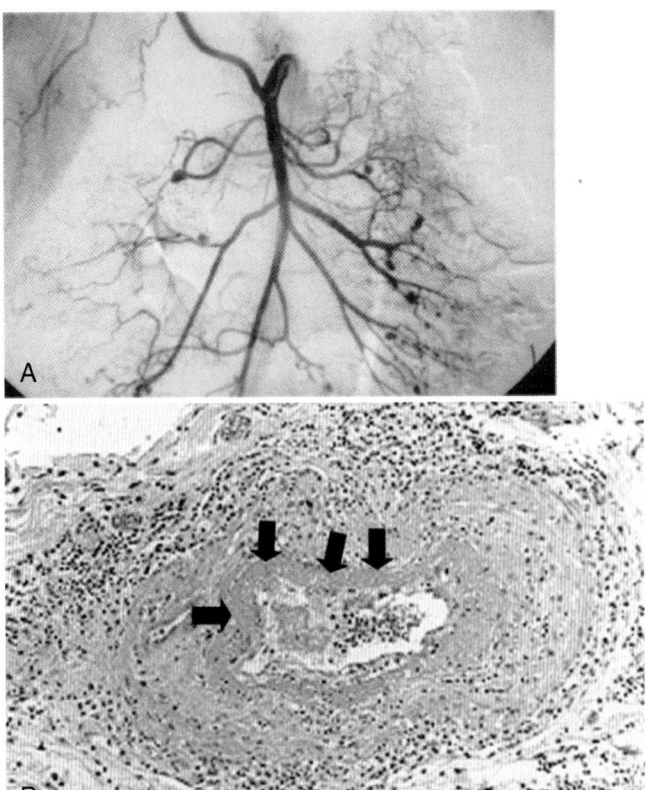

FIGURE 254-1. Vasculitis of medium-sized arteries in polyarteritis nodosa. **A,** Mesenteric angiogram showing numerous aneurysms in medium-sized arteries. **B,** Fibrinoid necrosis (*arrows*) in a jejunal artery from a patient who required surgical resection of necrotic bowel.

Kawasaki Disease

Kawasaki disease occurs exclusively in young children. Because of its striking mucocutaneous findings and lymphadenopathy, Kawasaki disease is also known as mucocutaneous lymph node syndrome. Features of Kawasaki disease include high fevers, cervical adenopathy, conjunctival congestion, buccal erythema, prominence of the tongue papillae ("strawberry tongue"), a polymorphous truncal rash, erythema of the palms and soles, and desquamation of skin from the fingertips occurring days to weeks into the illness.[7,8] In its acuity and severity, Kawasaki disease resembles toxic shock syndrome and scarlet fever, both of which are mediated by superantigens (see Pathophysiology).

In a small number of patients with Kawasaki disease, panvasculitis in the coronary vessels leads to acute cardiac complications. Coronary arteritis leads to narrowing of the vessel lumen by the migration of myointimal cells from the media through the fragmented internal elastic lamina. Direct complications include aneurysmal dilation and thrombosis of the coronary arteries, leading to myocardial infarction and possibly to death (in 1 to 2% of patients with Kawasaki disease during the acute illness). Late mortality from myocardial infarction may occur from the thrombosis of coronary artery aneurysms formed during the initial inflammatory stage. Such myocardial infarctions have been reported in middle-aged individuals who had febrile illnesses consistent with Kawasaki disease in childhood.

TREATMENT   Rx

The recommended therapeutic regimen in Kawasaki disease is the combination of intravenous immune globulin (IVIG; 400 mg/kg/day on 4 consecutive days) and acetylsalicylic acid (100 mg/kg/day, lowered to 3 to 5 mg/kg/day after resolution of the fever). IVIG prevents the formation of coronary aneurysms in most cases.[9] For patients who are predicted to be unresponsive to IVIG, the combination of IVIG plus cyclosporine (5 mg/kg for 5 days) is better than IVIG alone.[A3] Glucocorticoids are reserved for salvage therapy in patients whose treatment with IVIG and acetylsalicylic acid has failed.[A4]

Buerger Disease

Buerger disease, also known as thromboangiitis obliterans (Chapter 72), is not considered to be a primary form of vasculitis and was not included in the most recent consensus statement on nomenclature. Buerger disease has a remarkably strong yet poorly understood association with cigarette smoking. In short, it does not occur in the absence of exposure to tobacco. The vessels affected by Buerger disease are the distal medium-sized arteries and veins, particularly vessels at the levels of the ankles and wrists. The disease is characterized by thrombotic obliterations that begin distally and proceed proximally. Buerger disease tends to be segmental in nature, involving 5- to 10-cm lengths of blood vessels. Arterial obliteration leads to the development of collateral vessels with a "corkscrew" appearance on angiography. Vascular occlusion in Buerger disease often leads to the loss of digits and, if smoking persists, to loss of larger amounts of tissue (e.g., hands or feet). Despite the intense involvement of the extremities in Buerger disease, internal organ disease almost never occurs.

TREATMENT　Rx

Complete abstinence from tobacco is essential to the treatment of Buerger disease. Failure to stop smoking is associated with a dramatic increase in the risk of limb loss by amputation. No other therapeutic interventions, including glucocorticoids and anticoagulation, have dramatic effects on Buerger disease.

Small-Vessel Vasculitides

Antineutrophil Cytoplasmic Antibody–Associated Vasculitides

Granulomatosis with Polyangiitis

Classic GPA (formerly Wegener granulomatosis) involves the upper respiratory tract, lungs, and kidneys. Distinctive features may also occur in the eyes, ears, and other organs. The three pathology hallmarks of GPA are (1) granulomatous inflammation in the upper or lower respiratory tract, (2) necrotizing vasculitis affecting arteries or veins, and (3) segmental glomerulonephritis associated with necrosis and thrombosis of capillary loops, with or without granulomatous lesions.

Approximately 90% of patients with GPA have nasal involvement, including crusting, bleeding, and obstruction. Cartilaginous inflammation may lead to nasal septal perforation and collapse of the nasal bridge ("saddle nose" deformity). Erosive sinus disease and subglottic stenosis (narrowing of the trachea just below the vocal cords) are highly characteristic of GPA.

Both conductive and sensorineural hearing loss can occur in GPA, though conductive lesions caused by middle ear disease are more common. Orbital masses ("pseudotumors" that develop behind the eye), scleritis, and peripheral ulcerative keratitis are the most dangerous ocular lesions. Episcleritis and conjunctivitis also occur. Uveitis is rare. The clinical manifestations of GPA in the lung range from asymptomatic nodules to fulminant alveolar hemorrhage. The most common radiographic findings are pulmonary infiltrates, nodules, and cavitary lesions. Large-airway disease leading to bronchial narrowing is a challenging diagnosis to establish because patients present with few symptoms until advanced disease is present.

The clinical presentation of renal disease in GPA is usually rapidly progressive glomerulonephritis: hematuria, red blood cell casts, and proteinuria (usually non-nephrotic). Without appropriate therapy, end-stage renal disease may ensue within weeks.

Sixty percent of patients with GPA have musculoskeletal symptoms during their disease course. The presenting complaint is frequently arthralgias or an oligoarthritis that is migratory in nature. Skin lesions in GPA include the full panoply of lesions associated with cutaneous vasculitis, including purpura (Fig. 254-2). Cutaneous nodules over the extensor surfaces of joints, particularly the elbow, may mimic rheumatoid nodules. These lesions are known as cutaneous extravascular necrotizing granulomata or Churg-Strauss lesions. Meningeal inflammation, presenting with headaches, cranial neuropathies, and a clinical picture compatible with chronic meningitis, is perhaps the most common central nervous system (CNS) manifestation of GPA. Mononeuritis multiplex may affect the peripheral nervous system.

GPA is the prototype of conditions associated with ANCA.[10] Approximately 75 to 80% of GPA patients have antibodies directed against proteinase 3 (PR3), which lead to positive cytoplasmic (C-ANCA) staining on immunofluorescence testing of serum against human neutrophils. Another 10 to 15% have antibodies directed against myeloperoxidase (MPO), which cause perinuclear staining on immunofluorescence. An ANCA-negative assay sample does not exclude GPA, because a substantial minority of patients are ANCA-negative.

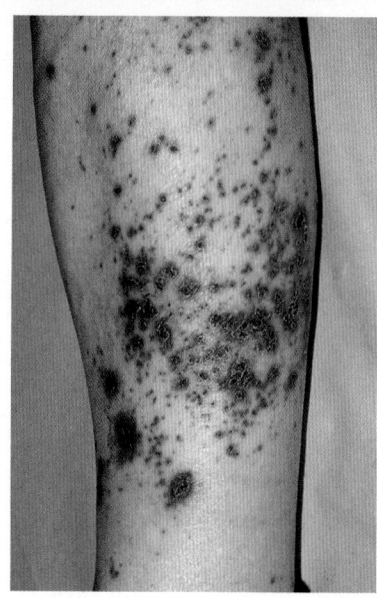

FIGURE 254-2. Cutaneous small-vessel vasculitis showing palpable purpuric lesions with necrosis and crusting.

ANCA titers do not correlate precisely with disease activity and, indeed, should generally not be used as the sole guide to treatment.

TREATMENT　Rx

Manifestations of GPA that constitute immediate threats either to the function of a vital organ or to the patient's life require treatment urgently.[11] From the late 1960s until 2010, the combination of cyclophosphamide (2 mg/kg orally daily) and high doses of glucocorticoids (prednisone 1 mg/kg orally daily, tapered during 6 to 12 months) was the standard of care for GPA. Intermittent administration of cyclophosphamide by IV infusion is also effective in remission induction. However, a multicenter clinical trial that compared rituximab to cyclophosphamide in patients with either GPA or microscopic polyangiitis demonstrated that rituximab (375 mg/m² weekly times four) is at least as effective as the conventional regimen.[A5][A6] Rituximab appears to be more effective for AAV patients who present with disease flares. An alternative dosing regimen of rituximab, 1 g times two separated by 2 weeks, may also be effective.[12] Limited forms of GPA may respond to the combination of methotrexate (up to 25 mg/week) and glucocorticoids, but rituximab is now often employed in this setting as well. Rituximab (e.g., 500 mg every 6 months) is more effective than azathioprine for maintaining remission in patients who demonstrate a tendency to flare.[A7] In patients with end-stage renal disease, renal transplantation can substantially reduce subsequent mortality.[13]

Microscopic Polyangiitis

Microscopic polyangiitis is characterized by (1) nongranulomatous necrotizing vasculitis with few or no immune deposits, (2) involvement of small (and possibly medium-sized) blood vessels in the arterial or venous circulation, and (3) tropism for the kidneys and lungs. Many cases of small-vessel vasculitis once regarded as polyarteritis nodosa are now classified more properly as microscopic polyangiitis. In contrast to polyarteritis nodosa, an ANCA-negative disorder, 70% of microscopic polyangiitis patients are ANCA positive. Thus, microscopic polyangiitis is considered to be a form of AAV. The ANCAs in microscopic polyangiitis are usually directed against myeloperoxidase, leading to a perinuclear pattern of staining on immunofluorescence testing (P-ANCA). Microscopic polyangiitis is not characterized by granulomatous inflammation, and upper respiratory tract symptoms, if present at all, are much milder than those associated with GPA.

TREATMENT　Rx

The approach to the treatment of microscopic polyangiitis is similar to the treatment of GPA. The combination of rituximab and glucocorticoids is the treatment regimen of choice for most patients with microscopic polyangiitis.

Eosinophilic Granulomatosis with Polyangiitis

EGPA (formerly named Churg-Strauss syndrome) is an eosinophil-rich form of granulomatous inflammation that involves the respiratory tract and other organs. The disease is associated with necrotizing vasculitis of small to medium-sized vessels. Two hallmarks of EGPA are asthma and eosinophilia. Several phases of EGPA are described:

- A prodromal phase characterized by the presence of allergic disease (typically asthma or allergic rhinitis), which may last months to many years
- An eosinophilia–tissue infiltration phase in which remarkably high peripheral eosinophilia may occur and tissue infiltration by eosinophils is observed in the lung, GI tract, and other tissues
- A vasculitic phase in which systemic necrotizing vasculitis afflicts a wide range of organs, ranging from the heart and lungs to peripheral nerves and skin

TREATMENT

Patients with mild disease may be treated with prednisone. The addition of mepolizumab, 300 mg subcutaneously each month, has also been shown to have an important glucocorticoid-sparing role. Patients with evidence of neurologic, cardiac, renal, or GI involvement should be treated with cyclophosphamide or rituximab[14] in addition to glucocorticoids. Although clinical remissions are obtained in more than 90% of patients with EGPA, the majority of patients are unable to discontinue glucocorticoids entirely (primarily because of asthma symptoms), and disease recurrences are seen in 25%. In most cases, relapses are heralded by the return of eosinophilia. Approximately 50% of cases of EGPA are associated with ANCA, usually directed against myeloperoxidase, but the percentage may be higher among untreated patients.

Immune Complex–Mediated Vasculitides

Anti–Glomerular Basement Membrane Disease

Anti–glomerular basement membrane (anti-GBM) disease is vasculitis affecting glomerular capillaries, pulmonary capillaries, or both, accompanied by the deposition of anti–basement membrane autoantibodies within basement membranes. Anti-GBM disease is discussed in detail elsewhere (Chapter 113).

Immunoglobulin A Vasculitis/Henoch-Schönlein Purpura

IgA vasculitis (IgAV) is characterized by nonthrombocytopenic purpura, arthritis, abdominal pain, and glomerulonephritis. The histopathologic findings are those of a leukocytoclastic vasculitis with IgA deposition. IgAV can develop at any age, but 80 to 90% of the cases occur in children. Although the cause is unknown, the disease's seasonal variation and the fact that two thirds of patients with IgAV experience antecedent acute upper respiratory illnesses suggest an infectious trigger in the majority of cases. The diagnosis of IgAV can be confirmed only by demonstration of IgA deposition within and around blood vessel walls.

The classic IgAV patient presents with the acute onset of fever, palpable purpura on the lower extremities and buttocks, abdominal pain, arthritis, and hematuria. The clinician must be alert to the possibility of IgAV even when only parts of the syndrome are present. Most patients with IgAV, especially children, have a self-limited disease that lasts an average of 4 weeks.

TREATMENT

Glucocorticoids ameliorate the GI, joint, and skin symptoms in many cases, but some patients respond surprisingly poorly to conventional doses of glucocorticoids, even in doses on the order of 40 to 60 mg/day. Anecdotal evidence suggests that pulse glucocorticoids (e.g., methylprednisolone 500 to 1000 mg/day times three doses) may abort persistent bouts of IgAV. The efficacy of glucocorticoids in the glomerulonephritis associated with this condition is controversial. Uncontrolled studies suggest that methylprednisolone pulses (1 g/day for three doses), followed by oral prednisone combined with azathioprine or mycophenolate mofetil may be useful in severe glomerulonephritis associated with IgAV.

Hypocomplementemic Urticarial Vasculitis

At least three subtypes of urticarial vasculitis are known: (1) normocomplementemic, a form that is generally idiopathic and benign (which may be viewed as a manifestation of cutaneous leukocytoclastic angiitis); (2) hypocomplementemic, a form that is often associated with a systemic inflammatory disease; and (3) hypocomplementemic urticarial vasculitis syndrome (HUVS), a potentially severe condition usually associated with autoantibodies to the collagen-like region of C1q. Most patients with the hypocomplementemic subtype have an underlying systemic disorder, such as systemic lupus erythematosus (Chapter 250) or Sjögren syndrome (Chapter 252). Many HUVS patients have C1q "precipitins," IgG autoantibodies to the collagen-like region of C1q that trigger the classical pathway of complement activation. The role of anti-C1q antibodies in disease pathogenesis remains unclear.

The lesions of urticarial vasculitis must be distinguished from the far more common chronic idiopathic urticaria (Chapters 237 and 411). Unlike idiopathic urticaria, the lesions of urticarial vasculitis last more than 48 hours, often have a purpuric component (i.e., they do not blanch), and resolve with postinflammatory hyperpigmentation. In urticarial vasculitis, lesions associated with vasculitis are often accompanied by stinging or burning. Urticarial vasculitis affects the capillaries and postcapillary venules, showing leukocytoclastic vasculitis on light microscopy. Direct immunofluorescence studies reveal both immunoglobulin and complement deposition in or around blood vessels of the upper dermis or the dermoepidermal junction.

TREATMENT

Patients with urticarial vasculitis whose serum complement levels remain normal during attacks often have self-limited disease and require little therapy. Other cases, especially HUVS, may cause life-threatening involvement of the lungs or other organs and require periods of intensive immunosuppression. Treatment decisions in HUVS must be individualized according to the patient's clinical status.

Cryoglobulinemia

Cryoglobulins are antibodies that precipitate from serum under conditions of cold and resolubilize on rewarming.[15] Cryoglobulins are classified into types I, II, and III on the basis of whether monoclonality and rheumatoid factor activity (the ability to bind to the Fc portion of IgG) are present. Type I cryoglobulins, which are monoclonal but lack rheumatoid factor activity, are associated with certain hematopoietic malignant neoplasms (e.g., multiple myeloma) and often lead to hyperviscosity rather than to vasculitis (Chapter 178). In contrast, type II and type III cryoglobulins may be associated with systemic vasculitis involving small (and often medium-sized) blood vessels. Vasculitis results from the deposition of cryoglobulin-containing immune complexes within blood vessel walls and the activation of complement.

Cryoglobulin types II and III are termed *mixed cryoglobulins* because they consist of complexes of both IgG and IgM antibodies. The IgM components in both type II and type III cryoglobulinemia possess rheumatoid factor activity (i.e., assays for rheumatoid factor are positive, indicating binding of the IgM antibody to the Fc portion of IgG). Whereas the IgM component in type II cryoglobulin is monoclonal, the IgM in type III cryoglobulin is polyclonal. Ninety percent of patients with vasculitis secondary to mixed cryoglobulins are hypocomplementemic, with C4 levels characteristically more depressed than C3. Infection with hepatitis C virus (HCV) accounts for at least 80% of the vasculitis cases associated with mixed cryoglobulins.[16]

TREATMENT

The optimal therapy for most cases of cryoglobulinemic vasculitis is successful treatment of the underlying HCV infection. For cryoglobulinemic patients with relatively mild disease (e.g., frequent purpuric lesions, shallow cutaneous ulcers), short courses of prednisone followed by the institution of effective therapy for HCV may be sufficient. For patients with severe cutaneous ulcers, mononeuritis multiplex, glomerulonephritis, or other manifestations of severe disease, glucocorticoids, rituximab, and possibly a short course of plasma exchange may be indicated.

Variable-Vessel Vasculitides

The variable-vessel vasculitides have no predominant type of vessel involved but rather can affect vessels of any size (small, medium, and large) and any type (arteries, veins, and capillaries).

Cogan Syndrome

The combination of inflammatory eye disease and vestibuloauditory dysfunction is the sine qua non of Cogan syndrome.[17] In addition to inflammatory disease of the eyes and ears, up to 15% of patients with Cogan syndrome have vasculitis involving medium-sized to large blood vessels. Although the ocular manifestations vary, the classic presentation is the combination of interstitial keratitis and sensorineural hearing loss. Cogan syndrome may appear first in either the eyes or the ears. Although intervals as long as 1 to 2 years have been described between the start of disease in one organ and the appearance of disease in the other, the time between disease manifestations in these organs is usually only a matter of months. Patients usually present with photophobia and blurry vision, sometimes accompanied simultaneously by auditory or vestibular dysfunction. The vascular disease associated with Cogan syndrome remains poorly described but typically involves the primary branches of the thoracic or abdominal aorta.

TREATMENT   Rx

Rapidly progressive sensorineural hearing loss requires early and aggressive therapy with high doses of systemic glucocorticoids. Some otolaryngologists also perform intratympanic injections of glucocorticoids. Cyclophosphamide, mycophenolate mofetil, and biologic agents such as tumor necrosis inhibitors or rituximab can be considered for patients with suboptimal responses to glucocorticoids who still have salvageable hearing. Nevertheless, attempts at treatment are begun too late in some patients, and it is important to realize when the risk of further immunosuppression outstrips the likelihood of long-term benefit. Many Cogan syndrome patients become candidates for cochlear implants.

Behçet Syndrome

Behçet syndrome may affect small, medium, and large vessels in either the venous or the arterial circulation.[18] The most typical lesions in Behçet syndrome are mucocutaneous, reflecting the involvement of small blood vessels. The triad of recurrent mouth ulcers, genital ulcers, and eye inflammation is the classic presentation. The criteria for diagnosis of the International Study Group for Behçet Syndrome consist of one required manifestation—recurrent oral ulceration—plus at least two of the following: recurrent genital ulceration, characteristic eye or skin lesions, or a pathergy reaction (see later). However, the spectrum of Behçet syndrome encompasses many manifestations not included in these criteria. In addition, oral ulcers are not invariably the first disease manifestation, so the diagnosis of Behçet syndrome must be considered in the occurrence of disease features otherwise highly characteristic (e.g., bilateral panuveitis).

Large-vessel complications of Behçet syndrome may include aneurysms in the pulmonary and systemic arterial systems. Venous complications include thromboses of the deep venous system, vena cava, portohepatic vein, and cerebral sinus. Pathergy—the development of pustules at the sites of sterile needle pricks—is a distinctive feature in many patients with Behçet syndrome, particularly those of Turkish origin. The arthritis of Behçet syndrome is a nondeforming, oligoarticular, asymmetrical arthritis of large joints. GI lesions in Behçet syndrome typically consist of ulcerations of the distal ileum or cecum. Crohn disease (Chapter 132), which can cause genital ulcers as well as GI tract disease, may be particularly difficult to distinguish from Behçet syndrome.

TREATMENT   Rx

Low-dose glucocorticoids are effective for intransigent mucocutaneous disease and may have a better side-effect profile than other medications used for this purpose (e.g., thalidomide). Intermittent courses of glucocorticoids during periods of particular mucocutaneous disease activity may be sufficient for patients with mild disease.[19] Apremilast, an oral phosphodiesterase 4 inhibitor, (at 30 mg twice daily for 12 weeks) has shown effectiveness in treating oral ulcers in a preliminary study.[A9] Colchicine is often considered for mucocutaneous disease, but its efficacy is doubtful.

Severe disease in any organ system always requires initial therapy with high doses of prednisone (e.g., 1 mg/kg/day). TNF inhibition with infliximab (5 mg/kg IV every 4 to 6 weeks) or adalimumab (40 mg every other week) is the treatment of choice for patients with the most severe forms of uveitis or meningoencephalitis.

Selected Single-Organ Vasculitides

Single-organ vasculitis is defined as vasculitis within the vessels of any type or size of a single organ, in the absence of any features (e.g., ANCA) suggesting one of the systemic forms of vasculitis.

Cutaneous Leukocytoclastic Angiitis

Cutaneous leukocytoclastic angiitis has also been termed *hypersensitivity vasculitis*. Cutaneous leukocytoclastic angiitis is the preferred name because no hypersensitivity or allergy is evident in many cases. Histories of exposure to new medications or to infections may be elicited. An immune complex deposition is central to the pathophysiologic process. Although it is occasionally associated with synovitis, other signs of systemic involvement are absent.

The skin lesions in cutaneous leukocytoclastic angiitis occur in "crops," coinciding with some period of elapsed time following exposure to the inciting antigen. The usual time between the exposure and the onset of clinically evident vasculitis is 10 to 14 days. The lesions typically occur first in dependent regions, such as on the lower extremities or buttocks. The rash may be asymptomatic but is usually accompanied by burning or tingling sensations.

TREATMENT   Rx

Keys to the management of cutaneous leukocytoclastic angiitis include (1) exclusion of any underlying form of vasculitis that may cause subclinical involvement of other organs and (2) removal of any agent (e.g., a medication) that may have triggered the vasculitis. For patients in whom a precipitant can be identified, elimination of the offending agent usually leads to resolution of the vasculitis within days to weeks. The type, intensity, and duration of therapy for cutaneous leukocytoclastic angiitis are based on the degree of disease severity. Mild cases may be treated simply with leg elevation, H_1 antihistamines, or low-dose prednisone. For persistent disease not associated with cutaneous gangrene, colchicine, hydroxychloroquine, or dapsone may be tried. For severe cases, high doses of glucocorticoids are indicated to suppress inflammation quickly and prevent skin ulceration.

Vasculitis of the Central Nervous System

CNS vasculitis[20] includes two major categories of disease, one of which is not a true vasculitis. These conditions are primary angiitis of the CNS (PACNS) and reversible cerebral vasoconstriction syndrome (RCVS). The diagnosis and management of these two conditions differ dramatically. The clinical, radiologic, and pathologic characteristics of PACNS and RCVS are shown in Table 254-5.

Primary Angiitis of the Central Nervous System

PACNS typically develops in a subacute fashion, with the evolution of multifocal strokes, encephalopathy, headache, and other clinical features over months. Headache is often the first symptom. As the condition progresses, most patients develop lethargy, confusion, and memory loss. Some patients develop multifocal strokes, seizures, evidence of increased intracranial pressure, or myelopathy. The results of routine laboratory tests (e.g., erythrocyte sedimentation rate) are often normal in PACNS. Lumbar puncture demonstrates abnormalities of the cerebrospinal fluid in approximately 80% of cases, usually a modest monocytosis and elevated protein. Lumbar punctures should be performed in all patients in whom the diagnosis of PACNS is considered seriously. Although the findings on lumbar puncture in PACNS patients are nonspecific, a normal lumbar puncture argues against PACNS, and the procedure frequently identifies important PACNS mimickers such as infection or malignancy.

Magnetic resonance imaging (MRI) is the critical imaging modality in PACNS. Because of the subacute nature of the disorder, MRI studies reveal multifocal CNS infarctions in most cases. Strokes, hemorrhagic lesions, and mass lesions typically occur in more than one vascular territory. A normal brain MRI argues strongly against the diagnosis of PACNS. Angiography is less helpful in the evaluation of patients with PACNS for two main reasons. First, the sizes of blood vessels involved in PACNS are often too small to be resolved adequately, even by conventional angiography. The false-negative rate of angiography in PACNS is on the order of 35%. Second, the "classic" string-of-beads abnormality on angiography, produced by segmental arterial narrowing alternating with dilations, is nonspecific and can be mimicked perfectly by a host of nonvasculitic conditions (the most common of which is RCVS). No angiographic pattern is pathognomonic for PACNS, and there

TABLE 254-5 PRIMARY ANGIITIS OF THE CENTRAL NERVOUS SYSTEM (PACNS) VERSUS REVERSIBLE CEREBRAL VASOCONSTRICTION SYNDROME (RCVS)

	PACNS	RCVS
Female-to-male ratio	1 : 1	2-3 : 1
Onset	Subacute (weeks to months)	Sudden (seconds to minutes)
Headache	Insidious, dull	Thunderclap
Typical lumbar puncture findings	Abnormal in 50-80%: lymphocytic pleocytosis; elevated protein	Normal
Typical MRI findings	Multifocal subacute infarctions	Normal Watershed infarcts in minority
Typical angiogram findings	Normal in up to 40% of cases Abnormal angiographic features when present cannot be distinguished from RCVS	Multifocal stenoses/ dilatations
Utility of brain biopsy	Reasonable sensitivity in appropriately selected patients Important for excluding disease mimickers	Little to no role Helpful if confusing clinical situation confounds differentiation from PACNS or PACNS mimickers

MRI = magnetic resonance imaging.

TABLE 254-6 MAJOR DISEASE CATEGORIES IN THE DIFFERENTIAL DIAGNOSIS OF VASCULITIDES

Other forms of vasculitis
Simultaneous occurrence of common medical problems in the same patient
Infections
    Bacterial, viral, mycobacterial, fungal
Occlusive processes
    Hypercoagulable states
    Livedoid vasculopathy (atrophie blanche)
    Atheroembolic disease
Malignant neoplasms
    Lymphoma (including lymphomatoid granulomatosis)
    Castleman disease
    Amyloidosis
    Paraproteinemias
Connective tissue disorders
    Systemic lupus erythematosus, mixed connective tissue disease
    Systemic sclerosis
    Rheumatoid arthritis
Miscellaneous
    Atrial myxoma
    Calciphylaxis
    Fibromuscular dysplasia
    Neutrophilic dermatoses
    Pyoderma gangrenosum
    Sarcoidosis
    Reversible cerebral vasoconstriction syndrome

is a significant tendency to overdiagnose "vasculitis" on angiographic grounds alone. A normal brain MRI in the setting of an abnormal angiogram suggests RCVS, not PACNS.

When employed in appropriately selected patients whose history and radiologic studies suggest PACNS, brain biopsy is associated with reasonable positive and negative predictive values and frequently identifies important PACNS mimickers.

TREATMENT   Rx

Prednisone and cyclophosphamide are appropriate for treatment of patients who have abnormal findings on brain biopsy. Treatment courses of 6 to 12 months are recommended.

Reversible Cerebral Vasoconstriction Syndrome

RCVS is probably far more common than PACNS. Overtreatment of patients with RCVS who are misdiagnosed as having PACNS leads to substantial morbidity. Eighty percent of patients with RCVS are women.

A careful history is the most important part of the evaluation. In contrast to the subacute course that typifies PACNS, RCVS usually begins in a more dramatic fashion with a "thunderclap" headache.[21] Compared with PACNS, the neurologic signs are less severe in RCVS (e.g., encephalopathy is less common). RCVS frequently occurs in the setting of precipitants associated with vasospasm, such as in the postpartum setting or following the use of vasoactive agents such as nasal decongestants and recreational drugs.

The lumbar puncture is usually normal in RCVS, and brain MRI usually does not show multifocal CNS infarctions, with the exception of watershed infarctions mentioned earlier. The typical angiographic findings in RCVS—vascular narrowing and beading—are generally indistinguishable from those of PACNS and conditions that mimic PACNS. Multifocal vascular narrowing is particularly characteristic of RCVS. The most distinctive angiographic feature of RCVS is that the abnormalities are completely reversible, usually within 4 to 8 weeks. These abnormalities in RCVS are caused by vasospasm rather than true vasculitis. In the evaluation of patients with potential RCVS, a diagnostic strategy that can clinch the diagnosis is a follow-up angiogram 4 to 8 weeks after the first. Angiographic abnormalities due to RCVS will resolve in this interval.

TREATMENT   Rx

Several approaches to the treatment of RCVS are reasonable. First, one may opt for watchful waiting. It is not clear that immunosuppression is either necessary or helpful. Moreover, attempts to treat vasospasm with calcium-channel blockers may lead to a vascular steal phenomenon, potentially causing harm. Second, because it is frequently difficult to do nothing for a patient with possibly serious CNS disease, calcium-channel blockers (e.g., nifedipine 30 mg three times daily) may be tried. Third, because of the frequent diagnostic uncertainty at the time of presentation, some clinicians opt to treat empirically with glucocorticoids (prednisone 1 mg/kg/day) for 1 month, followed by a taper over several weeks. Fourth, combinations of calcium-channel blockers and glucocorticoids are also reasonable. Cytotoxic therapy is not indicated in RCVS.

DIAGNOSIS
Differential Diagnosis

The major categories of diseases that can mimic vasculitis are displayed in Table 254-6. Certain features of a patient's case should raise the diagnostic suspicion for vasculitis. First, most cases of vasculitis do not begin suddenly but rather unfold subacutely during weeks or months. Second, pain is usually a prominent feature of vasculitis, resulting from arthritis or arthralgias, myalgias, headaches, neuropathy, testicular infarction, digital ischemia, sinusitis, otalgia, back pain (caused by aortic inflammation), postprandial abdominal pain (caused by mesenteric vasculitis), or other disease manifestations. Third, signs of inflammation such as fever, rash, weight loss, and elevated acute phase reactants are highly characteristic. Finally, multiorgan system involvement is the rule in vasculitis.

The diagnosis of vasculitis should be established through biopsy of an involved organ whenever possible. Diagnoses based on angiography alone have many potential pitfalls, as discussed in the sections on PACNS and RCVS. Angiographic findings that are "consistent with vasculitis" must be interpreted in the proper context. A diverse array of other diseases, ranging from atherosclerosis to vasospasm to pheochromocytoma, may mimic the angiographic appearance of vasculitis. Systemic vasculitis can also be mimicked by two or more common medical problems or treatment complications occurring simultaneously in the same patient. Finally, high on the differential diagnosis of any individual form of vasculitis are other forms of vasculitis. For example, digital ischemia and splinter hemorrhages may be secondary to idiopathic polyarteritis nodosa. They may also be caused by polyarteritis nodosa associated with HBV infection, GPA, EGPA, microscopic polyangiitis, cryoglobulinemia, Buerger disease, or some other form of vasculitis. Because the appropriate interventions for these conditions vary widely, careful distinction among these potential etiologies is essential.

TREATMENT   Rx

Current treatment approaches to specific vasculitides are described under their "Clinical Manifestations" for each disease. General points regarding therapy are addressed here.

The intensity of treatment in patients with vasculitis must be guided by the degree of disease activity. Specifically, the treatment of vasculitis should be predicated not only on abnormal laboratory test results but also on clear evidence of active disease. In addition, the intensity of treatment must be adapted to the type of vasculitis. Whereas giant cell arteritis responds to high doses of glucocorticoids in most cases, for example, GPA nearly always requires an additional agent (rituximab, cyclophosphamide, or methotrexate) for disease control. In contrast, despite the dramatic fashion in which they sometimes present, most cases of IgA vasculitis and cutaneous leukocytoclastic angiitis require no immunosuppressive treatment at all.

Conventional therapies such as glucocorticoids, immunomodulating agents, and cytotoxic drugs induce remissions and control vasculitis in most cases. Moreover, in some cases—a variable percentage, depending on the type of vasculitis—the disease is curable. Unfortunately, the treatments of vasculitis have enormous potential for toxicity. Regular monitoring of patients' bone marrow, renal, and hepatic function is essential to avoid treatment-induced toxicity. Prophylaxis against opportunistic infections, particularly *Pneumocystis* pneumonia (Chapter 321), is an important part of many vasculitis treatment regimens. During the tapering of immunosuppressive medications, disease flares are common in many forms of vasculitis.

A common error is treating patients with high doses of immunosuppressive agents for too long. The most appropriate use of medications such as cyclophosphamide and glucocorticoids is to induce remission as quickly as possible with early, aggressive treatment regimens, and then to convert patients to safer treatments for the maintenance of remission. Rituximab is replacing cyclophosphamide as the drug of choice for some forms of vasculitis, particularly AAV. Patients with AAV who demonstrate a tendency to flare are often retreated with rituximab (500 mg or 1 g) every 4 to 6 months, at least until lengthy periods of disease control are established.

PROGNOSIS

Assuming that the diagnosis is made before the patient has become catastrophically ill, the prognosis in systemic vasculitis is determined largely by the answers to four questions:

1. Was the diagnosis established before the occurrence of major irreversible organ damage?
2. Was aggressive (but appropriately dosed) treatment begun in a timely fashion?
3. Was there careful monitoring during treatment, and were specific steps taken to avoid drug-induced toxicity (e.g., opportunistic infection)?
4. Were the potentially toxic medications that induced remission stopped at an appropriate juncture and replaced with less dangerous medications (or was treatment stopped altogether)?

For most forms of vasculitis, the factors that determine long-term drug-free remissions remain poorly understood. The likelihood of achieving sustained remissions after discontinuation of all medications (or cures) varies according to the specific type of vasculitis.

FUTURE DIRECTIONS

Compelling laboratory and naturally occurring animal models of disease, combined with the known associations among HBV, HCV, and vasculitis in humans, suggest that additional links between infection and systemic vasculitis may be established in the future. Important strides have been made in the description of cytokine and chemokine pathways that are operative in vascular inflammation, but relevant anticytokine interventions remain to be defined for clinical therapies. B-cell depletion is emerging rapidly as the treatment of choice for some forms of severe vasculitis. IL-6 inhibition strategies also now play important roles in the large-vessel vasculitides. Additional studies are required to define the full spectrum of clinical utility of these and other biologic agents.

Grade A References

A1. Stone JH, Tuckwell K, Dimonaco S, et al. Trial of tocilizumab in giant-cell arteritis. *N Engl J Med.* 2017;377:317-328.
A2. Nakaoka Y, Isobe M, Takei S, et al. Efficacy and safety of tocilizumab in patients with refractory Takayasu arteritis: results from a randomised, double-blind, placebo-controlled, phase 3 trial in Japan (the TAKT study). *Ann Rheum Dis.* 2018;77:348-354.
A3. Hamada H, Suzuki H, Onouchi Y, et al. Efficacy of primary treatment with immunoglobulin plus ciclosporin for prevention of coronary artery abnormalities in patients with Kawasaki disease predicted to be at increased risk of non-response to intravenous immunoglobulin (KAICA): a randomised controlled, open-label, blinded-endpoints, phase 3 trial. *Lancet.* 2019;393:1128-1137.
A4. Wardle AJ, Connolly GM, Seager MJ, et al. Corticosteroids for the treatment of Kawasaki disease in children. *Cochrane Database Syst Rev.* 2017;1:CD011188.
A5. Stone JH, Merkel PA, Spiera R, et al. Rituximab versus cyclophosphamide for remission induction in ANCA-associated vasculitis. *N Engl J Med.* 2010;363:221-232.
A6. Specks U, Merkel PA, Seo P, et al. Efficacy of remission-induction regimens for ANCA-associated vasculitis. *N Engl J Med.* 2013;369:417-427.
A7. Guillevin L, Pagnoux C, Karras A, et al. Rituximab versus azathioprine for maintenance in ANCA-associated vasculitis. *N Engl J Med.* 2014;371:1771-1780.
A8. Wechsler ME, Akuthota P, Jayne D, et al. Mepolizumab or placebo for eosinophilic granulomatosis with polyangiitis. *N Engl J Med.* 2017;376:1921-1932.
A9. Hatemi G, Melikoglu M, Tunc R, et al. Apremilast for Behçet's syndrome—a phase 2, placebo-controlled study. *N Engl J Med.* 2015;372:1510-1518.

GENERAL REFERENCES

For the General References and other additional features, please visit Expert Consult at https://expertconsult.inkling.com.

255

GIANT CELL ARTERITIS AND POLYMYALGIA RHEUMATICA

ROBERT SPIERA

DEFINITION

Polymyalgia rheumatica (PMR) and temporal arteritis, also called giant cell arteritis (GCA), are companion systemic inflammatory disorders of unknown etiology that represent a spectrum from severe proximal aches and pains and constitutional symptoms to an occlusive granulomatous vasculitis of medium and large vessels that can lead to permanent blindness or other organ and tissue damage. These disorders occur primarily in patients older than 50 years, in women more than in men; they are propagated by antigen-driven, cell-mediated (T_H1) immune mechanisms that may be associated with specific genetic markers, and they are highly responsive to corticosteroids.

EPIDEMIOLOGY

In the United States, the average annual incidence of PMR is 52.5 per 100,000 patients aged 50 years and older and increases with age. The prevalence is about 0.5 to 0.7%. Internationally, the frequency varies, with the highest rates occurring in the Scandinavian countries.[1,2] The incidence and prevalence of GCA are approximately one third those of PMR.

PATHOBIOLOGY

The etiology of PMR and GCA are unknown, but both demonstrate familial aggregation and have a genetic association with human leukocyte antigen (HLA)-DR4 and a demonstrated sequence polymorphism encoded within the hypervariable region of the *HLA-DRβ1*04* gene. Other genetic associations have been suggested, including polymorphisms that may be seen in increased frequency in patients with the disease. Infectious triggers of GCA have been postulated. Varicella-zoster virus antigen has been detected in temporal artery biopsies of patients with GCA.[3] Abundant bacterial and viral DNA has been demonstrated in the arterial wall of patients with GCA using advanced DNA imaging techniques. Disease in genetically predisposed patients may also be triggered by endogenous antigens such as elastin, and the inflammatory manifestations are directed by specific patterns of cell-mediated, T_H1-associated cytokines. The cytokine production by the mononuclear cells in the involved tissues appears to influence the clinical phenotype.

In PMR, mononuclear cell inflammation can be found not only in the proximal joints, such as the shoulders, but also in the surrounding tendons, bursae, and soft tissues consistent with enthesitis. Although muscle pains may be present, no muscle inflammation is found.

CLINICAL MANIFESTATIONS

PMR and GCA are systemic inflammatory disorders that occur primarily in patients older than 50 years, in women more than in men (2:1), and in whites.

PMR and GCA are particularly uncommon in African Americans. Shared characteristics of the two disorders include significant cytokine-driven constitutional symptoms, such as fever, fatigue, and weight loss, as well as a markedly elevated erythrocyte sedimentation rate (ESR), anemia, and thrombocytosis. The musculoskeletal hallmark of PMR is proximal, severe, and symmetrical morning and even day-long stiffness, soreness, and pain in the shoulder, neck, and pelvic girdles. Fifty percent of patients with GCA share this characteristic proximal pain syndrome. Carpal tunnel syndrome and hand and knee synovitis may be seen in patients with PMR, but the overall presentation remains predominantly proximal, as opposed to rheumatoid arthritis, in which distal synovitis dominates. Whereas patients with PMR may appear to have proximal muscle weakness, this is invariably due to pain and not muscle inflammation (Table 255-1). Magnetic resonance imaging (MRI) and ultrasound studies[4,5] in patients with PMR have confirmed the presence of inflammation of extra-articular synovial structures, in particular subacromial and subdeltoid bursae in the shoulders.

Specific signs and symptoms of GCA are best appreciated in their anatomic and physiologic contexts. GCA preferentially affects certain blood vessels, including the branches of the external carotid artery, the ophthalmic artery and particularly its posterior ciliary branches, and the large arteries that arise from the aortic arch and abdominal aorta. Headache and scalp pain are probably the most frequent symptoms, occurring in 50 to 75% of patients. Headache is often the first manifestation of GCA and is described as boring, severe, and constant, unresponsive to simple pain medications and persisting through the night. Classically, patients complain of persistent and prominent temporal headaches, but occipital pains can also occur. Ear, pinna, or parotid gland pain may occur secondary to involvement of the posterior auricular artery. Jaw claudication and pain due to masseter muscle ischemia on chewing occur in 50% of patients. Lingual and maxillary artery involvement can lead to jaw or tongue pain on chewing or talking. The superficial temporal artery may become tortuous, prominent, nodular, or tender, but these findings are not invariable, and an abnormal temporal artery may be found on biopsy in vessels that appear normal. It is important to note that a dry, nonproductive cough can be a feature of the disease because this often may direct the clinician away from considering GCA and more toward consideration of an infectious or neoplastic respiratory cause of the symptoms. Rarely, mononeuritis multiplex or sensorineural hearing loss can occur but should lead the clinician to consider other possible vasculitides such as antineutrophil cytoplasmic antibody (ANCA)-associated vasculitis or polyarteritis nodosa.

TABLE 255-1 GIANT CELL ARTERITIS: CLINICAL FEATURES

INFLAMMATORY

Polymyalgia rheumatica: constitutional symptoms
   Fever
   Weight loss
   Fatigue
Laboratory abnormalities
   Hematologic: anemia, thrombocytosis
   Elevated sedimentation rate, C-reactive protein

ISCHEMIC

Ocular
   Diplopia
   Amaurosis fugax
   Fixed vision loss
   Complete blindness
Cranial symptoms
   Headache
   Jaw claudication
   Scalp tenderness
   Scalp or lingual necrosis (rare)
Cerebrovascular accidents
Large vessel disease
   Leg or arm claudication
   Diminished pulses, blood pressure asymmetry
   Aortic aneurysms

LATE COMPLICATIONS

Aortic aneurysms
   Thoracic aorta
   Abdominal aorta
Corticosteroid complications
   Osteoporosis
   Fractures
   Cataracts

Fixed or intermittent symptoms related to vasculitic involvement of the ophthalmic arteries and its branches are the most dreaded in this illness and demand immediate therapeutic intervention. These symptoms are related to vascular narrowing due to both active inflammation and endothelial injury–mediated vasospasm. Decreased vision secondary to arteritis is the most common serious consequence of GCA, occurring in 20 to 50% of patients who present to ophthalmologists. It is the presenting symptom in 60% of patients with GCA who develop visual loss. A careful history of most patients who present with "sudden" visual loss reveals that preceding headache, constitutional symptoms, and PMR occurred in approximately 40% of patients. Even the evolution of the visual loss is often staggered, with amaurosis fugax in 10% and a partial field defect progressing to complete blindness over days. If GCA remains untreated, the second eye may become involved within 1 to 2 weeks. The posterior ciliary arteries are the most frequently involved; thus, anterior ischemic optic neuropathy is the most common lesion, which can be easily defined by an ophthalmologist. Occlusion of the central retinal artery and its branches is uncommon; thus, exudates, hemorrhages, and frank vasculitis are infrequent. Five percent of patients with GCA may present with diplopia or ptosis, which may precede visual loss. The final visual abnormality can be a composite of many ischemic events occurring together in the optic nerve, the extraocular muscles, the chiasm, and the brain itself. Because GCA primarily involves arteries that contain elastica and the elastic lamina is lost as vessels pierce the dura, intracerebral lesions such as strokes are uncommon but not unheard of.

Large artery involvement most commonly presents as arm or leg claudication; rarer manifestations are stroke, subclavian steal syndrome, intestinal infarction, and symptomatic aortic aneurysm. Thus, a subclinical arteritis can exist and demands long-term monitoring. There is an emerging appreciation that some older patients classified as having GCA can present with large vessel disease resembling Takayasu arteritis clinically, with a paucity of cranial ischemic symptoms but often the presence of PMR-like symptoms. Conversely, in patients presenting with typical GCA with cranial symptoms and a positive temporal artery biopsy, large vessel disease with aortic wall thickening is markedly more frequent even early in the disease course.

Steroid-treated PMR and GCA are self-limited illnesses lasting 1 to 2 years in most patients. However, a subgroup of patients with both disorders can have active inflammatory disease as manifested by persistent symptoms and blood test signs of active inflammation for 7 to 10 years. Of note is the fact that thoracic aneurysms with giant cells in the tissue can develop as long as 15 years after the diagnosis, successful treatment, and discontinuation of steroids. Indeed, the incidence of thoracic and aortic aneurysms is markedly higher in patients with a prior history of presumably successfully treated GCA than in age-matched control subjects. In studies of repaired aortic aneurysms, pathologic findings consistent with GCA have been found in approximately 2 to 4% of specimens from individuals without previously recognized or suspected arteritis.

In most studies, survival rates for patients with PMR and GCA are similar to those of unaffected persons of the same age. However, one study did show that survival was decreased in a group of patients with GCA who had permanent visual loss and required more than 10 mg of prednisone per day at 6 months. This probably supports the experience that the morbidity and mortality are caused by steroid-related treatment complications in this high-risk, elderly group of patients possessing many comorbid conditions.

DIAGNOSIS

The diagnoses of PMR and GCA are based on clinical findings, with supporting but not diagnostic aid obtained from laboratory tests and temporal artery biopsy (Fig. 255-1).[6,7] No physician should await an abnormal finding on temporal artery biopsy or demand the presence of an elevated ESR before making the definitive diagnosis of GCA in the setting of a characteristic clinical picture. That said, the laboratory hallmark of PMR and GCA is an elevation in IL-6-stimulated acute phase reactants such as the ESR and C-reactive protein. The ESR is usually in excess of 50 mm/hour and may exceed 100 mm/hour. An ESR in the low 20s or 30s, however, does not exclude a diagnosis of PMR or GCA if other characteristic clinical features are present and especially if the patient is already taking steroids.

Normocytic, normochromic anemia and thrombocytosis occur in approximately 50% of patients with both disorders and are excellent guides to the state of inflammation. In both PMR and GCA, the frequency of rheumatoid factor, antinuclear antibody, ANCA, monoclonal proteins, and cryoglobulins is not higher than in age-matched control subjects, and complement is not reduced. Alkaline phosphatase activity may be elevated in one third of patients, primarily those with GCA. Although these tests are not indicated in PMR

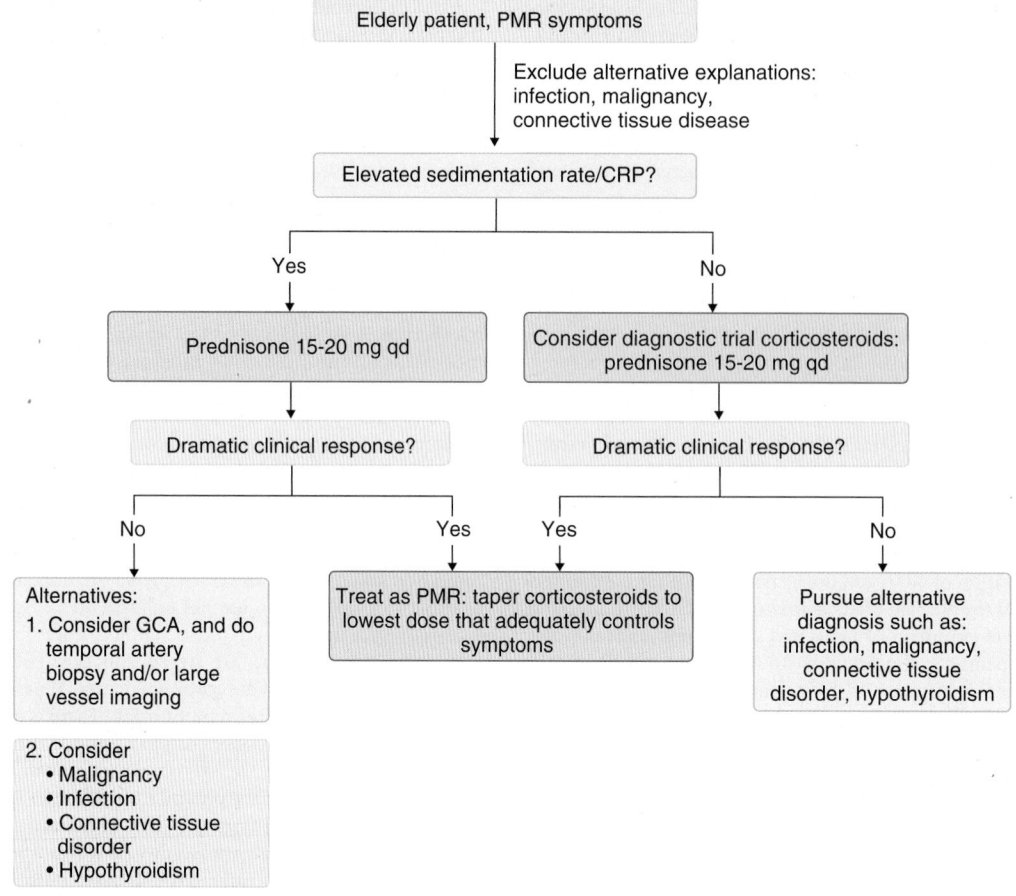

FIGURE 255-1. Diagnostic algorithm for polymyalgia rheumatica (PMR). CRP = C-reactive protein; GCA = giant cell arteritis.

and GCA, muscle enzymes and electromyography are normal, and muscle biopsy shows type II fiber atrophy but no inflammation.

Superficial Temporal Artery Assessment

Temporal artery tenderness, nodularity, and diminished pulsation are typical findings on physical examination in a patient with GCA. Color duplex ultrasonography has been used as an adjunctive noninvasive diagnostic tool in GCA. A hypoechoic halo around the superficial temporal artery has been reported in 73% of patients with biopsy-proven GCA. The halo, representing edema in the arterial wall, was observed bilaterally in a significant subset of patients and disappeared in a mean of 16 days after the initiation of steroids in one study. The presence of the halo in this study had a sensitivity of 73% and was 100% specific for GCA. Other groups have been unable to replicate this experience, however, finding Doppler ultrasonography to be no more sensitive or specific than physical examination in patients thought to have the disease. Findings of stenosis or occlusion of temporal arteries by Doppler ultrasound have also been recognized as being modestly sensitive and specific for the diagnosis of GCA in some studies. Operator dependency remains a challenge to the more widespread use of this modality diagnostically. [18F] Fluorodeoxyglucose–positron emission tomography (PET) may be helpful in identifying large vessel inflammation suggestive of GCA, but it is not helpful in assessing the temporal arteries themselves, given their relatively small size and high background uptake in that area. Conventional angiography is rarely used in the diagnosis of GCA. Some studies have suggested that MRI/magnetic resonance angiography (MRA) may be a helpful noninvasive diagnostic modality. Superficial cranial arteries can be visualized, and mural inflammatory changes and luminal narrowing can be identified. Large vessel involvement can also be assessed. Studies have suggested sensitivities and specificities of MRI/MRA similar to those of biopsy in the diagnosis of GCA. Nevertheless, temporal artery biopsy remains the diagnostic "gold standard" in GCA, and given the relatively easy accessibility of the artery and potentially significant morbidity of therapy in GCA, histologic confirmation is favored in most cases.

Although temporal artery biopsy continues to be an important diagnostic test for the presence of GCA, a few caveats must be stated. First, in a patient in whom the clinical diagnosis is likely, treatment with steroids should be instituted immediately without waiting for the biopsy results. Second, because of the skipped nature of the pathologic inflammatory lesions in the vessel wall, as many as 20 to 30% of biopsy specimens may be normal despite an overwhelming diagnostic likelihood of GCA. Because the biopsy is helpful in confirming the diagnosis of GCA, in which high doses of steroids are used, the following guidelines are given. Patients with pure PMR and no GCA signs or symptoms do not need a biopsy. However, because 10% of these patients may develop such clinical manifestations of GCA within the next year, they should be told to report such symptoms immediately. When GCA is likely, an outpatient biopsy should be performed on the symptomatic side of the head, preferably including inflamed areas with tenderness or nodularity and incorporating 2 to 3 cm of vessel. Multiple sections should be requested because of the segmental nature of the disease process. Some rheumatologists routinely request bilateral biopsies, which may increase the likelihood of obtaining an abnormal finding by up to 5%, whereas others perform a contralateral biopsy if the first specimen is normal. Diagnostic biopsy findings continue to be present for as long as 2 to 4 weeks after the clinical diagnosis is made and steroid treatment instituted, and may be seen even months into treatment.

Differential Diagnosis

The systemic nature of these disorders and the fact that they occur in elderly people demand careful diagnostic scrutiny to avoid missing a malignant neoplasm or major infection and possibly treating patients inappropriately with high-dose steroids. This is true in PMR because there is no diagnostic test and in GCA because the GCA biopsy finding may be normal in the face of active, vision-threatening vasculitis. Infections that must be considered and ruled out if clinically appropriate include tuberculosis, endocarditis, and hepatitis B and C. Malignant neoplasms such as lymphoma and multiple myeloma may mimic PMR, and an age-appropriate cancer evaluation is always indicated in this age group. Autoimmune disorders such as elderly-onset rheumatoid arthritis and systemic lupus erythematosus, as well as dermatomyositis and other types of vasculitis, must be considered in the differential diagnosis and sorted out by employing clinical information and serologic testing. There is support for the concept that elderly-onset rheumatoid arthritis is the same disorder as PMR with negative rheumatoid factor, a more proximal focus of joint inflammation, and a good response to low-dose prednisone. The distinction may be semantic because neither disorder tends to evolve into an erosive arthritis. A more protracted clinical course, however, is often seen in patients in whom distal synovitis is a prominent feature, and those patients are classified as having elderly-onset rheumatoid arthritis. PMR and GCA should always be thought of in the setting of a fever of unknown origin because symptoms and signs can be occult or the history incomplete.

TREATMENT Rx

Both PMR and GCA are highly responsive to corticosteroids, which are the treatment of choice.[8] This response is so characteristic that an immediate and dramatic improvement in PMR and GCA symptoms within 1 to 3 days after steroid institution supports the diagnosis. Conversely, a lack of rapid and significant improvement in signs, symptoms, and function within 5 to 7 days should lead the clinician to suspect the initial impression and consider an alternative diagnosis (e.g., tumor or infection) or the presence of GCA in PMR patients that might require a higher steroid dose. Because the inflammatory burden of the two disorders is different, different doses of steroids are employed at the start of treatment. Whereas PMR usually responds to 15 mg of prednisone daily, GCA usually requires 40 to 60 mg of prednisone per day in divided doses or higher doses if organ or tissue damage is present or threatened. In GCA, if visual symptoms are present as a fixed loss or amaurosis fugax, the patient often should be treated with high-dose intravenous methylprednisolone with doses ranging from 40 mg every 8 hours to 1 g/day for 3 days, followed by high-dose oral steroids in divided doses.

Within 2 to 3 days after the institution of steroids, most symptoms of PMR or GCA clear rapidly, and patients describe a miraculous improvement.[9] The steroid dose is then maintained for 2 to 3 weeks, during which the ESR, C-reactive protein, hemoglobin, and platelet counts normalize. Steroid taper is then instituted and guided by the clinical response. In PMR, taper is commonly by 1 mg every 7 to 10 days; in GCA, taper is by 5 to 10 mg every 7 to 10 days. In GCA, the use of alternate-day corticosteroid regimens to minimize steroid side effects is generally not recommended because randomized controlled trials have demonstrated higher rates of treatment failure with alternate-day dosing schedules. It is important that the taper be guided primarily by clinical findings (e.g., PMR stiffness, headache, fatigue) and that the level of ESR elevation be considered within that clinical context. One should never "chase the ESR" because the elderly patient would be subjected inappropriately to a dangerously high cumulative dose of steroids with their attendant side effects. An increased dose of prednisone should be based on a change in symptoms, not solely on an increase in the ESR. One possible exception is in a patient with a history of GCA and prior abrupt vision loss in one eye, in whom any further compromise of vision would be catastrophic. The effective dose demanded for a flare often can be as low as 5 to 10 mg/day of prednisone, and uncommonly up to 60 mg/day to control symptoms (e.g., visual abnormalities).

A persistently elevated ESR (>50 mm/hour) without PMR or GCA symptoms should alert the physician to look for alternative causes, such as infection. Treatment is a careful balancing act between disease control and avoidance of steroid-related toxicity. The overall goal of the patient and the physician is to attain the best disease control with the lowest dose of steroids. In most patients, prednisone can be tapered safely in 1 to 2 years. However, other patients may need to take low doses of steroids for 2 years or more. The higher the initial dose and cumulative dose, the greater the likelihood that the patient will develop a major steroid side effect such as sepsis, osteoporosis, osteonecrosis, diabetes, emotional lability, or myopathy (Chapter 32). Appropriate immunizations, osteoporosis regimens (calcium, vitamin D, and bisphosphonates), and metabolic monitoring are mandatory in all patients prescribed chronic steroid therapy.

The major feared outcome in GCA is ischemic complications of the disease, most often vision loss or, less frequently, cerebrovascular accident. Vision loss is usually irreversible, and although it is uncommon after the diagnosis is suspected and glucocorticoid therapy is instituted, it can occur early in the course of treatment. A meta-analysis of retrospective studies showed that antiplatelet or anticoagulant therapy has a marginal benefit when used together with corticosteroids in patients with established GCA. Although this has not been demonstrated in prospective randomized controlled trials, in most patients, adjunctive therapy with low-dose aspirin should be considered unless there is a strong contraindication to its use.

Alternative immunosuppressive agents have been tested in both PMR and GCA patients in an attempt to "spare steroids" and to control the inflammatory state. Studies examining the efficacy of methotrexate in GCA have yielded mixed results, with the largest, most recent study showing no incremental benefit from combined therapy. One individual patient meta-analysis of three randomized placebo-controlled trials suggested a modest benefit to methotrexate in GCA in terms of affording a steroid-sparing benefit and reducing likelihood of flares. Given the modest nature of the benefit demonstrated and the potential toxicities of methotrexate in this elderly population, methotrexate is not routinely incorporated as first-line therapy in GCA. In PMR, methotrexate has been shown in one study to afford a benefit in terms of steroid sparing and possibly reducing numbers of flares. The magnitude of the benefit appears modest, and no reduction in corticosteroid-related side effects was demonstrated. At present,

methotrexate is not routinely used in the management of either disease, but in individual patients with refractory disease or excessive corticosteroid morbidities, addition of weekly rheumatoid arthritis–level doses of methotrexate (7.5 to 20 mg/week) or azathioprine (2 mg/kg/day) is employed in selected instances. There have been case series suggesting cyclophosphamide may be of value in patients with refractory disease and/or unacceptable corticosteroid toxicity, but adverse events are common, and it is rare to use this agent in GCA.

Tocilizumab (TCZ), a humanized monoclonal anti-IL-6 receptor antibody, has been shown in 2 randomized trials to have efficacy in GCA.[A1][A2] TCZ use resulted in higher remission rates, less cumulative glucocorticoid use, and higher likelihood of sustained remission at 12 months than treatment with placebo.[10] Relatively rapid glucocorticoid tapers were utilized (tapered to off by month 6), without occurrence of cranial ischemic complications in these trials. Tocilizumab has recently been approved by the FDA for the treatment of GCA based on these findings. Two prospective open label trials have similarly suggested TCZ to afford a significant steroid sparing benefit in PMR, but this has not yet been tested in randomized blinded placebo-controlled trials.[11,12]

Randomized controlled trials of TNF inhibitors including infliximab and adalimumab in GCA have failed to demonstrate benefit in terms of preventing relapses or affording a steroid-sparing benefit.[A3] Treatment with abatacept, a costimulatory molecule blocker, has recently been shown in a randomized blinded placebo-controlled trial to result in a modest benefit in terms of relapse-free survival at 12 months[A4] and is presently being evaluated in a larger trial.

FUTURE DIRECTIONS

Better understanding of the disease-causing roles of immunologically active cells and their cytokine products, along with genetics and correlations with clinical subsets, will lead to more focused treatment modalities and the avoidance of the need for long-term treatment with steroids. A recently published cohort study revealed that GCA is associated with increased risks for myocardial infarction, stroke, and peripheral vascular disease,[13] suggesting that greater attention should be paid to cardiovascular risk reduction in patients with this disease.

Grade A References

A1. Villiger PM, Adler S, Kuchen S, et al. Tocilizumab for induction and maintenance of remission in giant cell arteritis: a phase 2, randomised, double-blind, placebo-controlled trial. *Lancet.* 2016;387:1921-1927.

A2. Stone J, et al. Tocilizumab for sustained glucocorticoid-free remission in giant cell arteritis. *N Engl J Med.* 2017;377:317-328.

A3. Yates M, Loke YK, Watts RA, et al. Prednisolone combined with adjunctive immunosuppression is not superior to prednisolone alone in terms of efficacy and safety in giant cell arteritis: meta-analysis. *Clin Rheumatol.* 2014;33:227-236.

A4. Langford CA, et al. A randomized double-blind trial of abatacept and glucocorticoids for the treatment of giant cell arteritis. *Arthritis Rheumatol.* 2015;67:3949-3951.

GENERAL REFERENCES

For the General References and other additional features, please visit Expert Consult at https://expertconsult.inkling.com.

256

INFECTIONS OF BURSAE, JOINTS, AND BONES

ERIC L. MATTESON AND DOUGLAS R. OSMON

INFECTION OF BURSAE
Septic Bursitis
DEFINITION

Bursae are the satellite structures that form to protect tissues from bony prominences. The superficial bursae, including the olecranon, prepatellar, infrapatellar, and bursae over the first metatarsophalangeal bunions, are more likely to become infected than are the deep bursae, such as the subacromial, trochanteric, and iliopsoas bursae.

EPIDEMIOLOGY

Olecranon bursitis may occur in as many as 10 in 100,000 persons. The majority of cases occur in men, and antecedent trauma to the skin is frequent.

PATHOBIOLOGY

Septic bursitis of superficial bursae is most commonly due to direct inoculation through the overlying skin; less commonly, it is secondary to overlying cellulitis. Most cases of deep septic bursitis are due to contiguous spread from adjacent infected joints or hematogenous seeding.

Predisposing risk factors for septic bursitis include trauma to the skin. For example, olecranon septic bursitis may occur in plumbers, athletes, and patients with chronic obstructive pulmonary disease (COPD) who frequently lean on their elbows; prepatellar or infrapatellar septic bursitis can occur in housecleaners, gardeners, and carpet layers. At least one third of patients with septic bursitis have an underlying comorbid illness such as diabetes mellitus, rheumatoid arthritis, gout, COPD, or alcoholism.

CLINICAL MANIFESTATIONS

In immune-competent patients, septic bursitis often but not always presents with fever and erythema and warmth of the overlying skin; there may be swelling of the bursae. In contrast to those with septic arthritis, patients with septic bursitis of superficial bursae have intact range of motion of the joints, which may be limited only at the extremes of flexion.[1] Pain on motion of the joint and restriction of joint range of motion are highly suggestive of septic arthritis. Acute phase reactants such as C-reactive protein, the sedimentation rate, and the white blood cell count (WBC) may be elevated.

DIAGNOSIS

Radiography should be performed to look for a foreign body and to evaluate the surrounding bones. Aspiration of bursal fluid is helpful in the diagnosis of patients who have pain, erythema, and/or swelling of an affected area. However, given the risk for contaminating the bursa if the aspiration occurs through cellulitic skin, many clinicians choose to aspirate a bursa only if empirical antimicrobial therapy has failed. Ultrasound or computed tomography (CT) guidance greatly enhances the successful aspiration of superficial bursae. Care must be taken not to violate the joint space when aspirating a bursa to avoid inoculating it.

The leukocyte count of the bursal fluid is generally lower than that seen in septic arthritis, with a mean of 13,500 cells/μL. Even in immune-competent hosts, cell counts can range from less than 1500/μL to greater than 100,000/μL. A leukocyte count greater than 2000/μL has a sensitivity of 94% and a specificity of 79% for superficial (olecranon or prepatellar) bursitis. Bacterial culture and in vitro susceptibilities must be obtained; if additional fluid is available, a Gram stain may be obtained, although its sensitivity may be as low as 15%. The presence of crystals does not exclude the possibility of septic bursitis (Chapter 257).

Staphylococcus aureus (Chapter 272) is the most common cause of septic bursitis, present in more than 80% of culture-proven cases, followed by β-hemolytic streptococci. Aerobic gram-negative bacilli, including *Escherichia coli, Campylobacter jejuni,* and *Pseudomonas* species, are rare causes of septic bursitis. Chronic bursitis may be associated with systemic infections due to *Brucella abortus,* atypical mycobacteria, or *Mycobacterium tuberculosis,* as well as fungi; the presence of these infections should raise the possibility of systemic infection.

Differential Diagnosis

In the immune-competent host, nonseptic bursitis (Chapter 247) may have a somewhat more indolent presentation than septic bursitis. The differential diagnosis includes gout, pseudogout, arthritis, and trauma with hemobursa. An overlying cellulitis may be confused with bursitis. Fever is usually not present in nonseptic bursitis because of mechanical or friction trauma.

TREATMENT   Rx

Treatment of septic bursitis is guided by knowledge of the putative underlying organisms, in most cases, *S. aureus.* Because the Gram stain is positive in less than two thirds of patients and cultures may be delayed, empirical therapy is guided by the clinical presentation. Most patients can be treated as outpatients, but those who are immunocompromised may require hospitalization for intravenous antibiotic therapy. Initial ambulatory treatment in patients without comorbidities may consist of an oral antistaphylococcal penicillin or first-generation cephalosporin. If community-acquired methicillin-resistant *S. aureus* (MRSA) is suspected, cotrimoxazole or minocycline may be added to one of these agents. In patients who are allergic to penicillin, oral clindamycin or linezolid may be used. Patients who have severe inflammation, are septic, or are immunocompromised may require hospitalization for initiation of treatment with intravenous nafcillin, oxacillin, or cefazolin; if methicillin-resistant *Staphylococcus aureus* (MRSA) is suspected, intravenous vancomycin, daptomycin, or linezolid should be used (Chapter 272). Vancomycin can also be used in patients who are allergic to penicillin.

The duration of antimicrobial therapy is guided by the clinical response and comorbid conditions. It should be continued until there is no longer bursal inflammation. This may require several weeks of intravenous or oral therapy and multiple aspirations. Failure of the septic bursitis to respond to initial antibiotic therapy mandates a second course of therapy; recurrence thereafter or inability to adequately drain the bursa with needle aspiration is an indication for surgical intervention.

PREVENTION

Because superficial septic bursitis is often associated with occasional or avocational activities involving kneeling or resting on the elbows, using protective padding may be helpful.

PROGNOSIS

The optimal duration of therapy is unknown, but prognosis of superficial bursitis is generally excellent. The presence of comorbid conditions, especially those associated with deep bursal infections, including septic arthritis, bacteremia, and osteomyelitis, is associated with more intractable and difficult disease.

INFECTION OF JOINTS
Septic Arthritis

DEFINITION

Septic arthritis refers to infection of a joint by a microorganism. It is associated with increased morbidity and mortality as well as loss of articular integrity and function.[2] Septic arthritis is usually caused by a bacterial infection. Other microorganisms can cause infections with clinical characteristics that differ from those of bacterial infections; these are reviewed separately.

NONGONOCOCCAL SEPTIC ARTHRITIS

EPIDEMIOLOGY

The incidence of septic arthritis affecting native joints is about 5 to 8 in 100,000 patient years. Among patients presenting with an acutely swollen and painful joint, the prevalence of bacterial arthritis ranges widely, from less than 10% to as high as 27%, depending on the source population. Nongonococcal septic arthritis is the most common form of septic arthritis and is somewhat more common in men than in women.

PATHOBIOLOGY

More than 90% of cases of septic arthritis are due to staphylococci or streptococci (Table 256-1). Septic arthritis can result from direct inoculation (e.g., accidents, bites, surgery) or by extension from infected bone into an adjacent joint space. Approximately 75% of cases are due to hematogenous spread, particularly in patients with indwelling catheters and immunocompromised patients. Septic arthritis due to needle arthrocentesis (<1 in 10,000 procedures) or arthroscopy (4 cases per 1000 to 10,000 procedures) is very rare.

Bacteria causing septic arthritis produce an acute inflammatory reaction in the synovial membrane. Synovial hyperplasia and inflammatory cell immigration with the release of pro-inflammatory and cartilage-destroying cytokines and proteases result in damage to cartilage and bone. Bacterial toxins and DNA and superantigens, such as those seen in staphylococcal toxic shock syndrome, also contribute to cartilage and bone damage.

Risk factors for the development of septic arthritis include penetrating trauma, diabetes, alcoholism, cutaneous ulcers, intravenous drug use, prosthetic joints, rheumatoid arthritis, osteoarthritis, and low socioeconomic status, as well as advanced age, skin infection, indwelling intravenous catheters, cancer, and immunosuppressive therapies, including biologic response modifiers used in the management of autoimmune diseases such as rheumatoid arthritis and inflammatory bowel disease.

TABLE 256-1 MICROORGANISMS RESPONSIBLE FOR ACUTE SEPTIC ARTHRITIS AND ACUTE AND CHRONIC OSTEOMYELITIS

SEPTIC ARTHRITIS		OSTEOMYELITIS: ACUTE AND CHRONIC	
MICROORGANISM	FREQUENCY (%)	MICROORGANISM	FREQUENCY (%)
Gram-Positive	*60-90*	*Gram-Positive*	*80-90*
Staphylococcus aureus	50-70	*Staphylococcus aureus*	60-80
Group A, B, C streptococci	15-30	Group A, B, C streptococci	10-20
Coagulase-negative staphylococci	6-20	*Staphylococcus epidermidis*	10-15
Streptococcus pneumoniae	1-3	*Streptococcus pneumoniae*	<1
Enterococcus sp	<1	*Enterococcus* sp	1-2
Corynebacterium sp	<1	*Corynebacterium* sp	1-2
Gram-Negative	*5-25*	*Gram-Negative*	*5-20*
Salmonella sp		*Salmonella* sp	
Pseudomonas aeruginosa		*Enterobacter* sp	
Escherichia coli		*Pseudomonas aeruginosa*	
Klebsiella pneumoniae		*Brucella* sp	
Enterobacter sp		*Pasteurella multocida*	
Kingella kingae		*Bartonella henselae*	
Haemophilus influenzae	<1-3*	*Propionibacterium* sp	
Anaerobes	*1-2*	*Anaerobes*	
Fusobacterium sp		*Bacteroides* sp	
Bacteroides fragilis			
Miscellaneous	*<5*	*Miscellaneous*	*5-7*
Mycoplasma		*Mycobacterium* sp	
Mycobacterium sp		Fungi (candidiasis, coccidioidomycosis, blastomycosis, histoplasmosis)	
Fungi			
Viruses			
Algae			

*Children.

CLINICAL MANIFESTATIONS

Most patients with bacterial arthritis feel ill and have fever. Immunocompromised and elderly patients may not have a marked febrile response. Most cases (>80%) of septic arthritis are monoarticular; the knee is involved in more than 50% of cases. Polyarticular joint sepsis may be seen in immunocompromised patients and those with rheumatoid arthritis or systemic lupus erythematosus. Such patients frequently lack typical signs and symptoms of infection and may not appear to be particularly ill at presentation, but they may have rapid cardiovascular decompensation. This is particularly true for patients who are taking glucocorticosteroids, other immunosuppressive agents, and biologic response modifiers, including tumor necrosis factor-α (TNF-α) inhibitors.

Patients with septic arthritis affecting nondiarthrodial joints, such as the acromioclavicular or sacroiliac joints, may have a history of intravenous drug use or may have intravenous catheters in place to treat other medical conditions. Infection of the symphysis pubis is associated with previous urinary tract or gynecologic surgery, pelvic malignancy, intravenous drug use, or vigorous weight-bearing physical activity, such as long-distance running, in female athletes.

A finding of microorganisms in the joint should lead to an appropriate history and physical examination to identify a source of hematogenous infection, such as cellulitis, pneumonia, or urinary tract infection. Staphylococci and β-hemolytic streptococci may enter directly through open wounds, whereas Gram-negative infection may be associated with bowel or bladder disease.

DIAGNOSIS

The diagnosis of septic arthritis is challenging because its signs and symptoms overlap those of other nonseptic inflammatory joint diseases (e.g., osteoarthritis, gout, rheumatoid arthritis, and juvenile rheumatoid arthritis), diseases that themselves can increase the risk for septic arthritis.[3] Plain radiography should be performed to evaluate the surrounding bones and joint space and to provide a baseline for comparison after therapy is completed. Imaging modalities such as magnetic resonance imaging (MRI), CT, and plain radiography are useful to determine whether there is associated osteomyelitis and in cases of diagnostic uncertainty.[4] Blood cultures are positive in up to 50% of patients with bacterial septic arthritis and should be obtained in all patients in whom this diagnosis is suspected. If septic arthritis is suspected, synovial fluid arthrocentesis is indicated,[5] and the fluid should be examined for bacterial culture and Gram stain; the latter is positive in only about 50% of patients. Specific cultures and stains for fungal and mycobacterial organisms should be done if there is a history of exposure or if antibacterial therapy has failed. Polymerase chain reaction (PCR) assays may be helpful for diagnosing less common joint infections such as *Borrelia,* but the value of PCR over standard culture for the diagnosis of staphylococcal or streptococcal joint infection has not yet been demonstrated. Other helpful examinations include leukocyte count and differential as well as evaluation of the synovial fluid for the presence of crystals (Chapter 257). The presence of gout or pseudogout crystals does not exclude the possibility of septic arthritis, particularly in patients whose WBC is above 50,000/μL.

A frequent clinical scenario is the patient who is anticoagulated. Because of the rapidly destructive nature of septic arthritis and the often profound systemic consequences, therapeutic anticoagulation is not a contraindication to arthrocentesis. The procedure may be assisted by ultrasound guidance, especially when only a small amount of joint fluid is present or when the joint is difficult to aspirate. CT-guided arthrocentesis is particularly useful for aspiration of deep joints such as the hips and nondiarthrodial joints.

The total WBC and differential in synovial fluid is helpful in distinguishing infected from noninfected joints in immunocompetent patients. A diagnosis of septic arthritis is present in 47% of patients with a synovial WBC greater than 50,000/μL and in 77% of patients with a WBC greater than 100,000/μL. It is important to realize that a WBC less than 50,000/μL, especially in immunocompromised patients, can be associated with septic arthritis, so the absolute WBC in synovial fluid is not, by itself, a reliable way to confirm or exclude a diagnosis of septic arthritis.

Differential Diagnosis

Symptoms of septic arthritis, such as acute joint pain, swelling, and even fever, with an increase in acute phase reactants, can be caused by crystalline arthritis (Chapter 257), especially pseudogout and gout, as well as psoriatic arthritis and reactive arthritis (Chapter 249). In patients who have preexisting inflammatory joint disease, such as rheumatoid arthritis, septic arthritis may be suspected if there is a sudden onset of acute or subacute monoarticular or pauciarticular joint swelling when the disease is otherwise well controlled. The presence or absence of fever is not a reliable indicator of an infected joint (Fig. 256-1).

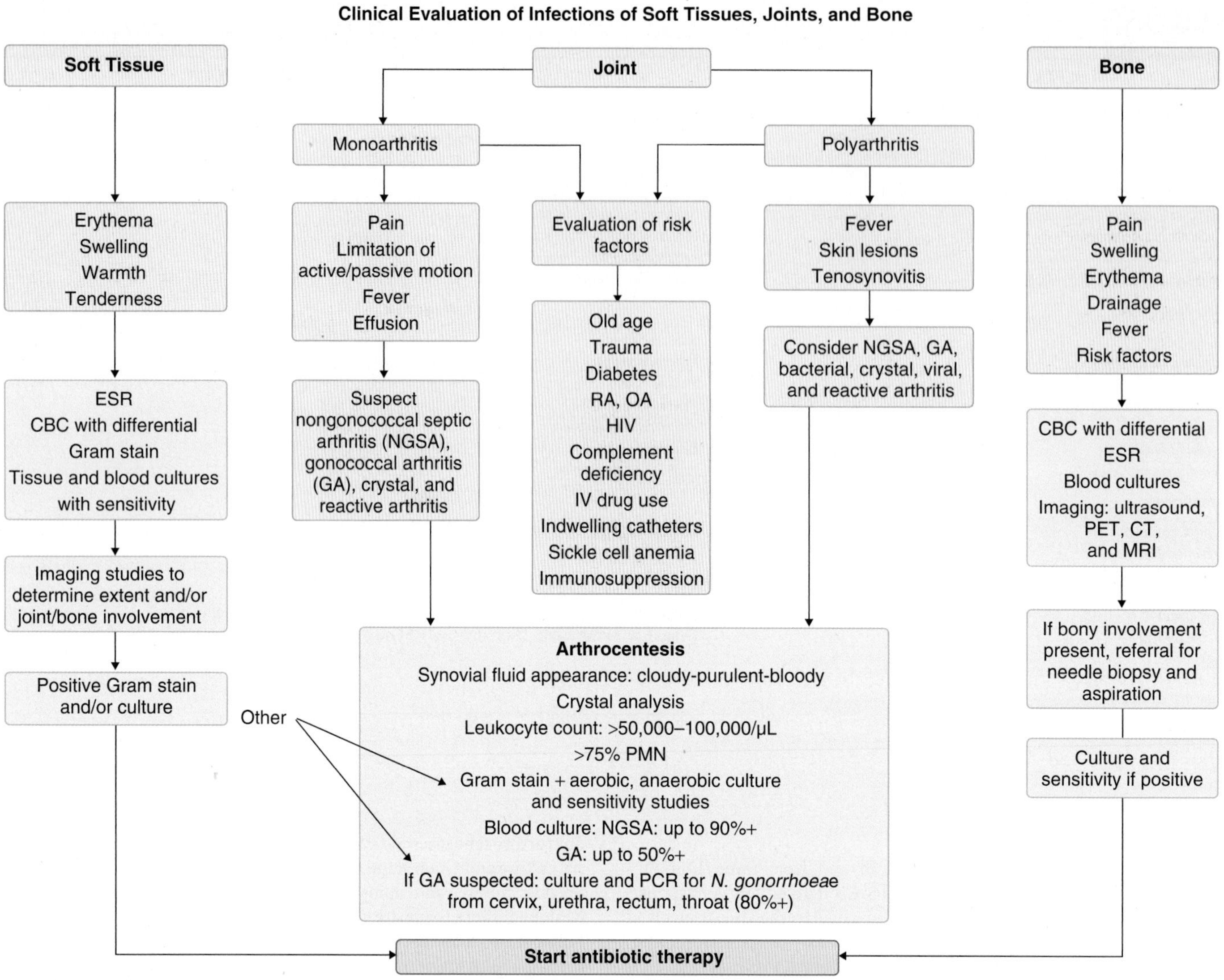

Clinical Evaluation of Infections of Soft Tissues, Joints, and Bone

FIGURE 256-1. Clinical evaluation of infections of soft tissues, joints, and bone. CBC = complete blood count; CT = computed tomography; ESR = erythrocyte sedimentation rate; GA = gonococcal arthritis; HIV = human immunodeficiency virus; IV = intravenous; MRI = magnetic resonance imaging; NGSA = nongonococcal septic arthritis; OA = osteoarthritis; PCR = polymerase chain reaction; PET = positron emission tomography; PMN = polymorphonuclear leukocyte; RA = rheumatoid arthritis.

TREATMENT   Rx

As soon as the joint has been aspirated and, ideally, after blood cultures have been obtained, prompt treatment with antibiotics must be instituted. Removal of purulent material and, where appropriate, débridement are essential. The choice of empirical antimicrobial therapy is based on which organisms are thought to be the likely cause of the septic arthritis and on the results of Gram stain and culture. No advantage of one antibiotic regimen over another has been demonstrated. If the initial Gram stain of the synovial fluid reveals gram-positive cocci, vancomycin is recommended, given the increasing frequency of infection due to MRSA and the need to initiate effective antimicrobial therapy as soon as possible. Daptomycin, linezolid, and ceftaroline are alternative agents. If the initial Gram stain reveals gram-negative bacilli, an agent with broad coverage, including activity against *Pseudomonas aeruginosa*, is recommended. Such agents include ceftazidime, cefepime, imipenem, meropenem, piperacillin-tazobactam, and intravenous ciprofloxacin. If the Gram stain is negative, vancomycin alone in immunocompetent patients or in those unlikely to have gram-negative infection based on history and examination, or vancomycin plus one of the gram-negative antibacterials listed, is reasonable. When culture and in vitro susceptibility results are available, therapy can be modified. The duration of antibacterial therapy usually ranges from 2 to 6 weeks, with data suggesting that one aspiration and 2 weeks of therapy are usually adequate, at least in children.

The role of arthroscopic versus needle versus open drainage of the joint remains unsettled.[6] Surgical management is appropriate for septic arthritis of the hip, for patients who fail to respond to serial needle aspiration and antibiotic therapy, and for patients who appear to be developing life-threatening complications such as necrotizing fasciitis. No studies have demonstrated the utility of lavage with or without synovectomy by arthroscopy versus arthrotomy or débridement. Patients should be mobilized as rapidly as possible to prevent joint contractures. The concomitant use of oral dexamethasone for 4 days can lead to more rapid symptomatic improvements in children,[A1] but no randomized trials have been reported in adults.

PREVENTION

In patients requiring immunosuppression or glucocorticosteroid therapy to manage their underlying diseases, every effort should be made to use the lowest possible dose of these medications.

PROGNOSIS

Up to one third of patients with septic arthritis have a poor functional outcome, particularly older patients, patients with preexisting diseases of the joints such as osteoarthritis or rheumatoid arthritis, and patients with prosthetic joints. Poor joint outcome is associated with *S. aureus* infection in more than 50% of patients; mortality may be as high as 10 to 15%, particularly in patients who are immunocompromised or have polyarticular sepsis.

GONOCOCCAL SEPTIC ARTHRITIS

EPIDEMIOLOGY

Neisseria gonorrhoeae (Chapter 283) is a common cause of polyarthralgias and arthritis as well as oligoarticular arthritis and tenosynovitis in young, healthy patients. Disseminated gonococcal infection occurs in 0.5 to 3% of patients with gonorrhea (Chapter 283). Many of these patients have arthritis. Disseminated gonococcal infection and septic arthritis due to *N. gonorrhoeae* occur two to three times more often in women than in men. Most patients do not have a recent history of a symptomatic genital infection. The incidence of gonococcal arthritis is 133 cases per 100,000 population per year. Predisposing factors for disseminated gonococcal infection with arthritis include pregnancy, recent menstruation, complement deficiencies (C5, C6, C7, or C8), and systemic lupus erythematosus.

CLINICAL MANIFESTATIONS

Patients with gonococcal arthritis usually present with one of two clinical syndromes. The first is a purulent arthritis without skin lesions; the second is the triad of tenosynovitis, dermatitis, and polyarthralgias without purulent arthritis. The latter patients may have bacteremia and fever as well as maculopapular, vesicular, necrotic, pustular skin lesions anywhere on the integument. The arthritis is usually asymmetrical and may involve large or small joints, typically the elbows and knees or joints distal to these.

DIAGNOSIS

A high degree of clinical suspicion is required for diagnosis because many patients are asymptomatic for the primary infection. A thorough joint evaluation is important, as is an evaluation of soft tissues, particularly for tenosynovitis affecting the hands and feet. Cultures of blood, endocervix, and urethra are essential; cultures of the pharynx and rectum may be very helpful. *N. gonorrhoeae* is isolated in less than 30% of patients with the tenosynovitis-dermatitis syndrome and in about 50% of those with monoarthritis. PCR may be used to detect the gonococcal DNA in synovial fluid, skin lesions, urine, and throat samples, which are culture negative. Cultures should be submitted on Thayer-Martin media. Patients with suspected gonococcal arthritis should be screened for other coexisting sexually transmitted infections (Chapter 269) such as syphilis, HIV, and chlamydia, as well as hepatitis B and C.

TREATMENT   Rx

Ceftriaxone is given for 2 to 4 days, followed by oral therapy to complete a minimum of 7 days of therapy, although up to 14 days of therapy is recommended. There is emerging resistance to fluoroquinolones, and unless specific in vitro susceptibility testing is available, their use is not recommended. Patients should also be treated for concomitant chlamydia with the regimens recommended by the U.S. Centers for Disease Control and Prevention (CDC). Most patients respond well to outpatient therapy, with complete resolution of the infection. Given emerging antimicrobial resistance, the most recent CDC guidelines for treating *N. gonorrhoeae* should be reviewed.

Viral Arthritis

Patients with viral syndromes may have polyarthralgias or inflammatory polyarthritis, which can mimic rheumatoid arthritis (Chapter 248). The most common viral infections associated with arthritis include hepatitis A, B, and C; cytomegalovirus; parvovirus B19; rubella; measles; and HIV. Other forms of viral arthritis are caused by adenovirus, echovirus, Epstein-Barr virus, and herpes zoster in North America and Europe; chikungunya (see later) and o'nyong-nyong viruses, especially in Africa; and Ross River virus in Australia. Arthritis related to viral infections is likely to be principally reactive in nature, rather than being caused by direct synovial infection.

Chikungunya (CHIK) virus infection (Chikungunya fever) is an arthropod-borne arbovirus infection that over recent decades has dispersed unexpectedly from tropical and subtropical regions of Africa and Asia to affect millions of people worldwide[7] as an emerging threat to global public health.[8] The illness occurs in two phases: an acute viremia followed by a chronic arthritis that can be accompanied by severe, incapacitating arthralgia. Attempts to isolate CHIK virus from synovial fluid have been unsuccessful,[9] and the chronic arthritis is now thought to be a postinfectious autoinflammatory disorder rather than persistent viral infection. It shares many clinical features with rheumatoid arthritis and responds variably to different disease-modifying antirheumatic drugs (DMARDs).

Other Forms of Infectious Arthritis
FUNGAL ARTHRITIS

Fungal arthritis is unusual and most commonly occurs in immunocompromised patients.[10] Treatment with high doses of immunosuppressants, anti-TNF agents, and possibly other biologic response modifiers used in the treatment of rheumatoid arthritis and other autoimmune diseases may increase the risk for fungal infections. The infections are often systemic and may be indolent. An understanding of the epidemiology of the organisms as well as the patient's risk factors, including occupational and avocational risk factors, is essential to the diagnosis. The most common fungi in the United States include *Blastomyces dermatitidis*, *Coccidioides immitis*, and *Histoplasma capsulatum*. *Sporothrix schenckii* fungal infections may be seen especially in gardeners. More unusual infections occur in immunocompromised patients, including *Aspergillus*, *Candida*, *Cryptococcus*, and *Nocardia*. The reader is referred to the specific chapters regarding these organisms for up-to-date antimicrobial recommendations.

LYME ARTHRITIS

Lyme disease (Chapter 305) usually causes oligoarticular arthritis, most commonly affecting the knee. Antibiotic treatment, as outlined in Chapter 305, is effective. Polyarticular disease affecting the small joints has been associated with HLA-DR4, which is found in greater frequency in patients with rheumatoid arthritis.

MYCOPLASMA ARTHRITIS

Mycoplasma hominis (Chapter 301) causes an oligoarticular or monoarticular arthritis. Risk factors include an immunocompromised state and hypogammaglobulinemia. The treatment of choice is tetracyclines, usually doxycycline; alternatively, clindamycin or fluoroquinolones can be used.

TUBERCULOUS ARTHRITIS

Most cases of tuberculosis (TB) (Chapter 308) in Canada, the United States, Western Europe, Australia, and New Zealand occur in immigrants. The arthritis is usually monoarticular or oligoarticular, affecting larger joints, and TB should be suspected in patients who have refractory monoarticular or pauciarticular arthritis thought to be secondary to another bacterial infection or to a systemic inflammatory disease such as rheumatoid arthritis.[11] TB screening is mandatory for all patients before beginning treatment with immunosuppressive drugs or biologic response modifiers.

The diagnosis of TB may be delayed by a lack of clinical suspicion because patients may not have pulmonary disease. Atypical mycobacterial infection may occur in fishermen and immunocompromised patients. Appropriate treatment for septic arthritis due to TB is based on guidelines and in vitro susceptibility testing, but it often includes isoniazid, ethambutol, or rifampin and pyrazinamide as empirical therapy (Chapter 308). Atypical mycobacteria are often not susceptible to traditional antituberculous agents, and infectious disease consultation is recommended. Patients with a history of TB in whom anti-TNF therapies are being considered should be appropriately treated for TB before these drugs are started. Patients with a positive purified protein derivative (PPD) test or QuantiFERON assay for TB without a history of diagnosed tuberculosis should be treated prophylactically for several months before starting anti-TNF therapy. Clinical suspicion and culture of synovial fluid or synovial membrane obtained at biopsy are essential to the diagnosis.

SYPHILIS

Musculoskeletal involvement by syphilis (Chapter 303) is manifold and includes monoarticular or oligoarticular arthritis, polyarthralgias, tenosynovitis, sacroiliitis, spondylitis, chondritis, osteitis, and periostitis. Charcot joints, osteitis, and chronic arthritis are typical of tertiary syphilis. Most patients with syphilis-related arthritis can be treated successfully. Arthritis may complicate congenital, secondary, and tertiary syphilis.

PROSTHETIC JOINT INFECTION

More than 1 million joint replacements (Chapter 260) are done each year in the United States, and this number continues to increase. Infection occurs in 0.3 to 1.7% of hip arthroplasties and 0.8 to 1.9% of knee arthroplasties, and the infection risk is two-fold to three-fold higher in patients with rheumatoid arthritis. Prosthetic joint infections are classified as (1) early infections, occurring within 3 months of joint replacement; (2) delayed infections, occurring 3 months to about 1 year after joint replacement; and (3) late infections, occurring more than 1 to 2 years after joint replacement. Infections occurring within the first year are usually related to the implantation surgery itself, and late infections are usually due to hematogenous spread.

The development of a bacterial biofilm on the prosthetic joint is characteristic of prosthetic joint infection, increasing the susceptibility to infection in experimental animal models with as few as 100 colony-forming units. These biofilms are formed by bacterial glycocalyx, which increases the organisms' resistance to antimicrobial agents and likely accounts for the difficulty in obtaining viable organisms from the infected joint. More than half of all prosthetic joint infections of hips and knees are caused by staphylococci. Other organisms, including gram-negative bacilli, anaerobes, and *Candida* species, may also cause infection. In particular, *Propionibacterium* species are associated with infected shoulder arthroplasties. About 20% of cases are polymicrobial, and in 7%, cultures are negative.

Risk factors associated with the development of prosthetic joint infection include wound healing complications, prior superficial surgical site infection, prior infection of the joint, previous surgery on the joint, rheumatoid arthritis, advanced age,[12] obesity, smoking, cancer, and diabetes mellitus. Other risk factors include simultaneous bilateral arthroplasty, prolonged operative time, requirement for blood transfusion, and infection occurring elsewhere in the body that can hematogenously seed the prosthesis.

Patients with early-onset infection may have classic symptoms and signs of septic arthritis, including joint pain, effusion, erythema, and fever. Patients with delayed infection may have only joint pain, with or without implant loosening, requiring a high degree of clinical suspicion for the presence of infection.

The definitive diagnosis of prosthetic joint infection is based on the recovery of organisms from multiple specimens of synovial fluid and periprosthetic tissue, sonication of the prosthesis itself, acute inflammation suggestive of infection on pathologic examination of periprosthetic tissue obtained at surgery, or the presence of a sinus track communicating with the prosthesis, even in the absence of microorganisms.[13]

An elevated sedimentation rate or C-reactive protein without another obvious cause, such as inflammatory arthritis or recent surgery, is very suggestive of infection in a patient with a painful, loose prosthesis.[14] Plain radiographs may show loosening, new bone formation, and lucencies along the implant margin but are often nonspecific. Technetium-based scintigraphy combined with indium-labeled white blood cell scanning is suggestive of established infection but is often not performed owing to the expense. MRI and CT have low utility in diagnosing prosthetic joint infection.

Surgical treatment of prosthetic joint infection typically consists of débridement with retention of the prosthesis for acute infection, resection arthroplasty with or without staged reimplantation for chronic infection, or amputation in a few limited instances. Systemic antibiotic therapy in a patient with a prosthetic joint infection is pathogen directed and driven by the surgical therapy used to manage the infection.[15] Following an attempt at salvage of the prosthesis with 2 to 6 weeks of effective intravenous antibiotic therapy, chronic suppressive therapy with oral antimicrobial agents is often used. In rifampin-susceptible staphylococcal infections, its addition to a companion intravenous or oral antimicrobial is recommended to avoid the emergence of resistance, to treat biofilm organisms, and to improve the chance of salvaging the prosthesis. Following resection arthroplasty, 4 to 6 weeks of pathogen-directed intravenous therapy is typical before an attempt at reimplantation several weeks later. The use of depot local antimicrobial therapy with antibiotic-impregnated polymethylmethacrylate spacers following resection arthroplasty is also very common. The reader is referred to recently released guidelines for more specific information on the diagnosis and management of prosthetic joint infection (Infectious Diseases Society of America guidelines).

PREVENTION

In addition to optimizing comorbidities such as diabetes mellitus and discontinuing tobacco use preoperatively, careful screening for infection, including asymptomatic urinary tract infection, is prudent when considering joint surgery. Perioperative antibiotic treatment with cephalosporin in patients undergoing prosthetic joint replacement reduces the risk for infection by approximately three-fold. Antimicrobial therapy should be given within 60 minutes of the initial incision, ideally before tourniquet application. Cefazolin or cefuroxime can be given to patients with normal renal function, and vancomycin can be used in patients who are allergic to penicillin.[16]

Whether an antirheumatic agent should be stopped before joint replacement surgery is unclear. The usual practice is to hold drugs such as methotrexate, anti-TNF agents, and other biologics including abatacept and tocilizumab for one to four half-lives before and after surgery. Published guidelines are available regarding the perioperative prescription of drugs used to manage rheumatic diseases when such patients undergo elective hip and knee arthroplasty.[17,18]

OSTEOMYELITIS

DEFINITION

Osteomyelitis is a bacterial infection of bone that causes destruction and can occur through a variety of mechanisms.[19]

EPIDEMIOLOGY

Osteomyelitis of the bones of the foot in adult patients with diabetes, neuropathy, and arterial insufficiency is very common.[20] Management of osteomyelitis in diabetic feet is discussed in Chapter 216. Hematogenous seeding of the spine also occurs, but less frequently. The incidence of osteomyelitis due to trauma and surgery is increasing.

PATHOBIOLOGY

Osteomyelitis can develop from (1) hematogenous seeding from a distant infection; (2) contiguous spread from nearby skin and joints; and (3) penetration of microorganisms into bone at the time of trauma or surgery. Unless there is trauma or the presence of a foreign body, bone is typically very resistant to infection. Organisms such as *S. aureus* cause disease more frequently because they colonize the skin in up to 30 to 40% of individuals, frequently cause cellulitis and bacteremia, and have the ability to bind to bone through the expression of receptors for fibronectin and collagen.[21]

Hematogenous causes of osteomyelitis typically present in the elderly; it usually involves two or more vertebrae and their intervening disc spaces. Bacteria gain access to these structures through the arterial and venous systems (Batson venous plexus). Bacteremia from any source can cause osteomyelitis of the spine, but cellulitis, urinary tract infection, and pneumonia are the most common sources.

Contiguous focus osteomyelitis is common in adults, typically occurring in the elderly. It results from the spread of infection from nearby skin, often in the feet of patients with diabetes, neuropathy, or vascular insufficiency, or in pelvic bones in patients with decubitus ulcers due to impaired sensation from spinal cord injury or disease. Alternatively, it can occur with orthopedic surgery, from contamination at the time of an open fracture, or from a human or animal bite.

Acute osteomyelitis has a duration of less than 10 days, whereas chronic infection has a duration of more than 10 days. *S. aureus* is the most common cause of hematogenous and contiguous osteomyelitis in adults. Osteomyelitis due to β-hemolytic streptococci and aerobic gram-negative bacilli is much less common, but it can occur if infections due to these organisms result in hematogenous seeding, if nosocomial contiguous osteomyelitis occurs due to surgical site infection, or if contamination occurs at the time of traumatic open fracture. Polymicrobial infection, including infection due to anaerobes, is very common in osteomyelitis of the bones of the feet associated with diabetes and vascular insufficiency. Coagulase-negative staphylococci can be pathogenic in patients with orthopedic implants.

CLINICAL MANIFESTATIONS

Localized pain over the affected bones is a hallmark of osteomyelitis. A sinus tract or swelling and erythema due to concomitant soft tissue infection or abscess may be present in osteomyelitis due to contiguous infection. Constitutional symptoms, including fever, are present in the minority of cases and more often in hematogenous osteomyelitis. If neurologic structures are involved, neurologic signs and symptoms may be present. Signs and symptoms due to a coexisting infection that has caused hematogenous osteomyelitis may be present as well. The differential diagnosis of osteomyelitis includes diseases that can cause acute and chronic bone pain in adults, including osteoarthritis, metastatic malignancy, fractures, and SAPHO (synovitis, acne, pustulosis, hyperostosis, and osteitis) syndrome, as well as postoperative pain and soft tissue infection without concomitant osteomyelitis.

DIAGNOSIS

The WBC is often elevated in hematogenous and acute osteomyelitis. Serum inflammatory markers such as the sedimentation rate and C-reactive protein are often abnormal, particularly in cases of hematogenous infection, but may be normal in chronic contiguous osteomyelitis. Blood cultures are positive in 25 to 50% of cases of hematogenous infection but are almost always negative in chronic osteomyelitis unless concomitant soft tissue infection is present. In the setting of chronic contiguous osteomyelitis, plain radiographs often show specific abnormalities; in vertebral osteomyelitis, they are often not helpful in confirming the diagnosis of infection.

The ability to probe percutaneously or to palpate bone with a probe (a sterile metal probe is inserted into the ulcer, and the test is positive if a hard, gritty surface is felt) is a simple, effective diagnostic test in patients with diabetes mellitus and possible contiguous osteomyelitis of the feet. For example, the probe-to-bone test has a sensitivity of 87% and a specificity of 83% for diagnosing foot osteomyelitis.[22]

MRI is the most sensitive and diagnostic imaging technique to identify osteomyelitis, except when orthopedic implants are present. Gallium scans are more sensitive and specific than three-phase technetium-99m (^{99m}Tc) bone scans or indium-labeled leukocyte scans for the diagnosis of vertebral osteomyelitis. Gallium scans may be used when spinal hardware is present that degrades the magnetic resonance images and in cases of skull bone osteomyelitis due to malignant external otitis.

Multiple specimens of involved bone, contiguous soft tissue, and purulence should be sent for Gram stain, aerobic and anaerobic culture, and pathologic examination at the time of bone biopsy or surgical débridement. If the history, examination, or imaging is suggestive of atypical infection, culture for fungi and mycobacteria or other unusual organisms should be performed.

TREATMENT   Rx

There are no large randomized studies comparing antimicrobial therapy for osteomyelitis. Antimicrobials for specific pathogens based on in vitro susceptibility testing are recommended, and examples of antimicrobials used to treat common pathogens causing osteomyelitis and septic arthritis are shown in Table 256-2. After 1 week of intravenous therapy, oral antibiotics can achieve adequate levels in bone,[23] and oral and parenteral therapies can achieve similar cure rates.[A2] Dalbavancin (1500 mg intravenously on days 1 and 8) may be an alternative for gram-positive infections.[A3] Although diabetic foot osteomyelitis

TABLE 256-2   ANTIMICROBIAL THERAPY FOR SELECTED MICROORGANISMS IN OSTEOMYELITIS OR SEPTIC ARTHRITIS IN ADULTS

MICROORGANISM	FIRST CHOICE*	ALTERNATIVE CHOICE
Methicillin/oxacillin/nafcillin–sensitive staphylococci	Nafcillin sodium or oxacillin sodium 1.5-2 g IV q4-6h for 4-6 wk or cefazolin 1-2 g IV q8h	Vancomycin 15 mg/kg IV q12h for 4-6 wk
Methicillin/oxacillin/nafcillin-resistant staphylococci (MRSA)	Vancomycin† 15 mg/kg IV q12h or daptomycin 6 mg/kg IV q24h	Linezolid 600 mg PO/IV q12h or daptomycin 6 mg/kg IV q24h† or 500-750 mg PO/IV daily
Penicillin-sensitive streptococci	Aqueous penicillin G 20 × 10⁶ U/24 hr IV either continuously or in six equally divided daily doses or ceftriaxone 1-2 g IV q24h or cefazolin 1-2 g IV q8h	Vancomycin 15 mg/kg IV q12h
Enterococci Penicillin and vancomycin susceptible	Aqueous crystalline penicillin G 20 × 10⁶ U/24 hr IV either continuously or in six equally divided daily doses or ampicillin sodium 12 g/24 hr IV either continuously or in six equally divided daily doses; the addition of gentamicin sulfate 1 mg/kg IV or IM q8h for 1-2 wk is optional	Vancomycin† 15 mg/kg IV q12h; the addition of gentamicin sulfate 1 mg/kg IV or IM q8h for 1-2 wk is optional
Enterobacteriaceae	Ceftriaxone 1-2 g IV q24h	Ciprofloxacin† 500-750 mg PO q12h
Pseudomonas aeruginosa	Cefepime 2 g IV q8-12h	Ciprofloxacin† 750 mg PO q12h or ceftazidime 2 g IV q8h

*Antimicrobial selection should be based on in vitro sensitivity data, as well as allergies, intolerances, and drug interactions in individual patients.
†Doses shown are based on normal renal and hepatic function and may need to be adjusted or serum levels monitored (vancomycin).
MRSA = methicillin-resistant *Staphylococcus aureus.*
Adapted from Berbari EF, Steckelberg JM, Osmon DR. Osteomyelitis. In: Mandell GL, Bennett JE, Dolin R, eds. *Mandell, Douglas, and Bennett's Principles and Practice of Infectious Diseases,* 7th ed. Philadelphia: Churchill Livingstone/Elsevier; 2010:1457-1467.

was once thought to require surgical resection, medical therapy is now recommended, provided that antibiotic sensitivity can be confirmed.[24]

The duration of antimicrobial therapy is almost always dictated by surgical therapy in chronic osteomyelitis. For example, if an amputation is performed, a short course of antimicrobial therapy may be required, whereas if an extensive débridement of chronic osteomyelitis is performed, prolonged intravenous antimicrobial therapy for 4 to 6 weeks is typically recommended. If the surgical therapy could lead to a worse outcome than no surgery, chronic oral antimicrobial suppression may be recommended. Acute hematogenous vertebral osteomyelitis in adults is typically treated with 6 weeks of intravenous antimicrobial therapy, which is as good as 12 weeks of treatment,[A4] without surgical intervention, after identification of the pathogen through percutaneous or open biopsy.[25] Hyperbaric oxygen therapy for chronic osteomyelitis is controversial. Medical management is the mainstay of treatment of spinal tuberculosis, with surgery indicated for specific situations.[26]

PREVENTION

Improving the control of diabetes and decreasing the incidence of peripheral vascular disease will reduce the incidence of diabetic foot bone infection. Optimal strategies to prevent surgical site infection after orthopedic procedures will prevent orthopedic implant infection after surgery and open fractures.

PROGNOSIS

The success of osteomyelitis management depends on the medical and surgical therapy employed and the ability to improve comorbidities such as arterial insufficiency. The ability of orthopedic surgeons to perform more extensive reconstructive surgery has allowed more extensive débridement and higher success rates, as well as restoration of function. Treatment failure can lead to relapse of infection or progression of infection to involve more of the affected bone. Long-standing osteomyelitis can be complicated by amyloidosis, squamous cell carcinoma of the skin in a chronic sinus tract, or primary bone malignancy.

Grade A References

A1. Qin YF, Li ZJ, Li H. Corticosteroids as adjunctive therapy with antibiotics in the treatment of children with septic arthritis: a meta-analysis. *Drug Des Devel Ther.* 2018;12:2277-2284.
A2. Li HK, Rombach I, Zambellas R, et al. Oral versus intravenous antibiotics for bone and joint infection. *N Engl J Med.* 2019;380:425-436.
A3. Rappo U, Puttagunta S, Shevchenko V, et al. Dalbavancin for the treatment of osteomyelitis in adult patients: a randomized clinical trial of efficacy and safety. *Open Forum Infect Dis.* 2019;6:1-8.
A4. Bernard L, Dinh A, Ghout I, et al. Antibiotic treatment for 6 weeks versus 12 weeks in patients with pyogenic vertebral osteomyelitis: an open-label, non-inferiority, randomised, controlled trial. *Lancet.* 2015;385:875-882.

GENERAL REFERENCES

For the General References and other additional features, please visit Expert Consult at https://expertconsult.inkling.com.

257

CRYSTAL DEPOSITION DISEASES

N. LAWRENCE EDWARDS

The destructive potential of intrasynovial crystals has been recognized for more than a century. The mechanisms by which certain crystals induce inflammation and joint destruction have become much better clarified over the past several decades. The three most common crystal-induced arthropathies are caused by precipitation of monosodium urate monohydrate, calcium pyrophosphate dihydrate, and basic calcium phosphate and are termed *gout, calcium pyrophosphate arthropathy,* and *basic calcium arthropathy,* respectively.

Basic calcium crystals are ultramicroscopic in size and are not detected by the compensated polarized microscopy used to identify monosodium urate and calcium pyrophosphate dehydrate crystals. Like monosodium urate and calcium pyrophosphate crystals, basic calcium phosphate crystals are biologically active and can accelerate atrophic changes in bone and cartilage. This chapter defines these separate crystalline arthropathies and describes their different pathogeneses and treatments.

GOUT AND HYPERURICEMIA

DEFINITION

Gout is a metabolic disorder resulting from the tissue deposition of monosodium urate crystals in or around joints and/or the crystallization of uric acid in the renal collecting system. Gout most commonly manifests as arthritis and is the most common inflammatory joint disease in men and in older women. Its incidence and prevalence are increasing worldwide. The metabolic derangement responsible for gout is the supersaturation of blood and body fluids with the urate ion to the point that crystal formation is possible. At physiologic pH and at normal body temperature, urate is considered to be supersaturated at concentrations of 6.8 mg/dL or greater. Therefore, from a biologic perspective, hyperuricemia is any serum urate level greater than 6.8 mg/dL in both men and women. Although hyperuricemia is a necessary prerequisite for developing gout, only 20% of all hyperuricemic subjects will ultimately develop gout.

EPIDEMIOLOGY

The incidence and prevalence of gout vary greatly throughout the world. In the United States, the United Kingdom, and much of Western Europe, the most recent estimates of the prevalence of gout have ranged from 3 to 6% in men and 1 to 2% in women. In developing countries the prevalence is much lower, typically less than 1%. At the same time, the highest prevalence has been noted in certain ethnic groups, especially in Oceanic populations, including Taiwanese Aborigines, Māori, and Pacific Islanders living in New Zealand, where prevalence estimates are more than 10%.[1,2] In Western societies, including the United States, the rate has more than doubled within the past three decades. A number of factors have been proposed to explain this dramatic rise. These include the overall increase in longevity; the increased prevalence of hypertension, metabolic syndrome, and obesity; the ubiquitous use of thiazide diuretics and low-dose aspirin; changes in dietary trends, including the greater use of high-fructose corn syrup as a sweetener; and finally, the increase in survival of patients with end-stage renal disease and organ transplantation.

There is a direct correlation between the degree of serum urate elevation and the likelihood of developing gout. The reported annual incidence of gout in subjects with baseline serum urate levels greater than or equal to 9 mg/dL is 4.9%, compared with only 0.5% in people with serum urate levels of 7.0 to 8.9 mg/dL.

PATHOBIOLOGY

Uric acid is the end product of purine metabolism in humans. In most mammals, purine catabolism is taken one step further through the enzyme uric acid oxidase or uricase, with the purine end product in these species being the very soluble allantoin. Humans and most other hominoids lost the ability to produce the enzyme uricase nearly 18 million years ago. As a result, uric acid accumulation is possible. Whether caused by overproduction of uric acid or its underexcretion by the kidneys, this accumulation leads to supersaturation of urate ion in blood and the precipitation of monosodium urate crystals in synovial fluid, soft tissues, and organs. Urate is produced by the conversion of a very soluble molecule, hypoxanthine, to the less soluble xanthine, which, in turn, is converted to the very insoluble uric acid by progressive purine ring oxidations catalyzed by the enzyme xanthine oxidase. Xanthine oxidase is present in several organs, but most activity in the body is found in the liver and intestines. Because of its potential for causing disease, urate elimination is very important. The total daily accumulation of uric acid from de novo synthesis, nucleotide degradation, and dietary consumption is normally balanced by renal excretion of approximately two thirds of the total urate turnover and intestinal elimination by the remaining one third.

Simply put, hyperuricemia occurs when urate production is not balanced by renal excretion. In 90% of all gout patients, the cause of this imbalance is renal underexcretion. The remaining 10% of gout cases are caused by purine overproduction or a combination of overproduction and underexcretion. The nongenetic causes of hyperuricemia include other medical conditions, dietary components, and medications (Table 257-1). These factors may result in either overproduction or diminished renal clearance of uric acid. Similarly, the genetic causes of hyperuricemia (Table 257-2) may affect either production or elimination of uric acid.[3]

Renal Urate Underexcretion

Because uric acid is small and not protein bound, it is completely filtered by the glomerulus. In normal persons, approximately 8 to 10% of the filtered

TABLE 257-1	NONGENETIC CAUSES OF HYPERURICEMIA

IMPAIRED URIC ACID EXCRETION

Clinical Conditions

- Reduced glomerular filtration rate
- Hypertension
- Obesity
- Systemic sclerosis
- Lead nephropathy

Drugs

- Diuretics
- Ethanol
- Low-dose salicylates (0.06-3.0 g/day)
- Cyclosporine
- Tacrolimus
- Levodopa
- Angiotensin-converting-enzyme inhibitors
- β-Blockers
- Nicotinic acid
- Pancreatic extract

EXCESSIVE URIC ACID PRODUCTION

Clinical Conditions

- Myeloproliferative and lymphoproliferative neoplasms
- Obesity
- Psoriasis

Diet Components

- Alcoholic beverages (especially beer)
- Red meat, organ meat, shellfish
- High fructose corn syrup

TABLE 257-2	GENETIC CAUSES OF HYPERURICEMIA

SYNDROME	PHENOTYPE
INBORN ERRORS OF PURINE METABOLISM	
Hypoxanthine-guanine phosphoribosyl transferase deficiency	Neurologic dysfunction, renal stones, early-onset gout
Phosphoribosyl pyrophosphatase synthetase overactivity	Neurologic dysfunction, early-onset gout
EXCESSIVE CELL DEATH AND URATE GENERATION	
Glycogen storage disease I	Growth restriction, lactic acidosis, early-onset gout
Glycogen storage disease III	Early-onset gout
Glycogen storage disease V	Early-onset gout
Glycogen storage disease VII	Early-onset gout
Fructose-1-phosphate aldolase deficiency	Growth restriction, liver failure, early-onset gout
Myoadenylate deaminase deficiency	Myopathy, gout
Carnitine palmitoyltransferase II deficiency (late onset)	Rhabdomyolysis, gout
REDUCED RENAL EXCRETION OF URIC ACID	
Medullary cystic kidney disease	Renal dysfunction, early-onset gout
Familial juvenile hyperuricemic nephropathy	Renal dysfunction, early-onset gout
Uric acid transportasome mutations	
GLUT-9	Familial gout
ABCG2	Familial gout
URAT1	Familial gout

load is ultimately cleared in the urine. The various renal tubular transporters that are responsible for determining how much of the filtered uric acid is actually excreted are located in the proximal convoluted tubules and are referred to collectively as the *transportasome* (Fig. 257-1). Both reabsorption and secretion occur in this segment through the actions of several organic acid transporters, with the net effect being the reabsorption of nearly 90% of the uric acid filtered at the glomerulus. These organic acid transporters are also responsible for eliminating organic acids other than uric acid as well as many commonly used medications. The most important tubular transporter of uric acid is URAT1. This transporter swaps urate ions for other monocarboxylate organic ions in both directions across the luminal membrane of proximal tubular cells.

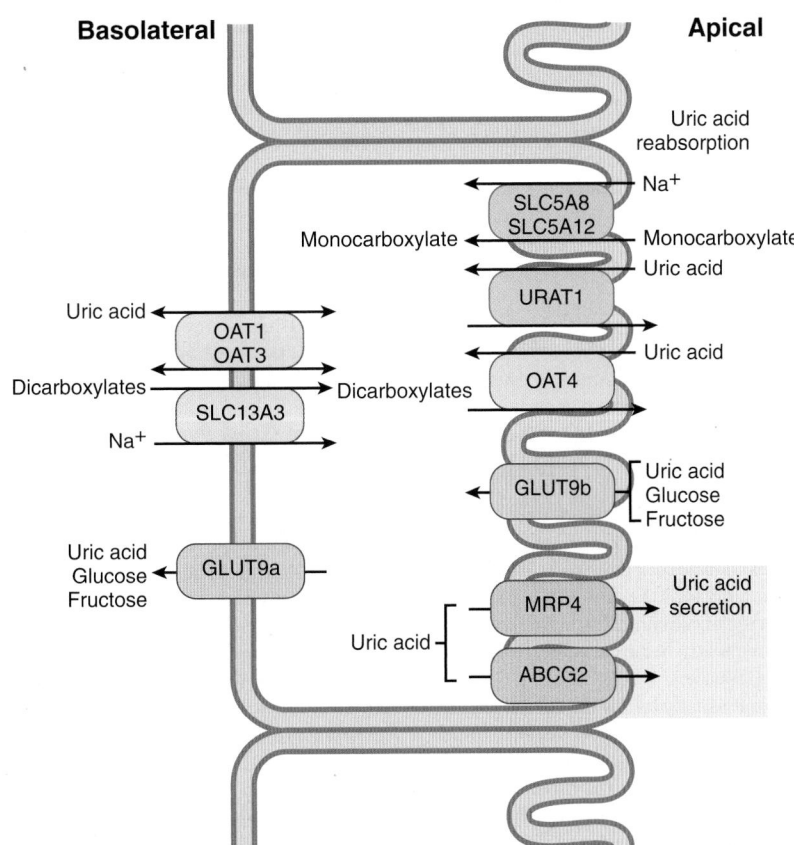

FIGURE 257-1. Renal transport of urate in proximal tubule of kidney. Serum urate reaches the tubule lumen by glomerular filtration and by secretion through the proximal tubular epithelium. Secretion of urate is facilitated in the luminal direction by MRP4, UAT, ABCG2, and NTP1, and at the basolateral membrane by OAT1 and OAT3. Reabsorption of urate from the tubular lumen is facilitated by URAT1, OAT4, OAT10, and the short isoform of GLUT (GLUT9b), and at the basolateral membrane by the long isoform (GLUT9a). ABCG2 = adenosine triphosphate–binding cassette transporter; GLUT = glucose transporter; MRP = multidrug-resistance-related protein; NTP = sodium phosphate transport protein; OAT = organic acid transporters; URAT = uric acid transporter.

This system can be driven to reabsorb more uric acid from the tubular lumen by raising tubular epithelial concentrations of lactate, pyruvate, or the ketoacids acetoacetate and β-hydroxybutyrate. Certain drugs, when present in the tubular lumen, can displace uric acid from the transporter, causing more uric acid to be lost in the urine. These compounds include lesinurad and probenecid.

When renal clearance of uric acid is compared between normal adult men and gouty men, the gouty subjects excrete only 70% as much uric acid as normal individuals at any given serum urate concentration. In general, gouty subjects required a serum urate concentration to be 1.7 mg/dL higher to obtain the same level of excretion as seen in normal subjects.

Most genetic polymorphisms associated with gout in genome-wide association studies encode for the various components of the uric acid transportasome (see Fig. 257-1). Polymorphisms in the glucose transporter GLUT-9 (encoded by the *SLC2A9* gene) are statistically the most significant determinants of serum urate. ABCG2 is a multifunctional transporter that belongs to the adenosine triphosphate (ATP)-binding cassette family found in the proximal tubule of the kidney as well as in the small intestine and liver. Polymorphisms in the gene encoding URAT1 may lead to either hypouricemia or hyperuricemia. A loss-of-function mutation results in familial renal hypouricemia.

The serum urate variance explained by these common genetic variants is only about 6% of the total variance observed between gouty and nongouty subjects. Similar risk-stratifying techniques demonstrate that 67% of the variance is caused by nongenetic factors such as serum creatinine, ethanol consumption, and the components of the metabolic syndrome.

Urate Overproduction

In approximately 10% of gouty subjects, hyperuricemia is caused by uric acid overproduction rather than reduced renal excretion. In most of these people, the hyperuricemia reflects accelerated cell turnover (e.g., lymphoproliferative and myeloproliferative diseases, psoriasis, chronic hemolytic states, polycythemia vera, and certain muscle glycogenoses) or by enhanced purine nucleotide breakdown (e.g., alcohol abuse or fructose ingestion). In addition to these secondary causes of urate overproduction, there are primary disease processes that are also responsible for urate overproduction. These are inborn errors of metabolism that result in increased de novo purine synthesis, as seen in phosphoribosyl pyrophosphate (PRPP) synthetase overactivity or decreased purine salvage as seen in the complete and partial hypoxanthine-guanine phosphoribosyltransferase (HPRT) deficiencies (Lesch-Nyhan syndrome and Kelley-Seegmiller syndrome, respectively). Regardless of the cause, urate overproduction is documented by a 24-hour urine collection showing greater than 1000 mg of uric acid while eating a standard Western diet.

Pathogenesis of Monosodium Urate Monohydrate Crystals and Inflammation

Monosodium urate crystals in joints, soft tissues, and organs are the cause of pain and destruction in gout. Urate crystals will form only when physiologic conditions permit. In plasma, urate becomes insoluble at concentrations of 6.8 mg/dL (408 μmol/L) with a pH of 7.40 and normal body temperature. A reduction in pH or temperature will lower the solubility threshold even further. Not all people who are hyperuricemic will form crystals, however. There appears to be an additional requirement of a "nucleation factor" that is still poorly defined.

Monosodium urate crystals form in joints and soft tissues of individuals long before they cause any symptoms of gout. They deposit in small lattice structures called *microtophi* on the surface of cartilage and synovial lining. These microtophi slowly grow but are generally stable as long as the environment surrounding them does not change drastically with regard to pH, urate concentration, or temperature. At the time of the first and subsequent flares, something does change in the joint environment to cause these crystal lattice structures to break apart and shed a massive number of crystals into the joint space. These newly released and nonopsonized crystals activate receptors on synovial macrophages and are then phagocytized by monocytes and macrophages, leading to interaction with the NLRP3 inflammasome. This results in the rapid production of interleukin-1β (IL-1β), which is responsible for all the cardinal features of the severe inflammation associated with acute gout.[4]

Although monocytes and macrophages are the major cellular sources of IL-1β, neutrophils predominate at the site of inflammation (e.g., joint), where monosodium urate crystals become extremely pro-inflammatory by activating neutrophils that then generate reactive oxygen species. However, neutrophils also have a major role in the resolution of acute gout through the formation of neutrophil extracellular traps (NETs). Neutrophil proteases are released into the NETs and cause the formation of cell aggregates that contain cellular debris and DNA. These cellular aggregates within NETs can rapidly degrade pro-inflammatory cytokines, thereby allowing for the spontaneous resolution of joint inflammation after 3 days (even in the absence of treatment). Therefore, neutrophils play a dual role in gouty inflammation, amplifying it initially but then mediating its resolution.[5]

CLINICAL MANIFESTATIONS

Classic Gout

The natural course of classic gout passes through three stages: asymptomatic hyperuricemia, acute intermittent gout symptoms, and chronic persistent gout symptoms.[6] The rate of progression from initial symptoms to persistent symptoms varies considerably from one person to another and is dependent on numerous factors, the most important being the degree of increase in serum urate levels.

Asymptomatic hyperuricemia refers to a state in which serum urate exceeds the level of solubility (6.8 mg/dL) but symptoms of crystalline deposition have not yet occurred. Only 15 to 20% of all hyperuricemic people are prone to develop monosodium urate crystals, and for this group, the period of asymptomatic hyperuricemia begins a stage of subclinical structural changes. In men, asymptomatic hyperuricemia frequently begins at puberty, whereas in women, it is usually delayed until menopause.

The initial clinical manifestations of gout usually follow decades of asymptomatic hyperuricemia. In men, the first flare usually occurs between the fourth and sixth decades of life. In women, the age of onset is older and varies with several factors, most importantly the age of menopause. The classic gout flare is hallmarked by the rapid development of warmth, swelling, erythema, and exquisite pain in one or occasionally two joints. The characteristically severe pain evolves from its faintest twinge to its most intense level over an 8- to 12-hour period. Initial episodes are usually monoarticular and involve lower extremity joints. The most common joint involved is the first metatarsal phalangeal joint (termed *podagra*), followed by the ankle, midfoot, and knee (Fig. 257-2). After years of recurrent gouty flares, upper extremity joints, including the wrists, elbows, and small joints of the hands, can also become involved. Systemic symptoms of fever, chills, and malaise may accompany gouty flares, along with an intense erythema extending beyond the area of the involved joint. This may lead to confusion with an infectious process.

Factors capable of provoking episodes of flare are those that cause fluctuations in serum urate levels, including trauma, surgery, starvation, overindulgence in certain high-purine foods, and the ingestion of any medication that raises or lowers serum urate.

Another characteristic of classic gout flares is their self-remitting nature for reasons discussed previously. For the first several acute flares, the duration of the attack is 5 to 8 days. The resolution of symptoms is gradual but complete, even if no anti-inflammatory therapy is administered. The periods between the flares are devoid of articular pain, although synovial fluid aspirates during this stage continue to show low-grade inflammation and the presence of monosodium urate crystals.

Eventually, the untreated patient will progress to persistent gouty arthritis, also referred to as *advanced gout*. This stage usually develops after 10 or more years of acute intermittent gout and is evident when the pain-free intercritical periods have disappeared. Gouty flares can continue to occur against this constantly painful background. The intensity of the chronic pain is not nearly as severe as that experienced with the acute flares.

The subcutaneous tophus is the most characteristic lesion of advanced gout. The development of tophaceous deposits of monosodium urate is a function of the duration and severity of hyperuricemia as well as the presence of proteinuria. Subcutaneous tophi may occur anywhere over the body but most commonly in the fingers, wrists, ears, knees, and olecranon bursa and at pressure points under the ulnar aspect of the forearm and Achilles tendon (Fig. 257-3). At this stage, gout can be confused with rheumatoid arthritis, especially if tophi are misdiagnosed as rheumatoid nodules.

Atypical Gout Presentations

Approximately 5% of patients with gout exhibit the onset of symptoms before age 25 years. Early-onset gout represents a special subset of patients who generally have a genetic component (see Table 257-2), with a more accelerated clinical course requiring more aggressive antihyperuricemic therapy.

In most large reviews, women account for no more than 5% of all gout subjects. This demographic is changing, with gout in older women becoming more common. Most women with gout are postmenopausal. Women who have premenopausal gout usually have renal insufficiency and hypertension and are taking thiazide diuretics, or they have a strong genetic predilection. Gout in older women may differ from classic gout in its propensity to occur in joints previously damaged by osteoarthritis such as the knees or the distal interphalangeal joints with Heberden nodes.

DIAGNOSIS

Hyperuricemia is an essential risk factor for developing gout, but it is not a reliable diagnostic test because many people with elevated serum urate levels will never develop gout. Serum urate levels during an acute flare of gout are also unreliable because they may be suppressed by as much as 1.5 to 2.0 mg/dL from baseline values. The definitive diagnosis of gout is made by polarized compensated microscopy of a synovial fluid aspirate from the affected joint. The presence of intracellular needle-shaped crystals with strong negative birefringence is the diagnostic "gold standard." Similar microscopic results from a tophus aspirate or spontaneously draining fluid would also confirm the diagnosis of gout.

Synovial fluid confirmation is obtained in as few as 10% of patients said to have gout. The presumptive diagnosis of gout is based on a pattern of acute joint symptoms coupled with the patient's own medical history or a family history. Key features include joint erythema, difficulty walking, time to maximal pain less than 24 hours, resolution by 2 weeks, presence of a tophus, and history of involvement of the first metatarsophalangeal joint.[7] The patient's medical history may reveal comorbidities frequently associated with gout or the use of medications associated with urate retention.

The characteristic clinical presentation is the rapid onset (over 8 to 12 hours) of severe pain in one or several lower extremity joints (especially the great toe, midfoot, and ankle). The presumptive diagnosis is given much greater

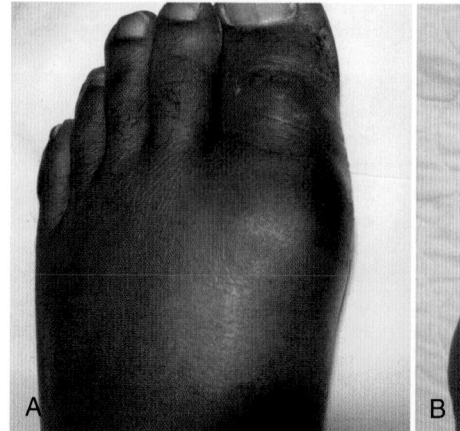
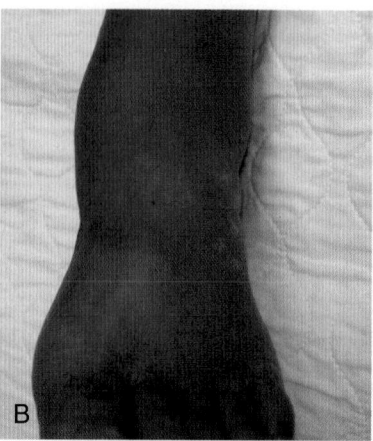

FIGURE 257-2. The intense inflammation of acute gouty arthritis. **A,** The marked swelling of the first metatarsophalangeal joint (podagra) is demonstrated. A dusky blue hue over an intense erythema is characteristic. **B,** Ankle swelling is shown with erythema extending beyond the area of the tibiotalar joint.

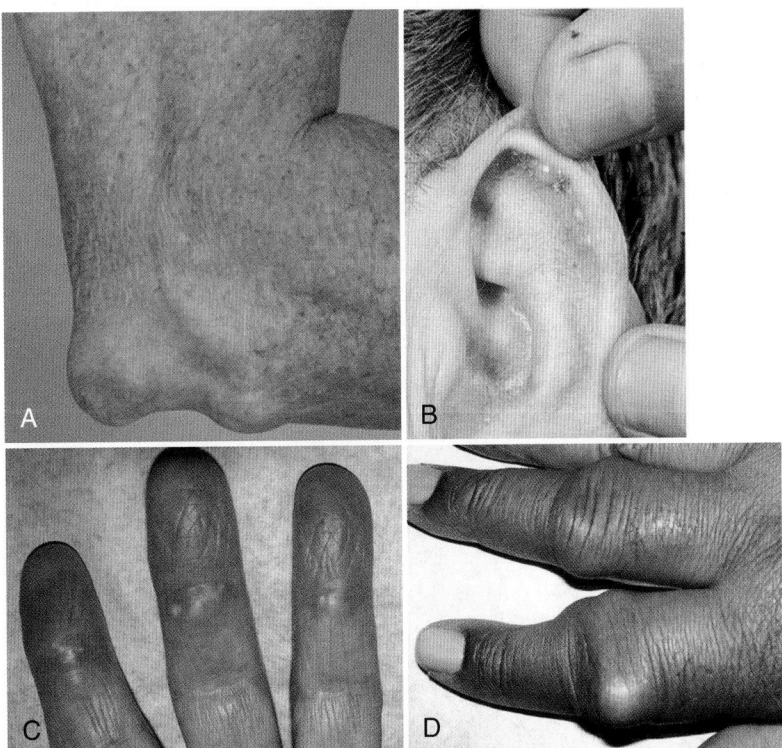

FIGURE 257-3. **Characteristic locations of gouty tophi. A,** At the elbow, tophi present as hard nodules along the ulnar ridge or as multiple nodules within the olecranon bursa. **B,** Ear tophi are uncommon but may be an easy source of crystal confirmation of gout when present. **C,** Small subcutaneous tophi can occur along the ventral creases of fingers. **D,** Tophi over the proximal interphalangeal or distal interphalangeal joints may be confused with Bouchard or Heberden nodes, respectively.

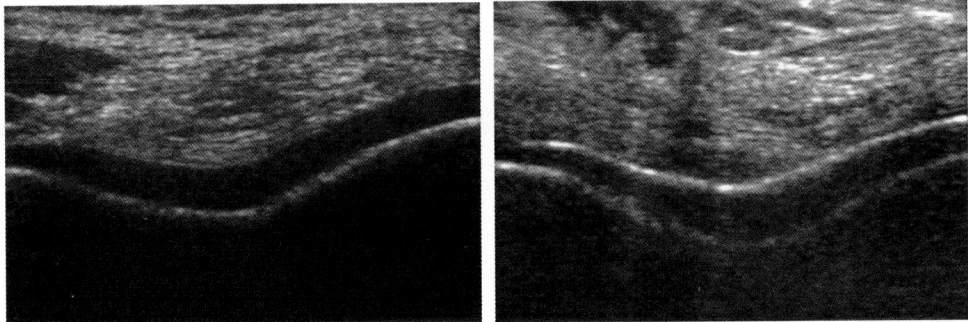

FIGURE 257-4. **Double contour sign.** Comparison of ultrasonographic appearance of normal (*left*) and gouty (*right*) knee with the probe in the suprapatellar, transverse orientation and the knee in flexion. The normal knee shows soft tissues overlying an anechoic (black) layer that represents hyaline cartilage. The single bright stripe represents the bony cortex of the anterior distal femur. The gouty knee demonstrated the "double-contour" sign composed of a layer crystals covering the hyaline cartilage and the lower bright contour being the femoral cortex.

credence if there have been similar previous attacks that spontaneously resolved to a symptom-free state.

Radiographic evaluation is not helpful in the early phase of gout except to rule out fracture. In advanced gout, affected joints may show punched-out periarticular erosions with classic overhanging edges. Ultrasonography can detect monosodium urate crystals layered over articular cartilage in early disease and may be diagnostic (Fig. 257-4). Magnetic resonance imaging is not part of a standard evaluation but will reveal soft tissue and intra-articular tophi long before they become clinically evident.

The differential diagnosis of acute gout includes bacterial infection, trauma, sarcoidosis, and calcium pyrophosphate arthropathy (pseudogout). Diseases occasionally confused with advanced gout include rheumatoid arthritis, reactive arthritis, and calcium pyrophosphate arthropathy.

TREATMENT AND PREVENTION   Rx

In the absence of definitive randomized trials, current practice guidelines for treatment diverge in some areas.[8,9] The American College of Rheumatology recommends a "treat-to-target" approach, using urate-lowering medications to lower serum uric acid levels to less than 6 mg/dL in patients with a history of two or more clinical flares, with close monitoring of uric acid levels. In contrast, the 2016 American College of Physicians guideline advocates a "treat-to-symptoms"

approach, emphasizing the use of anti-inflammatory medications (see later) to control flares and reserving urate-lowering medications for patients with frequent flares. This later approach is not evidence-based.

Regardless of which approach is selected, a heavy emphasis on patient education is needed to obtain an optimal treatment outcome.[10] Not only should patients be informed about dietary and other lifestyle changes, such as weight loss,[A1] that will lower their serum uric acid and lessen flares (Table 257-3), but they should also know that their disease is caused by an excessive burden of monosodium urate crystals already present in their joints and soft tissues. This understanding of the disease process underlying gouty arthritis will help shift the focus from symptoms to "urate burden" as the real target of treatment.

Gouty Flare

The treatment goal for gouty flare is to relieve pain and terminate the flare as quickly as possible. Resting the painful joint and applying ice are generally helpful, but pharmacologic intervention is usually necessary to alter the excruciatingly painful course that may last for several days to more than a week. The therapeutic options include nonsteroidal anti-inflammatory drugs (NSAIDs),[A2] oral colchicine,[A3] and corticosteroids. NSAIDs are widely used but may be inappropriate for patients with renal insufficiency or peptic ulcer disease. Oral colchicine administered as 1.2 mg (two tablets) at the time of flare onset followed in 1 hour by a third 0.6-mg tablet is the recommended dosing for the first 24 hours. This is followed by 7 to 10 days of once-daily or twice-daily colchicine depending on renal function. Corticosteroids can be administered orally (e.g.,

TABLE 257-3 SPECIFIC AMERICAN COLLEGE OF RHEUMATOLOGY RECOMMENDATIONS ON LIFESTYLE AND DIET FOR GOUTY PATIENTS

Weight loss for obese patients	Avoid: Organ meats High fructose corn syrup–sweetened drinks Alcohol overuse
Healthy overall diet	Limit: Beef, pork, lamb, shellfish Beer
Exercise to achieve fitness	Encourage: Low-fat dairy
Smoking cessation	
Stay well hydrated	

prednisolone, 30 mg once a day), intramuscularly, or intra-articularly for acute gout symptoms and is a valuable option in patients with poor renal function or intolerance to colchicine. A meta-analysis of double-blind, randomized, controlled trials indicates that oral prednisolone may be of similar efficacy and slightly safer than NSAIDs (naproxen or indomethacin) for the treatment of active, acute gout.[A4] Issues critical to treatment success for a gouty flare are the early initiation of treatment, ensuring adequate dosing of anti-inflammatory therapy, and continuing the treatment until the flare has completely resolved (usually 6 to 10 days). During the acute flare, subjects already taking urate-lowering therapy should continue the drug, whereas those not receiving this therapy should not be started.

Urate-Lowering Therapies

The principal goal of treating gout is to lower the serum uric acid below its saturation point so that the process of crystallization will cease and the accumulated urate burden will be gradually diminished. The 2012 American College of Rheumatology guidelines recommend a target serum urate of less than 6 mg/dL in all subjects, with an even lower target (<5 mg/dL) for patients with more advanced gout. Urate-lowering therapy is recommended for all patients with two or more gouty flares per year, patients with advanced disease, and those with kidney stones. Both allopurinol[A5] and febuxostat are xanthine oxidase inhibitors that are considered first-line urate-lowering therapy. The American College of Rheumatology guidelines recommend that the allopurinol starting dose be no greater than 100 mg/day. The dose is gradually escalated by 100 mg daily every 2 to 5 weeks, with serum urate monitoring until the target serum urate is achieved.[A6] The maximal U.S. Food and Drug Administration (FDA)-approved dose of allopurinol is 800 mg daily. In subjects with advanced chronic kidney disease, the initial dose should be reduced to 50 mg daily, with incremental dose escalations of 50 mg. Febuxostat is an alternative urate-lowering therapy and should be used in patients who have failed allopurinol treatment or have demonstrated sensitivity or intolerance to allopurinol.[11] The initial febuxostat dose of 40 mg daily can be increased to 80 mg daily after 2 weeks of therapy if the serum urate target is not achieved. In a randomized trial of gout patients with coexisting cardiovascular disease, overall rates of major cardiovascular events were similar in patients treated with febuxostat and allopurinol, but cardiovascular deaths or deaths from any cause were more frequent in the febuxostat group than in the allopurinol group for unclear reasons.[A7]

In patients who have gout but who have not attained the target serum urate despite maximal doses of either allopurinol or febuxostat, uricosuric agents (probenecid, up to 2 g daily)[A8][A9] can be added to the xanthine oxidase inhibitor. Pegloticase (8 mg by IV infusion every 2 weeks) is an intravenously administered monomethoxypoly(ethylene glycol)-conjugated recombinant uricase that dramatically lowers serum urate levels. It is approved by the FDA for the treatment of gout in patients for whom conventional therapy has been ineffective.

Before the initiation of any form of urate-lowering therapy, the patient should be placed on anti-inflammatory therapy to prevent or minimize the anticipated increase in flare activity that is associated with starting urate-lowering therapy.[A10] Background anti-inflammatory prophylaxis is in the form of colchicine once or twice daily or low-dose NSAIDs. Anti-inflammatory prophylaxis should be continued until the subject has been free of gout flares for 6 months or longer.

CALCIUM PYROPHOSPHATE DIHYDRATE CRYSTAL DEPOSITION DISEASE

DEFINITIONS

The heterogeneous group of clinical conditions associated with calcium pyrophosphate dehydrate crystals are collectively called *calcium pyrophosphate crystal deposition disease*. Within this spectrum is the common radiographic finding of chondrocalcinosis that is frequently asymptomatic. The acute synovitis associated with intra-articular calcium pyrophosphate crystals can closely mimic the findings of gout and is hence referred to as *pseudogout*. The more chronic changes associated with calcium pyrophosphate-induced bone and cartilage destruction is referred to as *pyrophosphate arthropathy*. These conditions are further classified as familial (genetic), metabolic, and sporadic.

EPIDEMIOLOGY

The true prevalence of calcium pyrophosphate crystal deposition disease is unknown, but it is generally thought to be underdiagnosed because of its confusion with other forms of arthritis.[12] The prevalence of radiographically appearing chondrocalcinosis has been studied extensively and is clearly an age-related phenomenon. Chondrocalcinosis of the meniscal and articular cartilage of the knee is seen in 4% of people between the ages of 55 and 59 years; in 18% of those 80 to 84 years; and in approximately 27% of those older than 85 years.

PATHOBIOLOGY

Clinical calcium pyrophosphate disease is divided into three categories based on the etiology of altered inorganic pyrophosphate metabolism. The categories are hereditary (familial), sporadic (idiopathic), and metabolic. All three types of calcium pyrophosphate disease are associated with extracellular inorganic pyrophosphate accumulation around chondrocytes, and extracellular inorganic pyrophosphate is necessary for the formation of calcium pyrophosphate crystals.

Hereditary forms of calcium pyrophosphate crystal deposition disease may be caused by increased transmembrane transport of chondrocyte intracellular inorganic pyrophosphate to its extracellular matrix by diminished activity of the protective pyrophosphate hydrolases, or because of altered influences of factors that lead to increased extracellular inorganic pyrophosphate, including transforming growth factor-β, bone morphogenic protein-2 and -4, ascorbic acid, and osteopontin.

Transporter mutations are rarely observed in the sporadic form of calcium pyrophosphate disease. Aging chondrocytes in culture produce considerably more inorganic pyrophosphate than do younger chondrocytes, although the exact mechanism for this is unclear.

The metabolic diseases that predispose to calcium pyrophosphate crystal deposition disease include hemochromatosis, hyperparathyroidism, hypomagnesemia (as in Gitelman syndrome), and hypophosphatasia. All of these metabolic conditions result in increased extracellular inorganic pyrophosphate or other alterations in the cartilage matrix that are permissive for calcium pyrophosphate crystal formation.

CLINICAL MANIFESTATIONS AND DIAGNOSIS

Calcium pyrophosphate crystal deposition disease presents in a variety of fashions. It is frequently asymptomatic (lanthanic) and recognized only by the appearance of chondrocalcinosis on radiographs. The most common clinical manifestation accounting for approximately 60% of calcium pyrophosphate disease is a polyarticular arthritis affecting joints not typically involved in primary osteoarthritis, including the wrists, shoulders, and metacarpophalangeal joints (particularly the second and third metacarpophalangeals).[13] This form of calcium pyrophosphate disease is called *pseudo-osteoarthritis* and may be associated with occasional inflammatory attacks. The acute monoarticular presentation is known as *pseudogout*. The pain and swelling of pseudogout can be similar to that seen in gout. The onset is usually not as abrupt as with gout, and the attacks tend to last longer—frequently months. Pseudogout occurs more often in the large joints than in small joints. Calcium pyrophosphate crystal deposition disease can occasionally present as a chronic polyarticular inflammatory disease that may mimic rheumatoid arthritis or polymyalgia rheumatica.

Calcium pyrophosphate disease is diagnosed by identifying chondrocalcinosis by radiography in a patient with a clinical history suggestive of the disease (Fig. 257-5). Definitive diagnosis is made by the finding of calcium pyrophosphate crystals by compensated polarized light microscopic examination of aspirated synovial fluid.[14]

PREVENTION AND TREATMENT   Rx

There are no specific therapies for calcium pyrophosphate crystal deposition disease.[15] In patients with metabolic disease–associated calcium pyrophosphate disease, treatment and control of the metabolic disease can afford some improvement in the arthritis, although this is not the case for phlebotomy-treated

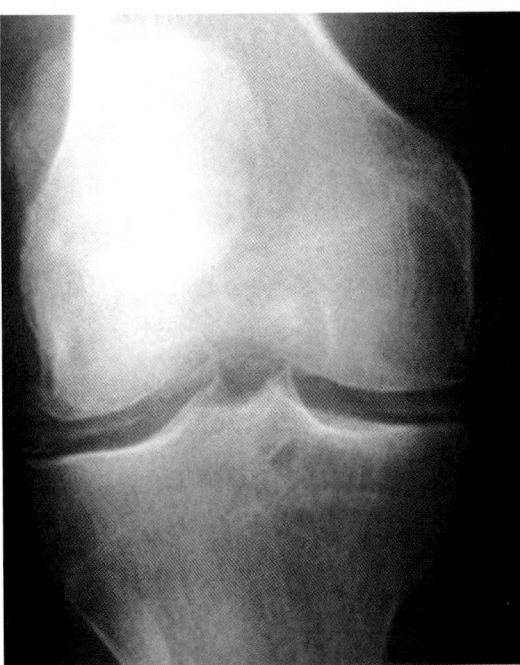

FIGURE 257-5. Calcium pyrophosphate dihydrate arthropathy of the knee. Radiographic evidence of chondrocalcinosis showing fibrocartilage calcification as thick, linear deposits parallel to and separate from subchondral bone.

hereditary hemochromatosis. For both the acute and chronic forms of calcium pyrophosphate crystal deposition disease, therapy is directed at symptoms. NSAIDs are the mainstay of treatment. Low-dose oral colchicine can be used in both acute and chronic settings. Intra-articular steroids have also been proved to be beneficial for symptomatic calcium pyrophosphate crystal deposition disease. The IL-1 inhibitor, anakinra, has been effectively used "off-label" for treating calcium pyrophosphate disease flares. On the other hand, intra-articular viscosupplementation (hyaluronic acid) may exacerbate joint symptoms.

APATITE (BASIC CALCIUM PHOSPHATE)-ASSOCIATED ARTHROPATHY

Basic calcium phosphate crystals include several different crystal species. The most common of these is hydroxyapatite. The basic calcium phosphate crystals are unlike monosodium urate or calcium pyrophosphate crystals in that they are not identifiable by polarized microscopy. These very tiny crystals are responsible for several important clinical conditions. Although basic calcium phosphate crystals are found in 50% of osteoarthritic synovial fluids, the incidence and prevalence of the individual apatite-associated clinical manifestations have not been established. This is especially true of the most severe and destructive apatite syndromes such as Milwaukee shoulder and tumoral calcinosis. The prevalence of the most common apatite-associated conditions, calcific periarthritis of the shoulder, was 3% in a large North American study.

PATHOBIOLOGY

Like monosodium urate and calcium pyrophosphate crystals, basic calcium phosphate crystals exert their pro-inflammatory effects by being phagocytized by resident synoviocytes and influxing leukocytes. Unlike monosodium urate and calcium pyrophosphate crystals, apatite crystals apparently do not act through the NLRP3 inflammasome. Rather, basic calcium phosphate crystals are dissolved in the acidic phagosome and raise intracellular calcium levels and then activate the calcium-dependent signaling pathways. The synoviocytes are stimulated by these pathways to increase production of tumor necrosis factor-α and IL-6, and influxing neutrophils are stimulated to increase pro-inflammatory oxygen radicals. The fibroblasts in the joint lining and surrounding soft tissues are stimulated to increase production of many of the matrix metalloproteinases, such as collagenase 1, collagenase 3, and stromelysin 1.

CLINICAL MANIFESTATIONS OF BASIC CALCIUM PHOSPHATE DEPOSITION

The clinical manifestations of basic calcium phosphate deposition can be acute or chronic, and their cause can be idiopathic, hereditary, or secondary to other

TABLE 257-4	CLINICAL MANIFESTATIONS OF BASIC CALCIUM PHOSPHATE DEPOSITION DISEASE

Osteoarthritis and basic calcium phosphate deposition
Acute inflammatory arthritis
Acute calcific periarthritis
Chronic noninflammatory arthropathy
Diffuse idiopathic skeletal hyperostosis (DISH)
Tumoral calcinosis
Calcifications associated with hypercalcemic states
   Hyperparathyroidism
   Hypervitaminosis D
   Sarcoidosis
   Metastatic cancer
   Myeloma
   Leukemia

diseases that cause hypercalcemia (Table 257-4). Basic calcium phosphate crystals can be found in 50% of synovial fluids from osteoarthritic knees. The presence of basic calcium phosphate crystals correlates with more severe radiographic changes secondary to more rapid deterioration in these osteoarthritic knees.[16] Acute inflammatory arthritis associated with basic calcium phosphate deposition is similar in many ways to that of gout and pseudogout and has been referred to as *pseudo-pseudogout*. The patients tend to be younger and usually have evidence of soft tissue basic calcium phosphate deposition elsewhere in the body. Periarticular calcifications are often asymptomatic. However, basic calcium phosphate deposition can cause an acute and severe inflammation of the ligaments, tendons, and bursae surrounding a joint, termed *acute calcific periarthritis*. This frequently occurs around the shoulders and hips but can also occur in fingers, toes, wrists, and ankles.

The most destructive basic calcium phosphate–associated arthropathy is Milwaukee shoulder, which is characterized by large, bloody noninflammatory effusions containing basic calcium phosphate crystals with or without calcium pyrophosphate crystals. The process results in the destruction of the rotator cuff leading to marked instability and glenohumeral cartilage dissolution. This process can also affect knees. Like the acute calcific periarthritis discussed previously, Milwaukee shoulder is observed in women four times more frequently than in men.

Diffuse idiopathic skeletal hyperostosis (DISH) is seen predominately in men and elderly people. The radiographic appearance of this condition is flowing ossifications along the anterolateral aspect of spinal vertebrae, especially in the thoracic spine. DISH is usually asymptomatic, but very large bridging osteophytes can cause pain; in the cervical spine, it can even result in dysphagia.

Idiopathic tumoral calcinosis is rare but most prevalent in young patients of African descent. These subjects have large irregular calcifying masses in the soft tissue surrounding the shoulders, hips, and elbows. Some cases show a familial occurrence and medical conditions associated with hyperphosphatemia.

Finally, metastatic calcifications can arise in any medical condition associated with hypercalcemia such as hyperparathyroidism, hypervitaminosis D, sarcoidosis, metastatic cancer, multiple myeloma, and leukemia.

TREATMENT AND PREVENTION   Rx

The treatment of most basic calcium phosphate–associated syndromes is conservative.[17] In acute inflammatory arthritis and periarthritis, low-dose oral colchicine and NSAIDs are the mainstay of a symptomatic therapy. The persistent large effusion seen in Milwaukee shoulder should be serially aspirated to decrease intracapsular pressure. The added effectiveness of corticosteroid injections in this setting is unproved. The calcinosis associated with abnormal calcium and phosphate metabolism is best managed by treating the underlying metabolic process.

Grade A References

A1. Nielsen SM, Bartels EM, Henriksen M, et al. Weight loss for overweight and obese individuals with gout: a systematic review of longitudinal studies. *Ann Rheum Dis.* 2017;76:1870-1882.

A2. van Durme CM, Wechalekar MD, Buchbinder R, et al. Non-steroidal anti-inflammatory drugs for acute gout. *Cochrane Database Syst Rev.* 2014;9:CD010120.

A3. van Echteld I, Wechalekar MD, Schlesinger N, et al. Colchicine for acute gout. *Cochrane Database Syst Rev.* 2014;8:CD006190.

A4. Yu J, Lu H, Zhou J, et al. Oral prednisolone versus non-steroidal anti-inflammatory drugs in the treatment of acute gout: a meta-analysis of randomized controlled trials. *Inflammopharmacology.* 2018;26:717-723.

A5. Seth R, Kydd AS, Buchbinder R, et al. Allopurinol for chronic gout. *Cochrane Database Syst Rev.* 2014;10:CD006077.

A6. Stamp LK, Chapman PT, Barclay ML, et al. A randomised controlled trial of the efficacy and safety of allopurinol dose escalation to achieve target serum urate in people with gout. *Ann Rheum Dis.* 2017;76:1522-1528.

A7. White WB, Saag KG, Becker MA, et al. Cardiovascular safety of febuxostat or allopurinol in patients with gout. *N Engl J Med.* 2018;378:1200-1210.

A8. Kydd AS, Seth R, Buchbinder R, et al. Uricosuric medications for chronic gout. *Cochrane Database Syst Rev.* 2014;11:CD010457.

A9. Perez-Ruiz F, Sundy JS, Miner JN, et al. Lesinurad in combination with allopurinol: results of a phase 2, randomised, double-blind study in patients with gout with an inadequate response to allopurinol. *Ann Rheum Dis.* 2016;75:1074-1080.

A10. Hill EM, Sky K, Sit M, et al. Does starting allopurinol prolong acute treated gout? A randomized clinical trial. *J Clin Rheumatol.* 2015;21:120-125.

GENERAL REFERENCES

For the General References and other additional features, please visit Expert Consult at https://expertconsult.inkling.com.

258

FIBROMYALGIA, CHRONIC FATIGUE SYNDROME, AND MYOFASCIAL PAIN

DANIEL J. CLAUW

DEFINITION

Fibromyalgia is the current term for individuals with chronic widespread musculoskeletal pain, for which no alternative cause can be identified. If fatigue rather than pain is the presenting complaint, individuals are often diagnosed with chronic fatigue syndrome.[1] Gastroenterologists often see the exact same patients and focus on their gastroenterologic complaints, and often use the terms functional GI disorder, irritable bowel syndrome (IBS), non-ulcer dyspepsia, noncardiac chest pain, or esophageal dysmotility to explain the patient's symptoms. Neurologists see these patients for their headaches or unexplained facial pain, urologists for pelvic pain and urinary symptoms (and use labels such as interstitial cystitis, chronic prostatitis, vulvodynia, and vulvar vestibulitis), dentists for temporomandibular disorders (TMD), and so on.

Until recently these unexplained pain syndromes perplexed researchers, clinicians, and patients, and went by terms such as idiopathic, functional, or somatization. However, it is now clear that:

- Individuals will sometimes only have one of these "idiopathic" pain syndromes over the course of their lifetime. But more often, individuals with one of these entities, and their family members, are likely to have several of these conditions. Many terms have been used to describe these co-aggregating syndromes and symptoms, including functional somatic syndromes, somatization disorders, allied spectrum conditions, sensory sensitivity syndromes, chronic multisymptom illnesses, and medically unexplained symptoms. The most recent term coined by the National Institutes of Health in the United States is probably the best accepted at present: chronic overlapping pain conditions.
- Some of these individuals have identifiable psychological or psychiatric comorbidities present, but many do not, and thus it is important to understand that the pathobiology of these processes is independent of, but sometimes overlaps with, that seen in mood disorders, post-traumatic stress disorder (PTSD), and others.
- Women are more likely to have these disorders than men (1.5 to 2 times as often), but the sex difference is much more apparent in clinical samples (especially tertiary care) than in population-based samples.
- Groups of individuals with these conditions (e.g., fibromyalgia, chronic fatigue syndrome, IBS, headache, TMD, etc.) typically display disturbances in pain and sensory processing including increased pain to normally painful stimuli or pain to normally nonpainful stimuli. This can be identified in the patient's history (e.g., by asking about sensitivity to bright lights, odors, drugs) as well as in research studies using quantitative sensory testing or functional neuroimaging. This suggests that these individuals have a central nervous system–mediated problem with augmented pain or sensory processing that is contributing to the pain and other somatic sensitivities the individual is experiencing, rather than simply a nociceptive focus confined to the region of the body where the person is currently experiencing pain.
- Similar types of therapies are efficacious for all of these conditions, including both pharmacologic (e.g., tricyclic compounds, serotonin norepinephrine reuptake inhibitors, and gabapentinoids) and nonpharmacologic treatments (e.g., education, exercise, cognitive behavioral therapy [CBT]). Conversely, individuals with these conditions typically do not respond to therapies that are effective when pain is caused by injury or inflammatory disorders of tissues (e.g., NSAIDs, opioids, local injections, surgical procedures).
- Subsets of individuals with any chronic pain condition (e.g., low back pain, osteoarthritis, autoimmune disorders, sickle cell disease, etc.) also have the same phenotypic features and underlying mechanisms as those seen in fibromyalgia. These individuals with sub-threshold fibromyalgia display the same pathologic features and differential responsiveness to peripherally directed versus centrally directed therapies.
- It is critical that clinicians seeing patients with chronic pain evaluate individuals for the presence of this phenotype because it can dramatically affect which treatments will work, or not work, for a given individual with chronic pain.

Until about a decade ago, these conditions were all on somewhat equal (and tenuous) scientific ground. But within a relatively short period of time, research methods such as experimental pain testing, functional imaging, and genetics have led to tremendous advances in the understanding of several of these conditions, most notably fibromyalgia, IBS, and TMD. Many in the pain field (Chapter 27) now feel that much chronic pain itself is a neural disease and that many of the underlying mechanisms operative in these heretofore considered idiopathic or functional pain syndromes may be similar no matter whether that pain is present throughout the body (e.g., in fibromyalgia) or localized to the low back, the bowel, or the bladder. Because of this, the more contemporary terms used to describe conditions such as fibromyalgia, IBS, TMD, chronic fatigue syndrome, vulvodynia, and many other entities include "centralized pain" or "central sensitization" to imply that the central nervous system is playing a prominent role in amplifying or causing the pain in most individuals with these syndromes (see Table 258-1). Many of these findings have also been noted in chronic fatigue syndrome but the various pathophysiologic theories of chronic fatigue syndrome vary widely, and are the source of considerable contention, so this chapter will focus where the evidence base is significantly stronger in fibromyalgia.

EPIDEMIOLOGY

Fibromyalgia and Chronic Widespread Pain

Epidemiologic studies of the historical component of the American College of Rheumatology (ACR) criteria for fibromyalgia, chronic widespread pain (CWP), have been extremely instructive. CWP is typically operationalized as pain above and below the waist, involving the left and right sides of the body, and also involving the axial skeleton. Population-based studies of CWP suggest that roughly 4 to 12% of the population has this symptom at any given point in time.[2] Chronic regional pain is found in 20 to 25% of the population. Both chronic widespread and regional pain occur about 1.5 times more often in women than in men. These findings are very similar in different countries, ethnicities, and cultures.

FIBROMYALGIA

The original 1990 ACR criteria for fibromyalgia required that an individual has both a history of CWP, and the finding of 11 or more of 18 possible tender points on examination. Tender points represent nine paired predefined regions of the body, often over musculotendinous insertions. If an individual reports pain when a region is palpated with 4 kilograms of pressure, this is considered a positive tender point. At the time the 1990 ACR criteria were published, it was thought that there might be some unique significance to the locations of tender points. Since then, we have learned that the tenderness in fibromyalgia extends throughout the entire body.

The tender point requirement in the 1990 ACR criteria not only misrepresents the nature of the tenderness in this condition (i.e., local rather than widespread), but also strongly influences the demographic and psychological characteristics of fibromyalgia. Women are only 1.5 times more likely than

TABLE 258-1 MECHANISTIC CHARACTERIZATION OF PAIN

	NOCICEPTIVE	NEUROPATHIC	CENTRALIZED
Cause	Inflammation or damage	Nerve damage or entrapment	CNS or systemic problem
Clinical features	Pain is well localized, consistent effect of activity on pain	Follows distribution of peripheral nerves (i.e., dermatome or stocking/glove), episodic, lancinating, numbness, tingling	Pain is widespread and accompanied by fatigue, sleep, memory and/or mood difficulties, as well as history of previous pain elsewhere in body
Screening tools		PainDETECT	Body map or FM Survey
Treatment	NSAIDs, injections, surgery, opioids	Local treatments aimed at nerve (surgery, injections, topical) or CNS-acting drugs	CNS-acting drugs, nonpharmacologic therapies
Classic examples	Osteoarthritis Autoimmune disorders Cancer pain	Diabetic painful neuropathy Post-herpetic neuralgia Sciatica, carpal tunnel syndrome	Fibromyalgia Functional GI disorders Temporomandibular disorder Tension headache Interstitial cystitis, bladder pain syndrome

Variable degrees of any mechanism can contribute in any disease.
CNS = central nervous system; FM = fibromyalgia; GI = gastrointestinal; NSAIDs = nonsteroidal antiinflammatory drugs.

TABLE 258-2 STRESSORS CAPABLE OF TRIGGERING FIBROMYALGIA AND RELATED CONDITIONS

- Peripheral pain syndromes
- Infections (e.g., parvovirus, EBV, Lyme disease, Q fever; not common upper respiratory infections)
- Physical trauma (automobile accidents)
- Psychological stress/distress
- Hormonal alterations (e.g., hypothyroidism)
- Drugs
- Vaccines
- Certain catastrophic events (war, but not natural disasters)

men to experience CWP, but are 11 times more likely than men to have 11 or more tender points. Thus, women are approximately 10 times more likely to meet 1990 ACR criteria for fibromyalgia than men. Yet, many men have the same symptoms, and this is one of many reasons that in 2010 new criteria for fibromyalgia were developed that did not require performing a tender point count, and more fully appreciated the other CNS-mediated symptoms that are seen commonly in fibromyalgia and related conditions, including fatigue, and sleep and memory issues.

The majority of patients with fibromyalgia develop their pain symptoms in multiple body regions early in life, frequently beginning in childhood or adolescence. Individuals who eventually go on to develop fibromyalgia are more likely to experience headaches, dysmenorrhea, temporomandibular disorders (TMD), chronic fatigue syndrome, myofascial pain, IBS and other functional gastrointestinal disorders, interstitial cystitis/painful bladder syndrome, endometriosis, and other regional pain syndromes (particularly with back and neck pain). In many cases, what may appear to a health care provider to be an entirely new type of acute or subacute pain is in fact only another region of the body involved with pain. The concept is evolving among pain specialists that these "centralized" pain disorders actually represent a single lifelong disease with a spectrum of symptoms in different regions of the body over time. The U.S. National Institutes of Health has recently used the term "chronic overlapping pain conditions (COPCs)" to denote the fact that these conditions often co-occur in the same individuals and share many pathogenic features.

Various types of environmental stressors, including but not limited to psychological factors, most likely trigger the development of fibromyalgia (Table 258-2). Fibromyalgia and related disorders are found at much higher than expected rates in individuals who have experienced specific infections (e.g., Epstein-Barr virus, Lyme disease, Q fever, viral hepatitis), trauma (such as motor vehicle accidents), and wartime military service. This is a contentious legal issue and not all would agree that all of these types of seemingly distinct entities can trigger or exacerbate fibromyalgia. Certainly assessing cause and effect in any given individual is almost impossible, because all individuals experience intermittent stressors of the variety that seemingly can trigger fibromyalgia. It is also likely that part of the reason these different stressors can seemingly lead to worsening of fibromyalgia or fibromyalgia symptoms is because of how these stressors affect activity level, sleep, or overall distress, any of which then can lead to worsening of pain and other symptoms.

Fibromyalgia is frequently found as a comorbidity in other chronic pain conditions such as osteoarthritis and autoimmune rheumatic diseases. As many as 25% of patients correctly diagnosed with generalized inflammatory disorders such as systemic lupus erythematosus (SLE), rheumatoid arthritis (RA), and ankylosing spondylitis will also fulfill ACR criteria for fibromyalgia. However, in clinical practice this co-expression often goes unrecognized, especially when the fibromyalgia develops after the autoimmune disorder or regional pain syndrome. In this setting when comorbid fibromyalgia goes unrecognized, patients are often unnecessarily treated more aggressively with potentially toxic biologics and immunosuppressive agents.

This comorbid form of fibromyalgia has been termed "secondary fibromyalgia." A more popular term to use for this phenomenon is that these individuals have "centralized" their pain. While peripheral nociceptive input might be involved for some of such a patient's pain, CNS factors are probably amplifying it, leading to other associated symptoms such as fatigue, memory problems, and disturbances of sleep and mood. The term "central sensitization" is also sometimes used to describe this phenomenon, but many feel that this term should be reserved for the more general disorder mediated by a multitude of different spinal and supraspinal mechanisms. Regardless of terminology, it is becoming increasingly important to identify the disorder because emerging evidence suggests that therapies that work best for peripheral, nociceptive pain (e.g., NSAIDs, opioids, injections, surgical procedures) are less likely to be effective in these patients.[3]

The "primary" form of fibromyalgia is also associated with serious comorbidities, with early life and ongoing stressors. Many if not most such patients have a lifetime history of a psychiatric disorder such as depression or anxiety. There is typically more psychiatric and psychological comorbidity noted in individuals who are refractory to treatment. The bidirectional relationship between fibromyalgia and psychiatric conditions is likely due at least in part to common triggers to both sets of conditions, as well as shared pathophysiology. Potentially modifiable risk factors for developing fibromyalgia or worsening its course include poor sleep, obesity, physical inactivity, and job or life dissatisfaction. Cognitive factors such as catastrophizing (irrational thinking that the pain is much worse or more serious than it actually is) or fear of movement have been found to be poor prognostic factors in fibromyalgia and other chronic pain states.

PATHOBIOLOGY

Animal Models of Fibromyalgia

Although few would purport that there is an animal model that mimics all of the key clinical features of fibromyalgia, nonetheless animal models can be very helpful in understanding the pathogenesis of this condition.[4] Animals develop the critical features of central sensitization or centralization of pain when exposed to swim stress, neonatal separation from their mothers, and many other nonpainful stressful stimuli.

Genetic Factors

The strong familial predisposition to fibromyalgia and other chronic pain conditions has led many to study specific genetic polymorphisms that may be associated with a higher risk of developing fibromyalgia. First, candidate gene studies showed that genetic findings such as the serotonin 5-HT2A receptor polymorphism T/T phenotype, serotonin transporter, dopamine 4 receptor, and COMT (catecholamine o-methyl transferase) polymorphisms all were noted in higher frequency in fibromyalgia patients than in controls. Subsequent studies confirmed some of these associations whereas others did not. Subsequent larger genome-wide linkage and candidate gene studies identified other putative targets. The linkage studies confirmed the strong genetic contribution to fibromyalgia, and suggested linkage of fibromyalgia to the chromosome 17p11.2-q11.2 region. The large candidate gene study identified significant differences in allele frequencies between cases and controls that were observed for three genes: *GABRB3*, *TAAR1*, and *GBP1*. In light of the fact that classic genetic studies have not yet identified strong, reproducible polymorphisms or haplotypes associated with fibromyalgia, and because there is clear evidence of environmental factors such as stress playing a prominent role in the pathogenesis, other groups have postulated that epigenetic findings might be important in fibromyalgia.[5] These are promising areas of inquiry that need further research.

Evidence of Central Nervous System Disturbances in Pain and Sensory Processing

The pathophysiologic hallmark of fibromyalgia is augmented central pain processing. Subsequent studies using more sophisticated measures of experimental pain testing showed that individuals with fibromyalgia are more tender everywhere in the body, not just in the 18 regions originally considered to be "tender points." Several potential mechanisms have been experimentally found to be potentially responsible for pain amplification in fibromyalgia, including a decrease in the activity of descending analgesic pathways, and a diffuse increase in the processing of all sensory stimuli (not just pain).

Brain Imaging Studies

Functional, chemical, and structural brain neuroimaging studies have provided the best "objective" evidence that the pain of fibromyalgia and related pain amplification syndrome is "real." Functional MRI (fMRI) studies have demonstrated that in individuals with fibromyalgia the application of mild pressure or heat stimulus that other individuals would sense as touch rather than pain, are experienced as pain. Individuals with or without fibromyalgia utilize similar brain activation patterns and brain areas involved in pain processing. The insula is a brain region that is consistently hyperactive and is likely to play a key pathogenic role in fibromyalgia and related conditions. This region has been noted to play a critical role in sensory integration, with the posterior insula serving a purer sensory role, and the anterior insula being associated with the emotional processing of sensations.

Patients with fibromyalgia have increased connectivity between brain regions involved in increasing pain transmission and neural networks not normally involved in pain. During a painful stimulus, connectivity is decreased between key antinociceptive regions and a region identified as a potential source of dysfunctional pain inhibition in fibromyalgia. Quantitative sensory testing studies have demonstrated that fibromyalgia patients are more sensitive to a number of sensory stimuli other than pain, and that machine learning paradigms can accurately distinguish fibromyalgia patients from individuals without fibromyalgia with over 90% accuracy.[6]

Imaging techniques have also been used to identify the neurotransmitter abnormalities that may be "driving" the pain amplification seen in fibromyalgia and other chronic pain disorders. Decreased *mu* opioid receptor availability (possibly due to increased release of endogenous *mu* opioids) has been reported in fibromyalgia. This finding, as well as previous studies showing increases in endogenous opioids in the cerebrospinal fluid (CSF) of fibromyalgia patients, has been suggested as evidence of why opioid analgesics appear to not be efficacious in fibromyalgia.

Using proton spectroscopy (H-MRS) to probe other neurotransmitters, fibromyalgia patients have been shown to have increases in brain concentrations of the body's major excitatory neurotransmitter, glutamate, in pain processing regions such as the insula. Drugs such as pregabalin and gabapentin are likely working in part in fibromyalgia by reducing glutamatergic activity. Individuals with fibromyalgia that had the highest pretreatment levels of glutamate in the posterior insula were those most likely to respond to pregabalin. When pregabalin led to improvement in symptoms in these individuals, there was normalization of functional MRI and connectivity findings, all suggesting that this neurotransmitter is playing a critical role in the pathogenesis of fibromyalgia at least in some individuals. These studies also help clarify why no single class of CNS analgesic is likely to be effective in every patient with pain of CNS origin.

DIAGNOSIS

A careful musculoskeletal history and examination remains the most important diagnostic test for individuals with chronic pain. There are a number of diagnostic criteria that can be used for fibromyalgia. For reasons noted above, the use of the original 1990 criteria is now being replaced by the more contemporary criteria proposed in 2010 and then modified in 2011 and 2016.[7] The advantage of these new criteria is that they are simple to use and acknowledge the nonpain symptoms of fibromyalgia and centralized pain. Finally, in addition to these criteria being used with a cut point to diagnose someone with fibromyalgia they also serve as a good measure of the presence and severity of fibromyalgia, or "fibromyalgianess." It has been shown that in individuals with conditions such as RA, low back pain, or osteoarthritis, an individual's fibromyalgia score, derived from measures very similar to the 2010/11/16 criteria, was typically more predictive of pain and disability than more objective measures of activity of these diseases, such as measures of inflammation or joint damage.

Because pain is a defining manifestation of fibromyalgia, its optimal management should be based on the features of the pain that can distinguish it from other painful disorders. The pain of fibromyalgia is typically diffuse or multifocal, is difficult to localize, often waxes and wanes, and is frequently migratory in nature. These characteristics of centralized pain are quite different from nociceptive pain, in which both the location and severity of pain are typically more constant. Patients may complain of discomfort when they are touched or when wearing tight clothing, and may experience dysesthesias or paresthesias that accompany the pain, as is seen with neuropathic pain.

There are no laboratory or imaging tests at this time that can distinguish the pain of fibromyalgia. The duration of time the patient has had symptoms should guide the intensity of the diagnostic work-up. If the patient's symptoms have persisted for several years, minimal testing is required, whereas a more aggressive strategy should be employed for acute or subacute onset of symptoms. Basic testing can be limited to complete blood count and routine serum chemistries, along with thyroid stimulating hormone (TSH) and erythrocyte sedimentation rate (ESR). Serologic studies such as ANA and rheumatoid factor assays are generally not needed unless there are clinical features that are not characteristic of fibromyalgia, or abnormalities are found on physical examination.

Aside from the many comorbid conditions already discussed, fibromyalgia may present similarly to a number of disorders or concurrently with other disorders that may confuse the diagnosis. Table 258-3 shows conditions that often mimic or present concurrently with fibromyalgia. Hypothyroidism and polymyalgia rheumatica can be differentiated from fibromyalgia by results of TSH and ESR. Sleep apnea and hepatitis C also simulate fibromyalgia, and tend to present more often in men than women.

The physical examination is generally unremarkable in individuals with fibromyalgia, but it is helpful to assess for diffuse tenderness. This is something that can be done in several ways that do not involve performing a tender point count. For example, individuals with fibromyalgia exhibit unusual sensitivity to the inflation of a blood pressure cuff. Assessing the pain thresholds in the hands and arms of any chronic pain patient can provide valuable diagnostic information. A rapid testing of this involves the application of firm pressure over several interphalangeal (IP) joints of each hand and also over the adjacent phalanges, and then more proximally to include firm palpation of the muscles of the forearm including the lateral epicondyle region. If the individual is tender in many of these areas, or in just the muscles of the forearm, they are likely to be diffusely tender and to have a low pain threshold. However, if the

TABLE 258-3	CONDITIONS THAT SIMULATE FIBROMYALGIA
COMMON	
Hypothyroidism	
Polymyalgia rheumatica	
Early in course of autoimmune disorders (e.g., rheumatoid arthritis or SLE)	
Sjogren syndrome	
LESS COMMON	
Hepatitis C	
Sleep apnea	
Chiari malformation	
Celiac sprue	

individual is only tender over the IP joints but not the other regions, and especially if there are additional inflammatory signs (e.g., swelling, erythema, warmth) associated with the tenderness, there should be more concern about a systemic autoimmune rheumatologic disorder. If tenderness is confined to only the bones, one might suspect a metabolic bone disease (Chapter 229) or condition causing periostitis (e.g., hyperparathyroidism).

Having ruled out other potential disorders in the differential diagnosis of the patient's pain, a somewhat important step in the management of fibromyalgia is asserting the diagnosis. Despite concerns that being "labeled" with fibromyalgia may in general cause more harm than good, nearly all existing studies suggest otherwise. The diagnosis of fibromyalgia is often a source of relief for the patient and leads to decreased health care utilization because of a reduction in referrals and diagnostic testing "looking for the cause of the pain."

TREATMENT   Rx

General Approach

Individuals diagnosed with fibromyalgia should receive some basic education regarding this disorder.[8] Clinicians can do this in the context of their practice (e.g., with nurse educators or other allied health professionals) or electronically using websites and videos (see Clauw YouTube patient videos). This education should stress the importance of the patients' active role in their own management. It should be explained at the outset that some of the most effective therapies are nondrug interventions such as exercise, improving sleep, and reducing stress. Although recent treatment guidelines favor the use of non-pharmacologic versus pharmacologic therapies,[A1] there are pragmatic factors in routine practice (lack of availability or reimbursement, patient is unwilling to try these therapies until their symptoms are somewhat better controlled)[9] that often make this impractical. Most patients will need some coordinated combination of pharmacologic and nonpharmacologic therapies to achieve meaningful improvement in symptoms and function. Table 258-4 outlines all of the evidence-based treatments for individuals with fibromyalgia.

Pharmacologic Therapy

There are a number of classes of drugs that can be of some benefit in fibromyalgia, but as in other chronic pain conditions, drugs only work well in a subset of patients, and the overall effect size of any of these therapies for any type of chronic pain is small to modest at best.

Tricyclic Agents

The earliest studied pharmacologic therapy for fibromyalgia was low doses of tricyclic compounds. The effectiveness of tricyclic antidepressants—particularly amitriptyline,[A2] cyclobenzaprine,[A3] and mirtazapine[A4]—in treating the symptoms of pain, poor sleep, and fatigue associated with fibromyalgia is supported by several randomized, controlled trials. Tolerability can be improved by starting with a very low doses (e.g., 10 mg of amitriptyline or 5 mg of cyclobenzaprine), giving the dose a few hours before bedtime, and then very slowly escalating the dose. Very-low-dose cyclobenzaprine has been shown to be quite effective in a subset of individuals with fibromyalgia with a specific sleep

TABLE 258-4 THERAPIES

PHARMACOLOGIC THERAPIES

- **Strong evidence:** tricyclics (amitriptyline, cyclobenzaprine); dual-reuptake inhibitors (SNRI/NSRI—venlafaxine, duloxetine, milnacipran); alpha-2-delta ligands (pregabalin, gabapentin)
- **Modest evidence:** tramadol; selective serotonin reuptake inhibitors (SSRIs); low-dose naltrexone; cannabinoids; gamma hydroxybutyrate (GHB)
- **Weak evidence:** growth hormone, 5-hydroxytryptamine, tropisetron, S-adenosyl-L-methionine (SAMe)
- **Not shown to be effective:** opioids, NSAIDs, corticosteroids, benzodiazepine and nonbenzodiazepine hypnotics, melatonin, guanifenesin, dehydroepiandrosterone

NONPHARMACOLOGIC THERAPIES

- **Strong evidence:** cardiovascular exercise, cognitive behavior therapy, patient education, multidisciplinary therapy
- **Modest evidence:** strength training, tai chi, yoga, mindfulness, hypnotherapy, biofeedback, balneotherapy
- **Weak evidence:** acupuncture, chiropractic, manual and massage therapy, electrotherapy, ultrasound
- **No evidence:** tender (trigger) point injections, flexibility exercise

pattern, with fewer side effects than seen in some of the earlier studies of higher doses.

Serotonin and Norepinephrine Reuptake Inhibitors

Because of a better side effect profile, newer antidepressants, such as selective serotonin reuptake inhibitors (SSRIs), are frequently used in fibromyalgia. The SSRIs fluoxetine, citalopram, and paroxetine have each been evaluated in randomized, placebo-controlled trials. The newer "highly selective" serotonin reuptake inhibitors (e.g., citalopram) appear to be less efficacious than the older SSRIs, which have some noradrenergic activity at higher doses.

Because tricyclic antidepressants and high doses of certain SSRIs such as fluoxetine and sertraline that have the most balanced reuptake inhibition had been the most effective analgesics in fibromyalgia and other chronic pain conditions, many concluded that dual receptor inhibitors such as serotonin-norepinephrine and norepinephrine-serotonin reuptake inhibitors (SNRIs and NSRIs) should be more effective than pure serotonergic drugs.[A5] The first available SNRI, venlafaxine, has data to support its use in the management of neuropathic pain. Retrospective trial data demonstrate that this compound is also effective in the prophylaxis of migraine and tension headaches. Two studies in fibromyalgia have reported conflicting results, with the one using a higher dose showing efficacy.

Two newer SNRIs, duloxetine and milnacipran, have undergone more recent multicenter trials and were shown to be effective in a number of outcome variables. They are both now approved in the United States for the treatment of fibromyalgia. These drugs seem roughly comparable in the overall efficacy profile, with studies generally noting modest improvement (although not reaching statistical significance in all studies) in clinical features such as pain, overall improvement, physical functioning, level of fatigue, and degree of reported physical impairment. For both compounds these effects appear to be unrelated to their effect on mood, suggesting that the analgesic and other positive effects of this class of drugs in fibromyalgia are not simply due to their antidepressant effects. The maximum approved dose of duloxetine is 60 mg per day, but it was studied in trials at doses up to 120 mg and shown to be safe. Likewise, the initial dose of milnacipran is 100 mg, but some patients benefit from increasing the dose to as high as 200 mg. Hypertension is more likely to be a problem with milnacipran, because it appears to be more noradrenergic; for these same reasons it might be slightly more likely to help with symptoms such as fatigue. Esreboxetine, a selective norepinephrine reuptake inhibitor, was also tested and shown to be efficacious in fibromyalgia, but this drug is not approved for use at this time.[A6] In summary, emerging evidence suggests that norepinephrine reuptake activity may be much more important than serotinergic reuptake for analgesic effects in patients with fibromyalgia.

Anticonvulsants

Placebo-controlled trials have shown that pregabalin is effective for pain, sleep disturbances, and fatigue in fibromyalgia. It became the first drug approved in the United States for this condition. Gabapentin has similar efficacy and adverse effects profile in fibromyalgia.[A7] These two drugs have the same mechanism of action, binding to the alpha-2-delta subunit of calcium channels, and both had been previously approved for treatment of neuropathic pain and other indications. The tolerability of these drugs can be enhanced by starting at a low dose, and giving either two thirds of the dose or the entire dose at bedtime. The maximally approved dose of pregabalin is 450 mg, but in trials it was studied at doses as high as 600 mg and shown to be safe and efficacious. For most patients, the dose of gabapentin needed for analgesic is often 1800 to 2400 mg/day. Two other drugs that likely work similarly to the gabapentinoids by counteracting the effects of increased glutamatergic activity are memantine[A8] and ketamine, both of which have some evidence of efficacy. Another antiepileptic compound, clonazepam, has demonstrated efficacy in treating temporomandibular disorder and associated jaw pain and is useful in the treatment of restless leg syndrome and thus may be of value in subsets of fibromyalgia patients with these comorbidities. In general, though, the risks associated with chronic benzodiazepine use likely outweigh the potential benefit.

Other CNS-Acting Drugs

Some reports have suggested that certain nonbenzodiazepine hypnotics, such as zopiclone and zolpidem can improve the sleep and, possibly, fatigue in fibromyalgia patients, but they have no significant effects on pain.

Gamma-hydroxybutyrate (also known as sodium oxabate), a precursor of GABA with powerful sedative properties, has been shown to be very efficacious in improving fatigue, sleep, as well as pain in patients with fibromyalgia. However, this drug is a scheduled substance in the United States because of its abuse potential, and was not approved by the U.S. FDA because of safety concerns. Other less-toxic GABA agonists may have an important role in the future for the treatment of fibromyalgia.

Cannabinoids are another class of drugs that has seen renewed interest in the management of chronic pain states. Two randomized controlled trials of synthetic cannabinoids in fibromyalgia (both with nabilone) have concluded that the drug is modestly efficacious (in one study for both pain and sleep, in the other study at lower dose for just sleep).[A9] There is increased recognition that this class of drugs may have utility in pain of neural origin.

Classic Analgesics

No adequate randomized controlled clinical trials have tested the efficacy of opioids for the pain of fibromyalgia. However, anecdotal experience indicates that this class of drugs is not effective in this setting. In fact, imaging studies of fibromyalgia patients who were studied with both functional MRI and PET with an opioid ligand suggested that the native state of fibromyalgia may be akin to that of opioid-induced hyperalgesia, and it is possible that, at least in a subset of individuals with fibromyalgia, opioids may make their hyperalgesia worse rather than better. Tramadol, a compound that has some opioid activity (weak μ-agonist activity) combined with serotonin/norepinephrine reuptake inhibition appears to be somewhat efficacious in the management of fibromyalgia, as both a single drug and in fixed-dose combination with acetaminophen.

A large number of fibromyalgia patients use nonsteroidal anti-inflammatory drugs (NSAIDs) and acetaminophen. Many studies have failed to confirm their effectiveness as analgesics in fibromyalgia when used as a single agent,[A10] but the combination of celecoxib and acyclovir has been found to be effective in fibromyalgia.[A11] It is not known whether the benefit came from one or both of these drugs. Patients may likewise experience enhanced analgesia when treated with combinations of NSAIDs and other agents.

Combination Therapy

Combining multiple classes of adjunctive pain medications has been a common practice. One study demonstrated that the combination of duloxetine and pregabalin was superior to either drug alone in treating fibromyalgia,[A12] consistent with other trials suggesting this is also the case in neuropathic pain.

Neurostimulatory Therapies

Transcutaneous electrical nerve stimulation (TENS) has been used for some time to treat musculoskeletal pain. A new group of neurostimulatory therapies is emerging that would be expected to be more effective for centralized pain, because these therapies all aim to stimulate the CNS to modulate pain transmission. These include noninvasive techniques such as repetitive transcranial magnetic stimulation (rTMS) and transcranial direct current stimulation (t-DCS). Outcomes with these therapies have yielded inconsistent results, but a trend is emerging suggesting that these treatments might be most effective in centralized rather than purely peripheral pain states. Furthermore, they have stimulation parameters that enable signals to travel into deeper cortical tissues than occurs with typical delivery of rTMS and tDCS. More invasive approaches such as spinal cord stimulation, deep brain stimulation, and vagal nerve stimulation show promise in refractory pain states.

Nonpharmacologic Therapies

Patients should be strongly encouraged to engage in nonpharmacologic therapies, especially exercise and mind-body practices. The best-studied nonpharmacologic therapies in fibromyalgia are CBT and exercise, both of which have been reported to be efficacious.[A13] These treatments can produce sustained (e.g., greater than one year) improvements, especially when an individual complies with the therapy.

For exercise, it is important to "start low, go slow." Exercise of different types (aerobic, stretching, strengthening) has been particularly well studied as a treatment of both chronic fatigue syndrome and fibromyalgia and has perhaps the strongest evidence base of any therapy. They typically improve fatigue, pain, and function for these conditions. In chronic fatigue syndrome this has been termed graded exercise therapy, and has been similarly shown to be helpful. Many fibromyalgia, chronic fatigue syndrome, and other chronic pain patients tend to be sedentary. In these individuals it might be more helpful to first focus on becoming more "active" rather than "exercising."

Among the different types of CBT, the one that has had increased attention has been a focus on using behavioral measures to treat the sleep disorders seen in conditions such as fibromyalgia. Preclinical and clinical research has shown the important role of sleep in pain transmission. There is a free website for patients (www.fibroguide.com) that allows patients to access these behavioral interventions over the internet rather than in person, and this website has been found to be effective in a randomized controlled trial. One study also suggested that adding emotional disclosure to standard CBT may be of benefit to a subset of patients.[A14]

As with other diseases, there is an increasing evidence base in fibromyalgia for a number of other nonpharmacologic, complementary and alternative therapies including mindfulness, tai chi, yoga, biofeedback, chiropractic manipulation, and acupuncture. There is some evidence that the use of alternative therapies gives patients a greater sense of control over their illness, so they should be encouraged to choose the nonpharmacologic therapy that best resonates with their beliefs and is locally accessible.

Trigger-point injections can be useful for the treatment of localized myofascial pain, but there is no evidence that adding corticosteroids or even local anesthetics adds anything to their beneficial effect.

Grade A References

A1. Macfarlane GJ, Kronisch C, Atzeni F, et al. EULAR recommendations for management of fibromyalgia. *Ann Rheum Dis*. 2017;76:318-328.

A2. Moore RA, Derry S, Aldington D, et al. Amitriptyline for neuropathic pain and fibromyalgia in adults. *Cochrane Database Syst Rev*. 2012;12:CD008242.

A3. Moldofsky H, Harris HW, Archambault WT, et al. Effects of bedtime very low dose cyclobenzaprine on symptoms and sleep physiology in patients with fibromyalgia syndrome: a double-blind randomized placebo-controlled study. *J Rheumatol*. 2011;38:2653-2663.

A4. Welsch P, Bernardy K, Derry S, et al. Mirtazapine for fibromyalgia in adults. *Cochrane Database Syst Rev*. 2018;8:CD012708.

A5. Welsch P, Uceyler N, Klose P, et al. Serotonin and noradrenaline reuptake inhibitors (SNRIs) for fibromyalgia. *Cochrane Database Syst Rev*. 2018;2:CD010292.

A6. Arnold LM, Hirsch I, Sanders P, et al. Safety and efficacy of esreboxetine in patients with fibromyalgia: a fourteen-week, randomized, double-blind, placebo-controlled, multicenter clinical trial. *Arthritis Rheum*. 2012;64:2387-2397.

A7. Derry S, Cording M, Wiffen PJ, et al. Pregabalin for pain in fibromyalgia in adults. *Cochrane Database Syst Rev*. 2016;9:CD011790.

A8. Olivan-Blazquez B, Herrera-Mercadal P, Puebla-Guedea M, et al. Efficacy of memantine in the treatment of fibromyalgia: a double-blind, randomised, controlled trial with 6-month follow-up. *Pain*. 2014;155:2517-2525.

A9. Walitt B, Klose P, Fitzcharles MA, et al. Cannabinoids for fibromyalgia. *Cochrane Database Syst Rev*. 2016;7:CD011694.

A10. Derry S, Wiffen PJ, Hauser W, et al. Oral nonsteroidal anti-inflammatory drugs for fibromyalgia in adults. *Cochrane Database Syst Rev*. 2017;3:CD012332.

A11. Pridgen WL, Duffy C, Gendreau JF, et al. A famciclovir + celecoxib combination treatment is safe and efficacious in the treatment of fibromyalgia. *J Pain Res*. 2017;10:451-460.

A12. Gilron I, Chaparro LE, Tu D, et al. Combination of pregabalin with duloxetine for fibromyalgia: a randomized controlled trial. *Pain*. 2016;157:1532-1540.

A13. Bidonde J, Busch AJ, Schachter CL, et al. Aerobic exercise training for adults with fibromyalgia. *Cochrane Database Syst Rev*. 2017;6:CD012700.

A14. Lumley MA, Schubiner H, Lockhart NA, et al. Emotional awareness and expression therapy, cognitive behavioral therapy, and education for fibromyalgia: a cluster-randomized controlled trial. *Pain*. 2017;158:2354-2363.

GENERAL REFERENCES

For the General References and other additional features, please visit Expert Consult at https://expertconsult.inkling.com.

259

SYSTEMIC DISEASES IN WHICH ARTHRITIS IS A FEATURE

STERLING G. WEST

Arthritis, arthralgias, and myalgias can be significant features of several systemic diseases and may be the presenting symptoms for some of these disorders (Table 259-1). Appropriate evaluation of these musculoskeletal symptoms, including selected laboratory tests and radiographs, can provide clues to the early diagnosis of these diseases. Synovial biopsies are rarely necessary but can be diagnostic. Brief descriptions of the arthritic manifestations of some of these systemic disorders follow; a more detailed discussion of each entity is found in the chapters devoted to these diseases. Because of the rarity of many of these diseases, evidence-based treatments with U.S. Food and Drug Administration–approved medications are lacking.

AUTOIMMUNE HEPATITIS

Patients with type I autoimmune hepatitis (Chapter 140) may present with a syndrome resembling systemic lupus erythematosus (SLE; Chapter 250).[1,2] Patients with the early-onset subset are frequently young and female, with complaints of polyarthralgia and occasionally fever. Laboratory examination may show leukopenia, a positive antinuclear antibody (70 to 90%), elevated erythrocyte sedimentation rate, polyclonal gammopathy, and elevated liver-associated enzymes. Hypocomplementemia and antibodies against double-stranded DNA are usually not seen, whereas antibodies against the smooth muscle antigen (F1 actin) support the diagnosis. Joint radiographs show soft tissue swelling without erosions or deformity. Joint pain resolves with corticosteroid therapy for the liver disease. Patients with autoimmune hepatitis have an increased risk for having a concurrent autoimmune disease, including Sjögren syndrome in about 7% of cases.

TABLE 259-1 SYSTEMIC DISEASES ASSOCIATED WITH ARTHRITIS

DISEASE	TEST*
GASTROINTESTINAL DISEASES	
Autoimmune hepatitis	Liver-associated enzymes, *ASMA*
Primary biliary cirrhosis	Alkaline phosphatase, *antimitochondrial Ab*
Pancreatitis-arthritis syndrome	Lipase, amylase, *abdominal CT scan*
Whipple disease	*Tissue biopsy, tissue immunohistochemical stain for Tropheryma whippelii, PCR for T. whippelii DNA*
Gluten-sensitive enteropathy	*Antitransglutaminase antibody, small bowel biopsy*
Inflammatory bowel disease	Stool guaiac, *colonoscopy*
Hepatitis B/hepatitis C	Liver-associated enzymes, *hepatitis serology, cryoglobulins*
Intestinal bypass arthritis	*Cryoglobulins*
HEMATOLOGIC DISORDERS	
Hemophilia	PTT, *factor VIII and IX levels*
Hemoglobinopathies	CBC, *hemoglobin electrophoresis*
Hypogammaglobulinemia	Low total protein, *SPEP, immunoglobulins*
Plasma cell dyscrasias	High total protein, *SPEP, UPEP, IEF*
ENDOCRINE DISORDERS	
Diabetes mellitus	Glucose, *hemoglobin A$_{1c}$*
Thyroid disorders	TSH, *thyroxine*
Parathyroid disorders	Calcium, phosphorus, *PTH*
Acromegaly	Radiographs, *growth hormone, IGF-I*
Hyperlipoproteinemia	Lipid panel
Paget disease	Bone-specific alkaline phosphatase, radiographs, *bone scan*
MALIGNANT DISORDERS	
Hypertrophic osteoarthropathy	Radiographs (hands, wrists, chest)
Leukemia and lymphoma	CBC, LDH, *bone marrow/tissue biopsy*
Carcinomatous polyarthritis	*Cancer screen*
Palmar fasciitis and arthritis	*CA-125, pelvic CT scan, cancer screen*
OTHER DISEASES	
Hemochromatosis	Iron studies, radiographs, *HFE gene*
Multicentric reticulohistiocytosis	Radiographs, *skin/synovial biopsy*
Sarcoidosis	Chest radiograph, *ACE level, tissue biopsy*
IgG4-related disease	Serum IgG4 level, *histopathology of biopsy specimens including IgG4 immunostaining*
Alkaptonuria	Radiographs, *urine homogentisic acid level*
Fabry disease	Angiokeratomas, *α-galactosidase A level or gene mutation*
Relapsing polychondritis	*Cartilage biopsy*
Cystic fibrosis	Chest radiograph, *sweat chloride, CFTR gene mutation*
Tenosynovial giant cell tumor: diffuse type (diffuse pigmented villonodular synovitis)	Synovial fluid analysis, *MRI, synovial biopsy*
Systemic infections	Cultures, serologies (RPR, HIV, EBV, parvovirus)

*Tests listed are common laboratory tests and radiographs that are frequently ordered; this information should provide a clue that a systemic disease is a possible cause of the patient's musculoskeletal symptoms. These tests, coupled with the history and physical examination, should be followed by more specific tests and biopsies (listed in italics) to confirm the diagnosis.
Ab = antibody; ACE = angiotensin-converting enzyme; ASMA = anti–smooth muscle antibody; CBC = complete blood cell count; CFTR = cystic fibrosis transmembrane conductance regulator; CT = computed tomography; EBV = Epstein-Barr virus; HIV = human immunodeficiency virus; IEF = immunoelectrophoresis; IGF-I = insulin-like growth factor-I; IgG4 = immunoglobulin G4; LDH = lactate dehydrogenase; MRI = magnetic resonance imaging; PCR = polymerase chain reaction; PTH = parathyroid hormone; PTT = partial thromboplastin time; RPR = rapid plasmin reagin; SPEP = serum protein electrophoresis; TSH = thyroid-stimulating hormone; UPEP = urine protein electrophoresis.

◉ PRIMARY BILIARY CHOLANGITIS (CIRRHOSIS)

Up to 50% of patients with primary biliary cholangitis (PBC) (Chapter 146) have other autoimmune disorders, including rheumatoid arthritis (RA), Sjögren syndrome, systemic sclerosis, systemic lupus erythematosus, and autoimmune thyroiditis. In addition to antimitochondrial antibodies, rheumatoid factor, antinuclear antibodies, and anticentromere antibodies are often present. More than 10% of patients with PBC have a symmetrical or asymmetrical small joint inflammatory arthritis. Unlike RA, it can involve distal interphalangeal joints and is rarely erosive or deforming. Other musculoskeletal manifestations

include osteomalacia related to vitamin D deficiency, osteoporosis related to renal tubular acidosis, and hypertrophic osteoarthropathy associated with liver disease.

◉ WHIPPLE DISEASE

An inflammatory arthritis occurs in 60 to 90% of patients with Whipple disease (Chapter 131) and may precede other clinical manifestations by years.[3] The joint involvement is typically an intermittent, migratory oligoarthritis affecting large joints more than small joints or the spine, lasting from several hours to days. The synovial fluid is inflammatory, with a predominance of mononuclear cells. Subcutaneous nodules are occasionally seen, contributing to an erroneous diagnosis of rheumatic fever or RA. However, patients consistently test negative for rheumatoid factor and antinuclear antibodies. Synovial biopsies show rod-shaped bacilli on electron microscopy, which have been identified as *Tropheryma whipplei*. Diagnosis is suspected when duodenal, synovial, or lymph node biopsies show periodic acid–Schiff–positive macrophages. Infection is confirmed by demonstration of the organism in tissue by immunohistochemical staining with antisera specific for *T. whipplei*. Quantitative polymerase chain reaction to detect *T. whipplei* DNA is used as a confirmatory test performed on tissue and body fluids.[4] Typically, the arthritis does not cause radiographic changes or deformities. Prolonged antibiotic therapy results in resolution of musculoskeletal as well as other symptoms of this disease. Relapses, especially neurologic, can occur in up to 35% of patients after cessation of antibiotic therapy.

◉ GLUTEN-SENSITIVE ENTEROPATHY (CELIAC DISEASE)

An asymmetrical oligoarthritis or symmetrical polyarthritis occurs in up to 25% of adults with celiac disease (Chapter 131). It may precede the enteropathic symptoms by months to years in up to 50% of cases. Large joints such as knees and ankles, more than hips and shoulders, are most commonly involved. Axial involvement is reported. The arthritis does not cause deformities or radiographic changes and resolves with a gluten-free diet in 40 to 50% of cases. Another musculoskeletal manifestation is osteomalacia related to vitamin D malabsorption, which may mimic diffuse fibromyalgia. Arthralgias due to gluten sensitivity without celiac disease are also reported.[5]

◉ PANCREATITIS-ARTHRITIS SYNDROME

Pancreatic panniculitis is a systemic syndrome occurring in some patients with pancreatic acinar cell carcinoma and less commonly in patients with pancreatitis or hematologic malignancies. This syndrome is characterized by tender red nodules, usually on the extremities; these are frequently misdiagnosed as erythema nodosum, but biopsy shows areas of lobular panniculitis with fat necrosis. Arthritis occurs in 60% of patients and usually involves the ankles and knees. Synovial fluid is typically noninflammatory and creamy in color. It contains multiple lipid droplets because of necrosis of fat in the synovial membrane. Other manifestations include osteolytic lesions (10%) from bone marrow fat necrosis, pleuropericarditis, fever, and eosinophilia. Magnetic resonance imaging (MRI) shows multifocal intraosseous fat necrosis and arthritis of the knees and feet.[6] The prominent fat necrosis is due to the release of lipase, amylase, and trypsin from the diseased pancreas. Another musculoskeletal manifestation resulting from pancreatic disease is osteomalacia from vitamin D deficiency related to malabsorption.

◉ HEMOPHILIA

Hemophilia A (factor VIII deficiency) and hemophilia B (factor IX deficiency) (Chapter 165) are associated with hemarthrosis.[7] Almost all patients with factor levels less than 1% of normal experience recurrent hemarthroses spontaneously or after minor trauma. Large joints (knees, elbows, ankles) are most commonly involved. Intramuscular hemorrhage can also occur. Recurrent hemarthrosis can lead to proliferative synovitis and cartilage degradation, resulting in both erosive and degenerative changes on radiographs. Physical examination shows bone enlargement, crepitus, atrophic muscles, and joint contractures. Treatment of acute monoarthritis consists of factor replacement to achieve a level of 30% or greater, given at the first sign of joint swelling. Patients with fever (temperature >38° C) or who fail to respond to factor replacement need joint aspiration to rule out septic arthritis, which occurs with an increased incidence in hemophilia. Chronic arthritis is treated with nonsteroidal anti-inflammatory drugs (NSAIDs), which do not inhibit platelet function; arthroscopic or radiation synovectomy for chronic synovitis; and total joint arthroplasty for end-stage joint disease. The regular prophylactic administration of factor replacement has reduced the risk for developing chronic arthropathy. Acute and chronic arthritis is less frequent and less severe in patients with hemophilia B compared with hemophilia A.

HEMOGLOBINOPATHIES

Patients with sickle cell anemia (Chapter 154) or the heterozygous states of sickle β-thalassemia and sickle hemoglobin C disease frequently experience polyarthralgia.[8] Local sickling of cells leads to obstruction of the microcirculation and to bone infarctions. Patients most commonly experience painful crises causing chest, back, and joint pain, which can be caused or worsened by glucocorticoid therapy. A painful large joint arthritis (usually in the knees), lasting days to 3 weeks, can also occur. Synovial effusions are usually noninflammatory but can be mildly inflammatory because of local phagocytosis of sickled cells. Infarcts in the metaphyses of bones are commonly found on joint radiographs. Vertebral bodies have a characteristic "Lincoln log" appearance or a central cuplike indentation ("codfish vertebrae"). Femoral and humeral head osteonecrosis can occur in up to 33% of sickle cell anemia and sickle hemoglobin C disease cases. Because of splenic autoinfarction, septic arthritis (*Staphylococcus aureus*) and osteomyelitis (50% caused by *Salmonella*) have been associated with sickle cell disease. In adults, gout has been reported. Treatment includes intravenous hydration, oxygen, and analgesics. Hydroxyurea can reduce the frequency of painful crises. In patients with β-thalassemia major (Cooley anemia; Chapter 153), significant expansion of bone marrow develops as a result of increased erythroid precursors, leading to osteoporosis and microfractures that affect primarily the lower extremities. Chelation therapy with deferiprone (to reduce iron overload) can cause arthralgias in 20% of patients.

HYPOGAMMAGLOBULINEMIA

Common variable immunodeficiency (CVID) and selective immunoglobulin A (IgA) deficiency are the most common immunodeficiencies[9] (Chapter 236). Adults with CVID can develop a nonerosive, noninfectious large joint oligoarthritis that responds to intravenous immunoglobulin therapy. However, septic arthritis caused by common pathogens or *Mycoplasma* can also occur and must be rigorously excluded. Autoimmune disorders occur in 30% of patients with CVID and may be the presenting manifestation. The most common are autoimmune cytopenias and pernicious anemia. Selective IgA deficiency (Chapter 236) is associated with various rheumatic manifestations, including positive autoantibodies, in the absence of clinical disease. Systemic autoimmune disorders, including SLE, juvenile idiopathic arthritis, and others, as well as organ-specific autoimmune disorders such as type 1 diabetes mellitus and myasthenia gravis, also occur in IgA-deficient individuals.

AMYLOIDOSIS

Primary amyloidosis and myeloma-associated amyloidosis are plasma cell disorders causing overproduction and tissue deposition of monoclonal immunoglobulin light chains (Chapter 179). Amyloid deposits in the synovium can lead to rheumatic symptoms. Amyloid arthropathy occurs in up to 5% of myeloma patients and may be the initial manifestation.[10] It affects both males and females at an average age of 60 years. The polyarthritis or oligoarthritis most commonly affects the shoulders, knees, wrists, and small joints of the hand. Subcutaneous nodules and carpal tunnel syndrome can be additional manifestations. It may be misdiagnosed as RA or polymyalgia rheumatica. Sedimentation rate is always elevated, but other serologies (rheumatoid factor, antinuclear antibodies) are negative. Synovial fluid is usually normal or minimally inflammatory. Congo red staining of spun synovial fluid can show amyloid deposits from synovial fragments. Joint radiographs are nonerosive but may show lytic bone lesions. The arthritic symptoms do not respond to glucocorticoids or other anti-inflammatory medications.

DIABETES MELLITUS

A causal relationship between arthritis in general and diabetes mellitus is not established.[11] However, certain specific musculoskeletal disorders are associated with diabetes.[12] Diabetic stiff hand syndrome of limited joint mobility[13] (diabetic cheiroarthropathy) occurs in more than 30% of patients with long-standing, poorly controlled type 1 or type 2 diabetes mellitus (Chapter 216). Patients present with the insidious development of flexion contractures and thickened skin of the fingers, which may be confused with scleroderma. These changes may be due to excess glycosylation of tendinous structures and accumulation of sugar alcohols, producing excess water content in the tissues leading to increased stiffness. Additionally, intracellular hyperglycemia causes oxidative stress and the formation of advanced glycation end products, which damage vascular endothelium and form cross-links with skin and tendon collagen

leading to biologic dysfunction. As a result of the inability to extend the fingers fully, the "prayer sign" is observed on physical examination. Unlike diabetic stiff hand syndrome, Dupuytren contractures[14] are due to a chronic thickening of the palmar aponeurosis, causing flexion deformities of the third and fourth digits. It is a frequent musculoskeletal complication, occurring in more than 20% of patients with type 2 diabetes. A less common manifestation is Charcot, or neuropathic, joints, occurring in less than 1% of all patients with long-standing diabetes. All patients have a diabetic peripheral neuropathy and typically present with painless swelling of the feet caused, most commonly, by destruction of the tarsometatarsal joints. Deformities can occur with midtarsal collapse ("rocker bottom" feet), predisposing to ulceration and infection of the skin over desensate bony prominences. Radiographs are diagnostic, and treatment should include supportive footwear and protected weight bearing.

Unlike Charcot joint, diabetic osteolysis and diabetic amyotrophy are unique to diabetes. The osteolysis is characterized by resorption of the distal metatarsal bone and proximal phalanges of the feet, giving radiographs a characteristic "licked candy" appearance. Pain is variable, and treatment is conservative because the process may terminate on its own. Diabetic amyotrophy is a lumbar polyradiculopathy (L2 to L4) that arises with severe pain, dysesthesias, and rapid atrophy of the proximal muscles of one or both thighs. Carpal tunnel syndrome (25%), adhesive capsulitis of the shoulder (frozen shoulder), flexor tenosynovitis (trigger finger) of the hands, diffuse idiopathic skeletal hyperostosis (DISH) (type 2 diabetes), osteopenia (type 1 diabetes), diabetic muscle infarction (usually of the thigh), osteomyelitis of the foot, and septic joints are all musculoskeletal conditions that occur with increased frequency in diabetic patients. Aggressive control of blood glucose helps prevent some of these musculoskeletal complications.

THYROID DISORDERS

Musculoskeletal symptoms occur in 33% of patients with clinical hypothyroidism (thyroid-stimulating hormone levels >20 μU/mL) (Chapter 213). Patients can present with carpal tunnel syndrome, Raynaud phenomenon, or muscle aching and stiffness similar to fibromyalgia and polymyalgia rheumatica. Patients with severe hypothyroidism can experience a noninflammatory myopathy with proximal muscle weakness and elevated creatine kinase, which may be confused clinically with polymyositis. Similarly, myxedematous patients can develop a symmetrical arthropathy of the large joints, especially the knees, associated with noninflammatory synovial fluid with increased viscosity. The association of hypothyroidism with chondrocalcinosis is controversial, but clearly patients beginning thyroid replacement therapy can experience an acute attack of pseudogout. Patients with hyperthyroidism can develop proximal myopathy (70%), adhesive capsulitis of the shoulder (10%), osteoporosis, or thyroid acropachy. Thyroid acropachy occurs in less than 1% of patients with Graves disease and consists of soft tissue swelling of the hands, digital clubbing, and periostitis, particularly involving the metacarpal and phalangeal bone shafts. Pain is usually mild, radiographs are characteristic, and there is no effective therapy. Patients with autoimmune thyroid disease have an increased prevalence of positive antinuclear antibodies and an increased association with systemic connective tissue diseases such as Sjögren syndrome.[15]

PARATHYROID DISORDERS

Primary hyperparathyroidism (Chapter 232) can develop with osteoporosis and fractures or with chondrocalcinosis and episodes of acute pseudogout. In severe hyperparathyroidism, which is rare, vague myalgias and arthralgias resembling fibromyalgia; a reversible, painless, proximal myopathy with normal creatine kinase; and osteitis fibrosa cystica with bone pain can be seen. Osteitis fibrosa cystica occurs primarily in patients with secondary hyperparathyroidism associated with renal failure and has a characteristic radiographic appearance, with subperiosteal resorption on the radial side of the phalanges, small erosions in the hands and distal clavicles, and discrete lytic bone lesions (brown tumors). Ectopic calcifications, joint laxity, and tendon ruptures have been reported in patients with severe hyperparathyroidism. Hypoparathyroidism has also been associated with myopathy and ectopic and perispinal ligament calcifications. Patients with type Ia pseudohypoparathyroidism and pseudopseudohypoparathyroidism have a shortened fourth metacarpal bone bilaterally.

ACROMEGALY

Up to 75% of patients with acromegaly (Chapter 211) develop an atypical form of osteoarthritis (OA). The knees, shoulders, hips, and lumbosacral and cervical spine are the most frequently symptomatic areas, although the hands reveal the most characteristic radiographic changes, with osteophytosis but, unlike primary OA, widened joint spaces due to cartilage hypertrophy. Carpal tunnel syndrome (50%), Raynaud phenomenon (33%), DISH (15%), and proximal muscle weakness with a normal serum creatine kinase can also occur.

HYPERLIPOPROTEINEMIA

Type IIa familial hyperlipidemia (Chapter 195) is associated with tendinous and tuberous-osseous xanthomas as well as episodic Achilles tendinitis. An acute migratory, inflammatory arthritis persisting up to a month and resembling rheumatic fever occurs in up to 50% of patients. Predominantly large joints are affected. In addition, a self-limited, acute monoarticular or oligoarticular arthritis involving the knee or ankle can occur. Patients with type III familial hyperlipoproteinemia can develop tendon and bone xanthomas. Patients with human immunodeficiency virus (HIV) infection taking protease inhibitor drugs can develop dyslipidemia leading to tendon xanthomas. In all hyperlipidemias, gout must be excluded before ascribing the symptoms to hyperlipoproteinemia. Therapy with NSAIDs and treatment of the underlying lipid disorder should be pursued. Notably, some of the therapies used to treat hyperlipidemia can cause musculoskeletal symptoms, including hyperuricemia and gout from nicotinic acid and myalgias (with or without elevated creatine kinase) or inflammatory myositis from statin therapy.

PAGET DISEASE

Paget disease (Chapter 233) can cause bone pain and deformity. An elevated bone-specific alkaline phosphatase and characteristic radiographic changes can help make the diagnosis. Joint pain caused by secondary OA in areas of bone involvement by Paget disease most commonly occurs in the hips, knees, or vertebrae. Spinal stenosis from Paget disease of the spine has been reported. Bisphosphonate therapy is highly effective.

HYPERTROPHIC OSTEOARTHROPATHY

Hypertrophic osteoarthropathy is a syndrome that includes clubbing of the fingers and toes, periostitis of long bones (distal tibia, femur, radius), and arthritis (Fig. 259-1). Hypertrophic osteoarthropathy is classified into primary (hereditary) and secondary forms. Between 80 and 90% of secondary hypertrophic osteoarthropathy is associated with intrathoracic neoplasms, especially non–small cell lung cancer.[16] Other causes include other neoplasms, chronic pulmonary infections, congenital heart disease, cirrhosis, HIV infection, medications (voriconazole), and inflammatory bowel disease. Patients with secondary hypertrophic osteoarthropathy can present with acute, severe, burning bone pain and a noninflammatory arthritis caused by periarticular periostitis. Pain is accentuated by dependency of the limbs. Pitting edema, warmth, and tenderness of the legs and forearms can be seen. Radiographs show diagnostic changes of periosteal elevation, new bone formation, or both along the distal ends of long bones. Therapy is symptomatic with NSAIDs, and hypertrophic osteoarthropathy improves with successful treatment of the underlying primary disease. In resistant cases, treatment with intravenous zoledronic acid or octreotide has been effective in modulating symptoms.

LEUKEMIA AND LYMPHOMA

Leukemia can arise as an asymmetrical or migratory polyarthritis, monoarthritis (rare), back pain (10%), or nocturnal bone pain. Articular manifestations occur in 14 to 50% of children and 4 to 16% of adults with acute leukemia and can precede the diagnosis by months.[17] Joint pain is attributed to leukemic synovial infiltration and usually involves the ankle or knee, but it can be polyarticular, resembling juvenile or adult RA. The joint pain is disproportionately more severe than the clinical findings. Synovial effusions are uncommon, and evidence of leukemic cells in the synovial fluid is rare. Bone pain due to subperiosteal leukemic cell infiltration occurs in up to 50% of patients, with long bone pain (lower extremities) more common in children and back pain more common in adults. Radiographs are normal in 50% of cases. The musculoskeletal symptoms are poorly responsive to NSAIDs but can resolve with successful therapy of the leukemia. Musculoskeletal symptoms occur in 25% of patients with non-Hodgkin lymphoma. Nocturnal bone pain is the most common presenting musculoskeletal complaint. A seronegative monoarthritis or polyarthritis can occur and should be suspected in patients with severe constitutional symptoms or lymphadenopathy out of proportion to the degree of arthritis. Patients with angioimmunoblastic T-cell lymphoma (Chapter 176) may occasionally develop a chronic, nonerosive polyarthritis with erythroderma.

CARCINOMATOUS POLYARTHRITIS

Polyarthritis can rarely (<2%) be the presenting manifestation of an occult malignancy; it may precede the discovery of the malignancy by several months. Breast, colon, lung, ovarian, and lymphoproliferative malignancies are the most commonly associated cancers. Clinical features suggesting carcinomatous polyarthritis include the explosive onset of a rheumatoid factor–negative, asymmetrical polyarthritis involving predominantly the lower extremities and sparing the hands and wrists in a patient older than 50 years. Another presentation is remitting seronegative symmetrical synovitis with pitting edema (RS3PE) of the hands and feet. Both presentations are associated with profound constitutional symptoms, elevated inflammatory markers, lack of erosions on radiographs, and poor response to glucocorticoids. Polymyalgia rheumatica and late-onset RA must be excluded. Treatment of the underlying malignancy results in improvement of the arthritis.

Immune checkpoint inhibitors targeting PD-1 and CTLA-4 can cause various immune-related adverse events (iRAEs) in 15 to 30% of treated patients.[18] Up to 5% can develop a rheumatologic iRAE, including an inflammatory arthritis resembling RA or reactive arthritis, sicca syndrome, myositis, polymyalgia rheumatica, or vasculitis. Patients may or may not respond to glucocorticoids and/or discontinuation of the cancer immunotherapy.

PALMAR FASCIITIS AND ARTHRITIS SYNDROME

Ovarian carcinoma (Chapter 189) is the most common malignancy found in patients (37%) with palmar fasciitis and arthritis. This musculoskeletal manifestation can also be seen in patients with breast, gastric, or pancreatic adenocarcinoma. Patients present with a severe, painful, symmetrical inflammatory

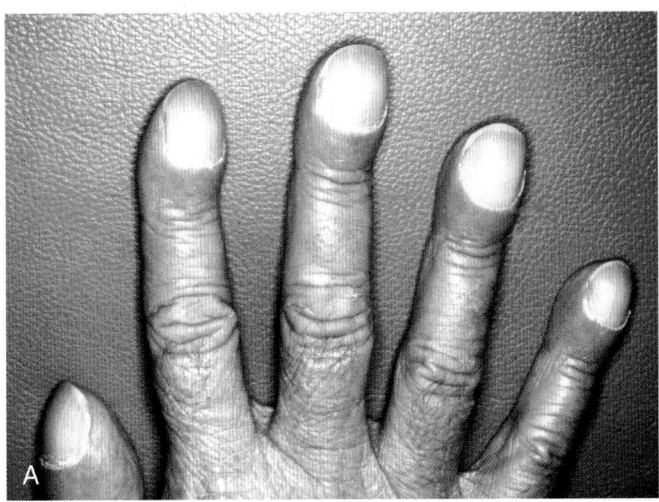
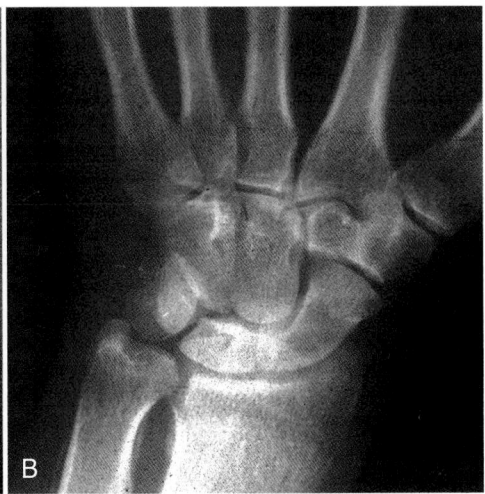

FIGURE 259-1. Hypertrophic osteoarthropathy. **A,** Severe clubbing of the nails. **B,** Radiograph demonstrating periosteal elevation of the distal radius and ulna.

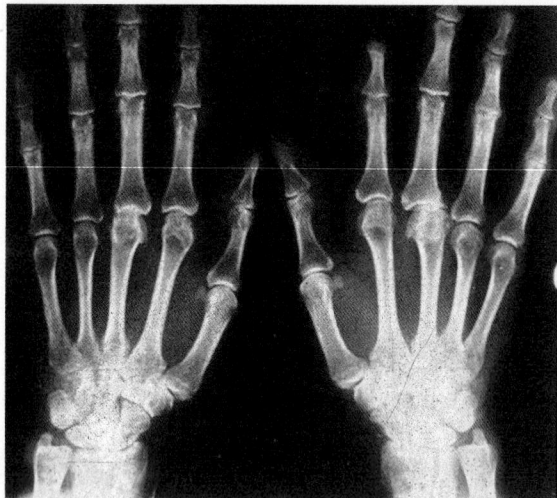

FIGURE 259-2. Hemochromatotic arthropathy. Radiograph demonstrating degenerative changes, with hooklike osteophytes of the second and third metacarpophalangeal joints bilaterally.

polyarthritis of the hands and wrists as well as a nodular fasciitis/tendonitis causing flexion contractures primarily of the fingers and, less commonly, the feet. Patients may have vasomotor instability, causing diagnostic confusion with complex regional pain syndrome or RA. This syndrome portends a poor prognosis because it typically manifests after tumor metastasis. Response to treatment is poor, although clinical improvement can occur with successful eradication of the underlying tumor.

HEMOCHROMATOSIS

Joint involvement occurs in 40 to 75% of patients with hereditary hemochromatosis (Chapter 201) and may be the presenting symptom (Fig. 259-2). The metacarpophalangeal (MCP) joints (especially the second and third MCP joints), wrists, knees, hips, shoulders, and ankles are most often involved in a symmetrical pattern. The arthropathy resembles OA, with joint swelling resulting from bone enlargement, but it is distinguished clinically by the involvement of atypical joints, such as MCP joints, wrists, and ankles. Radiographs show joint space narrowing, subchondral cysts, sclerosis, and osteophytes that are hooklike at the MCP joints. Chondrocalcinosis is present in up to 50% of patients. It is typically asymptomatic, but in some patients it leads to attacks of acute inflammatory synovitis (pseudogout), which may result in the misdiagnosis of RA. The prevalence of overt arthritis increases with age, and it may be only minimally symptomatic when the disease arises in other organs. However, it is not uncommon for articular pain to be the initial presenting complaint (33%). Consequently, all patients (especially Caucasian males) presenting with premature OA occurring in atypical joints, especially MCP joints and wrists, should be screened for hereditary hemochromatosis with iron studies. The mechanism whereby iron causes arthritis is unclear, but it may be related to hemosiderin deposits in the synovial membrane and chondrocytes activating degradative enzymes. Treatment is symptomatic with NSAIDs and, when severe, total joint arthroplasties. Phlebotomy for iron removal does not alter the course of the arthritis. Additional rheumatic manifestations in patients with hemochromatosis include osteoporosis related to hypogonadotropic hypogonadism, osteomalacia related to vitamin D deficiency when liver disease is severe, and an increased susceptibility to *Yersinia* septic arthritis.

MULTICENTRIC RETICULOHISTIOCYTOSIS

Multicentric reticulohistiocytosis (MRH) is a chronic, seronegative, symmetrical, inflammatory polyarthritis most commonly affecting the hands, shoulders, and knees.[19] It may resemble RA but can be differentiated by its prominent distal interphalangeal joint synovitis. The disease may also cause a spondylitis with axial involvement (50%). Joint involvement remits and relapses initially, but in 50% of cases it worsens into a severely deforming arthritis mutilans. Firm, nonpruritic, reddish brown or yellow papulonodular lesions ("coral beads") that wax and wane occur around the nail beds and on the face, hands, ears, and other areas predominantly above the waist. The skin lesions have a diagnostic histology. In 50 to 66% of patients, these diagnostic nodules follow the onset of arthritis by months to years.

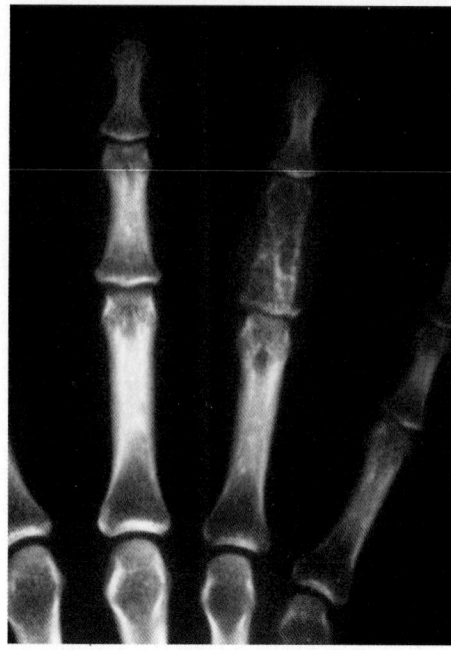

FIGURE 259-3. Sarcoid bone involvement. Punched-out lytic lesions of the middle phalanx, with soft tissue swelling.

Additional associations include xanthelasma (33%) and malignancies of various types (25%), which may precede or follow the onset of MRH. MRH usually remits spontaneously in 8 to 10 years but often leaves permanent cutaneous and joint damage. Treatment may include methotrexate or cytotoxic therapy if the arthritis is aggressive. Anti–tumor necrosis factor-α (anti-TNF-α) therapy and bisphosphonates are reportedly beneficial in resistant cases.

SARCOIDOSIS

Joint manifestations, including arthritis, periarthritis, and arthralgias, occur in 4 to 38% of patients with sarcoidosis (Chapter 89).[20] Rheumatic involvement is divided into acute and chronic types. The first consists of the triad of arthritis, erythema nodosum, and hilar adenopathy on chest radiographs (Löfgren syndrome), which may be accompanied by fever. Arthritis arises most often in the knees and ankles, and periarticular pain can be severe. Treatment is with NSAIDs, glucocorticoids, or both, and symptoms usually remit spontaneously over several weeks. The less common type of joint involvement (<5%) in sarcoidosis consists of synovitis that accompanies the slower onset, more chronic, systemic form of sarcoidosis. Polyarthritis, oligoarthritis, or monoarthritis can affect the small or large joints; it is typically nondestructive but in some cases can be aggressive. Dactylitis resulting from sarcoid bone and soft tissue involvement can occur (Fig. 259-3). In contrast to the acute type, chronic sarcoid arthropathy is characterized by mildly inflammatory synovial fluid and histologic granulomas on synovial biopsy. Treatment consists of NSAIDs, low-dose corticosteroids, hydroxychloroquine, and methotrexate or azathioprine. In refractory cases, anti-TNF-α therapy has been successful. Other musculoskeletal manifestations of sarcoidosis include lytic or sclerotic bone lesions (3 to 13%) and symptomatic acute or chronic myopathy (3%). Notably, asymptomatic lesions involving bone and muscle are much more common on MRI and tissue biopsies.

IMMUNOGLOBULIN G4–RELATED DISEASE

Patients with IgG4-related disease are typically men (70 to 75%) older than 50 years. Patients present with a variety of local and systemic manifestations, some of which can resemble several rheumatic diseases (Chapter 241).[21,22] For example, tumefactive lesions of the salivary glands can mimic Sjögren syndrome. Destructive sinus and middle ear lesions or periorbital masses can suggest granulomatous polyangiitis (GPA) (formerly Wegener granulomatosis). Furthermore, patients with IgG4-related disease frequently (40%) have allergic manifestations, including chronic sinusitis and pulmonary symptoms, which may add to the diagnostic confusion with GPA. IgG4-related disease can also cause an inflammatory aortitis with aneurysm formation that can be mistaken for giant cell arteritis. A fibrosclerotic presentation in the abdomen can mimic retroperitoneal fibrosis. Other organs that can be involved include the pancreas, biliary tree, kidneys, lymph nodes, meninges, thyroid, breast, prostate, pericardium, and skin. Although up to 70% of patients will have an elevated serum IgG4 level (>1.35 g/L), histopathologic analysis of biopsy specimens is the "gold standard" for diagnosis. The key pathologic features are a dense lymphoplasmacytic infiltrate organized in a storiform pattern, obliterative phlebitis, and a mild or moderate eosinophilic infiltrate. The plasma cell infiltrate will show more than 10 IgG4-positive cells per high-power field and a ratio of IgG4 to IgG positive cells that is higher than 40%. Glucocorticoids are effective in most patients. Several medications (azathioprine, mycophenolate mofetil, methotrexate) have been used as steroid-sparing agents to maintain remission. For refractory disease, B-cell depletion therapy with rituximab is effective.

ALKAPTONURIA (OCHRONOSIS)

Although an inherited disorder, alkaptonuria[23] is usually not diagnosed until the patient presents with progressive premature OA as a young adult (before age 30 to 35 years). The spine is initially involved, followed by the knees, shoulders, and hips. Small peripheral joints are spared. Radiographs show multiple vacuum discs, disc space ossification, and osteoarthritic changes in the spine. Nonarticular features include bluish brown discoloration of ear pinna, sclera, and nasal cartilage. Deposition of ochronotic pigment onto collagen fibers causes the articular cartilage to become brittle and fragmented. The noninflammatory synovial fluid may show tiny shards of pigmented cartilage ("ground pepper"). The diagnosis of alkaptonuria is suspected when fresh urine turns dark brown or black on standing or with alkalinization. The diagnosis is confirmed by quantitative measurement of increased homogentisic acid in urine. Testing for a mutation of the *HGD* gene that codes for homogentisate 1,2-dioxygenase can also be performed. There is no effective therapy for alkaptonuria, although nitisinone is currently under investigation. The arthritis is treated symptomatically with analgesics.

RELAPSING POLYCHONDRITIS

Relapsing polychondritis is an uncommon multisystem disorder characterized by recurrent episodes of inflammation of cartilaginous tissues.[24] Patients with relapsing polychondritis typically present with the sudden onset of pain and erythema involving the cartilage of the external ear, larynx, trachea, or nose. A nonerosive, seronegative polyarthritis or oligoarthritis affecting small, large, or parasternal joints (23 to 47%); ocular inflammation, including episcleritis or scleritis; and audiovestibular disturbances may also be presenting symptoms. The arthritis is typically acute, migratory, and episodic and resolves spontaneously over days to weeks. Rarely, it can become chronic. Tenosynovitis is also common. Relapsing polychondritis is presumably due to a cell-mediated and humoral immune response against cartilage components; biopsies showing acute and chronic inflammation destroying cartilage support the diagnosis. Late sequelae of relapsing polychondritis include deformity of the pinnae or nose, reduced vision or hearing, tracheal narrowing or collapse, and aortic insufficiency resulting from aortic ring dilation as well as other cardiovascular abnormalities. Patients with relapsing polychondritis frequently have associated coexisting diseases, such as systemic vasculitis, various connective tissue diseases (e.g., RA), myelodysplastic syndromes and other cancers, and thyroid disease. Treatment depends on the severity of the presentation and whether major organs are involved. Mild episodes of inflammation are treated with NSAIDs, colchicine, dapsone, and low-dose corticosteroids. Life-threatening or organ-threatening complications are treated with high-dose corticosteroids and immunosuppressive agents such as methotrexate or cyclophosphamide. Infliximab and tocilizumab have been anecdotally effective in treatment-resistant cases.

FUTURE DIRECTIONS

With the advances being made in immunology and genetics, there will be an increased understanding of the pathogenesis of many of these diseases. Treatments such as immunomodulating biologic agents or cartilage-preserving therapies will be developed on the basis of new discoveries elucidating the etiology of these unusual disorders. Because of the rarity of many of these diseases, the establishment of registries and international databases detailing clinical characteristics and response to therapies would be a valuable resource.

GENERAL REFERENCES

For the General References and other additional features, please visit Expert Consult at https://expertconsult.inkling.com.

260

SURGICAL TREATMENT OF JOINT DISEASES

C. RONALD MACKENZIE AND EDWIN P. SU

Estimates of the prevalence of arthritis and other rheumatic diseases demonstrate the enormous impact that these conditions have on the populace and the health care system in general. More than 21% of U.S. adults (46 million people) currently report physician-diagnosed arthritis. Although the majority of this burden arises as a consequence of osteoarthritis, the full span of the rheumatic diseases contribute to the impact of this class of conditions. Already the leading cause of disability in the nation, the number of people with arthritis and arthritis-attributable limitation in activity is anticipated to approach 67 million affected adults by the year 2030. Ultimately, surgical intervention is required in many of these individuals. Factors such as an increased patient awareness of the benefits of surgery, the desire for higher activity levels, and improvements in surgical techniques have, in concert with the increasing prevalence of chronic arthritis, fueled the growth in utilization of orthopedic surgery. By the year 2030, it is predicted that more than 500,000 hip replacements and 3 million knee replacements will be performed each year.

PATHOBIOLOGY

The pathobiology of joint arthritis leading to surgical intervention is essentially that of articular cartilage damage resulting in the loss of mechanical properties, accompanied by inflammation of the joint lining. With continued cartilage deterioration, stiffness and pain ensue. Without the protective layer of articular cartilage, the nociceptive and proprioceptive receptors in the periosteum are activated, leading to unremitting pain.

Osteoarthritis is the most common cause of end-stage arthritis. Osteoarthritis may be primary due to biochemical changes in the cartilage or secondary to systemic disease affecting the cartilage, joint damage from preexisting inflammatory joint disease, or trauma. Mechanical overload and imbalances lead to further cartilage degradation. Important adaptive processes such as subchondral sclerosis and osteophyte formation occur in response to joint overload, and, if chronically present, cyst formation in the subarticular bone may also result. Over time, the osteophytes or bone spurs will lead to restricted range of motion (Fig. 260-1).

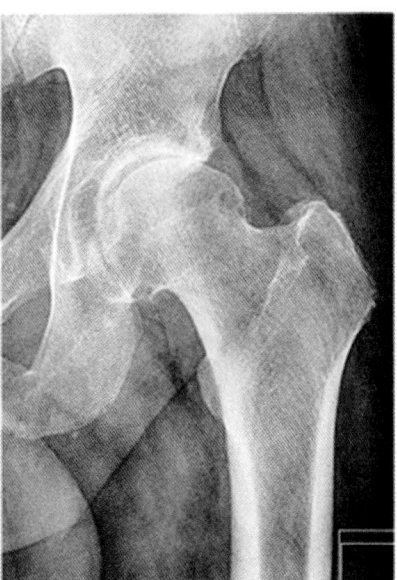

FIGURE 260-1. Radiograph of an osteoarthritic left hip. Note the asymmetrical joint space narrowing and subchondral sclerosis that are characteristic of a wear-and-tear pattern of joint deterioration.

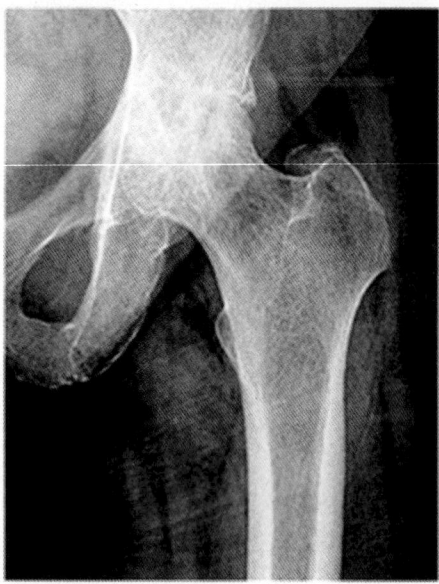

FIGURE 260-2. Radiograph of a left hip with end-stage inflammatory arthritis. Note the symmetrical pattern of cartilage loss and presence of osteopenia.

Inflammatory arthritis, by contrast, is a constellation of diseases involving the synovium. Included in this class of disorders are such important conditions as rheumatoid arthritis, psoriatic arthritis, and the seronegative spondyloarthropathies. On a pathologic level, all involve the release of inflammatory mediators in the adjacent synovium, leading to cartilage destruction. In contrast to osteoarthritis, there is no mechanical overload and no bone sclerosis or osteophyte formation. Rather, the inflammatory synovitis leads to characteristic loss of cartilage matrix, marginal bony erosions, and osteopenia (Fig. 260-2).

Trauma is another important cause of joint destruction. Post-traumatic arthritis is initiated by cartilage damage at the time of injury or by secondary mechanical imbalances that result from fractures of juxta-articular bone. Abnormal loading conditions will subsequently lead to a wear-and-tear form of cartilage arthritis.

Osteonecrosis is another entity that may lead to joint arthritis. In this process the blood supply to the bone is compromised, leading to necrosis of the bone supporting the articular surface. The most commonly affected joints are the hip, shoulder, and knee. As the disease progresses the necrotic bone may collapse, leading to the loss of articular integrity and progressive cartilage deterioration.

Other causes of arthritis that may lead to joint damage include metabolic disorders (chondrocalcinosis, gout), tumor (synovial chondromatosis), and infectious (post-septic) and bleeding disorders (hemophilia).

PREOPERATIVE CONSIDERATIONS

The indications for orthopedic surgery are refractory joint pain and disability. Ultimately, the patient and physicians need to agree that the possible benefits of surgery outweigh the risks. The decision to proceed with surgery therefore reflects the outcome of a partnership among the patient, the orthopedic surgeon, and the patient's primary physician or rheumatologist. Achieving the necessary decision-making balance may be complicated, especially given the increasing burden of comorbidity that accompanies the aging patient.

In the elective setting, joint replacement and spine surgery are the most common procedures under consideration. With the former, severe pain and functional limitation unrelieved by conservative treatment are the most common indications for surgical intervention. In the case of the spinal surgery, however, severe radiculopathy, nerve dysfunction (i.e., acute foot drop), and myelopathy are additional considerations. In contrast to elective surgery, there are circumstances when a deliberative approach is not possible because of the development of more urgent, occasionally life-threatening clinical problems. Examples include hip fracture, acute myelopathy, or the patient with an infected native or prosthetic joint. Because the patient's general health is at risk in these settings, the medical-surgical team must stabilize the patient as quickly as possible in order to optimize the outcome. Owing to the coupling of medical advances with increasing financial and resource constraints, a dominant trend toward the performance of surgery in the ambulatory setting has emerged. Indeed, the percentage of all surgical procedures performed on an outpatient basis in

the United States rose from 20% in 1982 to 60% in 1995, a phenomenon particularly relevant to the arthroscopic techniques of orthopedic surgery. Among the benefits of these developments has been the opportunity to move the preoperative medical evaluation to the outpatient arena. This practice allows time for discourse with the other physicians involved in the patient's care, for supplementary consultation and investigation, and the institution of therapy directed at optimizing the patient's medical status before the contemplated surgery. Approached in this manner, the preoperative evaluation becomes a focal point of communication among all members of the medical team, enhancing the collaborative nature of the consultative process and, ultimately, the patient's care.

Although the efficacy of preoperative assessment has not been definitively established, the aging and increasing complexity of modern-day surgical patients justifies this clinical practice. While no consensus exists regarding what constitutes the optimal preoperative medical evaluation, a growing literature pertaining to perioperative medicine supports various core principles that underlie effective medical consultation in this clinical setting.

ANESTHESIA IN THE ORTHOPEDIC PATIENT

Given the protean clinical features that accompany chronic arthritis and the connective tissue diseases, a variety of issues, including airway considerations, the surgical site (joint region), the anticipated duration of surgery, and comorbidities, are important determinants of the type of anesthesia to be employed, whether invasive monitoring will be necessary, and the length of time the patient will require intensive monitoring after surgery.

General and regional anesthesia are commonly used in the orthopedic patient. General anesthesia with endotracheal intubation may present a particular danger in patients with rheumatoid arthritis or ankylosing spondylitis. Patients with cervical spine instability or a rigid airway may require fiberoptic intubation. Regional anesthesia may involve local anesthesia or peripheral nerve block for minor procedures or epidural/spinal anesthesia for total joint arthroplasty.

Although the debate concerning the relative merits of regional versus general anesthesia endures, many procedures, particularly orthopedic surgery, are well suited for regional anesthetic techniques. Advantages of regional anesthesia include a reduction in blood loss, deep vein thrombosis and pulmonary embolism, adverse postoperative respiratory events, and death. Further postoperative pain, a significant problem for patients with painful rheumatic disease, may be best managed with regional anesthesia. For example, peripheral nerve blocks using longer acting anesthetics and infusion methodologies are often performed because they provide excellent intraoperative anesthesia and postoperative pain relief.

A number of options exist for the control of postoperative pain, including the traditional intravenous or intramuscular routes of narcotic medications (systemic), the use of epidural analgesia, and the local infiltration of anesthetics into the surgical site.[1] The direct administration of local mixtures of medications, including long-acting anesthetics and anti-inflammatory drugs, has become more popular because of the ease of use and excellent efficacy, particularly around the hip and knee joints. Patient-controlled analgesia (PCA) using an epidural route of administration is also an effective method of pain control after lower extremity surgery. Further, epidural PCA and local soft tissue injections facilitate postoperative physical therapy, which is important to the restoration of range of motion in patients undergoing orthopedic procedures. Both methods also reduce the systemic absorption of analgesics, thereby minimizing the problem of narcotic-induced respiratory depression. Parenterally administered nonsteroidal anti-inflammatory agents are also useful and can be used to reduce narcotic requirements after major surgery. However, the common contraindications to nonsteroidal anti-inflammatory drug (NSAID) therapy, such as peptic ulcer, renal, and ischemic heart disease, should be observed in the postoperative setting.

SURGICAL MANAGEMENT

Surgical treatment of joint disease is focused primarily on the relief of pain; secondary objectives are improvement in joint motion, swelling, return to function, and prevention of continued cartilage destruction. Realizing that surgical treatment has limitations and complications, the decision to move forward is one that must be individualized for each patient. Factors such as disease severity, the patient's desired activity level, and the anticipated longevity of the patient are all relevant to decision making. Typically, patients who are candidates for the surgical treatment of joint diseases have failed conservative measures (NSAIDs, physical therapy, intra-articular injections) and have daily pain that hinders their quality of life.

● ORTHOPEDIC PROCEDURES

Osteotomy

In circumstances in which a structural abnormality around a joint has led to mechanical overload, an osteotomy (bone cutting) may be an option to correct alignment problems. The most common sites for osteotomy are the hip, to treat acetabular dysplasia, and the tibia, to realign the knee. In acetabular dysplasia, the hip socket is excessively shallow, leading to abnormal stresses on the articular cartilage and premature osteoarthritis. An acetabular osteotomy can be performed in patients in whom cartilage still remains. By rotating the pelvic bones, a deeper socket can be formed, reducing stresses on the cartilage and thereby slowing down the arthritic process. With tibial osteotomy the knee joint can be realigned to direct forces away from the region of cartilage damage. Usually a varus (bow-legged) deformity indicates that the medial compartment of the knee is excessively worn, and, as such, a tibial osteotomy realigns the joint in such a way to direct forces to the uninvolved, lateral compartment. Typically, osteotomy is considered an option for younger patients (<40 years); beyond this age, the loss of cartilage is generally such that more reproducible results would be attained with total joint arthroplasty.

Arthroscopy

Arthroscopic surgery is performed by inserting a camera and specialized instruments into a joint through small, puncture-type incisions. Arthroscopic surgery is effective in the treatment of intra-articular pathology such as meniscal tears of the knee, labral tears of the hip, cartilage flaps, small chondral defects, and loose bodies. However, after the articular cartilage is significantly damaged, arthroscopic débridement is usually ineffective in the absence of mechanical symptoms such as locking and clicking.[A1-A4] In some instances, underlying joint arthritis may lead to tears in the meniscus or labrum; if such a tear results in new mechanical symptoms, then arthroscopic surgery may be helpful in selected cases. The benefit of arthroscopic subacromial decompression for shoulder impingement syndrome is variable but appears to be minimal overall.[A5,A6]

In the assessment of the hip there has been an increased focus on the femoral head and neck architecture as a cause of osteoarthritis. In certain patients, the anatomy of the femoral head and neck may lead to impingement of the femoral neck on the acetabular rim, typically in flexion and internal rotation.[2] This condition, known as femoroacetabular impingement, results in the repetitive contact between the femoral neck and acetabular rim and is believed to result in labral tears, cartilage damage, and eventual arthritis. Thus, there is currently much interest in reshaping the bones of the femur and acetabulum by so-called osteochondroplasty. This procedure is being performed as an open or arthroscopic procedure and provides good symptomatic relief in the short term. The long-term effects, specifically the impact on the future development of arthritis, have yet to be demonstrated for this procedure.[A7]

Synovectomy

Synovectomy refers to removal of the synovial lining of the joint, through either an open or arthroscopic approach. In conditions such as rheumatoid arthritis, in which the disease process involves an actively inflamed synovium, it follows that debulking the pathologic tissue may reduce symptoms and slow the destruction of cartilage.[3] In practice, synovectomy can be effective at relieving pain as long as there is remaining cartilage. However, the procedure has not been predictable in terms of regaining joint motion. Further, after the cartilage is completely worn through, the joint deterioration is too advanced for synovectomy to be helpful. Therefore, synovectomy is generally performed in patients with rheumatoid arthritis (or other forms of inflammatory arthritis) who have active synovitis in the presence of relatively preserved articular cartilage. The most common joints that benefit from synovectomy are the knee and elbow. However, synovectomy should be considered as "buying time" because the synovium will reappear.

Arthrodesis

Arthrodesis, or fusion of a joint, achieves the goal of pain relief by creating a nonmobile joint. Rather than have the arthritic joint surfaces elicit pain with movement, a surgical fusion (arthrodesis) of the articulating bones creates a construct that can bear weight and is stable. This is achieved by removing the articular surfaces from the joint and immobilizing the bones such that they heal in a solid union. This procedure was formerly the treatment of choice for hip and knee arthritis in young, active laborers because of its durability and avoidance of implants with their propensity to wear. However, creating stiffness at one joint will increase stresses on the joints above and below the fused joint.

Hip fusion may be performed in young patients to treat the sequelae of slipped capital femoral epiphysis, Legg-Calvé-Perthes disease, post-septic arthritis, or osteonecrosis of the femoral head. Fusion surgery can achieve a painless, supportive joint that is capable of bearing heavy loads while avoiding artificial implants. However, the gait mechanics are altered, requiring more energy for ambulation. Furthermore, the lack of motion at the hip increases stresses on the joints above and below the hip. Thus, the natural history of a hip fusion is the development of ipsilateral knee arthritis and low back pain after 20 to 25 years, necessitating much later the conversion of a fused hip to a hip replacement (fusion takedown). Although hip arthrodesis is still a viable option in the young arthritic patient, patients' desires for maintaining hip mobility in order to sit and drive have made this largely a treatment of the past.

Fusion of the knee joint is performed less commonly than hip fusion. In addition to the lack of motion that may make it difficult to sit or climb stairs, knee fusion cannot be converted to total knee replacement. Thus, knee fusion is generally considered a salvage procedure, mainly employed in situations in which replacement is not possible (e.g., lack of muscle function or persistent infection).

Ankle fusion is still commonly performed as the treatment of choice of tibiotalar arthritis.[4] Because the historical results of ankle replacement have not been durable, fusing the ankle is the best method of creating a pain-free joint. Furthermore, the ability of the knee and subtalar joints to compensate for a stiff ankle has made this procedure more tolerable.

Total Joint Arthroplasty

Joint arthroplasty is a term referring to the re-creation of congruent joint surfaces, typically with artificial parts. In certain patients and in non-load-bearing joints such as the elbow, interpositional arthroplasty can be performed by placing a tissue graft between the arthritic surfaces. In the case of weight-bearing joints such as the hip and knee, however, metal and plastic materials produce the most durable results. In such circumstances, the articular surfaces are replaced by shaped materials designed to re-create the joint kinematics; thus, the procedures are commonly called total hip, knee, and shoulder replacements.

In general, when the articular cartilage is completely worn or destroyed on both sides of the joint, arthroplasty is the most predictable option to relieve pain. After total joint arthroplasty, it is advisable to reduce stresses on the joint to promote implant longevity. This includes weight loss and avoidance of impact activities; walking, cycling, and gliding-type activities are permitted, but in general, running and jumping should not be performed. Because a total joint arthroplasty involves artificial, moving components, the replaced joints are subject to the same wear and tear as native joints. Thus, they have a finite lifespan that is dependent on a patient's weight and activity level and the implant materials. Subsequent revisions of joint replacements can be difficult and less durable, so it is wise to defer joint arthroplasty until there are no other options.

THR was first developed in the 1950s in the United Kingdom using metal and plastic components attached to the bone with cement. The early results were so predictable and reproducible that the technique rapidly spread worldwide. The National Institutes of Health, in 1994, published a consensus statement that THR "is one of the most successful surgical procedures and provides immediate and substantial improvement in a patient's pain, mobility, and quality of life. Compared to treatments for other chronic debilitating diseases, THR is highly cost effective."

THR is the treatment of choice for end-stage arthritis caused by any of the aforementioned pathobiologic processes.[5] It involves the exposure of the joint, removal of the arthritic femoral head at the level of the femoral neck, and removal of enough acetabular bone to place a prosthetic socket. The femoral implant is inserted into the intramedullary canal and anchored with bone-ingrowth techniques or bone cement. Any of the bearing materials for the hip are metal-on-polyethylene, ceramic on polyethylene, and ceramic-on-ceramic implants. These combinations of materials may be chosen based on the patient's age, activity level, and surgeon preference (Fig. 260-3). Metal-on-metal THR, popular for a time period in the early to mid-2000s, has now fallen out of favor because of findings of adverse local tissue reactions to the metal debris.

Using modern implant materials and surgical technique, the implant survival rates are 90 to 95% successful at 15 years; however, longevity will vary depending on patient factors such as weight and activity.[6] There have been cases in which THR implants have lasted more than 30 years. Because the current materials such as highly cross-linked polyethylene have only been in use for approximately 15 years, their ultimate durability is unknown.

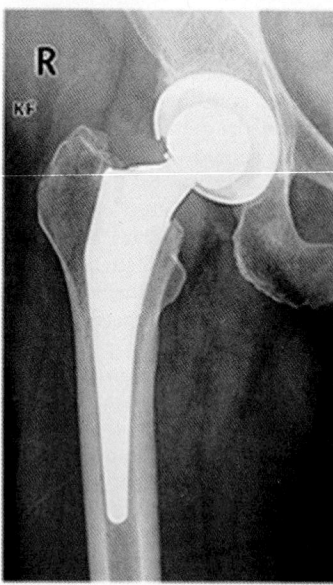

FIGURE 260-3. Radiograph of a total hip replacement consisting of uncemented acetabular and femoral components. The articulating materials are a metal ball and polyethylene liner.

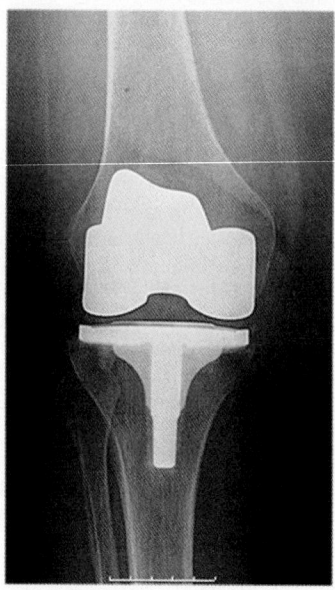

FIGURE 260-4. Radiograph of a total knee replacement. The components are metal, with a polyethylene insert between the tibial and femoral components.

A major cause of failure of THR has been wearing of the implant materials coupled with the body's reaction to the particulate debris shed into the joint space over time. In the process of immunologic uptake of the debris, inflammatory cytokines are released, causing osteoclasts to resorb periprosthetic bone. The end result of this osteolytic process is that the implant attachments to bone may be compromised, causing loosening of the prosthesis and pain. The hope is that the current generation of implant materials will reduce the amount of particulate wear debris, thereby extending longevity further.

TKR was developed in the United States shortly after THR. The surgery involves the removal of the arthritic surfaces of the tibia and femur followed by their replacement with a metal femoral implant and a metal and/or polyethylene tibial component (Fig. 260-4). It is termed "total" knee replacement to distinguish it from a unicompartmental or "partial" knee replacement.[7]

The recovery from TKR is more difficult than THR because of greater postoperative pain and the emphasis on regaining motion. Nonetheless pain relief and function are usually excellent after recovery is complete.[AB] Current studies demonstrate modern implant survival to be 90 to 95% at 15 years, again depending on patient factors.

Although less commonly performed than hip and knee replacement, total shoulder replacement is an excellent pain-relieving procedure for glenohumeral arthritis.[8] Developed from the experience gained from total hip and knee replacement, total shoulder replacement uses a stemmed humeral implant with a metal ball and metal and/or polyethylene glenoid socket. Total shoulder replacement requires an extensive rehabilitation protocol to regain range of motion and strength; however, 1 year after surgery, 95% of patients have pain-free use of the shoulder.

In general, smaller joints such as the wrist and ankle are better treated with arthrodesis because the implants necessary for arthroplasty in these joints have limited bone surfaces on which to attach the prosthesis. Additionally, the location of these joints allows the adjacent joints to compensate more effectively. However, there have been significant improvements in total ankle implant fixation that make this a viable option to treat tibiotalar arthritis, with preservation of ankle motion as the major benefit.

Surgical Innovations in Joint Arthroplasty
Minimally Invasive Surgery
As in all surgical subspecialties, there has been a movement toward minimally invasive surgery. This may be a misnomer because the actual work done inside the joint has not changed. Some surgeons have suggested the terminology be changed to "smaller incision surgery," or "less invasive surgery." In any case, the idea is that the smallest incision possible be used to perform the operation, resulting in less tissue trauma. The interest in this type of surgery has resulted in improvements in instrument design and surgical training. Until recently, a hip replacement was performed through a 10-inch incision but can now be done through a 4- to 5-inch incision. Similarly, knee replacement incisions are about one half of their former length. Despite these surgical advances,

even larger benefits have resulted from the increased attention to various nonsurgical modalities, all directed at more rapid surgical recovery. Examples include the increased use of peripheral nerve blocks, preemptive analgesia, and a more expeditious approach to rehabilitation. Such approaches have reduced the average hospital length of stay to 1 to 2 days after a THR and 2 to 3 days after a TKR. There is a growing trend in the United States to perform total joint arthroplasty as an outpatient procedure in a surgical center, with selected patients able to be discharged to home on the same day of the operation.

Improvements in Implant Technology
As the average age of patients undergoing hip and knee replacement decreases, while their activity levels increase, the number of revision surgeries is projected to grow. Therefore, much research is being performed to improve the longevity of implant materials. The "gold standard" of arthroplasty is to use a cobalt-chrome (metal) implant against a polyethylene (plastic) surface. Unfortunately, the harder metal surface will eventually wear away the softer plastic surface. Therefore, biomechanical engineers have developed a more resistant, "highly cross-linked" polyethylene that demonstrates greater wear resistance in laboratory simulators. Such highly cross-linked polyethylene has been in clinical use for about 15 years, and the early experience suggests significantly less wear compared with standard polyethylene. Other materials such as ceramics and metals are also being used in an attempt to improve longevity. Nonetheless, to date, there is no consensus concerning the optimal bearing surfaces.

Bone-preserving implants have also been developed in order to maintain more options when revision surgery becomes a necessity. Such procedures may require the removal of the implant and placement of a new prosthetic device; thus, with more bone available, surgical options are enhanced. One such bone-preserving implant is the hip-resurfacing device. This is discussed more fully later.

Unicompartmental knee replacement is a bone-preserving implant for the knee. As suggested by its name, it involves replacing only one of the three knee compartments with a prosthetic device (Fig. 260-5). Therefore, candidates for unicompartmental knee replacement must have arthritis limited to a single compartment. Because the surgical trauma and dissection are significantly reduced compared with TKR, patient recovery tends to be less painful and quicker. However, there remains a higher failure rate for unicompartmental knee replacement when compared with TKR because of the possibility of developing arthritic changes elsewhere in the joint.

Resurfacing Arthroplasty
Hip resurfacing is quickly growing as an alternative treatment to THR in the younger, active patient.[9] The primary benefit is the preservation of proximal femoral bone in the event that future (revision) surgery is necessary. Rather than removing the femoral head and portion of the femoral neck as in THR, the bone is sculpted to accept a metal resurfacing cap (like a tooth), preserving

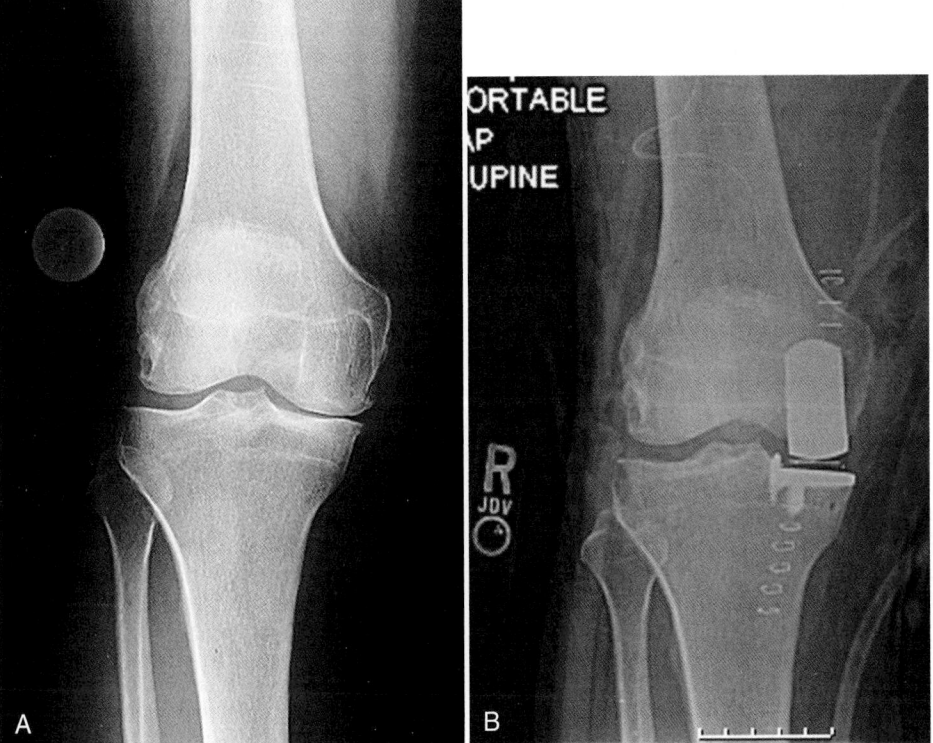

FIGURE 260-5. A, Radiograph of a knee with arthritis limited to the medial compartment. B, A medial unicompartmental knee replacement.

an additional 4 to 5 cm of bone (Fig. 260-6). The acetabulum is prepared to accept a metal socket, creating a metal-on-metal joint. There are currently no alternatives to the metal-on-metal articulation of a hip-resurfacing implant; however, in contradistinction to metal-on-metal THR, there appear to be fewer issues arising from the material in hip resurfacing. The likely explanation for this finding is that there are fewer pieces and junctions in a hip resurfacing compared with THR. The preservation of the proximal femoral bone raises an additional risk for failure (i.e., femoral neck fracture below the resurfacing implant), which is estimated to occur in 1% of cases. Although there are no defined age limits for hip resurfacing, the best candidates have been males younger than 55 years, likely because the bone quality in this demographic group is stronger and more robust. In this age group, the 10-year results of hip resurfacing in Australia have demonstrated a more than 94% rate of survival (free of revision), which is superior to THR. However, concerns regarding longevity, a greater short-term failure rate than THR, poorer results in women, and metal ion release have led to questions concerning the superiority of the procedure.

Computer Navigation and Robotic Surgery

An orthopedic surgeon relies on visualization, instrument jigs, and experience in order to recreate the proper joint mechanics. Although the surgeon may know exactly how the artificial components are to be placed, it may be difficult to achieve perfect alignment in every operation. Computer navigation is a tool that can be used to aid in the reproducible positioning of implants, where the information given by the navigation device is used by the surgeon to improve precision. Robotic surgery refers to the use of a machine that assists in the preparation of the bone and insertion of the implants; typically this is done through haptically guided limits imposed on the surgeon by a robotic arm. Although some errors are inherent in the precision of computer navigation and robotic surgery, such techniques have reliably diminished outlier results. It has yet to be determined whether the longevity of hip and knee replacements inserted with the aid of computer navigation differ from those inserted by conventional approaches. For this reason, as well as the expense and time associated with their use, computer navigation and robotic surgery are not universally practiced.

● ORTHOPEDIC PROCEDURES ON OTHER JOINTS

Elbow, Ankle, and Wrist

The elbow,[10] ankle, and wrist are less frequently replaced joints. With the exception of the rheumatoid wrist, these joints are less commonly afflicted

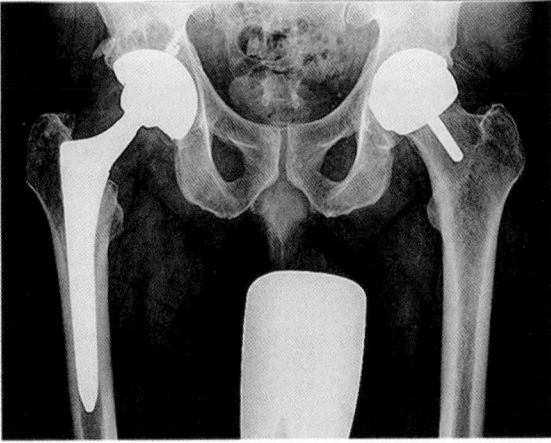

FIGURE 260-6. Radiograph of a patient with a right total hip replacement and a left hip resurfacing. The total hip replacement consists of a longer stem placed into the medullary canal of the femur. The hip resurfacing implant preserves the proximal femoral bone.

by chronic arthritis. Further, the smaller bones making up these joints also translate to a diminished surface area for implant fixation, thus lowering the durability of the surgical procedures. Although total joint arthroplasty can be successful at relieving pain in the short-term, 10-year results do not approach those of total hip or knee replacement. Synovectomy remains an effective surgical option in selected patients with inflammatory arthritis of the elbow, ankle, or wrist.

Spine

See Chapter 372.

● MANAGEMENT ISSUES IN PATIENTS WITH ARTHRITIS UNDERGOING SURGERY

Prevention of Postoperative Infection

Efforts to prevent and detect any infectious processes preoperatively and postoperatively are of utmost importance. The skin and urinary tract are sites of specific concern, and infection can be ruled out by a careful physical examination and routine preoperative urine culture. In addition, dental consultation may be appropriate in patients with poor oral hygiene and dentition.

Prophylactic antibiotic therapy for total joint arthroplasty patients should begin less than 2 hours before surgery and continue for 24 hours. A common protocol involves cefazolin (Ancef) 1 gram every 8 hours (total of three doses) or, in penicillin allergic patients, vancomycin 1 gram every 12 hours (total of two doses).

Peripheral Nerve Injuries

Peripheral nerve injuries arise more often after upper and lower extremity surgery because they generally result from excessive traction on the nerve or, alternatively, as a consequence of nerve compression resulting from prolonged positioning of the extremity during surgery or as a result of a cast. Early detection and intervention are critical to the outcome in these circumstances. Patients with chronic neurologic disease conditions, such as neuropathies in the setting of diabetes or spinal stenosis, are at increased risk for nerve injury.

Venous Thromboembolism

Prevention of venous thromboembolic phenomenon after orthopedic surgery is the most thoroughly studied of potential postoperative complications, and pulmonary embolism remains an important cause of mortality. The orthopedic literature has concentrated on lower extremity arthroplasty, although a recent study suggests that similar approaches should also be considered after total shoulder arthroplasty, when the risk for thromboembolism may be higher than generally appreciated.

After orthopedic surgery, a complicated balance exists between a possible life-threatening pulmonary embolus and the potential for postoperative bleeding. Numerous protocols have documented the effectiveness of prophylaxis, which should begin at the time of the procedure. Short intraoperative time reduces the risk for deep vein thrombosis, as does the type of anesthesia. Epidural anesthesia reduces the risk for proximal deep vein thrombosis following THR by two- to three-fold and also reduces the overall risk for deep vein thrombosis by at least 20%. Other intraoperative interventions, such as hypotensive anesthesia and intraoperative heparin administration, further reduce thrombogenesis. Mechanical methods also have proven efficacy at reducing risk for thromboembolism. These include compression methodologies such as stockings and various pneumatic devices, foot flexion-extension exercises, and early ambulation. These are safe, effective approaches that do not increase the risk for bleeding.

The mainstay of prevention is prophylactic anticoagulation, which should begin immediately after surgery. Regimes include low-molecular-weight heparin (see Table 76-2), and several new oral anticoagulants (see Table 76-5), often used in combination with various mechanical compression devices.

Fat Embolism Syndrome

Fat embolization (Chapter 74), a well-described complication of skeletal trauma, may also occur after procedures involving instrumentation of the femoral medullary canal. Although the embolization of fat is believed to occur in almost all patients who sustain hip or femoral fractures, 1 to 3% of patients undergoing joint replacement surgery (particularly simultaneous bilateral procedures) develop fat embolism syndrome.

The signs and symptoms of fat embolism syndrome involve the respiratory, neurologic,[11] and hematologic systems as well as the skin. Time of onset is variable, with hemodynamic instability developing almost immediately in some or insidiously over the first 2 to 3 postoperative days in others. In the latter, patients gradually become hypoxemic, may be hypotensive, and are often confused. Respiratory signs are the most common manifestation. Most patients develop mild to moderate hypoxemia or radiographic changes (mainly bilateral alveolar infiltrates), but only a minority will develop life-threatening adult respiratory distress syndrome. Neurologic manifestations range from mild drowsiness to acute confusional states or to severe obtundation and coma, all consequences of the hypoxemia and the direct effect of the embolization of fat on the brain. The skin eruption, which is rare in the total joint arthroplasty patient, takes the form of a petechial rash involving the folds of the neck and axillae, as well as petechiae in the subconjunctiva and oral mucosa. Retinal edema and hemorrhage are also commonly seen. Transient thrombocytopenia is common.

Although patients suspected to have developed fat embolism syndrome need to be closely monitored, in most instances after total joint arthroplasty the condition is relatively benign. Treatment is supportive and includes the administration of oxygen and the prevention of pulmonary hypertension (by fluid restriction and the use of diuretics and venodilators). Corticosteroids are not effective. In the majority of patients, the condition resolves within 3 to 7 days, although in severe cases the mortality rate has remained in the 5 to 15% range even with modern aggressive therapy.

Cervical Spine

In those rheumatoid patients who exhibit advanced destructive disease, cervical spine instability should be ruled out before surgery with flexion-extension films in patients with neck pain or crepitus on range-of-motion testing, radicular symptoms, or arm or leg weakness. Affected patients should wear a soft cervical collar to the operating room. When possible, epidural or spinal anesthesia should be employed.

Conversely, in the patients with ankylosing spondylitis, the rigid cervical spine may also present technical challenges for the anesthesiologist during intubation. Fiberoptic methods are often employed in this clinical setting.

Immunosuppressive and Anti-inflammatory Therapy

The anti-rheumatic disease medications are categorized as agents believed to modify disease activity (DMARDs), or as biologics, agents that target specific mediators (cytokines) of the inflammatory response. Corticosteroids, as well as other agents of uncertain mechanism of action, are also frequently employed. On a practical level the principle management questions are when a given medication should be stopped preoperatively and, in order to avoid postoperative disease flares, how soon can it be restarted afterward. In the case of the former, decisions are based on a medication's half-life, and with respect to the latter on the patient's postoperative course.

The literature on which treatment recommendations can be based is sparse, with no reported randomized controlled trials concerning this clinical problem. Nonetheless, a recent collaboration of the American College of Rheumatology and the American Association of Hip and Knee Surgeons derived evidence-based guidelines for the perioperative management of antirheumatic drug therapy, and their statement constitutes the most thoroughly considered assessment of this clinical issue[12] (E-Table 260-1).

 Grade A References

A1. Sihvonen R, Paavola M, Malmivaara A, et al. Arthroscopic partial meniscectomy versus placebo surgery for a degenerative meniscus tear: a 2-year follow-up of the randomised controlled trial. *Ann Rheum Dis.* 2018;77:188-195.

A2. van de Graaf VA, Wolterbeek N, Mutsaerts EL, et al. Arthroscopic partial meniscectomy or conservative treatment for nonobstructive meniscal tears: a systematic review and meta-analysis of randomized controlled trials. *Arthroscopy.* 2016;32:1855-1865.

A3. Sihvonen R, Englund M, Turkiewicz A, et al. Mechanical symptoms and arthroscopic partial meniscectomy in patients with degenerative meniscus tear: a secondary analysis of a randomized trial. *Ann Intern Med.* 2016;164:449-455.

A4. Abram SGF, Hopewell S, Monk AP, et al. Arthroscopic partial meniscectomy for meniscal tears of the knee: a systematic review and meta-analysis. *Br J Sports Med.* 2019. [Epub ahead of print.]

A5. Beard DJ, Rees JL, Cook JA, et al. Arthroscopic subacromial decompression for subacromial shoulder pain (CSAW): a multicentre, pragmatic, parallel group, placebo-controlled, three-group, randomised surgical trial. *Lancet.* 2018;391:329-338.

A6. Paavola M, Malmivaara A, Taimela S, et al. Subacromial decompression versus diagnostic arthroscopy for shoulder impingement: randomised, placebo surgery controlled clinical trial. *BMJ.* 2018;362:1-11.

A7. Griffin DR, Dickenson EJ, Wall PDH, et al. Hip arthroscopy versus best conservative care for the treatment of femoroacetabular impingement syndrome (UK FASHIoN): a multicentre randomised controlled trial. *Lancet.* 2018;391:2225-2235.

A8. Skou ST, Roos EM, Laursen MB. A randomized, controlled trial of total knee replacement. *N Engl J Med.* 2016;373:1597-1606.

A9. Caldeira D, Rodrigues FB, Pinto FJ, et al. Thromboprophylaxis with apixaban in patients undergoing major orthopedic surgery: meta-analysis and trial-sequential analysis. *Clin Med Insights Blood Disord.* 2017;10:1-8.

GENERAL REFERENCES

For the General References and other additional features, please visit Expert Consult at https://expertconsult.inkling.com.

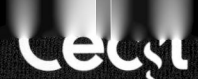

XXIV

INFECTIOUS DISEASES

261

INTRODUCTION TO MICROBIAL DISEASE: PATHOPHYSIOLOGY AND DIAGNOSTICS

W. MICHAEL SCHELD AND ROBIN PATEL

Infectious diseases have profoundly influenced the course of human history. The "black death" (caused by *Yersinia pestis*) changed the social structure of medieval Europe, in the process eliminating approximately a third of the population. The outcomes of military campaigns have been altered by outbreaks of diseases such as dysentery and typhus. Examples include Napoleon's retreat from Russia after typhus did more damage to his army than the opposition forces did; the decision by the French to sell the Louisiana Territory after French soldiers died from yellow fever in Cuba and the Gulf Coast; and the introduction of smallpox to the nonimmune population of the New World by Europeans, thus facilitating the "conquest" and the dawn of the colonial age. Malaria influenced the geographic and racial pattern and distribution of hemoglobins and erythrocyte antigens in Africa. The development of *Plasmodium falciparum* is inhibited by the presence of hemoglobin S, and Duffy blood group–negative erythrocytes are resistant to infection with *Plasmodium vivax*. Thus, populations with these erythrocyte factors are found in areas where malaria is common.

Infections are a major cause of morbidity and mortality in the world. Of the approximately 54 million deaths worldwide in 2016, at least one fourth overall were due to infectious diseases. In the United States, pneumonia is the fifth leading cause of death overall and the most common cause of death related to infection. Acquired immunodeficiency syndrome (AIDS) threatens to disrupt the social fabric in many countries of Africa and is severely distressing the health care system in the United States and other parts of the world. Approximately 36.7 million people worldwide are currently infected with human immunodeficiency virus (HIV), and since 1981, approximately 36 million have died (~700,000 in the United States alone). Deaths due to HIV/AIDS peaked at 1.9 million in 2005 and fell to 1.0 million in 2016. Global deaths due to malaria and pneumonia have also declined in recent years. Similarly, mortality rates for six common infectious diseases (accounting for ~96% of all infectious disease deaths) decreased 18% in the United States from 1980 to 2014,[1] although regional differences were striking by county, and diarrheal deaths actually increased, likely due to *Clostridioides* (*Clostridium*) *difficile*. Some of these recent global advances may be in jeopardy from rising temperatures.[2] The World Health Organization (WHO) predicts that climate change will result in 250,000 additional deaths per year between 2030 and 2050. Of this increase, about 108,000 will be related to malaria and diarrheal disease due to expansion of insect vector populations and distribution and in increased coastal flooding, respectively.

Infection can be defined as the multiplication of microbes (from viruses to multicellular parasites) in the tissues of the host. The host may or may not have symptoms. For example, HIV infection may cause no overt signs or symptoms of illness for years. The definition of infection should also include the multiplication of microbes on the surface or in the lumen of the host that causes signs and symptoms of illness or disease. For example, toxin-producing strains of *Escherichia coli* may multiply in the gut and cause a diarrheal illness without invading tissues. Microbes can cause diseases without actually coming in contact with the host by virtue of toxin production. *Clostridium botulinum* may grow in certain improperly processed foods and produce a toxin that can be lethal on ingestion. A relatively trivial infection, such as that caused by *Clostridium tetani* in a small puncture wound, can cause devastating illness because of a toxin released from the organism growing in tissues. It has now become apparent that multiple virulence factors of microorganisms can be carried in tandem on so-called pathogenicity islands of the genome (the "virulome").

We live in a virtual sea of microorganisms, and all our body surfaces have indigenous bacterial flora. In fact, we are a "super organism" as our native flora outnumbers our own human cells by a ratio of about 10 : 1. This normal flora actually protects us from infection. Reduction of gut colonization increases susceptibility to infection by pathogens such as *Salmonella enterica*. Bacteria that constitute normal flora microorganisms are thought to exert their protective effect by several mechanisms: (1) using nutrients and occupying an ecologic niche, thus competing with pathogens; (2) producing antibacterial substances that inhibit the growth of pathogens; and (3) inducing host immunity that is cross-reactive and effective against pathogens. These conclusions appear to be oversimplistic, however. For example, colonization of the gastrointestinal tract with *Bacteroides fragilis* expressing an immunodominant bacterial polysaccharide causes dendritic cell activation and induction of a T_H1-mediated response, leading to a splenic response characterized by normal numbers of $CD4^+$ T cells, lymphoid architecture, and systemic lymphocytic expansion. Thus, a single bacterial molecule in our gut is necessary to make us "immunologically fit." Indeed, it has become apparent that a healthy, diverse microbiome is vital to proper immune system function. The timing of changes in the microbiome can also be of crucial importance. For example, pregnant mice fed antibacterials pass along their altered gut microbiome to their offspring. The neonates, in turn, display decreased total numbers and composition of gut microbes that are associated with decreased numbers of circulating and bone marrow neutrophils. This disordered neutrophil homeostasis leads to impaired host defense and increased susceptibility to *E. coli* K1 and *Klebsiella pneumoniae* sepsis, classic neonatal pathogens in humans. Furthermore, because children are often prescribed multiple courses of antibacterials, one must wonder if these (often unnecessary) exposures later predispose them to epidemic disorders, such as asthma, autoimmunity, inflammatory bowel disease, and obesity.

Only a small proportion of microbial species can be considered primary or professional pathogens, and even among these species, a relatively small number of clones have been shown to cause disease. For example, epidemic meningococcal meningitis and meningococcemia are due to a small number of clones of *Neisseria meningitidis*, and the worldwide explosion of penicillin-resistant *Streptococcus pneumoniae* can be traced to a few clones originating in South Africa and Spain. This observation supports the concept that pathogenic organisms are highly adapted to the pathogenic state and have developed characteristics that enable them to be transmitted, to attach to surfaces, to invade tissue, to avoid host defenses, and thus to cause disease. In contrast, opportunistic pathogens cause disease principally in immunologically impaired hosts, and these organisms, which may be harmless members of normal flora in healthy persons, can act as virulent invaders in patients with severe defects in host defense mechanisms. Although opportunistic infection has traditionally been viewed as the exploitation of a weakened host through physiologic stress or immunocompromise (or both) by relatively "avirulent" pathogens, this is an oversimplification. For example, *Pseudomonas aeruginosa* recognizes host immune activation, specifically by binding interferon-γ to a cell surface protein OprF, which in turn, through a quorum-sensing signaling system, leads to the overexpression of virulence determinants such as PA-I (LecA) and pyocyanin. Thus, bacteria have developed a "contingency system" that recognizes immunologic perturbations in the host and counters this response by the expression of virulence factors.

Pathogenic organisms may be acquired by several routes. For example, direct contact has been implicated in the acquisition of staphylococcal disease. Airborne spread, usually by droplet nuclei, occurs in respiratory diseases such as influenza, in severe acute respiratory syndrome (SARS), and in the Middle East respiratory syndrome (MERS). Contaminated water is the usual vehicle in *Giardia* infection and typhoid fever. Food-borne toxic illnesses may be caused by extracellular toxins produced by *Clostridium perfringens* and *Staphylococcus aureus*. Blood and blood products may be vectors for transmitting hepatitis B and C viruses as well as HIV. Sexual transmission is also important for these agents and for a variety of other pathogens, including *Treponema pallidum* (syphilis), *Neisseria gonorrhoeae* (gonorrhea), and *Chlamydia trachomatis* (urethritis). The fetus may be infected in utero, and the infection may be devastating if the agent is rubella virus, cytomegalovirus, or parvovirus B19. Arthropod vectors may be important, as illustrated by mosquitoes for malaria and dengue, ticks for Lyme disease and ehrlichiosis, and lice for typhus.

Pathogens are able to cause disease because of a finely tuned array of adaptations, including the ability to attach to appropriate cells, often mediated by specialized structures, such as pili.[3] Microbes such as *Shigella* species have the ability to invade cells and cause damage. Toxins may act at a distance or may intoxicate only infected cells. Pathogens have the ability to thwart host defenses by a variety of ingenious maneuvers. The antiphagocytic coat of the pneumococcus is an example. Organisms may change their surface antigen display at an astonishingly rapid rate to outmaneuver the host immune system. Examples include influenza virus and trypanosomes. Certain pathogens (e.g., *Toxoplasma gondii*) have the ability to inhibit the respiratory burst of phagocytes, and others (e.g., *Streptococcus pyogenes*) can destroy phagocytic cells that have engulfed them. The environment plays an important role in infection, both in transmission and in the host's ability to combat the invader. The humidity and temperature of air may affect the infectivity of airborne pathogens. The sanitary state of food and water, woefully lacking in many areas of the developing world, is an important factor in the acquisition of enteric pathogens, one of the major causes of mortality, morbidity, and disability, such as physical and mental developmental delay leading to poor performance in school. That malaria was associated with the "bad air" of swamps was in fact due to the mosquitoes there, but the environmental association was appropriate. The nutritional status of the host is clearly a significant factor in certain infectious diseases. It is likely that micronutrient deficiency contributes to the invasion and multiplication of certain pathogens. A new concept is the possibility that infectious diseases cause malnutrition through a vicious cycle of diarrhea leading to dehydration and poor oral intake, resulting in secondary diarrhea with a propensity for "stunting" and delaying intellectual development. Establishment of infection is a complicated interplay of factors involving the microbe, the host, and the environment.

Host reaction to infection may result in illness. For example, previous infection with *Campylobacter jejuni* is responsible for about 40% of cases of Guillain-Barré syndrome. The mechanism is thought to be the production of antibodies against *C. jejuni* lipopolysaccharides that cross-react with gangliosides in peripheral nerves. Similarly, much of the damage resulting from meningitis is due to the host's response to invading bacterial pathogens.

With some exceptions, infectious diseases are treatable and curable. Thus, it is important to make an accurate etiologic diagnosis (see separate section later) and to institute appropriate therapy promptly. In acute infections such as pneumonia, meningitis, or sepsis, rapid institution of therapy may be life-saving; thus, a presumptive etiologic diagnosis should be established before a definitive diagnosis. This presumptive diagnosis is based on the history, physical examination, epidemiology of illness in the community, and rapid techniques such as microscopic examination of appropriate gram-stained specimens or techniques such as performance of antigen detection or a nucleic acid amplification test (NAAT). Antimicrobial therapy can then be instituted for the presumptive etiologic agents, but it must be reevaluated as more definitive diagnostic information becomes available.

The study, as well as the understanding, of infectious diseases is a dynamic process. A number of factors or themes of current interest contribute to this conclusion, including the following.

EMERGING INFECTIONS

The most obvious is AIDS, but recent examples with a major impact on public health in the United States include community-associated methicillin-resistant *S. aureus*, a hypervirulent strain of *C. difficile*, 2009 H1N1 influenza, and multidrug-resistant gram-negative bacteria, such as carbapenamase-producing Enterobacteriaceae. More than 400 new, emerging, or reemerging infectious diseases have been described in the past 70 years; approximately 60% are zoonoses associated with geographic "hot spots." Their emergence is driven largely by ecologic, socioeconomic, and environmental factors. Recent (2016-2018) outbreaks of new and/or reemerging infections include but are not limited to the following: *Candida auris* worldwide, cholera in Yemen (~1 million cases!), diphtheria in Bangladesh, H7N9 influenza in China, hepatitis A in the United States (e.g., San Diego, Louisville), listeriosis in South Africa (largest *Listeria* outbreak in history), plague in Madagascar, Kratom-associated salmonellosis in the United States, scarlet fever in England and Hong Kong, and yellow fever in Brazil (potential for worst outbreak since 1942 and the recent decision to vaccinate 78 million Brazilians by the end of 2018).

GENOMICS AND OTHER "OMICS"

The exact sequence of the genome of thousands of microbes relevant to humans has been determined. This new information, in concert with genomic information from multicellular organisms such as the *Anopheles* mosquito, offers promise for the development of new therapies and vaccines. Careful analysis of the genomes of pathogens will continue to yield important information about the pathogenesis of infection.[4] For example, genome sequencing of *S. pyogenes*, collected over time with relevant robust clinical information, has detected the acquisition of new determinants (often by prophage) responsible for increased virulence and resulting in toxic shock syndrome, necrotizing fasciitis, or both, even within a single patient with sequential samples. Proteomics, transcriptomics, metabolomics, and virulomics have transformed research on infectious

diseases and promise significant improvements in diagnostics and therapeutics in the future.

GENETIC FACTORS ALTERING SUSCEPTIBILITY TO INFECTION AND RESPONSE TO INFECTIOUS DISEASES

This field promises new and significant information relevant to the wide variety of responses to infectious diseases in humans. For example, an overvigorous response, with generation of tumor necrosis factor-α, may accentuate the development of cerebral complications in *falciparum* malaria. Analysis of single-nucleotide polymorphisms of the human genome could lead to an enhanced understanding of two fundamental issues in infectious diseases: why invasive, overt disease develops in only a small fraction of individuals challenged with a given microbe, and why infections are more severe in some people than others. Variants in genes that encode molecules that mediate attachment, pathogen recognition, inflammatory cytokine response, and innate and adaptive immunity are being identified at an astonishing rate.

INNATE IMMUNITY

This is an active field in the immunology of infectious diseases. The identification of pattern recognition receptors (e.g., toll-like receptors and nucleotide oligomerization domain–like receptors) that recognize pathogen-associated molecular patterns, as well as endogenous substances reflecting tissue injury (e.g., alarmins), has revolutionized our understanding of the early host response to infection. Agonists or antagonists of toll-like receptors have already entered clinical trials as adjuvant therapies or to improve the immunogenicity of vaccines. The other area that has exploded recently is the study of antimicrobial peptides (e.g., defensins, cathecidins, histatins, galectins) and their role in the early response to infectious disorders.

ANTIMICROBIAL RESISTANCE

The development of new antibacterial agents has slowed despite the burgeoning problem of antimicrobial resistance. This disconnect has been the focus of meetings among the pharmaceutical industry, the Infectious Diseases Society of America, the U.S. Food and Drug Administration and other government agencies, the American Society for Microbiology, and internationally. Multiresistant pneumococci, vancomycin-resistant *S. aureus* and enterococci, and, perhaps most important, multidrug-resistant gram-negative bacilli[5] are just a few examples. Not surprisingly, these drug-resistant bacteria can spread easily through international travel.[6] Perhaps somewhat counterintuitively, ingestion of non-antimicrobial agents (e.g., antipsychotics) may also contribute to resistance[7] and reduced gut microbiome diversity. Some multidrug-resistant gram-negative bacilli are susceptible to only a few agents of "last resort," such as colistin or tigecycline; others are truly untreatable. In 2014, the Wellcome Trust predicted that if current trends continue, antibacterial resistance will cost $100 trillion and cause 10 million deaths *annually* by 2050! The United Nations General Assembly held a special session on antibacterial resistance in late 2016, only the third time a health topic has been the subject of that format.

THE ROLE OF INFECTIOUS AGENTS IN CHRONIC DISEASES

Many so-called idiopathic diseases may in fact have an infectious basis. Conditions for which there is some evidence (but not conclusive proof) of an infectious basis include diabetes, atherosclerosis, acute leukemia, collagen vascular diseases, and inflammatory bowel disease. Detection of "uncultivatable" microorganisms by newer techniques, such as 16S ribosomal RNA gene or shotgun metagenomic analysis, may uncover agents responsible for "noninfectious" diseases or suggest a role in conditions that are considered infectious but in which the pathogen or pathogens are controversial. In addition, we know that hepatitis C virus, human papillomavirus, and *Helicobacter pylori* cause human cancers. Given the location in contact with the gut microbiota, colorectal cancers often contain bacteria. However, when the cancer metastasizes to the liver, the bacteria can hitch a ride! Further, mouse xenografts of human primary colorectal adenocarcinomas retain viable *Fusobacterium nucleatum* (and other microorganisms). Treatment of mice bearing a colon cancer xenograft with metronidazole reduces *Fusobacterium* load, cancer cell proliferation, and overall tumor growth.[8] The implications for cancer treatment could be substantial. Furthermore, changes in our own microbiome may lead to disease. Alterations in the gut microbiome are associated with obesity. Another recent example comes from experiments with mice lacking TLR5. These mice develop hyperphagia and hallmark features of the metabolic syndrome, including hyperlipidemia, hypertension, insulin resistance, and increased adiposity, associated with an altered gut microbiome. Further, transfer of this changed microbiota into germ-free wild-type mice induces most features of the metabolic syndrome in the recipients. The explosion of new knowledge on the role of the human microbiome in health and disease has been so rapid and profound in the last decade that we thought a separate chapter on this subject was warranted (Chapter 262).

LABORATORY DIAGNOSIS OF INFECTION

Introduction

Diagnostic testing for infectious diseases requires knowledge of appropriate test ordering as well as result interpretation. Because of advances in technology, specific infectious diseases are more often diagnosed today than in the past.[9] As clinical microbiology tests become increasingly complex, however, test ordering and result interpretation have become more difficult; consultation with infectious diseases specialists or clinical microbiologists is recommended for challenging situations. Microbiology testing involves more types of specimens (e.g., fluid, tissue, swab) and specimen sources (e.g., lung, gastrointestinal tract, bone, joint) than any other area of laboratory medicine. Infections can be caused by hundreds of species of organisms, ranging from bacteria to viruses, fungi, protozoa, parasites, and even algae. Simply detecting an organism does not necessarily mean that it is causing the patient's illness, because of the possibility of it being contaminating flora or from a prior infection. Testing methods, which include direct detection using visualization (often with specific stains), culture (which may be specialized, depending on the organism type), and molecular, proteomic, metabolomic, and immunologic methods, are ever-expanding and may vary from laboratory to laboratory. NAATs, which amplify microbial nucleic acid (DNA and/or RNA, depending on the organisms targeted) are increasingly used in clinical practice. The most common NAAT in clinical use is the polymerase chain reaction (PCR), but there are many other technologies available.[10] With PCR, a specific segment of DNA is amplified using a pair of primers (Fig. 261-1) (forward and reverse) in a reaction that includes the bases needed to synthesize DNA (deoxynucleotide triphosphates) and a heat-stable DNA polymerase. The reaction itself involves serial cycling of temperatures to anneal the primers, synthesize the DNA between them (a function of the enzyme, DNA polymerase), and then convert the DNA from double- to single-stranded

DNA to allow the reaction to recur. The upshot is that at the end of the temperature cycling, the targeted DNA segment, if present, has been exponentially amplified; the amplified DNA is detected using one of a variety of strategies, including fluorescently labeled probes that hybridize to amplified DNA during the course of the PCR reaction—so-called real-time PCR. Measurement of host response to infection, including traditional serologic testing, interferon-γ release assays, and more modern measurement of host transcriptional or proteomic responses, may be applied. Specialized testing not performed in a local laboratory may need to be sent to a reference laboratory. Organisms isolated in culture have historically been identified biochemically but today are increasingly identified using the proteomic technology, matrix-assisted laser desorption ionization time-of-flight mass spectrometry, which enables accurate identification of a myriad of bacterial and fungal isolates in minutes.

Quality of microbiology results depends not just on testing in the laboratory but also on proper selection, collection, and transportation of specimens for testing. Specimens for microbiology testing should be ideally, especially for culture-based tests, collected before administration of antimicrobial agents. It is important for those collecting the specimen to ensure proper specimen collection; specimens of poor quality may be rejected by the laboratory, but only if the laboratory can identify them as such (e.g., a putative sputum specimen that is really just oropharyngeal secretions). Certain types of tests are inappropriate for some specimen types (e.g., anaerobic cultures on sputum). Swabs hold minute volumes and are only recommended in limited situations (e.g., throat swab for *S. pyogenes* pharyngitis diagnosis); flocked swabs, which efficiently release their contents, are increasingly used. Still, if tissues or fluids can be collected, they are almost always preferred over swabs.

Three questions need to be answered with microbiology testing. The first is whether a patient's illness is microbial in nature. The second is to define the organism(s) causing the illness, and the third is to determine how the patient should be treated. If treatment is not directly evident from the nature of the organism detected, susceptibility testing is performed, typically on an organism recovered in culture. Common microbiology tests are presented next.

Blood Cultures

Conventional blood cultures, typically incubated for 5 days on modern continuous-monitoring blood culture instruments, allow recovery of most cultivable bacteria, along with most *Candida* species. Mycobacteria and dimorphic fungi ideally require specialized blood cultures and longer incubation

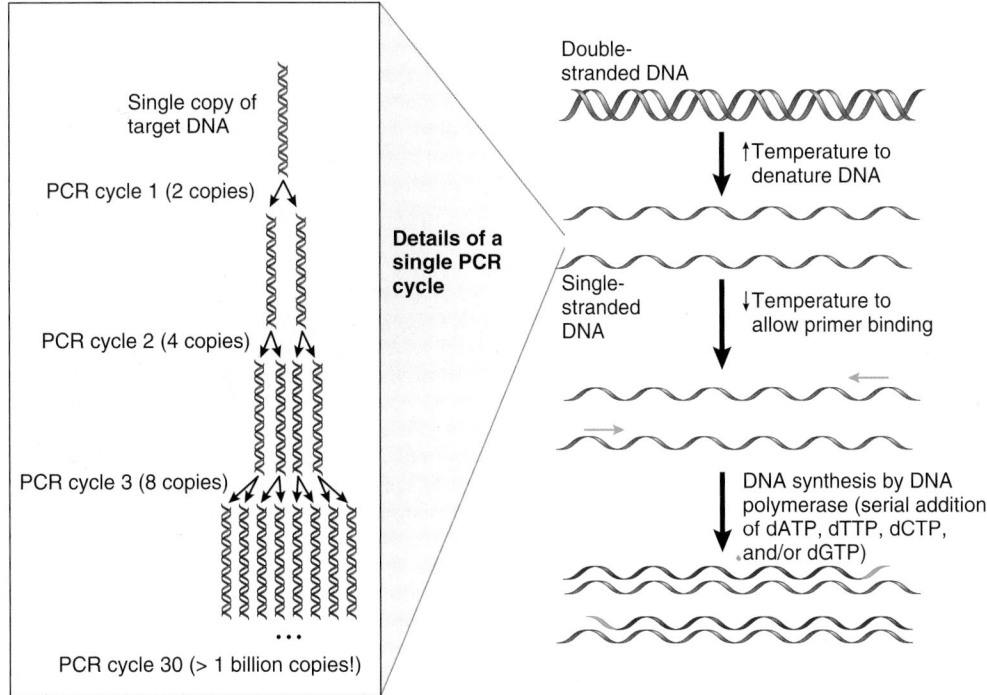

FIGURE 261-1. Polymerase chain reaction (PCR). dATP = deoxyadenosine triphosphate; dCTP = deoxycytidine triphosphate; dGTP = deoxyguanosine triphosphate; dTTP, thymidine triphosphate.

times. Collection of an optimal volume of blood and drawing blood cultures before administration of antibiotics are quality practices for conventional blood cultures. For adults, two culture sets or draws from separate venipuncture sites, each consisting of 20 to 30 mL of blood, inoculated into at least one aerobic and one anaerobic bottle per set, are recommended. There is no need to space blood culture draws over time. Single-draw blood cultures are strongly discouraged. Clinicians are notified when a blood culture becomes positive; at the time of notification, it may not be clear whether the organism represents a pathogen or a contaminant, a judgment that must be clinically made and refined as further results of testing of the positive blood culture bottle(s) become available. Contaminated blood cultures are common, with acceptable contamination rates as high as 3%, and can cause clinical confusion. Contamination can be recognized when blood cultures yield organisms such as coagulase-negative *Staphylococcus* species or *Corynebacterium* species from a single set. To minimize contamination, a dedicated phlebotomy team is ideal; the venipuncture site should be properly disinfected (e.g., with chlorhexidine or 2% iodine tincture). Many laboratories today use rapid methods, such as multiplex molecular panels, to identify bacteria and *Candida* species growing in positive blood culture bottles and to detect select antimicrobial resistance genes. These tests are ideally deployed in concert with an antimicrobial stewardship program.

Although catheter-drawn blood cultures are generally discouraged, a catheter-drawn blood culture set alongside a simultaneously collected peripherally drawn blood culture set may be helpful for diagnosis of catheter-associated bacteremia. If both grow the same organism and the blood culture collected from the intravascular catheter becomes positive more than 2 hours before the culture drawn peripherally (so-called differential time to positivity), there is a high likelihood of catheter-related bloodstream infection. In the case of multi-lumen catheters being assessed for catheter-associated bacteremia, consideration should be given to collection of blood through each lumen, along with a peripheral draw.

For infective endocarditis diagnosis, routine blood cultures are suggested; if negative, *Bartonella* and Q fever serology should be considered. Histopathology, stains, and molecular diagnostics (e.g., 16S ribosomal RNA gene PCR/sequencing, *Tropheryma whipplei* NAAT) may be applied to resected valves for the diagnosis of infective endocarditis.

Cerebrospinal Fluid Testing

Cerebrospinal fluid can be useful to diagnose meningitis and some cases of encephalitis (e.g., herpes simplex virus and enteroviral cases). Sufficient sample should be collected for all desired tests; it is helpful to collect extra fluid to be stored in the laboratory in case add-on tests are later desired (so as to avoid the need for a second lumbar puncture). Typically, three or four cerebrospinal fluid aliquots are collected in separate tubes. The first has the greatest potential for contamination and should therefore not be used for microbiology studies. Gram stain prepared after cytocentrifugation of cerebrospinal fluid and bacterial culture should be performed (along with conventional blood cultures), with cell count, differential, glucose, and protein, for diagnosis of bacterial meningitis. NAATs of cerebrospinal fluid are the tests of choice for diagnosis of enteroviral and herpes meningitis/encephalitis. Although a U.S. Food and Drug Administration–approved multiplex NAAT panel is available for diagnosing meningitis and encephalitis, it should not be considered a replacement for culture because it is not all-inclusive and because specificity issues have been reported.

The cryptococcal antigen test performed on cerebrospinal fluid should be used for rapid diagnosis of meningitis caused by *Cryptococcus neoformans/gattii*. For diagnosis of *Mycobacterium tuberculosis* meningitis, acid fast bacillus smear and culture of large volumes (≥5 mL) of cerebrospinal fluid, along with NAAT testing, are recommended.

Respiratory Specimen Testing

S. pyogenes pharyngitis is diagnosed by collecting a swab of the throat and tonsils (avoiding the teeth, gums, and cheeks), and testing it using culture, a rapid antigen test, or a NAAT. Negative rapid antigen tests for *S. pyogenes*, especially in children, should be confirmed by culture or a molecular assay. NAATs are ideally used for respiratory virus detection. A posterior nasopharyngeal swab submitted for *Bordetella pertussis* NAAT is the preferred approach for pertussis diagnosis. Multiplex NAAT panels are available; their ideal role in clinical practice is in the process of being defined.

For outpatient community-acquired pneumonia, specific testing is generally considered optional. For those with community-acquired pneumonia admitted to the hospital, however, pretreatment blood cultures, along with Gram stain and culture of sputum and, if disease is severe, urine antigen tests for *Legionella pneumophila* and *S. pneumoniae* are recommended. NAATs are choice diagnostics for pneumonia caused by *Mycoplasma pneumoniae* and, although it is a notably rare pathogen, *Chlamydophila pneumoniae*. For diagnosis of legionellosis, *Legionella* NAAT and culture of lower respiratory secretions can be performed, with the former being more sensitive than the latter. For diagnosis of hospital-acquired and ventilator-associated pneumonia, sputum, induced sputum, or nasotracheal aspirates can be tested on nonintubated patients, and endotracheal aspirates on intubated patients, using Gram stain and culture. A multiplex NAAT panel is available; its ideal role in clinical practice is being defined.

For diagnosis of pulmonary tuberculosis, expectorated sputum (or induced sputum or bronchoscopically obtained specimens) should be submitted for acid fast bacillus smear (three specimens), mycobacterial culture (three specimens), and *M. tuberculosis* NAAT (one specimen). In acid fast bacillus smear–positive patients, a negative *M. tuberculosis* NAAT makes a diagnosis of pulmonary tuberculosis unlikely. In acid fast bacillus smear–negative patients with an intermediate or higher level of suspicion for pulmonary tuberculosis, a negative *M. tuberculosis* NAAT cannot exclude pulmonary tuberculosis. Some NAATs for *M. tuberculosis* both detect the organism and provide rapid molecular drug susceptibility testing (rifampin with or without isoniazid). It should be noted that interferon-γ release assays and tuberculin skin tests do not differentiate latent from active tuberculosis and are not positive in all cases of active tuberculosis.

Stool Testing

Community-acquired diarrhea often resolves in less than a week in the absence of treatment; laboratory testing is not generally needed, unless the patient has fever, bloody diarrhea, dysentery, severe abdominal pain, or dehydration or is hospitalized or immunocompromised. For travel-related or community-acquired diarrhea lasting a week or longer, laboratory testing can be useful. The specimen of choice is diarrheal stool. Routine stool cultures typically evaluate for *Salmonella*, *Shigella,* and *Campylobacter* species and should also include evaluation for Shiga toxin–producing *E. coli* using a NAAT or antigen assay. *Vibrio* and *Yersinia* culture may be separate, specific requests using specialized media. Infection with *Giardia* species, *Cryptosporidium* species, or *Cyclospora cayetanensis* may present similarly to bacterial gastroenteritis, and these organisms are ideally identified using antigen detection or NAATs. Likewise, norovirus and other viral etiologies of gastroenteritis are ideally detected by NAATs; rotavirus can alternatively be detected using an antigen detection assay. Bacterial, parasitic, and viral gastroenteritis pathogens may be detected together in one test with commercial multiplex NAATs, some of which can yield results in as little as 1 hour.

C. difficile–associated diarrhea is often associated with antecedent antibiotic use or hospitalization, although community-acquired cases also occur; in suspected cases of *C. difficile*–associated diarrhea, specific testing is recommended by testing diarrheal stool using either a glutamate dehydrogenase antigen detection assay plus toxin A and B detection using an antigen detection assay (with or without arbitration by a NAAT for toxin-associated genes), or by performing a NAAT with toxin testing. Alternatively, a NAAT can be used alone, provided the patient being tested is likely to have *C. difficile*–associated diarrhea.

Urine Testing

Differentiation of asymptomatic bacteriuria, cystitis, and pyelonephritis requires clinical evaluation because Gram stain and culture findings may be similar for the three. Specimens submitted for bacterial urine culture should be collected in a way that minimizes contamination from perineal microbiota. The use of urine transport media or refrigeration after collection and specimen collection with straight "in-and-out" catheterization decreases the growth of small numbers of contaminating organisms, which can result in false-positive results. Urine specimens from patients who have urinary catheters in place for even a few hours frequently have colonizing microbiota due to biofilm formation on catheter surfaces; this may not represent a true urinary tract infection.

For diagnosis of acute bacterial prostatitis, the classic four-specimen "Meares and Stamey" approach, involving collection of the first 10 mL void, a midstream specimen, expressed prostate secretions, and a 10-mL post-prostate-massage urine may be used; this is considered positive if there is a 10-fold higher bacterial count in the expressed prostate secretions than the midstream urine. A two-specimen version, involving only the midstream urine and the expressed prostate secretions, can be alternatively applied.

Antimicrobial Susceptibility Testing

If treatment is not directly evident from organism detection/identification, antimicrobial susceptibility testing should be performed. Because of emerging resistance, antimicrobial therapy today needs to be informed by results of susceptibility testing more than in the past. This ensures that patients infected with resistant bacteria are readily identified and receive appropriate therapy, and also that those infected with susceptible bacteria are treated with appropriately narrow-spectrum antimicrobial agents. Bacteria may acquire resistance to antimicrobial agents through genetic exchange (e.g., acquisition of resistance plasmids) or mutation (e.g., acquisition of macrolide resistance through ribosomal RNA gene mutations). In some cases, resistance mechanisms for specific organism–antimicrobial agent combinations are so specific as to enable molecular susceptibility testing (e.g., *mecA* and *mecC* detection for diagnosis of methicillin-resistant staphylococcal infection). In other cases, molecular mechanisms of resistance are complex, precluding perfect prediction of phenotypic susceptibility with simplistic molecular approaches (e.g., ceftriaxone resistance in *E. coli*). The "gold standard" method for susceptibility testing is phenotypic susceptibility testing, which involves growing the organism with and without specific antimicrobial concentrations and comparing results. The traditional measurement of susceptibility is the minimum inhibitory concentration (MIC), which is the lowest concentration of the antimicrobial agent that inhibits the growth of the organism. Methods used to determine MICs are standardized, comprising use of uniform organism amounts and growth conditions including media, incubation conditions, and durations of incubation. To measure the MIC, the organism is grown in varying concentrations of an antimicrobial agent spanning a clinically significant range of concentrations. Dilutions can be prepared in wells of a microtiter well plate (or alternatively tested in test tubes or incorporated into agar plates) and, by convention, are doubled using a base of 1 μg/mL, for example, 0.5, 1, 2, 4, 8, and so on. An inoculum of the isolate is added, and after incubation for a defined time, wells are examined for turbidity produced by microbial growth. The first well in which visible growth is absent, indicated by clear broth, is the MIC of that organism. The MIC obtained is converted to "susceptible," "intermediate," "susceptible–dose dependent" or "resistant" categories by referring to an interpretative table. Use of the term "susceptible" implies that the MIC is at a concentration attainable in blood or other appropriate body fluid using usually recommended doses. "Resistant," the converse of "susceptible," implies that the MIC is not exceeded by normally attainable levels. As in all biologic systems, the MIC of some organisms lies between "susceptible" and "resistant" levels. Borderline results may be referred to as "intermediate" or "susceptible–dose dependent" because of technical variability and/or to indicate that the antimicrobial agent may still be used but at increased doses. Urine levels of some antimicrobial agents may be so high as to enable their use to treat urinary tract infections in the face of high MICs. Accordingly, for some antimicrobial agents, different interpretations of "susceptible" may apply to urinary versus nonurinary isolates. Likewise, for central nervous system infections (e.g., meningitis), there may be separate interpretations.

Susceptibility testing is automated using commercial systems, such as the Vitek system (bioMérieux) or the BD Phoenix Automated Microbiology System (BD Diagnostics). Using automated systems, organisms are incubated with multiple antimicrobial agents in specialized modules that are read automatically at regular intervals.

With disk diffusion testing, the inoculum is seeded onto the surface of an agar plate, to which disks containing defined amounts of antimicrobials are applied. While the plates are incubating, antimicrobial agents diffuse into the medium, producing a circular gradient around the disk. After incubation, the sizes of the zone of growth inhibition around the disks are used as an indirect measurement of the organisms' MICs. Such testing is influenced by microbial growth rate, how well the antimicrobial agent diffuses into the medium, and other technical factors. The diameter of the zone of inhibition obtained with the antibiotic being tested is converted to "susceptible," "intermediate," "susceptible–dose dependent" or "resistant" categories by referring to an interpretative table. Another diffusion procedure uses strips that contain gradient concentrations of antimicrobial agents that produce elliptical zones of inhibition that can be directly correlated with the MIC (e.g., ETEST®).

GENERAL REFERENCES

For the General References and other additional features, please visit Expert Consult at https://expertconsult.inkling.com.

262

THE HUMAN MICROBIOME

VINCENT B. YOUNG

The human microbiome has received considerable attention as a previously underappreciated factor in human health and disease.[1] In the past decade there has been an exponential increase in the number of articles published that even mention the word microbiome. With such an explosive increase in the interest of the role the microbial communities that live in and on us play in health, there is a need for physicians to understand what we actually mean when we use the term "microbiome," how this is studied, what associations exist between changes in the microbiome and disease, and how future therapies may specifically target the microbiome. This chapter will provide an introduction to this exciting new area of research and clinical focus.

DEFINITIONS

Physicians have traditionally referred to the "normal flora" when talking about the multitudes of microbes that live in and on the human body. While it is clear what this term refers to, our increased understanding of the evolution of life on earth divides all life into three main domains: the Bacteria, the Eukarya, and the Archaea. The term flora, taken from the Latin, refers to flowering plants. Initially, bacteria were thought to represent a branch of plants and hence were referred to as microflora or flora. However, now that we understand that plants are a small branch of the kingdom Eukarya and that bacteria actually represent a completely separate phylogenetic kingdom, this terminology is incorrect. Therefore, most scientists currently prefer the term *microbiota* (literally, "small life"). This term will be used in this chapter when specifically referring to the microbes that make up a given community. Although most of the attention has been paid to members of the Bacteria, we should note that this term can also encompass the Archaea as well as microbial Eukaryotes such as yeast and viruses. The term *microbiome* has had varied uses in the literature. Although some authors use the terms microbiota and microbiome interchangeably to refer to communities of indigenous microbes, we will reserve the term *microbiota* for when referring to the microbes themselves. The term *microbiome* will be used to refer to a specific community of microbes (i.e., microbiota) and the specific environment that they inhabit. This use reflects the incorporation of the term *biome*, which in ecologic terms refers to a community of organisms (plants and animals in the classical ecologic sense for which the term was coined) that occupies a distinct region with a specific environment. This distinction is important because the microbiome not only includes the microbiota but also the environment they inhabit. This environment is shaped not only by the microbes but also by the host. For example, the intestinal microbiome is composed of the microbes that inhabit this organ, and the intestinal content contains compounds derived from food as well as from the human host, such as digestive enzymes, mucin, and bile acids.

STRUCTURE AND FUNCTION RELATIONSHIPS OF THE MICROBIOME

The previous discussion of terminology is not meant as simply an academic exercise. The microbiome has been referred to as a "missing organ." As such, to understand what is meant by this concept, it is useful to think of the microbiome in terms of structure and function relationships. Medical students are taught about organ systems in terms of anatomy and physiology. Similarly, we can think about the anatomy and physiology of the indigenous microbiota. In terms of anatomy and structure of the microbiome, we can determine the range of microbial species and their relative abundance in a given community (i.e., the composition of the microbiota). To continue the anatomy and physiology analogy further, simply knowing the structure of the microbiota does not necessarily inform us about the specific function. The function of microbes in a specific environment can be ascertained by examining not only the community members but also determining the complete metabolic environment that these microbes inhabit. As noted earlier, this metabolic environment is defined not only by the microbes but also by the host. A specific example of this is the metabolism of bile acids found in the intestinal tract. Synthesized in the liver and excreted in bile in the form

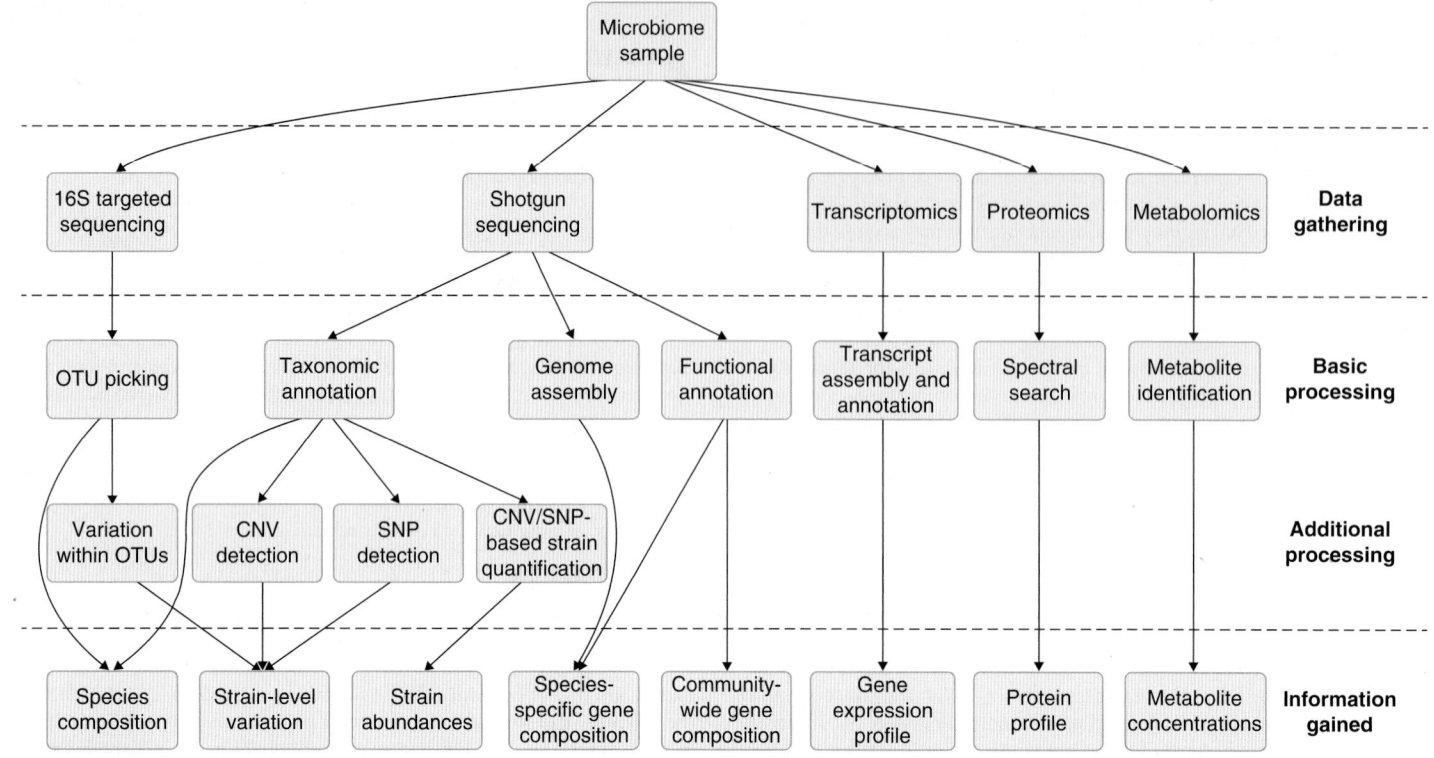

FIGURE 262-1. Schemes of microbiome analysis. Microbiome "omic" data can be processed and analyzed in various ways to address a diverse set of questions concerning the composition, capacity, and function of the microbiome. (From Noecker C, McNally CP, Eng A, Borenstein E. High-resolution characterization of the human microbiome. *Transl Res.* 2017;179:10-23.)

of bile salts conjugated to the amino acids taurine and glycine, these primary conjugated bile salts are further metabolized by members of the intestinal microbiota, which can remove these conjugated amino acids and further alter the chemical structure through enzymatic activities such as dehydroxylation. Secondary bile acids, which result from the microbe-mediated conversion of primary bile acids, have different chemical properties and thus influence host physiology in a differential manner. Bile acid receptors are differentially stimulated by various secondary bile acids, and thus metabolism of bile acids by the microbiota will have a direct influence on host physiology. Specific examples will be given later about how the microbiota can influence a wide variety of physiologic responses and how this can alter the health status of the host.

STUDYING THE MICROBIOME

A revolution in the study of communities of microbes arose through the pioneering work of Carl Woese, who redefined the "tree of life" through the study of the sequence of the RNA component of ribosomes. Subsequent work by Norman Pace and others allowed complex communities of microbes to be characterized through the culture-independent retrieval of rRNA-encoding gene sequences. Initially employed to study communities of microbes in environments such as soil and seawater, these techniques were initially extended to host-associated communities such as those found in association with invertebrates and the roots and leaves of plants. Subsequently, over the past two decades, microbial communities found in association with mammalian hosts have been studied using these techniques. The advances in nucleic acid sequencing technology that were developed in part due to the Human Genome Project have facilitated the advances in studying host-associated communities that were initially sponsored by efforts such as the National Institutes of Health Human Microbiome Project and the European MetaHIT efforts. Additionally, advances in mass spectroscopy have allowed functional characterization of communities by cataloguing and profiling the small molecules that are present in a given environment populated by microbes.

Although a detailed discussion of the specific techniques used to study the microbiome through the use of nucleic acid sequencing–based techniques and mass spectrometry analysis is beyond the scope of this chapter, it is useful to understand how these techniques can be used to gain specific information

about the structure and function of the microbiome (Fig. 262-1).[2] It is important to note that in some cases the information is limited to the structure (anatomy) of a microbial community in terms of the species composition and relative abundance of the microbes that are present. Functional data (physiology) can be gained by assaying metabolic potential or direct measurement of functional output in terms of gene expression and a catalog of the metabolites that are present in the microbiome. Overall, much of the work that is being done associating specific states of the microbiome with health and disease is being done in this "multi-omics" manner in which both the structure and the function of the microbiome are determined. A remaining question that often lingers in these studies is whether specific changes that are associated with a specific health state is positive or merely reflects the altered environment that is created by the presence of that state. Many of the current studies are endeavoring to determine whether there is truly a causal role for alterations in the microbiome and resultant disease. For conditions in which this is true, as will be discussed later, intentional alteration of the microbiome in either a preventive or therapeutic modality may represent a novel means to maintain health and treat disease.

ESTABLISHMENT OF THE MICROBIOME

One of the key questions that has been addressed with regard to the role of microbiome and human health concerns the means by which newborns establish their microbial communities at various body sites. It is generally accepted that the fetus is sterile in utero and that initial colonization occurs after birth. There has been some suggestion that the placenta may harbor a distinct microbial community, which may in turn play a role in the establishment of the neonatal microbiota, but this finding has not been widely confirmed. One point that has been established to a reasonable level of certainty is that birth mode can have at least a short-term effect on the composition of the microbiota of a newborn. Neonates who undergo vaginal birth have a distinct microbiome shortly after birth compared with children born by cesarean delivery. These distinctions resolve as the child grows older. What is unknown is whether these differences in early colonization have long-lasting effects on the health of the child. For example, these differences in initial microbiome establishment may underlie the known epidemiologic associations between cesarean birth and conditions such asthma and allergies.

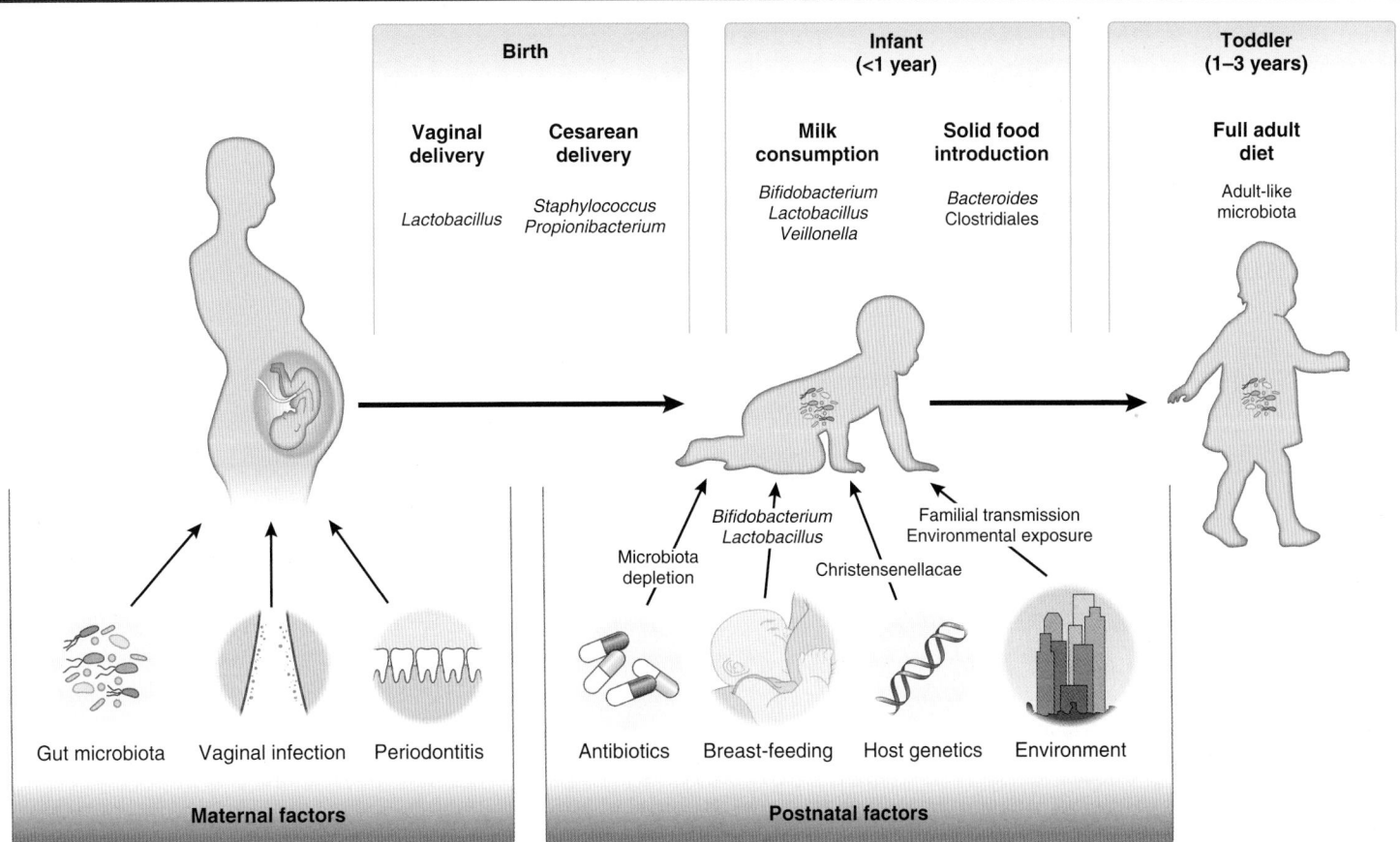

FIGURE 262-2. Factors shaping the neonatal microbiome. Maternal vaginal infections or periodontitis can result in bacteria invading the uterine environment. Delivery mode shapes the initial bacterial inoculum of the newborn. Postnatal factors such as antibiotic use, diet, genetics, and environmental exposure further configure the microbiome during early life. As diet diversifies with age, the microbiome gradually shifts toward an adult-like configuration, which is usually reached by age 3 years. (From Tamburini S, Shen N, Wu HC, Clemente JC. The microbiome in early life: implications for health outcomes. *Nat Med.* 2016;22:713-722.)

In addition to birth mode, a number of postnatal factors such as antibiotic use, breast-feeding, diet, and host genetics are thought to affect the developing microbiota of the child (Fig. 262-2).[3] After an "adult-like" microbiota is established, it is clear that there are regional differences in the composition of the microbiota (Fig. 262-3). However, although the distribution of the organisms present at each anatomic site represents an "average" composition, based on numerous surveys carried out by multiple laboratories, it is important to remember that there is significant variation in the specific composition of a given individual. The Human Microbiome Project, which characterized the microbiota of several hundred healthy individuals, further confirmed this variation in the species composition of the microbiota. However, when the high-level functional capacity of the microbiota at each anatomic site was examined by surveying the potential functions of the sum total of the genes present in the community (so-called metagenomic analysis), there was much less variation (Fig. 262-4). This has led to the belief that while the specific composition of the normal, healthy microbiota may vary from person to person, there are conserved functions that are present in a healthy community.

ALTERATION OF THE MICROBIOME

Given the apparent conservation of microbiome function in healthy individuals, it is not surprising that there is an extensive literature on the presence of altered microbiota in the setting of a variety of disease states. However, as noted previously, in many cases these were initially reports of altered microbiota in association with specific diseases. A causal role for changes in the microbiota leading to disease has only been demonstrated for a few conditions. In part this is because early cross-sectional studies simply compared individuals with and without disease. Since the presence of disease is often accompanied by altered host function, this can result in an altered environment for the microbiota. Therefore, whether observed differences in microbial community structure and function are along the causal path for disease cannot be discerned. In the following section, specific disease associations will be discussed. When

evidence is provided for a causal role for the microbiota in a condition, this will be highlighted.

Before we discuss specific disease associations with the microbiome, it is useful to consider how changes in the microbiota could play a role in the development of disease. To begin with, we can consider some of the potential functions that are normally supplied by the indigenous microbiota (Fig. 262-5). As noted earlier, the microbiota possesses a wealth of metabolic potential that can carry out a variety of catabolic and bioconversion activities.[4] Dietary substances such as carbohydrates and proteins can be metabolized by the indigenous gut microbiota. Additionally, host-derived biomolecules, including bile acids as discussed previously and compounds such as mucous and mucosal secretions, can be substrates for microbial metabolism. Xenobiotics, such as drugs and environmental toxicants, can also be subject to microbe-mediated conversion. In addition to catabolism and bioconversion, microbes can synthesize a wide range of compounds that can influence the physiology of the host. Microbial synthesis of vitamins and bioactive compounds, such as amines and neurotransmitters, has been demonstrated. Finally, host-microbe contact can directly alter the function of host tissues. Microbial contact with the immune system and mucosal surface, during both postnatal development and maturity, can influence gene expression and thus function of the host.

Given the breadth of functions attributed to the indigenous microbiota, it is clear that alteration of microbiota can lead to disruption of homeostasis. This disruption can be due to loss of a given function, inappropriate expression of a function in time or space, or introduction of maladaptive functions. All of these can lead to altered community function and resultant pathology. It is important to consider the mechanisms by which the normal indigenous microbiota can be altered (Tables 262-1 and 262-2). These mechanisms can involve the host, microbes (both resident and invasive), and environmental factors. The latter can importantly include iatrogenic factors such as medications, notably antibiotics, and surgical procedures that can alter anatomy or introduce foreign material. Although we commonly think of these as "disrupting" the microbiota, it is also important to note that many of the mechanisms

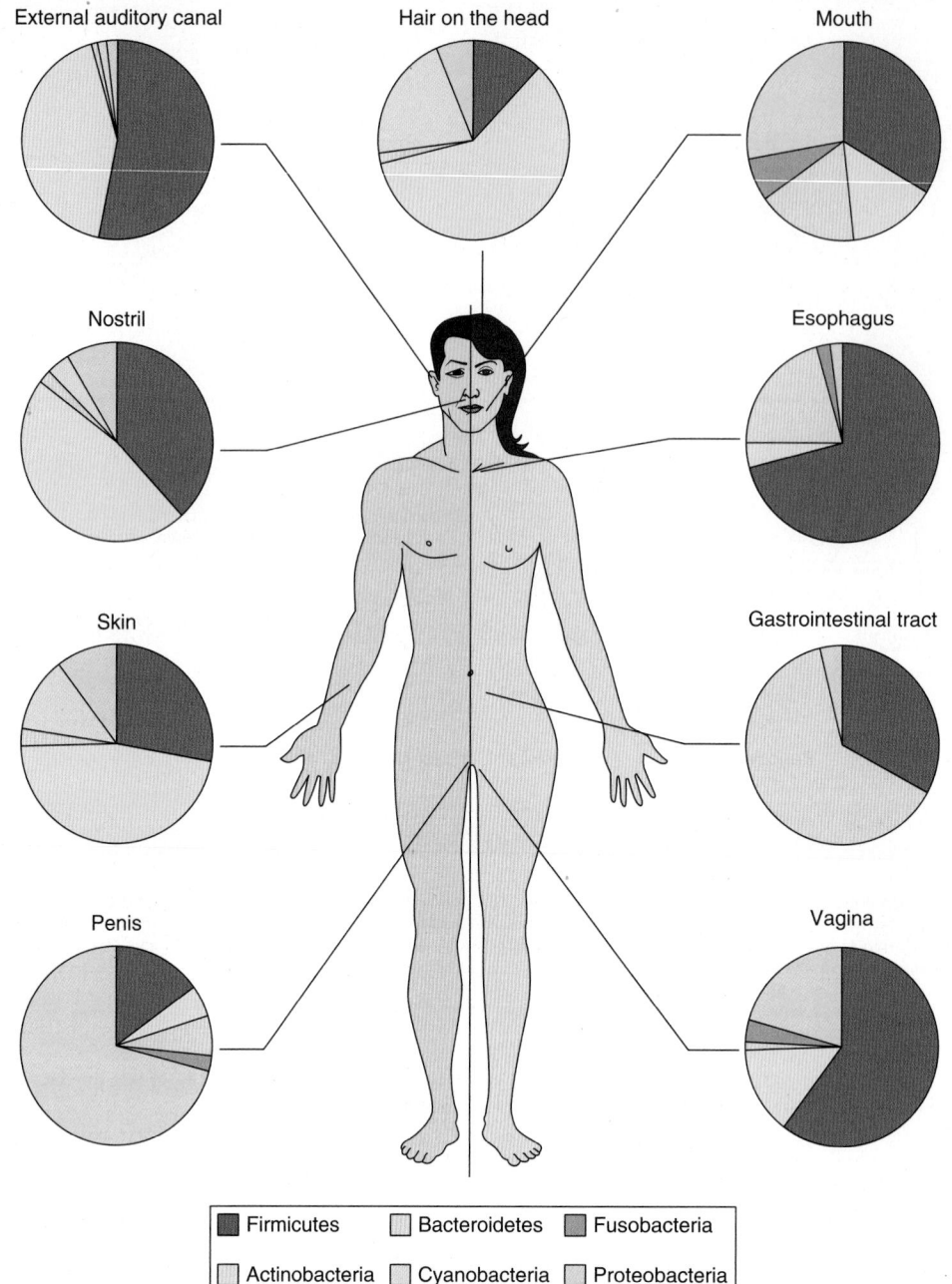

FIGURE 262-3. The relative abundances of the six dominant bacterial phyla in different body sites. Data are taken from multiple surveys of the microbiota. (From Spor A, Koren O, Ley R. Unravelling the effects of the environment and host genotype on the gut microbiome. *Nat Rev Microbiol.* 2011;9:279-290.)

are also being investigated as means to restore a disturbed microbiota to homeostasis. This will be discussed later.

🔵 DISEASE ASSOCIATIONS

The microbiome is being associated with a wide range of conditions, and it is likely that many more associations will be described in the coming years. This section will focus on specific conditions for which there is a depth of knowledge about the potential role of the microbiome in pathogenesis. It will also describe conditions that exemplify key mechanisms by which the microbiota can influence health.

Obesity

Given the broad metabolic capacity of the microbiota, it is tempting to think that these organisms can influence energy harvest from food. Early studies using culture-independent characterization of the microbiota showed that obesity in people and experimental animals was associated with an altered microbiota composition. Following up on these studies, studies involving the transfer of microbiota into germ-free mice was used to examine the causal

link between a specific microbiota and obesity. As mentioned earlier, it was initially thought that the gut microbiota, through its ability to ferment a variety of nondigestible carbohydrates, can increase the amount of energy harvested from the diet, but more recent data suggest that the relationship may be much more complex. The microbiota can directly influence the metabolism of its host through a variety of mechanisms (Fig. 262-6).[5] In addition to increased energy harvest, altered metabolic signaling and altered inflammatory tone combine with diet to allow the microbiota to modulate multiple pathways that can lead to obesity. The idea that disease is a product of the interaction between host, microbiota, and environment is one that is generalizable to all of the conditions where the microbiota is thought to contribute to pathogenesis.

Inflammatory Bowel Disease

It had long been theorized that alterations in the gastrointestinal microbiota were responsible for the initiation or persistence of inflammation encountered in inflammatory bowel disease (IBD). Evidence for this came from the clinical response of some patients to antibiotics and also from early culture-based studies in which potential pathogens were isolated from patients with IBD.

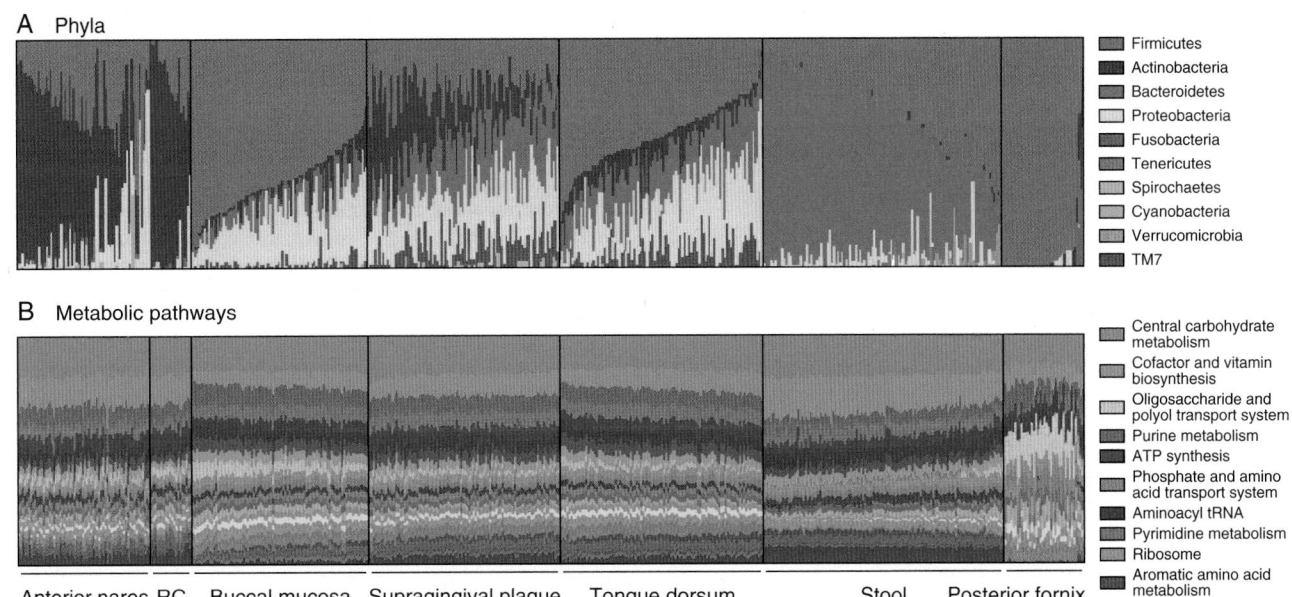

A Phyla

Firmicutes
Actinobacteria
Bacteroidetes
Proteobacteria
Fusobacteria
Tenericutes
Spirochaetes
Cyanobacteria
Verrucomicrobia
TM7

B Metabolic pathways

Central carbohydrate metabolism
Cofactor and vitamin biosynthesis
Oligosaccharide and polyol transport system
Purine metabolism
ATP synthesis
Phosphate and amino acid transport system
Aminoacyl tRNA
Pyrimidine metabolism
Ribosome
Aromatic amino acid metabolism

Anterior nares RC   Buccal mucosa   Supragingival plaque   Tongue dorsum   Stool   Posterior fornix

FIGURE 262-4. Comparison of the microbial composition (A) and predicted function (B) of the microbiota from seven different body sites of healthy individuals from the Human Microbiome Project. There is significant interindividual variation in the community composition, whereas the metabolic function is evenly distributed and prevalent across both individuals and body sites. ATP = adenosine triphosphate; RC = retroauricular crease. (From Human Microbiome Project Consortium. Structure, function and diversity of the healthy human microbiome. *Nature.* 2012;486:207-214.)

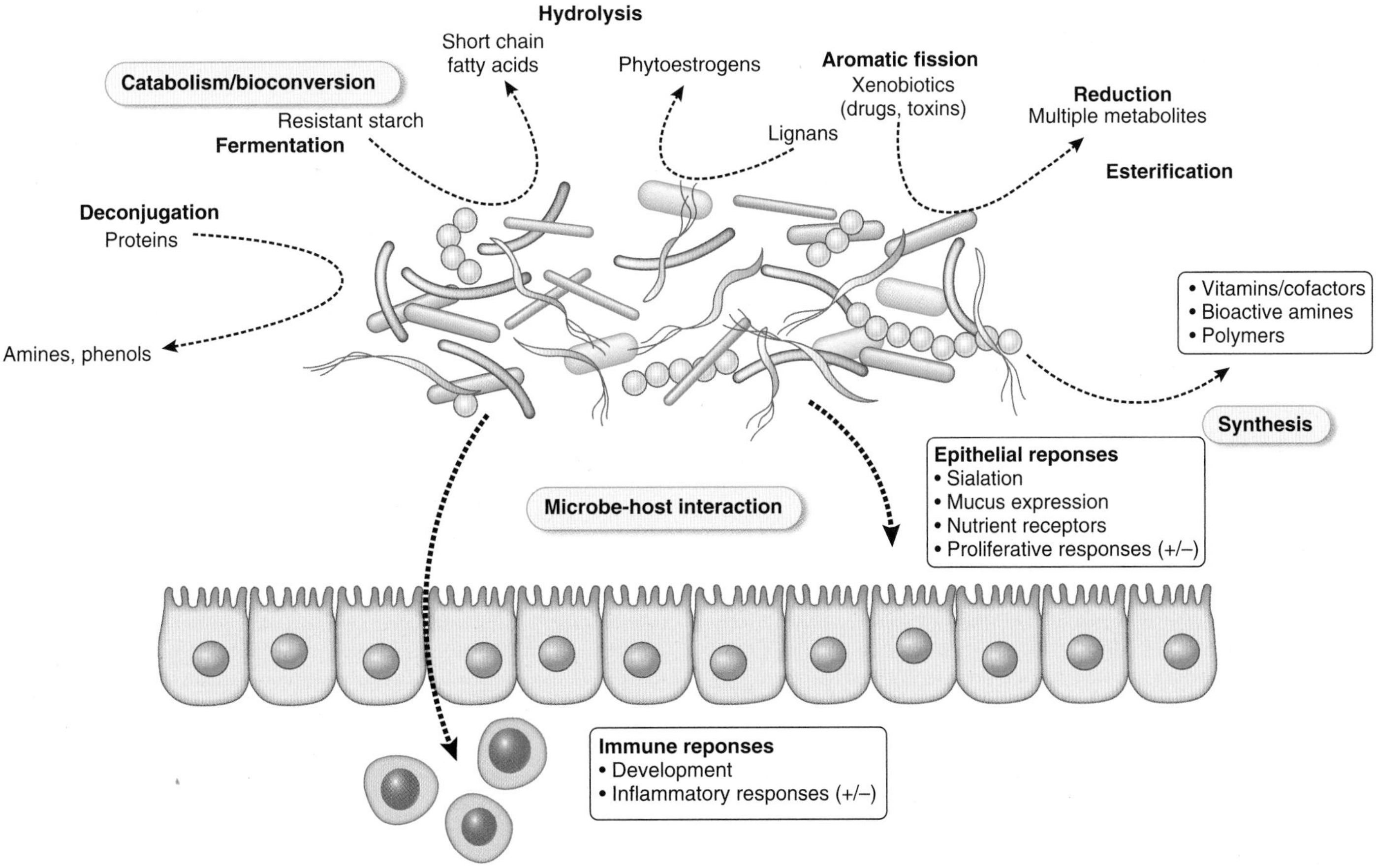

Hydrolysis

Short chain fatty acids

Phytoestrogens

Aromatic fission
Xenobiotics (drugs, toxins)

Catabolism/bioconversion

Resistant starch

Lignans

Reduction
Multiple metabolites

Fermentation

Esterification

Deconjugation

Proteins

• Vitamins/cofactors
• Bioactive amines
• Polymers

Amines, phenols

Synthesis

Epithelial reponses
• Sialation
• Mucus expression
• Nutrient receptors
• Proliferative responses (+/–)

Microbe-host interaction

Immune reponses
• Development
• Inflammatory responses (+/–)

FIGURE 262-5. Potential functions of the indigenous microbiota. The microbiota can have effects through the microbes' synthetic or catabolic metabolic activity or through direct host-microbe interactions. Catabolism and bioconversion of dietary or host-derived compounds can make nutrients more available to the host or alter the bioavailability of drugs. Some members of the microbiota can synthesize important cofactors or bioactive signaling molecules such as amines. Signaling between the microbiota and the host can trigger alterations in host function, such as altered expression of mucus or alteration of the immune response. (From Young VB. The role of the microbiome in human health and disease: an introduction for clinicians. *BMJ.*2017;356:j831.)

TABLE 262-1	FACTORS THAT CAN ALTER THE STRUCTURE AND FUNCTION OF THE MICROBIOTA

HOST FACTORS

Birth mode
Genetics
Gender
Immune status
Age
Preexisting disease
Anatomic disruption (e.g., gastrointestinal surgery, implantation of medical devices)

ENVIRONMENTAL/IATROGENIC FACTORS

Diet
Residence (urban vs. rural)
Animal exposure (including pets)
Environmental toxicants (naturally occurring or humanmade)
Antibiotics
Other drugs (e.g., chemotherapy, proton pump inhibitors, anti-inflammatory drugs)

MICROBIAL FACTORS

Infections (viral, bacterial, fungal, helminthic)
Ingestion of fermented foods (e.g., yogurt, kimchee, kefir)
Use of probiotic organisms

TABLE 262-2	STRATEGIES FOR TARGETING THE MICROBIOTA THERAPEUTICALLY

ADMINISTRATION OF MICROBES

Fecal microbiota transplantation
Single-agent probiotics
Designer microbial communities (multispecies probiotics)

MODULATION OF EXISTING MICROBES IN A COMMUNITY

Microbial nutrients (prebiotics)
Antibiotics

More recently, the recognition that polymorphisms in genes that are involved in sensing and responding to microbes, including the nucleotide-binding oligomerization domain-containing protein 2 (*NOD2*) are associated with increased risk for IBD provided further evidence for a microbial role in pathogenesis. The current thinking is that the microbiota plays a critical role in IBD, most likely through the role these microbes play in initiating and modulating mucosal immune responses.[6]

IBD is a condition in which the use of modern culture-independent methods for profiling the indigenous microbiota has demonstrated significant differences between patients with the disease and controls. As with many such cross-sectional studies, these types of association studies are unable to test causality directly. However, more recent studies have been designed that examine individuals before the onset of overt disease to examine more directly a role for the microbiota in initiating IBD. Early results are pointing to the idea that the microbiota itself can initiate the dysregulated inflammatory response that is seen in IBD, provided this occurs in individuals with a genetic predisposition to this type of response. Thus, IBD further emphasizes the idea that the microbiota is part of a complex system of interrelated factors, including the host, the indigenous microbes, and the environment, all of which intersect to influence the homeostasis of the entire system.

C. difficile Infection

Although the widespread use of antibiotics was hoped to initiate the end of infectious diseases, we are now only too aware that the unintended consequences of use of these drugs such as the rise and spread of resistant organisms has dashed these early hopes. Although antibiotic resistance was recognized early in the antibiotic era, it took longer for physicians to recognize that the "collateral damage" to the indigenous microbiota would also have negative health effects. As antibiotics with even broader spectra of activity became available, the development of antibiotic-associated colitis began to rise. In 1977, Koch's postulates were fulfilled, implicating *C. difficile* as the cause of the majority of cases of antibiotic-associated colitis.

Significant work has been completed that has defined some of the mechanisms by which disruption of the indigenous intestinal microbiota by antibiotics can lead to susceptibility to *C. difficile* infection (Fig. 262-7). The normal microbiota may be able to prevent colonization and disease by *C. difficile* through a variety of mechanisms, including competition for nutrients, stimulation of host responses, and altering key aspects of the physiology of the organism such as germination of spores and vegetative outgrowth with toxin production.[7] As noted later, *C. difficile* infection is also an area where there is currently a great deal of interest in treating this disease, in particular the recurrent form, by intentionally manipulating the microbiota to restore colonization resistance.

Colon Cancer

Because the gastrointestinal tract, in particular the distal portions, harbors the largest and densest population of microbes in the human body, it is not surprising that these microbes can profoundly affect colonic health. Owing to their extensive metabolic potential, the indigenous colonic microbes are able to carry out a large number of biotransformations that could alter susceptibility to the development of colorectal cancer.[8] The intestinal microbes play a key role in the metabolism of nitrosamines and polycyclic amines, both of which can have carcinogenic activity. On the opposing side, fermentation of nondigestible carbohydrates by the intestinal microbiota can lead to the production of short-chain fatty acids, such as butyrate, which has anti-inflammatory and antitumor activities. Thus, the microbiota can play both a potentiating and a protective role in the development of lower intestinal cancer. Furthermore, mucosal inflammation can play a key role in colon cancer development and given the relationship between the gut microbiota and intestinal inflammation as discussed with IBD, it is not surprising that this has been investigated as a mechanism by which the gut microbiome can influence colonic carcinogenesis.

In addition to studying the role of the microbiota in the mechanisms of colon cancer development, there has been interesting work that is investigating as to whether the microbiota can be used as a diagnostic or predictive tool for the detection of overt tumors. Although colonoscopy and the detection of fecal blood through techniques such as the fecal immunochemical test (FIT) are mainstays of colon cancer screening, many patients are hesitant to undergo the former invasive test while the latter has lower sensitivity. One group recently determined whether an assessment of the community structure of the microbiota could improve the performance of the FIT for the detection of various stages of colonic neoplasia.[9] Interestingly, these investigators reported that including an assessment of the microbiota markedly improved the sensitivity of FIT for early lesions such as adenomas. This work provides evidence for additional future roles for the assessment of the microbiota in clinical medicine.

Asthma

It was noted previously that birth mode and early childhood exposures such as breast-feeding and antibiotic use are associated with an altered risk for developing asthma and atopy. Cesarean delivery and early antibiotic exposures are associated with increased risk, whereas breast-feeding has a protective association. These observations suggest that the microbiota may be involved in a causal pathway because these neonatal and childhood exposures have been observed to be associated with variation in the bacterial microbiota. Furthermore, this represents evolution of the hygiene hypothesis, which posits that the development of a variety of diseases characterized by altered immune responses (including asthma, inflammatory bowel diseases, food allergy, and type 1 diabetes) stems from altered exposure to microbes (and helminths) during early life.

Neurologic Disorders

An exciting new area of investigation has examined how the central and peripheral nervous system may respond to cues from the microbiota, in particular the intestinal microbiota. This research suggests that the gut microbiota may play a key role in the long-observed "gut-brain axis." Changes in the gut microbiota have been associated with a variety of neurologic conditions ranging from autism, depression, and multiple sclerosis. Much of this work has yet to provide mechanistic links between the microbiota and these neurologic diseases, but as with the other associations, the potential mechanisms range from the production of bioactive microbial products to immunologic modulation by the microbiota.

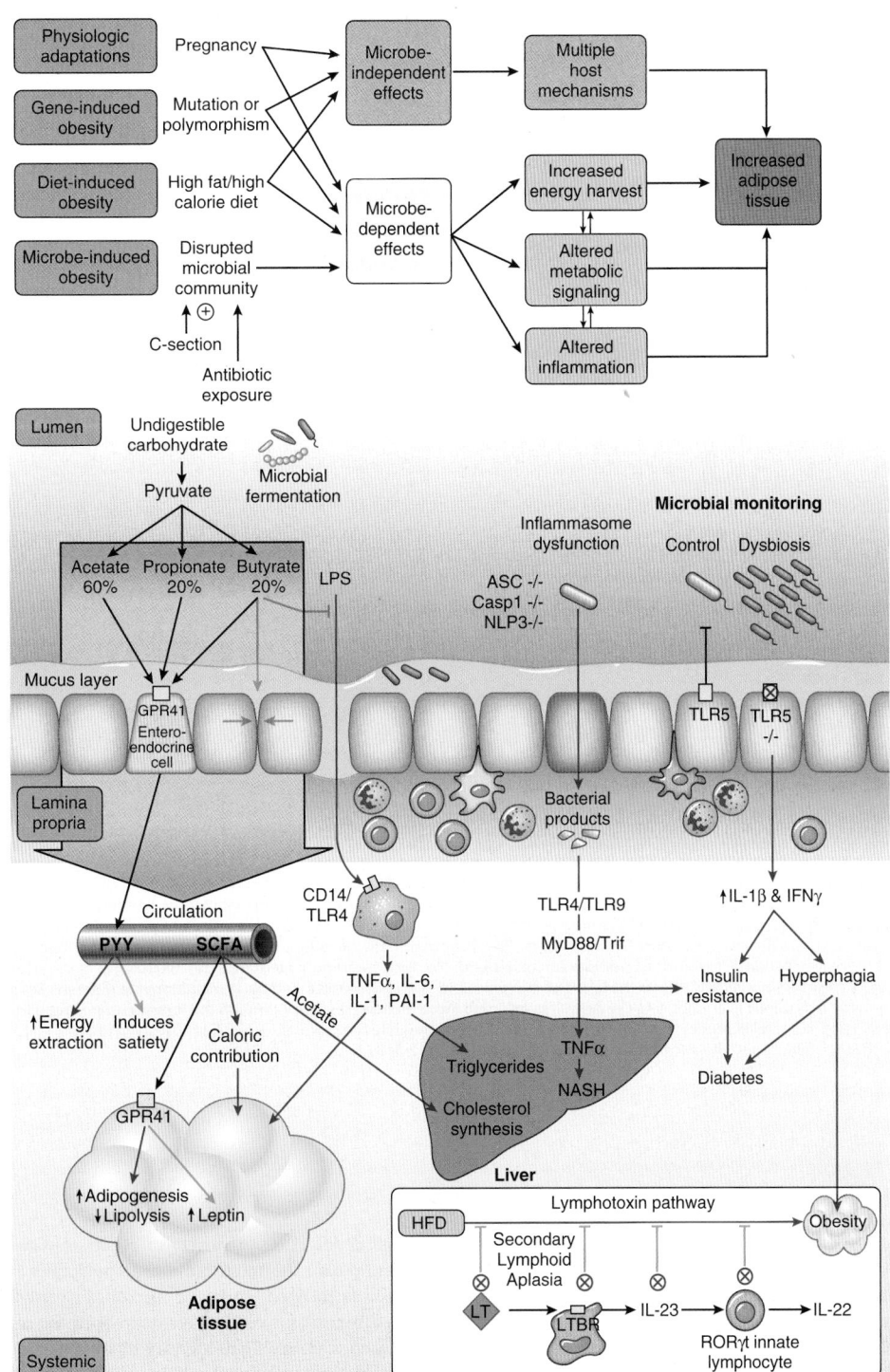

FIGURE 262-6. **Mechanisms by which the microbiota can influence host metabolism.** Undigested carbohydrates are fermented by the intestinal microbiota to short-chain fatty acids (SCFAs). SCFAs can signal to the host and modify metabolic activity. SCFAs are readily absorbed, contribute up to 10% of caloric intake, and can increase adipogenesis by binding GPR41 on adipocytes. Changes in inflammatory tone (e.g., via LPS stimulation) increase weight gain, total body and liver adiposity, and insulin resistance. (*Inset*) Deleting any component of the lymphotoxin pathway results in loss of control of the microbiome and blocks the ability of mice to gain weight on a high-fat diet. Cohousing lymphotoxin B receptor (LTBR)-deficient and wild-type (WT) mice restores diet-induced obesity and partially restores a WT/high-fat diet (HFD) microbiota. IFN = interferon; IL = interleukin; LT = lymphotoxin. (From Cox LM, Blaser MJ. Pathways in microbe-induced obesity. *Cell Metab.* 2013;17:883-894.)

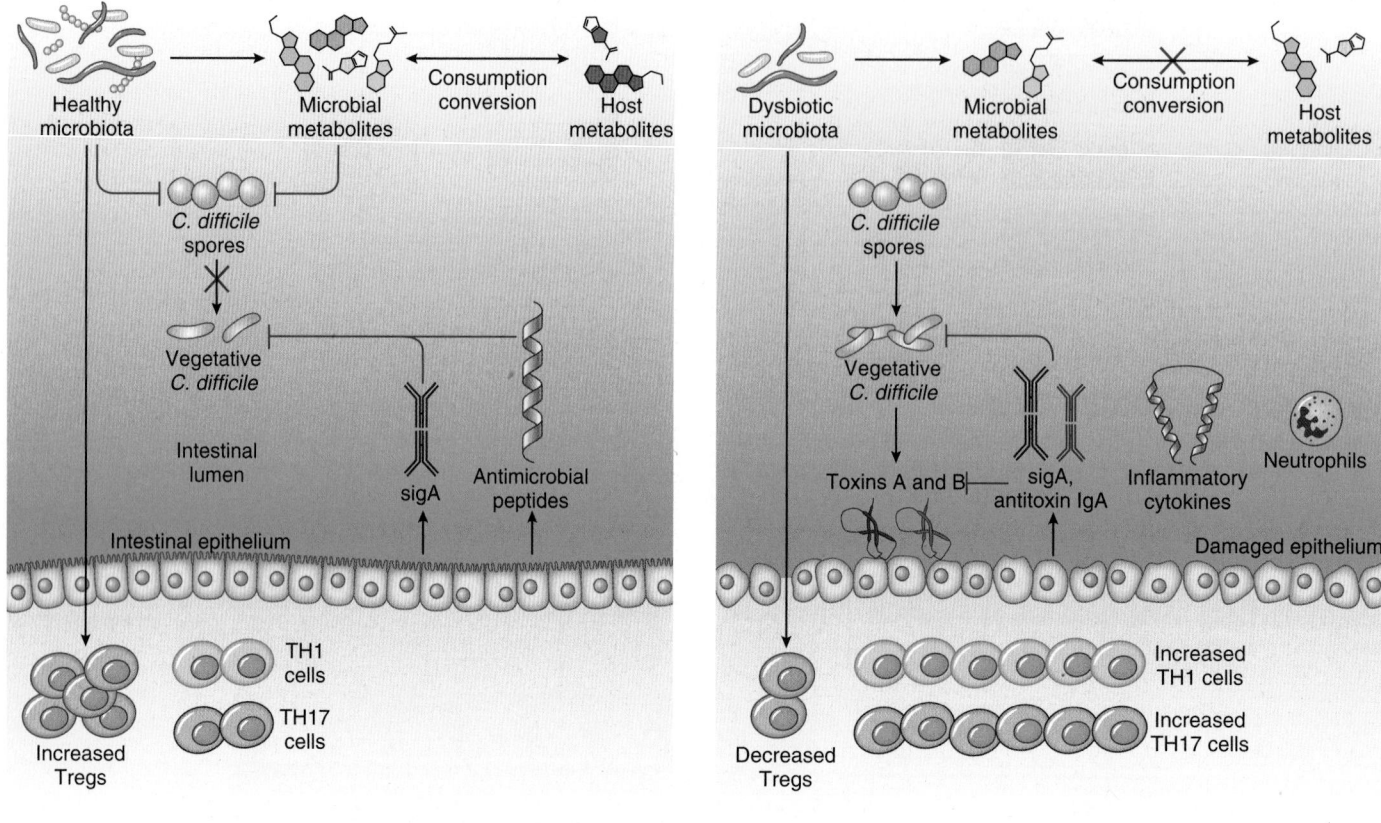

FIGURE 262-7. Proposed mechanisms of the microbiota on pathogen resistance and the host during *Clostridium difficile* infection. **(A)** Both microbial and host factors can inhibit germination and growth of *C. difficile*. A healthy microbiota is capable of consuming both microbial and host-generated metabolites, limiting the growth of *C. difficile*. Cross-talk between the microbiota and the host immune system results in a regulated immune response. Furthermore, the microbiota can stimulate production of antimicrobial peptides and secretory immunoglobulin A (sIgA), which can maintain the composition of the microbiota. **(B)** Disruption of the microbiota, due to factors such as antibiotic use, drugs, diet, or inflammation, can lead to the development of *C. difficile* infection. A dysbiotic microbiota can result in the loss of colonization resistance due to changes in the structural and/or metabolic environment. The loss of specific community members potentially affects the levels of microbial and host-generated metabolites, resulting in a different functional state that promotes spore germination and vegetative outgrowth. A dysbiotic microbiota may also result in an imbalanced immune response through the loss of immune regulation and a proinflammatory state, both of which may affect disease development. Toxin production by vegetative *C. difficile* can stimulate the production of inflammatory cytokines, neutrophils, and antitoxin antibodies. (From Seekatz AM, Young VB. *Clostridium difficile* and the microbiota. *J Clin Invest.* 2014:124:4182-4189.)

THERAPIES TARGETING THE MICROBIOME

Given the host of associations between an altered structure and function of the microbiota and disease, it is attractive to envision that intentional modulation of the indigenous microbiota could represent a novel strategy for disease prevention and treatment. This work is still in its infancy but has the potential to alter radically the practice of medicine. Many barriers exist before such treatment is commonplace, not the least of which is the fact that in many cases we still don't have causal links between the functional status of the microbiome and specific diseases. However, early work suggests that intentionally targeting the microbiota with therapeutic intent may have promise for selected conditions. One area that has been studied is in the setting of recurrent *C. difficile* infection.[A1] Even before *C. difficile* was demonstrated as the causative agent in antibiotic-associated colitis, it was recognized that transplanting feces from healthy patients to patients with severe or recurrent *C. difficile* infection could have remarkable efficacy. Subsequent work demonstrated diminished complexity of the gut microbiota in patients who were suffering from *C. difficile* infection and showed that fecal transplantation had clinical efficacy and that this was associated with an increase in community complexity through establishment of a portion of the transplanted microbes in the recipient's indigenous community.

Fecal transplantation has been attempted in preliminary studies in a number of other conditions, including inflammatory bowel disease, autism, and obesity. The results have been mixed to date, but work continues trying to determine whether this modality will have utility beyond recurrent

C. difficile infection. A variety of other strategies are also being investigated to manipulate the microbiota therapeutically.[10] Although probiotics in the form of fermented foods and microbes isolated from fermented foods such as lactobacilli and yeasts have been used for centuries, more contemporary approaches are trying to identify microbes that are present in the communities of healthy individuals and administer them as single agents or designer communities. Another strategy is to supply complex (nondigestible) carbohydrates to foster the growth and activity of preexisting microbes in a community. The use of such "prebiotics," either alone or in combination with probiotic microbes (so-called synbiotics) is another active area of research. Finally, directly targeting deleterious members of a microbial community, through antibiotics or potentially more targeted approaches such as bacteriophage or microbe-derived bacteriocins, is another potential strategy being investigated.

CONCLUSIONS

The microbiome is an exciting development in how we think about the role that microbes can play in health and disease. As we continue to understand how changes in the structure and function of our microbial symbionts affect our health, this can lead to novel methods for the prevention and treatment of a variety of health conditions. Assessment of the functional status of the indigenous microbiota and therapeutic manipulation of the microbiome is likely to be a key part of the developing paradigm of precision medicine (Fig. 262-8) that has the potential to alter the practice of medicine radically.

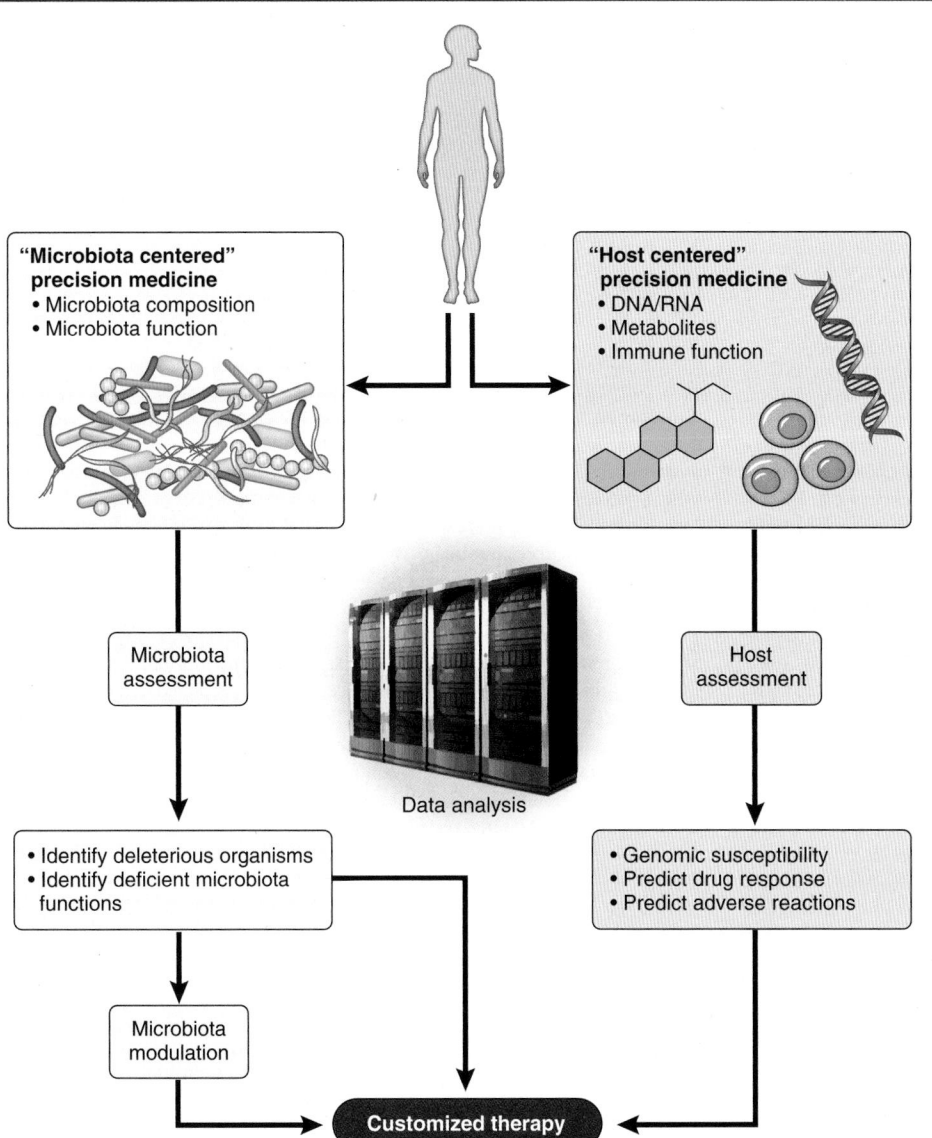

FIGURE 262-8. Incorporation of the microbiota into the developing precision medicine paradigm. As currently being developed, precision medicine proposes to determine responses to treatment according to the assessment of human genomics, metabolism, and immune function. On the basis of these data, susceptibility to disease, response to treatment, and potential adverse reactions can be predicted and a customized therapy designed. Because the microbiota can also influence this same susceptibility and response to treatment, we propose that assessment of the microbiota could also be incorporated into a complete precision medicine approach. (From Young VB. The role of the microbiome in human health and disease: an introduction for clinicians. *BMJ.* 2017;356:j831.)

 Grade A Reference

A1. Hui W, Li T, Liu W, et al. Fecal microbiota transplantation for treatment of recurrent *C. difficile* infection: an updated randomized controlled trial meta-analysis. *PLoS ONE.* 2019;14:1-14.

GENERAL REFERENCES

For the General References and other additional features, please visit Expert Consult at https://expertconsult.inkling.com.

263

PRINCIPLES OF ANTI-INFECTIVE THERAPY

M. LINDSAY GRAYSON AND GEORGE M. ELIOPOULOS

Among the most influential of all pharmaceutical agents ever developed, antimicrobials hold a critical place because the success of so many fields of medicine depends on their efficacy. Although the term *anti-infective agent* can be used more broadly to include substances that ameliorate infection by altering the virulence of the pathogen or modulating the host's response to infection, for purposes of this chapter, *anti-infective agent* and *antimicrobial agent* are used interchangeably to refer to drugs that inhibit the growth of microbial pathogens. Although this chapter focuses primarily on agents directed against bacterial pathogens, similar principles apply to antimicrobial agents that are active against fungal, viral, or parasitic infections. In all cases, selection of the most appropriate antimicrobial regimen depends on the susceptibility of the pathogen, the site of infection, the pharmacokinetic and pharmacodynamic characteristics of the agent (thereby affecting the selected dose), and the known characteristics of the affected host (age, gender, renal function, etc.). Some clinicians refer to the acronym MIND ME to assist with good antimicrobial prescribing (Table 263-1).

On the time scale of human history, the modern antibiotic era is short. Since the introduction of penicillin for general clinical use in the mid-1940s, the numerous antimicrobial agents developed for human use have saved countless lives and have led to amazing advances in health care. In fact, in the space of just one human lifetime, these compounds have been discovered, purified or synthesized for safe use, and then frequently misused in both human health and agricultural production, such that resistance has emerged very quickly in a manner that now threatens their efficacy and value—potentially returning us to a situation resembling the pre-antibiotic era. Any objective assessment of the past 80 years would likely conclude that the (mis)management of antimicrobials ranks as one of mankind's greatest wasted opportunities.

SELECTING ANTIMICROBIAL THERAPY TARGETING THE PATHOGEN

Empirical Antimicrobial Therapy

In most instances, selection of the initial antimicrobial therapy proceeds empirically, before a causative organism is identified or tested for susceptibility to

TABLE 263-1	APPROPRIATE PRESCRIBING ACRONYM—MIND ME
M	Microbiology guides therapy wherever possible.
I	Indications should be evidence based.
N	Narrowest spectrum of therapy is preferred.
D	Dosage is individualized to the patient and appropriate to the site and type of infection.
M	Minimize duration of therapy.
E	Ensure oral therapy is used when clinically appropriate.

Modified from Antibiotic Expert Group. Therapeutic Guidelines: Antibiotic. 15th ed. Melbourne: Therapeutic Guidelines Limited; 2014.

antimicrobial agents. The clinician's first decision is whether a patient's symptoms are likely to represent infection. Fever may result from neoplastic, rheumatologic, or other noninfectious processes and does not necessarily imply the presence of infection. Noninfectious causes of fever, such as deep vein thrombophlebitis, drug reaction, and vasculitis, may pose just as great a risk to the patient as infection and must not be overlooked. Additionally, serious infection can be present without the patient displaying a fever—especially if certain comorbidities are present, such as diabetes or immunosuppression.

Additional symptoms, signs, and laboratory or radiographic data usually help define whether infection is likely and, if so, localize the organ systems involved. This information allows an initial prediction about the organisms likely to be involved. For example, if the initial data cause one to suspect a diagnosis of community-acquired pneumonia in a previously healthy person who does not have any unusual exposures, *Streptococcus pneumoniae* and "atypical" bacteria such as *Mycoplasma pneumoniae* or *Chlamydophila pneumoniae* would be prominent on the list of potential pathogens to be targeted in selecting antimicrobial therapy. Examination of a gram-stained slide of expectorated sputum may provide valuable information. The prominent appearance of gram-positive cocci in clusters, for example, would alert the clinician to the possible presence of *Staphylococcus aureus,* many isolates of which are now methicillin resistant, and thus lead the clinician to select treatment options to include targeting of these organisms.

Guidance regarding the probable pathogens for site-specific infections and the susceptibility of these organisms to antimicrobial agents (which can vary depending on geographic location of the patient and the exposure) is available from a number of sources and national treatment guidelines. In some cases the susceptibility of suspected pathogens can be predicted with a high degree of certainty. For example, *Streptococcus pyogenes* remains uniformly susceptible to penicillin G. In other instances, resistance has emerged to antimicrobials previously considered to be highly active against a species. Resistance rates for a given organism may vary widely by region, by health care institution, or even by patient care area within a hospital. For this reason, access to periodically updated, cumulative antibiotic susceptibility profile data specific to an institution can be important. Typically presented in tabular form, these "antibiograms" describe the percentage of recently isolated bacterial pathogens that proved "susceptible" to the antibiotics tested and can help guide the selection of appropriate empirical regimens at that practice site.

There is mounting evidence that prompt initiation of appropriate empirical treatment results in improved clinical outcomes in those with serious infections. Thus selection of the most appropriate antimicrobial regimen depends on choosing the right drug (most effective considering the pathogen), at the right dose, via the right route (e.g., oral vs. intravenous, depending on absorption), for the right duration. To achieve this, a clear understanding of the most critical antimicrobials is required. For instance, published guidelines for the treatment of community-acquired pneumonia (Chapter 91) advise administration of the first dose of appropriate antimicrobial therapy while the patient is still in the emergency department.

Whenever possible, samples of purulent exudates, blood, or other body fluids suspected to be infected should be obtained for culture (and in some cases molecular analysis) before antimicrobial therapy is started. Identification and susceptibility testing of the microorganisms detected can be used to direct subsequent definitive treatment. At times, however, this principle must be overridden. For example, when bacterial meningitis is suspected, antibiotic therapy (often with adjunctive corticosteroids) must not be delayed when a lumbar puncture cannot be performed promptly to obtain spinal fluid for culture. In such instances, blood samples taken for culture before the administration of antibiotics often reveal the causative organism, or the pathogen may grow from spinal fluid even if lumbar puncture is delayed.

Definitive Antimicrobial Therapy

Identification of the causative pathogen and determination of its susceptibility to available drugs are the basis for optimizing definitive antimicrobial regimens. If selected wisely, the antibiotics used for empirical therapy are often appropriate for definitive therapy and can be continued. At other times, culture results allow one to change to a narrower spectrum, better tolerated, or less expensive antimicrobial. In some instances, test results indicate the need to broaden the spectrum of an anti-infective regimen by adding or substituting agents active against pathogens inadequately targeted by the initial empirical regimen. In all circumstances the choice of the most narrow-spectrum, but effective, agent is preferred to avoid unnecessary "collateral damage" to normal bacterial flora—especially in the gastrointestinal tract, where disruption of the routine microbiome can result in diarrhea and overgrowth with resistant bacterial and fungal species.

In almost all cases, it is desirable and useful to test an infecting organism's susceptibility to antimicrobials. Even for pathogens with relatively predictable susceptibilities, such as *S. pyogenes,* some isolates, although susceptible to penicillin G, are resistant to macrolide antibiotics (e.g., erythromycin, azithromycin) and other drugs, so the testing of alternative agents might be useful for patients who are intolerant of β-lactam antibiotics. Similarly, surveillance studies examining hundreds of *S. aureus* isolates have predicted that vancomycin or linezolid would inhibit virtually all clinical strains; therefore on statistical grounds, testing of these agents would not seem warranted. However, rare isolates resistant to these agents have now been encountered, and it is important to detect such isolates for both therapeutic and epidemiologic purposes. For most bacterial pathogens, resistance to commonly used agents is now sufficiently frequent that testing of antimicrobials being considered for definitive therapy is essential. This is especially the case for gram-negative pathogens such as Enterobacteriaceae, *Pseudomonas aeruginosa, Acinetobacter baumannii,* and *Stenotrophomonas maltophilia,* where multidrug-resistant isolates are now very common and often associated with transmissible (usually plasmid-borne) resistance genes, or are inherently resistant.

Susceptibility Testing

Several methods are available for determining the susceptibility of a bacterial isolate to antimicrobial agents being considered for therapy. Tests most frequently used in clinical microbiology laboratories today are variations of three methods: serial broth/agar dilution, disc diffusion, and gradient diffusion. The minimal inhibitory concentration (MIC) represents the lowest concentration of an antimicrobial tested that inhibits growth of the microorganism in test media.

In the dilution method, the antimicrobial is diluted in broth or agar to span a range of (usually) two-fold decreasing concentrations, and the medium is then inoculated with a standardized number of organisms. After incubation for a specified period (usually 16 to 24 hours) at 35° to 37° C, the series of dilution tubes or microtiter wells (for broth dilution) or agar plates (for agar dilution) is examined for growth. The MIC is determined by direct inspection as the lowest concentration that prevents turbidity of the broth or colony formation on agar. Modifications of this method allow the automation of many steps in the process, permitting more efficient test performance in clinical laboratories.

In the disc diffusion method, paper discs impregnated with a standardized amount of the antimicrobial are placed on an agar plate, the surface of which has been seeded with the bacterium to be tested. During incubation, the antimicrobial diffuses from the disc into the surrounding agar and inhibits growth of the seeded organism. After a specified period of incubation, the zone of growth inhibition around the disc is measured. By this method, the MIC is not determined directly. Instead, relying on accumulated data correlating inhibition zones with MICs, the measured zone is used to predict the susceptibility of the organism to the drug tested.

The gradient diffusion method is similar to the disc diffusion method, except that instead of using a round paper disc impregnated with a single concentration of the antimicrobial, this test uses a strip impregnated with the antimicrobial applied in a concentration gradient along its length (e.g., one commonly used brand is the Etest, previously known as the Epsilometer test). The strip is laid on the surface of an agar plate that has been inoculated with a suspension of the organism to be tested, and the plate is then incubated. By visually inspecting where the zone of growth inhibition on the agar surface intersects the strip (which is marked at intervals corresponding to MIC equivalents), it is possible to determine the MIC value directly.

To perform susceptibility studies and to interpret the results, it is necessary to identify the organism to be tested. This knowledge allows the selection of appropriate methods and interpretive criteria to determine whether an organism is "susceptible," "intermediate," or "resistant" to an antimicrobial on the basis of measurement of the MIC or the inhibition zone diameter. To illustrate this point, consider that an enterococcus is determined to be susceptible to penicillin if the MIC is less than or equal to 8 µg/mL, whereas for viridans streptococci, the corresponding "breakpoint" for susceptibility to penicillin is the MIC of 0.12 µg/mL. Thus knowledge that the MIC of penicillin against a gram-positive coccus growing in short chains is 2 µg/mL does not allow the determination of whether it is susceptible to penicillin unless the organism has been identified.

Additional tests are sometimes required to fully assess susceptibility to an antimicrobial. For oxacillin-susceptible *S. aureus,* a test for penicillinase production is performed to assess susceptibility to penicillin G. For erythromycin-resistant, clindamycin-susceptible *S. aureus,* the laboratory may perform a supplementary D-zone test or equivalent before reporting the clindamycin result. A positive D-zone test result (i.e., blunting of the inhibition zone around a clindamycin disc in proximity to an erythromycin disc) predicts the presence of *erm* genes. Their product, a ribosomal methylase, can confer resistance to clindamycin if it is expressed; however, clindamycin is a poor inducer of this resistance trait (in contrast to erythromycin, which is a good inducer). A positive test result thus implies the presence of inducible resistance traits. Mutants with constitutive production of methylase can be selected during treatment, resulting in the emergence of clindamycin resistance and an increased risk of clinical failure when this drug is used to treat serious staphylococcal infections caused by strains with the *erm* gene.

In principle, tests for the presence of resistance genes, their products, or both can be used in place of phenotypic resistance testing. Such methods have the potential to provide likely susceptibility information more rapidly than can be obtained with the usual susceptibility tests of growth inhibition, which generally require several hours of incubation. At present, these tests are not yet widely employed, with the exception of testing for methicillin resistance by detection of the *mecA* gene or its product, penicillin-binding protein 2a, or testing for rifampin resistance by detection of resistance mutations in *Mycobacterium tuberculosis.* Newer technologies, such as matrix-assisted laser desorption ionization–time of flight mass spectrometry (MALDI-ToF), are being explored as a means of providing not only more rapid identification of organisms but also their predicted susceptibility to antimicrobial agents.[1]

Bactericidal Activity

Antimicrobials can differ in terms of whether they substantially kill a pathogen (i.e., are "bactericidal") or whether they simply severely inhibit an organism's growth (i.e., are "bacteriostatic"). In vitro bactericidal activity is usually defined as a 99.9% reduction in the number of viable colony-forming units relative to the inoculum density at a specified incubation time, which is usually 20 to 24 hours; however, such testing is labor intensive and results can vary according to the exact methods and media used. In some clinical circumstances, agents that are bactericidal are theoretically preferable to a bacteriostatic alternative—for instance, in bacterial meningitis, where antimicrobial penetration through the blood-brain barrier may be limited and rapid, effective therapy is crucial to long-term outcome. Thus bactericidal agents have been generally preferred for serious infections such as endocarditis or meningitis, although the true clinical impact of this depends on the host, the agent, and the circumstances of the infection. For instance, bactericidal antibiotics have not been proven better than bacteriostatic antibiotics for abdominal, skin, or soft tissue infections or for pneumonia.[A1]

⬤ SELECTING ANTIMICROBIAL THERAPY APPROPRIATE TO THE INFECTION AND PATIENT

Nature of the Infection

Determination that a pathogenic microorganism is susceptible to an antibiotic in vitro does not ensure that treatment with that drug will result in a successful clinical outcome. The antimicrobial must reach the site of infection in adequate concentrations (generally multiple times the MIC), and it must demonstrate activity in the specific conditions associated with the infection (e.g., the milieu of an abdominal abscess is likely to be different from that of a cancellous bone infection). For some infections and antimicrobials, these requirements cannot easily be met.

For instance, a number of antimicrobials fail to penetrate into cerebrospinal fluid sufficiently well to permit their use for the treatment of bacterial meningitis in adults, such as first-generation cephalosporins and aminoglycosides, which, even when given intravenously, do not achieve adequate effective levels in the subarachnoid space. Aminoglycosides have been administered by intrathecal or intraventricular instillation when needed for the treatment of gram-negative meningitis, but the availability of newer β-lactams with broad activity, high potency, and reasonable cerebrospinal fluid penetration when administered intravenously has largely eliminated the need for direct instillation of antimicrobials. In other situations, antimicrobials may penetrate to the site of infection, only to be inactivated by local factors. For example, daptomycin is inactivated by interaction with pulmonary surfactant, so this antibiotic is not indicated for the treatment of bronchopneumonia, even though it is highly active against *S. pneumoniae* isolates in vitro. Antibiotics can also be inactivated by cellular debris or macromolecules present within abscesses, and some exhibit reduced potency at the low pH and reduced oxygen tensions prevailing at these sites. Finally, high densities of microorganisms within abscesses may produce sufficiently high concentrations of β-lactamases to inactivate some relatively labile β-lactam antibiotics. All these factors provide a critical rationale for the drainage of large abscesses as a fundamental adjunct to antimicrobial therapy.

Bacterial infections associated with foreign bodies such as artificial joints, cardiac pacemakers, or prosthetic heart valves can be particularly difficult to eradicate without removal of the foreign material. The reasons are not completely understood, but they relate, at least in part, to the presence of biofilm, which is composed of bacteria embedded within extracellular material that is adherent to the foreign body.[2] Bacteria recovered from biofilms are metabolically different from and less susceptible to antimicrobial agents than planktonic cells (i.e., those freely suspended in liquid medium) of the same organism. Some bacterial species, especially staphylococci, are a common cause of prosthetic device infections and readily produce biofilm on certain prosthetic materials, which makes effective antimicrobial therapy difficult. In some situations, a drug such as rifampin (an RNA polymerase inhibitor) is added to antimicrobial regimens for the treatment of such infections because it generally penetrates well into biofilms and displays relatively similar activity against both biofilm-associated and planktonic cells of a susceptible organism. However, because resistance to rifampin emerges rapidly if it is used as a single agent, it must be combined with a second active drug to minimize the risk that resistance will emerge. Thus treating such infections can be complex, require multiple antimicrobials in combination, and yet still be ineffective without removal of the infected biofilm-laden foreign material.

Host Factors

After consideration of the nature of the infection and the antimicrobials determined in vitro to be active against a bacterial isolate (or likely to be active against probable pathogens when an isolate is not yet available), the ultimate choice of an antimicrobial regimen must take into account a number of additional patient-specific factors.

Allergies

It is imperative to obtain a history of previous allergic reactions to antimicrobial agents (Chapter 239). Some reactions are by nature so severe and potentially life-threatening that one must avoid using the same agent or drugs within the same class for which cross-reactivity is likely to occur. Examples of such reactions include an immediate hypersensitivity reaction to penicillin (e.g., hives, lip swelling, laryngeal edema, circulatory collapse) and a mucocutaneous bullous eruption caused by a sulfonamide (e.g., Stevens-Johnson syndrome).

In cases in which the allergic reaction was mild, such as a faint, self-limited rash in a patient receiving penicillin, the clinician may elect to use a related antimicrobial, such as a cephalosporin, when the probability of cross-sensitivity and the risk for a severe adverse outcome if a reaction were to occur are both assessed to be low. In these instances, careful monitoring of the patient for adverse reactions is essential. Rarely, for patients with significant allergies to potentially life-saving antimicrobial agents for which no alternative exists, desensitization of the patient to the antimicrobial can be attempted so that the agent can be used. For example, desensitization protocols are available for penicillin and for trimethoprim-sulfamethoxazole. Because of the risks involved, these procedures may need to be performed in tightly monitored settings (e.g., intensive care unit).

Pregnancy

A number of antimicrobial agents have the potential to cause fetal harm if they are administered to a pregnant woman (Chapter 226). For example, tetracyclines can cause tooth discoloration and hypoplasia of dental enamel and are thus avoided in pregnant women and young children. Aminoglycosides (such as streptomycin) given during pregnancy can cross the placenta and can cause eighth nerve toxicity/damage in the neonate. The U.S. Food and Drug Administration (FDA) has established a new system of categorizing the risk of using various antimicrobials and other drugs during pregnancy and breast-feeding, in terms of risk to the mother, the unborn fetus, and the new neonate.[3] In designing antimicrobial regimens, the possibility of pregnancy should be considered in any woman of childbearing age so that the risks of candidate agents can be individually reviewed and the safest possible therapy selected. Similarly, many antibiotics used to treat lactating women can be found in breast milk. Thus it may be necessary to either suspend breast-feeding during treatment if exposure of the infant to the drug must be avoided, or choose an alternative agent that is safe for breast-feeding neonates.

Pregnant women may be particularly susceptible to certain antimicrobial-associated toxicities. Death resulting from hepatic failure has been described in pregnant women receiving large doses of tetracycline. Potentially life-threatening hepatic steatosis has been observed in patients treated with some older antiretroviral drug combinations (e.g., didanosine plus stavudine). Thus the metabolic changes associated with pregnancy can affect drug toxicity rates, even in patients where no such side effects would occur if they were not pregnant.

Age

Age-related metabolic differences and growth dynamics are important factors in drug choice, particularly at the extremes of age (childhood and the elderly). As noted earlier, tetracycline antibiotics should be avoided in children during tooth development to prevent discoloration and enamel hypoplasia of the permanent teeth. Similarly, because fluoroquinolone antimicrobials have been reported to cause erosion of cartilage and arthropathy in juvenile animals, they are generally best avoided in children, unless the condition is serious (e.g., complicated urinary tract infection and pyelonephritis) or there are no suitable effective alternatives.

Pediatric dosing regimens differ from those appropriate for adults. Some agents, such as linezolid, are eliminated much more rapidly in young children (excluding preterm neonates) than in older children and adults, so higher doses (per kilogram of body weight) may be required. In premature infants and neonates, renal function has not yet reached full capacity, and elimination of some antimicrobials may be delayed. Similarly, hepatic clearance activity is not fully developed in the very young, which can affect some drugs (e.g., cardiovascular collapse has been reported with chloramphenicol treatment in neonates). Absorption of oral antimicrobials may also differ with age if their absorption is dependent on gastric pH. The gastric pH of young children is higher than that of adults, and achlorhydria resulting in higher gastric pH is more common in adults older than 60 years than in younger adults. Thus in young children and older adults, the absorption of oral drugs that are unstable in acid, such as penicillin G, may be higher than that in younger adults. In contrast, antimicrobials such as ketoconazole require gastric acid for absorption and may be less bioavailable in persons with reduced gastric acid production.

A curious association between the appearance of a rash and the patient's age and sex was noted during development of the fluoroquinolone antimicrobial gemifloxacin. In clinical studies, rash was more common in young women than in men and older women, suggesting that there may be hormonal influences on the risk for development of a rash.

Renal and Hepatic Function

Renal excretion and hepatobiliary excretion are the major routes of elimination for most antimicrobial agents. Relatively few antibacterial agents can be administered without dosage adjustments in patients with renal dysfunction. Included among these drugs are nafcillin, ceftriaxone, doxycycline, azithromycin, and linezolid.

A number of antimicrobial agents require major dosage adjustments in the presence of renal dysfunction. The dosing interval for ceftazidime, usually administered every 8 hours in patients with normal renal function, is extended to once every 24 to 48 hours in persons with creatinine clearance below 10 mL/minute. Similarly, aminoglycoside dosing requires adjustment with impaired renal function to avoid toxicity. Vancomycin is also administered at substantially increased dosing intervals or at smaller doses as renal function declines. Because of the increased efficiency of newer hemodialysis membranes in removing vancomycin, dosages are usually based on measured serum drug concentrations, and dosing may be required after each dialysis session.

In some instances clearance of the antimicrobial agent is not affected by renal dysfunction, but excipients may accumulate, with the potential for toxic effects. For example, clearance of the antifungal agent voriconazole is not dependent on renal function. However, its intravenous preparation contains the solubilizing agent sulfobutyl ether β-cyclodextrin, which does accumulate in the presence of renal insufficiency. The intravenous preparation should generally be avoided in patients with moderate to severe renal dysfunction, but the oral formulation, which does not contain β-cyclodextrin, can be administered.

A number of other antimicrobials may accumulate in the presence of severe liver disease, with the possibility of an increased risk for adverse events. Antimicrobials requiring dose adjustments for various levels of hepatic insufficiency include metronidazole, chloramphenicol, tigecycline, caspofungin, and voriconazole. For ceftriaxone, dosage adjustments or careful monitoring may be required in patients with both hepatic and renal dysfunction.

Drug-Drug Interactions

One of the most important considerations in the selection of an appropriate antimicrobial regimen is to determine whether the drug(s) will interact with other medications the patient is taking. Some drug-drug interactions can have severe or even fatal consequences. Because there are too many potential interactions to list comprehensively here, clinicians should carefully check for interactions when addition of new antimicrobials is considered. Fortunately, resources are now available that allow the clinician to check for potential drug-drug interactions when an antimicrobial agent is ordered.

Nevertheless, there are some common themes to many drug-drug interactions. For instance, a large number of antimicrobials are eliminated through cytochrome P-450 pathways. As a result, they may interfere with the elimination of other drugs cleared by these pathways, leading to their accumulation to potentially dangerous levels. Several macrolide antibacterials, some fluoroquinolones, and human immunodeficiency virus protease inhibitors are among the most likely antimicrobials to inhibit the clearance of other drugs. For example, use of the protease inhibitor darunavir/ritonavir is contraindicated with several drugs, including ergot derivatives, the neuroleptic drug pimozide, certain sedative-hypnotic agents, and others. Macrolides may result in increased levels of some 3-hydroxy-3-methylglutaryl coenzyme A reductase inhibitors, which can lead to rhabdomyolysis.

In contrast, administration of rifampin induces the cytochrome P-450 system and may enhance the clearance of other drugs, some of which have narrow therapeutic windows. This may result in a number of important effects, including reduced effectiveness of oral contraceptives and increased warfarin requirements to maintain desired levels of anticoagulation. It is important to consider these potential interactions not only when starting rifampin therapy but also when *stopping* treatment. When rifampin is stopped, unless the previously increased dose of warfarin is adjusted downward accordingly, excessive anticoagulation and possibly serious bleeding can occur.

Numerous other drug interactions have been described. For instance, linezolid has weak monoamine oxidase inhibitor activity. As such, it has the potential to enhance the hypertensive effect of adrenergic agonists and has been associated with the development of serotonin syndrome in patients taking serotonergic antidepressants. Patients with this syndrome can exhibit a number of signs and symptoms, including fever, tachycardia, tremulousness, agitation, confusion, and clonus, occasionally with fatal results. Serotonin syndrome (Chapter 406) has been described in patients taking linezolid together with drugs other than selective serotonin reuptake inhibitors; in principle, it could occur when linezolid is combined with any of a large number of agents that increase serotonin concentrations in the central nervous system.

Other Host Factors

Several additional host factors may influence the choice of a suitable antimicrobial regimen. Some antimicrobials have the potential to induce hemolysis in persons with glucose-6-phosphate dehydrogenase deficiency (Chapter 152). Among the drugs that should be avoided in these individuals are primaquine, nitrofurantoin, and various sulfonamides.

Coexisting diseases should also be taken into account. Use of fluoroquinolones or linezolid has been associated with abnormalities in glucose homeostasis. Hyperkalemia has been observed in patients with renal insufficiency during treatment with trimethoprim-sulfamethoxazole because trimethoprim blocks the renal excretion of potassium in the distal tubule.

In some cases the patient's occupation might play a role in the selection of a treatment regimen. Antibiotics that can cause transient (minocycline) or permanent (streptomycin) dizziness or unsteadiness may create hazardous situations in those whose occupations require excellent balance. Antimicrobial agents with the potential to cause photosensitivity, such as tetracyclines, fluoroquinolones, trimethoprim, and sulfonamides, may be problematic in persons with significant sun exposure during outdoor employment or other activities such as travel in tropical areas.

⬤ ANTIMICROBIAL COMBINATIONS

Unfortunately it is often necessary for some hospitalized patients to require more than one antimicrobial agent simultaneously. There are a number of potential reasons for such combination therapy, but all too often the rationale is not always clearly defined or well considered and raises the possibility of potential disadvantages and toxicities, without any clear benefit. Nevertheless, there are a number of definable situations where combination therapy is beneficial; these broadly fall into five categories.

Improved Antimicrobial Spectrum during Empirical Therapy

A common reason for using more than one antimicrobial in hospitalized patients is to provide broader-spectrum therapy against potential pathogens and to maximize the likelihood of delivering an active antimicrobial agent as quickly as possible to seriously ill patients. When the pathogen is unknown, the antimicrobial regimen often includes an agent broadly active against gram-positive bacteria, especially staphylococci (and occasionally enterococci), as well as an agent active against aerobic or facultative gram-negative bacteria. Selection of the latter is strongly influenced by local patterns of antimicrobial resistance specific to the institution and might include an extended-spectrum cephalosporin, an aminoglycoside, a fluoroquinolone, a β-lactam–β-lactamase inhibitor drug, or a carbapenem—all depending on the clinical scenario. If intra-abdominal sepsis is likely, antibiotics with activity against gram-negative anaerobes also need consideration—these include metronidazole, clindamycin, β-lactam–β-lactamase inhibitor agents, and carbapenems. Because of the high frequency of antibiotic resistance in *P. aeruginosa* isolates, in settings in which that pathogen is encountered frequently, empirical use of two agents with antipseudomonal activity may be justified to maximize the likelihood that at least one of the agents will inhibit the organism.

Combination therapy is widely used in the initial treatment of hospitalized patients with community-acquired pneumonia (Chapter 91) to provide treatment for both typical (e.g., pneumococci) and "atypical" (e.g., *Legionella, Mycoplasma*) pathogens. Commonly used regimens include a third-generation cephalosporin such as ceftriaxone plus a macrolide, or occasionally penicillin G plus doxycycline. This cephalosporin provides broader-spectrum activity than penicillin G, including against *S. pneumoniae, Haemophilus influenzae, Moraxella catarrhalis,* and *K. pneumoniae;* but in many situations these latter pathogens are uncommon and penicillin G is adequate. The macrolide azithromycin is commonly added to provide activity against "atypical" bacteria that cause pneumonia, including *M. pneumoniae, C. pneumoniae,* and *Legionella* species. In the United States, but less frequently elsewhere, one of the respiratory fluoroquinolones may be used; however, although fluoroquinolones approved for respiratory tract infections are likely to treat most or all of the organisms targeted by the cephalosporin, isolates of *S. pneumoniae* resistant to fluoroquinolones do exist, so a number of guidelines recommend combination therapy in patients with severe pneumonia requiring hospitalization.

Treatment of Polymicrobial Infections

For many infections from which two or more pathogens are isolated, it is possible to provide adequate therapy with a single, broadly active antimicrobial agent. Switching to a single agent reduces the patient's exposure to potential antibiotic toxicities, is usually more convenient for nursing staff, and may be less expensive. However, in some situations the pathogen susceptibility profiles or patient's allergies to broad-spectrum agents justify the use of antibiotic combinations for the treatment of polymicrobial infections.

Avoidance of Drug Toxicity

In some circumstances the use of antibiotic combinations from different drug classes with additive antimicrobial activities and independent toxicities, each at modest doses, may be of benefit to achieve sufficient potency while avoiding toxicity. However, there are no situations in which subtherapeutic doses should be used. In the present era of rapidly emerging resistance, especially among some gram-negative pathogens, combination therapy is often required to achieve good efficacy while not requiring the use of extremely high doses of an individual toxic agent. In such situations, therapeutic monitoring of serum drug concentrations becomes especially important, so as to achieve the

appropriate tissue concentrations while minimizing toxicity. Thus therapeutic drug monitoring (TDM) is an important emerging field that all clinicians should understand.

Preventing the Emergence of Drug Resistance

The treatment of tuberculosis is a good example of using combinations of drugs to achieve good efficacy while also preventing the emergence of resistance to any one agent. The basis for this approach is that if resistance to two different agents occurs by independent mechanisms, the probability of resistance developing to both drugs is the product of the probability of resistance developing to each drug, which is likely to be very low, so resistance should not emerge.[4] Similar reasoning has justified the use of combination regimens when rifampin is required for the treatment of nonmycobacterial infections. Rifampin is rarely used alone because resistance to this agent can emerge quickly. However, the drug's activity against biofilm-associated bacteria responsible for foreign device infection is such that its combination with another active antimicrobial can be helpful in some circumstances. For example, rifampin plus vancomycin may be useful for coagulase-negative staphylococcal prosthetic valve endocarditis; similarly, rifampin plus a fluoroquinolone (e.g., ciprofloxacin) can be effective for some orthopedic device–related infections.

Despite these limited examples, there are other instances where combination therapy has not proven effective in preventing the emergence of resistance—especially when infections are related to gram-negative pathogens such as *P. aeruginosa* or *Enterobacter* species, which often display multiple resistance mechanisms (Chapter 289). In addition, there may be differential penetration of the two antimicrobials into the infected site or differences in activity at the site of infection, such that adequate concentrations of both agents are not achieved. Thus a more readily penetrating agent may be left relatively unprotected from resistance mechanisms in a "privileged" site of infection. Second, for some pathogens, resistance mechanisms against unrelated antimicrobial classes may not be truly independent. For example, some bacterial efflux pumps recognize chemically unrelated substrates, so upregulation of pump activity may confer resistance to several classes of antimicrobials simultaneously. In other instances, there may be coordinated upregulation of efflux mechanisms and downregulation of outer membrane protein channels (porins), again potentially conferring resistance simultaneously to two or more antimicrobial classes.

Achieving Synergy in Antibacterial Activity

Antibacterial synergy is the phenomenon where the activity of two antibiotics together is greater than the simple sum of each agent's activity alone. A good example of this is the recognition that using penicillin together with an aminoglycoside (e.g., streptomycin, gentamicin) for the treatment of enterococcal endocarditis is more effective than the expected efficacy of each drug individually. Penicillin alone usually inhibits but does not kill enterococci, and failure rates were high when penicillin G was used alone to treat enterococcal endocarditis. Alone, streptomycin has no significant activity against enterococci at clinically relevant concentrations. However, the combination results in bactericidal synergism in vitro and high cure rates in patients with enterococcal endocarditis. Detailed studies of this phenomenon demonstrated that in the presence of a cell wall–active antibiotic, uptake of the aminoglycoside into the bacterial cell increases substantially. Unfortunately, in recent years, increasing rates of high-level resistance to streptomycin (MIC >2000 µg/mL), gentamicin (MIC >500 µg/mL), or both have nullified the benefit of such combinations against a substantial number of enterococcal isolates.

Combinations of cell wall–active agents plus aminoglycosides have been shown to achieve synergistic killing against a broad range of gram-positive and gram-negative bacteria when tested in vitro. However, only in limited clinical scenarios has this in vitro observation translated into meaningful clinical treatment benefits—these include streptococcal and enterococcal endocarditis, where combination therapy is associated with improved cure rates and/or shorter treatment regimens. Modest clinical benefits have been noted when short courses of gentamicin were added to nafcillin for the treatment of *S. aureus* endocarditis, but at the cost of added nephrotoxicity. Against strains of viridans streptococci that are relatively insensitive to penicillin, the addition of an aminoglycoside for the first 2 weeks of a 4-week course of penicillin G can result in a higher likelihood of cure.

Although it was once considered important in the treatment of gram-negative bacterial infections, especially in immunocompromised (e.g., neutropenic) patients, the clinical value of a synergistic combination of a cell wall–active agent and an aminoglycoside has been difficult to prove in recent experience. To a large extent, the introduction of agents with potent activity against gram-negative bacteria has diminished the perceived value of synergistic combinations in such infections. Other examples include the combination of sulfamethoxazole and trimethoprim, where these agents block sequential steps in folic acid synthesis, such that bactericidal (or bacteriostatic) synergism is achieved against a number of important gram-positive and gram-negative pathogens. Similarly, quinupristin and dalfopristin are two streptogramin antibiotics that display bactericidal synergism activity against some gram-positive organisms, and for this reason the two drugs have been formally combined in a single commercial formulation.

β-Lactam–β-lactamase inhibitor antimicrobials represent another example of synergistic combinations. A growing number of such combinations are now available, and common examples include amoxicillin-clavulanate, ampicillin-sulbactam, ticarcillin-clavulanate, piperacillin-tazobactam, ceftazidime-avibactam, and ceftolozane-tazobactam. The β-lactamase inhibitors themselves, clavulanic acid, sulbactam, and tazobactam, lack significant antimicrobial activity; however, by inhibiting common β-lactamases that are sensitive to these agents, the inhibitors restore the activity of the hydrolyzable companion penicillins against many target pathogens elaborating these enzymes.

Rarely, antibiotic combinations can result in microbiologic antagonism, such that the combination may have *reduced* activity compared with the most active single agent of the treatment regimen. For example, antagonistic interactions against *S. aureus* between less bactericidal (linezolid) and more bactericidal (vancomycin) antimicrobials have been demonstrated in vivo in experimental endocarditis. Also, in vitro antagonism can be demonstrated when certain β-lactams are tested in combination against gram-negative bacteria with inducible β-lactamases. Here, exposure to one β-lactam can de-repress the synthesis of inducible β-lactamases, which then degrade the second antibiotic. Fortunately, however, it is uncommon to encounter clinically apparent antagonism between antibiotics in the patient care setting, and this drug interaction rarely needs consideration.

CONSIDERATIONS IN ANTIMICROBIAL ADMINISTRATION

Route of Administration

In almost all instances, antimicrobial therapy for infections of mild to moderate severity that are treated in the outpatient setting can be undertaken with oral agents, because most antimicrobial formulations are well absorbed by the gastrointestinal tract. There are notable exceptions, such as the use of intramuscular injections of benzathine penicillin for the treatment of syphilis or ceftriaxone for the treatment of otitis media or gonorrhea caused by strains resistant to oral agents.

Drugs such as doxycycline, metronidazole, chloramphenicol, some fluoroquinolones (e.g., levofloxacin, moxifloxacin), and linezolid demonstrate virtually complete bioavailability when administered by the oral route in persons with normally functioning gastrointestinal tracts, and they can often be used as an alternative to intravenous therapy in many patients with more serious infections. Even for these well-absorbed antimicrobials, however, treatment of seriously ill patients in the hospital is often initiated with intravenous formulations because of the uncertainty of gastrointestinal tract function under conditions of hemodynamic instability.

Antimicrobial therapy can be administered by other routes, including topical administration for the treatment of infected skin lesions (e.g., mupirocin ointments) and intravaginal administration for candidiasis (e.g., azole creams) or for bacterial vaginosis (e.g., metronidazole gel). Topical administration *onto* the eye is used to treat bacterial conjunctivitis or as adjunctive therapy for deeper infections; administration *into* the globe itself is a component of regimens for the treatment of endophthalmitis. Infections associated with peritoneal dialysis are frequently treated by intraperitoneal instillation of antimicrobials admixed with the dialysis solution. Rarely, direct administration into the thecal space or into the cerebral ventricles is necessary for the treatment of meningitis when the required antimicrobials do not achieve adequate concentrations in cerebrospinal fluid after systemic administration. For the treatment of *Clostridium difficile*–associated diarrhea, vancomycin reaches high concentrations in the intestine when it is given orally, but it is occasionally administered directly into the colon for the intraluminal treatment of severe infections.

Intravenous administration generally has the advantage of greater certainty regarding achieving adequate serum concentrations, but the need for intravenous access and its associated potential complications adds clinical complexity. The availability of long venous catheters, whether inserted centrally or peripherally, has made it possible to provide long-term courses of some antimicrobial agents that are not well absorbed orally. For example, infections

such as endocarditis, osteomyelitis, neuroborreliosis (Lyme disease), and other conditions such as deep abscesses can often be treated as outpatients, generally after an initial period of hospitalization for a full assessment of the infection, initiation of therapy, and stabilization of the medical condition. In addition to monitoring for adverse effects from the antibiotic itself, patients treated via indwelling intravenous devices require close observation for complications related to the catheter, such as thrombophlebitis, entry site infections, or line-related bloodstream infections.

Pharmacodynamic Considerations

The selection of an appropriate dosing regimen depends on both the pharmacokinetic characteristics of antimicrobial agents and their pharmacodynamic properties—namely, the antibiotic's concentrations after dosing, the observed antimicrobial effects against likely pathogens, and the potential adverse effects of the agent. Studies of the pharmacokinetic and pharmacodynamic properties of antimicrobial agents allow the prediction of their activities with various dosing regimens (Chapter 26).

For β-lactam antibiotics, the time during which the concentration of free drug (i.e., the non–protein-bound fraction) exceeds the MIC of the pathogen best relates to antimicrobial effectiveness in animal models. This provides the rationale for the frequent dosing schedules of β-lactams with short half-lives, such as penicillin G and the antistaphylococcal penicillins, and for the use of extended intravenous infusions when β-lactams are used to treat borderline-susceptible organisms.

In contrast, the aminoglycosides and fluoroquinolones demonstrate concentration-dependent killing of bacteria. For these drugs, animal models show that the ratio of either peak concentration to MIC or the area under the 24-hour drug concentration curve (AUC) to MIC better predicts effectiveness. With these agents, less frequent, higher dosing would generally be optimal. For the aminoglycosides, less frequent dosing may also allow more time for washout of the drug from the kidney, thus potentially minimizing the risk for nephrotoxicity.

For drugs such as daptomycin, the absorption of once-daily dosing largely mitigated the muscle toxicity that had been seen with more frequent dosing and allowed the use of this agent for serious gram-positive infections.

MONITORING ANTIMICROBIAL CONCENTRATIONS

Ideally, the concentrations of all antimicrobials should be monitored to ensure adequate therapeutic levels and avoidance of excessively high, potentially toxic concentrations. In practice, however, relatively few drug assays are readily available. Exceptions include commercial assays for the measurement of serum aminoglycoside concentrations, which, because of these agents' great potential for toxicity, are used frequently clinically. Commercial assays to measure vancomycin concentrations are also widely available, with monitoring of serum concentrations particularly important in patients with unstable renal function, those undergoing hemodialysis, patients at the extremes of body composition, or those with particularly serious infections in which high concentrations may be desirable. In some young adults, clearance of vancomycin may be so great that unexpectedly low concentrations result with the usual dosing regimens, hence levels should be monitored.

ADMINISTRATIVE ASPECTS OF ANTIMICROBIAL THERAPY

Formularies

In most practice settings today, the choice of antimicrobials is constrained in some way. For example, in hospitals and other facilities, institutional formularies may limit the choice of available antimicrobial agents, require special approval for the use of selected agents, or both. Such policies can, in principle, enhance efficiency by avoiding the need to stock and to dispense multiple agents with similar antimicrobial activities, minimize costs by allowing purchase of the most cost-effective alternatives, and potentially increase patient safety by encouraging clinical personnel to become familiar with a manageable number of agents. Although two drugs may have antimicrobial spectra that are so similar that only one need be included on a formulary, it is not always safe to assume that the activity of either agent can be predicted perfectly by susceptibility to the other. For example, for most bacterial species, the percentage of isolates susceptible to meropenem and imipenem will be roughly comparable. However, there are differences in mechanisms of resistance to these two carbapenems, so it is possible that a specific strain will be susceptible to one but resistant to the other. For serious infections, even when two drugs are considered interchangeable, one should determine susceptibility to the specific antimicrobial that is to be used. In the outpatient setting, oral agents are generally preferred for their convenience, as well as generally lower cost. In both health care settings, the practitioner must be familiar with the options available to patients under these constraints.

Antimicrobial Stewardship—Appropriate Prescribing to Limit Emergence of Resistance

In contrast to other medications, which almost always affect only the patient receiving them, antimicrobial use can also have a significant impact on the institutional environment and community in terms of overall emergence of resistance.[5] "Antimicrobial stewardship" programs should aim to ensure that the appropriate drug is used for the right indication, at the correct dose, for the correct duration. The purpose of such programs is to manage the use of antimicrobial agents on an administrative level in such a way as to avoid selective pressure leading to the spread of antibiotic resistance (Chapter 266). Antibiotic stewardship programs have been shown to significantly reduce the incidence of infections and colonization with antibiotic-resistant bacteria and *C. difficile* infection in hospital inpatients.[A2,6,7] Within institutions, antimicrobial-resistant organisms not only threaten the patient treated with the antimicrobial but also can be transmitted to other vulnerable persons, including those who have not been exposed to the drug. Such programs should also be interlinked with effective infection control programs to reduce the risk of cross-transmission of resistant strains. On a national and international level, appropriate antimicrobial stewardship can have major effects not only in health care settings,[8] but also on the environment, where high concentrations of antimicrobial-laden waste can have major environmental effects. In the United States and many other countries, more than 50% (in drug tonnage) of all antimicrobial usage is actually in agricultural production where waste control systems are often limited; hence appropriate use of antimicrobials is not simply a health care issue.

Grade A References

A1. Nemeth J, Oesch G, Kuster SP. Bacteriostatic versus bactericidal antibiotics for patients with serious bacterial infections: systematic review and meta-analysis. *J Antimicrob Chemother.* 2015;70:382-395.
A2. Baur D, Gladstone BP, Burkert F, et al. Effect of antibiotic stewardship on the incidence of infection and colonization with antibiotic-resistant bacteria and *Clostridium difficile* infection: a systematic review and meta-analysis. *Lancet Infect Dis.* 2017;17:990-1001.

GENERAL REFERENCES

For the General References and other additional features, please visit Expert Consult at https://expertconsult.inkling.com.

264

APPROACH TO FEVER OR SUSPECTED INFECTION IN THE NORMAL HOST

JAMES E. LEGGETT

We are constantly exposed to microorganisms through our skin or mucous membranes. Most microorganisms are adapted to niches in the environment that make them avirulent to humans or result in only transient or stable colonization. Infection can be defined by invasion of a pathogen that triggers an immune response, whether the infection is asymptomatic or symptomatic. Manifestations of infection are protean and are due as much to our immune response as to the attributes of the particular pathogen.

The inflammatory response that accompanies infection is usually marked by fever. Fever is a tightly controlled elevation in body temperature above the normal range in response to a central nervous system change in the set point. Normal oral temperature in 99% of the population ranges from 36.0° to 37.7° C, with a circadian variation of 1° C or more between the morning nadir and the evening peak. Mean oral temperature in healthy adults is 36.8° ± 0.4° C, with women exhibiting slightly higher values than men (36.9° vs. 36.7° C). Measured rectal temperatures are 0.4° C higher than oral and 0.8° C higher than aural (tympanic membrane) temperatures. Peripheral thermometers lack clinically acceptable accuracy compared with central thermometers.[1] Clinicians generally define significant fever as a temperature higher than 38.3° C (101.0° F). Despite historical claims, fever patterns are not especially helpful in establishing a specific diagnosis.

Acute febrile illnesses lasting less than 2 weeks usually have an infectious cause. These infections occur predominantly where body surfaces interact with the environment, such as the upper and lower respiratory tracts, gastrointestinal and genitourinary systems, and skin. The majority of acute respiratory and gastrointestinal infections are viral in nature. As the duration of the febrile illness lengthens beyond 3 weeks, other inflammatory illnesses become more prominent in the differential diagnosis. Most chronic febrile illnesses are not caused by infection.

● PATHOBIOLOGY OF INFECTION AND FEVER

Infection ensues when a pathogen overcomes innate and adaptive humoral and cellular immune responses. Normal indigenous microflora, host physical barriers (e.g., skin, mucous membranes, cilia), and soluble factors (e.g., cytokines, complement) provide important barricades to pathogen invasion. Disruption of these barriers by invading pathogens prompts adaptive immunity mediated by lymphocytes and macrophages. This inflammatory response plays an important role in containing infection, but an exaggerated response may worsen the clinical condition. A neutrophil response causes the damage seen in septic arthritis, and an unchecked immune response precipitates the systemic inflammatory response syndrome.

Body temperature is regulated both physiologically and behaviorally. Basal metabolic processes, governed by thyroid hormones, catecholamines, and growth hormone, are responsible for the normal resting body temperature. Thermogenesis may be increased up to 80% by hyperthyroidism and decreased as much as 50% by hypothyroidism. Moderate activity results in a transiently increased temperature until heat-dissipating processes are engaged. Each 1° F increase in temperature results in a 7% increase in the basal metabolic rate. Vaporization from the lungs and skin accounts for a third of basal body heat loss and for as much as all heat loss at ambient dry temperatures above 36° C. The elderly have a decrease in basal metabolism as well as blunted responses to thermogenic stimuli, but they have the same average core temperature as young people.

The hypothalamus contains temperature-sensitive neurons whose receptors for pro-inflammatory and anti-inflammatory cytokines maintain a homeothermic set point. Elevated body temperature prompts cutaneous vasodilation and sweating, and people may reduce activity and seek a cooler environment. In contrast, low body temperature prompts shivering, piloerection, cutaneous vasoconstriction, adding clothes, and seeking a warmer environment. Symptoms caused by fever may be due to the underlying disease or to the fever itself. Malaise is the rule, and many febrile patients experience myalgia secondary to the muscle contractions used to generate fever. Although it was once thought that the back and thigh pain related to rigors suggests bacteremia, any febrile stimulus can produce such symptoms. The chill associated with rigors may be related to the surface vasoconstriction that accompanies the increase in core temperature.

A complex physiologic process involving metabolic and immunologic responses produces fever (Fig. 264-1). Exogenous pyrogens cause fever largely mediated by endogenous pro-inflammatory pyrogenic cytokines (produced by phagocytic leukocytes, including interleukin-1, interleukin-6, tumor necrosis factor-α, and interferon-γ) that stimulate the immune responses of T and B cells, macrophages, and polymorphonuclear leukocytes. They activate toll-like receptors to induce prostaglandin synthesis. Feedback inhibitory responses (mediated by adrenocorticotropic hormone, arginine vasopressin, serotonin, dopamine, and other homeostatic mechanisms) emphasize the orchestrated nature of fever production and response to infection. Thermoregulatory mechanisms rarely allow fevers to exceed 41° C (106° F).[2] Temperatures exceeding 41° C are usually due to a drug-induced imbalance in these mechanisms and may cause direct cellular damage.

Failure of fever to develop during severe bacterial infection may be associated with higher morbidity and mortality. Whether this is due to the absence of fever or to associated conditions (e.g., chronic renal failure, corticosteroid use) has not been determined. Favorable effects of fever on host-microbe interactions are suggested by inhibited multiplication of some pathogens (e.g., *Streptococcus pneumoniae* and *Treponema pallidum*), reduced proliferation of pathogens in the presence of hypoferremia, augmented complement-mediated lysis, and increased neutrophil entry into inflammatory sites. Temperature-pulse dissociation,[3] in which there is relative bradycardia compared with the usual increase of 2.44 beats/minute per 1° F, has been described in typhoid

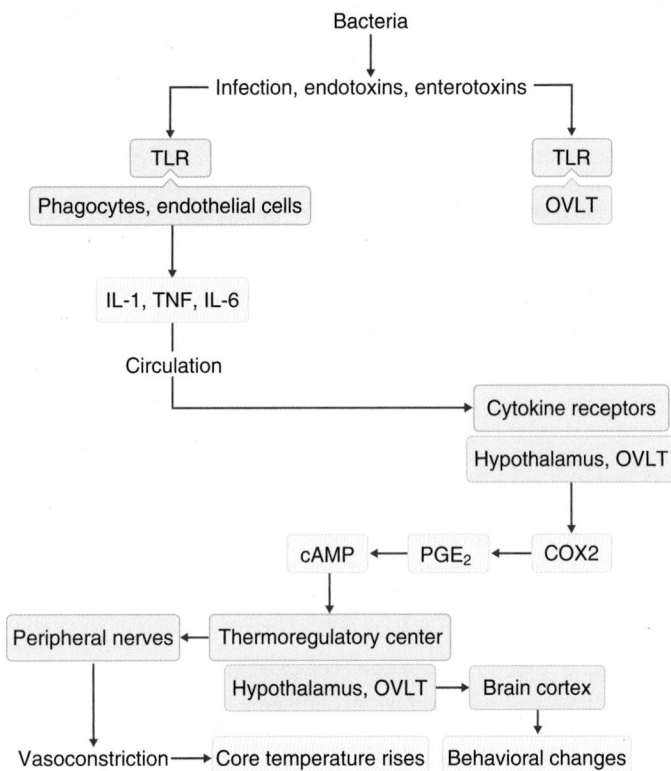

FIGURE 264-1. Pathways leading to the production of fever in bacterial infection, whether local or systemic. Bacteria release cell wall products such as peptidoglycans and endotoxin as well as enterotoxins, which bind to Toll-like receptors (TLRs) on phagocytes (neutrophils, macrophages) and endothelial cells. As a result, pyrogenic cytokines such as interleukin (IL)-1, IL-6, and tumor necrosis factor (TNF)-α are released into the circulation and bind to cytokine receptors in the hypothalamic organum vasculosum of lamina terminalis (OVLT). Bacterial products may also directly bind to TLRs on the OVLT. Activation of TLRs and cytokine receptors induces cyclooxygenase 2 (COX2), which leads to the production of prostaglandin E₂ (PGE₂) and elevates cyclic adenosine monophosphate (cAMP) in the brain. This, in turn, triggers neurons in the thermoregulatory center to raise the hypothalamic thermostatic set point. In addition, neuronal signals to the cortex prompt behavioral changes to conserve heat (e.g., posturing, adding clothing). The hypothalamus also triggers sympathetic peripheral efferent nerves that constrict peripheral blood vessels and conserve central heat until hypothalamic PGE₂ levels fall.

fever, leptospirosis, rickettsiosis, dengue, legionellosis, and babesiosis, for unclear reasons.

No laboratory abnormalities accompany typical benign acute viral infections. Leukocytosis (Chapter 158) of various lineages is usually seen in other infections in immunocompetent adults. Neutrophilia is the norm in most acute infections, whatever the cause. The elderly may not mount a neutrophilic response despite generally displaying bandemia during acute bacterial infection. Neutropenia (Chapter 158) may be seen in rickettsial, severe viral, and overwhelming bacterial infections. Eosinophilia (Chapter 161) is typical of invasive helminthic and some protozoal infections. Lymphocytosis may accompany viral and rickettsial infections and is common during convalescence from acute bacterial infection. Monocytosis may be seen in tuberculosis. Virtually all infections have an impact on the erythroid system. Given the long half-life of erythrocytes, usually only chronic infections or other inflammatory diseases result in anemia (Chapter 149). Few acute infections rapidly produce anemia. For instance, *Helicobacter pylori* may induce a bleeding ulcer, *Babesia* and *Plasmodium falciparum* may directly lyse erythrocytes, overwhelming clostridial and other bacterial infections associated with disseminated intravascular coagulopathy may cause hemolytic anemia, and *Mycoplasma pneumoniae* may induce immunologically mediated hemolysis.

APPROACH TO FEBRILE ILLNESS IN OUTPATIENTS AND INPATIENTS

Infectious disease epidemiology depends on the interaction among pathogens, susceptible hosts, and environmental conditions allowing exposure. Most infections are transmitted horizontally between people by contact (e.g., hands, fomites), a common vehicle (e.g., food, water), air (e.g., tuberculosis), or vectors (e.g., mosquitoes). Evaluation should determine whether the condition might be due to a transmissible agent and its source, whether the patient has done

TABLE 264-1	SELECTED EXAMPLES OF FEVER ASSOCIATED WITH RECENT TRAVEL	
	INCUBATION PERIOD	
DISEASE	**<2-3 WEEKS**	**>3-4 WEEKS**
COMMON		
Dengue	+	
Dysentery	+	
Entamebic liver abscess		+
Enteric fever	+	
Malaria	+	+
Pulmonary tuberculosis		+
Viral hepatitis		+
LESS COMMON		
Ehrlichiosis	+	
Leptospirosis	+	
Schistosomiasis		+
Viral (hemorrhagic, encephalitic)	+	
Visceral leishmaniasis		+

any recent traveling, whether there are secondary causes, and what measures need to be taken to contact health department officials and to prevent additional infections.

The patient's age influences which illnesses should be considered. Natural exposure or immunization generally limits certain illnesses, such as rubeola, rubella, and varicella. Waning of immunity may likewise lead to pertussis or mumps in young adults or reactivation of tuberculosis in the elderly. Other physiologic effects of aging, such as impaired bladder emptying, lead to increased rates of urinary tract infection in the elderly.

A patient's occupation and travel history should be noted. An abattoir worker is more likely to have been exposed to *Brucella* (Chapter 294) than is someone with another occupation. Indiana residents are more likely to be infected with histoplasmosis (Chapter 316), whereas those from the Southwest desert may have coccidioidomycosis (Chapter 316), despite having a similar febrile illness. Many other illnesses are likewise directly related to specific geographic exposure, with varying incubation times before their onset (Chapter 270). Typhoid fever should be manifested within a few weeks, whereas amebic liver abscess might not cause symptoms until months after a traveler's return from an endemic area (Table 264-1). The Centers for Disease Control and Prevention website (http://www.cdc.gov) and many others provide more specific information about prevalent infections in all parts of the world (Chapter 270).

Many travelers return home with fever after a variable incubation time, generally with other symptoms and signs as well. Most infections are unrelated to travel. Once routine infections have been ruled out, the differential diagnosis should include infections related to travel, whether within a region of the United States (e.g., babesiosis, ehrlichiosis, Colorado tick fever, hantavirus) or abroad (e.g., visceral leishmaniasis, tick-borne encephalitis in Europe)[4] (Chapter 270). For example, prompt evaluation of a patient who has traveled to a malaria-endemic area should be undertaken and blood tests performed to determine the presence of parasites.

The setting of febrile illness influences both the diagnostic approach and the differential diagnosis. In the ambulatory arena, with a generally healthy febrile patient, the clinician should not necessarily pursue a diagnosis as aggressively as with a hospitalized or chronically ill patient. Empirical treatment of a presumed urinary tract or respiratory infection is warranted in the outpatient setting, where the cost of a culture or rapid diagnostic test is often more than that of the antibiotic. However, the cost of diagnostic tests in a hospital setting is minimal in comparison to the daily cost of care, and accurate identification of the pathogen may speed hospital discharge. Pathogens commonly causing febrile illness in health care facilities, including nursing homes, may differ from those seen in ambulatory settings. Most patients in the ambulatory setting have noncritical, self-limited infections.

Fevers are usually due to invasive visceral disease, such as community-acquired pneumonia or pyelonephritis, but may be caused by cytomegalovirus. Common viral respiratory and gastroenteric infections as well as some cases of subacute bacterial endocarditis are accompanied by temperatures below 102°F. Moreover, many infections may not be associated with fever, (e.g., Lyme disease, osteomyelitis, and most sexually transmitted diseases). The clinician must always keep in mind that certain infections, such as sexually transmitted diseases (Chapter 269) including syphilis or herpes zoster, occur

TABLE 264-2 SELECTED CAUSES OF HOSPITAL-ASSOCIATED FEVER

COMMON	LESS COMMON
INFECTIOUS	**INFECTIOUS**
Clostridium difficile enterocolitis	Biliary tract disease
Pneumonia	Endometritis
Surgical wound	Intra-abdominal abscess
Urinary tract	Mediastinitis
Vascular catheter	Sinusitis
NONINFECTIOUS	**NONINFECTIOUS**
Drug-induced fever	Adrenal insufficiency
Hematoma	Gout
Immediate postoperative state	Myocardial infarction
Transfusion reaction	Organ infarction
Venous thromboembolism	Pancreatitis

TABLE 264-3 SELECTED INFECTIONS WITH FEVER AND RASH

ETIOLOGY	MACULES, PAPULES	VESICLES, BULLAE	PETECHIAE, PURPURA
BACTERIA			
Borrelia burgdorferi	+ (annular)		
Neisseria meningitidis			+
Rickettsia rickettsii	+		+
Treponema pallidum	+ (secondary)		
Vibrio vulnificus		+	
FUNGI AND MYCOBACTERIA			
Disseminated disease	+ (nodular)		
PROTOZOA			
Plasmodium falciparum			+
VIRUSES			
Chikungunya	+		
Enteroviruses	+	+	+
Epstein-Barr	+		+
Hemorrhagic fever			+
Herpes		+	
HIV	+		
Zika	+		

HIV = human immunodeficiency virus.

normally in immunocompetent hosts and may signal a higher risk for infection with human immunodeficiency virus (HIV) or an already established immunodeficiency.

Fever in Outpatients

In the ambulatory setting, an acutely febrile patient represents a common problem and only infrequently presents an enigmatic diagnostic challenge. In most instances, a febrile illness accompanied by localizing symptoms and signs suggests a specific diagnosis. For instance, leg erythema, pain, and fever in a patient with tinea pedis or a saphenous vein graft incision suggests streptococcal cellulitis.[5] If the patient has had a gradual onset and does not appear toxic, only clinical observation and follow-up are required. If the patient appears toxic, with tachypnea and apprehension or confusion accompanying localized findings, clinically focused diagnostic studies should be performed immediately, and hospitalization should be considered.[6] When a patient has fever and only nonspecific constitutional symptoms, it may be more difficult to address the problem in a single ambulatory clinic visit, requiring a balance between observation and investigation.

Fever in Inpatients

Fever and leukocytosis are the main clinical parameters for evaluating potential infections in hospitalized patients. However, about 10% of nosocomial bacteremias occur without fever, and health care–associated infections occur without fever in patients who are elderly or have significant comorbid conditions. Most cases of hospital-associated fever represent nosocomial infection, which typically involves the lower respiratory tract, urinary tract, or surgical wounds (Table 264-2). Some important causes of nosocomial fever may not exhibit easily discernible localizing symptoms or signs. Antibiotic-induced colitis secondary to *Clostridium difficile* (Chapter 280) is increasing in prevalence and may be characterized by little or no diarrhea. It is the most common cause of a leukemoid reaction in hospitalized patients. Other intra-abdominal processes involving the hepatobiliary system, bowel infarction, viscus perforation, or abscesses may have little in the way of localizing symptoms or signs.

Fever and infection are more frequent in severely ill comorbid patients in the intensive care unit (ICU) than elsewhere.[7] Infection was recently found to be present in more than 80% of febrile ICU patients, although both infectious and noninfectious causes of fever may coexist. Both ischemia and devitalization of tissue provoke an inflammatory response similar to that prompted by infection. About half of patients with acute myocardial infarction, deep vein thrombosis, or pulmonary embolism have a temperature between 38.0° and 38.5° C within 2 to 3 days after diagnosis. A third or more of patients with stroke demonstrate fever, which is also a common consequence of subarachnoid or intracerebral hemorrhage and subdural hematoma, especially within 72 hours of onset.[8] Fever and chills may be seen in up to a quarter of patients receiving platelet transfusions, although the frequency is much less with other blood products.

⬤ SYNDROMIC APPROACH

Fever and Rash

A syndromic approach narrows the many possible causes of a suspected infection. Two juxtaposed approaches are key to recognizing patterns. The clinician must be aware of (1) the differential diagnosis of the particular type of lesion observed and (2) the constellation of findings produced by individual pathogens. The variety of possible manifestations and the often overlapping symptoms and signs illustrate that both elements are key in arriving at a probable diagnosis. Moreover, fever and associated findings, such as exanthem, lymphadenopathy, or jaundice, may be due to noninfectious systemic diseases as well as infectious ones. For instance, leukocytoclastic vasculitis and fever may be found in meningococcemia, Rocky Mountain spotted fever, and hepatitis C, but they are also seen in noninfectious inflammatory diseases. Likewise, fever and adenopathy may be due to lymphoma or to cat-scratch disease.

A recognizable exanthem may lead to the immediate recognition of a particular pathogen (Chapter 412), but often a larger differential diagnosis must be entertained. The clinician must recognize the type or types of skin lesions present, the distribution of the exanthem, and the chronologic progression with respect to the onset of fever and other symptoms (Table 264-3). Morphologic variations in skin lesions help in the differential diagnosis. Maculopapular exanthems are frequently seen in viral illness, hypersensitivity drug reactions, and immune complex–mediated diseases. Erythema multiforme, a subset of maculopapular exanthem, can result from various viral infections or drug eruptions (Chapter 411). It may have a spectrum of disease that ranges from benign to the life-threatening Stevens-Johnson syndrome/toxic epidermal necrolysis complex. Herpes simplex virus is perhaps the most common cause of erythema multiforme. Although drugs, especially antibiotics, are the major precipitating factor in the Stevens-Johnson syndrome/toxic epidermal necrolysis complex, *M. pneumoniae* has been associated with it as well. Evolution of the cutaneous findings over time may give clues to the cause; for example, the initial blanching, erythematous, maculopapular lesions may later evolve into petechiae, as seen in meningococcemia, Rocky Mountain spotted fever, and dengue. Secondary syphilis may be manifested with a multitude of skin lesion morphologies. Sometimes, many different manifestations occur simultaneously in the same patient. Most vesiculobullous skin exanthems are immunologically mediated. The few infections associated with these eruptions include herpes simplex and varicella-zoster viruses and enteroviruses such as echovirus and coxsackievirus. The poxviruses, which can also cause such exanthems, are much rarer or are associated with bioterrorism. Pustules, or vesicles containing leukocytes, are usually associated with psoriasis or infections with *Pseudomonas*, *Staphylococcus*, or *Neisseria*. Bullous exanthems in the presence of sepsis suggest severe streptococcal cellulitis or necrotizing fasciitis, staphylococcal impetigo, or *Vibrio* infections.

Petechial and purpuric eruptions are due to the extravasation of red blood cells and should always lead to consideration of a potentially serious illness. Pathogens creating such lesions most commonly include *Neisseria meningitidis*, *Rickettsia*, and *Capnocytophaga canimorsus*, but these eruptions may be seen with a variety of other pathogens, including *Staphylococcus aureus*, group B streptococci, and other gram-negative bacilli. A petechial exanthem may also

TABLE 264-4	FEVER AND RASH INVOLVING THE PALMS AND SOLES

Erythema multiforme
Hand-foot-and-mouth disease
Neisseria infection
Rocky Mountain spotted fever
Streptobacillus moniliformis infection
Subacute bacterial endocarditis
Syphilis (secondary)
Toxic shock syndrome
Varicella-zoster infection

be seen with enteroviruses and viral hemorrhagic fevers. The most common causes of petechiae not attributable to infections include thrombocytopenia and vasculitis.

The presence of fever and rash involving the palms and soles allows considerable narrowing of the differential diagnosis (Table 264-4). In addition to the diffuse erythema associated with toxic shock syndrome, illnesses such as Rocky Mountain spotted fever, secondary syphilis, hand-foot-and-mouth disease, *Neisseria* infections, and rat-bite fever should be considered in patients with maculopapular exanthems involving these areas.

Nodular skin lesions may be either noninfectious, as seen in malignant disease or with certain drugs (e.g., sulfonamides), or infectious, as seen in a variety of inflammatory diseases. Atypical mycobacteria and disseminated fungi often produce skin nodules. The tender nodules of erythema nodosum usually occur in crops located pretibially, but they may be solitary or occur on other parts of the body. They do not typically suppurate, and they heal without scarring. Infectious agents are the most likely cause of erythema nodosum. Diffuse erythema may be seen with scarlet fever, toxic shock syndrome, Kawasaki disease, Stevens-Johnson syndrome, and toxic epidermal necrolysis, with desquamation occurring late in all these syndromes. Sweet syndrome, a febrile neutrophilic dermatosis, represents a hypersensitivity reaction often preceded by an upper respiratory tract infection.

Fever and Musculoskeletal Complaints

Fever and localized tenderness, swelling, or erythema generally accompany septic arthritis and are often associated with osteomyelitis (Chapter 256). Septic bacterial arthritis in adults usually is manifested acutely and involves a single large joint such as the knee, hip, or shoulder, unless the infection is directly inoculated by trauma or surgery. Septic oligoarthritis may be seen with endocarditis and rat-bite fever. Disseminated gonococcal disease is the usual cause of arthritis involving small joints of the wrist, ankle, and digits, often with tenosynovitis. Acute or subacute polyarthritis may be seen in several viral diseases, including chikungunya, dengue, parvovirus B19, hepatitis B, and Lyme disease. Hematogenous osteomyelitis in adults frequently involves the vertebrae and is almost always initiated by discitis with symmetrical involvement of vertical adjacent vertebrae (as opposed to malignant metastasis, which is asymmetrical and does not involve the disc).

Myositis secondary to clostridia, streptococci, or mixed aerobic-anaerobic infections usually causes an acutely septic picture with painful, edematous involvement of the limb or torso. Pyomyositis frequently involves deep muscles such as the psoas or gluteus and is usually due to *S. aureus*. Diffuse myositis may be seen with leptospirosis or toxoplasmosis, and rhabdomyolysis occurs with a variety of viral infections and legionellosis.

Fever and Lymphadenopathy or Hepatosplenomegaly

Fever and lymphadenopathy suggest a variety of illnesses, both infectious and noninfectious (Table 264-5). Lymphadenopathy (Chapter 159) may be regional or generalized. Local enlargement can occur with either a local infection or some systemic illnesses (e.g., posterior cervical lymphadenopathy with Epstein-Barr virus and other viral illnesses). Generalized lymphadenopathy suggests a systemic disorder, which may itself be either infectious or noninfectious. The combination of fever and lymphadenopathy secondary to infection is especially common during childhood, but it is also seen in adults. As in other syndromes, acute versus chronic adenopathy tilts the diagnosis toward different broad categories of illness. In chronic adenopathy, histopathologic evaluation of enlarged lymph nodes may point to a particular diagnosis. For instance, toxoplasmosis or cat-scratch disease can be easily differentiated from mycobacterial disease or sarcoidosis.

TABLE 264-5	COMMON CAUSES OF FEVER AND LYMPHADENOPATHY	
REGIONAL		**GENERALIZED**
Cervical		Cytomegalovirus
Streptococci		Epstein-Barr virus
Tuberculosis		HIV
Viral upper respiratory tract infection		Lymphoma
Peripheral		Sarcoidosis
Bartonella henselae		Syphilis (secondary)
Herpesviruses		Toxoplasmosis
Lymphoma		Viral hepatitis
Metastatic cancer		
Sporotrichosis		
Streptococci		
Inguinal		
Chancroid		
Herpes		
Lymphogranuloma venereum		
Syphilis (primary)		

HIV = human immunodeficiency virus.

TABLE 264-6	COMMON INFECTIOUS CAUSES OF FEVER AND JAUNDICE

Bacterial sepsis
Cholangitis
Hepatic abscess
Leptospirosis
Malaria
Viral hepatitis
Yellow fever

Fever and hepatosplenomegaly (Chapter 159) may provide an important clue to the cause of a febrile illness, which is typically either an infection or a malignant neoplasm arising from bone marrow or the reticuloendothelial system. Jaundice may also limit the differential diagnosis (Table 264-6). Aside from the viral hepatitides and other diseases affecting primarily the liver, many pathogens producing sepsis can cause hyperbilirubinemia.

APPROACH TO FEVER OF UNKNOWN ORIGIN

The majority of febrile illnesses are short-lived, but fever may persist for weeks or months as part of an infectious disease, inflammatory disorder, or occult neoplasm. When fever is caused by infection, the site is an area not easily controlled by host defenses, leading to the continued release of inflammatory cytokines. Likewise, macrophage and lymphocyte involvement in inflammatory disorders causes persistent cytokine production, as do certain neoplasms. Given this final common pathway, it is easy to understand why the majority of cases of classic fever of unknown origin (FUO), loosely defined as lasting longer than 3 weeks despite routine investigation, are found in these three broad categories.[9] Miscellaneous and undiagnosed illnesses round out the bulk of FUO cases (Table 264-7). The proportion of patients in each category varies by geographic locale, age, duration of fever, and immune status. As more effective molecular diagnostic methods of diagnosing viral and bacterial infections have become available, the proportion of patients with FUO in the miscellaneous and undiagnosed categories has increased to about a third of the total in developed countries. The longer a febrile illness persists without a diagnosis or appropriate therapy, the less likely it is to be due to an infection.

Bacterial species, particularly *Mycobacterium tuberculosis*, make up the largest category of infections that cause prolonged FUO. Other infections causing FUO may be localized in cryptic abscesses, especially intra-abdominally, or reside on heart valves, where the inflammatory response is blunted. Persistent viral infections constitute a small and shrinking subset of patients with FUO because modern techniques can more readily detect multiple viral infections including Epstein-Barr virus, cytomegalovirus, and others. Cytomegalovirus is the most common cause of mononucleosis in adults, and malaria is a common cause of fever in returning travelers.

Malignant disease may result in persistent fever due to the production of inflammatory cytokines, necrosis, or the presence of a complicating infection.

TABLE 264-7 FREQUENCY OF SELECTED CHRONIC FEBRILE ILLNESSES

INFECTION, 25-50%	MALIGNANT DISEASE, 20-30%	CONNECTIVE TISSUE DISEASE, 15-30%	MISCELLANEOUS, 10-20%	UNDIAGNOSED, 10-30%
Cytomegalovirus	Carcinomatosis	Polyarteritis nodosa	Drug-induced fever	
Endocarditis	Leukemia	Rheumatoid arthritis	Granulomatous hepatitis	
Intra-abdominal	Local tumor	Still disease	Inflammatory bowel disease	
Mycoses	Lymphoma	Systemic lupus erythematosus	Pancreatitis	
Occult abscess		Temporal arteritis	Pulmonary embolism	
Tuberculosis				

Malignant neoplasms manifesting as FUO include lymphomas, leukemias, and solid tumors with metastases to the liver. Connective tissue disorders may produce fever as a prominent feature of the illness, including adult Still disease (Chapter 245), the leading rheumatologic disorder manifesting as FUO. Temporal arteritis and polymyalgia rheumatica (Chapter 255) are seen almost exclusively in patients older than 50 years. Systemic lupus erythematosus (Chapter 250) is an occasional cause of FUO.

The miscellaneous category of FUO includes several disparate groups of diseases. Granulomatous diseases such as granulomatous hepatitis, Crohn disease, or sarcoidosis may incite cellular immune responses that result in fever. Granulomatous hepatitis was present in up to 6% of National Institutes of Health cases with fever lasting longer than 6 months. Chronic pancreatitis may occasionally cause FUO, as may recurrent pulmonary embolism.

Drug-induced fever (Table 264-8) may be the only manifestation of an adverse drug event in up to 5% of cases of drug hypersensitivity. The mechanisms by which drugs incite fever are not well understood in many cases. These events may result from hypersensitivity reactions, altered thermoregulatory homeostasis directly related to either drug administration or the drug's pharmacologic action, or idiosyncratic reactions. Hypersensitivity reactions usually cause an exanthem or enanthem and possible hepatic, renal, or pulmonary dysfunction in addition to fever. Antimicrobial agents appear to be the most common cause of drug-induced fever and are responsible for approximately a third of episodes in some studies. β-Lactams and sulfonamides account for most cases; they are also the most frequently administered antimicrobials. Anticonvulsants also commonly cause drug-induced fever. Altered thermoregulation is possible with a variety of drugs, including those with anticholinergic activity, such as phenothiazines and tricyclic antidepressants. Sympathomimetic agents, such as amphetamines and cocaine, may also cause fever. Drug administration itself may cause fever if the vehicle of the drug is contaminated with exogenous pyrogens or chemical phlebitis occurs. Some drugs have intrinsic pyrogenic properties, such as amphotericin B and bleomycin. Others cause fever as a result of their pharmacologic activity, such as interferon alfa or interleukin-2. With antibiotics, a form of drug-induced fever occurs with the rapid lysis of spirochetes or other bacteria, known as the Jarisch-Herxheimer reaction. Idiosyncratic drug-induced febrile reactions include malignant hyperthermia, neuroleptic malignant syndrome, and serotonin syndrome (Chapter 406). Drugs implicated in these reactions are inhaled anesthetic agents, central nervous system dopamine-depleting agents, and serotonin re-uptake inhibitors, among others. Drug-induced fever is a diagnosis of exclusion. The duration of drug exposure before the onset of fever, the clinical appearance of the patient, and the pattern of the fever are not particularly useful. Elimination of a single drug at a time, beginning with the one most likely to be implicated, is the usual means of identifying the causative agent. The fever abates once the drug has been eliminated from the body, usually within 3 to 4 days of discontinuing use of the drug.

In approaching a patient with fever of unknown origin, laboratory evaluation and diagnostic imaging studies should be chosen according to information derived from a detailed history and physical examination. These may initially include complete blood count and blood chemistry determinations, erythrocyte sedimentation rate or C-reactive protein, blood cultures, ferritin and antibody tests (antinuclear antibody, cytomegalovirus, Epstein-Barr virus, HIV), as well as a chest radiograph and computed tomography of the abdomen. 18-Fluoro-2-deoxy-D-glucose positron emission tomography (FDG-PET) may also be useful in difficult cases.[10-12] Despite the recent focus on "emerging" infectious diseases, the cause of FUO is still more likely to be a common pathogen presenting atypically.

TABLE 264-8 SELECTED AGENTS ASSOCIATED WITH DRUG-INDUCED FEVER

COMMON	LESS COMMON
ANTIMICROBIAL	
Amphotericin B	Clindamycin
β-Lactams	Fluoroquinolones
Sulfonamides	Rifampin
CARDIOVASCULAR	
Procainamide	Diltiazem
Quinidine	Hydralazine
CENTRAL NERVOUS SYSTEM	
Carbamazepine	Haloperidol
Phenytoin	Serotonin re-uptake inhibitors
MISCELLANEOUS	
Bleomycin	Allopurinol
Interferon alfa	Cimetidine
Interleukin-2	Tacrolimus

INITIAL MANAGEMENT OF SUSPECTED INFECTION IN THE AMBULATORY SETTING

An acutely febrile patient in the ambulatory setting presents a common but often demanding diagnostic problem. In most cases, the history and physical examination reveal diagnostic clues and may guide decisions about additional studies or therapy. More difficult to diagnose is a fever that occurs without localizing symptoms or is accompanied only by nonspecific symptoms, such as malaise or anorexia. Fortunately, most acute, undifferentiated febrile illnesses are benign and resolve spontaneously within 1 or 2 weeks without a specific diagnosis being made. In such cases, no further evaluation beyond the initial visit is warranted. If symptoms persist, the history and physical examination should be repeated, looking for previously unsought clues and new physical findings. Laboratory studies might be required.[13]

In patients with an illness involving cough of less than 3 weeks' duration, the evaluation should focus on ruling out a serious disorder. Normal vital signs and chest examination effectively rule out most cases of pneumonia. Such cough illnesses are caused by viral pathogens in more than 90% of cases. Antibiotics are ineffective in such patients, nor does antimicrobial therapy prevent bacterial pneumonia. The presence of sputum and its characteristics are not helpful in distinguishing bacterial from viral infections. Adults with prolonged coughing lasting longer than 3 weeks or with recurrent episodes should be evaluated for reactive airway disease, gastroesophageal reflux, and other illnesses. Infections rarely causing prolonged cough include *Bordetella pertussis*, *M. pneumoniae*, and *Chlamydophila pneumoniae*. Clinicians in this case should obtain a chest radiograph; treat for exacerbation of chronic obstructive pulmonary disease (fever, leukocytosis, purulent sputum), if present; treat a confirmed bacterial infection (Chapter 90); and direct therapy to a specific underlying cause or other causes.

Symptoms and signs of pharyngitis include fever, tonsillar exudates, tender anterior cervical lymph nodes, and absence of cough. If fewer than two of these criteria are present, the patient should be managed as though viral pharyngitis were the cause. Ninety percent of cases of pharyngitis in adults are viral in origin. With two or more of these criteria, one should consider obtaining a rapid streptococcal antigen test.[14] Because of the low incidence of streptococcal infection and acute rheumatic fever in adults, a negative rapid test result alone is sufficient to rule out infection with *Streptococcus pyogenes*. If the antigen test result is positive, the patient can be managed with a β-lactam antibiotic if not allergic. In a patient with symptoms of upper respiratory tract infection and a mucopurulent nasal discharge of less than 10 days' duration, purulent nasal secretions do not predict bacterial infection. Most cases of acute rhinosinusitis seen in the outpatient setting are caused by uncomplicated upper respiratory viral infection.[A1] If symptoms have been present for more than 10 days without improvement, or if there are specific symptoms of sinusitis of any duration (purulent nasal discharge lasting 3 to 4 days, unilateral facial pain and pressure, maxillary toothache, or worsening of symptoms after initial improvement), amoxicillin or another β-lactam should be considered, with other antimicrobial classes used in penicillin-allergic patients. Most clinical outcomes are not adversely affected by delayed antibiotics for upper respiratory infections.[A2]

Community-acquired pneumonia (Chapter 91) should be suspected in a patient with cough, sputum production, or dyspnea, especially if it is accompanied by fever and altered breath sounds. A chest radiograph should be performed to confirm the diagnosis. Determining where to care for the patient is the most important immediate decision. Outpatient care generally suffices for patients younger than 50 years with no cardiopulmonary disease; for patients with no comorbid conditions (including malignant disease, heart failure, diabetes, or hospitalization within the past year); and for patients with no physical examination findings, such as altered mental status, pulse of 125 beats/minute or greater, or respiratory rate of 30/minute or greater. Guidelines developed by the American Thoracic Society and the Infectious Diseases Society of America suggest a β-lactam, macrolide, or doxycycline. Among patients admitted to a non-ICU setting with clinically suspected community-acquired pneumonia, empirical β-lactam monotherapy is as good as β-lactam-macrolide combination therapy or fluoroquinolone monotherapy.[A3] Fluoroquinolones should be used for outpatients only when the patient has failed to respond to first-line therapy, has a significant comorbidity, or has a known allergy to a first-line agent.

Skin and soft tissue infections are caused, for the most part, by streptococci; a minority are due to *S. aureus* and, rarely, other bacteria whose presence may be suggested by epidemiologic considerations (e.g., swimming in fresh water, where *Aeromonas* may be the pathogen). Pain may be present for 12 hours or more before skin discoloration is noted. A furuncle or abscess formation should prompt consideration of *S. aureus* and, rarely, *Streptococcus anginosus* group. Incision and drainage may be sufficient for a skin abscess, although the rapidly expanding, virulent, community-acquired methicillin-resistant *S. aureus* phenotype may require antimicrobial therapy. Septic bursitis is nearly always due to *S. aureus*, and the infected bursa should be aspirated and drained, in addition to using antibiotics (Chapter 256).

Gastrointestinal infections may be due to ingested toxins, viruses, or, less commonly, bacteria, with or without associated toxin production. The appropriate approach depends on the epidemiologic setting, such as improper food storage, travel abroad, or contact with another ill person (Chapter 267). Symptoms of cystitis in a young, sexually active woman can be treated with empirical antibiotics, but when fever and flank pain are present and the patient is nauseated, consideration of a brief hospital admission or an initial intravenous dose of antibiotics may be necessary (Chapter 268). The possibility of pelvic inflammatory disease should also be entertained.

In the initial evaluation of a patient with a more chronic, persistent fever, a careful history and physical examination provide important diagnostic clues, directing further investigation. The initial goal is to characterize the illness accurately, in addition to eliciting important host and epidemiologic factors. A careful review of systems is necessary to understand the extent of involvement of various organ systems as well as to note previous medical conditions. The examination should be broader than for an acute febrile illness with localizing symptoms and signs. Laboratory tests may also play a more important role in guiding further investigation. Repeated evaluations are the norm rather than the exception in these cases.

Blindly initiating empirical therapy in febrile patients with no imminent risk of serious clinical harm or death should be discouraged because it may impede a timely diagnosis affording definitive care. Procalcitonin, which is a precursor of calcitonin, is an acute phase reactant that is more likely to be elevated with bacterial than with viral infections, and its use may reduce unnecessary antibiotics in some situations, such as patients with respiratory infections.[A4] However, procalcitonin distinguishes sepsis from nonseptic systemic inflammation poorly (71% sensitivity, 71% specificity, receiver operating characteristic curve 0.63), and it appears to be less useful in such

settings.[A5] Rapid multiplex polymerase chain reaction with templated comments from the laboratory can reduce treatment of blood culture contaminants and use of broad-spectrum antimicrobials.[A6]

● INITIAL MANAGEMENT OF SUSPECTED NOSOCOMIAL INFECTION

Determination of the nature of a febrile illness in a hospitalized patient must consider the host, the setting, and the timing of recent trauma or type and duration of surgery, in addition to the general approach taken for ambulatory patients. A classic mnemonic—the six *w*'s—may help guide the evaluation: wind, water, wound, walk, wonder drug, and what we did. "Wind" refers to fever within the first 24 hours of surgery, a fever is often thought to be related to the anesthetic agent, or surgical trauma. The only bacteria believed to cause significant infections within 24 hours of surgery are *S. pyogenes* and *Clostridium* species, both of which are unusual in the typical hospital patient. "Water" refers to a urinary tract infection occurring after the third day of urinary tract catheterization. Because nearly all nosocomial urinary tract infections occur in patients with indwelling urinary catheters or in those who have undergone urologic instrumentation, urinalysis or culture (or both) should be performed routinely only in febrile patients with such risk factors. There is a high prevalence of bacteriuria in patients who have been catheterized for 3 days or longer, and there is a low incidence of true infection attributable to bacteriuria. "Wound" infections commonly occur about 5 to 7 days postoperatively, whether they are surface wounds or complications of dehiscence of gastrointestinal anastomoses. Some of the highest rates of skin and soft tissue infections in the National Nosocomial Infection Surveillance database are seen with gastrointestinal procedures. Toxin-producing *C. difficile* is the only significant nosocomial gastrointestinal infection seen in hospitalized patients, so a routine bacterial stool culture is not necessary. "Walk" refers to possible deep venous thrombosis or pulmonary embolism in someone who has not received appropriate prophylaxis or who is otherwise at risk for thrombosis. Fever induced by a "wonder drug" is typically seen after approximately 7 to 10 days of use if the patient does not already have an allergy to that medication, in which case it recurs immediately. An exception to this rule is sulfamethoxazole, for which approximately half of hypersensitivity reactions occur within 3 days of initiation. Finally, "what we did" alerts the clinician to the possibility of an iatrogenic infection, such as intravenous catheter–related bacteremia.

● CONCLUSION

The initial management of patients with febrile illnesses requires three major considerations. First, is the illness more likely to be infectious or more likely to be related to some other process? Excessive antibiotic use when it is not warranted, such as for viral infections or collagen vascular disease, may cause an adverse reaction, in addition to contributing to the worldwide increase in antimicrobial resistance. However, an empirical antibiotic is appropriate in many cases of fever and localizing signs of bacterial infection. Second, the clinician must rapidly assess the severity of the illness and determine whether it is likely to cause significant organ damage or even death. In a febrile patient with signs of sepsis, the clinician must quickly decide which specific therapy is indicated because a delay in initiating antimicrobial therapy is correlated with increased morbidity and mortality. Finally, the clinician needs to determine whether supportive care alone, including antipyretic therapy, is warranted.

The nearly universal prevalence of febrile adaptive responses to microbial challenge suggests that fever has a net benefit to the host. In addition to clinical studies correlating elevated core temperature and improved prognosis during infection, investigations of principal endogenous mediators have provided evidence of a protective effect of pyrogenic cytokines. Although the use of antipyretic medications is a long-established and widespread practice, the actual benefit of temperature reduction in febrile patients is uncertain. Antipyretic therapy does not protect against the recurrence of childhood febrile seizures, nor has its risk-benefit ratio been determined in patients with cardiopulmonary and other underlying disorders. In summary, fever is usually not harmful, and antipyretics may confuse the clinical picture by dampening it, although their anti-inflammatory effects are often beneficial.[A7]

ᴳ°ᵃᵈᵉ Ⓐ Grade A References

A1. Lemiengre MB, van Driel ML, Merenstein D, et al. Antibiotics for clinically diagnosed acute rhinosinusitis in adults. *Cochrane Database Syst Rev.* 2012;10:CD006089.
A2. Spurling GK, Del Mar CB, Dooley L, et al. Delayed antibiotic prescriptions for respiratory infections. *Cochrane Database Syst Rev.* 2017;9:CD004417.

A3. Postma DF, van Werkhoven CH, van Elden LJ, et al. Antibiotic treatment strategies for community-acquired pneumonia in adults. *N Engl J Med.* 2015;372:1312-1323.

A4. Huang DT, Yealy DM, Filbin MR, et al. Procalcitonin-guided use of antibiotics for lower respiratory tract infection. *N Engl J Med.* 2018;379:236-249.

A5. Andriolo BN, Andriolo RB, Salomao R, et al. Effectiveness and safety of procalcitonin evaluation for reducing mortality in adults with sepsis, severe sepsis or septic shock. *Cochrane Database Syst Rev.* 2017;1:CD010959.

A6. Banerjee R, Teng CB, Cunningham SA, et al. Randomized trial of rapid multiplex polymerase chain reaction-based blood culture identification and susceptibility testing. *Clin Infect Dis.* 2015;61:1071-1080.

A7. Jefferies S, Weatherall M, Young P, et al. The effect of antipyretic medications on mortality in critically ill patients with infection: a systematic review and meta-analysis. *Crit Care Resusc.* 2011;13:125-131.

GENERAL REFERENCES

For the General References and other additional features, please visit Expert Consult at https://expertconsult.inkling.com.

265

APPROACH TO FEVER AND SUSPECTED INFECTION IN THE IMMUNOCOMPROMISED HOST

COSTI D. SIFRI AND KIEREN A. MARR

DEFINITION

Healthy individuals possess robust antimicrobial defense systems that include physical barriers in the form of skin and mucosal membranes, innate immune defenses that are conserved through evolution, and adaptive ("acquired") immune defense (Chapters 39 and 40). These systems are highly interconnected and work in concert through an array of defensive surfaces, cells, and soluble factors to protect a host from potential microbial assailants. The normal commensal microflora of the skin and mucosa protect the host by occupying body surface niches without activating the immune system and play an important role in immune system maturation and homeostasis. Nutritional status, multiorgan function, and age all contribute to normal immune function. Damage to any of these host defense components increases the risk for infection. While a wide assortment of conditions, including body surface burns, endocrine and metabolic disorders, and medications like glucocorticoids, can affect components of these defense systems and place an individual at increased risk for infection, the focus of this chapter will be on people with compromised immune systems due to treatment of neoplastic disease (with particular attention to hematologic disorders such as leukemia and lymphoma), recipients of solid organ or hematopoietic stem cell transplants, and those who take immunomodulatory medications for collagen vascular (immunologic) and rheumatologic conditions. Management of people with the acquired immunodeficiency syndrome (AIDS) is discussed in Chapter 364 and 365, and a more thorough discussion of primary immunodeficiency is provided in Chapter 236.

GENERAL CONCEPTS

The components of the immune system and other host defense mechanisms are represented in Table 265-1. The innate immune system is ancient (with origins that date back to the early single cell eukaryotes) and serves as the first line of host defense against pathogen attack. Components of the innate immune system include natural physical and chemical barriers, phagocytic cells, and germline-encoded signaling systems that recognize molecular components unique to microbes that are invariant because they are essential for survival of the microbe. These signaling systems rapidly (minutes to hours) distinguish "nonself" from "self," leading to the activation of protective phagocytic cells, proteolytic enzyme cascades, and antimicrobial peptides and other products (Chapter 39). The innate immune system also primes the adaptive immune system, which is more recent in evolutionary origin and is distinguished by the ability to create pathogen-specific responses and immunologic memory over several days. Like the innate immune system, the adaptive immune system is composed of both cellular and soluble factors (Chapter 40).

The risk for infection depends on the specific type of defect in host defenses. For example, impaired macrophage function as a consequence of tumor necrosis

TABLE 265-1 COMPONENTS OF THE IMMUNE SYSTEM

INNATE IMMUNE SYSTEM (IMMEDIATE, NON–PATHOGEN SPECIFIC, EVOLUTIONARILY ANCIENT, NO MEMORY)

Physical defense mechanisms	Skin
	Mucous membranes (e.g., oral mucosa, olfactory mucosa, gastric mucosa, intestinal mucosa, bronchial mucosa, genitourinary mucosa)
	Tears
	Mucus
	Ciliated respiratory epithelium
	Urine flow
Innate soluble and cellular defense mechanisms	Stomach acid
	Complement cascade
	Phagocytes (i.e., neutrophils, macrophages, dendritic cells)
	Mannose binding lectin
	Toll-like and Nod receptors
	Cytokines (e.g., IL-1, IL-4, IL-5, IL-6, IL-8, IL-10, IL-12, G-CSF, TNF-α, IFN-γ)
	Natural antimicrobial products (e.g., defensins, lactoferrin, lysozyme, reactive oxygen species)

ADAPTIVE IMMUNE SYSTEM (DELAYED, PATHOGEN SPECIFIC, EVOLUTIONARY ORIGIN WITH JAWED VERTEBRATES [~0.5 BILLION YEARS], MEMORY)

Cellular Adaptive Immune System	T lymphocytes
	• CD8$^+$ (cytotoxic)
	• CD4$^+$ (helper)
	• Γδ (alternative TCRs)
Humoral adaptive immune system	B lymphocytes
	• Immunoglobulins (IgM, IgG, IgA, IgE, IgD antibodies)

EFFECTORS OF IMMUNE FUNCTION

Effector	Resident microbial flora
	Organ function
	Age
	Stress
	Nutrition
	Metabolic homeostasis (e.g., pH, iron, uremia)

G-CSF = granulocyte colony-stimulating factor; IFN-γ = interferon-γ; IL = interleukin; TNF-α = tumor necrosis factor-α.

factor (TNF) therapy is a predisposing risk for infection due to intracellular pathogens such as *Mycobacterium tuberculosis* and *Histoplasma capsulatum*, while splenectomy and functional asplenism predispose to sepsis due to encapsulated bacteria, including pneumococcus and meningococcus. Detailed understanding of the nature of compromised host defense mechanisms and how the defect influences susceptibility to potential viral, bacterial, fungal, and parasitic pathogens allows one to pursue appropriate diagnostic evaluations, therapies, and prevention strategies (through vaccination, antimicrobial prophylaxis, pre-emptive monitoring, and lifestyle changes).

Determining whether an immunocompromised individual has a clinically significant infectious disease can be challenging. Several factors make it more difficult to identify infectious disease in individuals with compromised immune defenses. Potential etiologies of infection are diverse and range from typical, community-acquired pathogens to less common, opportunistic pathogens. Signs of inflammation, including fever, pain, and erythema, may be reduced, and laboratory markers of infection, such as changes in the white blood cell count and hepatic transaminase levels, may be subtle or difficult to interpret owing to the influence of baseline noninfectious processes (e.g., medications, organ dysfunction). Radiographic findings may also be blunted. Accordingly, infection may be advanced at the time of presentation. Furthermore, multiple infections or processes may occur simultaneously. Diagnosis can be challenging because serologic testing may not be useful. However, recent advances in the development and adoption of molecular diagnostic assays by clinical microbiology laboratories have proved especially useful tools in immunocompromised patients. Finally, numerous noninfectious causes of fever, including neoplastic disease, collagen vascular disease, allograft rejection, graft-versus-host disease, and medications (e.g., antibiotic-induced fever, cytokine release syndromes following monoclonal antibody therapies) may cause febrile illness that is indistinguishable from infectious processes. Consequently, significant and expedited efforts should be made to establish the etiology of fevers in a compromised host; invasive procedures, such as imaging guided biopsy, endoscopic procedures, and surgery may be required to establish a diagnosis.

APPROACH TO THE PATIENT

Broadly speaking, the factors that predispose immunocompromised patients to infection can be divided into two categories: intrinsic host factors as a consequence of illness and factors associated with medical treatment. Intrinsic host factors include underlying immunodeficiencies, medical comorbidities, past infections, metabolic derangements, and poor nutritional status. For patients with cancer, mechanical obstruction from tumors can predispose to organ dysfunction, infection, and abscess formation. Tumors of the head and neck, respiratory track, gastrointestinal tract, and female genitourinary tract predispose to infections in and adjacent to those anatomic spaces. Patients with chronic progressive organ dysfunction and failure are predisposed to infection as a consequence of their illness. Structural lung problems, such as cavitary lung disease, are a risk for colonization and superinfection by *Aspergillus* and nontuberculous mycobacteria. Progressive respiratory failure predisposes persons to pneumonia due to community-associated, healthcare-associated, and opportunistic pathogens. Progressive liver failure predisposes to fungal infections, including cryptococcosis. Immunodeficiency as a direct consequence of acquired immune system disorders, such as hematologic malignancies or bone marrow infiltration by metastasis of solid tumors, adds another layer of infection risk.

Medical treatment is the other major consideration that influences the risk for infection. Radiation therapy and cytotoxic chemotherapy of malignant disease directly or indirectly target cells of the immune system, leading to significant risk for infection. Physical and natural barriers, such as skin, mucosal membranes, uroepithelium, and ciliated respiratory epithelium, may be injured or impaired as a consequence of disease or treatment. Surgery and medical devices, such as central venous catheters, indwelling bladder catheters, and circulatory support devices, among others, predispose to infections from a range of nosocomial pathogens, including *Staphylococcus aureus*, coagulase negative staphylococci, the enterococci, enteric gram-negative bacteria, *Pseudomonas aeruginosa*, other multidrug-resistant gram-negative bacteria, and *Candida*. Bleeding and organ space collections such as urinomas and bilomas may become seeded and infected after surgery. Repeated surgery is a risk for both organ transplant recipients and patients with solid tumors. Patients with primary or metastatic lung cancer are susceptible to recurrent pneumonia. Patients with head and neck cancer and brain cancer are predisposed to aspiration pneumonitis and pneumonia. The use of immunosuppressive medications following allogeneic hematopoietic cell or organ transplantation is obviously a risk factor. The consequences of prior infections, empirical antibiotics, and treatment of infections lead to unbalanced changes in the composition of the gastrointestinal microbiome (termed *dysbiosis*) that may reduce barriers to colonization with drug-resistant pathogens and alter infection risk.

The approach to the immunosuppressed patient requires detailed information about the nature of the immunodeficiency and known related risks.[1] Table 265-2 outlines the specific immune defects in host responses that are associated with the types of conditions that characterize categories of medically immunosuppressed patients, including underlying condition and intervention. Especially in light of the great expansion of classes of immunomodulatory interventions currently available, knowledge of prior therapies received has become critically important in developing an informed approach to the compromised patient with suspected infection.

Patients with Neoplastic Disease

In patients with malignancies, the underlying condition contributes importantly to determining infectious risks. For example, absolute neutropenia or leukocyte dysfunction occurs in the setting of specific malignancies (e.g., acute or chronic leukemias). In such cases, the risk for bacterial infections is enhanced, even in the absence of chemotherapy. In other underlying conditions, such as chronic lymphocytic leukemia, there are frequently quantitative defects in humoral host defense products, such as decreased immunoglobulins and components of the complement cascade that are bactericidal. Other types of phagocytic cells include circulating monocytes and tissue macrophages, the fixed mononuclear cells of the reticuloendothelial system. These cells normally collaborate with helper T lymphocytes in defense against intracellular pathogens, such as mycobacteria, fungi, and some viruses and parasites. The spectrum of

---

TABLE 265-2 CONDITIONS, INTERVENTIONS, AND IMMUNE DEFECTS TYPICALLY ENCOUNTERED IN COMPROMISED HOSTS

UNDERLYING CONDITION	INTERVENTION	TYPE OF DEFECT
Treatment of neoplastic diseases (particularly hematologic malignant neoplasms)	Underlying disease (without intervention)	Defects in production of bone marrow cells associated with defects in cellular immunity and phagocytic function (e.g., cytopenias associated with bone marrow infiltration with malignant cells)
	Cytotoxic chemotherapies	Bone marrow suppression; defects in primary and secondary humoral and cellular immunity; breach in mucosal barriers (skin, gut); impairment in mucociliary clearance; defects in other organ function (e.g., kidney, liver)
Hematopoietic stem cell transplantation	Underlying disease, without intervention (e.g., hematologic malignant neoplasms)	Defects in primary and secondary humoral and cellular immunity; defects in phagocytic cell quantity and function
	Cytotoxic conditioning therapy (± total body irradiation)	Bone marrow suppression; defects in primary and secondary humoral and cellular immunity; breach in mucosal barriers; defects in organ function
	Stem cell manipulation (e.g., T-cell depletion)	Delay in cellular engraftment
	Prophylaxis and treatment of graft-versus-host disease (e.g., corticosteroids, calcineurin inhibitors, antimetabolites, TNF-α antagonists)	Defective function in phagocytic cells and dysfunction of primary and secondary humoral and cellular immunity
Solid organ transplantation	Underlying disease, without intervention (e.g., diabetes, end-stage liver disease)	Organ dysfunction and miscellaneous immune dysfunction
	Induction therapies (e.g., corticosteroids, antilymphocyte globulin, splenectomy, anti–interleukin-2 Ab, anti-CD52 Ab, calcineurin inhibitors	Depletion and impairment in primary and secondary cellular and humoral immunity
	Surgical intervention and altered anatomy	Breach in mucosal barriers; defects in organ function
	Acute and chronic rejection prophylaxis and treatment (e.g., corticosteroids, calcineurin inhibitors, antimetabolites and alkylating agents, plasmapheresis, antithymocyte globulin, monoclonal antibodies to B and T cells, anticytokine therapies, T-cell costimulation blockers)	Defective function in phagocytic cells, primary and secondary humoral and cellular immunity
Treatment of collagen vascular and autoimmune diseases	Anti-inflammatory and immunosuppressive agents (corticosteroids, nonsteroidal anti-inflammatory drugs, calcineurin inhibitors, sirolimus, mycophenolate mofetil)	Defective function in phagocytic cells, primary and secondary humoral and cellular immunity
	Antimetabolite and alkylating agents	Bone marrow suppression, defects in primary and secondary humoral and cellular immunity
	Biologic immune response modifiers (e.g., antithymocyte globulin, monoclonal antibodies to B and T cells, anticytokine therapies, T-cell costimulation blockers)	Defective function in primary and secondary humoral and cellular immunity

Ab = antibody; TNF-α = tumor necrosis factor-α.

infectious risks is further broadened and prolonged when patients with these underlying immune defects are treated with cytotoxic drugs. Chemotherapies can also be deleterious to the function of other organs that are critical to host defense, especially the integrity of the gastrointestinal tract mucosal barrier and airway innate clearance mechanisms, posing additional susceptibilities to bacterial and fungal pathogens. Thus, the underlying malignancy itself and the specific therapies that are used to treat it combine to create the profile of the types of infections to which the patient is at risk, both acutely and chronically.

Hematopoietic Stem Cell and Solid Organ Transplant Recipients

Hematopoietic stem cell transplantation (HSCT) (Chapter 168) exposes recipients to additional risks as a result of the agents used for conditioning therapy in preparation for the stem cell transplantation, variable rate and magnitude of cellular engraftment, and, in recipients of allogeneic HSCT, administration of additional agents to reduce risks for graft-versus-host disease (GVHD). GVHD itself and the treatments used to modulate it create additional risk for infection. Organ dysfunction, loss of natural barriers (skin and gut), and neutropenia dictate enhanced early risks for infection with bacteria and fungi that inhabit the gastrointestinal tract; impaired humoral and secondary immunity enhance late risks for infections caused by viruses, fungi, and encapsulated bacteria, especially in people treated aggressively for GVHD.

Immunodeficiency in solid organ transplant recipients is mostly caused by the initiation and chronic maintenance requirements of immunosuppressive therapies to suppress T- and B-lymphocyte function and to decrease risks for early and late graft rejection (Chapter 43). Additional factors that can exacerbate overall risks for infection include the altered anatomy preoperatively and postoperatively, the surgical intervention itself, and the potential of infection transmitted from the graft itself (i.e., donor-derived infection).

It is important to keep in mind that transplant recipients have increased risks both for acute infection and for reactivation of latent infections after initiation of immunosuppression. Hence, pretransplantation evaluation should be focused on detection of latent herpesviruses (e.g., cytomegalovirus [CMV]) and other pathogens (e.g., *M. tuberculosis*) that can be transferred or reactivated with transplantation and immunosuppression.

The overall risk for infection in organ transplant recipients is determined by interactions between the patient's (1) epidemiologic exposure and (2) "net state of immunosuppression."[2] Epidemiologic exposure to viral infections (both reactivation and disease) enhance risks for other infections. For example, CMV infection (Chapter 346) is known to be a risk for additional infections by other microorganisms in recipients of both hematopoietic stem cell and solid organ transplant grafts. The "net state of immunosuppression" is a conceptual measure of all factors contributing to an individual patient's risk for infection at any given time. Table 265-3 lists some of the clinical factors that influence the net state of immunosuppression. These include underlying medical conditions (e.g., diabetes mellitus, advanced age, malnutrition), the use of specific immunosuppressive therapies (and their potential synergisms), technical problems during surgery, post-transplantation organ dysfunction, the administration of broad-spectrum antibiotics, and prolonged airway intubation or use of urinary and vascular access. This concept, which originated from an understanding of solid organ transplantation, can perhaps be applied to the care of all immunosuppressed patients.

An ever-increasing number of types of immunosuppressive therapies are frequently administered to patients with active connective tissue diseases and autoimmune conditions. These are outlined in Table 265-2. This population of patients is growing in importance with increasing use of biologic immune response modifiers (Chapters 32 and 33) that enhance risks for both reactivation of latent infection (e.g., *M. tuberculosis* and *H. capsulatum*) and severe manifestations of acute infection. Infectious risks should be considered in balancing need for these therapies and designing preventive regimens.

⬤ FEVER IN THE COMPROMISED HOST

The onset of fever in an immunocompromised patient can be an ominous development. Depending on the nature and magnitude of the impaired host defenses, including comorbidities, a febrile response can indicate the onset of a life-threatening systemic infection. A diagnostic approach should be derived by careful consideration of the patient's signs and symptoms of infection, exact form(s) of immunocompromise, and whether the patient is at heightened risk for reactivation of latent infection. Because infection can progress rapidly, particularly in patients with absolute neutropenia (see later), empirical antimicrobial therapy is often indicated even before an infection is definitively identified.

CLINICAL MANIFESTATIONS AND DIAGNOSIS

In the setting of disease-associated or chemotherapy-induced neutropenia, fever is typically an important and often the only clinical indication of infection. Some patients with neutropenia and serious infection, especially those who are elderly, may be afebrile or even hypothermic on presentation. The risk for bacterial infection increases proportionally with the decline in neutrophil count, especially with prolonged durations of significant neutropenia.[3] Infection rates increase with neutrophil levels below 1000 cells/μL, progressively increasing as counts decline to less than 100 cells/μL. The duration of significant neutropenia is also an important determinant of the type of infection most likely to occur, with the risk for bacterial and fungal infections increasing with each successive week in which leukocyte counts are less than 500 cells/μL.

The most common causes of fever during neutropenia used to be gram-negative bacteria, usually originating in the gastrointestinal tract. In the 1990s, concurrent with the increased use of prophylactic and empirical antibiotics that covered gram-negative bacteria, especially quinolones and extended-spectrum β-lactams, rates of gram-negative bacteremias declined, and the rates of gram-positive bacteremias reciprocally increased. Studies have supported the liberal and prompt use of empirical antimicrobials in febrile neutropenic patients, selecting drugs that are active against the most likely pathogens, considering the patients' epidemiologic exposures and colonizing organisms, especially in the gastrointestinal tract.

The presentation of a febrile, neutropenic patient should immediately prompt the questions and considerations that are outlined in Table 265-4. The differential diagnosis of fever in these cases should be influenced by local and hospital exposures and the type of preventive antibiotics the patient might be receiving that would have likely altered the composition of the gastrointestinal microbiome. The type and duration of immunodeficiency (i.e., the "net state of immunosuppression") can alter overall risks. Specific organ dysfunction, such as underlying pulmonary disease or renal impairment, can predispose to unique infectious syndromes (see later). Epidemiologic exposures should be thoroughly explored. Current and previously administered antimicrobial drugs affect risks for specific infections. Especially for patients who are hospitalized in an acute care or chronic care facility or were recently hospitalized, it is useful to have information on colonizing organisms that may display complex resistance profiles, such as vancomycin-resistant enterococci and bacteria that express extended-spectrum β-lactamases or other resistance determinants (e.g., carbapenemases). Knowledge of recent colonization with these organisms or local institutional epidemiology should be considered when tailoring initial antibiotic management.

TABLE 265-3	FACTORS CONTRIBUTING TO THE "NET STATE OF IMMUNOSUPPRESSION"

Immunosuppressive therapy: type, temporal sequence, and intensity
Prior and current therapies (chemotherapy, radiation therapy, antimicrobial agents)
Integument barrier integrity (e.g., catheters, lines, drains)
Neutropenia, lymphopenia, hypogammaglobulinemia
Underlying immune defects (e.g., autoimmune disease, genetic polymorphisms)
Metabolic conditions: uremia, malnutrition, diabetes, cirrhosis, advanced age
Viral infection (e.g., herpesviruses [CMV, EBV], HBV, HCV, HIV, RSV, influenza)

CMV = cytomegalovirus; EBV = Epstein-Barr virus; HBV = hepatitis B virus; HCV = hepatitis C virus; HIV = human immunodeficiency virus; RSV = respiratory syncytial virus.
Adapted from Fishman JA. Infection in organ transplantation. *Am J Transplant.* 2017;17:856-879.

TABLE 265-4	APPROACH TO FEVER DURING CHEMOTHERAPY-INDUCED NEUTROPENIA

PAST AND CURRENT CLINICAL CONSIDERATIONS

What is the type and duration of immunologic deficiency?
Does the patient have any organ dysfunction that would predispose to particular infection?
Does the patient have any unique environmental or epidemiologic exposures?
What are the patient's prior infections and colonizing organisms?
What are the current and recently administered antimicrobial agents?
Are there any specific presenting signs or symptoms that suggest a particular type of infection or syndrome?

The onset of fever in a patient who is neutropenic or otherwise immuno-compromised requires a prompt and thorough bedside evaluation. Particularly neutropenic patients may not be able to mobilize a sufficient number of leukocytes to develop a clinically apparent inflammatory response. For example, they may not exhibit the expected brisk peritoneal signs of an acute abdomen, meningeal signs of a central nervous system (CNS) infection, or localized tenderness, swelling, and erythema for an abscess. This makes a careful and thorough physical examination and examination-guided imaging all the more important in these individuals. Beginning with examination of the head and neck, there should be a specific examination for evidence of CNS infection as well as a general evaluation of mental status. The oropharynx must be examined for evidence of pharyngitis and focal tenderness. Sinus membranes should be evaluated for the presence of erythema or necrosis. Complete examination of the heart, lung fields, and abdomen is critical, with attention to the potential presence of new murmurs, abnormal breath sounds, and intra-abdominal tenderness. The entire integument, including the perirectal area, should be examined. Severely neutropenic patients tend to get infections at either end of the gastrointestinal tract. Intravenous catheter exit sites and tunnels should be carefully inspected, and blood should be drawn through catheters for culture. Because classic signs of infection of catheter exit sites and tunnels can be absent or blunted in patients with neutropenia (with signs of infection present only after recovery of neutrophils), examination should be performed daily and with close scrutiny for evolving localized infection that may necessitate catheter removal.

Laboratory studies should be undertaken, with emphasis placed on procedures that can yield prompt results, such as Gram stain of body fluids, exudates, or aspirates. Blood cultures and cultures of other body fluids should be obtained promptly, preferably before initiating empirical antibiotics. Routine blood work should include a complete blood count with differential, serum creatinine concentration, and liver function studies. Chest radiograph should be part of the initial evaluation even if the chest examination is normal, as should routine urinalysis. Because routine radiographs are insensitive for detection of small nodular lesions, especially those caused by filamentous fungi, computed tomography (CT) should be performed in evaluating persistent fever, especially in the presence of airway symptoms. Noninfectious causes of fever (e.g., drug fever) cannot be overlooked in neutropenic patients even though they might often require less urgent intervention. No biomarker has yet to be proved reliable in discriminating between severe infection and other causes of fever during neutropenia, although the utility of lipopolysaccharide-binding protein, interleukin-6 and interleukin-8, procalcitonin, soluble TREM-1 (triggering receptor expressed on myeloid cells-1), and C-reactive protein, to name only a few, are being studied.

Multiple episodes of fever during prolonged hospitalization and neutropenia are not uncommon. Each episode requires comprehensive assessment. After a documented infection, it should not be assumed that a subsequent episode of fever is caused by recrudescence of the same pathogen.

TREATMENT   Rx

An initial consideration in the management of fever during neutropenia is whether the patient requires hospitalization for therapy.[4] Risk assessment is an integral part of early evaluation to determine whether outpatient therapy is feasible. Two risk assessment systems have been developed, and one, the Multinational Association of Supportive Care in Cancer (MASCC) risk index score (Table 265-5), has been validated as a useful predictor of outcome potentially assisting in identifying patients who can be treated with oral antibiotics and close monitoring at home rather than with inpatient therapy. However, other factors should be also considered in making this decision, such as the underlying disease, anticipated duration of neutropenia, other comorbidities, prompt patient access to a hospital, and the clinical judgment of the treating provider. Guidelines from the American Society of Clinical Oncology and the Infectious Diseases Society of America provide a framework for programmatic considerations and selection criteria for outpatient management of patients with febrile neutropenia (Fig. 265-1).[5,6]

Progression of infection can occur rapidly in neutropenic hosts. The very high mortality rates associated with bacteremia, especially that caused by gram-negative bacteria, prompted the introduction of routine empirical therapies. Initial antibiotic choice should be tailored to patient and institutional variables, as outlined in Table 265-2 and Figure 265-2. In low-risk patients who can be potentially treated with oral antibiotics,[A1] the combination of a fluoroquinolone such as ciprofloxacin with amoxicillin-clavulanate has been shown to be effective. In high-risk patients, admission for treatment and prompt administration

TABLE 265-5 THE MULTINATIONAL ASSOCIATION FOR SUPPORTIVE CARE IN CANCER (MASCC) INDEX

COMPONENTS OF THE MASCC INDEX

CLINICAL CHARACTERISTIC	SCORE*
Burden of illness (1 of the 3 options only):	
No or mild symptoms	5
Moderate symptoms	3
Severe symptoms	0
No hypotension (systolic BP >90 mm Hg)	5
No chronic obstructive pulmonary disease	4
Solid tumor or no prior fungal infection in patient with hematologic neoplasm	4
No dehydration (hydration with IV fluids not required)	3
Outpatient at onset of fever	3
Age <60 yr	2

*Maximum score: 26 (5 + 5 + 4 + 4 + 3 + 3 + 2). Low risk for complication = score ≥21; high risk for complication = score <21.
BP = blood pressure; IV = intravenous.
Data from Klastersky J, Paesmans M, Rubenstein EB, et al. The Multinational Association for Supportive Care in Cancer risk index: a multinational scoring system for identifying low-risk febrile neutropenic cancer patients. J Clin Oncol. 2000;18:3038-3051.

of a broad-spectrum intravenous antibiotic regimen is necessary. The international Surviving Sepsis Campaign recommends starting antibiotics as quickly as possible, preferably within an hour of recognition of fever during neutropenia. Some studies indicate that delays in administering antibiotics may lead to prolonged hospital stays.

Early studies demonstrated that the combination of an antipseudomonal β-lactam and an aminoglycoside is effective. However, a meta-analysis showed that monotherapy with one of the newer broad-spectrum β-lactams is associated with better outcomes compared with the combination therapy.[A2] Extended-spectrum agents, such as third- and fourth-generation cephalosporins (e.g., cefepime), antipseudomonal penicillins, and carbapenems (e.g., meropenem), have been subsequently shown to be effective options administered as monotherapy,[A3][A4] while the routine use of an aminoglycoside in combination may result in more toxicities and no better outcomes.

A controversial issue is if and when to start vancomycin in high-risk patients. While some advocates argue that resistant gram-positive infections (e.g., methicillin-resistant S. aureus) cause morbidity in neutropenic patients, several meta-analyses have shown that vancomycin does not reduce all-cause or infection-related mortality and may be associated with increased adverse effects, including nephrotoxicity and rash. Consequently, most guidelines do not support the routine administration of glycopeptides for febrile neutropenia. Nevertheless, empirical vancomycin use may be considered in specific clinical scenarios, such as documented or suspected catheter-related infection, gram-positive bacteremia pending final identification and susceptibility testing, colonization with methicillin-resistant S. aureus, sepsis with hemodynamic instability pending culture results, pneumonia, and soft tissue infection. Use of vancomycin should be reassessed within 2 to 3 days when initiated for one of these conditions; if cultures fail to identify a resistant gram-positive pathogen, intravenous vancomycin should be discontinued.

Clinical response to the first few days of therapy is a critical determinant of the course of extended antimicrobial therapy. The median time to defervescence is shorter in low-risk than high-risk patients (2 days vs. 5 to 7 days). If patients are stable yet still febrile during a period of prolonged and severe neutropenia, clinical judgment is required in deciding whether to maintain the initial regimen or to switch to an alternative one.[7] Even if patients become afebrile after 3 to 5 days of antibiotic therapy and cultures are negative, data are inconclusive.[A5] Some authorities recommend continuing the broad-spectrum intravenous coverage until recovery of the absolute neutrophil count, although this may not be possible in patients with an expectedly prolonged period of neutropenia. Others believe that a switch to oral treatment is justifiable (e.g., a fluoroquinolone possibly paired with a β-lactam) if a low-risk patient defervesces and appears to be clinically stable. If the neutrophil count recovers to above 500 cells/μL and fever persists, clinical judgment must be used to define ongoing need for antimicrobial therapy while a search for the cause of the fever is continued. Clinical deterioration should trigger consideration of infections resistant to the empirical regimen.

Causes of persistent fever can be either infectious or noninfectious. Noninfectious causes include drug reactions, transfusion reactions, pulmonary emboli, splenic infarcts, and the underlying malignant disease. Persistent fever may indicate infection by a microorganism that is resistant or not covered by the

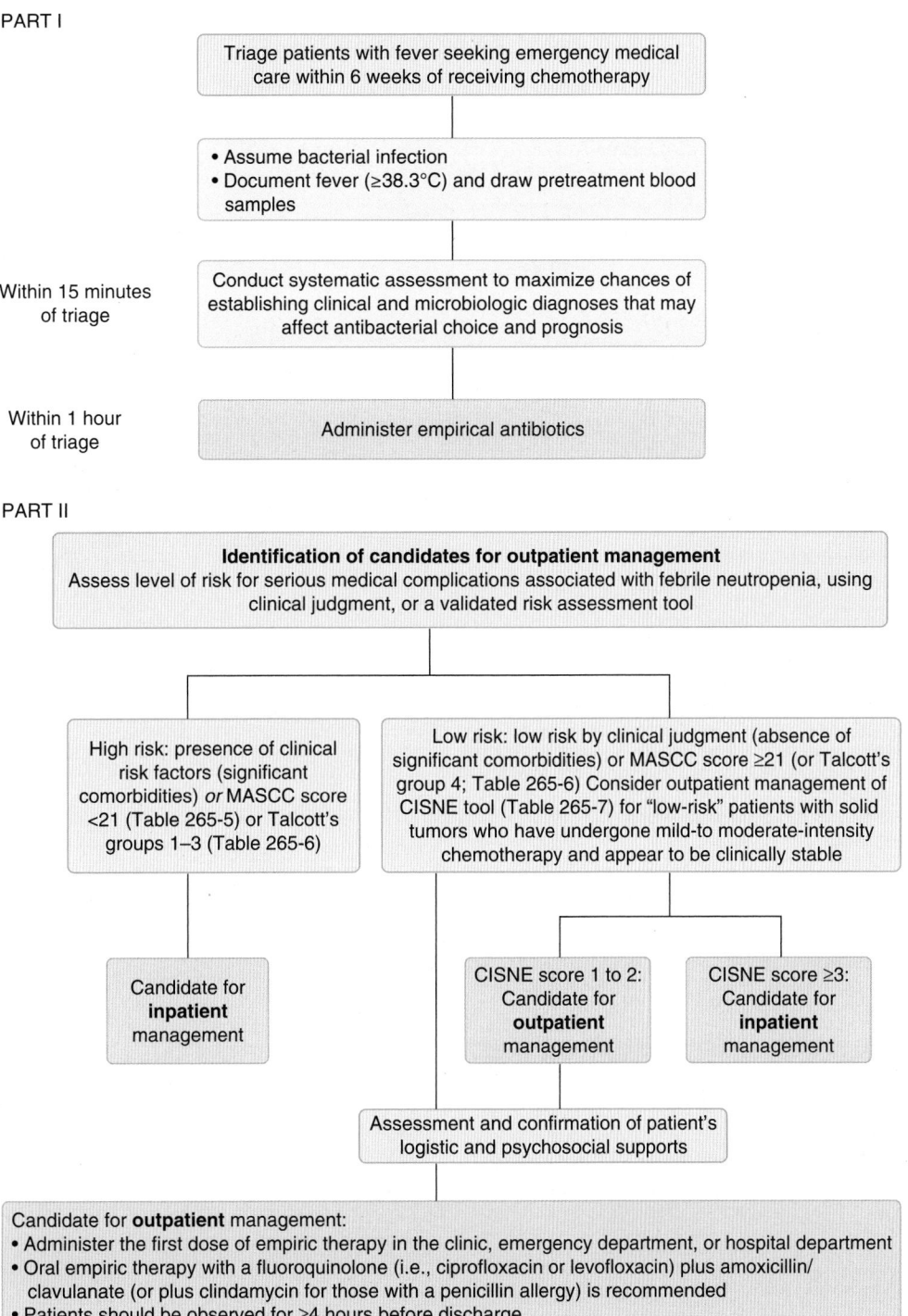

FIGURE 265-1. Summary of recommendations for outpatient management of fever and neutropenia in adults treated for malignancy. CISNE = Clinical Index of Stable Febrile Neutropenia; MASCC = Multinational Association for Supportive Care in Cancer. (Modified from Taplitz RA, Kennedy EB, Bow EJ, et al. Outpatient management of fever and neutropenia in adults treated for malignancy: American Society of Clinical Oncology and Infectious Diseases Society of America clinical practice guideline update. *J Clin Oncol.* 2018;36:1443-1453.)

empirical antibiotics chosen, or a loculated site of infection such as an abscess that also requires drainage for cure. Alternatively, nonbacterial pathogens should be considered, such as fungi (especially *Candida* and *Aspergillus* species), and should prompt evaluation and consideration of antifungal empirical therapies in the setting of fever that persists more than 4 to 7 days. Many drugs have been evaluated and shown to be effective in this setting, including azole drugs, echinocandins, and polyenes.[A6]

Persistently compromised hosts may remain febrile for weeks without identification of the cause. For a patient with persistent fever in whom no pathogen is identified, the duration of therapy should be based on integration of clinical data and the best estimate of the direction of the host's course. As indicated previously, therapy can be discontinued in stable, afebrile patients, assuming that the absolute neutrophil count exceeds 500 cells/μL. If broad-spectrum

antibacterial therapy is to be discontinued, the patient should be monitored carefully thereafter. For patients whose neutrophil counts remain at levels less than 500 cells/μL, particularly the subset with severe profound neutropenia of less than 100 cells/μL, it is prudent to continue empirical antibacterial and antifungal therapy, with reappraisal of all diagnostic measures. Proposed management algorithms for the use of empirical antimicrobials for febrile neutropenic patients after 2 to 4 days of empirical antimicrobial therapy and after 5 days of persistent fevers are shown in Figures 265-3 and 265-4, respectively.

The use of granulocyte colony-stimulating factors for the prevention of febrile neutropenia is discussed in Chapter 158. For the management of established fever in neutropenic patients and for the use of myeloid growth factors in patients with malignancies, evidence-based guidelines have been published by the American Society of Clinical Oncology and by the Infectious Diseases

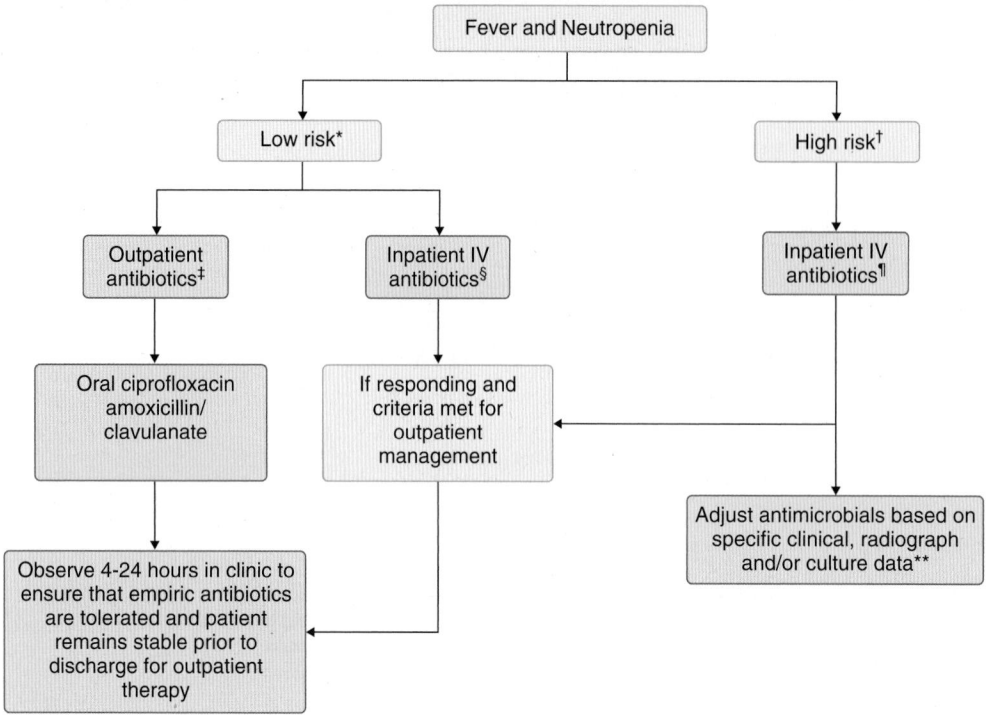

* Low Risk = anticipated neutropenia ≤7 days and clinically stable and no medical comorbidities.
† High Risk = anticipated neutropenia >7 days, *or* clinically unstable, *or* any medical comorbidities.
‡ If able to tolerate and absorb; caregiver, access, and transportation are available; patient and physician decide.
§ If there is documented infection requiring IV antibiotics; there is gastrointestinal intolerance; patient and physician decide.
¶ Empiric antibiotic monotherapy with any of the following: piperacillin/tazobactam, or carbapenem, or ceftazidime, or cefepime.
** For example: vancomycin and linezolid for cellulitis or pneumonia; add aminoglycoside and switch to carbapenem for pneumonia or gram negative bacteremia; metronidazole for abdominal symptoms of suspected *C. difficile* infection.

FIGURE 265-2. Initial management of fever (≥38.3° C) and neutropenia (≤0.5 × 10⁹ cells/mL). Limited data to support recommendation. IV = intravenous. (Modified from Freifeld AG, Bow EJ, Sepkowitz KA, et al. Clinical practice guideline for the use of antimicrobial agents in neutropenic patients with cancer: 2010 update by the Infectious Diseases Society of America. *Clin Infect Dis.* 2011;52:e56-e93.)

TABLE 265-6   TALCOTT'S GROUP CLASSIFICATION

GROUP	CHARACTERISTIC
I	Inpatients (at the time of fever onset)
II	Outpatients with acute comorbidity requiring, by itself, hospitalization
III	Outpatients without comorbidity but with uncontrolled cancer
IV	Outpatients with cancer controlled and without comorbidity

Adapted from Taplitz RA, Kennedy EB, Bow EJ, et al. Outpatient management of fever and neutropenia in adults treated for malignancy: American Society of Clinical Oncology and Infectious Diseases Society of America clinical practice guideline update. *J Clin Oncol.* 2018;36:1443-1453.

TABLE 265-7   THE CLINICAL INDEX OF STABLE FEBRILE NEUTROPENIA (CISNE)

EXPLANATORY VARIABLE	NO. OF POINTS
Eastern Cooperative Oncology Group performance status ≥ 2	2
Chronic obstructive pulmonary disease	1
Chronic cardiovascular disease	1
National Cancer Institute Common Toxicity Criteria mucositis of grade ≥ 2	1
Monocytes < 200/μL	1
Stress-induced hyperglycemia	2

The six variables are integrated into a score ranging from 0 to 8, which classifies patients into three prognostic classes: low risk (0 points), intermediate risk (1 to 2 points), and high risk (≥3 points). Adapted from Taplitz RA, Kennedy EB, Bow EJ, et al. Outpatient management of fever and neutropenia in adults treated for malignancy: American Society of Clinical Oncology and Infectious Diseases Society of America clinical practice guideline update. *J Clin Oncol.* 2018;36:1443-1453.

Society of America.[8,9] The guidelines generally agree, and they support the use of colony-stimulating factors in similar circumstances that indicate high risk for infection-associated complications and poor clinical outcomes, such as in patients with anticipated long and profound durations of neutropenia, advanced age, uncontrolled primary disease, hemodynamic compromise, pneumonia, and invasive fungal infections.

Table 265-8 summarizes some of the most common infectious and noninfectious syndromes that involve the skin, lungs, gastrointestinal tract, and nervous system in immunocompromised patients, and they are discussed next.

CUTANEOUS SYNDROMES

Cutaneous manifestations can provide a clue to bacteremia, and aspiration and culture of suspicious lesions can be as valuable as a blood culture. Ascending streptococcal or staphylococcal cellulitis can occur in both immunocompromised[10] and immunocompetent patients. Metastatic abscesses are a well-recognized complication of the *S. aureus* bacteremia syndrome. Necrotizing vasculitis is classically associated with *P. aeruginosa* infections; its cutaneous lesion of ecthyma gangrenosum is an erythematous, indurated target or "bull's-eye" lesion with an area of central necrosis that can appear in crops (Fig. 265-5 and Chapter 412). However, other gram-negative endotoxin-producing bacteria have been associated with similar cutaneous lesions.

Cutaneous mycobacterial infections can occur in patients with chronic T-cell deficiency and impaired cell-mediated immunity following HSCT or solid organ transplantation or as a consequence of treatment with TNF antagonists. Nontuberculous mycobacteria typically cause tender, erythematous nodular lesions that may ulcerate. They can arise either following direct inoculation (e.g., following trauma or cosmetic surgery) or, typically in immunocompromised

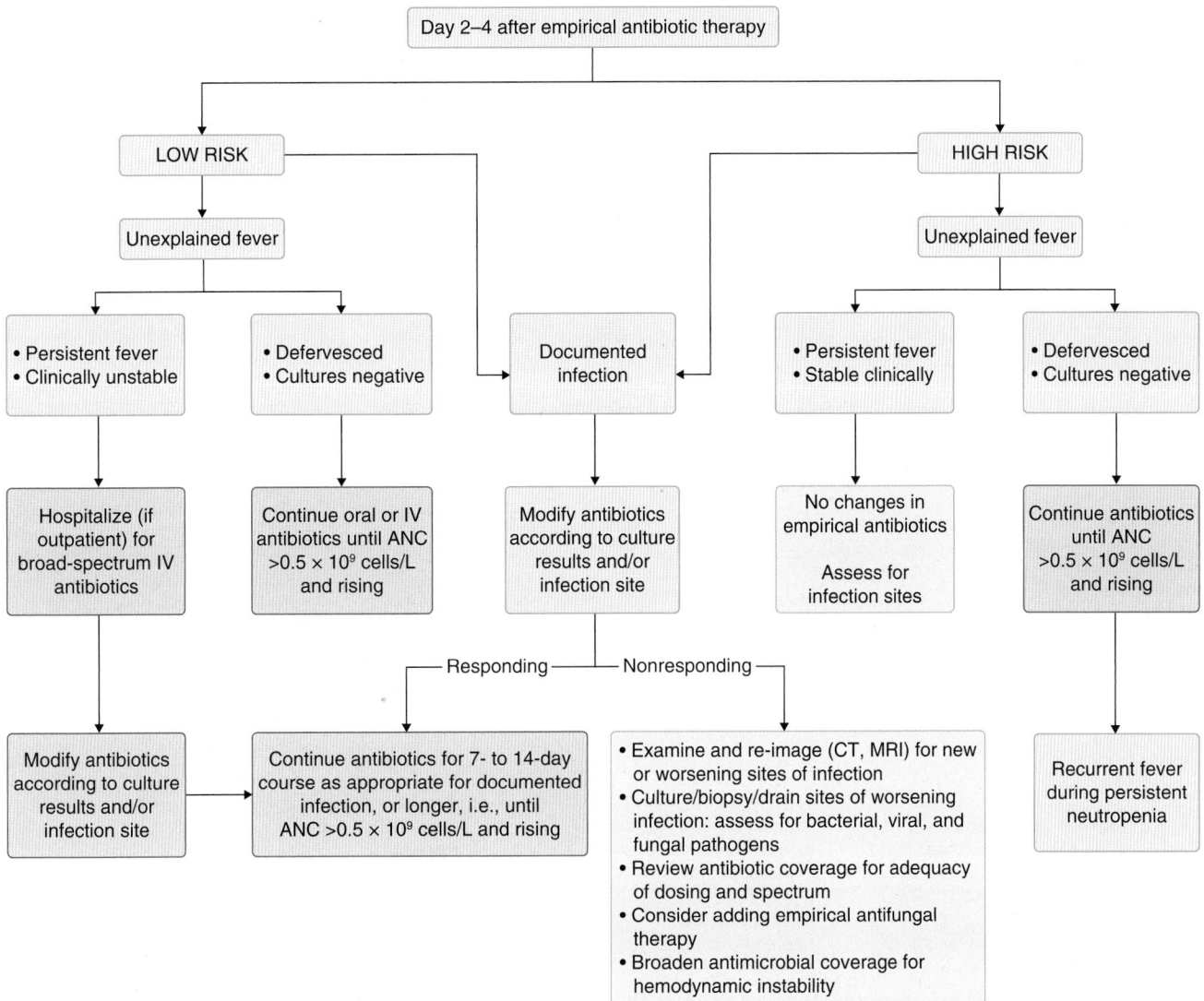

FIGURE 265-3. Reassessment after 2 to 4 days of empirical antibiotic therapy. ANC = absolute neutrophil count; CT = computed tomography; IV = intravenous; MRI = magnetic resonance imaging. (Modified from Freifeld AG, Bow EJ, Sepkowitz KA, et al. Clinical practice guideline for the use of antimicrobial agents in neutropenic patients with cancer: 2010 update by the Infectious Diseases Society of America. *Clin Infect Dis*, 2011;52:e56-e93.)

patients, as a consequence of disseminated disease and hematogenous seeding (Chapter 309). Important species include rapidly growing nontuberculous mycobacteria (i.e., *Mycobacterium chelonae, Mycobacterium abscessus,* and *Mycobacterium fortuitum*), *Mycobacterium haemophilum* often with concurrent pulmonary disease, and *Mycobacterium marinum* following fresh or salt water exposures (Fig. 265-6). *M. tuberculosis* is a rare cause of skin disease but should be considered with suggestive epidemiology; it can arise due to contiguous spread, for example, from an infected lymph node (e.g., scrofuloderma), or with disseminated infection (e.g., lupus vulgaris).

Nocardia species are another important cause of skin and subcutaneous infections in immunocompromised and noncompromised hosts (Chapter 314). *Nocardia* are environmentally ubiquitous saprophytes found in the soil and can cause local infection following direct inoculation; however, cutaneous nocardiosis may also be the first sign of systemic disease in immunocompromised hosts. Identification of *Nocardia* skin or soft tissue infection in immunocompromised patients, particularly in those with no history of penetrating trauma, should prompt evaluation of disseminated infection, including imaging of the lungs and brain. Cutaneous nocardiosis can be variable in presentation, including subcutaneous nodules (often with a sporotrichoid-like lymphocutaneous distribution), ulcers, abscesses, pyoderma, and cellulitis.

In the neutropenic host, disseminated fungal infections may be initially recognized by characteristic cutaneous lesions. Disseminated candidiasis in such individuals can present with diffuse maculopapular, erythematous, and sometimes tender lesions. The appearance of cutaneous lesions typically changes in character with engraftment of neutrophils (Fig. 265-7). Disseminated infections caused by filamentous organisms such as *Aspergillus* species cause similar

lesions, but usually fewer in number and more often with some component of central necrosis. Other filamentous fungi, namely, those with which infection is characterized by a high fungal burden, such as *Fusarium* species, typically cause more skin lesions in multiple stages of evolution, ranging from papules to larger erythematous lesions with central necrosis. Multiple filamentous fungi such as *Aspergillus* species and Zygomycetes can also cause primary cutaneous lesions, especially with a breech in skin integrity. Infection with *Cryptococcus neoformans* can be accompanied by cutaneous involvement, with manifestations ranging from molluscum-like lesions to primary cutaneous cellulitis, which may be especially common in solid organ transplant recipients. Cutaneous lesions are an opportunity to establish diagnosis through aspiration, biopsy, and culture.

Morbilliform eruptions or maculopapular exanthems are frequent in neutropenic patients and transplant recipients. They can be caused by drug reactions, GVHD, and numerous viral infections. Primary infection and reactivation with herpesviruses such as CMV and Epstein-Barr virus can be accompanied by rashes. Human herpesvirus 6, the primary cause of roseola infantum in childhood, leads to latency and can cause disease in immunocompromised hosts both by reactivation and by primary infection. Disease can be accompanied by fever, rash, myelosuppression, and involvement of other organ systems (e.g., CNS). In immunocompromised patients, adenovirus can be both primarily acquired, usually through the respiratory tract, and reactivated; it causes fever, rash, and potentially disease involving multiple organ systems (lungs, gastrointestinal tract, kidneys, liver, CNS). In HSCT recipients, the constellation of fever, rash, diarrhea, and hepatitis may be confused for severe GVHD. Parvovirus B19 infection can be severe in immunocompromised hosts and

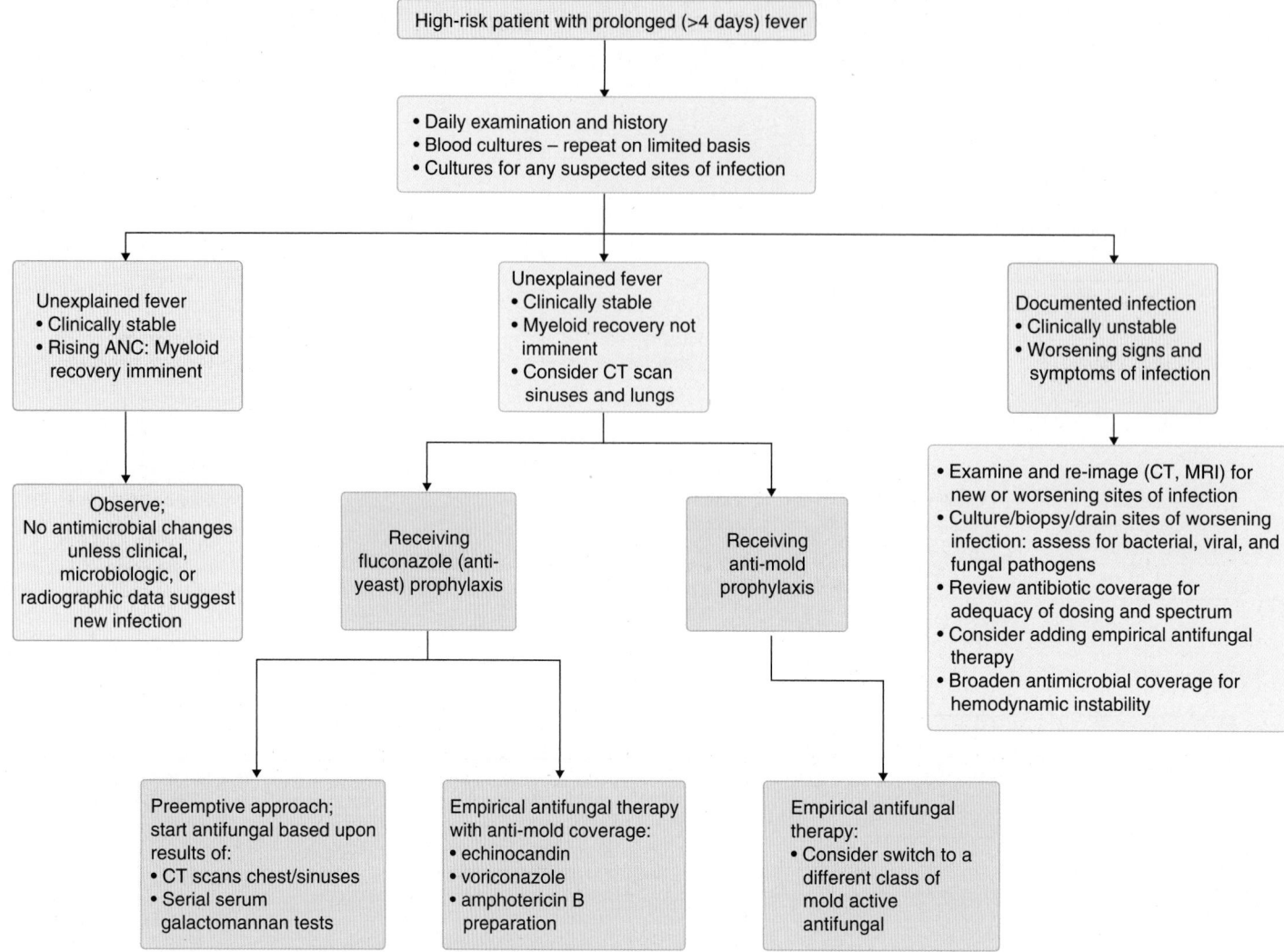

FIGURE 265-4. High-risk patient with fever after 4 days of empirical antibiotics. ANC = absolute neutrophil count; CT = computed tomography; IV = intravenous; MRI = magnetic resonance imaging. (Modified from Freifeld AG, Bow EJ, Sepkowitz KA, et al. Clinical practice guideline for the use of antimicrobial agents in neutropenic patients with cancer: 2010 update by the Infectious Diseases Society of America. *Clin Infect Dis.* 2011;52:e56-e93.)

associated with fever, rash, and manifestations of hemophagocytosis, although there are other infectious causes of hemophagocytic syndromes as well (Chapter 160). The characteristic vesicular rash of varicella reactivation is relatively frequent in stem cell and solid organ transplant recipients with chronic T-cell deficiencies, especially in the absence of antiviral prophylaxis. Disseminated disease in immunocompromised patients is associated with high mortality rates unless prompt antiviral therapy is initiated. Antivirals administered as prophylaxis in high-risk HSCT and solid organ transplant recipients can decrease both early morbidity and late mortality associated with herpes simplex virus (HSV), varicella-zoster virus (VZV), and CMV disease, although drug-related toxicities must be considered in risk-benefit calculations.

There are numerous noninfectious causes of rashes and lesions that are common in immunocompromised individuals, particularly drug-induced hypersensitivity syndromes that can be both mild and severe, and rarely progress to life-threatening toxic epidermal necrolysis.

Sweet syndrome, or acute febrile neutrophilic dermatosis, is characterized by skin lesions with neutrophilic infiltration in the dermis (see Fig. 411-23). It may appear during impending neutrophil recovery, treatment with granulocyte colony-stimulating factor, associated with numerous drugs, or as a paraneoplastic manifestation, particularly in hematologic malignancies (most commonly acute myelogenous leukemia). Biopsy with appropriate microbial stains and culture is essential to distinguish these lesions from infectious causes of ecthyma gangrenosum and other disseminated infections, such as those caused by mycobacteria, *Nocardia*, and fungi.

RESPIRATORY SYNDROMES

Pneumonia should be suspected in a patient who has respiratory symptoms as manifested by cough, shortness of breath, chest pain, and hypoxia, even in the absence of radiographic abnormalities initially. While opportunistic infections are always a consideration, pneumonia in immunocompromised patients is more often caused by community-acquired pathogens such as pneumococci and *Haemophilus influenzae* that can cause lobar or diffuse pneumonia. Patients on ventilators are at risk for secondary gram-negative bacillary pneumonia or staphylococcal pneumonia.

Opportunistic fungi have been increasingly recognized as causes of lung infection in immunocompromised neutropenic patients and transplant recipients. Epidemic mycoses such as blastomycosis, coccidioidomycosis, and histoplasmosis may be manifested as acute pneumonia after recent exposure in immunocompromised patients, making a travel history mandatory. Although *Candida* species commonly colonize indwelling vascular and urinary catheters, candidal pneumonia is unusual in the absence of systemic candidiasis. Although classically associated with an "interstitial pattern" of lung infiltration, *Pneumocystis* species pneumonia can be manifested as local consolidation or pulmonary nodules, exhibiting granulomatous inflammation on pathologic examination. Filamentous fungi, including *Aspergillus*, Zygomycetes, *Fusarium* species, and *Scedosporium* species, are challenging to treat. From an initial focus, *Aspergillus* infection can spread through the pulmonary vasculature, which sets the stage for localized hemorrhage, creating a halo sign on CT scan, and infarction and necrosis. This can progress to cavitary lesions. Invasive pulmonary aspergillosis is usually caused by *Aspergillus fumigatus* and can be very difficult to identify specifically by conventional methods for detecting fungal infections. Fluorescent in situ hybridization–based molecular methods will be a promising approach.[11] These organisms can also cause primary airway disease, presenting with features typical of tracheobronchitis, with or without findings apparent on CT scan. This infection is particularly well described in lung transplant recipients, who may also have involvement of the bronchial anastomosis.

TABLE 265-8 COMMON INFECTIOUS AND NONINFECTIOUS SYNDROMES IN IMMUNOCOMPROMISED HOSTS

PRIMARY ORGAN SYSTEM	BACTERIA	FUNGI	VIRUSES	PARASITES AND PROTISTS	NONINFECTIOUS
Cutaneous	Disseminated gram-positive and gram-negative bacteria, e.g., *Staphylococcus aureus* *Pseudomonas aeruginosa* *Mycobacterium* spp *Nocardia* spp	*Candida* spp. Filamentous fungi, e.g., *Aspergillus* spp *Zygomycetes* *Fusarium* spp *Scedosporium* spp *Cryptococcus* spp	Herpes simplex Varicella-zoster CMV HHV-6 Adenovirus Parvovirus B19	*Leishmania* spp Acanthamoeba *Naegleria fowleri* *Balamuthia mandrillaris*	Drug eruptions GVHD Sweet syndrome
Sinopulmonary	Gram-positive and gram-negative causes of sinusitis and pneumonia *S. aureus* *Streptococcus pneumoniae* *P. aeruginosa* *Haemophilus influenzae* Anaerobes *Legionella* *Nocardia* spp *Mycobacterium* spp	Filamentous fungi, e.g., *Aspergillus* spp *Zygomycetes* *Fusarium* spp *Scedosporium* spp *Cryptococcus* spp Endemic fungi, e.g., *Histoplasma capsulatum* *Coccidioides immitis* *Blastomyces dermatitidis* *Pneumocystis jiroveci*	Respiratory viruses, e.g., RSV Parainfluenza Influenza Adenovirus Reactivation herpes viruses, e.g., CMV, VZV	*Toxoplasma gondii* *Strongyloides stercoralis* hyperinfection syndrome	Drug-related pulmonary toxicities Pneumonitis (sirolimus) Diffuse alveolar damage Bronchiolitis obliterans syndromes
Gastrointestinal	Neutropenic enterocolitis ("typhlitis") Mixed gram-positive, gram-negative, anaerobes (*Bacteroides fragilis, Clostridium septicum*) *Clostridium difficile* colitis Enteric diarrheal pathogens *Salmonella* spp *Shigella* spp *Escherichia coli* *Campylobacter* spp	*Candida* spp. Microsporidia	CMV EBV-PTLD Adenovirus Coxsackievirus Rotavirus Norovirus	*Cryptosporidium* *Giardia lamblia* *Cystoisospora belli* *Cyclospora cayetanensis* *Strongyloides stercoralis*	Drug-related toxicities, e.g., MMF
Neurologic	Gram-positive and gram-negative bacteria *Listeria monocytogenes* Pneumococcus Meningococcus *Nocardia* spp *Mycobacterium tuberculosis* Syphilis	Filamentous fungi *Cryptococcus* spp	Herpes viruses HSV HHV-6 VZV JC virus West Nile virus Miscellaneous viral encephalitides	*Toxoplasma gondii* Acanthamoeba *Naegleria fowleri* *Balamuthia mandrillaris*	Drug-related toxicities, e.g., calcineurin inhibitor toxicity PRES carbapenem-related seizures voriconazole CNS toxicity Cefepime-induced encephalopathy

CMV = cytomegalovirus; EBV-PTLD = Epstein-Barr virus–post-transplantation lymphoproliferative disorder; GVHD = graft-versus-host disease; HHV-6 = human herpes virus 6; HSV = herpes simplex virus; MMF = mycophenolate mofetil; PRES = posterior reversible encephalopathy syndrome; RSV = respiratory syncytial virus; VZV = varicella-zoster virus.

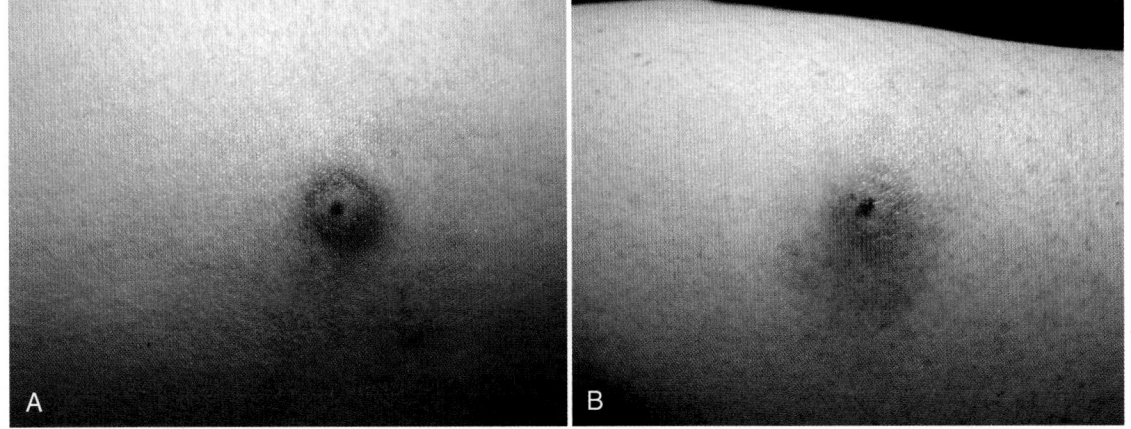

FIGURE 265-5. **Ecthyma gangrenosum.** A 28-year-old woman with fever and neutropenia while receiving chemotherapy for acute leukemia developed several tender edematous papules on her thighs. **A,** Central crust and surrounding erythema are shown. **B,** The papules became necrotic during 1 to 2 days, with the formation of black, well-demarcated eschar. Cultures from blood and the necrotic eschar grew *Pseudomonas aeruginosa*. (© DermAtlas; http://www.DermAtlas.org.)

There is a high risk for severe pulmonary infection caused by reactivation of *M. tuberculosis* in people who are treated with biologic immune response modifiers (Chapter 33), especially TNF antagonists, in the setting of autoimmune or other inflammatory diseases, such as rheumatoid arthritis, psoriasis, and inflammatory bowel diseases. The same patients are also at increased risk for invasive fungal infections, including reactivation of endemic infections such as histoplasmosis, warranting enhanced screening and a high level of suspicion for disease.

A particularly common concern is reactivation pneumonitis caused by members of the herpesvirus family, especially CMV, which occurs most frequently in the setting of chronic T-cell depression associated with transplantation. Respiratory viruses, which infect immunocompromised hosts with the

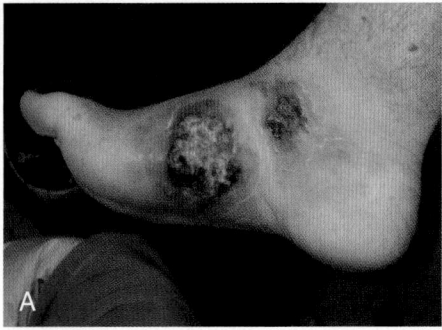
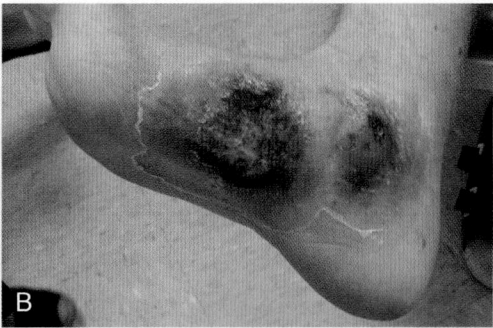
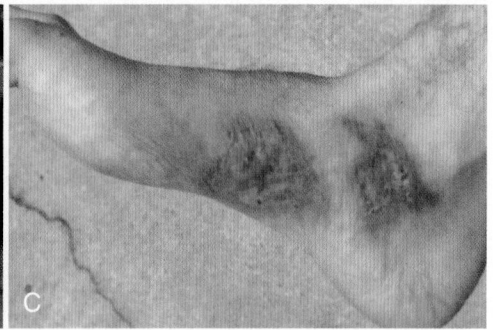

FIGURE 265-6. *Mycobacterium marinum.* A 20-year-old man with Crohn disease receiving infliximab developed progressively worsening nonhealing foot ulcers following trauma and exposure to brackish water 2 years earlier. Biopsy cultures of the ulcer grew *Mycobacterium marinum.* **A,** Two necrotic ulcers with central eschars, surrounding erythema, and pedal edema at the time of diagnosis. **B,** After 1 month of treatment, granulation tissue is evident in the base of the ulcer, and erythema and edema are reduced. **C,** After 10 months of treatment, the ulcers have closed with residual scars and hyperpigmentation.

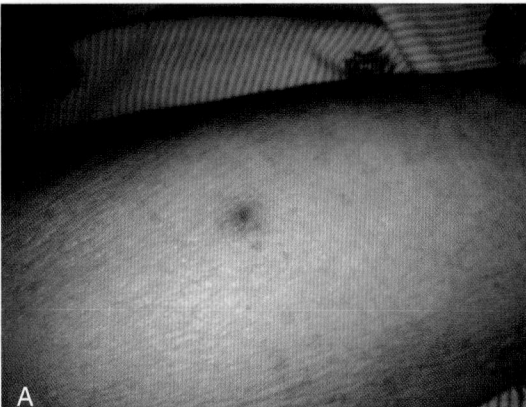
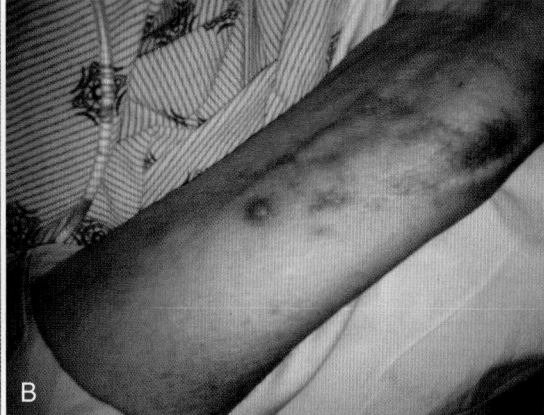

FIGURE 265-7. Disseminated candidiasis. A 60-year-old woman with fever during neutropenia that developed after receipt of therapy for acute leukemia developed tender papular lesions on her extremities, trunk, and back. **A,** Blood cultures returned positive for *Candida tropicalis.* **B,** After resolution of neutropenia, lesions developed a more pustular appearance.

same frequency as the general population, cause lower respiratory tract disease and pneumonitis more frequently in hosts with suppressed cellular immunity. Patients who have defects in cellular immunity typically exhibit higher viral loads and prolonged shedding, causing concern for the emergence of antiviral resistance and infection control.[12]

Noninfectious causes of pulmonary infiltrates in immunosuppressed hosts include early complications of chemotherapy administration (e.g., diffuse alveolar damage and hemorrhage) and late complications of GVHD and organ rejection (e.g., bronchiolitis obliterans syndromes). Certain drugs that are frequently administered in these populations of patients, like sirolimus, can cause direct lung toxicity.

GASTROINTESTINAL SYNDROMES

Diarrhea in an immunocompromised host can be caused by a wide variety of infectious and noninfectious etiologies,[13] including conventional enteric pathogens such as *Salmonella* (Chapter 292), *Shigella* (Chapter 293), and *Campylobacter* (Chapter 287). Currently and recently hospitalized patients who have received courses of antibiotic treatment are commonly infected with *Clostridium difficile* (Chapter 280). *C. difficile* colitis can be both severe and persistent in immunosuppressed hosts. More recently, norovirus has emerged as an important cause of chronic gastroenteritis in immunocompromised patients, in whom diagnoses have been commonly elusive and misapplied to noninfectious syndromes (e.g., GVHD), and outcomes can be poor (Chapter 356). Several intestinal protozoa are associated with diarrhea in compromised patients.[14] Three acid-fast staining protozoa, *Cryptosporidium* species, *Cystoisospora belli,* and *Cyclospora cayetanensis,* are associated with predisposing impairments in cell-mediated immunity (see Chapters 329 and 332). *Giardia lamblia* is classically associated with hypogammaglobulinemia. The Microsporidia are a family of eukaryotic obligate intracellular parasites once thought to be protozoa but more recently placed taxonomically closer to fungi. In addition to causing diarrhea in immune-suppressed patients, they are distinguished by the ability to cause extraintestinal disease in virtually any other organ.

Because acute and chronic diarrhea in immunocompromised patients can be caused by a wide array of bacterial, viral, and protozoal pathogens with broadly overlapping clinical presentations, multiplex molecular panels that have the capability of rapidly detecting one to two dozen potential gastrointestinal pathogens have become important diagnostic tools in recent years. Caution should be exercised in interpretation, however, because a positive result may reflect active infection or asymptomatic colonization. The small intestine is the primary location of calcineurin inhibitor (e.g., cyclosporine, tacrolimus) absorption and metabolism; elevated blood concentrations of calcineurin inhibitors to toxic levels may be a sign of enteritis, for example, due to rotavirus or *Cryptosporidium,* perhaps as a consequence of altered drug metabolism.

CMV is a major cause of gastrointestinal disease in transplant recipients and increasingly recognized in patients with impaired cell-mediated immunity not due to transplantation or AIDS (Chapter 352). It can involve the entire digestive tract from esophagus to anus, and patients typically present with signs and symptoms of disseminated disease, including fever, malaise, and bone marrow suppression (i.e., a mononucleosis-like syndrome). Symptoms of CMV gastritis, enteritis, and colitis include anorexia, nausea, abdominal discomfort, and diarrhea. CMV infection also causes mild elevations in hepatic enzymes and, rarely, fulminant hepatitis or pancreatitis, typically in the context of primary infection after liver transplantation or pancreas transplantation, respectively. Most laboratories use molecular assays (CMV nucleic acid amplification assays or CMV pp65 antigenemia assays) to establish a diagnosis of CMV gastrointestinal disease. However, sensitivity of these assays can occasionally be very low or undetectable because of tissue-invasive disease that is isolated ("compartmentalized") to the alimentary tract. In these cases, endoscopy is required to establish a diagnosis. Indeed, because colitis and diarrhea in immunocompromised patients can be caused by such a wide range of problems, including multiple infections, focal Epstein-Barr virus–associated post-transplantation lymphoproliferative disorder, GVHD, and drug-induced toxicity, uncertainty in diagnosis or failure of response to appropriate treatment requires further evaluation with endoscopy.

Individuals who have received long courses of chemotherapy, radiation, and antibiotics commonly experience *Candida* mucosal overgrowth in the mouth and esophagus. HSV and CMV can cause symptoms identical to those of *Candida* esophagitis. In severely neutropenic patients, anaerobic streptococci and gram-negative pathogens such as *P. aeruginosa* can cause severe mucositis and pharyngitis. In cancer patients, these organisms take advantage of the cytotoxic effects of chemotherapy, which promotes sloughing of mucosal surfaces and subsequently predisposes to infection. Neutropenic patients may also develop enterocolitis that can be of mixed anaerobic and aerobic bacterial origin. Neutropenic enterocolitis, also known as typhlitis or ileocecal syndrome, results from chemotherapeutic damage to the intestinal mucosa in the setting of neutropenia. Presentation usually includes fever, abdominal pain, nausea, vomiting, and diarrhea. Because neutropenic enterocolitis can rapidly progress to intestinal perforation, sepsis, and multisystem organ failure, prompt diagnosis and aggressive medical or surgical intervention are required.

NEUROLOGIC SYNDROMES

Brain abscess or meningitis can be caused in immunocompromised patients by gram-positive or gram-negative bacteria as well as by anaerobes.[15] *Listeria monocytogenes* is a particularly common cause of meningitis in these patients. Encapsulated bacteria such as pneumococci and staphylococci can cause metastatic CNS disease and meningitis. In patients with impaired cell-mediated immunity, *C. neoformans* is likewise a leading cause of CNS infection, usually presenting as cryptococcal meningitis or meningoencephalitis and sometimes as parenchymal mass lesions of the brain. *Aspergillus* species can infect the CNS both by direct sinus invasion and by hematogenous spread. Patients with impaired cellular immunity can develop CNS infection with *Toxoplasma gondii*, *M. tuberculosis*, *H. capsulatum*, or *Nocardia* species, either through severe infection by latent organisms or by reactivation. CNS syphilis should also be considered in patients with severe immunologic impairment.

Among the many viral etiologies of meningoencephalitis in immunocompromised individuals are enteroviruses, measles, neurotropic herpesviruses (HSV-1, CMV, VZV), and human herpesvirus 6. Progressive multifocal leukoencephalopathy caused by JC polyomavirus may occur in those with chronic CD4 lymphocytopenia and in recipients of hematopoietic stem cell or solid organ transplants as well as individuals treated with natalizumab, rituximab, and possibly other immunomodulatory monoclonal antibodies. Transplant recipients are also at increased risk for meningoencephalitis caused by West Nile virus. Patients with CNS symptoms presenting early after transplantation might be suspected of having severe infections acquired from the donor, including West Nile virus, rabies, HIV, lymphocytic choriomeningitis virus, or other viruses known to be transmitted through organ donation.

In addition to opportunistic infection, noninfectious causes of neurologic symptoms must be considered in immunocompromised patients, including drug toxicity, immunologic disorders, paraneoplastic syndromes, and Guillain-Barré syndrome. Posterior reversible encephalopathy syndrome (PRES) should be in the differential diagnosis of neurologic complications in transplant recipients, patients with autoimmune diseases, and those receiving high doses of cancer chemotherapy, particularly when the clinical presentation includes the sudden onset of severe "thunderclap" headache, seizures, confusion, and visual disturbance. PRES can be confirmed by characteristic CT or magnetic resonance imaging patterns of predominantly posterior cerebral edema and angiographic evidence of reversible vasoconstriction. PRES can be caused by endothelial injury, vasospasm, or edema associated with certain drugs such as calcineurin inhibitors (e.g., cyclosporine, tacrolimus).

Grade A References

A1. Vidal L, Ben Dor I, Paul M, et al. Oral versus intravenous antibiotic treatment for febrile neutropenia in cancer patients. *Cochrane Database Syst Rev.* 2013;10:CD003992.
A2. Beyar-Katz O, Dickstein Y, Borok S, et al. Empirical antibiotics targeting gram-positive bacteria for the treatment of febrile neutropenic patients with cancer. *Cochrane Database Syst Rev.* 2017;6: CD003914.
A3. Nakane T, Tamura K, Hino M, et al. Cefozopran, meropenem, or imipenem-cilastatin compared with cefepime as empirical therapy in febrile neutropenic adult patients: a multicenter prospective randomized trial. *J Infect Chemother.* 2015;21:16-22.
A4. Horita N, Shibata Y, Watanabe H, et al. Comparison of antipseudomonal beta-lactams for febrile neutropenia empiric therapy: systematic review and network meta-analysis. *Clin Microbiol Infect.* 2017;23:723-729.
A5. Stern A, Carrara E, Bitterman R, et al. Early discontinuation of antibiotics for febrile neutropenia versus continuation until neutropenia resolution in people with cancer. *Cochrane Database Syst Rev.* 2019;1:CD012184.

GENERAL REFERENCES

For the General References and other additional features, please visit Expert Consult at https://expertconsult.inkling.com.

266

PREVENTION AND CONTROL OF HEALTH CARE–ASSOCIATED INFECTIONS

DAVID P. CALFEE

THE BURDEN OF HEALTH CARE–ASSOCIATED INFECTIONS

The Centers for Disease Control and Prevention (CDC) defines health care–associated infections (HAIs) as infections that patients acquire during the course of receiving health care treatment for other conditions. *Nosocomial infection* is a term that refers specifically to an HAI that develops in association with hospital care. The development of infection during the course of health care is not, however, limited to the acute care hospital setting. Thus, *health care–associated infection* is the preferred term in referring to the broader spectrum of infections that develop during the course of health care, wherever that care may be provided, including acute care hospitals, long-term care facilities, rehabilitation facilities, dialysis facilities, and even the patient's home during the receipt of home care services.

The most extensive data regarding the incidence of and outcomes associated with HAIs come from the acute care hospital setting.[1] On the basis of a point prevalence study conducted in 183 U.S. hospitals in 2011, it was estimated that up to 1.4 million HAIs occur in hospital patients each year, with approximately 75,000 associated deaths (Table 266-1). By 2015, there was about a 16% decrease, from 4 to 3.2%, in prevalence.[2] Previous European studies have estimated that 4.1 million HAIs occur in European acute care hospitals each year. Thus, approximately one of every 14 to 20 patients admitted to U.S. and European hospitals develops an HAI, making HAI one of the most common complications associated with the receipt of health care. Moreover, these data indicate that HAIs are one of the top 10 causes of death in the United States. Whereas many of these HAI-associated deaths occur among patients who are already severely ill and who have a high likelihood of death due to their underlying disease, a substantial proportion of HAI-related deaths occur among persons who were otherwise expected to survive their hospitalization. In a single-center study, 31% of unexpected in-hospital deaths were determined to be possibly or probably related to an HAI. In addition to an increased risk of death, patients who develop HAI suffer a number of other adverse outcomes, including prolonged hospital stays, additional medical interventions and antibiotic treatment, discomfort, and loss of function and income. These statistics are particularly concerning when they are considered with the knowledge that many of these infections are preventable. In fact, a systematic review found that 55 to 70% of four of the most common types of HAIs are preventable through the use of currently available, evidence-based preventive strategies (see Table 266-1).

Although the majority of HAI statistics come from acute care hospitals, there are data to demonstrate that HAIs are significant problems in other health care settings as well. Point prevalence surveys conducted in European and the U.S. Veterans Affairs system long-term care facilities found that the prevalence of HAI among long-term care facility residents ranged from 2.4 to 5.2%. The overall burden of HAI among long-term care facility residents has been estimated to be 1.64 to 3.83 million infections per year in the United States and at least 2.6 million infections per year in Europe. Vascular access–related infections are the most common HAIs among patients requiring chronic hemodialysis for end-stage renal disease, with a reported incidence of 1.1 to 5.5 episodes per 1000 catheter days, and they are associated with increased morbidity, hospitalization, and death.[3] The magnitude of HAIs related to care provided in other settings, such as ambulatory surgery and endoscopy centers, has not been as thoroughly studied, but such infections have been well described.

TABLE 266-1 ESTIMATES OF THE BURDEN, COSTS, AND PREVENTABILITY OF COMMON HEALTH CARE–ASSOCIATED INFECTIONS IN U.S. HOSPITALS

TYPE OF INFECTION	NUMBER OF INFECTIONS PER YEAR[†]	AVERAGE ATTRIBUTABLE COST* PER INFECTION[‡]	CASE-FATALITY RATE[§]	PROPORTION PREVENTABLE[‖]
Urinary tract infection	28,100-176,700	$749-$1007	2.3%	65-70%
Catheter-associated urinary tract infection	19,024-119,626			
Surgical site infection	50,800-281,400	$11,087-$34,670	2.8%	55%
Pneumonia	50,800-281,400	$14,806-$28,508	14.4%	55%
Ventilator-associated pneumonia	19,863-110,027			
Blood stream infection	20,700-140,200	$6461-$29,156	12.3%	65-70%
Central line–associated blood stream infection	17,388-117,768			
C. difficile infection	23,700-155,000	$5682-$9124	2.9%	

*In 2007 U.S. dollars.
[†]Magill SS, Edwards JR, Bamberg W, et al. Multistate point-prevalence survey of health care-associated infections. *N Engl J Med.* 2014;370:1198-1208.
[‡]Scott RD. The direct medical costs of healthcare-associated infections in U.S. hospitals and the benefits of prevention. Centers for Disease Control and Prevention; 2009. Available at: http://www.cdc.gov/hai/pdfs/hai/scott_costpaper.pdf. Accessed August 14, 2017.
[§]Klevens RM, Edwards JR, Richards CL, Jr., et al. Estimating health care-associated infections and deaths in U.S. hospitals, 2002. *Public Health Rep.* 2007;122:160-166.
[‖]Umscheid CA, Mitchell MD, Doshi JA, et al. Estimating the proportion of healthcare-associated infections that are reasonably preventable and the related mortality and costs. *Infect Control Hosp Epidemiol.* 2011;32:101-114.

PATHOBIOLOGY

HAIs can be caused by organisms that are a part of the patient's normal flora (i.e., endogenous infection) or by pathogens acquired during exposure to health care (i.e., exogenous infection) through the contaminated hands of health care workers, the environment, contaminated medical equipment, other patients, or visitors. A variety of factors can contribute to the development of an HAI, and in many cases, HAIs are multifactorial in nature. These factors can be related to the pathogen, the host, the specific health care interventions that a patient receives, the setting in which health care is received, and the methods by which these interventions are made. HAI prevention strategies focus on eliminating, reducing, or modifying one or more of these risk factors.

Pathogen-Related Factors

A variety of pathogen-related factors contribute to the ability of an organism to cause infection. These factors include the organism's normal reservoir, mode of transmission (e.g., direct or indirect contact transmission, respiratory droplets, airborne particles), ability to survive on inanimate objects and surfaces, ability to produce biofilm, virulence factors, and resistance to antimicrobial agents and, for some organisms (e.g., *Clostridium difficile*), disinfectants.

Host-Related Factors

Many host-specific factors are associated with an inherent increased risk of one or more types of infection, regardless of the receipt of health care; however, when a patient with one or more of these risk factors enters the health care system, these factors contribute to an increased risk of HAI. Such risk factors include age (with neonates and older adults having an increased risk of infection because of incomplete development or senescence of the immune system, respectively), obesity, smoking, severity of illness, and certain medical conditions (e.g., burns, end-stage liver or renal disease, poorly controlled diabetes, some cancers, congenital or acquired immune deficiency). These factors reflect suppression of the immune system or breaches of other normal host defense mechanisms. Whereas many of these factors are not amenable to intervention or cannot be effectively modified in the short term, interventions that address remediable risk factors (e.g., obesity, smoking, poorly controlled diabetes mellitus) have the potential to reduce the risk of HAI during future episodes of health care.

Health Care–Related Factors

Health care–related HAI risk factors are those resulting from interventions that are intended to treat or otherwise provide benefit for a patient's existing medical conditions but that also introduce an increase in the risk of infection. These factors may disrupt normal host defenses or alter the patient's normal microbiologic flora. Health care–related risk factors include the use of invasive devices (e.g., central venous catheters, urinary catheters, endotracheal tubes), surgical procedures, exposure to antibiotics, receipt of immunosuppressive medications, and prolonged hospitalization. Because each of these interventions poses at least some degree of increased risk of infection, the risk-to-benefit

ratio of each intervention must frequently be reassessed so that patients are not exposed to unnecessary risk. For example, central venous catheters and indwelling urinary catheters are major risk factors for primary blood stream infection and urinary tract infection, respectively. In a patient who has a true medical need for one of these devices, the benefits of the catheter exceed the risk of infection. However, once the patient recovers from the condition that necessitated the catheter, the risks associated with the device then outweigh the benefits.

Exposure to antibiotics is a well-established risk factor for colonization and infection with multidrug-resistant organisms (MDROs) and development of *C. difficile* infection (CDI) through a mechanism known as antibiotic selection pressure. Antimicrobial use is common in acute care hospitals and other health care settings, such as long-term care and dialysis facilities and ambulatory care practices. A 2009 point prevalence survey of hospitals in 25 European countries found that 29% of hospitalized patients receive one or more antimicrobials during their hospital stay. In a 2011 study, the overall prevalence of antimicrobial use among patients in 183 U.S. hospitals was 49.9%. The prevalence of antimicrobial use, however, varied substantially among hospital locations, ranging from 2.9% in nursery wards to 77.3% in surgical critical care units. Even more important, studies have shown that 25 to 75% of antimicrobial use in acute care, long-term care, and hemodialysis facilities is unnecessary or inappropriate. Inappropriate and unnecessary antimicrobial use includes administration of antimicrobial regimens that are broader in spectrum or longer in duration than necessary, use of antibiotics that do not provide activity against the causative pathogen, treatment for test results that do not reflect the presence of infection (e.g., specimen contamination, asymptomatic colonization), use of antibacterial agents for treatment of conditions that are not due to bacterial infection (e.g., viral respiratory tract infections), and prescription of inappropriate doses of an antibiotic. Misuse and overuse of antimicrobial agents in the outpatient setting are also well-recognized problems in the United States and other countries, including many countries where antimicrobials can be obtained without a prescription. This inappropriate use of antimicrobial agents introduces unnecessary risk for the development of complications of antibiotic therapy, including CDI, MDRO infection, and toxicity, and represents an important target for intervention.

Health Care Delivery–Related Factors

This group of risk factors includes those that are introduced as a result of the way in which health care is delivered. These risk factors do not offer any potential benefit to patients but rather are associated only with risk. Health care delivery–associated risk factors include, among other things, failure to perform hand hygiene when indicated or to use aseptic or sterile technique during invasive procedures, unsafe injection practices (e.g., entering a multidose vial with a used needle), and failure to adequately clean and disinfect or sterilize the patient environment and medical equipment and instruments. These risks are all potentially modifiable and are thus important targets for HAI prevention initiatives. Antibiotic use, which has already been discussed as a patient-specific health care–related risk factor, can also be considered a health care delivery–related risk factor. Unlike with other types of drugs, use and misuse of antibiotics in one patient or population can introduce risks among the larger population through changes in microbial ecology (i.e., selection and increased prevalence of antimicrobial-resistant pathogens).

Many of these health care delivery–related factors are the result of poor adherence to recommended, evidence-based infection prevention practices. Despite recognition that poor hand hygiene practice is a leading cause of pathogen transmission, the existence of major national and international guidelines, and initiatives to improve hand hygiene practices among health care workers, compliance with recommended hand hygiene practices among health care personnel remains unacceptably low. In the United States, average rates of health care worker compliance with recommended hand hygiene practices have been reported to be less than 50%, with some individual studies reporting rates as low as 20% in some intensive care units (ICUs). Similarly, unsafe injection practices continue to be identified as the cause of health care–related transmission of blood-borne pathogens, such as hepatitis B and C viruses.

In recent years, there has been an increasing recognition of the role of environmental contamination in the transmission of health care–associated pathogens.[4] Environmental contamination with these organisms is common, and many of these organisms can persist in the health care environment for prolonged periods. For example, environmental contamination with *C. difficile* has been detected in up to 100% of hospital rooms occupied by patients with CDI, whereas methicillin-resistant *Staphylococcus aureus* (MRSA) has been detected on environmental surfaces in approximately 70% of hospital rooms housing patients infected and colonized with MRSA. Some but not all studies have identified similarly high rates of environmental contamination with multidrug-resistant gram-negative pathogens. This contamination can result in patient-to-patient transmission through transient contamination of health care workers' hands and equipment or by direct contact of the patient with the contaminated environment. Studies have shown that admission to a hospital room in which the prior occupant was colonized or infected with one of several MDROs is a significant risk factor for acquisition of that organism. Environmental contamination is, however, a potentially modifiable risk factor for HAI. Cleaning and disinfection of the environment and portable medical equipment that is shared among patients are often suboptimal. For example, one multicenter study conducted in 36 acute care hospitals in the United States found that at baseline, only 48% of high-risk environmental surfaces were cleaned during routine cleaning after discharge of the patient. Improvement in cleaning practices and other interventions to reduce the microbiologic burden in the health care environment has been shown to reduce the microbial burden of organisms in the environment and has been associated with a reduction in the risk of acquisition of MDROs and CDI. Identification of optimal strategies to reduce or eliminate the risk to patients that is posed by a contaminated health care environment is an area of active investigation, with study of methods to improve routine cleaning and disinfection as well as the study of novel methods of disinfection.[A1] Recent outbreaks of infection due to contaminated medical devices (e.g., duodenoscopes, heater-cooler devices used in cardiothoracic surgery procedures) highlight the critical role that cleaning and disinfecting or sterilizing of medical equipment plays in preventing health care–associated infections. In addition to cleaning and disinfection of environmental surfaces and disinfection or sterilization of shared medical equipment, environmental infection control interventions are important for preventing patients from acquiring pathogens due to exposure to water (e.g., *Legionella* species) and air (e.g., environmental fungi) within the health care setting.

Pathogens in Health Care–Associated Infections

The organisms most commonly identified in device- and procedure-associated infections (i.e., central line–associated blood stream infection, catheter-associated urinary tract infection, ventilator-associated pneumonia, and surgical site infection) vary somewhat among the different types and sites of infection. Overall, in the United States 10 pathogen groups accounted for more than 75% of pathogens identified in device- and procedure-related infections reported to the CDC through the National Healthcare Safety Network between 2011 and 2014.[5] These pathogen groups and the proportion of reported pathogens that they represented include *Escherichia coli* (15%), *Staphylococcus aureus* (12%), *Klebsiella* species (8.0%), coagulase-negative staphylococci (8%), *Enterococcus faecalis* (7%), *Pseudomonas aeruginosa* (7%), *Candida albicans* (7%), *Enterobacter* species (4%), *Enterococcus faecium* (4%), and other *Enterococcus* species (4%). Whereas many of these pathogens represent patients' endogenous flora, further discussion of several of the organisms that may be acquired during exposure to health care is warranted.

Multidrug-Resistant Organisms

An increasingly concerning problem is the emergence of acquired antimicrobial resistance among many of the bacterial pathogens that are common causes of HAIs (Table 266-2). MDROs represent a significant health threat because infections caused by many of these MDROs have been associated with worse outcomes than those caused by antimicrobial-susceptible strains of the same organism, including excess length of hospital stay, increased health care costs, and higher mortality, with mortality rates approaching 50% in some studies. Possible explanations for the observed increased rate of adverse outcomes associated with MDRO infections include the presence of more severe underlying disease, delays in initiating effective therapy, and the use of more toxic or less effective therapy for treatment of the infection. Regardless of their cause, the poor outcomes associated with MDRO infections highlight the critical need for effective preventive measures and development of new antibiotics with activity against these MDROs, particularly multidrug-resistant gram-negative bacilli (MDR-GNB).

Organisms can develop resistance to antimicrobial agents to which they were previously susceptible through a variety of mechanisms, including induction, genetic mutation, and acquisition of new genetic material (e.g., conjugation with cell-to-cell transfer of genetic material by plasmids or transposons). In the health care setting, however, patient-to-patient transmission of MDROs

TABLE 266-2 RATES OF ANTIMICROBIAL RESISTANCE AMONG PATHOGENIC ISOLATES FROM HEALTH CARE–ASSOCIATED INFECTIONS

		PROPORTION OF ISOLATES RESISTANT TO ANTIBIOTIC		
ORGANISM	**ANTIBIOTIC CLASS**	**United States (2011-2014)***	**ICUs in 43 Asian, African, European, and Latin American Countries (2007-2012)[†]**	**ICUs in 13 European Countries (2014)[‡]**
Staphylococcus aureus	Anti-staphylococcal penicillins (e.g., oxacillin, methicillin)	42-57%	36-62%	25%
Klebsiella species	Extended-spectrum cephalosporins	10-28%	63-71%	44%
	Carbapenems	3-13%	14-20%	8%
Pseudomonas aeruginosa	Carbapenems	8-28%	34-43%	28%
Enterococcus faecium	Glycopeptides (vancomycin)	58-86%	NR	NR
Acinetobacter baumannii	Carbapenems	33-69%	66-77%	64%
Escherichia coli	Extended-spectrum cephalosporins	13-24%	62-66%	17%
	Carbapenems	1-2%	5-8%	1%
	Fluoroquinolones	29-49%	64-70%	NR

ICUs, intensive care units; NR, not reported.

*Weiner LM, Webb AK, Limbago B, et al. Antimicrobial-resistant pathogens associated with healthcare-associated infections: summary of data reported to the National Healthcare Safety Network at the Centers for Disease Control and Prevention, 2011-2014. *Infect Control Hosp Epidemiol.* 2016;37:1288-1301.

[†]Rosenthal VD, Maki DG, Mehta Y, et al. International Nosocomial Infection Control Consortium (INICC) report, data summary of 43 countries, for 2007-2012. *Am J Infect Control.* 2014;42:942-956.

[‡]European Centre for Disease Prevention and Control. Annual Epidemiological Report 2016—Healthcare-associated infections acquired in intensive care units. Stockholm: ECDC;2016. Available at: https://ecdc.europa.eu/en/publications-data/healthcare-associated-infections-acquired-intensive-care-units-annual. Accessed August 12, 2017.

is more common than de novo development of resistance in a previously susceptible organism within the patient's existing microbiome. Identified risk factors for acquisition of MDROs include exposure to antibiotics, frequent or prolonged exposure to health care facilities (e.g., hospitals, nursing homes), poor infection control practices among health care workers, environmental contamination with MDROs, and prevalence of MDROs among other patients within a health care facility.

Among the pathogens reported to the CDC between 2011 and 2014 as causes of device-associated infections and surgical site infections, approximately 20% had antimicrobial susceptibility profiles that met the CDC's definition of multidrug resistance (see Table 266-2). Of note, 58 to 86% of *Enterococcus faecium* isolates were vancomycin resistant (VRE), and 42 to 57% of *S. aureus* isolates were resistant to methicillin (MRSA). These multidrug-resistant gram-positive pathogens have been recognized as significant health care–associated pathogens for several decades. More recently, the emergence of multidrug resistance among several gram-negative pathogens has been identified as a growing global health threat among persons receiving health care (Chapter 289). For example, approximately 55% of *Acinetobacter baumannii* isolates reported to the CDC in 2011-2014 demonstrated acquired resistance to at least one drug in three or more antibiotic classes. Such multidrug resistance definitions were also met by 13% of *Klebsiella* isolates and 14% of *P. aeruginosa* isolates. Antimicrobial resistance is an important problem in many regions of the world. For example, International Nosocomial Infection Control Consortium data from intensive care units in 43 countries in Asia, Africa, Europe, and Latin America collected between 2007 and 2012 demonstrated methicillin resistance in 61% of *S. aureus* isolates and extended-spectrum cephalosporin resistance in 66% of *Klebsiella pneumoniae* isolates and 63% of *E. coli* isolates. The lack of use of a standardized definition of multidrug resistance limits direct comparisons of resistance data from different populations. Standardized definitions for multidrug resistant, extensively drug resistant, and pandrug resistant have been proposed. Adoption of these or other standardized definitions is needed to allow a more thorough understanding of the global burden of antimicrobial resistance among health care–associated pathogens.

One example of the emergence and rapid dissemination of MDR-GNB is carbapenem-resistant Enterobacteriaceae (CRE), particularly *K. pneumoniae* (Chapter 289). Carbapenem resistance among these organisms was rare in the United States before the year 2000, at which time less than 1% of *K. pneumoniae* isolates reported to the CDC demonstrated such resistance. By 2009-2010, 8 to 13% of *K. pneumoniae* isolates from hospital-associated infections were resistant to carbapenems. In the United States, carbapenem resistance among the Enterobacteriaceae is most commonly due to the production of *K. pneumoniae* carbapenemase (KPC), a class A serine β-lactamase enzyme that hydrolyzes all β-lactam antibiotics. The KPC enzyme, which was first described in 2001, is encoded by the bla_{KPC} gene carried on a transmissible plasmid that also carries additional genes that confer resistance to several other classes of antimicrobial agents. Thus, in addition to carbapenem resistance, these organisms demonstrate resistance to other β-lactam antibiotics and to several other classes of antibiotics.

Asymptomatic carriage of MDROs is relatively common among persons with health care exposures. In fact, patients with clinically apparent MDRO infections represent a relatively small proportion of the total burden of these pathogens. Reported rates of MRSA carriage have ranged from 4.6 to 13.6% among hospital patients, 2 to 22% among U.S. ambulatory dialysis patients, and 10 to 100% among residents of long-term care facilities. The prevalence of VRE carriage among hospital patients and ambulatory dialysis patients has been reported to range from 6.3 to 67% and 0 to 16%, respectively. Studies that have included a variety of MDR-GNB have reported carriage rates of 19 to 32% in ICU patients and hospital patients with diarrhea, 25% among residents of long-term care facilities, and 16% among chronic hemodialysis patients. Studies that have focused specifically on carbapenem-resistant Enterobacteriaceae have demonstrated prevalence rates ranging from 2 to 5.4% among high-risk hospital patients in the United States and 2 to 49% among post–acute care facility patients in Israel. These asymptomatic carriers play an important role in the epidemiology of MDRO infections. First, they are at substantial risk of subsequent infection with the colonizing organism, with up to one third of carriers of MRSA, VRE, and MDR-GNB developing symptomatic infection within 12 months. Second, asymptomatic MDRO carriers can contribute to MDRO transmission within the health care system through contamination of their surrounding environment and of health care workers' hands, clothing, and medical equipment. In fact, several studies have demonstrated that the risk of acquiring an MDRO, such as MRSA, VRE, and MDR-GNB, during hospitalization is related to the prevalence, or colonization pressure,

of that MDRO among other patients. Finally, admission to a hospital room in which the prior patient was colonized or infected with the MRSA, VRE, or MDR-GNB has been associated with an increased risk of acquisition of those organisms.

There are, however, some encouraging data related to the incidence of some MDROs, particularly MRSA. In the United States, the incidence of hospital-onset invasive MRSA infections decreased 54% between 2005 and 2011. During the same time period, the incidence of invasive MRSA infections among dialysis patients, a group with a rate of invasive MRSA infection that is approximately 100 times greater than that of the general population, was also observed to have significantly decreased in the United States. These changes occurred despite the emergence of community-associated MRSA as a significant cause of skin and soft tissue infections among persons without typical health care–associated risk factors and the introduction of community-associated MRSA as a health care–acquired pathogen.[6] In England, an 86% reduction in the number of cases of MRSA bacteremia reported through a mandatory reporting system was observed between 2004 and 2012. The specific cause of these observed decreases in MRSA HAIs is uncertain and may be the result of improvements in basic infection control practices, introduction of specific MRSA prevention practices, or other changes in the epidemiology of this pathogen. There are also examples of successful containment of other MDROs. For example, the spread of CRE within Israeli hospitals has been substantially reduced with the introduction of a nationwide intervention.

Clostridium Difficile

C. difficile, the etiologic agent of pseudomembranous colitis, is the most common cause of health care–associated infectious diarrhea (Chapter 280). Although community-associated CDI occurs,[7] most cases are associated with receipt of health care. Analysis of CDC data from 2010 found that 94% of cases of CDI were associated with health care exposure but that 75% of cases had their onset outside of the hospital (e.g., in the community or in long-term care facilities). Clinical manifestations of CDI range from asymptomatic carriage to mild diarrhea to life-threatening colitis, toxic megacolon, and sepsis. The overall mortality associated with CDI has been reported to range from 2 to 6%, with substantially higher mortality among patients who develop toxic megacolon and other severe manifestations of the disease. Compared with patients without CDI, hospital patients who develop CDI experience an extended duration of hospitalization, and approximately 15 to 30% of these patients will experience at least one recurrence of the disease, typically within 1 to 2 months of the initial episode. Persons who experience one recurrence have a 50 to 60% chance of additional recurrences. Estimates of CDI-attributable hospital costs range from $5682 to $9124 per case (in 2007 U.S. dollars), amounting to a total cost of $1 billion to $4.8 billion per year.

More HAIs are now due to *C. difficile* than to MRSA. The incidence of CDI among hospitalized patients in the United States more than doubled between 2000 and 2009. Data from the CDC indicate that approximately 250,000 cases of *C. difficile* occur each year in the United States. In addition to an increased incidence of CDI, the rate of *C. difficile*–related deaths increased more than four-fold in the United States during the last decade, causing approximately 14,000 deaths per year. The observed increases in the incidence of and mortality associated with CDI were temporally associated with the emergence and dissemination of the 027/NAP1/BI strain of *C. difficile*, which has been associated with greater mortality and higher rates of recurrence than other circulating strains. Initially identified in North America, this epidemic strain has now disseminated globally.

The problem of *C. difficile* extends beyond the acute care hospital setting. For instance, data from Ohio indicate that 62% of CDI cases in 2006 occurred in nursing homes. Data from the CDC have shown that 20% of hospital-onset CDI occurs among persons with recent residence in a nursing home and that two-thirds of nursing home–onset CDI cases occur among residents who have been recently discharged from an acute care hospital. These findings demonstrate the complex epidemiology of CDI.

The development of CDI is a two-step process that first requires acquisition of *C. difficile* through fecal-oral transmission and then the presence or introduction of factors that allow progression to symptomatic disease. Although some healthy individuals without health care exposure are intestinal carriers of *C. difficile*, acquisition of the organism during contact with the health care system plays a critical role in the epidemiology of CDI. Transmission in the health care setting can occur as the result of exposure to organisms on health care workers' hands, environmental surfaces, or medical equipment. Hand contamination of health care workers is common after contact with the skin or environment of persons with CDI.[8] In the absence of effective hand hygiene practices, contaminated health care workers may transmit the organism to other patients. Contamination of the environment and medical equipment with *C. difficile* is also common. Testing performed in hospital rooms has identified *C. difficile* on environmental surfaces in up to 100% of rooms housing patients with active CDI and in as many as 33% of non-CDI patient rooms. Commonly contaminated surfaces include bed rails, bedside tables, telephones, call buttons, and blood pressure cuffs. *C. difficile* spores are resistant to killing by many common hospital disinfectants and can persist in the environment for long times, further contributing to the risk of exposure to a contaminated environment. Patients who are admitted to a hospital room in which the previous occupant had CDI have been found to be at greater risk for development of CDI than patients admitted to hospital rooms in which the previous occupant did not have CDI.

Once *C. difficile* has been ingested, several factors are known to be associated with development of symptomatic CDI. The major risk factor is receipt of antibiotics. Such exposures disrupt the normal intestinal flora and allow *C. difficile* to multiply to larger numbers and to produce toxins that result in disease. Although exposure to any antimicrobial agent may increase the risk for development of CDI, clindamycin, third-generation cephalosporins, penicillins, and fluoroquinolones may present the highest risk. Other factors that have been associated with an increased risk for development of CDI include receipt of cytotoxic chemotherapeutic agents and gastric acid suppressive medications such as proton pump inhibitors, failure to develop an antibody response to *C. difficile,* and older age (i.e., age older than 64 years).

Viruses
Respiratory Viruses
Common respiratory viruses, such as influenza, can be transmitted in the health care setting by health care workers, visitors, and patients, resulting in health care–acquired disease. Higher rates of morbidity and mortality have been observed among those who acquire infection during hospitalization, probably due to the presence of significant underlying medical illness. Despite several studies that have associated higher influenza immunization rates of health care workers with lower rates of nosocomial influenza transmission, the uptake of influenza vaccination among health care workers remains relatively low. This has led many public health agencies and professional societies to call for mandatory influenza vaccination policies for all eligible health care workers. The health care–associated transmission of newly emerged respiratory viruses, such as the severe acute respiratory syndrome coronavirus (SARS-CoV) in 2003, pandemic influenza in 2009, and the Middle East respiratory syndrome coronavirus (MERS-CoV) in 2013, highlights the importance of syndromic surveillance to allow rapid identification of patients with potentially communicable diseases and implementation of appropriate infection control precautions.

Blood-borne Viruses
Although routine screening of the blood supply for the blood-borne pathogens (BBPs) hepatitis B virus, hepatitis C virus, and human immunodeficiency virus has dramatically decreased the incidence of health care–associated BBP infections, transmission of these pathogens within health care settings continues to occur. Most health care–associated BBP transmission that occurs now is due to failure to adhere to recommended basic infection control practices. Unsafe injection practices (e.g., reuse of syringes, contamination of multidose vials, improper use and disinfection of blood glucose monitoring devices that are used for multiple patients) and inadequate cleaning, disinfection, and sterilization of medical equipment and the health care environment (e.g., dialysis facilities) have been identified in several recent outbreaks of patient-to-patient transmission of BBPs. A large proportion of documented health care–associated hepatitis B virus and hepatitis C virus transmission events has occurred in outpatient settings and long-term care facilities, highlighting the importance of infection prevention programs throughout the entire health care system. Transmission of BBPs from health care worker to patient is uncommon but can occur, typically in the setting of "exposure-prone" invasive procedures but also as a result of drug diversion by health care workers. Guidelines are available to assist health care workers and health care facilities in minimizing the risk posed to patients by a BBP-infected health care worker while allowing most such health care workers to remain involved in patient care activities (E-Table 266-1).

Fungi
Candida albicans and other *Candida* species accounted for approximately 9.3% of all pathogens reported to the CDC between 2011 and 2014 as causes of device-associated infections and surgical site infections, placing them among the most common pathogens implicated in HAIs. The recent emergence of multidrug-resistant *C. auris* as a cause of health care facility–associated outbreaks further highlights the importance of *Candida* species in HAI epidemiology. Exposure to environmental fungi, such as *Aspergillus* species, in the health care setting can result in HAI, particularly in immunocompromised hosts. Such exposure and resulting infection are most commonly associated with inadequate environmental control measures during construction, demolition, or water damage within the health care facility. A multistate outbreak of invasive fungal infections in the United States, mostly due to *Exserohilum rostratum* associated with contaminated methylprednisolone injections, demonstrates that contaminated medications and other medical products are additional potential sources of exposure to fungal pathogens during health care.

Device-Associated Infections
Central Line–Associated Blood Stream Infections
Central line–associated blood stream infections (CLABSIs) are blood stream infections that occur in patients with a central venous catheter and in whom there is no other identified source of the infection. Development of CLABSI has been associated with longer hospital stays, increased risk of death, and greater hospital costs than those observed among otherwise similar patients who do not develop CLABSI (see Table 266-1). Rates of morbidity and mortality, however, vary substantially, depending on the causative pathogen and characteristics of the patient in whom the infection occurs. Although CLABSIs are often thought of as a complication that occurs among ICU patients, the use of central venous catheters in non-ICU hospital wards has expanded substantially during the past few decades. Thus, the incidence of and the overall burden of CLABSI in some non-ICU wards now often exceeds that in ICUs. CLABSIs are also important problems among nonhospitalized persons with central venous catheters, such as persons receiving chronic total parenteral nutrition, chemotherapy, or dialysis in the outpatient or home care setting.

Blood stream infections due to central venous catheters are largely the result of contamination or colonization of the external surface or the intraluminal surface of the catheter. This contamination can occur either during catheter insertion or after insertion, related to a number of aspects of catheter use and care. Effective strategies have been identified to reduce the risk of catheter contamination during insertion and throughout the time that the catheter remains in situ.[9] This research has led to the development of evidence-based guidelines for prevention of vascular catheter–related infections (see E-Table 266-1). The "central line bundle" refers to a small number of evidence-based practices that, when used together, can reduce the risk of CLABSI even more than would be expected when the components are introduced individually. The central line bundle includes hand hygiene, maximal barrier precautions during insertion (i.e., use of sterile gown and gloves and a surgical cap and mask by the operator and covering the patient with a sterile, full-body drape), chlorhexidine skin antisepsis, optimal insertion site selection (i.e., avoidance of the femoral site in adult patients), and daily review of catheter necessity with immediate removal of catheters that are no longer necessary. Regarding the use of a cutaneous antiseptic prior to central venous catheter insertion, a recent randomized trial found that a chlorhexidine–alcohol skin antiseptic solution provided greater protection against short-term catheter-related infections than did a povidone iodine–alcohol solution.[A2] Other interventions that have been associated with reductions in CLABSI rates include covering of the insertion site with a sterile gauze or semipermeable transparent dressing, cleansing of the catheter insertion site with an antiseptic such as chlorhexidine, use of aseptic technique to access and to manipulate the catheter, scrubbing of the catheter hub with a disinfectant before accessing the catheter lumen for administration of medications or other products or for aspiration of blood, use of antimicrobial- or antiseptic-coated catheters, and use of chlorhexidine rather than regular soap and water for daily bathing of ICU patients. Widespread adoption of the central line bundle and other CLABSI prevention strategies has been associated with a substantial reduction in the incidence of CLABSI in U.S. hospitals. Data from the CDC demonstrate a 50% decrease in the incidence of CLABSI in U.S. hospitals between 2008 and 2014.

Catheter-Associated Urinary Tract Infections
A catheter-associated urinary tract infection (CAUTI) is a urinary tract infection that develops in a patient who has or who recently had an indwelling urinary catheter. Similar to the pathogenesis of catheter-related blood stream infections, CAUTIs develop by the introduction of pathogens into the bladder as a result of contamination and colonization of the internal or external surface of the catheter. Among patients with indwelling urinary catheters, the incidence

of bacteriuria is 3 to 8% per day, and 10 to 25% of those with bacteriuria will subsequently develop symptoms consistent with a urinary tract infection.

A number of basic practices, such as aseptic technique during insertion, maintenance of proper cleanliness and hygiene, securement of the catheter to avoid piston-like movement of the catheter within the urethra, and maintenance of a closed system with unobstructed flow of urine from the bladder into the collection system, are recommended to reduce the risk of CAUTI.[10] It has been estimated that with implementation of such practices, 65 to 70% of CAUTIs that occur in acute care hospitals could be prevented. Several studies have demonstrated that indwelling urethral catheters are often inserted for inappropriate reasons and that many catheters that were initially inserted for an appropriate indication remain in place even after the initial indication for catheterization has resolved. This may be due in part to lack of familiarity with appropriate indications for catheter insertion or with options that exist regarding alternatives to the use of indwelling urethral catheters. Additional studies have found that physicians are often unaware that their patient has a urinary catheter. Thus, perhaps the greatest opportunity for CAUTI prevention is avoidance of unnecessary catheter insertion and prompt removal of catheters that are no longer necessary. Development of protocols that explicitly define appropriate indications for insertion of urinary catheters, introduction of interventions that remind clinicians to reassess the appropriateness of a patient's urinary catheter, and nurse-driven protocols that allow nurses to remove unnecessary urinary catheters have been associated with reduced catheter use and lower rates of CAUTI.

Ventilator-Associated Pneumonia

In hospitalized patients, mechanical ventilation is one of the most common risk factors for the development of pneumonia. Mechanical ventilation and the interventions required to provide mechanical ventilation (e.g., endotracheal intubation, sedation) increase the risk of pulmonary infection through a variety of mechanisms, including an increased risk of aspiration of oropharyngeal and gastrointestinal secretions and impairment of the cough reflex. From both a clinical and epidemiologic standpoint, ventilator-associated pneumonia (VAP) is a difficult diagnosis to establish with certainty because of the subjective nature of many of the variables considered (e.g., chest radiograph findings, changes in the characteristics of respiratory tract secretions), alternative explanations for clinical and radiographic abnormalities (e.g., acute respiratory distress syndrome, atelectasis), and difficulty in determining whether the results of respiratory tract cultures represent true infection or colonization of the airway. To minimize subjectivity involved in making the diagnosis of VAP, a new surveillance classification has been proposed that characterizes all adverse ventilator-associated events (VAE) to replace the current VAP definition.[11]

Based on a point prevalence study, pneumonia is one of the two most common types of HAI and approximately 39% of cases are associated with mechanical ventilation. These infections are associated with mortality rates and health care costs that are among the highest observed among all HAIs (see Table 266-1). Studies suggest that at least 55% of VAP cases are preventable. As with other device-associated infections, avoiding the use of the device is the most effective means of preventing infection. For preventing VAP and other complications of mechanical ventilation, the use of noninvasive methods of ventilation, minimized use of sedation (e.g., manage patients without sedative if possible, daily sedation interruption and assessment of readiness to be extubated), and early mobilization can eliminate or at least reduce the duration of mechanical ventilation. For patients who do require mechanical ventilation, the following are routinely recommended for VAP prevention: proper cleaning, disinfection, sterilization, use, and maintenance of respiratory equipment; minimization of pooling of secretions above the endotracheal tube cuff; and elevation of the head of the bed (unless it is medically contraindicated). Routine oral hygiene, typically with an antiseptic such as chlorhexidine, is also a commonly used strategy that may be beneficial, but supporting data are limited. In some randomized, controlled trials, selective oropharyngeal or digestive decontamination has been associated with a significant reduction in VAP, but this approach has not yet been widely adopted as a standard of care in the United States, at least in part because of concerns that this intervention may lead to selection of antimicrobial-resistant organisms.

Other Device-Related Infections

With the advances that have occurred in medical technology in recent years, there have been substantial improvements in the capabilities of existing medical devices and the development of new implantable devices to treat and to manage a variety of medical conditions, particularly of the cardiovascular and nervous systems. These devices include cardiovascular implantable electronic devices

such as pacemakers and implantable cardioverter-defibrillators, ventricular assist devices, deep brain stimulators, and intrathecal pumps. The potential benefits that these devices may offer to patients come with at least some degree of risk of device-related infection.

Surgical Site Infections

Surgical site infections (SSIs) are infections that develop at the site of an operative procedure. Although only a relatively small proportion of patients who undergo surgery subsequently develop SSI and the overall mortality rate associated with SSI is relatively low, the absolute number of SSIs that occur and the overall cost and burden of morbidity and mortality associated with SSI are large because of the volume of surgical procedures performed each year (see Table 266-1). A number of factors contribute to the risk of SSI: the specific site and type of surgical procedure; duration of the procedure; tissue hypoxia at the surgical site; wound contamination with endogenous or exogenous organisms; surgical technique; perioperative infection prevention practices; environmental controls related to temperature, humidity, and air purity within the operating room; and the patient's underlying medical conditions, smoking status, and other factors that may increase the inherent risk of infection. Although some of these factors are not amenable to corrective intervention, many of them are, and a number of interventions have been proven to reduce the risk of SSI. In fact, it has been estimated that 55% of SSIs could be prevented by routine application of evidence-based preventive measures. The use of sterile technique, preoperative skin preparation with an antiseptic agent,[A3] administration of antimicrobial prophylaxis within 60 minutes before the surgical incision, maintenance of normothermia, and perioperative glucose control are practices that have been demonstrated to reduce the risk of infection associated with a wide variety of surgical procedures. There is also evidence that at least in some types of surgeries, the use of supplemental oxygen (e.g., 80% fraction of inspired oxygen) in the perioperative period may reduce the risk of SSI. Although substantial opportunities for improvement remain, surveillance data reported to the CDC's National Healthcare Safety Network by U.S. hospitals between 2008 and 2014 showed a 17% reduction in the incidence of SSI occurring in association with 10 common surgical procedures.

⬤ HEALTH CARE–ASSOCIATED INFECTION PREVENTION STRATEGIES

Many HAIs are preventable. This has been recognized since at least as early as the mid-1800s, when Semmelweiss demonstrated a dramatic reduction in sepsis-related deaths among maternity ward patients after an intervention to improve hand hygiene among health care workers. The degree to which HAIs are preventable was more clearly quantified in a multicenter study conducted in the 1970s. In that study, it was found that 32% of HAIs could be prevented through establishment of an effective infection control program. More recent estimates that take into account newer research and the technology that has been developed during the following three decades suggest that at least 55 to 70% of some of the most common HAIs can be prevented. Scientific research and clinical experience have led to the publication of evidence-based guidelines for the prevention of HAIs (see E-Table 266-1).

Antimicrobial Stewardship

Antimicrobial stewardship refers to interventions designed to improve the appropriateness of antimicrobial use by promoting the selection of an optimal antimicrobial regimen (i.e., the most appropriate drug, dose, duration, and route of administration) for a specific patient. The goals of an antimicrobial stewardship program are to optimize clinical outcomes (e.g., cure of infection related to antimicrobial use, minimize toxicity and other adverse events) and to limit the antimicrobial selection pressure that drives the emergence of antimicrobial-resistant strains. Multidisciplinary antimicrobial stewardship programs have been associated with several desirable outcomes, including significant reductions in antimicrobial use, reduced rates of antimicrobial resistance among health care–associated pathogens, reduced incidence of adverse outcomes associated with antibiotic use (e.g., toxicity, C. difficile infection), and significant reductions in hospital antimicrobial-associated costs.

A variety of approaches have been used by successful antimicrobial stewardship programs, and guidelines describing these strategies have been published (see E-Table 266-1).[12,13] One of the most commonly used and most effective strategies includes formulary restriction and requirement of preauthorization before prescribing certain antibiotics (e.g., antibiotics that are broad in their antimicrobial spectrum, are associated with significant toxicity, or are expensive). A second approach that has been considered to be a core strategy for antimicrobial stewardship activities is prospective audit of the appropriateness of prescribed antimicrobial therapy with provision of feedback to the prescribing clinician if opportunities for further optimization of therapy are available (e.g., narrowing or broadening spectrum of therapy, discontinuing antimicrobial therapy, or altering drug dose or dosing interval on the basis of available clinical data). Additional approaches that have been included in successful antimicrobial stewardship programs include education, development of guidelines and clinical pathways, computer-assisted decision support, and protocols to optimize conversion from the parenteral to the oral route of administration when appropriate. In addition to the standard challenges associated with implementation of interventions that require a change in human behavior and clinical practice, antimicrobial stewardship programs must also address the complex and constantly changing problems and issues associated with antimicrobial resistance.

Although an increasing proportion of acute care hospitals and long-term care facilities have introduced antimicrobial stewardship programs, many of these programs are not adequately resourced to reach their full potential. There is also a recognized need for development of such programs in other health care settings, such as long-term acute care hospitals, dialysis facilities, and outpatient practices.

Decolonization Therapy
Decolonization refers to the administration or application of antimicrobial or antiseptic agents to a person to eliminate or to reduce the burden of carriage of one or more pathogens. For example, selective oropharyngeal or digestive decontamination has been used for prevention of VAP and SSI after colorectal surgery, respectively. More recently, topical decolonization has been studied as a horizontal intervention for prevention of a variety of HAIs and prevention of transmission of a variety of pathogens. Several quasi-experimental, before-after studies have associated the use of chlorhexidine, compared with nonantimicrobial soap, for daily bathing of patients with significant reductions in rates of blood stream infections, including CLABSI, acquisition of MDROs, blood culture contamination, and contamination of the environment and health care workers. Thus far, two higher quality studies of daily chlorhexidine bathing have been published. A multicenter, cluster-randomized trial conducted in eight adult ICUs and one bone marrow transplant unit in the United States found that daily bathing with chlorhexidine, compared with nonmedicated soap, was associated with a 23% reduction in the combined outcome of MRSA and VRE acquisition.[A4] A similar study in pediatric ICUs showed a significant reduction in the incidence of bacteremia in the per-protocol analysis, although the difference observed in the intention-to-treat analysis did not reach statistical significance.[A5] A third cluster-randomized trial conducted in 74 adult ICUs in the United States found that providing all ICU patients with decolonization therapy that consisted of intranasal application of mupirocin for 5 days and daily chlorhexidine bathing significantly reduced the MRSA-positive clinical cultures attributable to the ICU by 37% and was associated with a lower incidence of all-cause blood stream infections compared with the use of active surveillance and contact precautions for MRSA-colonized patients without decolonization therapy.[A6] More recently published, single-center, randomized studies have yielded differing results. In one study, daily bathing with chlorhexidine was not associated with a reduction in the incidence of health care–associated infections in adult intensive care unit patients,[A7] while in another, every other day bathing with chlorhexidine was associated with a significant reduction in hospital-acquired infections.[A8] Thus, the role of routine chlorhexidine bathing as an HAI prevention strategy remains an unresolved issue. The inconsistent results obtained from clinical trials suggest that factors such as compliance and bathing technique as well as hospital-specific factors related to the epidemiology of HAI may influence the outcomes observed at the individual hospital and individual patient levels. In another cluster-randomized trial conducted in ICUs, selective decontamination of the digestive tract (SDD) and selective oropharyngeal decontamination (SOD) were compared for their impact on the prevalence of antimicrobial-resistant gram-negative bacteria, mortality, ICU-acquired bacteremia, and length of ICU stay. SDD was associated with a lower incidence of ICU-acquired bacteremia but was also associated with increased carriage of aminoglycoside-resistant gram-negative bacteria, thus raising concerns about long-term antimicrobial resistance risks with use of this strategy.[A9] Postdischarge MRSA decolonization with chlorhexidine and mupirocin can reduce subsequent MRSA infection by 30%.[A10]

Active Surveillance Testing
Active surveillance testing identifies asymptomatic carriers of a pathogen of interest (e.g., MRSA, VRE, MDR-GNB) with the intention to introduce additional interventions for identified carriers to prevent infection in the carrier or transmission to others. The interventions that may be applied to the identified carriers include transmission-based precautions (e.g., contact precautions), decolonization therapy (mostly applicable to *S. aureus*), and altered antimicrobial therapy (e.g., surgical antimicrobial prophylaxis). The role of active surveillance has long been the subject of debate and investigation. It is commonly used in outbreak control efforts in conjunction with other interventions. In the non-outbreak setting, there are numerous reports of use of active surveillance as part of a comprehensive program to reduce transmission of or infection with MDROs in individual hospitals, large hospital systems, and health care facilities within specific geographic regions, such as a number of northern European countries. A cluster-randomized trial conducted in U.S. ICUs found that there was not a significant difference in the incidence of colonization or infection with MRSA and VRE in ICUs that performed active surveillance testing with introduction of contact precautions for patients found to be carriers of MRSA or VRE compared with ICUs that did not conduct active surveillance testing.[A11] However, there was a delay in reporting the results of surveillance testing that was longer than would be anticipated in normal clinical practice, which may limit the ability to generalize the study findings to all settings.

Routine use of gowns and gloves for all patients is another intervention that has been used for its potential ability to reduce the risk of transmission of pathogens between patients by reducing contamination of health care workers' hands and clothing. A cluster-randomized study found that universal use of gowns and gloves for all patients in intensive care units was not associated with a reduction in the primary outcome of acquisition of either MRSA or VRE. There was, however, a significantly lower incidence of MRSA acquisition, a secondary study outcome, associated with universal gown and glove use.[A12] Thus, the utility of this strategy for preventing pathogen transmission remains uncertain.

GOALS AND INCENTIVES FOR HEALTH CARE–ASSOCIATED INFECTION PREVENTION
In addition to the obvious altruistic incentive of preventing patient harm, there are a number of additional incentives for health care providers and health care facilities to prevent HAIs. In the United States, the amount of attention given to HAIs and their prevention has greatly increased since the 1999 release of the Institute of Medicine report *To Err Is Human: Building a Safer Health System*. With this attention has come increasing pressure from the public, regulatory and accreditation agencies, and health care payers for the health care industry to improve its efforts and outcomes related to HAI prevention. The Centers for Medicare and Medicaid Services (CMS) Conditions of Participation list specific requirements for infection prevention and control processes in health care facilities that receive funding from CMS. Hospitals found to be deficient in the implementation of the requirements are at risk of losing the funding that they receive from the agency. Similarly, hospital accreditation agencies such as The Joint Commission have established standards for infection prevention programs and periodically survey hospitals to determine if such programs are in place. In addition, public reporting of hospital-specific HAI data by CMS and other agencies provides further incentive for hospitals to optimize their HAI prevention efforts.

Grade A References

A1. Anderson DJ, Chen LF, Weber DJ, et al. Enhanced terminal room disinfection and acquisition and infection caused by multidrug-resistant organisms and *Clostridium difficile* (the Benefits of Enhanced Terminal Room Disinfection study): a cluster-randomized, multicenter, crossover study. *Lancet.* 2017;389:805-814.

A2. Mimoz O, Lucet JC, Kerforne T, et al. Skin antisepsis with chlorhexidine-alcohol versus povidone iodine-alcohol, with and without skin scrubbing, for prevention of intravascular-catheter-related infection (CLEAN): an open-label, multicentre, randomised, controlled, two-by-two factorial trial. *Lancet.* 2015;386:2069-2077.

A3. Tuuli MG, Liu J, Stout MJ, et al. A randomized trial comparing skin antiseptic agents at cesarean delivery. *N Engl J Med.* 2016;374:647-655.

A4. Climo MW, Yokoe DS, Warren DK, et al. Effect of daily chlorhexidine bathing on hospital-acquired infection. *N Engl J Med.* 2013;368:533-542.

A5. Milstone AM, Elward A, Song X, et al. Daily chlorhexidine bathing to reduce bacteraemia in critically ill children: a multicentre, cluster-randomised, crossover trial. *Lancet.* 2013;381:1099-1106.

A6. Huang SS, Septimus E, Kleinman K, et al. Targeted versus universal decolonization to prevent ICU infection. *N Engl J Med.* 2013;368:2255-2265.

A7. Noto MJ, Domenico HJ, Byrne DW, et al. Chlorhexidine bathing and health care-associated infections: a randomized clinical trial. *JAMA.* 2015;313:369-378.

A8. Swan JT, Ashton CM, Bui LN, et al. Effect of chlorhexidine bathing every other day on prevention of hospital-acquired infections in the surgical ICU: a single-center, randomized controlled trial. *Crit Care Med.* 2016;44:1822-1832.

A9. Oostdijk EA, Kesecioglu J, Schultz MJ, et al. Effects of decontamination of the oropharynx and intestinal tract on antibiotic resistance in ICUs: a randomized clinical trial. *JAMA.* 2014;312:1429-1437.

A10. Huang SS, Singh R, McKinnell JA, et al. Decolonization to reduce postdischarge infection risk among MRSA carriers. *N Engl J Med.* 2019;380:638-650.

A11. Huskins W, Huckabee C, O'Grady N, et al. Intervention to reduce transmission of resistant bacteria in intensive care. *N Engl J Med.* 2011;364:1407-1418.

A12. Harris AD, Pineles L, Belton B, et al. Universal glove and gown use and acquisition of antibiotic-resistant bacteria in the ICU: a randomized trial. *JAMA.* 2013;310:1571-1580.

GENERAL REFERENCES

For the General References and other additional features, please visit Expert Consult at https://expertconsult.inkling.com.

267

APPROACH TO THE PATIENT WITH SUSPECTED ENTERIC INFECTION

HERBERT L. DUPONT AND PABLO C. OKHUYSEN

EPIDEMIOLOGY

Enteric infections are second only to respiratory tract infections as common infectious medical problems. In certain populations, enteric infections are hyperendemic: poorly nourished infants living in developing tropical countries showing excessive rates of mortality; infants in certain daycare centers; unhygienic residents of custodial institutions for persons with severe intellectual disabilities; immunosuppressed persons; and visitors from industrialized areas to developing regions with traveler's diarrhea.

ETIOLOGY

In approaching a patient with an enteric infection, epidemiologic (Table 267-1) and clinical (Table 267-2) features suggest a potential etiologic agent responsible for illness and a plan for evaluation (Table 267-3) and management (Table 267-4).[1]

Recent travel (Chapter 270) to mountainous regions or recreational lakes of North America should raise the suspicion of infection caused by *Giardia* species.[2] When diarrhea occurs during or after travel to a developing tropical region, a bacterial enteropathogen should be suspected.[3] The leading causes of traveler's diarrhea worldwide are the diarrheagenic *Escherichia coli* enterotoxigenic *E. coli* (ETEC) and enteroaggregative *E. coli* (EAEC). The invasive bacteria (*Shigella, Salmonella,* and *Campylobacter* species) cause diarrhea among travelers to all regions but are more common in Asia. Infection with *Cyclospora* species should be suspected when persistent or recurrent diarrhea follows

TABLE 267-1 EPIDEMIOLOGIC FEATURES IMPORTANT IN DETERMINING POTENTIAL CAUSE OF ENTERIC INFECTION IN A PERSON WITH DIARRHEA

EPIDEMIOLOGIC FEATURE	ETIOLOGIC AGENT TO SUSPECT
Travel to mountainous areas of North America	*Giardia* spp
Travel to Russia (especially St. Petersburg)	*Cryptosporidium, Giardia* spp
Travel to Nepal	*Cyclospora* spp
Travel to the developing tropical/semitropical world from an industrialized region	Enterotoxigenic *Escherichia coli,* enteroaggregative *E. coli; Shigella, Campylobacter, Salmonella* spp; other bacterial causes; *Giardia, Cyclospora, Cryptosporidium* spp and noroviruses
Presence of associated cases (an outbreak)	Use incubation period and clinical features to determine probable cause
Antibiotic, chemotherapy, or proton pump inhibitor use in the past 2 months, particularly with a history of recent or current hospitalization	*Clostridium difficile*
Contact with daycare centers	Any enteropathogen, often the low-dose organisms: *Giardia, Cryptosporidium, Shigella* spp or viral pathogens
Anal-genital, oral-anal, or digital-anal contact	Any organism spread by fecal-oral route; in those with proctitis, suspect *Neisseria gonorrhoeae, Chlamydia trachomatis,* herpes simplex, or *Treponema pallidum*
Immunosuppressed person	Any agent, especially *C. difficile,* norovirus, *Cryptosporidium, Cyclospora, Cystoisospora, Shigella,* and *Salmonella* spp; *C. jejuni, Mycobacterium avium-intracellulare,* microsporidia, herpes simplex virus, and cytomegalovirus
Recent or current cruise ship travel	Norovirus, less frequently enterotoxigenic *E. coli*

TABLE 267-2 CLINICAL FEATURES OF ENTERIC INFECTION

CLINICAL SYNDROME	ETIOLOGIC AGENTS SUSPECTED	SPECIAL CONSIDERATIONS
Sustained fever, often with systemic toxicity (enteric or typhoid fever)	*Salmonella typhi,* nontyphoid *Salmonella* spp, *Campylobacter* spp, *Shigella* spp, *Yersinia enterocolitica*	Stool and blood cultures; empirical antibiotics generally indicated. For this and other syndromes, multiplexed nucleic acid amplification tests are accurate and provide fast turn around. Confirmation with culture and sensitivity testing is recommended for bacterial agents of diarrhea
Acute watery (secretory) diarrhea	Any agent. Consider *Vibrio cholerae* (if water losses are major), enterotoxigenic or enteroaggregative *Escherichia coli, Shigella* spp, *Salmonella* spp, *Campylobacter jejuni,* viral or parasitic protozoal pathogen	Fluid and electrolyte therapy crucial for recovery in dehydration
Recurrent vomiting (gastroenteritis)	Viral agents (rotavirus or noroviruses) or preformed toxin (*Staphylococcus aureus* or *Bacillus cereus*)	In case of an outbreak, incubation period suggests the etiology
Bloody diarrhea (dysentery)	*Shigella* spp, *C. jejuni, Salmonella* spp, Shiga toxin–producing *E. coli* (e.g., O157:H7 or other serotype) or enteroinvasive *E. coli, Aeromonas hydrophila,* noncholera *Vibrio* spp, *Yersinia enterocolitica, Entamoeba histolytica,* or inflammatory bowel disease	Stool culture and occasionally parasite examination important to determining cause; hemolytic-uremic syndrome may complicate diarrheal disease caused by Shiga toxin–producing *E. coli* or rarely *Shigella dysenteriae*
Diarrhea lasting ≥2 weeks (persistent diarrhea)	*Giardia* spp and other protozoal parasites, bacterial overgrowth, *Tropheryma whipplei,* lactase deficiency, Brainerd diarrhea, postinfectious irritable bowel syndrome (PI-IBS), unmasked inflammatory bowel disease (IBD), or celiac sprue. Rarely due to conventional agents of bacterial diarrhea	Stool culture and parasite examination indicated; empirical anti-*Giardia* therapy may be useful; remove milk from diet; prior raw milk or untreated (well or surface) water consumption or international travel may predispose to Brainerd diarrhea; with illness lasting >30 days, consider Brainerd diarrhea, PI-IBS, celiac disease, or IBD

TABLE 267-3 LABORATORY TESTS AND PROCEDURES USEFUL IN THE DIAGNOSIS OF INFECTIOUS DIARRHEA

SPECIFIC TEST OR PROCEDURE	WHEN INDICATED	CLINICAL SIGNIFICANCE
Fecal leukocyte test	For moderate to severe cases	When present, indicates diffuse colonic inflammation, often due to *Shigella, Salmonella, Campylobacter* spp, Shiga toxin–producing *Escherichia coli*, or *Clostridium difficile*
Fecal lactoferrin	For moderate to severe cases to help identify inflammatory forms of enteric infection, to use in health care–associated diarrhea to help determine whether *C. difficile* toxin test should be performed	More sensitive test than fecal leukocytes and will pick up the same pathogens as fecal leukocytes but also pathogens associated with less striking degrees of inflammation (enteroaggregative *E. coli* and *C. difficile*)
C. difficile toxins A and B	Diarrhea associated with use of antibiotics, chemotherapy, or proton pump inhibitors, especially associated with current or recent hospitalization. Cases of community acquisition without health care exposure are increasingly being reported.	Most sensitive tests are culture and tissue culture toxin neutralization assay. Nucleic acid amplification tests are sensitive but lack specificity. Most specific tests are enzyme immunoassay for toxins A and B; a two-step procedure can be used: sensitive but nonspecific *C. difficile* glutamate dehydrogenase antigen test followed by toxin assay *or* nucleic acid amplification test followed by toxin immunoassay
Multiplexed nucleic acid amplification tests (NAAT)	Patients with persistent diarrhea, recent travel to developing countries, immunocompromised patients (HIV, solid organ transplant, hematopoietic stem cell transplant recipients)	Several platforms commercially available. Can detect up to 22 viral, bacterial, and protozoa targets. May detect incidental carriers or produce false positive results due to low target numbers or probe nonspecificity. The role of certain pathogens tested by these platforms such as enteropathogenic and enteroaggregative *E. coli* has not been validated in U.S. adults.
Stool culture for *Shigella, Salmonella, Campylobacter* spp, and Shiga toxin–producing *E. coli* (O157:H7 and others)	Moderate to severe diarrhea and when stools are positive for inflammatory markers or contain gross blood and mucus (dysentery)	The four mucosa-inflammatory bacteria are the only bacteria routinely sought by most laboratories. Culture offers the advantage of antimicrobial susceptibility testing and the study of outbreaks
Specialized stool culture for *Vibrio* spp	For cases of profuse watery diarrhea in cholera-endemic areas and outbreaks of seafood-associated diarrhea or dysentery	Cholera cases may need aggressive fluid therapy. Non–cholera vibrios can cause dysentery.
Parasite examination: (1) NAAT, (2) enzyme immunoassay for *Giardia* spp, *Cryptosporidium* spp, or *Entamoeba histolytica*; (3) acid-fast stain for *Cyclospora* or *Cryptosporidium* spp or *Cystoisospora*; or (4) trichome stain and microscopic examination	In any patient with persistent diarrhea and when diarrhea follows visits to mountainous or recreational lakes in North America, Nepal, Haiti, Peru, or Russia	NAATs are increasingly used for detection of *Cyclospora*, *Cryptosporidium* and *Giardia*. If microscopic evaluation is performed, experience of the laboratory personnel is important. The commercially available enzyme immunoassay tests are sensitive.
Esophagogastroduodenoscopy and flexible sigmoidoscopy	Persistent diarrhea in patients without evidence of cause of illness	Identified cause of diarrhea is treated; without diagnosis, subjects may be treated symptomatically.

TABLE 267-4 THERAPY FOR AND PREVENTION OF INFECTIOUS DIARRHEA

THERAPEUTIC OPTION	INDICATION	PHARMACOLOGIC AGENT
Oral fluid and electrolyte therapy	For infants, elderly patients, and anyone with profuse watery diarrhea	Soups, soft drinks, and saltine crackers are sufficient; formal oral replacement therapy may be needed with dehydrating forms of diarrhea
Diet: easily digestible foods	In all forms of diarrhea to facilitate enterocyte renewal and recovery	Soups and broth, saltine crackers, steamed vegetables, baked or broiled meats
Nonspecific therapy	For temporary (≤48 hours) control of diarrhea in older children and adults without evidence of severe diarrhea caused by an invasive or inflammatory bacterial or parasitic pathogen	Loperamide is the most effective symptomatic treatment and will decrease number of stools passed by 60%; bismuth subsalicylate is much less effective and will reduce number of stools by 40%; the antisecretory agent crofelemer is of value in HIV-associated diarrhea
Empirical antibacterial drugs	Enteric fever with toxicity Febrile dysenteric diarrhea Traveler's diarrhea	Fluoroquinolones for 7-10 days Azithromycin is recommended when fever or dysentery complicates illness Rifaximin 200 mg for 3 days, azithromycin 1000 mg in a single dose, or fluoroquinolone for 1-3 days when traveling to areas with low antibiotic resistance
Specific antibacterial therapy	Shigellosis, campylobacteriosis, cholera	See Chapters 286, 287, and 293
Antiparasitic drugs	Giardiasis, amebiasis, cryptosporidiosis, cyclosporiasis	See Chapters 329, 330, and 332
Prophylaxis in traveler's diarrhea	Persons traveling to developing areas on tight schedules, those with history of prior traveler's diarrhea, persons with unstable underlying medical disorders, and those interested in prophylaxis	Rifaximin, 200 mg twice daily with meals, while in a high-risk region

travel to Nepal, Haiti, or Peru or other regions of the developing world (travel-related infections are discussed in detail in Chapter 270).

A specific food or water vehicle cannot be suspected unless multiple cases of illness with a common exposure occur. All too frequently, persons assume that food consumed during their last meal before an illness onset is responsible for the symptoms. The highly variable incubation period for diarrheal disease, which may be as short as 2 hours after eating a food for preformed toxins, to a week or even longer for microbial enteropathogens, makes the determination of a specific food or beverage in a single case of illness impossible. When an outbreak of diarrhea results in multiple cases, a category of etiology (preformed toxin versus enteric infection) can be determined by calculating the incubation period after looking at timing of the common exposure and the time of first symptoms. Short incubation periods are characteristic of food poisoning associated with enterotoxins (2 to 7 hours for cases caused by *Staphylococcus aureus*, 2 to 4 hours for *Bacillus cereus* enterotoxin food poisoning). Longer incubation periods (usually 12 to 72 hours or longer) are associated with most cases of intestinal infection.[4]

The clinical expression of diarrheal illness will give clues to the etiologic agent involved in disease (see Table 267-2). In the patient with diarrhea who is receiving or recently has completed a course of an antimicrobial drug, a proton pump inhibitor, or an anticancer drug, particularly with recent or current hospitalization, *Clostridium difficile* infection (Chapter 280) should be suspected. An increasing number of cases of *C. difficile* diarrhea are occurring in the community without prior health care contact or antimicrobial use. When a person has close contact with an infant or infants attending a daycare center, a number of low–infectious dose pathogens are found in this setting (e.g., *Giardia*, *Cryptosporidium*, or *Shigella* species or viral pathogens, particularly norovirus) should be suspected. Persons practicing oral-anal, or digital-anal contact experience higher rates of enteric infection acquired through fecal-oral contamination, often associated with infection by multiple pathogens or through the practice of unprotected receptive anal intercourse leading to proctitis due to sexually transmitted organisms. When persons have advanced acquired immunodeficiency syndrome (AIDS) or other forms of severe immunodeficiency associated with chemotherapy, hematopoietic stem cell or solid organ transplantation, chronic use of immunosuppressive drugs, and depressed intestinal immunity may lead to enteric infection with a variety of parasitic, bacterial, or viral pathogens (see Table 267-1) (Chapter 265). Infants with malnutrition may develop persistent diarrhea and substantial long-term morbidity due to protozoal parasites, including *Giardia* and *Cryptosporidium*.

Enteric infection syndromes may be divided into at least five groups on the basis of the clinical presentation: (1) febrile systemic disease (enteric fever); (2) acute watery diarrhea (secretory diarrhea); (3) recurrent vomiting as the primary manifestation of enteric disease (gastroenteritis); (4) passage of many small-volume stools containing blood and mucus (dysentery); and (5) diarrhea lasting 2 weeks or longer (persistent diarrhea). Table 267-2 lists the major syndromes along with the expected cause.[5]

Noroviruses (Chapter 356) have become the major cause of food-borne gastroenteritis and the most commonly identified cause of waterborne enteric disease.[6] They have been identified as causes of persistent diarrhea in immunocompromised patients, especially in those undergoing hematopoietic stem cell transplantation. *Campylobacter* species (Chapter 287) is a commonly reported bacterial enteropathogen in industrialized countries and is the most important definable cause of Guillain-Barré syndrome (Chapter 392), often resulting in severe disease requiring assisted ventilation, intensive care unit confinement, and permanent neurologic sequelae. *E. coli* O157:H7 and other Shiga toxin–producing *E. coli* (STEC) (Chapter 288) are important causes of food-borne and waterborne colitis complicated by hemolytic-uremic syndrome in children and occasionally in elderly people.

The most commonly detected pathogens in endemic diarrhea in the United States in one study were noroviruses (26%), rotavirus (18%), and *Salmonella* species (5.3%). EAEC strains are being shown to be important causes of pediatric diarrhea in the United States as diagnostic methods improve. In May and June of 2011, there was a large outbreak of diarrhea and hemolytic-uremic syndrome reported from Germany and France due to an O104:H4 strain of enteroaggregative *E. coli* (EAEC) that had picked up the STEC phage controlling production of Shiga toxin. In the future, with improved diagnostic tools, we are likely to see more of these hybrid superpathogens with multiple virulence properties.

DIAGNOSIS
Laboratory Findings
Laboratory tests (Fig. 267-1; see Table 267-3) can be useful and are of particular value in the more severely ill patients, when subjects are forced by their illness to alter activities or are totally disabled and confined to bed or when

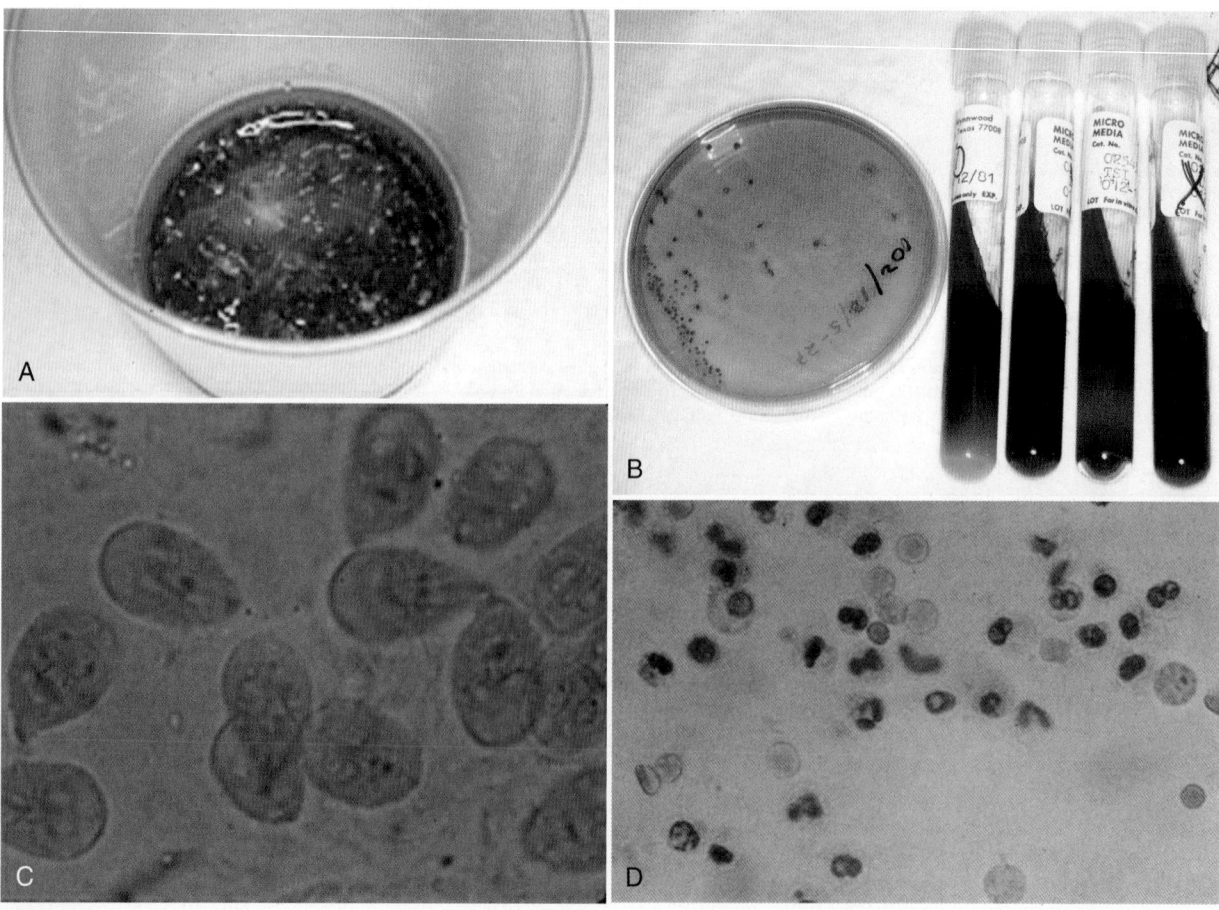

FIGURE 267-1. Laboratory tests to diagnose causes of diarrhea. A, Dysenteric stool. B, Stool culture and biochemical tests confirm *Salmonella*. C, *Giardia* trophozoites. D, Many leukocytes in diffuse colonic inflammation.

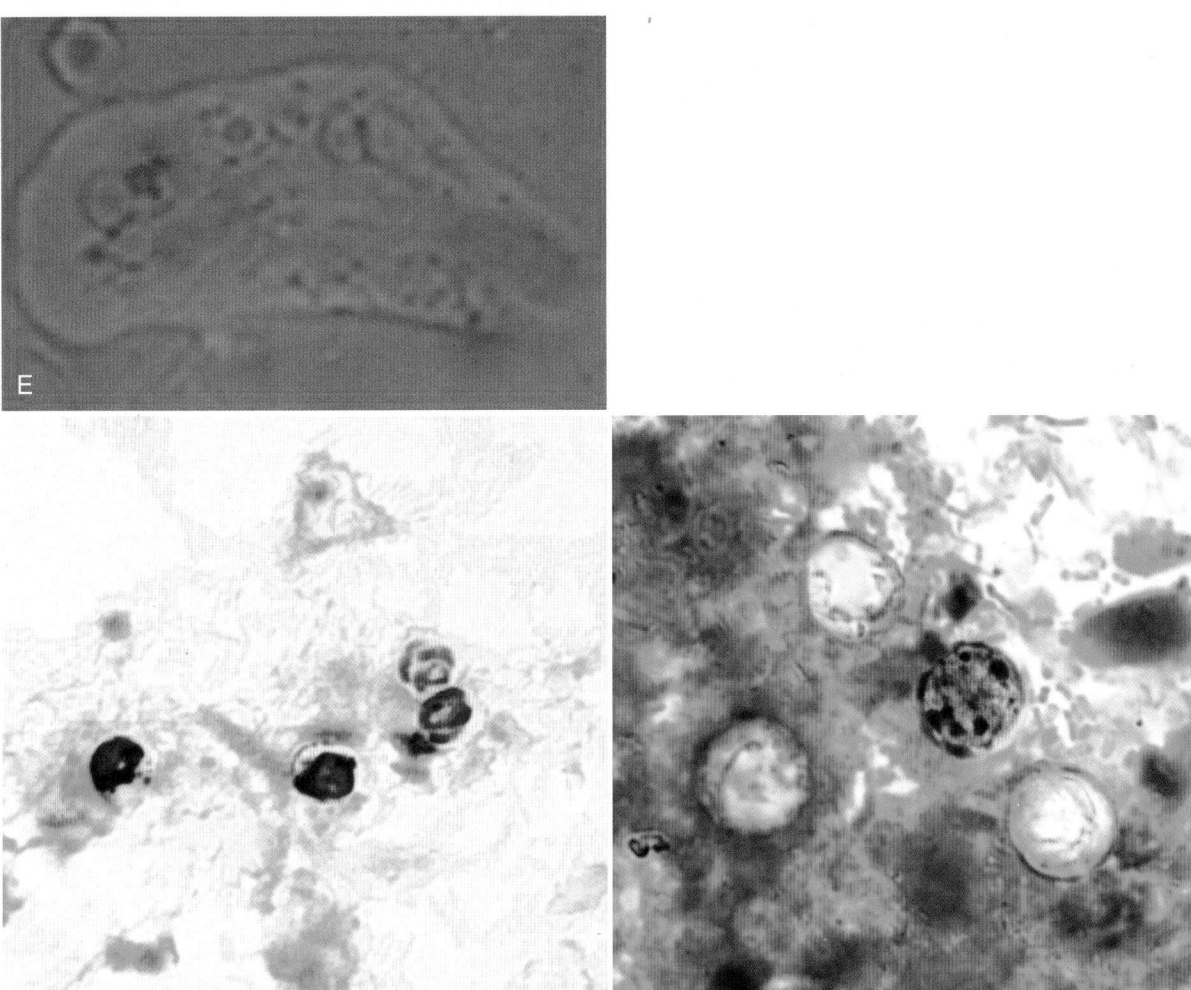

FIGURE 267-1, cont'd. E, *Entamoeba histolytica* trophozoite with ingested red blood cells. F, Oocysts of *Cryptosporidium* (*left*) and *Cyclospora* (*right*). (From the CDC Public Health Information Library. http://phil.cdc.gov/phil/home.asp: images 7829 and 7827.)

many patients are afflicted during an outbreak. In each of these situations, the laboratory may help establish cause and allow development of a proper plan of treatment (see Table 267-3). Standard laboratory tests include procedures looking for fecal inflammatory markers, such as microscopic detection of fecal leukocytes or the more sensitive, commercially available test, fecal lactoferrin or calprotein. These tests are particularly helpful to suggest the presence of the invasive bacterial pathogens *Shigella, Salmonella,* and *Campylobacter* species or the noninvasive but inflammatory *C. difficile.*

Enteropathogens associated with infectious diarrhea can be rapidly identified with new molecular methods, including real-time polymerase chain reaction, quantitation of pathogen load, and next-generation sequencing.[7-11] Stool culture is performed in more severe cases of sporadic diarrhea and in disease outbreaks and is carried out with blood culture in a patient with fever and systemic toxicity. Other indications for stool culture are presence of dysentery (passage of grossly bloody stools) and when fecal inflammatory markers are found. In dysenteric diarrhea, particularly in the presence of an outbreak, the laboratory should also be instructed to look for *E. coli* O157:H7 and other Shiga toxin–producing *E. coli.* Parasite examination is indicated by diarrhea and persistent (≥14 days) illness; evidence that the subject practices oral-anal sex or unprotected receptive anal intercourse; or associated immunosuppression. Other tests are indicated in special situations, including stool culture for *Vibrio cholerae* in a patient with severe watery diarrhea with excessive fluid losses in or returning from a cholera-endemic area and culture for *Mycobacterium avium* complex, herpes simplex virus, and cytomegalovirus in those with immunosuppression. For patients with persistent diarrhea without etiologic diagnosis when routine tests are employed, endoscopy (esophagogastroduodenoscopy and flexible sigmoidoscopy or colonoscopy) may be indicated in attempting to determine the nature and cause of illness.

TREATMENT Rx

Treatment of diarrhea should be tailored to the clinical syndrome. Oral rehydration therapy with fluids and electrolytes is used to treat acute watery diarrhea and gastroenteritis and all forms of enteric infection, especially when complicated with any degree of dehydration.[A1] Oral rehydration therapy is particularly important in infants; it can be life-saving in developing countries for infants with severe diarrhea. Patients with diarrhea should be fed easily digestible foods to facilitate enterocyte renewal and to speed up disease recovery. In afebrile, nondysenteric diarrhea, symptomatic drugs may allow older children and adults with illness to return earlier to school or work. Loperamide is the most active drug for improvement of symptoms. Bismuth subsalicylate can reduce diarrhea and is mildly effective in reducing nausea and vomiting associated with viral gastroenteritis.

For enteric fever, febrile dysenteric disease, and moderate to severe cases of traveler's diarrhea, empirical antimicrobial therapy is indicated (see Table 267-4). For outbreaks of dysenteric diarrhea, particularly in children in whom fever is not significant, antibacterial and antimotility drugs should be initially withheld while the etiology of the outbreak is being established to prevent patients infected by STEC strains from being predisposed to hemolytic-uremic syndrome. For bacterial and parasitic pathogen-specific diarrhea, antimicrobial therapy is often advised (see other chapters in the text for specific treatments). Because of the importance of diarrhea when persons travel from industrialized regions to developing countries, prophylaxis with the orally administered, poorly absorbed rifaximin can be employed for some groups (see Table 267-4), with expected protection rates exceeding 70%.

In sporadic cases of acute or persistent diarrhea, infectious agents are not always responsible. Table 267-5 offers a partial list of the noninfectious causes of diarrhea that should be considered.

TABLE 267-5 NONINFECTIOUS CAUSES OF DIARRHEA	
Running	Small bowel bacterial overgrowth
Fecal impaction	Systemic mastocytosis and eosinophilic
Drugs and laxatives	gastroenteritis
Enteral feeding	Tropical sprue
Irradiation	Celiac sprue
Pancreatic insufficiency	Dermatitis herpetiformis
Intestinal lymphangiectasia	Intestinal graft-versus-host disease
Foods (especially dietetic)	Thyrotoxicosis
Cirrhosis and biliary obstruction	Adrenal insufficiency
Diabetic diarrhea	Factitious
Alcoholism	Inflammatory bowel disease
Collagenous colitis	Food allergy
Microscopic colitis	Carcinoid
VIPoma	Villous adenoma
Ischemic bowel disease	Stress with autonomic stimulation
Irritable bowel syndrome	

PERSISTENT DIARRHEA

Persistent diarrhea for more than 2 weeks develops in about 3% of individuals who travel to developing countries. Common causes include parasitic infections (e.g., *Giardia* [Chapter 330], *Cryptosporidium* [Chapter 329]), and bacterial infections (e.g., enteroaggregative *E. coli* [Chapter 288]). The evaluation should include culture for bacterial pathogens and methods for detecting bacterial, viral, and protozoal infections (e.g., nucleic acid amplification tests), including multiplexed NAATs, as well as microscopy for protozoal infections. Antimicrobial therapy can be empirically given to patients who have recently returned from the developing world but should preferably be given based on the results of laboratory testing.[12] Therapy should be limited to the more severe cases to avoid post-antibiotic carriage of multidrug-resistant enterobacteriaceae, which has been shown to spread to family members and persist for as long as 12 months.

Grade A Reference

A1. Riddle MS, DuPont HL, Connor BA. ACG clinical guideline: diagnosis, treatment and prevention of acute diarrheal infections in adults. *Am J Gastroenterol.* 2016;111:602-622.

GENERAL REFERENCES

For the General References and other additional features, please visit Expert Consult at https://expertconsult.inkling.com.

268

APPROACH TO THE PATIENT WITH URINARY TRACT INFECTION

LINDSAY E. NICOLLE AND DIMITRI DREKONJA

DEFINITIONS

Urinary tract infection (UTI) is bacterial or fungal infection of urine with associated signs or symptoms. The clinical presentation varies from cystitis (bladder or lower tract infection), to pyelonephritis (renal or upper tract infection) and urosepsis (systemic inflammatory response syndrome or septic shock from a urinary source). Urethritis caused by *Chlamydia trachomatis, Ureaplasma urealyticum* (Chapter 269), or *Neisseria gonorrhoeae* (Chapter 283) and prostatitis (Chapter 120) and renal tuberculosis (Chapter 308) are addressed elsewhere in this text. Asymptomatic bacteriuria, although discussed here, is best considered as a state of colonization that requires treatment in only specific clinical circumstances.

Uncomplicated UTI occurs mainly in women with a normal genitourinary tract. Most episodes are manifested as cystitis; acute nonobstructive

TABLE 268-1 HOST FACTORS ASSOCIATED WITH COMPLICATED URINARY TRACT INFECTION	
	EXAMPLES
Obstruction	Urethral or ureteric strictures
	Tumor
	Diverticula
	Pelvicalyceal junction obstruction
	Prostate enlargement
	Urolithiasis
	Extrinsic compression
Functional	Neurogenic bladder
	Vesicoureteral reflux
	Anatomic defects
	Pregnancy
	Turbulent urethral urine flow
	Cystocele
Urologic interventions	Urethral or suprapubic catheters
	Urologic surgery
	Ureteric stents
	Nephrostomy tubes
	Cystoscopy
	Neobladders
Metabolic or congenital diseases	Urethral valves
	Polycystic kidneys
	Nephrocalcinosis
	Medullary sponge kidney
Immunologic abnormalities	Renal transplantation

pyelonephritis also occurs in these women, at a lower frequency. Complicated UTI refers to UTI occurring in patients with functional or structural abnormalities of the urinary tract. Complicating factors are host factors facilitating the establishment and persistence of bacteriuria or infection (Table 268-1). Uncomplicated UTI occurs rarely in young men. Men presenting with UTI should be assumed to have complicated infection until proven otherwise. Recurrent infection is typically considered a reinfection when it is caused by a new bacterial strain and relapse when the same strain that caused preceding infections is isolated, especially when the subsequent infection occurs within 30 days of completing therapy. It is clinically important to classify UTIs by site of infection, tendency to recur, and presence or absence of complicating factors.

EPIDEMIOLOGY

UTI is the most common bacterial infection. It is somewhat more common in boys than in girls in the newborn period because of the higher frequency of urethral malformations in boys. Later in childhood, UTIs are more common in girls, as is asymptomatic bacteriuria. More than half of all healthy women experience at least one symptomatic UTI in their lifetime, and each year, 2 to 10% of women experience at least one episode. UTI is uncommon in men with a normal genitourinary tract but increases after the age of 65 years, primarily attributable to prostate hypertrophy and prostatitis. The frequency of infection in patients with complicating factors varies by the abnormality promoting infection. For instance, patients with neurogenic bladder have continuing high rates of infection, but patients with abnormalities that can be corrected will no longer be at risk of infection. UTI is also one of the most common hospital-acquired infections; about 80% of these are a consequence of the use of an indwelling bladder catheter. However, many of these "cathether-associated" UTIs are asymptomatic bacteriuria detected via unnecessary urine cultures.

Asymptomatic bacteriuria is common. The prevalence increases from 1 to 2% of schoolgirls to 3 to 5% of sexually active premenopausal women, 10 to 20% of healthy postmenopausal women, and 40 to 50% of elderly women in nursing homes. It is infrequent in men until older ages, with 5 to 10% of elderly men in the community and 35 to 40% in nursing homes having bacteriuria. Some patients with genitourinary complications also have a very high prevalence. For instance, 50% of patients with a neurogenic bladder and without an indwelling catheter and 100% of patients with chronic indwelling catheters have bacteriuria.

PATHOBIOLOGY

Acute uncomplicated UTI follows ascension into the bladder or kidney of uropathogenic organisms from the normal gut flora that have colonized the vagina and periurethral mucosa. The ability of these organisms, usually *Escherichia coli*, to colonize and to persist within the urinary tract is dependent on an array of virulence factors that include adhesins, toxins, and iron-scavenging proteins. Organism virulence is a major determinant of whether symptomatic infection develops or is manifested as cystitis or pyelonephritis. Strains causing uncomplicated infection typically express the FimH adhesin, but this adhesin is not specific for UTI. *E. coli* isolated from uncomplicated pyelonephritis are characterized by the presence of the P fimbria adhesin Gal(α1-4) Galβ disaccharide globoside, which initiates mucosal inflammation. Adherence of organisms in the bladder or kidney activates the innate immune response leading to release of cytokines, particularly interleukin-6 and interleukin-8, and mobilizes leukocytes. This results in pyuria and local or systemic symptoms, including fever in patients with pyelonephritis.

The occurrence of acute uncomplicated UTI in healthy premenopausal women is determined by both genetic and behavioral factors. A genetic predisposition is supported by observations that a history of prior UTI is consistently one of the strongest associations with recurrent uncomplicated UTI, and women who experience these infections report a higher proportion of first-degree female relatives with recurrent UTI than do those without infection. One established genetic association is being a nonsecretor of the ABH blood group antigen (being unable to secrete blood type antigens into body fluids), with more avid binding of uropathogenic organisms to the vaginal epithelium in nonsecretors. Genetic polymorphisms affecting innate immunity are correlated with increased frequency of infection as well as with specific presentations. The strongest behavioral factors associated with uncomplicated UTI are sexual intercourse and spermicide use. For sexually active premenopausal women, 75 to 90% of episodes are attributed to intercourse. This is primarily attributed to ascension of periurethral organisms into the bladder with intercourse, but unprotected vaginal sex resulting in a reduction in endogenous anti–*E. coli* activity has also been reported.[1] The normal lactobacillus flora of the vagina maintains an acid environment that prevents colonization by potential uropathogens, and spermicide suppresses these organisms. Use of oral contraceptives or condoms, postcoital voiding, type of underwear, personal hygiene after voiding or defecating, and taking a bath rather than a shower are not associated with UTI recurrence, despite popular perceptions. Behavioral risk factors are similar for women for both cystitis and pyelonephritis, and even for asymptomatic bacteriuria. Sexual intercourse is not a major contributor to UTI in postmenopausal women. The most important determinants of infection in these women are having a history of UTI at a younger age and nonsecretory status (see above).

The risk of complicated UTI is determined by the underlying abnormality. Genitourinary abnormalities facilitate infection through increased entry of organisms into the bladder, such as intermittent catheterization or urologic procedures, and persistence of organisms within the urinary tract because of incomplete voiding or in biofilm on urologic devices. The determinants that promote symptomatic infection rather than asymptomatic colonization are not well characterized. However, obstruction and mucosal trauma with bleeding are well-recognized antecedents for bacteremia and sepsis in patients with preexisting bacteriuria. Although it is generally accepted that patients with diabetes have an increased incidence of UTI, this correlates more with long-term complications of diabetes, such as neurogenic bladder, than with the diabetes itself. Patients with poorly controlled diabetes, however, are at risk for more severe manifestations of infection.[2]

Acquisition of bacteriuria in individuals with indwelling urinary devices, including catheters, stents, and nephrostomy tubes, is primarily attributable to biofilm development along the device. Biofilm is composed of an extracellular polysaccharide material produced by the organisms that incorporates urine components including Tamm-Horsfall protein and magnesium or calcium ions. After insertion of the device, a conditioning layer composed of proteins and other host components immediately coats the device. Organisms adhere to this conditioning layer and initiate biofilm formation. Colonization usually begins at the urethral orifice or in the drainage bag, and the biofilm then ascends the catheter. Organisms growing in the biofilm persist in an environment relatively protected from antibiotics or host defenses. For patients with an indwelling catheter, the acquisition of bacteriuria occurs at a rate of 3 to 7% per day. Bacteriuria that follows indwelling catheter insertion is initially usually with a single organism, but polymicrobial flora is typical in mature biofilms on chronic indwelling devices. *Proteus mirabilis* is a particularly important organism for biofilm formation on chronic devices. These strains may produce copious biofilm, and urease production creates an alkaline environment leading to precipitation of calcium and magnesium ions. This creates a "crystalline biofilm" that is similar to the material causing infection stones and

may cause catheter obstruction. About 80% of episodes of urinary catheter obstruction are attributed to *P. mirabilis*.

ETIOLOGY

Table 268-2 summarizes the most common infecting organisms. In all types of UTI, *E. coli* is the dominant bacterial species, causing up to 85% of all symptomatic UTIs in women with community-acquired infections.[3] The second most common species causing uncomplicated cystitis is *Staphylococcus saprophyticus*, which is isolated more frequently in later summer and early fall. In patients with recurrent complicated UTI, species such as *Enterococcus faecalis*, *Enterococcus faecium*, *Klebsiella* species, *Proteus* species, *Providencia stuartii*, and *Morganella morganii* become more common. Patients with very frequent recurrences or with bladder catheters, particularly those in hospitals and nursing homes where antimicrobials are frequently used, may have *Pseudomonas aeruginosa*, *Acinetobacter baumannii*, *Serratia marcescens*, and *Stenotrophomonas maltophilia* isolated. In such patients, *E. coli* accounts for less than 50% of infections. Urolithiasis attributed to infection stones is associated with urease-producing organisms; the alkaline urine created facilitates struvite formation.[4] Repeated antimicrobial treatment administered to patients with recurrent complicated UTI often leads to increased antimicrobial resistance in the organisms isolated from recurrent infection. In health care facilities, the catheterized urinary tract is the most common site of isolation of multiply drug–resistant gram-negative organisms, including extended-spectrum β-lactamase–producing and carbapenemase-producing Enterobacteriaceae. *Candida* sp is the most common cause of fungal UTI. Patients with *Candida* infection are characterized by the presence of diabetes or of an indwelling urinary catheter and broad-spectrum antimicrobial exposure.

CLINICAL MANIFESTATIONS

Typical symptoms of cystitis, pyelonephritis, and urosepsis are listed in Table 268-3. The onset of cystitis is rapid, and symptoms usually develop within 24 hours.[5] Clinically, the lack of vaginal discharge differentiates cystitis from urethritis caused by chlamydia, ureaplasma, or gonococci. Women who experience recurrent episodes of acute uncomplicated UTI are more than 90% reliable for self-diagnosis.

Pyelonephritis may also have a rapid onset and may or may not be associated with cystitis symptoms. Bacteremia occurs in 10 to 30% of patients but does not have prognostic significance. The typical flank pain and tenderness, resulting from inflammation and edema of the renal parenchyma, may be masked by the intake of analgesic drugs such as acetaminophen, which may

TABLE 268-2	MICROBIAL ETIOLOGY OF URINARY TRACT INFECTIONS
ORGANISMS	**CLINICAL CHARACTERISTICS**
GRAM-NEGATIVE BACTERIA	
Escherichia coli	Typical
Klebsiella pneumoniae	Often reinfection
Enterobacter spp	Often reinfection or health care–associated infection*
Proteus spp	May indicate calculi; frequent with devices
Providencia stuartii	Often reinfection or health care–associated infection*
Morganella morganii	Often reinfection or health care–associated infection*
Serratia marcescens	Often health care–associated infection*
Acinetobacter baumannii	Often health care–associated infection*
Burkholderia spp	Often health care–associated infection*
Pseudomonas aeruginosa	Often health care–associated infection*
Stenotrophomonas maltophilia	Often health care–associated infection*
GRAM-POSITIVE BACTERIA	
Staphylococcus saprophyticus	Most common during late summer and fall
Staphylococcus aureus	May indicate focus outside the genitourinary tract
Enterococcus spp	Often reinfection
Other gram-positive bacteria	In most cases contaminants or colonizers
FUNGI	
Candida spp	May indicate focus outside the genitourinary tract

*Includes hospital and nursing home care.

TABLE 268-3	CLINICAL SYMPTOMS OF URINARY TRACT INFECTIONS
TYPE OF URINARY TRACT INFECTION	**TYPICAL SIGNS OR SYMPTOMS**
Cystitis	Frequency Dysuria Urgency Stranguria (difficulty in micturition) Suprapubic pain Hematuria
Pyelonephritis	Costovertebral angle pain or tenderness Fever Chills Cystitis symptoms (may be absent)
Urosepsis	Fever Chills, rigors Sepsis syndrome

TABLE 268-4	INTERPRETATION OF THE QUANTITATIVE URINE CULTURE
	QUANTITATIVE BACTERIAL COUNT
Asymptomatic bacteriuria	$\geq 10^5$ CFU/mL in two consecutive specimens for women
Acute uncomplicated cystitis	$\geq 10^2$ CFU/mL of *Escherichia coli* or *Staphylococcus saprophyticus*
Acute uncomplicated pyelonephritis	$\geq 10^4$ CFU/mL (95% have $\geq 10^5$ CFU/mL)
Complicated urinary tract infection	$\geq 10^5$ CFU/mL (lower counts may occur with diuresis)
Intermittent or in and out catheter collection	$\geq 10^2$ CFU/mL
Suprapubic or percutaneous aspiration	Any organisms isolated

also reduce the fever. An important differential diagnosis is renal calculus. This may have a similar location of pain but does not cause fever unless it is complicated by infection.

Complicated UTI is manifested across a clinical spectrum from minimal voiding abnormalities to symptoms consistent with cystitis, pyelonephritis, or severe sepsis. Urosepsis is a life-threatening condition, usually associated with bacteremia.[6] Obstruction or trauma to the mucosa from an indwelling catheter or with urologic surgery may precipitate bacteremia. Patients who present with urosepsis typically have complicated UTI rather than nonobstructive pyelonephritis.

DIAGNOSIS

Laboratory Findings

The hallmark of UTI diagnosis is demonstration of bacteriuria in a urine sample. A pretherapy urine culture specimen should be obtained for all patients presenting with pyelonephritis, urosepsis, or complicated UTI or when the diagnosis is uncertain. It is not generally recommended for acute uncomplicated cystitis because the clinical presentation is characteristic, and use of empirical short-course therapy means symptoms are often resolved by the time the culture is available. However, with increasing bacterial resistance culture results may be needed, and should certainly be obtained in the case of persistent symptoms despite empirical antimicrobial therapy or early recurrence post-therapy. The urine specimen must be collected in a manner that will limit contamination. The usual collection method is a midstream urine sample. Specimens collected from patients with indwelling catheters should be collected from the catheter port and not from the drainage bag. All specimens should be taken promptly to the laboratory to prevent growth during transportation. Urine specimens for culture must be collected before institution of antimicrobial therapy because the urine is rapidly sterilized after initiation of systemic antimicrobials.

Interpretation of the quantitative urine culture varies with the clinical presentation and collection method (Table 268-4). *Significant bacteriuria* is usually 10^5 CFU/mL or more, where one colony-forming unit (CFU) is one or more bacterial cells forming a colony when growing on an agar plate. In women

with symptoms of uncomplicated cystitis, 10^2 CFU/mL or more in midstream urine of *E. coli* or *S. saprophyticus* is consistent with infection. Other gram-positive organisms at any quantitative count should be interpreted as contaminants.

Pyuria is present in most patients with symptomatic UTI or asymptomatic bacteriuria. Many other abnormalities are, however, associated with pyuria, and the presence of pyuria does not diagnose infection or differentiate symptomatic from asymptomatic infection. The absence of pyuria has a high negative predictive value to exclude UTI for most patients. However, the absence of pyuria in a urine specimen from a woman with symptoms compatible with cystitis is not an indication to withhold empirical antimicrobial therapy.

For screening of bacteriuria, identification of nitrite in the urine may be useful. Gram-negative bacteria, with the exception of *P. aeruginosa*, will metabolize nitrate to nitrite, which can be demonstrated by a color reaction on a dipstick. Gram-positive bacteria and fungi do not metabolize nitrate. The technique is rapid (<1 minute) and inexpensive. It has a high degree of specificity but is insensitive because it does not detect infections caused by gram-positive organisms.

Conversely, some patients with evident pyuria will have negative urine cultures. Infectious causes of sterile pyuria include tuberculosis (Chapter 308), gonorrhea (Chapter 283), chlamydia (Chapter 302), mycoplasma (Chapter 301) and ureaplasma (Chapters 301 and 269), genital herpes (Chapter 350), trichomoniasis (Chapter 332), fungal infections (Chapter 322), and schistosomiasis (Chapter 334).[7]

Blood culture specimens should be obtained in all patients with suspected urosepsis. Patients with acute pyelonephritis, but not those with acute cystitis, have increased serum levels of C-reactive protein.

Imaging

Early imaging should be performed in any patient with urosepsis to identify abnormalities that require immediate source control. The optimal imaging modality is a computed tomography scan with intravenous contrast. Magnetic resonance imaging may not identify gas in tissues or small stones. Ultrasound may provide a rapid examination to exclude significant obstruction. Investigations are also indicated for patients with delayed response or failure to respond to appropriate antimicrobial therapy, or with early relapse of pyelonephritis after completion of therapy. The optimal management of complicated urinary infection requires characterization of underlying abnormalities and correction of these, whenever possible. Selected patients may require studies for diagnosis of vesicoureteral reflux or to characterize differential renal function.

Differential Diagnosis

Clinical manifestations will usually differentiate acute cystitis and acute pyelonephritis (Table 268-5). New-onset frequency, dysuria, and urgency without accompanying vaginal discharge or pain have a positive predictive value of 90% for acute cystitis. The differential diagnosis for women presenting with acute irritative lower tract symptoms includes sexually transmitted infections, vulvovaginal candidiasis, and noninfectious causes such as interstitial cystitis. Some patients who present with only lower tract symptoms may have renal infection, referred to as occult pyelonephritis. Patients with appendicitis and cholecystitis can present with flank pain similar to right-sided pyelonephritis, and pelvic inflammatory disease may be misdiagnosed as urinary infection.

TREATMENT   Rx

Symptomatic UTIs should be treated with antimicrobials to decrease the duration of symptoms and, for pyelonephritis, to limit damage to renal tissue. Antimicrobials selected for treatment should be excreted renally, so high antimicrobial concentrations are achieved in the renal parenchyma and urine.

Cystitis

Table 268-6 lists recommended choices for the antimicrobial treatment of cystitis. The shortest effective treatment duration for the antimicrobial should be used. Trimethoprim, trimethoprim-sulfamethoxazole, fosfomycin, pivmecillinam, and nitrofurantoin are recommended first-line treatments because they are effective with relatively short courses and since there is limited effect on normal flora, resistance emergence is less of a concern.[8] In a randomized trial, nitrofurantoin, 100 mg tid for 5 days, compared with single-dose fosfomycin, 3 grams, resulted in a significantly higher likelihood of clinical and microbiologic resolution at 28 days after completion of therapy for uncomplicated lower UTI in women.[A1] Trimethoprim or trimethoprim-sulfamethoxazole should be selected for initial empirical therapy only if the local prevalence of resistance to these

TABLE 268-5 DECISION PROCESS FOR DIAGNOSIS AND TREATMENT OF UPPER (PYELONEPHRITIS) VERSUS LOWER (CYSTITIS) URINARY TRACT INFECTIONS

	CYSTITIS	PYELONEPHRITIS
SIGNS AND SYMPTOMS		
Fever	No	Yes
Dysuria	Yes	May be present
Frequency	Yes	May be present
Flank pain	No	Yes
DIAGNOSIS		
Pyuria	Yes	Yes
Nitrite test result	Normally positive	Normally positive
Bacteriuria	Yes	Yes
C-reactive protein	Normal	Increased
Blood cultures	Negative	Positive in ≈10-30%
TREATMENT		
First line	Short-term oral therapy (Table 268-6)	Oral: fluoroquinolone for 7 days Parenteral: cephalosporin, fluoroquinolone, or aminoglycoside for 7-14 days (Table 268-7)
Second line	Fluoroquinolone for 3 days or cephalosporin for 7 days	Injectable cephalosporin until afebrile, followed by oral step-down for total of 2 weeks
Pregnant women	Nitrofurantoin or cephalosporin for 5-7 days	Injectable cephalosporin until afebrile, followed by oral cephalosporin for 14 days

TABLE 268-6 ANTIMICROBIALS USED TO TREAT CYSTITIS

ANTIMICROBIAL	DOSE* AND DURATION
FIRST-LINE THERAPY	
Trimethoprim	100-150 mg q12h for 3 days
Trimethoprim-sulfamethoxazole	160/800 mg q12 for 3 days or 320/1600 mg single dose
Nitrofurantoin	50-100 mg q8h for 5-7 days
Nitrofurantoin macrocrystals	100 mg bid for 5 days
Fosfomycin trometamol	3 g single dose
Pivmecillinam	400 mg bid for 3-5 days
OTHER	
Amoxicillin-clavulanate	500 mg (amoxicillin dose) q8h for 7 days
Amoxicillin	500 mg tid for 7 days
Cefpodoxime proxetil	100 mg bid for 3 days
Cefuroxime axetil	500 mg bid for 7 days
Cefixime	400 mg/day for 7 days
Ceftibuten	400 mg/day for 5-7 days
Norfloxacin[†]	400 mg q12h for 7 days
Ciprofloxacin[†]	250 mg q12h for 7 days (500 mg qd extended release)
Levofloxacin[†]	250-500 mg/day for 7 days
Doxycycline	100 mg bid for 7 days

*Doses given are for adults with normal renal function. The need to reduce dosages because of renal impairment related to infection in the kidneys, other renal diseases, or advanced age should always be considered.
[†]The FDA advises that the side effects of fluoroquinolones outweigh their benefits when patients with acute uncomplicated urinary tract infections have other options.

TABLE 268-7 ANTIMICROBIALS USED TO TREAT PYELONEPHRITIS

ROUTE OF ADMINISTRATION AND ANTIMICROBIAL	DOSE* AND DURATION
PARENTERAL	
First-Line Therapy	
Gentamicin	4.5 mg/kg/day × 10-14 days
Tobramycin	4.5 mg/kg/day × 10-14 days
Ciprofloxacin	400 mg q12h × 7 days
Levofloxacin	750 mg/day × 5 days
Cefepime	2 g q8-12h × 14 days
Cefotaxime	1 g q8h × 10-14 days
Ceftriaxone	1-2 g qd × 10-14 days
Other	
Ceftazidime	1 g q8-12h × 10-14 days
Ertapenem	1 g qd × 10-14 days
Meropenem	500 mg q6h × 10-14 days
Piperacillin-tazobactam	3.375 g q6h × 10-14 days
Doripenem	500 mg q8h × 10-14 days
Amikacin	15 mg/kg/day × 10-14 days
Trimethoprim-sulfamethoxazole	160/800 mg q12h × 14 days
ORAL	
First-Line Therapy	
Ciprofloxacin	500 mg q12h × 7 days
Levofloxacin	250-500 mg/day × 5-7 days
Other	
Amoxicillin-clavulanate	500 mg (amoxicillin dose) q8h × 14 days
Cefuroxime axetil	500 mg q12h × 14 days
Cefixime	400 mg/day × 14 days
Ceftibuten	400 mg/day × 14 days

*Doses given are for adults with normal renal function. The need to reduce dosages because of renal impairment should always be considered.

agents in community-acquired *E. coli* infections is less than 20%. Fluoroquinolones are not recommended for first-line therapy because of toxicity concerns and widespread use promoting emergence of resistance. β-Lactam antimicrobials are about 10% less effective than the first-line agents.[A2] Patients with recurrent cystitis can be effectively managed with a strategy of early self-treatment. Early empirical treatment usually leads to prompt improvement of symptoms. Nitrofurantoin and oral cephalosporins are preferred therapy for pregnant women because these are safe for the fetus.[9]

Pyelonephritis

For antimicrobial treatment of pyelonephritis, the initial decision is whether parenteral treatment is needed or whether oral treatment alone will suffice. Table 268-7 lists antimicrobials suitable for the treatment of pyelonephritis. After initial treatment with a parenteral drug, a transition to oral treatment that achieves adequate tissue levels (i.e., not nitrofurantoin or fosfomycin) is normally possible at 24 to 48 hours if the patient has clinically improved. The recommended treatment time is 7 to 14 days but 5 to 7 days is adequate for ciprofloxacin or levofloxacin.[A3-A5]

Complicated Urinary Infection

The antimicrobial regimen selected for treatment of complicated UTI is individualized on the basis of the site of infection, severity of the manifestations, new or presumed infecting organism and susceptibility, tolerance of the patient, and nature of the underlying abnormalities. When symptoms are mild, it is preferable to delay initiation of antimicrobial therapy until results of urine culture are available to allow optimal antimicrobial selection. Empirical antimicrobial therapy should be initiated when severe symptoms are present. Options include intravenous plazomicin (15 mg/kg once daily) or meropenem (1 g every 8 hours) for 4 to 5 days, followed by appropriate oral therapy for another 5 to 6 days.[A6] Other options include meropenem vaborbactam (2 g/2 g over 3 hours) or piperacillin tazobactam (4 g/0.5 g over 30 minutes) every 8 hours for 4 to 5 days, followed by 5 to 6 days of oral therapy.[A7] Plazomicin and meropenem vaborbactam are particularly useful for highly-resistant organisms where treatment options are limited. Oral or parenteral therapy is selected on the basis of the presentation and the likelihood of resistant organisms. Previous urine culture results from the patient and recent history of antimicrobial exposure are helpful to assess the likelihood of resistant organisms. Nitrofurantoin may be used for episodes of bladder infection but is not effective for renal infection and is contraindicated in individuals with renal failure. The empirical therapy selected should be reassessed after 48 to 72 hours, by which time the urine culture result should be available and the response to initial therapy can be assessed. If the organism isolated from a pretherapy urine culture specimen is resistant to the empirical antimicrobial therapy initiated, the antimicrobial regimen should be modified to an agent to which the organism is susceptible, irrespective of the clinical response. Antibiotic prophylaxis at the time of catheter removal to reduce the risk of subsequent symptomatic infection, remains controversial.

Asymptomatic Bacteriuria

Asymptomatic bacteriuria is increasingly recognized as a major driver of unnecessary antimicrobial use. Evidence supports treatment of asymptomatic bacteriuria before urologic procedures with anticipated trauma to the genitourinary mucosa. There is also evidence supporting treatment of asymptomatic bacteriuria in pregnant women.[A8] However, a recent study in low-risk pregnant women found that asymptomatic bacteriuria developed into pyelonephritis in only 2.4%, thereby raising the question of whether routine screening and treatment is indicated for all pregnant women,[10] especially with concern about promoting antibiotic-resistant organisms.[11]

For all other populations, including elderly women and men, treatment of asymptomatic bacteriuria has not been associated with improved outcomes but is consistently followed by reinfection with organisms of increasing antimicrobial resistance.[12] For some populations, evidence suggests that asymptomatic bacteriuria may protect subjects from symptomatic UTI. Bacteriuria in patients with indwelling catheters should not be treated unless the patient has symptoms attributed to urinary infection. Administration of antimicrobials to catheterized patients with asymptomatic bacteriuria inevitably results in reinfection with more resistant organisms. The optimal treatment for patients with nonspecific symptoms (fatigue, lethargy, poor concentration) and bacteriuria is unknown. Supportive care with observation versus a trial of antimicrobial treatment are potentially valid but unstudied options.

Infections in Elderly Men

Urinary tract infection is the leading cause of bacteremia in older men, almost always in the context of underlying prostate, bladder, or kidney abnormalities, including bacterial prostatitis (Chapter 120). For lower urinary tract infections, initial empiric therapy can be as for cystitis in women. However, culture-directed antimicrobial therapy is indicated as soon as possible, and antibiotics do not obviate the need for a urologic consultation and a full urologic evaluation,[13] which then guides further therapy. Treatment duration is typically longer than for women, but the minimum effective duration is unknown.[A9]

Urosepsis

The principles of management of urosepsis are similar to those for patients with severe sepsis from any site. Parenteral empirical antimicrobial treatment and supportive care should be initiated promptly.[14] The antimicrobials selected should provide broad-spectrum coverage for potential uropathogens, including resistant bacteria. Antimicrobial therapy should be reassessed when urine and blood culture results become available and the infecting organism and susceptibilities are identified.

Funguria

Funguria should be treated only when accompanied by symptoms of UTI. Symptomatic infection is treated with fluconazole 400 mg once daily for 1 day, followed by 200 mg once daily for 7 to 14 days. If *Candida* sp resistant to fluconazole is isolated, amphotericin B deoxycholate is the recommended alternative therapy because other antifungals have limited renal excretion.

Follow-up

Patients do not require follow-up urine cultures unless symptomatic infection persists or recurs. When there is early (<30 days) recurrence, the infecting organism should be re-evaluated to ensure that it is susceptible to the antimicrobial given.

PREVENTION

Premenopausal women with recurrent acute uncomplicated UTI should avoid spermicide use and may benefit from increasing their daily water intake to more than 1.5 L/day.[A10] For women with frequent recurrent acute uncomplicated UTI (more than two in 6 months or three in 12 months) presenting as cystitis or pyelonephritis, prophylactic antimicrobial therapy is effective, either as long-term low-dose prophylaxis[A11] or as postcoital prophylaxis

TABLE 268-8	PROPHYLACTIC REGIMENS TO PREVENT RECURRENT URINARY TRACT INFECTION IN WOMEN	
PREFERRED		**OTHER**
Long-term low dose		
Nitrofurantoin 50 mg od or 100 mg daily		Cephalexin 250-500 mg daily*
Trimethoprim-sulfamethoxazole, 40/200 mg daily or every other day		Norfloxacin 200 mg daily
		Ciprofloxacin 125 mg daily
Postcoital (single dose)		
Nitrofurantoin 50 or 100 mg*		Cephalexin 250 mg*
Trimethoprim-sulfamethoxazole 40/200 mg		Ciprofloxacin 125 mg
Trimethoprim 100 mg		Norfloxacin 200 mg

*Suitable for use in pregnancy.

(Table 268-8). The use of cranberry tablets or juice does not reliably decrease bacteriuria[A12] or the frequency of recurrent infection, and probiotics are not effective. For postmenopausal women, use of topical vaginal estrogens may decrease the frequency of infection.[A13] The use of systemic estrogen, however, is associated with an increased frequency of UTI. Prophylactic antimicrobial therapy is more effective than topical vaginal estrogen in these women.

Current recommendations suggest pregnant women should be screened for asymptomatic bacteriuria early in the pregnancy, usually at 12 or 16 weeks. If bacteriuria is present, these women should be treated and have subsequent follow-up culture specimens obtained monthly. If either asymptomatic colonization or recurrent infection occurs, prophylactic antimicrobial therapy with either cephalexin or nitrofurantoin should be considered through the duration of the pregnancy to decrease the risk for development of pyelonephritis in later pregnancy.

Prophylactic antimicrobial therapy has not been shown to be effective for patients with complicated UTI, including those with spinal cord injury or with chronic indwelling catheters. In these patients, the abnormality leading to impaired voiding means that bacteriuria is unavoidable, and antimicrobial therapy simply promotes bacteriuria with increasingly resistant organisms.

Infection control programs of health care facilities (Chapter 266) should include practices to prevent catheter-associated UTI.[15] Evidence-based guidelines provide clear recommendations for program components, including ongoing surveillance. The most important intervention is to avoid the use of an indwelling catheter wherever possible and, when there are clear indications for catheter use, to limit the duration to as short a time as possible. For adults who require intermittent self-catheterization, continuous antibiotic prophylaxis can reduce recurrent UTIs but at the risk of developing resistant organisms.[A14] The future development of biofilm-resistant materials may help reduce the problem of catheter-associated UTI.

PROGNOSIS

The prognosis of uncomplicated cystitis and pyelonephritis is good. Women with acute uncomplicated cystitis who do not receive antimicrobial therapy will usually have resolution of symptoms by 1 to 2 weeks. Women with even very frequent recurrent acute uncomplicated UTI experience no long-term adverse outcomes, such as renal impairment or hypertension. A small proportion of women with severe presentations of acute nonobstructive pyelonephritis develop renal scars, but these are not associated with impaired renal function. Patients with frequent recurrent complicated UTI may experience substantial morbidity with recurrent infections, but poor long-term medical outcomes are usually determined by the underlying abnormality rather than by infection. Patients with urosepsis have a fatality rate of about 10%. Factors increasing the risk of death are advanced age and significant underlying diseases as well as inadequate initial antimicrobial treatment.

Grade A References

A1. Huttner A, Kowalczyk A, Turjeman A, et al. Effect of 5-day nitrofurantoin vs single-dose fosfomycin on clinical resolution of uncomplicated lower urinary tract infection in women: a randomized clinical trial. *JAMA*. 2018;319:1781-1789.

A2. Hooton TM, Roberts PL, Stapleton AE. Cefpodoxime vs ciprofloxacin for short-course treatment of acute uncomplicated cystitis: a randomized trial. *JAMA*. 2012;307:583-589.

A3. Sandberg T, Skoog G, Hermansson AB, et al. Ciprofloxacin for 7 days versus 14 days in women with acute pyelonephritis: a randomised, open-label and double-blind, placebo-controlled, non-inferiority trial. *Lancet*. 2012;380:484-490.

A4. Dinh A, Davido B, Etienne M, et al. Is 5 days of oral fluoroquinolone enough for acute uncomplicated pyelonephritis? The DTP randomized trial. *Eur J Clin Microbiol Infect Dis.* 2017;36:1443-1448.

A5. Fox MT, Melia MT, Same RG, et al. A seven-day course of TMP-SMX may be as effective as a seven-day course of ciprofloxacin for the treatment of pyelonephritis. *Am J Med.* 2017;130:842-845.

A6. Wagenlehner FME, Cloutier DJ, Komirenko AS, et al. Once-daily plazomicin for complicated urinary tract infections. *N Engl J Med.* 2019;380:729-740.

A7. Kaye KS, Bhowmick T, Metallidis S, et al. Effect of meropenem-vaborbactam vs piperacillin-tazobactam on clinical cure or improvement and microbial eradication in complicated urinary tract infection: the TANGO I randomized clinical trial. *JAMA.* 2018;319:788-799.

A8. Widmer M, Lopez I, Gulmezoglu AM, et al. Duration of treatment for asymptomatic bacteriuria during pregnancy. *Cochrane Database Syst Rev.* 2015;11:CD000491.

A9. van Nieuwkoop C, van der Starre WE, Stalenhoef JE, et al. Treatment duration of febrile urinary tract infection: a pragmatic randomized, double-blind, placebo-controlled non-inferiority trial in men and women. *BMC Med.* 2017;15:1-9.

A10. Hooton TM, Vecchio M, Iroz A, et al. Effect of increased daily water intake in premenopausal women with recurrent urinary tract infections: a randomized clinical trial. *JAMA Intern Med.* 2018;178:1509-1515.

A11. Price JR, Guran LA, Gregory WT, et al. Nitrofurantoin vs other prophylactic agents in reducing recurrent urinary tract infections in adult women: a systematic review and meta-analysis. *Am J Obstet Gynecol.* 2016;215:548-560.

A12. Juthani-Mehta M, Van Ness PH, Bianco L, et al. Effect of cranberry capsules on bacteriuria plus pyuria among older women in nursing homes: a randomized clinical trial. *JAMA.* 2016;316:1879-1887.

A13. Beerepoot MA, Geerlings SE, van Haarst EP, et al. Nonantibiotic prophylaxis for recurrent urinary tract infections: a systematic review and meta-analysis of randomized controlled trials. *J Urol.* 2013;190:1981-1989.

A14. Fisher H, Oluboyede Y, Chadwick T, et al. Continuous low-dose antibiotic prophylaxis for adults with repeated urinary tract infections (AnTIC): a randomised, open-label trial. *Lancet Infect Dis.* 2018;18:957-968.

GENERAL REFERENCES

For the General References and other additional features, please visit Expert Consult at https://expertconsult.inkling.com.

269

APPROACH TO THE PATIENT WITH A SEXUALLY TRANSMITTED INFECTION

HEIDI SWYGARD AND MYRON S. COHEN

SEXUALLY TRANSMITTED INFECTIONS

DEFINITION

Sexually transmitted infections (STIs) include a wide variety of organisms that are transmitted through intimate contact involving skin or mucosal surfaces of the oropharynx, vagina, penis, and rectum. STIs can generally be divided into five broad categories (syndromes): urethritis, genital ulcers, epithelial cell disorders, female vaginal discharge, and ectoparasites (Table 269-1).

ETIOLOGY

The interaction between the host and the STI pathogen plays a critical role, and characteristic tissue changes offer exceptionally strong clues about etiology. Several STI pathogens cause local inflammation only (*Neisseria gonorrhoeae, Chlamydia trachomatis, Trichomonas vaginalis*), with the potential for local tissue invasion (*N. gonorrhoeae, C. trachomatis*) or systemic dissemination (*N. gonorrhoeae*). Some STI pathogens cause tissue ulceration (*Treponema pallidum, Haemophilus ducreyi*, herpes simplex viruses 1 and 2). Human papillomaviruses (HPVs) cause epithelial cell changes and predispose to neoplasm. Several STI pathogens (human immunodeficiency virus [HIV], hepatitis B and C viruses, cytomegalovirus) routinely use the genital tract for access without causing any local changes.

EPIDEMIOLOGY

STIs are among the most common infections worldwide, and most are never reported. The World Health Organization (WHO) estimates that nearly 1 million people worldwide become infected every day with any of four curable STIs: chlamydia, gonorrhea, syphilis, and trichomoniasis.[1] Each year there are almost 10 million new STIs reported among persons aged 15 to 24 years in the United States alone; many infections are subclinical and may escape detection, suggesting that these numbers are an underestimate. Of great

concern, STIs are generally transmissible whether they are symptomatic or asymptomatic.

The spread of STIs depends on the organism and the host, the length of time an infected person remains contagious, and the number of people exposed. These parameters have been reduced to the following formula:

$$R_o = B \times D \times C$$

where R_o is the basic reproductive rate of an infection, or the mean number of secondary cases a typical single infected person will cause in a population; B is the efficiency of transmission; D is the duration of infectiousness; and C is the number of sexual partners.

PATHOBIOLOGY

STI pathogens depend entirely on human-human transmission, although *T. vaginalis* may have some inanimate sources. The efficiency of transmission reflects the infectiousness of the index case (which depends on the concentration and phenotype of the organism in the genital tract) and the susceptibility of the sexual partner (which reflects the resistance of the host, whether it is hereditary, acquired, or innate). Because immunity to STIs is rare, reinfections are common, and vaccine development has been difficult; the only STI vaccines available target hepatitis B and HPV.

STIs produce syndromes precisely because each pathogen has a proclivity for one or more tissues and (when symptomatic) can evoke a predictable inflammatory response. For example, gonococci that infect the male urethra generally produce an intense neutrophil response that leads to a purulent discharge and pain with urination, whereas *C. trachomatis* is less likely to produce such a response in the same tissue and is more likely to produce a mild, watery discharge or no symptoms at all.

STIs serve as markers for sexual risk-taking behavior, so coinfections are common. Detection of an STI should lead to other tests. STI pathogens move together: gonorrhea and chlamydia cause urethritis; genital ulcers greatly increase the probability of HIV acquisition.

TABLE 269-1 SYNDROMES OF SEXUALLY TRANSMITTED DISEASES

SYNDROME	ORGANISM
URETHRITIS	
Gonococcal	*Neisseria gonorrhoeae*
Nongonococcal	*Chlamydia trachomatis*
	Trichomonas vaginalis
	Mycoplasma genitalium
	Ureaplasma urealyticum
	Neisseria meningitidis
	Herpes simplex (primary infection)
GENITAL ULCERS	
Syphilis	*Treponema pallidum*
Genital herpes	Herpes simplex
Chancroid	*Haemophilus ducreyi*
EPITHELIAL CELL INFECTIONS	
Genital warts	Human papillomavirus
Molluscum	*Molluscum contagiosum*
Cervical neoplasia	Human papillomavirus types 16 and 18
FEMALE GENITAL DISCHARGE	
Cervicitis	*Neisseria gonorrhoeae*
	Chlamydia trachomatis
	Trichomonas vaginalis
	Herpes simplex
Pelvic inflammatory disease	*Neisseria gonorrhoeae*
	Chlamydia trachomatis
Vaginitis	*Trichomonas vaginalis*
	Candida albicans
Bacterial vaginosis	*Gardnerella vaginalis*, anaerobes
ECTOPARASITES	
Pubic lice	*Phthirus pubis*
Scabies	*Sarcoptes scabiei*

DIAGNOSIS AND TREATMENT

Syndromic Strategies

Syndromic management means empiric treatment of the index case based on signs and symptoms and concomitant treatment of sexual partners is essential. This approach reflects the facts that the diagnostic accuracy of some tests is imperfect, coinfection demands combination therapy that overrides the search for individual pathogens, and patients who are not treated immediately may not return for therapy. The genital ulcer disease and urethral discharge syndromes (Chapter 283) have high sensitivity and specificity compared with laboratory diagnosis, and empirical therapy is so successful that follow-up care ("proof of cure") is usually unnecessary.[2] However, the vaginal discharge syndrome is far less sensitive or specific in terms of true STI diagnosis.[3] In addition, many women with endocervical or vaginal infection may be asymptomatic. In one study of South African women, almost 90% with a laboratory-confirmed STI diagnosis had no clinical symptoms and would therefore not have been treated without testing.

The syndromic approach is particularly critical in resource-constrained countries or in areas of the United States where laboratory tests are not available or their cost is prohibitive. In the United States, concomitant microbiologic diagnosis is preferred because it (1) confirms the choice of empirical therapy or redirects subsequent care; (2) permits the detection and monitoring of resistance to treatment; and (3) enables specific diagnoses to be reported to public health authorities, which is required by state law for many STIs. However, even when laboratory tests are ordered, the most appropriate treatment agent(s) should be provided empirically at the point of care to resolve infection and to reduce onward transmission.

Relationship of STIs to HIV Infection

Diagnosis of an STI demonstrates increased sexual risk-taking behavior and inconsistent condom use, and it serves as a marker for potential HIV infection. Any patient undergoing evaluation or treatment for an STI should be tested for HIV infection. Early diagnosis and treatment of HIV infection has major personal and public health benefits including reducing secondary HIV transmission.[A1]

In addition, STIs also contribute to HIV acquisition and hamper efforts at optimal prevention of HIV transmission. Genital ulcers disrupt the genital mucosal epithelium and allow the entry of HIV, and inflammation caused by ulceration recruits macrophages and lymphocytes, increasing the number of target cells for HIV and the number of receptors per cell.

⬤ SYNDROMES

Urethritis

Urethritis is characterized by some combination of urethral discharge and dysuria, but prostatitis can cause similar complaints. Urethritis is caused by a limited group of pathogens (see Table 269-1) that may be difficult to visualize microscopically or to grow in culture. Accordingly, empirical therapy is provided to treat a spectrum of potentially causative organisms.

Urethritis is diagnosed when one or more of the following are demonstrated: (1) mucopurulent or purulent urethral discharge, (2) Gram stain of urethral secretions demonstrating two or more leukocytes per oil immersion microscopic field, (3) positive leukocyte esterase test result on first-void urine, or (4) microscopic examination of first-void urine demonstrating 10 or more leukocytes per high-power field. If no urethral discharge can be expressed from the urethral meatus, a calcium alginate swab can be inserted 5 mm into the urethra; the material collected is transferred to a slide by rolling the swab along the glass.

A Gram stain of urethral discharge is a simple and rapid diagnostic test to document both urethritis and gonococcal infection (Chapter 283), characterized by the detection of leukocytes containing intracellular gram-negative diplococci. Confirmation of gonococcal urethritis does not rule out concomitant infection with Chlamydia or Mycoplasma. As culture and Gram stain have become less popular or less available, nucleic acid amplification tests (NAAT) that are highly sensitive and specific for the detection of organisms have been used routinely. Clinicians should use caution in relying solely on NAATs for gonorrhea; an outbreak of sexually transmitted Neiserria meningitidis in Atlanta was not easily evaluated because NAAT tests developed for gonorrhea could not detect this other Neisserial species.

Nucleic acid amplification tests for gonorrhea, Chlamydia, and Trichomonas can be applied to first-void urine samples (the meatus is intentionally not cleaned so that the urine is contaminated with these organisms) or urethral

---

TABLE 269-2 SYNDROMIC TREATMENT OF URETHRITIS
GONOCOCCAL*
Recommended
Ceftriaxone 250 mg injected intramuscularly once, *and* Azithromycin 1 g orally (single dose)
NONGONOCOCCAL
Recommended
Azithromycin 1 g orally (single dose), *or* Doxycycline 100 mg orally twice daily for 7 days
Alternative
Erythromycin base 500 mg orally four times daily for 7 days, *or* Erythromycin ethylsuccinate 800 mg orally four times daily for 7 days, *or* Ofloxacin 300 mg orally twice daily for 7 days, *or* Levofloxacin 500 mg orally once a day for 7 days
Recurrent or Persistent
If azithromycin was used for initial episode: moxifloxacin 400 mg orally once daily for 7 days. If doxycycline was used for initial episode: azithromycin 1 g orally (single dose) *PLUS* For men who have sex with women who live in areas where *T. vaginalis* is highly prevalent: metronidazole 2 g orally (single dose) *or* tinidazole 2 g orally (single dose)

*Uncomplicated anorectal and genital disease.
Adapted from Bachmann LH, Manhart LE, Martin DH, et al. Advances in the understanding and treatment of male urethritis. *Clin Infect Dis.* 2015;61 Suppl 8:S763-769.

---

swab material. NAATs are not approved for use in extra-genital testing; however, laboratories may opt to internally validate their use. Extra-genital testing among MSM is recommended since urine-based testing alone can miss a large proportion of infected individuals, contributing to ongoing transmission. Specific diagnosis may enhance the management of sexual partners, and the results from such tests should be reported to the health department. However, in practice, patients and (in most cases) sexual partners must be treated before the results of these tests are available.

Treatment for urethritis should be initiated as soon as possible after the clinical diagnosis and should be directly observed if feasible (Table 269-2). *N. gonorrhoeae* (Chapter 283) has become resistant to many antimicrobials, including quinolones and oral cephalosporins, which are no longer recommended. Thus, the choice of optimal therapies is limited. Dual therapy with azithromycin and ceftriaxone increases the cure rate of uncomplicated urogenital, anorectal, and pharyngeal gonorrhea and may help prevent the development of resistance.[A2]

In the past, azithromycin cured most cases of nongonococcal urethritis (NGU), including those caused by *Mycoplasma genitalium*, an increasingly recognized cause of NGU; now, however, reported cure rates are lower, sometimes in the 70% or so range.[4] Some studies suggest that doxycycline is more effective than azithromycin for NGU, but a longer course of treatment dependent on the patient's adherence must also be considered. Currently, there is no commercially available diagnostic test for *M. genitalium*, which complicates the treatment question. In some settings in which *M. genitalium* is a consideration, persistent or recurrent NGU should be treated with moxifloxacin for 7 to 10 days.[5,6] *T. vaginalis*, which is susceptible to metronidazole or tinidazole, also causes urethritis and should be considered in the face of NGU treatment failure.

Women with urethritis present with some combination of dysuria and pyuria, which must be differentiated from bacterial cystitis. Because treatment for urinary tract pathogens may also resolve sexually transmitted urethritis, the clinician treating a presumed bladder infection should consider an STI as well.

Genital Ulcers

In the United States, HSV-1 and HSV-2 (Chapter 350) and *T. pallidum* are responsible for virtually all the ulcers encountered, and HSV-1 and HSV-2 are by far the most common cause.

LYMPHOGRANULOMA VENEREUM

Lymphogranuloma venereum, caused by a serovar of *C. trachomatis* (Chapter 302), is characterized by local lymph node suppuration, ulceration and subsequent fibrosis, fistula formation, and distal edema. LGV can manifest as a syndrome mimicking proctocolitis with clinical findings of rectal discharge (mucoid or hemorrhagic in appearance), tenesmus, anal pain, constipation, and fever. Untreated, it can cause extensive local damage with fistulization and stricture formation. Secondary bacterial infections, some of which may be invasive, may occur. Outbreaks among MSM have been reported in the United States and Europe.

GENITAL HERPES

Genital herpes usually develops after an incubation period of less than 21 days and arises as clustered vesicles on an erythematous base. The vesicles become pustular and then rupture to form shallow, painful ulcers, which may coalesce. The ulcers heal by crusting over, and the process is usually completed 2 to 3 weeks after the initial lesions appear. Recurrences proceed through the same stages but generally last only about 5 to 7 days. The first (incident) episode of HSV-2 infection may be accompanied by systemic signs and symptoms including fever and headache, the latter reflecting the spread of HSV to the central nervous system. HSV-2 is the putative cause of Mollaret recurrent meningitis and may occur after a primary genital infection or as reactivation. It may also occur in the absence of genital lesions or a known diagnosis of HSV-2 infection.

About 20% of infected individuals manifest the classic genital presentation, 60% have mild and atypical signs and symptoms, and the remaining 20% are completely asymptomatic. Individuals who have acquired HSV-2 shed the virus approximately 3 to 4% of the time (even while asymptomatic), posing an ongoing risk to sexual partners. Serologic screening for genital herpes is associated with a high rate of false-positive test results and potential psychosocial harms. Evidence from randomized controlled trials does not establish whether preventive antiviral therapy for asymptomatic HSV-2 infection has benefit.[7]

SYPHILIS

The ulcerative lesion of syphilis (Chapter 303)—the chancre—is indurated and painless, and in many cases it escapes detection. Dark-field examination of scrapings suspended in saline from a genital ulcer may reveal motile spirochetes, and this finding is diagnostic. Secondary syphilis results when the spirochetes spread systemically, leading to a characteristic rash, alopecia, oral mucous patches, or condyloma latum. These skin manifestations should prompt testing for syphilis. The serologic screening test of choice for syphilis is based on the formation of antibodies to cardiolipin, a constituent of the spirochetal cell wall (e.g., rapid plasma reagin test, Venereal Disease Research Laboratory [VDRL] test, toluidine red unheated serum test [TRUST]). Confirmatory testing requires the search for an antitreponemal antibody (e.g., microhemagglutination assay–*T. pallidum*, fluorescent treponema antibody test). The anticardiolipin test provides a titer that must be used to monitor the response to treatment.

Some larger commercial laboratories have reversed the order of testing, using an antitreponemal test followed by an anticardiolipin test, which allows automation and may be cost-effective in areas of low syphilis endemicity. This represents a change in testing and interpretation and must be done with caution because such an approach cannot immediately separate old, treated infections from new infections (E-Fig. 269-1).

As syphilis rates have increased since 2000, so too have serious syphilis sequellae including congenital syphilis and ocular syphilis. Between 2014 and 2015, CDC identified 388 cases of ocular syphilis, occurring primarily in men, the majority of whom identified as MSM. Approximately half of the reported cases of syphilis met surveillance criteria for early syphilis (primary, secondary, or early latent). All patients diagnosed with syphilis should be questioned about ocular symptoms as well as symptoms suggestive of neurosyphilis. Neurosyphilis can occur at any stage of infection and should be suspected in any patient with a positive serologic test result who also has findings suggestive of nervous system involvement, including ocular and vestibular symptoms. Ocular and neurosyphilis are serious diseases requiring prompt evaluation and management; treatment of both requires 14 days of intravenous aqueous penicillin G. Later stages of syphilis may be identified only serologically or on pathologic specimens. Late latent syphilis and syphilis of unknown duration are managed with three weekly injections of intramuscular penicillin.

Worldwide, syphilis infection has been detected in a substantial number of people with recognized or unrecognized HIV infection, especially men who have sex with men. The U.S. Preventative Services Task Force recommends screening for syphilis infection in persons who are at increased risk of infection.[8,9] Screening HIV-positive men or MSM for syphilis every 3 months is associated with improved detection of syphilis.

CHANCROID

Chancroid (Chapter 285) infection with *H. ducreyi*, produces painful, ragged ulcers and tender inguinal lymphadenopathy, which may be fluctuant. Unlike the lesions of HSV infection, these genital ulcers are likely to vary in size.

Epithelial Cell Infections
HUMAN PAPILLOMAVIRUS

Sexually transmitted HPV infection (Chapter 349) is generally transient and asymptomatic, but some patients develop visible genital warts. These warts are painless, soft, moist, pink or flesh-colored swellings that vary in shape and can be raised or flat, single or multiple, small or large, and sometimes cauliflower shaped. Warts occur in the vulva, vagina, and anus; on the cervix; and on the penis, scrotum, groin, or thigh. Genital warts are diagnosed by visual inspection. Treatment is primarily with topical agents but is generally not curative.

Two oncogenic HPV genotypes (16 and 18) are responsible for almost all anogenital, cervical, and oropharyngeal cancers and precancerous lesions. HPV types 6 and 11 are responsible for most cases of genital warts and recurrent respiratory papillomatosis. Papanicolaou smears are recommended for sexually active women beginning at the age of 21 years, regardless of risk factor or age at coitarche; HPV testing, however, is not recommended for women younger than 30 years. Frequency of rescreening is influenced by age, previous screening results, and HPV results. Male gender, smoking, and HIV-positive status are significantly associated with prevalent oral HPV.[10]

Three HPV vaccines are currently approved by the Food and Drug Administration for use in males and females: a quadrivalent vaccine (protecting against HPV types 6, 11, 16, and 18), a bivalent vaccine (protecting against HPV types 16 and 18), and a 9-valent vaccine (6, 11, 16, and 18, 31, 33, 45, 52, and 58). Vaccination is recommended for males and females 26 years old and younger including previously unvaccinated, immunocompromised persons (e.g., HIV).

Female Genital Discharge

Infections of the female genitourinary tract produce several syndromes with overlapping symptoms (dysuria, vaginal discharge, vulvar irritation), the cause of which can usually be established with a careful history, examination, and laboratory tests. The initial approach depends on the primary anatomic site of infection—urinary tract, endocervix, or vagina. The columnar epithelium of the endocervix is susceptible to infection with *N. gonorrhoeae*, *C. trachomatis*, and *T. vaginalis*, and the vagina is susceptible to infection with *Candida albicans*, *T. vaginalis*, and the syndrome of bacterial vaginosis. The cervix may appear completely normal in women with cervical infection, but mucopurulence at the cervical os or mucosal friability suggests infection. Vaginitis is associated with a visible discharge, and the characteristics of the vaginal fluid offer diagnostic clues.

Female genital discharge is a condition in which syndromic management strategies generally lack sensitivity and specificity. In women with vaginal discharge, microscopic examination of a wet mount preparation may enhance the effectiveness of syndromic treatment, but interpretation of results is difficult and cannot exclude infection with several pathogens concurrently.

BACTERIAL VAGINOSIS

Bacterial vaginosis (BV) is the most common cause of vaginal discharge in the United States. Bacterial vaginosis is an anaerobic polybacterial dysbiosis of the vaginal microbiome (i.e., a vaginal microbiome not dominated by lactobacilli).[11] Women with bacterial vaginosis are often minimally symptomatic but may note mild vaginal discharge and vaginal odor (which is often increased after coitus).[12] The normal vaginal flora contains hydrogen peroxide–producing lactobacilli such as *Lactobacillus crispatus* and *Lactobacillus jensenii*, which probably help "defend" the vagina against a number of pathogens (an example of innate immunity). *Lactobacillus acidophilus* is rarely found in the normal vagina, which explains the failure of yogurt to serve as a remedy or a preventive. Bacterial vaginosis begins with the unexplained disappearance of the normal vaginal flora and its replacement with *Gardnerella vaginalis* and many species of anaerobic bacteria. The precise mechanism causing this shift in vaginal flora is poorly understood. Most recently, previously unrecognized anaerobic bacterial species (bacterial vaginosis–associated bacteria) have been described as potentially causative. In a study of 220 women with bacterial vaginosis, the vaginal milieu demonstrated great species diversity. African American women without bacterial vaginosis at the time of sampling had higher numbers of bacterial vaginosis–associated bacteria, which could contribute to an increased risk of bacterial vaginosis.

The discharge of bacterial vaginosis is homogeneous and may contain bubbles. Vaginal pH is elevated above the normal 4.0 to 4.5. Adding 10% potassium hydroxide to the vaginal discharge on the microscope slide or to the discharge present in the extracted speculum elicits an amine-like, fishy odor, yielding a positive "whiff" test result because of the elaboration of amines from the anaerobic flora. Examination of vaginal material as a wet mount reveals the absence of bacilli and their replacement with clumps of coccobacilli. Some vaginal epithelial cells are coated with coccobacilli, which may obscure their edges (clue cells) or the normally clear appearance of the cytoplasm, sometimes described as looking like a fried egg that has been salted and peppered. Relatively few polymorphonuclear leukocytes are observed; large numbers of leukocytes in the wet mount of a woman with bacterial vaginosis suggest a coincident infection, possibly trichomoniasis or bacterial cervicitis.

Bacterial vaginosis is not necessarily a benign change in flora. It is associated with an increased rate of upper tract infection (endometritis, salpingitis) and complications of pregnancy, including premature rupture of the membranes and preterm delivery. However, treatment of asymptomatic women with bacterial vaginosis who are not at high risk for preterm delivery appears to confer no benefit. Women with bacterial vaginosis may have increased risk for the acquisition of HIV; male partners may be at increased risk of HIV infection as well. Treatment is generally directed against the anaerobic flora and consists of metronidazole, tinidazole or clindamycin for 5 to 7 days. Alternative treatment regimens exist, but a single oral dose of metronidazole is not recommended for bacterial vaginosis because of the high failure rate. The bacterial vaginosis relapse rate is about 30%, and treatment of male sexual partners offers no benefit.

CANDIDIASIS

Vulvovaginal candidiasis (Chapter 318) is common and is seen most frequently in women taking antibiotics or using oral contraceptives when endogenous *Candida* species outgrow normal bacterial flora. Women usually complain of vulvar itching and discomfort and may or may not notice an accompanying discharge. The vagina generally maintains normal numbers of lactobacilli, so the vaginal pH is usually normal, which is helpful in discriminating between candidiasis and other vaginal infections. The labia and vaginal walls may be erythematous. Although classically described as "curdy," the discharge of candidiasis is frequently loose and is difficult to distinguish from other discharges. Vaginal material may be treated with 10% potassium hydroxide to destroy other cellular elements and to make the fungi easier to observe. Wet mount, however, has a sensitivity of only about 50%, and a woman with a classic clinical presentation should be treated even if fungal elements are not observed.

A wide range of topical antifungal medications are available (many without a prescription), and all these drugs are approximately equally effective, although the cure rate with some single-dose topical treatments appears to be lower than that with longer regimens. Fluconazole administered as a single oral dose of 150 mg is highly effective. Infection with yeasts other than *C. albicans* may require longer therapy.[13] Recurrent vulvovaginal candidiasis is a problem for many women, and optimal management has not been defined. Recurrent infection should lead the clinician to consider underlying diabetes mellitus or HIV infection. Treatment of sexual partners of women with candidiasis confers no benefit.

TRICHOMONIASIS

The estimated annual incidence of *Trichomonas vaginalis* worldwide exceeds that of chlamydia and gonorrhea combined.[14] Women with *T. vaginalis* infection may complain of purulent discharge and vulvar irritation. The vaginal walls are red, and the vagina may contain excessive yellow or green discharge that is bubbly or frothy appearing. The ectocervix may also be inflamed or have punctate microhemorrhages, causing the pathognomonic "strawberry cervix" (colpitis macularis). Vaginal pH is elevated, but the whiff test result is generally negative. Wet mount reveals large numbers of polymorphonuclear leukocytes as well as motile protozoa about the same size as the leukocytes, with visible flagella; motile organisms may be recognized in about two thirds of cases. Because of poor performance of wet mount microscopy, more sensitive testing is recommended; a variety of platforms are available (e.g., NAAT, DNA probe hybridization, and antigen detection). Therapy for trichomoniasis requires metronidazole or tinidazole, but resistant organisms are encountered with increasing frequency. A 7-day course of metronidazole (500 mg twice daily) is the preferred treatment in women,[A3] but a single 2-gram dose can be used in men.

TABLE 269-3   ANTIBIOTIC REGIMENS FOR THE TREATMENT OF PELVIC INFLAMMATORY DISEASE

OUTPATIENT (MILD-TO-MODERATE DISEASE)

Doxycycline (100 mg orally twice daily for 14 d) with or without metronidazole (500 mg orally twice daily for 14 d), *plus* one of the following:
Ceftriaxone (250 mg single dose IM)
or
Cefoxitin (2 g single dose IM concurrently with probenicid 1 g orally)

INPATIENT (MODERATE-TO-SEVERE DISEASE)

Cefotetan (2 g IV) *plus* doxycycline (100 mg orally or IV) q12h
or
Cefoxitin (2 g IV q6h) *plus* doxycycline (100 mg orally or IV q12h)
or
Clindamycin (900 mg IV q8h) *plus* gentamicin (3 to 5 mg/kg IV once daily)

Adapted from Brunham RC, Gottlieb SL, Paavonen J. Pelvic inflammatory disease. *N Engl J Med.* 2015;372:2039-2048.

CERVICITIS

The diagnosis of cervicitis is suggested by tenderness on bimanual examination, visible inspection revealing inflammation, or discharge. The specific diagnosis can be made only by detecting microorganisms from the cervix. *N. gonorrhoeae* and *C. trachomatis* have tropism for cervical tissue, whereas other pathogens (including HIV) can apparently infect the vaginal tissues as well.

PELVIC INFLAMMATORY DISEASE

Each year, more than 800,000 women develop pelvic inflammatory disease (PID) in the United States. The bacterial causes of PID are myriad and include *N. gonorrhoeae*, *C. trachomatis* (about 35% of cases),[15] and *Mycoplasma* (especially *M. genitalium*); other anaerobic and aerobic bacteria that colonize the vagina and CMV also have been implicated as causes of this infection that ascends from the cervix into the uterine cavity, producing endometritis, occasionally with extension to the fallopian tubes, causing salpingitis. Treatment should include therapy directed at anaerobes (Chapter 283; Table 269-3).[A4-16] A recent meta-analysis of 37 randomized clinical trials found no conclusive evidence that one regimen of antibiotics was safer or more effective than any other for the cure of PID, and there was no clear evidence for the use of nitroimidazoles (metronidazole) compared to use of other drugs with activity over anaerobes.[A5] Chlamydial salpingitis may be mild, and patients may not seek medical attention. Some intrauterine devices have been associated with an increased risk of salpingitis, and some data suggest that vaginal douching is a predisposing factor.

Adnexal tenderness on bimanual examination leads to the clinical diagnosis of salpingitis. Cervical tenderness, fever, leukocytosis, and an elevated sedimentation rate are sometimes observed. The clinical diagnosis is confirmed laparoscopically in only about 70% of cases, suggesting considerable error in diagnosis. Vaginal ultrasonography or computed tomography is often helpful in defining the cause of pelvic pain syndromes. Pregnant women with evidence of salpingitis should be hospitalized. Other indications for hospitalization include nonresponse to or intolerance of an oral regimen, presence of a tubo-ovarian abscess, and inability to rule out a surgical emergency, such as appendicitis.[17] Women should experience some clinical improvement within about 72 hours of initiation of therapy. Failure to do so is an indication for hospitalization. Infertility complicates approximately 15% of initial attacks of salpingitis and about 75% of women who suffer three or more attacks. Ectopic pregnancy, infertility, and tubo-ovarian abscess are complications of salpingitis.

⬤ PREVENTION

STIs are preventable. The Centers for Disease Control and Prevention recommends five strategies as the foundation for an effective prevention program: (1) education and counseling of persons at risk to motivate the adoption of safer sexual behavior; (2) identification of asymptomatic infected persons and symptomatic persons unlikely to seek diagnostic and treatment services; (3) rapid and effective diagnosis and treatment of infected persons; (4) evaluation, treatment, and counseling of exposed sexual partners; and (5) preexposure vaccination of persons at risk for vaccine-preventable STIs.

Behavioral Interventions

Abstaining from sexual intercourse or being in a long-term, mutually monogamous relationship with an uninfected partner is the most reliable way to prevent

STIs. Abstinence should be recommended during treatment for an STI and for anyone who wants to avoid STIs and unintended pregnancy. Both partners should be tested for STIs, including HIV infection, before initiating sexual intercourse.

Counseling is essential for people with STIs. Interactive counseling, video presentations, peer groups, and other formats that emphasize correct condom use have reduced the incidence of subsequent infections among STI clinic patients and adolescents. Randomized controlled trials demonstrate that structured risk reduction counseling can reduce the incidence of infections by 25 to 40% among some STI clinic populations.[A6] HIV testing is preceded by a counseling session, but there is little evidence of a preventive benefit from this communication.

Barrier Methods

When used consistently and correctly, male latex condoms are effective in preventing the sexual transmission of HIV infection and can reduce the risk of other STIs (gonorrhea, chlamydia, and trichomoniasis). However, because condoms do not cover all exposed areas, they are likely to be more effective in preventing infections transmitted by fluids from mucosal surfaces (e.g., gonorrhea, chlamydia, trichomoniasis, HIV infection) than in preventing those transmitted by skin-to-skin contact (e.g., HSV, HPV, syphilis, chancroid). Male condom failure usually results from inconsistent or incorrect use rather than from condom breakage. Non-latex condoms (those made of polyurethane or other synthetic material) can be used by persons with latex allergy. There is less information available on the effect of female condoms on the incidence of STIs. Although cervical caps and diaphragms cover the cervix, there is little evidence that they can prevent STIs or HIV infection.

Male Circumcision

Male circumcision reduces mucosal tissue susceptible to HIV and STI pathogens. Circumcision of adult men reduces the acquisition of HIV by more than 70% for up to 5 years after circumcision.[A7] Circumcision also appears to reduce the acquisition of other viral STI pathogens, including HSV-2 and HPV.

Partner Services

The detection of an STI demands consideration of the infected person's sexual partners, who may have undetected and serious disease. In addition, in the absence of partner treatment, reinfection of the index case can be expected. The probability that a sexual partner is also infected reflects the efficiency of transmission of the STI pathogen, as described earlier. For example, most men with gonococcal urethritis infect their partners, whereas only about half of patients with HIV infection have infected their partners at the time of outreach; partners who differ in terms of STI or HIV infection status are referred to as discordant.

Sexual partners can be notified directly by the infected person or by health care workers, sometimes through proactive contact tracing. In general, dependence on the infected person is a less reliable way to get partners treated. However, in many states it is legal to pursue expedited care by providing the infected patient with the appropriate treatment for his or her partners. Expedited partner care appears to work well for the treatment of gonorrhea and chlamydia infections.[A8]

Preexposure Interventions

Preexposure vaccination is the most effective method for preventing the transmission of certain STIs. For example, because hepatitis B virus is frequently transmitted sexually, hepatitis B vaccination is recommended for all unvaccinated persons being evaluated for an STI. In addition, hepatitis A vaccine is recommended for men who have sex with men and for drug users (both injection and noninjection). Vaccines for HPV are now available for both females and males (Chapter 349). The HPV vaccines now have more than 10 years of follow-up and demonstrate continued high rates of protection in women. HPV vaccination for males may reduce acquisition of genital warts and is protective against anal precancerous lesions, leading to vaccine recommendation for boys aged 9 to 26 years from the Advisory Committee on Immunization Practices.

Several studies have evaluated the effectiveness of antiretroviral agents for HIV preexposure prophylaxis. Results have indicated HIV prevention but only in the setting of high-level (>85%) medication adherence. Furthermore, because the only currently Food and Drug Administration–approved antiretroviral for HIV prevention is also a drug combination used for therapy, regular HIV screening is necessary to prevent the development of resistance should the patient become infected.[18] Although rare, HIV transmission in the setting of high levels of medication adherence have occurred. Topical HIV prevention by vaginal microbicides has been only partially successful, in large part because of poor adherence. Long-acting injectable drugs, vaginal rings, and coformulated options (i.e., contraceptive and antiretroviral agents) are under evaluation.

Postexposure Prophylaxis

After consensual or nonconsensual sexual exposure, a variety of STIs can be prevented with empirical antibiotics. Prevention of HIV infection requires antiretroviral agents used in combination (two nucleoside reverse transcriptase inhibitors and one integrase inhibitor) that must be initiated shortly after the exposure (<72 hours) and used for 28 days.

Contraception

All methods of birth control can influence the acquisition and outcome of an STI. In addition, pregnancy itself (in the absence of effective birth control) affects STI acquisition and the health of the pregnancy and the neonate. Accordingly, STI management demands consideration of the reproductive health of both partners as well as family planning issues. A systematic review suggested that there was no increased risk of HIV infection in oral contraceptive users; however, based on data for injectable hormonal contraceptives, progesterone-only injectable contraception may be associated with an increased risk of HIV; a trial comparing implants, injections, and IUDs is ongoing. Women using injectable hormonal birth control should be cautioned about consistent condom use for STI prevention until these relationships are better clarified.[19]

TOWARD A COMPREHENSIVE MANAGEMENT STRATEGY

Although most STIs are self-limited and readily treated, the comprehensive and proper management of the patient with an STI requires considerable skill. First, the correct syndrome must be recognized, and a decision about specific diagnostic tests must be made. Second, empirical therapy must be provided and must be sufficiently broad to promise cure or reduced duration of illness. Third, the clinician is obligated to search for other STIs of public health or personal significance. Fourth, the clinician must deal with the patient's sexual partners, through either referral or expedited partner therapy. Fifth, the patient needs counseling and adjunctive preventive measures, where appropriate. Such measures might include vaccination for hepatitis B or HPV or antibiotics to prevent another STI, such as incubating syphilis or HIV infection.

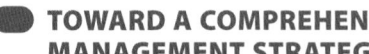 **Grade A References**

A1. Eshleman SH, Hudelson SE, Redd AD, et al. Treatment as prevention: characterization of partner infections in the HIV prevention trials network 052 trial. *J Acquir Immune Defic Syndr.* 2017;74:112-116.

A2. Workowski KA, Bolan GA. Sexually transmitted diseases treatment guidelines, 2015. *MMWR Recomm Rep.* 2015;64:1-137.

A3. Kissinger P, Muzny CA, Mena LA, et al. Single-dose versus 7-day-dose metronidazole for the treatment of trichomoniasis in women: an open-label, randomised controlled trial. *Lancet Infect Dis.* 2018;18:1251-1259.

A4. Creighton S. Gonorrhoea. *BMJ Clin Evid.* 2014;2:1-12.

A5. Savaris RF, Fuhrich DG, Duarte RV, et al. Antibiotic therapy for pelvic inflammatory disease. *Cochrane Database Syst Rev.* 2017;4:CD010285.

A6. Ross JD. Pelvic inflammatory disease. *BMJ Clin Evid.* 2013;12:1-28.

A7. Gray R, Kigozi G, Kong X, et al. The effectiveness of male circumcision for HIV prevention and effects on risk behaviors in a posttrial follow-up study. *AIDS.* 2012;26:609-615.

A8. Ferreira A, Young T, Mathews C, et al. Strategies for partner notification for sexually transmitted infections, including HIV. *Cochrane Database Syst Rev.* 2013;4:CD002843.

GENERAL REFERENCES

For the General References and other additional features, please visit Expert Consult at https://expertconsult.inkling.com.

270

APPROACH TO THE PATIENT BEFORE AND AFTER TRAVEL

DAVID O. FREEDMAN AND LIN H. CHEN

Prevention strategies and medical interventions for the traveler need to be individualized according to a risk assessment that considers both the itinerary and factors that are dependent on the prospective traveler.[1] A structured approach to patient interaction (Table 270-1) is the most efficient way to cover the necessary educational and preventive interventions. Because many of these measures will be initiated only much later at the traveler's destination, clearly printed instructions in lay language are advisable. The worldwide epidemiology of travel-related diseases is constantly changing. Special needs travelers, such as those who are immunocompromised, are pregnant, or have significant underlying disease, should be referred to a specialized travel medicine clinic.

Globally, approximately 100 million people travel from industrialized to developing countries each year. Several recent analyses have provided much needed new data on the profiles of travel-related illness determined by destination of travel.[2] Depending on destination, 22 to 64% of travelers report some illness; most of these problems are mild, self-limited illnesses, such as diarrhea, respiratory infections, and skin disorders. Infectious diseases account for up to 10% of the morbidity during travel but only 1% of the deaths, with malaria being the most common cause.

⬤ IMMUNIZATION

The choice of vaccines for an individual traveler is based on risk of exposure to vaccine-preventable diseases on the chosen itinerary, the severity of disease if it is acquired, and any risks presented by the vaccine itself. Travelers differ in their tolerance of risk. For the vaccine-preventable diseases, the monthly incidence for nonimmune travelers to developing countries is most significant for influenza at 1% and for symptomatic hepatitis A at 0.03% overall; the risk of symptomatic hepatitis B is most significant for long-stay travelers at 0.25% per month.[3] Enteric fever (typhoid and paratyphoid) has a risk of 0.03% per month on the Indian subcontinent and is 10 times lower in Africa and parts of Southeast Asia and Latin America. The risk of animal contact that presents rabies risk is also substantial, at about 1% per month. Risk of yellow fever may be as high as 0.1% per month of travel to an area with current epidemic transmission, but the risk varies greatly between destinations encompassed by the endemic area map. The risk of meningococcal meningitis, cholera, polio, varicella, and Japanese encephalitis in travelers is not known but is thought to be small (<0.0001%). Worldwide measles outbreaks and declining vaccination rates have led to a rise in travel-related measles.

Table 270-2 provides data on dosing, administration, need for boosters, and possible accelerated regimens for vaccines administered in the travel medicine setting. Details on vaccine composition, mechanism of action, use for routine adult and childhood primary vaccination, and adverse reactions can be found in Chapter 15. The following discussion focuses on indications for vaccines in the context of travel.

Verification and Update of Routine Immunizations

Because of the increased prevalence of many infections worldwide, routine adult immunizations need to be current.[4] If no adult doses of tetanus/diphtheria/acellular pertussis (Tdap) have ever been given, a dose of Tdap should be given regardless of the time elapsed since the last tetanus/diphtheria vaccination. Persons born in the United States before 1957 or born anytime in the developing world are considered immune to measles. Other adult travelers should have received at least two doses of live measles–containing vaccine during their life unless a history of measles infection can be documented. Unvaccinated persons who meet the accepted routine indications for influenza or pneumococcal vaccines (Chapter 15) should receive these during the pretravel consultation. Two doses of varicella vaccine spaced by at least 4 weeks should be considered for adult travelers without evidence of varicella immunity. Adults born before 1980 in the United States are considered immune.

Vaccines to Consider for All Developing World Travelers

A number of additional vaccines should be administered depending on the travel destinations.[5]

TABLE 270-1   THE PRETRAVEL CONSULTATION WITH A TRAVELER TO THE DEVELOPING WORLD—A STRUCTURED APPROACH

PERFORM RISK ASSESSMENT

The following must always be ascertained initially to determine appropriate preventive medical recommendations. Preprinted medical record forms may be used to record these.

Exact itinerary, including regions within each country to be visited

Dates of travel to assess risk of seasonal diseases

Age

Past vaccination history

Underlying illnesses

Current medications

Pregnancy status

Allergies

Purpose of trip

Risk exposures—blood, body fluids, adventure or extensive outdoor exposures

Urban versus rural travel

Type of accommodations

Level of aversion to risk

Financial limitations that may necessitate prioritization of interventions

ADMINISTER IMMUNIZATIONS

Administer routine vaccinations that are not up to date.

Administer indicated travel vaccines.

Provide to patient legally mandated Vaccine Information Statements from the Centers for Disease Control and Prevention (http://www.cdc.gov/vaccines/pubs/vis/).

Provide printed checklist to patient listing vaccines administered.

Record in the clinic record vaccines administered, lot number, and date.

Document vaccines offered to but declined by patient as well as nonrecommended vaccines administered at the patient's request.

PROVIDE MALARIA PREVENTION (IF INDICATED)

Determine whether malaria risk exists for the destination country. If yes:

Does the patient's itinerary within that country put him or her at risk? If yes:

Recommend malaria chemoprophylaxis. Several equally effective drugs of choice may be indicated. Ascertain which is best suited to the individual patient and itinerary.

Educate on personal protection against arthropods.

EDUCATE ON TRAVELER'S DIARRHEA

Recommend food and water precautions.

Educate on use of oral hydration and loperamide and prescribe standby therapy for severe diarrhea with azithromycin or a quinolone.

TEACH ESSENTIAL PREVENTIVE BEHAVIORS

Most travel-related health problems, including vaccine-preventable diseases, can be avoided through simple behaviors initiated by the traveler.

Educate on appropriate strategies in the following categories (some topics are not applicable to all destinations): blood-borne and sexually transmitted diseases, safety and crime avoidance, injury prevention, swimming safety, rabies, skin/wound care, tuberculosis, packing for healthy travel, obtaining health care abroad.

DISCUSS OTHER APPLICABLE HEALTH ISSUES

Advise and prescribe for altitude illness, motion sickness, or jet lag.

Discuss prevention of specific travel-related infections that are of some risk to the traveler and have a possible preventive strategy not included in strategies above.

Discuss any minimal-risk conditions (e.g., hemorrhagic fevers) that are a frequent cause of patient anxiety.

Hepatitis A

Hepatitis A vaccine is indicated for every nonimmune traveler to countries or areas with moderate to high risk of infection, which includes essentially everyone traveling outside the United States, Canada, Japan, Australia, New Zealand, Scandinavian countries, and developed countries in Europe. Because outbreaks also occur in developed countries, the vaccine is beneficial for all persons and has been incorporated into the routine childhood immunization schedule in the United States. A single dose of hepatitis A vaccine given any time before travel provides adequate protection. Persons with a history of hepatitis or who previously lived in an endemic country for a prolonged period may benefit from prevaccination serum antibody testing.

Hepatitis B

Pretravel hepatitis B vaccination is indicated for all nonvaccinated travelers with standard indications, such as health care workers, and all longer-stay travelers who will be visiting or residing in high- or moderate-risk areas. Transmission by routes such as sexual contact, blood transfusions, contaminated

TABLE 270-2 TRAVEL-RELATED VACCINES OF ADULTS

DISEASE	VACCINE	PRIMARY COURSE (A: ACCELERATED SCHEDULE)	ROUTE	FURTHER BOOSTERS
VACCINES TO CONSIDER FOR ALL DEVELOPING WORLD TRAVELERS				
Hepatitis A	Killed virus	0, 6-18 months	IM	None
Hepatitis B	Recombinant viral antigen	0, 1, 6 months	IM	None
		A: 0, 1, 2 months and 12 months	IM	
		A: 0, 1, 3 weeks and 12 months*	IM	
	Recombinant, adjuvanted	0, 1 month		
Hepatitis A/B	Combination of monovalent preparations	0, 1, 6 months	IM	None
		A: 0, 1, 3 weeks and 12 months	IM	
Typhoid	Capsular Vi polysaccharide	Single dose	IM	2-3 years
	Live attenuated Ty21a bacteria	0, 2, 4, 6 days	Oral	5 years
Influenza	Inactivated viral	Single dose	IM	Annual
	Live attenuated virus	Single dose (<50 years of age only)	Nasal	Annual
Varicella	Live attenuated virus	0, 4-8 weeks	SC	None
VACCINES FOR CERTAIN DESTINATIONS				
Yellow fever	Live attenuated 17D virus	Single dose	SC	10 years
Meningococcus	Quadrivalent conjugated polysaccharide (A, C, Y, W135)	Single dose	IM	5 years
Rabies	Inactivated viral cell culture	0, 7, 21-28 days	IM†	None routinely but two doses after each exposure
		0, 7 days per WHO but await national acceptance		
Japanese encephalitis (Vero cell)	Inactivated viral	0, 28 days	IM	1 year if at continued risk; no data on subsequent doses
		A: 0, 7 days†	IM	
Polio§	Inactivated viral	Single dose if adequate childhood series	SC; IM acceptable	None
Cholera‖	Live attenuated bacteria (CVD 103-HgR)	Single dose	Oral	3 months
	Killed bacteria + recombinant B toxin subunit¶	0, 1 week	Oral	2 years for cholera; 3 months for ETEC

*Regimen not approved by the U.S. Food and Drug Administration for monovalent hepatitis B vaccine but approved for combination hepatitis A/B vaccine containing the same quantity of hepatitis B antigen.
†Intradermal rabies preexposure vaccine is no longer produced, and the intramuscular 1.0-mL vials are not licensed for intradermal use in a 0.1-mL dose.
‡Regimen recently approved by the U.S. Food and Drug Administration following earlier approval by the European Medicines Agency.
§Oral polio vaccine is no longer produced in the United States.
‖Not available in the United States but available in Canada and most European countries.
¶Also licensed in some countries for traveler's diarrhea due to enterotoxigenic *Escherichia coli*.
A = accelerated regimen to be used for imminent departures; ETEC = enterotoxigenic *E. coli*; IM = intramuscular; SC = subcutaneous.

medical equipment, body piercing, tattooing, acupuncture, and sharing of bathroom facilities is difficult to control or to predict in the context of travel. Vaccination is advocated for some short-term travelers, especially younger travelers and those anticipating being in close contact with local populations, even if they have no specific risk factors. Adventure travelers (accident prone), backpackers, and those with underlying medical conditions are more likely to require contact with the medical system. Accelerated and hyperaccelerated schedules (see Table 270-2) are used widely in practice and are approved in many countries. These are helpful in administering all three primary doses necessary for high assurance of protection in the frequent circumstance in which the traveler is leaving in a very short time and is at risk of hepatitis B exposure. A recently-licensed adjuvanted 2-dose hepatitis B vaccine produces excellent rapid response.

Combination Hepatitis A and Hepatitis B Vaccine

The combined hepatitis A and hepatitis B vaccine provides convenience for travelers with an overlap of indications for use of the individual vaccines. A less well known accelerated 3-week schedule (see Table 270-2) is approved by the U.S. Food and Drug Administration.

Typhoid

Typhoid vaccine is indicated for all travelers to the Indian subcontinent and considered for those traveling to other endemic areas under all but the most deluxe and protected of conditions. Risk increases with trip duration, lodging and eating with local residents, and extent of travel off the usual tourist itineraries. Current typhoid vaccines do not protect against *Salmonella paratyphi*, which is emerging in many areas.[6] Adherence to the oral vaccine regimen may be as low as 70%.

Influenza

Influenza is transmitted year-round in the tropics. Recent data show that influenza is the most common vaccine-preventable illness in travelers. An increased

risk of influenza has been reported among cruise ship passengers. All travelers to destinations with current influenza virus circulation, not just those with the usual risk factors, should strongly consider influenza vaccination.[7]

Vaccines for Certain Destinations
Yellow Fever

The primary indication for yellow fever vaccination is to prevent infection in individuals at risk. A map of risk areas can be found at www.cdc.gov/travel. However, yellow fever is currently the only vaccine that falls under the International Health Regulations that may necessitate vaccination purely for regulatory reasons. A number of African countries and one in South America (French Guiana) require proof of yellow fever vaccination from all arriving travelers. Other countries, both within and outside the risk zone, have submitted more complex requirements to the World Health Organization. Current country-by-country yellow fever entry requirements are at www.who.int/ith/chapters/en/index.html. A Centers for Disease Control and Prevention–designated yellow fever vaccination center should be consulted for detailed requirements. Neither yellow fever vaccine nor any other vaccine is currently required for readmission to the United States. In general, all healthy adult travelers to areas with a risk of yellow fever transmission should be vaccinated. The true duration of immunity from yellow fever vaccination appears to be much longer than 10 years and may exceed 30 years.[8]

Meningococcus

Meningococcal vaccine is recommended for travelers to Africa's sub-Saharan "meningitis belt" during the dry season from December through June, especially if prolonged contact with the local populace is likely. Out-of-season epidemics have occurred in Ethiopia, Somalia, and Tanzania, indicating possible changes in epidemiologic trends. Muslims undertaking Hajj and Umrah pilgrimages in Saudi Arabia are at a higher risk of meningococcal disease, and proof of vaccination with quadrivalent vaccine within the past 3 years (for polysaccharide vaccine) or 5 years (for conjugate vaccine) is required to obtain pilgrimage visas. Polysaccharide vaccine is no longer produced in western countries.

Rabies

A preexposure rabies series is indicated for long-stay travel to endemic areas of Latin America, Asia, or Africa where the rabies threat is constant and where access to adequate postexposure rabies immune globulin and vaccine is likely to be limited. For short-term travel, risk groups for whom immunization should be considered include adventure travelers, bikers, hikers, cave explorers, and business travelers who travel for short but frequent trips and plan to go running outdoors on these trips.

Japanese Encephalitis

Japanese encephalitis is endemic to many rural farming areas of Southeast Asia and the Indian subcontinent. Sporadic cases with severe sequelae continue to occur in travelers.[9] In temperate regions, the transmission season is from May through October. In tropical or subtropical regions of Oceania and Southeast Asia, transmission may occur year-round. Vaccination is recommended for (1) long-stay travel to an endemic rural area; (2) expatriation to anywhere in an endemic country; (3) short-term travel to endemic rural areas with extensive outdoor exposure, such as with adventure travel; and (4) short-term travel in the face of a current local epidemic.

Polio

Because of eradication efforts, poliomyelitis remains in only a few countries, but complete control remains elusive. Adults traveling to countries that are currently polio endemic (updated information at www.polioeradication.org) and who have previously completed a primary vaccine series should receive a one-time single dose of inactivated polio vaccine as a booster.

Cholera

Cholera vaccination is no longer required by any country, and the risk to typical travelers is insignificant.[10] However, medical and aid workers staying for short periods in disaster areas or refugee camps may consider cholera vaccine. An oral live attenuated bacterial vaccine is available in the United States and an oral killed whole cell–B subunit vaccine is available widely outside the United States.

Sequence of Travel-Related Vaccines

All currently indicated immunizations can and should be given at the same time and in any combination (Chapter 15). If two live viral antigens are not administered on the same day, they must be spaced by a month. Minimum intervals between vaccine doses must be respected, although 4 days or fewer before the next interval are acceptable. Regimens that involve 1-week intervals (rabies, Japanese encephalitis, accelerated hepatitis) are exceptions. There is not a maximum interval between doses of a primary vaccine series; interrupted series (except oral typhoid and rabies) need not be restarted but can be resumed beginning with the dose that is overdue.

MALARIA CHEMOPROPHYLAXIS

An average of 1500 imported cases of malaria are reported annually in the United States. Estimates of risk in travelers not taking chemoprophylaxis vary widely by destination but range from 3.4% per month in West Africa to one tenth that on the Indian subcontinent and a further 10-fold reduction in South America. The majority of cases of imported malaria in the United States and Europe occur in immigrants visiting friends and relatives abroad.

Resources describing current country-specific malaria microepidemiology should be accessible immediately to those prescribing malaria prophylaxis. Dosing and pharmaceutical properties of antimalarial drugs are described in Chapter 324. In the limited number of countries where it is still effective, chloroquine, 500 mg salt (300 mg base) per week beginning the week before the first exposure to malaria and continuing for 4 weeks after the last exposure, is still the drug of choice. However, atovaquone/proguanil may still be used by short-stay travelers who prefer the shorter duration of that regimen.

For all other areas of the world, four drugs are equally effective, and the choice depends on both traveler and itinerary factors. Atovaquone/proguanil (250/100 mg) is a well-tolerated, once-a-day drug that should be started 1 day before arrival in the malarious area and continued for 7 days after the last exposure. The short period of postexposure use makes it convenient for the many travelers on typical 1- to 3-week itineraries. Medication cost and daily dosing make it difficult to use for extended periods. Weekly mefloquine (250 mg) is given 2 and preferably 3 weeks before the first exposure to malaria

and continued for 4 weeks thereafter. Weekly dosing and a long track record of efficacy make this drug the most effective for long-stay travelers. If contraindications to mefloquine exist for long-stay travelers, daily doxycycline (100 mg) beginning 1 day before exposure can be used; unlike atovaquone/proguanil, it must be continued for 4 weeks after exposure. Approximately 5% of individuals who take either mefloquine or doxycycline discontinue therapy because of side effects. Chemoprophylaxis may be started well before departure (3 to 4 weeks for mefloquine) in those concerned about possible intolerance to any drug. Tafenoquine, newly licensed by the U.S. FDA, can be used for chemoprophylaxis only after confirmation of adequate G6PD enzyme level. The dosing is 200 mg daily for 3 days prior to arrival in the malarious area, continued weekly during exposure, and 1 week after the last exposure.

Travelers should be reminded in writing to continue antimalarial drugs for the appropriate period after the last possible exposure, that malaria can still occur despite chemoprophylaxis, and that a malaria smear or malaria rapid diagnostic test is mandatory for any febrile illness occurring within 3 months after travel. Prevention of malaria in travelers residing in malarious areas for 6 months or more presents complex problems that have been reviewed elsewhere.

● DENGUE, CHIKUNGUNYA, ZIKA

An estimated 100 million cases of dengue fever and 250,000 cases of dengue hemorrhagic fever occur annually (Chapter 357). The past 20 years have seen a dramatic geographic expansion of epidemic dengue fever and dengue hemorrhagic fever.[11] Dengue accounts for up to 2% of all illness in returned travelers, and dengue is the most common systemic febrile illness in returned travelers from every region except sub-Saharan Africa, where malaria still predominates.

An outbreak of chikungunya virus infection (Chapter 358), caused by an alphavirus, emerged in 2004 in Kenya and has spread widely in Africa, Asia Pacific, and the Americas.[12] Similarly, Zika virus had been initially identified in Uganda in 1947 but remained relatively unknown until 2007, when an outbreak occurred in Yap. Subsequent dissemination with epidemics in the Americas led to the recognition of unfortunate consequences associated with intrapartum infection, now named congenital Zika syndrome. Zika infection can also cause Guillain-Barré syndrome (Chapter 392), which may not manifest until after the traveler has returned home.[13]

Dengue fever, chikungunya infection, and Zika virus infection are transmitted by day-biting *Aedes* mosquitoes, reinforcing the need to instruct travelers to the tropics in the need for both day and night use of repellents. Several candidate vaccines are in development, most advanced being dengue vaccines.

● TRAVELER'S DIARRHEA

The most frequent cause of traveler's diarrhea is enterotoxigenic *Escherichia coli* and in some locations enteroaggregative *E. coli*. *Salmonella*, *Shigella*, and *Campylobacter* each account for about 5 to 15% (Table 270-3).[14] In Asia, noncholera vibrios are significant.[15] Protozoa account for less than 5%. In adults, norovirus and rotavirus are increasingly detected. The mean duration of traveler's diarrhea, even if it is untreated, is 4 days.

All travelers to the developing world should be thoroughly educated in self-therapy for diarrheal disease and carry the appropriate agents while traveling (Table 270-4).[16,17] The majority of patients respond to loperamide. In severe or unresponsive cases, self-treatment with a single dose of azithromycin 1000 mg is usually sufficient, but patients may continue 500 mg daily for up to 3 days should the traveler's diarrhea persist. Other alternatives include single-dose levofloxacin 500 mg or rifaximin 1650 mg.[A1] Because of a significant increase in quinolone-resistant *Campylobacter* in Southeast Asia, India, and Nepal, the preferred antibiotic for self-treatment is azithromycin, although ciprofloxacin 500 mg/day for 3 days is an alternative.

For prevention of traveler's diarrhea, bismuth subsalicylate may be used. Most guidelines do not recommend antibiotic prophylaxis for the typical traveler because of potential adverse drug effects while away from medical care and because effective rapid-onset therapy is available for diarrhea should it occur. Exceptions include travelers with advanced human immunodeficiency virus (HIV) infection, those who have an underlying chronic medical problem that makes them more prone to adverse consequences from diarrhea, and travelers on a vital mission for a short period (less than 1 week) who cannot tolerate even a day of disability. If indicated, antibiotic prophylaxis can be carried out with rifaximin (200 mg) twice per day[A2]; prophylaxis should be used only for trips of 2 weeks or less.

TABLE 270-3	REGIONAL DIFFERENCES IN THE CAUSE OF TRAVELER'S DIARRHEA			
		APPROXIMATE %		
	LATIN AMERICA AND CARIBBEAN	SOUTH ASIA	SOUTHEAST ASIA	AFRICA
BACTERIA				
Enterotoxigenic *E. coli*	≥35	15-25	5-15	25-35
Enteroaggregative *E. coli*	25-35	15-25	Unknown	<5
Campylobacter	<5	15-25	25-35	<5
Salmonella	<5	<5	5-15	5-15
Shigella	5-15	5-15	<5	5-15
VIRUSES AND OTHER				
Norovirus	15-25	5-15	<5	15-25
Rotavirus	15-25	5-15	<5	5-15
Giardia	<5	5-15	5-15	<5

Adapted from Steffen R, Hill DR, DuPont HL. Traveler's diarrhea: a clinical review. *JAMA.* 2015;313:71-80.

TABLE 270-4	TREATMENTS FOR TRAVELER'S DIARRHEA	
PHARMACOLOGIC AGENT	RECOMMENDED DOSAGE	EFFECTIVENESS AND ADVERSE EVENTS
Bismuth subsalicylate	525 mg (1 oz liquid or 2 tablets chewed well) as needed up to 16 tablets in 24 hours	Moderately effective, turns stool and tongue black, may cause tinnitus from systemic salicylate absorption
Loperamide	4 mg then 2 mg after each unformed stool up to 8 mg/day	Rapid relief of diarrhea but must be combined with an antibiotic in patients with fever or dysentery
Azithromycin	500 mg daily for 3 days or single dose of 1000 mg	First choice for all severe diarrhea but nausea is frequent
Ciprofloxacin	500 mg or 750 mg daily for 1-3 days	Fluoroquinolones may be used for nonsevere diarrhea except for India and Southeast Asia where fluoroquinolone-resistant *Campylobacter* is common
Rifaximin	200 mg tid for 3 days	Ineffective against invasive pathogens (e.g., *Shigella, Salmonella, Campylobacter*)

Adapted from Steffen R, Hill DR, DuPont HL. Traveler's diarrhea: a clinical review. *JAMA.* 2015;313:71-80; and Riddle MS, Connor BA, Beeching NJ, et al. Guidelines for the prevention and treatment of travelers' diarrhea: a graded expert panel report. *J Travel Med.* 2017;24(Suppl 1):S2-S19.

PREVENTIVE BEHAVIORS

Most travel-related health problems, including many infectious diseases, can be significantly reduced through appropriate behavior by the traveler.

Mosquito Protection

Antimalarial chemoprophylactic drugs are less than 100% effective. Protection against arthropods will help prevent dengue, leishmaniasis, filariasis, and a number of important arboviral diseases. Travelers should be instructed to clothe themselves to reduce as much exposed skin as practicable and to apply a repellent containing DEET (concentration of 30 to 35%) to all exposed, nonsensitive areas of the body every 4 to 6 hours. More frequent application is required for agents containing lower concentrations of DEET. Travelers should sleep under a permethrin-impregnated bed net in malarious areas unless they are in a sealed air-conditioned environment. Although anopheline mosquitoes are night biters, *Aedes* spp mosquitoes are usually day biters, so vigilance at all times of day is necessary.

Food and Water Precautions

Travelers to developing countries should be diligent in washing their hands frequently; avoiding food from dubious eating places, markets, and roadside vendors; avoiding buffets where there are no food covers or fly controls; avoiding high-risk food such as shellfish, reef fish (ciguatera risk), undercooked meats and poultry, dairy products, unpeeled fruits, cold sauces, and salads; avoiding both tap water and drinks or ice made from tap water; and using sealed bottled water or chemically treated, filtered, or boiled water for drinking and brushing their teeth.

Sex

Education on the incidence of HIV infection and sexually transmitted diseases among professional sex workers abroad, on the use of condoms, and on the failure rate of condoms (3 to 5% breakage/slippage) should be given regardless of the apparent circumstances of the traveler. Unprotected sex even with fellow travelers is considered high risk. Travel is a disinhibiting experience in itself, and alcohol consumption tends to increase during travel. HIV pre-exposure prophylaxis has become more widely accepted and daily Truvada (200 mg emtricitabine plus 300 mg tenofovir) is an option to prevent HIV in persons at risk of exposure through sexual contact, including travelers.

Blood-borne Pathogens

Blood, blood products, syringes, and contaminated medical or dental instruments are a risk after accidents or trauma. Travelers should consider carrying an infusion set, needles, and a suture kit for high-risk areas. If possible, they should defer medical treatment and travel to a facility where safety can be ensured. Tattooing, acupuncture, and body piercing carry similar risks. Health care workers and others at risk in areas of high HIV prevalence without sophisticated medical infrastructure may consider carrying a 1- to 2-week supply of antiretrovirals to begin immediate postexposure prophylaxis, with the understanding that this is only an initial measure to allow time for travel to an adequate medical facility able to provide sophisticated testing and counseling. Two options are: (1) Descovy (emtricitabine 200 mg/tenofovir alfenamide fumerate [TAF] 25 mg) 1 tablet daily plus raltegravir 400 mg 1 tablet twice daily (or dolutegravir 50 mg 1 tablet daily); (2) Truvada (emtricitabine 200 mg/tenofovir 300 mg) 1 tablet daily plus docutegravir 50 mg 1 tablet daily.

Protection Against Skin Diseases

Infected mosquito bites are common. Practicing good hand hygiene in dirty environments and covering open wounds are preventive measures that all travelers should take. Scabies and lice infestations can be prevented by carrying out good personal hygiene. In Africa, all clothes dried outdoors should be ironed to avoid cutaneous myiasis due to the tumbu fly. Hats and sunscreen are mandatory in the tropics. Sunscreen should always be applied to skin before, and not after, an application of DEET.

Swimming and Water Exposure

Travelers should be instructed to avoid recreational (swimming, rafting, wading) or other exposure to fresh water in areas that are endemic for schistosomiasis. Hikers, bikers, and adventure travelers should consider prophylaxis with 200 mg of doxycycline once per week because of the significant risk of leptospirosis that exists in fresh water throughout the developing world. Walking barefoot in tropical areas predisposes to hookworm, *Strongyloides* infection, cutaneous larva migrans, and tungiasis.

Prevention of Tuberculosis

A predeparture baseline tuberculin skin test with annual retesting is indicated for long-stay travelers to developing countries. Aggressive treatment of skin test converters will prevent cases of active tuberculosis later. Travelers should avoid crowded public transportation or crowded public places and distance themselves immediately from anyone with a chronic or heavy cough. Expatriates should screen domestic help for tuberculosis.

NONINFECTIOUS TRAVEL PROBLEMS
Traveler's Thrombosis and Jet Lag

Travel-related immobility is associated with deep venous thrombosis and pulmonary embolism in otherwise healthy travelers. Risk of pulmonary embolus is essentially absent on flights lasting less than 6 hours. Those with clear, known risk factors are at highest risk. All travelers should avoid dehydration, avoid alcohol, and exercise the legs regularly in flight. Of many recommendations for prevention, only the use of graded 15 to 30 mm Hg compression stockings for those at higher risk is supported in trials,[A3] although prophylactic antithrombosis agents such as factor Xa inhibitor, direct thrombin inhibitor, and subcutaneous low-molecular-weight heparin are sometimes used in practice. Aspirin therapy is of no proven benefit in this setting.

Jet lag (Chapter 377) occurs after crossing three or more time zones. Melatonin (as little as 0.5 mg 30 minutes prior to targeted bedtime) may be useful for reducing the severity of jet lag,[A4] and zolpidem (5 mg) taken for a few nights at bedtime at the destination is generally effective.

Altitude Illness

Whether ascending by car or airplane, acute mountain sickness occurs in at least 25% of people who ascend rapidly to 2500 m or more and in most people who go quickly to 3000 m or more. Gradual ascent during days is rarely practiced by modern travelers. For prevention of altitude illness, acetazolamide, 125 mg twice a day beginning the morning of the day before ascent and continuing through the day after ascent, is effective.[A5][A6] If symptoms of mountain sickness, such as nausea, vomiting, anorexia, lightheadedness, fatigue, or insomnia, persist beyond the day after ascent, travelers may continue to take one tablet each evening. Other medications such as dexamethasone (4 mg twice daily) also can be used for prophylaxis or treatment (Chapter 88).[A7] Severe complications, such as pulmonary or cerebral edema, occur uncommonly under 3500 m and are best treated by oxygen and immediate descent. Those traveling above 3500 m for longer than a brief transit of a few hours should consult an expert.

POST-TRAVEL CARE

The approach to the patient requires knowledge of world geography, the epidemiology of disease patterns in 230 or so countries, and the clinical presentation of a wide spectrum of disorders. Most illnesses are mild, most are self-limited, and many are noninfectious. Based on 43,000 ill-returned travelers seen by the GeoSentinel Surveillance Network, specific travel destinations are associated with the probability of the diagnosis of certain diseases (E-Table 270-1). Diagnostic approaches and empirical therapies can be guided by these destination-specific differences. Important region-specific disease occurrence data indicate that (1) febrile illness[18,19] is most important from Africa and Southeast Asia; (2) malaria is one of the top three diagnoses from every region, yet during the past decade, dengue has become the most common febrile illness from every region outside of sub-Saharan Africa; (3) in sub-Saharan Africa, rickettsial disease is second only to malaria as a cause of fever; (4) respiratory disease is most important in Southeast Asia and sub-Saharan Africa; and (5) acute diarrhea is disproportionately from South Central Asia. Persistent diarrhea is a problem in up to 3% of people who return from developing countries, with parasites (especially *Giardia* and *Cryptosporidium*) and bacteria (especially enteroaggregative *E. coli* and *Shigella*) as the leading causes.

Fever in a traveler who has recently returned from the tropics is a potential emergency and must be evaluated immediately so that antimalarial or other definitive treatment can be initiated rapidly if it is indicated. Persistent gastrointestinal symptoms in a returning traveler require prompt evaluation and treatment (E-Table 270-2).[20] Certain long-term travelers should be evaluated by a travel or tropical medicine specialist when they return to be screened for conditions that may be asymptomatic, such as schistosomiasis or strongyloidiasis.

Travelers who become ill during or any time up to several months after a foreign trip will frequently associate that illness with a possible travel-specific

etiology. This may be the case, but often it is not. Routine things are common, and common things are common whether they are acquired during travel or at some time after the trip.

Grade A References

A1. Riddle MS, Connor P, Fraser J, et al. Trial evaluating ambulatory therapy of travelers' diarrhea (TrEAT TD) study: a randomized controlled trial comparing 3 single-dose antibiotic regimens with loperamide. *Clin Infect Dis.* 2017;65:2008-2017.
A2. Ng QX, Ho CYX, Shin D, et al. A meta-analysis of the use of rifaximin to prevent travellers' diarrhea. *J Travel Med.* 2017;24:1-5.
A3. Clarke MJ, Broderick C, Hopewell S, et al. Compression stockings for preventing deep vein thrombosis in airline passengers. *Cochrane Database Syst Rev.* 2016;9:CD004002.
A4. Tortorolo F, Farren F, Rada G. Is melatonin useful for jet lag? *Medwave.* 2015;15(suppl 3):1-9.
A5. Nieto Estrada VH, Molano Franco D, Medina RD, et al. Interventions for preventing high altitude illness: Part 1. Commonly-used classes of drugs. *Cochrane Database Syst Rev.* 2017;6:CD009761.
A6. Low EV, Avery AJ, Gupta V, et al. Identifying the lowest effective dose of acetazolamide for the prophylaxis of acute mountain sickness: systematic review and meta-analysis. *BMJ.* 2012;345:1-14.
A7. Simancas-Racines D, Arevalo-Rodriguez I, Osorio D, et al. Interventions for treating acute high altitude illness. *Cochrane Database Syst Rev.* 2018;6:CD009567.

GENERAL REFERENCES

For the General References and other additional features, please visit Expert Consult at https://expertconsult.inkling.com.

271
ANTIBACTERIAL CHEMOTHERAPY

ARNOLD LOUIE AND GEORGE L. DRUSANO

Antibiotics have been classified as "miracle drugs" because they have transformed our expectations regarding the outcomes of infections. More recently, they have been the backbone of modern interventional medicine. Barriers not meant to be breached have been. Catheters have been inserted into veins and arteries, the bladder, and the tracheal tree. These interventions support the seriously ill patient, but they also give bacteria access to normally sterile areas. Therapies for cancer and immune-mediated disease often leave patients severely immunosuppressed. Bacterial infections in such patients are serious and, when untreated or treated late, often result in death. Antibiotics provide critical life-saving support for such patients.

What is clear is that the overuse and poor use of antibiotics have allowed many pathogens to develop resistance to drugs. Multiresistant *Staphylococcus aureus* has become a plague both in the hospital and, of late, in the community. Extended-spectrum β-lactamases and *Klebsiella pneumoniae* carbapenemase enzymes have mediated resistance to many of our most potent and broad-spectrum β-lactam agents, including the carbapenems. Consequently, it is important to understand the principles of antibacterial chemotherapy to obtain the best clinical outcomes for our patients but also, in a broader sense, to lower the probability of the emergence of resistance and to maintain the potency of the drugs currently in our therapeutic armamentarium.[1,2] In this context, the significant decline in the use of antibiotics in the United States between 1999 and 2016 is a good sign.[3,4]

CHOICE OF ANTIBIOTIC, ANTIBIOTIC DOSE, AND SCHEDULE TO OPTIMIZE CLINICAL OUTCOME

As in all of clinical medicine, a well-done history and physical examination are central to proper decision making and to the achievement of optimal therapeutic outcomes in patients with infections. Key to choosing the correct drug, dose, and schedule of administration of an antibiotic is recognition that an infection exists. The next step is to document where the infection exists and then to identify the dominant organisms present at each site of infection. The next step is to determine whether there are any risk factors that might predict the presence of drug-resistant pathogens.

As an example, it is known that community-associated pneumonia is caused by certain traditional pathogens. *Streptococcus pneumoniae, Haemophilus*

TABLE 271-1	PRIMARY INFECTION SITES AND THE DOMINANT BACTERIAL SPECIES PRESENT

SITE	BACTERIA
Complicated skin or skin structure infection	*Staphylococcus aureus* and *Streptococcus* spp
Diabetic foot ulcer	Organisms above plus Enterobacteriaceae
Intra-abdominal infections	*Escherichia coli* and other Enterobacteriaceae plus anaerobes
Community-acquired bacterial pneumonia	*Streptococcus pneumoniae, Haemophilus influenzae, Moraxella catarrhalis,* "atypical" pathogens
Hospital-acquired pneumonia	*S. aureus, Klebsiella pneumoniae, Enterobacter* spp, *Pseudomonas aeruginosa, Acinetobacter* spp
Meningitis	*S. pneumoniae, H. influenzae* (nontypable), meningococci; in hospital settings, *S. aureus* and gram-negatives
Urinary tract infections	Enterobacteriaceae, particularly in sexually active women; multiresistant gram-negatives in patients with complicated urinary tract infections or those instrumented; enterococci, particularly in elderly men
Prostatitis	Enterobacteriaceae, enterococci, atypical pathogens

influenzae, and perhaps *Moraxella catarrhalis* are the "classic" bacterial pathogens associated with this entity. "Atypical" pathogens such as *Legionella* species, *Mycoplasma pneumoniae,* and *Chlamydophila pneumoniae* may also be seen. In contrast, intra-abdominal infections are dominated by *Escherichia coli* and other Enterobacteriaceae and anaerobic organisms such as *Bacteroides* species. Consequently, it is important to understand the dominant pathogens present at different infection sites so that the best drug or combination of drugs can be chosen to treat the infection.

Knowing the source of infection is also critical because drugs penetrate differently into different body sites. Classically, penetration is poorer into spaces where there are tight junctions, such as the central nervous system, the eye, and the prostate. In general, the penetration of many classes of antibacterial agents is good into complicated skin and skin structure infection sites. What is often not appreciated is the divergent penetrations of different agents and even agents within the same class into the lung to treat bacterial pneumonia. For instance, the penetration by macrolide antibiotics into skin infection sites is modest, but their penetration into the lung is good, with penetration ratios (area under the concentration-time curve [AUC] in lung epithelial lining fluid/AUC in plasma) ranging from 4 to 20. The penetration of β-lactam drugs can range from 15 to 100%, but there is no set of variables (at least to date) that explains such a range of penetrations. Table 271-1 presents a partial list of infection sites and their dominant pathogens. The point is not to have an encyclopedic knowledge of infection sites or of pathogens but to appreciate that different infection sites require different drugs to provide adequate coverage for the most likely pathogens present.

It is also important to understand other factors that increase the probability that a resistant organism is present at the primary infection site. An example is a patient who has recently taken antibiotics before acquiring the present infection. Other examples are the acquisition of an infection in the hospital or in an extended care facility and in a patient who is immunosuppressed. In such patients, the choice of antimicrobial agents must be carefully considered to cover more resistant pathogens.

CULTURE AND GRAM STAIN

Once the site of infection has been definitively identified or the most likely source of infection has been determined, it is critical to obtain culture specimens from that site as well as to obtain blood culture samples. Coordination with the microbiology laboratory is key to make sure that culture specimens are handled appropriately. Also of great importance is the performance and interpretation of a Gram stain on the specimen. This can be straightforward if the specimen is from a normally sterile space, or it may require considerable skill in interpretation if the specimen is from an area where mixed flora is normally present, such as expectorated sputum.

Although it is not possible to make a definitive diagnosis on the basis of the cellular morphology of the organism, it is possible to combine information

on the morphology, the organism's gram positivity or negativity, the infection site, and the most likely pathogens to make an initial antimicrobial choice with the highest probability of producing effective chemotherapy. The initial antibiotic chosen to cover organisms present at the primary infection site has a significant influence on the outcome of therapy. Initial choices should err on the side of caution. When definitive cultures are available, the chemotherapy can be "streamlined" to provide the most effective and least toxic antimicrobial for the patient. As the seriousness of the infection increases, providing the correct initial coverage becomes more important with regard to the ultimate outcome.

SUSCEPTIBILITY

Because infections occur at a specific place, it is important to have an understanding of the antimicrobial susceptibility patterns in one's particular hospital. Most frequently, the microbiology susceptibility patterns are different in the culture specimens taken from patients on the general wards as opposed to those in intensive care units (ICUs) because the former are generally (but not always) infected with pathogens derived from the community setting. In severely infected patients, particularly those whose infections were acquired in the ICU, it is critical to know the susceptibility patterns for these pathogens, which are likely to be multiply resistant to different classes of agents.

After the definitive culture, the identified pathogen must be examined in an antimicrobial susceptibility test. This can be automated, in which case the information returned is the minimal inhibitory concentration (MIC), or it can be reported from a disc diffusion test, where the results are typically reported as S (susceptible), I (intermediate), or R (resistant). The MIC is often misunderstood as the concentration of drug that prevents the pathogen from growing, but it is actually the concentration of drug that allows a tube (or well) containing the pathogen to remain clear by visual examination after 16 to 24 hours. If one starts with an organism concentration of 1 to 5×10^5 colony-forming units (CFUs)/mL, this criterion can actually allow almost a $1 \log_{10}$ (CFU/mL) increase in bacterial count over this time frame and still be read as the MIC. With all its limitations, the MIC provides critical information about drug choice. For several infections, such as meningitis, endocarditis, and perhaps bacteremia, knowing the minimal bactericidal concentration (defined as the concentration required to kill 99.9% of organisms during 16 to 24 hours) is valuable. In these cases, it is important to obtain multi-log killing of the organism to ensure a high probability of a good clinical outcome. For meningitis and endocarditis, there is also the confounding problem of penetration of the drug into the primary infection site. In other circumstances (e.g., ventilator-associated pneumonia) in which bacterial burdens are high, optimizing the probability of cure requires highly bactericidal therapy.

DETERMINING THE "CORRECT" DRUG DOSE

The correct drug dose is the one that produces a high likelihood of achieving a good clinical response with a low probability of causing a concentration-driven adverse event. Another consideration is that the optimal dose should have a high probability of suppressing the emergence of resistant mutants. To be confident that a drug dose has a high likelihood of producing a good clinical outcome requires an understanding of the relationship between the measure of drug exposure and infection outcome, that is, pharmacodynamics (Chapter 26).

When a drug is administered intravenously or orally, the drug concentration starts low, increases to a maximal value, then declines over time until another dose of the drug is given (in a multidose regimen). This drug concentration–time profile should be seen relative to a measure of drug potency against the pathogen in question: the MIC (or minimal bactericidal concentration). It is also critical to note that protein binding is important because in almost all cases, it is the free or non–protein-bound drug that kills the causative pathogen. So understanding the pharmacodynamics of a drug or class of agents first requires knowledge of the drug concentration–time profile, protein binding, and MIC (Fig. 271-1). For drugs that kill organisms much faster as their concentrations rise (e.g., fluoroquinolones, aminoglycosides), the free drug AUC/MIC ratio is most closely linked to drug effect. For other drugs (e.g., penicillins, carbapenems, cephalosporins, monobactams), the rate of organism kill rises with concentration and plateaus quickly, in which case the free drug time greater than MIC (T > MIC) is most closely linked to drug effect. On occasion, the free drug peak concentration/MIC ratio is linked to drug effect. This is seen when there is a rapid and frequent emergence of resistance and the peak concentration helps suppress the amplification of resistant mutant subpopulations.

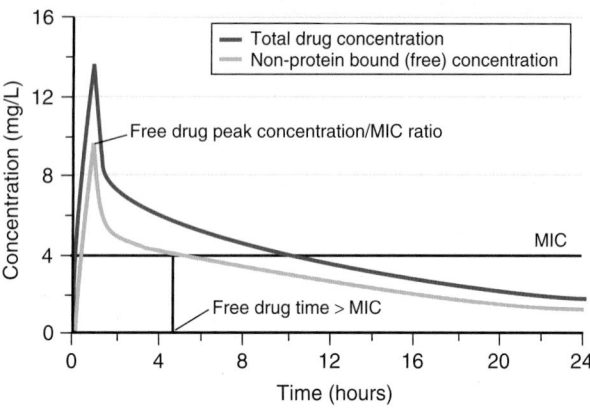

FIGURE 271-1. Three measures of drug exposure are important to the measure of potency, or the minimal inhibitory concentration (MIC). These measures are free drug peak concentration/MIC ratio, free drug time greater than MIC, and free drug area under the curve (AUC)/MIC ratio. AUC = area under the concentration-time curve.

These measures of drug exposure need to be linked to drug effect. There are a number of ways to do this, but two are most common. In the first and most valuable way, patients are studied during the course of a clinical trial. Multiple plasma samples are taken for documentation of the drug's pharmacokinetics and corrected for protein binding. The MIC of the infecting pathogen is determined for the drug being administered, and the three measures of drug exposure cited earlier are calculated. The outcome of the patient is then determined (usually success or failure, but in some instances, time to success or failure serves as the outcome measure). The appropriate measure of drug exposure is then linked to the outcome through logistic regression analysis. By creating such a relationship, it is possible to estimate the probability of a patient having a successful outcome if a certain measure of drug exposure is achieved. For example, if a patient receiving a drug that is a concentration-dependent killing agent achieves a free drug AUC/MIC ratio of 88, the logistic regression relationship allows the calculation that the probability of a good outcome is a specific number (perhaps 91%). During the past 10 years, such relationships have been generated for a great number of drugs and across drug classes. The most common relationships are for the fluoroquinolone antimicrobials, but examples can be found for the aminoglycosides, oxazolidinones, β-lactams, and glycylcyclines, among others.

The second way to link exposure to antibacterial effect is through preclinical animal models of infection. Here, the end point is most often microbiologic, although survivorship models have been employed. At the end of the experiment the drug concentration–time profile in the animals and the number of microbes at the infection site before and after therapy are quantified. Then the measure of drug exposure (as earlier) can be linked to the number of bacterial cells killed by a specific regimen. It is most often the case that drugs are administered to the animals in a "dose fractionation" fashion. For example, 400 mg/kg/day regimen of a β-lactam may be administered as the whole dose once-daily, half the dose every 12 hours, or one quarter of the dose every 6 hours. In this way, it can be determined whether free drug peak concentration/MIC ratio, free drug AUC/MIC ratio, or free drug time greater than MIC is the best measure of drug exposure for the class of drug being studied.

● EMERGENCE OF RESISTANCE

If the drug is properly chosen, the organism should have a high probability of being susceptible to it. However, during the course of therapy, the organism has many mechanisms available to make it less susceptible (the MIC increases) to the administered drug. This leads to less effect than was originally envisioned, which results in a lower probability of cure.

When are organisms likely to become resistant? There are many determinants, but five factors account for the majority of cases of resistance emerging during therapy. The first is the mutational frequency to resistance of the organism being treated. Because mistakes are made by the organism during replication, mutations occur in the genome at a specific rate, which is organism dependent. For antibiotic resistance, the mutational frequency rate is generally around 1 in 10^6 to 10^8 CFU. There are organisms, however—referred to as hypermutators—that have mutations in other places in the genome (often mutS) that alter their DNA replication error-checking mechanisms. These organisms' mutational frequencies are generally 10- to 100-fold higher than those of organisms without mutS mutations.

The second factor is related to the bacterial burden. As the bacterial burden increases and ultimately surpasses the inverse of the mutational frequency to resistance, it becomes more and more likely that a preexistent antibiotic-resistant mutant is already extant in the population. For instance, if the mutational frequency to resistance is 1 resistant organism per 10^7 CFU and the patient has a bacterial infection in which the total bacterial burden is 10^9 organisms, it is highly likely that a resistant organism is present in the population a priori. Antibiotic pressure provides these mutants with a selective advantage. They are amplified while the more susceptible bacteria are killed by the antibiotic. A calculation of the actual probability can be performed by a Poisson distribution, the bacterial burden, and the mutational frequency to resistance. Consequently, infections in which the bacterial burden is high are more likely to generate resistance during therapy. For example, in clinical trials of ventilator-associated pneumonia, single-agent β-lactam drugs or fluoroquinolones allow the emergence of resistance during therapy 33 to 50% of the time.

The third issue is drug penetration. There are circumstances (e.g., empyema) in which the bacterial burden is high but the drug's penetration to the infection site is reduced. In this case the emergence of resistance is more likely. In contrast, poor penetration with relatively low bacterial burdens (e.g., meningitis) generally does not result in a high probability of the emergence of resistance.

The fourth issue has to do with error-prone replication in bacterial pathogens. When resistance develops relatively late in therapy and the bacterial burden is modest, error-prone replication is often to blame. Antibiotics differ greatly with respect to their ability to induce the bacterial isolate to perform error-prone replication. Perhaps the best example is the fluoroquinolone antimicrobials because these drugs strike at the heart of DNA replication. The organism senses the attack of the antibiotic, and a whole cascade of events takes place, the most important of which is the induction of error-prone polymerases (e.g., pol V). These polymerases markedly increase the error rate in DNA replication. Most of these errors are lethal to the organism and therefore unhelpful to it. However, because this is a totally random process, by chance, a mutation can occur in a gene that provides protection from the onslaught of the antibiotic (e.g., a mutation in the DNA gyrase when the patient is receiving a fluoroquinolone). We perceive this as the organism's having a selective replication advantage (emergence of resistance), and we see an increase in the MIC of the mutant organism relative to the baseline organism.

The fifth factor has to do with mechanisms other than antibacterial target site mutations that allow the organisms to survive in the face of appropriate antibiotic chemotherapy. One extremely common mechanism seen in the majority of both gram-positive and gram-negative organisms is the upregulation of efflux pumps. These pumps are indiscriminate in their ability to pump molecules; they can eject multiple classes of antibacterials from the organism as well as natural substances that can harm it, such as metal ions. These pumps keep drug concentrations at their target sites much lower than they would be in the absence of the pumps. The pumps can be induced and then downregulated once the threat has passed, or occasionally, the organism can pick up a mutation in the part of the genome where expression of the pump is regulated, so the pump is always expressed (constitutive expression).

A similar process is seen with the production of β-lactamases. Often, these enzymes are situated on plasmids and are produced all the time. Sometimes, as with the efflux pumps, the bacteria sense the β-lactam, and their β-lactamase production is markedly increased (the phenomenon of induction, seen with ampC-type enzymes, which generally reside on the chromosome). Sometimes, also like the pumps, the organisms pick up a mutation in the part of the genome that regulates production of the β-lactamase. This is referred to as *stable de-repression*, and large quantities of the enzyme are made continuously. The enzyme hydrolyzes its substrate (the β-lactam drug), preventing this antibiotic from binding to the target sites, the β-lactam–binding proteins.

Finally, in gram-negative organisms, the drug must cross the diffusional barrier of the outer membrane before binding to β-lactam–binding proteins (if the drug is a β-lactam) in the periplasm of the organism, or it must cross the inner membrane if its target site is actually inside the organism. For many agents, particularly those that are water soluble, a large percentage of their influx is due to passage through porin proteins. These proteins are water-filled channels that pass through the entirety of the outer membrane of gram-negative bacteria. Part of their function is to provide access to nutrients for the organism and allow the easy diffusion of waste products. These channels are also used to obtain passage by water-soluble antibacterial agents. The organism has the ability to downregulate these channels, either temporarily or permanently (by mutation). An example is *Pseudomonas aeruginosa,* in which downregulation of the porin channel oprD markedly diminishes the penetration of carbapenem antibiotics (β-lactam agents), with a resultant two- to eight-fold rise in MIC. With all the mechanisms that can be brought to bear, it is no surprise that poor dosing and prolonged courses of therapy often lead to the emergence of resistance.

These mechanisms also interact. In the case of fluoroquinolone antimicrobials, where error-prone replication almost always occurs under pressure, the upregulation of efflux pumps relieves some of the antibiotic pressure, allowing the organisms to undergo more rounds of replication per unit of time, giving the error-prone replication mechanism more time to find a mutation that is not lethal and provides protection against the drug at the primary target site.

SUPPRESSING THE EMERGENCE OF RESISTANCE

Suppressing the emergence of resistance is an end point that is different from achieving a good clinical or microbiologic outcome. The antimicrobial exposure (free drug peak concentration/MIC ratio, free drug AUC/MIC ratio, or free drug time greater than MIC) necessary to suppress resistance is always at least as high as that required to attain maximal killing of bacterial cells, and in many instances, it is substantially higher.

Recently it has been shown experimentally that it is possible to identify doses and administration schedules of drugs that suppress the emergence of resistance as well as provide optimal killing of bacterial cells. Unfortunately, many of the exposures necessary to achieve such an outcome are high enough to increase the probability of drug toxicity. Nevertheless, as new agents are developed, it will become important to identify resistance-suppressive exposures and to ascertain whether they are too toxic to be used clinically, as a way of retaining the potency of the antibacterial therapeutic armamentarium.

The other way to help suppress the emergence of resistance is to employ combination chemotherapy. Combination therapy has major advantages, but there are significant disadvantages as well. Among the advantages are that combination therapy can improve the spectrum of coverage in the setting of empirical treatment as well as help suppress the emergence of resistance. This is best seen in the treatment of *Mycobacterium tuberculosis,* although there is growing evidence that this may also be true for difficult-to-treat pathogens such as *P. aeruginosa* and *Acinetobacter* species. Combination therapy can be effective against some pathogens in serious infections for which a single agent would not be adequate. Enterococcal endocarditis is the classic example; ampicillin or vancomycin is generally static and not up to the task of curing this disease, and the second agent (an aminoglycoside, streptomycin, or gentamicin) is somewhat resistant when it is used alone (MIC values <500 mg/L). Yet the combination produces excellent bacterial kill in the endocarditic vegetation, with a high probability of cure if the patient can tolerate the combination for the requisite time. Some authors have discussed reducing drug doses in combination as a way of ameliorating toxicity, but this theoretical advantage is difficult to demonstrate convincingly in the clinical setting.

The disadvantages of combination therapy are also well known. At full doses of each, there may be added toxicity, and there are certainly greater costs associated with combinations. Finally, combinations of agents may interact antagonistically instead of either additively or synergistically. For example, the combination of tetracycline and penicillin is somewhat antagonistic and caused a number of failures in the treatment of pneumococcal meningitis in the 1950s. However, there are circumstances in which weak antagonism is tolerable. It has been shown that isoniazid plus rifampin, part of the standard therapy for *M. tuberculosis,* is somewhat antagonistic with respect to cell killing, but the combination provides superb protection against the emergence of resistance. Consequently, in discussing drug interactions (synergy, additivity, antagonism), it is important to be specific about the end point to which one is referring.

MECHANISM OF ACTION

The search for new antimicrobials begins with the principle that the target that affects pathogens must not be in the human genome or must be sufficiently different that the agent in question does not cause appreciable human toxicity. β-Lactam antibiotics are a good example; the inhibition of peptidoglycan synthesis has no effect on humans because this target is simply not present. An example of differing susceptibility to inhibition because of poor sequence homology between bacteria and humans can be seen in the inhibitors of the bacterial ribosome. The bacterial ribosome is much smaller than that in humans

and has differing affinities for such drugs as aminoglycosides, tetracyclines, macrolides, and clindamycin. Consequently, such agents are an important part of the therapeutic armamentarium and cause only minor adverse effects related to their primary mode of action. In some cases, so-called off-target toxicity may take place. Again, an example is the β-lactams; a major toxicity is accelerated allergic reaction, even though the target for the agents is not present in humans. Table 271-2 lists the sites of action and the effects of many antimicrobial agents.

Often, antimicrobials are thought of as either *bacteriostatic* or *bactericidal,* for which there are standard definitions. An agent that causes a 1000-fold decline (3 $\log_{10}$ [CFU/mL] decrease) in an in vitro test system during 18 to 24 hours is defined as being bactericidal. Any agent that causes a smaller decline is defined as bacteriostatic. It is clear that these definitions are arbitrary; however, there is a clinical connection. Bacteriostatic and bactericidal antibiotics are equivalently effective for abdominal infections, skin and soft tissue infections, and pneumonia,[6] but data are not sufficient for meningitis, endocarditis, or neutropenia.[A1] Obviously, the more organisms the antimicrobial kills, the easier this is to accomplish. In other circumstances, such as multilobar pneumonia, it is critical to kill as many of the organisms as possible so as not to overwhelm the body's immunologic defenses. For these reasons, clinicians generally prefer bactericidal to bacteriostatic agents.

MECHANISMS OF RESISTANCE

Earlier, how to suppress the emergence of resistance was discussed. Here, the mechanisms by which organisms can become less susceptible to antimicrobial agents are examined. As stated earlier, in most cases, resistance is caused by an alteration in the target site; by an enzyme that alters the drug, resulting in a lack of activity; by the drug's being pumped out of the organism; or, in the case of gram-negative pathogens, by the loss or downregulation of a transmembrane porin protein. These mechanisms, along with error-prone replication, can interact to cause large increases in the MIC. For example, a gram-negative pathogen that acquired a mutation in its gyrase enzyme would generally have only a four-fold increase in its MIC value for a fluoroquinolone antimicrobial; however, if this isolate also had an efflux pump upregulated, the MIC could change 8- to 16-fold. Table 271-3 shows the mechanisms of resistance for multiple drug classes as well as the most common organisms in which these mechanisms are seen (also see Chapter 289 for Enterobacteriaceae and multidrug resistance).

EFFECTS OF PHARMACOKINETIC CHANGES

Whereas antimicrobial pharmacodynamics is the study of the effect of a drug on an infecting organism, pharmacokinetics is the study of the effect of the body's processes on the drug concentration–time profile and the drug's ability to penetrate to the infection site (or the toxicity site). It is a prime determinant of whether a drug will be able to kill or to inhibit the offending pathogen and, because many toxicities are concentration related, whether a serious drug-related toxicity will occur.

Earlier, the algorithm for identifying appropriate drug doses and administration schedules was outlined. Table 271-4 shows recommended doses and schedules of important antimicrobial agents as well as their protein-binding ability and whether alterations in renal or hepatic function generate major changes in the concentration-time profile. As in all chemotherapy, the aim is to generate a concentration-time profile in the plasma to generate a concentration-time profile at the infection site sufficient to inhibit or to kill the pathogen without causing toxicity.

Although there is almost always a guide to the concentration-time profile that results in an appropriate antimicrobial effect, it is more difficult to identify a linkage between drug exposure and the occurrence of toxicity. The association between aminoglycoside and daptomycin exposures and their toxicities have been elucidated.

For aminoglycosides, the relationships between drug exposure and the likelihood of a good clinical outcome and between drug exposure and the likelihood of nephrotoxicity have been determined. These are in the form of logistic regression functions, so the actual probability of both outcomes can be calculated. The one difference is that for the relationship with good outcome, the MIC value is part of the evaluation, whereas it does not figure in the toxicity relationship. Nevertheless, it is possible to derive appropriate information by making the outcome relationship MIC specific. Figure 271-2 illustrates the effect and toxicity relationships for aminoglycosides at three different MIC values. As shown, it is relatively easy to achieve a high probability of good clinical outcomes with aminoglycosides when the MIC is 0.25 mg/L, but it is virtually impossible to do so when the MIC rises to a value of 1.0 mg/L.

TABLE 271-2 MECHANISMS OF ACTION OF ANTIMICROBIAL AGENTS

AGENT	SITE OF ACTION	EFFECT	BACTERICIDAL	BACTERIOSTATIC
β-Lactams (penicillins, cephalosporins, carbapenems, aztreonam)	Cell wall: penicillin-binding proteins	Inhibit cross-linking of peptidoglycan (transpeptidation), impair cell wall synthesis	+	Occasionally (enterococci)
Vancomycin, teicoplanin, dalbavancin, telavancin, oritavancin	Cell wall: terminal D-alanyl-D-alanine of pentapeptide peptidoglycan precursor	Inhibit polymerization of disaccharide precursors to peptidoglycan (transglycosylation), impair cell wall synthesis	+	Occasionally (enterococci)
Daptomycin	Cell membrane	Rapid depolarization of membrane potential	+	Occasionally (enterococci)
Aminoglycosides	Protein synthesis: 30S ribosome subunit	Inhibit peptide elongation, cause misreading of genetic code, inhibit protein synthesis	+	
Tetracyclines, glycylcyclines	Protein synthesis: 30S ribosome subunit	Inhibit binding of transfer RNA, inhibit protein synthesis	Occasionally	+
Chloramphenicol	Protein synthesis: 30S ribosome subunit	Blocks attachment of aminoacyl transfer RNA, inhibits protein synthesis	Occasionally	+
Macrolides, azalides, ketolides	Protein synthesis: 50S ribosome subunit	Block transfer of amino acids to peptide chain, inhibit protein synthesis	Occasionally	+
Clindamycin	Protein synthesis: 50S ribosome subunit	Blocks transfer of amino acids to peptide chain, inhibits protein synthesis	Occasionally	+
Quinupristin-dalfopristin	Protein synthesis: 50S ribosome subunit	Block extrusion of peptide chains, inhibit protein synthesis	+	+ (with quinupristin resistance)
Linezolid and tedizolid	Protein synthesis: 50S ribosome subunit	Blocks formation of 70S initiation complex, inhibits protein synthesis	Occasionally	+
Rifampin	Nucleic acid synthesis: β-subunit of DNA-dependent RNA polymerase	Inhibits RNA synthesis	+	
Metronidazole	Nucleic acid synthesis	Damages nucleic acids, inhibits DNA synthesis	+	
Quinolones	Nucleic acid synthesis: DNA gyrase, topoisomerase IV	Impair supercoiling of DNA, prevent decatenation of DNA molecules after replication, inhibit DNA synthesis	+	
Sulfonamides	Folic acid synthesis: dihydropteroate synthetase	Competitive inhibition of synthesis of dihydrofolate from p-aminobenzoic acid, pteroate, and glutamic acid	Occasionally (when used with trimethoprim)	+
Trimethoprim	Folic acid synthesis: dihydrofolate reductase	Inhibits reduction of dihydrofolate to tetrahydrofolic acid	Occasionally (when used with sulfonamide)	+

The evaluation in the figure is based on twice-daily dosing; daily aminoglycoside dosing markedly improves this circumstance. Also, these relationships permit one to calculate the probabilities of effect and toxicity when, for example, aminoglycoside AUC is increased owing to renal dysfunction because these agents are largely eliminated renally.

When no toxicity relationship is available, there is still a drug exposure target for good clinical effect. Achievement of this target should be paramount, and alterations for renal or hepatic impairment should strive to maintain the high likelihood of effect seen in patients with a relatively normal clearance function. One can change the dose or schedule of a drug to decrease its accumulation in the presence of renal or hepatic impairment (depending on the drug) and then recalculate the impact on the likelihood of attaining a good clinical outcome. One can also calculate the amount of accumulation with the proposed dose reduction or extension of the dosing interval. For the increase in exposure (relative to that in normally clearing patients), there is no clear guidance, but one can accept a certain maximal amount of accumulation as long as the proposed dose adjustment maintains a high likelihood of a good outcome. The acceptability of the increased drug exposure after dosage adjustment is usually based on a combination of preclinical toxicology and the largest exposures seen in phase I and phase II clinical trials. However, the overarching issue is that the proposed dose or schedule alteration maintains a high probability of a good clinical outcome.

DRUG CLASSES AND THEIR PROPERTIES

During the past 75 years, a large number of different classes of antimicrobial agents have been developed. These classes differ in their mechanisms of action, mechanisms of emergence of resistance, and whether they kill substantial numbers of organisms or only inhibit bacterial growth. The following sections examine some of the properties of the major classes of antimicrobial agents in use today.

β-Lactam Agents

This class of drugs is arguably the most important group of antimicrobials. With chemical modification, they have an exceptionally broad spectrum of activity and, in general, an excellent safety profile. The major toxicity is related to allergic reactions to a degradation product of the drug. The β-lactams include the penicillins, cephalosporins, monobactams, and carbapenems.

These agents bind to their targets, bacterial β-lactam–binding proteins (also called penicillin-binding proteins). These binding proteins have an active site serine, and the drug forms a covalent bond with this site through the carbonyl of the β-lactam ring. Sometimes, the binding has direct effects on the organism's shape. For example, in gram-negative organisms, binding to penicillin-binding protein (PBP)-2 causes the organism to assume a spherical shape, whereas binding to PBP-3 causes the formation of long chains of organisms. In general, high-affinity binding to PBP-1 leads to the rapid death of the organism, sometimes accompanied by lysis. The classic response of *S. pneumoniae* to penicillin G is rapid lysis of the organism. Binding to PBP-1 (1a or 1b) leads to activation of *N*-acetylmuramic acid amidase, which destroys the bacterial cell wall, resulting in lysis.

The most common way for pathogens to protect themselves from β-lactams is by elaborating β-lactamases. The genes for these enzymes may be on plasmids or other bits of transmissible DNA, or they may reside on the

TABLE 271-3 MECHANISMS OF ANTIMICROBIAL RESISTANCE

ANTIBACTERIAL AGENT	MECHANISM	REPRESENTATIVE ORGANISM
β-Lactams (penicillins, cephalosporins, carbapenems, aztreonam)	Altered target (penicillin-binding proteins)	Methicillin-resistant *Staphylococcus aureus* (MRSA), penicillin-resistant *Streptococcus pneumoniae*, *Enterococcus faecium*
	Reduced permeability	*Enterobacter* spp, *Pseudomonas aeruginosa*, *Acinetobacter* spp
	Enhanced efflux	*P. aeruginosa*, *Acinetobacter* spp
	β-Lactamases	*S. aureus*, Enterobacteriaceae (includes ESBLs*), *Haemophilus influenzae*, *Moraxella catarrhalis*, *Neisseria gonorrhoeae*, *Enterococcus faecalis*, *P. aeruginosa*, *Acinetobacter* spp
Aminoglycosides	Inactivating enzymes (acetylation, adenylation, phosphorylation)	*S. aureus*, enterococci, *P. aeruginosa*, Enterobacteriaceae
	Reduced permeability	Enterobacteriaceae, *P. aeruginosa*, enterococci
	Enhanced efflux	*P. aeruginosa*
	Decreased ribosomal binding	*S. aureus*, *E. faecalis*, mycobacteria (streptomycin), gram-negative pathogens (aminoglycoside ribosomal methylase)
Chloramphenicol	Enhanced efflux	*H. influenzae*
	Reduced permeability	Enterobacteriaceae
	Inactivating enzyme (acetylation)	*S. aureus*, *S. pneumoniae*, enterococci
Daptomycin	Altered target	*S. aureus*
Glycylcyclines	Enhanced efflux	Enterobacteriaceae, especially *Proteus*
Macrolides, clindamycin, ketolide, quinupristin	Altered target (methylation of ribosomal RNA)	*S. aureus*, *S. pneumoniae* (not ketolide), streptococci, *Bacteroides fragilis*
	Enhanced efflux (not clindamycin or ketolide)	*S. pneumoniae*, streptococci
	Reduced permeability	Enterobacteriaceae
	Inactivating enzymes	*Escherichia coli*, *Klebsiella pneumoniae*, *S. aureus*
Oxazolidinones	Altered target	Streptococci, enterococci, *S. aureus*
Quinolones	Altered target (DNA gyrase, topoisomerase IV)	Enterobacteriaceae, *P. aeruginosa*
	Reduced permeability	Enterobacteriaceae, *P. aeruginosa*
	Enhanced efflux	*E. coli*, *P. aeruginosa*
Tetracyclines	Altered target (ribosome)	*N. gonorrhoeae*, streptococci
	Enhanced efflux	*E. coli*, *S. pneumoniae*
	Reduced permeability	Enterobacteriaceae
	Drug inactivation	*B. fragilis*
Rifampin	Altered target (β-subunit of polymerase)	*E. coli*, *S. aureus*, *Mycobacterium tuberculosis*
Sulfonamides, trimethoprim	Altered target (dihydropteroate synthetase or dihydrofolate reductase)	Enterobacteriaceae, *M. catarrhalis*
	Enhanced *p*-aminobenzoic acid production	*S. aureus*, *N. gonorrhoeae*
	Reduced permeability	*P. aeruginosa*, Enterobacteriaceae
Vancomycin and lipoglycopeptides	Altered target (peptidoglycan precursor binding site)	*E. faecium*, *E. faecalis*, *S. aureus*

*ESBLs = extended-spectrum β-lactamases.

bacterial chromosome. Some drugs, such as the carbapenems, are resistant to hydrolysis by many enzymes (but certainly not all of them, especially the metallo-β-lactamases and *K. pneumoniae* carbapenemase-type β-lactamases). The activity of β-lactams may be protected by administering these drugs in combination with a β-lactamase inhibitor. Examples include potassium clavulanate, sulbactam, tazobactam, and, most recently, avibactam and vaborbactam. These agents inhibit different types of β-lactamases, but only avibactams inhibit the ampC-type enzymes carried by *P. aeruginosa*, *Enterobacter* species, *Citrobacter* species, *Serratia marcescens,* and indole-positive *Protea* (SPICE organisms).

All β-lactams are relatively nonconcentration-dependent in their kill rate, and free (nonprotein bound) drug time greater than MIC (T > MIC) is the pharmacodynamic index linked with increased organism killing. The classes differ somewhat, with carbapenems requiring approximately 40% free drug T greater than MIC for near-maximal bacterial killing. For penicillins, this percentage is approximately 50%, and for cephalosporins and monobactams, it is 60 to 70%. When these agents need to penetrate to a site of infection, such as lung epithelial lining fluid or central nervous system, the pharmacodynamic target values may change somewhat.

Aminoglycosides

These important agents were discovered in the late 1940s for the treatment of *M. tuberculosis* (streptomycin). Screening of natural products identified a number of different aminoglycosides, such as kanamycin, neomycin, gentamicin (actually a combination of three congeners), and tobramycin. Other semisynthetic agents, such as amikacin, netilmicin, and arbekacin (among others), have been discovered and used for therapy in the United States and elsewhere.

Nephrotoxicity and middle ear toxicity (hearing loss or loss of balance) are the dose-limiting toxicities of aminoglycosides and resulted in their going out of favor in the 1990s and early in the first decade of the 21st century. It has now been recognized that most (but not all) of the nephrotoxic potential can be ameliorated by intermittent dosing of these drugs (usually once daily). Even with daily therapy, however, prolonged use can still result in nephrotoxicity or ototoxicity.

The recent rise in resistance, particularly among gram-negative bacteria, and new mechanisms mediating resistance to even the best β-lactam agents have resulted in renewed interest in existing aminoglycosides and a search for new ones that are more resistant to inactivation by the aminoglycoside-modifying enzymes, such as plazomicin. This aminoglycoside was recently approved for use for the treatment of complicated urinary tract infections. Due to structural modifications it remains active against many resistance mechanisms which render bacteria resistant to the other aminoglycosides.

These drugs are concentration-dependent in terms of their bacterial killing and are rapid killers.[7] Hence, the AUC/MIC ratio (or, as sometimes reported, peak concentration/MIC ratio) is the pharmacodynamic index most closely

TABLE 271-4 DOSAGE REGIMENS OF ANTIBACTERIALS, PHARMACOKINETICS, AND DOSE ADJUSTMENT IN PATIENTS WITH RENAL OR HEPATIC FAILURE

CLASS/AGENT	DOSE* FOR SYSTEMIC INFECTION	ORAL FORMULATION	PEAK SERUM CONCENTRATION (μg/mL)	PROTEIN BINDING (%)	NORMAL SERUM HALF-LIFE (hr)	HEPATIC FAILURE	RENAL FAILURE	SERUM LEVELS ALTERED BY DIALYSIS
AMINOGLYCOSIDES								
Amikacin	5-6.7 mg/kg q8h or 15-20 mg/kg q24h	—	35	0	2-3	No	Major	Yes (H, P)
Gentamicin	1.7 mg/kg q8h or 5 mg/kg q24h	—	7	0	2-3	No	Major	Yes (H, P)
Netilmicin	1.7 mg/kg q8h or 5 mg/kg q24h	—	7	0	2-3	No	Major	Yes (H, P)
Plazomicin	15 mg/kg q24h	—	74	0	3-4	No	Yes	Yes (H, P)
Tobramycin	1.7 mg/kg q8h or 5 mg/kg q24h	—	7	0	2-3	No	Major	Yes (H, P)
ANTITUBERCULOUS AGENTS								
Bedaquiline	400 mg q24h (PO) for 2 wk then 200 mg 3×/wk	Yes	5.5	99.9	3,960	No	No	No
Ethambutol	15 mg/kg q24h (PO)	Yes	2	10	3.3	No	Major	Yes (H, P)
Isoniazid	5 mg/kg q24h or 300 mg q24h (PO)	Yes	4.5	10	3	Yes	Major	Yes (H, P)
Pyrazinamide	10 mg/kg q8h (PO)	Yes	12	10	10	Yes	Yes	Yes (H)
Rifampin	10 mg/kg or 600 mg q24h (PO)	Yes	7	81-89	3	Yes	Minor	No (H)
CARBAPENEMS								
Doripenem	0.5-1.0 g q8h	—	23	<10	1	No	Yes	Yes (H)
Ertapenem	1 g q24h	—	155	95	4-5	Unknown	Yes	Yes (H)
Imipenem	0.5-1 g q6-8h	—	40	15	1	No	Avoid in severe renal dysfunction	Yes (H)
Meropenem	0.5-2 g q8h	—	50	<10	1	No	Yes	Yes (H)
Meropenem-vaborbactam	4 g q8h	—	50	<10	2.3	No	Yes	Yes (H)
FIRST-GENERATION CEPHALOSPORINS								
Cefadroxil	1000 mg q12h (PO)	Yes	16	20	1.5	No	Yes	Yes (H)
Cefazolin	0.5-2 g q8h	—	180	80	2	No	Major	Yes (H) No (P)
Cephalexin	250-500 mg q6h (PO)	Yes	18	15	1	No	Yes	Yes (H, P)
Cephradine	500-1000 mg q6-12h	Yes+	140	10	103	No	Yes	Yes (H, P)
SECOND-GENERATION CEPHALOSPORINS								
Cefaclor	250-500 mg q8h (PO)	Yes+	10	25	0.8	No	Yes	Yes (H)
Cefoxitin	1-2 g q6-8h	—	220	70	0.8	No	Yes	Yes (H) No (P)
Cefprozil	250-500 mg q12h (PO)	Yes	10	35	1.4	No	Yes	Yes (H)
Cefuroxime	750-1500 mg q8h	—	100	50	1.5	No	Yes	Yes (H, P)
Cefuroxime axetil	250-500 mg q12h (PO)	Yes	9	50	1.5	No	Yes	Yes (H, P)
THIRD-GENERATION CEPHALOSPORINS								
Cefdinir	300 mg q12h (PO)	Yes	2	65	1.7	Unknown	Minor	Yes (H)
Cefditoren pivoxil	400 mg q12h (PO)	Yes	4	88	1.6	No	Yes	Yes (H)
Cefixime	400 mg q24h (PO)	Yes	3-5	67	3	No	Yes	No (H, P)
Cefotaxime	1-2 g q6-8h	—	200	50	1.5	Minor	Minor	Yes (H) No (P)
Cefpodoxime proxetil	200-400 mg q12h (PO)	Yes	3	25	2.5	No	Yes	Yes (H)
Ceftazidime	1-2 g q8h	—	160	60	2	No	Major	Yes (H, P)
Ceftazidime-avibactam	2.5 g q8h	—	160	60	2	No	Major	Yes (H)
Ceftibuten	400 mg q24h (PO)	Yes	15	65	2.5	Unknown	Yes	Yes (H)

Drug	Dose							
Ceftizoxime	1-2 g q6-8h	—	130	30	1.3	No	Major	Yes (H) No (P)
Ceftriaxone	1-2 g q12-24h	—	250	90-95	8	No	No	No (H)
FOURTH-GENERATION CEPHALOSPORINS								
Cefepime	1-2 g q8h	—	193	20	2	No	Major	Yes (H, P)
Ceftaroline	600 mg q8-12h	—	21.3	20	2.6	No	Major	Yes (H)
Ceftolozane-tazobactam	1.5 g q8h	—	74	16-21	3.1	No	Yes	Yes (H)
PENICILLINS								
Amoxicillin	500 mg q8h (PO)	Yes	10	20	1	No	Yes	Yes (H) No (P)
Amoxicillin–clavulanic acid#	875/125 mg q8-12h	Yes	2.7	25	1.3	Unknown	Moderate	Yes (H, P)
Ampicillin	1 g q6h	Yes†	200	20	1	No	Yes	Yes (H) No (P)
Cloxacillin	500 mg q6h (PO)	Yes†	9	95	0.5	No	No	No (H, P)
Dicloxacillin	500 mg q6h (PO)	Yes†	18	97	0.5	No	No	No (H, P)
Nafcillin	1-2 g q4-6h	—	160	90	0.5	Yes	No	No (H, P)
Oxacillin	1-2 g q4-6h	—	200	90	0.5	Yes	No	No (H, P)
Penicillin G	3-4 million units q4-6h	Yes†	60	60	0.5	No	Yes	Yes (H) No (P)
Penicillin V	500 mg q6h (PO)	Yes	5	80	1	No	No	Yes (H) No (P)
Piperacillin/tazobactam	3.375-4.5 g q6-8h		240	50	1	Minor	Minor	Yes (H)
Ticarcillin/clavulanate	3.1 g q4-8h		220	50	1	Minor	Major	Yes (H, P)
MONOBACTAMS								
Aztreonam	1-2 g q8h	—	250	60	2	No	Major	Yes (H, P)
QUINOLONES								
Ciprofloxacin	400 mg q8-q12h 500-750 mg q12h (PO)	Yes†	2-3	30	4	No	Minor	No (H, P)
Delafloxacin	300 mg q12h	Yes	7.4	84	3.7	No	Minor	No (H)
Levofloxacin	250-750 mg q24h (IV or PO)	Yes	6-9	30	7	No	Yes	No (H, P)
Moxifloxacin	400 mg q24h (IV or PO)	Yes	4-5	50	10	No–minor	No	No (H, P)
TETRACYCLINES, GLYCYLCYCLINES								
Doxycycline	100 mg q12-24h (PO) after 200-mg loading dose	Yes	1.5-2.1	93	15-20	Avoid	No	No (H, P)
Minocycline	100 mg q12-24h (PO) after 200-mg loading dose	Yes	2.2	75	15	No	Avoid	No (H, P)
Tetracycline	500 mg q6h (PO)	Yes†	4	50	7	Avoid	Avoid	No (H, P)
Tigecycline	100 mg, then 50 mg q12h	—	0.6-0.9	70	37-38	Minor	No	No (H, P)
SULFONAMIDES								
Sulfadiazine	15 mg/kg q6h	Yes	30	50	3	Avoid	Avoid	Unknown
Sulfamethoxazole	0.5-1 g q6-8h (PO)	Yes	100	50	9	Avoid	Major	Yes (H) No (P)
Trimethoprim (with sulfamethoxazole)	3-5 mg/kg q6-8h (based on trimethoprim component)	Yes	3-9	60	10	No	Avoid	Yes (H) No (P)
MACROLIDES, LINCOSAMIDES, KETOLIDES								
Azithromycin	500 mg first dose, followed by 250 mg q24h or 500 mg × 3 days (PO) Single-dose therapy of 1-2 g for STIs	Yes†	0.4	25	12-50	Unknown	No	No (H, P)
Clarithromycin	500 mg q12h (PO)	Yes	2-3	70	7	No	Minor	Yes (H) No (P)
Clindamycin	0.3-0.9 g q8h	Yes	15	90	2.5	Minor	No	No (H, P)
Erythromycin	500 mg q6h (PO)	Yes†	1.8	70	2	Minor	No	No (H, P)
Telithromycin	800 mg q24h (PO)	Yes	2	65	10	No	No	No (H)

TABLE 271-4 DOSAGE REGIMENS OF ANTIBACTERIALS, PHARMACOKINETICS, AND DOSE ADJUSTMENT IN PATIENTS WITH RENAL OR HEPATIC FAILURE—cont'd

CLASS/AGENT	DOSE* FOR SYSTEMIC INFECTION	ORAL FORMULATION	PEAK SERUM CONCENTRATION (μg/mL)	PROTEIN BINDING (%)	NORMAL SERUM HALF-LIFE (hr)	HEPATIC FAILURE	RENAL FAILURE	SERUM LEVELS ALTERED BY DIALYSIS
OXAZOLIDONONES								
Linezolid	600 mg q12h	Yes	18	30	5	No–minor	No	Yes (H)
Tedizolid	200 mg q24h	Yes	2	70-90	12	No	No	No
OTHER AGENTS								
Chloramphenicol	0.25-1 g q6h Oral administration produces higher blood concentrations than IV administration.	Yes	8-14	60	1.5	Minor	No	Yes (H) No (P)
Daptomycin	4-6 mg/kg q24h	—	58-100	90	8-9	No	Minor	No (P) Minor (H)
Metronidazole	500 mg q6h (anaerobes) 250 mg q8h (trichomoniasis) 750 mg q8h (amebiasis) (IV or PO)	Yes	25	20	8	Yes	No	Yes (H) No (P)
Nitrofurantoin	100 mg q6h (PO)	Yes	Nil	60	0.3	No	Avoid	Yes (H)
Quinupristin-dalfopristin (30:70)	7.5 mg/kg q8-12h	—	3.2/8§	90/30	3/1§	Minor	No	No (P)
Spectinomycin	2 g/24 hr	Yes¶	100	0	2	No	Avoid	Unknown
Vancomycin	15 mg/kg q12h	Yes¶	35	50	6	No	Major	No (H, P)
Oritavancin	1200 mg once	—	138	85	245	No	Major	No (H)
Telavancin	10 mg/kg q24h	—	108	90	8	No	Major	No (H)
Dalbavancin	1500 mg once	—	287	93	346	No	Major	N0 (H)

*Dose in milligrams per kilogram body weight at hour intervals and/or oral dose in milligrams in patients with normal renal function; all doses are parenteral unless specified PO.

†Significant decrease or delay in absorption when administered with food.

‡Refers to information for clavulanic acid.

§Includes parent compound and active metabolites.

¶Oral vancomycin is not absorbed; it is used for intraluminal therapy only.

H = hemodialysis; P = peritoneal dialysis; STI = sexually transmitted infection.

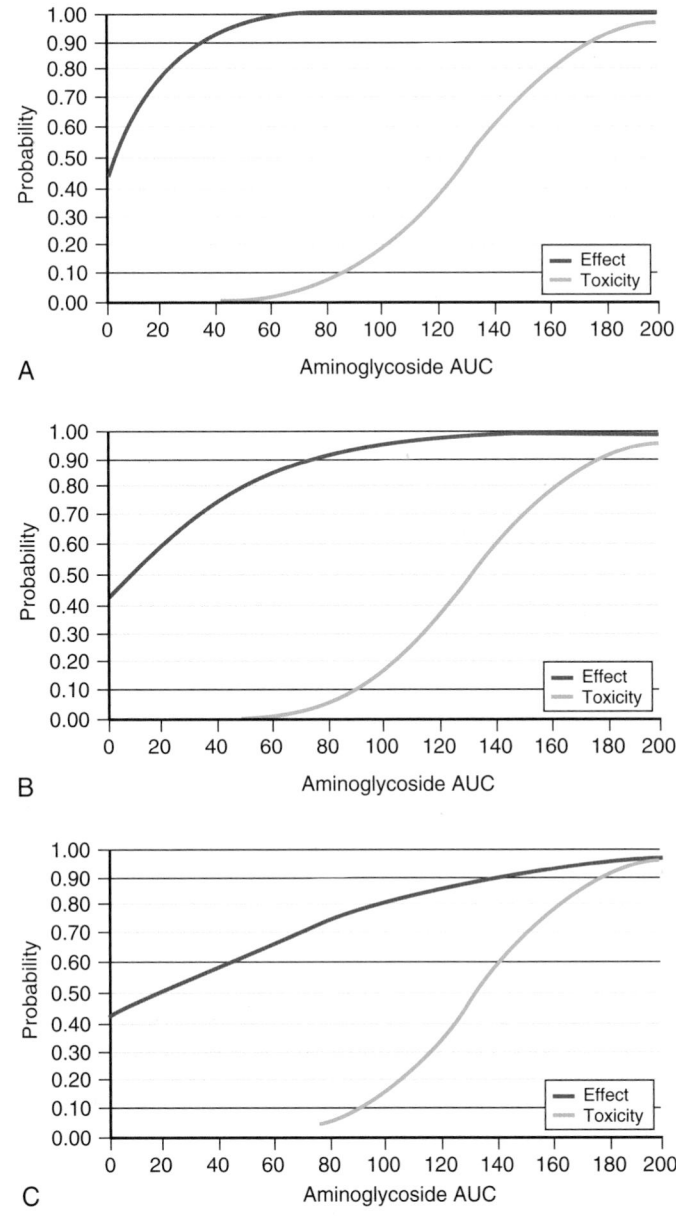

FIGURE 271-2. **Probability of clinical effect versus nephrotoxicity as a function of aminoglycoside area under the curve (AUC). A,** Minimal inhibitory concentration (MIC) = 0.25 mg/L. **B,** MIC = 0.5 mg/L. **C,** MIC = 1.0 mg/L.

substitution markedly enhanced the microbiologic activity of these drugs, making them useful for treating both community-associated infections (especially urinary tract infections and pneumonia) and hospital-associated gram-negative infections.

These drugs penetrate well into most body spaces and accumulate within mammalian cells. This makes them active against obligate intracellular pathogens such as *Chlamydophila, Legionella,* and *Mycoplasma.* They also penetrate well into body spaces with tight junctions (prostate, eye, central nervous system) and into the epithelial lining fluid of the lung.

Typically, the toxicities of these drugs are "off target." A number of these drugs were withdrawn from the marketplace or given black box warnings by health authorities because of the infrequent occurrence of tendon rupture and torsades de pointes (Chapter 59) or other serious and life-threatening toxicities, such as eosinophilic hepatitis. Recently, new black box warnings include hypoglycemia that may lead to coma and mental disturbances, including memory impairment and delirium. As a result, the Food and Drug Administration advises that the side effects of fluoroquinolones outweigh their benefits when patients with acute sinusitis have other options.

These agents are concentration-dependent bacterial killers, indicating that the free drug AUC/MIC ratio is best associated with a regimen's ability to kill bacteria. Of interest, particularly for a drug that is completely synthetic, there are a number of resistance mechanisms that allow bacterial escape from drug pressure. The combination of efflux pump overexpression and error-prone replication, resulting in target site mutants, as well as serious underdosing for some of the earlier drugs in the class, has resulted in the emergence of considerable resistance, particularly among gram-negative isolates and in the ICU setting.

Macrolides, Tetracyclines, Ketolides, Clindamycin, and Oxazolidinones

These agents bind to different places in the bacterial ribosome, making them inhibitors of protein synthesis and, for the most part, drugs with limited bactericidal activity. An exception may be their activity against *S. pneumoniae.*

Macrolides (particularly clarithromycin and azithromycin) are most useful for community-acquired respiratory tract infections, for two reasons. First, their spectrum is well suited to the classic and atypical bacteria encountered in these patients. Second, they concentrate well in lung epithelial lining fluid, with an accumulation that ranges from 6-fold to almost 20-fold that in plasma. This accumulation partially explains why these agents have fared much better in the respiratory tract setting than in the skin and skin structure setting. Telithromycin, a ketolide, retains activity against many (but not all) macrolide-resistant isolates.

The macrolides and telithromycin are free drug AUC/MIC ratio–driven drugs with respect to bacterial activity, but for different reasons. Telithromycin is somewhat concentration dependent with regard to its microbiologic activity, whereas classic macrolides are not. Telithromycin is more like aminoglycosides or quinolones in terms of the association between exposure indices and bacterial effect. Classic macrolides, especially azithromycin, induce a long persistent or post-antibiotic effect and are *not* concentration dependent in their bacterial effect. This post-antibiotic effect suppresses bacterial regrowth after the drug concentration declines below the MIC until the next dose of drug is administered. In this way, we perceive the linkage to be driven by the free drug AUC/MIC ratio but with a mechanism different from that of agents whose bacterial kill rate is concentration dependent.

Most of the toxicities seen are off target and gastrointestinal. There is also some prolongation of the QT interval (Chapter 48), which presumably explains why azithromycin has been considered to carry an increased risk of ventricular arrhythmia. However, a recent systematic review and meta-analysis of the cardiovascular safety of macrolides reported no association with arrhythmia or cardiovascular mortality.[8]

Tetracyclines have an exceptionally broad spectrum of activity, including both gram-positive and gram-negative pathogens, and are active against atypical pathogens. The latest incarnation of a tetracycline-type agent (tigecycline, a glycylcycline) has good activity against methicillin-resistant *S. aureus* (MRSA) as well. Tigecycline differs from previous tetracyclines (e.g., doxycycline, minocycline) in that its structure prevents many efflux pumps from removing the drug from the bacteria and also provides a degree of ribosomal protection.

The lincosamide antibiotic clindamycin has a spectrum that covers most clinically significant anaerobes, including many in the *Bacteroides* group (although some resistance is being seen). It is thus a useful agent for infections in which anaerobes play a prominent role, such as lung abscesses and

associated with bacterial killing. Therefore large doses administered daily to patients with normal renal function would be expected to optimize bacterial killing. As mentioned earlier, once-daily dosing also minimizes the probability of aminoglycoside nephrotoxicity.

The older aminoglycosides (streptomycin and gentamicin) have the best profile for synergizing with drugs active against gram-positive streptococci (particularly enterococci). Tobramycin generally has the most potent activity against *P. aeruginosa* (depending on the aminoglycoside-modifying enzymes present in a specific locale), and less resistance is generally seen with amikacin (again, depending on the locale). Streptomycin and amikacin, because of the number of amino groups carried, are usually about four-fold less potent than gentamicin or tobramycin. Consequently, their dosages are approximately three- to four-fold higher.

These agents should be thought of as components of combination regimens for seriously ill patients, particularly those thought to be infected by gram-negative organisms, in the empirical therapy setting.

Quinolones

These agents are completely synthetic and do not exist in nature. They are inhibitors (depending on the drug and the organism) of topoisomerases II and IV to block DNA replication, making them rapidly bactericidal. A fluorine intra-abdominal infections. In many areas of the country, it retains activity against MRSA, but this should be verified with a D-test (inducible macrolide-lincosamide-streptogramin resistance) in the microbiology laboratory. It also has good activity against many streptococci. Because it is a protein synthesis inhibitor, it may provide improved results when the staphylococcal or streptococcal isolate elaborates toxins.

Again, most toxicity is off target, with gastrointestinal symptoms being most frequent. Antibiotic-associated diarrhea and the more serious *Clostridium difficile* colitis can occur.

Linezolid and tedizolid are members of the oxazolidinone class of antibiotics and are protein synthesis inhibitors. They have excellent gram-positive activity, including robust activity against MRSA. Oxazolidinones penetrate well into skin as well as into the epithelial lining fluid. They are prescribed to treat skin and skin structure infections and currently only linezolid is licensed for treating streptococcal and staphylococcal (including MRSA) community-associated and nosocomial pneumonia. Intravenous and oral formulations of both drugs are available. Both drugs have high oral bioavailabilities.

The free drug AUC/MIC ratio is the pharmacodynamic index most associated with cell killing for the oxazolidinones. Bone marrow toxicity, including thrombocytopenia, neutropenia, and anemia, is linked to oxazolidinone dose and duration of therapy. Lactic acidosis, peripheral neuropathy, and optic neuritis have been reported. Resistance occurs rarely and is seen with enterococci more frequently than with *S. aureus*.

Vancomycin, Quinupristin-Dalfopristin, Daptomycin, and Lipoglycopeptides

Although structured differently, these agents (along with the oxazolidinones) are distinguished by having reliable activity against MRSA.

Vancomycin acts at the cell wall and alters cell membrane permeability. It is bactericidal. The free drug AUC/MIC ratio is the driver of antimicrobial effect. This glycopeptide drug has activity against many gram-positive pathogens and is active against *C. difficile* when it is administered orally. As with most drugs, wide use has caused the emergence of vancomycin resistance in both enterococci and *S. aureus* (although the latter is rare).

Although vancomycin has a reputation for being a somewhat slow killer, no new agent has significantly outperformed it, at least in trials of skin and skin structure infections. MIC creep has been documented. Although many *S. aureus* isolates were once susceptible with MIC values of 0.25 and 0.5 mg/L, these are now in the distinct minority; 1.0 mg/L represents the modal value, with a few isolates having values of 2.0 mg/L. The higher MICs make these isolates more difficult to treat reliably with standard dosing (1 g IV every 12 hours). Also, it has recently become clear that higher vancomycin doses are associated with a significantly higher risk of nephrotoxicity, even when the agent is administered alone. In addition to nephrotoxicity, vancomycin causes histamine release ("red man syndrome") when it is administered too quickly intravenously. Infusion times of approximately 1 hour are recommended for standard doses.

Oritavancin, dalbavancin, and telavancin are semisynthetic lipoglycopeptide derivatives of vancomycin that kill streptococci, enterococci, and staphylococci (including MRSA) in a concentration-dependent manner by the same mechanisms of action as vancomycin. They are licensed for treating skin and skin structure infections due to these microbes. Oritavancin and dalbavancin have long terminal half-lives and a single dose is given for treating these infections. Telavancin has an 8-hour serum half-life and is dosed once-daily. These drugs are not used for the treatment of colitis due to *C. difficile*.

Quinupristin-dalfopristin is a combination of streptogramin A and streptogramin B antibiotics. Although each is bacteriostatic, the combination can produce some cell killing because the two drugs are synergistic. The synergy is lost, however, with the emergence of resistance to either drug. Further, the amount of bacterial cell killing is modest because of the drugs' rapid half-lives and the imposition of a 12-hour dosing interval. This combination product has activity against resistant enterococci as well as MRSA. Its toxicity includes relatively severe muscle pain in some patients. It is also phlebitogenic and has to be administered with a central venous catheter, limiting its utility.

Daptomycin is a cyclic lipopeptide antibiotic discovered in the 1980s and resurrected in the 1990s with a greater understanding of the relationship between exposure and effect versus exposure and toxicity. It was discovered that the antibacterial effect against MRSA was driven by the free drug AUC/MIC ratio. Muscle effects were seen early in its development

that limited therapy. Trough concentrations of daptomycin drive this toxicity and can be ameliorated by once-daily dosing (thus minimizing trough concentrations).

This agent has been licensed for skin and skin structure infections and, of note, for complicated *S. aureus* bacteremia and right-sided endocarditis. It also has activity against enterococci. The drug is bound up in epithelial lining fluid by surfactant, excluding its use in the therapy for pneumonia.

Daptomycin may cause muscle toxicity, which is rare, but this may be preceded by the harbinger of an elevated creatine kinase level. The muscle damage is driven by daptomycin trough concentrations, generally above a concentration of about 25 mg/L. Monitoring of creatine kinase concentration is useful in the management of patients receiving daptomycin therapy.

⬤ TOXICITIES

All antimicrobials have toxicities. The most common observed toxicities for many antimicrobial agents are presented in Table 271-5.

⬤ DURATION OF THERAPY

Relatively little is known about the optimal duration of therapy. Some work has been done to define certain circumstances in which short courses of chemotherapy are effective. For instance, gonorrhea is highly likely to be cured by a single dose of drug (ceftriaxone, cefixime, fluoroquinolones), if the organism is susceptible to the drug.

For trimethoprim-sulfamethoxazole and fluoroquinolones, controlled trials have shown that 3 days of therapy is adequate for uncomplicated urinary tract infections. For β-lactam antimicrobials, a somewhat longer duration is required.

In community-acquired pneumonia, controlled trials with fluoroquinolones have demonstrated optimal results with 5 days of therapy. For bacterial sinusitis, direct sampling from the infected sinus has demonstrated that bacterial pathogens were eradicated by day 3 of therapy or earlier, particularly for *S. pneumoniae* infections.

In ventilator-associated pneumonia, a double-blind comparison of 8 versus 15 days of therapy demonstrated that, with a single exception, clinical outcomes were just as good, there was less emergence of resistance, fewer antibiotics were administered, and there was less toxicity with 8 days of therapy. The single exception was when a nonfermenting gram-negative rod was cultured (*P. aeruginosa* or *Acinetobacter* species). In this circumstance, there were significantly more relapses with 8-day versus 15-day treatment, but clinical outcomes were similar.

In some infections, the organisms are slow growing and require more time for control. Both endocarditis and osteomyelitis are examples. Therapy durations of 4 to 6 weeks and occasionally longer may be required for cure in this circumstance.

Finally, one of the longest durations of therapy is seen in the treatment of tuberculosis. In this case some organisms are in the "nonreplicative persister" (NRP) state, indicating that they are not growing or metabolically active. When recovered, they are still fully susceptible to the antimicrobials being used, but while in the NRP state, they are not readily killed with current chemotherapy (phenotypic, not genotypic resistance). Therapy durations of 6 months for wild-type organisms and 18 to 24 months for multidrug-resistant tuberculosis are required. Indeed, it is a major research goal to find drugs that will readily kill organisms in the NRP state and thus substantially shorten the therapeutic course for *M. tuberculosis*.

⬤ FAILURE OF ANTIMICROBIAL THERAPY

Antimicrobial therapy occasionally fails, with failure defined as the persistence of signs and symptoms of infection or the persistence of fever. When one is confronted with failure after what was thought to be adequate antimicrobial therapy, it should set off a sequence of investigations: Did resistance emerge, or did superinfection occur? Is there an obstructed hollow viscus (e.g., urinary or gastrointestinal tract)? Is there an undrained abscess or infected collection (e.g., empyema)? Is there an infected foreign body (e.g., intravenous catheter or prosthesis), or is there devitalized tissue (e.g., sequestrum in osteomyelitis)? Is the fever (if present) attributable to a drug being administered? Thoughtful reexamination should sort out the cause in many instances.

TABLE 271-5 DIVERSE TOXICITIES OF ANTIMICROBIAL AGENTS

AGENT	GENERAL	SKIN	GI TRACT	BLOOD CELLS	KIDNEY	NERVOUS SYSTEM	OTHER
Penicillins	Hypersensitivity, anaphylaxis, serum sickness	Rash, urticaria, erythema multiforme	Diarrhea (ampicillin, amoxicillin-clavulanate), hepatitis (oxacillin)	Coombs-positive hemolytic anemia, impaired platelet function (ticarcillin), leukopenia, thrombocytopenia	Nephritis (methicillin), hypokalemia (carboxy- and ureido-penicillins)	Seizures, twitching (high doses, renal failure)	Inactivates aminoglycosides when admixed; possible with concurrent therapy in renal failure
Cephalosporins	Serum sickness (cefaclor), hypersensitivity, anaphylaxis (rare)	Rash, urticaria	Diarrhea, hepatic dysfunction, precipitates in bile (ceftriaxone), mild increase in LFTs	Neutropenia, increased prothrombin time, bleeding (due to MTT side chain), positive Coombs test	Enhances aminoglycoside toxicity, acute renal failure (rare), interstitial nephritis		Disulfiram-like reaction with alcohol use (MTT side chain)
Carbapenems	Hypersensitivity	Rash, urticaria, erythema multiforme	Vomiting with rapid infusion (imipenem), abnormal LFTs	Bone marrow suppression, positive Coombs test	Renal dysfunction	Seizures, myoclonus	
Aminoglycosides	Fever	Rash			Reversible renal failure	Irreversible vestibular toxicity and/or auditory damage, muscle blockade (with anesthetics and myasthenia gravis)	
Vancomycin and lipoglycopeptides	Allergy, fever	Rash		Leukopenia, thrombocytopenia	Nephrotoxic	Decreased hearing, neuropathy	Histamine release with flushing and hypotension (infusion <1 hr, antihistamines can prevent)
Quinolones	Headache, allergy, anaphylaxis (rare)	Rash (gemifloxacin), urticaria, photosensitivity (lomefloxacin)	GI distress, abnormal LFTs			Dizziness, insomnia, nervousness, tremors, visual changes, seizures	Tendon rupture; arthropathy in young animals
Sulfonamides	Hypersensitivity, anaphylaxis, serum sickness, fever	Rash, Stevens-Johnson syndrome, photosensitivity	Hepatitis	Hemolysis (G6PD deficiency), agranulocytosis, marrow suppression	Crystalluria	Neuropathy	Vasculitis
Trimethoprim ± sulfamethoxazole	Fever	Rash, erythema multiforme, Stevens-Johnson syndrome, TEN	Hepatitis, pancreatitis	Marrow suppression	Hyperkalemia, acute renal failure		
Chloramphenicol	Fever			Marrow suppression (dose related), aplastic anemia	Optic neuritis, neuropathy	Circulatory collapse (gray baby syndrome in neonates)	
Tetracyclines	Hypersensitivity	Photosensitization (doxycycline)	GI discomfort, hepatotoxicity in azotemia or pregnancy		Antianabolic aggravation of azotemia (except doxycycline)	Vertigo (minocycline)	Deposition in bone (dysplasia) and teeth (staining)
Macrolides	Fever	Rash	GI discomfort			Reversible decreased hearing	Phlebitis (IV erythromycin), metallic taste (clarithromycin)
Clindamycin	Fever	Rash	Diarrhea, pseudomembranous colitis				
Metronidazole	Headache, hypersensitivity		Nausea, metallic taste, pancreatitis	Leukopenia		Peripheral neuropathy, ataxia	Mutagenic, carcinogenic in rodents, disulfiram-like reaction with alcohol

GI = gastrointestinal; G6PD = glucose-6-phosphate dehydrogenase; LFT = liver function test; MTT = methylthiotetrazole; TEN = toxic epidermal necrolysis.

Grade A Reference

A1. Nemeth J, Oesch G, Kuster SP. Bacteriostatic versus bactericidal antibiotics for patients with serious bacterial infections: systematic review and meta-analysis. *J Antimicrob Chemother.* 2015;70:382-395.

GENERAL REFERENCES

For the General References and other additional features, please visit Expert Consult at https://expertconsult.inkling.com.

272

STAPHYLOCOCCAL INFECTIONS

HENRY F. CHAMBERS AND GEORGE SAKOULAS

DEFINITION

Staphylococci are well adapted as commensals and as pathogens. Coagulase-negative species constitute a significant proportion of the normal human cutaneous microbiome. *Staphylococcus aureus*, a coagulase-positive species, is a nasopharyngeal colonizer in a third of individuals, most of whom will not become infected. As a pathogen, *S. aureus* is one of the most common causes of bacterial infections, which range in severity from relatively trivial skin infections to lethal invasive disease. Coagulase-negative species, intrinsically less virulent and less invasive than *S. aureus*, nevertheless are responsible for one in four health care–associated infections, particularly those involving indwelling medical devices. Prevalence of antibiotic-resistant strains of staphylococci has a profound impact on therapy.

The genus *Staphylococcus* consists of more than 30 distinct species. These organisms have coevolved as normal flora of mammals and birds. They are gram-positive spherical cells (i.e., cocci) 0.5 to 1.5 μm in diameter that divide in multiple planes to form clusters resembling grapes (*staphylo-* is derived from the Greek word for "bunch of grapes") when viewed under the microscope. Staphylococci are nonmotile, nonsporulating, hardy organisms. They are resistant to desiccation, extremes of pH, and high salt concentrations and are capable of growth under aerobic or anaerobic conditions. Staphylococci produce catalase, an enzyme that degrades hydrogen peroxide into water and oxygen, which definitively distinguishes them biochemically from streptococci and enterococci. The coagulase test is the basis for differentiating *S. aureus* from the numerous other nonpathogenic, coagulase-negative species. Coagulase is a secreted protein that, in the presence of a prothrombin-like plasma protein, converts fibrinogen to fibrin, forming a clot. *S. aureus* produces a variety of other species-specific surface proteins (e.g., protein A) that differentiate it from other species.

The staphylococcal chromosome is circular. Approximately 75% of the genes constitute a core genome common to all staphylococcal species. The remaining 25% contains species-defining elements and mobile genetic elements acquired by horizontal gene transfer. The *S. aureus* genome is abundant in genes encoding toxins, superantigens, and adhesins, whereas coagulase-negative species contain few adhesin and no toxin or superantigen genes. Genetically, *S. aureus* is sufficiently uniform to classify it as a single species; greater diversity among coagulase-negative species merits their classification as distinct species.

STAPHYLOCOCCUS AUREUS

EPIDEMIOLOGY

S. aureus is maintained in the human population primarily through asymptomatic colonization of the anterior nares, mucous membranes, and other moist areas of the body as well as of the groin, perineum, and perianal area in healthy children and adults. Infants become colonized by strains from their mothers within weeks of birth. Carriage rates are higher in children than in adults. Higher than average *S. aureus* carriage rates are associated with atopic dermatitis, eczema, chronic skin ulcers, and other acute and chronic skin conditions; insulin-dependent diabetes; dialysis; human immunodeficiency virus infection; and recreational injection drug use. Carriers have a several-fold higher risk for developing an *S. aureus* infection compared with noncarriers. The principal

mode of transmission of *S. aureus* is direct contact with an infected individual or an asymptomatic carrier, probably through transient hand carriage. *S. aureus* may also contaminate environmental surfaces, where it can persist for days. The role of environmental contamination in transmission is not well defined, but it may be important if heavily contaminated surfaces or materials are contacted. Droplet and aerosol transmission of *S. aureus* plays little if any role.

S. aureus is responsible for millions of infections in the United States each year, most of which are community-acquired skin infections. Approximately 5 to 10% of *S. aureus* infections are invasive, three fourths of which are associated with bacteremia. *S. aureus* also causes hundreds of thousands of health care–associated infections each year, about half of which are caused by methicillin-resistant *S. aureus* (MRSA) in the United States. Before the mid-1990s, MRSA strains were almost exclusively hospital or health care associated,[1] but they are now prevalent in the community. Although MRSA is now disseminated globally, there is marked geographic variation in MRSA burden that is due mainly to differences in local infection control practices and to pathogen-specific characteristics of the indigenously circulating clones.[2] Community-associated MRSA strains are distinct from classic health care–associated MRSA strains in several ways (E-Table 272-1).

PATHOBIOLOGY
Virulence Factors

S. aureus is highly adapted to humans through millions of years of coevolution with hominids. Well above 50 virulence factors, including adhesins, toxins, enzymes, surface-bound proteins, and capsule polysaccharides, may be produced (E-Table 272-2). Genes encoding virulence factors may be located on the chromosome as part of the core genome or within mobile genetic elements (or their remnants), including bacteriophages, pathogenicity islands, and cassettes, or on plasmids. Alpha-toxin, Panton-Valentine leukocidin, and phenol-soluble modulins, all of which provoke potentially deleterious host inflammatory response and cause host cell lysis, appear to be important virulence factors mediating disease severity, especially in community MRSA strains.[3] Protein A, a B-cell superantigen that promiscuously triggers B-cell proliferation and supraclonal expansion and apoptosis, interferes with host antibody-mediated adaptive immunity.

Virulence factors promote binding to host tissues; allow the organism to evade, circumvent, or disrupt host immune responses; and facilitate cell injury and tissue invasion. Variability in both the presence of virulence determinants and their expression among strains allows extreme diversity among clinical isolates, remarkable adaptability and versatility of *S. aureus* as a pathogen, and a wide spectrum of clinical syndromes. An extensive network of two component response systems, DNA-binding proteins and regulatory RNAs, controls the expression of virulence (and other) factors in response to environmental conditions. Principal among these is the accessory gene regulator *agr*, a two-component quorum sensing and global gene regulator that controls the expression of numerous surface and secreted proteins. Mutations in *agr* have been associated with loss of virulence.

Biofilm formation, a property of coagulase-negative species in particular, occurs in the presence of foreign material, such as vascular catheters or implanted devices. Biofilm is a complex network of extracellular polysaccharides, DNA, and protein in which bacterial cells become embedded, rendering them inaccessible to clearance by host defense mechanisms.[4] Organisms within biofilms tend to be metabolically inactive and tolerant to killing by antimicrobial agents.

Mechanisms of Disease

Pathogenesis of *S. aureus* disease occurs by two mechanisms: tissue invasion, which may be local or systemic, and toxin production. The typical lesion in tissues is the abscess, a focal collection of pus (liquefied and necrotic host tissue, blood, inflammatory cells, DNA, and cellular debris) and bacterial cells surrounded by an ill-defined layer of edematous and inflamed tissue infiltrated by acute and chronic inflammatory cells.

Host defenses against *S. aureus* infection primarily consist of an intact, normal skin barrier and the innate immune system.[5] Conditions in which these defenses are breached or impaired are associated with increased risk of *S. aureus* infection. Among these conditions are injection drug use, presence of vascular access devices, burns, chronic skin diseases, use of systemic steroids, traumatic wounds, minor skin abrasions or trauma, surgical procedures, insulin-dependent and non–insulin-dependent diabetes, peritoneal dialysis, hemodialysis, subcutaneous and intramuscular injections, acupuncture, prosthetic implants, and congenital or acquired neutrophil disorders (e.g., chronic granulomatous disease, Job syndrome), and advanced age. If the cutaneous barrier is breached, the next line of defense is the innate immune system. Neutrophils recruited to the site of infection ingest and kill staphylococci. Staphylococci elaborate numerous virulence factors specifically designed to thwart each step of the host response. If large numbers of organisms are present, the host response is overwhelmed, infection is not contained, and dissemination occurs. Endothelial cell injury and invasion can also occur. Intracellular organisms and small colony variants within phagocytes and endothelial cells may play a role in relapse and persistent bacteremia by acting as a protected sanctuary against the innate immune host response and antimicrobial therapy. High tissue burdens of organisms and bacteremia are usually but not always accompanied by fever, tachycardia, and other signs of the systemic inflammatory response syndrome, including frank septic shock.

The three toxin-mediated syndromes, which can occur in the absence of invasive disease, are staphylococcal food poisoning, staphylococcal toxic shock syndrome, and staphylococcal scalded skin syndrome. Staphylococcal food poisoning is caused by the ingestion of a preformed heat-stable enterotoxin. The emetogenic activity of enterotoxin is mediated by the intestinal release of 5-hydroxytryptamine and the stimulation of receptors present on afferent vagal neurons. Toxic shock syndrome is caused by a specific toxin, TSST-1, or other staphylococcal enterotoxins acting as superantigens that bind to major histocompatibility complex class II molecules of antigen-presenting cells and T-cell receptors, stimulating the massive release of cytokines from T cells and resulting in shock and death. Staphylococcal scalded skin syndrome and bullous impetigo are caused by either of two exfoliative toxins, A or B. These toxins are serine proteases that specifically cleave desmoglein 1, a desmosomal protein that anchors the overlying superficial epidermis to the stratum granulosum.

CLINICAL MANIFESTATIONS

Skin and Soft Tissue Infections

Skin and soft tissue infections are by far the most common infections caused by S. aureus; millions of cases occur annually in the United States (Chapter 412). Community MRSA strains have been associated with a marked increase in the rates of skin and soft tissue infections in the United States. This heterogeneous group of skin diseases includes impetigo, folliculitis, furuncle, abscess, erysipelas and cellulitis, mastitis (cellulitis of the breast), necrotizing fasciitis, and wound infections.

Impetigo, folliculitis, and furuncle are superficial infections; fever and other systemic signs of infection are not present. Impetigo is a focal infection of the epidermis that occurs most commonly in children (see Fig. 412-1). The typical lesion, which may be multiple or in clusters, is about 1 cm in diameter, with erythema surrounding a bulla or bullae (caused by the production of exfoliative toxin) containing cloudy fluid or with a crusty or scabbed-over appearance. Gram stain of the fluid or drainage from the lesion shows the organism. Folliculitis is a superficial infection with tender, erythematous, maculopapular or pustular lesions centered around hair follicles. Both impetigo and folliculitis readily respond to local measures, such as application of soap and water, topical antibiotics, or antiseptics; systemic antimicrobial therapy may be indicated for extensive or refractory infections.

A furuncle is simply a boil, a painful focal collection of pus with surrounding erythema measuring 1 to 2 cm or more in diameter that extends through the dermis into the subcutaneous tissue (see Fig. 412-2). It may drain spontaneously with application of hot compresses or can be surgically drained with simple incision and drainage. Antimicrobial therapy improves short-term cure rates and reduces rates of recurrence. The distinction between a furuncle and an abscess is somewhat arbitrary. Abscesses tend to be larger and deeper and may be associated with systemic signs of infection and bacteremia. Furuncles may extend to fascia or deeper tissues and coalesce into carbuncles, a more severe form of infection that may be accompanied by bacteremia. Large abscesses and carbuncles, particularly in the presence of fever and other systemic signs of infection, require surgical drainage and systemic antimicrobial therapy.

Erysipelas (see Fig. 412-4) and cellulitis, which are similar in appearance, are painful, warm, indurated, erythematous, nonlocalized infections that may be accompanied by lymphangitis. Cellulitis extends into the dermis and subcutaneous fat; erysipelas is more superficial. Cellulitis should be treated with systemic antimicrobial therapy. Cellulitis due to streptococci (Chapter 274) cannot reliably be distinguished from that caused by S. aureus owing to their similar appearance, although associated purulence suggests staphylococcal infection.

Necrotizing fasciitis is an infection of the deep layers of skin and subcutaneous tissues, extending to muscle and along fascial planes. It is associated with systemic toxicity, leukocytosis, and severe pain often out of proportion to the physical findings. The overlying skin may appear to be uninvolved, belying the serious nature of this infection, which requires immediate surgical intervention

for débridement of involved tissue. Necrotizing fasciitis, which is more typically caused by group A streptococci (Chapter 274) or mixed aerobic and anaerobic organisms, has been associated with community MRSA infection.

Pyomyositis (also termed tropical myositis) is a deep abscess or multiple abscesses within skeletal muscle. S. aureus is the most common cause. The patient presents with fever, pain, swelling, and induration that can be felt on deep palpation. The overlying skin and soft tissue may appear normal. There is often a history of trauma to the infected area. Although it can occur in otherwise normal children and adults, acquired immunodeficiency syndrome and other immunocompromising conditions are predisposing factors. This infection is thought to occur as a consequence of metastatic seeding from a subclinical bacteremia, although blood cultures may not be positive at the time of diagnosis. Computed tomography or magnetic resonance imaging should be obtained to identify lesions. The diagnosis is established by culture of pus collected by needle aspirate. Surgical or percutaneous drainage should be performed, and systemic antimicrobial therapy is indicated.

S. aureus causes 30% of surgical site infections overall in the United States, and approximately 50% of those follow neurosurgical or orthopedic procedures. These infections occur at the site of incision, typically after the second or third postoperative day.[6] Signs and symptoms are fever accompanied by erythema, edema, induration, drainage, pain, and tenderness at the surgical site. Superficial infections respond to removal of stitches, débridement of devitalized tissue, opening of the wound to allow drainage, and a short course of antimicrobial therapy. Deeper infections may require more extensive débridement and prolonged courses of therapy, particularly if bone or a prosthetic device is involved. Removal of infected prosthetic material or a foreign body greatly increases the chance of cure.

Bacteremia

Bacteremia, the presence of bacteria in the bloodstream, exemplifies the pathogenicity of S. aureus.[7] It is present in approximately 75% of cases of invasive infections. The most common sources of bacteremia are skin and soft tissue infections, central venous catheters and other intravascular devices, bone and joint infections, pneumonia, and endocarditis. Bacteremia can originate from any source, which may not be obvious in 25% of cases. Once organisms have invaded the bloodstream they can disseminate widely throughout the body, establishing multiple metastatic sites of infection and thereby perpetuating bacteremia. Fever is usually but not always present. Sepsis syndrome and septic shock are common, and death occurs in 10 to 20% of cases. Patients with occult S. aureus bacteremia have high rates of organ failure, septic shock, and high mortality.

The presence of bacteremia dictates the approach to the diagnosis, management, and therapy of S. aureus infection. When blood cultures are positive, even if the primary source is known, there is always the possibility of endocarditis or other secondary foci of infection. Echocardiography is generally recommended in cases of S. aureus bacteremia to look for valvular vegetations or other signs of endocarditis. An echocardiogram should be obtained in cases of complicated bacteremia, defined by the presence of any one of the following: positive blood cultures for 3 days or more, presence of an intracardiac device (e.g., pacemaker, prosthetic valve), presence of a secondary or metastatic focus of infection, relapse or recurrence of S. aureus bacteremia, or clinically suspected endocarditis. Transesophageal echocardiography, which is more sensitive than transthoracic echocardiography, is the preferred modality if the suspicion of endocarditis is moderate or high.[8]

Source control is the cornerstone of management and therapy. Both primary and secondary foci of infection should be identified and eliminated whenever possible because these may lead to treatment failure or relapse once antimicrobial therapy is discontinued. Computed tomography or magnetic resonance imaging should be considered if signs and symptoms point to deep tissue abscesses or osteomyelitis. Follow-up blood cultures should be obtained to document clearance. Persistent bacteremia is suggestive of endovascular infection, and failure to clear blood cultures after 3 to 4 days of appropriate therapy is a strong predictor of complicated bacteremia, necessitating a longer course of therapy. Antimicrobial therapy should always be administered. A shorter duration of therapy (i.e., 14 days) is appropriate for uncomplicated bacteremia (Table 272-1). Longer courses of 4 to 6 weeks are recommended for the treatment of endocarditis or bacteremia complicated by slow resolution or the presence of metastatic infection.

Endocarditis

S. aureus is the leading cause of both native valve and prosthetic valve endocarditis (Chapter 67), accounting for approximately 30% or more of all cases.

TABLE 272-1	CRITERIA FOR DIAGNOSIS OF UNCOMPLICATED *STAPHYLOCOCCUS AUREUS* BACTEREMIA*

Resolution of fever and systemic signs of infection by day 3 of therapy
Sterile blood cultures within 2 or 3 days of initiation of antimicrobial therapy
Presence of an identifiable and easily removable focus of infection
Prompt removal of the primary focus of infection
No echocardiographic or clinical signs of endocarditis
No osteomyelitis
No hematogenous secondary foci of infection
No preexisting valve abnormalities predisposing to endocarditis (e.g., prosthetic valve, rheumatic heart disease, bicuspid aortic valve)
No implanted prosthetic device (e.g., prosthetic hip)

*Uncomplicated *S. aureus* bacteremia can be treated with a shorter course of antibiotics (see text).

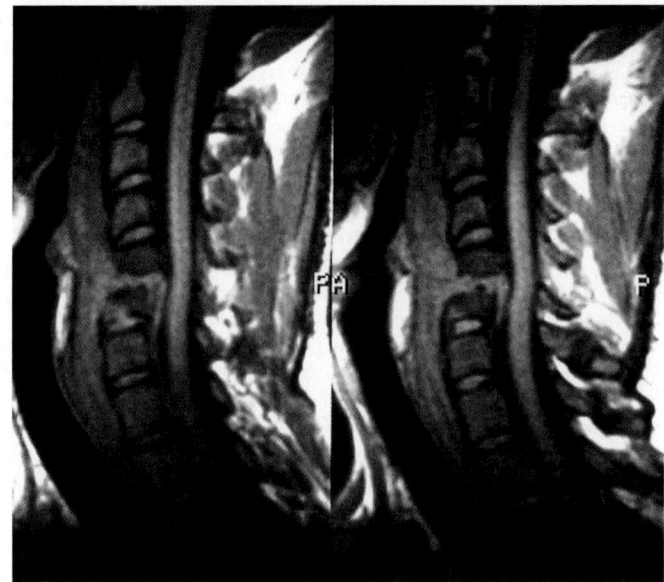

FIGURE 272-2. Noncontrast, non–fat-saturated, T1-weighted, sagittal sequence shows discitis, osteomyelitis, prevertebral and epidural abscess, and cord compression in a patient with *S. aureus* infection of the cervical spine.

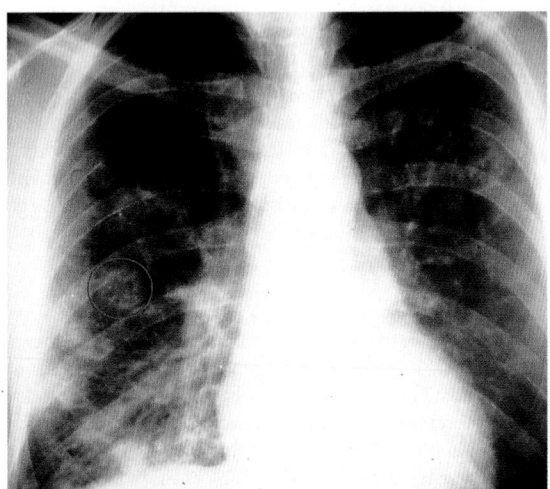

FIGURE 272-1. Chest radiograph shows multiple nodular pulmonary lesions, suggestive of septic embolization, in a patient with tricuspid valve *S. aureus* endocarditis. The red circle shows a lesion with signs of cavitation.

Endocarditis may be community acquired or, increasingly, health care associated. Risk factors include injection drug use, diabetes mellitus, hemodialysis, presence of a prosthetic valve or other implantable intracardiac device, and recent hospitalization. The presentation may be that of an acute febrile illness with high fever developing during a few days. The patient may appear toxic and septic, but some patients have surprisingly few acute symptoms, complaining only of protean symptoms such as shortness of breath, malaise, and weakness. The intracardiac source of infection may not be evident at first because a pathologic murmur may not be evident when the patient first presents. A quarter or more of patients have an associated infection of bone, joint, or skin and soft tissue. The aortic and mitral valves are most commonly involved in native valve infection except in injection drug users (discussed later). Systemic embolization to the brain, kidneys, spleen, gut, or other large vessels is clinically evident in about one third of cases. Peripheral manifestations, including Roth spots, Osler nodes, Janeway lesions, and petechiae, occur with a similar frequency. Morbidity and mortality are high, in part due to the occurrence of this infection in older patients, many of whom have medical comorbidities and impaired innate immunity. Strokes occur in approximately 20% of patients, and congestive heart failure occurs in 40 to 50%. Twenty-five percent to 30% of patients do not survive the initial hospitalization.

Native valve endocarditis in injection drug users involves the tricuspid valve in approximately three quarters of cases. Patients typically have fever, cough, hemoptysis, and pleuritic chest pain as a consequence of hematogenous seeding of the lung and septic emboli from the valve. The chest radiograph may show pulmonary infiltrates, signs of consolidation or pleural effusion, or multiple, often peripheral nodular pulmonary infiltrates with cavitation, hallmark features of septic embolization (Fig. 272-1). Patients tend to be young and otherwise healthy, so mortality is relatively low (≤5%). Injection drug users can also have aortic valve or mitral valve endocarditis, in which case the presentation is similar to that described earlier. Conversely, patients who are not injection drug users may have tricuspid valve endocarditis with pulmonary findings.

S. aureus prosthetic valve endocarditis is associated with a 40% or higher in-hospital mortality. Although prosthetic valve endocarditis can be managed medically in some cases, outcomes tend to be worse, and surgery and valve reimplantation are usually required to cure the infection or to manage its complications.

Pericarditis

S. aureus is the most common cause of purulent pericarditis in children and after cardiac surgery in adults. It may occur by contamination at the time of surgery; by bacteremic seeding from another site of infection; as a complication of endocarditis, paravalvular abscess, or myocardial abscess; or by direct extension of infection from pneumonia, lung abscess, or empyema. The presentation is that of acute pericarditis (Chapter 68), with fever and severe chest pain, tachycardia, and hemodynamic instability. The clinical course may be extremely rapid, terminating in septic shock or cardiac tamponade.[9] Immediate drainage of the infected pericardial space and administration of systemic antimicrobial therapy are indicated. Needle pericardiocentesis is useful for confirming the diagnosis and providing temporary decompression of the pericardial space, but definitive therapy requires surgical or continuous tube drainage.

Osteomyelitis

S. aureus is the most common cause of osteomyelitis, both acute and chronic (Chapter 256). The primary mode of infection is hematogenous seeding. Up to a quarter of cases of bacteremia are complicated by osteomyelitis, and concurrent bacteremia is present in 50% or more of osteomyelitis cases. Acute osteomyelitis—defined as an initial episode with a clinical course of days to weeks, but not months—is manifested with fever and pain at the site of infection. Long bones are more commonly infected in children, whereas vertebrae (most commonly lumbar and cervical) are more commonly infected in adults.[10] Adults can also have long bone osteomyelitis, usually from a contiguous focus of infection or at a site of fracture, prior trauma, or orthopedic hardware. Vertebral osteomyelitis is frequently accompanied by paravertebral or epidural abscess (Fig. 272-2). Back pain accompanied by signs of cord compression, such as radicular pain, sensory loss, lower extremity weakness, urinary retention, and bowel or bladder incontinence, is an emergency. Magnetic resonance imaging should be performed as soon as possible to define the location and extent of infection, and neurosurgical consultation should be obtained in anticipation of surgical decompression and drainage.

Septic Arthritis

S. aureus is the most common cause of septic arthritis (Chapter 256), usually as a consequence of bacteremic seeding, trauma, or a surgical procedure.[11] Risk factors include diabetes, recent joint surgery or joint prosthesis (Chapter 260), and rheumatoid arthritis (Chapter 248). Cardinal features are joint pain, history of joint swelling, and fever. The diagnosis is established by analysis of synovial fluid, in which the white blood cell count typically exceeds 25,000/μL, with 90% neutrophils. Blood cultures are positive in 30 to 50% of cases, organisms are seen on Gram stain of synovial fluid in about 50% of cases, and synovial fluid culture is almost always positive. Hip, knee, ankle, and wrist are most commonly affected. *S. aureus* also has a predilection for infecting the sternoclavicular, sacroiliac, and symphysis pubis joints. Multiple joints are involved in 5% of cases. Both antimicrobial therapy and drainage of the infected joint (by repeated needle aspiration, by arthrotomy, or arthroscopically) are required to prevent destructive arthritis.

Central Nervous System Infections

S. aureus is an uncommon cause of community-acquired central nervous system infections, such as meningitis, primary brain abscess, or subdural empyema. These infections are often associated with endocarditis or a contiguous focus of infection, such as cavernous sinus thrombosis. Mortality of these infections is as high as 30 to 50%. *S. aureus* is an important cause of nosocomial meningitis after head trauma, craniotomy, or implantation of intraventricular or extraventricular catheters.

Pulmonary Infections

S. aureus is an uncommon cause of community-acquired pneumonia (Chapter 91), accounting for 1 to 5% of cases, but with geographic and seasonal (i.e., increased during influenza season) variability. It may be a severe, often fatal, fulminant necrotizing pneumonia accompanied by evidence of cavitation on chest radiographs. Production of Panton-Valentine leukocidin has been associated with severe pneumonia. Community-acquired staphylococcal pneumonia should be considered, and coverage for MRSA strains should be included in the empirical regimen for severe pneumonia requiring admission to an intensive care unit (ICU) and pneumonia in a patient with prior or concomitant influenza.

Hospital-acquired and ventilator-associated pneumonias often are caused by *S. aureus* and MRSA. Patients with traumatic or medical brain injury (e.g., stroke, hemorrhage) are particularly prone to early colonization and subsequent pneumonia by this pathogen. Mortality can be as high as 40 to 50%, reflecting the virulence of the organism and the comorbid conditions that contribute to poor outcomes. The diagnosis is readily established by examination of a Gram stain and culture of sputum, tracheal aspirate, or lavage fluid (obtained to avoid oropharyngeal contamination), which typically shows organisms and numerous neutrophils. The culture is less specific than the Gram stain because it can be positive in colonized patients, but it is highly sensitive. Coverage for *S. aureus* can be discontinued if the organism is not isolated in culture.

Lung abscess and pleural empyema, infections most commonly caused by oral anaerobic bacteria, are occasionally caused by *S. aureus*. The clinical course may be subacute or even indolent. Empyema occurs as a complication of prior chest tube placement, surgery, trauma, staphylococcal pneumonia, or tricuspid valve endocarditis. These infections are treated with drainage and antimicrobial therapy.

Orthopedic Device–Associated Infections

Prosthetic joint and implant-associated infections occurring within the first 12 weeks of surgery are most commonly caused by *S. aureus*. *S. aureus* is second only to coagulase-negative staphylococci as a cause of these infections. The presentation may be acute, with joint pain, evidence of arthritis, fever, and systemic signs of infection. Alternatively, the infection may run a more chronic course, with pain and loosening of the prosthesis but little or no fever. Formation of biofilm makes treatment of these infections a particular challenge.[12] Intraoperative inspection, débridement, and hardware retention may be appropriate for infections of less than 3 weeks in duration or occurring within the first month of implantation. Otherwise, débridement and removal of the prosthesis or implant in conjunction with antimicrobial therapy offer the best chance of cure. This can be accomplished either as a one-stage procedure, in which the infected prosthesis or implant is removed and immediately replaced, or as a two-stage procedure, in which the device is removed and replaced after completion of a 6-week course of antimicrobial therapy.

Genitourinary Infections

Genitourinary infections arise by hematogenous dissemination or as an ascending infection, usually as a result of instrumentation, urinary catheterization, or surgery. These infections include cystitis, pyelonephritis, microabscess, perinephric abscess, prostatitis, and prostatic abscess. *S. aureus* can also be a contaminant introduced during the collection of urine from a patient with asymptomatic vaginal or perineal colonization. Contamination should be suspected if the urine colony counts are low, repeated urine cultures are negative, pyuria is absent, and there are no signs or symptoms of urinary tract infection. If contamination seems unlikely and there is no well-documented history of an event that could lead to ascending infection, hematogenous dissemination should be suspected. Blood cultures should be obtained to determine whether there is ongoing bacteremia and appropriate imaging studies performed to identify a deep focus of infection and the presence of renal and perinephric abscesses.

Toxin-Mediated Diseases

These diseases are caused by the ingestion of preformed toxin or the elaboration of toxin by *S. aureus* from a site of colonization or infection. Staphylococcal food poisoning is a gastroenteritis caused by the ingestion of enterotoxin produced in food contaminated with *S. aureus* from an infected or colonized food handler.[13] When contaminated food is kept at room temperature for several hours, organisms replicate and produce a heat-stable toxin that is not inactivated by cooking or digestive enzymes. Nausea, vomiting, abdominal pain, and diarrhea occur within 2 to 6 hours of eating the contaminated food. There is no fever, and the illness is self-limited, generally lasting about a day. Antibiotics have no role in therapy, which consists of fluid replacement to prevent dehydration. Infants, small children, and the elderly are more severely affected and may require intravenous fluids.

Toxic shock syndrome is caused by colonization or infection with a strain that elaborates a specific toxin, toxic shock syndrome toxin-1 (TSST-1), or another staphylococcal enterotoxin. TSST-1 is responsible for 100% of menstrual cases due to its ability to cross the vaginal mucosa and to achieve systemic concentrations.[14] TSST-1 and the staphylococcal enterotoxins SEA, SEB, and SEC are responsible for nonmenstrual toxic shock syndrome, which is characteristically associated with an identifiable focus of infection, usually of the skin. The diagnosis is clinical, defined by fever, erythroderma, hypotension, involvement of three or more organ systems (renal, hematologic, hepatic, pulmonary, gastrointestinal, muscle, central nervous system, mucous membranes), and desquamation, especially of the palms and soles, 1 to 2 weeks after the onset of illness. Bacteremia is present in only 5% of cases. The case fatality rate is about 5%. Treatment consists of systemic antimicrobial therapy, removal of the source of toxin production, and treatment of septic shock. Streptococcal toxic shock syndrome is discussed in Chapter 274.

Colonization or infection with an *S. aureus* strain that produces exfoliative toxin A or B may cause staphylococcal scalded skin syndrome, a disease primarily of infants but occasionally seen in adults (Fig. 272-3), and bullous impetigo, a pustular skin lesion. The appearance is that of a scald, burn, or blister. The differential diagnosis of staphylococcal scalded skin syndrome includes drug reaction (Chapter 411), toxic epidermal necrolysis (Chapter 410), Kawasaki disease (Chapter 410), and pemphigus foliaceus (Chapter 410).

DIAGNOSIS

S. aureus infection is diagnosed by isolating the organism in culture specimens of blood, tissue, or pus. Non–culture-based methods, such as nucleic acid amplification tests, are also available. Culture remains the "gold standard."

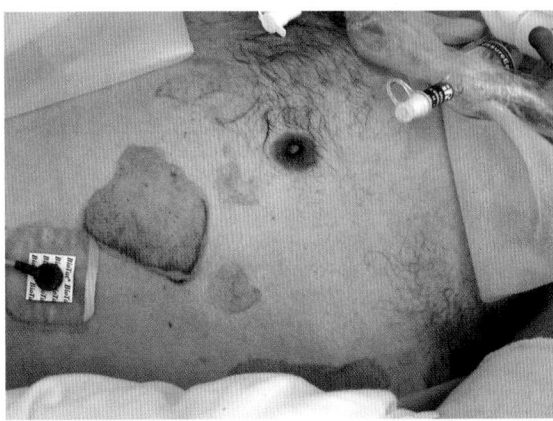

FIGURE 272-3. Scalded skin–type lesions with multiple ruptured bullae and desquamation in a patient with aortic valve endocarditis caused by an exfoliative toxin–producing strain of *S. aureus*.

Gram stain is useful for making a presumptive diagnosis of staphylococcal infection and should be performed whenever possible to look for gram-positive cocci in pus, bone or tissue samples, respiratory secretions, or body fluids such as cerebrospinal fluid, pleural or pericardial fluid, synovial fluid, or urine. Failure to isolate the organism in culture is strong evidence against *S. aureus* infection unless a patient is being actively treated with an antibiotic; even then, infected sites may remain culture positive for several days. The specificity of isolating *S. aureus* from blood or other sterile body sites is essentially 100%. Because of nasopharyngeal colonization in some uninfected individuals, isolation of *S. aureus* from culture of a respiratory specimen lacks specificity; however, if Gram stain also shows gram-positive cocci and many neutrophils, this is suggestive of *S. aureus* pneumonia.

Susceptibility Testing

Susceptibility testing should be performed for clinically significant isolates to guide antimicrobial therapy. The critical determination is whether the isolate is methicillin resistant (i.e., resistant to β-lactam antibiotics). Resistance to macrolides and fluoroquinolones is common, and these drugs should not be used to treat suspected staphylococcal infection without confirmation of in vitro susceptibility. Clindamycin is usually active against community strains, but less reliably so for hospital strains. Tetracyclines and trimethoprim-sulfamethoxazole are active against 80 to 90% of strains. Resistance to vancomycin, daptomycin, telavancin, or linezolid, although rare, may occur, particularly when there has been prior exposure to the drug, making susceptibility testing important for these antibiotics. Persistent endovascular infections are particularly prone toward reduced activity of vancomycin and daptomycin. This is due to relatively poor penetration of drug into vegetations, blunted bactericidal activity for slowly dividing organisms at high inocula, and, in the case of daptomycin, resistance of organisms to host antimicrobial peptides, which coselects for nonsusceptibility to daptomycin.

TREATMENT   Rx

The two principles of therapy for *S. aureus* infections are (1) source control by elimination of abscesses and infected foreign material whenever feasible and (2) administration of systemic antimicrobial therapy. For boils and uncomplicated cutaneous abscesses, incision and drainage may be all that is required, although adjunctive antimicrobial therapy improves cure rates even for simple abscesses.[A1][A2] Antimicrobial therapy is indicated if the infection is not amenable to removal (e.g., cellulitis, pneumonia), drainage is impossible or inadequate, systemic signs and symptoms of infection are present, or there is invasive disease (i.e., metastatic sites of infection; involvement of deep tissues, vital organs, sterile sites) and in all cases of bacteremia. Lack of adequate source control, such as an undrained focus of infection, retention of an infected foreign body, or endovascular infection, is the most common reason for unsatisfactory clinical response, treatment failure, or relapse.

The most important consideration in selecting an antibiotic is susceptibility of the *S. aureus* isolate to β-lactams. For invasive infections a penicillinase-resistant penicillin, such as nafcillin (1 to 2 g every 4 to 6 hours IV), oxacillin, flucloxacillin, or a cephalosporin (e.g., cefazolin 1 to 2 g every 8 hours IV) is the agent of choice for the treatment of methicillin-susceptible *S. aureus* (MSSA) infections; no other antibiotic, including vancomycin,[A3] is as safe or as effective as a β-lactam.[A4] Efficacy of β-lactams other than penicillinase-resistant penicillins and cefazolin for invasive staphylococcal infections is not well documented.

Recent retrospective studies have demonstrated that cefazolin is at least as effective as antistaphylococcal β-lactams in the treatment of *S. aureus* bacteremia, with fewer treatment-related adverse events. A recent U.S. nationwide cohort study showed a lower mortality rate in cefazolin-treated patients compared with those treated with nafcillin or oxacillin.[15] However, strains of *S. aureus* with class A β-lactamase are able to hydrolyze cefazolin in vitro, rendering them effectively resistant to the drug in high inocula. The clinical relevance and impact of this phenotype on outcome is not well defined.

An orally administered β-lactam (e.g., dicloxacillin 500 mg four times daily or cephalexin 500 mg four times daily) is appropriate for most cutaneous infections; a parenteral agent is recommended, at least initially, for invasive infections. Only if the patient is allergic or has a serious reaction is an agent other than a β-lactam preferred for the treatment of infection caused by an MSSA strain. The role of oral agents in step-down therapy of MSSA or MRSA bacteremia is unclear.

Methicillin-resistant strains are cross-resistant to all currently available β-lactams, except for ceftaroline (dose of 600 mg IV every 12 hours), which is indicated for treatment of skin and skin structure infections caused by methicillin-resistant strains. Otherwise, a β-lactam should not be used for treatment of infection known or suspected to be caused by a methicillin-resistant strain.

The prevalence of methicillin resistance in *S. aureus* isolates from hospital-acquired and health care–associated infections in the United States and in many European countries is 25 to 50% or higher. MRSA also causes a substantial proportion of community-onset infections in individuals lacking other risk factors, especially in the United States. Trimethoprim-sulfamethoxazole (one or two 80-/160-mg tablets twice a day), clindamycin (300 mg three times a day), and doxycycline or minocycline (100 mg twice a day) are active in vitro against most community-acquired MSSA and MRSA strains and are effective when administered orally for the treatment of skin and soft tissue infections in outpatients. Traditional fluoroquinolones should not be used because most methicillin-resistant strains are also fluoroquinolone resistant. However, the newest generation drug from this class, delafloxacin, was approved by the U.S. Food and Drug Administration in 2017 to treat skin infections, including those by MRSA, and has in vitro activity against strains that are resistant to early-generation fluoroquinolones.

For invasive infections caused by MRSA, vancomycin is still a drug of choice. It must be administered intravenously; doses of 30 to 60 mg/kg/day, adjusted on the basis of creatinine clearance, are recommended to achieve trough serum concentrations of 15 to 20 µg/mL for patients with bacteremia, endocarditis, or other serious infections. Treatment failures are not uncommon with bacteremia or endocarditis. Patients can remain persistently bacteremic (≥3 days or longer) or relapse, even when the strain is susceptible (minimal inhibitory concentration [MIC] ≤2 µg/mL) in vitro. Other than the presence of an undrained focus of infection, the reasons for this are unclear. Possible explanations include vancomycin's slowly bactericidal activity; tolerance, in which the isolate is inhibited at low concentrations but not killed; or so-called heteroresistance, in which a small fraction of the population of organisms has a higher MIC. Vancomycin MIC of 2 µg/mL has been associated with treatment failure in some retrospective studies but not in others.

Strains with intermediate susceptibility to vancomycin (MICs of 4 or 8 µg/mL), which account for 1 to 3% of MRSA isolates, should be considered resistant because this is highly predictive of vancomycin treatment failure. Vancomycin-resistant strains (MIC >8 µg/mL), which express the *vanA* gene, are rare.

Alternatives to vancomycin for MRSA include linezolid (600 mg every 12 hours, for pneumonia and skin and soft tissue infection), daptomycin (4 mg/kg once daily for complicated skin and soft tissue infections and 6 mg/kg once daily for bacteremia), telavancin (10 mg/kg once daily for skin and soft tissue infection and pneumonia when alternative treatments are not suitable), ceftaroline (skin and soft tissue infection), tedizolid (200 mg once daily for skin and soft tissue infection), oritavancin (1500 mg as a single dose for skin and soft tissue infection), and dalbavancin (1500 mg as a single dose for skin and soft tissue infection). These alternative agents have been shown to be noninferior to vancomycin in high-quality, randomized controlled trials, and none has demonstrated superiority.[A5-A7]

Some authorities recommend higher doses of daptomycin (e.g., 8 to 12 mg/kg/day) for treatment of bacteremia or endocarditis, particularly when the infection has failed to respond to vancomycin. Daptomycin should not be used to treat primary staphylococcal pneumonia because it is inactivated by pulmonary surfactant, although it is indicated for the treatment of hematogenous pneumonia, as occurs in tricuspid valve endocarditis or septic pulmonary embolization.

The role of combination therapy is ill defined. Aminoglycoside combination regimens are not recommended because of increased toxicity and adverse events without improved outcome compared with an effective single agent. Rifampin combination therapy is recommended for the treatment of osteomyelitis, device-related bone infection and prosthetic joint infection, or prosthetic valve endocarditis, particularly that caused by methicillin-resistant strains of staphylococci. Rifampin (300 to 450 mg twice daily) must always be administered in combination with a second active agent because resistance emerges rapidly during therapy. Rifampin combination therapy is not recommended for treatment of bacteremia or native valve endocarditis as outcomes are not improved compared with treatment with an effective single agent. In the randomized, double-blind, placebo-controlled ARREST trial for treatment of *S. aureus* bacteremia, adjunctive rifampicin (600 or 900 mg per day) provided no overall benefit over standard antibiotic therapy.[A8]

Case reports and case series have demonstrated successful clearance or refractory MRSA bacteremia utilizing combination therapy with daptomycin and either antistaphylococcal β-lactams or ceftaroline. The rationale is that the β-lactams enhance binding of daptomycin to the cell membrane. In addition, cell wall synthesized by MRSA in the presence of an antistaphylococcal β-lactam elicits stronger NLRP3 inflammasome activity from host macrophages, a phenomenon that may be lacking in some cases of persistent *S. aureus* bacteremia. The clinical benefit of these combinations beyond cases of persistent bacteremia salvage remains to be determined, especially in light of the high added treatment costs.

PREVENTION

The emergence of community MRSA and the large burden of hospital-acquired and health care–associated staphylococcal infections have stimulated renewed interest in prevention strategies. The organisms that cause these infections are usually resident flora (either *S. aureus* or coagulase-negative staphylococci), or they are acquired by direct contact with a contaminated source, such as a wound or dressing, the skin or hands of an asymptomatically colonized individual, or a contaminated health care provider. The most effective strategy is adherence to principles of basic infection control, the key component of which is hand hygiene, whether it is handwashing or use of an alcohol-based hand rub. This disrupts transmission of organisms by the hands of care providers, a well-documented source of bacterial contamination. Barrier precautions (gloves and gowns) are important for minimizing contact with infected wounds, contaminated secretions, and dressings. Isolation precautions and screening for asymptomatic carriage are more controversial and less well documented in terms of their efficacy. For patients undergoing surgical procedures, surgical hand and surgical site antisepsis, aseptic surgical technique, and antimicrobial prophylaxis are important preventive measures.

Another potentially effective means of preventing infection is screening and decolonization of *S. aureus* carriers.[16] Studies to determine whether screening, decolonization, and isolation actually prevent MRSA infection have had mixed results. In the ICU setting, universal decolonization with 2% chlorhexidine baths, mouthwash, or showers plus 2% intranasal mupirocin ointment was found to be more effective than targeted screening and decolonization or education alone in reducing MRSA rates.[A9][A10] In another trial, however, daily bathing with chlorhexidine did not reduce the incidence of health care–associated infections in critically ill adults in ICUs.[A11] This approach has yet to be widely adopted, and one concern is emergence of resistant strains.

Decolonization may be considered in two other settings: prevention of recurrent infection in individuals who have had several prior episodes and prevention of surgical site infections. The best-studied regimens are topically applied mupirocin nasal ointment (0.5 g twice daily in each nostril for 5 days), with or without bathing with chlorhexidine soap, and orally administered rifampin (600 mg in one or two divided doses) in combination with another active agent (e.g., a fluoroquinolone if the isolate is susceptible, trimethoprim-sulfamethoxazole, or doxycycline). In a randomized, double-blind, placebo-controlled, multicenter trial, the number of surgical site *S. aureus* infections acquired in the hospital was reduced by the rapid screening of nasal carriers by a real-time polymerase chain reaction assay and the decolonization of carriers with mupirocin nasal ointment and chlorhexidine soap.[A12]

Several antistaphylococcal vaccine candidates are currently in early phase clinical trials; the availability of an effective vaccine would be an important tool in preventing staphylococcal infections. A recombinant detoxified toxic shock syndrome toxin-1 variant vaccine has been shown to be safe and immunogenic,[A13] but its clinical benefit remains to be studied.

PROGNOSIS

Prognosis of *S. aureus* infections and outcomes depend on the site of infection, adequacy of source control, presence of comorbidities (e.g., diabetes; immunosuppression; underlying cardiac, renal, or liver disease), presence of bacteremia, presence of secondary foci of infection, presence of severe sepsis or septic shock, antibiotic effectiveness, and duration of therapy for complicated disease. Methicillin resistance is a risk factor for poorer outcome largely because of its health care association and occurrence in a population that is elderly and in which comorbid medical illnesses are prevalent, and possibly because less effective antibiotics (non–β-lactams) are used to treat these infections. Historically, untreated *S. aureus* bacteremia was lethal in 85% or more of cases. Antibacterial therapy, 4 to 6 weeks or longer for complicated bacteremia or infections of deep tissues, and recognition of the importance of source control have dramatically improved outcome. Mortality remains high, in the range of 20 to 40%, in patients with severe sepsis, septic shock, or endocarditis. Several studies have shown a strong link between elevated host interleukin-10 serum concentrations (>5 to 8 pg/mL) on clinical presentation and mortality in patients with *S. aureus* bacteremia, which may offer an opportunity for early identification of high-risk patients.

● COAGULASE-NEGATIVE STAPHYLOCOCCI

More than 30 different species of coagulase-negative staphylococci have been identified, and about half of these colonize humans. *Staphylococcus epidermidis* is the species that most commonly causes infection.[17] Coagulase-negative staphylococci infrequently cause infection unless there is a foreign body in

place, and although bacteremia occurs, metastatic seeding of secondary sites of infection is distinctly uncommon. Coagulase-negative staphylococci are typically resistant to methicillin and multiple other antibiotics, and they are an important reservoir of drug resistance elements that are horizontally transferrable to *S. aureus*. They are the most common cause of health care–associated infections overall in the United States (Chapter 266); they account for one third of central line–associated bloodstream infections; and they are the second most common cause of surgical site infections, particularly when a prosthetic device or other foreign material has been implanted. They also account for about 5 to 10% of cases of native valve endocarditis and about a third of cases of prosthetic valve endocarditis, particularly in cases with onset more than 2 months after valve implantation. Despite their relatively low virulence compared with *S. aureus*, mortality rates of patients with left-sided endocarditis caused by coagulase-negative staphylococci are similar to those caused by MRSA. Mortality is associated with β-lactam resistance (true for >80% *S. epidermidis*), again raising the concern of the inferiority of non–β-lactam drugs in the treatment of endovascular infections. Infections are often indolent, causing little in the way of fever or systemic signs of infection, but they may also be acute and life-threatening, as in the case of prosthetic valve endocarditis.

Coagulase-negative staphylococci are proficient biofilm producers. Consequently, débridement and removal of the infected prosthetic device or foreign body are paramount. Prosthetic joint infections occurring more than 1 month after device implantation are best managed with removal of the prosthesis and reimplantation in a one-stage or two-stage procedure. Antimicrobial therapy for these infections is similar to that for *S. aureus*, except that hematogenous seeding rarely occurs, so attention is focused primarily on source control.

Coagulase-negative staphylococci, because they are normal skin flora, are the most common blood culture contaminant. In approximately 75% of cases in which a blood culture is positive for coagulase-negative staphylococci, this reflects contamination rather than infection. Sorting out whether a positive culture represents contamination or true infection can be a challenge. A single positive blood culture or blood cultures in which more than one strain is present are likely to be due to contamination. Time to blood culture positivity, quantitative blood cultures, and the presence of multiple positive cultures can be useful in determining whether a positive blood culture represents true infection. Isolation of coagulase-negative staphylococci from the blood of a patient with a prosthetic valve, intravenous pacemaker, or vascular graft can be especially problematic because these patients are at high risk for true infection. Unless the patient is hemodynamically unstable or otherwise seriously ill, it is advisable to withhold antibiotics until additional culture specimens are obtained to document the presence of true bacteremia. Isolation of coagulase-negative staphylococci from culture specimens of deep tissue, bone, prosthetic devices, or other normally sterile sites, especially if multiple cultures are positive, strongly suggests true infection.

Staphylococcus lugdunensis causes infections that clinically resemble *S. aureus* infections and can occur in the absence of a foreign body and in otherwise normal hosts. These include prosthetic valve and native valve endocarditis, bacteremia, skin and soft tissue infection, septic arthritis, prosthetic joint infection, and osteomyelitis. It lacks free coagulase, but some strains produce a membrane-bound form that can lead to its misclassification as *S. aureus*. *S. lugdunensis* lacks protein A and is positive for ornithine decarboxylase and pyrrolidonyl arylamidase, differentiating it from *S. aureus*. *S. lugdunensis* is susceptible to most antibiotics, including penicillin (approximately 75% of isolates), and methicillin resistance is rare. Management of these infections is similar to that of *S. aureus* infections.

Grade A References

A1. Daum RS, Miller LG, Immergluck L, et al. A placebo-controlled trial of antibiotics for smaller skin abscesses. *N Engl J Med.* 2017;376:2545-2555.

A2. Talan DA, Mower WR, Krishnadasan A, et al. Trimethoprim-sulfamethoxazole versus placebo for uncomplicated skin abscess. *N Engl J Med.* 2016;374:823-832.

A3. McDanel JS, Perencevich EN, Diekema DJ, et al. Comparative effectiveness of beta-lactams versus vancomycin for treatment of methicillin-susceptible *Staphylococcus aureus* bloodstream infections among 122 hospitals. *Clin Infect Dis.* 2015;61:361-367.

A4. Bidell MR, Patel N, O'Donnell JN. Optimal treatment of MSSA bacteraemias: a meta-analysis of cefazolin versus antistaphylococcal penicillins. *J Antimicrob Chemother.* 2018;73:2643-2651.

A5. Wang Y, Zou Y, Xie J, et al. Linezolid versus vancomycin for the treatment of suspected methicillin-resistant *Staphylococcus aureus* nosocomial pneumonia: a systematic review employing metaanalysis. *Eur J Clin Pharmacol.* 2015;71:107-115.

A6. Corey GR, Wilcox MH, Talbot GH, et al; CANVAS 1 investigators. CANVAS 1: the first Phase III, randomized, double-blind study evaluating ceftaroline fosamil for the treatment of patients with complicated skin and skin structure infections. *J Antimicrob Chemother.* 2010;65(suppl 4): iv41-iv51.

A7. Rubinstein E, Lalani T, Corey GR, et al; ATTAIN Study Group. Telavancin versus vancomycin for hospital-acquired pneumonia due to gram-positive pathogens. *Clin Infect Dis.* 2011;52:31-40.

A8. Thwaites GE, Scarborough M, Szubert M, et al. Adjunctive rifampicin for *Staphylococcus aureus* bacteraemia (ARREST): a multicenter, randomised, double-blind, placebo-controlled trial. *Lancet.* 2018;391:668-678.

A9. Huang SS, Septimus E, Kleinman K, et al; CDC Prevention Epicenters Program; AHRQ DECIDE Network and Healthcare-Associated Infections Program. Targeted versus universal decolonization to prevent ICU infection. *N Engl J Med.* 2013;368:2255-2265.

A10. Huang SS, Singh R, McKinnell JA, et al. Decolonization to reduce postdischarge infection risk among MRSA carriers. *N Engl J Med.* 2019;380:638-650.

A11. Noto MJ, Domenico HJ, Byrne DW, et al. Chlorhexidine bathing and health care-associated infections: a randomized clinical trial. *JAMA.* 2015;313:369-378.

A12. Bode LG, Kluytmans JA, Wertheim HF, et al. Preventing surgical-site infections in nasal carriers of *Staphylococcus aureus*. *N Engl J Med.* 2010;362:9-17.

A13. Schwameis M, Roppenser B, Firbas C, et al. Safety, tolerability, and immunogenicity of a recombinant toxic shock syndrome toxin (rTSST)-1 variant vaccine: a randomised, double-blind, adjuvant-controlled, dose escalation first-in-man trial. *Lancet Infect Dis.* 2016;16:1036-1044.

GENERAL REFERENCES

For the General References and other additional features, please visit Expert Consult at https://expertconsult.inkling.com.

273

STREPTOCOCCUS PNEUMONIAE INFECTIONS

THOMAS MCDONALD FILE, JR.

DEFINITION

Streptococcus pneumoniae (*S. pneumoniae*) is a significant human bacterial pathogen and a major cause of community associated bacterial infections. It is the most common bacterial cause of community-acquired pneumonia (pneumococcal pneumonia), sinusitis, and bacterial meningitis. In children it is a common cause of otitis. This chapter will focus on pneumococcal pneumonia in adults; other infections due to *S. pneumoniae* are reviewed within other chapters. (See Chapter 384 for meningitis and Chapter 398 for sinusitis and otitis). Despite the availability of an effective vaccine, the burden of pneumococcal pneumonia is high particularly in older adults and those with underlying comorbidity.[1,2]

The Pathogen

S. pneumoniae (pneumococci) are lancet-shaped, encapsulated, gram-positive cocci. The cells are 0.5 to 1.2 μm in size and usually arranged end to end in pairs—often referred as diplococci (Fig. 273-1).[3] Colonies appear alpha

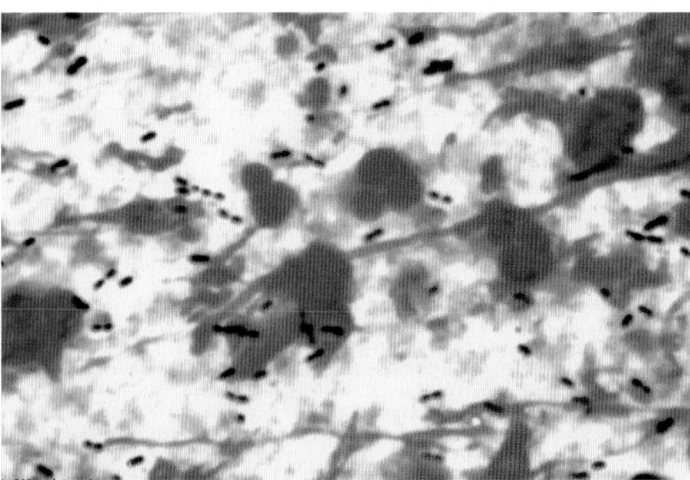

FIGURE 273-1. Gram stain of sputum from patient with pneumococcal pneumonia showing gram-positive diplococci aligned end to end.

hemolytic on standard blood agar when incubated in aerobic conditions. The major virulence factor is a polysaccharide capsule that covers the organism and inhibits phagocytosis. Strains of pneumococci are classified according to the type of capsule of which there are 97 known serotypes. Most *S. pneumoniae* serotypes have been shown to cause disease, but only a minority of serotypes produces the majority of pneumococcal infections. However, serotype patterns are slowly changing, in part because of the widespread use of polyvalent vaccine. Strains of *S. pneumoniae* can occasionally change capsular type via exchanging genes between different serotypes involved in capsule synthesis.[4] In addition, genetic mutations or deletions can result in emergence of nonencapsulated strains.[5] Such strains are less virulent but can be associated with noninvasive infection (e.g., conjunctivitis or otitis) and less commonly pneumonia. Another significant virulence factor, pneumolysin, is a cytolysin, which causes damage to host cells and interferes with host immunity.

EPIDEMIOLOGY

In 2005 the World Health Organization estimated that 1.6 million deaths occurred annually due to *S. pneumoniae*, mostly in infants and the elderly and most of those die from pneumonia.[6] It is estimated that about 900,000 U.S. adults develop pneumococcal pneumonia each year although this is likely an underestimate due to lack of identification of the pathogen in most cases of pneumonia; approximately 175,000 to 400,000 are estimated to require hospitalization. The incidence of pneumococcal pneumonia among adults requiring hospitalization in the United States ranges from 10 to 100/100,000 population with higher rates in the elderly and those with underlying medical conditions. Comparable data have been reported from Europe.[7] The number of cases is expected to increase as the population of the elderly increases. Pneumococcal pneumonia is associated with bacteremia in approximately 10 to 30% of cases. About 5 to 10% of patients with pneumococcal pneumonia will die, and the death rate is even higher in those age 65 years and older. Fewer people will develop pneumococcal meningitis, but the mortality rate for this infection is even higher (see Chapter 384 for meningitis).

S. pneumoniae is predominantly spread from direct person-to-person contact via airborne droplets. The spread of the organism is influenced by such factors as crowding, especially during the winter and in early spring when respiratory diseases are more prevalent. After transmission the organism commonly colonizes the nasopharynx from which it can spread to the lungs, paranasal sinuses, or middle ear.[8] It can also be transported in the blood to distal sites such as the brain, heart, and joints. Colonization in the pharynx is mediated by the binding of the bacteria to epithelial cells by means of surface protein adhesins. Strains with a smaller capsular size have increased exposure of adhesins, which correlates with enhanced colonization. Pneumococci may be isolated from the nasopharynx of 5 to 50% of healthy persons, depending on the population and setting, and carriage is most common in winter and early spring, especially in school-aged children.

From the nasopharynx, pneumococci can migrate to the lower respiratory tract by microaspiration of oropharyngeal secretions containing the organism. Contrary to previous concepts, the lower respiratory tract is not sterile. Pulmonary host defenses usually maintain the pulmonary microbiome at relatively low levels. The development of pneumonia indicates either a defect in host defenses, exposure to a particularly virulent microorganism, or an overwhelming inoculum.

S. pneumoniae has traditionally been the most common cause of community-acquired pneumonia (CAP) (See Chapter 91.). In the pre-antibiotic era, *S. pneumoniae* was responsible for more than 75% of cases of pneumonia. However, more recent studies have isolated the organism in only 5 to 15% of cases in the United States but in a higher proportion of cases in some other countries. Factors that are likely to have contributed to the decline in *S. pneumoniae* as a cause of CAP in the United States include the universal use of pneumococcal conjugate vaccines in children leading to herd immunity, the use of pneumococcal vaccines in adults, and a reduction in cigarette smoking. In addition, with standard diagnostic methods the etiology of CAP is only identified in a small minority of cases, and it is likely that *S. pneumoniae* is the cause of a significant number of unidentified cases.

Risk factors for pneumococcal pneumonia include prior or concurrent respiratory viral infection (especially influenza),[9] smoking, asthma, alcohol abuse, underlying chronic lung, liver, or heart disease, diabetes, cirrhosis, renal insufficiency, dementia, malnutrition, immunocompromise including HIV infection, intravenous drug use, and homelessness. Patients with immune defects (especially related to antibody production) are at significantly higher risk (see below in Pathogenesis).

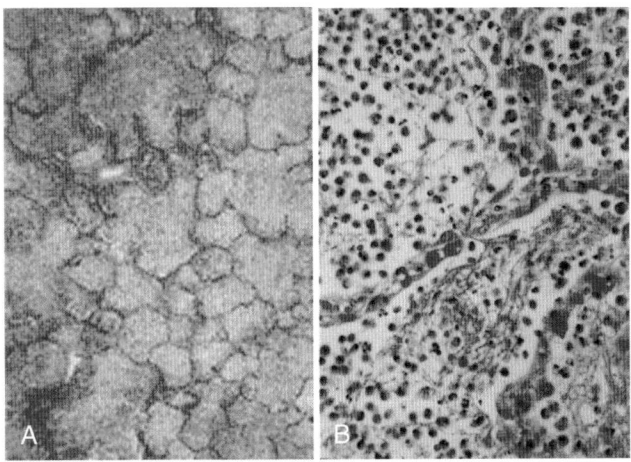

FIGURE 273-2. Pneumonia. A, Low-power magnification (×100) of hematoxylin and eosin (H&E) stain of tissue section from the left lower lobe of the lung. Note the intact alveolar walls and alveoli filled with edema and thick cellular exudates. B, Higher magnification (×500) H&E stain of the same section shown in A. Note the heavy infiltrate of polymorphonuclear cells and the intact alveolar walls.

PATHOBIOLOGY

The disease manifestations of *S. pneumoniae* are caused primarily by the host response to infection rather than the production of organism-associated toxins. The development of pneumococcal pneumonia becomes more likely when a more virulent strain or the amount of aspirated pneumococci overwhelms the host defense system in the respiratory tract (Fig. 273-2). Innate host defenses, which reduce development of pneumonia, include the physiologic removal of bacterial, which become enveloped within mucus and eliminated by the action of ciliated epithelial cells of the respiratory tract. Secretory IgA facilitates the trapping of bacteria in mucus by binding the bacteria to mucin; secretory IgA protease produced by *S. pneumoniae* can overcome this host defense. In addition, the polysaccharide capsule plays a role in reducing attachment to airway mucus.

S. pneumoniae resists phagocytosis in part because of the anti-phagocytic protection by its capsule. The virulence is directly related to the capsule. Antibodies directed against the specific type of capsular polysaccharide protect against disease caused by that specific strain by facilitating phagocytosis of the organism and killing of bacteria. Patients with abnormalities related to antibody production (e.g., asplenia, immunoglobulin deficiencies, multiple myeloma, chronic lymphocytic leukemia) or to phagocytic function (e.g., chronic granulomatous disease, hyperimmunoglobulin E syndrome [Job syndrome], myeloperoxidase deficiency, Chediak-Higashi syndrome) are therefore at higher risk for pneumococcal pneumonia and for worse outcomes when infection occurs.

CLINICAL MANIFESTATIONS

Clinical Presentation

The onset of clinical manifestations of pneumococcal pneumonia is variable depending on the virulence of the strain and host response factors. Disease may be mild, but there is a wide range in severity, including patients with overwhelming sepsis in whom the mortality rate may be greater than 50%. Classically, the onset is abrupt with fever, chills (often shaking), cough, and pain (often pleuritic). However, this constellation of manifestations presents in only a minority of cases. The presenting manifestations overlap with those associated with other causes of pneumonia; thus the etiology cannot be definitely established on the basis of clinical characteristics alone. Older patients may present with delirium as an initial manifestation. Other symptoms include vomiting, diarrhea, myalgias, and arthralgias. Patients with pneumococcal pneumonia often appear anxious. Most with pneumococcal pneumonia have fever; hypothermia is associated with increased mortality. In addition to fever, most patients have tachycardia, and tachypnea and shallow breathing is often present.

After the initial presentation, increasing systemic toxicity associated with hypoxia often follows. Auscultatory findings of crackling rales and bronchial breath sounds are localized to the involved segment or lobe. Confusion, obtundation, and stiff neck should lead to consideration of meningitis. The classic description of the sputum in lobar pneumococcal pneumonia is "rusty," due to mixed blood cells and hemoglobin in the sputum. Laboratory abnormalities

include leukocytosis with left shift. Leukopenia is found in a minority of cases and is associated with a poor prognosis. Severe infection may be associated with multiple organ dysfunction.

Chest radiogram typically reveals a homogenous lobar or segmental alveolar infiltrate. A small amount of pleural fluid is present in many cases. In addition to classic lobar infiltrate pneumococcal pneumonia can cause bronchopneumonia characterized by multiple opacities that tend to be patchy and/or confluent.

Complications

Potential complications of pneumococcal pneumonia include bacteremia with metastatic infection (septic arthritis, peritonitis, pericarditis, meningitis,[10] endocarditis[11]) and pulmonary complications of parapneumonic effusion, empyema, necrotizing pneumonia, and lung abscess. Risk factors for a complicated course include older age, preexisting lung disease, immunodeficiency or AIDS, and, importantly, acquisition of another nosocomial infection. The risk of overwhelming pneumococcal sepsis is increased in splenectomized patients, because the spleen is a principal site for clearance of this bacterium.

Up to one third of the patients hospitalized with pneumococcal pneumonia experience major cardiovascular events. In addition to the stress, hypoxemia, and inflammation associated with infection, pneumolysin may play a direct role in injury to the myocardium.

DIAGNOSIS

The utility of diagnostic studies to determine the etiology of community-acquired pneumonia has been controversial because of the lack of rapid, easily performed, accurate, cost-effective methods that provide immediate results for the majority of patients at the initial evaluation by a clinician in an office or acute-care setting. The etiology of CAP based on standard diagnostic methods is identified in a minority of cases. Nevertheless, there are good reasons for establishing an etiological diagnosis, namely to direct antibiotic management for an individual patient, to facilitate management of treatment failure, and, by de-escalation or narrowing of antibiotic therapy, to potentially decrease health care costs, drug side effects, and the selection pressure for antibiotic resistance. Diagnostic tests for pneumonia caused by *S. pneumoniae* include sputum Gram stain and culture, blood culture, immunochromatography, and molecular methods.

Sputum Gram Stain and Culture

The etiologic role of *S. pneumoniae* can be strongly implicated by the presence of gram-positive lancet-shaped diplococci on sputum Gram stain (Fig. 273-1) and isolation by culture. A Gram stain can be confirmed as *S. pneumoniae* by the Quellung reaction in which polyvalent capsular antibodies are added to the bacteria and then examined microscopically; swelling and increased refractiveness of the capsule is a positive reaction.

The value of routinely performing a Gram stain of the sputum and culture has been debated. These tests are limited by the fact that many patients cannot produce a good specimen, patients often receive antimicrobial agents before evaluation, and many specimens give inconclusive results. An additional limitation of the sputum Gram stain, especially as applied in the United States, is the notable decline in its use by house staff and attending physicians when initially evaluating patients with pneumonia. This is in part due to the Clinical Laboratory Improvement Act of 1988, which required that staff have credentials to interpret Gram stains of any specimens. Finally, outsourcing of specimens to laboratories outside the hospital leads to delays in processing and less direct communication between the microbiology laboratory and the clinician.

S. pneumoniae is recovered in a minority of sputum cultures in part because the organism has fastidious nutritional requirements and is often overgrown by contaminating oral bacteria. It is important that a good quality specimen be obtained for culture. A sputum specimen obtained by the examining clinician at the time of initial evaluation (often having the patient sit up if possible and applying percussion) is much more likely to provide a good quality sample than having a sputum collection container placed at the bedside by other health care providers. To be reliable the specimen should be actual sputum and not saliva, and therefore on microscopic exam should have high numbers of polymorphonuclear cells and few epithelial cells. On a blood agar plate *S. pneumoniae* can be identified by its susceptibility to an Optochin disk.

Blood Cultures

The yield of positive blood cultures for patients admitted with CAP are low, with usual rates of 5 to 15% depending on severity of disease; of these, *S. pneumoniae* accounts for approximately two thirds. Because *S. pneumoniae* is usually considered to be a likely pathogen, positive blood culture results have not clearly led to better outcomes or improvements in antibiotic selection. However, blood cultures can be valuable because, when positive, the microbial etiology is established, this may be the only diagnostic test performed, and it provides valuable information for tracking resistance data and evaluating serotypes for vaccine strategies. In part because of the relatively low yield in patients with CAP admitted to the general ward, the 2007 IDSA/ATS consensus guidelines recommend blood cultures for hospitalized patients with specific indications, including all patients who require admission to the intensive care unit for CAP, and consider them optional for other patients. Indications include cavitary infiltrates, leukopenia, active alcohol use, chronic severe liver disease, asplenia, positive pneumococcal urinary antigen, and large pleural effusion.

Immunochromatography

Urinary antigen tests are particularly attractive for detecting pneumococcal pneumonia when cultures cannot be obtained in a timely fashion or when antibiotic therapy has already been initiated. In serial specimens from known bacteremic cases, the pneumococcal urinary antigen detected by immunochromatographic assay was still positive in 83% of cases after 3 days of therapy. Studies in adults have shown a sensitivity of 50 to 80% and specificity exceeding 90%.[12]

Molecular Assays

Molecular assays for *S. pneumoniae* include nucleic acid amplification techniques, such as PCR and DNA hybridization. PCR is an attractive diagnostic tool for rapid diagnosis because it does not rely on bacterial growth or the viability of the organism. The interpretation of sputum PCR tests is complicated by the difficulty in differentiating between pneumococcal colonization and true infection. Multiplex PCR assays that include detection of *S. pneumoniae* from respiratory specimens are presently under late stage development.

TABLE 273-1	ANTIMICROBIAL THERAPY FOR PNEUMOCOCCAL PNEUMONIA	
	PREFERRED ANTIMICROBIALS	**ALTERNATIVE ANTIMICROBIALS**
ORAL AGENTS		
Penicillin susceptible (MIC ≤0.06 µg/mL*	Amoxicillin; penicillin	Oral cephalosporins (cefpodoxime; cefdinir; cefditoren; cefuroxime); Oral macrolides if susceptible in vitro[†] Clindamycin; doxycycline Respiratory fluoroquinolones (levofloxacin, moxifloxacin, gemifloxacin)
Penicillin resistant*	Fluoroquinolone; high-dose amoxicillin (3 g/day)	Clindamycin; linezolid; newer agents[§]
INTRAVENOUS AGENTS	Third generation cephalosporin (ceftriaxone, cefotaxime); ceftaroline[§]; penicillin[‡]; ampicillin[‡]	Fluoroquinolones; vancomycin; clindamycin; linezolid; broad-spectrum β-lactams[∥]; tigecycline

*Based on nonmeningitis breakpoint for oral penicillin; parenteral penicillin nonmeningitis breakpoint is ≤ 2.0 µg/mL; if concern for meningitis breakpoint for susceptible isolates is 0.06 µg/mL.
[†]High rate of resistance in U.S. and not recommended for empirical therapy without knowledge of the susceptibility results.
[‡]High dose (≥18 million units of penicillin or 12 g of ampicillin likely to be effective for most strains with elevated MICs).
[§]Ceftaroline more potent for *S. pneumoniae* than the third-generation cephalosporin (3rd gen Ceph) and often active even if resistance to 3rd Gen Ceph.
[∥]piperacillin/tazobactam, cefepime, ceftazidime, ertapenem, imipenem, meropenem.
[¶]Other antimicrobials in development.

TREATMENT   Rx

Overview

Antibiotic therapy for community-acquired pneumonia (CAP) is typically begun on an empiric basis because the causative organism is not identified in an appreciable proportion of patients (Chapter 91).[13] Antibiotics should be started as soon as possible once the diagnosis of CAP is considered likely and before leaving the emergency department or clinic. The majority of patients with CAP are treated empirically with a regimen that is likely to have activity against *S. pneumoniae*. However, when *S. pneumoniae* is identified by Gram stain and sputum culture, blood culture, pneumococcal urinary antigen, or molecular methods, narrowing therapy to target this organism should be based on available susceptibility data. The choice of initial therapy is complicated by the emergence of antibiotic resistance among *S. pneumoniae*.[14] Risk factors for drug-resistant *S. pneumoniae* (DRSP) in adults include:

- Age greater than 65 years
- β-Lactam, macrolide, or fluoroquinolone therapy within the past three to six months (an antimicrobial agent from an alternative class is preferred for a patient who has recently received one of these agents)
- Alcoholism
- Medical comorbidities
- Immunosuppressive illness or therapy
- Exposure to a child in a daycare center
- Exposure to the health care setting such as from prior hospitalization or from residence in a long-term care facility

Available data suggest that the impact of drug-resistant *S. pneumoniae* varies with antibiotic class and possibly with specific agents within a class.[15,16]

β-Lactam Resistance

Most studies suggest that current levels of β-lactam resistance do not cause treatment failures for patients with CAP when appropriate agents (i.e., amoxicillin, ceftriaxone, cefotaxime) and doses are used. However, therapy with cefuroxime has been associated with higher mortality rates in patients with bacteremic pneumococcal pneumonia.

Macrolide Resistance

In a global surveillance study of 1713 isolates of *S. pneumoniae* in 2014, 37.6% were resistant to azithromycin.[18] In a study from the same group in 2014 of 1926 pneumococcal isolates from adults in the United States, 43% were erythromycin resistant, with 20% having high-level resistance (MIC >16 µg/mL). Because the overall prevalence of macrolide-resistant *S. pneumoniae* is high in many parts of the world, including the United States, many experts recommend that a macrolide **not** be used as empiric monotherapy in such areas.

Fluoroquinolone Resistance

Although the United States prevalence rate of pneumococcal resistance to the newer fluoroquinolones (levofloxacin, moxifloxacin) remains low (below 3%), the rate of resistance has increased markedly in some countries. The administration of fluoroquinolones for CAP in patients with tuberculosis (TB) has been associated with a delay in diagnosis, increase in resistance, and poor outcomes; clinicians should perform appropriate diagnostic tests before prescribing fluoroquinolones to patients who are at risk for or have signs of TB.

Antibiotic Selection

In vitro activity for *S. pneumoniae* of frequently used antimicrobials is shown in E-Table 273-1. Recommendations for antimicrobial therapy of CAP to include effective coverage for *S. pneumoniae* are included in Table 273-1.

The selection of antimicrobials for suspected or confirmed pneumococcal pneumonia depends on site of care. Oral agents can usually be used for outpatient therapy. Most hospitalized patients are initially treated with an intravenous regimen. However, many patients without risk factors for severe pneumonia can be treated with oral therapy, especially with highly bioavailable agents such as the respiratory fluoroquinolones (levofloxacin, moxifloxacin, gemifloxacin). Additional factors that may affect the choice of antimicrobial regimen include the potential for inducing antimicrobial resistance, pharmacokinetic and pharmacodynamic properties, safety profile, and cost. In addition, if a patient has received an antimicrobial agent within the past 3 months there is greater likelihood of the causative strain of *S. pneumoniae* being resistant to that agent and an antimicrobial agent from an alternative class is preferred.

For patients with CAP who require admission to the hospital combination therapy with a β-lactam plus a macrolide or monotherapy with a respiratory fluoroquinolone are generally of comparable efficacy. However, the severity of adverse effects (including the risk for *C. difficile* infection) and the risk of selection for resistance in colonizing organisms are generally thought to be greater with fluoroquinolones. Furthermore, many observational studies have suggested that β-lactam plus macrolide combination regimens are associated with better clinical outcomes in patients with severe pneumococcal pneumonia, possibly due to the immunomodulatory effects of macrolides.[A1][A2]

Penicillin Allergy

For penicillin-allergic patients, the type and severity of reaction should be assessed. Individuals with a past reaction to penicillin that was mild (not Stevens/Johnson syndrome, toxic epidermal necrolysis, or drug reaction with eosinophilia and systemic symptoms [DRESS]) and did not have features of an IgE-mediated reaction can receive a broad-spectrum (third- or fourth-generation) cephalosporin or carbapenem safely. For penicillin-allergic patients, if a skin test is positive or if there is significant concern to warrant avoidance of a cephalosporin or carbapenem, an alternative regimen should be given.

Clinical Response to Therapy

With appropriate antibiotic therapy, some improvement in the patient's clinical course is usually seen within 48 to 72 hours. Although a clinical response to appropriate antibiotic therapy is seen relatively quickly, the time to resolution of all symptoms and radiographic findings is more prolonged. With pneumococcal pneumonia, for example, the cough usually resolves within eight days, and auscultatory crackles clear within three weeks. Patients who do not demonstrate some clinical improvement within 72 hours are considered nonresponders. Most common causes include severe disease, initial discordant therapy of resistant strains, extrapulmonary infection such as empyema, metastatic infection, instability of comorbid conditions, and noninfectious cause (pulmonary embolism, carcinoma, drug toxicity, immunologic disorder). Patients with bacteremic pneumococcal have higher in-hospital mortality and longer length of hospital stay.[19]

Duration of Therapy

The recommended duration for patients with good clinical response within the first two to three days of therapy is five to seven days total. Before stopping therapy, the patient should be afebrile for 48 to 72 hours, breathing without supplemental oxygen (unless required for preexisting disease), and have no more than one clinical instability factor (defined as HR >100 beats/min, RR >24 breaths/min, and SBP ≤90 mm Hg). A longer duration is needed for more complicated infections (e.g., empyema, extrapulmonary infection such as meningitis, endocarditis, septic arthritis).

The use of the serum biomarker procalcitonin (PCT) has been used as an aid in determining duration of antimicrobial therapy for CAP. PCT is a peptide precursor of calcitonin that is released by parenchymal cells in response to bacterial toxins and certain bacterial-specific proinflammatory mediators (e.g., interleukin [IL]-1β, tumor necrosis factor-α, and IL-6), leading to elevated serum levels in patients with bacterial infections. PCT shows a prompt increase upon initial infection within 6 to 12 hours and decreases rapidly when the bacterial infection is controlled by the host immune system and antimicrobial therapy. In contrast, PCT is downregulated in patients with viral infections because of release by cytokines typically associated with viral infections (interferon-γ). Serum PCT has been studied prospectively to facilitate the decision of whether to use antibacterial therapy[A3] and the duration of treatment in patients with pneumonia.[A4] PCT guidance has led to substantial reduction in duration of antibiotic use.

Adjunctive Therapy: Corticosteroids

Corticosteroids may be beneficial for serious pneumococcal pneumonia on the basis of a number of studies and meta-analyses.[A5][A6] The rationale for giving glucocorticoids as adjunctive therapy to antibiotics in hospitalized patients with CAP is to reduce the inflammatory response to pneumonia, which is likely to contribute to the morbidity of the disease. Patients most likely to benefit are those with severe infection (i.e., requiring intensive care unit admission) and associated with a high systemic inflammatory response. The potential advantage of adjunct corticosteroid therapy needs to be balanced against possible adverse effects such as hyperglycemia and an increase in CAP-related readmissions.[20]

receive PPSV23 until age 65 and then receive PCV13. When both PCV13 and PPSV23 are indicated, PCV13 should be administered first. If PPSV23 has previously been administered, PCV13 should be administered at least 1 year after PPSV23. When two or more doses of PPSV23 are indicated, the interval between PPSV23 doses should be at least 5 years. Supplemental information on pneumococcal vaccine timing for adults aged 65 years or older and adults aged 19 years or older at high risk for pneumococcal disease is available at www.cdc.gov/vaccines/vpd/pneumo/downloads/pneumo-vaccine-timing.pdf.

Influenza vaccine also reduces pneumococcal pneumonia because by reducing the morbidity of acute influenza the incidence of post-influenza bacterial pneumonia is lessened.

In addition to immunization, another consideration to lessen the burden of pneumococcal pneumonia is reducing the impact of comorbid conditions. Conditions associated with pneumococcal pneumonia include chronic pulmonary disease, chronic heart failure, diabetes, malnutrition, and swallowing disorders which increase the risk of aspiration. In addition to predisposing to infection, these conditions significantly worsen the outcome of pneumococcal pneumonia. Interventions to more intensively control such conditions should be employed. Because poor oral/dental hygiene is associated with increased bacterial colonization of oral secretions, attempts to improve dental hygiene may reduce the infectious consequences of aspiration. The relatively simple act of daily teeth brushing may help prevent pneumococcal pneumonia.

Grade A References

A1. Garin N, Genné D, Carballo S, et al. β-lactam monotherapy vs β-lactam-macrolide combination treatment in moderately severe community-acquired pneumonia: a randomized noninferiority trial. *JAMA Intern Med.* 2014;174:1894-1901.

A2. Nie W, Li B, Xiu Q. β-Lactam/macrolide dual therapy versus β-lactam monotherapy for the treatment of community-acquired pneumonia in adults: a systematic review and meta-analysis. *J Antimicrob Chemother.* 2014;69:1441-1496.

A3. Schuetz P, Wirz Y, Sager R, et al. Effect of procalcitonin-guided antibiotic treatment on mortality in acute respiratory infections: a patient level meta-analysis. *Lancet Infect Dis.* 2018;18:95-107.

A4. Pepper D, Sun J, Rhee C, et al. Procalcitonin-guided antibiotic discontinuation and mortality in critically ill adults: a systematic review and meta-analysis. *Chest.* 2019;155:1109-1118.

A5. Torres A, Sibila O, Ferrer M, et al. Effect of corticosteroids on treatment failure among hospitalized patients with severe community-acquired pneumonia and high inflammatory response: a randomized clinical trial. *JAMA.* 2015;313:677-686.

A6. Briel M, Spoorenberg SMC, Snijders D, et al. Corticosteroids in patients hospitalized with community-acquired pneumonia: systematic review and individual patient data meta-analysis. *Clin Infect Dis.* 2018;66:346-354.

A7. Vadlamudi NK, Parhar K, Altre Malana KL, et al. Immunogenicity and safety of the 13-valent pneumococcal conjugate vaccine compared to 23-valent pneumococcal polysaccharide in immunocompetent adults: a systematic review and meta-analysis. *Vaccine.* 2019;37:1021-1029.

GENERAL REFERENCES

For the General References and other additional features, please visit Expert Consult at https://expertconsult.inkling.com.

PROGNOSIS

The mortality rate for pneumococcal pneumonia varies by severity at presentation and host factors, ranging from 5 to 50%. Factors associated with increased mortality include older age, severity of disease, requirement for ventilation, shock, bilateral disease, amount and degree of underlying conditions, and renal failure.

PREVENTION

The best way to prevent pneumococcal pneumonia is through vaccination and stabilization of underlying conditions that predispose to infection (e.g., diabetes, congestive heart failure).

There are two types of pneumococcal vaccine recommended for adults: a pneumococcal conjugate vaccine (PCV13) and a pneumococcal polysaccharide vaccine (PPSV23). The conjugate vaccine contains antigens for 13 serotypes and is more immunogenic[A7] whereas the polysaccharide contains antigens of 23 serotypes.

Adults are recommended to receive 1 dose of PCV13 and 1, 2, or 3 doses of PPSV23 depending on indication (Chapter 15). All patients older than 65 years of age or who have immunocompromising conditions (e.g., HIV, immunosuppressive therapy, cancer chemotherapy) should receive PCV13. Patients with underlying conditions (e.g., chronic heart or lung disease, diabetes) should

---

274

NONPNEUMOCOCCAL STREPTOCOCCAL INFECTIONS AND RHEUMATIC FEVER

DENNIS L. STEVENS, AMY E. BRYANT, AND MELISSA M. HAGMAN

CLASSIFICATION AND IDENTIFICATION OF STREPTOCOCCI

Streptococci are gram-positive facultatively anaerobic, catalase-negative coccoid bacteria that grow in chains and colonize the skin and mucous membranes. When grown on blood agar plates, they may result in complete (β), incomplete (α), or no (γ) hemolysis. Using the Lancefield classification, hemolytic streptococci can be categorized into types A through G based on acid-extractable carbohydrate antigens of cell wall material. More modern classification schemes categorize hemolytic and nonhemolytic streptococci using modern biochemical and genetic techniques.

The major pathogenic β-hemolytic streptococci are group A (*Streptococcus pyogenes*) and group B (*Streptococcus agalactiae*). Although most of this chapter is dedicated to discussing these two pathogens and the clinical diseases that they cause, the remainder of the chapter includes discussions of *Streptococcus dysgalactiae* subspecies *equisimilis* (groups C and G streptococcus), viridans group streptococcus (no Lancefield group), and zoonotic streptococci (various Lancefield groups).

Streptococcus Pyogenes (Group A Streptococcus)

DEFINITION

S. pyogenes contains Lancefield group A antigen on the cell surface and thus is referred to as group A streptococcus. Group A streptococci are the most significant of the streptococcal human pathogens and cause an array of clinical infections ranging from pharyngitis, superficial skin infections, deep soft tissue infections, and toxic shock syndrome. Postinfectious sequelae include rheumatic fever, post-streptococcal glomerulonephritis, and reactive arthritis.[1]

EPIDEMIOLOGY

Human beings are the only known hosts for *S. pyogenes*. All group A streptococcal infections are more common in children younger than 10 years. The asymptomatic prevalence of the group A streptococcus carrier state is also higher in children (15 to 20%) than in adults (<5%). In addition to age, group A streptococcus epidemics are also associated with crowded conditions during the winter months in temperate climates. Per recent estimates from the U.S. Centers for Disease Control and Prevention (CDC), the incidence of invasive *S. pyogenes* infections in the United States in 2015 was 4.8 cases per 100,000 population per year.

PATHOBIOLOGY

The natural reservoirs for *S. pyogenes* are mucous membranes and skin. Group A streptococci adhere to host epithelium through complex interactions involving streptococcal factors such as M protein, lipoteichoic acid, fibronectin-binding protein, and fimbriae.[2] Although streptococci must adhere to the epithelium to cause most infections, such adherence is not sufficient to cause disease because patients may not develop symptomatic infection despite prolonged asymptomatic carriage of group A streptococcus.

The mode of transmission and portal of entry are usually obvious in clinical streptococcal infections. Pharyngeal and group A streptococci are transmitted from person to person through aerosolized microdroplets, and cutaneous acquisition is typically by direct contact. Epidemics of pharyngitis and scarlet fever can also be caused by the consumption of contaminated food or unpasteurized milk. Group A streptococcus infections frequently are seen during childbirth (puerperal sepsis), after surgery or burns (wound infection), and in war settings (epidemic gangrene)—thus, in most clinical streptococcal infections. In contrast, among patients with streptococcal toxic shock syndrome, the portal of entry is obvious in only 50% of cases.

Streptococci evade opsonophagocytosis through expression of antiphagocytic M protein, by use of immunoglobulin binding protein, by formation of a hyaluronic acid capsule, and/or by production of a C5a peptidase that destroys or inactivates complement-derived chemoattractants and opsonins.[3] At the focus of infection, the cytotoxic exotoxin streptolysin O (SLO) destroys approaching phagocytes. Distal to the infection, lower concentrations of SLO stimulate hyperadhesion of polymorphonuclear leukocytes to endothelial cells, thereby effectively preventing a tissue inflammatory response and promoting vascular damage. In a nonimmune host, SLO, streptococcal pyrogenic exotoxins (SPEs) A, B, C, MF, and SSA, and other streptococcal components drive the "cytokine storm" that causes hypotension and vascular leukostasis, thereby resulting in microvascular injury, shock, multiorgan failure, and even death.

CLINICAL MANIFESTATIONS AND DIAGNOSIS

Pharyngitis

Pharyngitis is the most common *S. pyogenes* infection, with peak incidence in children aged 5 to 15 years. Infection is characterized by an abrupt onset of fever, sore throat, and submandibular adenopathy. Chilliness is common, but frank rigors are unusual. Most patients report pain on swallowing, but cough and hoarseness are rare. On physical examination, the uvula is edematous, the tonsils are typically hypertrophied, the palate may have petechia, and the pharynx is usually erythematous with a punctate or confluent exudate (Fig. 274-1).

Acute pharyngitis induces antibodies against M protein, SLO, DNase, hyaluronidase, and if present, pyrogenic exotoxins. Even without treatment, the

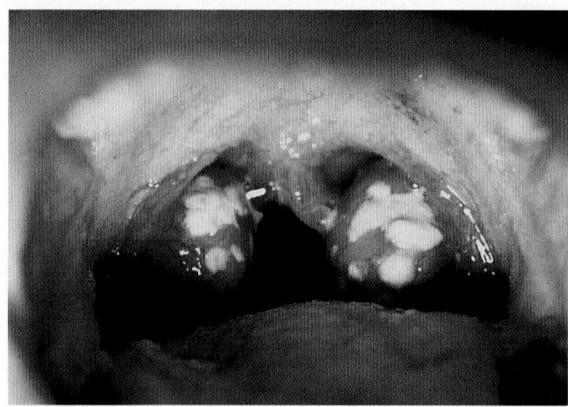

FIGURE 274-1. Acute streptococcal pharyngitis. Pus is present in the tonsillar crypts, and some palatal petechiae are seen. (From Forbes CD, Jackson WF. *Color Atlas and Text of Clinical Medicine*. 3rd ed. London: Mosby; 2003.)

TABLE 274-1	MODIFIED CENTOR CLINICAL DECISION RULE FOR DIAGNOSING GROUP A STREPTOCOCCAL PHARYNGITIS IN CHILDREN AND ADULTS

STEP 1—CALCULATE MODIFIED CENTOR SCORE

DIAGNOSTIC CRITERIA	POINTS
Temperature >38° C	+1
Absence of cough	+1
Swollen, tender anterior cervical lymph nodes	+1
Tonsillar swelling or exudate	+1
Age 3-14 years	+1
Age >44 years	−1

STEP 2—DETERMINE SUGGESTED MANAGEMENT

SCORE	RISK FOR STREPTOCOCCAL INFECTION	RAPID ANTIGEN TESTING AND/OR CULTURE	ANTIBIOTICS
≤0	1-2.5%	No	No
1	5-10%		
2	11-17%	Yes	If testing positive
3	28-35%		
≥4	51-53%	No	Yes, empiric

Adapted from: McIsaac WJ, Kellner JD, Aufricht P, Vanjaka A, Low DE. Empirical validation of guidelines for the management of pharyngitis in children and adults. *JAMA*. 2004;291(13):1587-1595.

pain, swelling, and fever of acute pharyngitis usually resolve spontaneously in 3 to 6 days. However, depending on the infecting strain, pharyngitis also can progress to suppurative head and neck infections, scarlet fever, bacteremia, rheumatic fever, or post-streptococcal glomerulonephritis. Streptococcal toxic shock syndrome is an uncommon sequela of symptomatic pharyngitis.

Although *S. pyogenes* is the most common cause of acute pharyngitis (20 to 40% of pediatric cases and 5 to 15% of adult cases), definitive diagnosis is difficult on purely clinical parameters. Even in older children or adolescents who have all the typical physical findings of streptococcal pharyngitis, the clinical diagnosis is correct in only about 75% of patients. The modified Centor score was designed to assist with diagnosis and to help reduce unnecessary use of antibiotics and streptococcal testing (Tables 274-1 and 401-2). If any one of the classic signs is absent, the likelihood of streptococcal pharyngitis is greatly reduced. Several societies suggest avoiding streptococcal testing and antibiotics if the modified Centor score is 0 or 1.[4] Providers can generally avoid testing in children younger than 3 years because of low rates of streptococcal infection complications in this age group.

Throat swabs for culture of *S. pyogenes* remain the diagnostic "gold standard." Rapid site-of-care antigen tests have sensitivities of 58 to 96%. Consistent with Infectious Diseases Society of America guidelines, a popular approach is to obtain two throat swabs from the tonsillar surface or posterior pharynx. Point-of-care polymerase chain reaction (PCR) testing may prove to be more accurate but still misses some culture-confirmed cases.[5] If a rapid streptococcal antigen test is positive on the first swab, the patient should be treated with antibiotics, and the second swab can be discarded. If the rapid test is negative in children and adolescents, the second sample should be sent for culture, and treatment should be withheld unless the result is a positive culture. In adults, the second sample usually need not be sent for culture because of the low incidence of group A streptococcal pharyngitis in adults and the low risk for subsequent acute rheumatic fever even if group A streptococcus pharyngitis is present. The delay in antibiotics for confirmed cases of group A streptococcus pharyngitis is reasonable because acute antibiotic treatment has limited effect on improving acute symptoms. Delaying treatment by several days, however, reduces unnecessary antibiotic use while still achieving the goals of preventing rheumatic fever and reducing spread of disease. Antibiotics, regardless of the timing, do not reduce the likelihood of post-streptococcal glomerulonephritis.

Scarlet Fever

Scarlet fever is the syndrome defined as streptococcal infection, most commonly pharyngitis, fever, and a characteristic rash. Ninety percent of cases of scarlet fever occur in children aged 2 to 8 years. Scarlet fever is most common during the winter months in temperate regions. The rash usually begins as small, flat, erythematous macules on the trunk 1 to 2 days after the illness begins. The rash then transforms into minute papules, giving a "sandpaper" feel to the skin as it spreads to the limbs, sparing the palms and soles. The rash can be accentuated in the skin folds and flexure creases as of the elbow (Pastia lines). Other features include flushed cheeks with circumoral pallor and enlargement of the papillae of the tongue (strawberry tongue). As the rash resolves over the course of 6 to 9 days, there is often desquamation beginning at the palms and soles. The pathogenesis of scarlet fever remains incompletely understood, but SPEs appear to play a role. Since the advent of penicillin treatment, scarlet fever has become uncommon, but recent outbreaks have been reported in England,[6] Australia,[7] and China.[8]

Impetigo and Ecthyma

Impetigo (Chapter 412) most commonly occurs in children aged 2 to 5 years. It may occur year-round in tropical areas but occurs predominantly in the summer in temperate climates. Risk factors for impetigo include poor hygiene and malnutrition. Unbroken skin is colonized, and then minor abrasions or other traumas lead to infection of the superficial keratin layer of the skin. Within 10 to 14 days, single or multiple thick-crusted, golden-yellow lesions appear. Ecthyma is an ulcerative form of impetigo characterized by erosions into the dermis. In the past, nonbullous impetigo as described here could be confidently diagnosed as streptococcal and differentiated from bullous impetigo caused by *Staphylococcus aureus*. More recently, however, *S. aureus* has been isolated with increasing frequency from nonbullous impetigo in the setting of penicillin treatment failure. Gram stain and culture of exudates from the skin lesions can help determine whether group A streptococcus or *S. aureus* is the cause.

Erysipelas

Erysipelas (Chapter 412), which is caused exclusively by *S. pyogenes*, is characterized by an abrupt onset of fiery red swelling of the face or extremities. The infection is most commonly seen in infants and elderly adults. Infection is confined to the upper dermis with prominent lymphatic involvement leading to well-defined margins raised above the level of the surrounding skin, particularly along the nasolabial fold, without the crusty lesions seen in impetigo with its involvement of the superficial keratin layer of skin. Other distinctive features of erysipelas include scarlet or salmon-red rash, intense pain, and rapid progression. Flaccid bullae may develop on the second to third day, but the infection rarely extends into deeper soft tissues.

Cellulitis

Cellulitis (Chapter 412) is infection of the subcutaneous tissues resulting in a pink hue to the skin and less defined borders than with erysipelas. Group A streptococcal cellulitis is usually nonpurulent. Purulent cellulitis is most commonly caused by staphylococcal species. Risk factors for streptococcal cellulitis include impaired lymphatic drainage, venous insufficiency, edema, obesity, and disruption of the cutaneous barrier as from wounds or dermatophyte infection (e.g., tinea pedis).

Severe Group A Streptococcal Infections
Bacteremia
Group A streptococcal bacteremia is relatively uncommon in the antibiotic era, and endocarditis is even less common. In contrast to pharyngitis, scarlet fever, and impetigo, bacteremia occurs more often in the elderly and in

neonates. The exceptions to these extremes of age are individuals with parenteral injection of illicit drugs and otherwise healthy middle-aged adults who develop bacteremia as part of a necrotizing soft tissue infection or streptococcal toxic shock syndrome. Uncomplicated bacteremia is treated with penicillin.

Puerperal Sepsis
Patients with *S. pyogenes* puerperal sepsis typically present with fever, abdominal pain, and hypotension without tachycardia or leukocytosis. Maternal mortality is highest when infection occurs within 4 days of delivery or during the late third trimester. The incidence is approximately six cases per 100,000 live births, and the case-fatality rate is about 3.5%. In the 1850s in Europe and the United States, nosocomial transmission was the rule. In modern times, nosocomial transmission still occurs, but because women are discharged home after 48 hours, acquisition may be from the home environment, particularly if young children at home have had recent streptococcal pharyngitis or are carriers of group A streptococcus.

Necrotizing Fasciitis/Necrotizing Soft Tissue Infection
Necrotizing fasciitis is an infection of the deep subcutaneous tissues and fascia that is characterized by extensive and rapidly spreading necrosis (gangrene) of the skin and underlying structures.[9] Streptococcal necrotizing fasciitis can begin at a site of trivial trauma (e.g., a burn, insect bite, or varicella lesion) or in an operative incision. Half of patients with necrotizing fasciitis, however, develop infection without a defined portal of entry. In these individuals, the "cryptic" infection begins in deep tissues at a site of muscle strain, bruise, or other nonpenetrating traumatic injury. In patients who have necrotizing fasciitis with a portal of entry, warmth, erythema, swelling, and tenderness develop and then rapidly spread both proximally and distally within 24 hours. During the second day, the erythema typically turns from red to purple and then to blue, and the patient develops blisters and bullae containing clear yellow fluid. Bacteremia is frequently present, and metastatic abscesses may occur. By the fourth to fifth day, frank gangrenous changes are evident in the affected skin, followed by extensive sloughing. The process may march inexorably over large body areas unless measures are taken to contain it. The patient with streptococcal necrotizing fasciitis appears perilously ill, with high fever and extreme prostration. Mortality rates are high (30 to 60%), even with appropriate treatment including antibiotics, aggressive fasciotomy, and surgical débridement.

In patients with cryptic *S. pyogenes* necrotizing fasciitis/myonecrosis who lack a discernible portal of bacterial entry, classical cutaneous signs of a necrotizing process are not initially apparent. In the absence of such clinical clues, the correct diagnosis is often missed or delayed until the patient manifests systemic shock and organ failure. This delay results in exceedingly high morbidity and mortality (70 to 85%). Pain out of proportion to the initial injury is usually an important clinical clue to the presence of the deep infection. Routine radiographs, computed tomography (CT) scanning, and magnetic resonance imaging (MRI) may show localized swelling of the deep tissues but characteristically do not show frank abscess or gas formation. Therefore, these are not definitive procedures. Unexplained tachycardia, a marked left shift, and an elevated creatine phosphokinase level can be important clues to the diagnosis of necrotizing soft tissue infections, and their presence should prompt surgical inspection of the deep tissues. Gram stains of aspirated fluid reveal chains of gram-positive cocci and few, if any, white blood cells. Similarly, a biopsy with frozen section may aid in the diagnosis of necrotizing fasciitis.

Myonecrosis
Myonecrosis is an invasive and destructive infection of the muscle and related structures. Among gram-positive organisms, *S. pyogenes* remains the most common etiologic agent. This is in contrast to myositis, which is strictly defined as a localized purulent infection of the muscle, where *S. pyogenes* is rarely involved. In myonecrosis, organisms are likely hematogenously translocated from the throat to the deep soft tissues, though antecedent or concomitant streptococcal pharyngitis is not a prerequisite for this infection. Systemic toxicity is common, and mortality is high (30 to 80%).

Streptococcal Toxic Shock Syndrome
Streptococcal toxic shock syndrome is more fully defined in Table 274-2, but simply stated it is any streptococcal infection that is associated with the sudden onset of shock and organ failure. Definite cases are those in which *S. pyogenes* is isolated from a normally sterile body site. The first cases of definitive streptococcal toxic shock syndrome were first described in the mid to late 1980s. Initial reports of streptococcal toxic shock syndrome were in adults, but children

TABLE 274-2 DEFINITION OF STREPTOCOCCAL TOXIC SHOCK SYNDROME

A. DEFINITION

Definite case	Illness fulfilling criteria B1 and C (1 and 2)
Probable case	Illness fulfilling criteria B2 and C (1 and 2) if no other cause for illness is found

B. ISOLATION OF GROUP A STREPTOCOCCI

1. From a normally sterile site (e.g., blood; cerebrospinal, pleural, or peritoneal fluid; tissue biopsy; surgical wound)
2. From a nonsterile site (e.g., throat, sputum, vagina, superficial skin lesion)

C. CLINICAL SIGNS OF SEVERE INFECTION

1. Hypotension (e.g., systolic blood pressure ≤90 mm Hg in adults or below fifth percentile for age in children)
2. Two or more of the following signs:
   Renal impairment (i.e., creatinine ≥2 mg/dL for adults, or ≥2 times the upper limit of normal for age, or ≥2 times baseline creatinine in persons with preexisting renal disease)
   Coagulopathy (i.e., platelets ≤100,000/µL or disseminated intravascular coagulation)
   Liver involvement (i.e., serum aspartate aminotransferase [AST], alanine aminotransferase [ALT], or total bilirubin levels ≥2 times the upper limit of normal for age, or ≥2 times baseline in persons with preexisting liver disease)
   Adult respiratory distress syndrome
   Generalized erythematous macular rash that may desquamate
   Soft tissue necrosis (e.g., necrotizing fasciitis, myositis, or gangrene)

Adapted from: The Working Group on Severe Streptococcal Infections. Defining the group A streptococcal toxic shock syndrome. Rationale and consensus definition. *JAMA.* 1993;269(3): 390-391.

can also be affected. Diabetes mellitus and alcoholism appear to be contributing factors, but many afflicted individuals have no underlying medical conditions and are not immunocompromised. This contrasts sharply with reviews of *S. pyogenes* bacteremia from several decades ago, which found that bacteremia occurred primarily in the very young, the very old, or patients with predisposing conditions, such as cancer, renal failure, severe burns, or iatrogenic immunosuppression. Streptococcal toxic shock syndrome rarely occurs secondary to symptomatic streptococcal pharyngitis and more often follows breaches in the skin and mucous membranes. The use of nonsteroidal anti-inflammatory drugs (NSAIDs) for pain associated with muscle strain, trauma, chickenpox, or childbirth has been suggested to predispose patients to increased risk and severity of infection. Clearly, NSAIDs may mask the early signs and symptoms of streptococcal infection, thus delaying diagnosis and treatment and increasing mortality. However, some experimental evidence suggests that nonselective NSAIDs (e.g., ibuprofen, ketorolac) actively accelerate the disease course and worsen outcomes. Investigations to resolve this issue are ongoing.

The first phase of streptococcal toxic shock syndrome begins with an influenza-like prodrome characterized by fever, chills, myalgias, nausea, vomiting, and diarrhea. Hypotension follows within 24 to 48 hours. Confusion develops in more than half of patients. Phase 2 is characterized by tachycardia, tachypnea, increasing pain, and persistent fevers. In children with varicella infection, toxicity or persistence of fever longer than 4 days should prompt careful evaluation for streptococcal toxic shock syndrome. In phase 3, shock and organ failure develop. Laboratory tests may show evidence of renal impairment and normal to mild elevations of white blood cell count with profound left shift, low albumin, and low calcium. Metabolic acidosis develops in phase 3 of disease. Because acute respiratory distress syndrome (ARDS) develops in 55% of patients with streptococcal toxic shock syndrome, blood gas levels can be helpful to evaluate the need for mechanical ventilation.

Pneumonia

Pneumonia caused by *S. pyogenes* is frequently associated with chronic pulmonary disease or with antecedent viral infections such as influenza, measles, or varicella. In one third or fewer of the cases, there is a history of preceding streptococcal upper respiratory infection. The onset is typically abrupt, and the disease is characterized by fever, chills, dyspnea, cough productive of blood-streaked sputum, and pleuritic chest pain. The pulmonary picture is one of bronchopneumonia, with consolidation being uncommon. Empyema develops in 30 to 40% of cases, tends to appear early in the disease, and typically consists of copious amounts of thin serosanguinous fluid. Bacteremia occurs in 10 to 15% of cases. Mortality has generally been low with penicillin therapy and adequate drainage of empyema but may be higher in older patients.

TREATMENT Rx

Antimicrobial Susceptibility

Group A streptococci continue to be susceptible to penicillin in vitro, and it remains the drug of first choice for treatment of infection. Cephalosporins are a reasonable alternative to penicillin in some cases because of ease of administration. Clindamycin should be used in addition to penicillin in serious group A streptococcal infection owing to the ability of clindamycin to prevent production of group A streptococcus exotoxins that mediate the clinical manifestations of disease. Treatment failures in patients with severe *S. pyogenes* infections have been described if clindamycin resistance is found. In the United States, clindamycin resistance is as high as 15%.[10] In other nations, resistance may be much higher. In China, for example, 95.5% of the strains of group A streptococci causing scarlet fever are clindamycin resistant. Clindamycin resistance can be constitutive or inducible. Inducible resistance develops after exposure to a macrolide and is identified in the laboratory using an erythromycin disk in the double-disk diffusion test.

In penicillin-hypersensitive patients, clindamycin or macrolides are the second-line drugs of choice. As with clindamycin, macrolide resistance is increasing. In a European study of *S. pyogenes* strains from 10 countries, the prevalence of erythromycin resistance had increased from 29.3% in 2002 to 2003 to 45.7% in 2004 to 2005. Those countries with higher erythromycin use had higher resistance rates. Fluoroquinolones can be used as an alternative for group A streptococcal skin and soft tissue infections in penicillin-hypersensitive patients in areas where clindamycin and macrolide resistance are high. Fluoroquinolone resistance is rare. Vancomycin is an option for intravenous therapy. Tetracycline resistance in group A streptococci is common, and therefore it should not be used unless sensitivities are known. Trimethoprim-sulfamethoxazole is not active against group A streptococci and therefore should not be used alone for infections in which group A streptococcus is the suspected pathogen.

Specific Infections

For *pharyngitis*, penicillin (either oral penicillin VK, 250 mg three times daily or 500 mg twice daily for 5 to 10 days, or injectable benzathine penicillin, 1.2 million units every 4 weeks) is the treatment of choice because it is cost effective, has a narrow spectrum of activity, and has long-standing proven efficacy (Chapter 401).[A1] Cefuroxime axetil (250 mg twice a day for 5 to 10 days) is also effective for primary treatment and for persistent infection. Patients with proven recurrent infections should receive clindamycin (300 mg orally three times a day for 10 days) or amoxicillin–clavulanic acid (875 mg orally twice a day, or 500 mg three times a day for 10 days). For patients who are allergic to penicillin, azithromycin (500 mg/day for 3 days or a single dose of 2 g) is another alternative.

For *scarlet fever*, the recommended treatment is 1.2 million units of benzathine penicillin G given intramuscularly or oral penicillin VK, 250 mg four times daily for 10 days. Most patients recover after 4 to 5 days, and the rash usually resolves completely over a period of several weeks.

For *impetigo* and *ecthyma*, topical 2% mupirocin[A2] or (retapamulin, a novel pleuromutilin antibacterial) is as effective as oral antibiotics and can reduce the likelihood of transmission of the streptococci to other individuals. Penicillin (penicillin VK 250 mg four times daily for 10 days) is first-line treatment for ecthyma or for impetigo present at multiple skin sites caused by streptococci. If *S. aureus* is contributing to infection, treatment should be with a penicillinase-resistant semisynthetic penicillin (e.g., dicloxacillin 250 mg orally four times daily) or a cephalosporin (e.g., cephalexin 250 mg orally four times daily) for methicillin-susceptible strains, or doxycycline (100 mg three times daily for 10 days) or clindamycin (300 mg three times daily for 10 days) for methicillin-resistant strains. None of these treatments prevents post-streptococcal glomerulonephritis.

For *erysipelas*, treatment is with oral penicillin (e.g., penicillin VK 250 four times daily for 10 days) or, if methicillin-sensitive *S. aureus* is of concern, oral dicloxacillin (500 mg four times daily) for a 10 day course. Surgical debridement is not indicated. Fever, pain, and the intense redness typically diminish promptly, but the swelling may progress temporarily despite treatment. About 5-10 days into the illness, the involved skin typically desquamates.

For cellulitis, oral antibiotic regimens are often as effective as intravenous regimens.[A3] Penicillin VK (250 to 500 mg four times daily for 10 days) is usually effective in treatment of streptococcal cellulitis. In situations where it is difficult to differentiate between streptococcal and staphylococcal skin and soft tissue infections, a penicillinase-resistant penicillin can be used. Options include oral cephalexin[A4] (500 mg four times daily for 10 to 14 days), clindamycin (300 to 450 mg four times daily for 10 days) or trimethoprim-sulfamethoxazole (160/800 mg twice daily for 10 days),[A5,A6] depending on the suspected pathogens, the host, and the severity of systemic toxicity. Intravenous vancomycin plus intravenous ceftazidime (15 mg/kg twice daily and 0.5 to 1 g three times daily, respectively, until clinical response allows transition to oral medications) can be reserved for severe cases. In penicillin-allergic patients, a first-generation cephalosporin may be used if hypersensitivity is not of the immediate type. Clindamycin, linezolid, or vancomycin may be used in patients who manifest anaphylactic hypersensitivity to β-lactam antibiotics. Penicillin (250 mg twice daily) is effective for preventing recurrent cellulitis.[A7]

Uncomplicated bacteremia is treated with intravenous penicillin (3 to 4 million units every 4 hours). Initial empiric antibiotic treatment for *necrotizing fasciitis* should be broad to cover for possible polymicrobial infection with vancomycin or linezolid plus piperacillin-tazobactam or a carbapenem, or plus ceftriaxone and metronidazole. Once a group A streptococcal necrotizing fasciitis is confirmed, antibiotics can be changed to penicillin plus clindamycin. Treatment recommendations for *myonecrosis* are the same as those for necrotizing fasciitis, including surgical intervention and antibiotics.

Pneumonia can be treated with amoxicillin-clavulanic acid (300-125 mg every 6 hours for 5 to 7 days) or levofloxacin (750 mg daily), moxifloxacin (400 mg daily), or gatifloxacin (320 mg daily) for 5 days. For hospital-acquired pneumonia, more aggressive regimens are required.

For *toxic shock syndrome*, management involves prompt and aggressive source control including surgical exploration and debridement of suspected deep-seated streptococcal infections. Fluid resuscitation and early antimicrobial therapy are mandatory. Empirical broad-spectrum antimicrobial coverage for septic shock should be initially instituted.[11] Once the etiology of *S. pyogenes* is confirmed, treatment with both IV penicillin G (3 to 4 million units every 4 hours) and IV clindamycin (600 to 900 mg every 8 hours for 10 to 15 days), followed by oral therapy is recommended. This recommendation is based largely on (1) studies in experimental animals and some reports in humans demonstrating clindamycin is more efficacious than penicillin in treating necrotizing fasciitis and myonecrosis and (2) the fact that, until recently, clindamycin resistance has rarely been reported. The superior efficacy of clindamycin has been attributed to its ability to suppress production of key *S. pyogenes* virulence factors and to the fact that, unlike penicillin, its mechanism of action is not dependent on the physiologic state of the organism. In addition, some reports show that clindamycin suppresses pro-inflammatory cytokine production by human mononuclear cells, and thus could mitigate the cytokine storm responsible for the systemic manifestations of toxic shock syndromes.[12] Penicillin is included in the current treatment recommendation largely because *S. pyogenes* remain universally susceptible *in vitro* and to cover potential clindamycin resistance. Routine secondary prophylaxis against streptococcal infection is not recommended for household contacts of index patients. Chemoprophylaxis can be considered in contacts with underlying host risk factors on a case-by-case basis.

Acute Rheumatic Fever and Rheumatic Heart Disease

Acute rheumatic fever (ARF) is a result of an autoimmune response to group A streptococcal infection. Rheumatic heart disease (RHD) is the long-term sequela of a single episode or repeated episodes of ARF (Chapter 66). The incidence of ARF and RHD is low in developed countries but continues to cause significant disease burden in resource-poor nations and in populations with crowded living conditions and poor access to health care. In these areas, untreated superficial *S. pyogenes* infections such as pharyngitis can lead to subsequent development of ARF. It is difficult to determine the incidence of ARF because diagnostic tools are lacking in many settings. In 2015, global estimates suggest that there were 33.4 million cases of RHD and 319,400 deaths; the highest prevalence of RHD and the highest age-standardized mortality due to RHD were found in Oceania, South Asia, and central sub-Saharan Africa.[13]

Acute Rheumatic Fever

ARF occurs most often in children 5 to 15 years of age.[14] Because RHD is often the result of recurrent infections and cumulative damage to heart valves, the peak prevalence of RHD is in the third and fourth decades of life. ARF occurs equally in men and women, but RHD is more common in women.

ARF develops approximately 2 weeks after the acute streptococcal infection, and symptoms usually last 2 to 4 weeks. Manifestations of ARF include fever (>90%), large-joint polyarthritis (75%), carditis (>50%), chorea (30%), subcutaneous nodules (<10%), and erythema marginatum (<10%). NSAIDs reduce arthritis pain rapidly, and the absence of symptomatic improvement with NSAIDs should prompt the clinician to think of other causes for the arthritis. The synovial fluid in ARF is sterile with a lymphocyte predominance. ARF can affect all parts of the heart, but the most clinically significant involvement is valvulitis of the mitral valve and, less frequently, of the aortic valve leading initially to valvular regurgitation (Chapter 66). Patients develop characteristic heart murmurs, and an echocardiogram should be considered to confirm clinical findings. The chorea (Sydenham chorea, St. Vitus dance) of ARF is characterized by involuntary, nonrhythmic, and purposeless movements of the body, limbs, and face. The chorea is usually more pronounced on one side of the body. The chorea stops during sleep. Erythema marginatum

---

TABLE 274-3	REVISED JONES CRITERIA FOR ACUTE RHEUMATIC FEVER

A. DEFINITION

Initial ARF	2 major or 1 major plus 2 minor criteria
Recurrent	2 major, or 1 major and 2 minor, or 3 minor

B. MAJOR CRITERIA

LOW-RISK POPULATIONS*	MODERATE- AND HIGH-RISK POPULATIONS
Carditis, clinical and/or subclinical echocardiographic valvulitis	Carditis, clinical and/or subclinical echocardiographic valvulitis
Arthritis, polyarticular	Arthritis, monoarticular or polyarticular
Chorea	Chorea
Erythema marginatum	Erythema marginatum
Subcutaneous nodules	Subcutaneous nodules

C. MINOR CRITERIA

LOW-RISK POPULATIONS	MODERATE- AND HIGH-RISK POPULATIONS
Polyarthralgia	Monoarthralgia
Fever ≥38.5° C	Fever ≥38.5° C
ESR ≥60 mm and/or CRP ≥3.0 mg/dL	ESR ≥30 mm and/or CRP ≥3.0 mg/dL
Prolonged PR interval (unless carditis is a major criterion)	Prolonged PR interval (unless carditis is a major criterion)

*Low-risk populations are those with an ARF incidence of <2 per 100,000 school-aged children per year or an all-age prevalence of rheumatic heart disease of ≤1 per 1000 population per year.
ARF = acute rheumatic fever; CRP = C-reactive protein; ESR = erythrocyte sedimentation rate.
Adapted from: Gewitz MH, Baltimore RS, Tani LY, et al. Revision of the Jones Criteria for the diagnosis of acute rheumatic fever in the era of Doppler echocardiography: a scientific statement from the American Heart Association. *Circulation.* 2015; 131(20):1806-1818.

---

is characterized by pink, nonpruritic, blanching macules or papules that spread in a serpiginous pattern on the trunk and proximal limbs. When subcutaneous nodules occur, they are usually 0.5 to 2 cm in diameter, painless, and present over bony prominences or extensor tendons. Rapid sleeping pulse rate and tachycardia out of proportion to fever are occasionally observed in ARF. Inflammatory markers are usually elevated, and the electrocardiogram may show a prolonged PR interval. Normochromic, normocytic anemia and leukocytosis are common.

There is no definitive test for ARF. Diagnosis relies on patients fulfilling a set of criteria, the most commonly used of which are the Jones criteria (Table 274-3).[15] These underwent a revision in 2015 to expand their applicability to low- and high-risk populations. For the purposes of the Jones criteria, low-risk populations were defined as those with an ARF incidence of less than 2 per 100,000 school-aged children per year or an all-age prevalence of RHD of less than or equal to 1 per 1000 population per year. In the Jones criteria for low-risk populations, the criteria focus on high specificity to avoid false-positive diagnosis. In populations with higher risk for ARF, the Jones criteria emphasize high sensitivity to reduce false-negative diagnoses.

The pathophysiology of ARF is not entirely understood. Tissue injury is mediated through an immune mechanism that is initiated by molecular mimicry. Similarities between the infectious agent and human protein lead to cross-activation of antibodies and T cells to human tissue. Carditis results from antibody-binding and T-cell infiltration of the heart; transient arthritis is due to immune complexes in the joints; chorea results from antibody binding to the basal ganglia; and skin manifestations are a result of delayed hypersensitivity reactions.

Management of ARF begins with careful assessment to rule out other causes of symptoms. ARF is a diagnosis of exclusion. Persons with ARF should be hospitalized. Eradication of group A streptococcus from the throat and secondary prophylaxis should be accomplished with intramuscular benzathine penicillin G every 4 weeks for a minimum of 10 years (and in some cases indefinitely). Other, less favorable and less effective options include oral penicillin, oral sulfadiazine, or an oral macrolide (for penicillin- and sulfa-allergic patients). First-line therapy for joint symptoms has traditionally been aspirin. Naproxen and ibuprofen have been used in small studies with success. Treatment with an NSAID should continue until all symptoms of ARF have resolved, not just the joint symptoms. This usually takes 1 to 2 weeks. Carditis is managed by treating the associated heart failure with diuretics, fluid restriction, and bed rest. In severe cases, some experts recommend use of systemic glucocorticoids even though high-quality evidence is lacking. Valve surgery is rarely needed for ARF, though it can be helpful in situations of acute rupture of a valve leaflet. Rheumatic chorea usually does not require treatment and resolves within weeks to months.

Rheumatic Heart Disease

Approximately 35 to 72% of patients with ARF develop clinical carditis, and another 18% have carditis present on echocardiogram without clinical symptoms.[16] Some individuals with carditis have complete resolution of cardiac abnormalities, and others go on to develop RHD. Resolution of carditis is most likely to occur in the first year after the acute carditis.

RHD, unlike ARF, which is a pancarditis, is almost exclusively a valvular pathology (Chapter 66).[17] RHD affects the mitral valve nearly 100% of the time and the aortic valve in 20 to 30% of cases. The pulmonic valve is rarely involved, and the tricuspid valve has histologic evidence of disease in 15 to 40% of patients, but the tricuspid valve disease is not usually clinically relevant. Echocardiography is used to evaluate for RHD. Mitral valve regurgitation is the most common valvular pathology in RHD. Mitral stenosis can also occur after progressive scarring of the mitral valve leaflets. RHD is the most common cause of mitral stenosis worldwide. When the aortic valve is involved, regurgitation is more common than stenosis. Persons with RHD should receive secondary prophylaxis as outlined previously with intramuscular benzathine penicillin G. Recurrent ARF can worsen RHD and is best avoided.

Pediatric Autoimmune Neuropsychiatric Disorders Associated with Streptococcal Infections

Group A streptococcal infections are hypothesized to be related to the acute onset of obsessive-compulsive disorder (OCD) and tics in children.[18] This phenomenon is termed pediatric autoimmune neuropsychiatric disorders associated with streptococcal infections (PANDAS). PANDAS is a subtype of pediatric acute-onset neuropsychiatric syndrome (PANS). PANS is OCD that presents with abrupt onset or the exacerbation of existing neuropsychiatric symptoms, including OCD, in children. Not all PANS cases are associated with streptococcal infection, but all PANDAS cases are associated, at least temporally, with streptococcal infection. Though controversial, PANDAS is defined as acute onset of OCD, tics, and piano-playing choreiform movements of the fingers and toes in children after streptococcal infection. Sometimes enuresis, separation anxiety, learning regression, and handwriting difficulties are also present. *S. pyogenes* infection appears to trigger development of antibrain autoantibodies to dopamine receptors, leading to neuropsychiatric symptoms in some individuals. There is no known treatment for PANDAS, but antibiotics for primary management and for secondary prevention of recurrent infections are under study.

Post-Streptococcal Glomerulonephritis

Post-streptococcal glomerulonephritis is a post-infectious, immune complex–mediated glomerulonephritis associated with prior skin or throat infection by group A streptococcus or occasionally groups C or G streptococcus. (Also see Chapter 113.) Immune complexes form in the glomeruli and invoke an inflammatory response, including activation of the complement system with reduction in circulating C3 levels. Historically, the typical patient with post-streptococcal glomerulonephritis is a child between ages 2 and 18 years with a male-to-female ratio of 2 : 1. The time between the initial streptococcal infection and nephritis is 7 to 10 days after throat infection and 2 to 4 weeks after skin infection. Post-streptococcal glomerulonephritis most commonly presents as nephritic syndrome with hematuria, edema, hypertension, and oliguria. Rarely, the presentation is of nephrotic syndrome or rapidly progressive crescentic glomerulonephritis. In typical cases, the symptoms resolve within 2 to 7 days. Asymptomatic disease is likely four to five times more common than clinically evident disease and manifests as microscopic hematuria and a fall in serum complement levels. In elderly individuals with post-streptococcal glomerulonephritis, azotemia, heart failure, and nephrotic-range proteinuria are more common than in children.

Post-streptococcal glomerulonephritis, like other postinfectious complications of streptococcal infection, is rare in developed countries. In developing countries, however, the annual incidence of disease is approximately nine cases per 100,000 population. The short-term prognosis in children is excellent, but adults have early mortality, in part owing to cardiovascular and other comorbid disease. Long-term development of end-stage renal disease is uncommon unless other contributors to renal disease (e.g., diabetes mellitus) are present.

Serologic assays for antibodies to *S. pyogenes* antigens such as SLO and DNase B are useful for retrospective diagnosis of antecedent *S. pyogenes*

infections in cases of suspected post-streptococcal glomerulonephritis. The rise in antibodies occurs 7 to 14 days after disease onset and peaks 3 to 4 weeks after infection. Renal biopsy is rarely necessary, but it should be considered when there is diagnostic doubt.

TREATMENT   Rx

If streptococcal infection is still present at the time of post-streptococcal glomerulonephritis diagnosis, the infection should be treated. In situations of post-streptococcal glomerulonephritis epidemics, preventative antibiotics for household contacts have been shown to reduce the number of cases of post-streptococcal glomerulonephritis. Otherwise, treatment of post-streptococcal glomerulonephritis is supportive, with treatment of volume overload and hypertension with loop diuretics, salt restriction, and antihypertensive agents.

STREPTOCOCCUS AGALACTIAE (GROUP B STREPTOCOCCUS)

DEFINITION

Streptococcus agalactiae contains Lancefield group B antigen on the cell surface and thus is referred to as group B streptococci. *S. agalactiae* was first identified as a cause of bovine mastitis. Group B streptococci colonize the genital tract, gastrointestinal tract, and occasionally the upper respiratory tracts of normal humans. In the laboratory, these organisms grow as gray-white colonies that are slightly larger than for group A streptococci but cause a narrower zone of hemolysis. They demonstrate a positive CAMP test and hydrolyze sodium hippurate, but they are not sensitive to bacitracin and do not hydrolyze bile esculin. Definitive bacteriologic identification requires group-specific antiserum or commercial kits. The polysaccharide capsule, which is the prime virulence factor in group B streptococcus, is critical for the organism to evade phagocytosis. Defined capsular polysaccharide types of group B streptococcus are designated Ia, Ib, Ic, and II through IX. Immunity is based on the development of opsonic type-specific antibody.

EPIDEMIOLOGY AND CLINICAL MANIFESTATIONS

Group B streptococci cause infection in neonates, pregnant women, and nonpregnant adults, especially the elderly and those with diabetes and other underlying medical disease.[19] In neonates, group B streptococci are the most common cause of pneumonia, sepsis, and meningitis in the United States and Western Europe. According to 2015 CDC estimates, the incidence of early and late-onset invasive group B streptococcus disease combined was 0.53 cases per 1000 live births. Group B streptococcus infection in neonates is caused by vertical transmission and classified by age at onset. Early-onset group B streptococcus infection usually presents at or within 24 hours of birth but can occur anytime in the first 6 days of life. Adults with group B streptococcus infections include postpartum women and patients who have risk factors such as diabetes, liver disease, peripheral vascular disease, or malignancy. The most common clinical manifestations are soft tissue infection, osteomyelitis, and septic arthritis. In 2015, the CDC estimated 8.9 cases of invasive group B streptococcus infection per 100,000 population in the United States, including neonates, children, and adults.

PREVENTION

Passive immunization (using intravenous immune globulin) and active immunization (using multivalent polysaccharide vaccine) have been promising in clinical trials[A8] and may eventually be clinically useful to prevent group B streptococcus neonatal sepsis and postpartum maternal infection. At this time, no licensed vaccine is available. In the interim, the current approach to the prevention of group B streptococcus infection is to provide intrapartum antimicrobial prophylaxis in women with prior delivery of an infant with invasive group B streptococcus infection, group B streptococcus bacteriuria during current pregnancy, culture evidence of vaginal or rectal group B streptococcus colonization, or unknown group B streptococcus status and either delivery before 37 weeks of gestation, duration of ruptured membranes of at least 18 hours, or intrapartum temperature of at least 100.4° F (≥38° C). All women at 35 to 37 weeks of gestation should be screened with rectal and vaginal swab for the presence of group B streptococcus unless some other indication for prophylaxis already exists. Prophylaxis is with penicillin or ampicillin. Both have been shown effective in reducing early-onset group B streptococcus infection. In persons with penicillin allergy, group B streptococcus susceptibility testing for clindamycin and erythromycin is recommended. When susceptibility testing is not available or if the group B streptococcus is resistant to clindamycin and erythromycin, vancomycin can be used.

TREATMENT Rx

Penicillin is the treatment of choice for group B streptococcus infections. Alternatives for penicillin-allergic patients include first-generation cephalosporins or vancomycin. Clindamycin or erythromycin can be used in penicillin-allergic patients when group B streptococcus susceptibility is known, but resistance is nearly 40% for clindamycin and 50% for erythromycin in some settings. Gentamicin can be used in addition to penicillin in persons with meningitis, endocarditis, bacteremia, and severe soft tissue infections until the infection is under control.

STREPTOCOCCUS DYSGALACTIAE SUBSPECIES *EQUISIMILIS* (GROUP C AND GROUP G STREPTOCOCCUS)

The group C and group G streptococci that colonize the human genital tract, gastrointestinal tract, upper respiratory tract, and skin belong to a single subspecies, *S. dysgalactiae* subspecies *equisimilis*. They produce streptolysin O and a disease spectrum that resembles group A streptococci, including bacteremia, septic arthritis, skin and soft tissue infection, and pharyngitis.

TREATMENT Rx

Treatment is with penicillin or other β-lactam antibiotics with or without concomitant low-dose gentamicin. As with group A streptococcal infection, clindamycin is used for *S. dysgalactiae* subspecies *equisimilis* infection for necrotizing fasciitis or streptococcal toxic shock syndrome. Clindamycin should not be used initially as a single agent, however, because some *S. dysgalactiae* subspecies *equisimilis* are resistant to clindamycin. *S. dysgalactiae* subspecies *equisimilis* may also be resistant to macrolides (15 to 25% of cases) or fluoroquinolones, limiting the utility of these antibiotics unless susceptibilities are known.

VIRIDANS GROUP STREPTOCOCCI (*STREPTOCOCCUS ANGINOSUS* GROUP/*STREPTOCOCCUS MILLERI* GROUP)

Viridans group streptococci include the *S. anginosus* group (also known as the *Streptococcus milleri* group). The *S. anginosus* group has three distinct species: *S. anginosus, Streptococcus constellatus*, and *S. intermedius*. Members of the *S. anginosus* group are nonmotile, facultative anaerobes that may be β-hemolytic but may also be α-hemolytic or nonhemolytic. *S. anginosus* group normally colonize the oropharynx, upper gastrointestinal tract, and appendix. Unlike *S. pyogenes* and *S. agalactiae*, *S. anginosus* group can cause abscess formation. Abscesses usually develop contiguous to the colonized mucosal surface as with dental or periappendiceal abscesses. Patients may develop primary bacteremia, with or without endocarditis, which then can seed metastatic abscesses of the lung, joints, bone, and spleen. *S. intermedius* has tropism to form abscesses in the brain and liver. In patients with oral, head and neck, and abdominal infections, *S. anginosus* group may present as part of a polymicrobial infection and should be considered a true pathogen. Empyema with *S. anginosus* group is usually the result of a surgical procedure involving the respiratory or gastrointestinal tract and in most cases requires thoracotomy due to loculation of the empyema and difficulty treating with antibiotics and chest thoracostomy alone. In reviewing Gram stains of pus from such infections, these organisms characteristically show 20 to 30 gram-positive cocci within neutrophils.

TREATMENT Rx

Treatment of *S. anginosus* group is typically drainage of any abscess and therapy with penicillin or another β-lactam antibiotic because most isolates are susceptible to β-lactam agents. A parenteral third-generation cephalosporin is recommended for brain abscesses and bacteremia. Vancomycin is a reasonable alternative for penicillin-allergic patients. Resistance to fluoroquinolones, if not present initially, may develop rapidly. Many strains are developing macrolide resistance, most are resistant to aminoglycosides, and sulfonamides have no activity against *S. anginosus* group strains. *S. anginosus* is a reservoir for antimicrobial resistance genes and has been shown to transfer resistance traits to other pathogenic organisms such as *S. pyogenes* and *S. pneumoniae*.

Other Viridans Group Streptococci

In total there are more than 30 recognized species of viridans group streptococci, including *Streptococcus mitis, Streptococcus oralis, Streptococcus sanguinis* (formerly *sanguis*), *Streptococcus mutans*, and *Streptococcus gordonii*. They are most commonly implicated in subacute bacterial endocarditis; catheter-related and neutropenia-related bloodstream infections; and purulent abdominal, hepatobiliary, brain, and dental infections. Penicillin resistance in these organisms is 30 to 50% in some areas, so empirical treatment usually begins with vancomycin and de-escalates to a β-lactam if the isolate is susceptible.

ZOONOTIC STREPTOCOCCUS
Streptococcus suis

Streptococcus suis (Lancefield groups R, S, and T) is a pathogen in pigs that can cause meningitis, sepsis, and arthritis in exposed humans. Most infections occur in individuals with extensive exposure to pigs, such as pig breeders, abattoir workers, and butchers. In this high-risk group of individuals, the annual risk for developing *S. suis* meningitis has been estimated at 1.2 to 3 cases per 100,000 population. *S. suis* is susceptible to penicillin, third-generation cephalosporins, and vancomycin. In persons with meningitis due to *S. suis*, steroid treatment in addition to antimicrobials may help reduce death and disability including hearing loss.[20] Wearing gloves for the handling of raw pork, good hand hygiene, and thorough cooking of pork should prevent most cases of *S. suis* infection.

Streptococcus canis

Streptococcus canis (Lancefield group G) is most commonly isolated from dogs, but it has been isolated also from cats, harbor porpoises, cows, mice, rats, and rabbits. Soft tissue infections and sepsis have occurred in humans, but infection is rare. Treatment is with a β-lactam antibiotic such as penicillin.

Streptococcus bovis/equinus Group (Including Streptococcus gallolyticus Subspecies gallolyticus and Streptococcus infantarius)

Streptococcus bovis/equinus complex bacteria are Lancefield group D nonenterococcal streptococci that colonize the intestines in 10% of healthy individuals. The *S. bovis/equinus* complex bacteria are associated with hepatobiliary disease, meningitis, and most infamously subacute endocarditis in the setting of colorectal carcinoma.[21] The *S. bovis/equinus* complex underwent reclassification in 2003 to *Streptococcus gallolyticus* subspecies *gallolyticus*, *S. gallolyticus* subspecies *pasteurianus*, *S. gallolyticus* subspecies *macedonicus*, and *S. infantarius*. Both *S. gallolyticus* and *S. infantarius* are highly sensitive to penicillin.

Streptococcus iniae

Streptococcus iniae is a β-hemolytic streptococcus without a Lancefield group antigen. It causes significant disease in fish, especially tilapia. Human infection results from the handling of live or killed fish. Skin and soft tissue infections are most common and often lead to bacteremia. Treatment is with a β-lactam antibiotic.

Grade A References

A1. van Driel ML, De Sutter AI, Habraken H, et al. Different antibiotic treatments for group A streptococcal pharyngitis. *Cochrane Database Syst Rev.* 2016;9:CD004406.

A2. Koning S, van der Sande R, Verhagen AP, et al. Interventions for impetigo. *Cochrane Database Syst Rev.* 2012;1:CD003261.

A3. Aboltins CA, Hutchinson AF, Sinnappu RN, et al. Oral versus parenteral antimicrobials for the treatment of cellulitis: a randomized non-inferiority trial. *J Antimicrob Chemother.* 2015;70:581-586.

A4. Pallin DJ, Binder WD, Allen MB, et al. Clinical trial: comparative effectiveness of cephalexin plus trimethoprim-sulfamethoxazole versus cephalexin alone for treatment of uncomplicated cellulitis: a randomized controlled trial. *Clin Infect Dis.* 2013;56:1754-1762.

A5. Miller LG, Daum RS, Creech CB, et al. Clindamycin versus trimethoprim-sulfamethoxazole for uncomplicated skin infections. *N Engl J Med.* 2015;372:1093-1103.

A6. Talan DA, Mower WR, Krishnadasan A, et al. Trimethoprim-sulfamethoxazole versus placebo for uncomplicated skin abscess. *N Engl J Med.* 2016;374:823-832.

A7. Thomas KS, Crook AM, Nunn AJ, et al. Penicillin to prevent recurrent leg cellulitis. *N Engl J Med.* 2013;368:1695-1703.

A8. Madhi SA, Cutland CL, Jose L, et al. Safety and immunogenicity of an investigational maternal trivalent group B streptococcus vaccine in healthy women and their infants: a randomised phase 1b/2 trial. *Lancet Infect Dis.* 2016;16:923-934.

GENERAL REFERENCES

For the General References and other additional features, please visit Expert Consult at https://expertconsult.inkling.com.

275

ENTEROCOCCAL INFECTIONS

PATRICE SAVARD AND TRISH M. PERL

DEFINITION

Enterococci, formerly called group D streptococci, are endogenous human gut flora that had been considered pathogens with low virulence in the past. However, more recently, they have emerged as increasingly important health care–associated pathogens. This emergence is primarily because of their inherent resistance to commonly used antimicrobials, acquisition of high-level resistance to vancomycin and aminoglycosides, persistence in the environment, and transmission from patient to patient by way of the contaminated hands of health care workers. Hence, the emergence of vancomycin-resistant enterococci (VRE) has limited therapeutic options in confirmed enterococcal infections and in empirical therapy for infections in severely ill hospitalized patients and represents a challenge for infection control in the health care setting. This chapter reviews the most important clinical manifestations of enterococci and their diagnosis and the importance of infection prevention.

The Pathogen

Members of the genus *Enterococcus* were long classified within group D of the genus *Streptococcus*. However, in the past 30 years, they have been reclassified based on new molecular and genetic analyses. Enterococci are catalase-negative gram-positive cocci that can appear singly or in pairs or short chains. They are facultative anaerobes that grow optimally at 35° to 37° C and are usually α-hemolytic or nonhemolytic on sheep blood agar. Enterococci can grow in broth containing 6.5% NaCl and hydrolyze esculin in the presence of 40% bile salts (bile-esculin medium) that can distinguish them from most streptococci. *Enterococcus faecalis*, the most common cause of enterococcal infections in humans, is the causative agent for 80 to 90% of the enterococcal infections followed by *Enterococcus faecium*, which is found in 5 to 10% of the infections. *Enterococcus casseliflavus*, *Enterococcus gallinarum*, and *Enterococcus raffinosus* are less frequently associated with infections, but clusters of infections have been reported. Other species isolated from different sources in humans include *Enterococcus avium*, *Enterococcus caccae*, *Enterococcus cecorum*, *Enterococcus dispar*, *Enterococcus durans*, *Enterococcus gilvus*, *Enterococcus italicus*, *Enterococcus hirae*, *Enterococcus malodoratus*, *Enterococcus mundtii*, *Enterococcus pallens*, *Enterococcus pseudoavium*, and *Enterococcus sanguinicola*.

EPIDEMIOLOGY

Enterococci are part of the normal human gut flora, and infections in both hospitalized and nonhospitalized patients can arise from either an endogenous or exogenous source. The proportion of infections caused by enterococci in hospitalized patients has been increasing over the past several decades. Overall, urinary tract infections (UTIs) are the most common clinical condition caused by enterococci. Based on data reported between 2011 and 2014 to the Centers for Disease Control and Prevention (CDC), enterococcal species are now the second most common isolates for any health care–associated infection and the single most common cause of central line–associated blood stream infections (CLABSIs). Enterococci are also a prominent cause of catheter-associated UTIs and surgical site infections, causing approximately 15% of these health care–associated infections in North America (Chapter 266). In the community setting, enterococci cause both complicated and uncomplicated UTIs and are involved in approximately 5 to 15% of all cases of infective endocarditis. Outside of the United States, these organisms are less common but increasingly important causes of infections.

In the 1970s, *E. faecalis* accounted for up to 95% of isolates and was associated with the introduction of third-generation cephalosporins. Increasingly, hospitalized patients, if they are colonized or infected with an *Enterococcus* species, tend to have a strain resistant to vancomycin and sometimes ampicillin (i.e., VRE).[1] *E. faecium* is the most common strain to acquire vancomycin resistance. VRE was first reported in Europe in 1986. Since the mid-2000s, the proportion of enterococcal strains resistant to vancomycin, primarily *E. faecium*, has risen steadily. According to the CDC's National Healthcare Safety Network (NHSN), 82.2% of *E. faecium* isolates and 9.2% of *E. faecalis* isolates from CLABSIs were resistant to vancomycin in 2014.[2] Also, according to a recent report by the CDC on antimicrobial resistance in the United States, 66,000 *Enterococcus* health care–associated infections are reported yearly, and 20,000 of them are caused by VRE. There are two major genotypes for acquired vancomycin resistance, VanA and VanB. The genes encoding the VanA phenotype result in high-level resistance to vancomycin and teicoplanin and are carried on a plasmid or a conjugative transposon that is transferable. VanA is mostly found in *E. faecium* and, less frequently, in *E. faecalis*. VanB is associated with variable resistance to vancomycin, but isolates are usually susceptible to teicoplanin. VanA and VanB are rarely found in other enterococci whereas VanC is intrinsically recovered from *E. casseliflavus* and *E. gallinarum*. Importantly, these genetic elements have been integrated into the genome of *S. aureus* that is resistant to vancomycin. The vancomycin-resistant *S. aureus* (VRSA) acquired a vancomycin resistance gene (*VanA*) from a VRE isolate that colonized a patient coinfected with methicillin-resistant *S. aureus*.

The epidemiology of VRE differs between Europe and North America. In Europe, VRE is often detected in farm animals, likely because of the use of the antibiotic avoparcin in animal feeds until it was banned in 1997. In the United States, avoparcin was never used in animal feeds, and therefore VRE is not usually found in farm animals or healthy humans. The proportion of VRE among enterococcal clinical isolates in hospitalized Europeans has been historically lower than in the United States; however, these rates are increasing. According to the European Centre for Disease Prevention and Control (ECDC), 8.3% of invasive isolates of *E. faecium* reported in 2015 in Europe were resistant to vancomycin, but the prevalence of VRE varies widely among the European countries. As reported by the ECDC in 2017, the proportion of enterococcal isolates from hospitalized European patients that are highly resistant to vancomycin varies by geographic region from less than 1% in France to up to 45.8% in Ireland.

Most VRE infections are associated with health care and result from an exogenous source, meaning transmission from the environment, another patient, or on the hands of a health care worker. Nearly all infections are preceded by a period of colonization, primarily in the gastrointestinal (GI) tract. A study of hospitalized patients found that the most sensitive predictor of VRE colonization was previous admission to an acute care hospital in the past year. Importantly, after being colonized with VRE, patients may harbor the strain in their GI tract for years. Similarly, a study among hemodialysis patients demonstrated that the primary risk factor for VRE colonization was hospitalization in the prior year. Although many colonized patients do not develop infections, they are still able to contaminate the environment and shed and transmit bacteria to other hospitalized patients. The organism has a predilection to contaminate the hospital environment and equipment and has been associated with outbreaks.

Apart from preexisting GI colonization, risk factors for enterococcal infections, particularly VRE infections, include severe underlying conditions such as renal failure, previous solid organ or bone marrow transplantation, solid and hematologic malignancy, diabetes mellitus, and neutropenia. Other factors associated with infection include prior surgical or GI procedures, presence of a vascular or urinary indwelling catheter, hospital factors such as location in the intensive care unit (ICU) or oncology ward, proximity to colonized patients, prolonged length of hospitalization, and recent antimicrobial exposure.

Numerous epidemiologic investigations have revealed that most classes of antimicrobials have been associated with VRE infections. In particular, vancomycin, cephalosporins, and drugs with anaerobic organism coverage use have been linked to VRE acquisition. However, measuring the attributable impact of a particular antibiotic on VRE acquisition is difficult. Increasingly, an association between VRE colonization and *Clostridium difficile* infection is reported in high-risk patients such as those with hematologic malignancies.

PATHOBIOLOGY

Enterococci are commensal organisms that colonize the human GI tract and female genital tract. They contaminate and can also be recovered from the environment. Although they are not as intrinsically virulent as other gram-positive pathogens, under certain conditions the commensal relationship is disrupted, and serious infections occur. Several adhesion factors have been identified, including aggregation substance, which allow binding to epithelial surfaces and enhance the ability for colonization. The ability to adhere to heart valves and urinary tract epithelium enables enterococci to cause endocarditis and UTIs. Enterococci are also known to secrete potential virulence factors. These include cytolysin–hemolysin, which is a bacterial toxin that is produced in a higher proportion of infecting strains compared with stool-colonizing strains. Infecting strains also possess the ability of intestinal translocation, although the exact mechanisms of this process have yet to be determined. In addition, some cell surface determinants that are encoded may mediate adherence to host tissues that may be important in this organism's role in endocarditis. To this point, little is known about the host defense mechanisms in enterococcal infections. In addition, the exact role of capsular polysaccharides in colonization or infection is unknown. Strains have been shown to survive within phagocytic cells, yet it is unclear whether this represents successful host defense or evasion by the enterococci. The intrinsic resistance to multiple antimicrobials (including cephalosporins, clindamycin, trimethoprim-sulfamethoxazole, and low-level aminoglycosides) that enterococci possess, along with their ability to acquire resistance to a wide range of antibiotics (including high concentrations of penicillins, fluoroquinolones, tetracycline, nitrofurantoin, and glycopeptides) through mutation or acquisition of new genes, enhances their ability to survive and multiply in the many hospitalized patients treated with broad-spectrum antimicrobials.

CLINICAL MANIFESTATIONS

No specific clinical manifestations can help distinguish enterococcal infections from infections caused by other bacteria. Enterococci are not thought to cause lower respiratory tract infections and, if found in this setting, likely represent colonization and not infection. Enterococci act as opportunistic pathogens in severely ill and compromised patients. They are known to cause UTIs, intra-abdominal abscesses, wound infection, bacteremia (including central line–associated blood stream infections), and endocarditis.

Urinary Tract Infections

Urinary tract infections are the most frequent type of infection caused by enterococci.[3] Most infections are nosocomial in origin and include uncomplicated cystitis, pyelonephritis, prostatitis, and perinephric abscess. These infections are typically secondary to urinary catheterization or instrumentation. In contrast to health care–associated UTI, enterococci cause fewer than 5% of uncomplicated cystitis or pyelonephritis cases in otherwise healthy non-hospitalized women. Patients with diabetes mellitus appear to be at increased risk for enterococcal UTI. Bacteremia is only infrequently associated with enterococcal UTI.

Bacteremia

Importantly, enterococci can cause infection or contaminate cultured blood via contaminated catheter hubs and contaminated skin. Determining a true bacteremia versus a blood culture that is not clinically significant can be a challenge. Given this backdrop, the incidence of bacteremia caused by enterococci continues to increase. Specific risk factors include prolonged hospitalization, preexisting urethral catheters or intravascular lines, recent surgery, malignancy, neutropenia, and biliary pathology. Secondary bacteremia without endocarditis usually arises from the urinary tract, hepatobiliary tract, or soft tissue infection. Bacteremia secondary to an intra-abdominal source carries a high mortality rate. Risk factors for VRE bacteremia parallel those mentioned previously but additionally include severe preexisting comorbid conditions, including hematologic malignancy, human immunodeficiency virus (HIV) infection, chronic renal insufficiency, and liver transplantation. Prior exposure to broad-spectrum antimicrobials, including those with antianaerobic activity

such as clindamycin or metronidazole, and exposure to multiple and prolonged antimicrobial therapy are consistent risk factors. Enterococcal bacteremia is frequently polymicrobial, and the clinical picture is often influenced by whether it is isolated alone or with other bacteria. When enterococci are isolated alone, the course is typically indolent, and frequently fever is the only sign. In contrast, polymicrobial bacteremia is more severe, often presenting with shock or disseminated intravascular coagulation. VRE bacteremia is associated with higher mortality rates than bacteremia caused by vancomycin-susceptible strains, and early treatment with an appropriate antibiotic within the first 48 hours of presentation has been associated with improved outcomes.

Endocarditis

Enterococci, particularly *E. faecalis,* are an increasingly frequent cause of endocarditis and represent approximately 10% of cases in non–intravenous drug users. Recent reports suggest that 50% of patients with *E. faecalis* endocarditis who undergo endoscopy have a colorectal neoplasm discovered.[4] The disease occurs most frequently in older patients, with a male predominance. Most cases appear to arise in the community. Patients with preexisting valvular heart disease, including prosthetic valves, are at highest risk, yet many patients lack underlying heart disease. Enterococci more commonly cause left-sided endocarditis primarily affecting the mitral valve. Clinically, these patients present with symptoms that closely resemble a subacute bacterial endocarditis caused by viridans streptococci. Many patients have symptoms for weeks or months before seeking medical care.

Intra-abdominal Infections

In intra-abdominal infections, enterococci are often detected as part of a polymicrobial process. These infections typically arise from a hepatobiliary source, including postoperative infection in liver transplantation, and are complicated by secondary bacteremia.

Skin and Soft Tissue Infections

Enterococci rarely cause cellulitis or other soft tissue infections alone but are often isolated in mixed surgical site infections, diabetic foot infections, and decubitus ulcers along with other gram-negative bacilli, gram-positive cocci, and anaerobic bacteria. Their clinical significance in these situations has not been adequately determined. Enterococci are not thought to be primary pathogens in chronic osteomyelitis. When they are identified, it is thought they may solely represent superinfection, and thus adequate therapy may not require antibiotics directed at enterococcal eradication.

DIAGNOSIS

The diagnosis of an *Enterococcus* infection is made by isolating the organism through culture of a sterile site, such as blood or urine. Recently, molecular techniques have been developed to identify *Enterococcus* more quickly. The diagnosis and differential diagnosis of specific conditions are the same as discussed for UTIs (Chapter 268) and endocarditis (Chapter 67).

TREATMENT   Rx

Therapy for enterococcal infections is complicated by the fact that strains exhibit inherent resistance to many commonly used antibiotics, including cephalosporins. In addition, enterococci can acquire resistance to a wide range of antibiotic classes, including aminoglycosides (high-level resistance), β-lactams, fluoroquinolones, and vancomycin. Thus, effective directed therapy for any severe enterococcal infection requires susceptibility testing by experienced microbiology laboratories, with therapy adjusted based on the results. Optimal therapy for most infections includes intravenous ampicillin, penicillin, or vancomycin. Given the resistance or tolerance to cell wall–targeting antibiotics, including penicillins and vancomycin, standard therapy with these antibiotics, except in UTIs, should include the addition of a synergistic aminoglycoside (i.e., gentamicin or streptomycin), as long as high-level resistance is not detected in the microbiology laboratory. Of note, neither tobramycin nor kanamycin showed synergistic activity against enterococci. This strategy of two-drug therapy has been associated with improved outcomes.[5] This is particularly important in the setting of suspected endocarditis. Recently, there has been increasing isolation of *E. faecium* strains with intrinsic resistance to penicillins. Still, most *E. faecalis* strains remain susceptible to ampicillin and the related piperacillin, in contrast to most *E. faecium* strains, which are resistant to ampicillin. Even when enterococcus appears susceptible to trimethoprim–sulfamethoxazole in vitro, it should not be used in therapy because clinical failures have been reported secondary to the ability of enterococci to use exogenous folate. Similarly, *E.*

faecalis is intrinsically resistant to quinupristin–dalfopristin, which therefore should not be used in therapy for infections caused by this species, as opposed to *E. faecium*, which remains susceptible to that drug. The recently FDA-approved lipoglycopeptide antibiotics (oritavancin and dalbavancin) are active against vancomycin-susceptible enterococci.

If the VRE strains are known to be susceptible, potential therapy in these infections includes linezolid, tigecycline, and daptomycin. Linezolid is commonly the drug of choice,[A1] although its use is associated with bone marrow suppression, including thrombocytopenia, and has only bacteriostatic activity against the enterococci. Linezolid, when used in combination with selective serotonin re-uptake inhibitors, can be associated with serotonin syndrome (Chapter 406). The newer oxazolidinone, tedizolid, showed activity against enterococci but clinical data are lacking. Although daptomycin is not approved by the U.S. Food and Drug Administration (FDA) to treat VRE, it treats skin and soft tissue infections and bacteremia.[6] Tigecycline is FDA approved to treat complicated skin and soft tissue infections and complicated intra-abdominal infections caused by vancomycin-susceptible isolates of *E. faecalis,* but a recent black box warning by the FDA limits its use. Nitrofurantoin remains an option for VRE UTIs. Given the complexity of enterococcal infections, an infectious disease consult should be considered for therapeutic guidance.

Urinary Tract Infections

A single agent can usually be used to treat enterococcal UTIs, including ampicillin, amoxicillin, penicillin, quinolones, fosfomycin, or vancomycin (E-Table 275-1). Vancomycin is typically reserved for penicillin-allergic patients or if the strain has high-level penicillin/ampicillin resistance. β-Lactam–β-lactamase inhibitor combinations are usually reserved for polymicrobial infections. Nitrofurantoin is also occasionally used because most strains remain susceptible. Fosfomycin is also indicated for UTIs caused by susceptible *E. faecalis.*

Bacteremia without Endocarditis

Many cases of enterococcal bacteremia are transient or self-limited, but antibiotic therapy with penicillin or ampicillin has been shown to improve outcomes (see E-Table 275-1), especially when instituted within 48 hours.[7] A prospective, observational, cohort study of daptomycin treatment of daptomycin-susceptible VRE blood stream infections showed that higher daptomycin doses (≥9 mg/kg) were associated with lower mortality than in those who received doses <7 mg/kg.[8] Unlike in endocarditis therapy, it is not known whether patients benefit from combination therapy (penicillin or ampicillin or vancomycin plus an aminoglycoside), except perhaps when an indwelling intravascular catheter is present. In the setting of an indwelling intravascular catheter, especially for VRE, removal of the catheter is indicated. If the bacteremia is secondary to another site such as an intra-abdominal abscess, drainage of the source is critical to cure.

Endocarditis

Combination therapy (intravenous penicillin, ampicillin, or vancomycin plus an aminoglycoside) with bactericidal activity to sterilize vegetations is the standard therapy for enterococcal endocarditis. Importantly, the aminoglycoside is used to provide synergistic killing of the organism. Another synergistic combination described for patients not tolerating aminoglycosides includes ampicillin plus ceftriaxone to treat *E. faecalis* endocarditis: it is hypothesized that complementary saturation of penicillin binding protein (PBP) by both antibiotics is a key mechanism. Cephalosporins bind to both PBP 2 and 3 at low concentrations whereas ampicillin binds to PBP 4 and 5, and the combination of ampicillin plus ceftriaxone is an attractive treatment option.[9] Also, in vitro studies suggest that ampicillin and ceftaroline show synergistic activity when combined with daptomycin compared to daptomycin monotherapy. Doses and durations are found in Chapter 67 and E-Table 275-1, but recent evidence suggests it is safe to switch from intravenous to oral medications after 10 days of therapy,[A2] and consultation with infectious diseases experts is generally indicated. The duration of therapy is typically 4 to 6 weeks with longer therapy given to patients who had prolonged symptoms before seeking therapy, prosthetic valve infection, or relapsed after initial treatment. If the causative enterococcal strain is highly resistant to both gentamicin and streptomycin, then alternative agents and durations must be explored, and surgery to excise infected valves should be considered. Optimal therapy of VRE strains that are resistant to ampicillin is not known but includes combination therapy under the guidance of an infectious diseases consultant. Several newly approved agents, including linezolid (not FDA approved for endocarditis treatment), and daptomycin (not FDA approved for enterococcal infections) could be considered if the strain is found to be susceptible. VRE endocarditis may require early surgery because outcomes with antibiotic therapy alone can be poor. Careful microbiologic and clinical assessment of all patients with enterococcal endocarditis and VRE in particular is helpful in deciding when surgery is necessary. If repeated blood cultures grow for more than 7 days after the initiation of medical therapy or other signs of uncontrolled infection (persistent fever or leukocytosis) are present, surgical repair of the valve or valve replacement should be considered early in the treatment course if there are no absolute contraindications for surgery. Detailed recommendations on the management of endocarditis can be found in the guidelines published by the American Heart Association and endorsed by the Infectious Diseases Society of America (IDSA) in 2016.[10]

Of note, linezolid resistance is increasingly reported even in patients without previous exposure to the antibiotic. Daptomycin resistance is also reported in both *E. faecalis* and *E. faecium* after prolonged courses of therapy.

PRIMARY PREVENTION

Optimal infection prevention for VRE, similar to many multidrug-resistant bacteria, includes proper use and compliance with hand hygiene, use of contact precautions, cohorting of colonized patients, proper management and timely removal of urinary and vascular catheters, reduction of antibiotic selective pressure through antimicrobial stewardship, and environmental cleaning of equipment and patient rooms. The latter is particularly important for VRE. A study in a U.S. hospital's medical ICU found that the number of patients already colonized with VRE in a defined geographic area ("colonization pressure") was the most significant variable in predicting new acquisition of VRE. Hence, decontamination of patients' skin, called source control, may broadly control transmission of resistant pathogens and reduce device-related infections such as central venous catheter–associated blood stream infections. Source control using daily bathing of patients with chlorhexidine gluconate (CHG)–saturated cloths has been associated with reduced VRE contamination of patients' skin and health care workers' hands. A multicenter cluster randomized, cross-over clinical study in ICUs found daily bathing with CHG solution reduced VRE acquisition by 25% and decreased the risk for VRE bacteremia in known VRE-colonized patients.[A3] Not all trials have reported comparable findings,[A4] but a recent prospective crossover pragmatic study in non–critical care inpatient units confirmed that daily bathing with chlorhexidine reduced hospital-associated VRE (and also MRSA) by 36% (and 55%, respectively), but sustained and appropriate application of chlorhexidine was a key component.[A5]

The methods for VRE-specific prevention are directed at preventing incident colonization in high-risk hospitalized patients. Nearly all enterococcal infections, including VRE infections, are preceded by GI colonization, and although most colonized patients do not develop infections, they are still able to shed and transmit bacteria to other hospitalized patients. At least with VRE, a colonization-to-infection ratio of 10 : 1 has been reported, suggesting for every one clinical infection in an ICU, there may be 10 colonized patients lurking undetected in the unit. Thus, the unrecognized colonized patients represent the target population for infection prevention and control efforts such as active surveillance. Active surveillance programs use rectal surveillance swabs to detect previously unrecognized colonized patients and isolate them to prevent further transmission. Currently, surveillance cultures or PCR are recommended at the time of hospital admission for patients at high risk for carriage of VRE, and colonized patients or infected patients should be placed in isolation using contact precautions. Contact precautions typically entail private rooms, dedicated equipment such as stethoscopes, and gloves and gowns for all patient contact, although in a recent randomized trial in medical and surgical ICUs, the use of gloves and gowns for all patient contact compared with usual care did not result in a difference in the acquisition of VRE (or methicillin-resistant *S. aureus*).[A6] Implicit in this is the continued use of standard precautions, which requires cleaning and disinfection of equipment that is used in patient rooms. Many hospitals do use active surveillance in the ICU and other wards with a high prevalence of VRE, although the overall adoption of this strategy has been hindered by the perceived high costs of surveillance programs and lack of available randomized control trial data.

PROGNOSIS

Enterococcal bacteremia is associated with prolonged hospitalization and added costs compared with similar patients without enterococcal bacteremia. Still, apart from enterococcal endocarditis, the attributable mortality of enterococcal infections is difficult to quantify owing to its predilection to infect patients with preexisting comorbid conditions and high levels of illness severity. In certain patient populations, including those with liver and bone marrow transplants, studies have suggested increased morbidity, length of stay, and mortality associated with vancomycin resistance. Furthermore, a recent meta-analysis reported that the odds of dying from a vancomycin-resistant enterococcal blood stream infection were 2.5 times higher than dying from an infection caused by a susceptible enterococcus. The unadjusted mortality in susceptible enterococcal bacteremia was 20%. It is unclear why resistance is associated with higher mortality, although it is thought that delayed adequate empirical therapy may play a role. These studies should be interpreted cautiously because the clinical impact of resistance in enterococci was assessed before the availability of newer antimicrobials with activity against VRE.

Grade A References

A1. Chuang YC, Wang JT, Lin HY, et al. Daptomycin versus linezolid for treatment of vancomycin-resistant enterococcal bacteremia: systematic review and meta-analysis. *BMC Infect Dis.* 2014;14:1-10.
A2. Iversen K, Ihlemann N, Gill SU, et al. Partial oral versus intravenous antibiotic treatment of endocarditis. *N Engl J Med.* 2019;380:415-424.
A3. Climo MW, Yokoe DS, Warren DK, et al. Effect of daily bathing with chlorhexidine on hospital acquired infection. *N Engl J Med.* 2013;368:533-542.
A4. Noto MJ, Domenico HJ, Byrne DW, et al. Chlorhexidine bathing and health care-associated infections: a randomized clinical trial. *JAMA.* 2015;313:369-378.
A5. Lowe CF, Lloyd-Smith E, Sidhu B, et al. Reduction in hospital-associated methicillin-resistant *Staphylococcus aureus* and vancomycin-resistant *Enterococcus* with daily chlorhexidine gluconate bathing for medical inpatients. *Am J Infect Control.* 2017;45:255-259.
A6. Harris AD, Pineles L, Belton B, et al. Universal glove and gown use and acquisition of antibiotic-resistant bacteria in the ICU: a randomized trial. *JAMA.* 2013;310:1571-1580.

GENERAL REFERENCES

For the General References and other additional features, please visit Expert Consult at https://expertconsult.inkling.com.

276

DIPHTHERIA AND OTHER *CORYNEBACTERIUM* INFECTIONS

LUCY BREAKWELL AND ROLAND W. SUTTER

DEFINITION

Diphtheria is an acute infectious disease caused by toxigenic *Corynebacterium diphtheriae,* a gram-positive bacillus. The hallmark of the disease is the presence of a thick, firmly adherent pseudomembrane at the site of infection. The organism primarily infects the mucosa of the nose, pharynx, tonsils, or larynx (respiratory diphtheria). Rarely, other mucosal sites may be infected (e.g., conjunctiva, genitals, or ear). In developing countries, a variety of indolent skin lesions (cutaneous diphtheria) are common. Absorption of toxin can result in severe complications such as life-threatening myocarditis or polyneuritis.

The Pathogen

C. diphtheriae is a member of a group of aerobic, nonmotile, unencapsulated, nonsporulating, pleomorphic gram-positive bacilli. Its name comes from the Greek *korynee* (meaning "club"), which describes the shape of the organism on stained smears, and *diphtheria* (meaning "leather hide"), for the characteristic adherent membrane. The genus *Corynebacterium* is characterized by bacilli that line up in parallel groups and bend when dividing to create "Chinese character" arrangements. Both nontoxigenic and toxigenic *C. diphtheriae* strains exist. Toxigenicity is conferred when a nontoxigenic organism is infected with a β-phage carrying the gene for the toxin (*tox*) and the *tox* gene is expressed. Nontoxigenic *tox* gene-bearing strains (NTTB), which have a mutation in the A-subunit of the gene that prevents expression, have been reported in Europe. *C. diphtheriae* has four biotypes—*gravis, mitis, intermedius,* and *belfanti*—that are distinguished by colonial morphology and varying biochemical and hemolytic reactions. Strains are distinguished by molecular techniques. Diphtheria toxin-producing strains of *Corynebacterium ulcerans* can also produce classic respiratory diphtheria-like disease, including distal toxic complications.

EPIDEMIOLOGY

Humans are the only natural reservoir of *C. diphtheriae,* although the organism has occasionally been isolated from a variety of domestic and other animals. Transmission occurs in close-contact settings through respiratory droplets or by direct contact with respiratory secretions or skin lesions. The organism may survive for weeks and possibly months on environmental surfaces and

in dust, and fomite transmission can occur. The majority of nasopharyngeal *C. diphtheriae* infections may abort or result in asymptomatic carriage, with clinical disease developing in only about one in seven individuals. However, asymptomatic carriers are key to sustaining transmission.

Respiratory diphtheria dominated in temperate climates in the prevaccine era, with a peak incidence during winter and spring seasons. Most individuals acquired natural immunity by their mid-teen years. Cutaneous disease is more common in tropical countries, but the contribution of cutaneous diphtheria to inducing immunity is unknown. Outbreaks of cutaneous diphtheria have occurred in the United States and Europe, but typically in homeless and alcoholic inner-city adult populations. There have been recent case reports from European countries of cutaneous diphtheria in the asylum-seeking and refugee populations.[1,2]

Diphtheria immunization with diphtheria toxoid (formalin-treated toxin) protects against disease but does not prevent carriage. After the introduction of the vaccine in the 1920s when the majority of older individuals had natural immunity, the incidence of respiratory diphtheria dropped dramatically as did the proportion of isolated toxigenic strains, presumably because the selective advantage of the *tox* gene—promotion of greater replication and spread of the organism—is lost in an immune host. Currently, respiratory diphtheria has virtually been eliminated from developed countries where childhood vaccination coverage is high. In the United States, reported cases fell from 147,991 in 1920, to 15,536 in 1940, to 6 from 2000 to 2016.[3] Since 2000, cases mostly occurred among unimmunized or inadequately immunized persons and were associated with importations of *C. diphtheriae* from other countries. The absence of reported respiratory diphtheria cases in the United States, however, does not indicate that circulation of toxigenic *C. diphtheriae* has ceased. Investigations among Native American communities in South Dakota and Ontario, Canada, indicated *C. diphtheriae* strains might have been circulating independently in these communities for more than 2 decades despite the lack of reported respiratory diphtheria cases. Toxigenic corynebacteria continue to be identified in other developed countries. For example, from 2007 to 2013, England reported 20 cases of toxigenic corynebacteria (60% due to *C. ulcerans* associated with animal contact and 40% due to *C. diphtheriae* associated with international travel and incomplete immunization).[4] Over half (55%) of the cases were among adults aged 45 years and older.

In the absence of natural environmental boosting, vaccine-induced immunity wanes with increasing age and duration since last dose, resulting in a potential increase in risk of acquiring infection among older adults. Serosurveys conducted in developed countries from 1994 to 2010 indicated that 13 to 60% of adults more than 40 years old had diphtheria antitoxin antibody levels below minimal protective levels.[5] A concentration of diphtheria antitoxin antibodies in the serum of 0.01 IU/mL is considered the lower limit of protection. Long-term protection against diphtheria requires a level of greater than 0.1 IU/mL. Many of the older adults in these surveys were born before the introduction of diphtheria toxoid into national immunization schedules and so may not have been fully vaccinated. In contrast, a serosurvey in the Netherlands (2010) found that, although diphtheria antitoxin antibody concentrations among vaccinated cohorts declined with age, they remained above minimal protective levels among all of those vaccinated 40 to 50 years previously.

Large outbreaks of diphtheria have occurred during the vaccine era. In the 1990s, there was a major resurgence of diphtheria in several countries of the former Soviet Union. In Russia, the number of reported cases rose from 593 in 1989 to 39,582 in 1994, with more than two thirds of cases occurring in adults. Large-scale vaccination campaigns to virtually the entire population in the affected countries reduced diphtheria incidence, from a peak of 50,449 cases in 1995, to 7197 cases in 1997, to preresurgence levels by the late 1990s (Fig. 276-1). However, diphtheria remains a public health concern in these countries. For example in Latvia, diphtheria immunization coverage among adults declined to less than 60% by 2014, and diphtheria incidence increased from 0.1 to 0.7 per 100,000 persons during 2010 to 2014.[6] More recently, large outbreaks have occurred in Brazil (2010),[7] Indonesia (2010 to 2012),[8] Thailand (2012), Lao PDR (2012 to 2013),[9] Haiti (2015 to 2016),[10] and Venezuela (2016),[11] as well as in the Rohingya refugee population of Bangladesh, and in Yemen due to war,[12] primarily among children younger than 15 years, and associated with non- or inadequate vaccination. In general, outbreaks of diphtheria may occur in a susceptible population caused by clonal spread of the organism or transfer of the *tox* gene-bearing bacteriophage to nontoxigenic strains of *C. diphtheriae*. Although reported diphtheria cases have declined globally from 11,625 cases in 2000 to 4530 cases in 2015, some countries (e.g., India) continue to have endemic foci (Fig. 276-1).

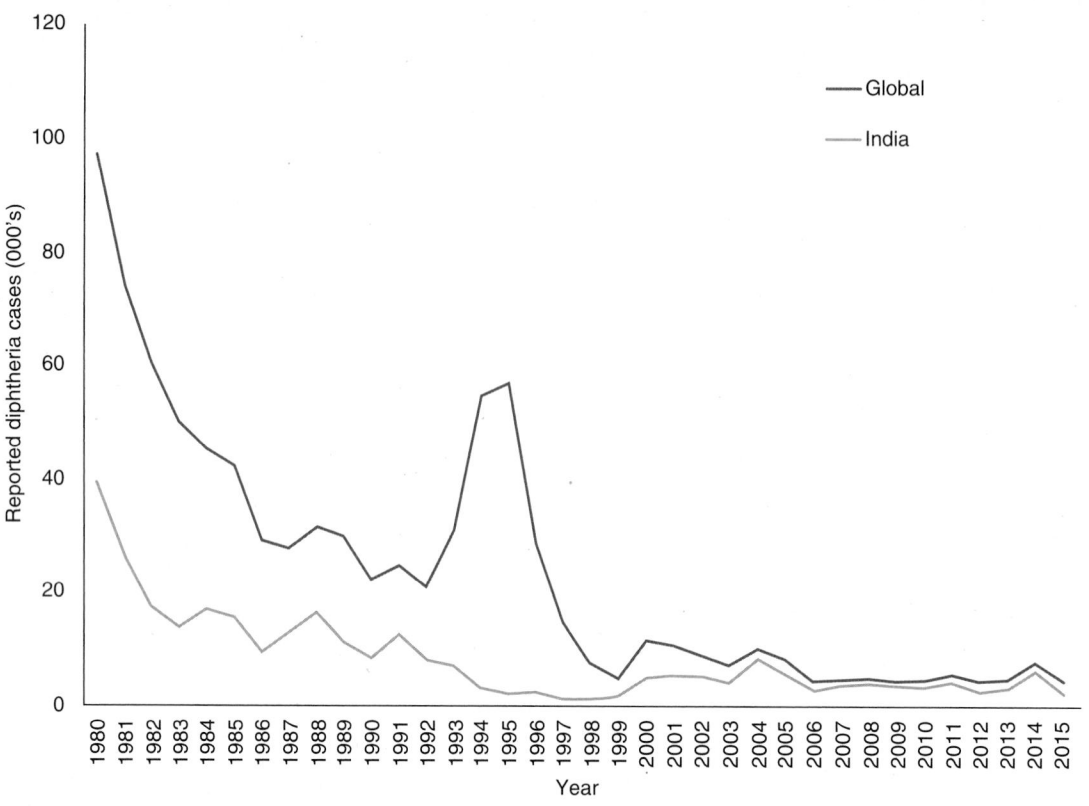

FIGURE 276-1. Reported diphtheria cases, worldwide, 1980 to 2015. (Data from the World Health Organization).

PATHOBIOLOGY

In classic respiratory diphtheria, *C. diphtheriae* colonizes the mucosal surface of the nasopharynx or larynx and multiplies locally without blood stream invasion. The symptoms and signs of diphtheria are attributable to toxin production. Diphtheria toxin is an extremely potent inhibitor of protein synthesis, and the estimated human lethal dose is 0.1 μg/kg. Released toxin causes local tissue necrosis with the formation of a tough pseudomembrane composed of a mixture of fibrin, dead cells, and bacteria that is firmly adherent to the underlying submucosal tissue. The membrane usually begins on the tonsils, on the posterior pharynx, or in the nose. In more severe cases, it progressively extends over the pharyngeal wall, fauces, and soft palate and into the larynx and may result in respiratory obstruction. Toxin entering the blood stream causes tissue damage at distant sites, particularly the heart (myocarditis), nerves (demyelination), and kidney (tubular necrosis). The extent of toxin absorption varies with the site of infection, being much less from the skin or nose than from the pharynx. Nontoxigenic strains mostly cause mild local respiratory disease and rarely produce a membrane, but have been associated with invasive infections such as endocarditis, septic arthritis, and osteomyelitis.[13]

CLINICAL MANIFESTATIONS
Respiratory Diphtheria

Infection limited to the anterior nares (nasal diphtheria) is manifested as a chronic serosanguineous or seropurulent discharge without fever or significant toxicity. A whitish membrane may be observed on the septum. The faucial (pharyngeal) form is most common. After an incubation period of 2 to 5 days, ranging from 1 to 10 days, the illness begins with a sore throat, malaise, and mild to moderate fever. Initially, there is mild pharyngeal erythema, usually followed by progressive formation of a whitish tonsillar exudate, which over 24 to 48 hours consolidates into a firmly adherent grayish membrane that bleeds on attempted removal. In more severe cases, the patient appears toxic and the membrane is more extensive. Cervical lymphadenopathy and soft tissue edema may occur and result in the typical bull neck appearance and stridor.[14] Laryngeal involvement (laryngeal diphtheria), which may develop on its own or as a result of membrane extension from the nasopharynx, is manifested as hoarseness, stridor, and dyspnea. The following clinical classification has been proposed by the World Health Organization: (1) catarrhal form (erythema of pharynx, no membrane), (2) follicular form (patches of exudate, no pharynx or tonsillar involvement), (3) spreading form (membranes covering the tonsils and the posterior pharynx), and (4) combined form (more than one anatomic site involved, e.g., throat and skin). The more severe clinical manifestations are associated with increasing toxin absorption levels.

The likelihood of toxic complications depends primarily on the interval between disease onset and administration of antitoxin. The severity of disease at initial evaluation closely predicts the likelihood of a severe clinical course, complications, and death. Myocarditis typically occurs in the first or second week after the onset of respiratory symptoms and develops either suddenly or insidiously with signs of low cardiac output and congestive heart failure. Conduction disturbances, which may occur without other signs of myocarditis, include ST-T wave abnormalities, arrhythmias, and heart block. Neurologic impairment is manifested as cranial nerve palsies and peripheral neuritis.[15] Palatal or pharyngeal paralysis (or both) occurs during the acute phase; peripheral neuritis, symmetrical and predominantly motor, occurs 2 to 12 weeks after onset of the disease. Motor deficit may range from minor proximal weakness to complete paralysis; in general, complete recovery from motor deficit is the rule. In fulminant, sometimes called "hypertoxic," diphtheria, toxic circulatory collapse with hemorrhagic features occurs.

Cutaneous Diphtheria

Cutaneous diphtheria lesions are classically indolent, deep, punched-out ulcers that may have a grayish-white membrane.[16] However, the lesions may be indistinguishable from impetigo, or *C. diphtheriae* may infect chronic dermatoses, resulting in a nontypical presentation. Coinfection with *Streptococcus pyogenes*, *Staphylococcus aureus*, or both occurs frequently. Toxic complications of cutaneous diphtheria alone are rare.

DIAGNOSIS

C. diphtheriae diagnosis should be based on clinical suspicion to allow treatment to start as soon as possible. Specimens for culture should be taken from beneath the membrane, the nasopharynx, and any suspicious skin lesions. Because special media are required, the laboratory should be alerted to the concern about diphtheria. Confirmation of infection is done by isolation through culture on selective media that inhibit the growth of other nasopharyngeal organisms; a medium containing potassium tellurite is generally used. Based on colonial morphology and Gram stain appearance, a presumptive diagnosis may be possible within 18 to 24 hours. Culture results may be negative if the patient previously received antibiotics. Toxigenicity testing should be performed on all *C. diphtheriae* isolates. Because both nontoxigenic and toxigenic strains may be isolated from the same patient, more than one colony should be tested. Traditional toxin testing methods include guinea pig inoculation and the modified Elek test. For the Elek test, the isolate and appropriate controls are streaked on a culture plate in which a filter strip soaked with antitoxin has been embedded; toxin production is confirmed by an immuno-precipitation line in the agar. Identification of the diphtheria *tox* gene allowed the development of polymerase chain reaction–based methods for identification of toxigenic strains.

Differential Diagnosis

The differential diagnosis includes streptococcal and viral tonsillopharyngitis, infectious mononucleosis, Vincent angina, candidiasis, and acute epiglottitis. Suspicion of diphtheria is increased if the patient has a history of travel to a region with endemic diphtheria, had contact with a recent immigrant from such an area, has a pre-antitoxin treatment serum antitoxin level of less than 0.01 IU/mL, or has not received diphtheria toxoid vaccination for many years. Previous animal contact may indicate toxigenic *C. ulcerans* infection.

TREATMENT   Rx

The decision to initiate therapy should be based on clinical suspicion because delayed treatment is associated with worse outcomes. The goals of treatment are to neutralize the toxin rapidly, eliminate the infecting organism, provide supportive care, and prevent further transmission (Table 276-1). The mainstay of therapy is equine diphtheria antitoxin. Because only unbound toxin can be neutralized, treatment should commence as soon as the diagnosis is suspected. Each day of delay in administration increases the likelihood of a fatal outcome. A single dose is given ranging from 20,000 units for localized tonsillar diphtheria to 100,000 units for extensive disease with severe toxicity. Children receive the same dose as adults. Antitoxin may be administered intramuscularly or intravenously; for more severe cases, the intravenous route is preferred. Tests for sensitivity to antitoxin should be performed before administering it and desensitization carried out if necessary.

Antibiotic therapy, by eliminating the organism, halts toxin production, limits local infection, and prevents transmission. Erythromycin orally or by injection (40 mg/kg/day; maximum 2 g/day) for 14 days, or parenteral procaine penicillin G (300,000 U if weight ≤10 kg or 600,000 U if weight >10 kg every 12 hours intramuscularly) until the patient can take oral medicine, followed by oral penicillin V (250 mg four times daily) for a total treatment course of 14 days or erythromycin (500 mg four times daily for 14 days) is the drug of choice. General supportive care includes ensuring a secure airway (with tracheotomy, if necessary), electrocardiographic monitoring for evidence of myocarditis, treating heart failure and arrhythmias, and preventing secondary complications of neurologic impairment such as aspiration pneumonia.

The patient should be in strict isolation until two consecutive negative cultures are obtained after therapy is completed. Natural infection does not confer immunity to the toxin, so persons recovering from diphtheria should complete active immunization during convalescence. Respiratory diphtheria infections are nationally notifiable, so the local health department must be notified. Close contacts, especially household contacts, should have cultures performed. Contacts should also be administered prophylactic antibiotics [benzathine penicillin G (600,000 U for persons <6 years old and 1,200,000 U for persons ≥6 years old) or a 7- to 10-day course of oral erythromycin (40 mg/kg/day for children and 1g/day for adults)] and be provided a booster dose of age-appropriate diphtheria toxoid-containing vaccine. A positive culture result in a contact may confirm the diagnosis if the patient is culture negative. All contacts without full immunization within the preceding 5 years should receive diphtheria toxoid.

The availability and access to diphtheria antitoxin has become problematic in recent years. At present, very few manufacturers exist worldwide. In the United States no FDA-licensed product is available because manufacturers discontinued diphtheria antitoxin production in 1997. However, diphtheria antitoxin can be obtained from the Centers for Disease Control and Prevention (770-488-7100) under an Investigational New Drug protocol, which describes in detail the procedures to follow when treating suspected diphtheria cases (https://www.cdc.gov/diphtheria/downloads/protocol.pdf). Given the scarcity of diphtheria antitoxin, there is an urgent need for alternative antitoxin preparations, such as human monoclonal antibodies.

TABLE 276-1	GOALS AND PROPOSED INTERVENTIONS FOR THE MANAGEMENT OF SUSPECTED DIPHTHERIA CASES
GOALS	**PROPOSED INTERVENTIONS**
Neutralize toxin as soon as possible to reduce severe complications, including death.	After a presumptive diagnosis of diphtheria, immediately obtain and administer antitoxin.
Eliminate the infecting organism and provide supportive care.	Initiate antimicrobial treatment, and arrange for appropriate supportive care.
Prevent further transmission of *C. diphtheriae* to close contacts, including hospital staff.	Isolate the patient as soon as suspected diphtheria is established; strictly observe respiratory barrier procedures. Notify the health department. Review the vaccination status of the family and other close contacts and initiate postexposure prophylaxis.
Confirm the diagnosis.	Collect appropriate specimens for culture (alert the laboratory to ensure that it can prepare specific culture media).
Induce long-term protection against *C. diphtheriae* in case and close contacts.	Complete the primary series with diphtheria toxoid containing vaccines as needed.

Currently in the United States, children are recommended to receive five doses of diphtheria toxoid (given with tetanus toxoid and pertussis vaccine as DTaP) at 2, 4, 6, 15 to 18 months, and a preschool booster dose at 4 to 6 years of age. For adolescents, a tetanus toxoid, reduced diphtheria toxoid, and acellular pertussis vaccine (Tdap) booster should be given between 11 and 12 years of age, mainly to provide additional protection against pertussis. Detailed recommendations for vaccination schedules can be obtained from the Advisory Committee for Immunization Practices (https://www.cdc.gov/vaccines/hcp/acip-recs/index.html).

Adults are recommended to receive tetanus toxoid, reduced diphtheria toxoid vaccine (Td) doses every 10 years. Adults who have not received a dose of Tdap, should receive one dose of Tdap as soon as feasible regardless of the interval since their last Td dose, then resume receiving a Td dose every 10 years (Chapter 15). The World Health Organization is currently reviewing available evidence on population diphtheria antitoxin seroprevalence and longevity of protection to reassess the necessity of the 10-year Td booster dose recommendation for adults to retain protection against diphtheria.[17] Since 2013, pregnant women are recommended to receive 1 dose of Tdap during gestational weeks 27 to 36 for each pregnancy, regardless of prior history of receiving Tdap. This recommendation was implemented to reduce pertussis morbidity and mortality in infants.

Only persons with a history of severe anaphylaxis to a vaccine component or after a prior dose should not receive additional doses of diphtheria toxoid. Vaccination should be deferred for persons with moderate or severe acute illness. Severe systemic adverse events after receipt of diphtheria toxoid are rare, and fever and other systemic symptoms are not common. However, local self-limited reactions, such as erythema and induration, are common.

Several countries have introduced glycoconjugate vaccines containing CRM_{197} (Cross Reactive Material 197), a genetically altered, fully immunogenic mutant of diphtheria toxin. Clinical trials have shown that CRM_{197} increased immunity to diphtheria; however, the role of CRM_{197} in contributing to or maintaining population immunity is unclear. In a guinea-pig model, receipt of CRM_{197}-conjugated meningococcal vaccines (with CRM_{197} concentration ranging from 3 µg to 44 µg) did not provide protection against a lethal challenge of diphtheria toxin.[18] However, given the different lengths, structures, and loads of the poly/oligosaccharides conjugated to CRM_{197} in different glycoconjugate vaccines, immunogenicity of CRM_{197} and ultimately protection against diphtheria toxin challenge would need to be assessed for each glycoconjugate vaccine.

PREVENTION

Immunization with diphtheria toxoid is the only effective means of primary prevention. The vaccine is approximately 95% effective, and protection is thought to last for at least 10 years.

PROGNOSIS

Diphtheria remains a serious disease associated with a high case-fatality rate. In the United States, the diphtheria case-fatality rate has remained virtually unchanged (5 to 10%) over recent decades.

TABLE 276-2 CORYNEBACTERIA AND RELATED ORGANISMS ASSOCIATED WITH HUMAN DISEASE

SITE OF INFECTION	PATHOGEN	CLINICAL SYNDROME	COMMENTS
Respiratory tract	Corynebacterium diphtheriae	Classic diphtheria	Toxin producing strains only
	Corynebacterium ulcerans	Diphtheria	Zoonotic infection; may produce diphtheria toxin
	Corynebacterium pseudodiphtheriticum	Pharyngitis. Rarely, pneumonia in patients with advanced AIDS	
	Arcanobacterium haemolyticum	Pharyngitis, tonsillar abscess, rash	Clinically indistinguishable from streptococcal pharyngitis
Skin and soft tissue	Corynebacterium pseudotuberculosis	Granulomatous lymphadenitis	Zoonotic infection, especially in sheep; occupational risk for veterinarians and butchers
	Corynebacterium minutissimum	Erythrasma	
	Corynebacterium kroppenstedtii, Corynebacterium striatum, and Corynebacterium amycolatum/C.xerosis	Granulomatous breast abscess	
Genitourinary tract	Corynebacterium diphtheria	UTIs in men; chronic prostatitis	More common in elderly, chronically ill, and immunosuppressed patients and in those with indwelling catheters
	Corynebacterium glucuronolyticum	Chronic and recurrent UTIs, encrusted cystitis	
	Corynebacterium urealyticum		
	Corynebacterium riegelli		
Health care–associated infections	Corynebacterium jeikeium and less commonly many others, including Corynebacterium amycolatum, Corynebacterium striatum, Corynebacterium urealyticum, and Corynebacterium aurimucosum	Catheter- and device-associated infections	C. jeikeium is the most common corynebacterial pathogen in hospitals and causes severe infections in immunosuppressed patients and those with indwelling devices
		Postprocedure wound and soft tissue infections	
		Prosthetic valve joint infections	C. striatum has been associated with infective endocarditis
		Nosocomial pneumonia	
		CSF shunt infections	

CSF = cerebrospinal fluid; UTI = urinary tract infection.

OTHER *CORYNEBACTERIUM* SPECIES

Corynebacteria other than *C. diphtheriae* are ubiquitous in the environment and are among the normal flora colonizing humans and animals. The pathogenic potential of many of these organisms was not appreciated in the past, but many are now known to be associated with specific and often serious infectious diseases,[19,20] especially in immunosuppressed, chronically ill, and hospitalized patients (Table 276-2). In general, these organisms remain susceptible to vancomycin, but resistance to other classes of antimicrobials is common and varies among species.

GENERAL REFERENCES

For the General References and other additional features, please visit Expert Consult at https://expertconsult.inkling.com.

277

LISTERIOSIS

HEATHER E. CLAUSS AND BENNETT LORBER

DEFINITION

Listeriosis is a food-borne infection caused by the gram-positive rod *Listeria monocytogenes*.[1] Most patients have impaired cell-mediated immunity and are seen with life-threatening bacteremia or meningitis. However, a self-limited, febrile gastroenteritis in healthy persons also occurs.

The Pathogen

Widely distributed in nature, *L. monocytogenes* may be found in soil, on vegetation, and in the stool of healthy mammals, including humans. It causes disease in animals, especially herd animals, and in humans. The organism has been isolated from many foods, including raw produce, raw milk, fish, poultry, and meat. Unlike most food-borne pathogens, *L. monocytogenes* can grow at refrigerator temperatures.

EPIDEMIOLOGY

Nonperinatal listeriosis is almost always the result of food-borne infection.[2] Listeriosis is a relatively rare food-borne illness (≈1% of U.S. cases) but is associated with a case-fatality rate of at least 16 to 20% (second only to *Vibrio vulnificus* at 35 to 39%) and causes approximately 19 to 28% of all food-borne disease–related deaths.[3] Outbreaks have been documented in association with coleslaw, milk, soft cheeses, ice cream, pâté, ready-to-eat pork products, deli counter meats,[4] hot dogs, smoked fish, butter, sprouts, taco or nacho salads, and cantaloupes. In 2011 *L. monocytogenes*–contaminated cantaloupes were responsible for the deadliest food-borne disease outbreak in U.S. history, with 28 states reporting illness in 146 persons and death in 30 (21% mortality). From 2017 to 2018, South Africa experienced the largest ever documented listeriosis outbreak, with more than 1000 laboratory-confirmed cases, more than 200 deaths, and a case-fatality rate of approximately 29%.[5]

Listeriosis is a nationally reportable disease in the United States. The Centers for Disease Control and Prevention has established PulseNet (http://www.cdc.gov/pulsenet/), a network of public health and food regulatory laboratories that use pulsed-field gel electrophoresis to subtype food-borne pathogens to detect promptly disease clusters that may have a common source. Presently, the annual incidence of listeriosis is 0.29 cases per 100,000 population, and it accounts for 1700 cases per year and about 350 deaths. Neonates and adults older than 60 years have the highest infection rates. Pregnant women represent 14% of all affected individuals; other adults at increased risk for invasive listeriosis (bacteremia, meningitis) include those with hematologic malignancies, advanced acquired immunodeficiency syndrome (AIDS), a solid organ transplant, iron overload, and anyone treated with corticosteroids or an anti–tumor necrosis factor (TNF) agent. Proton pump inhibitors increase infection risk.[6] However, as many as one fourth of all cases of invasive listeriosis occur in apparently healthy persons, particularly those older than 60 years.

PATHOBIOLOGY

L. monocytogenes enters the human body through the intestine, most often after the ingestion of contaminated food. The bacterium induces its own uptake by gastrointestinal cells and macrophages. Infectious or mechanical disruption of the GI tract occasionally may promote GI invasion.[7] Mother-to-child transmission occurs transplacentally or through an infected birth canal. Within the host cell, the bacterium is enclosed in a phagolysosome, but through the production of an exotoxin called listeriolysin O, it destroys the phagolysosome membrane and gains access to the cytoplasm. All pathogenic strains of *L. monocytogenes* produce listeriolysin O, the major virulence factor. Listeriae actively divide in the cytoplasm, migrate to the periphery of the cell by polymerization of host cell actin, and then push out the cell membrane to form pseudopods, which are taken up by adjacent host cells. The bacteria move from cell to cell in this fashion and repeat their life cycle without exposure to antibodies or complement.[8]

After invasion through the gastrointestinal tract, listeriae may disseminate hematogenously to any body site but show a particular tropism for the central nervous system (CNS). Less commonly, listeriae may spread intra-axonally through cranial nerves to reach the CNS; this mode of CNS invasion may result in rhombencephalitis (brain stem infection).

Immunity to listerial infection is handled chiefly through the cell-mediated arm of the immune system. *L. monocytogenes* infection induces a robust CD8 T-cell response, which plays a critical role in resolving the primary infection and providing protective immunity to reinfections.[9] Persons who have had splenectomy or have abnormalities solely of humoral immunity or leukocytes are not at increased risk for infection.

CLINICAL MANIFESTATIONS

The incubation period for invasive listeriosis (time from ingestion of contaminated food to illness) averages about 11 days; 90% is within 28 days.[10] Invasive listeriosis in an immunocompromised adult is most often manifested as bacteremia without an obvious focus. In such cases, patients have nonspecific complaints, such as fever, malaise, myalgia, and back pain. Bacteremia is the form of invasive listeriosis that complicates pregnancy; CNS infection in pregnancy is extremely rare in the absence of other risk factors. Listeriosis during pregnancy may lead to spontaneous abortion or neonatal sepsis, but early antimicrobial therapy may result in the birth of a healthy child. Endocarditis with *L. monocytogenes* can occur on both native and prosthetic valves and carries a high rate of septic complications.[11] Endocarditis, but not bacteremia per se, may be a clue to underlying colon cancer; colonoscopy should be considered in all cases of listerial endocarditis.

Persons in whom *L. monocytogenes* bacteremia develops may progress to CNS infection (neurolisteriosis), most commonly manifested as meningitis. *Listeria* has a predilection for infecting brain tissue as well as the meninges, and unlike other common bacterial causes of meningitis, it not infrequently causes encephalitis or brain abscess. Brain abscess as a result of infection by *L. monocytogenes* exhibits unusual features compared with other bacteria: listerial brain abscess coexists with bacteremia in nearly all cases and with meningitis in one fourth; in addition, abscesses are often subcortical.[12]

L. monocytogenes is the most common cause of bacterial meningitis in patients with lymphomas, organ transplant recipients, and patients treated with corticosteroids for any reason. Affected persons usually have the classic acute symptoms of meningitis, but the presentation is subacute (>24 hours) in 60% of cases. Nuchal rigidity is absent in 20%. Focal neurologic findings, including ataxia, tremors, myoclonus, and seizures, may be seen, consistent with the tropism of *Listeria* for brain parenchyma. Gram stain of cerebrospinal fluid (CSF) reveals small gram-positive rods in only about one third of cases. The glucose content in CSF is normal in more than 60% of cases; mononuclear cells predominate in 30%.

Listerial rhombencephalitis is an unusual form of listerial encephalitis that involves the brain stem and, unlike other listerial CNS infections, usually occurs in healthy adults. The typical clinical picture is one of a biphasic illness with a prodrome of fever, headache, nausea, and vomiting lasting about 4 days, followed by the abrupt onset of asymmetrical cranial nerve deficits, cerebellar signs, and hemiparesis or hemisensory deficits or both. Respiratory failure develops in about 40% of patients. Nuchal rigidity is present in about half, and CSF findings are only mildly abnormal, with a positive CSF culture in about 40%. Almost two thirds of patients are bacteremic. Magnetic resonance imaging is superior to computed tomography for demonstrating rhombencephalitis. Mortality is high, and serious sequelae are common in survivors.

Localized infection may occur after hematogenous seeding (e.g., liver abscess, septic arthritis) or, rarely, after direct inoculation (e.g., papulopustular rash, conjunctivitis). Osteoarticular listeriosis primarily involves prosthetic joints, occurs in immunocompromised patients, and requires implant removal for cure.[13]

Well-documented reports of food-borne outbreaks have demonstrated that ingestion of *L. monocytogenes* in a sufficiently large inoculum can result in a self-limited illness consisting of fever, chills, diarrhea, abdominal cramps, and sometimes nausea and vomiting. Symptoms follow exposure by 1 to 2 days and last for about 2 days.

DIAGNOSIS

Differential Diagnosis

Clinical situations in which a diagnosis of listeriosis should be considered include the following:

- neonatal sepsis or meningitis;
- meningitis or parenchymal brain infection in patients with subacute presentations, hematologic malignant neoplasms, AIDS, organ transplantation, corticosteroid immunosuppression, treatment with anti–tumor necrosis factor agents, or age older than 50 years;

- simultaneous infection of the meninges and brain parenchyma;
- subcortical brain abscess;
- fever during pregnancy;
- blood, CSF, or other normally sterile specimen reported to have "diphtheroids" on Gram stain or culture; and
- food-borne outbreak of febrile gastroenteritis when routine cultures fail to identify a pathogen.

The differential diagnosis of listerial CNS infection includes the more common causes of bacterial meningitis and brain abscess; indolent listerial meningitis or rhombencephalitis may mimic CNS tuberculosis.

Laboratory Findings

The diagnosis of listeriosis is made by routine bacterial culture of specimens from usually sterile sites, such as blood or CSF. The laboratory must exercise caution because *L. monocytogenes* may be mistaken for diphtheroids, streptococci, or enterococci. Specific stool culture is recommended only when routine stool cultures are negative in the setting of an outbreak of gastroenteritis; many people have enteric colonization with *L. monocytogenes* without invasive disease. The laboratory must be advised that listerial infection is suspected because the organism is unlikely to be identified with routine stool culture media.

Serologic testing (antibody to listeriolysin O) is not useful for invasive disease but may be helpful in the retrospective identification of food-borne outbreaks of febrile gastroenteritis when routine cultures are negative.[14] Real-time polymerase chain reaction analysis of CSF for the *hly* gene, which encodes listeriolysin O, has been useful in diagnosing CNS listeriosis, including cases in which routine bacterial cultures were negative, but this test is not yet commercially available. Whole genome sequencing has been used to enhance listeriosis outbreak detection and investigation.[15]

PREVENTION

Guidelines for preventing listeriosis are similar to those for preventing other food-borne illnesses. In general, one should thoroughly cook raw food from animal sources; wash raw vegetables thoroughly before eating; keep uncooked meats separate from vegetables and from cooked and ready-to-eat foods; avoid raw (unpasteurized) milk or foods made from raw milk; and wash hands, knives, and cutting boards after each handling of uncooked foods.

People at high risk for listeriosis (those immunocompromised by illness or medications, pregnant women, and the elderly) may choose to avoid soft cheeses such as feta, Brie, Camembert, blue veined, and Mexican-style cheese such as queso fresco. Hard cheeses, processed cheeses, cream cheese, cottage cheese, and yogurt are safe. Leftover foods or ready-to-eat foods such as hot dogs should be cooked until steaming hot. It is best to avoid foods from delicatessen counters, such as prepared salads, meats, and cheeses, or at least to reheat cold cuts thoroughly until they are steaming hot before eating.

Listeriosis is effectively prevented by trimethoprim-sulfamethoxazole given as *Pneumocystis* prophylaxis to organ transplant recipients, those receiving corticosteroid immunosuppression, or individuals infected with human immunodeficiency virus. Second episodes of neonatal listerial infection are virtually unheard of, and intrapartum antibiotics are not recommended for women with a history of perinatal listeriosis.

Except for transmission from infected mother to fetus, human-to-human transmission of listeriosis does not occur; patients do not need to be isolated. Novel biocontrol methods for *L. monocytogenes* biofilms are being investigated in food production facilities to prevent entry of the microorganism into the food production environments.[16]

TREATMENT

Recommendations for the treatment of infection with *L. monocytogenes* derive from in vitro data, animal models, and clinical experience with small numbers of patients. No controlled trials have been performed to prove the efficacy of one drug over another. Many antimicrobials show in vitro activity against *L. monocytogenes*. Clinical utility is more relevant than in vitro susceptibility test results because cephalosporins and other drugs to which the bacterium appears to be susceptible are inadequate to treat infection.

Twenty percent of cases of bacterial meningitis in those older than 50 years are due to *L. monocytogenes*. Therefore, empirical therapy for bacterial meningitis in all adults older than 50 years should include either ampicillin or trimethoprim-sulfamethoxazole, especially in the absence of associated pneumonia, otitis, sinusitis, or endocarditis, which would suggest a cause other than *L. monocytogenes*. Cephalosporins, commonly used for the treatment of bacterial meningitis, should not be used alone when *Listeria* is a diagnostic consideration.

Ampicillin is generally considered the drug of choice for treating confirmed cases of listeriosis. In cases of meningitis and endocarditis and in patients with severely impaired T-cell function, many authorities recommend the addition of gentamicin to ampicillin for synergy on the basis of in vitro testing and animal models. For meningitis, therapy should be continued for at least 3 weeks; bacteremic patients without CNS involvement may be treated for 2 weeks. Endocarditis and brain abscess should be treated for at least 6 weeks. Meningitis doses should be used to treat all cases of invasive listeriosis, even in the absence of CNS or CSF abnormalities.

In patients with penicillin hypersensitivity, trimethoprim-sulfamethoxazole is the preferred agent. It is bactericidal and appears to be as effective as the combination of ampicillin and gentamicin. Drugs that should be avoided because of treatment failure and relapse include cephalosporins, chloramphenicol, tetracycline, vancomycin, and erythromycin.

The French MONALISA national prospective cohort study has found significantly reduced survival in patients with neurolisteriosis who were treated with adjunctive dexamethasone.

Iron is a virulence factor for *L. monocytogenes*, and clinically, iron overload states are risk factors for listerial infection. Therefore, in patients with listeriosis and iron deficiency, it may be prudent to withhold iron replacement until antimicrobial therapy is complete.

PROGNOSIS

Listeria meningitis carries a mortality of about 25%, and mortality is higher in those with underlying malignant disease. Mortality from brain abscess and endocarditis is about 50%; survivors of brain abscess commonly have significant neurologic residua.

GENERAL REFERENCES

For the General References and other additional features, please visit Expert Consult at https://expertconsult.inkling.com.

278

ANTHRAX

DANIEL R. LUCEY AND LEV M. GRINBERG

DEFINITION

Anthrax is caused by *Bacillus anthracis*, a spore-forming, gram-positive rod that is aerobic or facultatively anaerobic. Although it is primarily a disease of animals (zoonosis), anthrax was developed as a biowarfare weapon by several nations in the 20th century and used for bioterrorism in the United States in 2001 when spores were mailed in letters.

The Pathogen

The bacterium is a large (1 to 1.5 by 3 to 5 μm), gram-positive rod. It has a ground-glass appearance of growth on sheep blood agar, with 2- to 5-mm, nonhemolytic, tenacious ("beaten egg white") colonies within 24 hours of culture; oval, central to subterminal spores; and a capsule that can be visualized by India ink staining.

EPIDEMIOLOGY

Human infection with *B. anthracis* is often linked to a zoonotic source, such as cattle, sheep, goats, water buffalo, and other animals. Meat, bones, hides, and hair have been reported to transmit infection. Spores can persist in soil for many years. Spores infect animals or humans, then germinate into the vegetative form of *B. anthracis* and cause disease. The World Health Organization provides an online global epidemiology database for anthrax along with guidelines for management of the disease in animals, humans, and the environment.

A systematic review of the worldwide medical literature found that between 1900 and 2005, at least 82 patients with inhalational anthrax were reported in clinical detail. These 82 cases included 18 patients from the United States with naturally acquired, animal-related disease in the 20th century and 11 patients with inhalational anthrax due to the bioterrorism-related events of 2001. In addition to these 82 cases, there were 41 cases confirmed by histopathology and microbiology of inhalational anthrax from the 1979 outbreak in Sverdlovsk that was linked to an accidental release of spores downwind from a military facility.

Naturally acquired human inhalational anthrax or gastrointestinal anthrax is exceedingly rarely diagnosed. Inhalational anthrax in recent years has been linked to exposure to spores contaminating drums made from animal hides. Gastrointestinal anthrax is linked to consumption of meat from infected animals.

Importantly, *B. anthracis* is not transmitted from person to person through the air. Only one quarter of autopsy-confirmed inhalational cases have had any evidence of pneumonia, specifically an acute hemorrhagic pneumonia.[1] All have had characteristic hemorrhagic mediastinal adenopathy, edema, and pleural effusions caused by the primary inhalation of spores. Infection by reaerosolization can occur even under outdoor conditions or within offices.

The most common form of anthrax is the cutaneous form. Direct contact with infected animals or contaminated animal products is the usual mode of transmission. Unexplained cutaneous anthrax cases could be an early clue to an intentional release of spores.

From 2009 to 2010, at least 80 confirmed or probable cases of anthrax occurred in persons who injected heroin in Europe, primarily in the United Kingdom.[2] From 2012 to 2013, at least another 14 cases occurred, again in the United Kingdom but also in Denmark, France, and Germany. A new term, *injection anthrax*, was applied to this novel route of infection and distinct clinical syndrome that involved severe soft tissue infection at the site of the injection and sometimes systemic disease. The single strain of *B. anthracis* in these outbreaks most closely matched that reported from a goat in Turkey, suggesting that heroin originating in Afghanistan or Pakistan and smuggled overland in an animal skin may have been the source of these spores in Europe.

PATHOBIOLOGY

Circulating encapsulated chains of *B. anthracis* are trapped in the lung capillary network, a phenomenon that may explain why the lung is always the terminal target of human infection regardless of the original route of infection in a murine model.[3] Major virulence factors of *B. anthracis* include its two binary toxins, edema factor and lethal factor, and also its antiphagocytic poly-D-glutamic acid capsule.[4] Edema toxin consists of edema factor bound to a third anthrax toxin component, protective antigen. Similarly, lethal toxin consists of lethal factor bound to protective antigen. These three toxin components, edema factor, lethal factor, and protective antigen, are encoded on one plasmid (pX-01). The antiphagocytic capsule is encoded on a second plasmid (pX-02). Both plasmids are necessary to cause disease.

The pathogenesis of anthrax has been attributed primarily to its two binary toxins. However, more recently, key roles for both nontoxin and toxin components have been implicated in the pathogenesis of the characteristic cardiac and endovascular abnormalities, bleeding, and shock. Nontoxin components include the peptidoglycan part of the bacterial cell wall and nontoxin metalloproteinases. Moreover, inhibition of both innate and adaptive immune responses occurs by the activities of both toxins and the antiphagocytic capsule.

Similarly, the sepsis model has been proposed to explain the high lethality of inhalational anthrax, rather than the toxin model. In this sepsis model, the primary role of anthrax toxin is to inhibit the immune response against the vegetative form of the bacteria, thus allowing the typically high levels of bacteremia to develop and subsequent shock, multiorgan failure, and death to occur.

Lethal toxin is a metalloproteinase and inhibitor of the mitogen-activated protein kinase intracellular signal transduction pathway. It contributes to the coagulation disorder, hemolysis, and hemorrhage seen with inhalational anthrax. Whether lethal toxin contributed to the vasculitis lesions reported in the 1979 outbreak in Sverdlovsk is uncertain. Edema toxin contributes to the typical "gelatinous" fluid in the mediastinum and abdomen as well as the marked edema seen in both cutaneous anthrax and injection anthrax. The mechanism is attributed to excessive production of cyclic adenosine monophosphate from adenosine triphosphate by edema toxin acting as an adenylate cyclase enzyme. The result is water and calcium dysregulation with marked edema.

CLINICAL MANIFESTATIONS

Major clinical manifestations of anthrax infection—inhalational, cutaneous, gastrointestinal, injection, and meningeal—are related to the routes through which *B. anthracis* can enter the body: inhalation, contact, ingestion, or injection (e.g., by contaminated heroin).

Inhalational anthrax almost always causes hemorrhagic mediastinitis, gelatinous edema, and mediastinal adenopathy, resulting in mediastinal widening, as well as pleural effusions due to blockage and reversal of normal lymphatic flow and drainage within the mediastinum. These pleural effusions can be large, bloody, and recurring unless repeatedly drained by thoracentesis or chest tube. Such effusions were found to contribute to respiratory failure in the 1979 outbreak in Sverdlovsk, in part due to compression of lung parenchyma and impaired gas exchange. During the outbreak, the pleural fluid was drained by thoracentesis, rather than by chest tube, and antibiotics were injected into the pleural space. Nevertheless, nearly every patient with inhalational anthrax who underwent autopsy in this outbreak was found to have large (average, 1776 mL) pleural effusions. Although it was not known in 1979 or in 2001, these pleural effusions can serve as a reservoir for toxin. Pleural fluid toxin levels were not tested until the two U.S. patients in 2006 and 2011. High levels of lethal factor were reported.

Radiography demonstrated pulmonary infiltrates in many cases. Thus, although inhalational anthrax has been stated by some not to cause pneumonia, these radiologic findings serve to emphasize the important diagnostic point for clinicians that not only mediastinal widening and pleural effusions but also pulmonary infiltrates are often seen. Thus, pulmonary infiltrates on radiologic imaging, whether or not interpreted as pneumonia, do not rule out the diagnosis of inhalational anthrax.

In 2005, a new three-part clinical staging system for inhalational anthrax (Table 278-1) was published, adding an intermediate progressive stage based on clinical, microbiologic, and radiologic information acquired from the 11 patients in 2001. Previously, these patients would have been included in the late stage, for whom death was considered almost certain. Importantly, all six of the patients who survived the anthrax attacks in 2001 had rapid therapy initiated, including pleural drainage, during this intermediate progressive stage. This three-part symptomatic clinical staging system is cited at www.cidrap.umn.edu/idsa/bt/anthrax/biofacts/anthraxfactsheet.html.

Although in 2001 none of the five patients in the late fulminant stage survived, the two U.S. patients in 2006 and 2011 both survived even though they required mechanical ventilation, placing them in the late fulminant stage. One additional treatment they received was anthrax antitoxin (see section on Treatment), which was not available in 2001.

The shortest incubation period that has been *documented* microbiologically or histopathologically is 4 days. The range is 4 to 43 days. Although shorter incubation periods may have occurred, none have been documented in the English or Russian literature by these laboratory criteria.

Cutaneous anthrax accounts for about 95% of patients with anthrax. The incubation period ranges from 1 to 12 days. Like the three clinical stages of symptomatic inhalational anthrax, three stages of cutaneous anthrax can be delineated: (1) an initial pruritic papule progressing to (2) a central vesicular or bullous lesion with surrounding nonpitting edema and finally, (3) a necrotic and hemorrhagic central lesion that evolves into the classic painless eschar with surrounding edema. Resolution can take up to 2 months. This three-stage progression can occur even if appropriate antibiotics are given. During the anthrax letter attacks of 2001, some of the cutaneous lesions were initially considered to be due to brown recluse spider bites. These lesions are usually painful, unlike the painless lesions of anthrax.

In contrast to cutaneous anthrax, injection anthrax described from Europe in persons injecting spore-contaminated heroin does not typically develop a black crusted eschar, can be painful, and can present with severe gastrointestinal or central nervous system manifestations that can rapidly lead to death. The 2011 official report from Health Protection Scotland on outbreaks of this novel form of anthrax advises physicians to suspect injection anthrax in heroin users who demonstrate any of three presentations: (1) severe soft tissue infection including necrotizing fasciitis and cellulitis/abscess, especially if marked edema is present (Fig. 278-1); (2) signs of sepsis even if no soft tissue infection is evident; and (3) meningitis or subarachnoid hemorrhage/intracranial bleed.

Gastrointestinal anthrax is divided into an oropharyngeal form and an intestinal form. The oropharyngeal form has painful cervical adenopathy and an incubation period between 2 hours and 6 days. The oral lesions can ulcerate. They also can progress to cause a white pseudomembrane with dysphagia and hoarseness. The intestinal form has been described to have three clinical phases, much like the three-part progressive clinical stages of inhalational anthrax and cutaneous anthrax: (1) a prodromal phase with fever, malaise, and sometimes syncope; followed by (2) a progressive phase with abdominal pain, nausea, vomiting, abdominal distention, ascites, and severe weakness; and finally (3) a fulminant phase with rapidly increasing abdominal girth and expanding ascites, paroxysmal abdominal pain, and shock. Of note, the U.S. patient with gastrointestinal anthrax in 2010 who survived had more than 50 liters of ascitic fluid drained as part of her therapy along with antibiotics and anthrax antitoxin.

Anthrax meningoencephalitis can occur in association with any of the other forms of anthrax, inhalation,[5] cutaneous, gastrointestinal, or injection, and rarely without a known portal of entry. Cerebral edema, parenchymal brain

TABLE 278-1	CLINICAL STAGING SYSTEM FOR INHALATIONAL ANTHRAX

I. EARLY PRODROMAL STAGE

Nonspecific illness sometimes described as "flulike" and including any of the following: fever, cough, headache, chills, nausea, chest pain, or abdominal pain. Laboratory tests and radiographs are nondiagnostic. The prognosis for cure is good with appropriate therapy, but the diagnosis is difficult to confirm acutely in this stage.

II. INTERMEDIATE PROGRESSIVE STAGE

Any of the following findings are defining inclusion criteria for this stage:
1. Positive blood cultures (typically positive in <24 hours)
2. Mediastinal adenopathy
3. Pleural effusions: bloody, often large, require drainage, and may recur

Findings in this stage may include high fever, dyspnea, confusion or syncope, or increasing nausea and vomiting. Exclusion criteria for this stage include the following:
1. Meningitis
2. Respiratory failure requiring intubation and mechanical ventilation or
3. Shock

Importantly, patients in the intermediate progressive stage can still be cured with appropriate antibiotics and drainage of pleural effusions by repeated thoracentesis or preferably chest tube to keep the pleural space dry to reduce the adverse mechanical effect on respiration by large-volume effusions and to remove potentially toxin-producing *Bacillus anthracis* from the pleural space.

III. LATE FULMINANT STAGE

Inclusion criteria include any one of the following findings:
1. Meningitis
2. Respiratory failure requiring intubation and mechanical ventilation
3. Shock: end-organ hypoperfusion

Findings in this stage may also include any of those from previous stages, so there are no exclusion criteria. The probability of survival is lowest in this stage. Novel therapeutics that safely and effectively neutralize anthrax toxin may be needed to increase survival.

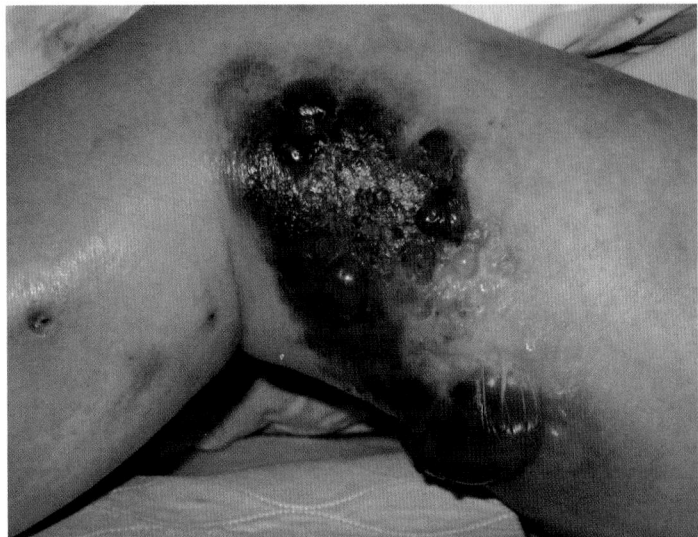

FIGURE 278-1. An example of the lesions due to injection anthrax.

hemorrhage, vasculitis, and subarachnoid hemorrhage can occur. The cerebrospinal fluid is often bloody with anthrax meningitis. At autopsy, the extensive bleeding gives a characteristic macroscopic appearance termed the cardinal's cap. This form of anthrax remains fatal in more than 95% of cases.

DIAGNOSIS

If anthrax is suspected,[6] blood should be obtained immediately before any antibiotics are given, primarily for microbiologic culture and possibly for newer assays for anthrax toxins whenever available. Notably, blood cultures from patients with inhalational anthrax will grow the large, gram-positive rods within 24 hours. Given such high levels of bacteremia, it is surprising that even one dose of an effective antibiotic has been reported to turn blood cultures negative, hence the need to draw blood culture samples before antibiotics are given. Toxin assays could still be positive after initial antibiotics, but these assays are still investigational at this time. Nasal cultures should not be performed as a routine clinical diagnostic test for individual patients because a negative result does not rule out inhalation of spores. Nasal cultures could be epidemiologically useful, however, as part of an investigation to help estimate the perimeter of exposure to spores.

In the microbiology laboratory, if the initial culture is suggestive of *B. anthracis*, three tests can be performed with a biosafety cabinet. These are assays for motility (nonmotile), catalase (positive), and hemolysis (negative). If these characteristics are found, identification is still not proved until a sample is sent to a reference laboratory where polymerase chain reaction analysis can identify *B. anthracis* and gamma-phage lysis of the encapsulated bacteria can provide confirmation. One or more antibody tests also are available, although results are unlikely to be positive during the earliest part of the disease. In contrast, a number of investigational anthrax toxin tests (e.g., for lethal factor, edema factor, or protective antigen) are being developed that should have positive results early in the disease, even if antibiotics have been given, and may also have prognostic value. These assays are available in the United States only through the Centers for Disease Control and Prevention (CDC).

A noncontrast computed tomography scan of the chest can be a valuable adjunctive diagnostic tool for inhalational anthrax. It is more sensitive than a chest radiograph for demonstrating the characteristic hyperattenuating mediastinal adenopathy causing the mediastinal widening and pleural effusions. The hyperattenuation is consistent with bleeding into lymph nodes and thus helps differentiate inhalational anthrax from tularemia, histoplasmosis, tuberculosis, sarcoidosis, and most other causes of mediastinal or hilar adenopathy.

Anthrax meningitis is typically neutrophilic and bloody. Very large gram-positive rods in the cerebrospinal fluid distinguish anthrax meningitis from other causes of gram-positive meningitis, such as the smaller *Listeria monocytogenes*. In the February 2014 *Emerging Infectious Diseases* online journal, the CDC published its first formal updated guidelines on anthrax since 2001, including diagnostic tests, prophylaxis, treatment, and monitoring. New diagnostic recommendations include a lumbar puncture at admission unless it is contraindicated because new treatment recommendations will be based in part on whether meningitis has been excluded.

TREATMENT   Rx

Treatment of symptomatic anthrax includes antibiotics and, in the case of inhalational anthrax, pleural fluid drainage. In addition, between 2012 and 2016 the Food and Drug Administration (FDA) licensed three anthrax antitoxins for treatment of inhalational anthrax. The CDC recommendations for prevention and treatment were updated in 2014, and the reader is referred to their webpage for complete details.[7]

Treatment with three intravenous antibiotics is recommended in the 2014 CDC recommendations if meningitis is possible or confirmed. These include a bactericidal fluoroquinolone (ciprofloxacin is the preferred drug), a bactericidal β-lactam (meropenem is the preferred drug), and a protein synthesis inhibitor (linezolid is the preferred drug). If meningitis is excluded, a bactericidal drug (ciprofloxacin is preferred) and a protein synthesis inhibitor (either clindamycin or linezolid) is preferred. In addition, CDC recommended that "an antitoxin should be added to combination antimicrobial drug treatment for any patient for whom there is a high level of clinical suspicion for systemic anthrax," based on their systematic review of the literature.

Although there is no conclusive evidence that the combination of anthrax antitoxin therapy and antibiotics provides a survival benefit in inhalation anthrax,[8] a total 60-day course of antibiotic therapy, of at least 2 weeks intravenously with more than one drug followed by the remainder with one oral drug, is

recommended for inhalational anthrax because of concern that spores may germinate into vegetative bacteria if therapy is stopped sooner.

An essential treatment modality for inhalational anthrax is pleural drainage. The CDC 2014 guidelines state: "Drainage of pleural fluid and ascites is believed to improve survival by reducing the toxin level and by decreasing mechanical lung compression. These data support the need for early and aggressive drainage of any clinically or radiographically apparent pleural effusions; chest tube drainage is recommended over thoracentesis because many effusions will require prolonged drainage. Thoracotomy or video-assisted thoracic surgery might be required to remove gelatinous or loculated effusions."

As of 2017, there are three types of anthrax toxin antibodies in the Strategic National Stockpile. One is polyclonal, called intravenous anthrax immune globulin, and is derived from the plasma of persons who have received the anthrax vaccine. Intravenous anthrax immune globulin has been given as adjunctive therapy to several patients, including three in the United States in 2006, 2009, and 2011 as well as several patients in the United Kingdom. Based on data in rabbits, it has recently been approved in the United States by the FDA for use in addition to antibiotics for inhalational anthrax. Another antitoxin is a humanized monoclonal antibody called raxibacumab that was licensed by the FDA in December 2012 for treatment of inhalational anthrax in both adults and children.[9] It had not been given to any patients with anthrax as of September 2017 but was licensed by the FDA on the basis of efficacy in animal models of inhalational anthrax plus human safety data in healthy volunteers. It does not cross the blood-brain barrier. It is given intravenously during 2 hours and 15 minutes, after a single dose of the antihistamine diphenhydramine. Another antibody, obiltoxaximab, is also FDA-approved to treat inhalational anthrax in combination with appropriate antibacterial drugs or to prevent inhalational anthrax based on its efficacy in rabbits and macaques, and safety in healthy human volunteers.[10]

PREVENTION

Clinical anthrax can be prevented by preexposure vaccination or by postexposure prophylaxis with antibiotics. Moreover, the monoclonal antibody antitoxin (raxibacumab) has been licensed by the FDA for postexposure prophylaxis in both adults and children "when alternative therapies are not available or not appropriate."

The current FDA-licensed anthrax vaccine contains protective antigen as the vaccine antigen and alum as an adjuvant. It requires five intramuscular injections, three primary and two booster, over 12 months when it is given before exposure. In contrast, postexposure prophylaxis requires only three injections given subcutaneously during a 1-month period. This vaccine is in limited supply and is dedicated primarily for use by the military; however, it is available to civilian populations through at least one commercial travel clinic.

Antibiotics that are approved by the FDA for postexposure prophylaxis include ciprofloxacin, doxycycline, and procaine penicillin G as well as levofloxacin. Either doxycycline or ciprofloxacin is recommended as the preferred drug by the CDC for initial prophylaxis when the antibiotic susceptibility of an anthrax strain is unknown. During pregnancy, however, ciprofloxacin is preferred to doxycycline according to 2014 CDC guidelines. The CDC website on anthrax (at http://www.bt.cdc.gov/agent/anthrax) has detailed recommendations regarding the choice of antibiotics, doses, and durations for both prevention and treatment of anthrax.

Prevention of anthrax due to bioterrorism remains a national priority. A suspicion of clinical anthrax or exposure to spores warrants immediate involvement of law enforcement authorities because of the possibility of a criminal act. Evolving approaches for detecting and responding to any future bioterrorism attacks with anthrax include the BioWatch system to detect aerosolized threats and the Autonomous Detection System in postal facilities. The Cities Readiness Initiative, as described by the CDC, is a program for multiple U.S. cities to help prepare for large-scale public health emergencies, including bioterrorism attacks (e.g., with aerosolized anthrax or another organism). Large volumes of medical supplies, including but not limited to antibiotics, can be delivered rapidly from the Strategic National Stockpile to one or more cities followed by local distribution. The 2012 Institute of Medicine report titled *Prepositioning Antibiotics for Anthrax* discusses the Strategic National Stockpile, Cities Readiness Initiative, BioWatch, and antibiotic issues including defining multidrug-resistant and extremely drug-resistant strains.

PROGNOSIS

The inhalational anthrax of all six patients who survived the attacks of 2001 was diagnosed during the intermediate progressive stage, and prompt therapy prevented progression beyond this stage. The 45% case-fatality rate in 2001 was much improved over the 88% rate seen in the United States from 1900 to 1976. Survival is more likely in patients who undergo pleural drainage, receive multidrug antibiotic regimens, do not require intubation or tracheotomy, and do not progress to anthrax meningoencephalitis. Of note, two patients with inhalational anthrax in the United States (in 2006 and 2011) with respiratory failure requiring mechanical ventilation have survived. Whether the addition of antitoxin to their intensive care, multiple antibiotics, and pleural drainage played a causal role in their survival is uncertain. Their survival emphasizes, however, that even patients in the late fulminant stage can sometimes survive.

The mortality from cutaneous anthrax is approximately 20% if it is untreated, particularly in patients in whom upper airway compression develops from a lesion on the neck or in whom secondary bacteremic anthrax meningitis develops. Anthrax meningitis remains fatal in more than 95% of victims, and thus better therapies are needed. The FDA licensure of the first anthrax antitoxin for both children and adults, as therapy and also as postexposure prophylaxis when alternative therapies are not available or not appropriate, may improve clinical outcome in systemic forms of anthrax. An antitoxin is still needed, however, that can treat anthrax meningitis.

FUTURE DIRECTIONS

A rapid test is still needed for the diagnosis of infection with *B. anthracis* in the early prodromal stage of the illness or in later clinical stages if the patient received antibiotics before blood culture samples were obtained. Such a test is likely to be based on a toxin or a toxin component. In 2015 the CDC reported a quantitative assay based on lethal toxin that met these criteria when tested in rhesus macaques infected with anthrax.[11] Ideally, such a rapid diagnostic clinical test should be available at the point of care.

Anthrax toxin inhibitors, in conjunction with antibiotics, could be particularly useful in treating patients who have progressed into the systemic stages of anthrax as a result of inhalational, gastrointestinal, or injection anthrax causing serious soft tissue infection. Timing of effective antitoxin use postexposure is uncertain, but has been estimated recently using models.[12] In addition, antitoxin could be useful in the setting of infection with an engineered form of multidrug-resistant or extremely drug-resistant anthrax. New anthrax vaccines are still being tested, but none have been FDA-licensed since 1970.

GENERAL REFERENCES

For the General References and other additional features, please visit Expert Consult at https://expertconsult.inkling.com.

279
ERYSIPELOTHRIX INFECTIONS

ANNETTE C. REBOLI

DEFINITION

Erysipelothrix rhusiopathiae causes three well-defined patterns of human infection: (1) erysipeloid, a cellulitis of the fingers and hands (also known as whale finger or pork finger), which is the most common manifestation of infection with *E. rhusiopathiae*; (2) a diffuse cutaneous form; and (3) a systemic or invasive form, with or without cutaneous involvement, usually manifesting as bacteremia which may be complicated by endocarditis.

The Pathogen

E. rhusiopathiae is a thin, pleomorphic, nonsporulating, microaerophilic gram-positive rod. It may be confused with other gram-positive bacillary organisms, particularly *Listeria monocytogenes* (Chapter 277) and *Corynebacterium* species (Chapter 276). It can be differentiated from *L. monocytogenes* by its lack of motility, lack of catalase and coagulase production, and resistance to neomycin. Most strains of *E. rhusiopathiae* produce hydrogen sulfide on triple sugar iron agar slants, a feature that distinguishes *E. rhusiopathiae* from *L. monocytogenes* and from corynebacteria. Because α-hemolysis may be seen after 48 hours of incubation of *E. rhusiopathiae*, confusion with streptococci may also occur. The term *erysipeloid* refers to cutaneous infection by *E. rhusiopathiae* and should

not be confused with erysipelas (see Fig. 412-4), which is a superficial cellulitis caused by streptococci or staphylococci.

EPIDEMIOLOGY

E. rhusiopathiae is found worldwide as a commensal or as a pathogen in a variety of wild and domestic animals, including swine, sheep, cattle, horses, dogs, cats, rodents, chickens, ducks, turkeys, penguins, and parrots, as well as in flies, ticks, mites, and lice. The greatest commercial impact of *E. rhusiopathiae* infection is due to disease in swine, but infection of sheep and poultry is also important economically. Environmental surfaces in contact with infected animals or their products are potential sources of *E. rhusiopathiae*. It can persist for prolonged periods in contaminated soil. *E. rhusiopathiae* is killed within 15 minutes by heating to 55° C and by several commercially available home disinfectants.

The incidence of cutaneous infection in humans seems to be decreasing because of technologic advances in animal industries. Infection is usually the result of contact with infected animals or their products. Persons at greatest risk for infection include fishers, fishmongers, farmers, butchers, slaughterhouse workers, and veterinarians.[1-3] The organism gains entry through cuts and abrasions on the skin and can result in infection from freshwater or seawater.[4] The seasonal incidence of erysipeloid parallels that of swine erysipeloid and is highest in the summer and early fall. The rare instances of systemic infection that do not have an occupational link tend to occur in immunocompromised hosts, suggesting that oropharyngeal or gastrointestinal colonization with the organism may occur. Chronic alcoholism has been acknowledged as a common underlying condition. Erysipeloid and erysipeloid with bacteremia have been reported rarely after cat and dog bites, suggesting that *E. rhusiopathiae* may be part of the oral flora of these animals.

PATHOBIOLOGY

The virulence of *E. rhusiopathiae* is associated, at least in part, with resistance to phagocytosis by polymorphonuclear leukocytes. This antiphagocytic ability results from the organism's possession of a capsule. In the absence of specific antibodies, *E. rhusiopathiae* evades phagocytosis, but even if it is phagocytosed, it is able to replicate intracellularly in these cells. Other virulence factors include enzymes (neuraminidase and hyaluronidase) and cell wall–associated proteins such as transporter and adhesion proteins.[5,6]

CLINICAL MANIFESTATIONS

Because of the mode of acquisition (contact with infected animals or their products, with organisms inoculating abrasions on the skin), lesions are usually confined to the fingers and hands (Fig. 279-1). A well-defined, slightly elevated, violaceous lesion accompanied by a very painful, throbbing, burning, or itching sensation develops within 2 to 7 days of traumatic dermal inoculation. The

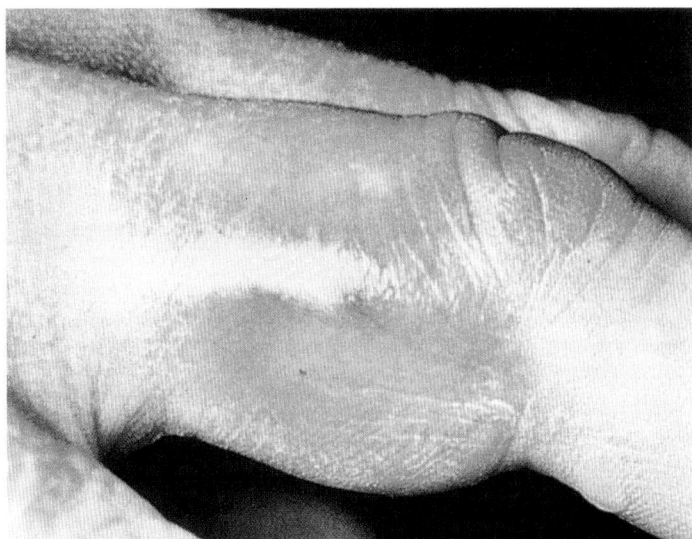

FIGURE 279-1. Erysipeloid with its characteristic purple, nonpurulent swelling of the finger. Also known as whale finger or pork finger, this form of cellulitis caused by *Erysipelothrix rhusiopathiae* should not be confused with streptococcal or staphylococcal erysipelas (see Fig. 412-4). (From Farrar WE, Wood MJ, Innes JUA, Tubbs H. *Infectious Diseases: Text and Color Atlas.* 2nd ed. New York: Gower Medical Publishing; 1992.)

infected area is swollen. Vesicles may be present, but suppuration is absent. The lesion spreads slowly to other fingers but rarely involves the fingertips or the skin above the wrist. As the lesion spreads peripherally, the central area clears. Systemic signs and symptoms are rare. There may be sterile arthritis of an adjacent joint. Regional lymphadenopathy or lymphadenitis occurs in about 20% of cases, and low-grade fever develops in approximately 10%. Lesions usually resolve within 3 weeks without treatment. Relapse occurs in 1% of cases.

The diffuse cutaneous form is rare. The cutaneous lesion progresses proximally from the site of inoculation or appears at remote areas. Patients often have fever and arthralgias, but blood cultures are generally negative.

Systemic infection with *Erysipelothrix* is uncommon. More than 100 cases of bacteremia have been reported; most of the patients had endocarditis.[7] This may be overestimated due to a reporting bias in case reports. Although cases of prosthetic valve endocarditis have been reported, most cases have involved native valves. In 60% of cases, infection developed on apparently normal heart valves. One third of patients had an antecedent or concurrent skin lesion of erysipeloid. The clinical manifestations of endocarditis secondary to *E. rhusiopathiae* and other microorganisms are similar. *E. rhusiopathiae* endocarditis correlates highly with occupation, exhibits a tropism for the aortic valve, affects more males than females, and is associated with high mortality. The high mortality may reflect a delay in appropriate therapy because of the empirical use of vancomycin, which is not an effective treatment of *E. rhusiopathiae*. Cases of *E. rhusiopathiae* endocarditis have been complicated by paravalvular and myocardial abscess formation, cerebral emboli, congestive heart failure, valve perforation, and acute renal failure. *E. rhusiopathiae* bacteremia without endocarditis occurs more frequently than was previously believed.[8] Bacteremia is occurring with increased frequency in immunocompromised patients, whereas endocarditis usually occurs in immunocompetent patients. Focal infections, including brain abscess, meningitis, endophthalmitis, osteomyelitis, septic arthritis, epidural and paravertebral abscesses, psoas abscess, liver abscess, necrotizing fasciitis, intra-abdominal abscess, and peritonitis, have been reported. Some of these infections were complications of bacteremia. Septic arthritis has occurred in native joints, in prosthetic joints, and after arthroscopic surgery.[9,10] Peritonitis has complicated peritoneal dialysis.

DIAGNOSIS

Diagnosis requires a high degree of suspicion in patients with exposures, usually work-related.[11] *E. rhusiopathiae* grows on routine laboratory media. Because *E. rhusiopathiae* is located only in deeper parts of the skin in cases of erysipeloid, biopsy of the entire thickness of the dermis from the edge of the lesion yields maximal recovery of the organism. Definitive diagnosis by skin biopsy is rarely necessary because of the classic clinical presentation and the rapid response to therapy. Routine blood culture techniques are adequate for growth and isolation of the organism in suspected cases of bacteremia or endocarditis. Various selective media have been used to improve the isolation of *E. rhusiopathiae* from contaminated specimens. Molecular techniques, such as polymerase chain reaction with primers specific for *E. rhusiopathiae*, have been developed and improve the efficiency of detection and identification. Matrix-assisted laser desorption ionization time-of-flight mass spectroscopy (MALDI-TOF MS) accurately and rapidly identifies *E. rhusiopathiae*.[12]

TREATMENT   Rx

Most isolates of *E. rhusiopathiae* are susceptible to penicillin, cephalosporins, imipenem, clindamycin, ciprofloxacin, ofloxacin, and daptomycin. Some resistance has been observed with erythromycin, tetracycline, chloramphenicol, and clindamycin.[13] *E. rhusiopathiae* is resistant to vancomycin, aminoglycosides, trimethoprim-sulfamethoxazole, and sulfonamides. Penicillin G is the treatment of choice. Uncomplicated cutaneous lesions generally respond well to a 5- to 7-day course of oral penicillin. Treatment hastens healing, although relapse may still occur. Bacteremia should be treated with intravenous penicillin; cases of endocarditis should be treated with 12 million to 20 million units of penicillin G daily or ceftriaxone 1 g daily for 4 to 6 weeks. Two weeks of intravenous therapy followed by 2 weeks of oral therapy has been successful. The use of quinolones or daptomycin may be considered for *Erysipelothrix* infections when the patient is allergic to β-lactams. Oral linezolid was used to complete therapy in a case of bacteremia complicated by endophthalmitis. Valve replacement may be necessary in patients with endocarditis. Infected prosthetic devices should be removed.

PREVENTION

Proper cleaning and disinfection of work surfaces and attention to hygienic work practices, including the use of gloves and hand hygiene, reduce the risk for infection. Vaccines are available for commercial use in animals only.

GENERAL REFERENCES

For the General References and other additional features, please visit Expert Consult at https://expertconsult.inkling.com.

280

CLOSTRIDIAL INFECTIONS

DALE N. GERDING AND STUART JOHNSON

Clostridial infections are characterized by disease produced by toxins. They include tetanus and botulism, both caused by neurotoxins, and clostridial myonecrosis or gas gangrene, caused by the toxins of *Clostridium perfringens* as well as those of other clostridial species. Although these clostridial infections remain important clinically, their frequency has declined markedly with the advent of vaccines and better public health measures. Several previously little known species of clostridia that produce very large clostridial cytotoxins (LCCs) varying in size from 250 to 308 kD have become increasingly prominent. They include, in particular, *C. difficile*, which is responsible for the most common health care–associated infections in the United States and for increasing mortality among elderly patients.[1] Another LCC-producing organism, *C. sordellii*, has caused devastating infections in young women in association with pregnancy and medical abortion, in injection drug users, and in patients with traumatic wounds. *C. novyi* type A is a third LCC organism that has also caused severe infections in injection drug users.

CLOSTRIDIUM DIFFICILE INFECTION

DEFINITION AND PATHOGEN

C. difficile infection (CDI) is a gastrointestinal infection characterized by diarrhea (three or more loose or unformed stools in ≤24 hours) and a positive test result for *C. difficile* toxin A or toxin B in stool, evidence of a toxin-producing strain of *C. difficile* in stool, or evidence of pseudomembranous colitis on direct visualization of the colon. *C. difficile* is a spore-forming, anaerobic, gram-positive organism that survives well in water, soil, and animals and has a worldwide distribution.

EPIDEMIOLOGY

CDI occurs most frequently in health care settings, particularly in long-term care facilities and acute care hospitals, and is most frequent and lethal among the elderly, especially those older than 75 years. Rates in U.S. hospitals have nearly tripled since 2000, and it is now estimated that there are 500,000 CDIs and nearly 30,000 CDI-associated deaths each year in the United States.[2] A specific strain of *C. difficile*—identified as the restriction endonuclease group BI, pulsed-field gel type NAP1, polymerase chain reaction ribotype 027 (BI/NAP1/027) strain—is thought to be responsible for much of the epidemic that has extended to Canada and Europe. Rates of community-onset CDI have also increased during the past decade, in association with the rising rates in hospitals and nursing homes. However, 94% of community-onset cases in a population-based study were associated with receiving some kind of recent health care, including outpatient visits, recently discharged patients, and nursing home residents. It is unlikely that community-associated cases (with no health care exposure) account for more than 10 to 15% of all CDIs. Risk factors for CDI include antimicrobial use, advanced age,[3] and stay in an acute or chronic care facility. Hospitals and nursing homes are considered a particularly high-risk environment because patients are elderly, antibiotic use is frequent, the environment is contaminated with *C. difficile* spores (which are difficult to eradicate), asymptomatic patients carry *C. difficile* in their stools, and health care workers carry *C. difficile* on their hands if they do not practice good hand hygiene.[4] *C. difficile* can be cultured from the stools of about 2 to 3% of healthy adults, but the frequency in asymptomatic hospitalized patients increases with the duration of hospitalization and may reach 20% or more. Exposure to nearly all antimicrobials has been associated with subsequent CDI, but those with the highest risk are clindamycin, the cephalosporins, and the fluoroquinolones. CDI is rare in children and young adults, despite their frequent exposure to antimicrobials. However, children younger than 1 to 2 years are commonly colonized with *C. difficile* while remaining asymptomatic, an observation that remains largely unexplained.

PATHOBIOLOGY

CDI risk appears to be minimal in the absence of antimicrobial therapy. When antimicrobials are administered, they have the unintended consequence of disrupting the normal protective bowel microbiota for days to weeks after the antimicrobial is stopped. If *C. difficile* is ingested during this time, the spores germinate in the gut, and the vegetative form of the organism multiplies and begins to make toxins. At this point, whether the patient will develop diarrhea is dictated by the status of his or her immunity to the toxins, which is best correlated with serum immunoglobulin G antibodies directed at toxin A and toxin B of *C. difficile*. Those with good antibody responses will be asymptomatic but will remain colonized with *C. difficile*, whereas those with little or no antibody response will develop diarrhea and CDI. Toxin A is primarily an enterotoxin, and toxin B is a cytotoxin. Both act by glucosylation of small GTPase proteins that cause disruption of the cell cytoskeleton, resulting in colonic epithelial cell rounding, fluid leakage, and cell death. In the presence of pseudomembranous colitis, the colon appears to be covered in yellow to white pseudomembranes that vary in size from punctate to completely confluent and covering the entire colon in advanced cases. On histologic evaluation, the colon demonstrates a marked neutrophil infiltration throughout its wall, with mucosal necrosis and volcano-like lesions from which the pseudomembrane is seen to "erupt." The pseudomembrane is composed of proteinaceous material and cellular debris.

CLINICAL MANIFESTATIONS

Clinical symptoms of CDI range from asymptomatic carriage to severe and sometimes life-threatening pseudomembranous colitis complicated by major fluid losses and systemic complications. With mild CDI, patients may simply have "nuisance diarrhea" that resolves when the implicated drug is discontinued. Others with more severe CDI have substantial fluid and protein losses combined with fever, cramps, hypoalbuminemia, leukocytosis, and hypotension. Leukocytosis is common (occurring in up to 50% of patients) and it is a marker of severe CDI when greater than 15,000/μL. Extremely high white blood counts (>50,000/μL) are an indication of fulminant and potentially fatal illness. Other factors that may be indicative of severe or late-stage disease include toxic megacolon, high fever, renal failure, hypotension, shock, and lactic acidosis with levels greater than 5.0 mmol/L.

DIAGNOSIS

The diagnosis should be suspected in any patient who has otherwise unexplained diarrhea (three or more loose or unformed stools in ≤24 hours) in association with recent or concurrent antibiotic use. Only about 10 to 20% of patients in this category actually have CDI, but this is the group of patients that should be tested. Episodes of CDI are often misdiagnosed, mainly due to lack of clinical suspicion or the use of inappropriate tests. The diagnosis of CDI is primarily based on the clinical signs and symptoms and is only confirmed by laboratory testing.[5]

The standard test to establish the diagnosis is to detect toxins A and B in stool or to detect a toxin-producing strain of *C. difficile* in stool. Tests that detect only toxin A are inadequate because about 1 to 3% of strains that cause CDI produce toxin B but not toxin A. The most common laboratory method has been an enzyme immunoassay, but its sensitivity is only 50 to 80%. Repeated testing does not improve the diagnostic accuracy because enzyme immunoassays also have specificity deficiencies that increase the rate of false-positive test results with repeated testing. Nucleic acid amplification tests (NAAT) of which polymerase chain reaction (PCR) is most commonly used for *C. difficile* in stool are widely available commercially and markedly improve test sensitivity to 90 to 95% (compared with the "gold standard" of culture for a toxigenic strain). NAAT tests are more expensive, but their use by clinical laboratories is widespread in the United States. They increase the sensitivity of CDI diagnosis, but some studies have shown that a positive test result for stool toxin should also be present to confirm the diagnosis, because patients with a positive molecular test but negative immunoassay have outcomes similar to patients without *C. difficile* by either test. The standard cell cytotoxin assay is little used but more sensitive than enzyme immunoassay. It has the disadvantages of a

24- to 48-hour turnaround and the requirement for tissue culture facilities. Stool culture for *C. difficile*, which is the most sensitive test available, is likewise slow and requires confirmation of toxin production by the organism before reporting. Testing of stools for glutamate dehydrogenase, or "common antigen," can be used as a rapid screening test, but it is only about 50% specific and requires confirmation with a toxin test, which can increase the turnaround time for reporting positive results. CDI can also be diagnosed by observing pseudomembranous colitis directly through sigmoidoscopy or colonoscopy or at surgery. When a negative test result does not confirm the diagnosis in a patient whose clinical symptoms are highly suggestive of CDI, empirical treatment of CDI should be given rather than repeating the test. The cause of infectious diarrhea in an adult patient with an onset longer than 48 hours after hospital admission is almost always CDI because other infectious enteric pathogens (with the exception of norovirus) are extremely rare in the hospital setting. Also common in the differential diagnosis are noninfectious causes of diarrhea, such as antibiotic or other drug-associated diarrhea, laxatives, ischemic colitis, and idiopathic inflammatory bowel disease. For patients with antibiotic-associated diarrhea and no evidence of colitis, the cause of diarrhea with a negative *C. difficile* toxin assay is usually not defined. New CDI guidelines in the United States recommend that NAAT testing alone be done only if patients are screened for documented diarrhea (3 or more loose or unformed stools in <24 hours and no laxative use) prior to submitting a stool for NAAT testing. If patients are not screened, a combination of tests that includes glutamate dehydrogenase (GDH) or NAAT and a confirmatory EIA test for toxin is recommended.[6]

PREVENTION

Two major prevention strategies are employed. The first is traditional infection control, in which barriers to transmission (gowns, gloves, isolation, hand hygiene, environmental cleaning) are used to prevent the spores of *C. difficile* from reaching the patient (Chapter 266). The second strategy is to reduce the likelihood of infection if the patient does encounter *C. difficile* while in the hospital. The most efficacious strategy, also known as antimicrobial stewardship, is to avoid or to minimize exposure to unnecessary antimicrobials, especially those with a high CDI risk,[7] such as clindamycin, cephalosporins, and fluoroquinolones. Interventions to restrict exposure to clindamycin and to cephalosporins have been highly effective in interrupting outbreaks of CDI in hospitals. Probiotics used prophylactically may also reduce CDI risk, but there is currently no consistent recommendation for their use.[8]

TREATMENT

Updated clinical practice guidelines for the diagnosis and treatment of CDI were published in 2018 by the Infectious Diseases Society of America (ISDA) and the Society for Healthcare Epidemiology of America (SHEA).[9] Treatment of CDI begins with discontinuation of the implicated antibiotic, supportive care, and avoidance of antiperistaltic agents.[10] Mildly ill patients may recover with these simple conservative measures, but most require specific treatment. Continuation of the offending antibiotics while CDI is being treated with vancomycin and other agents results in lower cure rates and higher CDI recurrence rates in patients. Metronidazole, at a dose of 500 mg orally three times a day for 10 to 14 days, has been the recommended treatment for patients with mild CDI because it is inexpensive. However, a large randomized prospective trial of vancomycin versus metronidazole has placed the recommendation into question because it showed vancomycin to be statistically superior to metronidazole for all patients with CDI.[A1] As a result, new U.S. guidelines no longer recommend metronidazole as first-line treatment of CDI of any severity. Patients with mild/moderate or severe CDI (variously defined as a white blood cell count >15,000 or a creatinine increase to >1.5-fold above baseline) should be treated with vancomycin 125 mg orally four times a day for 10 days or fidaxomicin 200 mg orally twice a day for 10 days. Fidaxomicin is a narrow-spectrum macrocycle antibiotic that is as efficacious as vancomycin and reduces recurrent infection.[A2] The anticipated response to these drugs is rapid defervescence, with gradual normalization of bowel habits. Mean time to resolution of diarrhea is about 3 days; if symptoms have not resolved by day 5 or day 6 of treatment, a change in therapy should be considered. However, there are no data to support the use of more than one drug at a time to treat CDI other than in fulminant disease. Failure to respond often means that either the disease has progressed too far or another condition is causing the symptoms. For patients with severe complicated or fulminant CDI, medical management includes vancomycin at a higher dose (500 mg four times a day) orally or by nasogastric tube; if ileus is present, metronidazole (500 mg IV every 8 hours) is added, with vancomycin also administered by enema. If symptoms progress with this therapy, colectomy may be life-saving and should be performed before the white blood cell count reaches 50,000/µL or lactate concentration reaches 5.0 mmol/L. A colon-sparing loop ileostomy procedure followed by infusion of polyethylene glycol and vancomycin has demonstrated reduced mortality compared with historic colectomy controls and may be a preferred procedure to colectomy.

Other antibiotic options include oral fusidic acid, teicoplanin, nitazoxanide, rifaximin, and bacitracin, but most of these drugs have been evaluated in only a small number of patients, and none (like metronidazole) has U.S. Food and Drug Administration (FDA) approval for the treatment of CDI. There is no convincing evidence that toxin-binding agents, such as cholestyramine and probiotics, are useful in treating CDI. About 20 to 25% of patients treated with either vancomycin or metronidazole have a recurrence of symptoms when treatment is stopped because of the persistence of *C. difficile* spores or acquisition of a new strain. Treatment of recurrent CDI with vancomycin, vancomycin plus taper and pulse, or fidaxomicin is recommended. Patients with multiple recurrences of CDI are extremely difficult to treat and may benefit from consultation with an infectious disease specialist or gastroenterologist. Actoxumab and bezlotoxumab[11] are human monoclonal antibodies against *C. difficile* toxins A and B, respectively. In patients receiving antibiotic treatment for primary or recurrent CDI, bezlotoxumab (infused at a dose of 10 mg per kilogram of body weight) was associated with a substantially lower rate of recurrent infection than placebo and had a safety profile similar to that of placebo. The addition of actoxumab did not improve efficacy.[A3]

Observational data and prospective randomized trials suggest that fecal microbiota transplantation can be an effective treatment for recurrent *C. difficile* infection.[A4][A5] Furthermore, frozen fecal microbiota transplantation is as effective as fresh microbiota for the clinical resolution of diarrhea in patients with recurrent *C. difficile* infection.[A6] In one randomized trial, donor stool administered via colonoscopy seemed safe and was more efficacious than autologous fecal microbiota transplantation in preventing further episodes of *Clostridium difficile* infection.[A7] Among adults with recurrent CDI, fecal microbiota transplantation via oral capsules was found to be not inferior to delivery by colonoscopy for preventing recurrent infection over 12 weeks.[A8] Among patients who have clinically recovered following treatment with metronidazole or vancomycin, oral administration of spores of nontoxigenic *C. difficile* strain M3 can colonize the gastrointestinal tract and significantly reduce recurrent CDI.[A9]

PROGNOSIS

The majority (≈80%) of patients respond to simple withdrawal of the implicated antibiotic combined with a single course of vancomycin or fidaxomicin. Some patients with fulminant disease eventually require colectomy. The attributable mortality rate is as high as 7% in large series, and the majority of lethal cases occur in patients older than 65 years. Patients with multiple recurrences require repeated courses of antibiotics, usually vancomycin with tapering and pulse-dose regimens, or fidaxomicin that may need to be continued for weeks to months, or may require resorting to fecal microbiota transplantation.

⬤ NECROTIZING CLOSTRIDIAL TISSUE INFECTION
Clostridium sordellii
DEFINITION AND PATHOGEN

C. sordellii is another clostridial species that produces large clostridial cytotoxins (LCCs), and it has become more common as a cause of septic shock and necrotizing fasciitis in association with trauma, childbirth, medical abortion, and injection drug use. *C. sordellii* antitoxin cross-neutralizes the cytotoxic effect of *C. difficile* toxins, indicating the similarity of these LCCs.

EPIDEMIOLOGY

The organism is commonly found in soil and in the feces of animals and occasionally transiently in the vagina or rectum of humans worldwide.[12] Soil contamination of wounds is the usual suspected route of infection. Infections have been described after traumatic wounds, childbirth, medical abortion, and intramuscular or subcutaneous injection drug use.

PATHOBIOLOGY

C. sordellii produces up to seven identified toxins; of these, hemorrhagic toxin (TcsH) and lethal toxin (TcsL), which are both LCCs and analogous to TcdA and TcdB of *C. difficile*, are considered major virulence factors. Both TcsL and TcsH are located on plasmids in *C. sordellii*. TcsL have been shown to be essential for virulence. The toxins produce local necrosis, progressive edema, and shock that results in high mortality. The toxins are glucosyltransferases that glucosylate the Rho, Rac, or Ras proteins, causing impaired cytoskeletal

organization and massive capillary leakage, leading to the progressive edematous state.

CLINICAL MANIFESTATIONS

Initial symptoms are nonspecific and include nausea, lethargy, dizziness, and tenderness at the infection site. Tachycardia and hypotension follow within hours. Laboratory tests show a marked leukocytosis or leukemoid reaction. Hypotension and tachycardia are refractory to treatment. Edema secondary to capillary leakage is prominent, resulting in hemoconcentration but little or no fever. Peritoneal and pleural effusions are common. White blood cell elevations greater than 75,000/µL are associated with a fatal outcome.

Infection Associated with Childbirth and Medical Abortion

This is a rare infection in which patients present 4 to 7 days after the administration of oral mifepristone and vaginal misoprostol for medical abortion with nausea, vomiting, weakness, abdominal pain, hypotension, and tachycardia but little or no fever and, often remarkably, a lack of findings on pelvic examination. The presentation is similar to toxic shock syndrome. There is rapid progression to vascular collapse and cardiac arrest. Leukocytosis is dramatic, with white blood cell counts near 100,000/µL in most patients. After delivery, the presentation is similar, but localized swelling and discoloration of the labia and perineum may be evident if the episiotomy site is infected. All patients to date have died.

Infection Associated with Injection Drug Use

Black tar heroin (a dark, gummy, less refined and cheaper form of heroin) has been associated with necrotizing fasciitis at the subcutaneous or intramuscular injection site, presumably a result of the contaminants mixed with the heroin. Patients present with 2 to 7 days of symptoms of necrotizing fasciitis of the upper or lower extremity where they injected heroin, in some cases accompanied by hypotension. Aggressive surgical débridement is required at the infection site, together with fluids and pressors. Cultures of débrided tissue reveal multiple organisms in addition to *C. sordellii*. Mortality in these patients is 50%.

DIAGNOSIS

Diagnosis is difficult because of the lack of specific symptoms, but it is usually made by identifying the likely source of infection and isolating *C. sordellii* from the infection site or blood cultures. Polymerase chain reaction analysis for *C. sordellii* in infected tissues may be required to make the diagnosis when cultures are negative. Other bacteria are also commonly found at the infection site. Computed tomography or magnetic resonance imaging may be helpful in identifying localized infections, which can then be excised or drained surgically, providing material for microbiologic diagnosis.

PREVENTION

C. sordellii infections are very rare, and the exact mechanism of infection, especially after medical abortion, is not known. However, careful attention to wound cleansing, avoidance of injecting drugs into skin or muscle, and good hygiene during childbirth are likely to help prevent *C. sordellii* infection.

TREATMENT

Definitive treatment information is lacking. The infection progresses so rapidly that therapeutic interventions are rarely successful. Surgery to remove necrotic sites of infection and administration of intravenous fluids and pressors to treat hypotension and tachycardia are supportive. Antibiotic susceptibility suggests that β-lactams, clindamycin, tetracyclines, and chloramphenicol are active, but no clinical treatment efficacy data are available. Theoretically, use of an antibiotic such as clindamycin to suppress toxin synthesis could be a useful adjunct to treatment. At present, there is no antitoxin available.

PROGNOSIS

Infections after childbirth or medical abortion have been uniformly fatal. Mortality in injection drug users or patients after trauma or surgery is about 50%.

Clostridium novyi Infection in Injecting Drug Users

C. novyi α-toxin causes an LCC-producing disease in humans. *C. novyi* has long been recognized as a cause of fatal toxemia in animals with contaminated wounds. An extended outbreak of human infections occurred in Scotland, Ireland, and elsewhere in the United Kingdom in 2000 to 2009 among persons injecting heroin extravascularly (skin or muscle popping). A localized necrotizing infection with painful edema, sepsis, and significant mortality was recognized. The findings include soft tissue inflammation, edema and necrosis at the injection sites, circulatory collapse, marked leukocytosis, and pleural effusions. Treatment usually involves débridement and antibiotic administration (gentamicin, flucloxacillin, penicillin, metronidazole, and clindamycin were used during this outbreak because infections are typically polymicrobial in origin).

Clostridial Myonecrosis (Gas Gangrene)

DEFINITION

Clostridial myonecrosis, or gas gangrene, can be caused by several *Clostridium* species, most commonly *C. perfringens* after trauma or tissue injury and *Clostridium septicum* after dissemination from a colonic source.

EPIDEMIOLOGY

Gas gangrene has historically been a complication of battlefield injuries and of trauma in noncombat settings. The estimated number of cases in the United States is about 1000 per year. Traumatic injuries account for about 50% of cases, with vehicular accidents accounting for the majority; the remaining cases develop in patients after crush injuries, industrial accidents, gunshot wounds, and burns. Minor injuries such as puncture wounds, intramuscular injections, simple lacerations, and subcutaneous injections with epinephrine may occasionally precipitate clostridial myonecrosis. Postoperative complications account for about 30% of cases and are most frequently associated with surgery on the appendix, biliary tract, or intestine. Approximately 20% are "spontaneous" or nontraumatic and are invariably associated with an occult colonic malignant neoplasm.

PATHOBIOLOGY

Clostridia are widely distributed in nature and can be cultured from nearly all soil samples, from environmental sites in the hospital, and from the human intestine. A critical factor is a physiologic state of the wound with conditions that support germination and toxin production by toxigenic clostridia. Particularly critical are a low oxidation-reduction potential, hypoxia, appropriate substrates, and calcium ions. The probability of infection is substantially increased by devitalized muscle and the presence of foreign material such as soil. *C. perfringens* elaborates at least 12 recognized toxins, most importantly α-toxin and θ-toxin of *C. perfringens* type A. Although the interaction is complex, good evidence supports a central role for α-toxin, a phospholipase C, and θ-toxin or perfringolysin O, a cholesterol-dependent cytolysin, in the extensive cell death and disruption of microvascular perfusion that are characteristic of clostridial myonecrosis. The vascular perfusion changes are likely mediated by toxin-induced platelet aggregation and leukocyte margination. The α-toxin of *C. septicum*, a pore-forming cytolysin unrelated to α-toxin of *C. perfringens*, also causes cell death and microvascular perfusion changes.

CLINICAL MANIFESTATIONS

Initial symptoms of traumatic myonecrosis usually occur 1 to 4 days after the precipitating event, although the range is 8 hours to 3 weeks. The initial symptom is pain that is often sudden and severe at the site of surgery or trauma. The involved skin has intense edema and is initially pale before progressing to a bronze or magenta color, followed by the formation of bullae. The bullae contain fluid that may be clear or hemorrhagic. The discharge has an odor that is described as "foul-sweet."

Circulatory collapse and hypotension unresponsive to fluid challenge are common and may reflect the effect of α-toxin, which suppresses cardiac contractility. About 15% of patients have bacteremia that is usually complicated by rapid hemolysis with a dramatic drop in the hematocrit, which may even decrease to 0%. Common complications include jaundice, hypotension, hepatic failure, and renal failure. The renal failure is often due to hemoglobinuria and myoglobinuria, but it may also be due to acute tubular necrosis from hypotension. Despite the severity of the illness, the patient's mental status is usually remarkably good until very late in the disease. Surgical intervention shows necrotic muscle that does not contract with stimulation. Deeper dissection reveals beefy red necrotic muscle that becomes black and extremely friable in the late stages.

Uterine gas gangrene, which was once common after septic abortions, is now rare but may complicate normal delivery, amniocentesis, cesarean section, or abortion. The onset is usually sudden, with fever, tachycardia, hypotension, renal failure, and jaundice. Radiography may show gas in the uterine wall. The urine is often "port wine" in color as a result of hemoglobinuria, and there is often jaundice because of massive intravascular hemolysis. The usual causes are *C. perfringens* and *C. sordellii*.

Spontaneous myonecrosis occurs in the absence of trauma and is usually caused by *C. septicum*. One distinctive association is with colon cancer and neutropenic enterocolitis, which represent portals of entry for hematogenous seeding of *C. septicum*. This infection is also seen with acute leukemia. The usual portals of entry are the terminal ileum, cecum, and ascending colon, hence the term *typhlitis* or neutropenic enterocolitis. Known or occult malignancy was associated in 71% of patients and mortality was 67% in one large recent review of spontaneous *C. septicum* myonecrosis.[13]

DIAGNOSIS

The diagnosis of gas gangrene is usually based on a constellation of characteristic clinical features, including myonecrosis of an extremity or abdominal wall, shock, and renal failure. The patient typically complains of severe pain. Early recognition is important because early institution of treatment may strongly influence the prognosis. The diagnosis is established by examination of skin and muscle, which shows putrid discharge, characteristic bullae, and crepitations. Gram stain demonstrates abundant gram-positive bacilli and no inflammatory cells. Histopathologic examination of the lesion shows myonecrosis without polymorphonuclear leukocytes, a finding that is remarkably different from most soft tissue infections, which do not feature necrosis and have abundant inflammatory cells. Gas is present in the tissue and may be detected by physical examination, radiography, or other imaging methods.

PREVENTION

The basic principle of prevention is adequate management of traumatic wounds—establishing adequate drainage, removing foreign bodies, draining hematomas, and ensuring good hemostasis.

TREATMENT   Rx

The most important facet of treatment is prompt surgical débridement. Many cases require extensive, often mutilating surgery. Penicillin and clindamycin are recommended but are rarely adequate without radical surgery, except in patients with neutropenic enterocolitis, who can often be managed with antibiotics. The rationale for penicillin combined with clindamycin is that some strains of clostridia are resistant to clindamycin, but clindamycin is probably the superior drug for reducing toxin formation. Other antibiotics that are generally effective include metronidazole and chloramphenicol. The use of hyperbaric oxygen is controversial, in part because the therapeutic trials have been either of poor quality or not convincing.

PROGNOSIS

Factors associated with a poor prognosis include advanced age, location on the trunk, association with severe underlying disease, leukopenia, renal failure, hemolysis, and shock. The best results are seen in young patients with involvement of a single extremity. Management plays an important role, particularly the use of early and aggressive surgery as well as antibiotics. The overall mortality rate of patients with traumatic gas gangrene in tertiary centers is about 25%.

● NEUROTOXIC CLOSTRIDIAL INFECTIONS

Botulism

DEFINITION

Botulism is a severe neuroparalytic disease characterized by a descending flaccid motor neuron paralysis. It is caused by botulinum toxin produced by *C. botulinum*.

The Pathogen

C. botulinum is a gram-positive, spore-forming obligate anaerobe that is widely distributed in nature and is frequently found in soil, marine environments, and agricultural products. Each strain produces one of eight toxins designated by the letters A to H. Botulinum toxin may also be produced by the related clostridial species *C. baratii* and *C. butyricum*. All these neurotoxins produce the same syndrome; the usual causes of disease in humans are types A, B, and E, with rare cases caused by type F.

EPIDEMIOLOGY

Botulism in humans is generally one of three types: food-borne botulism, infant botulism, or wound botulism. Rarely, botulism may be acquired as a result of iatrogenic misadventures with botulinum toxin, which is a potential bioterrorism agent if it is inhaled or ingested.

Food-borne botulism is the most common form of botulism in the world but is a distant second to infant botulism in the United States. Nevertheless, 31 cases from ingestion of prison-made alcohol (pruno),[14] and eight cases from ingestion of a commercially canned product (hot dog chili sauce) have occurred recently. Foods most frequently implicated are home-canned vegetables or fermented foods, and most cases are sporadic single cases occasionally involving two or three people. Commercially preserved and restaurant-prepared foods are also rare causes of food-borne botulism. Type A toxin is predominant in the United States. Alaska has the highest rate of any state, with approximately 35% of all cases; 80% of events and cases in Alaska are caused by type E and are most often associated with fermentation methods used to prepare fish and marine mammals by native Alaskans. Meat and meat products are frequently implicated in Europe, where the predominant toxin is type B. In China, the most frequent vehicle is a vegetable product, and type A predominates.

Infant botulism is the most frequently recognized form in the United States and is the most recently discovered type of botulism, first described in 1976. It is caused by production of botulinum toxin in the intestine after presumed spore ingestion and colonization in 2- to 36-week-old infants. Honey has been identified as a source of *C. botulinum* spores, but in most cases the source is never identified. Nearly all cases are caused by type A or type B toxin. The symptoms usually begin with constipation followed by poor feeding, weak cry, lethargy, and generalized weakness characterized as the "floppy baby syndrome" because of loss of head control. This form of botulism is rare in adults, occurring most often in patients with anatomic or functional abnormalities of the intestines.

Wound botulism, first described in 1943, is the least frequent form of the disease and is usually caused by either type A or type B toxin. Sporadic cases in traumatic wounds contaminated by soil are rarely reported. Outbreaks have been described in black tar heroin users in the western United States, particularly if they inject the drug intramuscularly or subcutaneously (skin popping).[15] These drug users also develop other clostridial infections, including necrotizing fasciitis caused by *C. sordellii* and *C. novyi* and tetanus caused by *C. tetani*.

Inhalation or ingestion of botulinum toxin is considered one of the top six bioweapon agents in terms of probability of use. The presumed method would be contamination of the food supply, water supply, or commercial beverages or aerosolization in a highly populated area to cause inhalational botulism. It is estimated that a point-source aerosol release of the toxin could incapacitate or kill 10% of people within a 0.5-km radius.

Iatrogenic botulism results from the misuse of botulinum toxin for cosmetic or therapeutic purposes. Cosmetic treatment doses are far too low to cause systemic disease, but the use of unlicensed products with high concentrations of botulinum toxin can cause systemic symptoms. Higher doses used for the management of muscle movement disorders have caused occasional cases with systemic botulism-like symptoms.

PATHOBIOLOGY

Pathologic findings are due to absorption of toxins from the intestine (ingested preformed toxin in foods or in situ production in the intestine in infants), inhalation (aerosol from bioterrorism), absorption from cutaneous infection sources (wounds), or iatrogenic injection. The toxin is disseminated by the systemic circulation and causes flaccid paralysis by binding presynaptic motor neuron terminals and blocking acetylcholine transmission across the neuromuscular junction. The estimated lethal doses of purified botulinum toxin A for a 70-kg human are 0.09 to 0.15 μg when given intravenously, 0.8 to 0.9 μg when inhaled, and 70 μg when given orally.

CLINICAL MANIFESTATIONS

In contrast to Guillain-Barré syndrome (Chapter 392), which is an ascending paralysis, botulism is characterized by generalized weakness and a descending paralysis. Symptoms are due to absorption of botulinum toxin from the gut, the lung, or a wound. Clinical symptoms consist of highly distinctive and usually symmetrical cranial nerve palsies, followed by a symmetrical descending flaccid paralysis. Prominently involved cranial nerves III, IV, and VI cause blurred vision and diplopia; involvement of cranial nerve VII causes

the characteristic expressionless facies and dysphagia; and involvement of cranial nerve IX causes dysarthria. Thus, the initial symptoms include the "four d's"—diplopia, dysarthria, dysphagia, and dysphonia—although the last is rarely reported, and blurred vision is reported more commonly than diplopia. These findings are followed by a descending upper extremity paralysis and respiratory paralysis. Neurologic examination shows bilateral cranial nerve VI paresis, ptosis, dilated pupils with a sluggish reaction, and diminished gag reflex, followed by descending involvement of motor neurons. Deep tendon reflexes are diminished or absent. Mentation remains clear, vital signs are normal, and the neurologic findings are symmetrical. The most common cause of death is respiratory failure. The tempo of the disease and the extent of paralysis in the absence of treatment are highly variable. The symptoms may be restricted to a few cranial nerves, or there may be complete paralysis of all voluntary muscles. Progression may occur during a period of hours or days. The timing and extent of neurologic deficits depend on the size of the botulinum toxin inoculum.

DIAGNOSIS

Botulism should be suspected in patients with an acute flaccid paralysis involving the cranial nerves, particularly in the presence of bilateral cranial nerve VI dysfunction, associated neurologic findings, and a 10-hour to 5-day history of consuming suspect food, such as preserved or home-canned foods. Nausea, vomiting, abdominal pain, and diarrhea are common early in the illness, with constipation present when paralysis develops. The finding of two or more cases that are epidemiologically linked is virtually diagnostic of food-borne botulism because other causes of paralysis are rare and sporadic. In the absence of a history of suspect food ingestion, potentially infected wounds should be sought, including injection sites in users of black tar heroin. With bioterrorism, the epidemiology may reflect a common source exposure, such as a local water supply or an aerosolized toxin, but it could also be widely distributed with a contaminated food source, such as the milk supply.

Laboratory tests for suspected food-borne botulism include analysis of serum, stool, gastric contents, or food for botulinum toxin and culture of stool and suspect food or wounds for *C. botulinum*. Toxin assay specimens should be collected before treatment with antitoxin. With wound botulism, recovery of *C. botulinum* from wound cultures or detection of toxin in serum is diagnostic. The toxin assays are generally available only at public health laboratories. The standard is a mouse bioassay for detection and quantification of toxin. Toxin type is determined by type-specific antibody neutralization. In general, adult patients with clinical evidence of food-borne botulism have detectable toxin in sera in a third of cases and detectable toxin in stool in a third of cases, but the organism is recovered from stool in about 60%.

The differential diagnosis includes myasthenia gravis, Guillain-Barré syndrome, tick paralysis, cerebrovascular accident, trichinosis, Eaton-Lambert syndrome, hypocalcemia, hypermagnesemia, organophosphate poisoning, atropine poisoning, and paralytic poisoning by shellfish or puffer fish. Electromyography using repetitive stimulation at 2 to 50/second may be helpful in distinguishing causes of flaccid paralysis. Electromyography patterns with slow and rapid supramaximal stimulation show similar responses in botulism and Eaton-Lambert syndrome. Findings on cerebrospinal fluid analysis and cranial imaging are normal in botulism.

PREVENTION

The disease can be prevented by destroying spores in the original food source, inhibiting germination, or destroying preformed toxin.

TREATMENT   Rx

Clinicians who suspect botulism should immediately seek clinical consultation, notify public health authorities, and administer antitoxin. The agency to contact in the United States is the state health department, which will contact the Centers for Disease Control and Prevention (CDC) if needed. Additional emergency consultation is available from the CDC botulism duty officer through the CDC Emergency Operations Center (telephone: 770-488-7100); similar public health agencies should be contacted in other countries. Treatment consists of supportive care and passive neutralization with equine botulinum antitoxin.

The standard treatment of adults since 2010 in the United States is heptavalent botulinum antitoxin (HBAT) through a CDC-sponsored FDA investigational new drug protocol. HBAT contains equine-derived antibody to the seven known botulinum toxin types (A to G) with the following nominal potency values: 7500 U anti-A; 5500 U anti-B; 5000 U anti-C; 1000 U anti-D; 8500 U anti-E; 5000 U anti-F; and 1000 U anti-G. BabyBIG (botulism immune globulin) is a human-derived treatment of infant botulism types A and B and is available for infant botulism through the California Infant Botulism Treatment and Prevention Program. The antitoxin should be given as early as possible and should not be delayed while awaiting microbiologic results. This treatment does not reverse paralysis or neutralize toxin already bound to nerve endings, but it does neutralize unbound toxin in the circulation to prevent progression. The HBAT antitoxin is derived from horses, and as a result, hypersensitivity reactions may occur.

Respiratory failure is a major risk, and patients must be monitored carefully with liberal criteria for ventilatory support. The requirement for mechanical ventilation varies from about 20% in adults with food-borne disease to 60% in patients with infant botulism. Other forms of supportive care include enteral or parenteral feeding and positioning in the reverse Trendelenburg position.

Toxin can be removed from the gastrointestinal tract by gastric lavage, cathartics, and enemas early in the course. Antibiotic treatment is unnecessary, except for wound botulism.

PROGNOSIS

The case-fatality rate for untreated food-borne botulism was once 60 to 70% but is currently 3 to 5% with treatment. Infant botulism in the United States now has a mortality rate of less than 1%; the use of human antitoxin has reduced the median duration of hospitalization from 6 to 3 weeks. Patients who survive any form of botulism generally have a complete recovery.

Tetanus

DEFINITION

Tetanus is a neurologic syndrome characterized by generalized rigidity and convulsive spasm of skeletal muscles caused by a neurotoxin elaborated at the site of injury by *C. tetani*.

The Pathogen

C. tetani is an anaerobic, gram-positive, slender, motile bacillus. When it sporulates, the terminal spore gives the organism a characteristic "drumstick" or "tennis racket" shape. The vegetative form produces tetanospasmin, a protein neurotoxin with a molecular mass of approximately 151 kD, including a heavy chain (100 kD) that binds neuronal cells and a light chain that blocks the release of neurotransmitters.

EPIDEMIOLOGY

C. tetani can be found in 2 to 23% of soil samples, with the highest yield in manure-treated soil. The organism can also be found in stool from a variety of domestic and farm animals and poultry. Tetanus is most common in warm climates and in highly cultivated rural areas. The greatest problem occurs in resource-limited countries because of high numbers of unimmunized mothers and unhygienic practices. The estimated annual toll from neonatal tetanus in developing countries is nearly 60,000, mostly secondary to inadequate passive immunity caused by absence of immunity in the mother.[16] In the United States, an average of 29 cases of tetanus were reported annually from 2001 to 2008 with a mortality of 13.2%, and almost all occurred in unimmunized or inadequately immunized persons. In the United States, patients 65 years of age and older constituted 31% of patients and had the highest mortality at 31%.

PATHOBIOLOGY

Tetanospasmin, also known as tetanus neurotoxin or TeNT, ranks with botulinum toxin as one of the most potent known microbial toxins; 2.5 ng/kg is a lethal human dose. Clinical tetanus usually results from entry of the organism into a wound and low oxygen conditions that allow spore germination and survival of the vegetative organism to produce toxin. Entry is usually through a traumatic or surgical wound, drug injection site, burn, skin ulcer, or infected umbilical cord. Tetanospasmin binds the peripheral nerve terminals and is then carried intra-axonally within membrane-bound vesicles to spinal neurons at a transport rate of approximately 75 to 250 mm/day. The light chain passes to the presynaptic terminals, where it blocks the release of neurotransmitters in inhibitory afferent motor neurons. Loss of the inhibitory influence results in sustained muscle contraction. Binding of the toxin is irreversible, so recovery requires the generation of new axon terminals.

CLINICAL MANIFESTATIONS

Forms of tetanus include generalized, local, cephalic, and neonatal. Generalized tetanus, which is the most common form, accounts for 80 to 90% of

reported cases in the United States. The usual incubation period is 3 to 21 days (mean, 8 days), depending largely on the distance between the site of injury and the central nervous system. A short incubation period is associated with more severe symptoms. Generalized tetanus is characterized by a persistent tonic spasm with brief exacerbations. The neck and jaw are almost always involved. Trismus (lockjaw) is the initial complaint in 75% of cases, so the patient is often initially seen by a dentist or oral surgeon. Other early features include irritability, restlessness, diaphoresis, and dysphagia with hydrophobia and drooling. Persistent spasm of the back musculature may cause opisthotonos. These early manifestations reflect involvement of the paraspinous muscles. With progression, all muscles contract, with stronger muscles overtaking weaker muscles. Noise or tactile stimuli may precipitate spasms and generalized convulsions. Involvement of the autonomic nervous system may result in severe arrhythmias, blood pressure oscillation, profound diaphoresis, hyperthermia, rhabdomyolysis, laryngeal spasm, and urinary retention. In most cases, the patient remains lucid and afebrile. The condition may continue for 3 to 4 weeks, despite antitoxin therapy, because of the time required for intra-axonal toxin transport. Complications include fractures from sustained contractions, pulmonary emboli, bacterial infections, and dehydration.

Local tetanus, in which the patient has persistent muscle contractions in the extremity involving a contaminated wound, is rare and shows considerable variation in severity. In mild cases, a patient may simply have spasms of the involved extremity; in more severe cases, local painful spasms progress to generalized tetanus. This relatively unusual form of tetanus has an excellent prognosis, with only about 1% mortality.

Cephalic tetanus is also rare and generally follows a head injury or occurs with *C. tetani* infection of the middle ear. Clinical symptoms consist of isolated or combined dysfunction of the cranial motor nerves, most frequently cranial nerve VII. This dysfunction may remain localized or progress to generalized tetanus. The incubation period is only 1 or 2 days, and the prognosis for survival is usually poor.

Neonatal tetanus is generalized tetanus resulting from *C. tetani* infection in neonates. It occurs primarily in underdeveloped countries, where it accounts for up to half of all neonatal deaths.

DIAGNOSIS

The diagnosis of tetanus is usually based on clinical observations. The putative agent, *C. tetani*, is recovered from wound culture only about 30% of the time. Results of cerebrospinal fluid analysis are entirely normal. Diagnostic testing is usually not necessary except in cases lacking an identified portal of entry. The differential diagnosis depends on the dominant clinical features and includes dystonic reactions as a result of neuroleptic toxicity, seizure disorders, hypocalcemic or alkalotic tetany, alcohol withdrawal, and strychnine poisoning. Strychnine also antagonizes glycine, and strychnine poisoning is the only condition that truly mimics tetanus. Strychnine levels in blood and urine establish the diagnosis. Dystonic reactions may resemble tetanus and are distinguished by rapid response to anticholinergic agents.

PREVENTION

Immunization with tetanus toxoid is virtually 100% effective, so nearly all cases of tetanus occur in unimmunized or inadequately immunized individuals. The Advisory Committee on Immunization Practices has recommended diphtheria and tetanus toxoids and acellular pertussis vaccine (DTaP) for active immunization of infants and children at 2 months, 4 months, 6 months, 15 to 18 months, and 4 to 6 years of age. Protective levels of serum antitoxin in persons who complete the primary series persist for at least 10 years. Td (tetanus and diphtheria toxoids adsorbed for adult use) is recommended every 10 years, but this recommendation has been modified because of concerns about waning adult pertussis antibody protection; as a result, the Advisory Committee on Immunization Practices recommends that all adults aged 19 years and older who have not yet received a dose of Tdap (tetanus toxoid, reduced diphtheria toxoid, and acellular pertussis) should receive a single dose regardless of the interval since last Td.[17] The recommended primary immunization series for unimmunized persons older than 7 years is Td at time 0, 4 to 8 weeks, and 6 to 12 months after the second dose, and then every 10 years. Nearly all states now require DTaP immunization for school enrollment. Immunization of childbearing women with Tdap confers protection to their infants through transplacental maternal antibody and is recommended during the third trimester of each pregnancy for optimal fetal passive antibody protection.

Prevention of tetanus after injury (Table 280-1) requires appropriate wound management, assurance of adequate immunity, and consideration of antibiotic

TABLE 280-1 GUIDE TO TETANUS PROPHYLAXIS IN ROUTINE WOUND MANAGEMENT

HISTORY OF ADSORBED TETANUS TOXOID (NO. OF DOSES)	CLEAN MINOR WOUNDS		ALL OTHER WOUNDS*	
	Tdap OR Td[†]	TIG[‡]	Tdap OR Td[†]	TIG[‡]
<3 or unknown	Yes	No	Yes	Yes
≥3	No[§]	No	No[¶]	No

*Such as (but not limited to) wounds contaminated with dirt, feces, soil, and saliva; puncture wounds; avulsions; and wounds resulting from missiles, crushing, burns, and frostbite.
[†]For children younger than 7 years, DTaP (pediatric diphtheria–tetanus toxoid plus acellular pertussis vaccine) is recommended; if pertussis vaccine is contraindicated, DT (pediatric diphtheria–tetanus toxoid) is given. For persons aged 7 to 9 years or 65 years or older, Td (adult tetanus–diphtheria toxoid) is recommended. For persons 10 to 64 years, Tdap (adult tetanus–diphtheria toxoid plus acellular pertussis vaccine) is preferred to Td if the patient has never received Tdap and has no contraindication to pertussis vaccine. For persons 7 years and older, if Tdap is not available or not indicated because of age, Td is preferred to TT (tetanus toxoid alone). Note that pediatric formulations (DT and DTaP) contain an amount of tetanus toxoid similar to that of adult Td, but they contain three to four times as much diphtheria toxoid. DTaP and Tdap vaccines do not contain thimerosal as a preservative.
[‡]TIG is human tetanus immune globulin. Equine tetanus antitoxin should be used when TIG is not available.
[§]Yes, if more than 10 years since the last dose.
[¶]Yes, if more than 5 years since the last dose.

prophylaxis. The aim of surgery is to eliminate necrotic tissue, purulent collections, and foreign bodies that promote the environmental conditions necessary for spore germination. Passive immunization with tetanus immune globulin (TIG) is recommended only for "tetanus-prone" wounds in patients with an inadequate or unknown primary immunization status. The determination of whether a wound is tetanus prone depends on the interval between injury and treatment, the degree of contamination, the extent of devitalized tissue or foreign bodies at the site of injury, and the depth of injury. Antimicrobial agents, such as penicillin and metronidazole, may be given to inhibit replication of the vegetative forms of *C. tetani*, but immunization and wound cleansing are considered more important.

TREATMENT   Rx

Patients with tetanus require intensive care with particular attention to respiratory support, treatment with benzodiazepines, autonomic nervous system support, passive and active immunization, surgical débridement, and antibiotics directed against *C. tetani*. There may be clinical progression for 2 to 4 weeks, despite antitoxin treatment, because of the time required to complete the transport of toxin. The severity of disease may be reduced by partial immunity; as a result, some patients have mild disease with minimal mortality, whereas others have mortality rates as high as 60% despite expert care.

Supportive Care
It is most important to assess airway function. Many patients require endotracheal intubation with benzodiazepine sedation and neuromuscular blockade; a tracheostomy should be placed if the endotracheal tube causes spasms. A feeding tube is usually required for nutritional support.

Control of Muscle Spasms
Benzodiazepines have become the mainstay of therapy to control spasms and to provide sedation. The most extensively studied is diazepam given in 5-mg increments; lorazepam and midazolam are equally effective. Patients with tetanus may have high tolerance for the sedative effects of these drugs and may require exceptionally high doses. When tetanus symptoms resolve, the drugs must be tapered during at least 2 weeks to prevent withdrawal reactions. If control of spasms cannot be achieved by benzodiazepines, long-term neuromuscular blockade is performed with vecuronium (6 to 8 mg/hour).

Passive Immunization
Human TIG should be given as soon as possible to neutralize toxin that has not entered neurons. The usual dose is 500 IU intramuscularly. Higher doses or intrathecal administration does not appear to be more effective. An alternative to TIG is pooled intravenous immune globulin. Equine TIG is equally effective, but the rate of allergic reactions is high because of the equine source; this preparation should not be used if human TIG is available.

Active Immunization
The standard three-dose schedule of immunization with tetanus toxoid should be given at an injection site separate from that used for immune globulin.

Antibiotic Therapy
C. tetani is susceptible in vitro to penicillins, cephalosporins, imipenem, macrolides, metronidazole, and tetracyclines. Clinical studies favor the use of metronidazole, which should be given in an intravenous dose of 2 g/day for 7 to 10 days.

Autonomic Nervous System Dysfunction
This complication generally reflects excessive catecholamine release and is usually treated with labetalol (0.25 to 1.0 mg/minute) for blood pressure control. Hypotension may require norepinephrine infusion. Bradycardia may require a pacemaker.

Surgery
Any wounds should be appropriately débrided.

PROGNOSIS

The overall mortality rate for generalized tetanus is 20 to 25%, even in modern medical facilities with extensive resources. Patients with moderate or severe generalized tetanus generally require treatment for 3 to 6 weeks. The highest mortality rates are at the extremes of age. The most frequent cause of death is pneumonia, but many patients have no obvious findings at autopsy, suggesting that death was directly due to the neurotoxin. Patients who recover usually recover completely.

OTHER CLOSTRIDIAL INFECTIONS
Clostridium perfringens Type C Enteritis

C. perfringens type C enteritis, also called enteritis necroticans, is a necrotizing disease involving the proximal small intestine caused by β-toxin–producing strains of *C. perfringens*. Enteritis necroticans occurs as sporadic cases or in outbreaks, most often in underdeveloped countries, most notably in Papua New Guinea in the 1960s and 1970s, where it was called pigbel because of its association with pork feasts by aboriginal people in the highlands. Outbreaks have also been reported among Khmer refugees in Thailand in the 1980s and in Sri Lanka in 2007. Enteritis necroticans also occurs rarely in isolated cases in the developed world, particularly among patients with diabetes mellitus.

PATHOBIOLOGY

Experimental and clinical evidence supports infection with *C. perfringens* type C and β-toxin as the causative agent of and key virulence factor in enteritis necroticans. The organism has been identified at the site of necrotic lesions, the disease can be reproduced in guinea pigs, isogenic β-toxin gene null mutants are avirulent, and vaccination with a toxoid preparation of β-toxin is protective. β-Toxin production is rapidly upregulated in the presence of Caco-2 enterocytes, and the toxin localizes to the endothelium in humans and piglets infected with *C. perfringens* type C. These findings may explain key histopathologic hallmarks of this disease, that is, deep small intestinal necrosis with vascular necrosis and hemorrhage in the lamina propria.

CLINICAL MANIFESTATIONS

In Papua New Guinea, affected patients usually develop severe abdominal pain 12 hours to several days after a ritual pork feast (or, presumably, other infected food). Vomiting and bloody diarrhea are frequently associated findings. The abdomen becomes distended, and thickened bowel loops are sometimes appreciated on palpation. Disease severity and whether the patient experiences spontaneous recovery or bowel perforation and death depend on the extent of intestinal involvement.

DIAGNOSIS

Recognition of the clinical syndrome is critical to making the diagnosis. Culture to identify specific β-toxin–producing strains of *C. perfringens* remains a research tool and is not helpful in the management of patients. Plain radiographs of the abdomen may show dilated small bowel loops and ileus.

PREVENTION

An effective toxoid vaccine was available and used in Papua New Guinea (where the disease is endemic) as well as in the Khmer refugee camp outbreak in 1986. Vaccination was discontinued in the mid-1990s, and the vaccine is no longer available. A 2002 survey of Papua New Guinea children in the highlands suggested that pigbel was responsible for 9 to 16% of acute abdominal cases and clustered in three close geographic regions.

TREATMENT Rx

Treatment is primarily supportive, including nasogastric suction and intravenous hydration. Surgical resection of the infected bowel is often required for those who do not initially respond to supportive measures. Antibiotics (penicillin, chloramphenicol, metronidazole) are almost always given empirically, but their role has not been defined. Prognosis depends on the extent of disease and the availability of surgery for those with more extensive intestinal involvement.

Clostridium perfringens Type A Diarrhea

C. perfringens type A is a well-recognized cause of food poisoning due to the ingestion of food, usually meat, heavily contaminated with enterotoxin-producing *C. perfringens* after storage at inappropriate temperatures. Enterotoxin production is associated with sporulation of ingested vegetative bacteria in the small intestine. The incubation period is 7 to 15 hours after ingestion, and the most prominent symptoms are diarrhea and abdominal pain. The syndrome is usually mild and self-limited.

In contrast to food poisoning due to *C. perfringens* type A, a more severe and protracted infectious diarrhea syndrome due to this organism has been recognized among hospitalized or institutionalized patients. These patients often have a history of prior or concomitant antibiotic use, and an enzyme immunoassay for *C. perfringens* enterotoxin is commercially available for investigative use. Metronidazole treatment is recommended for those with protracted diarrhea. As with CDI, diarrhea may recur after successful treatment.

Despite the self-limited nature of most food-associated diarrheal syndromes, *C. perfringens* type A has also been responsible for outbreaks of fatal illness in institutionalized mentally ill patients. A recent outbreak in a state psychiatric hospital linked to improperly prepared chicken was notable for three deaths (7% case-fatality rate) in patients taking antimotility agents and in whom necrotizing colitis was found at autopsy.

Grade A References

A1. Johnson S, Louie TJ, Gerding DN, et al. Vancomycin, metronidazole, or tolevamer for *Clostridium difficile* infection: results from two multinational, randomized, controlled trials. *Clin Infect Dis.* 2014;59:345-354.
A2. Cornely OA, Nathwani D, Ivanescu C, et al. Clinical efficacy of fidaxomicin compared with vancomycin and metronidazole in *Clostridium difficile* infections: a meta-analysis and indirect treatment comparison. *J Antimicrob Chemother.* 2014;69:2892-2900.
A3. Wilcox MH, Gerding DN, Poxton IR, et al. Bezlotoxumab for prevention of recurrent *Clostridium difficile* infection. *N Engl J Med.* 2017;376:305-317.
A4. van Nood E, Vrieze A, Nieuwdorp M, et al. Duodenal infusion of donor feces for recurrent *Clostridium difficile. N Engl J Med.* 2013;368:407-415.
A5. Hui W, Li T, Liu W, et al. Fecal microbiota transplantation for treatment of recurrent *C. difficile* infection: an updated randomized controlled trial meta-analysis. *PLoS ONE.* 2019;14:1-14.
A6. Lee CH, Steiner T, Petrof EO, et al. Frozen vs fresh fecal microbiota transplantation and clinical resolution of diarrhea in patients with recurrent *Clostridium difficile* infection: a randomized clinical trial. *JAMA.* 2016;315:142-149.
A7. Kelly CR, Khoruts A, Staley C, et al. Effect of fecal microbiota transplantation on recurrence in multiply recurrent *Clostridium difficile* infection: a randomized trial. *Ann Intern Med.* 2016;165:609-616.
A8. Kao D, Roach B, Silva M, et al. Effect of oral capsule- vs colonoscopy-delivered fecal microbiota transplantation on recurrent *Clostridium difficile* infection: a randomized clinical trial. *JAMA.* 2017;318:1985-1993.
A9. Gerding DN, Meyer T, Lee C, et al. Administration of spores of nontoxigenic *Clostridium difficile* strain M3 for prevention of recurrent *C. difficile* infection: a randomized clinical trial. *JAMA.* 2015;313:1719-1727.

GENERAL REFERENCES

For the General References and other additional features, please visit Expert Consult at https://expertconsult.inkling.com.

281
DISEASES CAUSED BY NON–SPORE-FORMING ANAEROBIC BACTERIA
ITZHAK BROOK

DEFINITION

Anaerobic bacteria are the predominant members of the indigenous, normal human flora, including the skin and the oral, gastrointestinal, and vaginal mucosa (Fig. 281-1; Table 281-1). However, the types of predominant anaerobes are different at each location.

The Pathogens

Advances in taxonomics have led to reclassification of many anaerobic species (E-Table 281-1). The genus *Bacteroides* is used only for species of the *Bacteroides fragilis* group. The "oral" *Bacteroides* and "pigmented" *Bacteroides* species have been reclassified as *Prevotella* (saccharolytic, pigmented species), *Porphyromonas* (asaccharolytic species), and other genera. Capnophilic organisms (which require an elevated concentration of carbon dioxide for growth), sometimes referred to as microaerophiles, are not true anaerobes and are often more related to *Campylobacter*, *Capnocytophaga*, and other genera. In addition, many new genera and several new species have been created to accommodate pathogens such as *Bilophila wadsworthia*, *Sutterella wadsworthensis*, *Centipeda periodontii*, and *Anaerobiospirillum thomasii*. *Fusobacterium nucleatum* is the predominant *Fusobacterium* species isolated from clinical specimens.

EPIDEMIOLOGY

Anaerobes are opportunistic pathogens that can cause serious infections, generally in synergistic infections in combination with aerobic bacteria. Because the microbiology of these infections is often complex and culture results may be delayed, awareness of the normal bacterial flora at the site of infection is an indispensable guide for selection and institution of empirical antimicrobial therapy.

PATHOBIOLOGY

Anaerobic bacteria range from those that cannot survive even a brief exposure to oxygen to those that can survive even in the presence of atmospheric oxygen (e.g., *B. fragilis*). Most anaerobes require an environment with a low oxidation-reduction potential (E_h gradient), which can be achieved in association with

TABLE 281-1	LOCATION OF VARIOUS GROUPS OF ANAEROBES AS NORMAL MICROFLORA IN HUMANS		
LOCATION	**NO. OF ORGANISMS PER GRAM**		**PREDOMINANT ANAEROBIC BACTERIA**
	AEROBES	**ANAEROBES**	
Skin	—	—	*Propionibacterium acnes* *Peptostreptococcus* spp
Mouth/upper respiratory tract (in saliva)	10^8-10^9	10^9-10^{11}	Pigmented *Prevotella* and *Porphyromonas* spp *Fusobacterium* spp *Peptostreptococcus* spp *Actinomyces* spp
Gastrointestinal tract (in fecal material)			
Upper	10^2-10^5	10^3-10^7	*Bacteroides fragilis* group *Clostridium* spp
Lower	10^5-10^9	10^{10}-10^{12}	*Peptostreptococcus* spp *Bifidobacterium* spp *Eubacterium* spp
Female genital tract (in vaginal secretions)	10^8	10^9	*Peptostreptococcus* spp *Prevotella bivia* *Prevotella disiens*

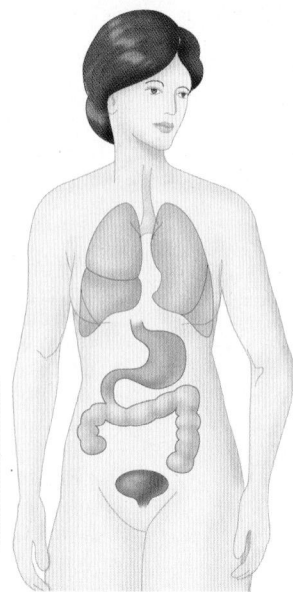

Skin
  Propionibacterium acnes
  Gram-positive cocci

Oral cavity and upper respiratory passages
  Prevotella melaninogenica
  Prevotella oralis
  Other *Prevotella sp*
  Porphyromonas sp
  Fusobacterium nucleatum
  Anaerobic cocci—pepto-
    streptococci, *Veillonella*,
    microaerophilic strepto-
    cocci
  Actinomyces

Female genital tract
  Prevotella melaninogenica
  Other *Prevotella*
  Other *Bacteroides*
  Peptostreptococcus
  Clostridium
  Porphyromonas

Colon
  Bacteroides fragilis group
  Anaerobic cocci—pep-
    tostreptococci,
    Veillonella
  Clostridium
  Eubacterium
  Bifidobacterium

FIGURE 281-1. Anaerobes as the predominant normal microflora of the human body by general anatomic location. (Modified from Finegold SM, Sutter VL. *Diagnosis and Management of Anaerobic Infections.* Kalamazoo, MI: Upjohn; 1976. Copyright by Dr. Finegold.)

TABLE 281-2 POTENTIAL VIRULENCE FACTORS IN VARIOUS ANAEROBES

FACTOR	SPECIES
ADHESION	
Capsule	*Bacteroides fragilis* group, *Prevotella melaninogenica*
Pili/fimbriae	*B. fragilis* group
	Porphyromonas gingivalis
Hemagglutinin	*P. gingivalis*
Lectin	*Fusobacterium nucleatum*
INVASION/TISSUE DAMAGE	
Proteases	*Fusobacterium necrophorum*
	Bacteroides spp
	Porphyromonas spp
Hemolysins	Many species
Endotoxin	*B. fragilis*
Fibrinolysin	*B. fragilis* group
	Porphyromonas spp
Heparinase	*B. fragilis* group
	Porphyromonas spp
Neuraminidase	*B. fragilis* group
	Porphyromonas spp
ANTIPHAGOCYTIC	
Capsule	*B. fragilis* group
	P. gingivalis
Lipopolysaccharide	*B. fragilis* group
	F. necrophorum, P. gingivalis
Metabolic products	Most anaerobes
TOXINS	
Endotoxin	*B. fragilis*
	F. necrophorum
Enterotoxin	*B. fragilis*

Modified from Duerden BI. Virulence factors in anaerobes. *Clin Infect Dis.* 1994;18(Suppl 4):253.

low pH, tissue destruction, byproducts from aerobic bacterial metabolism, or low oxygen content. Although they are not true anaerobes, some organisms, such as microaerophilic streptococci and other capnophilic or difficult-to-cultivate bacteria, are sometimes lumped together with anaerobes because of their fastidious nature. Some genera, such as *Lactobacillus* and *Actinomyces*, include both aerobic and anaerobic species.

Anaerobic bacteria possess a variety of virulence factors that are species specific (Table 281-2).

CLINICAL MANIFESTATIONS

Bacteremia

Transient anaerobic bacteremia occurs in about 85% of patients immediately after dental cleaning or manipulation. It is estimated that more than 200 cases of endocarditis from anaerobes are reported annually in the United States, usually in association with anatomic abnormalities or damaged cardiac valves (Chapter 67). Most anaerobic bacteremias are intermittent and associated with serious intra-abdominal or female genital tract, skin, and soft tissue infections, often proximal to the gastrointestinal tract. Which organisms are involved depends on their portal of entry and the underlying disease. The most common isolates are the *B. fragilis* group (60 to 75% of isolates). About 5 to 15% of bacteremias are caused by anaerobes, and they are the sole isolates in two thirds of these. The most commonly implicated anaerobes in bacteremia are *B. fragilis* and *Clostridium* spp.[1] Mortality associated with *B. fragilis* group bacteremia is 15 to 30%. Bacteremia with the *B. fragilis* group generally originates from a gastrointestinal source[2]; with pigmented *Prevotella, Porphyromonas,* and *Fusobacterium* spp, from oropharyngeal and pulmonary sources; with *Fusobacterium* spp, from the female genital tract; and with *Propionibacterium acnes,* from foreign body sources. Bacteremia with peptostreptococci is associated with all sources but especially with the oropharyngeal, pulmonary, and female genital tracts.

Central Nervous System Infections

Anaerobes can cause brain abscess, subdural empyema, epidural abscess, and meningitis. The main source of brain abscess is an adjacent, generally chronic infection in the ears, mastoids, sinuses, oropharynx, teeth, or lungs. Rarely, bacteremia of another origin or endocarditis can cause such infection.

Meningitis caused by anaerobes is uncommon and can follow respiratory or dental infection or develop as a complication of a cerebrospinal fluid shunt. The isolates usually cultured from brain abscesses that complicate respiratory and dental infections include *Prevotella, Porphyromonas, Bacteroides, Fusobacterium,* and *Peptostreptococcus* spp. Microaerophilic and other streptococci are also often isolated.[3] *Propionibacterium acnes* is common in shunt infections.

Head and Neck

Dental infections (Chapter 397) associated with a variety of oral anaerobes include periodontal disease, gingivitis, pulpitis, acute necrotizing ulcerative gingivitis, localized juvenile periodontitis, adult periodontitis, pericoronitis, endodontitis, periapical and dental abscesses, and postextraction infection. Peritonsillar, retropharyngeal, and parapharyngeal abscesses (Chapter 401) are deep-seated, potentially life-threatening infections that may spread into the various potential spaces of the neck or mediastinum and cause jugular vein thrombosis. Oral anaerobes can be recovered in more than 50% of such cases, usually mixed with aerobes. Other regional infections include cervicofacial actinomycosis (Chapter 313), Ludwig angina, *Fusobacterium necrophorum* sepsis with metastatic infection (Lemierre syndrome), suppurative sialoadenitis (including parotitis), neck space infections, thyroiditis and chronic sinusitis (Chapter 398), otitis media (Chapter 398), and mastoiditis. Management involves surgical drainage and appropriate antimicrobial therapy.

Pleuropulmonary

Anaerobes predominate in oral and upper respiratory tract normal flora, and most aspiration pneumonias[4] are due to this flora (Chapter 97). Aspiration can result from altered consciousness, dysphagia, or mechanical devices such as intubation equipment. Poor oral hygiene is associated with an increased anaerobic bacterial burden, and the presence of aerobes or necrotic tissue lowers the pH, which facilitates the growth of anaerobes. Anaerobes are involved in 90% of community-acquired aspiration pneumonia and in about a third of nosocomial aspiration pneumonia, empyema, lung abscess, and pneumonia associated with tracheostomy. If the anaerobic component of aspiration pneumonia is not treated, the anaerobes can cause a lung abscess. Management requires good pulmonary toilet and antimicrobial therapy.

Intra-abdominal

Because anaerobes outnumber aerobes by 1000 to 1 in the large intestine, they play a major role in almost all intra-abdominal infections. Most visceral abscesses (e.g., hepatic; Chapter 142), chronic cholecystitis (Chapter 146), perforated and gangrenous appendicitis (Chapter 133), postoperative wound infections and abscesses, diverticulitis (Chapter 133), and any infection associated with fecal contamination of the abdominal cavity involve both aerobes and anaerobes. *B. fragilis* group members predominate because they are encapsulated, resist phagocytosis, are often resistant to many antimicrobials, and promote abscess formation. They may also be associated with concomitant bacteremia and sepsis. Randomized controlled trials have found that prophylactic antibiotics covering both anaerobic and aerobic bacteria administered orally or intravenously before elective colorectal surgery reduce the risk of surgical wound infection by as much as 75%.[A1]

Obstetric-Gynecologic

A variety of obstetric-gynecologic infections involve anaerobes. These are polymicrobial and include bacterial vaginosis; soft tissue perineal, vulvar, and Bartholin gland abscesses; endometritis; pyometra; salpingitis; tubo-ovarian abscesses; adnexal abscess; pelvic inflammatory disease, which may include pelvic cellulitis and abscess; chorioamnionitis; vaginal cuff cellulitis; septic pelvic thrombophlebitis; intrauterine contraceptive device–associated infection; septic abortion; and postsurgical obstetric and gynecologic infections. Bacterial vaginosis has been associated with preterm labor or delivery, chorioamnionitis, low birthweight, postpartum endometritis, and postabortal pelvic inflammatory disease. Bacterial vaginosis can increase the risk for infection with human immunodeficiency virus type 1 and the development of other sexually transmitted diseases (Chapter 269).

Skin and Soft Tissue

Cutaneous infections include infected ulcers, cellulitis (including synergistic necrotizing cellulitis), pyoderma, paronychia, hidradenitis suppurativa, and a variety of secondarily infected sites. Such sites include secondarily infected gastrostomy or tracheostomy site wounds, subcutaneous sebaceous or inclusion cysts, eczema, psoriasis, poison ivy, atopic dermatitis, eczema herpeticum, scabies or kerion, and postsurgical wounds.

Subcutaneous infections include abscesses, decubitus ulcers, infected diabetic (vascular or trophic) ulcers, human and animal bite wounds, anaerobic cellulitis and gas gangrene, bacterial synergistic gangrene, Fournier gangrene, infected pilonidal cyst or sinus, and burn wounds. Anaerobic soft tissue infections that occur deeper are necrotizing fasciitis, necrotizing synergistic cellulitis, and gas gangrene. These infections can involve the fascia and can induce myositis and myonecrosis.

Cultures frequently yield isolates that are members of the normal flora of the region of the infection. In addition to oral and skin flora, human bite infections often contain *Eikenella* species, and animal bites harbor *Pasteurella multocida*.

The infections are generally polymicrobial, and some (e.g., decubitus ulcers, diabetic foot ulcers) are often complicated by osteomyelitis or bacteremia.

Deep tissue infections, such as necrotizing cellulitis, fasciitis, and myositis, often involve *Clostridium* species, *Streptococcus pyogenes*, or a polymicrobic aerobic and anaerobic flora. They are often associated with gas in the tissues and putrid-like pus with a gray, thin quality and have a high rate of bacteremia and mortality. Management of deep-seated soft tissue infection includes surgical débridement, drainage, and vigorous surgical management.

Osteomyelitis and Septic Arthritis

Anaerobes can be involved in osteomyelitis of the long bones after trauma and fracture, osteomyelitis related to peripheral vascular disease, decubitus ulcers, and osteomyelitis of the cranial and facial bones. Most of these infections are polymicrobial.

Cranial and facial bone osteomyelitis is generally caused by spread from a contiguous soft tissue source or from sinus, ear, or dental infection. Intestinal anaerobes originating from decubitus ulcers are involved in pelvic osteomyelitis. Osteomyelitis of long bones and septic arthritis are generally caused by hematogenous spread, trauma, or the presence of a prosthetic device.

The most commonly recovered anaerobes are peptostreptococci and *P. acnes* (often in prosthetic joint infection), *B. fragilis* group and fusobacteria (often of hematogenous origin), and clostridia (associated with trauma).

DIAGNOSIS

Anaerobic infections should be suspected in a number of specific clinical scenarios (Table 281-3). An appropriately collected microbiologic specimen (Table 281-4) is critical for accurate diagnosis.

TABLE 281-3 CLINICAL INDICATORS OF ANAEROBIC INFECTION

Infection adjacent to a mucosal surface
Foul-smelling discharge
Necrotic gangrenous tissue and abscess formation
Free gas or crepitus in tissue
Bacteremia or endocarditis with no growth on aerobic blood cultures
Infection related to the use of antibiotics effective against aerobes only (e.g., trimethoprim-sulfamethoxazole, aminoglycosides, older quinolones)
Infection related to tumors or other destructive processes
Infected thrombophlebitis
Infection after bites
Black discoloration of exudates containing *Prevotella melaninogenica*, which may fluoresce under ultraviolet light
"Sulfur granules" in discharges caused by actinomycosis
Clinical finding of gas gangrene or necrotizing fasciitis
Clinical condition predisposing to anaerobic infection (e.g., after maternal amnionitis, fistulous tracks, bites, dental infection, bowel perforation)

TABLE 281-4 SPECIMEN ACCEPTABILITY FOR ANAEROBIC CULTURE

SPECIMENS THAT SHOULD NOT BE CULTURED FOR ANAEROBES

Feces or rectal swabs
Throat or nasopharyngeal swabs
Sputum or bronchoscopic specimens
Routine or catheterized urine
Vaginal or cervical swabs
Material from superficial wounds or abscesses not collected properly to exclude surface contamination
Material from abdominal wounds obviously contaminated with feces, such as an open fistula

SPECIMENS APPROPRIATE FOR ANAEROBIC CULTURE

All normally sterile body fluids other than urine, such as blood, pleural fluid, and joint fluid
Urine obtained by suprapubic bladder aspiration
Percutaneous transtracheal aspiration, direct lung puncture, or double-lumen catheter bronchial brushing and bronchoalveolar lavage (both cultured quantitatively)
Culdocentesis fluid obtained after decontamination of the vagina
Material obtained from closed abscesses
Material obtained from sinus tracks or draining wounds

TABLE 281-5 GENERAL PRINCIPLES OF THERAPY FOR ANAEROBIC INFECTIONS

Decompression of closed spaces Débridement Drainage Relief of obstructions Irrigation Provision of adequate circulation when possible Removal of foreign bodies Antimicrobials	Activity against most likely pathogen or pathogens: location dependent, minimal effect on normal flora Absorption, appropriate route of administration (intravenous, oral) Penetration into site of infection Dosage appropriate for local tissue levels, body mass of patient, renal and liver function Duration appropriate for condition Susceptibility testing of isolate to guide specific therapy

TABLE 281-6 ANTIMICROBIAL SUSCEPTIBILITY PATTERNS FOR ANAEROBIC BACTERIA*

BACTERIA	PENICILLIN	β-LACTAMASE†	CEFOXITIN	CEFOTETAN	CARBAPENEMS, TIGECYCLINE	MOXIFLOXACIN	CLINDAMYCIN	METRONIDAZOLE
Bacteroides fragilis	−	+	+	+	+	+	V	+
Bacteroides thetaiotaomicron	−	+	V	V	+	V	V	+
B. fragilis group, other	−	+	V	V	+	+	V	+
Prevotella spp	V	+	+	+	+	+	+	+
Fusobacterium nucleatum	V	+	+	+	+	V	+	+
Fusobacterium necrophorum	+	+	+	+	+	V	+	+
Porphyromonas spp	+	+	+	+	+	+	+	+
Peptostreptococcus	+	+	+	+	+	+	+	V
Propionibacterium acnes	+	+	+	+	+	+	+	−
Veillonella	+	+	+	+	+	+	+	+
Actinomyces	+	+	+	+	+	+	+	−

*Based on a variety of in vitro susceptibility studies from different laboratories and using different techniques.
†β-Lactamase inhibitor–β-lactam combination (e.g., ticarcillin-clavulanate, ampicillin-sulbactam, piperacillin-tazobactam).
+= Susceptible; − = resistant; V = variable.

TREATMENT [Rx]

General principles of treatment (Table 281-5) include appropriate antimicrobial therapy coupled with prompt drainage, decompression of closed space infections, relief of obstructions, and surgical débridement. The various clinically important anaerobes can be characterized by reasonably predictable antimicrobial susceptibility patterns (Table 281-6).[5] However, some anaerobes have become resistant to antimicrobials, and many can develop resistance during therapy.[6] Reliable culture and sensitivity results should ultimately guide therapy.[7] The efficacy of hyperbaric oxygen is unproved, but its use in conjunction with other therapeutic measures is not contraindicated.

In choosing antimicrobials for the treatment of mixed infections, their aerobic and anaerobic antibacterial spectra and their availability in oral or parenteral form should be considered. Some antimicrobials have a limited range of activity. For example, metronidazole is active only against anaerobes and therefore cannot be administered as a single agent for the treatment of mixed infections. Others (i.e., carbapenems, a penicillin plus a β-lactamase inhibitor) have wide spectra of activity against aerobes and anaerobes.

Aside from susceptibility patterns, other factors influencing the choice of antimicrobial therapy include the pharmacologic characteristics of the various drugs, their toxicity, their effect on normal flora, and their bactericidal activity. Although identification of the infecting organisms and their antimicrobial susceptibility may be needed for selection of optimal therapy, the clinical setting and Gram stain preparation of the specimen may suggest the types of anaerobes present in the infection and the nature of the infectious process.

Even though the length of therapy for anaerobic infections is generally longer than that for aerobic and facultative infections, the length of treatment must be individualized, depending on the response. In some cases, treatment may require 6 to 8 weeks, but therapy may be shortened with proper surgical drainage. An anti–gram-negative enteric agent is generally added to treat Enterobacteriaceae in managing intra-abdominal infections.

The available parenteral antimicrobials for most infections are metronidazole, chloramphenicol, clindamycin, cefoxitin, a penicillin (e.g., ticarcillin, ampicillin, piperacillin) and a β-lactamase inhibitor (e.g., clavulanic acid, sulbactam, tazobactam), a carbapenem (e.g., imipenem, meropenem, doripenem, ertapenem), and tigecycline. Unfortunately, resistant strains are emerging.[8] In one randomized trial of adult patients with complicated intra-abdominal infections, including infections caused by multidrug-resistant pathogens, treatment with ceftolozane/tazobactam plus metronidazole was equivalent to meropenem.[A2]

An agent effective against gram-negative enteric bacilli (e.g., an aminoglycoside, fluoroquinolone) or an antipseudomonal cephalosporin (e.g., cefepime) is generally added to metronidazole and, occasionally, cefoxitin in the treatment of intra-abdominal infections. Penicillin can be added to metronidazole for the treatment of intracranial, pulmonary, or dental infections to cover microaerophilic streptococci and *Actinomyces* species. Penicillin is added to clindamycin to supplement its coverage against *Peptostreptococcus* species and other gram-positive anaerobic organisms. For *Chlamydia* and *Mycoplasma* species, doxycycline is added to most regimens in treatment of pelvic infections. Oral therapy is often substituted for parenteral therapy. The agents available for oral therapy are clindamycin, amoxicillin and clavulanate, and metronidazole.

Grade A References

A1. Nelson RL, Gladman E, Barbateskovic M. Antimicrobial prophylaxis for colorectal surgery. *Cochrane Database Syst Rev.* 2014;5:CD001181.
A2. Solomkin J, Hershberger E, Miller B, et al. Ceftolozane/tazobactam plus metronidazole for complicated intra-abdominal infections in an era of multidrug resistance: results from a randomized, double-blind, phase 3 trial (ASPECT-cIAI). *Clin Infect Dis.* 2015;60:1462-1471.

GENERAL REFERENCES

For the General References and other additional features, please visit Expert Consult at https://expertconsult.inkling.com.

282

NEISSERIA MENINGITIDIS INFECTIONS

DAVID S. STEPHENS

Neisseria meningitidis (the meningococcus) is the cause of epidemic bacterial meningitis, fulminant sepsis (meningococcemia), milder bacteremia, and, less commonly, focal infections (such as pneumonia, septic arthritis, purulent pericarditis, urethritis, and conjunctivitis).

The Pathogen

N. meningitidis is an aerobic, diplococcal gram-negative β-proteobacterium and a member of the family Neisseriaceae, which also includes *Neisseria gonorrhoeae* (Chapter 283), the cause of gonorrhea. The meningococcus is a frequent commensal of the human upper respiratory tract but can also cause local and devastating invasive human disease. Human mucosal surfaces, most commonly the nasopharynx but sometimes the rectum and urogenital tract, are the major reservoirs. There are 12 confirmed serogroups of *N. meningitidis*, based on different capsular polysaccharide structures, but only 6 serogroups (A, B, C, W, X, and Y) cause almost all invasive meningococcal disease globally (Fig. 282-1). Highly pathogenic meningococci are also distinguished by genetically defined clonal complexes and genotypes that can emerge and spread worldwide. Dissecting the basis of meningococcal disease has provided important scientific lessons about bacterial evolution and pathogenesis, antibiotic resistance mechanisms, innate and adaptive human immune responses, and vaccine development.

N. meningitidis has been recognized as a cause of rapid death, disability, and fear on disparate human populations for over 200 years. Beginning with the initial descriptions of outbreaks in Geneva in 1805 and New Bedford, Massachusetts in 1806, the meningococcus has been found to cause sporadic disease, case clusters, epidemics, and pandemics of meningitis and septicemia, and less commonly pneumonia and other local infections. An estimated 500,000 to 1 million cases have occurred worldwide each year, but the incidence is now being lowered by the widespread use of vaccines.[1] The greatest burden of disease has occurred in sub-Saharan Africa, where endemic rates of disease have been 3 to 10 per 100,000 population.[2] In addition, seasonal increases in disease and cyclic pandemics of serogroup A in sub-Saharan Africa occurred every 8 to 10 years since 1905. During epidemics and cyclic pandemics, the incidence can climb to 1 per 1000 population for weeks before the frequency of disease declines in the immediate outbreak area. The introduction in 2010 of a new meningococcal conjugate vaccine for serogroup A has eliminated serogroup A outbreaks in the region, but less severe outbreaks of serogroup C, X, and W continue.[3] Meningococcal epidemics, especially in developing countries, have been catastrophic and have contributed to a cycle of poverty and hence the disorganization of social structures.

Although overall incidence is declining, meningococcal disease remains sporadic with focal outbreaks/clusters in the United States, Canada, Mexico, Europe, Japan, Australia, China, Russia, South America (Chile, Brazil, Argentina), India, Southeast Asia, and other countries. Overall incidence in these countries is now less than 0.1 to 2 per 100,000 population. The introduction and widespread use of new meningococcal ACWY conjugate and serogroup B vaccines have helped to lower the overall incidence,[4] but slow declines in incidence began before new vaccine introductions. Outbreak-associated cases accounted for approximately 5% of all meningococcal disease cases in the United States between 2009 and 2013. Organization-based and university outbreaks were mostly caused by serogroup B, whereas serogroup C was the primary cause of community-based outbreaks.[5] Meningococcal disease has the highest incidence in children younger than 4 years (often serogroup B) and in adolescents, but in sporadic settings, half of all cases occur in adults.

N. meningitidis is transmitted among humans through close contact by large respiratory droplets or saliva. Colonization of the upper respiratory or other mucosal surfaces (e.g., nasopharynx) by *N. meningitidis* is the first step in establishment of a human carrier state of invasive meningococcal disease. Acquisition of meningococci through contact with secretions can be transient, lead to prolonged carriage, or result in invasive disease. The inoculum size needed for transmission is unknown. Invasive meningococcal disease usually occurs within 1 to 14 days of acquisition. Meningococci can be found in the urogenital tract and rectum and may be transmitted sexually.

Initial contact of meningococci with mucosal epithelial cells is mediated by type IV pili. These structures provide mobility ("twitching motility") to penetrate mucus and are the initial adhesins for human epithelial cells. Meningococci proceed to proliferate and form small microcolonies on the surface of human nonciliated epithelial cells. They can disseminate from colonies by post-translational glycan modifications of pili and migrate to adjacent cells by the pili-mediated motility. Meningococci can also spread from the nasopharynx to adjacent epithelial surfaces and infrequently cause local infections,

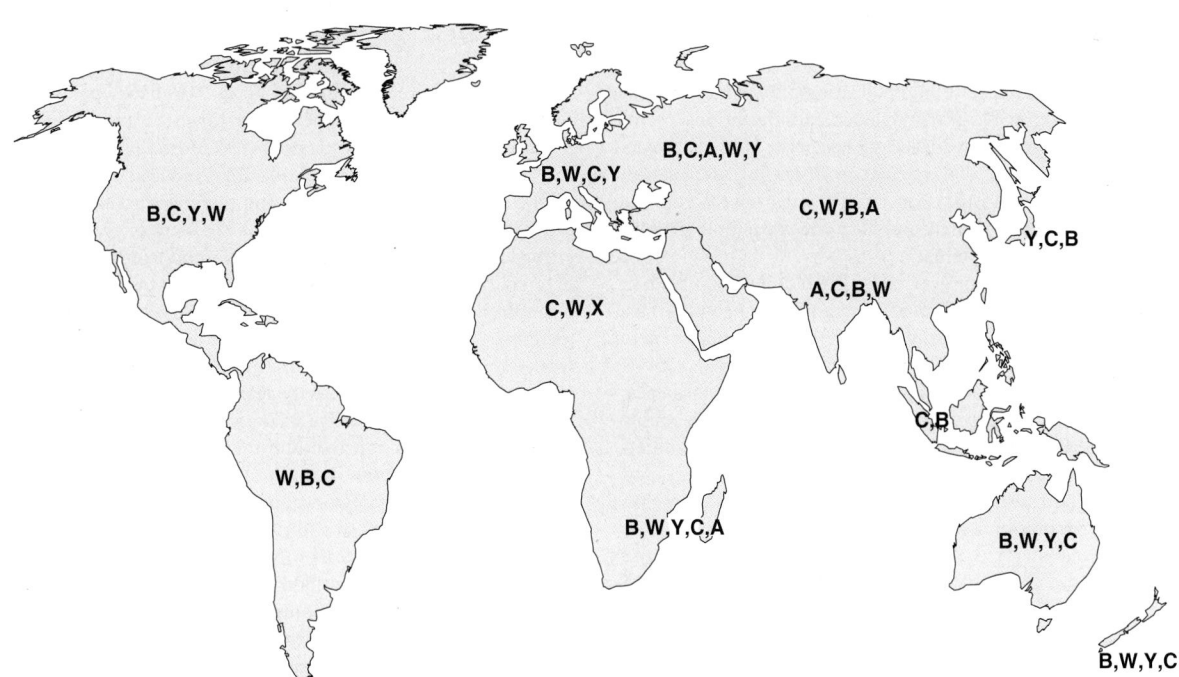

FIGURE 282-1. **Current epidemiology of meningococcal disease (global distribution of major serogroups causing disease by region).** (Modified from Stephens DS, Greenwood B, Brandtzaeg P. Epidemic meningitis, meningococcemia and *Neisseria meningitidis. Lancet.* 2007;369:2196-2210.)

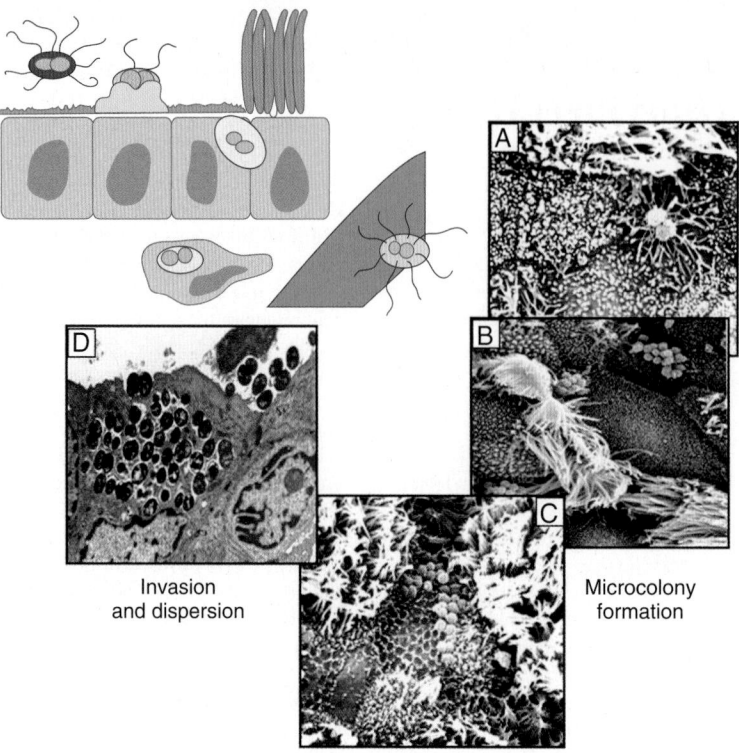

FIGURE 282-2. Steps in initiation of meningococcal colonization and invasion at the human nasopharynx. **A,** Adhesion and introduction of cell microvilli. **B,** Microcolony formation. **C,** Cortical plaque formation and close adherence. **D,** Human epithelial cell invasion. (Modified from Stephens DS. Biology and pathogenesis of the evolutionarily successful, obligate human bacterium *Neisseria meningitidis*. *Vaccine.* 2009;27S:B71-B77.)

including pneumonia, sinusitis, and otitis media. Other less common local infections include conjunctivitis, urethritis, and proctitis. Close adherence of meningococci to the host epithelial cells results in the formation of epithelial cell cortical plaques and leads to the recruitment of factors ultimately responsible for the formation and extension of host epithelial cell pseudopodia that can tightly bind the meningococcus. Intimate meningococcal association with the epithelial cell is mediated by the meningococcal surface components including opacity proteins Opa and Opc with CD66/carcinoembryonic antigen–related cell adhesion molecules and integrins, respectively, on the surface of the human cell. Other meningococcal epithelial cell mediators include the meningococcal adhesin NadA and meningococcal lipo-oligosaccharide. The formation of epithelial cell membrane protrusions and pseudopodia stems from the organization of specific molecular complexes involving the linkers ezrin and moesin along with the clustering of several membrane-integral proteins, including CD44, intracellular adhesion molecule 1, and cortical actin polymerization. These events can lead to internalization of *N. meningitidis* in epithelial cells (Fig. 282-2). Intracellular meningococci reside within a membranous vacuole and are capable of translocating through the epithelial layers within 18 to 40 hours. Meningococci are capable of intracellular replication (in part because of the protective capsule), can survive under microaerophilic conditions, use lactate as a carbon source, and have the capacity to acquire iron through specialized transport systems.

Meningococci can cross mucosal surfaces, enter the blood stream, and, in some individuals, produce systemic infections. Damage to the mucosal surface by coinfection, drying (e.g., very low humidity), or smoke exposure may increase this risk for meningococcal invasion. Similar molecular interactions noted for meningococci and epithelial cells also occur with endothelial cells, and meningococci can translocate across the blood-meninges barrier, possibly at the choroid plexus or by the opening of intercellular junctions, and proliferate in the subarachnoid space, causing meningitis. In the vasculature and cerebrospinal fluid (CSF), high levels of multiplying bacteria lead to an intense inflammatory response, with pronounced increases in concentrations of tumor necrosis factor-α, interleukins (1β, 6, 8, and 10), different chemokines, and other inflammatory mediators.

Meningococcal resistance to complement-mediated lysis or phagocytosis is due to the expression of the capsule, lipo-oligosaccharide, and several surface-exposed proteins (factor H–binding protein, NspA, Opc, NalP). Meningococcal endotoxin released in blebs plays a major role in the inflammatory events of meningococcemia and meningococcal meningitis. Meningococcal lipid A is responsible for much of the biologic activity and toxicity of meningococcal

endotoxin. The toll-like receptor 4 (TLR-4) is critical to the innate immune response to bacterial endotoxins, and meningococcal endotoxin is no exception. Activation of TLR-4 by endotoxin requires association with the accessory protein MD-2, an *N*-glycosylated 19- to 27-kD protein expressed in both a soluble and a membrane-bound form. Binding of endotoxin to MD-2 in association with TLR-4 leads to dimerization or oligomerization of two or more TLR-4s, subsequent cellular activation, and cytokine and chemokine release.

In contrast to invasive disease, an asymptomatic *N. meningitidis* carrier state is found in up to 8 to 25% of healthy individuals. Meningococcal carriage is affected by age, intimate personal contact, crowding (e.g., bars, dormitories), and vaccination or chemoprophylaxis interventions in the community. Variable carriage rates have been reported, even during epidemics. Meningococcal carriage is a dynamic process, is less common in young children (<3% and *Neisseria lactamica* predominates) than in older children, is highest in adolescents (7 to 37%), and increases in closed populations (e.g., military recruits, Hajj pilgrims).[6] Rates as high as 36 to 71% have been reported in military recruits. Damage to the upper respiratory tract by coinfections (e.g., mycoplasma, influenza, other respiratory viral infections), smoking, very low humidity, drying of mucosal surfaces, and trauma induced by dust particles predisposes to both meningococcal carriage and meningococcal disease. Meningococcal carriage has also been linked to status as a secretor of glycoprotein ABO blood group antigens, which are water soluble, and to ethnic background. In a large U.K. study, social behavior (e.g., attendance at pubs or clubs, intimate kissing, cigarette smoking, or exposure to passive smoke) was highly associated with the risk for meningococcal carriage. Carriage can be transient or last for days, weeks, or months and is an immunizing event leading to protective immunity (e.g., serum bactericidal activity against the meningococcus).

The absence of protective bactericidal antibodies is the most important predisposing factor for systemic meningococcal disease, but complement deficiencies (congenital or acquired such as with the complement inhibitor eculizumab), genetic polymorphisms, and other host cofactors can contribute to meningococcal disease and disease severity. Disappearance of protective maternal antibodies increases the risk in older infants and young children. Congenital and acquired antibody deficiencies also increase risk. Opsonization and phagocytic function do contribute to meningococcal host defense mechanisms, as shown by disease reduction after meningococcal vaccination in individuals with terminal complement deficiencies. Rapidly progressive, fatal meningococcemia can arise in patients without properdin, and there is a marked risk for recurrent meningococcal infections in those with defects in the terminal complement pathway (C5-C9) and C3 deficiency.

Polymorphisms in genes coding for the Fcγ-receptor II (CD32), Fcγ-receptor III (CD16), mannose-binding lectin, TLR-4, and β_2-adrenoceptor gene have been associated with increased risk. Mannose-binding lectin is a plasma opsonin that initiates complement activation; specific polymorphisms in the gene are identified more frequently in children with meningococcal disease than in controls in some studies. Plasminogen activator inhibitor 1 concentrations appear to affect the severity and mortality of meningococcal sepsis, suggesting that impaired fibrinolysis is an important factor in its pathophysiology. Meningococcal disease is also linked to immunosuppressive disorders, such as nephrotic syndrome, congenital or acquired hypogammaglobulinemia, splenectomy, and human immunodeficiency virus (HIV)/acquired immunodeficiency syndrome (AIDS) (about a 10-fold increased risk for sporadic meningococcal disease). However, there has been no documented increase in epidemic outbreaks of meningococcal disease in countries with very high rates of HIV infection.

Meningococci can multiply rapidly in the vascular compartment, with an estimated doubling time of 30 to 45 minutes in some patients, or in the CSF. The release of high levels of inflammatory mediators such as meningococcal endotoxin in the circulation or CSF triggers an exaggerated release of chemokines, cytokines, bradykinin, and nitric oxide. Vascular dilation, hypovolemia, capillary leak, and pronounced reduction in myocardial function are the result. At a later stage, substantial complement activation contributes to the altered endothelial barrier function and relaxation of the smooth muscles in the vessel wall through the generation of high levels of anaphylatoxins (C3a and C5a). The capillary leak syndrome results in an increased flux of albumin and water across the altered capillary wall to the extravascular space. A patient with fulminant meningococcemia accumulates a large amount of fluid in the extravascular tissue. Circulatory collapse and multiorgan dysfunction are the primary causes of death due to meningococcemia. In meningitis, morbidity and death are due predominantly to cerebral edema.

Unraveling the pathogenic mechanisms of this devastating, evolutionarily successful obligate human pathogen has significance for the understanding of human sepsis as well as for prevention through vaccines active at mucosal pathogens.

CLINICAL MANIFESTATIONS

Meningococcus causes meningitis (37 to 50% of cases), septicemia (meningococcemia, 10 to 18% of cases), or both (7 to 12% of cases). Less common presentations are a mild bacteremia or pneumonia (10% of cases) and, in less than 5% of cases, septic arthritis, pericarditis, chronic bacteremia, or conjunctivitis. Rarely, meningococci can cause urethritis or proctitis, although outbreaks of meningococcal urethritis have recently been reported in the United States and Europe. In endemic and epidemic disease outbreaks, hemorrhagic skin lesions (petechiae, purpura; Fig. 282-3) are present in 28 to 77% of patients

with invasive meningococcal disease on admission, but these lesions may be absent or difficult to see in patients with dark skin. Hemorrhagic lesions sometimes occur on mucous membranes and sclera, but they are especially prevalent on the limbs. The petechiae of meningococcemia are usually larger and bluer than the pinpoint petechiae caused by thrombocytopenia or leukocytoclastic vasculitis induced by other infections or drugs. A nonblanching macular rash can also be a manifestation of meningococcal bacteremia. Evolving ecchymoses and purpura (diameter >10 mm) are noted mainly in patients with meningococcemia and disseminated intravascular coagulation (Chapter 166), but they may not appear until 12 hours into the illness. In addition to vasculitis, other conditions in the differential diagnosis of meningococcemia include Rocky Mountain spotted fever (Chapter 311) and enteroviral infections (Chapter 355).

Meningitis is the most common clinical presentation of invasive meningococcal disease.[7] Headache, fever, and rash with meningismus and altered mental status are the characteristic features; however, the rash may be absent, and the presentation can resemble pneumococcal or bacterial meningitis of other causes, viral meningitis, or early-stage encephalitis. Bacteremic meningococcal pneumonia has been linked more often to serogroups Y and W and is more common in adolescents and adults, especially older adults (approximately one third of cases occur in those older than 65 years). Isolated septic pericarditis or septic arthritis can also be a presentation, and an autoimmune- or antibody-mediated polyarthritis can be seen in the recovery phase following invasive meningococcal disease. Chronic meningococcemia can be manifested with low-grade fever and a polyarticular arthritis that can be confused with rheumatoid arthritis.

DIAGNOSIS

The clinical diagnosis of meningococcal meningitis relies on the recognition of fever, rash, meningeal signs, and altered mental status. The early clinical diagnosis of meningococcemia is a challenge because a rash, meningeal signs, and high fever may not be present. The course can be fulminant (<24 hours), and the early stages of disease can mimic viral infections such as those caused by enterovirus or influenza. Thus, it can be difficult to identify and to treat the disease quickly. General symptoms of sepsis (nausea and vomiting, drowsiness, irritability, leg pains, cold hands and feet, abnormal skin color) are present. However, these symptoms (in contrast to fever and rash) are not likely to be specific markers. Parents and relatives should be instructed to undress and inspect a febrile child, adolescent, or adult for a rash, and physicians and other health care providers should be alert to the concerns of parents, relatives, or caregivers about the abrupt or rapid deterioration of a patient.

The definitive diagnosis of invasive meningococcal disease is based on bacteriologic isolation or antigen or DNA identification of *N. meningitidis* in a usually sterile body fluid, such as blood, CSF, synovial fluid, pleural fluid, urine,

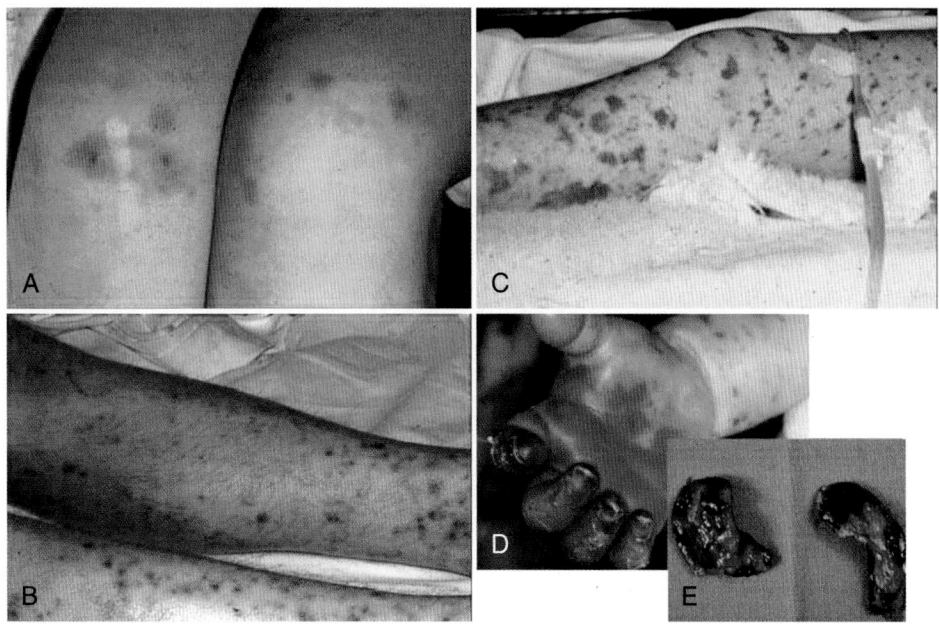

FIGURE 282-3. Clinical manifestations of meningococcal disease. **A** and **B,** Macular and petechial rashes of meningococcal bacteremia. **C,** Fulminant meningococcal sepsis with ecchymoses. **D,** Digital necrosis of meningococcemia sepsis. **E,** Hemorrhagic adrenals in fulminant meningococcal sepsis. (Modified from Stephens DS, Greenwood B, Brandtzaeg P. Epidemic meningitis, meningococcemia and *Neisseria meningitidis*. Lancet. 2007;369:2196-2210.)

or pericardial fluid. Blood and CSF are the most fruitful sources of positive cultures and for DNA identification by the polymerase chain reaction (PCR), but urine and skin lesions can also yield results in systemic meningococcal disease. The diagnosis of meningococcal meningitis is confirmed by CSF pleocytosis and Gram stain showing gram-negative diplococci (often inside neutrophils) and CSF culture, latex agglutination detecting meningococcal capsular polysaccharide in CSF, or PCR identifying *N. meningitidis* in CSF.

PCR is increasingly used for the diagnosis of meningococcal disease, including serogrouping and multilocus sequence typing, and has the potential to detect antibiotic resistance determinants. PCR techniques include real-time PCR of CSF, blood, and other sterile sites. Urine is a less sensitive fluid for PCR. An increasing number of patients are now diagnosed by PCR without culture, especially if they have received empirical prehospital antibiotic treatment. The sensitivity of PCR for the diagnosis of meningococcal meningitis is more than 90 to 95%; in contrast, the sensitivity of CSF or blood culture is less than 65%. In addition, whole genome sequencing is being increasingly used as an epidemiologic and organism confirmation tool.

TREATMENT   Rx

Early recognition and antibiotic administration (Table 282-1) are critical for effective treatment because effective antibiotics immediately stop the growth of *N. meningitidis*. Ceftriaxone and cefotaxime are the most effective antibiotics,[8] but penicillin, meropenem, and chloramphenicol also are effective in most cases. Fluoroquinolones and aztreonam are potential alternatives, but data on meningococcal disease are limited. Meningococci in CSF are killed within 3 to 4 hours after intravenous treatment with an adequate dose of a third-generation cephalosporin or penicillin, and concentrations of endotoxin in plasma fall by 50% within 2 hours. The concentrations of key cytokines and chemokines fall in parallel. Antibiotic treatment does not induce a large release of meningococcal endotoxin or lead to an increased inflammatory response.

Prehospital antibiotic treatment is advocated if the disease is suspected.[9] One goal is to reduce the case-fatality rate for patients with fulminant meningococcal sepsis or meningitis with rapidly increasing concentrations of meningococci and inflammatory mediators in the circulation or CSF. If antibiotic treatment is initiated before admission, ceftriaxone or another effective antibiotic can be injected intravenously or intramuscularly. During epidemics in developing countries, a single injection of ceftriaxone or long-acting chloramphenicol may be sufficient for patients with meningitis, and this simple treatment has saved many thousands of lives. The sensitivity of meningococci to penicillin is decreasing worldwide because of a reduced affinity for penicillin-binding protein 2, although high-level penicillin resistance remains rare in most countries. Fluoroquinolone resistance of meningococcal isolates, although rare, has also emerged. Ceftriaxone and cefotaxime can achieve CSF concentrations 45- to 8750-fold higher than the minimal inhibitory concentrations for meningococci. First-generation cephalosporins should not be used.

Patients with suspected bacterial meningitis of unknown cause are often given ceftriaxone or cefotaxime, often combined with vancomycin, until the causative agent has been identified. When *N. meningitidis* is identified, antibiotic treatment can be continued with a third-generation cephalosporin or possibly benzylpenicillin alone. Meropenem is also active clinically in the treatment of meningococcal meningitis, or chloramphenicol is a choice in penicillin- and cephalosporin-allergic patients. Traditionally, patients with meningococcal meningitis were treated for 7 days or longer, but 3 or 4 days of intravenous treatment can provide a cure without relapse.

TABLE 282-1 ANTIBIOTIC TREATMENT OF MENINGOCOCCAL MENINGITIS AND MENINGOCOCCEMIA

DRUG	AGE GROUP	DOSAGE
Ceftriaxone*	Children >3 months Adults	50 mg/kg IV q12h 1-2 g IV q12h
Cefotaxime	Adults	50-75 mg/kg q6-8h; maximum dose, 12 g/day
Penicillin G	Adults	50,000 U/kg IV q4h; up to 4 million U q4h
Meropenem	Adults	2 g IV q8h, 6 g/day
If penicillin and cephalosporin allergic, chloramphenicol†	Adults	25 mg/kg IV q6h, up to 1 g q6h

*Because of concerns in neonates from calcium/ceftriaxone precipitates and displacement of bilirubin from albumin by ceftriaxone, babies younger than 3 months should be started on cefotaxime 50 mg/kg q6-8h.
†Aztreonam or fluoroquinolones are potential alternatives.

Recognition of the different pathophysiologic processes associated with meningococcal meningitis (which causes death and morbidity predominantly by cerebral edema) and meningococcal septic shock (which causes death and morbidity predominantly through hypovolemia, capillary leak, respiratory distress, myocardial dysfunction, and multiorgan failure) has led to improved management strategies for these two different forms of disease. Early and aggressive management of shock through the use of volume expansion, oxygenation, intensive care monitoring, and inotropic support can reduce fatality rates of meningococcal sepsis from higher than 30% to 5 to 10%. In meningococcemia with hypotension, the primary goal is to increase the circulating blood volume by aggressive fluid treatment. Both colloids and crystalloids (saline 0.9%) can be used without a demonstrated difference in effectiveness. Adults are given saline starting with 1 L infused intravenously during 15 to 20 minutes, followed by several liters at a reduced rate. Some patients require two to three times their own blood volume during the first 24 hours. The total fluid volume needed per 24 hours is determined by response to treatment—tissue perfusion, blood pressure, urine output, and evidence of intravascular volume overload. The volume treatment may be combined with a vasopressor such as dopamine, norepinephrine, epinephrine, or dobutamine. It is important to monitor and correct acidosis, hypoglycemia, hypokalemia, hypocalcemia, and hypomagnesemia. Fluid treatment may be complicated in patients with reduced renal function. They may need dialysis or hemofiltration to compensate for renal failure and to reduce the substantial edema that accumulates.

Patients with meningitis without shock should be given the normal daily fluid requirement, supplemented with the volume lost before admission unless there is evidence of the syndrome of inappropriate antidiuretic hormone. Excessive volume treatment in patients with meningitis can induce fatal brain edema and herniation. Management of raised intracranial pressure (hyperosmolar solutions, diuretics, mechanical ventilation), seizures, and hyponatremia in neurointensive care is indicated.

Anticoagulant treatment of patients with meningococcemia and disseminated intravascular coagulation has not been documented to improve outcome. A phase III study of recombinant activated protein C in children with sepsis of all causes, including meningococcemia, was stopped because no benefit was noted, and recombinant activated protein C has been withdrawn from the market. The use of recombinant human tissue plasminogen activator does not appear to be beneficial. Randomized controlled clinical trials using hyperimmune serum, antibodies, or recombinant bactericidal or permeability-increasing protein (designed to inactivate *N. meningitidis* endotoxin) have not demonstrated a beneficial effect on survival. Blockade of other specific inflammatory mediators has not been adequately tested in meningococcal septic shock.

Patients with fulminant meningococcal septicemia can develop adrenal hemorrhage (Waterhouse-Friderichsen syndrome). The corticotropin concentration is higher, the cortisol concentration is lower, and the corticotropin-to-cortisol ratio is higher in patients with fatal meningococcal shock than in survivors. Adults with septic shock and indications of inadequate adrenal function are given low doses of steroids. Although the benefit has not been documented, many intensive care specialists use stress replacement doses of hydrocortisone in children with shock caused by *N. meningitidis*.

Plasmapheresis, blood exchange, and extracorporeal membrane oxygenation have been used in patients with meningococcemia; however, no controlled trials to assess the results have been done. Plasmapheresis and blood exchange appear to have little additive effect on the endogenous clearance of endotoxin and cytokines from the circulation. Extracorporeal membrane oxygenation has been used in several centers, with better results in children with acute pulmonary failure than in those with refractory septic shock. The use of insulin to control mild hyperglycemia in critically ill adults has not shown benefits (Chapter 100).

Pharmacologic doses of dexamethasone have been shown to reduce morbidity in pneumococcal and *Haemophilus influenzae* type b meningitis.[A1] However, the benefit of dexamethasone to reduce death caused by brain edema or to prevent sequelae such as deafness in patients with meningococcal meningitis remains unproven on the basis of large randomized controlled trials, even though trends toward reductions in hearing loss, mortality, and arthritis after meningococcal disease are reported. Many now recommend that dexamethasone (10 mg every 6 hours for the first 4 days and in children at a dose of 0.15 mg/kg every 6 hours for 4 days beginning before or with the first dose of antibiotics) be given early in suspected or confirmed bacterial meningitis. Other major life-threatening complications necessitating therapy include adult respiratory distress syndrome, neurologic sequelae ranging from coma to diabetes insipidus, pneumonia that is not necessarily meningococcal but may be secondary to aspiration during the obtunded state, and pericarditis.

Immune complex–mediated complications, such as arthritis, cutaneous vasculitis, iritis, episcleritis, pleuritis, and pericarditis, can first appear several days to 2 to 3 weeks after onset of illness, when the patient is otherwise improving. These complications, which can be multiple, are due to the deposition of antigen-antibody complexes composed of meningococcal capsular polysaccharide or other antigens, meningococcal-specific immunoglobulins, and C3. They complicate 6 to 15% of cases of meningococcal meningitis or septicemia. Treatment is with aspirin or nonsteroidal anti-inflammatory drugs, and resolution is complete, usually within 14 days from the onset and usually without residual sequelae.

TABLE 282-2 CHEMOPROPHYLAXIS AGAINST MENINGOCOCCAL INFECTION

DRUG	AGE GROUP	DOSAGE	DURATION AND ROUTE OF ADMINISTRATION*	CONSIDERATIONS
Rifampin	Children <1 month	5 mg/kg q12h	2 days, oral	
	Children >1 month	10 mg/kg q12h (maximum, 600 mg)	2 days, oral	
	Adults	600 mg q12h	2 days, oral	Rifampin can interfere with efficacy of oral contraceptives and some seizure prevention and anticoagulant medications; may stain soft contact lenses Not recommended for pregnant women
Ceftriaxone	Children <15 years	125 mg	Single IM dose	
	Children >15 years and adults	250 mg	Single IM dose	Ceftriaxone is recommended for prophylaxis in pregnant women.
Ciprofloxacin	Adults	500 mg	Single dose, oral	Not recommended routinely for persons <18 years of age, but use in infants and children (20 mg/kg) may be justified after careful assessment of the risks and benefits Not recommended for pregnant or lactating women Cases of ciprofloxacin resistance have been reported, and use for prophylaxis should be based on local sensitivity of the meningococcus to the drug.
Azithromycin		10 mg/kg (maximum, 500 mg)	Single dose, oral	Equivalent to rifampin for eradication of meningococci from nasopharynx, but data are limited

ANTIBIOTIC CHEMOPROPHYLAXIS FOR HOUSEHOLD OR INTIMATE CONTACTS
- Household contacts and persons sharing the same living quarters, particularly young children
- Daycare center, nursery school, or child-care contacts; frequent playmates of young children
- Close social contacts who were exposed to oral secretions in the week before onset, such as by kissing and sharing of eating and drinking utensils or toothbrushes
- For airline travel lasting more than 8 hours, passengers who are seated directly next to an infected person should receive prophylaxis.
- Routine prophylaxis is not recommended for health care professionals unless they have had intimate exposure to respiratory secretions.
- Because the risk for secondary cases is highest during the first few days after exposure, chemoprophylaxis should be initiated as soon as possible, ideally <24 hours after identification of the index patient.
- If more than 14 days have passed since the last contact with the index patient, chemoprophylaxis is not likely to be of benefit.
- Pharyngeal cultures are not helpful in determining the need for chemoprophylaxis and may unnecessarily delay the use of effective chemoprophylaxis.
- Chemoprophylaxis has also been recommended for patients given penicillin or chloramphenicol for treatment because pharyngeal carriage may not be eliminated with these antibiotics and the patient could remain colonized with a virulent strain.
- Ceftriaxone is recommended for pregnant women.
- May want to avoid ciprofloxacin or azithromycin in individuals at risk for QT-prolongation.

Recommended groups for chemoprophylaxis based on exposure to the case in the week before onset of illness.
*Administered orally unless otherwise stated.

PREVENTION

Chemoprophylaxis to eliminate meningococcal carriage is recommended for close contacts of patients to prevent further transmission and disease (Table 282-2).[10] The occurrence of meningococcal disease in household contacts is approximately 100-fold higher than in the general population. Secondary cases usually occur within 1 to 14 days of the primary case. Chemoprophylaxis can be helpful to control localized outbreaks, and a single dose of oral ciprofloxacin may be helpful in the epidemic setting.[AZ] Rifampin, ceftriaxone, azithromycin, and quinolones (but not penicillin) have the ability to eradicate meningococci in the nasopharynx. A majority of meningococcal isolates are now resistant to sulfonamides; resistance to rifampin can develop rapidly, and quinolone resistance in meningococci is reported.

Prevention through vaccination is the best option for the long-term control of meningococcal disease.[11] Capsular polysaccharide vaccines to decrease serogroup A, C, Y, and W meningococcal disease were introduced in the 1970s and 1980s. These vaccines are safe, with mild local adverse events, and are effective (>85%) in children older than 2 years and adults but are less immunogenic in younger children; immunity to the polysaccharide vaccines is limited to 3 to 5 years of protection, and immunologic hyporesponsiveness is induced by repeated doses of the polysaccharide. Also, meningococcal polysaccharide vaccines do not induce immunologic memory and have little or no effect on nasopharyngeal carriage. Although these vaccines were used extensively to control disease in military populations and in epidemics in the African meningitis belt, in the latter they were often deployed too late in the course of an outbreak. There was no evidence that widespread use of polysaccharide vaccines reduced the frequency of epidemics in Africa.

A major advance in the past 20 years has been the development and now widespread use of meningococcal polysaccharide-protein conjugate vaccines for A, C, Y, and W and their introduction first as a C conjugate into the United Kingdom and then with other conjugates in Europe, Canada, Australia, the United States, the African meningitis belt, and now globally.[12] These vaccines are safe and immunogenic in young children, induce immunologic memory, and can decrease nasopharyngeal carriage of meningococci. In the United

Kingdom, the introduction of the serogroup C conjugate meningococcal vaccine in 2000 to all children and young adults greatly reduced the rate of serogroup C disease (90% vaccine effectiveness at 3 years for patients aged 11 to 18 years). A major protective effect of the conjugate vaccines is mediated through herd protection. Rates of serogroup C carriage and disease in nonvaccinated individuals were reduced by more than 50% through herd protection. Polysaccharide-protein conjugate meningococcal vaccines containing serogroups A, C, Y, and W were introduced for adolescents in the United States in 2005 and subsequently extended to children aged 2 months to 10 years at increased risk for meningococcal disease. In addition to routine use in older children and adolescents (first dose at the age of 11 or 12 years with booster at 16 years), populations that benefit from the new conjugate vaccines are college freshmen, military recruits, patients with immunoglobulin or complement deficiencies (inherited or chronic deficiencies such as C3, properdin, factor D, or late complement components), patients with anatomic or functional asplenia, microbiologists who are routinely exposed to isolates of *N. meningitidis*, adults with HIV type 1 infections, and people who travel to or reside in countries where *N. meningitidis* is epidemic. An important example of a meningococcal conjugate vaccine development was the Meningitis Vaccine Program, a partnership between PATH, the World Health Organization, and the Global Alliance for Vaccines and Immunization for the development of a group A meningococcal conjugate vaccine for Africa, designated MenAfriVac, at less than $0.50 a dose. Because of the huge impact of herd immunity of the serogroup C conjugate vaccines in the United Kingdom, MenAfriVac was introduced as a mass vaccination strategy for those 1 to 29 years old. More than 284 million doses have been administered. To date, this has resulted in the virtual elimination of serogroup A meningococcal disease in the countries vaccinated.

The development of vaccines for serogroup B *N. meningitidis* has also shown significant progress. Serogroup B can cause prolonged outbreaks during many years, such as those seen in the 1990s in the Pacific Northwest (Oregon, parts of Washington), Brazil, Norway, and New Zealand and outbreaks in settings such as college campuses. The serogroup B capsule has an identical structure to polysialic structures expressed in fetal neural tissue and does not induce a protective bactericidal immunoglobulin G response. Thus, strategies have been focused on noncapsular antigens, such as outer membrane proteins containing vesicles (OMV) or conserved protein antigens. The diversity of major outer membrane structures in meningococci has limited OMV approaches for endemic disease but has been successful in controlling serogroup B epidemics that are strain specific (e.g., in New Zealand). Two new serogroup B vaccines, MenB4C (Bexsero)[13] and MenBFHbp (Trumenba),[14] based on surface protein antigens are now licensed. MenB4C contains three semiconserved surface protein antigens—a member of the factor H–binding protein family, neisserial adhesin A (NadA), and neisserial heparin-binding antigen—and a meningococcal serogroup B PorA-containing OMV preparation previously used to control the serogroup B clonal outbreak in New Zealand. Alum is the adjuvant. A second serogroup B vaccine, MenBFHbp (Trumenba) is based on two members of the factor H–binding protein family. The immunogenicity and safety of these vaccines have been demonstrated.[A3] The short-term prevention of serogroup B disease appears to be a significant step closer with these new vaccines that are now in use for treatment of outbreaks of serogroup B disease and in high-risk populations in several countries.

PROGNOSIS

Historically, the mortality of untreated systemic meningococcal disease was 70 to 90%. Despite highly effective antibiotics and aggressive supportive care, the mortality of invasive meningococcal disease remains at about 10%. The failure to recognize disease early, the very rapid development of disease (especially meningococcemia), and the time to administration of antibiotics remain the most significant challenges. The chance of surviving shock is directly correlated to plasma concentrations of endotoxin, and half the nonsurviving patients with shock die within the first 12 hours of hospital admission.

Long-term sequelae and morbidity after invasive meningococcal disease are significant. Neurologic impairment occurs in 7 to 10% with meningococcal meningitis, with palsies of the sixth, seventh, and eighth cranial nerves and hemiparesis and quadriparesis. Unilateral or bilateral sensorineural hearing loss occurs in 2 to 9% of cases, which is profound in 2% of affected individuals and necessitates cochlear implantation in 0.4%. Neurodevelopmental impairment, including behavioral and psychological problems, learning difficulties, memory deficits, executive function problems, decreased academic performance, spasticity, seizures, and focal neurologic signs, is seen in approximately 10%. Visual difficulties, seizures, and motor deficits are reported in 2 to 3%, with multiple neurologic disabilities occurring in 1 to 2% of affected individuals. Survivors of meningococcal sepsis in childhood have, in 5 to 20% as young adults, long-term behavioral and emotional problems, decreased intellectual functioning, and illness-related physical or social consequences.

Scarring of the skin, secondary to necrotic purpura, may vary from unnoticeable to requiring skin grafting. Multiple areas may be involved; the lower limbs are most frequently affected, followed by the arms, chest, and face. Amputations of the digits or limbs are frequently multiple; these result from necrosis of the skin, muscle, and bone of the affected parts (see Fig. 282-3D) and, depending on the site and extent, may require prostheses to improve function or appearance. Bone growth disturbances, stump overgrowth, scar contractures, and soft tissue and bone infections may complicate amputations. Limb-length discrepancies, which may result from the growth plate infarction, often necessitate further surgical intervention. Following acute renal failure at presentation, renal function recovers in the majority of individuals; however, evidence of renal dysfunction may persist for more than 4 years in both children and adults, with the risk being higher in those who required renal replacement therapy.

Meningococcal disease and its complications, often occurring rapidly in otherwise healthy individuals, also produce significant family, community, health care, and public health impact. The emotional toll on individuals who survive and on the families of those with meningococcal disease in intensive care units, of those who survive with complications and of those who die, is considerable and a global phenomenon. In communities, meningococcal disease may also create considerable fear and anxiety. Post-traumatic stress disorder occurs at a higher frequency in both patients and families, often months after the illness. In one study, post-traumatic stress disorder occurred in 15% of children, in half of the mothers, and in 19% of fathers at 3 months. Meningococcal disease and its complications also result in substantial hospital and long-term health care costs. Furthermore, delay in the diagnosis of meningococcal sepsis and meningitis and septicemia is a common reason for litigation.

If parents and health care professionals recognize the importance of fever and headache with or without a rash and seek treatment early, morbidity and mortality can be reduced with prehospital antibiotic treatment, rapid transportation to medical facilities, and stabilization in an intensive care unit. Prevention of meningococcal disease with new vaccines and vaccine strategies remains the major worldwide goal.

Grade A References

A1. Brouwer MC, McIntyre P, Prasad K, et al. Corticosteroids for acute bacterial meningitis. *Cochrane Database Syst Rev.* 2015;9:CD004405.
A2. Coldiron ME, Assao B, Page AL, et al. Single-dose oral ciprofloxacin prophylaxis as a response to a meningococcal meningitis epidemic in the African meningitis belt: a 3-arm, open-label, cluster-randomized trial. *PLoS Med.* 2018;15:1-19.
A3. Ostergaard L, Vesikari T, Absalon J, et al. A bivalent meningococcal B vaccine in adolescents and young adults. *N Engl J Med.* 2017;377:2349-2362.

GENERAL REFERENCES

For the General References and other additional features, please visit Expert Consult at https://expertconsult.inkling.com.

283

NEISSERIA GONORRHOEAE INFECTIONS

MATTHEW R. GOLDEN AND H. HUNTER HANDSFIELD

DEFINITION

Neisseria gonorrhoeae is a sexually transmitted organism that infects primarily the columnar epithelia of mucosal surfaces and causes urethritis in men and endocervicitis and urethritis in women. Other sites of primary infection include the rectum, pharynx, and conjunctiva, and vulvovaginitis can occur in prepubertal girls. The most common complication of gonococcal infection is pelvic inflammatory disease, which can lead to infertility, ectopic pregnancy, and chronic pelvic pain. Other much less common complications include epididymitis, posterior urethritis, urethral stricture, Bartholin gland abscess, and perihepatitis. Bacteremia may occur, with the production of characteristic cutaneous lesions, arthritis, and, rarely, endocarditis or meningitis. Neonatal conjunctivitis (ophthalmia neonatorum) was formerly a common cause of blindness. Gonococcal infections are also thought to increase the risk of human immunodeficiency virus (HIV) transmission from persons dually infected with HIV and *N. gonorrhoeae* and to increase the risk of HIV acquisition among persons with gonorrhea who are exposed to HIV.

The Pathogen

The gonococcal envelope is similar in its basic structure to that of other gram-negative bacteria and is composed of an inner cytoplasmic membrane, a middle peptidoglycan cell wall, and an outer membrane. The outer membrane contains several surface components that play a central role in the organism's interaction with the host and its pathogenicity. Pili, hairlike projections also referred to as fimbriae, are composed of several different protein subunits and, along with other outer membrane adhesins (i.e., opacity-related proteins), facilitate attachment and invasion of host cells. Gonococci vary the composition of these proteins and surface lipo-oligosaccharides over time, allowing the organism to elude host defenses. This phase variation has also been a barrier to successful vaccine development.

EPIDEMIOLOGY

Gonorrhea is the second most commonly reported infectious disease in the United States, with 555,608 cases reported to the Centers for Disease Control and Prevention (CDC) in 2017.[1] The incidence of gonorrhea in the United States in 2017 was 171.9 per 100,000 populational, though this number, which is based on cases reported to U.S. health departments, is undoubtedly an underestimate. The overall incidence of gonorrhea in the United States has increased 75% since 2009, the historic low in gonorrhea incidence, though it remains less than half the rate observed in the mid-1970s, the modern peak of gonorrhea incidence in the United States. The prevalence of gonorrhea among women tested through a population-based survey (the National Health and Nutrition Examination Survey) between 1999 and 2008 was 0.32%.

Like virtually all other sexually transmitted infections (STIs; Chapter 269), gonorrhea rates vary widely with age, geographic location, sexual orientation, and race or ethnicity. In the United States, the rate of reported infection is highest among 15- to 24-year-old women and 20- to 29-year-old men. Among women, rates are highest in the South and Midwest, whereas among men rates are highest in the South and West. These regional differences are, in part, a consequence of profound racial disparities and the explosive recent increase in gonorrhea rates among men who have sex with men.

Because national statistics do not consistently separate infections in men based on the gender of their sex partners, the heterosexual epidemic of gonorrhea is best understood by concentrating on the epidemiology of the infection among women. Among women, rates of reported gonorrhea among U.S. African Americans are almost 8.5 times higher than those among non-Hispanic whites, and rates among American Indians/Alaska Natives and Hispanics are 6 and 1.6 times higher, respectively, than those among non-Hispanic whites. Variations in reporting probably account for some of these observed differences because low socioeconomic status is associated with receiving care in public health clinics and other venues where there is more complete reporting than in the private health care sector. However, the marked disparity in reported rates is also apparent in population-based studies, clearly establishing that the different rates of infection in different racial and ethnic groups are not simply a result of reporting bias. The reasons for this profound disparity are certainly multifactorial and are not entirely clear. Different racial groups in the United States vary little in terms of their number of sex partners, so this cannot explain the different rates of STIs. Although inadequate access to medical care is likely to play a role in the racial disparities in STI rates, profound racial and ethnic disparities are also observed in the United Kingdom and the Netherlands, nations with nationalized health care systems in which access to care should be more uniform than it is in the United States. Research has highlighted the importance of concurrency (i.e., partnerships that overlap in time) and patterns of sexual mixing based on age, race, and level of sexual activity as critical determinants of a population's risk of STI. These factors are thought to be shaped by social factors (e.g., poverty, incarceration, joblessness, racism) that play a central role in defining the epidemiology of all STIs worldwide.

Numerous cities in the United States, western Europe, and Australia have reported increases in the rate and number of gonorrhea cases among men who have sex with men since the mid-1990s. There are no national data on gonorrhea rates in this population. However, well-documented trends in King County, Washington State are suggestive of what has occurred nationally and internationally. In 2017 the estimated incidence of reported gonorrhea in King County men who have sex with men was 4513 cases per 100,000, compared with 78 and 103 per 100,000 in men who have sex with women only and women, respectively. In part, the very high rate of gonorrhea among men who have sex with men in King County and elsewhere reflects high and probably increasing rates of testing, particularly screening for asymptomatic rectal and pharyngeal infections. However, the rate of urethral gonorrhea––an infection which is symptomatic in over 90% of cases––among men who have sex with men in King County was over 1400 per 100,000 (almost 14 times the rate observed in heterosexuals), demonstrating that disparities by sexual orientation are very large and not a consequence of differences in screening alone. Moreover, the rate of urethral gonorrhea among men who have sex with men in the area increased over 200% between 2008 and 2017, highlighting that rising rates reflect true increases in infections. Although it is not precisely defined, the risk of transmission from a man to a woman during a single episode of unprotected vaginal intercourse is thought to be 50 to 70%, and the risk of transmission from a woman to a man is 20%. The transmission risks associated with anal sex, fellatio, or cunnilingus are not well defined, but anal intercourse is probably a relatively efficient mode of transmission, and some data suggest that approximately one third of cases of urethral gonorrhea in men who have sex with men are transmitted through fellatio. Gonococci die rapidly on drying, and with the exception of occasional acquisition by laboratory personnel working with the organism, nonsexual transmission does not occur in adults. Perinatal transmission causing neonatal ophthalmitis or pharyngeal infection is now rare.

PATHOBIOLOGY

After attachment to host epithelial cells, gonococci are endocytosed into the cell in a process thought to be facilitated by Por (or protein 1). Gonococci then replicate within the host cell and are released into the subepithelial space.

Typical urethral infections result in prominent inflammation, probably as a result of the release of toxic lipo-oligosaccharide and peptidoglycan fragments as well as the release of chemotactic factors that attract neutrophilic leukocytes. The reasons that some gonococcal strains selectively cause asymptomatic genital infection are poorly understood, but this propensity may be related to differences in the organism's ability to bind complement-regulatory proteins that downregulate the production of chemotactic peptides. In particular, gonococcal strains that express PorB1A appear to bind factor H and complement-binding protein and have an increased propensity for causing disseminated gonococcal infections.[2]

Although the gonococcus is not highly mutable, many gonococci possess conjugative plasmids and are consequently able to efficiently transfer genetic material conferring resistance to penicillin and tetracycline. Gonococci are also capable of efficiently transferring naked DNA (transformation). These characteristics are important in the organism's ability to develop resistance to antimicrobials.[3,4] For example, recent evidence suggests that the gonococci with diminished susceptibility to oral cephalosporins possess genetic resistance mutations acquired from commensal *Neisseria* species commonly found in the oropharynx. Sustained clonal dissemination of antibiotic-resistant *N. gonorrhoeae* within a population is illustrated by the finding, through whole-genome sequencing, of a single clone of a high-level azithromycin-resistant strain being responsible for an outbreak of gonorrhea across England between 2014 and 2017.[5]

CLINICAL MANIFESTATIONS

Gonococcal infections can result in a number of specific clinical syndromes, each of which has its own manifestations, differential diagnosis, and recommended evaluation. The major clinical manifestations of gonococcal infection are discussed separately later. Gonococcal ophthalmia, now a rare complication, can result from direct contact or by autoinoculation in individuals with anogenital gonorrhea and is manifested as an acute, purulent conjunctivitis that can result in corneal ulceration if it is not treated promptly.[6]

DIAGNOSIS

Microscopy

Microscopy of a Gram-stained smear is positive when polymorphonuclear neutrophils are observed to contain intracellular gram-negative diplococci of typical morphology (Fig. 283-1). Gram-stained urethral smears are 90 to 98% sensitive in the diagnosis of symptomatic gonococcal urethritis in men and have a specificity greater than 95%. However, Gram stain is only approximately 50% sensitive for cervical or rectal infection and for asymptomatic urethral gonorrhea. Although Gram stain is often considered highly specific for such infections, the actual performance varies with the skill and experience of the examiner, and rectal and cervical smears are unreliable in many clinical settings. Smears are both insensitive and nonspecific for pharyngeal gonococcal infection and are not recommended.

Culture

Isolation of *N. gonorrhoeae* by culture, generally with antibiotic-containing selective media, is the historic mainstay of the diagnosis of gonorrhea.

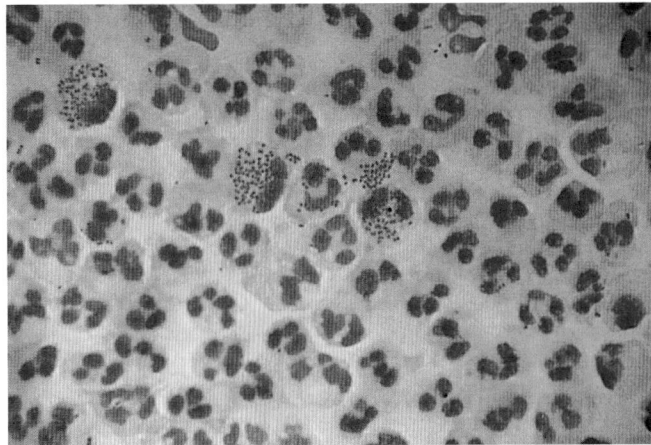

FIGURE 283-1. Gram stain in an acute case of gonococcal urethritis. This slide is used to demonstrate the nonrandom distribution of gonococci among polymorphonuclear neutrophils. Note that there are both intracellular and extracellular bacteria in the field of view.

Despite the proliferation of molecular diagnostic methods, culture retains important roles in surveillance for antimicrobial resistance and selected clinical settings. Ideally, growth media should be inoculated directly and placed promptly into a humid atmosphere with increased carbon dioxide, such as a candle extinction jar. However, standard transport systems (e.g., Culturette) are acceptable if specimens are kept moist, are not refrigerated, and are processed within 6 hours. In testing of specimens not likely to be colonized by competing flora (e.g., synovial fluid), nonselective chocolate agar should be used.

Nucleic Acid Amplification Tests

In most settings in the United States, nucleic acid amplification tests have now supplanted culture as the dominant laboratory test used to diagnose gonorrhea. Nucleic acid amplification tests approved by the Food and Drug Administration include polymerase chain reaction, transcription-mediated amplification, and DNA strand displacement. The advantages of nucleic acid amplification tests include increased sensitivity over culture, particularly for extragenital infections, the ability to test urine specimens and self-obtained vaginal swabs, and the fact that most nucleic acid amplification tests are now marketed as combination assays that allow simultaneous testing for *N. gonorrhoeae* and *Chlamydia trachomatis* (Chapter 302). The primary disadvantage of nucleic acid amplification tests is the inability to perform antimicrobial susceptibility testing. Many genes associated with antimicrobial resistance have been identified, and it is sometimes possible to identify resistant organisms using nucleic acid amplification. However, at present, no commercially available test for *N. gonorrhoeae* detects antimicrobial resistance, and for many drugs, the presence or absence of defined determinants of resistance are not sensitive and specific in defining whether an organism is susceptible to specific antimicrobials.

Although nucleic acid amplification tests have been approved by the Food and Drug Administration only for the testing of genital tract and urine specimens, increasing evidence suggests that at least some nucleic acid amplification tests are substantially more sensitive than culture in detecting *N. gonorrhoeae* in pharyngeal and rectal specimens and that these nucleic acid amplification tests are sufficiently specific to screen high-risk populations for rectal and pharyngeal gonorrhea. Given the decreasing availability of gonococcal culture, the poor sensitivity of culture on nongenital tract specimens, and the high prevalence of asymptomatic rectal and pharyngeal infections in some populations (particularly men who have sex with men), clinicians caring for patients at high risk for nongenital gonococcal infections should be able to use nucleic acid amplification tests. Recent studies suggest that self-obtained rectal and pharyngeal specimens yield accurate results and are acceptable to men who have sex with men.

⬤ CLINICAL SYNDROMES
Urogenital Gonorrhea in Males
▎CLINICAL MANIFESTATIONS AND DIAGNOSIS▕

Gonococcal urethritis in men is typically characterized by a purulent urethral discharge and dysuria. The usual incubation period is 2 to 6 days. A small minority of men who acquire urethral infection—generally estimated at 1 to 5%, and varying between specific strains of *N. gonorrhoeae*—remain asymptomatic.

Physical examination typically reveals purulent urethral exudate (Fig. 283-2); this is usually readily apparent, but compression of the urethra is sometimes required to express the exudate. Erythema of the meatus is sometimes present. Nongonococcal urethritis (Chapter 269) is typically characterized by less copious and less purulent discharge.

The diagnosis of gonococcal urethritis is usually suspected clinically, confirmed preliminarily by a Gram-stained smear showing leukocytes with intracellular gram-negative diplococci (see Fig. 283-1), and made definitively when *N. gonorrhoeae* is identified by culture or nucleic acid amplification testing. Despite the usual clinical differences between gonococcal urethritis and nongonococcal urethritis, substantial overlap exists, and microbiologic diagnosis should be routine even in clinically typical cases.

▎PROGNOSIS▕

With prompt treatment, urethral gonorrhea seldom results in significant long-term morbidity. Acute epididymitis complicates gonococcal urethritis in less than 1% of cases. Patients with epididymitis usually present with unilateral testicular pain and swelling, sometimes with fever. Posterior urethritis or prostatitis, typically manifested as pelvic or perineal pain and urinary

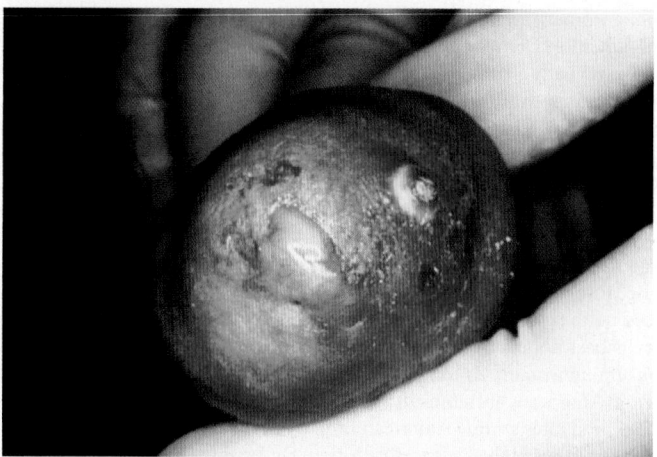

FIGURE 283-2. Male patient with a purulent penile discharge from gonorrhea and an overlying penile pyodermal lesion. Pyoderma involves the formation of a purulent skin lesion, which in this case is located on the glans penis.

retention, was once fairly common but is now rare. Urethral stricture, another formerly common complication, is now very rare. Gonorrhea is associated with an elevated risk of HIV infection, both directly and as an epidemiologic risk factor. Diagnosis of gonorrhea should alert clinicians to counsel such patients about sexual risks, test them for HIV infection, and encourage patients to seek frequent follow-up testing for HIV infection and other STIs.

Lower Genital Tract Gonorrhea in Females
▎CLINICAL MANIFESTATIONS, DIAGNOSIS, AND PROGNOSIS▕

The primary site of infection in women is the endocervical canal. The proportion of infected women who develop symptoms is not precisely known, but probably about 50% of incident infections are symptomatic. In any case, asymptomatic infections accumulate in populations, whereas many or most symptomatically infected women present for diagnosis and treatment. Therefore, most prevalent infections among women are asymptomatic or are associated with mild symptoms not perceived by patients as abnormal or important. Gonorrhea is sometimes associated with an abnormal vaginal discharge, but other lower genital tract infections, such as bacterial vaginosis, trichomonas vaginitis, and candidal vaginitis, are much more common causes of this symptom. Lower genital tract gonorrhea in women can be associated with abnormal vaginal bleeding, which typically is manifested as metrorrhagia, scant intermenstrual bleeding, or postcoital spotting. *N. gonorrhoeae* sometimes causes dysuria and can be isolated from the urethra in up to 80% of women with gonorrhea. However, the urethra is rarely the only infected site, except in women who have had hysterectomies. In a minority of women, physical examination is notable for a purulent or mucopurulent cervical discharge, cervical edema, or easily induced cervical bleeding, signs of mucopurulent cervicitis. In uncomplicated infections, purulent exudate can sometimes be expressed from a Bartholin gland duct, near the vaginal introitus laterally, or from Skene glands, adjacent to the urethral meatus.

Microbiologic diagnosis usually rests on identifying *N. gonorrhoeae* in cervical secretions by nucleic acid amplification test or culture. Gram-stained smears are insensitive and seldom used.

The most important common complication of lower genital tract gonorrhea in women is pelvic inflammatory disease (see later). Rarer complications include Bartholin gland abscess, which is manifested as a tender introital mass and may involve superinfection with facultative and anaerobic bacteria.

Pelvic Inflammatory Disease
▎CLINICAL MANIFESTATIONS▕

Pelvic inflammatory disease refers to an infection of the upper female genital tract and can involve the uterus (endometritis), fallopian tubes (salpingitis), and ovaries (oophoritis) as well as neighboring pelvic structures.[7] An estimated 10 to 40% of women with endocervical gonococcal infections develop pelvic inflammatory disease, and gonorrhea is thought to be the cause of approximately 5 to 30% of all diagnosed cases of pelvic inflammatory disease in the United States. However, this proportion varies with overall rates of gonorrhea and other causes of pelvic inflammatory disease in the population, such as chlamydial infection.

Low abdominal pain is the dominant symptom of pelvic inflammatory disease. Pain is variable in intensity and is often mild; it is usually bilateral, typically present for days to weeks before clinical presentation, and can be exacerbated by coitus. Approximately one third of women have abnormal vaginal bleeding. Fever, chills, anorexia, vaginal discharge, urethritis, and proctitis occur, but these symptoms are neither sensitive nor specific in identifying women with pelvic inflammatory disease. There is little if any difference in the severity of symptoms and signs of pelvic inflammatory disease associated with *N. gonorrhoeae, C. trachomatis*, or neither of these pathogens.

The physical examination is typically notable for diffuse abdominal tenderness that is greatest in the lower quadrants and for tenderness of the pelvic organs on bimanual examination, with or without manipulation of the cervix. Most women have signs of cervicitis or bacterial vaginosis. Fever is present in a minority of cases. Abdominal or adnexal signs are occasionally unilateral, and this finding can cause confusion with appendicitis, ectopic pregnancy, and other conditions. Right upper quadrant abdominal tenderness due to perihepatitis (Fitz-Hugh–Curtis syndrome) is sometimes present, which can mimic acute cholecystitis or viral hepatitis. Perihepatitis sometimes occurs in the absence of other abdominal or pelvic findings typical of pelvic inflammatory disease, especially when it is caused by *C. trachomatis*. Severe pelvic inflammatory disease may be accompanied by signs of generalized peritonitis.

DIAGNOSIS

The clinical diagnosis of pelvic inflammatory disease is imprecise. Published studies, which have used somewhat variable criteria in populations with different prevalences of the syndrome, have reported positive predictive values of 65 to 90% compared with the "gold standard" of laparoscopically defined pelvic inflammatory disease. Although nonspecific, the presence of neutrophils on a saline wet mount of vaginal secretions was 91% sensitive for endometritis in one study. The absence of white blood cells on a wet mount of vaginal secretions, particularly if mucopurulent cervicitis is also absent, should prompt the consideration of alternative diagnoses. The differential diagnosis of pelvic inflammatory disease includes ectopic pregnancy; appendicitis; rupture, bleeding, or torsion of an ovarian cyst; endometriosis; urinary tract infection or pyelonephritis; renal or ureteral stones; inflammatory bowel disease; and, rarely, viral hepatitis or cholecystitis.

Because of the potential seriousness of the infection and the relative simplicity, low cost, and low toxicity of treatment, clinical diagnostic criteria emphasize sensitivity at the cost of specificity. Clinicians therefore should maintain a low threshold for tentative diagnosis and presumptive treatment of pelvic inflammatory disease. The U.S. CDC recommends that all sexually active women with pelvic or lower abdominal pain and uterine, adnexal, or cervical motion tenderness be treated for possible pelvic inflammatory disease if no other cause of their symptoms and signs is readily apparent. Furthermore, screening of asymptomatic sexually active young women with nucleic acid amplification tests is recommended by the U.S. Preventive Services Task Force. Factors such as fever, an elevated erythrocyte sedimentation rate or C-reactive protein level, and concurrent bacterial vaginosis or mucopurulent cervicitis further support the clinical diagnosis, but these are frequently absent. Definitive diagnosis requires transvaginal ultrasound or other diagnostic imaging showing thickened or fluid-filled fallopian tubes or tubo-ovarian abscess or laparoscopy demonstrating purulent tubal exudate, erythema, or edema. Also, histologic evidence of plasma cell endometritis on endometrial biopsy has been associated with laparoscopic evidence of salpingitis, though biopsies are seldom performed in clinical practice.

PROGNOSIS

Fallopian tube scarring secondary to pelvic inflammatory disease often results in tubal factor infertility, ectopic pregnancy,[8] and chronic pelvic pain. Previous gonococcal and chlamydial infections are among the most common antecedents of these complications. Each episode of pelvic inflammatory disease, whether due to *N. gonorrhoeae, C. trachomatis*, or neither of these organisms, significantly increases the risk for recurrent salpingitis.

The natural history of clinically apparent pelvic inflammatory disease is well defined. In what is probably the best single study on the subject, tubal factor infertility occurred in 8% of women after a single episode of laparoscopically proved pelvic inflammatory disease, in 20% after two such episodes, and in 40% after three or more episodes. The first pregnancy after an episode of pelvic inflammatory disease was ectopic in almost 8% of women, and like tubal factor infertility, the risk of ectopic pregnancy increased with each successive episode of the syndrome. Chronic pelvic pain, sometimes disabling in its severity, occurs in almost 20% of women after one or more episodes of

pelvic inflammatory disease. Importantly, these outcomes were best studied in women with clinically apparent pelvic inflammatory disease, and the pertinent studies were undertaken at a time when clinical recognition and treatment were likely delayed. Many women suffer clinically mild or silent pelvic inflammatory disease. The risk of sequelae associated with silent pelvic inflammatory disease is not well defined, but more clinically severe pelvic inflammatory disease is associated with a higher risk of sequelae. Most women with tubal factor infertility deny a history of pelvic inflammatory disease, and it seems likely that silent pelvic inflammatory disease, particularly silent pelvic inflammatory disease associated with *C. trachomatis*, is responsible for most cases of STI-related reproductive tract sequelae. For example, *C. trachomatis* seropositivity is strongly associated with tubal factor infertility, independent of clinical or historical evidence of pelvic inflammatory disease.

Rectal Infection
CLINICAL MANIFESTATIONS

Gonococcal infection of the rectum is common in women and in men who have sex with men.[9] In women, infection is acquired either through perineal contamination with cervicovaginal secretions or by anal intercourse; the latter is thought to be the dominant route in men who have sex with men. In women with cervical gonorrhea and in men who have sex with men with gonorrhea at any anatomic site, about 40% have rectal infection. More than 80% of rectal infections are subclinical, but symptomatic proctitis sometimes is manifested as varying combinations of anal pruritus, mucopurulent discharge (often characterized by the patient as mucus-coated feces), pain, tenesmus, and bleeding. Symptomatic proctitis seems to be more common in men who have sex with men than in women with rectal gonorrhea, which suggests that the size of the infecting inoculum or trauma from anal intercourse may influence the clinical manifestations. Among men who have sex with men, rectal gonorrhea is a potent epidemiologic risk marker for the acquisition of HIV and may be a direct risk factor because anorectal inflammation enhances susceptibility to HIV infection.

DIAGNOSIS

Diagnosis of rectal gonorrhea depends on the identification of *N. gonorrhoeae*, usually by nucleic acid amplification testing. The Gram-stained smear is insensitive and nonspecific. The differential diagnosis of symptomatic proctitis includes other traditional STIs (herpes, syphilis, and chlamydial infection, including lymphogranuloma venereum) as well as ulcerative colitis, Crohn colitis, anal fissure, rectal lacerations, and proctocolitis caused by *Shigella, Campylobacter, Yersinia enterocolitica*, and other enteric pathogens. Recent studies using nucleic acid amplification testing among STI clinic patients suggest that approximately 5 to 10% of tested men who have sex with men and 1% of tested women have rectal infections without concurrent genital tract infections. Although less than 20% of women with gonorrhea have extragenital infections, more than half of men who have sex with men with gonorrhea have only extragenital infections, highlighting the importance of routine screening of men who have sex with men, but not women, for rectal gonorrhea.

Pharyngeal Infection
CLINICAL MANIFESTATIONS

Pharyngeal gonococcal infection results from orogenital exposure.[10] It is more efficiently acquired by fellatio than by cunnilingus and is found in approximately 8% of men who have sex with men evaluated in STD clinics, and in 3 to 7% of heterosexual men and approximately 30% of women and men who have sex with men with concurrent genital tract gonorrhea. Pharyngeal gonorrhea seldom causes symptoms, although rare cases may exhibit exudative pharyngitis and cervical lymphadenopathy. Isolated pharyngeal infection is common is men who have sex with men and may also be common in at least some populations of heterosexuals. Complications are infrequent, and most infections eventually resolve spontaneously or in response to therapy for genital or rectal infection. Therefore, although the modest morbidity associated with pharyngeal infections in and of itself does not justify extensive screening efforts, the oropharynx is an important reservoir for infection in some populations, particularly men who have sex with men, among whom approximately 30% of urethral infections result from exposure to pharyngeal infections. The oropharynx is also a site of gene exchange between *N. gonorrhoeae* and commensal Neisseria, and pharyngeal infections are thought to play a critical role in fostering the emergence of antimicrobial-resistant gonococci. Failure to identify and to eradicate pharyngeal infections helps sustain high levels of gonococcal transmission and may foster the spread of antibiotic-resistant gonococci. Accordingly, current guidelines suggest that men who have sex with men at risk for STIs be tested for pharyngeal gonorrhea.

Gonorrhea in Children

Gonococcal conjunctivitis may develop in infants born to mothers with gonorrhea, a condition termed ophthalmia neonatorum. Formerly a common cause of blindness, gonococcal ophthalmia is now rare in industrialized countries because of improved control of gonorrhea, routine use of neonatal ocular prophylaxis, and prompt antibiotic therapy. Neonates may also acquire pharyngeal or rectal infection and, rarely, gonococcal pneumonia or sepsis. Beyond the neonatal period, purulent vaginitis is the most common manifestation of gonorrhea or chlamydial infection in girls, and rectal or pharyngeal infection is the most common manifestation in prepubertal boys. Most cases are acquired through sexual abuse.

Disseminated Gonococcal Infection

CLINICAL MANIFESTATIONS

Disseminated gonococcal infection usually is manifested with various combinations of polyarticular tenosynovitis, dermatitis secondary to focal septic embolization, and septic arthritis. Studies undertaken in the 1960s and 1970s estimated that disseminated gonococcal infection occurred in 1 to 3% of adults with gonorrhea, but the risk depends on characteristics of the particular strains of *N. gonorrhoeae* circulating in the population. Today, disseminated gonococcal infection probably occurs in well under 1% of gonococcal infections in most geographic areas. Women may be somewhat more susceptible to disseminated gonococcal infection than men, and the onset often coincides with menstruation. Severity varies from a mild illness with slight joint discomfort, a few skin lesions, and little or no fever to a fulminant illness with overt polyarthritis, innumerable skin lesions, high fever, and prostration. Most persons with disseminated gonococcal infection have no symptoms of genital gonorrhea, probably because some strains of *N. gonorrhoeae* that are prone to disseminate are also associated with subclinical mucosal infections. The absence of clinical symptoms and signs of mucosal infection in these strains is probably due to their ability to bind complement downregulatory molecules, thereby diminishing the local inflammatory response.

The presentation of disseminated gonococcal infection can be divided into the clinical syndromes of tenosynovitis-dermatitis and monarticular or oligoarticular arthritis, although these presentations sometimes overlap. Tenosynovitis-dermatitis is thought to predominate early in the course of dissemination, and approximately 70% of disseminated gonococcal infection cases in published series present with this syndrome. These patients usually suffer migratory polyarthralgias without purulent arthritis. There is often tendon inflammation affecting the wrists, fingers, ankles, or toes. Skin lesions are typically painless, are few in number (5 to 30), affect predominantly the extremities, and are pustular or vesiculopustular (Fig. 283-3), although petechiae, hemorrhagic macules, papules, bullae, and nodules rarely occur (see Fig. 412-5). Axial skeletal involvement is uncommon, a feature that can help differentiate disseminated gonococcal infection from reactive arthritis (Chapter 249). The tenosynovitis-dermatitis syndrome often subsides spontaneously, or it may evolve during a period of several days into an overt septic arthritis with purulent synovial fluid, usually involving only one or two joints. Approximately 25 to 50% of persons with disseminated gonococcal infection present initially with purulent monarticular or oligoarticular arthritis, often without apparent sequential evolution from arthritis-dermatitis syndrome. This form of disseminated gonococcal infection typically affects the knee, ankle, elbow, or wrist, but any joint may be involved.

DIAGNOSIS

Sexually active young persons with arthritis, tenosynovitis, or papulopustular skin lesions should be tested for *N. gonorrhoeae* at all potentially exposed anatomic sites. The diagnosis of disseminated gonococcal infection is secure when gonococci are identified by culture or nucleic acid amplification testing in the blood, a skin lesion, or synovial fluid, but it is often made presumptively when genital, rectal, or pharyngeal gonorrhea is present in a patient with a compatible clinical syndrome that responds promptly to antibiotics.

Blood, synovial fluid, and mucosal tract cultures are positive in approximately 4 to 35%, 10 to 34%, and 80% of patients, respectively. However, the yield from culture varies with the clinical presentation. The performance of nucleic acid amplification test versus culture of blood, synovial fluid, or skin lesions has not been studied in patients with disseminated gonococcal infection. Patients with tenosynovitis-dermatitis more frequently have bacteremia, whereas patients with septic gonococcal arthritis are seldom bacteremic, and close to

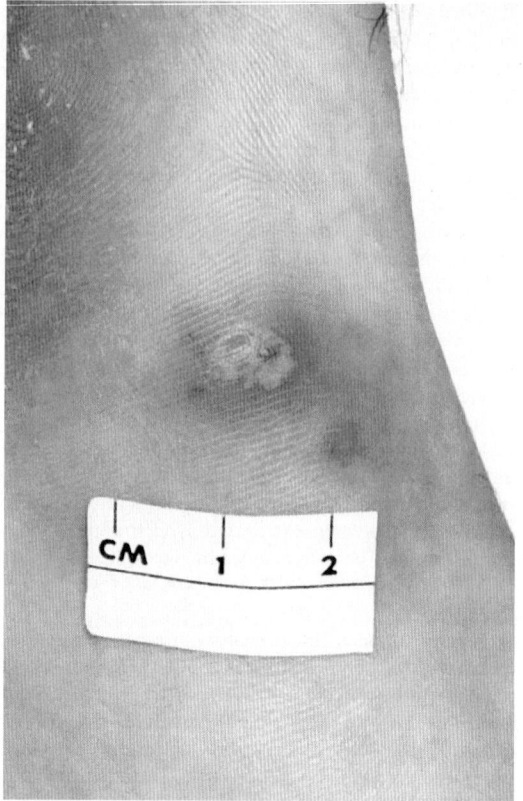

FIGURE 283-3. Cutaneous gonococcal lesion secondary to disseminated *Neisseria gonorrhoeae* infection. Although gonorrhea is a sexually transmitted disease, if it remains untreated, the *N. gonorrhoeae* bacteria responsible for the infection can disseminate throughout the body and form lesions in extragenital locations (also see Fig. 412-5). (From Handsfield HH. *Color Atlas and Synopsis of Sexually Transmitted Diseases.* 3rd ed. New York: McGraw-Hill; 2011.)

50% have positive synovial fluid cultures; it is reasonable to suspect that the yield might be higher with nucleic acid amplification testing. Because bacteremia is intermittent, clinicians should obtain more than one set of blood cultures to maximize the likelihood of isolating the organism. Similarly, nucleic acid amplification tests or culture specimens should be obtained from all potentially exposed anatomic sites (genital tract, pharynx, rectum). Cultures of skin lesions are generally negative despite demonstrable gonococci by fluorescent antibody, but nucleic acid amplification test results may be positive in persons with negative blood and mucosal site cultures. The peripheral blood leukocyte count is generally elevated but may be normal. The synovial fluid leukocyte count is usually 20,000 to 60,000/μL, with higher numbers of white blood cells seen in persons with clinically apparent arthritis than in those with tenosynovitis-dermatitis. Liver function tests often show elevations in aminotransferase levels, suggestive of mild hepatitis.

The differential diagnosis of disseminated gonococcal infection includes reactive arthritis (Chapter 249), meningococcemia (Chapter 282), other kinds of septic arthritis (Chapter 256), rheumatoid arthritis (Chapter 248), systemic lupus erythematosus (Chapter 250), acute HIV infection (Chapter 361), syphilis (Chapter 303), and other rheumatologic conditions and infectious diseases. Reactive arthritis, often triggered by sexually acquired chlamydial infection, is the principal consideration in young adults. The skin lesions of the two conditions, when present, are generally distinct and often pathognomonic for one syndrome or the other. In addition, conjunctivitis and involvement of the axial skeleton (e.g., sacroiliitis) are common in reactive arthritis and infrequent in disseminated gonococcal infection.

PROGNOSIS

Many cases of arthritis-dermatitis syndrome resolve spontaneously. With prompt treatment, few patients suffer sequelae of disseminated gonococcal infection, but untreated septic arthritis can lead to contiguous osteomyelitis or joint destruction. Endocarditis, meningitis, and myocarditis are occasionally seen, with or without a typical disseminated gonococcal infection syndrome. Gonococcal endocarditis usually involves the aortic valve and often progresses rapidly, leading to valve destruction and heart failure.

PREVENTION

Control of gonorrhea depends on prompt diagnosis and effective treatment of infected persons, screening of sexually active women and men who have sex with men in settings where gonorrhea is prevalent, treatment of patients' partners, rescreening of persons with a recent history of gonorrhea, and efforts to promote safer sexual behaviors (e.g., condom use, abstinence, fewer partners). Sexually active men who have sex with men outside of mutually monogamous relationships, including HIV-infected men, are at high risk for gonorrhea and should be tested at least annually for rectal and pharyngeal gonococcal infection as well as for chlamydial infection, syphilis, and HIV infection. Men who have sex with men with any of the following risks should be screened every 3 months: (1) gonorrhea, chlamydia, or syphilis diagnosis in the prior year; (2) use of methamphetamine or amyl nitrite (poppers); (3) more than 10 sex partners in the prior year; or (4) current use of HIV preexposure prophylaxis. In general, clinicians should perform syphilis testing on all HIV-infected men who have sex with men at every blood draw. The value of screening of asymptomatic men for urethral infection (by nucleic acid amplification testing of urine) is uncertain; the yield for gonorrhea is low in most settings, though such screening does sometimes identify men with asymptomatic chlamydial urethritis. Gonococcal screening criteria for woman are not well defined. However, because most nucleic acid amplification tests for *C. trachomatis* also test for *N. gonorrhoeae*, most chlamydia screening includes gonorrhea testing.

Public education and personal counseling of persons with gonorrhea or at risk of contracting it should emphasize the effectiveness of mutual monogamy and condoms for vaginal or anal sex for new or casual partnerships. Every patient with gonorrhea should be counseled about the risks for HIV infection and should be tested for HIV, *C. trachomatis*, and syphilis. Clinicians should recommend initiation of HIV preexposure prophylaxis to HIV-uninfected men who have sex with men they diagnose with gonorrhea. Because accurate epidemiologic data are essential to generate and to maintain resources for the prevention and control of STIs, all cases of gonorrhea, chlamydial infection, syphilis, and HIV infection should be promptly reported to the health department in accordance with local laws. Ultimate control of gonorrhea may require immunization, and some recent data suggest that the outer membrane vesicle meningococcal B vaccine may provide partial protection from gonococcal infection, though this finding requires confirmation. At present, no vaccine with proven efficacy against *N. gonorrhoeae* is available.

TREATMENT

Rx

Antimicrobial Susceptibility

The Centers for Disease Control and Prevention has identified antimicrobial resistant *N. gonorrhoeae* as one of the three greatest drug-resistant threats facing the United States. Gonococci with chromosomal or plasmid-borne mutations that confer relative or absolute resistance to the penicillins, tetracyclines, and sulfonamides are prevalent worldwide, and none of these drugs is acceptable as empirical therapy anywhere in the world. The prevalence of β-lactamase (penicillinase) plasmids, which confer absolute resistance to penicillin, ampicillin, and amoxicillin, varies from about 10% of gonococci in the United States and western Europe to almost 50% in some low and middle income nations.

In the United States, approximately 35% of gonococcal infections in men who have sex with men and 20% of infections in heterosexuals are caused by organisms that are resistant to ciprofloxacin and other fluoroquinolones. Resistant gonococci are more prevalent still in Europe (up to 50% in some countries). Fluoroquinolone-resistant gonococci are prevalent worldwide, and fluoroquinolones are no longer suitable for routine use unless recent local data demonstrate low levels of resistance or antimicrobial resistance testing from a patient's isolate demonstrates susceptibility.

Starting in 2014, the proportion of *N. gonorrhoeae* isolates with elevated minimum inhibitory concentrations to azithromycin has risen dramatically, and in 2016 3.6% of gonococcal isolates in the United States were no longer susceptible to azithromycin by the definition used in the United States (MIC ≥2 µg/mL), and over 11% were resistant by the definition used in the United Kingdom (MIC ≥1 µg/mL).[11] This change in gonococcal susceptibility has not yet resulted in changes in treatment guidelines in the United States or Europe, but raises concerns that macrolides may not be an effective part of gonorrhea treatment regimens in the future.

Perhaps the greatest concern related to gonococcal resistance is the emergence of resistance to extended spectrum cephalosporins. Strains with relative resistance to oral cephalosporins (e.g., cefixime, heretofore a mainstay of gonorrhea treatment) are thought to have emerged in Japan in the 1990s, becoming

commonplace during the first decade of the 21st century. A series of case reports subsequently described infections with ceftriaxone-resistant organisms, including a report describing a cluster of cases with high-level resistance to azithromycin and elevated minimum inhibitory concentrations to ceftriaxone in Hawaii in 2016. As of 2017, *N. gonorrhoeae* with elevated minimum inhibitory concentrations to cephalosporins were rare (<1% of cases). Nevertheless, ongoing surveillance for cephalosporin resistance remains a high priority, and decisions on how to treat gonorrhea need to incorporate strategies for diminishing the development of population-level antimicrobial resistance. Clinicians who treat patients for gonorrhea and other STIs should keep abreast of regional trends in resistance and be alert to modified therapeutic recommendations.

Principles of Treatment

Because of the need to curtail transmission, therapy is usually based on clinical or epidemiologic suspicion before the diagnosis is confirmed microbiologically.[12] Clinicians should presumptively treat all patients evaluated as contacts to persons with known gonococcal infections, all women with pelvic inflammatory disease or mucopurulent cervicitis, and, if Gram staining cannot be performed, all men presenting with a clinical syndrome of urethritis.[13] (Men with urethritis and no evidence of gonorrhea on Gram stain should be treated for nongonococcal urethritis.) Diagnosis by nucleic acid amplification testing precludes antimicrobial resistance testing, and even when *N. gonorrhoeae* is isolated by culture, susceptibility testing is rarely performed routinely. Accordingly, treatment of uncomplicated gonorrhea is dictated by national or local patterns of antimicrobial susceptibility, without knowledge of susceptibility in individual patients. However, susceptibility testing should be used to guide the treatment of gonococcal septic arthritis, endocarditis, or other serious complications, and clinicians should perform cultures with resistance testing whenever they suspect treatment failure following treatment with standard regimens.[14]

Dual treatment of uncomplicated gonorrhea, typically with both a cephalosporin and either azithromycin or doxycycline, has long been recommended to cover the possibility of simultaneous chlamydial infection, typically present in 5 to 10% of men who have sex with men, 15 to 25% of heterosexual men, and 35 to 50% of women with gonorrhea in North America. Some authorities have suggested that dual therapy with antibiotics with differing mechanisms of action may reduce selection pressure for antimicrobial resistance in *N. gonorrhoeae*. However, this hypothesis has not been proven and is increasingly questioned, with some experts now concerned that treatment with both ceftriaxone and azithromycin could promote azithromycin resistance in *N. gonorrhoeae* and in other sexually transmitted pathogens, such as *Mycoplasma genitalium*. At present, the CDC continues to recommend dual treatment. However, guidelines around the world are variable and in influx. British guidelines recommend treatment with 1 g of intramuscular ceftriaxone without a second drug, while Australian guidelines recommend 500 mg of intramuscular ceftriaxone with azithromycin 1 g PO.

Treatment Regimens

Despite concerns related to rising rates of azithromycin resistance, as of April 2019 ceftriaxone 250 mg intramuscularly plus azithromycin 1 g orally remains the preferred treatment regimen for uncomplicated gonorrhea in the United States (Table 283-1).[15] This regimen is highly effective against pharyngeal gonorrhea, which may be relatively resistant to oral therapies, and is designed to cover simultaneous chlamydial infection.[A1] Cefixime 400 mg orally (with azithromycin 1.0 g orally) remains appropriate when ceftriaxone therapy is not feasible (e.g., if a patient declines injection) or in expedited (unobserved) treatment of patients' sex partners. Clinicians should be mindful that ensuring that all patients and partners are treated is more important than always using intramuscular ceftriaxone. Persons with severe β-lactam allergies should receive azithromycin 2 g orally once, *plus* either a single dose of gentamicin 240 mg IM *or* a single dose of gemifloxacin 320 mg orally.[A2] Zoliflodacin, which inhibits DNA biosynthesis, appears to be effective as a single 2 to 3 g oral dose for treating uncomplicated urogenital and rectal gonococcal infections, but it is less effective for pharyngeal infections[A3]; FDA approval is pending.

Women with acute pelvic inflammatory disease should be treated with antibiotics active against *N. gonorrhoeae* and *C. trachomatis*. The role of anaerobic bacteria in pelvic inflammatory disease is uncertain, although it is not known whether anaerobic treatment is required for pelvic inflammatory disease. Most women can be treated as outpatients, but the following factors should prompt hospital admission: possible surgical cause of symptoms (e.g., appendicitis), pregnancy, failure to respond to oral therapy within 72 hours of initiation, inability to tolerate or to adhere to oral therapy, severe symptoms, and tuboovarian abscess.[16] The suggested outpatient regimen is ceftriaxone 250 mg IM plus doxycycline 100 mg PO twice daily for 14 days or cefoxitin 2 g IM plus probenecid 1 g PO as a single dose and doxycycline 100 mg twice daily for 14 days. Either regimen can be given with or without metronidazole (500 mg twice daily) for 14 days. For hospitalized patients or others who require parenteral therapy, the CDC recommends intravenous cefotetan or cefoxitin plus oral doxycycline or parenteral therapy with clindamycin plus gentamicin. Intravenous ampicillin-sulbactam plus oral doxycycline can also be used. Parenteral

TABLE 283-1	ANTIBIOTIC REGIMENS FOR THE TREATMENT OF GONORRHEA IN THE UNITED STATES*

UNCOMPLICATED GONORRHEA OF THE URETHRA, CERVIX, OR RECTUM

Preferred

Ceftriaxone 250 mg IM single dose *plus* azithromycin 1 g PO single dose

Alternatives

Cefixime 400 mg PO single dose *plus* azithromycin 1 g PO single dose
Or
Azithromycin 2 g PO single dose
plus gentamicin 240 mg IM single dose *or* gemifloxacin 320 mg PO as a single dose

PELVIC INFLAMMATORY DISEASE

Outpatient (Mild-to-Moderate Disease)

Doxycycline (100 mg orally twice daily for 14 d) with or without metronidazole (500 mg orally twice daily for 14 d), *plus* one of the following:
Ceftriaxone (250 mg single dose IM)
or
Cefoxitin (2 g single dose IM concurrently with probenecid 1 g orally)

Inpatient (Moderate-to-Severe Disease)†

Cefotetan (2 g IV) *plus* doxycycline (100 mg orally or IV q12h)
or
Cefoxitin (2 g IV q6h) *plus* doxycycline (100 mg orally or IV q12h)
or
Clindamycin (900 mg IV q8h) *plus* gentamicin (3 to 5 mg/kg IV once daily)

INFECTION OF THE PHARYNX

Ceftriaxone 250 mg IM single dose *plus* azithromycin 1 g PO as a single dose

CONJUNCTIVITIS (NOT OPHTHALMIA NEONATORUM)

Ceftriaxone 1 g IM single dose *plus* azithromycin 1 g PO as a single dose

DISSEMINATED GONOCOCCAL INFECTION

Preferred

Ceftriaxone 1 g IM or IV q24h‡
or
Ceftizoxime 1 g IV q8h
Plus
Azithromycin 1 g PO as a single dose

Alternative

Cefotaxime 1 g IV q8h

*Treatment of gonorrhea in adults should always include treatment of sex partners and advice to abstain from sex for 7 days.
†Parenteral therapy is continued until improvement is observed, after which oral therapy is prescribed to complete 14 days total treatment.
‡Treat with intravenous therapy until the patient has been clinically improved for 24 to 48 hours. Then switch to cefixime 400 mg orally twice a day to complete a 7-day course.

therapy is continued until improvement is observed, after which oral therapy is prescribed to complete 14 days' total treatment.

Most persons with disseminated gonococcal infection should be hospitalized and treated with a parenteral third-generation cephalosporin such as ceftriaxone, cefotaxime, or ceftizoxime. Joint irrigation or drainage appears to be unnecessary for septic arthritis, although repeated aspiration of synovial fluid may speed clinical improvement. Oral treatment (e.g., cefixime, cefpodoxime, or a fluoroquinolone) can usually be substituted after improvement begins and then continued to complete 7 days' therapy. More prolonged parenteral treatment and higher doses are indicated for the treatment of gonococcal meningitis or endocarditis, although modern data are lacking. Gonococcal epididymitis, bartholinitis, and other localized complications should generally be treated for 7 to 14 days with drugs active against both *N. gonorrhoeae* and *C. trachomatis*. Gonococcal conjunctivitis in adults can be managed with a single dose of ceftriaxone, 1 g IM, with optional saline lavage. The diagnosis of all forms of complicated gonococcal infection should be confirmed by culture with determination of antimicrobial susceptibility, which can guide completion of treatment after initial empirical therapy.

Management of Sex Partners

Failure to ensure treatment of patients' sex partners contributes to the continued transmission of gonorrhea and other bacterial STIs and often results in reinfection of the index case. For gonorrhea and chlamydial infection, all partners in the preceding 2 months should be treated; if the patient has not had sex in the preceding 2 months, the most recent partner should be treated. Very few U.S. health departments have the resources to attempt to ensure that sex partners receive treatment, and the responsibility to ensure partner treatment lies jointly with the patient and the diagnosing clinician. Optimally, the partners of persons with gonorrhea should undergo diagnostic testing for gonorrhea, chlamydial infection, syphilis, and HIV infection. However, clinicians should not wait to obtain the results of diagnostic testing before treating a potentially exposed sex partner; all partners of infected persons should be treated when they initially present for evaluation.

In most settings, approximately 50% of potentially exposed sex partners go untreated, risking ongoing transmission and reinfection of the original patient. In an effort to address this problem, the CDC and several state health departments in the United States recommend that clinicians offer heterosexual patients with gonorrhea or chlamydial infection medication to give to their sex partners. This practice, termed patient-delivered partner therapy (PDPT)—sometimes termed expedited partner therapy—is supported by three randomized controlled trials showing that treating sex partners without requiring attendance for care in person decreases the risk of reinfection and increases the proportion of partners treated. PDPT requires single-dose treatment, typically with cefixime plus azithromycin for gonorrhea or azithromycin alone for the partners of patients with chlamydial infection. PDPT currently is legal in most states of the United States and is likely to become permissible in other states, and clinicians should offer PDPT as an option for most heterosexual patients with gonorrhea or chlamydial infection. The CDC website maintains up-to-date information on the legality of PDPT in U.S. states and territories (http://www.cdc.gov/STD/ept/legal/default.htm). In addition to direct delivery of drugs to the patient for PDPT, it is often feasible to write or to telephone a prescription to a cooperating pharmacy. However PDPT is implemented, when practical, clinicians should provide written information about the medication and STI prevention as well as advice to seek clinical care in addition to taking the drugs provided. Examples of forms that can be dispensed with PDPT can be found at the following websites: http://www.doh.wa.gov/YouandYourFamily/IllnessandDisease/SexuallyTransmittedDisease/ExpeditedPartnerTherapy; http://www.cdph.ca.gov/HealthInfo/discond/Pages/SexuallyTransmittedDiseases.aspx. PDPT is generally not recommended for men who have sex with men with gonorrhea or chlamydial infection owing to potentially high rates of syphilis and HIV infection; the partners of such patients should be evaluated, treated in person, and in most instances be offered HIV preexposure prophylaxis.

Follow-up

The recommended treatment regimens cure 96 to 100% of uncomplicated cases of genital or rectal gonorrhea caused by susceptible strains and at least 90% of pharyngeal infections. Retesting of infected patients to document eradication of *N. gonorrhoeae* ("test of cure") is not recommended except in pregnant women, when adherence to therapy is in doubt, or when atypical treatment regimens are employed. When test of cure is indicated, culture can be performed a week after treatment is completed, but retesting by nucleic acid amplification should be delayed at least 2 weeks after treatment to reduce the possibility of detecting persistent gonococcal RNA or DNA despite the eradication of viable organisms.

Although test of cure is generally not advised, all persons diagnosed with gonorrhea should be rescreened 3 to 4 months after treatment. In prospective studies, 10 to 20% of both men and women with gonorrhea or chlamydial infection are infected when they are retested 3 to 4 months later. The likelihood of recurrent or persistent gonococcal infection among heterosexuals appears to be reduced by up to 70% when partners are managed with PDPT. Rescreening can be done with urine or self-obtained vaginal swab testing by nucleic acid amplification and does not require a second visit with a clinician.

Grade A References

A1. Creighton S. Gonorrhoea. *Clin Evid (Online)*. 2014;2:1-12.
A2. Kirkcaldy RD, Weinstock HS, Moore PC, et al. The efficacy and safety of gentamicin plus azithromycin and gemifloxacin plus azithromycin as treatment of uncomplicated gonorrhea. *Clin Infect Dis.* 2014;59:1083-1091.
A3. Taylor SN, Marrazzo J, Batteiger BE, et al. Single-dose zoliflodacin (ETX0914) for treatment of urogenital gonorrhea. *N Engl J Med.* 2018;379:1835-1845.
A4. Ferreira A, Young T, Mathews C, et al. Strategies for partner notification for sexually transmitted infections, including HIV. *Cochrane Database Syst Rev.* 2013;10:CD002843.

GENERAL REFERENCES

For the General References and other additional features, please visit Expert Consult at https://expertconsult.inkling.com.

284

HAEMOPHILUS AND *MORAXELLA* INFECTIONS

ADAM J. RATNER AND MICHAEL S. SIMBERKOFF

HAEMOPHILUS INFECTIONS

DEFINITION

The name *Haemophilus* is derived from the Greek nouns *haima*, meaning "blood," and *philos*, meaning "lover." *Haemophilus* species colonize the respiratory tract; cause infections of the respiratory tract, skin, or mucous membranes of humans; and from these sites can invade and cause bacteremia, meningitis, epiglottitis, endocarditis, septic arthritis, or cellulitis (Table 284-1).

The Pathogen

Haemophilus species are small, nonmotile, aerobic or facultative anaerobic, pleomorphic, gram-negative bacilli. The prototype of this genus, *Haemophilus influenzae*, was originally recovered from patients with influenza by Pfeiffer in 1893, and it was considered the cause of that disease for many years. Primary isolation of *Haemophilus* species is best accomplished on chocolate agar medium in a carbon dioxide–enriched atmosphere.

EPIDEMIOLOGY

The precise prevalence and incidence of *H. influenzae* infections are unknown. This organism can be detected in the nasopharynx of both children and adults. Before the introduction of an effective vaccine, between 3 and 5% of infants harbored *H. influenzae* type b in their nasopharynx. Children who have been immunized against *H. influenzae* type b are far less likely to be colonized and infected with this organism. However, the risk for infection in nonimmune household contacts of a patient with invasive *H. influenzae* disease is approximately 600-fold greater than the risk in the age-adjusted general population. Nontypeable *H. influenzae* can be detected in the nasopharyngeal cultures of more than 70% of young children, but infection occurs in only a small proportion of colonized individuals.

H. influenzae type b was the most common cause of meningitis in young children before effective vaccines were introduced in the 1980s. Vaccination has had a dramatic impact, with a reduction of more than 99% in invasive *H. influenzae* type b disease. A study covering the period from 1989 to 2008 from the U.S. Centers for Disease Control and Prevention's Active Bacterial Core surveillance system showed that the overall incidence of invasive *H. influenzae* infections fell from 4.39 cases per 100,000 population in 1989 (around the time of introduction of the *H. influenzae* type b conjugate vaccine in the United States) to 1.55 cases per 100,000 in 2008, and the percentage of invasive infections caused by *H. influenzae* type b fell from 87 to 3%, whereas the percentage caused by nontypeable *H. influenzae* strains increased from 16.8 to 68.4%. Because of the decrease in infections due to type b, the relative importance of nontypeable strains and serotypes a and f as causes of invasive *H. influenzae* disease has increased in the United States[1] and other countries where conjugate *H. influenzae* vaccines have been introduced, although the overall rate of invasive *H. influenzae* disease has been substantially decreased by vaccination.[2]

Patients with human immunodeficiency virus (HIV) infection are at increased risk for *H. influenzae* infection.[3] Rates of invasive *H. influenzae* infection in men aged 20 to 49 years with HIV infection and acquired immunodeficiency syndrome (AIDS) were 14.6 and 79.2 per 100,000, respectively. The majority of these infections were caused by nontypeable *H. influenzae* strains, although in a second study, 10 of 15 bacteremic *H. influenzae* type b infections observed in adults occurred in patients at risk for HIV infection, and AIDS was documented in seven of these patients.

Other factors also increase the risk for *H. influenzae* infection, including immunoglobulin deficiencies, sickle cell disease, splenectomy or functional asplenia, malignant disease, pregnancy, cerebrospinal fluid (CSF) leaks, head trauma, alcoholism, chronic obstructive pulmonary disease (COPD), and race. Eskimo, Navajo, and Apache children have *H. influenzae* type b infection rates that are significantly greater than those in comparable non-native populations. In addition, daycare attendance, crowding, the presence of siblings, prior hospitalizations, and previous otitis media have been shown to increase the risk for *H. influenzae* type b disease in young children, whereas breast-feeding decreases this risk.

PATHOBIOLOGY

H. influenzae consists of encapsulated (typeable) and nonencapsulated (nontypeable) forms. The encapsulated forms are responsible for most of the invasive infections in children and acute epiglottitis in both children and adults, whereas the nonencapsulated forms cause respiratory mucosal infections, conjunctivitis, female genital tract infections, and invasive disease in adults. Nontypeable *H. influenzae* is also an important cause of acute otitis media in children. The capsules of *H. influenzae* consist of polysaccharide antigens. Six capsular serotypes (a through f) exist and are important virulence factors that inhibit opsonization, clearance, and intracellular killing of the organisms. *H. influenzae* type b contains a pentose capsular polysaccharide consisting of polyribosyl ribitol phosphate (PRP). Other serotypes contain hexose polysaccharides. *H. influenzae* type b is more virulent than the other serotypes, probably because it is highly resistant to clearance once bacteremia has been initiated. Since the introduction of *H. influenzae* serotype b conjugate vaccines in the 1990s, most infections are caused by nontypeable strains and or non-b serotypes, (e.g., *H. influenzae* serotype a or f).[4-7]

Fimbriae are important virulence factors that enhance the adherence of *H. influenzae* to mucosal surfaces. Both typeable and nontypeable *H. influenzae* isolates contain fimbriae. The lipo-oligosaccharides of *H. influenzae* also contribute to their virulence. Phase variation of modifications to the *H. influenzae* surface lipo-oligosaccharide alters receptor tropism and evasion of innate immune defenses. Lipo-oligosaccharides appear to play a crucial role in facilitating the survival of *H. influenzae* on mucosal surfaces within the nasopharynx and in initiating invasive disease (blood stream invasion) from these sites.[8]

Outer membrane proteins also serve as virulence factors in *H. influenzae* disease. At least 15 different *H. influenzae* outer membrane proteins have been identified. One of these (P2, 39 to 40 kD) functions as a porin, and others are associated with iron binding. Successful scavenging of iron within the human host is crucial for multiplication of *H. influenzae*. *H. influenzae* produces a protease that specifically cleaves human immunoglobulin A1 (IgA1). This strategy is thought to facilitate mucosal carriage.

Antibodies have been recognized for decades as an important part of host defenses against *H. influenzae* diseases. The classic studies of Fothergill and Wright in 1933 demonstrated that most cases of *H. influenzae* meningitis occur in young children after they lose passively acquired maternal antibodies and before active humoral immunity to the organism develops. These protective antibodies function primarily to opsonize and to facilitate the clearance of *H. influenzae* rather than to kill virulent organisms directly.

Complement is also an essential component of host defenses against some *H. influenzae* diseases. Children with congenital deficiencies of C2, C3, and factor I have an increased incidence of *H. influenzae* infections. Patients who lack a functional spleen (e.g., those with sickle cell disease) or who have undergone splenectomy also are at risk for the development of overwhelming infection with *H. influenzae* type b. Shp2, an Src homology 2 domain-containing phosphatase, is required to coordinate macrophage function and innate immunity against H *influenzae* pulmonary infection.[9]

TABLE 284-1	SITES OF COLONIZATION AND INFECTIONS BY *HAEMOPHILUS INFLUENZAE*	
SPECIES	**NORMAL FLORA**	**ASSOCIATED DISEASES**
H. influenzae	Nasopharynx Upper respiratory tract	Meningitis Epiglottitis Sinusitis Otitis Pneumonia Cellulitis Arthritis Osteomyelitis Obstetric infections Endocarditis
H. influenzae, biogroup *aegyptius*		Purulent conjunctivitis Brazilian purpuric fever

CLINICAL MANIFESTATIONS

Meningitis

H. influenzae meningitis more commonly occurs in unvaccinated or undervaccinated children younger than 5 years, immunocompromised populations, and those with a history of skull trauma or CSF leaks. A surveillance study of bacterial meningitis in the United States from 1998 to 2007 demonstrated that *H. influenzae* caused 61 of 1083 (5.6%) cases of meningitis in adults, with more than 75% of these being due to nontypeable strains. In the same study, 42 of 587 (7.2%) of pediatric meningitis cases were due to *H. influenzae*, approximately 12% of which were type b.

H. influenzae meningitis is clinically indistinguishable from other forms of acute bacterial meningitis. Most patients with *H. influenzae* meningitis have CSF white blood cell counts greater than 1000/μL and hypoglycorrhachia. CSF Gram stain shows pleomorphic gram-negative bacilli in 60 to 70% of untreated cases. In some patients, however, the bipolar staining may result in a mistaken diagnosis of pneumococcal meningitis. Thus, Gram stain is neither sensitive nor specific for diagnosis of *H. influenzae* meningitis.

The diagnosis of *H. influenzae* type b meningitis is established by culture. Multiplex polymerase chain reaction panels targeting a range of CSF pathogens can detect *H. influenzae* nucleic acid, even in the setting of prior antibiotic treatment.

Epiglottitis

Before the availability of the conjugate vaccine, *H. influenzae* type b was the most common cause of acute epiglottitis, but it is rarely the cause in areas where vaccination has been introduced.[10] *H. influenzae* epiglottitis is a life-threatening infection in children that usually occurs in those younger than 5 years. The symptoms are fever, drooling, dysphagia, and respiratory distress or stridor, which appear during the course of hours. In adults, fever, sore throat, dysphagia, and odynophagia occur. Cervical tenderness and lymphadenopathy can be found at all ages. Laryngoscopy demonstrates a swollen, cherry-red epiglottis. However, this procedure should be avoided or undertaken only by experts because it may precipitate acute airway obstruction and thus make emergency tracheotomy necessary. A lateral radiograph of the neck may confirm the diagnosis of acute epiglottitis. The patient must be maintained in an upright position during this procedure, however, to avoid additional compromise of the airway. The cause is usually established by blood culture. Cultures of the pharynx and other mucosal surfaces are less useful because *H. influenzae* may be part of the normal flora. Vaccination has substantially decreased the overall incidence of epiglottitis.

Pneumonia

H. influenzae is a cause of pneumonia in both children and adults. These organisms can also cause nosocomial infections, including ventilator-associated pneumonia. The clinical features of *H. influenzae* pneumonia include fever, cough, and signs and radiographic findings of lobar consolidation. Parapneumonic effusions or empyema occur commonly in patients with *H. influenzae* pneumonia. Gram-negative bacilli in sputum suggest the diagnosis, but isolation of *H. influenzae* from sputum culture alone is inadequate to prove a cause because of the high frequency with which this organism colonizes the respiratory tract. A diagnosis can be established by isolating *H. influenzae* from either blood or pleural fluid. Most isolates are nontypeable.

Tracheobronchitis

Tracheobronchitis is a condition characterized by fever, cough, and purulent sputum that occurs in the absence of radiographic infiltrates suggestive of pneumonia. It frequently develops in patients with known chronic lung disease. Blood cultures are rarely positive. A combination of pleomorphic gram-negative bacilli predominating in purulent sputum, antibody titers to *H. influenzae* that rise after infection (although these are rarely performed in clinical settings), and a response, at least transiently, to treatment of *H. influenzae* infection strongly suggests this diagnosis.

Sinusitis

H. influenzae and *Streptococcus pneumoniae* are the most frequent bacterial isolates from antral punctures or surgical specimens of patients with acute sinusitis. Most *H. influenzae* isolates are nontypeable. Although patients may respond initially to treatment directed against *H. influenzae*, the response may be transient if sinus obstruction is not relieved.

Otitis Media

H. influenzae is an important cause of otitis media in young children. Nearly all of the *H. influenzae* isolates obtained by tympanocentesis are nontypeable. Patients with otitis media may have ear pain or exhibit irritability. Drainage can be present. An inflamed, opaque, bulging, or perforated tympanic membrane is usually demonstrated. The cause can be proved by Gram stain and culture of purulent fluid obtained by tympanocentesis. Otitis caused by *H. influenzae* type b may occur in association with bacteremia and meningitis.

Cellulitis

H. influenzae type b was formerly an important cause of cellulitis in children. Most of the infections occur on the face or neck. *H. influenzae* cellulitis is often described as causing a distinctive blue or violaceous discoloration of the skin. However, the fever, erythema, and tenderness observed may not be distinguishable from those attributable to other causes. The diagnosis is established by culture of blood or tissue aspirates from the involved area, or both.

Bacteremia without a Primary Focus of Infection

H. influenzae can cause primary bacteremia in both children and adults. In infants or children, occult meningitis or epiglottitis can be present in association with *H. influenzae* type b bacteremia. Rigorous clinical and laboratory evaluation is essential to avoid missing a diagnosis of life-threatening focal infection in these patients. In adults, primary *H. influenzae* bacteremia often occurs in those with underlying diseases, such as lymphoma, leukemia, or alcoholism.

Obstetric, Gynecologic, and Urologic Infection

Pregnancy is associated with a significant risk for *H. influenzae* infection. In one study, 7 of 47 adult *H. influenzae* invasive infections occurred in pregnant women. Nontypeable *H. influenzae* can cause tubo-ovarian abscess and salpingitis in women. A recent study of women in England and Wales showed that pregnancy was associated with an increased risk of invasive, mostly unencapsulated *H. influenzae* infection and that these infections were associated with poor pregnancy outcomes, including fetal loss and extremely premature births or stillbirths. In men, *H. influenzae* and *H. parainfluenzae* account for about 7% of cases of acute urethritis, perhaps related to unprotected oral sex.[11]

Pericarditis

Before routine immunization in the United States, *H. influenzae* type b was an important cause of primary bacterial pericarditis in children. It rarely causes this infection in adults; however, pericarditis can occur in association with pneumonia, probably as a result of contiguous spread of the infection.

Endocarditis

H. influenzae is an unusual cause of endocarditis in view of the frequency with which invasive disease occurs. Most infections occur in patients with preexisting valvular heart disease. Because of its slow initial growth in blood culture media, diagnosis of this infection may be delayed or missed. Patients with *H. influenzae* endocarditis are at high risk for arterial embolic phenomena.

Septic Arthritis

H. influenzae type b was a common cause of septic arthritis in young children before the introduction of the conjugate *H. influenzae* type b vaccine; it is rare in adults. *H. influenzae* type b arthritis is clinically indistinguishable from other causes of pyogenic arthritis.

Purulent Conjunctivitis and Brazilian Purpuric Fever

H. influenzae, biogroup *aegyptius* (Koch-Weeks bacillus), causes epidemic purulent conjunctivitis in children. This disease commonly occurs in hot climates or in the summer season.

The infection is characterized by conjunctival erythema, edema, mucopurulent exudate, and varying discomfort in the eyes. An unusually virulent clone of *H. influenzae*, biogroup *aegyptius*, causes an invasive infection called Brazilian purpuric fever, which is characterized by petechial or purpuric skin lesions and vascular collapse; it occurs days to weeks after an initial episode of conjunctivitis in infants and children younger than 10 years.

TREATMENT   Rx

Third-generation cephalosporins are considered the treatment of choice for invasive *H. influenzae* infections, such as meningitis or epiglottitis. Treatment with ceftriaxone (adult dose, 1 to 2 g intravenously every 12 hours) or cefotaxime (adult dose, 2 g intravenously every 6 hours) should be started in patients with proven or suspected *H. influenzae* infection, and it should be continued at least until full susceptibility data are available.

Ampicillin was effective treatment of all *H. influenzae* infections until the mid-1970s. Since the first reports of ampicillin-resistant *H. influenzae* isolates in 1972, however, the prevalence of resistance has increased dramatically. Most resistance is due to a plasmid-mediated, R-factor enzyme (TEM-1) β-lactamase, which can be detected rapidly in the laboratory. In addition, some isolates have altered penicillin-binding proteins that have decreased binding affinity to penicillin and other β-lactam antibiotics. Therefore, patients with proven or suspected *H. influenzae* infections should not be treated with ampicillin or second-generation cephalosporins until susceptibility to these antibiotics has been proved.

Oral antibiotics are commonly used to treat tracheobronchitis in patients with COPD and otitis media in children, in whom *H. influenzae* isolates are common. Because of resistance, ampicillin and amoxicillin cannot be recommended for the more serious of these infections unless the susceptibility of isolates is known. Most *H. influenzae* isolates are susceptible to amoxicillin-clavulanate, azithromycin, and clarithromycin. Fluoroquinolones, such as ciprofloxacin, ofloxacin, levofloxacin, and gatifloxacin, are usually active against these organisms.[12] Trimethoprim-sulfamethoxazole is also effective for most isolates.

PREVENTION

The first *H. influenzae* type b vaccines were licensed for use in the United States in 1985. They contained purified PRP antigens. However, post-licensing studies of PRP vaccines in the United States showed variable efficacy. The PRP vaccines elicit a type 2, thymus-independent B-cell response, generate few (if any) memory B cells, and fail to stimulate a response in neonates and infants.

Protein-conjugated PRP vaccines were developed to overcome the problem of lack of immune response in the most susceptible infants and some young children. Several are now licensed for use in infants. At present, protein-conjugated PRP vaccines are recommended for use in all infants older than 2 months but not earlier than 6 weeks of age. Studies have shown that protein-conjugated vaccines are effective in diverse populations, including adults with COPD.

Antibiotic prophylaxis is recommended if there is a nonimmunized or underimmunized household contact less than 4 years of age of a patient with invasive *H. influenzae* type b disease. In that setting, all household members should receive chemoprophylaxis. Rifampin is the treatment of choice. It should be given in a dosage of 10 mg/kg once daily for 4 days to infants younger than 1 month, 20 mg/kg (up to a maximum of 600 mg) once daily for 4 days to older children, and 600 mg/day for 4 days to adults. No prophylaxis is recommended for contacts of patients with nontypeable or non-type b *H. influenzae* disease, though clinicians may consider prophylaxis for invasive *H. influenzae* type a disease.

Other *Haemophilus* Species

Haemophilus parainfluenzae can be found as part of the normal microbiota of the mouth and pharynx (Table 284-1). It is a rare cause of meningitis in children and an even rarer cause of meningitis in adults. It may cause dental infections or dental abscesses. Cases of brain abscess, epidural abscess, liver abscess, osteomyelitis, pneumonia, empyema, epiglottitis, peritonitis, septic arthritis, and bacteremia have been reported to be caused by this organism. *H. parainfluenzae* also causes subacute endocarditis, often in young adults. Certain other species that can cause endocarditis were formerly grouped in the genus *Haemophilus*, including *H. aphrophilus*, *H. paraphrophilus*, and *H. segnis*. These are now considered members of the *Aggregatibacter* genus. *Haemophilus ducreyi* is the etiologic agent of the sexually transmitted infection chancroid, which causes genital ulcer disease.

⬤ *MORAXELLA* INFECTIONS

DEFINITION

Moraxella catarrhalis is most commonly associated with infections of the respiratory tract, including acute otitis media in children and exacerbations of chronic bronchitis in adults.

The Pathogen

Moraxella organisms are small, gram-negative bacteria that grow well on blood or chocolate agar. They are catalase and oxidase positive. These small diplococci

TABLE 284-2 SITES OF COLONIZATION AND INFECTION BY *MORAXELLA* SPECIES

SPECIES	NORMAL FLORA	ASSOCIATED DISEASES
M. catarrhalis	Oral cavity and upper respiratory tract	Chronic bronchitis exacerbation Otitis media Pneumonia Sinusitis Bacteremia, endocarditis Arthritis, osteomyelitis, epiglottitis (all extremely rare)
M. lacunata	Upper respiratory tract	Chronic conjunctivitis
Other *Moraxella*	Upper respiratory tract	Rare cases of bacteremia, endocarditis, arthritis, meningitis

are morphologically difficult to distinguish from *Neisseria*. Some *Moraxella* species are gram-negative coccobacilli. *M. catarrhalis* is the most important pathogen of this genus (Table 284-2).

PATHOBIOLOGY

M. catarrhalis is isolated exclusively from humans and is found predominantly in the respiratory tract. *M. catarrhalis* adheres to mucosal cells with the aid of pili. Infection is believed to result from contiguous spread of the organism from sites of colonization, possibly as a result of the introduction of new, more virulent strains to which the host lacks immunity. *M. catarrhalis* possesses multiple virulence factors that can be carried through biologically active outer membrane vesicles to contribute to the pathobiology of otitis media.[13]

M. catarrhalis can often be found in respiratory secretions together with *H. influenzae*. Although the mechanism for coexistence of these pathogens is not known, evidence suggests that the outer membrane vesicles of *M. catarrhalis* inactivate complement, thus enhancing survival of *H. influenzae*.

CLINICAL MANIFESTATIONS

M. catarrhalis is associated with exacerbations of chronic bronchitis. Studies indicate that this organism can be isolated from 0.2 to 8.1% of the sputum aspirates of patients with this disease. It is the third most common pathogen isolated from these patients behind *S. pneumoniae* and *H. influenzae*.

M. catarrhalis can cause pneumonia, particularly in elderly patients with COPD and other underlying conditions such as diabetes mellitus. Rare cases of bacteremic pneumonia have been reported. In addition, *M. catarrhalis* can cause nosocomial pneumonia with evidence of patient-to-patient spread of the organism.

M. catarrhalis is a common cause of otitis media in young children. Microbiologic studies indicate that this organism is present in approximately 15% of the aspirates from such patients. The organism also causes sinusitis and is a rare cause of bacteremia in children and adults.

Serious infections with other *Moraxella* species are uncommon. However, these organisms are associated with chronic conjunctivitis. Furthermore, case reports have documented the rare occurrence of invasive infections, including bacteremia, endocarditis, arthritis, pericarditis, and meningitis. Meningitis and other invasive infections may occur in patients with complement deficiency or other immune deficiencies.

TREATMENT ℞

Oral antibiotics are sufficient for the treatment of most noninvasive *M. catarrhalis* infections. β-Lactamases are present in many isolates. Therefore, treatment with amoxicillin-clavulanate (usual adult dose, 500 mg every 12 hours), a second- or third-generation cephalosporin, or a non–β-lactam antibiotic such as a fluoroquinolone should be initiated. Other than β-lactamase detection, susceptibility testing is rarely performed.

GENERAL REFERENCES

For the General References and other additional features, please visit Expert Consult at https://expertconsult.inkling.com.

285

CHANCROID

STANLEY M. SPINOLA

DEFINITION

Chancroid is a sexually transmitted disease characterized by painful genital ulcers and inguinal lymphadenitis caused by *Haemophilus ducreyi*. *H. ducreyi* recently emerged as a major cause of nonsexually transmitted cutaneous ulcers in children who live in yaws (Chapter 304)-endemic regions of the South Pacific and Africa. As described in Chapter 304, yaws is a nonsyphilitic treponematosis that causes a disfiguring and debilitating childhood infectious disease. *H. ducreyi* is a gram-negative coccobacillus that is not a true *Haemophilus* species. Within the Pasteurellaceae, *H. ducreyi* is grouped in a distinct lineage with *Mannheimia haemolytica* and *Actinobacillus pleuropneumoniae*. *H. ducreyi* is likely to have diverged from these animal respiratory pathogens to occupy its niche in the human epithelium.

EPIDEMIOLOGY

Chancroid is endemic in resource-poor regions of Africa and Asia and facilitates the transmission of human immunodeficiency virus (HIV-1). In the 1990s, the World Health Organization estimated the annual global prevalence of chancroid to be 4 million to 6 million cases. Because of the widespread use of syndromic management, which consists of treatment for syphilis and chancroid without diagnostic testing, the prevalence of chancroid has dramatically declined in endemic areas.[1] Chancroid can be maintained only in networks with high sex partner change rates; infected female sex workers play an important role in its epidemiology. Targeted treatment of sex workers leads to eradication of the disease in endemic areas. Despite these successes, reports of chancroid persist from many countries. Such reports imply a reservoir of untreated sex workers. Urban outbreaks of chancroid associated with sex work occurred in the United States in the 1980s and 1990s. Owing to contact tracing and treatment efforts, the number of domestic cases of chancroid has decreased steadily, with a 66-year low of six cases in 2014; such sporadic cases are likely to be imported after contact with infected persons in endemic areas.

The male-to-female ratio of chancroid is 3 : 1. The excess number of male cases is usually attributed to the infection of multiple partners by sex workers. However, human inoculation experiments indicate that men are twice as susceptible as women for development of pustules, suggesting that male gender is a risk factor for disease progression.

In yaws-endemic countries, *H. ducreyi* causes a chronic limb ulceration syndrome that occurs primarily in children. Close contact of family members with ulcer cases is implicated in transmission. In a cohort study done in yaws-endemic villages in Papua New Guinea, the prevalence of this syndrome was 3.2 cases per 100 persons. *H. ducreyi* is more common than *Treponema pallidum* subspecies *pertenue* in such settings.[2] The overall prevalence of *H. ducreyi* infection in children aged 5 to 15 years is an astoundingly high 7%. Similar data are reported from Ghana, the Solomon Islands and Vanuatu, which together with Papua New Guinea have the highest prevalence of "yaws." Whole genome sequencing suggests cutaneous ulcer strains diverged from multiple lineages of genital ulcer strains during the past 180,000 years.[3] Travelers to endemic areas can acquire limb ulcers following minor trauma; the first case of cutaneous ulcers caused by *H. ducreyi* in the Netherlands was reported in 2018 in a person who imported it from Indonesia.[4]

PATHOBIOLOGY

Much of what is known about the pathogenesis of *H. ducreyi* is derived from experiments in which bacteria are inoculated into the skin of the upper arm of human volunteers. Puncture wounds are required to initiate infection, and the estimated infectious dose is as low as one bacterium. Papules develop within 24 hours and either spontaneously resolve or evolve into pustules in 2 to 5 days. Neutrophils and macrophages surround the organism and form an abscess that erodes the epidermis. Below the abscess, there is a collar of macrophages and regulatory T cells and a dermal infiltrate of macrophages, CD4 and CD8 T cells, natural killer (NK) cells, and dendritic cells. This histopathology resembles a suppurative granuloma and is identical to that of natural ulcers. In both experimental and natural infection, *H. ducreyi* associates with neutrophils and macrophages, which fail to ingest the organism. Mutant

versus parent trials have revealed bacterial components that are required for infection; several are involved with adherence and resistance to serum killing and phagocytosis. In addition to gender, the human model has shown that there are host effects on disease progression. Differential host susceptibility is associated with distinct dendritic cell responses to the organism, which may shape T-cell and NK-cell responses that influence the ability of phagocytes to ingest the organism. There may be an immunogenetic basis for differential host responses.[5]

CLINICAL MANIFESTATIONS

To cause chancroid, *H. ducreyi* is thought to enter the skin through breaks in the epithelium that occur during intercourse. Papules form within hours to days and evolve into pustules in 2 to 3 days. After a few days to 2 weeks, the pustules ulcerate. Patients typically develop one to four painful ulcers (Fig. 285-1) but do not seek treatment until they have had ulcerative symptoms for 1 to 3 weeks. By this time, 10 to 40% have suppurative inguinal lymphadenopathy or buboes (see Fig. 285-1).

Natural ulcers are classically very painful and nonindurated, with ragged edges. The ulcer may be covered by a yellow or gray necrotic exudate and bleeds when scraped. However, this presentation occurs in a minority of patients; chancroid is frequently indistinguishable from syphilis and genital herpes. Lesions in men are usually on the foreskin, coronal sulcus, or penile shaft. Lesions in women are usually on the labia; but women may have internal vaginal and cervical ulcers that are painless. Lesions also occur on the thighs and buttocks or at distant sites; extragenital lesions are thought to be due to autoinoculation. Untreated, chancroid persists for months and causes giant ulcers, erosion of the infected area, or fibrosis, leading to phimosis in men.

Although cutaneous ulcers occur in adults, they primarily occur in children on the lower legs (Fig. 285-2). Ulcers due to *H. ducreyi* tend to be more tender, smaller, and less circular with less indurated edges than those due to yaws or dual infections. However, there is a great deal of clinical overlap. Up to 20% of asymptomatic children in endemic areas are colonized by *H. ducreyi* on their skin,[6] and it is likely that the organism enters and infects the skin via minor traumatic wounds.

DIAGNOSIS

Diagnosis of chancroid or cutaneous ulcers requires either a positive culture or a polymerase chain reaction (PCR) test. In research sexually transmitted disease clinics, PCR has a resolved sensitivity of 95 to 98% and a specificity of 99% for *H. ducreyi*. In comparison, the sensitivity for culture is approximately 75%, but clinical diagnosis is neither sensitive (range, 50 to 75%) nor specific (range, 50 to 75%). Unfortunately, PCR-based tests are not commercially

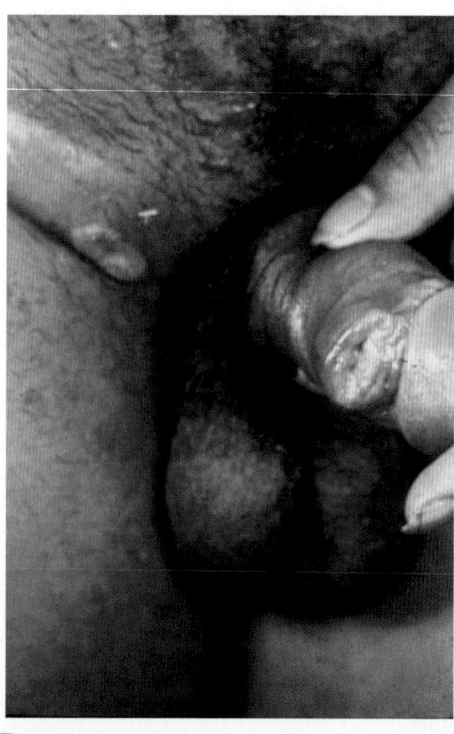

FIGURE 285-1. Typical chancroidal ulcer and lymphadenitis in a man. (From Herpes-Coldsores.com. http://www.herpes-coldsores.com/std/chancroid_pictures.htm.)

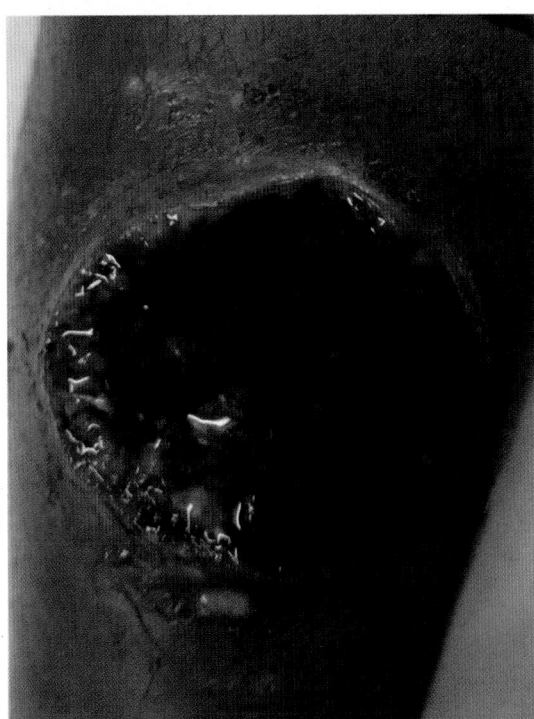

FIGURE 285-2. Cutaneous ulcer due to *Haemophilus ducreyi* in a child in Papua New Guinea. (Kindly provided by Oriol Mitja.)

available. Most sexually transmitted disease clinics do not routinely test patients for chancroid, and the diagnosis is typically made by the exclusion of genital herpes and syphilis. If patients with genital ulcers and lymphadenitis or treatment failure for primary syphilis appear in a community, public health authorities should be notified so that specific diagnostic testing can be initiated.

The differential diagnosis of chancroid includes syphilis, genital herpes, lymphogranuloma venereum, and granuloma inguinale. Mixed infections with herpes simplex virus or syphilis are common, occurring in approximately 17% of chancroid cases diagnosed by PCR. Patients with suspected chancroid should be tested for genital herpes and have serologic tests for syphilis and HIV-1 and a dark-field examination. The differential diagnosis of cutaneous ulcers includes yaws; but a significant number of cases are undiagnosed.

TREATMENT   Rx

Because of syndromic management, little is known about the current prevalence of antibiotic resistance in *H. ducreyi*, but most clinical isolates have had plasmid-mediated resistance to ampicillin, tetracyclines, and sulfonamides. The only reliable treatment regimens are macrolides, quinolones, and third-generation cephalosporins; there have been isolated reports of erythromycin and ciprofloxacin resistance. Owing to the propensity of *H. ducreyi* to acquire plasmids, the fact that some Enterobacteriaceae harbor plasmids that encode extended-spectrum β-lactamases and quinolone resistance is a concern. Current treatment recommendations for chancroid include single-dose azithromycin 1 g orally or ceftriaxone 250 mg intramuscularly, ciprofloxacin 500 mg orally twice a day for 3 days, and erythromycin base 500 mg orally three times a day for 7 days.[7] There are few data on the susceptibility of cutaneous isolates, but most children have responded to single dose azithromycin (30 mg/kg) orally.[A1] The 2017 European guidelines for management of chancroid have been published.[8]

Repeated aspiration of buboes may be required to effect a cure. In a randomized study comparing repeated aspiration versus incision and drainage, incision and drainage were considered preferable. However, incision and drainage may cause excessive scarring, especially in persons of African descent, and should be avoided according to some experts.

Initial reports of coinfection with HIV infection and chancroid suggest that such individuals have a greater number of ulcers that do not heal as readily after antibiotic treatment compared with patients infected with *H. ducreyi* alone and that single-dose regimens may not be effective in this setting. Antibiotic treatment failure is also associated with lack of circumcision. If close follow-up cannot be ensured, most experts recommend multidose regimens in HIV seropositives.

PROGNOSIS

Clinical cure correlates with a reduction in pain and purulence and re-epithelialization of the ulcer within 7 days. Patients who do not show improvement within 7 days should be regarded as treatment failures and given an alternative agent. Even if *H. ducreyi* is eradicated, ulcers may persist if genital herpes or syphilis is present and not treated. Most ulcers heal in 2 weeks; large ulcers may take 4 weeks to heal. The same principles seem to apply to cutaneous ulcers.

PREVENTION

Circumcision protects against chancroid in men. Condoms are likely to be protective. Although several antigens that may afford protection in animal models have been identified, there is no vaccine. Contacts of patients with chancroid should be treated with an approved regimen. Prevention of cutaneous ulcers is under investigation.

Grade A Reference

A1. González-Beiras C, Kapa A, Vall-Mayans M, et al. Single-dose azithromycin for the treatment of *Haemophilus ducreyi* skin ulcers in Papua New Guinea. *Clin Infect Dis.* 2017;65:2085-2090.

GENERAL REFERENCES

For the General References and other additional features, please visit Expert Consult at https://expertconsult.inkling.com.

286

CHOLERA AND OTHER *VIBRIO* INFECTIONS

EDUARDO GOTUZZO AND CARLOS SEAS

CHOLERA
DEFINITION

Cholera is a feared epidemic diarrheal disease caused by *Vibrio cholerae* serogroup O1 and, since 1992, by the new serogroup O139. The disease is characterized by acute watery diarrhea. In its more severe form, a person may be severely dehydrated and in hypovolemic shock; the patient may die in a matter of a few hours after contracting the infection if treatment is not provided. Cholera is endemic today in Africa, Asia, and Latin America. Seven pandemics have been registered in history since 1817; the most recent has lasted more than five decades since its recognition in Indonesia in 1961.[1]

The Pathogen

V. cholerae is a curved gram-negative bacillus that belongs to the family Vibrionaceae and shares common characteristics with the family Enterobacteriaceae. *V. cholerae* O1 can be classified into three serotypes according to the presence of somatic antigens and into two biotypes, classic and El Tor, according to specific phenotypic characteristics. There is no evidence of different clinical spectra among the three serotypes of *V. cholerae*. The classic biotype, responsible for the first six pandemics of cholera, causes an approximately equal number of symptomatic and asymptomatic cases, whereas the El Tor biotype causes more asymptomatic infections. The classic biotype is confined to the south of Bangladesh, and the El Tor biotype is responsible for the current pandemic. Variants of El Tor biotype, that share phenotypic features of both biotypes, are responsible for the current epidemics in Asia, Africa, and Latin America and may cause more severe disease. The O139 serogroup is composed of a variety of genetically diverse strains, both toxigenic and nontoxigenic; it is genetically closer to El Tor *V. cholerae*.

EPIDEMIOLOGY

Cholera has both a predisposition to cause epidemics with pandemic potential and an ability to remain endemic in all affected areas. People of all ages are at risk to contract the infection in epidemic settings, whereas children older than 2 years are mainly affected in endemic areas. *V. cholerae* lives in riverine, brackish, and estuarine ecosystems, where both O1 and non-O1 strains coexist, with non-O1 and nontoxigenic O1 strains predominating over toxigenic O1 strains. In its natural environment, *V. cholerae* lives attached to algae or to crustacean shells and copepods, with which it coexists in a symbiotic manner. Several conditions, such as temperature, salinity, and availability of nutrients, determine the survival of *V. cholerae*; when these conditions are adverse, vibrios survive in a viable but nonculturable state. More recent data suggest that cholera phages modulate the abundance of *V. cholerae* in the environment and determine the beginning and end of epidemics. Phages may also play a role in the emergence of new *V. cholerae* serogroups by transferring genetic material to nontoxigenic strains.

From its aquatic environment, *V. cholerae* is introduced to humans through contamination of water sources and food.[2] Once humans are infected, very high attack rates may take place, particularly in previously naïve populations. Acquisition of the disease by drinking contaminated water from rivers, ponds, lakes, and even tube well sources has been documented. Drinking unboiled water, introducing hands into containers used to store drinking water, drinking beverages from street vendors, drinking beverages to which contaminated ice has been added, and drinking water outside the home are risk factors; these factors contributed to the acquisition of cholera during the large Peruvian epidemic of 1991. Drinking boiled water, acidic beverages, and carbonated water and using narrow-necked vessels for storing water are protective measures. Epidemics of cholera associated with the ingestion of leftover rice, raw fish, cooked crabs, seafood, raw oysters, and fresh vegetables and fruits have been documented. Person-to-person transmission is less likely to occur because a large inoculum is necessary to transmit disease. High transmission rates (approximately 50%) are reported among household contacts of patients with cholera in endemic areas.

Epidemics of cholera tend to occur during the hot season. Factors affecting climate change and climate variability have an impact on the incidence of cholera. The El Niño–southern oscillation (ENSO), a periodic phenomenon representative of global climate variability, affects the transmission of cholera and vector-borne diseases. ENSO causes the warming of normally cool waters in the Pacific coastline of Peru, thereby promoting phytoplankton bloom, zooplankton bloom, and *V. cholerae* proliferation.[3]

Some host factors are important in the transmission of cholera. The chronic gastritis associated with *Helicobacter pylori* predisposes to cholera by inducing hypochlorhydria, which reduces the ability of the stomach to contain the infection. An unexplained predisposition to severe disease due to El Tor biotype in persons with the O blood group has been observed in Asia and more recently in Latin America. Innate predisposition has also been reported in endemic areas. Thus, complex associations among climatic, seasonal, bacterial, and human factors affect cholera transmission. Although for the most part cholera affects developing countries, several developed countries, such as the United States, Canada, and Australia, have reported indigenous and imported cases.[4] The most recent epidemics occurred in Haiti in 2010 and Yemen in 2016 and 2017.[5] Figure 286-1 shows the distribution of cholera in the world from 1989 to 2015.[6]

PATHOBIOLOGY

V. cholerae O1 and O139 cause clinical disease by secreting an enterotoxin that promotes the secretion of fluids and electrolytes by the small intestine. The infectious dose of bacteria varies with the vehicle. When water is the vehicle, more bacteria are needed to cause disease (10^3 to 10^8), but when the vehicle is food, lower amounts are needed (10^2 to 10^4). The incubation period varies from 12 to 72 hours; the median is 1.4 days. Cholera toxin (CTX) has two subunits, a pentamer B subunit and a monomer A subunit. The B subunit allows binding of the toxin to a specific receptor, a ganglioside (GM_1) located on the surface of cells lining the mucosa along the intestine of humans and certain suckling mammals. The active, or A, subunit has two components, A1 and A2, linked by a disulfide bond. Activation of adenylate cyclase by the A1 component results in an increase in cyclic adenosine monophosphate in intestinal epithelial cells, which blocks the absorption of sodium and chloride by microvilli and promotes the secretion of chloride and water by crypt cells. These events lead to the production of watery diarrhea with electrolyte concentrations similar to those of plasma, as shown in Table 286-1. A few other toxins have been isolated from pathogenic *V. cholerae*, but their roles in genesis of the disease are less clear.

CLINICAL MANIFESTATIONS

Cholera is characterized by watery diarrhea and dehydration, which ranges from mild to severe and life-threatening.[7] Patients with mild dehydration cannot be differentiated from those infected by other enteric pathogens causing watery diarrhea. In contrast, patients with severe dehydration secondary to cholera are easy to identify in that their stools have the appearance of rice water, and no other clinical illness produces such severe dehydration as quickly (in a matter of a few hours) as cholera. Onset of the disease is abrupt and characterized by watery diarrhea, vomiting, generalized cramps, and oliguria. Physical examination shows a feeble pulse, fever is rarely present, patients look anxious and restless, the eyes are very sunken, mucous membranes are dry, the skin has lost its elasticity and when pinched retracts very slowly, the voice is almost nonaudible, and intestinal sounds are prominent. Although watery diarrhea

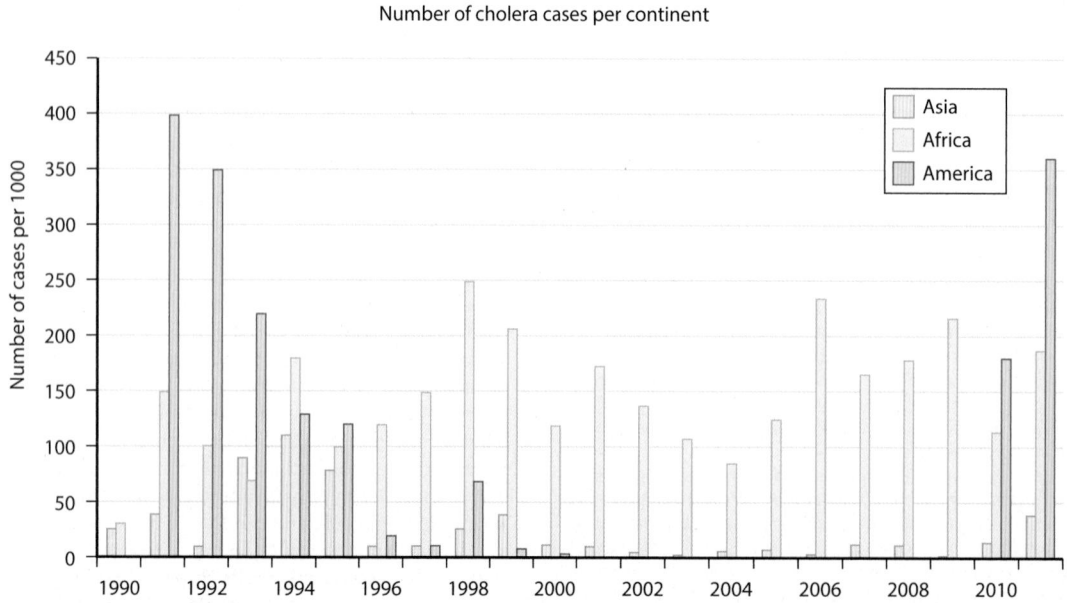

Number of cholera cases per continent

FIGURE 286-1. World distribution of cholera from 1989 to 2015 based on reports to the World Health Organization. (Reprinted with permission from the World Health Organization. Cholera, 2016. *Wkly Epidemiol Rec.* 2017;92:521-530.)

TABLE 286-1	ELECTROLYTE COMPOSITION OF CHOLERA STOOLS AND SOLUTIONS RECOMMENDED FOR TREATMENT						
		Na+	Cl−	K+	HCO3−	GLUCOSE	OSMOLARITY
Stools of adults with severe cholera		130	100	20	44		
Intravenous lactated Ringer solution		130	109	4	28*	0	271
Intravenous normal saline		154	154	0	0	0	308
Standard oral rehydration solution promoted by the WHO		90	80	20	10†	111	311
Reduced-osmolarity oral rehydration solution promoted by the WHO		75	65	20	10†	75	245
Rice-based oral rehydration solution		90	80	20	10†		270

*Lactated Ringer solution contains citrate instead of bicarbonate.
†Bicarbonate is replaced by trisodium citrate.
Glucose concentration is in mg/dL, electrolyte concentrations are in mEq/L, and osmolarity is in mOsm/L.
Cl− = chloride; K+ = potassium; Na+ = sodium; WHO = Word Health Organization.
Modified with permission from Seas C, DuPont HL, Valdez LM, et al. Practical guidelines for the treatment of cholera. *Drugs*. 1996;51:966-973.

is the hallmark of cholera, some patients do not have diarrhea but instead have abdominal distention and ileus, a relatively rare type of cholera called cholera sicca.

Laboratory findings in patients with severe dehydration consist of an increase in hematocrit, urine specific gravity, and total serum protein; azotemia; metabolic acidosis with a high anion gap; normal or low serum potassium levels; and normal or slightly low sodium and chloride levels. The calcium and magnesium content in plasma is high as a result of hemoconcentration. Leukocytosis is observed in patients with severe cholera. Hyperglycemia, caused by high concentrations of epinephrine, glucagon, and cortisol stimulated by hypovolemia, is more commonly seen than hypoglycemia. Acute renal failure is the most severe complication of cholera. Incidence rates of 10.6 cases per 1000 were reported in Peru during the first months of the 1991 epidemic. Patients with acute renal failure almost always have a history of improper rehydration. Cholera in pregnant women carries a poor prognosis. Pregnant women have more severe clinical illness, especially when the disease is acquired at the end of the pregnancy. Fetal loss occurs in as many as 50% of these pregnancies. Cholera in the elderly also carries a poor prognosis because of an increase in complications, particularly acute renal failure, severe metabolic acidosis, and pulmonary edema.

DIAGNOSIS

Chaotic movement under dark-field microscopy and a high number of bacteria in a stool sample from patients with diarrhea are characteristic of *V. cholerae* infection. Specific antisera against the serotype block the movement of vibrios and allow confirmation of the diagnosis. Under epidemic conditions, observing bacteria with a darting movement in a stool sample from a patient with suspected infection under dark-field microscopy is adequate to make the diagnosis. Definitive confirmation requires isolation of the bacterium in culture. Specific medium is needed to isolate *V. cholerae* from stool. Higher sensitivity and specificity have been reported with DNA amplification by polymerase chain reaction (PCR) for detection of vibrios in stool and environmental samples. A number of rapid tests have been developed, but few are suitable for public health purposes.

TREATMENT Rx

The objectives of therapy are to restore the fluid losses caused by diarrhea and vomiting, to correct the metabolic acidosis, to restore potassium deficits, and to replace continuous fluid losses. Treatment of patients with milder forms of dehydration is easy, but treatment of patients with severe dehydration requires experience and proper training. The intravenous route should be restricted to patients with some dehydration who do not tolerate the oral route, those who purge more than 10 to 20 mL/kg/hour, and all patients with severe dehydration. Rehydration should be accomplished in two phases: the rehydration phase and the maintenance phase. The purpose of the rehydration phase is to restore normal intravascular volume, and it should last no longer than 4 hours. Intravenous fluids should be infused at a total volume of 100 mL/kg during the rehydration phase in severely dehydrated patients. Lactated Ringer solution is preferred, but other solutions may be used as well (see Table 286-1). All signs of dehydration should have disappeared and the patient should pass urine at a rate of 0.5 mL/kg/hour or greater after the rehydration phase is finished. The maintenance phase follows immediately. During this phase, the objective is to maintain normal hydration status by replacement of ongoing losses. The oral

TABLE 286-2	RECOMMENDATIONS FOR TREATMENT OF CHOLERA PATIENTS

Determine the degree of dehydration on arrival.
Rehydrate the patient in two phases:
- Rehydration phase—lasts 2 to 4 hours
- Maintenance phase—lasts until the end of the diarrheal episode

Register and periodically review input and output in predesigned charts.
Use the intravenous route in the following situations:
- In all severely dehydrated patients, in whom the total volume to be infused during the rehydration phase is 100 mL/kg. For patients older than 1 year, 30 mL/kg should be infused in the first 30 minutes, the remaining 70 mL/kg should be infused in 2.5 hours. For children younger than 1 year, the first 30 mL/kg should be infused in 1 hour.
- Patients with some dehydration who are unable to tolerate the oral route
- Patients with high stool output (>10 mL/kg/hour) during the maintenance phase

Use oral rehydration solutions, glucose or rice based, during the maintenance phase to match ongoing losses. Volumes of 800 to 1000 mL/hour are usually required. Low-osmolarity solutions are not recommended.

Start an oral antimicrobial agent in patients with severe cholera when full rehydration has been achieved and oral tolerance is confirmed. Single-dose doxycycline, 300 mg, is the preferred regimen. Erythromycin or a quinolone is a suitable alternative.

Discharge patients only if oral tolerance is adequate (≥1000 mL/hour), urine output is satisfactory (≥40 mL/hour), and stool volume is low (≤400 mL/hour).

Modified with permission from Seas C, DuPont HL, Valdez LM, et al. Practical guidelines for the treatment of cholera. *Drugs*. 1996;51:966-973.

route is preferred during this phase, and the use of oral rehydration solutions is highly recommended. Oral rehydration therapy uses the principle of common transportation of solutes, electrolytes, and water by the intestine not affected by cholera toxin. People with diarrhea can undergo successful rehydration with simple solutions containing glucose and electrolytes. The World Health Organization recommends an oral rehydration solution with reduced osmolarity (245 mOsm/L) to treat all diarrheal diseases. This solution contains lower sodium than the standard oral rehydration solution promoted since 1975 (75 vs. 90 mEq/L). No more symptomatic hyponatremia is observed with the reduced-osmolarity solution than with the standard solution. The addition of L-histidine to rice-based oral rehydration solutions has been shown to reduce the volume and duration of diarrhea and the unscheduled use of intravenous therapy in adult cholera patients. Patients without severe dehydration who tolerate the oral route can be rehydrated with oral rehydration solutions exclusively and discharged promptly from the health center. Recommendations for treatment of cholera patients are shown in Table 286-2. Treatment of cholera caused by *V. cholerae* O139 is the same as described earlier.

Antimicrobial agents are not life-saving and always need to be accompanied by fluid therapy. Effective antibiotics in patients with severe dehydration decrease the duration of diarrhea and the volume of stool by nearly half.[A1] Oral tetracycline and doxycycline are the agents of choice in areas of the globe where sensitive strains predominate. A single dose of doxycycline (300 mg) is the preferred regimen. Pregnant women can be treated with erythromycin or furazolidone. Because of the emergence of resistance to tetracyclines and other antimicrobials in many endemic areas, the quinolones and, more recently, azithromycin have been tested in clinical trials. A single-dose regimen of azithromycin (20 mg/kg) showed clinical and bacteriologic results that were comparable to a 3-day regimen with erythromycin and to a single-dose regimen of ciprofloxacin in children and comparable to a single-dose regimen of ciprofloxacin (1 g) in adults, and 1 g azithromycin is equivalent to 3 days of norfloxacin (400 mg twice daily).[A2] The addition of oral zinc (30 mg/day) to an erythromycin regimen in children reduced the duration of diarrhea by 12%, with an additional 11% reduction in the volume of diarrhea in comparison to placebo. Antimotility agents such as loperamide or diphenoxylate, adsorbents, analgesics, and antiemetics are not recommended. Antisecretory drugs, including racecadotril, an enkephalinase inhibitor, are not useful in patients with severe cholera.

PREVENTION

Access to potable water and ensuring proper management of excreta to avoid contamination of other water sources are important measures to reduce transmission of cholera. Alternative ways to prevent cholera transmission are necessary in developing countries. Water can be made safer to drink by boiling, adding chlorine, or filtering it with cloth made of cotton. Chemoprophylaxis of household contacts of cholera cases is not routinely recommended.

An ideal vaccine against cholera should elicit a fast and long-lasting immune response with minimal side effects. Parenteral vaccines are no longer recommended. Two oral vaccines, the two-dose regimen of the inactivated vaccine WC-BS (whole cell plus B subunit) and a single dose of the live attenuated CVD 103-HgR vaccine, have been tested extensively in epidemic settings and in field trials in endemic areas, where they have safely elicited excellent immunogenicity.[A3][A4] Although the WC-BS vaccine showed good short-term protective efficacy (85% at 6 months), the results at 3 and 5 years were less impressive (40% or less).[A5][A6] A large effectiveness study in Mozambique confirmed the high short-term protection against cholera (80%) by this vaccine, especially against severe dehydration (90%). In Guinea, oral vaccine was 87% protective. In addition, reanalysis of data on this vaccine in field trials and in Zanzibar has shown that it may also confer herd protection in the unvaccinated population. Cost-effectiveness of interventions like this require prices of the oral vaccine below 1.3 USD. More recently, a single dose of the whole cell oral killed vaccine achieved 89.7% effectiveness during a cholera outbreak.[8] Complementary use of oral cholera vaccination, water sanitation, and hygiene interventions may have additive impact in endemic areas. A large field trial of the live attenuated vaccine in an endemic country showed no protective efficacy. However, this vaccine is immunogenic and effective in adult travelers and has been recently licensed in the United States.[9] Indications for use of the currently available cholera vaccines include travel to endemic areas and situations in which high attack rates of cholera are expected, such as after environmental disasters, in refugee camps, and in urban slums in highly endemic areas. Preemptive and reactive vaccination approaches should be thoroughly evaluated in epidemic settings. New oral vaccines, including both killed and live *Vibrio*, are being evaluated in endemic areas, with promising preliminary reports.

PROGNOSIS

Patients with severe cholera left untreated or improperly treated carry a poor prognosis, with mortality rates higher than 50%. However, case-fatality rates during epidemics may be reduced to values below 1% even in disaster situations, provided adequate access to health care centers and proper management of patients can be ensured. For example, mortality rates were extremely low during the Latin America epidemic in the 1990s, but rates of 19 to 35 deaths/1000 person-years were estimated during the epidemic in Haiti.[10] Lack of treatment, delay in treatment, and not being managed in an established treatment center were factors associated with mortality in a study in Cameroon.[11]

OTHER *VIBRIO* INFECTIONS

Noncholera vibrios have worldwide distribution and coexist in environments in which *V. cholerae* lives. They cause a spectrum of clinical syndromes, including acute diarrhea, soft tissue infections, and sepsis,[12] especially in immunocompromised hosts. The CDC estimates about 80,000 cases of vibriosis annually in the United States, about two thirds of which are food borne.[13] *Vibrio parahaemolyticus* predominates (about 45% of isolates) but is associated with a case-fatality rate below 1%. In contrast, *Vibrio vulnificus* accounts for about 20% of the isolates but is associated with a case-fatality rate of about 30%. *Vibrio* illnesses in the United States are seasonal and peak during the summer. The incubation period for noncholeragenic *Vibrio* infection is usually 12 to 72 hours but can be as long as 1 week.

Nontoxigenic *V. cholerae* causes gastroenteritis, but unlike toxigenic *V. cholerae* O1 or O139, nontoxigenic *V. cholerae* does not cause epidemics. Illness

ranges in severity from mild diarrhea to severe watery diarrhea. Fever and bloody diarrhea are unusual, but immunocompromised persons and those with liver disease can experience more severe illness, including fever, chills, and septic shock.

V. parahaemolyticus lives in marine environments and is a source of intestinal illness associated with the ingestion of contaminated shellfish. Certain serovars have shown pandemic spread (O3:K6 and O4:K68). It is not well known how this *Vibrio* causes infection in humans, but the clinical illness may mimic cholera, although most cases are milder and self-limited forms of acute watery diarrhea. Acute dysentery is reported rarely. Oral antibiotics, as used for traveler's diarrhea (Chapter 270), are usually efficacious, although local resistance patterns vary.

V. vulnificus is associated with wound infections in persons in contact with contaminated water as well as with primary sepsis in immunocompromised hosts. This pathogen is responsible for 95% of seafood related mortality in the United States. Wound infections follow trauma and are characterized by rapid progression of skin and soft tissue involvement, with necrosis and bulla formation occurring in more severe cases. Fever, chills, and sepsis syndrome may ensue rapidly. Primary sepsis with bacteremia and metastatic lesions on the skin, characterized by disseminated erythematous lesions that may evolve to necrotic lesions, is a distinctive clinical manifestation in patients with chronic liver illnesses or alcohol dependence and in patients with blood disorders such as thalassemia. A history of seafood ingestion, usually oysters, is typical. Patients are acutely ill with high fever and need to be managed aggressively with fluid resuscitation, surgical débridement, general supportive care, and antibiotic coverage. *V. parahaemolyticus* wound infections are generally less severe than those caused by *V. vulnificus*. However, in persons with liver disease or those who are immunocompromised, fatal infections can occur.

The recommended antibiotic approach is an intravenous combination of cefotaxime, 2 g four times a day, plus doxycycline, 100 mg two times a day. This combination is synergistic in vitro. Alternative antimicrobials are ceftazidime and ciprofloxacin.

Grade A References

A1. Leibovici-Weissman Y, Neuberger A, Bitterman R, et al. Antimicrobial drugs for treating cholera. *Cochrane Database Syst Rev.* 2014;6:CD008625.

A2. Bhattacharya MK, Kanungo S, Ramamurthy T, et al. Comparison between single dose azithromycin and six doses, 3 day norfloxacin for treatment of cholera in adult. *Int J Biomed Sci.* 2014;10:248-251.

A3. Lopez AL, Deen J, Azman AS, et al. Immunogenicity and protection from a single dose of internationally available killed oral cholera vaccine: a systematic review and metaanalysis. *Clin Infect Dis.* 2018;66:1960-1971.

A4. Desai SN, Akalu Z, Teshome S, et al. A randomized, placebo-controlled trial evaluating safety and immunogenicity of the killed, bivalent, whole-cell oral cholera vaccine in Ethiopia. *Am J Trop Med Hyg.* 2015;93:527-533.

A5. Bi Q, Ferreras E, Pezzoli L, et al. Protection against cholera from killed whole-cell oral cholera vaccines: a systematic review and meta-analysis. *Lancet Infect Dis.* 2017;17:1080-1088.

A6. Qadri F, Wierzba TF, Ali M, et al. Efficacy of a single-dose, inactivated oral cholera vaccine in Bangladesh. *N Engl J Med.* 2016;374:1723-1732.

GENERAL REFERENCES

For the General References and other additional features, please visit Expert Consult at https://expertconsult.inkling.com.

287

CAMPYLOBACTER INFECTIONS

BAN MISHU ALLOS

DEFINITION

Campylobacter jejuni is one of the most commonly recognized bacterial causes of diarrhea in developed and developing nations. More than 95% of campylobacters isolated in developed countries are *C. jejuni* or *C. coli*. However, other Campylobacter species are also associated with human disease.

The Pathogen

Campylobacters are motile, curved, gram-negative rods that are found in domestic and wild animals—especially poultry—all over the world. *C. jejuni* is microaerophilic, requires 3 to 15% oxygen for growth, and is oxidase and catalase positive. It grows best at 42° C; however, other Campylobacter species that may also be pathogenic grow best at 37° C. The whole genome sequences for multiple Campylobacter species have been determined.

EPIDEMIOLOGY

C. jejuni infections are endemic in young children in developing nations,[1] where it is among the three leading causes of childhood diarrhea along with norovirus and rotavirus (Chapter 356).[2] In developed nations, Campylobacter infections are among the most common bacterial causes of diarrhea in children and adults. The incidence of *C. jejuni* infection in the United States fell by more than 30% from 21.7 per 100,000 population in 1998 to 12.7 in 2008, but by 2012 the incidence had increased again to its highest level since 2000 and has remained stable since then. Indeed, by 2016, Campylobacter had become the most common reported cause of bacterial gastroenteritis.[3] The actual burden of disease caused by Campylobacter is probably much higher because even active surveillance systems substantially underreport the true incidence of infection. Epidemiologic studies have estimated that more than 2 million people in the United States are infected with *C. jejuni* each year. For reasons that are not clear, the incidence is highest in western states, such as California and Hawaii. Similarly high rates of infection are observed in Europe. In the United States, Europe, and Australia, *C. jejuni* infections show a substantial peak in warmer months.[4] Such seasonality is not observed in tropical developing countries, perhaps because of the absence of extreme temperature variations. PCR methods can now identify bacterial pathogens in most individuals with traveler's diarrhea (Chapter 270). Although *E. coli* remain the most commonly found pathogens in general, ciprofloxacin-resistant *Campylobacter* is commonly associated with traveler's diarrhea, particularly in Southeast Asia.[5]

The incidence of Campylobacter infections is highest in early childhood, an epidemiologic feature common to many food-borne bacterial pathogens. However, in the United States and other industrialized countries, the incidence of infections peaks again in early adulthood. Age-specific incidence of campylobacteriosis over time in Australia has recently shown declines in incidence in those aged less than 40 years combined with contemporaneous increases in older age groups, notably those aged 70 to 79 years.[6] The incidence of infection is also higher in men, a gender difference most pronounced in young adults.

Most human *C. jejuni* infections occur sporadically, with only a tiny fraction occurring as part of outbreaks. The dominant source of sporadic infections in both developed and developing countries is consumption or handling of poultry. Other sources of transmission in developed nations include foreign travel, contact with pets and other animals, contaminated drinking water, and consumption of unpasteurized milk. Cross-contamination within a kitchen (e.g., use of the same utensils or cutting boards to prepare uncooked chicken and to chop fruit) has led to a variety of foods being implicated as sources of human *C. jejuni* infection. In contrast to sporadic infections, the most common source of *C. jejuni* outbreaks is unpasteurized milk; large waterborne outbreaks occasionally occur. Transmission of *C. jejuni* infection from ill food handlers is uncommon. Even in households in which an individual has culture-proven *C. jejuni* gastroenteritis, secondary transmission to other family members is unusual.

PATHOBIOLOGY

Persons become infected with *C. jejuni* as a result of orally ingesting the organism, usually in food or water. Factors that affect whether Campylobacter infection leads to illness include the dose of bacteria ingested, the virulence of the organism, and the specific immunity of the host to the ingested organism. The minimum number of bacteria needed to cause illness varies between people, but it may be quite low; because *C. jejuni* is susceptible to gastric acidity, ingestion of very few organisms may cause illness if gastric pH is elevated as a result of illness or medication. The median incubation period is 2 to 4 days, although it may range from 1 to 7 days.

In early infection, *C. jejuni* multiplies in the bile-rich upper intestines; subsequently, tissue injury is seen in the jejunum, ileum, and colon. Gross inspection of the bowel shows a diffuse, bloody, edematous enteritis. Microscopic examination shows an inflammatory infiltrate consisting of neutrophils, mononuclear cells, and eosinophils in the lamina propria. The mucosal epithelium is ulcerated, and crypt abscesses may be seen. The pathologic appearance is nonspecific and may mimic ulcerative colitis or Crohn disease.

Invasion of the epithelium by *C. jejuni* appears to be central to its pathogenesis, and many factors influence how *C. jejuni* adheres to and invades intestinal tissues. A superficial conserved antigen, PEB1, appears to be a major adhesin and is a target of the immune response to *C. jejuni* infection. Other factors contributing to the invasiveness and pathogenicity of *C. jejuni* that may be encoded by a virulence plasmid include type IV secretion systems and mechanisms that disrupt microtubules in host cells. The presence of the plasmid pVir in clinical isolates is significantly associated with bloody stools. *C. jejuni* also may invade in an actin- and microtubule-independent manner. Glycolipids and glycoproteins on the surface of *C. jejuni* are important in the organism's survival in the intestinal lumen and in pathogenesis because they have an impact on cell-to-cell interactions as well as on the host's immune response to infection. The bacteria's flagella facilitate its ability to colonize the gastrointestinal tract by promoting the organism's motility and chemotaxis. *C. jejuni* may produce extracellular toxins, but their role in pathogenesis has not been confirmed, with the possible exception of the cytoskeletal distending toxin (cdt), which may facilitate intracellular activities that lead to apoptosis.

Regardless of the organism's virulence, host factors are pivotal in affecting the clinical outcome of infection. In healthy volunteers fed a fixed dose of a single *C. jejuni* strain, a spectrum of illnesses develops. Patients infected with *C. jejuni* excrete the organism in feces for 2 to 3 weeks. In developing nations, where the level of immunity to *C. jejuni* is higher because of recurrent exposure, the period of convalescent excretion of *C. jejuni* is shorter.

After recovery from Campylobacter infection, at least short-term immunity develops. The decreasing illness-to-infection ratio with age seen in developing nations also suggests that individuals are acquiring immunity. Specific immunoglobulin A, G, and M antibodies in serum and immunoglobulin A antibodies in intestinal secretions develop in patients infected with *C. jejuni*. Patients with congenital or acquired hypogammaglobulinemia are at risk for severe or recurrent *C. jejuni* infections. Because the incidence of *C. jejuni* infection is markedly higher in persons infected with human immunodeficiency virus (HIV), cell-mediated immunity might also play a role in preventing and terminating infection.

CLINICAL MANIFESTATIONS

The clinical consequences of Campylobacter infection range from complete absence of symptoms to fulminant sepsis and death. In most cases, however, illnesses are brief and do not require hospitalization. In developed nations, detection of *C. jejuni* in the stool of asymptomatic persons is rare. However, in developing nations, where infections are endemic and recurrent infections occur frequently, asymptomatic infections are more common. In both developing and developed nations, persons infected with *C. jejuni* typically contract a diarrheal illness that resolves within a week. The case-fatality rate associated with this infection is low, about 0.05 death per 1000 infections, and is not surprisingly highest among the elderly and persons with comorbid conditions.

The gastroenteritis that is caused by infection with *C. jejuni* is clinically indistinguishable from that caused by other bacterial enteric pathogens, such as *Salmonella* (Chapter 292), *Shigella* (Chapter 293), or *Escherichia coli* O157:H7 (Chapter 288). The most common symptoms are diarrhea, malaise, fever, and abdominal pain (Table 287-1). Campylobacterosis incubation periods vary considerably, ranging from 2.5 to 4.3 days, depending on subgroup.[7] Most patients with *C. jejuni* gastroenteritis experience at least 1 day with 10 or more

TABLE 287-1	CLINICAL FEATURES OF *CAMPYLOBACTER* ENTERITIS DERIVED FROM OUTBREAKS IN WHICH MORE THAN 50 PATIENTS WERE INFECTED

SYMPTOM	MEDIAN FREQUENCY (%)	RANGE (%)
Fever	50	6-75
Diarrhea	84	52-100
Headache	41	6-69
Abdominal pain	79	56-99
Myalgia	42	28-59
Vomiting	15	1-42
Blood in feces	15	0.5-32

Modified from Blaser MJ, Engberg J. Clinical aspects of *Campylobacter jejuni* and *Campylobacter coli* infections. In: Nachamkin I, Szymanski CM, Blaser MJ, eds. *Campylobacter*. 3rd ed. Washington, DC: ASM Press; 2008:99-121.

stools; the diarrhea may be loose, watery, or bloody. Nausea is reported by some patients, but vomiting is less common. More than half the patients describe subjective fever. The abdominal cramping may be severe and is sometimes the predominant symptom. Although in most patients the symptoms resolve within 7 days, symptoms may persist in 10 to 20% of patients, and another 5 to 10% may experience a relapse.

Almost regardless of the nature of the symptoms, fecal leukocytes are found in 75% of infected patients; gross or occult blood is seen in 50%. Peripheral white blood cell counts may be elevated, but liver function test results, the hematocrit, and serum electrolyte values are usually normal. Sigmoidoscopic examination reveals diffuse colonic inflammation, which is nonspecific.

Local complications of *C. jejuni* gastroenteritis are rare. In its most severe form, infection may lead to massive gastrointestinal hemorrhage or toxic megacolon. Infection of the biliary tract may result in obstructive hepatitis, cholecystitis (Chapter 146), or pancreatitis (Chapter 135). Other reported local complications include peritonitis (Chapter 133), splenic rupture, and exacerbations of inflammatory colitis. Bacteremia is detected in 1.5 per 1000 intestinal infections, with higher rates in persons who are immunocompromised or elderly, but transient bacteremia may be more common because blood cultures are infrequently obtained in patients with diarrhea and the bacteria are killed rapidly by normal human serum. Other extraintestinal complications, such as meningitis, endocarditis, osteomyelitis, and purulent arthritis, are rare.

Guillain-Barré syndrome (Chapter 392), which is a postinfectious complication of *C. jejuni* infection, occurs about once in every 2000 infections; between 30 and 50% of all cases may be triggered by a preceding *C. jejuni* infection.[8] Because the onset of neurologic symptoms occurs about 1 to 3 weeks after the onset of gastrointestinal symptoms, cross-reactivity between antibodies formed against the lipopolysaccharide and capsule of *C. jejuni* and proteins in peripheral nerve myelin or other glycolipids in peripheral nerves is probably the cause. Certain *C. jejuni* serotypes (O type 19, O type 41) are overrepresented in patients in whom Guillain-Barré syndrome develops after culture-documented *C. jejuni* infection. Other postinfectious complications of *C. jejuni* infection include reactive arthritis (seen mostly in persons with HLA-B27 histocompatibility antigens), uveitis, hemolytic-uremic syndrome, erythema nodosum, encephalitis, carditis, hemolytic anemia, and chronic gastrointestinal consequences such as irritable bowel syndrome, inflammatory bowel disease, and celiac disease.

DIAGNOSIS

The diagnosis of *C. jejuni* infection should be considered in any patient with an acute febrile diarrheal illness. The diagnosis is established by culturing the organism from stool or tissue. Primary isolation of Campylobacter species from blood may take up to 14 days. Culture-independent diagnostic tests are increasingly being used; however, such tests fail to provide antibiotic-susceptibilty data and also do not demonstrate if an isolate is part of a larger outbreak.

The presence of curved gram-negative rods on a Gram stain of stool is specific but only 50 to 75% sensitive for detecting *C. jejuni*. Examination of fecal specimens by dark-field microscopy is useful if it is done within 2 hours of passage; the characteristic darting motility of Campylobacter provides a presumptive diagnosis. Serum serologic studies of stool are currently available only as research tools. Use of polymerase chain reaction techniques for direct detection of organisms has been successful in research studies but has not yet been applied to the general clinical setting.[9]

Differential Diagnosis

In patients with acute colitis and bloody diarrhea, especially those whose symptoms last longer than 1 week, Campylobacter enteritis may be mistaken for ulcerative colitis or Crohn disease (Chapter 132). In such cases, it is critical to exclude infectious colitis before starting immunosuppressive therapy. In patients with severe abdominal pain, appendicitis may be suspected and unnecessary appendectomy may result (Chapter 133).

PREVENTION

Because the most common source of transmission of *C. jejuni* infection to humans in developed countries is by consumption and handling of poultry, interrupting this route of infection will probably have the greatest effect on reducing the burden of disease caused by Campylobacter. The nearly universal colonization of poultry flocks with *C. jejuni* makes eradication of the organism in chickens unlikely, but improvements in slaughtering plants appear to be reducing the level of contamination of products reaching humans. For the consumer, careful food preparation methods are critical; chicken must be cooked thoroughly. To avoid cross-contamination in the kitchen, cutting boards, knives, and other utensils used to prepare raw chicken should be washed with hot soapy water before being used to prepare foods eaten uncooked, such as fruits and vegetables. Person-to-person transmission of Campylobacter is not common; nevertheless, all persons with diarrhea, especially those who handle food, should wash their hands after using the bathroom. Travelers and campers should be cautioned against drinking untreated water. Many outbreaks of *C. jejuni* infection might also be avoided if persons abstain from drinking unpasteurized milk. Antibiotic prophylaxis for travelers is not advised. An effective anti-Campylobacter vaccine has not yet been developed.

TREATMENT   Rx

As is true for most patients with infectious or noninfectious diarrhea, the most important principle of treatment of Campylobacter gastroenteritis is restoration of proper hydration and electrolyte balance, typically with oral fluids. On occasion, intravenous fluids are needed, especially in elderly patients or young children. Most *C. jejuni* infections are self-limited and resolve without specific antibiotic treatment. Furthermore, treatment with antibiotics shortens the duration of illness by less than 48 hours. Prompt antimicrobial therapy is indicated for patients with high fever (>38.5° C), prolonged illness (>1 week), bloody stools, or worsening symptoms and for those who have relapsed. Antimicrobial treatment is also warranted in the elderly, infants, pregnant women, and persons who are immunocompromised, including those infected with HIV.

The current antibiotic of choice for treatment of *C. jejuni* gastroenteritis is azithromycin (500 mg daily for 3 days). For many decades, the antibiotic of choice for the treatment was erythromycin (500 mg twice daily for 5 days). Azithromycin and clarithromycin are as effective but are considerably more expensive. One concern with erythromycin, which is primarily metabolized by CYP3A4, is the risk of sudden cardiac death. The risk is increased five-fold when erythromycin is given with medications that inhibit CYP3A4.

Fluoroquinolones, carbapenems, aminoglycosides, and clindamycin may also be effective, but resistance to quinolones is now common in many parts of the world.[10] In general, rates of resistance to ampicillin, amoxicillin, and cephalosporins are too high for them to be useful in the treatment of *C. jejuni* infections.

Critically ill or septic persons with Campylobacter infection may benefit from carbapenems or aminoglycosides, agents to which campylobacters are exquisitely susceptible, with resistance rates consistently less than 1%. In contrast, persons with persistent or relapsing infection, especially those who are immunocompromised, may require prolonged use (sometimes months) of antibiotics. In the absence of continuing sepsis, oral agents may be used.

● OTHER *CAMPYLOBACTER* SPECIES

C. fetus may cause diarrhea and systemic illnesses, including meningitis,[11] in compromised hosts and diarrheal illnesses in normal hosts. Most *C. fetus* strains, unlike *C. jejuni*, are not susceptible to the lethal effect of normal human serum because they possess a protein capsule (S layer). In immunocompromised persons, *C. fetus* can cause extraintestinal illnesses such as bacteremia, vascular infections, and meningitis. *C. fetus* infection may also cause perinatal infection and fetal loss. Prolonged treatment with erythromycin plus either imipenem, meropenem, an aminoglycoside, or a third-generation cephalosporin is indicated for serious *C. fetus* infections.

C. upsaliensis may cause acute or chronic diarrhea in healthy or immunocompromised persons. The organism is frequently isolated from dogs with diarrhea, which could be a source for transmission to humans. Some *C. upsaliensis* strains are resistant to erythromycin, but most are susceptible to fluoroquinolones, doxycycline, third-generation cephalosporins, and amoxicillin-clavulanate.

C. hyointestinalis was first recognized as a cause of proliferative enteritis in swine; *C. lari* is most often cultured from gulls and other birds. Both organisms have now been identified as rare causes of watery diarrhea and abdominal cramping in immunocompetent children and adults. Most infected patients do not require antimicrobial therapy; all isolates studied in vitro have been susceptible to erythromycin.

C. concisus, long believed to be part of the microbiota of healthy persons, is now considered a possible cause of human gastrointestinal illness. An increasing body of evidence also has linked *C. concisus* infection with childhood Crohn disease.

Helicobacter cinaedi and *H. fennelliae*, once called *Campylobacter*-like organisms, are causes of proctocolitis or enterocolitis and have also been reported to cause bacteremia in immunocompromised patients. The organisms are frequently resistant to erythromycin; fluoroquinolones are considered the treatment of choice in patients who require antimicrobial therapy. The organisms are also susceptible to third-generation cephalosporins, aminoglycosides, and carbapenems.

Other Campylobacter or related species that have been associated with human illness include *C. mucosalis, C. doylei, C. curvus, C. insulaenigrae, C. rectus, C. helveticus, Arcobacter butzleri,* and *A. cryaerophila.* Illnesses include diarrhea and localized infections, presumably as a result of transient bacteremia from intestinal sources. Recently identified Campylobacter species that may be clinically relevant include *C. ureolyticus, C. troglodytis, C. lari* subspecies *concheus,* and *C. peloridis.* New pathogenic species of Campylobacter are being identified with some regularity.

PROGNOSIS

Even in critically ill patients, 1 week of therapy is generally sufficient to eradicate infection. Campylobacter infections in HIV-positive patients may be more severe, persist, recur, and be antibiotic resistant. More severe and extraintestinal illness is also more likely to occur in patients with acquired or congenital hypogammaglobulinemia. Most *C. jejuni* gastrointestinal infections in pregnant women are mild and self-limited, with no severe consequences for the mother or baby. However, if bacteremia develops in the mother, placental infection and fetal death may ensue. Infection during the third trimester can also cause neonatal sepsis and death if the woman is excreting Campylobacter in her stool at the time of delivery.

GENERAL REFERENCES

For the General References and other additional features, please visit Expert Consult at https://expertconsult.inkling.com.

288

ESCHERICHIA COLI ENTERIC INFECTIONS

THEODORE S. STEINER

DEFINITION

Bacteria belonging to the species *Escherichia coli* are a normal component of the intestinal microbiota (Chapter 262). The majority of *E. coli* are harmless commensals, but specific isolates have acquired pathogenicity genes that enable them to cause diseases, including urinary tract infections, bacteremia, meningitis, and diarrheal illness. One particular challenge to the clinician and microbiology laboratory is how to distinguish these pathogenic *E. coli* from harmless commensal strains to better guide diagnosis and treatment.

Enteric infections caused by *E. coli* may involve the small intestine, colon, or both, depending on the organism's genetic codes for virulence traits. These virulence traits include a variety of toxins, adherence factors, and secreted mediators that work together to perturb host intestinal physiology. Specific combinations of these factors produce six major pathotypes of diarrheagenic *E. coli*: enterotoxigenic, enteroinvasive, enterohemorrhagic, enteropathogenic, enteroaggregative, and diffusely adherent. In addition, these pathotypes can overlap; for example, some strains can express Shiga-like toxins that are characteristic of enterohemorrhagic *E. coli* without the usual associated adherence factors; these are collectively known as shigatoxigenic *E. coli*. Taken together, diarrheagenic *E. coli* not only constitute the major category of bacterial enteric pathogens but also provide important scientific models for the many ways in which enteric pathogens can cause disease.

The Pathogen

E. coli is a small catalase-positive, oxidase-negative, gram-negative bacillus in the family Enterobacteriaceae. It characteristically reduces nitrates, ferments glucose and usually lactose, and is either motile (with peritrichate flagella) or nonmotile. It exhibits a positive methyl red reaction and negative reactions with Voges-Proskauer, urease, phenylalanine deaminase, and citrate agents. *E. coli* is the predominant member of the Gammaproteobacteria in the intestinal tract of humans and other mammals, although it is greatly outnumbered by members of other bacterial phyla, which largely consist of strict anaerobes.

E. coli possess a complex envelope that consists of a plasma membrane, a peptidoglycan cell wall, and an outer membrane. The latter confers on the microorganism its mechanical properties of stiffness and strength.[1] The lipopolysaccharide cell wall of *E. coli* contains immunostimulatory lipid A attached to a core oligosaccharide chain. Most *E. coli* have immunogenic carbohydrate chains known as O antigens attached to this core glycolipid to produce over 170 O serogroups.[2] There are also at least 56 distinct flagellar (H) antigens based on variable domains of the flagellin gene. Some 80 variably heat-labile capsular (K) antigens have also been described. These O, H, and K antigen combinations have allowed serotyping of thousands of different strains, which historically was the simplest way to distinguish them. Whereas serotypes are sometimes useful in identifying specific pathotypes of *E. coli*, there are numerous adherence, enterotoxic, cytotoxic, and invasiveness factors that may be gained or lost by a particular serotype because they are characteristically encoded on transmissible genetic elements such as plasmids or bacteriophages. It is these factors that convey disease pathotype because they allow colonization and perturbation of host intestinal physiology. Indeed, molecular analysis available during the past decades has shown that commensal and pathogenic *E. coli* cluster into phylogenetic groups that are often independent of O:H serotype. Nevertheless, relatively few O serogroups tend to predominate in the normal human colon (O groups 1, 2, 4, 6, 7, 8, 18, 25, 45, 75, and 81), whereas others (Table 288-1) tend to be associated with specific virulence traits and thus different types of pathogenesis in the intestine.

Well-established mechanisms of *E. coli* pathogenesis include secretion of enterotoxins (enterotoxigenic *E. coli*), *Shigella*-like tissue invasion (enteroinvasive *E. coli*), and epithelial necrosis as a result of Shiga-like toxins (SLT-1/2 or Stx1/Stx2) causing food-borne hemorrhagic colitis (enterohemorrhagic *E. coli* and shigatoxigenic *E. coli*) (see Table 288-1). By comparison, the classically recognized enteropathogenic *E. coli* serotypes are neither enterotoxigenic nor invasive but rather attach to and efface the epithelium. Still other types of "enteroadherent" *E. coli* exhibit aggregating (enteroaggregative *E. coli*) or diffuse adherence (diffusely adherent *E. coli*) traits, and enteroaggregative *E. coli* in particular is associated with prolonged diarrhea in children in tropical developing areas, in patients infected with human immunodeficiency virus (HIV), and in acute diarrhea in outbreak settings and travelers from developed areas. Other *E. coli* strains possessing unique genetic traits (such as adherent-invasive *E. coli*)[3] may be involved in inflammatory bowel disease or other intestinal conditions. These strains are considered "pathobionts" rather than diarrheal pathogens, so they will not be discussed further in this chapter but are the subject of active research.

EPIDEMIOLOGY

Part of the challenge in studying the epidemiology of enteric *E. coli* infections is that, with the exception of enterohemorrhagic *E. coli*/shigatoxigenic *E. coli* strains, they are not identified in routine microbiology procedures in most clinical laboratories. In addition, the diagnostic methodologies have evolved, making it difficult to compare older and more recent studies. Nevertheless, several clear epidemiologic patterns have been revealed. In addition, specific single-nucleotide polymorphisms in several human genes encoding inflammatory mediators are associated with traveler's diarrhea caused by enterotoxigenic *E. coli*, enteroaggregative *E. coli*, or both.[4]

Enteric *E. coli* infections are acquired by the fecal-oral route, although the fecal sources and infectivity differ among the pathotypes. It is believed that a human reservoir is required for most recognized types of enteropathogenic *E. coli* and enterotoxigenic *E. coli*, although domestic dogs and cats can also harbor human pathogenic strains. Different enterotoxigenic *E. coli* strains can also be important veterinary pathogens, especially in calves and piglets, but the attachment and virulence traits of animal strains are different from those of strains that infect humans. The infectious dose of enterotoxigenic *E. coli* in volunteers is 10^6 to 10^{10} organisms, meaning that it usually requires multiplication in contaminated food or water vehicles for its transmission, rather than spreading directly from person to person. Heavy contamination with enterotoxigenic *E. coli* has been documented in foods prepared in homes and restaurants and by street vendors as well as in drinking water in many tropical areas. Contaminated water and food probably represent the major sources of their acquisition, primarily in warm or wet seasons.

As with most diarrheal illnesses, the highest age-specific attack rates of enterotoxigenic *E. coli* are found in young children, especially at the time of weaning, when enterotoxigenic *E. coli* accounts for anywhere from 3 to 39% (average, 13%) of acute diarrheal illnesses, depending on the population studied. Like

TABLE 288-1 DIFFERENT TYPES OF ENTERIC *ESCHERICHIA COLI* INFECTIONS

TYPE	MECHANISM	PREDOMINANT O SEROGROUPS	GENETIC CODE	DETECTION	CLINICAL SYNDROMES
ENTEROTOXIGENIC *E. COLI* (ETEC)					
Heat-labile toxin (LT)	Activates intestinal adenylate cyclase	6, 8, 11, 15, 20, 25, 27, 63, 80, 85, 139	Plasmid	Gene probe, PCR for LT	Watery diarrhea, traveler's diarrhea
Heat-stable toxin (STa: STh or STp)	Activates intestinal guanylate cyclase	12, 78, 115, 148, 149, 153, 155, 166, 167	Plasmid (transposon)	EIA, suckling mice, 6-hour ileal loop assay, gene probes, PCR	Watery diarrhea, traveler's diarrhea
ENTEROINVASIVE *E. COLI* (EIEC)					
	Cell invasion and spread	11, 28ac, 29, 124, 136, 144, 147, 152, 164, 167	Plasmid (140 MIa, pWR110)	Sereny test, gene probe, PCR for *ipaH*	Inflammatory dysentery
SHIGATOXIGENIC *E. COLI* (STEC)					
Enterohemorrhagic (EHEC)	Shiga-like toxins (SLTs/Stxs) and attaching/effacing ability	26, 39, 113, 121, 128, 139, 145, 157, occ 55, 111	STx phages and adhesin plasmids; type III secretion system	EIA or PCR for Stx1/2, serotype, cell adhesion with pedestal formation; Vero cell cytotoxicity; sorbitol agar; PCR for *eae*	Afebrile, bloody diarrhea; HUS in some cases
Non-EHEC STEC	Stx only without attaching/effacing; may carry other virulence phenotypes	26, 111, 103, 121, 45, 104, 145	Stx phage; may possess other virulence traits (e.g., O104:H4 EAEC)	Stx EIA or PCR; negative for *eae*	Hemorrhagic colitis, HUS, or benign watery diarrhea
ENTEROADHERENT *E. COLI*					
Typical enteropathogenic (EPEC)	Attach, then efface the mucosa	55, 86, 111, 114, 119, 127, 142	Bundle-forming pili on plasmid and chromosomal LEE	Serotype, focal HeLa cell adhesion, pedestal formation, gene probe or PCR for *eae*	Infantile diarrhea in developing areas
Atypical enteropathogenic (EPEC)	Attaching and effacing but different microcolony formation	26, 55, 86, 111, 119, 125, 128	Possess the LEE but not bundle-forming pili	Gene probe or PCR for LEE; cell adherence (variable)	Infantile and animal diarrhea in developed areas
Enteroaggregative (EAEC)	Colonize in aggregates; toxins (EAST, Pet), biofilm formation	3, 15, 44, 51, 77, 78, 91	Plasmid (AA); chromosome (Pic/ShET and type VI secretion)	Aggregative adherence to cells or strata; AA probe; PCR for *aggR* or other virulence genes; biofilm formation	Endemic persistent diarrhea, acute traveler's diarrhea, sporadic acute diarrhea
Diffusely adherent (DAEC)	Colonize (F1845 afimbriate adhesin)	86, 75, 15	Chromosomal/plasmid	HeLa cell adherence; DA gene probe/PCR	Persistent diarrhea in children >18 months old

AA = aggregative adherence; DA = diffuse adherence; EAST = heat-stable toxin; EIA = enzyme immunoassay; HUS = hemolytic-uremic syndrome; LEE = locus of enterocyte effacement; LT = heat-labile; PCR = polymerase chain reaction; SLT = Shiga-like toxin.

immunologically inexperienced young children, a traveler visiting tropical areas has a 30 to 50% chance of acquiring traveler's diarrhea (Chapters 267 and 270) during a 2- to 3-week stay unless untreated water or ice and uncooked foods such as salads are strictly avoided. The most commonly identified pathogen associated with diarrhea in most studies of travelers to tropical areas of the world is enterotoxigenic *E. coli*. A close second is enteroaggregative *E. coli*, now reported in 19 to 33% of affected travelers to India or Mexico.

Typical enteropathogenic *E. coli* strains have been recognized primarily in poor urban areas, especially among hospitalized infants in their first year of life, with apparent cross-infection in hospital nurseries. Although sporadic cases still occur, nosocomial outbreaks of enteropathogenic *E. coli* diarrhea during the summer appear to have become less common and less severe in industrialized countries in the past few decades. "Atypical" enteropathogenic *E. coli* strains lacking certain virulence factors have tended to predominate in developed areas but can be found in developing areas as well.[5] Although recent studies have found decreases in EPEC prevalence, it remains a common pathogen and "typical" EPEC is still generally associated with diarrhea rather than asymptomatic colonization.[6] There is emerging evidence that specific gene clusters may characterize diarrheagenic strains compared to nonpathogenic colonizers.[7]

Enterohemorrhagic *E. coli* frequently colonizes commercial livestock but does not infect them. Enterohemorrhagic *E. coli* (O157:H7 and others) infections were first attributed to eating undercooked hamburgers, but subsequent large outbreaks have been associated with contamination of unpasteurized apple juice, spinach, seed sprouts, flour,[8] and other vegetable items.[9] Approximately 600 people were infected in a large outbreak caused by contamination of the domestic water supply in Walkerton, Ontario, in 2000. A 2011 outbreak of shigatoxigenic/enteroaggregative *E. coli* strain O104:H4 associated with fenugreek sprouts sickened almost 4000 people in Europe. In 2016, a multistate outbreak of illness from enterohemorrhagic *E. coli* serogroup O121 and O26 strains, affecting 56 individuals was traced to contaminated flour from a large domestic producer in the United States.[10] In addition, the low

infectious dose of enterohemorrhagic *E. coli* O157:H7 means that person-to-person spread can occur, leading to secondary cases. Secondary cases of shigatoxigenic/enteroaggregative *E. coli* O104:H4 may also have occurred but appear to be very rare. Enterohemorrhagic *E. coli* and shigatoxigenic *E. coli* infections are especially alarming because of the risk of hemolytic-uremic syndrome (HUS) (Chapter 163). HUS can be fatal despite antimicrobial therapy, which in some instances may actually induce Shiga-like toxin production from bacteriophage carried within the organism and hence is generally not recommended. Patients who recover from HUS may also suffer chronic kidney injury as a result.

The natural reservoir of enteroaggregative *E. coli* is not known, but outbreaks have been traced to contaminated food, and live organisms can be found in drinking water, table salsa, and other consumable items in endemic tropical areas. Volunteer studies demonstrated that a high infectious dose is required for acquisition of enteroaggregative *E. coli*, suggesting that direct person-to-person spread may be difficult. In addition to its role in traveler's diarrhea, enteroaggregative *E. coli* is an important cause of both acute diarrhea and persistent diarrhea and malnutrition, especially in children in tropical areas and in patients with HIV/AIDS. It was also shown in several studies to be a major cause of sporadic diarrhea in the United States, Europe, and China, among other developed areas.

Limited data on enteroinvasive *E. coli* suggest that infectious doses are relatively high, but as with enterotoxigenic *E. coli* infections, adequate numbers of organisms have readily been spread in food with high attack rates in outbreak situations. This distinguishes enteroinvasive *E. coli* epidemiologically from *Shigella*, which is easily spread person to person as well as in contaminated food and water.

Diffusely adherent *E. coli* remains the least well understood pathotype and has not consistently been found more often in diarrheal cases than in controls. Nevertheless, some studies have shown a clear association with acute diarrhea in developing areas, particularly in children 1 to 4 years of age. Part of the difficulty is the heterogeneity of strains, some of which express different types of adhesins and different groups of virulence traits, leading to inconsistent pathogenicity.

PATHOBIOLOGY

The pathogenesis of enteric *E. coli* infection begins with ingestion of the organism in contaminated food or water or rarely direct person-to person spread, in the case of enterohemorrhagic *E. coli*. It then faces the normal gastric acid barrier. Both enterotoxigenic *E. coli* and enteroinvasive *E. coli* appear to be sensitive to gastric acid; neutralization of gastric acid reduces the infectious dose by 100- to 1000-fold. Hypochlorhydria increased the risk of enteropathogenic *E. coli* diarrhea in a volunteer study. Even though enterohemorrhagic *E. coli* expresses acid tolerance factors that may facilitate its survival in the stomach, hypochlorhydria was still shown to be a risk factor for HUS in one study.

After ingestion and passage through the stomach, enteric *E. coli* colonize the involved part of the intestinal tract using specialized adhesins and the coordinated expression of virulence traits. This can lead to toxin production, intracellular invasion, or other disruptions of host cell physiology. These virulence traits may be shared among different enteric *E. coli* as well as related enteric pathogens, and it is their combination that leads to the characteristic pathogenic and clinical features of infection. The incubation period between ingestion and symptom development varies from pathogen to pathogen. For example, it averaged 14 hours for enteroaggregative *E. coli* and 2 days for enterotoxigenic *E. coli* in volunteer studies; epidemiologic studies found an average incubation period of 3 to 4 days for enterohemorrhagic *E. coli* O157:H7 but 8 days for shigatoxigenic/enteroaggregative *E. coli* O104:H4.

Enterotoxigenic *E. coli* colonizes the upper portion of the small bowel using fimbriate or fibrillar surface proteins known as colonization factor antigens. The colonization factor antigens bind the organism to cell surface receptors on enterocytes. Whereas this colonization itself can lead to mild inflammatory changes in the epithelium, the majority of enterotoxigenic *E. coli* illness is due to its enterotoxins. Heat-labile toxin, with a molecular weight of about 86,000, consists of 5 binding "B" subunits and an enzymatic "A" subunit, and, like the closely related choleratoxin, binds to a monosialoganglioside (GM1) receptor. Also like choleratoxin (Chapter 286), the A subunit is an enzyme that ADP-ribosylates the regulatory subunit of adenylate cyclase, leading to constitutive production of cyclic adenosine monophosphate. The consequently increased chloride secretion and reduced sodium absorption combine to cause net isotonic electrolyte loss that can be as great as 1 liter/hour. Other human enterotoxigenic *E. coli* strains produce heat-stable toxin, which is a much smaller peptide than heat-labile toxin (18 to 19 amino acids) and activates intestinal particulate guanylate cyclase. Like cyclic adenosine monophosphate, the cyclic guanosine monophosphate thus formed also causes net secretion. The roles of other enterotoxins, such as LTII, EAST, EIET, and others seen in enterotoxigenic *E. coli*, enteroaggregative *E. coli*, and enteroinvasive *E. coli*, respectively, are unclear at present. Both the colonization traits and production of enterotoxin are encoded on transmissible plasmids. Besides the complications of dehydration, the only significant pathologic change with enterotoxigenic *E. coli* is depletion of mucus from intestinal goblet cells.

Enteroinvasive *E. coli*, like the closely related *Shigella*, can invade and multiply in epithelial cells, cause experimental conjunctivitis in guinea pigs (known as the Sereny test), and produce inflammatory colitis and dysenteric or bloody diarrhea. As seen with shigellosis, a striking inflammatory response occurs, with numerous polymorphonuclear leukocytes in stool. The colon shows patchy, acute inflammation in the mucosa and submucosa with focal denuding of the surface epithelium, usually without deeper invasion or systemic spread. Although epithelial cell invasiveness in both enteroinvasive *E. coli* and *Shigella* is encoded on a large 120- to 140-Md plasmid, several chromosomal determinants, including the O antigen, are crucial for full invasive virulence.

Typical **enteropathogenic** *E. coli* strains express plasmid-encoded genes conferring localized adherence to epithelial cells (through specialized bundle-forming pili) and chromosomal genes mediating attachment and effacement of microvilli. The latter is characterized by the formation of cellular pedestals that hold the bacteria intimately to the cell surface. These changes in the host epithelia are mediated through protein effectors injected directly into host cells by a specialized type III secretion system encoded on the chromosomal locus of enterocyte effacement. These secreted effectors cause cellular changes that lead to villous atrophy, mucosal thinning, inflammation in the lamina propria, and variable crypt cell hyperplasia. These morphologic changes are associated with a reduction in mucosal brush border enzymes and may contribute to the impaired absorptive function and diarrhea. Atypical enteropathogenic *E. coli* strains are generally defined as those expressing the locus

of enterocyte effacement but not the bundle-forming pili; they maintain the ability to attach/efface and cause epithelial injury.

Enterohemorrhagic *E. coli*, most notably serotype O157:H7 but also serogroups O26, O39, and others, cause type III secretion-dependent intimate adherence and microvillous effacement like enteropathogenic *E. coli*, but they also produce Shiga-like toxins that are responsible for the characteristic colonic mucosal disruption and hemorrhage as well as the complication of HUS. These toxins bind to the Gb3 surface ganglioside, leading to internalization and enzymatic inactivation of ribosomes, halting protein synthesis. Gb3 is highly expressed on vascular endothelial cells in the colon, kidney, and brain, which may explain the predilection for HUS to affect these organs. Organisms that produce Shiga-like toxins without intimate adherence and pedestal formation are known as shigatoxigenic *E. coli* or verotoxigenic *E. coli*, and often they lack the other virulence traits necessary for colonization and disease production. A notable exception was the shigatoxigenic/enteroaggregative *E. coli* O104:H4 that caused the 2011 European outbreak. The terms enterohemorrhagic *E. coli*, shigatoxigenic *E. coli*, and verotoxigenic *E. coli* were often used interchangeably in the older literature, until the important role of the attaching/effacing ability of true enterohemorrhagic *E. coli* strains like O157:H7 was understood.[11]

Enteroaggregative *E. coli* is defined by a characteristic aggregative adherence pattern to cells and the substrata associated with biofilm formation. This adherence requires a large plasmid known as the AA plasmid, which encodes specialized aggregative adherence fimbriae and other virulence genes, including a serine protease autotransporter toxin known as Pet and an antiaggregative protein called dispersin. Chromosomal virulence traits include a mucinase, Pic, and a second enterotoxin, ShET, as well as type VI secretion systems. Limited studies on human infections with enteroaggregative *E. coli* suggest that the organisms do not intimately adhere or invade but reside within a biofilm at the epithelial surface, where secreted factors contribute to a damaging host inflammatory response.

The fundamental pathogenesis of **diffusely adherent** *E. coli* is still an area of active investigation but appears to depend on direct interactions between specialized adhesins (Afa/Dr) and host membrane proteins such as CD55 (decay-accelerating factor) or carcinoembryonic antigen. Many diffusely adherent *E. coli* strains are closely related to uropathogenic *E. coli* with similar virulence traits. Some also express other virulence factors, including the serine protease autotransporter toxin SAT and a type III secretion system.

Host risk factors for diarrheogenic *E. coli* infection differ among the various bacterial pathotypes but in general include age, recent antibiotic use, and loss of gastric acid.

CLINICAL MANIFESTATIONS

The clinical manifestations of enteric *E. coli* infections differ among the pathotypes. Enterotoxigenic *E. coli* infections generally produce watery diarrhea, particularly in young children and travelers to tropical or developing areas. Diarrhea may range from mild to severe and cholera-like; it may be life-threatening, especially in small children and elderly individuals, who are particularly prone to dehydration, undernutrition, and electrolyte imbalance (especially hypokalemia and acidosis). Other characteristic symptoms include malaise, abdominal cramping, anorexia, and occasionally nausea, vomiting, or low-grade fever. The illness is generally self-limited to 1 to 5 days and rarely extends beyond 10 to 14 days. Infections with enterotoxigenic *E. coli* that produce both heat-stable toxin and heat-labile toxin or heat-stable toxin alone may be more severe than those caused by enterotoxigenic *E. coli* that produce only heat-labile toxin. The persistence of impaired mucosal absorptive capacity for 1 to 3 weeks may further compound the cycle of malnutrition that complicates diarrheal illnesses in children in developing, tropical areas.

Infection with enteroinvasive *E. coli* is characterized by inflammatory colitis, often with abdominal pain, high fever, tenesmus, and bloody or dysenteric diarrhea, essentially like that seen with *Shigella*. The incubation period is usually 1 to 3 days, with the duration generally self-limited to 7 to 10 days.

Outbreaks of enteropathogenic *E. coli* infection in newborn nurseries have ranged from mild transient diarrhea to severe and rapidly fatal diarrheal illnesses, especially in premature or otherwise compromised infants. The more severe illnesses appear to have been more common in industrialized countries before 1950. However, more recent outbreaks and sporadic cases are well documented. Endemic EPEC in infants can produce similar symptoms, including frequently profuse diarrhea.

Hemorrhagic colitis associated with enterohemorrhagic *E. coli* classically begins with watery diarrhea that quickly turns grossly bloody, with a conspicuous absence of fever or inflammatory exudate in stool but with significant abdominal pain. Although this diarrheal illness is self-limited, potentially fatal HUS or thrombotic thrombocytopenic purpura subsequently develops in a significant number of children and older adults (Chapter 163). Outbreaks of hemorrhagic colitis secondary to enterohemorrhagic *E. coli* in nursing homes or other institutions may be common and severe. The incubation period in two outbreaks has been 3 to 4 days (range, 1 to 7 days), and the illness is characteristically self-limited to 5 to 12 days (mean, 7.8 days). The clinical manifestations in the heat-stable toxin/enteroaggregative *E. coli* O104:H4 outbreak were similar, although rates of HUS were significantly higher (more than 20%) and women were disproportionately affected.[12]

Enteroaggregative *E. coli* has been associated with persistent diarrhea and malnutrition in children in developing areas, in HIV/AIDS patients, and in travelers who experience diarrhea (especially those genetically predisposed to greater inflammatory responses). Although infection is frequently asymptomatic, it may cause subclinical inflammation and lead to growth shortfalls.[13] No characteristic clinical features of enteroaggregative *E. coli* have been consistently identified, although some outbreaks were associated with bloody diarrhea and several studies suggest that elevated inflammatory markers in stool are fairly common. Diffusely adherent *E. coli* has also been associated with diarrhea with no particular identifying features in children older than 18 months.

DIAGNOSIS

With the exception of shigatoxigenic *E. coli*, definitive etiologic diagnosis of *E. coli* diarrhea requires documentation of a specific virulence trait or serotype, which requires specialized immunologic tests, tissue culture, animal bioassay, or molecular testing[14] that were historically available only in research and reference laboratories. Other than for shigatoxigenic *E. coli*, such tests are rarely cost-effective or clinically indicated, except in outbreak or research situations, because the infections are either self-limited without treatment (in endemic settings) or empirically treated with antibiotics (in the case of traveler's diarrhea). However, newer multiplex molecular testing platforms capable of identifying them are being introduced in clinical laboratories, which may lead to more frequent identification.

Enterohemorrhagic *E. coli* O157:H7 can be identified with reasonable accuracy by culture on sorbitol-MacConkey agar to identify nonfermenting colonies. However, it has long been recommended that any stool sample with visible blood should also be tested specifically for shigatoxins by enzyme immunoassay, polymerase chain reaction, or other molecular methods, which can identify non-O157 serotypes and rare sorbitol-fermenting O157 strains.[15] Many experts recommend that all stools submitted for culture be tested in this way. In hemorrhagic colitis due to enterohemorrhagic *E. coli*, sigmoidoscopy, which is rarely indicated, generally reveals only moderately hyperemic mucosa, and barium enema or CT scan may show a thumbprint pattern of segmental or diffuse colonic wall thickening. Some patients have superficial ulceration with mild neutrophil infiltration in the edematous submucosa. These changes are not pathognomonic.

Differential Diagnosis

Numerous other causes of diarrhea must be considered, depending on the clinical circumstances (Chapters 131 and 267). For example, self-limited, noninflammatory diarrhea in tropical, developing areas is most likely due to enterotoxigenic *E. coli*, enteroaggregative *E. coli*, rotaviruses (young children), or noroviruses (older children and adults) (Chapter 356). Noninflammatory diarrhea in older children or adults in temperate areas is more likely to be due to noroviruses (Chapter 356). *Vibrio* infections (Chapter 286) are common in areas endemic for cholera or in any coastal area where inadequately cooked seafood may be eaten. If noninflammatory diarrhea persists beyond a week, especially with weight loss, other possibilities include *Giardia lamblia* (Chapter 330), *Cryptosporidium* (Chapter 329), *Cyclospora* (Chapter 332), and microsporidial infection (Chapter 332). In outbreaks of food poisoning, *Staphylococcus aureus* (Chapter 272), *Clostridium perfringens* (Chapter 280), and *Bacillus cereus* should be considered.

Inflammatory colitis with high fever and tenesmus as well as leukocytes, mucus, and blood in the stool may well be due to enteroinvasive *E. coli* but should prompt a stool culture for more common invasive pathogens, such as *Campylobacter jejuni* (Chapter 287), *Shigella* (Chapter 293), *Salmonella* (Chapter 292), *Yersinia enterocolitica* (Chapter 296), or noncholera *Vibrio* (Chapter 286). Any patient with diarrhea and a history of recent antibiotic use, gastrointestinal surgery, or parturition should be screened for toxigenic *Clostridium difficile* (Chapter 280). Enterohemorrhagic *E. coli* should be strongly considered in any case of bloody diarrhea, particularly in the absence of fever; it is

recommended that laboratories now routinely screen for this pathogen in all stool cultures, and they should automatically screen any grossly bloody samples. Ischemic colitis and cytomegalovirus colitis can mimic enterohemorrhagic *E. coli* but should occur only in people at risk (vascular disease and immune compromise or inflammatory bowel disease, respectively).

TREATMENT   Rx

As with all diarrheal illnesses, the primary treatment for most *E. coli* diarrhea is replacement and maintenance of water and electrolytes, usually with a simple oral rehydration solution that uses the intact, sodium-coupled glucose or amino acid absorption (or both) to replace the fluid losses. Oral rehydration solution should be given ad libitum with free water, and in breast-fed infants, continued breast-feeding and early refeeding can compensate for the nutritional losses without an adverse effect on diarrhea output.[A1] Zinc supplementation is also recommended for diarrhea in children older than 6 months in developing areas where zinc deficiency is common because it significantly reduces diarrhea volume.[A2] The enkephalinase inhibitor racecadotril, which is available in Europe but not currently in North America, also reduces diarrheal volume in children with acute gastroenteritis and is as effective as loperamide in adults but less likely to cause constipation. Certain probiotic preparations have been shown in small studies to improve symptoms when they are added to oral rehydration solution in children with infectious diarrhea[A3] but are not yet universally recommended. Antimotility agents reduce the frequency of diarrheal stools but should not be used when fever or bloody diarrhea is present because they can increase the risk of mortality due to toxic megacolon or HUS. Bismuth subsalicylate may reduce symptoms in traveler's diarrhea but should be used with caution to avoid toxic doses of salicylate.[16]

Because most *E. coli* diarrhea is self-limited, the role of antimicrobial agents is debated and remains of secondary importance to rehydration. One situation in which treatment is generally favored is traveler's diarrhea (Chapter 270) because strong clinical studies have shown a benefit of antibiotics in reducing the duration of symptoms.[A4,A5] Unfortunately, rising antimicrobial resistance has narrowed the options for empirical therapy; currently, azithromycin, a fluoroquinolone, or rifaximin is recommended, with trimethoprim-sulfamethoxazole a somewhat less reliable alternative. Antimicrobials should not be used in enterohemorrhagic *E. coli* infection because of the possibility of increasing the risk of HUS and a lack of evidence of efficacy.

PREVENTION

Prevention of most *E. coli* enteric infections is ultimately related to basic economic development, adequate sanitary facilities, and sufficient availability of safe water. In the interim, especially in areas where adequate water supplies and sanitary facilities are not available, measures such as exclusive breast-feeding for at least 6 to 12 months and hand hygiene reduce the likelihood of acquiring *E. coli* enteric infections. Simple, portable water filters to reduce bacterial contamination are also in development.

Travelers to developing or tropical areas should avoid drinking untreated or unboiled water or ice and eating uncooked fruits or vegetables that may have been washed with highly contaminated water. Although a number of antimicrobial agents are effective during short periods when taken prophylactically, their effectiveness is ultimately limited by rapidly emerging resistance to antimicrobial drugs as well as by the potential side effects of their indiscriminate, widespread use. For example, although a number of studies suggested that rifaximin and fluoroquinolones are both effective at reducing incidence of traveler's diarrhea,[A6] resistance to the latter is now unacceptably high in many areas of the world to suggest their use. This, combined with the rapid effect of empirical antibiotics at the onset of diarrhea symptoms, has diminished enthusiasm for prophylactic antibiotics. Bismuth subsalicylate is modestly effective at preventing traveler's diarrhea, although with side effects. The killed *Vibrio cholerae*/cholera toxin B subunit vaccine (Dukoral), which is available in some countries, may provide transient, partial protection against enterotoxigenic *E. coli* in travelers although recent meta-analyses showed no overall benefit in prevention of traveler's diarrhea.[A7]

Sporadic enterohemorrhagic *E. coli* infections may be reduced by adequately cooking ground beef products, to an internal temperature of at least 160° F (71° C), and by careful handwashing and other hygienic measures in daycare centers and nursing homes. Unfortunately, large outbreaks due to contaminated produce continue to occur and are frequently associated with items meant to be eaten raw (such as sprouts). A vaccine composed from type III secreted effectors of enterohemorrhagic *E. coli* (Econiche) was developed to reduce colonization of livestock but is not currently available for use. Irradiation of meats and some produce to reduce viable bacterial contamination is approved in the United States, but these foods are not widely sold at the present time.

Antibiotics are still important in treating *E. coli*-associated travelers' diarrhea, but non-antibiotic strategies will be critical to limit the spread of antibiotic resistant strains and necessary for infections like enterohemorrhagic *E. coli* for which antibiotics are not recommended. Vaccine development appears to be the most promising strategy but at this time there is no effective licensed vaccine against intestinal pathogenic *E. coli*.[17]

PROGNOSIS

The greatest concern with enteric *E. coli* infections in developed areas is enterohemorrhagic *E. coli*/shigatoxigenic *E. coli*-associated HUS, which develops in 3 to 7% of sporadic cases and as high as 20% in outbreaks. Whereas most patients with HUS recover, they frequently require intensive medical care (including temporary hemodialysis), and as many as 30% of survivors have renal sequelae such as proteinuria, hypertension, reduced glomerular filtration rate, or, more rarely, dialysis dependence.[18]

On a global scale, the greatest impact of diarrheogenic *E. coli* is in children in poor, developing areas, who are prone to death from dehydration from these otherwise self-limited infections. Moreover, children who survive repeated episodes of infectious diarrhea (due to *E. coli* and other pathogens) may experience permanent deficits in growth and cognitive development, the full impact of which remains unknown. Lethal infections with typical enteropathogenic *E. coli* may also be associated with certain gene clusters, although it is too early to use such information for prognostic purposes.[19]

Grade A References

A1. Gregorio GV, Dans LF, Silvestre MA. Early versus delayed refeeding for children with acute diarrhoea. *Cochrane Database Syst Rev.* 2011;7:CD007296.

A2. Lazzerini M, Ronfani L. Oral zinc for treating diarrhoea in children. *Cochrane Database Syst Rev.* 2013;1:CD005436.

A3. Francavilla R, Lionetti E, Castellaneta S, et al. Randomised clinical trial: *Lactobacillus reuteri* DSM 17938 vs. placebo in children with acute diarrhoea—a double-blind study. *Aliment Pharmacol Ther.* 2012;36:363-369.

A4. Hu Y, Ren J, Zhan M, et al. Efficacy of rifaximin in prevention of travelers' diarrhea: a meta-analysis of randomized, double-blind, placebo-controlled trials. *J Travel Med.* 2012;19:352-356.

A5. Riddle MS, Connor P, Fraser J, et al. Trial evaluating ambulatory therapy of travelers' diarrhea (TrEAT TD) study: a randomized controlled trial comparing 3 single-dose antibiotic regimens with loperamide. *Clin Infect Dis.* 2017;65:2008-2017.

A6. Alajbegovic S, Sanders JW, Atherly DE, et al. Effectiveness of rifaximin and fluoroquinolones in preventing travelers' diarrhea (TD): a systematic review and meta-analysis. *Syst Rev.* 2012;1:1-10.

A7. Ahmed T, Bhuiyan TR, Zaman K, et al. Vaccines for preventing enterotoxigenic *Escherichia coli* (ETEC) diarrhoea. *Cochrane Database Syst Rev.* 2013;7:CD009029.

GENERAL REFERENCES

For the General References and other additional features, please visit Expert Consult at https://expertconsult.inkling.com.

289

INFECTIONS DUE TO OTHER MEMBERS OF THE ENTEROBACTERIACEAE, INCLUDING MANAGEMENT OF MULTIDRUG-RESISTANT STRAINS

DAVID L. PATERSON AND AMY J. MATHERS

DEFINITION

The Enterobacteriaceae are a family of gram-negative bacilli that are responsible for a broad range of infections in humans and in animals. They may be motile or nonmotile, depending on the species. They are aerobic or facultatively anaerobic in growth and have a predilection for inhabiting the gastrointestinal tract. Only

TABLE 289-1	SELECTED MEDICALLY IMPORTANT MEMBERS OF THE FAMILY ENTEROBACTERIACEAE
GENUS	**SOME IMPORTANT SPECIES**
Citrobacter	*C. freundii*
Enterobacter	*E. cloacae*
Escherichia	*E. coli*
Klebsiella	*K. pneumoniae, K. oxytoca*
Morganella	*M. morganii*
Plesiomonas	*P. shigelloides*
Proteus	*P. mirabilis, P. vulgaris*
Providencia	*P. stuartii*
Salmonella	*S. enterica*
Serratia	*S. marcescens*
Shigella	*S. sonnei*
Yersinia	*Y. pestis, Y. enterocolitica*

extragastrointestinal manifestations of disease are discussed in this chapter. Enteric infections caused by *Escherichia coli* are discussed in Chapter 288.

Members of the Enterobacteriaceae grow on a variety of solid media and are usually readily identified by clinical microbiology laboratories. Accurate speciation remains important in a clinical setting because of inherent differences in antibiotic susceptibility between species. Development of multidrug antimicrobial resistance in all gram-negative bacilli, including the Enterobacteriaceae, has been increasing in all parts of the world. Particular emphasis is placed in this chapter on epidemiology, treatment, and prevention of important multidrug-resistant strains.

Medically important members of the Enterobacteriaceae are listed in Table 289-1. Infections due to *Salmonella*, *Shigella*, and *Yersinia* are discussed in Chapters 292, 293, and 296, respectively.

EPIDEMIOLOGY

The Enterobacteriaceae are among the most common pathogens to infect humans worldwide. They are responsible for community-acquired, hospital-acquired, and health care–associated infections. Examples of the last category include infections acquired in nursing homes and those associated with outpatient management of cancers or hematologic malignant disease. As resident components of the flora of the gastrointestinal tract, isolates of Enterobacteriaceae may represent examples of colonization rather than true infection. This may apply to isolates from rectal swabs, urine, or respiratory secretions. In some regions, multidrug-resistant Enterobacteriaceae have become endemic, leading to substantial problems in the management of serious infections.[1,2] While multidrug resistance in the United States is still largely health care–associated, community-associated infections are beginning to emerge.[3,4]

E. coli is the most common cause of urinary tract infections (UTIs), accounting for more than 80% of isolates from urine in most clinical situations (Chapter 268).[5] Any of the remaining members of the Enterobacteriaceae can cause this infection; *Klebsiella* spp and *Proteus mirabilis* are among other common causes of UTI. The Enterobacteriaceae can cause uncomplicated cystitis in healthy women as well as acute pyelonephritis. UTIs frequently occur in patients with renal tract abnormalities or those who need frequent or chronic urinary catheterization. The presence of Enterobacteriaceae in urine does not always indicate infection because they may colonize the bladder or be found in contaminated, improperly collected samples.

There has been recent recognition of the spread of some successful strains of uropathogenic *E. coli* which account for a disproportionate amount of disease (see later under Pathobiology). In other words, *E. coli* isolates from unique patients with UTIs may be highly genetically related. Trimethoprim-sulfamethoxazole-resistant *E. coli* is notable for its spread in a clonal fashion in the United States (e.g., "clonal group A" and *E. coli* O15:K52:H1). A widely spread *E. coli* clone, defined by multilocus sequence typing as sequence type 131 (ST131), has been found to be associated with ciprofloxacin resistance and production of extended-spectrum β-lactamases (ESBLs). This clone is typically associated with community-acquired UTIs. It has been detected in every inhabited continent. While bacterial genetic background clearly plays an important role in determining antibiotic resistance, it is not sufficient by itself to result in infection with multidrug resistant uropathogenic *E. coli*.[6]

Given that the niche of most Enterobacteriaceae is in the gastrointestinal tract, it is not surprising that these bacteria are prominent as causes of peritonitis. *E. coli* ranks as the most common cause of both spontaneous bacterial peritonitis (occurring in cirrhotic patients) and bacterial peritonitis arising from visceral perforation. Pyogenic liver abscess and intra-abdominal abscess may also be due to *E. coli*. Other members of the Enterobacteriaceae may also cause these intra-abdominal infections, especially in patients with peritonitis occurring after prior surgery for intra-abdominal disease.

The Enterobacteriaceae may also be the causative pathogens of pneumonia. They are more frequently the cause of hospital- and health care–associated pneumonia than community-acquired pneumonia. *Klebsiella pneumoniae* was once renowned as a cause of community-acquired pneumonia in alcoholics but has declined in significance during the past few decades. Since the 1980s, a hypervirulent *K. pneumoniae* has emerged as a clinically significant pathogen. It has caused serious disseminated infections, typically involving pyogenic liver abscess, osteomyelitis, and/or endophthalmitis in immunocompetent and otherwise healthy people. Initial descriptions of hypervirulent *K. pneumoniae* were confined to East Asia but are now increasingly reported worldwide. Although mostly antibiotic-sensitive at this time, some cases of multidrug resistance have been identified.[7]

Hospital-acquired pneumonia due to the Enterobacteriaceae may be ventilator associated. The Enterobacteriaceae rank most common as causes of ventilator-associated pneumonia after *Staphylococcus aureus* and *Pseudomonas aeruginosa*.[8] The Enterobacteriaceae may also cause hospital-acquired pneumonia in non–mechanically ventilated patients, such as those with neurologic impairment from head injury or cerebrovascular accident.

Outbreaks of antibiotic-resistant *K. pneumoniae* infection in hospitals have been prominent for more than three decades. In the hospital setting, *K. pneumoniae* is usually the cause of peritonitis, pneumonia, or complicated UTI. Blood stream infection arising from another site of infection, from vascular catheters, or in association with neutropenia may also occur. In the 1970s, outbreaks due to gentamicin-resistant strains occurred. In the 1980s and 1990s, hospital outbreaks of ESBL-producing *K. pneumoniae* became commonplace. Finally, in the past decade, with carbapenems considered the last line of reliable therapy for invasive infections, *K. pneumoniae* carbapenemase (KPC)–producing *K. pneumoniae* became a substantial clinical and infection control issue in hospitals. The recent reported mortality is almost 50% among hospitalized patients who develop blood stream infections by carbapenem-resistant Enterobacteriaceae because of the lack of adequate treatment options. The KPC-producing organisms are discussed in detail in a subsequent section of this chapter.

PATHOBIOLOGY

The virulence factors associated with *E. coli* causing enteric infections are discussed in detail in Chapter 288. At least 40 different virulence genes have been described in *E. coli* causing extraintestinal infections. Among the virulence properties of these strains is the renowned ability of *E. coli* to adhere to uroepithelial cells. The ST131 *E. coli* clone is typically highly successful at causing extraintestinal infections. It belongs to "phylogenetic group" B2, which is known for extraintestinal pathogenic infections. In an evaluation of the ST131 clone, numerous extraintestinal virulence genes were found.

Mechanisms of Multidrug Resistance

Hard-to-treat and even untreatable infections with ESBL and carbapenem-resistant Enterobacteriaceae (CRE) have emerged worldwide and have become a serious threat to global public health.[9,10] The problem is compounded by travelers from high-income countries to low-income countries who frequently acquire multidrug-resistant Enterobacteriaceae infections, particularly in India where ESBL colonization is at 64% (Fig. 289-1). The global spread of drug resistance is further facilitated by migration of refugees and pilgrimages.[11] In short-stay acute care hospitals in the United States in 2015, the ESBL phenotype comprised 16.5% of all *Klebsiella* spp and *E. coli* isolates. The percentage of carbapenem-resistant *K. pneumoniae* was 3.1%, but this was a sharp decrease from 2007 when it was 10.6%.[12] The stabilization and even decrease in infections with ESBL and CRE phenotype Enterobacteriaceae in acute care facilities in the United States has been attributed to the implementation of the U.S. Centers for Disease Control and Prevention (CDC) containment strategy, the Antibiotic Resistance Laboratory Network (ARLN). Comparable initiatives to track drug resistance have been implemented by the Centers for Disease Dynamics, Economics and Policy, the Antibacterial Resistance Leadership Group, and in Europe by the European Centers for Disease Control and Prevention (eCDC) and the Combatting Bacterial Resistance in Europe project.

The molecular mechanisms of antibiotic resistance in the Enterobacteriaceae can be either intrinsic or acquired (Table 289-2) (also see Chapter 271). Intrinsic resistance occurs when bacteria possess properties that naturally resist the action of an antimicrobial often encoded in the chromosome of the wild-type population of a bacterial species (e.g., all *Klebsiella* spp produce a β-lactamase that hydrolyzes ampicillin). Acquired resistance occurs through mutations in the chromosome, change in gene expression, or acquisition of genes that confer resistance through horizontal gene transfer from other bacteria. From a molecular mechanism standpoint, bacteria resist antimicrobials in one of four ways: (1) alteration of antimicrobial uptake to the site of action (e.g., downregulating its expression of porins, nonspecific membrane channels, and thereby reducing its permeability to the antibiotic); (2) upregulating specific or multidrug resistance pumps to increase the efflux to expel the antibiotic; (3) altering the target site so that the antimicrobial cannot efficiently bind (e.g., by target site mutation, acetylation, phosphorylation); or (4) destruction of the antibiotic through enzymatic activity (e.g., β-lactamases and carbapenemases).[13] Acquired resistance can then proliferate through (a) proliferation of clonal lineages with antibiotic resistance gene mutations, including acquired β-lactamases and carbapenemases (i.e., clonal expansion) and/or (b) horizontal transfer of antibiotic resistance genes through mobile

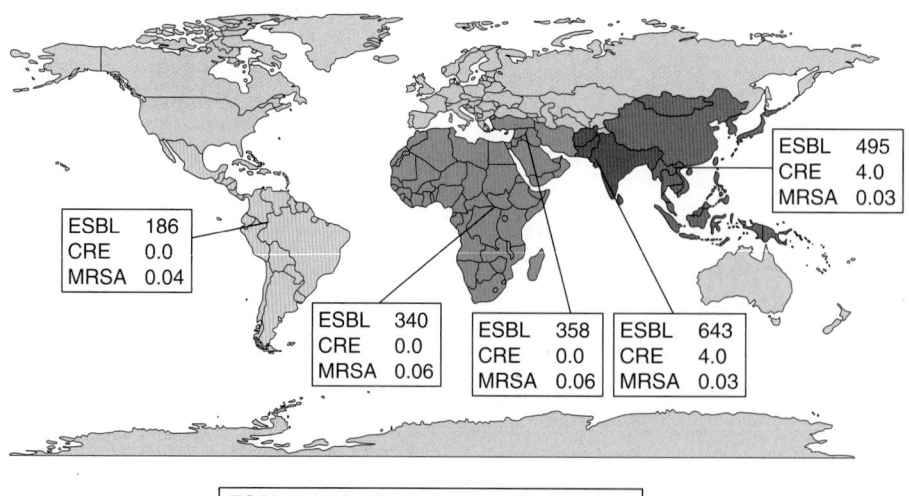

ESBL	186
CRE	0.0
MRSA	0.04

ESBL	495
CRE	4.0
MRSA	0.03

ESBL	340
CRE	0.0
MRSA	0.06

ESBL	358
CRE	0.0
MRSA	0.06

ESBL	643
CRE	4.0
MRSA	0.03

ESBL colonization rate per 1000 travelers
<200 200–400 400–600 >600

FIGURE 289-1. The number of drug-resistant organisms detected per 1000 healthy travelers. The risk for travelers returning from the countries indicated with drug-resistant bacterial organisms varies by region and type of microorganism. CRE = carbapenem-resistant Enterobacteriaceae; ESBL = extended-spectrum β-lactamase; MRSA = methicillin-resistant *Staphylococcus aureus*. (From Schwartz KL, Morris SK. Travel and the spread of drug-resistant bacteria. *Curr Infect Dis Rep.* 2018;20:29.)

TABLE 289-2 MECHANISMS OF ANTIBIOTIC RESISTANCE AND DRIVERS OF SPREAD OF MULTIDRUG-RESISTANT ENTEROBACTERIACEAE

1. MECHANISMS OF ANTIBIOTIC RESISTANCE

Intrinsic Resistance

Bacterial species with inherent properties that naturally resist the action of an antibiotic often encoded in the chromosome of the wild-type population of a bacterial species (e.g., all *Klebsiella* spp produce a β-lactamase that hydrolyzes ampicillin)

Acquired Resistance

Development of resistance to an antimicrobial through mutation, altered regulation, or acquisition of genes of antimicrobial resistance through horizontal gene transfer

2. MECHANISMS OF ANTIMICROBIAL RESISTANCE

Prevent Access to the Antibiotic Target

Reduce influx of the antibiotic (e.g., downregulate porins)
Increase efflux (e.g., overexpress specific or multidrug-resistance pumps)

Alter the Antibiotic Target

Change target structure through mutations to disable antibiotic binding
Modify and protect the target by mutation or post-translational modification

Inactivate the Antibiotic

Enzymatically hydrolyze the antibiotic (e.g., β-lactamases, carbapenemases)
Chemically alter the antibiotic to prevent antibiotic binding

3. DRIVERS OF SPREAD OF MULTIDRUG-RESISTANT BACTERIA

Clonal Expansion

Proliferation of clonal lineages with genes or mutations that can stably maintain antimicrobial resistance mechanisms

Horizontal Gene Transfer

Exchange of antimicrobial resistance genes between bacteria through mobile genetic elements, such as plasmids and transposons

genetic elements such as plasmids or transposons, which can spread across strains and species.

Another important development in antimicrobial resistance has been the rapid dissemination of colistin resistance through a resistance gene, *MCR*, which has quickly spread among bacteria through horizontal gene transfer. Originally identified in China, the *MCR* gene was most prevalent in livestock but also identified in retail meats as well as hospitalized patients.[14] This highlights the importance of antimicrobial use in animal husbandry as a driver of clinically relevant resistance dissemination and the importance of addressing areas outside of medicine to slow further development of bacterial drug resistance.

Narrow-Spectrum β-Lactamases

Ampicillin was introduced into clinical practice in the early 1960s. Within months of the release of ampicillin, a plasmid-mediated β-lactamase, called the TEM β-lactamase, was discovered leading to resistant of *E. coli*. Plasmids encoding resistance to ampicillin have now become widespread, with at least 40% of *E. coli* in most parts of the world now being TEM β-lactamase producers. Enterobacteriaceae such as *Klebsiella* and *Enterobacter* spp, with genes encoding β-lactamases inherent to their genome, are known to be intrinsically resistant to ampicillin.

Extended-Spectrum β-Lactamases

Third-generation cephalosporins (such as ceftriaxone) are intrinsically active against all Enterobacteriaceae. However, mutant genes encoding β-lactamases capable of inactivating third-generation cephalosporins were discovered in the 1980s. Some of the genes encoding these β-lactamases were identical to TEM, except for point mutations that led to an altered amino acid sequence. The subsequent structural change led to an ability to hydrolyze and thus to inactivate third-generation cephalosporins. In view of the extended spectrum of antibiotic-hydrolyzing abilities compared with the parent TEM (and SHV) enzymes, these β-lactamases were named ESBLs. In addition many new types of ESBLs have now been described, most notably the CTX-M type.

Frequently, the ST131 *E. coli* clone produces a CTX-M type of ESBL (especially CTX-M-15). Although ESBLs are typically susceptible to β-lactamase inhibitors (e.g., clavulanic acid), many ST131 *E. coli* isolates produce an additional β-lactamase (OXA-1) that confers resistance to β-lactamase inhibitors. The antibiotic resistance phenotype of the ST131-positive *E. coli* is that the organisms are typically resistant to ceftriaxone, cefotaxime, fluoroquinolones, trimethoprim, trimethoprim-sulfamethoxazole, penicillin-β-lactamase inhibitor combinations, and tetracyclines. Resistance to aminoglycosides is variable. The clone confers multidrug resistance by the presence of multiple antibiotic resistance genes. These are usually encoded on plasmids.

AmpC β-Lactamases

A number of genera within the Enterobacteriaceae have a chromosomally encoded β-lactamase capable of producing resistance to all penicillins and all cephalosporins except cefepime. In addition, these β-lactamases are not inhibited by β-lactamase inhibitors, such as clavulanic acid or tazobactam. These β-lactamases are known as AmpC β-lactamases or cephalosporinases. They are not derived from narrower spectrum parent β-lactamases, so it is not correct to call these ESBLs. These AmpC β-lactamases may be overproduced in the presence of certain antibiotics (i.e., the genes encoding the AmpC β-lactamases are "inducible"). *Enterobacter* spp, *Citrobacter freundii*, *Serratia marcescens*, and *Morganella morganii* have inducible, chromosomally encoded AmpC β-lactamases. AmpC β-lactamase genes have now been found on plasmids in *E. coli*, *Salmonella*, and other gram-negative bacteria and often lack regulation, resulting in high-level continuous expression.

KPC, NDM, and Other Carbapenemases

With the emergence of what we now call ESBLs, carbapenems became the antibiotics of last resort for treatment of patients with ESBL-producing Enterobacteriaceae infections. In 2001, a novel carbapenem-hydrolyzing β-lactamase from a carbapenem-resistant strain of *K. pneumoniae* was first described: the KPC. KPC-producing organisms are typically resistant to penicillins, cephalosporins, aztreonam, and carbapenems and are not inhibited by clavulanic acid or other commonly used β-lactamase inhibitors, such as sulbactam and tazobactam. CRE has been documented in *E. coli* and in many genera of the Enterobacteriaceae, such as *Enterobacter*, *Citrobacter*, and *Proteus* spp.

The original epicenter of KPC-producing *K. pneumoniae* was New York City. By 2004, approximately one fourth of *K. pneumoniae* isolates in a surveillance study in Brooklyn, New York, were KPC producing. Global spread is now well described. Another CRE produces the New Delhi metallo-β-lactamase (NDM) and has emerged in the past decade as a major cause of carbapenem resistance. Its epicenter is the Indian subcontinent. However, it has also been found to be endemic in some hospitals in the Balkan states as well as causing outbreaks in North America and Europe. Many outbreaks of NDM-producing organisms have been associated with interhospital transfers from hospitals in the Indian subcontinent. Worryingly, NDM-producing organisms have been found in drinking water in India and in food-producing animals in China. Other carbapenem-hydrolyzing β-lactamases seen in Enterobacteriaceae include the OXA-48-like, which is found in North Africa, the Middle East, and India and has since spread to other parts of the world, as well as a variety of other metallo-β-lactamases (such as of the IMP and VIM types). These enzymes all share the ability to render Enterobacteriaceae resistant to carbapenems and many other β-lactam antibiotics.

CLINICAL MANIFESTATIONS

The clinical manifestations of UTI, peritonitis, pneumonia, and blood stream infection due to the Enterobacteriaceae are described in other chapters.

DIAGNOSIS

Enterobacteriaceae is readily grown in clinical microbiology laboratories after collection of appropriate specimens. Examination of the Gram stain enables a rapid identification of gram-negative bacilli from gram-positive pathogens. However, it is frequently difficult on clinical grounds and by Gram stain results to differentiate Enterobacteriaceae from other gram-negative bacilli, such as *P. aeruginosa*.

When a member of the Enterobacteriaceae has been identified, it is important to ensure that appropriate speciation and antibiotic susceptibility testing have been performed. In some instances, specialized tests need to be performed by the clinical microbiology laboratory to detect ESBL or carbapenemase production. Increasingly, rapid molecular and phenotypic diagnostics are being introduced to expedite identification, susceptibility, and often common molecular mechanisms of resistance. Molecular epidemiologic assessment may need to be undertaken to determine whether an isolate belongs to an outbreak strain.[15]

TREATMENT Rx

Treatment depends on the site of infection and the extent of antibiotic resistance. Empirical antibiotic choices for orally administered therapy for UTI due to *E. coli* and the other Enterobacteriaceae may include fluoroquinolones, trimethoprim-sulfamethoxazole, amoxicillin-clavulanate, and nitrofurantoin. *P. mirabilis* is intrinsically resistant to nitrofurantoin. Empirical parenteral choices may include third-generation cephalosporins, penicillin–β-lactamase inhibitor combinations, aminoglycosides, fluoroquinolones, and carbapenems and should be based on local rates of resistance of the most commonly treated organisms.

The advent of antibiotic resistance in the Enterobacteriaceae has the potential to have a huge impact on treatment of common infections. UTI is a pertinent example. Orally administered choices such as fluoroquinolones, trimethoprim-sulfamethoxazole, and amoxicillin-clavulanate are typically inactive in the ST131 *E. coli* strain. There may be a need to now admit some patients to a hospital with simple UTI for initiation of parenteral antibiotics because of this antibiotic resistance. Worse still, some patients with hospital-acquired infection may need "last-line" antibiotics like colistin or polymyxin B with increased toxicity and less efficacy.

Treatment of Extended-Spectrum β-Lactamase-Producing Organisms

In vitro, the carbapenems (including imipenem, meropenem, doripenem, and ertapenem) have the most potent activity against ESBL-producing organisms. This is not surprising because these antibiotics are not inactivated by ESBLs. However, carbapenem-sparing strategies should be used, when feasible, for ESBL infections.[16] Carbapenems should be regarded as the drugs of choice for serious infections with ESBL-producing organisms on the basis of extensive positive clinical experience. No randomized trials have been completed comparing carbapenems with other antibiotic classes against ESBL producers. There is no evidence that combination therapy involving a carbapenem is superior to use of a carbapenem alone for ESBL producers. Observational data also suggest that quinolones or cefepime may be reasonable alternatives.[17]

Meropenem is generally the treatment of choice for serious infections due to ESBL producers.[A1] The ability to use ertapenem once daily makes it potentially useful in serious infections with ESBL producers in nursing home residents or patients continuing parenteral therapy out of the hospital. Ceftolozane/tazobactam plus metronidazole may be another alternative therapy to a carbapenem in patients with complicated intra-abdominal infections caused by ESBL-producing bacteria.[18] UTIs may be treated with orally administered fosfomycin, nitrofurantoin, cephalexin or amoxicillin-clavulanate if susceptible.

Treatment of Carbapenem-Resistant Organisms

Treatment of carbapenem-resistant organisms (e.g., due to KPC or NDM production) is difficult because they may lack susceptibility to all β-lactam antibiotics (including penicillins, cephalosporins, aztreonam, and carbapenems), fluoroquinolones, and aminoglycosides. Carbapenemase-producing organisms may sometimes appear susceptible to carbapenems such as meropenem and imipenem (although they are almost always recognized as resistant to ertapenem), but these antibiotics should not be relied on as monotherapy.

No randomized controlled trials have yet been performed evaluating different antibiotic options for carbapenemase producers. On the basis of observational studies, combination therapy appears to be superior to single-drug therapy. Combinations of a polymyxin, tigecycline, and meropenem have met with some success, but often high mortality is still reported. Most recently, two new agents with clinically effective carbapenemase inhibition have been approved by the U.S. Food and Drug Administration (FDA), which may help lower mortality: ceftazidime/avibactam and meropenem/vaborbactam. Ceftazidime/avibactam is active against KPC and OXA-48 producers,[19] although development of resistance is a concern, and combination therapy remains favored. Meropenem/vaborbactam was designed specifically to have activity against KPC-producing bacteria. Until more data are available, combination therapy likely will still be favored. Neither of these new agents has activity against metallo-carbapenemases (e.g., VIM and NDM).

Development of New Agents for Multidrug Resistance by Enterobacteriaceae

The developments that led to the current public health crisis of hard-to-treat or untreatable CRE are instructive.

Combination therapy is particularly indicated in CRE in high-risk patients, such as those in septic shock or with pneumonia.[20] Several new antibiotic combinations with a β-lactamase inhibitor are in development at this time, including cefepime/zidebactam (the latter being a non-β-lactam antibiotic); cefepime/tazobactam; cefepime/AAI101; meropenem-nacubactam; aztreonam/avibactam; and ceftaroline/avibactam. Non-β-lactam antibiotics in later phase clinical trials include the pathogen-specific anti-*Pseudomonas* drug murepavadin and the new fluoroquinolone finafloxacin. Several drugs are in the late stages of development, including cefiderocol, eravacycline, imipenem-cilastatin/relebactam, omadacycline, and plazomicin. Finally, delafloxacin and plazomicin were also recently approved agents with activity against gram-negative bacteria that produce ESBL.[21,22]

PREVENTION

Prevention of hospital-acquired outbreaks of ESBL, KPC, or NDM producers rests on a number of basic infection control principles. Also see Chapter 266. First, if a focus of infection exists in the hospital environment, it should be removed. Examples have included contamination of ultrasonography coupling gel and bronchoscopes. Outbreaks have been dramatically curtailed when these sources of contamination have been properly cleaned or removed from the hospital environment.

Present evidence suggests that transient carriage on the hands of health care workers is the most important means of transfer of ESBL-, KPC-, or NDM-producing Enterobacteriaceae from patient to patient. The hands of health care workers are presumably colonized by contact with the skin, stool, or bodily fluids of patients with colonization of the organism or by contact with a contaminated environment around the patient. Many patients may have asymptomatic colonization with ESBL-, KPC-, or NDM-producing organisms without signs of overt infection. These patients represent an important reservoir of organisms. In some hospital wards with ongoing issues with ESBL, KPC, or NDM producers, more than 30% of patients have gastrointestinal tract colonization with these organisms at any one time. These patients should be nursed with use of contact precautions. Hand carriage by health care workers is usually eliminated by hand hygiene with alcohol-based agents. Compliance with contact isolation precautions and hand hygiene needs to be high to maximize the effectiveness of these interventions.

Antimicrobial exposure is known to be a risk factor for ESBL *E. coli* and CRE carriage because it eliminates susceptible flora, thereby selecting for resistant bacteria. Changes in antibiotic policy may play a role in controlling outbreaks of ESBL, KPC, or NDM producers, but this concept remains controversial. In one reported outbreak of ESBL producers, no effort was made to change infection control procedures. Instead, at this hospital, ceftazidime use decreased and piperacillin-tazobactam was introduced into the formulary. This coincided with curtailment of the outbreak. In another institution, cephalosporins as an entire class were removed to exact control over endemic ESBL producers. The difficulty with this approach is that replacement of one antibiotic class with another may result in replacement of one antibiotic resistance issue with another. No study has demonstrated that removal of carbapenems from a hospital formulary leads to elimination of KPC or NDM producers. Because these organisms are resistant to multiple antibiotic classes, reduction of carbapenem exposure may not eliminate selection for CRE. Prudent use of all antibiotic classes with an emphasis on reducing duration of antibiotic use may be more useful than individual antibiotic class restriction.

PROGNOSIS

The prognosis of infection with the Enterobacteriaceae depends on multiple factors, such as site of infection, presence of underlying diseases, control of the infection source, and adequacy of empirical antibiotic therapy. At one extreme, inadequate orally administered antibiotic therapy for uncomplicated UTI due to an EXBL producer may have no impact on mortality, although it may have an impact on duration of symptoms and need for parenteral therapy for treatment failure. At the other extreme, patients in an intensive care unit with serious infections due to KPC or NDM producers may have an in-hospital mortality rate exceeding 70%. This may compare with in-hospital mortality rates of 20 to 30% in comparable patients without infection due to a KPC or NDM producer.

Grade A Reference

A1. Harris PNA, Tambyah PA, Lye DC, et al. Effect of piperacillin-tazobactam vs meropenem on 30-day mortality for patients with *E coli* or *Klebsiella pneumoniae* bloodstream infection and ceftriaxone resistance: a randomized clinical trial. *JAMA*. 2018;320:984-994.

GENERAL REFERENCES

For the General References and other additional features, please visit Expert Consult at https://expertconsult.inkling.com.

290

PSEUDOMONAS AND RELATED GRAM-NEGATIVE BACILLARY INFECTIONS

MATTHEW E. FALAGAS AND PETROS I. RAFAILIDIS

DEFINITION

Infections due to *Pseudomonas* spp are caused by members of the family Pseudomonadaceae. The Pseudomonadaceae is a group of gram-negative rods, including *P. aeruginosa*, the most frequently recovered human pathogen in the family. Other *Pseudomonas* spp include *P. putida, P. alcaligenes, P. fluorescens, P. luteola, P. mendocina, P. oryzihabitans, P. pseudoalcaligenes, P. stutzeri, P. chlororaphis, P. delafieldii, P. kingii, P. pertucinogena,* and *Pseudomonas* CDC group 1.

Related gram-negative bacillary infections include those due to *Stenotrophomonas maltophilia* (formerly known as *P. maltophilia* and *Xanthomonas maltophilia*) and members of the genus *Burkholderia* (*B. pseudomallei, B. mallei,* and *B. cepacia* complex [*B. cepacia* complex]).

The Pathogens

P. aeruginosa is a gram-negative, lactose nonfermenting, straight or slightly curved rod with a length ranging from 1.5 to 7 μm and a width of 0.5 to 1.0 μm. It is catalase positive, oxidase positive, and motile with one or more polar flagella. Most species oxidize glucose and reduce nitrate to nitrite or nitrogen gas. It has the ability to grow at 42° C. This pathogen is admirably armed on its exterior: a polysaccharide capsule along with lipopolysaccharides, pili, and flagella. Furthermore, the interior arsenal includes toxins such as exotoxin A, pyocyanin (blue or blue-green pigment), pyorubin (red or red-brown pigment), pyomelanin (black pigment), and pyoverdin (yellow-green pigment). *P. aeruginosa* is notorious for its ability to acquire resistance genes and to spread by horizontal transfer. The microorganism possesses a diversity of mechanisms that promote its survival, adaptation, and resistance to multiple classes of antibiotics that make it an emerging worldwide public health threat.[1]

Stenotrophomonas maltophilia is a gram-negative nonfermenting bacillus motile by polar flagella. It is also catalase positive; the majority of strains are oxidase negative, but some strains are oxidase positive. *B. cepacia* and *B. pseudomallei* are also motile gram-negative lactose nonfermenting bacteria. In contrast, *B. mallei* is nonmotile.

EPIDEMIOLOGY

P. aeruginosa is one of the most common pathogens in health care–associated infections. Ventilator-associated pneumonia, primary bacteremia associated with central venous catheters or secondary bacteremia due to infections present elsewhere in the body, urinary tract infections, and surgical site infections are the main types of infections associated with *P. aeruginosa* in the hospital setting. Data from the National Healthcare Safety Network at the Centers for Disease Control and Prevention indicate that in the United States during 2011 to 2014, *P. aeruginosa* was responsible for 7.3% of all health care–associated infections and was the sixth most frequent culprit among pathogens.[2] Approximately 2% of these strains are resistant to carbapenems, a powerful antibiotic against them. This organism is able to survive in environments that have only minimal nutritional components. *P. aeruginosa* can colonize moist surfaces of the axilla, ear, and perineum. It is also isolated from other moist, inanimate environments within the hospital, including water in sinks and drains, mechanical ventilation equipment, dialysis equipment, toilets, showers, hydrotherapy pools, mops, water for flowers, and even cleaning solutions.

Strains of *P. aeruginosa* resistant to multiple classes of antibiotics, including quinolones and β-lactams, are a major cause of morbidity and mortality worldwide. During a relatively short time, a multidrug-resistant *P. aeruginosa* strain can spread through neighboring countries. The use of broad-spectrum antibiotics is certainly a risk factor for the development of multidrug-resistant *P. aeruginosa*, as are deficiencies in infection control implementation.

A range of hosts are particularly prone to infections by this pathogen: patients with neutropenia, burns, cystic fibrosis (CF), chronic obstructive pulmonary disease (COPD), cancer, transplant recipients, diabetics, and patients with AIDS. Patients with compromised immunity due to treatment or by the disease, either humoral (hypogammaglobulinemia) or cellular (steroid treatment), as well as patients with foreign bodies (e.g., vascular grafts, orthopedic implants) are also more vulnerable to *P. aeruginosa* infections.

Community-acquired *P. aeruginosa* infection is related to exposure to water by the use of hot tubs, whirlpools, swimming pools, spas, and other types of baths as well as to the use of contact lenses, particularly the extended-wear variety. Puncture wounds including those through tennis shoes can give rise to *P. aeruginosa* infection. *P. aeruginosa* endophthalmitis after eye trauma can result in visual compromise, and *P. aeruginosa* endocarditis is frequently found in intravenous injection drug users. In addition, there is the possibility for drug-resistant *P. aeruginosa* in the community, and this risk has to be taken into account in prescribing antibiotic therapy.

S. maltophilia, once thought to be of limited virulence, is a significant emerging pathogen.[3] It is an environmental gram-negative, multidrug-resistant organism that mainly causes pneumonia and acute exacerbation of chronic obstructive pulmonary disease. Bacteremia, urinary tract infection, skin and soft tissue infections including cellulitis, osteomyelitis, endocarditis, and meningitis are among the infections caused by *S. maltophilia*.

Once isolated in the geographic setting of Southeast Asia and Australia with an incidence of approximately 50/100,000 in the general population, infections due to *B. pseudomallei* are of special interest because they are reported now more frequently also from the Indian subcontinent.[4] Fortunately, infection due to *B. mallei* is rare in humans.

B. cepacia belongs to the *B. cepacia* complex, which includes also *B. ambifaria, B. anthina, B. arboris, B. cenocepacia, B. contaminans, B. diffusa, B. dolosa, B. latens, B. lata, B. metallica, B. multivorans, B. pseudomultivorans, B. pyrrocinia, B. seminalis, B. stabilis, B. stagnalis, B. territorri, B. ubonensis,* and *B. vietnamiensis. B. cepacia* was previously reported under the name of *P. cepacia. B. cenocepacia, B. multivorans,* and *B. cepacia* are the predominant species of the *B. cepacia* complex that infect mainly patients with CF and chronic granulomatous disease. However, there are many reports of *B. cenocepacia, B. multivorans,* and *B. cepacia* infections (and of other *B. cepacia* complex species) in hospitalized patients without CF, such as patients with central venous catheters, manipulation of the urogenital tract (catheterization, instrument insertion, and biopsy), burns, and wounds (surgical and other).

PATHOBIOLOGY

The pathologic spectrum of *P. aeruginosa* infections depends on the site afflicted. Hemorrhage and necrosis may be present in severe *Pseudomonas* infections, such as in pneumonia and endocarditis. Notably, as regards the skin in the case of ecthyma gangrenosum, bacteria invade the arteries and veins of the skin, but there is little accompanying inflammation. This is reflected in the small quantity, if any, of pus present in these skin lesions. The pathology of *B. pseudomallei* infection is in sharp contrast, with intense inflammation leading to abscess formation and necrosis in the affected organs, as in the skin, liver, spleen, or lungs.

CLINICAL MANIFESTATIONS

A constellation of manifestations is included in the clinical spectrum of *P. aeruginosa* infections. There are no symptoms or signs to effectively discriminate *P. aeruginosa* infection from infections by other pathogens. Even ecthyma gangrenosum, which was once thought to represent a unique effect of *P. aeruginosa* infection, can be caused by other bacteria, such as *S. aureus* or *Citrobacter freundii*.

Febrile Neutropenia

P. aeruginosa infections during febrile neutropenia (Chapters 158 and 265) have a cardinal role. It is the organism against which empirical coverage must always be included. This principle remains unaltered over many decades. The importance of *P. aeruginosa* infection in neutropenic patients has not diminished, and the antimicrobial resistance of the bacterium has evolved to a painstaking therapeutic challenge. Mortality is high if infection is not appropriately treated by empirical therapy. The classic clinical syndromes in febrile neutropenic patients are bacteremia, pneumonia, and soft tissue infection, mainly manifested as ecthyma gangrenosum.

Bacteremia

Bacteremia due to *P. aeruginosa* remains one of the most difficult therapeutic challenges a physician may face. It is usually caused by primary infection at different sites, such as pneumonia, urinary tract infection, complicated intra-abdominal tract infection (peritonitis, abscess), and endocarditis.

Manifestations can include those of sepsis and septic shock, that is, fever, tachycardia, tachypnea, hypotension, and mental status changes ranging from confusion to coma (Chapter 100). Multiorgan failure with adult respiratory distress syndrome and acute renal failure along with coagulation defects (disseminated intravascular coagulation) may occur. In the ventilated patient, an increased index of suspicion for *P. aeruginosa* must be present in case of clinical deterioration.

Eye Infections

Keratitis is among the most frequent type of disease seen, and it is associated with contact lens wear, especially extended-wear lenses. However, any form of trauma may predispose to keratitis by direct inoculation into tissue, including surgery and burns. *P. aeruginosa* keratitis is a medical emergency because of the speed with which it can progress and lead to loss of vision. Pain and redness of the eye are cardinal manifestations of keratitis. The entire cornea is opacified, and sometimes perforation occurs.

Endophthalmitis is another fulminant *P. aeruginosa* eye infection that may result from penetrating injuries, surgery, perforation of a corneal ulcer, or seeding from bacteremia. Severe pain, chemosis, decreased visual acuity or even loss of vision, anterior uveitis, vitreous involvement, and panophthalmitis are manifestations of endophthalmitis.

Other rarer eye infections include blepharoconjuctivitis, corneal ulcer, scleritis, and canaliculitits (both primary and plug-related). In addition, *P. aeruginosa* may lead to orbital cellulitis in neutropenic patients and gangrene necrosis of the eyelids, both of which are metastatic foci of bacteremia.

Ear Infections

Acute otitis externa presenting with otalgia (ear pain) is commonly seen in children and results from infection of moist, macerated skin of the external ear canal. The source of the organism is likely to be hot tubs or swimming pools (swimmer's ear), particularly if they are not sufficiently chlorinated. The natural history is usually resolution without sequelae, but chronic drainage occurs in some patients. Chronic suppurative otitis media has been associated with *P. aeruginosa*. The main clinical manifestation is drainage of fluid. Cultures are usually polymicrobial, including *P. aeruginosa*. In a third of patients, it is found in isolation.

One of the most dramatic clinical manifestations of *Pseudomonas* infections is malignant otitis externa.[5] The diagnosis is made easily as long as there is a high index of suspicion, which should be the case in diabetics and patients with AIDS. Although literally a misnomer (because this is not a cancerous process), the fulminant evolution to death if it is not diagnosed and treated appropriately justifies this nomenclature. It usually afflicts the diabetic patient and is manifested with pain in the ear accompanied by fever (not always), drainage, and nerve palsies that may even be bilateral. Traction of the pinna will elicit pain in the majority of patients. Most commonly, cranial nerves VI to XII (in various combinations) may be involved, and thus hoarseness and dysphagia accompanying facial paralysis may be evident. Mental status may be affected (obtundation, coma) and signifies intracranial spread of the infection. A characteristic of the disease is the presence of granulation tissue at the junction of bone and cartilage in the meatus, in contrast with the generally intact tympanic membrane. Culture specimens should be taken from the external auditory canal. Computed tomography or magnetic resonance imaging findings include temporomandibular joint destruction, infratemporal fossa or nasopharyngeal soft tissue involvement, and evidence of meningitis or empyema.

Other types of ear infection include acute otitis media, chronic suppurative otitis media, perichondritis, and acute mastoiditis with its complications.

Acute Respiratory Tract Infections

The respiratory tract is among the most frequent sites of infection due to *P. aeruginosa*. This organism is a well-established and frequent cause of ventilator-associated pneumonia (VAP) and hospital-associated pneumonia.[6] The clinical manifestations may include fever, cough, production of purulent sputum, crackles, rhonchi, central cyanosis, tachypnea, use of accessory respiratory muscles, signs of septic shock, and multiorgan failure but cannot differentiate infection due to *P. aeruginosa* from other microorganisms as the pathogen. Identification of the bacterium can be based on culture of endotracheal tube aspirates as well as bronchoalveolar lavage fluid or even blood culture in the corresponding clinical setting. Ventilator-associated tracheobronchitis is usually far from innocuous, and treatment is needed to avoid progression to the more severe VAP. Obviously, for the ventilated patient, discontinuation of mechanical ventilation when feasible is a key management issue.

Pneumonia due to *P. aeruginosa* can also be community-acquired, particularly in patients with underlying structural lung disease, such as patients with COPD or bronchiectasis.

Chronic Respiratory Tract Infections

P. aeruginosa is responsible for chronic infections of the airways associated mainly with cystic fibrosis (CF)[7] and chronic obstructive pulmonary disease. A description and management of *P. aeruginosa* infection in patients with CF can be found in Chapter 83. Patients with advanced chronic obstructive pulmonary disease may become infected by *P. aeruginosa* and present with an exacerbation.

Another chronic infection of the respiratory tract associated with *P. aeruginosa* is diffuse panbronchiolitis, which affects mainly Asian populations. Nevertheless, forms of this disease have also been reported in white, Hispanic, and African American patients. Criteria have been established for diagnosis of this disease[8]:
1. persistent cough, sputum, and exertional dyspnea;
2. history of chronic paranasal sinusitis;
3. bilateral diffuse small nodular shadows on a plain chest radiograph or centrilobular micronodules on chest computed tomography images;
4. coarse crackles;
5. FEV_1/FVC <70% and PaO_2 <80 mm Hg; and
6. titer of cold hemagglutinin >64.

Criteria for definite diagnosis are a compilation of criteria 1 to 3 plus two criteria from 4 to 6. *P. aeruginosa* is isolated in advanced stages of the disease. It shows similarities to CF in terms of respiratory tract involvement, but it is characterized by the lack of affliction of other systems (pancreas, genital tract). Furthermore, the amount of sputum produced is usually at least 50 to 100 mL/day, and the genetic background is different, with associations to HLA-Bw52 and HLA-A11 reported.

Bone and Joint Infections

P. aeruginosa is among the main causative pathogens of bone infections when indwelling devices or prostheses used in orthopedic surgery or neurosurgery are present. Furthermore, *P. aeruginosa* is a significant cause of bone or joint infections (Chapter 256) in patients without foreign bodies. Such infections result from bacteremia, direct inoculation into bone, or spread from contiguous infection. Bacteremia secondary to either injection of contaminated illicit drugs or infective endocarditis in the population of intravenous drug users has been well documented to cause vertebral osteomyelitis, sacroiliac septic arthritis, and septic arthritis of the sternoclavicular joint. The clinical manifestations of vertebral *P. aeruginosa* osteomyelitis are more indolent than those of staphylococcal osteomyelitis. The duration of symptoms in the addict population with vertebral osteomyelitis is generally prolonged, ranging from weeks to months. Tenderness of the affected region has to be elicited, and there may be a decreased range of motion. Low-grade fever is more likely to be encountered than the high fever associated more classically with staphylococcal osteomyelitis. It may occur with or without endocarditis, but a primary site of infection is often not found. Its causative role seems to lag behind *S. aureus* in the affliction of the sternoclavicular joint.

Pseudomonas osteomyelitis of the foot most frequently follows puncture wounds through sneakers. The bacterium has been found between the rubber sole layers of sneakers in many cases. Most of these cases are reported in children, but it is also seen in adults. The main manifestation is pain in the foot, and there may be superficial cellulitis around the puncture wound and tenderness on deep palpation of the wound. Also, a group of patients that seems prone to *Pseudomonas* infections of bone and joints are those with Charcot arthropathy (neuropathic joint). Prolonged hospital stay and more surgical operations are associated with *P. aeruginosa* secondary bone infection in patients with Charcot arthropathy. *P. aeruginosa* also has the potential to cause bone and joint infections in patients with diabetic foot infections, especially when there is high local prevalence of the bacterium, warm climate, and frequent exposure to moisture.

Central Nervous System Infections

Involvement of the central nervous system is almost always secondary to a surgical procedure or penetrating head trauma and is rare after bacteremia. The entities seen most often are postoperative or post-traumatic meningitis, subdural empyema, and epidural infections resulting from initial contamination of access areas. Brain abscess secondary to embolic disease from endocarditis may be seen. Extension of the infection in necrotizing malignant otitis to the brain heralds an ominous clinical course. The cerebrospinal fluid profile of *P. aeruginosa* meningitis is that of pyogenic meningitis. Brain abscess and epidural and subdural empyema generally require surgical drainage in addition to antibiotics.

Urinary and Genital Tract Infections

P. aeruginosa urinary tract infections (cystitis, pyelonephritis, renal/perirenal abscess) usually occur as a complication of the presence of a foreign body, such as a catheter or stent in the urinary tract or an obstruction (mainly stone or malignant neoplasm) of the urinary system, or after instrumentation or surgery in the urinary tract. Notwithstanding the relationship between obstructive lesions and *P. aeruginosa* urinary tract infections, there have been descriptions of *P. aeruginosa* urinary tract infections in outpatient children and adults without relevant foreign bodies, stones, or other causes of evident obstruction. *P. aeruginosa* urinary tract infection frequently is associated with bacteremia. Genital tract infections due to *P. aeruginosa* include epididymitis, orchitis, epididymo-orchitis (with or without abscess), and prostatitis (with or without abscess).

Skin and Soft Tissue Infections, Including Burns

P. aeruginosa causes a variety of skin manifestations, including ecthyma gangrenosum in neutropenic patients. These are small, round lesions that occur either isolated or as aggregates. There is no skin site that is spared of their presence. More commonly, the limbs and the perineum are affected. The mouth may be involved as well. There is an evolution from vesicles to nodules that become hemorrhagic and necrotic and eventually ulcerate. Thus, they best fit in the vesiculonodular type of skin lesion description. Indeed, this evolution may lead to a spectacular increase from less than 1 to more than 10 cm in a period of less than 24 hours. One must not assume that ecthyma is only caused by *P. aeruginosa* as was thought in the past. This type of skin involvement can also be caused by other gram-positive or gram-negative bacteria (*S. aureus*, *S. pyogenes*, *Aeromonas* spp, *Serratia* spp, *S. maltophilia*) or fungi (*Candida* spp, *Aspergillus* spp, *Mucor* spp, and *Fusarium* spp).

Maceration of normal skin, such as from soaking in a hot tub, can lead to superficial infection and then potentially to soft tissue infection and even hematogenous dissemination. Folliculitis and other papular or vesicular lesions have also been attributed to *P. aeruginosa*. Other types of skin and soft tissue involvement are cellulitis, abscesses, toe web infection (webspace intertrigo), paronychia usually in association with green nail syndrome, and myositis. Secondary infection of chronic skin ulcers can also occur.

Burn wound infections by *P. aeruginosa* constitute one of the most significant problems caused by this organism. A distinct clinical picture of sepsis, in which high colony counts of *P. aeruginosa* exceed 10^5 organisms per gram of tissue, is the defining feature. Patients generally exhibit the progressive formation of a black necrotic eschar, with or without bacteremia. *P. aeruginosa* remains a major pathogen in settings in which burn patients have high rates of infection. The diagnosis may be made by culture of blood or by the pathognomonic clinical picture of an expanding burn lesion caused by infection with *P. aeruginosa*. Wound infection can also occur in pressure ulcers and surgical sites.

Endovascular Infections

P. aeruginosa may cause endovascular infections, including infective endocarditis mainly of native valves but also of prosthetic ones. Mycotic aneurysms may occur in the setting of endocarditis. In intravenous drug users, the source is generally contaminated material, needles, or other paraphernalia; in this population, *P. aeruginosa* may even lead to outbreaks of endocarditis. The manifestations of *P. aeruginosa* endocarditis resemble those of other forms of acute endocarditis in addicts except that it appears to be more indolent than *S. aureus* endocarditis. *P. aeruginosa* endocarditis occurs also in non–intravenous injection drug users. *P. aeruginosa* may also lead to septic thrombophlebitis.

Complicated Intra-abdominal Infections

P. aeruginosa is a pathogen involved in complicated intra-abdominal infections, usually as part of a polymicrobial infection. It is recovered in cases of secondary peritonitis, tertiary peritonitis, peritonitis associated with continuous ambulatory peritoneal dialysis, spontaneous bacterial peritonitis, and intra-abdominal abscesses.

Gastrointestinal Infections

Gastrointestinal infections due to *P. aeruginosa* include necrotizing enterocolitis in children and typhlitis in neutropenic patients (neutropenic enterocolitis).

Uncommon *P. aeruginosa* Infections

P. aeruginosa can cause a number of infrequently seen syndromes: noma neonatorum, a necrotizing mucosal and perianal infection of newborns; toe web infections; the "green nail syndrome" caused by *P. aeruginosa* paronychia as a result of diffusion of pyocyanin into the nail bed; and *Pseudomonas* hot-foot syndrome, which is manifested with tender plantar nodules. Shanghai fever is a sporadic community-acquired disease of previously healthy infants that is manifested as a necrotizing enteritis with fever and diarrhea and may lead to bowel perforation, seizures, and ecthyma gangrenosum. Laboratory parameters include leukopenia, thrombocytopenia, high C-reactive protein levels, coagulopathy, and hypoalbuminemia. The mortality is approximately 15%.

Infection due to *Pseudomonas* spp Other than *P. aeruginosa*

Infection due to other *Pseudomonas* spp may occur. *P. fluorescens* may lead to bacteremia associated with central venous catheters or transfusion-related bacteremia. Notably, a multistate outbreak due to contaminated heparinized saline flush occurred in the United States. Reports of *P. stutzeri* infections include peritonitis, meningitis, endocarditis, pneumonia, bacteremia, and endophthalmitis. *P. putida* has been reported as a causative pathogen in bacteremia, pneumonia, cholecystitis, cholangitis, and skin and soft tissue infections.

DIAGNOSIS

Diagnosis of *P. aeruginosa* rests on the culture of the pathogen from various human biologic samples or fluids (blood, urine, sputum, bronchoalveolar lavage, pleural, cerebrospinal fluid, wound, burn, pus) pertinent to the clinical presentation. A helpful interim pointer to the causative role of *P. aeruginosa* may be a consistent Gram stain performed in the pertinent biologic fluid or sample, pending the results of the corresponding culture. The usual investigational approach is followed initially to document the site(s)-specific infection coupled with the documentation of the bacterium on culture. For example, three sets of blood cultures in the time span of one hour and expeditious use of echocardiography are recommended for the diagnosis of endocarditis.[9] Computerized tomography of the brain, chest, abdomen, pelvis or magnetic resonance imaging of the brain, spine, or particular bony area, and transesophageal echocardiography are used to document the presence of infection but cannot corroborate *P. aeruginosa* as the potential pathogen. Currently, endotracheal aspiration with semiquantitative cultures to diagnose VAP is suggested rather than invasive sampling (performing bronchoscopy for bronchoalveolar lavage or obtaining samples through a protected specimen brush or blind bronchial sampling [mini-BAL]). In the setting of osteomyelitis, the acquisition of bone through fine-needle aspiration guided by CT or bone biopsy and culture through open biopsy may be necessary if blood cultures are sterile. Newer methods, including multiplex polymerase chain reaction tests, which are based on the detection of the bacterial DNA, have received clearance from the Food and Drug Administration (FDA) for use in clinical practice. They are especially of value in the setting of the intensive care unit, where speed is important in decreasing the mortality associated with delay in treatment of sepsis. Serology is not helpful in the diagnosis of *P. aeruginosa* infections. Pulsed-field gel electrophoresis, restriction fragment length polymorphism, multilocus sequence typing, and random amplified polymorphic DNA polymerase chain reaction are used mainly for epidemiologic purposes. The differential diagnosis lies between *P. aeruginosa* and pathogens that can lead to the same spectrum of diseases, especially in the hospital environment. External otitis, infection after a nail injury, or infection after immersion in water can provide some important clues that narrow the differential diagnosis spectrum in their respective settings. Nevertheless, diagnostic considerations have to include other pathogens as well. For example, fungal otitis has to be included in the differential diagnosis of external otitis as well as of other causes of earache.

In addition, the specific population of patients (e.g., neutropenic patients, patients with burns and wounds, CF patients, patients who have medically inserted equipment or foreign bodies) should be considered to have a high pretest probability of having a *P. aeruginosa* infection. Other types of infection in the hospital environment necessitate coverage for *Pseudomonas* until microbiologic data are available either from cultures or from molecular tests detecting the bacterium's DNA. A de-escalation protocol can then be performed to narrow the antibiotic spectrum.

At times, clinical acumen has to differentiate frank infection due to *P. aeruginosa* from colonization mainly on the basis of local symptoms and signs (pain, erythema, necrosis, exudate, edema, loss of function, dysuria, productive cough) or systemic symptoms and signs (fever, hypotension, tachycardia, dyspnea, hypoxia, rash, organ failure, radiologic change of previous imaging) of infection.

TREATMENT Rx

Treatment of *P. aeruginosa* Bacteremia

Guidelines from the Surviving Sepsis Campaign for patients with severe infections associated with respiratory failure and septic shock suggest combination therapy.[10] For the case of *P. aeruginosa* bacteremia this would include, for example, an antipseudomonal β-lactam and either an aminoglycoside or a fluoroquinolone. Nevertheless, combination therapy should not be routinely used for ongoing treatment of most other serious infections, including bacteremia and sepsis without shock or routinely for neutropenic sepsis/bacteremia. Time is of utmost importance and antibiotics should be commenced within an hour in the treatment of sepsis and septic shock. Current guidelines advise de-escalation in response to clinical improvement or infection resolution within the first few days (not specified currently but this was determined as 3 to 5 days in previous guidelines). De-escalation to the most appropriate single-agent therapy should be performed as soon as the susceptibility profile is known or clinical improvement is noted. Indeed, evidence-based data from meta-analyses suggest that a combination may not provide an advantage in terms of clinical outcomes, such as cure of the infection, or less emergence of resistance. Furthermore, a combination of a β-lactam and an aminoglycoside carries a higher rate of nephrotoxicity. There is therefore currently a trend that a β-lactam/β-lactamase inhibitor (piperacillin-tazobactam) or an antipseudomonal carbapenem (meropenem or imipenem-cilastatin) may be used alone as monotherapy without compromising patient outcomes. Nevertheless, monotherapy with an aminoglycoside or a quinolone is not suggested for the treatment of bacteremia because it is associated with poor clinical outcomes. Local in vitro antimicrobial susceptibility data regarding the level of resistance of local clinical isolates of *P. aeruginosa* to various antibiotics have to be taken into consideration.[11] The total duration of treatment of bacteremia was usually considered to be approximately 14 days in the non-neutropenic patient. However, the current guidelines for most serious infections associated with sepsis and septic shock recommend that 7 to 10 days are adequate in addition to source control for most infections (not applicable for endocarditis, osteomyelitis, abscesses of the brain or kidney), whereas longer courses are appropriate for patients with undrainable foci of infection, immunologic deficiencies including neutropenia, and patients with slow clinical resolution. Bacteremia in the non-neutropenic patient may be secondary to the presence of a central venous catheter or the presence of infection elsewhere (e.g., in the lungs, urinary tract, or cardiac valves). Removal of an infected central venous catheter may be necessary in addition to the systemic antibiotics provided for the treatment of bacteremia, while the duration of treatment of endocarditis should be protracted to reach 6 weeks in addition to potential cardiothoracic surgery. In the neutropenic patient at least 14 days are necessary and antibiotics are to be continued until the absolute neutrophil count is equal to or greater than 500 cells/μL. Bacteremia in the neutropenic patient may necessitate prolonged treatment of 4 to 6 weeks in the presence of endocarditis, deep-seated infection, septic thrombosis, or persistent bacteremia occurring more than 72 hours after catheter removal on appropriate antibiotics.

Removal of an infected vascular catheter or another infected foreign device (urinary catheter, implant) may be needed to control device-related infection due to *P. aeruginosa*. Source control of an infection nidus (drainage of an abscess or empyema, excision of necrotic tissue) is also of paramount significance.

Depending on the antibiotic susceptibility of *P. aeruginosa* isolates routinely found in a specific setting, one of the following regimens would be appropriate for *P. aeruginosa* bacteremia, provided renal function as assessed by creatinine clearance is relatively normal (>50 to 60 mL/minute): intravenous piperacillin-tazobactam, 3.375 to 4.5 g every 6 to 8 hours; ceftazidime, 2 g every 8 hours; cefepime, 2 g every 8 to 12 hours; meropenem, 1 to 2 g every 8 hours; imipenem, 0.5 to 1 g every 6 hours; doripenem, 0.5 g (1-hour infusion) every 8 hours; or aztreonam, 1.5 to 2 g every 6 to 8 hours (aztreonam has been used mainly for patients with β-lactam allergy). The addition of an aminoglycoside to the other regimens depends on the level of resistance to β-lactam antibiotics seen at any given institution. If administration of a second drug is indicated, amikacin 15 mg/kg every 24 hours may be added to the β-lactam antibiotic therapy. Addition of ciprofloxacin 400 mg every 8 to 12 hours IV (instead of an aminoglycoside) has been suggested to fare equally well.

Antibiotics that have to be considered if resistance to carbapenems with antipseudomonal spectrum is encountered include colistimethate sodium (polymyxin E or colistin parenteral form)[1] and polymyxin B. Two forms of colistin are commercially available: colistin sulfate and colistimethate sodium (also called colistin methanesulfonate, pentasodium colistimethanesulfate, and colistin sulfonyl methate). Colistimethate sodium is less potent than colistin sulfate. Colistin sulfate is administered orally (tablets or syrup) in bowel decontamination regimens and topically as a powder for the treatment of bacterial skin infections. Colistimethate sodium is available in parenteral formulations. The term *colistin* throughout this chapter refers to the formulation of colistimethate sodium, except if otherwise specified.

The suggested dosage of intravenous colistin for adult patients with normal renal function is different for manufacturers in the United States and the United Kingdom. Specifically, recommended dosage in the United States is 2.5 to 5 mg/kg/day of colistin base activity (75,000 to 150,000 IU/kg), divided into two to four equal doses (1 mg of colistin base activity, ≅30,000 IU; 1 mg of colistimethate sodium activity, ≈12,500 IU). However, further studies are needed to better clarify the appropriate dosing regimens of colistin, especially for patients with renal dysfunction or failure.

According to a colistimethate sodium (colistin) package insert in Europe, the following dosing recommendations are made: 9,000,000 international units (IU) daily in two to three divided doses, if creatinine clearance is above 50 mL per minute. In critically ill patients, a loading dose of 9,000,000 IU, followed by the maintenance dose of 4,500,000 IU every 12 hours daily. The interval from the loading dose until starting of the maintenance dose is not clarified by the manufacturer; it has been suggested to be 12 to 24 hours after the loading dose by an international consensus meeting. The following adjustment are suggested according to the package insert: for a creatinine clearance (CC) less than 10 mL per min: 3,500,000 IU daily in two divided doses administered 12 hours apart, CC 10 to less than 30 mL/min: 4,500,000 to 5,500,000 IU daily in two divided doses, CC 30 to less than 50 mL/min: 5,500,000 to 7,500,000 IU daily. Patients on hemodialysis: on days of hemodialysis 3,000,000 IU after the hemodialysis session. On days without hemodialysis sessions: 2,250,000 IU daily in two divided doses.

Recently, the following recommendations for the dosing of colistin methanesulfonate have been made by an international consensus meeting endorsed by various scientific societies (amongst others the American College of Clinical Pharmacists, Infectious Diseases of America, Society of Critical Care Medicine)[12]: for a creatinine clearance (CC) 70 to less than 80 mL/min: 9,000,000 (nine million) IU per day in two divided doses, administered 12 hours apart and infused over 30 to 60 minutes, CC of 60 to less than 70 mL/min: 8,350,000 IU daily in two divided doses, CC of 50 to less than 60 mL/min:7,400,000 IU daily in two divided doses, CC 40 to less than 50 mL per minute: 6,650,000 IU daily in two divided doses, 30 to less than 40 mL: 5,900,000 IU daily in two divided doses, CC 20 to less than 30: 5,300,000 IU daily in two divided doses, CC of 10 to less than 20 mL/min 4,850,000 IU daily in two divided doses, 5 to less than 10 mL/min 4,400,000 IU daily in two divided doses.

Regarding polymyxins B, according to the package insert of Polymyxin B, 15,000 to 25,000 units/kg body weight/day in individuals with normal kidney function. This amount should be reduced from 15,000 units/kg downward for individuals with kidney impairment. Infusions may be given every 12 hours and the total daily dose must not exceed 25,000 units/kg/day.

In contrast, an international consensus meeting suggests a loading dose for polymyxin B, based on total body weight (TBW) (equivalent to 20,000-25,000 IU/kg) over 1 hour. This loading dose is followed by a polymyxin B dose of 1.25 to 1.5 mg/kg (equivalent to 12,500-15,000 IU/kg TBW) every 12 hours, infused over 1 hour. Interestingly, they recommend that daily maintenance doses of polymyxin B should not be adjusted if the patient has renal impairment and propose that the package insert dose adjustment for renal impairment should be revised because it is not supported by modern pharmacokinetic data. However, the consensus concluded that larger pharmacokinetic studies in patients with renal insufficiency are needed to validate their recommendations. When dosing colistin, clinicians should be aware of the existing differences in dosage recommendations based on the specific formulation of colistin used. More recently, the parenteral formulation of fosfomycin sodium has been used in various European countries in combination with other antibiotics with an antipseudomonal spectrum.[13]

Another important consideration is the prolonged intravenous infusion of the antibiotics to exploit the pharmacodynamic properties of β-lactams in the treatment of *P. aeruginosa* and other infections. β-Lactam antibiotics have time-dependent antimicrobial activity, and thus their concentration in blood achieved by their prolonged intravenous administration is above the minimum inhibitory concentration for longer periods (proportion of the time between doses above minimum inhibitory concentration). A prolonged infusion of piperacillin-tazobactam during 4 hours may provide a survival benefit. Meropenem is usually infused in a relatively short infusion of 30 minutes; an extended meropenem infusion is one that extends to 3 hours. Doripenem should not be used in pneumonia according to an FDA warning based on a study comparing it with imipenem-cilastatin.

Despite the introduction of new broad-spectrum antibiotics in the antibiotic arsenal, one should remember that ertapenem, ceftaroline, and tigecycline do not possess antipseudomonal activity.

Treatment of Pneumonia

Patients with VAP and HAP due to *P. aeruginosa*, may have isolates resistant to many antibiotics, a problem that appears to be becoming progressively worse. Provided renal and liver function is normal, the following recommendations have been made by the Infectious Diseases Society of America and the American Thoracic Society regarding the treatment of VAP due to *P. aeruginosa* where double antipseudomonal coverage is appropriate: IV ceftazidime, 2 g every 8 hours; cefepime, 2 g every 8 to 12 hours; imipenem, 500 mg every 6 hours or 1 g every 8 hours; meropenem, 1 g every 8 hours; or piperacillin-tazobactam, 4.5 g every 6 hours or aztreonam 2 g IV q 8 hours **plus** a quinolone (levofloxacin 750 mg IV once daily **or** ciprofloxacin 400 mg IV every 8 hours) **or** an aminoglycoside (amikacin 15 to 20 mg/kg once daily, with a trough level of less than 4 to 5 μg/mL for amikacin, gentamicin 5 to 7 mg/kg IV every 24 h or tobramycin 5-7 mg/kg every 24 h) **or** a polymyxin. Dosing is based on colistin-based activity: 30 mg of colistin based activity (which corresponds to ≈80 mg of the prodrug colistimethate) is 1 million international units. In the absence of other options, use of aztreonam as an adjunct to another β-lactam is suggested for the treatment of VAP and for HAP to be acceptable because it has different targets within the bacterial wall.

For patients with VAP/HAP due to *P. aeruginosa* who are not in septic shock or at high risk for death and for whom the results of antibiotic susceptibility testing are known, current IDSA guidelines suggest monotherapy. Combination therapy is suggested for patients with shock and at high risk for death. For patients with *P. aeruginosa* who are susceptible only to polymyxins, intravenous polymyxins (colistin or polymyxin B) and inhaled colistin (administered promptly after being mixed with sterile water) are suggested.

A 7-day course of antibiotic therapy instead of 8 to 15 days is the current recommendation for VAP, depending on the rate of improvement of clinical, radiologic, and laboratory parameters. It is of particular importance that, regarding the subpopulation of VAP due to glucose non-fermenting gram-negative bacilli (that includes *P. aeruginosa*), no differences have been observed for mortality or recurrence of pneumonia compared to patients treated for a longer period.

Aminoglycosides are not optimally active in the lungs at concentrations used for intravenous administration. In contrast, the administration of aerosolized aminoglycoside may provide adequate drug levels in the tracheobronchial tree. Tobramycin (300 mg inhaled daily) and inhaled aztreonam lysine (75 mg three times daily for 28 days) have shown safety and efficacy for CF patients[A1] and have FDA approval only in patients with CF. Another antibiotic that has been used in different parts of the world, including the United States (FDA-approved for CF patients), for decades for the treatment of *P. aeruginosa* infections in patients with CF is the inhaled form of colistin. The effectiveness and safety of inhaled colistin in patients with CF has led to a revival of the use of the medication also in patients with *P. aeruginosa* infection in the critical care setting.[14] Inhaled colistin does not have FDA approval for patients without CF and is used on a compassionate basis.

Infections Caused by Organisms at One Time Classified as Pseudomonads

S. maltophilia causes a variety of organ afflictions. It is manifested as pneumonia, acute exacerbation of chronic obstructive pulmonary disease, bacteremia, soft tissue and skin infection, cellulitis, myositis, osteomyelitis, catheter-related bacteremia or septicemia, meningitis, endophthalmitis, keratitis, scleritis, dacryocystitis, endocarditis, urinary tract infection, and biliary sepsis. Whereas it has been regarded as a rare pathogen in the past, this is changing. Indeed, it is the 11th most frequently cultured microorganism in a U.S. multiple hospital study covering 1993 to 2004 (4.3% of 74,934 gram-negative bacilli). Furthermore, the prevalence of *S. maltophilia* in patients with CF has increased in a relevant study from 6 to 12.7% from 1995 to 2008. Selective media (vancomycin–imipenem–amphotericin B, gram-negative selective agar, BTB, and SM2i) have been developed to ease detection of *S. maltophilia*, especially because the pathogen is frequently co-cultured in samples of polymicrobial infections. Polymerase chain reaction amplification of 16 rRNA in blood has also been used.

TREATMENT ℞

The bacterium is usually susceptible to trimethoprim-sulfamethoxazole [TMP/SMX] (15 to 20 mg/kg/day trimethoprim component IV in 3 to 4 divided doses), which is regarded as the first-choice antibiotic. However, resistant strains are emerging. Other antibiotics that have been effective (rates of in vitro antimicrobial susceptibility varies) against *S. maltophilia* isolates include ciprofloxacin (400 mg IV every 12 hours/500 to 750 mg po every 12 hours), moxifloxacin (400 mg once daily IV), levofloxacin (750 mg once daily IV), ceftazidime (2 g every 8 hours IV), ticarcillin-clavulanate (3.1 g every 4 hours), tigecycline (100 mg IV loading dose followed by 50 mg IV every 12 hours), and minocycline (100 mg IV every 12 hours); sometimes these are used in combination with trimethoprim-sulfamethoxazole. Colistin or polymyxins B have also been used. Inherent resistance to carbapenems is a notable characteristic of this bacterium.

Melioidosis is an infection due to *B. pseudomallei* and occurs mainly in Southeast Asia and Australia.[17] A notable current addition to these geographic regions is the Indian subcontinent and Sri Lanka. One should also be aware of potential niduses in the Americas (Mexico and the northern part of South America) and Africa (Madagascar). Risk factors for acquisition of melioidosis include renal failure, diabetes mellitus, heavy alcohol consumption, chronic respiratory disease, thalassemia, glucocorticoid therapy, and cancer. It can also afflict immunocompetent travelers to the regions mentioned. Interestingly, there is a seasonal association with the rainy season in more than three quarters of cases. Clinical manifestations vary from asymptomatic infection to localized skin infection, pneumonia, and fulminant sepsis due to bacteremia. The formation of abscesses is a usual feature of the disease. Other manifestations include septic arthritis, osteomyelitis, prostatitis, neurologic manifestations such as brain stem encephalitis associated with cranial nerve palsies or myelitis with peripheral motor weakness, and kidney and spleen involvement. Suppurative parotitis, even bilateral in 10%, is a feature present in patients with melioidosis in Thailand and Cambodia. Parotitis afflicts mainly children. The bacterium may remain dormant and then reactivate. The portal of entry includes the respiratory system, the skin, and the gastrointestinal system. Indeed, recurrence of melioidosis is due to reactivation in approximately three quarters of cases.

TREATMENT ℞

There is a need for prolonged treatment of the bacterium that entails a 10 to 14 days regimen of intravenous antibiotic administration: ceftazidime, 2 g every 8 hours; meropenem, 1 g every 8 hours; or imipenem, 1 g every 6 hours. A switch from ceftazidime treatment to meropenem is warranted if the patient develops organ failure or a new focus of infection, or blood cultures remain positive at one week of treatment. In cases of ongoing septic shock, deep-seated or organ abscesses, extensive pulmonary disease, osteomyelitis, septic arthritis, melioidosis with neurologic manifestations, prolongation of this parenteral regimen to 4 or more weeks may be necessary. An extended course of oral eradication with TMP/SMX (first choice) for 12 to 20 weeks is necessary after initial intravenous antibiotics.[A2] The optimum duration for oral eradication is yet to be established. The dose of TMP/SMX is weight dependent: for patients more than 60 kg, 320 mg TMP/1600 mg SMX twice daily; for patients with weight from 40 to 60 kg, 240 mg TMP/1200 mg SMX every 12 hours; and for patients with a weight less than 40 kg, 160 mg TMP/800 mg SMX every 12 hours. In the case of allergy or adverse events, amoxicillin-clavulanate and doxycycline have been proposed as alternatives (second choice) to trimethoprim-sulfamethoxazole. The dose of amoxicillin/clavulanate is weight dependent: for patients 60 kg or more, three 500/125 mg tablets three times daily; and for patients less than 60 kg, two 500/125 mg tablets three times daily. Of note, *B. pseudomallei* is a bioterrorism factor B, and thus appropriate infection control and notification of authorities are mandatory. Postexposure prophylaxis may be necessary in this context with TMP/SMX or amoxicillin/clavulanate. Doses for TMP/SMX and for amoxicillin/clavulanate for postexposure prophylaxis are the same as those suggested for oral eradication treatment mentioned above but for a duration of only 3 weeks.

Glanders is an equine infection due to *B. mallei*. Humans acquire the disease from contact with horses or more rarely donkeys or mules in an occupational setting. It mainly is manifested with tracheobronchitis, pneumonia, skin lesions, or lymphadenopathy. The disease has been eradicated in many countries. Nevertheless, cases can occur especially in association with an occupational risk in veterinarians, veterinary students, farriers (hoof care workers), flayers (hide workers), transport workers, soldiers, slaughterhouse personnel, farmers, and horse fanciers. *B. mallei* remains a significant cause of zoonosis, and therefore appropriate veterinary surveillance is necessary, especially because *B. mallei* is also a significant bioterrorism agent (class B). Treatment of glanders in humans is based on limited data.

TREATMENT ℞

The approach to treatment is similar to that used for melioidosis, with intravenous meropenem, imipenem, or ceftazidime initially and then oral trimethoprim-sulfamethoxazole for 3 to 12 months.

B. cepacia is a plant and human pathogen. Its classification has evolved, as has its name. It was previously known as *P. cepacia* and then *Xanthomonas cepacia*. *B. cenocepacia*, *B. multivorans*, and *B. cepacia* belong to the *B. cepacia* complex and area pathogens mainly of patients with CF, chronic granulomatous disease, sickle cell disease, patients with burns, patients with bronchiectasis, and patients with malignancy. *B. cepacia complex* is implicated in infections of the lung, blood, and other sites in immunocompromised patients and even in immunocompetent patients and children in the hospital environment due to outbreaks. Aerosolized medications, chlorhexidine solutions, napkins, and prefabricated clothes along with horizontal transmission have led to significant morbidity and mortality. Patients with CF typically present initially with asymptomatic carriage. Nevertheless, pneumonia and progressive decline of lung function is associated with *B. cepacia* complex infections in patients with CF. The most dramatic presentation of the lung ailment is the cepacia syndrome, a fulminant necrotizing pneumonia often accompanied by bacteremia. Other types of infection include meningitis, endophthalmitis, pericarditis, endocarditis, burn wound infection, cholangitis, peritonitis, abscesses in the abdomen, perineum, or scrotum, and post-lung transplant pneumonia.

TREATMENT   Rx

High-quality data in the literature regarding the treatment of *B. cepacia* complex infections are scarce and suggested empiric treatment is further hampered by the variable antimicrobial resistance of the bacterium. Trimethoprim-sulfamethoxazole (10 to 15 mg/kg/day based on trimethoprim component) has been considered as first-line treatment (note that there are *B. cepacia* complex isolates resistant to TMP/SMX), but other first-line options are meropenem (1 to 2 g every 8 hours) or ceftazidime (2 g every 8 hours). Second-line options include minocycline (100 mg IV every 12 hours), ciprofloxacin, ticarcillin/clavulanate, and piperacillin/tazobactam. Although ciprofloxacin has also been used in the treatment of *B. cepacia* complex infections, the European Committee on Antimicrobial Susceptibility Testing (EUCAST) reports *B. cepacia* to be inherently resistant to ciprofloxacin. Furthermore, the Clinical and Laboratory Standards Institute reports intrinsic resistance to piperacillin/tazobactam and EUCAST reports intrinsic resistance for ticarcillin/clavulanate. Because of the variable resistance of *B. cepacia* complex, combinations of first- and second-line antibiotics (dual or even triple combinations) have been used for the treatment of critically ill patients.

PREVENTION

Primary prevention of *Pseudomonas* infections includes preventing pollution of water by *Pseudomonas*. This applies to both the public environment and the hospital environment. Outbreaks have been linked to aquatic environments such as whirlpools, swimming pools, and spas. Thus, control of growth of this organism in the recreational environment by proper antibacterial treatment of water is essential, comparable to the control practiced in hospitals. Contamination of various equipment and devices (i.e., breast implants, ocular implants, and sinus irrigation devices) must be avoided. Handwashing cannot be emphasized enough in the prevention of infections due to *P. aeruginosa*, *S. maltophilia*, and *B. cepacia*. Hospital point-of-use water filtration has also been employed in the battle against *P. aeruginosa* and *S. maltophilia* infections. Barrier nursing practices may decrease horizontal transmission, especially in the critical care environment. Isolation of patients infected with extensively drug-resistant and pandrug-resistant *P. aeruginosa* and strict infection control measures (dedicated personnel and equipment, use of gowns and gloves) may be needed to avoid intrahospital spread. Nevertheless, even antiseptic solutions may be contaminated by *P. aeruginosa*, *S. maltophilia*, and *B. cepacia*. Factors that shorten hospital length of stay and decrease the use of antibiotics are likely to decrease the incidence of these infections.

PROGNOSIS

P. aeruginosa infections carry a high mortality, even with treatment. Mortality rates of 30% have been reported for *P. aeruginosa* bacteremia.[18] Differences also exist between appropriately and inappropriately treated *P. aeruginosa* infections, with mortality rates even double when inappropriate antibiotics are used (usually for multidrug-resistant strains). Furthermore, *P. aeruginosa* infections are associated with increased length of hospitalization and medical costs. Loss of vision is the grave outcome of ophthalmic infection. Antibiotic resistance associated with *P. aeruginosa* will most likely continue to pose an enormous burden on human lives and financial resources in years to come.

S. maltophilia infections are associated with attributable mortality of up to about 37% if they are not appropriately treated. Melioidosis is associated with a 14% mortality rate in Australia and up to 40% in countries in Southeast Asia when it is treated. Fortunately, reports of glanders are rare in humans. Mortality of glanders with treatment is about 40 to 50%. *B. cepacia* has a predilection for CF patients and often signals impaired overall prognosis in these patients. Furthermore, *B. cepacia* seems to adversely affect transplantation. Indeed, in patients presenting with the cepacia syndrome, survival is unusual. Furthermore, many transplant centers do not support transplantation when *B. cepacia* is present because of the grave prognosis associated with the infection in the post-transplantation period.

Grade A References

A1. Smith S, Rowbotham NJ, Regan KH. Inhaled anti-pseudomonal antibiotics for long-term therapy in cystic fibrosis. *Cochrane Database Syst Rev*. 2018;3:CD001021.
A2. Chetchotisakd P, Chierakul W, Chaowagul W, et al. Trimethoprim-sulfamethoxazole versus trimethoprim-sulfamethoxazole plus doxycycline as oral eradicative treatment for melioidosis (MERTH): a multicentre, double-blind, non-inferiority, randomised controlled trial. *Lancet*. 2014;383:807-814.

GENERAL REFERENCES

For the General References and other additional features, please visit Expert Consult at https://expertconsult.inkling.com.

291

DISEASES CAUSED BY *ACINETOBACTER* AND *STENOTROPHOMONAS* SPECIES

KEITH S. KAYE AND ROBERT A. BONOMO

 ACINETOBACTER SPP

DEFINITION

The Pathogen

Acinetobacter species are gram-negative aerobic bacteria that are coccobacillary in shape and are generally described as aerobic, non–lactose-fermenting, non-fastidious, nonmotile, catalase positive, and oxidase negative. Unique among microbial pathogens, the appearance of *Acinetobacter* species visualized with a Gram stain is highly dependent on the life cycle. In the early growth phases, *Acinetobacter* spp appear rod shaped. In the stationary phase, they acquire a coccobacillary *Acinetobacter* spp morphology. Their description of being "nonmotile" is seriously being questioned.

In the context of this chapter, *Acinetobacter* spp refers specifically to *A. baumannii* and *A. baumannii-calcoaceticus* complex. A representative list of *Acinetobacter* species is provided in E-Table 291-1. Molecular methods used to identify and to classify *Acinetobacter* are listed in E-Table 291-2.

EPIDEMIOLOGY

Acinetobacter spp can colonize many body surfaces and cause infection in almost any organ system.[1] Consequently, there are a number of common clinical syndromes associated with infection by *Acinetobacter*. The most common infections are respiratory (pneumonia), blood stream (bacteremia), urinary tract, wound, skin and soft tissue, and burn infections; osteomyelitis secondary to trauma; and meningitis.[2] In general, infection is observed only in critically ill, immunocompromised, or injured hosts. Recently, infections by *Acinetobacter* spp are being described in patients without significant medical problems from the community setting.

During the past decade, *Acinetobacter* spp emerged in the United States from a pathogen that was primarily found in intensive care units (ICUs) to one that can affect patients in non-ICU wards, patients in long-term care settings,[3,4] and military personnel with combat injuries acquired in the Middle East. Overall, there are few distinguishing features of *Acinetobacter* spp infection except for, in some instances, skin manifestations. The frequency of *Acinetobacter* infections is often greater in the summer than in other seasons.

CLINICAL MANIFESTATIONS

Pneumonia

Because of colonization of the oropharynx and tracheostomy tubes in patients on ventilators, the upper respiratory tract is the most common site for infection by *Acinetobacter* species. The two distinct syndromes associated with respiratory tract infection due to *Acinetobacter* are community-acquired pneumonia (CAP) and health care–associated pneumonia (HCAP).[5] In tropical regions of China, Asia, Australia, and the South Pacific, CAP due to *Acinetobacter* species is increasingly recognized. In some locations, the incidence can exceed 15%. Reports have highlighted the emergence of *Acinetobacter* as a common cause of CAP in western China. In Saudi Arabia, *Acinetobacter* is the most common pathogen associated with late-onset and recurrent ventilator-associated pneumonia (VAP) in one adult ICU.

The common comorbid conditions predisposing to CAP due to *Acinetobacter* species are mainly chronic obstructive pulmonary disease (emphysema), renal disease, diabetes mellitus, and alcoholism.[6] CAP due to *Acinetobacter* species appears to be associated with a high incidence of bacteremia, acute respiratory distress syndrome, sepsis, and death (mortality rates in some reports are ≥50%). The reasons for these fulminant presentations are still unknown. Rarely, CAP due to *Acinetobacter* species can be manifested with consolidation and multiple lung abscesses.

More frequently, *Acinetobacter* spp are a cause of pneumonia in patients who have risk factors for antimicrobial resistant organisms, often manifested as VAP. In the United States, *Acinetobacter* species are a leading cause of VAP. HCAP due to *Acinetobacter* largely resembles the clinical spectrum of gram-negative pneumonias (bilateral infiltrates, pleural effusion, cavitations, hypoxemia, and bacteremia). Most cases are described in patients on ventilators. The main factors associated with HCAP due to *Acinetobacter* species are mechanical ventilation, previous antibiotic exposure, ICU stay, surgery, and underlying pulmonary disease. The major challenge complicating nosocomial pneumonia due to *Acinetobacter* species is the frequent recovery of multidrug resistant (MDR) and sometimes extensively drug resistant (XDR) strains. When isolates are MDR or XDR, the options for treatment are limited, and complications quickly arise.[7,8] HCAP due to MDR *Acinetobacter* has been associated with excess lengths of stay and mortality, although some studies have reported similar outcomes compared with control patients matched by severity of illness and duration of ICU stay.

Bacteremia

Blood stream infection due to *Acinetobacter* species is often a consequence of infection of intravenous catheters (i.e., central line–associated blood stream infection or CLABSI) or is secondary to HCAP due to *Acinetobacter*. Less commonly, wound infections can cause bacteremia. In most series, mortality associated with blood stream infection ranges from approximately 15 to greater than 50%.

Urinary Tract Infection

Urinary tract infections are most commonly caused by enteric gram-negative bacilli; only rarely are these infections caused by *Acinetobacter* species. The indwelling bladder catheter has been implicated as the major risk factor for urinary tract infection (cystitis and pyelonephritis) due to *Acinetobacter* species.

Wound, Burn, and Skin and Soft Tissue Infections

In many clinical series to date, traumatic or postoperative wounds, burns, and skin and soft tissue infections (SSTIs) are the most common causes of *Acinetobacter* infections. Most likely, the combination of antibiotic use, colonization, and compromised or devitalized tissues is responsible. The spectrum of infection can extend from cellulitis to necrotizing fasciitis.

Because of the outbreak of *A. baumannii* among military personnel in Iraq and Afghanistan, reports of severe wound infections and SSTIs caused by this pathogen are increasing in frequency. Necrotizing SSTI associated with *A. baumannii* occurs in hosts with underlying comorbidities (e.g., trauma, cirrhosis) and is often accompanied by bacteremia. *Acinetobacter* infection has become increasingly common among patients residing in burn units, sometimes resulting in unit-wide outbreaks. Multiple drug resistance and the presence of co-pathogens frequently complicate treatment. Most cases require surgical débridement and lead to substantial mortality. In addition, the use of central venous catheters and total parenteral nutrition is more common among patients with SSTIs. *Acinetobacter* species–associated SSTIs can be manifested with a peau d'orange appearance, with overlying tiny vesicles (Fig. 291-1), and, when

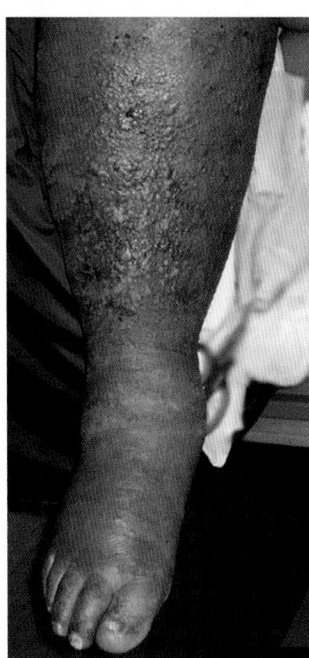

FIGURE 291-1. Cellulitis caused by *Acinetobacter baumannii*. There is characteristic edematous peau d'orange erythema, with associated vesicles that may coalesce to form nonhemorrhagic bullae. (From Guerrero DM, Perez F, Conger NG, et al. *Acinetobacter baumannii*–associated skin and soft tissue infections: recognizing a broadening spectrum of disease. *Surg Infect [Larchmt]*. 2010;11:49-57.)

untreated, can progress to necrotizing infection with bullae (hemorrhagic and nonhemorrhagic).

Osteomyelitis

The conflicts in Iraq and Afghanistan highlighted the first cases of osteomyelitis due to *Acinetobacter* species. Before this time, rare cases of osteomyelitis occurring in soldiers were reported during the Korean and Vietnam wars. Most of the initial reports from the Middle East described "contiguous focus" osteomyelitis. These patients had open fractures or exposed bone, with gross findings of infection: purulence, necrotic tissue, or environmental contamination with exposed bone; temperature higher than 38° C; leukocyte count greater than 12,000/μL; and *Acinetobacter* species identified from culture of deep wound tissue obtained intraoperatively. Frequently, these infections require multiple surgical débridements of necrotic bone.

Meningitis

Acinetobacter meningitis is occasionally found in the post-neurosurgical setting, with mortality exceeding 15 to 30%. Infection often involves intraventricular catheters.[9] Although *Acinetobacter* is an uncommon cause of meningitis from the community, the frequency is greater in cases of hospital-acquired meningitis, particularly among patients with meningitis involving an indwelling intraventricular catheter.

DIAGNOSIS

There are now more than 50 different species in the genus *Acinetobacter*, and their classification and identification remain problematic for clinicians. Automated and biochemical systems are sometimes inaccurate for the identification of *Acinetobacter* species. The introduction of matrix-assisted laser desorption/ionization time-of-flight into the clinical laboratory may facilitate better diagnosis.

TREATMENT   Rx

An increasing number of strains of *Acinetobacter* species are resistant to all antibiotics, and these strains are often responsible for outbreaks in large hospitals. These multidrug-resistant (MDR) or extremely drug-resistant (XDR) strains are resistant to three or more classes of antibiotics. Among the resistance genes found in *Acinetobacter* species are a large collection of genes encoding β-lactamases, aminoglycoside-modifying enzymes, and many efflux pumps. Even more concerning is the emergence of XDR strains of *Acinetobacter* that are resistant to carbapenems[10] and sulbactam, leaving few treatment options.

Unfortunately, resistance to "last-line" agents, such as the cationic antimicrobial peptides colistin (polymyxin E)[11] and its close relative polymyxin B, also occurs. Regrettably, colistin resistance is becoming more common as clinicians are forced to use this agent more frequently. In hospital environments, *Acinetobacter* species can withstand drying (desiccation) and may even be transmitted by aerosol/respiratory droplet. Combined with drug resistance, these characteristics create a formidable infection control challenge.

Increasing resistance to a variety of antimicrobial agents complicates the treatment of *Acinetobacter* species infections. In general, infections due to more resistant strains of *Acinetobacter* are associated with less favorable outcomes than are infections due to more susceptible strains. These worse outcomes are likely due in part to limited and suboptimal treatment options as well as delays in the time to implementation of effective antimicrobial therapy for patients with infections due to MDR and XDR *Acinetobacter* strains.

The treatment doses that follow all assume normal renal function; doses need to be adjusted based on the degree of renal insufficiency. When it is "susceptible," *Acinetobacter* is usually treated with sulbactam or a carbapenem. A commonly used dose of sulbactam (in the formulation of ampicillin-sulbactam in the United States) is 3 g IV every 6 hours. Some experts recommend a higher dose of ampicillin-sulbactam (3 g IV every 4 hours). Commonly used carbapenem regimens include imipenem 500 to 1000 mg IV every 6 hours or meropenem 500 to 1000 mg IV every 8 hours. Some experts recommend that higher doses of meropenem be used (1 g IV every 6 hours or 2 g IV every 8 hours). One must be cautious: susceptibility to imipenem does not always translate to susceptibility to meropenem, and susceptibility to ceftazidime does not always indicate that cefepime can be used. Aminoglycosides are an option for treatment of urinary tract infection and potentially for systemic infections. Unfortunately, the presence of ribosomal methyl transferases limits the use of plazomicin.

Treatment of infection with XDR *Acinetobacter* is challenging.[12] Tigecycline (100 mg loading dose, then 50 mg IV every 12 hours) and minocycline (200 mg IV or PO initially, followed by 100 mg IV or PO every 12 hours) have good in vitro activity against many strains of XDR *Acinetobacter*. Some experts recommend higher maintenance dosages of tigecycline (100 mg IV every 12 hours) and minocycline (200 mg IV or PO every 12 hours). These agents are appropriate for treatment of SSTI, but because of low serum concentrations and lack of clinical experience in the treatment of MDR and XDR *Acinetobacter*, monotherapy with these should for the most part be avoided for invasive infections such as bacteremia and pneumonia. Sometimes, there is no choice but to use tigecycline as it might be the only available agent with in vitro activity against infecting *Acinetobacter* strains. Eravacycline, a new synthetic fluorocycline, may have a role against *Acinetobacter* spp as MICs are better.

Invasive infections due to XDR strains, such as bacteremia, pneumonia, and deep wound infections, are often treated with a polymyxin antimicrobial, either colistimethate sodium (CMS, often referred to as colistin) or polymyxin B. If CMS is used, a loading dose of 300 mg colistin base activity should be administered, followed by maintenance dosing of 150 to 180 mg colistin base activity every 12 hours with subsequent renal dose adjustments made according to published guidelines.[13] If polymyxin B is used, a loading dose of 2.5 mg/kg × 1 should be administered intravenously, followed by a dose of 2.5 to 3.0 mg/kg/day by continuous IV infusion or in divided doses every 12 hours infused over a period of 60 minutes.[14]

Clinicians often treat invasive infections due to XDR *Acinetobacter* with combination therapy, although there is a lack of prospective controlled data demonstrating the superiority of combination therapy. Agents often combined with the polymyxins include rifampin (10 mg/kg/day, not to exceed 600 mg), imipenem or meropenem, sulbactam (ampicillin-sulbactam), tigecycline or minocycline, and aminoglycosides. In controlled trials, however, neither rifampin nor meropenem added measurable clinical benefit over colistin monotherapy for the treatment of serious infection due to MDR or XDR *Acinetobacter*.[A1][A2] The role of combination therapy in preventing the emergence of polymyxin resistance during therapy remains uncertain. A prospective clinical trial which included genotypic analysis of infecting *Acinetobacter* strains would be necessary to address the impact of combination therapy on the emergence of resistance. In addition, the benefit of aerosolized colistin has not yet been established.

The major adverse effect of polymyxin therapy is nephrotoxicity.[15] Current advances have improved our understanding of the pharmacokinetics, pharmacodynamics, and dosing of the polymyxins, but this is still an emerging and changing field. There is promising interest in the use of antioxidants (e.g., ascorbic acid) to prevent nephrotoxicity, but adequately powered randomized controlled studies have not been performed.

In cases of meningitis due to *Acinetobacter* species, treatment should be intravenous meropenem (2000 mg every 8 hours) plus the intraventricular/intrathecal administration of an aminoglycoside (gentamicin or amikacin, depending on susceptibilities). Intraventricular/intrathecal gentamicin is administered at a dose of 4 mg once daily every 1 to 3 days until clinical and microbiologic improvement occurs. Amikacin can be used in place of gentamicin at the dose of 30 mg once a day, if required. For cases of meningitis due to XDR *Acinetobacter*, intravenous colistin or polymyxin B should be supplemented with intraventricular or intrathecal administration of colistin 10 mg/day, or polymyxin B 5 to 10 mg/day.

PREVENTION

Infection prevention practices, including hand hygiene, use of contact precautions, maintenance of environmental cleanliness, and implementation of antimicrobial stewardship, can help prevent spread of *Acinetobacter* in the hospital. During outbreaks, cohorting of patients and use of dedicated staff to care for cohorted patients might be necessary to control spread. Removal of indwelling devices from patients, including vascular catheters and endotracheal tubes, can help prevent colonization and infection with *Acinetobacter*.

PROGNOSIS

Invasive infection due to *Acinetobacter* has been associated with crude mortality rates in excess of 50% and increases in duration of ICU stay of 6 days and duration of total hospital stay of more than 14 days, with data indicating that infection is a cause of, not a marker of, poorer prognosis.[16] Fatal *A. baumannii* infections in relatively immunocompetent patients appear to be related to clade B.[17] With appropriate early empiric therapy, however, the mortality rate for community-acquired infection can be as low as 11%.[18] By comparison, infections due to strains of MDR and XDR *Acinetobacter* are associated with increases in mortality and durations of hospitalization compared with more susceptible *Acinetobacter* strains.[19]

● *STENOTROPHOMONAS MALTOPHILIA*

DEFINITION

S. maltophilia has attracted significant attention because it is often MDR due to intrinsic and acquired factors. *S. maltophilia* contributes significantly to morbidity, but usually not mortality, in immunocompromised patients.

The Pathogen

S. maltophilia are gram-negative bacteria that need methionine for growth and, like *Pseudomonas aeruginosa* and *Acinetobacter* species, are non–lactose fermenters. *S. maltophilia* possess flagella that are multitrichous (more than one flagellum arising from the pole) and are distinguished from *P. aeruginosa* as oxidase negative. Colonies of *S. maltophilia* may appear pale yellow or lavender-green on blood agar plates. The organism emits a mild ammonia-like odor that is used for preliminary identification.

S. maltophilia can colonize inanimate surfaces in the hospital, including catheters, intravenous fluid, water supplies, and hospital equipment. This pathogen may also survive in hospital-grade disinfectant. Other health care–associated sources of *S. maltophilia* include contaminated intravenous fluids, hospital water and ice supplies, nebulizers, dialysis machines, ventilator circuits, thermometers, blood gas analyzers, intra-abdominal balloon pumps, and central venous or arterial pressure monitors.

EPIDEMIOLOGY

Despite its harboring many resistance genes, little is known about the virulence of *S. maltophilia*. Nevertheless, a number of risk factors are associated with infection by *S. maltophilia* (Table 291-1). Although *S. maltophilia* is regarded as primarily a nosocomial pathogen (it is the third most common nonfermenting gram-negative bacillus health care–associated pathogen), community-acquired infection can occur.[20] *S. maltophilia* infection primarily affects patients who are immunocompromised (including patients with hematologic malignant

TABLE 291-1	RISK FACTORS FOR INFECTION BY *STENOTROPHOMONAS MALTOPHILIA*

Prolonged hospitalization or intensive care unit stay
Intravascular catheters
Indwelling devices
Mechanical ventilation or tracheostomy
Neutropenia or cytotoxic chemotherapy
Solid organ transplantation
Immunocompromised state
Mucositis
Malignant disease
Chronic lung disease (especially cystic fibrosis and chronic obstructive pulmonary disease)
HIV infection
Hemodialysis
Antibiotic exposure (especially to carbapenems, extended-spectrum cephalosporins, and fluoroquinolones)
Exposure to other patients with *S. maltophilia*

neoplasms[21] and patients who underwent solid organ transplantation), patients cared for in ICUs who are mechanically ventilated, hemodialysis patients with intravascular catheters, neonates, and patients with cystic fibrosis. Colonization or infection with *S. maltophilia* among patients with cystic fibrosis (Chapter 83) has been associated with reduction in lung function.

CLINICAL MANIFESTATIONS

Respiratory Tract
The respiratory tract is the most common site of isolation of *S. maltophilia* in the hospital. Surveillance programs report a rate of culture-positivity of *S. maltophilia* from hospitalized patients with pneumonia of more than 3% in the United States. Nosocomial pneumonia due to *S. maltophilia* is often associated with significant pulmonary disease such as emphysema, bronchiectasis, lung transplantation, or endobronchial obstruction. In addition, many of these patients are on mechanical ventilators, have tracheostomy tubes in place, or are receiving broad-spectrum antibiotics. Among mechanically ventilated patients, it can be challenging to differentiate colonization due to *S. maltophilia* from infection. CAP due to *S. maltophilia* has been reported but is very rare.

The incidence of respiratory tract infection due to *S. maltophilia* in patients with cystic fibrosis (Chapter 83) is increasingly being reported. There may be clear links with resistance to antipseudomonal antibiotics (tobramycin, imipenem, ceftazidime) used to treat these patients. The presence of chronic *S. maltophilia* infection has been associated with increases in cystic fibrosis exacerbations, decline in lung function, hospitalizations, need for lung transplantation, and mortality. It remains unclear whether *S. maltophilia* has a causative association with poor outcomes or is merely a marker for severe underlying disease.[22]

Blood Stream Infection and Endocarditis
Bacteremia may be secondary to a respiratory, urinary, or gastrointestinal source but is most commonly due to infection of an indwelling intravascular device. In many cases, except for those involving intravenous catheters, the portal of entry is not apparent. Immunocompromised patients with indwelling intravascular catheters, including those with hematologic malignant disease, are at particularly high risk for CLABSI due to *S. maltophilia*. In these cases, removal of the infected catheter is an important component of management. On occasion, an environmental reservoir or contaminated vascular access device is linked to the presence of bacteremia. Intravenous drug users are at especially high risk for contaminating prosthetic valves with *S. maltophilia*. In the case of endocarditis, favorable outcomes are reported with antimicrobial therapy, but surgery may also be required.

Urinary Tract Infection
Although *S. maltophilia* is frequently recovered from urine specimens in patients with indwelling urinary catheters, the role of this organism as a pathogen in this setting is unclear.

Meningitis
Cases of central nervous system infection due to *S. maltophilia* are reported rarely. These are often associated with central nervous system devices or antecedent neurosurgery.

Skin and Soft Tissue Infection
S. maltophilia can be isolated from postoperative wounds, but its role as a pathogen in this setting is unclear. In contrast, *S. maltophilia* can cause burn wound sepsis, manifested as a syndrome very similar to ecthyma gangrenosum (Chapter 412) in immunocompromised oncology patients.

TREATMENT   Rx

As a pathogen that is an increasingly important cause of nosocomial infections, *S. maltophilia* exhibits intrinsic resistance to many antibiotics.[23] The complexity of resistance genes and mechanisms is summarized in Table 291-2. Resistance to imipenem, piperacillin-tazobactam, ceftazidime, and aminoglycosides is common. Despite significant resistance to many agents, trimethoprim-sulfamethoxazole remains the drug of choice (10 to 15 mg/kg/day IV, based on the trimethoprim component). Treatment duration is uncertain, but it is usually 7 to 14 days but might be longer for deep seated or endovascular infections. Although overall there is excellent susceptibility, resistance to trimethoprim-sulfamethoxazole has become more common, particularly in cystic fibrosis patients. In vitro studies indicate that ticarcillin-clavulanate (3.1 g every 6 hours), minocycline (200 mg followed by 100 mg every 12 hours, not to exceed 400 mg in 24 hours), some of

TABLE 291-2   MECHANISMS OF RESISTANCE IN *STENOTROPHOMONAS MALTOPHILIA*

DRUG	MECHANISM OF RESISTANCE
β-Lactams, including imipenem	L1 and L2 β-lactamases Outer membrane permeability/efflux
Aminoglycosides	Aminoglycoside-modifying enzymes, transport

the fluoroquinolones (particularly levofloxacin and moxifloxacin), and tigecycline may be useful agents. Polymyxin-based regimens may serve as alternatives in the face of resistance to trimethoprim-sulfamethoxazole, but susceptibility should be confirmed prior to administration (see earlier for details regarding polymyxin treatment). Aztreonam is effective against strains exhibiting resistance to β-lactams by metallo-β-lactamases, but can be compromised if the co-production of other β-lactamases, most notably the chromosomal L2 β-lactamase, is present. The addition of the β-lactamase inhibitor avibactam to aztreonam has been explored in an effort to preserve aztreonam activity in the setting of β-lactamase production.[24] In certain instances, ceftazidime combined with avibactam was added to aztreonam to restore susceptibility. Various combination regimens for invasive *S. maltophilia* infections have been studied and demonstrated synergy but their efficacy in clinical settings remains unclear. Inhaled antibiotics are a therapeutic option but their clinical effectiveness remains unknown.

PROGNOSIS
Among patients with VAP or bacteremia due to *S. maltophilia*, crude mortality rates in the range of 60% have been reported. Bacteremia has been associated with poor outcomes, particularly in patients with malignancy or severe immunocompromising conditions. The attributable mortality of invasive *S. maltophilia* infection has been reported to be between 12 and 37.5%, but patients who receive early appropriate antibiotic therapy appear to do better.

PREVENTION
Standard infection control practices including hand hygiene and thorough environmental cleaning can help prevent spread of *Stenotrophomonas* in the hospital. In outbreak settings, contact precautions and possibly cohorting of patients have been used to control spread.

Grade A References
A1. Durante-Mangoni E, Signoriello G, Andini R, et al. Colistin and rifampicin compared with colistin alone for the treatment of serious infections due to extensively drug-resistant *Acinetobacter baumannii*: a multicenter, randomized clinical trial. *Clin Infect Dis.* 2013;57:349-358.
A2. Paul M, Daikos GL, Durante-Mangoni E, et al. Colistin alone versus colistin plus meropenem for treatment of severe infections caused by carbapenem-resistant Gram-negative bacteria: an open-label, randomised controlled trial. *Lancet Infect Dis.* 2018;18:391-400.

GENERAL REFERENCES
For the General References and other additional features, please visit Expert Consult at https://expertconsult.inkling.com.

292

SALMONELLA INFECTIONS (INCLUDING ENTERIC FEVER)

JOHN A. CRUMP

DEFINITION
Many of the more than 2500 serovars (also called serotypes) of *Salmonella enterica* subspecies *enterica* infect humans and cause a range of clinical conditions from asymptomatic intestinal carriage to intestinal infection to invasive disease with extraintestinal complications. Each serovar designation follows the species name (e.g., *Salmonella enterica* subspecies *enterica* serovar Typhimurium) and is frequently abbreviated as simply *Salmonella* followed by the serovar name (e.g., *Salmonella* Typhimurium).

The Pathogen

Members of the family Enterobacteriaceae (also see Chapter 289), salmonellae are gram-negative, non-spore-forming bacilli. They can be differentiated into more than 2500 serovars by their somatic (O) antigens, which are composed of lipopolysaccharides and are part of the cell wall, and by their flagellar (H) and capsular (Vi) antigens. *Salmonella* serogroups were traditionally designated by letters based on O antigens (e.g., A, B, C1, C2). The growing number of serogroups then made it necessary to move to a numeric designation. During the transition, the traditional letter-based serogroup were retained in brackets after the numeric designation (e.g., O:2 [A], O:4 [B], O:6,7 [C1], O:8 [C2]). Some of the important serovars and their serogroups are Typhi (group O:9 [D1]), Choleraesuis (group O:7 [C1]), Typhimurium (group O:4 [B]), and Enteritidis (group O:9 [D1]). *Salmonella* Enteritidis and Typhimurium are the most common nontyphoidal serovars causing human disease. Today, serovar can be inferred by whole genome sequencing and subdivision within serovars, useful for epidemiologic investigations, is usually achieved by molecular or genomic subtyping methods.[1]

EPIDEMIOLOGY

Salmonella Typhi, *Salmonella* Paratyphi A, *Salmonella* Paratyphi B, *Salmonella* Paratyphi C, and *Salmonella* Sendai are either solely or almost exclusively pathogens of humans; they cause primarily enteric fever rather than diarrhea, and transmission is usually through water or food. As a result of modern sewage and water treatment facilities and improved food safety practices, typhoid fever and paratyphoid fever have become rare in high-income countries but remain a problem in countries that lack adequate sanitation and a safe water supply. There are usually fewer than 500 cases of typhoid fever each year in the United States, mainly acquired abroad[2]; in contrast, an estimated 10.9 million cases occurred globally in 2017.[3]

Other serovars of *Salmonella* (described here as nontyphoidal *Salmonella*) have reservoirs in warm-blooded animals and cause human illness after the consumption of contaminated meat or animal products, contamination of produce or water by animal feces or animal products, or exposure to animals and their environments. Some nontyphoidal *Salmonella* serovars appear frequently in particular animal species, and about 10% of *Salmonella* infections may be attributable to animal exposure, including small pet turtles.[4] *Salmonella* Enteritidis has a reservoir in chickens, and infection is often linked to the consumption of undercooked eggs and poultry products or exposure to live chicks. Such a relationship is less clear for some other nontyphoidal serovars (e.g., *Salmonella* Typhimurium). Foodborne nontyphoidal *Salmonella* was estimated to be associated with approximately 1.0 million domestically acquired illnesses and 378 deaths in the United States in 2006. In the United States, a disproportionate number of infections occur in July through October, probably related to warm weather. *Salmonella* infections are most common among infants and children younger than 5 years of age. Worldwide, nontyphoidal *Salmonella* was estimated to cause 153.1 million illnesses and 57,000 deaths in 2010, with 52% of these estimated to be foodborne.[5]

Antimicrobial Resistance

Salmonellae have become increasingly resistant to antimicrobial agents, often by acquiring resistance transfer factors (e.g., plasmid mediated). Mutations in the *waaY*, *phoP*, and *pmrB* genes also confer resistance to antimicrobial peptides.[6] It is thought that antimicrobial resistance in the human-restricted salmonellae (e.g., *Salmonella* Typhi) is driven primarily by antimicrobial use in humans, whereas antimicrobial resistance among the nontyphoidal salmonellae (e.g., *Salmonella* Typhimurium) is associated with the use of antimicrobial agents in farm animals. Among *Salmonella* Typhi isolated in the United States from 2008 through 2012, 10 to 13% were resistant to the traditional first-line antimicrobials ampicillin, chloramphenicol, and trimethoprim-sulfamethoxazole, whereas 69% showed decreased fluoroquinolone susceptibility. Resistance to extended-spectrum cephalosporins is emerging among *Salmonella* Typhi in south Asia but remains rare among *Salmonella* Paratyphi A. Among human nontyphoidal *Salmonella* bloodstream isolates in the United States from 2003 to 2013, resistance to three or more antimicrobial classes was common. In addition, 5.0% of human nontyphoidal *Salmonella* bloodstream isolates were resistant to ceftriaxone and 4.5% were resistant to ciprofloxacin.[7] Susceptibility breakpoints and interpretive criteria were established for azithromycin in 2015 in response to reports of *Salmonella* with elevated azithromycin minimum inhibitory concentrations.

PATHOBIOLOGY

Etiology

Salmonellae are transmitted by the ingestion of fecally contaminated food or water; contact with animals, their environments, and other fomites; and, rarely, close contact with infected persons (e.g., oral-anal intercourse). The ultimate sources of contamination are humans or animals that are acutely ill or are shedding the organism without symptoms.

Contaminated Animal Products

Salmonella infection in humans usually occurs from ingestion of contaminated animal food products, most often eggs, poultry, and meat. *Salmonella* Choleraesuis is associated with pig products, *Salmonella* Dublin with cattle and unpasteurized milk from cattle, and *Salmonella* Enteritidis with poultry and poultry products, including eggs. Fecal material on poultry and other animal carcasses can spread at slaughterhouses, such as when many poultry carcasses are placed in the same hot-water tank to remove feathers. *Salmonella* contaminating carcasses can multiply to high levels if meat or other animal products are not refrigerated. Human illness may result if such animal products are inadequately cooked or if utensils or other uncooked foods are cross-contaminated during preparation. A wide range of foods can be contaminated with animal or human feces, from production on the farm through consumption in the home. Reports of produce-associated *Salmonella* outbreaks, due to contamination by animal or human feces during production, are increasing.[8] *Salmonella* outbreaks have occurred from contaminated cheese, ice cream, vegetables, fruit, juice, and alfalfa sprouts.

Contaminated Food and Water
Contamination by Pets

Salmonella infections may be acquired after contamination of food or water with the feces of pet turtles, chicks, ducks, birds, dogs, cats, and many other species.

Contamination by Humans

Salmonella infection can also be acquired by eating food or by drinking water contaminated by human fecal shedders who have not adequately washed their hands. Infection has been spread by the fecal-oral route among children, by contaminated enema and fiberoptic instruments, by diagnostic and therapeutic preparations made from animal or insect products (e.g., pancreatic extract, carmine dye), and from intentional or unintentional contamination of restaurant salad bars. Outbreaks of salmonellosis may occur in institutionalized patients, who are probably more prone to the development of *Salmonella* infections for three reasons. First, within institutionalized populations, there is an increased prevalence of underlying diseases that decrease host defense mechanisms against salmonellae, such as disorders of gastric acidity and intestinal motility; second, the use of antimicrobial agents modifies the normal, protective intestinal flora; and third, institutional food prepared in bulk may be more likely to be contaminated than are individually prepared meals. Outbreaks in nurseries and among the elderly in nursing homes are associated with the highest case-fatality ratios (>5%).

Contact with Animals and Their Environments

Both healthy and sick animals may harbor and shed *Salmonella*. Transmission of *Salmonella* from animals and their environment to humans occurs primarily by the fecal-oral route. Animal hides and saliva often harbor fecal organisms, and transmission can occur when persons pet, touch, feed, or are licked by animals. Transmission has also been associated with contaminated animal bedding, flooring, barriers, other environmental surfaces, and clothing and shoes. Contact with calves, turtles and other reptiles, rodents, and young poultry and their environments has been associated with *Salmonella* outbreaks. Humans may also become infected when animals come into contact with their food or water. Infections can be prevented by education, supervision of animal contact, provision and promotion of handwashing facilities, and separation of food handling and consumption from animal areas.

Contact with Infected Persons

Close contact with persons shedding *Salmonella* is an occasional source of infection. Transmission has been documented among persons handling feces (e.g., parents changing the diapers of an infected infant) and is associated with certain sexual practices (e.g., oral-anal intercourse).

Pathophysiology

After the ingestion of organisms, the likelihood for development of infection, as well as the severity of infection, is related to the dose, the virulence of the *Salmonella* strain, and the status of host defense mechanisms. Usually at least 10^2 to 10^3 bacteria are required to produce clinical infection in a normal host. Higher inocula are associated with increased disease severity, whereas smaller inocula are more likely to result in transient intestinal carriage. Gastric acid serves as a host defense mechanism by killing many of the ingested organisms, and intestinal motility is probably another host defense mechanism. In the absence of or with a decrease in gastric acidity (e.g., in infants and the elderly; after gastrectomy, vagotomy, or gastroenterostomy; or with the use of drugs that reduce gastric acidity) and with decreased intestinal motility (e.g., the use of antimotility drugs), much smaller inocula can produce infection, and the infection tends to be more severe.

Administration of antimicrobial agents before the ingestion of salmonellae can markedly reduce the size of the inoculum needed to produce infection, presumably by reducing the concentration of protective bowel flora.

Although any *Salmonella* serovar can produce any of the *Salmonella* syndromes (transient asymptomatic carrier state, enterocolitis, enteric fever, bacteremia, and chronic carrier state), each serovar tends to be associated with certain syndromes much more frequently than with others. For example, *Salmonella* Anatum usually causes asymptomatic intestinal infection, whereas *Salmonella* Typhimurium generally causes enterocolitis. *Salmonella* Choleraesuis is more likely to produce bacteremia (often with metastatic infection) than asymptomatic infection or enterocolitis, and some serovars such as *Salmonella* Typhi and *Salmonella* Paratyphi A are most likely to cause enteric fever as well as the chronic carrier state. Fortunately, most *Salmonella* serovars are of relatively low pathogenicity for humans. Therefore, although food products are commonly contaminated, large outbreaks tend to involve the more virulent serovars.

To produce infection, invasion must occur across the mucosa of the intestine. When the organisms reach the lamina propria, an influx of polymorphonuclear leukocytes serves as a host defense mechanism to prevent invasion of the lymphatics. Certain serovars seem to have a greater ability than others to invade the lymphatics and subsequently to produce bacteremia (e.g., *Salmonella* Choleraesuis and *Salmonella* Dublin, which commonly produce bacteremia after intestinal infection). Both the small intestine and the colon are involved in the inflammatory process.

In the case of *Salmonella* Typhi and other causes of enteric fever, salmonellae invade the mononuclear phagocytes in Peyer patches in the ileum and mesenteric lymph nodes. Some intracellular salmonellae form a nonreplicating population of "persisters" that could provide a reservoir for relapsing infection; intracellular persistence is determined by conditions in the vacuolar environment of the infected cells. Others multiply intracellularly and are carried through the lymphatic system and blood stream to the liver, spleen, bone marrow, and other parts of the reticuloendothelial system. When in the reticuloendothelial system, they multiply intracellularly in mononuclear phagocytes and produce the systemic manifestations of enteric fever. The onset of fever is associated with bacteremia and the release of cytokines (e.g., tumor necrosis factor and interleukins) from mononuclear phagocytes. Ulcerations over Peyer patches are responsible for the intestinal manifestations of enteric fever, such as pain, perforation, and bleeding.

In *Salmonella* enterocolitis, the organisms remain localized in the intestinal mucosa, and diarrhea results from the inflammation produced by polymorphonuclear leukocytes. In addition, watery diarrhea may occur, apparently the result of the secretion of water and electrolytes by small intestinal epithelial cells in response to an enterotoxin secreted by some of the *Salmonella* strains or in response to tissue mediators of inflammation.[9]

Patients with diseases that impair host defense mechanisms seem to have an increased frequency of severe *Salmonella* infection. A striking association has been recognized between diseases producing hemolysis and *Salmonella* bacteremia. Specifically, *Salmonella* bacteremia is common in patients with sickle cell disorders, malaria, and bartonellosis. In fact, because of the frequency of *Salmonella* bacteremia in sickle cell diseases and the underlying bone disease in these patients to which salmonellae localize, these organisms are the most common cause of osteomyelitis in patients with sickle cell disorders (Chapter 154). Prolonged *Salmonella* bacteremia may occur in patients with hepatosplenic schistosomiasis, possibly related to localization on and in the intravascular schistosomes. Patients with lymphoma and leukemia are also more prone to the development of *Salmonella* bacteremia. A markedly increased frequency and severity of *Salmonella* infections in general have been observed in patients with human immunodeficiency virus (HIV) infection, particularly those with CD4+ T-lymphocyte counts less than 200 cells/μL. Prolonged and recurrent, refractory *Salmonella* bacteremia is common among these patients. Other risk factors that increase the frequency and severity of *Salmonella* infection are extremes of age, immunocompromised states (e.g., from immunosuppressive agents), malnutrition, and probably diabetes. Nontyphoidal *Salmonella* serovars are a leading cause of community-acquired blood stream infection in sub-Saharan Africa, where children younger than 3 years and HIV-infected adults carry most of the burden of invasive disease.

CLINICAL MANIFESTATIONS

Asymptomatic Intestinal Carrier State

The asymptomatic intestinal carrier state may result from inapparent infection (which is the most common form of *Salmonella* infection), or it may follow clinical disease (in which case the patient becomes a convalescent carrier). The carrier state is usually self-limited to several weeks to months, with the prevalence of positive stool cultures rapidly decreasing over time. By 1 year, far less than 1% of carriers still have positive stools. The main exception is *Salmonella* Typhi; about 3% of those infected excrete the organism for life. Women and older men are most likely to become chronic carriers of *Salmonella* Typhi, related to the presence of biliary tract disease, especially calculi. A patient who has had salmonellae in stool for 1 year (chronic carrier) is likely to become a lifelong carrier; the reservoir is in the biliary tree, usually in calculi in the gallbladder. Patients with *Schistosoma haematobium* infection are predisposed to become chronic urinary carriers of salmonellae.

Enterocolitis

After an incubation period of usually 12 to 48 hours, the illness starts suddenly with crampy abdominal pain and diarrhea. Nausea and vomiting may occur but are usually not prominent or persistent. The diarrhea may be watery and of large or small volume. Stools may contain mucus and are occasionally bloody. Polymorphonuclear leukocytes are present in the stool. Diarrhea may be mild or severe, with up to 20 to 30 stools a day. Fever is present in most patients, and the temperature may reach 40° C (104° F) or higher. The abdomen is tender to palpation. Transient bacteremia may occur and is most commonly seen in infants, the elderly, and patients with impaired host defense mechanisms.

Symptoms generally improve during a period of days, with fever lasting no more than 2 to 3 days and diarrhea lasting no more than 5 to 7 days. However, these symptoms occasionally persist for up to 14 days. More severe disease is seen with malnutrition, inflammatory bowel disease, and HIV infection. Reactive arthritis may follow enterocolitis in up to 7% of cases, especially among those with the HLA-B27 phenotype.

Enteric Fever

Enteric fever is produced by *Salmonella* Typhi (typhoid fever), *Salmonella* Paratyphi A, B, and C (paratyphoid fever), and occasionally other serovars. Sometimes it immediately follows classic enterocolitis caused by the same organism. The syndrome is characterized by prolonged, sustained fever and may be associated with relative bradycardia, splenomegaly, rose spots, and leukopenia.

Therapy aborts the course of the disease. The following is a description of untreated illness. After an incubation period of 5 to 21 days (generally 7 to 14 days), fever and malaise develop, often associated with cough. A small proportion of patients may have diarrhea during the incubation period. The fever tends to rise in a stepwise fashion during the first few days to a week and then becomes sustained, usually at 39.4° to 40.0° C (103° to 104° F) or higher. Relative bradycardia is seen in up to half of patients. Apathy, confusion, delirium, and even psychosis may occur. Abdominal distention, pain, and tenderness may occur in the first week and may be associated with diarrhea or constipation; these symptoms are generally more pronounced during the second week of fever. Most patients have abdominal tenderness during the course of the illness.

In about 30% of patients, rose spots develop on the abdomen or chest (or both) toward the end of the first week or during the second week of fever. These faint, salmon-colored maculopapular lesions are subtle and may be difficult to see, particularly in dark-skinned patients. Salmonellae can be cultured from punch biopsies of these lesions. Hepatosplenomegaly occurs in about half of patients. Leukopenia and neutropenia are seen in about 20%. Abnormal liver function test results are common.

After 2 weeks of illness, the severe complications of intestinal hemorrhage and perforation related to necrosis of Peyer patches may be observed in about 5% of patients. These perforations may require surgical as well as medical therapy and can occur even in a patient treated with antimicrobials. Intestinal perforation is the leading cause of death from enteric fever.

The illness usually resolves by the end of the fourth week in an untreated patient. Relapse may occur in untreated as well as in treated patients, but the illness is milder than the original episode.

Rarely, some of the following complications may occur: pancreatitis, cholecystitis, infective endocarditis, meningitis, pneumonia, hepatic or splenic abscess, orchitis, or focal infection at virtually any site.

Bacteremia

Patients with *Salmonella* bacteremia usually complain of fever and chills lasting days to weeks. Gastrointestinal symptoms are unusual, but in some patients *Salmonella* bacteremia follows classic enterocolitis. Other symptoms are nonspecific, such as malaise, anorexia, and weight loss. Metastatic infection of bones, joints, aneurysms (particularly of the abdominal aorta), meninges (mainly in infants), pericardium, pleural space, lungs, heart valves, cysts, uterine myomas, malignant neoplasms, and other sites is common, and symptoms may be related to the site of metastatic infection. Stool cultures are often negative for salmonellae, but blood cultures are positive.

Although any *Salmonella* serovar can produce bacteremia, *Salmonella* Dublin, *Salmonella* Choleraesuis, *Salmonella* Heidelberg, *Salmonella* Oranienburg, *Salmonella* Panama, and *Salmonella* Sandiego are associated with increased likelihood of bacteremia.[10]

Salmonella bacteremia occurs with increased frequency in infants, the elderly, and patients with diseases associated with hemolysis (e.g., sickle cell diseases, malaria, bartonellosis), HIV infection, lymphoma, leukemia, disseminated histoplasmosis, and perhaps systemic lupus erythematosus.[11] Localization to bone is common in patients with sickle cell diseases (Chapter 154). In Africa, the common symptoms of invasive nontyphoidal *Salmonella* disease, which is seen predominantly in patients with HIV infection, malaria, and malnutrition, are fever, hepatosplenomegaly, and respiratory symptoms; features of enterocolitis are often absent.

Prolonged *Salmonella* bacteremia lasting for months may occur in patients with hepatosplenic schistosomiasis. In patients with HIV infection, recurrent, relapsing *Salmonella* bacteremia may develop, which may be difficult to cure with antimicrobial agents.

DIAGNOSIS

Although *Salmonella* enterocolitis is an invasive disease, the differential diagnosis includes all causes of acute diarrhea, including invasive bacteria such as *Campylobacter jejuni*, *Shigella* species, invasive *Escherichia coli*, *Yersinia enterocolitica*, and *Vibrio parahaemolyticus*; toxigenic bacteria such as *Vibrio cholerae*, enterotoxigenic *E. coli*, enterohemorrhagic *E. coli* (e.g., *E. coli* O157:H7), *Staphylococcus aureus*, *Bacillus cereus*, *Clostridium perfringens*, and *Clostridium difficile*; viruses; and protozoa such as *Entamoeba histolytica*, *Giardia intestinalis*, and *Cryptosporidium* species. The invasive bacterial causes of diarrhea, enterohemorrhagic *E. coli* and *C. difficile* infection, are also associated with polymorphonuclear leukocytes in stool, whereas bacterial toxigenic causes (other than *C. difficile* and enterohemorrhagic *E. coli*), viruses, and protozoa generally are not. The bacterial toxigenic causes of diarrhea other than *C. difficile* and enterohemorrhagic *E. coli* do not produce fever.

Stool culture is definitive for the diagnosis of *Salmonella* enterocolitis, but by the time the results of stool culture are available, most patients are recovering. Culture-independent diagnostic testing is used increasingly, but positive results for *Salmonella* may require culture to yield an isolate for public health purposes. A stained smear of the stool usually demonstrates polymorphonuclear leukocytes. Serologic studies are of little clinical value in *Salmonella* enterocolitis, but they may be of use in epidemiologic studies. Culture-independent methods, including panel-based multiplex molecular diagnostics from stool specimens, are used increasingly by clinical laboratories.

The differential diagnosis of *Salmonella* bacteremia includes virtually all acute infectious and noninfectious causes of fever, including bacteremia caused by other organisms. The diagnosis is proved by isolation of the microorganism from blood or from another normally sterile site.

The differential diagnosis of enteric fever is broad and depends in part on the area of the world where the infection was acquired. All causes of sustained fever are in the differential diagnosis, including infective endocarditis, disseminated tuberculosis, brucellosis, tularemia, *Mycoplasma pneumoniae* infection, rickettsial infections, Q fever, and viral infections such as infectious mononucleosis. Depending on the site of acquisition, diseases such as malaria, amebic abscesses of the liver, and visceral leishmaniasis also enter into the differential diagnosis.

The diagnosis of enteric fever is best proved by isolation of the microorganism from blood, stool, or bone marrow.[12] During the first week of illness,

blood cultures are positive in about 90% of patients, but culture positivity decreases in the next 2 weeks to less than 50% during the third week of illness. Stool cultures are usually negative during the first week but are generally positive by the third week. Bone marrow cultures give the highest yield, with up to 95% being positive; they should be considered in suspected cases with negative blood cultures. Bone marrow cultures may be positive even after several days of antimicrobial treatment, when blood cultures have become negative. Urine cultures and cultures of punch biopsies of rose spots may also be positive. The string test to obtain samples of bile from the duodenum has likewise yielded positive cultures.

The peripheral leukocyte count is usually normal, but leukopenia, which occurs in about 20% of cases, may be suggestive of enteric fever. Fecal leukocytes are generally present.

The Widal and other serologic tests that detect serum antibodies against *Salmonella* Typhi are limited by shortcomings of both sensitivity and specificity and rarely provide useful information to guide management of the patient. Polymerase chain reaction and other molecular techniques lack sensitivity for diagnosis from blood and other specimens, but they have been used to determine the *Salmonella* serovar of bacterial isolates.

TREATMENT   Rx

Enterocolitis

The primary approach to the treatment of *Salmonella* enterocolitis is fluid and electrolyte replacement. Drugs with antiperistaltic effects, such as loperamide or diphenoxylate with atropine, can relieve cramps, but they should be used sparingly because they can prolong the diarrhea.

Salmonella enterocolitis is self-limited, and antimicrobial therapy is usually not indicated, except perhaps in groups of patients at high risk for invasive disease. Antimicrobial therapy reportedly has little effect on the clinical course, and in some studies, it has prolonged the duration of *Salmonella* excretion in stool. In addition, most patients are improving by the time salmonellae or other bacterial pathogens are isolated from stool.

The fluoroquinolones are active against virtually all bacterial pathogens that cause diarrhea (including salmonellae), except for *C. difficile* and many *Campylobacter* organisms. Thus, it is reasonable to use fluoroquinolones for patients with suspected or known *Salmonella* enterocolitis who are severely ill and suspected of being bacteremic. The threshold for antimicrobial treatment is also decreased in those at increased risk for severe illness (e.g., infants, the elderly, patients with sickle cell disease, immunosuppressed individuals). As an example, in adults, ciprofloxacin, 500 mg every 12 hours orally or 400 mg every 12 hours intravenously for 3 to 5 days, or until defervescence, has been widely used. An extended-spectrum cephalosporin such as ceftriaxone is an alternative. In the presence of gross bloody diarrhea, antimicrobial treatment should be withheld until the possibility of *E. coli* O157:H7 infection has been eliminated because antimicrobial therapy may increase the frequency of hemolytic-uremic syndrome.

Other agents, such as amoxicillin and trimethoprim-sulfamethoxazole, have also been widely used in severely ill adults. However, many strains of *Salmonella* are now resistant to these agents.

Enteric Fever

Resistance to the traditional first-line antimicrobial agents (ampicillin, chloramphenicol, trimethoprim-sulfamethoxazole) has emerged worldwide among the salmonellae causing enteric fever. Consequently, alternative antimicrobial agents are now preferred.

The fluoroquinolones remain agents of choice for the treatment of enteric fever in many parts of the world,[A1] but resistance has become sufficiently common in other areas for alternative antimicrobials to be used routinely. Fluoroquinolones can be administered orally and have high bioavailability, they concentrate in bile and the bowel, and they often retain activity against multidrug-resistant strains of *Salmonella* Typhi and other causes of enteric fever. Most important, the fluoroquinolones have proved to be effective in the treatment of enteric fever, even with short courses (e.g., 3 to 7 days). The proportion of patients cured exceeds 95%, and relapse and chronic fecal carriage after therapy are uncommon. Ciprofloxacin (500 mg orally twice a day) for 7 to 14 days has been the fluoroquinolone of choice for enteric fever. If a patient cannot tolerate oral therapy, the fluoroquinolones can be administered intravenously. Reduced susceptibility and resistance to fluoroquinolones are increasingly reported in *Salmonella* Typhi and *Salmonella* Paratyphi A strains both in the United States and elsewhere and are associated with treatment failure. If decreased fluoroquinolone susceptibility or resistance is suspected or demonstrated, alternative agents include extended-spectrum cephalosporins (e.g., intravenous ceftriaxone) and azithromycin.

Extended-spectrum cephalosporins such as ceftriaxone are recommended agents for the treatment of enteric fever in settings where fluoroquinolone resistance is common and where extended-spectrum cephalosporin resistance is rare.[A2][A3] Ceftriaxone dosed at 1 to 2 g every 12 to 24 hours for adults and 75 mg/kg/day for children, given intravenously or intramuscularly for 10 to 14 days, results in cure of 95% of patients. Outbreaks of extensively drug resistant, including ceftriaxone resistant, *Salmonella* Typhi are occurring in south Asia.

If the *Salmonella* isolate is shown to be susceptible by antimicrobial susceptibility testing, ampicillin, chloramphenicol, or trimethoprim-sulfamethoxazole may be considered. The ampicillin dose is 25 mg/kg intravenously every 6 hours. The use of chloramphenicol should be weighed against the risk for bone marrow toxicity. The chloramphenicol dose is 50 mg/kg/day orally, divided into four doses. Chloramphenicol can be given intravenously at the same dose if oral therapy is not possible. Trimethoprim-sulfamethoxazole (4/20 mg/kg intravenously or orally every 12 hours) is given for 10 to 14 days.

Azithromycin (10 mg/kg/day orally for 7 days) is effective in the treatment of patients with uncomplicated typhoid fever caused by multidrug-resistant and some extensively drug-resistant strains. The oral route of administration makes it a particularly attractive choice in settings where multidrug resistance is common and intravenous extended-spectrum cephalosporins are impractical, unavailable, or too expensive. Severe disease due to extensively drug-resistant *Salmonella* Typhi may require carbapenems.

Patients often require supportive care with intravenous saline, correction of electrolyte and acid-base disturbances, and, in the setting of intestinal bleeding, blood transfusion. If perforation is suspected, abdominal imaging should be performed to evaluate for free air. If perforation seems likely, laparotomy should be performed as soon as possible to repair the perforation. In the setting of perforation, antimicrobial therapy should be broadened to cover bowel flora. Two multicenter, international prospective cohort studies of 88 consecutive patients (adults and children) undergoing surgery for gastrointestinal typhoid perforation demonstrated high mortality and complication rates, with a 30-day mortality rate of 9.1%, surgical site infection in 67.0%, and organ space infection in 10.2% of patients.[13]

Steroid therapy is beneficial in some patients with severe enteric fever and coma, delirium, or shock. Dexamethasone is administered at doses of 3 mg/kg initially, followed by 1 mg/kg every 6 hours for 48 hours. Steroids can mask the signs and symptoms of abdominal perforation and should not be continued for more than 48 hours. Salicylates should be avoided.

Relapses of typhoid fever may be treated with the same antimicrobial regimen as the initial attack.

Bacteremia

The agents of choice to treat *Salmonella* bacteremia are the fluoroquinolones, such as ciprofloxacin, and the extended-spectrum cephalosporins, such as ceftriaxone. Typical doses are ciprofloxacin 400 mg every 12 hours intravenously and ceftriaxone 1 to 2 g every 12 to 24 hours intravenously. When the salmonellae are known to be susceptible, ampicillin 1 to 2 g intravenously every 4 to 6 hours or trimethoprim-sulfamethoxazole 8 mg/kg/day (of the trimethoprim component) intravenously can be used. Chloramphenicol is another option. Antimicrobial susceptibility testing is necessary because of the emergence of infections resistant to the fluoroquinolones or extended-spectrum cephalosporins and sometimes both.

In cases of sustained bacteremia, the possibility of endovascular infection should be investigated. For transient bacteremia or bacteremia without localization, therapy is continued for 7 to 14 days. With localization to bone, aneurysms, heart valves, and various other sites, antimicrobial therapy should be given for much longer periods (e.g., 6 weeks). Surgical drainage, removal of foreign bodies, or resection of an aneurysm is often necessary to cure localized infection. The possibility of schistosomiasis should be considered and treated, when present, in patients with sustained *Salmonella* bacteremia (Chapter 334). Patients with HIV infection tend to experience repeated relapses after treatment courses for *Salmonella* bacteremia. In this group, initial treatment with ciprofloxacin for 2 weeks or longer is recommended. Long-term suppressive therapy has been suggested for those experiencing frequent relapses.[14]

Carriers

Chronic carriers (i.e., >1 year) of salmonellae other than *Salmonella* Typhi are uncommon. Stools of convalescent carriers spontaneously become negative during a period of weeks to months, and no therapy should be given. The rare chronic carrier of *Salmonella* serovars other than Typhi (usually infected with *Salmonella* Paratyphi A, B, or C) may be treated with a fluoroquinolone, amoxicillin, or trimethoprim-sulfamethoxazole in the doses listed later for 4 to 6 weeks. Patients who experience relapse usually have gallbladder disease (most often calculi) and will not be cured with antimicrobial therapy alone. Cholecystectomy plus antimicrobial therapy may cure these patients, but it is doubtful that the carrier state is a sufficient indication for cholecystectomy.

Chronic carriers of *Salmonella* Typhi can be treated with ciprofloxacin (500 to 750 mg twice daily) for 6 weeks or with amoxicillin at doses of 6 g/day in three or four divided doses plus probenecid 2 g/day in divided doses for 6 weeks. Trimethoprim-sulfamethoxazole (160/800 mg twice daily) plus rifampicin (300 mg twice daily) for 6 weeks may be considered as an alternative regimen. Patients with persistent urinary carriage and *S. haematobium* infection should

be treated with praziquantel before eradication of *Salmonella* Typhi is attempted. For patients with persistent carriage and anatomic abnormalities (e.g., gallstones), cholecystectomy combined with antimicrobial therapy is often necessary. For patients with persistent carriage despite adequate antimicrobial therapy and without an identifiable anatomic abnormality, chronic suppressive therapy may be considered. Chronic carriers who do not prepare food and who practice adequate personal hygiene usually do not constitute a public health hazard. Therefore, after the institution of appropriate personal hygienic precautions, and in the absence of evidence of a chronic carrier infecting others, cholecystectomy is probably not indicated to eradicate the carrier state.

PREVENTION

Salmonella infection is best prevented by protecting the water supply, preventing fecal contamination during food production, cooking and refrigerating foods, pasteurizing milk and milk products, and handwashing before preparing foods. Travelers should judiciously avoid consuming untreated water (including ice), raw vegetables, and fruits. Food should be cooked or peeled, and drinks should be boiled, carbonated, or commercially bottled. The widespread presence of salmonellae in the animal kingdom means that reducing the risk for *Salmonella* infections requires a multifaceted approach.

There is no vaccine for *Salmonella* infection other than that for *Salmonella* Typhi. Travelers should be vaccinated before going to areas that are endemic for typhoid fever.[15] Two types of vaccines are available in the United States. One is the typhoid Vi capsular polysaccharide vaccine, which is administered as a single intramuscular injection, with booster doses given every 2 years if needed. This vaccine provides a degree of herd protection against typhoid fever when it is used at the population level. The other licensed typhoid fever vaccine type is the oral live attenuated Ty21a vaccine. Revaccination is necessary every 5 years, if indicated. Ty21a vaccine should not be used in immunocompromised persons or those receiving antimicrobials. Both types of vaccines confer greater than 75% protective efficacy. More recently, new Vi polysaccharide protein-conjugate vaccines have been developed for widespread use and show greater promise as routine health interventions.[A4] A typhoid Vi tetanus toxoid conjugate vaccine has been prequalified by the World Health Organization and is recommended for use as a single dose from age 6 months in typhoid endemic countries, but this vaccine is not yet licensed in the United States.[16]

Vaccines afford only partial immunity to typhoid fever. Persons who have been vaccinated should still restrict their diets to avoid potentially contaminated food and fluids. When cases of imported typhoid are identified in the United States, the local health department should be informed and will monitor stool cultures. Typhoid fever acquired in the United States is typically investigated by the public health department to identify potential sources and chronic carriers.

PROGNOSIS

Mortality in patients with *Salmonella* enterocolitis is rare; infants and the elderly are at greatest risk, with death occurring as a result of dehydration and electrolyte imbalance. Mortality from *Salmonella* bacteremia is not uncommon and is most likely to occur in the very young, the very old, the malnourished, and the immunocompromised.

Before the advent of antimicrobial therapy, typhoid fever had a case-fatality ratio of 15 to 20%. This has been reduced to less than 1% in industrialized countries. However, the case-fatality ratio remains high in some developing countries. The case-fatality ratio of invasive nontyphoidal *Salmonella* in Africa is approximately 20%. In treated patients, the temperature usually returns to normal after 3 to 5 days of therapy, but this may take longer in patients treated with extended-spectrum cephalosporins than in those treated with fluoroquinolones and in those infected with isolates with decreased fluoroquinolone susceptibility who are treated with ciprofloxacin.

In the era before antimicrobial therapy, 5 to 10% of patients who recovered from typhoid fever had relapses. Relapses continued to occur in 10 to 15% of patients treated with chloramphenicol, ampicillin, and trimethoprim-sulfamethoxazole, but this seemed to be much less frequent (<5%) among those treated with ceftriaxone and fluoroquinolones. Intestinal bleeding or perforation occurs in about 5% of patients. With perforation, case-fatality rates of 10 to 30% have been reported.

Up to 3% of patients recovering from *Salmonella* Typhi and nontyphoidal *Salmonella* infection become chronic carriers, persistently shedding the organism in their stool. Most persistently infected patients are immunocompetent, and about two thirds have relapsing diarrhea, indicating that they are not truly asymptomatic.[17]

Grade A References

A1. Effa EE, Lassi ZS, Critchley JA, et al. Fluoroquinolones for treating typhoid and paratyphoid fever (enteric fever). *Cochrane Database Syst Rev.* 2011;10:CD004530.

A2. Arjyal A, Basnyat B, Nhan HT, et al. Gatifloxacin versus ceftriaxone for uncomplicated enteric fever in Nepal: an open-label, two-centre, randomised controlled trial. *Lancet Infect Dis.* 2016;16:535-545.

A3. Thompson CN, Karkey A, Dongol S, et al. Treatment response in enteric fever in an era of increasing antimicrobial resistance: an individual patient data analysis of 2092 participants enrolled into 4 randomized, controlled trials in Nepal. *Clin Infect Dis.* 2017;64:1522-1531.

A4. Voysey M, Pollard AJ. Seroefficacy of Vi polysaccharide-tetanus toxoid conjugate vaccine (Typbar TCV). *Clin Infect Dis.* 2018;67:18-24.

GENERAL REFERENCES

For the General References and other additional features, please visit Expert Consult at https://expertconsult.inkling.com.

293

SHIGELLOSIS

GERALD T. KEUSCH AND ANITA K. M. ZAIDI

DEFINITION

Shigellosis is an acute infection of the large bowel due to four species of the genus *Shigella* (*dysenteriae, flexneri, boydii, soneii*), characterized by gut mucosal inflammation and fever.[1] Clinical disease ranges from watery diarrhea to bloody diarrhea or dysentery, a syndrome consisting of multiple small-volume bloody stools per day, abdominal cramping, and tenesmus, a painful straining with the urge to defecate.

The Pathogen

The genus *Shigella* consists of gram-negative bacilli within the family Enterobacteriaceae and tribe Escherichieae. It is, more accurately, a pathovar[2] of *Escherichia coli* (Chapter 288), but it remains a separate genus for historical reasons. Indeed, several *E. coli* serotypes cause *Shigella*-like illness and possess conserved virulence factors. *Shigella sonnei* is the most common species isolated in industrialized countries and, while *S. flexneri* continues to predominate in developing countries, there is an ongoing global spread of *S. sonnei* in industrializing countries in Asia, Latin America, and the Middle East.[3] *S. dysenteriae* type 1, responsible for multiyear outbreaks in Latin America, Asia, and Africa since 1969, has, for unknown reasons, been rarely identified since the late 1990s. *S. boydii* is found primarily in the Indian subcontinent. New serotypes, currently not identified by existing typing reagents, continue to evolve and in the future may contribute to the global disease burden of *Shigella*.[4]

EPIDEMIOLOGY

Shigella are pathogens for humans (and occasionally large nonhuman primates in captivity), with no other animal reservoirs, hence identifying sources of infection invariably tracks back to an infected human. The Centers for Disease Control and Prevention (CDC) maintains 5 different databases on *Shigella* infections in the United States, and another assessing antimicrobial resistance, each providing somewhat different estimates of disease burden. The incidence of culture-proven shigellosis, primarily due to *S. sonnei* (85%) and *S. flexneri* (9 to 10%), has been trending downward since 1970 (Fig. 293-1). It varies from year to year, driven by the number and size of outbreaks.

Transmission of *Shigella* infection occurs with a small inoculum, from 10 to 10,000 organisms, depending on the species involved, which explains why shigellosis is so frequently transmitted from person to person. Organisms are readily transferred from the stool of an infected person to a susceptible individual, often via the hands directly to the mouth (fecal-oral transmission), or indirectly through objects (fomites) previously handled by the infected person.

Approximately 50% of identified *Shigella* infections in the United States are transmitted by direct person-to-person transmission. *Shigella* is the second leading cause in these settings, although greatly exceeded by Norovirus.[5] Shigellosis incidence is highest in children 0 to 4 years of age, commonly associated with daycare centers, where hygiene is difficult to maintain, followed by children

5 to 9 years old. Children under 10 years collectively account for one third of all proven infections. Older individuals residing in long-term care facilities are another high-risk group because of the often poor hygiene in these facilities. *Shigella* can also be transmitted sexually, particularly among men who have sex with men (MSM).[6] The prevalence of *S. flexneri* infection is greater in this group compared to the general population, and is known to cause more severe illness than *S. sonnei*, including bloody diarrhea and dysentery. A recent outbreak among MSM uncovered coincident transmission among another previously unrecognized risk group, homeless persons, whose access to safe water and food, basic sanitation, and water for washing is limited.[7]

Shigella infection can also be transmitted via contaminated food or water. In 2016, *Shigella* was the third most common pathogen in food-borne gastroenteritis in the United States, with 2,913 confirmed cases, representing a 7% increase over the average from 2013 to 2015.[8] Such exposures are often due to an infected food handler with minimal or no symptoms who is still excreting the organism in stool. The result is a common source multiperson or multistate outbreak, which is more likely to be investigated and etiology determined. These outbreaks have identified new vehicles for exposure, for example fresh salsa or guacamole prepared in restaurants. Multicountry outbreaks of *S. sonnei* due to contaminated fresh foods shipped from Africa or Southeast Asia demonstrate how globalization of the food supply can also globalize infection with particular strains of *Shigella*. This has important implications for the importation of *Shigella* antimicrobial-resistant (AMR) strains from areas of the world where drug resistance is particularly high. Shigellosis among MSM also represents a documented mechanism for the intercontinental spread of AMR *Shigella*. Contamination of swimming pools or bathing areas, usually by young children carrying the organism who defecate in the water, can result in common-source outbreaks for susceptibles of any age. Outside of outbreaks, most cases of acute shigellosis in the United States are never reported because the predominant isolate is *S. sonnei* resulting in mild self-limited illness that is not microbiologically investigated. CDC estimates around 500,000 cases of *Shigella* infection occur each year in the United States, of which 130,000 are transmitted by contaminated food. Just a handful of deaths due to shigellosis are reported in the United States. Asymptomatic carriage of *Shigella* is typically limited to a few weeks; but because an etiologic diagnosis of *S. sonnei* is rarely made, convalescent carriers can return to their normal activities while they are still able to transmit infection.

Shigellosis in the developing world is a very different disease. Crowding facilitates person-to-person transmission, and limited availability of water, toilets, household hygiene, and refrigeration for food storage increases the ease of fecal contamination of food or water as the source. Due to the lack of latrines or toilets, open defecation remains common, providing an opportunity for flies to transfer pathogens to food or water, further spreading risk in communities. As a consequence, household transmission from an index case in Bangladesh was 44 times greater compared to a cohort of household contacts of uninfected matched controls.[9] An analysis of global food-borne shigellosis in 2010 estimated there were 849,468 illnesses and 2,621 deaths in 61 moderate-high income countries, and 188,000,000 cases and 64,993 deaths in the remaining 133 countries.[10] The rising prevalence of the less severe *S. sonnei* around the world, as well as *S. boydii* in the Indian subcontinent, and the disappearance of *S. dysenteriae* in recent years may partially account for the estimated 98% drop in mortality due to shigellosis in Asia. However other nonspecific interventions known to reduce *Shigella*-specific deaths, such as the use of measles vaccine, vitamin A or zinc supplements, improved general nutritional status, or access to better primary health care and antibiotics, undoubtedly play a significant role as well. Whereas *S. sonnei and S. boydii* usually cause mild infection, malnourished children exposed to high inocula of these organisms can develop severe, even lethal, disease similar to *S. flexneri*, even when they are hospitalized and receiving expert care. For these reasons, *Shigella* was the third leading cause of diarrheal disease deaths globally in 2015, resulting in an estimated 164,300 deaths, one third occurring in children under 5 years and the third leading cause in this age group, with 60% of deaths in those 15 and older in whom it was the leading cause of diarrheal deaths.[11]

Because of the small infectious inoculum, outbreaks readily occur during complex humanitarian emergencies such as floods, landslides, earthquakes, or the gathering of refugees of conflict into crowded camps with limited sanitary facilities. Recent outbreaks of *S. sonnei* and *flexneri* with antibiotic resistance have been identified in the makeshift camps in Europe for refugees and migrants streaming out of Syria and neighboring countries due to the ongoing civil war.[12]

In the United States, incidence is driven by outbreaks, does not exhibit marked seasonal variation, and is similar in males and females. *S. sonnei* is somewhat more common among females than males 10 to 39 years of age, presumably related to their greater exposure to infected young children, whereas severe shigellosis caused by *S. flexneri* is greatly increased in males compared

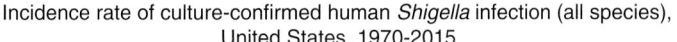

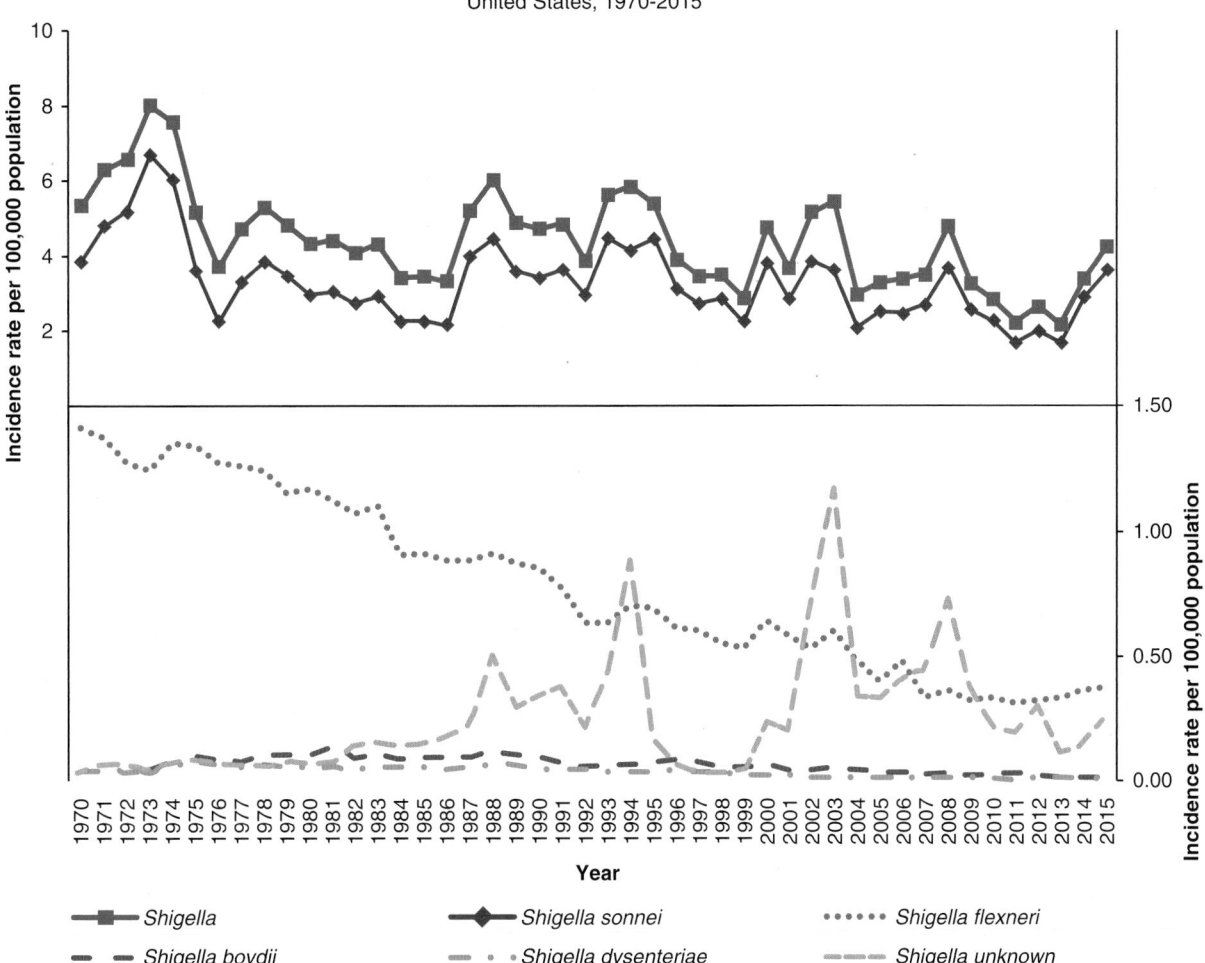

FIGURE 293-1. Incidence rate of laboratory-confirmed *Shigella* infection reported to the Centers for Disease Control and Prevention (all species), United States, 1970-2015. *Top panel,* The incidence rates of infection with *Shigella* (all species) and *Shigella sonnei*. Since 1970, the incidence rate of infection with *Shigella* (all species) has been driven by the incidence of infection with *Shigella sonnei*. *Bottom panel,* The incidence rate of infection with all *Shigella* species other than *Shigella sonnei,* including infections with an unspecified species. The incidence rate of infection with *Shigella flexneri* has been decreasing since the 1980s. Since the mid-1980s, the incidence rate of *Shigella* infection in which the species is not identified has fluctuated, likely representing, at least to some extent, outbreak situations in which public health laboratories did not characterize all outbreak-associated *Shigella* isolates to the species level. *Shigella boydii* and *Shigella dysenteriae* infections are rare in the United States.

to females, particularly among black men, in the age group 20 to 69 years,[13] probably related to transmission among the MSM population. In developing countries, shigellosis also occurs year-round, although discernible seasonal peaks may occur in the rainy season, when organisms from open defecation can be washed into drinking water sources, or in the dry season, when water for personal hygiene is scarce.

PATHOBIOLOGY

As a result of changes in gene expression, *Shigella* become resistant to acid pH as they multiply in the large bowel, providing protection for the bacteria when they transit the acidic environment of the stomach of a new susceptible host, accounting for the small inoculum required for transmission. Once past the stomach, *Shigella* turn off genes governing acid resistance and express other genes that allow them to invade the host's colonic epithelium through complex coordinated mechanisms.[14] There are two major barriers the organism must overcome; first, competitive inhibition of the normal intestinal microbiome in the colon by as yet unclear mechanisms, and second, penetration of the mucus layer overlying the epithelial cells, facilitated by expression and release of microbial mucolytic molecules. *Shigella* also downregulate the production of antimicrobial peptides by the intestinal mucosa, which might otherwise impair the initial invasion of M cells overlying lymphoid Peyer patches. The bacteria are then transcytosed to the lamina propria, where they are ingested by macrophages and induce the production of inflammatory cytokines, leading to macrophage death and the recruitment and migration of polymorphonuclear leukocytes into and through the mucosa. Together with *Shigella*-induced disruption of cell junction proteins, leukocyte migration forces open the tight junctions between epithelial cells. This allows many more organisms from the lumen to gain access to the basolateral membrane of colonic epithelial cells, where they induce the host cells to ingest them by

a mechanism resembling phagocytosis.[15] *Shigella* then lyse the phagocytic vesicle to enter the cytoplasm and multiply; although they are nonmotile, they use their capacity to cross-link actin in the cytoplasm to propel themselves to the host cell membrane. There, by the induced phagocytosis-like mechanism, they are transferred from one epithelial cell to another. The inflammation and death of contiguously invaded host epithelial cells results in mucosal ulcerations and further exudation of blood and leukocytes into the colonic lumen and ultimately in stool. At the same time, regulatory pathways are engaged to transmit alarm signals that activate the innate immune system in bystander cells to confine the invading organisms to the localized area of involvement.

CLINICAL MANIFESTATIONS

Infections due to *S. sonnei* or *S. boydii* typically are manifested after an incubation period of 1 to 3 days with fever and mild to moderate watery diarrhea (Table 293-1). They do not cause serious dehydration and generally resolve without specific treatment in 3 to 5 days. However, if the stool is examined under the microscope, white and red blood cells are observed, indicative of the underlying inflammation of the mucosa. When the inflammation is more severe, as with *S. flexneri*, the initial watery diarrhea may turn bloody and in some will progress to dysentery, with its characteristic small-volume bloody mucoid stool passed many (10 to >40) times per day, abdominal cramps, and tenesmus. The most severe infections are due to *S. dysenteriae* type 1 and progress rapidly from watery to bloody diarrhea and frequently to frank dysentery.

The severity of illness and variety of complications of *S. flexneri* and *S. dysenteriae* type 1 contributes to their importance as causes of death in children in developing countries. In this population, bacteremia with the infecting strain or other enteric flora can occur, and the intense mucosal inflammation can lead to toxic megacolon. Colonic perforation and pancolitis are rare complications that may require surgical intervention. In young children, in whom mesenteric

TABLE 293-1   CLINICAL SYNDROMES AND COMPLICATIONS OF SHIGELLOSIS

STAGE	TIME OF APPEARANCE AFTER ONSET OF ILLNESS	SYMPTOMS AND SIGNS	PATHOLOGY AND PATHOGENESIS
Prodrome	Earliest findings	Fever, chills, myalgias, anorexia	None or early colitis with cytokine response
Watery diarrhea	0-3 days	Fever, abdominal cramps, loose stools	Mild colitis with fecal leukocytes and erythrocytes
Bloody diarrhea	1-3 days	Frequent stools containing blood and mucus, abdominal cramps and tenderness, fever, anorexia	Colitis with fecal leukocytes and erythrocytes
Dysentery	1-5 days	Frequent small-volume stools consisting of blood, mucus, and pus; severe abdominal cramps; tenesmus	More extensive colitis with crypt abscesses and mucosal ulcerations
Acute complications	3-7 days	Seizures, obtundation, bacteremia, colonic obstruction, mucosal perforation, peritonitis	Severe colitis, terminal ileitis
Additional acute complications due primarily to infection with *Shigella dysenteriae* type 1	3-7 days	Toxic megacolon, leukemoid reaction, hemolytic-uremic syndrome	Severe colitis, expression of Shiga toxin
Postinfectious syndromes	1-3 weeks	Reactive arthritis, with or without urethritis and conjunctivitis	Autoimmune inflammatory response, most common in individuals expressing HLA-B27 antigen

support for the rectosigmoid colon is not fully developed, the intense proctitis results in straining to pass stool and may lead to rectal prolapse. A rapid rise in temperature can cause a seizure in this age group, distinguishable from typical febrile seizures by the older age of the child and the rarity of multiple seizures. Other central nervous system manifestations, such as obtundation, suggests the presence of hypoglycemia, due to poor food intake and inadequate gluconeogenesis, or hyponatremia, secondary to inappropriate secretion of antidiuretic hormone. Anorexia may be intense and prolonged, and combined with ongoing catabolism of host muscle protein associated with excessive pro-inflammatory cytokine production and protein-losing enteropathy due to colitis, results in some degree of protein-energy malnutrition that may progress to kwashiorkor and death (Chapter 203). *S. flexneri* infection is also associated with reactive arthritis and other autoimmune inflammatory manifestations, such as tendinitis, conjunctivitis, uveitis, urethritis, or erythema nodosum, a constellation of findings commonly termed reactive arthritis (formerly Reiter syndrome) (Chapter 249). This occurs primarily in individuals positive for HLA-B27 antigen and may be a consequence of molecular mimicry. *S. dysenteriae* type 1 infection may result in a leukemoid reaction associated with thrombocytopenia and microangiopathic hemolytic anemia, often followed by HUS (Chapter 163) and acute renal failure.

DIAGNOSIS

Shigellosis presenting with watery diarrhea is clinically indistinguishable from the many other causes of watery diarrhea, except for the frequency of fever in *Shigella* infections, unless the stool is examined microscopically to demonstrate the presence of red and white blood cells or infection is confirmed microbiologically or by molecular diagnostics (CIDT). Routine laboratory studies document leukocytosis with many immature "band" forms, especially in patients with bloody diarrhea or dysentery. In the developed world, these presentations are most commonly due to a Shiga toxin–producing *E. coli* (STEC), such as serotype O157:H7, or *S. flexneri* and less often *Campylobacter jejuni*, nontyphoidal *Salmonella* species, or rarely *Yersinia enterocolitica* or *Entamoeba histolytica*. In patients who have recently received antibiotics, bloody diarrhea is often the consequence of *Clostridium difficile* (Chapter 280). In contrast, a large multicountry study of moderate to severe pediatric diarrhea in low- and middle-income countries documented *S. flexneri* as the cause of most bloody diarrhea or dysentery, with no cases of *S. dysenteriae* detected among more than 10,000 individuals studied.[16] Syndromic diagnosis may fail to identify subjects with *Shigella* infection. In a study in Kenya, only 7 of 63 children with *Shigella* isolated from stool had clinically identified dysentery (sensitivity 11%, CI 4.6 to 21.6%).[17] Culture diagnosis not only takes days before results are available, but also often underestimates prevalence. False-negatives can be due to poor sample collection, delay in processing, or failure to use the best culture methods, as well as prior antibiotic administration which may limit detection of still viable but nonculturable organisms. In contrast, CIDT results can be available in hours, and for these reasons antigen capture or polymerase chain reaction diagnostic tests are becoming more attractive but may be more costly. In resource poor settings, the use of more than one selective culture medium and obtaining multiple specimens will increase the yield of positives. Initial screening is based on the failure of *Shigella* species to ferment lactose, with additional studies of lactose-negative colonies to detect anaerobic fermentation of glucose, and lack of motility or hydrogen

sulfide production to distinguish *Shigella* from *Salmonella* species. Specific diagnosis employs standard serologic methods for *Shigella* O antigens. This is why culture takes several days to confirm results. In the case of mild watery diarrhea due to *S. sonnei*, the patient is usually recovered by the time the laboratory results are available, so they are of little use in guiding treatment. Culture yields are maximized when only patients with bloody diarrhea or dysentery are studied. Results are valuable for selection of empirical treatment, and for epidemiologic purposes when antibiotic sensitivity is also determined to track the emergence of antibiotic resistance and help to select effective antibiotics when treatment is indicated.

TREATMENT

In healthy adults and children, most Shigella infections cause mild diarrhea, not requiring diagnostic work-up or antibiotic treatment. Clinical trial evidence supports the use of antibiotics to treat bloody diarrhea or dysentery due to *Shigella* to decrease the severity of symptoms and the duration of fever and diarrhea. 🅐 Over the years, successive antibiotics have been used to treat *Shigella* infections because of emerging drug resistance, including tetracycline, chloramphenicol, ampicillin, trimethoprim-sulfamethoxazole, nalidixic acid, pivmecillinam, ciprofloxacin, azithromycin, and ceftriaxone. For antibiotic susceptible strains, any of these antibiotics are effective for clinical and microbiologic cure and high-quality evidence regarding the superiority of one over the other is lacking. Single-dose or short-course treatment has shown promise but data remain limited and more studies are required. Some studies suggest that cefixime (an oral third-generation cephalosporin) is efficacious in children but is less effective in adults, and amoxicillin is less effective than ampicillin. Nonabsorbable antibiotics, such as oral furazolidone, rifaximin, and gentamicin possess in vitro activity against *Shigella* but are not recommended because optimal treatment requires therapeutic levels of the drugs in both the lumenal and the mucosal compartments, and these agents have shown variable efficacy in clinical use. Figure 293-2 illustrates the strategy for antibiotic therapy and recommended drugs for shigellosis in children and adults in high-income and low-income settings.

Therapeutic options for treating shigellosis are increasingly limited because of increasing and wide-spread resistance in both high-income and low-income countries.[18] In April 2017, the CDC issued guidance to limit antibiotic treatment of *Shigella* in the United States to patients who are immunocompromised or have severe illness, defined as requiring hospitalization, or suffering from invasive disease or complications.[19] Because identification of the etiologic agent for diarrhea can take 3 to 5 days, empiric therapy pending culture results is necessary in these severe cases. Local susceptibility data should guide antibiotic selection, and this is the rationale to systematically collect drug sensitivity information. The CDC advisory describes the emergence and spread of *Shigella* strains in the United with elevated minimum inhibitory concentration (MIC) values for ciprofloxacin of 0.12 to 1 µg/ml. Clinicians should be aware that laboratory standards may categorize these strains as susceptible to ciprofloxacin, yet they can harbor quinolone resistance genes known to confer reduced susceptibility and result in potential treatment failure or prolonged shedding, thereby increasing the risk of secondary cases. For these reasons, the CDC recommends that *Shigella* strains with an MIC of 0.12 µg/ml or higher should not be treated with fluoroquinolones. MSM populations are at increased risk of harboring antibiotic-resistant strains.

Resistance is more prominent in developing countries where both burden of infections and antibiotic use are high. As a consequence, oral therapy for shigellosis is becoming increasingly challenging, with severely limited therapeutic options. In South Asia, the majority of strains are now resistant to ciprofloxacin and resistance to azithromycin is rapidly emerging. It is possible that in

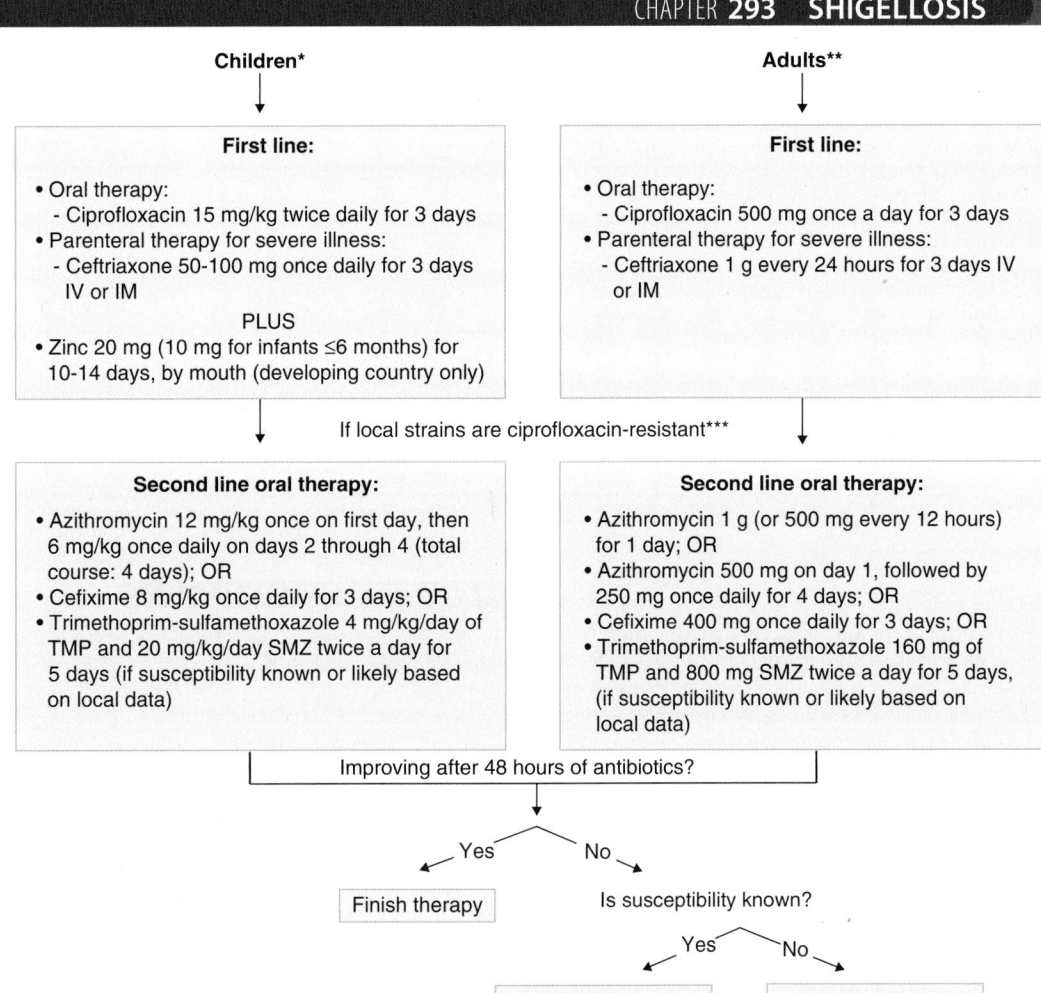

Children*

First line:

- Oral therapy:
  - Ciprofloxacin 15 mg/kg twice daily for 3 days
- Parenteral therapy for severe illness:
  - Ceftriaxone 50-100 mg once daily for 3 days IV or IM

PLUS

- Zinc 20 mg (10 mg for infants ≤6 months) for 10-14 days, by mouth (developing country only)

Adults**

First line:

- Oral therapy:
  - Ciprofloxacin 500 mg once a day for 3 days
- Parenteral therapy for severe illness:
  - Ceftriaxone 1 g every 24 hours for 3 days IV or IM

If local strains are ciprofloxacin-resistant***

Second line oral therapy:

- Azithromycin 12 mg/kg once on first day, then 6 mg/kg once daily on days 2 through 4 (total course: 4 days); OR
- Cefixime 8 mg/kg once daily for 3 days; OR
- Trimethoprim-sulfamethoxazole 4 mg/kg/day of TMP and 20 mg/kg/day SMZ twice a day for 5 days (if susceptibility known or likely based on local data)

Second line oral therapy:

- Azithromycin 1 g (or 500 mg every 12 hours) for 1 day; OR
- Azithromycin 500 mg on day 1, followed by 250 mg once daily for 4 days; OR
- Cefixime 400 mg once daily for 3 days; OR
- Trimethoprim-sulfamethoxazole 160 mg of TMP and 800 mg SMZ twice a day for 5 days, (if susceptibility known or likely based on local data)

Improving after 48 hours of antibiotics?

Yes → Finish therapy

No → Is susceptibility known?

Yes → Adjust therapy according to susceptibility results

No → Choose different 1st or 2nd line therapy not previously used

*The WHO expert committee on the use of essential medicines 2017[19] currently recommends no antibiotic treatment for non-bloody, non-febrile diarrheal episodes, including those due to *Shigella*.

**CDC recommends limiting antibiotic treatment of *Shigella* to patients who are immunocompromised or have severe illness, defined as requiring hospitalization, or suffering from invasive disease or complications.[18]

***CDC recommends that Shigella strains with an MIC of 0.12 µg/ml or higher should not be treated with fluoroquinolones.[18]

FIGURE 293-2. Treatment of shigellosis.

the near future there could be no oral antibiotics available to which *Shigella* are susceptible, making common community-acquired childhood infections very difficult to manage. The CDC and WHO have recently declared antibiotic resistant *Shigella* a serious public health threat requiring new interventions.

The WHO expert committee on the use of essential medicines 2017[20] currently recommends no antibiotic treatment for nonbloody, nonfebrile diarrheal episodes, including those due to *Shigella*. Ciprofloxacin is the first-choice antibiotic for bloody diarrhea or dysentery, with azithromycin, cefixime, and ceftriaxone among second-choice agents for ciprofloxacin-resistant strains. However, a recent large multicountry study has revealed a high residual mortality burden in children in developing countries in the 60- to 90-day period following clinically moderate-to-severe acute watery diarrhea, with a substantial proportion of these infections attributed to *Shigella*. Whether empiric antibiotic treatment of suspected nondysenteric shigellosis in children presenting with severe dehydration or malnutrition in developing countries confers survival benefit is unknown, and a current multicountry clinical trial is assessing whether children less than 2 years old with severe watery diarrhea or malnutrition in countries with a high child mortality burden might benefit from empiric antibiotic therapy with azithromycin.

In severe shigellosis, the prompt initiation of effective antibiotic treatment shortens the duration of illness and achieves a more rapid improvement in symptoms such as fever, cramps, and tenesmus. Evidence from Bangladesh demonstrates that prompt treatment of infections due to *S. dysenteriae* type 1 reduces the frequency of HUS and presumably other complications due to

colonic inflammation, such as megacolon, perforation, and rectal prolapse. Parenteral ceftriaxone has been most useful in severe or drug-resistant illness, children with immune deficiency including HIV, or inability to take oral medications due to vomiting or diminished consciousness. However, this requires hospitalization or outpatient administration and monitoring, and both decrease access to treatment and increase its cost. In addition, the increasing prevalence of extended spectrum β-lactamase (ESBL) isolates of *S. flexneri* and *S. sonnei* expressing the CTX-M type of β-lactamase that confers resistance to all β-lactam antibiotics except cephamycins and carbapenems is already compromising consideration of ceftriaxone as an effective treatment option.

In more severe infections, complications such as hypoglycemia or hyponatremia can be managed with appropriate glucose or saline given intravenously, but patients must be monitored by trained clinical staff. Colitis with toxic megacolon and intestinal perforation represent difficult problems, primarily associated with *S. dysenteriae* type 1 disease. To correct rectal prolapse in infants the mucosa should be kept moist with saline until manual reduction can be achieved. However, because of the recent disappearance of *S. dysenteriae* type 1 disease such complications are also diminishing in frequency. The prolonged anorexia and catabolic responses in shigellosis, require close attention to nutritional rehabilitation, especially in malnourished children in developing countries where the diet is often poor. Even with adequate protein-containing and energy-dense diets after infection, replacement of nutrient stores may take as long as four times the duration of the clinical illness and full nutritional recovery may not be possible before the next infection occurs, causing further nutritional deterioration. Administration of zinc is associated with a modest clinical benefit, including reduced duration of symptoms, as well as a reduction in subsequent diarrheal incidence. WHO guidelines recommend zinc supplementation in all children with diarrhea in resource-limited settings, where zinc deficiency is common.

Seizures can occur but are usually self-limited, and other neurologic complications respond to fluid and electrolyte management and correction of hypoglycemia and hyponatremia. Reactive arthritis is a greater problem because it is an autoimmune response that occurs primarily in genetically susceptible individuals positive for HLA-B27 antigen. Chronic destructive arthritis may require nonsteroidal anti-inflammatory agents, steroids, or inflammatory cytokine inhibitors, in addition to effective antibiotic treatment to eliminate the causative organism, as well as ongoing medical management.

Some evidence suggests that antimotility agents are contraindicated in shigellosis, particularly in cases of bloody diarrhea or dysentery in young children, because these drugs may slow peristalsis and prolong contact between the organisms and the mucosa, thereby increasing microbial invasion, pathologic changes, and severity, including toxic megacolon.

PREVENTION

Personal hygiene (in particular hand washing after handling the diapers of infected children and before food preparation), the sanitary disposal of feces, and protection of food and water sources from microbial contamination are essential to limit the spread of shigellosis. Preventing spread in daycare settings is a particular problem because it is so difficult to stop young children from constantly exploring their world, picking up bacteria on their hands, and bringing their fingers or contaminated fomites to their mouths. In such settings, it is particularly important for the adult caretakers to observe good personal hygiene and to supervise children in handwashing. Soap and water are sufficient, but hand sanitizers do work and may be more convenient. In environments where soap is unavailable, water used with sand or ash for scrubbing is helpful. Keeping infected children away from daycare until their stool is negative, if indeed cultures were done, or separating recently ill children from the susceptible has been recommended but is costly and not easy to accomplish. Household hygiene in the setting of an index case, including frequent handwashing, caution in the disposal of soiled diapers or underwear, regularly wiping down the area where these are collected with a disinfectant such as Lysol, and precautions in food preparation, can help limit intrahousehold spread. All of these measures are more difficult to implement in resource-limited environments without access to water for hygiene, let alone safe water for drinking or cooking, toilets or properly maintained latrines, ability to purchase disinfectants, or refrigeration to store food.

Vaccines, particularly for the more virulent species, would be useful. However, despite much effort and progress, a safe and effective vaccine has not been developed or approved for general use.[21] Vaccines against *Shigella* have been challenging to design because of the multiple species and serotypes, insufficient understanding of immunity and cross-protection, lack of a faithful animal model, and low commercial interest. In the United States populations for whom a *Shigella* vaccine could be recommended include travelers or military personnel who are deployed to high-risk locations. In low-income countries, a multivalent broadly protective vaccine against *S. flexneri* and *S. sonnei*, the two most common *Shigella* species in the last 20 years, would be extremely useful because shigellosis continues to account for a significant portion of the annual mortality due to diarrheal diseases. Our current understanding of immunity in shigellosis indicates that serotype-specific immunity is most important. Attenuated live oral vaccine candidates are probably most useful for travelers and military personnel deployed to high-risk areas; unfortunately, vaccines most effective in inducing immunity have also been the most reactogenic, causing fever and often mild diarrhea in recipients. For children in endemic areas current vaccines under clinical development are killed whole cells,[22] lipopolysaccharide (LPS) O antigen–protein conjugates, and subunit candidates. Newer-generation conjugate vaccines against LPS seem the most promising. Unless common protective antigens are identified, the most likely vaccine strategy will be based on a combination of serotype-specific antigens from the most prevalent and cross-protective *Shigella* isolates. Refinement of *Shigella* human challenge models offer promise for accelerating *Shigella* vaccine development.

PROGNOSIS

S. sonnei infection and most cases of *S. boydii* infection are mild and self-limited, with no sequelae. Infection with *S. flexneri* or *S. dysenteriae* responds to proper treatment with antibiotics. When treatment is not effective, either a drug-resistant strain or another etiologic agent should be suspected. In some instances, severe shigellosis with pancolitis has been misdiagnosed as inflammatory bowel disease. This can be a disaster if the patient is treated with steroids. Whereas early and effective treatment of *S. dysenteriae* type 1 reduces the risk of complications such as HUS and probably megacolon and bowel perforation, about 25% of those with HUS will have some permanent renal impairment, and a small percentage may progress to end-stage renal failure. Because of the autoimmune nature of reactive arthritis, usually associated with *S. flexneri*, early treatment might not prevent its occurrence but could mitigate its severity. Infection with one serotype of *Shigella* generally provides durable immunity to reinfection with the same strain but leaves the individual susceptible to other antigenically distinct strains and serotypes.

Grade A Reference

A1. Christopher PR, David KV, John SM, et al. Antibiotic therapy for Shigella dysentery. *Cochrane Database Syst Rev.* 2010;8:CD006784.

GENERAL REFERENCES

For the General References and other additional features, please visit Expert Consult at https://expertconsult.inkling.com.

294

BRUCELLOSIS

EDSEL MAURICE T. SALVANA AND ROBERT A. SALATA

DEFINITION

Brucellosis, previously known as Malta fever or undulant fever, is a zoonotic disease caused by bacteria of the genus *Brucella*. Human infection, which has protean manifestations, is acquired via direct contact, ingestion, or inhalation. Most disease is acquired by eating unpasteurized dairy products or undercooked meat. Occupational infection is typically inhalational or through contamination of exposed wounds and mucous membranes. Human-to-human transmission occurs but is rare. Brucellosis remains a significant public health and economic burden in many countries despite advances in detection, treatment, and prevention. In regions where the disease is endemic, brucellosis continues to have far-reaching deleterious effects on humans and animals alike.[1]

The Pathogen

Brucella is a slow-growing, small, aerobic, nonmotile, nonencapsulated, non–spore-forming, gram-negative coccobacillus. *Brucella abortus* (from cattle, bison, elk), *B. suis* (from pigs and feral swine), *B. melitensis* (from sheep, goats, and camels), and *B. canis* (from dogs) are the species that most commonly infect humans. Genetic analysis shows a high degree of homology among different species despite disparate preferred hosts, and virulence factors can vary between and within species. Whole genome sequencing can distinguish between genotypes at a higher resolution, and can provide clues to the organism's geographic origin.[2]

EPIDEMIOLOGY

Etiology

Brucella abortus is usually associated with mild to moderate sporadic disease. *B. suis* and *B. melitensis* infections are associated with suppurative or disabling complications and can have a prolonged course. Infection with *B. canis* has an insidious onset, relapses frequently, and has a chronic but relatively mild course. Two marine species, *B. pinnipedialis* (from seals) and *B. ceti* (from porpoises and dolphins) can cause neurobrucellosis in humans. *Brucella microti* (from common vole, red fox) has a high potential for pathogenicity, but no instances of human infection have been reported. Other *Brucella* species with known or potential human pathogenicity include *B. inopinata* (breast implant infection), *B. ovis* (sheep infection; no human cases), and *B. neotomae* (rodent infection; no human cases reported). BO2, a proposed species closely related to *B. inopinata*, has caused one human case of chronic destructive pneumonia.

Because of its pathogenicity and ability to remain viable in storage for long periods, *Brucella* spp. are potential agents for bioterrorism.[3]

Incidence and Prevalence

More than 500,000 cases of brucellosis are reported yearly to the World Health Organization (WHO) from 100 countries. *B. melitensis* infection accounts for most diagnosed cases, primarily from the Mediterranean region, Latin America, the Arabian Gulf, China, and the Indian subcontinent. *B. abortus* infection occurs worldwide but has been effectively eradicated in most northern and western European countries, Japan, and Israel. *B. suis* is found in the United States, South America, and Southeast Asia. *B. canis* infection occurs in North America, South America, Japan, and central Europe. High rates of *Brucella* seropositivity in African communities that keep livestock and consume unpasteurized milk have been reported, and undiagnosed African brucellosis likely represents a significant burden of infection. Returning travelers and immigrants from endemic countries continue to be diagnosed in otherwise low prevalence or nonendemic countries.

Brucellosis in animals is a chronic infection that can persist throughout life. Effective control programs in animals have decreased human brucellosis dramatically in the United States from more than 6000 cases in 1947 to fewer than 140 cases per year since 1993. Texas, California, Arizona, and Florida reported the most cases in 2010 (https://www.cdc.gov/brucellosis/resources/surveillance.html). *Brucella* infection in the United States occurs mostly through direct contact with animals or animal secretions in high-risk groups, including slaughterhouse workers, farmers, dairy workers, and veterinarians. Laboratory workers handling infected animals or *Brucella* cultures are also at risk. More than one half of reported cases are associated with meat processing, particularly from "kill areas." Many cases of *B. abortus* infection in veterinarians are from accidental exposure to live vaccines (which are pathogenic to humans) used to immunize livestock. Human infections in hunters of feral swine occur sporadically. Imported goat milk and cheese from Mexico (unpasteurized)[4] is an important source of *B. melitensis* infection. Brucellosis contracted abroad may not become symptomatic until the traveler returns. Human-to-human transmission has been documented in 45 cases, and has occurred through sexual transmission, breastfeeding, blood transfusion, bone marrow transplantation, nosocomial exposure, and perinatally.[5] Brucellosis in pregnancy has been associated with spontaneous abortions, congenital abnormalities, and neonatal infections. Childhood brucellosis, which occurs mostly in school-aged children, accounts for 3 to 10% of all reported cases worldwide. Human brucellosis incidence is epidemiologically linked to serious pregnancy complications.[6]

PATHOBIOLOGY

Pathogenesis

After penetrating the epithelial cells of human skin, conjunctiva, pharynx, intestine, or lung, *Brucella* organisms in naïve individuals induce a delayed inflammatory response (up to 48 hours) with polymorphonuclear leukocyte infiltration at the infection site. *Brucella* organisms are then ingested by dendritic cells, neutrophils, and tissue macrophages, and these subsequently spread to regional lymph nodes. If host defenses within the lymph nodes are overwhelmed or the burden of infection is high, bacteremia follows. The usual incubation period from infection to bacteremia is 2 to 4 weeks. Bacteremia is accompanied by phagocytosis of free *Brucella* organisms by macrophages, with localization primarily to the spleen, liver, and bone marrow. These form small, noncaseating granulomas which can serve as persistent sources of infection.

As an intracellular organism, *Brucella* has to avoid detection by the immune system and survive a hostile intracellular environment. *Brucella* organisms avoid initial detection by the host through multiple mechanisms. Its cell wall lipopolysaccharide (smooth LPS) differs significantly from regular bacterial LPS in two important ways: it has very little effect on Toll-like receptor type 4 (TLR4) activation, and it is resistant to complement activation. In addition, *Brucella* organisms deploy a protein that interferes with TLR signaling. Upon successful entry into the host, *Brucella* organisms in phagosomes are able to survive acidification and lysosome fusion through the induction of specific virulence factors such as the VirB type IV secretion system (T4SS) and urease (ure). To replicate, *Brucella* organisms intercept traffic between the endoplasmic reticulum and the Golgi apparatus. They also seem to inhibit apoptosis of infected cells, such as synoviocytes, thereby maintaining a persistent presence. A major role for the family of outer membrane proteins Omp25/Omp31 in pathogenicity has been elucidated. Omp22, omp25, and omp31 knockout mutants show substantially decreased virulence. Omp25 seems to inhibit TNF-α production by macrophages, and facilitates secretion of periplasmic proteins in acidic medium by modulating the permeability of the *Brucella*

membrane. Omp22 and omp25 are necessary for invasion and intracellular survival in host cells. Other known virulence factors that occur at high frequencies in pathogenic *Brucella* include integral membrane-bound protein (MviN), mannose-6-phosphateisomerase (ManA), mannosyl-transferase (WbkA), perosamine-synthetase (PerA), and outer membrane protein 19 (omp19).[7] Inflammation from the innate host immune response is likely the main driver of pathology, because no secreted proteolytic enzymes or bacterial toxins have been found. *Brucella* induces the production of host proinflammatory cytokines and metalloproteinases, which cause tissue damage.[8]

Immunity

Humoral factors play an important role in host defense against *Brucella* spp. Even in the absence of specific agglutinating antibody, normal human serum is bactericidal for *Brucella* organisms. The intracellular location of *Brucella* spp. within macrophages enables it to escape the lethal effects of serum to a certain extent. Specific serum agglutinating antibody has opsonic activity but does not correlate with the development of protective immunity.

A role for mononuclear phagocytes and cell-mediated immunity in brucellosis has been demonstrated. Prior infection with *Listeria monocytogenes* or *Mycobacterium tuberculosis*, both of which stimulate cell-mediated immune mechanisms, is protective against *Brucella* infection in animals. Skin testing with *Brucella* proteins elicits a typical delayed hypersensitivity response in infected individuals. Macrophages, activated with T helper 1 (T_H1)–type cytokines (including interferon-γ, tumor necrosis factor-α, interleukin-1, interleukin-12), kill *Brucella*. Despite high levels of T_H1 cytokine production, deficient effector phagocytic activity persists. Later in the course of infection, there is evidence of an unexpected inhibitory effect from neutrophils. Animal models have demonstrated more efficient killing of *Brucella* organisms in the absence of polymorphonuclear cells, which somehow dampen the immune response to this pathogen.

CLINICAL MANIFESTATIONS

Clinically, human brucellosis can be divided into subclinical illness, acute or subacute disease, localized disease, relapsing infection, and chronic disease (Table 294-1).

Subclinical Illness

Asymptomatic or clinically unrecognized human brucellosis often occurs in high-risk groups, including slaughterhouse workers, farmers, and veterinarians. The diagnosis is usually made through serologic means. More than 50% of abattoir workers and up to 33% of veterinarians have high anti-*Brucella* antibody titers but no history of recognized clinical infection. Children in endemic areas frequently have subclinical illness.

Acute and Subacute Disease

After an incubation period of several weeks or months, acute brucellosis may occur as a mild, transient illness (*B. abortus* or *B. canis*) or as an explosive, toxic illness with the potential for multiple complications (*B. melitensis* or *B. suis*). Approximately 50% of patients have an abrupt onset over days, but the remainder have an insidious onset over weeks. Symptoms in brucellosis are protean and nonspecific. More than 90% of patients experience malaise, chills, sweats, fatigue, and weakness. More than 50% of patients have myalgias, anorexia, and weight loss. Some patients complain of arthralgias, cough, testicular pain, dysuria, ocular pain, or blurring of vision. Few localizing physical signs are apparent. Fever, with temperatures often greater than 39.4° C (103° F), occurs in 95% of patients. An undulating or intermittent fever pattern is not unusual. A pulse–temperature deficit (i.e., relative bradycardia) may occur. Splenomegaly is present in 10 to 15% of cases, and lymphadenopathy occurs in about 14% of patients. Axillary, cervical, and supraclavicular lymphadenopathy are most frequent and may be related to hand wounds or oropharyngeal routes of infection. Hepatomegaly is less frequent. Other laboratory findings in acute or subacute disease may include mild anemia; lymphopenia; or neutropenia (especially with bacteremia); lymphocytosis; thrombocytopenia; or, in rare cases, pancytopenia. The majority of infected individuals recover completely without sequelae if diagnosed early with prompt initiation of therapy.

Localized Disease and Complications

Brucella organisms can localize to almost any organ but usually target the bones, joints, central nervous system, heart, lung, spleen, testis, liver, gallbladder, kidney, prostate, pancreas, thyroid, and skin. Disease may occur at multiple sites. About 47% of *Brucella* patients manifest osteoarticular complications. The most common manifestation is peripheral arthritis, particularly in the

TABLE 294-1   CLINICAL CLASSIFICATION OF HUMAN BRUCELLOSIS

CLASSIFICATION	DURATION OF SYMPTOMS BEFORE DIAGNOSIS	MAJOR SYMPTOMS AND SIGNS	DIAGNOSIS	COMMENTS
Subclinical		Asymptomatic	Positive (low-titer) serology, negative cultures	Occurs in abattoir workers, farmers, and veterinarians
Acute and subacute	Up to 2-3 mo and 3 mo-1 yr, respectively	Malaise, chills, sweats, fatigue, headache, anorexia, arthralgias, fever, splenomegaly, lymphadenopathy, hepatomegaly	Positive serology, positive blood or bone marrow cultures	Presentation can be mild, self-limited (*B. abortus*) or fulminant with severe complications (*B. melitensis*)
Localized	Occurs with acute or chronic untreated disease	Related to involved organs	Positive serology, positive cultures in specific tissues	Bone or joint, genitourinary, hepatosplenic involvement most common
Relapsing	2-3 mo after initial episode	Same as acute illness but may have higher fever and more fatigue, weakness, chills, and sweats	Positive serology, positive cultures	May be extremely difficult to distinguish relapse from reinfection
Chronic	>1 yr	Nonspecific presentation, but neuropsychiatric symptoms and low-grade fever most common	Low titer or negative serology, negative cultures	Most controversial classification; localized disease may be associated

acute setting, which typically affects wrists, knees, hips, and ankles. Sacroiliitis typically occurs in the acute setting and is a classical presentation that should prompt workup for brucellosis. Spondylitis and vertebral osteomyelitis, particularly in the lumbar area, are less common but also well-recognized complications and can be associated with paravertebral, epidural, and psoas abscesses. Prosthetic joint infections have been observed, with 24 reported cases mostly due to *B. melitensis* followed by *B. abortus*. These typically involve a hip or knee replacement, and one fourth responded to combination antimicrobial therapy while the rest required débridement or revision.[9]

Relapsing Infection
Up to 10% of patients with brucellosis relapse after antimicrobial therapy. The intracellular location of *Brucella* organisms predisposes to recurrence because these are relatively protected from host defense mechanisms, and antimicrobial agents may be unable to penetrate efficiently enough to kill all the bacteria. Intrinsic or acquired resistance to antibiotics is another factor that can lead to treatment failure. Relapses usually occur 3 to 6 months after completion of therapy but may be seen up to 2 years after initial treatment. Relapsing infection is difficult to distinguish from reinfection in high-risk groups with continued exposure. Relapses are associated with inappropriate or insufficient antimicrobial therapy, growth on blood cultures during the initial presentation, and an acute onset of disease.

Chronic Disease
Disease lasting more than 1 year is referred to as *chronic brucellosis*. A majority of patients classified as having chronic brucellosis really have persistent disease caused by inadequate treatment of the initial episode, or they have focal disease in bone, liver, or spleen. About 20% of patients diagnosed with chronic brucellosis complain of persistent fatigue, malaise, and depression; in many respects, this condition resembles chronic fatigue syndrome.

DIAGNOSIS

Culture
Many common illnesses mimic brucellosis, and a thorough history is essential, including occupation, travel to endemic areas, avocations, and ingestion of at-risk food and beverages. The most conclusive means of establishing the diagnosis of brucellosis is the recovery of the organism from a culture from normally sterile body fluid or tissue. Sensitivity of cultures range from 15 to 90%, depending on the methods used and the specimen type. Handling of *Brucella* cultures is potentially hazardous to laboratory personnel, and the laboratory should be informed if this organism is suspected, in addition to requesting them to extend the length of incubation because it may take more than 5 days for *Brucella* organisms to grow.

Blood cultures are positive in 10 to 30% of cases of acute brucellosis, although this can be as high as 85% with *B. melitensis*. The sensitivity of blood cultures decreases with increasing duration of illness. In *B. melitensis* infection, bone marrow cultures are more sensitive than blood cultures. In localized brucellosis (e.g., lymph nodes, spleen, liver, skeletal system), cultures of purulent material or tissues usually yield *Brucella* organisms. Culture of cerebrospinal fluid is positive in 45% of patients with meningitis. Antibodies against *Brucella* may be demonstrated in cerebrospinal fluid by enzyme-linked immunosorbent assay (ELISA).

Standard Tube Agglutination and Other Antibody Tests
In the absence of microbiologic confirmation, a presumptive diagnosis can be made by history and serology. The most frequently used test is the standard tube agglutination test (SAT), measuring antibody titers against *B. abortus* antigen. A fourfold or greater rise in titer over 2 weeks is considered significant. A presumptive case is one in which the agglutination titer is positive (1:160 in endemic areas; 1:80 in nonendemic areas) in single or serial specimens, with symptoms consistent with brucellosis. By 3 weeks of illness, more than 97% of patients demonstrate serologic evidence of infection. SAT detects antibodies to *B. abortus*, *B. suis*, and *B. melitensis* but not to *B. canis*. Serologic confirmation of *B. canis* infection requires *B. canis* or *B. ovis* antigen. After adequate antibiotic treatment, significant SAT titers can persist for up to 2 years in 5 to 7% of cases. Because of this, SAT titers are not useful in differentiating relapsing infection from other febrile illnesses in patients with a history of past *Brucella* infections. Individuals with subclinical infection may demonstrate significant SAT titers. In chronic brucellosis, antibodies which do not agglutinate at neutral pH increase and replace agglutinating antibodies, and so a complementary test that detects antibodies to smooth LPS, such as the *Brucella* Coombs test is recommended. A lateral flow immunochromatographic assay (LFA) using the purified antigen is another non–agglutination-based test. The Center for Disease Control uses a modified SAT known as the Brucella microagglutination test (BMAT). False-positive SAT titers have been associated with *Brucella* skin testing, cholera vaccination, or infection with *Vibrio cholerae*, *Francisella tularensis*, or *Yersinia enterocolitica*.[10]

Other Tests
Polymerase chain reaction with DNA sequencing offers highly accurate diagnosis of brucellosis in blood and other fluids or tissue samples. However, protocols still need to be standardized on a wider scale, and access to expertise and adequate laboratory facilities remains a significant limiting factor.

PREVENTION
The control of human brucellosis is directly related to prevention programs in domestic animals and the avoidance of unpasteurized milk and milk products. In slaughterhouses, important means of prevention include careful wound dressing, the use of protective glasses and clothing, the prohibition of raw meat ingestion, and the use of previously infected (immune) individuals in high-risk areas. Work is ongoing to find an effective vaccine for humans. Postexposure antimicrobial prophylaxis is controversial.

PROGNOSIS
Brucellosis treated appropriately within the first month of symptom onset is curable. Acute brucellosis often produces severe weakness and fatigue, and patients are frequently unable to work for up to 2 months. Immunity to reinfection follows initial *Brucella* infection in the majority of individuals. With early antimicrobial therapy, cases of chronic brucellosis or localized disease and complications are rare. Of the patients who die of brucellosis, 84% have endocarditis involving a previously abnormal aortic valve, often associated with severe congestive heart failure. Medical treatment alone is associated with a much higher risk of death compared to a combined medical and surgical approach for *Brucella* endocarditis.

TABLE 294-2	TREATMENT FOR BRUCELLOSIS	
	TREATMENT	**COMMENTS**
Acute, with no endocarditis or CNS involvement	Doxycycline (200 mg/day) for 6 weeks plus streptomycin (1 g/day) for 3 wk	Treatment of choice by WHO; widely used; low rate of relapse; IM administration of streptomycin may be difficult
Alternative agents: chloramphenicol, fluoroquinolones, TMP-SMX, imipenem	Combination therapy still preferred; ofloxacin (800 mg/day) plus rifampin (15 mg/kg/day) is the preferred alternative	
In children	TMP-SMX plus rifampin	
CNS	Doxycycline plus rifampin and TMP-SMX	Third-generation cephalosporin can be substituted if susceptible in vitro
Localized	Surgically drain abscesses plus antimicrobial therapy for ≥6 wk	
Brucella endocarditis	Bactericidal drugs; early valve replacement may be necessary	Possible aortic valve destruction and/or major arterial emboli

CNS = central nervous system; IM = intramuscular; TMP-SMX = trimethoprim–sulfamethoxazole; WHO = World Health Organization.

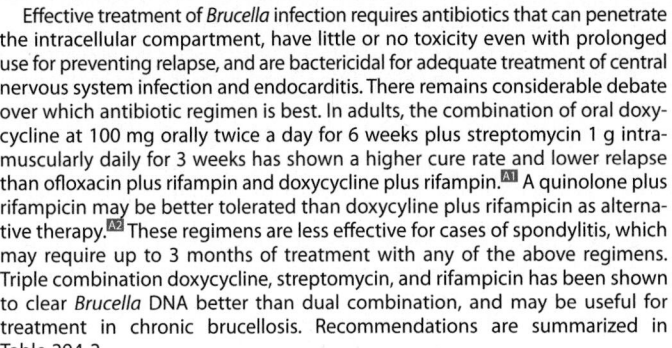

TREATMENT   Rx

Effective treatment of *Brucella* infection requires antibiotics that can penetrate the intracellular compartment, have little or no toxicity even with prolonged use for preventing relapse, and are bactericidal for adequate treatment of central nervous system infection and endocarditis. There remains considerable debate over which antibiotic regimen is best. In adults, the combination of oral doxycycline at 100 mg orally twice a day for 6 weeks plus streptomycin 1 g intramuscularly daily for 3 weeks has shown a higher cure rate and lower relapse than ofloxacin plus rifampin and doxycycline plus rifampin.[A1] A quinolone plus rifampicin may be better tolerated than doxycycline plus rifampicin as alternative therapy.[A2] These regimens are less effective for cases of spondylitis, which may require up to 3 months of treatment with any of the above regimens. Triple combination doxycycline, streptomycin, and rifampicin has been shown to clear *Brucella* DNA better than dual combination, and may be useful for treatment in chronic brucellosis. Recommendations are summarized in Table 294-2.

Grade A References

A1. Hashemi SH, Gachkar L, Keramat F, et al. Comparison of doxycycline-streptomycin, doxycycline-rifampin, and ofloxacin-rifampin in the treatment of brucellosis: a randomized clinical trial. *Int J Infect Dis.* 2012;16:e247-e251.
A2. Yousefi-Nooraie R, Mortaz-Hejri S, Mehrani M, et al. Antibiotics for treating human brucellosis. *Cochrane Database Syst Rev.* 2012;10:CD007179.

GENERAL REFERENCES

For the General References and other additional features, please visit Expert Consult at https://expertconsult.inkling.com.

295

TULAREMIA AND OTHER *FRANCISELLA* INFECTIONS

KAREN C. BLOCH AND WILLIAM SCHAFFNER

DEFINITION

Tularemia is an infectious zoonosis caused by *Francisella tularensis,* a small aerobic, pleomorphic, gram-negative bacillus. Many animal species harbor the organism, most prominently rabbits, squirrels, and muskrats. Humans acquire the infection through various means, including direct contact with infected animal tissues, ingestion of contaminated water or meat, the bite of an infected tick or deer fly, or breathing an aerosol of bacteria.[1] *F. tularensis* is highly infectious and is a well-recognized risk to laboratory personnel manipulating culture plates of the organism; paradoxically, the illness is not communicable from person to person. Edward Francis established that deer flies can transmit the infection from animals to humans and provided detailed descriptions of its clinical manifestations. Colloquially, the disease is often referred to as *rabbit fever* or *deer fly fever.*

The Pathogen

The organism occurs in two major subspecies (biovars). *F. tularensis* biovar *tularensis* (type A) is more virulent in animals and humans, has distinctive biochemical reactions (it produces acid from glycerol and has citrulline ureidase activity), and is the common North American biovar. In contrast, *F. tularensis* biovar *holarctica* (type B) is less virulent and occurs commonly in Europe and Asia.[2] Type B is most frequently isolated from rodent species, including muskrats (*Ondatra zibethicus*), mice (*Mus musculus*), beavers (*Castor canadensis*), voles (*Microtus* spp), and water voles (*Arvicola terrestris*), and has been associated with an outbreak of infection in wild-caught prairie dogs. Specific virulence factors for *F. tularensis* have not been identified.

EPIDEMIOLOGY

Tularemia has been reported in the United States, Canada, Mexico, Japan, and Europe (particularly Scandinavia).[3] In Iran, seroprevalence ranges from 6 to 14%.[4] It has not been reported in the United Kingdom or the Southern Hemisphere. In the United States, reported cases diminished during the second half of the 20th century from a high of 2291 cases in 1939 to the approximately 125 cases reported annually (E-Fig. 295-1). In 2015 the Centers for Disease Control and Prevention (CDC) reported 314 cases, driven by a 975% increase in the incidence of tularemia in Colorado, Nebraska, South Dakota, and Wyoming.[5] The increased incidence of tularemia in these states is notable, because although the disease has occurred in all the continental states, historically more than half of reported cases have been from Arkansas, Missouri, Oklahoma, and South Dakota. The island of Martha's Vineyard off the coast of Massachusetts is also a focus of tularemia.

In the United States, tularemia is usually acquired from tick bites or from contact with infected animals, especially rabbits. Tick-associated cases now constitute the most common route of transmission, and primarily occur during the summer.[6] The most common vectors in the United States are the wood tick (*Dermacentor andersoni*), the dog tick (*Dermacentor variabilis*), and the Lone Star tick (*Amblyomma americanum*). A smaller peak of autumn and winter cases is a consequence of rabbit hunters skinning and eviscerating their game. Public health education materials aimed at decreasing the hazards of handling wild animals have contributed to the reduction of tularemia in hunters. Mosquitoes are the common vectors in northern Europe. Occasional individuals acquire infection from the bite of an infected animal or, more likely, from the bite of an animal whose mouth was contaminated from recently eating a diseased animal. The latter likely explains most instances of cat-bite tularemia.

Males experience a higher incidence of disease than females in all age groups, probably as a consequence of their greater exposure to the outdoors and animal-related activities and less use of protective measures against tick bites. Persons in all age groups are affected, with children 5 to 14 years of age and older adults most prominently represented. In the United States, American Indians and Alaska natives experience the highest annual incidence (0.5 per 100,000); whites have a lower risk (0.04 per 100,000), and African Americans and Asians/Pacific Islanders have the lowest occurrence of tularemia (≤0.01 per 100,000).

Although tularemia is usually a sporadic infection, outbreaks of disease have been traced to laboratory exposure, contaminated groundwater, muskrat handling, dressing a dead hare, lawn mowing, and brush cutting. In the latter two cases, primary pneumonic tularemia apparently occurred when the affected individuals created an environmental aerosol by mowing grass and cutting brush that had been contaminated with *F. tularensis* excreted in the urine and feces of infected rodents. An outbreak of oropharyngeal tularemia in Turkey affecting 55 patients was ultimately traced to contaminated tap water. The organism can survive in water, mud, and straw for weeks to months.

Interest in tularemia has been enhanced because of its potential use as a bioterrorism agent.[7] Its high infectivity (as few as 10 organisms induces pneumonic disease), its ease of dissemination, and the difficulty of rapidly diagnosing acute illness are characteristics that merit its inclusion among threat agents. Thus tularemia must be reported immediately to local public health authorities. Unusual patterns of disease will be investigated for both conventional and bioterrorist sources.

PATHOBIOLOGY

F. tularensis can infect humans through several portals of entry, including the skin, mucous membranes, and gastrointestinal and respiratory tracts. It requires intracellular residence and can multiply within macrophages and other cells. A large, not completely understood secretion apparatus is found in *Francisella*, known as a type VI secretion system (T6SS). It is essential for *Francisella* to escape from their phagosomes and multiply within host macrophages to cause disease.[8] After inoculation into the skin and subcutaneous tissue, local bacterial multiplication occurs and evokes a suppurative necrotic reaction characterized by an initial polymorphonuclear response followed by an influx of macrophages and lymphocytes. These suppurative lesions evolve into granulomas. Bacteremia can occur both early and late during this process. The infection can disseminate to the lymph nodes, liver, spleen, lungs, and pleura. Viable *F. tularensis* can persist in tissues for long periods, contributing to the tendency to relapse after treatment.

CLINICAL MANIFESTATIONS

Classically, the clinical manifestations of tularemia have been separated into six categories: ulceroglandular, glandular, oculoglandular, typhoidal, oropharyngeal, and pneumonic.[9] Although this classification has historic roots, it should not be used rigidly because many patients have features of several types. The course of illness is determined by the portal of entry, the degree of systemic involvement, and the dose and virulence of the infecting strain of *F. tularensis*.

The general features of tularemia are similar regardless of the portal of entry. After exposure, the usual incubation period is 3 to 5 days (range, 1 to 21 days). The disease begins abruptly with the onset of fever (≥101° F), chills, malaise, and headache. Myalgia, vomiting, sore throat, and abdominal pain can also occur. Almost half the patients have a pulse rate that is substantially slower than would be anticipated based on the degree of fever (pulse-temperature dissociation). The fever may abate somewhat after 1 to 3 days, only to recur and continue along with other symptoms for 2 to 3 weeks. Untreated, weight loss, easy fatigability, and lymphadenopathy may persist for weeks longer.

Ulceroglandular Disease

Ulceroglandular disease is the form of infection most readily recognized by physicians. Along with fever and other constitutional symptoms, the patient calls attention to tender, swollen lymph nodes that drain an inoculation site. The nodes are usually axillary or inguinal, and a local lesion appears concurrently or 1 or 2 days before or after the lymphadenopathy. The lesions at the site of inoculation begin as small, red, tender, or painful papules that progress to pustules and then undergo necrosis to produce an ulcer with sharp, somewhat elevated edges and a flat base that becomes black (Fig. 295-1). Untreated, the ulcers heal over a period of weeks and leave scars.[10] Tick-induced infections produce lesions on the trunk, about the waist, and in the perineum, along with the expected local adenopathy. Children typically have occipital and cervical adenopathy from tick bites on the neck and in the hair. Animal exposure often produces lesions on the hands and forearms. Lesions may be multiple. Because the organisms evoke a localized granulomatous response, frank lymphangitis does not occur in uncomplicated tularemia, but an occasional patient manifests a chain of nodules in "sporotrichoid" fashion along the lymphatic drainage.

Patients with such apparently "localized" disease often have symptoms and findings indicating a more widespread infection. Sore throat with or without an erythematous pharynx occurs, as well as chest radiographic findings of patchy infiltrates in the lower lobes, pleural effusions, and hilar adenopathy.

Glandular and Typhoidal Disease

Glandular disease is essentially the same clinical syndrome as ulceroglandular disease but without the local lesion. Thus the patient has fever, constitutional symptoms, and lymphadenopathy. The local lesion may have been on a part of the body where it was not seen, or it may have been small and already healed

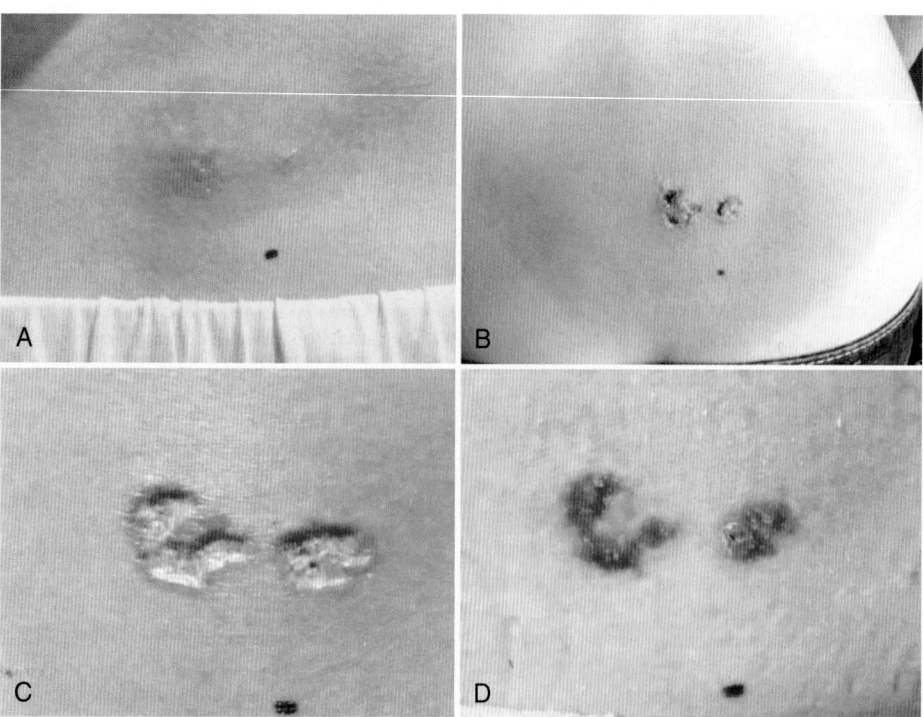

FIGURE 295-1. Ulcerative tularemia. (Source: Holland SD, Michelow IC. Tularemia masquerading as ecthyma. *J Pediatr.* 2016 Nov; 178.299. doi:10.1016/j.jpeds.2016.07.023. [Epub 2016 Aug 22.])

by the time the patient sought medical care. Glandular disease accounts for only 3 to 20% of cases. Typhoidal disease does not show evidence of lymphadenopathy and is essentially characterized by fever of unknown cause. These illnesses evade diagnosis unless the physician specifically considers the possibility of tularemia and inquires about tick or animal exposure. Occasionally, the diagnosis is made fortuitously when a positive blood culture is reported.

Oculoglandular Disease

Oculoglandular disease is rare (<5% of cases) and occurs when the conjunctival sac is the portal of entry via an aerosol, splash, or contaminated fingers. It is almost always unilateral and can have a dramatic manifestation with inflamed, swollen eyelids, chemosis, and painful conjunctivitis. The palpebral conjunctiva often shows small yellow nodules and ulcers, counterparts to the skin lesions of ulceroglandular disease. The affected regional lymph nodes are those of the head and neck.

Oropharyngeal Disease

Oropharyngeal disease is also uncommon in the United States and occurs when the mucous membranes of the mouth and pharynx are the portal of entry. Contaminated water or food (inadequately cooked game meat) is the source. Painful exudative pharyngitis and tonsillitis, pharyngeal ulcers, and swollen retropharyngeal and cervical lymph nodes are seen.

Pneumonic Disease

Although pneumonia may be one aspect of the other tularemic syndromes, *pneumonic tularemia* refers to an illness that manifests as a distinctive pneumonia.[11] It accounts for about 10% of reported cases and occurs from inhalational exposure. This is the form of the disease that would result from bioterrorism. In addition to fever and malaise, patients may have a dry cough, substernal discomfort, pleural pain, dyspnea, and sore throat. These pulmonary symptoms may not be very prominent in the context of the systemic illness. Hemoptysis is unlikely. The results of physical examination reflect the extent and distribution of the pneumonic process, which may range from barely evident to frank consolidation with pleural effusion. Radiographic findings range from modest peribronchial infiltrates early in the illness to distinctive bronchopneumonia with effusion. Hilar adenopathy is present in more than one third of cases. Sputum examination is not helpful. Pleural effusions generally contain more than 1000 lymphocytes/μL. Gram stain results are typically negative, and pleural biopsies occasionally contain granuloma, thus inviting confusion with tuberculosis. Without a suggestive history of tick or animal exposure, patients with tularemic pneumonia may be thought to have poorly responding community-acquired pneumonia. Fluoroquinolone antibiotics are commonly used as empirical therapy in this circumstance to treat some patients with undiagnosed tularemia pneumonia. Myocarditis is a rare complication.[12]

DIAGNOSIS

The diagnosis of tularemia involves serologic testing[13] with tube agglutination, microagglutination, or latex agglutination techniques. Antibody concentrations do not reach diagnostic levels until after the 11th day of illness. A single acute titer of 1 : 160 is considered presumptive; a confirmed diagnosis requires a four-fold rise in titer between acute and convalescent specimens. Titers of both immunoglobulin M and immunoglobulin G antibodies may remain elevated for many years after the illness. *F. tularensis* may be isolated from blood cultures and tissue specimens when media containing cysteine are used. Laboratory personnel should be notified when tularemia is suspected so that appropriate media can be used, incubation can be extended, and safeguards are in place to protect against the production of hazardous aerosols.[14]

Differential Diagnosis

The differential diagnosis of patients with tularemia is substantial. The local lesions can be confused with cat-scratch disease, brown recluse spider bites, *Mycobacterium marinum* infection, herpes simplex infection (Chapter 350), and even syphilis (Chapter 303) and chancroid (Chapter 285) when the lesions are in the perineum or on the penis. Pneumonic tularemia resembles common community-acquired pneumonia (Chapter 91), as well as less common infections such as psittacosis, legionellosis, and Q fever. The glandular and typhoidal forms can resemble typhoid fever (Chapter 292), brucellosis (Chapter 294), ehrlichiosis, and other illnesses accompanied by nonspecific fevers.

Routine laboratory studies do not provide specific results. Leukocyte counts may be within normal limits or elevated; thrombocytopenia, elevated liver enzymes, and sterile pyuria occur with some frequency.

TREATMENT Rx

Because tularemia is a relatively uncommon disease, therapeutic recommendations are based on a combination of in vitro studies and accumulated clinical experience. The preferred antimicrobials are streptomycin and gentamicin; either one is given for 10 days. Streptomycin is given at a dose of 1 g intramuscularly twice daily. Gentamicin may be more readily available and is administered at a dose of 5 mg/kg intramuscularly or intravenously once daily. Both chloramphenicol and the tetracyclines have been used in the past to treat tularemia; however, use of both these bacteriostatic agents has resulted in higher rates of relapse than treatment with streptomycin or gentamicin. Because chloramphenicol may produce bone marrow toxicity, it is rarely used today. Doxycycline is administered at a dose of 100 mg twice daily for 14 days. In recent years, ciprofloxacin has been used successfully in a growing number of patients; the dosage is 750 mg twice daily for 10 days.[15] Both of these drugs can be given orally at the same doses as soon as tolerated by the patient. There is a need to develop new therapeutic strategies to improve the management of patients with tularemia.

PREVENTION

Prevention of tularemia entails minimizing exposure to ticks and avoiding direct exposure to wild animals. Tick protection includes clothing that extends to the wrists and ankles, regular inspection for attached ticks, and the use of insect repellents containing diethyltoluamide (DEET). Gloves should be worn when skinning and dressing game animals, especially rabbits, and all wild rabbit and other game meats should be cooked thoroughly.

A live, attenuated vaccine has been used in the past to provide some protection to researchers working with *F. tularensis*. The vaccine is not available commercially, but another candidate vaccine is in preclinical testing.[16]

PROGNOSIS

Before treatment became available, acute tularemia often lasted as long as 1 month followed by several months of debility. The mortality rate approached 10%. When appropriately diagnosed and treated, the mortality rate from tularemia is now 1% or less.

GENERAL REFERENCES

For the General References and other additional features, please visit Expert Consult at https://expertconsult.inkling.com.

296

PLAGUE AND OTHER *YERSINIA* INFECTIONS

PAUL S. MEAD AND CHRISTINA A. NELSON

The genus *Yersinia* currently contains 19 species of which three are known to be important human pathogens, *Yersinia pestis*, *Y. enterocolitica*, and *Y. pseudotuberculosis*. The remaining species are generally considered nonpathogenic and are most frequently isolated from environmental sources. Two possible exceptions are *Y. intermedia* and *Y. frederiksenii*, which have been isolated from clinical samples, suggesting a possible role as rare human pathogens.

● PLAGUE

DEFINITION

Plague is a life-threatening flea-borne disease that is best known as the cause of the Black Death of the Middle Ages. The illness most often presents with regional lymphadenopathy but can also take the form of a primary pneumonia. Plague can be cured if treated promptly with appropriate antimicrobials.

The Pathogen

Plague is caused by *Y. pestis*, a microaerophilic, gram-negative, nonmotile, and nonsporulating coccobacillus belonging to the family Enterobacteriaceae.

Y. pestis can exist as a facultative intracellular pathogen and exhibits bipolar staining with Wayson, Giemsa, and Wright stains (Fig. 296-1). *Y. pestis* lacks a true capsule but has a carbohydrate-protein envelope comprised of the *capsular* or *fraction 1 antigen*. Although only one serotype is thought to exist, strains can be classified into biotypes. The three classic biotypes (*antiqua*, *mediaevalis*, and *orientalis*) differ in their ability to ferment glycerol and reduce nitrates. All three biotypes occur in Asia, which is generally accepted as the continent where plague originated. Two biotypes exist in Africa (*antiqua* and *orientalis*), but only the *orientalis* biotype occurs naturally in the Americas. All are highly virulent and appear to cause virtually identical signs and symptoms in humans.

EPIDEMIOLOGY

Plague is endemic in discrete areas of Africa,[1,2] Asia, and the Americas (Fig. 296-2), including the western United States (Fig. 296-3). In nature, *Y. pestis* is maintained through transmission cycles involving certain rodent species and their fleas, which act as vectors. Two general types of cycles have been postulated. Enzootic cycles involve low-level transmission among relatively resistant rodent species and are thought to pose little immediate risk to humans. Spread to more susceptible rodent species, however, can trigger an epizootic cycle in which the pathogen spreads rapidly through the rodent population, causing mass mortality. As rodent hosts die, infected fleas seek blood meals from nonrodent species, including humans. Although nonrodent mammals are typically dead-end hosts, some secondary transmission can occur, and rodent-consuming carnivores and raptors can potentially spread the disease to neighboring areas through the transport of infected rodent fleas. Recent work suggests a possible role for free-living ameba in maintaining *Y. pestis* in the environment.[3]

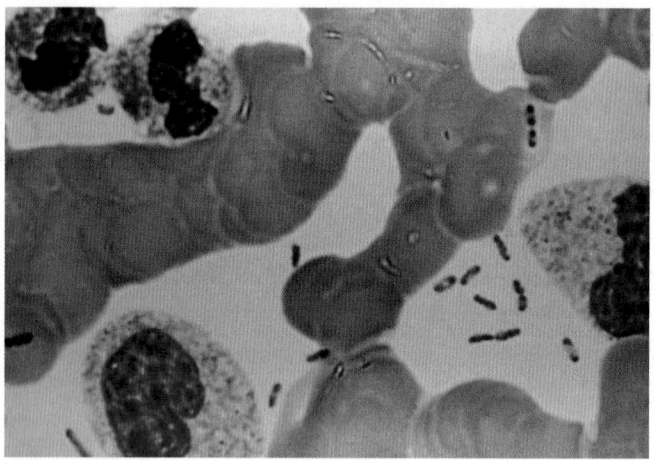

FIGURE 296-1. Wayson-stained blood smear from a fatal case of human septicemic plague. (Centers for Disease Control and Prevention.)

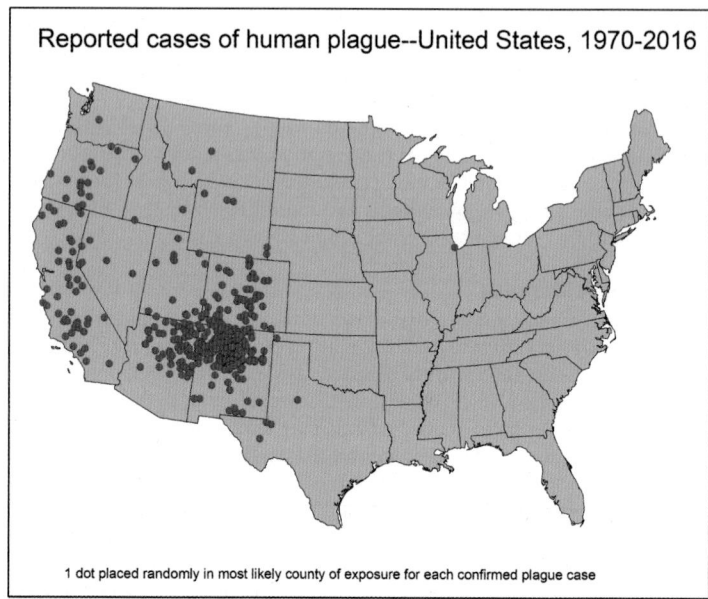

Reported cases of human plague--United States, 1970-2016

1 dot placed randomly in most likely county of exposure for each confirmed plague case

FIGURE 296-3. Distribution of human plague cases in the United States, 1970 to 2016. Case points were randomly placed within counties where exposures occurred to indicate the general distribution and clustering of cases by region. One dot placed in county of exposure for each plague case. (Centers for Disease Control and Prevention.)

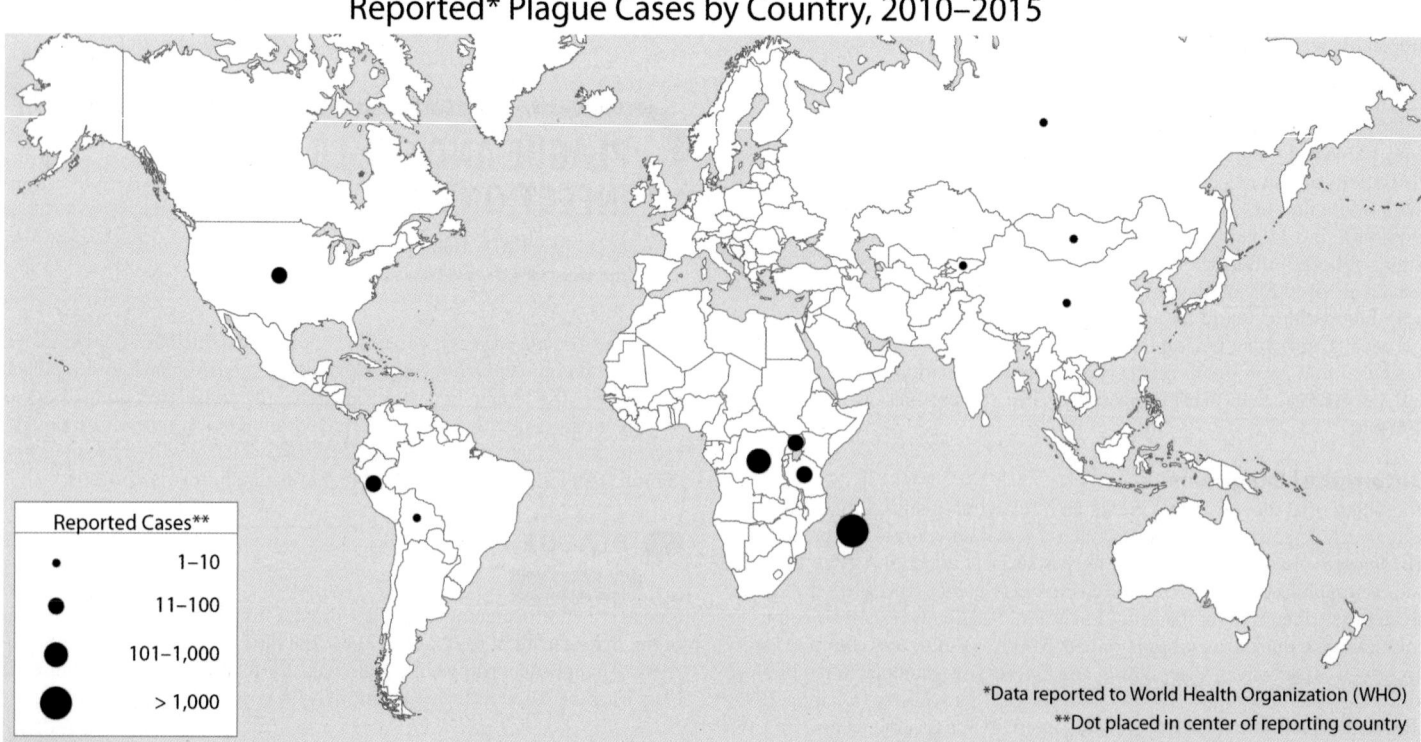

Reported* Plague Cases by Country, 2010–2015

Reported Cases**	
•	1–10
●	11–100
●	101–1,000
●	> 1,000

*Data reported to World Health Organization (WHO)
**Dot placed in center of reporting country

FIGURE 296-2. Worldwide distribution of plague in humans, 2010 to 2015. (Data compiled from the World Health Organization, Centers for Disease Control and Prevention, and other sources.)

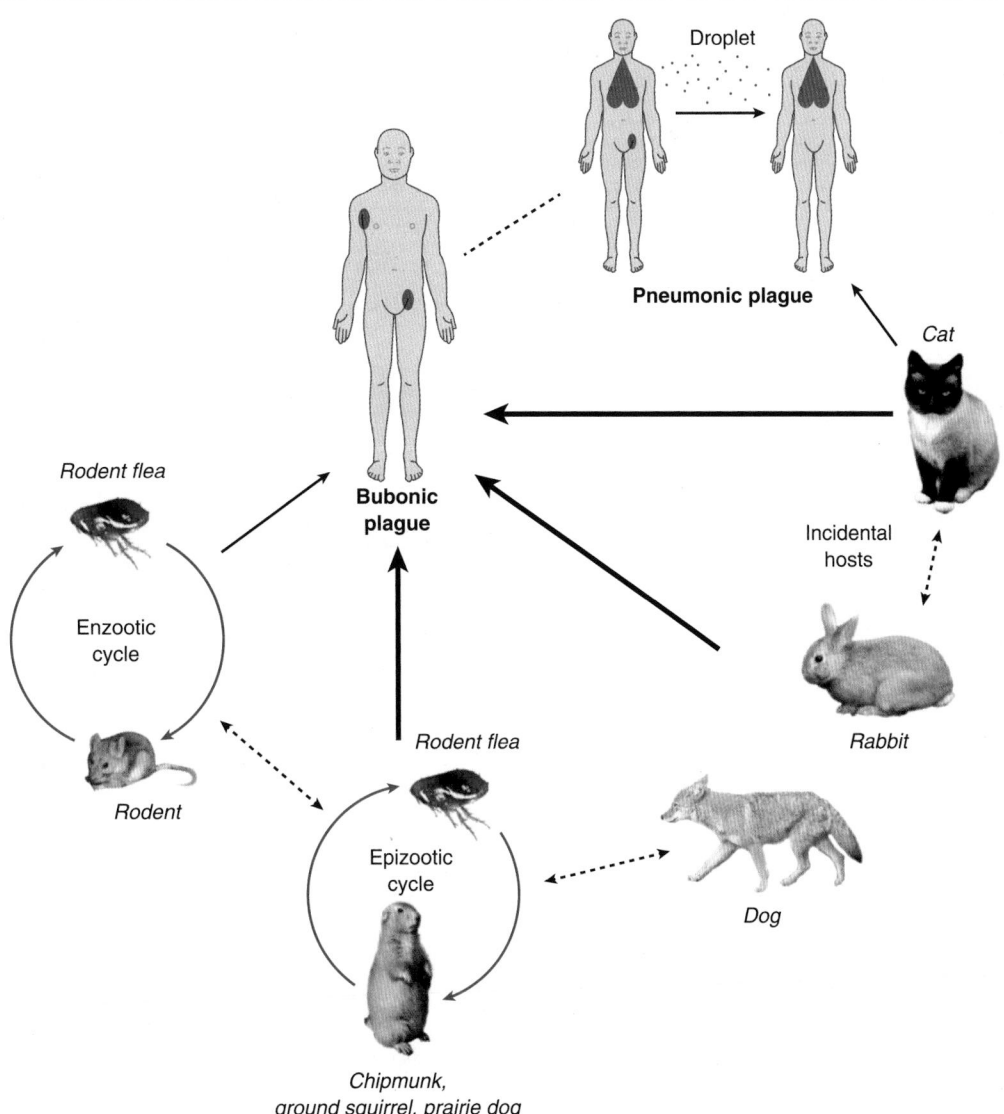

FIGURE 296-4. Ecology and transmission of plague. *Red circles* indicate zoonotic cycles. Common routes of transmission to humans indicated by *bold arrows* and uncommon routes by *thin arrows*. (Centers for Disease Control and Prevention.)

Humans can acquire plague through multiple routes, with the bite of an infected rodent flea being by far the most common (Fig. 296-4). Risk is greatest in endemic areas of the developing world where flea-infested commensal rats, especially *Rattus rattus* and *R. norvegicus*, live in close proximity to humans. The oriental rat flea, *Xenopsylla cheopis*, is a particularly efficient vector of *Y. pestis* and feeds readily on both rats and humans. In the United States, contact with commensal rats is less common and most cases result from the bites of fleas from other rodents, such as ground squirrels, prairie dogs, wood rats, and chipmunks. In this setting, flea bites are usually acquired during hiking, hunting, or other outdoor activities.[4] Allowing dogs to sleep in their owners' beds also appears to increase risk, presumably because these pets carry onto the bed fleas they acquired while roaming outside.

Although less common, humans can also become infected with *Y. pestis* through close contact with other infected mammals. Percutaneous exposure through direct contact with infected tissues, such as while skinning a rabbit or rodent for meat, or through the bites or scratches of infected carnivores such as cats, can transmit the organism. More concerning from a public health perspective is infection acquired though inhalation of infectious droplets. This usually occurs through exposure to animals or humans with pulmonary plague, and it results in primary pneumonic plague, a form of the disease that is often fatal and can spread from person to person under certain circumstances.

Despite the presence of plague-endemic areas on multiple continents, human infection is relatively uncommon. Prior to the discontinuation of routine notification in 2007, only 1000 to 6000 human plague cases were reported by the World Health Organization (WHO) each year. Over the last half century, the bulk of reported human cases has shifted from southeast Asia to sub-Saharan Africa. According to the most recently released WHO statistics covering the period 2010 through 2015, Madagascar, the Democratic Republic of Congo, Uganda, and other African countries accounted for 96.2% of the world's reported cases (Fig. 296-2). Asian countries accounted for only 0.5% of the total cases, and another 3.3% were reported from three countries in the Americas—Bolivia, Peru, and the United States. Much of the concern regarding plague stems not from the average case counts but from the potential for sudden outbreaks. In August 2017, a man in Madagascar died of pneumonic plague during a long bus ride, triggering an outbreak in which over 2,400 suspect cases were identified. Although it is likely that many of these patients did not actually have plague, the economic and social consequences were substantial.[5]

In the United States, plague is found in the continental states west of the 100th meridian. New Mexico accounts for the majority of human cases, followed by Arizona, California, and Colorado (Fig. 296-3). Since 2000, the annual number of cases has ranged from 1 to 17, with most cases occurring in the spring and summer. Cases are occasionally reported in other states, either due to travel to the west, as occurred in a Georgia resident in 2015, or due to laboratory exposure, as occurred in Illinois in 2009. Occupation-related infection has occurred among veterinary staff, biologists, and trappers, including cases of primary pneumonic plague among persons handling cats or dogs with signs of plague pneumonia, pharyngitis, or oral abscesses. Although human-to-human spread of primary pneumonic plague has not been confirmed in the United States since 1924, possible person-to-person transmission was identified in 2014 during an outbreak in Colorado. The overall case fatality rate for plague in the United States is typically less than 15%.[6]

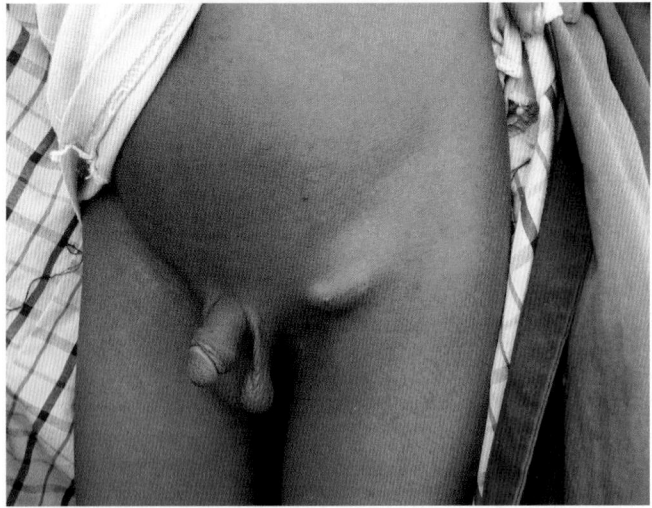

FIGURE 296-5. Young Malagasy boy with a bubo. (Courtesy Brook Yockey, Centers for Disease Control and Prevention.)

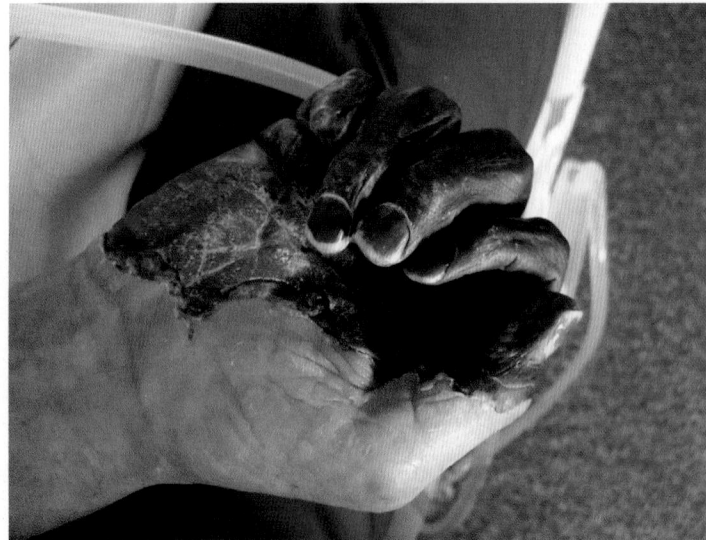

FIGURE 296-6. Hand of a patient with plague displaying acral gangrene, a manifestation that may have given rise to the term "black death." (Centers for Disease Control and Prevention.)

Concern has been raised that plague could be used as an agent of bioterrorism (Chapter 18). In most projected scenarios, bioterrorists would spread plague in an aerosol form, potentially resulting in numerous primary pneumonic cases, a high mortality rate, and widespread panic, especially if the *Y. pestis* strains released had been engineered to be resistant to antimicrobial agents commonly used to treat plague.

PATHOBIOLOGY

Few bacteria are more pathogenic for humans than *Y. pestis*. The organism's virulence reflects the need to achieve high levels of bacteremia in order to assure onward transmission to uninfected fleas. The process begins when *Y. pestis* enters the body, usually through the bite of an infected flea or other percutaneous exposure. Some bacteria are killed by polymorphonuclear leukocytes; however, others enter into mononuclear cells and are carried via lymphatics to the regional lymph nodes, where they replicate. Infected lymph nodes, termed *buboes* (Fig. 296-5), can appear edematous and congested early in the course of illness but exhibit little evidence of inflammatory infiltrates or vascular injury histologically. Within a few days, however, they contain massive numbers of *Y. pestis* and heavy neutrophil infiltrates, causing the substantial swelling and tenderness that are the hallmark of *bubonic plague*. As the illness progresses, hemorrhagic necrosis and vascular damage in the node become apparent; some nodes spontaneously rupture, and abscesses appear.

As the architecture of the infected lymph nodes break down, large numbers of *Y. pestis* enter the circulation, producing signs and symptoms typical of gram-negative sepsis. Disseminated intravascular coagulation (Chapter 166) can occur, triggering thrombosis within capillaries, vascular necrosis, ecchymoses, acral gangrene, and cutaneous, mucosal, and serosal petechiae (Fig. 296-6). Additional complications, seen in autopsy specimens, include diffuse hemorrhagic splenic necrosis, renal glomeruli containing fibrin thrombi, and multifocal necrosis in the liver. Of particular concern is hematogenous spread to the lungs, which can result in *secondary pneumonic plague*. Secondary pneumonic plague usually presents with scant sputum production and diffuse pulmonary infiltrates. Without prompt treatment, *Y. pestis* spreads from the interstitial spaces of the lung to the pulmonary alveoli; sputum increases in quantity and may become pink or blood tinged. At this point, a patient with secondary pneumonic plague can transmit infection to others through coughed respiratory droplets.

Inhalation of infectious droplets from patients with secondary plague causes primary pneumonic infection following an incubation period of 1 to 4 days. Patients with *primary pneumonic plague* experience a rapidly progressive lung infection that is initially lobular, then lobar, and finally multilobar, with large numbers of *Y. pestis* present in the alveoli and pulmonary secretions (Fig. 296-7). Primary pneumonic plague is also contagious and nearly always fatal in the absence of prompt antimicrobial treatment. It is important to note that a small percentage of patients with plague develop septicemia in the absence of recognized buboes, pneumonia, or other signs of localized infection, a condition referred to as *primary septicemic plague*. It is not clear why some

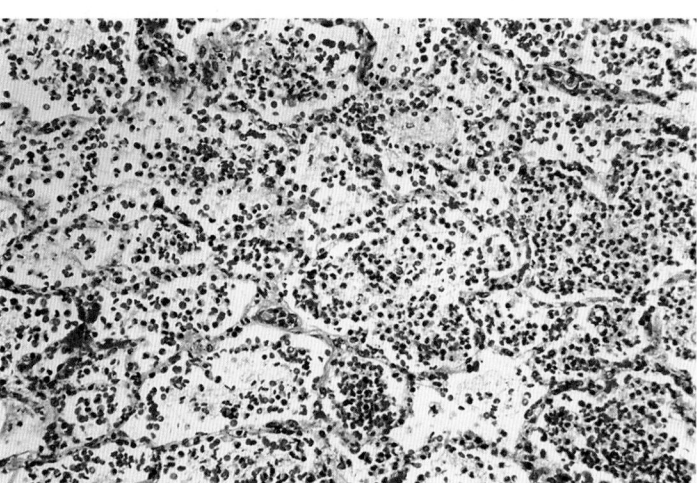

FIGURE 296-7. Photomicrograph of lung tissue from fatal case of primary pneumonic plague and septicemic plague. Note filling of alveolar spaces with inflammatory cells and debris. (Centers for Disease Control and Prevention.)

patients present without localizing symptoms, though notably abdominal pain is common. It is possible these cases reflect infection through the gastrointestinal tract or a flea bite on the trunk in a location where regional lymph nodes are mostly internal.

Multiple virulence factors have been shown to influence successful evasion of the host's immune system by *Y. pestis*, and it is likely that more will be recognized in the future.[7] The ability to escape from the host's innate immune defenses and disseminate to regional lymph nodes depends in part on a protease (Pla) encoded on the 9.5 kb plasmid that helps degrade fibrin clots and promote the production of excess plasmin, which can affect inflammatory exudates, break down extracellular proteins and basement membranes, and reduce levels of chemoattractants. Another virulence factor, YopM, is one of many *Yersinia* outer proteins (Yops), encoded by genes on the midsized (70 to 75 kb) plasmid of *Y. pestis*. Although most other Yops are degraded by the Pla protease, YopM is resistant to its activity and probably aids in the dissemination of *Y. pestis* by competing with platelets for thrombin, thereby reducing clotting, inhibiting the activation of platelets, and lowering local inflammatory responses. Initial invasion and dispersal to regional lymph nodes also depend on the ability of *Y. pestis* to survive for at least brief periods inside host phagocytes. Survival in such environments is promoted by other Yops that work in concert with a type III secretory apparatus to deliver into host phagocytes those Yops that act as intracellular effectors. These effector Yops disturb the cytoskeletal dynamics of phagocytic cells and block their production of proinflammatory cytokines. Affected phagocytes are rendered incapable of killing the invading *Y. pestis,* thereby allowing this bacterium to survive extracellularly in lymphoid tissues. Survival of *Y. pestis* in mammalian hosts also depends on its ability to acquire sufficient quantities of iron for growth. The most important means of iron uptake in *Y. pestis* is a siderophore (yersiniabactin) system that can effectively compete with host iron-binding molecules for this essential nutrient. The capacity of *Y. pestis* to survive within host phagocytes is complemented during later stages of infection by the expression of a glycoprotein capsular antigen (caf1 or fraction 1 antigen) that confers resistance to phagocytosis. Expression of caf1 is temperature dependent, being repressed at the cooler temperatures found in the flea vector and upregulated at mammalian host body temperatures.

CLINICAL MANIFESTATIONS

The three most commonly observed forms of plague (in order of decreasing occurrence) are bubonic, septicemic, and pneumonic. Unusual manifestations of plague include meningitis, pharyngitis, skin ulcers, and osteomyelitis. In rare instances, *Y. pestis* has been inoculated through the conjunctiva, resulting in oculoglandular plague. The incubation periods are 2 to 6 days for bubonic plague and 1 to 3 days for primary pneumonic plague.

The characteristic swollen and tender lymph nodes (buboes) of bubonic plague usually appear in the node or nodes located closest to the site of initial innoculation (Fig. 296-5). Most cases of bubonic plague in the United States are thought to be acquired from flea bites on the legs, as indicated by the appearance of inguinal or femoral lymph node involvement on the side where the flea bite occurred. Axillary buboes are also common, often indicating the handling of an infected animal or other flea-infested object. Cervical buboes are much less common in the United States than in many developing countries, perhaps because persons in the latter are more likely to sleep on dirt floors in flea-infested huts, thus increasing their chances of being bitten about the head and neck by infectious fleas. Occasionally, a skin lesion appears at the site of an infectious flea bite or other source of inoculation.

Symptoms of bubonic plague include fever, chills, myalgia, arthralgia, headache, malaise, and prostration. Untreated patients with bubonic plague become increasingly toxic, remain febrile, and experience tachycardia, agitation, confusion, delirium, and convulsions.

Septicemic plague manifests as a rapidly progressive, overwhelming endotoxemia. Patients often complain of gastrointestinal (GI) symptoms, including nausea, vomiting, diarrhea, and abdominal pain. Disseminated intravascular coagulation can also occur with the appearance of petechiae, ecchymoses, bleeding, and ischemia in the tips of the extremities. Later-stage septicemic patients are likely to experience refractory hypotension, renal dysfunction, obtundation, and other signs of shock. Patients with late-stage septicemic plague can also exhibit acute respiratory distress syndrome (Chapter 96), which has occasionally been confused with hantaviral pulmonary syndrome (Chapter 357) in the American Southwest. Because septicemic plague is likely to be fulminant and fatal, favorable outcomes depend on rapid diagnosis and prompt treatment with appropriate antimicrobials.

Pneumonic plague can be accompanied by fever, cough, chest discomfort that becomes increasingly painful, tachycardia, dyspnea, bacteria-laden sputum, chills, headache, achiness, weakness, and dizziness. As the illness progresses, patients may experience increasing respiratory distress, hemoptysis, cardiopulmonary insufficiency, and circulatory collapse. In the early stages of illness, patients with primary pneumonic plague may have signs of localized pulmonary involvement, beginning in a single lung and rapidly progressing to segmental consolidation and later bronchopneumonia, with death ensuing in as little as 1 to 3 days after the onset of symptoms. Localized infection is unlikely to be observed in the lungs of patients with secondary pneumonic plague because the lung tissues are infected initially through circulatory spread, which results in a diffuse interstitial pneumonitis. The appearance of sputum also differs in primary versus secondary pneumonic plague, being watery or mucoid, frothy, and perhaps tinged with blood in primary pneumonic cases but scanter, thicker, and more tenacious in secondary pneumonic cases.

DIAGNOSIS

Plague fatalities are typically related to delays in seeking treatment or misdiagnosis.[8] The differential diagnosis of plague in its various clinical forms includes staphylococcal (Chapter 272) or streptococcal adenitis (Chapter 274) or pneumonia (Chapter 91); cat-scratch disease (Chapter 299); tularemia (Chapter 295); chancroid (Chapter 285); acute filarial lymphadenitis (Chapter 335); mycobacterial infection (Chapter 309); septicemia caused by other bacteria; meningococcemia; mycoplasmal pneumonia and other community-acquired pneumonias; legionnaires disease (Chapter 298); Q fever; influenza pneumonitis (Chapter 340); hantaviral pulmonary syndrome (Chapter 357); viral pneumonia caused by respiratory syncytial virus (Chapter 338); cytomegalovirus (Chapter 352) or other viruses; and strangulated inguinal hernia.

Laboratory confirmation relies on bacterial culture accompanied by specific bacteriophage lysis tests or detection of a fourfold rise in antibody titer to the *Y. pestis* F1 capsular antigen over a period of 2 to 4 weeks. Preferred laboratory samples for culture include blood, bubo aspirates, sputum, bronchoalveolar fluid, and swabs of skin lesions or pharyngeal mucosa. Cerebrospinal fluid can also be collected from patients in whom plague meningitis is suspected. Although the procedures for confirming the laboratory diagnosis of *Y. pestis* infection are relatively simple, delays can occur because the relevant expertise and reagents are often limited to a few public health or reference laboratories. Automated bacterial identification systems frequently misidentify *Y. pestis* as a different organism (e.g., *Pseudomonas luteola*), which can also delay proper diagnosis. Because cases of plague can rapidly progress to a life-threatening illness and because culture of *Y. pestis* on bacteriologic media may require 48 hours or longer before colonies become visible, it is essential that patients suspected of having plague receive appropriate antimicrobial therapy immediately after samples have been taken. Direct fluorescent antibody assays can be used to identify *Y. pestis* bacteria in bubo aspirates, sputum samples, and tracheal washes; this procedure requires about 1 hour and provides strong presumptive evidence of infection. A presumptive diagnosis can also be obtained rapidly by detecting *Y. pestis* DNA in polymerase chain reaction (PCR) assays or *Y. pestis*–specific antigens in immunologic assays. In some developing countries, rapid immunochromatographic tests are used to detect plague antigen or antibodies. The potential advantages of these tests are that they require few laboratory resources, can be done in field settings, and yield results in less than 1 hour. The reliability and clinical performance of these tests are not well established, however, especially for testing samples such as sputum.

PREVENTION

No commercially available plague vaccine exists in the United States. Newer recombinant vaccines designed to stimulate immune responses to the F1 and V antigens of *Y. pestis* have yielded promising results and are effective in mice,[9] but they are unlikely to be available in the near future for general use.

Human plague risk can be reduced through the implementation of effective surveillance programs to rapidly identify human cases and evolving epizootics and allow effective intervention measures to be implemented. When appropriate, affected areas can be treated with insecticides to reduce the risk for flea bite exposure. Measures also should be taken to reduce the amount of food and shelter available to rodents. In rare instances, rodenticides can be used to reduce host numbers, but their use is not recommended before the implementation of effective flea control measures. Persons living in or visiting areas endemic for plague should avoid sick and dead animals and use insect repellents to reduce the risk for infectious flea bites. Dogs and cats should be prevented from roaming freely in rodent-infested areas, and these animals should be treated with flea control agents that safely and effectively kill fleas. Although most dogs appear to be somewhat resistant to plague, they can become infected and transmit infection directly to humans. Cats are highly susceptible, often experience severe illness, and can serve as sources of infection for their owners or veterinary staff. Cats that roam outside in endemic areas and suddenly become seriously ill should be taken to a veterinarian for evaluation.

Persons with pneumonic plague should be held in respiratory isolation for at least 48 hours after the initiation of appropriate antimicrobial therapy, and individuals caring for such patients should follow respiratory droplet precautions (masks, gloves, gowns, and eye protection). Although human-to-human transmission has not been confirmed in the United States for many decades, rare cases of primary pneumonic plague have occurred after face-to-face contact with infected cats that had oral lesions or symptoms of pneumonic plague. Veterinary staff from plague-enzootic areas should take appropriate precautions (masks, gloves, gowns, eye protection) when handling sick cats with illnesses suggestive of plague.

Prophylactic antimicrobial therapy is generally recommended for persons with possible plague exposure only in relatively high-risk situations, such as after close contact with patients with pneumonic plague, handling of *Y. pestis*–infected animals, or being bitten by rodent fleas in an area with a recent history of epizootic activity. The most recently recommended prophylactic antimicrobials are doxycycline and ciprofloxacin (Table 296-1).

TABLE 296-1	RECOMMENDATIONS FOR THE TREATMENT OF PATIENTS WITH PNEUMONIC PLAGUE IN CONTAINED AND MASS CASUALTY SETTINGS AND FOR POSTEXPOSURE PROPHYLAXIS*
PATIENT CATEGORY	**RECOMMENDED THERAPY**
CONTAINED CASUALTY SETTING	
Adults	Preferred choices: Streptomycin 1 g IM twice daily Gentamicin 5 mg/kg IM or IV once daily or 2 mg/kg loading dose followed by 1.7 mg/kg IM or IV 3 times daily Alternative choices: Doxycycline 100 mg IV twice daily or 200 mg IV once daily Ciprofloxacin 400 mg IV twice daily[†] Chloramphenicol 25 mg/kg IV 4 times daily[†]
Children[§]	Preferred choices: Streptomycin 15 mg/kg IM twice daily (maximum daily dose, 2 g) Gentamicin 2.5 mg/kg IM or IV 3 times daily[‖] Alternative choices: Doxycycline: if ≥45 kg, give adult dosage; if <45 kg, give 2.2 mg/kg IV twice daily (maximum, 200 mg/day) Ciprofloxacin 15 mg/kg IV twice daily[†] Chloramphenicol 25 mg/kg IV 4 times daily[‡]
Pregnant women[§]	Preferred choice: Gentamicin 5 mg/kg IM or IV once daily or 2 mg/kg loading dose followed by 1.7 mg/kg IM or IV 3 times daily[‖] Alternative choices: Doxycycline 100 mg IV twice daily or 200 mg IV once daily Ciprofloxacin 400 mg IV twice daily[†]
MASS CASUALTY SETTING AND POSTEXPOSURE PROPHYLAXIS	
Adults	Preferred choices: Doxycycline 100 mg PO twice daily[††] Ciprofloxacin 500 mg PO twice daily[†] Alternative choice: Chloramphenicol 25 mg/kg PO 4 times daily[‡‡]
Children[§]	Preferred choices: Doxycycline[††]: if ≥45 kg, give adult dosage; if <45 kg, give 2.2 mg/kg PO twice daily Ciprofloxacin 20 mg/kg PO twice daily Alternative choice: Chloramphenicol 25 mg/kg PO 4 times daily[‡‡]
Pregnant women[§]	Preferred choices: Doxycycline 100 mg PO twice daily[††] Ciprofloxacin 500 mg PO twice daily Alternative choice: Chloramphenicol 25 mg/kg PO 4 times daily[‡‡]

*In general, one antimicrobial agent should be selected, and therapy should be continued for 10 days. Oral therapy should be substituted when the patient's condition improves. These are consensus recommendations of the Working Group on Civilian Biodefense, updated to reflect approval by the U.S. Food and Drug Administration of specific fluoroquinolones for plague. Although animal and limited human studies support its use, gentamicin is not currently approved by the U.S. Food and Drug Administration (FDA) for treatment of plague in humans. Streptomycin, levofloxacin, ciprofloxacin, and moxifloxacin are FDA approved for treatment of plague.
[†]Other fluoroquinolones can be substituted at doses appropriate for age. The ciprofloxacin dosage should not exceed 1 g/day in children.
[‡]The concentration should be maintained between 5 and 20 μg/mL. Concentrations >25 μg/mL can cause reversible bone marrow suppression.
[§]In children, the ciprofloxacin dose should not exceed 1 g/day.
[‖]Aminoglycoside dosages must be adjusted based on renal function. Evidence suggests that gentamicin 5 mg/kg intravenously or intramuscularly once daily would be efficacious in children and may reduce adverse effects. Neonates up to 1 week of age and premature infants should receive gentamicin 2.5 mg/kg intravenously twice daily.
[§]In neonates, a gentamicin loading dose of 4 mg/kg should be given initially.
**The duration of treatment of plague in a mass casualty setting is 10 days. The duration of postexposure prophylaxis to prevent plague infection is 7 days.
[††]Tetracycline can be substituted for doxycycline.
[‡‡]Children younger than 2 years should not receive chloramphenicol. Chloramphenicol dose should not exceed 4 g/day. An oral formulation is available only outside the United States.
IM = intramuscular; IV = intravenous; PO = oral.
Adapted from Inglesby TV, Dennis DT, Henderson DA, et al. Plague as a biological weapon: medical and public health management. Working Group on Civilian Biodefense. *JAMA.* 2000;283:2281-2290.

TREATMENT Rx

The most commonly recommended agent for treating plague is streptomycin (see Table 296-1), but a randomized trial in Tanzania concluded that gentamicin and doxycycline are also effective for treating plague in adults and children with low rates of adverse events. A review of human cases treated in New Mexico also strongly suggests that gentamicin is effective and can be substituted for streptomycin. Tetracyclines are effective for treating uncomplicated cases of bubonic plague, and chloramphenicol is believed to be effective, particularly for plague meningitis. Although antimicrobial resistance is not believed to be a problem in the United States, strains resistant to tetracyclines and other agents have been described rarely, and resistance to streptomycin and chloramphenicol may also occur. Recently, the U.S. Food and Drug Administration approved levofloxacin, moxifloxacin, and ciprofloxacin to treat patients with plague under the agency's Animal Efficacy Rule, which allows evidence from animal studies, in this case those involving nonhuman primates, to be used to demonstrate the efficacy of a proposed treatment when it is not possible to conduct adequate trials in humans.

PROGNOSIS

Patients with uncomplicated bubonic plague respond quickly to appropriate antimicrobial therapy and typically defervesce, with relief from most other systemic manifestations within 2 to 5 days. Large buboes can remain swollen, however, for more than 1 week and may require incision and drainage if necrotic. In rare instances, ischemic necrosis in septicemic cases has resulted in the amputation of digits.

YERSINIOSIS

DEFINITION

The enteropathogenic *Yersinia, Y. enterocolitica* and *Y. pseudotuberculosis,* cause diarrheal illness and pseudoappendicitis. They differ substantially from *Y. pestis* in that they rarely cause death and are usually spread via the fecal–oral route.

The Pathogens

Y. enterocolitica is genetically quite distinct from *Y. pseudotuberculosis* and *Y. pestis.*[10] All three species, however, share an approximately 70-kb plasmid that encodes for various proteins (Yops) that are key virulence factors. Unlike *Y. pestis,* the enteropathogenic yersiniae are urease positive and motile at temperatures lower than 30° C. *Y. pseudotuberculosis* is rhamnose positive, thereby distinguishing it from the closely related *Y. pestis* and the more distantly related *Y. enterocolitica.* The enteropathogenic yersiniae are genetically more diverse than the more recently evolved plague bacterium. *Y. enterocolitica* contains six biogroups, five of which are known to be pathogenic for humans, and nearly 60 serogroups; *Y. pseudotuberculosis* has been classified into six distinct serogroups (O groups 1-6).

EPIDEMIOLOGY

Enteropathogenic yersiniae are transmitted via the fecal–oral route, with a relatively high median infectious dose of 10^8 to 10^9 bacteria. Typical sources of infection include inadequately cooked pork, dairy products, and certain vegetables. Both *Y. enterocolitica* and *Y. pseudotuberculosis* can survive and proliferate slowly at refrigerator temperatures. Although far less common, person-to-person transmission has been reported, as has transmission via blood transfusion. *Y. enterocolitica* frequently colonizes the oropharyngeal lymphoid tissues of pigs, explaining its particular association with pork products. Other species including rodents, rabbits, sheep, goats, cattle, horses, dogs, cats, and sometimes birds can serve as reservoirs. Most hosts act as asymptomatic carriers, but a few human cases have been associated with handling sick animals. Symptomatic patients shed large amounts of yersiniae for as long as 2 to 3 weeks. Untreated, infected persons can become carriers and shed for 2 to 3 months. Medical conditions associated with iron overload (e.g., hemochromatosis, thalassemia, cirrhosis) increase the risk of infection.

Yersiniosis is a reportable disease in many countries. Most cases result from *Y. enterocolitica* infection, and this agent reportedly accounts for 1% to 3% of all cases of acute enteritis in some areas. In 2015, the overall annual incidence in the United States was 0.28 cases per 100,000 persons, with rates approximately 3-fold higher among children younger than 5 years old and adults aged 70 years and older.[11] Although historically higher, rates among African Americans have decreased 10-fold since 1996, and are currently approximately half that of the overall rate. Previously high rates among African American populations were associated with the home preparation of chitterlings made from contaminated pork intestines. Exposure of contaminated pork products is also considered a likely source of infection for Asian Americans.

Y. enterocolitica serotypes O:3, O:8, O:9, and O:5,27 have been associated with human disease. Serotype O:3 (biotype 4) predominates in most countries and is found most commonly in swine. Serotype O:9 (biotype 2) has been isolated from sheep, cows, and goats. These last two serotypes are the most common causes of human infection worldwide but are considered less pathogenic than strains of the O:8 (biotype 1B) serotype, which are associated with the most severe outbreaks. Although serotype O:8 infections appear to be decreasing in incidence in the United States, they are becoming increasingly important in Japan, Italy, and France. In Europe, most cases involve serotype O:3 infections, although a few are associated with serotypes O:9 and O:5,27. Biotype 1A is generally considered nonpathogenic, and biotype 5 has been isolated only from hares. Strains pathogenic in humans are esculin, salicin, and pyrazinamidase negative.

Y. pseudotuberculosis has been isolated from rodents, cattle, sheep, cats, dogs, and birds. It occurs worldwide, but human infections are most commonly reported in northern Europe and in Asia, including Japan. O group 1, 2, and 3 strains are associated with human disease, with most cases being attributed to O:1 or O:2 strains. Infected animals serve as chronic carriers and sources for the infection of water and foods such as meat, dairy products, and stored vegetables. Some cases have been associated with the handling of kittens and puppies. Outbreaks of *Y. pseudotuberculosis* in Finland were traced to eating iceberg lettuce and carrots (serotypes O:3 and O:1, respectively). A large Canadian outbreak was associated with milk that had been pasteurized but nevertheless became contaminated. Outbreaks in the former Soviet Union have been associated with the consumption of root vegetables that were stored underground for winter consumption and presumably became contaminated with rodent excreta containing *Y. pseudotuberculosis*.

PATHOBIOLOGY

Y. enterocolitica possesses numerous virulence factors responsible for its persistence in the GI tract and ability to cause disease in susceptible hosts. Upon reaching the ileum, *Y. enterocolitica* adheres to the mucosa, where intracellular infections in Peyer patches, mucosal cells, and macrophages can occur. Invasion of the ileal mucosa, which is mediated by the presence of invasin, an outer membrane protein, and a 17-kD surface factor (Ail), affects intestinal barrier function.[12] An inflammatory response causes abdominal pain and diarrhea, as well as ulcerative ileitis, mesenteric adenitis, and necrosis within Peyer patches. Colonization of the oropharynx may cause an accompanying sore throat in up to 20% of patients. If the regional defenses are breached, the bacteria can disseminate and cause sepsis and hepatic and splenic abscesses. Polyarthritis can also occur later in the course of illness, particularly in human leukocyte antigen (HLA)-B27–positive individuals.

Similar to *Y. pestis,* the enteropathogenic yersiniae attack host lymphoid tissues. Invasion of these tissues and resistance against host defenses depend on the possession of the approximately 70-kb plasmid that is shared by each of the three pathogenic yersiniae and bears genes encoding for various Yops and the so-called V antigen. The products of this plasmid work in concert to inhibit phagocytosis and reduce inflammation, thereby suppressing the host immune response and favoring persistence of these microbes.

Patients with reactive arthritis (Chapter 249) are more likely to have fewer GI symptoms, lower T-cell proliferative responses to *Yersinia* antigens, lower initial immunoglobulin (Ig) M responses, higher and more persistent IgG and IgA responses, and increased levels of IgA with a secretory component. *Yersinia*-specific antibody responses are also more likely to persist in patients with reactive arthritis than in those with uncomplicated GI disease. *Yersinia* antigens thought to contribute to reactive arthritis include Yops and released proteins, which stimulate host CD4 cells, and heat shock protein 60, which has been hypothesized to work in conjunction with other antigens to modulate the host immune response. Evidence exists that hosts can maintain chronic *Y. enterocolitica* infections for years after the initial infection, a factor that may induce the inflammation associated with reactive arthritis (Chapter 249).

CLINICAL MANIFESTATIONS

After an incubation period of about 3 to 7 days, a gastroenteritis typically develops that can be difficult to distinguish from *Salmonella* (Chapter 292) or *Campylobacter* (Chapter 287) gastroenteritis. The most common clinical syndromes associated with *Y. enterocolitica* infection are acute enteritis with fever, diarrhea, vomiting, right lower quadrant pain suggestive of appendicitis (Chapter 133), erythema nodosum, and reactive arthritis. Other common symptoms include associated pharyngitis, rash, joint pain, and headache. Stool examination reveals leukocytes or erythrocytes, and one fourth of patients experience bloody diarrhea.

Y. pseudotuberculosis infections most commonly manifest as enterocolitis, pharyngitis, and pseudoappendicitis. Whereas enterocolitis is most likely to occur in young children, older children more frequently experience acute terminal ileitis, mesenteric adenitis, and systemic disease. Pseudoappendicitis has been reported in patients with mesenteric lymphadenitis. Sepsis is uncommon and is most likely to occur in persons with underlying conditions such as diabetes mellitus, cirrhosis, immunosuppression, older age, and hemochromatosis. Splenic abscesses, meningitis, or endocarditis can develop in septic patients, and the mortality rate can approach 50%. Erythema nodosum is identified in about one third of all patients and in 10% of adults.

DIAGNOSIS

Yersiniosis should be suspected in patients with abdominal pain and fever, especially if they live in high-incidence areas. The diagnosis is best accomplished by isolation of the bacterium from stool, blood, or other appropriate samples. Recovery of *Y. enterocolitica* and *Y. pseudotuberculosis* from clinical and environmental samples can be greatly complicated by the presence of other bacteria that are likely to predominate. The preferred selective medium for isolation from stool specimens is CIN (cefsulodin–irgasan–novobiocin) agar prepared with relatively low cefsulodin concentrations. Isolation of yersiniae is also helped by culture at 25° to 30° C, which results in better growth than when cultures are kept at 35° C and favors growth of the more cold-tolerant yersiniae over other bacteria that require higher temperatures. After being obtained, isolates can be confirmed as enteropathogenic *Yersinia* by biochemical tests. Biotyping and serotyping, which are often available only in research or reference laboratories, can provide useful epidemiologic information. Isolation difficulties and the reported low sensitivity (about 10^3 to 10^6 colony-forming units per gram of sample) of current isolation techniques have led some to suggest that PCR or other DNA-based methods are likely to result in the more rapid and sensitive detection of these bacteria. Data from the United States suggest a growing reliance on culture-independent methods of laboratory diagnosis.[13]

Tube or microagglutination tests can identify antibodies to the pathogenic *Y. enterocolitica* serogroups O:3, O:9, O:5,27, and O:8, but cross-reactivity can be a problem, particularly between *Y. enterocolitica* O:9 and *Brucella* spp. PCR for O genotyping of *Y. pseudotuberculosis* could eventually replace traditional serotyping methods. Immunologically mediated *Yersinia* illnesses, including reactive arthritis, are associated with the production of IgA antibodies that can be detected by enzyme-linked immunosorbent assay (ELISA) or immunoblotting. IgG antibodies can persist for many years, but persistence of IgA antibodies for more than a few months could indicate a chronic *Yersinia* infection.

PREVENTION

Prevention depends on measures intended to protect persons from contact with contaminated environments, foods, and wastes. These include using proper sewage disposal methods, protecting water supplies from contamination with human or animal wastes, following appropriate procedures for animal husbandry and slaughtering, thoroughly cooking meats (especially pork), avoiding long-term storage of meats at temperatures higher than 39° F, and consuming only pasteurized milk. Individuals should thoroughly wash their hands after handling potentially contaminated pork or other foods. Persons with diarrhea should not work in food-handling areas, care for young children, or work with patients, and hospital staff should follow enteric precautions. Vaccines are not available.

TREATMENT ℞

Antibiotics have not been shown to improve the course of uncomplicated enterocolitis or mesenteric adenitis, and the use of antimicrobial therapy is not generally recommended for intestinal forms of the disease. Such therapy is, however, recommended for immunocompromised patients, patients with septicemia, and those with systemic disease or extraintestinal foci of infection. It should be noted that in vitro susceptibility does not necessarily indicate efficacy in vivo.

Broad-spectrum cephalosporins, sometimes accompanied by aminoglycosides, have resulted in successful outcomes in patients with extraintestinal forms of yersiniosis, including septicemia. Ciprofloxacin, cefotaxime, and ceftriaxone are considered the most effective agents for treating *Y. enterocolitica* serogroup O:3 infection. *Y. enterocolitica* serogroup O:3 and O:9 isolates possess chromosomally determined β-lactamases that can confer resistance to ampicillin, carbenicillin, and cephalothin. Although serogroup O:8 strains, which produce type A β-lactamase, show resistance to the latter two agents, they are susceptible to ampicillin. It has yet to be determined whether antimicrobial therapy is useful for treating immunologically mediated forms of yersinial illness, including reactive arthritis.

PROGNOSIS

Cases of *Y. enterocolitica* enteritis are generally mild and self-limited after a 2- to 3-week course of illness. Sequelae most commonly include reactive arthritis and erythema nodosum. Glomerulonephritis and myocarditis have also been reported, particularly with serogroup O:3, biotype 4, phage type 8 infections. Other sequelae can include endocarditis, pericarditis, and osteitis. *Y. enterocolitica*–induced reactive arthritis, which can appear 1 to 3 weeks after infection, is oligoarticular, asymmetrical, and peripheral; it occurs most frequently in the lower limbs and eventually resolves over a period of a few weeks to months. HLA-B27–positive patients are more likely to experience severe and prolonged arthritis.

Y. pseudotuberculosis infections are also generally mild and self-limited. Reported complications include erythema nodosum, iritis, reactive arthritis, and nephritis. Although infection of the bloodstream by *Y. pseudotuberculosis* is rare, one review of 72 such cases reported that 26 (36%) were fatal.

GENERAL REFERENCES

For the General References and other additional features, please visit Expert Consult at https://expertconsult.inkling.com.

297

WHOOPING COUGH AND OTHER *BORDETELLA* INFECTIONS

CHRISTOPHER J. GILL AND ERIK L. HEWLETT

DEFINITION

Whooping cough, also known as "pertussis," is a respiratory illness that affects all age groups and is characterized by distinctive, violent, paroxysmal, coughing episodes, each of which may last several minutes and between which patients often feel entirely normal. In infants, pertussis may be manifested by spells of apnea and cyanosis, alone or in conjunction with coughing, which ends in the classic, inspiratory whoop that gives the disease its name. Severe and fatal disease is concentrated among infants. Whooping cough is primarily caused by infection with *Bordetella pertussis* or, much less frequently, *Bordetella parapertussis* or *Bordetella bronchiseptica*.[1,2]

The Pathogens

Including the classic species of *B. pertussis*,[3] *B. parapertussis*, and *B. bronchiseptica* (primarily a veterinary pathogen), there are now 16 known species of *Bordetella*, formally classified in the family Alcaligenacae.[4] In addition to the original three species listed previously, *B. holmesii* is recognized as a cause of pulmonary infections and whooping cough–like illnesses as well as invasive tissue infections. Other *Bordetella* species (E-Table 297-1) are associated with bacteremia and wound infections in patients with comorbid, immune-compromising conditions, such as diabetes and cancer/chemotherapy. *B. avium* (primarily a pathogen for poultry) and *B. hinzii* were named as subspecies of *Alcaligenes faecalis*, an environmental, gram-negative bacillus, which causes difficult-to-treat nosocomial infections, such as sepsis and ventilator-associated pneumonias.

Bordetella species are gram-negative coccobacilli and, contrary to earlier descriptions, *B. pertussis*, *B. parapertussis*, and likely others in addition to *B. bronchiseptica* are motile under specific conditions. *B. pertussis* was first isolated by Bordet and Gengou in 1906, and the medium most often used for isolation (Bordet-Gengou agar) still bears their names.

EPIDEMIOLOGY

Historically, pertussis was a childhood illness. Although children younger than 1 year are at the highest risk for death, more than 50% of reported cases in the United States now occur in those 10 years and older. Use of whole-cell pertussis vaccines (wPs), beginning in the 1940s, led to a 99% reduction in pertussis cases and established it as a "vaccine-preventable" disease.[5] In addition, pertussis vaccines have shifted the age-specific incidence of disease, as illustrated in Figure 297-1,[6] depicting the age distribution of pertussis cases in Sweden during 1989, when no pertussis vaccines were in use, and 2014, 17 years after the introduction of acellular pertussis vaccines (aPs). In the prevaccine era, pertussis was contracted in childhood; although resultant immunity was not lifelong, continued exposure maintained immunity with little or no clinical disease. Introduction of aPs for infants and children caused a marked reduction in cases in those age groups but shifted the burden of disease to adolescents and adults whose immunity was waning because of limited exposure.

In 2012, 48,277 cases of pertussis were reported in the United States, the highest number since 1959, and approximately 60% were in adolescents and adults. Concurrently, pertussis diagnosis transitioned from culture to polymerase chain reaction (PCR) testing, which is much more sensitive and relatively unaffected by antibiotics. Although this change likely resulted in detection of milder and atypical cases, severe/fatal disease in infants and overall number of cases have also increased and are not an artifact of detection bias. Pertussis is resurgent in the United States and elsewhere in the world, and the incidence is shifting toward a higher proportion of cases in older age groups.

Pertussis is endemic in the United States, with spikes in reported cases occurring in 3- to 5-year cycles, which are believed to reflect accumulation of susceptible subjects. Thus, prolongation of interepidemic cycle times strongly suggested that wPs have impaired transmission as well as a role in preventing disease.

Despite *B. pertussis* being fastidious and not easily cultured, pertussis is a highly contagious infection, with spread primarily by aerosol droplets. Furthermore, the long-held belief that there is no "carrier" state for pertussis (asymptomatic individuals harboring the organism) is challenged by data from experiments in primates. In contrast to animals convalescent from infection with *B. pertussis* and those that had received wP, aP recipients become infected with *B. pertussis* and transmit it to other animals, despite remaining without cough. Although not documented in humans, mathematical modeling suggests that transmission occurs by asymptomatic humans, consistent with current epidemiologic data.

PATHOBIOLOGY

B. pertussis produces a number of toxins, and pertussis was considered in the past to be a "toxin-mediated" disease. Although much is known about individual virulence factors, their roles in disease and an integrated understanding of the pathobiology are just beginning to develop.[7] Although a "cough toxin" has been postulated, mechanisms underlying the classic cough remain to be identified. The toxins and other virulence factors, elaborated at different times in the pathogen's life cycle and acting in different sites, allow pathogen persistence by modulating the host immune and inflammatory responses.[8]

Knowledge about individual toxins and adhesins is also important for their use as antigens in aPs. Filamentous hemagglutinin (FHA), pertactin (PRN), and fimbriae (FIM) are adhesins and are components in most aPs, all of which contain PToid. FHA interacts with the integrin CD11b/CD18 (also known as CR3 or Mac-1) and induces the functions of host myeloid cells to modulate inflammation.[9]

Pertussis toxin (PT) is an adenosine diphosphate (ADP)-ribosylating toxin that has Giα and several other guanosine triphosphate (GTP)-binding proteins as its targets.[10,11] It is a soluble toxin with local and systemic effects, most notable of which is induction of leuko-lymphocytosis. Early in infection, PT is immunomodulatory by inhibiting recruitment and function of alveolar macrophages and neutrophils. Its actions shift, however, during the course of infection, such that later, PT upregulates inflammatory responses, perhaps enhancing shedding and infectivity. Adenylate cyclase toxin (ACT) also binds CR3 to enter host cells and produce supra-physiologic levels of cyclic adenosine monophosphate (cAMP), which inhibits antibacterial functions of myeloid cells.

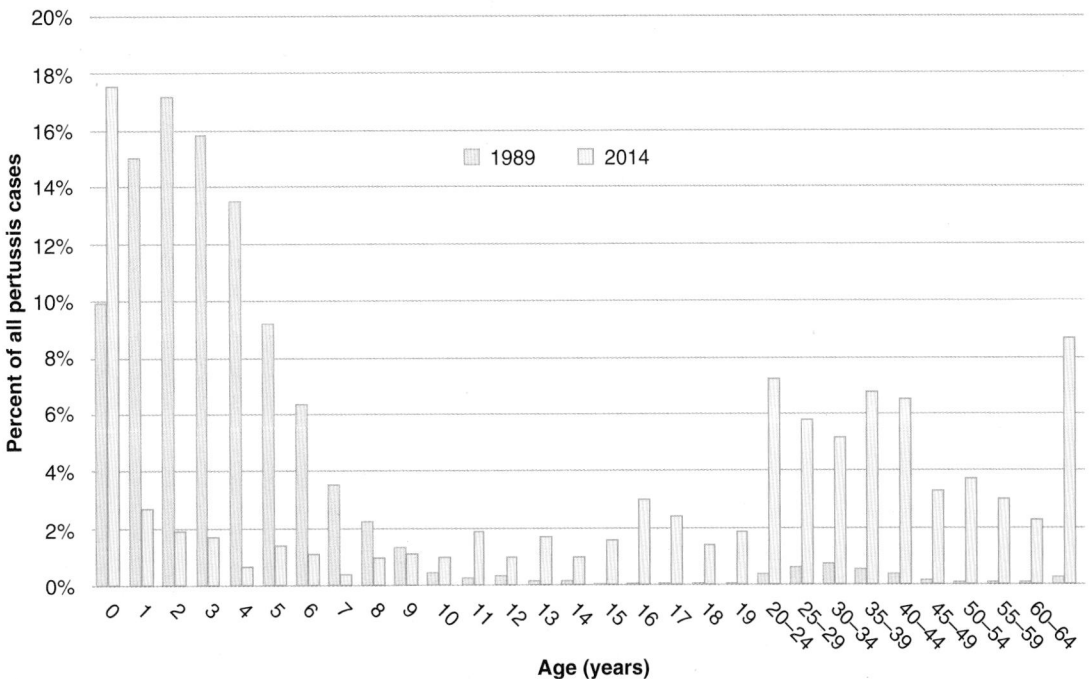

FIGURE 297-1. Distribution of whooping cough in Sweden by age ranges during a period when no pertussis vaccines were used (1989) and a period 17 years after the introduction of acellular pertussis vaccines (2014). (From Aronsson B vSK, Kallberg H, Bergstrom J, Lindstrand A, Uhnoo I, Tegnell A. *Pertussis Surveillance in Sweden: Seventeen Year Report.* Solna, Sweden: The Public Health Agency of Sweden; 2015.)

Although there are reports of bacteremia with *B. pertussis* and *B. parapertussis*, infections with these organisms are principally localized to the respiratory tract. Bacteria adherent to the cilia damage epithelial cells and stimulate mucus secretion. Intracellular *B. pertussis* organisms have been demonstrated, but the significance of these observations remains unknown.

CLINICAL MANIFESTATIONS

Although the paroxysmal cough of pertussis is striking and unforgettable, not all patients experience it.[12] Infants may have apnea, which only sometimes develops into paroxysmal cough. Furthermore, epidemiologic studies suggest that unrecognized pertussis may account for some sudden infant death syndrome (SIDS) cases. Following exposure to aerosol from a patient with pertussis, infected individuals develop nonspecific upper respiratory symptoms (mainly coryza) after 1 to almost 3 weeks. This long incubation period complicates epidemiologic tracking and outbreak control. Although infants are at greatest risk for morbidity and mortality, recent data show that clinically trivial infections, which resolve without classic cough, occur commonly in infants; thus, pertussis in this age group is not invariably typical in its presentation.

Importantly, clinical signs that indicate onset of the catarrhal phase (rhinorrhea, lacrimation, conjunctival injection, and sometimes low-grade fever) are nonspecific and do not suggest pertussis, except in the setting of an outbreak. This phase, which can last as little as a few days or as long as a week, may include a nonproductive cough. It is often not until a patient begins the paroxysmal phase with typical cough that a diagnosis of pertussis is considered. The striking cough, consisting of a series of uncontrollable expirations, followed by gasping inhalation, which is responsible for the "whooping" sound, is more frequent in children, may be associated with cyanosis, and may end with gagging and vomiting; in an infant, this can result in dehydration and malnutrition. The paroxysmal stage can last more than 4 weeks, and the development of fever or worsening pulmonary function suggests the possibility of secondary pneumonia. The paroxysmal cough occurs in at least 80% of adolescents/adults, but the whoop and post-tussive vomiting[13] are variable. In addition, adults may experience atypical symptoms, such as a scratchy throat and episodes of sweating.

Reduction in frequency and severity of cough marks transition to convalescent phase, which can last several months. It is often during this time that adults seek medical care for "chronic cough," leading to evaluation for conditions such as asthma, tuberculosis, chronic lung diseases, malignancies, and gastroesophageal reflux. After cough appears to have ended, patients may experience renewed coughing in conjunction with unrelated upper respiratory illnesses; this is often incorrectly interpreted as recurrence of pertussis. In 80% of adults, pertussis is at least 3 weeks in duration, and 27% are still coughing after 90 days.

Complications

In infants younger than 12 months who are hospitalized, about 25% have pneumonia, 1.1% experience seizures, and encephalopathy is seen in 0.3%, with an overall mortality rate of 1%. Pertussis in infants and small children can be complicated by pulmonary hypertension, which appears to be a direct consequence of the PT-induced lymphocytosis leading to pulmonary vascular congestion. Adolescents and adults may have some of these same complications with lower frequency, and adults can experience other problems related to their underlying medical conditions; cough syncope, herniated intervertebral disc, sudden-onset hearing loss, angina episodes, and even carotid artery dissection have been reported.[14] Paroxysmal cough and associated post-tussive vomiting can be severe enough to cause rib fractures, conjunctival hemorrhages, and other forms of tissue trauma.

DIAGNOSIS

Several methods have been used to detect *B. pertussis*, its products, and the host response to them, but each has its limitations. Culture is the "gold standard" (specificity approaching 100% in symptomatic patients), but even with specialized transport medium and a careful, interested laboratory, recovery rates are often less than 50% and are affected by duration of illness and use of antimicrobials before specimen collection. Cephalexin, which is ineffective against *B. pertussis*, is typically included in selective media such as Regan-Lowe but will inhibit growth of *B. holmesii*, potentially leading to false-negative culture results for this rare organism.

PCR-based diagnostic tests are much more sensitive than culture and can remain positive for days into antimicrobial treatment.[15] Appropriately designed PCR assays distinguish among *B. pertussis*, *B. parapertussis*, and *B. bronchiseptica*, depending on the target DNA sequence. Even with these precautions, there have been apparent "outbreaks" of pertussis that resulted from false-positive PCR assays. Ironically, several of these pseudo-outbreaks were due to pertussis vaccines: to note, a common acellular pertussis vaccine used in the United States includes *B. pertussis* DNA, which can contaminate clinical areas. Detection of serum antibodies to products of *B. pertussis* can be used to identify patients late in infection, but care must be taken to distinguish an acute response from residual antibodies to vaccine antigens; this is accomplished by higher thresholds for positive antibody responses.

Another concern is that PCR testing for *B. pertussis* has used an insertion sequence (IS481) found in abundance in its genome. This sequence is, however, found in *B. holmesii*, but not in *B. parapertussis*, resulting in *B. parapertussis* being overlooked and making it impossible to distinguish *B. pertussis* from *B. holmesii* based on the IS481 screening test alone. Use of additional primers to detect PT gene (not found in *B. holmesii*) and HIS1001 (only found in *B.*

holmesii) overcomes this problem. Multiplex PCR against each primer identifies all three species but may not be available in all laboratories.

In view of these diagnostic limitations, the World Health Organization has established a clinical case definition: 21 or more days of paroxysmal coughing with laboratory confirmation or epidemiologic linkage. Though useful for clinical trials, it is now clear that this definition misses cases of lesser severity, atypical presentation, or shorter duration.

Diagnosis of the very rare, environmental and nonrespiratory *Bordetella* species is difficult outside of research settings, and no standardized diagnostic tests exist. Some of the more recently discovered species were identified fortuitously using techniques such as whole-genome sequencing of soil samples or MALDI-TOF (matrix-assisted laser desorption/ionization—time of flight spectroscopy) techniques that are becoming more common in clinical microbiology facilities.

TREATMENT   Rx

Supportive Therapy

Because infants and young children have the highest risk for complications and death from pertussis, supportive therapy is often the most important component of their medical care. Close observation (preferably in the hospital) is essential to ensure adequate feeding, oxygenation, and hydration to minimize complications in this age group. Neither antibiotics (when administered after onset of paroxysmal cough) nor other pharmacologic interventions that have been tested for amelioration of cough have been found to be effective. Critically ill children with severe hypoxemia may benefit from extracorporeal membrane oxygenation (ECMO). The strong association of lymphocytosis with hypoxemia and pulmonary hypertension suggests that the lymphocytosis may participate in a causal pathway with the latter two. For this reason, leuko-reduction therapies, such as exchange transfusions or leukapheresis, have often been attempted in critically ill children but with uncertain benefit. This intervention has never been tested in a randomized controlled trial, but only in observational studies for which selection biases create an obvious barrier to estimating efficacy.

Antimicrobial Agents

There are two objectives in using antimicrobials in a patient with pertussis: first, to limit the course of illness in the treated patient; and second, to reduce transmission. Because individuals can remain culture positive and potentially transmit *B. pertussis* for several weeks after the onset of symptoms, it is appropriate to treat patients within that time frame. Antimicrobials do not, however, provide symptomatic relief or alter the course of illness in an infected individual unless initiated within the first week of symptoms (well before onset of paroxysmal cough).

The recommendation of the U.S. Centers for Disease Control and Prevention for the treatment of pertussis in adults is azithromycin (500 mg on day 1, followed by 250 mg/day on days 2 to 5) or clarithromycin (1 g/day in two divided doses for 7 days) or erythromycin (2 g/day in four divided doses for 14 days) or trimethoprim-sulfamethoxazole (trimethoprim, 320 mg/day, sulfamethoxazole, 1600 mg/day, in two divided doses for 14 days). Treatment with erythromycin for 7 days has now been shown to be as effective as 14 days.

PREVENTION

Immunization

Killed wPs were developed soon after isolation of *B. pertussis* in the early 1900s. Introduction of these into general use in the late 1940s had dramatic effects on the incidence of pertussis, with reported cases in the United States falling from more than 200,000 annually to less than 2000 in 1980.

In the 1970s and 1980s, increased recognition of adverse events in recipients of wPs led to public concern, which, in conjunction with bureaucratic pressure, was a factor driving development and adoption of alternative vaccines. Current aPs, which contain one or more purified protein antigen (PToid plus combinations of FHA, PRN, and FIM, types 2 and 3), are safe and cause significantly fewer adverse reactions than wPs. In recognition of the role for adolescents and adults in transmission to infants and small children, several aPs are licensed for administration to these groups.

Typically, pertussis vaccines (whether wP or aP) are delivered as part of multivalent combination vaccines. For example, in the United States, infants typically receive DTaP (diphtheria, tetanus, acellular pertussis), either combined with inactivated polio vaccine (IPV) and hepatitis B vaccine, or IPV plus *Haemophilus influenzae* type B (Hib) vaccine. Outside of the United States, wPs are similarly combined with other common injectable antigens in various combinations. Such vaccines are commonly referred to as "the pentavalent," even though the number of combination antigens may vary.

In addition, the strategy of "cocooning"—vaccination of all close contacts of a newborn—is being used as a means to prevent transmission to infants. Unfortunately, this approach has proved surprisingly ineffective in several randomized controlled trials.[16] One explanation for this seemingly paradoxical result is provided by studies in infant baboons, in which aP prevented symptomatic disease but failed to prevent infections and to render infected animals noncontagious.

By contrast, maternal Tdap (an adult/adolescent booster vaccine containing tetanus toxoid and reduced concentrations of diphtheria and pertussis antigens) is given later in pregnancy with the intent of providing passive immunity against pertussis to the infant. This approach has been highly effective at reducing infant pertussis in the United Kingdom and is now recommended in the United States for all pregnant women. Thus, any benefit of cocooning is likely due to vaccination of the mothers and other household contacts *before* delivery.

Unfortunately, in many countries, including the United States and the United Kingdom, pertussis rates began to increase 5 to 10 years after introduction of aPs. This is clearly due, in part, to the shorter duration of immunologic protection afforded by aPs. Furthermore, *B. pertussis* strains appear to be evolving to evade the specific alleles and antigens in aPs. A striking example of such evolutionary shifts is the near disappearance of pertactin-expressing *Bordetella* species in the United States.[17] Similar shifts have been reported for the vaccine alleles that code for FIM2, FIM3, and PT. However, none of these factors alone accounts fully for the epidemiologic patterns characterizing the pertussis resurgence.[18]

The failure of cocooning and the resurgence of pertussis despite high vaccine uptake rates have forced a reappraisal of aPs and a focus on the immunologic features that distinguish them from wPs. In a natural experiment, U.S. researchers examined age-specific pertussis incidence 20 years after the transition from wPs to aPs, with age as a proxy for which type of vaccine these individuals would have received; those younger than 11 years could only have received acellular pertussis vaccines, while those older than 15 years would have received wPs; and those in between, representing the transition years, likely received a blended schedule of the two types. While pertussis rates in the younger than 11 group increased steadily with age, consistent with the short duration of protection from aPs, in older children pertussis incidence fell dramatically, and among those 15 years and older, pertussis was almost completely absent. Thus, the duration of protection by wPs was greater that by aPs, and the overall benefit, reflecting, in part, herd protection, was also greater.

Interpretation of these epidemiologic data is supported by experimental infection of infant baboons with *B. pertussis*. Collectively, these studies established that wPs and aPs are both effective at preventing clinical illness, but they affect infection differently: wPs cut the duration of infection in half and reduce the peak bacterial burden,[19] whereas aPs have no impact on the magnitude or duration of infection. Moreover, animals receiving aP were easily infected by exposure to infected animals and transmitted *B. pertussis* to other animals, even in the absence of cough. Immunologically, wPs induce a helper T-cell response skewed toward T_H17 phenotypes, whereas aPs elicit T_H2 responses. Thus, available data suggest that much of the resurgence reflects differential immunologic responses to the two types of vaccine, with wPs having a greater impact on infection and transmission than aPs.

Such insights have renewed interest in pertussis vaccine development. While some have advocated for a return to wPs, or including them as part of a blended schedule with aPs, the lack of licensed wPs in the United States is a major barrier, and public acceptance could be challenging. Alternatives, including a live attenuated *B. pertussis* nasal vaccine (BPZE1) designed to optimize mucosal immune responses or a polysaccharide-protein conjugate vaccine linking *B. pertussis* capsule to PT are being examined.[20]

Chemoprophylaxis

Chemoprophylaxis with the aforementioned antimicrobial agents is an important mechanism for controlling outbreaks in hospitals or the community. This approach is effective when initiated before the onset of symptoms and is recommended for individuals exposed within the preceding 3 weeks, high-risk persons with underlying health problems, infants, and other individuals who have not been immunized.

PROGNOSIS

Most patients will eventually clear *B. pertussis*, even without antimicrobial treatment, but in a naïve host the clinical manifestations can persist for months, well beyond elimination of the causal organism. Furthermore, antimicrobials are of limited effectiveness in altering the course of the illness, unless started well before the paroxysmal phase begins. Infections with *B. bronchiseptica,* on the other hand, are often long-lasting and require antibiotic treatment for clearance.

GENERAL REFERENCES

For the General References and other additional features, please visit Expert Consult at https://expertconsult.inkling.com.

298

LEGIONELLA INFECTIONS

THOMAS J. MARRIE

DEFINITION

Legionellosis is the term for infection due to bacteria in the *Legionella* genus, of which there are two main manifestations—pneumonia (legionnaires disease) and Pontiac fever (named after Pontiac, Michigan, where it was first recognized). Pontiac fever is usually a mild febrile illness presumed to be a reaction to lipopolysaccharide of *Legionella* species.

The Pathogen

Legionellae are small, gram-negative, aerobic, non–spore-forming bacilli that measure 0.3 to 0.9 μm wide by 2 to 20 μm long (Fig. 298-1A to D). These organisms require special media for growth, and many laboratories are unable to isolate legionellae; thus, when laboratory expertise is uncertain, a negative culture is meaningless. They usually do not stain with Gram stain. In tissue specimens, Dieterle or Warthin-Starry stain may visualize these organisms. *Legionella micdadei* retains the modified acid-fast stain and can appear as acid-fast bacilli in clinical specimens. Legionellae are aquatic organisms that thrive in both natural and human-made waterways and distribution systems, especially hot-water pipes, water heaters (electrical more so than gas heaters), cooling

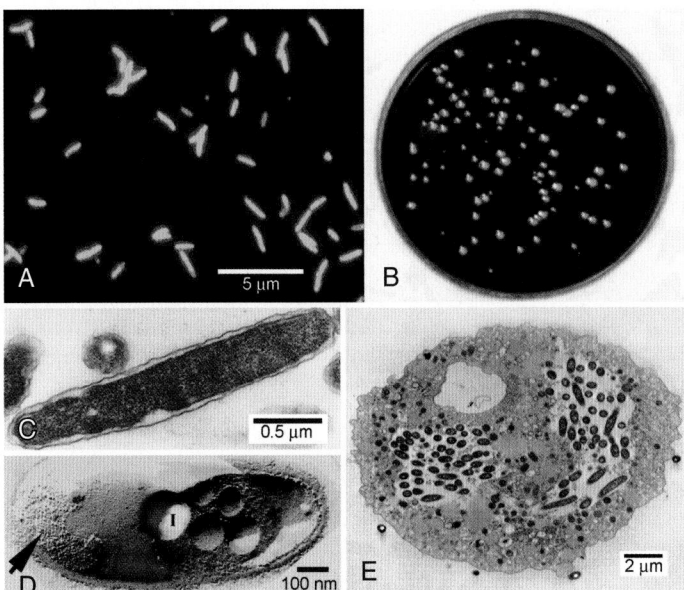

FIGURE 298-1. **A,** Direct fluorescent antibody stain of *Legionella pneumophila.* **B,** Colonies of *L. pneumophila* growing on a BCYE plate. **C,** Thin section of replicative form of *L. pneumophila.* **D,** Freeze-fracture replica of the mature infectious form obtained after growth in ameba. The latter shows prominent cytoplasmic inclusions (I) and a polar distribution of membrane proteins (*arrow*). **E,** Electron micrograph of *L. pneumophila* growing within *Acanthamoeba castellani.* (**A,** Courtesy Dr. Paul Hoffman, University of Virginia. **B,** Courtesy Dr. Sharon Berk, Tennessee Technical University. **C** to **E,** Courtesy Drs. Rafel Garduno and Gary Faulkner, Dalhousie University.)

towers, and water fountains. In these systems, they are found in biofilms that help confer resistance to biocides and chlorine. They are also found in moist soil and mud. They can survive in these environments for long periods and can tolerate temperatures of 0° to 68° C and a pH range of 5 to 8.5. In their natural environments, they are intracellular parasites of protozoa, such as the freshwater amebae *Acanthamoeba* and *Hartmannella* species (Fig. 298-1E). Indeed, legionellae can live in at least 20 species of ameba, two species of ciliated protozoa, and one species of slime mold. Free-living legionellae in biofilms are inactivated within a few weeks, whereas those residing in amebae survive for 6 months or more. Humans are accidental hosts who become infected by inhaling *Legionella* bacteria or amebae laden with these bacteria. Genomes of more than 500 different strains of *L. pneumophila* have been sequenced, and they range in size from 3.2 to 3.9 Mb. Legionellae have many eukaryotic-like proteins, which may help the intracellular growth of these organisms in human macrophages by mimicking host proteins. *Legionella* species have types I, II, IV, and V secretion systems, which allow the efficient and rapid delivery of molecules into the phagocytic host cell.

The number of new *Legionella* species continues to grow; there are now at least 59 *Legionella* species and 73 serogroups or more, including 15 serogroups of *L. pneumophila.* A variety of typing systems can be used to further refine the isolates so that individual strains can be identified, a factor that is important for determining the source of an outbreak or understanding the difference between environmental and clinical isolates. It is noteworthy that *L. pneumophila* and all its serotypes cause disease in humans (with serotype 1 predominant), whereas only about 50% of the remaining species of *Legionella* cause such disease.

Other *Legionella* spp that are more common causes of disease in humans are *L. micdadei, L. bozemanae, L. dumoffii,* and *L. longbeachae. L. longbeachae* is significantly more virulent than *L. pneumophila* in a mouse model of legionnaires disease, a finding that is substantiated clinically in that patients infected with *L. longbeachae* were more likely to require intensive care treatment than those infected with *L. pneumophila.*[1,2]

EPIDEMIOLOGY

The incubation period for legionnaires disease is most commonly cited as 2 to 10 days, with extremes of 1 to 28 days. Person-to-person transmission does not occur. Legionellosis is found worldwide, predominantly in developed countries owing to the frequent use of cooling towers and complex plumbing systems. Underdiagnosis may be a feature in developing countries because of the laboratory facilities required. In recent years, there has been an increase in *Legionella* cases in Japan from 56 cases in 1999 to 804 cases in 2011, reaching a rate of 1.15 per 100,000 population; in Europe, the rate in 2010 was 1.25 cases per 100,000, and in the United States, the rate increased from 0.42 to 1.62 per 100,000 between 2000 and 2014. Currently about 5000 cases are reported per year in the United States.[3] From 1990 to 2005, 23,076 cases of legionnaires disease were reported in the United States. Only 1.7% of these cases occurred in children, whereas 63% occurred in those aged 45 to 64 years. Males accounted for 61% of cases, and rates were highest in the eastern United States, where most cases occur in the summer or fall. The rate of legionnaires disease is 10 times higher in New York than it is in California. Also in the United States, the rate of legionnaires disease is higher in blacks than in whites, and it is 2.5 times higher in high-poverty areas compared with low-poverty areas. Eastern Canada also has higher rates of legionnaires disease than the rest of that country. The epidemiology of legionnaires disease in Europe is not dissimilar to that of the United States. The countries with rates of more than 2 per 100,000 were France, Denmark, Spain, Netherlands, and Italy. Twenty percent were travel associated, and the overall case-fatality rate was 11%. In the United States the case-fatality rate is 9%.

Accumulating international data have suggested that hot, wet weather is associated with *Legionella* risk. Using real-time polymerase chain reaction (PCR) assay on lower respiratory tract specimens in a routine practice over a decade show a seasonal pattern. Performing 44,000 *Legionella* PCR tests on Mayo Clinic and Mayo Medical Laboratories patients, positivity was highest in the summer and lowest in the winter (Fig. 298-2).[4] This seasonality observed with routine clinical PCR testing mirrors previous findings using culture in the greater Philadelphia area, the Netherlands, and Barcelona.

There is also an association between increased humidity and rainfall with cases of legionnaires disease. The connection may be aerosolization of *Legionella* from rain puddles on roads. In one study, 33 (47.8%) of puddle water samples were positive for *Legionella,* yielding 325 isolates. Among the 14 sequence types of the clinical isolates, 4 were present in puddle water isolates.

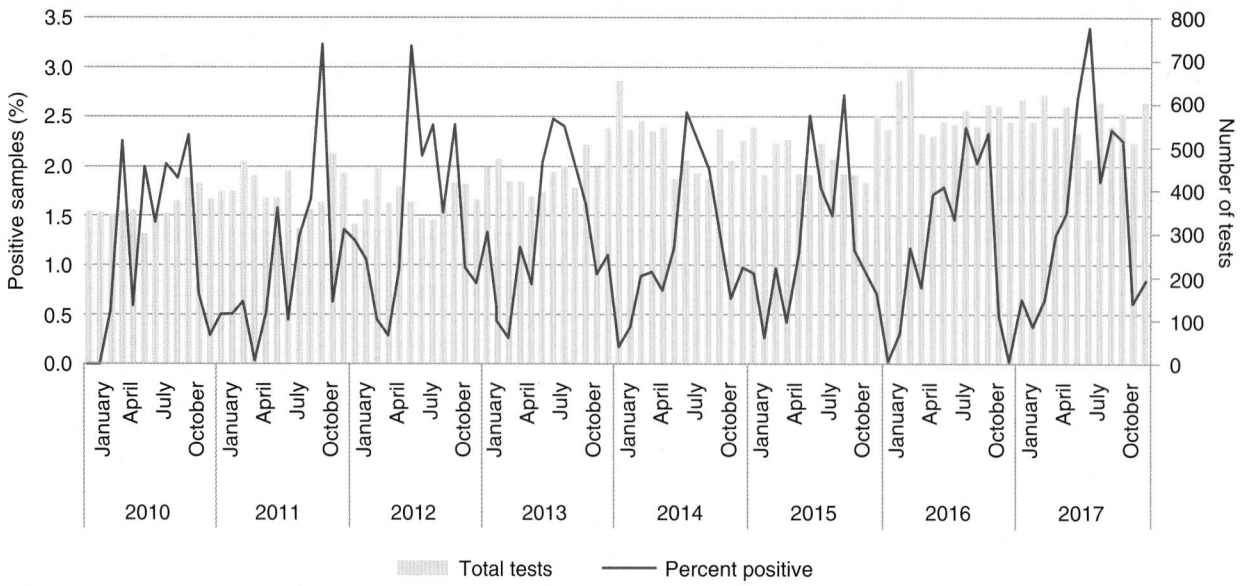

FIGURE 298-2. Seasonality of *Legionella* detection by real-time polymerase chain reaction (PCR). Data were obtained with PCR testing of more than 44,000 *Legionella* PCR tests on Mayo Clinic and Mayo Laboratories patients between January 2010 and December 2017. Average monthly *Legionella* PCR-positivity rates and test volumes over 8 years (2010–2017), The *dark-blue line* represents the mean monthly positivity, and the *light-blue bars* represent average monthly test volumes. (From Rucinski SL, Murphy MP, Kies KD, et al. Eight years of clinical *Legionella* PCR testing illustrate seasonal pattern. *J Infect Dis.* 2018 Apr 11. doi:10.1093/infdis/jiy201. [Epub ahead of print.])

TABLE 298-1 RISK FACTORS FOR LEGIONNAIRES DISEASE

RISK FACTOR	APPROXIMATE INCREASED RISK (-FOLD) OVER PERSONS WITHOUT THIS RISK FACTOR
HOST FACTORS	
Renal failure requiring dialysis	20
Corticosteroid therapy	5-10
Hairy cell leukemia	20
Lung or hematologic malignant neoplasm	7-20
Cytotoxic chemotherapy	5
>3 Alcoholic drinks/day	3-4
Cigarette smoking	2-10
Age >50 years	2
Diabetes mellitus	2
Solid organ transplantation (immunosuppression)	2
Anti–tumor necrosis factor treatment	16-21
Chronic heart or lung disease	>1
Splenectomy (non-*Pneumophila* strains only)	—
ENVIRONMENTAL FACTORS	
Travel	2
Recent plumbing work in home or at work	2
Hospitalization	—
Exposure to contaminated water sources—cooling towers, hot tubs, decorative fountains	—
Exposure to potting soil (Australia) for *Legionella longbeachae*	—

The most common risk factors for the acquisition of legionnaires disease are listed in Table 298-1.[5,6] *Legionella* species account for 1 to 5% of community-acquired pneumonia requiring admission to a hospital. In some areas, *Legionella* accounts for about the same percentage of pneumonia treated on an ambulatory basis. *Legionella* infections can be sporadic or occur in outbreaks. Outbreaks have been associated with exposure to a variety of aerosol-producing devices, including showers, a grocery store mist machine, cooling towers, whirlpool spas, decorative fountains, and evaporative condensers.[7] Other water sources implicated in transmission of legionnaires disease include water on trains, birthing pools, dental units, asphalt paving machines, and windscreen wiper fluid without added screen wash. Legionnaires disease can be acquired up to 10 to 11 km away from contaminated cooling towers. Aspiration of contaminated potable water by immunosuppressed patients is another mechanism by which *Legionella* is acquired. The U.S. Centers for Disease Control and Prevention (CDC) investigated 38 outbreaks of legionnaires disease from 2000 to 2014, 27 of which were land based. Median number of cases per outbreak was 10, ranging from 3 to 82. In 85% there was enough information to evaluate maintenance deficiencies.[8] These included process failures, human errors, equipment failures, and unmanaged external changes.[9] It was also noted that health care–associated outbreaks accounted for 57% of the cases and 85% of the deaths. Seven of the health care–associated outbreaks were in long-term care facilities.

Hotel travel–associated cases tend to be due to contaminated cooling towers and potable water, while ship travel–associated cases are usually due to contaminated hot tubs.

It is important to note that outbreak-associated cases account for the minority, only 5 to 10%, of cases of legionnaires disease.

Legionnaires disease in transplant recipients is frequently due to non-*Pneumophila* species, and hence urinary antigen cannot be relied on as a diagnostic tool in this setting. Only about 20% of the *Legionella* infections in this setting occur within the first 3 months after transplantation.

A number of biologic modifying agents used to treat cancer, autoimmune disease, multiple sclerosis, and other factors that compromise hosts seem to increase the risk for legionnaires disease. For example, treatment with infliximab results in a 15-fold increase in risk, and adalimumab with a 38-fold increase.[10]

Exposure to contaminated potting soil is a risk factor for *L. longbeachae* infection in Australia and New Zealand.

Pontiac fever occurs predominantly in outbreaks with very high attack rates. *L. pneumophila*, *L. micdadei*, and *L. anisa* have been implicated in outbreaks of Pontiac fever. Among residents of nursing homes, Pontiac fever has been associated with *L. pneumophila* concentrations of greater than 10^4 colony-forming units/L in shower water. Those receiving corticosteroid therapy have a six-fold higher risk for development of Pontiac fever.

PATHOBIOLOGY

After being inhaled, legionellae are phagocytosed in the lungs by alveolar macrophages. Only virulent strains of *Legionella* are capable of initiating organism-directed endocytosis when attachment to the alveolar macrophage through E-cadherin and β_1-integrin receptors occurs.[11] Legionellae abrogate phagosome-lysosome fusion and replicate in an endosome surrounded by the endoplasmic reticulum. Once it is intracellular, the bacteria-laden endosome recruits small vesicles, mitochondria, and ribosomes, and within 4 to 6 hours it becomes enveloped by the endoplasmic reticulum, thereby establishing the replicative endosome. After a latent period of about 12 hours, the bacteria start dividing. During this time, there is synthesis of up to 35 proteins and repression of 32 proteins. Iron must be available in the phagosome for growth. Growth continues in the macrophages for approximately 24 hours, at which time the macrophage dies and the bacteria are released. The released bacteria are often phagocytosed by other macrophages, dendritic cells, and epithelial cells, perpetuating the infection. Cell-mediated immunity is necessary for recovery from *Legionella* infection. Production of type 1 interferons has a protective effect by promoting the activation of macrophages. Activated macrophages limit the intracellular replication of legionellae by downregulating the expression of their transferrin receptors and limiting the availability of iron to the bacteria.

The pathogenesis of Pontiac fever is unclear. The onset of illness occurs within 12 to 36 hours after the inhalation of, presumably, endotoxin. This period is too short for bacterial multiplication to cause the symptoms.

CLINICAL MANIFESTATIONS

Most of our knowledge of the clinical features of legionnaires disease comes from studying patients who have been hospitalized with this illness, that is, those with the most severe manifestations. Fever (often high), malaise, and cough are present in most patients. Chills occur in about 75%, and dyspnea in just more than half the patients. Other features include myalgias, headache, chest pain, and diarrhea. The cough is nonproductive in 50% of patients; others have scant sputum production that is usually mucoid, rarely purulent, and very rarely bloody.[12] There are no clinical features that distinguish individual patients with legionnaires disease from those with pneumonia caused by other pathogens.[13] However, when patients with legionnaires disease are compared with those with community-acquired pneumonia due to other agents, the patients with legionnaires disease are more likely to have myalgias, headache, diarrhea, and a higher mean oral temperature at the time of presentation. They also present to the hospital sooner after the onset of symptoms, 4.7 days versus 7.7 days. When patients with legionnaires disease were compared with patients with bacteremic pneumococcal pneumonia, the following features were more associated with *Legionella* pneumonia: male sex, heavy drinking of alcohol, previous β-lactam therapy, temperature higher than 39° C, myalgias, and gastrointestinal symptoms. Pleuritic chest pain and purulent sputum were less likely to be present. In a young, otherwise healthy person with rapidly progressive pneumonia (especially if the progression occurs in the setting of β-lactam therapy), legionnaires disease should be strongly suspected. Mental confusion is common, and on occasion, the presentation is dominated by extrapulmonary manifestations such as reactive arthritis, cerebellar ataxia, seizures, myoclonus, or encephalitis. Rarely, extrapulmonary infection, such as prosthetic valve endocarditis, sinusitis, dialysis shunt infection, or abscess formation, occurs.

Physical findings include fever, tachypnea, relative bradycardia, and initially only a few crackles on chest examination. Later, the findings of pulmonary consolidation are not uncommon. Abdominal examination is usually unremarkable. Rash as a manifestation of legionnaires disease is very rare. Progression of the illness is not uncommon, even after the institution of antibiotic therapy. About half the patients with legionnaires disease who require hospitalization have a complicated course. The clinical presentations and outcomes of *Legionella* pneumonia in HIV-infected patients have been noted to be comparable to those without HIV infection.[14]

Survivors of legionnaires disease in one study had major sequelae persisting 17 months after diagnosis.

Pontiac fever has an incubation period of about 36 hours. Fever, severe myalgia, headache, and extreme fatigue are the dominant manifestations. The illness is of short duration, lasting, on average, 3 days.

DIAGNOSIS

It is most important to have a high index of clinical suspicion that a patient might have legionnaires disease.[15] Routine laboratory test results are nonspecifically abnormal. Leukocytosis is common; leukopenia, thrombocytopenia, and disseminated intravascular coagulation also occur. Other laboratory abnormalities may include hyponatremia (in about half the patients, sometimes severe), hypophosphatemia (also common, occurring early and resolving within a few days of the initiation of treatment), mild liver function test abnormalities (except for alkaline phosphatase, which is occasionally very elevated), elevated creatine kinase (occasionally with rhabdomyolysis), microscopic hematuria, and mild proteinuria. High procalcitonin levels exceeding 1.5 are associated with a higher rate of admission to intensive care units and death. Combinations of findings may be suggestive of legionnaires disease. These include high temperature, absence of sputum production, high lactate levels, increased C-reactive protein level, and low platelet counts.

There are a number of specific tests for the diagnosis of legionnaires disease. Tests to detect *L. pneumophila* SG 1 antigen in urine are available commercially.[16] These are easy to use, but there is a false-negative rate of up to 26%.

The sensitivity of the urinary antigen test in a review of published data was 0.74 (0.68 to 0.81), and the specificity was 0.991 (0.984 to 0.997). Rarely, the urinary antigen test result can remain positive for up to 1 year. Use of this test has allowed early diagnosis of legionnaires disease because of the very short time required to do the test. This may be a factor in the lower mortality rates from legionnaires disease compared with historical rates. If the urinary antigen test is positive for *Legionella*, it should be repeated after boiling the urine for 5 minutes and centrifuging it at 12,000 g for 5 minutes to avoid false-positive results. In hospitals with high numbers of immunosuppressed patients where legionellae other than serogroup 1 are more common, urinary antigen should not be relied on to make a diagnosis of legionnaires disease. Sputum culture has a low sensitivity but is 100% specific. It should be performed on all patients suspected of having legionnaires disease. Serologic tests are not useful in the immediate management of a patient because of the long time (6 to 12 weeks) required to seroconvert; however, they do have a role in the work-up of outbreaks of legionnaires disease. False-negative and false-positive serologic results do occur. A four-fold or greater increase in antibody titer between the acute and convalescent phase serum samples is diagnostic. A former criterion of a stable antibody titer of 1 : 256 or higher is no longer considered diagnostic. PCR can be used to amplify *Legionella* DNA in sputum, bronchoalveolar lavage fluid, pleural fluid, pulmonary tissue, or serum. PCR can detect 1 fg of *Legionella* DNA, equivalent to one microorganism. These tests have not yet gained widespread use clinically. In everyday use, PCR has a higher sensitivity than culture and is about 30% more sensitive than legionella urinary antigen.[17] *Legionella* can be isolated from the blood with special media or by subculturing onto BCYE (buffered charcoal–yeast extract) agar plates, but this is not used in practice.

A chest radiograph is necessary to establish a diagnosis of pneumonia. About half the patients with legionnaires disease have unilateral pulmonary involvement. The lower lobes are involved most commonly. About one third of patients have a pleural effusion. Dense opacification is common, but interstitial and nodular opacities also occur. Cavitation is uncommon; 70% of the 79 patients reported to date with lung abscess due to *Legionella* were receiving corticosteroids. Figures 298-3 to 298-6 illustrate some of the radiographic findings in legionnaires disease.

The diagnosis of Pontiac fever is based on demonstration of *Legionella* in water to which the patient was exposed, seroconversion to *Legionella*, and a compatible clinical course.

In patients who have died of legionnaires disease, the gross pathology examination shows focal or patchy lesions in about one third of cases, lobar pneumonia in about half, and focal hemorrhages in about one fourth. On microscopic examination, there is bronchopneumonia with diffuse alveolar damage and heavy infiltration of neutrophils, macrophages, desquamation of alveolar epithelial cells, and fibrin proteinaceous debris. On occasion, there is inflammation of blood vessels mimicking a vasculitis. Organisms can be visualized with Dieterle silver impregnation stain or by direct immunofluorescent staining (E-Fig. 298-1).

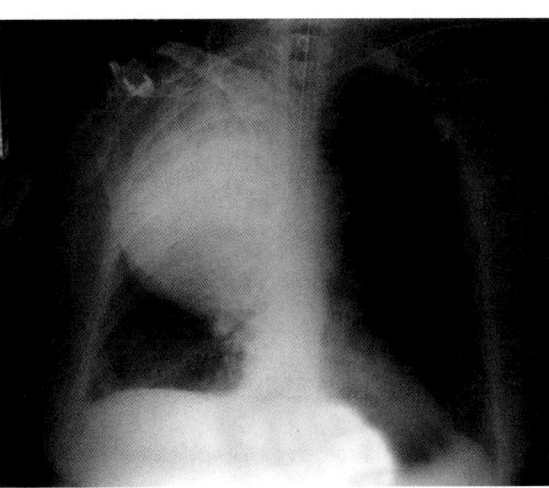

FIGURE 298-3. Posteroanterior chest radiograph of a patient with community-acquired pneumonia due to *Legionella pneumophila.* Note the dense consolidation of the right upper lobe, with bulging of the fissure. Such dense consolidation is a common radiographic appearance of legionnaires disease.

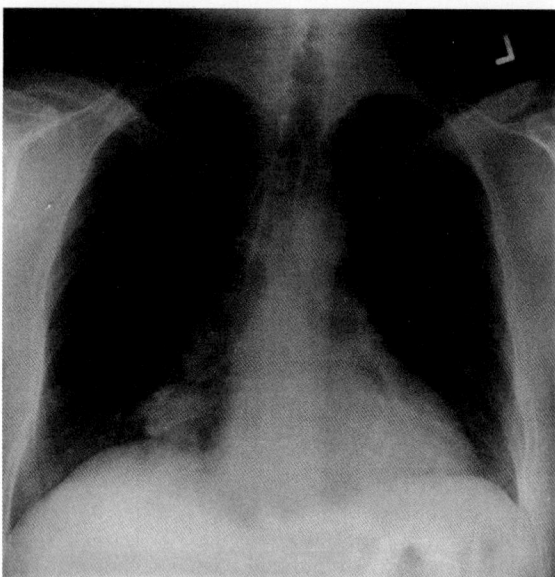

FIGURE 298-4. Posteroanterior chest radiograph of a patient with community-acquired legionnaires disease (*Legionella pneumophila*) manifesting as a right lower lobe nodular opacity.

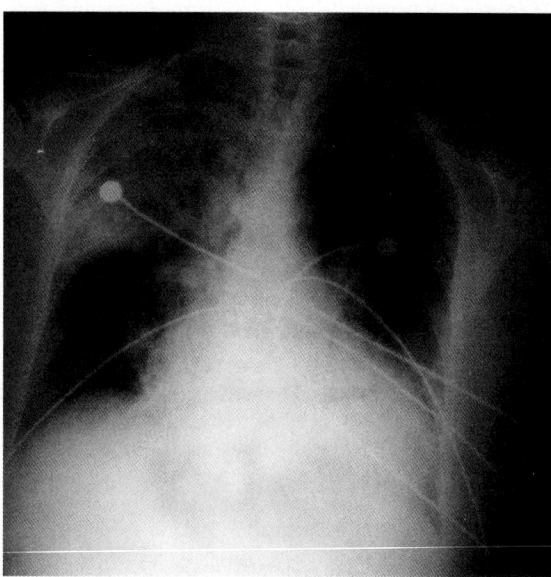

FIGURE 298-5. Posteroanterior chest radiograph of a patient with community-acquired *Legionella feeleii* pneumonia. There is patchy consolidation of the right upper lobe.

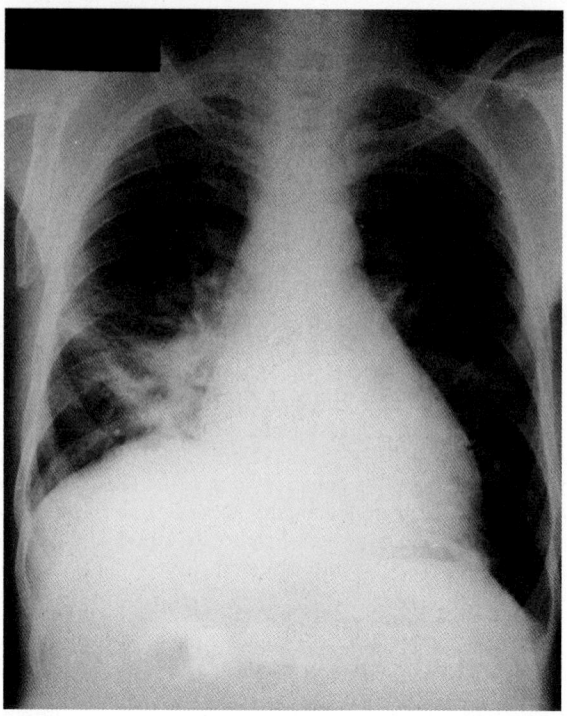

FIGURE 298-6. Posteroanterior chest radiograph of a patient with community-acquired pneumonia due to *Legionella pneumophila*. There is patchy consolidation at the right base, with subsegmental atelectasis and elevation of the right hemidiaphragm.

TABLE 298-2	TREATMENT FOR LEGIONNAIRES DISEASE	
SEVERITY OF *LEGIONELLA* PNEUMONIA	**DRUG**	**DOSAGE**
Mild pneumonia in a nonimmunocompromised person treated at home	Azithromycin	500 mg once daily for 3 days PO
	Clarithromycin	500 mg bid for 5-7 days
	Doxycycline	200 mg loading dose, then 100 mg bid for 5-7 days
	Levofloxacin	500 mg once daily for 5 days
	Moxifloxacin	400 mg once daily for 5 days
Pneumonia requiring hospitalization	Levofloxacin	750 mg once daily (IV initially) for 10 days
	Azithromycin	500 mg once daily (IV initially) for 10 days
	Moxifloxacin	400 mg once daily (IV initially) for 10 days
Pneumonia in immunocompromised host	Levofloxacin	750 mg once daily (IV initially) for 21 days
	Azithromycin	500 mg once daily (IV initially) for 21 days
	Moxifloxacin	400 mg once daily (IV initially) for 21 days

Differential Diagnosis

Legionnaires disease should be considered in any patient with pneumonia who is admitted to the hospital, especially those who require treatment in an intensive care unit. If *Legionella* is present in a hospital's water supply, legionnaires disease should be considered in all patients with nosocomial pneumonia.

TREATMENT AND PROGNOSIS Rx

The absence of data from randomized clinical trials limits the availability of high-grade evidence from which to make recommendations for the treatment of *Legionella* infections. However, the convergence of the results of data from animal experiments, large observational studies, and meta-analysis does provide guidance to current recommendations (Table 298-2). Before reviewing these data, it is important to understand that the mortality from *Legionella* infections in the United States had declined from 1980 through 1998. During that time, 6757 cases were reported to the CDC, and use of urinary antigen as a method of diagnosis increased from 0 to 69%. The case-fatality rate for community-acquired legionellosis declined from 26 to 10% and for nosocomial infections with *Legionella* from 46 to 14%. Although early diagnosis with *Legionella* urinary antigen may have played a role in this decrease, it is important to note that new therapeutic options such as levofloxacin were introduced in 1998 and may also have played a role in this reduction in mortality. In terms of recommending therapy, there are really three categories of *Legionella* infection: mild and moderate-severe community-acquired legionnaires disease and nosocomial legionnaires disease/immunocompromised host.

Review of the results of treatment of 446 patients with legionnaires disease, of whom 175 were treated with levofloxacin, 177 with azithromycin, and 58 with clarithromycin, showed that there were no significant differences in time to defervescence or time to clinical stability between those treated with levofloxacin or azithromycin.[18] Clarithromycin-treated patients had longer duration of intravenous antibiotic therapy and longer length of stay compared with levofloxacin-treated patients. The overall mortality rate was 4.3%.

The immunocompromised patient with legionnaires disease is a special case. In one study of 49 patients with legionnaires disease and cancer or hematologic malignancy, the case-fatality rate was 31%. The median time to a clinical response was 8 days. Thirty-five percent required prolonged treatment of 25 days, and two patients relapsed despite appropriate therapy. Twenty-seven percent who received combination therapy failed, and 34% who received monotherapy failed. None of the seven patients treated with clarithromycin or azithromycin failed. The addition of rifampin to a macrolide or a fluoroquinolone has to be carefully used in transplant patients because of interaction with immunosuppressive drugs. Thus, in this setting, azithromycin or a fluoroquinolone is considered first-line therapy.

The incidence of legionnaires disease is rising, and the mortality rate remains high, particularly for immunocompromised patients.[19] Cases of legionnaires disease should be reported to local health officials. An investigation is often required to determine the source of the *Legionella*.

GENERAL REFERENCES

For the General References and other additional features, please visit Expert Consult at https://expertconsult.inkling.com.

299

BARTONELLA INFECTIONS

JEAN-MARC ROLAIN AND DIDIER RAOULT

DEFINITION

Bartonella species belong to the alpha-2 subgroup of Proteobacteria and are closely related to the genera *Brucella*, *Agrobacterium*, and *Rhizobium*. Since 1993, the genus *Bartonella* has been reorganized by addition of the genera *Rochalimaea* and *Grahamella* to the family Bartonellaceae. Currently more than 40 known *Bartonella* species have been isolated from both animals and humans. These bacteria are considered emerging pathogens that are associated with zoonosis and human infections. Among them, 15 validated species have been implicated in human diseases: *B. henselae*, *B. quintana*, *B. bacilliformis*, *B. elizabethae*, *B. clarridgeiae*, *B. vinsonii* subsp. *arupensis*, *B. vinsonii* subsp. *berkhoffii*, *B. alsatica*, *B. tamiae*, *B. grahamii*, *B. washoensis*, *B. rochalimae*, *B.*

koehlerae, *B. mayotimonensis*, and *B. ancashensis* (Table 299-1). The other *Bartonella* species have been isolated only from the blood of animals, including rodents, felids, canids, dolphins, bats, and ruminants. The route of transmission of *Bartonella* species in mammals and humans is by fleas, ticks, mites, and lice (see Table 299-1).

Bartonella infections are emerging infectious diseases that lead to a wide spectrum of either acute or chronic diseases. The status of the host immune response plays an important role in the development of the different manifestations. Four different clinical syndromes may occur with *Bartonella* infections: (1) infection of red blood cells and erythrophagocytosis, (2) granulomatous disease controlled by the immune response, (3) blood culture–negative endocarditis and bacteremia, and (4) vasculoproliferative diseases.[1] A single *Bartonella* species can cause either acute or chronic infections and either vasculoproliferative or suppurative manifestations, but with different pathogenetic mechanisms that mainly depend on the patient's immune status. For example, *B. quintana* is responsible for trench fever as well as for endocarditis, bacteremia in the homeless population, and vasculoproliferative diseases, whereas *B. bacilliformis* is the agent of Carrión disease, which corresponds to either an acute intraerythrocytic bacteremic disease (Oroya fever) or a chronic vasculoproliferative disease (verruga peruana). Infection of red blood cells has been well established for *B. bacilliformis* (Oroya fever) and *B. quintana* (trench fever and bacteremia in the homeless), whereas *B. henselae* and *B. koehlerae* have been seen in erythrocytes of infected cats. *B. henselae* can cause granulomatous disease, that is, cat-scratch disease, which affects lymph nodes, but can also be responsible for other clinical manifestations or complications, such as endocarditis. Vasculoproliferative diseases include bacillary angiomatosis caused by *B. henselae* and *B. quintana*, peliosis hepatis caused by *B. henselae*, and verruga peruana caused by *B. bacilliformis*. The immune status of the host plays a critical role in the development of these different forms of the disease. *B. henselae* usually causes cat-scratch disease (a self-limited disease) in immunocompetent hosts, whereas it is responsible for bacillary angiomatosis in immunocompromised patients. In patients with a previous valvulopathy, any *Bartonella* infection may lead to endocarditis.

The Pathogen

Bartonella species are small, gram-negative, fastidious, pleomorphic coccobacilli or slightly curved rods (0.5 by 1 to 2 μm). Because of the slow growth of these bacteria and the lack of reproducible biochemical methods for their identification, they are usually identified by molecular methods. Matrix-assisted laser desorption/ionization time-of-flight mass spectrometry has emerged as a new technique for species identification and is an accurate and reproducible method for the rapid and inexpensive identification of *Bartonella* species. The

TABLE 299-1 *BARTONELLA* SPECIES CAUSING HUMAN DISEASE

BARTONELLA SPECIES	FIRST CULTIVATION		YEAR OF DESCRIPTION	RESERVOIR HOST/VECTOR	HUMAN DISEASE
	MAMMAL	COUNTRY			
B. alsatica	Wild rabbit (*Oryctolagus cuniculus*)	France	1999	Rabbit	Endocarditis, lymphadenopathy
B. ancashensis	Human	Peru	2013		Verruga peruana
B. bacilliformis	Human		1909	Human/sandfly	Carrión disease, Oroya fever, verruga peruana
B. clarridgeiae	Cat		1996	Cat/cat flea	Cat-scratch disease
B. elizabethae	Endocarditis patient	United States	1993	Rat	Endocarditis, neuroretinitis
B. grahamii	Woodland mammal (*Clethrionomys glareolus*)	United Kingdom	1995	Rat, insectivore	Neuroretinitis
B. henselae	Cat		1990	Cat/cat flea	Cat-scratch disease, endocarditis, bacillary angiomatosis, bacillary peliosis, Parinaud oculoglandular syndrome, neuroretinitis, osteomyelitis, arthropathy, bacteremia with fever
B. koehlerae	Domestic cat	United States	1999	Cat	Endocarditis
B. mayotimonensis	Endocarditis patient	United States	2009	Unknown	Endocarditis
B. quintana	Human		1920	Human/body louse	Trench fever, endocarditis, bacillary angiomatosis
B. rochalimae	Human	United States	2007		Bacteremia, fever, splenomegaly
B. tamiae	Human	Thailand	2008		Febrile illness
B. vinsonii arupensis	Cattle rancher	United States	1999	Dog, rodent/ticks	Bacteremia with fever
B. vinsonii berkhoffii	Dog	United Kingdom	1998	Dog	Endocarditis
B. washoensis			2000	Ground squirrel	Myocarditis

bacteria can grow on enriched blood-containing media with a 5% carbon dioxide atmosphere after 5 to 15 days to up to 45 days on primary culture. The optimal growth temperature ranges from 28° C for *B. bacilliformis* to 35° to 37° C for the other species. *Bartonella* species can also be cocultured with endothelial cells. *Bartonella* species are either flagellated or nonflagellated cells. *B. bacilliformis* uses flagella for binding and deforming into the surface of erythrocytes. Bacteria can either persist in the blood stream of the host as intraerythrocytic parasites or colonize human endothelial cells.

EPIDEMIOLOGY

Almost all *Bartonella* species are vector-borne bacteria (see Table 299-1). Some are limited geographically, such as *B. bacilliformis*, which is found only in the Andes Mountains in South America at high altitudes, where its principal vector, *Lutzomyia verrucarum*, is distributed; others have a worldwide distribution, such as *B. henselae* and *B. quintana*. Each *Bartonella* species is highly adapted to its mammalian reservoir, in which bacteria usually cause a long-lasting intraerythrocytic bacteremia that may be asymptomatic. Humans are the hosts and reservoirs for *B. bacilliformis* and *B. quintana*. *B. quintana* is transmitted by the human body louse by inoculation of arthropod feces through broken skin. Cats represent the main reservoir hosts for *B. henselae* infection; this pathogen is the agent of cat-scratch disease in humans, caused by cat bites or scratches. In the United States, about 12,000 outpatients and 500 inpatients are diagnosed annually.[2] *B. henselae* infection is transmitted from cat to cat by the cat flea. Cat fleas may also be infected by *B. quintana*. The role of dogs as reservoir hosts has been documented for several species, including *B. vinsonii* subsp. *arupensis*, *B. vinsonii* subsp. *berkhoffii*, and *B. henselae*. Wild rabbits are the reservoir hosts for *B. alsatica*, which is an agent of endocarditis and lymphadenopathy in humans in close contact with rabbits. For other *Bartonella* species known to cause diseases in humans, their pathogenic role and mode of transmission are not fully understood.

● INFECTION OF RED BLOOD CELLS: OROYA FEVER AND TRENCH FEVER

PATHOBIOLOGY

In Oroya fever, *B. bacilliformis* invades up to 80% of erythrocytes and produces their massive lysis, which results in severe hemolytic anemia, the major symptom of the disease. Similarly, trench fever is characterized by intracellular erythrocyte parasitism by *B. quintana*, with the percentage of infected red blood cells ranging from 0.001 to 0.005% (Fig. 299-1). Bacteria can also be seen extracellularly and in erythroblasts. This intracellular erythrocyte parasitism can presumably preserve the pathogens for efficient transmission by body lice, protect *B. quintana* from the host immune response, and contribute to decreased antimicrobial efficacy. During bacteremia in the homeless, *B. quintana* can also be seen in red blood cells.

CLINICAL MANIFESTATIONS

The main clinical manifestations of infection by *Bartonella* species are summarized in Table 299-2.

Oroya fever is the acute or hemolytic phase of Carrión disease, caused by *B. bacilliformis*[3]; it usually develops 3 to 12 weeks after inoculation. Oroya fever results from the massive invasion of erythrocytes by *B. bacilliformis*, and

without antibiotic treatment, it causes death in up to 85% of infected humans by hemolysis or when complicated by opportunistic infections such as salmonellosis. The onset is usually abrupt, with high fever, chills, headache, and anorexia. Patients have intense myalgias and arthralgias, abdominal pain, and jaundice. Complications are frequent, including meningoencephalitis, dyspnea, delirium, and superinfection leading to death. Asymptomatic persistent bacteremia may serve as the reservoir of the organism.

Trench fever is transmitted by lice and is the clinical manifestation of *B. quintana*. Trench fever affected more than 1 million people during World War I; more recently, *B. quintana* has been recognized in immunocompromised hosts, homeless people, and chronic alcoholics. Clinical manifestations of trench fever may range from asymptomatic infection to severe, life-threatening illness. After an incubation period of 2 to 3 weeks, there is a sudden onset of fever that lasts 1 to 3 days associated with headache, shin pain, and dizziness. Although fatal cases have not been reported, the disease may persist for 4 to 6 weeks and result in prolonged disability. Relapses may occur years later, and in some cases there may be bacteremia with no clinical signs.

● CAT-SCRATCH DISEASE

PATHOBIOLOGY

Little is known about the pathogenesis of the long-lasting lymphadenopathy in cat-scratch disease. Immunopathogenesis is assumed to play an important role in cat-scratch disease because bacteria have only rarely been isolated from affected lymph nodes. Thus, the disease is usually controlled by the host immune response, and there are few or no viable bacteria when lymph node biopsy specimens are analyzed; they are necrotic by pathologic examination.

CLINICAL MANIFESTATIONS

Typical cat-scratch disease is the most common manifestation of infection with *B. henselae* and usually is manifested as a self-limited regional lymphadenitis. Transmission from cat to human occurs directly by a cat scratch or cat bite or possibly by a cat flea or tick bite. A typical papule or pustule may be seen

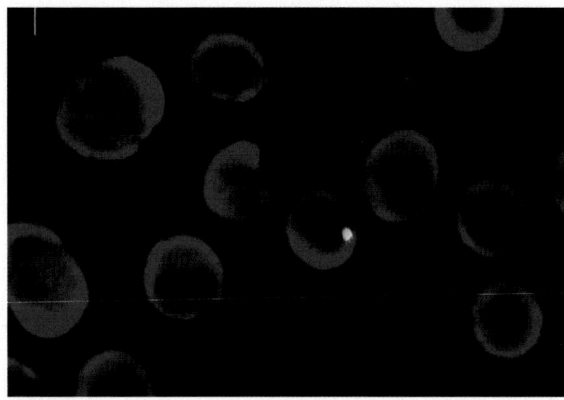

FIGURE 299-1. Section of human red blood cell infected with *Bartonella quintana* as viewed by confocal microscopy.

TABLE 299-2	CLINICAL MANIFESTATIONS ASSOCIATED WITH *BARTONELLA* SPECIES				
CLINICAL MANIFESTATION	**B. BACILLIFORMIS**	**B. QUINTANA**	**B. HENSELAE**	**B. ALSATICA**	**OTHERS**
Intraerythrocytic bacteremia	+	+			
Chronic bacteremia	+	+	+		+
Infective endocarditis		+	+	+	+
Verruga peruana	+				
Bacillary angiomatosis		+	+		
Peliosis hepatis			+		
Lymphadenopathy		+	+ (CSD)	+	+
SENLAT with skin lesion			+		
Meningoencephalitis			+		
Uveitis-retinitis		+	+		+

CSD = cat-scratch disease; SENLAT = scalp eschar and neck lymphadenopathy.

3 to 10 days after the scratch or bite at the site of inoculation and may last for 1 to 3 weeks. The subsequent lymphadenopathy is localized mainly to the axillary, cervical, or submaxillary nodes that drain the area where the cat scratch occurred. The enlarged lymph node is often painful and tender. Lymphadenopathy sometimes lasts for months, and in a few cases it can persist for as long as 1 to 2 years. In some cases, the lymph node may suppurate if it is not drained. Most patients are not febrile during the course of typical cat-scratch disease. Systemic or severe disease may occur in about 5 to 14% of patients, with most of them suffering severe systemic symptoms due to disseminated infection.[4] After exposure to *B. henselae*, patients may develop bacteremia with or without clinical signs of typical cat-scratch disease, and in patients with valvular lesions, this may result in infective endocarditis.[5,6] Thus, cat-scratch disease represents the primary infection of *B. henselae*, and endocarditis may follow in patients with heart valve lesions. It is a potential cause of "culture-negative endocarditis."

Approximately 10% of patients with cat-scratch disease have atypical clinical manifestations, including prolonged fever (>2 weeks), malaise, neuroretinitis, encephalitis, erythema nodosum, hepatitis, fatigue, weight loss, and splenomegaly. A recent clinical study showed that musculoskeletal manifestations (myalgia, arthritis, arthralgia, tendinitis, osteomyelitis, neuralgia) were present in more than 10% of patients with cat-scratch disease, demonstrating that these clinical manifestations are not as rare as might be expected from the cases reported in the past. In this series of 913 patients, myalgia and arthropathy were the most common manifestations, with an incidence of 5.8% and 5.5%, respectively. Moreover, these manifestations occurred primarily in adults whose ages ranged from 20 to 59 years. Myalgia had a mean duration of 4 weeks and was often severe. Arthropathy had a mean duration of 5.5 weeks, was more common in female patients older than 20 years, affected large and medium joints (half of those involved being weight-bearing joints), and was associated with symmetrical erythema nodosum early in the course of cat-scratch disease. These musculoskeletal manifestations are often severe and may evolve into chronic forms that persist for more than a year. Tendinitis, neuralgia, and osteomyelitis are less common, with incidences lower than 1%.

Ocular and Neurologic Manifestations

Parinaud oculoglandular syndrome is a self-limited conjunctivitis associated with preauricular lymphadenopathy. Other atypical manifestations include neurologic syndromes (meningoencephalitis, meningitis, neuroretinitis). Encephalopathy may occur in 2 to 4% of cat-scratch disease patients, mainly[7] adolescents and adults. Patients usually have persistent headaches with or without fever and may develop seizures. Acute neurologic disorders range from self-limited nuchal rigidity to pupillary dilation or aphasia and hemiplegia; they may last for several weeks to months. Neuroretinitis has been associated with cat-scratch disease in patients experiencing a sudden unilateral loss of visual acuity. The most common picture remains papilledema associated with macular exudates causing stellar retinitis. A few reports have now established that *B. henselae* can be responsible for uveitis, along with *B. grahamii* and *B. quintana*. Patients present with either nongranulomatous or granulomatous uveitis.[8,9]

Finally, tick-borne *B. henselae* infection has been described, including scalp eschar and neck lymphadenopathy after tick bites in three patients during the colder months in France. *B. henselae* was detected by molecular tools both in skin biopsy specimens (cervical and occipital) and in a *Dermacentor marginatus* tick removed from the scalp of one patient. All three patients had asthenia, but none had alopecia.

⬤ ENDOCARDITIS

PATHOBIOLOGY

B. quintana, B. henselae, B. alsatica, B. vinsonii subsp. *berkhoffii, B. elizabethae*, and "*Candidatus* Bartonella mayotimonensis" are common causes of blood culture–negative endocarditis, whereas *B. vinsonii* subsp. *arupensis* has been detected in a patient with fever and bacteremia; *B. washoensis* has been identified in one patient with myocarditis; *B. rochalimae* was reported in a patient with fever, bacteremia, and splenomegaly; and *B. tamiae* has been isolated in a patient with a febrile illness. Patients with endocarditis usually have preexisting heart valve disease that promotes the development of infective endocarditis and, in some cases, a definite risk factor for infection specifically with *Bartonella*. Endocarditis caused by *Bartonella* species exhibits slight inflammation, with a few inflammatory mononuclear cells and small vegetations; the bacteria are seen extracellularly in dense immunopositive clusters that are mainly included in vegetations and in neutrophil and macrophage cytoplasm.

CLINICAL MANIFESTATIONS

The most commonly identified agents of *Bartonella* endocarditis are *B. quintana*, followed by *B. henselae* and other *Bartonella* species. Patients appear to have chronic, blood culture–negative endocarditis, usually with fever (90%). Echocardiography reveals vegetations (in 90%).[10] Infections with *B. henselae* are epidemiologically linked to close contact with cats or cat fleas and previous valvular heart disease, whereas *B. quintana* endocarditis is frequently described in homeless and alcoholic patients with body lice infection and can be observed in patients without previous valve lesions. The onset is usually subacute, with some patients being afebrile at the time of admission. About half the patients have embolic phenomena. Interestingly, there is a north (Europe) to south (North Africa) gradient for the proportion of *Bartonella* endocarditis in humans; thus *Bartonella* is apparently a common cause of endocarditis in North Africa. Sporadic cases of endocarditis have also been associated with *B. koehlerae, B. vinsonii* subsp. *berkhoffii, B. vinsonii* subsp. *arupensis, B. elizabethae, B. alsatica*, and "*Candidatus* Bartonella mayotimonensis."

⬤ VASCULOPROLIFERATIVE DISEASE: VERRUGA PERUANA, BACILLARY ANGIOMATOSIS, AND PELIOSIS HEPATIS

PATHOBIOLOGY

Bartonella species have the ability to cause vasculoproliferative lesions through a process of pathologic angiogenesis resulting in the formation of new capillaries from preexisting ones.[11] These typical vasoproliferations can be expressed as skin lesions called bacillary angiomatosis, which are caused by *B. quintana* and *B. henselae*; there is also a cystic form in the liver and spleen called peliosis hepatis, which is caused only by *B. henselae*. Skin lesions are similar to those reported for verruga peruana, the chronic form of Carrión disease. Bacillary angiomatosis is a neovascular proliferation that has been reported most commonly in AIDS patients and involves the skin (Fig. 299-2) and lymph nodes; it occurs less frequently in patients with other causes of immunosuppression and only exceptionally in immunocompetent patients. In bacillary angiomatosis, lesions comprise proliferating endothelial cells, bacteria, and mixed infiltrates of macrophages/monocytes and polymorphonuclear neutrophils, leading to chronic inflammation. Bacteria are clustered as aggregates both surrounding and within endothelial cells, indicating that the vascular endothelium represents a target tissue for intracellular and extracellular colonization in vivo. On histologic evaluation, bacillary angiomatosis is a lobular proliferation of small blood vessels containing endothelial cells and bacteria, usually seen in clusters when stained with Warthin-Starry. As in bacillary angiomatosis, lesions of verruga peruana are characterized by lobular proliferations and atypical endothelial cells forming both relatively solid sheets and small, well-formed vessels with patent lumens. Lesions are typically infiltrated, indicating a chronic inflammatory process.

CLINICAL MANIFESTATIONS

As already noted, bacillary angiomatosis is seen most often in AIDS patients. Cutaneous lesions often arise in crops and can be subcutaneous or dermal nodules with red or purple papules millimeters to centimeters in diameter. When cutaneous lesions are absent, the diagnosis is often difficult and delayed because signs of visceral involvement are usually nonspecific. The potentially systemic nature of bacillary angiomatosis is reflected by the involvement of brain, bone, lymph node, bone marrow, skeletal muscle, conjunctiva, and

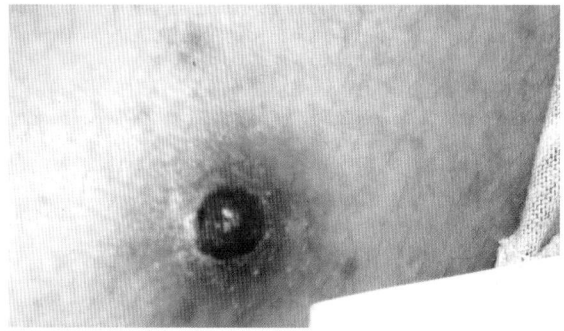

FIGURE 299-2. Skin lesion of bacillary angiomatosis.

TABLE 299-3 LABORATORY METHODS FOR THE DIAGNOSIS OF *BARTONELLA* INFECTIONS

CLINICAL MANIFESTATION	SEROLOGY	CULTURE	MOLECULAR METHODS	IMMUNOHISTOCHEMISTRY (WARTHIN-STARRY STAIN)	MICROSCOPY FOR INTRAERYTHROCYTIC ORGANISM (GIEMSA OR IF)
Oroya fever	−	+	+	−	+++
Verruga peruana	−	−	+	+	−
Trench fever	+/−	+	+	−	+
Chronic bacteremia	+/−	+++	+	−	−
Infective endocarditis	+++	+++	+++	+++	−
Bacillary angiomatosis	+/−	++	+++	+++	−
Peliosis hepatis	+/−	++	+++	+++	−
Cat-scratch disease	+	−	+++	+/−	+/−
SENLAT with skin lesion	+	+	+++	+	−
Meningoencephalitis	++	−	++	−	−
Uveitis-retinitis	++	−	++	+	−

The usefulness of these techniques varies according to the disease being tested.
IF = immunofluorescence; SENLAT = scalp eschar and neck lymphadenopathy.

mucosal surfaces of the gastrointestinal and respiratory tracts. Peliosis hepatis affects solid internal organs, primarily the liver, with reticuloendothelial elements; in the liver, it is defined as a vascular proliferation of sinusoidal hepatic capillaries resulting in blood-filled spaces. The spleen, abdominal lymph nodes, and bone marrow may also be involved.

Following acute Oroya fever, patients usually develop angioproliferative cutaneous tumors called verruga peruana after a latent period ranging from weeks to months. The infection is characterized by benign cutaneous vascular lesions typically consisting of round papules that are frequently pruritic and bleeding. The infection is accompanied by malaise and arthralgias. Skin lesions may change over time from miliary to nodular subcutaneous lesions to large mulaire lesions. These large lesions are often engorged with blood and prone to ulceration and bleeding. This eruptive phase clinically resembles Kaposi sarcoma or bacillary angiomatosis. However, it has a low morbidity, and there are no reports of mortality.

DIAGNOSIS OF *BARTONELLA* INFECTION

Methods used for the diagnosis of *Bartonella* infection include serology, microscopy, culture, molecular amplification of *Bartonella* species genes, direct immunofluorescence, and immunohistochemistry. The usefulness of these techniques may vary according to the disease involved (Table 299-3).

Serologic Tests

Serology remains the most widely used method for the diagnosis of cat-scratch disease and *Bartonella* endocarditis because culture and isolation are difficult and time-consuming, and molecular methods are not available in all laboratories. There are currently two classic serologic methods for the diagnosis of *Bartonella* infections: enzyme-linked immunosorbent assay and immunofluorescence assay. By immunofluorescence assay, an immunoglobulin G titer of 1 : 64 or greater should be considered positive for cat-scratch disease, whereas patients with endocarditis usually have higher antibody titers (≥1 : 800). In homeless patients, bacteremia has been associated with serologic tests that were positive for *B. quintana*. However, reported sensitivities of immunofluorescence assay vary considerably, from nearly 100% to less than 30%, depending on the nature of the antigens used and the selected patients.[12] Moreover, owing to cross-reactive antibodies between *Bartonella* species, the diagnosis of *Bartonella* infection at the species level is usually not possible. More sophisticated methods should be used, especially Western blot with cross-adsorption analysis. Western blot is also useful for the differential diagnosis of endocarditis because the profile obtained for endocarditis is specific compared with that for cat-scratch disease or chronic bacteremia.

Microscopy, Immunofluorescence, and Immunohistochemistry

The diagnosis of Oroya fever is based on examination of a peripheral blood smear stained by Giemsa; the percentage of infected red blood cells is sufficiently high so that bacteria are visible. Similarly, *B. quintana* can be seen within red blood cells with use of specific monoclonal antibody by immunofluorescence and confocal microscopy (see Fig. 299-1). Microscopic examination after Warthin-Starry silver staining or immunohistochemistry of a cardiac valve or skin biopsy specimen is also useful for the detection of *Bartonella* organisms in patients with endocarditis and bacillary angiomatosis.

Culture

Bartonella species can be recovered from the blood of bacteremic patients as well as from cardiac valves, skin and liver biopsy specimens, and, rarely, lymph nodes. Bacteria can be isolated directly from these specimens after plating onto blood agar solid media, blood culture in broth, and cocultivation in endothelial cells. Cultures are usually positive after 2 weeks of incubation, but up to 45 days may be necessary for primary isolation.

Molecular Detection Methods

Direct detection and final identification of *Bartonella* species from blood and tissue specimens, including lymph node, cardiac valve, skin, and liver, can be achieved by polymerase chain reaction (PCR) amplification and sequencing of various housekeeping genes.[13,14] PCR can also detect *Bartonella* at the species level from lymph nodes in cat-scratch disease, directly from cardiac valves in patients with endocarditis, and in patients with bacillary angiomatosis or peliosis hepatis. In one study, all cases of blood culture–negative *Bartonella* were diagnosed by real-time PCR.[15]

Differential Diagnosis

The differential diagnosis of bacillary angiomatosis is Kaposi sarcoma, but visualization of bacteria in the tissue specimen can help distinguish between these two entities. Trench fever may be confused mainly with typhus group rickettsiosis, relapsing fever, and malaria. Cat-scratch disease may be confused with tularemia, pyogenic lymphadenitis, mycobacterial infection, and neoplasia.

TREATMENT   Rx

Trench Fever

Before the advent of antibiotics, acetylsalicylic acid was the most effective drug for the pain caused by trench fever. However, a randomized clinical trial in homeless persons with episodes of bacteremia demonstrated that the combination of gentamicin and doxycycline is more effective in stopping bacteremia compared with no treatment or the use of β-lactams or doxycycline alone. Because the intraerythrocytic presence of *B. quintana* decreases antimicrobial efficacy, the duration of treatment is critical in trench fever. Patients with *B. quintana* bacteremia should be treated with gentamicin (3 mg/kg body weight/day IV for 14 days), in combination with doxycycline (200 mg/day PO) for 28 days.

Oroya Fever and Verruga Peruana

In Oroya fever, treatment with penicillin, streptomycin, fluoroquinolones, tetracycline, or erythromycin produces rapid defervescence and disappearance of the organisms from the blood, usually within 24 hours. As an alternative treatment, chloramphenicol can be used alone or in combination with a β-lactam. Treatment with chloramphenicol may also have the advantage of covering commonly associated *Salmonella* species. Patients with Oroya fever should be treated with chloramphenicol (500 mg PO four times a day) for 14 days in combination with another antibiotic (especially a β-lactam compound). Streptomycin (15 to 20 mg/kg/day for 10 days) was the traditional treatment for verruga peruana. However, its use is problematic, especially in children, and rifampin has become the drug of choice for the treatment of eruptive-phase bartonellosis. Failures of rifampin treatment have been reported in verruga peruana. Finally, ciprofloxacin (500 mg PO twice daily for 7 to 10 days) has been used successfully for the treatment of multiple eruptive-phase lesions in adults and has been proposed as an appropriate alternative. Doxycycline in association with gentamicin may be used to treat the eruptive phase of Carrión disease.

Cat-Scratch Disease

Typical cat-scratch disease is a self-limited illness that resolves within 2 to 6 months and usually does not respond to therapy because the bacteria within necrotic lymph nodes are not alive. In cases of long-lasting lymphadenopathy, patients should be reassured that it is benign and will probably subside spontaneously within 2 to 4 months. Management consists of analgesics for pain and prudent follow-up. However, azithromycin (500 mg PO on day 1 and 250 mg PO on days 2 to 5 as single daily doses) is an alternative for patients with large, bulky lymphadenopathy. If lymphadenopathy does not resolve, lymph nodes can be removed surgically. For atypical presentations of cat-scratch disease, there are no data regarding the benefit of specific antimicrobial therapy for immunocompetent patients. For neuroretinitis, the combination of doxycycline (100 mg PO or IV twice daily) with rifampin (300 mg PO twice daily) seems to promote disease resolution, to improve visual acuity, to reduce optic disc edema, and to decrease disease duration.

Endocarditis

Patients with *Bartonella* endocarditis have a higher death rate and undergo valvular surgery more frequently than patients with endocarditis caused by many other pathogens. Patients with suspected (but culture-negative) *Bartonella* endocarditis or proved *B. quintana* endocarditis should be treated with oral doxycycline 100 mg twice a day for 6 weeks in combination with gentamicin 3 mg/kg/day in one intravenous daily dose for 14 days.[16] The American Heart Association consensus on treating infective endocarditis is ceftriaxone plus gentamicin, with or without doxycycline, when *Bartonella* is suspected, and doxycycline plus gentamicin when *Bartonella* endocarditis is confirmed. However, there is direct evidence that patients receiving an aminoglycoside are more likely to fully recover, and those treated with aminoglycosides for at least 14 days are more likely to survive than those receiving a shorter duration of therapy. In the absence of any prospective study for the treatment of *Bartonella* endocarditis, the same regimen as for *B. henselae* and *B. quintana* should be used for endocarditis when another *Bartonella* species has been identified as the causative agent.

Bacillary Angiomatosis and Peliosis Hepatis

Without appropriate therapy, infection spreads systemically and can involve virtually any organ, and the outcome is sometimes fatal. Thus, antibiotic treatment is warranted in all cases of *Bartonella*-associated vasculoproliferative disease. On the basis of empirical clinical reports, erythromycin remains the treatment of choice and has been used successfully to treat many patients with bacillary angiomatosis. The response to treatment in bacillary angiomatosis can be dramatic in immunocompromised patients, with resolution of palpable subcutaneous lesions within hours. Erythromycin also has an antiangiogenic effect on microvascular endothelial cells that could explain this quick disappearance of lesions. Erythromycin (500 mg four times daily) for 3 months is first-line therapy. Doxycycline (100 mg PO or IV twice daily) is currently proposed as an appropriate alternative. In patients with serious infections, erythromycin or doxycycline can be used in combination with rifampin (300 mg PO twice daily). The duration of therapy is critical. We recommend that treatment be given for at least 3 months for bacillary angiomatosis and 4 months for peliosis hepatis. Peliosis hepatis responds slowly, and hepatic lesions continue to improve after several months of treatment, whereas cutaneous bacillary angiomatosis demonstrates improvement after 4 to 7 days of treatment and resolves after about 1 month of treatment. Relapses of peliosis hepatis and bacillary angiomatosis lesions after antibiotic treatment have been reported frequently, especially in immunocompromised patients with a shorter duration of therapy. Patients who relapse after the recommended treatment should probably be re-treated for 4 to 6 months with erythromycin (500 mg PO four times daily) or doxycycline (100 mg PO twice daily), and those with repeated relapses should receive antibiotic therapy as long as they are immunocompromised.

PREVENTION

Because arthropods play an important role in the transmission of feline *Bartonella* species to humans, rigorous arthropod control should be recommended by health care workers, particularly when advising immunocompromised individuals on the risks related to pet ownership. Cat fleas live on both cats and dogs and are best controlled by fumigating areas where these animals live.

PROGNOSIS

Mortality in those with Oroya fever was as high as 50% before the antibiotic era but is now limited by the use of antibiotics. Trench fever should be treated with antibiotics to avoid more severe disease, especially in patients with valvulopathy who are at risk for development of endocarditis. Cat-scratch disease usually resolves spontaneously without any treatment in immunocompetent patients. In the case of complications or in immunocompromised patients, antibiotic therapy should be given, and patients usually respond well to treatment. Finally, for vasculoproliferative diseases, antibiotics are usually effective if they are given for a long time, but cutaneous lesions in verruga peruana may benefit from surgery.

GENERAL REFERENCES

For the General References and other additional features, please visit Expert Consult at https://expertconsult.inkling.com.

300

GRANULOMA INGUINALE (DONOVANOSIS)

KHALIL G. GHANEM AND EDWARD W. HOOK III

DEFINITION

Granuloma inguinale, also known as donovanosis, is a slowly progressive ulcerative disease that involves principally the skin and subcutaneous tissues of the genital, inguinal, and anal regions.

The Pathogen

The causative organism is *Klebsiella granulomatis* (formerly *Calymmatobacterium granulomatis*), a gram-negative facultative intracellular parasite. The organism is challenging to cultivate but can sometimes be grown in yolk sacs, and successful cell culture has been reported from South Africa and Australia. Successful culture, in turn, has permitted the development of polymerase chain reaction assays, currently for research purposes.

EPIDEMIOLOGY

The organism is primarily transmitted sexually, but it can probably be transmitted by nonsexual contact as well. Transmission efficiency is relatively low, and multiple sexual contacts with an infected partner seem to be necessary for the transmission of infection. The disease is rarely encountered in the United States. Although still relatively rare, sporadic cases occur in India, Papua New Guinea, the Caribbean, Brazil, southern Africa, and parts of Australia.

CLINICAL MANIFESTATIONS

After an incubation period of up to 50 days, the initial lesion usually appears as a subcutaneous nodule that erodes through the surface and develops into a beefy, elevated granulomatous lesion (Fig. 300-1). The lesion is painless but tends to bleed easily, and it is not associated with systemic symptoms. Lesion exudate is often described as foul smelling. Secondary bacterial infection may cause a necrotic, painful, ulcerative lesion that may be rapidly destructive. A cicatricial form may also occur, with a depigmented elevated area of keloid-like scar containing scattered islands of granulomatous tissue. About 90% of lesions occur on the genitals and are commonly associated with pseudobuboes; these swellings usually are not due to involvement of the inguinal lymph nodes but rather are due to granulomatous involvement of subcutaneous tissue. Metastatic infection of bones or viscera (e.g., liver) is occasionally seen. Clinical experience suggests that secondary carcinomas (typically squamous cell carcinoma in patients with longstanding, chronic infection) may be a rare complication of granuloma inguinale.[1]

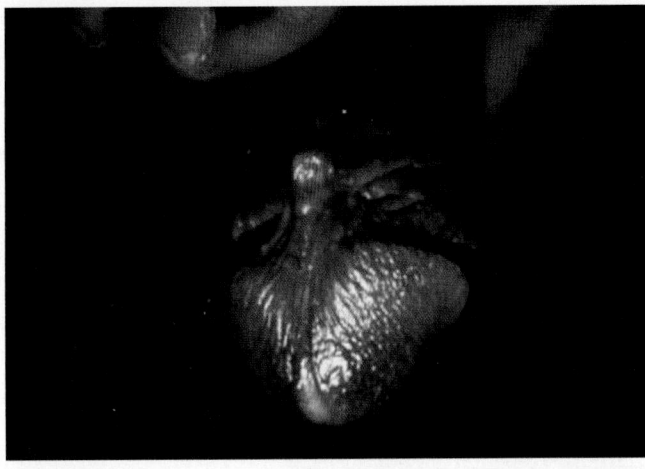

FIGURE 300-1. Typical primary lesion of granuloma inguinale. (Reproduced with permission from Herpes-Coldsores.com. http://www.herpes-coldsores.com/std/lympho-granuloma-pictures.htm.)

DIAGNOSIS

The diagnosis is made by demonstrating intracellular Donovan bodies in histiocytes or other mononuclear cells from lesion scrapings or biopsy samples. Wright stain and Giemsa stain of fresh impression smears or unfixed biopsy specimens usually demonstrate the bacilli relatively easily, although multiple biopsies may be necessary in chronic cases. Histologic examination of biopsy specimens shows plasma cells with some infiltration by polymorphonuclear leukocytes but no giant cells. In infected lesions, *K. granulomatis* is found primarily in histiocytes or other mononuclear cells. Cell culture and polymerase chain reaction methods are currently primarily research tools. No serologic test is clinically available.

Differential Diagnosis

The differential diagnosis includes squamous cell carcinoma, chancroid (Chapter 285), lymphogranuloma venereum (Chapter 302), syphilis (Chapter 303), and other ulcerative granulomatous diseases.[2] In the absence of therapy, patients may not present until lesions have been present for months, long after the lesions of syphilis and other ulcerative sexually transmitted diseases have resolved. Chancroid is usually differentiated by its irregular undermined borders, which are not seen in typical cases of granuloma inguinale. Dark-field examination and serologic tests should help distinguish syphilis. Biopsy of lesions may be necessary to distinguish granuloma inguinale from certain tumors.[3]

TREATMENT Rx

There are no high quality clinical trials of therapy for granuloma inguinale. Recommended treatment consists of azithromycin administered either as 1.0 g weekly or 500 mg daily or doxycycline 100 mg twice daily.[4] One double-strength trimethoprim-sulfamethoxazole tablet twice daily or erythromycin base 500 mg four times daily is recommended as alternative therapy. An aminoglycoside (e.g., gentamicin 1 mg/kg intravenously every 8 hours) may be added if these regimens do not result in clinical improvement within a few days. Treatment should be administered for at least 3 weeks and until lesions are completely healed.[5] Patients should be monitored for at least several weeks after treatment is discontinued because of the possibility of relapse. Although the risk of communicability appears to be low, sexual contacts should also be examined; at present, treatment of contacts is not indicated in the absence of clinically evident disease.

GENERAL REFERENCES

For the General References and other additional features, please visit Expert Consult at https://expertconsult.inkling.com.

301

MYCOPLASMA INFECTIONS

STEPHEN G. BAUM AND DAVID L. GOLDMAN

MYCOPLASMA PNEUMONIAE

DEFINITION

Mycoplasma organisms of the class Mollicutes are ubiquitous as pathogens and colonizing agents in the plant, animal, and insect kingdoms. They represent the smallest known free-living forms, but because they have fastidious growth requirements, they are difficult to culture. The presence of several species of *Mycoplasma* as commensals in animals and on human oral and genital mucosa frequently results in contamination of cell cultures. Such contamination led to the false implication of mycoplasmas as causative agents in many human diseases, both trivial and life-threatening. Of the human diseases that have proven to be due to mycoplasmas, pneumonia caused by *Mycoplasma pneumoniae* is by far the most clinically important.[1] This infection constitutes a significant proportion of cases previously classified as atypical pneumonia, a nonspecific term for patchy pneumonias that generally do not respond to β-lactam antibiotics and have etiologic agents that are not easily cultured or visible on Gram stain. The term *atypical pneumonia* persists despite our increasing ability to identify specific etiologic agents, such as viruses, *Legionella*, and *Chlamydophila*.

The Pathogen

Mycoplasmas are short rods (10×200 nm) that have no cell wall and are bounded by a sterol-containing membrane; thus, they are unaffected by cell wall–inhibiting antimicrobials such as β-lactams. In tissue culture, mycoplasmas are intracellular; but in vivo, infection is primarily extracellular and affects epithelial cells and their organelles, such as cilia. Attachment to respiratory epithelium is by way of terminal adhesin proteins in specialized tip organelles.

EPIDEMIOLOGY

M. pneumoniae infection is spread person to person by respiratory droplets produced by coughing. Relatively close association with the index case appears to be required. The disease is usually introduced into families by a young child; in some studies, most of the infected adults were the parents of young children. As opposed to most viral respiratory infections, which are manifested 1 to 3 days after infection, *Mycoplasma* has an incubation period of 2 to 3 weeks. Therefore, a careful history showing several weeks between cases within a family may be an important clue to the mycoplasmal etiology. Organisms can be cultured from the sputum of infected individuals for weeks to months after clinically efficacious treatment.

Most cases of *Mycoplasma* respiratory infection occur singly or as family outbreaks. However, in closed populations, such as military recruit camps and boarding schools, *Mycoplasma* can cause mini-epidemics and may be responsible for 25 to 75% of cases of pneumonia in such settings. Serologically based epidemiologic studies have documented the high incidence of *Mycoplasma* respiratory infection throughout the world. In the United States, it is estimated that each year at least one case of *Mycoplasma* pneumonia occurs for every 1000 persons, or more than 2 million cases annually. The incidence of *Mycoplasma* nonpneumonic respiratory infection may be 10 to 20 times greater. The highest attack rates are in individuals 5 to 20 years old, but *M. pneumoniae* infection can occur at any age and may cause particularly severe disease in neonates.

As opposed to viral respiratory infections that peak in winter in temperate climates, a few studies have reported a peak incidence of *M. pneumoniae* outbreaks in the fall. Most surveys, however, show little or no seasonal predominance in sporadic cases. Despite this, recurrent epidemic 4-year cycles have been described in several countries. There is an age-related relationship of upper versus lower respiratory tract infection caused by *M. pneumoniae*. In children younger than 3 years, primarily upper respiratory tract infection develops, whereas in those 5 to 20 years old, bronchitis and pneumonia tend to occur. In older adults, pneumonia predominates.

PATHOBIOLOGY

Because of the low fatality of most *Mycoplasma* infections, there is little human pathologic material. Inoculation onto animal tracheal organ cultures is

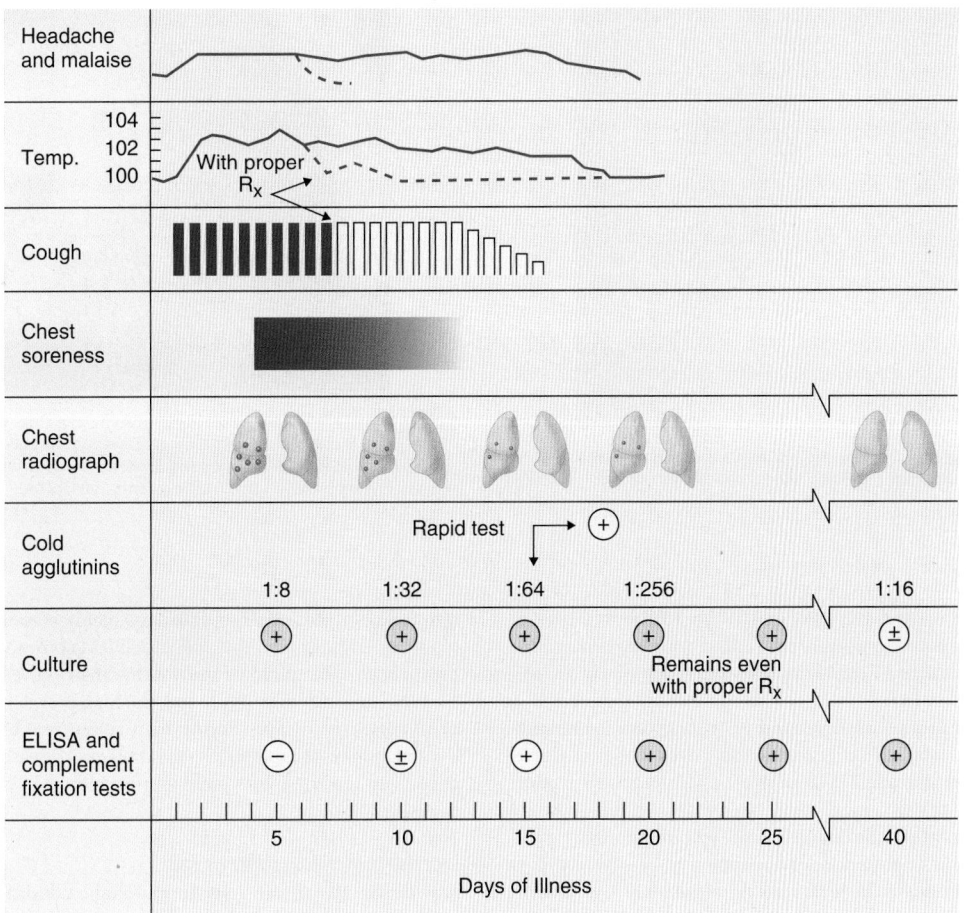

FIGURE 301-1. Major clinical and laboratory manifestations of mycoplasmal pneumonia. ELISA = enzyme-linked immunosorbent assay; R_x = treatment; Temp. = temperature. (Modified from Baum SG. Mycoplasmal infections. In: Wyngaarden JB, Smith LH Jr, eds. *Cecil Textbook of Medicine.*17th ed. Philadelphia: Saunders; 1985:1506.)

followed by ciliary damage and desquamation of surface epithelium. This latter effect is probably responsible for the hacking cough in *Mycoplasma* respiratory infection.

Several characteristics of *M. pneumoniae* probably play a direct role in the respiratory pathogenicity of this organism. The first is the affinity of *M. pneumoniae* for respiratory epithelial cells. Attachment appears to be between a terminal organelle at one end of the filamentous organism and a sialated glycoprotein (I-FI) on the surface of both respiratory epithelium and erythrocytes that acts as a receptor. *M. pneumoniae* attaches to ciliated epithelial cells at the base of cilia and appears to produce most of its physiologic and cytolytic changes while remaining extracellular. Hydrogen peroxide produced by *M. pneumoniae* (the only human mycoplasma to do so) may be responsible for some in vivo cell damage, as it is for the hemolysis seen when the organisms are grown on blood agar plates. *Mycoplasma* infection activates T and B cells and induces many pro-inflammatory and anti-inflammatory cytokines and chemokines that may play a role in inflammation-related cell destruction. *M. pneumoniae* also secretes a community-acquired respiratory distress syndrome (CARDS) toxin, which binds surfactant protein and dysregulates host adenosine diphosphate (ADP) ribosylation. High levels of CARDS toxin are produced during infection, and inoculation of this toxin in an animal model induces many of the pathologic features of *M. pneumoniae* infection, including vacuolization, cilostasis, and inflammatory changes.[2] Strain-specific elaboration of biofilms probably plays a role in protecting the organism from host immune cells and may decrease antimicrobial penetration.

In the course of *M. pneumoniae* infection, some patients produce cold agglutinins. These oligoclonal M-type immunoglobulins (IgM) cross-react with I antigens, one of the blood group antigens common to almost all mature human erythrocytes. High titers of the cold reactive antibody may cause hemolysis (presumably as a result of complement-activated, Coombs-positive erythrocyte destruction) and lead to some of the complications described in the Clinical Manifestations section. Like other IgM antibodies, the *Mycoplasma*-induced cold agglutinins (Chapter 151) develop early in the disease (7 to 10 days) and are often present by the time the patient seeks medical attention. The

titer of these agglutinins peaks at 2 to 3 weeks, and they persist for 2 to 3 months (Fig. 301-1).

CLINICAL MANIFESTATIONS

In view of the very high incidence of *Mycoplasma* respiratory infection when it is studied epidemiologically in large populations, versus the rarity of individual sporadic diagnoses, it appears that a specific, laboratory-confirmed diagnosis of this entity is seldom accomplished in routine clinical practice.[3] There are probably four reasons for this. First, *Mycoplasma* pneumonia is usually self-limited and rarely fatal. This fact dampens the zeal to establish the cause of infection. Second, mycoplasmas are relatively fastidious and slow growing; therefore, culture results, if obtained at all, often return only after the patient has recovered. Third, *M. pneumoniae* responds to the empirical antimicrobial therapy suggested for community-acquired pneumonia. Finally, knowledge of the epidemiology and clinical manifestations of infection is deficient, so the diagnosis is often not considered outside the classic age group.

Respiratory Infection

The majority of *M. pneumoniae* infections involve only the upper respiratory tract. After a 2- to 3-week incubation period, the disease has an insidious onset consisting of fever, malaise, headache, and cough (see Fig. 301-1). Cough is the clinical hallmark of *M. pneumoniae* infection. The frequency and severity of the cough increase during the next 1 to 2 days, and it may become debilitating. The gradual onset of symptoms is in contradistinction to the often fulminant manifestation of respiratory infection caused by influenza virus or adenovirus.[4]

In 5 to 10% of patients, depending somewhat on age, the infection progresses to tracheobronchitis or pneumonia. In these cases, the initial manifestations persist, and the cough becomes more severe. It is usually relatively nonproductive but may yield white or occasionally blood-flecked sputum. Gram staining of this sputum reveals inflammatory cells but no predominant bacterial species (part of the definition of atypical pneumonia). With continued cough, parasternal chest soreness may develop as a result of muscle strain, but true pleuritic

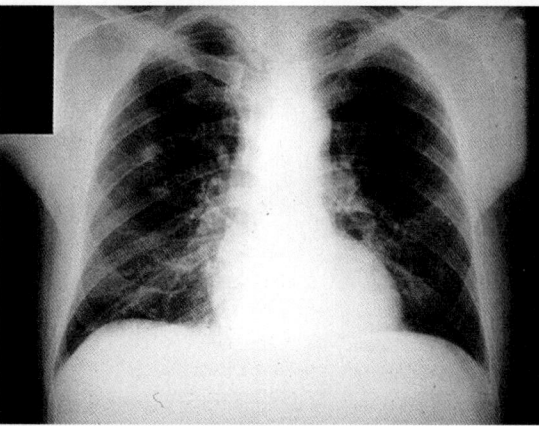

FIGURE 301-2. Chest radiograph showing moderate interstitial pneumonia due to *Mycoplasma pneumoniae* infection in a patient with a paucity of findings on chest auscultation.

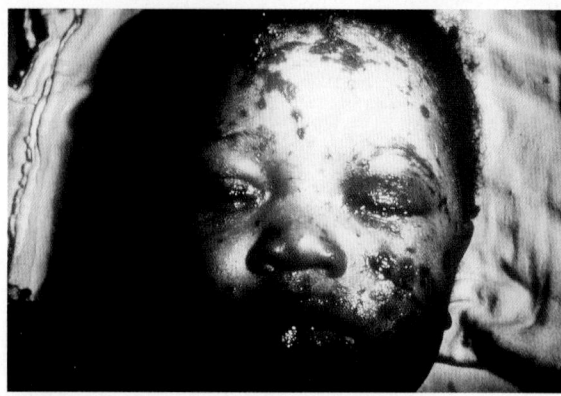

FIGURE 301-3. Stevens-Johnson syndrome in a child with *Mycoplasma* pneumonia. (From Baum SG. *Mycoplasma pneumoniae* and atypical pneumonia. In: Mandell GL, Bennett JE, Dolin R, eds. *Mandell, Douglas, and Bennett's Principles and Practice of Infectious Diseases.* 6th ed. Philadelphia: Churchill Livingstone; 2005:2274.)

pain is unusual. Fever is usually at the level of 101° to 102° F and may be associated with chills. As opposed to pneumonia caused by *Streptococcus pneumoniae* (Chapter 273), that caused by *M. pneumoniae* rarely produces true shaking chills. In comparison to influenza, which can also be manifested as an atypical pneumonia syndrome, myalgias and gastrointestinal complaints of nausea and vomiting are unusual. Diarrhea, sometimes a concomitant of adenoviral or *Legionella* pneumonia, is uncommon in *Mycoplasma* infection. Unfortunately, no clinical signs or symptoms can reliably differentiate *M. pneumoniae* infections from other community-acquired pneumonias.

On physical examination, the patient does not appear to be severely ill. In fact, this disease is the paradigm of the term *walking pneumonia*. The pharynx may be injected and erythematous, usually without the marked cervical adenopathy seen with group A streptococcal pharyngitis. *M. pneumoniae* is not a common cause of isolated pharyngitis in the pediatric or adult population. Much has been made of the finding of bullous myringitis in this disease. Although this abnormality was present in about 20% of volunteers with experimentally induced *M. pneumoniae* infection, true bullous myringitis in naturally occurring *Mycoplasma* disease is rare. In a study involving children, otitis was rarely associated with isolation of *Mycoplasma* and, on the contrary, was often associated with bacterial and viral upper respiratory tract pathogens. Thus, the absence of myringitis, bullous or otherwise, should not dissuade one from a diagnosis of *Mycoplasma* pneumonia.

Examination of the chest in patients with *Mycoplasma* pneumonia is often unrevealing, even in those with severe, productive cough. There may be no auscultative or percussive findings, or only minimal rales (crackles) may be present. The disparity between physical findings and radiographic evidence of pneumonia in this condition may be the greatest of any of the atypical pneumonia syndromes (Fig. 301-2). Although wheezing can occur in this disease, in one study of asthmatic patients, the presence of wheezing had a negative correlation with isolation of *M. pneumoniae* compared with isolation of viral respiratory pathogens such as respiratory syncytial virus (Chapter 338). *M. pneumoniae* does not seem to be a common pathogen in patients with preexisting chronic obstructive lung disease, either. Bacterial superinfection after *M. pneumoniae* respiratory infection is rare. The radiographic finding of interstitial or patchy alveolar pneumonia does not allow differentiation from any of the other causes of the atypical pneumonia syndrome.

Pleural effusion (usually small) occurs in 5 to 20% of patients with *M. pneumoniae* pneumonia. This low incidence of pleural inflammation is consistent with the rarity of pleuritic pain. If effusion is present, thoracentesis reveals serous fluid that is exudative, with minimal inflammatory reaction. The cell differential count in the fluid is variable, and bloody effusions are rare. It is unusual to isolate *M. pneumoniae* from effusions when they occur. Although the pneumonia is generally mild and self-limited, fulminant, severe, and lethal cases have been reported in normal young adults and may be underdiagnosed.

Extrapulmonary Involvement

Abnormalities in almost every organ system have been described as examples of the extrapulmonary manifestations of *M. pneumoniae* infection. The frequency of these extrapulmonary manifestations varies greatly from one report to another, and they are much less common when viewed as part of a prospective epidemiologic study rather than as the sum of isolated case reports. The conclusion appears to be that the high prevalence of *Mycoplasma* infection predisposes to the reporting of many concurrent but perhaps unrelated events as though they were part of the mycoplasmal disease. Several clinical syndromes have been reported with sufficient frequency to provide some support for a causal relationship.

Dermatologic Involvement

A wide variety of transient dermatologic conditions have been reported in conjunction with *Mycoplasma* pneumonia, including macular, morbilliform, and papulovesicular eruptions, as well as erythema nodosum and urticaria. Again, the variety and high incidence of these rashes in the absence of *Mycoplasma* infection make it difficult to define the relationships, if any, among these occurrences. Furthermore, the role of concurrent antibiotic therapy in the development of exanthems during *M. pneumoniae* infection is unknown. One skin condition that occurs often enough in concert with *M. pneumoniae* infection to provide some basis for relatedness is erythema multiforme majus, or Stevens-Johnson syndrome (Fig. 301-3). This rash has been reported in up to 7% of patients with *Mycoplasma* pneumonia and consists of erythematous vesicles, plaques, and bullae involving the skin, with particular localization at mucocutaneous junctions. The conjunctivae as well as organs of the gastrointestinal and genitourinary tracts and the joints may also be involved. Stevens-Johnson syndrome has been associated with isolated cases of many other infections, including some that can be manifested as atypical pneumonia syndrome, such as Legionnaires pneumonia, adenovirus respiratory-conjunctivitis syndrome, and influenza B infection. However, the association with *M. pneumoniae* infection is by far the most common. Stevens-Johnson syndrome tends to occur in younger patients with *Mycoplasma* pneumonia and has a definite male preponderance (2 : 1 to 4 : 1).

The pathogenesis of Stevens-Johnson syndrome is unclear. It has long been supposed that immunity plays a major role, but several reports have noted the culture of *M. pneumoniae* from the lesions. The relationship to the level of cold agglutinins in this disease is variable. It has been suggested that the development of Stevens-Johnson syndrome may be the result of augmented sensitivity to antibiotics in the presence of *M. pneumoniae* infection, but the syndrome develops in some patients even in the absence of previous or concurrent antibiotic therapy. Most patients clear the lesions in 1 to 2 weeks without scarring unless impetiginization supervenes.

A debilitating form of *M. pneumoniae*–associated mucositis without skin involvement has been described as an atypical Stevens-Johnson syndrome, but it is now increasingly recognized as a separate entity, termed *M. pneumoniae*–associated mucositis.[5,6]

Raynaud phenomenon (Chapter 72), a transient, reversible vasospasm of the digits that develops on exposure to cold, is not technically a dermatologic syndrome; however, it is manifested in the skin. This phenomenon occurs in many people, usually women, without any association with infection. Although the pathophysiologic mechanism of this condition in *M. pneumoniae* infection is unclear, it may be related to the in vivo action of cold agglutinins (see Diagnosis, later). Other vascular complications reported in *M. pneumoniae* infection include internal carotid artery occlusion and cerebral infarction.

Cardiac Complications

Cardiac abnormalities are among the most commonly reported extrapulmonary manifestations of *M. pneumoniae* infection. Signs and symptoms suggesting involvement of the heart are arrhythmia, congestive heart failure, chest pain, and electrocardiographic abnormalities, particularly conduction defects. Although cardiac abnormalities have been reported in as many as 10% of cases of *M. pneumoniae* infection, other reports indicate a much lower prevalence. Cardiac complications are more common with increasing age. They prolong the illness but rarely lead to death. The mechanism of heart damage is unknown, but *M. pneumoniae* has been isolated from the pericardial fluid of at least one patient.

Neurologic Complications

Neurologic complications are said to occur in about 0.1% of *Mycoplasma* infections, but proof of the cause of central nervous system involvement is somewhat tenuous. Central nervous system involvement is most common in children, with encephalitis the most common and most devastating.[7] Aseptic meningitis acute disseminated encephalomyelitis (ADEM), transverse myelitis, brain stem dysfunction, posterior reversible encephalopathy syndrome (PRES), Guillain-Barré syndrome, cerebral ataxia, and peripheral neuropathy have all been reported. Cerebrospinal fluid findings in these cases are variable, but the cellular response is usually minimal, with slightly elevated protein level and normal to slightly depressed glucose concentration. Most often, the diagnosis of *Mycoplasma*-related central nervous system involvement is based on the exclusion of other causes, the presence of an antecedent or intercurrent respiratory illness, and a rise in antibody titer to *M. pneumoniae* in serum. On occasion, *Mycoplasma*-specific antibodies have been demonstrated in cerebrospinal fluid, but these titers have paralleled serum antibody titers. Neurologic complications are usually reversible; however, mortality in patients with central nervous system involvement is higher than in those without such involvement. Although *M. pneumoniae* has been isolated from a few of these patients, polymerase chain reaction (PCR) failed to detect *M. pneumoniae* DNA in the cerebrospinal fluid of 11 patients deemed to have *M. pneumoniae*–related central nervous system disease on serologic grounds. Therefore, immune mechanisms of neural damage have been suggested. Some mycoplasmas elaborate a neurotoxin, but this has not been described for *M. pneumoniae*.

Musculoskeletal, Renal, and Hematopoietic Complications

Polyarthralgias are common in *Mycoplasma* pneumonia, but monarticular or migratory arthritis is rare. Immune mechanisms have been postulated, but there have been a few reports of the isolation of *M. pneumoniae* from joint fluid. Several of the cases of frank arthritis were reported in patients with hypogammaglobulinemia. Nonhuman mycoplasmas probably cause arthropathy in several animal species, and *Mycoplasma hominis* has been associated with human arthritis. Rhabdomyolysis has also been increasingly reported and may be associated with very high muscle enzyme, interleukin-18, and tumor necrosis factor-α levels.

Renal complications associated with immune complex deposition and high-titer cold agglutinins have been reported. There are several case reports of *M. pneumoniae*–associated aplastic anemia.

Conditions Leading to Increased Susceptibility

Several reports have emphasized the unusual severity of *M. pneumoniae* infection in patients with sickle cell disease or sickle-related hemoglobinopathies (Chapter 154). Large pleural effusions and marked respiratory distress may develop in these patients. *M. pneumoniae* is associated with acute chest syndrome, especially in children with sickle cell disease. Functional asplenia and its attendant opsonization deficiencies may contribute to overwhelming infection with *M. pneumoniae*, as they do with *S. pneumoniae* infection. Some patients with sickle cell disease and *M. pneumoniae* infection in whom extremely high cold agglutinin titers develop may experience digital necrosis, as they do with *S. pneumoniae* infection. Children with immunodeficiency syndromes have been the subjects of case reports of *M. pneumoniae* infection. Because *Mycoplasma* infections are so common in normal children, the contribution of immunodeficiency is unclear. *M. pneumoniae* is not a very common opportunistic agent in patients with acquired immunodeficiency syndrome (AIDS), but *M. fermentans* (*incognitus* strain) has been identified in these patients.

Unusually severe but nonlethal *M. pneumoniae* infection has also been reported in children with Down syndrome.

DIAGNOSIS

The diagnosis of *Mycoplasma* pneumonia is made primarily on clinical grounds. The organism can be grown in cell-free media, but most hospital diagnostic laboratories are not prepared to culture mycoplasmas. Because of this, there is considerable interest in developing rapid diagnostic tests with high sensitivity and specificity. These assays fall into three categories: detection of *M. pneumoniae*–specific immunoglobulins in serum and detection of *M. pneumoniae*–specific antigens or nucleotide sequences directly in clinical specimens. Diagnostically, the most useful *M. pneumoniae*–specific immunoglobulin to detect is IgM because it is most likely to indicate recent infection. Enzyme-linked immunoassays have been developed to detect IgM and IgG directed against *M. pneumoniae*. When used in patients with positive assays for complement-fixing antibodies, the enzyme immunoassay had a specificity of more than 99% and a sensitivity of 98%. Specificity was retained but sensitivity dropped to only 46% when IgG alone was the target. Variations on this theme detect IgM antibodies directed at specific *M. pneumoniae* antigens. The tests are simple to perform and have high sensitivity and specificity, but because all these tests are designed to detect IgM antibody, results may be negative early in the course of infection (<7 to 10 days). Therefore, they do not provide the desired confirmation early enough to guide initial therapy.

Detection of *M. pneumoniae* antigens directly in sputum specimens has been accomplished with the use of an antigen capture, indirect enzyme immunoassay. The specificity of the assay was high, the reagents reacting only with *M. pneumoniae* and *Mycoplasma genitalium*. Sensitivity was also relatively high (91%) when the assay was used on sputum and nasopharyngeal aspirates from patients who were shown by culture or serologically to have *M. pneumoniae* infection.

Detection of *M. pneumoniae*–specific nucleotide sequences directly in clinical material has been accomplished with the use of tests developed locally or by large reference laboratories. These tests, which can be completed in a few hours, detect either *M. pneumoniae* DNA (PCR) or ribosomal RNA (reverse transcriptase nucleic acid amplification). The high sensitivity and specificity of real-time PCR performed on sputum, nasopharyngeal aspirate, or throat swab material suggest that this test could serve as a specific and rapid diagnostic method.[8]

Compared with PCR as the "gold standard" of proven infection, very few of the available antibody assays have acceptable sensitivity and specificity. Nonetheless, potential limitations around these diagnostics relate to their nonquantitative nature and the unclear significance of positive results, which can occur in the context of colonization after acute infection has resolved. In such cases, the use of serology in addition to PCR technology may be helpful. Future assays are likely to utilize quantitative detection techniques, which should help to discern between colonization and infection.

TREATMENT ℞

Despite the number and variety of tests for the diagnosis of *M. pneumoniae* infection, most cases are encountered in the ambulatory setting, and the institution of antimicrobial therapy is empirical and based on clinical recognition of the syndrome.

Antimicrobial therapy is not necessary for mycoplasmal upper respiratory tract infection, and the mycoplasmal cause of this syndrome most often goes undiagnosed. The pneumonia caused by *Mycoplasma* is self-limited and not life-threatening in most cases. However, treatment with effective antimicrobials may shorten the duration of illness and, by reducing cough and the number of organisms per unit volume of sputum, may reduce the spread of infection to contacts. Because *Mycoplasma* pneumonia is sporadic, most of the studies of antimicrobial efficacy are directed not at this single agent but rather at the treatment of community-acquired pneumonia (Chapter 91), of which *Mycoplasma* makes up a variable percentage. Retrospective analysis of specific causes then allows microbe-specific efficacy.

As would be predicted by the lack of a cell wall, all mycoplasmas, including *M. pneumoniae*, are unaffected by β-lactam antibiotics such as the penicillins and cephalosporins. Aminoglycosides are effective in vitro but have not been evaluated for efficacy in vivo. The mainstays of treatment of *M. pneumoniae* respiratory tract infection have been macrolides and tetracyclines.[9] Use of either drug class significantly shortens the duration of illness. The radiographic findings may take a week or longer to resolve, even with appropriate therapy (see

Fig. 301-1), and organisms may continue to be cultured from sputum for several weeks after a complete course of clinically effective treatment. This may be a result of the fact that although *M. pneumoniae* causes respiratory disease as an extracellular parasite, it has the capacity to reside intracellularly as well, thus making it difficult to eradicate the organism in vivo as opposed to cell cultures. The effect of therapy on extrapulmonary manifestations is unknown. *M. hominis* is not sensitive to erythromycin.

Because of the adverse effects of erythromycin and tetracycline, there is considerable interest in the antimycoplasmal efficacy of other agents. Doxycycline is somewhat better tolerated than tetracycline and can be administered in two daily doses rather than three. In vitro, doxycycline is as effective as tetracycline against *M. pneumoniae*.

Several other classes of antimicrobials have significant in vitro and in vivo activity against *M. pneumoniae* and other *Mycoplasma* species, including the fluoroquinolones, broad-spectrum macrolides (azithromycin, clarithromycin), and members of the macrolide-lincomycin-streptogramin-ketolide (MLSK) class of antimicrobials. There are no good data on the optimal duration of therapy needed to minimize carriage and relapse with these agents.

The macrolides are more active in vitro than the tetracyclines are. Fluoroquinolones have adequate activity for the treatment of these infections. They are more active than the tetracyclines but are at least 100 times less active than the macrolides. The streptogramins are also less active than the macrolides but more active than the tetracyclines. There is a significant cost differential in the use of these drugs in the United States, even in generic form. Azithromycin is five to seven times more expensive than erythromycin or doxycycline, and levofloxacin is 12 times more expensive than erythromycin and 20 times the cost of doxycycline.

During the past decade, there have been increasing reports, first from Asia and later spreading to other areas including the United States,[10] describing decreasing susceptibility of *M. pneumoniae* isolates to the macrolides. By 2012, one study from China reported 95% macrolide resistance. In the United States, resistance was up to 13% by 2015. Taking all this into account, recommended therapy includes doxycycline 100 mg every 12 hours in older children and adults, or azithromycin 500 mg on day 1 and then 250 mg every 24 hours. Young children should be given azithromycin (10 to 12 mg/kg on day 1, followed by 5 mg/kg/day).[A1] Given its longer half-life, 10 days of azithromycin should be adequate therapy. Recently, the American Academy of Pediatrics has sanctioned short course of doxycycline in children less than 8 years of age, making doxcline a suitable alternative for younger children. The usual duration of doxycycline therapy is 14 days; shorter courses may lead to relapse. The addition of corticosteroids (e.g., prednisolone 1 mg/kg twice daily for 3 days then tapered over 1 week) has been reported to shorten the duration of symptoms in children with severe or refractory infections,[A2][11] especially when the serum lactate dehydrogenase level is above about 300 IU/L.

PREVENTION

Outbreaks of *M. pneumoniae* respiratory infection among military recruits have led to interest in producing a vaccine to protect against this organism. The resulting vaccines induced specific antibody responses, but protection was limited to no more than 50% of vaccine recipients. Live vaccines using attenuated wild-type and temperature-sensitive mutant mycoplasmas have proved no more effective. In one study, volunteers who received vaccine but did not mount an antibody response had more severe disease when rechallenged with wild-type *Mycoplasma* than did nonvaccinated personnel.

Although *M. pneumoniae* is perhaps the leading cause of atypical pneumonia syndrome in closed populations, the enthusiasm for developing a vaccine for this disease has waned. New technology involving DNA expression library immunization has proved successful in animal studies with nonhuman mycoplasmas, and these methods may breathe new life into *M. pneumoniae* vaccine development.

Secondary Prevention
Prophylactic antibiotic use in family members exposed to *Mycoplasma* decreases clinical disease in these patients, but seroconversion is not prevented. One study showed that azithromycin prophylaxis, given as a 500-mg loading dose and 250 mg/day on days 2 through 5, significantly reduced the secondary attack rate of *M. pneumoniae* infection in a long-term care facility.

● OTHER *MYCOPLASMA* SPECIES
Other proven *Mycoplasma* infections include those in the urogenital tract caused by *Ureaplasma* species, *M. hominis*, and *M. genitalium*; wound infections caused by *M. hominis*; and overwhelming systemic infection in

TABLE 301-1	SITES AND INFECTIONS RELATED TO HUMAN MYCOPLASMAS OTHER THAN *M. PNEUMONIAE*		
SUBGROUP	**SITES OF ISOLATION**	**DISEASES**	**OCCURRENCE**
M. hominis	GU tract (F > M)	Cervicitis, vaginitis, ?prostatitis	Common
	Conjunctivae (neonate)	Conjunctivitis	
	Blood (peripartum)	Peripartum sepsis	
	Surgical wounds, joints	Sternotomy infection, arthritis	
M. orale	Oropharynx	?	Common
M. salivarium	Oropharynx, gingiva	?Periodontal disease	Common
M. fermentans	GU tract, blood, tissues	Multisystem disease in AIDS	Uncommon
M. genitalium	GU tract	Urethritis, cervicitis, PID	Uncommon
Ureaplasma spp	GU tract	Urethritis, upper GU infection	Common

AIDS = acquired immunodeficiency syndrome; F = female; GU = genitourinary; M = male; PID = pelvic inflammatory disease; URI = upper respiratory tract infection.

immunocompromised patients caused by *Mycoplasma fermentans* (*incognitus* strain).

EPIDEMIOLOGY
Ureaplasma urealyticum, *Ureaplasma parvum*, *M. hominis*, and *M. genitalium* are spread venereally, are not well documented (Table 301-1), and are difficult to culture but can be better identified by nucleic acid amplification testing. Their true incidence and prevalence are uncertain, as is their public health impact.

PATHOBIOLOGY
The genital mycoplasmas attach to cells using an adhesion protein as well as lipid-associated membrane proteins that adhere by way of toll-like receptors. Once within the cell, *M. genitalium* has been shown to trigger elaboration of numerous cytokines that cause inflammation.

CLINICAL MANIFESTATIONS
Diseases attributed to *Ureaplasma* species include urinary tract infection with and without calculus formation. The organism has been implicated as a cause of low birthweight in neonates.

There is increasing evidence that chronic *M. genitalium* infection causes nongonococcal urethritis (Chapter 269) in males and cervicitis and pelvic inflammatory disease (Chapters 269, 283, and 302) in females, in whom it leads in some cases to tubal factor infertility (Chapter 223), preterm birth, and spontaneous abortion.[12,13] Chronic *M. genitalium* infection may enhance the acquisition of human immunodeficiency virus (HIV) through increased shedding, and prevalence of *M. genitalium* appears higher in patients with HIV than in the general population.

M. hominis is a common genitourinary and oral commensal as well and has been documented as a cause of endometritis and postpartum fever. *M. hominis* can also cause sternal wound infection after cardiothoracic surgery and has been implicated in arthritis in immunocompromised patients.

M. salivarium may be involved in periodontal disease. *M. fermentans, incognitus* strain, was identified about four decades ago as an infectious agent in immunocompromised patients, in whom it causes overwhelming multisystem involvement.

DIAGNOSIS
The development of nucleic acid amplification tests such as PCR has enhanced the ability to detect *M. genitalium* and other genital mycoplasmas in secretions. However, the sensitivity and specificity of these tests appear to vary. Some commercially available tests can detect several mycoplasmas and chlamydial organisms in a single panel, and the refinement and standardization of these tests should lead to additional clarity of the pathogenic role of these organisms.

TREATMENT Rx

M. hominis is not sensitive to macrolides, but it is sensitive to the other antimicrobials recommended for *M. pneumoniae* infection. Azithromycin (1-g single dose) achieves a significantly higher cure rate for *M. genitalium*–associated urethritis than does multidose doxycycline. The success rate for a single dose of 500 mg azithromycin is only about 60%, whereas moxifloxacin may be successful in close to 90% of cases.[14]

PROGNOSIS

Prognosis of early disease without scarring of the cervix and fallopian tubes is relatively good. However, treatment of all sexual partners of the index case is paramount to prevent reinfection. Prognosis also depends on the susceptibility of the offending organisms. It is highly likely that antimicrobial resistance will increase in the future, just as it has for azithromycin in the past.

Grade A References

A1. Mulholland S, Gavranich JB, Gillies MB, et al. Antibiotics for community-acquired lower respiratory tract infections secondary to *Mycoplasma pneumoniae* in children. *Cochrane Database Syst Rev.* 2012;9:CD004875.

A2. Huang L, Gao X, Chen M. Early treatment with corticosteroids in patients with *Mycoplasma pneumoniae* pneumonia: a randomized clinical trial. *J Trop Pediatr.* 2014;60:338-342.

GENERAL REFERENCES

For the General References and other additional features, please visit Expert Consult at https://expertconsult.inkling.com.

302
DISEASES CAUSED BY CHLAMYDIAE

WILLIAM M. GEISLER

DEFINITION

Chlamydiae are obligate intracellular bacteria that cause a variety of human and animal diseases and much morbidity. Chlamydiae were originally classified taxonomically into one genus, *Chlamydia*. On the basis of sequence analysis of 16S rRNA genes, it had been proposed that chlamydial taxonomy be revised to contain two genera: *Chlamydia* and *Chlamydophila*. However, on the basis of additional data on chlamydia genome sequences and meetings within the *Chlamydia* scientific community, it has been agreed that the family Chlamydiaceae will contain a single genus, *Chlamydia*. Within the family are now nine recognized species: *C. trachomatis, C. pneumoniae, C. psittaci, C. pecorum, C. muridarum, C. felis, C. abortus, C. suis,* and *C. caviae*. *C. trachomatis* is classified into a trachoma biovar and lymphogranuloma venereum (LGV) biovar. This chapter is limited to human diseases caused by chlamydiae.

The Pathogen

Chlamydiae have a gram-negative cell wall structure consisting of an outer membrane that contains lipopolysaccharide and an inner cytoplasmic membrane. The outer membrane contains a single 40-kD major outer membrane protein, OmpA (also known as MOMP), and two cysteine-rich minor outer membrane–associated proteins (OmcA and OmcB); through intermolecular and intramolecular disulfide bonding, these proteins form a complex that provides structural rigidity.

Chlamydiae grow only within intracellular membrane-bound vacuoles, termed inclusions,[1] that seclude the organism from extracellular and cytoplasmic environments. They share a distinct biphasic developmental cycle (Fig. 302-1) that includes an extracellular, metabolically inactive, infectious form (an elementary body) and an intracellular replicative form (a reticulate body). *In vitro* studies have shown that chlamydiae may enter a persistent state under certain conditions (penicillin treatment, challenge with certain cytokines, restriction of select nutrients) in which they have reduced metabolic activity and may be more refractory to antibiotic treatment; whether this occurs *in vivo* is unclear. Chlamydiae are unable to synthesize adenosine triphosphate and therefore depend on the host cell for nutrients to meet their energy requirements.

PATHOBIOLOGY

Macrophages are the principal host cells for *C. psittaci* and *C. trachomatis* LGV biovar, whereas the principal host cells for *C. trachomatis* trachoma biovar and *C. pneumoniae* strains are columnar epithelial cells at mucosal sites. Host cell tropism correlates with the type of inflammation elicited by chlamydiae. The LGV biovar and *C. psittaci* produce granulomatous inflammation, characteristic of delayed hypersensitivity reactions. The trachoma biovar produces neutrophilic exudate during acute infection and submucosal mononuclear infiltration with lymphoid follicle formation during later stages of infection.

Chlamydiae elicit both humoral and cellular immune responses. Infection can persist or recur even after an adaptive immune response develops, suggesting that the organism has evolved strategies for immune evasion. Persistent or recurrent infections can elicit inflammatory cellular immune responses that cause tissue injury.

CHLAMYDIAL DISEASES

Table 302-1 summarizes the diseases caused by chlamydiae in humans and the associated clinical and laboratory characteristics.

Chlamydia trachomatis

C. trachomatis infection is a common bacterial infection in humans and accounts for significant morbidity worldwide. *C. trachomatis* isolates have been differentiated into 18 major serovars (i.e., OmpA types) based on variations in OmpA that are identified on antigen cross-reactivity in the microimmunofluorescence test. The major diseases caused by *C. trachomatis* are trachoma, caused by serovars A, B, Ba, and C; sexually and perinatally transmitted diseases, caused by serovars D through K (and, rarely, serovars B and Ba); and sexually transmitted LGV, caused by serovars L1, L2, L2a, and L3. Sequencing of the *ompA* gene has led to the recognition of more OmpA variants, including L2b. Multilocus sequencing typing is a newer tool that has been used to further discriminate between *C. trachomatis* strains of the same OmpA genotype. Trachoma and LGV are endemic in developing areas of the world (although LGV outbreaks have also occurred in populations of men who have sex with men in developed countries), whereas sexually and perinatally transmitted non-LGV chlamydial infections occur worldwide.

TRACHOMA
EPIDEMIOLOGY

Trachoma is a chronic follicular conjunctivitis. The overall incidence is unknown, but it has been estimated by the World Health Organization (WHO) that 21.4 million people have active trachoma. Trachoma is endemic in more than 41 countries and is especially common in poor areas of sub-Saharan Africa, where the disease prevalence in children may exceed 40%. According to the WHO, there are 190.2 million people living in trachoma-endemic areas. Trachoma is a major public health problem because scarring from trachoma causes blindness, affecting 7.2 million people by WHO estimates. Trachoma is the most common preventable cause of blindness worldwide. Active trachoma often occurs in the first few years of life. The inflammation from recurrent or persistent trachoma can lead to conjunctival scarring, which can ultimately cause corneal damage and blindness later in life. The *C. trachomatis* serovars that produce trachoma are spread by direct contact with fingers or fomites (e.g., washcloths, handkerchiefs) contaminated with eye discharge from an infected person or by eye-seeking flies. Because of this mode of transmission, trachoma often clusters in households. Risk factors for trachoma include poor facial hygiene, limited access to water, poor sanitation, and proximity to other infected persons or to a heavy density of eye-seeking flies.

CLINICAL MANIFESTATIONS

There are two stages of trachoma disease, and they can overlap. Initially, trachoma begins as an inflammatory follicular conjunctivitis (i.e., active trachoma). On eversion of the upper eyelid, white to pale yellow lymphoid follicles can be visualized on the superior tarsal conjunctival surface, and papillae may be noted between follicles. Minimal watery or mucoid ocular discharge may also be seen. In more severe active trachoma, the conjunctiva can be thickened and edematous. Subsequently, conjunctival inflammation can progress to cause

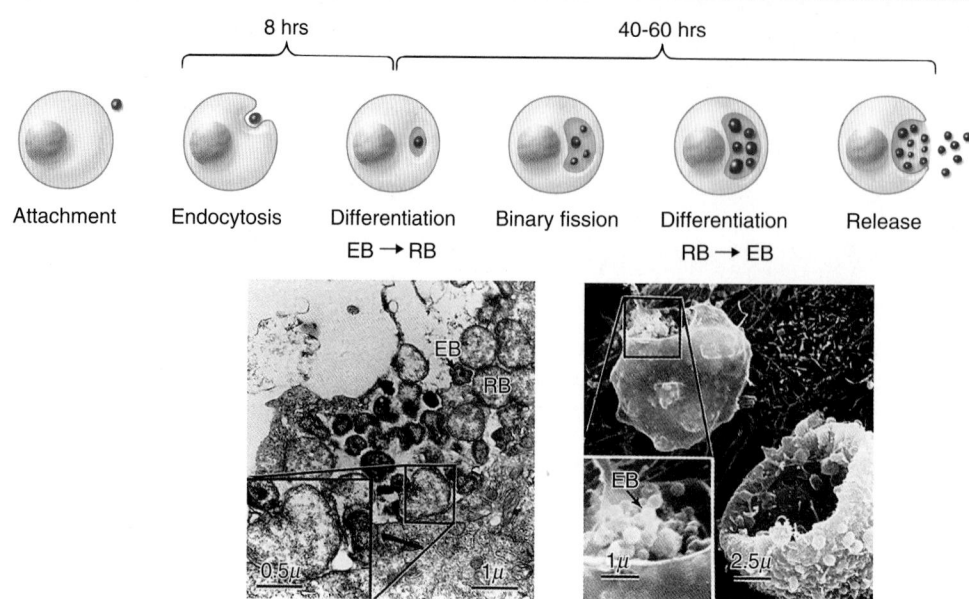

FIGURE 302-1. Developmental cycle of chlamydiae. The *top panel* shows the developmental cycle common to all chlamydiae. The *red dots* represent elementary bodies (EBs), and the *blue dots* represent reticulate bodies (RBs). Chlamydiae infect eukaryotic cells through multiple attachment mechanisms. After attachment, EBs enter the cell within a membrane-bound vacuole that remains unfused with lysosomes. EBs reorganize into RBs and asynchronously replicate 8 to 12 times, with a doubling time of 2 to 3 hours. At the conclusion of the growth cycle, RBs differentiate back to EBs, and each inclusion yields 100 to 1000 new infectious EBs. The *bottom left panel,* a transmission electron micrograph taken 40 hours after infection, shows the large RBs and the smaller EBs, which have a condensed nucleoid structure within their cytoplasm. The *bottom right panel,* a scanning electron micrograph taken 60 hours after infection, shows a membrane-bound vacuole containing many EBs exiting from an infected HeLa cell.

TABLE 302-1   MAJOR DISEASES CAUSED BY CHLAMYDIAE IN HUMANS AND ASSOCIATED CLINICAL AND LABORATORY FEATURES

SPECIES	SEROVAR	DISEASE	TRANSMISSION ROUTE	DIAGNOSIS	PREVENTION
C. trachomatis	A–C	Trachoma	Fomites, eye-seeking flies	Clinical criteria or culture/NAAT	SAFE strategy
	D–K	Urethritis, cervicitis, proctitis, epididymitis, PID	Sexual contact	NAAT	Abstinence or monogamy, education, condoms, partner treatment
	D–K	Inclusion conjunctivitis, infant pneumonia	Perinatal contact	Culture, DFA, NAAT, or serology (for pneumonia)	Prenatal chlamydia screening: treat infected mothers
	L1–L3	Lymphogranuloma venereum	Sexual contact	Serology or culture/NAAT plus OmpA typing	Abstinence or monogamy, education, condoms, partner treatment
C. pneumoniae	One	Upper respiratory infections, atypical pneumonia, asthma exacerbations	Respiratory droplet	Serology or culture/PCR	None
C. psittaci	Multiple	Psittacosis, atypical pneumonia, febrile illness	Aerosolized bird secretions, dust	Serology	Quarantine and chlortetracycline for imported birds, avoidance or precautions for at-risk subjects

DFA = direct fluorescent antibody test; NAAT = nucleic acid amplification test; PCR = polymerase chain reaction; PID = pelvic inflammatory disease; SAFE = World Health Organization's recommended strategy acronym for: surgery (for trichiasis), antimicrobials (periodic community-wide treatment), facial cleanliness, and environmental improvement.

scarring of the upper tarsal conjunctiva (the cicatricial stage of disease). Scarring deforms the eyelid and can lead to an inward turning of the eyelashes, which can result in corneal abrasion (trichiasis). Over time, trichiasis causes corneal edema, ulceration, vascularization (pannus), scarring, and opacification. The corneal damage leads to decreased vision or blindness, occurring mostly in young adults and middle-aged persons. Viral conjunctivitis (e.g., adenovirus) is manifested in a clinical fashion similar to active trachoma, but it is self-limited and usually resolves within a week. Trachoma can be complicated by superinfection with other bacterial pathogens (e.g., *Haemophilus influenzae*), which should be considered when purulent ocular discharge or significant inflammation of the bulbar conjunctiva is present.

DIAGNOSIS

Because the majority of trachoma cases occur in developing countries without access to laboratory testing or the necessary resources, trachoma is often diagnosed clinically on the basis of findings of active trachoma (follicles on the upper tarsal conjunctiva or pronounced inflammatory thickening of the tarsal conjunctiva) or cicatricial disease. When laboratories are available, detection of *C. trachomatis* provides definitive evidence of active trachoma and may identify infection in subjects with minimal clinical evidence of active trachoma. Isolation of the organism in cell culture is one means to detect *C. trachomatis*,

but the test's sensitivity is less than 50%, and the methods are labor-intensive. Nonculture tests have higher sensitivities in active trachoma. For instance, nucleic acid amplification tests (NAATs) are the most sensitive diagnostic tests, but they are not widely available in many trachoma-endemic areas. It is uncommon for adults with late scarring to have *C. trachomatis* detected by any of these assays.

TREATMENT   Rx

Active trachoma can be treated with a tetracycline eye ointment twice daily for 6 weeks or oral macrolide therapy.[2] The latter is preferred in part because extraocular sites such as the nasopharynx may be infected in young children. Single-dose oral azithromycin (20 mg/kg; maximum of 1 g) is as effective as tetracycline ointment and is more advantageous in terms of compliance and side-effect profile; tetracycline application can irritate the ocular surface.

Surgical intervention is the only effective management for trichiasis. Eyelid rotation surgery prevents the eyelashes from abrading the cornea, preventing blindness and other nonvisual symptoms.[3] Trichiasis recurrence after surgery is a major concern, and recurrence rates are highly variable across studies. Other concerns include accessibility to surgery and the patient's acceptance.

The WHO is committed to eliminating blinding trachoma by 2020 and recommends that all countries with endemic trachoma adopt the SAFE strategy: surgery (for trichiasis), antimicrobials (periodic community-wide treatment), facial cleanliness, and environmental improvement. Mass treatment of a community with single-dose oral azithromycin is safe and has dramatically reduced the prevalence of infection for up to 1 year after treatment; it has also been shown to reduce mortality in children.[A1] Annual azithromycin treatment is recommended for trachoma-endemic areas. Reintroduction of trachoma after mass treatment has been demonstrated, which may be due in part to decreased herd immunity. Repeated mass treatment (every few months) provides herd protection to the entire community.

Mass antibiotic treatment as the sole intervention for eliminating trachoma is unlikely to be successful if other factors that facilitate transmission are not addressed. Face-washing and good hygiene help reduce the risk for transmission through contact with fingers and flies. Although the promotion of facial cleanliness through educational campaigns may be one of the most important interventions, sustaining such behavioral changes can be challenging. Achieving better environmental conditions through measures that reduce household and community fly density and improve waste management and access to clean water can also limit transmission. Improvement in socioeconomic conditions in a community correlates with a decline in trachoma prevalence.

SEXUALLY AND PERINATALLY TRANSMITTED CHLAMYDIAL INFECTIONS

EPIDEMIOLOGY

Chlamydia is the most prevalent bacterial sexually transmitted infection in the United States. More than 1.7 million infections were reported to the Centers for Disease Control and Prevention (CDC) in 2017.[4] The number of reported cases is increasing each year; this could reflect increased chlamydia screening efforts rather than a true increase in infection burden,[5] but there is no strong evidence to support that screening rates are increasing, and thus it may be a true increase in the number of chlamydia cases. Taking into account underreporting and underscreening, it is estimated by the CDC that more than 2.8 million new chlamydial infections occur annually in the United States. Higher chlamydia prevalence rates have been associated with younger age (sexually active adolescents and young adults), select minority ethnic groups (especially African Americans), and new or multiple sexual partners. Chlamydia prevalence is higher in women than in men; it is unclear whether this is due to higher screening rates in women or whether women may be more susceptible to infection acquisition or persistence. Chlamydia prevalence is highest in the southeastern United States. The estimated total cost attributable to chlamydial disease in the United States exceeds $2.4 billion annually. From a global perspective, WHO estimates that there are approximately 131 million new cases of chlamydia annually. In addition to the adverse effects on the reproductive health of women, chlamydia has a substantial impact on prenatal and perinatal outcomes and facilitates the transmission of human immunodeficiency virus (HIV).

CLINICAL MANIFESTATIONS

Urethritis

C. trachomatis is the most common cause of nongonococcal urethritis in men,[6] being responsible for 20 to 50% of cases. Although the majority of men with chlamydial urethritis do not have symptoms, studies in high-prevalence venues (e.g., sexually transmitted disease clinics) have reported that 40 to 60% of men with chlamydial urethritis have symptoms. The most frequent symptoms are urethral discomfort (itching or pain) with urination and urethral discharge. On examination, a mild to moderate amount of clear or cloudy/mucoid (rarely purulent) urethral discharge may be visualized (Fig. 302-2A). Urethral discharge

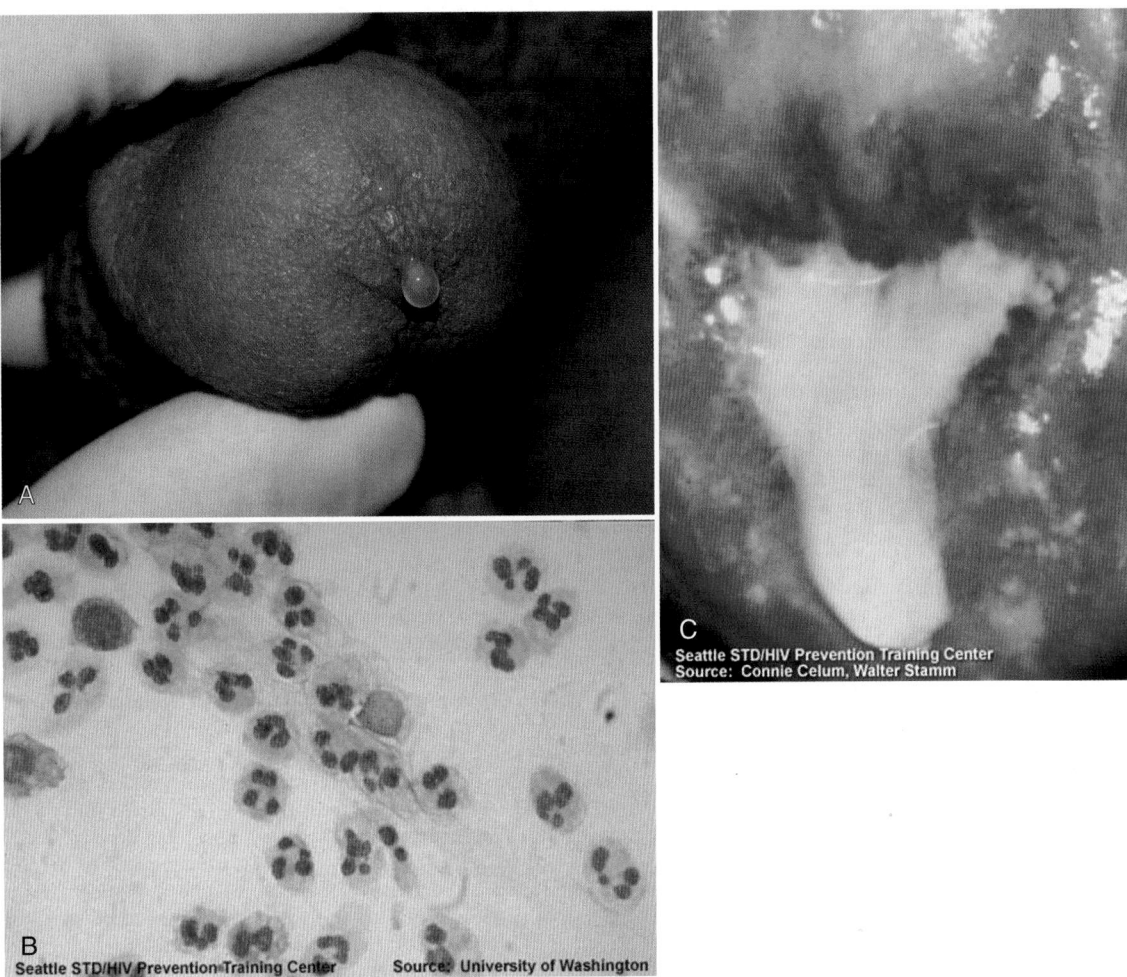

FIGURE 302-2. Clinical manifestations of genital *Chlamydia trachomatis* infection. **A,** Cloudy urethral discharge of urethritis. **B,** Urethral specimen Gram stain revealing nongonococcal urethritis findings: two or more polymorphonuclear cells per oil field (1000×) and the absence of intracellular gram-negative diplococci. **C,** Purulent endocervical discharge of mucopurulent cervicitis. **(A,** Courtesy James Sizemore, MD. **B** and **C,** From *Practitioner's Handbook for the Management of Sexually Transmitted Disease.* Retrieved from http://depts. washington.edu/handbook.)

sometimes becomes apparent only after stripping the urethra from the base of the penis to the glans; this should be considered in men reporting urethral symptoms but without urethral discharge on initial inspection. Gram stain from a urethral swab specimen demonstrates five or more polymorphonuclear leukocytes (PMNs) per oil field (1000×) in the majority of chlamydial infections (Fig. 302-2B). Chlamydial organisms cannot be visualized on Gram stain. Up to 20% of men with chlamydial urethritis have fewer than five PMNs per oil field on urethral Gram stain, reflecting the fact that minimal inflammation may be elicited in some cases of chlamydial urethritis. Urethral inflammation can also be detected by a positive urinary leukocyte esterase test result on unspun first-void urine.

C. trachomatis urethritis also occurs in women, who may have no symptoms or present with an acute urethral syndrome characterized by dysuria, urinary frequency, and/or pyuria. This acute urethral syndrome mimics a urinary tract infection, and chlamydia should be suspected in women with pyuria but negative urine nitrite and/or negative urine culture, especially in sexually active adolescents and young adults; many urinary tract infection treatments are not effective against chlamydia. Mild urethral discharge may be seen. Pelvic examination should be performed in women with suspected chlamydia urethritis to search for other clinical findings of chlamydia (e.g., cervicitis).

Epididymitis

Chlamydia can spread from the urethra to the epididymis, causing epididymitis in up to 1% of infected men.[7] Symptoms include testicular pain and scrotal erythema and swelling that are typically unilateral. On examination, there is palpable swelling and tenderness of the epididymis; accompanying findings may include testicular tenderness, scrotal erythema and swelling, urethral discharge, or hydrocele. In men younger than 35 years, *C. trachomatis* is the principal cause of epididymitis, whereas in men older than 35 years, complicated urinary tract infection with uropathogens is a more common cause, especially in those with prostate disorders. Up to 15% of epididymitis cases are complicated by chronic pain that is usually idiopathic and often unresponsive to antibiotics. Other complications include decreased fertility and, rarely, testicular abscess.

Cervicitis

C. trachomatis is the most common cause of cervicitis, being responsible for up to 50% of cases. The majority of women with endocervical chlamydial infection are asymptomatic. Symptoms, when present, are often mild and nonspecific for chlamydia and include the following: vaginal discharge, intermenstrual vaginal bleeding, dysuria, and pain during intercourse (dyspareunia). Up to 13% of women with asymptomatic cervical chlamydial infection have mucopurulent cervicitis detected on pelvic examination (Fig. 302-2C); this is characterized by a purulent or cloudy endocervical discharge visible in the endocervical canal or on the tip of an endocervical swab. A similar proportion may have endocervical bleeding that is easily induced with passage of a swab through the cervical os. Nonspecific findings may include vaginal discharge and edematous ectopy (a darker red area of columnar epithelium visible on the face of the cervix). A vaginal wet mount often shows more than 5 to 10 PMNs per 400× field.

Pelvic Inflammatory Disease

Chlamydia can spread from the cervix to the endometrium (causing endometritis), fallopian tubes (causing salpingitis), and peritoneum (causing peritonitis or perihepatitis). These upper genital tract infections are collectively referred to as pelvic inflammatory disease (PID; Chapters 269 and 283). Estimates of the proportion of cervical chlamydial infections that progress to PID vary greatly but are most commonly 10 to 35%.[9] The majority of PID cases are subclinical or silent. PID symptoms include pelvic or lower abdominal pain (especially during menses or the first 2 weeks of the menstrual cycle) and nausea. Fever is less common. Examination findings include cervical motion tenderness and tenderness of the uterus or adnexa. Although most cases of chlamydial PID are due to the natural progression of infection, they may also occur postpartum or after pregnancy termination. The long-term consequences of PID include infertility, ectopic pregnancy, and chronic pelvic pain.

Complications during Pregnancy

There is some evidence that genital chlamydial infection during pregnancy can lead to adverse outcomes, including preterm labor, low birthweight, miscarriage, and stillbirth.[10]

Reactive Arthritis

Reactive arthritis, characterized by the classic triad of trigger infection (e.g., chlamydia), conjunctivitis, and arthritis, can complicate chlamydial infection (Chapter 249). There is a male predominance in reactive arthritis cases triggered by chlamydia, and it has been estimated that reactive arthritis occurs in up to 1% of men presenting with chlamydial urethritis.

Proctitis

Proctitis caused by non-LGV *C. trachomatis* OmpA types is usually asymptomatic. Subjects with acute symptomatic proctitis may report rectal pain or bleeding, tenesmus, pruritus, rectal discharge, or diarrhea. Anoscopy or sigmoidoscopy may reveal friable mucosa and a mucoid or mucopurulent discharge. A rectal swab Gram stain often reveals many PMNs per oil field.

Conjunctivitis

An acute follicular conjunctivitis may rarely occur in adolescents or adults with genital chlamydial infection. The presumed mode of acquisition is autoinoculation with infected genital secretions. The typical clinical presentation is a subacute or indolent infection characterized by unilateral conjunctival redness, mucoid or mucopurulent ocular discharge, a foreign body sensation, and preauricular adenopathy.

Oropharyngeal Infection

C. trachomatis has been detected in the oropharynx of sexually active subjects and is asymptomatic in most instances. Recent evidence suggests that *C. trachomatis* can be transmitted from oropharyngeal sites to the genital tract, providing rationale for treatment of oropharyngeal chlamydia. However, because oropharyngeal chlamydia prevalence is very low in most populations and the clinical significance of *C. trachomatis* detected in the oropharynx is unclear, routine oropharyngeal chlamydia screening is not recommended.

Infant Inclusion Conjunctivitis and Pneumonia

Because the prevalence of chlamydia in pregnant adolescents and young adults in the United States can be high (>5%), the morbidity associated with perinatally transmitted chlamydia is considerable. Neonates exposed to *C. trachomatis* during passage through the birth canal may develop inclusion conjunctivitis (≈20 to 40%) or pneumonia (≈10 to 20%). The conjunctivitis, termed inclusion conjunctivitis because the cytoplasmic chlamydia inclusion bodies demonstrated in neonatal conjunctival scrapings are the same as those seen in genital scrapings from adults with genital chlamydia, usually develops 5 to 12 days after birth but may occur as long as 4 to 6 weeks after birth. Clinical manifestations include conjunctival injection and thickening, a clear or mucopurulent ocular discharge, and eyelid swelling. Chlamydia pneumonia in infants usually occurs subacutely between 1 and 3 months of age. Characteristic clinical features include a repetitive staccato cough and absence of fever. Other clinical findings may include tachypnea, crackles on auscultation of the lungs, nasal discharge, and eosinophilia. Chest radiographs may reveal bilateral diffuse infiltrates.

Lymphogranuloma Venereum

LGV is a sexually transmitted infection caused by invasive *C. trachomatis* LGV OmpA serovars. In contrast to infection with non-LGV strains, LGV is a more invasive systemic infection that involves lymphoid tissue (causing lymphadenitis) and can be ulcerative. LGV is endemic in Africa, India, Southeast Asia, South America, and the Caribbean. LGV had been uncommon in the United States. However, in recent years, developed countries have experienced a shift in LGV epidemiology and clinical presentation, and LGV has emerged in Europe and North America as a leading cause of proctitis and proctocolitis in men who have sex with men.[11]

Classically, the clinical manifestations of LGV differ in early versus later stages of infection. In the early stage (3 to 30 days after acquisition) of genital LGV, a primary skin lesion or lesions may develop on the genital mucosa or adjacent skin in the form of a papule, ulcer, or herpetiform lesion. The lesion is usually asymptomatic and goes unnoticed, but it may be erosive; it heals quickly without scarring. Early genital LGV may also be manifested as a nonspecific inflammatory syndrome (e.g., urethritis and cervicitis), similar to infection with non-LGV strains. Genital LGV can progress to an inguinal syndrome 2 to 4 weeks later, characterized by painful, erythematous inguinal lymphadenopathy (buboes) and systemic manifestations including fever, headache, arthralgias, myalgias, and leukocytosis. The buboes are commonly unilateral, and about one third spontaneously rupture and drain pus, which can be complicated by fistulas or sinus tracks; unruptured buboes usually heal. In later stages, genital tract fibrosis can lead to complications such as infertility, elephantiasis, strictures, fistulas, and subcutaneous sclerosis.

LGV may also be manifested as an anogenital syndrome with invasive proctitis. Symptoms include fever, tenesmus, anal pruritus, and a rectal discharge that may be mucoid or, less commonly, mucopurulent or bloody. Up to 20 to 30% of patients do not have symptoms. The rectal mucosa is friable, with multiple superficial ulcerations, and biopsy may reveal submucosal granulomas and crypt abscesses; these clinical and histopathologic findings resemble Crohn disease (Chapter 132). Late complications include rectal strictures, anal fistulas, and lymphorrhoids (perianal growths of lymphatic tissue).

Natural History

The natural history of untreated genital *C. trachomatis* infection has not been fully elucidated. Outcomes of untreated genital chlamydia include spontaneous resolution (i.e., immune-mediated clearance) and persisting infection; the latter may be subclinical or may progress to clinical manifestations (e.g., urethritis, cervicitis), which can remain uncomplicated or lead to a complication (e.g., PID). On the basis of limited evidence in subjects with chlamydia detected initially by a screening test who returned within weeks to months for treatment and were retested, anywhere from 10 to 40% of infections resolve spontaneously before treatment. Some patients with persisting infection develop clinical manifestations before returning for treatment, including a small proportion of females (up to 4%) who develop symptomatic PID. Other sparse data in females suggest that up to 50% of genital chlamydial infections resolve after a year, but a small percentage (<10%) could persist for several years. There is evidence to suggest that chlamydia resolution before treatment may lower the short-term risk for reinfection. An improved understanding of the natural history of chlamydia could have an impact on screening and treatment recommendations.[12]

DIAGNOSIS

C. trachomatis infections are difficult to diagnose clinically because the majority are asymptomatic, and even when symptoms or signs are present, they are nonspecific. Therefore, a definitive diagnosis relies on detecting the organism. Laboratory diagnosis confirms the clinical diagnosis in those with clinical manifestations and detects infection in symptom-free individuals (i.e., screening). The CDC recommends annual chlamydia screening for sexually active women younger than 25 years as well as for older women with risk factors (e.g., new or multiple sexual partners).[13] Select studies have demonstrated that chlamydia screening reduces the rate of PID. Surveillance data from the United States, England, and British Columbia during the past decade have demonstrated a steady decline in PID rates. Universal chlamydia screening in men is not recommended; selective chlamydia testing is appropriate in venues with high prevalences (e.g., STD clinics, correctional facilities), for high-risk men, or for men who have symptoms.

The reference standard for the detection of *C. trachomatis* has been isolation of the organism in cell culture. Development of nonculture tests was important because culture is technically demanding, expensive, and not widely available. Earlier nonculture tests included enzyme immunoassay, direct fluorescent antibody, and nucleic acid hybridization. These tests were less expensive and less technically demanding than culture but had lower sensitivities (lower limit of detection ≥10³ elementary bodies) and therefore detected fewer infections. These earlier tests have been replaced by NAATs, which are now the recommended diagnostic tests for chlamydia. NAATs have the highest sensitivity (detecting a small number of elementary bodies) and can be performed on genital swabs and on noninvasively collected specimens (first-catch urine and self-collected vaginal swabs and rectal swabs) with similar accuracy. The CDC's recommended specimens for screening with NAATs are first-catch urine in males and vaginal swabs in females. NAATs have not been cleared by the U.S. Food and Drug Administration for use with rectal, oropharyngeal, or conjunctival swab specimens; however, some laboratories have validated the assays to meet Clinical Laboratory Improvement Amendments (CLIA) requirements.

The role of serology in diagnosis of *C. trachomatis* infection is limited primarily to two indications: (1) infant pneumonia syndrome, the diagnosis of which is suggested by a *C. trachomatis* immunoglobulin M (IgM) antibody titer of 1 : 32 or greater with the microimmunofluorescence (MIF) assay; and (2) LGV, the diagnosis of which is suggested by a complement fixation (CF) antibody titer greater than 1 : 64 or MIF antibody titer greater than 1 : 256 in the appropriate clinical context. MIF has a higher specificity than CF. LGV can be more definitively diagnosed by demonstrating an LGV OmpA type on *C. trachomatis* DNA from infected material.

TREATMENT ℞

C. trachomatis is susceptible to tetracyclines, macrolides, and select quinolones (ofloxacin and levofloxacin, but not ciprofloxacin). The CDC's recommended treatment for uncomplicated chlamydia is either doxycycline 100 mg orally twice daily for 7 days or azithromycin 1 g orally in a single dose. A meta-analysis of urogenital chlamydia treatment trials that used primarily chlamydia culture revealed that these regimens are equally efficacious,[A2] with cure rates of about 97 to 98%, although one recent randomized trial that used the more sensitive NAAT found doxycycline to be slightly more efficacious than azithromycin for urogenital chlamydia.[A3] For rectal chlamydia, however, a recent meta-analysis of observational studies of rectal chlamydia treatments demonstrated that 1 week of doxycycline (100 mg twice daily) was significantly more efficacious than single-dose azithromycin (1 gram).[14] Randomized rectal chlamydia treatment trials are underway and should provide more definitive evidence of the efficacy of doxycycline and azithromycin for rectal chlamydia.

Treatment adherence is higher with azithromycin. Alternative treatment regimens include erythromycin base 500 mg orally four times a day for 7 days, ofloxacin 300 mg orally twice daily for 7 days, and levofloxacin 500 mg orally once a day for 7 days. Azithromycin is the recommended treatment for chlamydia-infected pregnant women. *C. trachomatis* epididymitis and PID should be treated with doxycycline for 10 and 14 days, respectively. Treatment of these syndromes is usually empirical before test results are available; therefore, ceftriaxone 250 mg intramuscularly in a single dose is added to doxycycline to cover gonorrhea. LGV should be treated with doxycycline for 3 weeks; some experts recommend azithromycin 1 g orally weekly for 3 weeks as an alternative.[15] Infant chlamydial infections are treated with erythromycin base 50 mg/kg/day orally divided into four daily doses for 14 days; data on other macrolides are limited, but a shorter treatment course with azithromycin 20 mg/kg/day orally may be effective.

A test of cure (approximately 3 weeks after completion of chlamydia treatment) is recommended only for pregnant women. Sexual partners (including current partners and those with contact in the preceding 60 days) and parents of chlamydia-infected infants should be evaluated and treated empirically. Expedited partner therapy, whereby chlamydia-infected patients are offered medication or a prescription to give to their sexual partners, or whereby clinicians provide medication to contacts without an examination, may reduce the risk for recurrent chlamydia. Patients and their partners should remain abstinent until treatment is completed.

PREVENTION

Education and the provision of condoms are preventive measures that should accompany chlamydia treatment. Recurrent chlamydia occurs in approximately 10 to 20% of chlamydia-infected subjects within a few months of treatment; therefore, repeated chlamydia testing is recommended approximately 3 months after treatment. Routine screening may reduce the risk for PID in sexually active young women. It has been recommended that all sexually active women younger than 25 years and older women at risk for chlamydia should be offered chlamydia screening annually. Sensitive testing can be done on vaginal swabs or urine samples collected by the patient, without need for pelvic examination.

Chlamydia pneumoniae

In 1986, a new chlamydial pathogen that caused acute respiratory tract infections was identified and designated *Chlamydia* strain TWAR. It was initially thought to be a novel *C. psittaci* strain but was later recognized as the species *C. pneumoniae*.[16] Pneumonia and upper respiratory tract infections (bronchitis, pharyngitis, laryngitis, and sinusitis) are the most frequently identified diseases caused by *C. pneumoniae*. However, *C. pneumoniae* may also contribute to exacerbations of chronic bronchitis and asthma. There is evidence suggesting that *C. pneumoniae* may contribute to atherosclerosis, although large *C. pneumoniae* treatment trials have not demonstrated benefit in preventing adverse cardiovascular events. Select central nervous system disorders (e.g., Alzheimer disease, multiple sclerosis) have been linked to *C. pneumoniae*, but a causal relationship has not been established.

EPIDEMIOLOGY

The majority of adults in the United States and other developed countries are seropositive for *C. pneumoniae*, up to 80% in some populations. Seroconversion often occurs during childhood or adolescence and may be subclinical. Studies incorporating culture or polymerase chain reaction (PCR) suggest that infection is not uncommon in children younger than 5 years. The CDC estimates there are 300,000 *C. pneumoniae* infections annually in the United States. *C. pneumoniae* causes an atypical pneumonia syndrome, with an estimated annual incidence of one case per 1000 population; epidemiologic studies suggest a 4-year cycle of increased pneumonia incidence. Up to 10% of community-acquired pneumonias are attributed to *C. pneumoniae*, and coinfection with other respiratory pathogens such as *Streptococcus pneumoniae* and *Mycoplasma pneumoniae* is not uncommon. The organism is believed to be acquired through the inhalation of infected respiratory droplets from persons with disease and possibly from symptom-free carriers. This mode of transmission can facilitate the spread of infection among household members and can cause epidemics in enclosed populations, such as persons in military barracks, nursing homes, and schools.

CLINICAL MANIFESTATIONS

Most *C. pneumoniae* infections occur in children, who often have mild clinical manifestations or do not have symptoms. Clinical manifestations are more evident in adults, especially the elderly, who have the highest incidence of *C. pneumoniae* pneumonia. *C. pneumoniae* causes an atypical pneumonia that is usually of mild to moderate severity. The incubation period may be several weeks, and the disease onset is gradual. A nonproductive cough is usually present and is often preceded or accompanied by nasal congestion, sore throat, and hoarseness. Headache may occur in up to half of patients. Fever and dyspnea occur less commonly. On examination, localized pulmonary crackles or rhonchi are often heard. Chest radiography shows pneumonitis, most often evident as a single subsegmental lower lobe infiltrate. The leukocyte count is usually normal. *C. pneumoniae* may also be manifested as isolated bronchitis, sinusitis, laryngitis, or nonexudative pharyngitis. The clinical course of these upper respiratory tract infections may be protracted for several weeks.

DIAGNOSIS

C. pneumoniae infection is usually diagnosed by serology or direct detection of the organism in respiratory specimens by cell culture or other nonculture methods. Serology is the test used in most clinical settings, with the MIF assay considered the reference standard for serodiagnosis. Acute infection is suggested by a four-fold rise in IgG from paired sera or a single high IgM (>1 : 16) or IgG (>1 : 512) titer. However, serology is limited by its specificity, reproducibility, and clinical correlation. *C. pneumoniae* can be isolated in cell culture, but culture is technically challenging and time-consuming. Antigen detection with use of fluorescent monoclonal antibodies has a lower sensitivity than culture and is also technically challenging. *C. pneumoniae* PCR is more sensitive than culture, and real-time PCR appears to have advantages over conventional PCR. Although there are still issues involving the standardization of PCR methods for *C. pneumoniae* detection, PCR is promising and will likely become the test of choice.

TREATMENT Rx

C. pneumoniae is susceptible to tetracyclines, macrolides, and fluoroquinolones. Treatment trials using culture have demonstrated that select macrolide and fluoroquinolone regimens eradicate *C. pneumoniae* in approximately 70 to 85% of subjects with pneumonia. The clinical response to treatment may be slow, and some patients may need retreatment. The suggested treatment duration for most regimens is typically 10 to 14 days, except that shorter courses may be effective for azithromycin (10 mg/kg on day 1, followed by 5 mg/kg during the next 4 days; up to 1.5 g orally during 5 days). Chronic *C. pneumoniae* infections may require even longer courses of treatment (e.g., 6 weeks), and macrolides are suggested in this setting. Protective immunity after *C. pneumoniae* infection may not occur, and therefore reinfection is common.

Chlamydia psittaci
EPIDEMIOLOGY

C. psittaci naturally infects a variety of mammals and birds. *C. psittaci* strains appear to be host specific, and most human infections are linked to contact with an infected bird.[17] *C. psittaci* infection in humans is termed psittacosis, in part because exposure to psittacine birds (parrots, parakeets, and budgerigars) is commonly implicated in infections. However, because human cases have been linked to exposure to finches, pigeons, pheasants, ducks, turkeys, chickens, seagulls, and other birds, ornithosis may be a more appropriate term. Psittacosis disease in birds ranges from an asymptomatic carriage state to a

mild symptomatic illness manifested by ruffled feathers, anorexia, shivering, dyspnea, diarrhea, or depression. Infected birds shed *C. psittaci* in urine, feces, or secretions from their beaks or eyes. Their feathers and surrounding environment become contaminated. Transmission to humans is primarily by inhalation of aerosolized bird secretions or dust. Infected birds may shed the organism for months. Person-to-person transmission rarely occurs.

Human psittacosis is a rare infection, due in part to antibiotic-laced bird feed and a mandated quarantine for imported birds. The number of cases of psittacosis in the United States has been stable for the past 10 years, with fewer than 50 confirmed cases reported annually; a larger number of cases are reported but not confirmed. An outbreak of psittacosis occurred in 2014 in New South Wales from a novel source, exposure to abnormal equine fetal membranes. This suggests that horse exposure may be a potential risk factor for psittacosis and highlights the potential for humans to acquire the infection from other infected mammalian hosts.

CLINICAL MANIFESTATIONS

Psittacosis initially involves the lungs and then spreads to the reticuloendothelial system. The clinical spectrum of infection ranges from asymptomatic to fulminant, and clinical manifestations may resemble several other nonspecific febrile systemic illnesses, including Q fever, typhoid fever, and legionnaires disease.[18] After an incubation period of 5 to 14 days, some patients may present with a nonspecific virus-like illness or a mononucleosis-like syndrome. The presentation most suggestive of psittacosis is an acute febrile atypical pneumonia.[19] Patients initially have an abrupt onset of shaking chills and a temperature as high as 40.5° C. Temperature-pulse dissociation (i.e., elevated temperature with a normal pulse) may occur. Constitutional symptoms, including headache, myalgias, and arthralgias, are prominent. A cough, usually nonproductive, appears early in the illness and may accompany chest pain, which is usually nonpleuritic. Auscultation may be normal or reveal bilateral crackles. Chest radiograph findings are usually more dramatic than lung examination findings; the most common finding is single lower lobe consolidation, but multiple localized bronchopneumonic patches, diffuse ground-glass changes, and a miliary pattern have been described. Small pleural effusions may be seen. In contrast to *C. pneumoniae* pneumonia, psittacosis is more severe, with high fever and absent or minimal upper respiratory complaints.

Extrapulmonary findings frequently occur in psittacosis. Splenomegaly is common. A faint erythematous, blanching, maculopapular rash (Horder spots), resembling the rose spots of typhoid fever, can occur, as can erythema nodosum. Signs of hepatitis, endocarditis (culture negative), pericarditis, myocarditis, meningoencephalitis, hemolytic anemia, or disseminated intravascular coagulation may be noted. *C. psittaci* infection has also been associated with nongastrointestinal extranodal marginal zone lymphomas of mucosa-associated lymphoid tissue, including ocular and central nervous system sites.

DIAGNOSIS

Psittacosis should be suspected in patients with a febrile illness (especially atypical pneumonia) who report exposure to sick or imported birds or who have regular exposure to birds, including bird owners, pet shop workers, veterinarians, zookeepers, and poultry processing plant workers. The diagnosis can be made with serology or by isolating the organism in cell culture. *C. psittaci* is a biocontainment level 3 agent because of its stability in the environment and aerosol transmission. Because laboratory-acquired *C. psittaci* infections are well documented, culture is discouraged and serology is preferred. If culture is attempted, laboratory staff should be notified in advance so that appropriate precautions can be taken. A serologic diagnosis of psittacosis is made by demonstrating (1) a four-fold or greater rise in CF or MIF antibody against *C. psittaci* to a titer of at least 1 : 32 from acute to convalescent sera collected at least 2 weeks apart (3 to 6 weeks is recommended) or (2) an IgM titer of 1 : 16 or greater against *C. psittaci* by MIF.

TREATMENT Rx

Untreated psittacosis can be fatal, but mortality is rare with prompt antimicrobial treatment. Because of the delay in laboratory diagnosis of psittacosis, empirical therapy should be provided on the basis of clinical suspicion. *C. psittaci* susceptibility has been demonstrated to tetracyclines, macrolides, and newer generation fluoroquinolones. The recommended treatment regimen, based on clinical experience, is either tetracycline 500 mg four times a day or doxycycline 100 mg twice a day for 10 to 21 days. Further studies on the clinical efficacy of azithromycin and fluoroquinolones are needed. The initial treatment response can be dramatic, with defervescence and marked clinical improvement within 24 to 48 hours. Full recovery may take several weeks, and relapse or reinfection can occur. Endocarditis treatment includes prolonged antibiotic therapy and consideration of valve replacement.

PREVENTION

Epidemic psittacosis is preventable by a 30-day period of quarantine for all imported psittacine birds and their treatment with feed containing chlortetracycline. The U.S. Department of Agriculture recommends extending treatment for an additional 15 days after quarantine. Prevention of epidemic and endemic psittacosis also relies on avoidance of or protection from exposure to dust or body secretions from birds or their living areas as well as avoidance of the handling of sick birds. Environmental sanitation is another important preventive measure, considering the organism's resistance to drying.

Grade A References

A1. Evans JR, Solomon AW. Antibiotics for trachoma. *Cochrane Database Syst Rev.* 2011;3:CD001860.
A2. Páez-Canro C, Alzate JP, Gonzalez LM, et al. Antibiotics for treating urogenital *Chlamydia trachomatis* infection in men and non-pregnant women. *Cochrane Database Syst Rev.* 2019;1:CD010871.
A3. Geisler WM, Uniyal A, Lee JY, et al. Azithromycin versus doxycycline for urogenital *Chlamydia trachomatis* infection. *N Engl J Med.* 2015;373:2512-2521.

GENERAL REFERENCES

For the General References and other additional features, please visit Expert Consult at https://expertconsult.inkling.com.

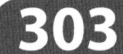

SYPHILIS

KHALIL G. GHANEM AND EDWARD W. HOOK, III

DEFINITION

Syphilis, which is a chronic infectious disease caused by the bacterium *Treponema pallidum* subspecies *pallidum*, is usually acquired by sexual contact with another infected individual. Syphilis is remarkable among infectious diseases for its large variety of clinical manifestations. If untreated, it progresses through primary, secondary, and tertiary stages. The early stages (i.e., primary and secondary), when lesions are present, are infectious. Spontaneous healing of early lesions occurs, followed by a long latent period. In about 30% of untreated patients, late disease of the heart, central nervous system (CNS), or other organs may develop years after the initial infection. Although the disease is less common now than previously, it remains a challenge to clinicians because of its protean manifestations, and it is of interest to biologists because of the prolonged, tenuous balance between the host and the invading spirochete.[1]

The Pathogen

The causative agent of syphilis, *T. pallidum* subspecies *pallidum*, is closely related to other pathogenic spirochetes (Chapter 304), including those causing yaws (*T. pallidum* subspecies *pertenue*) and pinta (*Treponema carateum*). *T. pallidum* is a thin, helical bacterium approximately 0.15 μm wide and 6 to 15 μm long. The organism has 6 to 14 spirals and is tapered on either end. It is too thin to be seen by ordinary Gram stain microscopy but can be visualized in wet mounts by dark-field microscopy or in fixed specimens by silver stain or fluorescent antibody methods.

Unlike most bacteria, which have protein-rich outer membranes, the *T. pallidum* outer membrane appears to be composed of predominantly phospholipids, with few surface-exposed proteins.[2] It has been hypothesized that because of this structure, syphilis can progress despite the brisk antibody response to non–surface-exposed internal antigens, which is the basis for serologic tests for the diagnosis and management of syphilis. Between the outer membrane and the peptidoglycan cell wall are six axial fibrils; three are attached at each end, and they overlap in the center of the organism. They are

structurally and biochemically similar to flagella and are in part responsible for the organism's motility.

It is possible to culture *T. pallidum*, but sustained *in vitro* cultivation is limited, and yields are very low. Culture is of no use in clinical practice. All isolates studied have been susceptible to penicillin and are antigenically similar. The only known natural hosts for *T. pallidum* are humans and certain monkeys and higher apes.

EPIDEMIOLOGY

With the exception of congenital syphilis, syphilis is acquired almost exclusively by intimate contact with the infectious lesions of primary or secondary syphilis (e.g., chancres, mucous patches, condylomata lata). Disease is usually acquired through sexual intercourse, including anogenital and orogenital intercourse. Health care workers are sometimes unexpectedly infected during examination of patients with infectious lesions. Infection by contact with fomites is extremely uncommon. Before the advent of modern blood banking techniques, syphilis was occasionally transmitted through the transfusion of blood from persons with *T. pallidum* bacteremia, and occasional parenteral transmission still occurs as a result of the sharing of contaminated needles.

Syphilis is most common in large cities among sexually active individuals. The highest rate is found in men between the ages of 20 and 29 years. In the United States, it is most prevalent in the West and in the South.[3]

Syphilis spares no class, race, or group. U.S. syphilis rates are about five-fold greater in African Americans than in non-Hispanic whites. In 2017, more than 85% of reported early syphilis occurred in men, and nearly 60% of total early cases occurred among men who acknowledged sex with other men. A traditional cornerstone of syphilis control has been the epidemiologic investigation and treatment of sexual contacts of patients with primary or secondary lesions and patients with early latent disease. Patients with primary and secondary syphilis name, on average, nearly three different sexual contacts within the previous 90 days. As syphilis has become associated with drug use and anonymous sex, epidemiologic investigations have become less efficacious.

The incidence of syphilis has generally declined worldwide for more than 100 years, with the exception of periods of war or social upheaval. With the introduction of penicillin, there was a rapid decline in primary and secondary syphilis, to approximately 4 cases per 100,000 people in 1957. This decline was followed by reductions in federal expenditures for syphilis control, which resulted in resurgence of infectious primary and secondary syphilis in the United States; peaks of more than 12 cases per 100,000 people were attained several times from 1965 through the mid-1990s.

During the past 40 years, syphilis epidemics have occurred serially in at least three U.S. population subgroups. In the 1970s and 1980s, men who had sex with other men accounted for a disproportionate number of the total cases of infectious syphilis. Similar trends occurred in other countries. Then, after a period of decline, U.S. syphilis rates nearly doubled from 1986 to 1990, with 50,578 cases reported in 1990 in an epidemic disproportionately affecting multiracial heterosexual men and women and occurring contemporaneously with an epidemic of crack cocaine use. After 1990, syphilis rates again declined; in 2001, there were 6103 cases of primary and secondary syphilis reported, one of the lowest numbers since 1959. Since 2001, syphilis rates have again begun to increase in men, and now especially men infected with HIV. Likewise, in the United Kingdom syphilis has been a resurgent sexually transmitted infection that is disproportionately diagnosed in patients with HIV, particularly in men who have sex with men.[4]

In 2017, the rate of reported primary and secondary syphilis in the United States was 9.5 cases per 100,000 population, more than triple the lowest-ever rate of 2.1 in 2000. During 2005 to 2017, primary and secondary syphilis rates increased among men of all ages, races, and ethnicities across all regions. Among women, rates increased during 2005 to 2008 and decreased during 2009 to 2013. From 2013 to 2017, rates among women increased 155.6% with a concomitant increase in cases of congenital syphilis.

Patients with clinically evident late syphilis, particularly those with cardiovascular or gummatous syphilis, are becoming less common, perhaps as a result of the effectiveness of penicillin therapy for early syphilis. However, surveys indicate that there are still significant numbers of patients with untreated neurologic syphilis, especially in older age groups.

Natural Course of Untreated Syphilis

The incubation period from the time of exposure to development of the primary lesion averages approximately 21 days (range, 10 to 90 days). Initially, a painless papule develops at the site of inoculation and soon breaks down to form a clean-based ulcer—the chancre—with raised, indurated margins (Fig. 303-1A).

The chancre persists for 2 to 6 weeks and then heals spontaneously. Several weeks later, a secondary stage characterized by low-grade fever, headache, malaise, generalized lymphadenopathy, and a mucocutaneous rash typically develops. There may be involvement of visceral organs. The secondary eruption may occur while the primary chancre is still healing or up to several months after disappearance of the chancre. Secondary lesions also heal spontaneously within 2 to 6 weeks, and the infection then becomes latent. In more than 20% of patients with untreated latent syphilis, relapsing lesions later develop, similar to those of the secondary stage; rarely, the relapse takes the form of recurrence of the primary chancre. In the era before antibiotics, late, destructive tertiary lesions involving the eyes, the CNS, the heart, and other organs, including the skin, eventually developed in about a third of untreated patients. These lesions may occur a few years to as long as 25 years after infection.

The incidence of late complications of untreated syphilis is currently unknown, but it seems to be less than that seen previously. Cases of gumma are now so rare as to be reportable.

PATHOBIOLOGY

T. pallidum may penetrate through normal mucosal membranes and minor abrasions on epithelial surfaces. The first lesions appear at the site of direct, primary inoculation. The minimal number of treponemes needed to establish infection is not known but may be as low as one. Multiplication of organisms is slow, with a division time in rabbits of approximately 33 hours. The slow growth of treponemes in humans probably accounts in part for the protracted nature of the illness, the relatively long incubation period, and the need for relatively long duration of therapy.

Syphilis is a systemic disease from the onset. Treponemes are capable of specific attachment to host cells, but it is not known whether attachment results in damage to the host cells. Most treponemes are found in the intercellular spaces, but they are occasionally seen within phagocytic cells. However, there is no evidence of prolonged intracellular survival of treponemes. *T. pallidum* is not known to produce toxins.

The primary pathologic lesion of syphilis is a focal endarteritis with an increase in adventitial cells, endothelial proliferation, and the presence of an inflammatory cuff around affected vessels. Lymphocytes, plasma cells, and monocytes predominate in the inflammatory lesion, and polymorphonuclear cells are seen in some cases. The vessel lumen is frequently obliterated. With healing, there is considerable fibrosis. Treponemes may be seen in most early lesions of syphilis and in some of the late lesions, such as the meningoencephalitis of general paresis.

Granulomatous reaction is common in secondary and late syphilis. The granulomas are histologically nonspecific, and cases of syphilis have been incorrectly diagnosed as sarcoidosis or other granulomatous diseases. Human inoculation studies suggest that the pathogenesis of the gumma, which is a granulomatous lesion, involves hypersensitivity to small numbers of virulent treponemes introduced into a previously sensitized host.

Intracutaneous inoculation of partially purified antigens of *T. pallidum* into patients with syphilis in various stages has shown that delayed cellular hypersensitivity develops only late in secondary syphilis but is uniformly present in latent syphilis. There may be temporary hyporesponsiveness of lymphocytes to treponemal antigens in patients with primary and secondary syphilis. It is possible that the waxing and waning of lesions in early syphilis depend on the balance between the development of effective cellular immunity and the suppression of thymus-derived lymphocyte function.

The host responds to infection by producing numerous antibodies; in some instances, circulating immune complexes may be formed as well. For example, nephrotic syndrome has occasionally been recognized in secondary syphilis, and renal biopsy specimens from such patients have shown membranous glomerulonephritis characterized by focal subepithelial basement membrane deposits containing immunoglobulin G, C3, and treponemal antibody.

CLINICAL MANIFESTATIONS
Primary Syphilis

The typical lesion of primary syphilis, the chancre, is a painless, clean-based, indurated ulcer (Fig. 303-1A). The chancre starts as a papule, but then superficial erosion results in ulceration. The borders of the ulcer are raised, firm, and indurated. On occasion, secondary infections change the appearance and cause a painful lesion. Most chancres are single, but multiple ulcers are sometimes seen, particularly when skinfolds are apposed (i.e., kissing chancres). An untreated chancre heals in several weeks and leaves a faint scar. The chancre is usually associated with regional adenopathy, which may be unilateral or bilateral. The regional nodes are movable, discrete, and rubbery. If the chancre

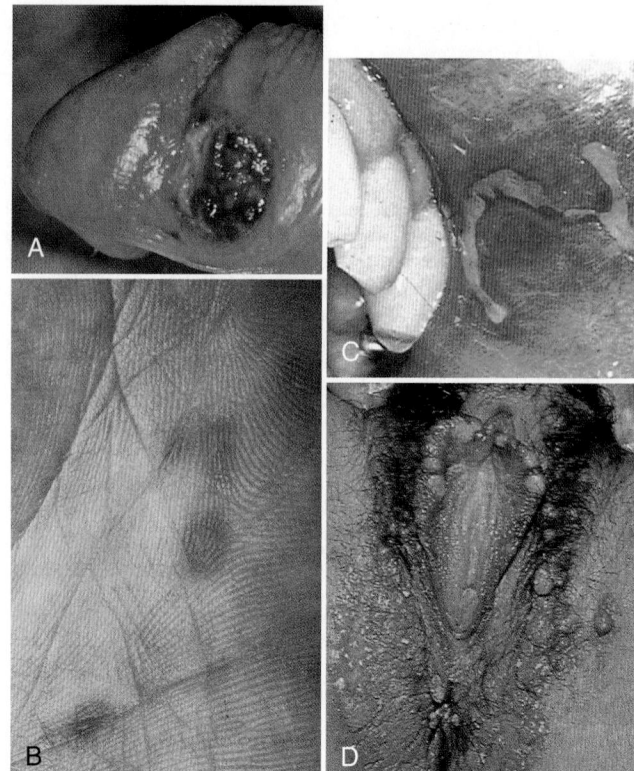

FIGURE 303-1. Syphilis lesions. **A,** Chancre in primary syphilis. **B,** Palmar lesions of a coppery color in secondary syphilis. **C,** Mucous patch in secondary syphilis. **D,** Condylomata lata in secondary syphilis. (**A, C,** and **D** from Forbes CD, Jackson WF. *Color Atlas and Text of Clinical Medicine.* 3rd ed. London: Mosby; 2003. **B** from Habif TP, Cambell JI, Quitadamo MJ, et al. *Skin Disease: Diagnosis and Treatment.* St. Louis: Mosby; 2001.)

occurs in the cervix or the rectum, the affected regional iliac nodes are not palpable.

Chancres can occur at any site of potential inoculation by direct contact, with most occurring in anogenital locations. Chancres may also be seen in the pharynx, on the tongue, around the lips, on the fingers, on the nipples, and in other diverse areas. The morphology depends in part on the area of the body where they occur and on the host's immune response. Chancres in previously infected individuals may be small and remain papular. Chancres of the finger may appear more erosive and can be quite painful. Chancres of the anal canal may be missed in men who have sex with men unless a careful examination is undertaken.

Secondary Syphilis

Between 4 and 8 weeks after the appearance of the primary chancre, signs and symptoms of secondary syphilis typically develop. Symptoms may include malaise, fever, headache, sore throat, and other systemic complaints. Most patients have generalized lymphadenopathy, including involvement of the epitrochlear nodes. Approximately 30% of patients have evidence of a healing chancre, although many patients (including a disproportionate number of women and of men who have sex with men) give no history of a primary lesion.

At least 80% of patients with secondary syphilis have cutaneous or mucocutaneous lesions at some point in their illness. The diagnosis is frequently first suspected on the basis of the cutaneous eruption. The rash is often minimally symptomatic, and many patients with late syphilis do not recall primary or secondary lesions. The rashes are varied in appearance but have certain characteristic features. The lesions are usually widespread, are symmetrical in distribution, and are frequently pink, coppery, or dusky red (particularly the earliest macular lesions). They are generally nonpruritic, although occasional exceptions have been reported, and they are rarely vesicular or bullous in adults. They are indurated, except for the very earliest macular lesions, and frequently have a superficial scale (i.e., papulosquamous lesions). The lesions tend to be polymorphic and rounded, and on healing, they may leave residual pigmentation or depigmentation. They may be faint and difficult to visualize, particularly on dark-skinned individuals.

The earliest pink macular lesions are typically seen on the trunk, with later spread to the rest of the body. The face is often spared, except around the mouth. Subsequently, a papular rash appears that is usually generalized but is marked on the palms and soles (Fig. 303-1B). These rashes are often associated with a superficial scale and may be hyperpigmented. When the rash occurs on the face, it may be pustular and resemble acne vulgaris. On occasion, the scaling may be so prominent that it resembles psoriasis. Ulceration may occur and produce lesions resembling ecthyma. In malnourished or debilitated patients, extensive and destructive ulcerative lesions with a heaped-up crust may occur, the so-called rupial lesions. Lesions around the hair follicles may result in patchy alopecia of the beard or scalp.

Ringed or annular lesions may occur, especially around the face and particularly on dark-skinned individuals. A lesion at the angle of the mouth or the corner of the nose may have a central linear erosion, the so-called split papule.

The palate and pharynx may be inflamed. In approximately 30% of secondary syphilis patients, so-called mucous patches (Fig. 303-1C) develop; these slightly raised, oval areas are covered by a grayish white membrane that, when raised, reveals a pink base that does not bleed. These lesions may be seen on the genitalia, in the mouth, or on the tongue.

In warm, moist areas such as the perineum, large, pale, flat-topped papules may coalesce to form condylomata lata (Fig. 303-1D). Papules may also be seen in the axilla and rarely occur in a generalized form. These papules are not to be confused with the common venereal warts (i.e., condylomata acuminata), which are small, often multiple, and more sharply raised than condylomata lata. Like mucous patches, condylomata lata are highly infectious.

Other manifestations of secondary syphilis include hepatitis, which has been reported in up to 10% of patients in some series. Jaundice is rare, but an elevated alkaline phosphatase level is common. Liver biopsy reveals small areas of focal necrosis and mononuclear infiltrate or periportal vasculitis. Spirochetes can often be visualized with silver stains. Periostitis with widespread lytic lesions of bone has been reported occasionally; bone scanning appears to be a sensitive test for early syphilitic osteitis. An immune complex type of nephropathy with transient nephrotic syndrome has been documented rarely. There may be iritis or an anterior uveitis. Between 10 and 30% of patients have pleocytosis in cerebrospinal fluid (CSF), but symptomatic meningitis is seen in less than 1% of patients. Symptomatic gastritis may occur.

Relapsing Syphilis

After resolution of the primary or secondary skin lesions, 20 to 30% of patients experience cutaneous recurrences. Recurrent lesions may be fewer or more firmly indurated than the initial lesions. Like the typical lesions of primary or secondary syphilis, they are infectious for exposed sexual partners.

Latent Syphilis

By definition, latent syphilis is the stage at which there are no clinical signs of syphilis. Latency, which begins when the first attack of secondary syphilis has passed and may last for a lifetime, is usually detected by reactive serologic tests for syphilis (see Diagnosis). Congenital syphilis must also be excluded before the diagnosis of latent syphilis can be made. Patients may or may not have a clinical history of earlier primary or secondary syphilis manifestations.

Latency has been divided into two stages: early and late. Most infectious relapses occur in the first year, and epidemiologic evidence shows that the most infectious period is during the first year of infection. Early latency is therefore defined as the first year after resolution of the primary or secondary lesions or as a newly reactive serologic test response for syphilis in an otherwise asymptomatic individual who has had a negative serologic test result within the preceding year. Late latent syphilis, or, more accurately, latent syphilis of unknown duration, is ordinarily not infectious, except for pregnant women, who can transmit infection to the fetus despite long-standing infection.

Late Syphilis

Late or tertiary syphilis (Table 303-1) is usually slowly progressive, although certain neurologic syndromes may have a sudden onset because of endarteritis and CNS thrombosis. Late syphilis is not infectious through sexual contact. Any organ of the body may be involved, but three main types of disease can be distinguished: late benign (gummatous), cardiovascular, and neurosyphilis.

Late Benign Syphilis

In the penicillin era, gummas are rare. They typically develop 1 to 10 years after initial infection and may involve any part of the body. Although gummas may be destructive, they respond rapidly to treatment and are therefore relatively benign. On histologic evaluation, the gumma is a granuloma.

TABLE 303-1	NEWLY DIAGNOSED TERTIARY SYPHILIS IN 105 PATIENTS IN DENMARK, 1961-1970
TYPE OF TERTIARY SYPHILIS	**NO. OBSERVED***
Neurosyphilis	72
Asymptomatic	45
Tabes dorsalis	11
General paresis	13
Meningovascular	1
Optic atrophy	2
Cardiovascular syphilis	44
Aortic insufficiency	16
Aortic aneurysm	13
Uncomplicated aortitis[†]	15
Late benign syphilis (gumma)	4

*Some patients had more than one form of late syphilis.
[†]Autopsy diagnoses only.

Gummas may be solitary or multiple and most often come to medical attention as space-occupying lesions. They are usually asymmetrical and are often grouped. Gummas may start as a superficial nodule or as a deeper lesion that breaks down to form punched-out ulcers. They are ordinarily indolent, slowly progressive, and indurated on palpation. Cutaneous gummas may resemble other chronic granulomatous ulcerative lesions caused by tuberculosis, sarcoidosis, leprosy, and other deep fungal infections. Precise histologic diagnosis may not be possible. However, syphilitic gummas are the only such lesions to heal dramatically with penicillin therapy.

Gummas may also involve deep visceral organs, particularly the respiratory tract, gastrointestinal tract, and bones. In addition, they may involve the larynx or the pulmonary parenchyma. Gummas of the stomach may masquerade as carcinoma of the stomach or lymphoma. Gummas of the liver were once the most common form of visceral syphilis and often manifested as hepatosplenomegaly and anemia and occasionally as fever and jaundice. Skeletal gummas typically produce lesions in the long bones, skull, and clavicle; a characteristic symptom is nocturnal pain. Radiologic abnormalities, when present, include periostitis and lytic or sclerotic destructive osteitis.

Cardiovascular Syphilis

The primary cardiovascular complications of syphilis are aortic insufficiency (Chapter 66) and aortic aneurysm (Chapter 69), usually of the ascending aorta. Less commonly, other large arteries may be affected, and involvement of the coronary ostia rarely results in coronary insufficiency. All these complications are caused by obliterative endarteritis of the vasa vasorum, with resultant damage to the intima and media of the great vessels. This damage results in dilation of the ascending aorta, but the valve cusps remain normal. An aneurysm occasionally is manifested as a pulsating mass bulging through the anterior chest wall. Syphilitic aortitis may also involve the descending aorta proximal to the renal arteries.

Cardiovascular syphilis usually begins within 5 to 10 years of the initial infection but may not be manifested clinically until 20 to 30 years later. Cardiovascular syphilis does not occur after congenital infection, a phenomenon that remains unexplained.

Asymptomatic aortitis is best diagnosed by visualizing linear calcifications in the wall of the ascending aorta by radiography. The signs of syphilitic aortic insufficiency are the same as for aortic insufficiency of other causes. In aortic insufficiency resulting from dilation of the aortic ring, the decrescendo murmur is often loudest along the right sternal margin. Syphilitic aneurysms may be fusiform but are more typically saccular and do not lead to aortic dissection. Between 10 and 20% of patients with cardiovascular syphilis have coexistent neurosyphilis.

Neurosyphilis

CNS involvement occurs throughout the natural history of syphilis. Neurosyphilis[5] can be divided into five groups: asymptomatic, syphilitic meningitis, meningovascular syphilis, tabes dorsalis, and general paresis. Asymptomatic neurosyphilis can occur at any time, whereas syphilitic meningitis is most common during the secondary stage of infection. Meningovascular syphilis, tabes dorsalis, and general paresis are typically manifestations of late syphilis. The divisions are not absolute, and overlap between syndromes is typical.

Syphilitic Meningitis

Acute to subacute aseptic meningitis can occur at any time after the primary stage, but it usually occurs within the first year of infection. It frequently involves the base of the brain and may result in unilateral or bilateral cranial nerve palsies. Mild aseptic meningitis may be relatively common in patients with early syphilis, but severe disease occurs in only about 1.5% of untreated patients. Syphilitic meningitis typically resolves without treatment.

Meningovascular Syphilis

Some patients have sufficient endarteritis and perivascular inflammation to result in cerebrovascular thrombosis and infarction, generally 5 to 10 years after the initial infection. However, case reports suggest that in syphilis patients with coexistent HIV infection, meningovascular syphilis may be manifested earlier or may be a manifestation of treatment failure. Patients frequently have associated aseptic meningitis. Most cerebrovascular accidents are not caused by syphilitic arteritis, even in patients with a reactive serologic test result for syphilis. However, syphilis should be considered a potential cause in relatively young patients with a history of syphilis and without other risk factors for cerebrovascular disease.

Tabes Dorsalis

Tabes dorsalis, which appears to be far less common than in the pre-penicillin era, is a slowly progressive, degenerative disease that involves the posterior columns and posterior roots of the spinal cord and results in progressive loss of peripheral reflexes, impairment of vibration and position sense, and progressive ataxia. Sensory changes may lead to chronic destructive changes in the large joints of the affected limbs in advanced cases (i.e., Charcot joints). Urinary incontinence and impotence are common. Sudden and severely painful crises of uncertain origin are a characteristic part of the syndrome. Severe, sharp abdominal pain may lead to exploratory surgery.

Optic atrophy is seen in 20% of cases. In 90% of patients, the pupils are bilaterally small and fail to constrict further in response to light, but they do respond normally to accommodation (i.e., Argyll Robertson pupils).

The onset of tabes dorsalis is usually first noticed 20 to 30 years after the initial infection. Its cause is unclear, and spirochetes cannot be demonstrated in the posterior column or dorsal root.

General Paresis

This form of neurosyphilis is a chronic meningoencephalitis resulting in the gradual and progressive loss of cortical function. It typically occurs 10 to 20 years after the initial infection. On pathologic examination, there is a perivascular and meningeal chronic inflammatory reaction, with thickening of the meninges, granular ependymitis, degeneration of the cortical parenchyma, and abundant spirochetes in tissues.

In its early stages, general paresis results in nonspecific symptoms of early dementia, such as irritability, fatigue, headaches, forgetfulness, and personality changes. Later, there is impaired memory, defective judgment, lack of insight, confusion, and often depression or marked elation. Patients may be delusional, and seizures sometimes occur. There may also be loss of other cortical functions, including paralysis or aphasia.

Physical signs are primarily those of the altered mental status. Cranial nerve palsies are uncommon, and optic atrophy is rare. The complete Argyll Robertson pupil is also uncommon, but irregular or otherwise abnormal pupils are not infrequent. Peripheral reflexes are often somewhat increased.

Ocular and Otic Syphilis

The eyes and ears may be affected during any stage of syphilis. Panuveitis is the most common ocular manifestation reported, but any portion of the eye may be affected.[6] Consequently, the clinical manifestations of ocular syphilis are broad. In half the cases, bilateral ocular involvement is noted. In 70% of cases, concomitant cerebrospinal fluid abnormalities consistent with neurosyphilis are detected. Otosyphilis presents with sudden fluctuating or persistent sensorineural hearing loss or vestibular symptoms. Common complaints, in addition to hearing loss, include tinnitus and vertigo. In half the cases, both ears are affected. Unlike ocular syphilis, over 90% of persons with otosyphilis will have a normal cerebrospinal fluid examination.

Syphilis-HIV Interactions

Syphilis, like other genital ulcer diseases, is associated with a three- to five-fold increased risk for acquisition of HIV infection. Presumably, genital ulcers act as portals of entry through which HIV may more readily infect exposed individuals. As a result, HIV serologic testing 3 months after a diagnosis of syphilis is recommended for all patients. Conversely, in individuals with HIV infection who acquire syphilis, the natural history of the infection may be modified.[7] HIV-infected syphilis patients are somewhat more likely than non–HIV-infected patients to present initially with secondary syphilis. HIV-infected secondary syphilis patients are also more likely than HIV-negative secondary syphilis patients to have coexistent chancres, suggesting that the healing of chancres is delayed or the appearance of secondary manifestations is accelerated in the presence of HIV coinfection. Coinfected patients may be at higher risk of developing neurologic complications, particularly early neurosyphilis.

Congenital Syphilis

Congenital syphilis results from the transplacental, hematogenous spread of syphilis from the mother to the fetus.[8] In 2017, 918 cases of congenital syphilis were reported in the United States with an estimated 660,000 annual cases worldwide.[9] A serologic test for syphilis should be performed in all expectant mothers at the beginning of pregnancy and should be repeated during the third trimester in women living in areas where syphilis is relatively common.[10,11]

The risk for fetal infection is greatest in the early stages of untreated maternal syphilis and declines slowly thereafter, but the untreated mother can infect her fetus during at least the first 5 years of her infection. Adequate treatment of the mother before the 16th week of pregnancy usually prevents clinical illness in the neonate. Later treatment may not prevent late sequelae of the disease in the child. Untreated maternal infection may result in stillbirth, neonatal death, prematurity, or syndromes of early or late congenital syphilis in surviving infants.

Manifestations of early congenital syphilis are often seen in the perinatal period but may not develop until the infant has been discharged from the hospital. The disease resembles secondary syphilis in adults, except that the rash may be vesicular or bullous. The child often has rhinitis, hepatosplenomegaly, hemolytic anemia, jaundice, and pseudoparalysis (i.e., immobility of one or more extremities) as a result of painful osteochondritis.

Late congenital syphilis is defined as congenital syphilis diagnosed more than 2 years after birth. The disease may remain latent, with no manifestations of late damage. Cardiovascular alterations have not been observed in patients with congenital syphilis. Neurologic manifestations are common and may include eighth cranial nerve deafness and interstitial keratitis. Periostitis may result in prominent frontal bones of the skull, depression of the bridge of the nose (saddle nose), poor development of the maxilla, and anterior bowing of the tibia (saber shins). There may be late-onset arthritis of the knees (Clutton joints). The permanent dentition may show characteristic abnormalities known as Hutchinson teeth; the upper central incisors are widely spaced, centrally notched, and tapered in the manner of a screwdriver. The molars may show multiple poorly developed cusps (mulberry molars).

DIAGNOSIS

Dark-Field Examination

The most definitive means of syphilis diagnosis is finding typical spirochetes in lesions of early acquired or congenital syphilis. Dark-field examination is often positive in cases of primary syphilis and in patients with the moist mucosal lesions of secondary and congenital syphilis. The result may occasionally be positive for aspirates of lymph nodes in secondary syphilis. False-negative results may occur in primary syphilis because of the application of soaps, antiseptics, or other compounds toxic to *T. pallidum* to the lesions. A single negative result is therefore insufficient to exclude syphilis. For high-risk individuals (e.g., drug users, men who have sex with men), it is appropriate to treat presumptively on the basis of suspicious lesions after performing serologic tests. Confusion may also arise because of the presence of spirochetes that are morphologically indistinguishable from *T. pallidum* organisms in the mouth, particularly around the gingival margins. Living *T. pallidum* organisms demonstrate gradual motion to and fro, rotational movement around the long axis, and rather sudden 90-degree flexing near the center of the organism.

Serologic Tests

Two basic types of serologic tests (Table 303-2) are widely used to diagnose infection with *T. pallidum:* (1) nontreponemal tests that detect antibodies reactive with diphosphatidylglycerol (cardiolipin), which is a normal component of many tissues; and (2) tests that detect antibodies to specific treponemal antigens.

Nontreponemal Tests

The standard tests to detect anticardiolipin antibody are the rapid plasma reagin (RPR) and Venereal Disease Research Laboratory (VDRL) tests, which

TABLE 303-2	SEROLOGIC TESTS FOR SYPHILIS
TYPE	**USE**
NONTREPONEMAL (ANTICARDIOLIPIN) ANTIBODIES	
VDRL (slide flocculation)	Screening, quantitation of response to treatment
RPR (circle card) (agglutination)	Screening, quantitation of response to treatment
SPECIFIC TREPONEMAL ANTIBODIES	
FTA-ABS (immunofluorescence with absorbed serum)	Confirmatory, diagnostic; not for routine screening
TP-PA (microhemagglutination)	Similar to FTA-ABS but can be quantified and automated
EIA and CIA	Confirmatory and increasingly used for screening; automated

EIA = enzyme immunoassay; CIA= chemiluminescence immunoassay; FTA-ABS = fluorescent treponemal antibody absorption test; RPR = rapid plasma regain test; TP-PA = *Treponema pallidum* particle agglutination; VDRL = Venereal Disease Research Laboratory.

TABLE 303-3	FREQUENCY OF POSITIVE SEROLOGIC TEST RESULTS IN UNTREATED SYPHILIS		
STAGE	**VDRL (%)**	**FTA-ABS (%)**	**TP-PA (%)**
Primary	70	85	50-60
Secondary	99	100	100
Latent or late	70	98	98

FTA-ABS = fluorescent treponemal antibody absorption test; TP-PA = *Treponema pallidum* particle agglutination; VDRL = Venereal Disease Research Laboratory.

are slide flocculation tests. The RPR and VDRL are readily quantified, so they are the tests of choice for monitoring patients' responses to treatment. The relative proportion of patients with a false-positive RPR result depends on the prevalence of syphilis in the community; the lower the prevalence of syphilis, the higher the proportion of reactive RPR test results from nonsyphilitic causes.

The RPR test result begins to turn positive less than 1 week after onset of the chancre; thus, a nonreactive RPR test result does not exclude primary syphilis, particularly if the lesion is less than 1 week old. The RPR test result is positive in 99% of patients with secondary syphilis (Table 303-3). Patients with advanced HIV infection may have negative test results, and some patients have such high titers of antibody that they are in antibody excess; dilution of their serum paradoxically results in conversion of a negative test result to a positive one, the so-called prozone reaction. RPR reactivity tends to diminish in later stages of syphilis, and only about 70% of patients with cardiovascular syphilis or late neurosyphilis have positive RPR test results.

The *quantitative titer* of the RPR or VDRL test is somewhat useful in diagnosis and is quite useful for monitoring of the therapeutic response. Most patients with secondary syphilis have titers of at least 1 : 16. Most patients with false-positive RPR test results have titers of less than 1 : 8. No single titer is diagnostic by itself. Significant rises (four-fold or greater) in paired sera, however, strongly indicate acute syphilis.

Treponemal Tests

Several types of treponemal tests are widely used. Treponemal enzyme immunoassays (EIAs) and chemiluminescence immunoassays (CIAs) using cloned treponemal antigens for treponemal antibody detection have become available from several manufacturers and have gained favor because of their low cost and ease of use. In addition to EIA and CIA tests, agglutination of particles to which *T. pallidum* antigens have been fixed is the basis of the widely used *T. pallidum* particle agglutination (TP-PA) test. The fluorescent treponemal antibody absorption (FTA-ABS) test has been widely used as well and is reported in terms of relative brilliance of fluorescence, from borderline to 4 plus; most laboratories report only test results with 2 plus or greater reactivity as positive. For patients lacking historical or clinical evidence of syphilis but with a reactive FTA-ABS test result, the test should be repeated. Use of another treponemal test may be helpful in problem cases. The TP-PA test is slightly

less sensitive than the RPR or FTA-ABS test in primary syphilis. Its sensitivity and specificity are otherwise nearly identical to those of the FTA-ABS test.

Because EIA and CIA serologic tests permit the screening of large numbers of sera and have performance characteristics (sensitivity, specificity, predictive values) similar to those of other treponemal tests, they have been increasingly used for syphilis screening. Persons with reactive treponemal antigen EIAs or CIAs should be tested with a quantitative nontreponemal test, such as the RPR or VDRL test, for confirmation and to permit the use of that test to evaluate the subsequent response to therapy. It is not unusual for patients to have a reactive EIA or CIA test result for syphilis and a nonreactive RPR or VDRL test result. A substantial proportion of these EIA or CIA-only positive test results are falsely positive or are detecting long-standing, often previously treated syphilis, but occasionally they may detect very recent infection before RPR or VDRL test results become positive.

When nontreponemal tests such as the RPR and VDRL are used for screening, treponemal tests are used to confirm that persons with reactive nontreponemal test results have antibodies to *T. pallidum*. Results of treponemal tests are not reliably quantified. They are sensitive and have a high degree of specificity, in that only approximately 1% of normal individuals have reactive treponemal test results. They are reactive in 85% of patients with primary syphilis, 99% with secondary syphilis, and at least 95% with late syphilis. They may therefore be the only test with a positive result in patients with cardiovascular or neurologic syphilis. For patients with late syphilis, treponemal test results often remain reactive for life, despite adequate therapy.

Point of care serologic tests for syphilis are currently available. These tests can detect treponemal antibodies, nontreponemal antibodies, or both. The performance characteristics vary, but in general, they are reasonably good.[12]

Differential Diagnosis

The differential diagnosis of a genital ulcer (Chapter 269) includes genital herpes (Chapter 350), chancroid (Chapter 285), lymphogranuloma venereum (Chapter 302), and a number of other ulcerative processes. Classically, herpetic ulcers are multiple, painful, superficial, and, if seen early, vesicular. However, atypical manifestations may be indistinguishable from a syphilitic chancre. Genital herpes is much more common than syphilis and is now the most common cause of a "typical chancre" in North America. Syphilitic chancres may also be coinfected with herpes simplex virus in about 15% of cases. The ulcers of chancroid are usually painful, often multiple, and frequently exudative and noninjured. Lymphogranuloma venereum may produce a small, papular lesion associated with regional adenopathy. Other conditions that must be distinguished include granuloma inguinale (Chapter 300), drug eruptions, carcinoma, superficial fungal infections (Chapter 409), traumatic lesions, and lichen planus (Chapter 409). In most cases, the final distinction is based on dark-field examination, which is positive only in syphilis, and on serologic test results.

The differential diagnosis of the skin lesions of secondary syphilis includes pityriasis rosea (Chapter 409), which can be differentiated by the occurrence of lesions along lines of skin cleavage and frequently by the presence of a herald patch. Drug eruptions, acute febrile exanthems, psoriasis, lichen planus, scabies, and other diseases must also be considered in some cases. A mucous patch may superficially resemble oral candidiasis (i.e., thrush). Infectious mononucleosis (Chapter 353) may appear similar to secondary syphilis, with sore throat, generalized adenopathy, hepatitis, and a generalized rash. Hepatitis (Chapter 139) may also cause confusion.

False-Positive Serologic Test Results for Syphilis

The RPR or VDRL test result is reactive in patients with other treponemal diseases, such as pinta, yaws, and endemic syphilis (Chapter 304). These test results may also be falsely reactive in persons who do not have treponemal infections based on a negative clinical history or negative results of serum treponemal tests.

The origins of false-positive results are better studied for nontreponemal tests than for treponemal tests. Acute (<6 months) false-positive RPR test results occur with low frequency in patients with atypical pneumonia, malaria, and other bacterial or viral infections, and they may occur after smallpox or other vaccinations as well. Chronic false-positive RPR test results (persisting >6 months) are relatively common in patients with autoimmune disorders such as systemic lupus erythematosus (Chapter 250), parenteral drug users, HIV-infected patients, patients with leprosy, and the aged. Between 8 and 20% of patients with systemic lupus erythematosus have false-positive RPR test results. Chronic false-positive RPR test results in female patients 20 years or younger indicate a significant risk for the future development of systemic

TABLE 303-4 PENICILLIN TREATMENT FOR SYPHILIS AS RECOMMENDED BY THE U.S. PUBLIC HEALTH SERVICE

INDICATIONS FOR SYPHILIS THERAPY*	DOSAGE AND ADMINISTRATION†	
	BENZATHINE PENICILLIN G	AQUEOUS BENZYLPENICILLIN G OR PROCAINE PENICILLIN G
Primary, secondary, and early latent syphilis (<1 year); epidemiologic treatment	Total of 2.4 million units; single IM dose of two injections of 1.2 million units in one session	Total of 4.8 million units IM in doses of 600,000 units/day for 8 consecutive days
Late latent (>1 year); cardiovascular syphilis, late benign (cutaneous, osseous, visceral gumma)	Total of 7.2 million units IM in doses of 2.4 million units at 7-day intervals during a 21-day period	Total of 9 million units IM in doses of 600,000 units/day during a 15-day period
Symptomatic or asymptomatic neurosyphilis	2-4 million units aqueous (crystalline) penicillin G IV q4h for at least 10 days	2-4 million units procaine penicillin IM daily and probenecid 500 mg orally four times daily, for 10-14 days
Congenital Infants	CSF normal: total of 50,000 units/kg IM in a single or divided dose at one session	CSF abnormal: total of 50,000 units/kg/day IM for 10 consecutive days‡
Older children	CSF normal: same as for early congenital syphilis, up to 2.4 million units	CSF abnormal: 200,000-300,000 units/kg/day aqueous crystalline penicillin IV for 10-14 days

CSF = cerebrospinal fluid.
*In pregnancy, treatment depends on the stage of syphilis.
†Individual doses can be divided for injection in each buttock to minimize discomfort.
‡For aqueous penicillin, give in two divided intravenous doses per day; for procaine penicillin, give as one daily dose intramuscularly.
Data from Workowski KA, Bolan GA. Sexually transmitted diseases treatment guidelines, 2015. *MMWR Recomm Rep.* 2015;64:1-137.

lupus erythematosus, thyroiditis, or other autoimmune disorders. As many as a third of parenteral drug users have false-positive RPR test results. More than 1% of persons 70 years old and 10% of those older than 80 years also have low-titer, false-positive RPR test results. In most cases of false-positive RPR test results, the titer is less than 1 : 8, although a few patients with lymphoma and other diseases have very high-titer, false-positive results.

Neurosyphilis

Asymptomatic neurosyphilis is diagnosed when there are CSF abnormalities, such as lymphocytic pleocytosis, protein elevation, or a reactive VDRL test result, in a syphilis patient in the absence of signs and symptoms of neurologic disease. Unlike serologic tests, the VDRL and RPR tests do not perform equally for CSF, and only the VDRL is recommended. Although numerous other processes can cause CSF pleocytosis or protein elevations, false-positive CSF VDRL test results are rare in the absence of a traumatic tap. If the CSF is normal 2 years or longer after the initial infection, a positive CSF finding is not likely to develop later. Routine lumbar punctures to examine CSF are not indicated in neurologically asymptomatic, immunocompetent patients with early syphilis. Lumbar puncture in HIV-infected persons with early syphilis is the subject of controversy.[13] Although HIV-infected persons, particularly those with a CD4 count less than 350 cells/μL or an RPR titer more than or equal to 1 : 32, may be more likely to have cerebrospinal fluid abnormalities consistent with neurosyphilis, there is no evidence that lumbar punctures in these asymptomatic patients leads to improved clinical outcomes. Although a nonreactive CSF FTA-ABS result may be useful to rule out the diagnosis, no diagnosis of neurosyphilis should be based solely on the CSF FTA-ABS test.

In syphilitic meningitis, the CSF shows a lymphocytic pleocytosis, with increased protein and usually normal glucose concentrations. The CSF VDRL test is often reactive. Rarely, the CSF glucose concentration is decreased. Without treatment, syphilitic meningitis generally resolves, similar to the course of other manifestations of early syphilis. This syndrome can mimic tuberculous or fungal meningitis or nonpurulent meningitis of various causes.

In tabes dorsalis, the VDRL test for serum is nonreactive in as many as 30 to 40% of patients, and 10 to 20% of patients (even before the advent of penicillin) have normal CSF VDRL results. The FTA-ABS test for serum is nearly always reactive. In general paresis, the CSF is nearly always abnormal, with lymphocytic pleocytosis and an increased total protein concentration. The VDRL test is usually reactive for CSF and serum.

Congenital Syphilis

Because many infants with congenital syphilis may be clinically normal at birth but develop serious, symptomatic disease some weeks later, it is important to determine whether a newborn with a reactive serologic test result for syphilis has passively transferred maternal antibody or is actively infected. If the mother has been adequately treated for syphilis during pregnancy and the infant is clinically normal at birth, one option is to monitor the infant carefully by serial examinations and RPR titers. If the reactive RPR result for the infant is caused by passively transferred maternal antibody, the titer will fall markedly in the first 2 months of life; a rising titer indicates active disease and the need for treatment. However, the risk of improper follow-up of RPR-positive but clinically normal neonates makes the immediate empirical administration of effective therapy an attractive alternative.

TREATMENT

T. pallidum is inhibited by less than 0.01 μg/mL of penicillin G. Because treponemes divide slowly and penicillin acts only on dividing cells, it is necessary to maintain serum levels of penicillin for many days (Table 303-4).[14]

Early Infectious Syphilis

Early syphilis (<1 year) can be treated with a single injection of 2.4 million units of benzathine penicillin G, which provides low but effective serum levels for about 2 weeks and cures approximately 95% of patients. It is not necessary to examine CSF at this stage because penicillin prevents the later development of neurosyphilis.

Individuals with other sexually transmitted diseases may have been exposed to syphilis at the time they became infected. Treatment with a single dose of β-lactam antibiotics (penicillins, cephalosporins), which provide relatively high serum levels for a brief period, is ineffective in established early syphilis but is curative if the disease is still in the incubating stage. The ceftriaxone regimen used for gonorrhea (Chapter 283) is probably curative for incubating syphilis, but careful follow-up is indicated if there is reason to suspect exposure to syphilis in a patient treated for gonorrhea with ceftriaxone. A multicenter, randomized trial in China showed that ceftriaxone (1.0 g intravenously once daily for 10 days) was noninferior to benzathine penicillin G (2.4 million units, intramuscularly, once weekly for 2 weeks) in nonpregnant, immunocompetent patients with early syphilis.[A1] Single-dose therapy with 2.0 g of azithromycin administered orally was as effective as benzathine penicillin therapy in several studies of early syphilis, but treatment failures have been reported in persons with coexistent HIV infection. Currently, azithromycin should not be used for the treatment of early syphilis unless close follow-up can be ensured. By comparison, the combination of oral amoxicillin 3 g plus probenecid is highly effective and tolerable for the treatment of syphilis in patients with HIV infection.[15]

For patients allergic to penicillin, 100 mg of doxycycline orally twice daily for 14 days is recommended. Particularly careful follow-up is necessary for patients treated with drugs other than penicillin because they may not be fully compliant with these prolonged courses of oral therapy and these regimens have been less fully evaluated clinically. Ceftriaxone, given in doses of 500 mg to 1.0 g intramuscularly daily for 10 days, may be effective but has been studied only in small numbers of patients with syphilis. Quinolone antibiotics have essentially no effect on syphilis.

Syphilis of More than 1 Year in Duration

Prolonged therapy with intramuscular injections of 2.4 million units of benzathine penicillin G weekly for 3 weeks is recommended for the treatment of late latent syphilis and latent syphilis of unknown duration. Limited evidence suggests that treatment of latent syphilis with a total dose of 7.2 million units of benzathine penicillin during a 3-week period is curative, even if the patient has asymptomatic neurosyphilis.

Although there is no evidence that therapy with antimicrobial drugs is clinically beneficial in patients with cardiovascular syphilis, treatment is recommended to prevent further progression of disease and because approximately 15% of patients with cardiovascular syphilis have associated neurosyphilis. If patients are allergic to penicillin, it is mandatory that the CSF be examined before therapy is undertaken; if the CSF is abnormal, desensitization to penicillin is generally recommended. With a normal CSF, tetracycline (500 mg orally four times a day) or doxycycline (100 mg orally two times a day) taken for 4 weeks is probably effective.

Neurosyphilis, Ocular Syphilis, and Otosyphilis

Larger doses of penicillin are recommended for persons with proven neurosyphilis (see Table 303-4). General paresis responds well to penicillin therapy if it is administered early, although progressive neurologic decline may develop later in as many as a third of treated patients. Carbamazepine in doses of 400 to 800 mg/day reportedly treats the lightning pains of tabes dorsalis effectively. While published studies show that a total of 6.0 to 9.0 million units of penicillin G results in a satisfactory clinical response in approximately 90% of patients with neurosyphilis who do not have HIV infection, current guidelines recommend higher doses of penicillin (up to 24 million units of intravenous penicillin G per day for at least 10 days) in all patients with neurosyphilis, ocular syphilis, and otosyphilis. Therapy for neurosyphilis can result in increased CSF pleocytosis for 7 to 10 days after treatment is started and may transiently convert a normal CSF to abnormal.

Syphilis in Pregnancy

Because of the risk to the fetus, evaluation and treatment of a pregnant RPR-positive patient must be rapid, particularly for those patients first seen in the later stages of pregnancy. If a confirmatory treponemal test result is positive and the patient has not been treated, penicillin should be administered in doses appropriate for early or late syphilis, as outlined earlier. For penicillin-allergic patients, penicillin desensitization is preferred; patients should not be treated with tetracycline or erythromycin because of toxicity (tetracycline) or lack of efficacy (erythromycin). For patients who are RPR positive but treponemal test negative and have no clinical signs of syphilis, treatment may be withheld; a quantitative RPR test and another treponemal test should be repeated in 4 weeks. If the treponemal titer has risen four-fold or more, or if clinical signs of syphilis have developed, the patient should be treated. If, after repeated examination, the diagnosis remains equivocal, the patient should be treated to prevent possible disease in the neonate. After treatment, a quantitative RPR titer should be monitored monthly; if it rises four-fold, the patient should be treated a second time.

Congenital Syphilis

Proper treatment of the mother usually prevents active congenital syphilis in the neonate. However, infected infants may be clinically normal at birth, and the infant may be seronegative if the mother's infection was acquired late in pregnancy. The infant should be treated at birth if the mother has received no treatment or inadequate treatment or has been treated with drugs other than penicillin, if the mother has not yet responded to possibly effective therapy, or if the infant cannot be carefully monitored for several months after birth. The infant's CSF should be examined before treatment. If the CSF is normal, the child can be treated with a single intramuscular injection of 50,000 units/kg (up to 2.4 million units) of benzathine penicillin G. If the CSF is abnormal, the infant should be treated with 50,000 units/kg of aqueous penicillin G given intramuscularly or intravenously twice daily for a minimum of 10 days. Alternatively, a single daily intramuscular injection of 50,000 units/kg of procaine penicillin may be given for 10 days. Antimicrobial agents other than penicillin are not recommended for treatment of congenital syphilis.

Jarisch-Herxheimer Reactions

Up to 60% of patients with early syphilis and a significant proportion of patients with later stages of syphilis experience a transient febrile reaction after therapy for syphilis. The pathogenesis is unclear, but it may be caused by the liberation of antigens from spirochetes.

This reaction usually occurs in the first few hours after therapy, peaks at 6 to 8 hours, and disappears within 12 to 24 hours of therapy. On occasion, Jarisch-Herxheimer reactions are mistaken for allergic reactions to syphilis therapy. Temperature elevation is usually low grade, and there is often associated myalgia, headache, and malaise. The skin lesions of secondary syphilis are frequently exacerbated during the Jarisch-Herxheimer reaction, and cutaneous lesions that were not visible may become visible. The reaction is generally of no clinical significance and in most cases can be treated with salicylates. Corticosteroids have been used to prevent adverse effects of the Jarisch-Herxheimer reaction, but there is no evidence that they are clinically beneficial (other than reducing fever) or necessary. Institution of treatment with small doses of penicillin does not prevent the reaction.

SCREENING AND PREVENTION

HIV-positive men or men who have sex with men should be screened for syphilis, some perhaps as often as every 3 months.[16] Screening is also recommended for other high-risk individuals, such as persons with previous syphilis infection, an infected sexual partner, or more than four sex partners in the preceding year.[17]

All patients with syphilis should be reported to public health authorities. In the absence of an effective vaccine, control of syphilis depends on finding and treating persons with infectious lesions of primary and secondary syphilis before they can transmit the disease as well as finding and treating individuals with incubating syphilis before infectious lesions develop. All patients with early syphilis (primary, secondary, or early latent) should be carefully interviewed by qualified persons to determine the nature of their recent sexual contacts. Approximately 16% of the named recent contacts of patients with early syphilis are found to have active, untreated syphilis on examination.

Treatment of the sexual contacts of patients with early syphilis with 2.4 million units of benzathine penicillin G intramuscularly is recommended even if the contacts are clinically and serologically normal on examination. This is because syphilis eventually develops in 30% of clinically normal contacts who are untreated. In general, preventive treatment is given to all sexual contacts in the past 90 days, although nearly all cases of syphilis in contacts develop within 60 days of exposure.

Roughly 1 million pregnant women are estimated to be infected with syphilis worldwide. Antenatal screening and treatment with a single dose of benzathine benzylpenicillin cures both maternal and congenital syphilis. Preventive strategies to eliminate mother-to-child transmission of syphilis are under study.[18]

PROGNOSIS
Follow-up Examinations

All HIV-seronegative patients with early or congenital syphilis should return for quantitative VDRL titers and clinical examination 6 and 12 months after treatment. For HIV-positive patients, serologic tests should be repeated at 3, 6, 9, and 12 months. Patients with late latent syphilis should also be examined 24 months after therapy.

In about 80 to 85% of patients with early (i.e., primary, secondary, or early latent) syphilis, quantitative RPR titers decline two or more dilutions (four-fold) by 6 and 12 months after therapy. In serofast patients (i.e., those whose titers do not decline appropriately), prolonged reactive RPR test results are associated with older age, lower initial RPR titers, prolonged infection, or more advanced stage (primary < secondary < early latent) infection. Re-treatment of patients with serofast RPR results at 6 months leads to serologic response to syphilis in a minority of patients. Chronic, low-titer RPR reactivity after therapy is much more common in cases of late syphilis and should not be viewed with alarm. Treponemal test results may remain positive for years despite adequate therapy. A four-fold or greater rise in RPR titer after therapy is sufficient evidence for repeated treatment. Patients with treated early syphilis are susceptible to reinfection, and many clinical and serologic relapses after therapy are probably reinfections.

Patients with neurosyphilis should be monitored with serologic tests for at least 3 years and with repeated CSF examinations at 6-month intervals. CSF pleocytosis is the first abnormality to disappear, but cell counts may not be normal for 1 to 2 years. Elevated CSF protein levels fall even more slowly, followed by a change in the positive CSF VDRL test result, which may take years to become negative. Rising CSF cell counts, protein level, and CSF VDRL titer obtained at follow-up are an indication for repeated treatment. Appropriate declines in serum nontreponemal antibody titers reflect improvement in CSF parameters.

Antibiotic therapy should ultimately cure essentially all patients with early or secondary syphilis, although treatment failures may occur in patients with concomitant HIV infection. In tabes dorsalis, penicillin usually arrests progression but does not reverse the symptoms. Meningovascular syphilis generally responds well, except for residual damage resulting from ischemic infarcts.

 Grade A References

A1. Cao Y, Su X, Wang Q, et al. A multicenter study evaluating ceftriaxone and benzathine penicillin G as treatment agents for early syphilis in Jiangsu, China. *Clin Infect Dis.* 2017;65:1683-1688.

GENERAL REFERENCES

For the General References and other additional features, please visit Expert Consult at https://expertconsult.inkling.com.

304

NONSYPHILITIC TREPONEMATOSES

KHALIL G. GHANEM AND EDWARD W. HOOK, III

DEFINITION

The nonsyphilitic treponematoses—yaws, endemic syphilis (previously known as bejel), and pinta—are the spirochetal diseases caused by *Treponema pallidum* subspecies (yaws and endemic syphilis) or by the closely related organism *Treponema carateum* (pinta). Like syphilis, the nonsyphilitic treponematoses are usually transmitted through direct contact with an infectious cutaneous or mucosal lesion. The natural history of the nonsyphilitic treponematoses also has a number of similarities to that of syphilis (Chapter 303).

The Pathogen

Yaws is caused by *T. pallidum* subspecies *pertenue*, endemic syphilis is caused by *T. pallidum* subspecies *endemicum*, and pinta is caused by *T. carateum*. The *T. pallidum* subspecies causing nonsyphilitic treponematoses are closely related to *T. pallidum* subspecies *pallidum*, which causes venereal syphilis; there is a high degree (more than 99%) of DNA homology, and they share unique pathogen-restricted antigens.[1] Analyses of recently described genetic sequence variations among *T. pallidum* subspecies promise the eventual clarification of pathophysiologic differences among the subspecies as well as answers to the age-old question of the origins of syphilis. Like *T. pallidum*, these treponemes are spirochetal bacteria with helical structures and measure about 0.2 μm in diameter and 10 μm in length. They are visible by dark-field microscopy but cannot be cultivated for prolonged periods in vitro.

EPIDEMIOLOGY

Worldwide, the nonsyphilitic treponematoses are rare. However, rates are increasing (particularly for yaws) in some regions where previous World Health Organization (WHO)–coordinated control programs had dramatically reduced disease prevalence. Yaws is prevalent in moist, humid regions, including rural areas of tropical Africa, the Americas, Southeast Asia, and the Western Pacific. Most cases are concentrated in three countries: Ghana, Papua New Guinea, and the Solomon Islands. The highest incidence occurs in children between 2 and 5 years of age. Endemic syphilis occurs in more arid climates, including Africa, eastern Mediterranean countries, the Arabian peninsula, central Asia, and Australia. Pinta occurs in rural areas of tropical Central and South America and affects mostly older children and adolescents. Humans are the only known carriers of the nonsyphilitic treponematoses, although *T. pallidum* strains associated with genital lesions have been described in African baboons, and serologic evidence of *T. pallidum* infection has been found in macaques.[2] The spirochete enters the skin only after it is broken, such as by a scratch or an insect bite. Transmission is believed to occur by contact of the skin directly or by indirect contamination through hands or fomites; it is facilitated by conditions of poor personal hygiene and crowding.

PATHOBIOLOGY

Primary nodular or ulcerative lesions typically develop at sites of inoculation after an incubation period of several weeks. Untreated primary lesions serve as a source for local spread through scratching or for hematogenous dissemination, which gives rise to a secondary stage of infection characterized by the development of widespread manifestations involving the skin, lymph nodes, and bone or cartilage. Without therapy, the primary and secondary manifestations of infection resolve, and the infection becomes latent, detectable only with serologic testing; however, periodic recurrent secondary manifestations may occur for several years. A proportion of persons with long-standing untreated infection are at risk for late sequelae, which may include bone deformity, destruction of nasal cartilage, or chronic skin changes. Unlike syphilis, the nonsyphilitic treponematoses are primarily diseases of children, are not transmitted across the placenta, and do not invade the central nervous system to cause clinical disease.

CLINICAL MANIFESTATIONS

Yaws, the most common nonsyphilitic treponematosis, produces a skin papule at the inoculation site after an incubation period of 3 to 4 weeks. The most common sites are the legs and buttocks. The papule enlarges, ulcerates, and forms a serous crust from which treponemes can be recovered. Regional lymphadenitis may accompany the papule, which heals spontaneously within 6 months. A generalized secondary rash occurs before or after the initial lesion heals; this rash is also papular and is often covered with brown crusts. Relapsing crops of lesions can occur. Papillomas may result, and the plantar surfaces of the feet are involved with hyperkeratotic lesions. Periostitis of the long bones leads to tenderness, and fever may be present. Relapsing lesions of early yaws may occur during a period of several years and result in chronic ulcerations and destructive gummatous lesions affecting the skin and bones.

Endemic syphilis produces patches on the mucous membranes of the oral cavity and pharynx and can cause split papules at the mucocutaneous junction of the oral angles. Anal, genital, and other intertriginous skin areas can be affected by lesions that resemble secondary syphilis. Regional lymphadenitis is common, and generalized rashes are rare. Healing of these early lesions is followed by latency, manifested as seropositivity, or by late lesions that resemble gummatous tertiary syphilis (Chapter 303). Lesions include nodular skin ulcers, bone deformities, and ulcerative lesions that can perforate the palate.

Pinta starts similarly as a cutaneous papule with regional lymphadenitis, followed by a generalized maculopapular eruption. One to 3 years after healing of the initial lesion, large hyperpigmented brown or blue macules develop; they subsequently lose their pigment and become white. The time required for lesions to pass through these stages varies, so the same patient may have coexisting areas of increased pigment and loss of pigment.

DIAGNOSIS

The clinical differentiation of cutaneous ulcers may be challenging, requiring the integration of epidemiologic features, clinical findings, and supportive but not diagnostic laboratory test results. The skin lesions of the endemic treponematoses may resemble other cutaneous processes, including impetigo (Chapter 410), scabies, cutaneous fungal infections (Chapter 409), and other diseases. By dark-field microscopy, the causative spirochetes from early skin lesions can be observed directly; however, dark-field microscopy is rarely available in settings where nonsyphilitic treponematoses are seen. There is no specific test for any of the nonsyphilitic treponematoses, but serologic tests for syphilis detect cross-reacting antibodies in these diseases. The rapid plasma reagin (RPR) test,[3] the Venereal Disease Research Laboratory (VDRL) test, and the specific treponemal tests give positive results if serum is obtained at least 2 weeks after the lesions initially appear. Point-of-care tests have been recently shown to have adequate performance characteristics for the serologic detection of yaws.

PREVENTION

The prevalence of these diseases was reduced dramatically in the 1950s by mass penicillin treatment campaigns. The WHO campaign reduced worldwide prevalence of yaws, for example, by 95% in the 1950s. These campaigns, however, were not adequate to eradicate the disease, and in recent years, the prevalence of yaws has increased. In 2012, the WHO launched a strategy for yaws eradication by 2020 using azithromycin rather than penicillin as preferred therapy for the infection. Current estimates are that as many as 2.5 million persons are infected worldwide, 75% of whom are younger than 15 years. Whereas penicillin is effective for both treatment and prevention of infection, requirements for cold chain transport, parenteral administration, and allergies sometimes compromise the utility of the drug. Recent studies of the etiology of cutaneous ulcers in children conducted in Papua New Guinea have demonstrated that *Haemophilus ducreyi*, the causative agent of chancroid, causes cutaneous ulcers among children in yaws endemic areas which are difficult to clinically differentiate from those of yaws.[4] Studies demonstrating the efficacy of single-dose oral azithromycin for both infections have simplified and expanded practical intervention strategies. For example, data from Papua New Guinea indicate that mass treatment with azithromycin can reduce the prevalence of active and latent yaws infection in endemic areas.[5]

TREATMENT AND PROGNOSIS ℞

Single-dose, long-acting benzathine penicillin G, 1.2 million units intramuscularly, has been the preferred treatment in patients with early lesions.[6] For patients with late manifestations, this therapy should be repeated twice at approximately 7-day intervals. The early lesions heal rapidly, and most seropositive cases convert to seronegative status. Late destructive lesions take longer to show improvement. A randomized trial demonstrated oral azithromycin, 30 mg/kg up to a maximal dose of 2.0 g, to be as effective as penicillin for yaws therapy, providing the first readily administered, single-dose alternative to penicillin for treatment and prevention of nonsyphilitic treponematoses.[A1] Since yaws and trachoma are co-endemic in several regions, and a lower dose of azithromycin (20 mg/kg) has been used for trachoma elimination, a randomized trial was conducted to compare the efficacy of standard-dose azithromycin (30 mg/kg) with low-dose azithromycin (20 mg/kg) in the treatment of active and latent yaws because the latter regimen could be given for yaws and trachoma simultaneously.[7] Low-dose azithromycin did not meet the prescribed noninferiority margin compared with standard-dose azithromycin in achieving clinical and serologic cure in polymerase chain reaction–confirmed active yaws.[A2] Since the margin was not attained because of a single participant who was a serologic failure, others have concluded that epidemiologic evidence would suggest that both dose regimens seem to be equally effective against yaws infections. Yaws eradication uses a single round of mass erythromycin treatment. However, long-term follow-up has shown that this strategy was not successful in achieving long-term elimination of yaws in high-endemic communities because of recurrent disease, in one case due to a mutation in the genes that confer resistance to azithromycin. Repeated mass treatment might be necessary to eliminate yaws.[8]

Grade A References

A1. Mitja O, Hays R, Ipai A, et al. Single-dose azithromycin versus benzathine benzylpenicillin for treatment of yaws in children in Papua New Guinea: an open-label, non-inferiority, randomized trial. *Lancet.* 2012;379:342-347.

A2. Marks M, Mitja O, Bottomley C, et al. Comparative efficacy of low-dose versus standard-dose azithromycin for patients with yaws: a randomised non-inferiority trial in Ghana and Papua New Guinea. *Lancet Glob Health.* 2018;6:e401-e410.

GENERAL REFERENCES

For the General References and other additional features, please visit Expert Consult at https://expertconsult.inkling.com.

305

LYME DISEASE

GARY P. WORMSER

DEFINITION

Lyme disease (also known as Lyme borreliosis) is a zoonotic infection that is transmitted by certain *Ixodes* tick species and caused by a group of related spirochetes referred to formally as *Borrelia burgdorferi* sensu lato, or more simply as Lyme borrelia.[1,2] Lyme disease was first described in 1977 after an investigation of a cluster of cases of arthritis among children living in the area of Lyme, Connecticut. With more than 300,000 cases estimated to occur annually,[3] it is the most common vector-borne infection in the United States; Lyme disease is also an infection of public health importance in both Europe and Asia. The most common clinical manifestation is a characteristic skin lesion called erythema migrans. This lesion is a result of inflammation associated with the centrifugal spread of the spirochete within the skin from the site where the tick deposited the microorganism. The spirochete may also spread hematogenously to other skin locations, resulting in secondary erythema migrans skin lesions, or to nonskin sites, such as the joints, nervous system, or heart, leading to a variety of extracutaneous clinical manifestations.[4]

The Pathogen

In the United States, the species of Lyme borrelia that causes the vast majority of human infections is *B. burgdorferi* (also referred to as *B. burgdorferi* sensu stricto). Although *B. burgdorferi* also causes Lyme disease in Europe, collectively other species of Lyme borrelia that can be distinguished genotypically account for the majority of infections there, especially *Borrelia afzelii* and *Borrelia garinii*. The fact that at least six species of Lyme borrelia may cause infection in Europe has created serodiagnostic challenges and accounts for a wider variety of possible clinical manifestations there than in the United States

(see later). *B. garinii* appears to be the most neurotropic and *B. burgdorferi* the most arthritogenic among the species of Lyme borrelia.

EPIDEMIOLOGY

In the United States, more than 95% of cases of Lyme disease are concentrated in just 14 states: 12 eastern states and two in the North Central region. The states with the largest number of cases are Pennsylvania, Massachusetts, New York, New Jersey, and Connecticut. *Ixodes scapularis* (also known as the deer tick or black-legged tick) is the tick vector in these states. *Ixodes pacificus* is the vector for cases that occur in the Northwest region. Lyme disease also occurs in limited areas of Canada. Cases of Lyme disease occur throughout the temperate regions of Europe and are especially common in Scandinavia and countries of central Europe such as Slovenia, Austria, and Germany. *Ixodes ricinus* transmits the infection in Europe, and *Ixodes persulcatus* is the vector in the Asian region of Russia, China, and Japan. Because Lyme disease is mainly prevalent in the northern part of the Northern hemisphere, it can be particularly misdiagnosed in travelers to southern parts of the world.[5]

The principal reservoirs for Lyme borrelia (i.e., source of infection for ticks) in the United States and Eurasia are small mammals such as mice and certain species of birds. Deer play an essential role in the life cycle of the *I. scapularis* tick species but are not a competent reservoir for *B. burgdorferi*.

The likelihood of acquiring Lyme disease is directly related to exposure to environments in which infected ticks are present. Of the three feeding stages in the life cycle of *I. scapularis*, the second or nymphal stage is the most important epidemiologically for transmission of infection to humans. The first or larval stage is uninfected and cannot transmit this infection. Although the third stage (i.e., the adult stage of the tick) is more likely to be infected with *B. burgdorferi* than the nymphal stage is, it is less important in transmission to humans because this stage is present in smaller numbers in the environment and because there is less human activity outdoors during the time periods in the spring and fall when this stage is seeking a blood meal. In addition, adult ticks are larger and their bites cause more skin irritation than bites of nymphal ticks do, thereby increasing the likelihood that they will be noticed and detached by a person who has been bitten. If they are not removed, *Ixodes* ticks will usually feed for at least 3 days (Fig. 305-1). Transmission of *B. burgdorferi* by *I. scapularis* or *I. pacificus* ticks is typically delayed for more than 36 hours from the start of the blood meal, providing the opportunity to prevent infection simply by finding and removing the tick.[5] Transmission of *B. afzelii* by the European tick *I. ricinus* is considerably faster, however, often occurring within the first 24 hours of feeding.

Most cases of erythema migrans in the United States occur during June through August. There is a bimodal age distribution, with the highest incidences in children 5 to 15 years old and in adults 45 to 55 years of age, but individuals of all ages are at risk. The reported incidence of Lyme disease in the United States is rising, partially as a result of expansion of the deer population and the spread of infected *I. scapularis* ticks to new geographic areas.[6]

Extracutaneous manifestations are somewhat less likely than erythema migrans to occur during June to August because the time from the tick bite

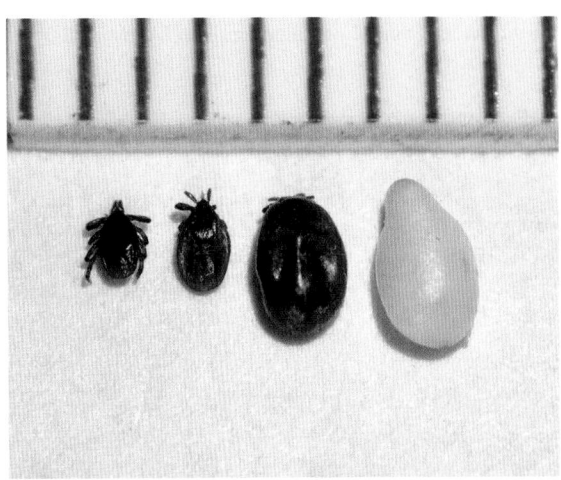

FIGURE 305-1. From left to right is an unfed nymphal stage *Ixodes scapularis* tick, a nymphal stage *I. scapularis* tick after about 48 hours of feeding, a nymphal stage *I. scapularis* tick after about 126 hours of feeding, and a sesame seed. The distance between the ruler marks is 1 mm. (Courtesy Kam Truhn of Fordham University.)

until the onset of these manifestations is longer. Because adult *I. scapularis* ticks may become active on warm days during the winter, cases of erythema migrans may occasionally occur even in the colder months.

B. burgdorferi is deposited by the tick into the skin rather than directly into the blood stream. Hematogenous dissemination seems to be an important mechanism responsible for spread of the spirochete to other sites. Alternatively, spread of the spirochete to other sites might occur through tissue planes. The likelihood of entry into the blood stream is affected by the strain of Lyme borrelia causing the infection. Unlike patients who are bacteremic with more conventional pathogens, patients with spirochetemia rarely appear "septic." In one study, only 5% of 93 spirochetemic patients were febrile when the blood culture specimen was obtained, and almost none was found to have leukocytosis. The lack of fever and other clinical signs of sepsis may be due to the absence of lipopolysaccharide within the borrelial cell wall.

Infection of humans or animals elicits innate and adaptive immune responses resulting in both macrophage and antibody-mediated killing of the spirochete. The inflammatory response in tissue typically shows an infiltration of lymphocytes, macrophages, and plasma cells, although granulocytes predominate in synovial fluid samples of Lyme arthritis patients. The potential for persistence of infection despite a robust humoral and cellular immunologic response is, however, typical of infection with Lyme borrelia, as it is with *Treponema pallidum* infection. The virulence factors responsible for persistence of infection include the spirochete's ability to downregulate expression of certain immunogenic surface-exposed proteins, including OspC, and to alter rapidly and continually by recombination of the antigenic properties of a surface lipoprotein known as variable major protein–like sequence expressed (VlsE). In addition, the spirochete's motility and ability to bind to various components of the extracellular matrix may also contribute to persistence.

All of the objective clinical manifestations of Lyme disease are thought to be due to an inflammatory response to live spirochetes or to their undegraded antigens. Obliterative endarteritis has been seen histologically in synovial tissue, but its importance in pathogenesis is unclear. Lyme borrelia are not known to produce toxins. In humans, the only role so far established for host genetic factors is in the development of antibiotic-refractory Lyme arthritis, which is seen most often in patients with certain HLA DR alleles, some of which coincide with those associated with rheumatoid arthritis.

The clinical manifestations are often categorized as follows:

- Early localized infection, typically manifested by a single erythema migrans (Fig. 305-2) skin lesion, with or without viral infection–like symptoms, but without objective extracutaneous manifestations
- Early disseminated infection, usually manifested by multiple erythema migrans skin lesions or by an objective manifestation of early neurologic Lyme disease or Lyme carditis
- Late disease, usually manifested by arthritis but may also include certain rare neurologic manifestations or the skin condition known as acrodermatitis chronica atrophicans (Fig. 305-3).

Children and adults have similar clinical manifestations. The expected frequency of the various clinical presentations is well illustrated by a study of 313 cases of Lyme disease diagnosed in Wurzburg, Germany, during a 12-month period. In this series, erythema migrans by itself was seen in 89% of cases, early neurologic manifestations in 3%, cardiac manifestations in less than 1%, borrelial lymphocytoma (see below under "Borrelial Lymphocytoma") in 2%, arthritis in 5%, and acrodermatitis chronica atrophicans in 1%. None of the patients had late neurologic Lyme disease. A similar distribution of cases has been seen in recent case series in the United States, except for the absence of borrelial lymphocytoma and acrodermatitis chronica atrophicans. In earlier studies in the United States from the 1980s, there was a much higher proportion of patients who had neurologic, cardiac, or joint manifestations. This may have been due to a bias of ascertainment in the older studies or to improved recognition and treatment of patients with erythema migrans more recently, thereby preventing the development of extracutaneous complications because they occur later.

Early Localized Infection
Single Erythema Migrans Skin Lesion

Erythema migrans is by far the most common clinical manifestation of Lyme disease. Although the appearance of the skin lesion is often distinctive (see Fig. 305-2), it is not pathognomonic for Lyme disease. Erythema migrans appears 7 to 14 days (range, 3 to 30 days) after tick detachment and is characterized by an expanding, flat to slightly raised, erythematous skin lesion (usually ≥5 cm in diameter) that is round or oval. The bite mark from the preceding tick bite can sometimes be identified at or near the center of the lesion and is called a punctum. Approximately 80% of patients in the United States with erythema migrans have just a single skin lesion. Nonspecific viral infection–like symptoms or signs, such as malaise, neck pain, headache, fatigue, migratory arthralgias, or chills and fever, may be present (Table 305-1) but are more common in patients infected with *B. burgdorferi* or *B. garinii* compared with *B. afzelii*. Prominent respiratory or gastrointestinal symptoms are highly atypical for Lyme disease. An acute febrile illness in the absence of a skin lesion or other objective clinical manifestation has been attributed to early Lyme disease, but the possibility of misdiagnosis is greater in this situation because of the potential for false-positive serologic test results.

Erythema migrans skin lesions can vary in appearance. Some (especially lesions of short duration) are nearly uniform in color, whereas others may show central clearing or a target-like appearance. About 5% have a vesicular-pustular center. Erythema migrans on the lower extremities may sometimes be purpuric. Lesions may be scaly when they are long-standing and fading or after topical corticosteroid creams have been applied. The most common locations include the thigh, back, shoulder, and calf. Lesions are often asymptomatic but can be mildly painful or pruritic, and tender regional lymphadenopathy may be present. The majority of U.S. patients with erythema migrans, as for all other clinical manifestations, do not recall a preceding tick bite.

Certain signs and symptoms that have been described in small numbers of patients with erythema migrans in early case series, such as hepatomegaly,

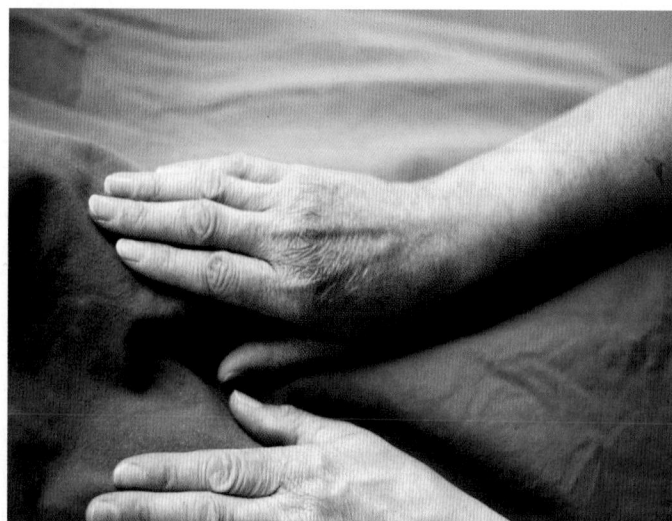

FIGURE 305-3. Acrodermatitis chronica atrophicans. This late cutaneous manifestation of Lyme borreliosis is characterized by slowly expanding red violaceous lesions that typically involve the dorsal surfaces of acral sites and do not heal spontaneously. The lesions are initially inflammatory and later on more and more atrophic. (Courtesy Dr. Franc Strle.)

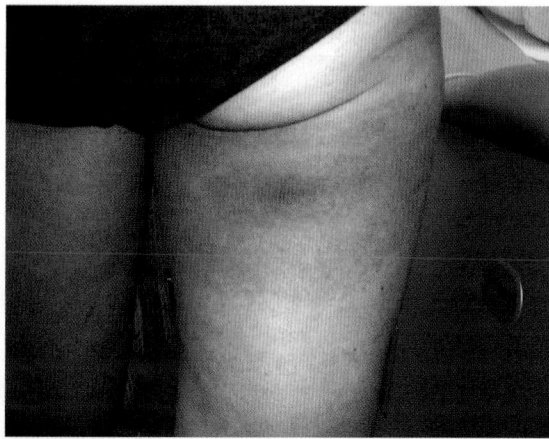

FIGURE 305-2. Erythema migrans skin lesion on the posterior aspect of the right thigh.

TABLE 305-1	CLINICAL SYMPTOMS AND SIGNS PRESENT IN AT LEAST 20% OF PATIENTS WITH ERYTHEMA MIGRANS
CHARACTERISTIC	**UNITED STATES (95% CI)**
Viral infection-like	65% (52-76%)
Fatigue	47% (37-58%)
Headache	36% (27-46%)
Myalgias	35% (26-45%)
Arthralgias	35% (25-46%)
Fever	33% (23-43%)
Stiff neck	31% (21-43%)
Lymphadenopathy	22% (13-33%)
Dysesthesia	20% (12-32%)
	EUROPE (95% CI)
Viral infection-like	37% (27-49%)
Dysesthesia	35% (25-47%)
Headache	20% (14-29%)

CI = confidence interval.
Modified from Tibbles CD, Edlow JA. Does this patient have erythema migrans? *JAMA.* 2007;297:2617-2627.

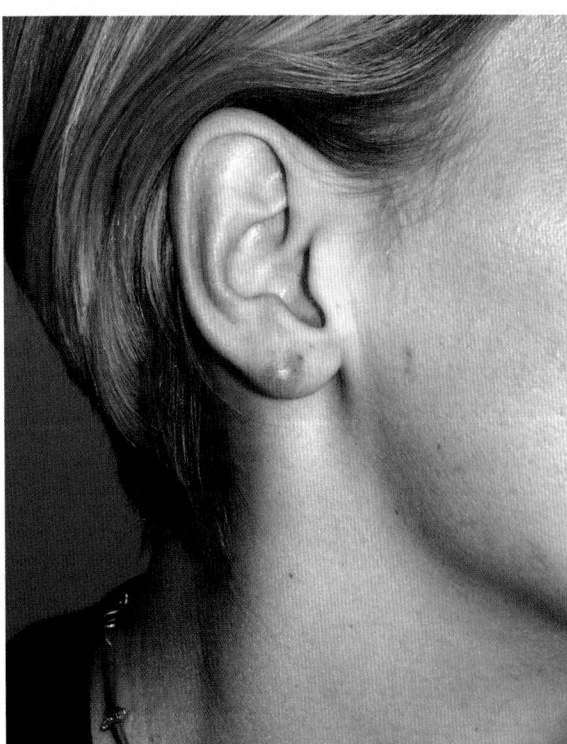

FIGURE 305-4. Borrelial lymphocytoma. A rare cutaneous manifestation of Lyme disease that is seen predominantly outside the United States, it is manifested as a solitary bluish red swelling most commonly on the earlobe of children and the breast in adults. (Courtesy Dr. Franc Strle.)

splenomegaly, sore throat, conjunctivitis, or testicular swelling, may have been coincidental findings. There has been no microbiologic confirmation of borrelia infection at these sites.

Borrelial Lymphocytoma

Borrelial lymphocytoma is a rare cutaneous manifestation of Lyme disease that almost never occurs in the United States. It often is manifested at or near a preceding tick bite as a solitary bluish red swelling with a diameter of up to a few centimeters. The most common locations are the earlobe in children and the breast in adults (Fig. 305-4). Histologic examination shows a dense infiltration of the cutis and subcutis by predominantly polyclonal B lymphocytes, frequently with germinal center formation. Histologic evaluation may be necessary to exclude malignant disease for patients with suspected borrelial lymphocytoma at a location other than the earlobe.

Early Disseminated Infection
Multiple Erythema Migrans Skin Lesions

In the United States, approximately 20% of patients with erythema migrans have multiple skin lesions at the time of presentation. Secondary erythema migrans skin lesions can be smaller than 5 cm, do not have a punctum, and are usually not tender or pruritic. They arise from hematogenous dissemination to the skin rather than from additional tick bites.

Early Neurologic Lyme Disease

Within weeks to several months after infection, patients may develop neurologic manifestations, the most common of which are cranial neuropathy (particularly peripheral seventh nerve palsy that may be bilateral), lymphocytic meningitis, and sensory (often painful) radiculopathy.[7,8] Less common manifestations include mononeuritis multiplex (multifocal involvement of anatomically unrelated nerves) and brachial or lumbosacral plexopathies. A pseudotumor cerebri–like picture has been reported occasionally in children. The presence of a concomitant erythema migrans lesion or the patient's recollection of a recent lesion consistent with erythema migrans may be helpful diagnostically. Studies suggest that approximately 90% of children with Lyme meningitis in the United States have at least one of the following three findings: concomitant erythema migrans, cranial nerve palsy, or papilledema.

Cardiac Lyme Disease

Weeks to months after infection, patients may develop cardiac manifestations of Lyme disease, most often fluctuating degrees of atrioventricular heart block or other manifestations of a myopericarditis, which may cause the patient to complain of lightheadedness, palpitations, dyspnea, chest pain, or syncope.[9] Heart block is typically at or above the atrioventricular node. Erythema migrans is often but not invariably present concurrently. Valvular dysfunction is not known to occur, and chronic cardiomyopathy has been reported only rarely in Europe.

Late Lyme Disease
Lyme Arthritis

If patients with erythema migrans in the United States are not treated with antibiotics, approximately 60% will develop a monoarticular or oligoarticular arthritis at a mean time of 6 months after disease onset (range, 4 days to as long as 2 years). In untreated patients, Lyme arthritis is characterized by intermittent attacks of synovitis that last for a few weeks to several months. One or two joints are involved at a time. Primarily large joints are affected,[10] but there may be involvement of the temporomandibular joint, small joints, and periarticular sites. The most commonly involved joint is the knee. Baker cysts may form and rupture. Joint swelling is often pronounced, but pain is usually relatively modest. Particularly in children, there may be concomitant fever, but adults are often minimally symptomatic aside from the arthritis.

In about 10% of adult patients with Lyme arthritis in the United States, involvement of a large joint (almost always the knee) may persist despite appropriate antibiotic treatment. Erosion of cartilage or bone may develop in such cases.

Late Neurologic Lyme Disease

After months to years of infection, late neurologic manifestations may develop. These include encephalomyelitis, peripheral neuropathy, and encephalopathy. Because most patients with Lyme disease are now diagnosed and treated early in the course of infection, these more indolent forms of neurologic Lyme disease are rare.

In untreated patients, encephalomyelitis has been monophasic and slowly progressive, mainly involving white matter. It is the most severe neurologic manifestation and, although infrequent, is probably more common in Europe than in the United States. Cerebrospinal fluid (CSF) examination typically shows a lymphocytic pleocytosis, a moderately elevated protein level, and a normal glucose level, with evidence of intrathecal production of antibody to borrelia. Magnetic resonance imaging of the affected part of the brain or spinal cord can demonstrate areas of inflammation, typically with increased signal on T2 and fluid attenuation inversion recovery imaging and enhancement after administration of contrast material.

In the United States, peripheral neuropathy typically is manifested as a mild, diffuse "stocking-glove" process. Patients may complain of intermittent limb paresthesias and sometimes radicular pain. The most common abnormality on neurologic examination is reduced vibratory sensation of the distal lower extremities. Electrophysiologic studies show a patchy axonal neuropathy. Nerve biopsy shows axonal loss and small perivascular collections of lymphocytes without spirochetes. The existence of this late onset peripheral axonal neuropathy, however, is controversial.[11]

Encephalopathy is an imprecisely defined clinical entity characterized by mild abnormalities of memory or other cognitive functions that are demonstrable on either a careful mental status examination or on formal neuropsychological testing. CSF examination findings may be completely normal or may show intrathecal antibody production, mild CSF protein elevation, or a mild pleocytosis. Cranial imaging studies may occasionally demonstrate focal areas of presumed parenchymal inflammation, but findings are most often normal.

Acrodermatitis Chronica Atrophicans

Acrodermatitis chronica atrophicans (Fig. 305-3) is a late skin manifestation of Lyme disease that is most commonly seen in women older than 40 years. This skin lesion develops insidiously several years after initial infection, usually on the extensor surfaces of the hands and feet. Early lesions are characterized by a slight bluish red discoloration and doughy swelling. Histologic examination shows lymphocytes and plasma cells in the skin and sometimes in the subcutis, with or without atrophy. Initially unilateral, the lesion may later become bilateral. Over time, there is resolution of the edema with development of skin atrophy. Nodules may develop over bone prominences. About two thirds of patients have an associated peripheral neuropathy, primarily of the affected extremity that is usually manifested as local sensory loss.

Although presumably any of the species of Lyme borrelia may cause acrodermatitis chronica atrophicans, by far the most common etiologic agent is *B. afzelii*. Therefore, this manifestation is rarely seen in the United States.

DIAGNOSIS
General Laboratory Testing

Blood counts are usually normal in Lyme disease, unless coinfection with *Anaplasma phagocytophilum*, *Babesia microti*, or a tick-borne encephalitis virus is present (see later). Lymphopenia, however, may be found in the absence of a recognized coinfection. In patients with erythema migrans, mild abnormalities of liver function tests (particularly elevations of aspartate and alanine aminotransferase levels) can be seen in approximately 35% of patients. The erythrocyte sedimentation rate may be modestly elevated in all stages of Lyme disease, but values greater than 80 mm/hour are distinctly uncommon.

CSF examination in Lyme meningitis typically shows a pleocytosis with more than 90% lymphocytes, a modestly elevated protein level, and a normal glucose level. Synovial fluid examination in Lyme arthritis typically shows approximately 25,000 white cells/µL (range, 500 to 110,000/µL) with a polymorphonuclear predominance.

Serologic Testing

Erythema migrans skin lesions may go unnoticed by the patient because of the absence of prominent local symptoms and occurrence on parts of the body that are difficult for the patient to visualize. Therefore, a complete skin examination should be performed for any patient thought to have early localized or disseminated Lyme disease. Erythema migrans is the only clinical manifestation sufficiently distinctive to allow a clinical diagnosis in the absence of a supporting laboratory test. Erythema migrans is diagnosed on the basis of recognition of the characteristic appearance of the skin lesion in persons who live in or have recently traveled to areas endemic for Lyme disease. Because of the short duration of infection at this stage, serologic assays for antibodies to Lyme borrelia are infrequently positive and thus should be obtained only in atypical cases, then in conjunction with convalescent-phase serologic testing 2 to 4 weeks after the acute sample is obtained (Table 305-2).

For non–erythema migrans presentations of Lyme disease, the mainstay of laboratory diagnosis is two-tier serologic testing in which the first tier test is usually a sensitive enzyme-linked immunosorbent assay (EIA). If the EIA result is positive or equivocal, separate IgM and IgG immunoblots are performed on the original serum sample. If symptoms have persisted for at least 4 weeks, then specifically the IgG immunoblot should be positive for the results to be interpreted as evidence of seropositivity. Untreated patients who remain seronegative for 6 to 8 weeks are unlikely to have Lyme disease, and other possible diagnoses should be pursued.

Omitting the first-tier EIA or interpreting the immunoblot with alternative criteria that are not evidence based will potentially decrease the specificity of testing and is not recommended. False-positive results on the IgM immunoblot may be due to cross-reactive antibodies that arise from polyclonal B-cell

TABLE 305-2	DIAGNOSIS OF LYME DISEASE	
DIAGNOSTIC MODALITY	**APPLICATION**	**COMMENT**
Visual inspection	Erythema migrans	Usually seronegative at time of presentation
Two-tier serology with a positive IgM and/or IgG immunoblot	Lyme carditis	Look for concomitant erythema migrans
	Early neurologic Lyme disease	Look for concomitant erythema migrans; intrathecal antibody may be detectable before serum antibody in Europe; PCR sometimes positive in CSF
	Borrelial lymphocytoma	Biopsy may be needed to exclude malignant neoplasm
Two-tier serology with a positive IgG immunoblot	Lyme arthritis	PCR often positive in synovial fluid
	Late neurologic Lyme disease	Intrathecal antibody positivity expected in Lyme encephalomyelitis
	Acrodermatitis chronica atrophicans	

CSF = cerebrospinal fluid; Ig = immunoglobulin; PCR = polymerase chain reaction.

stimulation. Probably the most common cause of false-positive results, however, is the overreading of nonspecific weak bands.[12] Background rates of seropositivity, which may exceed 4% in highly endemic areas of the United States with even higher rates than this in Europe, may also confound the interpretation of seroreactivity. Therefore, a positive serologic test result does not mean that the patient necessarily has active Lyme disease. The positive predictive value is most informative when the pretest probability based on the clinical features is at least 20%. Serologic testing is not indicated in routine follow-up of patients after treatment as either IgM or IgG borrelial antibodies may persist for many years in successfully treated patients.

Testing for borrelial antibody that is produced locally in the central nervous system (i.e., intrathecal antibody) may be helpful in the diagnosis of neurologic Lyme disease and has been reported to precede detection of serum antibody in a minority of European patients. Positive test results for intrathecal antibody may persist, however, for long periods after successful antibiotic treatment.

The European Society for Clinical Microbiology and Infectious Diseases (ESCMID) has summarized its recommendations for diagnosis: (1) typical erythema migrans should be diagnosed clinically and does not require laboratory testing; (2) the diagnosis of Lyme neuroborreliosis requires laboratory investigation of the CSF, including intrathecal antibody production; and (3) the remaining disease manifestations require testing for serum antibodies to *B. burgdorferi*.[13] Promising alternatives to two-tiered testing are under study.[14,15]

Other Diagnostic Modalities

Culture for Lyme borrelia is not routinely done or available to diagnose Lyme disease. It is unnecessary for patients with erythema migrans and too insensitive for patients with extracutaneous manifestations of Lyme disease. In contrast, polymerase chain reaction (PCR) for detection of borrelial DNA is positive on synovial fluid specimens in up to approximately 80% of untreated patients with Lyme arthritis, and a positive result lends support for this diagnosis in a patient who is IgG seropositive. The sensitivity of PCR in CSF tends to be much lower, however, and was only approximately 5% in a study of children from the United States with early neurologic Lyme disease. A negative PCR result on either type of fluid does not exclude Lyme disease.

Differential Diagnosis
Erythema Migrans

Tick-bite hypersensitivity reactions can be mistaken for erythema migrans, but these reactions occur within 48 hours of a tick bite, are usually pruritic, and tend to wane within a few days. In contrast, erythema migrans skin lesions in untreated patients will last for a median time of approximately 4 weeks in the United States and even longer in Europe. Bacterial cellulitis rarely occurs at the most frequent skin sites for erythema migrans and would not be expected to demonstrate central clearing or a target-like appearance. Erythema migrans, unlike erythema multiforme, does not involve the mucous membranes, palms, or soles. Southern tick-associated rash illness (STARI) is the most likely diagnosis in patients with erythema migrans–like skin lesions who were bitten by an *A. americanum* tick or developed this lesion in the southern United States (see under Pathobiology). Other considerations in the differential diagnosis of erythema migrans that usually can be readily distinguished include tinea (often pruritic with a thin, raised, scaly border), nummular eczema (symmetrical pruritic lesions with a tendency to scale and crust), granuloma annulare (acral location, especially on the dorsum of hands and feet, relatively fixed in size and <5 cm in diameter), contact dermatitis (pruritic with streaking along the area of contact and a vesicular component), urticaria (raised, pruritic, and usually <5 cm in diameter), fixed drug eruption (usually on genitals, hands, feet, or face and fixed in size), pityriasis rosea (multiple, moderately pruritic lesions with peripheral scale and relatively fixed in size), and spider bite (often very painful and necrotic with a central eschar).

Extracutaneous Lyme Disease

Included in the differential diagnosis of early neurologic Lyme disease is Bell palsy. Even in highly endemic areas of the United States, other causes of seventh nerve palsy outnumber Lyme disease by a margin of 3:1. Viral meningitis and mechanical radiculopathy can also potentially be confused with manifestations of early neurologic Lyme disease. Viral or other causes of myopericarditis may resemble cardiac Lyme disease. Many causes of synovitis might be considered in the differential diagnosis of Lyme arthritis, but the pattern of joint involvement, such as symmetrical small joint involvement in rheumatoid arthritis, is often distinctly different from that found in Lyme arthritis. Lyme encephalomyelitis may occasionally be confused clinically with a first episode of relapsing-remitting multiple sclerosis or primary progressive multiple sclerosis. Testing for borrelial antibody in serum (and CSF for the last condition) usually suffices to differentiate these conditions from Lyme disease.

TREATMENT   Rx

In vitro studies have shown that Lyme borrelia are highly susceptible to tetracyclines, most penicillins, and many second- and third-generation cephalosporins. B. burgdorferi is resistant to certain fluoroquinolones, rifampin, and first-generation cephalosporins. Whether macrolides are active in vitro depends on the borrelial strain tested and the assay technique used. Although most manifestations of Lyme disease will resolve spontaneously without treatment, antibiotic therapy may hasten resolution and prevent progression.

Oral antibiotic therapy is used to treat patients with erythema migrans (Table 305-3). Doxycycline, amoxicillin, and cefuroxime axetil are each highly effective[A1] and are the preferred agents for this indication. Macrolides such as azithromycin are somewhat less effective than other oral antibiotics and consequently are not recommended as first-line therapy.

Doxycycline alone among the first-line agents is effective against A. phagocytophilum coinfection and is the only agent for which a prospective clinical trial has demonstrated that just 10 days of treatment is effective. Doxycycline, however, may cause photosensitivity, which is a concern because early Lyme disease occurs most commonly during the summer months; in addition, this drug is relatively contraindicated in children younger than 8 years and in women who are pregnant or breast-feeding. When erythema migrans cannot be reliably distinguished from community-acquired bacterial cellulitis, either cefuroxime axetil or amoxicillin–clavulanate potassium (Augmentin) is preferred because these antimicrobials are generally effective against both types of infection.

Within 24 hours of initiation of antimicrobial therapy, up to 15% of patients treated for erythema migrans will experience a Jarisch-Herxheimer–like reaction characterized by an increase in the size or intensity of erythema in the skin lesion and more intense viral infection–like systemic symptoms. Fever, if present, should resolve within 48 hours and the skin lesion itself within 7 to 14 days. Other symptoms, such as fatigue or arthralgia, tend to improve but not invariably to resolve within this time frame, lasting for more than 3 months in one quarter of patients. Extending the initial course of treatment does not provide faster relief of symptoms. Oral antibiotic therapy is also used as first-line treatment for the other cutaneous manifestations of Lyme disease discussed elsewhere in this chapter and as initial treatment of patients with Lyme arthritis.

The preferred parenteral agent for Lyme disease is ceftriaxone because it is highly active against Lyme borrelia in vitro, crosses the blood-brain barrier well, and has a long serum half-life, allowing the convenience of once-daily administration. Alternative choices for parenterally administered antibiotics are cefotaxime and intravenous penicillin. Parenteral antibiotic therapy is recommended to treat patients with late neurologic Lyme disease and those with cardiac Lyme disease who are admitted to the hospital for monitoring (see Table 305-3). Parenteral antibiotics are often given to patients with Lyme arthritis who have failed to respond to one or more courses of oral antibiotic treatment.

In the United States, parenteral therapy has been the preferred management strategy for early neurologic Lyme disease, especially for meningitis and radiculitis, with oral therapy reserved for patients with uncomplicated seventh nerve palsy. Studies conducted in Europe, however, have provided convincing evidence that oral doxycycline is just as effective as ceftriaxone for any of the primary manifestations of early neurologic Lyme disease, and this agent is increasingly being used for this indication in the United States as well.[A2][A3] Other oral antibiotics, such as amoxicillin, have been used successfully to treat patients with uncomplicated seventh nerve palsy, but published data on efficacy are much more limited for these agents. Available data indicate that seventh nerve palsy will resolve, with or without antibiotic treatment, and that the rate of recovery is not accelerated by antibiotics. Therefore, the primary reason to treat such patients is to prevent the subsequent development of later complications, particularly Lyme arthritis.

The presence of either papilledema or sixth cranial nerve palsy may indicate the presence of increased intracranial pressure in patients with neurologic Lyme disease. The elevated pressure will typically fall in response to antibiotic therapy, but other measures conventionally used to lower pressure may need to be considered in individual cases.

Symptomatic patients with cardiac Lyme disease and those with high-grade first-degree atrioventricular heart block (PR interval of ≥300 msec) and second- or third-degree block should be hospitalized and closely monitored (Chapter 58). Temporary cardiac pacing may be required. In treated patients, complete heart block generally resolves within 1 week, and lesser conduction disturbances resolve within 6 weeks.

Lyme arthritis typically responds to antibiotic treatment. Patients whose arthritis is improved but not resolved after an initial course of oral therapy may be re-treated with a second course of oral antibiotics, with parenteral antibiotic therapy reserved for those without any significant clinical response. Approximately 10% of adult patients in the United States, however, do not respond clinically to antibiotic therapy and are said to have antibiotic-refractory Lyme arthritis; this condition has been defined as persistent synovitis for at least 2 months after completion of a course of intravenous ceftriaxone (or 1 month after completion of two 4-week courses of an oral antibiotic). Because these patients are no longer believed to be actively infected, they are customarily treated with nonsteroidal anti-inflammatory agents, intra-articular injections of corticosteroids, or a 6- to 12-month course of disease-modifying antirheumatic drugs.[16] Arthroscopic synovectomy has also been used successfully for patients with this condition.

Pregnant patients with Lyme disease are generally treated similarly to nonpregnant patients except that doxycycline has been considered to be relatively contraindicated. No published data convincingly support a congenital Lyme disease syndrome.

Post–Lyme Disease Symptoms and Syndrome

The outcome of treatment in most patients with erythema migrans is excellent. Studies show, however, that when questioned at 6 months or more after treatment of erythema migrans, approximately 10% of patients will report purely

TABLE 305-3	RECOMMENDED THERAPY FOR ADULT PATIENTS WITH LYME DISEASE*	
THERAPY	**MANIFESTATION**	**DURATION**
Doxycycline 100 mg PO bid *or* Amoxicillin 500 mg PO tid *or* Cefuroxime axetil 500 mg PO bid	Erythema migrans	10-14 days[†]
	Borrelial lymphocytoma	14 days
	Acrodermatitis chronica atrophicans	21-28 days
	Lyme arthritis	28 days
	Lyme carditis—mild	14-21 days
	Cranial neuropathy	14 days[‡]
Doxycycline 200 mg PO daily or 100 mg PO bid	Lyme meningitis or radiculopathy	14 days
Ceftriaxone 2 g IV daily	Lyme arthritis that failed to respond to oral therapy	14-28 days
	Late neurologic Lyme disease	14-28 days
	Lyme carditis requiring hospitalization	14-21 days
	Lyme meningitis or radiculopathy requiring hospitalization	14 days
Azithromycin 500 mg PO daily	Erythema migrans in a patient intolerant of doxycycline and β-lactam antibiotics	7 days

*Regardless of the clinical manifestations of Lyme disease, complete response to treatment may be delayed beyond the treatment duration. Relapse may occur with any of these regimens; patients with objective signs of relapse may need another course of treatment.

[†]10 days for doxycycline; 14 days for amoxicillin or cefuroxime axetil.

[‡]Although any one of first-line oral antibiotics appears to be effective in patients with cranial neuropathy, there is only limited experience in patients with a cranial neuropathy other than seventh nerve palsy or with agents other than doxycycline.

Modified from Wormser GP, Dattwyler RJ, Shapiro ED, et al. The clinical assessment, treatment, and prevention of Lyme disease, human granulocytic anaplasmosis, and babesiosis: clinical practice guidelines by the Infectious Diseases Society of America. *Clin Infect Dis.* 2006;43:1089-1134.

subjective symptoms such as fatigue or musculoskeletal pains.[17] These subjective symptoms are typically mild and may wax and wane in intensity. Patients who have them are referred to as having post–Lyme disease symptoms or syndrome, depending on the symptom duration and severity. The cause of these symptoms is currently unknown. Carefully done microbiologic evaluations in the United States have failed to find evidence of either persistent *B. burgdorferi* infection or a coinfection with a second *Ixodes*-transmitted pathogen. In patients with persistent symptoms attributed to Lyme disease, longer-term antibiotic treatment has been shown to have no additional beneficial effects on health-related quality of life beyond those with shorter-term treatment.[A4] Furthermore, retreatment has provided either no measurable benefit or a benefit so modest or ambiguous that it was outweighed by the risks associated with the antibiotic therapy. Therefore, symptomatic treatment is recommended for such patients.

Chronic Lyme Disease

The term *chronic Lyme disease* is poorly defined but widely used. In Europe, the term has been used to refer to the objective manifestations that most authorities prefer to call late Lyme disease. Others have used the term to refer to patients with post–Lyme disease subjective complaints. Most often, chronic Lyme disease is used as a diagnosis for patients with persistent pain, neurocognitive complaints, or fatigue, without objective clinical or serologic evidence of past or present *B. burgdorferi* infection. In this usage, the term is a misnomer and has become the latest in a series of postulated syndromes that attempt to attribute "medically unexplained symptoms" to particular infections.[18]

Coinfections

Ixodes ticks may be coinfected with and transmit Lyme borrelia along with other pathogens, such as *A. phagocytophilum*, *B. microti* (the primary cause of babesiosis), and a tick-borne encephalitis virus. The likelihood of coinfection is dependent on the particular species of *Ixodes* tick and on the geographic area. Thus, bites from *I. scapularis* ticks in certain areas may lead to the development of Lyme disease, human granulocytic anaplasmosis, or babesiosis as a single infection or less frequently as a coinfection. In addition, this tick species can potentially transmit the deer tick virus subtype of the Powassan virus, an *Ehrlichia* species referred to as *Ehrlichia muris eauclarensis*, and *Borrelia miyamotoi*.[19] In Europe, the most common coinfection is Lyme disease with tick-borne encephalitis virus infection.

Coinfection should be considered in patients from geographic areas endemic for these pathogens who present with more severe initial symptoms than are commonly observed with Lyme disease alone. In this situation, coinfection should be considered especially in those who have high-grade fever for more than 48 hours despite antibiotic therapy appropriate for Lyme disease; those who develop recurrent fever; and those who have unexplained leukopenia, thrombocytopenia, or anemia. Coinfection might also be considered in the situation in which there has been resolution of the erythema migrans skin lesion but either no improvement or worsening of the viral infection–like symptoms.

Reinfection

Patients treated for early Lyme disease do not appear to develop an immunologic response that is adequate to protect against reinfection with a different strain of *B. burgdorferi*. Therefore, patients with erythema migrans may become reinfected at a different skin site if they get a bite from another infected tick. Reinfection has been well documented only in patients who were treated for early infection (nearly always erythema migrans) and not after late manifestations of Lyme disease, such as Lyme arthritis. Clinical manifestations of reinfection appear to be similar to those of the primary infection.

PREVENTION

Lyme disease can be prevented by avoiding tick-infested environments and by covering bare skin and using tick repellents on skin and clothing when in such environments. The tick density around individual residences can be reduced by removing leaf litter, placing wood chips where lawns abut forests, and constructing fences to keep out deer. Applying acaricides to residential property can reduce the number of ticks but not necessarily to a level that will reduce household tick exposure or human diseases.[A5] Bathing within 2 hours of tick exposure has been shown to decrease the risk of Lyme disease. Daily inspections of the entire skin surface (including scalp) to remove attached ticks is recommended because of the grace period between the time of tick attachment and transmission of *B. burgdorferi*. Removal is accomplished by grasping the tick as close to its mouth parts as possible with a forceps (or tweezers) and then gently pulling it out. Clinical studies have demonstrated that without any other intervention, more than 96% of patients who find and remove an attached *I. scapularis* tick will remain free of Lyme disease, even in highly endemic geographic regions. If the tick is not found or removed, the probability of infection approaches the infection rate in the regional tick population (typically >20% of nymphal stage *I. scapularis* ticks are infected in highly endemic areas of the Northeast and Midwest United States).

Evidence shows that doxycycline chemoprophylaxis can further reduce the chance for development of Lyme disease after removal of an *I. scapularis* tick. A single 200-mg dose of doxycycline is about 90% effective in preventing erythema migrans at the tick bite site.[A6] Use of a single dose of doxycycline within 72 hours of tick removal should be considered for persons in highly endemic areas who are known to have been bitten by a nymphal or adult *I. scapularis* tick that was estimated to have been attached for at least 36 hours. Given the uncertain efficacy of a short course of amoxicillin in this situation, observation rather than chemoprophylaxis has been recommended for individuals for whom doxycycline is contraindicated. Topical azithromycin provides no prevention effect.[A7] No vaccine is currently available to prevent Lyme disease in humans.

Grade A References

A1. Torbahn G, Hofmann H, Rucker G, et al. Efficacy and safety of antibiotic therapy in early cutaneous lyme borreliosis: a network meta-analysis. *JAMA Dermatol.* 2018;154:1292-1303.

A2. Cadavid D, Auwaerter PG, Rumbaugh J, et al. Antibiotics for the neurological complications of Lyme disease. *Cochrane Database Syst Rev.* 2016;12:CD006978.

A3. Dersch R, Freitag MH, Schmidt S, et al. Efficacy and safety of pharmacological treatments for acute Lyme neuroborreliosis—a systematic review. *Eur J Neurol.* 2015;22:1249-1259.

A4. Berende A, ter Hofstede HJ, Vos FJ, et al. Randomized trial of longer-term therapy for symptoms attributed to Lyme disease. *N Engl J Med.* 2016;374:1209-1220.

A5. Hinckley AF, Meek JI, Ray JA, et al. Effectiveness of residential acaricides to prevent Lyme and other tick-borne diseases in humans. *J Infect Dis.* 2016;214:182-188.

A6. Warshafsky S, Lee DH, Francois LK, et al. Efficacy of antibiotic prophylaxis for the prevention of Lyme disease: an updated systematic review and meta-analysis. *J Antimicrob Chemother.* 2010;65:1137-1144.

A7. Schwameis M, Kündig T, Huber G, et al. Topical azithromycin for the prevention of Lyme borreliosis: a randomised, placebo-controlled, phase 3 efficacy trial. *Lancet Infect Dis.* 2017;17:322-329.

GENERAL REFERENCES

For the General References and other additional features, please visit Expert Consult at https://expertconsult.inkling.com.

306

RELAPSING FEVER AND OTHER *BORRELIA* INFECTIONS

WILLIAM A. PETRI, JR.

DEFINITION

Relapsing fever is a spirochetal infection with bacteria of the genus *Borrelia*. There are two modes of transmission: epidemic louse-borne and endemic tick-borne relapsing fever. Disease is characterized by recurrent bouts of fever and spirochetemia separated by short fever-free periods.[1]

The Pathogen

Members of the genus *Borrelia* are motile spirochetes that measure 0.5 μm in diameter and 5 to 40 μm in length. They are aerophilic and require long-chain fatty acids for growth. Louse-borne relapsing fever is caused by *Borrelia recurrentis*. Tick-borne relapsing fever organisms are named after their tick vector and include the closely related species *Borrelia duttonii* (Old World); *Borrelia hermsii*, *Borrelia turicatae*, and *Borrelia parkeri* (North America); and *Borrelia miyamotoi* (Old and New World).[2]

EPIDEMIOLOGY

Louse-borne epidemic relapsing fever is caused by *B. recurrentis* and is carried from person to person by the human body louse (*Pediculus humanus*). There is no animal reservoir. The spirochete lives in the louse hemolymph; infection is transmitted to humans when the louse is crushed on human skin and infective spirochetes penetrate the skin or mucous membranes. Epidemics have occurred during famines and at wartime when breakdown in sanitation favors the transmission of body lice. Louse-borne disease remains endemic in central and east Africa (Ethiopia, Somalia, Chad, and the Sudan) and in the South

American Andes (Bolivia and Peru). It is also being seen in recent refugees to western Europe.[3]

Tick-borne endemic relapsing fever occurs throughout the world and is transmitted to humans by *Ornithodoros* soft ticks. The ticks become infected by feeding on wild rodents (including mice, rats, squirrels, and chipmunks), which serve as natural reservoirs for the organisms. In the United States relapsing fever is limited to humid mountainous areas of the West at altitudes of 1500 to 8000 feet, where the tick vector *Ornithodoros hermsii* resides in forests of ponderosa pine and Douglas fir trees. A key diagnostic clue has been a history of sleeping in rodent-infested rustic cabins in western U.S. national parks. In Tanzania, where house infestation with *Ornithodoros* tick vectors can be very high, relapsing fever was identified in 11% of children seen at a clinic with fever. In the northeastern United States, the prevalence of antibodies to *Borrelia miyamotoi* is nearly 50%, as high as for *Borrelia burgdorferi* (Chapter 305).

PATHOBIOLOGY

Borrelia infection begins in the skin at the site of the louse or tick bite and is followed by rapid dissemination of the spirochetes through the bloodstream. Spirochetes are visible on Wright-stained peripheral blood smears during the initial febrile episode and during each febrile relapse in most patients. The spirochete burden in blood positively correlates with symptom severity. Clearance of spirochetes from blood is associated with the production of serotype-specific immune sera; anti-*Borrelia* antibodies have been shown in animal models to be the major mechanism of immune clearance of infection.

Relapses are associated with cyclic antigenic variation in the variable major proteins (VMPs), which are the abundant outer membrane proteins of the spirochete that carry the serotype-specific epitopes. Antigenic variation is the consequence of recombination events that occur between VMP genes at silent and expression sites on linear plasmids. A single *B. hermsii* bacterium may produce as many as 40 distinct serotypes.[4] Because spirochetes undergo one or several antigenic phases during infection, no specific or standard procedure has been developed for routine serodiagnosis of relapsing fever.

CLINICAL MANIFESTATIONS

An abrupt onset of fever (temperature >39° C in most patients), headache, myalgia, and shaking chills characterizes the onset of illness. Cough, nausea and vomiting, and fatigue are less frequent complaints. Signs include fever, tachycardia, lethargy or confusion, conjunctival injection, and epistaxis. Hepatosplenomegaly, jaundice, and often a truncal petechial rash are common signs in louse-borne relapsing fever. Neurologic findings may occur, including meningitis, meningoencephalitis, and facial palsy, although these entities are more common with tick-borne relapsing fever. Untreated louse-borne disease lasts 6 days, and relapses occur once after an afebrile period of 9 days. The initial illness of tick-borne relapsing fever lasts about 4 days without antibiotic treatment, with an average of two relapses (each after an average 10-day intervening afebrile period) before the diagnosis is made.[5]

Borrelia miyamotoi presents with high fever, chills, marked headache, and myalgia or arthralgia. Elevated liver enzyme levels, neutropenia, and thrombocytopenia are common.[6] Relapsing fever in pregnancy can cause placental damage and intrauterine growth retardation and results in miscarriage in a third of patients. Neonatal infection by both the tick- and louse-borne forms is accompanied by jaundice, hepatosplenomegaly, and often sepsis and hemorrhage. Fever and hepatosplenomegaly are also common signs in children. It has been also recognized in immunocompromised patients.

DIAGNOSIS

The diagnosis should be considered in patients with fever who are returning from a stay in cabins in the mountainous and high-elevation areas of the western United States.[7] Only a few patients will remember tick exposure, because *O. hermsii* is a night feeder, has a painless bite, and remains attached for only 15 minutes. Internationally, relapsing fever can occur sporadically wherever dwellings are infected with *Ornithodoros* ticks, as well as in epidemics with louse-borne disease.

Because the number of organisms in blood is extremely high, the diagnosis is most often made by direct visualization of the organism in a blood smear (Fig. 306-1), although the diagnosis can also be made with polymerase chain reaction and serodiagnostic tests. For *B. miyamotoi,* only 16% of patients are seropositive, but polymerase chain reaction testing is highly sensitive and specific.[8] Spirochetes can be demonstrated in peripheral blood smears taken during febrile episodes in 70% of patients. Additional sensitivity may be gained by examination of a buffy coat preparation of peripheral blood. Because of

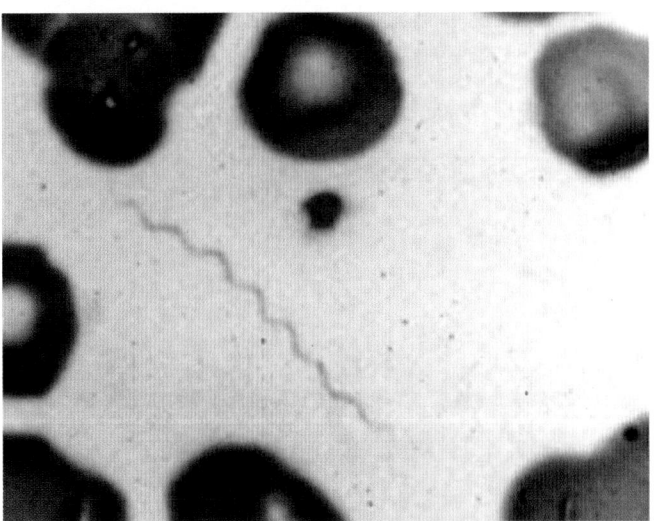

FIGURE 306-1. A single spirochete is seen in a Wright-stained thin blood smear from a patient with relapsing fever.

their characteristic locomotion, spirochetes can be readily detected by direct visualization of thick blood films under low-power microscopy. Culture of the organism requires a special medium and is not practical in a clinical laboratory setting. The white blood cell count is generally normal, but platelet counts of less than 50,000/μL occur in up to 90% of cases of louse-borne disease. Prothrombin and activated partial thromboplastin times are often prolonged. In louse-borne disease, elevations in liver function test results (serum aminotransferase and bilirubin levels) and blood urea nitrogen are common. Urinalysis may reveal proteinuria and microscopic hematuria. Examination of cerebrospinal fluid may show a lymphocytic pleocytosis, and spirochetes may be directly visualized.

TREATMENT ℞

Borrelia is generally quite sensitive to antibiotics, which has led to recommendations for single-dose treatments. Although this may be sufficient, especially for louse-borne disease, recent reports suggest that silent residual infections occur and may best be addressed by longer treatments. For tick-borne relapsing infection, treatment should extend for 7 days to reduce the risk for persistent infection. Tetracycline, doxycycline, ceftriaxone, and erythromycin are all effective antibiotics. Erythromycin should not be used in pregnant women and children younger than 7 years (in whom tetracyclines can stain the permanent teeth). Penicillin treatment has been reported to clear the spirochetemia more slowly than tetracycline does.

The Jarisch-Herxheimer reaction (typically characterized by a rise in body temperature of 1° C, rigors, a rise in blood pressure followed by a fall, and transient leukopenia) occurs 2 to 3 hours after treatment in many patients with louse-borne disease, less commonly in tick-borne disease, and should be anticipated and managed supportively. Death as a result of shock from the Jarisch-Herxheimer reaction occurs rarely. The Jarisch-Herxheimer reaction has been associated with accelerated phagocytosis of spirochetes by neutrophils and transient elevations in tumor necrosis factor–α (TNF–α), interleukin (IL)–6, IL-8, and IL-10. In small numbers of patients with louse-borne relapsing fever, anti–TNF-α antibodies have been effective in prevention.

PREVENTION

Prevention of louse-borne relapsing fever hinges on improving hygienic conditions, delousing affected areas, and antibiotic treatment of patients and close contacts. Tick-borne relapsing fever can be prevented by reducing the risk of contact with rodents and ticks, including repair of structural flaws in cabins and other residences so rodents cannot nest in or around them, as well as spraying infested indoor environments. Tick-bite screening and prophylactic treatment with doxycycline in highly endemic areas has been reported to be a practical, safe, and effective policy in preventing tick-borne relapsing fever.

PROGNOSIS

Epidemics of louse-borne relapsing fever have been reported, with mortality rates approaching 40%; as much as 5% of the mortality is related to

Jarisch-Herxheimer reactions with treatment. Mortality from tick-borne disease is less than 5%. Autopsies of patients with louse-borne disease have documented intracranial hemorrhage, brain edema, bronchopneumonia, hepatic necrosis, and splenic infarcts.

GENERAL REFERENCES

For the General References and other additional features, please visit Expert Consult at https://expertconsult.inkling.com.

307

LEPTOSPIROSIS

SHERIF ZAKI AND WUN-JU SHIEH

DEFINITION

Leptospirosis is a zoonotic disease caused by pathogenic *Leptospira* species spirochetes. Leptospirosis is distributed worldwide and is most prevalent in tropical developing countries. Leptospires frequently infect wild and domestic mammals. Humans are infected directly by contact with infected animals or indirectly through contact with soil or water contaminated by urine from infected animals. Disease severity ranges from mild and self-limiting to severe with life-threatening manifestations, including massive pulmonary hemorrhage and Weil disease (the triad of jaundice, acute renal failure, and bleeding).[1]

The Pathogen

Leptospires are thin, coiled, highly motile spirochetes in the *Leptospira* genus of the Leptospiraceae family. They measure 6 to 20 microns in length and 0.1 μm in diameter. One or both ends of the spirochete are usually hooked. They are obligate aerobes that can survive for several weeks in the environment. *Leptospira* is currently genetically classified into ten pathogenic species (*L. interrogans, L. kirschneri, L. borgpetersenii, L. santarosai, L. noguchii, L. weilii, L. alexanderi, L. alstoni, L. kmetyi, L. mayottensis*), five intermediate or opportunistic species, (*L. inadai, L. broomii, L. fainei, L. wolffii, L. licerasiae*), and

seven nonpathogenic species. Pathogenic leptospires are further classified into over 25 serogroups and 250 serovars that differ by geographic distribution and host specificity, which is useful information for outbreak and other epidemiologic investigations.

EPIDEMIOLOGY

Over 350,000 cases of leptospirosis are estimated to occur each year worldwide and are generally underreported. In the United States, leptospirosis is a nationally notifiable disease. The National Notifiable Diseases Surveillance System (NNDSS) began receiving case notifications for leptospirosis in 2014. In the first two years of notifications combined (2014 to 2015), the total case count for leptospirosis was 203 cases reported from 17 states, jurisdictions, and territories, with 114 total cases reported from Puerto Rico, 45 from Hawaii, and 11 from Guam.[2] The majority of infections are mild and self-limiting, but case fatality in reported cases may be as high as 10%. In endemic areas, up to 20 to 30% of cases with acute undiagnosed febrile illness may be due to leptospirosis,[3] and seroprevalence can range from 5 to 15%. Leptospirosis most often affects people who work outdoors or with animals, or those who take part in recreational activities involving water or soil, like swimming, boating, and gardening. After floods, heavy rains, or other natural disasters, anyone who has been in contact with floodwater, contaminated freshwater, or soil could be at risk for infection. The major groups at risk are slum dwellers, subsistence farmers, and animal workers, owing to exposure to rodent, domestic, and wild animal reservoirs. In both tropical and temperate climates, the urban poor are an underrecognized population at risk. Humans are considered accidental hosts; rare human-to-human transmission by transplacental infection and breast-feeding has been reported.

PATHOBIOLOGY

Leptospires can directly penetrate abraded skin and mucous membranes and spread hematogenously to target organs. The classic illness is biphasic, with the first phase characterized by leptospiremia and the second phase with organism clearance by agglutinating antibodies and an associated host response that can be immunopathogenic.[4] Leptospires can persist for a period of time in target organs. In asymptomatic reservoir animals, leptospires can reach massive densities within the renal tubules, resulting in continuous urinary excretion. Pathologic findings may include pulmonary hemorrhage, diffuse alveolar damage, mild to marked hepatocellular dissociation, mild portal hepatitis, lymphohistiocytic interstitial nephritis, renal tubular necrosis, and mild renal glomerular mesangial hyperplasia (Fig. 307-1).[5] Hemorrhage in other

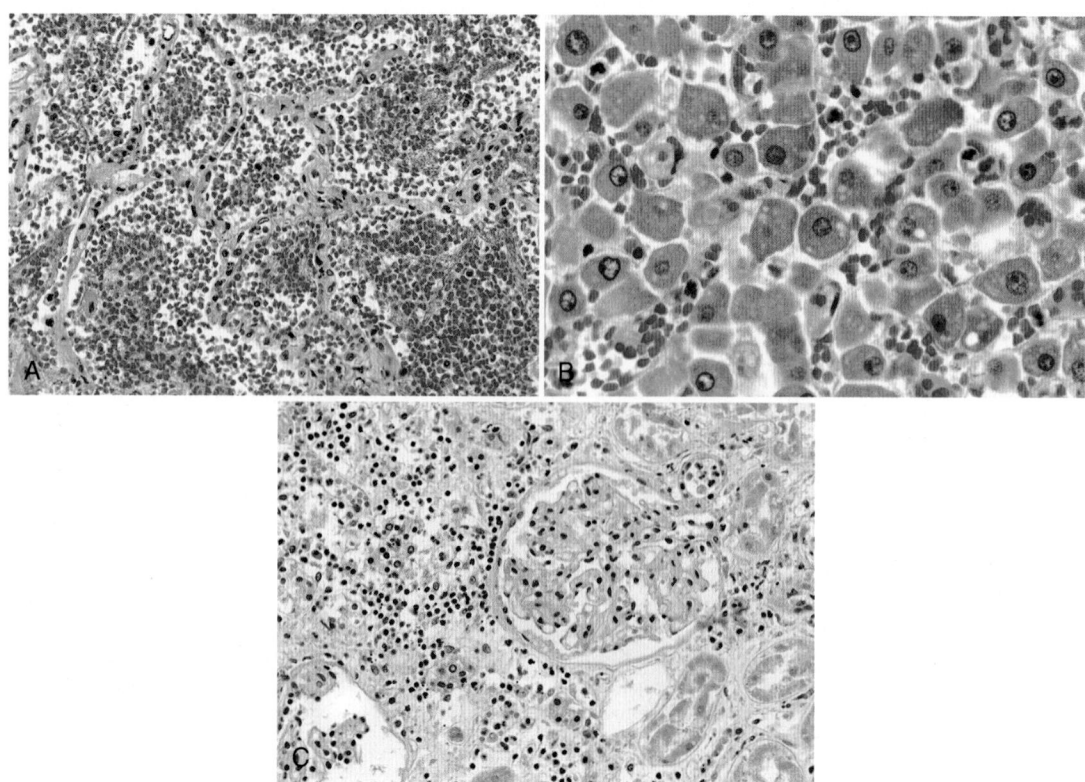

FIGURE 307-1. Pathologic features of severe leptospirosis. A, Pulmonary hemorrhage. B, Hepatocellular dissociation. C, Interstitial nephritis.

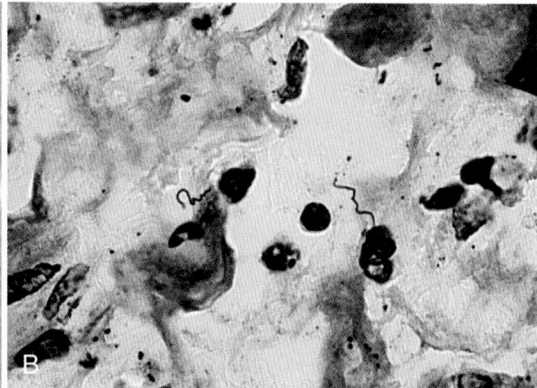

FIGURE 307-2. *Leptospira* in liver. Note the coiled nature of the spirochetes. **A,** Immunohistochemistry showing spirochetal and granular antigen staining. **B,** Warthin-Starry silver stain showing spirochetes.

organs, multifocal myocarditis, myositis, and hemophagocytosis may also be present. By immunohistochemistry or silver stains (Fig. 307-2), leptospires can be seen within the renal interstitium, hepatic parenchyma and sinusoids, and within the walls of small, medium, and large pulmonary blood vessels.

Leptospire tissue penetration may be mediated by a burrowing motion and secreted enzymes including collagenase and sphingomyelinase. Leptospiral proteins interact directly with host extracellular matrix components such as collagen, fibronectin, and laminins. Leptospires are resistant to the alternative pathway of complement-mediated lysis and can bind inhibitory complement factor H. Leptospiral lipopolysaccharides and lipopeptides have low endotoxic potency but can activate innate immune response through toll-like receptor (TLR)-2 signaling and are thought to generate a cytokine response.[6] Immunity is considered to be primarily humoral and serotype specific. Circulating immune complexes may contribute to renal damage and endothelial dysfunction. An expansion of γδ T cells occurs during infection. Leptospires may also directly activate plasminogen to plasmin, the main enzyme of the fibrinolytic system, which could promote hemorrhage. Genomic studies of pathogenic intermediate and saprophytic *Leptospira* species have revealed a relatively large genome that contains genes involved in environmental survival, chemotaxis, and motility that may be involved in pathogenesis. Little is known about host genetic risk factors, although the HLA-DQ6 allele has been associated with increased susceptibility to infection.

CLINICAL MANIFESTATIONS

The incubation period is typically 7 to 12 days (range, 2 to 30 days). During the early phase of illness (first 3 to 7 days), the majority of patients present with high fever (38° to 40° C) and myalgia. Cough, nausea and vomiting, diarrhea, headache, photophobia, and rash may be seen. Conjunctival suffusion is a characteristic finding (Fig. 307-3), but it is only seen in a third of patients near the end of early-phase illness. Myalgia may be pronounced and most frequently involves the calves and lumbar musculature, with creatine phosphokinase elevation. Severe cervical and abdominal myalgia may mimic nuchal rigidity or an acute abdomen, respectively. Rash occurs in 10 to 20% of patients and may be urticarial, maculopapular, or purpuric in a typically pretibial and truncal distribution. Hepatosplenomegaly and lymphadenopathy may also be present. Resolution of symptoms coincides with the presence of agglutinating immunoglobulin (Ig)M antibodies and reduction in leptospiremia. As a classic biphasic disease, fever may recur 3 to 4 days after remission. In this later immune phase, severe headache is often present and can be associated with photophobia, meningeal signs, and cerebrospinal fluid (CSF) pleocytosis.

Severe disease may occur progressively at initial presentation or during late-phase leptospirosis and result in 10 to 50% mortality. Life-threatening manifestations are renal failure, hypotension, hemorrhage, and respiratory failure. Jaundice occurs in 5 to 10% of patients, and serum bilirubin levels can be elevated up to 40 to 80 mg/dL, with only moderate and minor elevations in transaminase and alkaline phosphatase levels, respectively. Leptospirosis may present as acute cholecystitis. Long-term hepatic sequelae are typically not seen. Renal findings are typically of nonoliguric hypokalemic renal insufficiency and impaired tubular sodium reabsorption. Volume loss may result in oliguric renal insufficiency and acute tubular necrosis, and renal failure occurs in about half of severe cases. Common urinalysis findings are proteinuria, white blood cells, hematuria, and hyaline and granular casts.

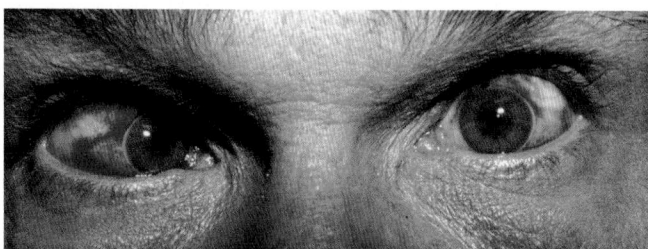

FIGURE 307-3. Conjunctival suffusion in a patient with severe leptospirosis. Conjunctival suffusion is a characteristic sign of leptospirosis and best seen along the right upper palpebral border above the subconjunctival hemorrhage. (Courtesy Antonio Seguro and Paulo Marotto, Hospital Emílio Ribas and Universidade de São Paulo.)

Pulmonary findings may include cough, dyspnea, and hemoptysis. Leptospirosis-associated pulmonary hemorrhage and acute respiratory distress syndrome is now recognized as a common clinical presentation.[7] The most frequent radiographic findings in patients with leptospirosis causing diffuse alveolar hemorrhage are ground-glass opacities, airspace nodules, ground-glass nodules, and consolidations.[8] Cardiac conduction abnormalities can be seen and tend to be nonspecific in mild disease. First-degree atrioventricular block and features of pericarditis are the most common findings in severe disease. Arrhythmias including ventricular fibrillation may also occur.

Thrombocytopenia is a frequent complication in leptospirosis, and this condition has been reported to be present in more than half of patients at the time of hospital admission. Lengthy disease and acute kidney injury are risk factors for thrombocytopenia. Prothrombin and partial thromboplastin times are typically normal or only mildly elevated. Petechiae, conjunctival hemorrhage, and purpura can be seen in addition to the more severe hemorrhagic manifestations.

Aseptic meningitis is the most frequent neurologic manifestation. Cerebrospinal fluid (CSF) findings include pleocytosis with neutrophil predominance in early disease, followed by lymphocyte predominance in later disease. Glucose is generally normal, and CSF pressure may be elevated. Less common are intracerebral hemorrhage, encephalitis, myelitis, and peripheral neuropathy. Ocular leptospirosis, including chronic uveitis, is thought to be primarily caused by an immunopathogenic mechanism and occurs late in the disease process.

DIAGNOSIS

Few clinical signs differentiate early-stage leptospirosis, and severe leptospirosis may be recognized in the form of Weil disease that is characterized by hepatorenal failure. Reference tests require specialized laboratories, and there is a need for point-of-care testing in tropical areas. Culture and serologic assays may provide false negatives.

Culture of the organism requires specialized media (Ellinghausen-McCullough-Johnson-Harris [EMJH] or Fletcher media), with often more than 4 weeks needed with observation under darkfield microscopy. Cultures generally have low sensitivity, with the best yield obtained from peripheral blood during days 1 through 4 of the acute illness; urine may be positive for up to day 10. Direct darkfield microscopy of clinical specimens can also be attempted but has low sensitivity and specificity.

The gold standard serologic test is the microagglutination test (MAT), available at the U.S. Centers for Disease Control and Prevention. MAT is considered positive if there is a four-fold rise in titer between acute and convalescent sera. This assay requires cultured *Leptospira*; it provides serotype data and has a very high specificity but lower sensitivity. U.S. Food and Drug Administration–approved IgM enzyme-linked immunosorbent assay (ELISA) and indirect hemagglutination assays are also available and appear to be as good as MAT. Multiple lateral flow rapid diagnostic "dipstick" tests are manufactured and used in other countries; however, their performance may not be well validated. Diagnostic polymerase chain reaction (PCR) assays are the most sensitive test overall, but combined PCR and MAT, supplemented by regionally validated ELISA testing, may be needed to maximize sensitivity.[9,10] Organisms within tissues can be detected by Warthin-Starry silver stain or immunohistochemistry.

Differential Diagnosis

As previously discussed, few clinical or laboratory findings differentiate leptospirosis from other causes of acute fever. Differential diagnosis depends on other concurrent diseases in the geographic area, most frequently malaria, dengue, typhoid fever, melioidosis, scrub typhus, and rickettsial diseases. Other diseases in the differential include influenza, acute viral hepatitis, yellow fever, bacterial and viral meningitis, bacterial sepsis, Zika virus, chikungunya virus, and hantavirus infection. A high index of suspicion is needed in endemic areas. Useful diagnostic clues are conjunctival suffusion, muscle tenderness, and pulmonary bleeding. Hypokalemia, elevated creatinine, elevated creatine phosphokinase, and thrombocytopenia are nonspecific but may also suggest leptospirosis.

TREATMENT   Rx

The World Health Organization guidelines and widespread clinical practice are to treat patients early with antibiotics for leptospirosis. Penicillin, doxycycline, or a cephalosporin appear to be equally efficacious, and doxycycline has the advantage of also treating rickettsial infections. Of note, a recent meta-analysis of five randomized trials concluded that the role of various antibiotics in treatment of leptospirosis is uncertain, and there is insufficient "grade A" evidence to recommend for or against the use of antibiotics to treat leptospirosis.[A1] Additional randomized controlled trials are needed.

Treatment regimens for mild leptospirosis include doxycycline (100 mg PO bid), ampicillin (500 mg PO q6h), amoxicillin (500 mg PO q8h), or azithromycin (1 g followed by 500 mg daily for 2 days); and for severe disease, intravenous (IV) penicillin (1.5 million units q6h), ceftriaxone (1 g daily), cefotaxime (1 g q6h), or doxycycline (100 mg IV q12h). Treatment duration is typically 7 days. The Jarisch-Herxheimer reaction (JHR), a febrile inflammatory reaction that occurs with initiation of treatment and results from clearance of the organism from the circulation, can occur in 20% of patients who receive antibiotics treatment.[11] Two risk factors have been independently associated with JHR occurrence: (1) *Leptospira interrogans* serogroup Australis as the infecting strain; and (2) starting antibiotics earlier than 3 days after symptom onset. Therefore, patients require monitoring at initiation of antibiotics.

Prompt triage of high-risk patients and aggressive supportive care are essential. Hypotension should be treated, and volume repletion is useful in limiting renal damage. Patients with nonoliguric hypokalemic renal insufficiency may be treated by intravenous volume and potassium repletion. Prompt dialysis is indicated for oliguric renal insufficiency, either by continuous hemofiltration or by peritoneal dialysis. Serial electrocardiograms are helpful to monitor for arrhythmia. Aggressive therapy may be needed to treat hemorrhage and respiratory failure.

PREVENTION

Preventive measures include sanitation to prevent population exposure to contaminated water, and limiting water contamination by animal reservoirs such as dogs, pigs, and cattle. Vaccination is available for domestic and livestock animals. Rodent control is important. Workers with occupational exposure to animals or contaminated water or soil are encouraged to use protective equipment such as gloves and boots. Travelers to endemic areas should be counseled on fresh water exposure. A vaccine is not available for human use within the United States. Vaccine trials have been performed in Cuba, Russia, and China; however, vaccine safety and efficacy are uncertain.

Prophylaxis with doxycycline (200 mg PO weekly) is widely used for persons with exposure to contaminated water or at high risk for leptospirosis. Prophylaxis may work better in reducing risk of clinical disease for short-term travelers with high risk, rather than residents in an endemic area. A single dosage of 200 mg doxycycline for prophylaxis might be effective for preventing leptospirosis among flood victims with laceration wounds after recent flood exposure[A2]; additional randomized controlled trials are needed.

PROGNOSIS

The majority of infections are self-limiting, and the median case fatality among patients who seek medical attention is about 2%. Severe leptospirosis is associated with a higher mortality: about 12% in patients with renal failure, about 20% in patients with jaundice, and about 60% in patients over age 60 years.[12] Death is more frequent during infection if there is oliguria, pulmonary hemorrhage, or respiratory insufficiency. Ocular disease, including chronic uveitis, may result in severe visual impairment.

Grade A References

A1. Charan J, Saxena D, Mulla S, et al. Antibiotics for the treatment of leptospirosis: systematic review and meta-analysis of controlled trials. *Int J Prev Med.* 2013;4:501-510.
A2. Schneider MC, Velasco-Hernandez J, Min KD, et al. The use of chemoprophylaxis after floods to reduce the occurrence and impact of leptospirosis outbreaks. *Int J Environ Res Public Health.* 2017;14:1-18.

GENERAL REFERENCES

For the General References and other additional features, please visit Expert Consult at https://expertconsult.inkling.com.

308

TUBERCULOSIS

JERROLD J. ELLNER AND KAREN R. JACOBSON

DEFINITION

Tuberculosis (TB) is a chronic granulomatous disease with a unique latent stage caused by the acid-fast bacillus (AFB) *Mycobacterium tuberculosis*. The lung is a site of disease in 75 to 80% of cases; frequent extrapulmonary sites are the lymph nodes, pleura, bones, and joints. TB is spread from person to person primarily by inhalation of infectious droplet nuclei aerosolized by patients with active pulmonary TB. TB is the leading infectious disease killer globally, with over 95% of cases and 99% of deaths occurring in resource-limited settings. The human immunodeficiency virus (HIV) pandemic led to a resurgence of TB worldwide and promoted explosive nosocomial outbreaks of multiple-drug resistant TB. The result was increased attention to TB as a global public health emergency and increased funding for TB control and research. The problems posed for TB control are compounded by increasing prevalence of drug-resistant disease that is expensive to treat and may be refractory to available drugs.[1]

The Pathogen

TB is caused by infection with one of four members of the *Mycobacterium tuberculosis* complex: *M. tuberculosis*, *M. africanum*, *M. orygis* or *M. bovis*. The causative organism is a slender, non-motile, non–spore-forming, non–toxin-producing bacillus that may be beaded in appearance and is approximately 2 to 4 µm in length. It is a slow-growing (doubling time of 18 to 24 hours) facultative aerobe that can persist intracellularly for prolonged periods. The organism is identified in clinical specimens as an acid-fast bacillus (AFB). *M. tuberculosis* can be stained with carbol fuchsin by either alkalinization (Kinyoun) or heat (Ziehl-Neelsen) methods. The waxy coat of *M. tuberculosis*, composed of mycolic acid and other complex lipopolysaccharides, precludes decolorization of the stain with a mixture of acid and alcohol.

DNA sequencing of *M. tuberculosis* and genetic manipulations have promoted basic understanding of the metabolism and virulence of the organism, its immunodominant antigens, and capacity to survive adverse conditions and persist intracellularly. Clinical isolates of *M. tuberculosis* differ in their virulence, potential for transmission in humans, and interaction with the host (immunopathology, induction of host cytokines, delayed-type hypersensitivity). For example,

TABLE 308-1 RISK FACTORS FOR TUBERCULOSIS			
RISK FACTOR	**INCREASED RISK OF RECENT INFECTION***	**INCREASED RISK OF PROGRESSION FROM INFECTION TO DISEASE**	**TST CUT POINT**
Household contact of PTB	X		>5 mm
Solid organ transplant recipients, immunosuppressive treatment (TNF inhibitors, prednisone >15 mg/day for >1 month), fibrotic lesions on chest radiograph consistent with prior TB		X	>5 mm
HIV infection	X	X	>5 mm
Foreign-born, injecting drug users, TST-positive children, adolescents, young adults	X		>10 mm
Residents or workers in hospitals, homeless shelters, correctional facilities, nursing homes, residences for the HIV-infected	X		>10 mm
Underweight (>15%), silicosis, diabetes mellitus (particularly insulin-dependent or poorly controlled), renal failure, hemodialysis, gastrectomy, jejuno-ileal bypass, carcinoma of the head and neck, lung cancer, lymphoma, leukemia		X	>10 mm
None			>15 mm

*Recent infection per se increases risk of progressing from infection to disease (12.9 cases per 1000 person-years in the first year compared to 1.6 per 1000 person-years in the subsequent 7 years).
HIV = human immunodeficiency virus; PTB = pulmonary TB; TNF = tumor necrosis factor; TST = tuberculin skin test.

the hypervirulent Beijing strain family overexpresses a phenolic glycolipid that inhibits innate immunity and may thereby contribute to its pathogenicity.

There are six main phylogeographic lineages of *M. tuberculosis*, each associated with a specific human population. The families differ in geographic distribution and in some cases the potential for transmission and pathogenesis. Strain typing is particularly useful in outbreak investigations and can be performed by several techniques, including restriction fragment length polymorphism of the insertional element IS 6110 or spoligotyping, and increasingly by deep DNA sequencing. The finding that multiple cases of TB are caused by the same strain and constitute a "cluster" suggests that they are epidemiologically linked although transmission may be recent or remote. Whole-genomic sequencing has emerged as a powerful tool to establish transmission even absent strong epidemiologic links.

TB caused by *M. africanum* is clinically identical to that caused by *M. tuberculosis*. *M. bovis* has greater than 95% DNA homology with *M. tuberculosis* and causes disease in humans, cattle, deer, badgers, and other animals. The main route of transmission of *M. tuberculosis* is person-to-person through respiratory aerosols generated by coughing. Bacilli in small droplet nuclei (1 to 5 μm in diameter) remain suspended in air for long periods and once inhaled can reach the airways, where only 1 to 5 organisms are sufficient to cause infection. Laryngeal involvement renders the patient highly infectious. Direct cutaneous inoculation ("prosector's wart") does occur. *M. bovis* can be transmitted by the gastrointestinal route, usually through ingestion of contaminated dairy products.

EPIDEMIOLOGY

The World Health Organization (WHO) estimates that in 2016 there were 10.4 million new cases of TB (10% in HIV-infected persons) and 1.7 million deaths (including 374,000 among people with HIV infection).[2] An estimated 40% of deaths in persons with HIV were due to TB. Fifty-six percent of TB cases were in five countries: India, Indonesia, China, the Philippines, and Pakistan. Worldwide, 65% of TB cases occur in males; the prevalence of disease peaks in young adults, with major economic consequence. Globally, both TB incidence (declining 2% per year) and case-fatality rates have been falling. However, TB incidence decline needs to accelerate to 4 to 5% annually to reach the WHO's 2020 *End TB Strategy* Milestones of 20% incidence reduction compared to 2015.

HIV infection has a profound effect on the epidemiology of TB, promoting and accelerating progression from infection to active TB, and on both reactivation and reinfection disease. Seventy-four percent of HIV-infected TB cases are in sub-Saharan Africa, resulting in TB case rates as high as 1% in South Africa and Swaziland.

In the United States in 2017 the incidence of TB was 2.8 per 100,000, with about 9000 new cases reported (about 6% were HIV-infected, 5% homeless, and 4.0% incarcerated).[3] The incidence rate in foreign-born individuals was 13-fold higher than in those born in the United States and foreign-born individuals accounted for 69% of new cases. Rates were 30-fold higher in non-Hispanic Asians than non-Hispanic whites. Of genotyped cases, 14% appear due to recent transmission versus 86% that appear to be reactivation of previous infection, which in foreign-born was due to acquisition in their country of origin whereas U.S.-born more likely acquired when TB was more common domestically. There is a corresponding shift of age-specific prevalence of TB in the United States towards older adults.

Country of origin is a large determinant of both the risk of latent TB infection and of TB disease. In a low-prevalence setting such as the United States, the prevalence of latent TB infection (defined as a positive tuberculin skin test or interferon-γ release assay [IGRA] but no active disease) is approximately 4%. An estimated 13 million people have latent TB in the United States.[4] Those infected are at markedly increased risk of disease compared to uninfected, a risk that is further increased by medical comorbidities and other factors shown in Table 308-1. The risk is not homogeneous within groups affected, for example, by extent of immunosuppression in HIV or duration, severity, and control of diabetes. Smoking and alcoholism also confer an increased risk for TB, although smaller than the conditions listed. In the United States in 2016, 16.4% of persons with TB had diabetes, 1.3% reported injecting drugs, 6.8% reported using noninjectable drugs, and 10% reported excessive alcohol use.

TB caused by drug-resistant organisms is a continuing threat.[5] Multidrug-resistant (MDR) TB (resistant to isoniazid [INH] and rifampin) and extensively drug-resistant TB (MDR plus resistance to fluoroquinolones [FQs] and to a second-line injectable [kanamycin, amikacin, or capreomycin]) are much more difficult and expensive to treat and in some cases may be incurable. In 2016, there were 600,000 new TB cases with rifampin resistance, the most effective first-line drug, of which 490,000 had MDR TB. Almost one-half (47%) of these cases were in India, China, and the Russian Federation. About 6.2% of MDR TB cases are extensively drug-resistant. Ninety-seven U.S. cases of MDR TB and one case of extensively drug-resistant TB were reported in 2016. Outcomes for drug-resistant TB remain poor, with only 54% of MDR TB patients and 30% of XDR TB patients successfully treated. This should improve with the introduction of more active drugs and drug regimens. The majority of cases of XDR TB in an area with a high TB burden were found to be probably due to transmission rather than to inadequate treatment, suggesting that control of the epidemic requires an increased focus on interruption of transmission.[6]

PATHOBIOLOGY

Typically the chain of transmission of TB begins with an infectious case of pulmonary TB (Fig. 308-1). Infectiousness of a patient is determined by sputum smear status (3 to 4+ AFB), cough strength and frequency, the presence of cavitary lung disease, and the characteristics of the physical space shared with the source (ventilation and air recirculation). However, not all strongly AFB smear–positive patients with pulmonary TB are equally infectious, and there may be high transmitters, owing to host or bacterial factors or both. Only about 50 to 60% of strongly sputum smear–positive persons with pulmonary TB generate aerosols that contain viable organisms. Certain strains of *M. tuberculosis* also may be transmission-prone.

In both low- and high-prevalence countries, exposure/infection may occur in the household. In this setting, where exposure may be intense and protracted, 50 to 75% of contacts become infected. The higher numbers result from studies in which repeated testing identifies all tuberculin skin test convertors. In

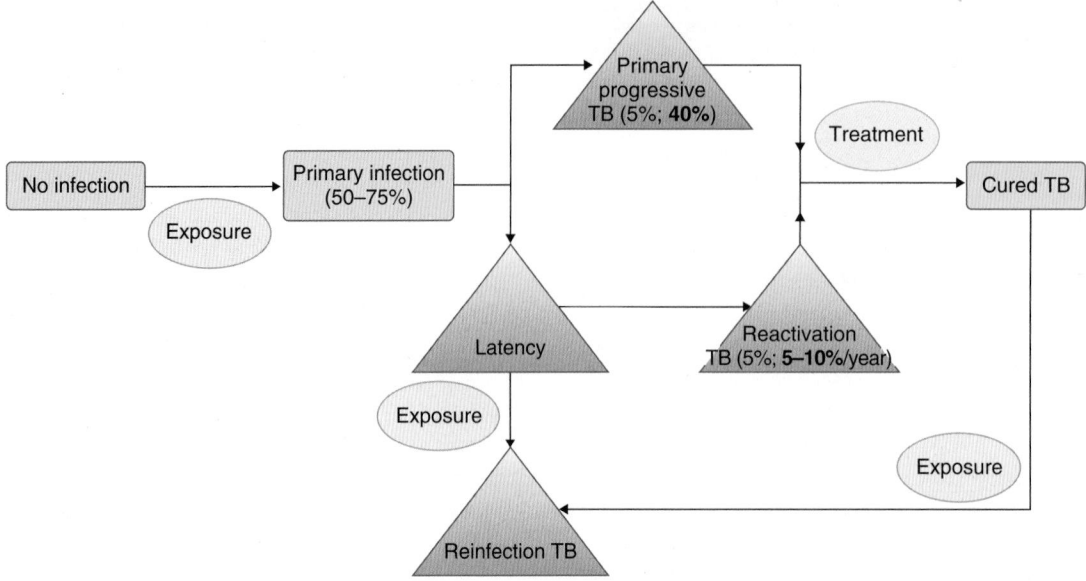

FIGURE 308-1. Natural history of TB. The proportion of individuals affected is shown in parentheses. Bolded figures are for HIV infection with severe immunosuppression. A number of medical risk factors besides HIV promote progression from *Mycobacterium tuberculosis* infection to disease (see Table 308-1).

outbreaks occurring in residential shelters, hospitals, and prisons, *M. tuberculosis* infection or disease also has been documented after brief exposure. Recent data suggest that in high prevalence settings, community transmission may be more common than household transmission, although the sites in the community may not be known. Important variables that may explain differences in transmission include virulence of the organism, innate immunity, and susceptibility of the exposed populations (e.g., HIV infected). Human genetic factors such as polymorphisms in expression or regulation of toll-like receptors (TLR), pattern recognition receptors important to innate immunity, may modulate risk and expression of infection (interferon gamma release assay [IGRA] or tuberculin skin test) as well as risk and expression of disease. Predisposition to disease is seen with defects in interferon (IFN)-γ and interleukin (IL)-12 receptors, consistent with their role in adaptive immunity. Polymorphisms that modify inflammation (e.g., by affecting leukotriene A$_4$ hydrolase) also may affect disease manifestations and response to therapy.

Two models of the natural history of TB are shown in Figures 308-1 and 308-2. There is increasing evidence that the natural history represents a continuum rather than distinct entities of latent and active TB. Diagnostic biomarkers that stratify risk of progression from latent TB infection to active TB would be of enormous value for targeting public health interventions. Host blood RNA signatures are currently being studied as predictors of those most at risk of developing active tuberculosis and therefore preferentially receive prophylaxis.

The lung is the site of most cases of reactivation TB. The hallmark of the pathology is granuloma formation with caseation necrosis and multinucleated Langerhans giant cells. The caseous material found in necrotic cavities contains AFB. *M. tuberculosis* multiplies exuberantly in the liquid caseum. Immunologically, expectorated sputum contains cytokines and both upregulators and downregulators of the immune and inflammatory response, the downregulation being dominant. Bronchoalveolar lavage shows a lymphocytic alveolitis, with an influx of immature macrophages representing monocytes attracted from blood. In sum, there is an active but well-regulated immune and inflammatory response concomitant with bacterial replication. As a consequence of the inflammation, extensive apoptosis occurs that might lead to the deletion of *M. tuberculosis*-responsive T cells, that may play a role in the requirement for a long duration of therapy. This is consistent with the recent finding of persistent areas of inflammation (by PET-CT scan) at the end of TB treatment, and in the susceptibility to reinfection TB. In HIV-infected persons with advanced immunosuppression, granulomas may be poorly formed or absent. Lung tissue is infiltrated with foamy epithelioid cells that are macrophages laden with AFBs. Caseation may or may not be present, but there is extensive inflammation and necrosis.

Extrapulmonary TB can involve any organ. Persistence of organisms in areas that are relatively well oxygenated may explain the more frequent sites of reactivation, such as the apices of the lung, cortices of the kidney, and vertebral bodies.

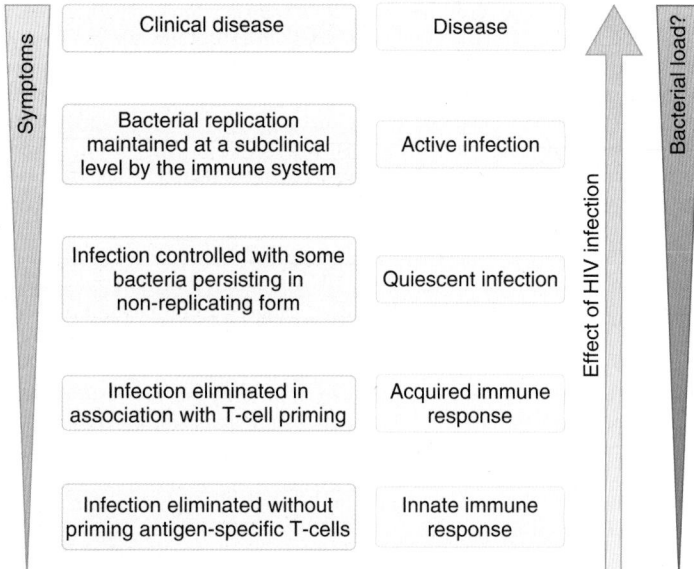

FIGURE 308-2. Tuberculosis infection as a spectrum. The outcome of infection by *Mycobacterium tuberculosis* is generally represented as a bimodal distribution between active tuberculosis (TB) and latent TB on the basis of the presence or absence of clinical symptoms. It is proposed that latent TB is usefully represented as part of a spectrum of responses to infection. One consequence of this model is that there may be a subpopulation within the group that is currently defined as having latent TB that should be preferentially targeted for preventive therapy. A second consequence is that efforts to develop drugs for effective treatment of latent TB would overlap the search for drugs that shorten treatment times for active TB. (From Barry CE 3rd, Boshoff HI, Dartois V, et al. The spectrum of latent tuberculosis. Rethinking the biology and intervention strategies. *Nat Rev Microbiol.* 2009;7:845-855, Figure 1.)

Several forms of extrapulmonary TB have a shared pathogenesis: discharge of a contiguous tuberculous focus into a serosal cavity, a brisk inflammatory reaction based on preexisting delayed-type hypersensitivity, fever, frequently negative smears of exudative fluid for AFBs, and sometimes a transiently negative tuberculin skin test. The site of infection that discharges may be a long-standing focus or one that was seeded during recent dissemination associated with primary infection. This basic scenario occurs in pleural TB, TB pericarditis, TB meningitis (the parameningeal focus is called a "Rich focus"), TB peritonitis, and TB arthritis.

Pleural TB represents an in situ delayed-type hypersensitivity reaction with activation of T$_H$1 helper T cells, abundant cytokines, including IFN-γ and tumor necrosis factor (TNF)-α, and apoptosis. In non–HIV-infected individuals,

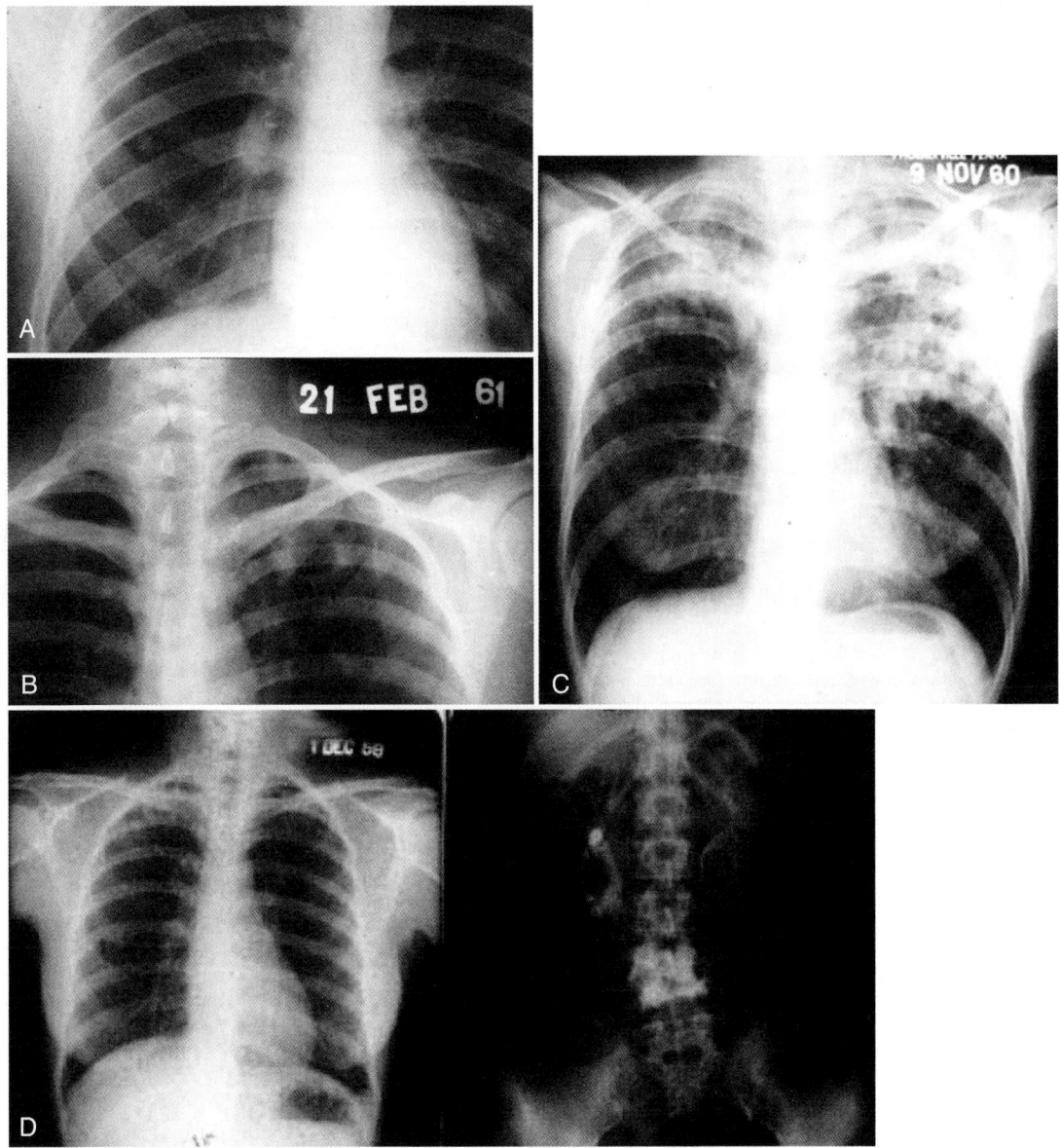

FIGURE 308-3. A, Ghon complex. B, Moderately advanced pulmonary tuberculosis (TB). C, Far advanced pulmonary TB. D, Pulmonary (*left*) and extrapulmonary (*right*) TB. (Radiographs courtesy Thomas M. Daniel, MD.)

organisms are sparse, which may be why self-cure of pleural TB can take place. However, in the absence of chemotherapy for TB, there is a high risk for TB recurrence, usually as pulmonary TB on the side contralateral to the effusion.

In addition to reactivation of a latent focus, reinfection with *M. tuberculosis* may occur and progress to disease. Reinfection is more likely if the host is immunosuppressed or if there is repeated or intense exposure. Treated cases of pulmonary TB also are predisposed to reinfection disease as discussed earlier. Latent TB infection is over 70% protective against reinfection TB.

CLINICAL MANIFESTATIONS
Primary Tuberculosis
Most cases of primary TB are unrecognized clinically except by conversion of the tuberculin skin test or IGRA. There may be fever, shortness of breath, nonproductive cough, and rarely erythema nodosum. Crepitations and focal wheezes may be present. Chest radiographs show small patchy opacities in the mid-lung fields, often with unilateral hilar lymphadenopathy. Upper or middle lobe collapse may also be seen as a result of bronchial compression by enlarged nodes or transient pleural effusion. Studies with positron emission tomographic computed tomography (PET-CT) scan show that most household contacts of infectious TB cases with a positive tuberculin skin test have mediastinal adenopathy that resolves with INH preventive therapy. HIV-infected and -uninfected persons with latent TB infection studied with this modality may show parenchymal uptake suggestive of subclinical disease. In most individuals (immunosuppression being the exception), the manifestations

of primary TB resolve without treatment, concurrent with the development of an adaptive immune response. During the subsequent period of clinical latency, evidence of the primary infection may be found as a small calcified parenchymal scar in the mid-lung fields (Ghon complex), sometimes associated with similar findings in the draining hilar nodes (Ranke complex) (Fig. 308-3A). A small scar caused by an arrested lesion in the apices of the lung is called a Simon focus.

Progressive Primary Tuberculosis
Failure to develop adaptive immunity is most common in young children, the elderly, and the immunocompromised. Progressive primary TB manifested as TB meningitis, miliary TB, or disseminated TB may develop in this setting. Primary infection also may progress to pulmonary TB within the first 1 to 2 years. In this case pulmonary TB usually is in the upper lobe and cavitary, distant from the site of primary infection. Recent data indicate that in high-prevalence areas most pulmonary TB cases represent progressive primary disease. Clinically, progressive primary and "post-primary" or reactivation TB are indistinguishable.

Reactivation (Post-primary) Tuberculosis
The terms *reactivation TB* and *post-primary TB* are used interchangeably to connote that primary TB is followed by a variable period of at least 2 years of clinical latency, after which TB develops in the setting of existing delayed-type hypersensitivity/adaptive immunity: existing sensitization to

mycobacterial antigens contributes importantly to the pathogenesis and clinical manifestations.

Pulmonary TB is the most common form of reactivation TB. Typical clinical findings in pulmonary TB consist of the insidious onset of a productive cough, night sweats, anorexia, and weight loss. Fever is present in approximately one half of those affected. Patients may be asymptomatic and the diagnosis suggested only by a chest radiograph obtained for other reasons (subclinical TB). The sputum may be purulent, blood streaked, or frankly bloody. Pleuritic chest pain may occur when there is subpleural inflammation. Dyspnea is not a hallmark of pulmonary TB, in part because thrombosis of vessels limits the perfusion of inflamed areas, so that hypoxemia is not a prominent clinical feature. Physical examination may show dullness to percussion, low-pitched amphoric (hollow-sounding) breath sounds, and occasionally crepitations that may be post-tussive. Chest radiographs often reveal more disease than suggested by physical examination (see Fig. 308-3B and C). Typically (>95% of cases), lesions are found in the apical and posterior segments of the upper lobes and the superior (dorsal) segment of the lower lobe. There is a progression from patchy opacities and consolidation to cavitation reflective of liquefaction and caseation. Advanced imaging with PET-CT shows a heterogeneity in metabolic activity of different lesions within the same patient (Fig. 308-4), which may be associated with variable response to treatment and may in some cases persist even after sterilization has been achieved. Rupture and discharge into bronchi and intrabronchial spread may lead to disease in multiple areas, including the other lung (so-called TB bronchopneumonia). There may be involvement of the larynx and middle ear. Early cavities are thin walled and evolve into characteristic chronic thick-walled cavities. Ten percent of all cavities have an air-fluid level. There may be an associated pleural effusion or rarely, with rupture of cavities into the air space, pyopneumothorax. If the disease is minimal, it may best be seen on apical lordotic chest radiographs or on CT scan. Rarely, chest radiographs are normal, and the accompanying symptoms and positive sputum smears may be the result of endobronchial lesions or rupture of a tuberculous node into the bronchi. Healing, fibrosis, and contraction obliterate small cavities, although large cavities may persist and even become the eventual nidus for an aspergilloma or a "scar" carcinoma.

In immunocompromised persons, the opacities may be located in the mid- and lower lung fields and be manifested as poorly resolving lobar or segmental pneumonitis, atelectasis, nodules, and cavities. In individuals with HIV whose CD4$^+$ count exceeds 200/μL, pulmonary TB may be typical in its manifestation. At lower CD4$^+$ counts, mid- and lower lung abnormalities are more common. At a CD4$^+$ count below 100/μL, the findings may be quite atypical, with prominent hilar and mediastinal adenopathy, pleural disease, interstitial or miliary opacities, or any combination of these manifestations. This picture resembles primary TB and, in fact, may represent progressive primary TB or reinfection disease. Chest radiographs are normal in up to 20% of persons with culture-confirmed TB, sometimes in the presence of a smear that contains AFB. In this CD4 strata, disseminated and extrapulmonary TB are the rule, with or without concurrent pulmonary TB.

Reinfection Tuberculosis

Reinfection TB is clinically indistinguishable from other forms and an important pathogenetic mechanism in high transmission settings. A documented change in the DNA fingerprint or sequence or occurrence in an outbreak setting, including among patients hospitalized in TB wards, may be the only evidence supporting the diagnosis of reinfection TB. In high TB burden settings, individuals previously successfully treated for TB may have as high as a five-fold risk compared to those with no history of developing TB disease, reflecting the high frequency of reinfection events that make up a high proportion of active cases.

Extrapulmonary Tuberculosis

Approximately 20% of cases of TB in non–HIV-infected populations are extrapulmonary (see Fig. 308-3D). In areas endemic for TB, extrapulmonary TB often occurs concurrently with pulmonary TB and is more common in children and young adults, in whom it represents progressive primary infection. By contrast, in low-prevalence areas, isolated extrapulmonary TB is more common, and there is a shift to the elderly that represents reactivation TB. HIV infection is associated with a higher frequency of extrapulmonary disease, including the more serious forms, disseminated TB and TB meningitis.

Pleural Tuberculosis

Pleural TB occurs by direct extension when a subpleural caseous focus discharges into the pleural space or through hematogenous seeding.[7] There may

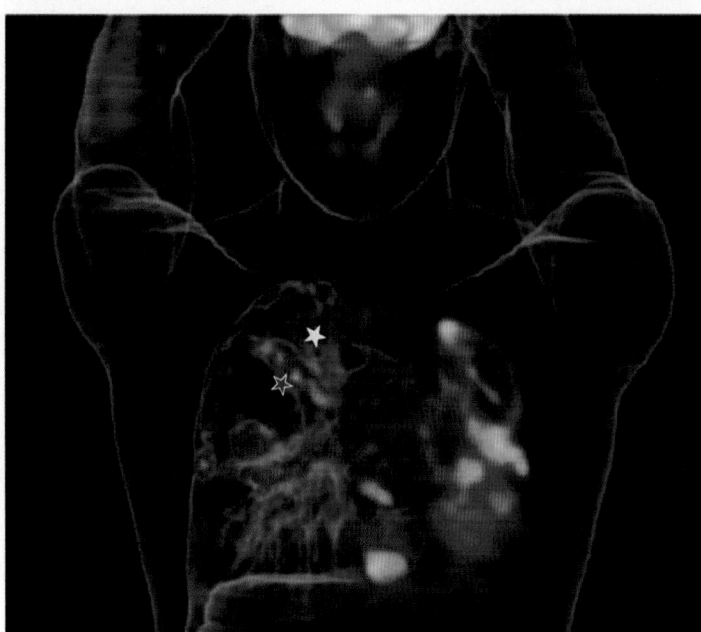

FIGURE 308-4. Positron emission tomographic computed tomography (PET-CT) imaging. An ^{18}F-fluorodeoxyglucose (FDG) PET-CT scan of a patient with tuberculosis with extensive bilateral disease and a complete collapse of the left lung. The right lung also shows extensive disease throughout and illustrates the variability of FDG-PET uptake among lesions within even a single infected patient. The yellow star illustrates one lesion that fails to take up FDG that lies immediately adjacent to a string of three lesions that take up label avidly (*red star*). These different types of lesions respond to chemotherapy with different kinetics, indicating that they represent distinct bacterial subpopulations in different microenvironments. (From Barry CE 3rd, Boshoff HI, Dartois V, et al. The spectrum of latent tuberculosis. Rethinking the biology and intervention strategies. *Nat Rev Microbiol.* 2009;7:845-855, Figure 2.)

be concurrent pulmonary TB. Its peak occurrence is 3 to 6 months after primary infection. The typical manifestation is abrupt onset of fever, pleuritic chest pain, and cough. Occasionally there is an insidious presentation consisting of fever, weight loss, and malaise. If the pleural effusion is large enough, shortness of breath may be seen. Physical examination shows dullness to percussion and decreased breath sounds. Above the area of dullness there may be true egophony. Chest radiographs typically show unilateral pleural effusion, more frequently in the right hemithorax. Bilateral disease occurs in 10% of cases. Pleural effusions may be medium-sized, large, or, uncommonly, massive.

Miliary Tuberculosis

Miliary TB usually has an insidious manifestation consisting of fever, weight loss, night sweats, and little in the way of localizing symptoms or signs. There may be concurrent TB meningitis with associated symptoms. Physical examination may show choroidal tubercles (raised white-yellow plaques on funduscopic examination, present in 15% of cases), lymphadenopathy, and hepatomegaly. Chest radiographs may show multiple bilateral small opacities termed *miliary infiltrates* because of their resemblance to millet seeds. The findings on initial chest radiographs are often subtle and may be clear-cut only in retrospect after 3 months of follow-up. Performance of CT or high-resolution CT is useful because of its increased sensitivity (Fig. 308-5). A variant of miliary TB is disseminated areactive TB, as may occur in HIV-infected patients or those treated with TNF inhibitors. In this entity, chest radiographic findings may be even more minimal or absent. In the HIV-infected individual with advanced immunodeficiency, blood cultures are positive for *M. tuberculosis* in 20 to 40% of patients and may be the only laboratory manifestation of TB.

Tuberculous Meningitis

TB meningitis is usually characterized by less than 2 weeks of fever, headache, and meningismus.[8] There may be depressed levels of consciousness, diplopia, and (rarely) hemiparesis. Physical examination shows a stiff neck and occasionally cranial neuropathy (VI, III, IV, VII in order of frequency) and long-tract signs. Chest radiographs may be consistent with pulmonary TB or miliary TB. CT of the head may show contrast enhancement over the basilar meninges, hypodense areas consistent with infarcts, hydrocephalus, and sometimes focal inflammatory lesions (tuberculomas). CT angiography may show entrapment of vessels or vasculitis.

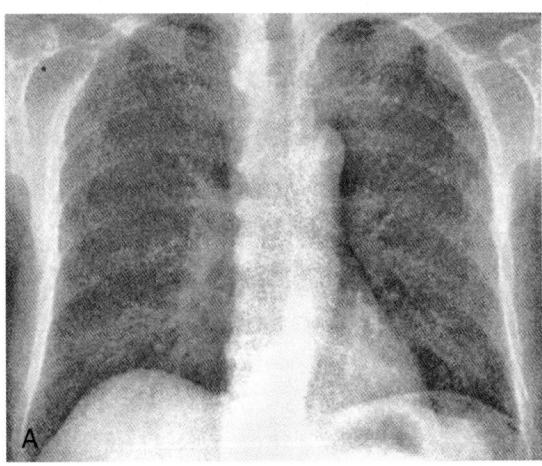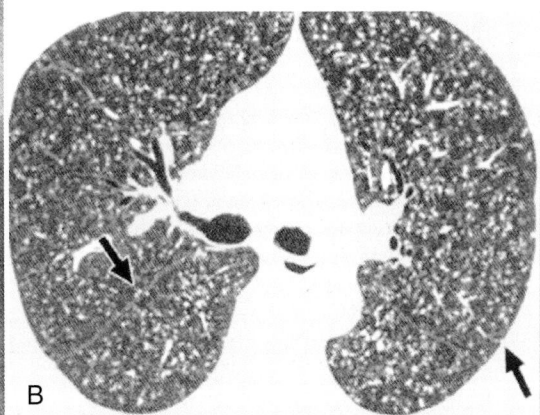

FIGURE 308-5. Miliary tuberculosis in a 70-year-old man. **A,** Posteroanterior chest radiograph shows evenly distributed, discrete, uniformly millet-sized nodular opacities in both lungs. **B,** High-resolution computed tomography (1.0-mm section thickness) at the level of the right upper lobar bronchus shows uniformly sized small nodules randomly distributed throughout both lungs. Note the subpleural and subfissural nodules (*arrows*). (From Jeong YJ, Lee KS. Pulmonary tuberculosis: up-to-date imaging and management. *AJR Am J Roentgenol.* 2008;191:834-844.)

Tuberculous Lymphadenitis

Lymphadenitis may be the sole manifestation of TB or, more frequently, particularly in the HIV infected, may accompany pulmonary TB. Patients with isolated lymph node disease may be afebrile. The supraclavicular and posterior cervical lymph nodes are most frequently involved, referred to as scrofula. This is in contrast to scrofula caused by atypical mycobacteria or *M. bovis* and often seen in children, in whom submandibular and high anterior cervical adenopathy predominates. The lymphadenitis is not usually painful although there may be tenderness and fluctuance, and aspiration of the lymph node with the finding of acid-fast bacilli (AFB) is an excellent approach to establish the diagnosis.

Tuberculous Pericarditis

The usual manifestation of TB pericarditis is chronic but may occasionally be subacute with fever, night sweats, chest pain, shortness of breath, pedal edema, and other signs of right heart failure.[9] Physical examination shows signs of pericardial disease, right-sided heart failure, and tamponade (in ≈10%). Pericardial aspiration and biopsy are the diagnostic procedures of choice. When the pericardial effusion is large or tamponade is present, a pericardial window can be both diagnostic and therapeutic.

Tuberculous Peritonitis

TB peritonitis may be accompanied by abdominal pain and fever, at times mimicking an acute abdomen. Alternatively, there may be an insidious presentation consisting of abdominal pain, swelling, night sweats, and weight loss. The clinical syndrome is caused by discharge of tuberculous lymph nodes into the peritoneal space. Exudative ascites is usually present unless TB is superimposed on preexisting transudative ascites, as in alcoholic liver disease. On physical examination, the abdomen has been described as "doughy," because matted loops of bowel may be palpable. A variant of this syndrome is perhaps best termed *abdominal TB*. In this case, the abdominal pain is subacute, the associated findings on physical examination less striking, and ascites less prominent or absent. The best method for diagnosis when ascites is present is laparoscopically guided peritoneal biopsy. In areas endemic for TB and HIV, the finding of intra-abdominal lymphadenopathy on abdominal ultrasound or CT is often used to support the diagnosis of abdominal TB.

Gastrointestinal Tuberculosis

Patients with gastrointestinal TB have fever, abdominal pain, diarrhea, and gastrointestinal bleeding or obstruction. Roentgenograms of the small bowel and abdominal CT show involvement of the terminal ileum, similar to Crohn disease. The diagnosis is made on clinical suspicion in areas endemic for TB and HIV or by the finding of TB elsewhere. Occasionally, intraluminal biopsy of the terminal ileum or other involved sites is used to establish the diagnosis.

Renal Tuberculosis

There may be few symptoms and signs associated with renal TB, although occasionally dysuria, hematuria, and flank pain are present. The diagnosis is often suggested by the finding of sterile pyuria or hematuria as initial abnormalities that trigger evaluation. Physical examination is usually unremarkable. CT shows renal cortical scarring, occasionally with mass or cavitary lesions, papillary necrosis with calyceal and ureteral dilation, or "beading" of the ureter because of ureteral strictures.

Vertebral Osteomyelitis

The initial site of disease is the subchondral region of the anterior portion of the vertebral body.[10] The lower thoracic and lumbar vertebrae are involved most commonly. The disc space is initially spared but becomes involved late with spread to adjacent vertebrae. Paravertebral "cold abscesses" may dissect through tissue planes. Patients have back and sometimes radicular pain. Occasionally and more often with cervical disease, there may be weakness of the legs and incontinence of stool and urine. Physical examination may show a gibbus deformity caused by anterior compression fractures or paraparesis. Radiographs of the spine, as well as CT and magnetic resonance imaging, may show abnormalities in adjacent vertebrae, with anterior compression (see Fig. 308-3D). Cold abscesses may be appreciated as well.

Other Forms of Extrapulmonary Tuberculosis

TB of the bone or joints may be manifested subacutely as a combination of synovitis and osteomyelitis. The joints involved may have sustained previous trauma. TB of the female genital tract may result in pelvic pain, menorrhagia, vaginal discharge, or infertility. Males may have an epididymal mass, sometimes seen in patients with miliary TB. TB also can cause granulomatous uveitis as well as phlyctenular keratitis.

DIAGNOSIS

Infection with *Mycobacterium Tuberculosis*

The diagnosis of latent TB infection (we will use the term LTBI because it still is standard, although a better term is MTB infection) is based on the finding of delayed-type hypersensitivity to mycobacterial antigens and the absence of clinically active TB. The tuberculin skin test has been used widely, and there is strong epidemiologic evidence supporting its interpretation. Tuberculin purified protein derivative (PPD) derived from autoclaved culture filtrates of *M. tuberculosis* is used to elicit delayed-type hypersensitivity. The response elicited by PPD is nonspecific because of broad cross-reactivity among tuberculous and nontuberculous mycobacteria and other organisms as well. The tuberculin skin test is performed by injecting 5 tuberculin units of PPD in 0.1 mL intradermally. The reaction is assessed as induration after 48 to 72 hours. Problems with the tuberculin skin test are legion. It is the only bioassay used in clinical medicine, and its accuracy depends strongly on correct user application and interpretation The sensitivity of the tuberculin skin test is less in immunosuppressed patients, such as those with HIV infection, and also less in the presence of active TB. The tuberculin skin test may revert to negative over time, and it may be boosted by the repeat application of PPD. On repeat testing the result is a "pseudoconversion" that does not represent new infection with *M. tuberculosis*. The greatest limitation of the tuberculin skin test is its nonspecificity. There has been uncertainty in its interpretation, particularly in the setting of previous vaccination with *M. bovis* bacille Calmette-Guérin (BCG). In fact, BCG administered once at birth has little effect on the tuberculin skin test beyond the first year. By 10 years of age, only 1% of positive tuberculin skin tests can be ascribed to previous BCG administration.

The tuberculin skin test remains of value in the diagnosis of latent TB infection in at-risk individuals who are candidates for treatment (preventive therapy). Interpretation of the tuberculin skin test is based on a "sliding scale" that takes into account an individual's a priori risk for *M. tuberculosis* infection (see Table 308-1). Changing the cut point for positives, in effect, modifies the sensitivity and specificity of the tuberculin skin test. Routine testing is not recommended for low-risk populations; however, testing may be performed because of employment. Certain populations should undergo annual testing, including staff or individuals living or working in congregate settings (hospital staff, incarcerated, homeless, HIV-infected, correctional facility staff), injection drug users, and others at risk because of sociodemographic factors. For individuals who will undergo an annual tuberculin skin test, a true baseline should be established by two-step skin testing. After the initial negative tuberculin skin test, the test is repeated in 1 to 3 weeks (there is no need to repeat the test if the first tuberculin skin test is positive). An increased reaction size on the second tuberculin skin test is known as "boosting" and may be due to previous infection with non-tuberculous mycobacteria or *M. tuberculosis* or vaccination with BCG. Tuberculin skin test conversion from negative to positive is the best indicator of intervening new infection with *M. tuberculosis* and is defined as an increase in reaction (induration) size of 6 mm or greater from less than 10 mm to 10 mm or greater. It also may be of value to perform a two-step tuberculin skin test on individuals older than 60 years and therefore at risk for tuberculin skin test reversion.

In HIV infection, the tuberculin skin test may be negative before administration of antiretroviral therapy (ART) and convert to positive with treatment. For this reason, it is recommended that the tuberculin skin test be repeated in tuberculin skin test–negative HIV-infected persons once their CD4$^+$ count reaches 200/μL and annually thereafter.

The sensitivity of the tuberculin skin test is decreased in individuals with active TB, more so in certain forms of extrapulmonary TB. Though insensitive for the diagnosis of active TB, the tuberculin skin test has another application in low-prevalence areas. If the differential diagnosis of a clinical condition includes TB, establishment of previous *M. tuberculosis* infection increases the likelihood that the clinical findings represent TB. The tuberculin skin test is of particular value in the evaluation of smear-negative patients with pulmonary disease suggestive of pulmonary TB and in patients suspected of having extrapulmonary TB. Confirmatory findings such as positive PCR, culture, or histology, response to therapy, and lack of an alternative diagnosis are necessary to establish the diagnosis of TB.

Interferon gamma releasing assays (IGRAs) (QuantiFERON-TB PLUS, T-test) have also been approved for the diagnosis of latent TB infection, and the CDC considers them interchangeable with the tuberculin skin test for individuals over 2 years of age. The assays represent in vitro cell culture in which blood cells are stimulated with a mix of antigens present in *M. tuberculosis* but not in BCG and most nontuberculous mycobacteria. The main advantage of IGRAs is specificity and ability to have interpretable results with only one patient visit. The disadvantages of IGRAs are expense, technical requirements, and controversy over test sensitivity in certain situations such as HIV infection and in household contacts of patients with pulmonary TB. Another issue has been instability of the result in individuals undergoing annual testing with IGRAs close to the cut point. That said, IGRAs have come to replace TST in many settings due to the single visit requirement, lack of need for operator experience, and higher specificity. Another factor is the current worldwide shortage of PPD.

Because treatment of latent TB infection is effective in tuberculin skin test–positive HIV-infected persons, and the risk for progression of infection is inordinately high in such individuals, it is important to perform tests with high negative predictive value. Therefore, both a tuberculin skin test and IGRA should be performed in HIV-infected persons and others at high risk of progression from *M. tuberculosis* infection to disease or of a poor outcome. Ideally the blood for IGRA should be drawn prior to TST placement to avoid false-positive IGRA from the PPD. If either the tuberculin skin test or the IGRA is positive, the individual is a candidate for treatment of latent TB infection. Recent studies indicate that IGRAs may be less sensitive than tuberculin skin test in household contacts recently infected with *M. tuberculosis*, a particularly high-risk group. This may be due to delayed conversion of IGRAs relative to tuberculin skin test. Mathematical modeling suggests IGRAs should replace

tuberculin skin test in immunocompromised and perhaps all individuals, and that despite their increased cost, they are cost-effective in the United States. Unfortunately, modeling currently is based on data that are quite variable between studies. A fourth-generation test, Quantiferon-Gold PLUS also contains CD8 stimulatory antigens and is supplanting earlier generations of this IGRA. Initial studies indicate similar performance to the Quantiferon-GOLD assay.

In high TB–prevalence areas, the World Health Organization (WHO) recommends preventive therapy for all HIV-infected persons because of the difficulty in implementing a tuberculin skin test program that would identify those who will achieve the greatest benefit of INH preventive therapy.

Active Tuberculosis

In countries with a high TB burden, the diagnosis of TB is often based on clinical symptoms and sputum microscopy. Clinical diagnosis without the benefit of culture confirmation or radiography is the norm in endemic countries where access to diagnostics is limited. The diagnosis is also made on clinical grounds alone when smears are negative and suspicion for TB is high. Clinical diagnosis is particularly important in HIV-infected persons because of the risk for rapid progression of the TB if left untreated, the more frequent occurrence of AFB smear–negative pulmonary TB, and in those with forms of TB that are "paucibacillary" (pediatric, meningeal, miliary, abdominal, pleural, pericardial), in which bacteria are few and AFB smears typically negative. The diagnosis of miliary, abdominal, pleural, and pericardial TB may be confirmed by the finding of AFBs in biopsied tissue or by culture. In the absence of bacteriologic confirmation, either because cultures (and GenXpert MTB/RIF) are unavailable or because they are negative, the final diagnosis often relies on response to therapy or establishment of an alternative diagnosis. It should be noted that the empirical approach, taken of necessity in resource-limited settings, leads to overdiagnosis and overtreatment of TB, which expends TB program resources and delays treatment of other infections. It is therefore preferable to attempt to establish a definite diagnosis based on the demonstration of *M. tuberculosis* by smears, cultures, or nucleic acid amplification tests in infected secretions or tissue specimens.

Sputum microscopy is the standard approach to the diagnosis of pulmonary TB. A smear requires 1000 to 10,000 bacilli/mL to be read as positive. Both hot and cold carbol fuchsin methods (Ziehl-Neelsen and Kinyoun) are used extensively. The use of fluorochrome stains such as auramine-rhodamine allows more rapid screening of sputum smears and improves sensitivity by about 10%. Three specimens, preferably early morning samples, should be examined to establish the diagnosis. Yield is higher in the presence of cavitary lung disease. Approximately one half of individuals with pulmonary TB are AFB sputum smear negative, and this proportion is higher in the HIV infected. The quantity of AFBs present in the sputum smear is a rough measure of the infectiousness of patients with pulmonary TB, and it is a convenient way to monitor response to treatment. On this basis, additional roles have evolved for the sputum smear as a tool to monitor the potential for transmission and response to therapy.

HIV-infected persons with pulmonary TB carry a particular risk for transmission to health care workers and have been documented as sources of nosocomial outbreaks. Therefore, in the United States, in areas of high prevalence of TB, HIV-infected persons with pulmonary symptoms should be placed into respiratory isolation until infectious TB can be reasonably excluded by three negative sputum smears for AFB on specimens separated by at least 8 hours.

The diagnosis of pediatric TB has always been problematic. Children do not produce sputum readily, and TB is often noncavitary, extrapulmonary, or both. Sputum samples may not be readily obtained from infants and children. Options in this case include sputum induction and gastric aspiration. The sensitivity of AFB smears of gastric aspirates and induced sputum is 25 to 30%. Recent studies indicate that induced sputum, culture of nasopharyngeal swabs, and GenXpert on stools have high enough yield so that gastric aspirates rarely are necessary. Nonetheless, the diagnosis often is based on clinical and epidemiologic features as well as response to therapy.

Bronchoscopy with bronchoalveolar lavage or transbronchial biopsy is another option for the diagnosis of TB and is useful in all severely ill individuals and the immunocompromised, in whom the diagnosis of TB or an alternative infection must be made quickly if treatment is to have an impact on patient outcome. Additionally, a post-bronchoscopy induced sputum has been shown to have higher yield.

AFB smears should be performed on normally sterile fluid obtained from all patients suspected of having TB. The yield of smears from pleural fluid, pericardial fluid, ascitic fluid, and cerebrospinal fluid (CSF) is low in patients with TB but may be higher in those with HIV coinfection, particularly if immunodeficiency is advanced. In TB meningitis, CSF may clot spontaneously, and AFB stains of the clot have increased yield. Rapid diagnosis of some forms of extrapulmonary TB may be made by biopsy of tissue (pleural, pericardial, peritoneal, synovial, terminal ileum); the presence of granulomas, particularly if necrotizing, virtually confirms the diagnosis. Necrotizing granulomas are seen in TB and fungal diseases (particularly histoplasmosis, blastomycosis, coccidioidomycosis, and sporotrichosis). AFBs may also be seen in tissue histology, and *M. tuberculosis* cultured from the specimen.

The diagnosis of miliary TB can be suggested by CT of the chest and confirmed by transbronchial lung biopsy (highest yield), as well as biopsy of the liver, bone marrow, or abnormal lymph nodes. If TB meningitis is suspected and the patient is immunosuppressed, it is particularly important to exclude cryptococcal meningitis by performing a cryptococcal polysaccharide antigen test, as well as an India ink preparation on CSF sediment.

The diagnosis of TB from specimens of normally sterile fluid can be difficult and is increased by culturing relatively large volumes. In addition, the yield of biopsy and culture of tissue (pleura, pericardium) is additive. There are particular diagnostic features for various forms of extrapulmonary TB. In TB meningitis, the initial CSF examination may show neutrophil predominance, but this evolves into a lymphocytic meningitis (100 to 500 cells/μL) with high protein and depressed glucose. TB of the pleura, pericardium, and peritoneum is associated with an exudative effusion, often with a lymphocyte predominance. Low glucose may be found in 20% of TB effusions but limits the differential diagnosis considerably. For example, malignancy, empyema, and rheumatoid arthritis are the other causes of pleural effusion with low glucose. Pericardial fluid in patients with TB pericarditis may be bloody. Eosinophilic meningitis and chylous pleural effusions or ascites may also be seen in TB.

Currently the gold standard for the diagnosis of TB is culture on solid (Löwenstein-Jensen) or in liquid (BACTEC MGIT 960 system) media. The mycobacteria growth indicator tube (MGIT) system is non-radiometric and based on oxygen quenching in the presence of replicating mycobacteria. When compared with solid media, culture with liquid media is more sensitive and growth is more rapid (1 to 3 weeks vs. 3 to 8 weeks for solid media). Once an isolate is available, drug susceptibility testing should be performed to guide therapy. This takes an additional 2 to 4 weeks on solid media, although isoniazid (INH) and rifampin susceptibility results are available in several days when the molecular line probe assay (described later) is used. Liquid medium can be inoculated with smear-positive specimens for direct drug susceptibility testing, which also accelerates the process. Once mycobacterial growth occurs, speciation is possible within hours with commercially available DNA probes. Nuclear acid amplification tests are approved and commercially available for use in TB diagnostics. Their sensitivity is somewhat higher than that of AFB smears, and their specificity is excellent. Expense precludes routine use of such tests, however.

The Xpert MTB/RIF has transformed TB diagnosis globally. Through in situ DNA amplification reaction, this test allows a specific diagnosis of TB and determination of susceptibility to rifampin within 90 minutes. After minimal processing, sputum is added to a cartridge. Gene amplification is done with primers based on the *rpoB* gene, which encodes the target of rifampin, and resistance-conferring mutations are detected. This method is capable of establishing the diagnosis of TB in 97% of patients with pulmonary TB, including 98% of AFB sputum smear–positive and 73% of smear-negative individuals, thus rivaling the sensitivity of solid culture. It does not require molecular expertise by the technician and is not subject to amplicon (DNA) contamination, because it is a closed system. The uptake of GenXpert has been remarkable. The government of South Africa has replaced sputum smear analysis with GenXpert for TB diagnosis. The government of Brazil is developing a similar policy. In Uganda, there will be a single reference laboratory for culture and drug susceptibility testing (DST). GenXpert will be available regionally and used mainly for the diagnosis of smear-negative cases. GenXpert is priced differently for low-income countries, but cost still may be prohibitive in some settings. The test allows more rapid diagnosis and initiation of treatment but has not led to more treated cases in high burden settings because many smear-negative patients were receiving empiric treatment if clinical suspicion was present. A new Xpert MTB/RIF Ultra cartridge was endorsed by the WHO as a replacement for the Xpert MTB/RIF cartridge in March, 2017. The cartridge has increased sensitivity, particularly among paucibacillary cases, but a slight decrease in specificity (from 98% to 96%). Encouraging is the test's reported increased capacity to detect TB meningitis, in which sensitivity for probable or definite infection was 70% (95% CI 47 to 87) for Xpert Ultra,

compared with 43% (23 to 66) for Xpert MTB/RIF, and 43% (23 to 66) for culture.

There are other candidate nucleic acid amplification tests (NAATs) about to undergo evaluation that are less expensive than GenXpert and may be truly point of care. [A1] For example, elevated blood levels of *BATF2* (basic leucine zipper transcription factor 2) are a sensitive biomarker for active TB.[11] Diagnostics for pediatric and extrapulmonary TB more sensitive than NAATs are likely to be based on host responses. As regards host-based diagnostics, there are promising data based on transcriptomics, proteomics, and metabolomics. For example, a three-gene transcriptional signature proposed for the diagnosis of TB is likely to be commercialized, and a 16-gene transcriptional signature of risk indicates increased risk of developing TB within a 2-year time frame. As host-based diagnostics become available, a new category of subclinical TB may become easier to diagnose, a category which has been challenging because by definition there are no symptoms and bacterial-based diagnostics are usually negative. The appropriate management of such patients is not clear because they may spontaneously resolve their minimal disease. If they are HIV infected there will be the risk of "unmasking TB" with the start of ART. Even HIV-uninfected patients they represent a high risk group with LTBI and probably should be treated as such.

TB in the HIV-infected patient poses particular diagnostic issues because of the increased likelihood of smear-negative pulmonary TB, and in advanced HIV, atypical presentation and extrapulmonary disease. The Alere Determine LAM TB test is a low-cost, rapid, lateral flow device (dipstick) that detects lipoarabinomannan, the major cell wall glycolipid of *M. tuberculosis*. Its use as a TB diagnostic test improved survival of HIV-infected patients admitted to hospital with low CD4 counts (<100). The WHO has endorsed the test for hospitalized HIV-infected individuals with CD4 lower than 100 and clinical suspicion for TB.

New diagnostics also target rapid determination of drug susceptibility. The Xpert MTB/RIF test described earlier detects the *rpoB* gene, where the majority of mutations that confer rifampin resistance occur. A new cartridge allows rapid detection of mutations for isoniazid, fluoroquinolones, and second-line injectables.[12] Similarly, the Hain Genotype MTBDR*plus* detects mutations for rifampin and for isoniazid (in *katG* and *inhA* promoter mutations) and more recently Genotype MTBDR*sl* detects mutations for fluoroquinolone and second-line injectables. The Genotype assays require the technician be trained in molecular methods, and results require several days. These molecular tests have been endorsed by the WHO for drug resistance detection. They allow drug susceptibility information to become available in many settings for more patients than has been available with culture-based methods.

TREATMENT   Rx

Comprehensive reviews of TB treatment provide complete information on drugs for TB, monitoring of therapy, management of adverse events, and treatment of pregnant women, children, and other special populations[13]:
https://www.cdc.gov/tb/publications/guidelines/pdf/clin-infect-dis.-2016-nahid-cid_ciw376.pdf

Treatment of TB is both a clinical and a public health issue. The goals are to cure the patient and minimize transmission. For that reason, the treating physician has the obligation to ensure that treatment is completed with good adherence to medications.[14] Because of the declining number of TB cases in the United States, with subsequent decline in expertise in TB management, treatment is more likely to occur in a public health clinic than in the private sector. The cornerstone of TB treatment is multidrug therapy. This is necessary because *M. tuberculosis* undergoes spontaneous mutation to drug resistance at a frequency such that most patients with cavitary lung disease—and therefore patients with a high burden of organisms—are likely to harbor resistant mutants.

For the treatment of TB caused by drug-susceptible organisms, there is an intensive phase of therapy for the first 2 months aimed at the rapidly dividing and metabolizing organisms and usually resulting in sterilization of sputum in those with pulmonary TB.[15] This is followed by a 4- to 6-month continuation phase that kills the slowly metabolizing persisting organisms. The four first-line anti-TB drugs (all orally administered)—INH, rifampin, ethambutol, and pyrazinamide—form the foundation of chemotherapy for TB. The precepts of therapy have been largely defined by controlled clinical trials. Standard short-course therapy for pulmonary TB requires a 2-month intensive phase of four drugs (INH, rifampin, ethambutol, and pyrazinamide), followed by a 4-month continuation phase with INH and rifampin. Pyridoxine should also be given to avoid peripheral neuropathy from INH. Linezolid (600 mg daily) may be substituted for ethambutol with equivalent results. [A2]

The use of intermittent dosing regimens increases the feasibility of directly observed therapy (DOT) but is controversial. Intermittent regimens may be slightly less effective than daily 5/7 regimens (5 weekdays observed, 2 weekend days self-administered). For patients with extensive cavitary disease and the severely immunosuppressed, daily therapy should be administered throughout the entire course. For HIV-infected persons with TB who are not severely immunosuppressed, treatment should be daily during the intensive phase and at least three times weekly during the continuation phase. Non–HIV-infected persons without extensive cavitary disease can be treated with intermittent regimens throughout. The problem of nonadherence has led to the directive to provide DOT.

The addition of pyrazinamide to the intensive phase allows for the so-called short-course chemotherapy; if pyrazinamide is not tolerated, comparable outcomes can be obtained with 9 months of INH-rifampin. Treatment of drug-susceptible TB with this standard regimen can be expected to cure approximately 90 to 95% of cases. Routine monitoring of liver function test results is not recommended unless there is preexisting liver disease. Patients should return to the clinic promptly with any signs of drug toxicity, particularly those of early hepatotoxicity (nausea, malaise, anorexia, upper abdominal discomfort). Visits should be scheduled monthly and include clinical assessment and sputum examinations. For those with pulmonary TB, sputum cultures are continued until two consecutive cultures are negative. In uncomplicated pulmonary TB, defervescence is expected within 2 weeks, and there should be weight gain and diminution of cough and chest pain. About 20% of patients with cavitary pulmonary TB remain sputum culture positive after 2 months of therapy. A positive sputum culture at 3 months or failure to improve on chest radiographs suggests nonadherence with therapy, low drug levels due to malabsorption or increased metabolism, drug-resistant TB, or an alternative or complicating diagnosis. The etiology of the persistent positive culture should be pursued. Positive sputum culture at 4 months is defined as treatment failure.

Extrapulmonary TB is usually associated with a smaller bacterial burden than is the case with pulmonary TB and can be treated with standard short-course regimens of 6 to 9 months' duration. However, because of the serious ramifications of treatment failure, more prolonged treatment of at least 9 to 12 months is recommended for miliary, meningeal, and skeletal TB. Adjunctive surgical débridement and stabilization may be necessary for skeletal TB. Adjunctive corticosteroids are indicated for TB pericarditis and severe pleurisy, as well as extensive pulmonary TB with clinical toxicity or respiratory failure. In TB meningitis, dexamethasone improves survival but has not had an impact on the proportion surviving with severe neurologic sequelae. Ventricular shunting may be necessary to relieve hydrocephalus.

HIV-TB Coinfection

HIV-TB coinfection creates additional management issues. Fortunately, the response to treatment of TB is comparable to that in HIV-uninfected individuals, except for higher early mortality in individuals with low CD4 counts at treatment initiation. Intermittent regimens have a tendency to lead to rifampin resistance; therefore, daily administration of drugs is recommended throughout. In a randomized trial among HIV-positive patients with pulmonary TB receiving antiretroviral therapy, a daily anti-TB regimen proved superior to a thrice-weekly regimen in terms of efficacy and emergence of rifampicin resistance.[A3] In resource-limited settings, the administration of cotrimoxazole prophylaxis is associated with improved survival. Integration of the treatment of TB and HIV rather than sequential treatment of first TB and then HIV is associated with a 56% reduction in mortality. The results of three randomized controlled trials support the current U.S. Department of Health and Human Services and Infectious Diseases Society of America guideline to start ART 2 weeks after initiation of TB treatment if CD4+ count is below 50 cells/µL.[A4] Early ART in HIV-infected adults with newly diagnosed TB improves survival in patients with CD4+ T-cell counts lower than 50 cells/µL, although treatment is associated with a 2-fold increased risk of TB-immune reconstitution inflammatory syndrome (TB-IRIS) (Chapter 367).[16] TB-IRIS is more likely to occur when the CD4+ count is low, the viral load is high, and the interval between starting TB drugs and ART is short. Immune reconstitution is associated with inflammation and transient exacerbation of disease mimicking progression of TB. There may, for example, be fever, lymphadenitis, and worsening parenchymal disease, including consolidation and new or progressing nodular opacities on chest radiographs. In about one third of dually infected patients, IRIS will develop within the first 2 months of treatment and often within the first 2 to 3 weeks of starting ART. TB-IRIS usually is not an important cause of mortality. A controlled trial has shown that corticosteroid therapy limits morbidity,[A5] although it is not useful for treating tuberculous pericarditis.[A6] More problematic is IRIS associated with respiratory failure or neurologic involvement. Initiation of ART in HIV-infected persons may also be associated with "unmasking TB," which occurs within 3 months. This may be due to a missed diagnosis of TB in screening, the development of inflammation at sites of mycobacterial replication in tissue, or progression of latent infection consequent to ART. Unmasking TB is common in countries endemic for TB (5 to 10% in Uganda, for example, but about 25% in South Africa) and associated with morbidity, mortality, and risk for nosocomial transmission.

In general, TB does not affect the response of HIV to ART. A major issue, however, is the interactions between rifamycins that induce CYP3A hepatic microsomal enzymes and protease inhibitors, integrase inhibitors, and some

non-nucleoside reverse transcriptase inhibitors (NRTIs). Because of its potency, simplicity, and proven clinical efficacy, efavirenz 600 mg with two NRTIs, along with rifampin-based TB regimens, is the preferred strategy for co-treatment of HIV and TB. Rifabutin is off-patent and available as a less potent inducer of cytochrome enzymes, but its own pharmacokinetics can be affected by certain ARTs. Rifampin is the preferred rifamycin for efavirenz-containing regimens, whereas rifabutin should be used at a dose of 150 mg daily with a boosted protease inhibitor. Rifampin can be used with dolutegravir at a doubled dose or rifabutin 300 mg daily can be used with daily dolutegravir. Patients should not be treated with tenofovir alafenamide (TAF) with rifamycins but switched to alternative HIV regimens. Guidelines for other drug combinations to avoid drug interactions were updated in September 2014[17] and are available at https://www.cdc.gov/tb/publications/guidelines/tb_hiv_drugs/recommendations02.htm.

Management of TB-HIV coinfection may be complicated for the clinician. For example, a new fever may be due to drug reaction, TB-IRIS, drug resistance, or a complicating opportunistic infection.

Drug-Resistant TB

Drug-resistant TB is more difficult to cure than drug-susceptible TB and in some instances may be incurable. Selection and monitoring of treatment for drug-resistant TB should be the responsibility of those experienced with the unique drug regimens and issues involved. It is clear that the addition of a single drug to a failing treatment regimen should never be done because it increases the risk of additional resistance development. A major problem is the lack of information on drug susceptibility at the time of initiation of treatment. In resource-limited settings, drug susceptibility testing may not be available at all. Although drug resistance can occur due to acquired resistance in an individual (the person is initially infected with a drug-susceptible strain that becomes drug resistant due to poor adherence to medications, low quality drugs, weak regimen), recent molecular and modeling data show up to 70% of drug-resistant strains occur due to transmission. Therefore, all individuals with TB disease would benefit from drug-susceptibility testing to ensure an effective regimen is given.

Monoresistance to INH has little effect on the outcome of TB treatment if identified early and adjustments to regimens are made. INH-monoresistant TB can be treated with rifampin, pyrazinamide, and ethambutol for 6 months. A recent individual patient data meta-analysis suggests that addition of a fluoroquinolone to 6 to 9 months of rifampin, ethambutol, and pyrazinamide may improve outcomes.[A7] However, in much of the world INH resistance is not detected unless an individual is failing a regimen, leading effectively to monotherapy (rifampin alone) during the continuation phase. Ideally, routine testing for all relevant drugs should be seen as a critical step to improve TB outcomes. Acquisition of additional drug resistance is more likely if the initial isolate was resistant to one drug (6%) or more than one drug (14%) versus being pansusceptible (0.8%).

MDR TB represents a more significant treatment challenge.[18] Not only is cure difficult and extremely expensive, but unrecognized MDR TB can lead to nosocomial outbreaks and rapid and high rates of fatality. In 2016, less than a quarter of the estimated 600,000 rifampin-resistant TB cases started MDR TB treatment and only 54% of those initiating care in 2014 had successful outcomes (cure or treatment completion). There is no substitute for performing drug susceptibility testing that includes all first-line and available second-line drugs on an initial specimen in order to ensure an effective regimen is given. MDR TB is not a homogeneous entity; some isolates are only resistant to INH and rifampin but half of MDR TB cases globally have resistance to pyrazinamide as well. Patients with resistance to additional first- and second-line drugs benefit from more individualized regimens with newer drugs.[19]

In October 2016, the WHO published updated guidelines for drug-resistant TB. The biggest modification is the availability of the shorter MDR TB regimen for adults and children, including those with HIV coinfection. The shorter regimen is 7 drugs (moxifloxacin, kanamycin, ethionamide, clofazamine,[A8] high-dose isoniazid, pyrazinamide, and ethambutol) for 4 to 6 months followed by 4 drugs (moxifloxacin, clofazamine, pyrazinamide, and ethambutol) for another 5 to 6 months, making the total course 9 to 12 months. This regimen is recommended in patients with rifampin-resistant or MDR TB who were not previously treated with second-line drugs and in whom resistance to fluoroquinolones and second-line injectable agents was excluded or is consider highly unlikely. If resistance to any drugs other than isoniazid in the regimen are known, then the short course is also not recommended.

For all other patients, the cornerstone of treatment of MDR TB is the traditional regimen which includes at least five drugs to which the isolate is susceptible. Typically, the regimen will include first-line drugs with retained activity, a fluoroquinolone (FQ), an injectable (amikacin, kanamycin, or capreomycin), and second-line drugs (ethionamide, cycloserine, PAS) with the goal of five effective drugs in the regimen. The duration of treatment is set at 18 to 24 months. Residual susceptibility to FQ treatment and capreomycin has been shown to be a determinant of treatment outcome. Surgical resection is a consideration if the disease is localized, sputum remains culture positive, medical therapy is not tolerated, or massive hemoptysis is present. Cure rates of 60 to 80% can be expected if therapy is targeted to drug susceptibility test results and MDR organisms remain sensitive to enough chemotherapeutic drugs that a reasonable regimen can be established. The U.S. Food and Drug Administration (FDA) also approved both bedaquiline and delamanid for the treatment of MDR TB, although bedaquiline is not yet recommended in children. Bedaquiline, a diarylquinoline, targets mycobacterial ATP synthase, and delamanid, a nitrodihydro-imidazooxazole, inhibits *M. tuberculosis* mycolic acid synthesis. Increasingly bedaquiline is being substituted for the aminoglycoside to avoid the injectable agent and its toxicity. These are the first new classes of TB treatment drugs to be approved by the FDA in 40 years. They are revolutionizing management of MDR TB.

The definition of extensively drug-resistant TB is an organism that is MDR with additional resistance to an FQ plus at least one of three injectables (amikacin, kanamycin, capreomycin). The outcome of treatment of extensively drug-resistant TB has been variable. The best reported results have been obtained in Peru, with a comprehensive approach that included therapeutic regimens that were tailored according to drug susceptibility testing. Effective regimens included cycloserine, capreomycin, and PAS. Moxifloxacin may be active even if the isolate is resistant to first-generation FQs. Adjunctive surgery should be considered. The newest drugs have become backbones for these regimens where they are available. Studies indicate that linezolid has remarkable activity against extensively drug-resistant TB,[A9] and other oxazolidinones are in development for TB treatment.

The emergence of drug resistance has emphasized the need for new drugs and new drug regimens. A drug regimen that shortens the course of TB would lessen the emergence of drug resistance, because adherence would increase and DOT would be simplified. Once MDR TB develops, particularly in the setting of extensively drug-resistant TB, new drugs are necessary to improve efficacy and shorten treatment.

There are promising developments with existing classes of drugs and with new classes about to enter or already in clinical trials. Rifapentine, a rifamycin with a longer half-life than rifampin, shows remarkable enhancement of sterilization of sputum at 2 months. Moxifloxacin has increased activity against *M. tuberculosis*, although data of its efficacy in 4-month regimens have been disappointing. Pretomanid, a nitroimidazole, is now being trialed with bedaquiline and linezolid as an all oral, short-course regimen for drug-resistant TB.

PREVENTION

The CDC guidelines for treatment regimens for latent TB infection, updated June 2017, include recommendations for HIV coinfected individuals, children, and pregnant women (https://www.cdc.gov/tb/topic/treatment/ltbi.htm).

The approach taken in a low-prevalence setting such as the United States is to target testing to those at high risk for recent *M. tuberculosis* infection and to those with comorbid conditions that predispose to progression from infection to disease. In either category, a positive test (IGRA or TST) becomes an indication for treatment of latent TB infection. Providers should only test individuals for TB infection as part of a work-up for active TB or if they plan to offer TB prophylaxis.

Latent TB infection can be treated with rifampin for 4 months, INH for 6 to 9 months, or INH plus rifapentine weekly for 3 months (12 doses), thereby decreasing the lifetime risk for development of TB by approximately 75 to 90%, depending on the level of adherence to treatment (Table 308-2).[20] These recommendations are consistent with an updated[A10] network meta-analysis of the best LTBI treatment options upon which these recommendations were originally based.[A11] Pyridoxine should be administered to prevent INH-induced peripheral neuropathy in those at risk. Monitoring of liver function is indicated in older individuals (the risk for hepatotoxicity increases beyond the age of 35 years) and in those with significant alcohol intake or underlying liver disease (or both). INH should be discontinued if symptoms develop (see Treatment) or hepatic transaminase levels rise to more than three to five times the upper limit of normal. Rifapentine plus INH once weekly for 3 months (12 doses) is as effective as 9 months of INH alone in preventing active TB in patients with latent infection.[A12] Administration of this regimen should be directly observed, although more recent research has shown that in the United States self-administration may be noninferior.[A13] Side effects from rifapentine, including hypersensitivity reaction, should be monitored. In HIV-infected persons in high TB burden settings, treatment of latent TB infection confers short-term efficacy (≈1 year), but this may be extended if ART is administered. Treatment for 3 years with isoniazid in HIV-infected persons confers an additional benefit that is most marked in the tuberculin skin test positives in high TB burden settings. Unfortunately, treatment of latent TB infection has not been applied broadly. This is in part due to the concern that if screening is inadequate, patients with active TB will be treated with a single drug and thereby acquire drug resistance. The available data do not support this concern. In a low-resource setting in the HIV infected, the absence of current fever, weight loss, or night sweats has a negative predictive value of 97%, may obviate the need for chest radiography if it is not routinely available, and identifies a group that should be treated with INH preventive treatment regardless of tuberculin skin test status. Although INH preventive therapy is the preferred regimen, there is renewed interest in the possibility that rifamycin-containing regimens may confer more sustained protection.

A recently completed study of HIV-infected individuals reports that daily isoniazid plus rifapentine for one month was noninferior to 9 months of isoniazid, had fewer adverse events, and was more likely to be completed.[A14] This ultra-short course may become the standard in the future. Currently no standard recommended treatment is available for contacts of MDR TB cases. Experts recommend considering fluoroquinolone-based preventive therapy. Three randomized controlled trials are planned to evaluate the effectiveness of preventive therapy for infected MDR TB contacts and include levofloxacin, isoniazid, or delamanid.

Secondary preventive therapy after completion of TB treatment is indicated in HIV-infected persons in the setting of intense exposure to *M. tuberculosis*. Data demonstrating efficacy of secondary prevention largely result from studies of adults in Congo and gold miners in South Africa.

A randomized controlled trial has demonstrated that in HIV-positive patients, early initiation of ART as compared with delayed treatment (where there was a decline in CD4 counts or AIDS-related illness had already occurred) led to a significant decrease in the development of TB.[A15]

Tracing of household contacts is a critical element of TB programs. The household is a major site of TB transmission, particularly in an area of low endemicity, so treatment of TST or IGRA converters is an important strategy for elimination of TB. In a high TB prevalence setting in Vietnam, a cluster-randomized, controlled trial found that household-contact intervention plus standard passive case finding was more effective than standard passive case finding alone for the detection of sputum smear-positive TB.[A16] It is essential that transmission be limited in hospitals and other settings in which infectious pulmonary TB patients may comingle with susceptible hosts. The risk of transmission to health care workers should be ascertained annually by skin testing. The finding of excessive risk for new TB infection should lead to focused measures for reducing transmission. All TB suspects should be placed in respiratory isolation in negative-pressure rooms with at least six air exchanges per hour and high-efficiency particulate air (HEPA) filtration or ultraviolet irradiation. N-95 personnel respirator devices that are fit-tested are necessary for individuals entering areas with a known high risk for exposure.

BCG vaccine is widely used and relatively safe except in the setting of immunosuppression. Unfortunately, efficacy has been variable by age and by latitude. A meta-analysis indicated an overall efficacy of 50%. It is approximately 80% effective in preventing the severe forms of TB in childhood, miliary TB, and TB meningitis. However, its failure to prevent adult TB, particularly at low latitudes that include the most endemic areas, means that BCG vaccine does not have an impact on the public health problem of TB. An experimental protective vaccine has shown promise in reducing cases of active pulmonary tuberculosis.[A17] However, the natural history of TB is such that large, lengthy, and expensive trials may be needed to establish protective efficacy.

PROGNOSIS

In the pre-chemotherapeutic era, minimal pulmonary TB stabilized in about 50% of cases. Pleural TB also self-cured, with a risk for reactivation as noted previously. With treatment, the prognosis of patients with TB depends on the extent of pulmonary TB, the sites of extrapulmonary TB, drug susceptibility of the isolate, and the presence of HIV infection and other comorbid conditions. With extensive pulmonary TB, respiratory failure may supervene with a poor prognosis. There is also increased risk for serious, sometimes

TABLE 308-2	TREATMENT OF LATENT TUBERCULOSIS
DRUG REGIMEN	**ADULT DOSE**
Isoniazid alone for 6 or 9 months	5 mg/kg (maximum 300 mg daily)
Rifampin alone for 4 months	10 mg/kg (maximum 600 mg daily)
Weekly rifapentine plus isoniazid for 3 months	Rifapentine, 15-30 mg/kg (maximum 900 mg); isoniazid, 15 mg/kg (maximum 900 mg)

Adapted from Getahun H, Matteelli A, Chaisson RE, et al. Latent *Mycobacterium tuberculosis* infection. *N Engl J Med.* 2015;372:2127-2135.

lethal, hemoptysis and pneumothorax. Miliary TB is associated with a high case-fatality rate, in part related to delays in diagnosis. TB meningitis is associated with serious neurologic residua, as well as high mortality. MDR TB and extensively drug-resistant TB are accompanied by high rates of treatment failure, morbidity, and mortality. TB in HIV-infected persons is associated with high early mortality that is poorly characterized. In the absence of ART, there is increased risk for other opportunistic infections and progression of HIV disease. The addition of ART, however, results in the morbidities associated with concurrent administration of TB and HIV medications and with TB-IRIS. Long-term outcomes of South African patients with extensively drug-resistant TB were poor irrespective of HIV status, and because of the scarcity of long-stay or palliative care facilities, substantial numbers of patients with extensively drug-resistant TB who had failed treatment and had positive sputum cultures were being discharged to likely transmit disease into the wider community.

Grade A References

A1. Theron G, Zijenah L, Chanda D, et al. Feasibility, accuracy, and clinical effect of point-of-care Xpert MTB/RIF testing for tuberculosis in primary-care settings in Africa: a multicentre, randomised, controlled trial. *Lancet.* 2014;383:424-435.

A2. Lee JK, Lee JY, Kim DK, et al. Substitution of ethambutol with linezolid during the intensive phase of treatment of pulmonary tuberculosis: a prospective, multicentre, randomised, open-label, phase 2 trial. *Lancet Infect Dis.* 2019;19:46-55.

A3. Gopalan N, Santhanakrishnan RK, Palaniappan AN, et al. Daily vs intermittent antituberculosis therapy for pulmonary tuberculosis in patient with HIV: a randomized clinical trial. *JAMA Intern Med.* 2018;178:485-493.

A4. Blanc F-X, Sok T, Laureillard D, et al. Earlier vs later start of antiviral therapy in HIV-infected adults with tuberculosis. *N Engl J Med.* 2011;365:1471-1481.

A5. Meintges G, Wilkinson RJ, Morroni C, et al. Randomized placebo-controlled trial of prednisone for paradoxical tuberculosis-associated immune reconstitution syndrome. *AIDS.* 2010;24:2381-2390.

A6. Mayosi BM, Ntsekhe M, Bosch J, et al. Prednisolone and *Mycobacterium indicus pranii* in tuberculous pericarditis. *N Engl J Med.* 2014;371:1121-1130.

A7. Fregonese F, Ahuja SD, Akkerman OW, et al. Comparison of different treatments for isoniazid-resistant tuberculosis: an individual patient data meta-analysis. *Lancet Respir Med.* 2018;6:265-275.

A8. Duan H, Chen X, Li Z, et al. Clofazimine improves clinical outcomes in multidrug-resistant tuberculosis: a randomized controlled trial. *Clin Microbiol Infect.* 2019;25:190-195.

A9. Lee M, Lee J, Carroll MW, et al. Linezolid for treatment of chronic extensively drug resistant tuberculosis. *N Engl J Med.* 2012;367:1508-1518.

A10. Menzies D, Adjobimey M, Ruslami R, et al. Four months of rifampin or nine months of isoniazid for latent tuberculosis in adults. *N Engl J Med.* 2018;379:440-453.

A11. Zenner D, Beer N, Harris RJ, et al. Treatment of latent tuberculosis infection: an updated network meta-analysis. *Ann Intern Med.* 2017;167:248-255.

A12. Sterling TR, Villarino ME, Borisov AS, et al. Three months of rifapentine and isoniazid for latent tuberculosis infection. *N Engl J Med.* 2011;365:2155-2166.

A13. Belknap R, Holland D, Feng PJ, et al. Self-administered versus directly observed once-weekly isoniazid and rifapentine treatment of latent tuberculosis infection: a randomized trial. *Ann Intern Med.* 2017;167:689-697.

A14. Swindells S, Ramchandani R, Gupta A, et al. One sent HIV-related tuberculosis. *N Engl J Med.* 2019;380:1001-1011.

A15. Grinsztejn B, Hosseinipour MC, Ribaudo HJ, et al. Effects of early versus delayed initiation of antiretroviral treatment on clinical outcomes of HIV-1 infection: results from the phase 3 HPTN 052 randomised controlled trial. *Lancet Infect Dis.* 2014;14:281-290.

A16. Fox GJ, Nhung NV, Sy DN, et al. Household-contact investigation for detection of tuberculosis in Vietnam. *N Engl J Med.* 2018;378:221-229.

A17. Van Der Meeren O, Hatherill M, Nduba V, et al. Phase 2b controlled trial of M72/AS01E vaccine to prevent tuberculosis. *N Engl J Med.* 2018;379:1621-1634.

GENERAL REFERENCES

For the General References and other additional features, please visit Expert Consult at https://expertconsult.inkling.com.

309

THE NONTUBERCULOUS MYCOBACTERIA

STEVEN M. HOLLAND

DEFINITION

Nontuberculous mycobacteria generally include the growing number of mycobacteria other than *Mycobacterium tuberculosis* and its close relatives (Chapter 308) and *M. leprae* (Chapter 310). Other names that have been used include *atypical mycobacteria, mycobacteria other than tuberculosis,* and *environmental mycobacteria.* The number of nontuberculous mycobacteria is growing rapidly

as a result of the advent of DNA sequence typing for determining criteria for speciation. Accordingly, the number of species of nontuberculous mycobacteria has increased to almost 170 and will continue to increase for the near future.

The Pathogens

Identification of any mycobacterium requires that the appropriate tests be thought of ahead of time and be performed, because routine microbiologic testing does not identify mycobacteria. Nontuberculous mycobacteria are typically first detected on acid-fast smears of sputum or other body fluids. When levels of organisms are high, mycobacteria may be seen on Gram stain as gram-positive beaded rods, but this finding is unreliable. The first step in identification is to request the appropriate smear (acid-fast or fluorochrome) and culture. Nontuberculous mycobacteria are broadly differentiated into rapidly growing (<7 days) and slowly growing (>7 days) forms. *M. tuberculosis,* by contrast, typically takes 2 or more weeks to grow. Formation of pigment in light (photochromogens) or dark (scotochromogens) and lack of pigment (nonchromogens) have also been used to help categorize nontuberculous mycobacteria. Current diagnostics use biochemical, nucleic acid, or cell wall composition on high-performance liquid chromatography for speciation (Table 309-1). For purposes of diagnosis, prognosis, and therapy, identification of nontuberculous mycobacteria should be taken to the species level.

EPIDEMIOLOGY

As a group, the nontuberculous mycobacteria are ubiquitous in soil and water and are often found in certain animals, but they rarely cause disease in humans. There are very few instances of human-to-human transmission of nontuberculous mycobacteria. However, *M. massiliense* has caused outbreaks of infection in cystic fibrosis centers. Because these infections are not reported to health agencies and their identification is sometimes problematic, reliable data on incidence and prevalence are lacking. In the United States, however, isolates of nontuberculous mycobacteria have exceeded those for *M. tuberculosis* for many years. In patients with cystic fibrosis (Chapter 83), for example, rates of clinical nontuberculous mycobacterial infection range up to 40%, but even more patients harbor the organism. Differentiating active disease from commensal harboring of the organism remains problematic. Other patient groups, such as those with bronchiectasis, also have elevated but undefined rates of nontuberculous mycobacterial infection.[1] The bulk of nontuberculous mycobacterial disease in North America is due to *M. kansasii, M. avium* complex (MAC),[2] and *M. abscessus.*

PATHOBIOLOGY

Because exposure is essentially universal and disease is rare, normal host defenses against nontuberculous mycobacteria must be highly effective. Therefore, otherwise healthy individuals in whom disease develops must have specific

TABLE 309-1	COMMON NONTUBERCULOUS MYCOBACTERIA
ORGANISM	**DISEASE**
RAPIDLY GROWING NONTUBERCULOUS MYCOBACTERIA	
M. abscessus	Lung, disseminated, lymph node
M. chelonae	Skin
M. fortuitum	Line infections, lung
M. smegmatis	Almost never associated with disease
SLOWLY GROWING NONTUBERCULOUS MYCOBACTERIA	
M. avium complex	Lung, disseminated, lymph node
M. kansasii	Lung
M. marinum	Skin, tendons (fish tank granuloma)
M. xenopi	Lung
M. simiae	Lung
M. szulgai	Lung
M. malmoense	Lung
M. scrofulaceum	Lymph node
M. haemophilum	Disseminated, skin
M. genavense	Disseminated
M. ulcerans	Skin (Buruli ulcer; toxin producing)
M. neoarum	Disseminated
M. celatum	Disseminated
M. gordonae	Almost never causes disease
M. terrae complex	Disseminated

M = *Mycobacterium.*

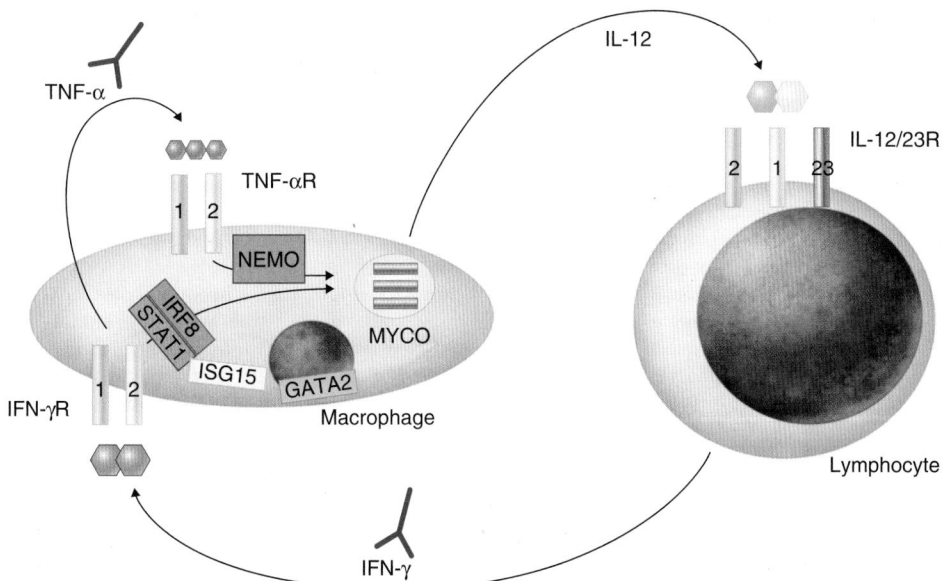

FIGURE 309-1. Schematization of the critical cytokine interactions between infected macrophages and T and natural killer lymphocytes. Organisms (MYCO) infect macrophages, which release heterodimeric interleukin (IL)-12. This acts on the IL-12/23 receptor complex and leads to the production of homodimeric interferon (IFN)-γ. IFN-γ acts on its receptor to stimulate the production of tumor necrosis factor (TNF)-α and kill intracellular organisms such as mycobacteria, salmonellae, and some fungi. Homotrimeric TNF-α acts on its own receptor and also contributes to killing of intracellular organisms. Both IFN-γ and TNF-α lead to upregulation of IL-12. TNF-α–blocking antibodies work either by blocking the ligand (infliximab, adalimumab, certolizumab) or by providing soluble receptor (etanercept). Mutations in both chains of IFN-γR, IL-12p40, and IL-12Rβ1, IL-12Rβ2, and signal elements for IFN-γR and TNF-αR have been identified through their predisposition to mycobacterial infections. IRF8 = interferon regulatory factor 8; ISG = interferon-stimulated gene; NEMO = nuclear factor kappa-B essential modulator; STAT1 = signal transducer and activator of transcription 1.

susceptibility factors that permit these infections to become established, multiply, and cause disease.

With the advent of human immunodeficiency virus (HIV) infection, CD4$^+$ T lymphocytes were identified as key effectors against nontuberculous mycobacteria. Much of the genetic basis of susceptibility to disseminated nontuberculous mycobacterial infection outside HIV infection has been found to be due to specific mutations in the interferon (IFN)-γ/interleukin (IL)-12 synthesis and response pathways. However, only about 70% of disseminated cases unassociated with HIV infection have a genetic diagnosis, and genetic causes of predisposition to nontuberculous mycobacterial lung disease are still very few.

Mycobacteria are typically phagocytosed by macrophages, which respond with the production of IL-12, a heterodimer composed of p35 and p40 moieties that together constitute IL-12p70 (Fig. 309-1). IL-12 activates T lymphocytes and natural killer (NK) cells through binding to its receptor (composed of IL-12Rβ1 and IL-12Rβ2/IL-23R) and results in phosphorylation of STAT4 (signal transducer and activator of transcription 4). IL-12 stimulation leads to production and secretion of IFN-γ, which activates neutrophils and macrophages to produce reactive oxidants and increase major histocompatibility complex display and Fc receptors. IFN-γ signals through its receptor (composed of IFN-γR1 and IFN-γR2), thereby leading to phosphorylation of STAT1, which in turn regulates IFN-γ–responsive genes such as those for the production of IL-12 and tumor necrosis factor (TNF)-α. Therefore, the positive feedback loop between IFN-γ and IL-12/IL-23 is pivotal in the immune response to mycobacteria and other intracellular infections (most importantly *Salmonella, Histoplasma, Coccidioides*). The advent of potent TNF-α inhibitors such as infliximab, adalimumab, certolizumab, etanercept, and golimumab (Chapter 33) has provided the ability to neutralize this critical cytokine, which has occasionally resulted in mycobacterial and fungal infections.

CLINICAL MANIFESTATIONS

Disseminated Disease

Disseminated nontuberculous mycobacterial disease secondary to MAC used to occur commonly in the setting of advanced acquired immunodeficiency syndrome (AIDS) but is now uncommon in North America because of MAC prophylaxis and improved treatment of HIV infection. The portal of entry was the bowel, with spread to bone marrow and the blood stream. Rapidly growing mycobacteria such as *M. fortuitum* sometimes infect deep indwelling lines. The severe disseminated infection seen with immune defects is typically associated with malaise, fever, and weight loss, and it is often accompanied by organomegaly and lymphadenopathy. Disseminated (two or more organs)

involvement in a child without an underlying iatrogenic cause should always prompt an investigation of the IFN-γ/IL-12 pathway.[3] Nontuberculous mycobacterial osteomyelitis is especially common with dominant negative mutations in IFN-γR1. A male with conical or peg teeth or an abnormal hair pattern and disseminated nontuberculous mycobacterial infection should be evaluated for defects in the pathway that activates nuclear factor (NF)κB. Some patients with disseminated rapidly growing infections (predominantly *M. abscessus*) have high-titer autoantibodies to IFN-γ.

Pulmonary Disease

Lung disease caused by nontuberculous mycobacteria is by far the most common form of the infection in North America. Predisposing factors include underlying lung disease, such as bronchiectasis (Chapter 84), pneumoconiosis (Chapter 87), chronic obstructive pulmonary disease (Chapter 82), primary ciliary dyskinesia, and cystic fibrosis.[4] The manifestations of *M. kansasii* infection can be very similar to those of tuberculosis (Chapter 308) and consist of hemoptysis, chest pain, and cavitary lung disease. MAC infection most commonly occurs in women in their sixth or seventh decade who have had months to years of nagging intermittent cough and fatigue, with or without sputum production or chest pain. Bronchiectasis and nontuberculous mycobacterial infection often coexist and progress in tandem, thus making causality difficult to determine. When compared with male smokers with upper lobe cavitary disease, who tend to carry the very same single strain of MAC indefinitely, nonsmoking females with nodular bronchiectasis tend to have several strains simultaneously and change them over the course of their disease process. Patients with pulmonary alveolar proteinosis (Chapter 85) are prone to pulmonary nontuberculous mycobacterial and *Nocardia* infections, likely reflecting their association with anti–granulocyte-macrophage colony-stimulating factor (anti–GM-CSF) autoantibodies and impaired alveolar macrophage function. Esophageal motility disorders such as achalasia (Chapter 129) have been associated with pulmonary disease, especially that caused by rapidly growing nontuberculous mycobacteria such as *M. abscessus*. It is important to note that lung disease rarely disseminates, illustrating that the defects leading to isolated pulmonary involvement are specific to the respiratory epithelium, whereas those defects leading to disseminated disease affect immune cells. Therefore, evaluation of isolated lung disease should focus on respiratory tract causes.[5]

Cervical Lymph Nodes

Isolated cervical lymphadenopathy, most frequently caused by MAC, is the most common form of nontuberculous mycobacterial infection in young children in North America. The organism is generally MAC, but other nontuberculous mycobacteria can also cause disease. The cervical swelling is often firm and relatively painless with a paucity of systemic signs. Because the differential diagnosis of painless adenopathy (Chapter 159) includes malignancy, many of these infections are incidentally diagnosed at biopsy. Local fistulas usually resolve completely with resection or antibiotic therapy or both.

Skin and Soft Tissue Disease

Mycobacterium marinum causes skin infections, usually papules or ulcers, associated with water exposure and is known as "fish tank granuloma."[6] Numerous outbreaks of skin infections caused by rapidly growing mycobacteria (especially *M. abscessus, M. fortuitum*, and *Mycobacterium chelonae*) have been due to skin contamination from instruments used for surgical procedures (especially cosmetic surgery), injections, and other procedures.[7] These infections are typically accompanied by painful, erythematous, draining subcutaneous nodules, usually without associated fever or systemic symptoms.

DIAGNOSIS

Nontuberculous mycobacteria are now the most common mycobacteria isolated from humans in North America.[8] The conventional tuberculin skin test (purified protein derivative [PPD]) evokes a cell-mediated response to secreted mycobacterial antigens. Unfortunately, the PPD test does not differentiate well between nontuberculous mycobacterial and tuberculosis infection, although large PPD reactions (>15 mm) more commonly signify tuberculosis. With the progressive decline in active tuberculosis in the United States, nontuberculous mycobacteria are likely to account for significant proportions of PPD reactivity. Newer IFN-γ release assays (IGRAs) incubate blood with relatively tuberculosis-specific recombinant proteins and elicit T-cell secretion of IFN-γ, thereby helping to clarify whether PPD reactivity is due to tuberculosis; however, *M. kansasii, M. szulgai*, and *M. marinum* cross-react in some IGRAs.

Isolation of nontuberculous mycobacteria from blood specimens is clear evidence of disease. However, because the slow-growing nontuberculous mycobacteria typically do not grow well in routine blood culture media, the diagnosis must be suspected to be made. Isolation of nontuberculous mycobacteria from a biopsy specimen is strong evidence of infection, but cases of laboratory contamination do occur. Identification of organisms on stained sections of biopsy material confirms the authenticity of the culture. Some unusual nontuberculous mycobacteria require lower incubation temperatures or special additives for growth (e.g., *M. haemophilum*).

The radiographic appearance of nontuberculous mycobacterial disease in the lung ranges from normal to nodules, bronchiectasis, air space disease, and extensive cavity formation, similar to that seen in tuberculosis (Fig. 309-2). Isolation of nontuberculous mycobacteria from respiratory samples presents special problems in both sensitivity and specificity. *M. gordonae* is often recovered from respiratory samples and is almost never thought to be a real pathogen. Many patients, especially those with bronchiectasis, will occasionally have nontuberculous mycobacteria recovered from sputum culture without such mycobacteria being seen on smear. Specific criteria for definitive diagnosis of

nontuberculous mycobacterial lung disease exist for MAC, *M. abscessus*, and *M. kansasii*, but they are probably good guidelines for other nontuberculous mycobacteria as well. A positive diagnosis requires that two of three sputum samples grow nontuberculous mycobacteria, regardless of smear findings; a positive bronchoscopic alveolar sample, regardless of smear findings; or a biopsy specimen of pulmonary parenchyma with granulomatous inflammation or mycobacteria found on section and nontuberculous mycobacteria on culture.

Once isolated, identification of nontuberculous mycobacteria is important because it will determine the broad class of antimycobacterial therapy to be used. Many laboratories now use DNA probes to identify MAC, *M. gordonae*, and *M. kansasii*.[9] Drug susceptibility testing is of limited and largely unproven value, although clarithromycin susceptibility testing for MAC and rifampin susceptibility testing for *M. kansasii* are indicated. Initial isolates of MAC that have not been exposed to macrolides are almost always susceptible to macrolides. Any nontuberculous mycobacteria that have resisted a course of antimicrobials should probably be tested for antibiotic susceptibility as well.

PREVENTION

Prophylaxis of MAC disease in patients infected with HIV is started when the CD4+ T-lymphocyte count is less than 50 cells/μL. Azithromycin 1200 mg weekly, clarithromycin 1000 mg daily, and rifabutin 300 mg daily are effective.

TREATMENT   Rx

It is rarely an emergency to initiate treatment of nontuberculous mycobacterial infections, which are relatively slow-growing chronic infections that evolve over a period of weeks to years, not hours to days. Therefore, empirical therapy is not usually needed, and identification of the species is advisable before starting complex, often poorly tolerated and potentially toxic regimens.[10] Similar to the case with tuberculosis, single-drug therapy is almost always associated with the emergence of antimicrobial resistance and is strongly discouraged.

MAC infection frequently requires complex multidrug therapy, the foundation of which is a macrolide (clarithromycin or azithromycin), ethambutol, and a rifamycin (rifampin or rifabutin). For disseminated nontuberculous mycobacterial disease in HIV-infected patients, the use of rifamycins poses special problems of drug interactions with protease inhibitors. For pulmonary MAC disease, three-times-weekly administration of drugs has been used successfully. The duration of therapy is prolonged, generally for 12 months after culture conversion and typically for a total of at least 18 months. Other drugs with activity against MAC include aminoglycosides, fluoroquinolones, and clofazimine. Adjuvant pulmonary resection is associated with a relatively high complication rate but also can provide a high level of success for selected patients who respond poorly to antibiotic treatment alone.[11]

M. kansasii lung disease is similar to tuberculosis in many ways and is also effectively treated with isoniazid (300 mg/day), rifampin (600 mg/day), and ethambutol (15 mg/kg/day). Treatment should continue until cultures have been negative for at least 1 year. Other drugs with very high activity against *M. kansasii* include clarithromycin, fluoroquinolones, and aminoglycosides. For skin ulcers caused by *M. ulcerans*, which is sensitive to temperatures above 37° C, local thermotherapy is highly effective and safe.[12]

Rapidly growing mycobacteria pose special therapeutic problems. Extrapulmonary disease in an immunocompetent host is usually due to inoculation (e.g., surgery, injection, trauma) or line infection and is often treated successfully with a macrolide and another drug (based on in vitro susceptibility), along with removal of the offending focus. By comparison, pulmonary disease, especially that caused by *M. abscessus*, is extremely difficult to eradicate, although repeated courses of treatment are usually effective in reducing the infectious burden and symptoms. Therapy generally includes a macrolide along with an intravenous agent such as amikacin, a carbapenem, cefoxitin, or tigecycline. Other oral agents used according to in vitro susceptibility testing and tolerance include fluoroquinolones, doxycycline, and linezolid. Inhaled amikacin may be an option for treatment-refractory pulmonary infections.[13]

Treatment of the other nontuberculous mycobacteria is less well defined, but macrolides and aminoglycosides are usually effective, with other agents added as indicated. Expert consultation is strongly encouraged for difficult or unusual nontuberculous mycobacterial infections.

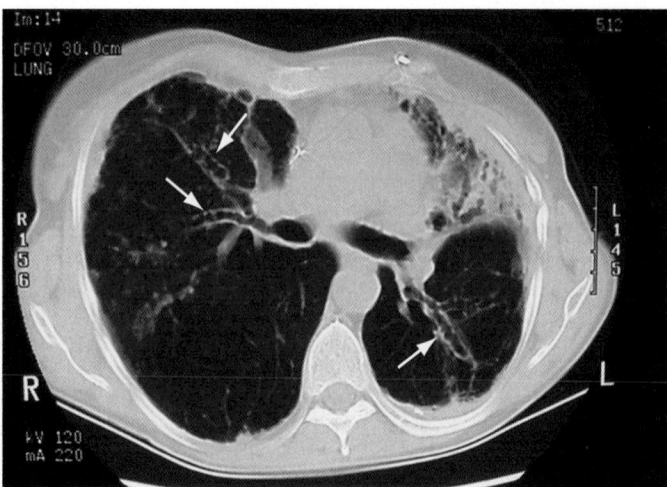

FIGURE 309-2. Chest computed tomography in a patient with severe pulmonary *Mycobacterium abscessus* infection. *Arrows* indicate bronchiectasis. Note the extensive left upper lobe destruction and diffuse pleural reaction. In addition, the left lung is smaller than the right as a result of extensive loss of lung parenchyma.

PROGNOSIS

The effect of nontuberculous mycobacterial infection on longevity is closely tied to the underlying condition (e.g., IFN-γ/IL-12 pathway defect, cystic fibrosis). With no or inadequate treatment, symptoms are intrusive, and the infections can lead to fatal complications, including overwhelming infection or severe lung destruction.

GENERAL REFERENCES

For the General References and other additional features, please visit Expert Consult at https://expertconsult.inkling.com.

310

LEPROSY (HANSEN DISEASE)

JOEL D. ERNST

DEFINITION

Leprosy (Hansen disease) is a chronic infection caused by *Mycobacterium leprae*, an acid-fast slowly growing bacterium that cannot yet be cultured in vitro. Leprosy is found worldwide, although three countries of high prevalence (India, Brazil, and Indonesia) currently account for more than 80% of reported cases.[1] The primary manifestations of infection with *M. leprae* occur in the skin and peripheral nerves. The skin lesions of leprosy are classically hypopigmented, hypoesthetic or anesthetic, and nonpruritic. Peripheral nerves can be damaged by direct infection with *M. leprae* or by the immune response to the infection; the result is loss of sensation and motor function. Additional morbidity is due to the peripheral nerve dysfunction, including painless traumatic and burn injuries, secondary bacterial infections, and muscle atrophy and contractures. Leprosy per se is not a cause of death, but the debility associated with leprosy contributes to the severity of poverty and the likelihood of death from malnutrition or other infections. Despite the low transmissibility of *M. leprae* and the ability of multiple-drug therapy to cure leprosy, it remains a stigmatized disease that can pose a challenge to diagnosis and therapy.

The Pathogen

M. leprae is an acid-fast bacillus that contains a mycolic acid–rich cell wall and a single membrane. Despite nearly 150 years of effort, *M. leprae* remains uncultivatible in vitro. For biochemical and structural characterization, *M. leprae* can be grown in large quantities in nine-banded armadillos (*Dasypus novemcinctus*), and inoculation of the footpads of athymic mice allows semi-quantitation of viable bacilli.

EPIDEMIOLOGY

Leprosy is found worldwide, although endemic leprosy is absent from northern Europe, where it was present in epidemic form as recently as the 19th century. The global prevalence of leprosy is about 175,000 known cases, and the current incidence is about 211,000. By definition of the World Health Organization (WHO) Strategic Plan for the Elimination of Leprosy, a newly diagnosed patient who has been treated with multidrug therapy is removed from the prevalence registry, which explains the lower prevalence than incidence of this chronic infection. Since initiation of the WHO Strategic Plan (whose goal is to eliminate leprosy as a public health problem, i.e., a prevalence of less than 1 in 10,000 in all regions), an estimated 16 million people have been cured of leprosy.

The success of multidrug therapy notwithstanding, leprosy remains a public health problem in 14 countries. India, Brazil, and Indonesia currently have the largest number of cases. Although domestic transmission of leprosy is extremely rare in the United States, 178 cases of leprosy were diagnosed in 2015, including cases in immigrants from India, Brazil, the Philippines, the Dominican Republic, and Mexico. Because leprosy is not highly transmissible, it is not considered a disease of travelers other than immigrants.

Inability to culture *M. leprae* in vitro has been a major hindrance to understanding the modes of transmission and reservoirs of the organism. Observational studies reveal a low frequency of leprosy in casual travelers or temporary residents of high-incidence regions, thus indicating that *M. leprae* is not highly transmissible. Even in areas of high incidence, clusters of leprosy are rare outside families or others with prolonged close contact. It is believed that transmission of *M. leprae* commonly occurs through the respiratory route, because nasal secretions of people with lepromatous leprosy may contain 10^7 viable bacilli per milliliter. In addition, transmission of *M. leprae* is thought to occur through contact with contaminated soil, although soil has not been found to be a reservoir for the bacilli.

PATHOBIOLOGY

Immunology

There is an inverse correlation between the number of lymphocytes and the number of acid-fast bacteria present in skin lesions. Tuberculoid lesions have abundant lymphocytes, well-formed granulomas, and few bacteria (hence this form of leprosy is also termed *paucibacillary*). In contrast, lepromatous lesions have very few lymphocytes, poorly organized or no granulomas, and large numbers of bacteria (also termed *multibacillary leprosy*). Between these polar extremes are intermediate forms that represent a continuum of the histopathologic and bacteriologic findings, termed *borderline tuberculoid, borderline,* and *borderline lepromatous* (Fig. 310-1). In addition to correlating with the number of bacteria in individual lesions, the polar forms of leprosy correlate with the total number of skin lesions in an individual patient: tuberculoid leprosy exhibits few (<five) lesions, whereas lepromatous leprosy is characterized by multiple lesions (≥five, up to hundreds).

Leprosy provides a paradigm for the effect of the cellular immune response to a bacterial pathogen on the clinical manifestations of the infection.[2] Individuals in whom a T helper 1 (T_H1) immune response (characterized by antigen-specific T cells that produce interferon [IFN]-γ, lymphotoxin [LTA], or interleukin [IL]-2 and no IL-4 or IL-5) develops to *M. leprae* exhibit few skin lesions and few bacteria within the lesions (paucibacillary leprosy).[3] In contrast, persons in whom a T_H2 immune response develops (T cells that produce little IFN-γ, lymphotoxin, or IL-2, but produce IL-4, IL-5, and IL-13) have larger numbers of skin lesions and large numbers of bacteria within lesions (multibacillary leprosy). Production of IL-17 is prevalent in persons with paucibacillary leprosy, whereas a predominance of regulatory T cells (Treg) and the cytokines that they produce (IL-10 and TGF-β) are associated with multibacillary leprosy. The primary determinant of the differential immune response to *M. leprae* is incompletely understood, although substantial evidence indicates that host genetic polymorphisms contribute to the likelihood of paucibacillary versus multibacillary leprosy. Complement activation is probably

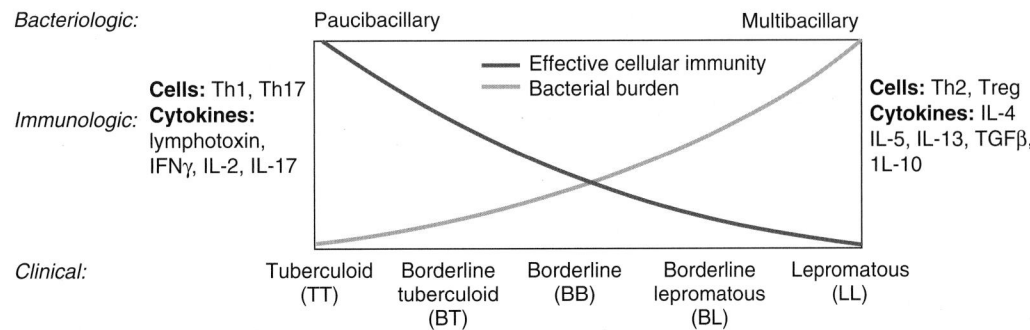

FIGURE 310-1. Bacteriologic, immunologic, and clinical spectrum of leprosy. Tuberculoid (paucibacillary) leprosy is characterized by Th1 and Th17 immune responses and few or no detectable bacilli in biopsy specimens of skin lesions or smears of skin slits. At the opposite pole of the spectrum, lepromatous (multibacillary) leprosy is accompanied by Th2 and Treg responses, numerous skin lesions, and numerous acid-fast bacilli on skin biopsy specimens or smears. The intermediate forms can be classified according to their resemblance to tuberculoid or lepromatous leprosy. IFN = interferon; IL = interleukin; TGF = transforming growth factor.

also involved in the pathogenesis of both the reversal reaction and erythema nodosum leprosum.

Pathogenesis of Nerve Damage

Peripheral nerve damage, the most important consequence of infection with *M. leprae,* occurs in all forms of leprosy and underlies the complications of the infection; multiple mechanisms contribute. *M. leprae* invades Schwann cells, the glial cells of peripheral nerves.[4] Schwann cells form a functional unit with peripheral nerve axons and are surrounded by laminin-2, a neural-specific extracellular matrix protein. The G domain of laminin-2 can bind simultaneously to *M. leprae* and to the Schwann cell laminin receptor α-dystroglycan. Once *M. leprae* is bound and internalized by Schwann cells, it can cause direct demyelination of peripheral nerves in the absence of an immune response, apparently by signaling through ErbB2 and Erk1/2.

In addition to direct damage to peripheral nerves by *M. leprae,* the immune response in leprosy also contributes to nerve damage. Pro-inflammatory cytokines such as tumor necrosis factor (TNF)-α, IL-1β, IL-17, and IFN-γ are especially prominent in lesions during reversal reactions, when irreversible nerve damage can occur. Because these molecules can contribute to inflammatory tissue damage and can induce apoptosis of Schwann cells in vitro, it is likely these mediators play an active role in nerve damage. Reversal reactions are also characterized by an increase in the number of CD4[+] T lymphocytes in lesions, and at least some of these CD4[+] cells exhibit a cytotoxic phenotype and kill *M. leprae*–infected Schwann cells through antigen- and major histocompatibility complex class II–dependent secretion of cytotoxic granule contents. Whether these mechanisms of nerve damage occur in chronic tuberculoid leprosy is not established, but similar cytokines and T lymphocytes are found in tuberculoid lesions.

CLINICAL MANIFESTATIONS

The most common manifestations of leprosy involve the skin and peripheral nerves and are determined by the polarity of the disease: paucibacillary (tuberculoid) or multibacillary (lepromatous).[5] The onset of leprosy is usually insidious. Depending on the form of leprosy, numbness may be an initial complaint or finding, and skin lesions may become apparent only months or years later. The classification of leprosy as tuberculoid, lepromatous, or one of the borderline forms is based on the combination of clinical examination, the number of bacteria seen on skin slit smears or skin biopsy specimens, and the histologic appearance. Because the nature of the potential complications and the specific course of chemotherapy are determined by the form of leprosy, accurate diagnosis and classification are essential.

Tuberculoid Leprosy

Tuberculoid leprosy is characterized by the presence of fewer than five skin lesions, which are typically hypopigmented or erythematous macules with raised erythematous borders and an atrophic center (Fig. 310-2). The skin lesions in tuberculoid leprosy are usually hypoesthetic or anesthetic; when multiple lesions are present, their distribution is asymmetrical. The skin lesions may be large and are most commonly found on the face, trunk, or extremities; however, they are not found in the axillae, groin, perineum, or on the scalp, presumably because of the preference of *M. leprae* for lower temperatures.

Local peripheral nerve involvement is common in tuberculoid leprosy and is asymmetrical. In addition to hypoesthesia or anesthesia of the skin lesions, nerve involvement in tuberculoid leprosy is manifested as enlargement or tenderness (or both) of the peripheral nerves that serve the region of the skin lesions. Superficial nerves such as the ulnar, superficial peroneal, or greater auricular nerves may be visibly enlarged, depending on the location of the skin lesions. Functional complications of nerve involvement, such as muscle atrophy and contractures, may be present at the time of diagnosis of tuberculoid leprosy. Tuberculoid leprosy is a stable form; it does not convert to borderline or lepromatous forms.

Lepromatous Leprosy

Lepromatous leprosy is characterized by multiple skin lesions that are smaller than those observed in tuberculoid leprosy (Fig. 310-3). Although the sites of skin lesions are similar to those of tuberculoid leprosy, the multiple lesions of lepromatous leprosy are often symmetrically distributed. Lepromatous macules may have poorly defined borders and no loss of sensation; local nerve enlargement is not characteristic. In addition to macules, lepromatous skin lesions may be nodules or plaques, or they may diffusely infiltrate the skin, especially on the face (which may cause loss of eyebrows and "leonine facies").

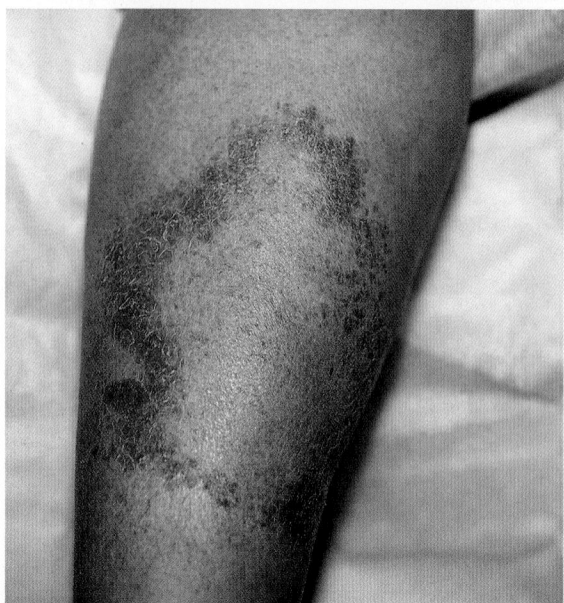

FIGURE 310-2. Tuberculoid leprosy. A single large lesion with irregular, raised, erythematous borders and a depressed, hypopigmented center is shown. These are usually hypoesthetic or anesthetic. (From Hansen's disease [leprosy]. In: James WD, Berger TG, Elston DM, eds. *Andrews' Diseases of the Skin.* 10th ed. Philadelphia: Elsevier; 2006.)

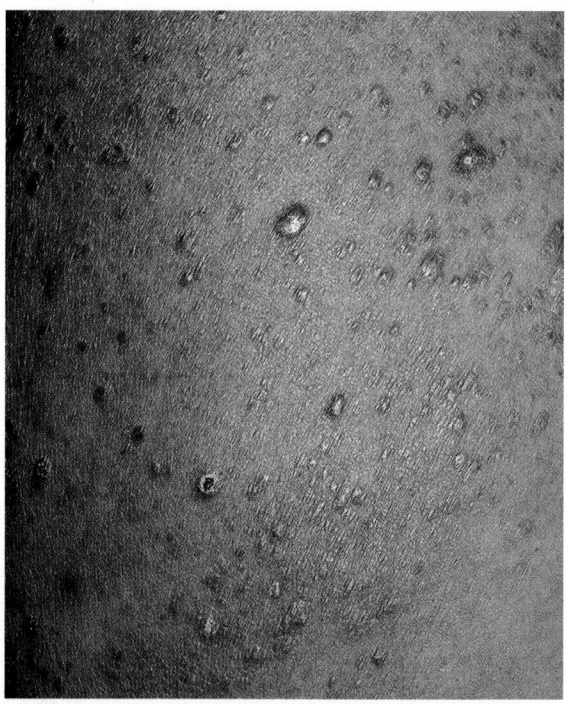

FIGURE 310-3. Lepromatous leprosy. Numerous papules and nodules are apparent. Lepromatous macules have ill-defined borders, with normal sensation usually maintained. Also see Figure 411-22 in Chapter 411. (From Hansen's disease [leprosy]. In: James WD, Berger TG, Elston DM, eds. *Andrews' Diseases of the Skin.* 10th ed. Philadelphia: Elsevier; 2006.)

Nerve involvement in lepromatous leprosy is characteristically symmetrical and exhibits a stocking-glove distribution unrelated to the location of skin lesions. Peripheral nerve involvement may initially be manifested as loss of temperature sensation, followed by loss of light touch, pain, and deep pressure sense. In addition, dysesthesia is common. Motor complications, including muscle weakness and atrophy of the muscles of the hands, feet, and face, develop in the absence of effective antileprosy chemotherapy. Autonomic dysfunction may be an early development in leprosy. Its manifestations may include anhidrosis, impaired sweating function, localized alopecia, and reduced heart rate variability. Involvement of the facial nerve may result in corneal exposure, ulceration, and blindness. Persons with lepromatous leprosy may also have rhinorrhea as a result of nasal mucosal involvement, and they may shed large numbers of *M. leprae* in their nasal secretions—one of the major sources of bacilli for transmission to other individuals. Like tuberculoid leprosy, lepromatous leprosy is stable; conversion to other forms does not occur.

Borderline Forms of Leprosy

Borderline tuberculoid leprosy is characterized by skin lesions similar to those of tuberculoid leprosy, but they are more numerous and may be accompanied by satellite lesions around large lesions. In borderline leprosy, skin lesions are numerous but remain asymmetrical. The lesions are usually plaques rather than macules and exhibit satellite lesions. Nerve involvement in borderline leprosy is manifested as thickening or tenderness of local nerves, but the skin lesions retain sensation. Borderline lepromatous leprosy is characterized by numerous symmetrical small macules, papules, plaques, and nodules but not the diffuse skin infiltration found in full-blown lepromatous leprosy. Unlike tuberculoid and lepromatous leprosy, the borderline forms are unstable and progress to the lepromatous form over time unless effective treatment is provided. Reactional states, including both reversal reactions and downgrading reactions, occur in those with borderline forms of leprosy.

Diffuse Lepromatous Leprosy (Lucio Leprosy)

A severe form of leprosy, characterized clinically by generalized and diffuse infiltration of the skin, and histopathologically by mycobacterial invasion of small vessel endothelial cells and vascular occlusion, has been observed in Mexico and the Caribbean region. Recent work has implicated a distinct species, *Mycobacterium lepromatosus,* as the cause of diffuse lepromatous leprosy. Comparison of genome sequences has revealed that *M. lepromatosus* and *M. leprae* shared a common ancestor, and have undergone distinct pathways of evolution, but it is not clear what forces account for this divergence. Likewise, it is not yet clear how the genomic differences account for the clinical and pathologic differences observed.

Reactional States

Individuals with leprosy may exhibit acute reactional symptoms and signs, even before they have been diagnosed with leprosy. Physicians in developed countries may encounter patients with reactional states in acute care settings.

Type 1 reactions, which are mediated by cellular immune responses to *M. leprae* antigens in skin lesions and nerves, occur in borderline tuberculoid, borderline, and borderline lepromatous leprosy. Type 1 reactions are frequently accompanied by worsening of peripheral nerve manifestations and may result in permanent nerve damage; they should be considered medical emergencies. Reversal reactions, which are type 1 reactions that occur after initiation of therapy for leprosy or for human immunodeficiency virus (HIV) infection, are associated with enhanced T_H1 immune responses that develop in patients with a large burden of *M. leprae;* they are most severe in those with borderline lepromatous leprosy. Downgrading reactions occur in association with the transition of borderline disease toward the lepromatous form. Although the immune mechanisms that underlie reversal reactions and downgrading reactions are believed to be distinct, their clinical manifestations are indistinguishable. Type 1 reactions may have an acute or insidious onset, and they are characterized by inflammation of preexisting skin and nerve lesions. Skin lesions, which become erythematous and edematous, may also become tender and thereby resemble cellulitis, but type 1 reactions are not accompanied by fever or other systemic symptoms or signs. Increased expression of TNF has been found in lesions during type 1 reactions and may contribute to the clinical and functional consequences. Moreover, type 1 reactions have been reported when TNF antagonist therapy has been withdrawn after diagnosis of borderline lepromatous leprosy. Transcriptomic analyses have also implicated the complement system in the pathogenesis of type 1 and type 2 leprosy reactions.

Type 2 reactions, also known as erythema nodosum leprosum (ENL), occur in persons with borderline lepromatous and lepromatous leprosy; they may be mediated by immune complexes rather than cellular immune responses. Type 2 reactions, which occur most often after initiation of antileprosy chemotherapy or during pregnancy, are generally accompanied by fever and arthralgias. Additional signs of systemic inflammatory disease may appear, including hepatosplenomegaly, lymphadenopathy, arthritis, nephritis, keratitis, and iritis. The skin lesions of ENL resemble those of classic erythema nodosum (Chapter 411 and Fig. 411-24), with widely distributed erythematous dermal and subcutaneous nodules whose location is unrelated to the leprosy lesions. Biopsy of ENL lesions shows neutrophilic infiltration of the deep dermis and subcutis, accompanied by other leukocyte populations, including T cells. Vasculitis can be present, but it is not a consistent finding.

Leprosy and Human Immunodeficiency Virus

CD4+ T-cell–mediated immunity is essential for control of *M. leprae,* and the extent of T_H1 immunity determines whether an individual will have tuberculoid or lepromatous leprosy. However, coinfection with HIV and depletion of CD4+ T lymphocytes does not affect the rate of progression of leprosy, nor does it cause conversion of tuberculoid leprosy to the lepromatous form. In contrast, type 1 reversal reactions may accompany immune reconstitution subsequent to initiation of effective antiretroviral therapy for HIV infection (Chapter 367). The manifestations of these reversal reactions are similar to those observed in patients who are not infected with HIV.

DIAGNOSIS

The diagnosis of leprosy should be considered in any patient with skin and peripheral nerve manifestations, especially those who have lived in countries where leprosy is endemic. Although leprosy is a chronic infection, its acute complications require prompt diagnosis and therapy to prevent irreversible peripheral nerve damage. It is also important to classify a patient's disease as tuberculoid, lepromatous, or one of the specific borderline forms, because correct classification is necessary for selecting optimal therapy and anticipating potential reactional states. Because *M. leprae* cannot be cultured in vitro and there is currently no reliable serologic test or other diagnostic biomarker for leprosy, diagnosis and classification of leprosy depend on the combination of clinical examination, histopathologic evaluation, and acid-fast staining of skin slit or biopsy specimens.[7]

Clinical Examination

Examination of an individual with possible or confirmed leprosy must include evaluation and documentation of the number, location, and characteristics of skin lesions. In addition to descriptions of the skin lesions, accurate classification of leprosy depends on whether the lesions are distributed symmetrically and whether they are hypoesthetic or anesthetic. The examination must also include a search for (1) enlarged and tender peripheral nerves; (2) the presence of sensory deficits (especially temperature sensation and pain) and skin ulcerations; and (3) the nature and distribution of motor deficits, muscle atrophy, and contractures. Because some medications used for the treatment of leprosy are contraindicated in pregnancy, women of childbearing age should be evaluated for pregnancy.

Skin Smears and Biopsies

In developing countries, classification of multibacillary or paucibacillary leprosy is made by the combination of clinical examination findings and bacterial counts as determined on acid-fast–stained smears made from skin slits of lesions and skin from cool areas of the body, such as the earlobes. In developed countries, skin biopsies are usually performed instead of skin slits. Skin specimens should be obtained from the active borders of lesions and should include subcutaneous tissue. On hematoxylin-eosin staining, tuberculoid leprosy is characterized by granulomas with giant cells, aggregates of epithelioid macrophages that are neither vacuolated nor foamy, and lymphocytes at the periphery. Although granulomas may be found in other skin diseases, selective destruction of nerve trunks and perineural fibrosis are specific features of leprosy. Acid-fast stains (preferably done with the Fite procedure) show rare or undetectable bacilli in tuberculoid leprosy. Lesions of lepromatous leprosy show poorly organized granulomas without giant cells or lymphocytes; macrophages are foamy and lipid laden. Acid-fast staining of lepromatous leprosy lesions reveals abundant bacilli that usually appear in large clumps ("globi"). The borderline forms of leprosy exhibit less well-organized granulomas with fewer giant cells and lymphocytes but more foamy macrophages and acid-fast bacilli as the spectrum varies from borderline tuberculoid to borderline lepromatous.

Specialized immunohistochemistry stains, such as for CD4+ T lymphocytes or cytokine expression, are useful in research studies but are not currently used for the clinical diagnosis or classification of leprosy. Polymerase chain reaction (PCR) amplification of mycobacterial genomic DNA from skin slits or skin biopsy specimens has not yet contributed to enhanced sensitivity of detection, but PCR can be used to distinguish *M. leprae* and *M. lepromatosus* in patients from regions where both pathogens may be found.[8]

Diagnosis of Reactional States

The diagnosis of type 1 reactions is based on clinical findings in a patient with borderline tuberculoid, borderline, or borderline lepromatous leprosy and acute inflammation of preexisting skin lesions, with or without worsening of nerve lesions. Type 1 reactions are not accompanied by systemic findings such as fever or arthritis. At highest risk for type 1 reactions are patients who have recently initiated antileprosy chemotherapy, although type 1 reactions can occur spontaneously. Diagnosis of a type 2 reaction (ENL) is also based on clinical findings of new erythematous subcutaneous or dermal nodules in a patient with borderline lepromatous or lepromatous leprosy. There are currently no diagnostic tests or biomarkers for ENL, and skin biopsy will not distinguish ENL from classic erythema nodosum.

TREATMENT   Rx

Agents to Treat Leprosy

The first-line antimicrobial agents for leprosy have been dapsone and rifampin. Clofazimine, minocycline, certain fluoroquinolones, and clarithromycin are also useful in specific contexts, including drug intolerance or resistance.

Dapsone is inexpensive and well tolerated, has a long serum half-life ($\approx$28 hours), and is safe for use during pregnancy. Glucose-6-phosphate dehydrogenase (G6PD)–deficient individuals (Chapter 152) are susceptible to dapsone-induced methemoglobinemia and hemolysis, and all patients should be screened for G6PD deficiency before starting dapsone. Patients with mild G6PD deficiency (the African type, caused by mutations that lead to instability of the enzyme) can begin dapsone at 25 mg/day but require close monitoring for hemolytic anemia. Dapsone can also cause bone marrow suppression and profound neutropenia. Other rare adverse effects of dapsone include hepatitis, cholestatic jaundice, and a hypersensitivity syndrome that usually occurs within 4 to 6 weeks of initiation of dapsone and is characterized by exfoliative dermatitis, generalized lymphadenopathy, fever, and hepatosplenomegaly. A study in China found that the presence of the HLA class I allele B*13:01 confers a seven-fold higher risk of the dapsone hypersensitivity syndrome, strongly implicating CD8$^+$ T cells in its pathogenesis.

Rifampin, the most bactericidal drug against *M. leprae,* is well absorbed after oral administration and has a serum half-life of approximately 3 hours. Rifampin should never be used as monotherapy because resistance can develop with single point mutations in its target, RNA polymerase II. Because rifampin is bactericidal and rapid release of components from dead bacteria can have pro-inflammatory effects, some experts withhold rifampin during reversal reactions. Adverse effects of rifampin include maculopapular rash, hepatotoxicity, an influenza-like syndrome (most frequent with intermittent therapy), and orange discoloration of tears, urine, saliva, and sweat. Thrombocytopenia occurs occasionally but is not usually severe. Rifampin also induces metabolism and decreases serum concentrations of other drugs, including antiretroviral protease inhibitors and non-nucleoside reverse transcriptase inhibitors, methadone, and oral contraceptives. Rifampin decreases serum concentrations of dapsone, but this effect is not clinically significant with a dapsone dose of 100 mg/day.

Clofazimine is a lipophilic dye that is bacteriostatic against *M. leprae.* It has a very long ($\approx$70 days) half-life and appears to have anti-inflammatory activity as well as direct bacteriostatic activity. Because of its anti-inflammatory activity, clofazimine is useful in the treatment of type 1 reactional states. Clofazimine is generally well tolerated; its major side effect is discoloration of the skin, which occurs in nearly all clofazimine-treated patients. The skin discoloration can range from reddish tan to bluish black and can be blotchy, but it is reversible within 6 to 12 months of discontinuation of the drug. In chronic reactional patients maintained with high doses of clofazimine (200 to 300 mg/day), enteropathy with crampy abdominal pain, mild nausea, or diarrhea (or both) and even bowel obstruction can develop.

Regimens to Treat Leprosy

Chemotherapy for leprosy involves the use of multiple drugs to optimize the rate of cure and prevent emergence of drug resistance.[9] The regimen currently recommended in the United States for paucibacillary (tuberculoid and borderline tuberculoid) leprosy in adults consists of dapsone, 100 mg, and rifampin, 600 mg, both given daily for 12 months. The U.S. recommended regimen for multibacillary leprosy in adults is dapsone, 100 mg, plus rifampin, 600 mg, and clofazimine, 50 mg, each given daily for 24 months (available at http://www.hrsa.gov/hansensdisease/diagnosis/recommendedtreatment.html). However, 6 months dapsone/rifampicin/clofazimine may be equally effective.[A1] Clofazimine is currently not commercially available, but it can be obtained in the United States through the National Hansen's Disease Program (1-800-642-2477). In resource-limited countries where the burden of leprosy is highest, the WHO regimen for paucibacillary leprosy is dapsone, 100 mg daily, plus rifampin, 600 mg once a month, for 6 months. The WHO regimen for adults for multibacillary leprosy (which differs from the U.S. recommendation) is dapsone, 100 mg daily, plus rifampin, 600 mg once a month, plus clofazimine, 50 mg daily, each given for 12 months, plus an additional dose of clofazimine, 300 mg once a month (available at http://www.who.int/lep/mdt/regimens/en/index.html). The monthly doses of rifampin and clofazimine should be administered under supervision. Alternative agents for patients with drug intolerance or drug resistance include clarithromycin (may be substituted for any of the first-line drugs), minocycline (may be substituted for dapsone or clofazimine), and ofloxacin (may be substituted for clofazimine, although it should be avoided in children).

Response to Therapy

Response to effective therapy for leprosy is seen clinically as flattening and resolution of the papules, nodules, or plaques, with or without improvement in nerve function. Clinical improvement may begin within the first months of therapy, but resolution of skin lesions is often delayed as long as 1 to 2 years after completion of therapy. Quantitation of the bacillary load to assess response to treatment is cumbersome, semiquantitative, and not recommended.

Patients who have been adequately treated may experience worsening of nerve and skin symptoms, perhaps because of a late reversal reaction or relapsed leprosy. If skin specimens do not reveal acid-fast organisms, a therapeutic trial of corticosteroids, which will ameliorate the symptoms of reversal reactions but not those of relapsed leprosy, can help make the distinction and assist in choosing subsequent therapy. Patients who experience relapse after treatment of paucibacillary disease should be treated for multibacillary disease, because the most likely cause of relapse is previous multibacillary disease that was misclassified. Patients with multibacillary disease who relapse should be retreated with a regimen containing dapsone and rifampin with the addition of at least two drugs that were not used in the initial treatment regimen, unless susceptibility testing is available and confirms that the organisms remain susceptible to dapsone and rifampin. The choices among additional drugs include minocycline, ofloxacin or moxifloxacin, and clarithromycin. Relapsed multibacillary patients may benefit from lifelong maintenance therapy after completing 2 years of a salvage regimen. Because susceptibility testing cannot be performed with in vitro assays, an alternative approach to determination of susceptibility by detecting mutations in the targets of dapsone and rifampin (*folP1* and *rpoB,* respectively) is beginning to be widely used and is commercially available. The mouse footpad assay has been used, but it is becoming less available.

Treatment of Reactional States

Type 1 reactions may develop before, during, or years after completion of antileprosy chemotherapy.[10] Type 1 reactions that involve worsening of nerve symptoms are medical emergencies because permanent nerve damage can occur. Type 1 reactions usually respond to prednisone at a daily dose of 60 to 80 mg, which can be tapered slowly once symptoms are controlled. Type 1 reactions can also respond to high-dose clofazimine (200 to 300 mg/day), although reactions with worsening nerve symptoms should be treated initially with prednisone. Patients who have type 1 reactions that occur before or during antileprosy chemotherapy and whose reactions include nerve involvement should have rifampin withheld until the worsened nerve symptoms resolve, because release of pro-inflammatory components from dying bacteria may contribute to inflammation and nerve damage. Dapsone and clofazimine should be continued during treatment of type 1 reactions.

The treatment of choice for severe type 2 reactions (ENL) is thalidomide, except in pregnant or potentially pregnant women. Thalidomide requires that patients and the prescribing physician be enrolled in the Risk Evaluation and Mitigation Strategy (REMS; http://www.thalomidrems.com/) program to avoid the drug's teratogenic effects. The mechanism of action of thalidomide is incompletely understood but is likely to include inhibition of TNF. The dose of thalidomide for ENL varies, depending on the severity of the reaction. In patients with ENL and high fever, frank arthritis, and large subcutaneous plaques, up to 100 mg four times daily may be required to achieve a clinical response. Once a clinical response is achieved, the dose of thalidomide may be tapered to a maintenance dose of 50 to 100 mg given once daily at night (because thalidomide is sedating). For milder cases of ENL, 50 to 100 mg per night may be sufficient to achieve and maintain control. ENL in women of childbearing age and thalidomide-unresponsive cases may respond to corticosteroids. Methotrexate may be efficacious in otherwise treatment-resistant ENL, but methotrexate has been assigned by the U.S. Food and Drug Administration to pregnancy category X (teratogenic risks "clearly outweigh" potential benefits) and is also contraindicated in nursing mothers. Antileprosy chemotherapy, including rifampin, should be continued in patients with ENL.

Other Therapy

Nerve damage in leprosy, which can result in muscle atrophy, contractures, and autoamputation, is the major cause of debility.[11] The benefit of therapies such as corticosteroids is uncertain.[A2] Supportive care, reconstructive surgery, physical and occupational therapy, and rehabilitation can be extremely valuable in allowing patients to achieve and maintain optimal function.

PREVENTION

There is currently no effective specific vaccine for leprosy, but several trials have observed a partial protective effect of bacille Calmette-Guérin (BCG) vaccination. It is likely that improved understanding of transmission of *M. leprae* will be generated by the use of DNA-based strain typing, so better preventive measures are likely to become available in the near future.[12]

PROGNOSIS

Multidrug chemotherapy cures a high proportion of people with paucibacillary and multibacillary leprosy. The currently recommended regimens provide high rates of response, with relapse rates of approximately 0.1% per year in paucibacillary cases and up to 5% per year in multibacillary cases. Some cases of paucibacillary leprosy may enter remission or even self-cure, but all cases of multibacillary leprosy are progressive. Because of its efficacy and low toxicity and to minimize long-term morbidity, multidrug chemotherapy should be used in all persons in whom leprosy is diagnosed.

Grade A References

A1. Penna GO, Buhrer-Sekula S, Kerr LRS, et al. Uniform multidrug therapy for leprosy patients in Brazil (U-MDT/CT-BR): results of an open label, randomized and controlled clinical trial, among multibacillary patients. *PLoS Negl Trop Dis.* 2017;11:1-19.
A2. Van Veen NH, Nicholls PG, Smith WC, et al. Corticosteroids for treating nerve damage in leprosy. *Cochrane Database Syst Rev.* 2016;2:CD005491.

GENERAL REFERENCES

For the General References and other additional features, please visit Expert Consult at https://expertconsult.inkling.com.

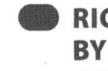

311

RICKETTSIAL INFECTIONS

PIERRE-EDOUARD FOURNIER AND DIDIER RAOULT

DEFINITION

Rickettsioses are emerging infectious diseases.[1] Because of better diagnostic tools and changes in tick exposure, many new rickettsial diseases have been described in the past two decades. Three families of diseases are grouped under this name: rickettsioses, ehrlichioses and anaplasmoses, and Q fever.

The Pathogens

The agents of rickettsial diseases (formerly grouped in the order *Rickettsiales*) are small gram-negative bacteria that grow within eukaryotic cells. Except *Coxiella burnetii*, the agent of Q fever, they have never been grown in axenic media thus far and for culture require living hosts such as cell cultures, embryonated eggs, or susceptible animals. With the exception of *Rickettsia prowazekii*, the agent of epidemic typhus, these bacteria infect humans incidentally and are mainly animal pathogens. On the basis of molecular phylogeny, the bacteria causing rickettsial diseases have been reclassified into three phyla (Table 311-1).

Because of their difficult growth in vitro, the main diagnostic tool for rickettsioses is serology. Serologic evaluation is frequently hampered by late positivity and cross-reactivity. The development of direct staining in blood smears or skin biopsy samples as well as polymerase chain reaction (PCR) amplification of DNA from blood samples, biopsy specimens, or cutaneous eschar swabs has considerably helped identification at the species level and led to the description of emerging pathogens.

RICKETTSIOSES (DISEASES CAUSED BY *RICKETTSIA* SPECIES AND *ORIENTIA TSUTSUGAMUSHI*)

DEFINITION

Rickettsia spp are small gram-negative bacteria that multiply freely in the cytoplasm of their host cells. The target cells in humans are vascular endothelial cells or monocytes, and vasculitis is the most prominent clinical manifestation. These bacteria invade cells by phagocytosis and escape the phagosome vacuole.

The Pathogens

The genome of *Rickettsia* is small, between 1.1 and 1.6 Mb; some have plasmids and potential for conjugation. These bacteria have a family of outer membrane proteins of the surface cell antigen family, including rOmpA (lacking in the typhus group) and rOmpB. These proteins are major antigens that help identify the rickettsial species, and their encoding genes are used for amplification and sequencing for diagnostic or taxonomic purposes. Among rickettsiae, two subgroups, the typhus and spotted fever groups, were identified on the basis of growth conditions and antigenicity. A specific group antigen, determined to be lipopolysaccharide, has been identified. The optimal growth temperatures are 37° C for the typhus group and 32° to 35° C for the spotted fever group. The complete genome sequencing of *R. prowazekii* (from the typhus group) showed that it is mainly a subset of *Rickettsia conorii* (a member of the spotted fever group).

Tick-Borne Rickettsioses
ROCKY MOUNTAIN SPOTTED FEVER
EPIDEMIOLOGY

Rocky Mountain spotted fever (RMSF), the most severe of tick-borne rickettsioses,[2] is caused by *Rickettsia rickettsii* (Table 311-2). It is the major tick-transmitted rickettsiosis recognized in America,[3] along with *Rickettsia africae* in the West Indies, *Rickettsia parkeri* in the southern states of the United States, and, perhaps, "*Rickettsia philipii.*" It was described first in the 19th century in the western United States. RMSF is prevalent in at least 44 states in the United States (Fig. 311-1) and in Central and South America (Argentina, Brazil, Colombia, Costa Rica, Mexico, and Panama).

R. rickettsii is transmitted transovarially to tick progeny from one generation to the next. The infecting ticks are mainly *Dermacentor andersoni* (a wood tick) in the western United States; *Dermacentor variabilis* (the American dog tick) in the East, the Midwest, and the South; and *Rhipicephalus sanguineus* in Arizona. In Central and South America, *Amblyomma cajennense* is the major vector. Humans are infected through infected saliva after a tick bite. The duration of attachment is critical in any tick-borne rickettsiosis, and transmission is unlikely when the tick feeds for less than 20 hours. The tick bite is painless and frequently unnoticed. Rarely, an eschar at the site of the tick bite is observed in RMSF. The epidemiology of RMSF undergoes largely unexplained yearly variations. This temporal repartition is determined by tick activity and human encounter. More than 500 cases occur each year, and more than 90% are reported from April to September. The disease is more prevalent in children younger than 10 years. A recent increase in spotted fever rickettsioses has been reported in the United States, but routine serologic assays do not allow discrimination between RMSF and other endemic rickettsioses.

CLINICAL MANIFESTATIONS

Two to 14 days after the tick bite, fever and headaches appear. The fever is high (temperature >102° F) and associated with nonspecific symptoms, including malaise, myalgias, nausea, vomiting, anorexia, and diarrhea. At this stage, RMSF is not frequently diagnosed, but during the "tick season," patients with high fever who live in or have a history of travel to an endemic location and, possibly, a history of tick bite should be considered as possibly having RMSF.

The most characteristic feature is a rash. However, the classic triad of fever, headache, and rash is present in only 44% of confirmed cases. A rash is found in 14% of cases on the first day of disease and in less than 50% in the first 3 days. The rash is macular; it appears first on the ankles and wrists and then generalizes. Spots are 1 to 5 mm in diameter and can evolve from pink to purpuric. A rash can appear later or even not at all; Rocky Mountain "spotless" fever represented 34% of cases in a series from the U.S. Centers for Disease Control and Prevention (CDC). Involvement of the palms and soles theoretically differentiates the typhus diseases (in which it is absent) from spotted fever rickettsioses.

Untreated patients worsen progressively. The disease is associated in various degrees with general manifestations related to vascular inflammation and increased vascular permeability and with multiple organ involvement that can lead to multiple organ dysfunction syndrome (MODS). In severe forms, patients suffer from edema, hypovolemia, hypoalbuminemia, and hypotension leading to shock. In very severe cases, necrosis and gangrene of the extremities occur. In some instances, noncardiogenic pulmonary edema develops; pulmonary involvement leading to respiratory distress can cause death. Renal failure can result either from hypovolemia and shock and be reversible or from acute tubular necrosis and require hemodialysis. The usual neurologic symptoms are confusion, lethargy, and stupor. In severe cases, delirium, coma, and seizures are observed. Cerebrospinal fluid (CSF) sampling exhibits meningitis in one third of cases; in general, a few mononuclear cells (10 to 100) are observed, along with increased protein but normal glucose levels. Heart involvement can cause arrhythmia. Liver involvement is manifested as an

TABLE 311-1   GENETIC CLASSIFICATION OF RICKETTSIALES

	GENUS	GROUP	SPECIES	SUBSPECIES	FIRST YEAR OF ISOLATION OR DISCOVERY
Rickettsiae	*Rickettsia*	Typhus	*R. prowazekii*		1916
			R. typhi		1920
		Spotted fever	*R. aeschlimannii*		2001
			R. akari		1946
			R. australis		1950
			R. conorii	*conorii*	1932
				israeli	1974
				caspia	1991
				indica	2001
			R. rickettsii		1919
			R. felis		2001
			R. helvetica		2000
			R. heilongjiangensis		1998
			R. honei		1991
			R. japonica		1992
			R. massiliae		2006
			R. monacencis		2007
			R. parkeri		2003
			"*R. philipii*"		1966
			R. raoultii		2008
			R. sibirica	*sibirica*	1946
				mongolotimonae	1996
			R. slovaca		1997
	Orientia	Scrub typhus	*O. tsutsugamushi*		1920
Ehrlichiae	*Ehrlichia*		*E. chaffeensis*		1991
			E. ewingii		1999
			E. canis		1996
			E. muris–like		2009
			Candidatus Neoehrlichia mikurensis		2007
	Anaplasma		*A. phagocytophilum*		1992
	Neorickettsia		*N. sennetsu*		1957
	Wolbachia		*W. pipientis*		2001
Coxiellae	*Coxiella*		*C. burnetii*		1931

TABLE 311-2   RICKETTSIAL DISEASES IN HUMAN BEINGS

DISEASE	ORGANISM	ARTHROPOD HOST	GEOGRAPHIC AREA	RASH	ESCHAR TACHE NOIRE	REGIONAL LYMPH NODE	HIGH FEVER	FATALITY RATE
TICK-TRANSMITTED SPOTTED FEVERS								
Rocky Mountain spotted fever	*R. rickettsii*	*Dermacentor andersoni* *Dermacentor variabilis* *Rhipicephalus sanguineus* *Amblyomma cajennense*	America (North, Central, and South)	Yes, may be purpuric	Very rare	No	Yes	High
Mediterranean spotted fever, Astrakhan fever, Indian tick typhus, Israeli spotted fever	*R. conorii*	*Rhipicephalus sanguineus*	Mediterranean, India, Caspian Sea, Africa	Yes, papular; may be purpuric	Yes	No	Yes	Moderate
African tick-bite fever	*R. africae*	*Amblyomma hebraeum* *Amblyomma variegatum*	Sub-Saharan Africa, West Indies	Yes, half of cases may be vesicular	Yes (frequently multiple)	Yes	No	Low
Queensland tick typhus	*R. australis*	*Ixodes holocyclus*	Eastern Australia	Yes, may be vesicular	Yes	?	Yes	Moderate
Siberian tick typhus	*R. sibirica*	*Dermacentor nuttallii*	Siberia, China, Mongolia	Yes	Yes	No	Yes	Low
Scalp eschar, neck lymphadenopathy after tick bite (SENLAT)	*R. slovaca* or *R. raoultii*	*Dermacentor marginatus* *Dermacentor reticulatus*	Europe, Pakistan	Very rare	Yes, may be erythematous	Yes (painful)	No	Low
Lymphangitis-associated rickettsiosis (LAR)	*R. sibirica mongolotimonae*	*Hyalomma asiaticum*	Mongolia, Africa, Europe	Yes	Yes	Yes	Yes	Low
Flinders Island spotted fever	*R. honei*	*Ixodes granulosus*	Flinders Island, eastern Australia	Yes	Yes	Yes	Yes	Low
Japanese spotted fever	*R. japonica*	*Ixodes ricinus*	Japan, Korea (China?)	Yes	Yes	No	Yes	Low

TABLE 311-2 RICKETTSIAL DISEASES IN HUMAN BEINGS—cont'd

DISEASE	ORGANISM	ARTHROPOD HOST	GEOGRAPHIC AREA	RASH	ESCHAR TACHE NOIRE	REGIONAL LYMPH NODE	HIGH FEVER	FATALITY RATE
Pacific coast tick fever	"R. philipii"	Dermacentor occidentalis	Northern California	Yes	Yes	No	Yes	Unknown
Unnamed	R. aeschlimannii	Hyalomma sp	Mediterranean, Africa	Yes	Yes	Yes	Yes	Unknown
	R. helvetica	Ixodes ricinus	Europe, Asia	No	Yes	No	No	Unknown
	R. massiliae	Rhipicephalus sanguineus	Europe, United States	Yes	Yes	No	Yes	Unknown
	R. monacencis	Ixodes ricinus	Europe	Yes	Yes	No	Yes	Unknown
	R. parkeri	Amblyomma maculatum	America	Yes	Yes	No	Yes	Unknown
FLEA-TRANSMITTED DISEASES								
Murine typhus	R. typhi	Xenopsylla cheopis Ctenocephalides felis (mosquitoes)	Worldwide	Yes	No	No	Yes	Low
Flea-borne spotted fever	R. felis	Ctenocephalides felis, Aedes mosquitoes	Worldwide	Sometimes	Sometimes	Unknown	Yes	Unknown
LOUSE-TRANSMITTED DISEASES								
Epidemic typhus	R. prowazekii	Pediculus humanus corporis Amblyomma ticks (?)	Worldwide	Yes	No	No	Yes	High
American sylvatic typhus	R. prowazekii	Flying squirrel ectoparasites	United States	Yes	No	No	Yes	Low
Brill-Zinsser disease (relapse of epidemic typhus)	R. prowazekii		Worldwide	Yes, could lack	No	No	No	Low
MITE-TRANSMITTED DISEASES								
Rickettsialpox	R. akari	Liponyssoides sanguineus	Worldwide	Yes, vesicular	Yes	Yes	Yes	Low
Scrub typhus	Orientia tsutsugamushi	Leptotrombidium sp (chiggers)	Central and eastern Asia, Australia	Yes	Yes	Yes	Yes	High, may relapse

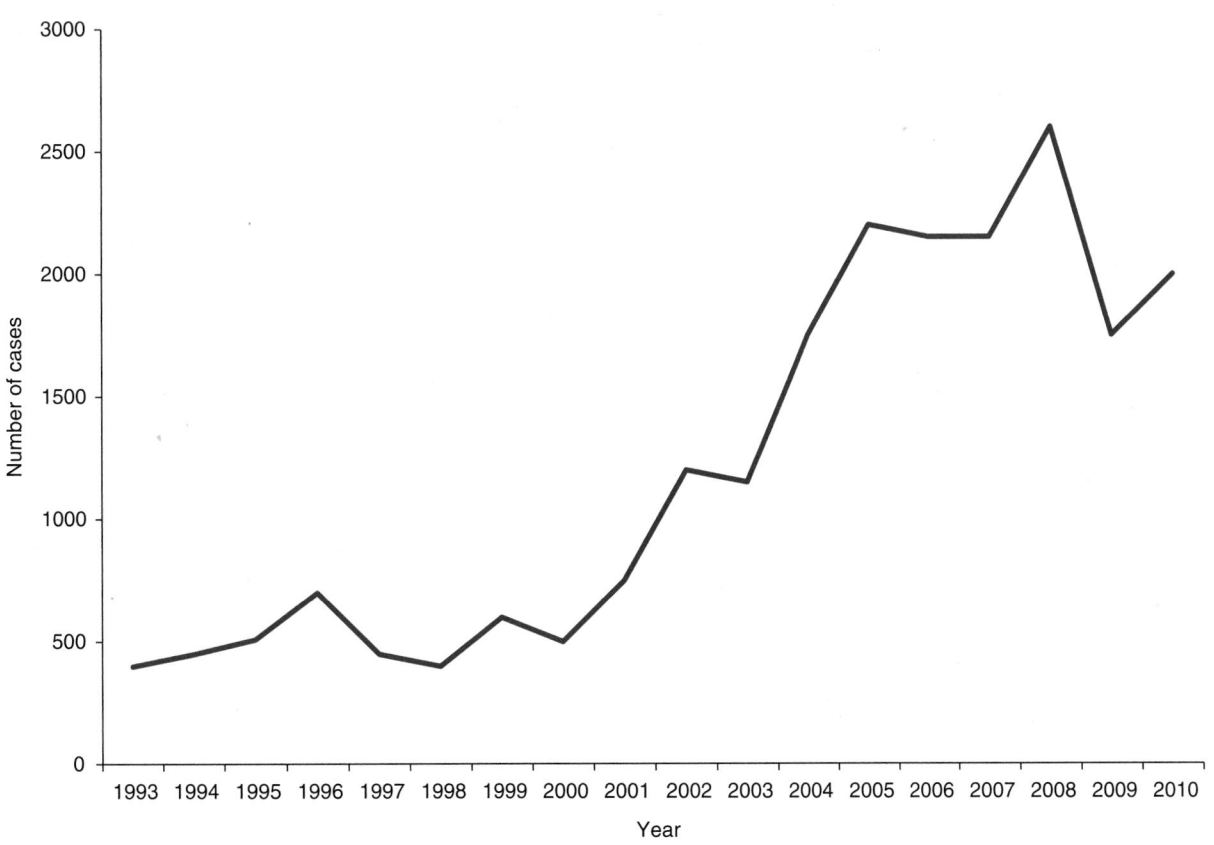

FIGURE 311-1. Number of reported cases of Rocky Mountain spotted fever in the United States, 1993 to 2010.

increase in transaminases in one third of patients and jaundice in 8%. Jaundice can also reflect hemolysis. Intestinal tract involvement is manifested as abdominal pain, diarrhea, vomiting, and severe bleeding (and upper gastrointestinal hemorrhage can cause death). Ocular involvement consists of conjunctivitis and retinal abnormalities, including hemorrhages, papilledema, and arterial occlusion.[4]

The blood cell count shows a normal number of white blood cells but often immature myeloid cells. Thrombocytopenia is observed in 30 to 50% of cases and may be marked in severe cases. Anemia develops in 30% of patients. Coagulopathy with decreases in clotting factors (including fibrinogen) and prolonged coagulation times may contribute to bleeding. There may be hypoalbuminemia, and proteins of the acute phase response are increased (C-reactive protein, ferritin, fibrinogen). Hyponatremia and hypocalcemia may be noted and correlate with severity, as does an increase in creatinine. Increased concentrations of serum liver and muscle enzymes such as aminotransferases (aspartate [AST] and alanine [ALT] aminotransferase), lactate dehydrogenase (LDH), and creatine kinase usually reflect the severity of organ involvement, including the lung, heart, liver, and rhabdomyolysis.

DIAGNOSIS

The diagnosis of RMSF should be based on clinical and epidemiologic findings and lead to early use of doxycycline. The most important clue is unexplained fever in a patient with a history of tick exposure in an endemic area. When a rash is present, RMSF should be suspected and the patient treated accordingly unless another cause is demonstrated. The differential diagnosis includes other rickettsioses (such as those caused by *R. parkeri* in southern states), meningococcemia, enterovirus infections, typhoid, leptospirosis, ehrlichiosis, gonococcemia, toxic shock syndrome, syphilis, rubella, measles, and Kawasaki syndrome. Drug hypersensitivity, especially after antimicrobial use for febrile illness, is sometimes confused with RMSF.

The main diagnostic test relies on serology, and treatment should never be delayed to obtain diagnostic confirmation. Criteria for laboratory confirmation include a fourfold or greater change in antibody titer determined by serology (measured by immunofluorescence antibody assay [IFA], complement fixation, or latex agglutination) and direct detection of the bacterium by demonstration of specific antigens by immunodetection, genomic amplification by PCR, or culture. A biopsy specimen of a skin lesion is the best sample for this purpose. Culture of rickettsiae takes 3 to 7 days and is restricted to specialized laboratories. It is performed on cell lines such as Vero, L929, or HEL cells in biosafety level 3 conditions. Immunodetection by IFA or immunohistochemistry is sensitive and specific. It can be performed with frozen or fixed and paraffin-embedded material and allows retrospective diagnosis. PCR amplification and identification is also a sensitive and specific detection method for rickettsioses in general but cannot replace IFA for the diagnosis of RMSF. Skin biopsy and direct detection in removed ticks yield the best results because blood contains inhibitors and only few copies of rickettsial DNA.

Two serum samples should be tested (early and convalescent). The early serum is usually negative because patients seroconvert between the 7th and 15th days. IFA can be used to detect either immunoglobulin G (IgG) or IgM antibodies. A cutoff value of 1 : 64 for total immunoglobulin and 1 : 32 for IgM antibodies is required for diagnosis. The latex agglutination cutoff is 1 : 64 or 1 : 128. Cross-reactive antibodies have been reported, mainly with infections caused by other rickettsioses, but also infections with *Ehrlichia, Bartonella, Legionella,* and *Proteus* spp. False-positive results, including IgM, may be observed when rheumatoid factor is present in serum and in patients with viral infection generating nonspecific B-lymphocyte proliferation (cytomegalovirus, Epstein-Barr virus). Complement fixation (which lacks sensitivity) and the Weil-Felix test (using antibodies that cross-react with *Proteus* strains) should not be used.

TREATMENT ℞

The prognosis for patients with RMSF depends on the timing of antimicrobial treatment. Doxycycline saves patients with RMSF.[5] The recommended dose is 100 mg two times a day, and treatment should be continued for at least 3 days after the fever resolves. Oral treatment is effective, but in patients with gastric intolerance or coma, the intravenous route is advised. Several antimicrobials are also effective in vitro against *R. rickettsii,* including fluoroquinolones, rifampin, and macrolide antimicrobials (azithromycin and clarithromycin but not erythromycin), but lack of clinical experience precludes their use for RMSF. β-Lactam antimicrobials, aminoglycosides, and cotrimoxazole are not effective.

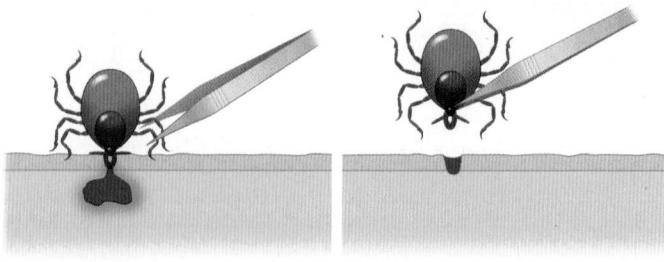

FIGURE 311-2. Tick removal technique.

Severely ill patients should be treated in intensive care units and fluid administration carefully monitored. Mechanical ventilation is used in case of respiratory distress, hemodialysis in patients with renal insufficiency, and antiseizure drugs in patients with seizures. Anemia and coagulation abnormalities may also be corrected. For patients with gangrene of the extremities, amputation may be necessary. Glucocorticoids have not proved useful.

PREVENTION

Prevention is based on avoidance of tick bites by use of repellents, protective garments, or both. To discourage tick attachment, repellents containing permethrin can be sprayed on boots and clothing and will last for several days. Repellents containing DEET (*N,N*-diethyl-*m*-toluamide) can be applied to the skin but will last only a few hours before reapplication is necessary. It is also useful to check for ticks after exposure. Careful examination of the scalp, groin, and axillae is recommended. The tick can be removed by forceps, and the skin should be disinfected (Fig. 311-2).

PROGNOSIS

The evolution of RMSF depends strongly on the timing of diagnosis and antimicrobial treatment. The current fatality rate is 2.4% on the basis of a 4-year national survey in the United States (27 deaths were attributable to RMSF during this period). This rate is currently declining, but this may result from reporting of confounding rickettsial diseases. No significant difference in outcome has been observed between blacks and whites, but the case-fatality rate was highest in people older than 70 years (9%). Patients with glucose-6-phosphate dehydrogenase (G6PD) deficiency are more susceptible to severe infection. Chloramphenicol has been associated with a poorer outcome than treatment with doxycycline. Recovery from RMSF is usually complete, but neurologic sequelae can remain, and amputation of extremities may be necessary after gangrene.

OTHER TICK-BORNE RICKETTSIOSES
EPIDEMIOLOGY

Like other tick-transmitted diseases, rickettsioses have a limited geographic distribution that is determined mainly by the tick vector ecology (Fig. 311-3). *R. parkeri* has recently been identified in the United States and South America. *R. conorii* is found in Europe around the Mediterranean and Caspian seas (*caspia* subspecies); *Rickettsia slovaca, Rickettsia raoultii,* and possibly *Rickettsia helvetica* in western and central Europe; and *Rickettsia sibirica mongolotimonae* in France and Greece. Elsewhere, a number of specific agents of rickettsial disease have been identified (see Table 311-2).

CLINICAL MANIFESTATIONS

R. conorii comprises different but closely related subspecies. Many names are given to the infection caused by *R. conorii:* Mediterranean spotted fever (MSF), boutonneuse fever, Marseilles fever, Kenya tick typhus (caused by the subspecies *R. conorii conorii*), Astrakhan fever (caused by *R. conorii caspia*), Israeli spotted fever (caused by *R. conorii israeli*), and Indian tick typhus (caused by *R. conorii indica*). *R. conorii* is closely related to *R. rickettsii,* with which it shares many common antigens that generate cross-reactive antibodies. MSF resembles RMSF but has some distinguishing features. The spontaneous evolution is milder, but a fatality rate of 1.5 to 2.5% in hospitalized patients is still observed. A malignant form of the disease that includes purpuric rash, shock, and MODS has been described in alcoholic, diabetic, human immunodeficiency virus (HIV)-infected, and old or debilitated patients. The typical clinical manifestation is that of a patient with fever, a rash, and a tache noire

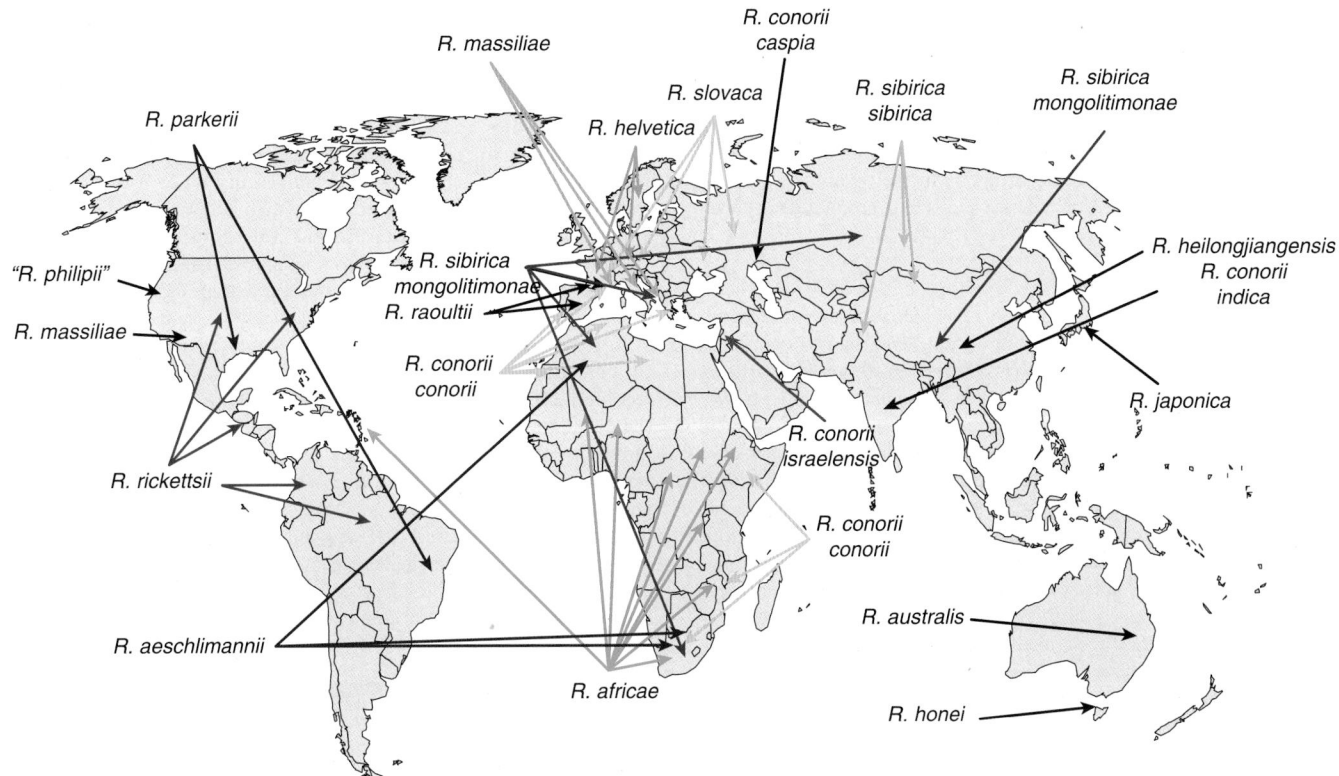

FIGURE 311-3. Geographic distribution of tick-borne rickettsioses.

(i.e., a black eschar at the site of the tick bite). A tache noire is found in 50 to 80% of cases. Multiple eschars are rare because the dog tick vector, *R. sanguineus,* seldom bites humans. The rash is frequently clearly papular, which led to one of the names of the disease, boutonneuse fever. Israeli tick-bite fever and Astrakhan fever appear to be milder than typical MSF, and a tache noire is usually lacking.

R. africae, which causes African tick-bite fever, may be responsible for most of the rickettsioses worldwide. It is extremely common in travelers visiting safari parks in southern Africa.[6] It is transmitted by African ticks, *Amblyomma hebraeum* and *Amblyomma africanum.* These ticks are often infected; as many as 60% can harbor *R. africae.* They usually feed on ungulates but attack human beings in groups and cause a high prevalence of infection in rural Africa (60% of tested patients exhibit antibodies) and in travelers. The tick attacks typically generate clusters of cases in safari tourists. The disease differs from MSF in that it is much milder, fever is frequently absent, a rash is observed in only half of patients, and the rash may be vesicular (which has never been reported in confirmed MSF). Moreover, several taches noires are frequently observed. They are prevalently found on the lower limbs and often associated with draining lymphadenopathy in the groin.

Japanese spotted fever (caused by *Rickettsia japonica*) and Siberian tick typhus (caused by *R. sibirica*) resemble MSF. Infections caused by *R. sibirica mongolitimonae* resemble MSF but in some cases exhibit distinguishing clinical features, including a tache noire, groin lymphadenopathy, and lymphangitis joining these two lesions. The disease has recently been named lymphangitis-associated rickettsiosis. *Rickettsia australis* (Queensland tick typhus) and *Rickettsia honei* (Flinders Island spotted fever) cause diseases resembling MSF, but their rash can be vesicular.

R. slovaca and *R. raoultii* cause a disease common in Europe named scalp eschar and neck lymphadenopathy transmitted by ticks (SENLAT, reported in the Czech Republic, France, Hungary, Germany, Italy, Lithuania, Romania, Spain). Its tick vectors, *Dermacentor marginatus* and *Dermacentor reticulatus,* preferentially bite in cold months and bite the scalp because they prefer hairy prey. In contrast to other tick-borne rickettsioses, the disease is more prevalent in children and women. It is rarely exanthematic; the typical clinical picture consists of an erythematous skin lesion at the site of the tick bite on the scalp that ranges from 2 to 8 cm in diameter and a draining neck lymphadenopathy (which may be painful). Rarely, patients may exhibit fever and a rash. Deep postinfectious asthenia and residual alopecia at the site of the tick bite can be observed. The occurrence of this rickettsiosis without rash may stimulate research on other new rickettsial diseases with only localized manifestations.

Other *Rickettsia* species have rarely been identified as causing SENLAT, including *Rickettsia massiliae, Rickettsia sibirica mongolitimonae,* and *Candidatus* Rickettsia rioja.

DIAGNOSIS

The diagnosis of other tick-borne rickettsioses is similar to that of RMSF, mainly by serology (IFA; see earlier). An exception is *R. slovaca* infection, in which the serologic response is weak, possibly because of its lack of general infection; in this case, PCR of a skin eschar sample by a swab or a lymph node aspirate provides the highest diagnostic yield. In *R. africae* infection, the serologic response occurs later than in RMSF and MSF, and late serum samples (i.e., 4 weeks after onset of symptoms) are therefore recommended.

TREATMENT Rx

Doxycycline (100 mg twice daily for adults or 4.4 mg/kg body weight per day in two divided doses for children under 45.4 kg [100 lb]) is the drug of choice for treatment. A single day of therapy usually suffices, but in adults with more severe disease, it should be administered until the patient is afebrile for 24 hours. In pregnant women, josamycin, a macrolide antimicrobial, has proved efficient at a dose of 3 g daily for 7 days for MSF; quinolones and newer macrolide antimicrobials give results comparable to those of doxycycline but require longer treatment courses.

Flea-Transmitted Diseases

Fleas (Chapter 104) can harbor two rickettsial species: *Rickettsia typhi,* the agent of murine typhus; and *Rickettsia felis,* the agent of flea-borne spotted fever. Both rickettsiae can be transmitted transovarially in the flea. Vectors are *Xenopsylla cheopis* and *Pulex irritans* but also *Ctenocephalides felis,* a cat flea. Rats, cats, opossums, and dogs can propagate infected fleas. These reservoirs and vectors are distributed worldwide, and thus these diseases have a global distribution. Fleas can be infected by both species at the same time.

MURINE TYPHUS
DEFINITION

Fleas are usually infected by *R. typhi* when feeding on apparently healthy rats that have blood-borne infection. Humans and other mammals are infected through autoinoculation by scratching a fleabite that is contaminated with feces from an infected flea. Murine typhus, because of its cycle, is more prevalent in hot and humid areas, when rats proliferate.

EPIDEMIOLOGY

In the United States, 50 to 100 cases are reported yearly, mainly in southern California and southern Texas. In California, a transmission cycle involving opossums and cat fleas has been demonstrated. Murine typhus is extremely common in Southeast Asia and North Africa and is a common cause of fever in travelers to those areas.

CLINICAL MANIFESTATIONS

On the basis of studies of infected volunteers, the incubation period is generally 8 to 16 days. The disease begins with abrupt fever, nausea, vomiting, myalgias, arthralgias, and headache. A rash is observed in 40 to 50% of patients about 6 days after the onset. It is detected even less frequently in patients with dark skin. The rash begins as pink maculae that can evolve to be maculopapular. It is often discrete, starting in the axilla; it generalizes to the trunk but does not usually involve the face, palms, and soles. In severe cases, it can become purpuric. The most frequently involved organ is the lung. One third of patients have a cough, and in one fourth, a nonspecific interstitial pneumonia develops that is sometimes associated with a pleural effusion. In severe forms, respiratory failure occurs. In patients with severe disease, neurologic symptoms range from confusion and stupor to coma and seizures. Cerebral hemorrhages may occur. Digestive involvement can be manifested as vomiting, abdominal pain, jaundice, and, in severe cases, hematemesis.

The white blood cell count shows leukopenia and then leukocytosis. Thrombocytopenia can be noted as well as anemia, specifically when hemolysis is observed (frequently in patients with G6PD deficiency). A moderate increase in serum liver enzymes is common. In patients with severe disease, hyponatremia and hypoalbuminemia are observed.

DIAGNOSIS

The diagnosis of murine typhus is based mainly on serology (IFA), with titers similar to those of RMSF. On serologic evaluation, *R. typhi* cross-reacts with *R. prowazekii*; it can be differentiated either by comparing titers (two dilutions or more if IgG and IgM titers are discriminative) or by cross-adsorption. In this technique, the serum is absorbed with either antigen and then retested, and the causative agent is that removing antibodies to both bacteria. Skin biopsies and blood samples for culture and PCR may be valuable.

TREATMENT   Rx

Treatment is the same as that for RMSF.

PROGNOSIS

The prognosis is usually favorable, but 10% of patients require intensive care and 1% die. Older patients and those with G6PD deficiency (Chapter 152) or chronic debilitating conditions are at higher risk.

FLEA-BORNE SPOTTED FEVER CAUSED BY *RICKETTSIA FELIS*

R. felis is mainly transmitted transovarially. Its genome comprises one or two plasmids, one being apparently conjugative. This is a new, incompletely defined disease. The bacterium is found in fleas in the Americas, Asia, Europe, Africa, and New Zealand. Isolated cases have been reported from Texas, Mexico, Brazil, France, and Germany. Reported cases all exhibited fever, a rash in six of seven cases, and inoculation eschar in some cases. The diagnosis can be based on serologic testing using specific *R. felis* antigen or PCR of blood or skin biopsy samples. Treatment has not been established, but the bacterium is highly susceptible to doxycycline and resistant to erythromycin. *R. felis* has been found at very high prevalence in the blood of febrile sub-Saharan Africans and is suspected to be transmitted by mosquitoes, as suggested by an animal model.

Louse and Mite Infections
EPIDEMIC LOUSE-BORNE TYPHUS
EPIDEMIOLOGY

The human body louse (Chapter 104) lives in clothes and multiplies rapidly when cold weather and lack of hygiene allow it to. The body louse transmits three bacterial diseases: trench fever (caused by *Bartonella quintana*) (Chapter 299), relapsing fever (caused by *Borrelia recurrentis*) (Chapter 306), and

exanthematic typhus (caused by *R. prowazekii*). The name *typhus* is derived from the Greek *tuphos*, which describes the neurologic condition associated with this disease and with typhoid. The body louse is prevalent during war, in poor countries, and in the homeless population of rich countries, including the United States and Europe. A 100,000-person outbreak of typhus was reported during the civil war in Burundi in 1997, and cases were reported in Russia, Peru, the United States, Algeria, and France in the 1990s. Louse-transmitted diseases killed more people than weapons did during central and eastern European wars in the 19th and 20th centuries.[7]

The epidemiology of *R. prowazekii* is mainly related to humans as reservoirs and lice as vectors. In the United States, the eastern flying squirrel (*Glaucomys volans volans*) is also a reservoir, and its fleas, lice, and mites can be infected.

R. prowazekii has also been found in *Amblyomma* ticks, but their role in the epidemiology of the bacterium is not known. The louse is infected when feeding on blood, which it does five times a day. *R. prowazekii* multiplies in the gut of the louse and is released in feces. After a few days, it destroys the intestinal epithelium, causing bright red blood to spread from the gut (typhus was also named the red louse disease). The patient is usually contaminated by infected feces (in which *R. prowazekii* survives for weeks), through aerosols, or by skin autoinoculation after scratching. Patients who recover from typhus may harbor the bacterium in a dormant form and suffer relapses under stressful conditions years later; this relapsing form is called Brill-Zinsser disease. During the relapse, a bacteremia occurs that may allow the start of a new outbreak if lice bite the patient.

CLINICAL MANIFESTATIONS

Typhus begins abruptly with fever, headaches, and myalgias, which may lead to the crouched posture termed *sutama*, as observed in the largest recent outbreak in Burundi. Cough and neurologic signs (stupor, confusion, or coma) are common.[8] A rash is observed in 20 to 80% of patients, depending on the population studied; it is probably commonly underobserved on dark skin. It generally starts in the axilla and then spreads. The rash is usually macular but can be papular or purpuric in severe cases. In some cases, diarrhea and jaundice are reported. Splenomegaly is infrequently found. In severe cases, shock occurs, and the fatality rate of epidemic typhus is 20 to 30% when untreated. Leukopenia, thrombocytopenia, and anemia, as well as an increase in serum hepatic enzymes, may be noted.

Sylvatic typhus in the United States is caused by an *R. prowazekii* variant and is a milder disease. The most prominent clinical features are neurologic. Few cases have been described, and nearly all occurred in areas where the eastern flying squirrel is found, east of the Mississippi.

Brill-Zinsser disease is difficult to diagnose because rash is rare and recent exposure to lice can be lacking. Interviewing the patient may reveal prior exposure to lice, associated or not with a diagnosis of typhus in previous years. The disease is mild, and the prognosis is good.

DIAGNOSIS

The diagnosis of typhus should be considered when grouped cases of high fever with confusion are observed in patients exposed to lice. The most common diagnostic error is to attribute the findings to typhoid (Chapter 292), which can have fatal consequences because the antimicrobials typically prescribed for that condition (β-lactams, cotrimoxazole, and quinolones) are ineffective treatment of typhus. In tropical countries, typhus is frequently confused with malaria, hemorrhagic fever, and dengue. In people with lice, it can be confused with trench fever and relapsing fever, but treatment for both can be prescribed.

The diagnosis of typhus should be clinical because the fatality rate is high and the treatment safe and efficient. Any outbreak of unexplained fever in unhygienic environments may suggest typhus, including outbreaks during civil wars, during social collapses, in jails, and in chronically poor and cold countries. The diagnosis is mainly based on serology, in which there is cross-reaction with *R. typhi* (see earlier). When the investigation is performed under difficult field conditions, a drop of blood applied on filter paper and sent to a reference laboratory is valuable for serologic testing. Culture and PCR are helpful and can be performed with a skin biopsy sample or blood. Lice are good diagnostic tools because they can be tested even when dry and can be sent in closed containers without specific temperature conditions.

TREATMENT

Treatment of typhus is extremely simple, cheap, and effective; 200 mg of doxycycline orally in two divided doses is life-saving. Comatose patients should be treated with doxycycline parenterally. In allergic patients, chloramphenicol is the only known alternative, prescribed at a dose of 2 g/day for 10 days. There is no current vaccination, and the fight against lice is the major prevention strategy. Because lice are fragile, changing and boiling clothes are efficient. When this is not possible, insecticides (primarily permethrin) or ivermectin orally should be used.

SCRUB TYPHUS (*ORIENTIA TSUTSUGAMUSHI*)

EPIDEMIOLOGY

Scrub typhus is a neglected tropical disease transmitted by the bite of trombiculid mite (Chapter 104) larvae infected by *O. tsutsugamushi*. These mites, also named chiggers, are vertically infected through their mother. Although rare cases have been reported in Chile, sub-Saharan Africa, and United Arab Emirates, scrub typhus distribution is mostly limited to a triangle extending between northern Japan, eastern Australia, and eastern Russia and includes the Far East, China, and the Indian subcontinent.[9] Altogether, 1 billion people may be exposed. Seasonality is determined by the emergence of larvae. It is one of the three most common causes of prolonged fever in rural Asia; in temperate zones, it occurs mainly in autumn and to a lesser extent in spring. *O. tsutsugamushi* species have a wide heterogenicity that may allow the definition of several species, but a single species is currently recognized with many serotypes. The more frequent are Kato, Karp, Gilliam, and Kawasaki.

CLINICAL MANIFESTATIONS

The disease occurs in patients exposed to rural or urban foci of scrub typhus after a delay of 10 or more days. The onset is usually sudden and includes fever, headache, and myalgias. Attentive examination may reveal an inoculation eschar at the site of the mite bite and tender draining lymph nodes. Most patients with scrub typhus present with relative bradycardia.[10] Generalized lymphadenopathy and rash may be observed. The symptoms vary according to organ involvement. Neuromeningeal symptoms are relatively common.[11] Severe forms can be manifested as septic shock. The lethality rate of untreated scrub typhus is 6%. Abortion commonly occurs in pregnant women.

Leukopenia, thrombocytopenia, and increased levels of hepatic enzymes can occur. Evolution depends on the hosts and strains, and the fatality rate ranges from 0 to 30%.[12] Scrub typhus is not more severe in HIV-infected patients, and surprisingly, HIV suppressive factors appear to be produced during infection. Relapses may occur in this disease.

DIAGNOSIS

Diagnosis may be difficult. Because the clinical features are frequently not specific, epidemiologic factors are critical. A diagnosis of infectious mononucleosis has erroneously been made in patients with scrub typhus. The bacterium can be detected by culture (in cells or mice) or by PCR in blood and biopsy specimens.[13] The serologic technique first used was agglutination of *Proteus mirabilis* serotype OXK in the Weil-Felix reaction. This test lacks sensitivity and specificity and should be replaced by IFA or enzyme-linked immunosorbent assay tests using the three or four major serotypes. Point-of-care testing for scrub typhus still lacks standardized methodology and reporting of diagnostic accuracy.[14]

TREATMENT   Rx

Chloramphenicol was the mainstay of treatment for many years, but now doxycycline is recommended. Single-day treatment with doxycycline is followed by relapses, and even repeated treatment for 2 days at a 7-day interval does not prevent all relapses. Hence, the currently recommended regimen is doxycycline, 100 mg orally twice a day, for 7 days. Cases resistant to doxycycline have been reported, and rifampin (600 mg orally daily) is a reasonable alternative. Quinolones should be avoided. Prophylaxis is based on the use of repellents.

RICKETTSIALPOX (*RICKETTSIA AKARI*)

EPIDEMIOLOGY

Rickettsialpox was first described in New York City, where it is still prevalent. *Rickettsia akari*, the causal agent, is transmitted by the bite of the mouse mite (*Liponyssoides sanguineus*). Its prevalence is probably underestimated; an active search revealed 13 cases in a New York hospital in the 1980s. Cases have been reported in Arizona, Utah, and Ohio. After the terrorist attacks of 9/11/01,

cases of black skin eschars were investigated for possible anthrax in New York but were in fact rickettsialpox. High seroprevalence was reported among intravenous drug users in Baltimore. Cases have also been reported from Russia, Ukraine, Slovenia, and Korea.

CLINICAL MANIFESTATIONS

Ten days after the mite bite, the beginning of the illness is marked by fever, headache, and myalgia. Careful examination reveals an inoculation eschar and draining lymphadenopathy that could be mistaken for cutaneous anthrax. Two to 6 days later, a rash appears and comprises 5 to 40 macular, then papular and vesicular, spots. This aspect led to the name of the disease. It is frequently mistaken for chickenpox. The disease is usually mild.

DIAGNOSIS

The diagnosis can be made by serologic testing with IFA. Specific antigens react with high titer, but antibodies to other *Rickettsia* may be detected. The diagnosis may also be made on skin specimens by culture, immunodetection, or PCR.

TREATMENT

Doxycycline is highly effective in these patients. Prevention is based on the control of mice.

● EHRLICHIOSES AND ANAPLASMOSES

DEFINITION

Ehrlichiae multiply exclusively in vacuoles of their eukaryotic cell host, where they form clusters known as morulae. The vacuoles are derived from phagosomes and help the organism escape bactericidal lysosomal fusion. In humans, ehrlichiae are associated with monocytes (*E. chaffeensis, E. canis, N. sennetsu*) or polymorphonuclear neutrophils (PMN) (*A. phagocytophilum, E. ewingii*).

Ehrlichioses can be acquired through tick bites, by ingestion of nematodes through contaminated water or animals (fish, snails), or as a consequence of filariasis.[15]

American Human Monocytic Ehrlichiosis (*Ehrlichia chaffeensis*)

EPIDEMIOLOGY

Human monocytic ehrlichiosis (HME) is caused by *E. chaffeensis*. This organism has been isolated or identified by PCR mainly in the United States, in the southeastern, south central, and mid-Atlantic states and California (Table 311-3). In the United States, *A. americanum* (Lone Star tick) is the vector

TABLE 311-3 EHRLICHIOSES AND ANAPLASMOSES

DISEASE	AGENT	VECTOR	GEOGRAPHIC REPARTITION
American monocytic ehrlichiosis	*Ehrlichia chaffeensis*	*Amblyomma americanum*	South central, southeastern, mid-Atlantic coastal states
Human granulocytic ehrlichiosis	*Anaplasma phagocytophilum*	*Ixodes ricinus*	Europe, China
		Ixodes scapularis	Northeast, upper Midwest, northern California
Japanese monocytic ehrlichiosis	*Neorickettsia sennetsu*	Helminth of the gray mullet?	Japan
Unnamed	*Ehrlichia canis*	*Rhipicephalus sanguineus*	Venezuela
	Ehrlichia ewingii	*Amblyomma americanum*	South central, southeastern, mid-Atlantic coastal states
	Ehrlichia muris–like	*Ixodes scapularis*	Indiana, Michigan, Minnesota, North Dakota, Wisconsin
	Candidatus Neoehrlichia mikurensis	*Ixodes ricinus*	Central and eastern Europe, northeastern China

(Chapter 104), and the white-tailed deer is the main mammalian reservoir. Immature ticks are infected by blood while feeding on persistently bacteremic reservoirs. *E. chaffeensis* is transmitted transstadially in the tick and infects its next host (deer or human) during its next blood meal. The disease epidemiology reflects the tick habitat and activity, with most cases being contracted in the southern United States, in rural areas, and from April to September. In highly endemic areas, the incidence can reach 100 cases per 100,000 inhabitants. The severity is age dependent, which may explain the lower incidence reported in children. Males are more often affected than females, with a sex ratio of 4 : 1.

CLINICAL MANIFESTATIONS

The incubation lasts for 7 to 10 days after an identified tick exposure in 80% of cases. Patients have fever, headache, malaise, nausea, and anorexia. Untreated patients worsen and may require intensive care. Digestive tract involvement consisting of nausea, vomiting, diarrhea, and abdominal pain is common. Central nervous system infection is manifested in many forms, ranging from confusion to coma. A rash is observed in one third of cases and lymphadenopathy in one fourth. In severe forms, sepsis syndrome and MODS may occur.

The white blood cell count typically shows leukopenia, caused by both lymphopenia and neutropenia. Thrombocytopenia is also frequently found; anemia may appear later. Coagulopathy may be observed in severe forms. Increases in serum enzymes, including AST, ALT, and LDH, may reflect organ involvement, as does creatininemia. CSF examination in patients with neurologic symptoms reveals pleocytosis and increased protein levels. Cells may be monocytic or PMN. The prognosis depends on early antimicrobial treatment, but the fatality rate is still high at 2.5%. In persons coinfected with HIV, it may be most severe; in one series, 6 of 13 patients died.

DIAGNOSIS

The diagnosis of HME should be considered in patients with a history of tick exposure and unexplained fever. HME resembles RMSF, but rash is less frequent. Later in the disease, it can be misdiagnosed as anything that causes severe sepsis.

Leukopenia associated with thrombocytopenia and an increase in liver enzyme levels may establish the etiology. Careful examination of blood and CSF smears may help identify typical morulae. Treatment should be started in any suspected case. The diagnosis can be confirmed by culture in specialized laboratories using a canine cell line, DH82. However, PCR is more practical; confirmatory PCR using a second target gene is useful. Most cases are currently diagnosed serologically by a four-fold or greater increase in antibody titer or by seroconversion. The reference technique is IFA. A single titer of 25 is indicative of the diagnosis. There are cross-reactive antibodies among *Ehrlichia* species and with *A. phagocytophilum*. Western blotting may be valuable to distinguish among these bacteria.

TREATMENT   Rx

Doxycycline (100 mg twice daily for adults) is the drug of choice for patients with ehrlichiosis. The optimal duration of therapy has not been established, but current regimens recommend continuation of treatment for at least 3 days after the fever subsides and until evidence of clinical improvement, for a minimum total course of 5 to 7 days. Severe or complicated disease may require longer treatment courses. Because tetracyclines are contraindicated in pregnancy, rifampin has been used successfully in a limited number of pregnant women with documented HME.

Human Granulocytic Ehrlichiosis (*Anaplasma phagocytophilum*)

EPIDEMIOLOGY

The first human case of *A. phagocytophilum* infection was recognized in 1990. The disease is found in America, Asia, and Europe (Fig. 311-4). It is transmitted by *Ixodes scapularis* (eastern North America), *Ixodes pacificus* (western North America), *Ixodes ricinus* (Europe), and *Ixodes persulcatus* (Asia), the vectors of Lyme disease (Chapter 305), and its epidemiology is similar.[16] Coinfection with the two diseases may occur. The temporal distribution of the disease parallels that of nymph tick activity, with two peaks in spring and autumn. Ticks are born free of *Ehrlichia* and are infected while feeding on bacteremic small mammals. Deer play a major role as hosts of adult ticks and reservoirs. In highly endemic areas, the incidence can reach 50 per 100,000 inhabitants per year. The mean age of diagnosed patients is high, and males are more frequently infected than females, with a sex ratio of 3 : 1.

CLINICAL MANIFESTATIONS

The incubation time is usually between 7 and 10 days, and 80% of patients report a history of tick exposure. Many infections may be asymptomatic or too mild to require a diagnostic procedure. The disease frequently begins abruptly, with fever, headache, malaise, and myalgias that may be particularly

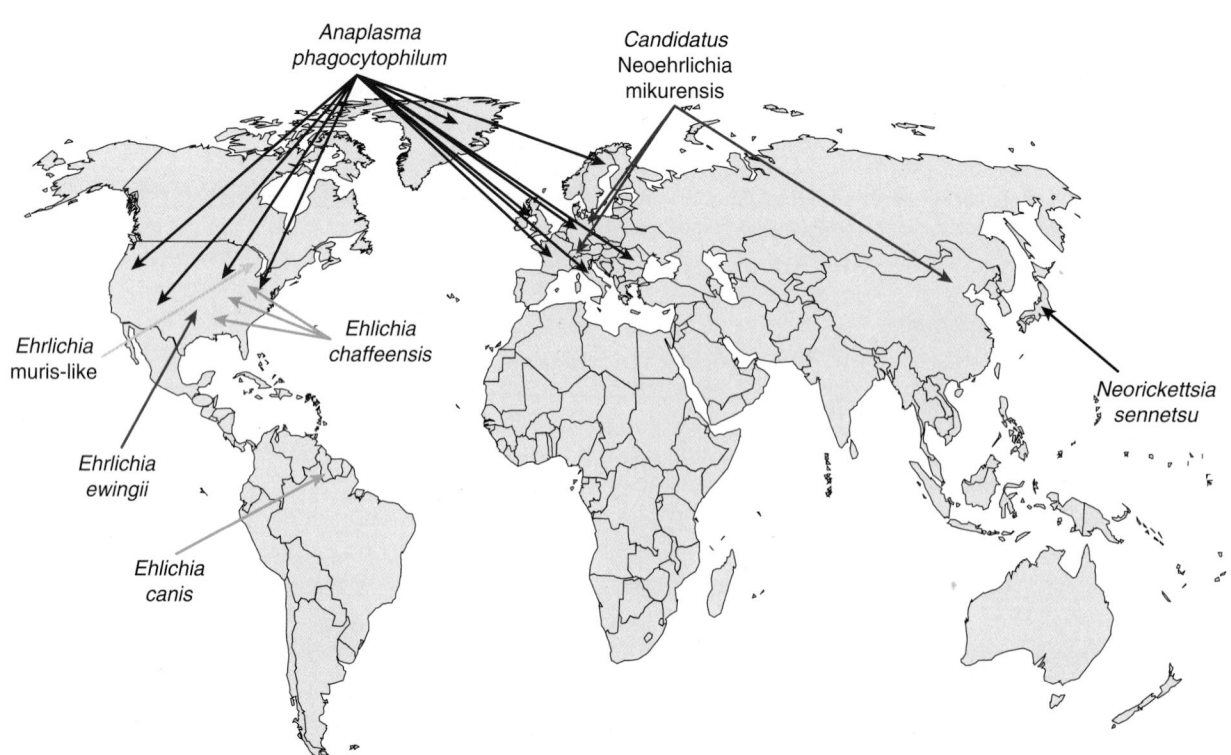

FIGURE 311-4. Geographic distribution of ehrlichioses.

severe. Rash is found in less than 10% of cases. Visceral involvement may be observed and includes digestive symptoms such as nausea, vomiting, and diarrhea. Neurologic symptoms may include confusion, meningitis, and meningoencephalitis.

The evolution of the disease is favorable in most cases, even without specific therapy, but the disease may progress to septic shock in some patients. Patients with underlying diseases are more at risk for dying. Most deaths are the consequence of *Anaplasma*-induced immunosuppression, and patients may experience invasive aspergillosis, candidiasis, cryptococcosis, and herpes esophagitis.

DIAGNOSIS

Laboratory findings consist of the association of thrombocytopenia and leukopenia (lymphopenia or neutropenia). An increase in serum transaminases is also frequent. The diagnosis can be made by careful examination of blood smears for morulae within PMN cells. Culture from blood is possible in appropriate cells (HL-60), and PCR is useful as for HME. Most cases are diagnosed by serologic testing with IFA, which is comparable to that in HME (see earlier).

TREATMENT   Rx

Treatment is similar to that of HME except that *A. phagocytophilum* is susceptible to fluoroquinolones in vitro, but these drugs have not been tested in patients.

Ehrlichia ewingii

Canine granulocytic ehrlichiosis, reported in the United States in 1972, is caused by *E. ewingii*. This bacterium was characterized by amplification and sequencing of the 16S ribosomal RNA gene. The vector of *E. ewingii* is *A. americanum*, which also transmits *E. chaffeensis*. Among 60 cases of ehrlichiosis in Missouri in 1999, 4 were caused by *E. ewingii*; 4 other cases have been reported since by the CDC. The disease has been prevalent in immunocompromised hosts coinfected with HIV or receiving immunosuppressive drugs. Patients who report tick exposure are noted to have fever, thrombocytopenia, leukopenia, and various symptoms, including meningitis. Morulae may be seen on blood smears in PMN cells. The evolution in reported cases was good; patients responded dramatically to doxycycline. Patients have antibodies to *E. chaffeensis*, and PCR has been shown to be useful when it is applied to blood samples. This diagnosis should be considered when ehrlichiosis is suspected in immunocompromised patients exposed to *A. americanum* ticks.

Ehrlichia canis

Canine monocytic ehrlichiosis was reported first in Algeria in the 1930s. It is caused by *E. canis* and transmitted by the dog tick *R. sanguineus*. This tick is found worldwide and is prevalent in temperate and hot areas. In 1996, a single case of infection was reported in an asymptomatic man from Venezuela who owned an infected dog. Recently, cases have been reported in patients in South America.

Ehrlichia muris–like Agent

Since 2009, more than 50 cases of an ehrlichiosis have been diagnosed in Wisconsin and Minnesota, caused by an *Ehrlichia* that is closely related to *E. muris*. The bacterium has also been cultured from *Ixodes scapularis* ticks in this area. Patients have fever, headache, myalgias, lymphopenia, thrombocytopenia, and transaminitis, and they recover with doxycycline treatment.

Candidatus Neoehrlichia mikurensis

Candidatus Neoehrlichia mikurensis, transmitted by *Ixodes* ticks, has been reported based on PCR testing of the blood of febrile immunocompromised patients in Europe and China.

Wolbachia Species

Wolbachia bacteria are endosymbionts of arthropods and nematodes. They were known to be present in filarial worms, but it was later shown that they may play a role in human disease. These bacteria manipulate the fertility of their host. Eradication of *Wolbachia* in filariae may lead to infertility and stop

the microfilariae from spreading. This effect was demonstrated by field treatment with doxycycline in patients with onchocerciasis. The patients improved when treated with this drug, which is effective on *Wolbachia* and subsequently on the worm's fertility but not on the worm itself. In 2001, it was shown that the adverse reactions observed after treatment of lymphatic filariasis may be caused by the release of *Wolbachia* from destroyed worms. Some authors suggested that eradicating *Wolbachia* before the anthelmintic prescription would avoid these reactions. For some reason, *Loa loa* (Chapter 335) do not harbor *Wolbachia*, and the genome of *Wolbachia* integrated in the *Brugia malayi* genome makes it inaccessible to therapy.

⬤ Q FEVER

DEFINITION

Q fever is a worldwide zoonosis caused by *Coxiella burnetii*. The name Q fever is derived from "query" to emphasize the surprising aspect of the disease first described in Queensland, Australia, in 1935 by Derrick. The infection in humans is variable in its severity, clinical expression, and natural course (i.e., acute or chronic). It is considered by the CDC to be a potential agent of bioterrorism. Ungulates (hoofed mammals) and pets are the major sources of human infection.

The Pathogen

C. burnetii is a gram-negative bacterium that naturally infects its host's monocytes. It multiplies in an acidic vacuole. Strains are heterogeneous genetically and antigenically and are associated with acute infections of variable severity. *C. burnetii* in vitro generates a deleted, avirulent mutant also named phase II. This mutant exhibits diagnostic antigens that are useful because they are more reactive during acute infection.

C. burnetii is incompletely eliminated after acute infection. In immunocompromised hosts and patients with cardiac valve lesions, *C. burnetii* continues to multiply despite high levels of antibodies and causes chronic infection. Control of the disease in acute Q fever is associated with the formation of a granuloma.

EPIDEMIOLOGY

C. burnetii infects a wide range of animals, including mammals, birds, and ticks. Ungulates and pets (cats and dogs) are the most common source of the disease. Mammals are infected through aerosols and may shed *Coxiella* in feces, urine, milk, and birth products. Humans are usually infected by aerosols or less frequently by exposure to milk products. Interhuman infections through sexual intercourse, during delivery, or by blood transfusion have been reported. *Coxiella* survives in the environment and can be spread far by the wind. In the past few years, major outbreaks were related to sheep and goats. The disease is partly seasonal and related to lambing time. Males have more severe disease but are not more often exposed to Q fever, and middle-aged people are more frequently affected and hospitalized. The number of reported cases recently increased dramatically in Europe and Asia. Many American soldiers were infected in Iraq. A giant outbreak was observed in the Netherlands from 2007 to 2010.[17]

CLINICAL MANIFESTATIONS

After contamination by *C. burnetii*, 60% of patients seroconvert without apparent disease, 38% experience a self-limited disease, and only 2% require diagnostic evaluation. Months to years after the primary infection, a chronic infection develops in 0.2 to 0.5% of patients, associated with an immunocompromised state, a cardiac valve lesion, or a vascular prosthesis or aneurysm.

Patients with diagnosed acute infection may have a variety of symptoms (Table 311-4). Isolated prolonged fever was observed in 14% of a series of more than 1000 patients. Pneumonia was found in 37% and was the only symptom in 17%. This percentage may vary according to the place of study and reach 90% of diagnosed cases. Some cases may be associated with respiratory distress.[18] Hepatitis is found in 60% of patients and is the sole manifestation in 40%. The association of fever and a moderate increase in transaminases is an important clue. Some hepatitides, specifically in middle-aged men, are associated with an inflammatory syndrome and autoantibodies and may be resistant to antimicrobial treatment. Liver biopsy, when it is performed, exhibits granulomas that may be typified by a lipid vacuole and surrounded by a fibrinoid ring in the form of a doughnut. Less frequently, in 1.5% of cases, patients exhibit a rash. Patients can have specific neurologic manifestations such as meningitis, encephalitis, meningoencephalitis, or peripheral neuropathy. In 1 to 2% of cases, patients have cardiovascular manifestations, such as

TABLE 311-4	SITUATIONS THAT SHOULD PROMPT SEROLOGIC TESTING FOR Q FEVER

ACUTE Q FEVER (PHASE II ANTIGEN AND IgG ≥200 AND IgM ≥50)

Fever in a patient in contact with ungulates (hoofed mammals)
Unexplained prolonged fever (>7 days)
Granulomatous hepatitis
Fever and thrombocytopenia
Meningoencephalitis
Myocarditis
Erythema nodosum
Fever during pregnancy
Fever in a patient in contact with a parturient pet
Unexplained atypical pneumonia
Fever and an increase in transaminases (2-5 times the normal level)
Aseptic meningitis
Guillain-Barré syndrome
Pericarditis
Spontaneous abortion

CHRONIC Q FEVER (PHASE I ANTIGEN AND IgG ≥800 AND IgA ≥100)

Blood culture–negative endocarditis
Patient with a valvulopathy and unexplained
    Fever
    Weight loss
    Fatigue
    Increased erythrocyte sedimentation rate
    Increased transaminases
    Thrombocytopenia
Patient with unusually rapid degradation of a prosthetic valve
Fever in a patient with a vascular aneurysm or prosthesis
Aseptic osteomyelitis
Chronic pericarditis
Multiple spontaneous abortions

pericarditis or more rarely myocarditis or acute endocarditis.[19] Rare cases of prosthetic joint infection have also been reported.

Evolution is usually favorable even without treatment, except in certain hosts. In pregnant women, symptomatic or not, Q fever compromises the pregnancy. When infected during the first trimester, the patient usually aborts spontaneously. When the patient is infected later, the disease can result in fetal death or prematurity, although in many the outcome may be normal. Chronic uterine infection may develop in half the patients infected during pregnancy, and these women may later experience multiple spontaneous abortions. Thirty percent to 50% of patients with heart valve or vascular lesions may experience chronic endocarditis within 2 years. This development is not prevented by regular treatment.

Patients with chronic Q fever endocarditis have a chronic infection with low-grade fever, progressive degradation of valve function, and progressive heart failure. Fever is intermittent, and vegetations are frequently absent on cardiac echocardiography. Endocarditis is therefore not frequently considered in the initial differential diagnosis. If it is not diagnosed, the disease progressively worsens, and emboli (mainly cerebral), as well as renal insufficiency, splenomegaly, and hepatomegaly, may be observed. Digital clubbing may also be seen. The main clue to the diagnosis in a patient with a valvulopathy is unexplained sickness (unexplained fatigue, weight loss, fever), a biologic abnormality (leukopenia, increased erythrocyte sedimentation rate, thrombocytopenia, increase in hepatic enzymes), or rapid degradation of a prosthetic valve. Chronic osteomyelitis, hepatitis, and infection of an aneurysm and vascular prosthesis have been reported.[20]

Leukopenia may be observed; thrombocytopenia is frequent, as are increases in hepatic enzymes. Lupus anticoagulant associated with antiphospholipid antibodies may be observed (Chapter 242), as may anti–smooth muscle antibodies. During endocarditis, antinuclear antibodies, microhematuria, and rheumatoid factor are frequently found.

DIAGNOSIS

The diagnosis is based mainly on serology (see Table 311-4). Direct detection by culture and PCR or immunochemistry in valve, liver, or blood samples is also useful, but serologic evaluation by IFA is the reference method. Two antigens (phase I and phase II) can be tested. Acute Q fever is diagnosed when seroconversion or a four-fold increase is obtained with phase II antigen.

A single serum test exhibiting IgG antibodies of 200 or greater and IgM of 50 or greater against phase II is also diagnostic. During chronic Q fever, antibodies are at higher titer and directed against both phase I and phase II. IgG against phase I at a titer of 800 or 1600 is diagnostic of chronic infection, as is IgA at 100 or greater. Serology is useful for follow-up of patients with acute Q fever and underlying disease and those with treated chronic Q fever. Culture may be performed in a BSL-3 laboratory. Although axenic culture has been reported, *C. burnetii* is most commonly grown in cell monolayers (notably, human lung endothelial cells).

In patients with vascular infection or prosthetic valve endocarditis, fluorodeoxyglucose (FDG)–positron emission tomography (PET)/computed tomography (CT) has proved useful.

TREATMENT Rx

Treatment is straightforward during acute Q fever. Doxycycline is the most efficient antimicrobial, and it should be prescribed for 2 weeks. Some patients with hepatitis do not respond well because of an excessive immune response. They rapidly improve with a short course of glucocorticoids. In pregnant women, cotrimoxazole during the entire pregnancy may decrease the chance of an unfavorable outcome. As for endocarditis, bactericidal treatment is necessary. In vitro, antimicrobial efficacy is impaired by the low pH of the intracellular host vacuoles within which *C. burnetii* resides. Hydroxychloroquine increases the pH of these vacuoles and restores the bactericidal effect of doxycycline. In patients with endocarditis, the recommended treatment is a combination of doxycycline (200 mg daily) and hydroxychloroquine (600 mg/day, then adjusted to reach a 1-mg/mL plasma concentration). This regimen is prescribed for 18 to 36 months based on serologic results. A more rapid favorable outcome can be obtained with doxycycline serum levels higher than 5 µg/mL. Some strains may be resistant to doxycycline, and new macrolides may be an alternative. The major adverse effect of this treatment is photosensitivity; sun exposure should be avoided. An alternative treatment is a combination of doxycycline and ofloxacin for 3 years or more.

PREVENTION

Prevention is based on veterinary control in animals. A vaccine is currently available in Australia.

Grade A Reference

A1. Kim YS, Kim DM, Yoon NR, et al. Effects of rifampin and doxycycline treatments in patients with uncomplicated scrub typhus: an open-label, randomized, controlled trial. *Clin Infect Dis.* 2018;67:600-605.

GENERAL REFERENCES

For the General References and other additional features, please visit Expert Consult at https://expertconsult.inkling.com.

312

ZOONOSES

J. STEPHEN DUMLER AND MEGAN E. RELLER

DEFINITION

Zoonoses, derived from the Greek words *zōio* (animal) and *nósos* (disease), are infectious diseases transmitted from animals, both wild and domestic, to humans or from humans to animals. Per the 2016 Global Burden of Disease Study, of 44 billion incident cases attributed to 328 diseases and injuries, 55% were caused by infectious or communicable diseases.[1] Critically important among communicable diseases are emerging or reemerging infectious diseases, 60 to 75% of which are zoonoses. Zoonotic pathogens or their toxins can be transmitted by several different routes: direct contact with animals or their products (e.g., tissue, urine, or excreta); animal bites and scratches; arthropod vectors; and consumption of contaminated food or water. Zika virus, *Borrelia burgdorferi*, *Babesia microti*, and *Plasmodium knowlesi* are well-recognized vector-transmitted zoonotic pathogens.[2] However, many arthropod vector–borne pathogens, such as *Plasmodium falciparum* or *Bartonella quintana*, are not zoonotic because they are transmitted from human to human through the vector and lack an animal reservoir. Similarly, many infections acquired from the environment are not zoonoses either; examples include melioidosis (*Burkholderia pseudomallei*) and histoplasmosis (*Histoplasma capsulatum*). Understanding the epidemiology and transmission of zoonotic versus non-zoonotic infections is critical for implementing control measures at local, regional, and international levels.

Implicit in the distinction of "zoonosis" from "anthroponosis" is the concept of spillover from animal host reservoirs.[3] Zoonotic spillover occurs when barriers that prevent a zoonotic agent from gaining access to and infecting a human are breached or fail. Unfortunately, the specific mechanisms are not always well-defined and can be difficult to predict, which impairs our ability to prepare for the emergence of new zoonoses. Such barriers include (1) factors related to the interaction between reservoir host and pathogens, including both the reservoir host distribution and density, as well as the prevalence of pathogens within hosts and the likelihood of release from the infected reservoir host; (2) the ability of the pathogen to survive and disseminate after release; and (3) human host-specific exposures and risk factors that affect the ability of the pathogen to enter and propagate within the human host, such as structural barriers, immunity to infection, and genetic predisposition to infection. Zoonotic infections, not surprisingly, are difficult to predict because distinct barriers are not equally shared for each pathogen/reservoir combination owing to the great genomic diversity of animals, humans, and microbes.[4]

EPIDEMIOLOGY

For many millennia, humans have associated themselves with wildlife and domestic animals, whether farm animals or companion pets. Dogs, sheep, goats, and other animals were domesticated as long as 10,000 to 30,000 years ago; in the United States today, approximately 60% of people own a pet. Dogs and cats are most frequent. However, other pets include fish, birds, reptiles, hamsters, guinea pigs, rabbits, and horses; exotic animals, including large cats, primates, and bears, are legal with or without permit in many (16 and 20, respectively) U.S. states. Wildlife-related recreation places more than 90 million U.S. residents at increased risk for zoonoses, and 72 million observe, feed, or photograph birds and other wildlife. Climate change is expected to increase the risk for zoonoses over the next 50 years because of extreme temperatures that precipitate increased rainfall and violent storms; rising sea level and floods that could impact zoonotic diarrheal disease; loss of biodiversity; collapse of ecosystems; an increase in pests; and the spread and increase in both neopteran (biting insect) and acarid (tick and mite) vectors of zoonotic pathogens.[5]

Most emerging zoonoses are acquired from contact with wildlife. In recent analytical models weighted for reporting bias, key factors predicting emergence of zoonoses are origin in tropical forest regions, increases in mammal biodiversity, and changes in anthropogenic land use related to agricultural practices[6,7] (Fig. 312-1). In unweighted models that do not account for reporting bias, urban residence or built-up land relating directly to human activity was by far the strongest predictor of risk. Detailed analyses using refined data pools such as these will increasingly help define general mechanisms such that attention can be focused in specific high-risk environments for early detection and implementation of interventions to minimize or abrogate risk and emergence of zoonoses.

Zoonoses are transmitted through one or more of several mechanisms: (1) direct contact with animals or infected materials and/or related inhalation; (2) animal bites and scratches; (3) bites or mechanical transmission by arthropod vectors; and (4) consumption of contaminated foods (Table 312-1). Direct contact with animals is a well-documented mechanism for acquiring viral, bacterial, protozoan, and fungal zoonotic pathogens. The risk is particularly high for those whose occupations or recreations involve contact with animals. For example, in a study of veterinarians in Oregon, contact-related ringworm was the most common zoonosis and rabies the most dangerous; cats were the most likely source of contact-related zoonoses. Significant risks also exist for farmers, abattoir workers, and others. Leptospirosis, likely one of the most neglected of all zoonoses worldwide with an estimated 1 million cases and nearly 60,000 deaths annually, is commonly acquired through direct contact with contaminated rodent urine; however, many wild and domestic animals can become colonized and excrete the spirochete in their urine.[8] *Coxiella burnetii* is distributed worldwide and acquired by inhalation of dust contaminated with excretions, such as milk, urine, and feces, and/or birth products, from infected animals.[9]

In addition to direct tissue injury, animal scratches and bites are a common cause of zoonotic infections. There are estimated 4.5 million dog bites annually in the United States alone, and 900,000 result in infection; therefore, approximately 1 in every 72 people is affected. Examples of pathogens include *Capnocytophaga canimorsus* from dog bites and *Pasteurella multocida* and *Bartonella henselae*, the etiologic agent of cat-scratch disease, from cat bites. In some regions of the world, endemic rabies is rampant.

Perhaps best known are zoonoses that are transmitted through arthropod bites, such as mosquitoes, flies, or ticks and mites. Vector-borne zoonotic viral infections include West Nile virus, Eastern equine encephalitis virus, Hendra virus, and others. *P. knowlesi*, *B. microti*, *Leishmania* spp, and *Trypanosoma* spp are examples of vector-borne zoonotic protozoal infections. *Leishmania* is associated with epidemics (799,000 cases in 2016) across southern Asia, northern Africa, and South America. *Trypanosoma brucei rhodesiense* and *T. brucei gambiense*, agents of African trypanosomiasis and human sleeping sickness, are transmitted by biting tsetse flies in Africa; nearly 11.5 million new cases occurred in 2016. Ticks and mites are the most important vectors of zoonotic disease in the developed world. In the United States from 2012 to 2016, 217,000 of 242,000 (90%) reported cases of vector-borne zoonosis were attributed to tick-borne infections, especially *B. burgdorferi* (Fig. 312-2); recent studies provide evidence that the actual number of *B. burgdorferi*

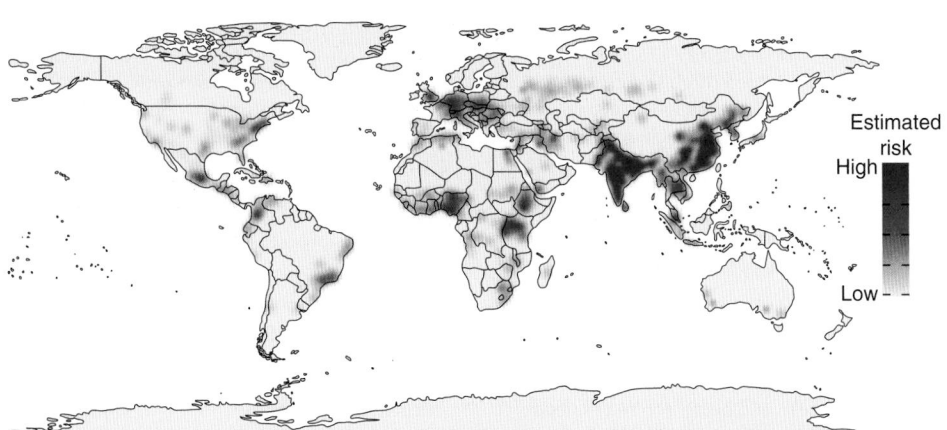

FIGURE 312-1. Heat map of predicted zoonotic emerging infectious disease estimated risk locations after factoring out reporting bias. Heat map estimated risk scale on right: highest risk is *blue*; lowest risk is *yellow*. (Adapted from Allen T, Murray KA, Zambrana-Torrelio C. Global hotspots and correlates of emerging zoonotic diseases. *Nat Commun*. 2017;8:1124.)

TABLE 312-1 EXAMPLES OF RECENTLY EMERGED AND REEMERGING ZOONOSES

DISEASE/ETIOLOGIC AGENT	TRANSMISSION	RESERVOIR HOST	CLINICAL MANIFESTATIONS
VIRUSES			
Bourbon virus	Ticks?	?	Fever, fatigue, rash, headache, myalgia, nausea, vomiting; leukopenia, thrombocytopenia
Heartland viruses	*Amblyomma americanum* tick bites	Deer?	Fever, headache, fatigue, anorexia, nausea, myalgia, arthralgia; thrombocytopenia, leukopenia
Zika virus	*Aedes aegypti* and *Aedes albopictus* mosquito bites	Nonhuman primates, sheep, bats, rodents	Rash, fever, arthralgia, conjunctivitis, myalgia, headache, retroorbital pain; congenital microcephaly, Guillain-Barré syndrome
Avian influenza (H5N1)	Inhalation	Poultry, wild and domestic waterfowl, other birds	Influenza-like illness, shortness of breath, difficulty breathing, viral pneumonia with or without acute respiratory distress syndrome, respiratory failure, multiorgan diseases
BACTERIA AND RICKETTSIAE			
Q fever *Coxiella burnetii*	Indirect (aerosol) exposure	Goats, sheep, cattle, wildlife	Acute: fever, fatigue, photophobia, headache; cough with pneumonia; hepatitis; chronic: endocarditis, immunosuppression, chronic renal insufficiency
Spotted fever rickettsiosis			
Maculatum rickettsiosis *Rickettsia parkeri*	*Amblyomma maculatum* ticks	Small mammals, cattle?	Fever, rash, eschar, myalgia, chills, fatigue, arthralgia, headache, lymphadenopathy
Pacific Coast tick fever *Rickettsia "philipii"* 364D	*Dermacentor occidentalis* ticks	Small mammals	Fever, headache, myalgia, arthralgia, malaise, lymphadenopathy (children), rash, eschar
Plague *Yersinia pestis*	Fleas	Small mammals	Fever, chills, headaches, carbuncles, lymphadenopathy with buboes, pneumonia, sepsis
PROTOZOA AND HELMINTHS			
Zoonotic malaria *Plasmodium knowlesi*	*Anopheles leucosphyrous* group mosquitoes	Macaques and monkeys	Fever, chills, headache, rigors, malaise, myalgia, cough, nausea, abdominal pain, vomiting, diarrhea
Babesiosis *Babesia microti*	*Ixodes scapularis* ticks	Small mammals	Fever, anemia, thrombocytopenia, elevated lactate dehydrogenase, hyperbilirubinemia, increased alanine aminotransferase and aspartate aminotransferase
Chagas disease *Trypanosoma cruzi*	Triatomine insects in *Triatoma, Rhodnius,* and *Panstrongylus* genera	Rodents, raccoons, skunks, coyotes	Chagoma (Romaña sign), fever, lymphadenopathy, edema, hepatosplenomegaly, myocarditis, meningoencephalitis; cardiomyopathy (arrhythmia, heart failure, atrioventricular/branch blocks, thromboembolism); gastrointestinal (dysperistalsis, megaesophagus, megacolon)
Baylisascariasis Baylisascaris spp.	Ingestion of contaminated materials	Raccoons, skunks, badgers	Larva migrans (visceral, neural); diffuse unilateral subacute neuroretinitis
FUNGI			
Talaromycosis *Talaromyces (Penicillium) marneffei*	Direct contact, indirect contact?	Bamboo rats	Fever, cutaneous or subcutaneous lesion(s), malaise, anemia, dyspnea, weight loss, lymphadenopathy, nonproductive cough, anemia

infections is more than 10 times that reported. Worldwide, ticks, lice, and mites are also significant, but underrecognized, causes of vector-borne bacterial zoonoses. Examples of neglected vector-borne bacterial zoonotic disease include tick- and louse-borne relapsing fever borreliosis; spotted fever group rickettsioses, transmitted principally by hard body (ixodid) ticks; and typhus group rickettsioses, transmitted by fleas and lice. Scrub typhus, caused by the rickettsia *Orientia tsutsugamushi* and transmitted by the larval stage (chigger) of a trombiculid mite, occurs across much of Asia and Oceania and is now emerging in Africa and South America; it is estimated to cause as many as 1,000,000 infections each year globally.[10]

Many important zoonotic infections are acquired through consumption of contaminated foods or water. The list of potential pathogenic agents is vast and includes viruses (such as hepatitis E virus); prions (such as bovine spongiform encephalopathy); bacteria (such as *Salmonella, Campylobacter, Listeria;* and *Brucella*); protozoa (such as *Cyclospora, Cryptosporidium,*[11] *Toxoplasma,* and *Giardia*); and helminths (such as *Taenia, Trichinella, Opisthorchis,* and *Clonorchis*).

CLINICAL MANIFESTATIONS

The clinical manifestations of zoonoses are as variable as those for nonzoonotic infections. Symptoms and signs may be referent to the skin, the gastrointestinal tract, the respiratory tract, the central nervous system, the musculoskeletal system, or major organs such as liver, kidneys, and heart; zoonotic infections can also present as undifferentiated fever, sepsis, or toxic shock–like syndromes. For the clinical manifestations with specific zoonotic agents or syndromes, the individual chapters that address each should be consulted. Although most

zoonoses are acquired locally, early identification requires taking a comprehensive history, including possible animal exposures and domestic and international travel.

DIAGNOSIS

The differentiation of zoonotic from nonzoonotic diseases is complex and challenging but often includes the same general diagnostic approaches. The key is to obtain sufficient historical details that might suggest a zoonotic exposure and which kind. Acquisition of information regarding potential exposure to animals must be thorough and should include occupation, travel, recreation, as well as pets (e.g., reptiles, exotic birds). One should enquire about travel to suburban and rural areas, where ticks are generally more prevalent, as well as international travel. One should ask about possible direct or indirect contact with animals, including bites and scratches, and exposure to vectors associated with zoonotic infection. Finally, one should ask about ingestion of specific food types associated with food-borne zoonoses, such as unpasteurized dairy products associated with *Brucella* and *Listeria.*

A careful physical examination, including a thorough skin evaluation of rashes, eschars, ulcers, or other lesions, is important. General laboratory and imaging studies as required can provide additional data. Depending on the specific suspected agent, confirmation of the etiology could require blood culture, blood smear, paired acute and convalescent serology to document a four-fold rise in antibody titer, and/or molecular testing. Mandatory reporting is required for some agents to protect the public's health.[12] Some tests are only available from large reference laboratories or at the U.S. Centers for Disease Control and Prevention.

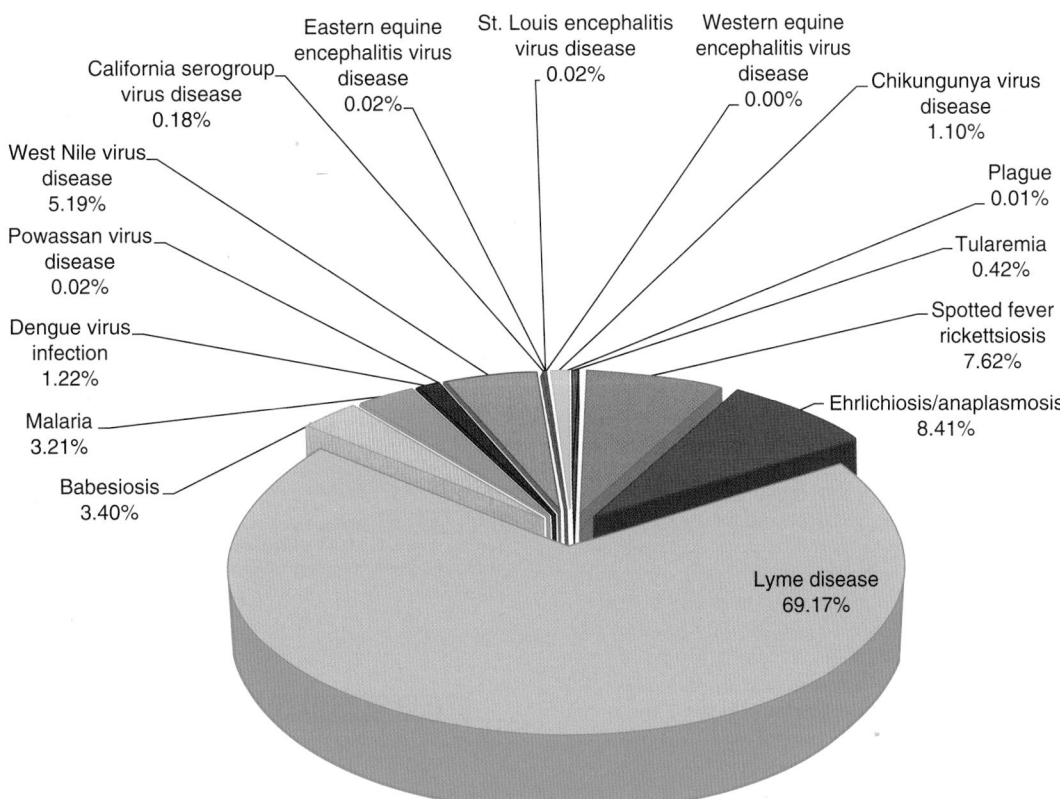

Vector-borne zoonotic disease, United States 2011-2016

California serogroup virus disease 0.18%

Eastern equine encephalitis virus disease 0.02%

St. Louis encephalitis virus disease 0.02%

Western equine encephalitis virus disease 0.00%

Chikungunya virus disease 1.10%

West Nile virus disease 5.19%

Powassan virus disease 0.02%

Dengue virus infection 1.22%

Malaria 3.21%

Babesiosis 3.40%

Plague 0.01%

Tularemia 0.42%

Spotted fever rickettsiosis 7.62%

Ehrlichiosis/anaplasmosis 8.41%

Lyme disease 69.17%

FIGURE 312-2. Proportion of vector-borne zoonoses by pathogenic agent as reported to the U.S. Centers for Disease Control and Prevention in the United States between 2011 and 2016; *N* = 286,017 cases. (Data from references 9-14).

TREATMENT ℞

As diverse as they are, zoonoses will have specific treatments based on identification of the causative agent. This information is supplied in detail in the relevant chapters of this textbook.

PREVENTION

Prevention of zoonotic diseases requires use of personal protection (frequent handwashing, gloves, and disinfectants) to avoid direct contact with infected animals; application of insect repellent to minimize exposure to vectors and their bites; and avoidance of consumption of undercooked meats, unpasteurized dairy products, uncooked seafood, and tap water in areas of the world where sanitation is inadequate. For some diseases, vaccines are available, and individuals at risk because of occupation (such as farmers, veterinarians, forestry workers, microbiology laboratorians), recreation, or travel to endemic areas should be vaccinated. When possible, pets and domestic farm animals should also be vaccinated. Immunocompromised individuals who are potential hosts must be particularly careful.

Finally, some pathogens warrant patient isolation to prevent spread. Historically, this list has included hemorrhagic fever viruses, Hantaviruses, rabies, severe acute respiratory syndrome (SARS) and Middle East respiratory syndrome (MERS) coronaviruses, and anthrax; however, the list has grown, and biocontainment units could be increasingly required in tertiary care referral hospitals.

It has been argued that more sophisticated analyses will be required to estimate the economic impact of emerging infectious diseases, most of which are zoonotic in etiology, in order to provide a rationale and justification for the global health policies and mitigation strategies that will have to be implemented in the future at considerable expense. Examples of such global strategies that have been proposed to have high impact on prevention of zoonotic infections include implementation of controls on wildlife trade and consumption; identification of land use conversions that most likely lead to emergence of zoonoses; and targeted global surveillance programs to identify novel pathogens of zoonotic potential before they emerge.[13]

PROGNOSIS

The prognosis of zoonoses is highly variable and dependent on the specific agent and disease. However, some zoonoses have high case fatality rates.

GENERAL REFERENCES

For the General References and other additional features, please visit Expert Consult at https://expertconsult.inkling.com.

313

ACTINOMYCOSIS

ITZHAK BROOK

DEFINITION

Actinomycosis is an uncommon, subacute to chronic bacterial infection that induces both suppurative and granulomatous inflammation. Localized swelling with suppuration, abscess formation, tissue fibrosis, and draining sinuses characterize this disease. The infection spreads contiguously and often forms draining sinuses that extrude characteristic but not pathognomonic "sulfur granules." Infections of the oral and cervicofacial regions are the most common, but any site in the body can be infected, including the thoracic region, abdominopelvic region, and central nervous system (CNS). Musculoskeletal, cutaneous, or disseminated disease is rare but does occur. Actinomycosis sometimes mimics other diseases, particularly malignancy.[1]

The Pathogen

Actinomycetes of the genera *Actinomyces, Propionibacterium,* and *Bifidobacterium* act as the principal pathogens. However, 98 to 99% of actinomycoses are caused by non–spore-forming anaerobic or microaerophilic bacterial species of the genus *Actinomyces,* family Actinomycetaceae, order Actinomyceta-les. Of the 30 *Actinomyces* spp, 8 may cause disease in humans: the strictly anaerobic *A. israelii, A. gerencseriae* (formerly known as *A. israelii* serotype II), *A. odontolyticus, A. naeslundii, A. meyeri, A. viscosus, A. pyogenes,* and *A. georgiae. A. israelii* is the most common species causing human disease. *P. propionicum* (formerly known as *Arachnia propionica*) and *B. dentium* (formerly known as *A. eriksonii*) also are associated with clinically indistinguishable infection.[2] The organisms are filamentous, branching, gram-positive, pleomorphic, non–spore-forming, non–acid-fast anaerobic, or microaerophilic bacilli. *Actinomyces* organisms are fastidious bacteria that require enriched culture media; 6 to 10% ambient CO_2 may aid in their growth, which takes up to 2 to 3 weeks in culture. Most actinomycotic infections are polymicrobial and involve other aerobic and anaerobic bacteria. The most common co-isolates depend on the infection site and are *Actinobacillus actinomycetemcomitans, Aggregatibacter aphrophilus, Eikenella corrodens, Bacteroides, Fusobacterium, Capnocytophaga,* aerobic and anaerobic streptococci, *Staphylococcus,* and Enterobacteriaceae.

EPIDEMIOLOGY

Actinomyces spp are members of the endogenous mucous membrane flora in the oral cavity, lower gastrointestinal tract, bronchi, and female genital tract. No external environmental reservoir, such as soil or straw, has been documented, nor has person-to-person transmission of pathogenic *Actinomyces* spp been demonstrated. Although infection can occur in all age groups, it is rarely seen in children or patients older than 60 years. Most cases are encountered in individuals in the middle decades of life. A male-to-female infection ratio of 3:1 is reported in most series. The explanation for this ratio is the higher prevalence of poor oral hygiene and oral trauma in men. The annual reported incidence in the United States is fewer than 100 cases. However, because of the fastidious nature of the organism, many cases are undiagnosed and the true incidence is probably much higher.

PATHOBIOLOGY

Actinomyces spp are agents of low pathogenicity and require mucosal barrier disruption to cause disease. Actinomycosis usually occurs in immunocompetent persons but may afflict those with diminished host defenses. Risk factors include steroids, bisphosphonates, leukemia with chemotherapy, human immunodeficiency virus (HIV), alcoholism, lung and renal transplant receipt, and local tissue damage caused by trauma, recent surgery, or irradiation. Oral and cervicofacial diseases are commonly associated with dental caries and extractions, gingivitis and gingival trauma, infection in erupting secondary teeth, chronic tonsillitis, otitis or mastoiditis, diabetes mellitus, immunosuppression, immunodeficiency, malnutrition, and neoplastic disease. Pulmonary infections generally arise after aspiration of oropharyngeal or gastrointestinal secretions and have been reported in patients with underlying lung disorders, such as emphysema, chronic bronchitis, and bronchiectasis. Gastrointestinal infection frequently follows loss of mucosal integrity, such as with surgery, trauma, foreign bodies, perforated appendix or diverticulitis, neoplasia, foreign bodies, and emergency colonic surgery. Extended use (>2 years) of intrauterine contraceptive devices (IUDs) increases risk for the development of actinomycosis of the female genital tract.

Other bacterial species that are frequently copathogens with *Actinomyces* spp may assist in the spread of infection by inhibiting host defenses and reducing local oxygen tension. Once the organism is established locally, it may spread progressively to surrounding tissues. The infection tends to spread without regard for anatomic barriers, including fascial planes and lymphatic channels. The end result is a chronic, indurated, suppurative infection (usually with draining sinuses and fibrosis, especially in pelvic and abdominal infection). The fibrotic walls of the mass before suppuration are "wooden" in nature and may be confused with a neoplasm. Hematogenous spread can be fulminant but is rare.

Actinomyces spp grow in microscopic or macroscopic clusters of tangled filaments surrounded by neutrophils. Plasma cells and multinucleated giant cells are often observed with lesions, as are large macrophages with foamy cytoplasm around purulent centers. When visible, these clusters are pale yellow and exude through sinus tracks; they are called sulfur granules (originally called drusen). These granules (1 to 2 mm in diameter) are made of aggregates of organisms and contain calcium phosphate. A central purulent loculation surrounds the granules. Their centers have a basophilic staining property, with eosinophilic rays terminating in pear-shaped "clubs." One to six granules can be present per loculation, and up to 50 loculations can be present in a lesion. Multicenter giant cells can be seen as well.

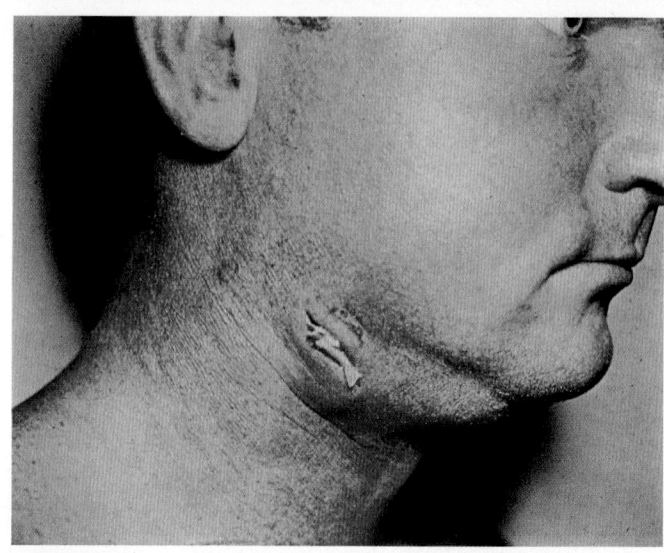

FIGURE 313-1. Actinomycosis of the jaw, observed at Letterman General Hospital, San Francisco, Calif., in a sergeant who had punctured the floor of his mouth while picking his teeth. (Courtesy Office of Medical History, Office of the Surgeon General, U.S. Army.)

CLINICAL MANIFESTATIONS

Physicians must be aware of typical clinical manifestations, such as cervicofacial actinomycosis following a dental focus of infection, pelvic actinomycosis in women with an intrauterine device, and pulmonary actinomycosis in smokers with poor dental hygiene.[3,4]

Cervicofacial

Cervicofacial infection is the most common manifestation of actinomycosis (Fig. 313-1).[5,6] It is generally odontogenic and evolves as a chronic or subacute, painless or painful soft tissue that is characterized as a slowly progressive, nontender swelling or mass involving the submandibular or paramandibular region. However, the submental and retromandibular spaces, temporomandibular joint, cheek, chin, and upper jaw can also be involved. The swelling may have a ligneous consistency caused by tissue fibrosis. Depending on the composition of the concomitant synergistic flora, the onset of actinomycosis may be acute, subacute, or chronic. When *Staphylococcus aureus* or β-hemolytic streptococci are involved, an acute painful abscess or a phlegmatous cellulitis may be the initial manifestation. Pain and trismus can be disproportionate to the degree of inflammation apparent. The chronic form of the disease is the most common presentation and is characterized by painless infiltration and bluish or reddish induration that generally progresses to form multiple abscesses and draining sinus tracts discharging pus that may contain sulfur granules in up to 25% of instances. Periapical infection, trismus, dyspnea, dysphagia, fever, pain, and leukocytosis may be present. The infection can extend to the carotid artery, tongue,[7] sinuses, ears, mastoid, orbit, salivary glands, pharynx, masseter muscle, thyroid, larynx, trachea, or thorax. Bone (most commonly the mandible) may be invaded from the adjacent soft tissue and results in periostitis or osteomyelitis. Cervical spine or cranial bone infection may lead to subdural empyema and invasion of the CNS. The differential diagnosis includes tuberculosis (scrofula), fungal infections, nocardiosis, suppurative infections by other organisms, and neoplasms.

Thoracic

Thoracic actinomycosis is an indolent, slowly progressive process involving the pulmonary parenchyma and pleural space. This form accounts for 15 to 30% of actinomycosis cases and is caused by aspiration of infective material from the oropharynx, as well as rarely after esophageal perforation, by extension into the mediastinum from the neck, by spread from an abdominal site, or by hematogenous spread to the lung. Infection can spread from a pneumonic focus across lung fissures to involve the pleura and the chest wall, with eventual fistula formation and drainage containing sulfur granules (Fig. 313-2). The mediastinum, endocardium, and pericardium also rarely can be affected. Granules are seldom present in sputum. The incidence of this complication, as well as the destruction of thoracic vertebrae and adjacent ribs, has declined in the antimicrobial era.

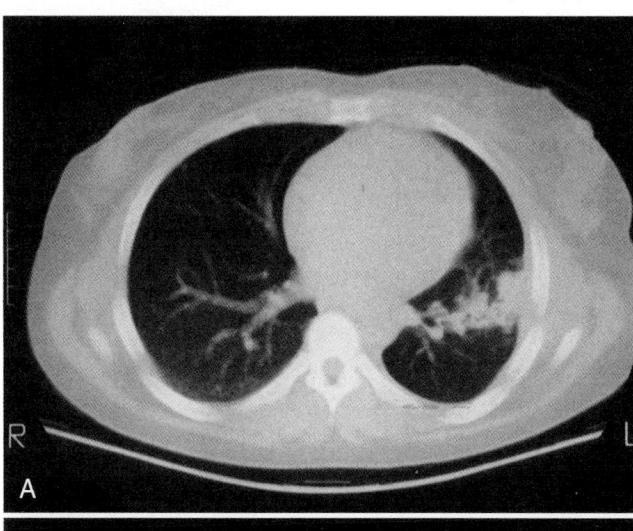

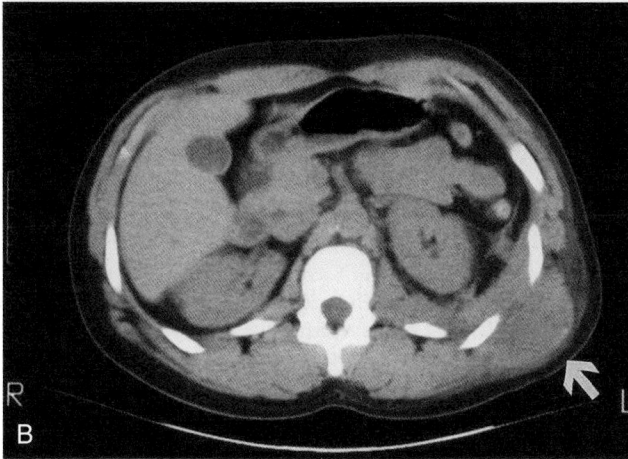

FIGURE 313-2. Thoracic computed tomography scan of a 43-year-old woman with pulmonary actinomycosis. **A,** There is consolidation of the lung with pleural thickening adjacent to the parenchymal disease. **B,** Abscess extended into the left breast and inferiorly to the costophrenic sulcus, to the retroperitoneum, and into the lateral abdominal wall (*arrow*).

The complaints of patients with thoracic actinomycosis are nonspecific. The most common are chest pain, productive cough, dyspnea, weight loss, and fever. Anemia, mild leukocytosis, and elevated sedimentation rate are relatively common. There is often a history of underlying lung disease, and patients are rarely initially seen in an early stage of infection. The pulmonary lesion is either a mass lesion or pneumonitis and may resemble tuberculosis, especially when cavity formation occurs, or blastomycosis, which may destroy ribs posteriorly but rarely forms sinuses. Nocardiosis, aspergilloma, bronchogenic carcinoma, cryptococcosis, aspiration pneumonia, and lymphoma also can mimic thoracic actinomycosis.[8] Pleural thickening, effusion, or emphysema is common.

Abdominal

Abdominal actinomycosis makes up approximately 20% of all cases of actinomycosis. It is a chronic, localized inflammatory process that can occur weeks, months, or years after the integrity of the gastrointestinal mucosa is breached by surgery, cancer, or trauma. Extension from the thorax or pelvis or through hematogenous dissemination also can occur.[9] The ileocecal region is involved most frequently (usually after a perforated appendix) with the formation of a mass lesion. The infection extends slowly to contiguous organs, especially the liver, and may involve retroperitoneal tissues, the spine, or the abdominal wall. Hepatic, renal, or splenic dissemination is an uncommon complication. Persistent draining sinuses may form, and those involving the perianal region can simulate Crohn disease (Chapter 132) or tuberculosis (Chapter 308). The extensive fibrosis of actinomycotic lesions, recognized by the examiner as a mass, often suggests tumor. A frequent finding on computed tomography (CT) is an infiltrative mass with dense inhomogeneous contrast medium enhancement. Constitutional symptoms and signs are nonspecific, the most common being fever, diarrhea or constipation, weight loss, nausea, vomiting, pain, and the sensation of a mass.

Pelvic

Pelvic infection is observed in patients with prolonged use of IUDs and also may occur from extension of intestinal infection, commonly from indolent ileocecal disease.[10] Manifestations may range from a chronic vaginal discharge to pelvic inflammatory disease with tubo-ovarian abscesses or pseudomalignant masses. Patients generally have abnormal vaginal bleeding or discharge, abdominal or pelvic pain, menorrhagia, fever, and weight loss.

Endometritis is the earlier form of the infection, followed by tubo-ovarian abscesses. Extension to the uterus, bladder, rectal area, abdominal wall, peritoneum, pelvic bones, thorax, and systemic circulation also can occur.

Central Nervous System

Infections of the CNS are very rare and generally manifest as single or multiple encapsulated brain abscesses[11] that appear as ring-enhancing lesions with a thick wall that may be irregular or nodular on contrast-enhanced CT scans. There are no features that readily distinguish actinomycosis from other causes of chronic brain abscesses. Rarely, solid nodular or mass lesions termed *actinomycetomas* or *actinomycotic granulomas* are found.[12] Headache and focal neurologic signs are the most common finding. Most actinomycotic infections of the CNS are seeded hematogenously from a distant primary site, but direct extension of cervicofacial disease also occurs. Sinus formation is not a characteristic of CNS disease. Meningitis caused by *Actinomyces* is chronic and basilar in location, and the cerebrospinal fluid pleocytosis is usually lymphocytic. Thus, it may be misdiagnosed as tuberculous meningitis. The meningitis of actinomycosis is characteristically a pachymeningitis that involves thickening of the dura mater.[13] Extension to the cranial epidural or subdural space and spinal epidural space also can occur from adjacent foci.

DIAGNOSIS

Appropriate microbiologic and pathologic studies are essential for diagnosis. A high index of suspicion should be communicated to the microbiology laboratory, along with material from draining sinuses, from deep-needle aspiration, or from biopsy specimens. CT or ultrasound needle aspiration can be used to obtain a biopsy specimen. It is important to avoid contamination of the specimen by normal flora and administration of antimicrobial therapy before a specimen is obtained. Anaerobic culture is required, and no selective media are available to restrict overgrowth of the slow-growing *Actinomyces* by associated microflora. The presence, in pus or tissue specimens, of non–acid-fast, gram-positive organisms with filamentous branching is suggestive of the diagnosis. The characteristic morphologic features of sulfur granules within are helpful. In tissue sections stained with hematoxylin-eosin, sulfur granules are round or oval basophilic masses with a radiating arrangement of eosinophilic terminal clubs. However, *Actinomyces* spp are infrequently visible in sections stained with hematoxylin-eosin; visualization is facilitated by special stains such as Gomori methenamine silver, *p*-aminosalicylic acid, McCallen-Goodpasture, and Brown-Brenn. Multiple biopsy sections from different tissue levels are recommended to improve the histopathologic diagnosis. The granules must be distinguished from similar structures that are sometimes produced in infections caused by *Nocardia, Monosporium, Cephalosporium, Staphylococcus* (botryomycosis), and others. *Actinomyces* and *Arachnia* can generally be differentiated from other gram-positive anaerobes by means of their growth rate (slow), by catalase production (negative, except for *A. viscosus*), and by gas-liquid chromatographic detection of the acetic, lactic, and succinic acids produced in peptone-yeast-glucose broth. Specific staining with fluorescent-conjugated monoclonal antibody testing, matrix-assisted laser desorption ionization time-of-flight mass spectrometry and molecular methods can be used, but these methods are not readily available to clinical microbiology laboratories.

Imaging methods such as conventional radiography, CT, and magnetic resonance imaging do not provide a specific diagnosis but allow more accurate definition of the dimensions and extension of the infection.

TREATMENT   Rx

Prolonged antimicrobial therapy (i.e., 6 to 12 months) has typically been recommended for patients with all clinical forms of actinomycosis to prevent disease recrudescence. However, individualization of courses of therapy is recommended because the duration of treatment depends on the initial burden of disease, the site of infection, and the clinical and radiologic response. Adequate drainage is indicated if abscesses are present.

Penicillin G is the drug of choice for treatment of an infection caused by any of the *Actinomyces*. It is given in high dosage during a prolonged period because the infection has a tendency to recur. Most deep-seated infections can be expected to respond to intravenous penicillin G, 18 to 24 million units/day given for 2 to 6 weeks, followed by an oral phenoxypenicillin in a dosage of 2 to 4 g/day. A few additional weeks of oral penicillin therapy may suffice for uncomplicated cervicofacial disease; complicated cases and extensive pulmonary or abdominal disease may require treatment for 12 to 18 months. Little evidence exists of acquired resistance to penicillin G by *Actinomyces* during prolonged therapy. The combination of a penicillin (i.e., amoxicillin, piperacillin) and a β-lactamase inhibitor (i.e., clavulanate, tazobactam) offers the advantage of coverage against penicillin-resistant aerobic and anaerobic copathogens.[14] Alternative first-line antibiotics include amoxicillin, tetracycline, erythromycin, and clindamycin. Ceftriaxone, imipenem, and fluoroquinolones have also been used successfully. Metronidazole, aminoglycosides, oxacillin, and cephalexin are not effective. In vitro antimicrobial susceptibility testing of *Actinomyces* is difficult, and the results may not be predictive of antimicrobial effects in vivo.

The need to use combination antimicrobial therapy to eradicate microorganisms that are isolated in association with *Actinomyces* has not been established. Clinical and microbiologic cure was achieved in more than 85% cases of cutaneous actinomycosis with amoxicillin/clavulanic acid 875/125 mg BID orally for up to 12 weeks in one series.[15] However, because many of these organisms are known pathogens, treatment is usually appropriate, especially with lower abdominal infections. Surgical removal of infected tissue also may be necessary in some cases, especially if extensive necrotic tissue or fistulas are present, if malignant disease cannot be excluded, and if large abscesses cannot be drained by percutaneous aspiration. When well-defined IUD-related symptoms and Papanicolaou smears demonstrate *Actinomyces* by specific fluorescence-labeled antibody, the IUD should be removed. Antimicrobial administration for a 2-week period may be indicated. More serious infections require prolonged therapy.

PROGNOSIS

The availability of antimicrobial treatment has greatly improved the prognosis for all forms of actinomycosis. At present, cure rates are high and neither deformity nor death is common.

GENERAL REFERENCES

For the General References and other additional features, please visit Expert Consult at https://expertconsult.inkling.com.

314

NOCARDIOSIS

FREDERICK S. SOUTHWICK

DEFINITION

Nocardiosis refers to infections caused by *Nocardia* spp. *Nocardia* most commonly causes pneumonia but also can infect the central nervous system (CNS) and the skin. Less commonly, this organism can disseminate throughout the body. These infections usually occur in patients with defective immunity.

Etiology

Nocardia spp are thin, aerobic, gram-positive bacilli that form branching filaments.[1] The bacteria stain irregularly and appear beaded on Gram stain. The speciation of *Nocardia* has been problematic. The original classification was based on the ability to use specific nutrients and decompose substrates such as adenine, casein, urea, gelatin, and xanthine. However, gene sequencing and DNA-DNA hybridization have now defined the true taxonomy.[2] The species called *N. asteroides* was previously reported to be the most common cause of human disease. However, the majority of these bacteria were misidentified by today's standards. The number of species causing human disease is large and includes *N. abscessus, N. brevicatena/paucivorans* complex, *N. nova* complex,

N. transvalensis complex, *N. farcinica, N. cyriacigeorgica, N. otitidiscaviarum, N. veterana, N. brasiliensis,* and *N. pseudobrasiliensis.*

EPIDEMIOLOGY

Nocardia spp are ubiquitous and primarily originate in soil. Despite being found throughout the environment, they rarely cause symptomatic infection in humans. Because nocardiosis is not a reportable disease, the frequency of this disease is mostly unknown. The annual incidence has been estimated to be 0.4 in 100,000. The risk for symptomatic *Nocardia* infection is greatly increased (estimated to be 140 to 340 times greater) in individuals who are immunocompromised, including patients who are receiving immunosuppressive agents following bone marrow or solid organ transplant,[3] and patients with acquired immunodeficiency syndrome (AIDS). Corticosteroids are the most frequent immunosuppressant associated with nocardiosis[4]; however, cases also have been reported in patients receiving anti–tumor necrosis factor-α antibody (infliximab) as well as other immunosuppressants.[5] It is important to keep in mind that trimethoprim-sulfamethoxazole prophylaxis does not always protect against *Nocardia.* Other risk groups include patients with cancer, Cushing disease, chronic granulomatous disease, and dysgammaglobulinemia. Patients with chronic pulmonary disorders, particularly alveolar proteinosis, are also more susceptible to this infection. In approximately one third of patients with nocardiosis, no predisposing condition can be identified.

PATHOBIOLOGY

Most *Nocardia* spp gain entry to the host via the respiratory tract or less commonly by skin inoculation. Invading bacteria elicit a neutrophil response that inhibits but does not kill the organism. The bacteria are phagocytosed by neutrophils and macrophages and become enclosed in a membrane-bound phagolysosome. In this closed environment neutrophils and macrophages can kill many species of bacteria by synthesizing superoxide and hydrogen peroxide. However, *Nocardia* can survive in this hostile environment by producing superoxide dismutase, an enzyme that inactivates these toxic oxygen byproducts. In addition *Nocardia* spp produce a mycolic acid called cord factor that inhibits the fusion of lysosomes with the phagolysosomal compartment, preventing toxic proteases and other antibacterial products from reaching the intracellular bacteria. Cell wall extractable lipids impair phagocytosis and inhibit bacterial killing. In addition to neutrophils and macrophages, cell-mediated and humoral immunity also play roles in protecting the host against *Nocardia* invasion, explaining the wide range of immunocompromised patients that are at increased risk for contracting nocardiosis.

CLINICAL MANIFESTATIONS

Nocardiosis has no pathognomonic characteristics, and delays in diagnosis are common.[6] Failure of a pulmonary or skin infection to respond to conventional antibiotic therapy should raise the possibility of a *Nocardia* spp infection. Nocardiosis always should be considered in the immunocompromised patient.[7]

Pulmonary Nocardiosis

Approximately two thirds of patients with nocardiosis present with pulmonary infection.[8] Pulmonary disease is usually subacute in onset, mimicking a fungal or mycobacterial infection, and is most commonly misdiagnosed as tuberculosis. The most common complaints are a persistent cough producing purulent sputum, fever, anorexia, and weight loss. Less commonly, patients may report pleuritic chest pain and dyspnea. Hemoptysis is rare but can develop in patients with large cavitary lesions. Acute onset of pneumonia has occasionally been reported in the immunocompromised host.

Central Nervous System Infection

Approximately 5% of patients with a *Nocardia* infection have CNS involvement. Multilocular brain abscess is the most common CNS manifestation and is usually the consequence of transient bacterial dissemination from the lung. Lesions can occur in any region of the brain, and symptoms depend on location. Headache is the usual initial complaint and frequently localized to the site of the abscess. Patients also may present with neurologic deficits and seizures. The combined findings of a lung nodule on chest x-ray and a ring-enhancing CNS lesion are often mistaken for metastatic lung carcinoma. Other diagnoses that should be considered when the immunocompromised host presents with both a lung and CNS focus are disseminated aspergillosis and toxoplasmosis. Meningitis is a less common CNS manifestation and is often associated with brain abscess (40% of meningitis cases). The CSF cell count

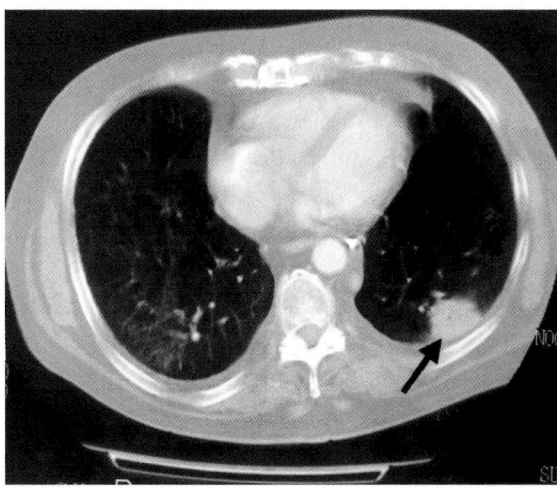

FIGURE 314-1. Chest computed tomography showing a peripheral nodular lung lesion (*arrow*) caused by *Nocardia* infection.

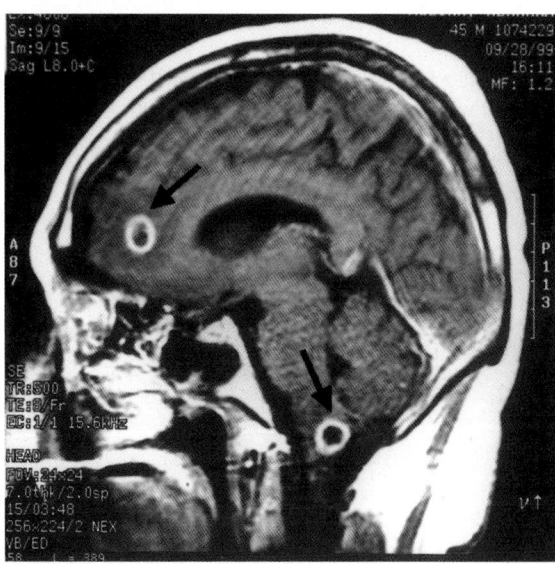

FIGURE 314-2. Multiple, gadolinium-enhanced brain lesions (*arrows*) caused by *Nocardia* infection.

usually reveals predominantly neutrophils and the CSF culture may be positive, particularly if the culture is held for a prolonged period.

Cutaneous Infection

Skin infection is usually caused by *N. brasiliensis* and typically follows a break in the skin that is contaminated by soil. Cutaneous disease has been reported in association with trauma, a postoperative wound, insect bites, thorn bush scratches, or even a cat scratch. Initially a pustule or a moderately erythematous, nonfluctuant nodule develops at the site of inoculation. Erythema can extend along the lymphatic system and is associated with tender lymphadenopathy. This form of cutaneous infection has been termed *lymphocutaneous* or *sporotrichoid* disease. Similar skin manifestations are seen with other etiologies, including cat scratch disease, tularemia, *Mycobacterium marinum,* and sporotrichosis. In the immunocompromised host, disseminated infection may be manifest by multiple erythematous raised nodules and is an ominous finding. In tropical regions of South and Central America *Nocardia* spp can cause ulcerations and large tumor-like lesions called *mycetomas* that are usually found on the lower legs.

DIAGNOSIS
Radiology

In pulmonary disease, chest x-ray findings are variable, with pulmonary nodules or mass lesions being seen most often (Fig. 314-1). Less frequently, consolidation, cavitary lesions with air-fluid levels, interstitial infiltrates, and pleural effusions are found. Chest CT often demonstrates areas of low attenuation within consolidations, multiple nodules, and chest wall extension of the infection. Patients with AIDS are more likely to have multiple pulmonary nodules, cavitary lesions, and upper lobe infiltrates. In some patients the infiltrate may resolve, particularly in patients with normal immune function. However, the patient may present with brain abscess several months later because of transient dissemination. In CNS infection CT or magnetic resonance imaging with contrast usually demonstrates one or more ring-enhancing lesions (Fig. 314-2). *Nocardia* brain abscess is more commonly multiloculated; otherwise the radiologic findings are like those in other bacterial causes of brain abscess. Positron emission tomography is not helpful in differentiating *Nocardia* brain abscess from tumor; both demonstrate increased uptake.

Histopathology

Invasive procedures are generally required for specific diagnosis. For pulmonary infection, bronchoscopy with transbronchial biopsy or skinny needle biopsy is recommended. CT-guided needle aspirate is the diagnostic procedure of choice for brain abscess. Histopathologic examination usually reveals an acute inflammatory response with a predominance of neutrophils. Micronodular abscesses with minimal capsular formation are usually found. Gram stain or Brown-Brenn stains reveal gram-positive, beaded, branching forms. The morphology is identical to that of *Actinomyces*; however, the high lipid content of its cell wall often renders *Nocardia* modified acid-fast positive, whereas *Actinomyces* spp are modified acid-fast negative. However, acid fastness may be variable when staining *Nocardia* colonies from cultures and is unreliable for direct clinical samples.

Culture

Isolation of the organism on culture provides a definitive diagnosis from needle aspirate samples of brain abscess, and a presumptive diagnosis when grown from respiratory and cutaneous samples. *Nocardia* grows best under aerobic conditions with 5 to 10% carbon dioxide. Because the organism grows slowly on blood agar, taking 3 to 5 days to form colonies, other organisms can overgrow. When *Nocardia* is suspected the clinical laboratory should be notified to allow the use of selective media and prolonged incubation.[9] 16S ribosomal RNA gene sequencing allows rapid speciation of isolates.[10] Antibiotic susceptibility testing always should be performed to guide the choice of therapy.[11]

TREATMENT

Because of the rarity of nocardiosis, no prospective treatment trials have been performed, and all recommendations are based on retrospective studies and in vitro sensitivity testing. Sulfonamides remain the treatment of choice for pulmonary and cutaneous disease. Trimethoprim-sulfamethoxazole given orally at a dose of 160/800 mg (one double strength) three times daily is the most commonly used adult regimen. When patients with disseminated and/or CNS *Nocardia* are treated with sulfonamides alone, survival has been less than 50%. One of the most common species to cause disseminated diseases, *N. farcinica,* is also one of the most common *Nocardia* spp to be resistant to sulfonamides. In these more serious conditions combination therapy is generally recommended,[12] the exact regimen being guided by antibiotic susceptibility testing. One recommended empirical regimen is trimethoprim-sulfamethoxazole 15 mg/kg/day IV of the trimethoprim component divided into 2 to 4 doses, amikacin (7.5 mg/kg every 12 hours), and either ceftriaxone (2 g twice daily) or imipenem (500 mg four times daily). In a retrospective study, patients failing trimethoprim-sulfamethoxazole responded to imipenem with or without amikacin. Linezolid (600 mg twice daily) has been used successfully in a small number of CNS infections. However, prolonged therapy with this agent can lead to bone marrow toxicity and warrants weekly monitoring of the peripheral blood cell counts. The newer fluoroquinolone moxifloxacin (400 mg/day PO) has been shown to have activity against several strains of *Nocardia,* including *N. farcinica* and *N. brasiliensis,* and this agent may prove useful in patients who cannot tolerate sulfonamides; however, relapse has been reported. Minocycline (100 mg PO twice daily) and amoxicillin-clavulanate (875/125 mg PO twice daily) are other potentially effective alternative treatments for *Nocardia.* Because of the intracellular nature of *Nocardia* and the slow rates of bacterial growth, antibiotic treatment for 6 to 12 months in the immunocompromised host and 4 to 6 months in the normal host is usually required to prevent relapse.[13]

In addition, for patients with brain abscess or subcutaneous abscesses, surgical drainage as well as antibiotics are required for cure.[14]

The overall mortality for nocardiosis is approximately 25%. In otherwise healthy individuals pulmonary nocardiosis has a better prognosis (15% mortality). The survival rate is worse in patients with bacteremia, patients with acute infection (symptoms for <3 weeks), patients receiving corticosteroids or cytotoxic agents, patients with disseminated disease involving two or more noncontiguous organs, and patients with meningitis.

GENERAL REFERENCES

For the General References and other additional features, please visit Expert Consult at https://expertconsult.inkling.com.

315

SYSTEMIC ANTIFUNGAL AGENTS

DAVID A. STEVENS AND DAVID W. DENNING

Methods for in vitro antifungal susceptibility testing are available as standardized tools. A variety of assays are available for therapeutic drug monitoring of serum and other body fluids. As more common mutations inducing resistance are uncovered, it becomes possible to develop molecular screening methods that can detect the resistance genes in clinical isolates, in advance of susceptibility test results. The increasing prevalence of drug resistance[1] requires careful antifungal stewardship programs.[2]

AZOLE ANTIFUNGAL AGENTS

Mechanism of Action

The azole ring confers antifungal activity on a variety of synthetic organic compounds. *N*-substitution of imidazoles has created a family of drugs called *triazoles* that have the same mechanism of action as imidazoles, a similar or broader spectrum of activity, and less effect on human sterol synthesis. Both imidazoles and triazoles inhibit C-14α demethylation of lanosterol in fungi; this leads to reduced concentrations of ergosterol, which is essential for a normal fungal cytoplasmic membrane. In some studies, the principal pharmacodynamic driver for response to the triazole antifungal agents has been the ratio of total drug exposure (area under the curve) to the minimum inhibitory concentration (MIC). Because of their interaction with the cytochrome P-450 (CYP) system and, in some cases, the P-glycoprotein pumps, the azoles as a class have a large number of drug-drug interactions, only some of which are covered here. In any patient in whom azole therapy is contemplated, package inserts for the drug should be consulted to determine which of the patient's other medications could result in a significant drug-drug interaction.

Newer triazoles have properties that make them preferable to ketoconazole.[3] These include not only less hormonal inhibition but also better distribution into body fluids, both parenteral and oral formulations, less hepatotoxicity, and a broader spectrum. Some have fewer drug interactions. Resistance to azoles in previously susceptible species is emerging.[4] Resistance mechanisms include increased drug efflux and altered or increased C-14α demethylase. Some of the common mutations in this demethylase in *Aspergillus* isolates from certain geographic areas, resulting in resistance, may have arisen owing to the widespread agricultural use of azole fungicides. All agents in this class have the potential for embryotoxicity and teratogenicity and should be avoided during pregnancy, particularly the first trimester.[5]

Itraconazole
Formulations and Pharmacology

Itraconazole is marketed as a capsule and as an oral suspension in cyclodextrin (an oligosaccharide ring). The ring entraps the hydrophobic, water-insoluble drug, thus making it soluble; it is then released at the lipid membrane of the enterocyte after oral administration. The solution can be delivered through a nasogastric tube in intubated patients, and it makes the dosing of infants and small children more convenient. Oral absorption of the capsule is significantly enhanced by food, whereas absorption of the solution is best on an empty stomach. Coadministration of a cola beverage with itraconazole capsules increases absorption. Peak levels with either preparation are achieved 4 to 6 hours after a dose. Steady state is achieved only after 13 to 15 days, at which time the β-elimination half-life is approximately 19 to 22 hours. Absorption of the capsule is markedly depressed in bone marrow transplant recipients, probably because of hypochlorhydria, mucositis, and graft-versus-host intestinal changes, and in patients with acquired immunodeficiency syndrome (AIDS) because of enteritis, but this problem can be alleviated by using the solution.

For deep mycoses, an initial itraconazole dose of 200 mg three times daily is recommended for the first 3 days to quickly achieve high serum and tissue levels. Hydroxyitraconazole, a metabolite of itraconazole, appears in the blood in amounts roughly twice that of the parent drug; it has antifungal activity and pharmacokinetics similar to those of the parent compound.

Bioassays of itraconazole yield much higher concentrations than measurement by high-pressure liquid chromatography; the difference results from the susceptibility of the bioassay organism to hydroxyitraconazole. Concentrations of itraconazole in tissue, pus, and bronchial secretions are generally higher than those in plasma. Ocular levels are low. Saliva concentrations persist for 8 hours after administration of the solution and may be beneficial in treating oral disease or eradicating oral colonization. The drug is metabolized in the liver and excreted in feces as metabolites. Of the liquid administered, less than 0.5% of the cyclodextrin is absorbed. No significant amount of bioactive itraconazole appears in urine. Plasma concentrations do not increase in patients with renal insufficiency or decrease with hemodialysis. The half-life is prolonged in those with cirrhosis.

Adverse Effects

The most common adverse effect is dose-related nausea and abdominal discomfort, but symptoms rarely necessitate stopping therapy. Dividing the dose and administering the drug twice daily can improve tolerance and raise blood levels. Hypokalemia and edema may occur at doses of 400 mg/day or higher. Allergic rash is seen occasionally. Itraconazole is rarely hepatotoxic. Diarrhea, nausea, and other gastrointestinal complaints are more frequent with the solution. A negative inotropic effect is rarely seen, manifested as subacute onset of cardiac failure.

Drug Interactions

Blood levels are reduced by about half in patients taking drugs that decrease gastric acidity. Some of the most notable drug interactions are rifampin, rifabutin, isoniazid, phenytoin, carbamazepine, and phenobarbital, all of which decrease itraconazole blood levels. Itraconazole decreases rifampin blood levels and increases blood levels of some antihistamines, potentially causing polymorphic ventricular tachycardia (torsades de pointes), as well as increasing levels of warfarin, benzodiazepines, hepatic hydroxymethylglutaryl–coenzyme A (HMG-CoA) reductase cholesterol-lowering agents, dihydropyridine calcium-channel blockers, digoxin, quinidine, cyclosporine, tacrolimus, methylprednisolone, human immunodeficiency virus (HIV) protease inhibitors (ritonavir, indinavir), and vinca alkaloids.

Uses

Itraconazole is useful for the treatment of invasive aspergillosis, allergic bronchopulmonary aspergillosis, chronic pulmonary aspergillosis, blastomycosis, histoplasmosis, meningeal and nonmeningeal coccidioidomycosis, paracoccidioidomycosis, sporotrichosis, phaeohyphomycosis, mucosal candidiasis, ringworm (including onychomycosis), and tinea versicolor. Itraconazole is also useful for the prevention of relapse of disseminated histoplasmosis in patients with AIDS. Itraconazole may be useful for prophylaxis against fungal infections during neutropenia and as empirical therapy for febrile episodes in neutropenia.

Fluconazole
Formulations and Pharmacology

Fluconazole is currently available in oral and vaginal tablets, as a powder for oral suspension, and as an intravenous formulation. Fluconazole is well absorbed from the gastrointestinal tract. Of the oral dose, 60 to 75% appears unchanged in the urine. Oral absorption is not decreased in patients with AIDS or patients taking H$_2$-blocking agents. Fluconazole penetrates into the brain, saliva, sputum, and urine.

The half-life increases with diminished renal function. Dose reduction has been recommended with reduced renal function, but as toxicity at high exposures is minimal, that should be weighed against undertreatment. The dose should be doubled in patients on hemofiltration because of rapid clearance.

Patients receiving hemodialysis should have one daily dose after each session.

Drug Interactions

Among other drug interactions, fluconazole can cause significant increases in the blood level of phenytoin, glipizide, glyburide, tolbutamide, warfarin, rifabutin, cisapride, quinidine, or cyclosporine. Rifampin lowers fluconazole blood levels by approximately one fourth.

Adverse Effects

Adverse effects are uncommon. Even with chronic therapy, including doses exceeding 400 mg/day, headache, hair loss, and anorexia were the most common symptoms; 10% of patients had rises in aspartate aminotransferase levels. Alopecia is reversible in most cases. Neurotoxicity has been described after heroic doses of 2000 mg/day.

Indications
Candidiasis (Chapter 318)

Provided the infection is not caused by fluconazole-resistant *Candida*, fluconazole is effective for the treatment of oropharyngeal and esophageal candidiasis. A single dose of 150 mg is approximately as effective as topical treatment of vulvovaginal candidiasis. For candidemia or deep-seated candidiasis in immunosuppressed patients or for rapidly progressing or severely ill patients, especially in initial therapy before susceptibilities are known, an echinocandin or an amphotericin preparation is preferred. It can be useful in prophylaxis (with premature neonates, some immunocompromised patients, in intra-abdominal surgery patients, and severe pancreatitis) and in oral continuation therapy at hospital discharge. Use of this drug for prophylaxis may result in shifts to less susceptible species in patient flora. In patients with *Candida* endocarditis, long-term fluconazole therapy has been used to prevent relapse after amphotericin B therapy.

Cryptococcal Meningitis (Chapter 317)

Clinical trials in AIDS have engendered the conventional practice of therapy with amphotericin B or amphotericin B plus flucytosine for at least the first 2 weeks. Therapy can then be changed to fluconazole 400 mg/day for 2 months if the patient is clinically stable. The propensity of patients with AIDS to relapse has led to maintenance therapy with fluconazole 200 mg/day, at least until antiretroviral therapy causes CD4 counts to approach normal. Itraconazole capsules are inferior to fluconazole for maintenance therapy. Relapse because of fluconazole resistance is rare. Fluconazole is effective for the eradication of genitourinary foci. For patients without AIDS, fluconazole is useful for those who have completed a course of amphotericin B and are at high risk for relapse.

Other Mycoses

Fluconazole is useful for coccidioidal meningitis and disseminated nonmeningeal coccidioidomycosis, but a direct comparison with itraconazole found a trend favoring itraconazole owing to its superior efficacy for skeletal infections. The two drugs were similarly efficacious for soft tissue and pulmonary infections. Cutaneous sporotrichosis, ringworm, histoplasmosis, and blastomycosis may respond to fluconazole, but the results are inferior to those with itraconazole.

Prophylaxis in Patients with Acquired Immunodeficiency Syndrome

Fluconazole has reduced the incidence of oral and vulvovaginal candidiasis and cryptococcosis in patients with advanced HIV infection, but it has negligible effects on other mycoses. Cost, lack of effect on survival, and the possibility of azole resistance have led the advisory committee of the Infectious Diseases Society of America to recommend against routine fluconazole prophylaxis in patients with AIDS.

Voriconazole
Formulations and Pharmacology

Voriconazole is marketed as tablets, oral solution, and as a solution in sulfobutyl ether β-cyclodextrin for intravenous administration. Voriconazole is cleared by hepatic metabolism, with less than 2% of the dose excreted unchanged in the urine. Voriconazole exhibits nonlinear pharmacokinetics in adults owing to saturation of the clearance pathways at higher doses, but linear kinetics in children, who usually clear the drug rapidly. The principal enzyme involved in clearance is hepatic CYP2C19 and CYP3A4. This enzyme has significant genetic polymorphisms that affect the metabolism of

this drug. Despite these differences in metabolism, the achieved plasma levels overlap, and an initial dose adjustment based on genotype or racial group is not necessary. Different studies have suggested that favorable outcomes correlate with serum concentrations greater than 1 to 2 μg/mL, and neurologic/psychiatric, hepatic, or cardiac side effects occur with levels greater than 5 μg/mL, so therapeutic drug monitoring is recommended, with dose adjustments as necessary.

Standard loading doses followed by maintenance doses that are 50% of normal are recommended for patients older than 75 years, or ones with mild-to-moderate hepatic cirrhosis. Dosage adjustments are not required for renal dysfunction, and voriconazole is not significantly cleared by hemodialysis. Because of potential nephrotoxicity from the cyclodextrin, the intravenous formulation should be used cautiously in patients with a creatinine clearance less than 50 mL/minute.

Drug Interactions

Voriconazole has many drug interactions. Rifampin, carbamazepine, long-acting barbiturates, glucocorticoids, and ritonavir induce the hepatic enzymes responsible for the clearance of voriconazole and thereby reduce voriconazole levels. Sirolimus levels are increased dramatically. Reduction in the clearance of pimozide, quinidine, and some antihistamines may be sufficient to place the patient at risk for QT prolongation. Cyclosporine, tacrolimus, warfarin, oral coumarins, lipid-lowering statin agents, benzodiazepines, calcium-channel blockers, sulfonylureas, methadone, and vinca alkaloids can be coadministered, but the dosages of these drugs may need to be reduced, and clinical or laboratory monitoring is suggested. Coadministration of voriconazole with omeprazole elevates the levels of both drugs. Voriconazole with rifabutin, phenytoin, or efavirenz results in lower voriconazole levels and elevated levels of the other drug. Other interactions have been documented, and any cytochrome P450 inhibitors, blockers, or inducers could have an interaction with voriconazole.

Adverse Effects

The most frequently reported adverse event is a transient, reversible visual disturbance beginning approximately 30 minutes after a dose. Patients should be advised to avoid activities that require keen visual acuity while experiencing visual changes. Hallucinations and confusion also have been reported, associated with higher blood levels. Liver enzyme abnormalities correlate with higher blood levels. Photosensitivity can be severe and has been associated with skin cancers in rare instances. Prolongation of the QT interval and tachyarrhythmias have been noted in patients with pro-arrhythmic risk factors, such as electrolyte abnormalities. Periostitis has been noted after prolonged therapy, apparently related to the fluoride atoms in the molecule. Leukoencephalopathy has been rarely reported.

Indications
Aspergillosis (Chapter 319)

Voriconazole was licensed for the treatment of invasive aspergillosis on the basis of a randomized, unblinded comparative trial in which, after 12 weeks, 53% of the patients randomized to voriconazole, but only 32% of those randomized to amphotericin B, had a successful outcome.

Other Mycoses

Voriconazole is also licensed for the treatment of invasive fusariosis and scedosporiosis, based on high response rates for these diseases. Infections by *Scedosporium apiospermum* complex may respond, but *Lomentospora (Scedosporium) prolificans* infections are commonly resistant. The drug is efficacious in esophageal candidiasis, invasive candidiasis, and refractory candidiasis. Although the drug has appeal for use in prophylaxis, there has been concern about breakthrough zygomycoses with long-term use.

Posaconazole
Formulations and Pharmacology

Posaconazole is available as an oral suspension and a tablet form. Absorption of the suspension is usually maximized by dividing the daily dose into four administrations and enhanced by taking the suspension with or after fatty food. Some commercial dietary supplements have the same effect as fatty meals and are better tolerated. The half-life is 20 to 35 hours. Clearance is primarily by fecal excretion, with only 13% excreted via renal clearance. Hepatic metabolism via uridine diphosphate glucuronidation plays only a small role in clearance, and CYP-mediated oxidation does not occur. The drug is concentrated in phagocytes. The dose is 800 mg/day for treatment of deep-seated mycoses, although 600 mg has been used successfully for prophylaxis, and 100 to 200 mg has been used for mucosal candidiasis. At steady state, 800 mg/day of the solution produces a peak concentration (C_{max}) of 4.2 μg/mL. Blood levels are unpredictable with the solution, and outcomes in the treatment of aspergillosis correlate with levels. Therapeutic drug monitoring is advisable, and levels greater than 0.7 μg/mL have correlated with efficacy in prophylaxis. Dosage adjustment is not needed for hepatic or renal failure or hemodialysis. The dosing for the 100-mg oral tablet is 300 mg twice daily as a first day loading dose, then 300 mg/day. Blood concentrations after administration of the tablets appear negligibly affected by food or by medications that affect gastric pH or motility. Side effects of the tablets that have been reported include somnolence, diarrhea, and flatulence. An intravenous formulation of posaconazole also provides reliable serum levels.

Drug Interactions

Although posaconazole has fewer interactions than itraconazole and voriconazole, there are many significant ones, including increased levels of calcium-channel blockers, cyclosporine, sirolimus, tacrolimus, quinidine, atazanavir, amiodarone, cisapride, corticosteroids, digoxin, benzodiazepines, methylprednisolone, and drugs for erectile dysfunction. Posaconazole levels are reduced by cimetidine, efavirenz, metoclopramide, rifampin, and, in some studies, with diarrhea and proton pump inhibitors. Posaconazole with phenytoin, carbamazepine, or rifabutin result in lower posaconazole levels and elevated levels of the other drug.

Adverse Effects

The paucity of side effects is similar to that of fluconazole. Gastrointestinal symptoms, headache, acneiform rashes of the face, and abnormal liver function are occasionally seen. Electrolyte abnormalities should be rectified before therapy to avoid arrhythmias.

Indications

Posaconazole has a very broad spectrum of activity against molds, including many zygomycetes, and the least cross-reactivity among the azoles to mutations in the ergosterol synthesis pathway that cause resistance. The main interest in the drug has been as prophylaxis and for salvage therapy of refractory mycoses. Efficacy in preventing opportunistic mycoses has been shown in patients at highest risk, transplant patients with graft-versus-host disease, and those with hematologic malignancies and neutropenia. Impressive results in salvage have been demonstrated in aspergillosis and coccidioidomycosis. Superficial candidiasis is also responsive.

Isavuconazole
Formulations and Pharmacology

Isavuconazonium is a water-soluble prodrug cleaved virtually completely by plasma esterases to isavuconazole. It is available for oral or intravenous use. The recommended dosing is to load with 372 mg (equivalent to 200 mg isavuconazole) thrice daily for 2 days, then switch to once daily. The pharmacokinetics are linear. The drug is highly protein bound. After oral administration, peak levels are reached in 2 to 3 hours. There is a long half-life, 60 to 130 hours. If given intravenously, the bottle should not be shaken, to avoid precipitation. Switching at any time from intravenous to oral dosing is facilitated by the fact that the pharmacokinetics are unchanged. There is a strong post-antifungal effect (inhibitory activity persisting long after drug is removed). The pharmacology is unaffected by meals, renal impairment, or patient age, race, or gender. Hepatic insufficiency produces small pharmacologic changes, and no dose alteration is recommended.

Adverse Effects and Drug Interactions

Although there are interactions with hepatic CYP 3A4 enzymes, the frequency of drug interactions appears lower than other triazoles. Methotrexate levels are increased. QT intervals are shortened, and the drug is contraindicated in patients with familial short QT intervals.

Side effects noted in clinical trials included nausea (26%), vomiting (25%), diarrhea (22%), with headache, hypokalemia, dyspnea, cough, and edema noted in 10 to 20% each. The overall frequency of serious side effects in comparative trials appeared less than voriconazole.

Uses

The enthusiasm for this drug relates directly to its activity in patients with zygomycosis or aspergillosis. The antifungal activity in vitro is broad, the biggest exceptions being *Fusarium* and *Wangiella* species. Notably, such activity

against species of zygomycetes is broad and probably less variable than posaconazole. In small series of patients, activity appears promising against cryptococcosis, paracoccidioidomycosis, coccidioidomycosis, histoplasmosis, and blastomycosis.

Ketoconazole

The main advantage of ketoconazole, an oral agent, was its lower cost compared with the cost of triazoles, although recent generic manufacture of triazoles has reduced that advantage. Although at a dose of 400 mg/day the drug is quite effective in many mycoses, usage has been supplanted by the triazoles, but least so in cutaneous mycoses. Elevating the dose in instances of poor response produced more evidence of increased toxicity than increased efficacy. It is of interest because it causes a dose-dependent depression in serum testosterone and cortisol that are profound enough to have prompted use in treatment of Cushing syndrome and prostate cancer. Although rare, the most serious side effect is hepatitis. Gastrointestinal symptoms and consequences of sex hormone impairment (e.g., menstrual irregularities, gynecomastia) are also sometimes seen. Oral absorption is impaired in the presence of hypochlorhydria.

● AMPHOTERICIN PREPARATIONS

Mechanism of Action

Amphotericin B is a lipophilic molecule that exerts its antifungal effect by insertion into the fungal cytoplasmic membrane. Amphotericin B causes membrane permeability to increase. Loss of intracellular molecules impairs fungal viability. The onset of action is rapid. Amphotericin B also has effects on oxidation that may enhance antifungal activity.

Spectrum of Activity and Mechanisms of Resistance

Amphotericin B is active against most fungi,[6] and its spectrum of activity is not influenced by the choice of formulation. When resistance occurs,[7-9] it is generally attributed to reductions in ergosterol biosynthesis and the synthesis of alternative sterols that lessen the ability of amphotericin B to interact with the fungal membrane; oxidant scavengers also may be produced. Primary resistance is common for *Scedosporium* and *Trichosporon* species. Among the *Candida* species, primary resistance is noted at meaningful frequencies most often for *C. lusitaniae*. Development of resistance in isolates of normally susceptible species is rare. In some studies, the principal pharmacodynamic driver of in vivo response has been the ratio of the peak serum concentration to the MIC.

Available Formulations

There have been four amphotericin B formulations available commercially in developed countries: amphotericin B deoxycholate (ABD) and three lipid-associated formulations—liposomal amphotericin B, amphotericin B lipid complex, and amphotericin B colloidal dispersion (ABCD). All formulations must be infused in 5% dextrose with no electrolytes added. Infusion bottles need not be protected from light. In attempts to produce less expensive lipid-associated formulations, some have advocated mixing ABD with a parenteral fat emulsion. Although less nephrotoxicity has been observed in adults given this preparation at a dose of 1 mg/kg/day compared with infusions of ABD in 5% dextrose, no advantage was found in children. Serum amphotericin B concentrations were also lower with the fat emulsion, raising the possibility that amphotericin B was simply aggregating in the fat emulsion, but the cloudiness could not be perceived in the milky-looking lipid. Use of such preparations should be reserved for investigational settings.

Amphotericin B Deoxycholate
Formulation

ABD for intravenous use is a colloidal suspension. If a filter with a 0.22-μm pore diameter is placed in the infusion line, considerable drug is removed by the filter. The addition of electrolyte aggregates the colloids, so the solution becomes cloudy; this is to be avoided. ABD is available from several generic manufacturers, and differences in the formulations may account in part for the intersubject variation in toxicities observed.

Pharmacology

Most of the drug leaves the circulation promptly, with only a small percentage being excreted in urine or bile. Amphotericin B is stored in the liver and other organs; the drug appears to reenter the circulation slowly. Blood levels are not influenced by hepatic or renal failure. Hemodialysis does not alter blood levels, except in an occasional patient with lipemic plasma who may be losing drug owing to its adherence to the dialysis membrane. Concentrations of amphotericin B in fluid from inflamed areas, such as pleura, peritoneum, joint, vitreous humor, and aqueous humor, are roughly two thirds of the nadir serum level. Amphotericin B penetrates poorly into either normal or inflamed meninges, saliva, bronchial secretions, brain, pancreas, muscle, bone, vitreous humor, and normal amniotic fluid. Urine concentrations are similar to serum concentrations. Peak serum concentrations with conventional intravenous doses are roughly 0.5 to 2 µg/mL; these concentrations fall rapidly and then slowly approach a plateau of roughly 0.2 to 0.5 µg/mL. The initial half-life is approximately 24 hours; the β-phase half-life is roughly 15 days. Serum concentrations can be detected for at least 7 weeks after the end of therapy, presumably reflecting release from cell membranes. The drug also has complex immunomodulatory properties that are potentially of clinical significance.

Nephrotoxicity

ABD causes a dose-dependent decrease in the glomerular filtration rate. The direct vasoconstrictive effect of amphotericin B on afferent renal arterioles results in reduced glomerular and renal tubular blood flow. Other effects on the kidney include potassium, magnesium, and bicarbonate wasting and decreased erythropoietin production. Loss of renal function is due to the destruction of renal tubular cells, disruption of tubular basement membrane, and loss of functioning nephron units. Saline loading, such as the infusion of 1 L saline before ABD, has been associated with reduced nephrotoxicity in some studies. Potassium wasting often requires supplemental oral or intravenous potassium. Renal tubular acidosis from bicarbonate wasting rarely requires base replacement, but other drugs and diseases that promote acidosis may act synergistically.

Azotemia caused by amphotericin B is often worse in patients taking other nephrotoxic drugs. Hypotension, intravascular volume depletion, and other preexisting renal disease all magnify the management problems associated with amphotericin B–induced azotemia. These toxicities are lessened by use of the lipid-associated formulations of amphotericin B.

Early in the course of therapy with ABD, azotemia may increase rapidly; it often improves a little and then stabilizes after several days. Adults with no other renal disease have an average serum creatinine level of 2 to 3 mg/dL at therapeutic doses, and therapy should not be withheld unless azotemia exceeds this level. Attempting to give ABD to an adult without causing azotemia usually leads to inadequate therapy.

Other Chronic Toxicity

Nausea, anorexia, and vomiting are common. Phlebitis occurs if peripheral vein catheters are used. Normocytic normochromic anemia occurs gradually. The hematocrit rarely falls below 20 to 25% unless other causes of anemia are present. Rarely, thrombocytopenia, modest leukopenia, elevated transaminases, arrhythmias, coagulopathy, hemorrhagic enteritis, tinnitus, vertigo, encephalopathy, seizures, hemolysis, or dysesthesia of the soles of the feet may be observed. Amphotericin B remains the first choice parenteral agent in pregnancy despite its potential toxicities.

Acute Reactions

Approximately 30 to 45 minutes after beginning the first few ABD infusions, chills, fever, and tachypnea may occur, peak in 15 to 30 minutes, and then slowly abate over 2 to 4 hours. A patient with underlying cardiac or pulmonary disease may have hypoxemia. These reactions are less common in young children or in patients receiving corticosteroids. Subsequent infusions of the same dose cause progressively milder reactions. Premedication with acetaminophen or the addition of hydrocortisone 25 to 50 mg to the infusion solution can diminish the reaction. Meperidine given early in a chill shortens the rigors but may induce nausea or emesis. Concern about this kind of reaction in an unstable patient has led some physicians to use a test dose of 1 mg given over a 15-minute period to assess the subsequent reaction over 1 hour before deciding whether to administer a full therapeutic dose. Patients with rapidly progressive mycoses should receive a full therapeutic dose within 24 hours. These reactions should not be mistaken for anaphylaxis or considered a contraindication to further amphotericin B. True allergic reactions are extremely rare.

Administration

ABD is infused over a 2- to 4-hour interval. Infusions 1 hour in duration generally appear to be safe for persons who have tolerated slower infusions.

Rapid infusion in patients with severely compromised renal function may lead to acute, marked hyperkalemia and ventricular fibrillation.

Patients receiving a stable daily dose can be changed to a double dose on alternate days to reduce the frequency of infusion-associated toxicity, particularly anorexia, and to make outpatient therapy more convenient. Doses above 1.5 mg/kg are generally not given on this schedule because the toxicity of such infusions is not well described. Continuous infusion of amphotericin B with doses up to 2 mg/kg/24 hours is another approach (based on limited data) to reducing toxicity, but this is not consistent with the observation that the principal pharmacodynamic driver of efficacy for amphotericin B is peak drug concentration.

Dosage

Daily ABD doses of 0.3 mg/kg often suffice for esophageal candidiasis. A dose of 0.5 mg/kg is appropriate for blastomycosis, disseminated histoplasmosis, and extracutaneous sporotrichosis. Patients with cryptococcal meningitis are generally given doses of 0.6 to 1 mg/kg; those with coccidioidomycosis may require doses of 1 mg/kg. Patients with mucormycosis or invasive aspergillosis are given daily doses of 1 to 1.5 mg/kg until improvement is clearly present. Doses of 0.5 to 1 mg/kg are often used in neutropenic patients receiving empirical amphotericin B. Local instillation of amphotericin B into cerebrospinal fluid (CSF), joints, or pleura is rarely indicated. One exception is coccidioidal meningitis, which may be treated with intrathecal ABD because it may produce superior results to systemic azole therapy, particularly in the long term, although with far greater toxicity. Intraocular administration for fungal endophthalmitis is occasionally used; doses of 10 µg appear to avoid retinal toxicity.

Lipid-Associated Formulations of Amphotericin B
Pharmacology and Toxicity

The three lipid-associated formulations have quite different pharmacokinetic patterns. When compared on the basis of equal dosages (milligram/kilogram), the lipid-associated formulations produce tissue amphotericin B concentrations that range from 90% lower to 500% higher than those seen with ABD, with the most consistent relative reduction seen in the kidney. The lipid-associated formulations are typically given at doses that are 3- to 12-fold higher than those used for ABD. All three formulations generally require higher doses in experimental animals to achieve the same therapeutic effect as ABD.

These higher but equipotent doses are notably better tolerated than ABD, with reductions in both the frequency and the severity of acute infusion-related reactions and chronic nephrotoxicity. An exception is ABCD, which generally induces acute infusion-related reactions similar to those for ABD.

Randomized clinical trials comparing ABD as therapy for a defined mycosis are limited to demonstrations that liposomal amphotericin B has a similar efficacy for cryptococcal meningitis and a greater efficacy for histoplasmosis. Randomized comparisons with ABD in persistently neutropenic and febrile cancer patients consistently demonstrate a better tolerability profile, but few data on differential antifungal effect. The aggregate open-label data on efficacy rates for the lipid-associated formulations are similar to those for ABD. Although the lipid-associated formulations are notably more costly than ABD, the purchase cost of the compound must be balanced against the morbidity of ABD-related nephrotoxicity and the financial costs of monitoring, treating, and managing it.

● ECHINOCANDIN ANTIFUNGAL AGENTS
General Features

The echinocandin antifungal agents act by inhibiting the synthesis of 1,3-β-D-glucan in the fungal cell wall. In studies, the principal pharmacodynamic driver of in vivo response has been the ratio of the peak concentration to the MIC. There are now three licensed echinocandins: caspofungin, micafungin, and anidulafungin. These agents are similar to one another, having very few drug interactions, an admirably low adverse event rate, and essentially identical antifungal spectra. Of the three drugs, caspofungin has the broadest array of approved indications and the most clinical data. Micafungin has the most detailed data on its use in neonates and children. Anidulafungin appears to have even fewer drug-drug interactions. All are cyclic lipopeptides that must be given intravenously.

They are fungicidal against all *Candida* species, including isolates resistant to other agents. Reduced activity against isolates of *Candida parapsilosis* and *Candida guilliermondii* and a paradoxical effect whereby high concentrations that permit growth in vitro have been noted in a minority of *Candida* isolates and do not appear to be clinically relevant. Resistance, though uncommon, is increasingly noted, and instances of resistance development on therapy have been described, especially in *C. glabrata*. All are active against *Aspergillus* species, but activity is limited to growing and dividing hyphal elements, so they are fungistatic. Their activity against other fungi is limited.

Caspofungin
Formulations and Pharmacology
The clearance of caspofungin is through a combination of spontaneous chemical degradation, hydrolysis, and *N*-acetylation. Dose adjustments are not required for impaired renal function or hemodialysis. The clearance of caspofungin is modestly reduced in subjects with moderate hepatic insufficiency, and a reduction of the usual daily dose is recommended. Penetration into infected tissues appears to be good.

Drug Interactions
Caspofungin has few meaningful drug interactions. Cyclosporine coadministration increases caspofungin exposure and has been associated with increased hepatic transaminase levels, so concomitant use requires caution. Caspofungin reduces tacrolimus exposure by approximately 20%, and dosage adjustments may be required. Rifampin reduces caspofungin blood levels by approximately 30%, so the daily dosage of caspofungin should be increased from 50 to 70 mg if these drugs are coadministered. Likewise, limited data on other inducers of drug clearance (efavirenz, nevirapine, phenytoin, dexamethasone, carbamazepine) suggest that reduced caspofungin levels are possible and that increasing the daily dose to 70 mg should be considered.

Adverse Effects
Overall, the adverse reactions with caspofungin have been infrequent and minor. Phlebitis, and symptoms possibly related to histamine release during rapid infusion, have been reported.

Indications
Caspofungin is indicated for the treatment of invasive candidiasis and esophageal candidiasis. Caspofungin is also indicated for invasive aspergillosis in patients who are refractory to or intolerant of other therapies. With its activity against these two major opportunistic pathogens, the use of caspofungin for empirical therapy in high-risk situations is logical and is supported by clinical trials.

Micafungin
Micafungin has an in vitro spectrum and properties similar to those of caspofungin. It is similarly cidal for *Candida* species and noncidal in vitro for *Aspergillus*.

Formulations and Pharmacology
The drug is light sensitive. After an intravenous infusion, the terminal half-life is approximately 15 hours. The recommended dose is 100 to 150 mg/day. Once-daily dosing produces steady state in 3 days. Metabolism appears to be mostly through fecal excretion; less than 1% is excreted in the urine. The drug appears to penetrate particularly well into the lungs, liver, kidneys, and gastric mucosa. No adjustment for hepatic or renal insufficiency is needed.

Drug Interactions
Micafungin has fewer drug interactions than caspofungin. There is no interaction with cyclosporine or rifampin.

Adverse Effects
Micafungin has an excellent safety profile. Histamine release, manifested most prominently by erythema over the body, can be avoided by slow infusion. Phlebitis has been reported.

Indications
Efficacy is good in invasive candidiasis and *Candida* esophagitis, similar to that of amphotericin or caspofungin. A trial of prophylaxis in neutropenic patients with hematopoietic stem cell transplant showed efficacy at 50 mg/day. Limited experience suggests comparable activity to caspofungin against invasive aspergillosis.

Anidulafungin
Formulations and Pharmacology
Anidulafungin is slowly degraded by the chemical opening of its ring structure. A 100-mg dose produces a C_{max} (peak concentration achieved) of 8.6 μg/mL at a time of peak concentration (T_{max}) of 6 to 7 hours. The half-life is 30 to 50 hours. Steady state is achieved in 3 to 10 days. Dose adjustments are not required for renal or hepatic insufficiency.

Drug Interactions
Anidulafungin has no meaningful CYP enzyme interactions. It is not an inducer, inhibitor, or substrate and has no interaction with drugs cleared by these pathways or drugs that induce these pathways. The lack of metabolism suggests this would be the best echinocandin to use in the presence of liver failure.

Adverse Effects
Histamine-mediated symptoms (e.g., rash, urticaria, flushing, pruritus, dyspnea, hypotension) have been noted on occasion, but they are infrequent when the rate of infusion does not exceed 1.1 mg/minute. Other adverse reactions to anidulafungin have generally been infrequent and minor (diarrhea, hypokalemia, elevated liver function tests, neutropenia, nausea, headache, dermatitis).

Indications
Anidulafungin is indicated for the treatment of invasive candidiasis and esophageal candidiasis. Randomized trials indicate that anidulafungin is at least as efficacious as fluconazole. Inefficacy against *C. parapsilosis* may be of greatest concern with this echinocandin.

⬤ FLUCYTOSINE
Formulation and Pharmacology
Flucytosine (5-fluorocytosine) is the fluorine analog of a normal body constituent, cytosine. Flucytosine is marketed as 250- and 500-mg capsules. Absorption from the gastrointestinal tract is rapid and complete, and approximately 90% is excreted unchanged in the urine. CSF concentrations are approximately 74% of simultaneous serum concentrations; the drug also penetrates well into aqueous humor, joints, bronchial secretions, peritoneal fluid, brain, bile, and bone, and it is readily cleared by hemodialysis and peritoneal dialysis.

The half-life of the drug in the serum of patients with normal renal function is 3 to 5 hours and is longer in newborns. Abnormal hepatic function has no influence, but decreased renal function prolongs the half-life.

Mechanisms of Action and Resistance
An MIC of 10 μg/mL or less is considered susceptible. Isolates of *Candida* species are usually susceptible, as are most isolates of *Cryptococcus neoformans*. Flucytosine is often active against isolates of *Aspergillus* species and against the melanin-pigmented molds that cause chromoblastomycosis. The mechanism of antifungal action appears to be deamination to 5-fluorouracil and then conversion through several steps to 5-fluorodeoxyuridylic acid monophosphate, a noncompetitive inhibitor of thymidylate synthetase, which interferes with DNA synthesis, or conversion to 5-fluouridine triphosphate, which is incorporated into RNA and causes aberrant transcription. In some studies, the principal pharmacodynamic driver of response was the proportion of time the blood level exceeded the MIC. Resistance may be due to loss of the cytosine permease that permits flucytosine to cross the fungal cell membrane or loss of any of the enzymes that lead to its conversion into forms that interfere with DNA or RNA synthesis.

Administration and Dosage
Flucytosine is administered orally, 100 to 150 mg/kg/day, in four divided doses. As an approximation, the total daily dose should be reduced to 75 mg/kg with a creatinine clearance of 26 to 50 mL/minute and to 37 mg/kg when the creatinine clearance is 13 to 25 mL/minute. Ideally, the blood level should be measured in azotemic patients 2 hours after the last dose and immediately before the next dose. These values should range between 10 and 100 μg/mL. Patients requiring hemodialysis can be given a single postdialysis dose of 37.5 mg/kg. Further doses are adjusted by blood level.

Flucytosine given alone to patients with normal renal, hematologic, and gastrointestinal function is infrequently associated with adverse effects, including rash, diarrhea, and hepatic dysfunction. In the presence of azotemia (such as that caused by concomitant amphotericin B), leukopenia, thrombocytopenia, and enterocolitis may appear. These complications seem to be far more frequent among patients whose flucytosine blood levels attain, and especially if they exceed, 100 to 125 μg/mL. Patients receiving flucytosine whose renal function is changing should have their serum flucytosine concentrations determined twice weekly, and the leukocyte count, platelet count, and liver function tests should be measured at a similar frequency. Patients in whom loose stools or dull abdominal pain suddenly develops or who have laboratory evidence consistent with flucytosine toxicity should have their flucytosine blood levels determined, and consideration should be given to withholding the drug until the situation is clarified. Patients with bone marrow and gastrointestinal toxicity from flucytosine often tolerate the drug at a reduced dosage. Uncommonly, vomiting, bowel perforation, confusion, hallucinations, headache, sedation, and euphoria have been reported. Flucytosine is contraindicated in pregnancy.

Conversion of flucytosine to 5-fluorouracil within the human body occurs to a sufficient degree to possibly account for the drug's toxicity to bone marrow and the gastrointestinal tract. It is likely that the drug is secreted into the gut, where flucytosine becomes deaminated by intestinal bacteria and is reabsorbed as 5-fluorouracil.

Flucytosine has a beneficial effect in patients with cryptococcosis, candidiasis, and chromoblastomycosis. It is not the drug of choice for any infection, however, because its clinical efficacy in the first two mycoses is inferior to that of amphotericin B, primary drug resistance is not uncommon in *Candida* infection, and secondary drug resistance is common in cryptococcosis and chromoblastomycosis.

Flucytosine and amphotericin B are at least additive in their effects. Flucytosine permits a lower dose of amphotericin B to be used to achieve the same therapeutic effect, and amphotericin B prevents the emergence of secondary drug resistance. These advantages have been confirmed in large multicenter studies of cryptococcal meningitis, and a more rapid antifungal effect has been shown.

Flucytosine therapy is more difficult to manage in patients with diminished bone marrow reserve. Intravenous flucytosine is no longer available in most countries, but it is used at the same dosage as the capsule formulation.

Flucytosine resistance has occurred, albeit uncommonly, during combination therapy. Use of combination therapy in such patients incurs the risk for toxicity without evidence that flucytosine adds to the therapeutic effect.

Use during Pregnancy

Amphotericin B, and lipid derivatives, appear to be safe during pregnancy. Fluconazole is teratogenic during the first trimester but safe if used as a single low dose. Itraconazole appears safe, but may be associated with increased fetal loss. Insufficient data are available regarding other antifungal agents.[10]

OTHER AGENTS

Combinations of antifungal agents are increasingly being used in an effort to improve the very poor response rates in some diseases and to combine drugs with different mechanisms of action. Although synergy in vitro may be relatively easy to demonstrate, there are few examples of synergy in animal model studies, and fewer in patients. The costs are high and the side effects are likely to be increased. The clinical advantages of the amphotericin-flucytosine combination in cryptococcosis have yet to be documented definitively in other situations.

Immunomodulators, particularly cytokines, hold promise, but insufficient clinical data exist to determine where and how these drugs might be used.[11] Granulocyte-macrophage colony-stimulating factor was shown to be effective in one trial when given prophylactically during induction therapy of patients with leukemia who are high risk.

Therapy of the various forms of tinea and of onychomycosis with systemic agents is discussed in Chapter 409. Although *Pneumocystis jiroveci* (formerly *Pneumocystis carinii*) is now classified among the fungi, the drugs used to treat it are not ones used to treat mycoses (Chapter 321).

GENERAL REFERENCES

For the General References and other additional features, please visit Expert Consult at https://expertconsult.inkling.com.

316

ENDEMIC MYCOSES

CAROL A. KAUFFMAN, JOHN N. GALGIANI, AND
GEORGE R. THOMPSON, III

BLASTOMYCOSIS

DEFINITION

Blastomycosis (North American blastomycosis) is an endemic mycosis that primarily causes infection of the lungs and skin and, less commonly, infection of the osteoarticular and genitourinary systems.[1]

The Pathogen

Blastomyces dermatitidis is a thermally dimorphic fungus. In the environment in the mold phase, the organism produces conidia, which when aerosolized and inhaled cause infection. At 37° C on culture media and in tissues, the organism is a distinctively appearing yeast that is 5 to 20 μm in diameter, has a thick refractile cell wall, and produces single broad-based buds (Fig. 316-1).

EPIDEMIOLOGY

B. dermatitidis exists in many diverse geographic areas worldwide, but most cases of blastomycosis are reported from the south central and north central regions of the United States[2] and the Canadian provinces surrounding the Great Lakes. The natural niche of *B. dermatitidis* is thought to be soil and decaying vegetation, especially in areas associated with rivers and lakes. Although most cases occur sporadically, several well-described outbreaks have occurred, often in association with activities along waterways. The typical patient in whom blastomycosis develops is a middle-aged man who has an outdoor occupation or hobby. The association of blastomycosis developing in both hunters and their dogs is well known in endemic areas.

PATHOBIOLOGY

After the inhalation of conidia, *B. dermatitidis* transforms into the yeast phase and causes pulmonary infection. Although many patients manifest only pulmonary symptoms, others have cutaneous lesions in the absence of other organ involvement or have disseminated infection. It is likely that most patients have asymptomatic hematogenous dissemination after the initial pulmonary infection. Thus, cutaneous lesions should be viewed as a manifestation of hematogenous spread of the organism. Except in rare instances, blastomycosis is not acquired by inoculation. Cellular immunity involving T lymphocytes and macrophages is an important component of the host response to infection with *B. dermatitidis*, but neutrophils also play a role. Most patients with blastomycosis are healthy hosts. Patients who are immunosuppressed are more likely to have severe disease. Infection in an immunosuppressed host can occur

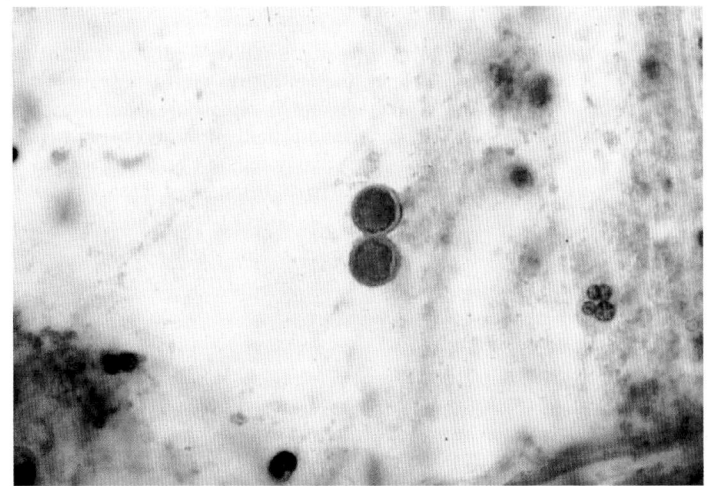

FIGURE 316-1. Papanicolaou stain of sputum showing a thick-walled yeast with broad-based budding typical of *Blastomyces dermatitidis*.

after new exposure to *B. dermatitidis* or, less often, from reactivation of a latent focus of infection acquired years earlier.

CLINICAL MANIFESTATIONS

Pulmonary

Most patients with acute pulmonary blastomycosis are asymptomatic or are thought to have community-acquired pneumonia. Patients with acute pneumonia have fever, malaise, a nonproductive cough, and a pulmonary infiltrate that shows lobar or multilobar patchy or nodular infiltrates on chest radiographs. Development of skin lesions is a strong clue for blastomycosis. Chronic pulmonary blastomycosis must be differentiated from tuberculosis, other fungal infections, and lung cancer. Fever, night sweats, weight loss, fatigue, cough, sputum production, hemoptysis, and dyspnea are commonly noted. On chest radiograph the lesions are cavitary, nodular, fibrotic, or masslike in appearance. Hilar and mediastinal lymphadenopathy and pleural effusions are not commonly seen. Overwhelming pulmonary disease with acute respiratory distress syndrome (ARDS) occurs infrequently but has a high mortality rate. Whether this is due to inhalation of a large number of conidia or to an exuberant host response is not known. Corticosteroids may provide benefit, and extracorporeal membrane oxygenation can sometimes be life-saving with severe disease.

Disseminated Infection

Cutaneous lesions are the most common manifestation of disseminated blastomycosis. The lesions can be single or multiple, usually well circumscribed, and painless. Papules, nodules, plaques, and ulcers can occur; often they are verrucous and develop multiple punctate draining areas in the center. The lesions clinically mimic those associated with nontuberculous mycobacteria, other fungal infections, pyoderma gangrenosum, and bromide use. An uncommon manifestation, seen in immunocompromised patients, is the appearance of hundreds of pustular lesions that readily reveal the organism when aspirated.

Another manifestation of disseminated blastomycosis is osteoarticular involvement. Osteomyelitis can be associated with contiguous skin lesions or can appear at sites distant from cutaneous lesions. It is helpful to obtain a bone scan in all patients with disseminated blastomycosis because of the propensity of the organism to infect bone. Genitourinary involvement may be asymptomatic or be associated with signs of prostatism and the presence of a nodule on digital examination. Infrequently occurring findings include laryngeal and oropharyngeal nodules; ocular lesions; central nervous system (CNS) involvement in the form of either meningitis or intracerebral mass lesions[3]; and dissemination to the liver, spleen, and lymph nodes.

DIAGNOSIS

The definitive diagnostic test for blastomycosis is growth of the organism from an aspirate, tissue biopsy specimen, sputum, or body fluid.[4] The mold phase takes several weeks to grow at room temperature. Once growth has occurred, the organism can be rapidly identified as *B. dermatitidis* with a highly specific and sensitive DNA probe. Histopathologic examination of cutaneous or pulmonary lesions, cytologic examination of sputum, bronchoalveolar lavage fluid, or other tissue fluids, and calcofluor fluorescent staining of sputum or purulent material from pustular lesions should be performed to look for the distinctive large, thick-walled yeast with a single broad-based bud. Identification of characteristic organisms allows a tentative diagnosis of blastomycosis and initiation of antifungal therapy before culture results are known.

An enzyme immunoassay for *B. dermatitidis* cell wall antigens is available for use on serum, urine, or BAL fluid. The sensitivity of this assay varies with different reports. Because *B. dermatitidis* and *H. capsulatum* share many cell wall antigens, this assay is often positive in patients with histoplasmosis, as well as in those with blastomycosis. Antibody tests for blastomycosis have been problematic, but a new assay appears to have increased sensitivity. Polymerase chain reaction on tissue samples has proved useful if histopathology and culture are not diagnostic.

TREATMENT   Rx

Guidelines for the treatment of blastomycosis have been published by the Infectious Diseases Society of America (IDSA).[5] With the exception of patients who have acute pulmonary blastomycosis that has totally resolved before the diagnosis is established, all patients with blastomycosis should be treated with an antifungal agent. Patients who have mild-to-moderate pulmonary or disseminated blastomycosis should be treated with itraconazole, 200 mg once or twice daily. The length of treatment is 6 to 12 months to achieve mycologic cure and prevent relapse. Fluconazole is not as effective as itraconazole. Voriconazole is effective in patients unable to tolerate itraconazole, and posaconazole has been effective in a few patients. The echinocandins are not active against *B. dermatitidis* and should not be used.

Patients who have severe pulmonary or disseminated blastomycosis, all patients with CNS infection, and most immunosuppressed patients should be treated initially with a lipid formulation of amphotericin B. The dosage is 3 to 5 mg/kg daily, except for CNS infection, for which 5 mg/kg daily should be used. After clinical improvement has occurred, usually within several weeks, therapy can be changed to itraconazole, 200 mg twice daily for a total of at least 12 months of therapy. For all patients who are treated with itraconazole, serum levels should be determined when steady state has been reached after 2 weeks of therapy to ensure adequate absorption. Serum concentrations should be greater than 1 µg/mL. Corticosteroids have been helpful as adjunctive therapy for patients with ARDS associated with blastomycosis, but this practice remains controversial.

PROGNOSIS

The prognosis for patients with pulmonary or disseminated blastomycosis is excellent; more than 90% are cured. Most reported deaths occur in patients with overwhelming pneumonia and ARDS.

HISTOPLASMOSIS

DEFINITION

Histoplasmosis is the most common endemic mycosis in the United States. Most infections are self-limited, but the organism has the ability to cause acute and chronic pulmonary infections and disseminated infection.[6]

The Pathogen

Histoplasma capsulatum var *capsulatum* is a thermally dimorphic fungus. In the environment and at temperatures lower than 35° C, it exists as a mold that produces conidia. It produces both tuberculate macroconidia, which are helpful for identification purposes in the laboratory, and microconidia, which are the infectious form. In tissues and at 35 to 37° C, *H. capsulatum* transforms into tiny 2- to 4-µm oval yeasts that reproduce by budding and parasitize macrophages. African histoplasmosis is caused by a different subspecies, *H. capsulatum* var *duboisii*, and has different disease manifestations, particularly involvement of skin, subcutaneous tissues, lymph nodes, and bone, and only rarely the lungs and other internal organs.

EPIDEMIOLOGY

Histoplasmosis, though found worldwide, is primarily a disease of North and Central America. *H. capsulatum* is endemic in the Mississippi and Ohio River valleys, with extension into the St. Lawrence basin; microfoci exist in discrete isolated areas in several eastern states. Soil, caves, and abandoned buildings containing high concentrations of bird or bat guano support luxuriant growth of the organism. Every year, thousands of individuals who live in areas endemic for *H. capsulatum* are infected. Most cases are sporadic and the exact source of exposure is unknown. Point source outbreaks have been well described in association with disruption of soil; cleaning attics, bridges, or barns; renovating or tearing down old structures laden with guano; and spelunking.

PATHOBIOLOGY

After inhalation of microconidia into the alveoli, a localized pulmonary infection ensues. Neutrophils and macrophages phagocytize the organism, now in the yeast phase; the organism is able to survive and travels within macrophages to the hilar and mediastinal lymph nodes and throughout the reticuloendothelial system by hematogenous dissemination. Such dissemination probably occurs in most persons who are infected and in normal hosts is associated with no symptoms. After several weeks, T cells specifically sensitized by *H. capsulatum* antigens activate macrophages, which are then able to kill the intracellular fungi. Histoplasmosis is a classic example of the pivotal importance of the cell-mediated immune system in containing intracellular pathogens.

The extent of disease is determined by both the number of conidia inhaled and the immune response of the host. A small inoculum can cause severe infection in immunosuppressed patients. Persons at greatest risk include those who have acquired immunodeficiency syndrome (AIDS), lymphoma, or are organ transplant recipients, and those taking corticosteroids or tumor necrosis factor inhibitors. As with some other endemic mycoses (see later under Coccidioidomycosis, Paracoccidiodomycosis), histoplasmosis can result from the more recently described "monogenic immunodeficiency disorders," including defects in the interleukin (IL)-12/interferon-gamma (IFN-γ) pathway and the T-helper IL-17 mediated response.[7] The latter includes the autosomal dominant "hyper-IgE syndrome" (also known as Job syndrome), which has been associated with cases of histoplasmosis.

Reactivation of latent infection takes place in patients who have deficient cell-mediated immunity, as evidenced by the occurrence of histoplasmosis in immunosuppressed persons who grew up in the endemic area but have not been back in that area for years.

CLINICAL MANIFESTATIONS

Acute Pulmonary Histoplasmosis

Infection is asymptomatic in most people infected with *H. capsulatum*. Those who do have symptomatic pulmonary infection usually have a self-limited illness that begins several weeks after exposure and is characterized by fever, chills, fatigue, nonproductive cough, anterior chest discomfort, and myalgias. A patchy lobar or multilobar nodular infiltrate is noted on chest radiograph.[8]

The differential diagnosis of acute pulmonary histoplasmosis includes pneumonia from *B. dermatitidis, Mycoplasma pneumoniae, Legionella* sp, and *Chlamydia pneumoniae*. When enlarged hilar or mediastinal lymph nodes are present, histoplasmosis should be strongly considered. The most difficult to differentiate is acute pulmonary blastomycosis because the endemic areas overlap, a comparable history of outdoor activities is often obtained, and radiographs show similar findings.

In patients who have experienced heavy exposure to *H. capsulatum,* as might occur during the demolition of old buildings or while spelunking in a heavily infested cave, and in those who are immunosuppressed, acute pulmonary histoplasmosis can be life-threatening. High spiking fevers, chills, prostration, dyspnea, and cough are prominent. Chest radiographs show diffuse reticulo-nodular pulmonary infiltrates, and acute respiratory distress syndrome (ARDS) can occur.

Chronic Pulmonary Histoplasmosis

Chronic cavitary pulmonary histoplasmosis is a progressive, often fatal form of histoplasmosis that develops almost exclusively in older patients who have chronic obstructive pulmonary disease. Symptoms include fever, fatigue, anorexia, weight loss, cough productive of purulent sputum, and hemoptysis. On chest radiography the usual findings are unilateral or bilateral upper lobe infiltrates with multiple cavities and extensive fibrosis in the lower lobes.[9] Chronic pulmonary histoplasmosis mimics tuberculosis, other fungal pneumonias (especially blastomycosis and sporotrichosis), and nontuberculous mycobacterial infections with regard to symptoms, signs, and radiographic findings.

Complications of Pulmonary Histoplasmosis

The mediastinal and hilar lymph nodes frequently calcify as the infection resolves; years later they can erode into bronchi and cause hemoptysis and expectoration of broncholiths. Granulomatous mediastinitis is an uncommon syndrome characterized by continuing inflammation and necrosis in the mediastinal lymph nodes. The enlarged nodes are readily apparent on chest radiographs, and computed tomography (CT) shows central necrosis and, in some cases, impingement on adjacent structures, including the esophagus, airways, and blood vessels. Although the symptoms usually resolve without treatment, obstructive syndromes can be severe and the nodes can persist for years.

Fibrosing mediastinitis is a rare complication of histoplasmosis in which the host responds to the infection with an inappropriate excessive fibrotic response. Obstruction of the airways, superior vena cava, or pulmonary arteries and veins can occur with resultant progressive right heart failure and respiratory insufficiency. Bilateral obstruction of the pulmonary vasculature is less common than unilateral involvement and carries a worse prognosis. Mediastinal widening is seen on chest radiographs, and CT and angiography define the extent of invasion and obstruction of mediastinal structures.

Pericarditis is a manifestation of a local inflammatory reaction to adjacent histoplasmosis. Patients respond promptly to anti-inflammatory medications without antifungal therapy. Hemodynamic compromise, though unusual, requires drainage of pericardial fluid; only rarely has progression to constrictive pericarditis been documented.

Disseminated Histoplasmosis

Symptomatic disseminated histoplasmosis occurs mostly in immunosuppressed patients, especially those with AIDS who have CD4+ counts lower than 150/μL and those who have a hematologic malignancy, have received an organ transplant, or are taking corticosteroids or tumor necrosis factor inhibitors. Symptoms and signs include chills, fever, anorexia, weight loss, hypotension, dyspnea, hepatosplenomegaly, and skin and mucous membrane lesions. Pancytopenia, diffuse pulmonary infiltrates on chest radiography and CT, findings of disseminated intravascular coagulation, and acute respiratory failure can be seen. This syndrome is indistinguishable from sepsis of any bacterial or viral cause. In patients with AIDS, the differential diagnosis includes cytomegalovirus, disseminated *Mycobacterium avium* complex infection, and tuberculosis.

Chronic progressive disseminated histoplasmosis is a fatal form of histoplasmosis that occurs mostly in middle-aged to elderly men who have no known immunosuppressive illness. The illness is characterized by fever, night sweats, weight loss, anorexia, and fatigue. Patients appear chronically ill, hepatosplenomegaly and mucocutaneous ulcerations are common, and adrenal insufficiency can develop. An increased erythrocyte sedimentation rate, elevated alkaline phosphatase, pancytopenia, and diffuse reticulonodular infiltrates on chest radiography and CT are typical. Patients with this form of histoplasmosis often have fever of unknown origin. Miliary tuberculosis, lymphoma, and sarcoidosis must be excluded.

Involvement of almost every organ system has been reported with disseminated infection. Adrenal insufficiency must be sought in any patient who has unexplained hypotension, hyponatremia, and hyperkalemia. Abdominal CT shows markedly enlarged adrenal glands. Central nervous system involvement manifests as either meningitis or focal lesions seen on magnetic resonance imaging and is more common in patients with AIDS. Skin lesions, also more common in patients with AIDS, can be papular, pustular, or ulcerated. *Histoplasma* endocarditis is a rare form of disseminated infection.

DIAGNOSIS

The definitive diagnostic test for histoplasmosis is growth of the organism in culture. Unfortunately, *H. capsulatum* may take as long as 6 weeks to grow in vitro. Tissue samples, bronchoalveolar lavage fluid, sputum, and blood are appropriate for culture. For patients who have evidence of dissemination, blood cultures are best performed with the lysis-centrifugation (Isolator tube) system; bone marrow and liver biopsy material often yield *H. capsulatum* in the setting of dissemination. If pulmonary histoplasmosis is a diagnostic consideration, the laboratory should be informed so that a special medium that decreases the growth of commensal fungi can be used for the culture of pulmonary samples. As soon as growth of a mold has been detected, highly specific DNA probes for *H. capsulatum* allow rapid identification of the organism.

If the patient is acutely ill, tissue biopsy should be performed to search for the distinctive 2- to 4-μm oval yeasts with single buds, which allows a tentative diagnosis to be made as quickly as possible. Routine tissue stains do not show the tiny yeasts; biopsy material must be stained with methenamine silver or periodic acid–Schiff stains. In patients with disseminated disease, bone marrow, liver, skin, and mucocutaneous lesions usually reveal many organisms. The organisms also can be seen within neutrophils in peripheral blood smears from patients with acute disseminated infection. In patients with chronic pulmonary histoplasmosis or granulomatous mediastinitis, biopsy of the lung or lymph nodes may reveal the organism.

Serology plays an important role in the diagnosis of both acute and chronic forms of histoplasmosis.[10] Complement fixation assays that use mycelial and yeast antigens and immunodiffusion tests are available. A four-fold rise in complement fixation titer or the appearance of an M band by immunodiffusion assay is very suggestive of histoplasmosis. A newer enzyme immunoassay has been shown to be positive in as many as 90% of patients with acute pulmonary histoplasmosis.[11] Serology is rarely helpful in immunosuppressed patients, who often cannot mount an antibody response. Because serologic tests are not definitive in patients with mediastinal lymphadenopathy, the results always should be confirmed by tissue biopsy.

An enzyme immunoassay for *H. capsulatum* polysaccharide antigen in urine and serum is extremely helpful in patients with disseminated infection and in those with acute pulmonary histoplasmosis. Almost 75% of patients who have experienced heavy exposure and demonstrate diffuse pulmonary infiltrates and more than 90% of patients who have disseminated histoplasmosis have a positive urinary antigen test. The assay is less useful for patients who have chronic cavitary histoplasmosis and not useful for granulomatous or fibrosing mediastinitis. False-positive reactions are seen routinely with blastomycosis. Antigen levels usually become undetectable with successful therapy. Polymerase chain reaction sometimes can be helpful if culture and serology are negative.

TREATMENT

Guidelines for the treatment of histoplasmosis have been published by the IDSA. Itraconazole is the drug of choice for mild-to-moderate histoplasmosis, and lipid formulations of amphotericin B should be used as initial therapy for severe, life-threatening infections.[12] Voriconazole and posaconazole have been used in fewer patients, but appear to be effective. Fluconazole is less active and should be considered a second-line agent. The echinocandins are not effective for histoplasmosis.

For all patients who are treated with itraconazole, serum levels should be determined when a steady state has been reached after 2 weeks of therapy to ensure adequate absorption. Serum concentrations should be greater than 1 µg/mL.

Pulmonary Histoplasmosis

Treatment is not usually given for acute pulmonary histoplasmosis; many times the diagnosis is not made until after the symptoms have resolved. However, if the patient remains symptomatic for at least 4 weeks, therapy with itraconazole, 200 mg once or twice daily for 6 to 12 weeks, should be given. All patients who have severe pulmonary histoplasmosis and all immunosuppressed patients should be treated with an antifungal agent. Lipid formulation amphotericin B, 3 to 5 mg/kg/day, is recommended for several weeks until a response is noted, at which time therapy can be changed to oral itraconazole, 200 mg three times daily for 3 days and then 200 mg twice daily. A short course of methylprednisolone is recommended for patients in whom respiratory distress develops in association with acute pulmonary histoplasmosis.

Antifungal therapy should be given to all patients with chronic pulmonary histoplasmosis. Itraconazole, 200 mg twice daily for 12 to 24 months, is recommended. A trial of itraconazole for 6 to 12 weeks is often given to patients with symptomatic granulomatous mediastinitis, although there are no data proving such therapy to be effective. Surgical resection of nodes causing obstructive symptoms may be beneficial. Antifungal therapy offers no benefit for patients with fibrosing mediastinitis. Surgery is not indicated and carries a high operative mortality rate. Intravascular stents have been used successfully in patients who have vascular obstruction.

Disseminated Histoplasmosis

All patients with symptomatic disseminated histoplasmosis should receive antifungal therapy. Patients who have only mild-to-moderate symptoms with acute disseminated disease and most patients with chronic progressive disseminated histoplasmosis can be treated with itraconazole, 200 mg twice daily after a loading dose of 200 mg three times daily for 3 days. A total of 12 months of therapy is generally adequate, but for those with chronic progressive disease, the duration of treatment may need to be longer.

Patients who have moderately severe to severe disseminated histoplasmosis should be treated with liposomal amphotericin B, 3 mg/kg/day. Therapy can be changed to itraconazole after the patient has responded to therapy, generally in a few weeks, and should continue for a total of 12 months. For those who are immunosuppressed, therapy with itraconazole, 200 mg/day, should continue until the immunosuppression resolves. For patients with AIDS, suppressive therapy can be safely stopped in those who have had a year of therapy, are receiving antiretroviral therapy, and have CD4+ counts greater than 150 cells/µL and undetectable HIV in the blood for at least 6 months.

Prevention of histoplasmosis is difficult because exposure can occur without the person's knowledge in highly endemic areas. Persons who are immunosuppressed should be advised to avoid demolition areas, spelunking, and cleaning of farm buildings or attics. A randomized, blinded, placebo-controlled trial in patients with AIDS found that itraconazole, 200 mg/day, was effective in preventing infection. Recommendations are to use prophylaxis only for patients whose CD4+ counts are lower than 150/µL and who live in a highly endemic area with a rate of histoplasmosis that is greater than 10 cases per 100 patient years. There are no recommendations for prophylaxis for other immunosuppressed patients.

PROGNOSIS

Acute pulmonary histoplasmosis is usually a self-limited disease. Patients who require treatment generally respond promptly to antifungal agents. However, the response of patients with chronic cavitary pulmonary histoplasmosis is often poor, primarily because of their severe underlying pulmonary disease. Mediastinal fibrosis has a poor prognosis, but intravascular stenting has led to improvement in many patients. Patients with disseminated histoplasmosis, even those with advanced AIDS, usually respond promptly to antifungal therapy; most deaths in immunosuppressed patients occur when the diagnosis is delayed. Older patients with chronic progressive disseminated histoplasmosis have a slower, but usually complete response to therapy.

TABLE 316-1	COCCIDIOIDOMYCOSIS: CLINICAL CHARACTERISTICS AND TREATMENT
CHARACTERISTIC	**DESCRIPTION**
Causative fungi	*Coccidioides immitis* and *Coccidioides posadasii*
Primary geographic distribution	Arid regions of the Western Hemisphere, including parts of Arizona, California, New Mexico, and Washington; western Texas; parts of Central and South America
Primary route of acquisition	Respiratory (inhalation of arthroconidia)
Principal site of disease	Lungs most common; spread to skin, bones, meninges, and other viscera uncommon but serious
Opportunistic infection in compromised hosts	Diffuse pneumonia and widespread infections common in patients with T-lymphocyte defects or during high-dose corticosteroid therapy or with TNF-α inhibitors
Drug of choice for most patients	No antifungal is required for uncomplicated pneumonia; fluconazole or itraconazole for progressive forms of infection
Alternative therapy	Amphotericin B (especially with diffuse pneumonia or rapidly progressive infections), voriconazole, posaconazole

COCCIDIOIDOMYCOSIS

DEFINITION

Coccidioidomycosis is a systemic fungal infection caused by *Coccidioides* spp endemic to some arid regions of the Western Hemisphere (Table 316-1).

The Pathogen

Coccidioides immitis and *C. posadasii* are dimorphic fungi classified as Ascomycetes by ribosomal gene homology. In their vegetative state, mycelia with true septations mature to produce arthroconidia, single cells approximately 2 to 5 µm in diameter. After infection, an arthroconidium enlarges to a spherule up to 75 µm in diameter and undergoes internal septation to produce scores of endospores. When the spherules rupture, packets of endospores are released and produce more spherules in infected tissue or revert to mycelia if removed from the body.

EPIDEMIOLOGY

Coccidioides organisms can be recovered from the soil of the low deserts of Arizona; Los Angeles County and the Central Valley of California; parts of other states, including New Mexico, Nevada, and Texas; and parts of Central and South America.[13] Isolated pockets of endemicity have been found unexpectedly elsewhere such as in Washington State. Endemic regions exist in arid regions, which are characterized by modest rainfall, mild winters, and low humidity. However, even in the most highly endemic areas, fungal colonies are sparse and occupy only a tiny fraction of the total acreage. Mycelia bloom beneath the surface during periods of rain, and arthroconidia develop as the earth dries. Rates of infection are highest during dry months, occasionally accentuated when soil is disturbed by windstorms or construction equipment. Exposure to contaminated bales of cotton or other fomites can rarely result in infection beyond the endemic regions. Person-to-person transmission of pulmonary infection has not been reported, and isolation precautions are unnecessary, even in acute care areas. As of 2013, *Coccidioides* spp are no longer listed and controlled by the Centers for Disease Control and Prevention as select agents.

Incidence and Prevalence

In general, the annual risk for infection within the most strongly endemic areas is 3%, resulting in approximately 150,000 new infections per year. Reported clinical illness following infection is increasing. For example, from 1998 to 2011, reported infections increased more than eight-fold. With unusually intense exposure, such as at archaeology sites or during military maneuvers within endemic regions, infections can develop in the majority of persons exposed for only a matter of days. Arizona and California contribute 66% and 31%, respectively, of all U.S. infections.

PATHOBIOLOGY

Inhaling even a single arthroconidium to the level of the terminal bronchiole initiates virtually all coccidioidal infections. Fungal proliferation engenders both granulomatous inflammation, which is associated with intact spherules, and acute inflammation, including eosinophils, which is associated with spherule rupture and proliferation. Focal pneumonia is often associated with ipsilateral hilar adenopathy; less frequently, infection enlarges the paratracheal, supraclavicular, and cervical nodes. Lesions occurring elsewhere are the result of hematogenous dissemination, and most become apparent within 2 years of the initial infection. Although progressive dissemination occurs in less than 1% of infections, as many as 8% of persons with self-limited infection manifest asymptomatic chorioretinal scars, suggesting that subclinical hematogenous spread may be frequent. Within weeks after infection, durable T-cell immunity normally arrests fungal proliferation, which allows the inflammation to resolve and prevents reinfection in the future. However, control of the infection occurs without sterilizing lesions, and reactivation of the dormant infection is possible even many years later in patients whose cell-mediated immunity becomes deficient. Monogenic immunodeficiency disorders of the IL-12/IFN-γ and the T-helper IL-17 mediated response can predispose to coccidioidomycosis, as they can to histoplasmosis and paracoccidioidomycosis.

CLINICAL MANIFESTATIONS

Two thirds of infections are asymptomatic and are detected only by finding dermal hypersensitivity to coccidioidal antigens. Those who become ill usually experience pulmonary syndromes that eventually are self-limited. However, some patients develop complications or progressive forms of infection that display a broad variety of manifestations and pose difficult management problems.

Primary Pulmonary Infections

Symptoms develop within 5 to 21 days after exposure. For residents of or recent visitors to southern Arizona, coccidioidomycosis accounts for approximately one third of cases of community-acquired pneumonia. Fever, weight loss, fatigue, dry cough, and pleuritic chest pain are common but nonspecific complaints. Arthralgia of multiple joints without significant effusion is also frequent and is referred to as "desert rheumatism." Occasionally, skin manifestations develop, including a short-lived nonpruritic maculopapular rash, erythema multiforme, or erythema nodosum. These arthritic and dermatologic manifestations are mediated by circulating immune complexes or other immunologic phenomena rather than by fungal dissemination and resolve without tissue destruction. Radiographs of the chest may not detect any abnormalities or may demonstrate pulmonary infiltrates that are either segmental or lobar. Hilar adenopathy is often a distinctive finding and may suggest lymphoma by its appearance. Peripneumonic pleural effusions may occur and generally resolve without intervention, although cultures of pleural biopsies usually yield *Coccidioides* spp. Eosinophilia may be a prominent finding in differential leukocyte counts of peripheral blood, and the erythrocyte sedimentation rate is generally elevated. Symptoms frequently persist for many weeks before improvement is clearly under way, and the illness, especially lassitude, may persist for months.

The primary pulmonary process produces a variety of sequelae. The most frequent is the development of a pulmonary nodule (Fig. 316-2), typically measuring 1 to 4 cm and lying within 5 cm of the hilum. Despite their harmless nature, coccidioidal nodules may cause concern because of their similarity to a malignant mass (Chapters 78 and 182). Positron emission tomography scans are typically positive. For these reasons, management usually requires percutaneous needle aspiration or resection.

Another consequence of pulmonary coccidioidomycosis is cavitation of the infiltrate, which occurs in approximately 5% of cases of pneumonia. Most cavities are solitary and thin walled and reside in an upper lobe, close to the pleura. Occasionally, they produce pain, hemoptysis, or adjacent infiltrates. Cavities may acquire mycetomas from either *Coccidioides* spp or some other colonizing mold. Infrequently, a cavity ruptures and forms a pyopneumothorax. Half of the time, this is the first symptom of coccidioidal infection and typically occurs in otherwise healthy young men. An air-fluid level in the pleural space, detectable by radiography, often helps differentiate this problem from a spontaneous pneumothorax. Prompt surgical resection of the cavity is the preferred treatment of this complication. The least common pulmonary complication is persistent fibrocavitary infection that progresses to involvement of both lungs.

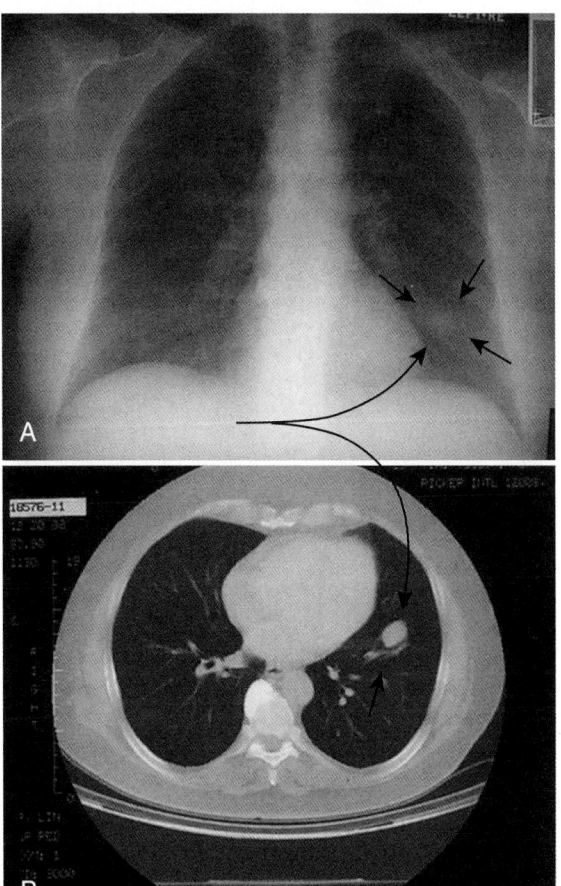

FIGURE 316-2. Coccidioidomycosis. **A,** Benign nodule secondary to coccidioidomycosis (*arrows*). **B,** Computed tomography scan of the nodule shown in **A** (*arrows*).

Extrapulmonary Dissemination

Coccidioidomycosis in patients with deficiencies in cellular immunity, such as solid organ recipients, patients receiving other immunosuppressive therapy, those with AIDS or lymphoma, and women during their third trimester of pregnancy, usually results in dissemination beyond the lungs. Mutations of the genes for γ-interferon or the interleukin-12 receptor also predispose persons to dissemination. However, disseminated infection occurs in some patients who have no underlying disease and do not manifest heightened susceptibility to other infections. Disseminated infection is more likely in men than in women and in persons of certain ancestry such as Africans, Filipinos, or Native Americans compared to Caucasians. The most common locations for disseminated lesions are the skin (cutaneous papules or subcutaneous abscesses), joints (especially the knee), and bones. Spinal coccidioidomycosis most frequently affects spinal segments (typically thoracic and lumbar) and can cause epidural and paravertebral abscesses.[14] In addition to azole therapy (see below), spinal instability and neurologic compromise are surgical indications for decompression and fusion. Such infections may produce one or many lesions and are frequently subacute or chronic in their manifestation. In broadly immunosuppressed patients, coccidioidal infections may be more fulminant, with fungemia detectable in blood cultures and the development of diffuse reticulonodular pulmonary infiltrates. Although the kidneys and the urinary bladder are rarely involved, *Coccidioides* may be recovered from concentrated specimens of urine, usually because of focal dissemination to the prostate. In contrast to histoplasmosis, the gastrointestinal tract is rarely involved in coccidioidomycosis.

DIAGNOSIS

Past infection with *Coccidioides* species can be detected by delayed-type hypersensitivity skin testing.[15] The diagnosis is definitively established by recovering *Coccidioides* spp from clinical specimens. On direct examination of respiratory specimens or tissue, spherules appear as large structures with refractile walls and internal organization; they are also seen on hematoxylin-eosin, silver, or periodic acid–Schiff stains of histologic preparations. Gram stain does not detect spherules. In culture, mycelial growth is often evident within the first week of incubation, and DNA probing with commercially available kits allows rapid genus identification. Recovery of *Coccidioides* spp from patients with only scant respiratory secretions associated with the initial pneumonia and from the cerebrospinal fluid of patients with meningitis may be difficult.

A presumptive diagnosis of coccidioidal infection is often based on the detection of specific antibodies in serum. Within the first weeks of the initial infection, a precipitin-type antibody is detected (IgM), usually by immunodiffusion techniques. Later, complement fixation–type antibodies (IgG) generally appear. However, these tests may be falsely negative as often as half the time during the first weeks of illness. When reported quantitatively, concentrations of complement fixation antibodies are usually highest in the most extensive infections and decrease in patients whose infections are controlled. An important means of diagnosing coccidioidal meningitis is the detection of *Coccidioides* antigen or complement fixation antibodies in cerebrospinal fluid, along with other abnormalities such as leukocytosis, elevated protein concentration, or low glucose concentration. Eosinophilia of the CSF can suggest coccidioidomycosis but is not always present. Newer enzyme immunoassay commercial kits are also available, are generally more sensitive than the older serologic tests, but occasionally produce falsely positive results. Coccidioidal antigens are sometimes found in the urine or serum of patients with widespread infection. A *Coccidioides* genus–specific, quantitative, real-time polymerase chain reaction assay has been developed for the early diagnosis of coccidioidomycosis. In 2014, a coccidioidal skin test became clinically available and, if positive, indicates past infection.

TREATMENT   Rx

The role of antifungal therapy for primary uncomplicated infections is unsettled because clinical trials have not been performed to determine whether treatment either shortens the course of symptoms or diminishes the chance of complications.[16] However, the value of treatment is clear for patients with progressive illness. Because many coccidioidal infections are chronic, initial treatment often consists of oral azole antifungal agents, such as fluconazole and itraconazole.[17] Responses to these two drugs are similar, but itraconazole is preferred in patients with skeletal infections. Doses of these azoles are 400 mg/day or higher, and treatment is usually continued for a year or more. Satisfactory responses are obtained in approximately two thirds of patients. Fluconazole is effective therapy for coccidioidal meningitis and has greatly reduced the number of patients treated with intrathecal amphotericin B. Unfortunately, cessation of azole therapy is often followed by a recurrence of symptoms, especially in those with coccidioidal meningitis. Therefore, many patients need protracted or even lifelong therapy to control disease activity. The limited evidence available for the newer azole antifungals (voriconazole, posaconazole) indicates that they are also effective in some patients and are sometimes useful for refractory infections. Amphotericin B remains a rational choice when treatment with azole antifungals has failed. Daily doses range from 0.4 to 1 mg/kg for the original deoxycholate formulation and up to 5 mg/kg per day for newer lipid formulations. Occasionally, in a patient with rapid disease progression, an amphotericin B formulation may produce a more rapid therapeutic response and is therefore the preferred initial therapy. In addition to antifungal agents, surgical removal of necrotic tissue may be essential to control the progressive damage from specific lesions.

PROGNOSIS

After resolution of the initial infection, most patients maintain lifelong immunity, and infections after re-exposure are rare. However, cessation of symptoms is frequently accomplished without eradicating *Coccidioides* completely, and recurrence of the original infection many years after the original episode is a well-recognized risk for intercurrent profound immunosuppression. Re-treating patients with rheumatic disease with biologic response modifiers or disease-modifying antirheumatic drugs after coccidioidomycosis appears to be safe in some patients. For patients in whom the initial infection cannot be resolved, the disease typically follows a protracted course. Although infection is more often debilitating than fatal, fulminant respiratory failure can occur, and, if untreated, coccidioidal meningitis is nearly always fatal within 2 years.

SPOROTRICHOSIS

DEFINITION

Sporotrichosis is a subacute or chronic infection that is usually localized to cutaneous and lymphocutaneous structures, but pulmonary, osteoarticular, and disseminated infection can occur in patients with varying states of immunodeficiency.

The Pathogen

Sporothrix spp are thermally dimorphic fungi. In the environment at temperatures lower than 35° to 37° C, the organism is a mold and produces conidia, the infectious form. In tissues and at 35° to 37° C, *Sporothrix* spp transform into the yeast phase.

EPIDEMIOLOGY

Sporothrix spp are found worldwide in climates ranging from temperate to tropical.[18] The organism exists in a variety of environmental niches, including soil, sphagnum moss, hay, decaying wood, and other vegetation. Infection is seen almost entirely in persons whose vocation, avocation, or living condition brings them into contact with the organism in the environment. Most cases of sporotrichosis are sporadic, but outbreaks have been described. An extensive outbreak extending over many years in Rio de Janeiro and occurring mostly in children and women has been traced to infected domestic cats.

PATHOBIOLOGY

Infection is almost always acquired by inoculation of conidia and remains localized to the immediate and contiguous cutaneous, subcutaneous, and lymphatic structures. Inhalation of conidia occurs less commonly and results in pulmonary and, rarely, disseminated sporotrichosis. The typical host response to infection with *Sporothrix* is a mixed neutrophilic and granulomatous reaction. Cell-mediated immunity is important in containing the infection. In individuals who have underlying illnesses, including alcoholism, diabetes mellitus, and chronic obstructive pulmonary disease, *Sporothrix* spp are more likely to involve osteoarticular structures and the lungs. Widespread dissemination develops in persons infected with human immunodeficiency virus (HIV) but is a distinctly unusual event in normal hosts.[19]

CLINICAL MANIFESTATIONS

Lymphocutaneous

Days to weeks after inoculation of *Sporothrix* spp conidia, a papular lesion develops at the inoculation site; the lesion becomes nodular and often ulcerates (Fig. 316-3). Drainage is not grossly purulent, and the lesion is not terribly painful. Similar lesions occur along the lymphatic distribution proximal to the primary lesion. Verrucous or ulcerative fixed cutaneous lesions do not exhibit lymphatic extension. The differential diagnosis of lymphocutaneous sporotrichosis includes *Nocardia* infections (Chapter 314), atypical mycobacterial infections (Chapter 309), especially *Mycobacterium marinum*; *Leishmania brasiliensis* infections (Chapter 327); and tularemia (Chapter 295).

Visceral and Osteoarticular

Pulmonary sporotrichosis occurs most often in middle-aged men who have chronic pulmonary disease and abuse alcohol. Fever, night sweats, weight loss, fatigue, dyspnea, cough, purulent sputum, and hemoptysis are common. Chest radiographs show unilateral or bilateral upper lobe cavities with variable amounts of fibrosis and nodular lesions. The disease mimics reactivation tuberculosis. Osteoarticular sporotrichosis is found most often in middle-aged men and occurs more frequently in alcoholics. The joints most commonly affected are the knee, elbow, wrist, and ankle. Isolated bursitis, tenosynovitis,

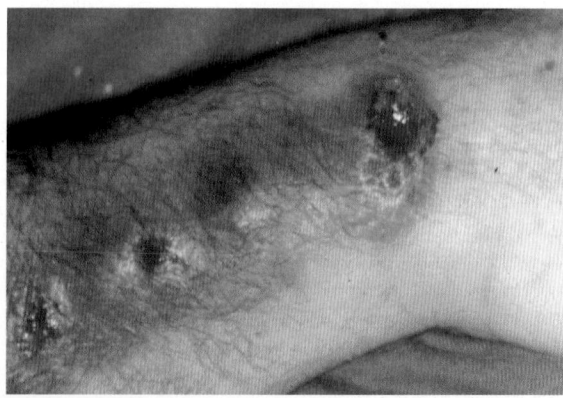

FIGURE 316-3. **Lymphocutaneous sporotrichosis.** The lesion at the inoculation site has ulcerated. (From Watanakunakorn C. Photoquiz. *Clin Infect Dis.* 1996;22:765.)

and nerve entrapment syndromes have been reported. Osteoarticular infection can follow local inoculation, but in most patients this occurs secondary to hematogenous spread. Disseminated sporotrichosis, manifested as widespread ulcerative cutaneous lesions with or without visceral involvement, is uncommon; most cases have been reported in patients with advanced HIV infection.

DIAGNOSIS

Growth of *Sporothrix* spp from culture of material aspirated from a lesion, a tissue biopsy specimen, sputum, or body fluid is the most effective method of establishing the diagnosis of sporotrichosis. Growth of the mold phase of the organism is usually evident within a few days. Histopathologic examination of biopsy material shows a mixed granulomatous and pyogenic process; the organisms are often present in small numbers and are frequently not seen. Serology is offered by some reference laboratories but is not standardized. Polymerase chain reaction testing obtained at a fungal reference laboratory has been used to confirm the diagnosis.[20]

TREATMENT — Rx

Because sporotrichosis is usually a localized subacute to chronic infection, oral antifungal agents are preferred; amphotericin B is reserved for severe visceral infections.[21] Guidelines for the management of sporotrichosis have been published by the Infectious Diseases Society of America. Itraconazole is the drug of choice for lymphocutaneous sporotrichosis. The usual dosage is 200 mg daily, and treatment should continue for several weeks after all lesions have disappeared, generally for a total of 3 to 6 months. Saturated solution of potassium iodide (SSKI) has been used to treat sporotrichosis for almost a century. The initial dose is 5 to 10 drops three times daily in water or juice, with the dose increasing over a period of several weeks to a maximum of 40 to 50 drops three times daily. SSKI has many side effects, including salivary gland swelling, metallic taste, rash, and fever; the only advantage is that it is inexpensive. Fluconazole is less effective than itraconazole but for occasional patients can be used at a dosage of 400 to 800 mg daily. Voriconazole is not active against *Sporothrix* spp and there is minimal experience using posaconazole.

Osteoarticular and pulmonary sporotrichosis are usually treated with itraconazole, 200 mg twice daily for 1 to 2 years. Other azoles are less effective, and SSKI is ineffective. In a seriously ill patient with pulmonary sporotrichosis, a lipid formulation of amphotericin B at a dosage of 3 to 5 mg/kg daily should be used as initial therapy. After the patient has shown improvement, therapy can be changed to itraconazole. A lipid formulation of amphotericin B, at a dosage of 3 to 5 mg/kg daily, is the drug of choice for disseminated sporotrichosis. Therapy can be changed to itraconazole, 200 mg twice daily, once the patient has stabilized. Patients with HIV infection and disseminated sporotrichosis should remain on lifelong maintenance therapy with itraconazole, 200 mg daily.

PROGNOSIS

The prognosis for patients with cutaneous and lymphocutaneous sporotrichosis is excellent. Almost all patients are cured. Extracutaneous forms of sporotrichosis do not respond well to therapy, partly because of delays in diagnosis and partly because of the underlying diseases that are frequently found in these patients. The outcome of disseminated sporotrichosis in patients with HIV infection has improved in recent years with effective antiretroviral therapy.

● PARACOCCIDIOIDOMYCOSIS

DEFINITION

Paracoccidioidomycosis (South American blastomycosis) is a subacute to chronic mycosis that is endemic in Central and South America. The disease is characterized primarily by pulmonary, mucous membrane, and cutaneous lesions, but disseminated disease also occurs.

The Pathogen

Paracoccidioides brasiliensis and *P. lutzii* are thermally dimorphic fungi. In the environment and at temperatures below 35° C, the organisms grow as a mold. In tissues and at 37° C in vitro, the organism assumes the yeast form with multiple narrow-based daughter cells attached to the mother cell.

EPIDEMIOLOGY

Paracoccidioides spp exist only in humid areas of Central and South America. More than 80% of cases are from Brazil. The presumed ecologic niche is in soil. The disease is most prevalent in middle-aged to elderly men from rural areas. Although the disease classically develops later in life, it is likely that initial exposure occurs many years earlier. Cases seen in areas outside Central and South America have all been linked to previous residence in the endemic area.

PATHOBIOLOGY

Paracoccidioidomycosis develops after the inhalation of aerosolized conidia encountered in the environment. Once in the alveoli, the mycelial phase converts to the yeast phase. In most patients, manifestations of disease do not develop at the time of the initial infection. The host defense mechanism against *P. brasiliensis* appears to be primarily cell-mediated immunity. The histopathologic picture includes both neutrophilic and granulomatous responses. Paracoccidioidomycosis in patients infected with HIV and in other immunosuppressed patients manifests as widespread disseminated infection. Like with histoplasmosis and coccidioidomycosis, patients with paracoccidioidomycosis may have an underlying monogenic immunodeficiency disorder involving the IL-12/IFN-γ pathway.[22] Reactivation of latent infection acquired years earlier is the presumed pathogenesis of most cases of the chronic adult form of paracoccidioidomycosis and cases that appear years after the patient has left the endemic area.

CLINICAL MANIFESTATIONS

Acute-Subacute (Juvenile) Paracoccidioidomycosis

The acute-subacute form of paracoccidioidomycosis occurs in less than 10% of patients. It is a disease of the reticuloendothelial system with widespread dissemination to the liver, spleen, lymph nodes, and bone marrow.[23] Patients younger than 30 years typically have this form of paracoccidioidomycosis; however, older adults, especially those who are immunosuppressed, also can manifest this type of rapidly progressive disease. In patients with HIV infection, rapid progression occurs with multiple cutaneous lesions, lymphadenopathy, hepatosplenomegaly, and severe pulmonary involvement with hypoxemia.

Chronic (Adult) Paracoccidioidomycosis

Chronic paracoccidioidomycosis is slowly progressive over many years and is the form seen in more than 90% of patients. Pulmonary involvement is prominent and clinically mimics tuberculosis and other chronic fungal pneumonias. Radiographically, nodular, interstitial, or cavitary lesions that tend to be in the middle and lower lung fields are seen. Many patients also have ulcerative or nodular mucous membrane lesions, primarily in the anterior nares, the oral cavity, and the larynx; these are slowly destructive and can lead to dysphonia and stenosis of the airway. Cutaneous lesions, particularly on the face, are also common and may be papular, nodular, ulcerative, or plaquelike. The mucocutaneous lesions must be differentiated from mucocutaneous leishmaniasis and squamous cell carcinoma.[24] Adrenal involvement has been reported in more than 90% of cases at autopsy, but adrenal insufficiency is only noted in about half of cases.

DIAGNOSIS

The definitive diagnosis of paracoccidioidomycosis is established by growth of *P. brasiliensis* in culture. The organism may take as long as 4 weeks to grow. For seriously ill patients, direct examination of body fluids, sputum, or purulent material treated with potassium hydroxide or calcofluor fluorescent stain or histopathologic examination of tissue biopsy samples can provide a presumptive diagnosis. The characteristic appearance of *P. brasiliensis* consists of thick-walled yeast cells that have multiple small, circumferentially attached, narrow-based budding daughter yeast cells—a distinctive morphologic picture likened to a ship's steering wheel.

A variety of immunodiffusion assays, enzyme immunoassays, and complement fixation assays are available in endemic areas, but sensitivity and specificity vary greatly. The immunodiffusion assay appears to be most useful. Polymerase chain reaction testing has been reported to have high sensitivity and specificity.

TREATMENT — Rx

The drug of choice for the treatment of paracoccidioidomycosis is itraconazole (200 mg/day for 6 to 12 months). Ketoconazole at a dosage of 200 to 400 mg daily for 1 year is effective and less expensive than itraconazole, but the incidence of side effects is greater and relapses occur more frequently than with itraconazole. Fluconazole is less effective and should not be used. Voriconazole has been shown to be as effective as itraconazole in a randomized open-label pilot study, and there are a few reports of the successful use of posaconazole and isavuconazole.[25] Sulfonamides have been used for years to treat paracoccidioidomycosis and are the most inexpensive form of treatment. However, relapse rates are higher than with the azoles. Amphotericin B is effective but rarely used, except in immunosuppressed patients with life-threatening disseminated disease. Most HIV-infected patients have been treated with amphotericin B as initial therapy, followed by lifelong suppressive therapy with either itraconazole or trimethoprim-sulfamethoxazole.

PROGNOSIS

Patients with paracoccidioidomycosis have an excellent response to antifungal therapy. Patients who have extensive pulmonary involvement at the time of diagnosis are at high risk for progressive fibrosis despite antifungal therapy.

GENERAL REFERENCES

For the General References and other additional features, please visit Expert Consult at https://expertconsult.inkling.com.

317

CRYPTOCOCCOSIS

CAROL A. KAUFFMAN AND SHARON C-A CHEN

DEFINITION

Cryptococcosis occurs most often in persons who are immunosuppressed, especially those infected with human immunodeficiency virus (HIV). Meningitis is the most common clinical manifestation, but pulmonary and other organ involvement occur as well.[1]

The Pathogen

Cryptococcus neoformans and, much less often, *Cryptococcus gattii* are the predominant *Cryptococcus* species causing infection in humans. In the environment, *Cryptococcus* species exist as yeasts that have minimal capsules and are easily aerosolized and inhaled. In tissues, the yeasts are enveloped by a large polysaccharide capsule that is a major virulence factor. *C. neoformans* is found in the soil and grows well in avian droppings that have high nitrogen content. *C. gattii* is more restricted geographically, but its distribution has increased in the last decade. Many cases still are seen in Australia and Southeast Asia, where the organism's ecologic niche is the eucalyptus tree, but cases also are reported from Brazil, the Pacific Northwest, and other areas of North America. Most of this chapter focuses on *C. neoformans*.

EPIDEMIOLOGY

Before the widespread availability of antiretroviral therapy (ART), cryptococcosis occurred in 5 to 10% of patients with acquired immunodeficiency syndrome (AIDS), and almost always in those with CD4 counts less than 50 cells/µL. Cryptococcosis is less commonly seen now in Europe and North America in this population but is extremely common in Africa, where it is estimated that the prevalence among HIV-infected patients is as high as 30%.[2]

In the non-AIDS population, cryptococcosis is a frequent opportunistic infection in patients who have received a solid organ transplant, have been treated with corticosteroids or other immunosuppressive therapies, or have underlying illnesses, such as diabetes mellitus, renal failure, cirrhosis, or chronic pulmonary disease. For some patients, the only risk factor appears to be older age. In every reported series, separate from those dealing only with HIV infection, approximately 20% of patients have no known underlying illness. *C. gattii* frequently causes illness in normal hosts.

PATHOBIOLOGY

The organism is inhaled from the environment and causes pulmonary infection initially. The primary host defense at this stage is complement-dependent macrophage and neutrophil phagocytosis and killing. Natural killer cells also

have the ability to kill the organism. Ultimately, however, T-cell immunity is the most important host determinant in limiting the replication of *C. neoformans*. In most normal hosts, the infection remains localized to the lungs and does not cause symptomatic infection. It is likely that a few organisms exist as walled-off subpleural granulomas in many who have had pulmonary infection. If the host becomes immunosuppressed, the organism can then reactivate and disseminate to other sites. *C. neoformans* is clearly neurotropic, and the primary disease manifestation is meningoencephalitis. However, dissemination to many organs is likely, especially in those with deficient T-cell immunity.

Virulence factors for *C. neoformans* include the capsule, which requires opsonization for efficient phagocytosis, and the production of melanin, which has been shown to occur in vivo and enables the organism to resist intracellular killing. Both of these factors may help explain the virulence of the organism once it has reached the central nervous system (CNS). Antibody and complement levels are low in the brain, and thus phagocytosis of the organism is minimal. Brain tissue provides high concentrations of substrates, such as catecholamines, for the phenol oxidase enzyme systems of *C. neoformans* that produce melanin, thereby aiding survival of the organism.

CLINICAL MANIFESTATIONS

Central Nervous System Infection

The most common manifestation of cryptococcosis is CNS infection. The typical picture is subacute to chronic meningoencephalitis. Patients usually have increasingly severe headaches over a period of several weeks, although some patients present over several days. Other symptoms and signs include nuchal rigidity, lethargy, personality changes, confusion, visual abnormalities (photophobia, diplopia, decreased visual acuity, papilledema, extraocular nerve palsies), and nausea and vomiting. Less commonly, hearing loss, ataxia, and seizures occur. Fever is present in only approximately half the patients. Elderly persons with cryptococcal meningitis may have just dementia, without other neurologic findings. AIDS patients often have subtle CNS symptoms but usually have fever and other constitutional symptoms and rapidly manifest signs of dissemination.[3]

Pulmonary Infection

In non–HIV-infected patients, the most common underlying risk factor for pulmonary cryptococcal infection[4] is chronic obstructive pulmonary disease, followed by corticosteroid use and receipt of a solid organ transplant. *C. neoformans* may merely be an airway colonizer in some patients; in others, symptomatic infection, manifested by fever, cough, and dyspnea, requires treatment with an antifungal agent. The typical lesion noted with pulmonary cryptococcosis is a pleural-based nodule. However, patchy pneumonitis, multiple nodular lesions, cavitary lesions, masslike lesions, and diffuse pulmonary infiltrates have all been noted with pulmonary cryptococcosis. Patients with advanced HIV infection are likely to have diffuse infiltrates that can progress rapidly to acute respiratory insufficiency. All immunosuppressed patients who have pulmonary cryptococcosis and all patients with any CNS symptoms should undergo lumbar puncture to be certain that meningitis is not present. Whether normal hosts with isolated pulmonary cryptococcosis and with negative serum antigen tests require lumbar puncture remains controversial.

Involvement of Other Organs

C. neoformans has been reported to infect most organs during the course of disseminated infection, especially in AIDS patients. Skin lesions are a prominent clue to dissemination, although isolated cutaneous cryptococcosis can occur in organ transplant recipients as well as in immunocompetent hosts. Papules that resemble molluscum contagiosum (Chapter 410) or an acneiform rash, nodules, ulcers, plaques, draining sinuses, and cellulitis have all been reported. Focal involvement can occur in the prostate and other organs of the genitourinary tract, in osteoarticular structures, in the breast, and in the eye, larynx, and other head and neck structures. The prostate, in particular, has been noted as a sanctuary from which persisting organisms can later disseminate.

DIAGNOSIS

The diagnosis of cryptococcosis is established when the yeast is grown in culture. Appropriate specimens for culture include cerebrospinal fluid (CSF), blood, sputum, material from skin lesions, and other body fluids or tissues that appear to be infected. The organism grows in several days on most standard agar media. Most automated blood culture systems allow rapid growth of *C. neoformans*. Visualization of the capsule and performance of a few simple tests differentiate *C. neoformans* from other yeasts. Tissue biopsy shows the 5- to 10-µm yeast surrounded by the capsule. Definitive diagnosis of cryptococcosis can be made by mucicarmine staining, which selectively stains the polysaccharide capsule a deep rose color. In CSF or other body fluids, an India ink preparation is useful in that it allows visualization of the budding yeast cells surrounded by the large capsule, but a negative test does not exclude a diagnosis of cryptococcosis (approximately 50% sensitivity in cryptococcal meningoencephalitis).

The latex agglutination assay for cryptococcal polysaccharide antigen (CRAG) is a highly sensitive and specific diagnostic test. CRAG is positive in CSF in almost 100% and in serum in about 75% of patients who have meningitis.[5] In AIDS patients, serum CRAG is almost always positive and is an excellent screening tool. In these patients, titers in both CSF and serum are exceptionally high because of the enormous burden of organisms. In non-AIDS patients who have pulmonary cryptococcosis, the CRAG assay is positive in only 25 to 50% of cases. False-positive results with the CRAG assay are uncommon but have been reported in patients with *Trichosporon asahii* infections because of cross-reacting antigens shared by both fungi.

A newer technique, lateral flow analysis (LFA) to detect cryptococcal polysaccharide antigen has been developed as a dipstick assay, similar to that of pregnancy tests, that can be performed in serum or CSF at the point of care by clinicians caring for the patient. This technique has been shown to be as sensitive and specific as the classic CRAG test.

The CSF of patients with cryptococcal meningitis typically has an increased number of white blood cells (but rarely >500/μL), a predominance of lymphocytes (although neutrophils are sometimes prominent early in the course), elevated protein, and decreased glucose. AIDS patients most often have normal or only mildly abnormal findings as a result of their markedly defective immune response. Despite normal CSF findings with regard to cells, protein, and glucose, every AIDS patient with a headache must have a CRAG or LFA test and culture performed on CSF. It is extremely important that an opening pressure be obtained when lumbar puncture is performed. Especially in AIDS patients, extremely high intracranial pressure (>350 mm H_2O) has been associated with poor outcomes and must be aggressively lowered.

All patients with cryptococcal meningitis should undergo computed tomography or magnetic resonance imaging of the brain to look for mass lesions and to assess ventricular size. Whether normal hosts with isolated pulmonary cryptococcosis require cerebral imaging should be considered in the context of the individual patient. Obstructive hydrocephalus is uncommon but requires a shunting procedure to decrease the pressure. More commonly, the increased intracranial pressure with cryptococcal infection is associated with normal-sized ventricles and is due to blockage at the arachnoid villi or increased brain edema (or both), perhaps related to the osmotic effect of the polysaccharide capsule. Different methods for reducing pressure are used in this situation.

TREATMENT Rx

Guidelines for the treatment of cryptococcal infection have been published by the Infectious Diseases Society of America (IDSA) and the World Health Organization.[6]

Central Nervous System Infection

Early multicenter randomized trials in non-AIDS patients showed superiority of the combination of amphotericin B and flucytosine for 6 weeks over amphotericin B alone for 10 weeks. Subsequent randomized trials in the azole era have been performed only in the AIDS population. They have confirmed the benefit of flucytosine added to amphotericin B for induction therapy and have shown that initial therapy with fluconazole alone or with amphotericin B alone is not as effective as therapy with amphotericin B and flucytosine. The combination of amphotericin B and flucytosine has been shown to be the most rapidly fungicidal regimen, and increasing numbers of reports have documented that rapid fungicidal activity that clears the organism from the CSF is associated with improved outcomes. Regimens using amphotericin B with fluconazole or flucytosine with fluconazole[A1] are less effective but reasonable alternatives when the preferred regimen of amphotericin B plus flucytosine is not available. Unlike bacterial meningitis, adjunctive dexamethasone is not beneficial and appears to be detrimental in HIV-infected patients.[A2]

Current recommendations for AIDS patients are to give induction therapy with intravenous amphotericin B deoxycholate, 0.7 to 1 mg/kg daily, combined with oral flucytosine, 100 mg/kg daily given in four divided doses for at least 2 weeks, followed by consolidation therapy with oral fluconazole, 400 mg daily for a minimum of 8 weeks, and then suppressive therapy with fluconazole, 200 mg daily. Lipid formulations of amphotericin B at daily dosages of 3 to 5 mg/kg daily are increasingly used because they are less nephrotoxic; however,

they are often not available in developing countries. Induction therapy with amphotericin B (1 mg/kg per day for 4 weeks) plus flucytosine (100 mg/kg per day for 2 weeks) is associated with improved survival among HIV-positive patients with cryptococcal meningitis compared with either amphotericin B alone or amphotericin B plus fluconazole (400 mg twice daily for 2 weeks).[A3]

Treatment strategies that could be more sustainable in underdeveloped areas of the world have been tested in a randomized trial of antifungal combinations to treat cryptococcal meningitis in Africa. One week of amphotericin B (1 mg per kilogram per day) plus flucytosine (100 mg per kilogram per day) and 2 weeks of fluconazole (1200 mg per day) plus flucytosine were found to be effective as induction therapy,[A4] and can be used to treat cryptococcal meningitis in resource-limited settings.

For patients who have undergone 12 months of antifungal therapy, who have CD4+ counts higher than 100/μL, and whose HIV viral load is undetectable on antiretroviral therapy, the suppressive therapy can be stopped. Suppressive therapy with fluconazole for transplant recipients is recommended for 6 to 12 months. The IDSA guideline recommendations for non–HIV-infected, non–transplant recipients are to treat with amphotericin B deoxycholate, 0.7 to 1.0 mg/kg daily, plus flucytosine, 100 mg/kg daily, in four divided doses for at least 4 weeks for induction therapy, followed by consolidation therapy with fluconazole, 400 mg daily for 8 weeks, and suppressive therapy with fluconazole, 200 mg daily for 6 to 12 months. Lipid formulations of amphotericin B may be used, and most physicians use a dose of 3 to 5 mg/kg daily, in the non-AIDS population.

Only one treatment trial used voriconazole in combination with amphotericin B, and there are case reports on the use of voriconazole and posaconazole for salvage treatment of cryptococcal meningitis. These are reasonable alternatives if no other azoles can be used. The echinocandins are not active against *C. neoformans* and should not be used.

A significant observation from the AIDS treatment trials was the role of increased intracranial pressure as a cause of early death from cryptococcal meningitis. An aggressive approach to the diagnosis and treatment of increased intracranial pressure in both AIDS and non-AIDS patients is mandatory and should include daily lumbar puncture or placement of a temporary lumbar drain or ventriculostomy until the opening pressure remains lower than 190 mm H_2O. Repeated lumbar punctures have been associated with improved survival rates. Treatment with corticosteroids, acetazolamide, or mannitol has not proved efficacious.

The development of immune reconstitution inflammatory syndrome (IRIS) can occur in patients with AIDS who are receiving effective ART that increases the CD4 count (Chapter 367). Symptoms of meningitis reappear and are due to the inflammatory response and not to a relapse of disease; IRIS is associated with an influx of CD4 lymphocytes and monocytes into the CSF.[7] In one randomized controlled trial, HIV-positive patients with cryptococcal meningitis who had not previously received ART were randomized to initiate either earlier ART (1 to 2 weeks after meningitis diagnosis) or deferred ART (5 weeks after diagnosis). Although the incidence of recognized cryptococcal IRIS did not differ significantly between the earlier and deferred ART groups, deferring ART for 5 weeks after diagnosis was associated with significantly improved survival, especially among patients with a paucity of CSF white cells.[A5] IRIS can also occur in transplant recipients in whom immunosuppressive therapy is decreased rapidly. Generally, no specific therapy is needed for mild IRIS, but sometimes corticosteroids are needed if increased intracranial pressure occurs and/or if there is evidence of cerebral edema.

Pulmonary and Other Nonmeningeal Infections

Treatment of nonmeningeal cryptococcosis depends on the severity of the infection. Many patients with isolated pulmonary or other focal infections are not severely ill, and oral fluconazole, 400 mg daily for 6 to 12 months, is recommended. For patients who are severely ill, therapy is the same as noted earlier for CNS infection.

PROGNOSIS

The outcome for both AIDS and non-AIDS patients with cryptococcal meningitis has improved markedly in the developed world.[8] In Africa, however, the mortality from cryptococcal meningitis in AIDS patients approaches 100% in some areas because of lack of access to specific therapy. Among patients with HIV, those with a predominant T_H1 cytokine profile in the CSF and blood at diagnosis appear to have a better survival.[9] Dementia, which usually occurs in older patients, hearing loss, and visual loss may not be reversed even though mycologic cure is achieved.

Fluconazole, 200 mg three times per week, is safe and effective as primary prophylaxis against cryptococcal disease in cryptococcal antigen-negative, HIV-infected adults with CD4 counts lower than 200 cells/μL, both before and during early antiretroviral treatment.[A6]

Grade A References

A1. Nussbaum JC, Jackson A, Namarika D, et al. Combination flucytosine and high-dose fluconazole compared with fluconazole monotherapy for the treatment of cryptococcal meningitis: a randomized trial in Malawi. *Clin Infect Dis.* 2010;50:338-344.
A2. Beardsley J, Wolbers M, Kibengo FM, et al. Adjunctive dexamethasone in HIV-associated cryptococcal meningitis. *N Engl J Med.* 2016;374:542-554.
A3. Day JN, Chau TT, Wolbers M, et al. Combination antifungal theory for cryptococcal meningitis. *N Engl J Med.* 2013;368:1291-1302.
A4. Molloy SF, Kanyama C, Heyderman RS, et al. Antifungal combinations for treatment of cryptococcal meningitis in Africa. *N Engl J Med.* 2018;378:1004-1017.
A5. Boulware DR, Meya DB, Muzoora C, et al. Timing of antiretroviral therapy after diagnosis of cryptococcal meningitis. *N Engl J Med.* 2014;370:2487-2498.
A6. Parkes-Ratanshi R, Wakeham K, Levin J, et al. Primary prophylaxis of cryptococcal disease with fluconazole in HIV-positive Ugandan adults: a double-blind randomised, placebo-controlled trial. *Lancet Infect Dis.* 2011;11:933-941.

GENERAL REFERENCES

For the General References and other additional features, please visit Expert Consult at https://expertconsult.inkling.com.

318

CANDIDIASIS

CAROL A. KAUFFMAN AND PETER G. PAPPAS

DEFINITION

Candidiasis encompasses a wide variety of clinical syndromes caused by yeasts of the genus *Candida.* Of the species that cause infection in humans, *Candida albicans* is the most common; *Candida glabrata, Candida parapsilosis,* and *Candida tropicalis* are responsible for most of the remaining infections. Organisms such as *Candida krusei, Candida lusitaniae,* and *Candida guilliermondii* are less common causes of infection.

The Pathogen

Candida species are 2- to 6-μm yeastlike organisms that reproduce by budding. Most species, with the exception of *C. glabrata,* form pseudohyphae (elongated buds that remain attached to the mother cell) and hyphae in tissues.

Candida species cause a wide spectrum of diseases ranging in severity from localized mucous membrane infection to life-threatening disseminated disease. The major determinant of the severity of infection is the host's immune response. Local infections are often related to overgrowth of *Candida* as a result of changes in the normal microbiota. Invasive infections that remain within an organ system, such as urinary tract infections, usually occur because of local anatomic abnormalities. In an immunosuppressed host, especially a patient with neutropenia, widespread visceral dissemination is common.

EPIDEMIOLOGY

Candida species reside normally in the gastrointestinal and genitourinary tracts and on the skin. As colonizers, *Candida* species do not cause infection unless there is a defect in host defense mechanisms or unless exogenous factors, such as antibiotic use or cutaneous disruption and/or maceration, have upset the ecology of the normal microbiota. *C. albicans* is the species most commonly found colonizing humans; *C. glabrata* is the second most common species, and *C. tropicalis, C. parapsilosis,* and others are found less often. The species of *Candida* colonizing and infecting patients has changed in recent decades in that *C. glabrata,* a species that is increasingly resistant to fluconazole, has become a prominent pathogen in many hospitals. In many parts of the world, the emergence of *C. auris,* a previously uncommon multidrug-resistant *Candida* species, has created new challenges in understanding the epidemiology, treatment, and prevention of this organism.

Though uncommon, acquisition of *Candida* from environmental sources has been noted. The *Candida* species most often associated with transmission from contaminated fluids or devices, especially central intravenous catheters, has been *C. parapsilosis.*

Candidiasis is the most common opportunistic fungal infection as a result of both the organisms' ubiquity and the increasing number of patients with risk factors for infection with these organisms.[1] The classic immunosuppressed host at risk for serious *Candida* infections is a neutropenic patient with a hematologic malignancy who has received cytotoxic agents and corticosteroids. Increasingly, however, candidiasis is seen in patients in intensive care units (ICUs). Risk factors for the development of serious *Candida* infections in ICU patients include diabetes,[2] the use of broad-spectrum antimicrobials, indwelling central venous catheters, previous surgical procedures, renal failure, parenteral nutrition, pancreatitis, any form of dialysis, and high Acute Physiology and Chronic Health Evaluation (APACHE) score. Certain ICU populations, especially very-low-birthweight neonates and burn victims, are at even higher risk for *Candida* infection than is the typical ICU patient.

The primary manifestation of *Candida* infection in patients with HIV/AIDS is mucocutaneous infection, primarily oropharyngeal candidiasis. The development of mucosal *Candida* infection is related to deficient T-cell immunity as reflected by a low CD4 lymphocyte count. With appropriate antiretroviral therapy, oropharyngeal candidiasis has become an uncommon opportunistic infection.

PATHOBIOLOGY

The usual mode of infection with *Candida* is egress from its normal niche into the bloodstream or other tissues; the source is usually the gastrointestinal tract, but the skin and genitourinary tract are other sources. The primary host defense in response to this event is phagocytosis and killing by neutrophils, monocytes, and macrophages. C-C chemokine receptor 2 (CCR2)-expressing inflammatory monocytes and their tissue-resident derivatives play an essential antifungal role, particularly in the first 48 hours after *Candida* infection. Phagocytosis is enhanced in the presence of specific anti-*Candida* antibody and complement. Several different mechanisms are operative within neutrophils and macrophages that allow the killing of yeasts. Thus, patients who are leukopenic, especially those with chemotherapy-induced disruption of the gut mucosa, are at great risk for invasion with *Candida* species. Once *Candida* gains access to the bloodstream, widespread hematogenous dissemination is the rule. Biopsy of involved organs shows multiple microabscesses composed of neutrophils (in a host who has these cells), budding yeasts, and often pseudohyphae or hyphae. Over time, the lesions show a mixed neutrophilic and granulomatous response.

T-cell immunity is an important host defense against infection with *Candida* at mucosal surfaces. In contrast to those with neutropenia, patients with deficient T-cell immunity are at risk for persistent and recurrent mucocutaneous candidiasis, but invasive infection rarely develops. The ubiquitin ligase, Casitas B lymphoma-b (CBLB), a T-cell activator and inducer of T-cell differentiation, is crucial for restraining the magnitude of the innate immune response against *C. albicans* infection but at the same time confers suboptimal protection to the host. CBLB therefore may be a potential drug target for systemic candidiasis.[3]

CLINICAL MANIFESTATIONS

Mucocutaneous Candidiasis
Oropharyngeal Candidiasis
Local mucous membrane and cutaneous lesions are the most common forms of *Candida* infection.[4] Oropharyngeal candidiasis, or *thrush* (Chapter 397), can be due to either local factors or T-cell dysfunction. Local factors include the use of broad-spectrum antimicrobials or inhaled corticosteroids, xerostomia, and radiation treatment of the head and neck. Denture stomatitis occurs frequently in persons who wear full upper dentures, especially those who do not remove their dentures at night.

Thrush secondary to T-cell dysfunction is most commonly seen in patients with HIV infection (Chapter 366) and is the most frequent opportunistic infection noted in patients with AIDS. The appearance of thrush in a previously healthy individual with no known risk factors should immediately raise suspicion of HIV infection.

Thrush manifests with white plaques on the buccal mucosa, palate, oropharynx, or tongue (Fig. 318-1). Scraping the lesions with a tongue depressor reveals an erythematous, nonulcerated mucosa under the plaques. Denture stomatitis almost always manifests as a painful erythematous palate without plaques. Angular cheilitis, or perlàche, which is the presence of painful cracks at the corners of the mouth, can occur with or without thrush.

Esophagitis
Esophagitis[5] may accompany oropharyngeal candidiasis or may occur independently of lesions in the oropharynx (Chapter 129). The development of

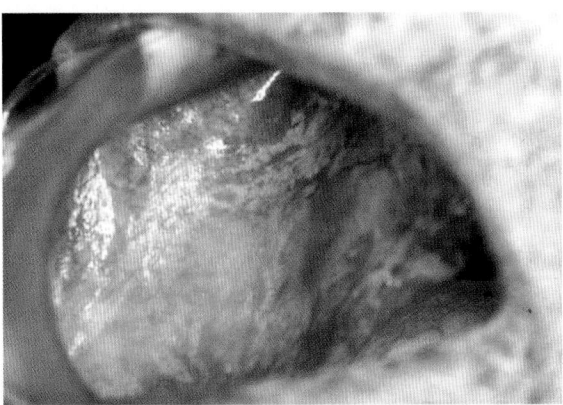

FIGURE 318-1. Thrush.

Candida esophagitis is almost always related to immune dysfunction and not simply to local factors. *Candida* esophagitis occurs in AIDS patients with low CD4 counts, patients with leukemia, and others taking immunosuppressive agents. *Candida* esophagitis occurs rarely in otherwise normal hosts. The classic symptom of *Candida* esophagitis is odynophagia localized to a discrete substernal area. The differential diagnosis includes ulcerations due to herpes simplex or cytomegalovirus and, in AIDS patients, idiopathic ulcers.

Vulvovaginitis

Candida vulvovaginitis is a common infection in women of childbearing age and is the most frequent mucocutaneous manifestation of *Candida* infection. Risk factors include conditions associated with increased estrogen levels, such as the use of oral contraceptives and pregnancy, diabetes mellitus, therapy with corticosteroids or broad-spectrum antimicrobials, and HIV infection. Symptoms include vaginal discomfort, discharge, and vulvar pruritus. The discharge is usually curdlike, but it can also be thin and watery. The labia are erythematous and swollen, and the vaginal walls show erythema and white plaques. Although most women have only a few episodes throughout their lives, a minority have frequent recurrences; in most of these patients, no discrete risk factor can be identified, and the cause is presumed to be local immune dysregulation.

Cutaneous Candidiasis

Candida infection of the skin (Chapter 412) occurs mostly in the intertriginous areas or under a large pannus or pendulous breasts. The lesions are erythematous, pruritic, and frequently pustular; have a distinct border; and are almost always associated with smaller satellite lesions, which helps distinguish candidiasis from tinea cruris or corporis. *Candida* onychomycosis results in thickened, opaque, and onycholytic nails. *Candida* can also cause paronychia, especially in those whose occupation involves frequent immersion of the hands in water.

Chronic Mucocutaneous Candidiasis

This uncommon syndrome usually begins in childhood and is characterized by recalcitrant and relapsing thrush, esophagitis, vaginitis, onychomycosis, and hyperkeratotic skin lesions on the face, scalp, and hands. Autosomal dominant chronic mucocutaneous candidiasis is associated with mutations in the CC domain of *STAT1* leading to defective T_H1 and T_H17 responses. Some patients have associated autoimmune endocrinopathies, including hypoparathyroidism, hypothyroidism, and hypoadrenalism (autoimmune polyendocrinopathy-candidiasis-ectodermal dystrophy [APECED], which is caused by a loss-of-function mutation of the autoimmune regulator gene, *AIRE*, and in these patients autoantibodies against interleukin-17 (IL-17) and IL-22 are found. (See Autoimmune Polyglandular Syndrome Type 1 in Chapter 218.)

Disseminated Infections
Candidemia

The most common manifestation of disseminated *Candida* infection is candidemia.[6] However, candidemia merely implies the presence of *Candida* in blood; it does not define the extent of visceral involvement. *Candida* obtained from a blood culture should never be considered a contaminant and should always prompt a search for the probable source and the extent of infection. Risk factors for candidemia include broad-spectrum antimicrobial therapy,

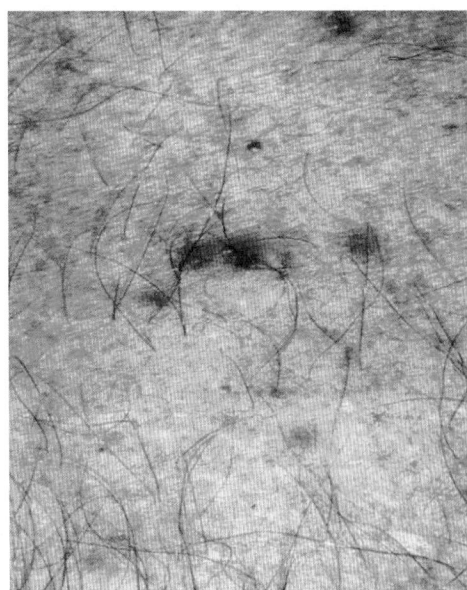

FIGURE 318-2. Skin lesions in invasive candidiasis.

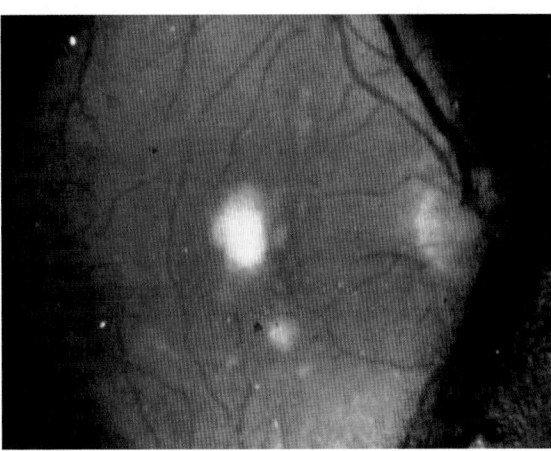

FIGURE 318-3. Retinal involvement.

central intravenous catheters, parenteral nutrition, renal failure, pancreatitis, any type of dialysis, surgical procedures involving the gastrointestinal tract, neutropenia, and corticosteroid therapy.[7] The attributable mortality from candidemia approaches 40%. Mortality is higher in elderly patients and neonates and among those with severe sepsis and poor source control.

Although candidemia is the most obvious manifestation of serious infection with *Candida* species, septic shock can occur, along with invasion of multiple viscera, in the absence of positive blood cultures. The clinical picture of invasive candidiasis is indistinguishable from that of bacterial infection. The characteristic histologic picture consists of multiple microabscesses in many organs. The eyes, kidneys, liver, spleen, and brain are the most commonly involved sites, but virtually all organs can be involved. Clinical clues to the diagnosis of invasive candidiasis include the appearance of skin and retinal lesions. The nonpainful, nonpruritic skin lesions are papular to pustular and surrounded by a zone of erythema (Fig. 318-2). Classical eye lesions appear as distinctive white exudates in the retina (Fig. 318-3); with extension into the vitreous body, the retina becomes obscured.

Endocarditis

Candida endocarditis is an uncommon and often fatal complication of candidemia. It occurs most often in intravenous drug users, patients who have prosthetic cardiac valves and intracardiac pacemaker devices, and those with central venous catheters in place. Blood cultures are usually persistently positive, and echocardiography reveals large vegetations that can readily embolize to major vessels.

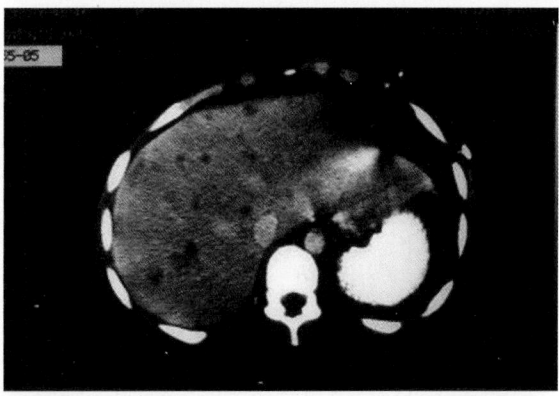

FIGURE 318-4. Computed tomography scan of a patient with chronic disseminated candidiasis (hepatosplenic candidiasis). Note the distinctive punched-out lesions in the liver.

Chronic Disseminated (Hepatosplenic) Candidiasis

This syndrome almost always occurs in leukemic patients who have had an episode of neutropenia. After the neutrophil count returns to normal, fevers that are often quite high, right upper quadrant tenderness, and nausea develop. The alkaline phosphatase level is generally elevated, and distinctive punched-out lesions are seen in the liver, spleen, and sometimes the kidneys on computed tomography (Fig. 318-4). Biopsy of these lesions shows microabscesses that may contain budding yeasts.

Focal Invasive Infections

These forms of candidiasis result from local inoculation, contiguous spread, or hematogenous spread. Hematogenous spread,[8] which often goes undetected, is probably the most common pathogenetic mechanism.

Urinary Tract Infections

Candiduria is a frequent finding in hospitalized patients and is related to factors such as diabetes mellitus, broad-spectrum antimicrobial treatment, indwelling urinary devices, and genitourinary tract structural abnormalities. Most patients with candiduria have only bladder colonization and not true infection. Urinary tract infection with *Candida* species can arise by two mechanisms. Patients with candidemia can develop multiple microabscesses secondary to hematogenous spread to the kidneys. Other patients, who have the risk factors noted earlier, can develop cystitis or ascending infection with pyelonephritis. Patients with cystitis or pyelonephritis have symptoms indistinguishable from those of bacterial infections. A fungus ball composed of fungal hyphae can develop at any level of the collecting system and lead to obstruction, with subsequent infection.

Osteoarticular Infections

Osteoarticular infections arise secondary to hematogenous seeding or exogenous inoculation during intra-articular injection, a surgical procedure, or trauma. Vertebral osteomyelitis is the most common manifestation of osteoarticular candidiasis. The symptoms of back pain and fever may occur many weeks after an episode of fungemia.

Endophthalmitis

Exogenous endophthalmitis occurs secondary to trauma or ophthalmic surgery. Most often, the procedure involved is cataract extraction, with or without lens implantation, and the most common infecting species is *C. parapsilosis*. Primary infection occurs in the anterior chamber, but ultimately the posterior chamber is also involved. Endogenous *Candida* endophthalmitis results from hematogenous seeding of the choroid and retina and is one of the most serious complications of candidemia. Characteristic white lesions are visible in the retina, and with progression of the infection, vitritis occurs; the risk for loss of vision is quite high.

Peritonitis

Candida peritonitis can follow bowel surgery or perforation. Symptoms are the same as those noted in bacterial peritonitis. Usually, this type of infection is polymicrobial, and abscess formation is common. In patients maintained on continuous ambulatory peritoneal dialysis, *Candida* peritonitis generally develops as a late infection after previous episodes of bacterial peritonitis. A cloudy dialysate, abdominal pain, and fever are typically noted.

Meningitis

Acute *Candida* meningitis occurs as part of disseminated infection, especially in low-birthweight neonates. Chronic meningitis, an uncommon manifestation of candidiasis, resembles cryptococcal or tuberculous meningitis with regard to symptoms and cerebrospinal fluid findings.

DIAGNOSIS

The diagnosis of mucocutaneous candidiasis is often made clinically. Culture is rarely indicated. Confirmation can be sought by scraping the lesions and performing either a potassium hydroxide preparation or a Gram stain to look for budding yeasts (Chapter 407). In cases in which the disease is recurrent or unresponsive to standard therapy, lesions should be cultured to establish whether a more resistant species, such as *C. glabrata* or *C. krusei*, is the causative agent. In the event of suspected esophagitis, endoscopy shows plaquelike lesions or ulcerations, and biopsy shows mucosal invasion with budding yeasts and pseudohyphae.

The diagnosis of invasive candidiasis is more difficult. Evidence of dissemination is usually sought by culturing blood or other sterile body sites. However, blood cultures are not sensitive enough for clinicians to rely on them to establish the diagnosis of invasive candidiasis in all cases or to rule out candidiasis as a diagnostic possibility. In addition, 1 to 4 days is required for growth to occur; in a desperately ill patient, this delay is problematic.

The tips of intravenous catheters that have been removed should be sent for culture. However, no studies have evaluated the number of yeasts that is indicative of infection, and many physicians accept the growth of any yeast as affirming infection that requires treatment. Many focal forms of candidiasis are indistinguishable from bacterial infection, and biopsy should be performed for histopathologic and culture studies.

In a seriously ill patient suspected of having candidiasis, the development of pustular skin lesions or typical retinal lesions can be helpful. Budding yeasts typical of *Candida* species should be sought by smearing material from a pustule on a slide and staining it with Gram stain or by performing a biopsy of a lesion and staining the tissue section with a silver stain. All patients who are candidemic or suspected of having disseminated *Candida* infection should undergo a dilated ophthalmologic examination, preferably by an ophthalmologist, to look for typical retinal lesions.

Imaging studies are invaluable for certain forms of candidiasis, especially chronic disseminated candidiasis, and they can be of major help in defining the extent of infection in other types of *Candida* infection, such as osteoarticular and urinary tract infections and endocarditis.

Non–culture-based techniques are increasingly used to aid in the diagnosis of invasive candidiasis,[9] including β-D-glucan, a cell wall component of many fungi, including *Candida* species. The β-D-glucan assay is not specific for *Candida* infections, but has moderately good sensitivity in patients at high risk for invasive candidiasis. PCR is not standardized, but some studies show that it is more sensitive than β-D-glucan and blood cultures. A more rapid technique can identify *Candida* species from whole blood by use of magnetic biosensor technology.[10]

TREATMENT

Guidelines for treatment of the various forms of candidiasis have been published by the Infectious Diseases Society of America (IDSA).[11] Mucocutaneous disease is obviously treated in a much different fashion than disseminated life-threatening infection. Because diagnostic tests are not sensitive, empirical therapy is indicated in some circumstances, and for patients at the highest risk for *Candida* infection, antifungal prophylaxis can decrease that risk (see below under "Prevention").

Mucocutaneous Infections

Most mucocutaneous infections should initially be treated with local creams, solutions, troches, or suspensions.[12] For thrush, clotrimazole troches (10 mg four or five times daily) are preferred to nystatin suspension (commonly given as "swish and swallow" four times daily). Patients with AIDS may not respond to local therapy, especially when their CD4 counts are low; in this situation, oral fluconazole 100 to 200 mg daily is given. For vaginitis, a variety of creams and vaginal tablets (miconazole, clotrimazole, and others) are effective, but many women prefer to take a single 150-mg fluconazole tablet orally. Recurrent vaginitis is a more complicated therapeutic issue and often requires chronic suppressive therapy with fluconazole.[13] Esophagitis should always be treated with a systemically absorbed agent; the usual treatment is fluconazole 200 mg/day for 14 days.

In patients with advanced AIDS and low CD4 counts, who are often taking fluconazole to prevent recurrent candidiasis, fluconazole-refractory disease may develop. For these patients, increasing the dosage of fluconazole or switching to itraconazole suspension 200 mg daily, voriconazole 200 mg twice daily, or posaconazole suspension 400 mg daily should be effective. If oral tablets and solutions are no longer effective, intravenous amphotericin B, caspofungin, anidulafungin, and micafungin are alternative agents that can be used. Patients with the syndrome of chronic mucocutaneous candidiasis require lifelong suppressive therapy with oral azole agents.

Candidemia and Invasive Candidiasis

All patients with candidemia should be treated with an antifungal agent, including patients who have only one blood culture that yields *Candida* and those with a vascular catheter tip that yields *Candida*. The rationale for this recommendation is related to the high rate of metastatic foci in major organs associated with hematogenously disseminated candidiasis. Randomized controlled trials have shown the effectiveness of the following antifungal agents for the treatment of candidemia: fluconazole 400 or 800 mg/day; the three echinocandins—caspofungin 50 mg/day, anidulafungin 100 mg/day, and micafungin 100 mg/day[A1]; voriconazole 3 mg/kg twice daily; amphotericin B 0.7 mg/kg/day; and a lipid formulation of amphotericin B 3 to 5 mg/kg/day. The IDSA guidelines recommend an echinocandin as initial therapy in both neutropenic and non-neutropenic patients. Fluconazole is an acceptable alternative, but only for patients who are not severely ill and who are considered unlikely to have an azole-resistant *Candida* species. Patients who have stabilized clinically and are found to have an isolate, such as *C. albicans*, that is likely to be susceptible to fluconazole can be transitioned to fluconazole from an echinocandin. Voriconazole can be used for step-down therapy if the organism is susceptible, but offers little advantage over fluconazole. Amphotericin B formulations are used infrequently, except for patients who are neutropenic and for neonates.

Vascular catheters should be removed if at all feasible because removal has been shown to help clear *Candida* from blood more quickly. Repeated blood cultures should be obtained to ascertain that the fungemia has resolved, and treatment should continue for 2 weeks after the date of the first negative blood culture. An individual patient-level quantitative review of seven randomized trials for the treatment of invasive candidiasis found an overall mortality in the entire data set of 31.4%. Significant predictors of mortality included increasing age; use of immunosuppressive therapy; and infection with *C. tropicalis*. Improved survival and clinical success was found with the use of an echinocandin and the removal of central venous catheters.

Because diagnostic tests are not sensitive, seriously ill patients who could have invasive candidiasis may need to be treated before culture confirmation. This approach is used frequently in neutropenic patients and is increasingly used in the ICU setting.[14] Liposomal amphotericin B, caspofungin, and voriconazole have been shown in randomized clinical treatment trials to be effective for empirical use in neutropenic patients. A placebo-controlled, randomized trial of fluconazole empirical therapy in ICU patients failed to show a benefit; however, there were acknowledged problems with the chosen end point, and the rate of candidemia was too low to allow a proper evaluation of empirical therapy. The IDSA guidelines recommend that empirical therapy be reserved for febrile, critically ill patients who have risk factors for invasive candidiasis. The preferred treatment is an echinocandin. In a randomized clinical trial of 260 non-neutropenic, nontransplanted, critically ill patients with ICU-acquired sepsis, *Candida* colonization, and multiorgan failure, on broad-spectrum antibiotics, empirical micafungin (100 mg daily for 14 days) decreased the rate of new invasive fungal infection but did not increase fungal-free survival at day 28.[A2] Compelling data for early treatment come from a study of 224 candidemic patients who had septic shock. Mortality rates as high as 98% were found in patients in whom there was a delay beyond 24 hours of the onset of shock in initiating antifungal therapy and in effecting source control, defined as draining abscesses and removing central venous catheters.

Endocarditis should be treated with a lipid formulation of amphotericin B, with or without flucytosine. Echinocandins are an acceptable alternative. Infected valves should be replaced. In a few patients for whom valve replacement was not an option, lifelong suppression with fluconazole appeared to be effective.

Chronic disseminated candidiasis generally requires months of therapy for cure. Most patients begin therapy with a lipid formulation of amphotericin B or an echinocandin and are then switched to fluconazole and treated until the lesions disappear on computed tomography scanning. This process of radiographic resolution may require several months.

Focal Invasive Infections

Treatment of focal infections depends on the organ system involved. Perhaps the simplest to treat are urinary tract infections. Most patients with candiduria are not infected but merely colonized; removing the selective pressure of antimicrobials and indwelling catheters eliminates candiduria in many of these patients. For those who have infection, oral fluconazole at a dosage of 200 mg/day for 2 weeks is recommended. Bladder irrigation with amphotericin B should

not be used because it eradicates only bladder colonization, requires that a catheter be placed in the bladder, and is associated with a high recurrence rate. None of the newer antifungal agents has a role in the treatment of urinary tract infections.

Osteoarticular infections require months of therapy; a lipid formulation of amphotericin B or an echinocandin can be given initially, followed by long-term therapy with an azole. Peritonitis associated with chronic ambulatory peritoneal dialysis can be treated with amphotericin B, fluconazole, or an echinocandin, depending on the species of *Candida* causing infection. Intraperitoneal administration of amphotericin B can be extremely irritating and should not be attempted. The dialysis catheter should be removed. Meningitis should be treated initially with a lipid formulation of amphotericin B and flucytosine; patients with more chronic disease can be switched to fluconazole for a longer duration of therapy.

Treatment of *Candida* eye infections varies with the extent of ocular involvement. Lesions discovered early at the stage of choroidal or retinal involvement perhaps can be treated effectively with systemic antifungal agents (amphotericin B, an echinocandin, fluconazole, or voriconazole) alone. Many experts prefer to use an agent, such as voriconazole or fluconazole, that achieves higher concentrations in the eye. Lesions extending into the vitreous require more aggressive therapy. The best results have been obtained with pars plana vitrectomy, injection of amphotericin B or voriconazole into the vitreous; and a systemic antifungal agent such as fluconazole or voriconazole for several weeks. Management must be individualized and performed in concert with an ophthalmologist experienced in the treatment of this infection. Treatment of endophthalmitis associated with an intraocular lens implant requires removal of the implant, vitrectomy, and local amphotericin B injections, as well as therapy with fluconazole or voriconazole.

PREVENTION

For certain populations at the highest risk for invasive fungal infection, prophylactic antifungal agents can prevent infection. The populations for whom prophylaxis is recommended include stem cell transplant recipients, patients with acute leukemia who are undergoing induction chemotherapy, high-risk liver transplant recipients, and pancreas and small bowel transplant recipients; in these groups, a variety of different agents are effective. In the ICU population, prophylaxis with fluconazole can be effective, but it is recommended only in units that have a high rate of invasive candidiasis, and only in those patients at the highest risk for infection. In a placebo-controlled trial of caspofungin as antifungal prophylaxis in adults who were in the ICU for at least 3 days, were ventilated, received antibiotics, had a central line, and had at least one additional risk factor, caspofungin was safe and tended to reduce the incidence of invasive candidiasis when used for prophylaxis, but the difference was not statistically significant.[A3] Restricting the use of prophylaxis to individuals at higher risk for candidiasis is essential to prevent the widespread use of azoles, with subsequent selection of resistant species. An experimental vaccine has shown promise in reducing recurrent symptomatic vulvovaginal candidiasis.[A4]

PROGNOSIS

The prognosis for patients with mucocutaneous infections is excellent. The prognosis for focal invasive infections depends on the organ involved and the patient's immune status. For example, whereas pyelonephritis may respond well to antifungal therapy, endocarditis and meningitis are more difficult to treat and have poor outcomes. Invasive candidiasis has a high mortality rate. Early treatment with an effective antifungal agent is extremely important for a favorable outcome.

Grade A References

A1. Kullberg BJ, Vasquez J, Mootsikapun P, et al. Efficacy of anidulafungin in 539 patients with invasive candidiasis: a patient-level pooled analysis of six clinical trials. *J Antimicrob Chemother*. 2017;72:2368-2377.
A2. Timsit JF, Azoulay E, Schwebel C, et al. Empirical micafungin treatment and survival without invasive fungal infection in adults with ICU-acquired sepsis, *Candida* colonization, and multiple organ failure. The EMPIRICUS randomized clinical trial. *JAMA*. 2016;316:1555-1564.
A3. Ostrosky-Zeichner L, Shoham S, Vasquez J, et al. MSG-01: a randomized, double-blind, placebo-controlled trial of caspofungin prophylaxis followed by preemptive therapy for invasive candidiasis in high-risk adults in the critical care setting. *Clin Infect Dis*. 2014;58:1219-1226.
A4. Edwards JE Jr, Schwartz MM, Schmidt CS, et al. A fungal immunotherapeutic vaccine (NDV-3A) for treatment of recurrent vulvovaginal candidiasis-a phase 2 randomized, double-blind, placebo-controlled trial. *Clin Infect Dis*. 2018;66:1928-1936.

GENERAL REFERENCES

For the General References and other additional features, please visit Expert Consult at https://expertconsult.inkling.com.

319

ASPERGILLOSIS

THOMAS J. WALSH

DEFINITION

Aspergillosis is a disease caused by one or more of the species of the genus *Aspergillus*. Sporelike structures called *conidia* are aerosolized from the mold form of the organism growing in the environment. When conidia reach tissue, they germinate to form invasive filaments called *hyphae*.

The Pathogens

The most common species infecting humans are *Aspergillus fumigatus*, *Aspergillus flatus*, *Aspergillus terreus*, and *A. niger*. The species are usually identified in culture by characteristic microscopic features of hyphae and the structures producing conidia. When some species are not readily identifiable, they may be reported by the clinical laboratory as "*Aspergillus* species" or "*Aspergillus* sp.*" *A. fumigatus* may be reported as "*A. fumigatus* species complex." Some species within *A. fumigatus* complex may be particularly drug resistant. *A. terreus* is resistant to amphotericin B. Aspergilli within tissue appear as dichotomously branched (Y-shaped) septate hyphae. *Scedosporium* and *Fusarium* species also may produce septate hyphae in tissue. The presence of septa and dichotomous branching differentiates *Aspergillus* species from the Mucorales, which are the causative organisms of mucormycosis (Chapter 320).

EPIDEMIOLOGY

Aspergillus species are ubiquitous organisms in the external environment, including soil, decaying matter, and air in temperatures as high as 40 to 50° C. Aspergilli are easily isolated from houses, particularly from basements, crawl spaces, bedding, humidifiers, ventilation ducts, potted plants, dust, condiments (e.g., pepper), and marijuana samples. Aspergilli cause abortion in cattle and are important pathogens of marine organisms, insects, and domesticated and wild birds. Aflatoxin, which is one of the most potent carcinogens known, is produced by strains of *Aspergillus flavus* at ambient temperature on stored grain, spices, and nuts. Foodborne ingestion of preformed aflatoxin may cause hepatic necrosis or hepatocellular carcinoma (Chapter 186) in animals and humans.

Aspergillus species may be acquired from airborne conidia in inpatient and outpatient health care settings. Nosocomial aspergillosis is associated with building renovation, new construction, unfiltered air, contaminated ventilation systems, and fireproofing materials. Hospital water, which may become aerosolized during activities such as showering, is a more recently described potential source of aspergilli. As human pathogens, *Aspergillus* species may cause acute invasive disease, chronic infection, or allergic symptoms.[1,2] A classification of aspergillosis is presented in Table 319-1.

Acute invasive aspergillosis develops in immunocompromised patient populations, particularly those with hematologic malignancies,[3] hematopoietic stem cell transplantation (HSCT), severe aplastic anemia, primary immunodeficiencies, and solid organ transplantation, especially of heart, lung, and liver. Genetic deficiency of the soluble pattern-recognition receptor called PTX3 (long pentraxin 3) caused by homozygous haplotype (h2/h2) in the *PTX3* gene of donor cells has been found to lead to impaired neutrophil antifungal capacity and increased risk for invasive aspergillosis in recipients of HSCT. Persistent neutropenia, corticosteroids, other immunosuppressive agents, graft-versus-host disease (GVHD), and cytomegalovirus (CMV) disease are the most frequently observed clinical risk factors. The mortality of acute invasive aspergillosis varies from as much as 100% with central nervous system (CNS) infection to approximately 65% with pulmonary infection in HSCT recipients. Early recognition of clinical manifestations followed by initiation of antifungal therapy may improve the ominous prognosis of acute invasive aspergillosis.

Invasive aspergillosis complicates the care of up to 13% of patients with immunocompromise. For the period of 2009 to 2013 in the United States, using propensity score matching, invasive aspergillosis was associated with increased hospital mortality and 30-day readmission rates, as well as excess duration of hospitalization and costs (attributable excess costs of up to $600 million annually).[4]

CLINICAL MANIFESTATIONS

Invasive Aspergillosis

The classic clinical manifestations of *invasive pulmonary aspergillosis* in immunocompromised hosts are fever and focal pulmonary infiltrates, nodules, or wedge-shaped densities resembling infarcts.[5] Cough, pleuritic pain, and hemoptysis also may be present. Focal pulmonary infiltrates may progress to a cavity on recovery from neutropenia. Pulmonary infiltrates may also present as bronchopneumonia in an immunosuppressed patient. The pulmonary pathology in all these entities is that of hemorrhagic infarction caused by the organism's capacity to invade blood vessel walls (angioinvasion). These processes lead to formation of a necrotic center surrounded by a ring of hemorrhage and edema, which correlates with a "halo sign" surrounding the nodular density. Concomitant pleural effusion may develop and represent *Aspergillus* empyema. Tracheobronchial aspergillosis in immunocompromised patients presents as ulcerative, pseudomembranous, or plaquelike large airway disease that may presage pulmonary parenchymal invasion.

Acute *Aspergillus* sinusitis may occur concomitantly or independently of invasive pulmonary aspergillosis. Although symptoms may include fever, localized pressure, and pain, they may be absent in severely immunocompromised patients. Eschar on the nasal septum and turbinates may be observed by speculum examination or endoscopy. Acute *Aspergillus* sinusitis of the ethmoid and sphenoid sinuses may progress to cavernous sinus thrombosis with symptoms referable to cranial nerves III, IV, $V_{1,2}$, and VI. *A. flavus* has a high propensity for causing acute sinus infection.

The tissue targets of *extrapulmonary* and *disseminated aspergillosis* most commonly include the CNS, where abscesses and infarcts are characteristic. Patients with CNS aspergillosis present with focal paresis, cranial nerve deficits, and seizures. The glucose level in cerebrospinal fluid (CSF) is usually normal, and cultures of CSF are negative. Other extrapulmonary manifestations include endophthalmitis, myocardial infarction, gastrointestinal disease, renal infarction, cutaneous lesions, and Budd-Chiari syndrome. Esophageal ulcers and mesenteric thrombosis may produce gastrointestinal bleeding. Renal infection may present as flank pain and hematuria.

Aspergillus endocarditis[6] usually begins as an isolated infection in intravenous drug users or after cardiac valvular surgery. *Aspergillus* endocarditis most commonly presents as major arterial emboli. Blood cultures, which are seldom

TABLE 319-1	CLASSIFICATION OF ASPERGILLOSIS
CATEGORY	**SPECIFIC FORMS OF ASPERGILLOSIS**

Acute invasive aspergillosis	Invasive pulmonary aspergillosis
	  Empyema
	  Tracheobronchial infection
	Extrapulmonary aspergillosis
	  Acute sinusitis
	  Focal rhinitis
	  Cerebral, cerebellar, or brain stem infarction
	  Endophthalmitis
	  Osteomyelitis
	  Epidural abscess
	  Cardiac aspergillosis
	    Myocarditis
	    Endocarditis
	    Pericarditis
	  Gastrointestinal aspergillosis
	  Renal infection
	  Cutaneous lesions (nodules, ulcers)
	Disseminated aspergillosis

Chronic aspergillosis	Aspergilloma Chronic necrotizing pulmonary aspergillosis Chronic cavitary pulmonary aspergillosis *Aspergillus* otomycosis
Allergic forms of aspergillosis	Allergic bronchopulmonary aspergillosis Extrinsic allergic alveolitis Allergic *Aspergillus* sinusitis

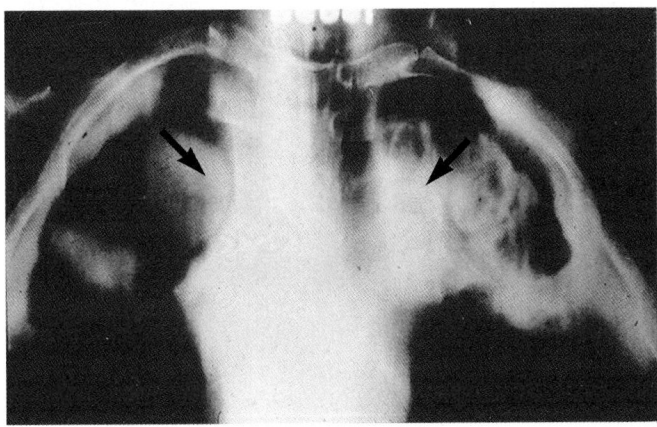

FIGURE 319-1. Tomogram of pulmonary aspergillomas (*arrows*).

positive, may be delayed in growth by as much as 14 to 21 days. Diagnosis is difficult, and despite valve replacement with antifungal therapy, mortality approaches 100%. *Aspergillus* pericarditis may arise from contiguous pulmonary lesions or through transmural infection from endocardial infection.

Locally invasive aspergillosis usually develops in immunocompromised patients as cutaneous ulcers, focal rhinitis, osteomyelitis, and septic arthritis.[7] Cutaneous ulcers have been associated with use of contaminated adhesive tape and arm boards. Blood-borne infection in illicit intravenous drug users may present as foci of dissemination in brain, lung, kidney, and bone. Keratitis, endophthalmitis, and infection of burn wounds may develop from traumatic inoculation in otherwise immunocompetent patients.

Chronic Pulmonary Aspergillosis

Aspergilloma appears on chest radiograph as a ball in a cavity. The fungus ball consists of matted hyphae and debris in a preformed cavity from previous pulmonary tuberculosis, histoplasmosis, or fibrocystic sarcoidosis (Fig. 319-1). Symptomatic patients present with cough, hemoptysis, dyspnea, weight loss, fatigue, chest pain, or fever. Sputum culture is typically positive for *Aspergillus* species, particularly *A. niger*. Pleural aspergillosis may complicate surgical resection of aspergilloma or develop spontaneously as a bronchopleural fistula or concomitantly with tuberculosis.

As a stage in the repair process of infarcted lung tissue in neutropenic patients, one or more apparent "aspergillomas" may develop in consolidated lesions during recovery from neutropenia. These apparent aspergillomas do not develop in preexisting cavities and create an "air-crescent sign," or Monod sign, during their formation.

Chronic necrotizing pulmonary aspergillosis and *chronic cavitary pulmonary aspergillosis* occur in patients with underlying chronic lung disease, chronic immunosuppression, such as that due to prolonged use of systemic corticosteroids, or both. Chronic necrotizing pulmonary aspergillosis characteristically causes a slowly progressive inflammatory destruction of lung tissue superimposed on chronic lung disease. Clinical manifestations of worsening pulmonary function, cough, and dyspnea in chronic necrotizing pulmonary aspergillosis may be indistinguishable from concomitant primary chronic respiratory disease.

Chronic cavitary pulmonary aspergillosis is defined as the presence of multiple *Aspergillus*-related cavities, which may or may not contain an aspergilloma. Patients with chronic cavitary pulmonary aspergillosis may have genetically mediated deficits in innate host defenses. Occurring in association with symptoms of cough, hemoptysis, and dyspnea, the progressive cavities of chronic cavitary pulmonary aspergillosis tend to coalesce with the loss of functional lung tissue.

Aspergillus otomycosis is a chronic infection that usually involves the external auditory canal with symptoms of pain, pruritus, hypoacusis, and otic discharge in patients with impaired mucocutaneous immunity, such as those with chronic eczema, hypogammaglobulinemia, diabetes mellitus, or HIV infection and those receiving corticosteroids. *Aspergillus* may involve the middle ear and extend into the mastoid sinus if the tympanic membrane has been perforated.

Allergic Forms of Aspergillosis

Allergic bronchopulmonary aspergillosis[8,9] develops most frequently in patients with a history of chronic asthma or cystic fibrosis. Occurring in genetically susceptible patients exposed to specific *Aspergillus* antigens, allergic bronchopulmonary aspergillosis is characterized by episodic airway obstruction, fever, eosinophilia, positive sputum cultures, mucous plugs containing hyphae, the presence of grossly visible brown flecks in sputum (hyphae), transient infiltrates and parallel "tramline" or ring markings on chest radiographs, proximal bronchiectasis, upper lobe contraction, and elevated levels of total immunoglobulins G and E (IgG and IgE). Eosinophilia may be present in blood, sputum, and lung tissue. Mucous plugs contribute to development of pulmonary infiltrates, atelectasis, and peribronchial inflammation. The parallel or ring markings are caused by thickened ectatic bronchi, whereas the upper lobe changes are due to progressive apical fibrosis. Pulmonary infiltrates in allergic bronchopulmonary aspergillosis may be nonsegmental and transient in association with eosinophilia and asthma; alternatively, they may be segmental and associated with bronchial obstruction by mucous plugs, wherein asthma and eosinophilia may be absent.

Extrinsic allergic alveolitis is an unusual allergic form of *Aspergillus* lung disease that has been most frequently associated with *Aspergillus clavatus* in malt workers. A hypersensitivity pneumonitis with dyspnea and fever develops approximately 4 hours after exposure. Diffuse reticulonodular interstitial infiltrates may be present at the time of symptoms. Patients have IgG precipitins and cell-mediated immune reactions against *Aspergillus* antigens. Granulomas are present in lung tissue. In contrast to allergic bronchopulmonary aspergillosis, eosinophilia is not a feature of *Aspergillus* extrinsic allergic alveolitis.

Allergic *Aspergillus* sinusitis is a noninvasive form of sinus disease that typically presents in patients with asthma, nasal polyps, sinus opacification, and eosinophilia. Sinus aspirate yields mucinous material containing eosinophils, Charcot-Leyden crystals (eosinophil-derived rhomboid crystals of lysophospholipase), and hyphal elements. Allergic *Aspergillus* sinusitis and allergic bronchopulmonary aspergillosis may coexist in some patients. Advanced forms of allergic *Aspergillus* sinusitis may present with proptosis and optic neuropathy, necessitating prompt surgical intervention.

DIAGNOSIS
Invasive Aspergillosis

Diagnosis of invasive pulmonary aspergillosis and disseminated aspergillosis is difficult. None of the aforementioned clinical manifestations are diagnostic for invasive aspergillosis. Advances in computed tomography (CT) have revealed characteristic features of nodules, halo signs, wedge-shaped infiltrates, and air-crescent signs during invasive pulmonary aspergillosis in immunocompromised patients (Fig. 319-2).[10] For example, infarct-shaped consolidations and smooth bronchial wall thickening are more frequent in invasive pulmonary aspergillosis, whereas mass-shaped consolidations and centrilobular nodules (<10 mm, clustered) are more frequent in tuberculosis.[11] However, infections caused by *Fusarium* species, *Scedosporium* species, the Mucorales, and *Pseudomonas aeruginosa* may be radiologically indistinguishable from invasive pulmonary aspergillosis. Microbiologic confirmation, where possible, is important to differentiate aspergillosis from other filamentous fungal infections. Bronchoalveolar lavage (BAL), percutaneous needle aspiration, videoassisted thoracoscopic (VATS) biopsy, and if necessary, open lung biopsy are standard procedures for establishing a microbiologic diagnosis of invasive aspergillosis. Specimens obtained from these procedures may demonstrate dichotomously branching septate hyphae by direct microscopy or grow *Aspergillus* species in culture. Each of these procedures is associated with falsenegative results, as well as with complications. Conversely, the presence of *Aspergillus* by direct examination or culture in an immunocompromised host with pulmonary nodules or well-circumscribed infiltrates carries a high probability for diagnosis of invasive aspergillosis.

Galactomannan, which is a heteropolysaccharide of the *Aspergillus* cell wall, is a useful biomarker that is released into the circulation and alveolar spaces during invasive pulmonary aspergillosis. Detection of galactomannan by enzyme immunoassay (EIA) in serum or BAL above certain thresholds is strong microbiologic evidence for a diagnosis of invasive aspergillosis in immunocompromised patients with characteristic clinical manifestations. Nonetheless, false-positive results have been reported in patients in which Plasmalyte was used for BAL, and in other deeply invasive mycoses such as blastomycosis and histoplasmosis. Serum galactomannan may be falsely negative in patients receiving antifungal prophylaxis or empirical therapy.

$(1{\rightarrow}3)$-β-D-Glucan is another *Aspergillus* cell wall polysaccharide that is detected in serum during invasive disease. The sensitivity of the *Limulus* spectrophotometric assay for detection of $(1{\rightarrow}3)$-β-D-glucan in patients with invasive aspergillosis appears to be comparable to that of the galactomannan EIA. However, because $(1{\rightarrow}3)$-β-D-glucan also is present in the cell wall of other medically important fungi, including *Candida* species, the specificity of $(1{\rightarrow}3)$-β-D-glucan for *Aspergillus* species is less than that of galactomannan.

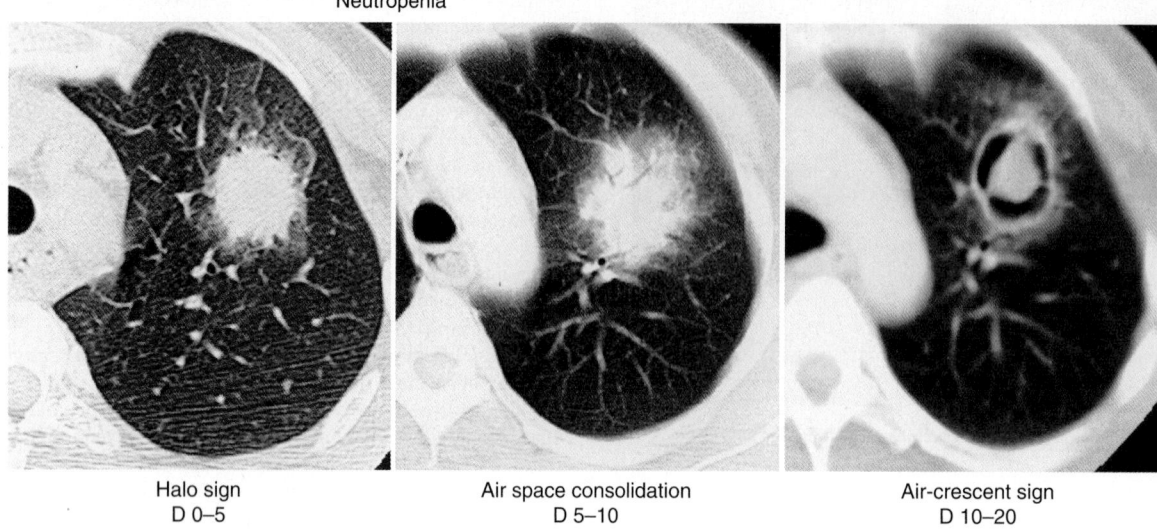

Neutropenia

Halo sign
D 0–5

Air space consolidation
D 5–10

Air-crescent sign
D 10–20

FIGURE 319-2. Evolution of radiography of invasive aspergillosis in an immunocompromised host. D = days after the lesion is first noted.

Molecular diagnostic tools, such as quantitative polymerase chain reaction (PCR), for diagnosis of invasive aspergillosis now appear to be equivalently accurate compared with EIA testing and β-D-glucan testing.[12,13] Ultimately, the combined use of improved diagnostic imaging, microscopy, culture methodology, cell wall biomarkers, and possibly PCR, in conjunction with careful bedside assessment of risk factors and clinical manifestations, will improve the diagnosis of invasive aspergillosis and early initiation of therapy. For example, the combination of galactomannan and PCR testing can diagnose aspergillosis earlier and reduce the incidence of invasive disease in high-risk hematology patients.[A1] Increasing data support monitoring serum galactomannan as a marker for therapeutic response.[14]

Diagnosis of locally invasive extrapulmonary aspergillosis causing mucocutaneous lesions, osteomyelitis, and septic arthritis is best accomplished with biopsy, direct microscopy, and culture. A diagnosis of *Aspergillus* keratitis is established by careful culture of corneal lesions by an ophthalmologist.

Allergic Forms of Aspergillosis

Diagnosis of allergic bronchopulmonary aspergillosis is based on the presence of a combination of clinical, biologic, and radiologic criteria (Fig. 319-3). The consensus criteria for establishing a diagnosis of allergic bronchopulmonary aspergillosis differ depending on the presence of cystic fibrosis. For patients with allergic bronchopulmonary aspergillosis without the presence of cystic fibrosis (Chapter 83), criteria for allergic bronchopulmonary aspergillosis include asthma, an immediate cutaneous reaction to *A. fumigatus* antigen, total serum IgE concentration higher than 1000 ng/mL, elevated *A. fumigatus*–specific serum IgE levels, precipitating serum antibodies to *A. fumigatus*, central bronchiectasis, peripheral blood eosinophilia, and characteristic pulmonary infiltrates. The latter two features (eosinophilia and pulmonary infiltrates) are considered nonessential because they only may be present during an acute phase of allergic bronchopulmonary aspergillosis.

Among patients with cystic fibrosis, distinguishing between allergic bronchopulmonary aspergillosis and an episode of clinical deterioration with colonization by *Aspergillus* species is challenging. The current criteria of the Cystic Fibrosis Foundation help to define allergic bronchopulmonary aspergillosis in that setting: clinical deterioration (coughing, wheezing, increased sputum production, exercise intolerance, and decrease in pulmonary function); immediate hypersensitivity to *A. fumigatus* (positive skin test or IgE response); total serum IgE concentration higher than 1000 ng/mL; precipitating antibodies to *A. fumigatus*; abnormal chest radiograph (central bronchiectasis); mucous plugs; or unexplained changes compared with previous chest radiograph).

A biphasic skin test response may assist in the diagnosis. A scratch test with *Aspergillus* antigens produces an immediate wheal-and-flare reaction that is mediated by IgE and blocked by antihistamines but not by corticosteroids. An intracutaneous test with the antigens produces a later (6 to 8 hours) reaction that is mediated by IgG and complement and blocked by corticosteroids.

An occupational history of exposure is critical to the diagnosis of *extrinsic allergic alveolitis*. A typical history of recurrent episodes developing within 24

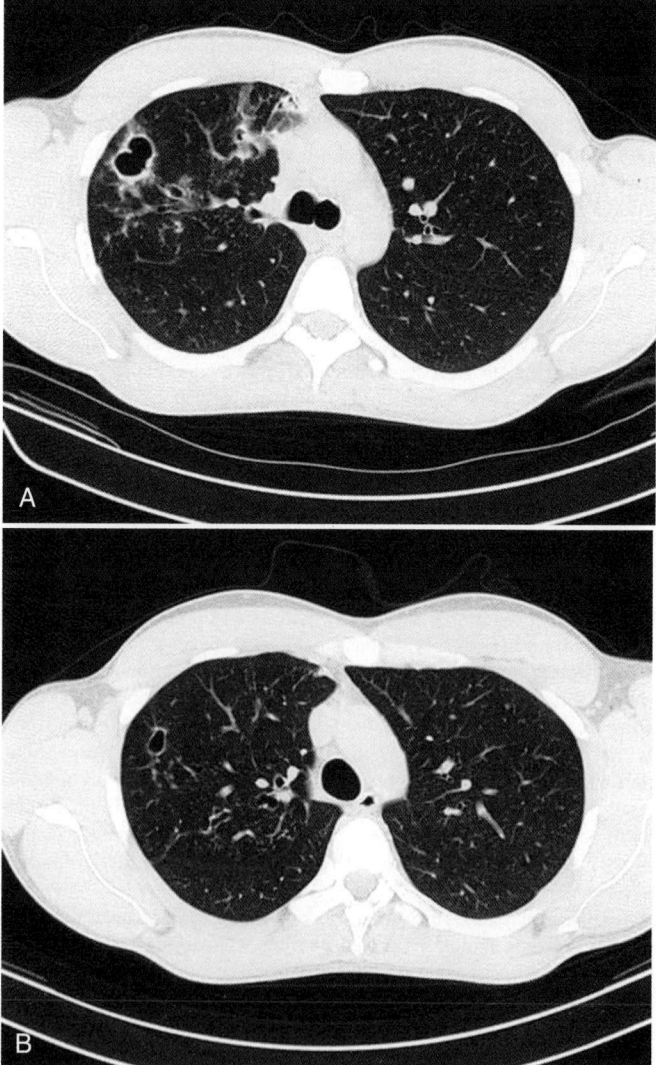

FIGURE 319-3. Allergic bronchopulmonary aspergillosis in a patient with a long history of asthma. **(A)** is a thin-slice CT image showing bronchiectasis with cystic changes in the right upper lobe. This patient had an underlying history of asthma and a markedly elevated immunoglobulin E level and other findings consistent with allergic bronchopulmonary aspergillosis. **(B)** The same patient after treatment with systemic steroids; the cystic bronchiectasis has markedly improved. (Courtesy of Anne E. O'Donnell, MD.)

hours after inhalation of conidial antigens in an agricultural environment, in conjunction with a negative scratch test, a positive intradermal test, and granulomas with immunoglobulins and complement in tissue, is diagnostically consistent with *Aspergillus* extrinsic allergic alveolitis.

Recurrent sinusitis in a patient with asthma, nasal polyps, eosinophilia, sinus opacification, and a sinus aspirate yielding mucinous material containing eosinophils, Charcot–Leyden crystals, and hyphal elements establishes a diagnosis of allergic *Aspergillus* sinusitis.

TREATMENT ⟨Rx⟩

Invasive Aspergillosis

The foundation of treatment of invasive aspergillosis consists of (1) antifungal medical therapy (Table 319-2), (2) reversal of immunosuppression, and where appropriate (3) surgical resection of infected lesions.[15,16] Dosages of antifungal agents are listed in Table 319-2. Voriconazole is recommended in most patients for the primary treatment of invasive aspergillosis, including pulmonary, disseminated, and extrapulmonary isolated infection. This recommendation is based on the randomized controlled trial showing that voriconazole is superior to deoxycholate amphotericin B (D-AmB) as primary treatment for invasive aspergillosis. However, not all patients are candidates to receive voriconazole. This includes patients with substantially elevated hepatic transaminases, hepatic dysfunction, and a history of intolerance of voriconazole. Such patients can be treated with isavuconazole, which may be equally effective with fewer drug-related adverse events, more predictable pharmacokinetics, and possibly becoming the treatment of choice.[A2] Another option is liposomal amphotericin B (L-AmB) as primary therapy. This recommendation is based on the randomized trial that demonstrated comparable efficacy of approximately 70% using dosages of 3 mg/kg/day and 10 mg/kg/day of LAmB in patients who had predominantly hematologic malignancies. L-AmB or isavuconazole is also indicated as primary therapy for patients in whom there is a suspicion for or documentation of concurrent mucormycosis. Recent emergence of resistance to voriconazole may threaten the future utility of this class of antifungal agents.[17]

Second-line or salvage antifungal therapy is indicated in patients who are intolerant of or whose infection is unresponsive to primary therapy. Among the antifungal agents used in this setting are a lipid formulation of amphotericin B, posaconazole, itraconazole, or an echinocandin (caspofungin is the only agent licensed for this indication). For patients who are already receiving voriconazole, a change of class to a lipid formulation, and use of another azole are alternative possibilities. Such decisions are complicated and warrant infectious diseases consultation with consideration of pharmacokinetic and host factors.

Antifungal therapy for invasive aspergillosis should be continued until lesions have resolved, cultures and biomarkers are negative, and reversible underlying predispositions have abated. Reinstating therapy in patients who have previously responded should be considered if immunosuppression is reinstituted or if neutropenia recurs.

Reversal of immunosuppression is a critical factor in the successful management of invasive aspergillosis. Recovery from neutropenia and decreasing the daily dosage or discontinuation of corticosteroids, where feasible, are two of the most important forms of improving host response. Depending on the protocol used, granulocyte transfusions may stabilize *Aspergillus* lesions until recovery from neutropenia. Granulocyte colony-stimulating factor (G-CSF) and granulocyte-macrophage colony-stimulating factor (GM-CSF) may accelerate recovery from neutropenia. The role of GM-CSF, G-CSF, or interferon-γ in immunocompromised non-neutropenic patients with invasive aspergillosis remains to be further defined.[18]

Surgical management of infected lesions is an important adjunctive component of primary therapy for several forms of invasive aspergillosis: endocarditis, pericarditis, osteomyelitis, epidural abscess, infected vascular catheters and prosthetic devices, and skin and soft tissue infection. Surgical management also is important for several conditions of invasive pulmonary aspergillosis: recurrent hemoptysis from a single cavitary lesion, invasion of a pulmonary lesion into the chest wall, and pulmonary lesions contiguous with great vessels or the pericardium. *Aspergillus* empyema requires closed chest tube drainage and possibly débridement of the infected pleural cavity. Débridement of sinus aspergillosis, particularly when the ethmoid and frontal sinuses are infected, may prevent extension into the orbit or into the cavernous sinus. Surgical resection of selected lesions of the CNS may be indicated for establishing a diagnosis, reducing increased intracranial pressure, and/or protecting critical neural centers. Location of CNS lesions and neurologic sequelae after resection are critical factors in neurosurgical management of aspergillosis.

Local infusion of antifungal agents, particularly intravitreal therapy for endophthalmitis, provides high concentrations to compartments that may not be reached by systemic therapy. Topical irrigation with voriconazole, amphotericin B, or if available, pimaricin is an important adjunct to management of *Aspergillus* keratitis.

Chronic Aspergillosis

Medical therapy has limited benefit in treatment of aspergilloma; however, some patients may benefit from extended use of an antifungal triazole. Lifelong commitment to an antifungal triazole should be balanced against the natural history of approximately 10% of aspergillomas resolving spontaneously. By comparison, medical therapy with itraconazole or voriconazole is the standard of treatment for chronic cavitary pulmonary aspergillosis. Patients with chronic cavitary pulmonary aspergillosis typically achieve improvement of symptoms and stabilization or improvement of radiologic changes. Patients with chronic necrotizing pulmonary aspergillosis also receive an antifungal triazole; however, assessment of response is more difficult because of the underlying chronic lung disease. The role of surgical resection in patients with solitary aspergilloma or chronic cavitary pulmonary aspergillosis is limited because of development of bronchopleural fistula, *Aspergillus* infection of the pleural space, and potentially further worsening of already compromised pulmonary function. However, surgical resection may have a more important role in treating patients with recurrent and severe hemoptysis, for which the benefits of removing the cavity usually outweigh the known risks. Bronchial artery embolization and transthoracic direct intracavitary instillation of antifungal agents for aspergilloma have only transient benefits but substantial risk.

Topical irrigating solutions of boric acid, acetic acid, or an antifungal azole cream may be effective in treating *Aspergillus* otomycosis. Voriconazole, posaconazole, or itraconazole may be necessary for refractory cases or perforated tympanic membranes.

Allergic Forms of Aspergillosis

Allergic bronchopulmonary aspergillosis is treated with a combination of corticosteroids and itraconazole. This recommendation is based on two double-blind, randomized, placebo-controlled trials for treatment of allergic bronchopulmonary aspergillosis. These studies demonstrated that itraconazole (200 mg twice daily orally for 16 weeks) resulted in significant amelioration of disease, as evidenced by improvement in exercise tolerance and pulmonary function, reduction in corticosteroid dose, increased interval between corticosteroid courses, and decreased eosinophilic inflammatory parameters and IgE concentration. A randomized trial of either oral itraconazole or prednisolone for 4 months to treat acute-stage allergic bronchopulmonary aspergillosis complicating asthma found prednisolone to be more effective in inducing response. However, itraconazole was also effective in a considerable number and with

TABLE 319-2	ANTIFUNGAL THERAPY OF INVASIVE ASPERGILLOSIS*
FIRST-LINE TREATMENT IN ADULTS†	
Drug of choice: Voriconazole	IV therapy: 6 mg/kg q12h for two doses, then 4 mg/kg q12h Oral therapy: 300 mg or 4 mg/kg bid
Alternate (see text for conditions): Liposomal amphotericin B	3-5 mg/kg IV daily
Isavuconazole	IV or oral therapy: 372 mg (isavuconazonium prodrug) q8h for 6 doses, then 372 mg q24h
SECOND-LINE OR SALVAGE TREATMENT IN ADULTS†	
Amphotericin B lipid complex *or*	5 mg/kg IV daily
Caspofungin *or*	70 mg IV daily for first dose, then 50 mg IV daily
Posaconazole	200 mg PO (suspension) qid or 400 mg PO bid 300 mg PO (delayed-release tablet) or IV bid day 1, then 300 mg PO or IV daily
or Itraconazole	400 mg PO (capsules) daily (in either one or two doses); or 2.5 mg/kg PO (solution) bid

*Refer to package insert for dosage modification of antifungal agents in liver disease or renal impairment.

†Duration of antifungal therapy depends on therapeutic response of documented lesions, burden of disease, host immunocompetence, and type of aspergillosis (e.g., acute invasive vs. chronic, vs. allergic). Guidelines of Infectious Diseases Society of America recommend at least 6 to 12 weeks for invasive pulmonary aspergillosis. Patients who are immunosuppressed continue treatment throughout the period of immunosuppression and until resolution of lesions. In patients previously diagnosed with invasive aspergillosis, antifungal therapy should be continued or reinitiated during subsequent periods of immunosuppression (e.g., chemotherapy, stem cell transplantation, graft-versus-host disease) to prevent recrudescence.

See reference 16 for more details.

fewer side effects than prednisolone.[A3] Although corticosteroid therapy is the mainstay of treatment of allergic bronchopulmonary aspergillosis, chronic administration of corticosteroids causes severe immunosuppression and multi-system metabolic abnormalities. Addition of itraconazole reduces organism burden, attenuates antigenic stimulus for destructive bronchial inflammation, and provides a corticosteroid-sparing effect. Intermittent use of corticosteroids or substantially raising the dose in patients receiving chronic therapy can produce rapid resolution of marked symptomatic episodes or deteriorating forced expiratory volume in 1 second (FEV$_1$). At this time there is a lack of evidence for the efficacy and safety of anti-IgE (omalizumab) therapy in patients with allergic bronchopulmonary aspergillosis and cystic fibrosis.[A4]

Extrinsic allergic alveolitis is best managed by removing patients from the allergenic environment. An accurate occupational and home environment history is critical to this intervention.

Allergic *Aspergillus* sinusitis is treated by endoscopic drainage to relieve obstruction by tenacious mucin. Itraconazole, nasal corticosteroids, and systemic corticosteroids, alone or in combination, may be beneficial in some patients with allergic *Aspergillus* sinusitis. Caution is warranted with chronic use of systemic or nasal corticosteroids. Itraconazole may have a corticosteroid sparing effect.

Combination Antifungal Therapy

Combinations of polyenes, triazoles, and echinocandins are being explored. The aggregate of well-conducted in vitro, in vivo, and clinical observational studies support the additive or synergistic interaction of a triazole and echinocandin in primary treatment of invasive pulmonary aspergillosis. In a randomized trial designed to study combination therapy for invasive aspergillosis, patients with hematologic malignancies and/or allogeneic HSCT were randomized at study entry to receive initial treatment with a combination of voriconazole and anidulafungin or voriconazole monotherapy.[A5] Combination therapy was associated with reduced all-cause mortality at 6 weeks compared with voriconazole monotherapy, but this difference did not reach statistical superiority. In patients with probable invasive aspergillosis, combination therapy was associated with a significant survival benefit.

PREVENTION

Several strategies may be used for prevention of invasive aspergillosis in immunocompromised patients: primary prophylaxis, empirical therapy, and secondary prophylaxis. Posaconazole is licensed for prophylaxis of invasive aspergillosis in patients with hematologic malignancies and in HSCT recipients. This recommendation in hematologic malignancies is based on a randomized clinical trial in patients undergoing chemotherapy for acute myelogenous leukemia or myelodysplasia. Posaconazole significantly prevented invasive fungal infections more effectively than did either fluconazole or itraconazole and improved overall survival. There were, however, more adverse events with posaconazole. Voriconazole also is used for this indication but with less evidence.[A6] A multicenter, randomized, double-blind trial comparing fluconazole versus voriconazole in HSCT recipients for the prevention of mycoses found nonsignificant trends of fewer *Aspergillus* infections with voriconazole. The study also demonstrated that in the context of intensive monitoring and structured empirical antifungal therapy, 6-month fungal-free survival did not differ in allogeneic HSCT recipients given prophylactic fluconazole or voriconazole. Empirical antifungal therapy provides early treatment for persistently febrile immunocompromised patients and systemic prophylaxis for high-risk hosts with or without pulmonary infiltrates. L-AmB, aerosolized amphotericin,[A7] caspofungin, and voriconazole have been used for this strategy. Secondary prophylaxis of invasive aspergillosis with voriconazole is used for patients with a history of previous aspergillosis who are scheduled for a subsequent cycle of immunosuppression that may increase the risk for recurrence.

Reduction of exposure to airborne conidia, such as by HEPA filtration of hospital air, avoiding activities that increase conidial aerosols (room maintenance, dust exposures, and contaminated materials [e.g., potted plants]), as well as providing clean water distribution systems, may reduce acquisition of *Aspergillus* by immunosuppressed or neutropenic patients.

For patients with allergic forms of aspergillosis, use of corticosteroids and itraconazole, alone or in combination, may prevent debilitating exacerbations. The toxicity of chronic administration of prednisone warrants strategies for intermittent administration of prednisone or corticosteroid-sparing use of itraconazole.

PROGNOSIS

Untreated invasive aspergillosis is associated with severe morbidity and high mortality in immunocompromised patients. Prognosis is improved by both early initiation of antifungal therapy, reversal of immunosuppression, and successful treatment of the underlying primary disease. For patients with chronic aspergillosis, multidisciplinary specialized supportive care may improve outcome and quality of life.

Grade A References

A1. Aguado JM, Vázquez L, Fernández-Ruiz M, et al. Serum galactomannan versus a combination of galactomannan and polymerase chain reaction-based *Aspergillus* DNA detection for early therapy of invasive aspergillosis in high-risk hematological patients: a randomized controlled trial. *Clin Infect Dis.* 2015;60:405-414.

A2. Maertens JA, Raad II, Marr KA, et al. Isavuconazole versus voriconazole for primary treatment of invasive mould disease caused by *Aspergillus* and other filamentous fungi (SECURE): a phase 3, randomised-controlled, non-inferiority trial. *Lancet.* 2016;387:760-769.

A3. Agarwal R, Dhooria S, Singh Sehgal I, et al. A randomized trial of itraconazole vs prednisolone in acute-stage allergic bronchopulmonary aspergillosis complicating asthma. *Chest.* 2018;153:656-664.

A4. Jat KR, Walia DK, Khairwa A. Anti-IgE therapy for allergic bronchopulmonary aspergillosis in people with cystic fibrosis. *Cochrane Database Syst Rev.* 2018;3:CD010288.

A5. Marr KA, Schlamm HT, Herbrecht R, et al. Combination antifungal therapy for invasive aspergillosis: a randomized trial. *Ann Intern Med.* 2015;162:81-89.

A6. Wingard JR, Carter SL, Walsh TJ, et al. Randomized, double blind trial of fluconazole vs. voriconazole for the prevention of invasive fungal disease after allogeneic hematopoietic cell transplantation. *Blood.* 2010;116:5111-5118.

A7. Xia D, Sun WK, Tan MM, et al. Aerosolized amphotericin B as prophylaxis for invasive pulmonary aspergillosis: a meta-analysis. *Int J Infect Dis.* 2015;30:78-84.

GENERAL REFERENCES

For the General References and other additional features, please visit Expert Consult at https://expertconsult.inkling.com.

320

MUCORMYCOSIS

DIMITRIOS P. KONTOYIANNIS

DEFINITION

Mucormycosis is the unifying term used to describe infections caused by fungi belonging to the order Mucorales. Zygomycosis, an alternative term used to describe these life-threatening infections, has become less accurate based on a recent taxonomic reclassification (using molecular methods) that abolished Zygomycetes as a class (and placed the order Mucorales in the subphylum Mucormycotina).[1] Mucorales typically cause aggressive, acute-onset, frequently fatal angioinvasive infections, especially in immunosuppressed hosts.

EPIDEMIOLOGY

Mucorales fungi are distributed worldwide and found in decaying organic substrates. The true incidence of mucormycosis is not known and probably is underestimated because of difficulties in antemortem diagnosis. The relative frequency of Mucorales families causing infection differs. In a review of more than 900 reported cases, the most common microbiologically confirmed infecting species were *Rhizopus* (47%), *Mucor* (18%), *Cunninghamella bertholletiae* (7%), *Apophysomyces elegans* (5%), *Absidia* (5%), *Saksenaea* (5%), and *Rhizomucor pusillus* (4%). Some Mucorales causing infection have specific geographic and host associations. For example, the thermophilic Mucorales *Saksenaea vasiformis elegans* have specific geographic distributions, as shown in victims of combat-related injuries from Afghanistan who developed necrotizing soft tissue infections. Also, major natural disasters have been associated with rapidly progressing necrotizing soft tissue infections by infrequently isolated species, such as those caused by *Apophysomyces elegans* in the Joplin tornado victims in 2011.

The classic risk factors for mucormycosis include hematologic malignancy, hematopoietic stem cell or solid organ transplantation,[2] poorly controlled diabetes mellitus, chronic acidemia, prematurity, profound chronic debilitation, trauma, burns, and very rarely intravenous drug use.[3] Nosocomial cutaneous infections can develop at surgical wound and intravenous catheter insertion sites. Finally, breakthrough mucormycosis has been increasingly observed in patients with leukemia and in recipients of hematopoietic stem cell transplants receiving *Aspergillus*-active drugs such as voriconazole (which has no anti-Mucorales activity). This association has been a topic of debate.

PATHOBIOLOGY

Mucorales species are saprophytic, rapidly growing fungi. Angioinvasive growth results in infarction and necrosis of surrounding tissue, which is the hallmark of mucormycosis. The major modes of transmission are inhalation, ingestion, and cutaneous inoculation, with inhalation of spores from environmental sources being the most common. Cutaneous or percutaneous transmission occurs with traumatic disruption of skin barriers, and it is the most important mode of transmission in immunocompetent hosts. Gastrointestinal acquisition, although less common, has occurred in patients with repeated ingestion of spores during severe malnutrition, non-nutritional substances (pica), contaminated herbal/homeopathic products, or allopurinol tablets.

Host immunity in healthy hosts prevents germination of fungal spores unless the inoculum is heavy.[4,5] To establish invasive infection, spores must overcome both innate and adaptive immune responses to germinate into hyphae. Defects in phagocytic activity caused by insufficient numbers (i.e., neutropenia) and functional defects caused by glucocorticoids, hyperglycemia, and/or acidosis allow unimpeded proliferation of fungi because of the absence of coordinated, effective host responses.[6] Mucormycosis is often disseminated in severely immunosuppressed patients, with high mortality rates.

Free iron is an essential component of the pathogenesis of mucormycosis, as suggested by the predisposition of patients with iron overload to such infections. These patients often receive iron chelator therapy. Both iron overload and the use of deferoxamine for iron chelation are risk factors for angioinvasive mucormycosis. *Rhizopus oryzae* can utilize deferoxamine as a xenosiderophore to form a ferrioxamine complex and to obtain more iron for use. Reassuringly, the newer iron chelator agents (e.g., deferasirox) are not associated with increased risk for mucormycosis; on the contrary, in preclinical models, deferasirox has exhibited direct fungicidal effects against Mucorales via iron starvation.

Historically, poorly controlled diabetes mellitus (types 1 and 2) has been a major predisposing factor, reported in 36 to 88% of all cases of mucormycosis. In particular, diabetic patients with ketoacidosis are susceptible to mucormycosis. Normal human serum cannot support the growth of *R. oryzae*, whereas serum in diabetic patients can do so. Acidosis disrupts the normal inhibitory activity of serum by attenuating the ability of transferrin to bind iron from the fungus. In addition, quantitative and qualitative neutrophil and phagocytic cell dysfunction occurs in diabetic patients with ketoacidosis and may play a role in the pathogenesis of mucormycosis.

CLINICAL MANIFESTATIONS

The clinical presentation of mucormycosis depends on the host's underlying immunological status and medical condition.[7] Hence, pulmonary mucormycosis is most common in neutropenic or corticosteroid-treated patients (e.g., hematopoietic stem cell and solid organ transplant recipients). In contrast, rhino-orbital or rhinocerebral mucormycosis is the characteristic presentation in patients with diabetic ketoacidosis. Finally, cutaneous mucormycosis in both immunocompetent and immunocompromised hosts is typically seen following local trauma or burns resulting in breakdown of skin integrity and/or subcutaneous tissue injuries. Infectious syndromes associated with Mucorales are grouped based on clinical presentation into one of six categories: (1) rhinocerebral, (2) pulmonary, (3) cutaneous, (4) gastrointestinal, (5) disseminated, and (6) unusual presentations, as follows.

Rhinocerebral Mucormycosis

Rhinocerebral mucormycosis describes an infection originating in the paranasal sinuses after inhalation of Mucorales spores and extending to the orbit (sino-orbital) or brain (rhinocerebral), particularly in patients with diabetic ketoacidosis or those with profound neutropenia.[8] Rhinocerebral mucormycosis is the most common manifestation. Early signs and symptoms of sinus invasion may be indistinguishable from common causes of sinusitis. Common symptoms include sinus pain, congestion, headache, mouth pain, otologic symptoms, and hypo-osmia/anosmia. Involved tissues become red and then violaceous and, finally, black due to thrombosis and tissue necrosis. Necrotic eschar of the nasal cavity and turbinates, facial lesions, and exophytic or necrotic lesions of the hard palate are signs of extensive, rapidly progressing infection. A painful black eschar on the palate or nasal mucosa is a classic diagnostic but late sign. Absence of this finding does not rule out rhinocerebral infection, as necrotic nasal or palate lesions are seen in only 50% of patients within 3 days of onset of infection. Extension into the periorbital region is not uncommon at presentation. Signs and symptoms of periorbital and orbital involvement include periorbital swelling, preseptal and/or orbital cellulitis, proptosis, chemosis, blurred vision or rapidly progressing external ophthalmoplegia, diplopia, eyelid gangrene, retinal detachment, and endophthalmitis. Also, patients with extensive rhino-orbital or rhinocerebral disease may present with trigeminal or other cranial nerve palsy, which is consistent with frequent histologic findings of perineural invasion. Infection can rapidly progress through the cavernous sinuses into the central nervous system, resulting in cavernous sinus and internal carotid artery thrombosis. A bloody nasal discharge may be the only sign indicating that the infection has invaded through the nasal turbinates and into the brain. Patients with advanced infection may have cranial neuropathies and/or altered consciousness; bone destruction; retinal artery, internal carotid artery, cavernous, and less often, sagittal sinus thrombosis; frontal lobe necrosis; epidural and subdural abscesses; and/or basilar artery aneurysm.

Plain films and cerebrospinal fluid findings lack sensitivity in diagnosing rhinocerebral mucormycosis. Computed tomography (CT) and magnetic resonance imaging (MRI) are more useful for revealing soft tissue involvement around the nerve sheaths and bone destruction. CT frequently shows mucosal thickening, air-fluid levels, and bony erosion. Orbital thickening may be detected earlier by using MRI. CT and MRI scans of the orbits may be unremarkable during the initial stages of mucormycosis, highlighting the importance of serial imaging in monitoring disease progression. Extraorbital muscle thickening is often the first sign of orbital involvement and should prompt empirical antifungal therapy followed by surgical exploration or biopsy.

Accurate diagnosis and prompt medical and surgical intervention are critical because of the rapid progression of the infection. Definitive diagnosis of necrotic lesions using biopsy and rapid histologic assessment of frozen sections should be performed as soon as possible because time to treatment directly affects outcome. In a review of 929 documented mucormycosis cases, the mortality rate was as follows: 62% in rhinocerebral mucormycosis, 24% in sino-orbital involvement, and 16% in isolated sinus disease. Isolated sinusitis is curable by following timely surgical intervention and systemic antifungal therapy.

Pulmonary Mucormycosis

The clinical manifestations of pulmonary mucormycosis are indistinguishable from those of invasive pulmonary aspergillosis (Chapter 319).[9] Patients may present with fever refractory to broad-spectrum antibiotics, nonproductive cough, and progressive dyspnea. Less commonly, pleuritic chest pain, hemoptysis, and pleural effusion are seen. If the major pulmonary blood vessels are invaded by fungal hyphae, massive, potentially fatal hemoptysis can occur. Pulmonary mucormycosis can progress and invade adjacent organs by traversing tissue planes, including the diaphragm, chest wall, and pleura (Fig. 320-1). Clues for distinguishing pulmonary mucormycosis from invasive pulmonary aspergillosis include the presence of pansinusitis, a history of prophylaxis with antifungals against *Aspergillus* but not Mucorales (e.g., voriconazole, echinocandins), and possibly continual absence of detectable *Aspergillus galactomannan* antigen in serum. In rare circumstances, pulmonary mucormycosis can present as an endobronchial or tracheal lesion with a less fulminant course, especially in diabetics. Tracheobronchial mucormycosis may cause airway obstruction or erosion of major pulmonary blood vessels and fatal hemoptysis. Fever, cough, dyspnea, and hemoptysis are the most common presenting symptoms.[10] In more immunocompetent hosts, pulmonary mucormycosis may present with more atypical, slowly progressing forms. Like *Aspergillus* species, Mucorales can form mycetomas in preexisting lung cavities and cause slowly necrotizing pneumonia and hypersensitivity syndromes. Investigators have also implicated *Rhizopus* species in allergic alveolitis among farm workers or sawmill workers (wood-trimmer's disease).

In most cases pathologic diagnosis is made via transbronchial biopsy. Because the first-line antifungal typically used for aspergillosis is voriconazole, which lacks activity against Mucorales, failure to achieve a timely diagnosis of pulmonary mucormycosis and delayed antifungal therapy (e.g., amphotericin B) rapidly worsens outcome.

Skin and Soft Tissue Mucormycosis

Cutaneous mucormycosis typically occurs in victims of severe skin or muscular injury.[11] It starts as erythema and a skin induration at a puncture site and progresses to necrosis with a black eschar. Cutaneous infections can quickly extend into the deep fascia and muscle layers. Necrotizing fasciitis is rare and has a poor prognosis. Neutropenic patients in particular are susceptible to lymphatic and blood vessel invasion, infarction, and necrosis with eventual dissemination. Interestingly, the skin appears to be a less common site of secondary involvement with disseminated mucormycosis than of infections

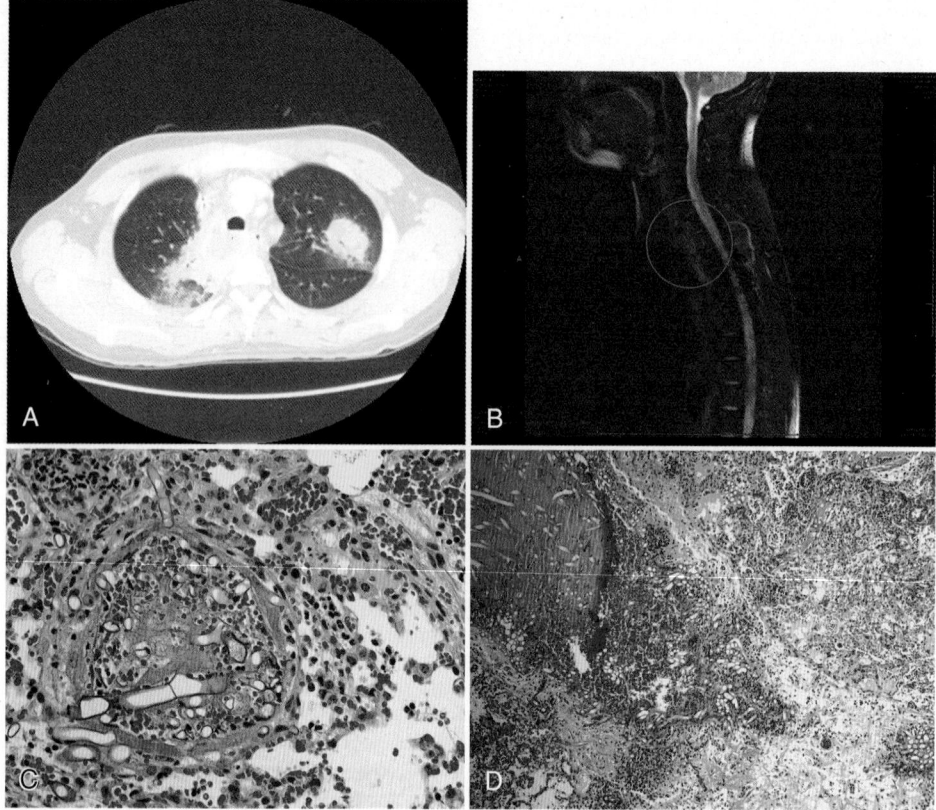

FIGURE 320-1. Extensive, progressive pulmonary mucormycosis in a patient with active leukemia and neutropenia. Characteristic extension of the infection across tissue planes to trachea (producing a fistula) and mediastinum (**A**) and adjacent spine (**B**) are shown. The histopathologic characteristics of profound necrosis and hemorrhage and pauciseptate, broad-based, ribbon-like Mucorales are also shown (**C** and **D**). Culture of a tissue biopsy specimen remained negative. The patient died 3 weeks after diagnosis, despite aggressive use of a high-dose lipid formulation of amphotericin B (AMB) and adjunct immune therapy.

by other hyaline molds such as *Fusarium* or *Scedosporium* species. Even so, skin lesions in patients with suspected mucormycosis should raise concerns about disseminated disease and prompt, careful clinical workup. Because the differential diagnosis of necrotic skin lesions is broad, especially in neutropenic patients, biopsy specimens should be obtained from the center of the lesion down to the subcutaneous fat. Excision and wide débridement of cutaneous lesions, coupled with systemic antifungal therapy and, on occasion, hyperbaric oxygen therapy, can further reduce mortality rates.

Gastrointestinal Mucormycosis

Primary gastrointestinal mucormycosis is rare. It can present as necrotizing enterocolitis and involve any part of the alimentary system with mortality rates of more than 85%. It occurs primarily in malnourished patients and premature infants, in which the stomach is the most commonly affected site, followed by the colon and ileum. The liver, spleen, and pancreas also can be involved. Physicians have described liver abscesses following ingestion of herbal products contaminated by *Mucor indicus*. Fungi can invade the bowel wall and blood vessels, resulting in bowel perforation, peritonitis, and massive gastrointestinal hemorrhage. In neutropenic patients, seeding of the gastrointestinal tract is likely more common than previously thought because 75% of gastrointestinal mucormycoses are diagnosed postmortem. Symptoms and signs of gastrointestinal mucormycosis include fever, abdominal distention, nausea, vomiting, abdominal pain, diarrhea, melena, hematemesis, hematochezia, and masslike appendiceal and ileal lesions. An increasing number of cases of gastrointestinal mucormycosis in immunocompetent hosts are being reported worldwide.[12]

Disseminated Mucormycosis

Disseminated mucormycosis is rarely apparent antemortem. Severely immunosuppressed patients (e.g., those with prolonged and profound neutropenia, allogeneic stem cell transplant recipients with severe graft-versus-host disease) and patients receiving deferoxamine iron chelation therapy are at the highest risk. Symptoms vary depending on the site of dissemination and degree of vascular infarction of the affected organs. The most common organ as source of dissemination is the lung, and the most common site of spread is the brain.

Diagnosis of disseminated mucormycosis is challenging and requires a high level of suspicion because the infection may present as an unexpected acute vascular event. Biopsy of suspected sites is critical because of the low yield of blood cultures and suboptimal recovery of the fungus from respiratory specimens. Without appropriate timely treatment, virtually all patients with disseminated mucormycosis die.

Rare Clinical Presentations of Mucormycosis

Mucormycosis has protean manifestations that involve any organ. Authors have reported isolated cases of tracheal, mediastinal, bone, heart, kidney, otitis externa, and corneal involvement. More recently, there have been reports of renal mucormycosis in patients with intravenous drug abuse and/or those receiving corticosteroids. Cerebral mucormycosis, often presenting as brain abscess involving the basal ganglia and in conjunction with infective endocarditis, has been typically observed in patients using illicit intravenous drugs.[13] Reports of peritonitis in patients undergoing continuous ambulatory peritoneal dialysis have been rare. In all cases of device-related mucormycosis, prompt removal of the device and several weeks of systemic antifungal therapy are essential for resolution of the infection.

DIAGNOSIS

The clinical signs and symptoms of mucormycosis are nonspecific. Therefore a high level of suspicion in susceptible patient populations is of paramount importance.[14] Biopsy analysis and culture from sterile sites remain critical. Tissue swabs and cultures of sputum, sinus secretions, and bronchoalveolar lavage fluid are usually nondiagnostic. For example, fungal contamination of clinical specimens occurs because the small size of sporangiospores (approximately 6 μm in width) allows easy dispersion via the airborne route. Particles of this size may remain airborne even with very slight movements in air and contaminate clinical samples. Therefore growth in culture may not represent clinically significant invasive mucormycosis. However, the value of Mucorales-positive cultures (especially repetitive cultures) as an important indication of infection in immunocompromised patients is quite high. The site of infection has a major impact on the likelihood of histopathologic diagnosis. With their ease of accessibility, sinuses are the major site of definite infection.

Histopathology

A variety of stains, including hematoxylin and eosin, Grocott-Gomori methenamine-silver nitrate, and periodic acid–Schiff, reveal characteristic hyphal elements in tissue. Histopathologic examination of infected tissue typically shows characteristic broad (3 to 25 μm in diameter), thin-walled, primarily aseptate hyphae; focal bulbous dilation; and nondichotomous irregular branching at occasional right angles accompanying tissue necrosis and fungal angioinvasion (see Fig. 320-1). Perineural invasion is found in 90% of tissues containing nerves. The inflammatory responses to mucormycosis can range from neutrophilic, granulomatous, and/or pyogranulomatous to minimal inflammation with hemorrhage. Also, fungal hyphae can be examined directly using a potassium hydroxide preparation of a tissue specimen or bronchial alveolar lavage fluid. Although contamination is always a possibility, discovery of fungal elements in a specimen obtained from an immunocompromised host is considered significant. Treatment with fluorescent stains such as Calcofluor White and Blankofluor may enhance detection of hyphal elements during microscopic examination. Improved staining procedures may be important when the number of organisms is small or the amount of tissue is limited.

Culture

Mucorales fungi characteristically produce large, ribbon-like hyphae with irregular diameters and only occasionally septa, resulting in characterization of these organisms primarily as aseptate fungi. Identification can be confirmed by observing the characteristic saclike fruiting structures (sporangia), which produce internally spherical yellow or brown spores (sporangiospores). Spores range from 3 to 11 μm in diameter and are easily aerosolized. Blood cultures are rarely positive for these pathogens despite their angioinvasive nature. Paradoxically, even when fungal hyphae are seen in histopathologic analysis, fungal cultures may not be positive because of the friability of nonseptated hyphae, making them more susceptible to damage during tissue manipulation. However, collection of several proper clinical specimens is important. Recovery of Mucorales from tissue can be improved by mincing (not homogenizing) tissue specimens and using culture techniques that simulate in vivo fungal growth, including incubation at 35° to 37° C under relatively semianaerobic conditions.

The importance of early differentiation of Mucorales from more common opportunistic molds such as *Aspergillus* species has generated considerable interest in development of culture- or histopathology-independent diagnostic tests such as detection of specific antigens or nucleic acids using polymerase chain reaction or in situ hybridization techniques. Molecular techniques for detecting Mucorales are few, not widely available, and investigational but promising.[15] This is an important unmet need for the management of mucormycosis.

TREATMENT   Rx

Approach to the management of suspected mucormycosis and assessment of treatment response are shown in Figure 320-2. Successful treatment of mucormycosis relies on a multifaceted strategy that includes (1) aggressive attempts at diagnosis and rapid initiation of effective antifungal therapy, (2) extensive surgical débridement, and (3) rapid control of underlying medical conditions.[16]

Again, early diagnosis is critical to the outcome. Small focal lesions can be surgically resected before they progress to involve critical structures or distal organs. Patients often have indolent clinical presentations until extensive invasion or dissemination of the infection occurs.

Antifungal Therapy

Delayed administration of systemic antifungal therapy increases the probability of patient death. Most of the knowledge about the activity of currently used antifungals comes from small case series, anecdotes, and animal models of infection. Therefore the optimal treatment approach is uncertain. Most of the clinical experience has been with amphotericin B. Previously, the recommended antifungal therapy for mucormycosis included amphotericin B deoxycholate at the maximum tolerated dosage, usually 1.0 to 1.5 mg/kg/day. The nephrotoxic and systemic toxic effects of regular amphotericin B led to the development of the lipid formulations of amphotericin B (liposomal amphotericin B, amphotericin B lipid complex, amphotericin B colloidal dispersion). These agents are less nephrotoxic than regular amphotericin B and can be given at higher doses (e.g., 5 to 10 mg/kg per day); however, there is no convincing evidence that this strategy is associated with improved outcomes.[17] Lipid formulations of amphotericin B are now considered the drugs of choice for mucormycosis. Furthermore, use of percutaneous or aerosolized amphotericin B in conjunction with concomitant systemic therapy has been successful in selected patients with pulmonary mucormycosis. Topical therapy with amphotericin B as well as other polyenes (natamycin) may be effective against primary cutaneous and ocular mucormycosis. Treatment of mucormycosis with amphotericin B–based combinations has been successful in small retrospective case series. In particular, a benefit has been suggested for echinocandin-liposomal amphotericin B combination in 41 diabetic patients with rhino-orbital mucormycosis compared with the ones who received amphotericin B lipid complex (ABLC) or liposomal amphotericin B alone. This benefit was most pronounced in patients with cerebral involvement. In contrast, there is no evidence that combination therapy is beneficial in patients with underlying hematologic cancer who develop mucormycosis.[18]

Although azoles traditionally have been inactive against Mucorales, the new broad-spectrum triazole posaconazole has demonstrated promising activity.

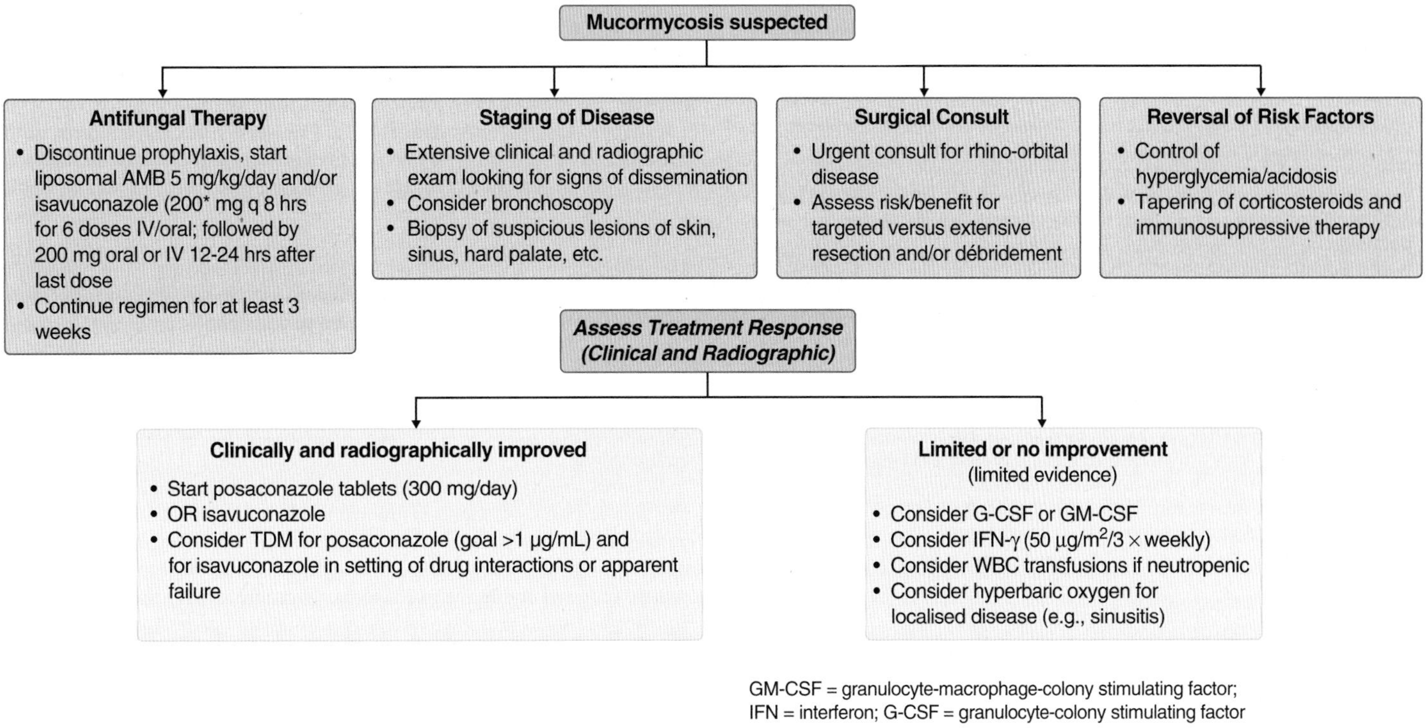

```
                        ┌─────────────────────────┐
                        │  Mucormycosis suspected │
                        └─────────────────────────┘
```

Antifungal Therapy
- Discontinue prophylaxis, start liposomal AMB 5 mg/kg/day and/or isavuconazole (200* mg q 8 hrs for 6 doses IV/oral; followed by 200 mg oral or IV 12-24 hrs after last dose
- Continue regimen for at least 3 weeks

Staging of Disease
- Extensive clinical and radiographic exam looking for signs of dissemination
- Consider bronchoscopy
- Biopsy of suspicious lesions of skin, sinus, hard palate, etc.

Surgical Consult
- Urgent consult for rhino-orbital disease
- Assess risk/benefit for targeted versus extensive resection and/or débridement

Reversal of Risk Factors
- Control of hyperglycemia/acidosis
- Tapering of corticosteroids and immunosuppressive therapy

Assess Treatment Response (Clinical and Radiographic)

Clinically and radiographically improved
- Start posaconazole tablets (300 mg/day)
- OR isavuconazole
- Consider TDM for posaconazole (goal >1 µg/mL) and for isavuconazole in setting of drug interactions or apparent failure

Limited or no improvement (limited evidence)
- Consider G-CSF or GM-CSF
- Consider IFN-γ (50 µg/m²/3 × weekly)
- Consider WBC transfusions if neutropenic
- Consider hyperbaric oxygen for localised disease (e.g., sinusitis)

GM-CSF = granulocyte-macrophage-colony stimulating factor; IFN = interferon; G-CSF = granulocyte-colony stimulating factor

FIGURE 320-2. Diagram of the management approach to patients with suspected mucormycosis. *200 mg of isavuconazole = 372 mg of isavuconazonium sulfate.

Among open-label studies and retrospective surveys evaluating posaconazole suspension as salvage therapy (800 mg/day) in patients with refractory mucormycosis, the agent showed a response rate approaching 70%. Furthermore, posaconazole has been well tolerated. Determining whether posaconazole alone or combined with a lipid formulation of amphotericin B or other agent (e.g., deferasirox) is of value requires further study. Posaconazole has limitations because absorption of the oral suspension is suboptimal in patients with mucositis, severe diarrhea, acid suppression therapy, or poor oral intake. Absorption of oral posaconazole is maximized when administered with high-fat foods in separate doses (four times daily). Finally, steady-state plasma concentrations of posaconazole are not reached until around 1 week of therapy. The new formula of posaconazole (posaconazole tablets 300 mg/daily) has not been studied adequately in mucormycosis. In a recent single-arm open-label trial of 37 patients with mucormycosis, the new triazole isavuconazole (loading dose 372 mg q 8 hrs for 6 doses IV/oral; followed by 372 mg oral or IV 12 to 24 hrs after last dose) was shown to have similar efficacy compared with amphotericin B in a matched case-control analysis.[19]

The duration of antifungal therapy should be determined on an individual basis. Near-normalization of radiographic imaging, negative follow-up biopsy specimens, and cultures from the affected site, as well as recovery from immunosuppression, are important indicators for stopping antifungal therapy.

Surgery

Surgical débridement of cutaneous lesions is crucial and must be done without delay because of the aggressively invasive nature of mucormycosis. A coordinated effort among all subspecialties involved (surgery, infectious diseases, head and neck, ophthalmology, pathology, clinical microbiology, and plastic surgery) is crucial, and the internist can play a vital role coordinating it.

Repeated removal of necrotic tissue or aggressive surgical measures such as enucleation of the eye may be required for control of the infection. Decisions regarding the extent of débridement are often made at the bedside. A CT scan or MRI before surgery and intraoperative frozen section analysis help determine the extent of tissue and tissue margin involvement. Low platelet counts, as may be seen in patients with underlying hematologic malignancies, must be corrected with transfusions before surgical intervention. Unfortunately, bleeding problems can limit surgical options. Surgery in conjunction with systemic antifungal therapy has been shown to significantly improve survival rates.

Management of Comorbidity and Adjunct Treatments

Adjunct measures have been proposed to improve host immunity and tissue viability, as well as to impede fungal proliferation. Rapid correction of underlying conditions, such as control of hyperglycemia, reversal of ketoacidosis,[20] rapid tapering of glucocorticoid therapy, and discontinuation of deferoxamine treatment, can influence outcomes. Hyperbaric oxygen is a beneficial adjunct therapy for mucormycosis, particularly in diabetic patients with rhinocerebral disease. Specifically, the increased oxygen pressure achieved seems to improve neutrophil activity and oxidative killing by polyene antifungals. Also, high concentrations of oxygen can inhibit growth of the organism in vitro and improve the rate of wound healing by increasing the release of tissue growth factors. However, this treatment has not been studied vigorously to determine efficacy and cannot be routinely recommended. Investigators have proposed several immune augmentation strategies as adjunct therapy, including administration of cytokines (e.g., granulocyte colony-stimulating factor [G-CSF], interferon). In refractory neutropenic patients, granulocyte transfusion may be beneficial until granulocyte recovery. These adjunct measures, although promising, are yet to be studied sufficiently. Finally, the new iron chelator deferasirox has been considered as an adjunct antifungal agent based on preclinical studies and very limited human experience with patients with refractory mucormycosis. Results of the small randomized, double-blinded DEFEAT Mucor trial were published in 2012.[A1] Twenty patients with proven or probable mucormycosis were randomized to treatment with liposomal amphotericin B plus deferasirox (20 mg/kg per day for 14 days) or liposomal amphotericin B plus placebo. Although reported adverse events were similar between the two study groups, significantly higher mortality rates were found in patients randomized to receive deferasirox at 30 days (45% vs. 11%) and 90 days (82% vs. 22%, P = .01). However, patients in the deferasirox arm were more likely than patients in the placebo arm to have active malignancy, neutropenia, and/or corticosteroid therapy, and less likely to have received additional antifungals, making the results of this pilot trial less conclusive. Nevertheless, currently available data do not support a role for initial deferasirox therapy for mucormycosis. Further knowledge of the unique virulence attributes of Mucorales based on genomic analysis might aid the development of novel therapeutic targets.

Grade A Reference

A1. Spellberg B, Ibrahim AS, Chin-Hong PV, et al. The Deferasirox-AmBisome Therapy for Mucormycosis (DEFEAT Mucor) study: a randomized, double-blinded, placebo-controlled trial. *J Antimicrob Chemother.* 2012;67:715-722.

GENERAL REFERENCES

For the General References and other additional features, please visit Expert Consult at https://expertconsult.inkling.com.

321

PNEUMOCYSTIS PNEUMONIA

JOSEPH A. KOVACS

DEFINITION

Pneumocystis jirovecii is a fungus that causes pneumonia almost exclusively in immunodeficient patients. *Pneumocystis* pneumonia (PCP) has been the most common life-threatening opportunistic infection in persons with HIV/AIDS. Although the frequency of PCP has decreased in HIV-infected patients first in association with the widespread use of anti-*Pneumocystis* prophylaxis and later with the introduction of effective combination antiretroviral therapy for HIV/AIDS, it continues to be seen with regularity in HIV-infected and other immunodeficient patients.[1] Over the past two decades, there has been a marked increase in outbreaks of PCP among renal transplant recipients, especially in Europe and Australia.

The Pathogen

Pneumocystis is an ascomycete fungus of the subphylum Taphrinomycotina, most closely related to *Schizosaccharomyces*, *Taphrina*, and *Saitoella* species of fungi. Molecular studies including whole genome sequencing have demonstrated that the genus *Pneumocystis* includes a group of closely related organisms that are unique species, each of which can infect only a single host species.[2] This has led to the application of species names to the group of organisms previously called *Pneumocystis carinii*, which now is reserved for a species that infects rats. The organism infecting humans has been renamed *P. jirovecii*. Despite the name change, the acronym PCP (for _P_neumocystis _p_neumonia) continues to be used to designate the disease in humans.

Pneumocystis species show a strict host specificity: attempts to transmit, for example, rat or human *Pneumocystis* to mice have been unsuccessful. Molecular evolutionary studies suggest that *Pneumocystis* species coevolved with their hosts, with rat and mouse *Pneumocystis* diverging an estimated 33 million years ago. Studies of *Pneumocystis* have been substantially hampered by an inability to grow any species in culture for a sustained period. Thus, the life cycle of *Pneumocystis* is unknown, although putative life cycles based on morphologic studies have been proposed; there is substantial evidence supporting a sexual phase in the life cycle. There are two easily recognized forms of the organism: trophic forms ($\approx$2 to 6 μm in diameter) and cysts (also called asci; $\approx$6 to 8 μm in diameter), which can contain up to eight intracystic bodies (ascospores); additional intermediate forms are also seen. Trophic forms, which have an amorphous shape, are estimated to outnumber cysts, which are spherical, by approximately 10:1 in an infected lung. The genome of *P. jirovecii*, approximately 8.2 million base pairs, is markedly contracted compared with other fungi and has lost multiple metabolic pathways, including enzymes needed to synthesize all amino acids de novo, enzymes needed for chitin synthesis and degradation, and carbonic anhydrase, an enzyme important for regulation of intracellular pH.[3] These findings suggest that that *Pneumocystis* lives exclusively in the mammalian host and cannot survive in the external environment.

Pneumocystis has evolved mechanisms to avoid host innate and adaptive immune responses. β-Glucans are masked by surface proteins, and enzymes needed to synthesize outer chain mannans have been lost; both can be recognized by host pattern recognition receptors. The most abundant surface protein of *Pneumocystis*, the major surface glycoprotein, is found on both cysts and trophic forms and is encoded by a multicopy gene family, only one of which is apparently expressed in a given organism; this provides *Pneumocystis* with the potential for antigenic variability. Although to date only a single *Pneumocystis* species has been found that infects humans, molecular typing techniques have demonstrated a high level of diversity among human *Pneumocystis* isolates.

EPIDEMIOLOGY

Pneumocystis has a worldwide distribution. Serologic studies show a high prevalence of anti-*Pneumocystis* antibodies in all populations studied to date. In America and Europe, serologic studies have demonstrated that most humans develop antibodies to *Pneumocystis* by an early age, suggesting that this is a ubiquitous organism. In support of this, an autopsy study in infants younger than 1 year with no major underlying medical problems identified *Pneumocystis* infection in lung tissue by polymerase chain reaction (PCR) in 100% of cases.

Animal studies have demonstrated that *Pneumocystis* is transmitted by the respiratory route and that cysts are required for transmission. Human infection appears to be transmitted in the same manner. There is no evidence that water or fomites play a role in transmission. A small number of animal studies and very limited human data suggest that transmission can occur transplacentally.

Given the strict host specificity of *Pneumocystis*, the source of organisms infecting humans is presumably other humans, by either direct or indirect exposure; *Pneumocystis* is not a zoonosis. PCR-based studies have identified *Pneumocystis* DNA in air sampled in close proximity to patients with PCP, and outbreaks, especially in renal transplant patients, have been linked to a single strain of *Pneumocystis*. These findings suggest that patients with PCP can transmit it to other susceptible patients.[4] Because clinically apparent PCP is rare, and given the high penetration of infection into healthy human populations at a young age, *Pneumocystis* infection is also likely acquired from apparently healthy humans, in whom subclinical infection (either asymptomatic or minimally symptomatic) must be quite common to allow such rapid and broad dissemination. The high frequency of detection in infants suggests an important role in transmission.

Although infection with *Pneumocystis* is widespread in immunocompetent hosts, it does not appear to cause significant disease. Clinically significant PCP occurs exclusively in patients with severe levels of immunodeficiency that are usually associated with a high risk for other opportunistic pathogens. Populations at risk include those with congenital immunodeficiencies (Chapter 236), especially severe combined immunodeficiency (SCID), hyper–immunoglobulin M (IgM) syndrome, and to a lesser extent, interleukin-21 (IL-21) receptor deficiency; patients with HIV infection (Chapter 361) and human T-lymphotropic virus-1–associated lymphoma (Chapter 176); patients receiving chemotherapy for the treatment of malignancies, especially lymphoma; transplant patients receiving immunosuppressive therapy; and patients being treated with prolonged courses of immunosuppressive drugs (Chapter 32), especially corticosteroids, including intermittent therapy, for diseases such as granulomatosis with polyangiitis (formerly Wegener granulomatosis), systemic lupus erythematosus, IgA nephropathy, certain dermatologic diseases, and breast cancer. Biologic agents (Chapter 33) such as alemtuzumab, rituximab, and those targeting tumor necrosis factor-α (TNF-α) are also associated with an increased absolute risk for PCP (e.g., 0.18 to 0.4% in patients receiving anti-TNF-α agents in Japan), as are idelalisib, ibrutinib, gemcitabine, and iguratimod (the latter is approved in China and Japan).[5,6]

Among patients with HIV infection, the best predictor of the risk for developing PCP is the CD4 count: patients with CD4 counts less than 200 cells/μL, and especially those with CD4 counts less than 100 cells/μL, are at greatest risk. Patients with a prior history of PCP and those with unexplained fever, weight loss, or thrush are also at increased risk. Among other patient populations, laboratory parameters are not as useful in quantifying risk, although non-HIV patients with CD4 counts less than 200 cells/μL also appear to be at increased risk.[7] Additional information on risk is provided in the section on prevention.

For many years, development of PCP was thought to result from a reactivation of latent infection by organisms that remained viable following infection at an early age, similar to tuberculosis. However, recent molecular epidemiologic studies based on the detection of mutations in the dihydropteroate synthase (DHPS) gene of *Pneumocystis*, as well as genotyping of isolates from outbreaks of PCP primarily in renal transplant patients, have provided compelling evidence that the infecting strain is often recently acquired. Molecular studies have further documented that in the majority of non-outbreak cases of PCP, multiple strains can be identified in respiratory samples. In patients who develop recurrent PCP, this recurrence can be due to relapse, especially for early recurrences, or to reinfection with a novel strain. Recurrent PCP occurs almost exclusively in HIV-infected patients, in whom the risk was greater than 50% early in the AIDS epidemic, before the availability of combination antiretroviral therapy (cART) and the broad use of anti-*Pneumocystis* prevention.

PATHOBIOLOGY

Animal studies have provided important insights into the pathogenesis of *Pneumocystis* infection. Exposure for as little as 1 day to a *Pneumocystis*-infected animal results in transmission of infection. In healthy animals, an adaptive immune response develops by approximately 5 to 6 weeks, which leads to control and clearance before the organism burden produces symptoms. CD4 cells are critical to this control, although other populations, including B cells and macrophages, also are important; B cells appear to have a major role in antigen presentation.[8,9] CD8 cells can contribute to the associated inflammation. In immunodeficient animal models, inability to control *Pneumocystis* replication leads to severe pneumonia by 2 to 3 months. Limited human data suggest a similar time course. Host inflammatory responses, in part attributable to organism-derived β-glucans, appear to play a critical role in the development of pulmonary symptoms.[10] This may account for the development of symptoms of PCP in patients in whom corticosteroids are being tapered, as well as the exacerbation of hypoxia that develops approximately 4 days after the initiation of anti-*Pneumocystis* therapy (in the absence of concomitant corticosteroid therapy).

The lung pathology in patients with PCP is characteristic. Staining with hematoxylin and eosin demonstrates an acellular, foamy, eosinophilic, intra-alveolar exudate associated with mild interstitial inflammation (Fig. 321-1). With disease progression, hyaline membrane formation and interstitial as well as intraluminal fibrosis develop. Although methenamine silver stain highlights cysts scattered throughout the eosinophilic exudate, based on Giemsa staining of thin sections as well as electron micrographs, this exudate is composed almost entirely of *Pneumocystis* organisms. Atypical pathology, including non-caseating granulomas and intrapulmonary cystic changes, can also be seen.

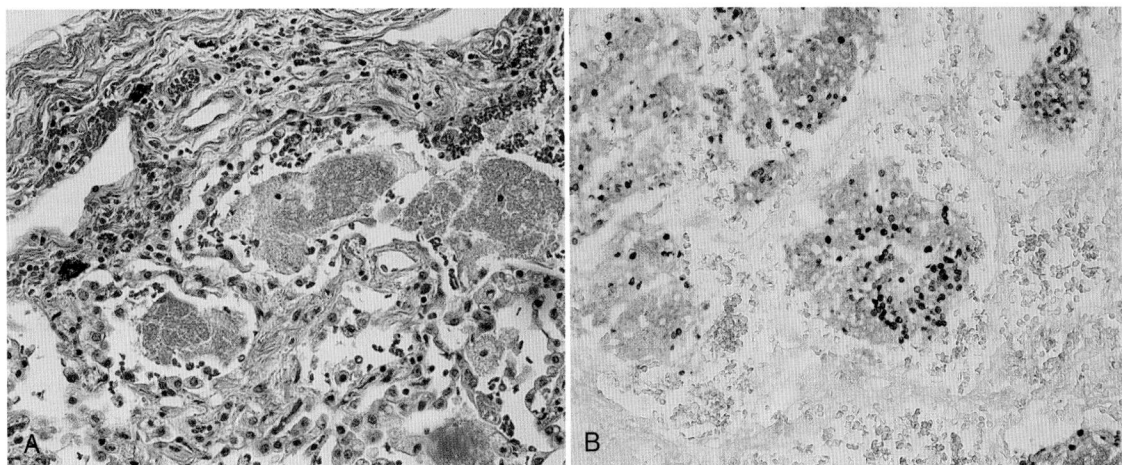

FIGURE 321-1. Histopathology of the lung of a patient who died from *Pneumocystis* pneumonia (PCP). **A,** The hematoxylin and eosin–stained section shows the characteristic acellular, eosinophilic, intra-alveolar exudate that is typical of PCP. **B,** Methenamine silver staining of lung tissue from the same patient demonstrates black-staining cysts scattered throughout the intra-alveolar exudates.

As noted earlier, patients with certain congenital immunodeficiencies, especially SCID patients, who have global T- and B-cell defects, and hyper-IgM syndrome patients, whose primary defect is in CD40-CD40L signaling, are at increased risk for developing PCP. Among HIV-infected patients, polymorphisms in the gene for FcγRIIa and in the chemokine receptor gene for CCRL2 were each associated with an increased risk for developing PCP in single studies.

CLINICAL MANIFESTATIONS

In nonimmunosuppressed humans, no well-defined clinical syndrome is associated with *Pneumocystis* infection. *Pneumocystis* has been identified in infants by PCR and may be associated with a mild respiratory syndrome, but a postulated association with sudden infant death syndrome has not been supported by data from well-controlled studies. *Pneumocystis* has been detected by PCR in pulmonary samples from patients with chronic obstructive pulmonary disease (COPD), and a history of PCP was associated with an obstructive pattern on spirometry in HIV-infected patients, but what role, if any, it plays in the development or progression of COPD (Chapter 82) remains to be elucidated.

Pneumonia is the primary clinical manifestation of *Pneumocystis* infection in immunosuppressed patients. PCP typically presents with a fever, nonproductive cough, and shortness of breath that initially occurs only on exertion but, without therapy, inevitably progresses to dyspnea at rest. Only one or two of these symptoms may be present initially. Development of symptoms may be insidious, over the course of a few weeks, as is common in patients with HIV infection[11]; a more rapid onset, over the course of only a few days, is more common in non-AIDS patients. Purulent sputum production is unusual, and chills and chest pain occur in a minority of patients. Patients with HIV infection may present with other manifestations of immunodeficiency, including weight loss and thrush.

In non-AIDS patients, corticosteroids are a common risk factor.[12] Clinical manifestations may develop as corticosteroids are being tapered, which presumably represents the unmasking of an inflammatory response to the infection as immunosuppression is decreased.

Rarely, extrapulmonary disease can involve the skin, eye (choroiditis), central nervous system, bone marrow, thyroid, spleen, liver, gastrointestinal tract, lymph node, or multiple organs in disseminated disease. Extrapulmonary disease can occur with or without concurrent pneumonia. Use of aerosol pentamidine for prophylaxis has been associated with an increased risk for extrapulmonary disease in HIV-infected patients, but even in that circumstance, it remains extremely rare. Symptoms are related to the particular site involved and may be nonspecific; diagnosis is often made at autopsy.

DIAGNOSIS

Given the nonspecific symptoms, especially early in the disease process, clinicians must have a high index of suspicion for PCP even in patients not known to be immunosuppressed; many patients with HIV infection are unaware of their status until they present with an opportunistic infection. Knowledge of the most recent CD4 count is helpful in assessing HIV-infected patients because PCP is rare in those whose CD4 counts are above 200 cells/μL.

Physical examination and routine laboratory tests are usually not helpful in making the diagnosis because many pulmonary processes, both infectious and noninfectious, can present in a similar manner. Moreover, even though patients may be tachypneic and appear to be in respiratory distress, those presenting early in the disease course may have an entirely normal lung examination. Lymphopenia is common but is a manifestation of the underlying disease rather than PCP. Lactate dehydrogenase levels may be elevated but have poor specificity.

The initial evaluation should include a chest radiograph and assessment of arterial oxygenation, either by blood gas measurement or by pulse oximetry. The chest radiograph typically shows perihilar or diffuse bilateral interstitial infiltrates that progress to a diffuse alveolar pattern (Fig. 321-2). However, PCP has been associated with unilateral disease, focal disease, consolidation, nodules, cavities, pneumothorax, and, rarely, pleural effusions. In up to 30% of patients with HIV infection, the chest radiograph appears normal; in this situation, a computed tomography (CT) scan of the chest, especially high-resolution CT, is invariably abnormal, usually showing a patchy or diffuse ground-glass pattern (see Fig. 321-2).[13]

Arterial oxygenation at rest is often abnormal, although in 30% or more of cases, it is within normal limits. Exercise testing induces desaturation and an increase in the alveolar-arterial oxygen (A-a O_2) gradient in the majority of patients with PCP, even those with normal oxygenation at rest or a normal chest radiograph. An abnormal resting diffusing capacity is also common. However,

although many of these tests have a high sensitivity for PCP, their specificity is poor because other respiratory processes show similar abnormalities.

Serologic tests are generally not helpful in diagnosing PCP. Although antibody titers against recombinant *Pneumocystis* proteins such as major surface glycoprotein may be increased in patients with PCP, such tests have not shown utility for diagnosis in individual patients. Although serum and bronchoalveolar lavage (BAL) β-D-glucan levels are elevated in many patients, this again is a nonspecific test because other fungal infections can also lead to elevations, and conditions unrelated to fungal infection can yield false-positive results. Thus, while it appears to have a high sensitivity, and PCP is less likely in patients with a low level, to date there are inadequate data from well-conducted prospective trials to support routine use of this assay for the definitive diagnosis of PCP.

Because *Pneumocystis* cannot be cultured, a definitive diagnosis of PCP requires detection of the organism in a pulmonary sample. This can be accomplished by any number of colorimetric or immunologic stains or by molecular techniques. Until the development of anti-*Pneumocystis* monoclonal antibodies in the 1980s, colorimetric stains were routinely used, and they continue to be used at many centers owing to cost considerations. Such stains include Gomori methenamine silver, toluidine blue O, Gram-Weigert, and cresyl echt violet, which stain the cyst wall of *Pneumocystis*, as well as Giemsa-type stains, including Diff-Quik, which can stain both trophic forms, the more abundant form of the organism, and intracystic bodies within cysts, but not the cyst wall. *Pneumocystis* can also be detected by Calcofluor white, Papanicolaou, periodic acid–Schiff, and, rarely, Gram stain. None of the colorimetric stains is specific for *Pneumocystis*. Cyst wall stains such as Gomori methenamine silver and toluidine blue O can stain other fungi, and Giemsa-type stains also stain background cells and cellular debris. The latter requires substantial expertise for correct interpretation.

Immunofluorescent assays using anti-*Pneumocystis* monoclonal antibodies provide a number of advantages over colorimetric stains.[14] They are specific for *Pneumocystis* and do not show cross-reactivity with other organisms, including fungi; they can be performed and interpreted rapidly; and they have increased sensitivity, especially when examining induced sputum samples (Fig. 321-3).

Molecular techniques, primarily PCR-based assays, have been extensively evaluated for diagnosing PCP. PCR assays are 10- to 100-fold more sensitive than stains for the detection of *Pneumocystis*; this may allow for diagnosis using samples such as oral washes, which have a lower organism burden than induced sputum or BAL.[15] This increased sensitivity, however, is associated with decreased specificity because it allows the detection of organisms in patients ultimately shown not to have PCP. The latter situation presumably reflects colonization or subclinical infection that does not require specific anti-*Pneumocystis* therapy. Quantitative PCR assays may help distinguish colonization from clinically significant infection.[16] PCR-based assays are being used with increasing frequency for definitive diagnosis but lack standardization among laboratories. The most commonly used gene targets for PCR amplification include the mitochondrial large subunit rRNA gene and the MSG gene family. Rare false-negative results can result from mutations in the targeted gene.[17] There is no U.S. Food and Drug Administration–approved commercial product available in the United States, although commercial kits are available in Europe.

As detection methods for *Pneumocystis* improved, there was a parallel improvement in sample acquisition. Before the AIDS epidemic, open lung biopsy was required for diagnosis. During the 1980s, bronchoscopy, initially with brushings and biopsy, and subsequently with BAL, was shown to have a greater than 90% sensitivity for diagnosing PCP; BAL continues to be the primary diagnostic modality at many centers today. Although expectorated sputum has a low diagnostic yield, induced sputum, especially when combined with immunofluorescent staining, can have a sensitivity approaching 90%. However, in many centers the diagnostic yield is much lower, likely due in part to variability in the methods used for induction and processing. Ideally, sputum induction should be the first step in diagnosis, followed by bronchoscopy with BAL (Fig. 321-4). Bronchoscopic or open lung biopsy is only rarely needed to make the diagnosis. PCR analysis of expectorated sputum, nasopharyngeal aspirates, oropharyngeal wash samples, and whole blood samples has been diagnostic in limited studies.

The differential diagnosis of pulmonary infiltrates in immunosuppressed patients is very broad and includes infections such as adenovirus, cytomegalovirus, tuberculosis, cryptococcosis, histoplasmosis, aspergillosis, and toxoplasmosis, as well as noninfectious processes such as tumor, congestive heart failure, pulmonary emboli, radiation- and chemotherapy-induced pneumonitis, and, especially in HIV-infected patients, nonspecific interstitial pneumonitis and Kaposi sarcoma.

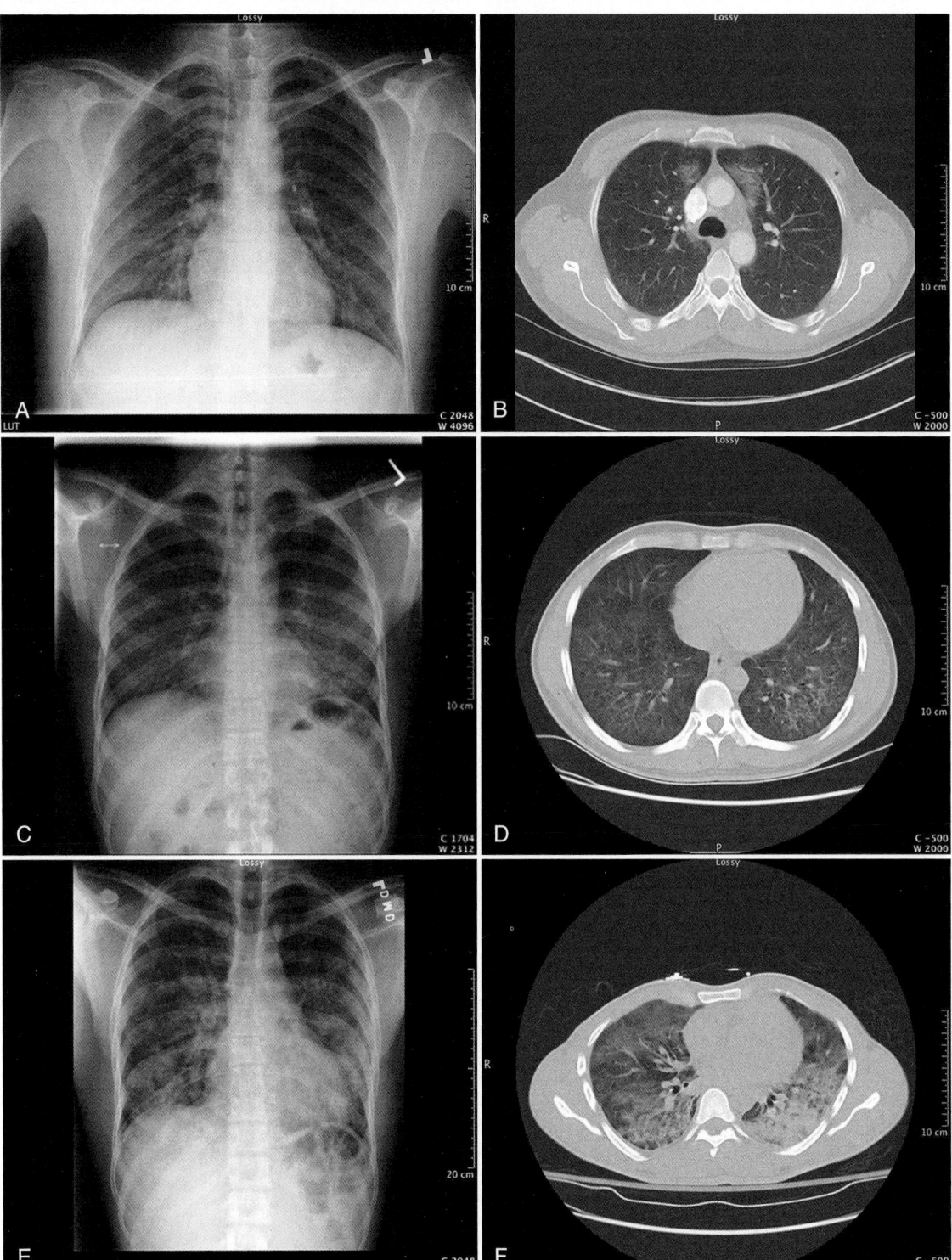

FIGURE 321-2. Chest radiographs (A, C, E) and corresponding computed tomography (CT) scans (B, D, F) from three HIV patients diagnosed with laboratory-confirmed *Pneumo-cystis* pneumonia. Patient 1 presented with no symptoms; had minimal abnormalities on an incidental chest radiograph (**A**), suggesting an interstitial process; and had focal infiltrates on CT (**B**). Patient 2 presented with fever and weight loss but no shortness of breath. Pulse oximetry demonstrated 99% saturation at rest, with a decrease to 89% with exercise. Chest radiograph (**C**) showed bilateral lower lobe infiltrates, and CT (**D**) showed bilateral lower lobe interstitial infiltrates with patches of ground-glass attenuation. Patient 3 presented with a 2-week history of fever, night sweats, shortness of breath, and weakness. His Pao$_2$ at diagnosis was 67 mm Hg, and his A-a O$_2$ gradient was 53 mm Hg. Chest radiograph (**E**) showed bilateral mid and lower lung field infiltrates, and CT (**F**) showed bilateral infiltrates with lower lung consolidation.

TREATMENT
Rx

Specific anti-*Pneumocystis* therapy should be initiated promptly when the diagnosis is suspected in a potentially susceptible patient.[18] Dosing regimens with documented efficacy are listed in Table 321-1. Although there are no controlled studies defining the optimal duration of therapy, HIV-infected patients should be treated for 21 days and non-HIV patients for at least 14 days.[19] For HIV-infected patients with moderate to severe disease (Pao$_2$ <70 mm Hg or A-a O$_2$ gradient >35 mm Hg), concomitant corticosteroid therapy should be administered.[A1] In contrast, the use of corticosteroids in non-HIV patients is not well defined, as discussed later. The diagnosis should be definitively confirmed by sputum induction or bronchoscopy as soon as possible; however, delaying such confirmation for a few days after the initiation of therapy will not decrease the diagnostic yield because organisms can be detected in clinical samples for more than 3 weeks after the initiation of therapy. Empirical therapy in the absence of a confirmed diagnosis runs the risk of delaying appropriate therapy for another infection, giving inappropriate therapy with known toxicities, and performing a definitive procedure such as bronchoscopy when the patient is failing therapy and consequently has more severe pulmonary compromise.

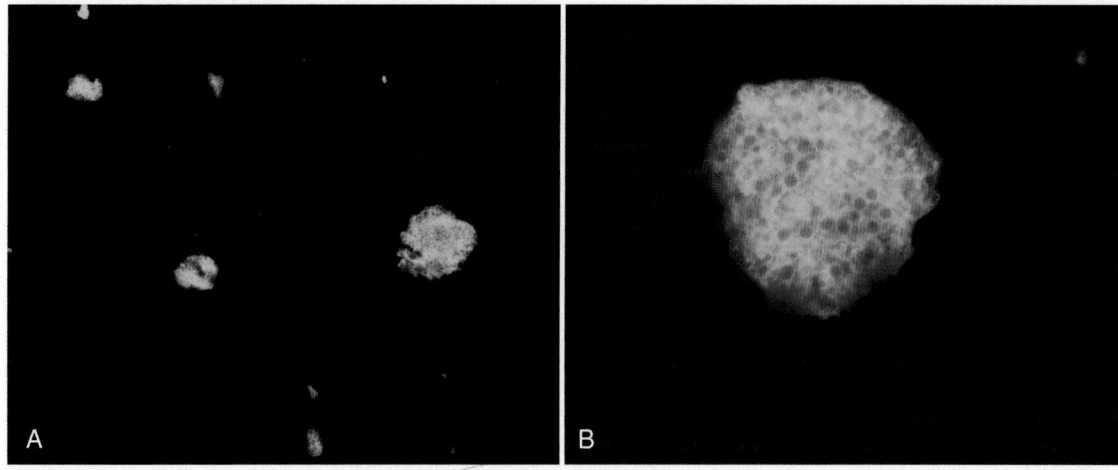

FIGURE 321-3. Immunofluorescent detection of *Pneumocystis* using a direct fluorescent antibody test to examine an induced sputum sample. A, Low power (100× original) allows visualization of multiple clusters of organisms staining bright green. B, With high power (400× original), individual organisms can be seen within a single cluster.

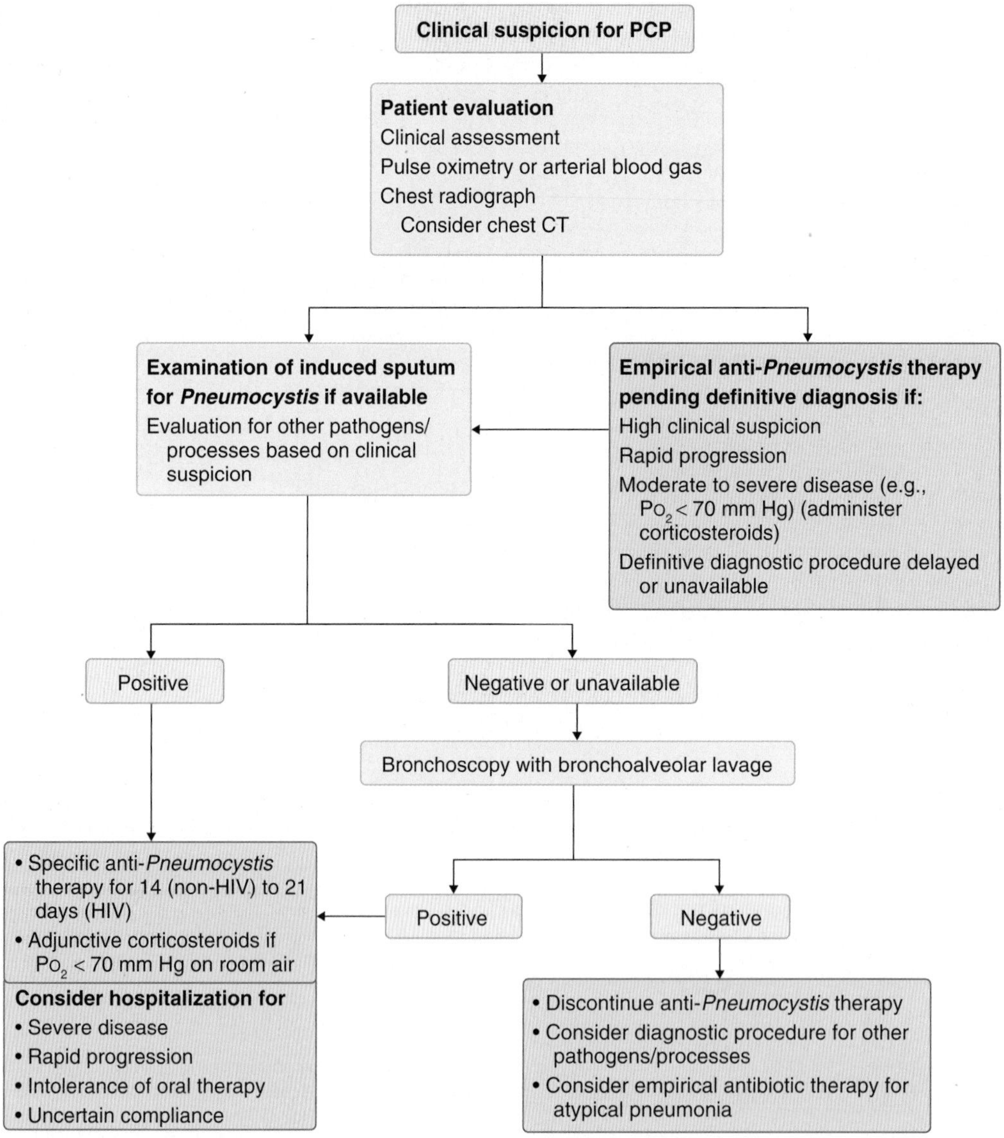

Clinical suspicion for PCP

Patient evaluation
Clinical assessment
Pulse oximetry or arterial blood gas
Chest radiograph
    Consider chest CT

Examination of induced sputum for *Pneumocystis* if available
Evaluation for other pathogens/processes based on clinical suspicion

Empirical anti-*Pneumocystis* therapy pending definitive diagnosis if:
High clinical suspicion
Rapid progression
Moderate to severe disease (e.g., $Po_2 < 70$ mm Hg) (administer corticosteroids)
Definitive diagnostic procedure delayed or unavailable

Positive

Negative or unavailable

Bronchoscopy with bronchoalveolar lavage

Positive

Negative

• Specific anti-*Pneumocystis* therapy for 14 (non-HIV) to 21 days (HIV)
• Adjunctive corticosteroids if $Po_2 < 70$ mm Hg on room air

Consider hospitalization for
• Severe disease
• Rapid progression
• Intolerance of oral therapy
• Uncertain compliance

• Discontinue anti-*Pneumocystis* therapy
• Consider diagnostic procedure for other pathogens/processes
• Consider empirical antibiotic therapy for atypical pneumonia

FIGURE 321-4. Algorithm for the evaluation of patients with suspected *Pneumocystis* pneumonia (PCP). CT = computed tomography; HIV = human immunodeficiency virus.

TABLE 321-1 DRUG REGIMENS FOR TREATMENT OF *PNEUMOCYSTIS* PNEUMONIA (PCP)

INDICATION	REGIMEN PREFERENCE	DRUG	ROUTE	DOSE	COMMENTS
Mild PCP: Pao_2 ≥70 mm Hg or A-a O_2 gradient ≤35 mm Hg	Preferred	Trimethoprim-sulfamethoxazole (TMP-SMX)	PO	2 double-strength (160 TMP + 800 SMX) tablets tid	
	Alternative	Trimethoprim plus	PO	5 mg/kg tid (15 mg/kg/d)	If possible test for G6PD deficiency before use
		Dapsone	PO	100 mg qd	
	Alternative	Clindamycin plus	PO	450 mg qid or 600 mg tid	If possible test for G6PD deficiency before use
		Primaquine	PO	30 mg (base) qd	
	Alternative	Atovaquone	PO	750 mg bid with food	
Moderate to severe PCP: Pao_2 <70 mm Hg or A-a O_2 gradient >35 mm Hg; moderate PCP (A-a O_2 gradient 35 to 45 mm Hg); can be treated with an oral regimen	Preferred	TMP-SMX	IV	5 mg/kg q8h TMP and 25 mg/kg q8h SMX (15 mg/kg/d TMP and 75 mg/kg/d SMX)	May switch to oral therapy following clinical improvement
	Alternative	Pentamidine	IV	3-4 mg/kg qd	Infuse over >60 min
	Alternative	Clindamycin plus	IV	600 mg q6h or 900 mg q8h	May switch to oral therapy following clinical improvement
		Primaquine	PO	30 mg (base) qd	No parenteral formulation is available
Adjunctive therapy for moderate to severe PCP: Pao_2 <70 mm Hg or A-a O_2 gradient >35 mm Hg	Preferred	Prednisone	PO	40 mg bid, days 1-5; 40 mg qd, days 6-10; 20 mg qd days 11-21	Begin as early as possible and within 72 hr; efficacy if started later has not been demonstrated
	Preferred	Methylprednisolone	IV	30 mg bid, days 1-5; 30 mg qd, days 6-10; 15 mg qd days 11-21	Use if parenteral therapy is necessary

Note: HIV-infected patients should receive 21 days of therapy; non-HIV patients should receive at least 14 days of therapy. G6PD = glucose-6-phosphate dehydrogenase.

The treatment of choice for PCP or extrapulmonary *Pneumocystis* disease, regardless of severity, is trimethoprim-sulfamethoxazole, which combines inhibitors of two enzymes in the folate synthetic pathway of *Pneumocystis*: sulfamethoxazole, an inhibitor of dihydropteroate synthase (DHPS), and trimethoprim, an inhibitor of dihydrofolate reductase (DHFR).[20] Trimethoprim-sulfamethoxazole is available in both oral and intravenous formulations. Oral therapy should be reserved for patients with mild to moderate disease in whom poor absorption is not a concern. Outpatient therapy should be reserved for patients with mild to moderate disease who will reliably return for follow-up.

The high incidence of PCP during the early years of the AIDS epidemic led to the identification of a number of new agents with anti-*Pneumocystis* activity, and these were extensively evaluated in randomized controlled trials, primarily in HIV-infected patients. In patients with mild to moderate disease (A-a O_2 gradient <45 mm Hg), trimethoprim-sulfamethoxazole has superior efficacy compared with atovaquone and similar efficacy compared with trimethoprim-dapsone and clindamycin-primaquine. In smaller, lower power studies, trimethoprim-sulfamethoxazole and pentamidine showed similar efficacy.

The major toxicities associated with trimethoprim-sulfamethoxazole include fever, rash, neutropenia, thrombocytopenia, nausea, vomiting, and transaminase elevations. Hyperkalemia and crystalluria have also been reported, and hyponatremia is seen primarily in association with intravenous administration. Toxicities usually appear after the first week of therapy. Toxicities are much more common in HIV-infected patients, occurring in about 50 to 60%; 15 to 35% of these patients discontinue therapy because of the adverse events. Although folinic acid can decrease the toxicities associated with some DHFR inhibitors such as pyrimethamine, it should not be administered with trimethoprim-sulfamethoxazole; in one placebo-controlled trial, it did not decrease side effects but was associated with an increased risk for therapeutic failure and death.

Alternative regimens for patients with mild to moderate disease include trimethoprim-dapsone, clindamycin-primaquine, and atovaquone. Like sulfamethoxazole, dapsone is an inhibitor of *Pneumocystis* DHPS. Adverse reactions to trimethoprim-dapsone include rash, fever, nausea and vomiting, transaminase elevations, methemoglobinemia, anemia, and mild hyperkalemia. Approximately 20 to 30% of patients with adverse reactions to trimethoprim-sulfamethoxazole experience adverse reactions to trimethoprim-dapsone. Toxicities associated with clindamycin-primaquine include fever, rash, diarrhea, anemia, neutropenia, transaminase elevations, and methemoglobinemia (Chapter 149). For both dapsone and primaquine and, to a lesser extent, sulfamethoxazole, glucose-6-phosphate dehydrogenase deficiency (Chapter 152) can increase the risk for hemolytic anemia and methemoglobinemia. In a randomized trial comparing trimethoprim-sulfamethoxazole, trimethoprim-dapsone, and clindamycin-primaquine in 181 HIV-infected patients with mild to moderate disease, response rates and toxicities were similar among the three arms, with an overall therapeutic failure rate of 9% by day 21 and a dose-limiting toxicity rate of 31%. Serious transaminase elevations were more common in the trimethoprim-sulfamethoxazole group, and serious hematologic toxicities were more common in the clindamycin-primaquine group.

Atovaquone is a hydroxynaphthoquinone with activity against *Toxoplasma* and malaria as well as *Pneumocystis*. Atovaquone (early tablet formulation) was less effective than trimethoprim-sulfamethoxazole in a randomized trial in

HIV-infected patients with mild to moderate disease and showed a trend toward lesser efficacy compared with pentamidine in another study. Low serum atovaquone levels and preexisting diarrhea were associated with therapeutic failure. The current formulation is a suspension that has approximately 50% greater bioavailability than the tablet formulation, which may result in improved responses. Atovaquone should be taken with food because this increases its bioavailability, and it should be avoided in patients with potentially decreased gastrointestinal absorption (e.g., diarrhea). Efavirenz can decrease atovaquone plasma concentrations. Toxicities of atovaquone include rash, fever, transaminase elevations, nausea, vomiting, diarrhea, neutropenia, and anemia.

Therapeutic alternatives to trimethoprim-sulfamethoxazole for patients with disease requiring parenteral therapy are limited to clindamycin-primaquine (but only clindamycin is available for intravenous administration) and pentamidine. Caspofungin and other echinocandins, which are β-1,3-glucan synthase inhibitors, cannot be recommended because there have been no clinical trials documenting their efficacy; β-1,3-glucan is present in the cyst but not in the trophic form of the organism.

Pentamidine was the first drug demonstrated to have anti-*Pneumocystis* activity. Available data suggest that trimethoprim-sulfamethoxazole and pentamidine have similar efficacy; trimethoprim-sulfamethoxazole is the preferred regimen because the toxicities associated with pentamidine are more frequent and potentially more severe. Intravenous pentamidine was originally associated with severe hypotension, but a slow (>1 hour) infusion is usually well tolerated. Toxicities associated with pentamidine, which occur in about 50 to 60% of patients and frequently result in discontinuation of the drug, include nephrotoxicity, hypoglycemia, hyperglycemia, fever, neutropenia, thrombocytopenia, hypotension, hyperkalemia, transaminase elevations, and pancreatitis. Hypoglycemia may be life-threatening and may precede the development of hyperglycemia; hyperglycemia may be irreversible. Torsades de pointes (Chapter 59) has also rarely been reported.

Adjunctive Corticosteroid Therapy

Initiation of specific anti-*Pneumocystis* therapy is associated with deterioration in oxygenation after approximately 3 to 4 days; this likely results from a host inflammatory response to organisms damaged by therapy. Randomized controlled trials have demonstrated that the early addition of corticosteroids to specific anti-*Pneumocystis* therapy in HIV-infected patients can prevent this deterioration and improve survival, without a significant increase in opportunistic complications other than localized herpes simplex infection.[A1] In the largest such study, corticosteroid therapy was associated with a 50% decrease in respiratory failure and mortality; this benefit was limited to patients with moderate to severe disease (E-Fig. 321-1). For HIV-infected patients, corticosteroids and specific anti-*Pneumocystis* therapy should be started at the same time. The addition of corticosteroids after 72 hours has shown no benefit, although it is reasonable to add them if patients exhibit deterioration after this time. Although the optimal regimen has not been defined by controlled trials, the tapering regimen from the largest study is most commonly used (see Table 321-1).

The optimal utilization of corticosteroids in non-HIV patients who are often receiving them as part of the treatment regimens for their underlying disease is less clear because data from randomized controlled trials are not available;

dosing may need to be individualized to balance the immunosuppressive effects that potentially contributed to the development of PCP against the anti-inflammatory effects that may ameliorate life-threatening pulmonary dysfunction.[21] One retrospective analysis of 31 patients suggested that increasing corticosteroids to a prednisone equivalent of 60 mg/day or more was associated with clinical benefit. However, a subsequent retrospective cohort study of 323 hospitalized patients with documented PCP without HIV concluded that the addition of early corticosteroids was not associated with improved respiratory outcomes.[22] At this point it would not be unreasonable to administer corticosteroids to non-HIV patients with moderate or severe disease if they were not receiving corticosteroids, using the same regimen as for HIV-infected patients; for patients already taking corticosteroids at lower doses, the dosage could be increased to those levels.

Initiation of Antiretroviral Therapy

Given that many patients with HIV infection who are diagnosed with PCP are not receiving antiretroviral therapy, an important issue is how soon to start cART after a diagnosis of PCP. Retrospective and prospective studies have suggested that, in general, it is safe to initiate cART while patients are being treated for PCP, and early cART may be associated with an improved outcome. In a randomized 282-patient trial that examined early versus late initiation of cART in patients with acute opportunistic infections, 63% of whom had PCP, the early initiation arm (cART started a median of 12 days after starting therapy for the opportunistic infection) had a decreased rate of AIDS progression or death. Similar findings for tuberculosis in developing countries have emphasized the benefit of early initiation of cART.

Major concerns about initiating cART include the risk for adverse drug reactions, which may be confused with adverse reactions to anti-PCP therapy; the risk for overlapping toxicities, which may complicate management; and the risk for immune reconstitution (Chapter 367), which has been rarely reported but can be life-threatening. Thus, many clinicians initiate cART during or immediately after completion of anti-*Pneumocystis* therapy, assuming the patient has shown clinical improvement, is able to tolerate oral medications, and accepts the commitment to lifelong therapy. However, the parameters for such an approach are difficult to define precisely. Patients who start cART early should be closely monitored for a recurrence of symptoms that may represent immune reconstitution.

Treatment Failure

The optimal approach to the management of patients who are failing therapy has not been well defined. In patients with progressive respiratory deterioration, it is critical that the diagnosis of PCP be confirmed rather than presumptive and that other concurrent processes (e.g., other infections, congestive heart failure, pulmonary emboli) have been ruled out; bronchoscopy should be considered to facilitate these determinations. Parenteral therapy should be used to eliminate absorption concerns, and corticosteroid medications should be added if this has not already been done. Because patients who will ultimately respond can show clinical deterioration at 3 to 4 days, as noted earlier, it is reasonable to wait 5 to 8 days before considering a change in drug therapy.

Only trimethoprim-sulfamethoxazole and pentamidine are available in parenteral formulations. Parenteral clindamycin is available, but primaquine is available only as a tablet. No randomized trials have examined the relative efficacy of these agents in patients who are failing therapy. For patients who have not received trimethoprim-sulfamethoxazole, this should be the first choice as an alternative agent, assuming the patient did not have a life-threatening adverse reaction previously. Rapid desensitization (similar to penicillin desensitization), ideally in consultation with an allergy specialist, can be considered in patients with prior adverse reactions; however, patients with a history of Stevens-Johnson syndrome or toxic epidermal necrolysis should not be rechallenged. Retrospective cohort studies and meta-analyses have found that clindamycin-primaquine is superior to pentamidine in patients failing a first-line regimen, but there are potential biases in such analyses (e.g., severity of illness or ability to take oral medications may have affected the choice of salvage regimen), although some studies attempted to correct for this. There are no data to recommend switching to an alternative agent rather than adding an alternative agent (if toxicity is not an issue); both approaches have been used.

Resistance

Although *Pneumocystis* cannot be cultured, molecular studies have identified mutations in genes that are the targets of anti-*Pneumocystis* therapy, and these mutations appear to represent the development of resistance by *Pneumocystis* to these agents. The best-characterized mutations have been identified in the DHPS gene of *Pneumocystis*, which is the target of sulfamethoxazole and dapsone. Two mutations at the active site of this enzyme, which can occur either individually or together, have been identified with greater frequency in patients receiving trimethoprim-sulfamethoxazole or dapsone for prophylaxis; in vitro studies suggest that these mutations confer resistance. The clinical relevance of these mutations remains uncertain; some studies have found worse outcomes in patients with these mutations, but others have found no such association. Most patients in whom these mutations were identified retrospectively were

successfully treated with sulfa-containing drugs. In contrast to DHPS, there are very limited reports suggesting that the DHFR gene of *Pneumocystis*, which is the target of trimethoprim and pyrimethamine, has developed potential drug-resistant mutations.

Atovaquone presumably binds to the mitochondrial bc₁ complex of *Pneumocystis* and thus inhibits electron transport. Multiple mutations have been identified in the cytochrome B gene of *Pneumocystis*, which presumably represent resistance in patients receiving atovaquone for prophylaxis; these mutations have not, however, been associated with clinical outcome.

Because the presence of these mutations has not been definitively associated with worsening prognosis, clinical decisions should not be based on their identification. Methods for identifying DHPS mutations are not readily available in the United States but are available in Europe through a commercial PCR kit[23]; their detection should remain a research tool until their clinical relevance can be better defined.

PREVENTION

Although *Pneumocystis* is transmitted by the airborne route, exposure to the organism appears to be ubiquitous in humans, suggesting that avoidance of exposure may be difficult. Currently, respiratory isolation of patients with active PCP is not required, although it is reasonable to avoid having a susceptible patient share a room with a PCP patient. Recent outbreaks in renal and liver transplant patients strongly suggest a common source of infection; a better understanding of the patterns of transmission in these settings may lead to improved guidelines for preventing the spread of infection. It is noteworthy that in these outbreaks, broad institution of anti-*Pneumocystis* prophylaxis was the intervention that terminated the outbreaks.

A major advance in the management of patients at risk for the development of PCP was the demonstration that trimethoprim-sulfamethoxazole was highly effective in preventing the disease in a susceptible pediatric population. Subsequent studies, primarily in HIV-infected patients, demonstrated that additional drug regimens were also effective. This has led to the broad use of anti-*Pneumocystis* prophylaxis in a wide range of susceptible populations.

Two important issues in administering prophylaxis are identifying populations at risk and defining the period of risk during which prophylaxis should be provided. AIDS patients are at especially high risk; before the use of prophylaxis or cART, the lifetime incidence of PCP in this population was estimated at 60 to 80%. The most recent CD4 count is a validated surrogate marker for HIV-infected patients: patients with CD4 counts below 200 cells/μL in the absence of cART are at substantially increased risk for developing PCP, and primary prophylaxis is recommended for this group. Although 10 to 15% of patients who develop PCP have higher CD4 counts, the incidence is very low in this population, given the large number of patients who fall in this category. Patients with CD4 counts greater than 200 cells/μL but a CD4 percentage of less than 14% or a history of an AIDS-defining illness are also candidates for prophylaxis. In addition, patients who develop PCP should be placed on prophylaxis after the treatment regimen is successfully completed (secondary prophylaxis). For pediatric patients with HIV infection, in whom the normal CD4 count changes with age, guidelines are based on current age. Prophylaxis is recommended for children older than 6 years with CD4 counts below 200 cells/μL or 15%; for children between 1 and less than 6 years old with CD4 counts below 500 cells/μL or 15%; and for all children younger than 12 months.[24]

Before the availability of cART, when patients with HIV infection initiated prophylaxis, they were committed to continuing it for life because immunologic decline was irreversible. With cART, however, control of HIV replication leads to an increase in the CD4 count, which is associated with a concomitant decrease in the risk for developing PCP. Multiple studies have shown that when the CD4 count has been above 200 cells/μL for at least 3 months (ideally in the setting of controlled HIV replication), prophylaxis can be safely discontinued because the risk for developing PCP is no greater than in patients whose CD4 counts never fell below 200 cells/μL. In most of these studies, the median CD4 count was greater than 300 cells/μL, and HIV viral loads were below detection limits in the majority of patients. Recent observational studies have suggested that prophylaxis can also be safely discontinued in patients with CD4 counts between 100 and 200 cells/μL who have virologically suppressed HIV, but specific criteria for discontinuation (e.g., duration of viral suppression) were not defined in these studies. A reasonable approach would be to discontinue primary or secondary prophylaxis in such patients if the viral load remains below detection limits for 3 to 6 months. In patients with CD4 counts less than 100 cells/μL, prophylaxis should be maintained regardless of the viral load.

Among non–HIV-infected patients, the CD4 count is not routinely measured, and it has not been shown to have the same predictive value for the development of PCP as in HIV-infected patients; however, CD4 counts below 200 cells/μL do appear to increase their susceptibility. In a meta-analysis of PCP prophylaxis in a variety of types of non-HIV immunocompromised patients, trimethoprim-sulfamethoxazole prophylaxis was found to be overall highly effective,[A2] with one half-strength dose per day appearing to be as efficacious and less toxic than higher doses.[A3] Recommendations for PCP prophylaxis in these populations are based on clinical parameters, including empirical identification of periods of risk and estimation of levels of immunosuppression.[25] Very broad prophylaxis has not been implemented because of the side effects associated with these regimens; for example, there is concern that trimethoprim-sulfamethoxazole can cause bone marrow suppression that would interfere with engraftment or cause nephrotoxicity that would damage a transplanted kidney.

Risk factors for non–HIV-infected patients include underlying disease, older age, use of immunosuppressive drugs, radiation therapy, graft-versus-host disease, and concomitant cytomegalovirus infection (Chapter 352). Patients with malignancies, especially hematologic malignancies, but increasingly solid tumors as well, are at risk for PCP primarily owing to the therapies they receive; the incidence can range from 1 to 43% in the absence of prophylaxis and is highly dependent on the intensity and duration of immunosuppression. In the absence of prophylaxis, the risk for developing PCP in transplant patients, whether hematopoietic stem cell transplantation (HSCT) (Chapter 168) or solid organ transplantation (Chapter 43), is reportedly about 5 to 15%, although lung and heart-lung transplant patients appear to have a higher incidence (up to 43%). Among patients with collagen vascular disease, the reported risk is less than 2% without prophylaxis, although patients with granulomatosis with polyangiitis (formerly Wegener granulomatosis) (Chapter 254) reportedly have a risk up to 12%, presumably because of the use of more immunosuppressive treatment regimens. In patients with inflammatory bowel disease (Chapter 132), the incidence in one large retrospective cohort study was about 1% per year, with a greater risk for Crohn disease compared with ulcerative colitis. The current risk for developing PCP in non-HIV populations is difficult to quantify because of the widespread use of prophylaxis and because immunosuppressive regimens are evolving. In a recent cohort study of HSCT patients, the risk for PCP in the setting of widely used prophylaxis was 0.28 to 0.63%, with approximately ¼ of cases occurring greater than 270 days after transplantation.[26]

To facilitate the management of prophylaxis in at-risk, non-HIV populations, a number of guidelines have been developed by expert panels that have made recommendations based on the strength of the available data.[27] For allogeneic stem cell transplant recipients, prophylaxis is recommended from the time of engraftment to at least 6 months after transplantation, and longer for patients who continue receiving immunosuppressive therapy or who have chronic graft-versus-host disease. For autologous stem cell transplant recipients, who have a lower risk for PCP, prophylaxis for 3 to 6 months should be considered if the degree of immunosuppression is substantial owing to

underlying disease or therapy (e.g., patients with leukemia or lymphoma receiving intensive conditioning or immunosuppressive therapy). Cancer patients meeting the following conditions should receive prophylaxis as indicated: acute lymphocytic leukemia, throughout therapy; therapy with alemtuzumab, for 2 months after completion and until CD4 is greater than 200 cells/μL; therapy with idelalisib with or without rituximab, or with prolonged corticosteroids, or temozolomide combined with radiation therapy, at least through active therapy; therapy with purine analogues or other T-cell-depleting regimens, consider until CD4 is greater than 200 cells/μL.

For solid organ transplant patients, prophylaxis has not been universally adopted; it has been used primarily in centers with a known incidence greater than 3%. Guidelines recommend the administration of prophylaxis for 6 to 12 months in most solid organ transplant patients, with longer periods, up to lifelong, in heart, lung, liver, and intestine transplant recipients.

As noted earlier, a number of outbreaks of PCP have recently been reported in renal transplant patients, and many developed disease more than 1 year after transplantation. Given this, some authors are suggesting that lifelong prophylaxis may be needed in this population.[28] Risk factors identified in case-control studies have included older age, recent or concurrent cytomegalovirus infection, and treatment for rejection. Specific immunosuppressive drugs, such as mycophenolate mofetil and cyclosporine, have not been consistently implicated. Rare outbreaks have also been reported in liver transplant patients.

For patients with inflammatory bowel disease (Chapter 132), who appear to be at increased risk as newer immunosuppressive agents are used, data are limited; however, consensus-based guidelines recommend prophylaxis for patients receiving triple immunomodulators that include either a calcineurin inhibitor or an anti-TNF agent. No consensus has been reached for less intensive regimens. For patients with connective tissue disorders or vasculitis, there are currently no consensus guidelines.

Corticosteroid therapy (Chapter 32) is a well-described risk factor in non–HIV-infected patients, with approximately 90% of patients receiving such therapy before developing PCP in some studies. Higher dose and longer duration increase the risk. Not all patients who receive corticosteroids are at risk, however; for instance, asthmatic patients receiving corticosteroid therapy are at low risk. Although there are no consensus guidelines on the use of prophylaxis for patients receiving corticosteroids, one reasonable approach is to provide prophylaxis to patients with an underlying immunosuppressive or inflammatory disease who receive at least 20 mg of prednisone or equivalent for longer than 1 month. Other immunosuppressive agents (Chapter 32), such as calcineurin inhibitors, sirolimus, TNF antagonists, and rituximab, also appear to increase the risk for developing PCP, primarily in the patient populations noted earlier.

Trimethoprim-sulfamethoxazole is the first-line agent for prophylaxis in all populations (Table 321-2). Alternatives include dapsone alone or combined with pyrimethamine plus leucovorin, atovaquone, and aerosol pentamidine administered by the Respirgard II nebulizer. In a randomized trial of 843 HIV-infected patients comparing trimethoprim-sulfamethoxazole with dapsone and aerosol pentamidine, no significant differences were seen on an intent-to-treat basis, but

TABLE 321-2 DRUG REGIMENS FOR PREVENTION OF *PNEUMOCYSTIS* PNEUMONIA (PCP)				
INDICATION	**DRUG**	**ROUTE**	**DOSE**	**COMMENTS**
Preferred	Trimethoprim-sulfamethoxazole (TMP-SMX)	PO	1 double-strength tablet (160 mg TMP + 800 mg SMX) or one single-strength tablet (80 mg TMP + 400 mg SMX) qd	Also active in preventing toxoplasmosis
Alternative	TMP-SMX	PO	1 double-strength tablet (160 mg TMP + 800 mg SMX) three times weekly	Also active in preventing toxoplasmosis
Alternative	Dapsone	PO	100 mg qd or 50 mg bid	Test for G6PD deficiency before use
Alternative	Dapsone plus	PO	50 mg qd	Also active in preventing toxoplasmosis
	Pyrimethamine plus	PO	50 mg once weekly	
	Leucovorin	PO	25 mg once weekly	Should be administered with pyrimethamine to minimize toxicity
Alternative	Atovaquone	PO	1500 mg qd with food	Likely active in preventing toxoplasmosis; efavirenz can decrease concentrations
Alternative	Pentamidine	Aerosol	300 mg via the Respirgard II nebulizer once monthly	Not active in preventing toxoplasmosis
	Pentamidine	IV	4 mg/kg administered over >1 hr	Limited observational data primarily in pediatric populations; not active in preventing toxoplasmosis

Note: Patients receiving pyrimethamine-sulfadiazine and atovaquone therapy for toxoplasmosis do not appear to need additional prophylaxis for PCP; patients receiving clindamycin-pyrimethamine therapy for toxoplasmosis will need additional prophylaxis for PCP. G6PD = glucose-6-phosphate dehydrogenase.

the lowest failure rates were seen while patients were receiving trimethoprim-sulfamethoxazole. Conversely, trimethoprim-sulfamethoxazole was superior to aerosol pentamidine in another randomized study. In other large randomized trials in HIV-infected patients, the following regimens showed similar efficacy: atovaquone suspension and dapsone, atovaquone suspension and aerosol pentamidine, and dapsone-pyrimethamine and aerosol pentamidine. No randomized trials of these regimens have been conducted in non–HIV-infected populations, but clinical experience suggests that they are effective in these populations as well. Observational studies primarily in non-HIV pediatric populations suggest that monthly intravenous pentamidine is also effective. Patients receiving pyrimethamine plus sulfadiazine plus leucovorin for treatment of toxoplasmosis do not require additional anti-*Pneumocystis* prophylaxis because this regimen also prevents PCP.

Although the combination of sulfadoxine and pyrimethamine is also efficacious, it is contraindicated in patients with sulfonamide allergies. Moreover, because Stevens-Johnson syndrome and other potentially life-threatening cutaneous reactions are more common with this combination than with trimethoprim-sulfamethoxazole, and because its long half-life results in slow clearance after the drug is discontinued, sulfadoxine plus pyrimethamine should probably not be used in sulfa-tolerant patients if trimethoprim-sulfamethoxazole is available.

HIV-infected patients with a prior history of a mild sulfa allergy (e.g., mild rash, excluding those with prior Stevens-Johnson syndrome or toxic epidermal necrolysis) can often be safely rechallenged with trimethoprim-sulfamethoxazole. Randomized trials have demonstrated that dose escalation over a 6- to 13-day period is associated with better tolerance than direct rechallenge with full-dose trimethoprim-sulfamethoxazole, and that up to 75% of patients can continue to receive trimethoprim-sulfamethoxazole for at least 6 months.

PROGNOSIS

Mortality for untreated PCP approaches 100%. With therapy, the survival rate for HIV-infected patients with confirmed PCP is now as high as 95%, but a poorer survival rate of 75% has been reported in patients without HIV infection. Risk factors for death in HIV-infected patients include more severe hypoxia, older age, recurrent episodes of PCP, low hemoglobin, and the presence of comorbid conditions. Although mortality for patients admitted to an intensive care unit is high, survival for HIV-infected patients has improved in recent years, now approaching 75%.

Grade A References

A1. Ewald H, Raatz H, Boscacci R, et al. Adjunctive corticosteroids for *Pneumocystis jiroveci* pneumonia in patients with HIV infection. *Cochrane Database Syst Rev.* 2015;4:CD006150.
A2. Stern A, Green H, Paul M, et al. Prophylaxis for *Pneumocystis* pneumonia (PCP) in non-HIV immunocompromised patients. *Cochrane Database Syst Rev.* 2014;10:CD005590.
A3. Utsunomiya M, Dobashi H, Odani T, et al. Optimal regimens of sulfamethoxazole-trimethoprim for chemoprophylaxis of *Pneumocystis* pneumonia in patients with systemic rheumatic diseases: results from a non-blinded, randomized controlled trial. *Arthritis Res Ther.* 2017;19:1-10.

GENERAL REFERENCES

For the General References and other additional features, please visit Expert Consult at https://expertconsult.inkling.com.

322

MYCETOMA AND DEMATIACEOUS FUNGAL INFECTIONS

PETER G. PAPPAS AND DIMITRIOS P. KONTOYIANNIS

DEFINITION

Dematiaceous fungi represent a large group of fungal organisms characterized by the presence of abundant melanin in the cell wall, which gives rise to a brown-black coloration on artificial culture media and which can be seen on histopathologic specimens. A related term, *phaeohyphomycosis*, refers broadly to infection by these pigmented fungi. The two terms are often used

interchangeably. Dematiaceous fungal infections generally fall into three broad categories: mycetoma (e.g., Madura foot), chromomycosis (also known as chromoblastomycosis), and phaeohyphomycosis.[1,2] Mycetoma (a tumor produced by fungi) is a disease of historical interest and was first described in 1842 in the Madura district of India, hence the terms "Madura foot," "maduromycosis," and "maduromycetoma."

The Pathogens

More than 100 dematiaceous fungi have been identified as causes of disease in humans. The most common organisms and their related conditions are listed in Table 322-1. The taxonomy of the dematiaceous fungi is somewhat confusing because these agents belong to different classes, including Hyphomycetes, Ascomycetes, Basidiomycetes, Coelomycetes, and Zygomycetes. The most common agents of phaeohyphomycosis include species in the following genera: *Alternaria, Bipolaris, Curvularia, Exophiala, Cladosporium, Cladophialophora, Fonsecaea, Exserohilum, Ochroconis, Phialophora, Phaeoacremonium,* and *Chaetomium.* These agents are ubiquitous saprophytes of soil and decaying matter, and some are important plant pathogens. In tissue, these organisms exist as yeastlike cells, septated hyphae, or a combination of yeast and hyphae. Most of these organisms demonstrate melanin pigmentation (brownish coloration) in the cell walls on microscopic examination.

Most cases of chromomycosis are caused by three species: *Fonsecaea pedrosoi, Cladosporium carrionii,* and *Phialophora verrucosa.* The distinctive histologic appearance is characterized by the presence of thick-walled, dark brown bodies known as *sclerotic cells* or *copper pennies,* which represent individual organisms and may be seen in clusters or as single cells. The etiologic fungi causing chromomycosis are indistinguishable on histologic examination of tissue.

Mycetoma is caused by two groups of organisms: (1) the filamentous aerobic actinomycetes (actinomycetoma) and (2) a wide range of saprophytic soil and woody plant fungi (eumycetoma). Eumycetoma accounts for about 50% of cases of mycetoma.[3] A variety of *Nocardia* species (e.g., *Nocardia brasiliensis, Nocardia asteroides*), *Actinomadura* species (e.g., *Actinomadura pelletierii, Actinomadura madurae*), and *Streptomyces* species (e.g., *Streptomyces somaliensis*) cause actinomycetoma. Most cases of eumycetoma are due to *Madurella* species

TABLE 322-1	DEMATIACEOUS FUNGI AND ASSOCIATED DISEASES
CLINICAL CONDITION	**COMMON ETIOLOGIC AGENTS**
Chromomycosis	*Fonsecaea pedrosoi* *Cladophialophora carrionii* *Phialophora verrucosa*
Cutaneous or subcutaneous disease	*Exophiala jeanselmei* *Exophiala dermatitidis* *Phialophora* spp *Bipolaris* spp *Alternaria* spp
Sinusitis	*Bipolaris* spp *Curvularia* spp *Exserohilum* spp *Alternaria* spp
Central nervous system	*Cladophialophora bantiana* *Verruconis (Ochroconis) gallopava* *Rhinocladiella mackenziei* *Chaetomium atrobrunneum* *Exophiala dermatitidis*
Health care associated	*Exserohilum rostratum* *Exophiala* spp
Disseminated	*Exophiala dermatitidis* *Exophiala jeanselmei* *Bipolaris* spp *Verruconis (Ochroconis) gallopava* *Phialophora* spp *Lomentospora (Scedosporium) prolificans*
Eumycetoma	*Madurella mycetomatis* *Exophiala* spp *Curvularia* spp *Leptosphaeria senegalensis*
Non-dematiaceous fungi	*Pseudallescheria boydii* *Acremonium* spp *Fusarium* spp

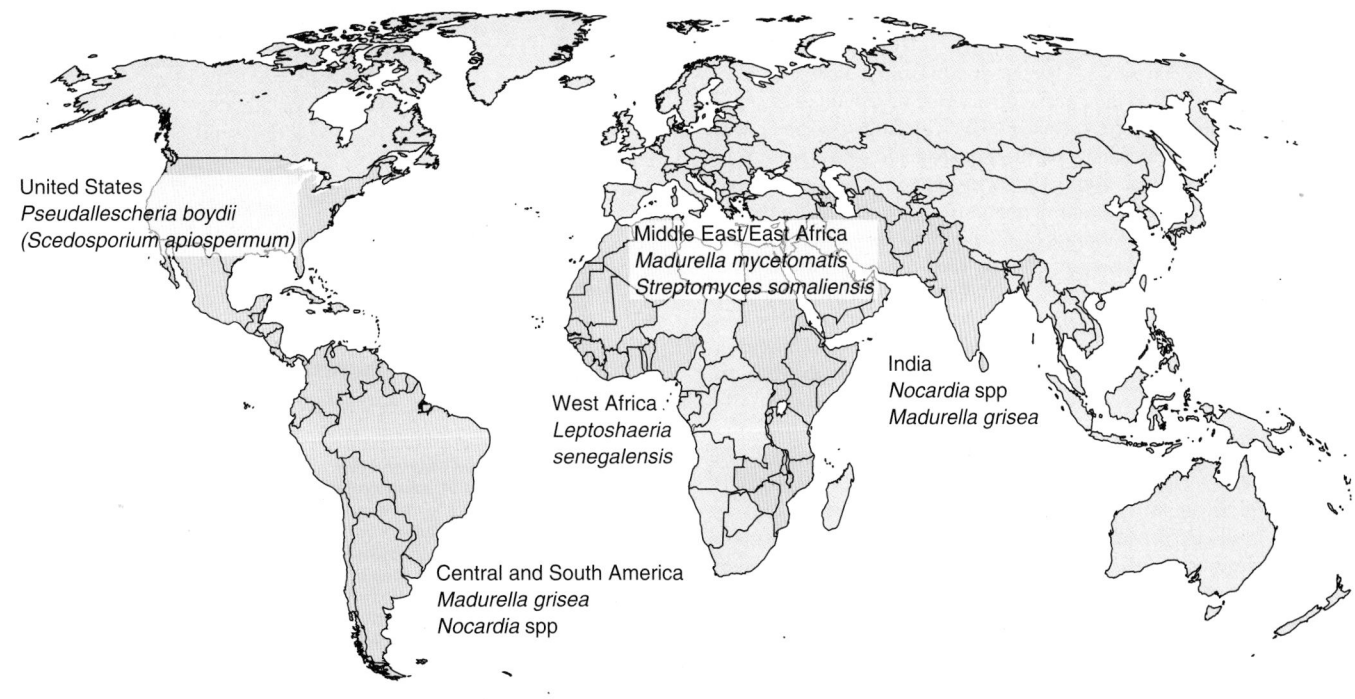

United States
Pseudallescheria boydii
(Scedosporium apiospermum)

Middle East/East Africa
Madurella mycetomatis
Streptomyces somaliensis

India
Nocardia spp
Madurella grisea

West Africa
Leptoshaeria
senegalensis

Central and South America
Madurella grisea
Nocardia spp

FIGURE 322-1. Predominant agents of mycetoma according to region.

(e.g., *Madurella mycetomatis* causes 70% of all cases of eumycetoma worldwide). Other causes of eumycetoma include some nondematiaceous fungi such as *Fusarium* species, *Acremonium* species, *Pseudallescheria boydii,* and several phaeohyphomycetes including *Exophiala* and *Curvularia* species. Eumycetoma is further characterized on the basis of the color of the granular drainage: white- to yellow-grain mycetomas (white piedra) are typically caused by hyalohyphomycetes (e.g., *P. boydii, Fusarium* species, *Acremonium* species), and black-grain eumycetomas are caused by *Madurella* species and other less common fungi.[4]

EPIDEMIOLOGY

Dematiaceous fungi are found in the environment worldwide. Although there is no unique endemic area for most of these infections, some observations are relevant. Allergic fungal sinusitis associated with dematiaceous fungi appears to be more common in the southern United States. Chronic infections of the lower extremities are more commonly seen in men and in tropical areas. Chromomycosis are more prevalent in rural populations in the tropics and are hyperendemic in certain geographic areas such as Madagascar, India, Brazil, and other poorer countries in Africa and South America. Cutaneous infections usually occur as a result of minor skin trauma and direct inoculation of the organism.

Phaeohyphomycosis is an important emerging fungal infection in medically advanced regions, particularly among immunocompromised patients such as solid organ and hematopoietic stem cell transplant recipients, patients with prolonged neutropenia, and other immunocompromised individuals.[5,6] Risk factors for extracutaneous infection include intravenous drug abuse, chronic sinusitis, freshwater immersion, and chronic immunosuppression. Phaeohyphomycosis is reported in human immunodeficiency virus (HIV)-infected patients but is far less common than other opportunistic fungi. Extracutaneous invasive disease can also occur in otherwise normal patients but is much less common. Recent data suggest subtle host immune abnormalities, including *CARD*-9 mutations and other disorders associated with TH-17 deficiency, in a subset of these previously "normal" individuals.[7,8]

In the United States, an epidemic of fungal meningitis, epidural abscess, sacroiliitis, vertebral osteomyelitis, discitis, and peripheral arthritis involved over 750 persons and was caused by *Exserohilum rostratum* following injection of contaminated methylprednisolone acetate from a single compounding pharmacy; this is a dramatic example of the risk for dematiaceous fungal infections following invasive procedures in the health care setting.[9] Previous reports of infection due to *Exophiala* species following contaminated steroid injections, infected breast implants, other prosthetic materials, and, rarely, contaminated intravascular catheters and intravenous fluids further underscore the importance of these organisms as potential health care–associated pathogens.

Mycetoma has a global distribution, but it occurs primarily in the tropical zones. The disorder is quite prevalent in India, Latin America, the Middle East, and sub-Saharan Africa (the "mycetoma belt"). Sudan has a particularly high burden of mycetoma.[10] Indigenously acquired mycetoma is sporadic in North America and Europe. Moreover, the relative frequency of actinomycetoma and eumycetoma differs among geographic areas. Eumycetoma is more common in India and Africa, and actinomycetoma is more common in Central and South America. Furthermore, the causative agents of mycetoma differ in their geographic distribution. For example, *P. boydii* is the most common agent of mycetoma in North America, and *Actinomadura* and *Nocardia* species are predominant in Central and South America. *Leptosphaeria senegalensis* and *M. mycetomatis* are predominant in sub-Saharan Africa and India (Fig. 322-1).

The ratio of male to female patients with mycetoma is 5 : 1. The disease is typically seen in rural areas and in persons susceptible to local trauma and contamination from soil. Hence, farmers, gardeners, woodcutters, herders, and people who work outside while barefoot are more susceptible to this infection.

Local trauma (e.g., wood splinters) introduces a mycetoma-causative organism into the skin and subcutaneous tissues and initiates a chain of events that leads to chronic, suppurative granulomatous inflammation, tumefaction, formation of multiple fistulous tracts and sinuses, deep abscesses, fibrosis and scar formation, and extension to adjacent connective tissue across the lines of least resistance (fascia) and ultimately to bones, muscles, nerves, and tendon sheaths, leading to gross anatomic distortion of the affected site.

The genetics and immunopathogenesis of mycetoma are not well defined, but it appears that there are differences in host susceptibility as some infected persons have impaired or delayed hypersensitivity reactions or polymorphisms in genes encoding for chemokines (e.g., CCL50) and cytokines (e.g., interleukin-10). Mycetoma does not appear to be more common in immunocompromised hosts.

CLINICAL MANIFESTATIONS

Chromomycosis is manifested as a cutaneous or subcutaneous lesion that may range in size from a small papule to a large confluent plaque involving a major portion of an extremity.[11] Single or multiple lesions are seen; ulceration may occur. Lesions may remain unchanged in size and consistency for months or years, although most tend to progress in the absence of specific therapy. Chronic lesions may become dry and crusted with a raised border, which may be smooth or irregular, and which may take on a verrucous, warty appearance. Multiple lesions can coalesce to form larger plaques in which central scarring may develop. Cutaneous lesions usually remain confined to one anatomic site, although nodular lymphangitis and multifocal cutaneous disease from autoinoculation may occur. Common complications include local disfigurement due to scarring and extensive tissue involvement. Disseminated disease involving visceral organs is rare.

Superficial phaeohyphomycosis is characterized by tinea nigra and black piedra.[12] Tinea nigra is a darkening of the skin caused by growth of *Phaeoannellomyces werneckii* in the stratum corneum. Black piedra is associated with the development of focal thickening on the hair shaft and results from colonization of the shaft by *Piedraia hortae*. *Cutaneous phaeohyphomycosis* involves deeper skin structures and results in dermatomycosis and onychomycosis; this is frequently due to agents such as *Scytalidium* and *Phyllosticta* species.

Subcutaneous phaeohyphomycosis may be confused clinically with chromomycosis. Patients have discrete subcutaneous nodules or cysts that result from direct inoculation or penetrating trauma. The most common organisms are *Exophiala jeanselmei*, *Exophiala dermatitidis*, *Alternaria alternans*, and *Phialophora* species. *Mycotic keratitis* as a result of infection with *Curvularia*, *Exophiala*, and *Exserohilum* species may occur after corneal trauma or surgery.

Foreign body–related infections are seen in patients undergoing chronic ambulatory peritoneal dialysis in whom fungal peritonitis develops, in patients with indwelling intravenous catheters, and in other devices such as breast implants.

Fungal sinusitis[13] is commonly associated with dematiaceous fungi and can be manifested as allergic fungal sinusitis, a fungus ball in a sinus cavity, and invasive fungal sinusitis associated with extension into bone, soft tissue, and the central nervous system. This last destructive process is indistinguishable from rhinocerebral zygomycosis or invasive *Aspergillus* sinusitis. *Bipolaris*, *Curvularia*, *Exserohilum*, and *Alternaria* species are the most common organisms causing invasive fungal sinusitis.

Systemic phaeohyphomycosis may result from direct extension from a colonized area or dissemination from a distant source. Most patients with systemic disease have significant underlying immunosuppression, and the organisms have a proclivity for involvement of the brain, lungs, endocardium, and other visceral organs. Among patients with primary central nervous system disease, *Cladophialophora bantiana*, *Rhinocladiella mackenziei*, and *Chaetomium atrobrunneum* are the most common etiologic agents, and the majority of these are otherwise healthy patients with little or no underlying immunodeficiency. Among immunocompromised patients, *Verruconis* (*Ochroconis*) *gallopava*, *Bipolaris* species, and *Exophiala dermatitidis* are seen more commonly.

In severely immunocompromised patients, especially those with hematologic malignancies or stem cell transplant recipients with or without prolonged and profound neutropenia, infection due to *Lomentospora* (*Scedosporium*) *prolificans* can present as multiorgan dissemination. Infection due to this multidrug-resistant pathogen is associated with an exceptionally high mortality rate.

Mycetoma is a chronic, slowly progressive infection that starts in the subcutaneous tissue and spreads across tissue planes to contiguous structures. The lesion is usually confined to one anatomic site. The clinical manifestations and natural history of mycetoma are variable and, to some degree, related to the pathogenic agent involved. For example, the progression of eumycetoma tends to be slower than that of actinomycetoma. In addition, eumycetoma lesions tend to be more confined and have less inflammation and fewer granulomas and fistulas but more fibrosis compared with actinomycetoma lesions. The foot is the most common site involved in mycetoma (Fig. 322-2), followed by the hands, but any other part of the body may become involved. Painless nodular and/or papular swelling is a common early manifestation of mycetoma, followed by a slow evolution to painless, fixed woody induration. This infection typically runs a chronic, relentless course, sometimes spanning several decades. It is characterized by recurring cycles of suppuration, draining sinuses, bacterial superinfection, and scar formation. Old sinuses close, and new ones occur. Satellite lesions are common. Constitutional symptoms are rare. The presence of fever often indicates bacterial superinfection. Substantial bone involvement mimicking chronic osteomyelitis with cavitary bone lesions, periosteal reaction or sclerosis (seen with radiography, computed tomography, or magnetic resonance imaging [MRI] studies), osteoporosis, and reactive periosteal bone formation may occur. However, pathologic fractures are rare. Because nerves are relatively spared from involvement, neuropathic manifestations are uncommon. Inexorable limb deformity and misuse because of destruction of deeper tissues may be seen in chronic, refractory, and advanced cases.[14] Mycetoma does not spread hematogenously; thus, visceral dissemination is not seen, although regional lymphadenitis may occur.

DIAGNOSIS

The diagnosis of a dematiaceous fungal infection is suggested by direct examination of a clinical specimen with a 10% potassium hydroxide preparation or special stains to demonstrate pigmentation in the cell walls of these organisms. For patients with chromomycosis, the finding of sclerotic cells or copper

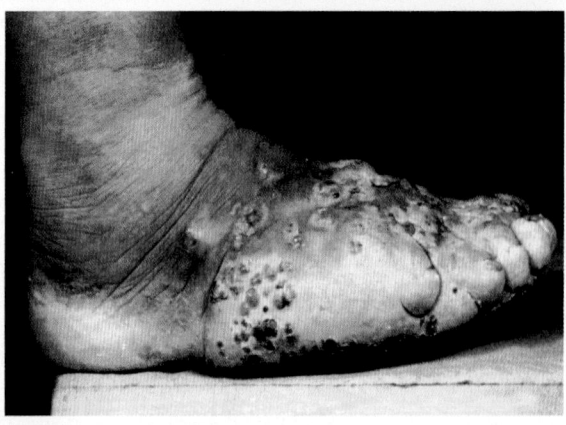

FIGURE 322-2. Clinical presentation of mycetoma. A 40-year-old farmer from rural Venezuela with a 10-year history of foot edema and slowly progressive deformity following an injury caused by being struck by a hammer presented with chronic crusted plaques, multiple confluent tender abscesses with fistulization, and release of black grains. The range of motion of the patient's ankle and foot joints was limited, but the joints were not painful. A deep skin biopsy with hematoxylin and eosin staining, periodic acid–Schiff staining, foot radiography, sampling of black grain smears, and a mycology culture were performed. The foot radiograph showed osteofibrosis, destruction of articular surfaces, osteoporosis, and ankylosis, and *Madurella* spp grew in the culture. (Courtesy of Dr. M. Mendoza, Instituto De Biomedicina, Laboratorio de Micología, San Jose Caracas, Venezuela.)

pennies on skin biopsy is characteristic, and special stains are usually unnecessary. For patients with other forms of phaeohyphomycosis, the Fontana-Masson stain is useful in distinguishing organisms with significant melanin content. Culture remains the means by which a specific etiologic diagnosis is established, and the identity of the organism is largely based on colony and microscopic morphology.[15] A polymerase chain reaction–based diagnostic assay for *Exserohilum rostratum* was developed in the context of the fungal meningitis outbreak and serves as a reliable marker of infection among exposed patients. Otherwise, serologic studies and molecular diagnostics for other organisms are not generally available.

The diagnosis of mycetoma is complicated by the fact that nonfungal organisms are frequent etiologic agents. The diagnosis is suspected in the presence of granular drainage from a characteristic skin lesion. However, grains in tissue alone may be difficult to culture because they may be composed of dead organisms. Furthermore, grains may be contaminated by surface bacteria or fungi. Thus, a deep-tissue biopsy specimen is ideal for staining (hematoxylin and eosin, Gram stain, modified Ziehl-Neelsen stain, Gomori methenamine silver, periodic acid–Schiff) and appropriate selective bacterial and fungal cultures. Alternatively, aspiration of grains from unopened sinus tracts can provide suitable material for culture. The culture should be maintained for several weeks because some of the causative agents of mycetoma (e.g., *Nocardia* and *Streptomyces* species) may require 4 to 6 weeks for detection by culture methodology.

Differential Diagnosis

The specific manifestations of chromomycosis, cutaneous and subcutaneous phaeohyphomycosis, and mycetoma are often confused with other entities. It is important to consider benign or malignant skin tumors, other chronic granulomatous lesions (e.g., thorn granuloma), and verrucous leishmaniasis. Deep skin and subcutaneous infections due to other fungi (e.g., blastomycosis, sporotrichosis, cryptococcosis, and coccidioidomycosis), and higher-order bacteria (e.g., nocardiosis, mycobacteriosis), must be considered. Skin lesions without fistulas can occasionally resemble unusual forms of sporotrichosis (mycetomatous lymphatic sporotrichosis) and granulomatous dermatophyte infections. The latter infection, which is typically seen in Africans and sometimes called pseudomycetoma (Majocchi granuloma), is a painless granulomatous induration of the skin and subcutaneous tissues caused by dermatophytes that may be associated with grains consisting of fungi. Unlike mycetoma, pseudomycetoma is confined to the skin and subcutaneous tissue and does not spread to deeper tissues. Chronic severe botryomycosis (typically caused by *Staphylococcus aureus*) with purulent exudates, grains, and draining sinus tracts may be confused with mycetoma. Actinomycosis (Chapter 313), which is caused by endogenous microaerophilic actinomycetes, also has a propensity for grains and formation of draining sinus tracts, but its location is characteristic in the neck, chest, abdomen, and pelvis. Differentiation between mycetomas with bone involvement and chronic osteomyelitis or osseous tumors may be challenging. Ultrasonography has been used to reliably differentiate mycetoma from either tumor or osteomyelitis. The dot-in-circles sign seen on MRI (tiny hypodense foci, representing grains, within high-hyperintensity spherical lesions, representing granulomas, scattered by areas of fibrosis) may provide an early and specific diagnostic clue for mycetoma.

TREATMENT   Rx

For chromomycosis, surgical excision of a cutaneous or subcutaneous lesion is often curative,[16] although antifungal therapy is usually given in conjunction with surgery. There is only anecdotal evidence and a few small trials that have examined the efficacy of antifungal therapy for this condition. Further details about systemic antifungal agents are found in Chapter 315. Historically, oral 5-flucytosine (5-FC, 150 mg/kg/day in four divided doses) has been advocated for the oral treatment of chromomycosis based on moderate in vitro activity and clinical experience. Because of limited availability, cost, and potential toxicity, 5-FC is rarely used for this purpose. The triazoles, including itraconazole (200 mg orally twice daily), voriconazole (200 mg twice daily), and posaconazole (300 mg daily), demonstrate the best in vitro activity, although clinical studies with these agents are very limited. Terbinafine (500 mg orally twice daily) has been used successfully for the treatment of chromomycosis and is an effective alternative. Duration of therapy, with or without surgical excision, is generally 3 to 12 months, depending on clinical response.

For phaeohyphomycosis, the expanded-spectrum triazoles, including itraconazole, voriconazole, posaconazole, and isavuconazole, demonstrate excellent in vitro activity against the most common pathogenic dematiaceous fungi. Amphotericin B has modest in vitro activity against most of these fungi and is usually reserved for patients with life-threatening or disseminated disease. Most patients with epidemic *Exserohilum rostratum* infections have been treated successfully with voriconazole (intravenous, then oral), with or without a lipid formulation of amphotericin B, for severe central nervous system involvement. Posaconazole has been used as salvage therapy for those intolerant to voriconazole or in whom voriconazole has failed. Among the triazoles, posaconazole probably offers the most potential in this clinical setting based on anecdotal experience from patients with central nervous system infection. The length of antifungal therapy for any of the systemic phaeohyphomycoses is unclear, but therapy should probably be continued for at least 4 to 6 months or until 1 month after resolution of all signs and symptoms of disease.

Therapy for mycetoma should be individualized. Optimal management is not well defined, and the literature provides only heterogeneous and uncontrolled studies. As such, there is no "gold standard" therapy for mycetoma. Successful treatment is dependent upon distinguishing actinomycetoma from eumycetoma, identification of the causative pathogen, and the extent of tissue invasion.

For actinomycetoma, treatment consists of chronic antimicrobial therapy (at least 9 to 12 months) in conjunction with limited debulking surgery in selected cases.[17] Several regimens (trimethoprim-sulfamethoxazole, tetracyclines, dapsone, streptomycin) have been used in different sequences and combinations depending on the organism (e.g., trimethoprim-sulfamethoxazole with or without dapsone for *Nocardia* species, streptomycin with dapsone for *A. madurae*). Parenteral streptomycin is usually reserved for refractory cases not responding to oral therapy. Response to therapy is slow (usually within 4 weeks), and relapse is common. Several cycles of therapy may be necessary for chronic recurrent disease.

The best treatment results for eumycetoma have been achieved with prolonged use (at least 9 to 12 months) with an imidazole such as ketoconazole 200 to 400 mg daily or itraconazole 200 to 400 mg daily, combined with appropriate surgery. In vitro activity and clinical experience with the newer azoles (voriconazole, posaconazole, and isavuconazole) and terbinafine are promising, but data are very limited.[18] Clinical results with amphotericin B for refractory cases have been generally disappointing, and many of the causative agents demonstrate in vitro resistance to this compound.

Surgery often plays a pivotal role in eumycetoma because most disease is refractory to antifungal therapy alone. The need and extent of surgery depend on the specific agent and the degree of tissue invasion. Wide-margin surgery for localized lesions is usually curative. Extensive débridement and disfiguring surgery are reserved for severe and refractory cases.

The prognosis for mycetoma depends on the anatomic site and degree of tissue involvement. Extension into bony structures is associated with the worst long-term consequences. Thus, early diagnosis and intervention are critical in optimizing outcomes. Finally, mycetoma is a frequently ignored infection, causing significant socioeconomic burden in many impoverished regions of the world. As such, it is notable that mycetoma is now recognized as a *neglected tropical disease* by the World Health Organization.[19] It is hoped that in gaining this status, there will be greater efforts toward education, prevention, specific therapies, and research.

GENERAL REFERENCES

For the General References and other additional features, please visit Expert Consult at https://expertconsult.inkling.com.

323

ANTIPARASITIC THERAPY

RICHARD D. PEARSON

Although substantial progress has been made in reducing the impact of protozoal and helminthic infections, including a major reduction in deaths due to malaria and the near eradication of the guinea worm, *Dracunculus medinensis,* parasitic diseases remain a major cause of morbidity and mortality worldwide, particularly in impoverished tropical regions. In the United States, parasitic diseases are most often encountered among immigrants and international travelers to endemic areas and among a growing number of persons with compromised immunity due to human immunodeficiency virus/acquired immunodeficiency syndrome (HIV/AIDS), organ transplants, immunosuppressive medications, neoplasms, or other causes. A number of drugs are available to treat protozoal and helminthic diseases, but physicians practicing in industrialized countries may not be familiar with their use. This chapter focuses on their therapeutic indications, pharmacology, and major side effects. Generalizations emerge that help in organizing an otherwise vast array of information.

In considering the chemotherapy of parasitic diseases, it is helpful to group infections into those caused by protozoa, single-celled organisms that can multiply by cell division, and helminths, multicellular worms with complex internal structures. Protozoa multiply in their human hosts. They can be grouped into those that live aerobically in the blood stream or tissues, and those that reside under anaerobic conditions in the gastrointestinal tract or vagina. The most important systemic protozoal infections are attributable to members of the phylum Apicomplexa, which are responsible for malaria, babesiosis, toxoplasmosis, and cryptosporidiosis, and to members of the order Kinetoplastida, which are responsible for Chagas disease, human African trypanosomiasis (sleeping sickness), and leishmaniasis. Amoeba and other types of protozoa can also cause disease.

Helminths are subdivided into nematodes, or roundworms, which can be grouped into those that live in the gastrointestinal tract and those found elsewhere in the body, and platyhelminths, or flat worms, which are subdivided into cestodes, or tapeworms, and trematodes, or flukes.

Detailed information about the diagnosis and treatment of specific parasitic diseases can be found in the chapters to follow, the U.S. Centers for Disease Control and Prevention (CDC) (see A-Z Index; https://www.cdc.gov/az/a.html),[1] and textbooks of tropical diseases. Many antiparasitic drugs are commercially available in the United States, whereas others can only be obtained directly from the manufacturer, special pharmacies, or the CDC Drug Service. Some are available through investigational new drug protocols. Major challenges in recent years have arisen from a shortage of some antiparasitic drugs and, in the United States, massive increases in the cost of others. A number of drugs used to treat bacterial or fungal pathogens are also effective in the treatment of parasitic diseases. They are discussed elsewhere (Chapters 271 and 315).

PROTOZOAL DISEASES

Malaria (Plasmodium species): Treatment and Prevention

A number of drugs are available for the treatment and prophylaxis of malaria. Most act on *Plasmodium* species within erythrocytes. The antimalarial drug of choice depends on the infecting species and the likelihood of resistance (Chapter 324). Resistance to chloroquine is now widespread among *Plasmodium falciparum* in most regions of the world and well documented in *Plasmodium vivax* in some areas. Artemisinin-based combination therapy (ACT), including the fixed drug combination **artemether-lumefantrine,** is the treatment of choice for acute malaria acquired in areas with chloroquine resistance. The fixed drug combination **atovaquone-proguanil** or the antibiotic **doxycycline** is commonly used for prophylaxis in travelers to areas with chloroquine-resistant *Plasmodium* species. Chloroquine is used for treatment and prophylaxis in areas where *Plasmodium* species are sensitive. Only primaquine and tafenoquine kill hypnozoites of *P. vivax* and *Plasmodium ovale* in the liver. Country-specific recommendations for prophylaxis and treatment are provided by the CDC (www.cdc.gov/travel/) and in "CDC Health Information for International Travel 2018."[2]

Artemisinins are the most rapidly acting drugs available for the treatment of malaria.[3] They are sesquiterpene lactone derivatives of the wormwood plant *Artemisia annua,* from which qinghaosu, the Chinese herbal medication for fever, is derived. They are endoperoxide-containing compounds. In the presence of intraparasitic iron, they are converted into free radicals and other intermediates that alkylate specific malarial proteins and act rapidly to kill intraerythrocytic parasites. The artemisinins are administered with a second antimalarial drug having a different mechanism of action and longer half-life to prevent the development of resistance.[4] The route of administration of artemisinins varies; some are well absorbed orally, whereas others must be administered intravenously, intramuscularly, or by suppository. Their short half-lives preclude their use for prophylaxis. Side effects in humans are common, but seldom result in discontinuation of treatment. Delayed hemolysis up to 4 weeks after treatment has been observed in persons treated with artesunate[5] or some other artemisinins. Neurologic toxicity and cerebellar dysfunction have been observed in dogs receiving chronic, high-dose artemisinin therapy, but have not emerged as a problem in humans treated for acute malaria.

Artemether-lumefantrine, a fixed drug combination, is used throughout the world (including the United States) to treat chloroquine-resistant malaria. It is taken with food, but grapefruit juice should be avoided. Common adverse reactions in adults are headache, anorexia, dizziness, asthenia, arthralgia, and myalgia. The most common in children are fever, cough, vomiting, anorexia, and headache. These side effects do not usually result in discontinuation of therapy. Of greater concern, lumefantrine can result in prolongation of the QT interval and is contraindicated in persons with abnormal QTc. It also inhibits CYP206 and can thereby reduce the metabolism of other medications including those that prolong the QTc. It can also decrease the effectiveness of birth control pills. Care must be taken in reviewing the recipient's medication list for potential interactions.

Artesunate is available from the CDC under an expanded access investigational new drug protocol for the intravenous treatment of severe malaria (contact the CDC Malaria Hot Line for information). Quinidine gluconate is no longer available in the United States. Artesunate is rapidly hydrolyzed to dihydroartemisinin, which is responsible for the antimalarial effect. Studies in malaria-endemic regions suggest that parenteral artesunate has a higher success rate and lower adverse event rate than quinidine. In addition to the side effects with artemether described previously, artesunate has been associated with delayed hemolysis (unrelated to glucose-6-phosphate dehydrogenase [G6PD] deficiency) up to 4 weeks after therapy.

Atovaquone-proguanil, a fixed drug preparation, is used for the treatment of uncomplicated, chloroquine-resistant and -sensitive malaria, as well as prophylaxis. Atovaquone is a highly lipophilic compound with low aqueous solubility. Administration with food enhances its absorption two-fold. Plasma concentrations do not increase proportionately with dose. Atovaquone is highly protein bound with a half-life exceeding 60 hours. It undergoes extensive enterohepatic cycling and is eventually excreted unchanged in feces. Atovaquone selectively inhibits electron transport in the mitochondria of susceptible *Plasmodium* at the level of the cytochrome bc_1 complex, which results in collapse of the mitochondrial membrane potential. It also affects pyrimidine biosynthesis, which is obligatorily coupled to electron transport in *Plasmodium.* Resistance develops rapidly when atovaquone is used alone to treat malaria. Atovaquone is generally well tolerated but can cause nausea, vomiting, diarrhea, rash, and pruritus.

Proguanil is absorbed slowly after oral administration. The serum level falls to zero within 24 hours, so it must be administered daily. Its triazine metabolite, cycloguanil, inhibits dihydrofolate reductase in susceptible *Plasmodium* species. Resistance is well documented when proguanil is used alone. In addition, proguanil acts synergistically with atovaquone to collapse the mitochondrial membrane potential in susceptible *Plasmodium* species.

The combination of atovaquone-proguanil is the best tolerated of the options for prevention of chloroquine-resistant malaria. It is begun 1 to 2 days before departure and continued during the time of exposure and for 7 days thereafter. Higher doses of atovaquone-proguanil, administered over a 3-day period, are used to treat acute, uncomplicated malaria. Potential side effects include abdominal pain, nausea, vomiting, diarrhea, headache, pruritus, and rash. Asymptomatic, transient elevations in liver enzymes have been observed with treatment doses.

Chloroquine was once the mainstay of malaria treatment and prevention, but widespread resistance among *P. falciparum,* and in some locations, especially Papua New Guinea and Indonesia, *P. vivax,* now limits its use. Chloroquine, a 4-aminoquinoline, has a bitter taste but is well absorbed from the gastrointestinal tract. Its half-life, which varies among persons, averages 4 days, thus permitting once-weekly administration for prophylaxis. Chloroquine is concentrated in the hemoglobin-containing digestive vesicles of asexual intraerythrocytic parasites. It inhibits the parasite's heme polymerase that incorporates ferriprotoporphyrin type IX complexes, which are potentially toxic to the parasite, into insoluble, nontoxic, crystalline hemozoin. Chloroquine-resistant strains of *P. falciparum* actively transport chloroquine out of the intraparasitic compartment. Hydroxychloroquine (Plaquenil), which is used for rheumatologic diseases, is also effective against chloroquine-sensitive *Plasmodium* species.

Chloroquine is generally well tolerated when used at the doses recommended for the prophylaxis and treatment of malaria. Side effects include headache, nausea, vomiting, blurred vision, dizziness, and fatigue. Some persons with African ancestry experience pruritus, which responds to antihistamines. Rare side effects include depigmentation of hair, exacerbation of psoriasis, blood dyscrasias, seizures, neuropsychiatric effects, and reactions in persons with porphyria. Retinal damage has occurred in persons receiving chloroquine at high doses for the treatment of rheumatologic disorders, but it has not been documented as a problem in those taking it weekly over a period of many years for malaria prophylaxis. Cardiopulmonary collapse and death can occur after accidental overdose and in adults attempting suicide. As little as 5 g of chloroquine can be fatal unless treatment is promptly initiated with mechanical respiration, anticonvulsants, and blood pressure support.

Doxycycline 100 mg taken daily by adults provides effective prophylaxis against all *Plasmodium* species. It is begun 1 to 2 days before exposure and continued during the time of exposure and for 4 weeks after departure from a malaria-endemic area. Doxycycline or tetracycline is also often administered with quinine for the treatment of acute chloroquine-resistant malaria, but neither doxycycline nor tetracycline acts rapidly enough to be used alone for treatment. Doxycycline is generally well tolerated, although it can cause gastrointestinal symptoms and "pill" esophagitis. To avoid the latter, it should be taken with a full glass of water, and the recipient should remain upright for an hour or more after ingestion. Other important potential side effects include photosensitivity dermatitis, *Candida albicans* vaginitis, and *Clostridium difficile* colitis. Finally, doxycycline and tetracycline should not be used in children younger than 8 years or in women who are pregnant or breast-feeding unless the potential benefits outweigh the risks.

Mefloquine, a quinoline methanol compound derived from quinine, was once commonly used for prophylaxis, and occasionally for the treatment of chloroquine-resistant *P. falciparum* malaria. Concern about neuropsychiatric and other toxicities and the availability of better alternatives now limit its use.

Mefloquine is available for oral administration only. Slowly and incompletely absorbed, it is 99% protein bound. It has a variable half-life ranging from 6 to 23 days with a mean of approximately 14 days. It is metabolized and excreted slowly through bile and feces. It is associated with nausea, dizziness, vivid dreams, fatigue, and lassitude. Less common side effects, but of greater concern, are anxiety, depression, acute psychosis, and seizures. Mefloquine is contraindicated in persons with a history of epilepsy or psychiatric disorders. It also depresses atrioventricular conduction and should not be used in persons taking β-blockers for cardiac indications. Mefloquine now carries a U.S. Food and Drug Administration (FDA) black-box warning. Although not approved for use during pregnancy or in children weighing less than 15 kg, mefloquine has been used in these situations when its potential benefits are judged to outweigh its risks. It has been reported to have no adverse effects on pregnancy outcomes (such as stillbirths and abortions) and no effects on low birth rate and prematurity.[6]

Primaquine, an 8-aminoquinoline, and **tafenoquine,** an analogue, kill the hypnozoite stage of *P. vivax* and *P. ovale* in the liver. Primaquine is used as a 14-day course at the end of treatment or prophylaxis to prevent late relapses in persons who are or may have been infected with these *Plasmodium* species. It is also an alternative for daily primary prophylaxis for *P. vivax* and other species. In that case, it is begun 1 or 2 days before exposure and continued during and for 7 days after a traveler leaves a malaria-endemic area. Tafenoquine is administered as a single 300 mg dose following treatment of acute malaria due to *P. vivax* and *P. ovale* to prevent relapse. It can also be used for primary prophylaxis in travelers; 200 mg daily for 3 days before travel, then once weekly while in the malarious region, then in the week following exit, a final dose 7 days after the previous dose in the malarious region.

Primaquine is absorbed orally and rapidly converted to carboxyprimaquine, which has a half-life of approximately 7 days. It is generally well tolerated, although some recipients experience abdominal cramps, epigastric distress, and nausea. Tafenoquine is better absorbed, has a half-life of approximately 15 days, and is less likely to cause gastrointestinal problems. The major concern with primaquine and tafenoquine is hemolysis in persons with glucose-6-phosphate dehydrogenase (G6PD) deficiency (Chapter 152). The G6PD status of the recipient must be determined before it is administered. Rarely, primaquine causes neutropenia, methemoglobinemia, hypertension, or arrhythmias. Both drugs are contraindicated during pregnancy and in breast-feeding mothers because life-threatening hemolysis may occur if the fetus or baby is deficient in G6PD. Tafenoquine can cause severe psychiatric reactions and is contraindicated in persons with a history of psychosis or schizophrenia.

Quinine sulfate, a cinchona alkaloid, is the oldest of the antimalarials. It has a very bitter taste. It is rapidly absorbed after oral administration and has a half-life of 16 to 18 hours in persons with malaria. Quinine has the poorest therapeutic to toxicity ratio of any antimalarial drug. The side effects, known collectively as cinchonism, include tinnitus, decreased hearing, headache, nausea, vomiting, dysphoria, and visual disturbances. They are dose related and reversible. Quinine has also been associated with severe hypoglycemia in persons with heavy *P. falciparum* infections as a result of the utilization of glucose by intraerythrocytic *Plasmodium* and release of insulin from the pancreas. Hypoglycemia can be treated and prevented by the intravenous administration of glucose. Rare complications with quinine include massive hemolysis in patients with heavy *P. falciparum* infection resulting in hemoglobinuria and renal failure (blackwater fever), cutaneous hypersensitivity reactions, agranulocytosis, and hepatitis. Quinine can cause respiratory paralysis in persons with myasthenia gravis. It stimulates uterine contractions during pregnancy and can result in abortion, but it has saved the lives of many pregnant women with *P. falciparum* malaria. Quinine dihydrochloride given intravenously can cause myocardial depression, peripheral vascular collapse, respiratory depression, and potentially death.

Quinidine gluconate, the stereoisomer of quinine, is no longer available in the United States. It is used for the intravenous treatment of patients with complicated malaria and in those who cannot take antimalarials orally. Quinidine gluconate was once widely used for the treatment of ventricular ectopy, but it has been replaced by newer antiarrhythmic agents, which has decreased its availability in many hospitals. Side effects include prolongation of the QT interval, arrhythmias, and hypotension, particularly if it is infused too rapidly. Persons receiving intravenous quinidine should be monitored in an intensive care setting. Therapy should be switched to an oral antimalarial medication as soon as possible.

Toxoplasmosis, Babesiosis, and Amoebic Encephalitis

Toxoplasma gondii (Chapter 328) and *Babesia* species (Chapter 332) are other important pathogens of the phylum Apicomplexa. **Pyrimethamine** and **sulfadiazine** are used for the treatment of toxoplasmosis. They inhibit sequential steps in the folic acid metabolic pathway. Pyrimethamine preferentially inhibits dihydrofolate reductase. It is well absorbed orally. The major side effect is macrocytic anemia, which can be prevented by the concurrent administration of **leucovorin.** Sulfonamides reduce the activity of dihydropteroate synthetase and the binding of *p*-aminobenzoic acid to it. In ocular toxoplasmosis with macular involvement, corticosteroids are used along with anti-*Toxoplasma* therapy to minimize the local inflammatory response. **Clindamycin** and **pyrimethamine** or **atovaquone** and **pyrimethamine** are therapeutic options in sulfonamide-intolerant patients. Persons with AIDS, CD4+ counts less than 100/μL, and serologic evidence of *T. gondii* infection should receive prophylaxis with one of the following regimens: daily **trimethoprim-sulfamethoxazole, pyrimethamine** and **dapsone, pyrimethamine** and **atovaquone,** or **atovaquone** alone. **Spiramycin,** a macrolide, is used for the treatment of toxoplasmosis during pregnancy. Pyrimethamine is currently in short supply. Trimethoprim-sulfamethoxazole is a potential alternative when it is not available. Two therapeutic regimens are available for babesiosis. The combination of **clindamycin** and **quinine** is usually used in persons with severe babesiosis, but side effects are common. Long-term treatment (≥6 weeks) is often necessary for those who are immunocompromised. **Atovaquone** and **azithromycin** is better tolerated and used for less severe babesiosis (Chapter 332). Finally, the addition of **miltefosine,** an FDA-approved antileishmanial drug,[7] to multidrug regimens has improved the likelihood of survival in persons with granulomatous amebic encephalitis due to *Acanthamoeba* or *Balamuthia.* It is now recommended as part of multidrug regimens to treat granulomatous amebic encephalitis as well as primary amebic meningoencephalitis due to *Naegleria.*[8]

Intestinal and Vaginal Protozoa

Several major luminal pathogens, including *Entamoeba histolytica* (Chapter 331), *Giardia lamblia* (Chapter 330), and *Trichomonas vaginalis* (Chapter 332), live in anaerobic conditions in the intestine or vagina. The 5-nitroimidazoles, metronidazole and tinidazole, are first-line therapy for them, but refractory giardiasis and trichomoniasis are documented. Tinidazole has more favorable pharmacodynamics and is generally better tolerated. Because neither metronidazole nor tinidazole reliably eradicates cysts of *E. histolytica* in the colon, either paromomycin, a poorly absorbed aminoglycoside, or iodoquinol, both of which are active in the lumen of the bowel, is administered as well. Either one of these drugs or diloxanide furoate is used alone to treat persons with asymptomatic cyst excretion.

Giardiasis can also be treated with nitazoxanide. It is well tolerated, and a liquid formulation is available for children. Nitazoxanide is the only drug effective in the treatment of cryptosporidiosis (Chapter 329). It can cure immunocompetent persons, but not those with AIDS. Trimethoprim-sulfamethoxazole, which inhibits successive steps in the folic acid pathway, is the drug of choice for *Cystoisospora* (*Isospora*) *belli* and *Cyclospora cayetanensis.* Ciprofloxacin is a second-line alternative for the former. Either tetracycline, metronidazole, or nitazoxanide can be used to treat symptomatic *Balantidium coli* infection.

Metronidazole, a 5-nitroimidazole, is rapidly absorbed after oral administration and has a half-life of 8 hours. More than half of each dose is metabolized in the liver. The metabolites and remaining parent drug are excreted in urine. Metronidazole is activated by reduction of its 5-nitro group through a sequence of intermediate steps involving microbial electron transport proteins of low redox potential. It is concentrated in susceptible anaerobic organisms and serves as an electron sink. Nausea, vomiting, diarrhea, and a metallic taste are often associated with the use of metronidazole. They are less common with the lower doses recommended for the treatment of giardiasis than with the higher doses used for amebiasis. Other untoward effects include headache, dizziness, vertigo, and numbness. Potentially severe disulfiram-like reactions occur in patients who ingest alcohol while taking metronidazole.

Tinidazole, another 5-nitroimidazole, has a similar mechanism of action and spectrum of activity as metronidazole, but more favorable pharmacodynamics, and it is generally better tolerated. It has been used widely around the world for the treatment of giardiasis, intestinal amebiasis, and trichomoniasis. In comparison with metronidazole, it has a longer half-life, a shorter and less complicated dosing regimen, and fewer gastrointestinal side effects. It, too, can cause severe disulfiram-like reactions after alcohol ingestion.

Nitazoxanide, a nitrothiazolyl-salicylamide derivative thiazolide, has a broad spectrum of activity against protozoa and helminths. It is formulated as a liquid for children. Nitazoxanide is well absorbed orally and hydrolyzed to its active metabolite tizoxanide, which undergoes conjugation to tizoxanide glucuronide. The parent compound is not detectable in serum. Maximum concentrations of the metabolites are observed in 1 to 4 hours. They are excreted in urine and bile. Tizoxanide is highly protein bound. Although its antiparasitic mechanism of action is uncertain, nitazoxanide inhibits pyruvate : ferredoxin oxidoreductase–dependent electron transport reactions essential for the metabolism of susceptible anaerobic organisms. It is very well tolerated in children and adults.

● AFRICAN TRYPANOSOMIAIS (SLEEPING SICKNESS), CHAGAS DISEASE, AND LEISHMANIASIS

The Kinetoplastida, *Trypanosoma brucei rhodesiense* and *Trypanosoma brucei gambiense,* which cause human African trypanosomiasis (sleeping sickness); *Trypanosoma cruzi,* the etiology of Chagas disease; and *Leishmania* species, which cause cutaneous, mucosal, and visceral leishmaniasis often pose substantial therapeutic challenges.[9]

African Trypanosomiasis (Sleeping Sickness)

Suramin, pentamidine, eflornithine, and **melarsoprol** are used for the treatment of human African trypanosomiasis (Chapter 325). Suramin or pentamidine is recommended for the hemolymphatic stage of *T. brucei rhodesiense* and *T. brucei gambiense,* respectively. Both drugs are associated with potentially serious side effects, and suramin can cause severe reactions in persons co-infected with Onchocerca volvulus. **Eflornithine,** which is much better tolerated, is effective against both the hemolymphatic and central nervous system (CNS) stages of *T. brucei gambiense* infection. It does not have activity against

T. brucei rhodesiense. Unfortunately, eflornithine is costly and supplies are limited. It is available in the United States from the CDC. It can be used alone, but eflornithine is often co-administered with nifurtimox for CNS *T. brucei gambiense* infection. Melarsoprol is used for persons with CNS involvement due to *T. brucei rhodesiense* and *T. brucei gambiense* when eflornithine is not available. Melarsoprol can result in severe toxicity, including life-threatening encephalopathic reactions.

Chagas Disease
Benznidazole or **nifurtimox** orally is used to treat *T. cruzi* infections (Chapter 326). Benznidazole has been the drug of choice in endemic areas of Latin America and nifurtimox in the United States.[10] Both drugs are available from the CDC. They lower mortality and shorten the duration of acute Chagas disease. Treatment is recommended for persons with recent infection as well as asymptomatic children and adults through middle age with indeterminate-stage *T. cruzi* infection. The percentage of those who are parasitologically cured by treatment has been debated. Neither benznidazole nor nifurtimox can reverse the cardiac or gastrointestinal manifestations of chronic Chagas disease. Side effects are common with both drugs and increase in frequency and severity with age. Benznidazole is administered daily for 1 month and is associated with allergic dermatitis, peripheral neuropathy, insomnia, and gastrointestinal symptoms, including anorexia and weight loss. Nifurtimox is administered daily for 3 months and is associated with anorexia, nausea, vomiting, weight loss, headache, dizziness or vertigo, paresthesias, weakness, and polyneuropathy.

Leishmaniasis (Cutaneous, Mucosal, and Visceral)
Treatment of cutaneous leishmaniasis depends on the size, number, complexity, and location of skin lesions, their cosmetic impact, the infecting *Leishmania* species, and its propensity to cause mucosal disease.[11] Uncomplicated lesions acquired in Europe, Africa, and Asia, where mucosal involvement is rare, can be followed without therapy if they appear to be healing spontaneously. Lesion-directed treatment options include cryotherapy; heat therapy, which requires a specialized delivery system; or intralesional injection of **stibogluconate sodium,** which is not available in the United States. Topical therapy with direct application of **paromomycin** is another option. An ointment containing 15% paromomycin and 12% methylbenzethonium chloride in white paraffin developed in Israel has been used. A U.S. Army formulation of topical paromomycin also appears promising.

Parenteral or oral antileishmanial therapy is used for persons with complicated cutaneous leishmaniasis and for those who are or may be infected with *Leishmania braziliensis* or related New World species potentially associated with mucosal leishmaniasis.[12] **Miltefosine** is FDA approved for the oral treatment of cutaneous leishmaniasis due to *Leishmania braziliensis*. The efficacy with other *Leishmania* species varies. **Liposomal amphotericin B** and **amphotericin B deoxycholate** are effective, but more toxic, parenteral alternatives. **Stibogluconate sodium** and **meglumine antimoniate** were once widely used, but their toxicity, the requirement for parenteral administration, and increasing resistance have limited their use. Fluconazole and other imidazole antifungals have activity against some *Leishmania* species.

Mucosal leishmaniasis is less responsive to treatment than cutaneous leishmaniasis, and relapses are common.[13] Therapeutic options include liposomal amphotericin B, miltefosine, amphotericin B deoxycholate, stibogluconate sodium, or meglumine antimoniate.

Visceral leishmaniasis is a potentially fatal disease. The drug of choice is liposomal amphotericin B. Miltefosine and amphotericin B deoxycholate are alternatives. Sodium stibogluconate or meglumine antimoniate are used in some geographic areas where resistance has not yet emerged.

Liposomal amphotericin B was the first drug approved by the FDA for treatment of visceral leishmaniasis (Chapter 327) in the United States. Liposomes deliver amphotericin to macrophages where leishmania reside. Liposomal amphotericin B is better tolerated than amphotericin B deoxycholate, which is an alternative. Other lipid-associated amphotericin B preparations appear to be effective, but they have been less extensively studied and are not FDA approved for this indication.

Miltefosine, an alkylphospholipid and phosphocholine analog, initially developed as an antineoplastic drug, is FDA approved for the treatment of visceral leishmaniasis and cutaneous leishmaniasis due to *L. braziliensis*. A major advantage is oral administration.[14] The pharmacokinetics are characterized by a long elimination half-life and extensive drug accumulation. The mechanism of action is uncertain, but miltefosine induces apoptosis-like changes in the parasite. Side effects are frequent, but typically mild to moderate. Dose-dependent gastrointestinal toxicity can result in nausea, vomiting, and diarrhea, which tend to decrease with continued administration of the drug. Elevations in liver enzymes and creatinine are common but usually transient. Miltefosine is embryotoxic and is thus contraindicated during pregnancy. Contraceptive cover is mandatory in women of childbearing years during and for 4 months after therapy. Relapses have been reported after the treatment of visceral leishmaniasis. They are frequent in persons with concurrent AIDS.

Stibogluconate sodium and **meglumine antimoniate,** pentavalent antimony drugs, were used to treat visceral leishmaniasis in the past, but resistance is now common among *Leishmania donovani* isolates in India, adjacent countries, and some other areas of the world. Pentavalent antimony drugs require parenteral administration. Side effects increase with age and include gastrointestinal symptoms, pancreatitis, myalgias, headache, malaise, elevated liver enzyme levels, and occasionally bone marrow suppression. Nonspecific ST-T wave changes are common. Sudden death has been reported in older persons and in those receiving more than the recommended dose.

⬤ HELMINTHIC DISEASES
The treatment of helminthic diseases is discussed based on their taxonomy and the site of infection. A number of anthelminthic drugs are available. Several have multiple indications. Information about their pharmacology is provided at the end of this section.

Intestinal Roundworms (Nematodes)
Intestinal roundworms (Nematodes) (Chapter 335) are among the world's most prevalent parasites. *Ascaris lumbricoides,* the hookworms *Ancylostoma duodenale* and *Necator americanus,* and *Trichuris trichiura* each infect millions of people worldwide. *Strongyloides stercoralis* is less common, but can progress to life-threatening hyperinfection in immunocompromised persons. Many residents of impoverished areas harbor more than one of these species. A number of drugs are available to treat them for *Enterobius vermicularis* (pinworm) and other intestinal roundworms. Albendazole, mebendazole, pyrantel pamoate, and ivermectin have replaced older anthelmintics that were more toxic, such as piperazine and thiabendazole, or less effective.

Albendazole has a broad spectrum of activity. It is active against *A. lumbricoides,* the hookworms, and *T. trichiura.* Administered as a single 400-mg dose, it has been widely used in mass treatment programs in areas where these soil-transmitted roundworms are prevalent.[15] However, reinfection is common, and treatment is often repeated at 3- to 4-month intervals. The CDC recommends presumptive treatment of immigrants from endemic regions with a single dose of albendazole before arrival in the United States. Daily doses of albendazole for 3 days are recommended for persons with heavy *T. trichiura* infection. Albendazole, 400 mg twice daily for 7 days, is used as an alternative to ivermectin for the treatment of *Strongyloides stercoralis* infection. Failures can occur with either drug, and they are often used together for longer periods to treat those with disseminated hyperinfection. Albendazole is effective against *Enterobius vermicularis,* the pinworm, in a single dose that is repeated in 2 weeks. It can be used for cutaneous larva migrans, which is caused by migrating stages of *Ancylostoma braziliense* and other intestinal roundworms of animals. It is the drug of choice for trichinosis, and it has been used for the treatment of *Trichostrongylus* species and *Capillaria philippinensis.* There has been a massive increase in the cost of albendazole in the United States.

Mebendazole, 100 mg orally twice daily for 3 days, has a similar spectrum of activity as albendazole against *A. lumbricoides,* hookworms, and *T. trichiura.* In this regimen, it is more effective than a single dose of albendazole and is considered the treatment of choice for heavy *T. trichiura* infections. A single 500-mg dose of mebendazole has been used in mass treatment programs. Mebendazole is effective in treating pinworms when given at 100 mg orally in one dose followed by a second dose after 2 weeks. It is an alternative to albendazole for the treatment of trichinosis. Mebendazole is poorly absorbed and ineffective against *S. stercoralis.*

Pyrantel pamoate is a relatively safe, poorly absorbed, over-the-counter drug with activity against *A. lumbricoides,* hookworms, and pinworm, but it is not effective against *T. trichiura* or *S. stercoralis.* When used for pinworm infection, it is administered as an oral suspension at a dose of 11 mg/kg (to a maximum of 1 g), which is repeated after 2 weeks.

Ivermectin at an oral dose of 200 µg/kg daily for 2 days is considered the treatment of choice for uncomplicated *S. stercoralis.* In immunocompromised persons with hyperinfection, daily doses are given until stool and sputum exams are negative for larvae for 2 weeks. It is also effective against cutaneous larva migrans and *A. lumbricoides* but not hookworms. It is an alternative to mebendazole for the treatment of *T. trichiura.*

Systemic Roundworms (Nematodes)

Diethylcarbamazine is the drug of choice for the treatment of lymphatic filarial infections (Chapter 335) caused by *Wuchereria bancrofti, Brugia malayi,* and *Brugia timori,* as well as for tropical pulmonary eosinophilia. It promotes the host's killing of microfilariae of these species and also damages or kills adult worms. Inflammatory side effects are common. They are due in part to the release of lipopolysaccharide from endosymbiotic *Wolbachia* bacteria within dying filaria. *Wolbachia* are necessary for filarial development and are a potential drug target. Long-term therapy with doxycycline results in their elimination and has been used for therapy. Diethylcarbamazine is also used for *Loa loa* infections in persons with acceptably low levels of microfilaremia (<8000/mL). Encephalopathy may result from treatment of those with more. In that case, apheresis or treatment with albendazole is used first to reduce the number of microfilaria. Diethylcarbamazine should not be used for onchocerciasis. It kills the microfilariae of *O. volvulus* rapidly, and the release of parasite and *Wolbachia* antigens can result in severe ocular and systemic inflammatory responses. The latter, known as the Mazzotti reaction, can be life threatening and is characterized by fever, urticaria, lymphadenopathy, tachycardia, hypotension, arthralgias, peripheral edema, and abdominal pain. Diethylcarbamazine has also been used prophylactically to prevent loiasis.

Ivermectin is the treatment of choice for onchocerciasis. It is administered as a single dose of 150 µg/kg. It does not kill adult *Onchocerca volvulus,* but it decreases ova production and reduces microfilariae in the skin and eyes. Retreatment is usually necessary at 6- to 12-month intervals until the patient is free of symptoms. For *Onchocerca volvulus,* biannual treatment leads to substantial reductions in community infection rates after four or five rounds of therapy. Ivermectin has activity against the microfilariae of *W. bancrofti* and *Brugia* species, but it does not kill adult worms and is not recommended for treatment of these organisms. Ivermectin should not be given to persons with heavy concurrent *Loa loa* infections because it kills *Loa loa* microfilaria rapidly and can result in encephalopathy.

Tapeworms (Cestodes)

Praziquantel has a broad spectrum of activity against tapeworms (Chapter 333) and flukes. It is the drug of choice for adult tapeworms in the human intestinal tract. It is effective against *Taenia solium* (pork tapeworm), *Taenia saginata* (beef tapeworm), *Taenia asiatica* (Asian tapeworm), *Diphyllobothrium latum* (fish), and *Hymenolepis nana* (dwarf tapeworm) when administered as a single dose. Niclosamide, which is not absorbed, is an effective alternative for the treatment of *T. saginata* and *D. latum.* It also kills adult *T. solium,* but disintegration of the worm and release of viable ova into the intestinal lumen raise the theoretical possibility of autoinfection. In the case of *H. nana,* a dose of nitazoxanide, 500 mg twice daily for 3 days, provides an alternative to praziquantel. Nitazoxanide also has activity against *T. saginata* and potentially other tapeworm species.[16]

Neurocysticercosis caused by the larval or tissue stage of *T. solium* is a major cause of seizures and other CNS abnormalities in residents and immigrants from endemic areas of Latin America and other endemic regions. Symptoms can result from the physical presence of cysticerci, but inflammation elicited by the release of antigens from dying cysticerci is often more important. Both albendazole and praziquantel are capable of killing cysticerci in the brain; albendazole has superior pharmacokinetics. Their use depends on the clinical syndrome.[17] Concurrent administration increases the parasiticidal effect in patients with multiple brain cysticerci without increased side effects.[A1] Corticosteroids are administered with anthelmintic therapy to reduce the inflammatory response. The CDC recommendation for albendazole is 15 mg/kg/day in 2 divided doses for 15 days, and for praziquantel 50 mg/kg/day for 15 days.[18] The concurrent use of corticosteroids increases the serum level of albendazole but decreases that of praziquantel. Neither albendazole nor praziquantel should be used in persons with cysticerci in the eye or spinal cord because the release of antigens from dying cysticerci can trigger a locally destructive inflammatory reaction.

Surgery or PAIR (percutaneous aspiration, injection of chemicals, and reaspiration) is the preferred approach for *Echinococcus granulosus* cysts. Albendazole is used for inoperable *E. granulosus* and *Echinococcus multilocularis* disease and in persons in whom medical treatment is preferred for other reasons. Administered at a dose of 400 mg twice daily for adults, generally for 1 to 6 months, albendazole may cure approximately one third of uncomplicated *Echinococcus granulosus* liver cysts. Albendazole is also administered before

ultrasound-guided PAIR or surgery to prevent seeding of the peritoneum should the cyst's contents spill. Potentially fatal bone marrow suppression and hepatitis are concerns in persons receiving high-dose, prolonged albendazole therapy.

Flukes (Trematodes)

Praziquantel is the drug of choice for the treatment of all forms of schistosomiasis (Chapter 334), as well as intestinal, lung, and liver flukes (Chapter 334), with the exception of *Fasciola hepatica.* For schistosomiasis, two or three doses of praziquantel are given in 1 day depending on the species. Oxamniquine is an alternative for *Schistosoma mansoni,* but it is more toxic and less effective. Either praziquantel or albendazole can be used to treat the liver fluke *Clonorchis sinensis.* *F. hepatica* is usually treated with triclabendazole. Bithionol, which is more toxic, and nitazoxanide are alternatives.

Pharmacology of Drugs Used for Helminthic Diseases

Albendazole is poorly soluble in water, but it is well absorbed when administered with a fatty meal. It undergoes rapid first-pass metabolism in the liver to albendazole sulfoxide, which has excellent anthelmintic activity. The serum half-life of albendazole sulfoxide is 8 to 9 hours. Elimination of albendazole sulfoxide and other metabolites is primarily through the kidney. Albendazole binds to tubulin in susceptible parasites, inhibits microtubule assembly, and decreases glucose absorption. It does not affect human tubulin. It also inhibits fumarate reductase in helminths. Concurrent administration of dexamethasone, which is frequently given to prevent cerebral edema in persons with neurocysticercosis, increases serum levels by approximately 50%. The cerebrospinal fluid (CSF) concentration of albendazole is approximately 40% that in serum.

Albendazole is generally well tolerated when given as a single dose for the treatment of intestinal roundworm infections, although gastrointestinal discomfort may develop or patients may experience migration of adult *A. lumbricoides* from the nose or mouth or see them in their stool. Albendazole at higher doses and for longer duration is used for persons with neurocysticercosis. Corticosteroids are administered concurrently to reduce intracranial inflammation and increased intracranial pressure. Albendazole is contraindicated in persons with cysticerci in the eye or spinal cord. High-dose, prolonged therapy with albendazole, such as that recommended for echinococcal disease, can be complicated by alopecia, hepatitis, or bone marrow suppression, which is not always reversible after discontinuation of the drug. Albendazole is embryotoxic in animals and contraindicated during pregnancy.

Diethylcarbamazine, a piperazine derivative, is well absorbed orally and has a half-life of 8 hours. The parent drug and its metabolites are excreted through the kidney. Although the mechanism of action is uncertain, the piperazine moiety may result in paralysis of sensitive helminths. Diethylcarbamazine also alters the surface membranes of susceptible microfilariae, thereby resulting in destruction by the host's immune system. Side effects include those caused by the drug and those that result from release of the parasite antigens and lipopolysaccharide from filaria-harbored, endosymbiotic *Wolbachia.* Adverse effects include nausea, vomiting, anorexia, headache, malaise, weakness, arthralgias, and rarely, acute psychotic reactions. In patients with lymphatic filariasis, localized swelling or nodules may develop along the lymphatics during treatment and transient lymphedema or hydrocele may develop.

Ivermectin is a macrocyclic lactone produced by *Streptomyces avermitilis.* It has a broad spectrum of activity against helminths and arthropods, including *Sarcoptes scabiei,* the cause of scabies. It is well absorbed after oral administration. Ivermectin is highly protein bound, has a serum half-life of 12 hours, and accumulates in adipose tissue and the liver. It is subject to enterohepatic recirculation and ultimately eliminated in stool. Ivermectin activates the opening of gated chloride channels in susceptible helminths and arthropods. The result is an influx of chloride ions and paralysis of the pharyngeal pumping mechanism of helminths. Ivermectin is generally well tolerated in humans, although inflammatory reactions can develop in response to antigens released from dying parasites.

Mebendazole is only slightly soluble in water and is relatively poorly absorbed from the gastrointestinal tract. This is advantageous for the treatment of intestinal parasites but limits its effectiveness against tissue-dwelling helminths. Absorbed drug is metabolized in the liver and excreted in urine. Mebendazole selectively binds to helminthic tubulin, blocks its assembly into microtubules, and inhibits glucose uptake. This leads to depletion of glycogen stores and ultimately death of the parasite. Mebendazole is relatively well tolerated in the doses used to treat intestinal helminths. Transient abdominal pain and diarrhea occur in a small number of recipients. Mebendazole is contraindicated during pregnancy.

Praziquantel is well absorbed after oral administration. It undergoes extensive first-pass metabolism, and the metabolites, which are inactive, are excreted in urine. Praziquantel is approximately 80% protein bound, with a serum half-life of 4 to 6 hours. It is rapidly taken up by susceptible cestodes and trematodes. In the case of schistosomes, praziquantel damages the tegument, which results in intense vacuolation and increased permeability to calcium. Adult schistosomes are paralyzed and translocated to the liver through the portal circulation. Sequestered antigens are exposed on their surface, permitting binding of antibodies and phagocytes resulting in immune destruction. Praziquantel is an alternative to albendazole for the treatment of neurocysticercosis. The concurrent administration of corticosteroids, which are necessary to decrease inflammation and edema in the brain, reduces the serum concentration of praziquantel. The concentration in CSF is approximately 15 to 20% that of serum.

Praziquantel is frequently associated with mild, transient side effects, including headaches, lassitude, dizziness, nausea, vomiting, and abdominal discomfort, but they are seldom severe enough to interrupt therapy. Untoward reactions attributed to release of parasite antigens have been reported in patients treated for schistosomiasis and pulmonary paragonimiasis. Increased intracranial pressure resulting from release of cysticercal antigens is a potentially life-threatening consequence in patients receiving praziquantel for neurocysticercosis. Corticosteroids should be administered concurrently. Praziquantel is contraindicated in persons with cysticerci in the eye or spinal cord.

 Grade A Reference

A1. Garcia HH, Gonzales I, Lescano AG, et al. Cysticercosis Working Group in Peru. Efficacy of combined antiparasitic therapy with praziquantel and albendazole for neurocysticercosis: a double-blind, randomised controlled trial. *Lancet Infect Dis.* 2014;14:687-695.

GENERAL REFERENCES

For the General References and other additional features, please visit Expert Consult at https://expertconsult.inkling.com.

324

MALARIA

PHILIP J. ROSENTHAL AND MOSES R. KAMYA

DEFINITION

Malaria is caused by infection with protozoan parasites of the genus *Plasmodium,* all of which are transmitted by bites of infected anopheline mosquitoes.[1,2] Malaria is typically characterized by an acute febrile illness, with parasites infecting large numbers of erythrocytes, and classically entails recurrent episodes of fever and chills. It was first described thousands of years ago and is named on the basis of the belief that it was caused by the bad air of the marshes surrounding Rome. Malaria is common, causing hundreds of millions of illnesses each year throughout most of the tropics. Severe disease can occur, primarily with *Plasmodium falciparum* infection, with the acute development of serious organ dysfunction or when chronic and repeated infection leads to severe anemia. *P. falciparum* malaria has killed about half a million people per year in recent years, mostly children in sub-Saharan Africa.

The Pathogen

P. falciparum is responsible for most episodes of severe malaria. It is endemic in most malarious areas and is by far the predominant species in Africa. *Plasmodium vivax* is about as common as *P. falciparum,* except in Africa, but causes severe disease much less commonly. However, studies suggest that severe illness associated with *P. vivax* infection is more common than had previously been appreciated.[3] *Plasmodium ovale* and *Plasmodium malariae* are much less common causes of disease and generally do not cause severe illness. A fifth parasite causing human infections is *Plasmodium knowlesi,* a parasite of macaque monkeys that is a fairly common zoonosis in parts of Southeast Asia and has been responsible for malarial illnesses, including severe disease, in individuals exposed to macaque-biting vectors in forested areas.

EPIDEMIOLOGY

Malaria in Endemic Countries

Malaria is the most important parasitic disease of humans, causing hundreds of millions of illnesses and hundreds of thousands of deaths each year. The disease is endemic in most of the tropics, including many parts of South and Central America, Africa, the Middle East, the Indian subcontinent, Southeast Asia, and Oceania. Transmission, morbidity, and mortality are greatest in Africa, where infection with *P. falciparum* predominates. In most other endemic areas, disease caused by both *P. falciparum* and *P. vivax* is common. In highly endemic areas, the group at greatest risk is young children, who experience most episodes of disease and the most deaths. A second high-risk group is pregnant women, with high risks of maternal and fetal morbidity from *P. falciparum* malaria, including many deaths secondary to low birthweight. In highly endemic areas, in addition to extensive mortality, malaria exerts a massive toll through adverse effects on child development; contributions to school and work absenteeism; and, overall, billions of dollars in lost income among the poorest citizens of the poorest countries of the world. In areas of developing countries with lower levels of malaria transmission, malaria can be epidemic, with intermittent increases in transmission that cause major morbidity in relatively nonimmune populations. Although the burden of malaria remains enormous, with increased control activities worldwide mortality was estimated to decrease 57% between 2000 and 2015, with 446,000[4] or 631,000[5] deaths in 2015 reported using different modeling approaches. However, after marked gains, morbidity and mortality appear to have stabilized, with World Health Organization (WHO) estimates essentially unchanged since 2015.

Malaria in Travelers

Malaria is also common in travelers of any age from nonendemic areas to the tropics and may be manifested in those who have returned to nonendemic areas up to many months after travel. Indeed, malaria is the most common documented cause of febrile illness in travelers returning from the tropics to developed countries. Malaria is also rarely transmitted in areas considered nonendemic, including the United States, when imported parasites are transmitted by local anopheline mosquitoes, by blood products, or through congenital spread of infection.

Malaria Transmission

Malaria is transmitted by multiple species of mosquitoes of the genus *Anopheles,* which vary in geographic distribution, ecologic preferences, and susceptibility to mosquito control measures. Anopheline mosquitoes bite at night, so personal mosquito control measures focus on avoidance of mosquito bites during sleep. Levels of malaria transmission in endemic areas vary greatly, from areas where residents experience only rare infectious bites to regions of Africa where individuals may receive hundreds of infectious bites each year.

Recent Changes in the Epidemiology of Malaria

A major effort to eradicate malaria after World War II led to elimination of the disease in many areas, including the United States and Europe, but eventually failed to control the disease in most of the tropics. During the ensuing decades, improvements in malaria control were few, and malarial morbidity worsened in many areas, driven by the loss of enthusiasm for vector control; increasing resistance of mosquitoes to insecticides; and, in particular, resistance of parasites to commonly used antimalarial drugs. More than 50 years later, a new large effort to control and eventually to eradicate malaria has been initiated.[6] Key control measures include indoor residual spraying of insecticides, distribution of insecticide-impregnated bed nets, prompt provision of effective drugs to those with malaria, and targeted administration of drugs to prevent infection in high-risk groups. Recent efforts have led to documented decreases in levels of malarial morbidity and mortality in some areas, notably parts of Africa, Asia, and Oceania with relatively low levels of transmission intensity. It is of great interest to learn whether recent advances due to intensified control efforts can bring sustained improvements to those parts of the world most affected with malaria, in particular, highly endemic regions of Africa and Asia.

Malaria and Human Immunodeficiency Virus Infection

Malaria does not differ as markedly between those with human immunodeficiency virus (HIV) infection and others as is the case with typical opportunistic infections. However, several interactions between malaria and HIV infection have been established. First, HIV infection appears to disrupt the acquired immune response to malaria and thereby increases the incidence and severity of malaria. Second, acute malaria elevates HIV viral load and so may increase the risk of HIV transmission. Third, HIV infection may be associated with reduced efficacy of antimalarial treatment, especially in the setting of severe immune suppression. Fourth, therapies for each infection may have an impact on the other, leading to unanticipated effects on drug efficacy or toxicity. Fifth, routine interventions for HIV infection may affect the incidence of malaria; notably, daily trimethoprim–sulfamethoxazole, a routine regimen in HIV-infected patients, offers partial protection against malaria. Because both HIV infection and malaria are common in many areas, in particular sub-Saharan Africa, even modest associations are important. Thus, malaria coinfection in HIV-infected individuals may be an important factor in promoting the spread of HIV infection in Africa. However, increasing implementation of insecticide-treated bed nets, prophylaxis against opportunistic infections with trimethoprim–sulfamethoxazole, and antiretroviral therapy will likely substantially lessen malaria risk in HIV-infected patients, such that the risk in those receiving optimal management will not be substantially greater than that in the general population.

PATHOBIOLOGY
Parasite Life Cycle

Malaria is transmitted by the bite of infected female anopheline mosquitoes. During feeding, mosquitoes inject sporozoites, which circulate to the liver and infect hepatocytes, causing asymptomatic liver infection (Fig. 324-1). Merozoites are subsequently released from the liver, and they rapidly infect erythrocytes to begin the asexual erythrocytic stage of infection that is responsible for human disease. Multiple rounds of erythrocytic development, with production of merozoites that invade additional erythrocytes, lead to large

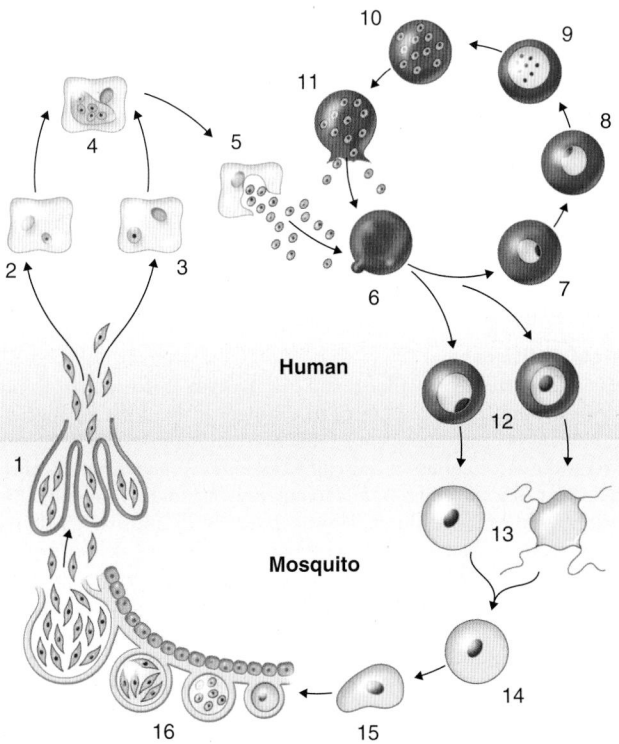

FIGURE 324-1. Life cycle of the malaria parasite. The *upper* and *lower halves* of the diagram indicate the human and anopheline mosquito parts of the cycle, respectively. Sporozoites from the salivary gland of a female *Anopheles* mosquito are injected under the skin (1). They then travel through the blood stream to the liver (2) and mature within hepatocytes to become tissue schizonts (4). Up to 30,000 parasites are then released into the blood stream as merozoites (5) and produce symptomatic infection as they invade and destroy red blood cells. However, in *Plasmodium vivax* and *Plasmodium ovale* infection, some parasites remain dormant in the liver as hypnozoites (3), which can later develop to tissue schizonts and merozoites, leading to relapse. Within the blood stream, merozoites (5) invade erythrocytes (6) and mature to the ring (7, 8), trophozoite (9), and schizont (10) asexual stages. Mature schizonts lyse their host erythrocytes and release the next generation of merozoites (11), which invade previously uninfected cells. Some erythrocytic parasites differentiate to sexual forms (male and female gametocytes) (12). When taken up by a mosquito, the gametocytes mature to male and female gametes (13), fuse to form zygotes (14), and then develop into ookinetes that invade the gut of the mosquito (15) and develop into oocysts (16). Mature oocysts produce sporozoites, which migrate to the salivary gland of the mosquito (1) to allow another human infection. (From Krogstad DJ: Blood and tissue protozoa. In: Schaechter M, Medoff G, Eisenstein BI, eds. *Mechanisms of Microbial Diseases.* 2nd ed. Baltimore: Williams & Wilkins; 1993:600.)

numbers of circulating parasites and clinical illness. Each erythrocytic cycle lasts approximately 24 hours for *P. knowlesi*; 48 hours for *P. falciparum, P. vivax,* and *P. ovale;* and 72 hours for *P. malariae.* Some erythrocytic parasites also develop into sexual gametocytes, which are taken up by mosquitoes. In the mosquito, gametocytes mature to gametes, and after fusion of male and female gametes to produce zygotes, parasites develop into ookinetes, oocysts, and then salivary gland sporozoites that are infectious for humans, allowing completion of the life cycle and infection of others. *P. vivax* and *P. ovale* also cause a chronic liver infection, in which hypnozoites persist in hepatocytes in a dormant state not eradicated by most therapies for acute disease and subsequently can progress to erythrocytic infection and a relapse of clinical illness.

Pathogenic Features of Malaria Parasites

The most common clinical feature of malaria is fever. Fever coincides with rupture of large numbers of schizont-infected erythrocytes at the completion of the erythrocytic cycle and with high circulating levels of tumor necrosis factor (TNF). Severe falciparum malaria is associated with very high levels of TNF and other inflammatory cytokines, but the specific roles of cytokines in pathogenesis are not well understood. *P. falciparum* infects erythrocytes of all ages, so it is capable of routinely causing high parasitemias, with infection of more than 1% of erythrocytes and more than 10^5 infected erythrocytes per microliter of blood. Non–*P. falciparum* parasites infect smaller numbers of erythrocytes, limiting the extent of infection and morbidity. Non–*P. falciparum* parasites are more likely to cause highly synchronous infections, leading if untreated to regular cycles of fever every 48 (*P. vivax* and *P. ovale*) or 72 (*P. malariae*) hours, often with minimal symptoms between fever episodes.

The contribution of parasite virulence determinants to the severity of malaria is poorly understood. A key biologic feature of *P. falciparum* infection is the ability of parasites to mediate the adherence of infected erythrocytes to a number of ligands on endothelial cells. By this mechanism, erythrocytes infected with the more mature stages of erythrocytic parasites do not circulate but rather adhere within small blood vessels in the brain and other organs. This phenomenon, termed cytoadherence, allows parasites to avoid passing through the spleen, where abnormal erythrocytes would be cleared. Cytoadherence is also likely to play a major role in mediating severe manifestations of *P. falciparum* malaria, with local inflammatory changes mediated by large numbers of adherent parasites leading to organ dysfunction. In particular, *P. falciparum* malaria can progress to cerebral malaria, including coma; noncardiogenic pulmonary edema, including severe respiratory compromise; and renal failure, severe anemia, acidosis, hypoglycemia, and other syndromes of organ dysfunction. Pregnancy selects for a subset of *P. falciparum* strains that specifically bind to ligands in the placenta. Pregnant women in endemic areas, in particular those in their first pregnancy who lack antibodies specific for placenta-binding parasites, are at high risk of morbidity, including anemia, from high parasite loads in the placenta and of poor fetal outcomes, including intrauterine growth retardation, spontaneous abortion, and low birthweight.

A common cause of death from *P. falciparum* malaria, in particular in children in endemic areas, is severe anemia. Anemia is caused by destruction of infected and uninfected erythrocytes, decreased hematopoiesis, and bleeding. In many endemic areas, most asymptomatic young children are infected with *P. falciparum,* with chronic infection causing chronic anemia. Other factors contributing to anemia are nutritional deficits and intestinal roundworm infections. With frequent malarial infections and chronic anemia, children are ill equipped to manage acute worsening of the anemia caused by acute malarial illness. With limited access to health care, children often present for medical care late in the course of illness if at all, and many deaths result.

P. falciparum parasites use antigenic variation to evade the host immune response. The principal protein that mediates the cytoadherence of infected erythrocytes to endothelial cells, *P. falciparum* erythrocyte membrane protein-1 (PfEMP-1), is transported to the erythrocyte surface and is a target of host immune responses that limit infection. The PfEMP-1 family comprises about 60 proteins, but only one PfEMP-1 variant is expressed on the surface of an infected erythrocyte at a time. During the course of an infection, parasites frequently vary the expression of PfEMP-1s to stymie host responses. This factor and the high variability in sequence of many PfEMP-1 molecules present a broad repertoire of antigens and probably help explain the slow acquisition of protective antimalarial immunity. Antigenic variation and other aspects of immunologic diversity are not clearly understood for non–*P. falciparum* malaria parasites, but each species appears capable of repeated infections.

Plasmodial parasites other than *P. falciparum* do not cause cytoadherence of infected erythrocytes, infect lower numbers of erythrocytes, and are much less commonly responsible for complicated and severe disease. However, recent reports suggest that *P. vivax* can cause severe disease, in particular respiratory compromise, more commonly than has previously been appreciated. *P. vivax* is also particularly prone to cause splenic rupture, although this complication can be seen with all malarial species. *P. malariae* most commonly causes a mild febrile illness, but chronic or repeated infection has been associated with an immune complex–mediated glomerulonephritis with nephrotic syndrome (Chapter 113). Recent reports indicate that *P. knowlesi* can cause severe illness, including deaths. The short (24-hour) erythrocytic cycle of *P. knowlesi,* which allows more rapid replication of these parasites compared with others, may partly explain the propensity of this zoonotic parasite to cause severe illness.

Host Immunity and Genetics

The nature of human immune responses to malaria remains not well characterized, but protective responses require multiple infections and apparently humoral and cell-mediated responses. Where *P. falciparum* malaria is common, disease occurs primarily in children. After some protection during the first few months of life, probably because of protective effects of maternal antiplasmodial antibodies and fetal hemoglobin, young children are infected frequently, experience repeated febrile malaria illnesses, and are at high risk of severe disease. With repeated episodes of malaria, children develop partial immunity. Immunity develops gradually, with some protection against severe malaria after only a few infections, increasing protection against symptomatic illness, and eventually strong protection against infection. Thus, in highly endemic areas, young children experience frequent episodes of malaria, especially at about age 6 months to 5 years; older children are frequently infected but uncommonly symptomatic; and adults experience identifiable malarial parasitemia less commonly. However, antimalarial immunity is not complete; malaria can occur in individuals of any age. In addition, immunity requires boosting by repeated infections, so adults are at increased risk of disease if they return to a highly endemic site after an extended stay in a nonendemic area.

A number of human genetic polymorphisms offer protection against malaria. The best characterized is sickle hemoglobin (Chapter 154). Hemoglobin S heterozygotes are partially protected against severe *P. falciparum* malaria, leading to a balanced polymorphism in which the survival advantage of the polymorphism allows persistence of sickle cell disease in homozygotes. Other erythrocyte polymorphisms that also are likely to offer protection against malaria include hemoglobin C and E, thalassemias (Chapter 153), glucose-6-phosphate dehydrogenase deficiency (Chapter 152), and ovalocytosis (Chapter 152). The Duffy antigen, an erythrocyte chemokine receptor of uncertain function, is the principal receptor on human erythrocytes for attachment and subsequent invasion of *P. vivax*. Most Africans lack the erythrocyte Duffy antigen, explaining the uncommon prevalence of *P. vivax* in most of Africa.

CLINICAL MANIFESTATIONS

Uncomplicated Malaria

Most malarial episodes, even with *P. falciparum* infection, are uncomplicated. The incubation period after an infectious bite is usually 10 to 14 days for *P. falciparum* and about 2 weeks for other species, but this can be much longer, especially in non–*P. falciparum* malaria and in individuals with prior immunity. The hallmark of malaria is fever, often with a nonspecific influenza-like prodrome including headache and fatigue followed by a classic malarial paroxysm including chills, high fever, and then sweats. Patients may be remarkably well between febrile episodes. Fevers are typically irregular early in the illness but without therapy may become regular, with 48-hour (*P. vivax* and *P. ovale*) or 72-hour (*P. malariae*) cycles, especially with non–*P. falciparum* disease. Headache, malaise, myalgias, arthralgias, rigors, confusion, cough, chest pain, abdominal pain, anorexia, nausea, vomiting, and diarrhea are common. Seizures are often simple febrile convulsions, especially in young children, but they also may represent evidence of severe neurologic disease. Physical findings may be absent or include signs of anemia, jaundice, splenomegaly, and mild hepatomegaly. Rash and lymphadenopathy are not typical in malaria and thus are suggestive of another cause of fever. Laboratory studies commonly show anemia, thrombocytopenia, and liver and renal function abnormalities.

Severe *P. falciparum* Malaria

Severe malaria can be defined as presentation with signs of severe illness or organ dysfunction (including prostration, impaired consciousness, convulsions, respiratory distress, shock, acidosis, severe anemia, excessive bleeding, hypoglycemia, jaundice, hemoglobinuria, and renal impairment) or a high parasite load (generally peripheral parasitemia >5% or >200,000 parasites/μL). Cerebral malaria,[7] the most common severe complication in children, is generally defined as altered consciousness in the setting of *P. falciparum* malaria. Seizures are common, and deep coma, abnormal posturing, focal neurologic findings, and abnormal respiratory patterns can be seen. The mortality rate is 15% to 25%, with about 10% with persistence of neurologic sequelae, but many patients do remarkably well with appropriate therapy.

Severe anemia is a common presentation, particularly in young children. Transfusions are avoided when possible but play a key role in the management of those with severe anemia. Respiratory failure is caused by noncardiogenic pulmonary edema and is more common in adults than in children. Mechanical ventilation can be life saving, if available. Acute renal failure is also more common in adults and generally due to hypoperfusion and acute tubular necrosis; hemofiltration and hemodialysis are valuable, if available. Blackwater fever, including intravascular hemolysis and hemoglobinuria, has an uncertain etiology but can be caused by quinine. Hepatic dysfunction, including jaundice, can be seen; jaundice may also be caused by hemolysis. Splenic enlargement is common, and splenic rupture can occur. Hypoglycemia is common because of glucose consumption by parasites, increased demand, impaired gluconeogenesis, and quinine-induced insulin secretion; blood glucose levels should be observed closely, with glucose replacement as needed. Metabolic acidosis, particularly lactic acidosis, is common; the value of specific therapies for acidosis or aggressive fluid resuscitation is uncertain. Electrolyte derangements can be seen. Coagulopathy, caused by consumption of clotting factors, and marked thrombocytopenia, caused by increased platelet turnover, can lead to significant bleeding. Bacterial infection and sepsis can coexist with malaria; presumptive use of antibiotics is warranted when signs of sepsis are noted.

Complications of Non–*P. falciparum* Malaria

The large majority of infections with non–*P. falciparum* parasites are uncomplicated both in endemic areas and in nonimmune travelers. Nonetheless, *P. vivax* infection is common in many areas, and studies from a number of sites in Asia and Oceania have shown that it makes up about a quarter of children hospitalized with severe malaria, with a mortality rate of about 1%. Important features of severe *P. vivax* malaria include severe anemia and respiratory distress. All malarias, but in particular *P. vivax* infection, can be complicated by splenic rupture. Chronic malaria infections can be complicated by hyperreactive malarial splenomegaly, with massive splenomegaly and findings of hypersplenism. Chronic infections can also lead to the nephrotic syndrome, particularly with *P. malariae* infection.

DIAGNOSIS

Clinical Features

In individuals with febrile illness and malaria risk, it is essential to make a diagnosis promptly and important to distinguish the different species that infect humans because management differs according to the infecting species. Malaria is the most common cause of febrile illness in many areas, and with limited diagnostic capabilities, it is frequently diagnosed based only on presentation with a febrile illness. However, formal diagnosis is preferred. In travelers returning from endemic areas with fever, historical details can aid in the diagnosis. Malaria is most likely in individuals who failed to use measures to prevent infection and in travelers to the most highly endemic areas, such as rural sub-Saharan Africa. *P. falciparum* malaria generally has a fairly short incubation period in nonimmune individuals, so it presents within 1 to 2 months of return in more than 90% of travelers. Infection with the other malarial species can present in a number of months and uncommonly more than 1 year after exposure.

Blood Smears

The standard means of diagnosis in malaria-endemic areas is by thick blood smear. In this procedure, 1 drop of blood is allowed to dry on a slide, erythrocytes are lysed, and parasites are then stained with Giemsa. Parasites are easily identified by trained microscopists, and parasite density can be estimated on the basis of counts relative to those of leukocytes. However, thick blood smears do not allow identification of erythrocyte morphology, which is helpful in species diagnosis, and are difficult for those with limited training. Giemsa-stained thin blood smears offer an improved means of characterizing parasite morphology, but the process is much less efficient than for thick smears. Thus, thick smears are the standard means of diagnosis in highly endemic areas, and thin smears are preferred where malaria is uncommon and where laboratory personnel have ample time to examine multiple microscopic fields. It is important to distinguish infecting species of malaria parasites. In *P. falciparum* infection, generally only ring-form asexual parasites are seen. Trophozoites of

P. vivax and *P. ovale* are present in enlarged (and ovoid in the case of *P. ovale*) erythrocytes that contain inclusions known as Schüffner dots. Intraerythrocytic *P. malariae* and *P. knowlesi* trophozoites are often elongate in shape. Sexual stage gametocytes (which have a characteristic oblong shape in *P. falciparum*) are also seen on blood smears; most treatments do not eradicate gametocytes, so persistence of these forms for a few weeks is not a sign of treatment failure.

Antigen Detection

An important new means of malaria diagnosis is antigen detection. Multiple simple tests are now available, incorporating colorimetric detection of one or two antigens in an assay that requires limited training and only a few minutes.[8] The most used assays in Africa use histidine-rich protein-2 (HRP2), a protein that is abundant and long-lived but expressed only by *P. falciparum*. Other assays identify plasmodial lactate dehydrogenase and aldolase, which are produced by all human malarial species. Some tests use two antigens to separately identify *P. falciparum* and all-species plasmodial infection. Rapid diagnostic tests have become a standard component of many malaria control programs. One test is approved in the United States. However, with many different tests available around the world, standardization is not optimal, and the specific role of rapid antigen tests for the diagnosis of malaria in different epidemiologic settings is not yet established. In addition, there is increasing evidence of *P. falciparum* lacking HRP2 in some areas, including parts of South America and other regions, leading to concern that HRP2-based diagnostic tests may miss some cases of falciparum malaria.

Other Diagnostic Tests

Serologic tests are available to identify prior malaria infection, but responses develop slowly and persist for an extended period, so these tests have limited value for acute diagnosis. Malaria parasites can be identified with molecular amplification assays using primers encoding genus- and species-specific sequences. These tests are highly sensitive and convenient for research purposes because they can be conducted on DNA extracted from blood spotted onto filter paper in field settings. Quantitative polymerase chain reaction assays are most sensitive, but loop-mediated isothermal amplification and related assays are highly sensitive and more practical for many field settings. Molecular assays are not practical for routine diagnosis, however, because of the time required, the uncertain significance of a positive result in endemic areas where low-level parasitemia may be clinically insignificant, and cost and logistical requirements.

TREATMENT   Rx

The treatment of falciparum malaria has been challenged by drug resistance for many years.[9,10] Artemisinin-based combination therapy (ACT) is recommended in nearly all countries endemic for *P. falciparum* malaria (Table 324-1).[11] Non–*P. falciparum* malaria is still generally treated with chloroquine, although chloroquine resistance is increasing in *P. vivax*; resistant vivax malaria can be treated with other drugs used to treat falciparum malaria.

Chloroquine and Other Aminoquinolines

Chloroquine has been widely used to treat malaria for more than 70 years. It remains the treatment of choice for non–*P. falciparum* malaria and *P. falciparum* malaria in the few areas where resistance has not been seen (Central America and the Caribbean) and is generally rapidly effective and well tolerated. For *P. vivax* and *P. ovale* infections, primaquine or tafenoquine must also be given to eradicate dormant liver forms and thereby prevent subsequent relapse. Chloroquine remains effective as weekly chemoprophylaxis to prevent malaria in areas without resistance. Amodiaquine and piperaquine probably share mechanisms of action with chloroquine, but they are routinely active against chloroquine-resistant parasites because of increased potency compared with chloroquine and some differences in mechanisms of resistance; each is now a component of a leading ACT (Table 324-2). Amodiaquine is somewhat less well tolerated than other aminoquinolines. It is generally safe with short-term use but can cause rare serious hepatic and bone marrow toxicity, especially with chronic use, and so it is not recommended for chemoprophylaxis. The ACT dihydroartemisinin-piperaquine has shown excellent efficacy in most regions, but frequent failures, mediated by resistance to both components of the regimen, have recently been seen in Southeast Asia.

Mefloquine and Lumefantrine

Mefloquine offers effective therapy and chemoprophylaxis for most chloroquine-resistant strains of *P. falciparum* and for other species. Resistance to mefloquine is uncommon but has been seen in parts of Southeast Asia,

TABLE 324-1	TREATMENT OF MALARIA*
CHLOROQUINE-RESISTANT *PLASMODIUM FALCIPARUM*, RESISTANT *PLASMODIUM VIVAX*, OR SPECIES UNIDENTIFIED	
UNCOMPLICATED DISEASE	
Coartem (artemether 20 mg, lumefantrine 120 mg)	4 tablets orally twice daily for 3 days
or	
Malarone (atovaquone 250 mg, proguanil 100 mg)	4 tablets daily for 3 days
or	
Quinine	650 mg quinine sulfate 3 times daily for 3-7 days
plus	
Doxycycline	100 mg twice daily for 7 days
or plus	
Clindamycin	600 mg twice daily for 7 days
or	
Mefloquine	750 mg followed by 500 mg in 6-8 hours; can also be given as a single 1250-mg dose, although this is less well tolerated than the divided dose
COMPLICATED *P. FALCIPARUM* MALARIA OR UNABLE TO TOLERATE ORAL MEDICATIONS†	
IV artesunate‡	2.4 mg/kg every 12 hr on day 1; then daily for 2 additional days
or	
IV quinidine gluconate§,‖	10 mg/kg over 1 to 2 hr; then 0.02 mg/kg/min *or* 15 mg/kg over 4 hr; then 7.5 mg/kg over 4 hr every 8 hr
or	
IV quinine dihydrochloride§,‖	20 mg/kg over 4 hr; then 10 mg/kg every 8 hr
or	
IM artemether‖	3.2 mg/kg IM; then 1.6 mg/kg/day
CHLOROQUINE-SUSCEPTIBLE *P. FALCIPARUM* AND OTHER SPECIES	
Chloroquine phosphate	1 g, followed by 500 mg at 6, 24, and 48 hr *or* 1 g at 0 and 24 hr; then 0.5 g at 48 hr
plus (for *P. vivax* and *P. ovale* only)	
Primaquine¶	30-mg base (52.6 mg primaquine phosphate) daily for 14 days
or	
Tafenoquine¶	300 mg single dose

*Dosages refer to salts unless indicated and are for adults. For pediatric dosing and full Centers for Disease Control and Prevention (CDC) recommendations, see http://www.cdc.gov/malaria/pdf/treatmenttable.pdf.
†IV regimens should be given until the patient can tolerate oral agents and then followed by a course of oral therapy (doxycycline, clindamycin, or full treatment courses of other drugs, as listed) when patients can tolerate this.
‡Available in the United States on an investigational basis through the CDC.
§Cardiac monitoring should be in place during IV administration of quinidine or quinine.
‖Not available in the United States.
¶Use primaquine only after demonstrating normal levels of glucose-6-phosphate dehydrogenase.
IM = intramuscular; IV = intravenous.

with failures of the ACT artesunate-mefloquine. Mefloquine is one of three drugs recommended for chemoprophylaxis against *P. falciparum* by the Centers for Disease Control and Prevention (CDC). Tolerability of chemoprophylactic and especially treatment doses of mefloquine is often limited by neurologic and gastrointestinal (GI) toxicity. Lumefantrine is only used in combination and offers effective therapy with artemether as Coartem, the most widely used ACT to treat falciparum malaria.

Quinine and Quinidine

Quinine has been used to treat malaria for hundreds of years. It offers rapid action against all species, with limited known resistance except in Southeast Asia, where failures against *P. falciparum* malaria are fairly common. Quinine can be used to treat uncomplicated malaria, but GI and other nonspecific

TABLE 324-2　RECOMMENDATIONS FOR THE TREATMENT OF *PLASMODIUM FALCIPARUM* MALARIA IN DEVELOPING COUNTRIES*

REGIMEN	NOTES
Artemether–lumefantrine (Coartem, Riamet)	First-line therapy in many countries; FDA approved
Artesunate–amodiaquine (ASAQ)	First-line therapy in many African countries
Artesunate–mefloquine	Standard therapy in parts of Southeast Asia
Dihydroartemisinin–piperaquine	Recently limited by resistance in SE Asia, but highly effective elsewhere

*Recommendations modified from World Health Organization. Guidelines for the Treatment of Malaria. Geneva: World Health Organization; 2015.
FDA = U.S. Food and Drug Administration.

toxicities lead to difficulty in tolerating a full 7-day treatment course. This problem is circumvented by combining a 3-day course of quinine with other agents. For severe disease, intravenous (IV) quinine has been a standard therapy for many years but offers inferior efficacy compared to IV artesunate. In the United States, IV quinine and quinidine are now unavailable, and IV artesunate is the standard treatment for severe malaria.

Primaquine and Tafenoquine

Primaquine (typically 30 mg daily for 14 days)[A1] and tafenoquine (a single 300 mg dose)[A2][A3] are related aminoquinolines that are the only available drugs to eradicate dormant liver forms of *P. vivax* and *P. ovale*. These forms can lead to relapses after therapy with chloroquine and other agents. Primaquine and tafenoquine are also alternative agents for chemoprophylaxis against *P. falciparum* and other species. Both drugs can cause hemolysis or methemoglobinemia (Chapter 149) in individuals with deficiency in glucose-6-phosphate dehydrogenase (G6PD) (Chapter 152). Testing for deficiency should be performed before use of the drugs. As a new strategy to lower transmission, a single low dose of primaquine in conjunction with artemisin-based combination therapy is a well-tolerated treatment for uncomplicated falciparum malaria and can lower transmission to mosquitoes in subjects with normal G6PD levels.[12]

Inhibitors of Folate Metabolism

Inhibitors of dihydrofolate reductase and dihydropteroate synthase are used in fixed-dose combination regimens for the treatment and prevention of malaria. For treatment, sulfadoxine–pyrimethamine (Fansidar) was heavily used to treat uncomplicated *P. falciparum* malaria, but resistance has increased markedly in most endemic areas. The dihydrofolate reductase inhibitor proguanil is combined with atovaquone in Malarone (see later). For chemoprophylaxis, sulfadoxine–pyrimethamine is no longer recommended because of drug resistance and rare life-threatening dermatologic toxicities. However, less frequent dosing in intermittent preventive therapy regimens has been well tolerated and has decreased malaria in high-risk African groups, particularly pregnant women and young children, although efficacy is limited by drug resistance. Seasonal malaria chemoprevention with monthly combined sulfadoxine–pyrimethamine and amodiaquine during the transmission season is now recommended for malaria control in areas of Africa with highly seasonal transmission and limited drug resistance. Daily trimethoprim–sulfamethoxazole, a common prophylactic to prevent opportunistic infections in individuals with HIV infection, has offered some protection against malaria in Africa.

Artemisinins

Artemisinin, the active component of an herbal medicine from China, and a number of its analogues offer rapid elimination of circulating malaria parasites and activity against gametocytes to limit disease transmission. The drugs are all short-acting, leading to frequent recrudescences of infection after short-course monotherapy. For this reason and to limit selection of resistance, artemisinins are now used in combination with longer acting drugs to treat malaria in 3-day regimens. A number of these combinations have become the standard therapies for *P. falciparum* malaria in most endemic countries (see Table 324-2). Leading regimens are fixed-dose combinations of artemether–lumefantrine (Coartem; the only ACT approved in the United States), artesunate–amodiaquine, artesunate–mefloquine, and dihydroartemisinin–piperaquine. All these regimens have demonstrated excellent treatment efficacy in Africa in children[A4-A6] and pregnant women[A7]; different regimens have had optimal efficacy in different regions. ACTs have also shown excellent efficacy for the treatment of vivax malaria.[A8] Other ACTs that are not currently recommended by the WHO but are available for the treatment of malaria in some countries and have also shown good efficacy include artesunate–pyronaridine,[A9] arterolane–piperaquine,[A10] artemisinin–piperaquine, and artemisinin–naphthoquine.[A11] Resistance to artemisinins is a recent concern, with

evidence for prolonged times to parasite clearance in Southeast Asia suggestive of diminished drug responsiveness of *P. falciparum*.[13] Of great concern, treatment efficacies of ACTs have recently waned in parts of Southeast Asia, most notably for dihydroartemisinin–piperaquine, with resistance to both components of the regimen leading to high clinical failure rates.[A12]

Artemisinins also have a key role for the treatment of severe malaria. IV artesunate has been shown to be superior to quinine for the treatment of severe malaria in a mostly adult population in Asia and in African children,[A13] notably with survival advantages over quinine in both populations. For settings with limited infrastructure, intramuscular artemether[A14] and intramuscular[A15] or intrarectal artesunate have also shown excellent efficacy. IV artesunate should now be considered the first-line therapy for severe malaria in the United States, where it is not routinely available, but can be readily obtained from the CDC for this indication. Artemisinins are generally very well tolerated, with minimal toxicity, although delayed hemolysis can occur after therapy, in particular with IV artesunate.[14]

Atovaquone–Proguanil (Malarone)

This fixed-dose combination of a dihydrofolate reductase inhibitor and atovaquone, which has a unique antimalarial mechanism, has excellent efficacy against most *P. falciparum* infections. It is approved for both treatment and chemoprophylaxis of *P. falciparum* malaria and other species in the United States, where it is now widely used for both indications. Malarone offers excellent efficacy with minimal toxicity. Adverse effects may include GI symptoms, elevations in liver enzymes, headache, and rash. Widespread use in developing countries is limited by high cost and concerns about resistance because resistance to each component drug is readily selected, but it has been suggested that atovaquone-resistant parasites cannot complete development in mosquitoes, preventing transmission of these parasites.[15]

Antibiotics

A number of antibacterials are slow-acting antimalarials. Tetracyclines and clindamycin should not be used alone to treat malaria but are combined with quinine to allow a shorter duration of therapy with that drug. In addition, doxycycline is effective in chemoprophylaxis of most *P. falciparum* malaria and is recommended for this purpose by the CDC, in particular for travelers to regions of Southeast Asia with high-level resistance to other drugs.

Treatment of Severe Malaria

Severe malaria is a medical emergency and requires parenteral therapy. With appropriate prompt therapy and supportive care, rapid recoveries may be seen even in very ill individuals. Standard therapy for severe malaria is IV artesunate, which must be obtained from the CDC. If acquisition is delayed, short-term therapy with an oral agent is appropriate until IV artesunate is available. Appropriate care of severe malaria includes close nursing care; maintenance of fluids, electrolytes, and glucose; respiratory and hemodynamic support; and consideration of blood transfusions, anticonvulsants, antibiotics for bacterial infections, and hemodialysis or hemofiltration. Aggressive fluid resuscitation, blood transfusion for moderate anemia, exchange transfusion, and specific treatment of acidosis are of uncertain value. After the acute illness, IV artesunate should be followed by oral longer acting drugs, typically a full course of an oral ACT, Malarone, mefloquine, or quinine plus doxycycline or clindamycin.

PREVENTION

Key malaria control interventions in malaria-endemic regions are control of mosquito vectors by indoor residual spraying of insecticides; personal protection against mosquito bites with insecticide-impregnated bed nets; routine use of artemisinin-based combination therapies, which offer prompt control of malaria infections and activity against gametocytes to limit transmission to mosquitoes; and selected use of intermittent preventive therapies to decrease malarial incidence in high-risk groups. A long-lasting piperonyl butoxide-treated insecticidal net and pyrethroid indoor residual spraying interventions have shown improved control of malaria transmission compared with standard long-lasting insecticidal nets.[A16][A17]

Ivermectin, which is used to treat some helminth infections, is also mosquitocidal and can reduce malaria transmission when provided in addition to standard malaria therapy.[A18]

No vaccine to prevent malaria is yet available, but extensive research on potential vaccines is under way. RTS,S, which is based on an immunogenic sporozoite antigen, is the most advanced vaccine candidate. Multiple clinical trials showed protection in children immunized with RTS,S, with about 25% to 50% protection against malaria in the year after immunization, but lower levels of protection in very young children, in areas of highest malaria exposure, and over longer periods of time.[A19-A21] Based on these results, a new concept is seasonal malaria immunization, with provision of short-acting vaccines

TABLE 324-3	CHEMOPROPHYLAXIS OF MALARIA*

AREAS WITH CHLOROQUINE-RESISTANT *PLASMODIUM FALCIPARUM*

Malarone	1 tablet (250 mg artesunate/100 mg proguanil) daily
Mefloquine	250 mg weekly
Doxycycline	100 mg daily
Primaquine[†]	30 mg daily during exposure (chemoprophylaxis) or 30 mg daily for 14 days (terminal prophylaxis against *P. vivax* and *P. ovale*)
Tafenoquine[†]	200 mg daily for 3 days prior to travel, then 200 mg weekly during travel

AREAS WITHOUT CHLOROQUINE-RESISTANT *P. FALCIPARUM*

Chloroquine phosphate	500 mg weekly

*Recommendations may change on the basis of drug resistance patterns. For additional details and pediatric dosing, see Centers for Disease Control and Prevention guidelines (http://www.cdc.gov). Begin 1 to 2 weeks before travel for mefloquine and 2 days before for doxycycline, Malarone, and primaquine; continue for 4 weeks after leaving the endemic area (1 week for Malarone and tafenoquine; 2 weeks for primaquine). All doses refer to salts unless indicated.
[†]Use primaquine only after demonstrating normal levels of glucose-6-phosphate dehydrogenase.

during the high transmission season.[16] Controlled human malaria infection was prevented in 9 out of 9 (100%) malaria-naïve, healthy adult volunteers who ten weeks earlier were immunized with radiation-attenuated *Plasmodium falciparum* sporozoites inoculated by mosquitoes.[17] Other approaches under study include vaccines containing erythrocytic, liver-stage, and sexual-stage antigens.

Preventive Measures for Travelers to Malaria-Endemic Regions

It is important for nonimmune travelers (Chapter 270) to endemic areas to be protected against potentially lethal malaria. Travelers should decrease exposure to night-biting anopheline mosquitoes by use of insecticide repellents and sleeping in rooms that are screened or equipped with insecticide-impregnated bed nets. Standard advice for travelers to endemic areas is also to use low doses of preventive drugs chosen on the basis of the resistance profile of the particular region. Chloroquine is still recommended for malaria-endemic regions of Central America and the Caribbean. For nearly all other areas, the CDC recommends use of daily Malarone, weekly mefloquine, or daily doxycycline; details of dosing vary, but it is important to continue therapy after return from travel to eliminate parasites as they emerge from the liver (Table 324-3). Primaquine and tafenoquine (FDA approved in 2018) offer alternative chemoprevention regimens. For areas with high risk of *P. vivax* malaria, some authorities recommend a full treatment course of primaquine after travel to eliminate dormant liver stages. For all chemoprophylaxis, it is important to appreciate that no mosquito avoidance methods or drug regimens are fully protective, so consideration of malaria as a cause of fever in returned travelers is essential (Chapter 270).

PROGNOSIS

Patients with malaria caused by *P. vivax*, *P. ovale*, or *P. malariae* generally respond well to chloroquine and make an uneventful recovery. Chloroquine-resistance is increasing with *P. vivax* from many areas; failures of initial treatment are usually not dangerous but should be followed by treatment with another regimen, such as an ACT, Malarone, or mefloquine. Patients with *P. falciparum* malaria also generally respond well to prompt therapy as long as the disease is not overly advanced at presentation. The mortality rate in those with uncomplicated *P. falciparum* malaria is about 0.1%. Key contributing factors to most deaths from *P. falciparum* malaria are probably a delay between the appearance of symptoms and presentation for definitive therapy and the use of suboptimal therapies. Presentation with high-level parasitemia (>200,000 parasites/μL or >5% parasitemia) or signs of severe malaria are predictive of a poor outcome. However, with aggressive support, even individuals with severe disease can often experience complete recoveries.

Grade A References

A1. Lacerda MVG, Llanos-Cuentas A, Krudsood S, et al. Single-dose tafenoquine to prevent relapse of *Plasmodium vivax* malaria. *N Engl J Med*. 2019;380:215-228.
A2. Llanos-Cuentas A, Lacerda MVG, Hien TT, et al. Tafenoquine versus primaquine to prevent relapse of *Plasmodium vivax* malaria. *N Engl J Med*. 2019;380:229-241.

A3. Graves PM, Choi L, Gelband H, et al. Primaquine or other 8-aminoquinolines for reducing *Plasmodium falciparum* transmission. *Cochrane Database Syst Rev*. 2018;2:CD008152.
A4. Four Artemisinin-Based Combinations (4ABC) Study Group. A head-to-head comparison of four artemisinin-based combinations for treating uncomplicated malaria in African children: a randomized trial. *PLoS Med*. 2011;8:1-16.
A5. Yeka A, Kigozi R, Conrad MD, et al. Artesunate/amodiaquine versus artemether/lumefantrine for the treatment of uncomplicated malaria in Uganda: a randomized trial. *J Infect Dis*. 2016;213:1134-1142.
A6. Sirima SB, Ogutu B, Lusingu JPA, et al. Comparison of artesunate-mefloquine and artemether-lumefantrine fixed-dose combinations for treatment of uncomplicated *Plasmodium falciparum* malaria in children younger than 5 years in sub-Saharan Africa: a randomised, multicentre, phase 4 trial. *Lancet Infect Dis*. 2016;16:1123-1133.
A7. PREGACT study group. Four artemisinin-based treatments in African pregnant women with malaria. *N Engl J Med*. 2016;374:913-927.
A8. Gogtay N, Kannan S, Thatte UM, et al. Artemisinin-based combination therapy for treating uncomplicated *Plasmodium vivax* malaria. *Cochrane Database Syst Rev*. 2013;10:CD008492.
A9. Pryce J, Hine P. Pyronaridine-artesunate for treating uncomplicated *Plasmodium falciparum* malaria. *Cochrane Database Syst Rev*. 2019;1:CD006404.
A10. Toure OA, Valecha N, Tshefu AK, et al. A phase 3, double blind, randomized study of arterolane maleate-piperaquine phosphate vs artemether-lumefantrine for falciparum malaria in adolescent and adult patients in Asia and Africa. *Clin Infect Dis*. 2016;62:964-971.
A11. Laman M, Moore BR, Benjamin JM, et al. Artemisinin-naphthoquine versus artemether-lumefantrine for uncomplicated malaria in Papua New Guinean children: an open-label randomized trial. *PLoS Med*. 2014;11:1-18.
A12. Amaratunga C, Lim P, Suon S, et al. Dihydroartemisinin-piperaquine resistance in *Plasmodium falciparum* malaria in Cambodia: a multisite prospective cohort study. *Lancet Infect Dis*. 2016;16:357-365.
A13. Dondorp AM, Fanello CI, Hendriksen IC, et al. Artesunate versus quinine in the treatment of severe falciparum malaria in African children (AQUAMAT): an open-label, randomised trial. *Lancet*. 2010;376:1647-1657.
A14. Esu E, Effa EE, Opie ON, et al. Artemether for severe malaria. *Cochrane Database Syst Rev*. 2014;9:CD010678.
A15. Kremsner PG, Adegnika AA, Hounkpatin AB, et al. Intramuscular artesunate for severe malaria in African children: a multicenter randomized controlled trial. *PLoS Med*. 2016;13:1-22.
A16. Tiono AB, Ouedraogo A, Ouattara D, et al. Efficacy of Olyset Duo, a bednet containing pyriproxyfen and permethrin, versus a permethrin-only net against clinical malaria in an area with highly pyrethroid-resistant vectors in rural Burkina Faso: a cluster-randomised controlled trial. *Lancet*. 2018;392:569-580.
A17. Protopopoff N, Mosha JF, Lukole E, et al. Effectiveness of a long-lasting piperonyl butoxide-treated insecticidal net and indoor residual spray interventions, separately and together, against malaria transmitted by pyrethroid-resistant mosquitoes: a cluster, randomised controlled, two-by-two factorial design trial. *Lancet*. 2018;391:1577-1588.
A18. Ouédraogo AL, Bastiaens GJ, Tiono AB, et al. Efficacy and safety of the mosquitocidal drug ivermectin to prevent malaria transmission after treatment: a double-blind, randomized, clinical trial. *Clin Infect Dis*. 2015;60:357-365.
A19. Olotu A, Fegan G, Wambua J, et al. Four-year efficacy of RTS,S/AS01E and its interaction with malaria exposure. *N Engl J Med*. 2013;368:1111-1120.
A20. RTS,S Clinical Trials Partnership. Efficacy and safety of RTS,S/AS01 malaria vaccine with or without a booster dose in infants and children in Africa: final results of a phase 3, individually randomised, controlled trial. *Lancet*. 2015;386:31-45.
A21. Olotu A, Fegan G, Wambua J, et al. Seven-year efficacy of RTS,S/AS01 malaria vaccine among young African children. *N Engl J Med*. 2016;374:2519-2529.

GENERAL REFERENCES

For the General References and other additional features, please visit Expert Consult at https://expertconsult.inkling.com.

325

AFRICAN SLEEPING SICKNESS

WILLIAM A. PETRI, JR.

DEFINITION

Human African trypanosomiasis, commonly known as sleeping sickness, is a vector-borne parasitic disease transmitted to humans and animals by the bite of the tsetse fly (genus *Glossina*). Infection is caused by protozoa of the genus *Trypanosoma* and species *brucei*.[1] In humans, there are two forms of illness caused by two distinct subspecies that are morphologically identical but differ in their geographic range and clinical presentations. *Trypanosoma brucei gambiense* is typically found in west and central Africa and *Trypanosoma brucei rhodesiense* in east Africa. *T. b. gambiense* has a more chronic course, and *T. b. rhodesiense* causes a rapid disease course; both have late stages marked by meningoencephalitis, resulting in coma and death if untreated. There is a third subspecies, *Trypanosoma brucei*, known to cause chronic infection called nagana in cattle; however, humans are not susceptible to this organism. Chagas disease, or American trypanosomiasis, is covered in Chapter 326.

The Pathogen

As an extracellular microbe, the parasite must evade immune clearance to establish a persistent infection. The surface of the trypanosome is covered by a dense, homogeneous coat of variant surface glycoproteins (VSGs), which are immunodominant. Each individual trypanosome expresses only one VSG at a time but possesses more than 1000 different silent copies of the VSG gene, and switching to a new VSG occurs at a frequency of about 1×10^{-6} parasites. Hence, the trypanosomes expressing a given VSG will eventually be cleared by the host antibody response, but any individual trypanosome that has switched to a new VSG will evade immune clearance, resulting in a new peak of parasitemia. Recombination between VSG alleles ensures a virtually limitless repertoire of new VSGs; therefore antibody-mediated parasite eradication is impossible.

EPIDEMIOLOGY

Human African trypanosomiasis is relatively less of a problem now than it was in the prior century, partly because of cyclic epidemics in the past, as well as recent increases in public health efforts for control.[2] However, it remains a looming threat to an estimated 60 million people living in tsetse fly–inhabited areas among 36 countries of sub-Saharan Africa and causes significant morbidity, accounting for 1.5 million disability-adjusted life-years in Africa as a whole.[3]

The first epidemic occurred in the Congo basin and Uganda between 1896 and 1906, driven in part by natural disasters that decimated populations of livestock and regional droughts, as well as changes in population distribution influenced by colonialism. The second epidemic occurred in numerous endemic countries in the 1920s; control was achieved after major efforts to systematically screen and treat individuals followed by extensive vector control programs, including bush clearing and insecticide spraying. These acts were nearly successful in halting transmission by the 1960s; however, the independence of many African nations around this time hindered the sustainability of prevention and control programs. The incidence began to rise by the 1970s and surged a decade later, leading to the third epidemic of the 20th century. However, in the past 15 years, increased access to at-risk populations for diagnosis and treatment has led to a 68% reduction in the incidence of reported cases.

Despite increased surveillance efforts during the past 15 years, there are still at-risk areas that lack active monitoring programs, and many people are thought to die of human African trypanosomiasis without an accurate diagnosis. The World Health Organization (WHO) reported an annual incidence of 12,000 cases in 2007, a dramatic decrease from the estimated incidence of 300,000 cases a decade earlier. It is estimated that 300,000 to 500,000 people are infected, contributing to approximately 100,000 deaths each year. More than 90% of reported cases are due to *T. b. gambiense,* the majority being from the Democratic Republic of the Congo.

The geographic distribution includes areas where the vector, parasite, reservoir hosts, and human hosts cohabit (Fig. 325-1). In general, these include focal areas on the African continent within 15 degrees North and 15 degrees South latitude, with a predilection for rural areas. Humans at greatest risk for infection are those who rely on animal husbandry, agriculture, fishing, and hunting for their livelihoods. Often, disease is concentrated among foci of rural areas, having significant socioeconomic impact on affected villages. With a few exceptions, this infection is never found in urban areas. There have been fewer than 50 cases reported annually outside of Africa, usually the result of travel by North Americans or Europeans to African game reserves.

T. b. gambiense is transmitted by tsetse flies from the *Glossina palpalis* group, the annotated genome sequence of which has been reported. Tsetse flies are typically found along riverbanks among wooded areas in the more tropical regions of central and West Africa. The reservoir hosts for *T. b. gambiense* and the focus of public health campaigns are mainly humans. Because of this, *T. b. gambiense* is not generally considered a zoonotic disease; the role of the animal reservoir for this organism remains undetermined, although natural infections have been reported in domestic animals such as dogs, sheep, cattle, and pigs.

T. b. rhodesiense is transmitted by tsetse flies belonging to the *Glossina morsitans* group, which are commonly found among woodland and savannah areas of east and central Africa. *T. b. rhodesiense* is a zoonotic disease with numerous wild and domestic species of animals acting as reservoirs. With this infection, the animal reservoir serves an important role in the cycle, sustaining parasite transmission and human infections. Domestic species, especially cattle, have the potential to drive outbreaks and, not surprisingly, have served as the focus of successful prevention campaigns.

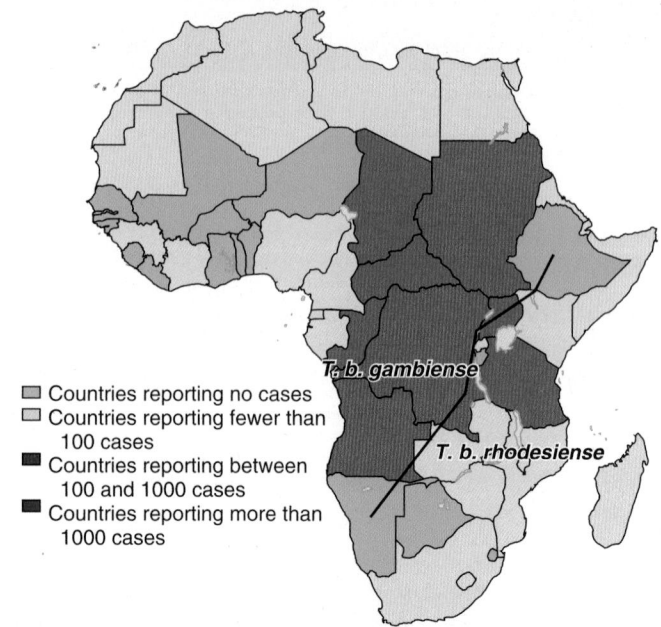

Countries reporting no cases
Countries reporting fewer than 100 cases
Countries reporting between 100 and 1000 cases
Countries reporting more than 1000 cases

T. b. gambiense

T. b. rhodesiense

FIGURE 325-1. Map of human African trypanosomiasis. These 36 sub-Saharan African countries are considered endemic for human African trypanosomiasis. *Shaded areas* represent the reported incidence from 1997 to 2006. The *black line* roughly represents the dividing line for the two parasites, although some overlap may already occur.

PATHOBIOLOGY

After the bite of a tsetse fly carrying metacyclic trypomastigotes, a local reaction (chancre) may form at the inoculation site. This symptom is seen with *T. b. rhodesiense* infection and is more frequently observed in travelers but is rarely seen with *T. b. gambiense* infection. Parasites subsequently disseminate into the blood and lymphatic systems in what is considered stage I of the disease. Spread of the parasites into the central nervous system (CNS) defines stage II of the disease, which is invariably fatal if untreated. The parasite appears to remain extracellular throughout the course of infection.

Peaks and waves of parasitemia occur during stage I disease and result in the classic symptom of intermittent fever. These bouts of fever correspond to a type 1 inflammatory response (Chapter 42), in which classically activated macrophages produce high levels of tumor necrosis factor (TNF) and nitric oxide. This helps in the control of parasitemia but also contributes to tissue damage. Type 2 inflammatory responses with high interleukin-10 production may subsequently occur, which limit TNF and nitric oxide production after initial parasitemia has been controlled. Antibody responses are directed to VSGs and other trypanosome antigens (e.g., antigens from lysed parasites), but autoantibodies are also produced. Generalized febrile episodes are observed together with lymphadenopathy and myocardial and pericardial inflammation. Cardiac involvement is typically more severe with *T. b. rhodesiense* infection. Anemia, thrombocytopenia, disseminated intravascular coagulation, and renal disease may also be observed.

In stage II of the disease, parasites cross the blood-brain barrier and invade the CNS. Acute meningoencephalitis develops, with a variety of inflammatory cells infiltrating the brain, including macrophages, lymphocytes, plasma cells, Mott cells (plasma cells with spherical cytoplasmic inclusions composed of immunoglobulin), and morular cells (plasmacytoid cells with transparent hyaline vesicles in the cytoplasm). These inflammatory cells are found in the meninges, which become thickened, as well as in the perivascular spaces and neuropil. Edema, hemorrhage, and granulomatous lesions are often present; thrombosis and neuronal degeneration may also be observed.

Genetic resistance to African sleeping sickness is due to a common (in individuals of African descent) polymorphism in the *APOL₁* gene, a component of high-density lipoprotein. This gene product mediates serum resistance to the parasite. An untoward consequence of this polymorphism is that individuals with two copies of the variant allele (15% of African Americans) are at increased risk of chronic kidney disease.

CLINICAL MANIFESTATIONS

The clinical manifestations of human African trypanosomiasis differ on the basis of the infecting organism. *T. b. gambiense* is more of a chronic disease, with an estimated average duration of 3 years; infection with *T. b. rhodesiense* progresses much more rapidly, leading to coma and death within weeks to months. However, infection with *T. b. gambiense* has been known to also cause a rapid decline. Other similarities exist, including an early hemolymphatic stage (stage I) and a late stage characterized by prominent CNS disease including meningoencephalitis (stage II).[4]

West African Sleeping Sickness

Infection starts after the bite of a fly infected with *T. b. gambiense*. At the site of inoculation, a painful, indurated, and erythematous trypanosomal chancre may develop 1 to 2 weeks after the bite and resolves spontaneously after several weeks. On occasion, the chancre may ulcerate. However, these features are rarely seen at the time of clinical presentation and sometimes are not known to have occurred on history; thus many develop disseminated disease without awareness of a localized infection.

The hemolymphatic stage, when parasites disseminate throughout the body, may not be manifested clinically until weeks or months after the initial bite. Typical symptoms include intermittent spiking fevers, occasionally accompanied by headaches and malaise. These features may persist for weeks or months because of the cyclic nature of parasitemia and antibody production against the various antigens sequentially expressed by the parasite.

Lymphadenopathy (Chapter 159) is a common finding in West African sleeping sickness. Whereas regional lymphadenopathy may develop after the initial bite, generalized lymphadenopathy around the head and neck is often found as chronic illness develops. Enlargement of nodes in the posterior cervical triangle, commonly known as Winterbottom sign, is the classic finding, but other cervical and supraclavicular nodes may also be involved. Affected nodes are discrete, movable, rubbery nodes that are nontender to palpation; over time, they may become more indurated because of fibrosis.

Other symptoms reported include pruritus, occasionally accompanied by rash, arthralgias, and periarticular swelling, as well as by transient edema of the extremities and face. Less common symptoms include features consistent with neuroendocrine dysfunction, including loss of libido and impotence, amenorrhea and infertility, alopecia, and gynecomastia. Signs of disease include hepatomegaly and splenomegaly; cardiac dysfunction, including tachycardia; electrocardiographic abnormalities such as prolonged QTc intervals and repolarization changes; and, less commonly, pericarditis or myocarditis. Hemolytic anemia and derangements in liver function test results may occur.

Months or even years after the initial infection, stage II disease develops and is characterized by headaches, daytime somnolence, and neuropsychiatric features. Behavioral changes, including irritability, confusion, inability to concentrate, and lassitude, are among the first signs of CNS disease; psychosis has also been described. Neurologic findings are numerous and include a variety of motor and sensory disturbances, including extrapyramidal features, dysesthesias, and visual impairment. These symptoms have given the infections its common name of sleeping sickness and are manifested by daytime somnolence and nocturnal irritability. Late-stage disease is marked by cerebral edema and meningoencephalitis. Progressively, a loss of neurologic function can lead to paralysis, and many may succumb to aspiration pneumonias or malnutrition; otherwise, coma leads to death in the absence of treatment.

East African Sleeping Sickness

Compared with Gambian sleeping sickness, East African sleeping sickness is more rapidly progressive. The infective bite is more frequently associated with the development of a chancre, although some studies report this in only 20% of patients. An incubation period lasting days to weeks is needed before symptoms are demonstrated. Initial symptoms include severe intermittent fevers that may resemble those found with malaria. Lymphadenopathy is not as common with this infecting organism; the Winterbottom sign is typically absent. Skin changes are more prominent, and rashes in the early stage of infection are particularly common in expatriates with the infection. In addition, cardiac manifestations are more commonly and clinically relevant; tachycardia, arrhythmias, myocarditis, and congestive heart failure have been documented and may be severe enough to cause death before the development of severe CNS disease. CNS disease mirrors that of West African sleeping sickness, but the onset occurs earlier and the rate of deterioration is more rapid. Hematologic abnormalities include anemia,[5] thrombocytopenia, and disseminated intravascular coagulation. Death may ensue after weeks or months without treatment.

DIAGNOSIS

Epidemiologic clues and clinical findings may together suggest the diagnosis of human African trypanosomiasis, but definitive diagnosis relies on demonstration

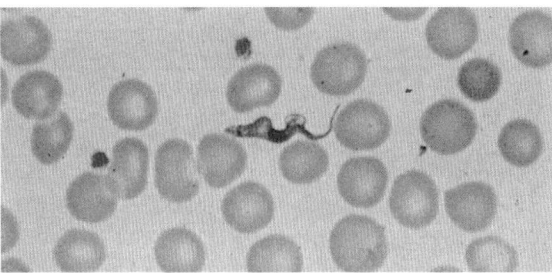

FIGURE 325-2. *Trypanosoma rhodesiense* in peripheral blood. It has a nucleus, posterior kinetoplast, undulating membrane, and flagellum (×1500).

of the parasite. In the early stage of disease, light microscopy and Giemsa stain may be used to visualize the highly motile parasites directly from fresh specimens of fluid expressed from chancres or lymph node aspirates. Peripheral blood smears, including Giemsa-stained thick and thin smears and bone marrow aspirates, have been successful. Blood smears have increased sensitivity when they are performed during stage I disease, when parasitemia is high (Fig. 325-2); the threshold for visualization of parasites by thick smear is approximately 5000 parasites/mL. Performance is superior with *T. b. rhodesiense* infection, given the higher parasite load. If the initial smear analysis is negative, subsequent examinations should be pursued. Concentration techniques, including buffy coat examination, should be used when technically feasible. Culture of any of these fluids may yield higher sensitivity than smear preparations.

Cerebrospinal fluid (CSF) must also be analyzed to determine the most appropriate treatment. Abnormalities in CSF analysis often start with increased cell counts and progress to include an elevated opening pressure and total protein levels with an increased polyclonal immunoglobulin M (IgM). Stage II disease is defined by the presence of more than 5 white blood cells/μL, the presence of trypanosomes, or an elevated total protein (>370 mg/L) in the CSF. Newer diagnostic methods, including polymerase chain reaction analysis of CSF and a latex-agglutination test for CSF IgM, hold promise but require validation to determine outcomes after treatment of patients with positive test results.

Allocation of resources to this neglected tropical disease in recent years has allowed slow but exciting progress in the field of human African trypanosomiasis diagnostics. The genomes of *T. brucei* species have been mapped, and molecular assays have been developed that can distinguish among species of human African trypanosomiasis with a single polymerase chain reaction test. Novel uses of mass spectrometry have been developed that use proteomic signature analysis to identify specific fingerprints of human African trypanosomiasis with the host.

In contrast to these highly technical and expensive methods, other tests suitable for the field are being validated, including the dot-ELISA test, which would be able to provide information on stage of disease. Serology tests are also available for diagnosis of *T. b. gambiense* infection. The card agglutination test for trypanosomiasis with *T. b. gambiense* (CATT) is commonly used by screening programs; the sensitivity ranges from 87% to 98%, depending on the population under study, and the specificity may be as high as 95%. No serology tests are available for *T. b. rhodesiense* infection. Rapid serologic tests for infection with *T. b. gambiense* include human African trypanosomiasis Sero-Strop (which uses a dipstick method) and the human African trypanosomiasis Sero + K SeT test (which uses a lateral flow device) for testing blood or plasma, respectively. The WHO Collaborating Centres for human African trypanosomiasis are important resources for clinical diagnostic tests.

TREATMENT   Rx

Very few drugs have been available for treatment of human African trypanosomiasis, and those that have been commonly used are quite toxic (Table 325-1). Treatment depends on the infecting organism and the stage of disease. Distribution of drugs is through the WHO in Geneva. For stage I disease with *T. b. gambiense* infection, pentamidine is the drug of choice.[A1] The standard regimen consists of daily parenteral administration for 1 week; however, studies are ongoing to determine the efficacy of shortening therapy to three doses.

Suramin is also used for stage I disease with *T. b. rhodesiense*. This medication is complex to mix and to administer. The drug must be administered in a slow intravenous infusion periodically during 3 weeks. Although anaphylaxis is rare

TABLE 325-1	DRUGS USED TO TREAT HUMAN AFRICAN TRYPANOSOMIASIS				
DRUG	**CLASS**	**STAGE**	**ROUTE**	**ADULT DOSE**	**ADVERSE EFFECTS**
TRYPANOSOMA BRUCEI GAMBIENSE					
Pentamidine	Aromatic diamidine	I	IM or IV	4 mg/kg daily for 7 days	Pain, GI symptoms, hypoglycemia or hyperglycemia, electrolyte abnormalities, leukopenia, thrombocytopenia
Eflornithine	Ornithine carboxylase inhibitor	II	IV	100 mg/kg q6hr for 14 days	GI symptoms, bone marrow toxicity, seizures
Eflornithine plus nifurtimox				Nifurtimox 15 mg/kg per day orally in three doses × 10 days; eflornithine 400 mg/kg per day intravenously in two 2-h infusions (each dose diluted in 250 mL of water for injection) × 7 days	
TRYPANOSOMA BRUCEI RHODESIENSE					
Suramin	Polysulfonated naphthylamine derivative of urea	I	IV	1 g IV on days 1, 3, 7, 14, and 21 (after test dose of 100-200 mg)	Anaphylaxis, nephrotoxicity, fever, rash, pruritus, arthralgias, reversible peripheral neuropathy, and bone marrow toxicity
Melarsoprol	Trivalent arsenical	II	IV	1.2 mg/kg q8hr for 3 consecutive days each week for 3 weeks (maximum daily dose, 180 mg)	Encephalopathic syndromes, peripheral neuropathy, paralysis, cardiac dysrhythmias, GI symptoms, rash, pruritus, thrombophlebitis

GI = gastrointestinal; IM = intramuscular; IV = intravenous.

(approximately 1 in 20,000 patients), a test dose is recommended before full treatment is initiated. A number of side effects require close monitoring, the most important being nephrotoxicity. Urinalysis is recommended before each dose, and the drug should be discontinued if proteinuria persists and casts are seen in the urine sediment.

The first choice for treatment of stage II *T. b. gambiense* is the combination of nifurtimox and eflornithine.[A2] Nifurtimox is administered orally, whereas eflornithine requires frequent intravenous administration. Melarsoprol remains the only agent available for the treatment of stage II *T. b. rhodesiense* infection. It is a highly effective but impressively toxic drug used for stage II disease with either organism. The side effects are numerous, but the most important is the life-threatening encephalopathy that may develop from the arsenic (highly fatal) or as an inflammatory reaction. Concomitant steroid use is helpful in reducing the risk of encephalopathy and death without compromising the efficacy of melarsoprol. Gradual increase in the first round of treatment between 2 and 3.6 mg/kg in divided doses three times daily during 3 days has also been shown to reduce the risks of encephalopathy. Melarsoprol resistance is widespread. The mechanism of resistance to this drug has been pinpointed to mutations affecting an aquaglyceroporin (AQP2), a parasite solute and drug transporter.[6]

Tafenoquine, which is an oral antimalarial drug belonging to the 8-amino-quinoline family, has in vitro activity against *T. brucei*. Whether it will become a clinically useful alternative is unknown at this time.[7] Another potential new alternative, oral pafuramidine (100 mg twice a day for 10 days), can provide an overall cure rate of about 90% at 12 months but has been discontinued because of late renal toxicity.

Few therapeutic options are available to treat the late stage of African trypanosomiasis. However, oral fexinidazole,[8] given once daily orally, has been found to be effective and safe for the treatment of *T. b. gambiense* infection compared with nifurtimox eflornithine combination therapy in late-stage infection.[A3]

PREVENTION

To date, there is no vaccine against human African trypanosomiasis. The mainstays of prevention include active case finding with early treatment and vector control.[9] Given the nature of each infection, active case surveillance is more suitable for infection with *T. b. gambiense*, but vector control is more effective for prevention of infection with *T. b. rhodesiense*. The goal of active case finding is to identify infected individuals who may still be in the asymptomatic stage or early stage. This approach, which is more suited for disease from *T. b. gambiense*, typically consists of a screening examination for lymphadenopathy followed by a CATT test. If results are positive for both, the patient should undergo further evaluation with lymph node aspirate and blood testing. If trypanosomes are found, the patient should be treated. Vector control measures include tsetse fly traps and insecticide-impregnated screens; the traps are easily maintained by locals, but the screens require regular retreatment and thus are more labor intensive and costly to maintain. Mass spraying, once a successful method until the 1960s, is no longer practiced. However, if an epidemic does occur, ground or aerial spraying combined with disruption of the animal reservoir's habitat may be the most effective method of achieving rapid vector control.

Travelers to endemic areas should be aware of this disease and should use basic protective measures. Protective clothing of at least medium weight should be worn; neutral colors are most effective because flies are attracted to bright and dark colors. Tsetse flies are attracted to moving vehicles but rest in the shade or bushes. Although use of insect repellant is prudent for other vector-borne illnesses that may be endemic in these areas, it has not been proven to substantially reduce the risk of tsetse fly bites. There is no recommended chemoprophylaxis for travelers.

Grade A References

A1. Pohlig G, Bernhard SC, Blum J, et al. Efficacy and safety of pafuramidine versus pentamidine maleate for treatment of first stage sleeping sickness in a randomized, comparator-controlled, international Phase 3 clinical trial. *PLoS Negl Trop Dis*. 2016;10:1-17.
A2. Kansiime F, Adibaku S, Wamboga C, et al. A multicentre, randomised, non-inferiority clinical trial comparing a nifurtimox-eflornithine combination to standard eflornithine monotherapy for late stage *Trypanosoma brucei gambiense* human African trypanosomiasis in Uganda. *Parasit Vectors*. 2018;11:1-11.
A3. Mesu VKBK, Kalonji WM, Bardonneau C, et al. Oral fexinidazole for late-stage African *Trypanasome brucci gambiense* trypanasomiasis: a pivotal multicentre, randomised, non-inferiority trial. *Lancet*. 2018;391:144-154.

GENERAL REFERENCES

For the General References and other additional features, please visit Expert Consult at https://expertconsult.inkling.com.

326

CHAGAS DISEASE

LOUIS V. KIRCHHOFF

DEFINITION

Chagas disease, or American trypanosomiasis, is caused by the protozoan parasite *Trypanosoma cruzi*. The terms *Chagas disease*, *American trypanosomiasis*, and *T. cruzi infection* are synonyms.

The Pathogen

Several dozen species are included in the genus *Trypanosoma*, but only the African trypanosome *Trypanosoma brucei* (subspecies *T. b. gambiense* [West

African] and *T. b. rhodesiense* [East African]) (Chapter 325) and the American trypanosome *T. cruzi* cause disease in humans. Many species of triatomine insects, also called kissing bugs, act as vectors for *T. cruzi*, and many species of wild and domestic mammals, as well as humans, are involved in the complex life cycle of this fascinating organism. The vectors become infected by ingesting blood from mammals that have parasites in their blood stream. The parasites then multiply in the gut of the insects and are ultimately discharged in the feces of the vector. Transmission to a new mammalian host occurs when parasite-laden vector feces contact vulnerable surfaces such as the mucosae of the mouth or nose, the conjunctivae, or breaks in the skin. When in contact with tissues of the new host, the contaminating parasites enter local cells and multiply intracellularly, and as parasitized cells rupture, they are released into the lymphatics and blood stream. The circulating organisms enter new cells at distant sites and in this manner maintain an endless process of asynchronous multiplication. The life cycle is completed as parasites are swept up in blood meals taken by vectors. In addition to vector-borne transmission, *T. cruzi* can be transmitted by blood or organs donated by infected persons, from mother to unborn child, by the ingestion of contaminated food or drink,[1] by infected persons to sexual contacts,[2] and in laboratory accidents.

EPIDEMIOLOGY

Epizootiology of *T. cruzi*

The triatomine vectors that transmit *T. cruzi* are found in the Americas from southern Argentina through the southern half of the United States. The parasite has been isolated from more than 100 species of domestic and wild mammals, which for the most part likely become infected when they eat infected vectors or through congenital transmission. Armadillos, wood rats, raccoons, and opossums are typical wild mammalian reservoirs, and these and other species that harbor *T. cruzi* can be found in large numbers in the southern and southwestern parts of the United States.

Typically, humans acquire *T. cruzi* infection, which is lifelong, when they live in houses in enzootic areas where the sylvatic cycle of transmission is active. The process begins when vector species adaptable to living in human dwellings take up residence in niches in the primitive wood, mud, and stone houses that are typical in many endemic regions. These vectors become domiciliary, and they then take blood meals, mostly at night, from the humans who occupy the dwellings that they have invaded, as well as from domestic animals that sleep there, particularly dogs. Thus, Chagas disease is primarily a public health problem among poor people who live in rural areas.

Epidemiology of Chagas Disease in the Endemic Countries

Chagas disease is a zoonosis that is endemic in Mexico and all countries of Central and South America. None of the Caribbean islands are endemic. In 2014, the Pan American Health Organization estimated that in the 21 endemic countries, 6 million people are chronically infected with *T. cruzi*, 30,000 new cases occur each year, and up to 14,000 deaths result from Chagas disease annually.[3] Since 1991 a major international vector control program in the southern cone countries of South America (Chile, Argentina, Paraguay, Brazil, Bolivia, and Uruguay) has achieved a marked reduction in vectorial transmission of *T. cruzi* through housing improvement, education of people at risk for acquiring the infection, and spraying of residual insecticides. Substantial reductions in prevalence rates in school-aged children and in blood donors constitute clear evidence of the success of the program. Uruguay, Chile, and Brazil were certified as being free of vector transmission in 1997, 1999, and 2006, respectively. Marked reduction in transmission has been achieved in Argentina as well. Similar programs have been initiated in Central America and the Andean countries. In parallel with the vector control programs, donor screening has been implemented throughout almost the entire endemic range, and with the notable exception of Mexico, transmission of *T. cruzi* by transfusion has largely been eliminated.

Epidemiology of Chagas Disease in the United States

As noted, the sylvatic cycle of *T. cruzi* exists in much of the southern and southwestern regions of the United States, but only six cases of autochthonous (disease spread from one individual and acquired in another individual in the same place) acute Chagas disease have been reported: three in Texas and one each in Tennessee, Louisiana, and California. Moreover, in the first 4 years of blood donor screening that started in January 2007, in which approximately 29 million units were tested, only 16 *T. cruzi*–infected donors, who appeared to have acquired the infection autochthonously, were identified. In the past 30 or more years, fewer than 30 laboratory-acquired and imported cases of acute Chagas disease have been reported to the U.S. Centers for Disease Control

and Prevention (CDC). Only one of the latter infections occurred in a tourist returning to the United States, but three such instances have been reported in Europe as well as one in Canada. Thus, acute Chagas disease is extremely rare in the United States, and there is no indication that its incidence is increasing.

A recent estimate puts the number of *T. cruzi*–infected persons currently living in the United States at about 240,000 to 300,000.[4] Several studies done before blood donor screening began in 2007 identified *T. cruzi*–infected persons in the donor pool, and nine instances of transmission by transfusion in the United States and Canada were described. Since screening began in 2007, more than 50 million units have been screened, and more than 3,000 *T. cruzi*–infected donors have been identified and permanently deferred from donation. The confirmed rate of *T. cruzi* infection in donors is about 1 in 13,300. With the goal of reducing the enormous cost of universal screening ($100 to $200 million per year), a U.S. Food and Drug Administration (FDA)-approved selective screening protocol based on previous negative test results has been implemented.

In Europe, infection is seen primarily in Latin American immigrants to Spain, Italy, France, the United Kingdom, and Switzerland. The pooled seroprevalence among such immigrants is about 4%, with an 18% seroprevalence among immigrants from Bolivia.[5] The transplantation in the United States of organs from three persons with undiagnosed chronic *T. cruzi* infection resulted in acute Chagas disease in five recipients, one of whom died of the infection. To date, two instances of congenital transmission of *T. cruzi* here have been reported. A reasonable estimate of the number of babies born in the United States each year with congenital Chagas disease puts it in the range of 63 to 315. The fact that most babies with congenital Chagas disease are asymptomatic and the low level of knowledge about Chagas disease among caregivers likely underlie the dearth of reported cases.

PATHOBIOLOGY

In acute Chagas disease, an inflammatory lesion, called a chagoma, may appear at the site of entry of the parasites. Local histologic changes include intracellular parasitism of muscle and other subcutaneous tissues, lymphocytic infiltration, interstitial edema, and hyperplasia of lymph nodes that drain the area. As the parasites spread systemically through the lymphatics and blood stream, muscles, including the myocardium, are the most heavily parasitized tissues, but the organisms can invade essentially any tissue. Myocarditis may develop in association with focal areas of infected cardiomyocytes, inflammation, and necrosis. The characteristic pseudocysts seen in sections of *T. cruzi*–infected tissues are actually host cells filled with multiplying forms of the parasite (Fig. 326-1). In some patients, parasites can be seen in cerebrospinal fluid (CSF).

In persons with chronic Chagas disease, the heart is the organ most commonly affected. Hearts obtained at autopsy from patients who died of Chagas cardiomyopathy usually have a global appearance reflecting biventricular enlargement and thinning of ventricular walls (Fig. 326-2). Mural thrombi are frequently present, and an apical aneurysm of the left ventricle is typical in patients with advanced disease. At the cellular level, the process that underlies these gross pathologic abnormalities is a chronic inflammation with mononuclear

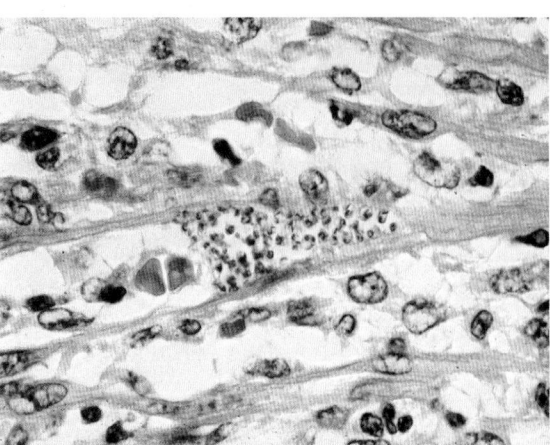

FIGURE 326-1. *Trypanosoma cruzi* in cardiac muscle of a child who died of acute Chagas myocarditis. An infected myocyte containing several dozen *T. cruzi* amastigotes is in the center of the field (hematoxylin-eosin staining, ×900).

cell infiltration, diffuse interstitial fibrosis, and atrophy of myocardial cells. The chronic inflammation affects the conduction system as well and causes a variety of rhythm disturbances, including atrial bradyarrhythmias and fibrillation; premature ventricular contractions; bundle branch blocks, often of the right bundle; ventricular tachycardia; and third-degree atrioventricular block. Parasites are rarely seen in diseased tissues by conventional histologic methods, but several studies using polymerase chain reaction (PCR) assays found a correlation between the intensity of inflammation and the presence of parasites. Evidence accumulated to date implicates the persistence of parasites and the resulting chronic inflammation in affected tissues—rather than autoimmune mechanisms—as the basis for the pathogenesis in patients with chronic *T. cruzi* infection.

The dilation and hypertrophy observed on gross examination of the esophagus or colon of a patient with chronic Chagas disease of the digestive tract (megadisease) can be striking. Focal inflammatory lesions with lymphocytic infiltration are seen on microscopic examination of affected tissues. In addition, the number of neurons in the myenteric plexus is reduced, and periganglion and intraganglion fibrosis with Schwann cell proliferation and lymphocytosis is present. In most patients, the clinical consequences of this parasympathetic denervation are limited to the esophagus or colon (or to both), but the ureters, biliary tree, and other hollow viscera can be affected as well.

CLINICAL MANIFESTATIONS
Acute Chagas Disease
Acute Chagas disease is usually an illness of children but can occur at any age. Symptoms are typically mild and nonspecific (Table 326-1).[6,7] When the parasite has entered through a break in the skin or the site of a vector's

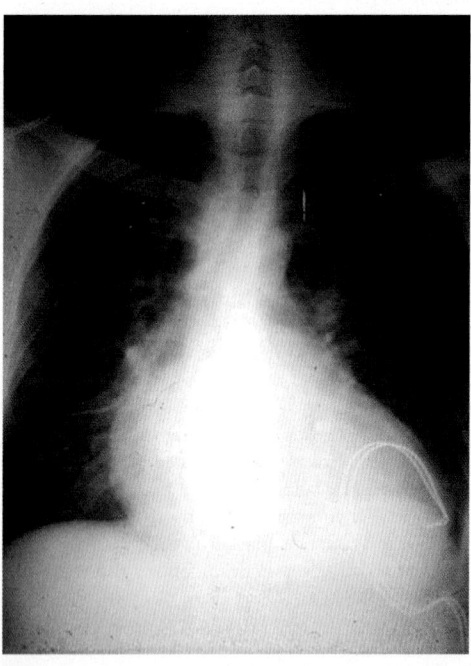

FIGURE 326-2. Chest radiograph of a patient from Bolivia with chronic *Trypanosoma cruzi* infection, rhythm disturbances, and cardiomyopathy. Pacemaker wires can be seen in the area of the left ventricle.

puncture, as noted, a chagoma may appear with local lymphadenopathy. The Romaña sign, the classic finding in acute Chagas disease, consists of painless edema of the palpebrae and periocular tissues and may appear when the conjunctiva is the portal of entry. These initial local signs can be followed by fever, malaise, anorexia, and edema of the face and lower extremities. Generalized lymphadenopathy and hepatosplenomegaly may also be present. Severe myocarditis may develop as well, and most deaths are caused by the resulting congestive heart failure. Meningoencephalitis is a rare complication. In untreated patients the acute illness resolves spontaneously over a period of 6 to 8 weeks as the patient enters the indeterminate phase of Chagas disease, which is characterized by subpatent parasitemia, absence of associated signs and symptoms, and easily detectable antibodies to *T. cruzi*.

Chronic Chagas Cardiopathy
In only 10 to 30% of persons chronically infected with *T. cruzi* does clinically manifested disease develop. It most often involves rhythm disturbances or cardiomyopathy.[8] Symptoms of cardiac Chagas disease can develop insidiously over years and often decades after the initial infection. Clinical findings reflect the rhythm disturbances, congestive heart failure, and thromboembolism that characterize the illness. Dizziness, syncope, and even seizures can result from a wide variety of arrhythmias. The cardiomyopathy often leads to biventricular failure, and right-sided heart failure can predominate in patients with advanced disease. Chronic Chagas disease is an independent risk factor for stroke.

Chronic Gastrointestinal Chagas Disease (Megadisease)
The esophagus and colon are the segments of the gastrointestinal (GI) tract most commonly affected in persons with chronic *T. cruzi* infection. In patients with megaesophagus, the symptoms are similar to those of idiopathic achalasia (Chapter 129) and may include cough, dysphagia, odynophagia, and regurgitation. Hypersalivation and consequent salivary gland hypertrophy develop in some patients with advanced esophageal dysfunction. Aspiration can occur, especially during sleep, and in untreated patients, repeated episodes of aspiration pneumonitis are common. Weight loss and even cachexia in patients with severe megaesophagus can combine with pneumonitis to cause death. Patients with chagasic megacolon have intermittent abdominal pain and chronic constipation and in advanced cases can go for several weeks between bowel movements. Rarely, acute obstruction, occasionally with volvulus, can lead to perforation, sepsis, and death.

IMMUNOSUPPRESSION AND TRANSPLANTATION IN PATIENTS INFECTED WITH *T. CRUZI*
When persons with chronic carriage of *T. cruzi* become immunosuppressed, reactivation of the infection can occur, sometimes with an intensity that is atypical of acute Chagas disease in immunocompetent persons.[9] The overall incidence of reactivation in immunosuppressed persons who harbor the parasite chronically is not known. Reactivation after renal transplantation has been reported, and in rare instances central nervous system abscesses and skin lesions were involved. The consensus view is that Chagas disease should not be a contraindication to kidney transplantation. In *T. cruzi*–infected patients who do undergo the procedure, periodic monitoring for signs and symptoms of acute Chagas disease should nonetheless be carried out, including careful neurologic evaluation, and parasitologic testing should be performed when acute illnesses occur postoperatively.

Reactivation of *T. cruzi* infection can also occur in persons coinfected with the parasite and human immunodeficiency virus (HIV). Dozens of such patients have been described. It is striking that in many of these patients *T. cruzi* brain

PHASE OR FORM	CLINICAL MANIFESTATIONS	DIAGNOSIS	TREATMENT SUCCESS
Acute infection	Usually nonspecific mild symptoms	Wet prep of blood or PCR	80-100%
Congenital infection	Asymptomatic or nonspecific mild symptoms	Wet prep of blood or PCR	80-100%
Chronic infection	Asymptomatic, without ECG change	Positive serology	May decrease progression to cardiomyopathy
Cardiomyopathy	Arrhythmias, syncope, left ventricular dysfunction, heart failure, ECG conduction abnormalities	Positive serology	Benefit not established
Gastrointestinal	Dilation of esophagus, colon, or both	Positive serology	Benefit not established
Reactivation in immunosuppressed hosts	Acute myocarditis, CNS abscesses, skin chagomas	Wet prep of blood or PCR	Suppression of acute symptoms and parasitemia, but long-term benefit not clear

TABLE 326-1 CLINICAL MANIFESTATIONS AND DIAGNOSIS OF CHAGAS DISEASE

CNS = central nervous system; ECG = electrocardiogram; PCR = polymerase chain reaction.
Adapted from Bern C. Chagas disease. N Engl J Med. 2015;373:456-466.

abscesses developed, which do not occur in immunocompetent patients with chronic Chagas disease. It has been shown that HIV viral loads increase in the context of reactivated acute Chagas disease. Calculations based on the overlapping epidemiologies of HIV and *T. cruzi* infections in the endemic countries suggest that the incidence of reactivation of the latter in coinfected persons is low.

DIAGNOSIS

Acute Chagas Disease

The first step in considering the diagnosis of acute Chagas disease is establishing that a person is at risk for *T. cruzi* infection. Risk factors include recent residence or blood transfusion in an endemic area, birth to a mother with geographic- or transfusion-associated risk in the case of a newborn, or a laboratory accident involving the parasite. Definitive diagnosis of acute Chagas disease can be made only by detecting parasites. Serologic assays for *T. cruzi*–specific IgM are not accurate enough to justify their use. In immunocompetent persons suspected of having acute Chagas disease, the most productive approach is examination of wet preparations of anticoagulated blood or buffy coat for the highly motile blood stream parasites. They can be seen in Giemsa-stained smears as well. In infected immunocompromised patients. Moreover, parasites can sometimes be found in other specimens such as lymph node aspirates, biopsy specimens of skin lesions, bone marrow, endomyocardial tissue, CSF, and pericardial fluid.

When these direct methods fail to detect organisms in an at-risk person, samples should be tested with a PCR assay (see later).[10] PCR assays have been shown to be more sensitive than the direct methods described earlier for detecting *T. cruzi*. Another method is to culture blood or other samples in specialized liquid medium, but the usefulness of this approach is limited by low sensitivity (50 to 70% for hemoculture) and by the fact that cultures take a minimum of 2 weeks before turning positive. In newborns whose blood is negative both by direct examination and in a PCR assay right after birth, serologic evaluation for *T. cruzi*–specific IgG should be performed 6 to 9 months later, by which time maternal antibodies will have disappeared.

Chronic Chagas Disease

Chronic *T. cruzi* infection is usually diagnosed by detecting IgG antibodies that specifically bind to parasite antigens, and in almost all instances isolation of the organism is not necessary. There is no credible evidence that "seronegative chronic Chagas disease" exists. More than 30 serologic assays for diagnosing Chagas disease are currently available commercially in endemic countries, where they are used widely for testing clinical specimens and screening blood donors. Even though these tests generally have high sensitivity and specificity, false-positive reactions do occur, typically with specimens from people who have other infectious diseases or autoimmune conditions. The World Health Organization has recommended that testing be done with two assays based on different formats. In the United States, the Ortho *T. cruzi* ELISA Test System (Ortho-Clinical Diagnostics, Raritan, NJ) and the Abbott Prism Chagas Assay (Abbott Laboratories, Abbott Park, IL) are approved by the FDA for screening donated blood. The Abbott ESA Chagas and the Chagas RIPA have both been cleared by the FDA for confirmatory testing of donor samples that are positive in the screening tests.

In human studies, the sensitivity of the PCR assays has ranged from 44.7 to 100%, with most being higher than 90%. It is generally accepted that the level of sensitivity of these assays is not high enough to justify their use for confirmatory testing of serologically positive donor samples. In contrast, PCR assays may be useful in persons who have borderline serologic results, in patients suspected of having congenital or acute Chagas disease in whom parasites are not detected microscopically, and in infected patients who have received specific treatment. In all such persons, because of the sensitivity issue, only positive PCR results can be taken as being truly indicative of infection status.

TREATMENT ℞

Antiparasitic Drugs

The two drugs currently available for treating Chagas disease (benznidazole and nifurtimox) are unsatisfactory, and the need for a parasitologically curative drug regimen is the most important current challenge in Chagas disease research (also see Chapter 323).[11] Benznidazole is considered the drug of choice by most Latin American experts.[12]

Benznidazole is a nitroimidazole derivative. Cure rates are similar or perhaps a bit higher than those achieved with nifurtimox. A cure rate higher than 90%

in babies with congenital infection has been observed with benznidazole. Side effects can include rash, peripheral neuropathy, and granulocytopenia. The recommended oral dosage of benznidazole is 5 to 10 mg/kg body weight per day for children and 5 mg/kg body weight per day for adults, in both cases for 60 days.[13]

Nifurtimox is a nitrofuran derivative that has been used for more than three decades. Nifurtimox reduces symptoms and decreases mortality rates in patients with acute Chagas disease, approximately 70% of whom are cured parasitologically. Nifurtimox also can cure a substantial portion of children in the indeterminate phase, but unfortunately, cure rates may be less than 10% in adults with long-standing chronic *T. cruzi* infection. Disadvantages of nifurtimox include its long course of treatment and occasionally bothersome side effects, including GI complaints such as anorexia, nausea, vomiting, weight loss, and abdominal pain. Patients taking the drug may also have neurologic symptoms such as insomnia, restlessness, paresthesias, twitching, polyneuritis, and even seizures. For adults, the recommended oral dosage is 8 to 10 mg/kg body weight per day. For adolescents, the dose is 12.5 to 15 mg/kg/day, and for children 1 to 10 years of age, it is 15 to 20 mg/kg/day. The drug should be given each day in four divided doses, and treatment should be continued for 90 to 120 days. In the United States, nifurtimox can only be obtained from the CDC Drug Service (404-639-3670).

There is broad agreement among experts that treatment is indicated in all patients with acute or congenital infections, as well as in chronically infected children up to 18 years old. This recommendation is supported by several studies suggesting that a majority of such patients appear to be cured parasitologically. By extension, it would be reasonable to treat anyone 18 years or older known to have acquired *T. cruzi* infection within the past 17 years. There is also broad agreement that persons with advanced symptomatic *T. cruzi* infection should not be given specific treatment. The remaining question, then, is whether adults with long-standing indeterminate-phase infections, who by far constitute the largest group of *T. cruzi*–infected persons, should be treated. This is a thorny question because the burden of taking a full course of either drug can be substantial and because parasitologic cure rates are so low. In asymptomatic patients, benznidazole can convert up to 90% of PCR-positive patients who are able to tolerate the drug to negative for a year,[A1][A2] but there is no clear evidence that such therapy delays the onset of symptoms, slows disease progression, or reduces mortality rates. In a randomized trial of benznidazole in 3000 patients ages 18 to 75 years with Chagas disease and incipient cardiac disease, PCR positivity was significantly suppressed in the subjects treated with benznidazole through 5 years of follow-up, but there was no significant reduction in clinical cardiac deterioration or in deaths.[A3] One area of hope in this dreary landscape of drugs for Chagas disease relates to whether treatment before pregnancy reduces the likelihood of subsequent congenital transmission of *T. cruzi*. In a handful of studies done in Argentina and Spain now involving a total of more than 250 babies born to women who had been or during the study were treated with benznidazole or nifurtimox, either when they were younger than 18 years or as adults, not a single baby was found to have congenital Chagas disease.[14] This outcome compares with historical rates of congenital transmission of 2 to 10%, as well as a rate of 16% in one of the trials in which there was an untreated arm. The fact that under current perspectives regarding the efficacy of treatment, a substantial proportion of the girls and women treated would not have been cured parasitologically, makes this outcome unexpected. In any event, the results suggest that all girls of any age, as well as all women of childbearing age, who have geographic or maternal risk for Chagas disease should be screened serologically. Those determined to be positive, after ruling out pregnancy, should be treated with a full course of benznidazole with the goal of reducing the rate of congenital transmission to babies they may have, even years later.

Management of Symptomatic Chagas Disease

An algorithm for the evaluation of persons with newly diagnosed Chagas disease has been developed (Fig. 326-3). *T. cruzi*–infected patients in whom symptomatic cardiac or GI disease develops should be referred to appropriate subspecialists. Beyond the possible use of nifurtimox or benznidazole, treatment of acute and chronic Chagas disease is symptomatic (Chapter 54). In patients with symptomatic chronic Chagas cardiac disease, treatment should be directed at managing symptoms with the anticoagulants and cardiotropic drugs used in patients with cardiomyopathy of other causes.[15] Some data suggest that carvedilol (up-titrated to 25 mg twice daily) may reduce mortality in Chagas cardiomyopathy.[A4] Pacemakers are useful in patients with ominous arrhythmias. Implantable cardioverter-defibrillators may be useful in selected patients with dysrhythmias due to Chagas heart disease, but this issue needs further investigation in prospective randomized trials.[16]

Heart transplantation (Chapter 53) is an option in patients with end-stage Chagas cardiac disease, and more than 150 such patients have undergone the procedure in Brazil and the United States.[17] As is the case with other *T. cruzi*–infected patients who are immunosuppressed, reactivation is a risk but is manageable. The usefulness and side effects of long-term prophylaxis for reactivation with either benznidazole or nifurtimox in *T. cruzi*–infected patients after heart

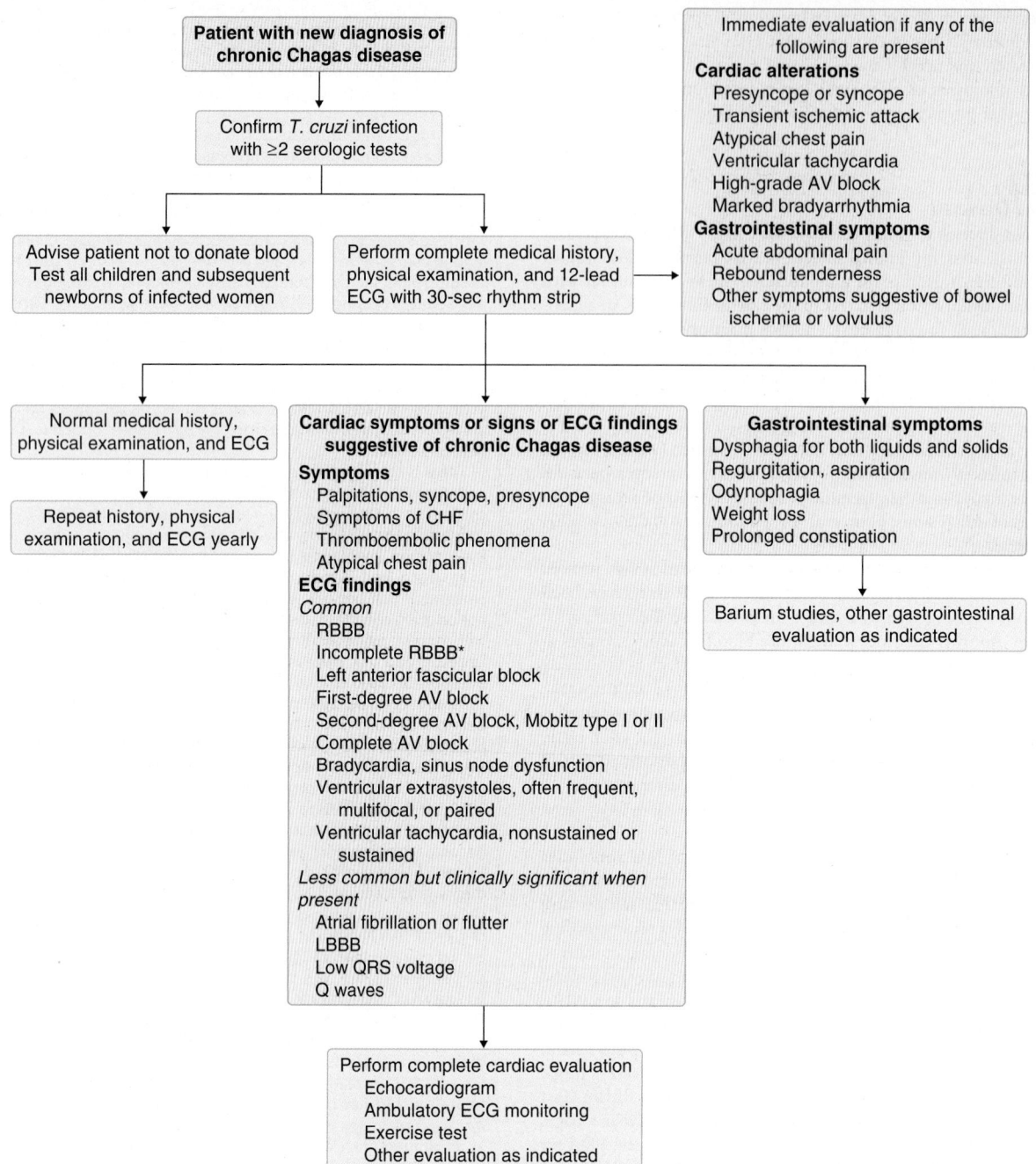

*QRS interval of 0.10 to 0.11 seconds in adults. Criteria based on the *Minnesota Code Manual of Electrocardiographic Findings* with modifications from Maguire et al. Different criteria may be required for ECGs in children.

FIGURE 326-3. Algorithm for baseline evaluation of a patient with newly diagnosed chronic *Trypanosoma cruzi* infection. AV = atrioventricular; CHF = congestive heart failure; ECG = electrocardiogram; LBBB = left bundle branch block; RBBB = right bundle branch block. (From Bern C, Montgomery SP, Herwaldt BL, et al. Evaluation and treatment of Chagas disease in the United States: a systematic review. *JAMA.* 2007;298:2171-2181.)

transplantation have not been evaluated. The long-term survival of Chagas patients with heart transplants appears to be longer than that of patients undergoing cardiac transplantation for other reasons, probably because the lesions of *T. cruzi*–associated pathology affect mostly the heart.

Chagas megaesophagus should be treated as normally done for idiopathic achalasia (Chapter 129), which usually responds to balloon dilation of the lower esophageal sphincter when symptoms are mild. Surgical treatment may be required in patients who do not respond to repeated attempts at balloon dilation. Laparoscopic myotomy is being used with increasing frequency to treat Chagas megaesophagus, as is the case with achalasia.

Chagas megacolon in its early stage can be treated with a high-fiber diet and occasional laxatives or enemas. Fecal impaction requiring manual disimpaction can occur, and toxic megacolon requires surgery. In patients with advanced megacolon, volvulus (Chapter 133) can develop when an enlarged and lengthened sigmoid colon twists and folds on itself; volvulus causes a constellation of symptoms and in many cases requires immediate surgery. Even if the symptoms associated with volvulus are resolved without operative

intervention, however, surgical treatment is usually ultimately necessary because the volvulus tends to recur. Several surgical procedures are used to treat advanced Chagas megacolon, all of which include resection of the sigmoid and removal of part of the rectum.

PREVENTION

Reducing human contact with triatomine vectors through education of at-risk persons, housing improvement, and spraying of residual insecticides in endemic countries has resulted in reduction or elimination of vector transmission of *T. cruzi* in a major part of the endemic range, and progress in this regard is expected to continue.[18] Serologic screening of donated blood has essentially eliminated transfusion-related transmission of the parasite in most endemic areas. Outbreaks of acute Chagas disease through oral transmission can be avoided by the implementation of better food safety standards. Drug treatment

TABLE 326-2	PREDICTING DEATH IN CHAGAS HEART DISEASE	
CHARACTERISTIC		**POINTS**
Male sex		2
Functional class III or IV		5
Low QRS voltage on electrocardiography		3
Cardiomyopathy on chest radiography		5
Left ventricular systolic dysfunction on echocardiograph		3
Nonsustained ventricular tachycardia on Holter monitoring		3
10 year mortality:	0-6 points	9%
	7-11 points	37%
	12-20 points	85%

Adapted from Rassi A, Jr., Rassi A, Little WC, et al. Development and validation of a risk score for predicting death in Chagas' heart disease. *N Engl J Med.* 2006;355:799-808.

of *T. cruzi*–infected women before pregnancy reduces the likelihood of congenital transmission. No protocols have been defined and validated for preventing reactivation of *T. cruzi* infection in chronically infected persons who are immunosuppressed iatrogenically or by HIV. A treatment regimen that reliably results in parasitologic cure is needed to prevent the onset or progression of chronic symptomatic Chagas disease.

PROGNOSIS

The prognosis for patients with acute Chagas disease is generally excellent because most acutely infected persons have only mild symptoms that resolve spontaneously, even without specific treatment. The occasional patient who has symptomatic acute Chagas myocarditis should generally do well if treated early. In persons with chronic *T. cruzi* infection, the lifetime risk for the development of related cardiac or GI dysfunction is only 10 to 30%. A validated risk score assessment tool can estimate prognosis in the absence of heart transplantation (Table 326-2).

Grade A References

A1. Molina I, Gomez I, Prat J, et al. Randomized trial of posaconazole and benznidazole for chronic Chagas' disease. *N Engl J Med.* 2014;370:1899-1908.
A2. Morillo CA, Marin-Neto JA, Avezum A, et al. Randomized trial of benznidazole for chronic Chagas' cardiomyopathy. *N Engl J Med.* 2015;373:1295-1306.
A3. Morillo CA, Waskin H, Sosa-Estani S, et al. Benznidazole and posaconazole in eliminating parasites in asymptomatic *T. cruzi* carriers: the STOP-CHAGAS Trial. *J Am Coll Cardiol.* 2017;69:939-947.
A4. Martí-Carvajal AJ, Kwong JS. Pharmacological interventions for treating heart failure in patients with Chagas cardiomyopathy. *Cochrane Database Syst Rev.* 2016;7:CD009077.

GENERAL REFERENCES

For the General References and other additional features, please visit Expert Consult at https://expertconsult.inkling.com.

327

LEISHMANIASIS

PIERRE A. BUFFET AND SIMON L. CROFT

DEFINITION

Leishmaniasis is caused by protozoan parasites of the genus *Leishmania* that are generally transmitted between mammalian hosts by female phlebotomine sandflies. The parasite exists as an extracellular flagellated form, the promastigote, in the sandfly gut, and as an intracellular form, the amastigote, that survives and multiplies in a phagolysosomal compartment of macrophages in the mammalian host. The disease in humans affects either the skin/mucosae or internal organs and ranges in severity from a single, self-curing, limited skin lesion to widespread multilesional cutaneous involvement, and from a single nodule to potentially fatal visceral disease affecting spleen, liver, and bone marrow.

This disease complex is caused by 20 species of *Leishmania*, which are widely distributed in Europe, Asia, Africa, and South and Central America, with limited foci in Southeast Asia.[1] The characteristics of the main *Leishmania* species are summarized in Table 327-1. There are an estimated 1.5 to 2.0 million new cases each year, with up to 70,000 deaths, although this is probably an underestimate because leishmaniasis is not a reportable disease in many of the 101 countries and territories in which it is known to occur. Many *Leishmania* infections are either asymptomatic or diagnosed several months after the onset of symptoms.

Clinical aspects are considered under separate sections for visceral leishmaniasis (VL) and cutaneous/mucosal leishmaniasis (CL, ML).

EPIDEMIOLOGY

Infection is established in the mammalian host following a bite of the female sandfly belonging to either *Phlebotomus* spp in Europe, Asia, and Africa or *Lutzomyia* spp in the Americas. Different species of sandfly are associated with transmission of different *Leishmania* species. Most species that cause CL have a zoonotic (acquired from another mammal) transmission cycle, with the exception of *Leishmania tropica*, which is frequently anthroponotic (transmitted between human beings). VL is either normally anthroponotic (in the case of *Leishmania donovani*) or zoonotic (in the case of *Leishmania infantum*). The predominant mammalian hosts (the reservoirs) are associated with different *Leishmania* species in diverse ecosystems (Fig. 327-1).

VL is caused by either *L. donovani* or *L. infantum* (which is identical to *Leishmania chagasi* in South America). These species have different geographic distributions, with the highest incidence found in the poorest communities in seven countries (Bangladesh, Nepal, India, Sudan, South Sudan, Ethiopia, and Brazil), and it is potentially fatal if untreated. An estimated 1 in 5 to 1 in 50 infections are symptomatic, depending on the parasite species and host immunity. Since 2005, there has been a regional program to eliminate VL, during which time there has been a reduction of annual incidence by more than 90% on the Indian subcontinent. Nevertheless, the economic burden of infection remains enormous.[2]

CL, which undergoes self-cure in 20 to 90% of patients within 3 to 18 months (depending on infecting species and geographic location), is widely distributed, but its prevalence is difficult to estimate because of underreporting. Prevalence is associated with age, possibly related to the acquisition of immunity and risk factors, including the presence of domestic animals, rodents, or other mammalian hosts. Ecologic conditions for sandflies, including shaded and humid habitats in crevices and mammal burrows, have been identified. Urbanization, deforestation, and migration have resulted in changing patterns of disease, with transmission occurring in peridomestic cycles. Other forms of transmission, such as through organ transplantation, intravenous needles shared by drug users, or laboratory exposure, have been reported.

PATHOBIOLOGY

The infection is initially established in the skin after the inoculation of infective metacyclic promastigotes by the sandfly. These infective forms have a glycoprotein coat (a lipophosphoglycan) that enables them to resist complement and attach to and invade host cells. Peptides in sandfly saliva (e.g., maxadilan) cause vasodilation and erythema and help establish infection in the dermal layer of the skin. Early responses to infection involve neutrophil infiltration and invasion of resident macrophages. Progress of the disease depends on the parasite species and host responses. For both VL and CL, disease progression depends on the maintenance of a parasite-specific immunosuppressive state. During established disease, host cell macrophages are in a deactivated state but become activated either spontaneously or after treatment. They are then able to kill the parasites, which are sensitive to nitric oxide and oxygen radicals, in the phagolysosomal compartment. Resolution of disease, following the activation of macrophages, is enhanced by a helper T-cell type 1 (T_H1) response after interaction between antigen-presenting cells (e.g., dendritic cells) with CD4$^+$ and CD8$^+$ T cells and subsequent secretion of pro-inflammatory cytokines (e.g., interleukin-1 [IL-1], interferon-γ, tumor necrosis factor-α). However, in clinical forms such as active VL or diffuse CL, a T_H2 cell response predominates, whereby downregulation of macrophage activity follows the production of cytokines such as IL-4, IL-10, IL-13, and transforming growth factor-β. This profile has been defined in experimental models, mainly inbred mice, and clinical studies support the notion of a generally similar profile in typical, polar infections in humans. Immunologic patterns may be more complex in some clinical forms, with

TABLE 327-1   CHARACTERISTICS OF THE MAIN *LEISHMANIA* SPECIES

LEISHMANIA SPP	*LEISHMANIA* SUBGENUS	DISTRIBUTION: OLD WORLD	DISTRIBUTION: NEW WORLD	PRIMARY FORM	SECONDARY FORMS	ANTHROPONOTIC: AREAS OF TRANSMISSION	ZOONOTIC: RESERVOIR	ALTERNATIVE NAME
L. donovani	*Leishmania*	Indian subcontinent E. Africa		VL	PKDL CL, ML OIVL	Indian subcontinent E. Africa		Kala-azar
L. infantum (L. chagasi)	*Leishmania*	Europe Asia	S. & C. America	VL	CL, ML OIVL		Canid	
L. major	*Leishmania*	Asia N. & E. Africa Europe		CL			Rodent	
L. tropica	*Leishmania*	Asia Europe		CL	Recidivans	Syria Afghanistan	Rodent	Aleppo boil
L. aethiopica	*Leishmania*	Ethiopia		CL	DCL		Hyrax	
L. mexicana	*Leishmania*		C. America	CL			Rodent	Chiclero ulcer
L. amazonensis	*Leishmania*		C. & S. America	CL	DCL		Rodent	
L. braziliensis	*Viannia*		S. America	CL ML	DissCL Lymph		Rodent, marsupial	ML-espundia
L. panamensis	*Viannia*		C. & S. America	CL	ML Lymph		Edentate rodent	Ulcera de bejuco
L. guyanensis	*Viannia*		S. America	CL	ML Lymph		Rodent, edentates	Pian bois
L. peruviana	*Viannia*		S. America	CL			Canid	Uta
L. martiniquensis/ siamensis	*Leishmania?*	South East Asia/ West Indies		CL, VL	DCL			

CL = cutaneous leishmaniasis; DCL = diffuse cutaneous leishmaniasis; DissCL = disseminated cutaneous leishmaniasis; Lymph = nodular lymphangitis; ML = mucosal leishmaniasis; OIVL = opportunistic infection with VL in HIV-infected patients; PKDL = post–kala-azar dermal leishmaniasis; VL = visceral leishmaniasis.

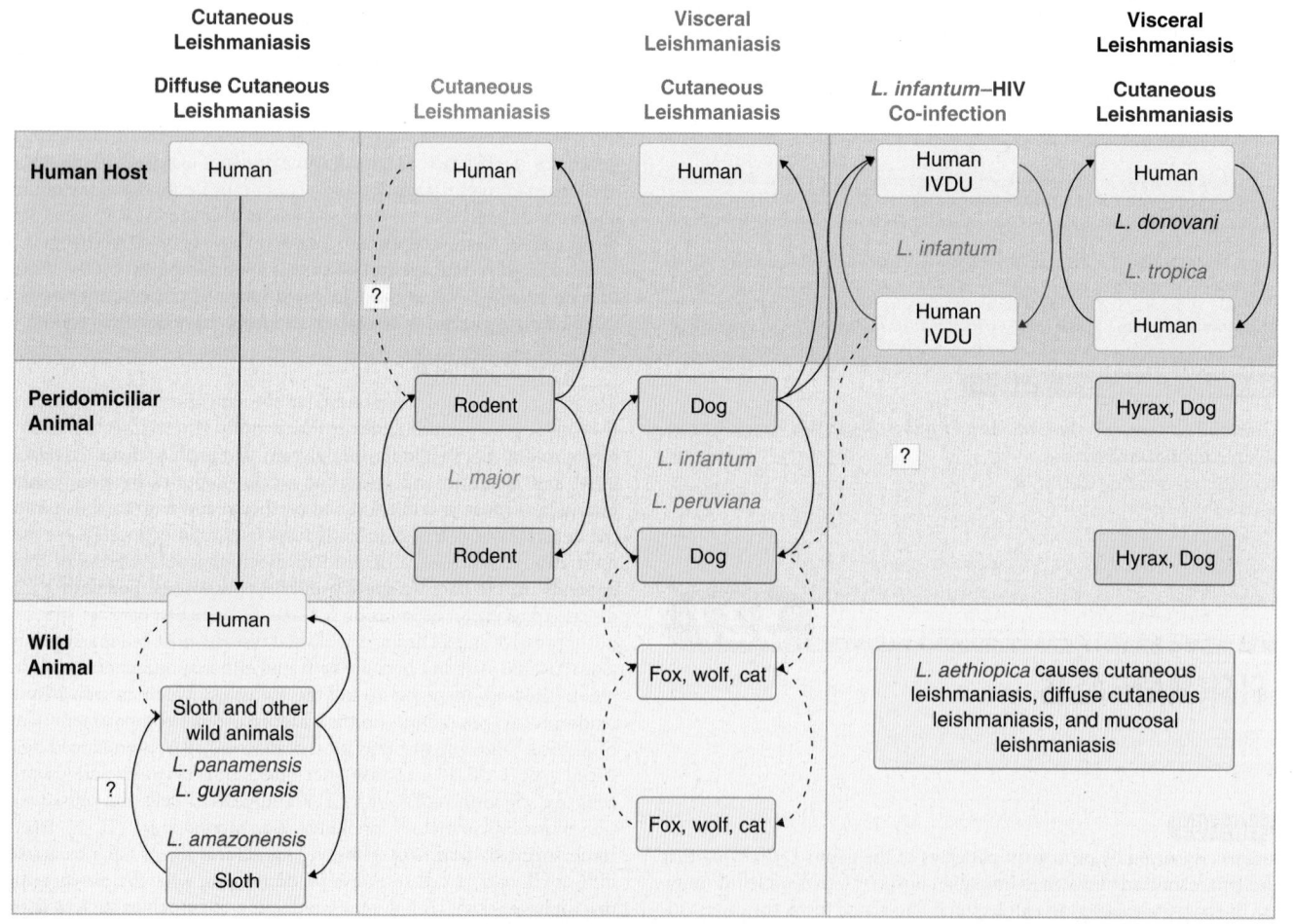

FIGURE 327-1. Old World and New World zoonotic and anthroponotic life cycles of the main species of *Leishmania*. Leishmaniasis is often referred to as a "disease complex" because different forms of disease can be caused by the same parasite species and similar forms of disease can be caused by different parasite species. IVDU = intravenous drug use.

antiparasitic immunity also playing a pathogenic role and contributing to tissue damage

In patients with VL, the absence of a T-cell-specific immune response to leishmanial antigens is associated with uncontrolled progression of infection. This is linked to elevated levels of IL-10 and decreased production of interferon-γ. Genetic susceptibility to *L. donovani* in Sudan has been associated with a solute carrier family (formerly NRAMP1) that regulates macrophage activation and with a polymorphism in the IL-4 gene. In localized simple CL, patients show a T_H1-type response and a delayed-type hypersensitivity (DTH) response. DTH is frequently measured by a Montenegro skin test, which can also be used in epidemiologic prevalence studies. Chronic infections show a T_H2-type response, most predominantly in patients with diffuse CL, in whom there is complete anergy to leishmania antigen and no DTH response. Patients with ML have a T_H1 or T_H2 cell response or both and have a strong or weak DTH response. Post–kala-azar dermal leishmaniasis (PKDL), a rare sequela to cure from VL, is poorly understood. The roles of $CD4^+$ and $CD25^+$ T cells appear to be different in Indian and Sudanese forms of PKDL.

 VISCERAL LEISHMANIASIS

CLINICAL MANIFESTATIONS

The onset of VL, often referred to as kala-azar when caused by *L. donovani*, occurs weeks to months after the initial infection. Clinical signs and symptoms, such as fever, splenomegaly, and hepatomegaly, do not distinguish VL from hyperreactive malarial splenomegaly or other infectious or hematologic conditions. Moderate to severe anemia, mild to moderate leukopenia, thrombocytopenia, systemic inflammation, and polyclonal hypergammaglobulinemia, either isolated or combined, suggest but do not confirm the diagnosis. Parasitologic tests are therefore indispensable before making a therapeutic decision.[3]

DIAGNOSIS
Parasitology

Microscopic visualization of amastigotes in samples from the lymph nodes, bone marrow, liver, spleen, or other organs was usually the first step in diagnosis. Because spleen aspiration causes life-threatening complications in approximately 0.1% of patients, it should be performed only in trained facilities and only if other, lower risk methods cannot be used. It is still used in the field because of the higher cost, logistic constraints, and lower sensitivity of bone marrow aspiration. Polymerase chain reaction (PCR) is more sensitive than microscopic examination and has become the first-line test in several referral hospitals and research centers.[4] Quantitative PCR with validated thresholds allows accurate diagnosis with venous blood samples, thereby avoiding bone marrow aspiration.

Serology

Serologic tests based on indirect fluorescent antibody (IFA), enzyme-linked immunosorbent assay (ELISA), or Western blot display high performance but require equipment that is poorly adapted to field settings. The direct agglutination test (DAT) and immunochromatography (dipstick) using the rK39 antigen have high diagnostic accuracy and can be used in peripheral health centers. Whatever the serologic test used, specific antibodies remain detectable for several years after cure or asymptomatic infection.

Antigen Detection Tests

A latex agglutination test that detects a heat-stable, low-molecular-weight carbohydrate antigen in the urine of patients with VL showed good specificity but low to moderate sensitivity in East Africa and the Indian subcontinent. Further development of antigen-based tests is leading to new products.[5]

Complex Manifestations of Visceral Leishmaniasis
VISCERAL LEISHMANIASIS–HUMAN IMMUNODEFICIENCY VIRUS COINFECTION

Although the clinical manifestations in VL patients infected with human immunodeficiency virus (HIV) without severe immunosuppression are generally similar to those in immunocompetent patients, atypical clinical features can be found in patients with low $CD4^+$ T-cell counts ($<200/\mu L$). In the latter group, physicians may order investigations for VL even in the absence of classic signs (e.g., lack of splenomegaly). A substantial proportion of patients coinfected with leishmaniasis and HIV may have other opportunistic infections that complicate the clinical diagnosis. The parasitic load is usually higher, and parasites may be found in tissues other than spleen, liver, bone marrow, or lymph nodes (e.g., gut or lung), especially in severely immunosuppressed

patients. Therefore, the sensitivity of microscopic examination, culture, or PCR of blood (plain blood or buffy coat) or bone marrow aspirates is generally higher than that in immunocompetent VL patients. Limited data have also shown high sensitivity of the latex agglutination test in the urine of patients coinfected with leishmaniasis and HIV. In contrast, the sensitivity of serologic tests is decreased in coinfected patients, although study results are equivocal and depend on several factors, such as the test format, region of endemicity, and level of immunosuppression. For example, the DAT has shown high sensitivity in Ethiopia. Increased sensitivity can be achieved by using a sequential combination of different serologic tests.

POST–KALA-AZAR DERMAL LEISHMANIASIS

After successful treatment of visceral disease due to *L. donovani*, a proportion of patients progress to disseminated cutaneous disease.[6] This was reported in up to 20% of patients in Sudan and 0.5% in India and Bangladesh, although recent studies show an increase in the proportion of PKDL cases in these countries. In a small proportion of patients with PKDL, uveitis occurs with poor visual prognosis. Studies in India have shown that smears are more likely to show amastigotes if taken from nodular lesions rather than papular or macular lesions of PKDL. Serologic tests such as the DAT, ELISA, and rK39 immunochromatography are of limited value because a positive finding may be the result of persistent antibodies following the past episode of VL. Nevertheless, serology can be helpful when a previous history of VL is uncertain.

TREATMENT

General Principles

The therapeutic management of patients with VL requires renutrition, broad-spectrum antibiotics if bacterial superinfection is suspected, transfusion in cases of severe anemia, and proper hydration, especially when amphotericin B is used for the specific antileishmanial treatment.

The clinical response to antileishmanial agents depends on the clinical form and the infecting species or even the subspecies (zymodeme). Many antileishmanial agents are either toxic, expensive, or difficult to administer in field conditions. No single satisfactory option for treating most of the clinical forms or species has been validated. Although therapeutic decisions and follow-up have become relatively simple for the treatment of VL in nonendemic and some endemic countries based on the powerful, well-tolerated agent liposomal amphotericin B,[7] more complexity persists for the treatment of VL in East Africa and in endemic countries where liposomal amphotericin B is not available.[8] Deciding on treatment for relapsing VL in immunocompromised patients and for CL or ML often requires expert advice.

Visceral Leishmaniasis in Immunocompetent Patients
Single-Agent Therapies

Liposomal amphotericin B achieves high cure rates in India, with a single course of treatment of 10 mg/kg now recommended in the national program for VL elimination. In East Africa, the doses of liposomal amphotericin B required to cure VL (30 to 50 mg/kg cumulatively) are markedly higher than those used in India, and the drug fails in about 20% of patients, even with these higher doses.[A1] It also is effective for treating PKDL.[9] Liposomal amphotericin B is associated with less infusion-related fever and chills, less renal toxicity, and a reduction in the number of infusions and length of hospitalization compared with conventional amphotericin B deoxycholate. The better renal tolerance of liposomal amphotericin B is especially beneficial in patients with renal failure or a kidney graft and in those with an increase in serum creatinine during amphotericin B deoxycholate therapy. Liposomal amphotericin B is the antileishmanial agent with the best risk-to-benefit ratio. It is now the first-line option in most nonendemic countries, both in children and in adults. The high cost of liposomal amphotericin B has reduced its use in endemic countries, and wider implementation is greatly facilitated by donation. In India, 100% of patients with VL in the liposomal therapy group and 98% in the conventional therapy group had apparent cure responses at day 30. Cure rates at 6 months were similar: 95.7% with liposomal therapy and 96.3% with conventional therapy.[A2] *Amphotericin B* (cumulative dose of 7 to 15 mg/kg) cures more than 98% of patients in India, whereas treatment of visceral infection with *L. infantum/chagasi* requires at least 14 mg/kg (generally 21 mg/kg cumulative dose over 10 days).

Pentamidine is efficient in treating VL only when high doses (more than seven injections of 4 mg/kg) are used. These are toxic, and pentamidine is no longer used for the initial treatment of VL. Lower doses (fewer than four injections of 4 mg/kg) induce much fewer adverse events and are still used for the secondary prophylaxis of VL in HIV-infected patients (fortnightly to monthly injections).

Pentavalent antimonials (sodium stibogluconate, meglumine antimoniate) are still prescribed as first-intention drugs in many areas. In the Indian subcontinent (mainly in northern Bihar), *L. donovani* is resistant to pentavalent antimonials. Their efficacy has decreased from 90% to less than 40% over the past 40 years. In other VL foci, failure rates of initial treatment do not exceed 10% as long as the dosage is respected (20 mg/kg/day of pentavalent antimony for 28 days). In an endemic country, mortality in treated patients may exceed 10%, with toxicity positively correlating with age. Pentavalent antimonials are contraindicated in patients with heart, kidney, or liver disease or advanced age and in pregnant women. Generic formulations have generally but not constantly demonstrated activity and tolerance identical to that of sodium stibogluconate.

Miltefosine is an alkyl phosphocholine. The oral form (2.5 mg/kg/day for 28 days) is very effective for VL in India. In Ethiopian patients with VL (28% with HIV infection), there was significantly higher mortality with sodium stibogluconate (generic) than with miltefosine (9.7 vs. 2.1%), despite the lower parasitologic efficacy of miltefosine (92.1 vs. 99.3%). Miltefosine is contraindicated in pregnant women and those who may become pregnant. Because of persistent levels of the drug, contraceptive measures must be observed for more than 3 months after therapy. Compared with a decade ago, substantial increase in the failure rate of oral miltefosine has been noted in the treatment of visceral leishmaniases in India and Nepal since 2012.

Paromomycin (aminosidine sulfate) (15 mg/kg in sulfate form equivalent to 11 mg of base per kilogram intramuscularly for 21 days) is highly effective in India, where it was registered in 2006. In East Africa, its efficacy is significantly lower. Similar to the situation with miltefosine, the longevity of the product would probably be better preserved in combination than as a single-agent therapy.

Combinations/Coadministration

To limit extension of the resistance to pentavalent antimonials and prevent the emergence of resistance to paromomycin or miltefosine, shorter courses of combined therapy are being investigated. Because only miltefosine may be administered orally, this approach is based at least partly on products administered parenterally. The combination of antimony and paromomycin is approved for use because high cure rates have been reported in East Africa, but this treatment still requires many injections. Combinations of amphotericin with oral miltefosine (sequential) and intramuscular paromomycin with miltefosine can achieve cure rates of up to 98% with 7- to 10-day courses of therapy. A single infusion of liposomal amphotericin B followed by oral miltefosine has been highly effective in India, but confirmation studies are required there and elsewhere.

Visceral Leishmaniasis in Immunodeficient Patients
Leishmania infantum–HIV Coinfection

As with other major opportunistic infections during HIV infection, treatment may be subdivided into initial course and secondary prophylaxis. With initial treatment, the efficacies of meglumine antimoniate and amphotericin B are similar. The severe adverse effects of antimony derivatives are more common in this context. Doses of liposomal amphotericin B administered to immunodeficient patients are higher (40 mg/kg in cumulative dose) than those administered to immunocompetent patients. When therapeutic immunosuppression may not be reduced or optimization of highly active antiretroviral therapy is not possible, secondary prophylaxis is often proposed. Amphotericin B lipid complex moderately reduces the frequency of recurrences. Discontinuous administration of liposomal amphotericin B is generally used, but a progressive reduction in its efficacy sometimes leading to complete unresponsiveness has been reported. Miltefosine is another option, especially if the reduction in parasitic load is backed up by quantitative PCR with a validated threshold (low residual load probably being associated with a lower risk for resistance). Administration of pentamidine once or twice a month is another potentially interesting option because drug levels persist for weeks or months after a single administration. Pancreatic tolerance should be monitored closely.

Leishmania donovani–HIV Coinfection

Patients should benefit from effective antiretroviral treatment. The experience with *L. infantum*–HIV coinfection is in part transposable. The potential risk for the emergence of resistance to antileishmanial agents is still more significant in this context because *L. donovani* (but not *L. infantum*) can be transmitted by sandflies from human to human. Liposomal amphotericin B 30 mg/kg plus miltefosine achieved a higher initial cure rate than liposomal amphotericin B alone (40 mg/kg) in East Africa,[A3] but defining the best strategy to reach sustained cure without relapse and preventing unresponsiveness to drugs will require further research, including the identification of an affordable, effective drug regimen for secondary prophylaxis.

CUTANEOUS LEISHMANIASIS

CLINICAL MANIFESTATIONS

Although the signs and symptoms of CL vary considerably (Fig. 327-2)—from pure nodular lesions to developing ulceration through dry crusty lesions and squamous plaques—there are some fairly constant features. First, firm

infiltration is almost constant (the exception being the initial macule of PKDL). Second, the evolution is subacute. A lesion reaching its maximum size in less than a week is most likely not due to CL. Finally, except in patients with numerous satellite papulopustules, the lesion or lesions are sharply defined. Colonization of the CL ulceration with bacteria may give the lesion a purulent appearance, whereas patent superinfection adds an erythematous ring distinctly overflowing the infiltrated edge of the ulceration and making a usually cold and painless lesion feel hot and painful. Several dermatologic conditions such as staphylococcal or streptococcal infection, mycobacterial ulcer, leprosy, fungal infection, cancer, sarcoidosis, and tropical ulcer mimic CL or ML lesions (see Fig. 327-2).[10] Because treatment is costly and potentially toxic, diagnostic confirmation is necessary.[11]

DIAGNOSIS
Parasitology

Scraping, fine-needle aspiration, or biopsy of lesions provides appropriate samples in which amastigotes can be identified (Fig. 327-3). Scraping should be performed at both the center and edges of the lesion with a curved scalpel blade. Local anesthesia considerably reduces patients' discomfort and increases sensitivity. Using an adrenaline-containing local anesthetic (contraindicated for lesions on extremities) or pinching the lesion between the thumb and finger until blanching appears helps obtain a bloodless scraping, thus optimizing microscopic examination. The 2- to 4-mm skin fragment obtained by punch biopsy provides abundant material, which facilitates the search for scarce parasites and for an alternative diagnosis by culture (e.g., mycobacteria, fungi) as well as histopathologic examination. Culture of a biopsy sample requires homogenization in saline or culture medium under sterile conditions.

The material obtained by any of these methods can be used for microscopic examination, culture, and PCR. Microscopic examination of Giemsa-stained material is the most widely available method.[12] Culture of the parasite in specific media (such as fetal calf serum–supplemented Schneider's or Novy-Nicolle-McNeal media) allows identification, characterization, and storage of the isolate. Detection of parasitic nucleic acids by molecular diagnosis (mainly PCR) increases sensitivity and allows identification of the *Leishmania* species. This is particularly useful in regions (e.g., New World) where several *Leishmania* species, with various clinical outcomes and responses to treatment, coexist. Both culture and molecular-based identification of species, now including mass spectrometry, require substantial laboratory infrastructure and technical expertise.

Serology

Serologic diagnosis is of limited use for CL because of low sensitivity and variable specificity. The leishmanin (or Montenegro) skin test (LST) evaluates the cell-mediated response against *Leishmania* spp. The LST requires culture and fixation of—preferentially—local species of *Leishmania* and therefore lacks standardization. The production of commercial formulations of the LST lacks sustainability. Like serologic tests, the LST does not distinguish between past and present infections.

Complex Manifestations of Cutaneous Leishmaniasis
MUCOSAL LEISHMANIASIS

A proportion of CL infections (about 1 to 10% in Brazil, Bolivia, and Peru) caused by *Leishmania braziliensis* or *Leishmania guyanensis* progress to a metastatic infection of the mucosa of the oral/nasal cavity or larynx, often 1 to 5 years after healing of the initial simple cutaneous lesion. Mucosal *Leishmania braziliensis* infection has also been reported in travelers returning from endemic countries.[13] Immunopathology shows extensive destruction of local tissue. Allergic rhinitis, paracoccidioidomycosis or other deep mycosis, cancrum oris, leprosy, and sarcoidosis may mimic the lesions of ML. Positive serology (e.g., IFA, ELISA) or LST indicates possible ML. Parasites are scarce in mucosal lesions. Therefore, a search for parasites in mucosal samples—obtained by scraping or biopsy—by microscopic examination or by culture lacks sensitivity. PCR has proved to be the most sensitive approach to confirm ML.

DIFFUSE CUTANEOUS LEISHMANIASIS

Patients with diffuse CL have an anergic response to *Leishmania* antigens, and nonulcerative nodules, loaded with parasites, disseminate from the initial site of infection to multiple skin sites. There is no self-cure, and treatment is difficult. This form of the disease is found in South America and East Africa, often associated with *Leishmania amazonensis* and *Leishmania aethiopica* infection.

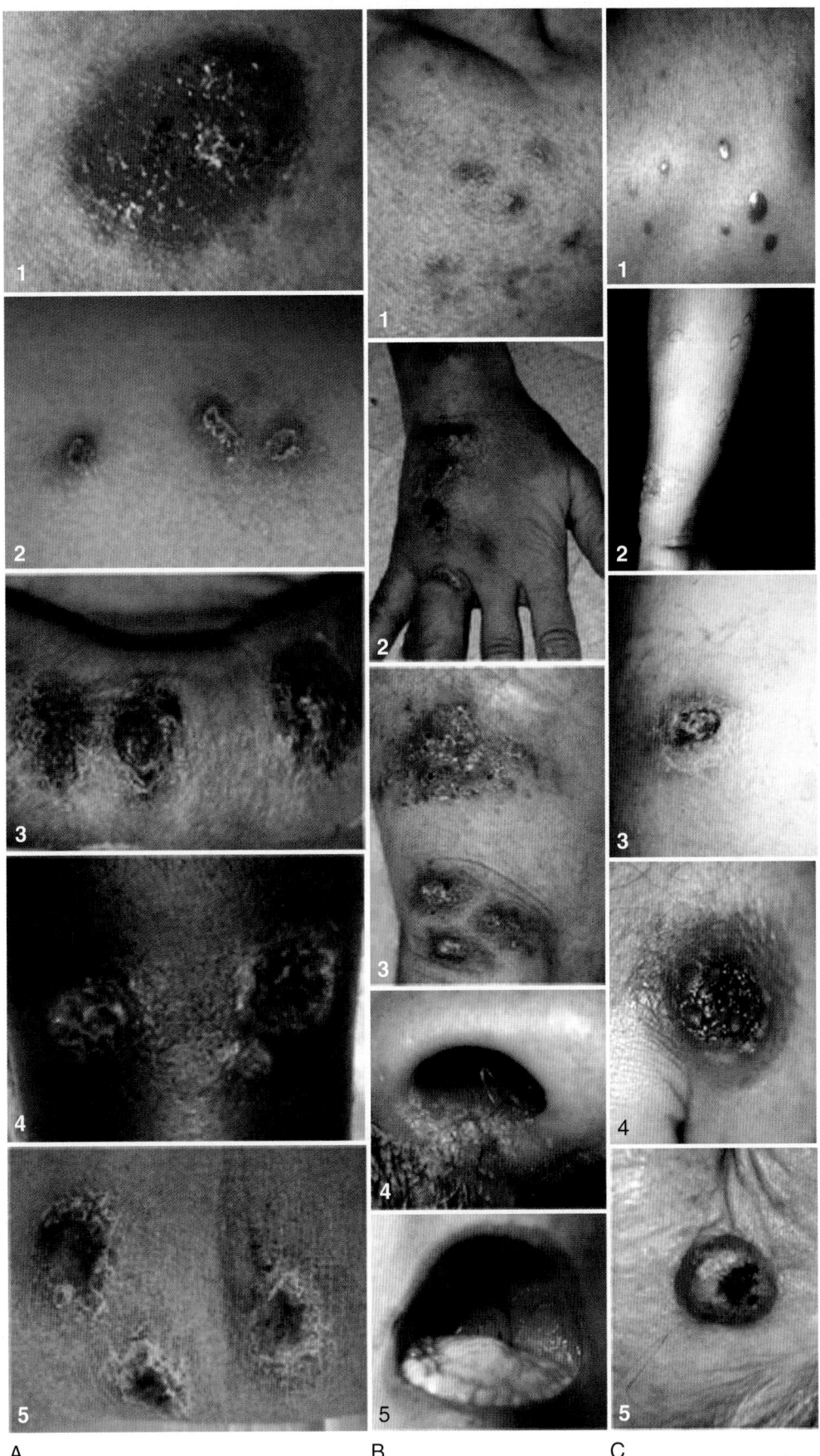

FIGURE 327-2. **Clinical features of cutaneous leishmaniasis (CL). A,** Typical forms of CL. **A1,** Papular-nodular. **A2,** Squamous. **A3,** Crusty. **A4,** Ulcerated. **A5,** Superinfected lesions. **B,** Atypical forms of CL and mucosal leishmaniasis. **B1,** Multiple papules on the face (*L. infantum,* Balearic islands). **B2,** Nodular lymphangitis (*L. braziliensis,* Brazil). **B3,** Multiple lesions with numerous peripheral papules (*L. major,* Tunisia). **B4,** Initial spread to the nasal mucosa (anterior septum, *L. braziliensis,* Bolivia). **B5,** Infiltration and ulceration of the tonsils (*L. infantum,* France). **C,** Clinical manifestations that are not CL. **C1,** Multiple papules (late secondary syphilis) (Chapter 303). **C2,** Nodular lymphangitis (sporotrichosis) (Chapter 316). **C3,** Single crusty ulceration (*Mycobacterium ulcerans* infection) (Chapter 309). **C4,** Ulcerated acute *Staphylococcus aureus* infection (Chapter 272). **C5,** Ulcerated nodule keratoacanthoma (Chapter 193).

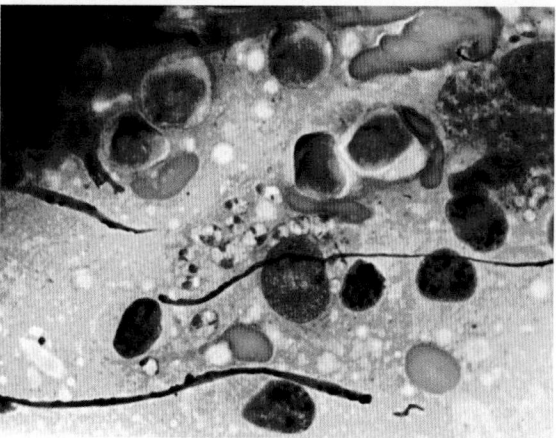

FIGURE 327-3. Amastigotes of *Leishmania major* in scrapings from a skin ulcer.

RECIDIVANS CUTANEOUS LEISHMANIASIS

Recidivans CL is characterized by the development of lesions containing granulomatous tissue. The lesions often take many years to heal and may arise years after healing of a simple localized lesion. New ulcers and papules may form over the edge of the old scar. Infections are normally associated with *L. tropica* infection and are difficult to treat.

TREATMENT   Rx

The clinical consequences of CL are dermatologic; concomitant visceral impairment is exceptional. The intensity of the discomfort, related to one or several oozing or unsightly lesions, and the impact of atrophic, hypopigmented, or hyperpigmented scars depend on the lesions' topography. In the New World, mucosal impairment may affect up to 1 to 15% of patients, with greater incidence in Bolivia. The risk for metastasis (initially nasal and then affecting the entire otorhinolaryngeal zone) has strongly influenced therapeutic decisions. Systemic treatment of any New World CL has been recommended, but recent data indicate that a different strategy should probably be considered.[14] Inadequate surgical excision and pentavalent antimonials or systemic pentamidine administered in excessive doses or without sufficient follow-up may paradoxically be a major risk for patients with CL.[15]

Local therapy with intralesional injections of pentavalent antimonials[16] (preferentially following a brief application of liquid nitrogen),[A4] photodynamic therapy, and thermotherapy are attractive options to avoid potentially toxic, expensive, or impractical systemic schedules.[17] However, implementation of these methods is hampered by logistic constraints and requires skilled health care providers. An efficient topical ointment or simple, painless physical methods would resolve most of these issues. An ointment containing paromomycin has shown efficacy with acceptable local tolerance in patients with CL caused by several species in North Africa and Central America and in travelers.[A5][A6] An algorithm for therapeutic decisions is proposed in E-Figure 327-1. When local treatment cannot be administered or has failed, systemic therapy is used. Oral therapy with relatively nontoxic drugs (high-dose fluconazole,[A7] miltefosine) would be the simplest option, but no optimal drug regimen has been solidly validated so far.[18] Oral miltefosine monotherapy has been successful in Brazil and in travelers with complex forms.[A8] In CL caused by *L. guyanensis* or *Leishmania panamensis,* low doses of pentamidine 1 to 3 injections generally cure more than 75% of patients.[A9] The efficacy of liposomal amphotericin B in CL is variable.[19]

There are no vaccines for human disease and no prophylactic drug regimens. Leishmanization, or inoculating people with live virulent parasites to cause a local limited lesion and provide protection, was used for CL (e.g., in Iran) but is not recommended by the World Health Organization.[20] Sandflies are sensitive to most insecticides, and attempts to control transmission has been made with residual spraying in houses. Insecticide-impregnated bed nets and dog collars (to prevent transmission of zoonotic CL) have been investigated. The high incidence of vertical and venereal transmission in dogs may cause elimination programs to fail in *L. infantum* foci, while long-term asymptomatic carriage of *L. donovani* in humans threatens elimination efforts in the Indian subcontinent.

PROGNOSIS

Most untreated patients with established VL ultimately die. VL has an excellent prognosis with less than a 2% death rate in patients treated soon enough with liposomal amphotericin B. Mortality increases when bleeding (mainly from the digestive tract or lung) or secondary bacterial infection occurs, usually after prolonged untreated evolution or unresponsiveness of VL to first-line agents. Post-therapeutic relapse is very frequent in HIV-coinfected patients with low initial or persistently low CD4$^+$ counts. In immunosuppressed patients, VL contributes to a fatal outcome. A proportion of *L. donovani*–infected patients experience PKDL weeks to years after the initial episode, and this may rarely lead to severe ocular involvement. CL caused by *L. braziliensis* may metastasize to the nose and other mucous membranes with variable frequency in different areas. CL caused by *L. tropica* often relapses (recidivans CL). A small proportion of patients infected with *L. amazonensis* and *L. aethiopica* experience diffuse CL. Even when treated, many CL lesions leave disfiguring, hypotrophic, hypopigmented, hyperpigmented scars, and stigmatization.

Grade A References

A1. Khalil EA, Weldegebreal T, Younis BM, et al. Safety and efficacy of single dose versus multiple doses of AmBisome for treatment of visceral leishmaniasis in eastern Africa: a randomised trial. *PLoS Negl Trop Dis.* 2014;8:1-9.

A2. Sundar S, Chakravarty J, Agarwal D, et al. Single-dose liposomal amphotericin B for visceral leishmaniasis in India. *N Engl J Med.* 2010;362:504-512.

A3. Diro E, Blesson S, Edwards T, et al. A randomized trial of AmBisome monotherapy and AmBisome and miltefosine combination to treat visceral leishmaniasis in HIV co-infected patients in Ethiopia. *PLoS Negl Trop Dis.* 2019;13:1-19.

A4. Saghafipour A, Mozaffari E, Rezaei F. The evaluation of intralesional glucantime and cryotherapy plus intralesional glucantime therapeutic efficacy on zoonotic cutaneous leishmaniasis: a randomized clinical trial. *J Clin Pediatr.* 2017;5:6689-6697.

A5. Ben Salah A, Ben Messaoud N, Guedri E, et al. Topical paromomycin with or without gentamicin for cutaneous leishmaniasis. *N Engl J Med.* 2013;368:524-532.

A6. Soto J, Soto P, Ajata A, et al. Topical 15% paromomycin-aquaphilic for Bolivian *Leishmania braziliensis* cutaneous leishmaniasis: a randomized, placebo-controlled trial. *Clin Infect Dis.* 2019;68:844-849.

A7. Galvão EL, Rabello A, Cota GF. Efficacy of azole therapy for tegumentary leishmaniasis: a systematic review and meta-analysis. *PLoS ONE.* 2017;12:1-24.

A8. Chrusciak-Talhari A, Dietze R, Chrusciak Talhari C, et al. Randomized controlled clinical trial to access efficacy and safety of miltefosine in the treatment of cutaneous leishmaniasis caused by *Leishmania (Viannia) guyanensis* in Manaus, Brazil. *Am J Trop Med Hyg.* 2011;84:255-260.

A9. Gadelha EPN, Ramasawmy R, da Costa Oliveira B, et al. An open label randomized clinical trial comparing the safety and effectiveness of one, two or three weekly pentamidine isethionate doses (seven milligrams per kilogram) in the treatment of cutaneous leishmaniasis in the Amazon Region. *PLoS Negl Trop Dis.* 2018;12:1-13.

GENERAL REFERENCES

For the General References and other additional features, please visit Expert Consult at https://expertconsult.inkling.com.

328

TOXOPLASMOSIS

JOSÉ G. MONTOYA

DEFINITION

Toxoplasma gondii is a protozoan parasite that infects most species of warm-blooded animals, including humans, and can cause toxoplasmosis. The term *toxoplasmosis* is reserved for the disease, when clinical manifestations are present, whereas *Toxoplasma infection* is preferred for the asymptomatic presence of the parasite. Toxoplasmosis may result in significant morbidity and mortality of the fetus, newborn, and immunocompromised patient. However, toxoplasmosis can also manifest in immunocompetent patients as chorioretinitis, lymphadenopathy, pneumonia, brain abscesses, myositis, myocarditis, and hepatitis. In animal models and epidemiological studies in humans, *Toxoplasma* infection has been associated with behavioral changes, mental illness, and neurocognitive impairment, although compelling, conclusive evidence for these associations has not yet been produced.

A more aggressive form of congenital and adult toxoplasmosis appears to occur in certain geographic locales in Latin America, where pneumonia, fever of

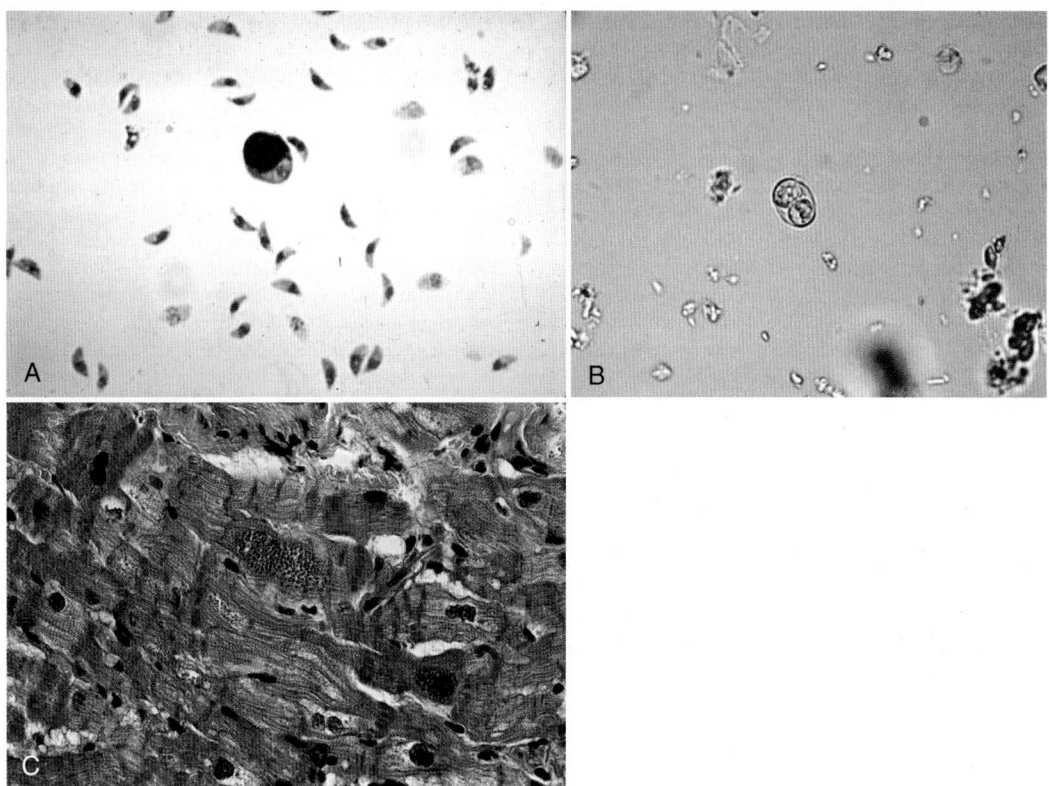

FIGURE 328-1. *Toxoplasma gondii* exists in nature primarily in three forms. **A,** Tachyzoites are bow shaped, measure 2 to 3 μm wide and 5 to 7 μm long, and can be stained with Wright-Giemsa stain. **B,** Oocysts isolated from cat's feces are subspherical to spherical and measure 10 × 12 μm in diameter. **C,** Tissue cyst observed in human myocardial tissue stained with hematoxylin and eosin. Tissue cysts vary in shape and size and may reach more than 100 μm.

unknown origin, brain abscesses, and death have been reported in HIV-negative and otherwise immunocompetent individuals. Recent epidemiologic studies have established the role of novel risk factors for the acquisition of the acute infection, including the ingestion of untreated water, oysters, mussels, or clams.

The Pathogen

T. gondii is an intracellular parasite with a high capacity for host cell invasion due to a motile invasive form with capacity for rapid replication (tachyzoite or trophozoite) that is equipped with an evolutionarily unique apical complex and a mechanism of actin-based gliding motility.[1] The sexual cycle of the parasite only takes place in the small intestine of animals belonging to the feline family, the definitive host. The asexual cycle takes place in tissues and cells of its intermediate hosts (e.g., humans).

In nature, the parasite exists in several forms, including the tachyzoite (Fig. 328-1A), the oocyst that contains sporozoites (Fig. 328-1B), the tissue cyst that contains bradyzoites (Fig. 328-1C). The tachyzoite is the rapidly proliferating form of the parasite responsible for the clinical manifestations of toxoplasmosis observed in the setting of the acute infection or reactivation of a latent infection. The tissue cyst is the slower metabolic form of the parasite responsible for chronic infection and for its transmission through meat consumption in humans and animals. It has been thought that tissue cysts persist in tissues for the life of the host and cannot be eradicated by currently available drugs, but the notion of persistence of the parasite for the life of the host has been recently challenged.[3,4] Tissue cysts vary in shape and size from younger ones that contain only a few bradyzoites to older tissue cysts that may contain several thousand bradyzoites and may reach more than 100 μm in size. The central nervous system (CNS), eye, and skeletal, smooth, and heart muscles appear to be the most common sites of tissue cyst formation (i.e., latent infection). Oocysts are primarily responsible for the worldwide and large-scale spread of the parasite among different populations of other animals and humans. Domestic and feral animals belonging to the Felidae family shed oocysts after they ingest any of the infectious forms of the parasite: tachyzoites, tissue cysts, and oocysts. As many as 10 million oocysts may be shed in the feces of an infected animal in a single day for periods varying from 7 to 20 days. Oocysts may remain viable for as long as 18 months in moist soil; this results in an environmental reservoir from which incidental hosts may be infected.

EPIDEMIOLOGY

The prevalence of *T. gondii* infection varies significantly according to geographic locale and the socioeconomic status of the population. It can be as low as 7% in England and as high as 78% in Brazil. Seroprevalence increases with age because of increasing length of exposure with age, and it is inversely associated with socioeconomic status because of the strong influence of hygienic and alimentary habits in the transmission of the parasite. The overall age-adjusted seroprevalence of *T. gondii* infection in the United States has been recently reported at 11%, but it may be higher in certain geographic areas, ethnic, and socioeconomic groups. The seroprevalence of the parasite has declined during the past 30 years in the United States and several other countries[5] but appears to be stable or increasing in certain geographic locales, such as in the tropics (e.g., Latin America).

Humans and nonfelid animals are incidental hosts and become infected primarily by the ingestion of infected meat containing tissue cysts or of contaminated food, water, or soil material containing oocysts. They can also become infected during gestation by vertical transmission of the parasite from the mother to her offspring. In addition, humans can become infected through organ transplantation and, more rarely, in the setting of laboratory accidents. Ingestion of raw or undercooked meat contaminated with tissue cysts, untreated water, food, or soil contaminated with oocysts are the major routes of infection of humans with the parasite. Untreated water has been found to be the source of large epidemics of toxoplasmosis in Canada and Brazil.

The main risk factors for *T. gondii* infection in the United States include eating raw ground beef, rare lamb; eating locally produced cured, dried, or smoked meat; eating raw oysters, clams, or mussels; working with meat; drinking unpasteurized goat's milk; and having three or more domestic kittens. Untreated water as a potential vehicle for the transmission of *T. gondii* has been established in several large epidemiologic studies and was found to have a trend toward increased risk for acute infection in the United States.

In up to 50% of individuals acutely infected with *T. gondii,* it is not possible to identify the presence of a known risk factor for their acute infection. Thus, attempting to establish whether a patient is at risk for toxoplasmosis solely on the basis of the epidemiologic history is a futile task. The possibility of toxoplasmosis should not be excluded from the differential diagnosis of patients presenting with syndromes suggestive of the disease solely on the basis of a negative epidemiological history.

The seroprevalence of *T. gondii* infection in immunocompromised patients reflects the seroprevalence of the particular population from which they come. Latent *T. gondii* infection can reactivate in these patients, particularly in those with the acquired immunodeficiency syndrome (AIDS) and in hematopoietic stem cell, kidney, heart, and liver transplant recipients. In these patients, it is important to establish whether they have been infected with the parasite before severe immunosuppression ensues or their transplant procedure because serologic testing in severe immunosuppression or after transplantation may be unreliable. Approximately 30% of AIDS patients who are infected with *T. gondii* will develop toxoplasmosis by reactivation of their chronic infection if their CD4 count falls below 200 cells/μL and they are not taking anti-*Toxoplasma* primary prophylaxis. The advent of highly active antiretroviral therapy, in addition to the use of primary anti-*Toxoplasma* prophylaxis, has clearly contributed to the decline in the incidence of toxoplasmosis in AIDS patients. Among hematopoietic stem cell transplant (HSCT) patients, those recipients who are *Toxoplasma* seropositive before allogeneic transplantation and then develop graft-versus-host disease have the highest risk for reactivation.

For solid organ transplants, the highest risk for toxoplasmosis is observed when an allograft from a *Toxoplasma*-seropositive donor (D⁺) is transplanted into a seronegative recipient (R⁻). In D⁺/R⁻ patients, there is a 25% risk for development of potentially life-threatening toxoplasmosis if effective anti-*Toxoplasma* prophylaxis is not instituted. It is highly advised that the *Toxoplasma* serologic status of the donor and the recipient be established before transplantation. Serologic test results are less reliable in the post-transplantation period, and they may significantly vary without any clinical relevance.

Transmission of *T. gondii* to the fetus can occur during pregnancy when a woman acquires her primary infection during gestation. The incidence of seroconversion for pregnant women in the United States has been estimated at 0.27%. The overall rate of transmission of the parasite (prevalence of congenital toxoplasmosis) in seroconverting women has been estimated between 50 and 60% before spiramycin was instituted as an attempt to decrease vertical transmission and 25 to 30% thereafter. The transmission rate increases with the gestational age at which maternal infection is acquired. In women who have been treated for toxoplasmosis during gestation, it can be as low as 4.5% during the first trimester, 31.7% during the second trimester, and as high as 63% during the third trimester. The likelihood of severe disease is inversely proportional to the gestational age at which maternal infection was acquired. Although objective data are lacking on the prevalence of congenital toxoplasmosis in the United States, it has been estimated that among the approximately 4.0 million live births per year, congenital *T. gondii* infection occurs in 400 to 5000 newborns. The global annual incidence of congenital toxoplasmosis[6] has been estimated to be 190,100 cases. This is equivalent to a burden of 1.2 million disability-adjusted life years. Particularly high burdens are seen in South America and in some Middle Eastern and low-income countries. Toxoplasmosis also causes significant morbidity and mortality in the United States.[7]

PATHOBIOLOGY

Pathogenesis

After oral infection with tissue cysts (e.g., contaminated meat) or oocysts (e.g., contaminated soil, water, or food), the wall of both infectious forms is disrupted by the digestive juices of the gastrointestinal tract. Bradyzoites (from cysts) and sporozoites (from oocysts) are released and converted to the rapidly replicating tachyzoite form. Tachyzoites have the capacity to infect contiguous cells or distant tissues by hematogenous and lymphatic spread. Tachyzoites appear to actively and rapidly migrate across epithelial cells and may traffic to distant sites while they are extracellular (acute infection) or within infected immune cells subverted by the parasite to facilitate its own spread (i.e. Trojan horse hypothesis).[8] The formation of the parasite vacuole within infected cells appears to be an important mechanism for *Toxoplasma* survival and subversion.[9] The histologic hallmark of tachyzoites is necrosis surrounded by inflammation.

In immunocompetent individuals, the immune system controls the proliferation of the tachyzoite and induces its conversion to bradyzoites, facilitating the final formation of tissue cysts (chronic infection). Tissue cysts persist for the life of most infected individuals, and *T. gondii* can be isolated from tissues of individuals who have died from causes other than toxoplasmosis.

Pathology

Most of the data on the pathology of toxoplasmosis come from studies of congenitally infected babies and immunosuppressed patients. CNS lesions of patients with toxoplasmosis are characterized by significant necrosis and surrounding inflammation. In congenitally infected cases, necrotic areas may calcify and lead to typical radiographic findings suggestive but not diagnostic of toxoplasmosis. Hydrocephalus may result from obstruction of the aqueduct of Sylvius or foramen of Monro by very high protein concentrations (e.g. >1000 mg/dL). Tachyzoites and tissue cysts may be visualized near necrotic foci, near or in glial nodules, in perivascular regions, and in cerebral tissue uninvolved by inflammatory changes.

Formation of multiple brain abscesses is relatively common in patients with AIDS. In the areas around the abscesses, edema, vasculitis, hemorrhage, and cerebral infarction secondary to vascular involvement may also be present. Important associated features in toxoplasmic encephalitis are arteritis, perivascular cuffing, and astrocytosis. A "diffuse form" of toxoplasmic encephalitis has been described with histopathologic findings of widespread microglial nodules without abscess formation in the gray matter of the cerebrum, cerebellum, and brain stem.

Pulmonary involvement by *T. gondii* in the immunodeficient patient can lead to interstitial pneumonitis, necrotizing pneumonitis, consolidation, pleural effusion or empyema, or all of these. Chorioretinitis in AIDS patients is characterized by segmental panophthalmitis and areas of coagulative necrosis associated with tissue cysts and tachyzoites.

Toxoplasmic lymphadenitis in immunocompetent individuals may result in patterns of findings that are often diagnostic of the disease: a reactive follicular hyperplasia; irregular clusters of epithelioid histiocytes encroaching on and blurring the margins of the germinal centers; and focal distention of sinuses with monocytoid cells.

CLINICAL MANIFESTATIONS

Toxoplasmosis should be entertained in the differential diagnosis of several clinical syndromes in immunocompetent, unborn, newborn, infant, pediatric, adult, and immunocompromised patients (Table 328-1). Symptoms result from the primary infection or reactivation of the parasite due to T-cell-mediated or severe B-cell-mediated immunodeficiency. Primary infection can be asymptomatic in a significant number of individuals, and conventional risk factors for the acute infection may not be present in a particular patient. Thus, the possibility of acute toxoplasmosis or *T. gondii* infection should not be ruled out because of the absence of epidemiologic risk factors (e.g., exposure to cats or undercooked meat) or symptoms in a given patient. For this reason, if the goal is to detect each case of primary *T. gondii* infection in a population of patients (e.g., pregnant women), only systematic and universal screening methods can achieve such an objective; testing of only symptomatic patients or those with conventional epidemiologic risk factors will miss a significant number of acute cases.

Severity of toxoplasmosis due to primary infection or reactivation in a given patient or population may be influenced by the infecting strain, size of the inoculum, infectious form (e.g., oocyst vs. cyst), genetics of the host (e.g., presence of HLA-DQ3), or net state of immunosuppression. Patients infected in certain geographic locales (e.g., South America) have more aggressive clinical presentations, including a more severe primary infection and disease due to reactivation. These observations need to be kept in mind on seeing ill travelers returning from those endemic areas or patients who were born in those areas and in whom toxoplasmosis by reactivation has been included in their differential diagnosis.

Lymphadenopathy due to toxoplasmosis may be completely asymptomatic or be accompanied by other symptoms, such as fever (temperature as high as 104° F), headache, general malaise, and fatigue. It can be localized or generalized. A solitary, occipital, and painlessly enlarged lymph node can be the sole manifestation of toxoplasmosis in a child, pregnant woman, or adult. However, more generalized cervical, axillary, and abdominal lymphadenopathy has also been reported. Lymph nodes are usually 1 to 3 cm in size, nonsuppurative, and nontender on palpation. They usually regress within 12 weeks, but a mild relapse of the lymphadenopathy has been observed between months 3 and 6. Recurrence of toxoplasmic lymphadenopathy beyond the sixth month is extremely rare.

Ocular disease due to *T. gondii* can be asymptomatic or symptomatic and can be the result of congenital or postnatally acquired infection.[10] In both settings (congenitally and postnatally acquired), toxoplasmic chorioretinitis can be discovered at the time of the diagnosis of the infection or as a reactivation of the subsequent latent infection months to years later. Up to 17% of patients acutely infected with the parasite in Brazil and in a Canadian outbreak of toxoplasmosis presented with concurrent symptomatic toxoplasmic chorioretinitis at the time their acute infection was diagnosed. Similar cases have

TABLE 328-1	CLINICAL MANIFESTATIONS OF TOXOPLASMOSIS IN HUMANS
CLINICAL CATEGORIES	**CLINICAL MANIFESTATIONS AND SYNDROMES**
Primary infection	
Immunocompetent individuals and pregnant women	Most patients are asymptomatic. However, in ≈10% of patients, the following symptoms or syndromes, alone or in various combinations, have been reported: fever, lymphadenopathy, headache, myalgias, arthralgias, sore throat, stiff neck, nausea, abdominal pain, anorexia, rash, confusion, earache, eye pain, general malaise, fatigue.
Chorioretinitis resulting in blurred vision, eye pain, decreased visual acuity, floaters, scotoma, photophobia, or epiphora
Hepatitis; myositis; myocarditis
Disseminated disease, pneumonia, brain abscesses, and even death have been observed in immunocompetent individuals infected with atypical strains of *Toxoplasma gondii* (e.g., in Latin America).
Congenital toxoplasmosis	
Fetus	Ultrasound study can be normal or reveal hydrocephalus, brain or hepatic calcifications, splenomegaly, ascites, pericarditis. Fetal death can also result from overwhelming infection.
Newborn	Newborn can be entirely normal, have a nonspecific illness, or have abnormal findings on physical examination including chorioretinitis, strabismus, blindness, seizures, encephalitis, abnormal cephalic perimeter (microcephaly or hydrocephalus), psychomotor or mental retardation, hepatosplenomegaly, pneumonitis, diarrhea, hypothermia, jaundice, petechiae, rash. Intracranial calcifications can be present in brain imaging studies. Newborns can also die as a result of overwhelming infection.
Children and adults	Children can continue to suffer the chronic sequelae of the congenital disease. However, children may be born apparently normal and become symptomatic for the first time during childhood, adolescence, or adulthood, primarily in the form of reactivation of congenitally acquired chorioretinitis.
Chronic infection	Asymptomatic. However, some investigators have proposed a role of chronic infection in individuals with schizophrenia, bipolar disease, and behavioral issues including a higher incidence of motor vehicle accidents.
Chorioretinitis can occur as a reactivation of congenital or postnatally acquired disease in otherwise immunocompetent individuals.
Reactivation of chronic infection in immunocompromised patients	Multiple brain abscesses, diffuse encephalitis, seizures, chorioretinitis, fever of unknown origin, pneumonia, myocarditis, hepatosplenomegaly, lymphadenopathy, rash

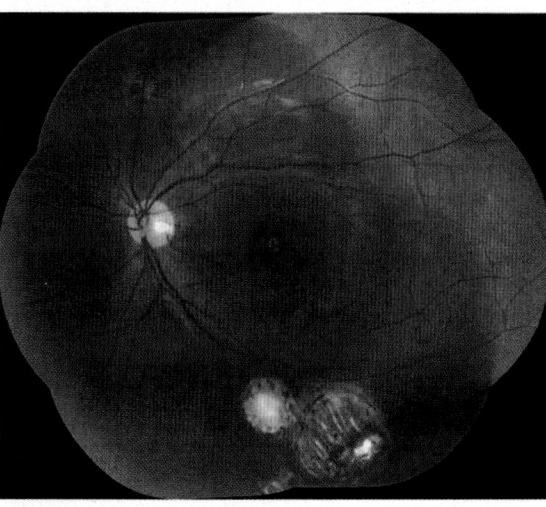

FIGURE 328-2. The morphology of the retinal lesions on funduscopic examination believed to be characteristic of toxoplasmic retinochoroiditis. An active whitish infiltrate is usually attached to the darkly pigmented border of an older scar.

Congenital disease can be asymptomatic in the fetus, newborn, child, or adult. However, most of the infected offspring will eventually develop signs and symptoms of toxoplasmosis (see Table 328-1). The classic triad of chorioretinitis, hydrocephalus (Fig. 328-3A and B), and brain calcifications is highly suggestive of toxoplasmosis and is primarily seen in babies whose mothers have not been treated against the parasite during gestation. Eye examination by an experienced pediatric ophthalmologist may reveal active or inactive toxoplasmic chorioretinitis. New lesions have been reported in up to 30% of congenitally infected children observed up until 11 years of age when their mothers have been treated but in up to 70% when their mothers have not.

Chronic infection is believed to be asymptomatic. However, several studies have recently suggested the possibility that chronic infection may play a role in the predisposition of infected individuals to have a higher frequency of traffic accidents, mental illness (e.g. schizophrenia, bipolar disease), and behavioral abnormalities. Neurocognitive impairment has been associated with latent *T. gondii* infection in HIV-positive patients whose HIV infection has been successfully controlled with antiretroviral therapy.[11]

Overt reactivation of the chronic infection is usually observed in patients with significant impairment of T-cell-mediated immunity or severe impairment of B-cell-mediated immunity. Toxoplasmosis by reactivation can cause brain abscesses, diffuse encephalitis, seizures, chorioretinitis, fever of unknown origin, pneumonia, myocarditis, hepatosplenomegaly, lymphadenopathy, and rash. Although multiple brain abscesses (Fig. 328-3C) are commonly described in patients with toxoplasmic encephalitis, diffuse encephalitis without space-occupying lesions by magnetic resonance imaging has been reported with a very high mortality. Fever with pneumonia can be the sole manifestation of toxoplasmosis in immunocompromised patients, including hematopoietic stem cell transplant (HSCT) and solid organ transplant recipients. Toxoplasmic pneumonitis can be manifested by cough, dyspnea, hypoxia, and diffuse bilateral or localized infiltrates. Most patients with toxoplasmic pneumonia have been reported to have bilateral ground-glass opacities that can be confused with *Pneumocystis* pneumonia, viral etiologies, atypical pneumonia, or strongyloidiasis. Fever alone has frequently been described in patients with allogeneic HSCT and liver transplant patients. Reactivation in heart tissue causing congestive heart failure, arrhythmias, and pericarditis has been described.

DIAGNOSIS

Laboratory methods for the diagnosis of *T. gondii* infection and toxoplasmosis include serologic tests, polymerase chain reaction (PCR), microscopic examination of tissue and body fluids, and attempts to isolate the parasite (Table 328-2).[12]

The first step is to establish whether the patient has never been infected with *Toxoplasma* or has an acute or latent *T. gondii* infection; this can be accomplished by serologic testing. Serologic tests can determine this infection status regardless of the presence or absence of symptoms. Available serologic tools include methods to detect *T. gondii*–specific immunoglobulin G (IgG)-, IgM-, IgA-, IgE-, and IgG-based avidity and differential agglutination (AC/HS).

been described in Europe and the United States. *T. gondii* strain type appears to be a contributing factor determining severity and recurrence of ocular toxoplasmosis. Symptomatic ocular disease primarily consists of a retinochoroiditis that can result in blurred vision, eye pain, decreased visual acuity, floaters, scotoma, photophobia, or epiphora. The morphology of the retinal lesions on funduscopic examination is thought to be characteristic of toxoplasmosis. An active whitish infiltrate is usually attached to the darkly pigmented border of an older scar (Fig. 328-2). However, retinal lesions tend to be less typical in older or immunocompromised patients.

Other less common but well-documented syndromes have been associated with the acute infection, including hepatitis, myositis, myocarditis, and skin lesions. More aggressive disease, including pneumonia, brain abscesses, and death, has been observed in immunocompetent patients in Latin America.

Primary infection can be observed in solid organ transplant patients when an allograft from a seropositive donor is transplanted into a seronegative recipient (D^+/R^-). Disseminated and localized toxoplasmosis has been reported in this setting, including myocarditis, pneumonia, fever of unknown origin, and encephalitis.

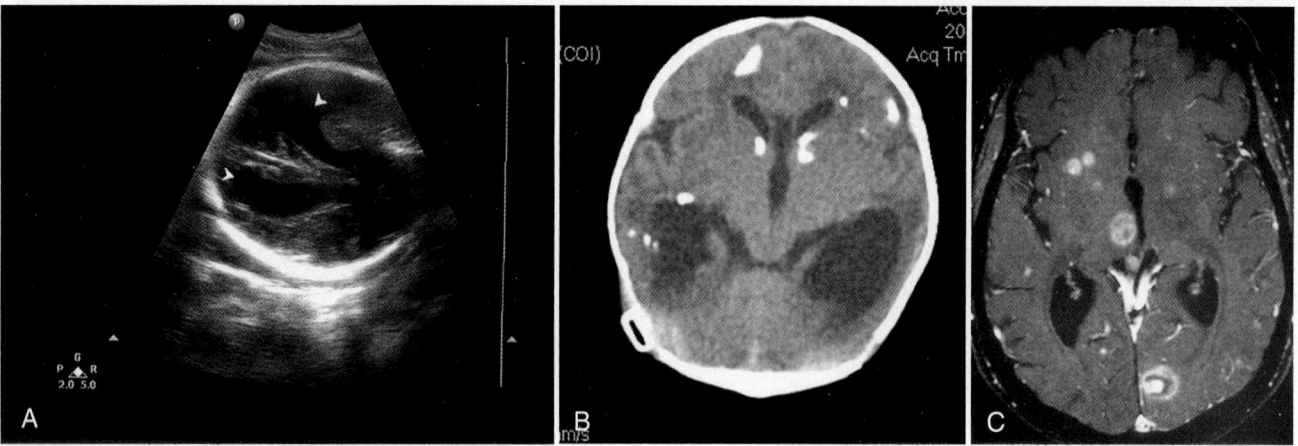

FIGURE 328-3. Radiologic manifestations of central nervous system toxoplasmosis. **A,** Fetal ultrasound of a fetus congenitally infected with *Toxoplasma gondii* in the United States reveals hydrocephalus. **B,** Computed tomography scan of the brain of a newborn congenitally infected with *T. gondii* in the United States reveals hydrocephalus and calcifications. **C,** Magnetic resonance image of the brain of an AIDS patient revealing multiple ring-enhancing brain lesions.

TABLE 328-2 LABORATORY METHODS FOR THE DIAGNOSIS OF *TOXOPLASMA GONDII* INFECTION AND TOXOPLASMOSIS* IN HUMANS

METHOD	CLINICAL INTERPRETATION
Serologic tests	
IgG	A positive test result establishes that the patient has been infected with *T. gondii*. However, a negative test result can be seen in patients infected within 4 weeks before serum sampling or in patients unable to produce IgG (e.g., immunocompromised hosts).
IgM	A positive test result suggests but is not necessarily diagnostic of an acute infection.
	Sera with positive IgM test results should be sent to a reference laboratory for confirmatory testing that includes a more specific IgM assay and additional tests, including avidity, acetone (AC)-fixed versus formalin (HS)-fixed (AC/HS) differential agglutination test of tachyzoites, and IgA and IgE.† Positive IgM test results can be seen in chronically infected patients because of persistence of the IgM response or false-positive results observed in certain commercial kits.
Confirmatory testing for positive IgM test results	IgG avidity test; differential agglutination (AC/HS); IgA, IgE performed at a reference laboratory.† At PAMF-TSL, a high IgG avidity test result‡ or a nonacute AC/HS test result indicates that the patient has been infected for more than 4 mo (avidity) or 12 mo (AC/HS).
Polymerase chain reaction (PCR)	The B1 gene and the 529-bp repetitive element are the most commonly used gene targets for amplification.
	PCR test can be performed in any body fluid, including amniotic fluid, peripheral blood, cerebrospinal fluid, bronchoalveolar lavage fluid, vitreous fluid, aqueous humor, peritoneal fluid, pleural fluid, ascitic fluid, and urine. PCR can also be performed in any tissue.
	A positive test result in any body fluid establishes that the patient has either acute or reactivated toxoplasmosis. However, a positive PCR test result in tissue is more difficult to interpret because it does not differentiate symptomatic toxoplasmosis from a latent infection.
	Although DNA extraction is more cumbersome, it can be attempted in paraffin-embedded tissue.
Direct visualization of the parasite	Identification of tachyzoites in any body fluid or tissue is diagnostic of toxoplasmosis due to acute infection or reactivation of a chronic infection. Tachyzoites can be identified by hematoxylin and eosin or cytologic studies but are better visualized with Wright-Giemsa and immunoperoxidase stains.
	Identification of cysts by hematoxylin and eosin or immunoperoxidase stains confirms the presence of *T. gondii* in the host but does not necessarily establish that the patient has toxoplasmosis.
	However, a strong inflammatory response surrounding the cysts is highly suggestive of toxoplasmosis, possibly explaining the patient's symptoms.
Attempts to isolate the parasite	A positive isolation study in any body fluid establishes the diagnosis of toxoplasmosis.
	Isolation of *T. gondii* in cell cultures or peritoneal cavity of mice can be attempted at reference laboratories. These studies can be important in trying to establish a correlation between the genetics of the parasite and its clinical manifestations.
Histology of the lymph node	Classic histologic triad is considered diagnostic: follicular hyperplasia, epithelioid histiocytes impinging on the margins of the germinal centers, and monocytoid cells focally distending sinus walls.

*T. gondii infection = asymptomatic presence of the parasite. Toxoplasmosis = active symptoms and signs are present.
†For example, Palo Alto Medical Foundation Toxoplasma Serology Laboratory (PAMF-TSL), Palo Alto, Calif; www.pamf.org/serology; 650-853-4828; toxolab@pamf.org.
‡The window of exclusion for acute infection varies for different avidity kits (usually between 3 and 5 months).

With the use of commercial kits for the detection of IgG and IgM, most hospital-based or commercial laboratories can reliably diagnose the absence of *T. gondii* infection (negative IgG/negative IgM) and the presence of chronic infection (positive IgG/negative IgM). However, the diagnosis of acute infection is more challenging. A positive IgM test result is observed during the acute infection, but it may remain positive for months to years in certain individuals without any apparent clinical relevance. In addition, commercial IgM kits have been designed to be extremely sensitive so that an acute infection will be rarely missed; as a consequence, their specificity is somewhat sacrificed. Of patients who are found to be IgM positive at hospital-based or commercial laboratories, 78% are found to be chronically infected when their serum is tested at the national reference laboratory for the study and diagnosis of toxoplasmosis in the United States (Palo Alto Medical Foundation Toxoplasma Serology Laboratory [PAMF-TSL], Palo Alto, Calif; www.pamf.org/serology; 650-853-4828; toxolab@pamf.org).[13] At PAMF-TSL, a battery of confirmatory tests (avidity, differential agglutination, IgA, IgE) are performed in addition to the "gold standard" dye test for IgG and the "double" sandwich capture enzyme-linked immunosorbent assay for IgM for confirmatory testing of positive IgM test results obtained at hospital-based or commercial laboratories. These tests are used in various combinations, depending on the clinical scenario of each patient and the questions of the treating physician. For an appropriate interpretation of the serologic test results obtained at PAMF-TSL, it is also crucial to have relevant clinical information available for the medical consultant. (For instance, low positive IgG and positive IgM test results with a high IgG avidity test result will mean no risk for congenital toxoplasmosis for a 16-week pregnant woman, but the same results can be highly supportive of the diagnosis of toxoplasmic encephalitis for an AIDS patient with multiple brain lesions.) At PAMF-TSL, three interpretations can be given to final serologic test results: (1) acute, results are consistent with a recently acquired infection; (2) chronic, consistent with an infection acquired in the distant past; and (3) equivocal, cannot exclude a recently acquired infection—an earlier or subsequent sample is required to attempt to establish whether the infection is acute or chronic. For serologic test results consistent with an acute infection, an attempt is made by the medical consultants at PAMF-TSL to establish the approximate date that the infection was acquired.

The definitive diagnosis of toxoplasmosis (due to primary infection or reactivation of a chronic infection) requires the identification of tachyzoites in tissues or body fluids or the amplification of parasite DNA in any body fluid (see Table 328-2). Tachyzoites can be visualized in histologic sections stained with hematoxylin and eosin or in cytologic preparations without any specific staining, but they are better visualized with Wright-Giemsa (see Fig. 328-1A) and *T. gondii*–specific immunoperoxidase stains. Real-time PCR (in any body fluid including cerebrospinal) has become a useful method for the diagnosis of toxoplasmosis in immunocompromised patients and for the prenatal diagnosis of congenital toxoplasmosis (in amniotic fluid). Isolation of the parasite in any body fluid is also diagnostic of toxoplasmosis and can be attempted at reference laboratories. The diagnosis of toxoplasmosis can be indirectly supported by the use of serologic tools, demonstration of cysts in tissues (see Fig. 328-1C) surrounded by an inflammatory response, and attempts to isolate the parasite (see Table 328-2).

Immunocompetent Patients, Pregnant Women, and Patients with Lymphadenopathy

The first diagnostic goal in these patients is to establish whether they have ever been infected with *T. gondii*. If *T. gondii*–specific IgG and IgM test results are negative, the possibility that the patient's symptoms are due to the parasite can be ruled out. During pregnancy, these results confirm that the mother has not been exposed to *T. gondii* but that she is at risk, if exposed, to acquire the primary infection during pregnancy and therefore can potentially transmit *T. gondii* to her offspring. In attempting to determine whether the patient is infected with *T. gondii*, it is important to perform both IgG and IgM tests because during the first 4 weeks of the acute infection, the IgG can still be negative while the IgM will be positive. In these cases, seroconversion can be diagnosed by having a new positive IgG test result in a subsequent serum sample. In rare instances, infected patients may be IgG negative because of their incapacity to produce IgG.

If the patient is found to be IgG positive, the next goal is to determine whether the patient is having an acute infection or has been chronically infected (e.g., >6 months). If the IgG titer is low (e.g., a dye test at PAMF-TSL ≤512) and the IgM test result is negative, the patient has essentially been infected for more than 6 months. With these results, a patient whose symptoms or lymphadenopathy had a date of onset within 6 months of serum sampling will be considered unlikely to have toxoplasmosis. For a pregnant woman whose serum was obtained within 6 months of gestation, these results will mean that her infection was acquired before conception and that the risk for congenital toxoplasmosis is essentially zero.

If the patient is found to have a positive IgM test result confirmed to be indicative of a recently acquired infection at a reference laboratory and the onset of symptoms or lymphadenopathy diminishes within the time predicted by the serologic test results for the acquisition of *T. gondii*, the patient will be diagnosed as having acute toxoplasmosis. For a pregnant woman, if the predicted time for when the infection was acquired falls within her gestational age, she will be diagnosed with toxoplasmosis during pregnancy and at risk for transmitting the parasite to her baby.

In patients with lymphadenopathy, the histologic examination of the lymph node tissue obtained by excisional biopsy can be diagnostic or pathognomonic of toxoplasmic lymphadenitis (see earlier under Pathology).

Prenatal and Postnatal Diagnosis of Congenital Toxoplasmosis

After the diagnosis of acute toxoplasmosis or *T. gondii* infection has been confirmed or is highly suspected in the mother, the next step is to attempt to establish whether her offspring has been infected. Consultation with reference centers for the study and diagnosis of congenital toxoplasmosis is highly recommended.

Ultrasound abnormalities can be consistent with or suggestive of congenital toxoplasmosis (see Fig. 328-3A), but they are not diagnostic. The method of choice for the prenatal diagnosis of congenital toxoplasmosis is a PCR in amniotic fluid obtained at 18 weeks of gestation. Attempts to diagnose congenital toxoplasmosis from amniotic fluid obtained before 18 weeks of gestation

should be avoided because the studies reported to date have included only pregnant women whose gestational age was 18 weeks or more. In addition, false-negative results have been reported in women whose amniocentesis was performed before 18 weeks of gestation. The overall sensitivity of the amniotic fluid PCR has been reported between 64 and 92% and is highly dependent of the gestational age at which the mother acquired the infection.

In the newborn, congenital toxoplasmosis can be confirmed by positive *T. gondii*–specific serologic test results or PCR. Samples for serology should be obtained in the peripheral blood of the baby. Cord blood should be avoided because of the high rate of maternal blood contamination. However, there is still a small degree of maternal blood contamination in newborn blood obtained by peripheral venipuncture, during the first 5 days of life for IgM antibodies and the first 10 days of life for IgA antibodies. A positive IgM immunosorbent agglutination assay (after 5 days of life) or IgA enzyme-linked immunosorbent assay (after 10 days) is diagnostic of congenital disease. Congenitally infected babies can be positive for both; positive for either one, but negative for the other test; or negative for both.[14] A positive *T. gondii*–specific IgM in cerebrospinal fluid (CSF) is diagnostic of congenital disease, but testing of the CSF by PCR rather than for IgM is strongly recommended because of the higher sensitivity of the PCR test. The diagnosis can also be made by a positive PCR in peripheral blood, CSF, or urine. The CSF of infected infants may exhibit very high levels of protein (e.g., ≥1000 mg/dL). Cellular response in CSF is characterized by lymphocytosis, and eosinophilia may be present. Brain imaging studies may reveal calcifications or hydrocephalus; computed tomography scan is superior to ultrasound examination in the detection of these CNS abnormalities (see Fig. 328-3B).

Ocular Disease

Serologic and PCR testing can be helpful in the diagnosis of toxoplasmic chorioretinitis. An IgG-negative/IgM-negative patient is unlikely to have ocular disease due to toxoplasmosis. However, patients should be tested at reference laboratories (e.g., PAMF-TSL) because their *T. gondii*–specific IgG can be present but at very low levels such that only a gold standard method like the dye test can detect it. In patients with eye lesions typical of toxoplasmic chorioretinitis (see Fig. 328-2), a positive IgG test result at a relatively low titer (e.g., a dye test at PAMF-TSL ≤512) and a negative IgM test result are diagnostic of ocular disease due to the parasite reactivation. If the serologic test reveals a positive IgM result and confirmatory testing at PAMF-TSL establishes the diagnosis of an acute infection in patients 1 year of age or older, the eye disease is most likely the result of eye involvement in the setting of a recent and postnatally acquired infection.

In patients with atypically appearing lesions or in whom the response to anti-*Toxoplasma* drugs is atypical or absent, a *T. gondii*–specific immune load (aqueous humor) or PCR in ocular fluids (vitreous fluid is preferable to aqueous humor because of probable higher sensitivity, but it is riskier to obtain) should be considered.

Immunocompromised Patients

It appears that acute infection rarely occurs in immunocompromised patients. However, life-threatening disease can occur when the patient's latent infection is reactivated by AIDS, HSCT, solid organ transplantation, or other diseases characterized by severe T-cell or B-cell deficiency.

Toxoplasmosis can also develop when *T. gondii* is transmitted from a seropositive donor to a seronegative recipient through an infected allograft (e.g., heart, liver, kidney). Therefore, to establish the risk for toxoplasmosis and to have a high index of suspicion when patients develop illnesses suggestive of toxoplasmosis, all immunocompromised patients should be tested for *T. gondii*–specific IgG as soon as they have been diagnosed with the underlying disease or it has been established that they will be subsequently immunosuppressed. In addition, serologic testing may not be reliable when immunosuppression is advanced or severe. Post-transplantation serologic test results for IgG antibodies may remain positive or may rise, decrease, or even become negative. Thus, pretransplantation *Toxoplasma* serologic studies are critical for interpretation of subsequent test results and clinical evaluation. Solid organ donors should also be tested for *T. gondii*–specific IgG as their allograft has the potential to transmit the parasite to the transplanted patient (e.g., heart, heart-lung, kidney, kidney-pancreas, liver, liver-pancreas). Toxoplasmosis in solid organ transplant recipients causes substantial morbidity, including disseminated disease, and mortality.

In AIDS patients suspected of having toxoplasmic encephalitis with the presence of multiple brain-occupying and ring-enhancing lesions (see Fig. 328-3C), a CD4 count below 200 cells/μL, and a positive *T. gondii*–specific

IgG, the response to anti-*Toxoplasma*-specific treatment is considered an additional "diagnostic" criterion of toxoplasmic encephalitis. In these patients, invasive diagnostic tests (e.g., lumbar puncture, brain biopsy) are considered unnecessary unless they do not respond to treatment within a 7- to 10-day period. This diagnostic paradigm should not be applied to other populations of immunosuppressed patients (e.g., transplant patients) because their differential diagnosis often includes other pathogens, such as invasive mold infections. In those patients, examination of the CSF by PCR or brain biopsy should be attempted at the outset of the central nervous system illness.

The definitive diagnosis of toxoplasmosis in immunosuppressed patients relies on PCR, direct visualization of the parasite, and attempts for isolation of the organism (see Table 328-2). PCR testing in body fluids is the diagnostic method of choice for immunosuppressed patients at risk for toxoplasmosis who develop unexplained fever (e.g., in whole blood), pneumonia (e.g., in bronchoalveolar lavage fluid), brain lesions (e.g., in CSF), or other compatible syndromes. Theoretically, PCR can be performed in any body fluid or tissue, and laboratories have validated its use in most fluids and some tissues. Attempts to identify the tachyzoite or tissue cyst in tissues by microscopy can be enhanced with the use of the *T. gondii*–specific immunoperoxidase stain. CSF examination by PCR or brain biopsy should be initially considered in AIDS patients who have a low likelihood of having toxoplasmic encephalitis, such as those who have a single lesion by magnetic resonance imaging examination, have tested seronegative for *T. gondii* infection, have a CD4 count of more than 200 cells/μL, or who are not responding to an appropriate anti-*Toxoplasma* regimen.

TREATMENT   Rx

Principles of antiparasitic therapy are discussed in Chapter 323. Treatment of toxoplasmosis is indicated for immunocompetent patients with acute infection in the setting of ongoing fever, myocarditis, myositis, hepatitis, pneumonia, brain lesions or skin lesions, and lymphadenopathy accompanied by severe or persisting symptoms. Treatment is indicated as well for patients with active chorioretinitis due to primary infection or reactivation of a latent infection (Table 328-3). In immunocompetent patients, treatment is prescribed for 3 to 4 weeks or until symptoms have subsided, whichever is longer. For toxoplasmic lymphadenitis, trimethoprim-sulfamethoxazole (TMP-SMZ) (8 mg TMP/40 mg SMZ per kilogram per day divided into two doses for 1 month) increased the cure rate to 65% compared with a 13% resolution rate with placebo.[A1] Treatment is also often recommended for all pregnant women suspected of having or diagnosed with primary infection during gestation (Table 328-4) in an attempt to prevent transmission of the parasite to the fetus (spiramycin) or, if congenital infection has occurred, to start treatment of the fetus in utero (pyrimethamine, sulfadiazine, and folinic acid). During pregnancy, treatment regimens are prescribed for the duration of the gestation. There was a worldwide controversy about the efficacy of spiramycin to decrease the incidence of congenital toxoplasmosis and of pyrimethamine, sulfadiazine, and folinic acid to decrease the frequency of clinical signs in infected offspring. Although no definitive studies ever disproved their efficacy, several epidemiologic studies erroneously concluded that there was no evidence of benefit. However, since 2006, several studies have reported a strong association between prenatal treatment of women infected during gestation (with spiramycin or pyrimethamine, sulfadiazine, and folinic acid) and decreases in the incidence of congenital toxoplasmosis and frequency of clinical signs in infected offspring. Spiramycin is recommended for pregnant women who have been definitively diagnosed to have or are highly suspected of having an acute infection during pregnancy that was acquired before 18 weeks of gestation. Spiramycin should be given throughout pregnancy unless fetal infection is suspected or documented. Fetal infection should be investigated with amniotic fluid PCR at 18 weeks of gestation to see whether *Toxoplasma* DNA is amplified and with monthly follow-up ultrasound examinations. Therapy with pyrimethamine, sulfadiazine, and folinic acid is recommended for pregnant women who have been definitively diagnosed to have or are highly suspected of having an acute infection during pregnancy that was acquired after 18 weeks of gestation, whose amniotic fluid PCR is positive for the presence of *Toxoplasma* DNA, or whose follow-up ultrasound examinations are suggestive of fetal congenital toxoplasmosis in the setting of acute *Toxoplasma* infection during gestation. In addition, newborns and infants diagnosed with or suspected of having congenital toxoplasmosis should also be treated during their first year of life (see Table 328-4).

Treatment at higher doses is urgently indicated for all immunocompromised patients with toxoplasmosis due to reactivation of their latent infection or primary infection acquired by natural exposure to the parasite or by solid organ transplantation (see Table 328-3). If untreated, toxoplasmosis in these patients has a very high rate of morbidity and mortality.

TABLE 328-3	TREATMENT REGIMENS FOR PATIENTS WITH ACUTE OR PRIMARY TOXOPLASMOSIS AND IMMUNOCOMPROMISED PATIENTS WITH TOXOPLASMOSIS DUE TO REACTIVATION*

	IMMUNOCOMPETENT PATIENTS WITH ACUTE INFECTION[†]	IMMUNOCOMPROMISED PATIENTS
Pyrimethamine (PO)	50 mg every 12 hr for 2 days, followed by 25 to 50 mg daily	200 mg loading dose, followed by 50 mg/day (<60 kg) to 75 mg/day (>60 kg)
plus Folinic acid[‡]	10-20 mg daily (during and 1 week after therapy with pyrimethamine) *plus either sulfadiazine or clindamycin or atovaquone as follows:*	10-20 mg daily (up to 50 mg/day; during and 1 week after therapy with pyrimethamine) *plus either sulfadiazine or clindamycin or atovaquone as follows:*
Sulfadiazine (PO) *or*	75 mg/kg (first dose), followed by 50 mg/kg every 12 hr (maximum 4 g/day)	1000 mg (<60 kg) to 1500 mg (>60 kg) every 6 hr
Clindamycin (PO or IV) *or*	300 mg every 6 hr	600 mg every 6 hr (up to 1200 mg every 6 hr)
Atovaquone (PO)	1500 mg orally twice daily	1500 mg orally twice daily
Trimethoprim-sulfamethoxazole (PO or IV)	10 mg/kg/day (trimethoprim component) in two or three doses	10 mg/kg/day (trimethoprim component) in two or three doses (doses as high as 15-20 mg/kg/day have been used)
Pyrimethamine and folinic acid *plus*	Same doses as above	Same doses as above
Clarithromycin (PO) *or*	500 mg every 12 hr	500 mg every 12 hr
Dapsone (PO) *or*	100 mg/day	100 mg/day
Azithromycin (PO)	900 to 1200 mg/day	900 to 1200 mg/day

After the successful use of a combination regimen during the acute or primary therapy phase, the same agents at half-dose are usually used for maintenance or secondary prophylaxis.
*Preferred regimens: pyrimethamine, sulfadiazine, and folinic acid or trimethoprim-sulfamethoxazole. Assistance is available for the diagnosis and management of patients with toxoplasmosis at the Palo Alto Medical Foundation Toxoplasma Serology Laboratory (PAMF-TSL), Palo Alto, Calif; www.pamf.org/serology; 650-853-4828; toxolab@pamf.org.
[†]Particularly in the setting of myocarditis, myositis, hepatitis, pneumonia, brain or skin lesions, and lymphadenopathy accompanied by severe or persisting symptoms. Also indicated for those with active ocular disease due to primary infection or reactivation.
[‡]Folinic acid = leucovorin; folic acid must not be used as a substitute for folinic acid.

PREVENTION
Primary Infection

Because approximately 50% of patients may inadvertently become infected with the parasite without having a recognized risk factor for acute infection, only systematic serologic testing can establish whether a patient has been exposed to *T. gondii*. Thus, each pregnant woman and immunocompromised patient should be screened for *T. gondii*–specific IgG and IgM regardless of their epidemiologic history. Seronegative pregnant women and immunocompromised individuals should be counseled on how to maximize their prevention efforts to avoid infection with *T. gondii*. In addition, seronegative pregnant women should be tested serially during gestation in an attempt to diagnose seroconversion at the earliest time possible. In some countries, such as France, seronegative pregnant women are mandated by law to be tested every month for *T. gondii*–specific IgG and IgM.[15] Women who seroconvert are offered spiramycin (if infected before 18 weeks of gestation) or pyrimethamine, sulfadiazine, and folinic acid (if infected after 18 weeks). Mothers whose amniotic fluid is found to be positive by PCR or those in whom fetal ultrasound study is highly suggestive of congenital toxoplasmosis are offered pyrimethamine, sulfadiazine, and folinic acid. Although infection often occurs in the absence of known risk factors for the acute infection, educational interventions to avoid exposure to the parasite have been shown to be effective in decreasing the incidence of seroconversion during gestation.

TABLE 328-4	TREATMENT REGIMENS FOR PREGNANT WOMEN WHO HAVE LIKELY ACQUIRED *TOXOPLASMA GONDII* INFECTION DURING GESTATION AND INFANTS SUSPECTED OF HAVING OR CONFIRMED TO HAVE CONGENITAL TOXOPLASMOSIS	
	DURING PREGNANCY	**IN CONGENITAL DISEASE**
Spiramycin (oral)	Recommended for pregnant women suspected of having or confirmed to have acquired the infection during gestation and before 18 weeks of gestation. Spiramycin should be administered until delivery in those with negative amniotic fluid PCR test results and normal follow-up ultrasound studies or low suspicion of fetal infection. Spiramycin is not teratogenic, and it is available in the United States only through the Investigational New Drug (IND) process at the Food and Drug Administration (301-796-1400). Prior medical consultation is required.* Dosage: 1 g (3 million units) every 8 hr (for a total of 3 g or 9 million units per day)	Not recommended during pregnancy if the fetus has been documented to be or suspected to have been infected. In the setting of fetal infection, pyrimethamine, sulfadiazine, and folinic acid should be instituted (see below)

Pyrimethamine (oral)
  plus sulfadiazine (oral)
  plus folinic acid[†] (oral)
	Recommended for women ≥18 weeks of gestation in whom it is suspected or confirmed that the acute infection has been acquired at or after 18 weeks of gestation or who have a positive amniotic fluid PCR test result or an abnormal ultrasound study suggestive of congenital toxoplasmosis
	
	Pyrimethamine is teratogenic and should not be used during pregnancy before week 18 (in some centers in Europe, it is used as early as week 14).
	
	Sulfadiazine should not be used alone.
	
	Dosages:
	  Pyrimethamine: 50 mg every 12 hr for 2 days followed by 50 mg daily
	  Sulfadiazine: 75 mg/kg (first dose) followed by 50 mg/kg every 12 hr (maximum 4 g/day)
	  Folinic acid[†] (leucovorin): 10-20 mg daily (during and for 1 week after pyrimethamine therapy)
		Infant (treatment regimen is usually recommended for 1 year):
		  Pyrimethamine: 1 mg/kg every 12 hr for 2 days; followed by 1 mg/kg/day for 2 or 6 months; followed by 1 mg/kg/day every Monday, Wednesday, Friday
		  Sulfadiazine: 50 mg/kg every 12 hr
		  Folinic acid[†] (leucovorin): 10 mg three times weekly
		  Prednisone (if CSF protein ≥1 g/dL or severe chorioretinitis): 0.5 mg/kg every 12 hr (until CSF protein <1 g/dL or resolution of severe chorioretinitis)
		Older children with active disease (usually 1-2 weeks beyond resolution of clinical manifestations):
		  Pyrimethamine: 1 mg/kg every 12 hr (maximum 50 mg) for 2 days followed by 1 mg/kg/day (maximum 25 mg)
		  Sulfadiazine: 75 mg/kg (first dose) followed by 50 mg/kg every 12 hr
		  Folinic acid[†] (leucovorin): 10-20 mg three times weekly
		  Prednisone (severe chorioretinitis):
		    1 mg/kg/day, divided bid, maximum 40 mg/day, rapid taper

*Palo Alto Medical Foundation Toxoplasma Serology Laboratory (PAMF-TSL), Palo Alto, Calif; www.pamf.org/serology; 650-853-4828; toxolab@pamf.org; or U.S. (Chicago) National Collaborative Treatment Trial Study (NCCTS), 773-834-4152.

[†]Folic acid should not be used as a substitute for folinic acid.

CSF = cerebrospinal fluid; PCR = polymerase chain reaction.

The majority of epidemiologic studies worldwide have recognized contaminated and undercooked meat as one of the main risk factors for the transmission of the parasite. This appears to be the case in Europe, North America, and Latin America. Tissue cysts in meat are rendered nonviable by γ-irradiation (0.4 kGy), heating throughout to 67° C, or freezing to −20° C for 48 hours and then thawing.[16] Cured, dried, or smoked meat has been associated with the acute infection and should not be considered *Toxoplasma* free. Soil exposure and soil-related activities have been reported to play a more prominent role in transmission in certain geographic areas, such as Latin America.

In seronegative recipients of a solid organ from a seropositive donor, TMP-SMZ for at least 6 months or pyrimethamine for at least 6 weeks has been reported to be effective in the prevention of primary infection in the newly immunosuppressed patient.

Reactivation of Latent Infection in Immunocompromised Patients and Those with Ocular Disease

Drugs used to prevent reactivation of the latent infection in immunosuppressed hosts include TMP-SMZ (e.g., single strength or 80 mg TMP and 400 mg SMZ, 1 tablet per day) and atovaquone (1500 mg/day). Dapsone-pyrimethamine and sulfadoxine-pyrimethamine have been also reported to be effective, but their use appears to be limited because of potential hematologic toxicity.

Prophylaxis against reactivation of latent infection has been successful in AIDS patients dually infected with HIV and *T. gondii* (*Toxoplasma* IgG seropositive) and whose CD4[+] T-cell counts are below 200 cells/μL. For prophylactic purposes, TMP-SMZ should probably not be used below a minimum dose of 160 mg TMP/800 mg SMZ orally twice a day on a thrice-weekly regimen or 80 mg TMP/400 mg SMZ once a day. In AIDS patients, 100 mg of dapsone plus 50 mg of pyrimethamine orally twice weekly or atovaquone (1500 mg/day) has also been effective in preventing toxoplasmic encephalitis. Findings in these studies have been extrapolated to non-AIDS immunosuppressed patients because of the absence of data in this population of patients.

Toxoplasma-seropositive recipients of an allogeneic HSCT (Chapter 168) who develop graft-versus-host disease represent a unique challenge. Reactivation of toxoplasmosis can be manifested by a nonspecific illness (e.g., fever

or pneumonia) and be life-threatening. The disease is often not recognized. Atovaquone prophylaxis has been proposed as an alternative regimen in these patients, given the potential bone marrow toxicity of TMP-SMZ. Some investigators have proposed a preemptive strategy in which *Toxoplasma*-seropositive patients who receive an allogeneic HSCT are monitored on a routine basis (e.g., weekly for the first 100 days) with *T. gondii* PCR.[17] Those found positive would receive preemptive prophylaxis with TMP-SMZ or atovaquone.

Discontinuation of prophylaxis against toxoplasmic encephalitis has proved safe in AIDS patients receiving highly active antiretroviral therapy who demonstrate an increase in their CD4[+] T-cell counts to at least 200 cells/μL and whose viral load has been undetectable for at least 6 months.

In patients with ocular toxoplasmosis who experience frequent relapses (e.g., more than two episodes per year), 80 mg TMP/400 mg SMZ daily for at least 1 year has been shown to be effective in the prevention of their recurrences.[A2]

PROGNOSIS

The primary infection has a wide spectrum of manifestations in humans, from asymptomatic in most individuals to pneumonia or life-threatening disease if it is acquired in certain areas of the world. Primary infection can also be fatal in the fetus and in immunocompromised individuals. Early diagnosis and treatment can make a significant difference in the prognosis of these patients.

It is not clear at this time whether chronic infection in immunocompetent individuals is clinically irrelevant. Several investigators have proposed that latent infection with the parasite may play a significant role in mental illness (e.g., schizophrenia) or in the propensity of the infected individual to incur motor vehicle crashes. Immunocompetent patients can reactivate chronic infection in their retina, and the prognosis is influenced by the proximity of the lesions to the macula, involvement of one or both eyes, and number of relapses. It is believed that treatment can slow the progression of these lesions and expedite their healing.

Reactivation of latent infection in immunosuppressed individuals with significant defects in their T-cell-mediated or B-cell-mediated immunity, if untreated, is 100% fatal. Even when treated in an intensive care unit, disseminated toxoplasmosis in immunocompromised patients has a mortality rate of about 80%.

Grade A References

A1. Alavi SM, Alavi L. Treatment of toxoplasmic lymphadenitis with co-trimoxazole: double-blind, randomized clinical trial. *Int J Infect Dis.* 2010;3:e67-e69.
A2. Felix JP, Lira RP, Zacchia RS, et al. Trimethoprim-sulfamethoxazole versus placebo to reduce the risk of recurrences of *Toxoplasma gondii* retinochoroiditis: randomized controlled clinical trial. *Am J Ophthalmol.* 2014;157:762-766.

GENERAL REFERENCES

For the General References and other additional features, please visit Expert Consult at https://expertconsult.inkling.com.

329

CRYPTOSPORIDIOSIS

CIRLE A. WARREN AND ALDO A.M. LIMA

DEFINITION

Cryptosporidiosis is the disease in humans and animals caused by protozoal parasites of the genus *Cryptosporidium* (Apicomplexa).[1] *Cryptosporidium* spp are major waterborne parasites worldwide, and more than 14 species have been documented to infect humans.[2] Two named species, *C. hominis* and *C. parvum* "bovine genotype" (*C. pestis*), are considered of major public health significance. Four (*C. cuniculus, C. meleagridis, C. viatorum,* and *C. felis*) and eight (*C. parvum, C. fayeri, C. canis, C. suis, C. ubiquitum, C. scrofarum, C. muris,* and *C. andersoni*) of 14 named species are considered of moderate and minor public health significance, respectively. There are nine species of 30 that are shared between humans and cattle.

The Pathogen

The family Cryptosporidiidae has a hidden sporocyst and undergoes monoxenous completion of its cycle in one host, where it can cause predominantly intestinal, cloacal, and gastric infections.

The life cycle begins with ingestion of *Cryptosporidium* oocysts (2 to 5 μm) by the vertebrate host, with subsequent excystation within the lumen of the small intestine to release four sporozoites (Fig. 329-1). The sporozoites attach to and enter the host's epithelial cells to form intracellular but extracytoplasmic parasitophorous vacuoles, where they develop into trophozoites and subsequently type 1 meronts (schizonts). By asexual nuclear division, they multiply and release six to eight type 1 merozoites that invade neighboring host cells and develop into type 2 meronts, or trophozoites, to complete the asexual reproductive cycle. Type 2 meronts undergo two nuclear divisions and release four type 2 merozoites that can infect the host's cells and further develop into male (microgamont) or female (macrogamete) forms. Microgametes released from the microgamont can penetrate the macrogametes to form zygotes. Approximately 20% of the zygotes develop into thin-walled autoinfectious oocysts; some 80% become thick-walled oocysts, which are excreted in stool.

Cryptosporidium oocysts have at least five characteristics that make this organism a common problem and that help define the potential risk for person-to-person spread and for waterborne and food-borne disease outbreaks. First, *Cryptosporidium* oocysts are resistant to many chemical disinfectants, such as chlorine. Second, the organism is highly infectious, with the median *C. parvum* infectious dose being 132 or fewer oocysts. Third, the size of the oocysts, 2 to 5 μm, allows them to pass through many conventional filters. Fourth, the monoxenous life cycle allows infectious oocysts to be excreted in large numbers in feces, which can easily spread. Fifth, the organism is associated with geographic, seasonal, and socioeconomic differences in the distribution of *Cryptosporidium* spp.

EPIDEMIOLOGY

Cryptosporidiosis is seasonal and related to precipitation and temperature fluctuations worldwide. Excystation of *C. parvum* increases in water temperatures up to 46° C (natural sunlight for 12 hours). Two waterborne outbreaks in recent times brought cryptosporidiosis to public health attention. In January 1989, an increased number of cases of cryptosporidiosis were reported in Swindon and Oxfordshire, United Kingdom, with a peak reached in March. Mapping of the addresses of early cases showed associations with water supplies. This outbreak resulted in 516 cases and thus ignited public interest and led to an official inquiry. The second outbreak occurred in early spring 1993 in Milwaukee, Wisconsin, and was the largest documented outbreak of waterborne disease ever in the United States, with an estimated 403,000 people having acute watery diarrhea and potentially 112 deaths. Findings from this outbreak indicated that *Cryptosporidium* oocysts passed through the filtration system of one of the city's water treatment plants. Swimming pool contamination, especially of bigger pools, pools with more heterogeneous mixing such as municipal pools, and pools catering to young children (wading pools), is associated with more cases.[3,4] Food-borne outbreaks have also been reported in association with contaminated apple cider, unpasteurized milk, chicken salad, vegetables, raw produce, and shellfish.[5]

The prevalence of cryptosporidiosis varies by geographic region, with the highest rates seen in developing countries[6] in children. Pathogen-specific burden of community diarrhea in developing countries was evaluated in a multisite birth cohort study. *Cryptosporidium* spp was one of the five pathogens, including norovirus GII, rotavirus, *Campylobacter* spp, and astrovirus, that exhibited the highest attributable burdens of diarrhea in the first year of life.[7] In the Global Enteric Multicenter Study (GEMS) of moderate to severe diarrhea and using quantitative molecular assay, *Cryptosporidium* spp was found as one of the most common causes of diarrhea in children younger than 5 years in Africa and Asia.[8] In children younger than 5 years, rotavirus, *Cryptosporidium* spp, and *Shigella* spp were shown to be responsible for most deaths associated with diarrheal diseases.[9] Cryptosporidiosis continues to be a significant cause of intestinal infection among individuals with human immunodeficiency virus (HIV) and acquired immunodeficiency syndrome (AIDS) who are not on effective antiretroviral therapy.[10] In resource-sufficient settings, cryptosporidiosis has emerged as an important cause of diarrhea among HIV-negative individuals who are either solid organ or hematopoietic stem cell transplant recipients.[11]

PATHOBIOLOGY

Cryptosporidium oocysts and sporozoites interact with host cells, in the processes of excystation, gliding motility, attachment, invasion, parasitophorous vacuole formation, intracellular maintenance, and host cell damage. Oocysts of *Cryptosporidium* spp use their cysteine and serine proteases and aminopeptidase for excystation in the upper part of the small bowel and release infective sporozoites that invade the mucosal epithelium and occasionally Peyer patch M cells, often extending to the terminal ileum and colon. The sporozoites secrete proteins from the apical organelles for locomotion and attachment. In immunocompromised patients, the organisms can be found throughout the gut, biliary tract, pancreas, and respiratory tract. As noted earlier, trophozoites undergo asexual reproduction by merogony to form type 1 and then type 2 meronts. Sporozoites and merozoites are internalized by similar invasion machinery and actin reorganization. Two classes of proteins, mucin-like glycoproteins and thrombospondin-related adhesive proteins, mediate adhesion of the parasite. The parasite uses proteases for the proteolytic processing of surface and apical complex proteins for invasion and for egress from the host cells. Entry into the host's cell occurs within 30 seconds and is dependent on the parasite's actomyosin cytoskeleton to enter host-derived bimembrane parasitophorous vacuoles in a unique intracellular but extracytoplasmic niche. Dense polymerized actin forms at the base fusion of the host-parasite bimembranes. Invasion of cells of the host leads to displacement of the microvillous border, villous atrophy, blunting and crypt cell hyperplasia, and marked infiltration by lymphocytes, plasma cells, and some neutrophils into the lamina propria, with apoptosis of infected cells and significant alteration in intestinal permeability. Upregulation of nuclear factor κB and the pro-inflammatory cascade causes secretory and mildly inflammatory diarrhea. Pro-inflammatory cytokines, such as tumor necrosis factor-α, interleukins-1β and -8, and lactoferrin, are significantly increased in murine and human infections. Interleukins-1β and -8 both upregulate cyclooxygenase 2, which results in prostaglandin synthesis in the epithelial cells and production of substance P by the inflammatory cells; these products together decrease net sodium absorption and

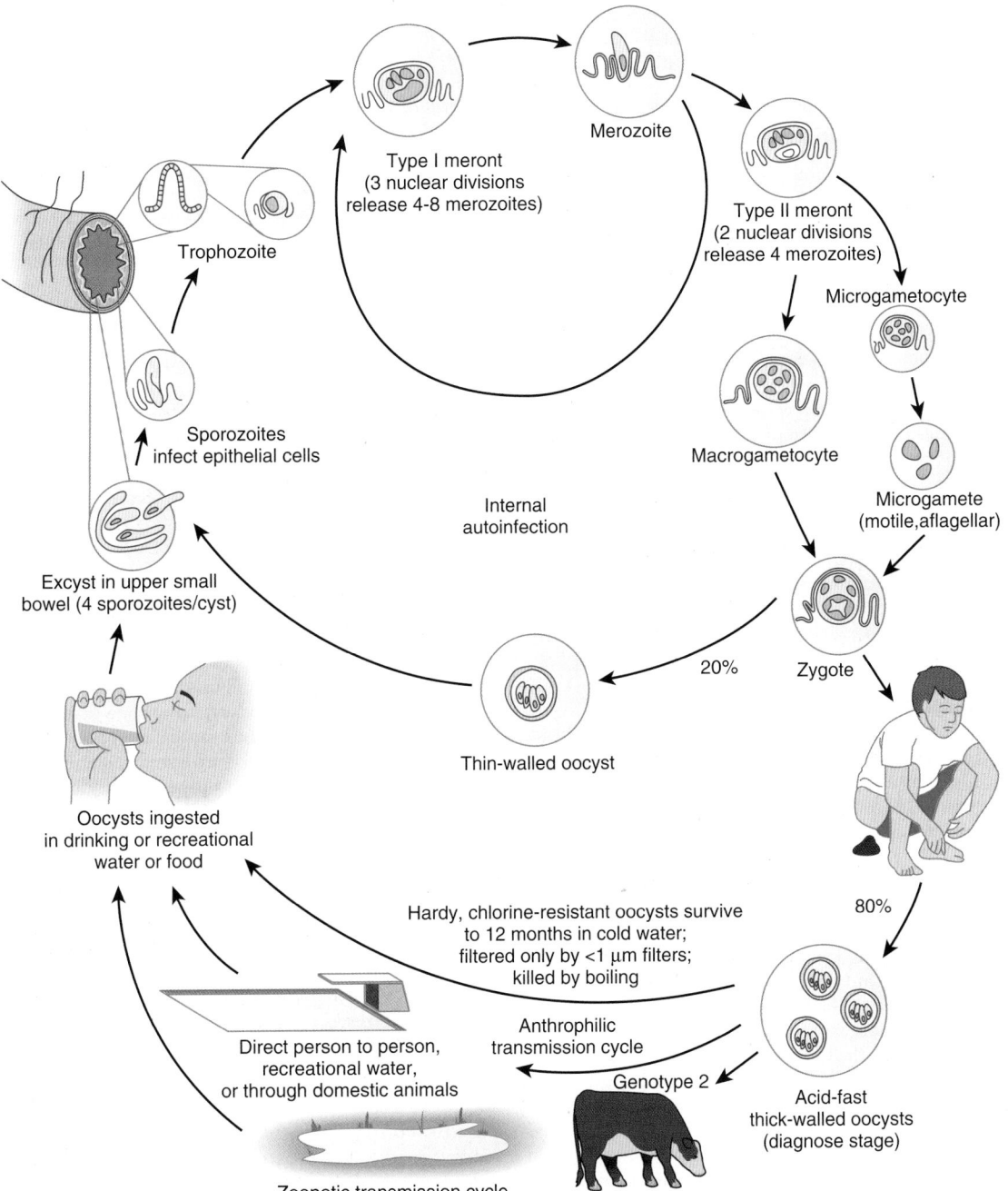

FIGURE 329-1. Life cycle of *Cryptosporidium* spp. (Redrawn with permission from Kosek M, Alcantara C, Lima AAM, et al. Cryptosporidiosis: an update. *Lancet Infect Dis.* 2001;1:262-269.)

increase net chloride secretion, which causes the secretory diarrhea often seen with this infection.

CLINICAL MANIFESTATIONS

Cryptosporidiosis is a cosmopolitan, self-limited infection in immunocompetent hosts that affects all age groups and both sexes. In developing countries, the disease occurs most frequently in children younger than 5 years because of high rates of fecal-oral exposure and the development of partial immunity in older children and adults. In developed countries, the disease occurs at all ages, and most cases are associated with small waterborne outbreaks, frequently with contamination of recreational water. Patients from developed countries are more often adults. The incubation period is approximately 1 week, with a range of 1 to 30 days. The diarrhea can have a sudden onset, frequently with voluminous watery stools, abdominal pain, nausea or vomiting, bloating, malaise, fatigue, weight loss, and occasional fever. In young children at risk in developing countries, it may have a long-term impact on physical activity, school performance, and development of cognitive function. Rarely, respiratory infection and cough have been reported. In normal hosts, the disease usually lasts 1 to 3 weeks but sometimes for more than a month. Oocyst

shedding typically lasts 1 to 2 weeks but can occur for up to 2 months. Patients with T-cell immune deficiency, such as those with hematologic malignant neoplasms (particularly children), primary T-cell deficiencies (severe combined immunodeficiency and CD40 ligand deficiency), and HIV/AIDS, are at high risk for the development of more severe disease and have an increased risk for death.

Immunocompetent Host

Data on the natural history of cryptosporidiosis in immunocompetent hosts have been obtained mostly from developed countries, and such data are derived from waterborne outbreaks, patients seeking medical assistance, travelers, animal workers, children in daycare, and their contacts. Most patients in outbreaks and travelers are adults and usually have diarrhea with a median duration of 14 days and a range of 1 to 100 days. The duration and severity of diarrhea appear to be similar for *C. parvum* and *C. hominis* infections. Recurrence of diarrhea is common and occurs in 30 to 41% of patients. Reports from the United Kingdom describe abdominal pain (96%), vomiting (65%), fever (59%), and bloody diarrhea (11%). The clinical manifestations in 285 people surveyed with a confirmed laboratory diagnosis of *Cryptosporidium* infection in the massive outbreak in Milwaukee showed a median duration of 9 days (range, 1 to 55 days), with watery diarrhea in 93%, abdominal cramps in 84%, fever in 57%, and vomiting in 48%. Patients may continue to shed oocysts for 7 months despite being asymptomatic.

Childhood Cryptosporidiosis in Developing Countries

In developing countries, cryptosporidiosis is associated with prolonged (7 to 13 days) or persistent (≥14 days) diarrhea, increased overall burden of diarrhea, risk for malnutrition, and infant mortality. A nested case-control study from a cohort of children in Brazil has shown that children younger than 1 year with cryptosporidiosis have subsequent increased diarrheal burdens and growth shortfalls. These findings have been extended in a shantytown in Peru, where cryptosporidiosis has been associated with growth faltering and stunting. This was also true for children with asymptomatic infections, which are even more common in endemic areas. The long-term impact of childhood diarrhea and cryptosporidiosis has also been evaluated in a cohort study in Brazil, in which it was shown that children with more diarrhea morbidity or cryptosporidiosis early in life (0 to 2 years) have reduced fitness and impaired cognitive function at 6 to 9 years of age. Several studies have now shown that oocysts are shed longer and the number of oocysts is higher with *C. hominis* than with *C. parvum* infection. In Brazil, a birth cohort study demonstrated that children with *C. hominis* infection have higher fecal lactoferrin and delayed growth in comparison to those with *C. parvum* infections. Diarrhea, nausea, vomiting, and general malaise are more frequently associated with *C. hominis* infection. Subtype family analysis of *C. hominis* (Ia, Ib, Id, and Ie) has indicated that Ib is more commonly associated with nausea, vomiting, and general malaise.

Immunocompromised Hosts

Low CD4$^+$ lymphocyte counts in HIV-infected patients are associated with severe cryptosporidial diarrhea. For example, patients with CD4$^+$ counts higher than 180/μL usually have transient or self-limited disease, whereas those with CD4$^+$ counts lower than 50/μL often have severe disease with more than 2 L of stool per day. Asymptomatic carriage of the parasite is common in individuals with HIV/AIDS in resource-limited settings. The introduction of highly active antiretroviral therapy (HAART) heralded reduced rates of cryptosporidiosis in patients with HIV/AIDS. HAART may also directly inhibit sporozoite development and invasion in the host's cells. Patients with other immune disorders, such as T-cell immune deficiency (severe combined immunodeficiency and CD40 ligand deficiency) or hematologic malignant neoplasms, particularly children, are at higher risk for more severe, prolonged, or extensive disease, with infection occasionally extending to the gallbladder, the pancreatic duct, and even the bronchial tree. Several complications in these patients have been described, including pancreatitis, cholecystitis, sclerosing cholangitis, papillitis, and terminal bile duct stenosis with subsequent biliary cirrhosis. More recently, *Cryptosporidium* spp infection has been recognized as one of the causes of diarrhea in transplant recipients. In a nationwide collection of cases among solid organ transplantation patients in France, it occurred at a median time of 3.4 (0 to 19.8) years after transplantation.[12] Coinfection with other pathogens, extraintestinal involvement (biliary tract and lungs), and relapse were reported in this immunocompromised group.

DIAGNOSIS

The clinical manifestations and physical examination findings in patients with cryptosporidiosis are not unique. The differential diagnosis should include other causes of infectious gastroenteritis, such as *Giardia, Cyclospora, Isospora,* microsporidia, *Escherichia coli* pathotypes (enteropathogenic [EPEC], enteroaggregative [EAEC], diffusely adherent [DAEC], enterohemorrhagic [EHEC], enteroinvasive [EIEC], and enterotoxigenic [ETEC]), *Campylobacter, Salmonella, Shigella,* rotavirus, norovirus, and others. Definitive diagnosis of *Cryptosporidium* enteric infection is made by stool examination.[13] Up to three fecal samples with fixation and concentration before permanent staining or polymerase chain reaction analysis may increase detection rates. Oocysts are stained with the acid-fast stain, modified Ziehl-Nielsen stain, fluorescence staining with auramine-phenol, or immunofluorescent stains. Acid-fast staining requires around 500,000 oocysts per gram for detection in formed stools, whereas immunofluorescence is at least 10 times more sensitive, and commercially available enzyme-linked immunoassays have a sensitivity and specificity approaching 100% for *Cryptosporidium*. Polymerase chain reaction testing can detect as few as 50 to 500 oocysts per milliliter of liquid stool and can be used to differentiate or even to quantify *Cryptosporidium* species and genotypes.

TREATMENT   Rx

Nitazoxanide has emerged as the only promising candidate for treatment of cryptosporidiosis. It is licensed in the United States for treatment of cryptosporidiosis in nonimmunodeficient children and adults and has reportedly reduced the duration of diarrhea and oocyst shedding in several double-blind, placebo-controlled clinical trials. A clinical trial of nitazoxanide in Egypt in adults (500 mg twice daily for 3 days) and children (200 mg for 4- to 11-year-olds and 100 mg for 1- to 3-year-olds, twice daily for 3 days) with cryptosporidiosis showed that 80% exhibited resolution of diarrhea versus 41% of the placebo group. A second clinical trial of a 3-day course of treatment showed resolution of symptoms at 4 days in 96% of the patients receiving nitazoxanide tablets (500 mg twice daily for 3 days) versus only 41% of those receiving placebo tablets.

There is no evidence of a reduction in the duration or frequency of diarrhea with nitazoxanide, but nitazoxanide has resulted in significantly greater oocyst clearance than has placebo in immunocompetent individuals according to a meta-analysis. In patients with HIV/AIDS, HAART has emerged as the most important therapy to prevent and reduce the severity and frequency of cryptosporidiosis. In transplant recipients, prolonged courses of antiparasitic treatment and/or reduction of immunosuppression have been reported to yield anecdotal success.[14] Oral rehydration therapy or intravenous fluid replacement for more severe disease is key to preventing dehydration and risk for immediate death.

PREVENTION

Prevention of person-to-person spread should be achieved with personal hygiene guidelines such as frequent handwashing after using or cleaning the toilet, changing diapers, and caring for a person with diarrhea. It is recommended that people with cryptosporidiosis be excluded from the workplace setting until 48 hours after the last diarrheal episode. Handwashing facilities should be available and used at farms to facilitate personal hygiene. Because most outbreaks of cryptosporidiosis are linked to oocysts in source water, routine survey of treated water for this parasite is key to preventing major spread of this disease. Optimization of multibarrier approaches, including chemical treatment and water filtration and treatment systems, is highly recommended. Ultraviolet irradiation and ozone are effective in inactivating *Cryptosporidium* and *Giardia* cysts in water and may prove useful in controlling the transmission of waterborne protozoa. In a systematic review of literature, the availability and use of sanitation facilities and water treatment was found to be associated with lower odds of protozoal infections in general, although only water treatment significantly decreased *Cryptosporidium* spp infections.[15]

PROGNOSIS

Cryptosporidiosis is usually a self-limited disease. Nevertheless, gastrointestinal and joint symptoms can persist for several months after the initial infection with *Cryptosporidium*.[16] In epidemics, the mortality rate may be as high as 3 per 10,000 in symptomatic people in the general population. Children in the developing world often have stunted growth, whether as a reflection of the disease itself or the conditions that led to infection. For severely immunocompromised AIDS patients, cryptosporidiosis can be difficult to eradicate and is associated with a poor prognosis.

GENERAL REFERENCES

For the General References and other additional features, please visit Expert Consult at https://expertconsult.inkling.com.

330

GIARDIASIS

THEODORE E. NASH AND DAVID R. HILL

DEFINITION

Giardia lamblia (*Giardia duodenalis, Giardia intestinalis*) is a ubiquitous, small intestinal protozoan parasite of humans and other mammals. It is the most common parasitic infection of the gastrointestinal tract in the United States as well as worldwide and is responsible for outbreaks of diarrhea and sporadic endemic disease.[1,2]

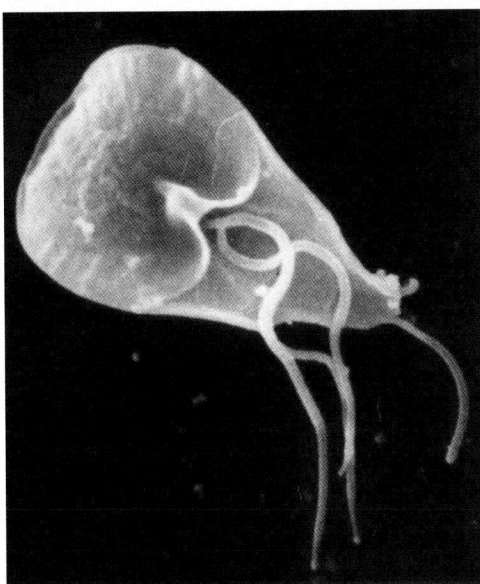

FIGURE 330-1. *Giardia lamblia.* This scanning electron micrograph reveals some of the external ultrastructural details displayed by a flagellated *G. lamblia* protozoan parasite.

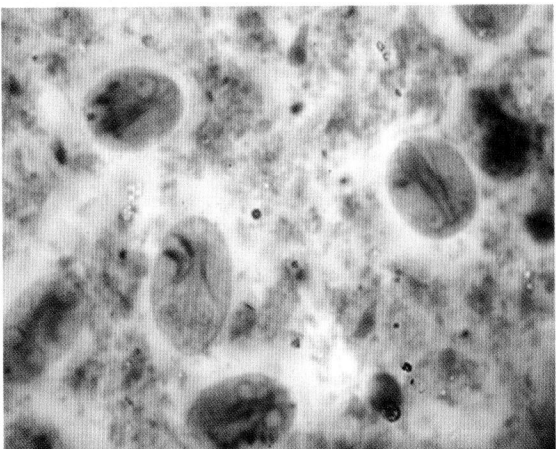

FIGURE 330-2. Iron hematoxylin stain of *Giardia lamblia* cysts from stool.

The Pathogen

Giardia has a simple life cycle. The trophozoite, which is 9 to 21 μm long, 5 to 15 μm wide, and 2 to 4 μm thick (Fig. 330-1), resides in the small intestine and is responsible for manifestations of disease. It has four pairs of flagella, two nuclei, and a ventral sucking disc by which it may adhere to intestinal epithelial cells. The dorsal surface is pear shaped and bilaterally symmetrical, with the two highly characteristic nuclei best visualized after staining. In the lower small intestine, the trophozoite develops into an environmentally resistant cyst. Detection of soluble cyst wall proteins in the feces forms the basis of many stool antigen assays.

Excreted cysts are mature and infectious. They are oval and about 8 to 12 μm in length and 7 to 10 μm in width (Fig. 330-2). After ingestion and exposure to acid and proteases in the stomach and intestines, they excyst in the small intestine, yielding two trophozoites from each cyst, which quickly divide again. In vitro, trophozoites double in number every 6 hours for the fastest growing isolates.

A number of morphologically identical but genetically distinct *Giardia* infect humans and animals that are now divided into eight assemblages. Humans, as well as some animals, are typically infected with either assemblage A or B. These two assemblages are genetically and biologically diverse and appear to be two separate species.[3]

Giardia is well adapted to its existence as a parasite. It has two equal functioning nuclei and lacks mitochondria and peroxisomes. It has a simplified metabolism and is dependent on the host for nutrients such as purines, pyrimidines, cysteine, and cholesterol. The WB isolate, assemblage A, has a compact genome (11.7 Mb) with unusually short promoters. The parasite's rigid cytoskeleton is composed of unique families of structural proteins and carbohydrates.

Giardia is the only bowel-dwelling parasite that undergoes antigenic variation. Only one of a family of about 250 variant-specific proteins (VSPs) is expressed on the surface of the trophozoite at a time.[4] Both immune and biologic selection of trophozoites that express specific VSPs occurs in humans and animals with giardiasis. Expressed VSPs must be compatible with the host's intestinal environment and are probably not recognized by the host's immune system because antibodies to VSPs are inhibitory or cytotoxic. Whereas all VSPs are transcribed, all but one of the transcripts are eliminated by RNA interference–based mechanisms, resulting in expression of a single VSP surface protein. Exactly how selection and switching occur is unclear.

EPIDEMIOLOGY

Giardia is among the most common parasitic infections of humans; it is highly infectious, and cysts are frequently excreted in large numbers (as high as 10^7 cysts per gram of feces), especially in young children. Cysts can survive for months in cold water, are relatively resistant to chlorination, but are intolerant of desiccation and heat in comparison to the relatively resistant ova of cryptosporidia and helminths. Experimentally, between 10 and 100 cysts is sufficient to establish infection nearly all of the time. Consequently, ingestion of water or food that contains small levels of contamination can result in infection. Approximately 20,000 infections are reported annually in the United States, but because of underreporting, actual infections are estimated at more than 1 million cases per year.

Infections are most common in young children and are more frequent in summer and fall months. Giardiasis is acquired after ingestion of contaminated water or food or through person-to-person contact. In past decades, large outbreaks in high-income countries such as the United States occurred after ingestion of contaminated drinking water obtained from surface sources such as reservoirs, lakes, and mountain streams.[5] However, with improved water treatment measures, ingestion of contaminated recreational water from pools or lakes is now a more common source of outbreaks. Backpackers who ingest untreated surface water remain at risk of infection. In 2011 and 2012, 1 to 2% of giardiasis cases were associated with a detected outbreak. The overall incidence rate is about 6 per 100,000 population in the United States.[6]

Although outbreaks from contaminated food or infected food handlers are well described, they are less frequently documented. Worldwide, person-to-person transmission may be the most frequent mode of infection and is the primary way children are infected in daycare centers, where infection can be common. Person-to-person spread occurs among family members with infected children and following sexual practices that lead to fecal-oral contact.[7] In low-income, highly endemic regions, almost all children are infected by 2 to 3 years of age, many of them persistently.[8] Although partial immunity can develop in previously exposed adults, reinfection of children after treatment is common in highly endemic regions. Longer-term travel, particularly to South Asia, increases the risk of giardiasis. For the returned traveler with intermittent or persistent diarrhea, giardiasis should be ruled out.

The understanding of immunity in humans is based mostly on animal models that have limited applicability to human infection and disease. In addition, some of the findings are conflicting. In the classic human experimental infections reported by Rendtorff and colleagues in the 1950s, self-cure occurred in about 84% of the persons. In a more recent experimental human challenge study, in which the infecting parasite was well characterized and the inoculum known, rechallenge with the same isolate after treatment resulted in brief, asymptomatic infections in two persons, suggesting development of partial immunity. Humans with hypogammaglobulinemia are susceptible to *Giardia* and have more severe disease that is resistant to treatment. Studies in animals support a major role of intestinal antibodies (particularly immunoglobulin A [IgA]) in protective immunity and an essential role of T-cell immunity and interleukin-17 (IL-17) in the control of *G. lamblia* infection.

Giardia infections are neither more severe nor more common in most other immunosuppressed states and in persons with selective IgA deficiency. Even though most human immunodeficiency virus–infected patients respond to usual treatment, a subset develop recurrent or repeated infections that are difficult to treat.

PATHOBIOLOGY

Giardia infections involve complex interactions between host and parasite. The two assemblages (A and B) that infect humans are composed of genetically distinguishable isolates, which may vary in infectivity, antigenicity, and virulence. Isolates of assemblage B are particularly heterogeneous compared with assemblage A. In addition, human hosts vary in susceptibility to infection and disease and in the response or tolerance to infection. Pathogenic mechanisms need to explain the varied clinical manifestations as well as the contrasting situation in which there are high rates of infection and disease seen in water-borne outbreaks of giardiasis in regions where infections are sporadic, as in the United States, compared with the mostly asymptomatic infections in children in highly endemic low-income regions. In addition, infection with *Giardia* can lead to malabsorption, weight loss, and nutritional deficiencies in some settings and little effect on nutritional parameters in other settings.

Giardia is strictly an intraluminal parasite that adheres to the epithelium by way of an adhesive or sucking disc. Invasion of the epithelium either does not occur or is rare. The number of trophozoites in the intestine can be so large that adherent organisms cover much of the epithelial surface. This could disrupt the epithelial brush border and contribute to disaccharidase deficiency seen in some patients. A number of studies demonstrate direct epithelial cell barrier dysfunction in vitro and in vivo in humans. There is no evidence of production of a classic enterotoxin, although it is possible that secreted or surface proteins may be injurious to cells or stimulate an immune response. Of patients with persistent giardiasis after treatment, nearly half exhibited inflammation on small bowel biopsy specimens, supporting the view that chronic inflammatory responses contribute to disease at least in this subset.

CLINICAL MANIFESTATIONS

The clinical manifestations, course, and duration of *Giardia* infections are variable. Infections may be self-limited or persistent, asymptomatic or symptomatic.[9] In general, patients are not as sick as those with bacterial diarrheas. Acute disease manifestations occur commonly in travelers and in outbreaks and are characterized by diarrhea, nausea, anorexia, dehydration, flatulence, eructation, foul-smelling stools, distention, abdominal cramping, and weight loss. Malabsorption is more commonly seen in chronic infection. Fever and vomiting are uncommon. Blood, mucus, and polymorphonuclear cells in the stool, which are not usual features of small bowel infections, should suggest an alternative or additional diagnosis. Dehydration, although uncommon, may be severe and require hospitalization; hospitalization for giardiasis does occur in the United States. On occasion, nausea and vomiting will predominate and suggest other causes.

In experimental infections using inoculated cysts, presence of cysts in the stool occurred 6 to 15 days (mean, 9 days) after inoculation. In more recent experimental infections, *Giardia* antigen was detected 1 day before cyst excretion. In one well-documented food-borne outbreak, 74% became ill, with an incubation period of 2 to 19 days and peak symptoms at 5 to 6 days. Symptoms continued for a median of 18 days.

Acute symptoms can resolve, wax and wane, or settle into a chronic phase, which can be prolonged and last weeks to months. Long-lasting symptoms should prompt a search for the parasite. Lactose deficiency is common and can persist for some weeks after treatment, and it needs to be distinguished in symptomatic patients from relapse or reinfection. In extreme cases, malabsorption and weight loss are severe and mimic sprue.

A typical scenario is a mildly to moderately ill person who complains of an increased number of urgent loose stools, with flatus, cramping, anorexia, and weight loss. There may be periods when the person feels better only to relapse and become noticeably worse. After days to several weeks, the individual will seek medical help. Similar to other causes of infectious diarrheas, symptoms can continue after successful treatment. Some patients will develop irritable bowel syndrome (Chapter 127). Uncommonly, *Giardia* is found in biliary and pancreatic ducts and can cause cholecystitis and pancreatitis. Extraintestinal manifestations and long-term consequences are uncommon, but a series of sporadic cases documented them in a third of the patients. The manifestations can include rash, reactive arthritis, eye complaints, and cognitive deficiencies.

In highly endemic regions, infection is almost universal by 2 to 3 years of age, and prevalence rates remain high throughout childhood, commonly above 20%. In these settings, despite high prevalence and constant reinfection, *Giardia* is an uncommon cause of acute diarrhea compared with agents such as rotavirus, enterotoxigenic *Escherichia coli, Shigella, Campylobacter,* and *Cryptosporidium.* However, *Giardia* has been associated with longer lasting diarrhea (≥14 days), and chronic infection has been associated in multiple study sites with stunting.[10,11] Persistent diarrhea as a result of infection with *Giardia* is a cause of malnutrition.[12] In contrast, *Giardia*-naïve visitors frequently develop

symptomatic giardiasis while visiting or working in highly endemic regions.[13] Some studies suggest that giardiasis may protect against other enteric pathogens.

DIAGNOSIS

The diagnosis of giardiasis is based on detection of cysts, trophozoites, parasite-specific antigens, or specific DNA in fecal samples. Because excretion of cysts may be variable or in low concentrations, a single-stool microscopy for ova and parasites is only 50 to 80% sensitive, and multiple-stool examinations may be necessary. In most laboratories stool antigen tests are standard; they are more sensitive compared with microscopy. They detect about 80% of the infections compared to molecular tests, but it is unclear whether these missed infections are clinically relevant. Molecular detection methods are superior to stool antigen detection.[14] Neither antigen- nor molecular-based tests require a trained microscopist. Examination of small intestine biopsies or intestinal contents for trophozoites was the previous "gold standard" for diagnosis but is now uncommonly needed to establish or to confirm the diagnosis. In low-intensity infections, testing methods can be falsely negative and require repeated testing.

Other laboratory findings are nonspecific. The white blood cell count and liver function test results are usually normal. Electrolyte disturbances can be present if diarrhea and vomiting are severe. White blood cells, lactoferrin, blood, and mucus are not found in the stool. Immunoglobulin levels are usually normal but abnormally low or absent in susceptible hypogammaglobulinemic individuals.

TREATMENT   Rx

Details of antiparasitic therapy in general are provided in Chapter 323. Tinidazole (Tindamax), a Food and Drug Administration (FDA)–approved nitroimidazole drug similar to metronidazole (Flagyl) and albendazole, have been the treatments of choice[A1][A2]; other nitroimidazoles (e.g., ornidazole and secnidazole) that are not approved in the United States are also effective. Tinidazole is given as a single dose, and compared with metronidazole it has fewer side effects and greater efficacy. In adults, the dose is 2 g orally; in children, the dose is 50 mg/kg as a single dose with a maximum of 2 g. Metronidazole has been used to treat giardiasis for decades but has never been approved by the FDA for this indication; it requires multiple dosing at 250 mg orally three times a day for 5 to 7 days for adults and 15 mg/kg/day in three divided doses for 5 to 7 days for children. Gastrointestinal side effects of metronidazole are relatively common, and alcohol should not be taken concomitantly because of the possibility of a disulfiram-like reaction with both drugs. Albendazole (400 mg/day for 5 days), not presently approved by the FDA for treatment of giardiasis, may be an acceptable alternative to metronidazole, with fewer side effects; however, there is limited experience with this drug. Nitazoxanide has broad activity against protozoa, helminths, and bacteria and is FDA approved for the treatment of giardiasis. It is given at a dose of 100 mg orally every 12 hours for 3 days for children ages 12 months to 3 years, 200 mg orally every 12 hours for 3 days for children 4 to 11 years of age, and 500 mg orally every 12 hours for 3 days for persons older than 12 years. Because it is available in a liquid suspension as well as in a 500-mg tablet, it may be easier to give to young children. It should be given with food. Most of the side effects are gastrointestinal symptoms and headache.

Paromomycin, a nonabsorbable aminoglycoside, has been used in pregnant women to avoid the theoretical fetal adverse events of nitroimidazoles, particularly during the first trimester. It is given to adults at a dose of 500 mg three times a day for 5 to 10 days and to children at 25 to 35 mg/kg/day orally in three divided doses for 5 to 10 days. Quinacrine and furazolidone (FDA approved but not usually available) are also active against *Giardia* but should be reserved for use in particular situations.

Patients usually experience relief of symptoms on treatment. Failure of treatment is frequently heralded by a return of symptoms days to weeks after cessation of therapy and requires either re-treatment with an alternative class of drug or an increased dosing of the initial therapy. Clinical cases of nitroimidazole-resistant infections are increasingly seen, particularly in returned travelers from South Asia.[15,16] They usually respond to combination treatment; quinacrine and metronidazole have been most effective, with metronidazole plus albendazole also showing efficacy.[17]

PREVENTION

Infection is prevented by scrupulous personal hygiene, proper disposal of sewage, removal or killing of cysts from water supplies, and preventing contamination of food and water. Cysts are relatively labile and are susceptible to heating and filtration with small water volume filters of 0.2 to 1 μm. Heating (bringing water to a boil) is preferred because other pathogens found in feces are also inactivated. Cysts are not reliably susceptible to chlorination because the concentrations of chlorine, water temperatures, turbidity, and pH present when treating commercial water supplies are suboptimal. Four drops of 5.25% bleach to 1 liter for 1 hour at room temperature is sufficient for killing. At lower temperatures, inactivation may not be complete.

Grade A References

A1. Pasupulet V, Escobedo AA, Despande A, et al. Efficacy of 5-nitromidazoles for the treatment of giardiasis: a systematic review of randomized controlled trials. *PLoS Negl Trop Dis.* 2014;8:1-11.

A2. Escobedo AA, Ballesteros J, Gonzalez-Fraile E, et al. A meta-analysis of the efficacy of albendazole compared with tinidazole as treatments for *Giardia* infections in children. *Acta Trop.* 2016;153:120-127.

GENERAL REFERENCES

For the General References and other additional features, please visit Expert Consult at https://expertconsult.inkling.com.

331

AMEBIASIS

WILLIAM A. PETRI, JR.

DEFINITION

Amebiasis is due to infection with the enteric protozoan parasite *Entamoeba histolytica*. Amebiasis can cause asymptomatic colonization, diarrhea, dysentery, and colitis, as well as spread extraintestinally to cause liver and rarely brain abscess (Fig. 331-1).

The Pathogen

E. histolytica has a low infectious dose (<100 organisms), is resistant to chlorine, and is environmentally stable. These properties make it a threat to food and water supplies, as the 1998 municipal water outbreak of amebic liver abscess in Tbilisi, Georgia, demonstrated. Its tissue-destructive properties are the reason for the parasite's being named *histolytica*.

EPIDEMIOLOGY

Most *E. histolytica* infections occur in the developing world, including the Indian subcontinent, Southeast Asia, sub-Saharan Africa, and Central and South America, as a result of fecal-oral transmission. A national serologic survey in Mexico demonstrated antibody to *E. histolytica* in 8.4% of the population. In an urban slum of Fortaleza, Brazil, 25% of the population tested carried antibody to *E. histolytica*, and the prevalence in children 6 to 14 years of age was 40%. In Dhaka, Bangladesh, where diarrheal diseases are the leading cause of childhood death, the annual incidence of *E. histolytica* infection in a cohort of preschool children was 40%. The annual incidence of amebic liver abscess was 21 cases per 100,000 inhabitants in Hue City, Vietnam. The best current estimate by the World Health Organization is that *E. histolytica* infection results in 34 to 50 million symptomatic cases each year worldwide and as many as 100,000 deaths.

In the United States, amebiasis is the third most common parasitic infection after giardiasis and cryptosporidiosis (1.2 cases/100,000 U.S. population). Most cases in industrialized countries occur in travelers to and immigrants from endemic regions as well as in institutionalized individuals. In returning travelers, diarrhea is the predominant reason for a patient to visit a physician, and amebiasis is the second most common cause of diarrhea in returning travelers. Previously reported high rates of *E. histolytica* infection in homosexual men in the United States actually reflect a high prevalence of *Entamoeba dispar* infection in this population. In contrast, in Asia, amebiasis is more frequently an initial symptom of human immunodeficiency virus (HIV) infection and acquired immunodeficiency syndrome because of the common risk for acquisition of both HIV infection and amebiasis through the sexual practices of men who have sex with men. The typical patient with an amebic liver abscess

in the United States is a 20- to 40-year-old Hispanic male immigrant. Several groups are at increased risk for severe amebiasis, including the very young or old, malnourished persons, pregnant women, and patients treated with corticosteroids.

PATHOBIOLOGY

Killing of host cells is required for invasion of the intestine by the parasite. The process of host cell destruction has been experimentally separated into sequential steps of adherence, a nibbling-like process termed *amebic trogocytosis*, contact-dependent cytotoxicity, followed finally by phagocytosis of the host cell corpse.[1] The initial contact of parasite to host is mediated by the parasite's galactose and *N*-acetyl-D-galactosamine (Gal/GalNAc)–specific lectin, which binds to carbohydrate determinants on the host's intestinal epithelium. Human cells die by apoptosis induced by *E. histolytica*, a process that requires attachment of the Gal/GalNAc lectin to a host cell's receptor, as well as the parasite's acid intracellular vesicles, which may serve as delivery vehicles for an amebic pore-forming protein. *E. histolytica* initiates apoptosis in host cells by directly activating the host cell's distal apoptotic machinery; caspase 3 is activated within minutes of *E. histolytica* adherence, a caspase 3 inhibitor blocks *E. histolytica* killing, and caspase 3–deficient or bcl-2–overexpressing mice are resistant to amebic infection. Recognition and ingestion of the apoptotic host cell's corpse are required for colonic infection by the parasite, and multiple ligands and receptors are involved, including the Gal/GalNAc lectin, a phosphatidylserine receptor, serine-rich *E. histolytica* protein, and collectins. After ingestion of the corpse of the host cell, additional parasitic factors participate in invasion into the intestinal mucosa. For example, *E. histolytica* encodes at least 44 cysteine proteinase genes that have been implicated in degradation of colonic mucin glycoproteins; digestion of extracellular matrix, hemoglobin, and villin; and inactivation of interleukin-18 (IL-18).

The innate immune response to amebic infection includes activation of the alternative complement pathway, with C3a and C5a recruiting neutrophils to the site of infection but with amebae resisting killing by the membrane attack complex through the Gal/GalNAc lectin. In the murine model of intestinal amebiasis, innate resistance is conferred by nonhematopoietic cells, thus suggesting the importance of epithelial production of cytokines such as tumor necrosis factor–α (TNF-α), IL-1α, IL-6, IL-8, growth-related oncogene–α (GRO-α), and granulocyte-macrophage colony-stimulating factor. Granulocytes are the earliest innate cellular immune response (within 1 to 2 days) for both intestinal and hepatic amebiasis. Depletion of neutrophils or eosinophils in a murine model results in exacerbated amebic hepatic and intestinal disease.[2] Macrophages and T lymphocytes are also recruited by day 3 of an infection. Macrophages acquire amebicidal activity after in vitro stimulation with interferon-γ (IFN-γ), TNF-α, or colony-stimulating factor 1. Natural killer cells may be important in part as a source of IFN-γ, as well as infiltrating mast cells for their ability to contribute to the innate immune response by the production of IL-6 and TNF-α.

The acquired immune response reflects the opposing roles of IL-4 and IFN-γ in persistence and clearance of amebic infection, respectively. Inbred mice of the CBA strain are susceptible to intestinal amebiasis and develop a rapid T_H2 phenotypic immune response, and this response is deleterious insofar as inhibition of IL-4 can convert the response to a healing IFN-γ response. Effective acquired immunity in humans is associated with both a systemic IFN-γ and a mucosal IgA response directed at the Gal/GalNAc lectin. Children with mucosal IgA against the Gal/GalNAc lectin were found to have 86% fewer new *E. histolytica* infections in the following year. Similarly, the risk for amebiasis was 50% lower in children who were in the 50th percentile and above for the production of IFN-γ by peripheral blood mononuclear cells stimulated with soluble amebic antigen. The composition of the gut microbiome is associated with symptomatic amebiasis likely through induction of an inflammatory immune response.[3]

CLINICAL MANIFESTATIONS
Asymptomatic Intraluminal Amebiasis

The asymptomatic cyst-passing carrier state is the most common type of amebic infection. All *Entamoeba moshkovskii* and *E. dispar* infections and as many as 80% of *E. histolytica* infections are asymptomatic.[4] Asymptomatically infected individuals represent a risk to the community because they are a source of new infections and a risk to themselves because 1 in 10 to 20 colonized individuals progress to symptomatic infection. The host has a bearing on whether infection is asymptomatic in that children heterozygous for the HLA class II DQB1*0601/DRB1*1501 haplotype have been found to be protected from

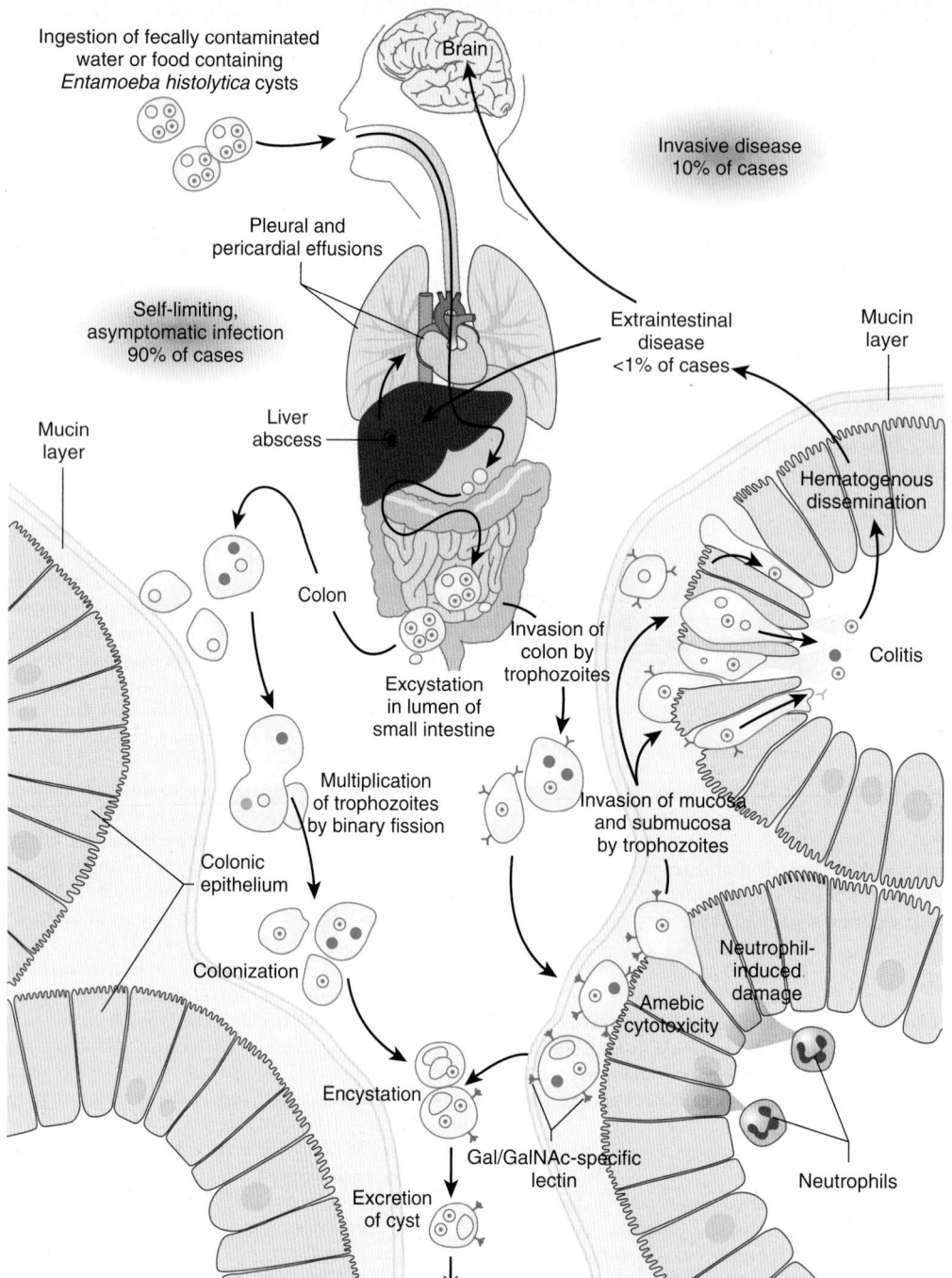

FIGURE 331-1. Life cycle of *Entamoeba histolytica*. Infection is normally initiated by the ingestion of fecally contaminated water or food containing *E. histolytica* cysts. The infective cyst form of the parasite survives passage through the stomach and small intestine. Excystation occurs in the bowel lumen, where motile and potentially invasive trophozoites are formed. In most infections, the trophozoites aggregate in the intestinal mucin layer and form new cysts, which results in a self-limited and asymptomatic infection. In some cases, however, adherence to and lysis of the colonic epithelium, mediated by the galactose and *N*-acetyl-D-galactosamine (Gal/GalNAc)–specific lectin, initiates invasion of the colon by trophozoites. Neutrophils responding to the invasion contribute to cellular protection at the site of invasion. Once the intestinal epithelium is invaded, extraintestinal spread to the peritoneum, liver, and other sites may follow. Factors controlling invasion, as opposed to encystation, probably include parasitic "quorum sensing" signaled by the Gal/GalNAc-specific lectin, interactions of amebae with the bacterial flora of the intestine, and innate and acquired immune responses of the host. (Redrawn with permission from Haque R, Huston CD, Hughes M, et al. Current concepts: amebiasis. *N Engl J Med.* 2003;348:1565-1573.)

symptomatic infection with amebiasis. In addition, certain genotypes of *E. histolytica* appear to be associated with the propensity for colonization as opposed to invasion.

Amebic Diarrhea

Amebic diarrhea without dysentery is the most common amebic disease.[5] It is defined as diarrhea in an *E. histolytica*–infected individual. There is no requirement for the presence of mucus or visible or microscopic blood in stool for the diagnosis of amebic diarrhea. In one community-based study of a cohort of preschool children in Bangladesh, the annual incidence of amebic infection, diarrhea, and dysentery was 45%, 9%, and 3%, respectively. The mean duration

of amebic diarrhea was 3 days in one study. It causes approximately 2% of cases of diarrhea severe enough to warrant hospital evaluation in developing countries such as Bangladesh.

Amebic Dysentery or Colitis

Diarrhea with mucus or visible or microscopic blood in a patient with *E. histolytica* infection is the definition of amebic dysentery or colitis. Approximately 15 to 33% of patients with *E. histolytica* diarrhea also have amebic dysentery. The onset of symptoms is typically gradual during a period of 3 or 4 weeks after infection, with abdominal tenderness and increasingly severe diarrhea being the primary complaints. Patients with bacterial causes of dysentery usually

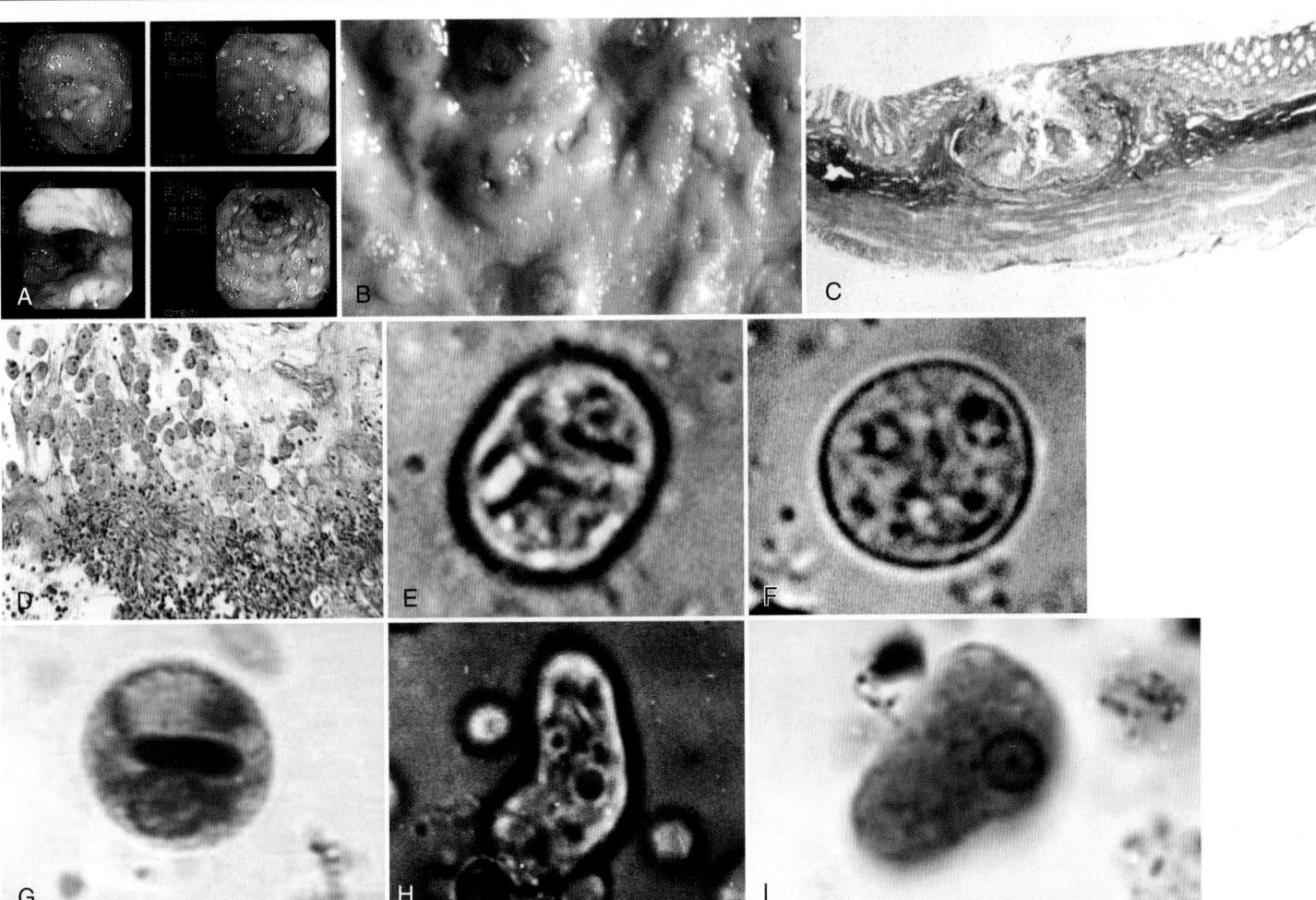

FIGURE 331-2. Endoscopic and pathologic features of intestinal amebiasis. **A,** Colonoscopic appearance of intestinal amebiasis. **B,** Colonic ulcers averaging 1 to 2 mm in diameter on gross pathologic examination. **C,** Cross section of a flask-shaped colonic ulcer (hematoxylin-eosin stain, magnification ×20). **D,** Inflammatory response to intestinal invasion by *Entamoeba histolytica* (hematoxylin-eosin stain, magnification ×100). **E and F,** *E. histolytica* cysts in a saline preparation (magnification ×1000). **G,** Iodine-stained cyst from stool (magnification ×1000). **H,** *E. histolytica* trophozoite with an ingested erythrocyte in a saline preparation from stool (magnification ×1000). **I,** Trophozoite from stool stained with trichrome (magnification ×1000). (*B–D,* From the slide collection of the late Dr. Harrison Juniper.) (From Haque R, Huston CD, Hughes M, et al. Current concepts: amebiasis. *N Engl J Med.* 2003;348:1565-1573.)

have only 1 or 2 days of symptoms. Surprisingly, fever is present in only a minority of patients with amebic colitis. In young children, intussusception, perforation, peritonitis, or necrotizing colitis may develop rapidly (Fig. 331-2). Unusual manifestations of amebic colitis include toxic megacolon (0.5% of cases, usually requiring surgical intervention) and ameboma (granulation tissue in the colonic lumen mimicking colon cancer in appearance).

Amebic Liver Abscess

Amebic liver abscess is 10 times as common in men as in women and is unusual in children. The typical patient with an amebic liver abscess in the United States is an immigrant from an endemic area, a man age 20 to 40 years with fever, right upper quadrant pain, leukocytosis, abnormal serum transaminase and alkaline phosphatase levels, and a defect seen on hepatic imaging studies.[6] Among travelers, the average interval between exposure and clinical presentation can be up to 18 months.[7] Most patients have 2 to 4 weeks of prior fever, cough, and abdominal pain in the right upper quadrant or epigastrium. Involvement of the diaphragmatic surface of the liver may lead to right-sided pleural pain or referred shoulder pain and an elevated right hemidiaphragm seen on chest radiography (Fig. 331-3). Hepatomegaly with point tenderness over the liver, below the ribs, or in the intercostal spaces is a typical finding.

If a space-filling defect in the liver is observed, the differential diagnosis includes (1) amebiasis (most common in men with a history of travel to or residence in a developing country), (2) pyogenic or bacterial abscess (particularly suspected in women, patients with cholecystitis, the elderly, individuals with diabetes, and patients with jaundice), (3) echinococcal abscess (which would be an incidental finding because echinococcal abscess should not cause pain or fever), and (4) cancer. Most patients with amebic liver abscess will

have detectable circulating antigen in serum as well as serum antiamebic antibodies.

In children, abdominal pain is reported infrequently with amebic liver abscess. More commonly, high fever, abdominal distention, irritability, and tachypnea are noted. Some of these children are admitted to the hospital with fever of unknown origin. Hepatomegaly occurs frequently, but elicitation of hepatic tenderness is not well documented. In one report, four of five children younger than 5 years died of amebic liver abscess because the diagnosis was not suspected.

Unusual extraintestinal manifestations of amebiasis include direct extension of the liver abscess to the pleura or pericardium and brain abscess. Death usually results from rupture of the liver abscess into the peritoneum, thorax, or pericardium, but it may also be caused by extensive hepatic damage and liver failure.

Other Extraintestinal Infections

Thoracic amebiasis is the most common type of extra-abdominal amebiasis after liver abscess and occurs in about 10% of patients with amebic liver abscess. It develops by direct extension from the liver. Pericardial amebiasis is the next most common form of extraintestinal involvement and may result from rupture of a liver abscess in the left lobe of the liver into the pericardium or from extension of the right-sided pleural amebiasis. Cerebral amebic abscesses have been found in about 0.5 to 5% of patients with amebic liver abscess. In one series of 18 patients with proven cerebral amebiasis, findings on the initial neurologic examination were normal in 13. Other foci of infection are rare, but amebic rectovesical fistula formation and involvement of the pharynx, heart, aorta, and scapula have been reported. Cutaneous infection may arise from trophozoites emerging from the rectum.

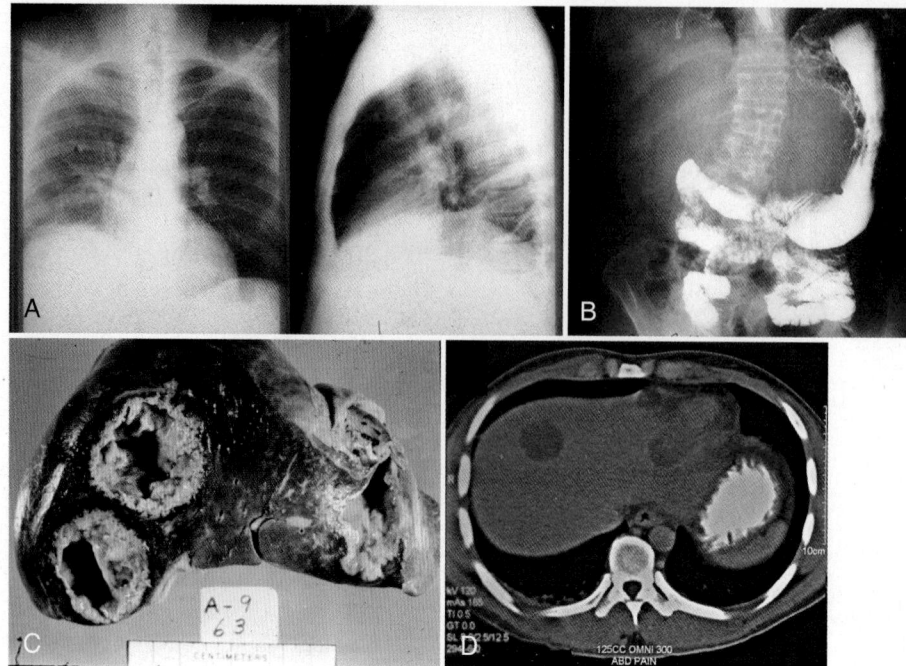

FIGURE 331-3. Radiographic and pathologic features of extraintestinal amebiasis. **A,** Left posteroanterior and right lateral chest radiographs in a patient with amebic liver abscess. The findings include an elevated right hemidiaphragm and evidence of atelectasis. **B,** Luminal narrowing revealed by barium enema examination in a patient with an ameboma. **C,** Two abscesses in the right lobe and one abscess in the left lobe of a patient with amebic liver abscess. **D,** Abdominal computed tomography showing one abscess in the right lobe and one abscess in the left lobe in a patient with amebic liver abscess. (From Haque R, Huston CD, Hughes M, et al. Current concepts: amebiasis. *N Engl J Med.* 2003;348:1565-1573.)

TABLE 331-1 SENSITIVITY OF TESTS FOR DIAGNOSIS OF AMEBIASIS

TEST	COLITIS	LIVER ABSCESS
Microscopy: stool	25-60%	10-40%
Stool antigen detection	80%	≈40%
Serum antigen detection	65%	>95%
Microscopy: abscess fluid	N/A	≤20%
Real-time PCR	>95%	>95%
Serologic testing (indirect hemagglutination)		
Acute	70%	70-80%
Convalescent	>90%	>90%

N/A = not available; PCR = polymerase chain reaction.
Modified from Haque R, Huston CD, Hughes M, et al. Current concepts: amebiasis. *N Engl J Med.* 2003;348:1565-1573.

DIAGNOSIS

Diagnosis of amebiasis is best accomplished by the combination of serology and identification of the parasite in feces or at extraintestinal sites of invasion by PCR or antigen detection (such as pus obtained by fine needle aspiration of a liver abscess).[8] Examination of stool for ova and parasites should *not* be used to diagnose amebiasis (Table 331-1). The most sensitive diagnostic approach is the combined use of *E. histolytica*–specific antigen detection or polymerase chain reaction plus serology.[9] Amebic colitis can also be diagnosed by colonoscopy, which can show characteristic discrete ulcers or erosions with white or yellow exudates, especially in the cecum, and can identify trophozoites in about 90% of patients.[10]

TREATMENT   Rx
(also see Chapter 323)

Therapy for invasive infection differs from that for noninvasive infection, which may be treated with paromomycin (Table 331-2). Invasive infections require treatment with nitroimidazoles, particularly metronidazole, tinidazole, secnidazole, or ornidazole. For amebic colitis, tinidazole reduces treatment failure

TABLE 331-2 DRUG THERAPY FOR TREATMENT OF AMEBIASIS

DRUG	ADULT DOSAGE	SIDE EFFECTS
AMEBIC LIVER ABSCESS		
Metronidazole	750 mg PO tid × 10 days	Primarily GI side effects: anorexia, nausea, vomiting, diarrhea, abdominal discomfort, or unpleasant metallic taste Disulfiram-like intolerance reaction to alcoholic beverages Neurotoxicity, including seizures, peripheral neuropathy, dizziness, confusion, irritability
or		
Tinidazole	2 g PO once daily × 5 days	Primarily GI side effects and disulfiram-like intolerance reaction to alcoholic beverages as for metronidazole
Followed by a luminal agent		
Paromomycin	30 mg/kg/day PO in 3 divided doses per day × 5-10 days	Primarily GI side effects: diarrhea, GI upset
or		
Diloxanide furoate	500 mg PO tid × 10 days	Primarily GI side effects: flatulence, nausea, vomiting Pruritus, urticaria
AMEBIC COLITIS		
Metronidazole	750 mg PO tid × 5-10 days	Same as for amebic liver abscess
Plus a luminal agent (same as for amebic liver abscess)		
ASYMPTOMATIC INTESTINAL COLONIZATION		
Treatment with a luminal agent as for amebic liver abscess		

GI = gastrointestinal; PO = per os (by mouth); tid = three times a day.
Modified from Haque R, Huston CD, Hughes M, et al. Current concepts: amebiasis. *N Engl J Med.* 2003;348:1565-1573.

TABLE 331-3 FREE-LIVING AMEBAE

ORGANISM	DISEASE	EPIDEMIOLOGY	DIAGNOSIS	CLINICAL COURSE	THERAPY
Naegleria fowleri	Primary amebic encephalitis	Warm freshwater exposure	CSF wet mount for amebae, PCR	Death within 1-2 weeks of onset	Combination therapy with amphotericin B, miltefosine, rifampin, fluconazole, and azithromycin
Acanthamoeba spp	Keratitis	Corneal trauma, usually from contact lens	Corneal scraping for amebae and cysts	Subacute	Polyhexamethylene biguanide, chlorhexidine, propamidine, hexamidine
Acanthamoeba spp	Granulomatous amebic encephalitis	Immunodeficient (organ transplants, HIV/AIDS)	Biopsy of brain or skin abscess—IFA or PCR	Subacute	Combination therapy with miltefosine, pentamidine, an azole (fluconazole or itraconazole), and/or sulfadiazine
Balamuthia mandrillaris	Granulomatous amebic encephalitis	Immunodeficient but also immunocompetent	Biopsy of brain	Subacute	Combination therapy with miltefosine, pentamidine, fluconazole, and sulfadiazine plus either azithromycin or clarithromycin
Sappinia	Amebic encephalitis	Single patient was not immunodeficient			Azithromycin, pentamidine, itraconazole, flucytosine

AIDS = acquired immunodeficiency syndrome; CSF = cerebrospinal fluid; HIV = human immunodeficiency virus; IFA = indirect fluorescent antibody; PCR = polymerase chain reaction.
Modified from Visvesvara GS, Moura H, Schuster FL. Pathogenic and opportunistic free-living amoebae: *Acanthamoeba* spp, *Balamuthia mandrillaris*, *Naegleria fowleri*, and *Sappinia diploidea*. *FEMS Immunol Med Microbiol*. 2007;50:1-26.

rates and adverse effects compared with metronidazole.[A1] In the rare case of fulminant amebic colitis, it is prudent to add broad-spectrum antibiotics to treat intestinal bacteria that may spill into the peritoneum. Parasites persist in up to half of the patients who are treated with a nitroimidazole, so treatment should be followed with paromomycin or the second-line agent diloxanide furoate to cure luminal infection. High-throughput drug screening has identified auranofin, a U.S. Food and Drug Administration–approved drug used for treatment of rheumatoid arthritis, as a potentially active agent against *E. histolytica*. Drainage of a liver abscess should be considered in patients who do not show a clinical response to drug therapy within 5 to 7 days or in those with a high risk for rupture of the abscess, as defined by a cavity with a diameter of greater than 5 cm or by the presence of lesions in the left lobe. Percutaneous needle aspiration or catheter drainage is the procedure of choice for drainage of a liver abscess. Surgical intervention is occasionally required for drainage of a liver abscess, acute abdomen, gastrointestinal bleeding, or toxic megacolon.

PREVENTION

The feasibility of prevention by vaccination with the parasite's Gal/GalNAc lectin is supported by substantial data from human, animal model, and in vitro studies.[11] This vaccine is in the late stages of preclinical development for the prevention of amebiasis in infants and children in the developing world. Provision of sanitation and clean water and safe sexual practices to prevent fecal-oral transmission are of great importance but not universally effective because of the low infectious dose and chlorine resistance of the cyst.[12]

PROGNOSIS

Therapy for amebiasis is highly effective. Drug resistance is not reported.

FREE-LIVING AMEBAE

Rare infections of the central nervous system can be seen with infection by free-living amebae of the genera *Naegleria*, *Balamuthia*, *Acanthamoeba*, and *Sappinia*. *Naegleria fowleri* is the agent of primary amebic meningoencephalitis, which occurs in previously healthy children and young adults who have swum in fresh water 2 to 5 days before the onset of meningoencephalitis. Cerebrospinal fluid has a polymorphonuclear predominance, and motile amebae can be seen in a wet mount of cerebrospinal fluid. The disease is relentlessly progressive to death in most patients. In one case of successful treatment, a combination of intrathecal and intravenous amphotericin B and miconazole and oral rifampin was used. *Acanthamoeba* can cause keratitis[13] in individuals with corneal injuries (usually from contact lens use), as well as granulomatous amebic encephalitis in the immunocompromised. Granulomatous amebic encephalitis is caused by Acanthamoeba, *Balamuthia*, and *Sappinia*[14]; it is usually associated with focal neurologic findings and has a subacute course. Miltefosine should be part of combination therapy (Table 331-3).

Grade A Reference

A1. Pandey S, Gupta GK, Wanjari SJ, et al. Comparative study of tinidazole versus metronidazole in treatment of amebic liver abscess: a randomized control trial. *Indian J Gastroenterol*. 2018;37: 196-201.

GENERAL REFERENCES

For the General References and other additional features, please visit Expert Consult at https://expertconsult.inkling.com.

332

BABESIOSIS AND OTHER PROTOZOAN DISEASES

SAM R. TELFORD, III, AND PETER J. KRAUSE

BABESIOSIS

Babesiosis is a tick-borne, malaria-like disease caused by sporozoan parasites of the genus *Babesia*.

EPIDEMIOLOGY

With few exceptions, *Babesia* spp are transmitted by ixodid ticks. Thus, wherever humans are intensely exposed to hard-bodied ticks, babesiosis should be part of the differential diagnosis for a patient presenting with fever and hematologic abnormalities.

Three worldwide epidemiologic patterns are apparent. The first involves the rodent-maintained *Babesia microti*, which is a species complex distributed across the Holarctic. A median of 1400 cases of *B. microti* babesiosis were reported each year from the northeastern United States and upper Midwestern states from 2011 through 2014, the first 4 years that human babesiosis has been designated as a notifiable infectious disease by the Centers for Disease Control and Prevention (CDC). By comparison, about 30,000 Lyme disease cases are reported each year in the United States, although both babesiosis and Lyme disease are thought to be underreported. The vector for *B. microti* is the same as that for Lyme disease (Chapter 305), the deer tick, *Ixodes dammini*, also known as northern populations of *I. scapularis*.[1] Indeed, concurrent babesiosis and Lyme disease is common. Immunocompetent as well as immunocompromised individuals are at risk. Within the last decade, *B. microti* has been increasingly reported in an expanded distribution in the United States from the original foci in coastal New England and the Upper Midwest, and it is possible that babesiosis cases eventually may be found wherever Lyme disease is intensely zoonotic. In addition, cases of *B. microti* or *B. microti*–like babesiosis have been reported from Australia, Canada, China, Germany, Japan, Poland, Spain, South Africa, and Taiwan; the vectors for these have not been definitively identified. The second pattern is represented by cases of babesiosis due to *Babesia divergens*, *B. divergens*–like, or closely related species (e.g., *Babesia venatorum*) that have been reported from Asia and Europe. Almost all cases in Europe have been in splenectomized patients residing in sites where castor bean ticks (*Ixodes ricinus*) and deer are common. *Babesia venatorum* recently has been found to be endemic in northeastern China. A few cases of *Babesia divergens*–like infections (referred to as MO-1) have been described in the United States. The third pattern of babesiosis involves sporadic cases due to diverse *Babesia* spp. These include *Babesia duncani* (WA-1) and CA-type parasites of the western United States; a *Babesia motasi*–like infection (KO-1) in Korea; and unidentified or poorly characterized *Babesia* spp from China, Colombia, Egypt, India, Mexico, Mozambique, and South Africa.

Although the known zoonotic tick vectors (*I. dammini, I. ricinus*) have marked seasonal periods of activity (May to August) and the majority of reported cases are acquired during these times, babesiosis may be diagnosed at any time of the year. More than 230 cases of transfusion-acquired babesiosis due to *B. microti* and three due to *B. duncani* have been reported. The actual number of cases is thought to be much greater. Babesiosis is currently the most commonly reported transfusion-transmitted disease in the United States, and the number of such cases is increasing, including those ending in death (Chapter 167). Cases occur throughout the year, and about 10% of cases occur in nonendemic areas because *Babesia*-infected blood is exported to nonendemic areas or persons become infected in endemic areas and subsequently donate blood in nonendemic areas. A few cases of transplacentally transmitted babesiosis have been reported.

PATHOBIOLOGY

The pathophysiology of *Babesia* infection is directly related to the development of parasitemia. Peripheral blood parasitemias of 70% or greater have been reported, although most cases sustain parasitemias on the order of 0.5 to 5%.

Excessive production of pro-inflammatory cytokines seems to best explain the most common clinical manifestations, which include fever, sweats, chills, headache, myalgia, nausea, vomiting, diarrhea, and pallor. Such findings are not seen when erythrocyte lysis is due to noninfectious causes, which suggests that the release of merozoites serves as a trigger for the pro-inflammatory cascade. Elevated serum concentrations of TNF as well as of interferon-γ, interleukins 2 and 6, E-selectin, vascular cell adhesion molecule 1, and intracellular cell adhesion molecule 1 are detected during the acute phase of human *B. microti* infection and return to baseline within 3 months after resolution of infection.

Severe illness caused by infection with *Babesia* includes a complex array of metabolic abnormalities and organ dysfunction. Pulmonary disease is the most common complication in people experiencing severe *Babesia* infection, with up to 20% of patients suffering from noncardiogenic pulmonary edema. Pro-inflammatory cytokines appear to mediate the pulmonary complications of *Babesia* infection, at least in part. It is also likely that lung and other end-organ disease is mediated, at least in part, by vascular stasis.

CLINICAL MANIFESTATIONS

About a quarter of *B. microti* infections in adults and half of those in children are subclinical.[2] This estimate is derived from an epidemiologic study that determined the frequency of people who seroconverted during the course of the summer transmission season but reported no illness, coupled with a careful accounting of symptomatic cases. Most people experience a mild to moderate illness lasting about a week. There is a gradual onset of malaise, anorexia, fatigue, fever (temperature as high as 40° C), sweats, and myalgia. Nausea, vomiting, headache, shaking chills, emotional lability, depression, hemoglobinuria, and hyperesthesia also have been reported. Findings on physical examination consist of fever, pallor, splenomegaly, and hepatomegaly. Laboratory abnormalities include anemia, thrombocytopenia, and leukopenia. Parasitemia generally ranges from barely detectable on blood smear to 5% in previously healthy people but may reach 85% in asplenic and other immunocompromised patients. Serum lactate dehydrogenase, bilirubin, and transaminase levels may be elevated in more severe cases. Persistent relapsing illness may occur in highly immunocompromised people who fail to clear the infection for months or more than a year despite multiple courses of antibiotics. The case-fatality rate for *B. microti* babesiosis has been estimated to be 6 to 9% in hospitalized patients but may be as high as 20% in immunocompromised hosts, including those who acquire the infection through blood transfusion. Review of the Medicare database (2006-2013) demonstrated that about 1%

of 10,000 cases in patients older than 65 years of age died within 30 days of diagnosis. Severe babesiosis usually occurs only in people with asplenia, malignant disease, coinfection with human immunodeficiency virus (HIV), organ transplants, immunosuppressive treatment, or age younger than 2 months or older than 50 years. About a third of treated asplenic babesiosis patients without history of autoimmune disease may suffer warm autoimmune hemolytic anemia that requires immunosuppressive treatment.[3]

Cases of babesiosis caused by *B. divergens* tend to be severe, at least in part because they are primarily reported in immunocompromised patients. Virtually all European patients experiencing *B. divergens* infection have been splenectomized, and about a third of the patients died. In these patients, there is an acute onset of illness with hemoglobinuria, a persistent nonperiodic high fever (temperature of 40° to 41° C), shaking chills, intense sweats, headaches, and myalgia, as well as lumbar and abdominal pain. Vomiting and diarrhea may occur. Pulmonary, renal, or liver failure may develop rapidly. In fatal cases, patients become comatose with multiorgan failure. *B. duncani, B. venatorum,* and *B. divergens*–like infections also have often been reported in immunocompromised hosts with a similarly severe course of illness. In contrast, *B. venatorum* infection in 48 immunocompetent patients in northeastern China was similar to that of *B. microti* infection, with full recovery of all patients, including seven patients who were admitted to hospital.

DIAGNOSIS

The diagnosis of babesiosis is based on epidemiologic and clinical findings and confirmed by laboratory testing. It should be considered in patients who live or travel in *Babesia* endemic regions or who have received a blood transfusion within the previous six months and whose clinical findings are consistent with babesiosis. The diagnosis may be confirmed by examination of a Giemsa-stained thin blood smear for the presence of parasites within erythrocytes. In immunocompromised patients, parasitemias are likely to exceed one infected cell per oil immersion field and thus are quickly detected. For *B. microti* babesiosis (Fig. 332-1), examination of a slide for 10 minutes or as many fields as needed to tally 200 leukocytes (that are not infected but serve as a marker for effort) and repeated smears performed twice a day may be required. Standard Romanowsky stains (Giemsa, Wright) using malaria protocols are optimal. Artifactual inclusions are limited mainly to stain precipitates (which can be determined by their presence in the plasma spaces between cells), Howell-Jolly or Heinz bodies (Chapter 148), or platelets superimposed on erythrocytes, which always have a light-colored halo when visualized this way. *Babesia* spp have clearly defined chromatin with a lighter-colored cytoplasm (Fig. 332-2A). They may be mistaken for early malarial trophozoites. Neither malarial nor babesial rings have hemozoin (malarial pigment), so this is not a good feature to distinguish between the two. Paired piriform parasites, arranged in a *v*, are suggestive of *B. divergens* or *B. divergens*–like infection (Fig. 332-2B). Rings of all sizes may be seen in all species. Multiple parasites may frequently be seen in single erythrocytes, as well as clumps of extracellular parasites. Tetrad forms (Fig. 332-2C) and Maltese cross forms (Fig. 332-2D) are diagnostic but are rarely seen in *B. microti* babesiosis. They seem to be more common with *B. duncani* or CA-type infections.

Polymerase chain reaction (PCR) assays are more sensitive than blood smears in cases in which parasitemias are sparse and may be as good as or better than a blood smear for making the diagnosis in clinical practice. Real-time PCR

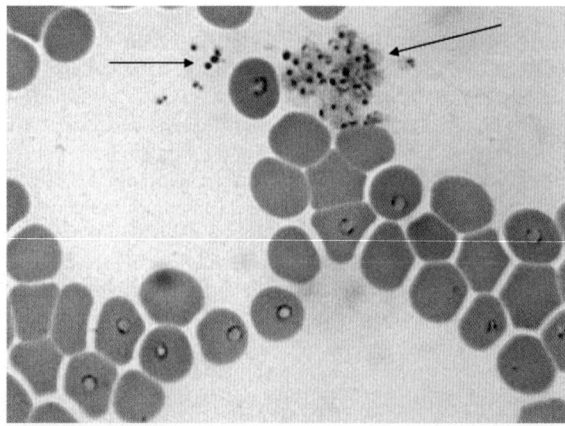

FIGURE 332-1. *Babesia microti.* Human infection, Nantucket Island. Predominance of ring forms with a cluster of extraerythrocytic parasites (*arrow*) free in the plasma.

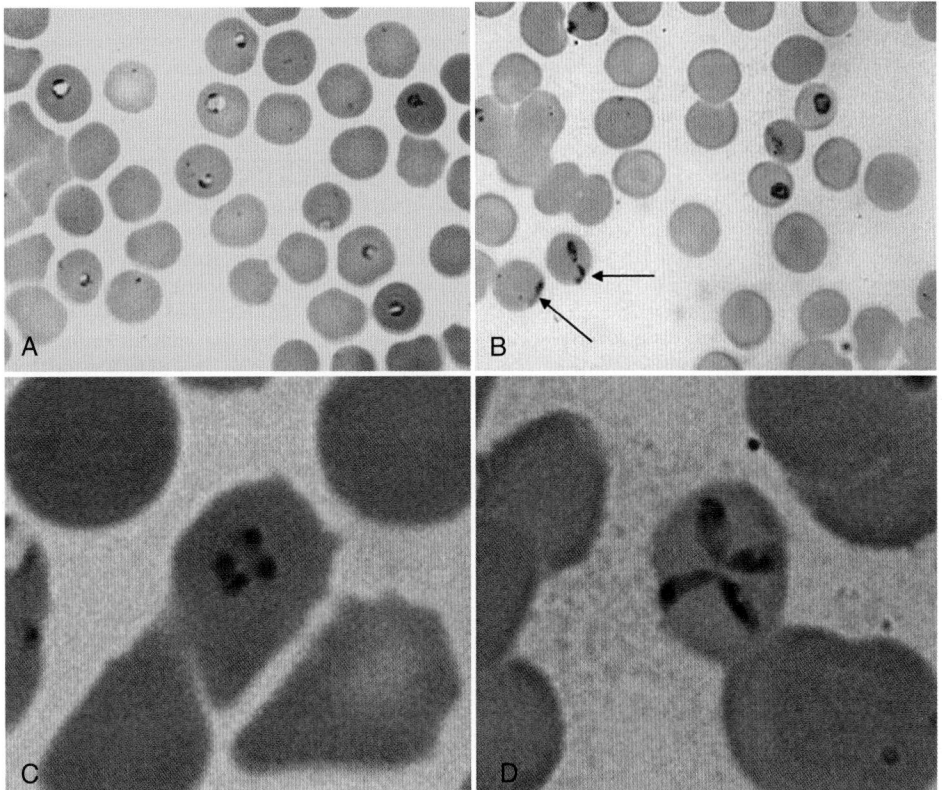

FIGURE 332-2. Diagnosis of *Babesia* infection. **A,** Typical thin-film field demonstrating ring forms of *B. microti* with vacuole or "whitish" cytoplasm demarcated by a dark-staining, defined chromatin. **B,** *B. Divergens*–like (MO-1) with robust rings; accolé form and paired piriform parasites are marked by *arrows*. **C,** Tetrad forms of *B. microti*. **D,** MO-1, classic Maltese cross. (Microscope slide from human case of MO-1 kindly provided by Dr. J. F. Beattie, Department of Pathology, The Medical Center, Bowling Green, Ky.)

assays performed in-house would provide confirmation nearly as quickly as microscopy with the added advantage of increased sensitivity.[4]

Serologic testing is useful for confirming *B. microti* infection. The indirect immunofluorescence test (IFAT), using antigen from infected hamster red cells, is sensitive and specific and is currently the serologic method of choice. Analysis of paired acute and convalescent serum samples is most useful for a confirmation of *B. microti* infection. The presence of parasite-specific IgM may indicate that the patient has an acute infection even in the absence of readily demonstrable parasitemia. Serology is not generally useful for *B. divergens* babesiosis (although the IFAT is generally sensitive and specific), given its fulminant natural history. Because parasitemia occurs before an antibody response and the doubling time of *B. divergens* can be as short as 8 hours, treatment needs to be initiated immediately on the basis of clinical suspicion and initial laboratory results. Serology for *B. duncani* is complicated by a high rate of false positives, and specificity depends on carefully establishing a diagnostic threshold dilution. Antigens for other of the *Babesia* spp infecting humans are not available.

The known vectors for human babesiosis are ticks that also transmit the agents of Lyme disease, human granulocytic anaplasmosis, *Borrelia miyamotoi* infection, *Ehrlichia muris*–like infection, and tick-borne encephalitis virus. Thus, coinfections should be considered in all patients with babesiosis. Acute illness in patients coinfected with Lyme disease and babesiosis is more severe and more persistent than in patients experiencing Lyme disease alone.

TREATMENT   (Rx)

Mild to moderate *B. microti* infection typically occurs in immunocompetent people. Therapy for these individuals should consist of the combination of atovaquone (750 mg orally twice daily for 7 to 10 days) and azithromycin (500 to 1000 mg initial dose followed by 250 mg orally daily for 7 to 10 days). For immunocompromised hosts, the azithromycin dose should be increased to 600 to 1000 mg orally daily for 7 to 10 days.[5,6] A prospective randomized trial demonstrated that patients treated with atovaquone and azithromycin cleared parasitemia as effectively as did those receiving clindamycin and quinine and with fewer side effects.

Severe babesiosis usually occurs in immunocompromised hosts, including premature infants, those over 50 years of age, people who have asplenia,

malignancy, HIV infection or who are on immunosuppressive medications. For severe babesiosis, a 7- to 10-day course of the combination of atovaquone (750 mg orally twice daily) and azithromycin (500 mg intravenously once a day) is recommended. An alternative combination is clindamycin (300 to 600 mg every 6 hours intravenously) and quinine (650 mg orally every 8 hours).

An incidental finding of parasites (e.g., during a manual CBC, or at a blood donation center that proactively performs screening) in an otherwise healthy individual would not require treatment.

Treatment may occasionally fail in high-risk patients or in those who must discontinue quinine because of side effects, such as severe tinnitus and gastrointestinal distress, or because of the rare occurrence of antibiotic resistance with atovaquone and azithromycin. A prolonged course of treatment may be required to clear parasitemia in certain immunocompromised patients, including those with B-cell lymphoma or other conditions treated with rituximab, patients with malignancy who also are asplenic, patients with organ or stem cell transplantation, and patients with HIV/AIDS. In such cases, combination therapy should be used that may include two or more of the following antimicrobials: artemisinin, atovaquone, azithromycin, clindamycin, doxycycline, atovaquone-proguanil (Malarone), pentamidine, quinine, and trimethoprim-sulfamethoxazole. Once an effective combination is identified, it should be continued for at least 6 weeks and 2 weeks beyond the time when *Babesia* can no longer be visualized on blood smear or blood samples become PCR negative. Other drugs have been demonstrated to be effective against *B. microti* in laboratory models (e.g., robenidine, primaquine, artesunate, and endochin-like quinolones) but await clinical trials.

Exchange transfusion should be considered in severely ill patients with parasitemias in excess of 10%, evidence of severe hemolysis, or organ compromise. In particularly severe babesiosis cases, partial or complete blood exchange transfusion (1 to 3 blood volumes) should be undertaken, in addition to treatment with atovaquone and azithromycin. Apheresis may help reduce circulating factors (e.g., inflammatory products liberated by the parasite) that contribute to pathology.

PREVENTION

Prevention depends on reducing the risk for tick bites. Immunocompromised individuals should be especially careful to use personal protection and may even consider avoiding highly endemic sites such as coastal New England and Long Island in the United States during May through July, when risk is the greatest. Use of repellants such as DEET or application of permethrin to clothing will greatly reduce tick attachment. Such products should be applied to shoes, socks, and trouser cuffs. Wearing light-colored long pants and tucking the cuffs into socks will also help prevent ticks from gaining access to attachment sites. Daily examination for attached ticks should be performed; the best way to do this is to feel for new bumps on a soapy body in the shower. Any attached ticks should be promptly removed by simple traction, which is best accomplished with the use of tweezers, as illustrated in Figure 311-3 in Chapter 311. As with the agent of Lyme disease, ticks must be attached at least 36 to 48 hours before a sufficient inoculum of *Babesia* sporozoites is delivered. Community-level prevention should focus on public education about the risks of tick-borne infection, reducing habitat for ticks (brush removal and landscaping around yards), or reducing the reproductive hosts for the tick. Deer reduction will reduce the abundance of the deer tick vector for *B. microti* babesiosis. Screening blood donations for *B. microti* antibodies and *B. microti* DNA (using PCR) can decrease the risk of transfusion-associated babesiosis.[7,8]

PROGNOSIS

Death may occur in patients with severe babesiosis, but other long-term sequelae have not been reported for patients who have been adequately treated. In most patients who complete a full treatment regimen, *B. microti* DNA becomes undetectable by PCR within 3 months. Infection does not imply protective immunity based on laboratory rodent models, although subsequent infections are limited in duration and intensity. Recrudescent infections have been reported, mainly in immunocompromised individuals.

MISCELLANEOUS ENTERIC PROTOZOA

The gastrointestinal and urogenital tracts may contain representatives of the four major groupings of protozoa (amebae, sporozoa, flagellates, and ciliates). Diarrhea and other lower gastrointestinal signs and symptoms may be caused by diverse protozoa. Specific clinical diagnosis is difficult because expert clinical parasitology support is required to determine whether an agent that has been detected in a stool sample is a pathogenic species. However, new point-of-care antigen detection tests, or nucleic acid amplification tests (NAAT) are sensitive and specific when they can be used. Identification is necessary because treatment options differ by the agent. With the exception of *Trichomonas vaginalis* infection (sexually transmitted), all of the enteric protozoa are acquired by the ingestion of food or materials contaminated by human feces; a small subset may have extraintestinal manifestations. Given a shared mode of transmission (fecal-oral), demonstrating the presence of any one of these protozoa within a stool sample from a patient is justification for an intensified search for those that are recognized as clinically significant pathogens (*Entamoeba histolytica*, *Giardia lamblia/intestinalis*, *Cyclospora cayetanensis*, *Cystoisospora belli*, and *Cryptosporidium parvum/hominis*). Other protozoa, many of which morphologically resemble true pathogens, are commonly detected within stools of patients with lower gastrointestinal disturbances, but support for their role as etiologic agents is weak.

Cryptosporidiosis (Chapter 329), giardiasis (Chapter 330), and amebiasis (Chapter 331) are discussed in separate chapters. Trichomoniasis and coccidian enteritis are discussed here because they are relatively common infections.

Trichomoniasis
EPIDEMIOLOGY

Trichomonas vaginalis is among the most prevalent of all pathogenic protozoa and is one of the most common sexually transmitted infections in the United States and likely worldwide.[9] As many as 30% of female college students and 40% of pregnant Nigerian women were found to be infected. The highest incidence of infection occurs in women with multiple sexual partners and those with other sexually transmitted diseases (Chapter 269): 24% of HIV-positive South African women presenting for their first antenatal screening were infected by *T. vaginalis* and 4.5% of 10,000 women presenting to U.K. STD clinics for chlamydia and gonorrhea testing by NAAT were found to be infected by *T. vaginalis*. *T. vaginalis* also can be passed from infected mothers to their newborn daughters, but it is seldom symptomatic in girls before menarche. The parasite is able to survive for some time in moist environments, and nonvenereal transmission, although uncommon, can occur. Trichomoniasis, like other sexually transmitted diseases, may increase the likelihood of transmission of HIV.

PATHOBIOLOGY

T. vaginalis, known colloquially as a flagellate, is classified in the phylum Metamonada and class Parabasalia, along with another human pathogen,

Dientamoeba fragilis (previously thought to be an ameba). The 10- to 15-μm-long trophozoites multiply by longitudinal binary fission on the epithelial surface of the vagina or urethra as well as in vaginal or urethral secretions and are thereby transmitted by sexual intercourse. No cyst form is known, and the trophozoites are easily killed by drying.

CLINICAL MANIFESTATIONS

Trichomoniasis is one of three common causes of vaginitis or vaginosis (along with bacterial vaginosis and vulvovaginal candidiasis).[10] It is characterized by a thin gray to yellowish green frothy discharge; vulvovaginal erythema; ectocervical erythema or "strawberry cervix," observable mainly by colposcopy; pH higher than 4.5; increased presence of polymorphonuclear leukocytes; and a positive result of the whiff test, in which a foul fishy odor is intensified on addition of potassium hydroxide. The incubation period for trichomoniasis is 5 to 28 days. In addition to a frothy discharge, vaginitis can be accompanied by vulvovaginal irritation, dyspareunia, abdominal pain, and dysuria. Symptoms may worsen during menstruation. Population-based studies indicate that as many as half of *T. vaginalis* infections in women and the majority in men are asymptomatic. *T. vaginalis* can frequently be isolated from the male partners of infected women and can produce symptomatic urethritis. Urethral discharge is generally scant in these cases. Pharyngitis with positive *T. vaginalis* NAAT has been reported. Rarely, *T. vaginalis* is associated with epididymitis, superficial penile ulcerations that are usually located under the prepuce, or prostatitis. *T. vaginalis* infection is not associated with a greater risk of advancement of prostate cancer.

DIAGNOSIS

The CDC guidelines (http://www.cdc.gov/std/treatment/2010/vaginal-discharge.htm#a2) state that all women with a sexually transmitted infection should be specifically tested for evidence of *T. vaginalis* infection, and HIV-positive women should be tested annually. The WHO vaginal discharge syndromic management/vaginal discharge flowchart for diagnosis of trichomoniasis has 99.93% positive predictive value.[11] In women, vaginal and urethral secretions should be examined. *T. vaginalis* is seen in wet mounts of vaginal secretions in approximately 60% of infected women, thus confirming the diagnosis. Live *T. vaginalis* have a twitching or tumbling motion in wet mounts, and polymorphonuclear leukocytes are usually present. Direct immunofluorescent antibody staining is more sensitive than wet mounts but technically more difficult. Culture is an even more sensitive method of diagnosis; commercial kits for culture are available, but the results are not available for 3 to 7 days. *T. vaginalis* is occasionally identified in Papanicolaou-stained smears; Giemsa stain may also be used (Fig. 332-3). For men, a wet mount of material from a platinum loop scraping of the anterior urethra reveals the organism in approximately half the cases. Prostatic massage before collection of urine for *Trichomonas* culture is a more sensitive diagnostic approach. *T. vaginalis* is not found in the gastrointestinal tract, and the presence of trichomonads in wet fecal mounts or stained fixed fecal smears (iron hematoxylin or trichrome) most likely represents the commensal *Pentatrichomonas* (formerly *Trichomonas*) *hominis*. Serology has limited clinical use because of issues of sensitivity and specificity and because evidence of exposure does not imply current disease.

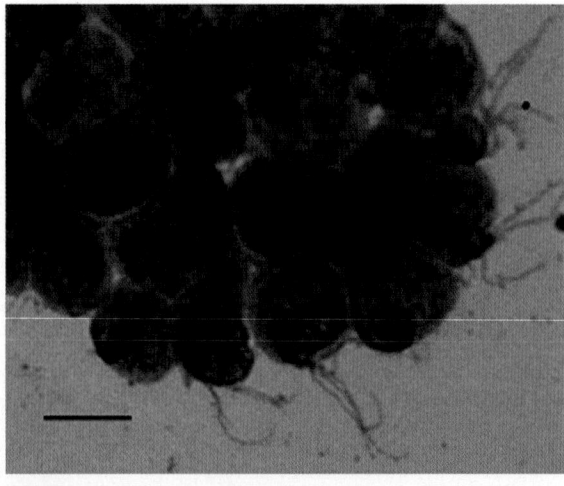

FIGURE 332-3. *Trichomonas vaginalis,* Giemsa-stained smear of cultivated trophozoites. (Bright-field microscopy, ×630. Scale bar is 15 μm.)

Diverse CLIA-waived, CLIA moderate level, or FDA-approved rapid point-of-care tests are now available, as are NAAT through commercial clinical laboratories, all of which have excellent sensitivities and specificities[12] and almost always outperform the classical microscopy based tests.

TREATMENT Rx
(also see Chapter 323)

Tinidazole, a single 2-g oral dose in adults, or metronidazole, either as a single 2-g oral dose or 500 mg twice daily for 7 days, is the treatment of choice with 7-day treatment providing a higher cure rate.[A1] Tinidazole is the better tolerated of the two. Single-dose therapy (metronidazole or tinidazole) ensures compliance of the patient but can produce nausea and a metallic taste, particularly with metronidazole. Both tinidazole and metronidazole have a disulfiram-like effect, and patients who consume alcohol within 24 hours of metronidazole or 72 hours of tinidazole may experience severe nausea, vomiting, and flushing. The use of tinidazole and metronidazole is relatively contraindicated during pregnancy, given the lack of well-controlled studies. Treatment failures with metronidazole are uncommon but well documented. HIV-positive women should be treated for 7 days with 500 mg per day of metronidazole because of frequent recrudescence with the single-dose therapy. Some instances of treatment failure in immune-intact women result from reinfection, others from poor compliance, but some are caused by metronidazole-resistant parasites. A repeated course of metronidazole (2 g orally daily for 5 days) may be tried. If patients remain refractory to appropriate treatment, metronidazole sensitivity can be tested by the CDC (available at www.dpd.cdc.gov/dpdx/HTML/DiagnosticProcedures.htm). Metronidazole gel delivered intravaginally does not achieve therapeutic levels but clinical improvement has been documented with intravaginal boric acid.

PREVENTION

Condoms (male or female) reduce risk of acquiring trichomoniasis. Sexual partners should be treated concurrently to prevent reinfection because nearly 20% of male partners are coinfected.

PROGNOSIS

Rare complications include pelvic inflammatory disease. Infection during gestation may lead to fetal growth retardation. There is no natural or acquired immunity, so reinfection may be common.

Coccidian Enteritis
EPIDEMIOLOGY

The coccidia, with 43 genera and more than 1700 recognized species, are well-known veterinary pathogens. At least two of the coccidia, *Cyclospora cayetanensis* (an eimeriid) and *Cystoisospora belli* (a sarcocystid), are causative agents of enteritis in humans. Despite their ubiquity (nearly 100 species have been described), *Sarcocystis* spp have been rare causes of human enteritis and an even less common cause of myositis,[13] although *Sarcocystis nesbitti* caused a disease comprising fever, myalgia, headache, and myositis in 89 college students who had traveled to Malaysia. *C. cayetanensis* may have both an animal and human reservoir, but *C. belli* is thought to be an anthroponosis. Cyclosporiasis is a cause of gastroenteritis in tropical and subtropical areas, with Peru, Mexico, Haiti, Caribbean countries, and Nepal commonly reporting such cases. During 1996 to 2016, 595 cases of cyclosporiasis were reported through FoodNet [https://wwwn.cdc.gov/foodnetfast/] but this surveillance program comprises only 10 states (15% of the U.S. population). Outbreaks involving hundreds of cases are common and invariably traced to contaminated fresh produce such as raspberries, basil, snow peas, or mesclun. Such outbreaks have a distinct seasonality, with most cases presenting during June and July. Cyclosporiasis is commonly diagnosed in international travelers, and large outbreaks have been reported from cruise ships.

Isosporiasis/cystoisosporiasis remains understudied despite it being described in military patients during World War I. It is mainly reported from AIDS patients.

PATHOBIOLOGY

Oocysts are passed in feces and must sporulate for at least a day (*C. belli*) or 5 to 11 days (*C. cayetanensis*) before attaining infectivity. Sporozoites are liberated in the small bowel, penetrating enterocytes (for *C. cayetanensis*, mainly in the jejunum). *C. cayetanensis* appears to have a complicated developmental cycle with at least two merogonic cycles in the bowel, leading to the formation of gametes. The gametes fuse within the enterocyte cytoplasm, and an oocyst

wall is deposited around the zygote. The sexual cycle begins about a week after infection, with oocysts sloughing into the bowel lumen and subsequently out of the body through feces. Biopsy specimens from infected patients demonstrate mononuclear and eosinophilic infiltrates in the lamina propria as well as alterations to the morphology of villi. Humans appear to be intermediate hosts for certain *Sarcocystis* spp, with sporozoites liberated in the small bowel, entering the vasculature, and forming cysts in muscle.

CLINICAL MANIFESTATIONS

After an incubation period of approximately 1 week, either organism produces watery diarrhea, nausea, vomiting, abdominal pain, myalgias, anorexia, and fatigue. Illness is usually self-limited, but symptoms can be prolonged (10 to 12 weeks) and associated with steatorrhea, flatulence, and substantial weight loss in persons who are immunocompromised, especially those with AIDS. Infections may also be asymptomatic. With *S. nesbitti*, fever and prominent myalgias are the dominant presentation. Cystoisospora has been detected in the gallbladder and apparently causes a subclinical infection in immunocompetent individuals, but is associated with acalculous cholecystitis in immunosuppressed patients.[14] Sarcocystosis may comprise infection with zoonotic species or with those that have humans as definitive hosts. With the former, diverse species cause aberrant infection with a tropism to muscle; myalgias and edema may result. The latter usually colonize the intestinal epithelium but are not associated with disease. Rarely, a diarrheal disease may result. Both kinds of sarcocystosis are acquired by ingesting poorly cooked meat.

DIAGNOSIS

The diagnosis is confirmed by identifying coccidia in stool samples stained with modified acid-fast or modified safranin preparations or by phase contrast microscopy or bright-field microscopy (using iodine as a contrast medium) of wet mounts (Fig. 332-4). *C. cayetanensis* and *C. belli* may be sensitively detected by fluorescent microscopy of wet mounts. The CDC can help confirm the identification of these enteric protozoa by telediagnosis (sending a digital image of suspicious microscopy findings). PCR is specific and can be sensitive, depending on the mode of DNA extraction, but there are no FDA-approved assays available; PCR support may be requested from the CDC through state public health departments. *S. nesbitti* and likely other zoonotic *Sarcocystis* spp appear to undergo an aberrant asexual cycle only within humans and may not produce oocysts to be liberated into the bowel; therefore, diagnosis has required muscle biopsy and demonstration of sarcocysts by histology or detection of the agent's DNA by PCR.

TREATMENT Rx

Rehydration is important, as it is for any severe diarrheal disease. Both infections may respond to treatment with 160 mg trimethoprim and 800 mg sulfamethoxazole taken twice daily for 7 to 10 days. HIV-infected patients may require a longer course of therapy. The widespread use of trimethoprim-sulfamethoxazole (Bactrim) prophylaxis for *Pneumocystis* has reduced the incidence of coccidial diarrhea in patients with HIV infection. No specific treatment has been recommended for sarcocystosis.

PREVENTION

At the community level, preventing the contamination of water and food (mainly vegetables and fruits) by animal or human feces reduces the risk of transmission. Washing vegetables and fruits in water will reduce the potential inoculum but does not eliminate all risk. Sarcocystosis may be prevented by ensuring that meat is well cooked.

PROGNOSIS

Reactive arthritis, Guillain-Barré syndrome, Reiter syndrome, cholecystitis, and cholangitis have been reported as complications of either coccidian enteritis, mainly in patients with AIDS. Otherwise, treatment appears to eradicate the organism. Whether reinfection may occur is not known. Reports of extraintestinal development of *C. belli* and *C. cayetanensis* suggest the possibility of reinvasion of the bowel with ensuing recrudescence of signs and symptoms.

Other Enteric Protozoans

A number of other protozoa transmitted by fecal-oral contamination have been associated with enteric disease (Table 332-1). Microsporidia have classically been considered to be protozoa but are now known to be obligately

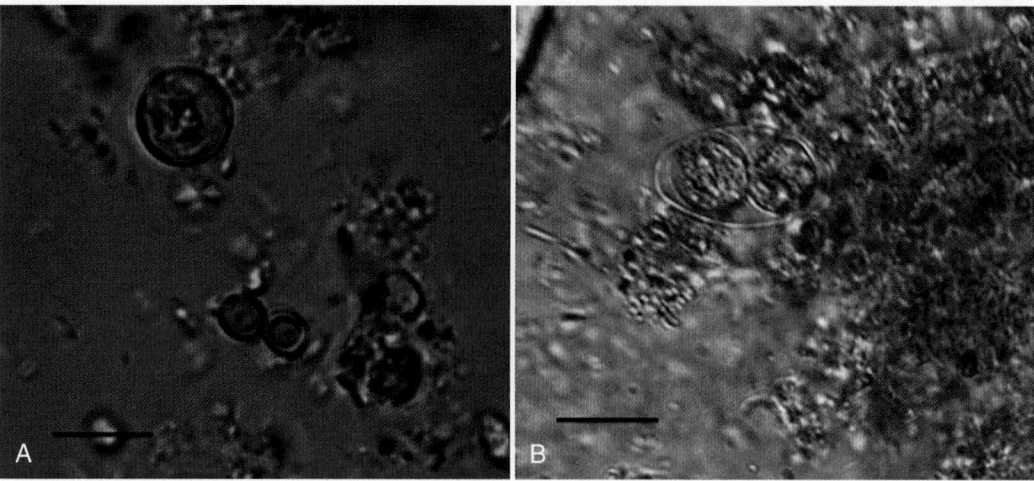

FIGURE 332-4. Diagnosis of coccidian enteritis. **A,** *Cyclospora cayetanensis*, seen on formalin-fixed human feces, unsporulated. (Bright-field microscopy, ×1000 with green contrast filter. Scale bar is 10 μm.) Note the doublet of yeast cells in lower right of the photomicrograph. **B,** *Cystoisospora belli*, seen on formalin-fixed human feces, partially sporulated. (Bright-field microscopy, ×400. Scale bar is 15 μm.)

TABLE 332-1　OTHER ENTERIC PROTOZOA

ORGANISM	EPIDEMIOLOGY	MANIFESTATIONS	THERAPY*
Balantidium coli	Primarily an infection of animals, especially pigs, but also affects humans	Asymptomatic or mild and self-resolving; occasionally more severe with abdominal pain, blood, and mucus in stool	Tetracycline (500 mg qid for 10 days) Alternative: metronidazole (750 mg tid for 5 days) or iodoquinol (650 mg tid for 20 days)
Blastocystis hominis	Probably worldwide, including North America; often found concomitantly with *Giardia lamblia*	Pathogenicity is debated	The need for treatment is debated, but symptomatic improvement has been reported with metronidazole (750 mg tid for10 days), or trimethoprim-sulfamethoxazole (160 mg TMP/800 mg SMX bid for 7 days)
Dientamoeba fragilis	Worldwide distribution; frequently found concomitantly with the pinworm *Enterobius*	Often asymptomatic; diarrhea reported	Paromomycin (25-35 mg/kg body weight per day in 3 doses for 7 days), metronidazole (500-750 mg tid for 10 days), or iodoquinol (650 mg tid for 20 days)
Microsporidia[†] (*Enterocytozoon bieneusi, Encephalitozoon intestinalis, Anncaliia* sp, *Tubulinosema* sp, *Nosema* sp, *Pleistophora* sp, *Vittaforma* sp)	Apparent worldwide distribution	AIDS patients with persistent diarrhea and wasting; self-limited cases in immunocompetent persons; ocular disease is increasingly recognized	Oral fumagillin (20 mg tid) has been effective for *E. bieneusi*, but it has been associated with thrombocytopenia. Albendazole (400 mg bid) has been effective for *E. intestinalis*. Treatment with HAART may lead to clinical response in HIV-infected patients with microsporidial diarrhea.
Sarcocystis species	Worldwide distribution, more commonly in sites of cattle or swine production	Often asymptomatic; nausea, vomiting, abdominal pain, and diarrhea may occur; eosinophilic necrotizing enteritis has been reported. Infection is usually asymptomatic for *S. hominis* and *S. suihominis* for which humans are definitive hosts (parasites undergo sexual reproduction); zoonotic *Sarcocystis* spp cause aberrant infection with muscle tropism, causing myalgias and edema.	No specific therapy

*Based on CDC recommendations, www.cdc.gov/parasites/az/index.html. Accessed May 9, 2019. The dosages and durations are for adults.
†Associated with persistent, severe diarrhea in persons with AIDS.
AIDS = acquired immunodeficiency syndrome; HAART = highly active antiretroviral therapy; HIV = human immunodeficiency virus.

intracellular fungi[15]; they are a diverse group and at least 7 genera have been implicated as human pathogens. They are discussed here because diagnostic parasitology laboratories continue to confirm diagnoses of these agents. *Dientamoeba, Blastocystis, Balantidium*, and some of the microsporidia reside in the lumen of the bowel, and others invade and multiply within enterocytes; heavy infection may result in diarrhea. Some of the microsporidia cause conjunctivitis or other ocular disease. Enteric protozoa should be considered in the differential diagnosis of patients with persistent diarrhea and abdominal symptoms, particularly those with a history of recent international travel. A clinical diagnosis is rarely possible; laboratory tests, mainly for ova and parasites in stools, establish the diagnosis. Expert microscopists are required because these parasites may be confused with fecal debris. Pathogenic protozoa must also be differentiated from commensals such as *Entamoeba coli, Endolimax nana, Iodamoeba bütschlii, Pentatrichomonas hominis*, and *Chilomastix mesnili*. Therapy includes administration of the appropriate antiprotozoal drug and rehydration, as listed in Table 332-1 (also see Chapter 323).

Grade A Reference

A1. Kissinger P, Muzny CA, Mena LA, et al. Single-dose versus 7-day-dose metronidazole for the treatment of trichomoniasis in women: an open-label, randomised controlled trial. *Lancet Infect Dis.* 2018;18:1251-1259.

GENERAL REFERENCES

For the General References and other additional features, please visit Expert Consult at https://expertconsult.inkling.com.

333

CESTODES

A. CLINTON WHITE, JR., AND ENRICO BRUNETTI

DEFINITION
The Pathogens

Cestode parasites are members of the animal kingdom, subphylum Cestoda. The organisms are characterized by several life cycle stages, which typically develop in distinct hosts. The adult stage is the tapeworm, which is acquired by ingestion of uncooked tissues harboring larval forms. After ingestion, the larvae excyst and the scolex attaches to the intestines. Segments, termed *proglottids*, develop at the base of the scolex and are displaced from the scolex by new proglottids to form a chain or tapeworm. The host in which the tapeworm develops is termed the *definitive host*. The proglottids contain male and female sexual organs and produce large numbers of ova. The proglottids or their ova are shed in stools. Humans are the definitive hosts for a number of different tapeworms, including the *Taenia* species, *Diphyllobothrium* species, and *Hymenolepis nana*. Humans can also be an accidental host for the dog and cat tapeworms of the genus *Dipylidium* (Table 333-1).

The intermediate hosts harbor the larval form of the parasite. Infection follows ingestion of the ova. Under the influence of gastric and intestinal fluids, the ova hatch, releasing the invasive larvae (oncospheres), which migrate to tissues, forming tissue forms. The forms in tissue vary between organisms and may include the cysticercus (a bladder containing a single invaginated scolex), the coenurus (a bladder with multiple scolices), the hydatid (a cystic structure with a germinal layer, which forms numerous protoscolices), or the plerocercoid (a solid form seen in *Spirometra* species). Humans can harbor the intermediate forms of *Taenia solium* (cysticercosis), *Echinococcus granulosus* group (cystic hydatid disease), *Echinococcus multilocularis* (alveolar hydatid disease), and rarely other organisms (Table 333-2). Humans can serve as both the definitive host and an intermediate host for two species, *T. solium* and *H. nana*. In the case of *T. solium*, humans are the obligate host for the tapeworm stage (pork tapeworm) but can also harbor the cystic form (cysticercosis). In the case of *H. nana*, both stages typically develop in a single person, with the cysticercoid form in the intestinal wall and the tapeworm in the lumen.

INTESTINAL TAPEWORM INFECTIONS
Diphyllobothrium Species (Fish Tapeworm)

Diphyllobothrium tapeworms are large segmented parasites that are acquired by ingestion of undercooked or pickled freshwater fish dishes (sushi, sashimi, ceviche, carpaccio, gefilte fish). The tapeworms develop within a few weeks and can live for more than 10 years.

EPIDEMIOLOGY AND PATHOBIOLOGY

Diphyllobothrium species are found worldwide, including foci in Europe, North and South America, and Asia. Perhaps 20 million people are thought to be infected worldwide. Major foci include Russia, Japan, and South America. Disease was formerly highly endemic in Scandinavia, where it is now rarely diagnosed.

In most cases, infection has little impact on the host. However, one species, *Diphyllobothrium latum*, contains vitamin B_{12} receptors on the surface of the tapeworm, which can out-compete the host, leading to vitamin B_{12} deficiency (Chapter 155). This manifestation has been described only in Scandinavia.

CLINICAL MANIFESTATIONS AND DIAGNOSIS

In most of those infected, *Diphyllobothrium* species produce few or no symptoms. Some may complain of gastrointestinal symptoms (abdominal discomfort, nausea, weight loss). The main clinical manifestation is the observation of proglottids being passed in stool. Pernicious anemia with symptoms of anemia or peripheral neuropathy may develop with *D. latum* infection. The diagnosis depends on observation of the characteristic operculated eggs in stool.

TREATMENT AND PREVENTION   Rx

A single oral dose of praziquantel (5 to 10 mg/kg) is usually adequate for therapy (Table 333-3). Niclosamide can be used as an alternative (2 g [adults] or 50 mg/kg [children] in a single dose chewed and swallowed), but it is not available in the United States. Parasites in fish can be killed by cooking (>56° C, >5 minutes) or freezing (−20° C, 24 hours). Infected fish may also be identified by inspection.

Hymenolepis nana

Hymenolepis nana is the human dwarf tapeworm. *Hymenolepis diminuta*, a rat tapeworm, can also cause human infection.

EPIDEMIOLOGY AND PATHOBIOLOGY

H. nana is prevalent worldwide, with estimates of at least 50 to 75 million people infected. Infection follows ingestion of ova. The larvae are released, invade, and develop into cysticercoid forms in the intestinal villi. After a few days, the cysticercoids mature, invade the lumen, and are transformed into a scolex, forming small tapeworms (up to 5 cm long), which begin producing eggs within 2 to 3 weeks. Autoinfection either in the intestines or by the fecal-oral route can lead to heavy infection.

CLINICAL MANIFESTATIONS AND DIAGNOSIS

Most infections are asymptomatic. However, some children may be infected by hundreds or thousands of worms, which can cause abdominal pain, loose stools, diarrhea, and malabsorption. Diagnosis depends on observation of the characteristic eggs in stool. More than one specimen may be required.

TABLE 333-2 HUMAN LARVAL CESTODE INFECTIONS

ORGANISM	COMMON NAME	ORGANS INVOLVED
Taenia solium	Cysticercosis	Brain, spinal fluid, eye, muscle
Echinococcus granulosus group	Cystic hydatid disease	Liver, lung, other
Echinococcus multilocularis	Alveolar hydatid disease	Liver
Taenia multiceps, Taenia spp	Coenurosis	Brain, eyes
Spirometra species	Sparganosis	Subcutaneous tissue, viscera

TABLE 333-1 COMMON HUMAN TAPEWORM INFECTIONS

ORGANISM	INTERMEDIATE HOST	COMMON NAME	CLINICAL PRESENTATION	TREATMENT
Diphyllobothrium spp	Fish	Fish tapeworm	Passing segments, pernicious anemia	Praziquantel, niclosamide
Hymenolepis nana	Humans	Dwarf tapeworm	Asymptomatic, diarrhea	Praziquantel, niclosamide
Taenia saginata	Cattle	Beef tapeworm	Asymptomatic, passing segments	Praziquantel, niclosamide
Taenia asiatica	Pigs	Asian tapeworm	Asymptomatic, passing worms	Praziquantel, niclosamide
Taenia solium	Pigs	Pork tapeworm	Asymptomatic, passing segments	Praziquantel, niclosamide
Dipylidium caninum	Fleas	Dog tapeworm	Passing segments	Praziquantel, niclosamide

TABLE 333-3 THERAPY FOR INTESTINAL TAPEWORM INFECTIONS

	PRAZIQUANTEL	NICLOSAMIDE	NITAZOXANIDE
Dosage			
Adults	5-10 mg/kg for all age groups (25 mg/kg for *Hymenolepis nana*)	2 g (4 tablets)	500 mg
Children >34 kg		1.5 g (3 tablets)	200 mg
Children 11-34 kg		1 g (2 tablets)	100 mg
Administration	Taken as a single dose	Taken as a single dose; tablets must be chewed and swallowed	Taken twice a day for 3 days
Side effects	Mild but frequent, including dizziness, myalgias, nausea, vomiting, diarrhea, abdominal pain	Nausea, vomiting, abdominal pain, diarrhea, drowsiness, dizziness, headache, pruritus	
Pregnancy		No known mutagenic effects; considered safe if indicated	

TREATMENT AND PREVENTION

Praziquantel (15 to 25 mg/kg as a single oral dose) is usually effective in treating *H. nana* infection,[1] but it may need to be repeated in heavy infection (see Table 333-3). Nitazoxanide (100 mg by mouth twice daily for 3 days for children 1 to 3 years of age, 200 mg by mouth twice daily for 3 days for children 4 to 11 years of age, and 500 mg by mouth twice daily for 3 days for older children) is a reasonable alternative therapy; efficacy is about 75 to 82%. Niclosamide also can be used as an alternative, but must be continued for 7 days. Transmission is by the fecal-oral route and could be prevented by improved hygiene. Mass chemotherapy has been used to control infection in some populations.

Dipylidium caninum

Dipylidium caninum is a common tapeworm of dogs and cats. Dogs are infected by ingestion of fleas, which carry the cysticercoid form in their body cavities. The tapeworms can also develop in children who have ingested the fleas. It is widespread worldwide, but human infections are unusual.

CLINICAL MANIFESTATIONS AND DIAGNOSIS

Infection may be asymptomatic. In some cases, the motile proglottids may be noted in stool. The proglottids are similar in size and shape to rice grains. Diagnosis depends on identification of the ova in stool or identification of the proglottids.

TREATMENT AND PREVENTION

There are no controlled trials of treatment for *Dipylidium* infection, but infection is likely to respond to regimens used for other tapeworms (see Table 333-3). The main measure for prevention is treatment of pets for fleas and tapeworms.

Taenia saginata

Taeniasis refers to infection with the tapeworm form of one of three *Taenia* species. *Taenia solium* and *Taenia asiatica* are acquired from ingestion of undercooked pork. *Taenia saginata*, called the beef tapeworm, is a common intestinal infection worldwide. Cattle are the intermediate hosts, harboring the tissue cysticerci in their muscle. Humans are the obligate definitive host, harboring the tapeworm form.

EPIDEMIOLOGY AND PATHOBIOLOGY

T. saginata is common worldwide in areas where cattle are raised and human fecal material contaminates the pastures. Approximately 45 to 60 million people are thought to be infected. It is found on most continents. Very high rates (>20% of the population) have been noted in east Africa, Bali, and Tibet. It is likewise endemic in the Middle East, the Americas, and Europe. *T. saginata* is also common in other parts of Asia, but many of the epidemiologic studies did not differentiate *T. saginata* from *T. asiatica*.

T. saginata tapeworms are acquired by ingestion of undercooked beef. The scolex attaches to the intestinal wall, and proglottids form at the base of the scolex. The proglottids gradually enlarge as they are displaced from the scolex by newer proglottids. The chain of proglottids can reach a length of up to 30 feet. The terminal proglottids are shed periodically in the stool. Terminal proglottids are typically off-white, 2 to 3 cm long, 0.5 to 1 cm wide, and 1 to 2 mm thick.

CLINICAL MANIFESTATIONS AND DIAGNOSIS

Mild symptoms (e.g., nausea, abdominal discomfort, anorexia, and pruritus) may be noted. The motile proglottids may cause discomfort as they exit the anus or may be noted in stool.

Ova may be noted in stool. The ova are 40 μm in diameter, surrounded by brown radial striations, and the embryos have six hooks. However, the ova of the three *Taenia* species are morphologically indistinguishable. The proglottids can be distinguished from those of *T. solium* by counting the number of uterine branches (≥14 branches suggests *T. saginata*). However, the proglottids of *T. saginata* cannot be readily distinguished from *T. asiatica*.

TREATMENT, PREVENTION, AND PROGNOSIS

Taeniasis can be treated with praziquantel in a single dose (see Table 333-3). Single doses of niclosamide are also effective. Nitazoxanide has also been used for *T. saginata*. Taeniasis can be prevented by inspection of beef. Also, cooking to 56° C for 5 minutes or freezing at −20° C for 7 to 10 days destroys the infective larvae. Only minor symptoms are noted and are eventually self-limited with or without treatment.

Taenia asiatica

T. asiatica is a cause of taeniasis in Asia, termed *Asian taeniasis*. Infection is acquired by ingestion of undercooked pork. Pigs are infected by ingestion of the ova from tapeworm carriers. *T. asiatica* has been widely described in China, Taiwan, Korea, Indonesia, and Southeast Asia. The clinical manifestations, diagnosis, treatment, and prevention of *T. asiatica* infection are similar to those noted for *T. saginata* infection.

Taenia solium

T. solium, also known as the pork tapeworm, can cause both tapeworm infection and larval infection termed *cysticercosis*. *T. solium* tapeworm infections are caused by ingestion of infected undercooked pork. The scolex evaginates and attaches to the intestines, forming proglottids. The proglottids gradually mature as they are separated from the scolex by new proglottids. The adult worms are often 10 to 20 feet long. Within the mature proglottids, thousands of microscopic ova develop. The ova are either excreted into the stool or shed with the proglottids. By contrast, ingestion of the ova results in development of larval infection, termed cysticercosis (see later). Thus, the tapeworm carrier poses risk of self-infection as well as infection to other people.

EPIDEMIOLOGY AND PATHOBIOLOGY

T. solium is common worldwide in areas where pigs are raised and where pigs have access to human fecal material. Only a few million people are thought to harbor the tapeworm form. Pork tapeworm infection is highly endemic in Latin America, sub-Saharan Africa, south, east, and southeast.

T. solium tapeworms are acquired by ingestion of undercooked pork. The scolex attaches to the intestinal wall and proglottids form at the base of the scolex. The proglottids gradually enlarge as they are displaced from the scolex by newer proglottids. The terminal proglottids are shed periodically in the stool. Terminal proglottids are typically off-white, 2 cm long, 0.5 to 1 cm wide, and 1 to 2 mm thick.

CLINICAL MANIFESTATIONS AND DIAGNOSIS

Mild symptoms (e.g., nausea, abdominal discomfort, anorexia, and pruritus) may be noted. The proglottids may be noted in stool. Diagnosis is made by the finding of ova in stool. The ova are 40 μm in diameter, surrounded by brown radial striations, and embryos have six hooks and are morphologically indistinguishable from the other *Taenia* species.

TREATMENT AND PREVENTION Rx

Taeniasis can be treated with praziquantel in a single dose. However, praziquantel should be used with caution in areas where cysticercosis is prevalent, because it can precipitate symptoms such as seizures. Single doses of niclosamide are also effective. Taeniasis can be prevented by inspection of pork. Also, cooking to 56° C for 5 minutes or freezing at −20° C for 7 to 10 days destroys the infective larvae. Current control measures include mass chemotherapy for entire populations with praziquantel (see below in the section on cysticercosis)

● TISSUE CESTODE (CYST) INFECTION
Taenia solium (Cysticercosis)

DEFINITION

T. solium is the cause of human larval infection termed cysticercosis. The normal hosts for the larval (cysticercus) forms are pigs. When ingested by pigs, the ova hatch, releasing the invasive larvae (termed *oncospheres*), which invade the intestines, migrate to tissues (especially muscle), and mature into cysticercus forms within the tissues. The cysticercus consists of a thin translucent bladder containing an invaginated scolex, which is poised to form a tapeworm after being ingested by a human host. The ova are also infectious to people, including the tapeworm carrier. The sticky ova attach to the hands of the tapeworm carrier and are transmitted by the oral route to the carrier or close contacts. After ingestion, the ova can migrate to tissues and form cysts (cysticercosis). The presence of cysticerci in the central nervous system is termed *neurocysticercosis*. Neurocysticercosis includes cysticerci in the brain parenchyma (parenchymal neurocysticercosis) and cysticerci in the ventricles, subarachnoid space, spine, and eye (extraparenchymal neurocysticercosis).

EPIDEMIOLOGY

Cysticercosis is found in all regions of the world where pigs are raised with access to human fecal material.[2] However, exact data on incidence and prevalence are available from only a limited number of studies because of the requirement for neuroimaging studies to make a diagnosis. In the 19th century, infection was highly endemic in Europe. However, with improving standards of living, local transmission is now limited to a few rural areas in southern and eastern Europe. Cysticercosis is widespread in rural areas of Latin America. In endemic villages, more than 10% of the population may have abnormalities on neuroimaging studies consistent with neurocysticercosis.[3] Studies have highlighted the importance of cysticercosis in sub-Saharan Africa. Cysticercosis is widespread in India, Nepal, Southeast Asia, and parts of China. In India, the most common manifestation of neurocysticercosis is seizures and a single enhancing lesion. In the United States, over 2000 cases are diagnosed each year. Most cases are in immigrants from pig-raising villages in Mexico and Latin America. However, there are also imported cases from Asia and a few locally acquired infections.

PATHOBIOLOGY

For cysticercosis, the pathogenesis and pathophysiology vary with the location of the cysticerci and the host inflammatory response. Cysticerci in the brain parenchyma initially suppress the host inflammatory response. After a silent period, estimated to be several years, the cysticerci lose the ability to suppress the host inflammatory response, leading to parenchymal inflammation, which typically is manifested by seizures. The cysticerci induce a granulomatous response, which gradually degrades the parasites. In some cases, the lesions resolve. However, in others, degradation leads to formation of calcified granulomas. These calcified lesions may intermittently become inflamed (as evidenced by edema or contrast enhancement on magnetic resonance imaging [MRI] scan) and may cause recurrent seizures during a period of years. In some cases, cysticerci develop within the ventricles of the brain and can mechanically cause obstructive hydrocephalus. Cysticerci in the subarachnoid space may cause a chronic arachnoiditis, which can be manifested by vasculitis and stroke,

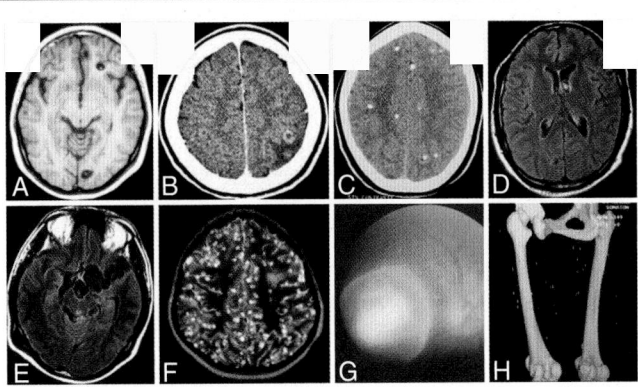

FIGURE 333-1. Human neurocysticercosis can be classified on the basis of neuroimaging studies. **A,** Multiple cystic lesions. **B,** Single enhancing lesion. **C,** Multiple calcifications. **D,** Intraventricular cysticerci. **E,** Subarachnoid cysticerci. **F,** Diffuse infection with cerebral edema, termed cysticercal encephalitis. **G,** Ocular cysticerci. **H,** Diffuse muscle calcifications. (Reprinted from Garcia HH, Del Brutto OH. Neurocysticercosis: updated concepts about an old disease. *Lancet Neurol.* 2005;4:653-661.)

communicating hydrocephalus, basilar meningitis, and, in some cases, mass effect. Cysticerci can also develop in the spine (manifested as radiculitis), eye, subcutaneous tissue, and muscle.

CLINICAL MANIFESTATIONS

The clinical manifestations vary with the location of the cysticerci and the associated host response (Fig. 333-1).[4] All forms of disease may be associated with headaches. In general, parenchymal cysticerci are associated with seizures, whereas ventricular and subarachnoid cysticercosis are associated with hydrocephalus.

Single Enhancing Lesion

A single enhancing lesion is the most common manifestation of cysticercosis in India and the United States. Patients typically present with seizures, which can be focal or focal with secondary generalization. Many will have a single seizure or a few seizures during the period when the cysticercus is degenerating, but the duration of seizures is eventually self-limited in most cases. However, a few go on to develop calcified lesions, which are a risk factor for recurrent seizures.

Multiple Parenchymal Cysticerci

In patients with multiple lesions, the main presentation is with seizures, associated with parenchymal inflammation. In contrast to those with single lesions, seizures are more likely to recur.

Calcified Lesions

Many patients do not present until after they have calcified lesions. Patients with calcified lesions may develop recurrent seizures during a period of years. Some cases are associated with the development of mesiotemporal sclerosis and refractory epilepsy (Chapter 375).

Ventricular Cysticerci

The cysticerci typically are manifested by obstructive hydrocephalus. The patient may present with headache, nausea and vomiting, dizziness, altered mental status, or papilledema with altered vision. This is a medical emergency and can be fatal if it is not treated.

Subarachnoid Cysticerci

Cysticerci in the basilar cisterns are often accompanied by cysticerci in other locations, including parenchymal cysticerci or calcifications, ventricular cysticerci, and spinal or ocular cysticerci; patients may present with disease attributable to cysticerci at these sites. Cysticerci in the basilar cisterns are particularly prone to cause arachnoiditis. Manifestations of arachnoiditis may include vascular involvement (large- or small-vessel strokes), meningeal signs, or communicating hydrocephalus (headaches, nausea, vomiting, dizziness, and altered mental status).

DIAGNOSIS

The major clinical manifestations of neurocysticercosis (e.g., seizures and hydrocephalus) are not specific, and it is difficult to identify the parasites. The main tools used to diagnose neurocysticercosis are neuroimaging studies. Computed tomography (CT) scans are sensitive for identification of parenchymal calcifications, which appear as 2- to 5-mm nodules. CT may also reveal parenchymal cysticerci or obstructive hydrocephalus. MRI scans are more sensitive for identification of the cysticerci, especially in the subarachnoid space and ventricles. Three-dimensional sequences such as fast imaging employing steady-state acquisition (FIESTA) are particularly effective for ventricular and subarachnoid cysticerci. The cysticerci are typically round, 1 to 2 cm in diameter. The cyst fluid is usually isodense with spinal fluid. In uninflamed cysticerci, the walls may not be visible. However, most cases demonstrate enhancement of the cyst walls or surrounding tissues and associated edema. In some cases, the scolex may be visible as a 1- to 2-mm solid nodule, cylinder, or spiral on the side of the cystic lesions. Serologic tests are useful to confirm the diagnosis. Assays using crude antigen, including enzyme-linked immunosorbent assay, are associated with poor sensitivity and specificity and are not reliable. An immunoblot assay using semipurified membrane glycoproteins is highly specific for the diagnosis. The sensitivity is excellent in cases with extraparenchymal or multiple parenchymal cysticerci. However, the sensitivity is poor in those with single enhancing lesions or just calcifications. Antigen detection assays are sensitive and more specific for viable cases and are increasingly available in the United States. Revised diagnostic criteria published recently have defined neurocysticercosis as a "definitive diagnosis" or only a "probable diagnosis."[5]

TREATMENT   Rx

Treatment varies with the clinical manifestations and form of infection.[6,7] Seizures should be treated with antiepileptic drugs (Chapter 375). Phenytoin and carbamazepine are typically used and can control the seizures. Newer antiepileptic drugs may be more effective. There are no viable parasites in those with just calcified lesions, so the main measure is to control symptoms (e.g., antiepileptic drugs for those with seizures). In patients presenting with hydrocephalus, surgery to reestablish cerebrospinal fluid flow is the critical initial step in management. The role of antiparasitic drugs (Chapter 323) varies with the form of infection. Randomized controlled trials have demonstrated more rapid resolution of parenchymal cystic lesions with fewer generalized seizures in those treated with corticosteroids and albendazole (15 mg/kg/day in two daily doses) compared with those treated with placebo.[A1] Praziquantel (50 to 100 mg/kg/day in three daily doses) can be used as an alternative. There are emerging data on the use of the two drugs in combination, which may have greater cysticidal activity in those with more than 2 parenchymal cysticerci.[A2] A number of clinical trials in subjects with single enhancing lesions have demonstrated a slightly more rapid radiologic resolution and fewer seizures in those treated with steroids and antiparasitic drugs.[A3][A4] Higher-dose steroids may decrease seizures near the time of antiparasitic treatment, but the differences are not dramatic. For patients with cysticerci in the ventricles, management usually involves removal of the cysticerci. This can be best achieved by neuroendoscopy for lateral and third ventricular cysticerci. However, the main alternative approach is placement of a ventriculoperitoneal shunt. Chronic steroids and antiparasitic drugs may decrease the rate of shunt failure, which usually results from clogging of the shunts by the cysticerci or proteinaceous debris. There are no controlled trials on the management of subarachnoid cysticercosis. However, expert opinion supports treatment of subarachnoid cysticercosis with prolonged courses of antiparasitic drugs (e.g., albendazole for months), higher doses of albendazole, or combinations of albendazole and praziquantel. Chronic anti-inflammatory medications (e.g., prednisone 1 mg/kg/day, or 24 mg/day of dexamethasone) are also critically important. Patients who will be treated with chronic steroids should be screened for *Mycobacterium tuberculosis* and *Strongyloides* infections before initiation of steroid therapy. Methotrexate is increasingly recommended as a steroid-sparing agent. Patients with hydrocephalus should be treated by cerebrospinal fluid diversion (e.g., ventriculoperitoneal shunting). Before treatment with antiparasitic drugs, patients should undergo a funduscopic examination. Intraocular parasites may develop brisk inflammatory responses after treatment with antiparasitic drugs. Because this inflammation could lead to blindness, most authorities recommend extraction of the parasites before antiparasitic therapy. However, there are also reports of treatment of intraocular parasites with antiparasitic drugs.

PREVENTION

Although transmission of *T. solium* is potentially preventable, population-wide eradication efforts have proved very difficult. Recently, however, transmission of *T. solium* infection was interrupted in a highly endemic region of Peru by a program emphasizing mass antiparasitic treatment of the human population

with niclosamide, treatment of pigs with oxfendazole, plus vaccination of piglets.[A5]

PROGNOSIS

The prognosis varies significantly between the different forms of neurocysticercosis. Parenchymal enhancing lesions and parenchymal cystic lesions will eventually resolve, but this may take months to years. Patients who have or develop calcifications are at lifelong risk for recurrent seizures. Patients with ventricular or subarachnoid disease are at high risk for morbidity and mortality. However, a recent case series noted no deaths with optimal management.

Cystic Hydatid Disease (*Echinococcus granulosus* group)

DEFINITION

Cystic echinococcosis, also called cystic hydatidosis, is caused by the larval stage of cestodes of the *Echinococcus granulosus* complex. All of these parasites were initially thought to be a single species, *E. granulosus*. However, molecular studies demonstrate that *E. granulosus* comprises a number of different species and genotypes. In humans, the clinical manifestations range from asymptomatic infection to severe, potentially fatal disease.

Echinococcal cysts consist of a periparasitic host tissue (pericyst or adventitia), which encompasses the larval endocyst, and the endocyst itself. The endocyst has an outer, acellular laminated layer and an inner, or germinative, layer that gives rise to brood capsules and protoscolices. The cyst is filled with clear fluid, numerous brood capsules, and protoscolices. Some cysts may also harbor daughter cysts of variable size. The protoscolices convert to tapeworms in the canine definitive hosts but can also form new cysts when released in mammalian tissues.

EPIDEMIOLOGY

E. granulosus species occur on all continents and in circumpolar, temperate, subtropical, and tropical zones. The highest prevalence of the parasite is found in parts of Eurasia, Africa, Australia, and South America. Within the endemic zones, the prevalence of the parasites varies from sporadic to high, but only a few countries can be regarded as being free of *E. granulosus*.

It is difficult to determine the true incidence of cystic echinococcosis because of the slow rate of growth and variable clinical presentation. Most epidemiologic reports are based on hospital- and surgery-based surveys that greatly underestimate the actual rates of infection, especially in low socioeconomic groups with limited access to diagnosis and treatment.

Since the mid-1980s, however, mass community-based surveys using portable ultrasound scanners have been conducted in many remote, rural areas of the world. The sensitivity and specificity of ultrasound have been shown to be superior to those of serology in prevalence surveys.[8] These studies showed the real burden of disease, uncovering population infection rates of up to 6.6%.

E. granulosus exists as a complex of species and strains that differ in a variety of criteria that may have an impact on the epidemiology, pathology, and control of cystic echinococcosis. To date, 10 distinct genotypes (G1 to G10) have been identified. Some distinct species have been identified (*Echinococcus equinus*, *Echinococcus ortleppi*). The great majority of *E. granulosus* isolates from human patients thus far have been of the sheep genotype (G1).

CLINICAL MANIFESTATIONS

The presentation of human cystic echinococcosis is protean. Patients seek medical attention when a large cyst has some mechanical effect on organ function or rupture of a cyst causes acute hypersensitivity reactions. The cyst is often diagnosed incidentally during ultrasound examination, chest radiography, or body scanning performed for other clinical reasons. The liver is the most frequent location of echinococcal cysts, representing approximately 70% of cases.[9] The lungs are the second most common location. However, cystic echinococcosis can occasionally occur in virtually any other organ.

Common symptoms are upper abdominal discomfort and pain, poor appetite, and a mass in the abdomen. Physical findings are hepatomegaly, a palpable mass on the surface of the liver or other organs, and abdominal distention. Other manifestations include jaundice, colic-like pains, portal hypertension, ascites, and compression of the inferior vena cava. If cysts in the lung rupture into the bronchi, symptoms may include intense cough, a salty taste in the mouth, or vomiting of hydatid material and cystic membranes. Patients may present with a chest mass, chest pain, chronic cough, pneumothorax, eosinophilic pneumonitis, pleural effusion, parasitic lung embolism, hemoptysis, or biliptysis. Cysts in the heart can cause a cardiac mass, pericardial effusion, and embolism. Cysts in the breast must be differentiated from neoplasms.

Cysts located in the spine and in the brain can cause serious neurologic symptoms, including paralysis and seizures.

DIAGNOSIS

The diagnosis of cystic echinococcosis is based on imaging methods and on serology, but serology has only a confirmatory role. Routine laboratory tests are nonspecific. Cyst rupture into the biliary tree may cause elevation of alkaline phosphatase, sometimes in association with hyperamylasemia and eosinophilia (up to 60%). Unless the cyst has ruptured, eosinophilia is low grade or absent.

Imaging

Modern imaging tools (ultrasound, CT, and, to a lesser extent, MRI) are central to the diagnosis and clinical management of cystic echinococcosis. Ultrasound is the procedure of choice for diagnosis of asymptomatic cystic echinococcosis.[10] Ultrasound is also useful for longitudinal studies, such as monitoring the response of cysts to treatment and recording cyst growth rate. In 2003, the World Health Organization (WHO) Informal Working Group on Echinococcosis proposed a standardized ultrasound classification (Fig. 333-2). This classification defines six cyst stages that are assigned to three clinical groups. The active group comprises developing cysts, which may be unilocular (CE1) or multivesicular with daughter cysts (class CE2) and are usually found to be viable. The transitional group (class CE3) contains cysts that are usually starting to degenerate. There are two types of CE3: the "water lily sign" for floating membranes, which is now known as subclass CE3a; and predominantly solid cysts with daughter cysts, or subclass CE3b. This subdivision is based on their different response to percutaneous treatment (see later) and albendazole, which is generally good for CE3a and poor for CE3b. A study using nuclear magnetic resonance spectroscopy has found that CE3a and CE3b may have different metabolic characteristics. The inactive group (classes CE4 and CE5) exhibits involution and signs of solidification of cyst content with increasing degrees of calcification and is nearly always found to be nonviable.

CT scanning has the advantage of inspecting any organ, detecting smaller cysts located outside the liver, locating cysts precisely, and sometimes differentiating parasitic from nonparasitic cysts. MRI may have some advantages over CT scanning in the evaluation of postsurgical residual lesions, recurrences, and selected extrahepatic infections, such as cardiac infections. Furthermore, a study has shown that MRI reproduces the ultrasound-defined features of cystic echinococcosis better than CT does. If ultrasound cannot be performed because of cyst location or patient-specific reasons, MRI with heavily T2-weighted series is preferable to CT. Plain radiographs are used for cysts in the lungs, bone, and muscle and for detection of calcified cysts.

Serology

Serologic tests are useful for confirmation of presumptive imaging diagnoses. However, many tests are available, and they are not standardized. Their sensitivity varies with the location of the cysts. Hepatic cysts are more likely to elicit an immune response than are pulmonary, brain, or splenic cysts. Serologic test results are usually positive when the endocyst is detached (CE3a) and in active (CE2) and transitional (CE3b) stages. Serologic test results are generally negative in patients with inactive cysts (CE4 and CE5). Titers tend to slowly decrease when a cyst becomes inactive (CE4, CE5) and after radical surgery. Titers may remain positive after conservative surgery in which the antigen source (the germinal layer) is not completely removed. Antibody titers usually increase immediately after medical or percutaneous treatments because of the mobilization of the antigen following disruption of cyst integrity.

Other Diagnostic Procedures

Fine-needle aspiration of the cyst performed under ultrasonographic guidance, with a transhepatic approach, under anthelmintic coverage, is useful for differentiation of cystic echinococcosis, malignant neoplasms, abscesses, and nonparasitic cysts. The procedure must be carried out in the presence of an anesthesiologist ready to manage the rare but possible anaphylactic reaction.

TREATMENT Rx

The appropriate treatment depends on factors of the individual patient, the characteristics of the cyst, the therapeutic resources available, and the physician's preference.[11] There are few randomized clinical trials evaluating treatment options, so a low level of evidence supports one therapeutic modality over another.[12]

Surgery

Surgery has long been the only option in the treatment of cystic echinococcosis. However, in the past two decades, medical treatment, percutaneous procedures, and a "watch and wait" approach have been successfully introduced and replaced surgery as the treatment of choice in selected cases. Surgery remains the main therapy in complicated cysts (i.e., those with rupture, biliary fistula, compression of vital structures, superinfection, or hemorrhage), cysts at high risk of rupture, or large cysts with many daughter vesicles that are not suitable for percutaneous treatments. Surgery can be performed as an open procedure, with either radical or conservative techniques, or laparoscopically, but there are controversies as to the safest and most effective technique and in which cases it should be applied. In all hepatic cases, perioperative albendazole prophylaxis, from 1 week before surgery until 4 weeks postoperatively, is recommended as a cautionary measure to minimize the risk of fluid spillage and consequent secondary echinococcosis from seeding of protoscolices in the abdominal cavity. Some authorities treat with praziquantel as well. Most experts recommend avoiding preoperative antiparasitic drugs for lung and intracranial disease.

Percutaneous Treatments

Percutaneous techniques provide an alternative to surgery and benzimidazole derivatives. These treatment modalities aim either to destroy the germinal layer with scolicidal agents or to evacuate the entire endocyst. The most popular method aimed at destroying the germinal layer is PAIR (puncture, aspiration, injection of a scolicidal agent, and reaspiration). Many modified catheterization techniques are used to evacuate the endocyst and are generally reserved for cysts that are difficult to drain or tend to relapse after PAIR, such as multivesiculated cysts or cysts with predominantly solid content and daughter cysts.

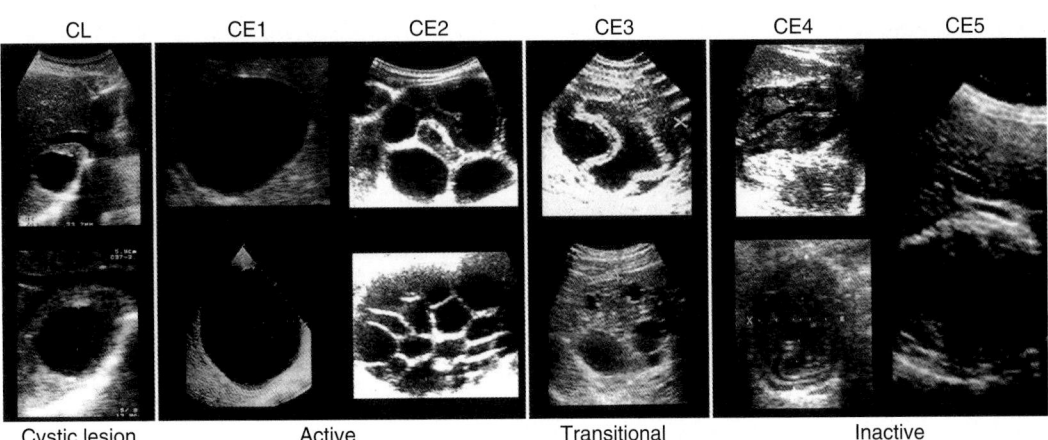

| CL | CE1 | CE2 | CE3 | CE4 | CE5 |

| Cystic lesion | Active | Transitional | Inactive |

FIGURE 333-2. WHO Informal Working Group on Echinococcosis standardized ultrasound classification of cystic echinococcosis. CL lesions are cystic lesions lacking a distinct wall and may have other diagnoses. CE1 lesions are cystic lesions with a visible wall that may demonstrate protoscolices ("hydatid sand"). CE2 lesions include internal septation. CE3 lesions may be detached from the wall (CE3a, top row) or have daughter cysts with internal thickening (CE3b, bottom row). CE4 lesions are heterogeneous lesions with degeneration. CE5 lesions show thick calcification.

A growing number of articles have reported its safety in treating abdominal, especially liver, echinococcal cysts. In a study on 5943 percutaneous punctures of echinococcal cysts, lethal anaphylaxis occurred in 0.03% of procedures, whereas reversible allergic reactions complicated 1.7% of procedures. Prophylactic administration of albendazole for at least 30 days after puncture is a cautionary measure that should always accompany PAIR. PAIR is generally successful at inducing permanent solidification in CE1 and CE3a cysts. A few reports with long-term follow-up indicate that multivesicular cysts (i.e., CE2 and CE3b) tend to relapse repeatedly after PAIR.

Chemotherapy

Albendazole (Chapter 323) is the antiparasitic drug of choice for cystic echinococcosis. It is administered orally at a dosage of 10 to 15 mg/kg/day; administration should be continuous without treatment interruptions. However, the optimal dosage and optimal duration of treatment with albendazole have not been formally assessed, and data from the small clinical trials generally fail to take into account the cyst's characteristics. A recent systematic review on the effect of albendazole showed that the efficacy of the drug may have been overstated in previous retrospective, nonrandomized studies. Albendazole induces solidification in small and medium-sized CE1 and CE3a cysts, whereas it has generally little effect on giant (diameter >10 cm) CE1 and CE3a cysts. It has no effect on most cases of CE2 and CE3b cysts.

Adverse effects of benzimidazoles (Chapter 323) include hepatotoxicity, leukopenia, thrombocytopenia, and alopecia. Increases in aminotransferases may be due to drug-related efficacy or real drug-related toxicity. Whereas teratogenic risks are theoretical, it is nonetheless good practice to avoid use during pregnancy when possible and to delay treatment until after delivery unless it is absolutely necessary.

Watch and Wait

Inactive liver cysts that are free of complications, such as compression on neighboring organs, are increasingly monitored without being treated.[13] Prospective studies need to be carried out to confirm the safety of this option.

Follow-up

Follow-up is crucial to evaluate the efficacy of treatment. Long-term follow-up, generally more than 5 years, is required to evaluate local recurrences, which have been reported up to 10 years after apparently successful treatment. When the combination of imaging and serology is inconclusive, fine-needle aspiration should be performed to ascertain the viability of the cyst contents.

Alveolar Hydatid Disease (*Echinococcus multilocularis*)

Alveolar hydatid disease is caused by the tissue forms of *Echinococcus multilocularis*. In tissues, typically the liver, *E. multilocularis* grows as a budding mass rather than as a large cystic lesion. The tissues resemble lung tissues, hence the name "alveolar." The normal definitive hosts are canines, including wolves and foxes. The normal intermediate hosts are rodents. Humans are accidentally infected by contact with soil containing the ova.

EPIDEMIOLOGY

E. multilocularis is endemic in arctic and alpine areas of the Northern Hemisphere. It is highly endemic in western China, Tibet, and central Asia. In recent years, *E. multilocularis* has emerged as an important problem in Alpine areas of central Europe and adjacent forested areas.[14]

CLINICAL MANIFESTATIONS AND DIAGNOSIS

Human *E. multilocularis* infection almost invariably involves the liver, in which it is manifested as a tumor-like mass that gradually expands during decades. The main symptoms are liver discomfort and swelling. Diagnosis is by demonstration of a characteristic mass on imaging studies, with the etiology confirmed by serologic tests.[15]

TREATMENT AND PROGNOSIS   Rx

Surgery remains the mainstay of treatment of *E. multilocularis*. When feasible, all infected tissues should be removed. Apparently curative therapy should be followed by a 2-year course of albendazole to decrease the risk of relapse. In some cases, resection is feasible only when it is accompanied by liver transplantation. In cases that are not amenable to surgical resection, prolonged courses of albendazole can suppress growth of the lesion. After treatment with benzimidazoles, mortality is similar to that of the age- and sex-matched general population.

Other Larval Cestode Infections

Sparganosis is caused by infection with the larval (plerocercoid) stage of *Spirometra mansonoides*. Infection is acquired by ingestion or application of infected meat (frogs, birds, fish) or exposure of skin to infected flesh (e.g., poultices of infected tissues). After infection, plerocercoids develop in the tissues, typically presenting as subcutaneous or central nervous system nodules or occasionally larva migrans symptoms. Treatment usually involves removal of the nodule.

Coenurosis is a rare larval cestode infection caused by human infection with the larval stage of the dog tapeworms *Taenia multiceps* and *Taenia serialis*. In the tissue, the larva forms a cystic lesion containing multiple scolices (the coenurus). The cystic lesion is usually single and most frequently identified in brain, eye, or soft tissues. Treatment usually involves removal.

Echinococcus oligarthrus and *Echinococcus vogeli* have been associated with polycystic hydatid disease in northern South America. *Taenia crassiceps* has been identified in the eye and in tissues of compromised hosts. *Hymenolepis*-like organisms have also been identified in tissues of AIDS patients.

Grade A References

A1. Baird A, Wiebe S, Zunt JR, et al. Evidence-based guideline: treatment of parenchymal neurocysticercosis: report of the Guideline Development Subcommittee of the American Academy of Neurology. *Neurology.* 2013;80:1424-1429.
A2. Garcia HH, Gonzales I, Lescano AG, et al. Efficacy of combined antiparasitic therapy with praziquantel and albendazole for neurocysticercosis: a double-blind, randomised controlled trial. *Lancet Infect Dis.* 2014;14:687-695.
A3. Zhao BC, Jiang HY, Ma WY, et al. Albendazole and corticosteroids for the treatment of solitary cysticercal granuloma: a network meta-analysis. *PLoS Negl Trop Dis.* 2016;10:1-15.
A4. Garcia HH, Gonzales I, Lescano AG, et al. Enhanced steroid dosing reduces seizures during antiparasitic treatment for cysticercosis and early after. *Epilepsia.* 2014;55:1452-1459.
A5. Garcia HH, Gonzalez AE, Tsang VC, et al. Elimination of *Taenia solium* transmission in northern Peru. *N Engl J Med.* 2016;374:2335-2344.

GENERAL REFERENCES

For the General References and other additional features, please visit Expert Consult at https://expertconsult.inkling.com.

334

TREMATODE INFECTIONS

EDGAR M. CARVALHO, ALDO A.M. LIMA, LUIS A. MARCOS, AND EDUARDO GOTUZZO

SCHISTOSOMIASIS

DEFINITION

Schistosomiasis is one of the most important parasitic diseases of humans and is a global public health problem in the developing world. The disease is caused by trematodes of the genus *Schistosoma*, and it is estimated that 250 million people are infected and 779 million are at high risk for infection. Mortality from schistosomiasis is estimated at 13,000 deaths per year and the burden of disease at 3.3 million disability-adjusted life-years lost per year.[1]

The Pathogen

Six major species of *Schistosoma* affect humans: *S. mansoni, S. haematobium, S. japonicum, S. intercalatum, S. mekongi,* and *S. guineensis,* and the sequencing of the *S. mansoni, S. haematobium,* and *S. japonicum* genome has been determined. These species differ biologically from one another and in their geographic distribution and the type of disease that they produce. The schistosomes are digenetic parasitic trematodes. Although they are morphologically distinct, the species of *Schistosoma* that infect humans share some common features. The large male (0.6 to 2.2 cm × 2 to 4 mm) has a ventral gynecophoric canal in which the female (1.2 to 2.6 cm × 1 to 2 mm) is held during copulation.

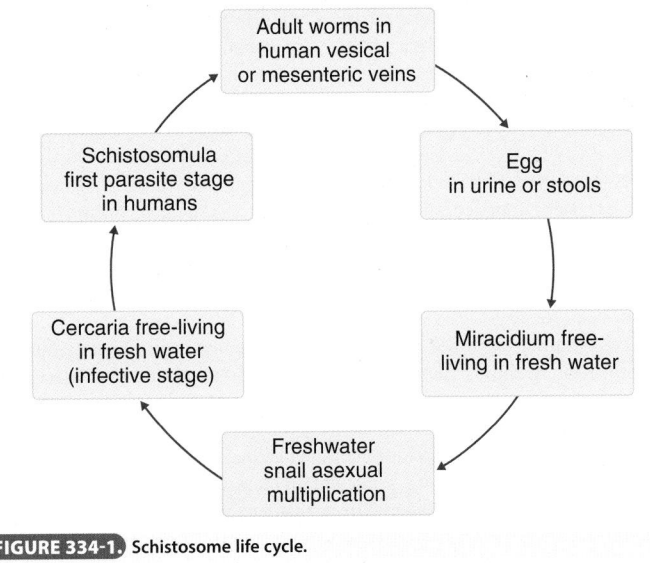

FIGURE 334-1. Schistosome life cycle.

EPIDEMIOLOGY

Schistosomiasis occurs mainly in rural agricultural and periurban areas. Programs for schistosomiasis control are advancing and helping in disease reduction.[2] However, schistosomiasis is still endemic in 78 countries. *S. mansoni* is found in the Arabian Peninsula, Egypt, Libya, Sudan, most countries in sub-Saharan Africa, Brazil, Suriname, and Venezuela. *S. haematobium* is endemic in the Middle East and most of the African continent, including the islands of Madagascar and Mauritius. *S. japonicum* is endemic in China, Indonesia, and the Philippines; it has also been reported from Thailand. *S. intercalatum* has been reported from 10 countries in Africa. *S. mekongi* is found in Cambodia and Laos.

The endemicity of schistosomiasis depends on the urban disposal of urine (*S. haematobium*) and feces (*S. mansoni, S. japonicum, S. intercalatum, S. mekongi, S. guineensis*), the presence of suitable snail hosts, and human exposure to cercariae. The freshwater snail intermediate hosts are *Biomphalaria* species in Africa and *Biomphalaria glabrata* (*Australorbis*) and *Tropicarbis* in South America and the West Indies. In some cases, the endemicity of schistosomiasis may be maintained by animal reservoirs. Such is the case with *S. japonicum,* which infects dogs and cows.

Etiology and Life Cycle

Adult worms live in the mesenteric veins (*S. mansoni, S. japonicum, S. mekongi, S. intercalatum,* and *S. guineensis*) or in the venous plexus around the lower ends of the ureters and the urinary bladder (*S. haematobium*) (Fig. 334-1). In these sites, they start their sexual reproduction by releasing eggs. Once deposited in the host, eggs may stay in the mesenteric vein, be trapped in the intestines, escape to the intestinal lumen, and migrate by portal blood to the liver (*S. mansoni, S. japonicum*). Eggs of *S. haematobium* may be trapped in the intestines and bladder and may escape to the intestinal or bladder lumen. After being excreted with feces or urine into fresh water, the eggs hatch and release ciliated motile miracidia that penetrate into the snail intermediate host. Following asexual multiplication in the snail, the development of cercariae, the infective forms for humans, takes 4 to 7 weeks. After leaving the snails, the cercariae can survive in fresh water for almost 72 hours. When penetration of the skin in the human host occurs, the cercariae lose their tails and change into schistosomula. Schistosomula migrate to the lungs and, in about 6 weeks, mature to adult worms and descend to their final habitat. Viable eggs can be seen in excretions (i.e., stool or urine) 5 to 9 weeks after cercarial penetration. The lifespan of the worms ranges from 5 to 10 years.

PATHOBIOLOGY

The pathogenesis of acute human schistosomiasis is mainly related to egg deposition, liberation of antigens of adult worms and eggs, and an exaggerated inflammatory response characterized by high levels of pro-inflammatory cytokines such as interleukin-1 (IL-1), IL-6, and tumor necrosis factor (TNF).

In chronic schistosomiasis, tissue injury is mediated by egg-induced granulomas and the subsequent appearance of fibrosis. In *S. haematobium,* infected eggs induce granuloma formation in the urinary tract. Because the habitat of *S.*

mansoni, S. japonicum, S. mekongi, S. guineensis, and *S. intercalatum* worms is the mesenteric blood vessels, the intestines are involved primarily, and egg embolism results in secondary involvement of the liver. Host genetics, immunologic response, and parasite load measured by egg count in the stool are associated with a greater chance for hepatosplenic involvement. IL-4, IL-13, and IL-17 have been associated with granuloma formation and liver fibrosis. Enzymes and antigens released from eggs sensitize host lymphocytes, which migrate to areas of egg deposition and recruit other cell types, such as macrophages, eosinophils, and fibroblasts. The size of these granulomas and the resulting fibrosis lead to most of the characteristic chronic fibro-obstructive lesions in schistosomiasis. In the liver, the granulomas result in perisinusoidal obstruction of portal blood flow, portal hypertension, splenomegaly, esophageal varices, and portosystemic collateral circulation. Liver cell perfusion is not reduced; consequently, liver function test results remain normal for a long time.

In schistosome-infected populations, the intensity of infection increases during the first 2 decades of life as children accumulate worms, and then declines. Although there is a decrease in exposure with age, the lower intensities of infection in older individuals are due in part to acquired resistance. There is an association between parasite-specific IgE, eosinophila, and resistance to reinfection. In the *S. haematobium*–infected population, IgE increases progressively with age, and IgE antibodies directed against adult worm antigens are associated with subsequent low intensities of reinfection. Similar associations between high IgE levels or a high IgE/IgG4 ratio and resistance to reinfection have been found among Brazilian and Kenyan subjects exposed to *S. mansoni.* In contrast, susceptibility to reinfection has been associated with IgG4, which may serve as blocking antibody, inhibiting the action of IgE. A major codominant gene, called *SM1,* in the human host's genome controls the intensity of infection by *S. mansoni.*

Modulation of the immune response is a characteristic of chronic schistosomiasis, and *S. mansoni* antigens downmodulate the immune response by increasing their production of regulatory cytokines such as IL-10 and the frequency of regulatory T cells.[3] *S. mansoni* infection attenuates the clinical manifestations of type 1 diabetes and experimental autoimmune encephalitis in mice. In humans, *S. mansoni* attenuates the clinical manifestations of asthma and is inversely associated with the development of myelopathy related to human T-cell leukemia virus type 1 (HTLV-1) infection. *S. mansoni* infection may impair immunologic response to vaccines and change manifestations of other infectious diseases.

CLINICAL MANIFESTATIONS

Clinical manifestations of schistosomiasis are divided into schistosome dermatitis, acute schistosomiasis, and chronic schistosomiasis.[4] Schistosome dermatitis, or swimmer's itch, is seen mainly when avian cercariae penetrate the skin and are destroyed. Schistosome dermatitis is a sensitization phenomenon occurring in previously exposed persons. The cercariae evoke an acute inflammatory response with edema, early infiltration of neutrophils and lymphocytes, and later invasion of eosinophils. A pruritic papular rash occurs within 24 hours after the penetration of cercariae and reaches maximal intensity in 2 to 3 days.

Acute schistosomiasis occurs usually 20 to 50 days after primary exposure. Though asymptomatic in endemic areas, acute schistosomiasis is becoming a frequent and major clinical problem in nonimmune individuals from urban regions who are exposed for the first time to a heavy infection in an endemic area. The clinical syndrome (i.e., fever, chills, liver and spleen enlargement, and marked eosinophilia) originally described for *S. japonicum* infection, and still common for this species, is increasingly being diagnosed in Brazil and Africa in individuals with *S. mansoni* infection. Malaise, diarrhea, weight loss, cough, dyspnea, chest pain, restrictive respiratory insufficiency, and pericarditis are also documented in this phase. High levels of TNF and circulating immune complexes are found in the patient's blood in this phase of illness, and they coincide with the development of abdominal pain, diarrhea, and weight loss and with respiratory and pericardial manifestations, respectively. Acute disease is not observed in individuals living in endemic areas for schistosomiasis.

In chronic schistosomiasis, abdominal pain, irregular bowel movements, and blood in the stool are the main symptoms of intestinal involvement. Colonic polyposis secondary to schistosomiasis may occur, especially in Egypt.

Hepatosplenic involvement is the most important cause of morbidity with *S. mansoni* and *S. japonicum* infection. Patients may remain asymptomatic until the manifestation of hepatic fibrosis and portal hypertension develops. Hepatic fibrosis is caused by a granulomatous reaction to *Schistosoma* eggs that have been carried to the liver. Although the intensity of infection is clearly linked directly to liver damage, the immune response, extent of collagen deposition, and genetic factors can potentiate disease in some individuals with only moderate infections or inhibit disease in others with heavy infections.

Hematemesis from bleeding esophageal or gastric varices may occur. Anemia and decreasing levels of serum albumin are observed. A few patients have severe hepatosplenic disease with decompensated liver disease. Jaundice, ascites, and liver failure are then observed. Concomitant infection by *Salmonella* species and, to a lesser extent, other gram-negative bacteria with *S. mansoni* or *S. haematobium* leads to a picture of prolonged fever, hepatosplenomegaly, and mild leukocytosis with eosinophilia. Coinfection with *S. mansoni* and hepatitis B or C virus exacerbates liver pathology. Glomerulonephritis and hypersplenism are other complications associated with hepatosplenic schistosomiasis. Pulmonary hypertension is increasingly recognized with the use of more advanced diagnostic technology. Pulmonary hypertension has been detected in 10.7% of patients with liver fibrosis. In countries endemic for *S. mansoni* up to 30% of all cases of pulmonary hypertension are due to schistosomiasis. Cerebral schistosomiasis is observed in patients with *S. japonicum* infection. It may occur as early as 6 weeks after infection, and its most common manifestation is focal seizures. Signs and symptoms of generalized encephalitis may occasionally be found. In *S. mansoni* infection, neurologic involvement is mainly characterized by transverse myelitis. An association between *S. mansoni* or *S. haematobium* and human immunodeficiency virus (HIV) infection has been documented in areas where both infectious agents are found. Although the immune response of patients with schistosomiasis is altered by HIV, it has not been reported to be associated with any clear changes in the degree of infection or severity of manifestations of schistosomiasis.

In *S. haematobium* infection, the main organ system involved is the urinary tract. The acute granulomatous response to parasite eggs in the early stages causes urinary tract disease, such as urethral ulceration and bladder polyposis. In chronic disease, usually in older patients, granulomas at the lower ends of the ureters obstruct urinary flow and may cause hydroureter and hydronephrosis. Bladder fibrosis and calcification are also seen in this phase. Up to 70% of infected individuals have hematuria, dysuria, or urinary frequency. Radiologic findings include hydronephrosis, hydroureter, ureteral strictures, dilation or distortion, ureteral calcifications, ureterolithiasis, calcified bladder, polyps, reduction in bladder capacity, irregular contraction of the bladder wall, or a dilated bladder because of bladder neck fibrosis. An increased incidence of squamous cell carcinoma of the bladder (Chapter 187) has been reported in endemic areas of *S. haematobium* infection, but the mechanism of carcinogenesis is unknown. *S. haematobium* eggs have occasionally been found in the lungs, with subsequent focal pulmonary arteritis and pulmonary hypertension.

DIAGNOSIS

A definitive diagnosis of schistosomiasis can be made only by finding schistosome eggs in feces, urine, or a biopsy specimen, usually from the rectum (Table 334-1).[5,6] A history of contact with contaminated water and appropriate clinical manifestations are important steps in establishing the diagnosis. Because schistosome eggs may be few, concentration by sedimentation should be performed. All eggs from feces, urine, or tissues should be examined under high power to determine their viability by visualizing the activity of cilia of the excretory flame cells of the enclosed miracidium. Dead eggs may persist for a long time after successful therapy or natural death of the worms. The presence of only dead eggs does not necessarily require treatment. Because the intensity of infection is associated with morbidity, quantitative techniques are recommended. For *S. mansoni* and *S. japonicum*, the Kato-Katz thick smear method is used. In patients with chronic *S. mansoni* and *S. japonicum* infection and liver disease, the diagnosis is sometimes made by documentation of eggs in liver specimens. Ultrasonography allows determination of the degree of liver fibrosis. *S. mekongi* and *S. intercalatum* infection is diagnosed by examining the stool for eggs.

Urine examination for *S. haematobium* eggs can be performed by direct or concentration methods. Samples should be obtained at midday, when excretion of eggs is maximal. After *S. haematobium* infection is diagnosed, assessment of urinary tract pathology by ultrasonography is recommended. Because of an increased incidence of carcinoma of the bladder, cancer surveillance should be performed in patients with *S. haematobium* infection (Chapter 187).

Molecular and immunodiagnostic assays are helpful in the diagnosis of acute infection and in diseases associated with light infection as in schistosomal myeloradiculopathy associated with *S. mansoni* and *S. haematobium* infection. Serologic assays have proven useful clinically for diagnosis by detection of antibodies to *Schistosoma mansoni* antigens. However, serologic tests cannot distinguish between active and past exposure. Quantification of circulating cathodic antigen (CCA) in urine has a higher sensitivity than the Kato-Katz method and has also been used to monitor the efficacy of antischistosome chemotherapy.[7] A significant decrease in antigen levels or negativity of the test is observed as early as 10 days after therapy. Molecular techniques for schistosoma DNA detection in fecal, urine, and blood specimens also increase sensitivity.[8]

TREATMENT AND PREVENTION Rx

Chemotherapy is the principal modality for prophylaxis, control, and cure of schistosomiasis. Several compounds are in use, including metrifonate, oxamniquine, praziquantel, and artemisinin derivatives (artesunate and artemether) for prophylaxis, control, and treatment of schistosomiasis. Praziquantel, a pyrazinoisoquinoline derivative, is the drug of choice for the treatment of schistosomiasis for four reasons: high efficacy against all schistosome species and against cestodes, lack of serious short-term and long-term side effects, administration as a single oral dose, and competitive cost. A recent review confirmed that a single dose of praziquantel (40 mg/kg) is an effective treatment for *S. mansoni* infection.[A1] Lower doses may be less effective and there is no additional benefit for higher doses. Oxamniquine (40 mg/kg) is also effective, and based on limited evidence to date it is uncertain which intervention is more effective. Further research will help optimize the doses for young children. A meta-analysis also confirmed that artemisinin derivatives, different from oxamniquine, used in combination with praziquantel increase the cure rates in schistosomiasis treatment, but not artemisinin derivatives or oxamniquine alone.[A2]

TABLE 334-1	DIAGNOSIS OF SCHISTOSOMIASIS	
SCHISTOSOME	**EGGS**	**DIAGNOSIS**
S. haematobium	Mainly found in urine but may be found in stools or rectal biopsy specimens Eggs: 143 × 50 μm; spindle shaped: rounded anterior, conical posterior, tapering to a terminal delicate spine	Obtain urine sample at midday (when eggs are excreted); more than one sample may be needed Examine urine directly or by filtering 10 mL of urine through a Nuclepore membrane Urine-circulating antigen test for diagnosis of light infection and serologic test to diagnose of early or light infection Rectal biopsy in suspected cases with negative urine for egg and for circulating cathodic antigen
S. mansoni	Found in stool eggs: 155 × 66 μm; oval with lateral, long spine	Examine stool for eggs Use the Kato-Katz thick smear method for quantification purposes Urine-circulating cathodic antigen test, serologic testing, or rectal biopsy to diagnose stool-negative cases, particularly in lightly infected patients
S. japonicum	Found in stool Eggs: 89 × 67 μm; oval or rounded with a lateral, short, sometimes curved spine	Examine stool for eggs Kato-Katz thick smear (for quantitative assessment) Urine-circulating cathodic antigen test, serologic test or rectal biopsy for those with light infections, especially with less common manifestations (e.g., cerebral schistosomiasis)
S. mekongi	Found in stool Eggs: 60 × 32 μm; smaller than eggs of S. japonicum	Examine stool for eggs
S. intercalatum	Found in stool Eggs: 180 × 65 μm; terminal spine	Examine stool for eggs

TABLE 334-2 CLINICAL MANIFESTATIONS, DIAGNOSIS, AND TREATMENT OF LIVER, INTESTINAL, AND LUNG FLUKE INFECTIONS IN HUMANS

FLUKE, NUMBER OF PEOPLE INFECTED, AND GEOGRAPHIC DISTRIBUTION	CLINICAL MANIFESTATIONS OF ACUTE AND CHRONIC PHASES	DIAGNOSIS*	TREATMENT[†]
LIVER FLUKES			
Fasciola spp 17 million Cosmopolitan	Acute [‡]Hepatomegaly, eosinophilia, fever, abdominal pain, metastatic-like lesions on liver CT Chronic [§]Biliary obstruction, gallstones, fibrosis, cholangitis	Stools are negative Serology (Fas2 ELISA) Eggs in stool Fas2 ELISA	TCZ
Opisthorchis spp 11.2 million Asia	[‡]Fever, malaise, arthralgia, lymphadenopathy, and rash [§]Jaundice, cholangitis, cholangiocarcinoma	Serology Eggs in stool	PZQ
Clonorchis spp 35 million Asia, Eastern Europe	[‡]Fever, rash, malaise, and RUQ abdominal discomfort [§]Choledocholithiasis, cholangitis, cholecystitis, liver abscess, and possible cholangiocarcinoma	Serology Eggs in stool	PZQ
INTESTINAL FLUKES			
Fasciolopsis buski and others[§] 50 million Asia and North Africa	Small bowel inflammation, ulceration, mucus secretion, protein-losing enteropathy, malabsorption	Eggs in stool	PZQ
LUNG FLUKE			
Paragonimus spp 23 million Asia, Americas, Africa	[‡]Abdominal pain, pleuritic pain, cough, eosinophilia [§]Hemoptysis, cough, chronic pleural effusions, pulmonary cysts	Abscess serology Eggs in sputum or stool	PZQ or TCZ

*For egg morphology and size, refer to text in the Diagnosis section.
[†]For drug regimens, refer to text in the Treatment section.
[‡]Acute.
[§]Chronic. For chronic infection, a sedimentation technique is preferred (suggested technique: rapid sedimentation technique or Kato-Katz technique).
[¶]Diagnosis and treatment also apply for other intestinal flukes.
CT = computed tomography; ELISA = enzyme-linked immunosorbent assay; PZQ = praziquantel; RUQ = right upper quadrant; TCZ = triclabendazole.

The standard recommended treatment consists of a single dose of praziquantel, 40 mg/kg, for *S. mansoni*, *S. haematobium*, and *S. intercalatum* infection. In *S. japonicum* infection, a total dose of 60 mg/kg is recommended, split into two or three doses in a single day. Although no significant difference was found in the overall cure rates between single-dose (40 mg/kg) and double-treatment (40 mg/kg with 2-week interval) regimens of praziquantel for *S. haematobium*, the effect of double treatment resulted in significant reduction in infection intensity and microhematuria, which may have an impact in reducing morbidity. *S. mekongi* may require two treatments at 60 mg/kg body weight. With these dosages of praziquantel, recorded cure rates are 75 to 85% for *S. haematobium*, 63 to 85% for *S. mansoni*, 80 to 90% for *S. japonicum*, 89% for *S. intercalatum*, and 60 to 80% for double infections with *S. mansoni* and *S. haematobium*. A decrease in the efficacy of praziquantel has been observed in patients coinfected with HTLV-1.

Praziquantel is well tolerated and effective in patients of all ages and for different clinical forms of schistosomiasis, including advanced hepatosplenic cases (*S. mansoni*), cerebral schistosomiasis (*S. japonicum*), and neurologic syndromes (*S. mansoni* and *S. haematobium*), possibly in association with corticosteroids. However, praziquantel has a low prophylactic effect, which reduces its efficacy in areas of high transmission. There have been several reports of persistent schistosome egg shedding after treatment, raising concern about the emergence of drug resistance. A systematic review and meta-analysis showed that either artesunate or artemether has confirmed prophylactic effect across different trials performed in China. Further studies will be necessary to examine the combination of antischistosome chemotherapy for *S. haematobium* infection in which repeated standard treatment fails to clear the infection.

The most common adverse events observed with praziquantel or oxamniquine are related to the gastrointestinal tract: abdominal pain or discomfort, nausea, vomiting, anorexia, and diarrhea. These symptoms can be observed in up to 50% of patients but are usually well tolerated. Other side effects are related to the central nervous system (e.g., headache, dizziness, drowsiness) and the skin (e.g., pruritus, eruptions) or may be nonspecific (e.g., fever, fatigue). In general, the cumulative experience from many studies allows the conclusion that praziquantel is an extremely well-tolerated drug that requires minimal medical supervision and is therefore particularly suitable for mass chemotherapy programs. Mass drug administration with praziquantel has been used as the mainstay of programs for the control and prevention of schistosomiasis morbidity. However, this approach alone is not sufficient to eliminate or interrupt transmission of this disease. The development of anti-*Schistosoma* vaccines is necessary.[9] Additional measures such as provision of clean water, use of molluscicides, adequate sanitation, and improvement of socioeconomic conditions should also be implemented to control the disease.[10,11]

LIVER FLUKES

The geographic distribution, clinical manifestations, diagnosis, and treatment of liver, intestinal, and lung fluke infections are summarized in Table 334-2.

Fascioliasis

Fascioliasis is a zoonosis caused by *Fasciola hepatica* (adult: 30×13 mm) or *F. gigantica* (adult: 75×20 mm). The most common natural hosts are cattle, sheep, and goats.

EPIDEMIOLOGY

The infection is distributed globally. An estimated 2.6 million people are infected by this parasite, mainly from South America, Africa, and Asia. The highest prevalence rates (>60%) have been reported in Peru and Bolivia.

PATHOBIOLOGY

The life cycle begins when the parasite's eggs in stool are deposited in water; miracidia appear, develop, and hatch in 9 to 14 days and invade many species of freshwater snails (*Lymnaea* spp), in which they multiply as sporozoites, rediae, and cercariae during a period of 4 to 7 weeks. They then leave as free-swimming cercaria that subsequently attach to watercress, water lettuce, alfalfa, mint, parsley, or khat. The main source of infection is consumption of raw vegetables or water contaminated with metacercariae. Women have a higher incidence of the disease, with more severe infections and complications than seen in men.

CLINICAL MANIFESTATIONS

After consumption of contaminated vegetables, the larvae excyst in the duodenum and then migrate through the bowel wall to the liver through the peritoneal cavity. In 4 weeks they reach the liver, penetrate the Glisson capsule, and cause inflammation and pain. An acute diarrhea of 2 to 5 days' duration may occur before liver invasion. During their migration through the liver, the ongoing inflammatory process is accompanied by fever, pain, and eosinophilia. In a few cases, intense hemorrhage manifested as subcapsular liver hematoma may develop. Computed tomography (CT), magnetic resonance imaging, or ultrasonography can detect these initial lesions. Furthermore, migration of the parasite leaves a trail or track that can be observed in histologic sections or by imaging (CT). The flukes sometimes die and leave cavities filled with necrotic debris that are eventually replaced by scar tissue and then become calcified. After 3 to 5 months of migration in the liver, the juvenile larvae finally reach the bile ducts. During this invasive, migratory, or acute phase the clinical manifestations are prolonged fever, hepatomegaly, abdominal pain, and eosinophilia. Multiple hypodense lesions are seen on CT, similar to metastases, but they change in position, attenuation, and shape in time because the parasites are still migrating. Acute fascioliasis is clinically similar to acute cholecystitis but with the addition of significant eosinophilia. It can occur in travelers with acute subcapsular hematoma or "metastatic-like lesions" seen on CT of the liver. Hyperbilirubinemia is notably absent in this phase. Other manifestations are anorexia, weight loss, nausea, vomiting, cough, diarrhea, urticaria, lymphadenopathy, and arthralgias. Occasionally, the juvenile larvae reach other ectopic or extrahepatic locations, such as subcutaneous tissue, the pancreas, the eye, the brain, and the stomach wall, among others. In endemic areas, the acute phase manifestations can be superimposed on chronic infection.

Arrival of the parasite in the bile ducts marks the beginning of the chronic phase. Mature flukes consume hepatocytes and duct epithelium and reside for years in the hepatic and common bile ducts and sometimes in the gallbladder. In this chronic phase, the liver contains large dilated, thick-walled, and calcareous bile ducts with yellowish-brown bile. The bile ducts have a thickened hyperplastic wall with marked fibrosis. Symptoms usually reflect biliary obstruction with colicky pain in the right upper quadrant and epigastric area. Eosinophilia is absent in half of the chronic cases. Bacterial superinfection of these cysts and consequent cholangitis can develop. Other complications are hemobilia and liver fibrosis. Alkaline phosphatase is commonly elevated because of biliary obstruction, which sometimes requires surgical intervention. On imaging, the initial lesions may be often confused with hepatic metastases. Other findings on CT are hepatomegaly, tracklike hypodense lesions in subcapsular locations, multiple hypodense nodular areas (abscess-like lesions), or low-density, serpiginous, tortuous, tunnel-like branching lesions ranging from 2 to 10 mm. CT also can show subcapsular hematoma, enhancement of the Glisson capsule, necrotic granuloma, and cystic calcifications. After maturation, the adult flukes start laying eggs, which are passed from the sphincter of Oddi to the intestines and evacuated to the environment along with stool. Adult parasites can live in the bile ducts for up to 13 years. In endemic populations, chronic infection has been reported as mildly symptomatic, whereas in travelers or temporary residents, it has been reported to cause biliary obstruction, with adult parasites being seen on endoscopic retrograde cholangiopancreatography (ERCP).[12,13]

In summary, the typical clinical presentation of acute fascioliasis must be differentiated from cholecystitis; "liver metastasis" with fever and eosinophilia should raise the possibility of this infection; and in children and adolescents, systemic toxocariasis will be in the differential diagnosis.

Clonorchiasis and Opisthorchiasis

Clonorchiasis is the disease caused by *Clonorchis sinensis*, also called the Chinese or oriental liver fluke (adult: 10 to 25 mm × 3 to 5 mm). Opisthorchiasis is caused by *Opisthorchis viverrini* (adult: 5 to 10 mm × 1 to 2 mm) and *Opisthorchis felineus* (adult: 7 to 12 mm × 2 to 3 mm). The most common natural hosts are dogs, cats, pigs, and some small wild mammals.

EPIDEMIOLOGY

The global estimate for the number of people infected with both infections is 46.2 million, 35 million for *C. sinensis* (15 million in China), 10 million for *O. viverrini* (8 million in Thailand and 2 million in the Lao People's Democratic Republic), and 1.2 for *O. felineus*. There are 601 million and 79.8 million people at risk of infection with *Clonorchis* and *Opisthorchis*, respectively. Both infections are endemic in the Far East, Southeast Asia, and Eastern Europe. *C. sinensis* is endemic in northeast China, southern Korea, Japan, Taiwan, northern Vietnam, and the far eastern part of Russia, and *O. viverrini* is endemic in Laos, Thailand, Vietnam, and Cambodia. *O. felineus* infection is prevalent in Russia, Ukraine, and Kazakhstan.[14]

PATHOBIOLOGY

The life cycle starts when the adult worm deposits fully developed eggs, which are then passed to the environment through feces. They hatch in water and the miracidia infect their first intermediate host, a freshwater snail (*Bithynia* spp or *Parafossarulus* spp), where they transform into sporocysts, rediae, and cercariae. Cercariae are released from the snail and then penetrate freshwater fish, which are the second intermediate host (*Cyclocheilichthys* spp, *Puntius* spp, *Hampala dispar*); the cercariae encyst as metacercariae in the muscles or under the scales. In general, the infection is acquired by eating raw or

uncooked cyprinoid fish products in rural areas or dishes such as koi-pla, a salad made with raw fish. The metacercariae pass through the stomach and reach the small intestine unharmed. Then, through the ampulla of Vater, they reach the bile ducts, where they mature into adult worms within 4 weeks and deposit yellow, operculated eggs. The parasites may live for up to 45 years in a human host.

CLINICAL MANIFESTATIONS

Clonorchiasis as an acute infection caused by *C. sinensis* is usually asymptomatic, but some patients may have fever, rash, malaise, and right upper quadrant abdominal discomfort.[15] Chronic infections may be manifested as recurrent pyogenic cholangitis, cholecystitis, obstructive jaundice, hepatomegaly, cholecystitis, multiple hepatic tumors, cholelithiasis, or pancreatitis. In chronic carriers with a high load of parasites, cholangiocarcinoma may develop, especially in Thailand.[16]

Opisthorchiasis as an acute infection caused by *O. viverrini* can cause right upper quadrant abdominal pain, flatulence, fatigue, and a hot sensation over the abdomen. In the chronic phase, mild hepatomegaly occurs, mainly in more heavily infected patients (egg counts >10,000/g). Jaundice and splenomegaly are not observed. Intrahepatic duct stones and recurrent suppurative cholangitis are common manifestations of opisthorchiasis. Whenever jaundice and ascending cholangitis are detected, fluke-related cholangiocarcinoma should be suspected.

In opisthorchiasis caused by *O. felineus*, infestation usually follows the consumption of raw, slightly salted, and frozen fish ("stroganina"), and acute symptoms occur 2 to 4 weeks later, including high-grade fever, nausea, vomiting, abdominal pain, malaise, arthralgias, lymphadenopathy, and rash. Peripheral eosinophilia is a common finding, especially during the initial 2 to 6 weeks of the infection, together with raised liver enzyme levels. In chronic infection, the eosinophilia is usually milder. Patients may have suppurative cholangitis and liver abscesses because of biliary obstruction. Ultrasonography or CT demonstrates the pathologic changes in the liver, including intrahepatic duct dilation and periductal changes.

The pathologic and clinical consequences of these flukes are related to the intensity and duration of cumulative infestations. In general, they cause inflammation around the biliary tree, severe hyperplasia of epithelial cells, metaplasia of mucin-producing cells in the mucosa, and progressive periductal fibrosis. There are clear associations between *O. viverrini* infection and cholangiocarcinoma.[17] Several *N*-nitroso compounds and their precursors occur at low levels in fermented food, such as preserved mud fish paste (*pla ra*), a condiment that is a ubiquitous component of the cuisine of northeastern Thailand and Laos.

● INTESTINAL FLUKES

The most common human intestinal trematode is *Fasciolopsis buski* (adult: 20 to 75 mm × 8 to 20 mm). It is found mainly in the central and southeast parts of Asia. *F. buski* is a common parasite in pigs. Others are *Heterophyes* (adult: 1 to 2 mm in length), *Metagonimus yokogawai* (adult: 1 to 2.5 mm × 0.4 to 0.75 mm), and *Echinostoma* spp (adult: 6.5 × 1 to 2 mm).

EPIDEMIOLOGY

More than 50 species of intestinal trematodes from the Far East, Middle East, and North Africa have been reported to cause human infection. *H. heterophyes* also can be found in the Nile delta region of Egypt. An estimated 40 to 50 million people are infected with one or several species of intestinal flukes. Their life cycles are similar. The adult worm, attached to the intestinal wall of humans, produces eggs that are passed in feces. The eggs reach water, and miracidia develop and penetrate the first intermediate host—snails. During the course of 6 to 7 weeks inside the host snails, they develop into sporocysts, rediae, and cercariae. The cercariae leave the snails to encyst in the second intermediate host, which can be freshwater snails, fish, tadpoles, or vegetables. Humans are infected by the ingestion of raw stems, leaves (especially bamboo shoots), watercress, or water chestnuts with encysted metacercariae. In the human duodenum, the metacercariae attach to the walls and become adult worms in approximately 3 months.

PATHOBIOLOGY AND CLINICAL MANIFESTATIONS

Despite the fact that the majority of intestinal fluke infections are asymptomatic, they may cause inflammation, ulceration, and mucus secretion at the site of attachment, particularly in the duodenum and jejunum. In fact, gastrointestinal hemorrhage, perforation, and abscesses have been observed. The differential diagnoses include typhoid fever, intestinal tuberculosis, and amebiasis. In these endemic cases, ulcerative colitis and other inflammatory diseases of the bowel are uncommon. In heavy infection, intestinal obstruction, protein-losing enteropathy, malabsorption, impaired vitamin B_{12} absorption, hypoalbuminemia, and anasarca have been reported. The adult worm causes traumatic, toxic, and obstructive damage to the intestinal mucosa. Some cases have been diagnosed by direct visualization of the adult parasite via esophagogastroduodenoscopy.

PULMONARY FLUKES

Paragonimiasis is a zoonosis caused by *Paragonimus* species (adult size: 10 × 5 mm). Reservoir hosts include felids, canids, viverrids, mustelids, some rodents, and pigs. At least 10 species of *Paragonimus* are known to cause human disease; of these, *Paragonimus westermani* is the most common.

EPIDEMIOLOGY

An estimated 23 million people are infected worldwide with *Paragonimus* species, and 293 million are at risk. Human paragonimiasis is distributed mainly in Southeast Asia, Japan, Korea, China, and the Philippines, where *P. westermani* is the main species. In other areas of low endemicity, other species have been reported, such as *Paragonimus mexicanus* in Latin America, *Paragonimus kellicotti* in North America, *Paragonimus heterotremus* in India, and *Paragonimus africanus* and *Paragonimus uterobilateralis* in West Africa.[18]

PATHOBIOLOGY

The life cycle starts when the eggs are excreted unembryonated in sputum, or alternatively they can be swallowed and passed in stool. In the external environment the eggs become embryonated, and miracidia hatch; seek the first intermediate host, a snail (families Pleuroceridae and Thiaridae); and penetrate its soft tissues. Within the snail, asexual reproduction occurs for several weeks, with transformation into sporocysts, rediae, and cercariae; the last emerge from the snail and invade the second intermediate host, a crustacean such as a crab or crayfish, where they encyst and become metacercariae. This is the infective stage for the mammalian host. Human infection occurs by eating inadequately cooked or pickled crab or crayfish that harbor metacercariae of the parasite. The metacercariae excyst in the duodenum, penetrate the intestinal wall, and migrate through the peritoneal cavity toward the lungs. During migration through the peritoneum and diaphragm, the inflammatory process causes abdominal pain and dry cough. When invading the lungs, they become encapsulated and develop into adults. Infections may persist for 20 years in humans.

CLINICAL MANIFESTATIONS

Paragonimiasis typically results from the consumption of raw or improperly cooked crustaceans, especially crabs. Recently in the United States, some autochthonous cases have been reported in the Midwest in people who consumed raw crayfish while camping during the summer. Most of the infected people are asymptomatic and have subclinical disease. During the first month of infection, abdominal pain may represent the juvenile larvae migrating through the abdominal cavity before reaching the lungs. Irritation of the diaphragm or pleura may cause dry cough. Fever, chest pain, fatigue, and urticaria may follow, as well as eosinophilia. Pleural effusions may be seen at this stage, with significant eosinophilia noted on analysis of pleural fluid, which can be the first clue to the diagnosis. In fact, pleural manifestations predominate early in the disease process, whereas lesions of the pulmonary parenchyma predominate later in the course of disease. Moreover, pneumothorax and mild eosinophilia may occur only 1 month after the initiation of infection. The migrating worms may cause bronchiectasis, interstitial pneumonitis, transient hemorrhage, or bronchopneumonia. Again, pulmonary lesions and eosinophilia raise the possibility of paragonimiasis. Cough and recurrent hemoptysis are common clinical findings in this phase. The chronic stage occurs when the worms are paired in a cyst in the pulmonary parenchyma. Eggs are produced 6 weeks after infection, and if there is communication with the bronchial tree, eggs may be seen in a sputum sample under microscopy, or they can be swallowed and passed with stool. The rusty discoloration of sputum is caused by the presence of the tan- to brown-pigmented *Paragonimus* eggs; the sputa of these patients have been classically described as resembling "iron filings." Charcot-Leyden crystals can be seen.

Peripheral blood eosinophilia and elevated total serum IgE levels are observed in approximately 80% of patients. Common findings on chest CT are pleural effusion, hydropneumothorax, pulmonary nodules or consolidation of air spaces, and cysts. The most common ectopic form is cerebral paragonimiasis, which is manifested as eosinophilic meningitis or meningoencephalitis,[19] brain tumor, or just residual calcifications from a past infection.

MANAGEMENT OF LIVER, INTESTINAL, AND LUNG FLUKE INFECTIONS

DIAGNOSIS

In general, transmission of food-borne trematodiases is restricted geographically, and distribution is one of the most important factors in suspecting this diagnosis. In the appropriate clinical setting, laboratory and imaging data can add information to narrow the differential diagnosis. Acute fluke infections require a high level of suspicion. Serologic tests, direct visualization of the migrating larvae, or empirical therapy with a significant clinical response (including reduction of eosinophilia) are major criteria to confirm the diagnosis. In the chronic phase, the diagnosis is usually made by visualization of the eggs in stool or, in the case of *Paragonimus*, in sputum. A sedimentation technique must be performed on a series of at least three stool specimens from alternate days or even weeks. Immunodiagnostics is an excellent tool, particularly for patients who do not have demonstrable eggs in clinical specimens.

If acute fascioliasis is strongly suspected, serology would be the next step. Cathepsin L1–based antibody enzyme-linked immunosorbent assay (ELISA) has a sensitivity of 92% and a specificity of 84%. If negative, the diagnosis is unlikely. If serology is not available, CT of the liver can visualize the characteristic tracklike lesions. However, because the parasitic lesions are very similar to metastases, liver biopsy may be necessary. If serology or CT is not available, a trial of triclabendazole with clinical (including eosinophilia) resolution is the major criterion for diagnosis. In chronic fascioliasis, the Lumbreras rapid sedimentation technique is the method of choice to detect the eggs in stool. At least three stool examinations are preferred. If negative, serology can be helpful. Ultrasonography and CT have low sensitivity in this phase. ERCP usually finds the adult parasites in the bile duct when performed for other reasons. Nonetheless, ERCP can be useful to eliminate the adult parasites causing biliary obstruction.

In opisthorchiasis, serology or stool examinations can be performed to approach the diagnosis. The Ov-CP-1–based ELISA has a sensitivity of 95% and a specificity of 96%. For *C. sinensis*, ELISA has a sensitivity between 81.3 and 96% and a specificity between 92.6 and 96.2%. For detection of eggs and to measure the intensity of infection, the Kato-Katz technique is preferred. Intestinal fluke eggs can be detected by performing a sedimentation stool technique, preferably in consecutive stool samples.

For paragonimiasis, an immunoblot assay performed with a crude antigen extract of *P. westermani* has been in use at the U.S. Centers for Disease Control and Prevention; the sensitivity of the test is 96%, and its specificity is 99%. This would be the ideal first step to confirm the diagnosis. In the acute phase, the precise location of the migrating larva is unknown and a biopsy may not necessarily target the parasite. When serologic findings are negative (or not available), a trial of praziquantel or triclabendazole with a positive clinical response in 48 to 72 hours is a major criterion for diagnosis. In the chronic phase, several sputum samples have to be examined by a sedimentation technique to increase sensitivity. Stool examinations are complementary because the eggs can be swallowed by the host and then passed through stool. If a pulmonary cyst contains adult parasites with eggs but they do not have communication to the main bronchi, serologic examination is indicated to confirm the diagnosis. If not available, biopsy is warranted.

Under the light microscope, the morphologic characteristics and size of the eggs may be sufficient to identify the specific fluke.

TREATMENT AND PREVENTION ℞

For fascioliasis, 10 mg/kg of triclabendazole once or twice has a cure rate higher than 90%, and it is the treatment of choice, but failures have been reported. Cure is achieved if stool examinations remain negative for at least 3 months. Serology usually can take more than a year to resolve. In treatment of the chronic phase, the dead parasites can occasionally cause biliary obstruction, which may need surgical consultation. In case of failure, some experts recommend at least double doses of triclabendazole for 2 days, and even multiple rounds are needed to resolve the infection.

For *O. viverrini*, a single dose of praziquantel (40 to 50 mg/kg) has a cure rate of 91 to 97%. For clonorchiasis, the recommended dose of praziquantel is 25 mg/kg three times for 1 day (total dose of 75 mg/kg), which has a cure rate of 83 to 85%. Tribendimidine has been found to be comparably effective as praziquantel in the treatment of *C. sinesis* infection with fewer adverse events in an open-label randomized trial.[A3] Tribendimidine (100 to 600 mg orally) is an efficacious alternative to praziquantel for treating *O. viverrini*[A4] but may or may not be quite as efficacious.[A5]

For intestinal flukes, praziquantel, 25 mg/kg by mouth three times daily for 1 day, is recommended.

For paragonimiasis, praziquantel, 25 mg/kg by mouth three times daily for 3 days, or triclabendazole, 10 mg/kg by mouth once or twice, is highly effective. For ectopic cases, surgery may be necessary. In follow-up, negative stool examinations in the ensuing weeks can confirm cure. However, because the rate of reinfection is high in individuals from endemic areas, a suddenly positive stool examination is highly suggestive of a new infection rather than failure to respond to treatment.

Prevention of infection with these flukes depends on several factors, including recognizing their geographic distribution and avoiding consumption of raw vegetables, fish, crayfish, or contaminated water in endemic areas. Proper medical advice must be given to individuals traveling to or planning to reside in endemic areas, not only to prevent flukes' infection but also risk for coinfections with other parasites. Control of these flukes in animals is impractical because of wild animal reservoirs, but in human infections it is challenging. It involves changing long-established cultural, dietary, and sanitary habits. Massive chemotherapy to highly endemic populations may reduce the infection in humans and in selected animals.

Grade A References

A1. Danso-Appiah A, Olliaro PL, Donegan S, et al. Drugs for treating *Schistosoma mansoni* infection. *Cochrane Database Syst Rev.* 2013;2:CD000528.

A2. Pérez del Villar L, Burguillo FJ, López-Abán J, et al. Systematic review and meta-analysis of artemisinin based therapies for the treatment and prevention of schistosomiasis. *PLoS ONE.* 2012;7:1-15.

A3. Xu LL, Jiang B, Duan JH, et al. Efficacy and safety of praziquantel, tribendimidine and mebendazole in patients with co-infection of *Clonorchis sinensis* and other helminths. *PLoS Negl Trop Dis.* 2014;8:1-10.

A4. Sayasone S, Odermatt P, Vonghachack Y, et al. Efficacy and safety of tribendimidine against *Opisthorchis viverrini*: two randomised, parallel-group, single-blind, dose-ranging, phase 2 trials. *Lancet Infect Dis.* 2016;16:1145-1153.

A5. Sayasone S, Keiser J, Meister I, et al. Efficacy and safety of tribendimidine versus praziquantel against *Opisthorchis viverrini* in Laos: an open-label, randomised, non-inferiority, phase 2 trial. *Lancet Infect Dis.* 2018;18:155-161.

GENERAL REFERENCES

For the General References and other additional features, please visit Expert Consult at https://expertconsult.inkling.com.

335

NEMATODE INFECTIONS

DAVID J. DIEMERT

DEFINITION

Nematode infections are highly prevalent worldwide, affecting millions. Nematodes are complex, nonsegmented roundworms with specialized organs that include a protective outer coating or cuticle, a complete and functional gastrointestinal tract, and muscular, nervous, and reproductive systems. Most species are free-living in soil or water, but a few parasitize humans.

Nematodes of medical importance can be categorized into those that primarily affect the gastrointestinal tract, where adult worms become established and cause disease, and those that affect other tissues and organ systems. The former group includes the roundworm *Ascaris lumbricoides*, the hookworms *Ancylostoma duodenale* and *Necator americanus*, the pinworm *Enterobius vermicularis*, the whipworm *Trichuris trichiura*, and the threadworm *Strongyloides stercoralis*. Zoonotic intestinal nematodes such as *Trichostrongylus* and *Anisakis* also occasionally infect and cause disease in humans. Nematodes that invade and cause disease primarily in tissues outside the gastrointestinal tract include those that cause lymphatic filariasis (*Wuchereria bancrofti*, *Brugia malayi*, and *Brugia timori*), *Onchocerca volvulus*, *Loa loa*, the guinea worm *Dracunculus medinensis*, and *Trichinella* and *Angiostrongylus* species.

Nematodes that infect humans measure from several millimeters to more than a meter in length and often survive for months to years within their host.

With the exception of *S. stercoralis* and *Capillaria philippinensis*, adult worms cannot complete their life cycle within a human host. Instead, sexually mature adult worms mate and produce eggs or larvae that must have at least one stage of development outside the host, either in the environment or in an intermediate host.

Nematode infections are rarely fatal; they more commonly result in chronic morbidity such as iron deficiency anemia caused by hookworm or blindness due to onchocerciasis. For most nematodes, the severity of the clinical manifestations of infection is proportional to the number of worms harbored by a given host; although light infections with only a few worms are usually asymptomatic, pathologic features appear with heavier worm burdens.

Nematode infections are prevalent in the temperate and tropical regions of Africa, Asia, and Latin America. They are transmitted by the oral ingestion of embryonated eggs or by penetration of infective larvae through the skin, either by direct contact with contaminated soil or by the bite of an arthropod vector. Nematode infections are most common in areas with poor sanitation, where the environment is contaminated by human feces, and in climates that support survival of the insect vector if one is involved in the life cycle.

INTESTINAL NEMATODE INFECTIONS

Ascariasis

The Pathogen

A. lumbricoides, colloquially known as roundworm, is acquired by oral ingestion of embryonated eggs. In the stomach, the egg's protective outer shell is dissolved by gastric acid, releasing larvae into the small intestine, where they penetrate the intestinal wall and enter the portal circulation. The larvae migrate to the pulmonary vasculature, where they penetrate into the alveoli, ascend the bronchial tree, and are swallowed back into the intestinal tract where they develop into adult worms 9 to 11 weeks after egg ingestion. Adult worms (Fig. 335-1) range in length between 15 and 50 cm and survive in the host for approximately 18 months. Female adult *Ascaris* worms release more than 200,000 eggs per day that are expelled in feces. Fertilized eggs (Fig. 335-2)

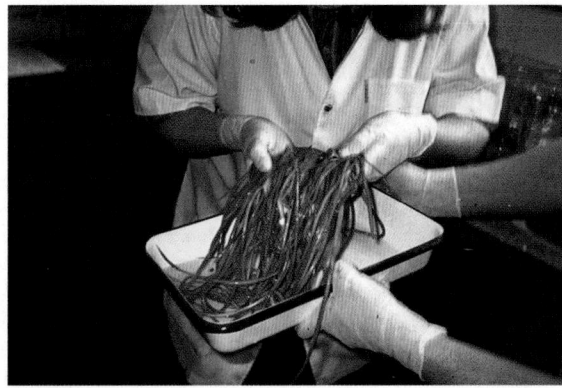

FIGURE 335-1. Mass of adult *Ascaris lumbricoides* worms recovered from a child after the administration of mebendazole. (Reproduced with permission from Dickson Despommier.)

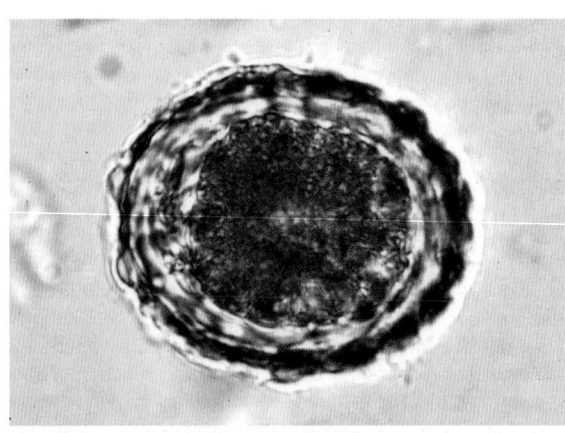

FIGURE 335-2. Fertilized, unembryonated egg of *Ascaris lumbricoides*. (Reproduced with permission from Dickson Despommier.)

become infectious after embryonating in warm, moist, shady soil. Eggs are resistant to extreme temperatures and desiccation and can survive up to 15 years in the environment.

EPIDEMIOLOGY

A. lumbricoides is the most prevalent nematode infection worldwide, affecting approximately 800 million people in sub-Saharan Africa, south and Southeast Asia, and Latin America, primarily in rural areas of high population density that lack adequate sanitation or treatment of sewage or where untreated human feces are used as fertilizer.[1] Climate is an important determinant of disease in that warm temperature and adequate moisture are required for embryonation of eggs in soil. In endemic areas, the prevalence and intensity of infection increases dramatically during the first 2 to 3 years of life, remains high between the ages of 4 and 15 years and then declines during adulthood.

CLINICAL MANIFESTATIONS

Low-intensity *A. lumbricoides* infections are usually asymptomatic. Clinical manifestations are associated with heavy worm burdens and result from larval migration through the lungs and from parasitism of the gastrointestinal tract by adult worms. During pulmonary migration, *A. lumbricoides* larvae can induce an intense reaction that is due to both physical disruption and a hypersensitivity response to secreted antigens. This phenomenon is more common in areas in which transmission is seasonal, such as on the Arabian Peninsula, where outbreaks of pneumonitis typically follow the rainy season because of resumption of transmission. Symptoms include sudden onset of wheezing, dyspnea, paroxysmal nonproductive cough, and high fever and may last for 2 to 3 weeks before resolving spontaneously. Respiratory symptoms may coincide with or be preceded by urticarial rash, angioedema, abdominal pain, and vomiting.

With moderate or heavy infections, obstruction can be caused by a mass of worms in the small intestine or migration of worms to the biliary tree, pancreatic duct, or appendix. Intestinal obstruction is more common in young children because of the smaller lumen size and is characterized by colicky abdominal pain and vomiting that may progress to signs of intestinal perforation. Hepatobiliary and pancreatic ascariasis are more common in adults. Chronic intestinal infection can manifest as abdominal pain and distention, diarrhea, and nausea. More insidious effects, especially in children, include decreased protein and fat absorption, development of vitamin A and C deficiencies, and lactose intolerance, which together lead to stunted growth and impaired cognitive development.

DIAGNOSIS

The diagnosis of ascariasis is usually made by microscopic examination of a sample of feces for characteristic thick-shelled eggs.[2] However, during the pulmonary phase of infection, ova will not be detectable in feces because adult worms have not yet matured and begun producing eggs; instead, larvae, as well as eosinophils or Charcot-Leyden crystals (formed from the breakdown of eosinophils), may be visualized on microscopic examination of sputum. Pulmonary disease is also usually characterized by peripheral eosinophilia and transient infiltrates on chest radiographs. The diagnosis of intestinal or biliary obstruction caused by *A. lumbricoides* is usually made by ultrasound examination or endoscopic retrograde cholangiopancreatography (ERCP).

TREATMENT

Intestinal ascariasis is usually cured with a single oral dose of albendazole (Table 335-1).**A1 A2** Alternatives include mebendazole, ivermectin, or pyrantel pamoate. No specific treatment is recommended for symptoms of pulmonary ascariasis because the condition is self-limited. In severe cases of biliary obstruction, including cholangitis, ERCP with or without resection of the ampulla of Vater is highly successful and may preclude the need for surgery.[1]

PREVENTION

The definitive means of preventing *Ascaris* infection is improvement of hygiene and proper disposal of human waste.[3] In endemic communities where this is not feasible, morbidity control consists of regular (usually annual) mass administration of an anthelmintic medication such as albendazole or mebendazole to preschool- and school-aged children.[4]

TABLE 335-1	TREATMENT OF INTESTINAL NEMATODES
NEMATODE	**TREATMENT**
Ascaris lumbricoides	Albendazole, 400 mg once. Alternatives: mebendazole, 500 mg once or 100 mg bid for 3 days, ivermectin 150-200 µg/kg once, or pyrantel pamoate, 11 mg/kg once with the maximum daily dose not to exceed 1 g
Hookworm (*Necator americanus* and *Ancylostoma duodenale*)	Albendazole, 400 mg daily for 3 days. Alternatives: mebendazole, 500 mg daily or 100 mg bid for 3 days, or pyrantel pamoate, 11 mg/kg for 3 days with the maximum daily dose not to exceed 1 g. Tribendimidine, 400-mg single dose alone or in combination, comparable to albendazole
Trichuris trichiura	Albendazole, 400 mg daily for 3 days. Alternative: mebendazole, 100 mg bid for 3 days, ivermectin 200 µg/kg daily for 3 days
Enterobius vermicularis	Pyrantel pamoate, 11 mg/kg once, with a second dose 2 wk later; maximum dose of 1 g. Alternatives: mebendazole, 100 mg once, or albendazole, 400 mg once, repeated in 2 wk
Strongyloides stercoralis	Uncomplicated infection: ivermectin, 200 µg/kg daily for 2 days.* Alternative: albendazole, 400 mg bid for 7 days
Trichostrongylus spp	Pyrantel pamoate, 11 mg/kg once; maximum dose of 1 g. Alternatives: albendazole, 400 mg daily for 10 days, or mebendazole, 500 mg daily for 10 days
Capillaria philippinensis	Albendazole, 400 mg bid for 10 days. Alternative: mebendazole, 500 mg daily for 20 days

*Treatment may need to be extended in immunocompromised patients with disseminated disease.

Hookworm
The Pathogen

Hookworm infection in humans is due almost exclusively to two species: *N. americanus* and *A. duodenale*. However, incidental infection with the zoonotic hookworms *Ancylostoma caninum*, *Ancylostoma braziliensis*, *Bunostomum phlebotomum*, and *Uncinaria stenocephala* can cause self-limited dermatologic lesions known as cutaneous larva migrans (Fig. 335-3). Additionally, *Ancylostoma ceylanicum*, normally a hookworm infecting cats, has been reported to cause intestinal hookworm disease in humans, especially in Asia, whereas *A. caninum* has been implicated as a cause of eosinophilic enteritis in Australia.

Infection occurs when exposed skin comes in contact with infective filariform larvae in fecally contaminated soil or grass. Larvae penetrate the skin, enter the afferent circulation, and are transported to the pulmonary vasculature, where they penetrate the alveolar wall, ascend the bronchial tree to the larynx, and are swallowed into the gastrointestinal tract. Larvae mature into sexually mature adult worms 5 to 9 weeks after skin penetration. Adult hookworms reside in the lumen of the small intestine, where they attach to the mucosa by means of cutting teeth (*A. duodenale*) or a rounded cutting plate (*N. americanus*). After mating in the host intestinal tract, female adult worms produce eggs that are expelled from the body in feces; *A. duodenale* female worms lay approximately 28,000 eggs daily, whereas the output from *N. americanus* worms averages around 10,000 a day. Hookworm eggs hatch in warm, moist, sandy soil and release larvae that can infect another host. Humans are the only major definitive host for these two parasites, and there are no intermediate or reservoir hosts. *A. duodenale* survives on average for 1 year in the human intestine, whereas *N. americanus* lives for 3 to 5 years.

EPIDEMIOLOGY

More than 450 million people are infected with hookworms worldwide.[5] *N. americanus* is widespread, whereas infection with *A. duodenale* is more geographically restricted. The highest prevalence of infection occurs in rural areas of tropical and less developed countries, where environmental and socioeconomic conditions favor transmission. Climate is an important determinant of transmission, with adequate moisture and warm temperature being essential for larval development in soil. Equally important determinants of infection are poverty and lack of access to adequate sanitation and clean water. In children living in endemic areas, prevalence increases with age until it plateaus by about 10 years of age, whereas intensity of infection rises at a slower rate during childhood, reaches a plateau by around 20 years, and then increases again in the elderly. Whether such age dependency reflects

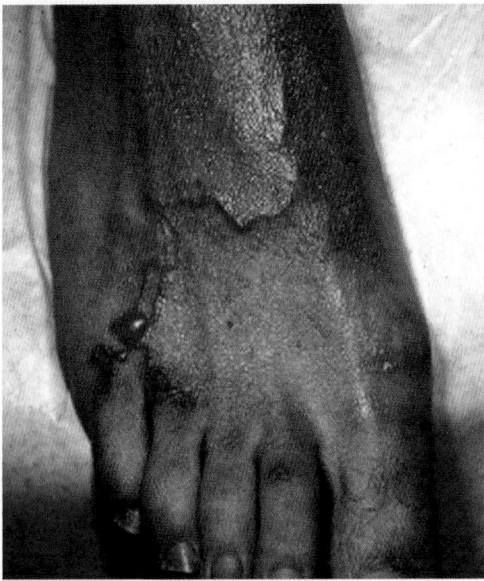

FIGURE 335-3. Typical lesion of cutaneous larva migrans. An erythematous, serpiginous track caused by intradermal migration of a dog (*Ancylostoma caninum*) or cat (*Ancylostoma braziliense*) hookworm larva is apparent. (Reproduced with permission from Gregory L. Zalar.)

differences in exposure, acquired immunity, or a combination of both is controversial.

Although cutaneous larva migrans is found throughout the tropics, in the United States it is diagnosed primarily in travelers who have recently returned from a vacation to a tropical beach destination, especially in the Caribbean, Brazil, Mexico, and Southeast Asia. Occasionally, autochthonous cases (originating where found) have been reported in the United States, usually from southeastern coastal states such as Florida and South Carolina. Cutaneous larva migrans occurs when exposed skin comes in contact with the larval stages of the dog or cat hookworms *A. caninum* or *A. braziliense*, respectively, present in moist soil or sand contaminated with animal feces. Other animal hookworms such as *U. stenocephala* and *B. phlebotomum* are less common causes.

PATHOBIOLOGY

The major pathology of hookworm infection is due to the associated gastrointestinal blood loss and the resulting iron deficiency anemia. Hookworms attach to the intestinal mucosa and secrete enzymes that enable them to invade submucosal tissues and ingest villous tissue and blood. Hemoglobinases within the hookworm's digestive canal degrade host hemoglobin for use as an essential nutrient source. The amount of blood loss is directly related to the total worm burden. *A. duodenale* causes more blood loss than *N. americanus*: each *N. americanus* worm results in a daily blood loss of 0.03 to 0.1 mL, whereas the corresponding figure for *A. duodenale* is between 0.15 and 0.26 mL.

CLINICAL MANIFESTATIONS

The clinical features of hookworm infection are due to the acute manifestations associated with larval migration through the skin and other tissues or acute and chronic manifestations resulting from parasitism of the gastrointestinal tract by adult worms. Repeated skin exposure to hookworm larvae can result in a hypersensitivity reaction known as "ground itch," a pruritic erythematous and papular rash that appears most commonly on the hands and feet. In contrast, when zoonotic hookworm larvae penetrate the skin to produce cutaneous larva migrans, most commonly on the feet, thighs, and buttocks, they are unable to complete their life cycle in the human host and eventually die after causing a typical clinical syndrome of intensely pruritic, erythematous serpiginous tracks (see Fig. 335-3). Tracks appear after an incubation period of a few days, can be single or multiple, and advance by millimeters to a few centimeters each day. Vesiculobullous or papular lesions may develop along the tracks, as can secondary bacterial infection as a result of scratching. Untreated, lesions usually heal spontaneously within weeks to months following death of the larvae in the skin.

Migration of hookworm larvae through the lungs may induce mild and transient pulmonary symptoms consisting of dry cough, sore throat, wheezing, and low-grade fever. Uncommonly, acute symptomatic disease may follow

the oral ingestion of *A. duodenale* larvae, known as Wakana syndrome, which is characterized by nausea, vomiting, pharyngeal irritation, cough, dyspnea, and hoarseness.

Abdominal symptoms and signs caused by hookworm infection are rare. Instead, the manifestations of hookworm disease occur when intestinal blood loss exceeds the nutritional reserves of the host and results in iron deficiency anemia. Usually only moderate- and high-intensity (≥2000 eggs per gram of feces) hookworm infections produce clinical disease, which resembles that of iron deficiency anemia secondary to other causes (Chapter 150). In addition, the protein losses associated with heavy hookworm infection can result in hypoproteinemia and anasarca. As iron deficiency anemia develops and worsens, weakness, palpitations, fainting, dizziness, dyspnea, lassitude, and headache may result. Uncommonly, there may be constipation or diarrhea with occult blood in the stool or frank melena, especially in children; there may also be an urge to eat soil (pica). Overwhelming hookworm infection may cause listlessness, coma, and even death, especially in infants. Because children and women of reproductive age have reduced iron reserves, they are at particular risk for symptomatic disease. Severe iron deficiency anemia caused by hookworm during pregnancy can result in adverse consequences for the mother, her unborn fetus (miscarriage, intrauterine growth restriction), and the neonate (anemia, failure to thrive). In children, the anemia and protein malnutrition associated with chronic intestinal parasitism cause long-term impairments in physical and cognitive development.

DIAGNOSIS

The diagnosis of hookworm infection is made by microscopic identification of characteristic eggs in the stool. The eggs of *N. americanus* and *A. duodenale* cannot be distinguished because both are colorless and have a single thin hyaline shell with blunted ends; they range in size from 55 to 75 μm by 36 to 40 μm. Egg concentration techniques, such as the formalin–ethyl acetate sedimentation method, can be used to detect even light infections, although a direct wet mount examination is adequate for detecting moderate to heavy infections. In addition, eosinophilia is a common finding in chronic infection and also during larval migration through the lungs.

TREATMENT   Rx

Three daily oral doses of albendazole, 400 mg, is the recommended treatment of intestinal hookworm infection (see Table 335-1). Tribendimidine, at a single oral dose of 400 mg, alone or in combination, has been found to have a similar, noninferior efficacy profile as albendazole.[A3] Less effective alternatives include mebendazole, pyrantel pamoate, and single-dose albendazole. Iron supplementation should be considered in those with significant or symptomatic anemia. For cutaneous larva migrans, although the disease is self-limited and will resolve spontaneously within weeks to a few months, treatment with a single dose of ivermectin will lead to more rapid resolution of symptoms and skin manifestations. Albendazole is an alternative treatment of cutaneous larva migrans.

PREVENTION

The ideal method for preventing hookworm infection is improvement in hygiene and proper disposal of human waste. Until this occurs, in endemic communities control of disease consists of regular (at least annual) mass administration of an antihelmintic medication such as albendazole or mebendazole. For cutaneous larva migrans, tourists should be advised to wear shoes or sandals when walking to and on beaches and to avoid beaches frequented by stray cats and dogs.

Trichuriasis
The Pathogen
T. trichiura, or whipworm, does not have a tissue migratory phase like *A. lumbricoides* and hookworm, and its entire life cycle in the host is confined to the gastrointestinal tract. After embryonated eggs are ingested orally, larvae are released into the small intestine where they undergo a series of molts before being carried passively to the transverse and descending colon. The adult worm's narrow anterior end embeds in the columnar epithelium, while the posterior portion protrudes into the lumen, thereby allowing eggs to be released into feces, which are then passed into the environment where they must embryonate in warm, moist soil to complete the life cycle. Adult worms

can measure up to 50 mm in length and survive in the host for approximately 1.5 to 2 years. The period between ingestion of eggs and detection of eggs in feces is about 90 days.

EPIDEMIOLOGY

The estimated worldwide prevalence of trichuriasis is 477 million, most commonly in poor, rural areas of the tropics and subtropics where disposal of human waste is inadequate. Children are more frequently infected than adults and more likely to have higher worm burdens. Humans are the only host.

CLINICAL MANIFESTATIONS

Most *T. trichiura* infections are asymptomatic. Symptomatic disease occurs primarily in children because the majority of heavy infections (>10,000 eggs per gram of feces) occur in this age group. Heavy infections can be accompanied by acute dysentery or chronic colitis resembling inflammatory bowel disease and result in abdominal pain and diarrhea. Chronic mucosal inflammation and edema of the colon and rectum can lead to protracted tenesmus that results in rectal prolapse. Chronic *Trichuris* colitis can also lead to malnutrition, impaired growth, and anemia.

DIAGNOSIS

Infection is diagnosed by microscopic identification of the typical barrel-shaped eggs with bipolar plugs in direct or concentrated smears of fecal specimens.

TREATMENT   Rx

Although *T. trichiura* responds less effectively than *A. lumbricoides* or hookworm to treatment with albendazole or mebendazole, a 3-day course of one of these two benzimidazole drugs is the recommended therapy, as listed in Table 335-1. The addition of ivermectin (200 μg/kg) to either drug increases the response rate significantly.[A4]

PREVENTION

As for *A. lumbricoides* and hookworm, control of trichuriasis in endemic areas consists of regular mass anthelminthic drug administration, primarily to preschool- and school-aged children, although single doses of albendazole or mebendazole are poorly effective for this intestinal nematode.

Enterobiasis
The Pathogen

E. vermicularis, or pinworm, is transmitted by the fecal-oral route. Embryonated eggs on fingernails, bedding, or clothing are ingested and hatch in the small intestine, where larvae develop into adult worms measuring between 2 and 5 mm. Adults migrate to the large intestine, where they mate. Gravid female worms emerge nightly from the anus to deposit large numbers of eggs (11,000 per worm) on the perianal and perineal skin, where they rapidly embryonate within 6 hours. If they are still on the skin, infective larvae are released that can migrate back through the anus into the rectum (retroinfection); alternatively, autoinfection occurs when eggs are transferred to the mouth via scratching skin on which eggs have been deposited, commonly in children. In infected females, larvae may also migrate into the genital tract and establish an ectopic infection.

EPIDEMIOLOGY

E. vermicularis is found worldwide and is the most prevalent nematode infection in temperate climes. Transmission is especially frequent in primary schools and daycare centers where children are in close contact.

CLINICAL MANIFESTATIONS

Although pinworm infections may be asymptomatic, perianal pruritus is the most common symptom and is caused by an allergic response to worm proteins. The pruritus can be intense and result in chronic sleep deprivation. Rarely, adult *E. vermicularis* may precipitate appendicitis. When hatched larvae migrate into the female genital tract, vulvovaginitis, salpingitis, or peritonitis may develop.

DIAGNOSIS

Pinworm infection is diagnosed by identifying eggs through microscopic examination of a piece of cellophane tape applied to the perianal region

immediately after waking and before bathing. Characteristic *E. vermicularis* eggs are oval and slightly flattened on one side. It is unusual to find eggs in feces or adult worms in the perianal area. Repeated examination may be necessary.

TREATMENT   Rx

Pinworm infection is treated with a single dose of pyrantel pamoate, mebendazole, or albendazole, which must be repeated 2 weeks later because the drugs do not kill eggs or developing larvae (see Table 335-1). Given the high rate of transmission, all household members and individuals in close contact with the patient (e.g., other children attending the same daycare center) should also be treated. Bedding and underclothes should be thoroughly laundered in hot water followed by a hot dryer to kill remaining eggs.

Strongyloidiasis
The Pathogen

S. stercoralis, or threadworm, is endemic in warm climates worldwide, including parts of the United States. Infection occurs when exposed skin comes in contact with free-living filariform larvae in soil contaminated with human feces. Similar to hookworm, larvae penetrate the skin, enter the vasculature, and migrate to the pulmonary capillaries, where they penetrate into the alveoli, ascend the bronchial tree to the pharynx, and are swallowed into the gastrointestinal tract. Further development into adult worms occurs in the upper small intestine, where parasites live embedded in the mucosa. Unlike most nematodes, *S. stercoralis* reproduces by parthenogenesis, with no apparent parasitic male worm present in the human host. Female worms begin laying eggs within 25 to 30 days after infection. The embryonated eggs hatch rapidly in the intestinal lumen and release non-infectious rhabditiform larvae that migrate to the colon and are excreted in feces. Alternatively, larvae may directly penetrate the colonic mucosa or perianal skin after migrating out of the anus and enter the circulation directly, a mechanism known as autoinfection. This phenomenon can lead to maintenance of parasitism in the host for decades.

Infectious filariform larvae develop in the soil by direct transformation from rhabditiform larvae or indirectly from eggs produced by free-living adult worms that have developed from rhabditiform larvae in warm, moist, sandy soil.

Swollen belly syndrome, a less common type of strongyloidiasis seen in infants living in central Africa and Papua New Guinea, has been attributed to infection with *Strongyloides fuelleborni*, normally a zoonosis of nonhuman primates.

EPIDEMIOLOGY

S. stercoralis infection is endemic in the tropical and subtropical regions of sub-Saharan Africa, Asia, Latin America, and areas of eastern and southern Europe, with a worldwide prevalence of up to 100 million.[6] In the United States, infection is diagnosed most frequently in immigrants, commonly from Southeast Asia, although strongyloidiasis is still endemic in parts of rural Appalachia. *S. stercoralis* can also be transmitted sexually through oral-anal contact, most often among men who have sex with men. Transmission via transplantation of solid organs from infected donors has also been reported.

PATHOBIOLOGY

In the immunologically competent, infection does not usually result in symptomatic disease. Serious complications of infection, however, may occur in individuals with cell-mediated immunodeficiency such as those chronically taking corticosteroids, solid organ transplant recipients, patients with Hodgkin disease and other lymphomas, leukemic patients, and those infected with human T-cell lymphotropic virus type 1. In these patients, the *S. stercoralis* autoinfection cycle can become amplified and lead to a hyperinfection syndrome with a large increase in the total worm burden in the infected person. Hyperinfection can lead to life-threatening dissemination of larvae and adult worms to aberrant sites such as the brain, pancreas, and kidneys. For unknown reasons, acquired immunodeficiency syndrome has not been associated with hyperinfection syndrome or with disseminated strongyloidiasis. Disseminated strongyloidiasis is frequently accompanied by bacterial sepsis due to translocation of enteric organisms carried by migrating larvae.

Most *S. stercoralis* infections, especially in immunocompetent hosts, are asymptomatic or are associated with only mild gastrointestinal manifestations such as abdominal pain, bloating, and watery diarrhea. Gastrointestinal bleeding, manifested by hematochezia or melena, occurs in less than 20% of those infected. Rare causes of morbidity include small bowel obstruction, paralytic ileus, and a malabsorption syndrome (especially in children).

During the migratory phase of larvae through the lungs, symptoms are rare in immunocompetent patients, although there may be peripheral eosinophilia. However, pulmonary signs and symptoms in immunocompromised persons with hyperinfection syndrome can be severe and resemble those of adult respiratory distress syndrome with acute onset of dyspnea, productive cough, and hemoptysis accompanied by fever, tachypnea, and hypoxemia.

Migration of filariform larvae from the anus can lead to a dermatologic manifestation known as larva currens, which is characterized by migratory serpiginous erythematous maculopapular tracks, primarily on the skin of the buttocks, groin, and lower abdomen.

Autoinfection leading to exceptionally high worm loads (i.e., hyperinfection) and disseminated strongyloidiasis can occur in persons with deficient cell-mediated immunity. Because asymptomatic infection with *S. stercoralis* may persist for decades after initial infection, it is important to remember that a change in immune status associated with conditions such as the administration of immunosuppressive drugs following solid organ transplantation may result in hyperinfection syndrome even though the infection was previously asymptomatic. Massive increases in the number of *Strongyloides* larvae because of hyperinfection can present as acute enteritis with severe diarrhea and ulcerative disease of the small and large intestine. During disseminated infection, larvae and sometimes adult worms penetrate the intestinal mucosa, migrate to aberrant sites, including the central nervous system, and result in metastatic abscesses and gram-negative meningitis due to enteric bacteria being carried by the migrating parasites. Less common complications of disseminated disease include glomerulonephritis and minimal-change nephrotic syndrome, acute respiratory distress syndrome, and alveolar hemorrhage.[7] Mortality from hyperinfection and disseminated disease can be high, although early diagnosis and prompt initiation of treatment are associated with improved outcomes.

Infants with swollen belly syndrome caused by *S. fuelleborni* are often seen acutely with abdominal ascites that is not accompanied by diarrhea or fever. The ascites is due to gastrointestinal protein loss; it can be significant enough to cause respiratory impairment and is associated with a high rate of mortality.

Definitive diagnosis of *S. stercoralis* infection relies on microscopic identification of larvae in feces or other fluids (such as sputum) or tissues. Intestinal strongyloidiasis can be diagnosed by identification of larvae in direct smears of freshly passed stool, although the sensitivity of a single fecal sample examination is as low as 30%. Sensitivity can be increased by examining multiple fecal specimens, by using concentration techniques, and by plating feces on an agar plate and inspecting for tracks of colonies created by bacteria being dragged by migrating larvae.

Hyperinfection syndrome and disseminated strongyloidiasis can be diagnosed by detection of filariform larvae in duodenal fluid obtained by endoscopy, in sputum, or in bronchoalveolar lavage specimens. Larvae have also been recovered from cerebrospinal fluid, urine, peritoneal washings, skin, and the brains of immunocompromised persons.

Fluctuating eosinophilia is common with uncomplicated intestinal strongyloidiasis, especially during the pulmonary migration phase of initial infection. However, eosinophilia may be absent in patients with hyperinfection and dissemination. In fact, those with hyperinfection and eosinophilia have a better prognosis than do those without eosinophilia.

Serologic diagnosis using an enzyme-linked immunosorbent assay (ELISA) that detects antibodies to filariform larvae is very sensitive, even in immunocompromised hosts with disseminated strongyloidiasis, although false-positive results may occur in cases of coinfection with other nematodes, particularly filaria. Specificity is improved by using the newer luciferase immunoprecipitation system (LIPS) assays that incorporate *Strongyloides*-specific recombinant antigens. LIPS assays have the additional advantage of rapid reversion to seronegative after treatment compared with the slow decline in ELISA titers.

Uncomplicated intestinal strongyloidiasis can be treated effectively with ivermectin (200 µg/kg body weight daily for 2 days), with cure rates, defined as the absence of larvae by parasitologic methods 1 year after treatment, exceeding 90%.[A5] Albendazole is an alternative treatment (see Table 335-1).[8] Decreases in antibody titer and eosinophil count indicate a treatment response in the absence of continued exposure. After 6 months, ELISA titers should decrease significantly, whereas LIPS assays should revert to negative. However, more recently reported long-term follow-up studies for up to 4 years after ivermectin treatment showed that larvae were detected again in 14 of 21 patients, observed as early as 30 days after treatment, and *S. stercoralis* DNA was detected in all patients, both in their 30-day posttreatment and subsequent stool samples. These data suggest that long-term parasitologic cure is unlikely, and strongyloidiasis must be considered a chronic infection for which ivermectin administration schedules should be re-evaluated.[9]

In immunocompromised patients with hyperinfection or disseminated disease, daily treatment with ivermectin should be extended. Some experts recommend continuing treatment until 2 weeks after fecal examinations have become negative (i.e., for one autoinfection cycle). For severely ill patients who are unable to tolerate oral therapy, parenteral veterinary and enema ivermectin preparations have been used. Combination therapy with ivermectin and albendazole may also be used to treat disseminated strongyloidiasis, but data on whether this improves prognosis over monotherapy are lacking.

In endemic areas, the risk for infection can be reduced by minimizing skin contact with contaminated soil, although elimination of this infection will occur only with improvements in sanitation and treatment of human waste. To prevent hyperinfection in individuals already infected, diagnosis should be attempted before the onset of immunosuppression if possible, such as before organ transplantation or cancer chemotherapy. Anyone who has resided in or traveled to an endemic area should undergo screening for asymptomatic infection, preferably by serology or, if not possible, by microscopic examination of at least three fecal samples for the presence of larvae. Patients with positive screening test results should be treated empirically with ivermectin. Individuals with negative screening test results but unexplained eosinophilia and a history of exposure should also be considered for empirical treatment. In those undergoing hematopoietic stem cell transplantation, documentation of response with at least three consecutive negative fecal examinations or a negative LIPS assays is recommended before proceeding with transplantation.

UNCOMMON INTESTINAL NEMATODIASES

Humans may serve as incidental hosts for some nematodes that ordinarily parasitize the intestines of other mammals.

Trichostrongylus

Human infections with various species of the genus *Trichostrongylus* have been reported in Iran, the Far East, and Australia. Humans become infected when larvae are ingested with leafy vegetables that have been contaminated with soil containing the feces of herbivorous animals. *Trichostrongylus* worms are similar to hookworms in their morphology, appearance of their eggs on fecal examination, and the pathology that they induce. Heavy infections may be accompanied by diarrhea and anemia. Drugs recommended for treatment are pyrantel pamoate, albendazole, or mebendazole (see Table 335-1).

Anisakiasis

Anisakiasis results from ingestion of the larvae of nematodes that normally infect sea mammals such as dolphins, whales, and seals. Larvae of the genera *Anisakis*, *Phocanema*, and *Pseudoterranova* infect the flesh of a number of saltwater fish species as intermediate hosts. Consumption of raw or undercooked fish, often in the form of sushi or sashimi, results in release of the infective larvae into the stomach, followed by invasion of the stomach or duodenal wall, which causes upper abdominal pain that can be intense. Anisakid worms cannot further develop in humans and die within a few days; an eosinophilic granulomatous reaction may result that mimics a gastric tumor. Diagnosis and treatment are accomplished by endoscopic removal of the parasite. Infection is prevented by cooking or freezing seafood before consumption. Of note, salting, smoking, and marinating fish do not kill anisakid larvae.

Capillaria philippinensis

C. philippinensis can cause a serious intestinal infection that has been reported primarily in the Philippines and Thailand, although it has also been observed in Japan, Taiwan, Korea, and Egypt. Adult worms resemble those of *Trichinella spiralis*, although biologically they mimic *S. stercoralis* in that they have an autoinfectious cycle of reproduction in which larvae can develop into adult worms without leaving the host. Even though the life cycle has not been completely elucidated, this nematode probably parasitizes waterfowl that feed on fish and crustaceans, which serve as intermediate hosts. Humans become infected by eating raw or undercooked infected shrimp or fish. Adult worms travel to the mucosal crypts of the small intestine, where they deposit larvae, sometimes resulting in overwhelming infection. Clinical disease consists of severe diarrhea associated with anorexia, vomiting, and weight loss. Mortality rates as high as 10% have been reported, with death resulting from severe malabsorption and protein-losing enteropathy. Diagnosis depends on visualizing eggs or larvae in feces. The treatment of choice is albendazole or mebendazole (see Table 335-1).

TISSUE NEMATODES

The tissue nematodes can be divided into those for which humans are the principal host (the filariases) and those that usually infect animals but can incidentally infect humans. Several zoonotic nematodes, such as *Toxocara*, *Trichinella*, and *Angiostrongylus*, infect humans following accidental oral ingestion of eggs or larvae but are unable to complete their life cycle in the host. Clinical manifestations are primarily due to the aberrant migration of larvae through various tissues.

Toxocariasis

DEFINITION

Accidental ingestion of embryonated eggs of the dog roundworm *Toxocara canis*, or less frequently of the cat ascarid *Toxocara cati*, can lead to the clinical syndromes of visceral larva migrans and ocular larva migrans. Symptoms are caused by the migration of larvae through the organs of the body, resulting in serious disease and even death.

EPIDEMIOLOGY

Toxocara infections in animals are ubiquitous throughout the world. In humans, children are most frequently infected, probably by exposure to soil contaminated with dog or cat feces when playing outside. Visceral larva migrans occurs most commonly in children younger than 5 years, whereas ocular larva migrans typically affects older children between the ages of 5 and 10 years.

PATHOBIOLOGY

The life cycle of *Toxocara* in the animal host resembles that of *A. lumbricoides* in humans; larvae penetrate the intestinal wall after being released from ingested eggs, migrate through the vasculature to the lungs, enter into the alveolar space, and ascend the bronchial tree until they are swallowed back into the gastrointestinal tract, where they develop into adult worms that can produce eggs. However, when embryonated *Toxocara* eggs are ingested by humans, the released larvae migrate throughout the body (most commonly to the lungs, the liver, the central nervous system [CNS], and occasionally the eyes) but cannot develop into adult worms. Ultimately, the larvae die, inducing significant immediate-type and delayed-type hypersensitivity reactions that result in eosinophilic granuloma formation. Visceral larva migrans and ocular larva migrans seem to be mutually exclusive, suggesting that different *Toxocara* strains may have different tissue tropisms. Alternatively, visceral larva migrans may result from repeated infections, whereas ocular larva migrans may be a manifestation of infection in children who have not been previously sensitized.

CLINICAL MANIFESTATIONS

Most *Toxocara* infections in humans are asymptomatic. Visceral larva migrans is characterized by low-grade fever, pulmonary symptoms including cough and wheeze, and less frequently hepatosplenomegaly accompanied by right upper quadrant pain.[10] Symptoms appear gradually and resolve over 4 to 8 weeks. Myocarditis, nephritis, and CNS disease are less common. CNS involvement can result in seizures, encephalopathy, neuropsychiatric symptoms, or an eosinophilic meningoencephalitis.

Ocular larva migrans typically presents as unilateral visual impairment that is sometimes accompanied by strabismus. The degree of vision loss is dependent on the particular ocular structure involved, and permanent blindness can occur. Ocular larva migrans involving the retina can be difficult to distinguish from other causes of focal intraretinal lesions, such as retinoblastoma or tuberculosis.

DIAGNOSIS

Toxocariasis can be presumed on the basis of a compatible clinical presentation and history of exposure to dogs or cats. Eosinophilia and hypergammaglobulinemia are often present. Serologic testing using an ELISA in combination with immunoblot to detect anti-*Toxocara* antibodies may be informative, although this does not distinguish between active infection and past exposure. Recent development of ELISAs incorporating recombinant *T. canis* antigens has improved assay sensitivity and specificity. Biopsy of tissues to document the presence of larvae is not recommended because of low sensitivity.

Computed tomography and fluorescein angiography may be helpful in the diagnosis of ocular larva migrans, especially to differentiate it from retinoblastoma and other causes of intraocular space-occupying lesions. Elevated levels of anti-*Toxocara* antibodies in aqueous and vitreous humor fluid relative to serum are also suggestive of this diagnosis.

TREATMENT Rx

Albendazole (400 mg given twice daily for 5 days) is the treatment of choice for acute toxocariasis (Table 335-2). Mebendazole is not recommended because of its poor oral bioavailability. In patients with severe pulmonary, cardiac, or neurologic involvement, corticosteroids may reduce the severity and duration of symptoms. Ocular larva migrans is treated by vitrectomy, corticosteroids, albendazole, or a combination of these.
See also Chapter 323.

PREVENTION

Visceral larva migrans and ocular larva migrans may be prevented by periodic anthelminthic treatment of dogs and cats, proper disposal of pet feces, covering sandboxes, washing hands after playing with dogs or cats, and keeping children from playing in areas where pets have defecated.

TABLE 335-2 TREATMENT OF TISSUE NEMATODE INFECTIONS

NEMATODE INFECTION	TREATMENT
Toxocariasis	Albendazole, 400 mg bid for 5 days
Trichinellosis	Albendazole, 400 mg bid for 8-14 days*
Angiostrongyliasis	Treatment with albendazole or mebendazole is controversial but may relieve symptoms.
Gnathostomiasis	Albendazole, 400 mg daily for 3 wk Alternative: ivermectin, 200 µg/kg/day for 2 days +/− Surgical removal
Lymphatic filariasis	Diethylcarbamazine, 6 mg/kg/day divided in three doses for 12 days†, plus doxycycline, 100-200 mg/day for 6 wk
Onchocerciasis	Ivermectin, 150 µg/kg once (alternative: moxidectin 8 mg once), repeated every 6-12 mo until resolution of symptoms, plus doxycycline, 200 mg/day for 6 wk‡
Loiasis	Diethylcarbamazine, 8-10 mg/kg/day divided in three doses for 21 days†‡
Mansonella perstans	Doxycycline, 200 mg/day for 6 wk
Mansonella ozzardi	Ivermectin, 200 µg/kg once
Mansonella streptocerca	Diethylcarbamazine, 6 mg/kg/day divided in three doses for 12 days Alternative: ivermectin, 150 µg/kg once
Dracunculiasis	Extraction of the adult worm

*Treatment is effective only if it is initiated during the intestinal phase of infection.
†Start at a dose of 50 mg on the first day, 50 mg three times/day on the second, 100 mg three times/day on the third, and then 8-10 mg/kg/day on day 4 onward.
‡Repeated treatment after 6 months is often necessary if symptoms and eosinophilia persist.

Baylisascariasis

Baylisascariasis is a rare zoonosis caused by infection with *Baylisascaris procyonis,* an ascarid parasite of raccoons and other small carnivores. In North America, infection is most commonly associated with contact with raccoons or environments contaminated with their feces and occurs predominantly in infants and young children who ingest the embryonated eggs while playing with soil. Clinically, disease is manifested as neural larva migrans due to larval invasion of the CNS after release from ingested eggs in the gastrointestinal tract. Characteristic findings include fever, altered mental status, focal neurologic deficits, and seizures. Examination of the cerebrospinal fluid (CSF) reveals eosinophilic meningitis. *B. procyonis* has also been associated with ocular larva migrans. Infection can be fatal or result in permanent neurologic or visual impairment. When neural larva migrans is present, response to treatment with anthelmintics is poor, although corticosteroids may be helpful. Successful use of laser photocoagulation in ocular larva migrans has been reported. Prophylactic albendazole (25 mg/kg/day for 20 days) started within days of an exposure may prevent clinical disease.

Trichinellosis

DEFINITION

Trichinella infects a range of mammalian hosts, with the domestic pig serving as the most important reservoir worldwide. Humans are infected through eating raw or undercooked pork or other meats of domestic or wild animals that are contaminated with larvae that are encysted in muscle tissue.[11] Although larvae develop into adults in the human intestinal tract, mate, and produce offspring larvae, clinical disease is characterized not so much by the intestinal infection as by the newborn larvae that penetrate the intestinal wall and disseminate throughout the body.

EPIDEMIOLOGY

Several different species of *Trichinella* can cause disease in humans, although *Trichinella spiralis* is the most common. *T. spiralis* is enzootic throughout the world in omnivorous and carnivorous wild animals, including bears, boars, and rats. *Trichinella nativa* affects predominantly carnivores (e.g., walruses, polar bears, and seals) living in the Arctic and subarctic regions of North America, Europe, and Asia. *Trichinella* is introduced into domestic animal populations, usually pigs or horses, by feeding them unprocessed meat scraps of infected animals, most commonly rats. Because of regulations banning this practice in the United States, Canada, and the European Union, human infection by consumption of undercooked or smoked pork products or beef contaminated with the encysted larvae has been virtually eliminated,[12] although it still occurs throughout the rest of the world. Instead, ingestion of poorly cooked wild game, especially bear or boar meat, is now the most common source of infection in these places. An important source of infection with *T. nativa* in Alaskan and Canadian Arctic native populations is eating of uncooked walrus meat.

PATHOBIOLOGY

Trichinellosis, also called trichinosis, results from ingestion of striated muscle containing encysted infective larvae. Larvae are released from muscle tissue by digestive enzymes in the stomach and then migrate to the upper small intestine, where they rapidly develop into sexually mature adult worms after only 2 days. Adults live embedded in the columnar epithelium, where they grow to a length of 3 mm (females) or 1.5 mm (males). Females begin producing newborn larvae within 5 days of mating. Adult worms remain viable for an additional 3 to 5 weeks, after which acquired immunity develops that leads to their expulsion from the host.

Newborn larvae possess a swordlike stylet in their oral cavity that permits them to penetrate the lamina propria and enter the lymphatic and blood vessels of the host, allowing them to migrate throughout the body. Larvae enter all types of cells, where they usually die, with the exception of striated skeletal and cardiac muscle cells. Unique among nematodes, mature *Trichinella* larvae have an intracellular phase, developing and transforming muscle cells into "nurse cells" that support larval growth and development (Fig. 335-4). In nurse cells, *Trichinella* larvae can survive for decades. Although nurse cells do not result in any disease in most mammals, they can induce an eosinophilic granulomatous reaction in humans that may result in significant tissue damage and dysfunction.

CLINICAL MANIFESTATIONS

Clinical disease in humans can be divided into an initial intestinal phase followed by a systemic or muscle phase. The initial phase of infection that occurs within days after ingestion of larvae may be associated with mild diarrhea,

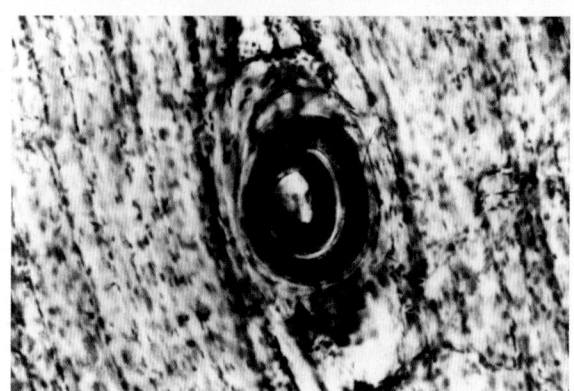

FIGURE 335-4. Nurse cell in muscle tissue containing a larva of *Trichinella spiralis.* (Courtesy of Dr. I. Kagan, Centers for Disease Control and Prevention.)

abdominal pain, and vomiting. This phase is self-limited and usually resolves spontaneously within 10 days.

The systemic dissemination of *Trichinella* larvae can result in myocardial, pulmonary, and focal neurologic manifestations, although usually only in the most heavily infected persons. This systemic phase of infection usually begins 2 to 3 weeks after ingestion of infective larvae and may persist for several weeks. Clinical manifestations typically include fever, periorbital or facial edema, a diffuse inflammatory myositis (Chapter 253) that is characterized by myalgias and muscle tenderness, and petechial hemorrhages most easily observed in the subungual skin and conjunctivae. Larval invasion of the myocardium[13] can lead to myocarditis (Chapter 54) that may result in heart failure or arrhythmias.

As with most nematodes, the severity of symptoms is related to the total worm burden. Because adult worms are incapable of reproducing within the host, the number of encysted larvae ingested is the most important determinant of the number of larvae that invade muscle and other tissues.

DIAGNOSIS

A diagnosis of trichinellosis should be suspected in individuals with a compatible clinical presentation, a history of eating raw or undercooked meat, eosinophilia, and increased muscle enzymes such as creatine kinase and lactate dehydrogenase. Definitive diagnosis depends on visualization of nurse cells in a muscle biopsy specimen or detection of *Trichinella*-specific DNA by the polymerase chain reaction (PCR) technique, although this tool is not widely available. Findings on muscle biopsy may be normal even in heavily infected patients because of sampling error. Detection of anti-*Trichinella* antibodies can be very useful in making a diagnosis; ELISA is the most commonly used method. Antibodies can be detected as early as 12 days after initial infection.

TREATMENT (Rx)

During the intestinal phase of infection, albendazole is recommended at a dosage of 400 mg given twice daily for 8 to 14 days to kill the adult worms and prevent release of newborn larvae (see Table 335-2). Although it is not known if albendazole is effective against newborn larvae, administration of this drug during the systemic phase of infection could potentially worsen symptoms by exacerbating the host inflammatory response to dying larvae. Treatment of severe systemic disease, including myocarditis and neurologic disease, should be directed toward reducing inflammation, most commonly with corticosteroids, although albendazole should also be given in such cases as corticosteroids may delay expulsion of adult worms from the intestine thus increasing the number of newborn larvae that may be released. Symptomatic treatment with antipyretics and analgesics should also be considered.

See also Chapter 323.

PREVENTION

Trichinella infection is prevented by thoroughly cooking meat to kill encysted larvae. Freezing meat solid at −20° C for at least 3 days will kill *T. spiralis* but not all other species of *Trichinella*. Of note, curing and smoking techniques do not reliably kill this nematode.

Angiostrongyliasis

DEFINITION

Angiostrongylus cantonensis and *Angiostrongylus costaricensis* are nematodes that normally infect rodents, primarily rats. The adult worms of *A. cantonensis*, or rat lungworm, inhabit the pulmonary arteries of rodents; larvae are produced that migrate to the pharynx, are swallowed, and then are passed in the feces. Mollusks such as snails, slugs, and prawns serve as intermediate hosts until they are ingested by definitive hosts. Released larvae migrate to the brain, where they develop into immature adult worms before traveling to the pulmonary vasculature to become sexually mature adults. Humans are incidentally infected after eating raw or poorly cooked mollusks or fresh vegetables contaminated with parts of infected mollusks; larvae can migrate to the CNS but cannot develop further. As opposed to *A. cantonensis*, the larvae of *A. costaricensis* can develop into sexually mature adult worms in the local lymphatics and mesenteric arterioles of humans and release eggs and larvae into the intestinal tissue, causing an intense eosinophilic granulomatous reaction.

EPIDEMIOLOGY

Human infections with *A. cantonensis* occur mainly in Southeast Asia and the South Pacific and less frequently in Brazil, the Caribbean, and Louisiana.[14] Abdominal angiostrongyliasis due to *A. costaricensis* has been reported mainly in Latin America, mostly in young children.

CLINICAL MANIFESTATIONS

After ingestion, *A. cantonensis* larvae penetrate the intestinal wall and migrate to the brain, the meninges, and less commonly the spinal cord and eye. Fever, severe headache, meningismus, nausea, vomiting, seizures, and focal neurologic deficits may develop. *A. costaricensis* infection can mimic appendicitis with right-sided abdominal pain, vomiting, and fever. Less frequently, gastrointestinal bleeding may occur.

DIAGNOSIS

Diagnosis of *A. cantonensis* infection is based on a history of ingestion of potentially contaminated food, the presence of peripheral eosinophilia, and detection of eosinophils and rarely larvae in the CSF. In neither CNS nor intestinal angiostrongyliasis are larvae or eggs found in the feces, although both may be seen in tissue specimens for *A. costaricensis*. Serology is not commercially available.

TREATMENT AND PREVENTION (Rx)

Most patients infected with either species of *Angiostrongylus* recover completely after approximately 2 weeks. The use of anthelmintics (Chapter 323) is controversial, with only a few reports of benefit with albendazole or mebendazole, usually administered in combination with analgesics and corticosteroids to relieve symptoms. Serial lumbar punctures to remove CSF can relieve symptoms of raised intracranial pressure caused by infection with *A. cantonensis*. Proper cooking of food and washing of vegetables can prevent this infection.

Gnathostomiasis

Gnathostoma spinigerum is an intestinal nematode of dogs and cats; intermediate hosts include tiny crustaceans (copepods), amphibians, freshwater fish, and birds. Human infection occurs throughout the Far East, Thailand, and Latin America, particularly Mexico, through eating raw or undercooked invertebrate hosts harboring larvae. Larvae are released in the intestine and subsequently migrate through the body but are unable to reach sexual maturity in humans. The most common clinical presentation is migrating painful and pruritic subcutaneous swellings. Eosinophilic meningitis and ocular larva migrans may also occur, with potentially devastating results, including paralysis, subarachnoid hemorrhage, and permanent visual loss. Peripheral eosinophilia, often significant, is usually present; with meningitis, eosinophils are also present in the CSF. Although serologic testing is not available in the United States, laboratories in Thailand and Japan can perform it. Treatment of cutaneous disease with either a 3-week course of albendazole or a 2-day course of ivermectin is recommended (see Table 335-2); for neurologic or ocular involvement, anthelminthics are not advised because they may worsen manifestations. Gnathostomiasis may be prevented by thoroughly cooking fish.

Filariases

DEFINITION AND PATHOBIOLOGY

The filariases are arthropod-borne nematode infections that are endemic mostly in tropical areas of the world, in which mature adult worms live in the lymphatics or in connective tissue (Table 335-3). Eight filarial species infect humans: *Wuchereria bancrofti*, *Brugia malayi*, *Onchocerca volvulus*, *Brugia timori*, *Loa loa*, *Mansonella streptocerca*, *Mansonella perstans*, and *Mansonella ozzardi*. The first three are the most common filariases worldwide. Although not usually fatal, these infections can result in significant disability and disfigurement, such as irreversible limb lymphedema (*W. bancrofti* and *B. malayi*) or blindness (*O. volvulus*). Most of the filariases require prolonged exposure for disease to be manifested and are therefore uncommon in short-term travelers to endemic areas.

For all of the filarial nematodes, infection begins with the bite of an infected arthropod vector that deposits infective larvae called microfilariae into the skin or blood. During several months, microfilariae mature into adult worms capable of mating to produce microfilariae that can be ingested by another arthropod vector to complete the life cycle. Adult worms can survive for 5 to 17 years in the human host; microfilariae live for between 5 months and 5 years. For most of the filarial nematodes except *B. malayi* and *M. perstans*, humans are the only definitive host.

CLINICAL MANIFESTATIONS

Clinical manifestations of infection are varied. Severity of disease is in most cases proportional to the worm burden harbored by an individual, with relatively light infections commonly being asymptomatic. For several of the filariases, the host inflammatory response to infection becomes apparent only on the death of the adult worms or microfilariae. This may be triggered by exposure to filarial antigens that were previously hidden from the immune system or by release of bacterial endosymbionts of the genus *Wolbachia* that live inside several of the filariae. *Wolbachia* are of the order Rickettsiales and are found in the hypodermis of adult worms and in oocysts, embryos, and microfilariae; they play a critical role in worm viability and fertility.

DIAGNOSIS

Diagnosis of filarial infections usually depends on the microscopic examination of either blood or skin specimens for characteristic microfilariae (see Table 335-3). Microfilariae of the different filarial species measure between 170 and 320 μm in length and can be distinguished on the basis of the tissue source of the specimen, the presence or absence of a sheath, and the arrangement of nuclei in the tail. For some filarial species, microfilariae are present in the blood only during certain periods of the day to coincide with biting habits of the arthropod vector, which must be taken into account in timing blood collection for microscopy. Serology is not useful in endemic areas because a positive result does not distinguish between previous and current infection, and there is considerable antigenic cross-reactivity between the filariae and other nematodes. Detection of antifilarial antibodies may, however, be useful in returned long-term travelers or expatriates who are not originally from endemic areas.

TREATMENT (Rx)

Diethylcarbamazine (DEC), ivermectin, and albendazole are the principal antifilarial drugs, although they have varying efficacies against the different filarial species (see Table 335-2). DEC is macrofilaricidal (active against the adult worm) for *W. bancrofti*, *Brugia* species, and *L. loa*, although prolonged or repeated courses are required for this effect. More commonly, the goal is to suppress microfilaria production by adult female worms, which can be achieved by single doses of antifilarial drugs administered alone or in combination annually or biannually. Reduction of microfilariae in the blood or skin can in some cases ameliorate symptoms or prevent progression of disease as well as interrupt transmission. Furthermore, targeting the *Wolbachia* endosymbionts of some filarial species with extended courses of antibiotics such as doxycycline can be macrofilaricidal.

LYMPHATIC FILARIASIS

DEFINITION

The three etiologic agents of lymphatic filariasis, *W. bancrofti*, *B. malayi*, and *B. timori*, are transmitted to humans through the bite of an infected mosquito. Microfilariae deposited at the bite wound subsequently migrate through the subcutaneous tissue to the lymphatic system, where adult worms develop

TABLE 335-3 FILARIAL PARASITES OF HUMANS

SPECIES	DISTRIBUTION	VECTOR	MICROFILARIAE		
			PRIMARY LOCATION	PERIODICITY	PRESENCE OF SHEATH
Wuchereria bancrofti	Tropics worldwide	Mosquitoes	Blood	Nocturnal, subperiodic	+
Brugia malayi	India, Southeast Asia	Mosquitoes	Blood	Nocturnal, subperiodic	+
Brugia timori	Indonesia	Mosquitoes	Blood	Nocturnal	+
Onchocerca volvulus	Africa, South America	*Simulium* blackflies	Skin, eye	None or minimal	−
Loa loa	West and Central Africa	*Chrysops* flies	Blood	Diurnal	+
Mansonella perstans	Africa, South America, Caribbean	Midges	Blood	None	−
Mansonella ozzardi	Central and South America, Caribbean	Midges, *Simulium* blackflies	Blood	None	−
Mansonella streptocerca	West and Central Africa	Midges	Skin	None	−

after approximately 4 to 12 months. The worms reside coiled in lymph nodes and may extend into afferent lymph vessels and surrounding subcutaneous tissue. The lymphatics of the lower and upper extremities and male genitalia are most commonly affected. After mating, females, which measure between 4 and 10 cm in length, twice the length of males, release more than 10,000 microfilariae a day that migrate into the blood stream until ingestion by biting mosquitoes. In most endemic areas, microfilariae are present in the peripheral blood only at night, when mosquito vectors are most likely to bite. Adult filariae live between 5 and 8 years within the host, although infections lasting for decades have been reported.

EPIDEMIOLOGY

An estimated 70 million people are affected by lymphatic filariasis worldwide; most cases are caused by *W. bancrofti,* and less than 5 million are due to *B. malayi. B. timori* is of minor importance, being restricted to southeastern Indonesia. *W. bancrofti* is widely distributed in the tropics, especially in Southeast Asia, the Indian subcontinent, Africa, South America, the Caribbean, and the South Pacific. The major vectors of bancroftian filariasis are *Culex* mosquitoes in urban areas, anopheline mosquitoes in rural areas of Africa, and *Aedes* species in the Pacific.

Humans are the only definitive host for *W. bancrofti. B. malayi,* however, can be zoonotic, with both monkey and feline species serving as reservoir hosts. Brugian filariasis is found primarily in India, Malaysia, and other areas in Southeast Asia.

PATHOBIOLOGY

The pathology of filarial infections is primarily due to obstruction of the lymphatic circulation resulting from damage induced by adult worms, specifically a local inflammatory lymphangitis with components of the innate and adaptive immune response leading to vessel wall hypertrophy. This inflammatory response can be triggered by release of antigens from dead or dying worms, although evidence suggests that it is also induced by living worms and *Wolbachia* antigens that are excreted or secreted into the surrounding milieu. Inflammatory damage is also exacerbated by secondary bacterial and fungal infections.

The initial inflammatory response leads to endothelial and connective tissue proliferation and vessel dilation, which impairs normal lymphatic function and results in lymphedema that is initially reversible. However, worm death results in a granulomatous reaction to released worm and *Wolbachia* antigens. The infiltration of giant cells as well as plasma cells, eosinophils, and neutrophils can completely occlude the lumen of the lymphatic vessel. Over time, progressive fibrosis and obstruction of lymph flow result in irreversible edema. Although recanalization and collateralization of lymph vessels may occur, lymphatic function remains compromised.

CLINICAL MANIFESTATIONS

The clinical manifestations of lymphatic filariasis cover a wide spectrum from asymptomatic infection to severe chronic lymphatic obstruction accompanied by lymphedema and enlargement of the affected limb or body part (referred to as elephantiasis). Other common clinical outcomes include acute episodic lymphadenitis (also called filarial fever) and tropical pulmonary eosinophilia. Most infected individuals living in endemic regions are clinically asymptomatic, although microfilariae can be observed in their blood. Despite the absence of a significant inflammatory response, these individuals may nevertheless exhibit dilation of the affected lymphatics on ultrasound, which precedes the onset of clinically apparent disease.

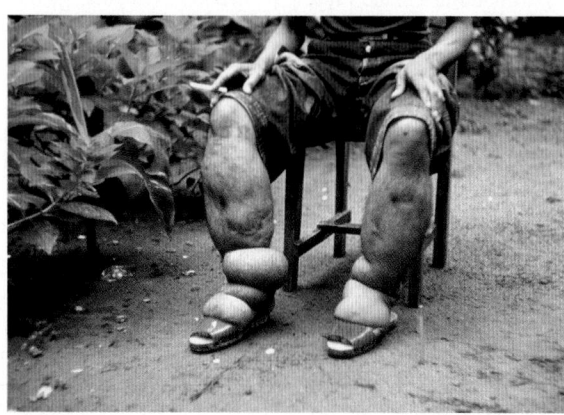

FIGURE 335-5. Elephantiasis, or chronic lymphedema due to infection with *Wuchereria bancrofti.* (Courtesy of the Centers for Disease Control and Prevention.)

For unknown reasons, newly exposed individuals may develop acute inflammatory reactions that can rapidly progress to chronic or irreversible changes compared with those born in endemic areas. Severe episodes of lymphadenitis, often with genital involvement, may lead to the relatively rapid development of lymphedema and elephantiasis within a year of presentation. Findings usually resolve quickly if the individual is promptly removed from the endemic area. Microfilariae are usually not detected in these patients.

Acute Lymphadenitis

Acute episodes of retrograde lymphadenitis occur most commonly in adolescents in endemic areas, often in response to dying adult worms. Painful, erythematous enlargement of an affected lymph node, most commonly inguinal, precedes the onset of lymphangitis and is accompanied by fever and chills. Episodes usually last for about a week, frequently recur, and can be incapacitating. Defervescence is abrupt and associated with desquamation of the overlying skin. In men, inguinal lymphadenitis can be complicated by epididymitis and orchitis. Patients with filarial fevers may be microfilaremic but often are not.

Elephantiasis

Repeated episodes of lymphadenitis eventually lead to dilation of the lymphatic vessels, resulting in chronic lymphedema over the course of months to years (Fig. 335-5). The extremities, breasts, and genitalia are most commonly affected, although with *B. malayi* infection, usually only the lower parts of the legs are involved. The edema is initially pitting in nature, but the subcutaneous tissue eventually loses its elasticity, resulting in woody edema with thickening of subcutaneous tissue and hyperkeratosis. Secondary bacterial or fungal infection contributes significantly to the chronic pathologic process of elephantiasis.

In bancroftian filariasis, hydrocele is a common manifestation of chronic filariasis in men and can sometimes become massive and debilitating; lymphedema of the vulva is less commonly seen in women. Involvement of the retroperitoneal lymphatics can lead to their rupture to produce intermittent chyluria or chylocele.

Tropical Pulmonary Eosinophilia

Tropical pulmonary eosinophilia (Chapter 161) develops in a small minority of individuals with filarial infections. The syndrome is most commonly seen in young men living in southern India, although it also occurs in Pakistan, Sri Lanka, Southeast Asia, and Brazil. Characteristic clinical findings include nocturnal paroxysmal cough, wheeze, and low-grade fever that are accompanied by weight loss and eosinophilia. Levels of total immunoglobulin E (IgE) and antifilarial antibodies are typically high. Chest radiographs may show diffuse interstitial infiltrates or mottled opacities. Without treatment, chronic restrictive lung disease may develop.

DIAGNOSIS

Definitive diagnosis usually relies on microscopic examination of a Giemsa-stained blood smear for microfilariae. Although thick blood smears are relatively insensitive except in cases of high microfilaremia, concentration or filtering techniques can increase the diagnostic yield. Characteristic microfilariae are 250 to 320 μm in length. Collection of blood should be timed according to the known periodicity of the microfilariae.

A rapid immunochromatographic card test is available for *W. bancrofti* (there is no equivalent test for *Brugia* infections) and has the advantage of not requiring nocturnal collection of blood because it detects circulating antigen of the adult worm and not microfilariae. PCR methods have been developed to detect filarial antigens in blood, but these are not widely available. Serologic detection of antifilarial antibodies is of limited value because of extensive antigenic cross-reactivity with other nematodes. Furthermore, actively infected individuals cannot be distinguished from those previously infected, and those merely exposed but not infected may also have positive serologic test results.

Ultrasound examination of the lymphatic vessels of the spermatic cord of men can be used to visualize the "filarial dance sign," which is pathognomonic for a nest of filarial parasites.

Individuals with elephantiasis may be amicrofilaremic. Diagnosis therefore depends on a compatible clinical history and physical examination in the context of the appropriate epidemiology, and it may be supported by a positive antigen test or, in men, by a suggestive scrotal ultrasonogram. It should be distinguished from podoconiosis, a tropical lymphedema that results from long-term barefoot exposure to red-clay soil derived from volcanic rock and that may be a T-cell-mediated inflammatory disease.

TREATMENT   Rx

Management of lymphatic filariasis differs according to whether the aim is disease control or cure of an individual patient. In endemic areas, annual mass drug administration with a combination of antifilarial drugs can reduce transmission by decreasing the number of microfilariae in the blood available to biting mosquitoes. These programs use different two-drug combinations of single-dose DEC, ivermectin, and albendazole, administered at least annually, although a recent study showed sustained reduction in microfilaremia for 3 years after single-dose coadministration of all three drugs.[A6] DEC is administered with albendazole except in areas where onchocerciasis or loiasis is also endemic, in which case ivermectin plus albendazole is used.

All individuals with active infection by a lymphatic filarial parasite, whether symptomatic or asymptomatic, should be treated with an antifilarial medication (see Table 335-2). The treatment of choice is DEC (6 mg/kg/day for 12 days). In the United States, DEC is available only through the Centers for Disease Control and Prevention (CDC) drug service (http://www.cdc.gov/laboratory/drugservice/formulary.html). For patients with high levels of microfilariae in the blood, treatment can be started at a low dose of 50 mg daily and scaled up during the first 3 days to reduce side effects of treatment such as fever, headache, dizziness, nausea, vomiting, rash, myalgias, and arthralgias. These normally resolve after a few days of treatment and can be treated with antipyretics, antihistamines, and, if symptoms are severe, corticosteroids.

DEC is both microfilaricidal and partially macrofilaricidal. In individuals who will not be returning to endemic areas, repeated treatments with DEC are often attempted to kill the adult worms instead of just reducing the levels of microfilariae in the blood. Typically, courses of DEC are repeated every 6 to 12 months. Although the adult worm burden is reduced in most treated individuals, all parasites are eliminated in less than one fourth. In men with live adult worms visible by ultrasound in the scrotal lymphatics, serial studies may be performed to monitor the effects of therapy.

Unfortunately, lymphedema due to lymphatic filariasis is usually not reversible with DEC treatment, except in the very early stages. Nevertheless, the chronic sequelae of lymphatic filariasis can be limited by prevention of secondary bacterial and fungal infection through meticulous hygiene and prompt treatment of suspected infections with antimicrobials. Limb elevation, physiotherapy, and use of elastic stockings may slow the worsening of lymphedema. Surgery is usually not indicated except for cases of hydrocele.

Interestingly, treatment directed against the *Wolbachia* endosymbiont has been shown to be effective in killing adult *W. bancrofti* and *Brugia* worms. Doxycycline, 100 or 200 mg daily for 4 to 8 weeks, reduces female worm fertility with a resulting suppression of microfilaremia for up to a year and reduces the number of live adult worms. Given the duration of treatment, these regimens are not ideal for disease control programs in endemic countries.

DEC is highly effective in the treatment of tropical pulmonary eosinophilia. Treatment with a dose of 6 mg/kg/day for 14 to 21 days results in resolution of symptoms within a week, although relapse may occur even after an interval of years.

See also Chapter 323.

PREVENTION

Annual mass treatment with single doses of two antifilarial drugs can significantly reduce the prevalence of infection within a community. In some areas, DEC-fortified table salt has been used to reduce the levels of microfilaremia in affected communities to interrupt transmission. Vector control through the use of insecticide-treated bed nets and residual indoor spraying of insecticides may have some efficacy.

ONCHOCERCIASIS
DEFINITION

Onchocerciasis, or river blindness, caused by the nematode *O. volvulus*, is transmitted to humans by *Simulium* blackflies. Infective microfilariae develop into male and female adult worms over a period of several months and live for 9 to 14 years coiled within subcutaneous fibrous nodules (onchocercomas). Adult females measure between 20 and 70 cm in length and remain confined to the nodules; males are only 3 to 5 cm long and freely migrate through the subcutaneous tissues between nodules to inseminate females. Mature female worms produce up to 1500 microfilariae per day, which leave the nodule to migrate primarily through the skin and ocular tissues. Microfilariae live within the host for 12 to 18 months.

EPIDEMIOLOGY

Onchocerciasis is endemic in equatorial Africa, with small foci in Yemen and an area on the border between Brazil and Venezuela. Approximately 18 million people are estimated to be infected, while 270,000 are blind due to this parasite. More than 99% of cases occur in sub-Saharan Africa, with Nigeria being the most highly endemic country. Because *Simulium* blackflies require fast-flowing, well-oxygenated water for egg laying and reproduction, cases are concentrated around streams and rivers, often in the most fertile farming areas.

Blindness caused by *O. volvulus* results in significant morbidity, long-term disability, and reduced economic productivity. In addition, onchocerciasis has been associated with a reduced life expectancy of at least 10 years compared with uninfected individuals in the same area, an effect that appears to be independent of the blindness that develops.

PATHOBIOLOGY

The pathologic changes of onchocerciasis are primarily due to an inflammatory reaction to microfilariae, mostly in the skin, eyes, and lymph nodes. Adult worms contained in nodules are relatively isolated from the host immune response. Tissue damage results from a cell-mediated immune response to dying microfilariae, which becomes more pronounced as infection persists. The degree of tissue damage is directly related to the intensity of infection as well as the magnitude of the host response. Sclerosing keratitis, the major cause of blindness, results from an inflammatory reaction to dying intraocular microfilariae that is dependent on helper T-cell type 2 (T_H2) cytokines. With time, neovascularization and scarring of the cornea lead to corneal opacification and eventual blindness. In the skin, similar immune responses result in pruritus and angioedema. Ongoing low-grade inflammation in the skin eventually leads to loss of elasticity and atrophy. Chronic inflammatory changes and fibrosis are also seen in lymph nodes.

Like the nematodes responsible for lymphatic filariasis, *O. volvulus* adult worms contain endosymbiotic *Wolbachia* bacteria that are obligatory for the development, survival, and fertility of these worms. Pro-inflammatory *Wolbachia* proteins released by dying microfilariae may be responsible for a significant part of the immunopathology associated with onchocerciasis. For example, *Wolbachia* antigens have been shown to interact with the innate immune system through a toll-like receptor 2–mediated mechanism.

CLINICAL MANIFESTATIONS
Onchodermatitis

Onchocerciasis commonly presents with a diffuse papular dermatitis that is intensely pruritic.[15] In heavily infected individuals in endemic areas, the pruritus is intractable, leading to scratching and excoriation to the point of bleeding and even suicide. Hypersensitivity reactions, scabies, insect bites, and atopic or contact dermatitis should be considered in the differential diagnosis of the acute papular dermatitis seen with onchocerciasis. The skin of affected areas becomes edematous and thickened, loses its elasticity, and takes on an orange-peel texture. A lichenified dermatitis (referred to as sowda) may occur; it consists of an intensely pruritic eruption limited to one extremity, usually a leg, with hyperpigmented papules and plaques accompanied by edema of the entire limb. Over time, the skin will atrophy and fine wrinkles appear, especially over the buttocks. Pruritus is uncommon at this point. Areas of depigmentation may occur most commonly over the shins, a phenomenon called leopard skin.

Subcutaneous Nodules

Subcutaneous onchocercomas containing adult worms are most often palpable over bony prominences. In Africa, the nodules are most commonly found over the hips and lower limbs; in South America, they are usually located on the head and upper part of the body. Nodules measure between 0.5 and 3 cm in diameter and are freely mobile. In lightly infected individuals, such as expatriates, nodules are usually not detectable.

Ocular Lesions

Initial ocular involvement is characterized by conjunctivitis, excess tearing, and photophobia in response to dying microfilariae. At this point in the course of disease, punctate keratitis or snowflake corneal opacities are present. During 20 to 30 years, this progresses to sclerosing keratitis, neovascularization, and corneal opacification. The anterior chamber of the eye may also be involved, with iritis, iridocyclitis, and secondary glaucoma. Posterior ocular disease can be manifested as chorioretinitis, optic neuritis, and optic atrophy.

Lymphadenopathy

Lymphadenopathy is frequently found in the inguinal and femoral areas in Africa and in the head and neck in South America. Advanced disease in the inguinal region can result in the so-called hanging groin, with elongated atrophic skin containing nontender and fibrotic lymph nodes.

DIAGNOSIS

Definitive diagnosis has traditionally been made by observing unsheathed motile microfilariae measuring 200 to 300 μm in length that are released from superficial skin snips. To take a skin snip, a thin piece of skin overlying a bone prominence that has been tented up with a needle is sliced with a scalpel blade, or a corneal-scleral punch instrument is used to obtain a small piece of skin. Avoidance of blood contamination is critical so as to avoid confusion with blood-borne microfilariae in cases in which patients are coinfected with other filariases. Typically, six snips are taken, one from over each scapula, iliac crest, and lateral aspect of each calf, and then incubated with warm physiologic saline and examined microscopically for motile microfilariae after incubating for up to 24 hours. PCR amplification of filarial DNA directly from skin snips is far more sensitive than direct visualization but is not widely available. With ocular disease, free microfilariae may be visible by slit lamp examination in the anterior chamber or aqueous humor.

Subcutaneous nodules can be sampled or examined by ultrasound to demonstrate the presence of adult worms. Serologic tests are usually positive for antifilarial antibodies but are not specific because of considerable antigenic cross-reactivity with other nematodes. Eosinophilia is a common but inconsistent finding.

In the past, the Mazzotti test was used to diagnose onchocerciasis. In this test, a challenge dose of DEC was administered to patients suspected of having onchocerciasis; with *O. volvulus* infection, an intense pruritic skin reaction would develop within hours. However, in patients with high-intensity infections, the Mazzotti reaction could be severe and even worsen ocular disease, resulting in permanent visual loss. Therefore, this test is no longer recommended, although some instead suggest the application of a small amount of DEC-containing cream to the skin to provoke a localized Mazzotti reaction.

TREATMENT   Rx

Ivermectin or moxidectin are the treatments of choice for onchocerciasis (see Table 335-2). Administration of a single dose of ivermectin (150 μg/kg) or moxidectin (8 mg [age >12 yrs]) is effective in ameliorating ocular and dermatologic disease by destroying microfilariae and suppressing their release from female worms. Because neither ivermectin nor moxidectin is active against adult worms, treatment must be repeated every 6 to 12 months, probably for at least 10 years in those without further exposure. For unknown reasons, pruritus in lightly infected expatriates may require more aggressive and frequent treatment for the first 2 years. Within 24 hours of treatment, fever and pruritus may occur in reaction to the dying microfilariae or released *Wolbachia* antigens, especially in those with high pretreatment levels of microfilariae. Another potential agent is moxidectin (8 mg single oral dose), which appears to be as effective, or even more effective, compared with ivermectin.[A7]

Use of ivermectin or moxidectin in areas where *L. loa* (see later) is coendemic should be undertaken with caution because treatment may precipitate severe reactions including encephalopathy in those with high *L. loa* microfilaremia. The LoaScope is a mobile-telephone-based videomicroscope that, with the use of a smartphone coupled to a simple optical device, provides a rapid, point-of-contact, field-friendly, and accurate method to quantify *L. loa* microfilariae. It has enabled a test-and-not-treat strategy to identify individuals with high blood levels of circulating *L. loa* microfilariae who are at particular risk for serious adverse events and should be excluded from mass drug administration strategies for the elimination of lymphatic filariasis and onchocerciasis.[16] DEC should never be used for treatment of onchocerciasis because of frequent serious reactions to dying microfilariae ranging from urticaria and angioedema to hypotension and death. Although the drug suramin (available from the U.S. CDC drug service) is active against adult *O. volvulus* worms, because of its excessive toxicity, it is used only in rare situations. Nodulectomy successfully resolves the infection in some cases.

Doxycycline, 200 mg/day administered for 4 to 6 weeks, followed by single-dose ivermectin, has been shown to deplete *Wolbachia* endosymbionts from adult worms, resulting in a significant macrofilaricidal effect and suppression of embryogenesis and microfilaria production for up to 18 months in the remaining adult worms.[A8] Increasingly, this regimen is recommended for patients with onchocerciasis who have left an endemic area and will not be re-exposed.

See also Chapter 323.

PREVENTION

Regular mass administration of ivermectin to affected communities forms the core of the global eradication strategy for onchocerciasis. Implementation of this program has been made easier because the drug is donated by the manufacturer. In addition to benefiting infected individuals, mass drug administration reduces the microfilariae available to vectors and thus interrupts the transmission cycle. For travelers to endemic areas, use of insect repellent may be beneficial.

LOIASIS
DEFINITION

Loiasis is caused by infection with the filarial nematode *L. loa*, otherwise known as the African eye worm. *L. loa* are transmitted by flies of the genus *Chrysops* during a blood meal. Adult worms develop during a period of 1 to 4 years and live for up to 17 years. They migrate freely in the subcutaneous tissue, including the subconjunctiva or sclera of the eye. Adult females measure between 40 and 70 mm in length; males are shorter, measuring between 25 and 35 mm. After mating, females release microfilariae into the blood. *L. loa* microfilariae exhibit a diurnal periodicity coinciding with the feeding habits of *Chrysops*, with microfilaremia peaking around midday.

EPIDEMIOLOGY

Loiasis is endemic in the rain forest regions of central and west Africa, with the highest prevalence in Gabon, Cameroon, the Democratic Republic of the Congo, Nigeria, and the Central African Republic.[17] Loiasis requires a shorter period of exposure than other filarial infections and can be seen in returning travelers or expatriates who have spent extended periods in Africa.

PATHOBIOLOGY

Neither adult *L. loa* worms nor microfilariae have any direct pathologic effects. In a subset of infected individuals, a hypersensitivity response, termed a *Calabar swelling*, develops to secretions from adult worms or released microfilariae, resulting in recurrent localized angioedema that often precedes the migrating worm. These patients have high serum levels of IgE antibodies and eosinophilia. This reaction is more commonly observed in visitors to endemic areas than

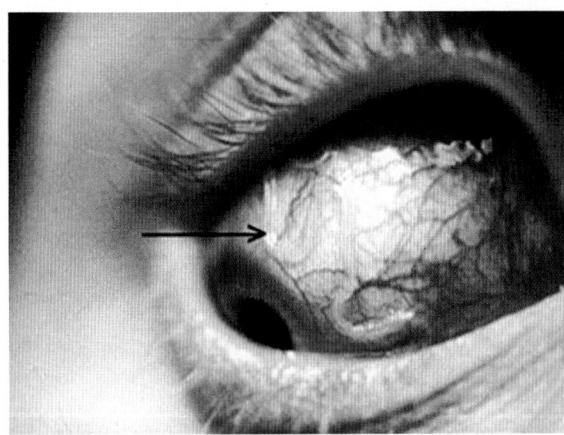

FIGURE 335-6. Adult *Loa loa* worm migrating across the eye (*arrow*).

in native residents. Unlike other filariae, *L. loa* does not contain *Wolbachia* endosymbionts.

CLINICAL MANIFESTATIONS

Most individuals with loiasis are asymptomatic despite being microfilaremic. Clinical manifestations of infection are more common in long-term visitors to endemic areas than in people native to the regions. Recurrent Calabar swellings are the most common finding in these individuals, who are not usually microfilaremic. They are nonerythematous swellings measuring 5 to 20 cm in diameter that typically occur on the extremities and the face and last for a few days. The onset is often preceded by pruritus and pain. On occasion, adult worms may migrate across the subconjunctiva or sclera of the eye, causing severe pain and inflammation (Fig. 335-6). Rare complications of infection include nephropathy and encephalitis, which usually develop in those with high levels of microfilariae after receiving DEC or ivermectin treatment for other filarial infections. Endomyocardial fibrosis resulting from eosinophilic infiltration of the myocardium has been reported in association with loiasis.

DIAGNOSIS

Diagnosis depends on microscopic examination of a Giemsa-stained blood film for characteristic sheathed microfilariae. Blood should be collected between 10 AM and 2 PM because of the diurnal periodicity of the microfilariae. Because individuals who are not native to endemic areas are usually not microfilaremic, diagnosis relies on a compatible history, clinical findings, peripheral eosinophilia, and elevated antifilarial antibody levels. Adult worms can sometimes be surgically removed while migrating across the eye or through subcutaneous tissues. Calabar swellings must be distinguished from onchocercomas and other causes of angioedema.

TREATMENT   Rx

DEC (8 to 10 mg/kg/day for 21 days) is active against both adult *L. loa* worms and microfilariae (see Table 335-2). Treatment is usually increased from a dose of 50 mg/day on the first day to the full dose on the fourth day to minimize the likelihood of treatment-associated complications, the most serious of which are glomerulonephritis and a potentially fatal encephalopathy. Treatment-associated complications are more common with high pretreatment microfilarial levels and result from host allergic reactions to dying microfilariae. Antihistamines and corticosteroids may be employed to reduce allergic side effects. Alternatively, apheresis can be used to remove circulating microfilariae before initiation of DEC. Albendazole, which is microfilaricidal but has no activity against adult worms, has been used to reduce microfilaria levels before treatment with DEC. Repeated courses of DEC may be necessary in about half of patients before clinical manifestations completely resolve. Persistent or increasing eosinophilia or levels of antifilarial antibodies 6 months after treatment should also prompt re-evaluation for repeated treatment. Adult worms in the eye may be surgically removed.

Ivermectin is microfilaricidal but has no macrofilaricidal effect and may cause toxic encephalopathy in individuals with high microfilaria levels. In areas where onchocerciasis is coendemic, this infection should be ruled out and treated before initiation of DEC to prevent toxicity from dying *O. volvulus* microfilariae.

See also Chapter 323.

PREVENTION

Weekly chemoprophylaxis with DEC administered as a 300-mg dose is effective in preventing loiasis in long-term residents of endemic areas.

LESS COMMON FILARIAL INFECTIONS

Mansonella perstans

M. perstans infection occurs throughout west and central Africa, in northeastern South America, and in parts of the Caribbean. Microfilariae are transmitted by *Culicoides* midges and develop into adult worms that live in serous body cavities, such as the pleural, pericardial, and peritoneal spaces, as well as in mesenteric and retroperitoneal tissues. Most infections are asymptomatic, although painless conjunctival nodules with eyelid edema have been reported. Transient angioedema and Calabar-like swellings, fever, headache, arthralgias, and neurologic manifestations may also occur. Microfilariae do not exhibit periodicity and can be observed on stained blood films. Eosinophilia is common. *M. perstans* harbor *Wolbachia* endosymbionts, and treatment with doxycycline, 200 mg/day for 6 weeks, has been shown to be highly effective in suppressing microfilaremia for up to 3 years, suggesting that the treatment is macrofilaricidal.

Mansonella ozzardi

Infections with *M. ozzardi* occur in Central and South America and parts of the Caribbean, especially Haiti. Vectors include *Simulium* blackflies and midges. Adult worms locate to the peritoneal and thoracic cavities or the lymphatics; microfilariae circulate in the blood without periodicity. Infection usually results in asymptomatic eosinophilia, although arthritis and allergic symptoms such as urticaria and lymphadenopathy may occur in response to dying worms. Administration of ivermectin as a single dose of 200 μg/kg has been reported to provide long-term suppression of microfilaremia and improvement of symptoms. Neither DEC nor the benzimidazoles are effective.

Mansonella streptocerca

M. streptocerca is endemic in the tropical forest zone of west and central Africa and is transmitted by biting midges. Similar to *O. volvulus*, adult worms live in the subcutaneous tissues, as do microfilariae. In contrast to onchocerciasis, microfilariae do not invade the eye. Infection is usually asymptomatic, although a pruritic dermatitis with depigmentation similar to onchodermatitis can affect the trunk and upper extremities. Associated axillary or inguinal adenopathy is common. Microfilariae have characteristic hooked tails and can be visualized in skin snips. In areas where onchocerciasis is coendemic, skin specimens must be stained to differentiate *M. streptocerca* from *O. volvulus*. DEC is microfilaricidal and macrofilaricidal and is given as 6 mg/kg/day for 12 days. Ivermectin is effective against microfilariae but not adult worms.

Zoonotic Filarial Infections

A rare accidental filarial infection of humans with the dog heartworm *Dirofilaria immitis* occurs worldwide. Transmitted by mosquitoes, *D. immitis* microfilariae cannot reach maturity in humans but embolize to the lung after dying in the right ventricle. Most infections are asymptomatic, but some people experience cough, chest pain, and hemoptysis consistent with lung infarction. Chest radiographs demonstrate typical coin lesions that may be mistaken for carcinoma. Other animal filariae, including *Dirofilaria repens* of dogs and *Dirofilaria tenuis* of raccoons, can infect humans and result in subcutaneous nodules that may be migratory. Eosinophilia and antifilarial antibodies are not usually present in zoonotic filarial infections. Surgical removal of lesions is both diagnostic and curative.

Dracunculiasis

Dracunculiasis is a disfiguring disease caused by the nematode *Dracunculus medinensis,* or Guinea worm. Although previously found in the Indian subcontinent and Latin America, it is now endemic in only four countries in sub-Saharan Africa (South Sudan, Chad, Mali, and Ethiopia) due to concerted eradication efforts. In 2017, fewer than 50 cases were identified. Transmission to humans occurs through ingestion of copepods, tiny crustacean intermediate hosts that harbor infective larvae. Released larvae penetrate the intestinal wall and migrate to the subcutaneous tissues, where they develop into adult worms. After approximately a year, female worms induce vesicular skin lesions, usually on the lower extremities, that eventually ulcerate. On direct contact with fresh water, the female worm releases thousands of motile larvae that can then complete the transmission cycle by infecting copepods in the water. Adult worms measure up to a meter in length. Fever and allergic symptoms, including wheezing and urticaria, may precede rupture of the blister or occur upon attempted extraction of the worm. Secondary bacterial infection of the skin lesions is frequent. Although not commonly fatal, dracunculiasis can result in significant disability.

Traditionally, emerging worms are extracted by slowly winding a few centimeters of the parasite on a stick each day, taking care not to break it. Surgical removal can also be attempted but may exacerbate allergic symptoms. There is no effective chemotherapy for this infection. Prevention efforts have been highly successful in interrupting transmission and have led to eradication of the parasite from many countries. Strategies include filtering of drinking water through finely woven cloth, education of infected individuals not to enter fresh water, treatment of water sources with larvicides, and provision of safe drinking water from wells.

Grade A References

A1. Moser W, Schindler C, Keiser J. Efficacy of recommended drugs against soil transmitted helminths: systematic review and network meta-analysis. *BMJ.* 2017;358:1-10.

A2. Adegnika AA, Zinsou JF, Issifou S, et al. Randomized, controlled, assessor-blind clinical trial to assess the efficacy of single-versus repeated-dose albendazole to treat *Ascaris lumbricoides, Trichuris trichiura,* and hookworm infection. *Antimicrob Agents Chemother.* 2014;58:2535-2540.

A3. Moser W, Coulibaly JT, Ali SM, et al. Efficacy and safety of tribendimidine, tribendimidine plus ivermectin, tribendimidine plus oxantel, pamoate, and albendazole plus oxantel pamoate against hookworm and concomitant soil-transmitted helminth infection in Tanzania and Côte d'Ivoire: a randomised, controlled, single-blinded, non-inferiority trial. *Lancet Infect Dis.* 2017;17:1162-1171.

A4. Knopp S, Mohammed KA, Speich B, et al. Albendazole and mebendazole administered alone or in combination with ivermectin against *Trichuris trichiura:* a randomized controlled trial. *Clin Infect Dis.* 2010;51:1420-1428.

A5. Suputtamongkol Y, Premasathian N, Bhumimuang K, et al. Efficacy and safety of single and double doses of ivermectin versus 7-day high dose albendazole for chronic strongyloidiasis. *PLoS Negl Trop Dis.* 2011;5:1-7.

A6. King CL, Suamani J, Sanuku N, et al. A trial of a triple-drug treatment for lymphatic filariasis. *N Engl J Med.* 2018;379:1801-1810.

A7. Opoku NO, Bakajika DK, Kanza EM, et al. Single dose moxidectin versus ivermectin for *Onchocerca volvulus* infection in Ghana, Liberia, and the Democratic Republic of the Congo: a randomised, controlled, double-blind phase 3 trial. *Lancet.* 2018;392:1207-1216.

A8. Abegunde AT, Ahuja RM, Okafor NJ. Doxycycline plus ivermectin versus ivermectin alone for treatment of patients with onchocerciasis. *Cochrane Database Syst Rev.* 2016:CD011146.

GENERAL REFERENCES

For the General References and other additional features, please visit Expert Consult at https://expertconsult.inkling.com.

336

ANTIVIRAL THERAPY (NON-HIV)

JOHN H. BEIGEL AND SHYAMASUNDARAN KOTTILIL

Although some viral infections are self-limited, others can cause significant morbidity and mortality. Effective therapy is available for many of these infections. This chapter reviews currently available antiviral agents for the treatment of infections caused by viruses other than human immunodeficiency virus (HIV). Not all agents discussed are licensed in all countries.

Currently available agents can be classified into those that directly inhibit viral replication at the cellular level (antivirals), those that modify the host response to infection (immunomodulators), and those that directly inactivate viral particles (microbicides/virucides). Antiviral agents can be classified based on their mechanism of action. For example, nucleic acid analogues inhibit viral DNA or RNA synthesis by competing with endogenous nucleic acids and block the viral DNA polymerase or RNA transcriptases. By comparison, protease inhibitors prevent viral replication by binding to the enzymes that cleave viral protein precursors into active proteins.

Antiviral strategies that are not covered in this chapter include local destructive measures that destroy both host tissues and virus simultaneously, such as cryotherapy, laser, and podophyllin treatment of warts. Although effective, such measures are useful only for discrete or localized mucocutaneous infections.

ANTIVIRALS FOR HEPATITIS B VIRUS INFECTIONS

Acute hepatitis B virus (HBV) infection (Chapter 139) generally does not require antiviral treatment. Currently approved antivirals for chronic hepatitis B (Chapter 140) include six nucleic acid analogues (adefovir, entecavir, lamivudine, telbivudine, tenofovir disoproxil fumarate (TDF), and tenofovir alafenamide [TAF]), as well as two immune modulators (interferon-alfa-2b and pegylated [PEG]-interferon-alfa-2a) (Tables 336-1 to 336-3).[1] Treatment may be initiated with any approved antiviral medications, but tenofovir, TAF, entecavir, and PEG-interferon-alfa-2a are generally the preferred agents. Tenofovir or entecavir is preferred for patients with compensated cirrhosis (Chapter 144). The goal of antiviral treatment is to suppress HBV replication and reduce the progression of liver disease and its complications.

Patients with chronic hepatitis B (hepatitis B surface antigen [HBsAg] positive for >6 months, detectable serum HBV DNA >20,000 IU/mL, and an alanine aminotransferase [ALT] level more than twice the normal level) should be evaluated for treatment. Patients with clinically decompensated hepatitis B (e.g., icterus or other signs) generally require antiviral treatment. Therapy in hepatitis B e antigen (HBeAg)-positive chronic hepatitis B should be continued until the patient has achieved HBeAg seroconversion and serum HBV DNA is undetectable, followed by at least 6 months of additional treatment after the appearance of anti-HBe. Therapy in HBeAg-negative chronic hepatitis B should continue for at least a year. Patients with decompensated cirrhosis or recurrent hepatitis B after liver transplantation should receive lifelong treatment.

TABLE 336-1 ANTIVIRALS FOR HEPATITIS VIRUS INFECTIONS

VIRAL INFECTION	DRUG	ROUTE	USUAL ADULT DOSAGE
Chronic hepatitis B	Tenofovir disoproxil fumarate	PO	300 mg/day
	Tenofovir alafenamide	PO	25 mg/day
	Entecavir		
	Naïve virus	PO	0.5 mg daily; optimal duration of therapy unknown
	Lamivudine-resistant virus	PO	1 mg daily; optimal duration of therapy unknown
	Interferon-alfa-2b	SC	6 MU/m² (up to 10 MU) three times weekly for 16-24 wk
	PEG-interferon-alfa-2a	SC	180 µg weekly for 48 wk
	Adefovir	PO	10 mg/day
	Lamivudine	PO	100 mg/day
	Telbivudine	PO	600 mg/day
Chronic hepatitis C	Ledipasvir/sofosbuvir	PO	90 mg/400 mg once daily for 12-24 wk
	Sofosbuvir/velpatasvir	PO	400 mg/100 mg/day for 12 wk
	Sofosbuvir/velpatasvir/voxilaprevir	PO	400 mg/100 mg/100 mg/day for 12 wk
	Daclatasvir/sofosbuvir	PO	60 mg/400 mg/day for 12-24 wk
	Grazoprevir/elbasvir	PO	100 mg/50 mg/day for 12-16 wk
	Glecaprevir/pibrentasvir	PO	300 mg/120 mg/day for 8-16 wk
	Ombitasvir/paritaprevir/Ritonavir + dasabuvir	PO	12.5 mg/75 mg/50 mg (two pills once daily) + dasabuvir 250 mg twice daily for 12-24 wk (+RBV for genotype 1a)
	Daclatasvir/asunaprevir	PO	60 mg/400 mg/day for 24 wk
	Sofosbuvir	PO	400 mg once daily for 12-24 wk
	Simeprevir	PO	150 mg once daily for 12 wk
	PEG-interferon-alfa-2a	SC	180 µg weekly for 48 wk
	or PEG-interferon-alfa-2b	SC	1.5 µg/kg weekly for 48 wk
	plus ribavirin	PO	800-1200 mg/day, depending on weight

TABLE 336-2 MECHANISMS OF EXCRETION AND THRESHOLDS FOR DOSE ADJUSTMENT

	MAJOR ROUTE OF ELIMINATION	THRESHOLD FOR ADJUSTMENT IN RENAL INSUFFICIENCY OR FAILURE	ADJUSTMENT FOR HEPATIC FAILURE	SPECIAL ADJUSTMENT FOR ELDERLY
Adefovir	Renal	CrCl <50 mL/min	No adjustment	
Entecavir	Renal	CrCl <50 mL/min	No adjustment	
Lamivudine	Renal	CrCl <50 mL/min	No adjustment	
Ledipasvir/sofosbuvir	Renal	CrCl <30 mL/min/1.73 m^2	No adjustment	
Sofosbuvir/velpatasvir	Renal	CrCl <30 mL/min/1.73 m^2	No adjustment	
Voxilaprevir	Hepatic	CrCl <30 mL/min	No adjustment	
Ombitasvir/paritaprevir/ Ritonavir + Dasabuvir	Renal	No adjustment	Contraindicated	
Ribavirin	Renal	CrCl <50 mL/min	No adjustment	
PEG-interferon-alfa-2a	Renal	CrCl <50 mL/min	Progressive rise in alanine transaminase	>60 yr, consider reduction
Telbivudine	Renal	CrCl <50 mL/min	No adjustment	
Sofosbuvir	Renal	CrCl <50 mL/min	No adjustment	
Simeprevir	Hepatic	No adjustment	No adjustment	
Boceprevir	Hepatic	No adjustment	No adjustment	
Daclatasvir	Hepatic	No adjustment	No adjustment	
Asunaprevir	Hepatic	No adjustment	Contraindicated	
Glecaprevir/pibrentasvir	Hepatic	No adjustment	Contraindicated	
Grazoprevir/elbasvir	Hepatic	No adjustment	Contraindicated	

TABLE 336-3 SIGNIFICANT ADVERSE EFFECTS (U.S. FDA BLACK BOX WARNING)

DRUG	BLACK BOX SYNOPSIS
Adefovir	Severe acute exacerbations of hepatitis B may occur with cessation of therapy. Nephrotoxicity may occur in patients at risk for renal dysfunction. Lactic acidosis and severe hepatomegaly with steatosis
Entecavir	Severe acute exacerbation of hepatitis B may occur with cessation of therapy. Lactic acidosis and severe hepatomegaly with steatosis
Grazoprevir/elbasvir	Hepatitis B virus reactivation in patients with HCV and HBV
Interferon-alfa	May cause or aggravate neuropsychiatric, autoimmune, ischemic, and infectious disorders
Lamivudine	Severe acute exacerbations of hepatitis B may occur with cessation of therapy. Lactic acidosis and severe hepatomegaly with steatosis
Ledipasvir/sofosbuvir	Hepatitis B virus reactivation in patients with HCV and HBV
Ombitasvir/paritaprevir/ ritonavir plus dasabuvir	Hepatic failure in patients with decompensated liver cirrhosis
Voxilaprevir	Hepatic failure in patients with decompensated liver cirrhosis
Glecaprevir/pibrentasvir	Hepatic failure in patients with decompensated liver cirrhosis
Ribavirin	Monotherapy is not effective. Hemolytic anemia Teratogenic and embryocidal
Sofosbuvir	Life-threatening bradycardia when administered with amiodarone Hepatic failure in patients with decompensated liver cirrhosis
Telbivudine	Severe acute exacerbation of hepatitis B may occur with cessation of therapy. Lactic acidosis and severe hepatomegaly with steatosis
Tenofovir plus TAF	Severe acute exacerbations of hepatitis B may occur with cessation of therapy.

Tenofovir Disoproxil Fumarate

Tenofovir, a nucleotide analogue of adenosine monophosphate, was first approved for the treatment of HIV infection. TDF is an ester prodrug of tenofovir, with an effective tenofovir bioavailability of 25%. Administration following a high-fat meal increases the oral bioavailability.

Clinical Uses

Tenofovir is approved for the treatment of chronic hepatitis B in adults with evidence of active viral replication and either persistent elevations in serum aminotransferase levels or histologically active disease. Treatment with tenofovir is more effective than adefovir or entecavir in producing histologic improvement and viral suppression in patients with HBeAg-negative or HBeAg-positive chronic hepatitis B.[A1] Tenofovir also has demonstrated efficacy in patients with lamivudine-resistant HBV.

Toxicity

Tenofovir is generally safe and well tolerated for up to 5 years. The most common side effects are nausea, diarrhea, vomiting, and anorexia. Lactic acidosis with hepatic steatosis has been reported, primarily when it is used in combination with other nucleoside analogues. Acute exacerbations of hepatitis B have been reported after discontinuation of tenofovir in patients who are coinfected with HIV and HBV.

Antiviral Resistance

Mutations in HBV polymerase that confer reduced susceptibility to tenofovir occur during prolonged use (>12 months). In vitro studies showed that adefovir-resistant HBV mutations are associated with three- to five-fold decrease in response to tenofovir, though clinical implications are not known.

Tenofovir Alafenamide

TAF, which is a new prodrug of tenofovir, is a successor of TDF. TAF is converted intracellularly to tenofovir. Its active diphosphate metabolite is targeted at the RNA-dependent DNA polymerase of either HBV or HIV. TAF is even licensed to treat hepatitis B infection. TAF accumulates in lymphatic tissue and in the liver, and it enters cells more efficiently than TDF. For these reasons, TAF can be given at a lower dose, thereby resulting in lower plasma tenofovir levels and a much lower risk for kidney toxicity or bone density changes.

Clinical Uses

In clinical trials, TAF was noninferior to TDF in achieving HBV DNA levels below 29 IU/mL.[A2] TAF-treated patients had significantly smaller decreases in bone mineral density at the hip and spine in both HBeAg-positive and HBeAg-negative patients, and HBeAg-positive patients also had smaller mean increases in serum creatinine levels. Patients treated with TDF for 96 weeks and then switched to TAF had improvements in renal function and bone mineral density 24 weeks after switching.

Toxicity

TAF, compared with TDF, has been shown to have less adverse effects in kidney (glomerular and tubular) function and bone mineral (spine, hip) density.

Antiviral Resistance

TAF leads to little or negligible emergence of drug resistance (to tenofovir). Clinical observations show a very low incidence of TFV genotype resistance in treatment-naïve patients treated either with TAF or TDF. In patients treated with elvitegravir, cobicistat, and emtricitabine combined with either TAF or TDF, emergence of drug resistance did not exceed 1% for either HIV and HBV.

Entecavir

Entecavir, which is a deoxyguanosine nucleoside analogue with specific antiviral activity for hepadnaviruses, is more potent than lamivudine and retains some activity against lamivudine-resistant HBV variants. It is well absorbed after oral administration, and its prolonged half-life (128 to 149 hours) allows once-daily dosing.

Clinical Uses

Entecavir is approved for the treatment of chronic hepatitis B in adults with evidence of active viral replication and either persistent elevations in serum aminotransferases or histologically active disease. Compared with lamivudine or telbivudine, entecavir is more efficacious in reducing HBV DNA levels and normalizing serum aminotransferases, as well as in improving histologic abnormalities. Like tenofovir, entecavir can be used for lamivudine-resistant HBV infections, but higher doses and longer durations of therapy are needed.

Toxicity

Adverse effects reported during entecavir therapy include headache, fatigue, dizziness, nausea, abdominal pain, rhinitis, fever, diarrhea, cough, and myalgia. Lactic acidosis and severe hepatomegaly with steatosis have been reported. Severe exacerbations of hepatitis B have been observed after cessation of therapy.

Antiviral Resistance

Virologic breakthrough can occur in up to 4% of patients but is usually not indicative of resistant virus. True entecavir resistance, which is caused by specific mutations in HBV polymerase, is uncommon (1.2% after 5 years of treatment). In vitro studies show that entecavir-resistant mutations are susceptible to adefovir and tenofovir, but there is very little supportive clinical data.

Interferons

Interferons are glycoprotein cytokines with a complex array of antiviral, immunomodulating, and antineoplastic properties. Interferons are currently classified as α, β, or γ. The natural sources of these classes in general are leukocytes, fibroblasts, and lymphocytes, but they now can be produced by recombinant DNA technology. Although the full mechanism of interferon's action is not defined, interferons generally induce synthesis of new cellular RNA and proteins that mediate antiviral effects through multiple different mechanisms.

Interferons generally must be administered daily or several times per week. However, the combination of interferon with polyethylene glycol to form PEG-interferon significantly prolongs absorption and provides higher, more sustained plasma levels that enable once-weekly administration.

Clinical Uses

In chronic active hepatitis B, treatment with interferon-alfa leads to loss of HBV DNA and biochemical and histologic improvement in about 25 to 40% of patients. Administration of PEG-interferon-alfa-2a or PEG-interferon-alfa-2b for 48 weeks converts about 30% of patients to seronegative status after 6 months of treatment. Whether combination therapy with interferons and antivirals confers an additional benefit compared with monotherapy for treating chronic hepatitis B is not known.

Adefovir

Adefovir, an acyclic analogue of adenosine monophosphate, is administered orally as a prodrug, adefovir dipivoxil, which is rapidly converted enzymatically to adefovir in intestinal epithelium.

Clinical Uses

In chronic hepatitis B, prolonged administration of adefovir is effective in improving histologic abnormalities of the liver, decreasing HBV DNA levels, and normalizing biochemical (ALT) markers in patients with HBeAg-positive and HBeAg-negative chronic hepatitis B. Adefovir is a slightly weaker antiviral and therefore not considered first-line therapy, but it is useful for resistant viruses (effective against chronic hepatitis B resistant to lamivudine) and HIV/HBV coinfection (see later).

Toxicity

The major adverse effect is nephrotoxicity, which is manifested by increased serum creatinine levels and sometimes hypophosphatemia, both of which are usually reversible with discontinuation of the drug. Common side effects include asthenia, headache, nausea, vomiting, and diarrhea. In addition, severe exacerbations of hepatitis B have been observed after cessation of therapy.

Antiviral Resistance

Adefovir resistance due to point mutations in HBV polymerase develops in about 6% of patients after 3 years of therapy. Lamivudine generally retains activity against adefovir-resistant variants.

Lamivudine

Lamivudine is a deoxycytidine nucleoside analogue active against retroviruses and hepadnaviruses. The triphosphate inhibits HBV polymerase, and its incorporation into viral DNA results in termination of the DNA chain.

Clinical Uses

Lamivudine suppresses hepatitis B viral replication, improves histologic abnormalities of the liver, reduces progression of fibrosis, and decreases the risk for late complications. Monotherapy with lamivudine appears to be inferior to the newer antivirals, as well as monotherapy with interferon, for sustained control of HBV replication. Combination therapy with lamivudine and interferon has shown inconsistent benefit compared with either drug alone. The dosing for HBV is lower than for HIV.

Toxicity

Adverse effects of lamivudine include diarrhea, headache, and elevated liver enzymes. Severe post-treatment exacerbations of hepatitis B, including fatalities, have occurred after discontinuation of lamivudine, especially in patients who are coinfected with HBV and HIV.

Antiviral Resistance

Lamivudine resistance caused by mutations in HBV polymerase is common during prolonged treatment of hepatitis B and emerges in about 20% of treated patients annually. Resistance is associated with increases in viral replication and aminotransferases.

Telbivudine

Telbivudine is a synthetic thymidine nucleoside analogue with activity against HBV, including some lamivudine-resistant variants. The triphosphate form competitively inhibits the HBV DNA polymerase (reverse transcriptase).

Clinical Uses

In comparative trials against lamivudine or adefovir, telbivudine demonstrated greater virologic response at week 52 (60 vs. 40% of subjects had HBV DNA negative by polymerase chain reaction analysis). The development of resistance with telbivudine is up to 5% after 1 year and 25% after 2 years. Telbivudine-resistant viruses are cross-resistant with lamivudine. Owing to the high development of resistance and cross-resistance, telbivudine is not considered a first-line treatment for hepatitis B.

Toxicity

Common side effects include headache, nausea, and vomiting. Severe acute exacerbations of hepatitis B have been reported in patients who have discontinued anti-HBV therapy. Myopathy, manifested by muscle aches or weakness with increased serum creatine kinase levels, has rarely been reported.

Special Considerations—HIV/HBV Coinfection

Lamivudine, entecavir, tenofovir, and TAF have activity against both HIV and HBV. Monotherapy treatment of HBV with these agents should not be used in HIV coinfected patients, owing to the development of HIV resistance.

Emtricitabine is licensed only for the treatment of HIV but is also weakly active against HBV. Withdrawal of this medication, like withdrawal of tenofovir or lamivudine, may cause acute, sometimes fulminant, exacerbations of hepatitis B in HIV/HBV coinfected patients.

If concurrent treatment of HBV and HIV is warranted, tenofovir plus emtricitabine, tenofovir plus lamivudine, or TAF plus emtricitabine should be considered as the nucleoside backbone of a fully suppressive antiretroviral regimen.[2] If tenofovir or TAF cannot be used, entecavir is an alternative as part of an antiretroviral regimen. In coinfected patients who require treatment for HBV but not HIV or who are already well controlled on anti-HIV viral therapy but now need hepatitis B treatment, PEG-interferon-alfa-2a monotherapy should be considered. If the antiretroviral regimen must be changed owing to HIV virologic failure and the HBV is adequately suppressed, antiviral drugs active against HBV should be continued for HBV treatment.

ANTIVIRALS FOR HEPATITIS C VIRUS INFECTIONS

Treatment of *acute* hepatitis C remains symptomatic, and antiviral therapy generally is not indicated. For *chronic* hepatitis C (Chapter 140), however, the goal of therapy is sustained virologic response (absence of hepatitis C virus [HCV] RNA for at least 12 weeks after completion of therapy) to prevent the morbidity and mortality associated with liver disease and long-term complications, such as hepatocellular carcinoma, liver failure, transplantation, and death. Treatment has been shown to decrease liver inflammation and cirrhosis as well as reduce the risk for hepatocellular carcinoma.

Interferon-free regimens are preferred over interferon-based regimens (see Table 140-5 in Chapter 140 and Tables 336-1 to 336-3).[3] Ledipasvir/sofosbuvir, sofosbuvir plus simeprevir, or ombitasvir/paritaprevir/ritonavir plus dasabuvir are preferred regimens for HCV genotype 1.[A3] Sofosbuvir and weight-based ribavirin are preferred for HCV genotypes 2 and 3. Ledipasvir/sofosbuvir and sofosbuvir plus simeprevir are preferred regimens for HCV genotype 4. Sofosbuvir/velpatasvir and ledipasvir/sofosbuvir are considered primary regimens for HCV genotype 5 or 6.

Interferon-based regimens now are generally reserved for patients who do not have access to interferon-free regimens. Sofosbuvir in combination with ribavirin and pegylated interferon has good efficacy for all genotypes. Simeprevir plus ribavirin and pegylated interferon may be used as alterative regimens for genotypes 1 and 4. Retreatment after failure of the initial regimen generally requires expert consultation.

Ledipasvir/Sofosbuvir

Ledipasvir is an HCV NS5A inhibitor. Sofosbuvir is a nucleotide prodrug that, when triphosphorylated, inhibits HCV NS5B, an RNA-dependent RNA polymerase. Both NS5A and NS5B are important for HCV viral replication. Ledipasvir/sofosbuvir is available as a combination fixed-dose once-daily oral tablet.

Clinical Uses

Ledipasvir/sofosbuvir is currently licensed in the treatment of genotypes 1, 4, 5, and 6 chronic HCV without cirrhosis and genotypes 1 and 4 with decompensated cirrhosis. For treatment-naïve patients with or without cirrhosis, treatment should continue for 12 weeks. This regimen has been associated with a sustained virologic response of 99% at 12 weeks, and the duration of treatment may be reduced to as low as 8 weeks without significant changes in efficacy.[A4] For treatment-experienced patients, 12 weeks of treatment is recommended for those without cirrhosis and 24 weeks for those with cirrhosis; the sustained virologic response is also 94 to 99%.[A5] Ledipasvir/sofosbuvir has also been recommended in the treatment of genotype 4 chronic HCV.

Toxicity

The most common side effects are headaches and fatigue. Significant drug interactions may occur with medications such as rifampin or St. John's wort.

Resistance

Resistance to the individual component drug may occur but is rare. Ledipasvir is active against sofosbuvir-resistant viruses, and sofosbuvir retains activity against ledipasvir-resistant viruses, so the clinical significance of resistance mutations is not known.

Sofosbuvir/Velpatasvir

Velpatasvir is a potent pangenotypic HCV NS5A inhibitor that is approved to treat hepatitis C patients in combination with sofosbuvir, an NS5B inhibitor. Sofosbuvir/velpatasvir is available as a fixed dose combination tablet.

Clinical Uses

Sofosbuvir/velpatasvir is currently licensed in the treatment of adult patients with chronic hepatitis C genotype 1, 2, 3, 4, 5, or 6 infection with any degree of liver damage, including decompensated cirrhosis. The addition of ribavirin is recommended when treating patients with decompensated cirrhosis. The duration of treatment is 12 weeks, which is associated with sustained virologic response in more than 99% of patients.[A6]

Toxicity

The most common adverse reactions associated with 12 weeks of sofosbuvir/velpatasvir treatment are fatigue and headaches. Significant bradycardia can occur with concomitant use of sofosbuvir/velpatasvir and amiodarone, which is contraindicated.

Antiviral Resistance

Preexisting NS5A mutants do not seem to influence the outcome of sofosbuvir/velpatasvir treatment. NS5A-resistant variants that confer in vitro resistance to velpatasvir have been isolated from the blood of the few patients who relapse. The significance of these mutants is not completely understood.

Sofosbuvir/Velpatasvir/Voxilaprevir

Velpatasvir is a potent pangenotypic HCV NS5A inhibitor to treat hepatitis C patients in combination with sofosbuvir, an NS5B inhibitor. Voxilaprevir is a second-generation HCV serine protease inhibitor. A single fixed-dose combination tablet of sofosbuvir, velpatasvir, and voxilaprevir is approved by the U.S. Food and Drug Administration (FDA) for treatment of HCV patients who have been previously treated with other direct acting antivirals.

Clinical Uses

Sofosbuvir/velpatasvir/voxilaprevir is currently licensed in the treatment of adult patients with chronic hepatitis C genotype 1, 2, 3, 4, 5, or 6 infection with any degree of liver damage without cirrhosis or compensated cirrhosis who have been previously treated with an HCV direct-acting antiviral agent regimen. The duration of treatment is 12 weeks, which is associated with sustained virologic response in more than 99% of patients.[A7]

Toxicity

The most common adverse reactions associated with 12 weeks of sofosbuvir/velpatasvir/voxilaprevir treatment are fatigue, headaches, nausea, and diarrhea. Significant bradycardia can occur with concomitant use of sofosbuvir/velpatasvir/voxilaprevir and amiodarone, which is contraindicated.

Antiviral Resistance

Preexisting NS5A or NS3 mutants do not seem to influence the outcome of sofosbuvir/velpatasvir/voxilaprevir treatment. NS5A-resistant variants that confer in vitro resistance to velpatasvir have been isolated from the blood of few patients who relapse. The significance of these mutants is not completely understood.

Glecaprevir/Pibrentasvir

A fixed-dose combination of glecaprevir, an NS3/4A protease inhibitor, and pibrentasvir, an NS5A inhibitor, is approved for the treatment of patients with chronic HCV genotype 1, 2, 3, 4, 5, or 6 infection without cirrhosis and with compensated cirrhosis (Child-Pugh A). The combination is available as a single pill.

Clinical Uses

Glecaprevir/pibrentasvir is currently licensed in the treatment of adult patients with chronic hepatitis C genotype 1, 2, 3, 4, 5, or 6 infection with all degrees of liver damage without cirrhosis or compensated cirrhosis (Child-Pugh A). The duration of treatment, which is 8 weeks for those without cirrhosis and 12 weeks for those with cirrhosis, is associated with sustained virologic response in more than 99% of patients.[A8] The combination pill is also indicated for the treatment of adult patients with HCV genotype 1 infection, who previously have been treated with a regimen containing an HCV NS5A inhibitor or an NS3/4A protease inhibitor, but not for those who failed both. For treatment-experienced genotype 1 patients, who have failed a previous NS5A inhibitor (but not NS3)-containing HCV regimen, 16 weeks of treatment is recommended. For treatment-experienced genotype 1 patients, who have failed a previous NS3 inhibitor (but not NS5A) containing HCV regimen, 12 weeks of treatment is recommended. For HCV genotype 1, 2, 4, 5, or 6 patients who have failed previous HCV regimens that did not include either an NS3 or

NS5A inhibitor, either 8 weeks (those without cirrhosis) or 12 weeks (with cirrhosis) is recommended. For HCV genotype 3 patients who have failed previous HCV regimens that did not include either an NS3 or NS5A inhibitor, 16 weeks is recommended. Glecaprevir/pibrentasvir is the only interferon-free regimen shown to be effective in patients with stage 4 or 5 chronic kidney disease and all genotypes of HCV.[A9]

Toxicity

The most common adverse reactions associated with 12 weeks of glecaprevir/pibrentasvir treatment are fatigue and headaches in about 10% of all patients.

Antiviral Resistance

Preexisting NS5A or NS3 mutants do not seem to influence the outcome of glecaprevir/pibrentasvir treatment. NS5A- and NS3-resistant variants that confer in vitro resistance to both drugs have been isolated from the blood of few patients who relapse. The significance of these mutants is not completely understood.

Daclatasvir

Daclatasvir is an NS5A inhibitor that can be used in combination with either sofosbuvir or asunaprevir for treatment of hepatitis C infection.

Clinical Uses

Daclatasvir is approved by the FDA to treat adult patients with HCV genotype 1 or 3 infection in combination with sofosbuvir. The treatment duration is for 12 weeks. The treatment is approved for patients with or without cirrhosis, but the response rate is reduced in patients with cirrhosis. Daclatasvir is metabolized through CYP3A, so the dose must be reduced with strong CYP3 inhibitors and increased with CYP3A inducers.

Toxicity

The most common adverse reactions associated with 12 weeks of sofosbuvir/daclatasvir treatment are headaches, fatigue, and nausea. Significant bradycardia can occur with concomitant use of sofosbuvir and amiodarone, which is contraindicated.

Antiviral Resistance

Preexisting NS5A mutants do not seem to influence the outcome of sofosbuvir/daclatasvir treatment. NS5A-resistant variants that confer in vitro resistance to daclatasvir have been isolated from the blood of few patients who relapse, but the significance of these mutants is not completely understood.

Daclatasvir/Asunaprevir

Asunaprevir is an HCV NS3 (serine protease) inhibitor, and daclatasvir is a potent HCV NS5A inhibitor. The combination is licensed to treat patients with hepatitis C in Europe and Japan.

Clinical Uses

The combination is approved for treatment of adults who have hepatitis C genotype 1 infection with compensated cirrhosis, who are ineligible or intolerant to interferon-based therapy, and who have failed to respond to interferon-based therapy. The combination has resulted in high response rates for both genotype 1a and 1b patients when treated for 24 weeks.[A10]

Toxicity

Nasopharyngitis, headaches, and fatigue are the most common adverse events.

Antiviral Resistance

Preexisting NS5A and NS3 polymorphisms can lead to reduced response rates with daclatasvir/asunaprevir combination, and hence these patients are treated for an extended period of time (24 weeks).

Grazoprevir/Elbasvir

Grazoprevir is a second-generation HCV NS3/4A (serine protease) inhibitor, and elbasvir is a potent HCV NS5A inhibitor. The combination is available as a fixed-dose combination single tablet and licensed to treat patients with hepatitis C.

Clinical Uses

The combination grazoprevir/elbasvir is indicated with or without ribavirin for treatment of chronic HCV genotypes 1 or 4 infection in adults. For genotype 1a patients, testing of NS5A-resistant-associated polymorphisms

before treatment is indicated. For treatment-naïve adult patients with hepatitis C genotype 1a (without polymorphisms), genotype 1b, and genotype 4, a total duration of 12 weeks is recommended. For treatment-experienced patients with hepatitis genotype 1, addition of ribavirin and treatment for 12 weeks is recommended. For HCV patients with genotype 1a and with the NS5A polymorphisms, addition of ribavirin for a total duration of 16 weeks is recommended. A major advantage of this combination over sofosbuvir-based combination is use in patients with significant renal impairment, including patients in hemodialysis,[A11] because both drugs are metabolized by the liver. Conversely, this combination is contraindicated in patients with decompensated liver disease. Grazoprevir/elbasvir may be used in patients with stage 4 or 5 chronic kidney disease and HCV genotypes 1 or 4.

Toxicity

The most common adverse reactions associated with 12 weeks of grazoprevir/elbasvir treatment are headaches, fatigue, nausea, and diarrhea. Anemia is also associated with concomitant use of ribavirin.

Antiviral Resistance

Presence of five preexisting NS5A-resistant-associated polymorphisms (M28A/G/T, Q30H/K/R/Y, L31F/M/V, H58D, Y93H/N/S) in HCV genotype 1a is associated with lower response rates when treated with grazoprevir/elbasvir alone, but results in high response rates when ribavirin is added and total treatment duration is extended to 16 weeks. Hence, resistant-associated polymorphism testing is recommended for patients with HCV genotype 1a.

Ombitasvir/Paritaprevir/Ritonavir plus Dasabuvir

Ombitasvir is an HCV NS5A inhibitor, and paritaprevir is an inhibitor of the HCV NS3/4A protease. Ritonavir has no activity against HCV, but it is an inhibitor of hepatic CYP3A and is added to increase paritaprevir levels. These three drugs are co-formulated into one tablet that is packaged with dasabuvir, an inhibitor of the HCV NS5B polymerase.

Clinical Uses

Ombitasvir/paritaprevir/ritonavir plus dasabuvir is currently licensed for the treatment of genotype 1 chronic HCV. In patients without cirrhosis, treatment for 12 weeks has been associated with a sustained virologic response of 97 to 99%. For genotype 1a, the addition of ribavirin may decrease virologic failures.[A12]

Toxicity

The many drug interactions that are due to the ritonavir inhibition of CYP3A should be closely evaluated before initiation of therapy. The most common side effects include nausea and diarrhea, as well as rash, headache, and fatigue.

Resistance

Treatment-emergent mutations were observed in patients with virologic failure, though the clinical significance of this is not known.

Sofosbuvir
Clinical Uses

Sofosbuvir is currently licensed as a component of a combination antiviral treatment regimen for HCV genotypes 1 to 4. For genotypes 1 and 4, sofosbuvir is used in combination with PEG-interferon and ribavirin for 12 weeks. This regimen has been associated with a sustained virologic response of about 90% at 12 weeks. In genotypes 2 and 3, sofosbuvir in combination with ribavirin for 12 or 24 weeks also has been associated with about a 90% sustained virologic response. For patients who cannot tolerate an interferon-based regimen (autoimmune disorders, decompensated hepatic disease, leukopenia, thrombocytopenia, anemia, or preexisting cardiac disease), sofosbuvir may be used with simeprevir or ribavirin for 24 weeks.

Toxicity

Common side effects include headache, fatigue, anemia, and diarrhea. Severe pancytopenias and severe depression have been reported. Sofosbuvir is a substrate of drug transporter P-gp, and drugs that are potent P-gp inducers (e.g., rifampin or St. John's wort) may decrease sofosbuvir's plasma concentration.

Resistance

The emergence of resistance while on sofosbuvir treatment is extremely rare.

Simeprevir

Simeprevir is a protease inhibitor that binds to the NS3/4a of hepatitis C.

Clinical Uses

Simeprevir is currently licensed for the treatment of chronic hepatitis C genotype 1 as either initial therapy or for use after failure of prior interferon-based therapy. Simeprevir is given for 12 weeks in combination with PEG-interferon-alfa and ribavirin, followed by PEG-interferon-alfa and ribavirin for an additional 12 weeks (treatment naïve) or 36 weeks (prior nonresponse). In naïve patients, virologic response is about 80%. Although not as effective as sofosbuvir, simeprevir is superior to other protease inhibitors and has become second-line therapy in genotype 1 (FDA approved) and genotype 4 (not FDA approved) hepatitis C.

Toxicity

Dermatologic (including rash, pruritus, and photosensitivity) and gastrointestinal side effects are the most common adverse reactions.

Resistance

Intrinsic resistance of the NS3 to simeprevir can be caused by the Q80K polymorphism. Patients should be screened for baseline mutation of this gene before initiation of therapy.

Boceprevir

Boceprevir is a protease inhibitor that binds to the NS3/4a of hepatitis C.

Clinical Uses

Boceprevir is currently licensed only for the treatment of genotype 1 in patients with compensated liver disease. It is used in combination with PEG-interferon and ribavirin in treatment-naïve patients as well as in patients who have not responded adequately to PEG-interferon and ribavirin. Boceprevir should not be used as monotherapy. Boceprevir is started 4 weeks after initiation of therapy with PEG-interferon and ribavirin, and combination therapy is continued for an additional 24 to 44 weeks based on virologic response. Subjects with undetectable HCV RNA level at weeks 8 and 24 may be considered for a shorter duration of treatment (28 weeks in total). In patients with evidence of virologic failure (HCV RNA level is >100 IU/mL at treatment week 12 or detectable at treatment week 24), treatment with all three drugs should be stopped. Because of its inferior efficacy, boceprevir is not considered a first-line therapy for hepatitis C.

Toxicity

Common side effects include fatigue, nausea, shivering, alopecia, and dysgeusia. Patients should be monitored for serious side effects such as anemia and neutropenia, which occasionally can be dose-limiting. Patients who develop anemia on combination therapy including boceprevir may be managed by reducing the ribavirin dose. Boceprevir is a strong inhibitor of cytochrome P450 3A4/5, so drug-drug interactions (including over-the-counter and oral contraceptives) must be considered.

Resistance

Resistance to boceprevir can occur on therapy. Because boceprevir and telaprevir are structurally similar, cross-resistant mutations may emerge, and patients should not be retreated with another protease inhibitor.

Telaprevir

Telaprevir was previously licensed for the treatment of chronic HCV but was withdrawn from the market in 2014.

Pegylated Interferon-2b and Ribavirin
Clinical Uses

Neither ribavirin nor interferon should be used as monotherapy for hepatitis C. In genotype 1, the combination of PEG-interferon and ribavirin may be considered in treatment-naïve subjects who cannot be given interferon-free regimens, although sustained virologic response rates are significantly inferior. Longer durations of treatment, up to 72 weeks, may improve virologic response. PEG-interferon and ribavirin should be administered for 24 weeks for HCV genotypes 2 and 3 and for 48 weeks for HCV genotypes 4, 5, and 6.

Toxicity

Common side effects of interferon administration include influenza-like symptoms (fever, chills, headache, malaise), but these symptoms usually become less severe with repeated treatments. Major toxicities include bone marrow suppression, especially granulocytopenia and thrombocytopenia, which are generally reversible when therapy is discontinued. Neuropsychiatric disturbances may be manifested by depression, anxiety, somnolence, confusion, and behavioral changes. Other side effects include profound fatigue and anorexia, weight loss, hypothyroidism or hyperthyroidism, alopecia, and cardiotoxicity with arrhythmias and reversible cardiomyopathy. Some side effects (e.g., hypothyroidism) can present a year or longer after therapy has finished.

Systemic ribavirin is frequently associated with hemolytic anemia (in up to 60% in some series) and sometimes with electrolyte abnormalities, including hypocalcemia and hypomagnesemia. Arrhythmias, pruritus, rash, nausea, and myalgia have been reported, as have neurologic side effects, including insomnia and irritability. Ribavirin may be gonadotoxic and teratogenic in humans.

Special Considerations—HIV/HCV Coinfection

Initial treatment regimens for HCV/HIV-coinfected patients are the same as those recommended for individuals without HIV infection. However, when treating both HCV and HIV, drug-drug interactions and additive toxicities must be considered.[4] Ledipasvir can increase tenofovir levels, and HIV regimens without tenofovir or TAF should be considered. Ombitasvir/paritaprevir/ritonavir plus dasabuvir will have interactions with many antiretroviral drugs. This regimen can be used with most nucleoside inhibitors and raltegravir, but use of other protease inhibitors, especially ritonavir-boosted regimens, requires expert consultation.

The HIV antivirals didanosine (DDI) and zidovudine (AZT) [Chapter 364]) should not be used with ribavirin. DDI levels and its active metabolite are increased when administered with ribavirin and can cause hepatic failure, severe peripheral neuropathy, pancreatitis, and lactic acidosis. AZT administered with ribavirin can cause severe neutropenic anemia, and the combination should not be used. If ribavirin is the preferred therapy, discontinuation of DDI and AZT should be considered before initiation of ribavirin.

⬤ ANTIVIRALS FOR HERPESVIRUS INFECTIONS

Acyclovir and Valacyclovir

Acyclovir, which is an acyclic analogue of the nucleoside guanosine, is converted to its active form through initial monophosphorylation by a virus-encoded thymidine kinase (TK). Although normal human cells possess TK, the affinity of acyclovir for viral TK is approximately 200 times greater than for human TK. The monophosphate then undergoes two additional host cell enzyme-mediated phosphorylations to acyclovir triphosphate (acycloguanosine triphosphate), which preferentially inhibits viral DNA polymerase. The higher concentrations of the activated form in infected cells and its affinity for viral polymerases result in low toxicity to normal host cells.

Valacyclovir is the L-valyl ester prodrug of acyclovir. Addition of the L-valyl ester fosters greater oral absorption, after which valacyclovir is converted to acyclovir; the prodrug provides three to five times greater bioavailability than oral acyclovir.

Clinical Uses

Acyclovir and valacyclovir (Tables 336-4 to 336-6) are used principally to treat infections caused by herpes simplex virus (HSV [Chapter 350])[5] and varicella-zoster virus (VZV [Chapter 351]). Depending on the country, acyclovir is available in a topical ointment and cream, oral capsules, and intravenous and ophthalmic formulations. Valacyclovir is available only as an oral capsule.

Oral acyclovir or valacyclovir decreases the duration of symptoms by approximately 50% and reduces the duration of viral shedding by about 90% in initial episodes of genital herpes. Two or 3 days of therapy appear to be sufficient for recurrent genital herpes. Chronic suppression is highly effective in reducing clinical and viral recurrences, and valacyclovir reduces the risk for transmission of genital HSV between heterosexual partners by 48%. For herpes labialis (cold sores), 1 day of therapy with oral valacyclovir improves time to healing and reduces pain, whereas acyclovir ointment has no consistent clinical benefit.

Parenteral acyclovir is indicated for the initial treatment of mucosal or cutaneous HSV infection in immunocompromised patients, neonatal HSV infections, and disseminated or organ-invasive infections in immunocompetent patients. A subsequent switch to oral valacyclovir is possible in some circumstances. High-dose parenteral acyclovir is the therapy of choice for treatment of HSV encephalitis.

Acyclovir and valacyclovir are indicated for acute VZV (chickenpox) in adults. Parenteral acyclovir should be used for severe acute VZV, including

TABLE 336-4 ANTIVIRALS FOR HERPESVIRUS INFECTIONS

VIRAL INFECTION	DRUG	ROUTE	USUAL ADULT DOSAGE
HERPES SIMPLEX VIRUS			
Genital herpes			
First episode	Acyclovir	PO	400 mg tid or 200 mg five times/day for 7-10 days
	Famciclovir	PO	250 mg tid for 7-10 days
	Valacyclovir	PO	1 g bid for 7-10 days
Recurrent	Acyclovir	PO	800 mg tid for 2 days, or 400 mg tid or 200 mg five times/day for 5 days
	Famciclovir	PO	1000 mg bid for 2 doses
	Valacyclovir	PO	500 mg bid for 3 days or 1 g/day for 5 days
Suppression	Acyclovir	PO	400 mg bid or 200 mg tid
	Famciclovir	PO	250 mg bid
	Valacyclovir	PO	500 mg/day or 1 g/day (10 or more episodes/yr)
Orolabial herpes	Penciclovir 1%	Topical	Apply cream every 2 hr while awake for 4 days
	Acyclovir 5%	Topical	Apply cream five times/day for 4 days
	Docosanol 10%	Topical	Apply cream five times/day until healing
	Valacyclovir	PO	2 g q12h × 2 doses
	Acyclovir	PO	400 mg five times/day for 5 days
	Famciclovir	PO	1500 mg single dose
Mucocutaneous disease	Acyclovir	IV	5 mg/kg/8 hr for 7-14 days
	Acyclovir	PO	400 mg five times/day for 7-14 days
	Valacyclovir	PO	500 mg or 1 g bid for 7-10 days
Encephalitis	Acyclovir	IV	10 mg/kg/8 hr for 10 days
Neonatal	Acyclovir	IV	10-20 mg/kg/8 hr for 14-21 days
Keratoconjunctivitis	Trifluridine	Topical	1 drop of 1% solution q2h up to 9 drops/day
	Vidarabine	Topical	½-inch ribbon of 3% ointment five times daily
Acyclovir-resistant HSV	Foscarnet	IV	40 mg/kg q8-12 h until healed
CYTOMEGALOVIRUS			
CMV retinitis	Ganciclovir	IV	5 mg/kg/12 hr for 14-21 days (maintenance: 5 mg/kg/day)
	Valganciclovir	PO	900 mg bid for 21 days (maintenance: 900 mg/day)
	Cidofovir	IV	5 mg/kg once weekly × 2 weeks (maintenance: 5 mg/kg q2wk)
	Foscarnet	IV	60 mg/kg/8 hr or 90 mg/kg q12h for 14-21 days (maintenance: 90-120 mg/kg daily)
	Fomivirsen	Intravitreal	330 μg q2 weeks × 2 weeks (maintenance: 330 μg every month)
HIV infection, CMV colitis or esophagitis	Ganciclovir	IV	5 mg/kg/12 hr for 14-28 days (until symptoms resolved)
Prophylaxis (transplantation)	Valganciclovir	PO	900 mg daily
	Ganciclovir	IV	5 mg/kg/12 hr for 7-14 days, then 5 mg/kg IV once a day
Prophylaxis (stem cell transplantation)	Letermovir	PO or IV	480 mg/day through 100 days post-transplant
Prophylaxis (advanced HIV infection)	Ganciclovir	IV	5 mg/kg daily
VARICELLA-ZOSTER VIRUS			
Varicella	Acyclovir	PO	800 mg qid for 5 days
Varicella in immunocompromised hosts	Acyclovir	IV	10 mg/kg/8 hr for 7-10 days
Herpes zoster in immunocompromised hosts	Acyclovir	IV	10 mg/kg/8 hr for 7-10 days
Herpes zoster in normal hosts	Acyclovir	PO	800 mg five times daily for 7-10 days
	Valacyclovir	PO	1 g tid for 7 days
	Famciclovir	PO	500 mg tid for 7 days

TABLE 336-5 MECHANISMS OF EXCRETION AND THRESHOLDS FOR DOSE ADJUSTMENT

	MAJOR ROUTE OF ELIMINATION	THRESHOLD FOR ADJUSTMENT IN RENAL INSUFFICIENCY OR FAILURE	ADJUSTMENT FOR HEPATIC FAILURE	ADJUSTMENT FOR OBESITY
Acyclovir IV	Renal	CrCl <50 mL/min	No adjustment	Dose by ideal body weight
Acyclovir PO	Renal	CrCl <25 mL/min/1.73 m²	No adjustment	Dose by ideal body weight
Valacyclovir	Renal	CrCl <50 mL/min	No adjustment	Unknown
Famciclovir	Renal	CrCl <60 mL/min	No adjustment	Unknown
Foscarnet	Renal	CrCl <1.4 mL/min/kg	No adjustment	Unknown
Ganciclovir IV	Renal	CrCl <70 mL/min	No adjustment	Unknown
Valganciclovir	Renal	CrCl <60 mL/min	No adjustment	Unknown
Letermovir	Hepatic	Avoid IV if CrCl <50 mL/min	No adjustment in mild or moderate impairment	Unknown
Cidofovir	Renal	CrCl <55 mL/min	No adjustment	Unknown

TABLE 336-6	SIGNIFICANT ADVERSE EFFECTS (U.S. FDA BLACK BOX WARNING)
DRUG	**BLACK BOX SYNOPSIS**
Cidofovir	Renal impairment, including renal failure; prehydrate and use probenecid Neutropenia May be carcinogenic and teratogenic and may cause hypospermia or aspermia
Foscarnet	Nephrotoxicity; prehydrate Seizures related to minerals and electrolyte disturbances
Ganciclovir	Neutropenia, anemia, thrombocytopenia May be carcinogenic and teratogenic and may cause hypospermia or aspermia
Valganciclovir	Neutropenia, anemia, thrombocytopenia May be carcinogenic and teratogenic and may cause hypospermia or aspermia

pneumonia, encephalitis, thrombocytopenia, and severe hepatitis, or in immunocompromised hosts. Acyclovir is also indicated in VZV reactivation (zoster). In adults treated within 24 hours of the development of a varicella rash, acyclovir decreases the severity of disease and number of lesions, but oral valacyclovir may be more effective than oral acyclovir. Intravenous acyclovir is warranted for zoster in immunocompromised hosts. Both acyclovir chemoprophylaxis and valacyclovir chemoprophylaxis reduce the incidence of recurrent HSV in recipients of stem cell and solid organ transplants, but valacyclovir is superior for prevention of cytomegalovirus (CMV) disease.

Toxicity
Acyclovir and valacyclovir have excellent safety profiles and are generally well tolerated. Common side effects include nausea, vomiting, and headaches. Major adverse effects include renal dysfunction and central nervous system (CNS) toxicity. Dehydration and preexisting renal dysfunction predispose to the development of renal impairment. Neurologic side effects include tremor, myoclonus, confusion, lethargy, agitation, and hallucination. Renal dysfunction predisposes to the development of neurotoxicity. Neutropenia and other signs of bone marrow toxicity have also been reported rarely.

Antiviral Resistance
Despite widespread use of acyclovir, the development of HSV resistance in immunocompetent subjects is uncommon (prevalence <1%). However, antiviral resistance is higher in immunocompromised subjects, including those with HIV infection (prevalence of 5%) or bone marrow transplants (prevalence of up to 30%). Drug-resistant refractory VZV infections can occur in highly immunocompromised patients. Intravenous foscarnet or cidofovir may be effective for infections caused by acyclovir-resistant viruses.

Penciclovir and Famciclovir
Penciclovir is an acyclic guanine analogue that unlike acyclovir is not an obligate chain terminator and may be incorporated into DNA. Penciclovir is phosphorylated by viral TK to penciclovir monophosphate, which is then converted to penciclovir triphosphate. Penciclovir demonstrates in vitro activity against VZV and HSV comparable to that of acyclovir. The bioavailability of penciclovir after oral administration is less than 2%. In contrast, famciclovir is an oral prodrug that is deacetylated and oxidized in the liver to form penciclovir; the bioavailability of penciclovir averages 77% after administration of famciclovir.

Clinical Uses
Penciclovir and famciclovir are used to treat HSV and VZV infections. Penciclovir is available as a topical cream and in some countries as an intravenous formulation. Famciclovir is available as a capsule.

Topical penciclovir, which is approved for the treatment of recurrent HSV labialis, reduces pain and lesions by about 1 day. Famciclovir is approved for the treatment of recurrent HSV labialis and genital infections and for herpes zoster, and its effectiveness is similar to valacyclovir or acyclovir. Famciclovir may also be used for suppressive therapy.

Toxicity
Topical penciclovir is well tolerated; the majority of adverse reactions are local irritation and mild erythema. Adverse effects of oral famciclovir include headache, dizziness, nausea, and diarrhea.

Antiviral Resistance
Penciclovir resistance in HSV has been uncommon in immunocompetent subjects but, like acyclovir resistance, more frequent in immunocompromised hosts (2.1%). Most acyclovir-resistant HSV isolates are cross-resistant to penciclovir.

Ganciclovir and Valganciclovir
Ganciclovir is an acyclic deoxyguanosine analogue with antiviral activity against multiple herpesviruses, including HSV, VZV, CMV (Chapter 352), Epstein-Barr virus (EBV [Chapter 353]), and human herpesvirus 8. Ganciclovir has activity against HSV and VZV, but it has more adverse reactions compared with acyclovir. It is much more active than acyclovir against CMV and EBV. The bioavailability of oral ganciclovir is less than 10%. Valganciclovir, the L-valyl prodrug of ganciclovir, increases the bioavailability of ganciclovir to approximately 60% after oral administration.

Clinical Uses
Ganciclovir is available as an oral capsule, a parenteral injection, and an ocular implant; valganciclovir is available only as a tablet. Ganciclovir and valganciclovir are effective for treatment of CMV retinitis, for which they are comparably active. In the absence of immune reconstitution, long-term suppression therapy is necessary. They are also used for life-threatening CMV diseases in patients with acquired immunodeficiency syndrome (AIDS) and other immunocompromised conditions and for prevention of CMV disease in transplant patients. For immunocompromised patients with organ-invasive CMV infections, intravenous ganciclovir provides clinical response rates of 70 to 90%, although response rates are lower for CMV pneumonitis after stem cell transplantation or CMV encephalitis in patients with AIDS. Oral valganciclovir provides long-term outcomes similar to those of intravenous ganciclovir for the treatment of CMV disease.

Long-term prophylaxis with ganciclovir or valganciclovir reduces the incidence of CMV disease after solid organ and stem cell transplantation, but this therapy has substantial side effects, including bone marrow suppression. These drugs can also be used as preemptive therapy for patients who have CMV viremia or antigenemia. In the prevention of CMV disease, preemptive valganciclovir therapy may be equally effective to chronic valacyclovir prophylaxis.

Toxicity
The most common adverse effect with ganciclovir and valganciclovir is bone marrow suppression, particularly neutropenia and thrombocytopenia, which occur in up to 50% of patients given intravenous ganciclovir. Fever, edema, phlebitis, headache, neuropathy, disorientation, nausea, anorexia, rash, and myalgias have also been reported with ganciclovir therapy. Intravitreal ganciclovir implants may cause vitreous hemorrhage and retinal detachment.

Antiviral Resistance
Ganciclovir resistance secondary to mutations in CMV kinase and sometimes DNA polymerase is related to the length of ganciclovir exposure and the degree of immunosuppression. Resistance may be associated with progressive disease during continued ganciclovir use; foscarnet and cidofovir are alternative treatments.

Letermovir
Letermovir is the first agent in the non-nucleoside 3,4 dihydro-quinazoline class of antivirals that inhibits the CMV DNA terminase complex. This enzyme is required for viral DNA processing.

Clinical Uses
Letermovir use is indicated for a very specific population—prophylaxis of CMV infection and disease in CMV seropositive recipients of an allogeneic hematopoietic stem cell transplant. Although ganciclovir and valganciclovir are effective in preventing CMV infection, their use is limited by myelosuppression. Prophylaxis with letermovir prevents significantly more CMV infections compared with placebo. The use of letermovir for treatment of active CMV disease or in other indications has not been evaluated and therefore cannot be recommended until additional data are available.

Toxicity

The most common side effects are nausea, vomiting, and diarrhea, but they occur at similar rates as with placebo. The cardiac adverse event rate (primarily tachycardia and atrial fibrillation) is higher in patients receiving letermovir than placebo (13% vs. 6%). Letermovir is an inhibitor of OATP1B1/3 transporters and has numerous drug-drug interactions, including with immunosuppressants and antimicrobial agents. Consultation with an experienced clinical pharmacologist is highly recommended. In patients with CrCl less than 50 mL/min and receiving IV letermovir, accumulation of the intravenous vehicle, hydroxypropyl betadex, could occur.

Antiviral Resistance

The emergence of resistance while on letermovir is rare. Letermovir is fully active against CMV viruses that are resistant to cidofovir, foscarnet, or ganciclovir.

Foscarnet

Foscarnet is a pyrophosphate analogue that acts as a noncompetitive inhibitor of many viral RNA and DNA polymerases. When a nucleotide is incorporated into a DNA or RNA strand by a polymerase, pyrophosphate is released. Foscarnet directly inhibits viral polymerases without phosphorylation, so TK-deficient acyclovir-resistant HSV and VZV are susceptible to this agent.

Clinical Uses

For extraretinal CMV disease, foscarnet has demonstrated efficacy similar to that of ganciclovir. Foscarnet is as effective as ganciclovir for the treatment of CMV retinitis in patients with AIDS, and combination therapy with ganciclovir may be superior to monotherapy with either agent for recalcitrant retinitis. The choice of agent may be dictated by the side-effect profile. Foscarnet is also effective for the treatment of acyclovir-resistant HSV and VZV infections.

Toxicity

Nephrotoxicity with azotemia and proteinuria is dose limiting and occurs in more than one third of patients. A slow infusion rate and saline hydration reduce the risk. Other common side effects include anemia (30 to 50% of patients), granulocytopenia, diarrhea, nausea, vomiting, fever, seizures, paresthesias, headache, and genital ulcers. Marked electrolyte disturbances may develop, including hypophosphatemia, hypocalcemia, hypokalemia, and hypomagnesemia. Foscarnet can prolong the QT interval and be associated with cardiac arrhythmias, including ventricular tachycardia, ventricular fibrillation, and torsades de pointes.

Antiviral Resistance

The development of CMV resistance to foscarnet as a result of mutations in viral DNA polymerase is uncommon except after prolonged administration. In AIDS patients with retinitis, foscarnet resistance is detectable in 13% of patients at 6 months and in 37% at 12 months.

Cidofovir

Cidofovir, which is an acyclic phosphonate derivative of cytosine, is phosphorylated to its active diphosphate form by host cellular enzymes. Cidofovir diphosphate competitively inhibits viral DNA polymerase and viral DNA synthesis. Despite a short serum half-life, the antiviral effects are protracted because of prolonged intracellular concentrations of the phosphorylated metabolite.

Clinical Uses

Cidofovir is commercially available as an intravenous infusion, and investigational formulations have included topical gel and intravitreal and intralesional injections. Intravenous cidofovir is licensed for the treatment of CMV retinitis. Because of its toxicities, it is generally reserved for when ganciclovir or foscarnet therapy is failing. Limited data suggest that intravenous cidofovir may be effective in other CMV infections (pneumonitis, gastroenteritis), acyclovir- or foscarnet-resistant HSV infections, certain forms of human papillomavirus disease, invasive adenoviral infections in transplant recipients, and possibly BK virus infection in renal transplant patients. In addition, in vivo and animal data suggest efficacy of cidofovir against smallpox, vaccinia, and monkeypox infections.

Toxicity

Dose-related nephrotoxicity, characterized by increased serum creatinine, proteinuria, and tubular dysfunction, is the main side effect of intravenous cidofovir. Adequate hydration and concomitant oral probenecid reduce the risk. Other common side effects include diarrhea, asthenia, nausea, vomiting, neutropenia, fever, and rash. Iritis, intraocular pressure changes, loss of visual acuity, and uveitis have been reported with intravenous cidofovir. Intravitreal cidofovir is effective but locally toxic.

Antiviral Resistance

Sustained exposure to cidofovir does not easily induce resistance, although resistance has infrequently been described in HSV and CMV.

Fomivirsen

Fomivirsen, which is an antisense oligonucleotide that inhibits CMV replication, is currently available as an intravitreal injection that is effective for both newly diagnosed CMV retinitis and CMV retinitis failing usual therapies, although direct comparisons with other agents are lacking. Intravitreal administration of fomivirsen may cause increased intraocular pressure, iritis, vitreitis, and cataracts in 10 to 20% of patients. Topical corticosteroids may be useful for treating inflammatory changes.

Docosanol

Docosanol, which is a 22-carbon saturated fatty alcohol that inhibits intracellular penetration of lipid-enveloped viruses, is approved as an over-the-counter cream for the treatment of herpes labialis. Frequent topical applications have shown reductions in time to cessation of pain and healing, but direct comparison to other agents is lacking. Local reaction, rash, and pruritus are common side effects.

● ANTIVIRALS FOR INFLUENZA VIRUS INFECTIONS

Currently approved antivirals for the treatment of influenza include two neuraminidase inhibitors (oseltamivir and zanamivir), one endonuclease inhibitor (baloxavir marboxil), and two adamantanes (amantadine and rimantadine) (Tables 336-7 and 336-8). The choice of treatment for influenza should be dictated by circulating strains, antiviral resistance within those strains, and side-effect profiles.

Oseltamivir, Zanamivir, and Peramivir (Neuraminidase Inhibitors)

Oseltamivir, zanamivir, and peramivir are sialic acid analogues that inhibit influenza virus by competitively interacting with the neuraminidases of influenza A and B viruses. Influenza neuraminidase cleaves terminal sialic acid residues and destroys the receptors recognized by viral hemagglutinin. By this mechanism, the drugs inhibit the release of virus from infected cells, thereby preventing viral aggregates and spread within the respiratory tract.

Oseltamivir is administered orally as the phosphate prodrug, which is rapidly absorbed and hydrolyzed to the active form oseltamivir carboxylate. Bioavailability exceeds 75%. Conversely, the oral bioavailability of zanamivir is poor, so it is delivered as an orally inhaled powder. Peramivir is available only as a parenterally infused solution.

Clinical Uses

Oseltamivir and zanamivir are effective for the treatment and prophylaxis of acute influenza A and B infections. Early treatment in adults decreases the duration and severity of illness and reduces lower respiratory tract complications, antibiotic use, and, with oseltamivir, hospitalizations. In low-risk ambulatory subjects, oseltamivir alleviates symptoms faster than placebo, and it also decreases the risk for lower respiratory complications. In cohort studies of hospitalized subjects, treatment with oseltamivir has been associated with a significant reduction in death. Zanamivir is also effective in alleviating

TABLE 336-7	ANTIVIRALS FOR INFLUENZA VIRUS INFECTIONS		
VIRUS	**DRUG**	**ROUTE**	**USUAL ADULT TREATMENT DOSAGE**
Influenza A and B virus	Oseltamivir	PO	75 mg bid for 5 days
	Peramivir	IV	600 mg single IV dose
	Zanamivir	Inhalation	10 mg bid by inhaler for 5 days
	Baloxavir marboxil	PO	40 to ≤80 kg: 40 mg single dose >80 kg: 80 mg single dose
Influenza A virus	Amantadine	PO	100 mg bid or 200 mg daily for 5 days
	Rimantadine	PO	100 mg bid for 5 days

TABLE 336-8 MECHANISMS OF EXCRETION AND THRESHOLDS FOR DOSE ADJUSTMENTS				
	MAJOR ROUTE OF ELIMINATION	**THRESHOLD FOR ADJUSTMENT IN RENAL INSUFFICIENCY OR FAILURE**	**ADJUSTMENT FOR HEPATIC FAILURE**	**SPECIAL ADJUSTMENT FOR THE ELDERLY**
Amantadine	Renal	CrCl <50 mL/min/1.73 m²	No adjustment	>65 years: 100 mg daily
Rimantadine	Hepatic and renal	CrCl <10 mL/min/1.73 m²	100 mg daily	100 mg daily
Oseltamivir	Renal	CrCl <60 mL/min	No adjustment	
Peramivir	Renal	CrCl <50 mL/min	No adjustment	
Zanamivir	Renal	No adjustment	No adjustment	
Baloxavir marboxil	Hepatic	Not evaluated on CrCl <50 mL/min	No adjustment in mild or moderate impairment	Not evaluated in patients >65 years of age

symptoms and decreasing the risk for lower respiratory complications. Both zanamivir and oseltamivir are also highly effective for the prevention of influenza. Peramivir is licensed as a single-dose intravenous infusion for uncomplicated influenza. However, as a once- or twice-daily infusion in patients hospitalized with influenza, its efficacy is similar to oseltamivir.[A13] Combining oseltamivir with other antivirals (amantadine and ribavirin) does not improve efficacy over oseltamivir alone.[A14]

Toxicity

The most common side effects with oseltamivir are nausea and vomiting. They also may be associated with headache, rash, and possibly abnormal aminotransferase levels. Zanamivir is generally well tolerated, but severe bronchospasm has been reported primarily in patients with underlying airway disease. The most common side effects of peramivir are nausea, diarrhea, and mild neutropenia.

Antiviral Resistance

Oseltamivir resistance can be preexisting (widespread or local) or can emerge during therapy. In the immunocompromised host and possibly in individuals with H5N1 or H1N1, the development of resistance is associated with treatment failure. Zanamivir resistance is rare, and zanamivir retains clinical effectiveness against the most common oseltamivir-resistant variants.

Baloxavir Marboxil

Baloxavir marboxil is a prodrug that is converted by hydrolysis to baloxavir. Baloxavir, which is among a novel class of antivirals for influenza, inhibits the endonuclease activity of the polymerase acidic (PA) protein, which is an influenza-specific enzyme in the viral RNA polymerase complex and is responsible for viral gene replication.

Clinical Uses

Baloxavir marboxil is indicated for the treatment of acute influenza A and B infections in adults and children older than 12 years of age. Clinical efficacy is similar to oseltamivir, but baloxavir marboxil is unique in that it is administered as a single dose.[A15] Currently, there are no data available to support its use in pregnant women, children younger than 12 years of age, or for prophylaxis.

Toxicity

Baloxavir marboxil is well tolerated with few side effects. The most common side effects are diarrhea and bronchitis and occurred in similar rates as placebo.

Antiviral Resistance

Circulating resistance to baloxavir is currently rare, although treatment-emergent resistance was 20 to 23% in patients 1 to 11 years of age and 3 to 11% patients 12 to 64 years of age.

Amantadine and Rimantadine (Adamantanes)

Currently circulating H1N1 and H3N2 viruses are highly resistant to adamantanes. Unless circulating strains are documented as susceptible, these compounds should not be used. Amantadine and rimantadine are symmetrical tricyclic amines with activity against many influenza A viruses (Chapter 340). By inhibiting the ion channel function of the M2 protein of influenza A, they interfere with uncoating of the virus and release of the viral genome.

Clinical Uses

Amantadine and rimantadine decrease the length and severity of uncomplicated influenza A virus infection by susceptible strains if they are initiated within the first 2 days after the onset of symptoms, but it is uncertain whether they reduce the risk for complications. Both drugs are formulated for oral administration, and amantadine also has a pediatric syrup formulation. In recent years, marked increases in antiviral resistance in community isolates have limited the utility of these drugs.

When adamantine-susceptible viruses are circulating, both rimantadine and amantadine are effective when they are used for prophylaxis (overall 66% average for rimantadine and 74% for amantadine). Despite prophylaxis, subclinical infections may still develop and elicit immune responses that are protective against antigenically related viruses.

Toxicity

Amantadine causes CNS side effects in 10 to 30% of healthy young adults who take the standard adult dose; the frequency is significantly lower with rimantadine. Neuropsychiatric side effects include anxiety, nervousness, insomnia, and, particularly in the elderly or those with renal insufficiency, hallucinations, confusion, disorientation, and psychosis or coma. Amantadine (or less often rimantadine) is associated with an increased risk for seizures. Both drugs cause gastrointestinal side effects. Orthostatic hypotension occurs in 1 to 5%. Anticholinergic side effects, including dry mouth, occur in amantadine recipients.

Antiviral Resistance

Single point mutations in M2 confer high-level resistance to these drugs and make them ineffective. Such resistant variants emerge commonly during treatment and are transmissible.

⬤ OTHER ANTIVIRALS

Ribavirin

Ribavirin is a purine nucleoside with antiviral activity against some DNA viruses and many RNA viruses, including influenza A and B, parainfluenza, coronaviruses including Middle East respiratory syndrome (Chapter 342), measles (Chapter 343), respiratory syncytial virus (RSV [Chapter 338]), retroviruses (Chapter 354), arenaviruses such as Lassa virus (Chapter 357), and some hantaviruses (Chapter 357) and hepatitis C virus (Chapter 140).

Clinical Uses

Aerosol administration of ribavirin has been used to treat RSV bronchiolitis and pneumonia in children and to treat influenza A and B infections. Limited benefit has been seen with oral ribavirin in uncomplicated influenza. Aerosol ribavirin combined with intravenous immune globulin, particularly with the anti-RSV monoclonal antibody palivizumab, appears to reduce the mortality of RSV infection in bone marrow transplant and other highly immunocompromised patients.

Systemic ribavirin reduces the mortality associated with Lassa fever and Asian (Korean) hemorrhagic fever with renal syndrome (Chapter 357), although not mortality in patients with hantavirus-associated cardiopulmonary syndrome. It appears to have activity in Congo-Crimean hemorrhagic fever and in Nipah virus infections. Ribavirin is often recommended as treatment of hemorrhagic fevers of unknown etiology or secondary to arenaviruses or bunyaviruses in the event these viruses are used as biologic weapons.

Given the breadth of ribavirin's activity against many viruses, it is often used for emerging infectious diseases (e.g., severe acute respiratory syndrome [SARS] and Middle East respiratory syndrome). However, the concentrations needed to show efficacy in cell cultures and animal models may be significantly higher than can be obtained in humans. Caution is therefore urged when ribavirin is suggested for treating these diseases.

Ribavirin can improve the sustained virologic response for chronic hepatitis C infection when used with pegylated interferons, but the new directly acting antiviral agents are used without ribavirin. However, ribavirin is still used in patients with viral resistance to grazoprevir/elbasvir and in patients with cirrhosis (combined with ombitasvir/paritaprevir/ritonavir plus dasabuvir, and with sofosbuvir plus ledipasvir for treatment-experienced patients).

Imiquimod

Imiquimod and the related compound resiquimod are topical immune response modifiers that lack direct antiviral effects. Instead, these agents induce activation of immune cells (monocytes, macrophages, natural killer cells) to produce antiviral cytokines, particularly interferon-α and tumor necrosis factor-α.

Topical imiquimod cream is approved for the treatment of condyloma acuminatum (Chapter 349). In immunocompetent patients, imiquimod leads to complete clearance of warts in 37 to 52% of patients. It is administered as a topical cream three times weekly for a maximum of 16 weeks and is washed off 6 to 10 hours after application.

Side effects are primarily local and include erythema, irritation, tenderness, and (less often) erosion. The side effects usually resolve with cessation of the drug.

 ## Grade A References

A1. Han Y, Zeng A, Liao H, et al. The efficacy and safety comparison between tenofovir and entecavir in treatment of chronic hepatitis B and HBV related cirrhosis: a systematic review and meta-analysis. *Int Immunopharmacol.* 2017;42:168-175.

A2. Abdul Basit S, Dawood A, Ryan J, et al. Tenofovir alafenamide for the treatment of chronic hepatitis B virus infection. *Expert Rev Clin Pharmacol.* 2017;10:707-716.

A3. Zhu GQ, Zou ZL, Zheng JN, et al. Systematic review and network meta-analysis of randomized controlled trials: comparative effectiveness and safety of direct-acting antiviral agents for treatment-naive hepatitis C genotype 1. *Medicine (Baltimore).* 2016;95:1-10.

A4. Kowdley KV, Gordon SC, Reddy KR, et al. Ledipasvir and sofosbuvir for 8 or 12 weeks for chronic HCV without cirrhosis. *N Engl J Med.* 2014;370:1879-1888.

A5. Afdhal N, Reddy KR, Nelson DR, et al. Ledipasvir and sofosbuvir for previously treated HCV genotype 1 infection. *N Engl J Med.* 2014;370:1483-1493.

A6. Feld JJ, Jacobson IM, Hezode C, et al. Sofosbuvir and velpatasvir for HCV genotype 1, 2, 4, 5, and 6 infection. *N Engl J Med.* 2015;373:2599-2607.

A7. Bourliere M, Gordon SC, Flamm SL, et al. Sofosbuvir, velpatasvir, and voxilaprevir for previously treated HCV infection. *N Engl J Med.* 2017;376:2134-2146.

A8. Kwo PY, Poordad F, Asatryan A, et al. Glecaprevir and pibrentasvir yield high response rates in patients with HCV genotype 1-6 without cirrhosis. *J Hepatol.* 2017;67:263-271.

A9. Gane E, Lawitz E, Pugatch D, et al. Glecaprevir and pibrentasvir in patients with HCV and severe renal impairment. *N Engl J Med.* 2017;377:1448-1455.

A10. Tamori A, Hai H, Uchida-Kobayashi S, et al. Outcomes for cirrhotic patients with hepatitis C virus 1b treated with asunaprevir and daclatasvir combination. *Ann Hepatol.* 2017;16:734-741.

A11. Bruchfeld A, Roth D, Martin P, et al. Elbasvir plus grazoprevir in patients with hepatitis C virus infection and stage 4-5 chronic kidney disease: clinical, virological, and health-related quality-of-life outcomes from a phase 3, multicentre, randomised, double-blind, placebo-controlled trial. *Lancet Gastroenterol Hepatol.* 2017;2:585-594.

A12. Ferenci P, Bernstein D, Lalezari J, et al. ABT-450/r-ombitasvir and dasabuvir with or without ribavirin for HCV. *N Engl J Med.* 2014;370:1983-1992.

A13. Ison MG, Hui DS, Clezy K, et al. A clinical trial of intravenous peramivir compared with oral oseltamivir for the treatment of seasonal influenza in hospitalized adults. *Antivir Ther.* 2013;18:651-661.

A14. Beigel JH, Bao Y, Beeler J, et al. Oseltamivir, amantadine, and ribavirin combination antiviral therapy versus oseltamivir monotherapy for the treatment of influenza: a multicentre, double-blind, randomised phase 2 trial. *Lancet Infect Dis.* 2017;17:1255-1265.

A15. Hayden FG, Sugaya N, Hirotsu N, et al. Baloxavir marboxil for uncomplicated influenza in adults and adolescents. *N Engl J Med.* 2018;379:913-923.

GENERAL REFERENCES

For the General References and other additional features, please visit Expert Consult at https://expertconsult.inkling.com.

337

THE COMMON COLD

BRUCE BARRETT AND RONALD B. TURNER

DEFINITION

The common cold is a clinical syndrome characterized by rhinorrhea and nasal obstruction, which are frequently accompanied by sore throat, sneezing, cough, and general malaise. The common cold syndrome is among the most prevalent of illnesses, and it is very costly, especially considering the resulting absenteeism from school and work. Common cold is both a clinical and a cultural construction. Although it presumably is always caused by a virus, it is not defined by the specific etiologic agent.

The Pathogens

Human rhinoviruses are RNA viruses that infect the upper respiratory epithelium. Rhinoviruses, which have long been known as common cold viruses, cause up to half of all common cold illnesses.[1] The more than 150 rhinovirus genotypes are classified as species A, B, or C based on sequence homology. Rhinoviruses are important causes of exacerbations of chronic bronchitis (Chapter 82) and asthma (Chapter 81). Rhinovirus infection can cause bronchiolitis in infants and young children, and it is the predominant cause of an exacerbation of childhood asthma. Among elderly patients, especially those with lung disease, rhinovirus infection is an important cause of hospitalization, pneumonia, and death.

The common cold illness syndrome can also be caused by coronaviruses (Chapter 342), parainfluenza viruses (Chapter 339), respiratory syncytial virus (Chapter 338), metapneumoviruses (Chapter 91), adenoviruses (Chapter 341), bocaviruses (Chapter 347), and influenza viruses (Chapter 340; Table 337-1).[2] Bacterial pathogens such as *Mycoplasma pneumoniae* (Chapter 301), *Bordetella pertussis* (Chapter 297), group A streptococcus (Chapter 274), *Streptococcus pneumoniae* (Chapter 273), and *Haemophilus influenzae* (Chapter 284) are sometimes the only identifiable pathogen in a person who is experiencing the common cold syndrome, but the role of these organisms, which colonize the upper respiratory tract in healthy individuals, is not clear. Co-detection of more than one virus, or of a virus plus a bacterial pathogen, is fairly common.

EPIDEMIOLOGY

The incidence of common cold decreases with age, from about six symptomatic episodes per year in young children, to approximately two episodes per year in adults. Asymptomatic infections are also common. The incidence of illness is higher in adults who have occupational or household exposure to children, and in young children who are cared for in child-care centers. Common cold illnesses occur year-round in temperate climates but have a substantially increased incidence between the early autumn and late spring. Reasons for the seasonality of rhinovirus (and other respiratory viruses) are poorly understood.[3] In tropical climates, colds can occur year-round without defined seasonality.

PATHOBIOLOGY

Respiratory pathogens are spread from person to person by direct contact with either infected individuals or contaminated objects in the environment, by large-particle aerosols, or by small-particle aerosols. The rhinoviruses may be primarily spread by direct contact, but recent data suggest a role for other mechanisms. For example, respiratory syncytial virus (Chapter 338) may be spread by either direct contact or large-particle aerosols, and influenza (Chapter 340) may be spread more by small-particle aerosols.

The common cold syndrome is initiated by viral infection of the epithelial cells in the nasal passageways or upper pharynx. Influenza and adenovirus

TABLE 337-1	VIRUSES ASSOCIATED WITH THE COMMON COLD	
VIRUS GROUP	**ANTIGENIC TYPES**	**PERCENTAGE OF CASES**
Rhinoviruses	>150	30-60
Coronaviruses	5	10-15
Parainfluenza virus	5	5
Respiratory syncytial virus	2	5-10
Influenza virus	3	5-15
Adenovirus	47	5
Metapneumovirus	2	5
Bocavirus	2	5-20

From Byington CL, Ampofo K, Stockmann C, et al. Community surveillance of respiratory viruses among families in the Utah Better Identification of Germs-Longitudinal Viral Epidemiology (BIG-LoVE) study. *Clin Infect Dis.* 2015;61:1217-1224; Monto AS. Epidemiology of viral respiratory infections. *Am J Med.* 2002;112(Suppl 6A):4s-12s; Szilagyi PG, Blumkin A, Treanor JJ, et al. Incidence and viral aetiologies of acute respiratory illnesses (ARIs) in the United States: a population-based study. *Epidemiol Infect.* 2016;144:2077-2086.

produce obvious damage to the respiratory epithelium. Rhinovirus and respiratory syncytial virus, in contrast, have little or no detectable impact on the epithelium. Regardless of the histopathology, all of these viruses stimulate a nonspecific host inflammatory response that appears to be responsible for many of the symptoms associated with the common cold.

The nasal obstruction of the common cold appears to result primarily from increased nasal blood flow and pooling of blood in the capacitance vessels of the nasal passageway. Sympathetic and parasympathetic pathways are involved. The increase in nasal secretion associated with the common cold may also contribute to the nasal obstruction. Rhinorrhea is primarily a result of increased vascular permeability, with leakage of serum into the nasal secretions, producing both transudates and exudates. Increased mucus production contributes to the secretions during the later stages of the illness.

Cough (Chapter 77) occurs in the majority of colds and tends to last longer than other symptoms. Multiple factors may play a role in the pathogenesis of cough. Cough may be related to infection of the lower airway, irritation of upper airway receptors with neurologically mediated airway reactivity, or postnasal drip with pharyngeal or tracheal irritation.

The risk for infection after exposure to the respiratory viruses is primarily dependent on the presence of specific neutralizing antibodies. Antibody responses to the rhinoviruses, adenoviruses, and influenza viruses are protective against subsequent infection. The frequency of infection with these viruses is a result of the large number of distinct serotypes of rhinovirus and adenovirus and the ability of the influenza viruses to behave as though there are multiple virus serotypes by virtue of the rapid mutation of surface antigens. The parainfluenza viruses, respiratory syncytial viruses, and metapneumoviruses do not produce protective immunity, so reinfection is common, although preexisting antibodies can moderate the severity of illness.

Susceptibility to and pathogenesis of the common cold are multifactorial processes, with innate and adaptive immune mechanisms influenced by genetic predisposition,[4] by previous antigen exposure, and by general health. Polymorphisms of mannose-binding lectin and various toll-like receptors may confer susceptibility or partial protection. Inflammatory cytokines associated with the severity of disease include various interferons, interleukins, and other factors, which rise markedly in nasal secretions but usually do not change much in the serum. Recent research suggests that the respiratory microbiome may be involved. Specific genes and epigenetic influences on the expression of those genes may predispose toward higher levels of inflammatory cytokines and more severe respiratory illness.

Although specific mechanisms are not well understood, several decades of research have shown that susceptibility to common cold is influenced by mental health. Risk factors include perceived stress, social isolation, negative emotional style, and a history of stressful life events.[4,5] Observational studies suggest that people who engage in regular exercise experience fewer and milder common cold episodes than those who do not.

CLINICAL MANIFESTATIONS

The incubation of common cold illness is generally short, ranging from 2 to 8 days, although adenoviruses may have an incubation of as long as 13 days. The common cold illness syndrome generally persists for 5 to 10 days, but about 25% may persist for as long as 2 weeks. A sore or scratchy throat is frequently reported as the first symptom. Sneezing is also a common early symptom. Nasal obstruction and rhinorrhea develop rapidly and, by day 2 or 3 after the onset of illness, are often the most bothersome symptoms. Cough generally develops later in the illness and frequently is the most bothersome symptom as the cold resolves.[6] Postviral cough may persist for several weeks. When asked to rate what bothers them most about their colds, people tend to identify general malaise or interference with daily activities as more important than severity of specific symptoms.

Physical findings are generally restricted to the upper respiratory tract. Swelling of the nasal epithelia and increased nasal secretion may be obvious to the examiner. A change in the color or consistency of nasal secretions is common during the course of the illness and is not indicative of sinusitis or bacterial superinfection. The posterior pharynx may show signs of inflammation similar to streptococcal pharyngitis. Paroxysmal cough or wheezing may occur.

DIAGNOSIS

The differential diagnosis of the common cold includes noninfectious disorders as well as other upper respiratory tract infections. Allergic rhinitis (Chapter 398) has a symptom complex similar to that of the common cold, although the presence of nasal or conjunctival itching suggests allergic disease. Most patients can reliably differentiate these illnesses.

Sinus involvement is present in uncomplicated cold illnesses, and superimposed bacterial sinusitis (Chapter 398) is often difficult to differentiate from an uncomplicated cold. Sinonasal symptoms that persist without improvement for more than 10 days and that are accompanied by unilateral maxillary sinus pain and purulent discharge may suggest the presence of bacterial sinusitis that may respond to antibiotics.[7]

When symptoms are more severe—with rapid onset, feverishness, and headache or muscle aches, accompanied by sore throat or cough—an "influenza-like illness" may be diagnosed. Although influenza-like illness is more likely to be produced by influenza infection than other pathogens, any of the common cold viruses can produce this more severe variant of common cold.[8,9]

Routine laboratory studies are not helpful for the diagnosis or management of the common cold. Although the viral pathogens associated with the common cold may be detected, especially by polymerase chain reaction, these studies are of little clinical value. White blood counts and differentials, as well as radiographic or computed tomographic imaging of the lungs or sinuses, also have no proven clinical value. For patients with pharyngeal exudates, swollen cervical lymph nodes, and feverishness, a rapid test for streptococcal pharyngitis (Chapter 274) may be useful.

TREATMENT   Rx

No treatments are proved to reduce the duration of common cold illness or to have a substantive impact on overall severity. Several treatments, however, may confer limited symptomatic benefit, which must be balanced against the potential for side-effects.

Antivirals and Antibiotics

Specific antiviral therapy is generally not useful for the treatment of common cold. The neuraminidase inhibitors oseltamivir and zanamivir (Chapter 336) have a modest effect on influenza virus infections, but the difficulty of distinguishing influenza from common cold, and the need to start treatment very early in the illness, are practical limitations to the use of these agents. Antibacterial therapy is of no benefit. Despite decades of efforts to reduce antibiotic prescribing for common cold, this practice remains disturbingly common.

Nasal Congestion

Both topical and oral adrenergic agents (Table 337-2) have limited efficacy as nasal decongestants.[A1] Although direct comparison has not been performed, it is generally accepted that topical over-the-counter agents, such as intranasal xylometazoline or oxymetazoline, are more effective than oral drugs for nasal congestion. Prolonged use of the topical adrenergic agents should be avoided to prevent the development of an apparent rebound effect when the drug is discontinued (rhinitis medicamentosa). Systemic absorption of oxymetazoline and xylometazoline have rarely been associated with bradycardia, hypotension, and coma. The systemic side effects of the oral adrenergic agents such as pseudoephedrine include central nervous system stimulation, which can cause insomnia, jitteriness, or palpitations. Adrenergic decongestants should probably be avoided by patients with hypertension or heart disease. Nasal saline is an inexpensive and safe treatment for nasal congestion, but research to date has not demonstrated substantive benefit in common cold.

Rhinorrhea

The treatment of rhinorrhea is primarily by blockade of cholinergic stimulation of glandular secretion. Intranasal ipratropium bromide reduces rhinorrhea

TABLE 337-2	TREATMENTS FOR THE COMMON COLD	
DRUG	**DOSE AND DURATION**	**SIDE EFFECTS**
Topical adrenergic agents: oxymetazoline	2-3 sprays of 0.05% solution every 12 hr as needed for up to 3 days	Rebound nasal congestion with prolonged use Nasal stinging or burning
Oral adrenergic agents: pseudoephedrine	60 mg every 4-6 hr up to 240 mg/day as needed for nasal congestion	Insomnia Agitation
Antihistamines: chlorpheniramine	4 mg orally every 4-6 hr up to 24 mg/day as needed for rhinorrhea or sneezing	Sedation
Anticholinergics: ipratropium bromide	2 sprays per nostril of 0.06% solution every 6-8 hr as needed for rhinorrhea	Nasal dryness

in colds by 22 to 31% compared with placebo.[A2] The most common side effects of intranasal ipratropium are nasal irritation and bleeding, which are twice as common in those receiving intranasal ipratropium compared with placebo.[A3] First-generation (sedating) antihistamines, owing to their anticholinergic properties, may have mild beneficial effects on rhinorrhea. The major side effects associated with antihistamines are sedation and drying of the eyes, mouth, and nose.

Cough

Cough during colds is produced by several different mechanisms, so treatment should be directed at the most likely underlying cause (Chapters 77 and 401). If cough is caused by nasal obstruction or postnasal drip, it may respond to treatment with an antihistamine or antihistamine-decongestant combination. If a more persistent cough is the result of virus-induced reactive airway disease or viral infection of the lower airways, patients may benefit from bronchodilator therapy (Chapter 81). Nonspecific cough suppression with codeine, dextromethorphan, or moguisteine are not useful for treatment of cough associated with colds. Expectorants such as guaifenesin are not antitussive agents and are not useful for treatment of cough in colds.

Pain-Related Symptoms

Headache and body aches are experienced very frequently among people with colds, especially among people with symptoms qualifying them for an influenza-like illness diagnosis. Acetaminophen (e.g., 750 to 1000 mg every 4 to 6 hours) and nonsteroidal anti-inflammatory agents (e.g., ibuprofen 200 mg every 4 to 6 hours) are effective for pain, including the sore throat, headache, ear pain, and myalgias that can accompany common cold. These analgesics do not, however, relieve nasal congestion, rhinorrhea, or cough.

Combination Therapies

Combination cold therapies available without a prescription (e.g., analgesics, decongestants, antihistamines, and/or antitussives) may have modest benefits over placebo, but any symptomatic benefits should be weighed against potential side effects.[A4] Therapies specifically targeted to an individual's symptoms of nasal obstruction, rhinorrhea, or sore throat are preferable to avoid the side effects of unnecessary medications.

Other Remedies

Zinc lozenges (e.g., zinc acetate or zinc gluconate, dosed at ≥75 mg/day of elemental zinc) can improve common cold recovery rates by 20 to 40%.[A5] However, zinc lozenges may be associated with sore mouth and occasional nausea, and intranasal zinc may cause nasal irritation or nosebleeds. Echinacea formulations are of uncertain benefit for treating the common cold.[A6]

PREVENTION

Chemoprophylaxis or immunoprophylaxis is generally not available for the common cold.[A7] Immunization or chemoprophylaxis against influenza (Chapter 340) may be useful for prevention of colds caused by this pathogen, but influenza is responsible for only a small proportion of all colds. Vitamin C (ascorbic acid) has at most limited effectiveness for either prevention or treatment of the common cold.[A8] Echinacea may have a very modest benefit as a preventive therapy.[A9] Several randomized trials also suggest that exercise may help to prevent common cold illness.[A10] Other nonpharmacologic interventions touted as effective prophylaxis for the common cold but of unproven benefit include zinc, vitamin E, ginseng, and handwashing. Handwashing has undeniable benefits for public health and can be recommended despite the limited evidence specific to common cold prevention. The other interventions named here, although probably safe, have no demonstrable benefit and may simply contribute to the unnecessary health care expenditures related to the common cold.

PROGNOSIS

The common cold usually has little medical significance because complete recovery can be expected. However, these illnesses are often complicated by otitis media (Chapter 398), sinusitis (Chapter 398), or pneumonia (Chapter 91) that may be a direct result of the viral infection or may be due to bacterial superinfection. Exacerbations of asthma (Chapter 81) and chronic bronchitis (Chapter 82) are important complications of the common cold. For elderly who are frail or have advanced lung disease, common cold can lead to hospitalization or death. Rhinovirus infection within a family also appears to facilitate within-family transmission of *S. pneumoniae*, which may then result in pneumonia.[10]

Grade A References

A1. Deckx L, De Sutter AI, Guo L, et al. Nasal decongestants in monotherapy for the common cold. *Cochrane Database Syst Rev.* 2016;10:CD009612.
A2. AlBalawi ZH, Othman SS, Alfaleh K. Intranasal ipratropium bromide for the common cold. *Cochrane Database Syst Rev.* 2013;6:CD008231.
A3. De Sutter AI, Saraswat A, van Driel ML. Antihistamines for the common cold. *Cochrane Database Syst Rev.* 2015;11:CD009345.
A4. De Sutter AI, van Driel ML, Kumar AA, et al. Oral antihistamine-decongestant-analgesic combinations for the common cold. *Cochrane Database Syst Rev.* 2012;2:CD004976.
A5. Hemilä H, Fitzgerald JT, Petrus EJ, et al. Zinc acetate lozenges may improve the recovery rate of common cold patients: an individual patient data meta-analysis. *Open Forum Infect Dis.* 2017;4:1-6.
A6. Karsch-Völk M, Barrett B, Kiefer D, et al. Echinacea for preventing and treating the common cold. *Cochrane Database Syst Rev.* 2014;2:CD000530.
A7. Simancas-Racines D, Franco JV, Guerra CV, et al. Vaccines for the common cold. *Cochrane Database Syst Rev.* 2017;5:CD002190.
A8. Hemilä H, Chalker E. Vitamin C for preventing and treating the common cold. *Cochrane Database Syst Rev.* 2013;1:CD000980.
A9. Karsch-Völk M, Barrett B, Linde K. Echinacea for preventing and treating the common cold. *JAMA.* 2015;313:618-619.
A10. Grande AJ, Keogh J, Hoffmann TC, et al. Exercise versus no exercise for the occurrence, severity and duration of acute respiratory infections. *Cochrane Database Syst Rev.* 2015;6:CD010596.

GENERAL REFERENCES

For the General References and other additional features, please visit Expert Consult at https://expertconsult.inkling.com.

338

RESPIRATORY SYNCYTIAL VIRUS

H. KEIPP TALBOT AND EDWARD E. WALSH

DEFINITION

Respiratory syncytial virus (RSV), which causes yearly winter outbreaks in temperate climates, is the most important cause of bronchiolitis and pneumonia in young infants, a common cause of illness in older children and young adults, and can be severe in elderly persons, adults with underlying cardiopulmonary disease, and the severely immunocompromised.

The Pathogen

RSV is a single-stranded RNA-enveloped virus of the family Paramyxoviridae, genus *Pneumovirus*; it is related to human metapneumovirus. Two major transmembrane glycoproteins (G, attachment protein; F, fusion protein) carry neutralizing epitopes, and two nonstructural proteins (NS1 and NS2) block the antiviral activity of type I interferons, whereas a secreted form of G bearing a CX3C chemokine motif may modulate immune responses. Two major virus groups (A and B), each with multiple genotypes, are distinguishable.

EPIDEMIOLOGY

In the United States epidemics begin in the south in late fall, move steadily north, and peak in February and March in colder climates.[1] In tropical areas, RSV may occur throughout the year, with peaks during the rainy season. RSV annually causes approximately 100,000 hospitalizations and accounts for 60% of bronchiolitis and 25% of pneumonia cases in infants. Mortality is rare in the United States (<400 deaths annually), but deaths are substantially greater in underdeveloped countries.[2] About half of infants become infected in their first winter and all by age 2. RSV is transmitted principally by direct contact with large-particle fomites of respiratory secretions rather than by small-particle aerosolization.

Between 1 and 3% of primary infections result in hospitalization, but lower socioeconomic status, crowding, underlying prematurity, congenital cardiac abnormalities, bronchopulmonary dysplasia, and immunosuppression are each associated with increased risk for serious disease. Severe disease is also associated with specific polymorphisms in the promoter regions of cytokine genes. Hospitalization is most frequent between the ages of 1 and 6 months, peaking at 2 months of age with a rate of 25.9 per 1000 children. However, the majority of hospitalized infants are normal healthy infants without identifiable risk factors. The overall burden of RSV in infants 0 to 6 months of age is 132 office visits, 55 emergency department visits, and 17 hospitalizations per 1000. Reinfection occurs frequently throughout life, although subsequent illness is less severe and hospitalization infrequent for most older children and young adults, but can cause severe disease and hospitalization in persons with underlying cardiac or pulmonary conditions.

Though often not considered in adults, RSV infection is common and may be severe in the elderly. RSV accounts for 15 to 20% of medically attended outpatient respiratory illnesses in persons older than 45 years, and RSV-associated mortality among persons age 65 and older is about 90% as high as influenza A and greater than double that of influenza B. RSV infection is implicated in 6 to 15% of hospitalizations for acute pulmonary symptoms in the winter among community-dwelling elderly persons, numbers that are similar to those for influenza.[3,4]

RSV infection has been documented in up to 10% of bone marrow transplant recipients (Chapter 168), patients with acute leukemia (Chapter 173), and heart/lung transplant recipients (Chapters 53 and 93) during the winter months. In this setting, in-hospital outbreaks can develop quickly if patients are not adequately isolated.

PATHOBIOLOGY

Virus most commonly enters through the nose or eye and then spreads from the upper to the lower respiratory tract. Pathologic findings include a lymphocytic peribronchiolar infiltration with edema, obstruction, and necrosis. Bronchiolitis with multiple areas of atelectasis, and pneumonia with interstitial infiltration of mononuclear cells, as well as alveoli filled by edema and necrosis, develop in infected patients.

CLINICAL MANIFESTATIONS

Infants experience upper respiratory symptoms of conjunctival injection, mucopurulent nasal discharge, cough, and low-grade fever after an incubation period of 2 to 8 days. Otitis media (Chapter 398) is often associated with secondary bacterial infection. After several days, lower respiratory tract symptoms appear in 25 to 50% of infants, with cough, wheezing, tachypnea, and use of accessory muscles as the disease progresses. Expiratory wheezes, rhonchi, and fine rales are the most common findings on lung examination. Sudden apnea may develop in the youngest infants. Hyperinflation and diffuse interstitial pneumonitis are the most frequent radiographic findings. High-titer virus shedding lasts 7 to 10 days, although immunocompromised infants may excrete virus for a month or longer, even when asymptomatic. Coinfection with other respiratory viruses occurs in up to 30% of patients, but it usually is neither clinically discernible nor definitively associated with more severe illness.

Adults with RSV typically begin with upper respiratory symptoms, but many patients have lower respiratory symptoms, especially wheezing. Low-titer virus shedding often persists for 10 days or longer. In elderly persons, RSV attack rates are 3 to 5% annually; wheezing is more common than with influenza (Chapter 340),[5] whereas fever is less common. Symptoms can progress to respiratory failure. In frail elderly persons or in patients with underlying chronic obstructive pulmonary disease or heart failure severe disease can develop. Attack rates in nosocomial nursing home outbreaks average 10 to about 90%, with crackles and wheezes evident in a third of patients and radiographically confirmed pneumonia in approximately 10%. The incidence of bacterial superinfection in hospitalized adults with RSV is about 30%, similar to that of other common respiratory viruses, including influenza.[6]

In bone marrow transplant recipients, RSV usually presents initially with upper respiratory symptoms.[7] In about 30% of patients, lower respiratory tract disease follows, often with severe symptoms.

DIAGNOSIS

In infants, a presumptive diagnosis is suggested by typical symptoms during the epidemic season, but the diagnosis often is not considered in adults. Diagnosis can be made by reverse transcription–polymerase chain reaction (RT-PCR), which is the test of choice and has high sensitivity and specificity. Viral culture, which can take up to 10 days, has a sensitivity of only about 75%.

In adults, viral culture has poor sensitivity (30%), whereas RT-PCR detects infection in three quarters of culture-negative cases that are seropositive, using acute and convalescent serum. Owing to very poor sensitivity, antigen detection by immunofluorescence and enzyme immunoassay are not useful in adults, even if immunocompromised. In immunocompromised patients, chest radiographs demonstrate diffuse interstitial and alveolar infiltrates. A useful clinical clue to the presence of RSV is the frequent presence of radiographically proven sinusitis. Upper respiratory tract symptoms distinguish this illness from cytomegalovirus pneumonia (Chapter 352).

TREATMENT Rx

Therapy for most infants is symptomatic and generally is limited to hydration and supplemental oxygen. Bronchodilators have not been demonstrated to be effective, although they are occasionally used. Similarly, glucocorticosteroids have not been shown to have benefit in most studies. Inhaled ribavirin (2 g administered by aerosol three times daily for 3 to 5 days) may be beneficial for infants at high risk for serious disease and those who are severely ill, although clinical trials have not demonstrated benefit for most infants.

No placebo-controlled studies of the effect of inhaled ribavirin have been conducted in adults with severe RSV disease, but the evidence suggests potential benefit in immunocompromised adults with RSV pneumonia (2 g every 8 hours for 5 to 10 days), especially if begun before development of lower respiratory symptoms.

Some studies using antibody therapy (the monoclonal antibody palivizumab, 15 mg/kg once, or polyclonal immunoglobulin) combined with inhaled ribavirin suggest benefit in the treatment of RSV pneumonia in immunosuppressed adults, although conclusive randomized studies have not been performed. An experimental oral RSV-entry inhibitor and an oral nucleoside analog have shown promise in reducing the viral load in experimental human challenge models of RSV infection and are currently in clinical trials.[8-10] A number of other antiviral approaches are being studied actively. Bacterial superinfection can develop, with *Streptococcus pneumoniae* (Chapter 273) and *Haemophilus influenzae* (Chapter 284) being the most frequent organisms. For such patients, appropriate antimicrobial treatment (Chapter 91) is mandatory.

PREVENTION

Adherence to standard infection-control principles (e.g., gloves, gowns, frequent handwashing) substantially reduces nosocomial spread. A vaccine is not yet available.[11] RSV F nanoparticle vaccines have been immunogenic and well tolerated but have not been shown to protect older adults against RSV infections.[12] Parenteral humanized RSV monoclonal antibody (palivizumab, 15 mg/kg monthly during the RSV season) has demonstrated benefit when administered prophylactically to specific high-risk infant groups. Palivizumab prophylaxis in healthy late-preterm infants (32 to 35 weeks' gestation) also can reduce subsequent wheezing by 50% during the first year of life.[A1]

PROGNOSIS

RSV infection in severely immunocompromised adults such as bone marrow transplant recipients (Chapter 168) and those with acute leukemia (Chapter 173) undergoing cytotoxic chemotherapy can carry a 60% mortality rate when pneumonia develops. Lymphopenia (<100/μL) and high-dose total body irradiation are associated with more severe disease, but progression to pneumonia is very unusual in patients with an absolute lymphocyte count above 1000/μL. In lung transplant recipients, bronchiolitis obliterans syndrome may occur in 10 to 50% of patients as a late sequela of RSV infection.

Mortality is rare in otherwise healthy infants but can reach 37% in infants with cardiac disorders. In children, a link between severe bronchiolitis and subsequent asthma remains unresolved. In normal infants and healthy adults, the outcome is generally good, but the risk of mortality in adults is higher with RSV than with influenza.[13] Hospitalized older adults can have mortality rates of about 10%.

Grade A Reference

A1. Blanken MO, Rovers MM, Molenaar JM, et al. Respiratory syncytial virus and recurrent wheeze in healthy preterm infants. *N Engl J Med.* 2013;368:1791-1799.

GENERAL REFERENCES

For the General References and other additional features, please visit Expert Consult at https://expertconsult.inkling.com.

339

PARAINFLUENZA VIRAL DISEASE

GEOFFREY A. WEINBERG AND KATHRYN M. EDWARDS

DEFINITION

Human parainfluenza viruses (hPIVs) are important causes of a wide spectrum of respiratory illnesses. In infants and young children, they produce acute upper and lower respiratory tract infections ranging from the common cold (Chapter 337) and otitis media (Chapter 398) to severe croup, bronchiolitis, and pneumonia (Chapter 91). In older children and adults, hPIV infections are usually limited to the upper respiratory tract (Chapter 90), although immunocompromised individuals may develop fatal respiratory failure.[1]

The Pathogen

The hPIVs are enveloped, single-stranded, nonsegmented RNA viruses that belong to two genera in the family Paramyxoviridae. Members of this family also include respiratory syncytial virus (RSV [Chapter 338]), human metapneumovirus (Chapter 337), measles virus (Chapter 343), mumps virus (Chapter 345), Hendra and Nipah viruses, and the pathogenic animal viruses of Newcastle disease, canine distemper, and rinderpest. The hPIV genome encodes six structural proteins. The hemagglutinin-neuraminidase (HN) and fusion (F) proteins, which are exposed on the bilayered lipid envelope surrounding the helical nucleocapsid–RNA complex, mediate both attachment to host sialic acid–containing glycoproteins and penetration of the virus into susceptible mammalian cells. These proteins have retained their antigenic stability for many years, unlike the "drift and shift" of the hemagglutinin and neuraminidase of influenza viruses. The four serotypes of hPIV are called types 1 to 4, including two subgroups (A and B) of type 4 virus.

The hPIVs replicate in the ciliated epithelial cells that line the respiratory tract on its luminal surface. This selective tropism is consistent with the absence of invasive disease or viremia in the immunocompetent host. Syncytium formation, which is noted in viral cell cultures and in the lungs of immunocompromised patients with severe pneumonia, is not thought to be important in typical infections of previously healthy individuals.

EPIDEMIOLOGY

The hPIVs are ubiquitous, with a worldwide geographic distribution.[2,3] Their transmission is principally by large-particle fomites via close person-to-person contact. Parainfluenza virus activity displays both endemic and epidemic patterns, with each serotype favoring different age groups and distinct clinical syndromes but with enough overlap to preclude specific diagnosis based solely on clinical and epidemiologic grounds.

Primary infection with hPIV occurs early in childhood. Of the parainfluenza viruses, type 3 (hPIV-3) generally infects infants first, such that 50 to 67% of infants demonstrate serologic evidence of infection by 1 year of age. Parainfluenza viruses 1 and 2 (hPIV-1 and hPIV-2, respectively) then most commonly infect children between 2 and 5 years of age. Parainfluenza virus 4 (hPIV-4) less commonly causes symptomatic respiratory infections; in some studies hPIV-4 is found more often in viral coinfection with other pathogens.[4]

Until the early 1960s, hPIV-1 caused endemic annual disease in the United States. For the past several decades, however, hPIV-1 has been associated with biennial outbreaks in the fall of odd-numbered years. Infections with hPIV-2 largely follow this same curious pattern but occur much less commonly than hPIV-1 infections. Infections with hPIV-3 have remained endemic throughout the year, with peaks in the late spring. The incubation period for all serotypes of hPIV is between 3 and 6 days in experimentally infected adults, but natural infections in children have incubation periods of 2 to 4 days.

The hPIVs are second only to RSV as the cause of acute upper and lower respiratory tract infections in young children in the United States. In a population-based study of children younger than 5 years hospitalized with fever or acute respiratory tract infection, 7% of children had laboratory-confirmed hPIV infection (by cell culture and molecular amplification techniques), compared with 19% with RSV and 6% with influenza A or B virus infections.[5] The hospitalization rate for hPIV infection in children younger than 5 years was 1.02 per 1000 children per year. Extrapolating to the entire U.S. population, these data suggest that approximately 23,000 hPIV annual hospitalizations occur in children younger than 5 years. The rates of emergency department and outpatient health care visits attributable to hPIV infections in young children are 10- to 50-fold greater than hospitalization rates. Further, immunity to hPIV infection is neither complete nor durable, so older children and adults can exhibit symptomatic infection, sometimes leading to office visits and hospitalization.

CLINICAL MANIFESTATIONS

Primary Infection

Illness associated with primary hPIV infection varies by age and viral serotype. Underlying medical conditions such as cardiopulmonary compromise and immune disorders increase the severity of disease. Large cohort and longitudinal family studies have shown that hPIV infections are responsible for about 65% of croup, 20 to 40% of lower respiratory infection, and 20% of upper respiratory infection in young children. The majority of children have experienced primary hPIV infection by the time they enter elementary school. Thus, although hPIV also causes upper respiratory infections in adults, these are reinfections rather than primary infections (see later). In general, hPIV-1 and hPIV-2 are most commonly associated with croup, whereas hPIV-3 infection often presents as undifferentiated febrile illness, bronchiolitis, or pneumonia.

Infection typically begins with upper respiratory signs and symptoms, notably coryza, rhinorrhea, pharyngitis without cervical adenopathy, and low-grade fever. Symptoms typically persist for 3 to 5 days. About 15 to 25% of infected children develop signs of croup or progress to lower respiratory tract disease (e.g., bronchiolitis, pneumonia) indistinguishable from RSV infection.

Croup is characterized by a raspy barking cough with notable inspiratory stridor, dyspnea, and respiratory distress. These symptoms, which are generally spasmodic, result from subglottic inflammation and edema. On occasion, severe stridor may develop and make differentiation from epiglottitis caused by Haemophilus influenzae type b (Chapter 284) difficult, although epiglottitis is much less common in the United States since universal Hib vaccination became routine in 1990.

Croup is very rare in adults but has been associated with hPIV in isolated case reports. Epiglottitis is seen more often in adults, but it is more commonly associated with staphylococcal or streptococcal infection. Epiglottitis is a medical emergency for patients of all ages and must be distinguished from croup to allow proper therapy, including emergent intubation of the airway. For patients who are judged to have a stable enough airway to permit urgent radiography rather than emergent tracheostomy, the differences between these two entities are clearly shown in lateral neck radiographs, on which subglottic edema and narrowing are seen with croup, and swelling of the epiglottis is seen with epiglottitis (Figs. 339-1 and 339-2). Children with bronchiolitis or pneumonia caused by hPIV have cough, rales, and wheezing associated with hypoxia, and their chest radiographs often exhibit air trapping.

Reinfection

Reinfection with hPIV is less severe and typically causes rhinorrhea in normal children and adults. Reinfection with hPIV is estimated to account for 1 to 15% of all acute respiratory illnesses in adults, the majority of whom present with simple upper respiratory tract infections. However, as with RSV, some adults may develop severe disease that requires hospitalization and even ventilatory support.[6,7] In such patients, fever, cough, dyspnea, and wheezing are common. Radiographic changes, primarily lobar or interstitial infiltrates, are seen in more than 50% of adults hospitalized with hPIV infection.

Elderly and Immunocompromised Patients

Nursing home outbreaks of hPIV infection may include a high incidence of pneumonia, just as hPIV infections often cause severe pneumonia in immunocompromised children and adults. Among healthy elderly residents of long-term care facilities, hPIV infections are as common as infections caused by influenza A virus, influenza B virus, or RSV. Ten percent of children and 2 to 7% of adults with leukemia or hematopoietic stem cell or solid organ transplant recipients develop hPIV infections, with about 90% of those due to hPIV-3. Although 80 to 90% of hPIV infections among patients with malignancy are community acquired, nosocomial outbreaks have occurred even in stem cell transplant units.

Approximately 25% of hPIV-infected stem cell transplant recipients develop lower respiratory disease, mostly in the first 100 days after transplantation, when lymphopenia and neutropenia are most pronounced. The strongest identified risk factors for hPIV infection in this setting are neutropenia, lymphopenia, more severe disease, and the use of corticosteroids, especially at

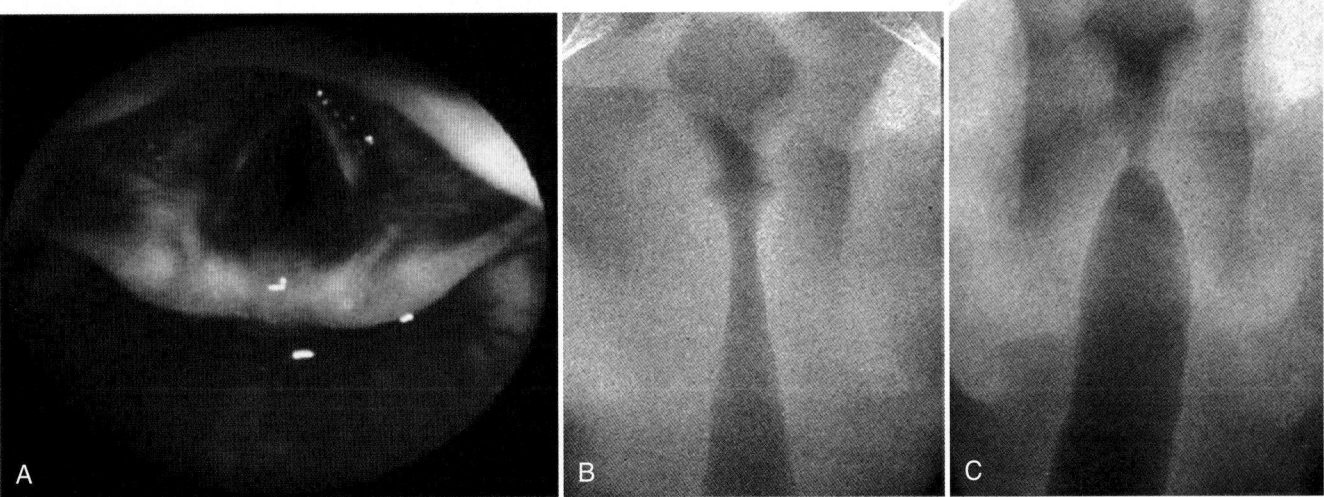

FIGURE 339-1. Subglottic edema. **A,** Endoscopic view of subglottic edema in viral croup. **B,** Radiologic presentation of subglottic edema in viral croup, causing narrowing ("steeple sign") of the tracheal air shadow, compared with (**C**) a normal tracheal air shadow. (From Hammer J. Acquired upper airway obstruction. *Paediatr Respir Rev.* 2004;5:25-33.)

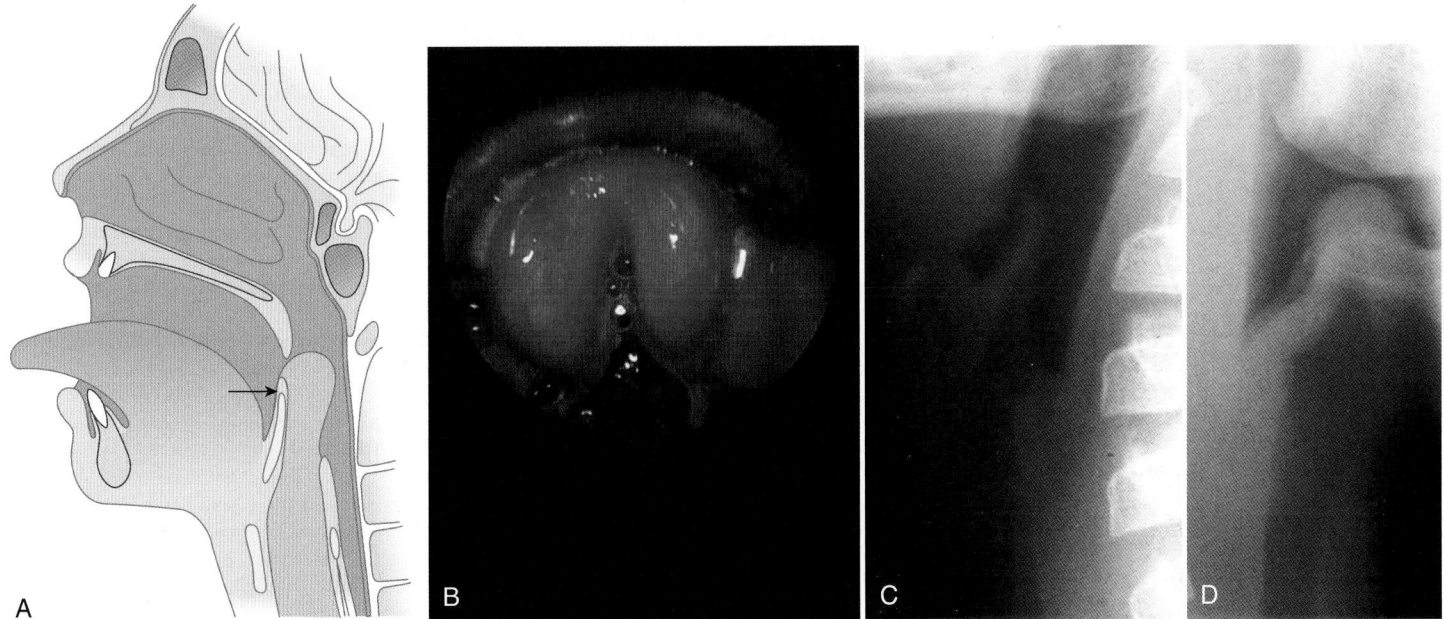

FIGURE 339-2. Epiglottitis. Schematic (**A**) and endoscopic view (**B**) of epiglottitis. **C,** The typical lateral neck radiographs of a normal child and (**D**) a child with epiglottitis ("thumb sign" of swollen epiglottis) are displayed. (From Hammer J. Acquired upper airway obstruction. *Paediatr Respir Rev.* 2004;5:25-33.)

higher doses.[8] Fever, cough, dyspnea, and sputum production are the most common symptoms. Coinfection with *Aspergillus* (Chapter 319) and other pathogens has been reported in hematopoietic stem cell transplant recipients with pneumonia as well.

DIAGNOSIS

Although hPIV may be suspected on clinical and epidemiologic grounds, specific diagnosis requires isolation of the virus or detection of viral antigen or RNA in respiratory secretions. Reverse transcription–polymerase chain reaction (RT-PCR) assays are highly sensitive and specific for diagnosis. Alternatively, cultures of monkey kidney or human embryonic kidney cells can be used to grow the virus, with cytopathic effects detected in 5 to 10 days (except for hPIV-4, which requires up to 3 weeks). Rapid direct or indirect immunofluorescence tests are less sensitive and specific than culture or PCR but still are used in some clinical laboratories.

Definitive diagnosis of parainfluenza infection in adults, even by RT-PCR, may be more difficult than in children, presumably because less virus is shed in partially immune adults. However, virus can usually be recovered from the nasopharyngeal secretions or bronchoalveolar lavage fluid in hematopoietic stem cell transplant recipients with pneumonia.

TREATMENT Rx

Specific antiviral treatment of hPIV infection is currently unavailable. Aerosolized ribavirin has in vitro activity against hPIV and is approved for use in RSV infection. Although it has shown few benefits in immunocompromised children and adults with severe hPIV pneumonia, even when administered with concomitant intravenous immunoglobulin, some experts will offer aerosolized or intravenous ribavirin, with or without intravenous immunoglobulin, to immunocompromised patients with severe disease.

For previously healthy children with croup, general comfort, which usually means sitting in the lap of a parent or caregiver, is widely recommended. Humidified air (mist) repeatedly has been shown to have no benefits and actually is associated with adverse effects, including anxiety, difficulty with cardiorespiratory monitoring, and bacterial and fungal contamination of both hot and cold mist humidifiers. Oxygen may be given by holding the end of the tubing near the nose and mouth ("blow-by" oxygen).

Children with mild to moderate croup (i.e., without stridor or significant chest wall indrawing at rest, or with stridor and indrawing but without agitation) may be given oral dexamethasone, 0.6 mg/kg body weight, and observed; if they improve, they may be discharged to home.[A1] Children with severe croup (stridor, chest wall indrawing, and agitation) may benefit from blow-by oxygen, inhaled racemic epinephrine (0.05 mL/kg body weight of a 2.25% solution of racemic epinephrine for nebulization, up to a maximum dose of 0.5 mL) or nebulized L-epinephrine (0.5 mL/kg of 1:1000 L-epinephrine, up to a maximum dose of 5 mL), and concomitant dexamethasone.[A2] Children should be admitted to the hospital if no significant clinical improvement is seen after several hours of observation and therapy.

Oral dexamethasone is as effective as intramuscular dexamethasone or nebulized budesonide and easier to administer. Corticosteroids decrease the need for hospitalization and return visits, decrease length of stay both in emergency departments and after hospital admission, and decrease the need for intubation. In general, there are no reasons to institute either antibiotic therapy or short-acting bronchodilator therapy in children with croup.

Investigational therapies for hPIV infection include both nonspecific and specific measures. Inhalation of heliox (helium-oxygen mixture) may decrease the work of breathing and improve gas exchange in children with moderate to severe croup, but adequately controlled clinical trial data are not yet available. The novel antiviral agent DAS181, a sialidase fusion protein with activity against both influenza and parainfluenza viruses, has shown beneficial effects in a small number of adults and children with severe hPIV infection and is undergoing clinical trials.[9]

PREVENTION

Clinical trials of live attenuated hPIV vaccines are ongoing. Two approaches have been taken to produce live-attenuated intranasal hPIV-3 vaccines. One approach has been to attenuate an hPIV-3 isolate by repeated cold-temperature passage and manipulation by recombinant technology. A second has been to use a related but nonvirulent bovine PIV-3 as a backbone in which to insert hPIV-3 genes to produce an attenuated chimeric vaccine virus. Another vaccine candidate under study uses the chimeric bovine-human PIV-3 virus, but with an additional RSV gene inserted into the vaccine virus genome in an attempt to prevent both of these common infections in young children. Vaccines against hPIV-1 infection (with or without RSV components) also are under development.

PROGNOSIS

In otherwise healthy children, mortality after hPIV infection is less than 0.1%. By comparison, mortality after hPIV pneumonia in patients undergoing stem cell transplantation is as high as 10 to 30%.

Grade A References

A1. Fernandes RM, Oleszczuk M, Woods CR, et al. The Cochrane Library and safety of systemic corticosteroids for acute respiratory conditions in children: an overview of reviews. *Evid Based Child Health.* 2014;9:733-747.
A2. Bjornson C, Russell K, Vandermeer B, et al. Nebulized epinephrine for croup in children. *Cochrane Database Syst Rev.* 2013;10:CD006619.

GENERAL REFERENCES

For the General References and other additional features, please visit Expert Consult at https://expertconsult.inkling.com.

340

INFLUENZA

MICHAEL G. ISON AND FREDERICK G. HAYDEN

DEFINITION

Influenza is an acute febrile respiratory viral illness that usually occurs in annual outbreaks of varying severity and occasionally causes worldwide epidemics (pandemics). Increasingly, sporadic zoonotic infections, sometimes associated with limited human-to-human transmission, are being documented. Influenza viruses infect the respiratory tract, are highly contagious, and classically produce prominent systemic symptoms early in the illness. Influenza infection causes various clinical syndromes in adults, including nonfebrile common colds (Chapter 337), pharyngitis (Chapters 274 and 401),

tracheobronchitis (Chapter 90), pneumonia (Chapter 91), and a range of nonrespiratory complications. Conversely, infections with other respiratory viruses, such as respiratory syncytial virus (RSV [Chapter 338]) or adenovirus (Chapter 341), may produce influenza-like illness. Influenza A viruses have caused five pandemics of varying severity within the past 120 years (E-Table 340-1). The 1918–1919 pandemic caused at least 500,000 deaths in the United States and more than 40 million worldwide, whereas the 2009 H1N1 pandemic was associated with substantially less mortality. Seasonal epidemics may cause enormous morbidity, economic loss, and often substantial mortality. Each year in the United States, seasonal influenza epidemics are associated with an estimated 4.3 to 16.7 million medical visits, 140,000 to 710,000 hospitalizations, and 12,000 to 56,000 respiratory and circulatory deaths.

The Pathogen

Influenza viruses belong to the family Orthomyxoviridae and are divided into four types (A, B, C, and D) based on their protein composition and other properties (E-Table 340-2). The virion (E-Fig. 340-1) is a medium-sized enveloped pleomorphic particle covered with two types of surface glycoprotein spikes, the trimeric hemagglutinin (H or HA) and the tetrameric mushroom-shaped neuraminidase (N or NA). The envelope is composed of a lipid bilayer overlying the matrix (M1) protein that surrounds the viral genome, which consists of eight segments of single-stranded negative sense RNA in influenza A and B viruses. Influenza C viruses have seven segments and only a single surface glycoprotein. Genomic replication occurs in the nucleus of infected cells, and multiple cellular proteins and pathways are involved during the infection of host cells.

Whereas influenza B and C viruses are principally human pathogens, influenza A viruses primarily infect aquatic birds and sometimes establish lineages that circulate in other animal hosts, including other avians, swine, horses, marine mammals, and dogs. Influenza D appears to be pathogenic in cattle and perhaps other domestic animals. Influenza A viruses are further classified into subtypes on the basis of their HA and NA glycoproteins. Sixteen HA and nine NA subtypes are currently recognized in avians, and two others are recognized in bats. Only three HAs (H1, H2, and H3) and two NAs (N1 and N2) have been documented thus far in epidemic and pandemic human influenza A viruses, although other HAs (e.g., H5, H6, H7, H9, H10) and NAs (e.g., N4, N7, N8, N9) have been found in zoonotic infections. Each strain is identified by type, subtype if influenza A, site, sample number, and year of isolation.

EPIDEMIOLOGY

Antigenic and Genetic Variation

Influenza viruses are unique among the respiratory viruses with regard to their extent of genetic and antigenic variation, epidemic behavior, and frequent association with excess mortality during community outbreaks—characteristics and pathogenicity that exemplify human influenza virus's efficient host-to-host transmissibility. The changing antigenicity of the surface glycoproteins largely accounts for repeated influenza epidemics. Antibody to HA can neutralize viral infectivity and is thus the major determinant of immunity. Current vaccines are based largely on inducing hemagglutination-inhibition (HAI) or neutralizing antibodies to HA. Anti-NA antibody limits viral replication and probably reduces the severity of infection. Variation involves either relatively minor (antigenic drift) or major (antigenic shift) changes in antigenicity. Significant antigenic variation is much less frequent with influenza B or C than with influenza A.

Antigenic drift results from point mutations in the HA gene segment that cause amino acid substitutions in at least one of five key antigenic sites on HA. Drift can also occur in NA and in T-cell epitopes on internal proteins. Antigenic variants emerge frequently (every year or every few years) within an influenza A or B virus. For example, the original H3N2 variant, A/Aichi/68, has undergone successive drifts resulting in epidemic strains that include the recent circulation of A/Kansas/14/2017 (H3N2)-like virus. Immunologic selection favors transmission of the new variant over the old because of the less frequent presence of antibody to the new virus in the population.[1]

Antigenic shift results from the appearance of a novel influenza A virus with HA or HA and NA glycoproteins that are new to humans or that reappear after decades of absence. Because of the lack of population immunity, a new strain that is efficiently transmitted from person to person can cause pandemic disease. The origins of new pandemic strains and the basis for their possible recirculation remain incompletely understood. Avian influenza viruses have most frequently served as the reservoir of new genes for pandemic viruses. Reassortment of gene segments may occur when two influenza viruses simultaneously infect a single cell, and reassortment events in which human viruses acquired avian genes led to both the 1957 and 1968 pandemic viruses. Because swine can support replication of both human and avian viruses, they have been postulated to serve as a mixing vessel for the generation of new strains or as the host in which avian viruses can adapt to mammals. The 2009 H1N1 pandemic virus arose as a quadruple reassortant that derived gene segments from Asian and North American swine lineage viruses that harbored genes derived from swine, avian, and human viruses.

Multiple reassortment events may occur over a period of years before a pandemic virus emerges. For example, the 1918 pandemic virus appears to have been composed primarily of avian genes that underwent adaptation in a mammalian host before causing the pandemic. Frequent intra-subtypic reassortment also occurs among seasonal human influenza A viruses and sometimes leads to new antigenic variants and sometimes to altered virulence.

Epidemic or Interpandemic Influenza

An epidemic is an outbreak of influenza confined to one geographic location. In temperate climates, community epidemics of influenza A virus infection often have a characteristic pattern, typically reaching a sharp peak in 2 or 3 weeks after initial recognition and persisting for 6 to 10 weeks. Increased numbers of schoolchildren with febrile respiratory illness are often the first indication of influenza in a community, soon followed by illnesses in adults and, 1 to 2 weeks later, by increased hospital admission of patients with influenza-related complications. Hospitalization rates in high-risk persons increase two- to five-fold during major epidemics. School and employment absenteeism increases, as does mortality from pneumonia and underlying conditions, especially in older adults during A/H3N2 epidemics. Epidemics occur almost exclusively during the late autumn and winter months in temperate areas, but activity may extend into spring months. Influenza activity may occur year-round in the tropics or display other patterns.[2] The reasons for the distinct seasonality of influenza in temperate climates are uncertain but may include the school calendar, increased close indoor contact, and low absolute humidity, which affects airborne transmissibility. Winter holidays delay the peaks of seasonal epidemics and shift the risk of infection toward adults.[3] Outbreaks sometimes occur in tour groups (land or ship) and in chronic care facilities during summer months, particularly after the appearance of a drift variant. Regional differences in the timing, magnitude, and causative viruses of influenza outbreaks are common. During epidemics, overall attack rates typically range from 5 to 20% in adults. Attack rates of 40 to 50% may occur in semiclosed populations, such as on hospital floors and chronic care facilities, as well as in highly susceptible age groups such as children. Influenza A and B viruses, two different influenza A subtypes, two different influenza B lineages, or two different strains within a single subtype may co-circulate or occur sequentially during one season in a given location. In addition, simultaneous outbreaks of influenza A virus and RSV or other respiratory viruses occur. Strains circulating at the end of one season's epidemic are sometimes responsible for the next season's outbreak (the so-called herald wave phenomenon).

Pneumonia- and influenza-related deaths fluctuate annually, with peaks in the winter months in temperate climates. When such deaths exceed the expected threshold, the cause is typically influenza A, but influenza B virus or RSV can occasionally be responsible. Influenza A/H3N2-dominant seasons are associated with two to three times higher mortality rates than are H1N1 and B-dominant seasons. Although mortality is usually greatest during pandemics, substantial mortality occurs with epidemics. During seasonal influenza, more than 85% of pneumonia- and influenza-related deaths occur in persons aged 65 years and older. Mortality risk is especially high in those aged 85 years and older. Cardiovascular events (e.g., myocardial infarction) and worsening of other chronic diseases contribute substantially to the increased mortality during influenza epidemics.

Pandemic Influenza

Pandemics of influenza A result from the emergence of a new virus capable of sustained person-to-person transmission and to which the population contains no or limited immunity. The virus spreads worldwide, often circulating outside of the usual influenza season, and usually infects persons of all ages. Preexisting immunity due to prior infection with antigenically related viruses can provide partial protection, as occurred in older adults during the 2009 H1N1 pandemic. Pandemics are associated with high morbidity rates, especially in children, and sometimes notably increased mortality rates in pregnant women and young and middle-aged adults. For example, more than 90% of deaths in the 1918 and 2009 pandemics occurred in persons younger than 65 years. In the 2009 pandemic, adults hospitalized with H1N1 were

more likely to have severe pneumonia, shock, sepsis, and organ failure and to require intensive care unit (ICU) care than were patients with seasonal influenza.

The interval between pandemics is variable (10 to 40 years) and unpredictable. The most severe pandemics have been associated with major antigenic alterations in both major surface glycoproteins. Depending on population susceptibility and perhaps changes in the virus, one or more waves, sometimes with increased severity, may follow the initial one. As the level of immunity in the population increases, antigenic drift within the subtype may cause repeated epidemics in subsequent years, and excess mortality in persons younger than age 65 may continue for some years. For example, the pandemic 2009 H1N1 virus has continued to cause fatal infections at least ten years after its initial emergence.

Zoonotic Influenza

Zoonotic infections may be acquired from swine, poultry, or rarely other animals. Although most avian influenza viruses do not cause infections directly in humans, zoonotic infections due to avian H5, H7, H9, and rarely other subtypes continue to represent potential pandemic threats.[4] Initially recognized by a cluster of human cases in Hong Kong in 1997, an epizootic of avian H5N1 infections has affected poultry in many areas of Asia, the Middle East, Europe, and Africa and continues to cause sporadic human illnesses with high mortality and occasional instances of nonsustained human-to-human transmission. Since 2013, repeated waves of zoonotic avian H7N9 infections in China have been associated with case-fatality rates of approximately 35% in hospitalized patients.[5] The outbreaks have included limited family clusters, nosocomial transmission, many milder illnesses in the community, and increasing geographic spread in poultry and humans. This virus continues to evolve genetically, thereby leading to variants with altered antigenicity and recently with increased virulence for birds (high-pathogenicity) and possibly humans; as a result, it currently is considered to be a high pandemic threat. Closure of live bird markets and perhaps seasonal decreases in avian infections have been associated with rapid reductions in the number of affected persons. Mass poultry immunization was associated with marked decrease in human cases during the 2017–2019 winter seasons.

In the United States infrequent zoonotic infections have been recognized for decades in people exposed to swine. Since 2012, reassortant swine H3N2 viruses that acquired the M gene and sometimes other genes from the pandemic 2009 H1N1 virus (designated variant H3N2, or H3N2v) have caused hundreds of sporadic infections, particularly in the context of agricultural fairs, sometimes followed by limited human-to-human transmission and serious infections. Other variant swine-origin viruses (H1N1v, H1N2v) have also caused zoonotic infections.

PATHOBIOLOGY

Influenza virus infection is transmitted from person to person by virus-containing respiratory secretions. Large-droplet and small-particle aerosols over short distances (1 to 2 meters) both appear to contribute, but transmission by other routes, including hand contamination from secretion-laden fomites followed by self-inoculation into the eye or nose, may also occur. Infection by avian viruses can occur after direct contact with infected birds or their excreta, exposure to contaminated environments and infectious aerosols, ingestion of inadequately cooked food, and sometimes by inoculation into the conjunctiva.

The cellular receptor binding patterns and tissue tropism of influenza viruses are key determinants in transmissibility and pathogenesis. Efficient virus transmission between humans depends on virus attachment to and replication in cells bearing α-2,6-linked sialosaccharides in the upper respiratory tract and tracheobronchial tree. By comparison, the α-2,3-linked sialosaccharides, which are the preferred receptors for avian viruses, are concentrated on cells in the distal bronchioles, alveoli, and conjunctiva. Once the virus initiates infection of the respiratory tract epithelium, successive cycles of viral replication infect large numbers of cells and result in destruction of respiratory epithelium and sometimes pneumocytes through direct cytopathic effects or apoptosis. Virulence, which is a multigenic characteristic with contributions from HA, NA, NS, and polymerase proteins, varies widely among strains and is not necessarily linked to transmissibility.

The incubation period averages 2 days and varies from about 1 to 4 days for seasonal influenza but may be up to 1 week and possibly longer in infections caused by avian viruses. The quantity and duration of virus replication in the respiratory tract generally correlate with the severity of illness and levels of host pro-inflammatory cytokine-chemokine responses. Rapid innate cellular responses are induced through toll-like receptors and retinoic acid inducible gene I (*RIG-1*) that detect viral RNA and lead to the production of cytokines and interferons (IFNs). Elevated levels of mediators such as IFN-α, interleukin (IL)-6, and tumor necrosis factor (TNF)–α occur in blood and respiratory secretions and contribute to systemic symptoms and fever. Deficient IFN responses have been associated with severe influenza.

The duration of viral replication depends on age, immune status, underlying conditions, viral strain, and assay method. In seasonal influenza, upper respiratory viral detection generally continues for 3 to 5 days in adults but is longer in the elderly and hospitalized patients and may persist for weeks to months in immunocompromised hosts. Higher level and more prolonged viral replication, sometimes for weeks, occurs in the lower respiratory tract of patients with viral pneumonia, including patients with pandemic 2009 H1N1 or avian H5N1 and H7N9 infections. This course typically occurs in association with high plasma pro-inflammatory cytokine-chemokine responses, particularly IL-6, IL-8, and macrophage inflammatory protein (MIP)–1β, which likely reflect production in the infected lung. Viremia or extrapulmonary dissemination is rarely detected in human influenza, but both occur in some patients with avian H5N1 infections, in whom gastrointestinal replication may also occur, and with severe infection caused by pandemic or seasonal strains. Detection of viral RNA in the blood is associated with worse prognosis, particularly in immunocompromised patients.

Nasal and bronchial biopsy specimens from persons with uncomplicated influenza reveal desquamation of the ciliated columnar epithelium and loss of cilia. The lungs in fatal influenza may show necrotizing bronchitis, diffuse alveolar damage with epithelial necrosis, alveolar edema and hemorrhage, and hyaline membrane formation, followed later by squamous metaplasia and fibrosis. Secondary bacterial infections develop as a result of altered bacterial flora, damage to bronchial epithelium with depressed mucociliary clearance, decreased polymorphonuclear and alveolar macrophage functions, accumulation of alveolar fluid, and suppression of other host immune responses.

Humoral immunity to influenza appears to be largely subtype specific and durable for a particular strain. A child's first influenza A virus infection results in immune memory for the virus and its subtype, and subsequent infections or immunizations reinforce the antibody responses, perhaps contributing to protection against related HA subtypes (e.g., initial H3N2 infection reducing risk of H7N9 illness).[6] Neutralizing, hemagglutination-inhibiting (HAI), anti-NA, complement-fixing, enzyme-linked immunosorbent assay and immunofluorescent antibodies begin to develop in the sera of persons with primary influenza virus infection during the second week after infection and reach a peak by 4 weeks.[7] Secretory antibodies develop in the upper respiratory tract and consist predominantly of immunoglobulin A (IgA) antibodies. Antibody responses are brisker in subsequent infections or following immunization in adults. Protective immunity against influenza virus infection is mediated by neutralizing antibodies, and protection against illness is generally associated with serum HAI titers of 1:40 or greater, serum-neutralizing antibody titers of 1:8 or greater, or nasal-neutralizing antibody titers of 1:4 or greater, although protective titers vary with the strain, as well as with the patient's age and overall immune status. Non-neutralizing antibodies to other viral proteins, including anti-NA antibodies, can inhibit viral replication by antibody-dependent cellular cytotoxicity, complement-dependent cytotoxicity, and other mechanisms, such as preventing the release of virus from cells.

Type-specific cell-mediated immune responses usually develop by 1 week after infection and are considered important for termination of viral replication. Memory lymphocytes from previous infections can limit the severity of disease even in the absence of specific antibodies and may confer some degree of heterosubtypic immunity. Both virus-specific CD4+ and CD8+ T-lymphocyte responses to conserved epitopes on internal proteins appear to contribute.

An increasing number of host genetic factors are being recognized as increasing the risk of severe influenza. One allele in the IFN-induced transmembrane 3 (*IFITM3*) gene has been linked to both severe pandemic H1N1 and avian H7N9 illness.

CLINICAL MANIFESTATIONS
Influenza Syndrome

An abrupt onset of feverishness, chilliness, rigors, headache, myalgia, and malaise is characteristic of influenza but occurs in less than two thirds of cases. Systemic symptoms predominate initially, and prostration occurs in more severe cases. Myalgia, arthralgia, malaise, and headache are usually the most troublesome early symptoms, and their severity is generally related to the level of fever. Ocular symptoms, including photophobia, tearing, burning, and pain on moving the eyes, are sometimes present. Conjunctivitis is

characteristic in some avian H7 virus infections, although not in recent zoonotic H7N9 cases. Respiratory symptoms, particularly dry cough and nasal discharge, are typical early in the illness but are overshadowed by the systemic symptoms. Nasal obstruction, hoarseness, and sore throat are likewise common. Pandemic 2009 H1N1 and avian influenza illness are associated with nausea, vomiting, and diarrhea in some adults. As systemic illness diminishes, respiratory complaints and findings become more apparent. Cough is the most frequent and troublesome symptom and may be accompanied by substernal discomfort or burning. Cough, lassitude, and malaise may persist for several weeks before full recovery. Among immunosuppressed patients, particularly recipients of stem cell and solid organ transplants, fever and clinical symptoms initially may be minimal to absent. Despite the paucity of presenting symptoms, however, such patients may progress to severe lower respiratory tract disease.

Fever is the most common initial physical finding, but it may be minimal or absent, especially in elderly patients or immunocompromised hosts. The temperature usually rises rapidly to a peak of 38° to 40° C within 12 hours of onset, concurrently with systemic symptoms. Fever is usually continuous but may be intermittent, especially if antipyretics are administered. Typically, the duration of fever in adults is about 3 days, but it may last only 1 to 5 or more days. Early in the course of illness, the patient appears toxic, the face is flushed, and the skin is hot and moist. The eyes are watery and reddened. Clear nasal discharge is common. The mucosa of the nose and throat is hyperemic, but exudate is not observed. Small, tender cervical lymph nodes are often present. Transient scattered rhonchi or localized areas of rales are found in less than 20% of cases.

The same pattern of illness occurs with any strain of influenza A or B virus. Illness is more frequent and severe in smokers. In children, maximum temperatures are often higher, cervical adenopathy may be more frequent, and nausea, vomiting, and abdominal pain are more common than in adults. Older adults, especially the infirm elderly, develop fever, muscle aches, sore throat, and headache less often but have higher rates of altered mental status and pulmonary complications. In zoonotic infections due to avian H5N1 or H7N9 viruses, upper respiratory complaints are less frequent, gastrointestinal complaints are more common, and progressive viral pneumonia with high mortality is much more likely. Influenza C virus generally causes sporadic upper respiratory tract illness or febrile bronchitis.

Persons at higher risk for influenza-associated complications and hospitalization (Table 340-1) include pregnant women (especially during the second and third trimesters or early postpartum period), morbidly obese patients, immunosuppressed persons, and patients with various comorbid diseases. Most adults hospitalized with seasonal influenza have exacerbations of any underlying cardiopulmonary (e.g., myocardial ischemia, heart failure, chronic obstructive pulmonary disease) or metabolic (e.g., diabetes) conditions, and about one third have pneumonia.

Respiratory Complications

Three pneumonic syndromes have been described—primary influenza viral pneumonia, secondary bacterial pneumonia, and mixed viral and bacterial pneumonia (Chapter 91)—but their clinical presentations and courses overlap considerably. Influenza A and B virus infections are often associated with other respiratory tract complications, including exacerbations of chronic bronchitis, asthma, or cystic fibrosis; croup and bronchiolitis in young children; and otitis media, sinusitis, and rarely parotitis or bacterial tracheitis. Apparently uncomplicated influenza frequently causes tracheobronchitis and is often accompanied by abnormal tracheobronchial clearance, airway hyperactivity, and dysfunction of small airways lasting weeks. A syndrome mimicking pulmonary embolism with transiently altered perfusion scans has also been described.

Severe primary influenza viral pneumonia and associated acute respiratory distress syndrome (ARDS [Chapter 96]) is uncommon during epidemics but accounts for 20 to 50% of pneumonias in hospitalized patients during pandemics. ARDS also has been the principal manifestation of severe pandemic 2009 H1N1 or avian H5N1 and H7N9 illness. Severe viral pneumonia occurs predominantly in persons with underlying pulmonary and cardiac disorders, pregnancy, or immunodeficiency states, although up to 40% of reported cases and most patients with H5N1 have no recognized underlying disease. After a typical onset of influenza, patients often have progressive cough, dyspnea, sometimes hemoptysis, and even cyanosis within 3 to 7 days. Bilateral pulmonary infiltrates and hypoxemia, often indicative of ARDS, may evolve rapidly. Gram staining of sputum may show abundant polymorphonuclear leukocytes but scant bacterial flora. Sputum and endotracheal aspirates usually yield high titers of influenza virus, but upper respiratory samples are sometimes negative, even by viral RNA detection assays.

TABLE 340-1 USE OF INFLUENZA VACCINE IN SPECIAL POPULATIONS AND SITUATIONS

When vaccine supply is limited, vaccination efforts should focus on delivering vaccination to persons at higher risk for influenza-related complications listed below as well as these persons:

POPULATIONS AT HIGHER RISK FOR MEDICAL COMPLICATIONS ATTRIBUTABLE TO SEVERE INFLUENZA
- All children aged 6 through 59 months;
- All persons aged ≥50 years;
- Adults and children who have chronic pulmonary (including asthma) or cardiovascular (except isolated hypertension), renal, hepatic, neurologic, hematologic, or metabolic disorders (including diabetes mellitus);
- Persons who are immunocompromised owing to any cause (including immunosuppression caused by medications or by HIV infection);
- Women who are or will be pregnant during the influenza season;
- Children and adolescents (aged 6 months through 18 years) who are receiving aspirin- or salicylate-containing medications and who might be at risk for experiencing Reye syndrome after influenza virus infection;
- Residents of nursing homes and other long-term care facilities;
- American Indians/Alaska Natives; and
- Persons who are extremely obese (BMI ≥40).

PERSONS WHO LIVE WITH OR CARE FOR PERSONS AT HIGHER RISK FOR INFLUENZA-RELATED COMPLICATIONS
- Health care personnel, including physicians, nurses, and other workers in inpatient and outpatient care settings, medical emergency-response workers (e.g., paramedics and emergency medical technicians), and employees of nursing home and long-term care facilities who have contact with patients or residents, and students in these professions who will have contact with patients;
- Household contacts (including children) and caregivers of children aged ≤59 months (i.e., aged <5 years) and adults aged ≥50 years, particularly contacts of children aged <6 months; and
- Household contacts (including children) and caregivers of persons with medical conditions that put them at high risk for severe complications from influenza.

IMMUNOCOMPROMISED PERSONS
- LAIV should be avoided in immunocompromised patients.
- Studies suggest improved immunogenicity with the use of high dose influenza vaccine.

PERSONS WITH A HISTORY OF GUILLAIN-BARRÉ SYNDROME FOLLOWING INFLUENZA VACCINATION
A history of Guillain-Barré syndrome within 6 weeks following a previous dose of any type of influenza vaccine is considered a precaution to vaccination. Persons who are not at high risk for severe influenza complications and who are known to have experienced Guillain-Barré syndrome within 6 weeks of a previous influenza vaccination generally should not be vaccinated. Seasonal chemoprophylaxis is an option in such persons. However, the benefits of influenza vaccination might outweigh the risks for certain persons who have a history of Guillain-Barré syndrome and who also are at high risk for severe complications from influenza.

PERSON WITH A HISTORY OF EGG ALLERGY
For persons who report a history of egg allergy:
- Persons with a history of egg allergy who have experienced only urticaria (hives) after exposure to egg should receive influenza vaccine. Any licensed, recommended, and age-appropriate influenza vaccine (i.e., any IIV, RIV4, or LAIV4) that is otherwise appropriate for the recipient's health status may be used.
- Persons who report having had reactions to egg involving symptoms other than urticaria (hives), such as angioedema, respiratory distress, lightheadedness, or recurrent emesis; or who required epinephrine or another emergency medical intervention, may similarly receive any licensed, recommended, and age-appropriate influenza vaccine (i.e., any IIV, RIV4, or LAIV4) that is otherwise appropriate for their health status. The selected vaccine should be administered in an inpatient or outpatient medical setting (including, but not necessarily limited to, hospitals, clinics, health departments, and physician offices). Vaccine administration should be supervised by a health care provider who is able to recognize and manage severe allergic reactions.
- A previous severe allergic reaction to influenza vaccine, regardless of the component suspected of being responsible for the reaction, is a contraindication to future receipt of the vaccine.

A vaccine recipient should be observed for 15 minutes following administration of any vaccine.

BMI = body mass index; HIV = human immunodeficiency virus; IIV = inactivated influenza vaccine; LAIV = live-attenuated influenza vaccine; RIV = recombinant influenza vaccine.

Modified from Grohskopf LA, Sokolow LZ, Broder KR, et al. Prevention and control of seasonal influenza with vaccines: recommendations of the Advisory Committee on Immunization Practices—United States, 2018-2019 influenza season. *MMWR Recomm Rep.* 2018;67:1-20.

In patients with classic bacterial superinfection, transient improvement for 1 to 4 days may be followed by recrudescence of fever, increased cough, sputum production, pleuritic chest pain, and a localized area of consolidation. Some patients develop fulminant pneumonia. Gram staining and culture of sputum or blood cultures most often reveal *Streptococcus pneumoniae* (Chapter 273), *Staphylococcus aureus* (Chapter 272) including community-acquired methicillin-resistant *S. aureus, Haemophilus influenzae* (Chapter 284), or *Streptococcus pyogenes.* Such patients usually respond to specific antibiotic therapy, although staphylococcal infections may be particularly virulent and cause destructive pulmonary lesions. Secondary pneumonias caused by a range of nosocomial bacterial pathogens are common in patients who are hospitalized with influenza, particularly patients who require mechanical ventilation. Use of high-dose corticosteroids appears to be a risk factor for bacterial suprainfection, invasive aspergillosis, and increased mortality (Chapter 319).

In addition, during an outbreak of influenza, many less distinct syndromes are observed; patients may have viral tracheobronchitis (Chapter 90), milder forms of localized viral pneumonia, or mixed viral and bacterial infection. Many such patients respond to antibiotics. Immunocompromised hosts, including transplant recipients and acute leukemia patients undergoing chemotherapy, may have high rates of pneumonia and associated mortality after influenza if they are not treated with appropriate antiviral and antimicrobial medications.

Nonrespiratory Complications

Severe influenza, including both pandemic 2009 H1N1 and avian H5N1 or H7N9 disease, may be associated with sepsis syndrome (Chapter 100), acute renal insufficiency (Chapter 112), and multiorgan failure. Lymphopenia and thrombocytopenia are common in severe influenza; the hemophagocytic syndrome and disseminated intravascular coagulation (Chapter 166) can occur. A wide variety of extrapulmonary complications have been recognized in association with influenza.[8] Myositis with tender leg muscles and elevated serum creatine kinase levels is uncommon in adults, but rhabdomyolysis (Chapter 105) can be severe and cause myoglobinuria. Pregnant women have increased risk of premature labor and spontaneous abortion. Toxic shock syndrome (Chapter 272) caused by respiratory tract infection with toxin-bearing *S. aureus* or *Streptococcus pyogenes* can occur, and outbreaks of meningococcal infection (Chapter 282) have been associated with both influenza A and B virus infections. Myocarditis (Chapter 54) or pericarditis (Chapter 68) occurs uncommonly but can result in severe disease. Neurologic complications include aseptic meningitis (Chapter 384), myelitis (Chapter 383), encephalopathy (Chapter 386), necrotizing encephalitis, postinfluenzal Guillain-Barré syndrome (Chapter 392), or immune-mediated encephalitis or cerebellitis. Reye syndrome (Chapter 141), which is a well-recognized hepatic and central nervous system complication of influenza A and B virus infections in children and rarely in adults, is associated with salicylate use. Possible associations with late-onset Parkinson syndrome or with neuropsychiatric disorders in the offspring of women experiencing intrapartum infection remain uncertain.

DIAGNOSIS
Clinical

In an individual case, influenza often cannot be distinguished from infection with a number of other viruses or nonviral pathogens that produce similar clinical manifestations (Chapters 90 and 401). Conversely, when public health authorities report an epidemic of influenza in a given community and an adult patient is seen with typical febrile respiratory illness, it is highly likely that these symptoms are caused by an influenza A or B virus infection. In such circumstances, the presence of fever and cough has a positive predictive value of about 80% for laboratory-proven influenza in ambulatory adults and children. However, the predictive value of influenza-like illness in hospitalized patients is much lower.

Patients should be asked about recent travel and exposures to ill persons, poultry, swine, and their environments. A positive travel history should prompt a review of the potential presence of novel or emerging respiratory viruses in the region. If risk factors for zoonotic influenza are present, specific laboratory testing is available through most health departments.

Laboratory

Currently, molecular methods have supplanted culture as the gold standard in the diagnosis of influenza. Detection of viral RNA by rapid (20 minutes or less) nucleic acid amplification testing (NAAT) can provide reliable results (92 to 95% sensitivity and >98% specificity) at the point of care and is the test of choice for patients who have suspected influenza infection and who are hospitalized, are in special risk groups (e.g., immunocompromised hosts), or are candidates for antiviral treatment.[9] This linkage of NAAT testing to the decision regarding antiviral use is acceptable, provided that such testing does not cause a significant delay in initiating treatment. Commercial assays that detect influenza and a variety of other respiratory viruses can be completed within 1 to 2 hours.

Older rapid influenza diagnostic tests can detect influenza viral antigens in less than 15 minutes but have low sensitivity (<20 to 70%) in adults, so negative results should not guide individual treatment decisions. However, such tests may be helpful in investigating outbreaks while awaiting more definitive test results. The limited specificity (generally 90 to 95%) of some rapid tests makes their predictive value low outside the influenza season, although optical readers appear to enhance their reliability. Changes in FDA regulations now limit rapid influenza diagnostics to tests with sensitivities of at least 80%.

Viral culture of nasal, sputum, or tracheal secretions during the first 2 or 3 days of illness is less sensitive than NAAT and usually takes 48 hours or longer. Serologic methods are less useful clinically because they require convalescent serum obtained 14 to 21 days after the onset of infection. Antiviral drug–resistant variants may emerge during therapy or may rarely be circulating in the community, and clinical progression despite 5 to 7 days of antiviral therapy should prompt studies for antiviral resistance.

Detection of secondary bacterial infections generally relies on standard microbiologic studies (e.g., blood culture, sputum Gram stain and culture, urinary antigen testing). In hospitalized patients, a low serum procalcitonin level may help discriminate viral from mixed influenza-bacterial pneumonia and reduce antibiotic use (Chapter 91).[A1]

PREVENTION

Vaccination

Annual influenza immunization is recommended for all persons aged 6 months or older in the United States (Chapter 15).[10,11] Persons at higher risk for influenza-related complications or who care for or are exposed to them remain particular priorities of immunization efforts (see Table 340-1), especially when vaccine delays or shortages occur. Influenza vaccine policies differ across countries. Because influenza immunization benefits both mother and infants, the WHO has ranked pregnant women as the highest priority, followed (in no particular order) by health care workers, children 6 to 59 months of age, the elderly, and individuals with high-risk conditions. Maternal immunization benefits both mother and child.[12]

Seasonal vaccine should be given each year in the fall as soon as available, preferably by October before the influenza season in northern temperate areas. Quadrivalent vaccines with two A (H1N1, H3N2) and two B lineage (Yamagata, Victoria) antigens are preferred over trivalent vaccines because of their better breadth of coverage.

Egg-grown, intramuscularly administered inactivated influenza vaccines for persons 6 months of age and older, a high-dose inactivated vaccine and an MF-59 adjuvanted inactivated vaccine for persons aged 65 years and older, and a live-attenuated intranasal vaccine for otherwise healthy persons aged 2 to 49 years are currently licensed in the United States (E-Table 340-3). A mammalian cell culture–grown inactivated vaccine, and a recombinant DNA–produced HA vaccine, particularly useful in those with severe egg allergy, are also approved for seasonal use. Racial and ethnic disparities in influenza

vaccination rates persist, and rates for key target groups, including pregnant women and health care workers, remain suboptimal. Immunization of health care personnel, which represents an important patient safety issue, can be enhanced by strategies to improve access, and especially by employer mandates.

Inactivated vaccines (Chapter 15) given by intramuscular injection provide about 50 to 70% protection against seasonal influenza illness in healthy adults, albeit with substantial year-to-year variations in effectiveness,[A2] and reduce work absenteeism, use of health care resources, and antibiotics when the vaccine is well matched to the epidemic strain. On average, the effectiveness of the vaccination seems to decline by about 7% per month for at least 6 months after vaccination.[13]

Immunogenicity and hence protection rates with inactivated seasonal vaccines are lower in elderly persons, particularly infirm nursing home residents, and in immunosuppressed patients. The effectiveness of influenza vaccine for prevention of medically attended acute respiratory illness among the elderly in nursing homes is estimated to average 20 to 40%. In ambulatory high-risk patients, immunization reduces hospitalizations from pneumonia, influenza, and major cardiovascular events,[A3] as well as all-cause mortality during the influenza season. Both higher-dose inactivated vaccines (four-fold or three-fold more HA per strain) and adjuvanted inactivated vaccine are more immunogenic and protective than standard vaccine against seasonal influenza illness in older ambulatory adults and are the preferred vaccine for these individuals.[A4] High dose vaccine also results in improved protection among kidney transplant patients.[A5] Immunization of children appears to reduce respiratory illness in household and community contacts.[A6] Immunization of health care providers reduces the risk of transmission to patients as well as their own risk of infection.

Because protection is greatly reduced or absent in some seasons and some patient groups, new vaccines with improved immunogenicity are being developed. Oil-in-water adjuvants (e.g., MF-59, AS03) are immunogenic at lower HA doses and appear to be especially effective for inducing adequate immune responses to novel influenza viruses. For H5 and H7 vaccines, two doses with an oil-in-water adjuvant appear to be necessary for adequate immunogenicity. An AS03-adjuvanted H5N1 vaccine (containing only 3.75 µg HA antigen) was approved for adults in the United States in 2013. A virosome-adjuvanted vaccine is approved in Europe.

With inactivated vaccine, fever and systemic symptoms occur at rates comparable to those of adults given placebo but are more common in young children. Among adults, 25% or more may have mild local reactions at the site of injection. Injection site reactions and systemic complaints (headache, fatigue, myalgia, arthralgia) are more frequent after the high HA content or oil-in-water adjuvanted inactivated vaccines. Intranasal vaccine causes coryza and sore throat in adults.

Hypersensitivity reactions to residual egg proteins or other vaccine components occur rarely, and vaccine is contraindicated in persons with chicken egg anaphylactic hypersensitivity unless the patient has been desensitized. Inactivated vaccine does not cause exacerbation of asthma but may be rarely associated with Guillain-Barré syndrome in older adults.

Medications

Oral oseltamivir and inhaled zanamivir are effective for chemoprophylaxis of both influenza A and B virus infections, including postexposure prophylaxis in households (Table 340-2), with each reducing the risk of symptomatic influenza infections by about 60 to 80%. Because of widespread resistance in circulating strains, rimantadine and amantadine are no longer effective for prophylaxis or treatment. When an outbreak develops, unimmunized high-risk persons can be given chemoprophylaxis and inactivated vaccine simultaneously, with cessation of chemoprophylaxis after 14 days. Alternatively, if vaccine is not available or contraindicated, is a poor match, or if the patient is highly immunosuppressed, chemoprophylaxis may be continued for the duration of the community outbreak. When given to patients and staff alike, these drugs are helpful in managing nosocomial outbreaks.[14] Therapeutic doses (i.e., twice daily) should be considered for postexposure prophylaxis in immunocompromised hosts and in individuals exposed to novel influenza viruses to increase effectiveness and possibly reduce antiviral resistance emergence.

Most public health authorities do not advise routine use of antiviral chemoprophylaxis, largely because of concerns regarding promotion of antiviral resistance and drug availability. In the community setting, close monitoring and early initiation of antiviral treatment is an alternative approach after suspected influenza exposures. Chemoprophylaxis is generally not recommended if more than 2 to 3 days have elapsed since exposure to a person with seasonal influenza.

TABLE 340-2 ANTIVIRAL DOSE RECOMMENDATIONS IN ADULTS

DRUG	ROUTE	TREATMENT	PROPHYLAXIS	DOSE REDUCTIONS	COMMENT
Oseltamivir	Oral	75 mg bid	75 mg once daily†	CrCl ≤60 mL/min	Gastrointestinal and (very uncommonly) CNS side effects
Zanamivir	Inhaled	10 mg bid	10 mg once daily†	Avoid in those with underlying airways disease	Training in use of the inhaler device is important
Peramivir*	Intravenous	600 mg single IV dose in uncomplicated illness	Not studied	CrCl <50 mL/min	Single dose approved for uncomplicated influenza in adults in the United States
Laninamivir*	Inhaled	40 mg once in uncomplicated illness (Japan)	20 mg once daily for 2 days (Japan)	Avoid in those with underlying airways disease	Currently investigational in the United States; approved in Japan
Zanamivir*	Intravenous	600 mg q12h	Not studied	CrCl <80 mL/min	Currently investigational in the United States
Favipiravir*	Oral	1600 mg twice on day 1; 1600 mg bid (Japan) on days 2-5	Not studied	Avoid in pregnancy	Approved in Japan but investigational in the United States; inhibitory for NAI- and adamantane-resistant viruses; teratogenic
Pimodivir	Oral	600 mg q12h	Not studied		Currently investigational in the United States; inhibitory for NAI- and adamantane-resistant viruses
Baloxavir	Oral	80 or 40 mg single dose in uncomplicated illness	Not studied	Weight-based dosing	Approved 2018 in the United States; inhibitory for NAI- and adamantane-resistant viruses
Amantadine	Oral	100 mg bid	100 mg bid	Age >64 yr, CrCl <50-80 mL/min	Gastrointestinal and CNS side effects Currently circulating strains are resistant
Rimantadine	Oral	100 mg bid	100 mg bid	Age >64 yr, CrCl <10 mL/min, or severe hepatic dysfunction	Lower risk of CNS side effects than with amantadine Currently circulating strains are resistant

*Oral favipiravir is approved in Japan but only for treating novel or reemerging influenza infections when other drugs are ineffective or not sufficiently effective; higher dose regimens are being studied in the United States.

†Full therapeutic doses for postexposure prophylaxis (i.e., twice-daily dosing) are appropriate for infections due to novel influenza viruses and in immunocompromised hosts.
The standard duration of treatment in uncomplicated illness is 5 days, except for baloxavir or IV peramivir, for which single doses suffice. A longer treatment duration (e.g., 10 days) should be considered for infections in seriously ill patients, immunosuppressed hosts, or infections caused by novel viruses. Higher doses (e.g., 150 mg or 225 mg twice daily) of oseltamivir have been used in patients with serious lower respiratory illness, immunocompromise, or infections by novel viruses. The duration of prophylaxis depends on the epidemiologic setting; durations of 2 weeks after immunization or 7 to 10 days for postexposure prophylaxis are appropriate. Antiviral prophylaxis may interfere with response to intranasal live-attenuated vaccine but not to intramuscular inactivated vaccine.
CNS = central nervous system; CrCl = creatinine clearance; NAI = neuraminidase inhibitor.

Precautions

On entry to a health care facility, source control (e.g., facemask placement) and instruction in respiratory hygiene and cough etiquette should be implemented for symptomatic patients. Patients hospitalized with suspected or proven influenza should be managed with standard and droplet precautions and, when possible, private rooms. Facemasks likely provide some degree of protection for health care workers during routine patient care, but compliance with a properly fitted N95-type respirator provides better protection. An N95-type respirator should be used with other precautions (including gloves, gown, and eye protection with face shield or goggles; an airborne infection isolation room) during aerosol-generating procedures. Other strategies for preventing nosocomial influenza include influenza vaccination of both health care providers and patients, appropriate management of ill health care providers and visitors, and engineering measures (e.g., adequate air exchanges). Early implementation and compliance with masks and hand hygiene appears to reduce the risk of secondary infections somewhat in household contacts.

The risk of zoonotic infections can be reduced by avoiding exposure to potentially infectious poultry or swine and their environments. Although the highly pathogenic H5N1 virus causes lethal poultry outbreaks, the low pathogenic H7N9 virus does not cause discernible illness in affected birds. Travelers to affected countries should avoid visiting live bird markets, practice frequent hand hygiene, and not eat inadequately cooked poultry products. Avoiding farms, live animal markets, and agricultural fairs, especially for at-risk persons, may reduce risk of swine influenza virus infections.

TREATMENT ℞

Hospitalized Patients

Antiviral treatment (see Table 340-2) is recommended as soon as possible for patients who have proven or suspected influenza and who manifest severe, complicated, or progressive illness; are hospitalized; or have underlying conditions that increase the risk for complications (see Table 340-1), including adults older than age 64 years and children younger than age 5 years.[15] In patients who have serious illness or high-risk conditions, decisions about initiating antiviral therapy should not wait for laboratory confirmation of influenza.

Fulminant influenza viral pneumonia, particularly following pandemic 2009 H1N1 or avian influenza infection, requires intensive care including ventilatory support (Chapter 97), often renal replacement therapy, and sometimes extracorporeal membrane oxygenation. Adults admitted with community-acquired pneumonia (Chapter 91) during the influenza season should initially receive both early antiviral therapy[16] and antibiotics, with subsequent therapy guided by microbiologic study results. ICU complications, including ventilator-associated pneumonia, are common. Early neuraminidase inhibitor therapy appears to reduce mortality in patients if it is initiated before onset of respiratory failure. Intravenous formulations of peramivir and zanamivir provide reliable delivery of high drug levels in seriously ill persons,[A7] and zanamivir is available for compassionate use in a very limited number of countries. However, intravenous zanamivir is no more effective than oral oseltamivir in hospitalized patients with influenza.[A8]

Double-doses of oseltamivir and combinations of oseltamivir, amantadine, and ribavirin do not appear to be more clinically effective than standard doses, although they may clear influenza viruses more rapidly.[A9] Longer courses (e.g., 10 days) and perhaps higher doses are warranted in critically ill patients and immunocompromised hosts, in whom monitoring for virologic clearance is warranted.[17] A single dose of peramivir[A10] appears to be as effective as a 5-day regimen of oseltamivir in treating uncomplicated influenza. If intravenous peramivir is used in hospitalized patients, daily dosing is advisable.

Adding sirolimus to oseltamivir may have accelerated viral clearance and clinical recovery in mechanically ventilated pandemic 2009 H1N1 patients,[A11] and adding 2 days of naproxen and clarithromycin to oseltamivir may reduce mortality compared with oseltamivir alone in hospitalized adults.[A12] Systemic corticosteroids given for influenza-associated pneumonia or ARDS have been associated with prolonged viral replication, adverse effects, and increased mortality, so their routine use should be avoided.

During therapy, the emergence of oseltamivir resistance is infrequent but is more common in children and immunocompromised hosts, and it highlights the need for ongoing susceptibility monitoring in high-risk patients with persistent symptomatic viral shedding after 5 to 7 days of treatment. Zanamivir is inhibitory for most oseltamivir-resistant variants, and intravenous zanamivir is currently preferred for treating severe infections that are suspected or proven to be oseltamivir resistant. Polymerase inhibitors baloxavir and pimodivir are undergoing studies in combination with neuraminidase inhibitors in hospitalized influenza patients.

Outpatients

Treatment within 2 days of the onset of symptoms also may be considered in low-risk outpatients with uncomplicated febrile illness, in whom therapy reduces the duration of symptoms by 1 to 2 days, the time to functional recovery, and the risk for respiratory complications that lead to antibiotic use.[A13] Early oseltamivir therapy also decreases the risk for pneumonia and hospitalization, and even delayed use appears to reduce mortality in hospitalized patients.[A14] Although initiation of therapy is most effective if started within 2 days of the onset of symptoms, later initiation of therapy appears to reduce mortality. Recently baloxavir has been approved for the treatment of uncomplicated influenza A illness. Single-dose baloxavir shows similar clinical efficacy but greater antiviral effects than oseltamivir in outpatient adolescents and adults, including those with co-morbidities[A15]; baloxavir appears more effective than oseltamivir in influenza B. Emergence of influenza A viruses with reduced susceptibility to baloxavir occurs in some treated patients.

Oral rimantadine or amantadine shortens the duration of fever and symptoms in uncomplicated influenza A caused by susceptible strains (see Table 340-2), but these drugs are not currently recommended because of widespread antiviral resistance.

Inhaled zanamivir may be infrequently associated with bronchospasm, sometimes severe, and nebulization of the lactose-containing commercial form is contraindicated in intubated patients. Oseltamivir is associated with nausea, vomiting, rash, and possibly rare neuropsychiatric symptoms.

Symptomatic measures include antipyretics and cough suppressants. Salicylates should not be used, especially in children younger than age 16 years, because of their association with Reye syndrome.

PROGNOSIS

Most influenza patients make a full recovery, but they may require several weeks to return to their premorbid functional status. The risk of acute myocardial infarction is increased more than 6-fold in the first 7 days after diagnosis.[18] Influenza in elderly persons can cause prolonged loss of function and impairment of activities of daily living.

The mortality rate from seasonal influenza or pandemic 2009 H1N1 illness has been low (approximately 1 in 10,000 persons), but the mortality impact differs across age and risk groups. Although approximately 90% of seasonal influenza-related deaths occur in persons who are older than 65 years or at high risk because of comorbid conditions, most pandemic 2009 virus deaths have been in patients younger than 65. Mortality occurs in about 5 to 10% of adults hospitalized with seasonal influenza but is as high as 40 to 60% in zoonotic H5N1 and H7N9 infections. Bacterial infections (Chapter 91) were associated with more than 90% of fatal pneumonias in the 1918 pandemic and about 20 to 40% in the 2009 H1N1 pandemic. Detection of viral RNA in the blood is a poor prognostic finding that may reflect high viral burden in the lower respiratory tract. Once viral pneumonia progresses to respiratory failure, the mortality rate is often 50% or higher, but the risk is reduced by early antiviral therapy and high-quality intensive care support.

Grade A References

A1. Schuetz P, Wirz Y, Sager R, et al. Effect of procalcitonin-guided antibiotic treatment on mortality in acute respiratory infections: a patient level meta-analysis. *Lancet Infect Dis.* 2018;18:95-107.

A2. Demicheli V, Jefferson T, Ferroni E, et al. Vaccines for preventing influenza in healthy adults. *Cochrane Database Syst Rev.* 2018;2:CD001269.

A3. Udell JA, Zawi R, Bhatt DL, et al. Association between influenza vaccination and cardiovascular outcomes in high-risk patients: a meta-analysis. *JAMA.* 2013;310:1711-1720.

A4. Dunkle LM, Izikson R, Patriarca P, et al. Efficacy of recombinant influenza vaccine in adults 50 years of age or older. *N Engl J Med.* 2017;376:2427-2436.

A5. Kumar D, Campbell P, Hoschler K, et al. Randomized controlled trial of adjuvanted versus non-adjuvanted influenza vaccine in kidney transplant recipients. *Transplantation.* 2016;100:662-669.

A6. Yin JK, Heywood AE, Georgousakis M, et al. Systematic review and meta-analysis of indirect protection afforded by vaccinating children against seasonal influenza: implications for policy. *Clin Infect Dis.* 2017;65:719-728.

A7. Nakamura S, Miyazaki T, Izumikawa K, et al. Efficacy and safety of intravenous peramivir compared with oseltamivir in high-risk patients infected with influenza A and B viruses: a multicenter randomized controlled study. *Open Forum Infect Dis.* 2017;4:1-8.

A8. Marty FM, Vidal-Puigserver J, Clark C, et al. Intravenous zanamivir or oral oseltamivir for hospitalised patients with influenza: an international, randomised, double-blind, double-dummy, phase 3 trial. *Lancet Respir Med.* 2017;5:135-146.

A9. Beigel JH, Bao Y, Beeler J, et al. Oseltamivir, amantadine, and ribavirin combination antiviral therapy versus oseltamivir monotherapy for the treatment of influenza: a multicentre, double-blind, randomised phase 2 trial. *Lancet Infect Dis.* 2017;17:1255-1265.

A10. Whitley R, Laughlin A, Carson S, et al. Single dose peramivir for the treatment of acute seasonal influenza: integrated analysis of efficacy and safety from two placebo-controlled trials. *Antivir Ther.* 2015;20:709-719.

A11. Wang CH, Chung FT, Lin SM, et al. Adjuvant treatment with a mammalian target of rapamycin inhibitor, sirolimus, and steroids improves outcomes in patients with severe H1N1 pneumonia and acute respiratory failure. *Crit Care Med.* 2014;42:313-321.

A12. Hung IFN, To KKW, Chan JFW, et al. Efficacy of clarithromycin-naproxen-oseltamivir combination in the treatment of patients hospitalized for influenza A(H3N2) infection: an open-label randomized, controlled, phase IIb/III trial. *Chest.* 2017;151:1069-1080.

A13. Dobson J, Whitley RJ, Pocock S, et al. Oseltamivir treatment for influenza in adults: a meta-analysis of randomised controlled trials. *Lancet.* 2015;385:1729-1737.

A14. Venkatesan S, Myles PR, Leonardi-Bee J, et al. Impact of outpatient neuraminidase inhibitor treatment in patients infected with influenza A(H1N1)pdm09 at high risk of hospitalization: an individual participant data metaanalysis. *Clin Infect Dis.* 2017;64:1328-1334.

A15. Hayden FG, Sugaya N, Hirotsu N, et al. Baloxavir marboxil for uncomplicated influenza in adults and adolescents. *N Engl J Med.* 2018;379:913-23.

GENERAL REFERENCES

For the General References and other additional features, please visit Expert Consult at https://expertconsult.inkling.com.

341

ADENOVIRUS DISEASES

MICHAEL G. ISON

DEFINITIONS

Human adenoviruses, which are members of the *Adenoviridae* family and the *Mastadenovirus* genus, are divided into seven species (A, B, C, D, E, F, and G; Table 341-1). Modern sequencing and molecular diagnostics have identified over 80 serotypes. Adenoviruses are double-stranded DNA, nonenveloped viruses that code for 20 early and 15 late proteins. The knobbed fiber protrudes from the fiber base (Fig. 341-1).

EPIDEMIOLOGY

Adenoviruses cause a range of infections from mild self-limited respiratory viral infections, conjunctivitis, and diarrhea to severe disseminated disease. Adenoviruses have a worldwide distribution, and infections occur throughout the year without significant seasonal variability. Most infections occur as sporadic events, although local or regional epidemics have been described. Asymptomatic respiratory infection is common and is associated with prolonged carriage, particularly in feces and tonsillar tissue. Most patients with adenovirus infection are children, generally younger than 5 years, and most individuals have serologic evidence of exposure to adenovirus by age 10. Only about 25% of symptomatic cases occur in adults.[1] Adenoviruses 1, 2, and 5 are most

TABLE 341-1 CORRELATION OF ADENOVIRUS SUBGROUP AND SEROTYPE WITH MAJOR SITES OF INFECTION

SUBGROUP	SEROTYPE	MAJOR SITE OF INFECTION
A	12, 18, 31,* 61	Respiratory, urinary tract, gastrointestinal (GI)
B1	3, 7, 16, 21, 50, 68, 66, 68	Respiratory, eye (including pharyngoconjunctival fever), GI
B2	11,† 14,‡ 34,† 35,† 55,‡ 66	Urinary tract, respiratory
C	1, 2, 5, 6, 57	Respiratory, urinary tract, GI (especially hepatitis)
D	8§-10, 13, 15, 17, 19§, 20, 22-30, 32-33, 36, 37§-39, 42-49, 51, 53-54, 58, 56, 60, 62, 63-65, 67, 69, 70-71	Eye, GI
E	4	Upper respiratory tract infection, pneumonia
F	40,* 41*	GI
G	52	GI

*Associated with infantile gastroenteritis.
†Associated with hemorrhagic cystitis and interstitial nephritis.
‡Associated with epidemic pneumonia with high mortality rate.
§Associated with epidemics.

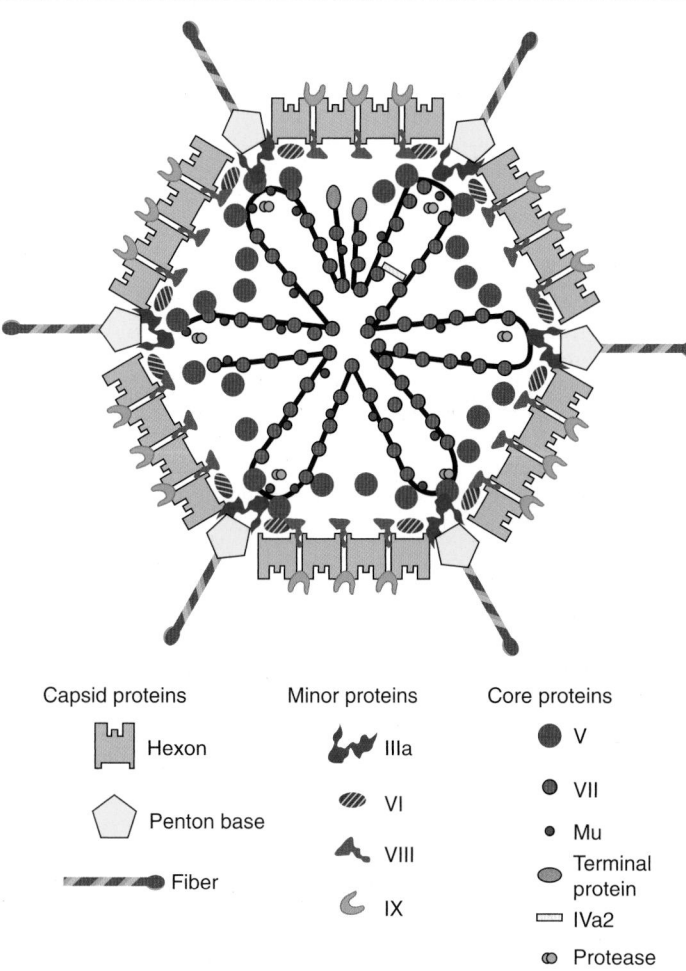

Capsid proteins
Hexon
Penton base
Fiber

Minor proteins
IIIa
VI
VIII
IX

Core proteins
V
VII
Mu
Terminal protein
IVa2
Protease

FIGURE 341-1. Adenovirus.

common among children, whereas adenoviruses 3, 4, and 7 are more common in adults.

Recent severe outbreaks in the United States have resulted in cases requiring hospitalization, and nosocomial transmission can cause severe infections in health care workers. Adenovirus is the leading cause of respiratory viral infections among military recruits. Unlike the year-round circulation of adenovirus in civilians, peaks of disease are recognized within the first 4 weeks of training exercises among military recruits. Rates of adenovirus among military recruits declined significantly with widespread use of an oral live-attenuated vaccine in 1971, increased after supplies of vaccine were depleted by 1999, then declined again after an oral live-attenuated adenovirus type 4 and 7 vaccine was approved in 2011 (E-Fig. 341-1).[2]

PATHOBIOLOGY

Adenoviruses enter susceptible hosts by the mouth, nasopharynx, or ocular conjunctiva. The fiber protein of the virus binds to a cellular receptor that varies by serotype. On initial infection, local replication can induce considerable cellular damage owing to tissue invasive infection. Necrotizing bronchitis, bronchiolitis, interstitial pneumonia, and fibrin and hyaline membranes are seen within the alveoli during pulmonary infections. In ocular infections, exudative and mononuclear infiltrates develop beneath the epithelium. Replication results in desquamated epithelial cells, which induce hypertrophy in regional lymphatic tissue and active proliferative germinal centers. This reaction can cause swollen adenoids or intussusception (Chapter 133) associated with enlarged mesenteric lymph nodes, particularly in children.

Components of both the innate and adaptive immune responses are important for the control of adenovirus replication. Alveolar macrophages and Kupffer cells help eliminate adenovirus from the lung and liver and also secrete inflammatory cytokines such as tumor necrosis factor (TNF), interferon (IFN)–γ, interleukin (IL)–1β, IL-6, IL-8, and IL-12. CD4+ and CD8+ T lymphocytes play a particularly important role in the control and clearance of replicating adenovirus in humans, and the absolute lymphocyte and CD4+ T-lymphocyte

levels correlate inversely with adenovirus infection and the risk for developing disseminated adenoviral infections in immunosuppressed transplant patients.

Both group- and type-specific neutralizing and non-neutralizing antibodies are produced in response to infection and also play a role in limiting infection. Group-specific antibodies do not neutralize the virus but can confirm infection. Neutralizing antibodies may protect against disease manifestations in the previously infected host or against reinfection with the same serotype, but they do not eliminate the carrier state.

CLINICAL MANIFESTATIONS

Adenovirus infections have a wide range of clinical manifestations that are linked to the virus type (see Table 341-1) as well as to the age and immunocompetence of the host. Common syndromes include infections of the respiratory tract, eye, gastrointestinal tract, genitourinary tract, and central nervous system (CNS). Disseminated infection also occurs, especially in immunosuppressed patients. Associations with adenovirus and obesity have been proposed as well.

Respiratory Tract Infections

About 10% of pneumonias in childhood and up to 5% of community-acquired pneumonias in some series of adults[3,4] may be attributable to adenovirus. Typical symptoms include nasal congestion, coryza, and cough, which may mimic pertussis infections (Chapter 297). Generalized malaise, fever, chills, myalgia, headache, and abdominal pain are common systemic symptoms. Exudative tonsillitis and cervical adenopathy are also seen. If conjunctivitis accompanies these signs and symptoms, the disease is designated as pharyngoconjunctival fever. Otitis media is a common presentation, particularly among infants under 1 year of age. Cases in children and in adults, especially military recruits, are indistinguishable from other viral respiratory infections such as influenza (Chapter 340), parainfluenza (Chapter 339), and respiratory syncytial virus (Chapter 338). Recent outbreaks of sometimes severe and fatal adenovirus pneumonia have been described and should be kept in the differential in patients with severe pneumonia.[5]

Ocular Infections

The two most common manifestations of ocular adenovirus infection are pharyngoconjunctival fever and epidemic keratoconjunctivitis. Pharyngoconjunctival fever is typically a mild form of acute follicular conjunctivitis that accompanies febrile pharyngitis or cervical adenitis following a 6- to 9-day incubation period and may affect both eyes. Both bulbar and palpebral conjunctival involvement may occur. Swimming pools or lakes are a common source of infection. Symptoms typically resolve without treatment and without sequelae.

Epidemic keratoconjunctivitis is a more serious disease, with edema of the eyelids, pain, lacrimation, and photophobia.[6] Painful corneal opacities may occur, although they typically resolve over time. The disease typically involves just one eye and is self-limited. However, it may rarely result in permanent corneal damage, and large corneal epithelial full-layer detachment can also occur. Recovery may take up to 4 weeks. The disease is highly contagious, including nosocomial transmission to members of the health care team; as a result, diligent infection control is required even in suspected cases.

Gastrointestinal Tract Infection

Adenovirus can infect any part of the gastrointestinal tract and cause fever, nausea, vomiting, and diarrhea. Up to 10% of pediatric cases of diarrhea are caused by adenovirus, often with symptoms persisting for 8 to 12 days. Some adenoviruses can also cause mesenteric adenitis, which may clinically mimic appendicitis and rarely result in intussusception (Chapter 133). Adenovirus inclusions are seen in about one third to one half of appendices removed at surgery.

Genitourinary Tract Infections

Hemorrhagic cystitis, which typically manifests as microscopic or macroscopic blood in the urine and pain and cramping of the bladder, has been reported in children with adenoviruses 11 and 21 infection. Adults can present with urethritis with or without cystitis due to adenoviruses 19 and 37. Both diseases typically resolve over time without intervention.

Other Manifestations of Adenovirus

Meningitis (Chapter 384) and encephalitis (Chapters 359 and 386) have been reported occasionally in association with adenovirus infection. Adenovirus infection also can cause myocarditis and dilated myocardiopathy (Chapter 54).

A number of studies have found an association between detection of adenovirus in amniotic fluid associated with abnormal fetuses. In particular, echogenic liver lesions with or without hydrops and neural defects in fetuses were more common with patients with adenovirus detected in the amniotic fluid.

Adenovirus Diseases in Immunocompromised Patients

Primary adenovirus infection or reactivation of infection causes a wide range of infectious syndromes in immunocompromised children and adults. In the hematopoietic stem cell transplantation population (Chapter 168), the incidence of disease ranges from 3 to 47%.[7] Risk factors include an allogeneic transplant, T cell–depleted grafts, use of alemtuzumab, and acute graft-versus-host disease. Severe respiratory disease, hepatitis, colitis, hemorrhagic cystitis, and adenoviral keratoconjunctivitis can occur. Severe lymphopenia (<300 cells/μL) is associated with disseminated disease. Although disseminated disease only affects 1 to 7% of hematopoietic stem cell transplantation recipients, it is associated with a significant risk of mortality (8 to 26%).

Among various solid organ transplant recipients, asymptomatic adenovirus viremia is common.[8] However, progression to symptomatic disease is more common in small bowel and liver transplant recipients, pediatric transplant recipients, patients who receive antilymphocyte antibodies, and patients with donor-positive/recipient-negative adenovirus status. Adenoviral hepatitis, typically caused by adenoviruses 1, 2, or 5, is most common among liver transplant recipients and can be diagnosed by detection of viremia or visualization of viral intranuclear inclusions on biopsy. Adenovirus enterocolitis occurs in small bowel transplant recipients and may mimic rejection. Adenoviral pneumonia is associated with graft loss, death, or progression to obliterative bronchiolitis for lung transplant recipients. Adenovirus causes hemorrhagic cystitis with or without interstitial nephritis in kidney transplant recipients. Such patients typically present with fever, hematuria, and new-onset renal dysfunction. Adenovirus DNA in biopsy specimens is associated with worse outcomes among pediatric heart transplant patients.

Primary adenoviral infections can cause severe, frequently fatal disease in children with primary immunodeficiency syndromes, including severe combined immunodeficiency disease (Chapter 236). Fatal cases have been reported in patients with acquired immunodeficiency syndrome (AIDS), but most are self-limited, particularly in patients on highly active antiretroviral therapy or without significant CD4 lymphopenia.

DIAGNOSIS

Diagnosis of adenovirus depends on isolation of the virus from infected tissue and either histopathologic evidence of local replication or clinical symptoms consistent with infection. Detection of virus alone is not diagnostic of an adenovirus disease, because the virus can be latent in some tissues and can be intermittently shed from the throat or in the stool for months to years after primary infection. Quantitative polymerase chain reaction (PCR) has a higher diagnostic yield than culture or direct fluorescent antigen detection. Quantitative PCR assays are also useful to predict progression to disseminated disease in pediatric and, to a lesser extent, adult hematopoietic stem cell transplantation recipients and to determine response due to therapeutic interventions. It is critical to recognize that, particularly in immunocompromised patients and in patients with nonpulmonary disease, use of nasal swabs for detection of adenovirus using one of the many commercially available respiratory viral panel assays may fail to detect adenovirus infection. Testing of relevant specimens (e.g., stool for gastrointestinal disease, urine for urinary tract disease, blood for systemic or disseminated disease, and ocular swabs or fluid for ocular disease) is required for accurate detection of adenovirus.

TREATMENT Rx

No antiviral agents are specifically approved for the treatment of adenovirus. Ribavirin has not been helpful. Cidofovir, which is a potent inhibitor of adenovirus in cell culture, has been used (preferably at 1 mg/kg three times a week), but data suggest that its ratio of efficacy to toxicity, predominantly nephrotoxicity, is too narrow to be clinically useful, except for severe infections.[9]

Brincidofovir, an experimental drug, is not nephrotoxic and is under active study in pediatric and adult hematopoietic stem cell transplantation patients,[10] in whom it has been generally well tolerated and shown to suppress adenovirus compared with placebo.[A1][A2] Further trials are ongoing. A newer approach using adenovirus- and multivirus-specific T cells is also being studied in prospective trials.[11]

PREVENTION

Strict attention to contact and droplet precautions can prevent health care–associated and institutional outbreaks of adenovirus infections, including epidemic keratoconjunctivitis. An oral live-attenuated adenoviruses 4 and 7 vaccine is well tolerated, with a vaccine efficacy of 99.3%.[A3] Currently, the vaccine is only indicated and available to U.S. military personnel, ages 17 to 50 years.

PROGNOSIS

Prognosis is strongly linked to immune competence. Immunocompetent patients typically have self-limited illnesses that generally can be managed with symptomatic care, although some epidemics, including adenoviruses 7 and 14 epidemics, have resulted in high case-fatality rates. In immunocompromised adults, persistent or rising adenovirus viremia predicts progressive infection; in such cases, a reduction of immunosuppression and institution of antiviral therapy are associated with better outcomes. By comparison, patients with ongoing or predicted recovery of their lymphocyte counts may clear their viremia without specific intervention.

Grade A References

A1. Hiwarkar P, Amrolia P, Sivaprakasam P, et al. Brincidofovir is highly efficacious in controlling adenoviremia in pediatric recipients of hematopoietic cell transplant. *Blood.* 2017;129:2033-2037.

A2. Grimley MS, Chemaly RF, Englund JA, et al. Brincidofovir for asymptomatic adenovirus viremia in pediatric and adult allogeneic hematopoietic cell transplant recipients: a randomized placebo-controlled phase II trial. *Biol Blood Marrow Transplant.* 2017;23:512-521.

A3. Kuschner RA, Russell KL, Abuja M, et al. A phase 3, randomized, double-blind, placebo-controlled study of the safety and efficacy of the live, oral adenovirus type 4 and type 7 vaccine, in U.S. military recruits. *Vaccine.* 2013;31:2963-2971.

GENERAL REFERENCES

For the General References and other additional features, please visit Expert Consult at https://expertconsult.inkling.com.

342

CORONAVIRUSES

SUSAN I. GERBER AND JOHN T. WATSON

DEFINITION

Human coronaviruses were, until 2003, recognized as a frequent cause of common cold symptoms, occasionally a cause of lower respiratory tract disease, but rarely if ever a cause of serious disease. In 2003 a novel coronavirus was recognized in humans as the etiologic agent of the outbreak of severe acute respiratory syndrome (SARS).[1,2] The SARS outbreak demonstrated that coronaviruses can be serious human pathogens and led to discovery of other novel human coronaviruses as well as multiple novel coronaviruses in bats, the likely reservoir for SARS coronavirus. Furthermore, in 2012 the Middle East respiratory syndrome (MERS) coronavirus emerged and provided another example of coronavirus's ability to cause severe human disease.[3,4]

The Pathogens

Coronaviruses are members of the family Coronaviridae, which includes two subfamilies, Coronavirinae and Torovirinae. Coronaviruses are single-stranded positive-sense RNA viruses with a genome of approximately 30 kb, the largest genome among RNA viruses. These viruses were named coronaviruses because by electron microscopy they have club-shaped surface projections that give them a crown-like appearance. The genome encodes four or five structural proteins (a spike protein [S], a small envelope protein [E], a membrane protein [M], a nucleocapsid protein [N], and sometimes a hemagglutinin-esterase protein [HE]), a varying number of open reading frames scattered among the structural genes, and a polyprotein that is processed into multiple (usually 16) nonstructural proteins. These nonstructural proteins participate in virus replication but are not incorporated into the virion. Coronaviruses have also been isolated from a variety of animals and birds and, in their respective species, cause a wide range of respiratory, gastrointestinal (GI), neurologic, and systemic illnesses. The coronaviruses are divided into four genera: alpha, beta, gamma, and delta. The 229E and NL63 viruses are alphacoronaviruses, whereas OC43 and HKU1 are betacoronaviruses. SARS coronavirus and MERS coronavirus are both betacoronaviruses but belong to different lineages. Detection and characterization of novel coronaviruses in bats has greatly expanded our understanding of diversity among coronaviruses and will likely continue to do so.

EPIDEMIOLOGY

The common human coronaviruses—229E, OC43, NL63, and HKU1—appear to be transmitted through close contact that probably includes contamination of hands from person-to-person contact or from fomites, followed by auto-inoculation to the mucosal surfaces of the mouth, nose, or eyes or inhalation of infectious droplets and possibly aerosols. Symptoms occur 2 to 4 days after infection. These coronaviruses are detected in patients with acute respiratory illnesses, most often a mild upper respiratory tract illness (i.e., common cold) but also in patients with more serious respiratory illnesses, including pneumonia, bronchiolitis, and croup. Coronavirus infections are detected early in childhood, and repeated infections can occur throughout life. About 50% of children have antibodies against OC43 by 3 years of age, and about 70% of adults have such antibodies. Up to 75% of children have antibodies against NL63 and 229E by 3 to 4 years of age. Studies looking for 229E- and OC43-like infections suggest that coronaviruses are associated with about 15% of cases of the common cold and with up to 10% of cases of acute respiratory illnesses in children and adults. Individually, 229E, OC43, HKU1, and NL63 are detected in less than 1 to 4% of cases, and their individual contributions will vary by location and year. Serious illness has been reported in outbreaks among elderly patients in nursing homes. In one outbreak associated with OC43 infection, for example, 23 residents and 24 staff reported influenza-like illness, and three residents died. However, some reports have found rates of detection of coronaviruses among hospitalized children with acute respiratory illness and/or fever to be similar to the rates of asymptomatic controls, thereby raising questions about the virus's role in more severe disease and hospitalization. The 229E, OC43, NL63, and HKU1 coronaviruses can be detected throughout the year, but peak detection is often during fall and winter months in temperate climates. A second respiratory viral pathogen can be detected in 20 to 60% of specimens positive for one of these coronaviruses.

Most documented SARS coronavirus infections in humans occurred in persons ill with a SARS-like illness during the 2002–2003 global outbreak. It is likely that wild animal markets in Guangdong Province, China, played a key role in amplifying and introducing the virus into humans, but the original source of the outbreak virus was likely bats. Detection of multiple SARS-like and other coronaviruses in bats suggests that they are a rich source of coronaviruses. A coronavirus recently isolated from bats has 95% nucleotide sequence identity to the SARS viruses and can infect humans via the ACE2 receptor. Although animals were the original source of human infections, global spread of SARS coronavirus occurred through human-to-human transmission and involved droplet, fomite transmission, and, in some instances, probably small-particle aerosol transmission. Most transmission occurred within households, hospitals, or other health care facilities; little transmission occurred in the community.

More recently, MERS coronavirus was first recognized in the Arabian Peninsula in 2012. Coronaviruses similar to the MERS coronavirus have been detected in bats, suggesting that bats may be a source of this virus. Dromedary camels, however, appear to act as a reservoir for the virus and a vehicle for human transmission. Dromedary camels in the Middle East and Africa may harbor live MERS coronavirus, and young camels in these areas nearly universally have antibody titers detected by the age of 2 years. Furthermore, in humans without known preillness exposure to other human MERS cases, direct exposure to dromedary camels during the prior 2 weeks is independently associated with developing MERS.[5] Person-to-person spread occurs within health care settings and is associated with the majority of reported transmission. For example, an outbreak of 186 cases in the Republic of Korea in 2015 resulted from a single infected traveler who returned from the Arabian peninsula.[6] Transmission among household family members also has been reported, but so far there has been no evidence of sustained community transmission. The incubation period is estimated at just over 5 days (range, 2 to 14 days), and sporadic human cases and clusters of MERS coronavirus infections continue to be reported.

PATHOBIOLOGY

The human coronaviruses characterized to date infect humans through the respiratory tract. The sites where the virus then replicates is determined at least in part by which cells express the respective receptors. The receptors for 229E and NL63 coronaviruses are aminopeptidase N and angiotensin-converting enzyme 2 (ACE2), respectively. The receptors for OC43 and HKU1 coronaviruses have not yet been determined, but OC43 may use several cell surface molecules as receptors, including 9-O-acetylated neuraminic acid. The primary receptor for SARS coronavirus is ACE2, but the virus also binds to two C-type lectins expressed on dendritic cells, DC-SIGN and L-SIGN. Aminopeptidase N is expressed in various cells, including respiratory, GI, kidney epithelial, and myeloid cells, but 229E is known to infect only respiratory epithelial cells. ACE2 is found in various tissues, including the lung, GI tract, heart, and kidneys. The SARS coronavirus has consistently been detected in pneumocytes in the lung and enterocytes in the GI tract and is occasionally found in other cells, including distal tubular cells in the kidney and macrophages in various tissues. Autopsy studies suggest that infection in the lung leads initially to diffuse alveolar damage and later may lead to a repair process that includes fibrosis in the alveolar walls. It is not known whether NL63, which also uses ACE2 as its receptor, infects sites other than the respiratory tract. The MERS coronavirus receptor is the exopeptidase dipeptidyl peptidase 4 (DPP4), also known as CD26. DPP4 is found on many different cell types including nonciliated bronchial epithelial cells, bronchiolar epithelial cells, alveolar epithelial cells, endothelial cells, and lung ex vivo organ cultures. In addition, DPP4 is expressed on the epithelial cells in kidney, small intestine, liver, and prostate as well as in activated leukocytes.

It is likely that the illness associated with coronavirus infections results from both the cytopathic effect of the virus and the host immune and inflammatory response to the viral infection. How this interplay contributes to disease, however, is not understood. The biphasic course of SARS in some patients, with the onset of severe disease in the second week of illness and the decrease in lymphocyte numbers, suggests a role for the host response and virus-induced immune suppression in the disease process. Similarly, it appears that the host response and virus-induced immune suppression may also contribute to MERS coronavirus disease.

CLINICAL MANIFESTATIONS

229E, OC43, NL63, and HKU1 coronavirus infections are commonly associated with acute respiratory illnesses that are usually mild and consistent with the common cold (Chapter 337) but can also result in the full range of acute respiratory illnesses, including pneumonia (Chapter 91), croup (Chapter 401), bronchiolitis, and bronchitis (Chapter 90). The best studied of these coronaviruses, human coronaviruses 229E and OC43, cause respiratory symptoms (e.g., rhinorrhea, nasal congestion, sore throat, cough) as well as systemic symptoms (e.g., fever, headache, malaise) when they are inoculated intranasally into adult volunteers. Symptoms develop 2 to 4 days after inoculation, but about 30% of volunteers who excrete virus have no associated illness. Symptoms usually persist for about 1 week but sometimes for as long as 3 weeks. Previous infection does not induce high levels of protective immunity. Humans can be reinfected with respiratory coronaviruses throughout life, and human volunteers can be symptomatically reinfected with the same strain of coronavirus 1 year after the first infection. As with other infections, the severity of disease varies among individual patients during the same outbreak and among groups of patients during different outbreaks in the same community.

In contrast to the mild illness associated with 229E and OC43, SARS coronavirus infection nearly always results in a serious illness that requires hospitalization, often in an intensive care unit (ICU), and a high fatality rate. Radiologic evidence of pneumonia was seen in nearly all SARS coronavirus–infected persons, and acute respiratory distress syndrome (Chapter 96) requiring admission to an ICU and mechanical ventilation developed in 20% or more of patients. The initial clinical manifestation of SARS was often systemic symptoms of fever, malaise, and myalgias from 2 to 10 days (rarely >10 days) after exposure. Several days after the onset of systemic symptoms, lower respiratory tract symptoms of nonproductive cough and shortness of breath were noted. Unlike patients with other respiratory virus infections, the majority of patients never experience upper respiratory tract symptoms such as rhinorrhea, sore throat, or nasal congestion (Table 342-1). During the course of their illness, most SARS coronavirus–infected patients had elevated liver enzyme levels and lymphopenia, including a substantial drop in numbers of both $CD4^+$ and $CD8^+$ T cells. In general, children had less severe illness than adults.

The clinical spectrum of MERS coronavirus illness ranges from asymptomatic infection to severe illness.[7] Symptoms include cough, fever, malaise, chills, arthralgias, rigors, and dyspnea. Approximately 25% of patients have GI symptoms that include diarrhea, vomiting, and abdominal pain. Patients who are

TABLE 342-1	PERCENTAGE OF HOSPITALIZED SARS AND MERS CORONAVIRUS–INFECTED PATIENTS WITH SELECTED CLINICAL AND LABORATORY FEATURES OF SARS AND MERS CORONAVIRUS INFECTIONS	
	SARS	**MERS**
CLINICAL OR LABORATORY FINDING	**AT HOSPITAL ADMISSION**	**AT PRESENTATION**
Fever	90-100%	≈90-100%
Cough or shortness of breath	40-75%	83%
Diarrhea	20-30%	26%
Chest radiograph abnormalities	65-90%	100%
Lymphopenia*	50-90%	34%

*Both CD4+ and CD8+ lymphocyte counts are decreased.
MERS = Middle East respiratory syndrome; SARS = severe acute respiratory syndrome.
From Assiri A, Al-Tawfiq JA, Al-Rabeeah AA, et al. Epidemiological, demographic, and clinical characteristics of 47 cases of Middle East respiratory syndrome coronavirus disease from Saudi Arabia: a descriptive study. *Lancet Infect Dis.* 2013;13:752-761.

severely ill have pneumonia that sometimes progresses to acute respiratory distress syndrome.

Laboratory findings include leukopenia and lymphopenia, and some patients have thrombocytopenia and abnormal liver enzymes. Chest radiographic findings have included patchy infiltrates, lobar opacities, and similar to the SARS coronavirus, a ground-glass appearance.

DIAGNOSIS

Because illness is usually mild and there is no effective treatment, the diagnosis of 229E, OC43, NL63, and HKU1 coronavirus infections has not been important to the management of patients. The accurate diagnosis of SARS and MERS coronavirus infections is, however, critical for the management of individual patients and to mount an appropriate public health response.

229E, OC43, HKU1, and NL63 Coronavirus Infections

Coronavirus polymerase chain reaction (PCR) assays are the assays of choice for diagnosis of infection. Most coronavirus PCR assays are type specific—that is, specific to MERS coronavirus, SARS coronavirus, 229E, OC43, HKU1, or NL63 RNA. Coronavirus diagnostic assays are becoming more generally available and are sometimes part of a PCR panel designed to detect respiratory viruses. Presence of the virus can also be inferred by electron microscopy and confirmed by in situ or immunohistologic assays of affected tissues. Positive immunohistologic and in situ hybridization studies document the site of infection and help support a link between the virus and the disease process. A variety of enzyme or fluorescent immunoassays for antibodies have been used successfully to detect infection. Most assays detect immunoglobulin G (IgG) antibodies, but virus neutralization antibody assays are more specific. Serologic tests to detect a diagnostic rise in antibodies between acute and convalescent serum specimens for 229E, OC43, HKU1, and NL63 coronavirus infections are not helpful for managing an acute illness but can be helpful for epidemiologic studies.

SARS

Three features of SARS cases help guide approach to its diagnosis. First, SARS has been documented only in persons who have some potential exposure—that is, to patients with SARS, to a location with SARS transmission, to a laboratory working on SARS coronavirus, or to a setting where SARS-infected animals might be located (e.g., southern China). Second, nearly 100% of infected patients develop chest radiographic abnormalities by day 10 of their illness. Finally, SARS nearly always develops within 10 days of exposure. Thus a suspicion of SARS and a diagnostic evaluation can be limited to patients who have a severe lower respiratory tract illness and some potential exposure to SARS within 10 days before the onset of illness.

Laboratory confirmation of SARS coronavirus infection early in the illness proved to be difficult even with sensitive real-time PCR assays. Unlike in most respiratory viral infections, the highest titer of virus or viral RNA was found in clinical specimens from the beginning of the second week of illness. During the first week of illness, the best way to detect infection is by a sensitive PCR assay or a sensitive enzyme immunoassay for N protein antigen applied to respiratory and serum specimens. During the second week of illness, respiratory and stool specimens are most likely to be positive for viral RNA. Antibodies were sometimes detected early in the second week of illness but at times were not detected until 4 weeks into the illness. Because antibodies to SARS coronavirus were rarely present before the 2003 outbreak, a single positive antibody test result from an ill person could be considered diagnostic of an acute SARS coronavirus infection. However, because the reemergence of SARS coronavirus will have substantial public health, social, and economic impact, and because of occasional cross-reacting antibodies induced by other coronaviruses, a neutralization antibody test and confirmatory testing by a reference laboratory are required to confirm the diagnosis. Public health departments should be consulted for questions about SARS diagnostic tests.

MERS

A diagnosis of MERS coronavirus infection should be considered in patients with severe acute respiratory infection of unknown cause and a possible exposure or epidemiologic link to the Arabian Peninsula.[8] PCR assays have been used to detect RNA in upper respiratory tract specimens (nasopharyngeal, oropharyngeal) and preferably in lower respiratory tract specimens (sputum, tracheal aspirate, and bronchoalveolar lavage fluid have the highest viral loads), as well as in serum, stool, and urine. A confirmed case of MERS coronavirus infection requires a positive PCR on at least two specific gene targets or a single positive target with sequencing on a second.

A number of serologic assays can detect antibodies to the nucleocapsid and spike proteins. The sensitivity and specificity of these assays for diagnosing current or past MERS coronavirus infection have not yet been determined. Public health departments should be consulted for questions about MERS diagnostic tests.

TREATMENT ℞

There is no virus-specific treatment for 229E, OC43, HKU1, and NL63 coronavirus infections, but the illnesses are mild and usually resolve in a few days to a week. Patients require symptomatic therapy or, uncommonly, management of complications of infection.

Treatment of SARS and MERS coronavirus infections is more complex. Currently, no antiviral drug has proved to be effective for either. With the high death rate associated with both of these viruses and the lack of clinical or in vitro data to guide treatment, supportive measures, including mechanical ventilation and oxygenation regimens (Chapter 96), are used. In the SARS coronavirus outbreak, in vitro data showed little if any antiviral effect with ribavirin and suggested that interferon alfa, SARS convalescent phase immune globulin, and lopinavir plus ritonavir might have been useful. Although many people were treated during the outbreak, lack of control groups makes it impossible to determine which if any therapies were beneficial. For MERS coronavirus, in vitro data and animal models demonstrate inhibitory effects for a number of antiviral agents, including interferons, ribavirin, and lopinavir/ritonavir. Immunotherapeutic options undergoing evaluation include convalescent plasma and monoclonal and polyclonal antibodies. However, no consensus is currently available regarding their efficacy for treating human infection.

PREVENTION

Handwashing and other infection-control measures probably decrease the spread of coronaviruses in the home, health care facilities, and other settings. These strategies focus on reinforcing the need for patients with respiratory illnesses to cover the nose and mouth when coughing or sneezing, to use tissues to contain respiratory secretions, and to wash the hands after contact with respiratory secretions. Staff should use good infection-control practices.

Within 4 months of the initiation of the 2003 SARS outbreak, the outbreak was contained and human-to-human transmission stopped without a vaccine or effective antiviral therapy but thorough implementation of the classic public health tools of early case detection, isolation, and contact tracing and management, including quarantine of contacts. For MERS, the effectiveness of these measures in interrupting transmission also has been repeatedly demonstrated, most notably for outbreaks associated with health care facilities.

The cases of laboratory-acquired SARS coronavirus infection and the subsequent transmission of disease to others after one such case reinforces the importance of strict attention to safe laboratory practices. Because the reemergence of SARS could lead to global spread, the local, national, and global public health and health care communities must be alerted quickly and updated regularly about new cases and the status of transmission.

Strict attention to standard contact and airborne precautions is recommended for SARS and MERS coronavirus–infected patients within hospital settings. MERS coronavirus infections continue to occur in the Middle East, and local, national, and global public health and health care communities should be immediately notified of a case. Vaccine development is underway for both SARS and MERS coronaviruses.

PROGNOSIS

Patients with typical community-acquired coronavirus infections typically recover completely. However, patients with compromised cardiac, pulmonary, or immune systems are at increased risk of more serious lower respiratory tract illness, and outbreaks of human coronavirus infections in elderly patients in chronic care facilities can cause severe lower respiratory illnesses and deaths. In the SARS outbreak, nearly 10% of patients died. The death rate was especially high, approaching 50%, in elderly patients and patients with underlying illnesses. Although most survivors of SARS coronavirus infection appeared to achieve full recovery, as many as 25% had abnormal pulmonary findings such as ground-glass opacities on chest radiograph or abnormal pulmonary function test results (e.g., decreased diffusing capacity) 6 months or more after their illness. The MERS fatality rate initially was reported to be about 40%, but is now lower as less severe cases and seropositive persons without obvious infection have been identified.[9]

GENERAL REFERENCES

For the General References and other additional features, please visit Expert Consult at https://expertconsult.inkling.com.

343

MEASLES

MARTIN G. OTTOLINI

DEFINITION

The term *measles* is applied most appropriately to "rubeola" (also known as "morbilli"), an extremely contagious, prolonged respiratory and systemic viral illness characterized by high fever, an erythematous maculopapular rash, cough, coryza, and conjunctivitis. A member of the family Paramyxoviridae, within the genus *Morbillivirus*, the measles virus exhibits at least 24 distinct genotypes but behaves as a single serotype because natural infection or adequate immunization confers broad protection against all types.[1]

EPIDEMIOLOGY

In the 1950s and early 1960s, measles was ubiquitous in the United States, with more than 500,000 cases reported annually, and nearly everyone was infected by adulthood. By 2000, a two-dose, live-attenuated vaccine led to endemic measles being declared "eliminated" from the United States.[2] Between 2009 and 2014, however, the annual incidence has ranged from 55 to 667 cases, with an average of 10 annual outbreaks. Recent increases may be related to a surge in global travel to and from countries with endemic measles or outbreaks, combined with local vulnerability owing to reduced immunization rates.

The global incidence of measles has decreased from an estimated 29 million cases in 2000 to approximately 7 million in 2016, with a reduction in annual measles deaths from about 650,000 in 2000 to 90,000 by 2016.[3] However, global protection with at least one immunization has stagnated since 2010, at rates of about 85%, with only about 60% of individuals receiving the required two immunizations.[4] In 2015, only 16% of low-income countries achieved the goal of greater than 90% first-dose coverage, a goal that was met by 91% of high-income countries.[5]

Multiple factors challenge the "theoretically possible" goal of measles elimination: the financial constraints of the two-dose schedule, high population density, increased mobility, regions with weak health care infrastructure periodically worsened by armed conflict or natural disasters, and the emergence of elective vaccine avoidance, particularly in developed nations.[6] Difficulty

remains in reaching children in India, Nigeria, Pakistan, Ethiopia, Indonesia, and the Democratic Republic of the Congo. In 2014, a nearly 10-fold increase in measles cases occurred in the Philippine Islands and Southeast Asia after a typhoon devastated health care infrastructure in late 2013. That natural disaster converged with regionally lower U.S. immunization rates to enable the 2014-15 outbreak associated with an amusement park in Southern California, with molecular epidemiology implicating the same B3 genotype in both outbreaks.[7]

Measles may be the most contagious pathogen known to humans, and it has no other reservoir. Its basic reproduction number, the R_0, which represents the number of naïve contacts potentially infected by exposure to one contagious individual, has been estimated to be 12 to 18,[8] an R_0 far higher than the R_0 of two to three for Ebola (Chapter 357) and influenza (Chapter 340). Travel-related measles most often occurs in young adult males traveling to and from Asia for tourism, business, or social visits. Of travelers seen at 24 sites in the U.S. Global TravEpiNet network, 16% were eligible for an additional dose of measles-mumps-rubella (MMR) vaccine, yet more than half did not receive the vaccine.[9] Unfortunately, even two doses of vaccine does not guarantee protection against infection on exposure to an active case, despite evidence of a good antibody response.[10]

PATHOBIOLOGY

Measles virus is spread very effectively by contact with large droplets or inhalation of aerosolized small droplets, which can remain suspended for hours after an infected individual has exited.[11] Unlike other paramyxoviruses, which primarily infect and inflame respiratory epithelia, measles virus targets the immune system. Measles virus initially infects dendritic cells in the respiratory tract or conjunctiva, which migrate to regional lymph nodes where they infect CD150(SLAM)-expressing T and B cells. Infected lymphocytes then travel to other lymphoid tissues, including the spleen, tonsils, and other lymph nodes to propagate infection. Virus may enter the central nervous system (CNS) through infected lymphocytes. Infection of the gastrointestinal (GI) system, kidney, liver, and skin occurs by circulation of infected immune cells. Measles virus later infects the respiratory epithelium through the Nectin-4 receptor, spreads from cell to cell to cause damage and sloughing, and then is expelled as infectious droplets by coughing to repeat the cycle.

Measles virus evades immune recognition by inhibiting type 1 interferons, so extensive viral replication and systemic spread precede clinical disease. The buccal mucosal lesions (Koplik spots) and the classic rash result from infection of capillary endothelium by measles virus, with syncytial cell formation as well as local production of nitrous oxide and tumor necrosis factor-α. Measles virus–specific T-cell host-immune responses lead to eventual necrosis of infected cells with viral clearance. Poor measles virus–specific T-cell responses are observed in individuals who are severely malnourished and immunocompromised, with reduced cellular necrosis and delayed viral clearance, thereby explaining their less obvious but prolonged skin changes.

The most dramatic aspect of measles virus infection may be its transient yet profound suppression of the immune system, possibly by targeting CD150(SLAM)-expressing cells. While inducing a cytotoxic T-cell response that clears infected cells and induces measles virus–specific memory B cells, measles virus concurrently depletes subsets of both regional and circulating T and B cells, with a loss of immune memory. The depletion of lymphocytes in gut and respiratory epithelium leads to increased morbidity and mortality from other infections and explains the increase in all-cause mortality after measles infection.

CLINICAL MANIFESTATIONS

Measles should be suspected in the presence of fever and a maculopapular (nonvesicular) rash. Measles has a 7- to 21-day incubation period, with onset of fever and malaise (prodrome), as well as the more specific combination of a "croupy or brassy" cough, coryza, conjunctivitis, and photophobia beginning about 10 days after exposure (Fig. 343-1).[12] Koplik spots (Fig. 343-2),[13] which are raised bluish-white papules inside both cheeks, may appear at this time; though pathognomonic, they are often missed or misdiagnosed as thrush, and they fade as the rash emerges. The classic erythematous blanching maculopapular rash begins on the face, spreads down the body, and becomes confluent and darker in color over days (Fig. 343-3A). The rash is more subtle in dark-skinned patients (Fig. 343-3B), in whom the diagnosis may be delayed. In the malnourished and immunosuppressed individuals, a prolonged desquamating dermatitis is commonly seen (Fig. 343-3C). Body temperature is high, 39-40.5° C, beginning with the prodrome and continuing at least 4 days into the rash. Patients are contagious to others from 4 days prior until 4 days after onset of

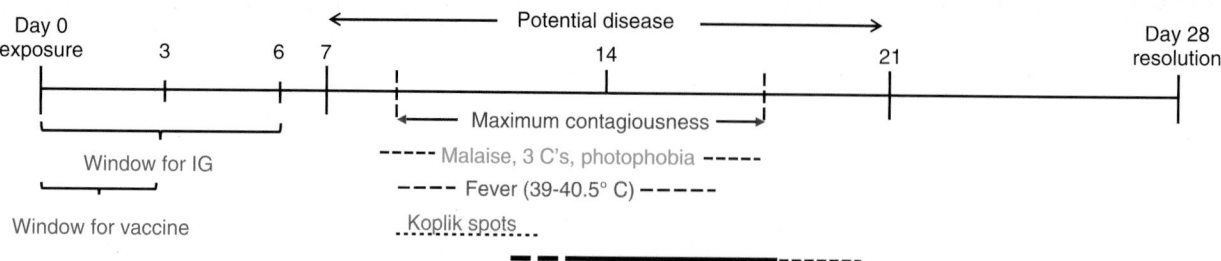

FIGURE 343-1. Clinical progression of measles. 3 C's = cough, coryza, conjunctivitis; IG = immunoglobulin.

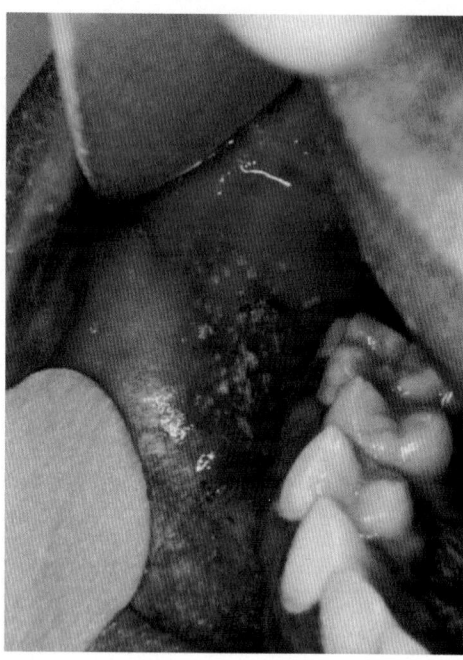

FIGURE 343-2. Typical Koplik spots.

the rash. As the rash darkens and fades, the skin will often flake and peel. In individuals with waning or incomplete postimmunization protection,[14] the rash and clinical symptoms may be more mild.

Complications

Before its elimination in the United States, common complications of measles infection included primary viral or secondary bacterial pneumonia (6%), otitis media (7%), and diarrhea (8%). Rare severe complications include GI bleeding and disseminated intravascular coagulation (Chapter 166). Immunosuppressed individuals may develop a fatal giant cell viral pneumonia.

DIAGNOSIS

Many diseases in children and adults have morbilliform rashes and systemic findings, so clinicians must use experience and judgment to decide if there is substantial risk that a patient's illness may be measles and represent the index case of a potential outbreak (Table 343-1). Patients may have marked leukopenia and lymphopenia, but suspected measles infection must be confirmed by reverse transcription–polymerase chain reaction (RT-PCR) testing of samples obtained from sites of shedding, including the nasopharynx, oropharynx, conjunctiva, and even urine; or confirmatory serology.[15] Virus recovery by PCR or culture allows epidemiologists to genotype the isolate and to help control outbreaks. Unvaccinated infected individuals may develop an elevated measles-specific immunoglobulin M antibody as soon as the first day of rash, whereas acute and convalescent serologies can detect a four-fold or greater rise in measles-specific antibody. Clinicians should confer with regional or national public health experts if a case of measles is confirmed.

TABLE 343-1 DIAGNOSING MEASLES

CLINICAL PRINCIPLE	QUESTIONS TO ASK
Measles is acquired only from a person with measles	Travel to endemic areas or regions with outbreaks? Warnings from health department/CDC of local measles? Suspicious ill contacts with risk factors?
The individual must be susceptible	Natural immunity (born before 1957, history of infection)? Is the patient inadequately immunized or immunosuppressed?
Most patients are ill-appearing	Ill enough to consider "admission" to a hospital (a rash in an otherwise well individual is rarely measles)?
There is a predictable evolution of systemic findings	Croupy cough, coryza, and conjunctivitis (3 Cs)? Relentless high fever for several days? Did Koplik spots precede the rash? (often unrecognized)
The rash is impressive, with a few exceptions	Previously healthy patient with lighter skin color—is there a distinct rash (see Fig. 343-3A)? Hard to distinguish due to darker skin color in this previously healthy infant (see Fig. 343-3B)? "Head-trunk-limb" progression, increasing confluence? Is patient malnourished/immunosuppressed (rash can be absent/atypical; see Fig. 343-3C)
Other diagnoses are much more common	Enterovirus (Chapter 355), parvovirus (Chapter 347), roseola (Chapter 410), rubella (Chapter 344), EBV (Chapter 346), streptococcal/staphylococcal (Chapters 272 and 273), toxin? Risk for rickettsial illnesses (Chapter 311) in region, outdoor exposure? Kawasaki disease (Chapter 254), other vasculitis, or immunologic disease? Risks for drug toxicity—new medications (Chapter 239)?
The experience of the examining clinicians is critical	Clinicians from the 1960s–1980s, or with global experience? Team consensus? This will be a public health emergency! Ability to confirm rapidly by acute IgM serology or PCR?

CDC = Centers for Disease Control and Prevention; EBV = Epstein-Barr virus; IgM = immunoglobulin M; PCR = polymerase chain reaction.

TREATMENT   Rx

Treatment is supportive, with control of fever, hydration, nutrition, and observation for the serious complications of pneumonia and encephalitis (see Prognosis). Clinicians who rarely see measles may be alarmed by the prolonged high fever and malaise. Hospital admission for hydration or other concerns must be weighed against the challenge of infection control.

Vitamin A supplementation is recommended to reduce overall mortality, and potentially reduce the risk for xerophthalmia, corneal scarring, and blindness as well as the debilitating prolonged diarrhea of measles, especially in populations with vitamin A deficiency or malnutrition.[A1] Dosing is 50,000 units for infants younger than 6 months, 100,000 units for children aged 6 to 11 months, and 200,000 units for patients older than 12 months on both days 1 and 2 of presentation. A second course can be given 4 to 6 weeks later to patients with ophthalmic findings of vitamin A deficiency.

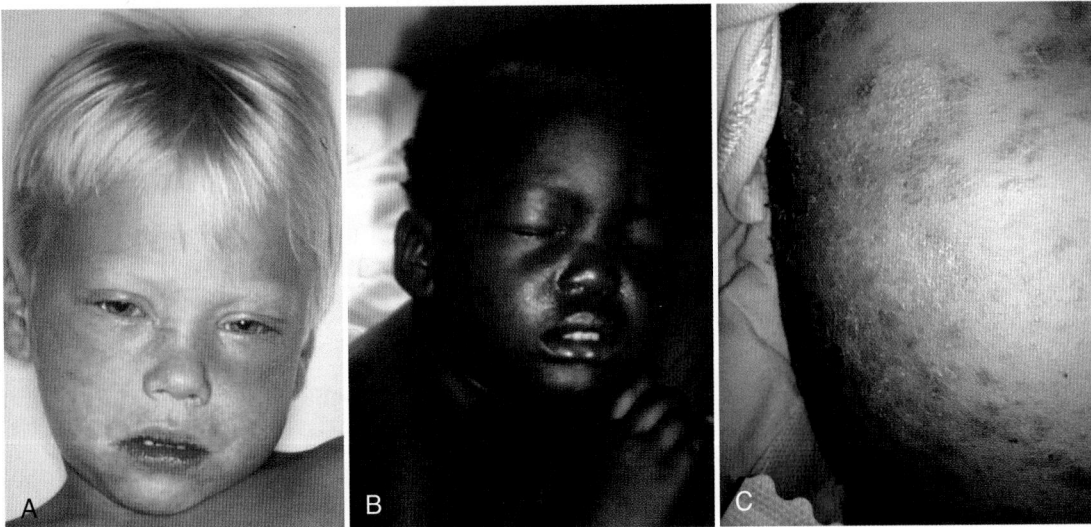

FIGURE 343-3. The variable rash of measles. **A,** Classic erythematous rash, conjunctivitis, and coryza. **B,** Rash is difficult to perceive on dark skin, but patient has typical conjunctivitis and coryza. **C,** Prolonged desquamating dermatitis in a malnourished child with measles.

Immunization with Live Virus Vaccines

Immunization with live-attenuated measles virus vaccine, often as MMR and sometimes with varicella (MMRV), stimulates long-acting antibodies and cellular immunity. Immunization strategies are designed both to protect the individual and to ensure that least 89 to 94% of a population is protected, a level required to diminish measles propagation within the population, termed "herd immunity."

Two immunizations should be delivered, at least 1 month apart, when the protective yet also vaccine-inhibitory effects of passively transferred maternal antibody diminish (Chapter 15).[16] The first dose is routinely administered at 9 to 12 months of age and can be given as early as 6 months if the infant is born during an outbreak or high-risk situation or is traveling to such a region. If it is given before 9 months of age, a third dose is needed to ensure that two are given after the loss of maternal antibody. However, an additional early dose given at 5 to 6 months of age provides no incremental benefit in reducing subsequent hospitalizations or mortality.[A2] The second dose can be given from 1 month to years later, often at entry to formal schooling. As the world's population shifts to relying on vaccine immunity, further doses during adulthood may be required. For example, only 82% of recent U.S. military recruits had detectable measles titers, lower than the level desired for herd immunity, and recruits older than 30 years had even lower rates, possibly suggesting waning titers.

An experimental aerosolized vaccine might become an appealing option, especially in developing countries. Although aerosolized vaccine is immunogenic, it is not as good as regular subcutaneous vaccination (85 vs. 95% subsequent seropositivity).[A3]

Vaccine Safety

Measles vaccine is highly safe, with minimal side effects. Common reactions include fever 7 to 12 days after immunization in less than 15% of cases and transient rashes or lymphadenopathy in less than 5% of children and 20% of adults. Up to 25% of naïve postpubertal females have transient arthralgia, which rarely persists or recurs, 1 to 3 weeks after immunization. Febrile seizures occur in 1 per 3000 to 4000 infants 6 to 14 days after immunization, and very rare occurrences of anaphylaxis or thrombocytopenia have occurred. No evidence supports any causal relationship between receipt of measles vaccine and autism-spectrum disorders or autoimmune disorders, including Guillain-Barré syndrome, inflammatory bowel disease, or type 1 diabetes.

Immunization is encouraged for individuals with early-stage human immunodeficiency virus (HIV) who are successfully managed with antiviral therapy, and reimmunization should be considered for children who have immune reconstitution later in life. MMR vaccines are avoided in pregnant women or those who may become pregnant in the subsequent 28 days, primarily to avoid exposure to the rubella component, although vaccine-associated problems for any component are extraordinarily rare. MMR or MMRV vaccine should be avoided in patients with primary or acquired immunodeficiency (Chapters 236 and 360), including late-stage HIV or ongoing systemic immunosuppressive therapy, and in patients who have recently received antibody-containing blood products (immunoglobulin or whole blood), which might inhibit the vaccines. Measles and other immunizations should be planned around the timing of induction and recovery from immunosuppression for the growing group of patients who receive targeted immunotherapies.

Isolation of Suspected Infected Individuals and Postexposure Prophylaxis

Immediate isolation of suspected cases and quarantine of any contacts without presumptive immunity are standard practices. Hospitalized patients are ideally managed in negative-air-pressure isolation rooms using airborne precautions.

If a risk for exposure has been identified early, contacts can be screened for natural immunity or adequate immunization; if indicated, a dose of measles vaccine can be delivered within 72 hours of exposure.[17] Passive immunoprophylaxis with human immunoglobulin preparations can achieve protective levels of antimeasles antibody in patients who were exposed between 3 and 6 days earlier, are pregnant, have late-stage HIV infection, or have other contraindications to vaccine.[A4]

Vaccine Avoidance

Voluntary avoidance or delay of measles immunization is a growing problem, with 3% of surveyed U.S. parents refusing MMR for their children and another 25% reporting delaying immunization, often because of missed opportunities or limited health care resources, but sometimes because of concerns about too many vaccines or potential side effects. The global challenge remains to eliminate barriers to timely measles immunization for all populations.

Fatality rates are 2 to 3 per 1000, mostly in infants or adults older than 30 years, but fatality rates rise to 6 to 30% in populations with malnutrition and vitamin A deficiency. CNS complications take several forms, most commonly an acute encephalitis with infection of neuronal tissues in 1 to 3 cases per 1000, with a 10% fatality rate and permanent sequelae in 25% of survivors. An early postinfectious encephalitis, perhaps related to a host immune response to molecular mimicry by the virus, can occur even in the absence of a rash and can lead to relapsing symptoms and fatal outcomes in approximately 1 per 1000 infected children and 1 to 2 per 1,000,000 immunized children. A persistent infection of neurons called *measles inclusion-body encephalitis* is a progressively fatal disease that may occur in very young or otherwise immunosuppressed individuals.[18] The most dramatic long-term complication of measles is subacute sclerosing pan-encephalitis (SSPE; Chapter 346), which occurs in 1 per 25,000 individuals years after measles infection (not immunization), more often in children infected at a young age. SSPE reflects slow spread of a possibly mutated virus from neuron to neuron, with progressive neuronal loss and death within 1 to 3 years.[19]

Grade A References

A1. Bello S, Meremikwu MM, Ejemot-Nwadiaro RI, et al. Routine vitamin A supplementation for the prevention of blindness due to measles infection in children. *Cochrane Database Syst Rev.* 2016;8:CD007719.

A2. Schoeps A, Nebié E, Fisker AB, et al. No effect of an additional early dose of measles vaccine on hospitalization or mortality in children: a randomized controlled trial. *Vaccine.* 2018;36:1965-1971.

A3. Low N, Bavdekar A, Jeyaseelan L, et al. A randomized, controlled trial of an aerosolized vaccine against measles. *N Engl J Med.* 2015;372:1519-1529.

A4. Young MK, Nimmo GR, Cripps AW, et al. Post-exposure passive immunisation for preventing measles. *Cochrane Database Syst Rev.* 2014;4:CD010056.

GENERAL REFERENCES

For the General References and other additional features, please visit Expert Consult at https://expertconsult.inkling.com.

344

RUBELLA (GERMAN MEASLES)

SUSAN E. REEF

DEFINITION

Rubella, also known as German measles, is an acute viral illness that usually presents with a generalized maculopapular rash of 1 to 3 days' duration, low-grade or no fever, and associated clinical symptoms such as lymphadenopathy, arthropathy, and conjunctivitis. However, about 20 to 50% of persons infected with rubella may present without a rash or other symptoms.

The Pathogen

Rubella virus is a member of the Togaviridae family and the genus *Rubivirus*. Rubella virus is a single-stranded enveloped RNA with a single antigenic type. It measures 50 to 70 nm in diameter and has two envelope proteins (E1, E2) and a core protein (c). The core protein is surrounded by a single-layer lipoprotein envelope with spikelike projections that contain the two glycoproteins, E1 and E2. Humans are the only known reservoir.

EPIDEMIOLOGY

In the prevaccine era, rubella epidemics occurred approximately every 6 to 9 years in the United States. The last major American epidemic, which occurred in 1964 to 1965, resulted in an estimated 12.5 million cases and approximately 20,000 cases of congenital rubella syndrome. In 1969, live attenuated rubella vaccines were licensed in the United States and were introduced into the routine childhood immunization program. In 1979, the RA 27/3 rubella virus vaccine replaced prior rubella virus vaccines. Since 2003, 18 or fewer cases have been reported annually in the United States, and rubella is no longer endemic in the United States.[1]

By 2015, endemic rubella and the congenital rubella syndrome were eliminated in the Americas, and the number of rubella cases reported globally decreased to about 22,000 in 2016. However, rubella and congenital rubella syndrome continue to be of global public health importance, and the global incidence is probably substantially underestimated because rubella cases in many countries may be misidentified as measles cases. The true current annual incidence of the congenital rubella syndrome is unknown, but now only 9% of pregnant women worldwide are estimated to be seronegative for rubella.[2] Nevertheless, the entry of asylum-seekers from Africa and Asia into Europe and the United States poses a continuing challenge.[3]

In 2016, 78% of World Health Organization member countries included rubella in national childhood immunization schedules. By the end of 2017, four of six World Health Organization regions (Americas, European, western Pacific, southeast Asia)[4] had established rubella control and congenital rubella syndrome prevention or elimination goals.

PATHOBIOLOGY

Rubella

Rubella virus is transmitted through person-to-person spread by droplets shed from the respiratory secretions of infected persons. The first point of entry is the nasopharynx, where replication occurs and then spreads to the lymph nodes. Subsequent viremia may seed multiple organs, including the placenta. Viremia occurs between 8 and 9 days after exposure and peaks at 10 to 17 days, just before the onset of the rash, which usually occurs 16 to 18 days after exposure. Although individuals with rubella are considered to be only moderately contagious, they may shed virus from 7 days before the onset of the rash to approximately 5 to 7 days or more after its disappearance. Persons with both clinical and subclinical infections are considered contagious.

Congenital Rubella

Rubella virus viremia can infect the placenta of pregnant women, and viral replication can infect all fetal organs. In tissue specimens, infections with rubella virus have diverse effects, ranging from small foci of infected cells in apparently normal tissue to hypoplasia, generalized vasculitis, and cell destruction. The hallmark of fetal infection is chronic infection that persists throughout fetal life, with shedding of virus up to 1 year of age.

Infants with congenital rubella syndrome may shed large quantities of virus from body secretions, particularly from the throat. Rubella virus can be found in the nasopharyngeal secretions of more than 80% of infected infants during the first month of life. Rubella virus is found in 11% of infected infants between 9 and 12 months of age and in only 3% in the second year of life. Viral shedding by infants with congenital rubella syndrome can result in nosocomial outbreaks, so only individuals immune to rubella virus should be in contact with infants with congenital rubella syndrome or with congenital infection even in the absence of clinical signs of congenital rubella syndrome.

CLINICAL MANIFESTATIONS

Postnatally Acquired Rubella

Acquired rubella, which occurs in 50 to 80% of persons infected with rubella virus, is characterized by a generalized maculopapular rash that usually persists for 1 to 3 days (Fig. 344-1). The rash usually starts on the face and neck and progresses downward. The rash is fainter than the rash of measles (Chapter 343) and does not coalesce. Because of the mildness of the rash, it may be difficult to detect in persons with darker skin. Children usually have few or no prodromal symptoms, so the rash is usually the first sign of illness. However,

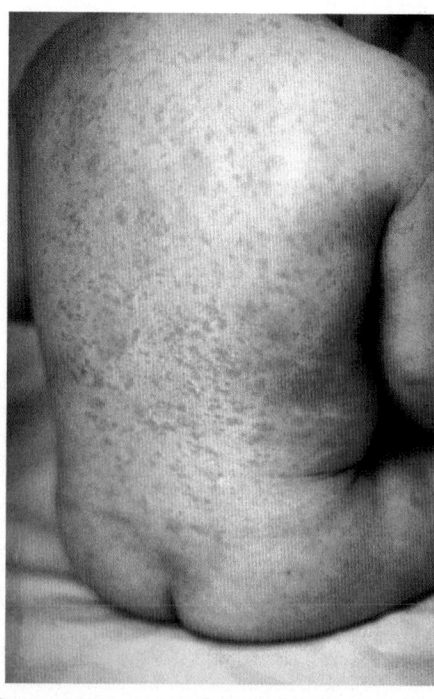

FIGURE 344-1. Rash of rubella on the skin of a child's back. The distribution is similar to that of measles, but the lesions are less intensely red. (From the Centers for Disease Control and Prevention Public Health Image Library, ID #: 712.)

in older children and adults, a 1- to 5-day prodrome of low-grade fever, malaise, and upper respiratory symptoms often precedes the rash. The incubation period is 14 days, with a range of 12 to 23 days. Lymphadenopathy, particularly occipital and postauricular, may be noted during the second week after exposure.

Rubella disease is usually mild and results in few complications. Arthralgia and arthritis are commonly observed in infected adults, particularly in postpubertal females. Other less common complications are thrombocytopenia (one in 3000 rubella cases) and encephalitis (one in 6000 rubella cases).

Congenital Rubella Syndrome

The most serious consequences of rubella virus infection occur when a woman becomes infected during pregnancy, particularly during the first trimester.[5] Complications can include miscarriage, fetal death, or a live birth with a constellation of congenital defects known as congenital rubella syndrome. The most common defects of congenital rubella syndrome affect the eyes (e.g., cataracts, pigmentary retinopathy, microphthalmos, congenital glaucoma), the ears (e.g., sensorineural hearing impairment), and the heart (e.g., patent ductus arteriosus, pulmonary arterial stenosis). Other clinical manifestations of congenital rubella syndrome may include microcephaly, developmental delay, and purpura, including dermal erythropoiesis (blueberry muffin syndrome).

Among pregnant women infected with rubella virus during the first 10 weeks of gestation, up to 90% of their live born infants may have congenital rubella syndrome. Among women infected during the first 20 weeks of pregnancy, the rate of congenital rubella syndrome in live born infants is 20%. Infants who are born with rubella virus infection but who do not have any apparent signs or symptoms of congenital rubella syndrome are referred to as infants with congenital rubella infection only.

DIAGNOSIS

Postnatally Acquired Rubella

Because many rash illnesses may mimic rubella virus infection and because 20 to 50% of rubella virus infections may be subclinical, laboratory testing is the only way to confirm the diagnosis. Some illnesses with clinical presentation similar to that of rubella include scarlet fever (Chapter 410), roseola (Chapter 410), fifth disease (Chapter 347), and measles (Chapter 343).

During the first 4 days after the onset of the rash, rubella RNA detection by reverse transcription–polymerase chain reaction (RT-PCR) is the most sensitive way to make the diagnosis.[6] For later diagnosis, serologic immunoglobulin M (IgM) antibodies are generally detectable for up to 6 weeks after the onset of the rash. Late diagnosis also can be made on the basis of a significant rise in the IgG antibody titer in paired acute and convalescent specimens. The acute serum specimen should be collected within 7 to 10 days after the onset of the rash, and the convalescent serum specimen should be collected 14 to 21 days after the first specimen.

Rubella virus can be isolated from the nasopharynx (i.e., nasal, throat), blood, urine, and cerebrospinal fluid specimens of persons with rubella and congenital rubella syndrome. The most frequently positive results are from throat swabs. Rubella virus can be isolated during the prodromal period and up to 2 weeks after onset of the rash. For viral cultures, specimens should be obtained during the time of maximum virus secretion—up to 4 days after the onset of rash.

Diagnosis in Pregnant Women

In the United States, all pregnant women should be screened for rubella IgG antibodies as part of routine prenatal care. Pregnant women who have a positive serologic test result for IgG antibody to rubella virus are considered to be immune if they do not have a recent history of exposure to rubella virus. Susceptible pregnant women should be vaccinated postpartum. Pregnant women exposed to rubella virus should be evaluated for evidence of acute infection by testing for presence of IgM antibodies in sera or a significant rise of IgG antibodies in acute and convalescent sera. Pregnant women with evidence of acute infection should be monitored clinically and evaluated for gestational age at infection to assess the risk for fetal infection.

Congenital Rubella

Diagnosis of congenital rubella syndrome in infants can be confirmed by either serologic or virologic methods. Serum IgM antibodies may be present in an infant with congenital rubella syndrome for up to a year after birth; however, IgM antibody may not be detectable during the first month of life. Thus, infants who are younger than 1 month and who have symptoms consistent with congenital rubella syndrome should be retested at 1 month of age. Congenital rubella syndrome also can be confirmed by documentation of a persistent rubella serum IgG titer beyond the time expected from passive transfer of maternal IgG antibody (i.e., a rubella titer that does not decline at the expected rate of a two-fold dilution per month).

Rubella virus from congenitally infected infants can be isolated most commonly from throat swabs and less commonly from urine and cerebrospinal fluid specimens. Infants with congenital rubella may excrete virus for up to 1 year, but specimens for virus isolation are most likely to be positive if they are obtained within the first 6 months after birth. Rubella virus in infants with congenital rubella syndrome also can be detected by RT-PCR with use of the same specimens as for viral isolation.

TREATMENT ℞

There is no specific treatment of rubella or congenital rubella syndrome. For persons with rubella, symptomatic treatment may be warranted for clinical manifestations such as arthralgias, myalgias, and fever. Infants with congenital rubella syndrome should be evaluated and treated by specialists for their specific clinical manifestations.

PREVENTION

Passive Immunization

Administration of immune globulin after exposure to rubella virus will not prevent infection or viremia but might modify or suppress symptoms. Therefore, immune globulin is not recommended for routine postexposure prophylaxis of rubella in any circumstance.

Active Immunization

One dose of live attenuated rubella vaccine (RA 27/3, RCV) induces rubella IgG antibody seroconversion in 95% or more of persons. Immunity is considered long term, probably lifelong. RCV is available as a monovalent formulation or in combination with measles-mumps (MMR) and measles-mumps-varicella (MMRV) vaccines (Chapter 15).

In the United States, the routine rubella vaccination policy is to immunize children with the first dose of MMR at 12 to 15 months of age and to provide a second dose at 4 to 6 years of age. The MMRV vaccine also can be given to children up to age 12 years. Persons who were born in 1957 or later and who do not have a medical contraindication (e.g., pregnancy) should receive at least one dose of MMR unless they have documentation of one dose of live rubella virus vaccine or laboratory evidence of immunity or laboratory confirmation of disease. A third vaccination in early adulthood can seroconvert the majority of individuals who were seronegative despite earlier vaccination.[7] High-risk groups who should be targeted for vaccination include health care personnel, persons attending post–high school educational facilities, the military, international travelers, and nonpregnant women of childbearing age.

In follow-up studies of more than 2700 susceptible women who were unknowingly pregnant and who received a live attenuated rubella vaccine, none of their infants was born with congenital rubella syndrome. Nevertheless, because of the theoretical risk for congenital rubella syndrome in infants born to pregnant women vaccinated with RCV, the vaccine should not be given to pregnant women, and pregnancy should be avoided for at least 28 days after receipt of vaccine. Receipt of RCV during pregnancy is not generally considered to be an indication for termination of pregnancy.

PROGNOSIS

Because rubella is usually a mild disease, the prognosis is excellent, with complete recovery in almost all persons. Deaths are seen in 0 to 50% of patients who develop rubella encephalitis. The prognosis for infants with congenital rubella syndrome is dependent on their clinical manifestations and access to quality medical care.

GENERAL REFERENCES

For the General References and other additional features, please visit Expert Consult at https://expertconsult.inkling.com.

345

MUMPS

MANISHA PATEL AND JOHN W. GNANN, JR.

DEFINITION

Mumps is an acute systemic viral infection that occurs most commonly in children, is usually self-limited, and is clinically characterized by nonsuppurative parotitis.

The Pathogen

Mumps virus is a member of the family Paramyxoviridae. Mumps virions are pleomorphic, roughly spherical enveloped particles with an average diameter of 200 nm. Glycoprotein spikes project from the surface of the envelope. A helical nucleocapsid composed of nucleoproteins and of linear, nonsegmented, single-stranded, negative-sense RNA approximately 15.3 kilobases in size encodes seven major proteins as well as several minor proteins. Humans are the only natural hosts for mumps virus, although infection can be induced experimentally in a variety of mammalian species. In vitro, mumps virus can be cultured in many mammalian cell lines and in embryonated hens' eggs. Though mumps is considered a monotypic virus, 12 genotypes of mumps have been designated based on sequence heterogeneity within the viral genome.

EPIDEMIOLOGY

During the pre-vaccine era, mumps was primarily a disease of school-aged children (5 to 9 years), with 90% of urban children infected by age 14 years. Although the reported incidence in the United States peaked in 1942 with 251 cases per 100,000 population, mumps was an endemic disease with seasonal activity highest between January and May, resulting in millions of cases annually. Following licensure of live mumps vaccine in 1967, the incidence of mumps decreased to 88 cases per 100,000 population in 1968. In 1985, only 2982 cases of mumps were reported, an incidence of 1.3 per 100,000 population, which represented a 98% decline from the number of cases reported in 1968. A resurgence occurred from 1986 to 1987 during which 20,621 cases were reported, with more than half among older children and adolescents 10 to 19 years of age, thereby suggesting an immunity gap from either lack of vaccination or disease exposure. Following the resurgence, sporadic outbreaks of mumps in secondary schools were attributed to vaccine failure among one-dose recipients. After 1989, when the Centers for Disease Control and Prevention (CDC) Advisory Committee on Immunization Practices (ACIP) issued a recommendation that all children receive a second dose of the measles-mumps-rubella (MMR) vaccine at the time of school entry to improve measles control, the incidence of mumps was again reduced to 1.0 per 100,000 population by 1992. Rates continued to decline until 2006, when a second resurgence in the central United States increased the incidence to 2.2 cases per 100,000 population, primarily in college students vaccinated with two doses. In response to this resurgence, ACIP recommended two doses of MMR for high-risk adults, including health care workers, international travelers and students at post–high school educational institutions. In 2010, another mumps outbreak resulted in 3500 cases in New York and New Jersey, with the highest rate among boys 13 to 17 years of age who attended tradition-observant Jewish schools; about 90% of cases had received at least two doses of a mumps-containing vaccine, thereby suggesting their illness was because of intense exposure, particularly among boys in school. In another outbreak in New York City, 90% of cases had received at least one dose of vaccine, with 77% having received two doses. The effectiveness of a two-dose regimen for preventing mumps was 86%. In an outbreak in Guam during 2009 and 2010, 287 of 505 mumps cases occurred among school-aged children, even though 93% had received two doses of vaccine; crowding at home and high student contact rates were identified as risk factors for transmission. A third resurgence occurred in 2016 to 2017 due to outbreaks in settings where prolonged, close personal contact was common, such as college campuses.[1] The highest incidence was among young adults 18 to 24 years of age; more than 80% of cases with known vaccination status had received at least 2 doses.[2] Although primary vaccine failure (insufficient initial protective immune response) does occur, secondary vaccine failure (waning immunity) is a risk factor when exposure to infection is high, such as in outbreaks occurring in close contact settings.[3] These findings suggest the need for a novel mumps vaccine with a longer duration of protection.

PATHOBIOLOGY

Mumps is highly contagious and can be transmitted experimentally by inoculation of virus onto the nasal or buccal mucosa, suggesting that most natural infections result from droplet spread of upper respiratory secretions. The mean incubation period for mumps is 18 days. Primary viral replication takes place in epithelial cells of the upper respiratory tract, followed by spread of virus to regional lymph nodes and subsequent viremia. Because virus can be isolated from saliva for 5 to 7 days before and up to 9 days after the onset of clinical symptoms, an infected individual is potentially able to transmit mumps for up to 2 weeks.

Transient IgM antibody responses are detected early in the course of mumps infection, followed by the appearance of IgG antibody and cytotoxic T lymphocytes. Mumps-specific IgG can be detected during the first week of acute infection, peaks at 3 to 4 weeks, and persists for decades.

CLINICAL MANIFESTATIONS

During the pre-vaccine era, an estimated 30% of mumps infections in children were subclinical or associated only with nonspecific upper respiratory infection symptoms; rates of subclinical infection among highly vaccinated populations are unknown but are likely higher.

Parotitis

Mumps usually begins with a short prodromal phase of low-grade fever, malaise, headache, and anorexia.[4] Young children may complain of ear pain initially. The characteristic parotid tenderness and enlargement, in which the earlobe is lifted forward and obscures the angle of the mandible, then develops (Fig. 345-1). The parotid glands are involved most commonly, although other salivary glands may occasionally be enlarged. Parotitis may initially be unilateral, with swelling of the contralateral parotid gland occurring 2 to 3 days later in 90% of cases. Painful parotid gland enlargement progresses for a period of about 3 days, followed by defervescence and resolution of the parotid pain and swelling within about 7 days.

Aseptic Meningitis

Symptomatic meningitis occurs in up to 10% of cases; about 50% of patients with mumps parotitis have cerebrospinal fluid (CSF) pleocytosis without clinical evidence of meningitis. Signs and symptoms of meningeal inflammation (headache, neck stiffness, vomiting, and lethargy) plus high fever usually develop 4 to 5 days after the onset of parotitis, although the meningitis may occasionally precede the parotitis. Indeed, 40 to 50% of all cases of documented mumps meningitis occur in patients who never exhibit clinical parotitis. For unexplained reasons, symptomatic central nervous system (CNS) involvement with mumps is two to three times more common in boys than in girls. Examination of CSF usually reveals normal opening pressure and a mononuclear cell pleocytosis with an average cell count of 450/μL. Polymorphonuclear leukocyte predominance in CSF may be seen in some patients early during the course of mumps meningitis. CSF protein is generally normal or mildly elevated (<100 mg/dL). Hypoglycorrhachia, which is not usually seen in viral meningitis, may be present in 10 to 30% of patients with mumps meningitis.

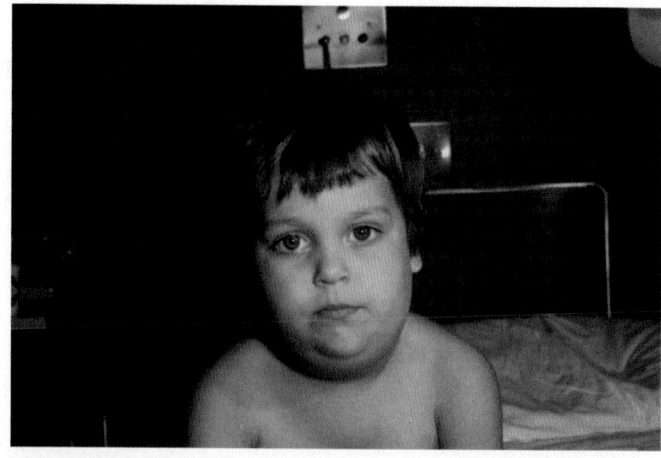

FIGURE 345-1. Mumps. Child with submandibular swelling due to mumps parotitis. (From the Centers for Disease Control and Prevention Public Health Image Library, ID #: 4491.)

Mumps virus can be recovered from CSF. Whereas the symptoms of mumps meningitis typically resolve within 7 to 10 days, the CSF abnormalities may persist for up to 5 weeks.

Encephalitis

The spectrum of mumps-induced CNS disease ranges from mild "aseptic" meningitis (which is common) to severe encephalitis (which is rare). Some cases of encephalitis develop concurrently with the parotitis and are thought to result from direct extension of viral infection from the choroid plexus ependyma into parenchymal neurons. Other cases of mumps encephalitis occur 1 to 2 weeks after the onset of parotitis and may represent a demyelinating postinfectious encephalitis. Clinical findings in mumps encephalitis include obtundation (and less commonly delirium), generalized seizures, and high fever. Other neurologic findings can include focal seizures, aphasia, paresis, and involuntary movements.

Orchitis

Epididymo-orchitis is rare in young boys with mumps, but it occurs in 15 to 35% of postpubertal males with mumps. Orchitis is most often unilateral (bilateral involvement occurs in 17 to 38% of cases) and results from replication of mumps virus in the seminiferous tubules, with resulting lymphocytic infiltration and edema. Orchitis typically develops within 1 week of the onset of parotitis, although orchitis, like mumps meningitis, can develop before or even in the absence of parotitis. Mumps orchitis is characterized by marked testicular swelling and severe pain accompanied by fever, nausea, and headache. The pain and swelling resolve within 5 to 7 days, but residual testicular tenderness can persist for weeks. Testicular atrophy may follow orchitis in 35 to 50% of cases; however, sterility is an uncommon complication, even in men with bilateral orchitis.

Other Manifestations

Mumps can cause inflammation of other glandular tissues, including pancreatitis and thyroiditis. Oophoritis and mastitis have been reported in postpubertal women with mumps. Transient renal function abnormalities are common in mumps, and virus can be isolated readily from urine; significant renal damage is rare, however. Other infrequent manifestations of mumps include sensorineural deafness (either transient or permanent), arthritis, myocarditis, and thrombocytopenia. Whether maternal mumps infection during the first trimester of pregnancy results in an increased frequency of spontaneous abortions is unclear, and no evidence has linked maternal mumps to congenital malformations.

DIAGNOSIS

The diagnosis of mumps is usually based on clinical findings in a child with fever and parotitis, particularly if the individual is known to be susceptible and has been exposed to mumps during the preceding 2 to 3 weeks. An atypical clinical presentation (e.g., meningitis or orchitis without parotitis) requires laboratory confirmation. Culturing for mumps virus has largely been replaced by reverse transcription-polymerase chain reaction (RT-PCR) assays. Detection of mumps virus by RT-PCR or a positive mumps virus culture is confirmatory. Serologic demonstration of mumps immunoglobulin M (IgM) can also aid in the diagnosis of mumps, although false negatives can occur, particularly in previously vaccinated persons. IgM is detectable during the first week of illness and persists for at least 6 weeks but may be more transient in vaccinated persons. Detection of IgM is improved if serum specimens are collected longer than 3 days after the onset of symptoms. Seroconversion or a significant rise in IgG antibody titer in acute and convalescent sera can also be diagnostic but can be more challenging to detect in vaccinated persons whose IgG titers may already be high. About 30% of patients have an elevated serum amylase level that may be due to parotitis or pancreatitis.

The differential diagnosis of a mumps-like syndrome includes infections caused by other viruses, such as Epstein-Barr virus (Chapter 353), human herpesvirus type 6, adenovirus (Chapter 341), influenza A virus (Chapter 340), parainfluenza virus (Chapter 339), coxsackievirus (Chapter 355), or lymphocytic choriomeningitis virus. Among 101 sporadic cases of parotitis assessed in the United States in 2009 to 2011, for example, the most commonly detected viruses were Epstein-Barr virus (23%) and human herpesvirus type 6 (10%); mumps virus was not detected in any specimens, although 17% of cases demonstrated positive mumps IgM. More recently, several hundred cases of influenza A (H3N2)-associated parotitis were reported during the 2014-2015 influenza season.[5] Bacteria such as *Staphylococcus aureus* can cause suppurative parotitis. Parotid gland enlargement can also occur in patients

with AIDS, particularly children. Parotid gland enlargement can also be associated with Sjögren syndrome (Chapter 252), sarcoidosis (Chapter 89), amyloidosis (Chapter 179), thiazide ingestion, iodine sensitivity, tumor, or salivary duct obstruction. Careful examination should distinguish parotitis from lymphadenopathy.

TREATMENT

Management of a patient with mumps consists of conservative measures to provide symptomatic relief, adequate hydration, and nutrition. Treatment of orchitis includes bed rest, scrotal support, analgesics, and ice packs. Patients with significant CNS involvement require hospitalization for observation and supportive care. There is currently no established role for antiviral drugs, interferon, corticosteroids, or passive immunotherapy in the treatment of mumps.

PREVENTION

The cornerstone of mumps prevention is active immunization with the live attenuated mumps vaccine (Chapter 15). In the United States, mumps vaccine is administered in combination with the measles and rubella vaccines (MMR) to children at 12 to 15 months of age, with a second dose at 4 to 6 years of age.[6] The median vaccine effectiveness is estimated to be 78% (range 49 to 91%) for 1 dose of MMR and 88% (range 31 to 95%) for 2 doses. Most adults (>90%) born in the United States before 1957 were naturally infected and are therefore immune, but the mumps vaccine is indicated for susceptible adults. High-risk adults such as health care personnel, international travelers, and students attending colleges or other post–high school educational institutions should receive two doses of MMR if they do not have other evidence of presumptive immunity. Administration of the live mumps vaccine is contraindicated in pregnant women. Vaccination is also not recommended in persons who have received immunoglobulin therapy, which might interfere with the immune response to the vaccine, within the preceding 3 months or in persons with severe systemic immunosuppression caused by disease or medical therapy.

The Jeryl-Lynn (JL) strain of attenuated mumps virus used in the United States since 1967 is a very well-tolerated vaccine, although rare instances of fever, parotitis, and possibly aseptic meningitis have been reported after immunization. Beginning in 1988, an increased frequency of cases of vaccine-related mumps meningitis was recognized in other countries. These cases occurred after the administration of MMR vaccines containing other mumps strains, such as Urabe AM9 or Leningrad 3. This problem has not been seen in the United States, where the JL mumps vaccine strain continues to be used. Despite genotypic differences in the JL mumps vaccine strain (genotype A) and the currently predominant circulating strain in the United States (genotype G), sera from persons vaccinated with the JL mumps vaccine strain effectively neutralize genotype G mumps strains.

Questions about prevention often arise when an individual with no history of mumps disease or vaccination is exposed to a patient with active mumps. Presumptive immunity of the exposed individual can be determined by serologic testing (mumps IgG by ELISA). However, neither the presence nor the level of mumps-specific IgG can fully predict protection against mumps disease, although sera from cases tend to have lower preexposure neutralizing antibody titers and lower mumps-specific IgG concentrations compared with sera from noncases. Further, only moderate correlation is seen between the level of mumps-specific IgG serum antibodies and virus-neutralizing antibody responses. It is possible that the level of immunity required to protect against classic clinical mumps illness depends on the initial inoculum of virus, so that protection at a particular antibody titer may not be absolute.

In intense exposure settings, in which outbreaks occur with evidence of ongoing transmission despite high two-dose vaccination coverage, a third dose of measles-mumps-rubella vaccine is beneficial and is recommended by the U.S. Centers for Disease Control and Prevention for groups determined by public health to be at risk for mumps and its complications.[7-9] Mumps vaccine can be safely administered to an individual of unknown immune status, although the efficacy of postexposure vaccination for preventing mumps has not been determined.

For infection control purposes, patients with mumps require both standard precautions and droplet precautions for at least 5 days after the onset of parotitis. In the outpatient setting, a patient with suspected mumps should wear a mask and be isolated from other potentially susceptible persons. When a patient with mumps is hospitalized, a private room is required; caregivers should wear masks, and the patient should wear a mask while being transported.

PROGNOSIS

Long-term sequelae of mumps parotitis are uncommon. Complications and hospitalization rates are lower among vaccinated patients compared with unvaccinated persons. Mumps meningitis is generally benign, and significant neurologic complications are rare. Recovery from mumps encephalitis is generally complete, although complications such as aqueductal stenosis with hydrocephalus, seizure disorders, and psychomotor retardation have been reported. The overall mortality rate from mumps encephalitis is 1.5%. Lifelong immunity follows natural infection, although symptomatic reinfection can occasionally occur.

GENERAL REFERENCES

For the General References and other additional features, please visit Expert Consult at https://expertconsult.inkling.com.

346

CYTOMEGALOVIRUS, EPSTEIN-BARR VIRUS, AND SLOW VIRUS INFECTIONS OF THE CENTRAL NERVOUS SYSTEM

JOSEPH R. BERGER AND AVINDRA NATH

● CYTOMEGALOVIRUS INFECTION

Human cytomegalovirus (CMV) is a ubiquitous herpesvirus that is acquired throughout life (Chapter 352). In children, CMV is an important[1] and relatively common cause of congenital neurologic deficits. In the United States, seroprevalence rates are 40% in adolescents and 60 to 90% in adults. Primary infection is usually asymptomatic in young, healthy adults but may be associated with a transient mononucleosis-like syndrome. CMV results in major neurologic disability in the setting of immunosuppression, particularly in transplant recipients, in persons with acquired immunodeficiency syndrome (AIDS), and in those with hematologic malignant neoplasms. CMV may involve the meninges, brain, spinal cord, peripheral nerves, and muscle. Additionally, as with some other herpes viruses, notably, varicella zoster virus (VZV) and herpes simplex virus 1 and 2 (HSV), CMV is a cause of retinitis and acute retinal necrosis.

Cytomegalovirus Encephalitis

In patients with AIDS, CMV encephalitis generally occurs only in the presence of profound immunosuppression (CD4 T lymphocyte counts <100 cells/μL). The most typical presentation in patients with AIDS is a subacute, diffuse encephalopathy evolving over a period of weeks and characterized by headache, impaired cognition and sensorium, apathy, and social withdrawal. Virtually all patients with CMV encephalitis have systemic CMV infection. Neurologic examination reveals abnormal mentation and variable motor features, including hyperreflexia, ataxia, and weakness. CMV ventriculitis is characteristically present, and progressive ventricular enlargement may be observed. Other features may suggest brain stem encephalitis, including internuclear ophthalmoplegia, nystagmus, cranial nerve palsies, gaze paresis, ataxia, and quadriparesis. Cerebral infarction resulting from CMV vasculitis, acute subarachnoid hemorrhage, and intracerebral hemorrhage may be observed. CMV myelitis, polyradiculitis, and multifocal neuritis may also occur with CMV encephalitis. Distinctive retinal lesions may be seen ophthalmoscopically (Chapter 352) and serve as a useful diagnostic clue. CMV can also be vertically transmitted and cause a congenital infection in the fetus resulting in the classic triad of chorioretinitis, microcephaly, and cerebral calcifications.

Cerebral imaging studies are of limited sensitivity and low specificity in patients with CMV encephalitis. Ependymal or meningeal enhancement as well as areas of focal infarction or necrosis may be visualized. Magnetic resonance imaging (MRI) may show restricted diffusion and high T2 signal intensity lesions lining the ependyma of the lateral ventricles. Progressive ventricular enlargement is suggestive of CMV ventriculitis. Rarely, CMV infection may be manifested as a cerebral mass lesion.

Cerebrospinal fluid (CSF) findings are variable. Most patients have elevated protein levels and a CSF pleocytosis, but leukocytes may be absent and glucose levels may be normal or decreased. In contrast to other viral infections that usually cause a lymphocytic predominance in the CSF, a marked pleocytosis with a polymorphonuclear leukocyte preponderance may occur in patients with CMV ventriculoencephalitis. CMV can rarely be cultured from CSF. CSF real-time polymerase chain reaction (PCR) for CMV has a high sensitivity and specificity; nonetheless, the diagnosis is often difficult and relies on a high index of clinical suspicion. CMV serology is not helpful for diagnosing an active infection. Histopathologic examination reveals multinucleate cells with intranuclear cytomegalic inclusions (Fig. 346-1).

Myelitis

CMV transverse myelitis, which may be seen in both immunocompetent and immunosuppressed patients, is indistinguishable neurologically from other forms of transverse myelitis (Chapters 372 and 383).[2] A severe necrotizing CMV myelitis, which is usually longitudinally extensive and involves several spinal segments, may occur in the immunosuppressed host, particularly with human immunodeficiency virus (HIV) infection, and is commonly associated with polyradiculitis. Some cases of necrotizing myelitis in the absence of a typical polyradiculitis syndrome have been described, with patients displaying acute or progressive paraplegia and disturbances in urinary and rectal sphincter function. Reflexes are preserved or enhanced in the legs unless concurrent

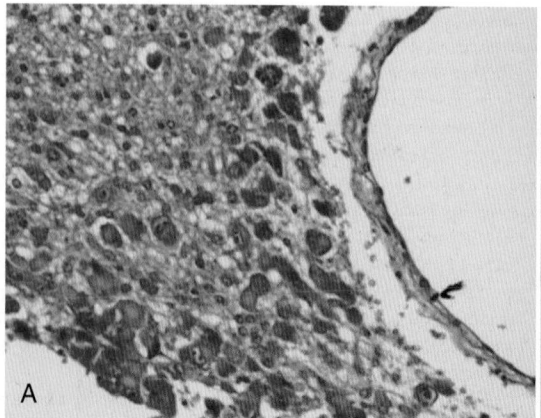
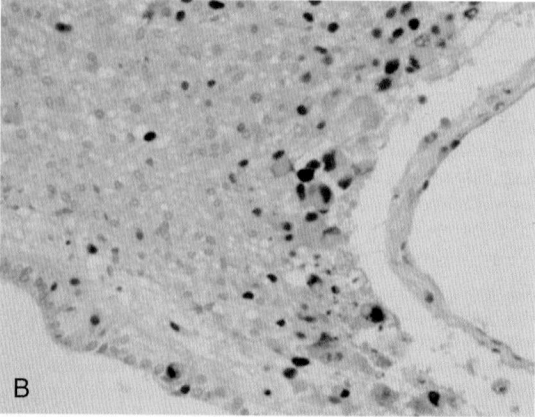

FIGURE 346-1. Pathology of CMV encephalitis. **A,** Large cells are seen in the perivascular region, some are multinucleated. **B,** The cytomegalic inclusions are present in the nucleus and stain with an antibody to CMV (brown). Magnification is 40×. (Courtesy Martha Quezado, National Institutes of Health, Bethesda, MD.)

neuropathy is present. A sensory level may be demonstrable. The combination of radicular complaints and a CSF polymorphonuclear pleocytosis may serve as a clue to the diagnosis. As with CMV encephalitis, the diagnosis is best established by CSF PCR for CMV.

Polyradiculomyelitis

Before the era of highly active antiretrovirals, as many as 25% of patients dying of AIDS had neuromuscular disease from CMV, predominantly localized to the perineurial and epineurial regions. CMV polyradiculomyelitis in HIV-infected patients is manifested subacutely during a period of days to weeks. Initial symptoms of paresthesias or dysesthetic pain localized to the perineum and lower extremities are followed by rapidly progressive paraparesis with hypotonia and diminished or absent lower extremity reflexes. Urinary retention is characteristic, and rectal sphincter incontinence is common. Variable sensory findings are typically overshadowed by weakness. Babinski signs and diminished sensation below a discrete level across the trunk are evidence of an associated myelitis. With time, symptoms progress by ascending to involve the upper limbs and sometimes the cranial nerves. CSF examination generally shows polymorphonuclear pleocytosis, prominent elevation of protein levels, and a low glucose level. Spinal magnetic resonance imaging (MRI) may be normal or show enhancement of the conus medullaris, cauda equina, meninges, and nerve roots. Electrophysiologic studies reveal axonal neuropathy with evidence of acute denervation. Variable slowing of nerve conduction may occur.

The appearance of acute cauda equina syndrome in a patient with AIDS or in a solid organ or bone marrow transplant recipient is suggestive of CMV infection, particularly when a polymorphonuclear pleocytosis is present in CSF; however, the syndrome is not pathognomonic. Other conditions that may produce a cauda equina syndrome in AIDS patients include lymphomatous meningitis, syphilis, toxoplasmosis, other herpesvirus infections, and cryptococcal or bacterial meningitis. Progressive multifocal motor and sensory neuropathy that evolves during a period of weeks to months has also been seen in patients with CMV infection. Paresthesia and dysesthesia are quickly followed by prominent motor weakness involving both the upper and lower limbs asymmetrically. Neurogenic atrophy may be prominent. Nerve biopsy reveals necrotizing neuritis with mononuclear and polymorphonuclear infiltrates and cytomegalocytes localized around endoneurial capillaries in the nerve trunks and roots. Some patients may have necrotizing arteritis. As with CMV encephalitis and myelitis, PCR for CMV in CSF is the most helpful diagnostic measure.

TREATMENT   Rx

CMV neurologic complications should be treated with ganciclovir (5 mg/kg intravenously every 12 hours) plus foscarnet (60 mg/kg intravenously every 8 hours or 90 mg/kg intravenously every 12 hours until symptomatic improvement), followed by maintenance therapy with oral valganciclovir (900 mg daily) and intravenous foscarnet (90 to 120 mg/kg intravenously during 2 hours, every 24 hours); however, evidence of efficacy in these conditions is limited chiefly to case reports and small series. Neither drug penetrates the CNS well. Cidofovir is a second-line agent (5 mg/kg by intravenous infusion during 1 hour once a week for 2 consecutive weeks, with saline hydration and probenecid, 2 g orally 3 hours before the dose and 1 g orally at 2 hours and 8 hours after the dose). CMV strains resistant to these agents have emerged, and CMV encephalitis has developed in the presence of maintenance ganciclovir therapy for CMV retinitis. Combination therapy (foscarnet and ganciclovir) or different drugs should be considered in patients already undergoing suppressive monotherapy or in those with persistent CSF pleocytosis. Maintenance therapy, which is the same regimen given every other week, is required unless the patient experiences immune reconstitution, such as after highly active antiretroviral therapy (HAART) in an AIDS patient or discontinuation of immunosuppressive regimens in a transplant or cancer patient. Intravitreal treatment of CMV retinitis permits higher targeted concentrations of the antiviral agent. Ganciclovir implants have demonstrated effective long-term local control of the retinitis. Other agents (foscarnet, cidofovir, and fomivirsen) require weekly intravitreal injections.

PROGNOSIS

The prognosis for long-term survival, especially with AIDS, is very poor, and most patients have only limited neurologic recovery.

● EPSTEIN-BARR VIRUS INFECTION

Epstein-Barr virus (EBV), the major cause of infectious mononucleosis (Chapter 353), is distributed worldwide. Individuals in areas of high population density

and lower social strata acquire the virus in early childhood. However, sero-epidemiologic studies indicate that more than 90% of people are infected by EBV by 30 years of age.

Neurologic manifestations occur in 1 to 5% of patients with primary EBV infection and may be the predominant clinical finding. The most common neurologic disorder associated with infectious mononucleosis is meningoencephalitis, which is rare in early childhood and is most often observed in persons between the ages of 15 and 25 years. Its onset may be gradual during a span of several days or be explosive. Fever, headache, mild stiff neck, confusion, lethargy, seizures, and hyperreflexia are the most typical features. Some patients may present predominantly with ataxia, cerebellitis, or other focal neurologic features, including hemiparesis, focal seizures, and brain stem findings. Hyperintense signal abnormalities on T2-weighted and fluid attenuated inversion recovery (FLAIR) cranial MRI are frequently observed but are nondiagnostic. PCR for EBV in CSF and comparison of levels of antibody to EBV in the serum and CSF may be diagnostically useful.

Ganciclovir treatment (10 mg/kg/day intravenously for 3 weeks followed by 1000 mg/day orally for another 3 weeks or until the virus is cleared) has been used in some cases but is of unproven value. The prognosis for patients with EBV meningoencephalitis is excellent, often with complete resolution in 1 to 2 weeks.

Another neurologic consequence of EBV observed in immunosuppressed patients, especially in AIDS, is primary central nervous system lymphoma. As many as 90% of primary central nervous system lymphomas in this population are associated with EBV, although they are very rarely observed in immune-competent individuals.

● SLOW VIRUS INFECTIONS OF THE CENTRAL NERVOUS SYSTEM

Human T-Lymphotropic Virus Type 1 and Human Immunodeficiency Virus

These viruses and their neurologic sequelae are considered in Chapters 354 and 366, respectively.

Subacute Sclerosing Panencephalitis

EPIDEMIOLOGY AND PATHOBIOLOGY

Subacute sclerosing panencephalitis (SSPE), which is caused by the measles virus (Chapter 343), usually affects children, but can present in young adulthood.[3] Patients generally have a history of measles within the first 2 years of life, and it is speculated that such early host exposure allows the emergence of persistent but defective virus replication because the SSPE virus genome, particularly the matrix gene, differs from wild-type measles. SSPE occurs after a latency period of months to years following acute measles infection. As a result of effective vaccination strategies against measles virus, the incidence of SSPE has decreased markedly to about 4 to 5 cases per year in the United States. However, the disease still persists in certain areas of the world (e.g., the Indian subcontinent and the Middle East) owing to low rates of measles vaccination.

Gray matter is most prominently involved. The pathologic features of SSPE include gliosis, loss of myelin, and perivascular infiltrates of lymphocytes and plasma cells in white and gray matter. Neuronal cell loss is seen in later stages of the illness. Intranuclear Cowdry type A inclusions containing viral nucleocapsids are identified in neurons and glia.

CLINICAL MANIFESTATIONS AND DIAGNOSIS

SSPE usually begins with cognitive and behavioral changes such as irritability and emotional lability; cortical blindness is often an early feature. Macular retinitis may also be an early manifestation. Progression is associated with motor dysfunction, including prominent myoclonus with prominent axial musculature involvement, cognitive decline, choreoathetosis, dystonia, and rigidity. Its course progresses during a period of 1 to 3 years to rigid quadriparesis and a vegetative state, frequently accompanied by autonomic features, such as hyperthermia, excessive sweating, and altered pulse and blood pressure. The condition affects boys more often than girls. Retinal changes such as macular retinitis and pigmentary changes can precede the neurologic manifestations by several months.

The electroencephalogram typically reveals unilateral or bilateral periodic complexes with synchronous bursts of two or three high-amplitude slow waves per second, with recurrence at regular intervals of 5 to 8 seconds and a 1 : 1 relationship with myoclonic jerks. MRI of the brain shows high signal intensity lesions that are diffuse in the subcortical and periventricular white matter with cortical atrophy, but also rarely may involve the basal ganglia and brain stem. In early stages of the illness, the MRI may be normal. Computed tomography (CT) of the brain shows generalized atrophy. CSF protein, glucose, and cell levels are usually normal; CSF is characterized by a high immunoglobulin concentration, oligoclonal bands, and intrathecal synthesis of antibody to measles virus antigens. Serum measles antibody titers are also high. These findings are usually sufficiently characteristic for diagnosis, but measles RNA can be detected in the brain by PCR. Rarely, brain biopsy is needed for definitive diagnosis in atypical cases. Measles virus may also cause subacute encephalitis in an immunocompromised host. The prominence of cognitive and motor dysfunction in these patients resembles that of SSPE, but in the clinical setting, its subacute onset and more rapid evolution and the presence of generalized seizures rather than myoclonus are distinctive. Brain abnormalities include abundant intranuclear inclusions, but inflammation is minimal, and neither serum nor CSF antibody titers against measles virus are high. For this reason, brain biopsy is generally needed for diagnosis.

TREATMENT AND PROGNOSIS Rx

There is no established, unequivocally effective treatment of SSPE, but arrest of the disease has been reported in some patients with SSPE after long-term treatment with intrathecal interferon-α with intravenous ribavirin or oral inosine pranobex. About 5% of patients remit spontaneously, but SSPE progresses inexorably to coma, brain stem involvement, and death in 2 to 5 years in the remainder of patients. In immunosuppressed children, such as those with HIV infection, SSPE may be fulminant and may result in death over weeks to 3 to 4 months.

Progressive Rubella Panencephalitis

Rubella infection during pregnancy can cause a congenital rubella syndrome. Manifestations include microcephaly, cataracts, glaucoma, congenital heart defects, and sensorineural hearing impairment. Progressive rubella panencephalitis is a rare disorder resembling SSPE but caused by rubella virus (Chapter 344). It occurs as a complication of congenital rubella syndrome or, more typically, after childhood rubella. With the advent of widespread rubella immunization, this disorder has been nearly eliminated in the United States, but is still seen in as many as 100,000 cases[4] in regions of the world where children are not universally vaccinated.

A hiatus of years separates early infection from the onset of neurologic deterioration, which is characterized by behavioral changes, cognitive impairment, cerebellar ataxia, spasticity, and sometimes seizures. Myoclonus is a less prominent feature than it is in SSPE. CSF shows mild pleocytosis and oligoclonal bands. Intrathecal CSF antibodies to rubella virus or isolation of the virus from brain or peripheral blood lymphocytes confirms the cause. Pathologic changes include perivascular inflammation and microglial nodules; the white matter is generally more involved than gray matter, and axons are preserved, in contrast to SSPE where gray matter abnormalities predominate. There is no effective treatment, and the prognosis is similar to that for SSPE.

Progressive Multifocal Leukoencephalopathy

DEFINITION

This demyelinating disease is associated with infection of oligodendrocytes by JC virus, a papovavirus that is widely distributed in humans and must undergo genetic rearrangements in its noncoding control region to enable it to replicate efficiently in glial tissue. Progressive multifocal leukoencephalopathy (PML) was the first demyelinating disease to be unequivocally associated with a viral infection.

EPIDEMIOLOGY

Serologic studies indicate that the infection predominantly occurs during childhood, and more than half of the population has been infected by age 20 years. Lesser increments of JC virus seropositivity are observed in each decade thereafter. Despite the wide dissemination of JC virus infection, PML is rarely observed in the absence of underlying cellular immunosuppression, and even then it is not very common. It is also rarely observed in childhood. Until the AIDS epidemic, PML was most commonly observed in patients with lymphoproliferative disorders (62% of cases) and less commonly with myeloproliferative diseases (7%), carcinomatous diseases (2%), other immunodeficiency states, and granulomatous disorders such as tuberculosis and sarcoidosis. The

prevalence of PML has increased dramatically during the AIDS pandemic: as many as 5% of AIDS patients developed PML in the pre-HAART era. Even with the profound reduction in the incidence of AIDS-related PML following the introduction of HAART, AIDS remains the most common underlying disorder associated with the disorder. Although PML has been observed with a variety of immunomodulatory/immunosuppressive agents, there is a unique association between PML and the monoclonal antibody, natalizumab, an α4β1 and α4β7 integrin inhibitor used in the treatment of multiple sclerosis (Chapter 383) and Crohn disease (Chapter 132).[5] In certain populations treated with natalizumab, the incidence rate of PML equals or exceeds that observed with AIDS.[6] In general, the risk of PML with other agents is orders of magnitude lower than that with natalizumab.

PATHOBIOLOGY

The cardinal feature of PML is demyelination, which is typically multifocal but occasionally unifocal (Fig. 346-2). These lesions may occur in any location in the white matter. The lesions range in size from 1 mm to several centimeters; larger lesions may reflect the coalescence of multiple smaller lesions. The other histopathologic hallmark of PML is the presence of hyperchromatic, enlarged oligodendroglial nuclei and enlarged bizarre astrocytes with lobulated hyperchromatic nuclei. Electron microscopic examination reveals the JC virions, which are 28 to 45 nm in diameter and appear singly or in dense crystalline arrays in oligodendroglial cells and, less frequently, in reactive astrocytes. Inflammatory infiltrates are typically absent, except in patients who have reconstitution of their immune system, such as HIV-infected patients being treated with HAART, in whom macrophages and lymphocytes may be found.

CLINICAL MANIFESTATIONS

The clinical hallmark of PML is the presence of focal neurologic symptoms and signs associated with radiographic evidence of white matter disease in the absence of a mass effect. The most common initial symptoms include weakness, speech and language abnormalities, and behavioral and cognitive disturbances. Gait disturbances, sensory loss, and visual impairment all occur in approximately 20 to 30%. Seizures and brain stem symptoms are less common. Signs noted on physical examination parallel the reported symptoms, with weakness, typically a hemiparesis, detected in more than half of patients at initial evaluation. Gait abnormalities, cognitive problems, and speech and language disorders (i.e., dysarthria and dysphasia) are observed in about 25% as heralding manifestations. Limb and trunk ataxia, which typically reflects cerebellar involvement, is detected in as many as 10% of patients. Neuro-ophthalmic symptoms occur in 50% of patients with PML and are often the initial manifestation of the disorder. The most common visual deficit is homonymous hemianopia or quadrantanopia secondary to lesions of the optic radiations. Cortical blindness may develop. Other neuro-ophthalmic manifestations include optic agnosia, alexia without agraphia, and oculomotor abnormalities. Sensory disturbances occur with PML, but are distinctly less common than impairment of strength or visual function.

DIAGNOSIS

The diagnosis of PML may be strongly suggested by the clinical manifestations and the radiographic imaging. A clinical presentation and a brain MRI consistent with PML, in the absence of other disorders that may explain the findings, coupled with a positive CSF PCR for JC virus is regarded as diagnostic of PML. Brain biopsy with demonstration of the characteristic histopathologic triad of PML coupled with immunohistochemical or electron microscopic evidence of JC virus remains the "gold standard" for diagnosis.

CT of the brain reveals hypodense lesions of the affected white matter that generally have a "scalloped" appearance because of involvement of the subcortical arcuate fibers lying directly beneath the cortex. Cranial MRI shows a hyperintense lesion on T2-weighted or FLAIR images in the affected regions (Fig. 346-3) and usually shows a hypointense lesion on T1-weighted images. Faint contrast enhancement, typically at the periphery of lesions, is seen in approximately 5 to 10% of pathologically confirmed cases of AIDS-associated PML and in 40 to 50% of natalizumab-associated PML on MRI. Contrast enhancement is typically a feature observed in association with immune reconstitution inflammatory syndrome (Chapter 367). Frontal and parieto-occipital lobe lesions predominate, but the lesions may be observed in other sites, including the basal ganglia, the internal and external capsules, and the posterior fossa structures (i.e., cerebellum and brain stem).

The results of routine analysis of CSF are not diagnostic, but CSF protein may be elevated. Ultrasensitive quantitative PCR for JC virus in the CSF is not only highly sensitive but also specific.

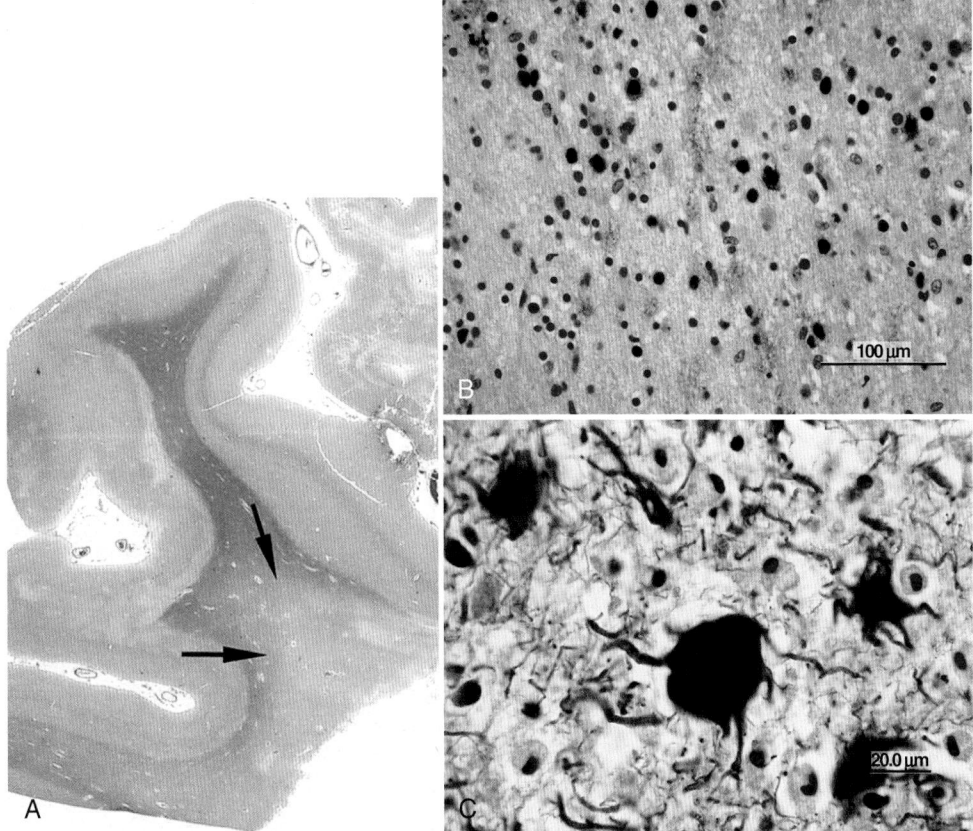

FIGURE 346-2. Pathology of progressive multifocal leukoencephalopathy. **A,** An area of demyelination is seen in the white matter that fails to stain with Luxol fast blue dye. **B,** Immunohistochemical staining with antibody to papovavirus shows brown-staining nuclei in oligodendrocytes, indicative of JC virus infection. **C,** Immunohistochemical staining for glial fibrillary acidic protein shows large bizarre astrocytes. (Courtesy Dr. Carlos Pardo, Johns Hopkins University, Baltimore, MD.)

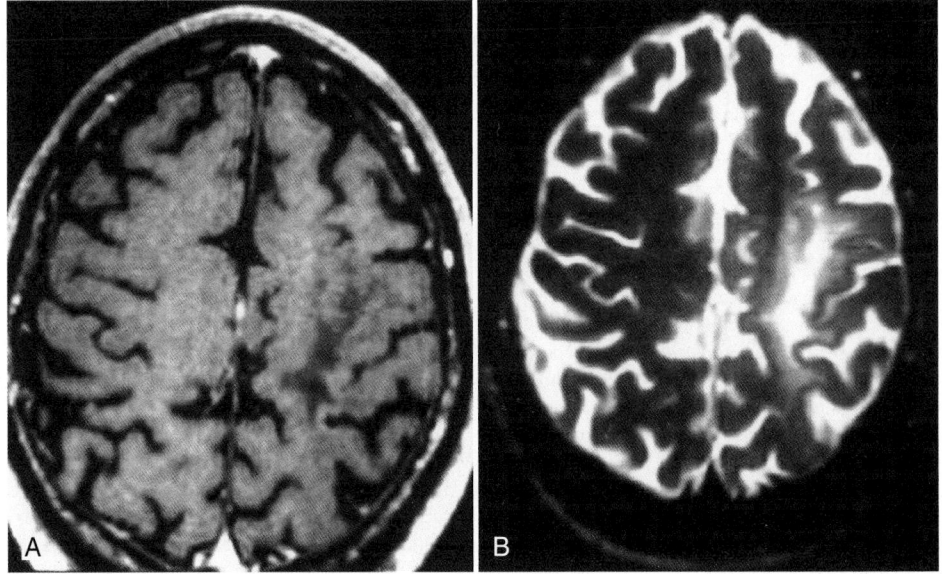

FIGURE 346-3. Cranial magnetic resonance images of progressive multifocal leukoencephalopathy. **A,** A T1-weighted image shows a hypointense signal abnormality of the left frontal lobe white matter. **B,** On T2-weighted imaging, the lesion is hyperintense.

TREATMENT ⟨Rx⟩

Although a number of compounds can prevent JC viral replication in vitro, there currently is no effective medication for PML. The best treatment is restoration of a normal immune system by treating the underlying cause. Cell-based therapy directed against BK virus[7] and the PD-1 inhibitor, pembrolizumab, show promise in the treatment of PML,[8] but additional studies are warranted before their widespread adoption. In AIDS-related PML, an effective antiretroviral regimen improves prognosis. In natalizumab-associated PML, plasma exchange can hasten the drug's elimination. When the immune system recovers, patients may develop a PML immune reconstitution inflammatory syndrome, in which a paradoxical clinical and radiographic worsening accompanies the return of a robust immune response.

PROGNOSIS

Previously, PML was regarded as a fatal illness, with survival averaging 3 to 4 months in the typical patient. After the introduction of HAART, approximately

50% of patients with AIDS-associated PML survive for more than 12 months, often with partial or nearly complete clinical and radiographic recovery.[9] Factors associated with a more benign course include the presence of PML as the heralding manifestation of AIDS, high or climbing CD4+ T-lymphocyte counts, contrast enhancement of the lesions on radiographic studies, and any clinical or radiographic evidence of recovery. JC virus–specific T lymphocytes appear to be critical for control of the infection.

GENERAL REFERENCES

For the General References and other additional features, please visit Expert Consult at https://expertconsult.inkling.com.

347

PARVOVIRUS

NEAL S. YOUNG

DEFINITION

B19 parvovirus, which was discovered in the mid-1970s by electron microscopic observation of an anomalous precipitin reaction of a normal blood donor's serum (occupying position 19 in plate B), was first linked to human disease by the observation of virus-specific immunoglobulin M (IgM) antibody or the virus itself in the sera of sickle cell disease patients suffering transient aplastic crisis (Chapter 154). The common illness caused by the virus was identified later during outbreaks of fifth disease, a highly contagious rash illness of childhood long suspected of having a viral etiology. The ability of parvovirus to persist and to be manifested as an isolated hematologic syndrome was demonstrated by the presence of the virus in fetal liver at autopsy of hydropic newborns and in immunosuppressed patients with chronic pure red cell aplasia (Chapter 156).[1]

The Pathogen

The parvoviruses form small icosahedral capsids of about 25 nm. They have a limited genome of single-stranded DNA. The approximately 5600 nucleotides of B19 parvovirus show remarkably little sequence variation among isolates; two variants, V9 and A6, are of uncertain clinical significance.

The Parvoviridae family contains many pathogenic animal viruses: feline panleukopenia virus, the cause of a fatal agranulocytosis in cats; canine parvovirus, which probably arose from the cat virus as a host range variant in the 1970s to produce a global pandemic and can cause fatal myocarditis in puppies; Aleutian mink virus infection, a model of immune complex disease; and porcine parvovirus, responsible for fetal wastage in pig litters. Antibodies to human adeno-associated viruses, which are dependoparvoviruses that are used as gene therapy vectors, occur naturally in humans, but B19 is the only parvovirus known to be pathogenic in humans.

EPIDEMIOLOGY

B19 infection is global; infectivity rates, inferred from the presence of anti-parvovirus IgG antibody in sera, are similar worldwide. Only isolated populations, such as Amazonian tribesman and residents of remote islands off the coast of Africa, have escaped exposure. B19 parvovirus infection is common in childhood, and half of 15-year-old adolescents have specific antiparvovirus B19 antibodies. Infection continues throughout adult life, and most elderly people are seropositive. In temperate climates, most infections occur in the spring, with small epidemics every few years being typical. Transmission is respiratory by droplet spread, and secondary infection rates among household contacts are high. Nosocomial infection can occur, and B19 parvovirus has been transmitted in blood products, especially pooled components such as factor VIII and IX concentrates. Producers of plasma derivatives now voluntarily screen by quantitative measurement of B19 DNA to reduce the risk for iatrogenic transmission. The lack of a lipid envelope and the stable DNA genome make parvoviruses notoriously resistant to heat inactivation and solvent detergents.

PATHOBIOLOGY

The biology of the Parvoviridae makes them especially dependent on helper function from host cells or other viruses. The autonomous parvoviruses propagate in actively dividing cells; the family Parvoviridae includes disease-causing animal parvoviruses. Adeno-associated viruses grow in tissue cultures infected with adenoviruses and herpesviruses and are popular vectors for gene transduction and therapy. B19 is the type member of the *Erythrovirus* genus, which includes very similar simian viruses, all of which are best propagated in the erythroid progenitor cells that are responsible for red blood cell production in the bone marrow. Active replication of virus can be detected by the presence of double-stranded intermediate forms by simple DNA hybridization methods. The transcription map of the erythroviruses differs markedly from that of other Parvoviridae. Only three genes produce proteins of known function. Many antigenic determinants recognized by the host immune system are located in helical loops that form the surface of each capsomere. Most of the capsid is composed of a major structural protein, called VP2, but about 5% of the capsid is the minor structural protein, VP1, which differs from VP2 only by an additional 226 amino acids at the amino terminus; this VP1 unique region is located external to the capsid surface and contains linear epitopes recognized by neutralizing antibodies.

The only known natural host cell of B19 parvovirus is the human erythroid progenitor. The tropism of the virus for an erythroid cell host results from its cellular receptor, globoside, a neutral glycolipid also known as erythrocyte P antigen. Rare individuals with the p phenotype, who congenitally lack globoside on their erythrocytes, are genetically insusceptible to B19 parvovirus infection; they show no serologic evidence of previous infection, and their marrow erythroid progenitors proliferate normally in the presence of high concentrations of virus. Parvovirus kills erythroid progenitors by expression of its nonstructural protein, and it is possible that some cells, such as megakaryocytes, may be lysed by restricted expression of viral proteins in the absence of viral propagation. B19 can be efficiently propagated in tissue culture of primary human hematopoietic cells in which erythropoietic differentiation is stimulated by erythropoietin. There is evidence that parvovirus DNA can integrate into the genome of erythroid precursor cells in tissue culture.[2]

The humoral immune response is dominant in B19 parvovirus infection. Levels of the chemokine CXCL-10 rise with acute viremia.[3] Natural antibody production correlates with disappearance of the virus from blood, and the presence of IgG appears to confer lasting protection against a second infection. Parvovirus infection can persist if immunoglobulin production is defective such that antibody fails to neutralize the virus; reactivity of antibodies to the unique amino-terminal region of VP1 is especially important.

CLINICAL MANIFESTATIONS

Fifth Disease

Most B19 parvovirus infections are asymptomatic. The most common clinical manifestation of infection is erythema infectiosum, or fifth disease, a rash illness of childhood characterized by a "slapped cheek" appearance (Fig. 347-1). In adult volunteers inoculated intranasally with B19, nonspecific influenza-like complaints occurred early along with viremia; the cutaneous eruption a week later corresponded to the appearance of antiviral antibodies. These more specific symptoms of B19 parvovirus infection are secondary to immune complex formation and deposition. Serologic testing generally shows seroconversion, IgM antibody or the appearance of IgG antibody to parvovirus. The rash of fifth disease may be evanescent, and recurrences can be provoked by sunlight, heat, emotion, or exercise. Fifth disease can be confused with rubella. In adults, the rash is less characteristic, can present as palpable purpura, may be associated with pruritus in up to 50% of patients, and can be difficult to visualize in dark-skinned individuals.[4]

B19 Arthropathy

In contrast to the mild course in children with fifth disease, acute parvovirus infection in adults, particularly immunocompetent middle-aged women, may cause significant arthropathy. Not only arthralgia but also a true inflammatory arthritis can occur in older patients. Symmetrical joint involvement of the hands, ankles, knees, and wrists can resemble rheumatoid arthritis (Chapter 248), and the test result for rheumatoid factor may be positive. B19 arthropathy usually resolves within a few weeks; joint destruction does not occur. Parvovirus is not the cause of rheumatoid arthritis, but case reports suggest that B19 infection may mimic, precipitate, or worsen a variety of rheumatologic diseases, including juvenile rheumatoid arthritis, systemic lupus erythematosus,

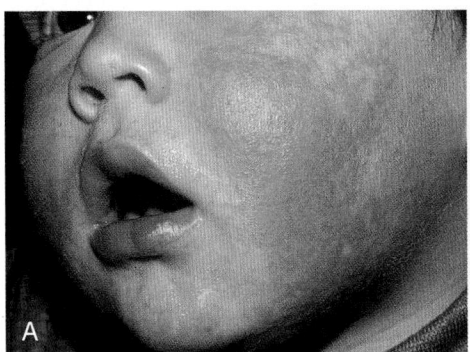

FIGURE 347-1. Erythema infectiosum. In this infection by parvovirus B19, a child will develop prominent erythema of the cheeks, "slapped cheeks" **(A)**, followed by a lacelike erythema on the extremities **(B)** and buttocks. It is also known as fifth disease.

and fibromyalgia. Autoantibodies that can appear during infection may be the link between the virus and its immune-mediated manifestations.

Transient Aplastic Crisis

In patients who have hematologic malignancies, have recent hematopoietic stem cell transplants, have underlying hemolysis, or have a high demand for production of circulating erythrocytes, acute B19 parvovirus infection causes transient aplastic crisis, an abrupt cessation of red blood cell production that exacerbates or, in previously compensated states, provokes severe anemia.[5,6] Erythropoiesis is temporarily suppressed in all B19 parvovirus infections, but hemoglobin levels remain stable because of the long lifespan of erythrocytes. The anemic crises associated with low or absent reticulocytes in hereditary spherocytosis and sickle cell disease are virtually always secondary to B19 parvovirus infection. Parviremia is present in patients with transient aplastic crisis, and red cell production resumes once antibodies to the virus are produced and the infection is cleared. Transient aplastic crisis is generally a unique event in the patient's life, thus suggesting induction of long-lasting protective immunity. Although it is self-limited, aplastic crisis often requires transfusion and can lead to severe, occasionally fatal anemia that precipitates congestive heart failure and cerebrovascular accidents. Transient aplastic crisis is associated with a stereotypical bone marrow morphology, absence of maturing erythroid precursors, and the presence of "giant pronormoblasts" (Fig. 347-2) that are the cytopathic effect of parvovirus infection.

White blood cell and platelet counts may fall modestly during transient aplastic crisis, especially in patients with functioning spleens. Occasional cases of agranulocytosis may be due to B19; thrombocytopenia and pancytopenia have been reported, and B19 can precipitate a benign virus-associated hemophagocytic syndrome.

Persistent Infection

In patients who cannot mount an appropriate host antibody response, B19 parvovirus persists in the circulation, often at extremely high levels ($>10^{12}$ genome copies per milliliter). Patients do not develop the clinical features of fifth disease but instead have an entirely hematologic syndrome of pure red cell aplasia. The anemia is severe and requires transfusion; reticulocytes are absent from blood, as are erythroid precursors from marrow. Observation of giant pronormoblasts in the marrow may lead to the diagnosis. The failure to produce neutralizing antibodies to B19 parvovirus occurs in patients with congenital immunodeficiency (Nezelof's syndrome), with iatrogenic immunodeficiency (chemotherapy or immunosuppressive drugs), and with acquired immunodeficiency. Pure red cell aplasia secondary to parvovirus may be the first manifestation of the acquired immunodeficiency syndrome (AIDS), but this presentation is less common in the era of highly active antiretroviral therapy.

Hydrops Fetalis

B19 parvovirus infection of the pregnant mother followed by transplacental transmission to the fetus can lead to an adverse outcome, either miscarriage or hydrops fetalis.[7] Parvovirus infects the fetal liver, the site of erythrocyte production during early development. Hydrops is the result of severe anemia as well as perhaps myocarditis, contributing to congestive heart failure. Prospective studies have estimated a 30% risk for transplacental infection and 9% risk for fetal loss in women who are exposed to B19 during pregnancy. Infection during the second trimester poses the greatest risk for birth of a hydropic infant; B19 parvovirus accounts for 10 to 20% of all cases of nonimmune

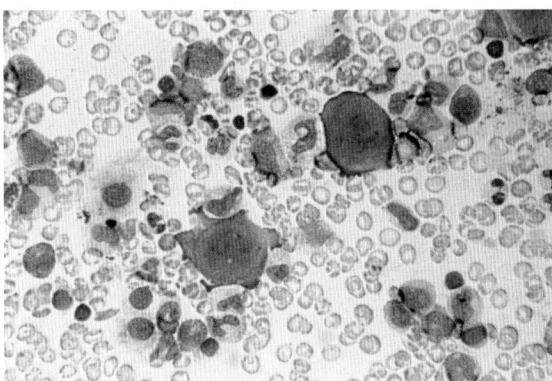

FIGURE 347-2. Bone marrow aspirate of a patient with chronic pure red cell aplasia secondary to persistent B19 parvovirus infection. Mature erythroid precursors are absent, and the prominent giant pronormoblasts are typical of B19 infection.

hydrops fetalis. The risk for spontaneous abortion resulting from first-trimester infections has been more difficult to quantitate. The likelihood of an infection increases in epidemic years and correlates with the level of contact of the pregnant woman with children. Although most B19 infections during pregnancy probably do not lead to either loss of the fetus or congenital anomalies, B19 infection is a cause of fetal death. Congenital malformations have not been consistently associated with intrauterine parvovirus infection. However, severe anemia at birth with bone marrow histology consistent with either constitutional pure red cell aplasia (Diamond-Blackfan anemia) or congenital dyserythropoietic anemia has occurred in infants salvaged by in utero blood transfusions or exchange transfusion at birth.

Other Syndromes

Elevated hepatic aminotransferase levels can accompany fifth disease, and parvovirus infection has been associated with severe but usually self-limited hepatitis in some children. The presence of B19 genetic sequences in cardiac tissue has led to a diagnosis of parvovirus myocarditis. Serologic and DNA evidence of B19 infection implicated parvovirus in some patients with necrotizing vasculitis, Kawasaki disease, Henoch-Schönlein purpura, and giant cell arteritis. Glove-and-sock syndrome, an exanthem localized to the hands and feet and consisting of edema, erythema, paresthesia, and pruritus, has been linked to B19. Chronic fatigue syndrome may follow parvovirus infection. Meningitis, encephalitis, and a variety of neurologic complications may occur with fifth disease and parvovirus infection.

Subtle late effects of viral infection, not related to persistent infection, may include a worsening of the manifestations of malaria (Chapter 324), especially the severity of anemia. Previous viral infection also has been linked to cerebral infarctions in patients with sickle cell diseases[8] and to arterial ischemic strokes in pediatric populations.[9]

However, false-positive results arise when the diagnosis of infection rests on detection of amplified B19 genome by polymerase chain reactions. Furthermore, B19 parvovirus can persist at low levels in various tissues of normal individuals for many months after infection. For example, whole genome sequencing has detected B19 in 0.12% of individuals without apparent infectious disease, usually but not always at relatively low viral abundance.

TABLE 347-1	DIAGNOSIS OF PARVOVIRUS B19				
DISEASE	**IgM**	**IgG**	**B19 DOT BLOT***	**B19 PCR**
Fifth disease	+++	++	−	+
Polyarthropathy syndrome	++	+	−	+
Transient aplastic crisis	+/−	+/−	++	++
Persistent anemia	+/−	+/−	++	++
Hydrops/congenital infection	+/−	+	+/−	++
Previous infection	−	++	−	+/−

*Sensitivity about 106 genome copies per milliliter.
Ig = immunoglobulin; PCR = polymerase chain reaction.

DIAGNOSIS

Laboratory diagnosis relies on serologic and DNA tests[10] (Table 347-1). Virus-specific antibodies are measured in standardized commercial solid-phase enzyme-labeled immunoassays, generally using recombinant capsid proteins. "Capture" formats are preferred to detect serum IgM, which is first bound to a solid phase coated with anti-μ-chain antibodies, followed by the addition of viral antigen and an antiviral monoclonal antibody. IgM antibodies are diagnostically positive in almost all cases of fifth disease at initial evaluation and appear within a few days of the onset of transient aplastic crisis; IgM may persist for months after acute infection. IgG is usually assayed in conventional indirect assays. IgG circulates later than IgM, generally at the end of the first week of illness. Although titers of IgG are generally highest in the year after an acute infection, substantial interindividual variation and the presence of IgG in a large proportion of the population make measurement of IgG less helpful than other tests for diagnosis of parvovirus. DNA assays are required for persistent B19 infection, in which antibody production is absent or minimal. Parvovirus can also be found in the sera of patients with early transient aplastic crisis. Direct hybridization methods are reliable, and they detect clinically relevant viral titers of greater than 10^6 international units (orders of magnitude below levels present in both acute and persistent infection). Gene amplification methods are more sensitive but less reliable because of false-positive results. Virus can be detected in amniotic fluid, and both virus and IgM antibody to B19 are found in umbilical cord blood; the mother's serum will show seroconversion during pregnancy, but maternal IgM may be absent at the onset of hydrops fetalis.

PREVENTION

Effective vaccines exist for animal parvoviruses, and human B19 infection can also probably be prevented. A recombinant immunogen in development for the human virus lacks DNA and is therefore noninfectious; the empty capsids have been engineered to overexpress the highly immunogenic minor structural protein VP1, and a single 2.5-μg dose of empty capsids elicited excellent neutralizing antibody responses in normal volunteers. Vaccination could prevent transient aplastic crisis in patients with sickle cell disease and other hemolytic anemias, pure red cell aplasia in some immunodeficient individuals, and hydrops if seronegative mothers were inoculated early in pregnancy. Unfortunately, there has yet to be commercial interest in developing a vaccine.

TREATMENT   Rx

Most parvovirus infections in normal children and adults do not require specific therapy. Isolation of infected individuals is impractical, with the exception of hospitalized cases. Pure red cell aplasia and the underlying persistent B19 parvovirus infection can be dramatically terminated by discontinuation of immunosuppressive therapy or institution of effective antiretroviral drugs in patients with AIDS. Commercial immunoglobulins are a good source of antibodies to parvovirus, and persistent B19 infection responds to a 5- or 10-day course of IgG at 0.4 g/kg with a prompt decline in serum viral DNA, as measured by hybridization methods, accompanied by reticulocytosis and increased hemoglobin levels. This regimen has been curative in congenital immunodeficiency, but parvovirus in AIDS patients can persist at lower levels, and relapses of anemia may require repeated IgG administration. Immunoglobulin therapy can precipitate fifth disease rash and arthralgia. Hydrops fetalis may resolve spontaneously, but intrauterine blood transfusions have been used with apparent success. Chronic arthropathy has been treated symptomatically with anti-inflammatory drugs, and there is not a role for the administration of immunoglobulin. As

important as recognizing parvovirus infection is avoiding misinterpretation of laboratory studies, such as positive IgG serology or borderline IgM and DNA test results, and misguided maneuvers that delay appropriate alternative treatments.

GENERAL REFERENCES

For the General References and other additional features, please visit Expert Consult at https://expertconsult.inkling.com.

348

SMALLPOX, MONKEYPOX, AND OTHER POXVIRUS INFECTIONS

BRETT W. PETERSEN AND INGER K. DAMON

DEFINITION

Human illness caused by a poxvirus is characterized by a cutaneous manifestation; illness may be localized or systemic, depending on the particular poxvirus and the route of introduction. DNA-based assays, including DNA sequencing, are the most precise methods for identification and differentiation of poxvirus genera, species, strains, and variants. The guanosine plus cytosine content of orthopoxviruses, yatapoxviruses, molluscum contagiosum virus, and parapoxviruses is approximately 33%, 32%, 60%, and 63%, respectively.

The Pathogens

All poxviruses described in this chapter (Table 348-1) belong to the family Poxviridae, subfamily Chordopoxvirinae.[1]

EPIDEMIOLOGY

Recognition of the epidemiologic characteristics of poxvirus diseases is valuable in assessing the potential etiologic agent of a particular suspected poxvirus lesion. Knowledge of zoonotic reservoirs, geographic localizations, and capacity for epidemic transmission is critical for clinical assessment and control measures. All human poxvirus infections are zoonotic in nature, with the exception of molluscum contagiosum and variola, which are solely human pathogens. Transmission of virus to humans and to animals is through direct contact with lesions, by fomites, or by inhalation of respiratory droplets.

Parapoxvirus and molluscipoxvirus infections are endemic worldwide; orthopoxvirus and yatapoxvirus infections are geographically restricted, probably by the distribution of competent reservoir hosts. Variola virus (the causative agent of smallpox, a disease declared eradicated in 1980) is the only poxvirus required to be reported to public health systems under the International Health Regulations. In addition to variola virus, Congo Basin clade monkeypox viruses are considered to be select agents by the U.S. government; they must be reported and appropriately handled if discovered and if samples are maintained in the United States. Furthermore, because the availability of laboratory diagnostic testing is limited in many parts of the world, the true incidence and prevalence of poxvirus infections are uncertain.

Orthopoxvirus

The epidemiology of smallpox, caused by *orthopoxvirus variola*, is understood through detailed studies conducted during the end of the eradication campaign. Interhuman transmission of variola virus generally occurred through the inhalation of large airborne respiratory droplets of infectious virus. Transmission usually required prolonged face-to-face or other close contact, although airborne transmission over longer distances had been reported.[2] Transmission by fomites or contact with infectious material from the rash also occurred. Aggregate data, collected during the smallpox eradication campaign, suggest a secondary attack rate of 58.4% in unvaccinated close or household contacts and a secondary attack rate of 3.8% in previously vaccinated close or household contacts. Case-fatality rates for variola major varied with the type of disease manifested,

TABLE 348-1	TAXONOMY OF POXVIRUSES KNOWN TO INFECT HUMANS
GENUS	**SPECIES**
Orthopoxvirus	Variola virus, vaccinia virus, cowpox virus, monkeypox virus, putative novel species from Georgia and Alaska
Parapoxvirus	Orf virus, milker's node virus, bovine papular stomatitis virus, sealpox virus
Yatapoxvirus	Tanapox virus (Yaba-like disease virus), Yaba monkey tumor virus
Molluscipoxvirus	Molluscum contagiosum virus

but aggregate rates of 10 to 30% in various outbreaks have been recorded. Severity of disease correlated with rash burden and was also more severe in children and pregnant women. Variola alastrim minor, a variant of variola with a case-fatality rate of less than 1%, had similar human-to-human disease transmission characteristics.

Monkeypox has a more complex epidemiology. The virus is zoonotic, and two genetically discrete virus clades have been described, each with apparent distinct clinical and epidemiologic parameters. Human infections in western and central Africa were first identified in 1970. Investigations in the Congo basin country Zaire, now the Democratic Republic of Congo, demonstrated that human-to-human transmission of monkeypox was less prevalent than that of smallpox. The secondary attack rate in unvaccinated contacts of monkeypox cases was calculated to be 9.3% versus 37 to 88% for smallpox. Previous smallpox vaccination (administered 3 to 19 years prior) appeared to be 85% protective in preventing disease acquisition in contacts and also ameliorated the severity of disease. Overall, most identified cases acquired disease from presumed animal exposure; only 28% of cases were ascribed to person-to-person transmission. A case-fatality rate of approximately 10% was observed in unvaccinated persons, and the majority of fatalities and the most severe disease manifestations were observed in children younger than 5 years. Serosurveys suggested that subclinical infection may have occurred in up to 28% of close contacts of monkeypox patients in some communities; this relatively low rate may contribute to the rarity of sustained generations of human-to-human transmission in household and other close-contact situations. However, more recent studies of household attack rates in an outbreak setting suggest that up to 50% of infections may be transmitted from human to human, and the seroprevalence of anti-orthopoxvirus antibodies in unvaccinated individuals is about 20 to 25% in central and western Africa.[3,4]

Among primary cases, recent close contact—through hunting, skinning, killing, cooking, or playing with carcasses—was identified with *Cercopithecus*, *Colobus*, and *Cercocebus* (primate); *Cricetomys* (terrestrial rodent); and *Funisciurus* and *Heliosciurus* (squirrel species). Samples of animals collected in areas of western and central Africa surrounding human cases have demonstrated orthopoxvirus-specific seroprevalence in various members of these species, and the virus itself has been isolated from a rope squirrel (*Funisciurus anerythrus*) and a sooty mangabey (*Cercocebus atys*). The prevailing hypothesis is that one or more squirrel or rodent species is the probable reservoir of disease.

The disease reemerged in 1996 in the Democratic Republic of Congo, this time with 88% of cases derived from secondary human-to-human contact presumed to be because of the cessation of routine smallpox vaccination in 1980 after the eradication of smallpox. Mortality was only 1%. Ecologic serosurveys showed orthopoxvirus seroprevalence in terrestrial rodents (*Cricetomys emini*) and in one domestic pig (*Sus scrofa*).

Monkeypox virus was introduced to the United States in 2003 through a consignment of animals from the West African country of Ghana. The virus was identified as belonging to a distinct clade of monkeypox that included previous West African monkeypox isolates as well as isolates derived from earlier outbreaks in primate colonies. The U.S. cases had a less pronounced rash and a less severe illness, with no mortality or human-to-human transmission. When cases in the United States (2003) were compared with cases in Congo Basin (1980 to 1986), disease in the United States was less severe based on clinical criteria, the extent of the rash, and the case-fatality rate after controlling for age and vaccination status. These data, along with animal model studies and comparisons of the genomes of West African and Congo Basin monkeypox viruses, suggest at least two populations or clades of monkeypox virus. The apparent decreased pathogenicity and transmissibility of West African

clade monkeypox virus infection led, in part, to its declassification as a U.S. select agent in 2013.

Cowpox virus is found in Europe and Asia and is maintained in rodents; in Britain, the reservoirs are bank voles and wood mice. Human infection is a zoonosis. The domestic cat has been a common source of human infection, which probably explains the occurrence of cases in children; 26% of 54 cases occurred in children younger than 12 years. Most feline and human cases occur between July and October, with only occasional cases between January and June. Recent outbreaks in Europe have documented pet rats, or feeder rats, to be a source of transmission to humans. Cowpox virus also is prevalent in European zoos, where cheetahs, lions, anteaters, rhinoceros, elephants, and okapi have occasionally transmitted infection to animal handlers. No case of bovine cowpox has been detected since 1976, but two cases of a novel orthopoxvirus infection were recently reported in the country of Georgia in men who were exposed to ill cows.[5] Another novel orthopoxvirus infection with a clinical presentation similar to cowpox was reported in a patient in Alaska, but the source of infection was unclear.[6]

Vaccinia is the live virus contained in preparations of the smallpox vaccines used to eradicate smallpox. In the United States, the vaccine is recommended for laboratory personnel who use replication-competent orthopoxviruses and for selected military personnel. Contacts of vaccinees occasionally develop vaccinia infections. The origin of vaccinia is unknown, and no natural host for the virus is known. Recent studies have further distinguished cowpox and vaccinia viruses, both of which have been used as smallpox vaccines, and suggest that vaccinia viruses may have descended from horsepox virus.[7] Vaccinia "variants" have been described, including buffalopox from contact with infected animals in India and vaccinia viruses in dairy cattle workers in Brazil and Colombia.

Parapoxvirus

Human infection is an occupational hazard of farm workers, abattoir workers, veterinary surgeons, students, and persons who participate in animal slaughter associated with religious observances (e.g., Eid al-Adha). It is most common in the lambing and calving seasons and among sheep workers. Recently, a novel poxvirus with 88% similarity to *Parapoxvirus* viruses was reported in one patient in Tennessee and one in Missouri, both of whom had regular contact with horses.[8]

Factors responsible for ongoing transmission have been attributed both to the environmental stability of orf virus in scab material and to the manifestation of chronic infections in some animals. A new parapoxvirus has been identified in deer hunters found to have cutaneous lesions after hunting and field-dressing deer.

Molluscipoxvirus

Molluscum contagiosum virus occurs worldwide, and increasing reports of the disease have paralleled the number of reported cases of acquired immunodeficiency syndrome (AIDS). Traditional modes of transmission are associated with mild skin trauma such as abrasions, direct contact with a lesion, and fomites (e.g., shared towels) in some cases. However, the disease appears to be sexually transmitted, and genital lesions are more common than lesions elsewhere on the body. Children in daycare or school situations may transmit the disease to other children. Secondary spread of lesions may occur by autoinoculation (excoriation of primary lesions and spread to areas of normal skin) as well as by shaving. No known animal reservoir exists.

Yatapoxvirus

Tanapox virus is restricted to Africa, principally to Kenya and the Democratic Republic of Congo, and probably has a simian reservoir. Direct primate-to-human transmission through a break in skin has rarely been described in animal handlers, but an insect or arthropod intermediary may be involved in the transmission of tanapox virus to humans. No human-to-human transmission has been reported. Yaba monkey tumor virus causes localized infections after contact with infected primate lesions. Little is known about the epidemiology of this virus.

PATHOBIOLOGY

The majority of smallpox infections were initiated by inhalation of respiratory droplets and implantation of virus on the oropharyngeal and respiratory mucosa. No primary localized site of infection was evident if the route of exposure was by inhalation. Disease could also be introduced through suspensions of virus obtained from scabs of patients that were introduced percutaneously and constituted the practice of variation. In these cases (when skillfully administered), illness was usually less virulent, a localized primary infectious lesion was present, and the asymptomatic incubation period was truncated. Lastly, transmission by fomites, such as soiled clothing or bed linens, was infrequently reported.

After entry, virus moves to local lymph nodes and then disseminates to the reticuloendothelial system to replicate further. At this time, the individual is asymptomatic. In 10 to 14 days, secondary viremia occurs and heralds the prodrome of symptomatic illness. During this time, virus seeds the oropharynx and epidermis. The absence of a keratinized structure in the mucosa of the oropharynx leads to ulceration and release of virus in saliva; virus replicates in the epidermis to cause the characteristic macular, papular, vesicular, and pustular eruptions of smallpox.

In experiments in monkeys, high levels of type I interferons, interleukin-6, and interferon-γ are seen; D-dimers and thrombocytopenia suggest disseminated intravascular coagulation. Apoptosis with loss of T cells in lymphoid organs was also observed. Of note, tumor necrosis factor-α (TNF-α) levels were minimal in the infected animals, with a notable decrease in the expression of genes regulated by nuclear factor κB and TNF-α.

In humans, the viral lesions characteristic of illness primarily develop in the epidermis, where the cells of the malpighian layer swell and vacuolate to undergo ballooning degeneration. The cytoplasm continues to enlarge, loss of nuclear material is noted, and coalescence of vacuoles through cell rupture creates reticulating degeneration of the middle and upper layers of the stratum spinosum. In the next stages, the vesicle is formed. High titers of virus are found within the lesions. In mucosal surfaces, the absence of a horny layer allows the necrosis caused by proliferation of virus within the epithelium to create ulcers and leads to liberation of large quantities of virus into the oropharynx. Evaluation of other organs in human smallpox has been done only in select autopsy cases. Mild pathologic changes are seen in the lungs.

CLINICAL MANIFESTATIONS
Orthopoxvirus
Smallpox

Naturally acquired variola virus infection is characterized by fever and a distinctive rash, with several different clinical presentations (Table 348-2). When the disease still existed, an asymptomatic incubation period of 10 to 14 days (range, 7 to 17) was followed by a fever that quickly rose to about 103° F (38° to 40° C), sometimes with dermal petechiae. Associated constitutional symptoms included backache, headache, vomiting, and prostration. Within a day or two after incubation, a systemic rash with a characteristic centrifugal distribution (i.e., lesions present in greater numbers on the oral mucosa, face, and extremities than on the trunk) appeared. The fever typically abated as the rash developed. Lesions commonly appeared on the palms and soles. The rash lesions were initially macular and then advanced to the papular stage, at which point they enlarged and progressed to a vesicle by day 4 or 5 and a pustule by day 7. When lesions became pustular, the fever typically returned. Lesions became encrusted and scabbed by day 14 and then sloughed off. Skin lesions in the vesicular and pustular stages were deep-seated and in the same stage of development in any one area of the body (Fig. 348-1). The

ordinary disease type was subgrouped into three categories based on the extent of rash on the face and the body: confluent, semiconfluent, and discrete. In *ordinary confluent disease*, no area of skin was visible between vesiculopustular rash lesions on the trunk or the face. In *ordinary semiconfluent* and *discrete disease*, patches of normal skin were visible between rash lesions on the trunk and face, respectively. Less severe manifestations (modified smallpox or variola sine eruptione) occurred in both unvaccinated and, more commonly, vaccinated individuals. The mortality rate correlated with the rash burden.

Four main clinical types of variola can be subgrouped according to the World Health Organization (WHO) classification schema: *ordinary smallpox* (≈90% of cases) produced viremia, fever, prostration, and rash, and mortality rates were generally proportional to the extent of rash and ranged as described earlier; *(vaccine) modified smallpox* (5% of cases) produced a mild prodrome with few skin lesions in previously vaccinated people and had a mortality rate well below 10%; *flat smallpox* (≈5% of hospitalized cases) produced slowly developing lesions that were difficult to ascertain because they appeared flush with the (edematous) skin at the vesicular stage, and it was almost always fatal; and *hemorrhagic smallpox* (<1% of cases) induced bleeding into the skin and the mucous membranes and was invariably fatal. A discrete type of the ordinary form, with a typical febrile prodrome and rash, resulted from alastrim variola minor infection. Individuals with this form of disease were not nearly as moribund or "toxemic" as individuals with variola major infection. Previous vaccination was not necessarily protective against the hemorrhagic forms of disease but seemed to be protective against flat forms of disease.

In flat smallpox, illness was heralded by the abrupt onset of fever with temperatures of 38.3° to 38.9° C and the appearance of the rash after 3 to 4 days. The oral enanthem was often confluent, and sloughing of rectal mucosal membranes was also reported. At the papulovesicular stage of disease, lesions appeared as small indentations (day 6) with hemorrhages in the bases and were surrounded by an erythematous ring. By day 7 or 8, the lesions appeared flat. Bullous lesions that would slough were reported. Fever persisted throughout the disease course, and respiratory complications were often observed by day 7 or 8 of illness. Thrombocytopenia, neutropenia, and lymphocytosis were reported.

In hemorrhagic forms of smallpox, illness began with fever and typical prodromal symptoms; the fever never abated. Early after the onset of fever, petechiae and purpuric rashes became apparent; subconjunctival hemorrhages, hematuria, and vaginal bleeding were also seen. Patients usually died by day 6 of illness, well before any classic vesiculopustular rash was evident. In late hemorrhagic disease, after the onset of fever, typical maculopapular lesions developed, but the fever did not abate. The lesion evolved slowly, and areas of hemorrhage were evident at the base of the lesions. Bleeding occurred in

TABLE 348-2	WORLD HEALTH ORGANIZATION SMALLPOX TYPES
WHO SMALLPOX TYPE	**CLINICAL DEFINITION**
Variola sine eruptione	Fever, no rash
Modified	Like ordinary, with an accelerated course
Ordinary discrete	Fever, rash; areas of normal skin between pustules, even on the face
Ordinary semiconfluent	Fever, rash; pustules confluent on the face, discrete elsewhere
Ordinary confluent	Fever, rash; pustules confluent on the face and forearms
Flat	Fever, erythema, and edema of the skin; vesicles soft, flat, and bullous
Hemorrhagic, early	Fever (persistent), hemorrhages and petechiae, purpuric rash at illness onset
Hemorrhagic, late	Fever (persistent), rash, hemorrhage into the base of vesicles late in illness

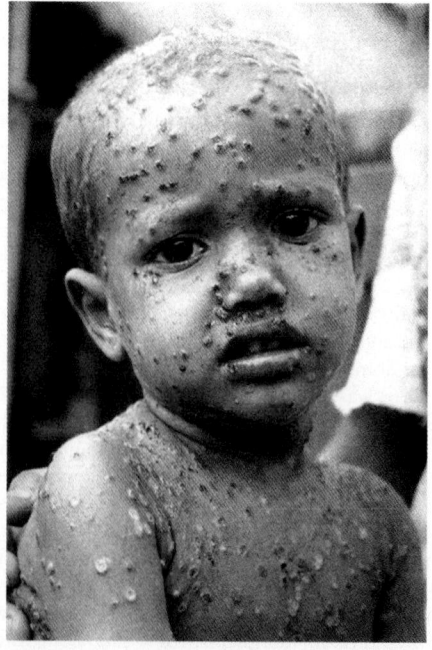

FIGURE 348-1. Pustular lesions of smallpox and beginning of scarring on the face and upper part of the torso. (From the Centers for Disease Control and Prevention Public Health Image Library, ID #: 7055. Photograph by Stan Foster.)

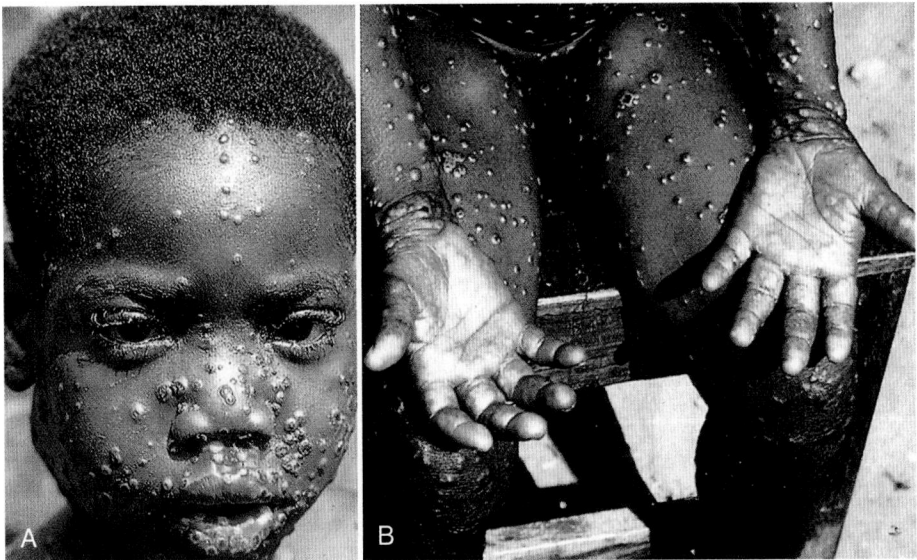

FIGURE 348-2. Rash of monkeypox of the head (A) and extremities (B) in a 7-year-old girl in central Zaire. (From Peters W, Pasvol G. *Tropical Medicine and Parasitology*. 5th ed. New York: Mosby; 2002:238.)

the mucous membranes, thrombocytopenia was profound, and death occurred between days 8 and 10 of illness.

Monkeypox

After an incubation period of 7 to 17 days (mean, 12 days), a prodrome of fever, headache, backache, and fatigue begins.[9] The cutaneous eruption evolves similar to that of smallpox. Lesions evolve in the same stage in any one part of the body from macules, papules, and vesicles to pustules, and then they crust and scar (Fig. 348-2). After resolution of the rash, hypopigmentation is followed by hyperpigmentation of the scarred lesions. Pronounced cervical, postauricular, submandibular, and inguinal lymphadenopathy clinically distinguishes monkeypox from smallpox.

Vaccinia

Multiple-puncture vaccinia virus infection by a bifurcated needle is the current smallpox vaccination regimen used for laboratory personnel working with orthopoxviruses, health care personnel, and military in the United States. Most commonly, the infection progresses through a standard course of events from vesicle to pustule. ACAM2000, which is the only smallpox vaccine currently licensed in the United States, is expected to have a similar safety profile to historical smallpox vaccines. Major complications include progressive vaccinia, eczema vaccinatum, generalized vaccinia, postvaccinial encephalitis, accidental infection, and myopericarditis.

Progressive vaccinia, which is a rare and often fatal vaccine complication in persons with severe deficiencies in cellular immunity, occurs in about 1 per million vaccines, with a case-fatality rate of about 35%. Progressive vaccinia is characterized by frequently painless growth and spread of the vaccine virus beyond the inoculation site, often leading to necrosis and sometimes metastases to other body sites. The possibility of progressive vaccinia should be considered if vaccinia virus infection continues to progress and expand without apparent healing more than 15 days after vaccination.

Eczema vaccinatum can occur in people with a history of atopic dermatitis (eczema), irrespective of its severity or activity, owing to local spread or dissemination from the primary vaccination site or contact with the unscabbed vaccination site of another person. A localized or generalized papular, vesicular, or pustular rash can develop anywhere on the body or be localized to previous eczematous lesions. Systemic illness with fever, malaise, and lymphadenopathy may occur. In the 1968 national U.S. surveillance of smallpox vaccination, there were 66 cases (no deaths) of eczema vaccinatum among 14.5 million vaccinees (4.6 cases/million) and 60 cases (1 death) among their several million contacts.

Generalized vaccinia describes the vesicular rash that develops after vaccination. Excluding dissemination associated with eczema vaccinatum and progressive vaccinia, it has been extremely rare to document virus in these lesions. True generalized vaccinia is believed to represent the end product of viremic spread of virus, and no predisposing factors have been identified. Generalized vaccinia was estimated to occur in about 242 of every million primary vaccinations. Studies done during the vaccination program in 2002 in the United States indicate that the majority of cases previously reported to be generalized vaccinia likely were generalized rashes caused by inflammatory or allergic responses to the vaccine, and not true generalized vaccinia, thereby leading to the coining of the term "postvaccinal nonviral pustulosis."

Postvaccination encephalomyelitis is a rare but serious complication that usually occurs only in primary vaccinees. Patients have variably displayed clinical and diagnostic features suggestive of a postimmunization demyelinating encephalomyelitis or direct viral invasion of the nervous system. This postvaccination reaction typically occurs 11 to 15 days after vaccination. Symptoms include fever, headache, vomiting, confusion, delirium, disorientation, restlessness, drowsiness or lethargy, seizures, and coma. Cerebrospinal fluid can demonstrate elevated pressure but generally has a normal cell count and chemistry profile. The diagnosis is one of exclusion, and no specific tests are available to confirm it. However, a few cases have been demonstrated to have anti-orthopoxvirus immunoglobulin M (IgM) or IgG responses in their cerebrospinal fluid.

Accidental infection occurs when virus from the vaccination site is transferred to another site or to another person through intimate skin contact. This complication generally occurs with primary vaccinees rather than revaccinees. Accidental self-inoculation, which most commonly occurs on the face, mouth, lips, or genitalia, is not usually serious and requires no specific treatment. Inoculation of the eye or eyelid is more serious and can be sight threatening if it is not evaluated and treated appropriately (Fig. 348-3). Between 1963 and 1968, ocular vaccinia was observed in 348 persons, including 22 who had evidence of corneal involvement and 11 who experienced permanent defects.

With bovine-associated vaccinia virus infections (e.g., buffalopox viruses in India and vaccinia viruses in Brazil and Colombia), up to 10 lesions have been described on the hands or arms of exposed farmworkers; fever, lymphadenopathy, backache, and fatigue are also associated symptoms.[10] Transmission is believed to occur by unprotected contact with active lesions present on animal teats and udders. Interhuman transmission of bovine-associated vaccinia virus to family members has been reported to occur through contact with lesion exudates.

Cowpox

Cowpox lesions are generally restricted to the hands and face; most patients (72%) have only one lesion. Multiple lesions may be caused by multiple primary inoculations, by autoinoculation, and very infrequently by lymphatic or viremic spread. The cowpox lesion passes through macular, papular, vesicular, and pustular stages before forming a hard black crust. The lesion is generally very painful, and erythema and edema are common at the late vesicular and pustular stages. Patients usually have lymphadenitis, fever, and general malaise. These features are generally severe in children, and absence from school or work is common. About 30% may be hospitalized. Most patients take 6 to 8 weeks to recover, but up to 12 weeks may be required. On occasion, a very severe infection and death may occur, typically in immunosuppressed individuals

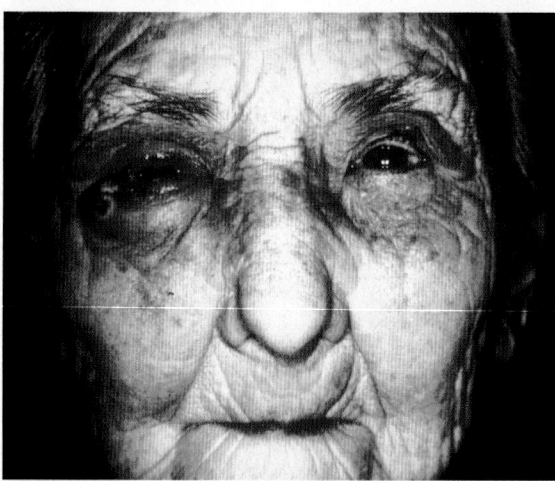

FIGURE 348-3. Vaccinia autoinoculation of an eye. (From the Centers for Disease Control and Prevention Public Health Image Library, ID #: 3322.)

and patients with skin conditions such as atopic dermatitis. Scarring is usually permanent.

Parapoxvirus

Lesions, such as from the orf virus,[11] start as erythematous papules and progress in 1 to 2 weeks to target lesions with a red center surrounded by a white halo and an outer inflamed halo. Lesions then progress to a nodular and then a papillomatous stage, which often has a "weeping" surface. In some patients, lesions may enlarge and persist for weeks before resolving by a crusting stage, which also may persist for weeks. Very large granulomatous lesions may occasionally require surgical débridement or removal.

Most patients have only one lesion, but multiple primary lesions may develop. Systemic reaction is relatively uncommon, and the lesion is often not particularly painful. Lymphadenopathy is present in some patients, and lymphangitis is relatively uncommon. Erythema multiforme (Chapter 411) can develop in up to one third of patients.

Molluscum Contagiosum Virus

Molluscum infection occurs when molluscum contagiosum virus comes into contact with nonintact skin. The characteristic lesion begins as a small papule and, when mature, is a discrete, 2- to 5-mm-diameter, smooth, dome-shaped, pearly or flesh-colored nodule that is often umbilicated (see Fig. 411-9 in Chapter 411).[12] A cheesy, off-white or yellowish material is easily expressed from lesions. Most patients have 1 to 20 lesions, but hundreds of lesions may occasionally be present. Because of multiple simultaneous infections or mechanical spread, the lesions may become confluent along the line of a scratch, and satellite lesions are sometimes seen.

In children, molluscum lesions occur mainly on the trunk and proximal ends of the extremities; in adults, lesions tend to occur on the trunk, pubic area, and thighs. In all cases, however, infection can be transmitted to other areas by autoinoculation. In men infected with human immunodeficiency virus (HIV), molluscum lesions can occur along the beard line and result in ocular involvement.

Individual lesions persist for about 2 months, but the disease usually persists for 6 to 9 months. Individuals with impaired cell-mediated immunity, including persons with HIV infection, tend to have more severe and prolonged infection.

Yatapoxvirus

Tanapox infection begins with a short febrile (38° to 39° C) illness that persists for 2 to 4 days and is sometimes accompanied by headache, backache, or prostration. The eruption of a lesion is frequently heralded by pruritus at the site of the outbreak. The lesion appears as a hyperpigmented macule, which often has central elevation and evolves to a papule with palpable induration. About 80% have a solitary nodule, but as many as 10 lesions can occur. Most lesions (72%) occur on the lower extremities, and the fewest occur on the face and areas normally covered by clothing.

Fever and systemic symptoms wane as the lesion erupts. The papule then becomes more "pocklike" but contains no fluid; umbilication or a pseudocrust may develop. Typically, the papule evolves into a firm, deep-seated, elevated

nodule. At the end of the first week, the lesion is surrounded by erythema and indurated skin, and regional lymphangitis is common. Lesions then either ulcerate or become larger nodules (up to 2 cm in diameter) within about 2 weeks, after which the local inflammatory response wanes and the lesions began to granulate. Resolution of lesions occurs within 6 weeks. Infection appears to confer lifelong immunity.

DIAGNOSIS

Before its eradication, smallpox was relatively easy to recognize. Chickenpox (Chapter 351) produces a centripetally distributed rash and rarely appears on the palms and soles; in chickenpox, prodromal fever and systemic manifestations are mild, the lesions are superficial in nature, and lesions in different developmental stages may be present in the same area of the body. Other diseases and conditions that could be confused with vesicular-stage smallpox include monkeypox, generalized vaccinia, disseminated herpes zoster or herpes simplex virus infection (Chapters 350 and 351), drug reactions (eruptions), erythema multiforme (Chapter 411), enteroviral infections (Chapter 355), scabies (Chapter 104), insect bites, impetigo (Chapter 412), and molluscum contagiosum. Diseases confused with hemorrhagic smallpox included acute leukemia (Chapter 173), meningococcemia (Chapter 282), and idiopathic thrombocytopenic purpura (Chapter 163). The Centers for Disease Control and Prevention have developed a protocol for evaluation of patients for potential smallpox (available at https://www.cdc.gov/smallpox/clinicians/algorithm-protocol.html) and an algorithm for laboratory assessment of the vesiculopustular stage of rash (available at https://www.cdc.gov/smallpox/lab-personnel/laboratory-procedures/rash-testing.html).

Orthopoxvirus

Nucleic acid–based tests and polymerase chain reaction (PCR) assays are currently the first approach to the diagnosis of orthopoxvirus infections. Serologic tests are largely genus specific, detect IgG, and usually cannot differentiate among species, although IgM levels can help differentiate recent orthopoxvirus infection from remote vaccination. Viral culture and electron microscopic evaluation of virion particles from clinical rash specimens are other options. If the diagnosis of smallpox is being considered, viral culture requires a biosafety level 4 (BSL-4) containment facility that is sanctioned by the WHO to use variola virus.

Parapoxvirus

The differential diagnosis of parapoxvirus lesions can include ecthyma gangrenosum as a result of a *Pseudomonas aeruginosa* infection (Chapter 290), vaccinia or cowpox infection, cutaneous anthrax (Chapter 278), erysipeloid (Chapter 279), tularemia (Chapter 295), and tumor. Farm workers recognize the infection and tend not to seek medical attention for routine cases, so about 45% of reported cases may have no known contact with infected animals, and the clinical diagnosis of such cases may be difficult. With negative-stain electron microscopy, virions with the characteristic morphology of parapoxviruses are usually seen easily in lesion extracts, thereby providing a rapid, certain diagnosis of the genus. The virus can be grown in cell culture, and PCR detection can be performed. Species-specific and species-generic protein-based diagnostics have also been developed for parapoxviruses.

Molluscum Contagiosum Virus

The clinical appearance of molluscum lesions usually is sufficiently characteristic to permit a clinical diagnosis. Brick-shaped virions typically can be seen in large numbers if the cheesy material expressed from the lesion is examined by electron microscopy. The virus has not been cultured in standard tissue culture systems. The characteristic histopathology of these lesions is diagnostic, but PCR methods can also identify molluscum contagiosum.

Yatapoxvirus

The limited geographic distribution of tanapox virus and the patient's travel history help with the diagnosis of tanapox infection. Unique clinical features that differentiate tanapox from other orthopoxvirus infections are the nodular nature of the rash lesion, the paucity of lesions, the benign disease course, and the protracted resolution of the rash. The solid nodular and ulcerated lesions are larger and develop more slowly than those of monkeypox, but they are smaller and develop more rapidly than those of tropical ulcers.

Tanapox virus can be detected by electron microscopy, but the appearance of the virions cannot exclude infection with other morphologically similar brick-shaped poxviruses. Nucleic acid testing or cell line culture can make the definitive diagnosis.

TREATMENT AND PREVENTION Rx

Orthopoxvirus

Vaccination with smallpox vaccine is the mainstay for prevention of ortho-poxvirus infection and was the primary method used to eradicate smallpox. Stockpiles of vaccine are available should smallpox recur, and clinical guidance for their use in an emergency have been developed (available at https://www.cdc.gov/mmwr/preview/mmwrhtml/rr6402a1.htm).[13] In the United States, however, smallpox vaccine is currently recommended only for laboratory personnel who work with infectious orthopoxvirus, certain health care personnel, and certain members of the military. In part because of stringent prescreening procedures, recent adverse events are rare with vaccination, but myopericarditis is estimated to occur at a rate of 5.7 per 1000 primary vaccinees based on clinical trial data with ACAM2000. A replication-deficient smallpox vaccine (MVA-BN) developed for use in persons with HIV infection and atopic dermatitis has also been stockpiled.

Early administration of vaccinia immune globulin (VIG) may reduce the mortality of eczema vaccinatum from 30 to 40% to 7%, and VIG may also be useful for other complications (e.g., progressive vaccinia, severe generalized vaccinia, or contact infection) of vaccinia (smallpox) vaccine administration and for other orthopoxvirus infections. However, VIG alone has no clear benefit for treatment of smallpox infection itself.

Antiviral compounds (Chapter 336) with in vitro and in vivo activity against poxviruses include specifically 5-iodo-2′-deoxyuridine, adenine arabinoside, and trifluorothymidine. Because of their systemic toxicity, these compounds have been used topically for the treatment of orthopoxvirus ocular infections. In vitro, cidofovir is active against cowpox, vaccinia, monkeypox, and variola; in vivo, it protects challenged animals when it is given prophylactically or early in the evolution of disease. Cidofovir has known renal toxicity and is administered with hydration and probenecid. Brincidofovir has been effective in treatment of systemic rabbitpox infection in rabbits and was used as part of a multidrug regimen to treat a case of progressive vaccinia.[14]

Tecovirimat is an effective small-molecule antiviral in animal models of systemic orthopoxvirus infection[15,16] and has been used successfully as part of a multidrug regimen to treat a human case of eczema vaccinatum and a case of progressive vaccinia. It is part of the U.S. Strategic National Stockpile and was licensed by the FDA for treatment of human smallpox disease in July 2018.

Parapoxvirus

Most workers at risk for parapoxvirus become infected, and reinfection also occurs. The vaccine used to control orf in sheep is fully virulent and has caused human infection. Treatment options are limited; anecdotal reports have described the use of topical and intralesional cidofovir, and other options may be topical formulations of interferon-modulating compounds such as imiquimod.

Molluscum Contagiosum Virus

Molluscum contagiosum infection is benign, and recovery is usually spontaneous, but treatment may be sought for cosmetic reasons, particularly for facial or multiple lesions. Options include cryotherapy, mechanical curettage, and chemical treatments such as podophyllin or podofilox, cantharidin, iodine, and tretinoin.[17] Irritation has been a side effect of many of the chemical treatments. Topical application of a 3% cidofovir antiviral cream or suspension has been reported to be beneficial, as has the use of potentially immune-modulating cimetidine or topical imiquimod therapy. However, no therapy is documented to be beneficial by well-controlled randomized trials,[A1] although topical 10% potassium hydroxide solution, applied twice daily, is sometimes recommended. Covering of lesions and the use of proper hand hygiene after contact with lesions should prevent transmission in most situations. For individuals with AIDS and molluscum, highly active antiretroviral therapy with a resulting improvement in the CD4+ cell count appears to be efficacious.

PROGNOSIS

Monkeypox and smallpox both cause human illness, with mortality rates ranging from 10 to 40%; variola minor variants, however, have mortality rates of less than 1%. Vaccinia virus and cowpox virus infections usually cause self-limited disease but can be severe and fatal in persons with immunosuppression or certain skin conditions such as atopic dermatitis. Yatapoxvirus infections are self-limited, and the illness resolves in the course of a few weeks. Parapoxvirus infections are manifested chiefly by localized symptoms, and the lesions resolve within a month or so in nonimmunocompetent hosts. Molluscum contagiosum infection is benign, usually with a spontaneous recovery, but the infection can persist for months.

Grade A Reference

A1. van der Wouden JC, van der Sande R, Kruithof EJ, et al. Interventions for cutaneous molluscum contagiosum. *Cochrane Database Syst Rev.* 2017;5:CD004767.

GENERAL REFERENCES

For the General References and other additional features, please visit Expert Consult at https://expertconsult.inkling.com.

349

PAPILLOMAVIRUS

WILLIAM BONNEZ AND JOHN M. DOUGLAS, JR.

DEFINITION

Human papillomaviruses (HPVs) are a group of small DNA viruses that cause a variety of benign and malignant lesions of the skin and mucous membranes. The most commonly recognized HPV-associated diseases include warts (Chapter 411) at anogenital sites (condyloma acuminatum), other skin surfaces (common wart or verruca vulgaris, as well as flat wart or verruca plana), and the plantar surface of the foot (verruca plantaris). In addition, HPV infection causes squamous intraepithelial lesions, or incipient cancers, of the cervix, also known as cervical intraepithelial neoplasia, and of other anogenital sites. It is considered the etiologic agent of a variety of cancers, especially cervical cancer.

The Pathogen

HPV is a member of the family Papillomaviridae. Like all papillomaviruses, HPV is nonenveloped, measures 55 nm in diameter, and has a double-stranded circular DNA genome of approximately 7900 base pairs enclosed by an icosahedral capsid. The HPV genome contains three functional regions: early genes (six total—E1, E2, E4, E5, E6, E7), which are expressed soon after infection and control replication, transcription, and cellular proliferation; late genes (two total—L1, L2), which are expressed in later stages of infection and encode the structural capsid proteins; and the long control region, which contains regulatory sequences that control the replication and transcription of early and late genes. Papillomaviruses complete their life cycle only in terminally differentiated epithelial cells and thus cannot be grown in monolayer cell cultures. Papillomavirus taxonomy is based on a genotyping system involving the use of DNA sequence relatedness of the gene encoding L1, the major capsid protein, with different types defined as having less than 90% homology.

Papillomaviruses are classified taxonomically by genus (Greek letters) and species (numbered), each containing one or more types. Most HPV types are included in three large genera: alpha (primarily mucosal or genital types), beta, and gamma (both of which cause cutaneous lesions). Currently, 230 types of HPV have been identified, over 40 of which infect genital skin and mucosa [http://pave.niaid.nih.gov/#explore/reference_genomes/human_genomes]. Of the genital types, approximately 15 are considered high risk because they are associated with high-grade squamous intraepithelial lesions and cancers of the cervix, anus, penis, vulva, vagina, and oropharynx, whereas others are considered low risk because they are largely associated with genital warts and low-grade squamous intraepithelial lesions.

EPIDEMIOLOGY

HPV infections are primarily transmitted by direct contact of skin or mucous membranes with an infected lesion. Genital HPV infection is typically contracted through sexual intercourse, although nonpenetrative genital contact, oral-genital contact, and manual-genital contact are also possible routes of transmission. In addition, genital HPV infection can be transmitted to the mouth and upper respiratory tract perinatally from infected mothers to newborns. For nongenital HPV infection, personal skin-to-skin contact also plays a primary role, although for plantar warts, fomite transmission from moist surfaces could be an important source of infection. Both genital and nongenital infection can be transmitted to new sites by autoinoculation.

Regarding genital HPV, an estimated 45% or so of the United States male and female population aged 18 to 69 years, or about 84 million persons, are infected and about 14 million new infections occur annually, thereby making genital HPV the most common sexually transmitted infection.[1] The prevalence of anogenital warts is estimated to be approximately 1% in the sexually active adult population. Acquisition of infection begins shortly after sexual debut, with an estimated 40 to 60% incidence of at least one type within 2 years of initiation of sex. Risk factors for infection include variables related to probable exposure (e.g., younger age at onset of sexual activity, increased number of recent and lifetime partners, and number of partners of the sex partners), susceptibility (e.g., lack of circumcision for men), and absence of prevention factors (e.g., lack of consistent condom use or immunization). Most infections are asymptomatic and clear without treatment; only 10% are estimated to persist longer than 2 years.[2,3] The incidence and prevalence of genital HPV infection and genital warts are declining most drastically in the countries with the most successful immunization programs, including a 60 to 70% decrease in U.S. women under age 25 years.[4,5]

Oral HPV infection is usually asymptomatic, but when symptomatic it takes the appearance of warts or papillomas. Its prevalence in U.S. adults is lower than genital infection—approximately 5 to 7% in women and nearly 12% in men,[6] almost half of which are due to high-risk types. Newly acquired oral oncogenic HPV infections are rare in healthy men, and most infections are cleared within 1 year. Cutaneous HPV infection is most typically recognized as common and plantar warts, especially in children, in whom annual incidence rates of up to 30% have been reported.

All types and manifestations of HPV infection are more common in persons with impaired cell-mediated immunity, such as those infected with human immunodeficiency virus (HIV) or receiving immunosuppressive therapy. Among HIV-infected women or men who have sex with men, the prevalence of anal high-grade squamous intraepithelial lesions is about 13% and 30%, respectively; relative to the general population, these anal cancer incidences are increased 7- and 30-fold, respectively. Whether genital HPV infection may increase susceptibility to HIV infection remains debated.

Cervical cancer has declined in developed countries since the initiation of cytologic screening programs, although about 13,000 cases and 4,200 deaths still occur in the United States annually.[7] Cervical cancer is the fourth most common and lethal cancer in women worldwide, and 85% of the 530,000 annual cases occur in the less developed world. Considering all anatomic sites, over 31,500 HPV-associated cancers (1.7% of all cancers) occur in the U.S. each year, about 60% among females.[8] The sharp rise in the incidence of HPV-associated oral cancers in men is of concern.[9]

PATHOBIOLOGY

HPV infections cause disease by inducing proliferation of the epithelium of the skin and mucous membranes. In benign lesions, such as warts and condylomas, all epithelial layers are involved, except for the basal layer of replicating keratinocytes. The proliferation of the stratum spinosum is called acanthosis, that of the stratum granulosum parakeratosis, and that of the stratum corneum hyperkeratosis. The overall growth is called papillomatosis because it typically occurs mostly above the tissue surface but is also associated with a deepening of the rete ridges of the basement membrane. It is also accompanied by large cells with a hyperchromatic, shrunken nucleus (or nuclei) surrounded by a halo (called koilocytes) in the stratum acanthosum. For the cytopathologist, koilocytosis is the hallmark of HPV infection.

Epidermodysplasia verruciformis is an uncommon autosomal recessive disease with diffuse warts that result from the mutation of one of two adjacent genes, EVER1/TMC6 and EVER2/TMC8, each coding for proteins involved in the transcription factor NF-κB that participates in the control of cell-mediated immunity.

For precancerous or cancerous lesions, dyskaryosis is caused by the proliferation of the basal layer cells, which also exhibit abnormal mitoses. This dyskaryosis progresses by replacing the upper layers of the stratified epithelium, thereby causing increasing grades 1 to 3 of intraepithelial neoplasia, according to how many thirds of the epithelium are involved. Full-thickness involvement defines carcinoma in situ. The breach of the basement membrane indicates invasive cancer. The intraepithelial neoplasias (IN) of the cervix, vagina, vulva, penis, and anus also go by the acronyms of CIN, VAIN, VIN, PIN, and AIN, respectively. For the cervix, low-grade squamous intraepithelial lesion (LSIL) is the equivalent of flat condyloma and CIN1, whereas high-grade squamous intraepithelial lesion (HSIL) regroups CIN2 and 3. To parallel these changes, low and high cervical intraepithelial neoplasia (LCIN and HCIN, respectively) are now terms also used in histology. The higher the cytologic or histologic grade of neoplasia, the higher the intralesional relative prevalence of high-risk HPV types.

At the cellular level, infection begins in the lowest and least differentiated layer of the epithelium, the basal cells, when they are exposed by microtrauma. Transcription and protein expression are highly coordinated with the level of cellular differentiation. In the basal layer, the viral genome becomes established in the nucleus as an episome that replicates in tandem with cellular replication,

thus maintaining a stable copy number of viral genomes. As basal cells migrate up and differentiate in the superficial layers of the epithelium, full vegetative viral DNA replication and expression of structural proteins occur, with assembly of infectious virions in the most superficial layer of the epithelium. Virions are released with the sloughing of dead cells during normal cellular turnover.

Persistent infection with various high-risk types of genital HPV is firmly established as the cause of squamous cell carcinoma and adenocarcinoma of the cervix, and HPV 16 in particular plays a causal role in other anogenital and oropharyngeal squamous cell cancers. There are also associations of beta-HPV types with squamous cell cancer of the skin. HPV DNA can be detected in more than 99% of cervical cancer cases, with 70% of cancers caused by the two most common high-risk types, HPV 16 and 18. The pathogenesis of HPV-induced cancer involves viral integration into the host genome with resulting disruption of the E2 transcription regulatory gene and increased expression of E6 and E7 proteins. These proteins have oncogenic activity and affect cell growth by binding with tumor suppressor proteins, E6 with p53 and E7 with the retinoblastoma tumor suppressor protein, thereby disrupting apoptosis and cell cycle regulation.

The oncogenic risk of HPV varies not only by type, with HPV 16 being the most oncogenic, but also according to variants (i.e., sharing between 95 and 98% of DNA homology) within a given type. A high viral load may also contribute to the risk. Although a persistent infection with a high-risk type is "necessary" for the development of cervical cancer, it is not considered "sufficient" because cancer does not develop in the majority of persistently infected women. Possible cofactors include cigarette smoking, prolonged hormonal contraceptive use, multiparity, micronutrient deficiency, immunodeficiency (e.g., HIV infection), and possibly other infections, (i.e., Chlamydia trachomatis and herpes simplex virus type 2). In addition, data supporting a familial risk for cervical cancer point to possible genetic factors, including genes controlling the immune response (e.g., HLA, TNF) and cell cycle (e.g., p53).

The squamous epithelium of the ectocervix and columnar epithelium of the endocervix form a squamo-columnar junction that, from birth through life, recedes towards the endocervix, traveling an area called the transformation zone where cervical cancers (Chapter 189) arise. Squamo-columnar junctions, but without a transformation zone, also exist in the anus and larynx, and HPV benign or malignant lesions often arise in epithelium that is in close proximity (see Chapter 136 for anal cancer).

The immune response to HPV infection is less robust than for most viral infections. Viral proteins and infectious virions develop in superficial cells with limited contact with the immune system, and there is no cell lysis or viremia to trigger an inflammatory response. In addition, HPV suppresses several components of the immune response, including the interferon pathway and the expression of inflammatory cytokines and MHC I. Antibody to HPV develops in only an estimated 60% of infected individuals, often as long as 6 to 12 months after infection. In contrast, the dynamics of the immune response are quite different after immunization, with almost 100% seroconversion within several months and antibody levels many-fold higher than those after natural infection. The high prophylactic efficacy of papillomavirus vaccines is due to humoral immunity and the intense production of neutralizing antibodies. Once papillomavirus infection is established, cellular immunity appears to be critical for clearance of infection.

CLINICAL MANIFESTATIONS

The clinical manifestations of HPV infection vary by anatomic site and viral type. Common warts are exophytic, hyperkeratotic papules that typically occur on the hands but can appear on any skin surface, occasionally including the genital skin; they are most commonly caused by HPV types 1, 2, 4, 27, and 57. Plantar warts, which are caused by similar types of HPV, are hyperkeratotic papules. They may present as deep plantar warts that often are very painful and endophytic in growth. They are typically associated with HPV types 1 or 63. More superficial and painless mosaic warts are typically caused by HPV types 2 or 4. In contrast, flat warts (verruca plana), which are small flat-topped papules that occur more commonly on the face, hands, and legs, are caused by a different group of nongenital HPV types (e.g., types 3, 10, 28, 38, 42, 49, 75, 76).

Epidermodysplasia verruciformis is usually manifested in childhood as diffuse warts that respond poorly to treatment. The diffuse warts of epidermodysplasia verruciformis can be associated with two types of lesions: flat warts caused by the same HPV types as in normal hosts, and scaly tinea versicolor–type lesions caused by epidermodysplasia verruciformis–associated types. The latter are associated with the development of squamous cell cancers in sun-exposed areas in 30 to 70% of persons of age 30 years and older. Similar skin lesions and, rarely, associated skin cancers can develop in other patients with acquired defects in cell-mediated immunity or who are immunosuppressed.

Anogenital warts are papillomatous growths that occur throughout the anogenital skin and mucosa, typically at sites of genital friction. HPV types 6 or 11 are found in about 85% of cases, with approximately half of infected persons developing warts. Perianal warts (Chapter 136) are most common in persons with a history of anal intercourse and are often associated with intra-anal warts, but they also can occur without such contact, such as through autoinoculation when wiping. Anogenital warts can range from flat or papular lesions to the classic pedunculated, cauliflower-shaped condyloma acuminatum. Warts are typically asymptomatic, noticed either by the patient as a "bump" or inadvertently during a genital examination, although they can cause itching, burning, pain, or, rarely, bleeding. In pregnant women mechanical obstruction of the birth canal has been reported.

The most common clinical manifestations of oral HPV infection include oral squamous cell papillomas and condylomata acuminata, caused by HPV types 6 and 11. Less frequent, and differentiated by histology, are common skin warts caused by cutaneous HPV. Focal epithelial hyperplasia is an uncommon disorder with a predilection for Native Americans and South Africans. It presents as round, flat papules that can be confluent and are mostly associated to HPV types 13 and 32. Warts caused by genital types can also rarely occur in the upper respiratory tract, where they produce a serious recurrent respiratory papillomatosis that can cause hoarseness and even compromise the airway. Squamous intraepithelial lesions or intraepithelial neoplasias are most commonly found on the cervix as a result of screening for cervical cancer by cytology (Papanicolaou [Pap] test) or HPV molecular testing, with confirmation by colposcopy and biopsy. These potential precursors of cancer and resulting cancers also can occur at other anogenital sites (vulva, vagina, anus,[10] and penis[11]). Most squamous intraepithelial lesions are not visible on mucosal surfaces without the application of 3 to 5% acetic acid and magnification. On the external genitalia, they can appear as flat hyperpigmented papules.

Bowenoid papulosis combines hyperpigmentation, intraepithelial neoplastic histology, and the cytoarchitecture of a condyloma. It can transform into Bowen disease, which is a carcinoma in situ.

DIAGNOSIS

Both cutaneous (Fig. 349-1) and genital (Fig. 349-2) warts generally present an easily recognized clinical picture and can be diagnosed by history and physical examination without laboratory testing. The application of 3 to 5% acetic acid on the genital or anal mucosa or the skin causes whitening of HPV lesions and greatly facilitates the examination, especially when combined with magnification with loupes or a colposcope. Oral lesions are also generally recognized by history and physical examination.

The differential diagnosis of cutaneous warts includes seborrheic and solar keratoses, nevi, irritated acrochordons, corns (also called calluses or clavi), and squamous cell carcinoma (Chapters 193 and 411). Lichen planus (Chapter 409) can mimic flat warts and corns of the foot, but plantar warts can be distinguished from corns when shaving of the lesion reveals dark red punctations, which are small thrombosed blood vessels. Genital warts must be distinguished from the condylomata lata of secondary syphilis (Chapter 303), which are typically flat-topped, moist, and kissing lesions. Genital warts are often confused with molluscum contagiosum, which presents as smooth, pale or inflamed, dome-shaped papules, typically with a central dimple (Chapter 411). Biopsy for histopathologic examination may be helpful for lesions at all anatomic sites that are atypical or not responsive to therapy, those suggestive of high-grade squamous intraepithelial lesions or cancer (e.g., pigmented, indurated, fixed, bleeding, or ulcerated), or lesions in immunocompromised patients.

Cervical squamous intraepithelial lesions have traditionally been detected by cervical cytology through Pap tests, with assessment of abnormal results by colposcopy and biopsy for histopathologic examination. However, HPV testing is more sensitive than Pap tests for detecting cervical intraepithelial neoplasia 2/3 and more effective in prevention of cervical cancer.[A1] HPV DNA testing in combination with cytology (co-testing) can enhance the sensitivity of screening in women older than age 30 years and permit the interval between screening to increase from every 3 years to every 5 years.[12] HPV tests are also recommended for triage of women whose Pap test results show atypical squamous cells of undetermined significance, which is an equivocal test

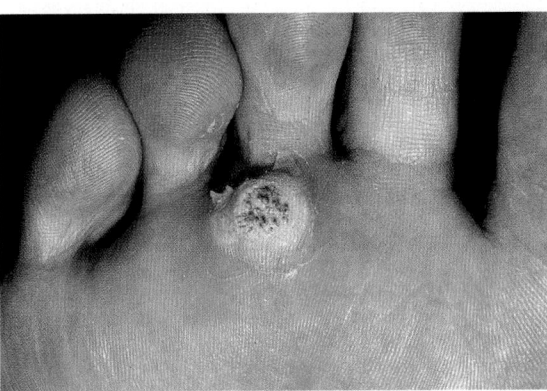

FIGURE 349-1. Plantar wart. A hyperkeratotic, verrucous papule or plaque beneath a pressure point on the sole of the foot is characteristic. HPV types 1 (myrmecia), 2 (mosaic), and 4 are most common. Because plantar warts are driven into the skin by the pressure of walking or standing, they are usually the most treatment resistant.

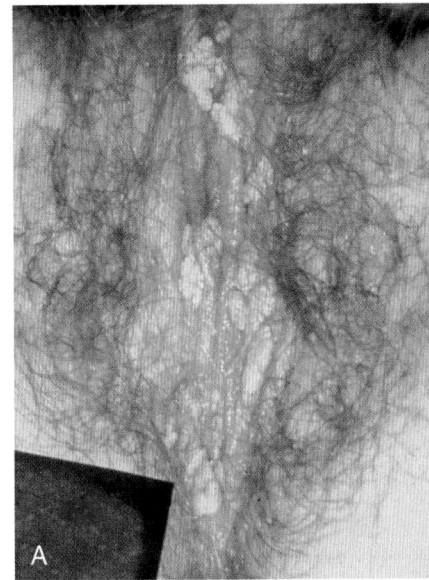
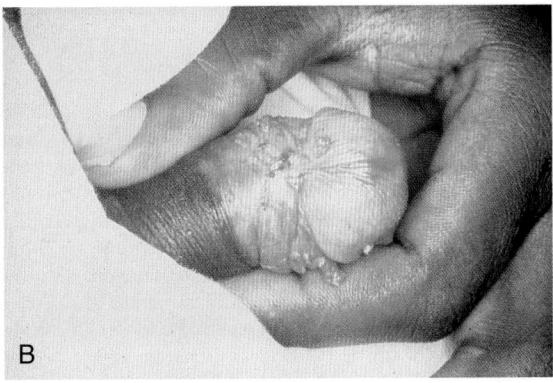

FIGURE 349-2. Genital human papillomavirus (HPV) infection. A, Vulvovaginal HPV infection. B, Penile HPV infection. (From Vermund SH, Bhatta MP. Papillomavirus infections. In: Cohen J, Powderly WG, eds. *Infectious Diseases,* 2nd ed. St Louis: Mosby; 2004.)

TABLE 349-1 RECOMMENDED TREATMENT OF GENITAL WARTS

PATIENT APPLIED

Podophyllotoxin (podofilox) 0.5% solution or gel; to be applied in up to 4 weekly cycles (bid for 3 days, followed by 4 days without treatment)

Imiquimod 3.75% cream (to be applied once daily at bedtime) or 5% cream (to be applied once at bedtime 3 times per week) for 6-10 hours for up to 16 weeks

Sinecatechins 15% ointment; to be applied 3 times daily for up to 16 weeks

PROVIDER ADMINISTERED

Cryotherapy with liquid nitrogen or cryoprobe; to be applied once every 1-2 weeks*

Trichloroacetic or bichloroacetic acid 80-90% solution; to be applied once weekly*

Office surgery* (excision, electrocautery, curettage)

*Safe for use in pregnancy.

---

result. HPV testing has not been validated and is not recommended for screening for infection at other sites (e.g., anus, oropharynx).

TREATMENT Rx

Management of HPV infection is directed toward diagnosis and treatment of the lesions themselves because there are no virus-specific therapies. Many lesions resolve spontaneously, so the goal of treatment is amelioration or prevention of symptoms or, in the case of high-grade squamous intraepithelial lesions, prevention of progression to cancer. Treatment involves destruction of lesions by physical techniques or topically applied or injected cytotoxic agents. Because treatment does not eradicate infection in surrounding tissues, recurrent lesions are common.

Treatment of warts depends on their location and size, the patient's preferences, and the provider's experience. Recommended first-line treatment of common and plantar warts is the application of topical salicylic acid; second-line treatment of recalcitrant lesions includes cryotherapy,[A2] which also can be used for flat warts, intralesional bleomycin, pulsed dye laser therapy, and surgical excision. Recommended treatment of genital warts (Table 349-1) includes patient-applied podophyllotoxin (0.5 or 0.15% solution or gel applied twice a day for 3 days, repeated weekly for four cycles), imiquimod, or sinecatechins, as well as provider-administered cryotherapy, trichloroacetic acid, or surgical excision; alternative treatments include laser surgery, infrared coagulation, and electrosurgery.[13] Oral lesions can be treated by locally destructive physical techniques (cold-blade excision, cryotherapy, or laser surgery), whereas options for laryngeal papillomas include microdébridement, laser surgery, or photodynamic laser therapy.

For cervical lesions, treatment depends on histologic staging after colposcopy and biopsy and clinical context (see http://www.asccp.org/Guidelines-2/Management-Guidelines-2). The general principles are as follows. Because cervical intraepithelial neoplasia grade 1 usually regresses spontaneously, follow-up (by cytology, HPV test, or colposcopy) without treatment is recommended. Treatment is generally recommended for all cervical intraepithelial neoplasia grade 2/3 lesions, except in pregnant women, who have higher rates of spontaneous regression and a greater risk of reproductive tract complications after treatment, and in young woman with cervical intraepithelial neoplasia grade 2. Treatment options include a variety of ablative and excisional techniques such as cryosurgery, loop electrosurgical excision procedure, and laser surgery. Treatment is 90 to 95% effective in preventing the recurrence of lesions, and comparative clinical trials have shown similar efficacy for different treatment modalities.

PREVENTION

Primary Prevention

Primary prevention of HPV infection depends on avoidance of contact with infectious lesions and reduction of susceptibility through immunization. For example, the use of footwear in locker rooms may prevent plantar warts. For genital HPV infection, correct and consistent condom use can reduce the risk for both HPV infection and the HPV-associated diseases of genital warts, cervical squamous intraepithelial lesions, and cervical cancer. Condom use also assists in the clearance of existing cervical HPV lesions. Male circumcision may reduce the prevalence of genital HPV infection in men, but whether it affects the transmission or clearance of these infections is unclear.[A3]

Of greatest importance for prevention are HPV vaccines (Chapter 15), which are composed of virus-like particles assembled from the major capsid protein, L1 (Table 349-2). Gardasil-9 is a nonavalent vaccine that extends Gardasil coverage (types 6, 11, 16, and 18) to five additional high-risk HPV

TABLE 349-2 U.S. ADVISORY COMMITTEE ON IMMUNIZATION PRACTICES RECOMMENDATIONS FOR HPV VACCINATION*

WHOM TO VACCINATE

Immunocompetent population
- At age 11-12 years (but may start as early as age 9; it should start at age 9 in children with a history of sexual assault)
- Men aged 13-21 years. It can be considered in heterosexual males aged 13-26 years

Immunocompromised subjects (with B- and T-cell alterations, HIV, malignancy, transplantation, autoimmunity, or using immunosuppressive drugs) of both sexes
- Vaccination is recommended as early as possible between the ages 9 and 26 years

HOW TO VACCINATE

Recommended dosage and schedule: 0.5 mL intramuscularly
- If vaccination is initiated before age 15 years, give 2-dose schedule: 0 and 6-12 months
- If vaccination is initiated at age 15 years or older, give 3-dose schedule: 0, 1-2 months, and 6 months

SPECIAL CONSIDERATIONS

Schedule modifications: if doses are missed, series does not need to be restarted, but second and third doses should be given as soon as possible

Cervical cancer screening: no change in recommended interval

Special situations: females with genital warts, abnormal Pap test results, or positive HPV test results are unlikely to be infected with all vaccine types and should be immunized per other recommendations; males with genital warts should also be immunized per other recommendations

Pregnant and lactating women: not recommended for use in pregnancy based on lack of data; may be used in lactating women

Immunocompromised persons: no safety concerns because vaccine is noninfectious, but immune response and effectiveness might be reduced

Not recommended for females or males <9 and >26 years of age

*These recommendations have been adapted to reflect that (Gardasil-9) is the only available HPV vaccine in the U.S.

Modified from:

Petrosky E, Bocchini JA, Jr., Hariri S, Chesson H, Curtis CR, Saraiya M, et al. Use of 9-valent human papillomavirus (HPV) vaccine: updated HPV vaccination recommendations of the Advisory Committee on Immunization Practices. *MMWR Morb Mortal Wkly Rep.* 2015;64:300-304.

Meites E, Kempe A, Markowitz LE. Use of a 2-dose schedule for human papillomavirus vaccination—updated recommendations of the Advisory Committee on Immunization Practices. *MMWR Morb Mortal Wkly Rep.* 2016;65:1405-1408.

National Center for Immunization and Respiratory Diseases. Recommended Immunization Schedule for Adults Aged 19 Years or Older, United States, 2017. Atlanta, GA: February 6, 2017. https://www.cdc.gov/vaccines/schedules/hcp/imz/adult-conditions.html.

---

types (31, 33, 45, 52, 58). In addition to protecting against cervical intraepithelial neoplasia, cervical adenocarcinoma in situ, and cancer, it also protects against vulvar intraepithelial neoplasia, vaginal intraepithelial neoplasia, and cancers of the vulva or vagina in females, as well as against anal intraepithelial neoplasia[A4][A5] and anal cancer in males. In addition, vaccination protects both males and females against genital warts. Cervarix is bivalent (types 16 and 18) and is approved for the prevention of cervical intraepithelial neoplasia, cervical adenocarcinoma in situ, and cancer of the cervix associated with these two HPV types. Gardasil-9 is now the only vaccine available in the United States. HPV vaccination has no therapeutic benefit against existing infections or lesions but may lower the rate of disease recurrence after successful treatment. Because effective protection develops only in the subjects without present or past infection, it is important to administer the vaccine before the onset of sexual activity to have the fullest benefit.

Other than transient local side effects at the site of intramuscular injection, mostly related to the adjuvant, the HPV vaccines have been very safe.[14] The longevity of protection is not yet established but has reached at least 10 years with the 3-dose regimen. Two-dose regimens are now recommended for some individuals because of the excellent and durable antibody response.[A6][A7] The HPV vaccine does not contain any live virus and can be given safely to immunocompromised persons.

HPV vaccination status currently does not alter recommendations regarding screening for cervical cancer. This recommendation could change in the future, however, if high vaccine coverage continues to lower the prevalence rates of cervical HPV infections.[15] For example, in countries in which the vaccine has been used in females, the prevalence of female genital warts has declined substantially; and when vaccine coverage exceeds 50%, this protection (herd immunity) can extend to unvaccinated men and women. Evidence also suggests

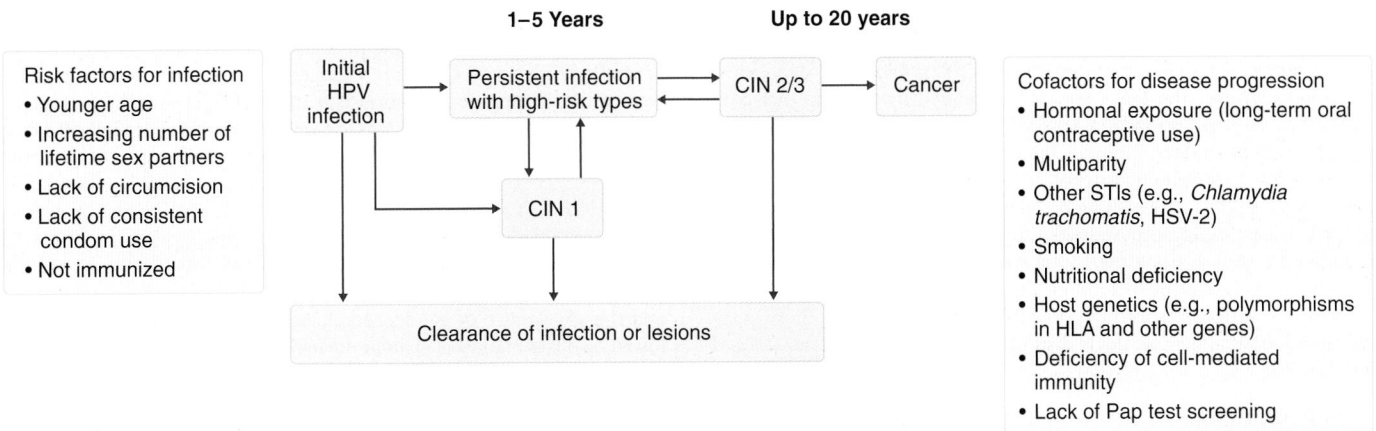

1–5 Years   Up to 20 years

FIGURE 349-3. Natural history of genital human papillomavirus (HPV) infection and cervical cancer. CIN = cervical intraepithelial neoplasia; HSV = herpes simplex virus; STIs = sexually transmitted infections.

that HPV vaccination has reduced the incidence of cervical intraepithelial neoplasia and abnormal Pap smears, and in Finland, the incidence of HPV-associated cancers. The vaccine has been effective in reducing the prevalence of oral HPV[16] but has not been effective in preventing anal infection or anal high-grade squamous intraepithelial lesions in HIV-infected men.

Secondary Prevention
Screening plus treatment of high-grade cervical squamous intraepithelial lesions is one of the most successful of all cancer prevention strategies (see Chapter 189). The value of cytologic screening for anal intraepithelial lesions (Chapter 136) in HIV-positive men who have sex with men is controversial but not currently recommended because of limited data on the natural history of these precursor lesions, the reliability of screening methods, and the safety and effectiveness of treatment.

PROGNOSIS
Although the natural history of HPV infection is not fully characterized, the large majority of infections and premalignant lesions are self-limited in most immunocompetent patients. Whether infections no longer detectable have been cleared by the immune system or remain latent in the basal layer of the epithelium with the potential for reactivation is not clear, but the higher prevalence of detectable infection in advanced than in early HIV infection, as well as in immunosuppressed individuals, supports the possibility of long-term infection. Many if not most clinical lesions resolve spontaneously after the patient develops cell-mediated immunity. Spontaneous regression within a year is estimated to occur in 25% of genital warts and more than 50% of common warts in children.

The natural history of cervical intraepithelial neoplasia has been most intensively studied because of its relationship to cervical cancer, although many questions remain unanswered. Estimates of the likelihood of regression versus the risk of progression to invasive cancer are 90% and 1%, respectively, for cervical intraepithelial neoplasia grade 1, 40% and 5% for cervical intraepithelial neoplasia grade 2, and 32% and 30% for cervical intraepithelial neoplasia grade 3. Low-grade and high-grade squamous intraepithelial lesions may represent a continuum of the same process or distinct processes, in which low-grade lesions represent a usually transient infection characterized by production of capsid protein (and probably infectious virions) and only minor cellular abnormalities, whereas high-grade lesions represent proliferation of immature cells as a result of the activity of oncogenic proteins of high-risk types (Fig. 349-3). Initial infection frequently leads to a transient low-grade squamous intraepithelial lesion, with persistent infection in less than 10% of cases. Persistent infection can, however, lead directly to high-grade squamous intraepithelial lesions within several years and can progress to invasive cancer after several decades. The natural history of squamous intraepithelial lesions at other anogenital sites is less well defined, but they may be associated with higher rates of spontaneous regression.

The majority of patients with HPV infection have an excellent prognosis, with cancer occurring infrequently among the large number of persons infected. Treatment can hasten the resolution of cutaneous and genital warts and is highly effective for cervical lesions. Among women with cervical intraepithelial neoplasia grade 3, long-term studies indicate that the 30% risk of cancer in untreated women can be reduced to less than 1% with treatment.

Grade A References

A1. Melnikow J, Henderson JT, Burda BU, et al. Screening for cervical cancer with high-risk human papillomavirus testing: updated evidence report and systematic review for the US Preventive Services Task Force. *JAMA*. 2018;320:687-705.

A2. Bertolotti A, Dupin N, Bouscarat F, et al. Cryotherapy to treat anogenital warts in nonimmunocompromised adults: systematic review and meta-analysis. *J Am Acad Dermatol*. 2017;77:518-526.

A3. Zhu YP, Jia ZW, Dai B, et al. Relationship between circumcision and human papillomavirus infection: a systematic review and meta-analysis. *Asian J Androl*. 2017;19:125-131.

A4. Arbyn M, Xu L, Simoens C, et al. Prophylactic vaccination against human papillomaviruses to prevent cervical cancer and its precursors. *Cochrane Database Syst Rev*. 2018;5:CD009069.

A5. Huh WK, Joura EA, Giuliano AR, et al. Final efficacy, immunogenicity, and safety analyses of a nine-valent human papillomavirus vaccine in women aged 16-26 years: a randomised, double-blind trial. *Lancet*. 2017;390:2143-2159.

A6. Iversen OE, Miranda MJ, Ulied A, et al. Immunogenicity of the 9-valent HPV vaccine using 2-dose regimens in girls and boys vs a 3-dose regimen in women. *JAMA*. 2016;316:2411-2421.

A7. D'Addario M, Redmond S, Scott P, et al. Two-dose schedules for human papillomavirus vaccine: systematic review and meta-analysis. *Vaccine*. 2017;35:2892-2901.

GENERAL REFERENCES

For the General References and other additional features, please visit Expert Consult at https://expertconsult.inkling.com.

350

HERPES SIMPLEX VIRUS INFECTIONS

RICHARD J. WHITLEY AND JOHN W. GNANN, JR.

DEFINITION
The Pathogen
Ancient Greek writings contain descriptions of spreading cutaneous lesions that we now recognize as disease caused by herpes simplex virus (HSV), a member of the family Herpesviridae. In 1968, well-defined antigenic and biologic differences were demonstrated between HSV type 1 (HSV-1) and HSV type 2 (HSV-2). Among the herpesviruses, HSV-1 and HSV-2 are most closely related, with approximately 60% genomic homology. Historically, HSV-1 was more frequently associated with nongenital infection and HSV-2 with genital disease, but that distinction is becoming blurred with the recognition that HSV-1 causes more than half of genital infections in some populations. These two viruses can be distinguished most reliably by DNA restriction enzyme analysis or genomic sequencing, but differences in antigen expression and biologic properties also serve as methods for differentiation.

Inclusion in the family Herpesviridae is based on the structure of the virion (E-Fig. 350-1). HSV contains double-stranded DNA at its central core, has a molecular weight of approximately 100 million, and encodes at least 80 polypeptides. The DNA core is surrounded by a capsid that consists of 162 capsomers arranged in icosadeltahedral symmetry. The capsid is 100 to 110 nm in diameter. Tightly adherent to the capsid is the tegument, which consists of amorphous material. Loosely surrounding the capsid and tegument is a lipid bilayer envelope derived from host cell membranes. The envelope consists of polyamines, lipids, and glycoproteins. These glycoproteins confer distinctive properties to the virus and provide unique antigens, which are the targets of host immune responses. Notably, glycoprotein G (gG) provides antigenic specificity to HSV, thereby resulting in an antibody response that allows serologic distinction between HSV-1 (gG-1) and HSV-2 (gG-2).

EPIDEMIOLOGY

HSV infections are very common worldwide in both developed and developing countries. Animal vectors for human HSV infections have not been described, and there is no seasonal variation in the incidence of HSV infections. HSV is transmitted from infected to susceptible individuals during close personal contact, and the virus must come in contact with mucosal surfaces or abraded skin for infection to be initiated. Because approximately half of the world's population has HSV infections and because such infections are rarely fatal, a large reservoir of HSV exists in the community to perpetuate person-to-person transmission.

Seroprevalence studies have demonstrated that acquisition of HSV-1 infection is related to socioeconomic and behavioral factors. Antibodies, which indicate past infection, are found early in life among individuals of lower socioeconomic groups, presumably a consequence of crowded living conditions that provide a greater opportunity for direct contact with infected individuals. Antibodies develop in as many as 75 to 90% of individuals from lower socioeconomic populations by the end of the first decade of life. In contrast, only 30 to 40% of persons in the middle and upper socioeconomic groups are seropositive by the middle of the second decade of life.

Because infections with HSV-2 are usually acquired through sexual contact, antibodies to this virus are rarely found until the onset of sexual activity. There is a progressive increase in infection rates, with HSV-2 in all populations beginning in adolescence. Overall, about 15 to 20% of Americans have genital HSV-2 infection. Rates of HSV-2 infection are highest among women, non-Hispanic blacks, men who have sex with men, and immunocompromised persons. Genital herpes infection has been found to be an important risk factor for the transmission of human immunodeficiency virus (HIV; Chapter 362).

Genital HSV disease during gestation can result in transmission of HSV to the fetus, most frequently related to shedding of the virus in genital secretions at the time of delivery. The incidence of cervical shedding in pregnant women with asymptomatic HSV-2 infection is approximately 1%. Most infants in whom neonatal disease develops are born to women who are completely asymptomatic for genital HSV infection at the time of delivery and who have neither a known history of genital herpes nor a sexual partner reporting a genital vesicular rash. These women account for 60 to 80% of all women whose children acquire neonatal HSV infection. Women who experience a symptomatic or asymptomatic primary infection in the third trimester of gestation have a 30 to 50% risk for transmitting infection to the child.

PATHOBIOLOGY

Replication of HSV is a multistep process (E-Fig. 350-2). After binding of the virion to the host cell and release of the nucleocapsid into the cytoplasm, DNA is uncoated and transported to the nucleus. This release is followed by transcription of immediate-early genes, which encode the regulatory proteins, and is followed by the expression of proteins encoded by early and then late genes. These proteins include enzymes necessary for viral replication and structural proteins.

Assembly of the viral core and capsid takes place within the nucleus. Envelopment at the nuclear membrane and transport out of the nucleus occur through the endoplasmic reticulum and the Golgi apparatus. Glycosylation of the viral membrane occurs in the Golgi apparatus. Mature virions are transported to the outer membrane of the host cell inside vesicles. Release of progeny virus is accompanied by cell death.

A critical factor for transmission of HSV is intimate contact between a person who is shedding virus and a susceptible host. With inoculation onto skin or mucous membranes, HSV replicates in epithelial cells; the incubation period is 4 to 6 days (E-Fig. 350-3). As replication continues, cell lysis and local inflammation ensue, resulting in the formation of characteristic vesicles on erythematous bases. During primary infection, lymph nodes in the area of viral replication may become enlarged. Viremia may result in visceral dissemination in immunocompromised patients. In all hosts, the virus generally ascends peripheral sensory nerves to reach the dorsal root ganglia. Replication of HSV within neural tissue is followed by spread of the virus to other mucosal and skin surfaces by means of peripheral sensory nerves. HSV replicates further in epithelial cells and reproduces the lesions of the initial infection until infection is contained through host immune responses.

The histopathologic changes induced by HSV replication are similar in both primary and recurrent infection, including ballooning of infected cells and the appearance of condensed chromatin within the nuclei of cells, followed by degeneration of cellular nuclei. Cells lose intact plasma membranes and form multinucleated giant cells. They may also demonstrate intranuclear inclusions known as Cowdry type A bodies, which are suggestive, but not diagnostic, of HSV infection. With cell lysis, clear vesicular fluid containing large quantities of virus accumulates between the epidermis and dermal layer. The dermis reveals an intense inflammatory response, more so with primary infection than with recurrent disease. As healing progresses, the clear vesicular fluid becomes pustular with the accumulation of inflammatory cells. The pustule ruptures, resulting in an ulcer, which then forms a scab; scarring is uncommon.

Vascular changes in the area of infection include perivascular cuffing and hemorrhagic necrosis. These changes are particularly prominent when organs other than skin are involved, as is the case with herpes simplex encephalitis or disseminated neonatal HSV infection. Local lymphatics can show evidence of infection with intrusion of inflammatory cells because of draining of infected secretions from the area of viral replication. As host defenses are mounted, an influx of mononuclear cells can be detected in infected tissue.

A unique characteristic of all herpesviruses is their ability to establish latent infection, that is, to persist in an apparently inactive state for varying lengths of time, and then to be reactivated (E-Fig. 350-4). The latent viral genome may be either extrachromosomal or integrated into host cell DNA, depending on the virus.

Latency is established when HSV reaches the dorsal root ganglia after retrograde transmission through sensory nerve pathways. Latent virus may be reactivated and enter a replicative cycle at any point in time. Reactivation of latent virus is a well-recognized biologic phenomenon, but not one that is clearly understood from a molecular standpoint. Stimuli associated with the reactivation of latent HSV have included stress, fever, menstruation, and exposure to ultraviolet light. Precisely how these factors interact at the level of the ganglia remains to be defined. Reactivation may be clinically asymptomatic, or it may produce life-threatening disease.

CLINICAL MANIFESTATIONS

Gingivostomatitis

Gingivostomatitis (usually caused by HSV-1) occurs most frequently in children younger than 5 years. Illness is characterized by fever, sore throat, pharyngeal edema, and erythema, followed by the development of vesicular or ulcerative lesions on the oral and pharyngeal mucosa. Recurrent HSV-1 infections of the oropharynx are most frequently manifested as herpes simplex labialis (cold sores or fever blisters) and usually appear on the vermilion border of the lip (Fig. 350-1). Recurrences are triggered by fever, stress, and exposure to ultraviolet light as well as by other factors. Intraoral lesions as a manifestation of recurrent disease are uncommon.

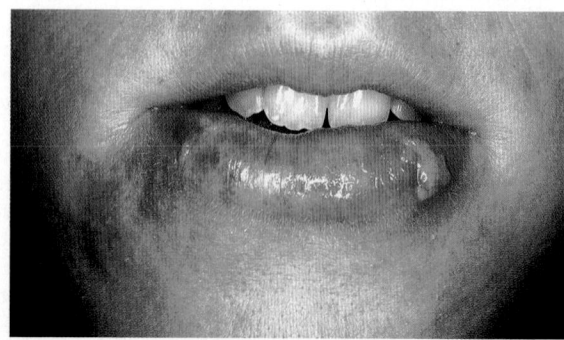

FIGURE 350-1. Herpes labialis, classic grouped blisters.

Genital Herpes

Genital herpes was historically attributed to HSV-2, but at least 50% of all new primary cases in young adults are caused by HSV-1.[1] Notably, well over half of initial episodes of genital herpes caused by either HSV-1 or HSV-2 are subclinical. Symptomatic primary infection in women usually involves lesions on the vulva, vagina, and cervix. In men, symptomatic primary infection is most often associated with lesions on the glans penis, prepuce, or penile shaft. In individuals of either gender, primary disease is associated with fever, malaise, anorexia, and bilateral inguinal adenopathy. Women frequently have dysuria and urinary retention as a result of urethral involvement. Aseptic meningitis develops in as many as 10% of individuals with primary infection. Sacral radiculomyelitis may occur in both men and women and results in neuralgias, urinary retention, or obstipation. Complete healing of primary infection may take several weeks. The first episode of genital infection is less severe in individuals who have previously had HSV-1 infections at other sites. Antibodies to HSV-1 appear to ameliorate the severity of initial HSV-2 clinical disease.

Recurrent genital infections in either men or women can be particularly distressing. The frequency of recurrences varies significantly from one individual to another but is always less frequent with HSV-1 genital disease than with HSV-2. In the first year after initial genital herpes caused by HSV-2, the median number of symptomatic recurrences is four.

Only 10 to 25% of persons with serologically confirmed HSV-2 infection are aware that they have genital herpes. Investigations using polymerase chain reaction (PCR) sampling have shown that 80 to 90% of HSV-2-infected individuals have transient episodes of asymptomatic viral shedding from the genital tract on 10 to 20% of days. Asymptomatic viral shedding from undiagnosed patients is the most common source of new transmissions.

Herpetic Keratitis

Herpes simplex keratitis (Chapter 395) is usually caused by HSV-1 and is often accompanied by conjunctivitis. It is considered the most common infectious cause of blindness in the United States. The characteristic lesions of HSV keratoconjunctivitis are dendritic ulcers best detected by fluorescein staining of the cornea. Deep stromal involvement has also been reported and may result in visual impairment.

Other Cutaneous Manifestations

HSV infections can occur at any skin site. Common among health care workers are lesions on the fingers, known as herpetic whitlow. Similarly, in wrestlers, disseminated cutaneous lesions known as herpes gladiatorum may develop as a result of physical contact.

Herpes Meningitis

HSV can cause lymphocytic meningitis.[2] HSV-2 meningitis, associated with symptomatic or asymptomatic genital herpes, can cause recurrent episodes of meningitis. Symptoms include fever, meningismus, and headache, which can be severe. HSV meningitis is usually self-limited and does not progress to herpes encephalitis.

HERPES SIMPLEX VIRUS INFECTIONS IN IMMUNOCOMPROMISED HOSTS

HSV infections in immunocompromised hosts, including patients with acquired immunodeficiency syndrome, are usually due to reactivation of latent infection and are clinically more severe, may be progressive, and require a longer time to heal. Manifestations of HSV infections in this population of patients include pneumonitis,[3] esophagitis, hepatitis, colitis, disseminated cutaneous disease, and central nervous system (CNS) infections. Individuals suffering from HIV infection may have extensive perineal or orofacial ulcerations. HSV infections are also noted to be of increased severity in individuals with extensive burns.

DIAGNOSIS

Definitive diagnosis of HSV infection requires detection of viral DNA by PCR testing or isolation of virus. DNA amplification has become the diagnostic method of choice in assessing cerebrospinal fluid (CSF) specimens for evidence of HSV infection of the central nervous system.[4] PCR is now widely used for confirmation of HSV as the cause of mucocutaneous or ocular infections. Viral culture is no longer frequently used but is essential when an HSV isolate is required to assess possible resistance to antiviral drugs.

In the absence of PCR or diagnostic virologic facilities, cytologic examination of cells scraped from a clinical lesion may be useful in making a presumptive diagnosis of HSV infection (Tzanck prep). Staining the preparation with HSV-specific monoclonal antibodies improves the sensitivity of the technique.

Type-specific serologic assays that reliably establish whether an individual is infected with HSV-1 or HSV-2 (or both) are commercially available. These tests are based on antigenic differences between HSV-1 and HSV-2 glycoprotein G.

TREATMENT Rx

For *immunocompromised* patients with extensive cutaneous HSV disease or with visceral organ disease, the treatment of choice is intravenous acyclovir (5 to 10 mg/kg every 8 hours for 5 to 7 days, dose adjusted for renal function). Caution must be exercised when acyclovir is administered intravenously because it may crystallize in the renal tubules when it is infused too rapidly. Valacyclovir (500 to 1000 mg two or three times daily) and famciclovir (250 to 500 mg three times daily) are orally administered antiviral drugs that have improved pharmacokinetic profiles compared with oral acyclovir. These drugs are effective alternatives for non-life-threatening HSV infection.

High-risk immunocompromised hosts are at risk for developing infection due to acyclovir-resistant HSV. Resistance is usually due to a mutation resulting in altered or deficient thymidine kinase enzyme that is essential for activation of acyclovir. Such patients can be managed with intravenous foscarnet or cidofovir, although both of these drugs can have significant adverse effects. (see Tables 336-4 and 336-5 in Chapter 336).

In *immunocompetent* hosts with mucocutaneous infections, oral acyclovir (200 mg five times daily for 5 days) reduces lesions and speeds recovery.[A1] Oral valacyclovir (1 g/day for 5 days or 500 mg twice daily for 3 days) and oral famciclovir (1 g twice daily for 1 day) are equally effective and more convenient.[5] Topical acyclovir is minimally efficacious and is not recommended.[A2] Immunocompetent patients with HSV meningitis typically improve with or without specific antiviral therapy. Their treatment can focus on rehydration and analgesia rather than intravenous acyclovir therapy.

HSV has been used for experimental gene therapy. By removal of the $\gamma_1 34.5$ gene, both neurovirulence and the propensity to establish latency are ablated. These engineered viruses are being experimentally tested in patients with glioblastoma multiforme and metastatic colorectal cancer.

PREVENTION

Secondary Prevention

Screening of asymptomatic patients for genital herpes simplex is not recommended.[6] All patients with symptomatic genital HSV recurrences should be considered candidates for chronic suppressive antiviral therapy. Potential regimens include oral acyclovir 400 mg twice daily, oral valacyclovir 500 mg or 1 g/day, and oral famciclovir 250 mg twice daily.[A3] Such regimens are approved by the U.S. Food and Drug Administration for genital herpes but not for herpes labialis, for which the benefit of viral suppression is small with oral agents and not proved with typical agents. However, antiviral suppressive therapy does not reliably prevent recurrent HSV-2 meningitis.

Primary Prevention

At present, experimental vaccines for HSV-1 and HSV-2 remain under investigation; however, none are currently in phase III clinical trials. In a recent randomized trial, pericoital use of tenofovir gel, an antiviral microbicide, reduced HSV-2 acquisition in women by about 50%.[A4] Acyclovir, valacyclovir, and famciclovir are given to recipients of solid organ and bone marrow transplants in the immediate post-transplantation period in an effort to prevent reactivation of latent disease. Valacyclovir (500 mg daily) can decrease person-to-person transmission of HSV-2 when taken by the infected partner in a discordant couple. Suppressive therapy of an HSV-2-infected but HIV-seronegative person does not prevent HIV acquisition from HIV-seropositive partners.

HERPES SIMPLEX ENCEPHALITIS

Herpes simplex encephalitis[7] is characterized by hemorrhagic necrosis of the temporal lobe (Chapter 386). Disease begins unilaterally and can spread to the contralateral temporal lobe (Fig. 350-2). It is the most common cause of focal, sporadic encephalitis in the United States today and occurs in approximately 1 in 150,000 to 500,000 individuals per year. More than 90% of cases in adults are caused by HSV-1. The actual pathogenesis of herpes simplex encephalitis requires further clarification, although it has been speculated that primary or recurrent virus can reach the temporal lobe by ascending neural pathways, such as the trigeminal tracts or the olfactory nerves. HSV-1 encephalitis is associated with defects in genes in the toll-like receptor 3 pathway.[8]

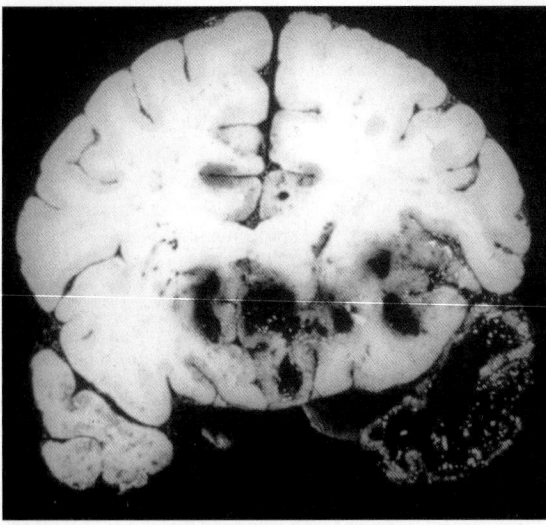

FIGURE 350-2. Hemorrhagic temporal lobe necrosis in herpes simplex encephalitis.

CLINICAL MANIFESTATIONS AND DIAGNOSIS

Clinical manifestations of herpes simplex encephalitis reflect temporal lobe involvement and include headache, fever, altered consciousness, behavioral changes, aphasia, and other focal neurologic abnormalities. Seizures are also common. CSF findings in these patients are variable but usually reveal a lymphocytic pleocytosis (25 to 75 WBC/μL, 75 to 90% mononuclear cells). The protein concentration is mildly elevated (65 to 85 mg/dL), and the glucose level is usually normal. Magnetic resonance imaging (which is more sensitive than computed tomography) can suggest the diagnosis by demonstrating abnormalities of the temporal lobe, which are unilateral in the early stages of the disease. Diagnosis can be confirmed detection of HSV DNA by PCR in the CSF.

TREATMENT AND PROGNOSIS   Rx

Without effective antiviral therapy, mortality is higher than 70%, and less than 10% of patients return to baseline neurologic function. With appropriate therapy using intravenous acyclovir (10 mg/kg every 8 hours for 14 to 21 days), the mortality rate can be reduced to 10 to 25%, with 40 to 55% of patients able to resume their activities of daily living. There is no benefit to long-term oral valacyclovir administration following acyclovir treatment.[A5]

Instances of recurrent HSV encephalitis have been reported, but many cases of relapsing neurologic symptoms are now thought to be due to postinfectious autoimmune phenomena, especially anti-*N*-methyl-D-aspartate receptor antibody encephalitis (Chapter 386).[9]

● NEONATAL HERPES SIMPLEX VIRUS INFECTION

Neonatal HSV infection is estimated to occur in approximately 1 in 3500 deliveries in the United States each year.[10] Approximately 70% of cases are caused by HSV-2 and usually result from contact of the fetus with infected maternal genital secretions at the time of delivery. Manifestations of neonatal HSV infection can be divided into three categories: skin, eye, and mouth disease; encephalitis; and disseminated infection. As the name implies, skin, eye, and mouth disease consists of cutaneous lesions and does not involve other organ systems. Involvement of the CNS may occur with encephalitis or disseminated infection and generally results in diffuse encephalitis. CSF analysis characteristically reveals elevated protein levels and mononuclear pleocytosis. Disseminated infection involves multiple organ systems and can cause disseminated intravascular coagulation, hemorrhagic pneumonitis, encephalitis, and cutaneous lesions. Diagnosis is difficult in the absence of skin lesions, which occurs in as many as 36% of cases. The mortality rate for each disease classification varies from zero for skin, eye, and mouth disease to 5% for encephalitis and 25% for neonates with disseminated infection, even with appropriate antiviral treatment. In addition to the high mortality associated with these infections, morbidity is significant in that children with encephalitis or disseminated disease develop normally in only 40% of cases, even with appropriate antiviral therapy (acyclovir, 20 mg/kg every 8 hours for 14 days

for skin, eye, and mouth infections and 21 days for central nervous system or disseminated disease). Six months of suppressive acyclovir therapy (300 mg three times daily) can significantly improve neurologic outcome.

Grade A References

A1. Hollier LM, Eppes C. Genital herpes: oral antiviral treatments. *BMJ Clin Evid*. 2015;2015:1-17.
A2. Chi CC, Wang SH, Delamere FM, et al. Interventions for prevention of herpes simplex labialis (cold sores on the lips). *Cochrane Database Syst Rev*. 2015;8:CD010095.
A3. Le Cleach L, Trinquart L, Do G, et al. Oral antiviral therapy for prevention of genital herpes outbreaks in immunocompetent and nonpregnant patients. *Cochrane Database Syst Rev*. 2014;8:CD009036.
A4. Abdool Karim SS, Abdool Karim Q, Kharsany AB, et al. Tenofovir gel for the prevention of herpes simplex virus type 2 infection. *N Engl J Med*. 2015;373:530-539.
A5. Gnann JW Jr, Skoldenberg B, Hart J, et al. Herpes simplex encephalitis: lack of clinical benefit of long-term valacyclovir therapy. *Clin Infect Dis*. 2015;61:683-691.

GENERAL REFERENCES

For the General References and other additional features, please visit Expert Consult at https://expertconsult.inkling.com.

351

VARICELLA-ZOSTER VIRUS (CHICKENPOX, SHINGLES)

JEFFREY COHEN

DEFINITION

Primary infection with varicella-zoster virus results in the rash of varicella (chickenpox). The varicella-zoster virus establishes a latent infection in the nervous system and can reactivate later in life to cause zoster (shingles).

The Pathogen

Varicella-zoster virus is a member of the alpha herpesvirus family and has a DNA core surrounded by a nucleocapsid, which is in turn surrounded by a viral envelope that is studded with glycoproteins. Antibody to viral glycoproteins is important for neutralizing the virus's infectivity and for protecting against primary infection. The virus encodes a thymidine kinase, which phosphorylates acyclovir, which in turn inhibits viral DNA replication by inhibiting the varicella-zoster virus DNA polymerase.

EPIDEMIOLOGY

Before the advent of an effective vaccine, more than 95% of children in temperate climates were infected with varicella-zoster virus. By comparison, infection is usually delayed until adulthood in tropical climates. Varicella usually occurs in children younger than 5 years. Zoster is less common in tropical areas, probably because of a delay in acquisition of varicella. Varicella is more common in the winter and spring, whereas zoster has no seasonal predilection.

Primary varicella infection can occur after exposure to either chickenpox or zoster. The virus is spread by droplets and aerosols from patients or by contact with vesicular lesions. Persons are infectious beginning about 2 days before the rash appears and continuing until all lesions have crusted. Although 60 to 90% of susceptible household contacts develop varicella, only 20 to 30% of susceptible persons exposed to zoster become infected. More than 95% of primary infections result in the symptoms of varicella, and second episodes of varicella are rare. Varicella is more severe in persons with impaired cellular immunity, including patients with acquired immunodeficiency syndrome (AIDS) and infants whose mothers present with varicella 5 days before to 2 days after delivery.

About 50% of persons who have had varicella and live to age 85 years will develop zoster. The risk for zoster rises with increasing age (especially 50 years and older) and with increasing impairment of cellular immunity. Perhaps because of advanced medical care and recognition by physicians, the reported incidence of zoster has increased by four-fold over the past six decades,[1] although hospitalizations for zoster have decreased in adults since 2008, apparently related to the herpes zoster vaccine.[2] Men with AIDS have a 20-fold higher risk for development of zoster than age-matched controls. Less than 5% of persons have a second episode of zoster, but recurrent zoster is more common in persons with impaired cellular immunity.

PATHOBIOLOGY

Varicella is transmitted by the respiratory route. The virus is thought to infect epithelial cells and lymphocytes in the oropharynx and upper respiratory tract or in the conjunctiva, and then infected lymphocytes subsequently spread the virus throughout the body. The virus then enters the skin through endothelial cells in blood vessels and spreads to epithelial cells, where it causes the vesicular rash of varicella. Lesions initially are vesicular but become pustular after the infiltration of inflammatory cells. Later the lesions break open and dry to form crusts that usually heal without scarring. During primary infection, neurons in cranial nerve ganglia and dorsal root ganglia become latently infected with the virus.

If varicella-zoster virus–specific cellular immunity declines, the virus can reactivate from a ganglion, travel down the axon, and replicate in epithelial cells to cause dermatomal zoster. In highly immunocompromised persons, high-grade viremia during reactivation causes disseminated zoster.

Antibodies, which usually are present at the time varicella presents clinically, persist for life. Antibody is important for protection against varicella, as evidenced by the ability of varicella immune globulin to attenuate the disease. Cytotoxic T cells are present within 2 to 3 days after the onset of varicella and limit its severity. Varicella is more severe in persons with impaired cellular immunity but not in patients with hypogammaglobulinemia. Cellular immunity, not antibody, is required to prevent reactivation of virus and zoster.

CLINICAL MANIFESTATIONS

Varicella

Varicella begins with fever and malaise followed 1 to 2 days later by a disseminated, pruritic, vesicular rash (Fig. 351-1).[3] The usual incubation period for varicella is 2 weeks (range, 10 to 21 days) after exposure to an infected person. The lesions begin as papules that become vesicles, followed by pustules and then crusts. Lesions appear on the head and then spread to the trunk and then to the extremities; the mucosa can also be involved. There are typically 200 to 500 lesions in different stages on the skin. New lesions occur for up to 5 days in normal hosts, and crusting is complete within 2 weeks.

The most common complication of varicella is bacterial superinfection of skin lesions. Group A streptococcus (Chapter 274) or *Staphylococcus aureus* (Chapter 272) infections can cause cellulitis, bacteremia, and necrotizing fasciitis. Other complications include cerebellar ataxia, viral pneumonitis, hepatitis, and thrombocytopenia. Less frequent complications include viral meningitis, encephalitis, vasculopathy (which presents as a stroke), disseminated intravascular coagulopathy (Chapter 166), and Reye syndrome (more common in children receiving aspirin) (Chapter 141). Complications involving the lungs and liver are more common in children with impaired cellular

immunity, including those receiving systemic steroids, children with chronic pulmonary or skin disease, adults, and pregnant women during the third trimester. The fetal varicella syndrome, which occurs in fetuses infected during the first trimester, is characterized by atrophy of limbs with scarring of skin, chorioretinitis or cataracts, and central nervous system abnormalities. Patients with AIDS and moderately reduced CD4 cell counts may develop recurrent varicella lesions in the absence of new exposures, and patients with CD4 cell counts below 200/μL may develop progressive varicella with new lesions occurring for at least 1 month or chronic verrucous lesions.

Zoster

In healthy persons, zoster presents with localized pain and increased sensation for 1 to 3 days before the development of a dermatomal vesicular rash that does not cross the midline (Fig. 351-2).[4] Zoster most frequently presents in the dermatomes innervated by trigeminal or thoracic ganglia. The rash is usually accompanied by itching, tingling, or pain. The lesions evolve from vesicles to pustules, and crusting is usually complete by 10 days. In normal hosts, a few lesions may develop outside of the dermatome owing to low-grade viremia. Some patients with zoster sine herpete never develop a rash. In persons with very impaired cellular immunity, reactivation is often associated with high-grade viremia with dissemination to large areas of the skin and involvement of multiple organs. As a result, patients with underlying malignancies are more likely to develop serious complications from their zoster infections, and zoster is occasionally associated with an occult hematologic malignancy.[5]

A dreaded complication of zoster is post-herpetic neuralgia (Chapter 27), with pain persisting for at least 1 month after the rash has resolved. Risk factors include older age and severe immunosuppression.[6] Patients may have allodynia (sensation of pain after nonpainful stimuli), paresthesias, dysesthesias, or severe neuropathic pain. Post-herpetic neuralgia is more common in persons older than 50 years. Other complications of zoster include bacterial superinfection; ocular disease, involving any of the structures of the eye, due to reactivation in the ophthalmic branch of the trigeminal ganglia; facial palsy caused by reactivation in the VII cranial nerve; Ramsay Hunt syndrome, with pain and vesicles in the ear, numbness of the anterior tongue, and ipsilateral facial palsy due to reactivation in the geniculate ganglion of the VII cranial nerve; motor neuropathy; and meningitis.[7] Zoster vasculopathy, occurring at the time of zoster or a few months later, can present with stroke due to inflammation of the cerebral arteries.

Progressive outer retinal necrosis, with few inflammatory ocular cells, occurs when varicella-zoster virus reactivates in the eye of severely immunocompromised persons, including patients with AIDS and low CD4 cell counts. In contrast, acute retinal necrosis with a marked inflammatory response occurs when the virus reactivates in otherwise healthy persons. Patients with AIDS or recipients of hematopoietic stem cell transplants can have pancreatitis, hepatitis, and pneumonitis in the absence of or preceding a rash. In one study, varicella-zoster virus antigen was found in 74% of temporal artery biopsies of patients with giant cell arteritis (Chapter 255) compared with just 8% of controls.[8]

DIAGNOSIS

Most cases of varicella and zoster are diagnosed on the basis of their clinical presentation. A disseminated vesicular rash with lesions in various stages of

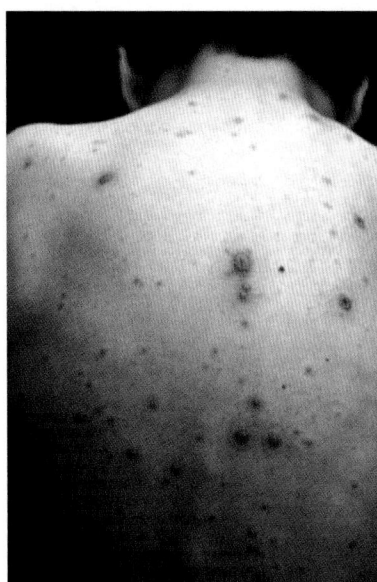

FIGURE 351-1. Child with varicella. (Courtesy of Centers for Disease Control and Prevention.)

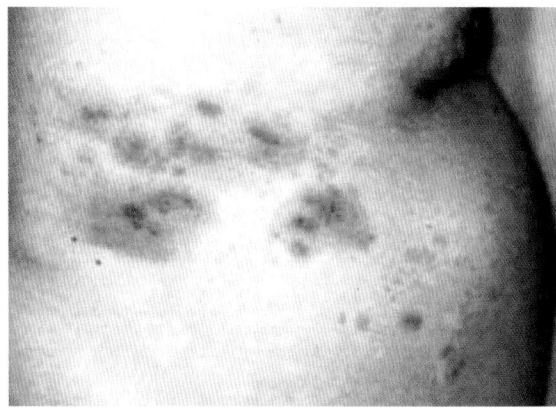

FIGURE 351-2. Dermatomal zoster. (Courtesy of Centers for Disease Control and Prevention.)

evolution is usually sufficient for a diagnosis of varicella. The differential diagnosis includes impetigo (Chapter 412), enterovirus infections (Chapter 355), herpes simplex (Chapter 350), Stevens-Johnson syndrome (Chapter 411), and guttate psoriasis (Chapter 409). A dermatomal vesicular rash that does not cross the midline in a patient with a prior history of pain in the area is usually diagnostic of zoster. Herpes simplex is the most common disease that resembles zoster.

When the diagnosis of varicella or zoster must be confirmed definitively, polymerase chain reaction (PCR) for varicella-zoster virus from vesicular fluid is the most sensitive and specific test.[9] PCR for varicella-zoster virus in the blood can be useful for diagnosis of visceral zoster in highly immuno-compromised persons before the onset of rash. PCR for varicella-zoster virus in the cerebrospinal fluid and intrathecal synthesis of varicella-zoster virus–specific antibody is useful for diagnosis of varicella-zoster virus neurologic diseases. Culture is less sensitive than PCR because the virus is very labile. Direct fluorescent antibody testing of vesicle fluid is rapid but less sensitive than PCR. Detection of multinucleated giant cells (Tzanck smear) is less specific because lesions of herpes simplex virus have a similar appearance. Biopsy specimens show eosinophilic intranuclear inclusion bodies and multinucleate giant cells.

Serology for varicella-zoster virus is useful to determine the need for postexposure prophylaxis in persons who are at high risk for disease after exposure to varicella or zoster. Enzyme-linked immunosorbent assay tests are less sensitive than latex agglutination assays and may not detect antibodies in vaccinees.

TREATMENT Rx

Varicella

Symptomatic treatment includes acetaminophen for fever and lotion or baths for pruritus. Although acyclovir is licensed for the treatment of varicella, the drug is not recommended for otherwise healthy children because it only modestly decreases symptoms by about 1 day. Acyclovir reduces visceral dissemination in immunocompromised persons, in whom intravenous acyclovir (500 mg/m^2 every 8 hours for children, 10 mg/kg every 8 hours for adults) is recommended for 7 to 10 days or until all lesions have crusted. Oral acyclovir (20 mg/kg four times daily for children or 800 mg five times daily for adults) given within 24 hours after the onset of rash reduces the duration of symptoms and is recommended for treatment of adolescents, adults, newborns whose mothers developed varicella near the time of delivery, immunocompromised persons, children with chronic pulmonary or skin disease, and persons with complications of varicella. Acyclovir also should be considered for household contacts of persons with varicella or for pregnant women in the third trimester; these patients often have more severe disease. Oral valacyclovir is also approved for treatment of children ages 2 years to younger than 18 years with varicella (20 mg/kg three times daily with a maximum dose of 1 g). Oral valacyclovir (1 g three times daily) or famciclovir (500 mg three times daily) results in higher antiviral drug levels than does oral acyclovir and can be used in nonpregnant adults.

Zoster

Acyclovir, valacyclovir, and famciclovir (for 7 days at the same doses as for varicella) are licensed for the treatment of zoster. Oral valacyclovir and famciclovir result in higher levels of antiviral activity than oral acyclovir does. Although therapy should be started within 3 days of the rash, therapy may still be of benefit if new lesions continue to occur after this time. Because patients younger than 50 years usually have little pain associated with zoster, antiviral therapy is often not used in these patients unless they have moderate to severe pain, have disease involving the eye, have other complications, or are immunocompromised. Antiviral drugs (see earlier) reduce the duration of lesions and zoster-associated pain but not the incidence of post-herpetic neuralgia.[A1] In severely immunocompromised persons, intravenous acyclovir (7 to 10 days or until all lesions have crusted) reduces the risk for visceral dissemination. Oral valacyclovir or famciclovir may be used in persons who are less severely immunocompromised.

Corticosteroids (e.g., prednisone, 60 mg/day and tapered over 21 days), in combination with acyclovir, reduce acute pain and improve the quality of life in persons older than 50 years but do not reduce the risk for post-herpetic neuralgia. Patients with moderate to severe pain often require narcotics.

Treatment of post-herpetic neuralgia is challenging.[10] Gabapentin (initiated at a dose of 300 mg at bedtime and titrated to a maximum dose of 1200 mg three times daily) or pregabalin (initiated at a dose of 75 mg at bedtime and titrated to a maximum dose of 300 mg twice daily) may reduce pain.[A2] Additional agents include nortriptyline (initiated at a dose of 25 mg at bedtime and titrated to a maximum dose of 150 mg daily), lidocaine patches, and topical capsaicin (which itself causes pain that is not tolerated in up to one third of patients). Opioid analgesics (see Table 27-4 may be needed, but there are concerns about long-term efficacy and safety.

Treatment of Varicella-Zoster Virus Complications and Acyclovir-Resistant Varicella-Zoster Virus

Intravenous acyclovir is recommended for persons with acute retinal necrosis. Corticosteroids (e.g., prednisone, 1 mg/kg per day for 3 to 5 days) and intravenous acyclovir (10 to 15 mg/kg every 8 hours for 14 days) are recommended for nonimmunocompromised persons with varicella-zoster virus vasculopathy. Zoster involving the eye should be evaluated by an ophthalmologist to assess the potential value of topical or intraocular therapy, such as the need to reduce intraocular pressure to treat glaucoma or to use mydriatics to prevent synechiae.

Acyclovir-resistant varicella-zoster virus infections are rare and are limited almost exclusively to patients with AIDS or recipients of transplants. Foscarnet (40 mg/kg every 8 hours) for 2 weeks or until all lesions have crusted is the treatment of choice for acyclovir-resistant varicella-zoster virus.

PREVENTION

Varicella

Patients with varicella or zoster are considered infectious until all lesions have completely crusted. Airborne and contact precautions are recommended for varicella, whereas only contact precautions are necessary for immunocompetent persons with localized zoster.

The live attenuated varicella vaccine is recommended for children aged 1 to 12 years and for persons 13 years and older without immunity to the virus. The vaccine is 92% effective in protecting against symptomatic varicella and more than 95% effective in protecting against severe disease.[A3] Two doses of vaccine are given subcutaneously. The varicella vaccine is also given as part of a combined measles, mumps, rubella vaccine (MMRV) for children 1 to 12 years of age in the United States. The rate of disease due to varicella declined by 90% in the United States during the first 13 years after the vaccine was licensed.

The most common complications of varicella vaccination are pain at the injection site, fever, and a mild rash within 2 weeks after vaccination. The rash is often localized to the area of vaccination and is often papular; in some healthy persons, the rash can be disseminated, although there are fewer lesions and symptoms are much less severe than with wild-type virus. In persons with severely impaired cellular immunity, rash is more common, can be extensive, and may be accompanied by organ dysfunction. The varicella vaccine establishes latency and can cause shingles, although this complication occurs less commonly with vaccine virus than with wild-type virus. The vaccine strain of varicella has been transmitted to third parties only by vaccinees who developed a rash. Varicella vaccine is contraindicated in pregnant women and persons receiving high-dose immunosuppressive therapy (e.g., ≥2 mg/kg of prednisone daily) or with hematologic malignant neoplasms. Vaccination should be considered for human immunodeficiency virus (HIV)–infected children with age-specific CD4$^+$ T cells of 15% or more and adolescents and adults with CD4$^+$ T-cell counts of 200 cells/µL or higher. Serologic testing to verify immunity is not recommended for health care workers who have received two doses of vaccine because the currently available commercial antibody assays are not sensitive enough to detect protective levels of antibody.

Zoster

Two intramuscular doses of a subunit vaccine containing varicella-zoster virus glycoprotein E and the AS01$_B$ adjuvant system (called HZ/su) were 97% effective against herpes zoster for all age groups,[A4] with a 90% efficacy in persons over age 70 years.[A5] This vaccine is approved by the FDA and is preferentially recommended over the live attenuated zoster vaccine by the Advisory Committee for Immunization Practices for prevention of zoster and its complications in persons 50 years of age or older. This vaccine is recommended for immunocompetent adults, including those who previously received the live attenuated zoster vaccine,[11] because of its improved efficacy despite more local and sometimes systemic side effects. A live attenuated zoster vaccine is also approved by the U.S. Food and Drug Administration (FDA) for persons 50 years of age or older and recommended by the Advisory Committee on Immunization Practices for persons 60 years of age or older (Chapter 15). The vaccine is about 50% protective in preventing zoster and 66% effective in preventing post-herpetic neuralgia, although the vaccine's efficacy against zoster declines somewhat after 3 years.[12] Transient pain and erythema at the injection site are not uncommon, but serious complications attributable to the vaccine have not been reported. The vaccine also can be given safely to adults with a prior history of zoster. The vaccine is contraindicated in persons with hematologic malignant neoplasms, AIDS, or HIV infection with CD4 count of 200/μL or lower and in persons receiving high-dose immunosuppressive therapy (e.g., ≥20 mg of prednisone daily) or anti–tumor necrosis factor-α therapy.

Postexposure Prophylaxis

In persons exposed to varicella, three options are available. Varicella vaccine is preferred if exposure occurred within the prior 3 days and the patient is not immunocompromised. Vaccine is estimated to be 70 to 90% effective in healthy persons. VariZIG (formerly available as varicella immune globulin) prevents or attenuates varicella in 90% of susceptible persons if it is given within 4 days of exposure. The FDA has approved VariZIG for use within 10 days of exposure, but it should be given as soon as possible after exposure. VariZIG (given intramuscularly at 125 units/10 kg body weight, up to a maximum of 625 units) is indicated for susceptible persons at risk for severe varicella (e.g., pregnant women, preterm infants, neonates whose mothers have varicella between 5 days before and 2 days after delivery, immunocompromised persons) who are in close contact with patients with varicella or zoster. VariZIG has no effect in the treatment of zoster.

Oral acyclovir (40 to 80 mg/kg daily in four divided doses for 1 week beginning 7 to 9 days after exposure) is estimated to be 80 to 85% effective as postexposure prophylaxis. It is often used when the exposure occurred too long ago for vaccination or VariZIG.

PROGNOSIS

Before vaccination, about 200 children died of varicella each year in the United States. Now varicella is the underlying cause of death in an average of less than three Americans younger than 20 years annually.

Grade A References

A1. Chen N, Li Q, Yang J, et al. Antiviral treatment for preventing postherpetic neuralgia. *Cochrane Database Syst Rev.* 2014;2:CD006866.
A2. Wang SL, Wang H, Nie HY, et al. The efficacy of pregabalin for acute pain control in herpetic neuralgia patients: a meta-analysis. *Medicine (Baltimore).* 2017;96:1-9.
A3. Marin M, Marti M, Kambhampati A, et al. Global varicella vaccine effectiveness: a meta-analysis. *Pediatrics.* 2016;137:1-12.
A4. Lal H, Cunningham AL, Godeaux O, et al. Efficacy of an adjuvanted herpes zoster subunit vaccine in older adults. *N Engl J Med.* 2015;372:2087-2096.
A5. Cunningham AL, Lal H, Kovac M, et al. Efficacy of the herpes zoster subunit vaccine in adults 70 years of age or older. *N Engl J Med.* 2016;375:1019-1032.
A6. Macartney K, Heywood A, McIntyre P. Vaccines for post-exposure prophylaxis against varicella (chickenpox) in children and adults. *Cochrane Database Syst Rev.* 2014;6:CD001833.

GENERAL REFERENCES

For the General References and other additional features, please visit Expert Consult at https://expertconsult.inkling.com.

352

CYTOMEGALOVIRUS

W. LAWRENCE DREW AND GUY BOIVIN

DEFINITION

Cytomegalovirus (CMV) is a member of the herpesvirus family and shares, with the other members, the ability to establish a long-lived latent infection. Most of the clinical diseases caused by this virus result from reactivation of latent virus in immune-impaired patients, although primary infection in such patients can also be devastating.

The Pathogen

CMV has a linear, double-stranded DNA genome with about 250,000 base pairs that encode about 160 proteins. On microscopic examination, the hallmark of CMV infection is a large (cytomegalic), 25- to 35-μm cell containing a large central, basophilic intranuclear inclusion (Fig. 352-1), referred to as an owl's eye.

EPIDEMIOLOGY

Multiple mechanisms account for the spread of this virus, including vertical (in utero, during vaginal delivery, and by breast milk) and horizontal (saliva, genital, urine, blood) contact. These routes of transmission lead, collectively, to a 15 to 20% seroprevalence by 15 years of age in developed countries, with a higher seroprevalence in lower socioeconomic settings. From that age on, there is a steady upward trend of 1 to 2% per year that is due in part to sexual transmission. As a result, approximately 50% of the general population of the United States is antibody positive by 35 years of age, and a 1% per year rate of increase occurs thereafter. In underdeveloped countries, up to 90% of persons may be seropositive by 2 years of age.[1] Presumably, crowded living conditions permit spread of the virus through close contact with body fluids. A recent study showed that CMV was viable on metal and wood for up to 1 hour, glass and plastic up to 3 hours, and rubber, cloth, and crackers up to 6 hours. CMV was more likely to be isolated from wet, highly absorbent surfaces. These considerations were felt to be particularly important because children may actively shed CMV in saliva and urine for months to years, and exposure to bodily fluids from young children poses substantial risk for CMV exposure among women of reproductive age. Two additional mechanisms of transmission are blood transfusion and organ transplantation. A final important epidemiologic fact is that reinfection with a different strain of CMV may occur in CMV-seropositive persons, especially those who are immunocompromised, pregnant, or sexually promiscuous.

PATHOBIOLOGY

In fully immunocompetent individuals, CMV rarely causes clinically evident end-organ disease. When immune mechanisms are deficient, especially those mediated by CD4+ and CD8+ lymphocytes, latent virus replicates and causes both direct and indirect effects. Examples of direct virally mediated diseases are necrotizing CMV retinitis and esophagitis. In contrast, CMV pneumonitis is frequently manifested as subtle histologic alterations accompanied by limited viral replication, thus suggesting that immune-mediated injury may be the primary pathologic mechanism. Such injury may result from the upregulation and release of cytokines, including tumor necrosis factor-α, interferon-γ, and interleukin-2. Immune-mediated tissue injury may also be effected by CD8+ cytotoxic T lymphocytes directed against CMV-infected target cells. The clinical manifestations of CMV infection, including meningoencephalitis, retinitis, enteritis, vasculitis, pneumonitis, myocarditis, lymphadenitis, hepatitis, adrenalitis, and pancreatitis, reflect the range of cell types that CMV is capable of infecting. The indirect effects of CMV include increased risks of some bacterial infections and invasive fungal diseases, reactivation of other herpesviruses, immunosenescence, rejection, graft loss, and death.

The immune response to CMV infection involves both the humoral and cell-mediated arms, but the CD8+ cytotoxic T-cell response appears to be the most important. The CMV envelope glycoproteins that participate in viral entry are gB, gH/gL, and gCII. Humoral immunity directed at gB has been detected in convalescent phase sera and has been shown to block viral entry, cell-to-cell transmission, and syncytium formation in CMV-infected cells. Not surprisingly, gB is the primary target of experimental vaccines.

Fundamental to the pathogenesis of CMV is latency, or persistence of the viral genome in host cells without evidence of productive viral replication. It

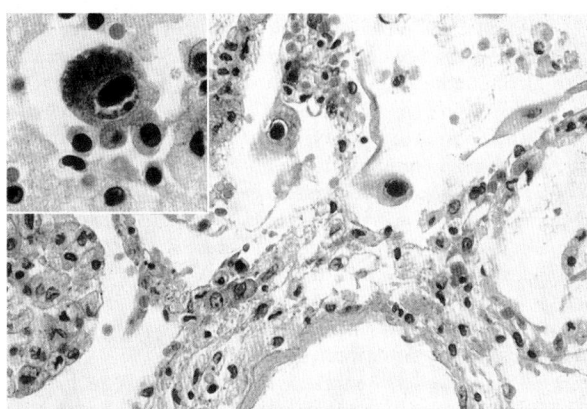

FIGURE 352-1. Cytomegalovirus (CMV) pneumonia. A lung biopsy specimen was stained with hematoxylin and eosin and magnified 250-fold. The **inset** shows a CMV "owl's eye" inclusion.

is thought that monocytes and bone marrow progenitor cells are sites of human CMV latency. Reactivation from the latent state has classically been associated with immunosuppression. Exposure to a rich milieu of cytokines and growth factors results in the activation of signal transduction pathways, generation of increased levels of intracellular transcription factors, and production of viable virus.

CLINICAL MANIFESTATIONS
Congenital and Neonatal Infection
In the developed world, congenital infection occurs in approximately 0.2 to 0.7% of newborns. Thus in the United States each year, approximately 40,000 infants are born excreting CMV, and about 4000 (or ~10%) of these newborns show clinical evidence of congenital disease, such as microcephaly, intracerebral calcification, hepatosplenomegaly, and rash. About 90% of these clinically infected newborns will survive, but half of the survivors will have unilateral or bilateral hearing loss, mental retardation, or both. Mothers of most infants with these stigmata had a primary infection during pregnancy, although it is now well known that clinically evident congenital infection also occurs in infants born to mothers with past CMV infection. In mothers with a primary infection, a negative amniocentesis markedly reduces the likelihood of hearing impairment and makes more serious sequelae very unlikely.[2] In newborns who are born to women with primary CMV infection but are initially asymptomatic, a CMV DNAemia at birth of 12,000 copies/mL or greater increases the likelihood of CMV-related sequelae, with the risk of a hearing deficit increased if the viral load in blood is 17,000 copies/mL or greater. Up to 14% of asymptomatic infected babies at birth will eventually develop learning problems or hearing loss.[3]

Infection in Immunocompetent Persons
Virtually all CMV infections occurring in immunocompetent persons are asymptomatic. In some patients, a clinical illness resembling infectious mononucleosis may develop (Chapter 353), but with minimal pharyngitis and lymphadenopathy. Atypical lymphocytosis develops in these patients, similar to Epstein-Barr virus infection, but they have a negative heterophil antibody test result. CMV reactivation is more common in elderly and frail individuals[4] and is especially common (33%) in critically ill immunocompetent patients, in whom it is associated with prolonged hospitalization and mortality, but whether it causes these effects is unclear.[5]

Infection in Transplant Recipients
When a CMV-seronegative recipient receives a solid organ from a CMV-seropositive donor, the resulting illnesses include the "CMV syndrome," characterized by fever, neutropenia, atypical lymphocytes, and often hepatosplenomegaly. CMV disease may also develop in the transplanted organ. For example, CMV hepatitis in liver transplant recipients is associated with fever, hyperbilirubinemia, and elevated liver enzymes; liver failure may ensue and necessitate retransplantation.[6] Recipients of a solid organ transplant may develop CMV disease by reactivation of latent infection, reinfection by an exogenous strain, or transmission of CMV from a seropositive donor to a seronegative individual (primary infection). Disease in CMV-seropositive recipients is, fortunately, less severe than that resulting from primary infection. CMV infection occurs more commonly in recipients of lung or liver transplants than in recipients of kidney transplants.

CMV pneumonia may occur after solid organ transplantation but is most common after stem cell transplantation.[7] Fever, nonproductive cough, and dyspnea can progress rapidly. The diagnosis is suggested by interstitial to nodular infiltrates rather than by alveolar densities on chest radiographs. In contrast to solid organ transplantation, CMV disease after stem cell transplantation usually results from reactivation of latent CMV in a seropositive recipient rather than from a new, primary infection.

CMV may cause disease throughout the gastrointestinal tract. Colitis, which is a common syndrome in transplant recipients, is manifested as diarrhea, weight loss, and fever. It is characterized by diffuse submucosal hemorrhages and ulcerations.

Infection in Patients with Acquired Immunodeficiency Syndrome
In the era before highly active antiretroviral therapy, CMV retinitis occurred in approximately one third of patients with acquired immunodeficiency syndrome (AIDS), most often in those with CD4 counts below 50/μL. It usually begins unilaterally with visual blurring, floaters, decreased acuity, and loss of visual fields and progresses to blindness if it is untreated. The retinal

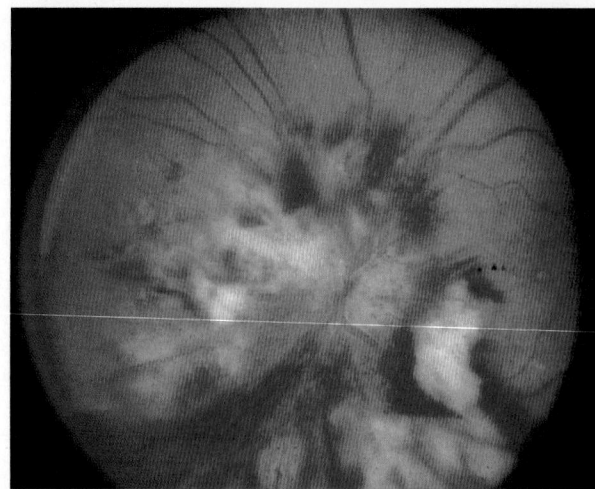

FIGURE 352-2. Cytomegalovirus retinitis as seen by direct ophthalmoscopic examination.

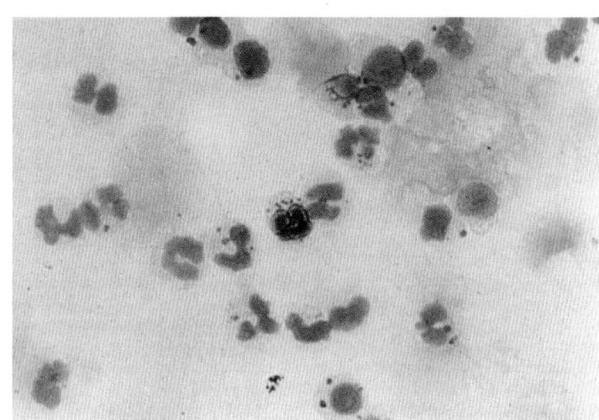

FIGURE 352-3. Peripheral blood leukocytes stained with monoclonal antibody to cytomegalovirus pp65 antigen by the immunoperoxidase technique (magnification ×500).

examination is abnormal, and the finding of apparent hemorrhages and exudates is the best diagnostic test (Fig. 352-2). CMV colitis is similar to that seen in transplant recipients, but esophagitis is also common and characterized by distal ulceration, which may be single but extensive. CMV neurologic disease occurs in multiple forms, including encephalitis and a polyradiculopathy/myelitis syndrome. With the efficacy of combination antiretroviral therapy, the incidence of all of these CMV syndromes has decreased dramatically, but they are still seen before human immunodeficiency virus (HIV) treatment or when such treatment is interrupted or ineffective. Even in the current era of HIV treatment, evidence of immunoglobulin G–positive CMV infection is associated with an increased risk of severe non–AIDS-defining events and non–AIDS-related death, especially cardiovascular and cerebrovascular events, thereby suggesting a role for CMV coinfection in vascular/degenerative organ disorders in HIV-infected patients.[8]

DIAGNOSIS
Assay of viral DNA by the polymerase chain reaction (PCR) is more sensitive than viral culture and is the best assay for the early detection of CMV disease. This assay, mainly performed on whole blood or plasma, can provide quantification that is especially helpful in supporting the diagnosis of CMV disease, enacting preemptive antiviral intervention, and monitoring therapy. Monoclonal antibodies can also be used to quantify viremia by counting CMV antigen–positive cells directly in peripheral blood leukocytes (antigenemia) (Fig. 352-3). The antigenemia test is less sensitive than PCR assays and not suitable for large-volume testing.

Viral culture, which was the prior "gold standard" for diagnosing CMV, has been supplanted by the assays described previously. Routine culture may require at least 4 to 6 weeks, whereas the newer methods described previously yield results within a day. The clinical significance of positive CMV cultures may be difficult to ascertain, particularly in immunosuppressed patients. For example, CMV may be present in the saliva or urine of up to 60 to 90% of transplant recipients and patients with AIDS, and virus in these sites does not prove that CMV is the cause of a patient's illness. Cytologic and histologic abnormalities are not sensitive measures of CMV infection, but they are specific and indicative of CMV disease.

PREVENTION

A nonviable CMV vaccine, containing the gB antigen with MF59 adjuvant, decreases primary infection in young women by about 45%[A1] but is not commercially available. Other vaccine candidates are being developed but remain experimental, including a new vaccine strategy based on the pentameric gH complex.

Because CMV is transmitted by exchange of secretions or excretions, infection can be diminished by reducing exposure to body fluids. For example, transmission by both vaginal and anal intercourse, which are bidirectional risks, can be diminished by "safe sex." Similarly, limiting the contact of seronegative pregnant women with the secretions and excretions of children, especially preschoolers in daycare, can decrease primary infection and, in turn, congenital disease.

The risk for acquiring CMV disease can be reduced in seronegative, immunosuppressed patients through the use of blood products or organ grafts from CMV-seronegative donors. Valganciclovir and ganciclovir provide effective prophylaxis in solid organ transplantation, and they are commonly administered for a 3- to 6-month period after transplantation.[A2] However, late-onset CMV end-organ disease may occur when the antiviral drug is eventually discontinued. Prophylaxis has been uncommon for stem cell transplant recipients, and these patients typically have been monitored weekly (from day 10 to day 100 after transplantation) for CMV DNA or antigenemia, with antiviral therapy introduced preemptively if viremia occurs.[A3] With this strategy, infection is not prevented, but end-organ disease is avoided. More recently, letermovir, a CMV terminase substitute, at a dose of 120 or 240 mg daily, has been shown to reduce the incidence of CMV infection in such patients,[A4] and it has become an important addition to modern therapy.[9] CMV-specific hyperimmune globulin (CMVIG) is not effective in treating pregnant women with primary CMV infection and preventing congenital infection.[A5] CMVIG has been used prophylactically in high-risk seronegative organ transplant recipients, in whom it reduced CMV disease and CMV mortality. It is very expensive, however, and antivirals are more commonly used alternatives. Valacyclovir or valganciclovir can also be used to prevent CMV reactivation in critically ill patients,[A6] but it is not clear that such therapy reduces mortality.

TREATMENT   Rx

Oral valganciclovir, intravenous ganciclovir, intravenous ganciclovir followed by oral valganciclovir, intravenous foscarnet, intravenous cidofovir, and ganciclovir intraocular injection coupled with valganciclovir are all effective treatments of established CMV diseases (Table 352-1). These drugs (especially ganciclovir/valganciclovir) can also be used preemptively (i.e., when the viral load reaches a predetermined level even before the development of clinical disease).

Ganciclovir (dihydroxypropoxymethylguanosine [DHPG], Cytovene) is a nucleoside analogue given intravenously, 5 mg/kg two times daily during initial induction (2 to 3 weeks); maintenance therapy consists of 5 mg/kg once daily (Chapter 336). Valganciclovir (an oral prodrug of ganciclovir) achieves levels comparable to intravenous ganciclovir at 5 mg/kg when it is given orally in a 900-mg dose. Initial response in retinitis (improvement or stabilization of vision or ophthalmoscopic appearance) occurs in approximately 75% of patients treated with ganciclovir or valganciclovir. CMV retinitis can also be treated locally by intraocular ganciclovir injection, but this approach should be accompanied by valganciclovir to treat and/or prevent extraocular end-organ disease. Ganciclovir together with CMV hyperimmune globulin may reduce the mortality of CMV pneumonia after stem cell transplantation from approximately 85 to 40%, although the benefit of the antibody is unproved. Ganciclovir resistance may occur as a result of mutations in the protein kinase gene (UL97) and/or in the DNA polymerase gene (UL54). Granulocyte colony-stimulating factor may be needed to offset neutropenia.

Foscarnet, or phosphonoformic acid, blocks the pyrophosphate-binding site of viral DNA polymerase, thereby preventing cleavage of pyrophosphate from deoxynucleotide triphosphate. The recommended initial therapy with foscarnet is 60 mg/kg intravenously every 8 hours or 90 mg/kg every 12 hours. The maintenance dose ranges from 90 to 120 mg/kg daily. Adverse effects include renal impairment, anemia, hypocalcemia (especially ionized calcium), hypomagnesemia, and hypophosphatemia. Resistance to foscarnet can develop because of mutations in the DNA polymerase gene. Although it is effective for treating

TABLE 352-1   TREATMENT OF CYTOMEGALOVIRUS DISEASE

	PREFERRED THERAPY	ALTERNATIVE THERAPY
Cytomegalovirus (CMV) retinitis* Sight-threatening lesions	Valganciclovir 900 mg bid PO ± ganciclovir intraocular injection	Ganciclovir IV; foscarnet IV; plus ganciclovir intraocular injection
Peripheral lesions	Valganciclovir 900 mg bid PO	Ganciclovir IV or foscarnet IV
Maintenance therapy	Valganciclovir 900 mg qd PO	Ganciclovir IV or foscarnet IV
Relapsing	Reinduction with ganciclovir IV or valganciclovir 900 mg bid PO ± ganciclovir intraocular injection	
Ganciclovir resistant	Foscarnet IV ± ganciclovir intraocular injection	Cidofovir (if only UL97 mutation)
CMV gastrointestinal disease	Ganciclovir IV for 3-6 wk or valganciclovir 900 mg bid PO for 3-6 wk	Foscarnet IV for 3-6 wk
CMV neurologic disease	Ganciclovir IV + foscarnet IV	
CMV viremia syndrome	Valganciclovir 900 mg bid PO or ganciclovir IV until viremia clears	Foscarnet IV
Ganciclovir resistant	Foscarnet IV	

*If not already begun, antiretroviral therapy should be initiated concurrently with anti-CMV therapy, except possibly when treating central nervous system disease. For retinitis, anti-CMV therapy should be continued until the CD4 count has exceeded 100-150 cells/µL for ≥6 months and the retinitis is inactive. If anti-CMV therapy is discontinued, regular monthly eye examinations should be continued. Early relapses of CMV retinitis in patients treated systemically are usually due to inadequate drug penetration, and reinduction with the same drug is often effective. Drug resistance may occur in patients treated for ≥3 months. Therapy of these patients may be guided by genotyping.
bid = twice daily; IV = intravenously; PO = orally; qd = once daily.
Adapted from Drew WL, Erlich KS. Management of herpesvirus infections (cytomegalovirus, herpes simplex virus, and varicella-zoster virus). In: Volberding PA, Greene WC, Lange J, et al., eds. *HIV/AIDS Medicine Medical Management of AIDS 2012.* Philadelphia: Saunders Elsevier; 2012:433.

CMV retinitis, its toxicity and the absence of an oral formulation make foscarnet a second choice for treatment of CMV disease. It is sometimes used in combination with ganciclovir for infections such as central nervous system disease or for treatment of ganciclovir-resistant virus.

Cidofovir, or 3-hydroxy-2-phosphonomethoxypropyl cytosine (HPMPC), is a nucleotide analogue that does not require phosphorylation by virus-encoded enzyme. It is therefore active against ganciclovir-resistant CMV strains that have resistance mutations only in UL97, the protein kinase gene. When DNA polymerase (UL54) mutations occur in ganciclovir-treated patients, cross-resistance to cidofovir is frequent. These resistance mutations also occur in patients treated with cidofovir alone. The drug has an extremely long half-life that permits intravenous administration as infrequently as every 2 weeks during maintenance treatment.

Cidofovir is nephrotoxic, especially to the proximal renal tubule, but this side effect appears to be diminished by prehydration and concomitant probenecid therapy. Cidofovir toxicities make it a second- or third-line agent for CMV. Other drugs under investigation include brincidofovir, maribavir, and letermovir.[10]

PROGNOSIS

In immunocompetent patients, the mononucleosis-like CMV syndrome resolves spontaneously. Infections in immunocompromised patients are much more serious and may result in failure of a transplanted solid organ and/or systemic CMV disease. For CMV pneumonia, death often occurs even with antiviral therapy, especially after stem cell transplantation. In AIDS patients, CMV infection generally resolves when CD4 counts exceed 100/µL, but it is a grave prognostic sign if counts do not recover to those levels.

Grade A References

A1. Bernstein DI, Munoz FM, Callahan ST, et al. Safety and efficacy of a cytomegalovirus glycoprotein B (gB) vaccine in adolescent girls: a randomized clinical trial. *Vaccine.* 2016;34:313-319.

A2. Mumtaz K, Faisal N, Husain S, et al. Universal prophylaxis or preemptive strategy for cytomegalovirus disease after liver transplantation: a systematic review and meta-analysis. *Am J Transplant.* 2015;15:472-481.

A3. Boeckh M, Nichols WG, Chemaly RF, et al. Valganciclovir for the prevention of complications of late cytomegalovirus infection after allogeneic hematopoietic cell transplantation: a randomized trial. *Ann Intern Med.* 2015;162:1-10.

A4. Chemaly RF, Ullmann AJ, Stoelben S, et al. Letermovir for cytomegalovirus prophylaxis in hematopoietic-cell transplantation. *N Engl J Med.* 2014;370:1781-1789.

A5. Revello MG, Lazzarotto T, Guerra B, et al. A randomized trial of hyperimmune globulin to prevent congenital cytomegalovirus. *N Engl J Med.* 2014;370:1316-1326.

A6. Cowley NJ, Owen A, Shiels SC, et al. Safety and efficacy of antiviral therapy for prevention of cytomegalovirus reactivation in immunocompetent critically ill patients: a randomized clinical trial. *JAMA Intern Med.* 2017;177:774-783.

GENERAL REFERENCES

For the General References and other additional features, please visit Expert Consult at https://expertconsult.inkling.com.

353

EPSTEIN-BARR VIRUS INFECTION

ROBERT T. SCHOOLEY

DEFINITION

Epstein-Barr virus (EBV), a member of the gamma human herpesvirus family, is the etiologic agent of infectious mononucleosis and of a diverse assortment of neoplastic syndromes.

EPIDEMIOLOGY

Ubiquitous in the human population, EBV is found in 90 to 95% of adults throughout the world. As in the case of other herpesviruses, infection with EBV is lifelong. The virus resides in B lymphocytes and is intermittently shed asymptomatically in oropharyngeal secretions, which accounts for the bulk of its transmission in the human population. The virus is not contagious by casual contact and is usually acquired during early childhood by sharing of saliva-bearing fomites or during adolescence by kissing, although it can be acquired at any decade of life. In addition to oropharyngeal spread, the virus can be transmitted by blood transfusion or through organ donation.

Most childhood EBV infections are clinically silent, but infection of adolescents and adults results in the clinical syndrome of infectious mononucleosis between 25 and 50% of the time, depending on the setting. The incidence of infectious mononucleosis is highest in the 15- to 24-year-old age group. Incidence rates in men and women are equal, but the peak incidence is 2 years earlier in women than in men. Incidence rates are lower in lower socioeconomic populations, in which the likelihood of acquisition is greater in childhood than in adolescence.

PATHOBIOLOGY

EBV enters B lymphocytes through the CD21 molecule on the surface of B cells or nasopharyngeal epithelial cells.[1] Once inside the cell, the virus expresses several nuclear proteins (termed *Epstein-Barr nuclear antigens* [EBNAs]) that activate EBV-encoded latent membrane proteins and other gene products responsible for regulation of B-cell growth. These events are associated with the transformation or immortalization of the B cell that is the phenotypic hallmark of B-cell infection. EBV-transformed B cells proliferate vigorously and maintain EBV DNA within progeny cell nuclei in an episomal state. During acute EBV infection, up to 20% of peripheral blood B cells express EBNA.

The host response to acute EBV infection consists of a vigorous and coordinated cellular and humoral immune response. The humoral immune response includes IgM and IgG antibodies directed at the viral capsid (VCA) and to EBNA, as well as "heterophile" antibodies to surface antigens of sheep red blood cells. Heterophile antibodies are useful diagnostically and are present at some point in up to 90% of cases. These antibodies are an epiphenomenon in host defense and are not cross-reactive with any known viral antigens.

The cellular immune response includes both natural killer and EBV-specific CD4$^+$ and CD8$^+$ T lymphocytes. The expansion of the CD8$^+$ subset of T lymphocytes during acute EBV infection includes a subset of large, activated cells demonstrable on standard peripheral blood smears as "atypical" lymphocytes. This vigorous cellular immune response is associated with an outpouring of cytokines, including tumor necrosis factor, interleukin-1, and interleukin-6, that are responsible for many of the symptoms and signs of infectious mononucleosis. Over a period of 4 to 6 weeks after initial evaluation in most patients, adaptive immune mechanisms gain control of the EBV-driven B-cell proliferation and the virus enters into a lifelong period of symbiosis with the host. The virus is asymptomatically shed approximately 15% of the time in the oropharyngeal fluids of healthy human immunodeficiency virus type 1 (HIV-1)–seronegative adolescents and adults and is shed even more often in individuals with T-cell defects, such as occur with HIV-1 infection or immunosuppression associated with organ allografts.

CLINICAL MANIFESTATIONS

Most cases of acute EBV infection are clinically silent. The syndrome of infectious mononucleosis consists of the clinical triad of fever, sore throat (Chapter 401), and lymphadenopathy, in association with an atypical lymphocytosis and the transient appearance of heterophile antibodies.[2]

The incubation period between exposure and the onset of symptoms is generally 30 to 50 days. The onset of symptoms may be abrupt, or it may be heralded by a several-day nonspecific prodrome of malaise and low-grade fever. Although the classic syndrome includes fever, sore throat, and adenopathy, the findings may be dominated by only one or any combination of these symptoms.[3] Other common clinical manifestations include headache, malaise, and anorexia. On physical examination, patients are usually febrile. Pharyngeal erythema, tonsillar enlargement (see Fig. 401-4 in Chapter 401), and cervical adenopathy are generally present. Mild periorbital edema may also be observed. Abdominal findings may include splenomegaly or hepatomegaly, or both. Splenomegaly can be demonstrated by ultrasonographic examination in virtually all patients with infectious mononucleosis, although palpable splenomegaly is only present in about 20% of patients. Splenic enlargement is usually maximal in the second or third week of illness and might not be detectable at the initial presentation. Adenopathy may be observed in noncervical regions, but it is usually much less prominent than in cervical regions.

More serious primary infections can occur in individuals over age 30 years.[4] Approximately 5% of patients will exhibit a rash that may be macular, scarlatiniform, or urticarial in nature. Ampicillin or its derivatives evoke a pruritic maculopapular eruption in 15 to 30% of patients with acute EBV infection in recent series, compared with a reported 80 to 100% in earlier reports.[5] Patients with an ampicillin-induced rash during acute EBV infection generally tolerate the drug and other penicillin products when administered later in life.

DIAGNOSIS

Because clinical manifestations of acute EBV infection are variable and other organisms may cause similar clinical syndromes, laboratory tools are required to confirm an etiologic diagnosis. Heterophile antibodies to sheep red blood cells are classically used to diagnose EBV-induced infectious mononucleosis. Although ultimately demonstrable in approximately 90% of symptomatic acute EBV infections, these antibodies are present in only about two thirds of patients at initial encounter. If antibodies are negative at the outset and clinical suspicion is high, repeat testing in the second or third week of the illness is warranted. EBV-specific antibodies remain the "gold standard" for the diagnosis of acute EBV infection, but if heterophile antibodies are demonstrated in a straightforward case of infectious mononucleosis, EBV-specific serologic studies are not generally required. IgM antibodies to the EBV capsid antigen (VCA) are the most useful serologic study in the diagnosis of acute EBV infection.[6] Relatively high titers of IgG antibodies to VCA persist for life after initial infection and are not useful in making the diagnosis of acute EBV infection. Antibodies to EBNA are slower to arise than those to capsid antigens, and acute infection may be diagnosed by demonstration of seroconversion to this antigen.

Among pathogens causing clinical syndromes that can be mistaken for acute EBV infection, cytomegalovirus (Chapter 352) is the most frequent. Patients with cytomegalovirus infection are less likely to have an acute onset of illness, and pharyngitis is less frequently a prominent manifestation of the illness. *Toxoplasma gondii* (Chapter 328) infection can also present as a nonspecific febrile illness that can be confused with infectious mononucleosis. Streptococcal pharyngitis (Chapter 274) and primary herpes stomatitis (Chapter 350) may occasionally cause symptoms that are mistaken for acute EBV infection. None of these syndromes is associated with heterophile antibodies or with other serologic evidence of acute EBV infection. The differential diagnosis is generally made by serologic studies directed at these organisms or by culture.

Nonetheless, physicians should be cognizant that organisms such as group A β-hemolytic streptococci (Chapter 274) and herpes simplex virus are also common in the human population and may be demonstrated in people whose symptoms are nonetheless due to acute EBV infection.

PREVENTION AND TREATMENT

Because the virus is usually transmitted by asymptomatic oral shedders and is so common in the human population, epidemiologic interventions directed at patients with acute infection are not warranted to prevent spread. No vaccine yet has been developed. The clinical course is generally self-limited and does not usually require specific therapeutic intervention beyond the use of aspirin or acetaminophen for antipyresis and mild pain relief, except in the presence of specific complications such as when lymphadenopathy threatens the airway or in certain cases of autoimmune hemolytic anemia (Chapter 151) or thrombocytopenia (Chapter 163). Short courses of corticosteroids have been used to hasten symptomatic recovery in cases in which the symptoms are severe or refractory.[A1] Corticosteroids should not, however, be used routinely and should consist of no more than a 10- to 14-day tapering course that begins at a dose equivalent of 0.5 mg/kg of prednisone.[7] Although EBV replication can be inhibited in vitro or in vivo by acyclovir and related antiviral agents, the symptoms of infectious mononucleosis are primarily driven by the immune response to the virus and follow the time of maximal viral replication. Antiviral agents have not been demonstrated to significantly accelerate resolution of symptoms or prevent complications of the disease.[A2]

PROGNOSIS

Most patients recover uneventfully from the acute symptoms and signs of infectious mononucleosis over a 2- to 3-week period, although many patients may have a variable period of malaise and fatigue that can last for another 3 to 4 weeks. Some patients may take longer to make a full recovery and experience fatigue and difficulty concentrating for up to 6 months after diagnosis. Symptoms often wax and wane and can be extremely troublesome. Reassurance is usually the best approach to these patients. Corticosteroids are not of benefit in this setting. Recovery may be less straightforward in patients with certain specific complications of acute EBV infection (outlined in the next section). Death from infectious mononucleosis is rare. When it does occur, it is most frequently associated with neurologic complications, splenic rupture, or the X-linked lymphoproliferative syndrome (discussed later).

Complications

Although most patients recover spontaneously from acute EBV infection, a number of complications may arise. In some patients, these complications dominate the clinical findings, and seroconversion to EBV may be the only evidence of acute EBV infection. The most serious complication of acute EBV infection arises in individuals with the X-linked lymphoproliferative syndrome. This syndrome occurs in males with mutations in the signaling lymphocyte activation molecule (SLAM)–associated protein (SAP) that regulates T cells and natural killer (NK) cells. These otherwise healthy individuals have severe clinical symptoms, a pronounced lymphocytosis consisting of T and B cells, and severe hepatitis. If patients survive the acute infection, the syndrome may evolve into progressive agammaglobulinemia or lymphoma in the following months. The genetic defect associated with this syndrome can be diagnosed in utero, and early bone marrow transplantation has been recommended for the prevention of the devastating clinical syndrome associated with the acquisition of EBV infection.

A number of less severe, organ system–specific complications are seen substantially more frequently than the X-linked lymphoproliferative syndrome. Patients should be specifically warned about splenic rupture, a complication attributable to splenomegaly (Chapter 159) and associated stretching of the splenic capsule that occurs most frequently in the second or third week of the illness, when other symptoms of the disease are abating. It may be accompanied by trauma but may also occur without an obvious antecedent event. Patients should be counseled against activities that might result in abdominal trauma for 6 to 8 weeks after the onset of symptoms. Left upper quadrant pain, especially pain radiating to the subscapular region, should raise this diagnostic consideration. As with other complications of acute EBV infection, splenic rupture may occur occasionally in patients without other prominent clinical manifestations of acute EBV infection. Other hematologic complications include autoimmune hemolytic anemia (Chapter 151), thrombocytopenia (Chapter 163), and neutropenia (Chapter 158). These complications usually arise from a combination of self-reactive antibodies and hypersplenism, are generally self-limited, and resolve with resolution of the illness. Corticosteroids

may be of benefit in more severe cases of autoimmune hemolytic anemia or thrombocytopenia.

Neurologic complications can also occur during acute EBV infection. EBV DNA has been detected in brain tissue from rare patients with clinical manifestations compatible with herpes simplex encephalitis (Chapter 386). Although these patients have a much better prognosis than those with herpes simplex encephalitis, they should receive parenteral acyclovir or ganciclovir. Other neurologic complications include aseptic meningitis (Chapter 384), cerebellitis, mononeuritis multiplex (Chapter 392), Bell palsy (Chapter 392), Guillain-Barré syndrome (Chapter 392), and transverse myelitis (Chapters 372 and 383). These complications may be clinically dramatic but are usually self-limited and associated with full recovery in 85% of patients without specific antiviral therapy.

Mild hepatomegaly is common in acute infectious mononucleosis, and biochemical evidence of hepatitis (Chapter 139) is to be expected in virtually every case of acute infection. More severe hepatic complications are uncommon, however. Renal, cardiac, pulmonary, and skeletal muscle complications are rare.

OTHER CLINICAL MANIFESTATIONS

In addition to infectious mononucleosis, EBV is also associated with neoplasia and lymphoproliferative disorders, which are seen most frequently in patients with defects in cellular immunity but are not restricted to such patients.

Post-transplant Lymphoproliferative Disease

EBV-driven B-cell proliferation that is insufficiently regulated in the presence of prolonged periods of severe T-cell immunodeficiency may result in a polyclonal proliferation of B cells that is initially similar to that seen in acute infectious mononucleosis. Although most frequently occurring in the setting of organ transplantation, especially when patients are immunosuppressed with agents directed specifically at T lymphocytes, this syndrome can be seen in other conditions with similar levels and durations of immunodeficiency such as HIV-1 infection. Post-transplant lymphoproliferative disease (PTLD)[8] is often but not invariably EBV driven. EBV-associated PTLD is seen earlier in the post-transplant course than non–EBV-associated cases and is seen more often when the donor is EBV seropositive and the recipient is seronegative. PTLD is more common in association with graft-versus-host disease, in patients who undergo splenectomy before transplantation, in patient/donor pairs with higher degrees of human leukocyte antigen (HLA) mismatch, and in transplantation of organs requiring more severe immunosuppression, including multiple-organ transplants, as well as lung, pancreas, liver, and heart transplants.

Patients with PTLD often present with fever, adenopathy, and splenomegaly. If the immunodeficiency persists, these disorders often proceed from a polyclonal stage, which can be reversed with restoration of immunity, to a monoclonal or oligoclonal stage that is progressive despite restoration of cellular immunodeficiency. These tumors are less frequently seen in the current era in which allograft-associated immunosuppression is better targeted and less intense.

The diagnosis is not generally difficult to make in the appropriate clinical setting and should be confirmed histopathologically. Elevated plasma levels of EBV DNA are associated with an increased risk of PTLD, but preemptive monitoring of EBV DNA has not been shown to be clinically useful. The predictive value of elevated EBV DNA for PTLD is less well established after solid organ transplantation than after bone marrow transplantation.

There is some evidence that PTLD may be less frequent in patients who have received acyclovir or ganciclovir after transplantation, but these agents are less useful once the syndrome develops. Successful management depends on the extent to which the immunosuppressive condition can be reversed before the evolution of restricted clonality. Therapy with anti-CD20 antibodies, with or without chemotherapy, is the treatment of choice for PTLD. Radiation therapy is also used in some patients.

Burkitt Lymphoma

EBV was initially described in patients with African Burkitt lymphoma. The tumor is composed of small, noncleaved B cells and, unless aggressively treated, is rapidly fatal.[9] This aggressive B-cell lymphoma with a predilection for the head and neck is endemic in equatorial Africa and is geographically linked to *Plasmodium falciparum* malaria. EBV DNA is readily demonstrable in tumor biopsy specimens, and high titers of antibodies to EBV structural antigens are found in plasma. Sporadic cases of abdominal B-cell lymphomas with a histologic appearance compatible with Burkitt lymphoma are also observed but are associated with EBV only about 25% of the time. The tumor is likewise seen in patients with HIV-1 infection.

Although the risk for HIV-associated Burkitt lymphoma increases with advancing immunodeficiency, it may be seen in patients with relatively preserved CD4 cell counts. Antiretroviral therapy reduces but does not eliminate the risk for Burkitt lymphoma in HIV-1–infected persons. Despite the high-grade clinical behavior of the tumor, it should be vigorously treated because it is usually quite responsive to combination chemotherapy with or without radiation therapy (Chapter 176).

Hodgkin Lymphoma

EBV is also associated with a subset of Hodgkin lymphomas (Chapter 177),[10] especially those of the lymphocyte-depleted or mixed-cellularity histologic subtypes. EBV DNA and proteins are detected in the Reed-Sternberg cells that are characteristic of Hodgkin lymphoma. Therapy for EBV-associated Hodgkin lymphoma is directed at the tumor. The specific approach used is based on the histology and extent of disease (Chapter 177) and is not determined in a given patient by its relationship to EBV.

Central Nervous System Lymphoma

EBV is also associated with central nervous system (CNS) lymphoma (Chapter 176).[11] This tumor was most frequently observed in the post-transplant setting before the HIV epidemic but is now the most frequent CNS neoplasm in HIV-1–infected individuals. The major differential diagnostic challenge is with *T. gondii* infection (Chapter 328). Although a tissue-based diagnosis is definitive, noninvasive neurodiagnostic approaches coupled with the demonstration of EBV DNA in cerebrospinal fluid by polymerase chain reaction can strongly support the diagnosis of lymphoma over that of *T. gondii* infection. Radiation therapy may be used but its effects are generally palliative.

Nasopharyngeal Carcinoma

EBV has also been associated with certain cases of nasopharyngeal carcinoma (Chapter 181).[12] This tumor is rare in Western countries, but it is much more frequent in southern China and in the Inuit population of Alaska. EBV-associated cases are generally less histologically differentiated than sporadic forms of nasopharyngeal carcinoma. EBV DNA is demonstrable in tumor tissue, and high titers of IgA and IgG antibodies to the EBV capsid antigens are found in plasma.[13] The prognosis for this tumor is poor, although it is often treated with radiation therapy (Chapter 181).

Other EBV-Associated Neoplasms

EBV collaborates with another human gamma-herpesvirus, human herpes virus type 8, to cause primary effusion lymphoma in the HIV-1–infected population. These aggressive tumors present in body cavities such as the pleural, peritoneal, and pericardial spaces. EBV DNA may also be found in moderate to slowly progressive destructive midline facial angiocentric tumors of T- and NK-cell phenotypes. This neoplasm presents clinically as a syndrome that was previously known as lethal midline granuloma (Chapter 176). EBV also plays a key role in the pathogenesis of an angiocentric EBV-associated B-cell tumor, which presents clinically as lymphomatoid granulomatosis and hemophagocytic lymphohistiocytosis (Chapter 160).[14]

Oral Hairy Leukoplakia

This clinical manifestation of EBV infection is characterized by a corrugated or "hairy" plaquelike lesion that extends around the lateral aspects of the tongue (Chapter 397). Oral hairy leukoplakia is most often observed in individuals with chronic forms of cellular immunodeficiency, especially those with HIV-1 infection and CD4 cell counts less than 200/μL. It is most often clinically confused with mucocutaneous candidiasis (Chapter 318) but can be differentiated because its distribution is restricted to the lateral surface of the tongue. Unlike thrush, it does not involve the buccal mucosa, palate, or pharynx and is not readily removed by superficial scraping. Biopsies demonstrate a characteristic histopathologic pattern, as well as the presence of EBV antigens and DNA within squamous epithelial cells. Although the lesions may be cosmetically troublesome, they are not generally painful. In the case of HIV-1–associated oral hairy leukoplakia, the lesions resolve with successful antiretroviral chemotherapy (Chapter 364).

Chronic Active EBV Infection

Infrequent patients with no apparent defect in cellular immunity have been described in which chronic EBV infection has been associated with persistent or intermittent hepatitis or interstitial pulmonary disease (or both).[15] These

rare patients with bona fide organ system disease should not be confused with individuals who have chronic fatigue syndrome or fibromyalgia rheumatica (Chapter 258). This nonspecific clinical syndrome, which is seen most frequently in young and middle-aged women, is characterized by malaise and difficulty concentrating without objective physical findings. Although an etiologic or contributing role for EBV had been posited, there is no evidence that the virus plays a role in this condition.

Grade A References

A1. Rezk E, Nofal YH, Hamzeh A, et al. Steroids for symptom control in infectious mononucleosis. *Cochrane Database Syst Rev.* 2015;11:CD004402.

A2. De Paor M, O'Brien K, Fahey T, et al. Antiviral agents for infectious mononucleosis (glandular fever). *Cochrane Database Syst Rev.* 2016;12:CD011487.

GENERAL REFERENCES

For the General References and other additional features, please visit Expert Consult at https://expertconsult.inkling.com.

354

RETROVIRUSES OTHER THAN HUMAN IMMUNODEFICIENCY VIRUS

CHARLES R.M. BANGHAM AND WILLIAM A. BLATTNER

DEFINITION

There are now four members of the human T-lymphotropic virus (HTLV) family: HTLV-1, discovered in 1979; HTLV-2, discovered in 1982; and HTLV-3 and HTLV-4, discovered in 2005. HTLV-1 has been causally linked to adult T-cell leukemia/lymphoma and to several chronic degenerative conditions, most notably HTLV-1-associated myelopathy/tropical spastic paraparesis (HAM/TSP),[1] whereas disease associated with HTLV-2 is rare, and no disease associations have been established with HTLV-3 or HTLV-4.

The Pathogens

Within the taxa of RNA reverse transcribing viruses, the HTLV viruses, along with bovine leukemia virus, are classified in the subfamily Retroviridae within the genus *Deltaretrovirus* (formerly termed *Oncovirus*). The molecular structure of these viruses distinguishes them from the other group of complex human retroviruses, the human immunodeficiency retroviruses HIV-1 and HIV-2 (Chapter 362), which are members of the genus *Lentivirus*. Both deltaretroviruses and lentiviruses are capable of prolonged asymptomatic infection. In vitro, however, HIV-1 and HIV-2 have cytopathic effects on human T cells, whereas HTLV-1 and HTLV-2 are capable of transforming T cells into immortalized cell lines. The HTLVs are diploid single-stranded RNA viruses that replicate through cDNA, a proviral intermediate, by reverse transcriptase, a viral polymerase.

EPIDEMIOLOGY

HTLV-1 is widely disseminated worldwide and is estimated to infect 5 to 10 million persons, with the aggressive T-cell malignant neoplasm adult T-cell leukemia/lymphoma developing in 2 to 6% and chronic inflammatory diseases, mainly HAM/TSP, developing in another 1 to 5% in their lifetime.[2] Similar to HIV, molecular epidemiology suggests that the four major subtypes of HTLV identified in humans arose from separate interspecies transmission from simians to humans. The discovery of HTLV-3 and HTLV-4 was made in Cameroon, where closely related viruses in nonhuman primates led to their discovery in humans with exposure as bushmeat hunters. Related to such interspecies transmission, there are four major geographic subtypes of HTLV-1: cosmopolitan subtype A; central African subtype B; Australo-Melanesian (Papua New Guinea, Melanesia, and Australian aborigines) subtype C; and central African/Pygmies subtype D. Central Africa also carries a few rare subtypes (E, F, G). Within the cosmopolitan group are four subgroups: transcontinental; Japanese; West African; and North African. The virus from Australo-Melanesia differs molecularly from the Japanese and African strains by 5 to 10%, the result of independent evolution of the virus in these populations separated for tens of thousands of years. The genetic stability of HTLV-1 in comparison with HIV-1 reflects the observation that HTLV persists in the host mainly through proliferation of proviral DNA-harboring cells rather than infection of new cells. The HTLV subtypes differ phylogenetically by approximately 30 to 40% among each other.

HTLV-1 is not present in all human populations but rather clusters geographically: southern Japan; Melanesia; Australia (in aboriginal peoples); western, central, and southern Africa and, by the slave trade from Africa, the Caribbean and the United States in African Americans; Central and South America; and the Mashhad region of Iran. HTLV-1 infection in western Europe is predominantly linked to migration patterns, but the high prevalence of HTLV-1 infection in Romania remains unexplained. HTLV-1 is found in some indigenous populations of North America as well as in persons who migrate from the endemic regions. There is increasing evidence of HTLV-1 infection in the Indian subcontinent and China, but the extent is uncertain. HTLV-2 is found in Native American people throughout North, Central, and South America and in West Africa. HTLV-2 infections also occur in the United States and Europe in injection drug users, in whom the virus is spread by needle sharing and other injection practices as well as by sexual contact. HTLV-3 and HTLV-4 were originally detected in Cameroon and have been detected in only a few persons, but their extent in West Africa is not yet known.

Routes of Transmission

HTLV, like HIV-1, is transmitted sexually, perinatally, and by transfusion or injection drug use (Table 354-1).

Sexual Transmission

Sexual transmission of HTLV-1 from male to female, female to male, and male to male has been documented. HTLV-1 is almost exclusively cell-associated: transmission between individuals requires transfer of infected lymphocytes, and cell-free blood products are not infectious. Coincidental infection with other sexually transmitted diseases, particularly those associated with ulcerative and inflammatory genital lesions, amplifies the risk for transmission. In HTLV-1 infection, elevated viral load is linked to heightened transmission. In regions endemic for the virus, there is a characteristic age-dependent rise in HTLV-1 seroprevalence. This increase first becomes evident in the adolescent years; it is steeper in women than in men and continues in women after 40 years of age, whereas rates in men plateau around the age of 40 years. This pattern reflects more efficient male-to-female transmission. For HTLV-2, the rates for both genders are equal, thus suggesting that there may be differences in the kinetics of transmission between the two viruses.

Perinatal Transmission

Transmission of HTLV-1 through breast-feeding is more efficient than in utero or perinatal transmission. Major risk factors that increase the efficiency of transmission include high proviral loads and increased duration of breast-feeding (>6 months). On average, 20% of infants breast-fed by HTLV-1-positive mothers seroconvert to HTLV-1, whereas only 1 to 2% of bottle-fed infants become infected. In contrast, in utero and perinatal transmission accounts for virtually all mother-to-child HIV-1 transmission in the West, and breast-feeding accounts for an additional 15 to 20% of infant HIV infection in Africa. HTLV-2 is detectable in breast milk, and, as with HTLV-1, breast-feeding accounts for many childhood infections.

Transfusion and Injection Drug Use

Parenteral transmission, through either transfusion or injection drug use, is a major source of HTLV infection. Among U.S. blood donors who are confirmed to be HTLV positive, the major risk factors are intravenous drug use, birthplace in parts of the Caribbean or Japan where the virus is endemic, and sexual contact with a person with this profile.

In the United States, more than 50% of HTLV infections among screened potential blood donors are due to HTLV-2, and effective screening can eliminate transfusion-related infection. By comparison, HTLV-1 predominates in other countries where HTLV infections are present. Among injection drug users, most HTLV infections also are due to HTLV-2.

Both HTLV-1 and HTLV-2 are transmitted only by direct cell-to-cell contact, through a specialized structure called a virologic synapse, whereas HIV-1 is transmitted either through a virologic synapse or by plasma or plasma products. Approximately 50% of the recipients of HTLV-1- or HTLV-2-positive blood seroconvert, compared with more than 95% for HIV-1.

The only documented illness linked to HTLV-1 or HTLV-2 transfusion-associated transmission is the HTLV-associated demyelinating neurologic syndrome HAM/TSP. Leukemia has not been associated with transfusion of HTLV-positive blood. Solid organ transplantation from HTLV-1-infected donors is associated with a high rate of transmission and rapid onset and progression of HAM/TSP.

Other Means of Infection

"Casual contact," without sexual contact or exposure to cellular blood contents, is not a source of infection. There are limited data on health care and laboratory workers who experience a needlestick or skin or mucous membrane exposure. However, the risk for infection should be assessed by the clinical history, in particular of sexual contacts and blood transfusions, and potential seroconversion should be monitored.

Coinfection with HIV

Coinfection with HTLV-1 and HIV-1 appears to increase the progression to acquired immunodeficiency syndrome (AIDS) through unexplained mechanisms, possibly related to the cell-proliferative effects of HTLV-1 on HIV-1-infected T cells and/or coreceptor expression modulating CD4 cell permissiveness. Elevated CD4 counts due to HTLV-1 in patients with HIV/HTLV-1 coinfection can underestimate the degree of immune suppression. HAM/TSP and adult T-cell leukemia/lymphoma can occur in coinfected patients, but the clinical manifestations of HIV/HTLV coinfection in the era of early and fully suppressive antiretroviral therapy are poorly understood.

PATHOBIOLOGY
Virology

The HTLV viruses, which are single-stranded RNA viruses that contain a diploid genome, replicate through a DNA intermediary that integrates into the genome of the target T cell as a provirus, thereby resulting in lifelong infection. HTLV-1 is approximately 100 nm in diameter and has a thin, electron-dense outer envelope and an electron-dense, roughly spherical core. The total provirus genome contains 9032 nucleotides with two identical sequences termed *long terminal repeats* (LTRs) at the 5′ and 3′ ends of the genome, which contain regulatory elements that control virus expression and virion production. The retroviral structural genes (*gag* and *pol*) code for large overlapping polyproteins that are later processed into functional peptide products by virally encoded protease and cellular proteases. The viral genes are *gag* (group-specific antigen), *pol* (polymerase/integrase/protease), and *env* (envelope). In addition, HTLV-1 has a series of regulatory genes, *tax* and *rex*, and several smaller gene products that regulate infection and virus expression. A single viral gene (basic leucine zipper factor [*HBZ*]) is encoded by the minus strand of the HTLV-1 provirus

TABLE 354-1 TRANSMISSION OF HTLV-1 AND HTLV-2		
MODE OF TRANSMISSION	**HTLV-1**	**HTLV-2**
MOTHER TO INFANT		
Transplacental	Yes	Not known
Breast milk	Yes	Probable
SEXUAL		
Male to female	Yes	Yes
Female to male	Yes	Yes
Male to male	Yes	Not known
PARENTERAL		
Blood transfusion	Yes	Yes
Injecting drug use	Yes	Yes
COFACTORS		
Ulcerative genital lesions	Yes	Not known
Cellular transfusion products	Yes	Yes
Sharing of "works"**	Yes	Yes
ELEVATED VIRUS LOAD		
Mother to infant	Yes	Not known
Heterosexual	Yes	Not known

*Intravenous paraphernalia, such as needles.

and transcribed from the 3′ LTR. Tax protein plays a central role in enhancing the transcription of viral and cellular gene products that promote viral replication and transformation of human T lymphocytes. Through binding to transcription factor complexes, Tax promotes transcriptional activation of the viral genome, and by binding to key regulatory proteins of the NF-κB signaling pathway, Tax promotes cell activation and disease pathogenesis. Through binding to regulatory enhancers of the cell and through abrogation of key suppressor genes, Tax initiates the immortalization of the infected T cells. However, the *tax* gene is susceptible to genetic mutations and is expressed in only about 60% of adult T-cell leukemia/lymphoma cases. The viral protein Rex stabilizes viral mRNA and is essential for export of full-length Gag/Pol and single-spliced Env mRNA from the nucleus to the cytoplasm. *HBZ*, the only viral gene consistently expressed in all adult T-cell leukemia/lymphoma patients, appears to be essential for persistent HTLV-1 infection. HBZ inhibits the Tax-mediated activation of viral gene transcription through the 5′ LTR, which ultimately represses expression of viral proteins while simultaneously promoting the proliferation and survival of infected cells. A typical person infected with HTLV-1 carries between 10,000 and 100,000 infected T-cell clones, which appear to survive for the lifetime of the host. Most (95%) infected cells are helper (CD4$^+$) T cells; 5% of the load is carried in cytotoxic (CD8$^+$) T cells. The proviral load (the percentage of infected mononuclear leukocytes in the blood), which frequently exceeds 5%, is limited by the host's cytotoxic T-lymphocyte response. Most HTLV-1-specific cytotoxic T lymphocytes recognize the Tax protein, but it is recognition of the HBZ protein that is associated with efficient control of the virus. An individual with an efficient cytotoxic T-lymphocyte response to HBZ has a lower proviral load and consequently a lower risk for both the inflammatory and malignant diseases caused by HTLV-1.

Viral Life Cycle

The initial stage of HTLV infection involves transmission from an infected lymphocyte in contact with an uninfected cell, through a specialized structure called the virologic synapse. After infection, the viral life cycle involves membrane fusion, followed by reverse transcription from an RNA template to a circular DNA provirus that is transported to the cell nucleus and integrated into the host genome. During the long chronic phase of infection, viral replication is primarily achieved through proliferation of proviral DNA-harboring cells rather than through repeated cycles of cell-to-cell infection. For viral entry, HTLV-1 utilizes three distinct molecules for infection of activated T cells: heparan sulfate proteoglycans, neuropilin 1, and glucose transporter 1. HTLV-2, which infects almost exclusively CD8$^+$ T cells, also uses neuropilin 1 and glucose transporter 1 for entry into the cell. After uptake and uncoating, viral RNA is transcribed into double-stranded DNA by reverse transcriptase, an RNA-dependent DNA polymerase complexed to the RNA in the core of the virus particle. This double-stranded viral DNA is integrated into the host cell nucleus by the virally encoded integrase, thereby resulting in lifelong cell infection. The viral LTR elements are essential for integration and regulation of viral genome expression, which is controlled mainly by Tax and HBZ.

Pathogenesis of Adult T-Cell Leukemia

HTLV-1 causes adult T-cell leukemia/lymphoma through a multistage process.[3] The clonal pattern of integration of HTLV-1 in the host genome in adult T-cell leukemia/lymphoma cells indicates that the disease is derived from a single transformed tumor cell that evolved from a virus infection *before* transformation rather than afterward as a passenger virus. The integrated HTLV-1 genome is incomplete in some cases of adult T-cell leukemia/lymphoma, but it always includes an intact *HBZ* gene. Tax is an oncoprotein that interacts with numerous cellular proteins to reprogram cellular processes to alter transcription, cell cycle regulation, DNA repair, and apoptosis, thereby allowing cells with potential carcinogenic mutations to survive and to escape cell death. HBZ is also a key oncogenic protein involved in modulating cellular pathways related to cell growth and survival, immune response, and T-cell differentiation.

In some healthy carriers, oligoclonal T-cell proliferation can later progress to malignant transformation or may disappear spontaneously. Morphologically abnormal "flower cells" (Fig. 354-1), which represent T cells with deeply lobulated nuclei resembling adult T-cell leukemia/lymphoma cells, are seen on peripheral blood smears of healthy carriers, and increased numbers are detected in persons with high HTLV viral loads.

Pathogenesis of Myelopathy/Spastic Paraparesis

Viral overproduction, as measured by high viral loads, appears to result from defective host immune responses. Local pathologic changes in neuronal tissue are thought to result from the toxic effects of cytokines released by HTLV-1-infected cells and by the local antiviral T cells. Intense mononuclear (mainly T-cell) infiltrates are associated with progressive neuronal loss. Lesions are found scattered throughout the central nervous system (CNS) but are particularly frequent in the spinal cord, where they cause most of the signs and symptoms of HAM/TSP.[4]

⬤ ADULT T-CELL LEUKEMIA/LYMPHOMA

EPIDEMIOLOGY AND PATHOBIOLOGY

The cumulative lifetime incidence of adult T-cell leukemia/lymphoma in persons infected with HTLV-1 is between 2 and 6%, with about 2500 to 5000 cases per year in the approximately 5 to 10 million infected persons worldwide.

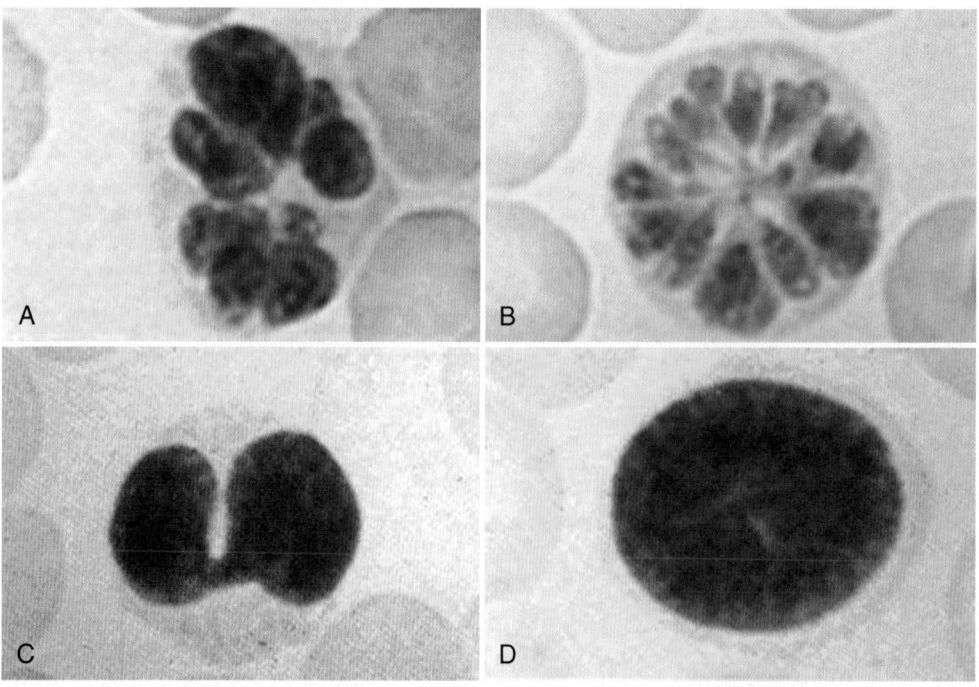

FIGURE 354-1. Photomicrographs demonstrating the morphologic features of leukemic cells observed in different subtypes of adult T-cell leukemia/lymphoma (ATL). A and B, Polylobulated morphology of the acute type, with the highly characteristic "flower cell" shown in B. C, Typical cleaved cell seen in chronic-type ATL. D, Typical morphology of smoldering ATL. (Courtesy of K. Yamaguchi and K. Takatsuki.)

TABLE 354-2 HTLV-ASSOCIATED DISEASES

DIAGNOSIS	NATURE OF SYNDROME	STRENGTH OF ASSOCIATION
HTLV-1-ASSOCIATED DISEASES		
Adult T-cell leukemia/lymphoma	Aggressive lymphoproliferative malignant disease of mature T lymphocytes	Strong
HTLV-associated myelopathy/tropical spastic paraparesis (HAM/TSP)	Chronic progressive demyelinating syndrome of long motor tracts of spinal cord	Strong
Polymyositis (Chapter 253)	Degenerative inflammatory syndrome of skeletal muscles	Probable
Sporadic inclusion body myositis (Chapter 253)	Recently described HTLV-associated inflammatory muscle disease	Possible
Infective dermatitis	Chronic generalized eczema in adults and children; potential for preleukemia and immunodeficiency	Strong
Uveitis (Chapter 395)	Inflammatory infiltration of the uvea of the eye	Strong
Sjögren syndrome/keratoconjunctivitis sicca (Chapter 252)	Loss of tear production and dry eyes and dry mouth	Probable
Pulmonary lymphocyte alveolitis/cryptogenic fibrosing alveolitis	Pulmonary infiltrate involving T lymphocytosis in lungs of patients with HAM/TSP and HTLV uveitis	Possible
Bronchiectasis (Chapter 84)	Associated with repeated or chronic pulmonary infections	Probable
HTLV-associated arthritis	Large-joint polyarthropathy; rheumatoid factor positive, with HTLV-1-positive cells infiltrating the synovia	Probable
Immunodeficiency (Chapter 236)	Subclinical (e.g., decreased PPD response) or clinical (e.g., association with clinical tuberculosis and poor response to therapy for symptomatic strongyloidiasis; association of HTLV-1 with disseminated strongyloides infection [strongyloidiasis]); schistosomiasis	Probable
Miscellaneous clinical conditions	Case reports of small cell lung cancer with monoclonal HTLV-1 integration and invasive cervical cancer	Uncertain
HTLV-2-ASSOCIATED DISEASES		
HTLV-associated myelopathy	Increased numbers of cases among blood donors	Definite but rare

HAM = HTLV-1-associated myelopathy; PPD = purified protein derivative; TSP = HTLV-1-associated topical spastic paraperesis.

Nearly all patients who develop this disease are infected in infancy because the disease has a long latency period.[5]

The disease typically presents in the fifth to seventh decade[6]; the risk is slightly higher in HTLV-1-infected males. The age-adjusted incidence rate of adult T-cell leukemia/lymphoma in the United States is 0.05 cases per 100,000 for men and 0.03 per 100,000 for women. In areas endemic for HTLV-1, such as southern Japan and the Caribbean Islands, adult T-cell leukemia/lymphoma accounts for half or more of adult lymphoid malignant neoplasms. Adult T-cell leukemia/lymphoma is rarely seen in children; but in one pediatric series, four of the eight patients shared a homozygous deletion in the *p16* gene locus, and deletion of exons 7 and 8 of *p53* was detected in another child, thereby suggesting that a genetic predisposition interacts with viral infection to accelerate the progression of the disease.

CLINICAL MANIFESTATIONS

The most common disease caused by HTLV-1 is adult T-cell leukemia/lymphoma (Table 354-2), which is a high-grade lymphoma (Chapter 176), usually of large, medium, or pleiotropic cell morphology and advanced clinical stage.[7] The acute form of adult T-cell leukemia/lymphoma, which accounts for about 55% of cases, is characterized by an aggressive, mature T-cell leukemia that presents with a high white blood cell count, hypercalcemia, and frequent cutaneous involvement. The lymphoma type (about 20% of cases) shares all the same features except for peripheral blood involvement. Other cases resemble T-prolymphocytic leukemia and are termed *chronic adult T-cell leukemia/lymphoma* (about 20% of cases). A subset of chronic cases with high serum levels of lactate dehydrogenase (LDH) and blood urea nitrogen (BUN) and low levels of albumin share the survival characteristics of the more aggressive acute and lymphoma types of adult T-cell leukemia/lymphoma, including a poor response to treatment. Smoldering adult T-cell leukemia/lymphoma (about 5%) may clinically resemble mycosis fungoides/Sézary syndrome (Chapter 176), with cutaneous involvement manifested as erythema or as infiltrative plaques or tumors (Fig. 354-2).[8] A long prodrome of signs (e.g., cutaneous rashes) and symptoms (e.g., fevers) is sometimes noted in chronic and smoldering adult T-cell leukemia/lymphoma before transformation to an acute or lymphoma type that is rapidly fatal.

DIAGNOSIS

The diagnosis should be considered in any adult who has a mature T-cell lymphoma and hypercalcemia or cutaneous involvement (or both) with

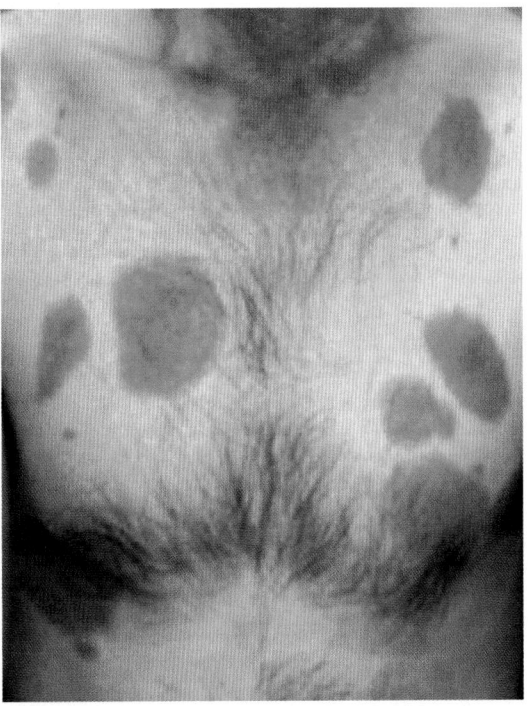

FIGURE 354-2. Cutaneous involvement in adult T-cell leukemia/lymphoma. (From Tomita H, Fumihide O, Kuwatsuka S, et al. Attenuation of an adult T-cell leukemia lesion after treatment of a concomitant simplex infection: a case study. *Virol J*. 2012;9:224. http://www.virologyj.com/content/9/1/224. Creative Commons Attribution License.)

characteristic "flower cells" (see Fig. 354-1). The diagnosis is established by testing of serum for HTLV-1 antibodies. Polymerase chain reaction (PCR) can detect infection, identify the type of virus, and quantify the proviral load. The cytologically distinct flower cell (a sine qua non of adult T-cell leukemia/lymphoma) is also seen in apparently healthy carriers. Occasional cases with characteristic clinical features are HTLV-1-antibody negative but provirus positive as detected by PCR in blood cells or in biopsy specimens. C-C chemokine receptor 4 (CCR4) is expressed on adult T-cell leukemia/lymphoma cells in more than 90% of cases.

TREATMENT   Rx

Treatment is based on the type of adult T-cell leukemia/lymphoma and its natural history, but it is also influenced by the patient's age and the presence of certain biomarkers.

Smoldering and Chronic Adult T-Cell Leukemia/Lymphoma

Watchful waiting has traditionally been recommended for patients with smoldering disease and some patients with chronic disease with a favorable biomarker profile (normal LDH, BUN, and albumin levels) because cytoablative therapy increases the risk for lethal opportunistic infections. Observational data suggest, however, that 5-year survival can be improved by treating smoldering and selected chronic adult T-cell leukemia/lymphoma with high doses of the antiviral agent zidovudine (500 to 1000 mg/day in divided dosage) in combination with interferon-α (6 to 9 million units). In the absence of controlled trials to define the optimal dose and duration of treatment, zidovudine and interferon are continued indefinitely, or as long as they are tolerated.

Acute, Lymphoma, and Aggressive Chronic Adult T-Cell Leukemia/Lymphoma

A regimen of three successive drug combinations (vincristine, cyclophosphamide, doxorubicin, and prednisone [VCAP], doxorubicin, ranimustine, and prednisone [AMP], and vindesine, etoposide, carboplatin, and prednisone [VECP] [Chapter 176]) provides a 28% rate of progression-free survival at 1 year, a median survival time of 13 months, and a 3-year overall survival rate of 24%, but it is associated with hematologic and infectious complications. Retrospective case series report a long-term survival rate of 20 to 40% after allogeneic hematopoietic stem cell transplantation (Chapter 168) but with significant treatment-related mortality.[9] Current standard of care for patients with aggressive forms of adult T-cell leukemia/lymphoma and favorable prognostic factors is VCAP-AMP-VECP alone. For patients with an unfavorable prognostic profile (thrombocytopenia, eosinophilia, bone marrow involvement, elevated LDH levels, high interleukin-5 serum level, CCR4 expression, lung resistance–related protein, *p53* mutation, and/or *p16* deletion), VCAP-AMP-VECP chemotherapy followed by allogenic stem cell transplantation is recommended.

Mogamulizumab (a humanized anti-CCR4 monoclonal antibody) has shown modest benefit in patients who did not respond or relapsed after conventional therapy.[A1] Other therapies, such as lenalidomide and histone deacetylase inhibitors, have shown some promise but need further study. Whether chimeric antigen receptor T-cell (CART) therapy will be helpful remains unknown.

PROGNOSIS

The prognosis of adult T-cell leukemia/lymphoma is little changed in the past 25 years. Smoldering adult T-cell leukemia/lymphoma has a relatively good prognosis, with a 5-year survival rate of 70%. In the chronic subtype, 5-year survival is only 20%, even including the more favorable subset of patients with normal LDH, BUN, and albumin levels. In the aggressive forms of acute and lymphoma-type disease, median disease-free survival is 0.6 years and overall survival is only 0.8 years because of mortality linked to rapid tumor growth, infectious complications, and metabolic complications, especially hypercalcemia. Significant negative prognostic factors[10] also include poor performance status at diagnosis, older age, advanced stage, and elevated serum LDH levels, as well as adverse genetic tumor profiles.[11] Death usually results from rapid growth of tumor cells, hypercalcemia, bacterial sepsis, and opportunistic and other infectious complications.

● HTLV-ASSOCIATED MYELOPATHY/TROPICAL SPASTIC PARAPARESIS

EPIDEMIOLOGY AND PATHOBIOLOGY

HTLV-1 causes a chronic inflammatory neurologic syndrome known as HAM/TSP. The lifetime incidence is approximately half the rate for adult T-cell leukemia/lymphoma, with approximately 1 to 2% of carriers affected. HAM/TSP is approximately two times more likely to develop in females. The majority of adult cases occur in the 30- to 50-year age group, but cases have occurred in children as young as 3 years. The mean latency period before onset of HAM/TSP is shorter than that for adult T-cell leukemia/lymphoma, and

both early-life and adult exposure can cause HAM/TSP. More than a dozen cases of myelopathy associated with HTLV-2 have been reported, but the occurrence is very infrequent compared with HTLV-1 carriers.

The pathogenesis results from trafficking of infected T cells into the perivascular areas and parenchyma of the spinal cord, where they cause astrocytosis. Chronic inflammation of spinal gray and white matter results in a progressive degeneration of the lateral and posterior columns, followed over time by loss of both myelin and axons in the anterior columns.

CLINICAL MANIFESTATIONS

Symptoms include stiff gait, spasticity, lower extremity weakness, back pain, urinary incontinence, impotence, and (rarely) ataxia. Patients typically present with a stiff gait that progresses (usually slowly) to increasing spasticity and weakness, with incontinence and impotence developing later, although bladder symptoms and low back pain may have been noted for months or years. In contrast to classic multiple sclerosis (Chapter 383), in which remissions may be seen, HAM/TSP is characterized by a relentlessly progressive course. Although lesions may occur anywhere in the CNS in HAM/TSP, degeneration of long motor neurons in the spinal cord accounts for the great majority of the signs and symptoms. Progression of the disease is usually slow, but some cases are acutely progressive, especially those associated with transfusion of HTLV-1-positive blood or transplantation-associated infection. Other manifestations of HTLV-1-associated "autoimmune" disease may be observed coincident with the neurologic syndrome.

DIAGNOSIS

The diagnosis is suspected in patients with unexplained loss of pyramidal tract functions and is confirmed by testing of sera for HTLV-1 antibodies. Oligoclonal immunoglobulin bands in the cerebrospinal fluid (CSF) of patients with HAM/TSP react to HTLV-1 antigens, and the CSF-to-serum ratio of HTLV-1 antibodies is greater than 1. PCR quantification of the HTLV-1 cell-associated provirus in the CSF is also diagnostic. Spinal cord lesions often appear hyperintense on T2-weighted magnetic resonance imaging.

TREATMENT   Rx

Few randomized controlled trials on the therapy of HAM/TSP have been conducted. The International Retrovirology Association has drawn up guidelines for the management of HAM/TSP, using the internationally agreed GRADE system (https://htlv.net/HAMpdf). The strongest evidence of benefit is for corticosteroids: 1 g/day intravenous pulsed methylprednisolone for 3 to 5 days, followed by long-term low-dose (e.g., 5 mg daily) oral prednisolone as maintenance. Higher doses of oral steroids may be required. A range of steroid-sparing therapies have been used, notably cyclosporin 2.5 mg/kg/day in divided doses, azathioprine 25 to 100 mg daily, salazopyrine 1000 to 1500 mg daily, and methotrexate 7.5 mg to 12.5 mg weekly with folate recovery, but further studies are required to determine long-term efficacy. To date, there is no evidence to support the use of antiretroviral therapy alone, although the HTLV reverse transcriptase and integrase enzymes can be inhibited in vitro. There also is insufficient evidence to support the use of other therapies, although the recent study of mogamulizumab is promising.[12]

PROGNOSIS

The prognosis of HAM/TSP is poor, with inexorable progression of neurologic deterioration. By 20 years, about 50% of patients are confined to a wheelchair.

● OTHER HTLV-ASSOCIATED CONDITIONS

HAM/TSP is the archetype of a series of HTLV-1-induced inflammatory syndromes characterized by a high viral load and mononuclear cell infiltration into the tissues. Examples include skeletal muscle polymyositis, sporadic inclusion body myositis, uveitis (30 to 40% of cases in areas endemic for HTLV),[13] lung involvement (pulmonary lymphocytic alveolitis, cryptogenic fibrosing alveolitis, bronchiectasis), Sjögren syndrome/keratoconjunctivitis sicca, and infective dermatitis, which is a pediatric syndrome characterized by inability to clear bacterial skin infections (see Table 354-2). Carriers of HTLV-1 also have elevated rates of invasive cervical cancer, tuberculosis, parasitic infestations (especially strongyloidiasis), scabies, and refractory generalized eczema associated with infective dermatitis. One prospective study of HTLV-2-positive drug users showed an excess of asthma-related deaths and an increased frequency of skin and soft tissue infections.

Patients often seek medical attention when confronted with a positive HTLV test result based on blood bank screening. Confirmation with Western blot or PCR is needed. Confirmed positive patients should be told that complications related to HTLV-1 infection are uncommon and that HTLV-2 hardly ever causes disease. Second, it should be emphasized that these viruses are not easily transmitted, but the patient should be advised how transmission can be prevented. Third, the patient should be counseled concerning the distinction between HTLV and HIV because the greatest fear that patients may experience is that they have the "AIDS virus." Other guidelines for prevention include the following:

- Blood for donation should be screened before transfusion, and positive donors should be excluded from donating. All solid-organ transplant donors should be screened for HTLV-1 infection and the use of such organs carefully considered with the potential recipient, given the high rate of HAM/TSP.
- HTLV-1/HTLV-2–positive mothers should be discouraged from breast-feeding to prevent mother-to-infant transmission, except in settings where diarrheal disease in non-breast-fed infants presents an even higher risk for morbidity and mortality.
- Condoms should be used by discordant couples. However, given the relatively low frequency of sexual transmission per sexual encounter, couples who desire a pregnancy could time unprotected sexual intercourse to coincide with periods of maximal fertility. Such decisions require careful discussion between the physician and the patient.

Unlike HIV, postexposure prophylaxis (sexual exposure) is not routinely recommended because the efficacy of such prophylaxis for HTLV infection in humans has not been established. Vaccines containing whole virus and recombinant HTLV-1 envelope antigens have successfully prevented HTLV-1 infection in monkeys and in a rabbit model. However, a vaccine for humans is unlikely to be a high priority because of the relatively low incidence of clinical disease.

Grade A Reference

A1. Phillips AA, Fields P, Hermine O, et al. Mogamulizumab versus investigator's choice of chemotherapy regimen in relapsed/refractory adult T-cell leukemia/lymphoma. *Haematologica*. 2019;104: 993-1003.

GENERAL REFERENCES

For the General References and other additional features, please visit Expert Consult at https://expertconsult.inkling.com.

TABLE 355-1 CLASSIFICATION OF ENTEROVIRUSES

SPECIES	SEROTYPES
Enterovirus A	CV- A2-A8, A10, A12, A14, A16 EV- A71, A76, A90-A92, A114, A119-121
Enterovirus B	CV- A9 CV- B1-B6 E- 1-7, 9, 11-21, 24-27, 29-33 EV- B69, B73-B75, B77, B78, B79-B88, B93, B97, B98, B100, B101, B106, B107, B110-113
Enterovirus C	PV- 1-3 CV- A1, A11, A13, A17, A19-A22, A24 EV- C95, C96, C99, C102, C104, C105, C109, C113, C116-C118
Enterovirus D	EV- D68, D70, D94, D111, D120

TABLE 355-2 THE 13 MOST COMMON ENTEROVIRUS SEROTYPES REPORTED BY NATIONAL ENTEROVIRAL SURVEILLANCE SYSTEM LABORATORIES TO THE CDC, 2009–2013

ENTEROVIRUS SEROTYPE	PERCENTAGE
Coxsackievirus A6	12.3
Echovirus 11	7.9
Echovirus 18	5.6
Coxsackievirus A9	5.1
Coxsackievirus B4	5.0
Echovirus 30	5.0
Echovirus 6	5.0
Enterovirus D68	4.3
Coxsackievirus B5	4.1
Coxsackievirus B3	4.1
Echovirus 9	4.0
Coxsackievirus B1	3.5
Coxsackievirus A16	2.9
Total	69.1

From Centers for Disease Control and Prevention (CDC). Enterovirus and parechovirus surveillance—United States, 2009-2013. *MMWR Morb Mortal Wkly Rep.* 2015;64:940-943.

355

ENTEROVIRUSES

JOSÉ R. ROMERO

DEFINITION

The enteroviruses belong to the genus Enterovirus in the family Picornaviridae. With the advent of molecular virology, the more than 100 recognized strains are classified on the basis of phylogenetic analysis of the nucleic acid sequence of VP1, the major enteroviral capsid protein (Table 355-1).

The Pathogens

Enteroviruses are small (30 nm in diameter), nonenveloped, icosahedral-shaped viruses. The viral capsid is composed of four viral proteins (VP1 to VP4). The enteroviruses possess an approximately 7.4-kilobase positive-sense single-stranded RNA genome. The 5′ end of the genome is covalently linked to a small protein, VPg. The genome is organized into a long (about 740 nucleotides) 5′ nontranslated region that precedes a single continuous open reading frame measuring about 6.63 kilobases. The open reading frame, which is followed by a short 3′ nontranslated region and a terminal polyadenylate tail, yields a single large polyprotein that is post-translationally modified to produce four capsid proteins, seven nonstructural proteins, and several functional protein intermediates. The 5′ and 3′ nontranslated regions of VPg participate in replication of the viral genome. The 5′ nontranslated region of the enterovirus is essential for translation and contains determinants of neurovirulence in the polioviruses.

EPIDEMIOLOGY

Worldwide, an estimated 1 billion or more enteroviral infections occur annually. In the United States about 30 to 50 million annual infections result in approximately 10 to 15 million symptomatic cases, with coxsackievirus A6, echovirus 11, echovirus 18, coxsackievirus A9, coxsackievirus B4, echovirus 30, echovirus 6, and enterovirus D69 accounting for approximately 50% of enteroviral infections.[1]

Humans are the only known reservoir for enteroviruses. Enteroviral infections are seasonal, and the majority of infections occur during the summer and early autumn in temperate regions. For example, more than 80% of infections occur in the United States from June through October. However, winter outbreaks highlight their panseasonal occurrence. In tropical and subtropical regions, infections continue year-round, with an increased incidence during the rainy season.

Globally, the dominant circulating enterovirus serotypes may vary annually by geographic region. In the United States 13 serotypes accounted for nearly 70% of all isolates reported (Table 355-2).

More than 80% of infections occur in individuals younger than 20 years, with the highest incidence in infants and children 4 years and younger. Nearly

45% of all infections occur in infants younger than 1 year. Among household members of infected children, clinical or serologic evidence of secondary infection can be seen in more than 50% of susceptible individuals. A male preponderance is noted in persons younger than age 20 years (male-to-female ratio of 1.4 : 1) but not in older individuals.

Localized enteroviral outbreaks have been reported in neonatal units, nurseries, daycare centers, schools, camps, sports teams, and military facilities. Community-wide outbreaks are common. Extensive regional outbreaks of EV-A71 have occurred in the Asia-Pacific region. Occasional pandemics, such as acute hemorrhagic conjunctivitis caused by EV-D70 and CV-A24, also have occurred.

Effective antipolio immunization programs have eradicated wild-type poliovirus serotype 2 worldwide. Serotype 3 was last detected in 2012 but has not yet been declared eradicated. Cases of serotype 1 now appear to be restricted to Afghanistan, Pakistan, and Nigeria, where unfortunately it remains endemic.[2] Despite greater than 95% polio vaccine rates, wild-type 1 genotype polioviruses have persistently circulated in southern Israel and intermittently in other areas, fortunately without any paralytic cases, as determined by intensified surveillance.

The use of live attenuated poliovirus vaccines has led to the problem of vaccine-derived polioviruses (VDPVs) as a result of the excretion of neurorevertant vaccine (Sabin) strains from individuals who have primary humoral immunodeficiencies, but not secondary humoral or other immunodeficiencies, or as a result of natural recombination between Sabin strains and members of the Enterovirus C species.[3] VDPVs that can circulate in the environment with evidence of person-to-person transmission have been termed *circulating vaccine-derived polioviruses* (cVDPVs). A third group of VDPVs, designated ambiguous VDPVs, are clinical isolates from individuals without known immunodeficiency or sewage isolates whose ultimate source is unknown. Similar to wild-type poliovirus, cVDPVs can cause acute flaccid paralysis in unimmunized or incompletely immunized individuals and have caused multiple outbreaks worldwide. To eliminate the risk for polio owing to VDPVs, all use of oral live attenuated poliovirus vaccines would have to cease. As an initial step toward that goal, a global synchronized switch from the trivalent oral polio vaccine to a bivalent vaccine containing only types 1 and 3 attenuated polioviruses was undertaken in 2016.[4]

PATHOBIOLOGY

The polioviruses and the majority of the nonpolio enteroviruses are transmitted through a fecal-oral route. Notable exceptions include CV-A21 and EV-D68, which are spread by the respiratory route, and EV-D70, which may spread by contaminated fomites or ocular and respiratory secretions. Evidence also supports transplacental transmission of the enteroviruses.

Ingestion of the enteroviruses results in infection of cells of the pharynx and, because the virus is acid resistant, the lower gastrointestinal tract. Initial viral replication, which is thought to occur in the mucosal tissues of the nasopharynx and intestinal tract (i.e., tonsils and Peyer patches), leads to seeding of the deep cervical and mesenteric lymph nodes. Further replication at these sites results in a minor viremia with seeding of multiple organs, including the liver, lungs, heart, and central nervous system (CNS). Viral replication at these sites causes many of the clinical manifestations of infection and is followed by a major viremia that may infect the CNS if it was spared during the initial viremia. The virus is cleared by type-specific neutralizing antibodies directed at the capsid proteins by day 7 to 10 after infection. IgA antibodies appear in the respiratory and gastrointestinal tracts 2 to 4 weeks after infection.

The host humoral immune response is pivotal in the prevention and eradication of enteroviral infections. Congenital or acquired B-cell immunodeficiencies may result in chronic or prolonged infection. Experimental evidence suggests that the interferons are important in limiting the spread of poliovirus once infection has occurred. Natural killer cells and gamma or delta T cells may play roles in regulating the host T-cell response.

Histopathologic findings in patients who died of poliomyelitis reveal neuronal necrosis in association with mononuclear and polymorphonuclear infiltrates that are initially perivascular in distribution but are later found diffusely within the gray matter of the anterior horns of the spinal cord, the reticular formation of the hindbrain, the vestibular nuclei, and the roof nuclei of the cerebellum. In nonpolio enterovirus CNS infections in immunocompetent hosts, findings include edema of the meninges and cerebral parenchyma, with microscopic perivascular lymphocytic infiltration, increased numbers of oligodendrocytes, and focal areas of necrosis and hemorrhage. In cases of enteroviral myocarditis (Chapter 54), a mononuclear cell inflammation is associated with widespread myocardial necrosis followed by fibrosis, which may be focal but results in myocardial damage.

CLINICAL MANIFESTATIONS

The incubation period for enterovirus infections is generally 3 to 6 days, with a range of 2 days to 2 weeks. Depending on serotype and the age of the patient, as many as 90% of infected individuals may have subclinical infections.[5] The enteroviruses are responsible for a wide array of clinical syndromes affecting nearly every organ system, and no enterovirus serotype is uniquely associated with a single disease or clinical syndrome (Table 355-3).

The most frequent enteroviral syndrome, seen in about 50 to 80% of cases, is nonspecific febrile illness, which occurs most commonly in infants, toddlers, and young children. The onset of illness is abrupt, with fever, poor appetite, lethargy, irritability, emesis, diarrhea,[6] and upper respiratory tract symptoms. Physical findings are minimal and consist of mild pharyngeal and conjunctival injection and lymphadenopathy. Exanthems may be present in about 25% of cases.

DIAGNOSIS

Nucleic acid amplification techniques (e.g., reverse transcription–polymerase chain reaction [RT-PCR] and nucleic acid–based sequence amplification) are the preferred methods for detection and identification of all enteroviruses.[7] Multiple studies have documented that nucleic acid amplification techniques are more sensitive and rapid than cell culture for the detection of enteroviruses in cerebrospinal fluid (CSF). RT-PCR can detect enteroviruses in CSF, blood, tissue, stool, and other body fluids within hours, and the results can shorten hospitalizations, decrease the use of antibiotics, and reduce health care costs.

Serologic testing is of limited use, although a four-fold change in antibody titer to a specific serotype of enterovirus in paired acute and convalescent sera can establish the diagnosis. Cell culture is not recommended because of limited sensitivity, prolonged positivity even after the related clinical syndrome may have resolved, and the several days required for viral detection.

TREATMENT AND PROGNOSIS Rx

Nonspecific febrile enteroviral infections generally resolve in less than 5 days without sequelae. Because of concern for possible occult bacterial infection, however, significant numbers of young infants and children are hospitalized for evaluation and empirical therapy. After infection, virus may be shed into the nasopharynx for 2 to 6 weeks and in feces for several months.

SPECIFIC CLINICAL SYNDROMES
Central Nervous System Infections

ACUTE FLACCID PARALYSIS
CLINICAL MANIFESTATIONS AND DIAGNOSIS

During poliovirus epidemics, 90 to 95% of infections are subclinical. In another 4 to 8% of patients, infection results in fever, fatigue, headache, anorexia, myalgia, and sore throat, which resolve in 2 to 3 days. Paralytic polio develops in less than 1 to 2% of infected individuals.

Sporadic cases of acute flaccid paralysis can also be seen with other enteroviruses, especially coxsackievirus CV-A7 and enterovirus EV-A71, and EV-D68.[8] EV-A71 recently caused an outbreak of paresis in Australia, with 95% of patients having enteroviral RNA in their feces; about 90% of cases resolved by 1 year.[9] In a recent outbreak of flaccid paralysis among children in Colorado, preceding or concurrent EV-D68 infection was documented in 12 of 25 cases and thought to be the probable cause in the other 13. In Japan, however, only 9 of 58 cases of acute flaccid paralysis could be linked to EV-D68, and the virus was detected in the CSF in only one case.[10] Among 59 cases of acute flaccid myelitis of unknown etiology in California between 2012 and 2015, 54 were preceded by or concurrent with a respiratory or gastrointestinal illness, but only one third of patients had culture or serologic evidence of enteroviral infection.[11] With the exception of EV-A71 and EV-D68, the paralysis associated with nonpolio enteroviruses tends to be milder, and fever is absent at the time of onset of the paralysis. The upper extremities, face, and cranial nerves are more commonly involved. Sensory pathways remain intact.

CSF may reveal a normal cell count or a mild lymphocytic pleocytosis (<100 cells/μL) in association with mildly increased protein and normal glucose concentrations. Neuroimaging is not generally useful, but increased signal may be seen on T2-weighted magnetic resonance imaging in the anterior horn regions of the spinal cord in patients whose acute flaccid paralysis is caused by poliovirus and nonpolio enteroviruses.

TABLE 355-3 CLINICAL MANIFESTATIONS OF NONPOLIO ENTEROVIRUS INFECTIONS*

CLINICAL SYNDROME	GROUP A COXSACKIEVIRUSES†	GROUP B COXSACKIEVIRUSES	ECHOVIRUSES	ENTEROVIRUSES
Asymptomatic infection	All serotypes	All serotypes	All serotypes	All serotypes
Undifferentiated febrile illness ("summer grippe") with or without respiratory symptoms	All serotypes	All serotypes	All serotypes	D68, D70, A71
Aseptic meningitis (often associated with an exanthem)	1, 2, 3, 4, 5, 6, 7, 8, 9, 10, 11, 14, 16, 17, 18, 22, 24	1, 2, 3, 4, 5, 6	1, 2, 3, 4, 5, 6, 7, 8, 9, 10, 11, 12, 14, 16, 17, 18, 19, 20, 21, 25, 30, 31, 33	D70, A71
Encephalitis	2, 4, 5, 6, 7, 9, 10, 16	1, 2, 3, 4, 5	2, 3, 4, 6, 7, 9, 11, 14, 17, 18, 19, 25, 30, 33	D70, A71
Acute flaccid paralysis (poliomyelitis-like)	4, 5, 6, 7, 9, 10, 11, 14, 16, 21, 24	1, 2, 3, 4, 5, 6	1, 2, 4, 6, 7, 9, 11, 14, 16, 17, 18, 19, 30	D68?, D70, A71
Myopericarditis	1, 2, 4, 5, 7, 8, 9, 14, 16	1, 2, 3, 4, 5, 6	1, 2, 3, 4, 6, 7, 8, 9, 11, 14, 16, 17, 19, 25, 30	
Pleurodynia	1, 2, 4, 6, 9, 10, 16	1, 2, 3, 4, 5, 6	1, 2, 3, 6, 7, 8, 9, 11, 12, 14, 16, 19, 25, 30	
Herpangina	1, 2, 3, 4, 5, 6, 7, 8, 9, 10, 16, 22	1, 2, 3, 4, 5	6, 9, 11, 16, 17, [22], 25	A71
Hand-foot-and-mouth disease	4, 5, 6, 7, 9, 10, 16	2, 5	7	A71
Exanthems	2, 4, 5, 6, 7, 9, 10, 16	1, 2, 3, 4, 5	2, 4, 5, 6, 9, 11, 16, 18, 25	A71
Common cold	2, 10, 21, 24	1, 2, 3, 4, 5	2, 4, 8, 9, 11, 20, 25	
Lower respiratory tract infections (bronchiolitis, pneumonia)	7, 9, 16	1, 2, 3, 4, 5	4, 8, 9, 11, 12, 14, 19, 20, 21, 25, 30	D68, A71, C104
Acute hemorrhagic conjunctivitis§	24			D70
Generalized disease of the newborn	3, 9, 16	1, 2, 3, 4, 5	3, 4, 6, 7, 9, 11, 12, 14, 17, 18, 19, 20, 21, 30	

*A great many enterovirus serotypes have been implicated in most of these syndromes, at least in sporadic cases. The serotypes listed are those that have been clearly or frequently implicated. Serotypes with a strong association are underlined.
†Because detection of many of the group A coxsackieviruses originally required suckling mouse inoculation, they are likely to be underreported as causes of illness.
§Conjunctivitis without hemorrhage is frequently seen in association with other manifestations in patients infected with many group A and group B coxsackieviruses and echoviruses, especially coxsackieviruses A9, A16, and B1 to B5 and echoviruses 2, 7, 9, 11, 16, and 30.
From Modlin JR. Enterovirus. *Cecil Textbook of Medicine*. 23rd ed. Philadelphia: WB Saunders; 2008, with minor changes.

TREATMENT AND PROGNOSIS Rx

No specific therapy exists. Efforts should focus on monitoring for the development of respiratory failure or airway compromise as well as control of pain associated with muscle spasms.

The mortality rate associated with spinal poliomyelitis is about 5%. The mortality rates for enteroviruses associated with nonpolio enteroviral acute flaccid paralysis are not known. Before modern methods of respiratory and cardiovascular support, mortality rates higher than 50% were common in patients with bulbar or medullary poliomyelitis. The ultimate outcome of the paralysis is highly variable and can range from complete resolution to lifelong persistence. The greatest gains in recovery of strength occur during the first 6 months of convalescence. Paralytic limbs become atrophic, thereby leading to skeletal deformities. Patients with nonpolio enteroviruses usually have a more rapid recovery and less atrophy than do those with classic polio. However, in the recent Colorado outbreak of EV-D68, about 75% of patients had limited or no improvement of their flaccid paralysis at 30 days, and the other 25% had only partial recovery by that time.

A syndrome of postpoliomyelitis muscle atrophy, which may be seen in 25 to 85% of individuals 2 to 3 decades after recovery from paralytic disease, is characterized by the gradual development of weakness, pain, and atrophy. Possible mechanisms include aging and neuronal dropout in compromised neuromuscular connections or, less likely, reactivation/ongoing poliovirus infection.

MENINGITIS

The enteroviruses, especially those within the Enterovirus B species, are the dominant cause of viral meningitis (Chapter 384) in all ages. In a recent survey, almost 52% of all cases of meningitis and encephalitis in the United States from 2011 to 2014 were documented to be enteroviral infections.[12]

CLINICAL MANIFESTATIONS AND DIAGNOSIS

The clinical picture varies with age. The predominant symptoms of meningitis in neonates are nonspecific fever, irritability, lethargy, and poor feeding, often with a full fontanelle and a generalized rash. In neonates with meningoencephalitis, clinical findings may consist of fever, lethargy, seizures, full fontanelle, and focal neurologic abnormalities. Hepatitis, myocarditis, or pneumonitis, singly or in combination, may be present in severe cases.

In older infants and children, an abrupt onset of fever is the most frequent initial symptom. The fever may persist for 1 to 5 days and may exhibit a biphasic pattern. Irritability or lethargy is common. Other nonspecific symptoms include poor feeding, vomiting, diarrhea, and rash. Headache is present in nearly all children old enough to report it. Rash, malaise, sore throat, abdominal pain, and myalgia are common, and photophobia may be reported. Seizures occur in less than 5% of cases. Examination may reveal a full fontanelle. Signs of meningeal irritation (i.e., nuchal rigidity, Brudzinski and Kernig signs) occur in less than 10% of infants younger than 3 months and increase with age.

In adolescents and adults, headache is nearly always present and severe enough to require narcotic analgesics for control. Some patients report temporary relief of headache after lumbar puncture. Fever is not universal, but photophobia, signs of meningeal irritation, nausea, emesis, and neck stiffness occur in more than two thirds of patients. Myalgia is reported in 20 to 90% of patients. Less frequent findings include rash and abdominal pain.

CSF analysis generally reveals a mild to moderate lymphocytic pleocytosis (<500 cells/μL).[13] Some patients, however, may have lymphocyte counts higher than 1000 or have neutrophilic pleocytosis early in the course of illness and then progress to a predominance of lymphocytes hours to days later. In a small percentage of patients, particularly infants, no pleocytosis is present even though enterovirus can be detected. The protein concentration may be increased. Although the glucose concentration is generally normal, hypoglycorrhachia may occur, particularly in association with group B coxsackievirus meningitis. Neuroimaging in cases of meningitis is generally unrevealing. Nucleic acid amplification testing can detect enteroviruses in CSF. The serotypes most frequently identified from CSF specimens are from the enterovirus B species.

TREATMENT AND PROGNOSIS Rx

Treatment is supportive, with control of fever and pain. Currently available antiviral agents are not helpful. Hospitalization may not be necessary in adolescents and adults who appear well if a bacterial cause can be confidently excluded. In children and infants or when bacterial infection cannot be confidently excluded in adults, hospitalization and initial empirical antimicrobial therapy are advisable (Chapter 384) while awaiting the results of bacterial cultures of blood and CSF. Intravenous fluids may be required to prevent dehydration. Control of headache pain may require narcotic analgesics. Uncommon complications in all ages include coma, increased intracranial pressure, and inappropriate secretion of antidiuretic hormone.

The overwhelming majority of patients recover fully. The duration of illness in infants and children is generally less than 1 week. In adults, full recovery may take up to 3 weeks.

ENCEPHALITIS

The enteroviruses are responsible for up to 22% of identifiable causes of viral encephalitis (Chapter 386). In the single largest report of enterovirus-related encephalitis, 73% of confirmed cases occurred in individuals younger than 20 years, including about 40% of cases in patients younger than 10 years.

CLINICAL MANIFESTATIONS AND DIAGNOSIS

The onset of neurologic findings may be abrupt or be preceded by fever, headache, malaise, myalgia, upper respiratory symptoms, rash, nausea, emesis, or diarrhea. Somnolence, lethargy, and altered consciousness are common. Patients may exhibit irritability, changes in personality, or hallucinations. Generalized or focal seizures occur in up to 30% of patients, and a minority of patients may progress to coma. Neck stiffness and ataxia are frequent physical findings. Focal neurologic findings such as hemiplegia, hemichorea, and paresthesias are reported in nearly 30% of patients. The focal nature of the seizures and abnormal neurologic findings may be reminiscent of herpes simplex virus encephalitis (Chapter 350).

Among enteroviral encephalitides, EV-A71 is uniquely associated with severe brain stem encephalitis (rhombencephalitis), primarily in children. The initial manifestation may be a prodrome of either hand-foot-and-mouth disease or herpangina, which is followed by myoclonus that may be associated with ataxia, tremors, or cranial nerve abnormalities and a rapid onset of neurogenic pulmonary edema, shock, coma, and apnea.

Evaluation of CSF may reveal mild to moderate lymphocytic pleocytosis (<500 cells/μL), but the CSF white cell count may be normal. The protein concentration may be increased and may be the sole abnormality. The glucose concentration is generally normal. Enteroviruses may frequently be detectable by nucleic acid amplification testing of CSF.

TREATMENT AND PROGNOSIS   Rx

Management is supportive, with monitoring for the development of respiratory failure or airway compromise. Nearly 50% of patients require intensive care. In patients with focal neurologic findings, empirical acyclovir (10 to 15 mg/kg every 8 hours) is warranted until herpes simplex virus is excluded.

The median duration of hospitalization is less than 1 week, and mortality is below 10%. For severe EV-A71 rhombencephalitis, however, mortality may approach 70%. Long-term sequelae after rhombencephalitis include myoclonus, abducens nerve palsy, facial diplegia, ataxia, dysarthria, internuclear ophthalmoplegia, and central apnea.

Myopericarditis

Members of the Enterovirus B species and especially the group B coxsackieviruses are responsible for approximately a third of cases of acute myocarditis (Chapter 54). The majority of cases occur in young adults.

CLINICAL MANIFESTATIONS AND DIAGNOSIS

An upper respiratory tract infection may precede the onset of cardiac symptoms by 1 to 2 weeks. Fever may be present, and common initial symptoms include dyspnea, chest pain, and fatigue. Physical examination may reveal a gallop rhythm or a pericardial friction rub.

Cardiomegaly may be seen on the chest radiograph. Electrocardiographic findings vary and include low-voltage QRS complexes, ST segment depression, T wave inversion, pathologic Q waves, ventricular arrhythmias, and heart block. Echocardiographic findings include a decreased ejection fraction, ventricular dilation, and pericardial effusion. Blood troponin levels are frequently elevated. Cardiac magnetic resonance imaging may help localize areas of myocarditis. Myocardial biopsy is recommended in selected patients who have refractory heart failure or suspected giant cell myocarditis (Chapter 54); enterovirus can be detected by nucleic acid amplification tests.

TREATMENT AND PROGNOSIS   Rx

Supportive treatment includes bed rest and management of heart failure (Chapter 53), arrhythmias (Chapters 58 and 59), and pericarditis with or without pericardial effusion (Chapter 68). Immunosuppressive therapy is not generally recommended (Chapter 54). In approximately a third of patients with acute myocarditis, chronic dilated cardiomyopathy develops. In patients with pericarditis, recurrent pericardial effusions or chronic constrictive pericarditis may develop in the future.

Exanthems and Enanthems

Enterovirus infections may result in a wide spectrum of febrile exanthems and enanthems, including macular, papular, maculopapular, morbilliform, rubelliform, vesicular, urticarial, papulopustular, and scarlatiniform types. Exanthems are more commonly observed in children 15 years or younger. Any serotype is capable of causing several different rashes. With the exception of CV-A16, no serotype is associated with a unique rash. Echovirus 9 and CV-A9 can cause petechial or purpuric rashes reminiscent of meningococcemia (Chapter 282).

Hand-Foot-and-Mouth Disease and Herpangina

Hand-foot-and-mouth disease is typically associated with Enterovirus A species, particularly CV-A16, CV-A6, and EV-A71.[14,15] Herpangina is also most commonly caused by the group A coxsackieviruses in the Enterovirus A species, but it has also been associated with group B coxsackieviruses, echoviruses, and enteroviruses from the Enterovirus B species.

CLINICAL MANIFESTATIONS AND DIAGNOSIS

Hand-foot-and-mouth disease begins with low-grade fever, malaise, anorexia, and oral soreness. In 1 to 2 days, oral macules appear and then rapidly vesiculate and ulcerate. Oral lesions are typically distributed on the buccal mucosa and tongue, but they may also occur on the palate, uvula, anterior pillars, and gums. In approximately two thirds of patients, the enanthem is accompanied by an exanthem, with tender 3- to 7-mm vesicles on the dorsum of the hands and feet, frequently involving the palms and soles. Lesions may appear on the buttocks but tend not to be vesicular. Hand-foot-and-mouth disease associated with CV-A6 has a wider distribution of skin lesions that enlarge and vesiculate. Onychomadesis (loss of fingernails) can occur 1 to 2 months after the infection.

Herpangina begins with high fever, particularly in young patients. Additional findings include sore throat, mild cervical lymphadenopathy, sialorrhea, anorexia, dysphagia, abdominal pain, and emesis. Examination of the mouth and throat reveals 1- to 2-mm papulovesicular, grayish white lesions with an areola of erythema, primarily located on the anterior pillars of the tonsillar fauces. The soft palate, uvula, and tonsils may also be involved. Rarely, the posterior buccal surfaces and dorsal tip of the tongue may be involved. During a period of 2 to 3 days, the lesions increase to 3 to 4 mm in size. On average, five lesions are present.

TREATMENT AND PROGNOSIS   Rx

Hand-foot-and-mouth disease usually resolves in less than 1 week and herpangina generally resolves in 10 days, both typically uneventfully, without the need for hospitalization and without sequelae. Infants and young children may require hospitalization for administration of parenteral fluids. Disease associated with CV-A6 has a higher rate of hospitalization. Hand-foot-and-mouth disease due to EV-A71 may precede the development of life-threatening rhombencephalitis (see Encephalitis). Experimental EV71 vaccines are greater than 90% effective against EV71-related hand-foot-and-mouth disease and greater than 80% effective against EV71-associated serious diseases, but do not protect against coxsackievirus A16 infections.

Acute Hemorrhagic Conjunctivitis

Acute hemorrhagic conjunctivitis (Chapter 395) is associated with EV-D70 and CV-A24. The illnesses caused by the two serotypes are indistinguishable from each other. However, acute hemorrhagic conjunctivitis caused by CV-A24 may be more commonly accompanied by upper respiratory and systemic symptoms and may be associated with less severe conjunctival hemorrhage. High secondary attack rates within households are common. Other enteroviruses can cause acute conjunctivitis or keratoconjunctivitis but generally without hemorrhagic manifestations.

CLINICAL MANIFESTATIONS

An incubation period of about 1 to 2 days precedes the rapid onset of palpebral swelling associated with lacrimation, photophobia, blurring of vision, and severe ocular pain. The hallmark subconjunctival hemorrhages vary in size from petechiae to large blotches. Although transient keratitis occurs frequently, it seldom results in subepithelial opacities. Preauricular adenopathy is common, but fever is not. An ocular mucopurulent discharge may occasionally be present.

TREATMENT AND PROGNOSIS · Rx

Management is supportive. The illness usually persists for 1 to 2 weeks, but complete recovery is generally the rule. A transient lumbar radiculomyelopathy and acute flaccid paralysis–like illness may develop in some patients.

Respiratory Tract Syndromes

The enteroviruses may cause upper and lower respiratory tract syndromes, alone or accompanying other syndromes. As determined by nucleic acid amplification testing, enteroviruses are responsible for up to 15% of upper respiratory tract syndromes. They also cause 18% of lower respiratory tract syndromes in hospitalized children and 25% of hospitalizations in patients with acute wheezing. EV-D68 and EV-C104 are being increasingly recognized as causes of respiratory tract disease.

CLINICAL MANIFESTATIONS AND DIAGNOSIS

The enterovirus "summer cold" (Chapter 337) consists of nasal congestion, rhinorrhea, and sneezing. Malaise and cough may be present. Fever and sore throat are typically absent or minimal.

Pharyngitis, tonsillitis, or pharyngotonsillitis begins abruptly with fever and sore throat. The nasopharynx, tonsils, uvula, and soft palate demonstrate erythema and inflammation. Petechiae may be present, and cervical lymphadenitis is common. Other syndromes associated with the enteroviruses include bronchitis (Chapter 90) and bronchiolitis.

Enteroviral pneumonias begin gradually with coryza, anorexia, and low-grade fever. A nonproductive cough, tachypnea, retractions, nasal flaring, and wheezing may be present. In severe cases, cyanosis may develop. The chest radiograph may demonstrate perihilar infiltrates, patchy consolidation, air trapping, and atelectasis. EV-D68 has become a cause of significant respiratory disease, primarily in young children and infants but also in adolescents and adults. An underlying pulmonary condition such as asthma or wheezing has been reported in up to 70 to 80% of cases. EV-D68–associated respiratory syndromes include pneumonia, bronchiolitis, asthmatic bronchitis, asthma exacerbation, and wheezing. Signs and symptoms include cough, wheezing, dyspnea, tachycardia, and inter- and subcostal retractions. Acute flaccid paralysis is a rare complication. Interestingly, fever may be absent, but hypoxia is common. The chest radiograph may show infiltrates and atelectasis.

TREATMENT AND PROGNOSIS · Rx

Treatment is supportive and consists of control of fever and pain. In older children and adults, hospitalization is not usually required. Resolution occurs in 7 days or less. Hospitalization and admission to an intensive care unit may be required for respiratory support of EV-D68 infection. Death is uncommon but does occur.

Myositis
PLEURODYNIA

The group B coxsackieviruses are the major cause of sporadic and epidemic pleurodynia, but the syndrome may also be caused by a limited number of echoviruses and group A coxsackieviruses within the Enterovirus A and B species.

CLINICAL MANIFESTATIONS AND DIAGNOSIS

The onset of illness is abrupt in approximately 75% of patients. In the remainder, the onset of pleuritic chest pain is preceded by a prodrome of headache, malaise, anorexia, and vague myalgia lasting up to 10 days. Pain may be referred to the lower ribs or the sternum, and it can radiate to the shoulders, neck, or scapula. Pain is exacerbated by deep breathing, coughing, sneezing, or movement. During paroxysms, patients tend to be tachypneic and to have shallow breathing. Additional findings can include abdominal pain, headache, cough, anorexia, nausea, vomiting, and diarrhea. Fever may be biphasic.

Physical examination does not generally reveal muscle tenderness, obvious myositis, or muscle swelling. A pleural friction rub may be present in 25% of patients. The chest radiograph is typically normal.

TREATMENT AND PROGNOSIS · Rx

Treatment is supportive, with an emphasis on nonsteroidal analgesics (e.g., ibuprofen, 200 to 400 mg per dose every 4 to 6 hours) or hydrocodone (5 to 10 mg four times per day) alone or in combination with acetaminophen to control pain. The symptoms may persist for 1 to 14 days (mean of 3.5 days) and resolve without sequelae, although recurrent symptoms may occur in 25% of patients.

INFLAMMATORY MYOSITIS

Multiple enteroviral serotypes are associated with focal or generalized myositis. In patients with B-cell immunodeficiencies, a dermatomyositis-like syndrome may develop.

CLINICAL MANIFESTATIONS AND DIAGNOSIS

Nonspecific findings include fever and chills. Involved muscles may be weak, tender, and edematous. Chemical evidence of myositis may be evidenced by elevated serum levels of creatine kinase, myoglobinemia, and myoglobinuria.

TREATMENT AND PROGNOSIS · Rx

Treatment is supportive. With the exception of patients with B-cell immunodeficiencies, recovery is complete and rapid.

Enterovirus Infections in Special Populations
PATIENTS WITH B-CELL IMMUNODEFICIENCIES

Nonpolio enteroviruses and polioviruses may result in chronic or prolonged infections in patients with congenital or acquired B-cell immunodeficiencies (Chapter 236), such as those with X-linked agammaglobulinemia, hyper-IgM syndrome, severe combined immunodeficiency syndrome, or common variable immunodeficiency, or in patients receiving chemotherapy or immuno-modulatory therapies, especially rituximab and obinutuzumab, who are undergoing bone marrow or solid organ transplantation.

CLINICAL MANIFESTATIONS AND DIAGNOSIS

Meningoencephalitis, pulmonary infections, and severe gastroenteritis can occur. The initial symptoms may consist of only persistent headaches and lethargy. As the disease progresses, additional neurologic findings develop and may include ataxia, loss of cognitive skills and memory, dementia, emotional lability, paresthesias, weakness, dysarthria, and seizures. Non-CNS manifestations include a dermatomyositis-like syndrome, edema, exanthems, and hepatitis. CSF demonstrates a persistently elevated protein concentration and pleocytosis. Enterovirus is detectable in CSF by RT-PCR.

TREATMENT AND PROGNOSIS · Rx

Children with humoral immunodeficiency (Chapter 236) should receive lifelong immunoglobulin replacement therapy in an attempt to prevent chronic infection. However, chronic meningoencephalitis develops in some patients and is usually ultimately fatal. Severe or fatal enteroviral infections have been reported in individuals receiving rituximab.

Handwashing is the primary method for the prevention of enteroviral infections. Only poliovirus infections are currently preventable through vaccination. Successful trials of inactivated EV-71 vaccines have been completed in China.[A1][A2] Their efficacy in other regions of the world will depend on their ability to protect from disease caused by the different genotypes found worldwide.

Grade A References

A1. Zhu FC, Meng FY, Li JX, et al. Efficacy, safety, and immunology of an inactivated alum-adjuvant enterovirus 71 vaccine in children in China: a multicentre, randomised, double-blind, placebo-controlled, phase 3 trial. *Lancet.* 2013;381:2024-2032.
A2. Zhu F, Xu W, Xia J, et al. Efficacy, safety, and immunogenicity of an enterovirus 71 vaccine in China. *N Engl J Med.* 2014;370:818-828.

GENERAL REFERENCES

For the General References and other additional features, please visit Expert Consult at https://expertconsult.inkling.com.

356

ROTAVIRUSES, NOROVIRUSES, AND OTHER GASTROINTESTINAL VIRUSES

MANUEL A. FRANCO AND HARRY B. GREENBERG

DEFINITION

Viruses are a principal cause of acute infectious gastroenteritis, a syndrome of vomiting, watery diarrhea, or both that begins abruptly in otherwise healthy persons. Two distinct viruses account for much of these cases. Before rotavirus vaccines were widely introduced over the last 15 years, rotaviruses accounted for over 400,000 deaths annually. Rotaviruses remain the most frequent cause of sporadic, severe gastroenteritis in young children and are currently responsible for the death of approximately 600 children daily worldwide,[1] mainly in developing countries that have not yet implemented widespread rotavirus vaccination. Noroviruses are the primary cause of epidemic infectious gastroenteritis in both infants and adults in developed countries. For example, outbreaks of gastroenteritis in closed settings, such as cruise ships and nursing homes, are a typical manifestation of norovirus infections. However, noroviruses are also an increasingly common cause of sporadic, severe gastroenteritis in young children and adolescents.[2]

The Pathogens
Noroviruses

Noroviruses, which are one of the five genera of the Caliciviridae family, are nonenveloped, icosahedral viruses with a relatively small, positive-sense, single-stranded RNA genome. The norovirus genus is further classified into five genogroups (GI to GV), only three of which (GI, GII, and GIV) are known to infect humans. GIII and GV viruses infect bovines and mice, respectively, and to date these animal viruses have not been shown to infect humans. Viruses in each genogroup are further divided into genotypes (more than 25 have been described) and subgroups. Norwalk virus is a prototype genogroup I genotype 1 (GI.1) virus. The norovirus genome is approximately 7.7 kilobases in size and consists of three open reading frames, the first of which encodes the nonstructural proteins that are essential for virus replication. The second open reading frame encodes the major capsid protein, viral protein 1 (VP1). When VP1 is expressed as a recombinant protein, 180 molecules autoassemble into virus-like particles (VLPs) that closely resemble authentic virions and that have proven to be critical to the study of noroviral epidemiology and immunity. Human noroviruses have only recently been reproducibly cultured in vitro in human enteroids,[3] so diagnosis generally depends on amplification of virus genes by the polymerase chain reaction (PCR; see later) or use of VLPs as recombinant antigens for serologic analysis.

Rotavirus

Rotaviruses, which belong to the family Reoviridae, are large, icosahedral, nonenveloped viruses with a segmented, double-stranded RNA genome and a triple-layered protein coat. Rotaviruses are classified into groups A through G on the basis of the presence of cross-reactive antigenic epitopes and their overall genetic relatedness. Group A rotaviruses are the most commonly encountered viral enteric pathogens of young humans and many other mammalian species. Group B viruses have been identified sporadically in outbreaks of adult diarrheal illness in China and more recently in studies of children with sporadic gastroenteritis, principally in India. Group C rotaviruses are primarily veterinary pathogens and are infrequently associated with diarrheal disease in humans and animals around the world compared with group A rotaviruses. Groups D through G rotaviruses have been isolated only from animals, primarily avian species. Rotaviruses are 100-nm particles that have three concentric layers of proteins: the core is composed of VP1, VP2, and VP3 and the segmented, double-stranded RNA genome; the intermediate layer is formed by VP6, the most abundant and antigenic structural viral protein; and the external layer is composed of VP7 and VP4. The genome, which is composed of 11 segments of double-stranded RNA that together are approximately 18 kilobases in length, encodes six structural and six nonstructural proteins. As is the case among virtually all other RNA viruses, the rotavirus RNA polymerase is error prone and, along with selective pressure such as the evolution of immunity, drives viral diversity. For rotaviruses, gene reassortment, which is the mixing of gene segments from different parental viruses in cells coinfected by two or more strains, and rearrangement of the viral genome also contribute to genetic diversity. Reassortment of gene segments between animal and human rotavirus strains also occurs in natural settings, especially in less developed countries. Recently an efficient and practical helper virus–free method was developed to recover recombinant rotaviruses, and this method will certainly lead to improved understanding of rotavirus biology as well as enhance the possibility of developing improved vaccines.[4]

Other Agents

Other viral agents that cause human acute infectious gastroenteritis that is difficult to distinguish from disease caused by rotaviruses and noroviruses include the sapovirus (like norovirus, a member of the Caliciviridae family), enteric adenoviruses (Chapter 341) belonging to types 40 and 41, and astroviruses (Table 356-1). The frequency of detection (by PCR assays) of these viruses in individuals with acute gastroenteritis depends on the setting, but they are almost always detected much less frequently than are rotaviruses and noroviruses. Coronaviruses (Chapter 342), toroviruses, picobirnaviruses, picornavirus (Chapter 355), bocavirus, parechoviruses, and pestiviruses have also been isolated occasionally from persons with acute gastroenteritis, but their roles as causative agents of enteric disease remain unproven. Among patients with acute gastroenteritis, no etiologic agent is found in approximately 25 to 50% of cases.

EPIDEMIOLOGY
Norovirus

Over time, noroviruses appear to undergo antigenic drift in response to the acquisition of immunity in the general population, much like influenza viruses.[5] At present, gastroenteritis cases around the world are most frequently caused by the GII.4 norovirus strain, but new strains generally evolve every 2 to 4 years owing to antigenic drift. Outbreaks frequently take place in settings of close human contact, such as military establishments, cruise ships, nursing homes, and schools, especially in cold and dry weather (see Table 356-1). Viral spread is enhanced by the very high level of infectivity of noroviruses, as data suggest that 1 to 10 particles constitute an infectious dose.

Noroviruses of genotypes GII.4 and GII.3 also are responsible for about 12 to 20% of sporadic gastroenteritis in children younger than 5 years in both developed and developing countries.[6] In the United States, where rotavirus vaccination is now widespread, noroviruses have recently surpassed rotavirus as the principal cause of medically attended visits for gastroenteritis in children younger than 5 years. In a birth cohort study from eight sites in South America, Africa, and Asia, rotavirus had the highest attributable burdens for sites without rotavirus vaccination.

Rotavirus

The incidence of rotaviral disease is similar in children in both developed and developing countries, suggesting that public hygiene measures such as access to clean water do not replace the need for an effective vaccine. In developed

TABLE 356-1 EPIDEMIOLOGIC AND CLINICAL FEATURES OF NOROVIRUS AND ROTAVIRUS

	NOROVIRUS	ROTAVIRUS	ASTROVIRUS
Epidemics	Occurs year-round; outbreaks tend to peak in cold weather	Year-round in equatorial countries; winter peak in others	Winter epidemics in children and endemic year-round
Key driver of epidemics	Antigenic drift strains promoted by population-based immunologic pressure	Size of the susceptible birth cohort	Unknown
Transmission	Fecal-oral, water, and food-borne outbreaks	Fecal-oral	Fecal-oral
Severity of diarrhea in children	Mild to moderate but can be severe	Most severe	Milder than rotavirus or norovirus
Reservoir	Humans are the only known reservoir of noroviruses that infect humans	Mostly humans, but rotaviruses from farm animals and pets (especially in developing countries) can infect humans but rarely spread	Humans are the only known reservoir of astroviruses that infect humans
Prevention	Viral protein 1–based vaccine in development	Several live attenuated vaccines available	No vaccine in development
Age predisposition	All ages	Primarily children <5 years; disease transmission in older family contacts is relatively low (<25%)	Generally children, but adults may also get disease

countries, before the implementation of highly effective vaccines, rotavirus was a major economic burden but rarely the cause of fatal disease; after the implementation of vaccines, the epidemiology of rotavirus disease has changed, with, for example, the peak incidences in nonvaccinated children in Finland now occurring between 6 and 16 years of age and in the elderly over 70 years of age.[7]

In the temperate zones of the world, rotaviral illness occurs primarily during epidemic peaks in the cooler months of the year (see Table 356-1). This pattern is not seen, however, in countries within 10 degrees of the equator, where disease occurs in an endemic fashion year-round. Before the introduction of rotavirus vaccination, a yearly wave of rotaviral illness spread across the United States and Europe following highly specific and recurrent spatiotemporal patterns. In the United States this pattern of spread has been correlated with variation in birth rates, thereby suggesting that the number of babies experiencing their first infection is one of the primary drivers of rotavirus epidemics. The high birth rates in developing countries may also influence their differential epidemiologic distribution of rotaviruses. The widespread use of rotavirus vaccine has greatly reduced or eliminated this spatiotemporal spread of rotavirus in the United States and Europe.

Antibodies against the two outer capsid proteins are the basis of serotypic classification of rotaviruses into G (glycoprotein, VP7) and P (protease-sensitive, VP4) serotypes. For technical reasons, P serotyping reagents are infrequently available, and classification is based on the P genotype (provided in brackets). Worldwide, most human infections are caused by just five types of group A rotavirus; P[8]G1 is by far the most common (approximately 53% of strains), followed by P[8]G3, P[4]G2, P[8]G9, and P[8]G4. In some developing areas such as India, Brazil, and Africa, P[6]G9, G5, and G8 rotaviruses, respectively, are also frequently encountered. Some human rotavirus strains may have arisen after reassortment with bovine or porcine rotaviruses. A high prevalence of G12 viruses has recently been observed in several countries, suggesting that this serotype may be an emerging rotavirus strain. Results from a large multicenter study in sub-Saharan Africa and south Asia, where most of the gastroenteritis deaths in children younger than 5 years of age occur, confirmed that rotavirus is the most common etiologic agent of this syndrome and causes an important nutritional burden in children.

PATHOBIOLOGY

Norovirus

Histo–blood group antigens (HBGAs) are the receptors for noroviruses and determine susceptibility to disease in a strain-specific manner. The HBGAs are complex carbohydrate oligosaccharides linked to proteins or lipids that are expressed on the mucosal epithelia of the digestive tract. All three major families of HBGA, the ABO, Lewis, and secretor families, are involved in binding noroviruses. The secretor status of a person is controlled by the fucosyltransferase 2 (FUT2) gene. Secretor-negative individuals are specifically resistant to infection with the Norwalk virus (GI.1) and some GII viruses as well.

Although norovirus RNA has been detected in the bloodstream of up to 15% of patients with norovirus gastroenteritis, the site of primary viral replication is most probably in the gastrointestinal tract. Recently human noroviruses have been successfully cultivated and passaged in vitro in differentiated human stem-cell–derived intestinal epithelial cell enteroid cultures. Consistent with the strong association of vomiting with norovirus disease, gastric emptying is delayed. Proximal jejunal biopsy specimens show blunting of the villi with crypt cell hyperplasia and cytoplasmic vacuolation, sometimes with an increase in epithelial cell apoptosis. A functional alteration of the epithelial barrier is likely to occur. Unknown at present is the effectiveness and persistence of long-term immunity in the context of natural infection, in which the infectious dose is generally quite low. The recent successful cultivation of noroviruses suggests that the role of neutralizing antibody as a determinant of protection can finally be carefully examined.

Rotavirus

For rotaviruses, HBGAs have also been recently proposed as receptors that determine susceptibility to disease in a strain-specific manner. Rotaviruses replicate in the villus tip cells of the small bowel, where the pathologic process includes shortening and atrophy of the villi, vacuolization of enterocytes, mononuclear infiltration in the lamina propria, and distention of the cisternae of the endoplasmic reticulum. However, the severity of clinical disease has not been directly related to the extent of intestinal disease; rather, it is related to levels of viral RNA in stool.

During the initial phases of the disease, altered intestinal secretion, motility, and permeability contribute to the pathophysiologic mechanism of diarrhea. Later during disease, malabsorption can occur. Rotaviral NSP4, encoded by rotavirus gene 10, is a viral enterotoxin that mediates, at least in part, the early secretory components of the diarrhea. It has also been postulated that viral infection increases intestinal motility by stimulating the enteric nervous system, possibly through NSP4. Whether and to what degree the enterotoxic effect of NSP4 is clinically relevant in children or other animal species remains to be determined. Infected individuals have a short period of viremia, but its clinical consequences are unclear other than correlating with the level of fever. However, most rotavirus-infected children have mild elevations in hepatic enzymes, thereby suggesting that low-level hepatitis is a common occurrence.

Rotavirus serum IgA levels measured shortly after natural infection in children generally correlate with intestinal IgA levels and appear to also correlate with protection. One explanation for recurrent rotavirus (and norovirus) infections is that protection from reinfection is mediated by intestinal IgA, which is not long-lasting in humans. Another explanation is that protection is dependent on neutralizing antibodies to one or both highly variable outer-capsid rotaviral proteins. However, a monovalent P[8]G1 vaccine induces significant protection against strains with different serotypes, thereby supporting the conclusion that protective immunity to rotavirus infection is, in large part, heterotypic. Recently an analysis of human monoclonal antibodies directed at either VP4 or VP7 demonstrated that heterotypic immunity to these proteins was, in fact, quite common.[8]

CLINICAL MANIFESTATIONS

Norovirus

The clinical manifestations of norovirus infection are variable and depend in part on the age of the individual infected. About one third of infections are asymptomatic, but symptoms include diarrhea, nausea, vomiting, abdominal cramps, fever, and malaise that generally persist for 1 to 3 days. In children younger than 11 years, disease typically begins with the sudden onset of vomiting and can last 4 to 6 days. Virus can be shed in low titers for up to 8 weeks from otherwise healthy individuals and for more than a year in patients with severe immunodeficiency syndromes. In neonates and premature infants, vomiting often is not a symptom, and infection has been associated with necrotizing enterocolitis. To support the diagnosis of norovirus outbreaks, the following four criteria have been proposed: (1) vomiting in more than half of affected persons; (2) mean (or median) incubation period of 24 to 48 hours; (3) mean (or median) duration of illness of 12 to 60 hours; and (4) absence of bacterial pathogens in stool culture.

Rotavirus

Rotavirus diarrhea and dehydration tend to be more severe than illness caused by the other childhood enteric pathogens. Rotavirus diarrhea is watery, persists for approximately 5 days, is often preceded by the sudden onset of vomiting, and is frequently accompanied by fever and dehydration. The incubation period of rotavirus is estimated to be less than 48 hours. Viral excretion in feces persists for 10 days in most children and can persist for up to 57 days. Excretion times are longer on examination by sensitive PCR-based assays rather than solid-phase immunoassay. By the age of 5 years in an unvaccinated setting, virtually all children have naturally acquired immunity to rotavirus, and very severe disease after this age is uncommon.

DIAGNOSIS

Norovirus

Reverse transcription–PCR (RT-PCR) is currently the procedure of choice to detect norovirus in clinical specimens, in food, and in water. Although enzyme-linked immunosorbent assays (ELISAs) to detect noroviruses are available in Europe, their sensitivity is genotype dependent, and diagnostic specificity and sensitivity vary based on the diversity of the circulating strains in the population. Moreover, these immunoassays are not easily adaptable for detection of new strains. Norovirus RNA is detected by RT-PCR in stool samples of up to 16% of healthy individuals, a finding that complicates the diagnosis of norovirus gastroenteritis. Although the relationship between disease symptoms and viral load has not been fully established, a quantitative real-time RT-PCR has been proposed to establish a relative threshold of positivity for attributing disease to norovirus.

Rotavirus

Before the introduction of the rotavirus vaccine in developed countries, well above 50% of the moderate to severe diarrheal episodes in young children during the rotavirus "season" were due to rotavirus. In tropical countries, the presence of other enteric pathogens and the absence of seasonal occurrence of rotaviral disease make it more difficult to determine which diarrheal episodes are caused by rotavirus without a diagnostic assay. Numerous ELISAs for rotavirus are commercially available, and these are generally sensitive, specific, and easy to use under most conditions. PCR has increased sensitivity for detection of rotavirus and has permitted easy typing of viruses. With PCR-based methods, however, up to 29% of healthy children younger than 1 year may be rotavirus positive, so it is difficult to associate the detection of the virus RNA with gastroenteritis. Thus ELISA or quantitative RT-PCR (using a threshold level as for norovirus) is preferable for diagnosis of rotavirus gastroenteritis.

PREVENTION

Norovirus

The development of a norovirus vaccine for humans is likely to be a challenge owing to the antigenic heterogeneity among circulating strains, the propensity of noroviruses to undergo antigenic drift, waning immunity, and the lack of well-established correlates of protection.[9] Nevertheless, a new VLP-based vaccine candidate has recently shown promising efficacy in the experimental viral challenge setting.[A1]

High percentage alcohol-based sanitizers (99.5% ethanol) and 10% povidone-iodine antiseptics are superior to other alcohol-based sanitizers at reducing norovirus contamination. Simple household antimicrobial hand soap and handwashing with tap water also decrease viral contamination.

Rotavirus

The first vaccine (RotaShield [Wyeth-Lederle]), which was a quadrivalent mixture of rhesus-human rotavirus reassortants, each containing a G protein from a common human rotavirus serotype, was licensed for use in the United States but subsequently withdrawn from the market because of its association with intussusception. Subsequently, two second-generation vaccines were shown in large studies to be safe, effective, and cost-effective in developed

and developing countries. These two current rotavirus vaccines have been based on two different approaches. One type of vaccine (RV5, RotaTeq [Merck]) uses a modified pentavalent vaccine made of a mixture of bovine and human reassortant rotaviruses. Another approach (RV1, Rotarix [GlaxoSmithKline]) is a monovalent attenuated human virus vaccine. Neither type of vaccine prevents subsequent rotavirus infection or mild illness, but both types effectively prevent severe illness, especially in developed countries.

Protection rates in developed and middle-income countries for these two rotavirus vaccines are very similar,[10] varying from 70 to 80% against any rotavirus disease and 90 to 100% against severe gastroenteritis. In resource-poor settings, vaccination can safely and successfully be accomplished in neonates.[A2] Although both licensed vaccines may slightly increase the risk of intussusception,[11] their persistent benefits[12] far outweigh this low-level risk. Even in the United States, where the burden of severe disease from rotavirus is lowest, the rotavirus vaccine has significantly reduced health care utilization and expenses for diarrhea in children.

In the United States vaccination also has had an unexpected effect on rotavirus-induced diarrhea among unvaccinated persons, thereby suggesting the induction of herd immunity. The U.S. Advisory Committee on Immunization Practices (Chapter 15) and the World Health Organization now recommend the routine use of these vaccines.

Currently several other rotavirus vaccine formulations are becoming available, mostly to reduce costs, but like current vaccines are only about 50% efficacious against severe diseases in the poorest developing countries.[A3] Even with this reduced effectiveness, however, the two licensed vaccines are still cost-effective in the less developed world.

TREATMENT　

Because both norovirus and rotavirus disease resolves within days without treatment, the basic therapeutic goal is to prevent acute dehydration. The recommended oral rehydration salts solution, which now has an osmolarity of 331 mmol/L, is as effective as higher osmolarity solutions. After rehydration, rapid age-appropriate refeeding is recommended. Rotavirus disease induces self-limited intestinal lactase deficiency, but lactose-containing products, particularly maternal milk, should not be withheld.

Passive oral immunotherapy with diverse preparations of immunoglobulins can shorten the duration of rotavirus infection but probably is economically feasible only for immunodeficient patients or low-birthweight infants in the developed world. Recently in Bangladesh, a llama-derived, heavy-chain antibody fragment specific for rotavirus was able to reduce stool output in male infants with severe rotavirus-associated diarrhea.[A4] *Lactobacillus,* a bacterium present in yogurt, is safe and, in limited studies, appears moderately effective for treatment of acute rotavirus gastroenteritis. Nonetheless, different preparations of lactobacilli vary greatly in dose of bacteria, and a general recommendation on their use has not been issued. Several studies in developing countries have shown that zinc supplementation (10 mg/day for infants younger than 6 months and 20 mg/day for older children) is useful for the treatment and prevention of diarrhea, but further studies are needed to determine whether treatment will be useful in all developing and developed countries.

At present, no pharmacologic treatment of rotavirus or norovirus diarrhea is recommended. Racecadotril (4.5 mg/kg per day), an enkephalinase inhibitor that acts on the enteric nervous system, has been shown to be useful as an adjunct to treat rotaviral diarrhea in some but not all studies. Ondansetron (0.15 mg/kg per day), a serotonin antagonist, is effective in reducing the emesis from gastroenteritis during the phase of oral rehydration.[A5] In several small studies, nitazoxanide (15 mg/kg per day) was helpful in the treatment of rotavirus gastroenteritis.[A6] More studies are needed before any of these various preparations can be generally recommended for treatment of rotavirus diarrhea.

Grade A References

A1. Leroux-Roels G, Cramer JP, Mendelman PM, et al. Safety and immunogenicity of different formulations of norovirus vaccine candidate in healthy adults: a randomized, controlled, double-blind clinical trial. *J Infect Dis.* 2018;217:597-607.

A2. Bines JE, At Thobari J, Satria CD, et al. Human neonatal rotavirus vaccine (RV3-BB) to target rotavirus from birth. *N Engl J Med.* 2018;378:719-730.

A3. Isanaka S, Guindo O, Langendorf C, et al. Efficacy of a low-cost, heat-stable oral rotavirus vaccine in Niger. *N Engl J Med.* 2017;376:1121-1130.

A4. Sarker SA, Jakel M, Sultana S, et al. Anti-rotavirus protein reduces stool output in infants with diarrhea: a randomized placebo-controlled trial. *Gastroenterology.* 2013;145:740-748.

A5. Marchetti F, Bonati M, Maestro A, et al. Oral ondansetron versus domperidone for acute gastroenteritis in pediatric emergency departments: multicenter double blind randomized controlled trial. *PLoS ONE.* 2016;11:1-15.

A6. Mahapatro S, Mahilary N, Satapathy AK, et al. Nitazoxanide in acute rotavirus diarrhea: a randomized control trial from a developing country. *J Trop Med.* 2017;2017:1-5.

GENERAL REFERENCES

For the General References and other additional features, please visit Expert Consult at https://expertconsult.inkling.com.

357

VIRAL HEMORRHAGIC FEVERS

DANIEL G. BAUSCH

DEFINITION

Viral hemorrhagic fever is an acute systemic illness classically involving fever, a constellation of initially nonspecific signs and symptoms, and a propensity for bleeding and shock. It may be caused by more than 30 different viruses from four taxonomic families, Filoviridae, Arenaviridae, Bunyaviridae, and Flaviviridae (Table 357-1),[1] although not every virus in these families causes the syndrome. All are single-stranded lipid-enveloped RNA viruses with small genomes (10 to 19 kilobases) that can be relatively easily inactivated in the environment. Virtually all hemorrhagic fever viruses are zoonotic, maintained in nature by a variety of mammalian reservoirs, usually with a tight pairing between the virus and the specific reservoir species. Depending upon the virus, primary transmission to humans may be from contact with infected animal excreta or the bite of an arthropod vector. Transmissibility between humans and pathogenicity vary with the specific virus and sometimes even among strains of the same virus. Many of the hemorrhagic fever viruses are considered potential bioterrorist threats (Chapter 18).

EPIDEMIOLOGY

Maintenance in Nature and Transmission to Humans

With the exception of dengue virus, for which humans can now be considered the reservoir, hemorrhagic fever viruses are zoonotic, maintained in nature in mammalian reservoirs (see Table 357-1). Although viral hemorrhagic fevers collectively can be found worldwide, the endemic area of any given hemorrhagic fever virus is usually smaller than the extent of its natural reservoir or arthropod vector. With the exception of dengue and some hantaviruses, human infection is generally infrequent. Humans are dead-end hosts.

Hemorrhagic fever viruses may be transmitted to humans by usually inadvertent, direct exposure of mucous membranes or broken skin to the infected blood or excreta of its animal reservoir or, in the case of the flaviviruses and most of the bunyaviruses, by the bite of an arthropod vector. The infectious dose for most hemorrhagic fever viruses appears to be low, sometimes on the order of just a few virions. Aerosol transmission is not a predominant mode of spread, if it occurs at all, but studies in nonhuman primates show that transmission of many hemorrhagic fever viruses is possible through artificially created aerosols, thereby raising the possibility of their potential use as bioweapons (Chapter 18).

Bat-Borne Viruses

The filoviruses (from the Latin *filo,* "thread," referring to their filamentous shape), Marburg and Ebola, are perhaps the most feared of all hemorrhagic fever viruses.[2] Fruit bats appear to be the filovirus reservoir, with transmission to humans likely from exposure to infected bat excreta or saliva. Nonhuman primates, especially gorillas and chimpanzees, and other wild animals may become infected, presumably from similar bat exposure, and transmit filoviruses to humans through contact with blood and body fluids of these animals, usually in association with hunting. Nonhuman primates, which are also dead-end hosts who develop severe and usually fatal disease similar to that seen in humans, may be easier prey for hunters when sick. Because hemorrhagic fever viruses are rapidly inactivated by heating, infection probably occurs by exposure during butchering and preparation, rather than by consumption of cooked meat. In the Philippines, Ebola Reston virus has been isolated from pigs that were presumably infected from exposure to bats. The 2013 to 2016 outbreak of Ebola virus disease in West Africa dwarfed all prior Ebola outbreaks combined, with a reported 28,616 cases and 11,310 deaths, but a 2018 to 2019 outbreak in northeastern Democratic Republic of the Congo has resulted in more than 1500 reported cases and over 1000 deaths.[3]

Rodent-Borne Viruses

Arenaviruses (from the Latin *arena,* "sand," referring to their sandy appearance on electron microscopy) are divided into Old World (or lymphocytic choriomeningitis/Lassa) and New World (or Tacaribe) complexes.[4] Lassa virus and Lujo virus are found in Africa, whereas Junín, Machupo, Guanarito, Sabiá, and Chapare viruses are found in South America. Although there may be subtle differences among the syndromes produced by the New World arenaviruses, they are usually grouped together simply as the South American hemorrhagic fevers.

The genus Hantavirus of the Bunyaviridae family is similarly divided into Old and New World complexes. The Old World hantaviruses, such as Hantaan, Seoul, and Puumala, among many others, cause hemorrhagic fevers with prominent renal involvement across Europe and Asia. New World hantaviruses, such as Sin Nombre and Andes, among many others, cause a viral hemorrhagic fever named hantavirus pulmonary syndrome, sometimes also called hantavirus cardiopulmonary syndrome to emphasize the significant cardiogenic component of this disease.

Pathogenic arenaviruses and hantaviruses are maintained in nature through chronic asymptomatic infection in rodents of the Muridae family, with a strict pairing between the specific virus and rodent species. Transmission between rodents may be by vertical or horizontal transmission or both, depending on the specific virus. Transmission to humans occurs through exposure to rodent excreta, either from aerosols produced when rodents urinate or by direct inoculation to the mucous membranes, although the precise modes of transmission remain to be elucidated. Secondary aerosol generation is notoriously inefficient, so disturbing shed urine is a less likely mechanism of infection. In West Africa, Lassa virus is sometimes contracted when rodents are trapped and prepared for consumption or, more rarely, through a rodent bite. Experimental data suggest that humans may be infected with arenaviruses by the oral route. Lassa virus transmission[5] seems to be increasing across West Africa, with epidemic-level spread in Nigeria in 2018 and 2019.

The rodents that transmit Lassa, Machupo, and many of the Old World hantaviruses commonly invade the peridomestic environment, thereby putting housewives, children, and others who spend time at home at risk. In contrast, the reservoirs for Junín, Guanarito, and most of the New World hantaviruses typically inhabit agricultural fields, wood lots, or other rural habitats, thereby putting outdoor workers, campers, and hikers at risk.

Mosquito-Borne Viruses

Rift Valley fever virus is maintained in domestic livestock, such as cattle, buffalo, sheep, goats, and camels, in which it often provokes spontaneous abortion. The virus may be transmitted to humans by direct exposure to these animals, especially during parturition, or by mosquitoes. Farmers, abattoir workers, and veterinarians are at particular risk.[6]

Yellow fever virus is maintained in a cycle between monkeys and forest canopy mosquitoes. Sporadic cases occur when humans are bitten by these mosquitoes. Larger outbreaks occur when humans bring the virus back to more settled environments, where the urban mosquito *Aedes aegypti* can spread the virus directly between humans. *Ae. aegypti*, which typically lay eggs in artificial containers around the home and bite during the day, become infective a few weeks after feeding on a viremic monkey or human. A yellow fever outbreak in Angola and the Democratic Republic of the Congo in 2016,[7] and increased transmission in Latin America in 2017 to 2018, especially in Brazil, resulted in thousands of cases and prompted mass vaccination campaigns of millions of people.

Although nonhuman primates are also a reservoir for sylvatic strains of dengue, the virus is now adapted and maintained in humans, with a regular transmission cycle akin to that of urban yellow fever. Despite the presence of dengue virus in the tropics worldwide, less than 10% of infected persons develop hemorrhagic fever, primarily children between the ages of 4 and 12 years.

Tick-Borne Viruses

The viruses that cause Crimean-Congo hemorrhagic fever,[8] Omsk hemorrhagic fever, Kyasanur Forest disease, and Alkhumra hemorrhagic fever are maintained

TABLE 357-1   PRINCIPAL VIRUSES CAUSING HEMORRHAGIC FEVER

VIRUS	DISEASE	GEOGRAPHIC DISTRIBUTION OF DISEASE	PRINCIPAL RESERVOIR/VECTOR	ANNUAL ESTIMATED CASES	CASE-TO-INFECTION RATIO	HUMAN-TO-HUMAN TRANSMISSIBILITY
FILOVIRIDAE*						
Ebolavirus†	Ebola virus disease†	Sub-Saharan Africa	Fruit bat?	—†	1:1	High
Marburgvirus	Marburg virus disease†	Sub-Saharan Africa	Fruit bat: Egyptian fruit bat (*Rousettus aegyptiacus*), perhaps others	—†	1:1	High
ARENAVIRIDAE§‖						
Old World Group						
Lassa	Lassa fever	West Africa	Rodent: Natal mastomys or multimammate rat (*Mastomys natalensis*)	50,000-100,000	1:5-10	Moderate
Lujo§	Lujo HF	Zambia	Unknown, presumed rodent	Unknown	Unknown	Moderate to high
New World Group						
Junín	Argentine HF	Argentine pampas	Rodent: corn mouse (*Calomys musculinus*)	≈100	1:1.5	Low
Machupo	Bolivian HF	Beni department, Bolivia	Rodent: large vesper mouse (*Calomys callosus*)	≤50	1:1.5	Low
Guanarito	Venezuelan HF	Portuguesa state, Venezuela	Rodent: cane mouse (*Zygodontomys brevicauda*)	≤50	1:1.5	Low
Sabiá**	Proposed name: Brazilian HF	Rural area near São Paulo, Brazil?	Unknown, presumed rodent	Unknown	1:1.5	Low?
Chapare††	Chapare HF	Cochabamba, Bolivia	Unknown, presumed rodent	Unknown	Unknown	Unknown
BUNYAVIRIDAE§						
Old World Group						
Hantaan, Seoul, Puumala, Dobrava-Belgrade, others	HF with renal syndrome	Hantaan: northeast Asia Seoul: urban areas worldwide Puumala and Dobrava-Belgrade: Europe	Rodent Hantaan: striped field mouse (*Apodemus agrarius*) Seoul: brown or Norway rat (*Rattus norvegicus*) Puumala: bank vole (*Clethrionomys glareolus*) Dobrava-Belgrade: yellow-necked field mouse (*Apodemus flavicollis*)	50,000-150,000	Hantaan: 1:1.5 Others: 1:20	None

New World Group

Disease	Distribution	Source/Vector	Estimated cases/yr	Ratio	Nosocomial transmission
Sin Nombre, Andes, Laguna Negra, others Hantavirus pulmonary syndrome	Americas	Rodent Sin Nombre: deer mouse (*Peromyscus maniculatus*) Andes: long-tailed colilargo (*Oligoryzomys longicaudatus*) Laguna Negra: little laucha or small vesper mouse (*Calomys laucha*)	50,000-150,000	Sin Nombre: 1:1 Others: up to 1:20	None, except for Andes virus
Rift Valley fever	Sub-Saharan Africa, Madagascar, Saudi Arabia, Yemen	Domestic livestock/mosquitoes (sylvatic *Aedes* and others)	100-100,000[‡,‡‡]	1:100	None
Crimean-Congo HF	Africa, Balkans, southern Russia, Middle East, India, Pakistan, Afghanistan, western China	Wild and domestic vertebrates/tick (primarily *Hyalomma* species)	≈500	1:1-2	High
FLAVIVIRIDAE					
Yellow fever	Sub-Saharan Africa, South America up to Panama	Monkey/mosquito (*Aedes aegypti*, other *Aedes* and *Haemagogus* species)	5,000-200,000[§§]	1:2-20	None
Dengue	Tropics and subtropics worldwide	Human/mosquito (*Ae. aegypti* and *albopictus*)	100,000-200,000,000[§§]	1:10-100, depending on age, previous infection, genetic background, and infecting serotype	None
Omsk HF	Western Siberia	Rodent/tick (primarily *Dermacentor* and *Ixodes* species)	100-200	Unknown	Not reported
Kyasanur Forest disease	Karnataka state, India; Yunnan Province, China; Saudi Arabia	Vertebrate (rodents, bats, birds, monkeys, others)/tick (*Haemaphysalis* species and others)	≈500	Unknown	Not reported, but laboratory infections have occurred
Proposed name: Alkhumra HF[||||]	Saudi Arabia, Egypt	Ticks?	≤50	Unknown	Not reported

*Five species or subtypes of Ebolavirus are recognized with varying associated case-fatality ratios (see Table 357-2). All are endemic to sub-Saharan Africa, with the exceptions of Reston ebolavirus, which is found in the Philippines.

†Increasing recognition that hemorrhage is seen a minority of patients with filovirus infection has prompted preference for the terms "Ebola/Marburg virus disease" rather than "Ebola/Marburg hemorrhagic fever."

‡Although some endemic transmission of the filoviruses (Ebolavirus > Marburgvirus) and Rift Valley fever virus occurs, these viruses have most often been associated with outbreaks.

§The virus families Arenaviridae and Bunyaviridae are serologically, phylogenetically, and geographically divided into Old World (i.e., Africa and Asia) and New World (i.e., the Americas) complexes.

||In addition to the arenaviruses listed in the table, Flexal and Tacaribe viruses have caused human disease as a result of laboratory accidents. Another arenavirus, Whitewater Arroyo, has been noted in sick persons in California, but its role as a pathogen has not been clearly established.

¶Only five cases (four of them fatal) from one outbreak in 2008 have been noted. The index case came to South Africa from Zambia.

**Only three cases (one fatal) have been noted, two of them from laboratory accidents.

††Discovered and recognized to date only from a small outbreak in 2003 from which blood was obtained from one fatal case and Chapare virus isolated. Few other details have been reported.

‡‡Although Rift Valley fever virus can be found throughout sub-Saharan Africa, large outbreaks usually occur in East Africa's Rift Valley region.

§§Based on estimates from the World Health Organization. Significant underreporting occurs. Incidence may fluctuate widely in place and time.

||||Alkhumra is considered by some to be a variant of Kyasanur Forest disease virus. Disagreement exists over the proper spelling of the virus, written as Alkhurma in some publications.

HF = hemorrhagic fever.

in small mammals, such as rodents, hares, and hedgehogs, among which the viruses are spread by ticks. Humans are infected either by tick bites or by exposure to contaminated blood or excreta of the reservoir animals. Ticks also spread Crimean-Congo hemorrhagic fever virus to large mammals, including cattle and other domestic livestock, whose transient and asymptomatic viremia puts farmers, abattoir workers, and veterinarians at risk.

Human-to-Human Transmission

Secondary human-to-human transmission occurs with many of the hemorrhagic fever viruses (see Table 357-1). Secondary attack rates for hemorrhagic fever viruses are generally low (less than 15% for Ebola Zaire virus),[9] probably because transmission between humans requires direct contact with contaminated blood or body fluids. However, as evidenced by the 2013 to 2016 events in West Africa, the risk of transmission can increase significantly in large outbreaks when many sick patients overwhelm fragile health systems and infection prevention and control measures break down, especially when health care workers are insufficiently trained and equipped.[10] Human-to-human infection probably usually occurs through oral or mucous membrane exposure, most often in the context of providing care to a sick family member (community) or patient (nosocomial transmission). Funeral rituals that entail the touching of the corpse were a major source of infection during the West Africa Ebola virus outbreak. Infection through fomites cannot be excluded. In some cases, highly infectious "super spreaders" have been suspected, but there is no evidence for natural aerosol transmission between humans. Despite modern-day travel, imported cases of viral hemorrhagic fever remain rare and usually do not result in secondary transmission because of the more routinely maintained infection prevention and control practices in resource-rich countries.

With the exception of hantaviruses and some of the flaviviruses, infectivity parallels the clinical state. Persons are most infectious late in the course of severe disease, when viral loads are high and patients shed virus into the environment through vomiting, diarrhea, and bleeding. The risk of transmission during the incubation period or from asymptomatic persons is negligible, although a case of Argentine hemorrhagic fever occurred from blood transfusion from an asymptomatic donor.

PATHOBIOLOGY

Microvascular instability and impaired hemostasis are the pathobiologic hallmarks of viral hemorrhagic fever. With the exception of disease caused by the hantaviruses and some of the flaviviruses, the pathogenesis of viral hemorrhagic fever appears to be related to unchecked viremia, with most fatal cases failing to mount a significant antibody response. By comparison, infectious virus is cleared rapidly from the blood in survivors. In dengue, yellow fever, and hantavirus infections, in which viremia is usually cleared before the most severe phase of the disease, the host immune response may play a detrimental role. The unique process of antibody-mediated immune enhancement,[11] in which secondary infection with a different dengue virus serotype is more severe than the primary one, may play a role in the pathogenesis of dengue hemorrhagic fever. Data from animal models suggest that cardiac inotropy may also be directly or indirectly inhibited in some viral hemorrhagic fevers, especially Lassa fever.

After inoculation, virus first replicates in dendritic cells and other local tissues, with subsequent migration to regional lymph nodes and then dissemination through the lymph and blood monocytes to a broad range of tissues and organs, including the liver, spleen, lymph nodes, adrenal glands, lungs, and endothelium. Migration of tissue macrophages results in secondary infection of permissive parenchymal cells. During the acute illness, virus can be found in a wide variety of body fluids, including blood, saliva, stool, and breast milk.

The interaction of virus with immune cells, especially macrophages and endothelial cells, results directly or indirectly (through soluble mediators) in cell activation and the unleashing of an inflammatory and vasoactive process consistent with the systemic inflammatory response syndrome. The synthesis of cell surface tissue factor triggers the extrinsic coagulation pathway. Impaired hemostasis may entail endothelial cell, platelet, or coagulation factor dysfunction. Disseminated intravascular coagulopathy (DIC) is frequently noted, especially with Ebola, Marburg, and Crimean-Congo hemorrhagic fever viruses.

Inflammatory cell infiltrates, which are usually mild, consist of a mix of mononuclear cells and neutrophils. In some viral hemorrhagic fevers, such as Ebola, virus replication and dissemination are facilitated by virus-induced suppression of the host adaptive immune response. Failure of the immune response to adequately respond appears to be a major determinant of severity in Lassa fever.

Tissue damage may be mediated through direct necrosis of infected cells or indirectly through apoptosis of immune cells, as seen in other forms of septic shock. The most affected organs vary with the virus (Table 357-2). For example, renal tubular necrosis and retroperitoneal edema are seen in hemorrhagic fevers with renal syndrome, whereas interstitial pneumonitis and myocardial depression are the hallmarks of hantavirus pulmonary syndrome. The liver is particularly affected in yellow fever, with fatty degeneration, coagulative midzonal necrosis of hepatocytes, and the presence of Councilman bodies. The brain and meninges are particularly affected in Kyasanur Forest disease and Omsk hemorrhagic fever and often in the South American hemorrhagic fevers as well. Reticuloendothelial proliferation is seen in Kyasanur Forest disease, with marked erythrophagocytosis in the spleen.

CLINICAL MANIFESTATIONS

Viral hemorrhagic fever is seen in both genders and all age groups, with a spectrum from relatively mild or even asymptomatic infection to severe vascular permeability resulting in shock, multiorgan system failure, and death. Although the clinical presentation may differ for each viral hemorrhagic fever as disease progresses, the limited data do not permit clear distinctions in most cases, especially in the early phases of disease. Dengue and Rift Valley fever viruses cause a range of syndromes, including rash and central nervous system involvement (Chapters 358 and 359). Hemorrhagic fever occurs in a minority of infections with these viruses. After an incubation period ranging from days to weeks, most patients present with nonspecific signs and symptoms difficult to distinguish from a host of other febrile illnesses (see Table 357-2),[12] including fever, general malaise, anorexia, headache, chest or retrosternal pain, sore throat, myalgia, arthralgia, and lumbosacral pain. Conjunctival injection or hemorrhage is frequent but is not accompanied by itching, discharge, or rhinitis (Fig. 357-1). Relative bradycardia (Faget sign) and orthostatic hypotension may be noted, especially in yellow fever and dengue virus infections. The pharynx may be erythemic or, less frequently, exudative, especially in Lassa fever, and incorrectly lead to a diagnosis of streptococcal pharyngitis or mononucleosis. Hiccups are often seen in Ebola virus disease, although the pathogenesis of this manifestation is unclear.

After the first few days, gastrointestinal signs and symptoms readily ensue, including nausea, vomiting, epigastric and abdominal pain, abdominal tenderness, and nonbloody diarrhea or constipation. A misdiagnosis of appendicitis or other acute abdominal emergency (Chapter 133) sometimes prompts potentially hazardous surgical interventions.

Neck pain and stiffness, retro-orbital pain, photophobia, and other meningeal signs are common in Rift Valley fever, Kyasanur Forest disease, and Omsk hemorrhagic fever. A dry cough, sometimes accompanied by a few scattered rales on auscultation, is common, but prominent pulmonary symptoms are uncommon early in the course of the disease, except with hantavirus pulmonary syndrome. With the exception of yellow fever, jaundice is not typical except in patients with underlying Gilbert syndrome, drug reactions, or coinfection. Hepatosplenomegaly is frequent, but whether it is specific to the viral hemorrhagic fever or simply represents the high underlying prevalence of hepatosplenomegaly in populations in sub-Saharan Africa is unknown.

Various forms of rash, including morbilliform, maculopapular, petechial, and ecchymotic, may be seen (see Table 357-2). A maculopapular rash on the torso or face may be one early and relatively specific but insensitive indicator of Ebola or Marburg virus disease. Rash almost always occurs in fair-skinned persons with Lassa fever but, for unclear reasons, rarely in blacks.

In severe cases, patients progress after 7 to 10 days of illness to vascular instability, which may be manifested by conjunctival injection and hemorrhage, facial flushing, edema, bleeding, hypotension, shock, and proteinuria. Facial swelling and neck swelling are classic and relatively specific signs of Lassa fever and Lujo hemorrhagic fever. The likelihood of clinically discernible hemorrhage varies with the infecting virus (see Table 357-2) and may be manifested as hematemesis, melena, hematochezia, metrorrhagia, petechiae, purpura, epistaxis, and bleeding from the gums and venipuncture sites (Fig. 357-2). Hemoptysis and hematuria are infrequent. Hemorrhage is almost never present in the first few days of illness. Large ecchymoses are characteristic of Crimean-Congo hemorrhagic fever. Central nervous system manifestations, including delirium, tremor, gait anomalies, convulsions, and hiccups, may be noted in end-stage disease, especially in Kyasanur Forest disease, Omsk hemorrhagic fever, and the South American hemorrhagic fevers, particularly Argentine hemorrhagic fever. Nevertheless, the cerebrospinal fluid findings are usually normal, with the exception of patients who have meningoencephalitis

TABLE 357-2 PATHOBIOLOGIC AND CLINICAL ASPECTS OF VIRAL HEMORRHAGIC FEVERS

DISEASE	INCUBATION PERIOD (DAYS)	ONSET	BLEEDING	RASH	JAUNDICE	HEART	LUNG	KIDNEY	CENTRAL NERVOUS SYSTEM	EYE	CASE-FATALITY RATIO	CLINICAL MANAGEMENT
FILOVIRIDAE												
Ebola virus disease	3-21	Variable	++	+	+	+	+	+	+	++*	40-85%[†]	Supportive
Marburg virus disease	3-21	Abrupt	++	+	+	+	+	+	+	++	22-85%[‡]	Supportive
ARENAVIRIDAE												
Lassa fever	5-16	Gradual	+	+[§]	0	++	+	++	+	0	20%	Ribavirin
Lujo HF	9-13	Abrupt	++	+	0	?	+	+	+	0	80%	Ribavirin
South American HF[‖]	4-14	Gradual	+++	+	0	++	+	0	+++	0	15-40%	Ribavirin, convalescent plasma
BUNYAVIRIDAE												
HF with renal syndrome	9-35	Abrupt	+++	0	0	++	+	+++	+	0	<1-50%, depending on specific virus	Ribavirin
Hantavirus pulmonary syndrome	7-35	Gradual	0 (except for Andes virus infection)	0	0	+++	+++	+	+	0	<1-50%, depending on specific virus	Supportive, ECMO?
Rift Valley fever[¶]	2-5	Abrupt	++	+	++	+?	0	+	++	++	Up to 50% in severe forms	Ribavirin?
Crimean-Congo HF	1-12**	Abrupt	+++	0	++	+?	+	0	+	0	15-30%	Ribavirin?
FLAVIVIRIDAE												
Yellow fever	3-6	Abrupt	+++	0	+++	++	+	++	++	0	20-50%	Supportive
Dengue HF	3-15	Abrupt	++	+++	+	++	+	0	+	0	Untreated: 10-15% Treated: ≤1%	Supportive
Omsk HF	3-8	Abrupt	++	0	0	+	++	0	+++	+	1-3%	Supportive
Kyasanur forest disease	3-8	Abrupt	++	0	0	+	++	0	+++	+	3-5%	Supportive
Alkhumra HF[††]	3-8	Abrupt	++	+	+	+	+	0	++	+	20-25%	Supportive

*Potentially sight-threatening uveitis, early cataract formation, and other ocular sequelae are noted in up to one third of survivors.

[†]Five species or subtypes of Ebolavirus are recognized with varying associated case-fatality ratios during outbreaks: Zaire, 85%; Sudan, 55%; Bundibugyo, 40%; Tai Forest (also called Côte d'Ivoire), 0% (only one recognized case, who survived); Reston, 0% (not pathogenic to humans).

[‡]The case-fatality ratio was 22% in the first recognized outbreak of Marburg virus disease in Germany and Yugoslavia in 1967 but has been consistently above 80% in outbreaks in central Africa, where the virus is endemic. Possible reasons for this discrepancy include differences in quality of care, strain pathogenicity, route and dose of infection, underlying prevalence of immunodeficiency and comorbid illnesses, and genetic susceptibility.

[§]A morbilliform or maculopapular rash almost always occurs in persons with lighter skin, who are usually expatriates, but for unclear reasons is rarely present in darker-skinned Africans from the endemic area.

[‖]Data are insufficient to distinguish between the syndromes produced by the various arenaviruses found in the Americas. They are thus frequently grouped as the South American hemorrhagic fevers.

[¶]Hemorrhagic fever, encephalitis, and retinitis may be seen in Rift Valley fever independently of each other.

**The incubation period of Crimean-Congo HF varies with the mode of transmission: typically 1 to 3 days after tick bite and 5 to 6 days after contact with infected animal blood or tissues.

[††]Based on preliminary observations. Fewer than 100 cases have been reported.

ECMO = extracorporeal membrane oxygenation; HF = hemorrhagic fever; 0 = sign not typically noted/organ not typically affected; + = sign occasionally noted/organ occasionally affected; ++ = sign commonly noted/organ commonly affected; +++ = sign characteristic/organ involvement severe.

due to Kyasanur Forest disease and Omsk hemorrhagic fever, in which an elevated protein level is common. Renal insufficiency or failure is common, especially in hemorrhagic fever with renal syndrome and in Lassa fever, and it is associated with a poor prognosis.

Biphasic illnesses are classically noted for the flavivirus hemorrhagic fevers, in which a quiescent period of days (yellow fever, dengue hemorrhagic fever, and Rift Valley fever) to weeks (Kyasanur Forest disease and Omsk hemorrhagic fever) precedes the most severe manifestations, including hemorrhage, shock, renal failure, and meningoencephalitis. Distinct progressive phases of disease and recovery are classically described for hemorrhagic fever with renal syndrome (prodrome, hypotension, oliguria/renal failure, diuresis, and convalescence) and yellow fever (infection, intoxication, recovery) but are not seen in all cases. The initial manifestations for hantavirus pulmonary syndrome may be mild and nonspecific, but the disease may progress to require mechanical ventilation and pressor support within 24 hours; sinus bradycardia and ventricular tachycardia or fibrillation may occur. Encephalitis and retinitis may develop in Rift Valley fever independently of the presence or absence of viral hemorrhagic fever.

Bilateral noncardiogenic interstitial pulmonary edema consistent with the adult respiratory distress syndrome (ARDS) is the hallmark of hantavirus pulmonary syndrome, although chest radiographs may be normal early in the disease even when the patients complain of shortness of breath. Only about 30% of patients with hantavirus pulmonary syndrome have radiographic evidence of pulmonary edema on initial evaluation, although it develops in virtually all persons within 48 hours.

Pregnant women with viral hemorrhagic fever usually present with severe disease, including spontaneous abortion and vaginal bleeding. However, initially mild symptoms that nevertheless progress to severe and even fatal disease have been noted, perhaps because the immune tolerance of pregnancy dampens the initial inflammatory clinical manifestations.

DIAGNOSIS

Because of their associated severity, risk of secondary spread, high degree of public scrutiny, and unfamiliarity to most physicians, consultation with a specialist who has experience with viral hemorrhagic fevers should be sought as soon as the diagnosis is considered. When to "sound the alarm" of viral hemorrhagic fever is a case-by-case decision left to the treating physician in consultation with experts in the field. Most viral hemorrhagic fevers are rare, and routinely practiced universal precautions are protective in most cases, at least in the early phases of disease.

The early nonspecific presentation of viral hemorrhagic fevers makes them extremely difficult to diagnose clinically, especially outside of the setting of a recognized outbreak, which is usually detected when clusters of cases occur, especially when they involve health care workers. The differential diagnosis includes a broad array of febrile illnesses that varies by geographic region (Table 357-3). A complete epidemiologic history (including details of travel,

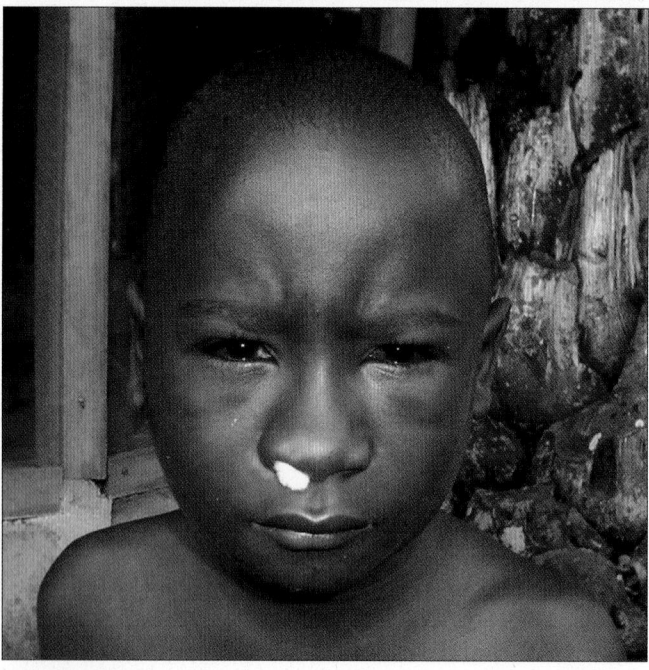

FIGURE 357-1. Subconjunctival hemorrhage and facial swelling in a boy with Lassa fever in Sierra Leone.

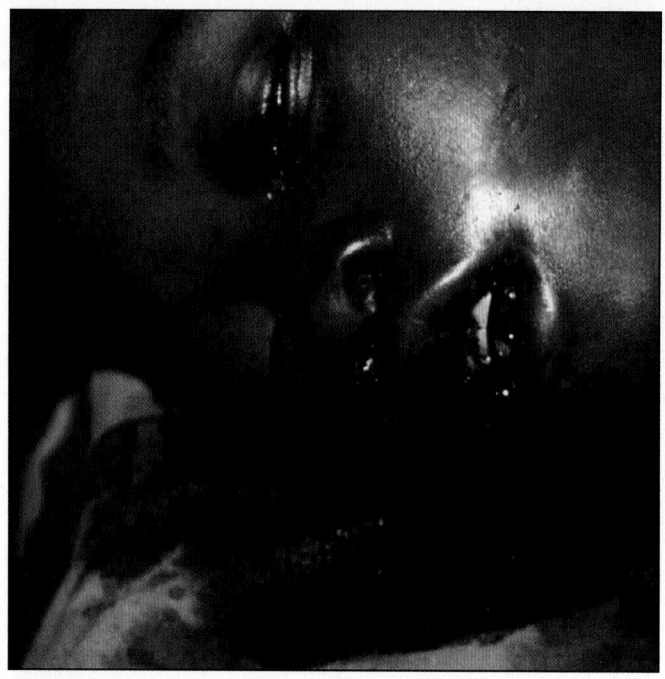

FIGURE 357-2. Bleeding in a patient with Ebola virus disease. (From Bausch DG. Viral hemorrhagic fevers. In: Schlossberg D, ed. *Clinical Infectious Disease*. New York: Cambridge University Press; 2008.)

TABLE 357-3	DIFFERENTIAL DIAGNOSIS OF THE VIRAL HEMORRHAGIC FEVERS
DISEASE	**DISTINGUISHING CHARACTERISTICS AND COMMENTS**
PARASITES	
Malaria	Classically shows paroxysms of fever and chills; hemorrhagic manifestations less common; malaria smears or rapid test result usually positive; coinfection (or baseline asymptomatic parasitemia) common; responds to antimalarials
Amebiasis	Hemorrhagic manifestations other than bloody diarrhea generally not seen; amebic trophozoites identified in the stool by microscopy or antigen assays; responds to antiparasitics
Giardiasis	Positive stool antigen test result or identification of trophozoites or cysts in stool; responds to antiparasitics
African trypanosomiasis (acute stages)	Especially the East African form; examination of peripheral blood smear/buffy coat may show trypanosomes
BACTERIA (INCLUDING SPIROCHETES, RICKETTSIA, EHRLICHIA, AND COXIELLA)	
Typhoid fever	Hemorrhagic manifestations other than bloody diarrhea generally not seen; responds to antibiotics
Bacillary dysentery (including shigellosis, campylobacteriosis, salmonellosis, and enterohemorrhagic *Escherichia coli* and others)	Hemorrhagic manifestations other than bloody diarrhea generally not seen; responds to antibiotics
Capnocytophaga canimorsus	Associated with dog and cat bites, typically in persons with underlying immunodeficiency, notably asplenic patients; responds to antibiotics
Meningococcemia	Bacterial-induced DIC may mimic the bleeding diathesis of VHF; bleeding within the first 24-48 hours after onset of illness and rapidly progressive illness typical; large ecchymoses typical of meningococcemia are unusual in the VHFs except for Crimean-Congo HF; rapid serum latex agglutination tests can be used to detect bacterial antigen in meningococcal septicemia; may respond to antibiotics (critical to administer early)
Staphylococcemia	Bacterial-induced DIC may mimic the bleeding diathesis of VHF; may respond to antibiotics
Septic abortion	History of pregnancy and positive pregnancy test
Septicemic or pneumonic plague	Bacterial-induced DIC may mimic the bleeding diathesis of VHF; large ecchymoses typical of plague are unusual in the VHFs except for Crimean-Congo HF; pneumonic plague may mimic hantavirus pulmonary syndrome; may respond to antibiotics
Streptococcal or Epstein-Barr virus pharyngitis	May mimic the exudative pharyngitis sometimes seen in Lassa fever
Tuberculosis	Hemoptysis of advanced pulmonary tuberculosis may suggest VHF, but tuberculosis generally has a much slower disease evolution
Tularemia	Ulceroglandular and pneumonic forms more common; responds to antibiotics
Acute abdominal emergencies	Appendicitis, peritonitis, and bleeding upper gastrointestinal ulcer
Pyelonephritis and post-streptococcal glomerulonephritis	May mimic HF with renal syndrome
Anthrax (inhalation or gastrointestinal)	Prominent pulmonary manifestations and widened mediastinum on chest radiograph in inhalation form; responds to antibiotics
Atypical bacterial pneumonia (*Legionella*, *Mycoplasma*, *Chlamydophila pneumoniae* and *C. psittaci*, others)	May mimic hantavirus pulmonary syndrome; exposure to birds; symptoms often not present until late in the illness in psittacosis; responds to antibiotics

TABLE 357-3 DIFFERENTIAL DIAGNOSIS OF THE VIRAL HEMORRHAGIC FEVERS—cont'd

DISEASE	DISTINGUISHING CHARACTERISTICS AND COMMENTS
Relapsing fever	Recurrent fevers and influenza-like symptoms, with direct neurologic involvement and splenomegaly; spirochetes visible in blood while febrile; responds to antibiotics
Leptospirosis	Jaundice, renal failure, and myocarditis in severe cases; responds to antibiotics
Spotted fever group rickettsiae (including African tick bite fever, boutonneuse fever, Rocky Mountain spotted fever)	Incubation period of 7-10 days after tick bite, compared with 1-3 days in Crimean-Congo HF; necrotic lesions (eschar) typically seen at site of tick bite in some rickettsial diseases, whereas there may be only slight bruising at the bite site in Crimean-Congo HF; rash (if present) of rickettsial infection classically involves palms and soles
Q fever (*Coxiella burnetii*)	Broad spectrum of illness, including hepatitis, pneumonitis, encephalitis, and multisystem disease with bleeding; responds to antibiotics
Ehrlichiosis	Diagnosis by serology and PCR; blood film may be useful; responds to antibiotics
VIRUSES	
Influenza	Prominent respiratory component to clinical presentation; no hemorrhagic manifestations; influenza rapid test result may be positive; may respond to anti-influenza drugs
Arbovirus infection (including dengue and West Nile fever)	Encephalitis unusual but when present may mimic the VHFs with significant neurologic involvement (Kyasanur Forest disease, Omsk HF); usually less severe than VHF; hemorrhage not reported
Viral hepatitis (including hepatitis A, B, and E; Epstein-Barr; and cytomegalovirus)	Jaundice atypical in HF except yellow fever; test results for hepatitis antigens positive; fulminant infection resembling VHF may be seen in persons with underlying immune deficiencies
Herpes simplex or varicella-zoster	Fulminant infection with hepatitis (with or without vesicular rash); elevated transaminases and leukopenia typical; disseminated disease may be noted in otherwise healthy persons; poor response to acyclovir drugs unless recognized early
HIV/AIDS	Seroconversion syndrome or HIV/AIDS with secondary infections, especially septicemia
Measles	Rash may mimic that seen in early stages of some VHFs and may sometimes be hemorrhagic; prominence of coryza and upper respiratory symptoms in measles should help differentiate; vaccine preventable
Rubella	Rash may mimic that seen in early stages of some VHFs; usually a mild disease; vaccine preventable
Hemorrhagic or flat smallpox	Diffuse hemorrhagic or macular lesions; in contrast to the VHFs, the rash may involve the oral mucosa, palms, and soles; smallpox in the wild has been eradicated
Alphavirus infection (including chikungunya and o'nyong-nyong)	Joint pain typically a predominant feature
FUNGI	
Histoplasmosis	Pulmonary disease may mimic hantavirus pulmonary syndrome; recent entry into mines or caves
NONINFECTIOUS ETIOLOGIES	
Heat stroke	History for extreme heat exposure; absence of sweating; bleeding not typical, but DIC may occur
Idiopathic and thrombotic thrombocytopenic purpura (ITP/TTP)	Presentation usually less acute than in VHF; may have prominent neurologic symptoms in TTP; coagulation factors normal and DIC absent; often respond to corticosteroids (ITP) or plasma exchange (TTP)
Acute glaucoma	May mimic the acute ocular manifestations of Rift Valley fever
Hematologic malignant neoplasms (leukemia, lymphoma)	May resemble leukemoid reaction occasionally seen in HF with renal syndrome
Drug sensitivity or overdose	Stevens-Johnson syndrome and anticoagulant (warfarin) overdose
Industrial and agricultural chemical poisoning	Especially anticoagulants, although other symptoms of VHF absent
Hematoxic snake bite envenomation	History of snake bite

DIC = disseminated intravascular coagulopathy; HF = hemorrhagic fever; PCR = polymerase chain reaction; VHF = viral hemorrhagic fever.

possible exposures, and occupational risks), details of the evolution of symptoms, physical examination, and preliminary basic laboratory results (Table 357-4) are critical. A diagnosis of viral hemorrhagic fever should be considered in patients with a clinically compatible syndrome who, within the incubation period for the particular viral hemorrhagic fever in question, (1) reside in or traveled to an endemic area (see Table 357-1); (2) had potential direct contact with blood or body fluids of someone who was ill with an acute viral hemorrhagic fever, such as health care workers, persons caring for family members at home or preparing bodies for burial, and laboratory personnel; (3) had contact with live or recently killed wild animals (especially nonhuman primates) in or recently arriving from an area where a viral hemorrhagic fever is endemic (although direct contact with the animal reservoir is not usually reported even in confirmed cases); (4) worked in a laboratory or animal facility where hemorrhagic fever viruses are handled; or (5) had unprotected sex with a male who recovered from a viral hemorrhagic fever in the last year.

The index of suspicion should be especially high for persons in specific high-risk occupations, including health care workers, abattoir workers, veterinarians, farm workers, hunters, taxidermists, and travelers who have recently returned from endemic areas.[13,14] ARDS (Chapter 96) or other respiratory compromise in a person living in an endemic area for New World hantaviruses should prompt consideration of hantavirus pulmonary syndrome. Risk of tick infection, including physical examination for an eschar, should be assessed if

a tick-borne viral hemorrhagic fever is suspected. However, most viral hemorrhagic fevers are rare even in persons possessing one of the risk factors, so alternative diagnoses should always be aggressively sought, especially malaria and typhoid fever in areas where they are endemic. Acts of bioterrorism (Chapter 18) must be considered if viral hemorrhagic fever is strongly suspected in a patient without any of the aforementioned risk factors, especially if clusters of cases occur. All cases should be immediately reported to local, state, and federal health authorities.

Laboratory Testing

Prompt laboratory confirmation, preferably using polymerase chain reaction (PCR) assays, is imperative.[15] PCR assays generally have sensitivities and specificities greater than 90%. False-negative results may occur when a patient is tested very early in the course of disease when virus levels may still be below the threshold of detection. If viral hemorrhagic fever is still suspected despite a negative test, the patient should be monitored, treated empirically as needed, and, if still ill, retested a few days later when, with the exception of flavivirus infections, the viral load would normally have risen to a detectable level.

Enzyme-linked immunosorbent assays for viral antigen and immunoglobulin M antibody, virus culture, and immunohistochemistry on postmortem tissues also generally have sensitivities and specificities greater than 90%, although serologic diagnosis of flavivirus infection is often complicated by cross-reactions. The sensitivities and specificities of newly developed rapid diagnostic tests

TABLE 357-4 INDICATED CLINICAL LABORATORY TESTS AND CHARACTERISTIC FINDINGS IN PATIENTS WITH VIRAL HEMORRHAGIC FEVER

TEST	CHARACTERISTIC FINDINGS AND COMMENTS
Leukocyte count	Early: moderate leukopenia (except for hantavirus infection, in which early leukocytosis with immunoblasts is classically noted) Later: leukocytosis with left shift; granulocytosis more suggestive of bacterial infection
Hemoglobin and hematocrit	Hemoconcentration (especially noted in hemorrhagic fever with renal syndrome and hantavirus pulmonary syndrome)
Platelet count	Mild to moderate thrombocytopenia
Electrolytes	Sodium, potassium, and acid-base perturbations, depending on fluid balance and stage of disease
BUN/creatinine	Renal failure may occur late in disease
Serum chemistries (AST, ALT, amylase, γ-glutamyltransferase, alkaline phosphatase, creatinine kinase, lactate dehydrogenase, lactate)	Usually increased, especially in severe disease; AST > ALT A lactate level >4 mmol/L (36 mg/dL) may indicate persistent hypoperfusion and sepsis. Lactate dehydrogenase is typically markedly increased in hantavirus pulmonary syndrome
Sedimentation rate	Normal or increased
Blood gas	Metabolic acidosis may be indicative of shock and hypoperfusion
Coagulation studies (PT, PTT, fibrinogen, platelets, D-dimer)	DIC common in Ebola, Marburg, Lujo virus, Crimean-Congo HF, and New World arenavirus infections
Urinalysis	Proteinuria common; hematuria may be occasionally noted. Sediment may show hyaline-granular casts and round cells with cytoplasmic inclusions
Blood culture	Useful early to exclude VHF and later to evaluate for secondary bacterial infection. Blood should be drawn before antibiotic therapy is instituted
Stool culture	Useful to exclude VHF (in favor of hemorrhagic bacillary dysentery)
Thick and thin blood smears	May aid in the diagnosis of blood parasites (malaria and trypanosomes), bacterial sepsis (meningococcus, *Capnocytophaga*, and anthrax), and ehrlichiosis. All negative in VHF unless coinfection
Rapid test, PCR, or other assay for malaria	Negative in VHF unless coinfection with malaria

ALT = alanine aminotransferase; AST = aspartate aminotransferase; BUN = blood urea nitrogen; DIC = disseminated intravascular coagulation; HF = hemorrhagic fever; PCR, polymerase chain reaction; PT = prothrombin time; PTT = partial thromboplastin time; VHF = viral hemorrhagic fever.

are still being evaluated. In the United States, viral hemorrhagic fever testing can be arranged through the Centers for Disease Control and Prevention (phone 470-312-0094; email spather@cdc.gov).

TREATMENT Rx

The rarity of most viral hemorrhagic fevers and their typical occurrence in remote and resource-poor settings make controlled studies on treatment difficult. Treatment guidelines generally follow those recommended for septic shock (Chapter 100). Consensus guidelines for supportive care for Ebola virus include isolation in an intensive care unit where close monitoring and critical supportive care can be provided.[16,17]

Clinical Management Guidelines
Fluid and Electrolyte Management
Severe microvascular instability, often complicated by vomiting, severe and sometimes voluminous diarrhea, and decreased fluid intake, typically requires aggressive fluid replacement and or vasopressor support to prevent shock, while avoiding serious electrolyte imbalances. Although the optimal fluid management strategy is not known, overaggressive and unmonitored rehydration may lead to significant third-spacing and pulmonary edema, especially in hantavirus pulmonary syndrome.

TABLE 357-5 RIBAVIRIN THERAPY FOR VIRAL HEMORRHAGIC FEVER

INDICATION	ROUTE	DOSE*	INTERVAL
Treatment	IV[†]	30 mg/kg (maximum 2 g)[‡]	Loading dose, followed by:
	IV[†]	15 mg/kg (maximum 1 g)[‡]	every 6 hours for 4 days, followed by:
	IV[†]	7.5 mg/kg (maximum 500 mg)[‡]	every 8 hours for 6 days
Prophylaxis	PO	35 mg/kg (maximum 2.5 g)[‡]	Loading dose, followed by:
	PO	15 mg/kg (maximum 1 g)[‡]	every 8 hours for 10 days

*Pharmacokinetic and sensitivity testing for ribavirin has not been extensively performed for each viral hemorrhagic fever. The intravenous dose used is derived from that found efficacious in Lassa fever. Oral ribavirin has also been reported to be efficacious in many viral hemorrhagic fevers, especially for Crimean-Congo hemorrhagic fever, but few controlled data are available. Intravenous administration is strongly suggested whenever possible.
[†]The drug should be diluted in 150 mL of 0.9% saline and infused slowly.
[‡]Reduce the dose in persons known to have significant renal insufficiency (creatinine clearance of less than 50 mL/minute).
IV = intravenous: PO = oral.

Blood Products and Management of Disseminated Intravascular Coagulation
Although bleeding may be profuse in some viral hemorrhagic fevers, especially Crimean-Congo hemorrhagic fever and Ebola and Marburg virus disease, blood products should not be given empirically but only to meet defined clinical and laboratory parameters in the face of clinically significant hemorrhage. Transfusions, preferably with packed red blood cells, should be used to maintain a hemoglobin concentration above 7.0 g/dL while avoiding volume overload, taking into account that chronic anemia due to malaria and malnutrition may be frequent in patients in certain geographic areas. Whole blood is a reasonable alternative if packed cells are not available.

The possibility of DIC (Chapter 166) should be assessed by the relevant laboratory parameters (see Table 357-4), such as D-dimer levels. Platelet transfusions are generally not given to patients with DIC unless serious hemorrhage is present. When given, the platelet count should generally rise by at least $5\text{-}10 \times 10^3/\mu L$ per unit of platelets transfused, although the response may be less if there is ongoing DIC and platelet consumption. Impaired platelet aggregation may promote hemorrhage in some viral hemorrhagic fevers, especially Lassa fever, even when platelet counts are not drastically low. Transfusion of fresh-frozen plasma (FFP) (15 to 20 mL/kg) should be considered when bleeding is present and fibrinogen levels are less than 100 mg/dL. Fibrinogen concentrate (total dose of 2 to 3 g) or cryoprecipitate (1 U/10 kg) may be administered instead of FFP, although FFP has the theoretical advantage of containing all coagulation factors. Vitamin K (10 mg intravenously or orally on 3 consecutive days) may be given, especially if underlying malnutrition or liver disease is suspected. Folic acid has also sometimes been added to prevent the detrimental effect of acute folate deficiency on platelet production, especially in malnourished patients, although the efficacy of this treatment is unknown.

Oxygenation and Ventilation
In the early phases of disease and in the absence of iatrogenic pulmonary edema, most patients can be supported with oxygen administered by nasal cannula or face mask. The exception is hantavirus pulmonary syndrome, for which early endotracheal intubation and mechanical ventilation (Chapter 97) are often life-saving. In neurologically intact patients with hypoxemia, noninvasive positive-pressure ventilation may be a useful adjunct to passive oxygenation. When mechanical ventilation is required, lung-protective tidal volumes of 6 mL/kg of ideal body weight should be employed. Extracorporeal membrane oxygenation has been used with apparent benefit in hantavirus pulmonary syndrome.

Antibiotics and Secondary Infection
Until a diagnosis of viral hemorrhagic fever can be confirmed, patients should be immediately covered with appropriate antibacterial or antiparasitic therapy, with specific consideration of malaria (Chapter 324) and tick-borne rickettsial diseases (Chapter 311). Since translocation of gut bacteria to the bloodstream is a concern, regimens should cover enteric organisms. These drugs should then be stopped unless there is evidence of coinfection. Secondary bacterial infection should be suspected when patients have persistent or new fever after about 2 weeks of illness, a time when most viral hemorrhagic fevers either have resulted in death or are resolving.

Antiviral Therapy
The only currently available specific antiviral therapy for any viral hemorrhagic fever is ribavirin, although this off-label use is not approved by the U.S. Food and Drug Administration (Table 357-5). The best data are for hemorrhagic fever with renal syndrome. Although long considered the standard of care for Lassa

fever, more studies are needed to confirm its efficacy for this disease. Anecdotal data suggest efficacy in other arenavirus hemorrhagic fevers, but results are mixed and consensus is lacking regarding the drug's use in Crimean-Congo hemorrhagic fever. In vitro data generally show activity of ribavirin against dengue, yellow fever, Rift Valley fever, and Omsk hemorrhagic fever viruses, but clinical studies have not been performed. The main side effects of intravenous ribavirin are a mild to moderate hemolytic anemia, which infrequently necessitates transfusion and disappears with cessation of treatment, and rigors when the drug is infused too rapidly. The Chinese drug chongcao shenkang has been reported to be efficacious in hemorrhagic fever with renal syndrome.

In a clinical trial conducted during the West Africa Ebola virus outbreak, the monoclonal antibody cocktail ZMapp reduced mortality from 37 to 22%, although patient recruitment was insufficient to reach targeted statistical endpoints.[A1] The RNA polymerase inhibitor favipiravir showed efficacy only in milder cases of Ebola virus disease. During the outbreak, a survival benefit was noted in patients who received artesunate-amodiaquine rather than artemether-lumefantrine for empirical treatment of possible malaria, but this association must be further investigated. A randomized clinical trial of four drugs is ongoing in the Democratic Republic of the Congo.

Transfusion of appropriately titered convalescent plasma within the first 8 days of illness has been reported to reduce the case-fatality of Argentine hemorrhagic fever from 15 to 30% to less than 1%. However, this therapy has been associated with a convalescent phase neurologic syndrome characterized by fever, cerebellar signs, and cranial nerve palsies in 10% of treated patients. Animal studies show convalescent plasma to be efficacious in Lassa fever as well, but only if it contains a high titer of neutralizing antibody and if there is a close antigenic match between the infecting viruses of the donor and recipient. Convalescent plasma also appears to be efficacious for Crimean-Congo hemorrhagic fever and Rift Valley fever, but there are no controlled data. A clinical trial of convalescent plasma for Ebola virus disease did not show efficacy.

Various immune modulators, including ibuprofen, corticosteroids, anti–tumor necrosis factor-α, nitric oxide inhibitors, statins, and interleukins, have not shown conclusive benefit in the treatment of sepsis. In a small study, recombinant interleukin-2 reduced the degree of acute renal insufficiency in hemorrhagic fever with renal syndrome, but further studies are needed before it can be considered the standard of care. Clinical trials of corticosteroids in hemorrhagic fever with renal syndrome have shown mixed results. Corticosteroids (e.g., 200 mg intravenous hydrocortisone per day, divided into two to four daily doses or administered by continuous infusion) are recommended only when adrenal insufficiency is strongly suspected, the target blood pressure is not maintained despite adequate fluid repletion and vasopressors, or cerebral edema is suspected.

Management of Pregnancy

Uterine evacuation in pregnant patients appears to lower maternal mortality and should be considered, given the extremely high maternal and fetal mortality associated with viral hemorrhagic fever. However, this procedure must be performed with extreme caution because it can be considered high risk with regard to potential nosocomial transmission. Although it is technically contraindicated in pregnancy (Food and Drug Administration Category X), considering the very high maternal and fetal mortality, ribavirin should nevertheless be considered as a life-saving measure for the mother who has a viral hemorrhagic fever for which the drug is efficacious (see Tables 357-2 and 357-5). Recent experience following this approach in the management of patients with Lassa fever in Nigeria has resulted in favorable outcomes.

Pain Management and Other Considerations

Oral or parenteral acetaminophen, tramadol, opiates, or other analgesics should be used as needed for pain control (see Table 27-4), adjusting as necessary for hepatic insufficiency. Use of salicylates and nonsteroidal anti-inflammatory drugs should be avoided because of the risk of bleeding. Prophylactic therapy for gastrointestinal stress ulcers with proton pump inhibitors or histamine H_2-receptor antagonists is recommended (see Table 129-1). Antiemetics, such as the phenothiazines, are frequently warranted. Seizures can usually be managed with standard medications (Chapter 375).

Discharge and Monitoring

Because the patient's clinical status and infectivity generally correlate with the level of viremia, patients who have recovered from their acute illness can safely be assumed to have cleared their viremia and can be discharged without concern of subsequent transmission, with the exception of the risk of sexual transmission (see later) and possible transmission to infants through breast milk in women infected during pregnancy. Negative PCR testing is often used as a criterion for discharge, but PCR testing does not assess for infectious virus.

PREVENTION

Infection Prevention and Control

It is prudent to place the patient in a negative airflow room if it is available, but hermetically sealed isolation chambers are not required. Insecticide-treated bed nets and room screens should be used in open-air settings to prevent transmission of arthropod-borne hemorrhagic fever viruses. Access to the patient should be limited to a small number of designated staff with specific instructions and training regarding guidelines for infection prevention and control. Although normal barrier nursing precautions to prevent parenteral and droplet exposure to blood and body fluids are usually adequate to prevent infection, specific enhanced protection measures, including personal protective equipment, are warranted if the diagnosis of viral hemorrhagic fever is suspected.[18] Other essential components of infection prevention and control include proper staff-to-patient ratios, waste disposal, and disinfection procedures. Small-particle aerosol precautions should be used when procedures such as endotracheal intubation may generate aerosols.

Contact Tracing

The early nonspecific presentation of the viral hemorrhagic fevers poses a serious challenge to effective epidemiologic surveillance. Fortunately, the low secondary attack rates afford a measure of reassurance even when cases go unrecognized as long as proper barrier nursing is maintained. Furthermore, because mild cases, which may be still more difficult to recognize, are usually not very infectious, missed or delayed diagnosis of these patients is unlikely to pose a problem from an infection control standpoint.

Persons with unprotected direct contact with a patient during the symptomatic phase of a human-to-human communicable viral hemorrhagic fever should be monitored daily for evidence of disease for the duration of the longest possible incubation period, starting after their last contact (see Table 357-2). Given the generally low secondary attack rates, especially outside of caretakers, widespread contact tracing, laboratory testing, and postexposure prophylaxis are not indicated for casual contacts. Close contacts should check their temperature daily and record the results in a log. Despite lack of evidence for transmission during the incubation period, it is usually recommended that exposed persons avoid close contact with household members that might result in exposure to body fluids, such as sex, kissing, and sharing of utensils for the duration of the incubation period. Confinement of asymptomatic persons is not warranted, but persons who develop fever or other signs and symptoms suggestive of viral hemorrhagic fever should be immediately isolated until the diagnosis can be ruled out.

Vaccines

Vaccines for viral hemorrhagic fevers are at various stages of development. The 17D live attenuated yellow fever vaccine has a generally excellent protection and safety profile despite recognition of rare serious adverse events in elderly persons.[A2] Confirmed previous vaccination with 17D should essentially exclude the diagnosis of yellow fever unless the patient was immunocompromised at the time of vaccination.[19]

A highly efficacious live attenuated vaccine, Candid 1, also exists for Argentine hemorrhagic fever, although it is licensed only in Argentina. Candid 1 may also be effective in Bolivian hemorrhagic fever but does not protect against other arenavirus infections.

A phase III trial of a recombinant, replication-competent vesicular stomatitis virus-based vaccine expressing a surface glycoprotein of Zaire Ebolavirus showed 100% vaccine efficacy and has increasingly been deployed in outbreaks on a clinical trial basis.[A3][A4] Adverse effects were frequent but mostly minor, although vaccine-induced arthritis, dermatitis, and vasculitis were reported. Various other vaccines for Ebola virus are under development.[20]

Although a tetravalent vaccine for dengue virus showed initial promise and has been adopted by a number of countries,[A5] dengue may be more severe in dengue-naïve persons who were vaccinated but subsequently contract the disease. Experimental vaccines for hemorrhagic fever with renal syndrome,[21] Rift Valley fever, Omsk hemorrhagic fever, and Kyasanur Forest disease may be efficacious, although most have not been widely tested and are not widely approved or available. A number of vaccine candidates have been shown to be efficacious in animal models of Marburg and Lassa virus infections.

Postexposure Prophylaxis

Postexposure prophylaxis should be considered only in persons with distinct high-risk exposure, defined as follows: (1) penetration of skin by a contaminated sharp instrument (e.g., needlestick injury); (2) exposure of mucous membranes or broken skin to blood or body secretions (e.g., blood splashing in the eyes or mouth); (3) participation in emergency procedures without appropriate personal protective equipment (e.g., resuscitation after cardiac arrest, intubation, or suctioning); and (4) prolonged (i.e., hours) and continuous contact in an enclosed space without appropriate personal protective equipment. The most infectious patients are those with severe clinical conditions, usually late in the course of illness. Prophylaxis should not be used when the only exposure was during the incubation period or after acute disease has subsided.

Postexposure prophylaxis with oral ribavirin has been recommended for Lassa fever, other arenavirus infections, and Crimean-Congo hemorrhagic fever, although no systematic data are available on its efficacy, and the frequent minor adverse events sometimes can be mistaken for the early signs of disease. When used, oral ribavirin should be started immediately after the exposure, but not before counseling between the patient and the physician. The drug should be taken with food. Baseline hemoglobin, hematocrit, bilirubin, and creatinine levels should be determined, and therapy should be adjusted or reconsidered if significant anemia or renal insufficiency develops.

Convalescent plasma is given as postexposure prophylaxis for Argentine hemorrhagic fever. Numerous experimental vaccines, monoclonal antibodies, and other compounds have shown efficacy as postexposure prophylaxis in animal models, especially for filovirus infections, but reliable data on their efficacy in humans are not available.[22]

Reservoir and Vector Control
Avoiding contact with bats, primarily by avoiding entry into caves and mines in endemic areas, is a key prevention measure for Ebola and Marburg viruses. Personal protective equipment may be indicated for miners and other persons who work in these environments. Humans should also avoid exposure to fresh blood, body fluids, or meat of wild animals, especially nonhuman primates.

For rodent-borne viruses, whose reservoirs often colonize human dwellings, improved "village hygiene" is recommended, such as eliminating unprotected storage of garbage and foodstuffs and plugging holes that allow rodents to enter homes. Prevention of the mosquito-borne hemorrhagic fever viruses hinges on controlling *Aedes* mosquitoes in and around the home, primarily by elimination of clean standing water containers that serve as larval habitats and by use of screened windows and doors, insecticide-treated bed nets, protective clothing, mosquito repellent, and aerosol bomb insecticides in enclosed spaces. Analogous measures can help protect against tick bites.

PROGNOSIS
The clinical course of viral hemorrhagic fever unfolds quite rapidly. In fatal cases, death usually occurs within 7 to 10 days after the onset of hemorrhagic fever symptoms in filovirus infection and in about 2 weeks with the arenaviruses and some of the other viruses. Mortality usually does not result directly from exsanguination, and external bleeding is seen in a minority of cases of viral hemorrhagic fever. Most deaths are thought to result from a process akin to septic shock (Chapter 100) when insufficient effective circulating intravascular volume leads to hypotension, cellular dysfunction, and multiorgan system failure. Meningoencephalitis, renal failure, respiratory failure, rhabdomyolysis, and cardiac arrhythmias may contribute to death in some patients. Thrombotic coronary or cerebrovascular accidents related to thrombocytosis and a hypercoagulable state have been documented during early recovery after Ebola virus disease.

Common indicators of a poor prognosis include shock, bleeding, neurologic manifestations, high levels of viremia (or surrogate measurements of antigen or genome copies),[23] elevated levels of aspartate aminotransferase (>150 IU/L), and pregnancy, especially during the third trimester, in which maternal and fetal mortality may be above 90%.

However, mild and even asymptomatic cases have been reported for what are considered the most virulent viral hemorrhagic fevers. Reasons for this heterogeneity are largely unknown, although differences in route and dose of infection, underlying comorbid illness, and host genetic predisposition have been postulated.

During the West Africa Ebola virus outbreak, the case fatality rate in the 27 patients who received care in the United States and Europe was only 18.5%, compared with 31 to 76% reported from West Africa.[24] It is unknown whether this difference relates to use of experimental therapies, better intensive care, genetic predisposition, or fewer comorbid conditions.

Sequelae
Convalescence from Ebola virus disease is prolonged, often with a year or more of persistent arthralgia, ocular complications (including potentially sight-threatening uveitis that may result in early cataract formation),[25] abdominal pain, extreme fatigue, anorexia, and mental health sequelae. Ebola virus can persist for months or even years in immunologically protected tissue compartments, including the testes/semen, chambers of the eye, central nervous system,

and in the fetus, placenta, and amniotic sac/fluid of women infected during pregnancy. Ebola virus RNA has been detected in the semen over a year after acute disease, with rare evidence of male-to-female sexual transmission over a year after recovery.[26] Consequently, abstinence or safe sex with condoms is recommended for at least 1 year after recovery or until virus clearance from the semen can be confirmed through laboratory testing.

Two cases of Ebola virus recrudescence have been noted in persons cared for in high-resource settings with prolonged viral persistence—uveitis at 14 weeks after recovery and meningitis with seizures at 9 months after recovery. Ebola virus was isolated from the anterior chamber fluid of the eye and the cerebrospinal fluid, but both patients eventually cleared the virus and recovered.

Hearing loss, which may be permanent, is noted in up to 30% of survivors of Lassa fever[27] and also after Venezuelan hemorrhagic fever. It first appears during convalescence, may be unilateral or bilateral, and is not associated with severity of the acute disease or treatment with ribavirin. Optic retinopathy with vision loss has been noted in survivors of Rift Valley fever. Management of the sequelae of viral hemorrhagic fever is generally supportive,[28] with the exception of uveitis, for which urgent treatment with topical steroids and atropine may be sight-saving.

Breast-feeding should be avoided during convalescence unless there is no other way to support the baby. Proper infection prevention and control precautions should be taken when attending all births to women who were infected with filoviruses during pregnancy.

Grade A References

A1. Davey RT Jr, Dodd L, Proschan MA, et al. A randomized, controlled trial of ZMapp for Ebola virus infection. *N Engl J Med.* 2016;375:1448-1456.
A2. Gotuzzo E, Yactayo S, Cordova E. Efficacy and duration of immunity after yellow fever vaccination: systematic review on the need for a booster every 10 years. *Am J Trop Med Hyg.* 2013;89:434-444.
A3. Regules JA, Beigel JH, Paolino KM, et al. A recombinant vesicular stomatitis virus Ebola vaccine. *N Engl J Med.* 2017;376:330-341.
A4. Henao-Restrepo AM, Camacho A, Longini IM, et al. Efficacy and effectiveness of an rVSV-vectored vaccine in preventing Ebola virus disease: final results from the Guinea ring vaccination, open-label, cluster-randomised trial (Ebola Ça Suffit!). *Lancet.* 2017;389:505-518.
A5. Hadinegoro SR, Arredondo-Garcia JL, Capeding MR, et al. Efficacy and long-term safety of a dengue vaccine in regions of endemic disease. *N Engl J Med.* 2015;373:1195-1206.

GENERAL REFERENCES

For the General References and other additional features, please visit Expert Consult at https://expertconsult.inkling.com.

358

ARBOVIRUSES CAUSING FEVER AND RASH SYNDROMES

STANLEY J. NAIDES

COLORADO TICK FEVER

DEFINITION
Colorado tick fever (mountain fever, American mountain fever) is an acute, often self-limited, typically biphasic febrile illness that is seen in the Rocky Mountain areas, the Sierra Nevada and Wasatch ranges, and the Black Hills mountain areas. The virus is transmitted through the bite of the hard-shelled tick *Dermacentor andersoni* (Rocky Mountain wood tick), and the disease's range corresponds to the vector's range. Other coltiviruses, such as the Salmon River, Eyach, Banna, Beijing, and Gansu viruses, have also been implicated in human disease.

The Pathogen
The causative agent, Colorado tick fever virus, is a member of the genus Coltivirus, family Reoviridae. Coltiviruses have a genome consisting of 12

double-stranded RNA segments. Colorado tick fever virus is the prototype member.

EPIDEMIOLOGY

D. andersoni is found at elevations of 4000 to 10,000 ft. Seasonal temperatures tend to influence the range, with the vector being found at higher elevations in warmer seasons and at lower elevations in colder seasons. Human exposure usually occurs during outdoor recreational activities in these areas. Occasional exposure occurs in nonendemic areas from ticks exported out of the endemic region in clothes, hiking equipment, or baggage. Infections generally take place between March and September, when the adult tick is most plentiful. Ticks are most abundant in south-facing dry and rocky slope habitats that favor small rodents (e.g., chipmunks, ground squirrels, marmosets), with underbrush cover, burrows, and humidity for the ticks. Colorado tick fever virus is found in nymphal and adult ticks that overwinter on the rodent host, in which viremia persists for weeks to months. In the endemic area, as many as 14% of *D. andersoni* ticks carry Colorado tick fever virus. Humans are an incidental host. Colorado tick fever is not a federal reportable disease in the United States, but a total of 83 cases were reported from 2002 through 2012 in Arizona, Colorado, Montana, Oregon, Utah, and Wyoming.[1] The actual number of cases is probably significantly larger and includes subclinical, mild, and unreported cases.

The geographic range of Colorado tick fever may be larger than the well-recognized endemic mountain areas. Serologically confirmed cases in California have been attributed to the Colorado tick fever–related virus S1-14-03, which is transmitted by *D. variabilis* (American dog tick). Salmon River virus causes a Colorado tick fever–like illness in rafters on the Salmon River in Idaho. Another similar virus, Eyach virus, has been implicated in neurologic illness in France and Germany and has been isolated from the deer ticks *Ixodes ricinus* and *I. ventalloi*. Colorado tick fever has been reported rarely in mainland China.

PATHOBIOLOGY

Colorado tick fever virus replicates in CD34+ stem cells in bone marrow and leads to mild to moderate leukopenia and thrombocytopenia. The virus also replicates in committed erythrocyte precursors and may be detected in circulating erythrocytes up to 4 weeks after infection.

CLINICAL MANIFESTATIONS

Patients report a tick bite or exposure in 90% of cases, but there is no notable local reaction to the tick bite. After a mean incubation of 3 to 4 days (range, 0 to 14 days), sudden-onset fever develops in association with malaise, chills, myalgia, weakness, headache, photophobia, retro-orbital pain, and cutaneous hyperesthesia. Conjunctival and oropharyngeal injection, palatal enanthem, lymphadenopathy, and splenomegaly may be present. The absence of prominent respiratory and gastrointestinal symptoms helps exclude other febrile illnesses. A petechial or maculopapular exanthem, found in 15% of patients, may be confused with the rash of Rocky Mountain spotted fever (Chapter 311). The illness has a "saddleback" fever pattern consisting of resolution of the initial fever within 1 week and recrudescence after a 2- to 3-day hiatus. A third fever episode may occur.

Leukopenia develops 5 to 6 days after onset of the illness. Mild thrombocytopenia and anemia may occur.

Myocarditis, pneumonitis, hepatitis, orchitis, and epididymitis may complicate adult infection, and aseptic meningitis or encephalitis may occur in up to 10% of childhood infections.

DIAGNOSIS

Clinical diagnosis is confirmed by demonstration of the Colorado tick fever viral genome or specific acute phase IgM antibody. The viral genome may be detected up to 6 weeks after infection by nucleic acid–based methods such as reverse transcription–polymerase chain reaction (RT-PCR) on blood or stored blood clots. Virions in circulating erythrocytes may be detected by immunofluorescent antibody labeling. Anti–Colorado tick fever virus IgM antibody is detected by antibody capture enzyme-linked immunosorbent assay (ELISA) or complement fixation. Neutralization assays using Vero or BHK-21 cells have been helpful.

Differentiating Colorado tick fever from Rocky Mountain spotted fever (Chapter 311) may be difficult before the appearance of the typical rash of the latter. However, Rocky Mountain spotted fever does not have a saddleback fever pattern and is 20 times less common than Colorado tick fever in the western endemic area.

TREATMENT Rx

Treatment is supportive. Aspirin is contraindicated to avoid complicating thrombocytopenia.

PROGNOSIS

Extreme weakness and malaise may persist for weeks to months after final resolution of the fever. Older patients have a prolonged recovery. Seventy percent of patients older than 30 years may still have fatigue 3 weeks after the fever, whereas children and adolescents may recover completely within a week. Rare instances of maternal-fetal transmission have been reported. Full recovery eventually occurs, except when the disease course is complicated by neurologic insult. Patients should refrain from donating blood for 6 months.

● DENGUE

DEFINITION

Dengue is an acute febrile illness characterized by severe muscle and joint pain, rash, malaise, and lymphadenopathy. The severity of the musculoskeletal complaints gave rise to the sobriquet *breakbone fever*. Dengue occurs in the tropical and subtropical climes of the Caribbean, Central and South America, Asia, and Africa. The mosquito range extends into the southeastern part of the United States, where dengue reemerged in the 1980s. After World War II, a spreading global pandemic has been associated with erosion of mosquito control programs, human population spread into rural settings, increased air travel, deterioration in public health infrastructure, and global warming. Each year, more than 200 million people worldwide are infected with dengue.[2]

The Pathogen

Dengue virus is a member of the Flaviviridae family, which consists of single-stranded RNA viruses with a lipid envelope approximately 50 nm in diameter. There are four serotypes of dengue: DEN-1, DEN-2, DEN-3, and DEN-4. No cross-protection is seen among the serotypes, so dengue can develop after infection with another serotype. Infection with a second serotype places the individual at risk for the development of hemorrhagic fever (Chapter 357).

EPIDEMIOLOGY

Dengue is transmitted to humans by the bite of female *Aedes aegypti* and *A. albopictus* mosquitoes. *A. albopictus* has become the dominant pest mosquito in many urban centers. Members of the two mosquito species acquire dengue virus by biting humans, typically during the day. The mosquitoes nest in stagnant water around human dwellings; they are not typically encountered in the forest. In the human host, dengue virus may reach a titer of greater than 10^8 median infectious doses per milliliter. The mosquito becomes infected when taking its meal from a viremic host. The virus continues replication in the midgut epithelium and salivary glands of female mosquitoes, which remain infectious for life. Within 8 to 12 days of the initial infection, the mosquito's salivary glands become infected, and virus is shed with saliva during the next blood meal. A given mosquito may infect multiple individuals, especially in view of its skittishness during feeding—slight movement of the host interrupts its meal, after which it returns to the original or another host. Zoonotic life cycles involving nonhuman primates (i.e., chimpanzees, gibbons, and macaques) and canopy-dwelling forest *Aedes* species have been demonstrated in western Africa and Malaysia.

The incubation period is typically 4 to 7 days but may range from 3 to 14 days.[3] During outbreaks in the southeastern United States and Puerto Rico, the risk for infection may be as high as 79% in naïve hosts, and clinical disease may develop in up to 20%. Immunity against the infecting serotype is probably lifelong, but individuals remain susceptible to the remaining serotypes. Peak transmission occurs after increased rainfall, when rainwater collected in household containers allows expansion of mosquito populations. Epidemics tend to occur in 3- to 5-year cycles, but interepidemic cases occur regularly.

Dengue is a particular risk to visitors to the tropics and is a leading cause of pediatric morbidity and mortality in endemic areas. Globalization and climate change have contributed to expansion of the geographic range. In one study of people who now live in the United States but who were born, lived in, or traveled to dengue-endemic countries, 19% had IgG antibodies to dengue, but 85% of these individuals had no clinical history of dengue. Dengue accounts for approximately 2% of the febrile illnesses in travelers returning to the United States.

PATHOBIOLOGY

Dengue hemorrhagic fever (Chapter 357) and dengue shock syndrome are forms of dengue reinfection characterized by capillary leakage and hemorrhage. Previous infection with an alternative serotype allows antibody to the previously encountered serotype to combine with the newly infecting serotype. Although the first exposed serotype antibody is not neutralizing, it does allow enhanced antibody-mediated macrophage uptake, thereby leading to macrophage activation and increasing viral replication and viral load. Excretion of vasoactive inflammatory mediators by macrophages results in vascular leakage; severe vascular leak causes shock. Endothelial cell swelling and perivascular edema may occur. Rarely, dengue shock syndrome may occur with primary infection. Variation in a strain's ability to generate enhancing antibody, as well as differences in virulence, may account for differences in clinical behavior.

CLINICAL MANIFESTATIONS

Dengue infection is often subclinical. When it is symptomatic, dengue may be manifested as classic dengue, dengue hemorrhagic fever, or dengue shock syndrome. Patients may also have mild illness characterized by nonspecific fever, anorexia, and headache.[4]

Classic dengue, which typically occurs in nonindigenous older children and adults, is characterized by sudden-onset fever, severe frontal headache, retro-orbital pain, myalgia, and, in many cases, nausea, vomiting, rash, lymphadenopathy, and arthralgia. During outbreaks, loss of appetite and thirst may be early symptoms whose recognition can shorten the time to case identification. Patients may experience generalized weakness, altered taste, rigors, and cutaneous hyperesthesia. Classic dengue is self-limited, but some patients progress to dengue hemorrhagic fever or dengue shock syndrome, which is characterized by capillary leakage, hypotension, narrowed pulse pressure, and shock. Dengue in pregnancy may be severe.[5]

Physical examination demonstrates fever, relative bradycardia, scleral injection, ocular pressure tenderness, and pharyngeal injection. A transient macular rash appears on days 1 or 2 of illness. On days 2 and 3 of illness, fever and other symptoms may improve. The fever is typically but not consistently biphasic. After a hiatus of typically 2 days, fever and other symptoms recrudesce, although less severely. Generalized, nontender lymphadenopathy of the posterior cervical, epitrochlear, and inguinal regions may develop. Rash also recurs and appears as 2- to 5-mm speckles of pallor surrounded by erythema and occasionally accompanied by burning dysesthesia of the palms and soles. The rash may desquamate.

DIAGNOSIS

An adequate travel history and knowledge of occurrence of disease in the community can lead to consideration of dengue in the differential diagnosis. Point-of-care diagnostic testing for a dengue virus nonstructural protein 1 and dengue-specific IgM is helpful but not always conclusive.[6] Serotype-specific PCR-based assays are available. Specific IgM antibody appears 3 to 5 days after infection. IgG antibody appears 9 to 10 days after infection. Cross-reactivity with other flaviviruses prevents serotype-specific diagnosis. Neutralization testing with hemagglutination inhibition is more specific, and complement fixation testing for IgG in paired sera is helpful. Viremia is of adequate intensity in infections with DEN-1, DEN-2, and DEN-3 to allow viral isolation. Viremia in DEN-4 infections is often less intense and more difficult to detect through inoculation of mosquito cells in vitro.

Leukopenia develops by the second day of fever, falling to a low of 1000 to 2000 cells/mL by day 5 or 6, and is associated with granulocytopenia. In dengue hemorrhagic fever, thrombocytopenia of less than 100,000 cells/mL and a prolonged prothrombin time are characteristic. Mild to moderate proteinuria and a few casts may be detected.[7] Aspartate transaminase levels may be increased.

TREATMENT, PREVENTION, AND PROGNOSIS Rx

Classic dengue resolves abruptly in 5 to 7 days, but fatigue and depression may linger for weeks; survival is uniform. The prognosis of patients with dengue hemorrhagic fever (Chapter 357) and dengue shock syndrome depends on early diagnosis and the introduction of supportive measures. Treatment is supportive and consists of antipyretics and analgesics. Initial resuscitation of patients with shock syndrome (Chapter 98) with crystalloid and colloidal solutions is indicated in those with moderately severe dengue shock syndrome. Fresh-frozen plasma and blood products are used as necessary, but their benefit is unclear.[8] Most infected patients recover fully, but the overall mortality rate is about 1% because of the poorer outcome of dengue shock and hemorrhagic fever (Chapter 357).

A new tetravalent dengue vaccine can prevent about two thirds of cases of dengue and about 95% of severe cases. A1 A2 The vaccine is approved for use in the United States and Mexico, but concern over antibody-dependent enhancement of postvaccination infection[9] has led to caution in widespread deployment.

● WEST NILE FEVER VIRUS

DEFINITION

West Nile fever is an acute febrile illness associated with malaise, rash, headache, myalgia, and lymphadenopathy. Infection involves a bird-mosquito-human cycle. Viremia develops in all varieties of birds. Bats, cats, chipmunks, domestic rabbits, horses, skunks, squirrels, dogs, sheep, llamas, and alpacas may be infected.

The Pathogen

West Nile fever virus, which is the most widely distributed flavivirus, is transmitted by a variety of mosquito species. The mosquito vector varies: *Culex univittatus, C. pipiens,* and *C. molestus* in the Middle East and Africa; *Mansonia metallicus* in Uganda; and *C. tritaeniorhynchus* in Asia. After introduction into the New York City area in 1999, *C. pipiens* became the most important vector in the United States. Other mosquito species may carry the virus.

EPIDEMIOLOGY

Viral transmission involves mosquitoes and wild birds, with mammals, including humans, being incidental end-stage hosts. In endemic areas, more than 60% of young adults have antibodies, thus suggesting a high prevalence of inapparent or undifferentiated febrile illness in children. There is no gender predominance. Between 0.5 and 1% of infected individuals experience a more severe illness. Incubation is typically 3 to 15 days but may be as short as 1 day. West Nile virus emerged in the United States in New York and has spread throughout the continental United States, Canada, Mexico, the Caribbean, and Central and South America. In America, birds of the Corvidae family (e.g., crows, jackdaws, ravens) are often infected, and recognition of increased death in crow populations continues to serve as a sentinel for the presence of West Nile virus. In addition to mosquito transmission, the virus has been transmitted by a transplanted organ, through blood transfusion, transplacentally, and in the laboratory. In 2016, 2150 cases of West Nile disease were reported to the U.S. Centers for Disease Control and Prevention, and 61% of these cases were neuroinvasive.[10]

PATHOBIOLOGY

West Nile virus grows in a variety of cells in vitro and produces cytopathic effects in *A. albopictus* cells. Individuals in whom encephalitis develops show evidence of diffuse brain inflammation and neuronal degeneration, with virus detected early in multiple sites. The virus initially replicates in keratinocytes and skin-resident dendritic cells, which then migrate to local lymph nodes, where replication generates viremia and organ dissemination. Either immune cell trafficking or disruption of the blood-brain barrier allows neuroinvasion.

CLINICAL MANIFESTATIONS

Approximately 80% of infections are asymptomatic, and most of the remaining infections are mild and manifested by fever, malaise, headache, nausea, anorexia, generalized lymphadenopathy, and myalgia after an incubation period of 1 to 6 days.[11] Like Colorado tick fever and dengue, West Nile fever may be biphasic. Nonpruritic, maculopapular, or roseolar rash occurs on the chest, back, and arms in half the patients, beginning during or with resolution of the fever. The rash persists for up to 1 week and then resolves with desquamation. Patients may experience vomiting, diarrhea, abdominal pain, and pharyngitis. Aseptic meningitis or encephalitis (Chapter 359) may occur in the elderly and, less commonly, in the very young. Severe neurologic disease, including meningitis, myelitis, encephalitis, and flaccid paralysis of the limbs and respiratory muscles, resembling poliomyelitis (Chapter 355),[12] can develop. Anterior myelitis or hepatitis may also occur. Disease is usually milder in children than in adults.

DIAGNOSIS

West Nile virus may be isolated from up to 77% of patients with West Nile fever on the first day of illness, but viral isolation is less common in patients with encephalitis (Chapter 359). Low-titer viremia may persist for the first 5 days of illness. Tests in acute and convalescent phase serum for virus-specific antibody using ELISA or immunofluorescence are diagnostic. However, virus-specific IgM may persist in the serum at 1 year after infection in a minority of patients. Cerebrospinal fluid examination may reveal a lymphocytic pleocytosis (1800 cells/μL) with some increase in protein but a normal glucose concentration. Viral RNA is detected in cerebrospinal fluid by RT-PCR in about 50% of cases, but detection of West Nile virus–specific IgM in cerebrospinal fluid is more sensitive and is diagnostic of neuroinvasion because IgM normally does not cross the blood-brain barrier. Neutralization assays help distinguish cross-reactive antibodies to other flaviviruses. RT-PCR may detect viral RNA in human samples and in avian and insect specimens.

TREATMENT AND PREVENTION Rx

Treatment is supportive. Licensed antiviral agents are not available. Infection is controlled by the endogenous development of neutralizing antibodies to protein E, the viral envelope protein. A live-attenuated vaccine has been shown to be safe and immunogenetic but is not currently available.[13]

PROGNOSIS

Illness generally persists 3 to 6 days before rapid recovery. In patients with neurologic disease during the acute illness, about 50% have long-term sequelae, including fatigue, depression, weakness, tremor, headache, and difficulties with memory and word finding. Mortality rates of 10% or higher occur in patients with encephalitis (Chapter 359).

⬤ ZIKA VIRUS

Zika virus (Chapter 359) can cause fever, rash, arthralgia, and conjunctivitis—generally resembling dengue and chikungunya, but usually milder. Its most serious manifestations are neurologic: Guillaine-Barré syndrome (Chapter 392) and fetal microcephaly. Zika virus is discussed in Chapter 359.

⬤ PHLEBOTOMUS FEVER

DEFINITION

Phlebotomus fever (i.e., sandfly fever, pappataci, and 3-day fever) is an acute, mild, self-limited febrile illness transmitted through the bite of *Phlebotomus* flies.

The Pathogen

Phlebotomus fever viruses are members of the genus Phlebovirus, family Bunyaviridae. The latter consists of a group of single-stranded RNA viruses that are 80 to 120 nm in diameter, possess a lipid envelope, and have three segments in the genome. A related virus, the Toscana virus hosted by *Phlebotomus perniciosus* and *P. perfiliewi*, causes a similar illness in countries surrounding the northern Mediterranean basin and is emerging in western Europe. The related Punique, Granada, and sandfly fever Turkey viruses may cause similar febrile illnesses, acute meningitis, or meningoencephalitis. In 2009 a novel phlebovirus causing severe fever, thrombocytopenia, and a case fatality rate up to 30% emerged in Asia.[14]

EPIDEMIOLOGY

The virus's distribution parallels the distribution of *Phlebotomus* flies found throughout the Mediterranean basin, Middle East, and western India and Pakistan. In Central America, *Lutzomyia* fly species may transmit the virus. These tiny sandflies pass through mosquito netting to feed in the early evenings. Virus is maintained by transovarial and transstadial transmission. During outbreaks, humans may serve as a reservoir. Human infection is more common in rural areas during the summer months.[15] The incubation period is 2 to 6 days. Sandflies spread by hopping, thus limiting their travel range. Use of insect sprays locally is effective in decreasing risk.

CLINICAL MANIFESTATIONS

Sandfly fever virus causes an acute febrile illness associated with malaise, headache, photophobia, ocular pain, altered taste, myalgia, and arthralgia. The myalgias may be localized to specific regions (e.g., the chest) and simulate regional syndromes such as pleurodynia. A macular or urticarial rash may appear. Examination may show relative bradycardia after the first day, conjunctival injection, mild papilledema, or small palatal vesicles. Fever lasts 2 to 4 days and then subsides. Weakness and malaise may persist during convalescence. About 15% of patients experience recrudescence in 2 to 12 weeks. Aseptic meningitis may occur with mild cerebrospinal fluid pleocytosis. Peripheral leukopenia and lymphopenia may be present early in the illness. However, leukopenia may be delayed in some patients until the third day of illness, and a rebound relative lymphocytosis may be encountered.

DIAGNOSIS

The diagnosis of phlebotomus fever is confirmed by isolation of virus after intracerebral inoculation of suckling mice, detection of the viral genome by RT-PCR, or detection of specific IgM antibody by ELISA.

TREATMENT AND PROGNOSIS Rx

Treatment is supportive, and recovery is complete. Ribavirin (Chapter 336) has been proposed as a therapeutic option.

⬤ RIFT VALLEY FEVER

Rift Valley fever, which is an acute-onset, febrile illness, is often associated with epizootic waves of spontaneous abortion in livestock.[16]

DEFINITION

The Rift Valley fever virus is a member of the family Bunyaviridae, genus Phlebovirus, but unlike other members of the genus, it is transmitted by *Aedes* mosquitoes.

EPIDEMIOLOGY

Rift Valley fever occurs throughout most of Africa, with the majority of epizootic outbreaks occurring in eastern and southern Africa, although outbreaks occurred in Saudi Arabia and Yemen in 2000 and Mauritania in 1998, 2003, 2010, and 2012. The principal initial vectors are probably the *Aedes* species associated with flooding, although *Stomoxys* flies have been shown to transmit virus as well. Shallow pools along rivers and streams play an important role as mosquito breeding sites. Feeding on nearby livestock allows a local epizootic outbreak and amplification of the virus in local mosquito populations, including *C. pipiens* in Egypt and *C. theileri* in eastern Africa. Exposure to aborted livestock increases human risk of infection.

Hemorrhagic fever in humans is typically seen 1 to 2 weeks after a wave of abortion in livestock. Initial human cases usually occur in those who have close contact with livestock. The virus is highly transmissible through aerosolization of cattle fluids. Although the risk for severe human infection is less than 1%, the extensive exposure associated with outbreaks can lead to significant morbidity and mortality. For example, in the 1977–1978 Egyptian outbreak associated with movement of camels from Sudan, an estimated 200,000 people were infected, with 600 deaths. Zinga virus, isolated in central Africa and Madagascar and shown to be responsible for mild human illness, is a strain of Rift Valley fever virus.

PATHOBIOLOGY

Rift Valley fever virus grows well in a variety of cell cultures and has cytopathic effects. After infection by a mosquito bite, virus is transported through the lymphatics to regional lymph nodes, where replication allows amplification of the input inoculum and development of viremia with systemic spread. Viral replication in liver, spleen, lymph node, adrenal, lung, and kidney tissues is highly cytopathic. In severe cases, hepatic necrosis and, rarely, focal brain necrosis may occur. Encephalitis is not associated with viremia, thus suggesting that this sequela is immune mediated rather than a direct viral effect. Inflammatory cell infiltration is associated with focal necrosis in the brain. Spontaneous abortion is common in livestock, but fetal loss in humans is not clearly correlated with viral infection.

CLINICAL MANIFESTATIONS

Most human infections are mild, with an abrupt onset of fever, chills, malaise, and arthralgia following a 2- to 6-day incubation. Despite the development of neutralizing antibodies, however, about 1 to 2% of infections progress to more severe disease, including a severe hemorrhagic fever associated with hepatic necrosis and disseminated intravascular coagulopathy. Recovery is complicated by retinal vasculitis or encephalitis, which occurs in less than 0.5% of patients 1 to 4 weeks after recovery and is associated with recurrent fever. In severe cases, focal brain necrosis and encephalitis may lead to hallucinations, stupor, coma, and death.

DIAGNOSIS

Intense viremia allows detection of virus by quantitative real-time RT-PCR. Specific IgM and IgG are detectable by ELISA applied to acute and convalescent (after 1 to 2 weeks) paired sera.

TREATMENT, PREVENTION, AND PROGNOSIS   Rx

Treatment is supportive. Ribavirin (see Table 357-5 and Chapter 336) exhibits limited penetration of the blood-brain barrier, but has shown promise in combination with favipiravir, a selective inhibitor of RNA-dependent RNA polymerase, in animal studies. In endemic areas, vaccination of livestock is the most effective preventive measure.

The prognosis is good in the absence of retinitis or encephalitis. A high viral load at initial evaluation is a prognostic indicator for a poor outcome.

CHIKUNGUNYA FEVER

DEFINITION

Chikungunya fever is a febrile arthritis that occurs in sporadic cases and in epidemics.

The Pathogen

Chikungunya, an enveloped, single-stranded RNA virus 60 to 70 nm in diameter, is a member of the family Togaviridae, genus Alphavirus. Chikungunya virus is transmitted by mosquitoes, principally *Aedes* species, but also by *Mansonia africana* and other genera. Known animal reservoirs are monkeys, baboons, and, in Senegal, *Scotophilus* bat species. During outbreaks, humans are the major reservoir.

EPIDEMIOLOGY

Chikungunya, which is endemic in sub-Sahara Africa, India, the Philippines, and Southeast Asia, spread in 2004–2005 to the Seychelles, Mauritius, and Mayotte islands with a genotype better adapted to *A. albopictus*. This genotype then spread to India, where the outbreak continues with millions being affected. The global emergence of this disease is exemplified by outbreaks in Réunion Island, Bhutan, Papua New Guinea, Italy, India, and several Caribbean islands. Non–travel-related cases have been reported in Florida, United States.[17] Outbreaks typically develop after heavy rains. In urban settings, outbreaks are explosive. In endemic areas, seroprevalence rates may be as high as 90%, thus suggesting that time required for loss of herd immunity is the reason for the prolonged absence of cases in a region after an outbreak. Globalization may contribute to increasing propensity for spread. After inoculation, the incubation period is typically 2 to 3 days but ranges from 1 to 12 days.

PATHOBIOLOGY

Intense viremia develops within 48 hours of the mosquito bite and wanes 2 to 3 days later. Onset of hemagglutination inhibition and neutralizing antibodies clears the viremia. Superficial capillaries in rash-involved skin demonstrate erythrocyte extravasation and perivascular cuffing. The virus adsorbs to human platelets and causes them to aggregate. Synovitis probably results from direct chikungunya viral infection of synovium.

CLINICAL MANIFESTATIONS

Chikungunya fever is characterized by an explosive onset of fever and severe arthralgia.[18] Constitutional symptoms, fever (temperature to 40° C), rigors,

headache, photophobia, retro-orbital pain, conjunctival injection, pharyngitis, anorexia, nausea, vomiting, abdominal pain, tense lymphadenopathy, and myalgia are common. A maculopapular rash located on the torso, extremities, and occasionally the face, palms, and soles occurs in most patients 1 to 10 days after onset of the illness. Appearance of the rash is often associated temporally with initial defervescence; the rash may recur with fever and may be pruritic. Isolated petechiae and mucosal bleeding may occur, but significant hemorrhage is rare. Desquamation may take place when the rash resolves. The initial acute illness may last 2 to 3 days (range, 1 to 7 days). Fever may recrudesce after a 1- to 2-day hiatus. The polyarthralgia is migratory and predominantly affects the small joints of the hands, wrists, feet, and ankles, with less prominent involvement of the large joints.[19] Previously injured joints may be more severely affected. Stiffness and swelling may occur, but large effusions are uncommon. Synovial fluid shows decreased viscosity with poor mucin clot and 2000 to 5000 white blood cells per milliliter. Symptoms, including arthralgia, arthritis, and tenosynovitis, may persist for months to years. Maternal-fetal transmission may result in severe neonatal infection. Chikungunya virus can also cause central nervous disease symptoms, including encephalitis, especially in the very young or very old.

DIAGNOSIS

Chikungunya fever must be differentiated from dengue and o'nyong-nyong fever. Chikungunya virus may be isolated from blood during the initial 2 to 4 days of illness. In some patients, viral antigen may be detected in acute sera by hemagglutination assay as a result of the intensity of the viremia. Commercially available real-time RT-PCR assays on acute phase serum may be used to confirm the diagnosis. Specific IgM antibody may be detected for 6 months or longer. Hemagglutination inhibition and neutralization antibodies develop as the viremia is cleared. Complement fixation antibodies are positive by the third week and slowly decrease during the subsequent year.

Chronic chikungunya arthritis must be differentiated from rheumatoid arthritis (Chapter 248). At least one rheumatoid factor isotype is present in about 25% of patients with chikungunya arthritis. Citrullinated cyclic peptide antibody is uncommon. Serum levels of the synovial protein 14-3-3η are elevated in only 10% of patients with chikungunya arthritis compared with a 64% positivity rate in early rheumatoid arthritis.

TREATMENT AND PROGNOSIS   Rx

Treatment is supportive. Nonsteroidal anti-inflammatory agents are useful. During the acute arthritis, range of motion exercises lessen the stiffness. In most cases, mild joint symptoms may persist for months. Following the outbreak on Réunion Island in 2006, 70% of affected patients had episodic arthralgia, typically symmetrical and incapacitating, with joint swelling in 63% at 3 years after infection. Destructive arthropathy is rare, but higher initial viral loads portend more joint destruction and residual disability.[20] Encephalitis can result in a mortality rate of about 15%, with some degree of permanent disability in 30 to 45% of survivors. A safe, immunogenic vaccine is currently under investigation.[21]

O'NYONG-NYONG FEVER

DEFINITION

O'nyong-nyong means "joint breaker" in the Acholi dialect of northwestern Uganda, where o'nyong-nyong fever first appeared in February 1959.

The Pathogen

O'nyong-nyong fever is clinically similar to chikungunya fever, and the viruses share antigenic similarity. O'nyong-nyong virus is also a member of the family Togaviridae, genus Alphavirus.

EPIDEMIOLOGY

Within 2 years of its appearance in 1959, the o'nyong-nyong fever virus spread through Uganda and eastern Africa and affected 2 million people. Serologically determined attack rates ranged from 50 to 60%, with case rates of 9 to 78%. Disease spread at a rate of 2 to 3 km daily. After the epidemic, the virus was not detected again until it was isolated from *Anopheles funestus* mosquitoes in Kenya in 1978. *A. gambiae* also serves as a vector. Serologic surveys suggested that o'nyong-nyong virus is endogenous, but cases were not detected again until 1996–1997, during an outbreak in south central Uganda. An outbreak in western Côte d'Ivoire occurred in 2003. The nonhuman vertebrate reservoir for o'nyong-nyong virus is not known. The incubation period lasts at least 8 days. O'nyong-nyong fever virus vectors include *A. funestus, A. gambiae,* and other species.[22]

Igbo-ora (meaning "the disease that breaks your wings") virus is a variant of o'nyong-nyong, with 98.5% homology between the two at the genomic level. Igbo-ora is serologically similar to the chikungunya and o'nyong-nyong viruses. In 1984 an epidemic of fever, rash, arthralgia, and myalgia occurred in four villages on the Ivory Coast. The virus was isolated from *A. funestus* and *A. gambiae* mosquitoes and from affected individuals.

PATHOBIOLOGY

Little is known about the pathobiology of o'nyong-nyong fever.

CLINICAL MANIFESTATIONS

Illness begins with a sudden onset of polyarthralgia and polyarthritis. Between 4 and 7 days later, rash begins with improvement in joint symptoms. The rash is uniform in nature, begins on the face, and then spreads to the torso and extremities and occasionally to the palms. The rash lasts 4 to 7 days before fading. Fever is not prominent, but postcervical lymphadenopathy may be marked. Arthralgia is incapacitating in most patients for up to a week, but residual joint pain may persist for months.

DIAGNOSIS

O'nyong-nyong fever is difficult to differentiate from chikungunya fever and may also be mistaken for measles. Specific hemagglutination inhibition and complement fixation tests are available. Mouse antisera raised against chikungunya virus react equally well with o'nyong-nyong virus, but o'nyong-nyong antisera do not react well with chikungunya virus. O'nyong-nyong–specific RT-PCR is available in reference laboratories.

TREATMENT AND PROGNOSIS

Treatment is symptomatic. Although residual joint pain often persists, there do not appear to be any long-term sequelae.

● MAYARO FEVER

DEFINITION

Mayaro fever is an acute febrile illness characterized by fever, rash, arthralgia, and arthritis. Mayaro virus was first recognized in Trinidad in 1954. It has caused recorded outbreaks in Bolivia and Brazil and is endemic in the rain forest region where Bolivia, Brazil, and Peru share borders. Mayaro virus has a monkey reservoir and is transmitted to humans by *Haemagogus* mosquitoes dwelling in the tropical rain forest canopy.

The Pathogen

Mayaro virus is a member of the family Togaviridae, genus Alphavirus.

EPIDEMIOLOGY

Mayaro virus was responsible for an outbreak in Belterra, Brazil, in 1988. Eight hundred of 4000 exposed latex gatherers became infected, with a clinical attack rate of 80%. Forest workers and hunters continue to be at greatest risk. Serologic surveys demonstrate inter-outbreak background cases. Cases of imported Mayaro virus infection have been documented in the United States and in Europe after travel to the endemic Brazil-Bolivia-Peru interborder region. The virus has been isolated from a bird in Louisiana, thus raising the specter of emergence in North America.

PATHOBIOLOGY

Viremia occurs during the first 1 to 2 days of illness.

CLINICAL MANIFESTATIONS

Illness is characterized by a sudden onset of fever, headache, dizziness, chills, and arthralgia in the small joints of the hands and feet. About 20% of patients have joint swelling. Unilateral inguinal lymphadenopathy is seen occasionally. Leukopenia is common. Fever resolves after 3 to 7 days, but a maculopapular

rash then develops on the trunk and extremities of about two thirds of patients and lasts about 3 days.

DIAGNOSIS

RT-PCR with ELISA is available and is the diagnostic test of choice.[23] Mayaro virus may be isolated from blood by growth in Vero or C6/36 cells. A specific IgM is also available as an antibody capture ELISA.

TREATMENT AND PROGNOSIS

Treatment is supportive. Recovery is complete, although some patients have persistent arthralgia 6 months later.

● ROSS RIVER FEVER VIRUS (EPIDEMIC FEBRILE POLYARTHRITIS)

Ross River fever virus causes an acute-onset, febrile illness characterized by rash and arthralgia. Ross River virus is a member of the family Togaviridae, genus Alphavirus.

EPIDEMIOLOGY

Epidemics of fever and rash have been observed in Australia since 1928. Isolation of Ross River virus from mosquitoes, its serologic association with epidemic polyarthritis, and isolation of the virus from epidemic polyarthritis patients in Australia confirmed Ross River virus as the etiologic agent of epidemic polyarthritis. Seroprevalence has been observed in endogenous populations in Papua New Guinea, western New Guinea, the Bismarck Archipelago, Rossel Island, and the Solomon Islands. An outbreak in the Fiji Islands affected more than 40,000 individuals in 1979 to 1980. A similar epidemic occurred in the Cook Islands early in 1980. Antibodies to Ross River virus are not found in individuals west of Weber's line, a hypothetical line separating the Australian geographic zone from the Asiatic zone. Endemic cases and epidemics occur in tropical and temperate regions in Australia. Queensland and New South Wales have a particularly high annual incidence associated with higher rainfall. High rainfall usually precedes epidemic periods, with cases subsequently occurring from spring through fall. Seroprevalence may reach just 6 to 15% in temperate coastal zones but is 27 to 39% in the plains of the Murray Valley river system. In Queensland, annual rates of disease range from 31.5 to 288.3 per 100,000 person-years. From 1992 to 2006, 55,000 cases of Ross River virus infection were reported in Australia.

A. vigilax is the major vector on the eastern coast of Australia and *A. camptorhynchus* in the salt marshes of southern Australia. *C. annulirostris* is a freshwater breeding vector. Other Australian *Aedes* species and *Mansonia uniformis* may also serve as vectors. In outbreaks on the Pacific islands, *A. polynesiensis, A. aegypti, A. vigilax,* and *C. annulirostris* may have contributed to transmission. Domestic animals, rodents, and marsupials may serve as intermediate hosts. Virus may persist in *Aedes* mosquitoes.

There is a predominance of women among infected individuals. Children have a case attack rate ratio lower than that of adults. The incubation period is 7 to 11 days.

Barmah Forest virus, another alphavirus found in Australia in 1986, may be manifested in a fashion similar to epidemic febrile polyarthritis. The number of cases reported annually has been increasing since its initial discovery.

PATHOBIOLOGY

Ross River viral antigen may be detected in monocytes and macrophages early in infection, but intact virus is not identifiable by electron microscopy or cell culture. Dermal vessels show mild perivascular mononuclear cell infiltrates, mostly T lymphocytic, in erythematous and purpuric areas. Vessels in purpuric areas also show erythrocyte extravasation. Antigen can be demonstrated in epithelial cells in erythematous or purpuric skin and in the perivascular zone in erythematous skin. However, viral antigens have not been found in normal skin. Synovium undergoes lining cell hypertrophy and sublining vascular proliferation and mononuclear cell infiltration. Viral RNA can be identified by RT-PCR. Synovial fluid cell counts range from 1500 to 13,800 cells/mL and consist of monocytes, vacuolated macrophages, and a few neutrophils. Animal models of infection indicate that Ross River virus targets bone, joint, and skeletal muscle and elicits an inflammatory response mediated by the innate immune system.

CLINICAL MANIFESTATIONS

Arthralgia typically occurs abruptly, followed in 1 to 2 days by a macular, papular, or maculopapular rash that may be pruritic.[24] Three fourths of patients have severe, incapacitating arthralgia in an asymmetrical and migratory distribution. Commonly affected joints are the metacarpophalangeal joints, finger interphalangeal joints, wrists, knees, and ankles. The shoulder, elbow, toe, spine, hip, and temporomandibular joints may also be affected. Arthralgias are worse in the morning and after periods of inactivity. A third of patients have synovitis. Polyarticular swelling and tenosynovitis are common. Up to a third of patients have paresthesias or palm or sole pain. Classic carpal tunnel syndrome may occur.

In some individuals, rash may precede or follow the joint symptoms by 11 or 15 days, respectively. On occasion, vesicles, papules, or petechiae are seen. The trunk and extremities are typically involved, but the palms, soles, and face may also be affected. The rash resolves by fading to a brownish discoloration or by desquamation. Fever tends to be mild to moderate and lasts 1 to 3 days. Headache, nausea, and myalgia are common. Mild photophobia, respiratory symptoms, and lymphadenopathy may occur.

DIAGNOSIS

In the Australian epidemics before 1979, patients were antibody positive at the time of initial evaluation. However, in the Pacific island epidemics of 1979 to 1980, patients remained viremic and serologically negative for up to a week after the onset of symptoms. Virus in serum is stable for up to a month at 0° to −10° C. Current testing in Australia is performed with an indirect ELISA. The presence of specific IgM or evidence of seroconversion to IgG positivity supports the diagnosis of a recent infection.

TREATMENT AND PROGNOSIS   Rx

Treatment is supportive. Nonsteroidal anti-inflammatory drugs provide relief of joint pain. Half of all patients return to activities of daily living within 4 weeks despite residual polyarthralgia. Joint symptoms may recur, but episodes gradually resolve. In some patients, joint symptoms may persist for up to 3 years. Mild exercise tends to improve the joint symptoms.

SINDBIS

Sindbis virus causes a sudden-onset, febrile illness associated with arthralgia and rash. It is known as Ockelbo disease in Sweden, Pogosta disease in Finland, and Karelian fever in the Karelian Isthmus of Russia. *Aedes, Culex,* and *Culiseta* mosquitoes transmit the virus to humans, with birds serving as intermediate hosts.

EPIDEMIOLOGY

The virus was first isolated from *Culex* mosquitoes in the Egyptian village of Sindbis in 1952. Outbreaks frequently occur in the forested areas of Sweden, Finland, and the Karelian Isthmus, but sporadic cases and small outbreaks have occurred in Uganda, South Africa, Zimbabwe, central Africa, and Australia. Individuals involved in outdoor activities or occupations are at greatest risk. In northern Sweden, 2.9% of the population has Sindbis virus–specific serum IgG positivity indicative of prior infection.

PATHOBIOLOGY

Skin lesions show perivascular hemorrhage, lymphocytic infiltrates, edema, and areas of necrosis. Virus has been isolated from skin lesions. Antiviral IgM may persist for years, thus raising the possibility that Sindbis virus arthritis is associated with viral persistence and a direct viral effect on the synovium. Autophagy, an evolutionarily conserved intracellular mechanism for recycling cytoplasmic material to lysosomes for degradation during times of stress, may be disrupted in neurons by Sindbis virus infection, thereby leading to programmed cell death or apoptosis.

CLINICAL MANIFESTATIONS

Arthralgia and rash are the initial symptoms, although one may precede the other by a few days. Arthralgia and arthritis involve the small joints of the hands and feet, wrists, elbows, ankles, and knees.[25] On occasion, arthralgia affects the spine. Tendinitis is common and often involves the Achilles and hand extensor tendons. Fever, if present, tends to be mild to moderate. Constitutional

---

symptoms, headache, fatigue, malaise, nausea, vomiting, pharyngitis, and paresthesias may be present but are not usually severe. Macular rash typically begins on the torso and then involves the arms, legs, palms, soles, and occasionally the head. Macules evolve to papules that have a tendency to vesiculate. Vesiculation is prominent on pressure points, including the palms and soles. As the eruption fades, a brownish discoloration is left. Vesicles on the palms and soles may become hemorrhagic. Rash may recur during convalescence.

DIAGNOSIS

Specific IgM detected by enzyme immunoassay supports a diagnosis of Sindbis virus infection. IgM titers may wane during a period of 3 to 4 years.

TREATMENT AND PROGNOSIS   Rx

Treatment is supportive. Nonerosive chronic arthropathy is common in Sweden and Finland, with up to half of all patients having joint symptoms 2.5 years after infection. In a few cases, symptoms may persist for up to 6 years.

Grade A References

A1. Villar L, Dayan GH, Arredondo-Garcia JL, et al. Efficacy of a tetravalent dengue vaccine in children in Latin America. *N Engl J Med.* 2015;372:113-123.

A2. Hadinegoro SR, Arredondo-Garcia JL, Capeding MR, et al. Efficacy and long-term safety of a dengue vaccine in regions of endemic disease. *N Engl J Med.* 2015;373:1195-1206.

GENERAL REFERENCES

For the General References and other additional features, please visit Expert Consult at https://expertconsult.inkling.com.

359

ARBOVIRUSES AFFECTING THE CENTRAL NERVOUS SYSTEM

THOMAS P. BLECK

Arboviruses, which are also termed *arthropod-borne viruses,* can affect the central nervous system (CNS). These viruses share a number of clinical and epidemiologic similarities and have an RNA genome, but they do not form a formal virologic taxonomic group. Arboviruses generally have avian or small mammalian reservoirs and are transmitted to humans and other large mammals incidentally when an infected mosquito or other arthropod obtains a blood meal.

EPIDEMIOLOGY

Most human disease is subclinical; a few patients have a brief febrile illness resembling influenza, and a small percentage, usually at the extremes of age, suffer meningitis or encephalitis.[1] The diseases (Table 359-1) reflect the quotidian and seasonal characteristics of their insect vectors. Other viruses of the same genera cause hemorrhagic fever (Chapter 357), and other less frequently encountered arboviruses are also capable of producing encephalitis (Chapter 386).

Many of these agents cause notifiable disease in the United States: St. Louis, West Nile, Powassan, eastern equine, western equine, and the California serogroup encephalitis viruses. Case definitions and additional information are available at http://www.cdc.gov/ncidod/dvbid/arbor/index.htm.

The diseases described here are zoonoses (Chapter 312), that is, illnesses caused by viruses transmitted from animals to humans. They are more prevalent in the tropics and subtropics and are usually localized because of ecologic restrictions on their transmission. Recent studies confirm that most arboviruses, including dengue and chikungunya,[2] also cause encephalitis; they are discussed in Chapter 358.

TABLE 359-1 ARTHROPOD-BORNE VIRUSES ASSOCIATED WITH HUMAN ENCEPHALITIS

VIRUS	INSECT VECTOR	COMMON VERTEBRATE HOSTS	GEOGRAPHIC DISTRIBUTION
TOGAVIRIDAE			
Alphaviruses	Mosquitoes		
Eastern equine encephalitis	*Culiseta* spp, *Aedes* spp, *Coquillettidia* spp		Eastern United States and Gulf Coast, Caribbean region, South America
Western equine encephalitis	*Culiseta* spp, *Culex* spp		Western United States, Canada
Venezuelan equine encephalitis	*Aedes* spp, *Culex* spp, *Psorophora* spp, and *Mansonia* spp		South America, Central America, Florida and southwestern United States
FLAVIVIRIDAE			
Japanese serocluster	Mosquitoes		
Japanese encephalitis	*Culex* and *Aedes* spp		East and Southeast Asia, India, Australia
West Nile encephalitis	*Aedes* spp, *Culex* spp, and others		Africa, Middle East, North America
St. Louis encephalitis	*Culex* spp		Western Hemisphere
Murray Valley encephalitis	*Culex* spp		Australia
Zika	*Aedes* spp		Worldwide
Tick-borne encephalitis complex			
Central European encephalitis	*Ixodes* spp	Goats, sheep	Europe, Russia
Russian spring-summer encephalitis	*Ixodes* spp		Europe, northern and central Asia
Kyasanur Forest disease	*Haemaphysalis spinigera*	Rodents, insectivores	India
Omsk hemorrhagic fever	*Dermacentor reticulatus*	Rodents	Central Asia
Powassan	*Ixodes* spp	Squirrels, groundhogs	North America, Russia
Louping ill	*Ixodes ricinus*	Small mammals, sheep, birds	British Isles
Langat	*Ixodes* spp	Rodents	Malaysia, Thailand, parts of former Soviet Union
BUNYAVIRIDAE			
California encephalitis	*Aedes melanimon, Aedes dorsalis*	Rodents, rabbits	California
La Crosse encephalitis	*Aedes triseriatus*	Chipmunks, squirrels	Eastern and Midwestern United States

TABLE 359-2 FEATURES OF ARBOVIRAL ENCEPHALITIDES IMPORTANT IN THE UNITED STATES

	EASTERN EQUINE ENCEPHALITIS	WESTERN EQUINE ENCEPHALITIS	VENEZUELAN EQUINE ENCEPHALITIS	WEST NILE ENCEPHALITIS	ST. LOUIS ENCEPHALITIS	CALIFORNIA SEROGROUP ENCEPHALITIS
Annual U.S. cases of symptomatic disease	10	0-2 cases, mostly infants and children	Rare, mostly children	Up to 3000, mostly >40 years	0-2000, mostly >50 years	10-50, mostly children
Time of year	Late summer, early fall	Early and mid summer	Summer	Summer, fall	Mid to late summer	July-September
Case-fatality rate	50-70%, highest in children <15 years and adults >55 years	3-5% in children	35% in children, <10% in older persons	14-19%, 30% in adults >70 years	9% overall; 0% <20 years, 30% >65 years	<1%
Residual damage	30-50%, especially in children	33% in infants	Frequent in children	50%, more frequent in elderly	Frequent in elderly	Probably rare
Cerebrospinal fluid findings (cells/μL)	500-2000 cells, predominantly neutrophils	<500 cells, predominantly lymphocytes	<500 cells, predominantly lymphocytes	<500 cells, predominantly lymphocytes	<500 cells, predominantly lymphocytes	<500 cells, predominantly lymphocytes

PATHOBIOLOGY

Two pathologic processes are common to the arboviral encephalitides: neuronal and glial damage mediated by intracellular viral infection; and migration of immunologically active cells into the perivascular space and brain parenchyma. Endothelial cell swelling and proliferation, destruction of myelin sheaths in deep white matter areas, and vasculitis are present in some arboviral encephalitides.

After a bite by an infected arthropod, viral replication occurs in local tissues and regional lymph nodes. Viremia, which seeds extraneural tissues, occurs and persists depending on the extent of replication in extraneural sites, the rate of viral clearance by the reticuloendothelial system, and the appearance of humoral antibodies. The sites of extraneural infection vary among the viruses. Many alphaviruses and flaviviruses involve striated muscle and endothelium, whereas Venezuelan encephalitis virus is associated with myeloid and lymphoid tissue invasion. During viremia, the neural parenchyma may be invaded, but the mode of penetration of virus across the blood-brain barrier is not completely understood. Possible mechanisms include passive movement of virus across vascular membranes and viral replication in the cerebral capillary endothelium. Factors that increase vascular permeability or disrupt the blood-brain barrier promote invasion of the nervous system. Infected monocytes may also bring the virus into the CNS. In experimental animal infection, flaviviruses enter the CNS through the olfactory epithelium.

The immune response to flaviviruses starts with an innate interferon response to viral replication. Neurons then produce chemokines that recruit various components of the cellular immune response. The induced T-cell and monocyte trafficking is needed to clear the virus from the CNS, but it can also damage neurons.

The immature brain is more susceptible to damage by western equine, Venezuelan equine, and California serogroup encephalitis viruses (Table 359-2). St. Louis encephalitis and West Nile encephalitis principally affect the elderly, whereas Japanese encephalitis and eastern equine encephalitis have a bimodal incidence and strike both children and elderly persons. In endemic areas, immunity accumulated with increasing age may reduce the incidence of disease in older persons for some viruses; however, the reasons for the increased severity of illness with other viruses remain unknown.

CLINICAL MANIFESTATIONS

Clinical symptoms and signs vary among the viral causes (see later), although all share common signs and symptoms of encephalitis (Chapter 386).

DIAGNOSIS

Diagnosis depends on a careful history that includes exposure to vertebrate animals and arthropod vectors, age, season, and travel, including the geographic site of exposure. Laboratory confirmation of infection is essential. The virus may be isolated from acute phase serum or whole blood in laboratory animals or in tissue culture. Neutralization, complement fixation (CF), hemagglutination inhibition (HI), fluorescent antibody, and enzyme-linked immunosorbent assay (ELISA) of acute and 3-week convalescent sera can also produce the correct diagnosis. Antigen detection and IgM capture ELISA often permit diagnosis on initial evaluation and within a week of the onset of illness in most cases. Sensitive nucleic amplification assays using reverse transcription–polymerase chain reaction (RT-PCR) are under development for a number of the arboviruses and may lead to earlier diagnosis.

Differential Diagnosis

The most important initial consideration is to differentiate arboviral encephalitides from other acute CNS infections, including infections other than encephalitis (Chapters 384 and 385), treatable causes of encephalitis (Chapter 386), and paraneoplastic and autoimmune encephalitis (Chapters 384 and 386). Anti–N-methyl-D-aspartate (NMDA) receptor encephalitis, which is as common as most viral causes of encephalitis in parts of the United States (Chapter 383),[3] is an important part of the differential diagnosis, particularly in young women and especially because—unlike arboviral infections—it often responds to immunosuppressive treatment.

The early prodrome resembles influenza (Chapter 340). Bacterial meningitis (Chapter 384; especially early or partially treated), infective bacterial endocarditis (Chapter 67), brain abscess (Chapter 385), subdural empyema (Chapter 385), and cerebral thrombophlebitis may mimic viral encephalitis, and the cerebrospinal fluid (CSF) profile is sometimes similar. Other infections that occasionally cause meningoencephalitis that may resemble arthropod-borne viral encephalitis include tuberculosis (Chapter 308), cryptococcosis (Chapter 317), histoplasmosis (Chapter 316), coccidioidomycosis (Chapter 316), Rocky Mountain spotted fever (Chapter 311), leptospirosis (Chapter 307), falciparum malaria (Chapter 324), trichinosis (Chapter 335), Naegleria meningitis (Chapter 384), typhoid fever (Chapter 292), Lyme disease (Chapter 305), and Mycoplasma pneumonia (Chapter 301).

Acute meningoencephalitis may result from infections with other viruses, including herpesviruses (Chapter 350), human immunodeficiency virus (Chapter 362), mumps virus (Chapter 345), enteroviruses (Chapter 355), lymphocytic choriomeningitis virus (Chapter 384), rabies (Chapter 386), influenza (Chapter 340), and the exanthematous viral infections of childhood (Chapters 343 and 344). The exposure history, the presence of similar disease in the community, and the summer-fall occurrence are principal clues to an arboviral etiology. Enteroviruses (Chapter 355) also cause summer-fall outbreaks, but the predominant syndrome is aseptic meningitis, and the concomitant occurrence of rash or pleurodynia is a helpful clue. Herpes simplex encephalitis (Chapter 386) presents an important diagnostic consideration because effective therapy is available and should be started quickly. The presence of localizing neurologic signs, localizing findings on computed tomography (CT) or magnetic resonance imaging (MRI), and detection of herpes simplex DNA in CSF by PCR help distinguish herpes simplex encephalitis from the arboviral encephalitides.

Noninfectious diseases of the CNS, such as stroke (Chapter 379), may rarely be confused with viral encephalitis. Subarachnoid hemorrhage (Chapter 380) produces meningismus, fever, headache, and neurologic signs that mimic an infectious etiology. Metabolic encephalopathies occasionally have features suggesting infectious encephalitis. Neoplastic or granulomatous diseases involving the CNS and a variety of diseases of uncertain etiology (Behçet disease [Chapter 254], Reye syndrome, acute multiple sclerosis [Chapter 383], and systemic lupus erythematosus [Chapter 250]) must be considered in the differential diagnosis as well.

PREVENTION

Control can be achieved by interruption of the cycle, including vaccination of reservoir animals, vector control, and education on vector avoidance. Practical measures include wearing long-sleeved clothing, using insect repellents, limiting outdoor activities during peak mosquito season, and eliminating standing pools of water. Vaccines are currently available for Japanese encephalitis.

TREATMENT ℞

Treatment is symptomatic and may include bedrest, antipyretics, and analgesics. Early empirical treatment of herpes simplex encephalitis (Chapter 350) may be appropriate while the diagnostic evaluation to document arboviral encephalitis proceeds. To date, no immunologic therapy has demonstrated a useful effect in humans.

● EASTERN EQUINE ENCEPHALITIS

EPIDEMIOLOGY

Human disease is relatively rare, with fewer than 10 cases occurring each year in the Gulf Coast and Atlantic states, usually in association with an equine epizootic involving 100 to 300 animals. Outbreaks generally occur during the late summer and early fall. The occurrence of equine cases or outbreaks of fatal encephalitis in penned exotic birds precedes the appearance of human cases by several weeks or more. Epizootics of eastern equine encephalitis have been reported in the Caribbean (Hispaniola) and South America.

In temperate areas, eastern equine encephalitis virus circulates between wild birds and Culiseta melanura mosquitoes in a freshwater swamp habitat. Equine epizootics and associated human cases result from extension of the transmission cycle to involve Aedes and Coquillettidia mosquitoes, which feed on horses and humans.

PATHOBIOLOGY

The brain is grossly edematous and congested, and the inflammatory response is predominantly polymorphonuclear. The areas most affected are the basal ganglia, thalamus, hippocampus, and frontal and occipital cortices. Focal vasculitis, endothelial cell swelling, intravenous and arteriolar thrombus formation, demyelination, necrosis, neuronolysis, and neuronophagia are prominent. Eastern equine encephalitis virus appears to make use of host micro-RNAs to limit replication in myeloid cells, thereby restricting the host immune response and causing more severe neurologic damage.

CLINICAL MANIFESTATIONS

Onset is abrupt, with high fever, vomiting, and somnolence. Stupor, coma, myoclonus, and generalized convulsions appear within 24 hours to as long as 10 days later.[4] Autonomic disturbances (sialorrhea) may be prominent, and respiratory difficulty and cyanosis are frequent. In children, facial, periorbital, or generalized edema may be present.

A striking peripheral leukocytosis with immature neutrophils occurs frequently in patients with eastern equine encephalitis. CSF examination reveals 500 to 2000 white blood cells/μL (predominantly neutrophils). As the total cell count falls, neutrophils may persist as a significant fraction. Red blood cells may be present, protein concentration is elevated, and the glucose level is normal.

DIAGNOSIS

Brain CT and MRI are frequently abnormal and reveal lesions in the basal ganglia, thalami, and brain stem. The virus can rarely be isolated from blood or CSF. Serologic diagnosis by demonstration of a rise in antibody titer in appropriately timed paired sera is the most practical and available test. Because of the rapid course of the clinical disease, sera should be obtained at 2- to 3-day intervals during the acute phase of illness.

PREVENTION

An experimental formalin-inactivated chick embryo cell culture vaccine is used to protect laboratory and field workers. Reduction of mosquito populations by appropriate use of insecticides may be effective in threatened or established outbreaks.

TREATMENT ℞

Treatment is supportive. Control of fever, intracranial pressure, seizures, fluid and electrolyte disturbances, and the airway is critical. Although attempts at immunologic therapy have been reported, no controlled data are available.

PROGNOSIS

The case-fatality rate is 50 to 70%. Mortality, like incidence, is highest in children younger than 15 years and in persons older than 55 years, with no gender predilection. Death usually occurs during the first week; in surviving patients, recovery begins during the second week and may progress rapidly. Good functional recovery is associated with a long prodromal course and absence of coma. Residual damage, found in 30 to 50% of patients, is often severe, especially in children, and is characterized by mental retardation, spastic paralysis, and radiographic evidence of brain atrophy.

WESTERN EQUINE ENCEPHALITIS

EPIDEMIOLOGY

Few cases of western equine encephalitis have been reported in recent decades; the most recent epidemic occurred in Colorado in 1987. Epidemics occur in early or mid summer and may follow heavy snow melt or flooding, conditions favorable for breeding of mosquitoes. Cases of encephalitis in equines often precede the appearance of human disease. The illness principally affects residents of rural communities, and the incidence is higher in males than in females.

The ratio of inapparent to apparent infection is also age dependent and ranges from about 1 : 1 in infants younger than 1 year, to 58 : 1 in children 1 to 4 years old, to more than 1000 : 1 in persons older than 14 years. Western equine encephalitis virus also occurs in South America. Equine epizootics in Argentina have been associated with human cases.

Western equine encephalitis virus circulates between wild birds and *Culex tarsalis* mosquitoes. *C. tarsalis* is responsible for infection of humans and equines, which have low or undetectable viremia and do not perpetuate the chain of transmission. In temperate areas, transmission ceases during the winter months.

PATHOBIOLOGY

Pathologic examination of the brains of infants reveals massive parenchymal destruction; children dying months or years after the acute insult often have large cystic lesions in many areas of the brain. In older children and adults, acute western equine encephalitis is characterized by focal necrosis and perivascular cuffing, predominantly in the basal ganglia and thalami but also in deep cerebral white matter.

CLINICAL MANIFESTATIONS

The disease usually begins with an influenza-like illness consisting of fever, headache, malaise, and myalgia lasting 1 to 4 days. Somnolence, lethargy, photophobia, vomiting, and neck stiffness may follow; neurologic involvement may rapidly progress to stupor, coma, and seizures. Pareses, cranial nerve deficits, tremors, and abnormal reflexes may be present. In fatal cases, patients die 1 to 2 days after coma develops. Congenital infections have been documented and result in severe and progressive neurologic deterioration.

Leukocytosis and a shift to the left are common. The CSF contains fewer than 500 white blood cells/μL (at first polymorphonuclear, then mononuclear) and an elevated protein concentration (usually 90 to 110 mg/dL).

DIAGNOSIS

Viral isolation from blood or CSF is almost never successful. Diagnosis is achieved by demonstration of a rise in HI, fluorescent antibody, CF, ELISA, or neutralizing antibody titers in appropriately timed (10 to 14 days apart) paired sera. Demonstration of IgM antibodies in serum or CSF by ELISA provides a presumptive diagnosis.

PREVENTION

An experimental formalin-inactivated vaccine grown in chick embryo cell culture has been used to protect laboratory workers but is not indicated for others. In threatened or ongoing epidemics, residents should be advised to use protective clothing, insect repellents, and window screens and to restrict outdoor activity in the early morning, late afternoon, and evening (times of greatest mosquito activity). Public health measures include spraying insecticides aimed at the adult *C. tarsalis* vector.

TREATMENT

There is no specific therapy for western equine encephalitis. Supportive therapy is similar to that discussed earlier for eastern equine encephalitis.

PROGNOSIS

Western equine encephalitis is most severe in infants and young children. The case-fatality rate is between 3 and 5%. Survivors generally experience sudden and rapid recovery. However, about a third of surviving infants suffer mental retardation, cerebellar damage, choreoathetosis, and spastic paralysis. Children with protracted illnesses in whom convulsions develop during the acute stage are more likely to suffer long-term neurologic sequelae. Adults may have a prolonged convalescent syndrome, but objective residua are rare.

VENEZUELAN EQUINE ENCEPHALITIS

Six antigenic subtypes of Venezuelan equine encephalitis virus (I to VI) with several antigenic variants of subtypes I and III are recognized serologically. Subtypes IAB and IC are responsible for epidemics involving humans and equines. In Florida, subtype II is enzootic and produces sporadic human disease. Methods of transmitting Venezuelan equine encephalitis virus as a biologic warfare agent were developed in the 1960s; an epidemic of Venezuelan equine encephalitis, especially if humans and horses become ill simultaneously, could represent an attack rather than naturally occurring illness.

EPIDEMIOLOGY

Before 1973, large equine epizootics occurred at 5- to 10-year intervals in Venezuela, Colombia, Ecuador, and Peru and involved many thousands of animals with mortality rates as high as 40%. Associated human morbidity was also great (up to 32,000 clinical cases). The disease was quiescent for several years but has reemerged in the Gulf Coast region of Mexico in the past decade. The last major outbreak occurred in Venezuela and Colombia in 1995, with more than 85,000 human cases. Laboratory infections are common in unvaccinated persons who work with the virus or infected animals.

A large variety of mosquito vectors, including species of the genera *Aedes*, *Psorophora*, and *Mansonia*, transmit subtypes IAB and IC during epizootic epidemics.[5] Equines are the principal viremic hosts. Virus may be present in the pharyngeal excretions of human patients; contact or aerosol person-to-person spread, although possible, is not epidemiologically important.

The other members of the Venezuelan equine encephalitis viral complex, including subtype II in Florida, have enzootic transmission cycles involving *Culex* mosquitoes and small forest rodents and marsupials. Human disease is sporadic and relatively uncommon.

PATHOBIOLOGY

Pathologic changes in the CNS include edema, congestion, meningeal and perivascular inflammation, intracerebral hemorrhage, neuronal degeneration, and vasculitis. In addition, hepatocellular degeneration and necrosis, widespread lymphoid depletion and follicular necrosis, and interstitial pneumonitis are frequent. Congenitally infected fetuses demonstrate massive and widespread necrosis of brain tissue, hemorrhage, and resorption of brain material resulting in hydranencephaly.

CLINICAL MANIFESTATIONS

The predominant syndrome is a self-limited influenza-like illness; encephalitis develops in only about 4% of infected persons, principally children younger than 15 years. Subclinical infections are rare.

After an incubation period of 2 to 5 days, there is a sudden onset of fever, chills, malaise, and headache, followed by myalgias, nausea, vomiting, and occasionally diarrhea. Physical examination reveals fever, tachycardia, conjunctival injection, and, in some cases, nonexudative pharyngitis. The acute illness generally subsides in 4 to 6 days, and convalescent symptoms may last up to 3 weeks. A biphasic course has sometimes been noted; acute symptoms can reappear after a brief remission, within a week after initial onset.

When it occurs, severe encephalitis is characterized by meningeal signs, seizures, tremor, stupor, coma, spastic paralysis, abnormal reflexes, cranial nerve palsies, and central respiratory failure. Residual neurologic damage occurs in severe cases. Infections of pregnant women acquired during the first and second trimester may result in fetal encephalitis and death.

The peripheral leukocyte count is often low, with a decrease in both lymphocytes and neutrophils, or normal with relative lymphopenia. In patients with CNS signs, the CSF contains up to 500 cells/μL, predominantly lymphocytes. Serum lactate dehydrogenase and aspartate aminotransferase concentrations may be elevated.

DIAGNOSIS

In contrast to the other arboviral encephalitides, Venezuelan equine encephalitis virus can be isolated from blood or from throat swabs or washings during the first 3 or 4 days of illness. Serodiagnosis is usually more practical and is achieved by testing appropriately timed paired sera by HI, CF, ELISA, neutralization, or IgM immunoassay.

PREVENTION

An experimental live attenuated vaccine made from subtype IAB is used for adult laboratory personnel. It provides solid immunity to subtypes IAB and IC but incomplete protection against heterologous Venezuelan equine encephalitis viruses. A phase 1 trial of a DNA vaccine suggests that it is safe and immunogenic. Epidemics and epizootics can be prevented by effective vaccination of equines. Spraying insecticides to reduce adult (infective) mosquito populations is the only means of immediate control in the face of an ongoing epidemic. Individual protection against mosquitoes is advised.

TREATMENT   Rx

No specific therapy is available, and treatment of encephalitis cases is supportive.

PROGNOSIS

The case-fatality rate in children 5 years or younger with encephalitis is approximately 35%, but it is less than 10% in older persons.

JAPANESE ENCEPHALITIS

EPIDEMIOLOGY

Japanese encephalitis virus is a flavivirus that causes epizootics of clinical encephalitis in equines. The disease occurs throughout Asia, including Japan, China, the Korean peninsula, Taiwan, Okinawa, Vietnam, the Philippines, Burma, Malaysia, Bangladesh, east and south India, Sri Lanka, Thailand, and Indonesia. More than 30,000 clinical cases occur annually, about one third of which are fatal. Japanese encephalitis is a summertime disease in temperate areas but occurs sporadically year-round in the tropics. Several species of *Culex* mosquitos can transmit the virus, most notably *C. tritaeniorhynchus*.

Epidemics are most frequent at the northern fringe of the tropical zone, with a high incidence noted in southern China. It is a predominantly rural disease, and the incidence in males is often higher than in females. In hyperendemic areas, more than 70% of adult populations surveyed have antibodies, and children younger than 15 years are principally affected by the disease. In areas without a high prevalence of background immunity (e.g., northern India), however, all age groups are affected. In Japan, where schoolchildren have been protected by vaccination campaigns targeted at this age group, encephalitis has become prominent in the elderly. The ratio of clinically inapparent to apparent infection is higher than 500 : 1 in children and decreases with age; in Korea, the ratio in American servicemen was estimated at 25 : 1.

PATHOBIOLOGY

Neuropathologic changes and the distribution of lesions are similar to those described for St. Louis encephalitis (see later).

CLINICAL MANIFESTATIONS

Manifestations of Japanese encephalitis include abrupt fever, headache, and gastrointestinal symptoms. Meningeal irritation develops within 24 hours and is followed on the second or third day by the appearance of irritability, impaired consciousness, seizures (especially in children), muscle rigidity, parkinsonian findings, ataxia, coarse tremor, involuntary movements, cranial nerve deficits, paresis, hyperactive deep tendon reflexes, and pathologic reflexes.[6] Weight loss and dehydration are often striking findings. In mild cases, fever subsides after the first week, and neurologic signs resolve by the end of the second week after onset. In severe cases, hyperpyrexia, progressive neurologic dysfunction, and coma result in death, usually between the seventh and tenth days. About 25% of patients undergo a prolonged recovery, with permanent sequelae often remaining. The occurrence of such sequelae correlates with severity of the acute stage of illness, and young children are most susceptible. Cardiorespiratory complications are frequent during the acute stage in these patients. A poor prognosis is associated with protracted high fever, frequent or prolonged seizures, high protein content in CSF, Babinski signs, and early respiratory depression. Fetal death from transplacental Japanese encephalitis infection has been reported.

DIAGNOSIS

Moderate peripheral leukocytosis and neutrophilia occur early in the disease. Pleocytosis (predominantly lymphocytic), protein elevation, and normal glucose concentration in CSF are usual findings.

MRI in Japanese encephalitis reveals edema in the basal ganglia, thalami, and focal areas of the cerebral cortex; evidence of hemorrhage in these areas may likewise be present. Enhancement may also be noted in the meninges, brain stem, and spinal cord.

Virus is rarely isolated from blood. Virus is also rarely recovered from the CSF of patients who live but may be recovered from the CSF of a third of patients who die. HI and neutralizing antibodies appear during the first week, and CF antibodies appear during the second week. Cross-reactions with other flaviviruses make serodiagnosis difficult. Specific IgM antibodies in serum or CSF are detectable by immunoassays in more than three fourths of patients at the time of hospital admission.

PREVENTION

Newer inactivated Vero cell culture–derived vaccines, including IC51 (marketed as Ixiaro and Jespect), CC-JEV (marketed as Encevac), and Jenvac, are available for use in persons older than 17 years and have been shown to be safe in children.[A1] They are more immunogenic than the older inactivated mouse brain–derived vaccine. In children who receive the vaccine plus one booster, about 98% continue to have evidence of seroprotection at 5 years.[7] A combined yellow fever–Japanese encephalitis vaccine (ChimeriVax-JE) is available in Australia and Thailand. A chimeric vaccine, which is effective when it is administered concomitantly with measles-mumps-rubella vaccine, holds promise for children in endemic areas.[A2] In China, a live attenuated vaccine (SA14-14-2) is commonly used.

Ixiaro is licensed in the United States for individuals aged 2 months and older traveling to high-risk areas. Generalized urticaria and angioedema may occur in 0.3%. Because two doses of the inactivated vaccine are used and approximately 1 month is required to confer protection, vaccination is not a practical measure in the event of an ongoing epidemic.

Reduction of vector mosquito populations by the application of insecticides may help abort outbreaks. Immunization of swine is an ancillary control strategy.

TREATMENT   Rx

Treatment is supportive (see Eastern Equine Encephalitis). A randomized trial of interferon alfa showed no benefit.

PROGNOSIS

The case-fatality rate is probably about 25%. Sequelae such as mental impairment, emotional lability, choreoathetosis, tremor, parkinsonism, autonomic disturbances, paralysis, and psychiatric disturbances have been reported in up to 75% of patients.

WEST NILE FEVER AND ENCEPHALITIS

The majority of people infected with West Nile virus are asymptomatic, with fever and sometimes a rash developing in about 20% of cases. CNS manifestations, potentially serious and disabling, occur in less than 1% of patients, although this percentage is higher in the elderly. West Nile virus is discussed in Chapter 358.

ZIKA VIRUS

Zika virus (Chapter 358) is a flavivirus related to West Nile virus (Chapter 358) and dengue (Chapter 358). Although the reported cases have been transmitted by *A. egypti*, especially in Oceania, Brazil, and the Caribbean, the virus has also been found in *A. albopictus*, which has a much broader distribution in North America.[8] Symptoms, including fever, rash, arthralgia, and conjunctivitis, often resemble dengue (Chapter 358) and chikungunya (Chapter 358), but are usually milder. In one study in Yap, nearly 75% of the population had been infected based on antibody surveys, but none had been hospitalized or died.

Zika can cause meningoencephalitis, acute demyelinating encephalomyelitis, and myelitis resembling that associated with West Nile virus.[9] Guillain-Barré syndrome (Chapter 392) can occur in up to 1 in 750 cases.[10]

Diagnosis can be confirmed by the detection of viral nucleic acid by RT-PCR within the first week of clinical illness or by the detection of IgM antibodies by IgM-capture enzyme-linked immunosorbent assay (MAC-ELISA) in the first week after the onset of symptoms and persisting for several months. During a Zika outbreak in Colombia about 40% of Guillain-Barré cases were associated with immunologic evidence of recent Zika infection.

Most concerning, however, is the risk to the developing fetus.[11] Zika increased the risk of fetal microcephaly to an absolute risk of about 7% in French territories in the Americas[12] and the risk of gross neurologic abnormalities to

42% in Rio de Janeiro.[13] Rates were above 50% for first- or second-trimester infections and 30% for third-trimester infections.

TREATMENT AND PREVENTION Rx

No proven treatment is available. Zika virus vaccines under development appear to be safe and immunogenic, but their clinical efficacy is uncertain.[14]

ST. LOUIS ENCEPHALITIS

ETIOLOGY

St. Louis encephalitis virus, a member of the family Flaviviridae, shares close antigenic relationships with Japanese encephalitis, Murray Valley encephalitis, and West Nile viruses and is related to yellow fever (Chapter 357) and dengue (Chapter 358) viruses. Strains associated with *Culex pipiens*–borne epidemics in the northern United States are distinct from endemic strains transmitted by *C. tarsalis* in the western states.

EPIDEMIOLOGY

The virus is present in all parts of the Western Hemisphere, but epidemics occur only in North America and some Caribbean islands. During epidemic years, the virus has been responsible for up to 80% of all reported cases of encephalitis of known etiology in the United States. Epidemics of up to 2000 cases have taken place, mainly in urban-suburban localities of the Ohio-Mississippi River basin and in eastern and central Texas and Florida. Small outbreaks have also occurred in the western United States.[15] Epidemics generally take place between July and September but may arise later in the year in warm areas such as Florida. Previous exposure and immunity to dengue may provide a degree of cross-protection against clinical St. Louis encephalitis. The ratio of inapparent to apparent infection is 800:1 in children up to 9 years of age, 400:1 in persons aged 10 to 49 years, and 85:1 in persons older than 60 years.

In most of the eastern United States, St. Louis encephalitis virus circulates between wild birds and *C. pipiens* mosquitoes, which breed in polluted water. In Florida and in parts of the Caribbean, *C. nigripalpus* is the principal vector. The cycle in the western United States also involves wild birds, but the vector is *C. tarsalis,* also that of western equine encephalitis. Because of the similar ecology of St. Louis encephalitis and western equine encephalitis viruses in the West, mixed outbreaks occur, mostly in rural, agricultural areas.

Above-average summer temperatures and conditions such as deficient rainfall, which create stagnant pools suitable for *C. pipiens* breeding, are associated with epidemics in the eastern United States. St. Louis encephalitis in the western states is favored by warm spring temperatures, heavy snow melt, and flooding.

PATHOBIOLOGY

Pathologic changes in fatal cases are limited to microscopic findings. Leptomeningitis is characterized by lymphocytic inflammation. Parenchymal changes consist of lymphocytic perivascular cuffing, cellular nodule formation, and neuronal degeneration.

CLINICAL MANIFESTATIONS

Three clinical syndromes are recognized: febrile headache, aseptic meningitis, and encephalitis. After an incubation period of 4 to 21 days, a variable period of nonspecific symptoms, including fever (temperature of 38° to 41° C), headache, malaise, drowsiness, myalgia, and sore throat, may be followed by an acute or subacute onset of meningeal or encephalitic signs, or both. Nausea, vomiting, and photophobia are common.

Neurologic abnormalities occur in up to 25% of patients. Extrapyramidal abnormalities and altered consciousness are the most significant findings. Other findings include meningismus, cranial nerve deficits (particularly the facial nerve), abnormal reflexes, tremors, myoclonic twitching, nystagmus, and ataxia. Motor abnormalities are infrequent, and sensory changes are extremely uncommon. Seizures occur in 10% of patients and are a poor prognostic sign, as is a persistent high temperature of 40° to 41° C. Signs of markedly increased intracranial pressure are unusual. A Guillain-Barré–like syndrome (Chapter 392) has occasionally been associated with St. Louis encephalitis, both as an acute manifestation and during the convalescent period.

In uncomplicated cases of St. Louis encephalitis, a moderate peripheral neutrophilic leukocytosis and shift to the left are noted. CSF pressure is elevated, protein level is mildly elevated, and glucose concentration is normal; a pleocytosis of up to 500 cells/μL is present, with an early neutrophilia predominance changing to lymphocytes within days. Serum creatine kinase, aspartate aminotransferase, and aldolase levels are frequently elevated. The electroencephalogram typically shows polymorphic delta activity, most prominently in the frontal and temporal regions; electrographic seizures are common. CT scans are normal, but MRI may show edema involving deep structures such as the substantia nigra. Hypo-osmolality, presumably as a result of the syndrome of inappropriate antidiuretic hormone secretion (Chapter 212), is noted in a third of patients.

Genitourinary tract symptoms (urgency, frequency, incontinence, and retention), microscopic hematuria, pyuria, proteinuria, and elevated blood urea nitrogen are frequent. St. Louis encephalitis viral antigen in cells of the urinary sediment has been detected by fluorescent techniques, and virus-like particles have been detected in urine by immunoelectron microscopy.

DIAGNOSIS

St. Louis encephalitis virus is rarely isolated from blood or CSF obtained during the acute phase of illness. Serologic diagnosis is achieved by demonstration of changing antibody titers; the HI, fluorescent, ELISA, and neutralizing tests demonstrate antibody within the first week after onset, and titers rise during the ensuing 2 weeks. CF antibodies appear 10 to 20 days after onset. Rapid, early diagnosis is possible by detection of IgM antibodies by ELISA in serum and CSF. Serologic cross-reactions may occur in persons with previous exposure to dengue, West Nile, and other related flaviviruses. RT-PCR provides a more specific diagnosis, but its sensitivity is uncertain.

PREVENTION

No vaccine is available for St. Louis encephalitis. Surveillance of viral activity in vectors and avian hosts is used to define the risk for human infection and to initiate vector control efforts. In an established outbreak, avoidance of mosquito bites and spraying to reduce infected adult mosquitoes are the only effective means of control.

TREATMENT Rx

Treatment is supportive.

PROGNOSIS

A convalescent syndrome characterized by weakness, fatigue, nervousness, tremulousness, sleeplessness, irritability, depression, difficulty concentrating, and headaches occurs in 30 to 50% of older persons and clears in 80% of them within 3 years. The overall case-fatality rate is approximately 9%. Mortality is negligible in persons younger than 20 years but rises steeply after 55 years to approximately 30% in patients older than 65 years. Approximately 50% of the deaths occur during the first week, and 80% occur within 2 weeks after onset.

MURRAY VALLEY ENCEPHALITIS AND ROCIO ENCEPHALITIS

Murray Valley encephalitis and Rocio encephalitis, which are similar to Japanese encephalitis in their pathogenesis and clinical features, are caused by closely related flaviviruses. Murray Valley encephalitis has occurred in small epidemics in the Murray and Darling River valleys of Victoria and New South Wales, Australia. The virus is endemic in northern Australia and New Guinea, where it is maintained in a bird-mosquito cycle. Rocio encephalitis has caused epidemics of 1000 or more cases in São Paulo State, Brazil.

TICK-BORNE ENCEPHALITIS

PATHOGENS

A complex of six antigenically related tick-borne flaviviruses cause encephalitis: Powassan, tick-borne encephalitis, louping ill, Kyasanur Forest disease, Omsk hemorrhagic fever, and Langat viruses. The predominant syndrome is hemorrhagic fever (Chapter 357), but meningoencephalitis may be a component of the disease spectrum. Two subtypes of tick-borne encephalitis virus (central European encephalitis and Russian spring-summer encephalitis) are distinguished by serologic tests, are ecologically distinct, and differ in virulence for humans. Powassan and louping ill viruses are rare causes of encephalitis in North America and the British Isles, respectively. These viruses are easily distinguished serologically from mosquito-borne flaviviruses but induce cross-reactions within the complex.

EPIDEMIOLOGY

Tick-borne encephalitis occurs in Europe (including eastern Europe and Ukraine), southern Scandinavia, and far eastern Russia during the summer months, which corresponds to peak tick vector populations. Several hundred to more than 2000 cases are reported annually, with morbidity rates of up to 20 per 100,000 inhabitants. Adults older than 20 years are mainly affected, and persons frequenting wooded areas that are heavily tick infested are at highest risk. In Europe, the disease is relatively mild (case-fatality rate of 1 to 2%), but in the Far East, it is severe (20 to 25%).

The vector of tick-borne encephalitis is *Ixodes ricinus* in Europe and *Ixodes persulcatus* in the Far East. The tick vector also serves as a reservoir for the virus. Larval ticks parasitize small rodents, which serve as amplifying viremic hosts during the spring and summer. Large vertebrates (goats, sheep, cattle) are hosts for nymphal and adult ticks. Outbreaks have occurred in families or groups of individuals ingesting unpasteurized milk or cheese from goats or sheep.

CLINICAL MANIFESTATIONS

Inapparent infections are common. Symptomatic tick-borne encephalitis in Europe typically (but not invariably) has a biphasic course beginning 7 to 14 days after exposure with an influenza-like illness that lasts 1 week, followed by a period of clinical remission for several days and then an abrupt onset of aseptic meningitis or meningoencephalitis. The meningoencephalitis is usually benign, although severe paralytic illness, myelitis, myeloradiculitis, and bulbar forms may occur.

In the Far East, tick-borne encephalitis begins suddenly with fever, headache, and gastrointestinal symptoms, followed rapidly by the appearance of depressed sensorium, coma, convulsions, and paralysis. Bulbar paralysis and cervical myelitis are frequent findings. In fatal cases, death occurs in the first week after onset. Aseptic meningitis and milder forms of encephalitis also occur. Chronic forms of tick-borne encephalitis have been described, with active clinical and pathologic abnormalities present a year or more after onset.

DIAGNOSIS

Brain MRI in patients with tick-borne encephalitis shows evidence of edema in the basal ganglia, thalami, and brain stem in about 20% of cases. MRI of the spinal cord may show anterior horn cell lesions corresponding to lower motor neuron weakness on examination.

Isolation of virus from blood is also possible during the early phase of illness. Serologic diagnosis is achieved by the HI, CF, neutralization, or ELISA techniques.

PREVENTION

In eastern Europe and the former Soviet Union, vaccines are used in high-risk groups (forestry and agricultural workers, military personnel).[16] In Austria, immunization of the general population has resulted in a marked decline in incidence. Avoidance of tick exposure by wearing of protective clothing and use of repellents may be recommended in areas of high tick-borne encephalitis activity.

TREATMENT   Rx

Treatment is supportive (see Eastern Equine Encephalitis).

PROGNOSIS

In European tick-borne encephalitis, convalescence is often prolonged, and residual paralysis may follow in severe cases. In the Far East, survivors frequently have residual paralysis, especially lower motor neuron paralysis of the upper extremities or shoulder girdle as a result of spinal cord involvement.

Louping III Encephalitis

Louping ill causes encephalitis in sheep (rarely in cattle, horses, and swine) in Scotland, northern England, and Ireland. Sporadic human cases have been recognized. Louping ill virus is maintained in nature by *I. ricinus* ticks and a variety of hosts, including small mammals, ground-dwelling birds (grouse), and probably sheep. The clinical features of louping ill resemble the European form of tick-borne encephalitis.

Powassan Virus Encephalitis

Powassan virus encephalitis has been documented in an increasing number of cases in the northeastern United States and eastern Canada in recent years.[17] The virus is not associated with animal disease. The transmission cycle of Powassan virus involves *Ixodes cookei, I. marxi,* and possibly other tick species along with mammals, particularly rodents and carnivores. Powassan encephalitis is characterized by fever and nonspecific symptoms, followed by encephalitic signs, which are frequently severe. Peripheral blood and CSF changes are similar to those described for other forms of flaviviral encephalitis. The case-fatality rate is about 50%, and residual paralysis may persist in survivors.

CALIFORNIA SEROGROUP ENCEPHALITIS

At least four members of the California serogroup of the Bunyaviridae family (Bunyavirus genus)—La Crosse, California encephalitis, Jamestown Canyon, and snowshoe hare viruses—cause encephalitis. California encephalitis virus occurs in the western United States (California, New Mexico, Utah, Texas) and has been implicated only rarely in human infections. In contrast, La Crosse virus, distributed more widely in the eastern half of the United States and southern Canada, is a major human pathogen. Jamestown Canyon and snowshoe hare viruses have also been implicated in sporadic cases of human encephalitis in the north central United States and Canada. California serogroup viruses have been implicated in human disease in China and the former Soviet Union.

EPIDEMIOLOGY

California serogroup encephalitis occurs as an endemic rather than an epidemic disease, with individual or small clusters of cases scattered across affected areas. Seventy to 120 cases are reported each year, generally between July and September, with a peak incidence in August. The virus primarily affects persons younger than 15 years living in rural and suburban areas characterized by deciduous hardwood forests. It is most prevalent in the north central states, where it is responsible for as many as 20% of cases of acute CNS infection in children. Focal "hot spots" (communities, even backyards) of recurrent summertime viral activity are recognized. The ratio of inapparent to apparent infection has been estimated variably at between 26 : 1 and 157 : 1.

The vector of La Crosse virus is *Aedes triseriatus,* which breeds both in forest tree holes and in artificial containers, notably discarded tires. This vector also serves as a reservoir for La Crosse virus. Wild rodents (squirrels, chipmunks) contribute to the cycle of transmission as viremic hosts. Humans acquire the disease by being bitten by an infected mosquito. *Aedes communis, A. stimulans, A. triseriatus,* and possibly anopheline mosquitoes are involved in transmitting Jamestown Canyon virus, and deer are the principal vertebrate hosts.

PATHOBIOLOGY

Histopathologic features in the CNS are qualitatively similar to those of other viral encephalitides. However, absence of inflammatory lesions in the cerebellum, medulla, and spinal cord may be a distinguishing feature of La Crosse infection.

CLINICAL MANIFESTATIONS

The clinical spectrum of California serogroup virus infection includes nonspecific febrile illness, aseptic meningitis, and meningoencephalitis. The disease begins with fever, headache, sore throat, and gastrointestinal symptoms. In mild cases, CNS signs appear on the third day after onset and subside within 7 to 8 days. In the more severe form, neurologic signs appear within 24 to 48 hours of onset, usually in the form of generalized seizures, elevated intracranial pressure, and altered consciousness, and persist longer. Encephalitis may be severe in the acute stage, but the disease is almost always self-limited; death is extremely rare.

The peripheral white blood cell count is elevated, with a predominance of polymorphonuclear cells and a shift to the left. CSF contains up to 500 lymphocytes/μL; the protein level is normal or mildly elevated, and the glucose concentration is normal. The electroencephalogram reveals generalized slowing in the delta and theta range; focal delta wave activity related to cortical destruction and focal seizures are also common findings.

DIAGNOSIS

In contrast to the other arboviral encephalitides, brain MRI in patients with California serogroup encephalitides may show lesions involving the temporal lobe in a pattern similar to that of herpes simplex encephalitis. The virus cannot be recovered from blood or CSF obtained during the acute phase. Diagnosis is best achieved by counterimmunoelectrophoresis, HI, CF, fluorescent, ELISA, and neutralization tests for antibody in paired acute and convalescent sera. The most practical, sensitive, and reliable methods are the HI test with La Crosse viral antigen and IgM antibody capture ELISA. Viral RNA can be detected in CSF or brain tissue by RT-PCR, although the sensitivity of the test remains to be determined.

PREVENTION

There is no vaccine for California encephalitis, although research involving DNA-based vaccines appears promising. Vector control methods are of uncertain usefulness in this disease. In defined hot spots of recurrent viral activity, breeding sites for *A. triseriatus* should be eliminated, particularly by draining or eliminating standing water (e.g., discarded tires or birdbaths) and filling holes in trees. Parents should protect children by limiting exposure and using mosquito repellents.

TREATMENT Rx

Treatment is supportive.

PROGNOSIS

The case-fatality rate is less than 1%. The risk for permanent neuropsychiatric sequelae is unclear, but hemiparesis and persistent seizure disorders have been reported.

Grade A References

A1. Dubischar KL, Kadlecek V, Sablan B Jr, et al. Safety of the inactivated Japanese encephalitis virus vaccine IXIARO in children: an open-label, randomized, active-controlled, phase 3 study. *Pediatr Infect Dis J.* 2017;36:889-897.

A2. Huang LM, Lin TY, Chiu CH, et al. Concomitant administration of live attenuated Japanese encephalitis chimeric virus vaccine (JE-CV) and measles, mumps, rubella (MMR) vaccine: randomized study in toddlers in Taiwan. *Vaccine.* 2014;32:5363-5369.

GENERAL REFERENCES

For the General References and other additional features, please visit Expert Consult at https://expertconsult.inkling.com.

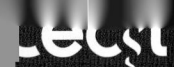

XXV

HIV AND THE ACQUIRED IMMUNODEFICIENCY SYNDROME

360

EPIDEMIOLOGY AND DIAGNOSIS OF HUMAN IMMUNODEFICIENCY VIRUS INFECTION AND ACQUIRED IMMUNODEFICIENCY SYNDROME

LARRY W. CHANG AND THOMAS C. QUINN

GLOBAL STATISTICS

Since the HIV epidemic began in the first half of the 20th century, more than 76 million people have been infected with HIV and 35 million people have died of HIV.[1] In 2016, according to estimates by the Joint United Nations Program on HIV/AIDS (UNAIDS), 36.7 million people were living with HIV (Table 360-1 and Fig. 360-1). Adults constituted the majority of those infected; children (persons less than 15 years of age) accounted for 2.1 million infections. Globally, people living with HIV were evenly divided by gender, although there was substantial regional variation. For example, women accounted for 59% of adults living with HIV infection in sub-Saharan Africa compared with 35% outside of this region. Sub-Saharan Africa continued to have the majority of persons living with HIV and the highest HIV prevalence rates, but large epidemics are present worldwide (Fig. 360-2 and see Table 360-1). The continuing rise in the population of people living with HIV infection reflects the combined effects of continued HIV transmission and the beneficial impact of antiretroviral therapy, resulting in fewer deaths.[2]

In 2016, 1.8 million people became newly infected with HIV globally, which has been a decline of 16% since 2010 and a marked decline from the more than 3 million infections per year experienced during the peak of the epidemic in the 1990s (see Fig. 360-1B and Table 360-1). These declines have been most prominent among children, in whom new infections have decreased by 47% since 2010; decreases in adults have occurred more slowly, 11% since 2010. Despite this progress, declines remain well short of the pace needed to meet United Nation's 2020 targets of 500,000 infections per year. Progress has been uneven across regions, with the steepest declines in new HIV infections in eastern and southern Africa (29%) compared with a troubling 60% rise in new infections in eastern Europe and central Asia. Low- and middle-income settings constitute more than 90% of new infections, and sub-Saharan Africa alone accounts for 64% of all new HIV infections globally.

The major mode of HIV transmission globally in 2016 was heterosexual transmission, although infections continue to spread at high rates among key populations such as men who have sex with men (MSM) and people who inject drugs (PWID). These and other key populations continue to play important roles in all major regional epidemics (E-Fig. 360-1). Outside of sub-Saharan Africa, key populations and their partners accounted for 80% of new HIV infections in 2015. Overall, women acquire new HIV infections at roughly the same rate as men. However, new infections in young women aged 15 to 24 years were 44% higher than in men, which is a particular concern because this age group accounted for 34% of all new HIV infections in 2016 and is part of an ongoing demographic youth bulge.

HIV continues to be a major source of global morbidity and mortality, although significant progress has been made in scaling up treatment. Deaths from HIV have declined from a peak of 1.9 million deaths in 2005 to 1.0 million in 2016 (Fig. 360-1C), likely owing to increased HIV treatment access and fewer new HIV infections. Gender disparities in mortality are substantial, with deaths 27% lower among women compared with men, likely because of higher HIV treatment uptake among women. There have been even sharper declines in child mortality due to HIV, with 120,000 deaths in 2016 compared with 210,000 in 2010, a 43% decline. Similar to reductions in new HIV infections, declines in deaths due to AIDS-related illnesses have been most pronounced in eastern and southern Africa. In contrast, there have been concerning increases in AIDS-related mortality in the Middle East and North Africa and eastern Europe and central Asia (E-Fig. 360-2).

GLOBAL IMPACT AND RESPONSE

For the first two decades of the epidemic, fatality rates from AIDS steadily increased, and the average life expectancy in some countries in sub-Saharan Africa declined from 62 to 47 years of age. For example, in Haiti, life expectancy was nearly 6 years less than it would have been in the absence of AIDS. Cambodia experienced a reduction in life expectancy of more than 4 years. In 1995 in the United States, AIDS was the leading killer of Americans aged 25 to 44 years. Globally, HIV has now claimed an estimated 35 million lives.

Beginning in 1996 in high-income countries, the advent of combination antiretroviral therapy for HIV infection led to dramatic declines in HIV-associated mortality. However, low-income and most middle-income countries (with the notable exception of Brazil) were initially not able to access these medications widely. At an unprecedented 2001 special session of the United Nations General Assembly on AIDS, 189 nations agreed that AIDS was a national and international security issue of the highest priority. The Global Fund for AIDS, Tuberculosis, and Malaria was subsequently founded in 2002 and raised funds from private donations and industrialized countries to help support access to care and treatment in low-income countries. This new organization was joined by the U.S. President's Emergency Plan for AIDS Relief (PEPFAR), which began in 2004 and continues to provide treatment and care for HIV-infected individuals globally, as well as additional resources for enhancing prevention efforts to prevent further transmission. PEPFAR has become the single largest global health commitment in United States history.

As of 2016, an estimated 70% of people living with HIV globally are aware of their HIV status. Among those who know their status, an estimated 77% are on treatment, meaning that among all people living with HIV, about 53% are on treatment (Figs. 360-3 and 360-4). Of people on treatment, an estimated 82% are virally suppressed. Thus, in 2016, about 44% of all people living with HIV are currently virally suppressed (Fig. 360-4). While this represents remarkable progress from the early 2000s, significant gaps in testing and care remain. There is also considerable regional variation, with progress on 90-90-90 targets well advanced or met in countries in western and central Europe and North

| **TABLE 360-1** | REGIONAL HUMAN IMMUNODEFICIENCY VIRUS AND ACQUIRED IMMUNODEFICIENCY SYNDROME STATISTICS AND FEATURES AT THE END OF 2016 |

REGION	ADULTS AND CHILDREN LIVING WITH HIV/AIDS	ADULTS AND CHILDREN NEWLY INFECTED WITH HIV	MAIN MODES OF TRANSMISSION FOR ADULTS LIVING WITH HIV/AIDS
Eastern and southern Africa	19,400,000	790,000	Hetero
Western and central Africa	5,100,000	270,000	Hetero
North Africa and Middle East	230,000	18,000	Hetero, IDU
Asia and the Pacific	5,100,000	270,000	Hetero, IDU
Latin America	1,800,000	97,000	MSM, IDU, Hetero
Caribbean	310,000	18,000	Hetero, MSM
Eastern Europe and central Asia	1,600,000	190,000	IDU, Hetero, MSM
Western and central Europe and North America	2,100,000	73,000	MSM, IDU, Hetero
Total	36,700,000	1,800,000	

AIDS = acquired immunodeficiency syndrome; Hetero = heterosexual transmission; HIV = human immunodeficiency virus; IDU = transmission through injection drug use; MSM = sexual transmission through men who have sex with men.

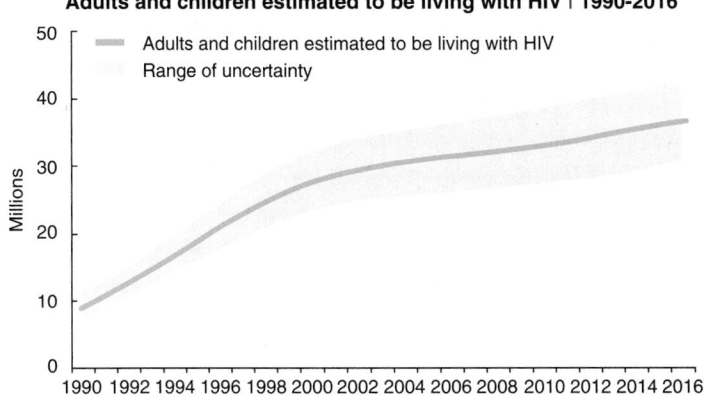

Adults and children estimated to be living with HIV | 1990-2016

A

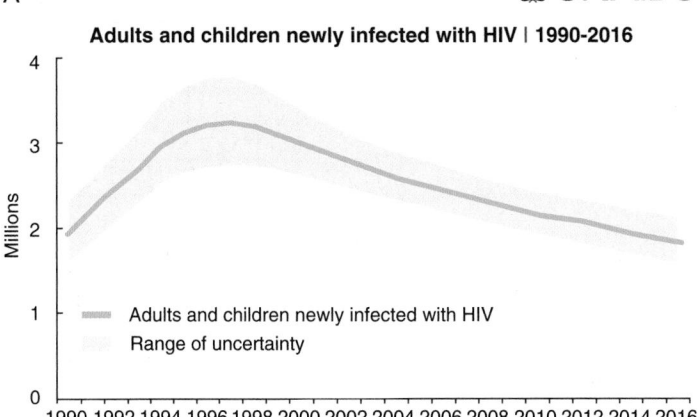

Adults and children newly infected with HIV | 1990-2016

B

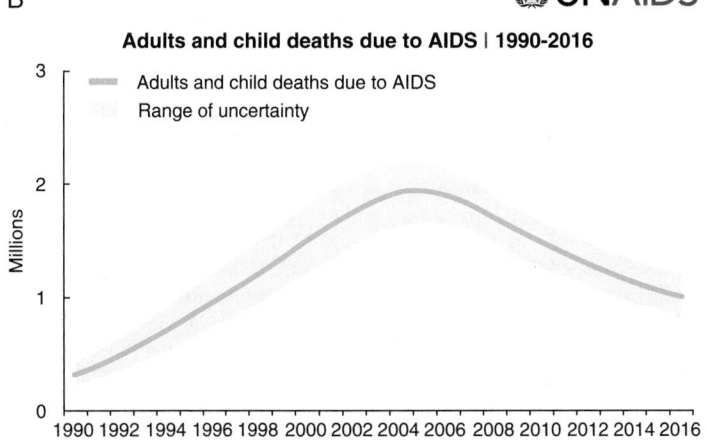

Adults and child deaths due to AIDS | 1990-2016

C

FIGURE 360-1. **A total of 36.7 million people were living with HIV infection in 2016. Global HIV trends in number of people living with HIV (A), new infections (B), and fatalities (C), from 1990 to 2016. (Data from WHO 2017.)**

America, but less so in eastern Europe and central Asia, the Middle East, and North Africa (E-Fig. 360-1). There is also large variation within regions. For example, Botswana is the first country in Africa to have already reached 90-90-90 targets.[3]

Specifically regarding HIV treatment access, in 2016, an estimated 19.5 million people were on treatment, a 35-fold increase since 2005 (see Fig. 360-4). The trajectory of treatment access has been consistently upward for the past decade and a half and is on target to reach 2020 UNAIDS goals of 30 million people on antiretroviral therapy. People living with HIV also appear to be accessing antiretroviral therapy earlier after initial HIV infection, although 29% of people globally still initiate treatment with CD4$^+$ T-cell counts less than 200 cell/μL. The rapid expansion of antiretroviral therapy is one of the most remarkable achievements in recent public health history. As a result of the

rapid increases in treatment, life expectancy losses have been largely reversed in many countries (E-Fig. 360-2).[4] Modeling and early empirical evidence suggest that treatment scale-up to 90-90-90 targets in conjunction with other HIV prevention interventions will have substantial impact on reducing HIV incidence.[5] Expanded treatment access to pregnant women living with HIV has already resulted in large declines in mother-to-child transmission of HIV.

While progress in HIV prevention and treatment service access has been impressive, numerous challenges remain. These include significant gender disparities, with men globally having lower coverage of antiretroviral therapy (47%) compared with women (60%). Men are also less likely to have suppressed HIV viral loads. Young people living with HIV are less likely to know their HIV status, be on treatment, and have suppressed viral loads compared with older age groups. Key populations, sex workers, MSM, people who inject drugs (PWID), transgender people, and prisoners have additional barriers to testing and care, which have led to disproportionate gaps in the HIV prevention and care cascade. HIV viral load testing access has increased rapidly: 8.1 million people living with HIV had access to HIV viral load testing in 2016 compared with 4.4 million a year prior, but more than half of persons on treatment remain without periodic viral load testing. In almost all target countries, global uptake of voluntary medical male circumcision, which has been found to reduce the risk for HIV acquisition among heterosexual men by about 55% and among MSM by about 20%,[A1] remains well below World Health Organization targets of 90%. Condoms, an effective HIV prevention tool, remain underused. Globally, comprehensive harm reduction programs for PWID, including needle-syringe programs and opioid substitution therapy, are also infrequently implemented. Finally, stigma, discrimination, and HIV criminalization laws hinder HIV service uptake and retention, particularly among key populations.

Numerous strategies are being used in the continuing global response to overcome existing challenges across the continuum of care. These include the expansion of relatively new interventions such as pre-exposure prophylaxis (PrEP), either on-demand[A2] or daily[A3] among high-risk HIV-negative persons (E-Fig. 360-3)[A4] and HIV self-testing and community-based testing to increase awareness of HIV serostatus. Differentiated care, a client-centered approach to HIV service delivery, is another approach being implemented that attempts to simplify and adapt HIV services to individual patient circumstances (e.g., stable people living with HIV on antiretroviral therapy with undetectable viral loads may need fewer provider visits, or a group of people living with HIV may form community-based treatment and support groups). New, cheaper, and improved antiretroviral therapy in many global settings may also improve access and patient outcomes. Linkage of people living with HIV into care and retention when they are in care are also critical areas needing strengthening to reach global targets. In the years to come, additional resources will be required to reach the additional millions of HIV-infected people who require treatment and millions of HIV-negative persons who would benefit from HIV prevention services.

● REGIONAL EPIDEMICS AND RESPONSES

Eastern and Southern Africa

The 19 countries that make up eastern and southern Africa represents the epicenter of the global HIV/AIDS pandemic (see Table 360-1).[6] In the first half of the 20th century in sub-Saharan Africa, humans initially became infected from a similar, related retrovirus in chimpanzees and sooty mangabey monkeys. This retrovirus then evolved within the human host into what we now know is HIV. For years, the infection remained limited to remote rural regions of Africa, but with urbanization, infected individuals migrated to major urban centers, where transmission was amplified, and HIV spread to thousands of individuals within a relatively short period and eventually into a global pandemic.

Today, more than half of all people living with HIV are in eastern and southern Africa. HIV prevalence overall was 7.0% in 2016 but varied widely across countries, a modest decline from regional rates as high as 9% around the turn of the century. The highest HIV prevalence rates in the world are found in Swaziland (27.2%). South Africa, the most populous country in this region, has an HIV prevalence of 18.9%. The main mode of transmission is heterosexual sex (see Table 360-1). The number of new HIV infections in eastern and southern Africa has dropped from 1.1 million in 2010 to 790,000 in 2016, a 29% decline. However, some countries, such as Ethiopia and Madagascar, experienced increases in the number of new infections over the same time period. Notably, South Africa alone accounted for one third of new HIV infections in 2016. A key intervention to prevent HIV, voluntary medical male circumcision, has only increased modestly in this region (E-Fig. 360-4).

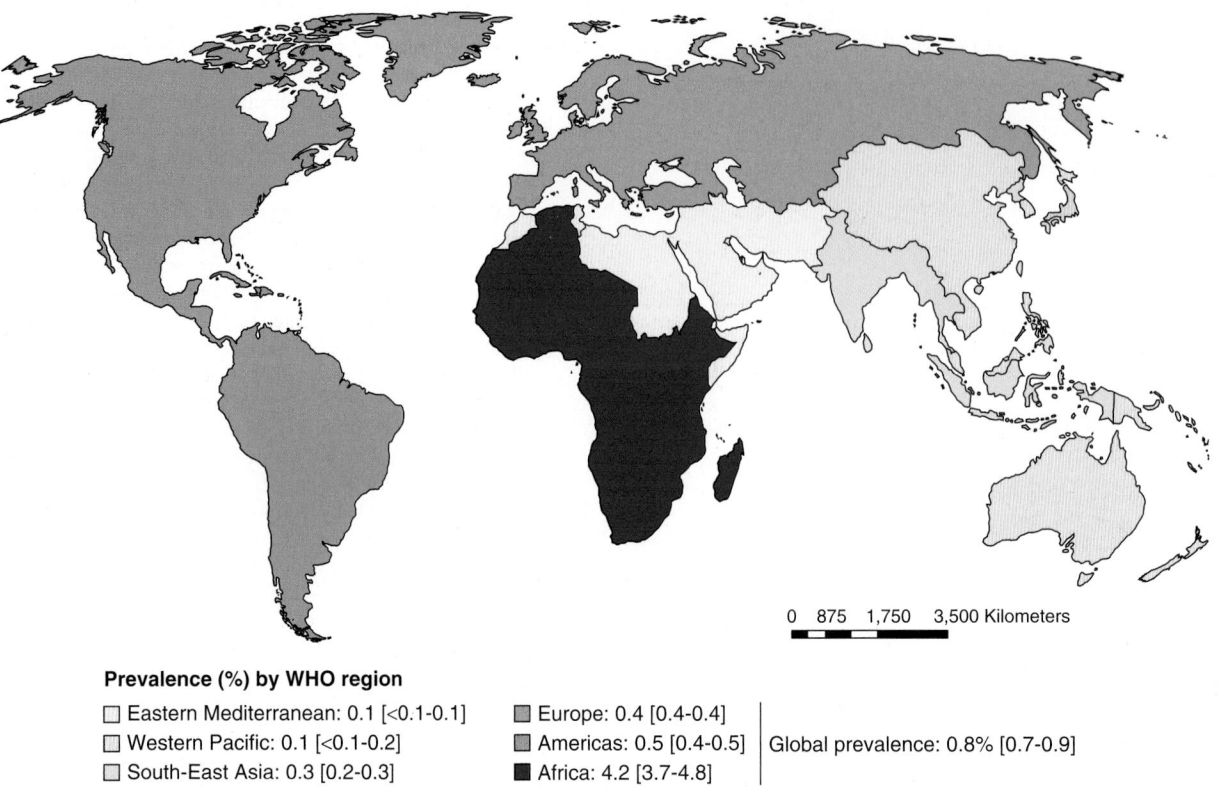

Prevalence of HIV among adults aged 15 to 49, 2016
By WHO region

0   875   1,750   3,500 Kilometers

Prevalence (%) by WHO region

☐ Eastern Mediterranean: 0.1 [<0.1-0.1]   ☐ Europe: 0.4 [0.4-0.4]
☐ Western Pacific: 0.1 [<0.1-0.2]   ☐ Americas: 0.5 [0.4-0.5]   Global prevalence: 0.8% [0.7-0.9]
☐ South-East Asia: 0.3 [0.2-0.3]   ■ Africa: 4.2 [3.7-4.8]

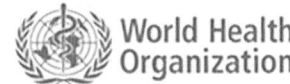 World Health Organization

FIGURE 360-2. Prevalence of HIV among adults aged 15-49 years, 2016, by World Health Organization (WHO) region. The boundaries and names shown and the designations used on this map do not imply the expression of any opinion whatsoever on the part of the World Health Organization concerning the legal status of any country, territory, city or area of its authorities, or concerning the delimitation of its frontiers or boundaries. (Data from WHO 2017.)

Knowledge of HIV status in eastern and southern Africa has risen steeply over the past decade. Currently, about 75% of all people living with HIV in this region are aware of their HIV status (E-Fig. 360-5), 60% are on treatment, and an estimated 50% are virally suppressed, still well short of the 73% viral suppression goals of the 90-90-90 targets for 2020. Nevertheless, significant progress has been made with treatment scale-up, with an estimated 11.7 million people on treatment in eastern and southern Africa in 2016, triple the number in 2010 (see E-Fig. 360-5). As a result, mortality from AIDS-related deaths in this region has dropped by 42% since 2010 to a still substantial 420,000 deaths in 2016. Continued support of treatment and prevention services will be needed if this region is to maintain and build on recent advances.

Western and Central Africa

This region includes 24 countries and accounts for 17% of people living with HIV globally. Overall HIV prevalence was 2.0% in this region, with prevalence ranging from 6.2% in Equatorial Guinea to 0.4% in Niger. The main mode of transmission is heterosexual sex (see Table 360-1). The number of HIV infections in this region declined modestly by 9% from 2010 to 2016, 400,000 to 370,000. In countries such as Congo, Ghana, and Liberia, the number of new infections increased by more than 15%. Of note, Nigeria accounted for 59% of new HIV infections in this region in 2016 because of its large population; however, the number of new infections decreased in Nigeria by 6% from 2010 to 2016.

Knowledge of HIV serostatus remains suboptimal in this region, with only 42% of people living with HIV being aware of their status, 35% being on treatment, and an estimated 25% being virally suppressed (E-Fig. 360-6), well below UNAIDS goals. Not surprisingly, AIDS-related mortality remains substantial in this region, with 310,000 deaths in 2016, a smaller decrease than has been seen in eastern and southern Africa (see E-Fig. 360-6). HIV testing, prevention, and treatment programs will need to be expanded in this region to better address the ongoing epidemic.

North Africa and the Middle East

This region includes 21 countries and contains 230,000 people living with HIV. HIV prevalence averages less than 0.1% in countries in this region. The number of new HIV cases in North Africa and the Middle East has remained stable between 2010 and 2016 at around 18,000 cases annually. Certain countries have had drops in new cases during this time, such as Morocco (42%) and Iran (14%). In contrast, Egypt (76% increase) and Yemen (44% increase) have moved in the opposite direction. Three countries—Iran, Sudan, and Somalia—accounted for 65% of all new HIV infections in this region. The epidemic in this region is driven primarily by a combination of injection drug use and heterosexual transmission.

Knowledge of HIV status in this region in 2016 was 58% (E-Fig. 360-7). Access to antiretrovirals among all people living with HIV was 24%, which is very far off global goals but does represent a doubling of access since 2010. Viral suppression among all people living with HIV was 16%, dramatically short of the UNAIDS goal of 73% viral suppression. In contrast to most other regions, AIDS-related deaths in North Africa and the Middle East rose from 3600 deaths in 2010 to 11,000 deaths in 2016, a staggering 205% increase. This region still needs substantial additional efforts to close major gaps in treatment and prevention cascades.

Asia and the Pacific

After sub-Saharan Africa, Asia and the Pacific, home to 30 countries and 60% of the world's population, have the second largest number of HIV-infected individuals in the world, estimated at 5.1 million, which is 14% of the global total.[7] With the exception of Thailand, where HIV prevalence is 1.1%, national HIV prevalence levels remain comparatively low, less than 1%, in most countries of Asia and the Pacific. However, low prevalences in large population bases can result in substantial HIV burdens. For example, India's national adult HIV prevalence rate of 0.3% offers little indication of the serious situation facing the country, where an estimated 2.1 million people were living

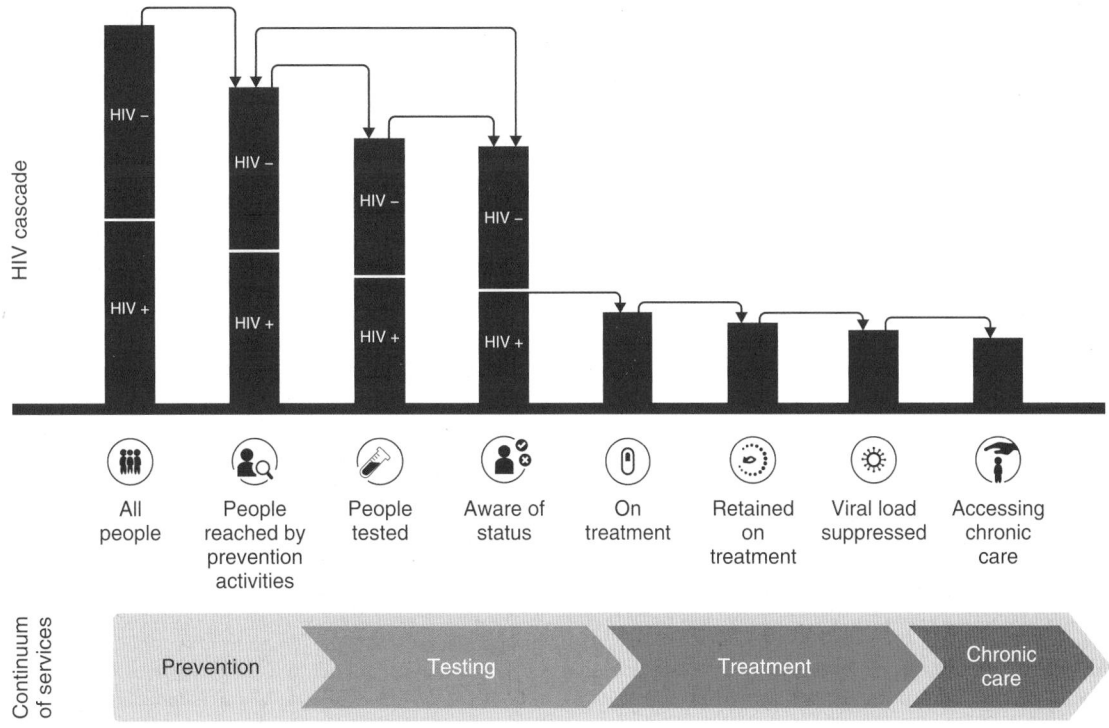

Source: Global Health Sector Strategy on HIV, 2016-2021.

World Health Organization

FIGURE 360-3. HIV prevention and care cascade describes the continuum of services for preventing and treating HIV. (Data from WHO Global Health Sector Strategy on HIV, 2016-2021. Geneva: WHO; 2016.)

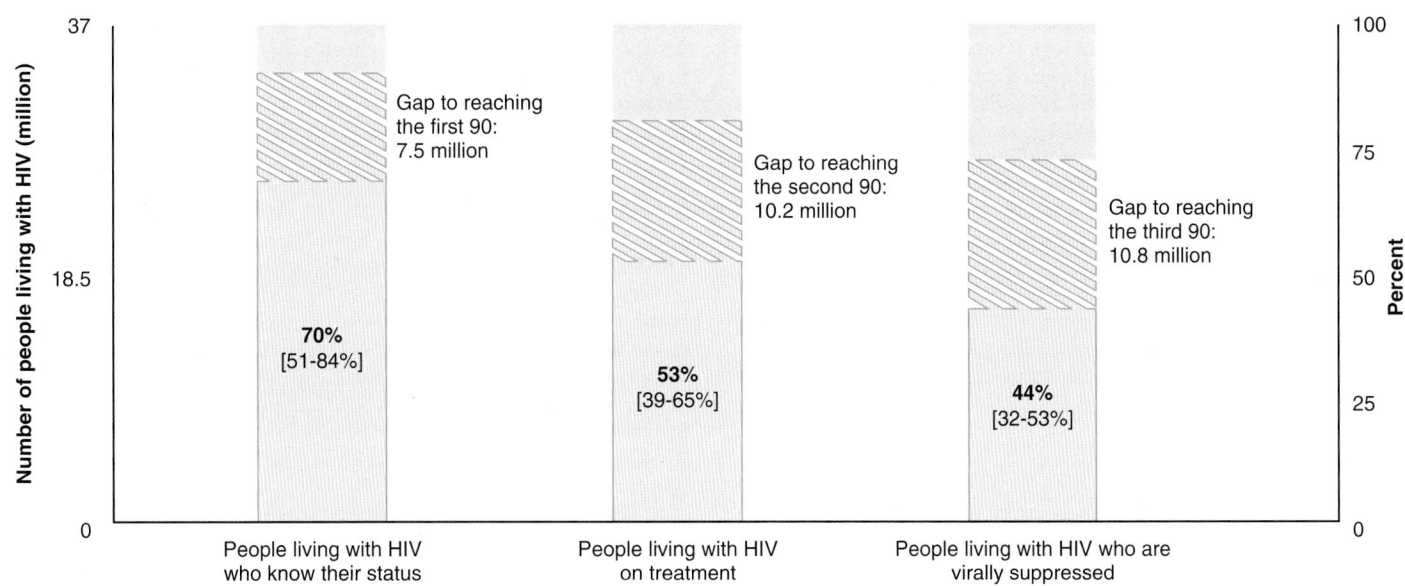

The HIV testing and treatment cascade

Knowledge of HIV status, treatment coverage, and viral load suppression, global, 2016

Source: UNAIDS special analysis, 2017.

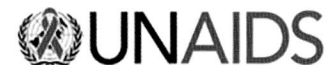

FIGURE 360-4. Global trends in number of people living with HIV on antiretroviral therapy and 2020 target. (Data from UNAIDS. UNAIDS Data 2017. Geneva: UNAIDS; 2017.)

with HIV at the end of 2016—one of the highest figures in the world after South Africa. In 2016, there were 270,000 new infections in this region, a decline of 13% from 2010; however, there was significant variation by country (e.g., Thailand experienced a 50% decrease, whereas annual new infections increased in Pakistan by 39% and in the Philippines by a remarkable 141%).

Throughout the region, the epidemic is one that continues to primarily involve key populations, although more recently the epidemic in many parts is steadily expanding into lower risk populations through transmission to the sexual partners of key populations. For example, in China, where the epidemic was previously driven by transmission through injection drug use, heterosexual transmission has become the predominant mode of HIV transmission. To compound the tragedy of the epidemic in China, reports from Henan province in central China demonstrate that tens of thousands and possibly more rural villagers became infected by selling their blood to collecting centers that did not follow basic blood donation safety procedures.

Knowledge of HIV serostatus in Asia and the Pacific has increased steadily and in 2016 was at 71% (E-Fig. 360-8). Awareness was particularly high in Malaysia (96%) and Thailand (91%) but quite low in certain countries such as Indonesia (35%). About 2.4 million people living with HIV in this region on are on antiretroviral therapy, representing 47% of this population, a remarkable increase from just 19% coverage in 2010, although still well short of UNAIDS 90-90-90 goals. Viral suppression rates are estimated at 39% of all people living with HIV, a very significant gap. With increased treatment access, mortality has declined to 170,000 deaths in 2016, a 29% decrease from 2010. Although some progress has been made in this region, substantial additional efforts are needed to reach key populations, address disparities in service and treatment access, and reach 90-90-90 goals.

Eastern Europe and Central Asia
The 17 countries that make up this region contain 1.6 million people living with HIV. HIV prevalence averages 0.9%, but, in contrast to other regions, the HIV epidemic in many countries of Eastern Europe and central Asia is growing.[8] An estimated 190,000 new cases of HIV occurred in 2016, a remarkable 60% increase from 2010 when there were 120,000 new cases. The HIV epidemic in this region is strongly driven by PWID, who accounted for 42% of all new infections in 2015, and is dominated by two countries, Russia and Ukraine. Russia accounted for 81% of all new HIV infections in this region in 2016; Ukraine accounted for 9%. In recent years, the Russian Federation has experienced an exceptionally steep rise in reported HIV infections, about half of which are attributed to injection drug use and half to heterosexual sex. The number of new HIV cases in Russia increased by 108% between 2010 and 2016.

Knowledge of HIV status in this region has improved slowly, with 63% aware in 2016 (E-Fig. 360-9). Antiretroviral therapy access has improved from 2010 when only 12% of all people living with HIV were on treatment, with 28% now accessing antiretrovirals. However, the coverage rates remain woefully low when compared with global goals. Among those on treatment, viral suppression is good, but because of the low treatment access rates, only 22% of all people living with HIV in this region are virally suppressed. Injection drug users, the population most at risk for HIV in Eastern Europe and central Asia, are often least likely to receive treatment when they are medically eligible. Not surprisingly, AIDS-related deaths in this region have continued to rise. In 2016, there were 40,000 AIDS-related deaths, a 25% increase from 2010. If more resources are not brought to bear and effective interventions are not implemented in the more severely affected countries in this region, it is likely that the epidemic in these countries will continue to worsen over the next decade.

Latin America
An estimated 1.8 million adults and children are living with HIV in the 17 countries that make up the Latin America region. Overall HIV prevalence is 0.5% in this region. Brazil, with its large overall population, accounts for 830,000 people living with HIV. In 2016, the number of new HIV infections was 96,000, an unappreciable change from 2010 when there were 94,000 new infections. Although certain countries experienced significant decreases of more than 20% in new infections since 2010 (e.g., Colombia, El Salvador, Nicaragua, and Uruguay), other countries experienced increases, including Chile (34%) and Guatemala (23%). Because of its size, Brazil accounted for about half of all new HIV infections in this region. HIV transmission in Latin America is predominantly through heterosexual or homosexual transmission. Key populations in certain areas continue to be disproportionately affected by the epidemic.

Latin America has overall done well with increasing HIV testing service access, with 81% of people living with HIV aware of their HIV status (E-Fig.

360-10). In 2016, there were 1.0 million people living with HIV on antiretroviral treatment in this region, nearly double the number from 2010, representing 58% of all people living with HIV. Viral suppression was estimated at 46% of all people living with HIV in 2016, well short of 90-90-90 goals. Countries such as Bolivia, Paraguay, and Guatemala have, in particular, struggled to increase access to antiretrovirals, with only roughly one third of people living with HIV accessing antiretrovirals in these countries. Mortality from AIDS has modestly decreased in Latin America. From 2010 to 2016, there was a decrease of 12% down to 36,000 annual deaths. Certain countries did particularly well, such as Peru, Honduras, and Colombia, which all had mortality declines greater than 45%. Conversely, Bolivia, Guatemala, Paraguay, and Uruguay all had increases in the number of AIDS-related deaths. Increased resources, price reductions in antiretroviral therapy, and other strategies will be needed to move this region toward epidemic control goals.

Caribbean
The 16 countries in the Caribbean region accounted for 310,000 people living with HIV in 2016. Overall HIV prevalence was 1.3%. In several Caribbean countries, adult HIV prevalence rates are surpassed only by the rates experienced in sub-Saharan Africa, which makes this region the second most affected in the world. Haiti and the Bahamas remain the worst affected, with an estimated national prevalence of 2.1% in Haiti and 3.3% in the Bahamas. The number of new cases in 2016 remained largely the same as years prior. Four countries—Cuba, the Dominican Republic, Haiti, and Jamaica—accounted for the majority of new infections. New infections doubled in Cuba between 2010 and 2016, while Haiti and Trinidad and Tobago experienced declines approaching 25%. Homosexual and heterosexual transmission continues to be the major mode of transmission throughout the region, although there is evidence that spread of HIV is increasing through sharing of infected drug equipment.

Knowledge of HIV status in this region stands at 64%. Of all people living with HIV, 52% are on antiretroviral treatment, about double from 2010, and 34% are suppressed, which remains well short of UNAIDS goals (E-Fig. 360-11). With increasing access to treatment, AIDS-related deaths have declined. In 2016, 9400 AIDS-related deaths are estimated to have occurred, a 55% decrease from 2010. Resources for HIV treatment and prevention in this region remain limited, and additional measures and support will be needed to reach 90-90-90 goals.

Western and Central Europe and North America
Forty countries make up this high-income region spread across two continents where 2.1 million people living with HIV reside. Overall HIV prevalence is 0.3%, with no country having a prevalence higher than 0.5%. The number of new HIV infections has declined modestly (9%) from 2010 to 2016, with an estimated 79,000 new infections in 2016. The United States (see later) accounted for about half of all these new infections. Certain countries have experienced substantial declines over the same time period, such as the Netherlands (55% decrease). However, the Czech Republic (80% increase), Serbia (70% increase), and Slovakia (60% increase) have moved in the opposite direction.

The HIV epidemic in western Europe is a result of a multitude of epidemics that differ in their timing, scale, and effects on populations. Unsafe sex between men remains the most important factor for spread in North America and most countries in western Europe. A large proportion of new HIV diagnoses in this region also occur through heterosexual intercourse. Injection drug use remains a major mode of transmission, particularly in the Baltic countries (Estonia, Latvia, and Lithuania). Most data from high-income countries demonstrate that the epidemic has shifted to the poor and marginalized sections of society. Recent introduction of PrEP has likely resulted in decreasing HIV transmission among MSM in certain settings.

In 2016, this well-resourced region had 85% of people living with HIV aware of their status (E-Fig. 360-12). In 2016, 76% of all people living with HIV were on treatment, an increase of 46% from 2010. Of all people living with HIV, an estimated 64% are virally suppressed, within reach of the 73% UNAIDS targets for viral suppression. As a result of the expanded testing and treatment, AIDS-related deaths have decreased by about 58% from 2000 to 2016 with a current rate of 18,000 annual deaths. Despite significant successes, marginalized populations continue to disproportionately share in the burden of new infections and mortality. New efforts and strategies will be needed to reach UNAIDS targets.

The United States
The first five cases of HIV in the United States were reported in 1981. In 2015, an estimated 1.1 million people were living with HIV in the United States.[9]

Nationally, the adult HIV prevalence was estimated to be about 0.5%. This increase in people living with HIV reflects mixed results in the United States' efforts to combat its epidemic. More people infected with HIV are living longer because of antiretroviral therapy, but unfortunately, the early major gains made in prevention have not been sustained. Of those people living with HIV, about 162,500 (15%) were not yet aware that they are infected with HIV in 2015. Of the 973,000 who had been diagnosed, about 76% were men. Of the men, about 36% were black/African American, 35% were white, and 23% were Hispanic/Latino. Of the women, 59% were black/African American, 17% were white, and 19% were Hispanic/Latino. Of the men, most (71%) acquired infection attributable to male-to-male sexual contact,[10] with 10% due to heterosexual contact and 10% due to injection drug use. In contrast, among women, 75% of infections were attributable to heterosexual contact and 22% to injection drug use. Of note are the tremendous regional and state-by-state differences in HIV prevalence (Fig. 360-5). The highest rates of diagnosed HIV infection are found in southern states, the mid-Atlantic, and California.

The number of newly recorded HIV cases in 46 states with confidential name–based reporting has varied only slightly since the late 1990s, although there has been a recent modest trend downward. In 2016, there were an estimated 40,300 new HIV infections, down by about 6% from 2011. About 70% of these new infections in 2016 occurred in MSM; 24% were among heterosexuals; and 6% were among PWID without male-to-male sexual contact. Men accounted for 81% of all new diagnoses. Since 2011, there have been modest declines in new HIV infections among heterosexuals, PWID, and white homosexual and bisexual men (about 10 to 15%). In contrast, there were no declines among black/African American homosexual and bisexual men, and infections actually increased among Hispanic/Latino homosexual and bisexual men by about 14%. As a result, black male-to-male sexual contact and Hispanic/Latino male-to-male sexual contact represent increasingly large shares of all new HIV infections in the United States.

In the United States, more than 700,000 people with AIDS have died since the epidemic began. Mortality peaked in 1995 and has steadily declined since then with the use of increasingly effective antiretroviral therapy, although the slope of decline has been modest or flat for more than a decade now (Fig. 360-6). In 2015, there were 15,800 deaths of persons with diagnosed HIV infection, a rate of 4.9 per 100,000. Marked racial/ethnic disparities were evident, with death rates among black/African Americans (17.5) much higher compared with Hispanic/Latinos (4.4) and whites (2.5); black/African Americans accounted for 45% of all deaths of persons with diagnosed HIV infection, Hispanic/Latinos 16%, and whites 32%.

Further declines in mortality will require greater success in encouraging timely diagnosis of HIV infection and entry into care. An estimated 15% of people living with HIV in the United States are unaware of their HIV status. Moreover, in 2014, 38% of people living with HIV have not accessed HIV care, and only 49% of all people living with HIV are virally suppressed in the United States (Fig. 360-7). Viral suppression was particularly low in those aged 13 to 24 years (27%) compared with 55 to 57% suppression in persons older than 45 years. Black/African Americans also had the lowest rates of viral suppression (43%) compared with other races. New resources and strategies will be needed to close these disparities and gaps in the HIV care continuum.

With such a long-standing epidemic, complacency has increased, and many prevention efforts have dwindled as a result of declining mortality. The increasing uptake of PrEP by mostly MSM offers hope but is tempered by increasing rates of sexually transmitted infections (STIs) among MSM and uneven access to PrEP for other high-risk groups. Renewed efforts to enhance treatment and prevention efforts will be needed to drive down rates of new HIV infections and HIV-associated mortality.

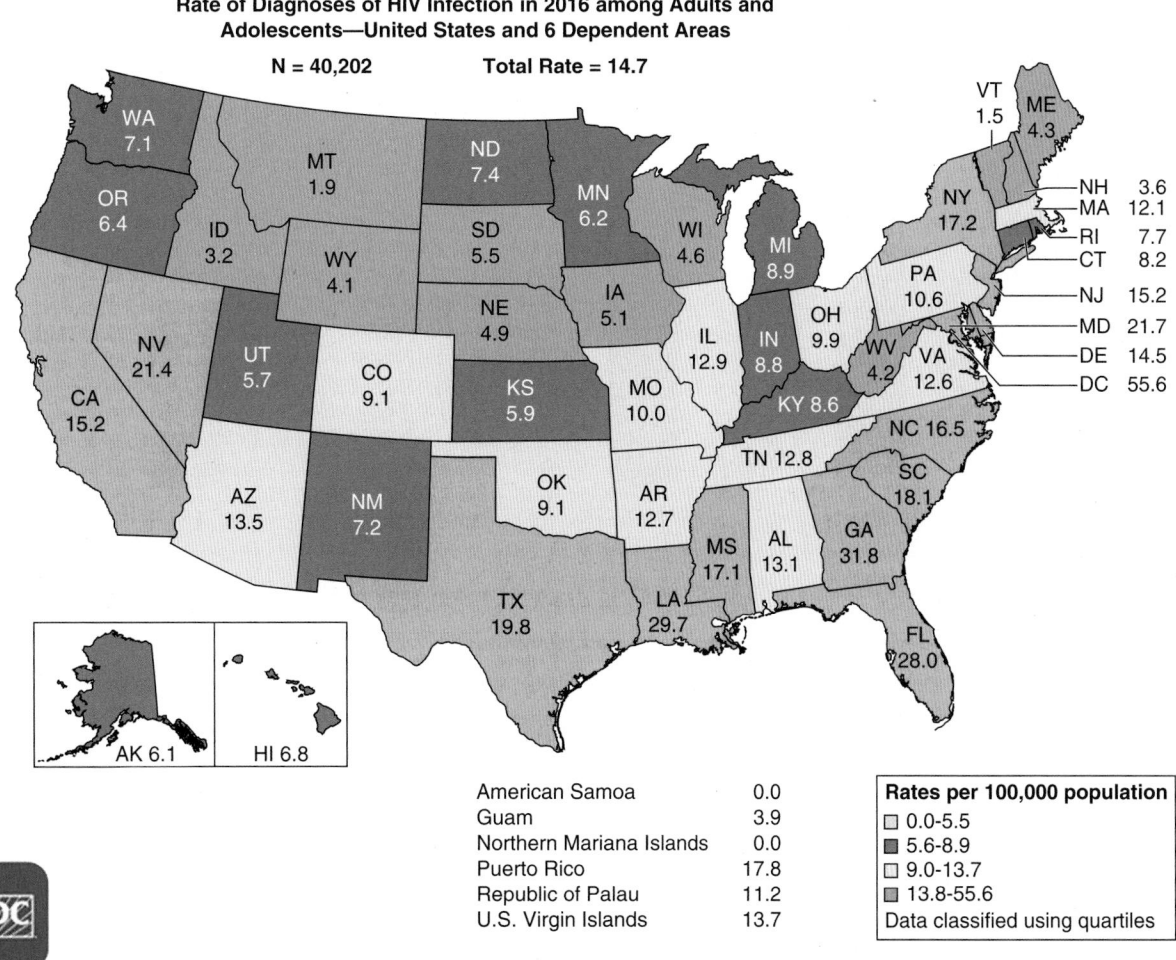

Rate of Diagnoses of HIV Infection in 2016 among Adults and Adolescents—United States and 6 Dependent Areas

N = 40,202   Total Rate = 14.7

American Samoa	0.0
Guam	3.9
Northern Mariana Islands	0.0
Puerto Rico	17.8
Republic of Palau	11.2
U.S. Virgin Islands	13.7

Rates per 100,000 population
- ☐ 0.0-5.5
- ■ 5.6-8.9
- ☐ 9.0-13.7
- ■ 13.8-55.6

Data classified using quartiles

FIGURE 360-5. New HIV diagnoses in the United States for the most-affected subpopulations, 2016. Note: Data for the year 2016 are preliminary and based on 6 months reporting delay. (Data from Centers for Disease Control and Prevention. HIV Surveillance Report, 2016.)

Stage 3 (AIDS) Classifications and Deaths of Persons with Diagnosed HIV Infection Ever Classified as Stage 3 (AIDS), among Adults and Adolescents, 1985–2015 United States and 6 Dependent Areas

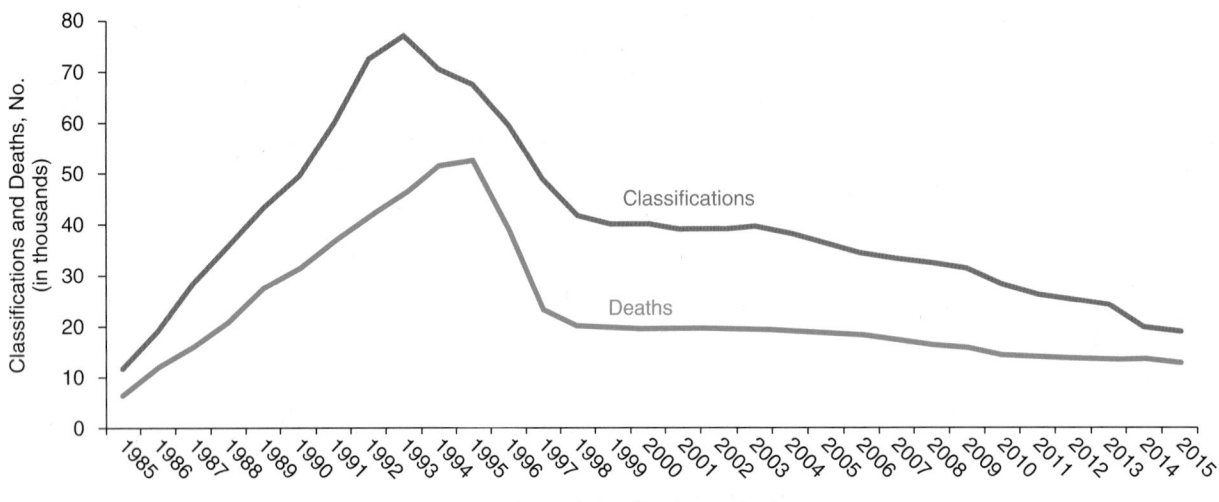

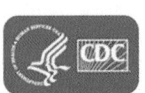

Note. Deaths of persons with HIV infection, stage 3 (AIDS) may be due to any cause.

FIGURE 360-6. Trends in AIDS classifications and deaths among adults and adolescents in the United States and dependent areas, 1985-2015. (Data from Centers for Disease Control and Prevention. HIV Surveillance Report, 2016.)

Persons Living with Diagnosed or Undiagnosed HIV Infection HIV Care Continuum Outcomes, 2015—United States

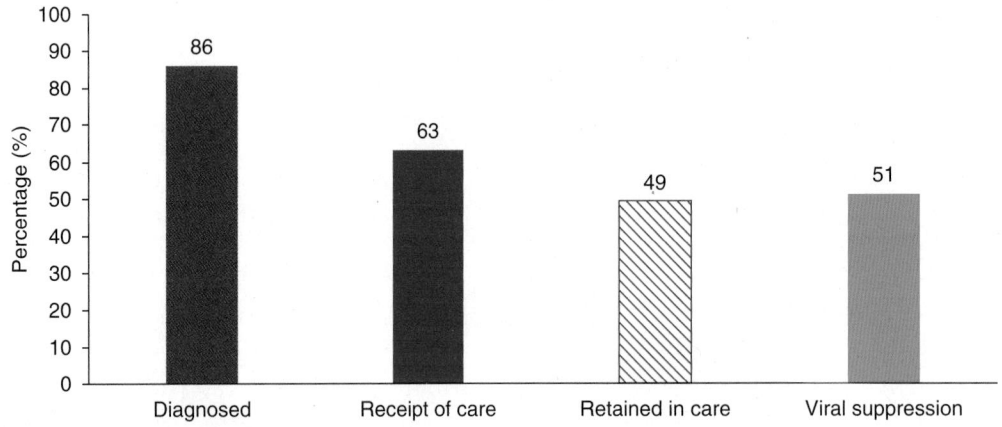

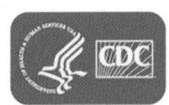

Note. Receipt of medical care was defined as ≥1 test (CD4 or VL) in 2015. Retained in continuous medical care was defined as ≥2 tests (CD4 or VL) ≥3 months apart in 2015. Viral suppression was defined as <200 copies/mL on the most recent VL test in 2015.

FIGURE 360-7. HIV care continuum in the United States in 2015. (Data from Centers for Disease Control and Prevention. HIV Surveillance Supplemental Report, 2016.)

DIAGNOSIS

Screening for HIV Infection

Although patients with acute HIV infection may have symptoms such as fever, headache, or malaise or signs such as lymphadenopathy—most commonly about 2 weeks after infection when viral counts peak—an estimated 10 to 60% of patients will have neither signs nor symptoms.[11] Findings that most increase the likelihood of early HIV infection include genital ulcers, weight loss, vomiting, and lymphadenopathy. However, because the history and physical examination are of very limited value in making the diagnosis of early HIV infection, laboratory testing is key to making the diagnosis.[12]

The U.S. Preventive Services Task Force on HIV screening recommends that clinicians screen for HIV infection in all adolescents and adults aged 15 to 65 years. Younger adults and older adults who are at increased risk also should be screened. In addition, they recommend that clinicians screen all pregnant women for HIV, including those who present in labor who are untested and whose HIV status is unknown. These recommendations are based on increasing evidence of the benefits of early antiretroviral therapy for

HIV-infected persons and its effectiveness in preventing HIV transmission. Also supporting these recommendations for screening are the facts that about 15% of HIV-infected individuals in the United States are unaware of their infection and that identification and treatment of HIV infection are associated with a markedly reduced risk for progression to AIDS, AIDS-related events, and death in individuals with immunologically advanced disease. A randomized trial (HPTN 052) clearly demonstrated that the use of antiretroviral therapy is associated with substantially decreased risk for transmission from HIV-positive persons to uninfected sexual partners.[A4] Furthermore, evidence also demonstrates that the identification and treatment of pregnant women dramatically reduces rates of mother-to-child transmission. The overall benefits of screening for HIV infection in adolescents, adults, and pregnant women are therefore substantial.

On the basis of HIV prevalence data, MSM and people who are actively injecting illicit drugs are at very high risk for new HIV infection and would qualify for increased HIV screening.[13] Behavioral risk factors for HIV infection include having unprotected vaginal or anal intercourse; having sexual partners who are HIV-infected, bisexual, or injection drug users; or exchanging sex for drugs or money. Other persons considered at high risk include those who have acquired or request testing for other STIs. Patients may request HIV testing in the absence of reported risk factors. Individuals not at increased risk for HIV infection include persons who are not sexually active, those who are sexually active in exclusive monogamous relationships with uninfected partners, and those who do not fall into any of the previously mentioned categories. It is recognized that these risk categories are not mutually exclusive, the degree of sexual risk is a continuum, and individuals may not be aware of their sexual partners' risk factors for HIV infection. For patients younger than 15 years and older than 65 years, it would be reasonable for clinicians to consider HIV risk factors on an individual basis, especially those with new sex partners. However, clinicians should bear in mind that adolescent and adult patients may also be reluctant to disclose having HIV risk factors.

The evidence is insufficient to determine optimum time intervals for HIV screening. One reasonable approach would be a one-time screening of adolescents and adult patients to identify persons who are already HIV positive, with repeated screening of those who are known to be at risk for HIV infection, those who are actively engaged in risky behaviors, and those who live or receive medical care in a high-prevalence setting (HIV seroprevalence >1%). High-prevalence settings include STI clinics, correction facilities, homeless shelters, tuberculosis clinics, clinics serving MSM, and adolescent health clinics with high prevalence of STIs. Currently, a reasonable approach may be to rescreen groups at *very high* risk for new HIV infection at least annually and individuals at *increased risk* at slightly longer intervals (3 to 5 years). Women screened for HIV during previous pregnancies should be rescreened for HIV at all subsequent pregnancies. The U.S. Centers for Disease Control and Prevention (CDC) also recommend that all persons aged 13 to 65 years be screened for HIV in health care settings located in areas where the prevalence of undiagnosed HIV infection is greater than 0.1% and that persons with increased risk for HIV be retested at least annually.

Laboratory Assays

Diagnosis of HIV infection is usually based on a combination of serologic detection of immunoglobulin antibodies to HIV-specific proteins, detection of HIV antigens such as p24, or detection of HIV RNA. The preferred testing algorithm in the United States uses a fourth-generation HIV-1/HIV-2 combination immunoassay, which detects HIV p24 antigen and HIV antibodies, followed by confirmatory testing with an HIV-1/HIV-2 antibody differentiation immunoassay and HIV RNA testing as needed for indeterminate cases.[14] The combined tests are highly accurate, with sensitivity and specificity greater than 99.5%. Results are typically available within 1 to 2 days for most commercial laboratories. In resource-limited settings, different algorithms are recommended, typically using a combination of two different rapid antibody tests.

The diagnostic accuracy of HIV infection has improved with each generation of serologic assays. Whereas the first-generation tests were based on whole viral lysate and an indirect enzyme immunoassay, second-generation tests use synthetic and recombinant peptide antigens that have improved sensitivity and specificity. Third-generation assays have used "sandwich" assay formats that allow simultaneous detection of immunoglobulin M (IgM) and IgG antibodies. Now, fourth-generation assays combine antibody and antigen testing within the same diagnostic test format. With increasing sensitivity of these diagnostic assays, the "window period" wherein HIV antibodies may not be detected because of acute or very recent infection has gradually shortened from 6 weeks to less than 3 weeks. This shortening of the window is particularly important when acute infection may not be suspected. In patients with symptoms and signs of acute HIV infection or potential recent exposure to HIV, direct testing with sensitive assays such as nucleic acid testing for HIV RNA is warranted.

Rapid tests represent a major advance in HIV serologic testing. Rapid HIV testing may use either blood or oral fluid specimens and can provide results as quickly as 5 minutes. The sensitivity and specificity of the rapid tests are also greater than 99.5%; however, initially positive results require confirmation with conventional methods. Rapid testing can be offered on site in a variety of settings, including clinics, mobile vans, health fairs, and places of worship. Rapid testing is becoming the test of choice for all patients who request screening for immediate feedback and opportunities for quick intervention and counseling. Rapid tests are particularly important in management decisions of occupational or nonoccupational exposures, when patients are unlikely to return for results and seroprevalence rates are high, such as STI clinics or emergency departments, and when patients with an acute illness in which HIV-related complication is being considered and serostatus is not known.

In 2012, the U.S. Food and Drug Administration (FDA) approved the first in-home HIV test (OraQuick), which allows for self-administration of an HIV test detecting antibodies to both HIV-1 and HIV-2. This test is available for consumers in drugstores or can be ordered online, and individuals may obtain test results within 20 to 40 minutes after collecting an oral fluid sample by swabbing the upper and lower gums inside the mouth and placing the sample into a developer vial provided as part of the kit. As with all rapid HIV assays, positive test results are preliminary and need to be confirmed with a standard HIV antibody test. In clinical trials, self-testing with this rapid HIV assay had a sensitivity of 92% and a specificity of 99.98% compared with the standard enzyme immunoassay (EIA) screening assay. Another home testing option is kits that allow finger-prick blood samples to be taken at home, which are then mailed to a laboratory for screening and confirmation. Results are obtained by phone using an individual identifier code or online.

Other methods to establish HIV infection include viral isolation or qualitative or quantitative detection of HIV nucleic acid through polymerase chain reaction (PCR) techniques, branched-chain DNA testing, or nucleic acid sequence–based amplification. Limitations of these assays include cost, the requirement for venipuncture and more laboratory technology, and the time interval between sample collection and test results. None of these tests is considered superior to routine serologic testing. However, viral detection is useful in specific situations, such as diagnosis of neonatal HIV infection when maternal antibody is passively transferred to the fetus, potentially providing a false-positive serologic result in an uninfected infant, in patients with indeterminate serologic results, or in those who may be in the window period before HIV seroconversion.

In 2014, the CDC evaluated and offered an updated testing algorithm for the diagnosis of HIV infection in the United States (Fig. 360-8). In this algorithm, all initial testing of serum is performed by an FDA-approved fourth-generation HIV-1/HIV-2 immunoassay. Specimens that are reactive on the fourth-generation assay should be retested/confirmed with an FDA-approved second-generation antibody assay that differentiates HIV-1 antibodies from other HIV antibodies, providing a definitive diagnosis of either HIV-1 or HIV-2. Seropositive individuals should initiate medical care that includes additional laboratory tests such as viral load, CD4 determination, and antiretroviral resistance assays to stage HIV disease and for the selection of initial antiretroviral drug regimens. Specimens that are reactive on the fourth-generation assay but negative on the HIV-1/HIV-2 antibody differentiation assay should be retested with an FDA-approved nucleic acid test for HIV-1 RNA. Under these circumstances, a reactive nucleic acid test indicates the presence of acute HIV infection, although RNA levels of less than 1000 copies/mL may indicate a rare false-positive result. A negative result would indicate the absence of HIV-1 and either a false-positive result on the initial fourth-generation assay or, rarely, recent HIV-2 infection. If HIV-2 infection is a possibility, an HIV-2-specific antibody or real-time PCR test for HIV-2 DNA/RNA can be considered.

The previously described algorithm emphasizes high sensitivity during initial testing with the fourth-generation immunoassay, in which false-positive antibody-negative test results might occur, but these can be resolved during subsequent laboratory testing as recommended. The new diagnostic algorithm replaces the previous most commonly used algorithm consisting of the Western blot with an HIV-1/HIV-2 antibody differentiation assay as the supplemental test and includes an RNA test to resolve reactive immunoassays with negative supplemental test results. In retrospective studies, this algorithm performed better than Western blot at identifying HIV antibody-positive persons, detecting acute HIV infections, and diagnosing unsuspected HIV-2 infections.

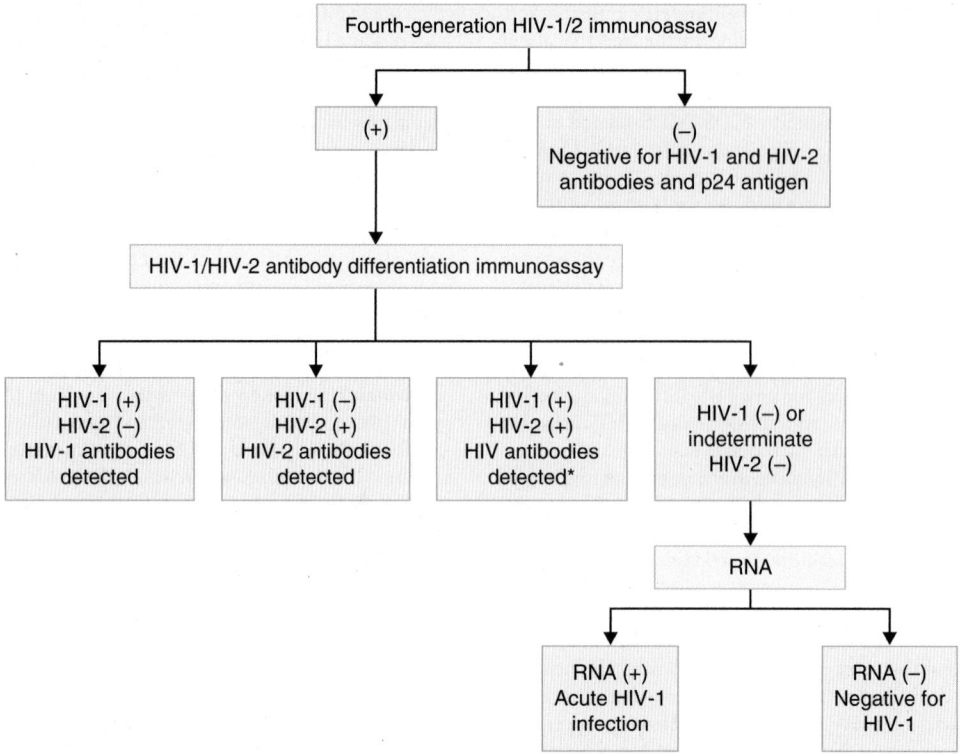

FIGURE 360-8. HIV diagnostic testing algorithm evaluated in the United States. *Additional testing required to rule out dual infection with HIV-1 and HIV-2. (Modified from Centers for Disease Control and Prevention and Association of Public Health Laboratories. Laboratory Testing for the Diagnosis of HIV Infection: Updated Recommendations. Published June 27, 2014.)

Grade A References

A1. Sharma SC, Raison N, Khan S, et al. Male circumcision for the prevention of human immunodeficiency virus (HIV) acquisition: a meta-analysis. *BJU Int.* 2018;121:515-526.

A2. Molina JM, Capitant C, Spire B, et al. On-demand preexposure prophylaxis in men at high risk for HIV-1 infection. *N Engl J Med.* 2015;373:2237-2246.

A3. Riddell J 4th, Amico KR, Mayer KH. HIV preexposure prophylaxis: a review. *JAMA.* 2018;319:1261-1268.

A4. Severe P, Juste MA, Ambroise A, et al. Early versus standard antiretroviral therapy for HIV-infected adults in Haiti. *N Engl J Med.* 2010;363:257-265.

GENERAL REFERENCES

For the General References and other additional features, please visit Expert Consult at https://expertconsult.inkling.com.

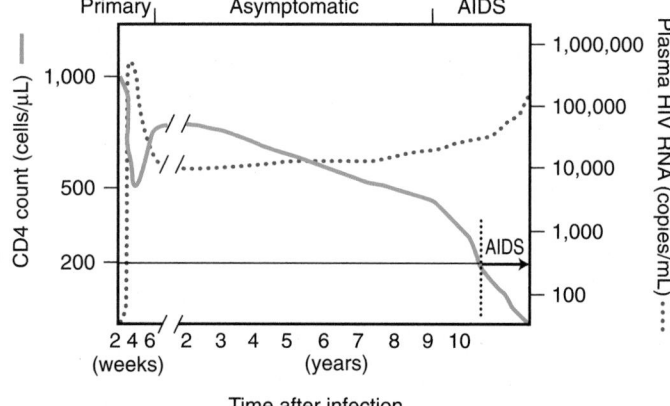

FIGURE 361-1. Natural history of human immunodeficiency virus type 1 (HIV-1) infection. CD4 counts and viral load are shown in the three phases of infection. AIDS = acquired immunodeficiency syndrome.

361

IMMUNOPATHOGENESIS OF HUMAN IMMUNODEFICIENCY VIRUS INFECTION

JOEL N. BLANKSON AND ROBERT F. SILICIANO

PRIMARY INFECTION

The natural history of human immunodeficiency virus type 1 (HIV-1) infection is illustrated in Figure 361-1. Peak viremia appears about 2 weeks after the first detection of HIV in blood, followed by reduction to a viral load set point at about 1 month after infection.[1] During acute HIV-1 infection, massive viral replication occurs in CD4+ T lymphocytes in the absence of an adaptive immune response. CD4+ T cells in the gut-associated lymphoid tissue and other mucosal sites express high levels of the HIV coreceptor CCR5 and are thus particularly prone to infection and depletion by the commonly transmitted R5 variants of HIV-1. In animal models, approximately 30% of memory CD4+ T cells are infected and depleted by 4 days after infection. This is in contrast to chronic infection, in which less than 1% of all CD4+ T cells are productively infected at any given time. As a result of this massive early infection, plasma levels of virion-associated HIV-1 RNA of more than 1 million copies per milliliter are typically seen in plasma within 2 weeks of infection, and patients tend to experience a constellation of signs and symptoms known as the *acute retroviral syndrome.*[2] There can be significant declines in peripheral CD4+ T-cell counts in primary infection resulting in opportunistic infections. Within several weeks, the development of an effective HIV-1–specific cytolytic T-lymphocyte response results in the partial control of viral replication, and the plasma HIV-1 RNA level (commonly known as the "viral load") falls and reaches a steady-state level known as the *set point.* The magnitude of the set point viral load during the second asymptomatic phase of the infection reflects a dynamic equilibrium between viral replication and the HIV-1–specific immune response. This set point determines the rate of progression to the final phase, clinical acquired immunodeficiency syndrome (AIDS). The median set point is approximately 30,000 HIV-1 RNA copies per milliliter, and most patients who have this level of viremia will develop AIDS in a 5- to 10-year period if they are left untreated. Patients with much higher set point viral loads will tend to be rapid progressors who develop AIDS much more quickly; conversely, patients with much lower viral loads tend to be long-term nonprogressors.

Elite controllers, who represent less than 1% of HIV-infected individuals, spontaneously suppress HIV viremia but also demonstrate chronic inflammation that may increase the risk of comorbid conditions. In these individuals, HIV-specific resident memory T cells are abundant in lymphoid tissues, and they exhibit distinct functional properties.[3] One of the most common findings in elite controllers is the presence of human leukocyte antigen (HLA)-B*27 and or HLA-B*57 alleles. Overall, elite controllers are hospitalized almost twice as frequently as persons with medically controlled HIV possibly because of residual immune activation, and cardiovascular hospitalizations are an important contributor.[4]

SPECIFIC IMMUNITY FOR HUMAN IMMUNODEFICIENCY VIRUS

The host mounts a vigorous immune response to HIV-1 infection. The virus is thought to activate plasmacytoid dendritic cells through toll-like receptors, resulting in the secretion of type I interferons and other inflammatory cytokines. Whereas type I interferons have direct antiviral properties and enhance the HIV-1–specific immune response, excessive secretion may play a key role in pathogenic immune activation of CD4+ and CD8+ T cells (Fig. 361-2). Natural killer (NK) cells are important effector cells in the innate immune response that become activated when infection of target cells by HIV-1 or other viruses results in the downregulation of HLA molecules or the expression of specific ligands.[5] Patients expressing certain NK receptor alleles are more likely to become long-term nonprogressors, suggesting that these cells may play a protective role possibly by controlling early HIV-1 replication, leading to the development of an effective adaptive immune response. Myeloid dendritic cells play a key role in the presentation of HIV-1 antigens to HIV-1–specific CD4+ and CD8+ T cells, which results in initiation of the adaptive immune response. They express CD4 molecules and have been shown to bind HIV-1. It is thought that in the process of presenting antigen, these cells may inadvertently transmit HIV-1 to clusters of activated CD4+ T cells.

The role of the humoral response in HIV-1 infection is not clear. HIV-1–specific antibodies, which are used to diagnose HIV-1 infection, do not develop until after peak viremia occurs. There is thus a window period in primary HIV-1 infection during which viremia is present in the absence of detectable antibodies. A subset of the antibodies that eventually appear is capable of preventing infection by blocking the interaction of the HIV-1 envelope protein gp120 with CD4 and coreceptor proteins on the surface of target cells. These so-called neutralizing antibodies are present at relatively low titers and have limited access to the critical regions of gp120. Studies suggest that the most effective neutralizing antibodies do not develop until 2 to 3 years after infection. These broadly neutralizing antibodies may eventually form the basis of a vaccine by preventing new infections.[6] However, although neutralizing antibodies in general can exert significant selective pressure on the virus, immunologic escape through rapid viral evolution is common, and the bulk of evidence suggests that these antibodies do not play a major role in the control of viral replication in most long-term nonprogressors.

The selective depletion of CD4+ T cells is the main reason that HIV-1 infection results in such profound immunosuppression. These so-called helper T cells play a major role in every facet of the adaptive immune response. The ability of HIV-1–specific CD4+ T cells to proliferate and to secrete key cytokines such as interleukin-2 (IL-2) is lost shortly after primary infection, setting up the entire HIV-1–specific response for failure.

CD8+ T cells contribute to the control of HIV-1 infection by the direct lysis of infected cells and by the secretion of soluble factors such as macrophage inflammatory protein 1β that bind to chemokine receptors, thereby preventing HIV-1 entry into target cells. However, the HIV-1–specific CD8+ T-cell response that partially controls HIV-1 replication after peak viremia in primary infection does not achieve sterilizing immunity,[7] partly because of a reservoir of latent virus in resting memory CD4+ T cells that develops shortly after infection. These quiescent cells probably do not make HIV-1 proteins and thus are not recognized by cytolytic T lymphocytes. Furthermore, the cytolytic T-lymphocyte response in patients with progressive disease is of poor quality with limited proliferative capacity. Furthermore, the low fidelity of HIV-1 reverse transcriptase results in the development of mutations with each round of replication. Mutations that lead to escape from cytolytic T-lymphocyte responses have a selective advantage and are thus selected for rapidly.

THE EFFECT OF HUMAN IMMUNODEFICIENCY VIRUS-1 REPLICATION ON THE IMMUNE SYSTEM

Whereas the HIV-1–specific immune response helps limit the rate of viral replication, sterilizing immunity is not achieved, and ongoing viral replication has a negative impact on the immune system. Continuous viral replication results in chronic immune activation (see Fig. 361-2). The mechanism is not understood. The chronic immune response to the virus may lead to nonspecific inflammation, and microbial translocation resulting from the depletion of CD4+ T cells in the gut-associated lymphoid tissue also may be important. Whatever the mechanism, immune activation appears to drive the depletion of CD4+ T cells. The level of immune activation markers on CD8+ T cells correlates better with the rate of CD4 decline than does the magnitude of the viral load in untreated patients.

Increased levels of activation markers are seen on NK cells, B cells, CD4+ T cells, and CD8+ T cells. Activation is accompanied by an increase in the turnover rate of these cells. The function of NK cells is compromised, which may predispose to the poor control of other viruses. B-cell defects result in hypergammaglobulinemia and the production of autoantibodies. Poor antibody responses to vaccines are also seen as CD4+ T cells decline.

Studies of viral dynamics make it clear that most productively infected cells live only a short time (~1 day) before succumbing to viral cytopathic effects

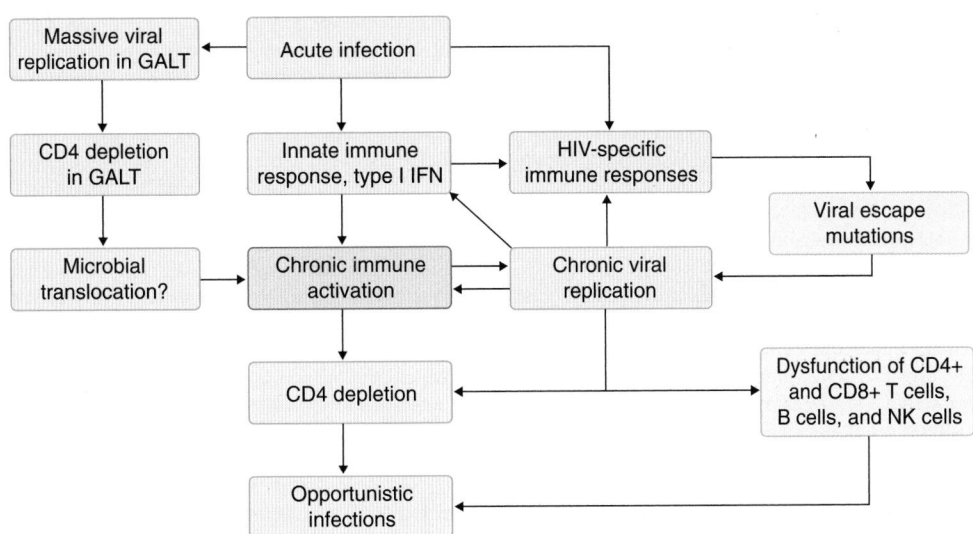

FIGURE 361-2. Parameters involved in chronic immune activation and CD4+ T-cell depletion. GALT = gut-associated lymphoid tissue; HIV = human immunodeficiency virus; IFN = interferon; NK = natural killer.

or host cytolytic T lymphocytes or NK cells. Although the loss of infected CD4⁺ T cells contributes to CD4 depletion, there is marked depletion of CD4⁺ T cells even though at any given time during chronic infection only 1% or less of these cells is productively infected. However, more recent studies have suggested that non-productively infected CD4⁺ T cells are also susceptible to cell death by a pro-apoptotic and pro-inflammatory host response. Thus, it is currently thought that death of non-productively infected CD4⁺ T cells and chronic immune activation leading to the death of noninfected CD4⁺ T cells are the principal mechanisms for CD4 depletion. Support for this idea comes from studies of the closely related simian immunodeficiency virus that replicates in natural simian hosts without causing immune activation or CD4 depletion. In addition to the quantitative loss of CD4⁺ T cells in HIV-1 infection, marked skewing of the CD4 T-cell repertoire is seen, and there is a diminished qualitative memory response to recall antigens long before the CD4⁺ T-cell count drops to 200 cells/μL. The chronic activation and high turnover rate of these cells eventually result in the progressive CD4 decline that is characteristic of HIV-1 infection.

There is evidence of immune exhaustion for both CD4⁺ and CD8⁺ T cells, and there is decline in the qualitative features of the CD8⁺ T-cell response to other chronic viruses such as cytomegalovirus and Epstein-Barr virus. This may be the result of anergy or depletion of the CD4⁺ T cells that are needed to sustain functional CD8⁺ T-cell responses.

● CLINICAL CONSEQUENCES OF HUMAN IMMUNODEFICIENCY VIRUS INFECTION

Clinical immunodeficiency is associated with the late stages of HIV-1 infection, when profound CD4⁺ T-cell depletion has occurred.[8] However, some level of immunodeficiency may be present shortly after infection because of qualitative changes in the immune response related to ongoing viral replication. As a result, patients are more susceptible to infections such as *Mycobacterium tuberculosis* infection (Chapter 308) before the CD4 count reaches the 200 cells/μL threshold that defines AIDS. Patients are also much more susceptible to malignant neoplasms such as non-Hodgkin lymphoma (Chapter 176) at any CD4⁺ T-cell count. Other opportunistic infections arise at fairly predictable CD4⁺ T-cell counts. *Pneumocystis jiroveci* infections (Chapter 321) occur at CD4 counts of lower than 200 cells/μL, *Cryptococcus neoformans* (Chapter 317) and *Toxoplasma gondii* infections (Chapter 328) occur at CD4 counts of lower than 100 cells/μL, and *Mycobacterium avium* complex (Chapter 309) and cytomegalovirus infections (Chapter 346) occur at CD4 counts below 50 cells/μL. Whereas these infections are a consequence of diminished cellular immunity, there is also a marked increase in invasive pneumococcal infections (Chapter 273) in HIV-1–infected patients, possibly because of defects in humoral immunity.

The Response to Antiretroviral Therapy

Treatment with selected combinations of antiretroviral drugs, known as active antiretroviral therapy (ART), suppresses viral replication to below the limits of detection of current commercial assays (20 copies of HIV-1 RNA per milliliter of plasma). Current evidence suggests that ART produces a complete or nearly complete arrest in viral replication in adherent patients, but trace amounts of viremia persist because of stable viral reservoirs, including the latent reservoir in resting CD4⁺ T cells. This suppression of viral replication is usually accompanied by a substantial increase in CD4⁺ T-cell counts. The initial rise in CD4⁺ T-cell counts occurs mostly as a consequence of migration of cells from lymph nodes (where 98% of all CD4 T cells reside) to the peripheral blood as inflammation diminishes in lymphoid tissue. Subsequently, there is an increase in the production of memory CD4⁺ T cells in most individuals. Naïve T-cell production is also sometimes seen at lower levels. Clinical studies have shown that patients who experience significant immune reconstitution can safely discontinue prophylactic therapy for opportunistic infections. However, it is not clear whether patients who maintain undetectable viral loads while receiving ART yet do not achieve significant CD4 T-cell immune reconstitution are still at risk for opportunistic infections. Two large studies have shown that although the use of IL-2 treatment in conjunction with ART will cause a significant increase in CD4⁺ T-cell counts in these patients, the enhanced immune reconstitution is not associated with any clinical benefit.

Just as a decline is seen in the functional CD4⁺ T-cell response shortly after primary infection, there is a qualitative improvement in CD4⁺ T-cell function shortly after ART is initiated. In some cases, there are exaggerated immune responses to opportunistic infections leading to the immune reconstitution inflammatory syndrome (IRIS; Chapter 367), particularly when there is rapid control of viral replication after the initiation of ART. IRIS usually presents

as a paradoxical worsening of a disease process a few weeks after ART is started and can occur even before there are significant changes in the absolute CD4⁺ T-cell counts. IRIS has been reported for virtually all known opportunistic infections, and in some cases it can occur in response to previously unrecognized infections. There have not been clinical trials looking at treatment of this condition, but nonsteroidal anti-inflammatory drugs and corticosteroids have been routinely used with varying degrees of success (Chapter 367).

GENERAL REFERENCES

For the General References and other additional features, please visit Expert Consult at https://expertconsult.inkling.com.

362

BIOLOGY OF HUMAN IMMUNODEFICIENCY VIRUSES

FRANK MALDARELLI

Human immunodeficiency virus (HIV) causes progressive immune deficiency and death from opportunistic infections or neoplastic diseases. Developments in diagnosis, prevention, and treatment that have reduced morbidity and mortality from HIV emerged from identification and characterization of HIV.[1] Groundbreaking discoveries of the retrovirus causing AIDS (1983 to 1985) were followed by characterization of HIV gene products and elucidation of virus replication, leading to identification of critical antiviral targets and directly to development of effective combination antiretroviral therapy (cART) in 1995 to 1996. As described (Chapter 364), introduction of cART has tipped the balance of epidemic spread, with fewer deaths than new infections. This transformed landscape of the HIV epidemic presents new challenges. The expanding size of the HIV-infected population undergoing therapy, elevated mortality in infected individuals despite cART, and emergence of antiviral drug resistance make the discovery of strategies to eradicate or control HIV in the absence of cART a public health imperative. Here we summarize basic concepts of HIV biology, but our understanding of HIV remains incomplete; new and ongoing studies that characterize host-virus interactions will continue to identify novel antiviral targets and lead to innovative strategies to eradicate HIV.

● CLASSIFICATION AND ORIGIN

HIV belongs to the *Lentivirus* genus of the Orthoretrovirinae subfamily of Retroviridae; all retroviruses are defined by the presence of a specific enzyme, reverse transcriptase, that catalyzes the synthesis of DNA from an RNA template, the central and unique event in retrovirus replication permitting integration of the viral DNA into the host genome. Retroviridae is a large family of viruses infecting diverse vertebrate hosts, mostly mammals and birds. Retroviruses are responsible for a spectrum of diseases, including immunodeficiencies and neoplastic, neurologic, hematologic, encephalitic, and inflammatory disorders. Members of the *Lentivirus* genus cause chronic, recurrent, or progressive diseases, including immunodeficiencies, in various mammalian species.

Following the development of the first tools for laboratory diagnosis of HIV infection, additional analysis identified individuals with symptomatic AIDS who did not have serologic responses characteristic of HIV, leading to the identification of a second distinct immunodeficiency virus, denoted HIV-2. HIV-2 had a distribution restricted largely to West Africa and to countries having economic, political, or cultural ties to West Africa.

HIV is genetically diverse, and the origin and spread of HIV variants currently circulating in humans has been traced by analyzing nucleic acid sequences of HIV and closely related viruses in primates; these analyses strongly indicate that HIV emerged from zoonotic transmissions from primates to humans, likely during the period of 1890 to 1930 in Central and West Africa. Zoonotic transmission requires close contact of blood and body fluid; scratches, bites, and butchery of captured infected animals provide ready mechanisms for transmission. Opportunities for zoonotic transmission have likely taken place for thousands of years, and the reasons that an epidemic spread did not occur until recently are unclear. A number of factors may have contributed to

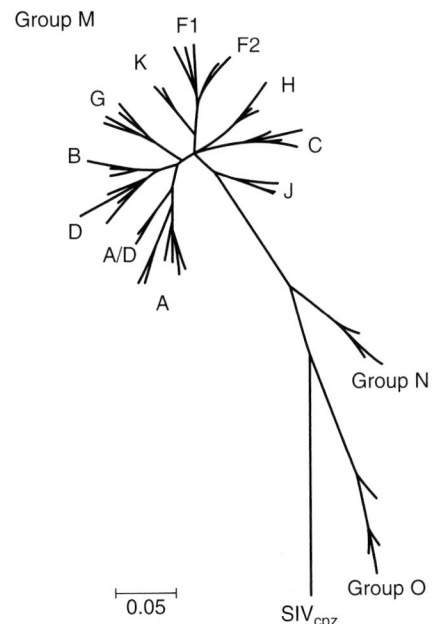

FIGURE 362-1. Phylogenetic relationships of HIV-1 groups and subtypes. Reference sequences of HIV RT were aligned in maximum likelihood phylogenetic trees constructed and rooted on the distant ancestor, SIV chimpanzee sequence (SIV$_{cpz}$). Group M viruses radiate in a starlike fashion, consistent with a common ancestor. An example of recombinant sequences (A/D) containing portions of parental subtypes A and D are identified as intermediate between the parental subtypes. Groups O and N are distantly related to group M and likely represent independent zoonotic events. Marker = genetic distance depicting percent difference. (HIV Sequence Database, http://www.hiv.lanl.gov/.)

epidemic spread during the late 19th and 20th centuries, including profound increases in human population density, malnutrition contributing to underlying immunodeficiency, population shifts due to political upheaval, and infrastructure development, such as roads, facilitating human travel and potential spread over long distances.

Further genetic analysis and sampling of nonhuman primate species shed new light on sources of the HIV epidemic. The relatively high genetic variability of HIV has been useful, both for classification purposes and for characterizing the source and spread of HIV. Currently, four distinct groups have been identified: a large group of viruses found throughout the world (M, for "main"), a relatively small group of viruses in central Africa (O, for "other"), and two small groups in individuals with West African origin, denoted N and P (c. 20 and 2 infections, respectively). Phylogenetic reconstructions demonstrate distinct lineages for HIV-1 groups, indicating that each is the result of a distinct zoonotic event (Fig. 362-1). M viruses are closely related to a similar simian immunodeficiency virus present in chimpanzee species (denoted SIV$_{cpz}$ simian immunodeficiency virus, cpz to indicate the specific animal reservoir). Group O is most closely related to the SIV present in western lowland gorillas and in chimpanzees. In contrast, HIV-2 is highly related to SIV$_{smm}$, a lentivirus commonly present in the sooty mangabey monkey, which has a native range including West and Central Africa, where HIV-2 was identified.

Group M viruses represent the great majority of infections in humans and are quite diverse, with at least nine subtypes, denoted A to D, F to H, J, and K. Analysis of the relationships of the nucleic acid sequences reveals an overall "starlike" phylogeny (see Fig. 362-1), indicating that, in general, all the current variants emerged from a common ancestor. Studies of the earliest viral sequences identified revealed it is likely that HIV underwent diversification early after transmission from animal reservoirs. Recombination among these subtypes may occur (see Fig. 362-1, *A/D*; and see later), yielding new recombinant viruses that are classified as circulating recombinant forms.

After AIDS emerged, HIV spread rapidly throughout the world; while Africa maintained a highly diverse group of viruses, founder effects resulted in spread of one or a limited number of subtype viruses in countries outside Africa. The epidemic in the United States began with subtype B virus; although initially attributed to single case reports of individuals, careful and exhaustive analyses traced the HIV epidemic from Africa to the United States through Haiti, and early expansions in major metropolitan areas, with New York City as a critical nexus.

All current laboratory methods that detect HIV identify *all* HIV-1 and HIV-2 variants. In individuals from relevant geographic origin, especially West Africa, it is of paramount importance to characterize the infection precisely to target therapy appropriately; HIV-2 and group O HIV-1 are naturally resistant to non-nucleoside reverse transcriptase inhibitors and to fusion inhibitors. Because dual HIV-1/HIV-2 infections are possible, it is imperative that all individuals from endemic areas for these two viruses (especially West Africa) be tested for *both* HIV-1 and HIV-2.

● STRUCTURE AND MOLECULAR BIOLOGY
Genome Structure and Organization
Like all retroviruses, HIV replicates through a DNA intermediate. The virion contains two copies of single-stranded (+) sense RNA (denoted viral RNA), and the stably infected cell contains double-stranded viral DNA integrated into the host genome (denoted the provirus). As shown in Figure 362-2 and E-Figure 362-1, viral RNA and the provirus have distinct genomic organization in untranslated 3′ and 5′ regions. Untranslated regions at each end of the genome contain a short terminal repeat as well as unique sequences at the 5′ (U5) and 3′ (U3) regions that are duplicated during replication, generating a longer duplicated sequence termed the *long terminal repeat* at each end of the provirus.

HIV encodes nine genes whose products are required for structural, enzymatic, regulatory, and innate immune neutralization functions (see E-Fig. 362-1). By convention, HIV genes are denoted in lower italics (*gag, pol,* etc.) with names that broadly reflect their function, location in the virion, or a historical vestige of prior viral classification (e.g., *gag,* "group antigen"). Additional genes were characterized that function in regulation or replication (*tat, rev, vpr*) or in blocking immune responses to HIV (*vif, vpu, nef*); all are critical for HIV infection in vivo.

Virion Structure
The HIV virion contains viral gene products and cellular components essential to transmit infection and establish the proviral state.[2] HIV virions are roughly spherical particles with a diameter of 80 to 120 nm and are composed of a viral core enveloped by a lipid membrane (Fig. 362-3).

The core of the mature virion is a conelike structure composed of the HIV p24 capsid (CA), which encapsidates components necessary for replication: two copies of HIV genomic RNA template complexed with HIV p6 nucleocapsid (NC); tRNA^{lys} primer; HIV enzymes reverse transcriptase, protease, and integrase; and HIV Vif. The viral envelope, which is derived from the plasma membrane of the host cell as HIV undergoes budding, contains viral proteins Gp120 (SU) and Gp41 (TM) as well as a structural matrix protein, MA.

Replication Cycle
Early Events in Replication
Attachment and Fusion
Virus replication is initiated by direct contact of virions or infected cells with susceptible host cells (Fig. 362-4).[3] Productive infection requires specific and essential interactions mediated by surface Env glycoprotein trimeric complexes consisting of HIV sp120 SU noncovalently bound to HIV gp41 TM. The attachment phase is mediated exclusively by the SU envelope glycoprotein, which engages two distinct cell surface proteins for attachment, a receptor and a coreceptor (see Fig. 362-4). HIV initially binds CD4, resulting in conformational change in Env, which facilitates coreceptor binding. Typically, SU proteins use either the human chemokine receptor 5 (CCR5) or the human chemokine receptor 4 (CXCR4) to infect CD4$^+$ T cells, but CCR5/CXCR4 dual tropic viruses circulate as well. Although virus infection can be propagated with either CCR5 or CXCR4 as coreceptor, initial infection likely requires CCR5 tropic virus.[4] Human populations have a significant population of individuals encoding a mutant CCR5 gene, who do not synthesize functional CCR5. HIV infection of individuals homozygous for CCR5 mutation is exceedingly rare, suggesting that initiation of infection virtually always requires interactions with CCR5.[5] Inhibition of SU-coreceptor interactions has been achieved pharmacologically, and the U.S. Food and Drug Administration (FDA)-approved coreceptor inhibitor maraviroc has potent anti-HIV activity. Unfortunately, HIV can mutate to use the CXCR4 receptor and thus no longer be effectively treated with maraviroc.[6] A newly developed monoclonal antibody, ibalizumab, directed against an extracellular CD4 domain, interrupts Env-CD4 binding without blocking CD4 immune function; ibalizumab has shown promising results in clinical trials and is FDA-approved for multi-drug resistant HIV.[7]

Engaging both receptor and coreceptor results in conformational change in Gp41, which reorganizes its structure and provides sufficient energy to

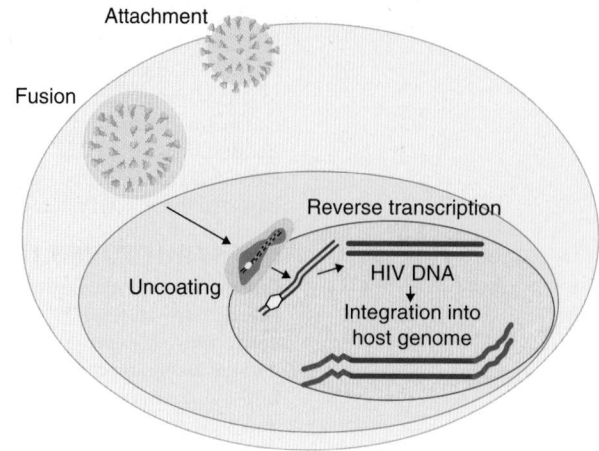

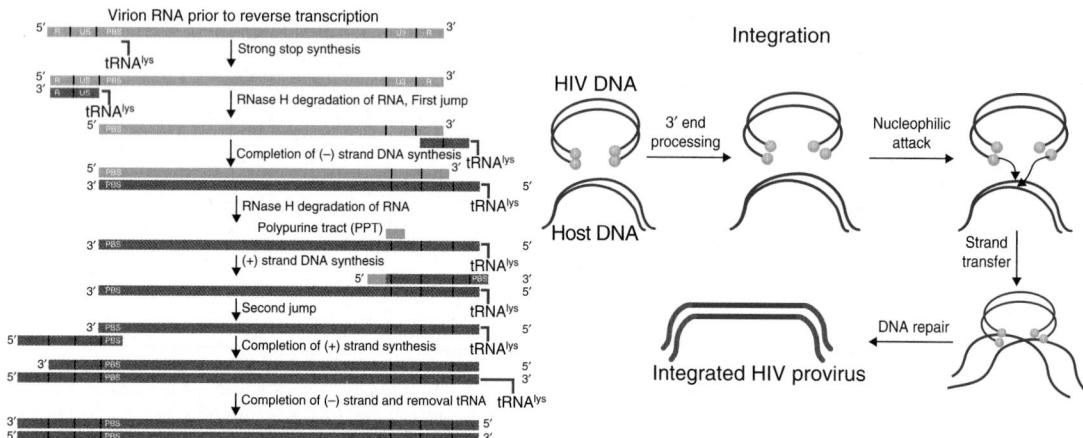

FIGURE 362-2. Early events in HIV replication include attachment, fusion, uncoating, reverse transcription, and integration into the host genome. Details of HIV reverse transcription and integration are depicted.

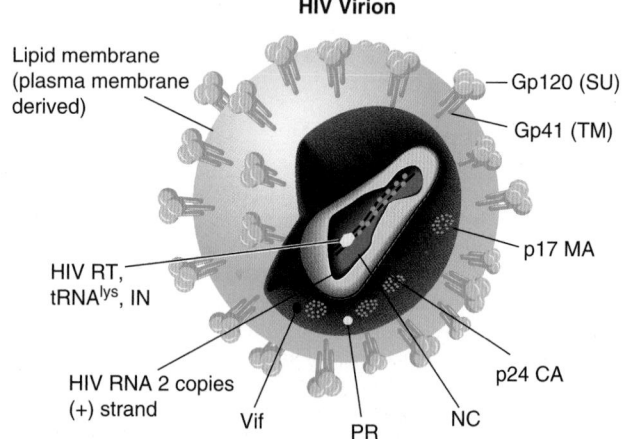

FIGURE 362-3. **The HIV virion.** HIV is an enveloped virus consisting of two (+) sense copies of viral RNA, enzymes required for replication contained in a viral core enveloped in a membrane derived by budding from the infected cell.

drive membrane fusion. TM-mediated membrane fusion can be inhibited using specific peptide inhibitors that bind to Gp41; one such peptide fusion inhibitor, enfuvirtide, is in clinical practice.

Uncoating

Following entry into CD4 cells, HIV cores undergo uncoating (see Fig. 362-4).[8] Uncoating represents a critical checkpoint for innate antiviral activity that can strongly restrict infectivity. An interferon-inducible host protein, TRIM5-alpha, can block uncoating of a number of viruses through interactions with the viral core; unfortunately, TRIM5-alpha cannot restrict either HIV-1 or HIV-2. TRIM5-alpha is under substantial genetic selection, with one of the fastest rates of positive selection of any human gene. Studies suggest that the current version of TRIM5-alpha present in human populations may have been selected during a previous epidemic to protect against an ancient retroviral infection. In this model, simply summarized as "generals are always fighting the last war, especially if they have won it," the current TRIM5-alpha was selected in the past to prevent a retroviral infection. Unfortunately, the current TRIM5-alpha is unable to restrict HIV, and uncoating takes place unabated in human cells. The requirements, precise intracellular location, and kinetics of HIV uncoating remain poorly understood, but pharmacologic disruptors of the process (PF74) are currently under study.

Reverse Transcription: Viral Genome Replication

Following uncoating, HIV has fresh access to nucleoside triphosphates, permitting reverse transcription to take place. Although traditionally thought to occur in the cytoplasm (see Fig. 362-4), reverse transcription is not required for nuclear import, and the process may occur in the nucleus. The (+)-strand template strands of HIV RNA are complexed with reverse transcriptase and a specific tRNA^{lys} that functions as a primer located at a specific primer binding site (see E-Fig. 362-1) near the 5′ end of the template RNA and HIV RNA. Reverse transcription is a multistep process (see Fig. 362-2) that first synthesizes a DNA copy of the RNA genome and then excises the RNA from the RNA-DNA hybrid using an RNase H function of reverse transcriptase.[9] RNA removal is incomplete, and residual RNA in a region denoted the polypurine tract (see Fig. 362-2) then serves to prime the next round of DNA synthesis. During reverse transcription, a number of strand transfer events occur, permitting opportunities for frequent recombination. Reverse transcriptase is highly prone to error, with only a rudimentary editing function. As a result, complete reverse transcription yields approximately one mutation per virion synthesized per replication cycle. The replication cycle for HIV, estimated as 1 to 2 days, is relatively short, and the replicating population size is substantial. The combination of rapid and error-prone synthesis in a large replicating population results in a genetically diverse population that can respond rapidly to

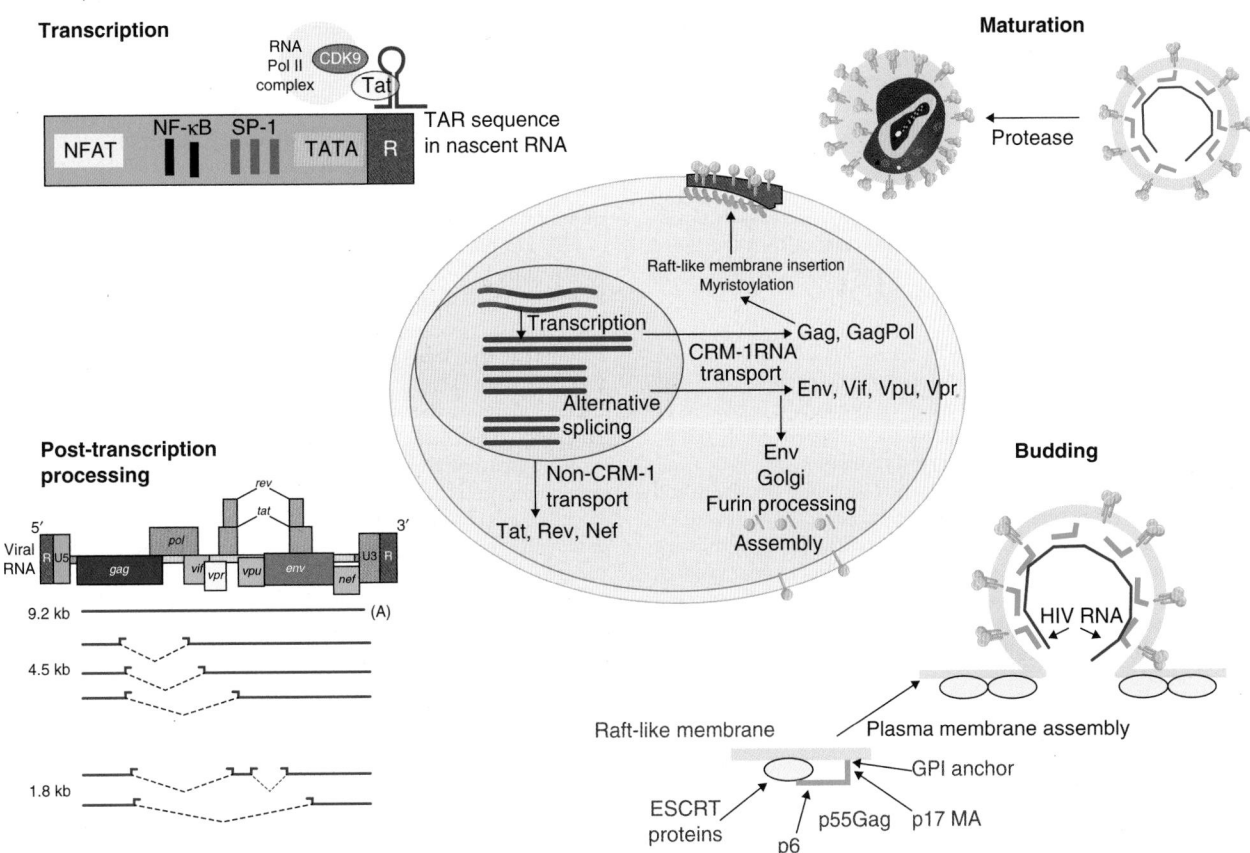

FIGURE 362-4. Late events in HIV replication. After establishment of the provirus, transcription, post-transcriptional processing translation, virion assembly, budding, and virion maturation take place by co-opting cellular processes.

immune- or drug-selective pressure. Thus, rapid error-prone replication, combined with recombination, represents an important pathogenic determinant for HIV.

Reverse transcription was the first target for antiretroviral therapy, and a number of direct and allosteric inhibitors of reverse transcription have been developed. All reverse transcription inhibitors inhibit RNA-dependent DNA synthesis or DNA-dependent DNA synthesis. Nucleoside and nucleotide reverse transcriptase inhibitors are dideoxy analogues of deoxynucleotides that are incorporated as the template is copied and act as chain terminators, blocking additional nucleic acid synthesis. Non-nucleoside inhibitors of reverse transcription bind to reverse transcriptase in a hydrophobic domain proximal to the active site, deforming the enzyme structure and disrupting nucleic acid synthesis.

Nuclear Transport and Integration
Newly synthesized HIV DNA undergoes integration into the host genome. A complex of the HIV protein integrase, newly synthesized HIV DNA, and associated proteins has been labeled an *intasome*.[10] Structural studies have revealed a multimer of integrase molecules bound to the ends of the retroviral DNA, bringing the DNA ends in close proximity, poised for integration into the genome in a multistep process (see Fig. 362-2). Integration is a highly successful target for antiretroviral therapy, and inhibitors that block the transfer of HIV DNA strand into the host genome are now first-line antiretroviral choices in clinical practice (Chapter 364).

Early Evasion of Intracellular Immunity: Vif and Vpu
HIV infection triggers a complex set of immune responses, and several viral factors function to counteract innate and adaptive immunity. As described earlier, HIV is able to infect human cells because an otherwise effective restriction mechanism blocking uncoating by TRIM5-alpha is unable to detect the incoming virus. Infection results in activation of two additional interferon-induced genes, the ABOBEC family (apolipoprotein B mRNA editing enzyme, catalytic polypeptide-like) of nucleic acid editing enzymes and BST-2 (tetherin). HIV in turn encodes specific functions to counteract such antiviral mechanisms.

The interferon-induced APOBEC family of proteins are nucleic acid editing enzymes capable of catalyzing the removal of amino groups from the cytosine

portion of cytidine; on copying, these deaminated cytidines base pair with adenosine, not guanine, and the net result is the introduction of multiple G-to-A mutations, resulting in hypermutation and complete viral inactivation. APOBEC can, in the absence of viral factors, be incorporated into new virions. As a result, during the next round of infection, after HIV enters a new host cell, APOBEC proceeds to hypermutate the newly reverse-transcribed HIV genome. To block APOBEC-mediated inactivation of HIV, a viral gene product, Vif (see E-Fig. 362-1), directly binds to APOBEC proteins, redirecting it to degradation by ubiquitination pathways. Redirecting APOBEC for elimination rather than virion incorporation effectively neutralizes a potent innate immune response.

A second product of interferon induction is the bone marrow stromal antigen 2 (BST-2), CD317, or tetherin. BST-2 is tethered to the plasma membrane at both its amino and carboxy termini and is enriched at virion budding. Tetherin can block the budding process directly. Newly budding virions may contain one end of the tetherin molecule in the virion membrane, while the other end of tetherin remains on the cellular membrane, thereby effectively blocking virion release. To counter this host mechanism, the HIV-encoded protein Vpu effectively blocks tetherin by a number of mechanisms, including direct binding and redirecting the protein to intracellular degradation.

Late Steps in Replication
Transcription and Translation: Exploiting Cellular Processes to Balance Production of Viral Gene Products
After the proviral state is established, HIV produces viral RNA and proteins using viral factors in concert with cellular mechanisms of transcription and translation. Thus, HIV replicates not by dismantling cell functions but rather by employing specific interactions between host factors, which ensures a balanced abundance of viral gene products.

Transcription
The integrated provirus is expressed in the context of host chromatin. The U3 portion of the HIV long terminal repeat contains binding sites for transcription factors common in lymphocytes and in macrophage-monocyte lineages, including activator protein 1 (AP-1), specificity protein 1 (SP-1), nuclear factor kappa B (NF-κB), and nuclear factor of activated T cells (NFAT)

binding sites. The presence of the viral transcription factor transactivator of transcription (Tat) markedly stimulates transcription through binding to a specific RNA enhancer, denoted the transactivating region (TAR), and recruiting additional transcription factors (see Fig. 362-4).

Post-transcriptional Processing

Retroviruses transcribe all of their genes from a single promoter. Full-length HIV RNA is processed for expression of all nine gene products and encapsidated as the viral genome into virions. To provide sufficient mRNA species to express all HIV proteins, RNA processing is highly regulated by alternative splicing and differential RNA transport (see Fig. 362-4).

Translation of mRNA

All HIV RNAs are translated by cellular ribosomes on either smooth or rough endoplasmic reticulum. Abundance of several HIV proteins is regulated by translational mechanisms and post-translational modifications mediated by host mechanisms that are critical for viral protein function.

Full-length HIV RNA serves as RNA for encapsidation into the virion and for Gag/Pol synthesis. Gag is synthesized as a 55-kd polyprotein precursor in relatively abundant amounts. Gag protein is N-myristoylated, permitting the protein to bind cellular membranes. The *pol* gene products are translated though frameshifting mechanisms. Frameshifting is relatively inefficient, and the relative abundance of *pol* enzyme gene products is substantially lower than Gag proteins, effectively controlling the levels of enzymes in favor of an abundance of structural proteins.

HIV Vpu and Env proteins are translated from a 4.5-kb bicistronic mRNA, permitting effective production of both Vpu and Env proteins. As Vpu sequesters CD4 by direct protein-protein interactions on intracellular membranes (see later), it prevents CD4-Env interactions that would arrest Env within the cell. Thus, the coordinated expression of Vpu with Env ensures efficient expression of Env. Env is synthesized as a gp160 precursor of Env SU and TM, cotranslationally inserted into the lumen of rough endoplasmic reticulum membranes and glycosylated predominantly at a number of canonical N-glycosylation sites.

Multiply spliced mRNA species encoding *tat, rev,* and *nef* are translated earliest after infection; Tat and Rev are transported to the nucleus, where they activate transcription and transport (see earlier). Nef serves a number of cytoplasmic functions in evasion of host immunity by binding MHC-1 and CD4, redirecting them away from plasma membranes. Thus, at an early time in the infectious cycle, immune molecules that help identify and target virus-infected cells are downregulated from the cell surface of infected cells, facilitating virus replication.

Transport and Assembly of Virion Components: An Elegant Dance

The late steps in virus replication are complex, but dissecting the individual steps has identified a number of critical interactions between host and virion components that represent active areas for development of useful therapeutics.

HIV virion proteins and virion RNA species traffic to the plasma membrane, where virion assembly takes place. Nascent Gag and GagPol polyprotein precursors undergo cotranslational modifications that target Gag to membranes.[11] Gag has self-assembly properties, but correct initial assembly of the virion core into a hexagonal lattice includes incorporation of virion RNA and additional factors. Virion RNA undergoes dimerization largely through direct RNA-RNA interactions that require specialized RNA sequences, denoted psi sequences, at the 5′ region of the genome favoring incorporation of only unspliced HIV RNA species. Gag polyprotein precursor can bind HIV RNA directly, providing a potential mechanism for transport to the cell membrane. Gag also accumulates in specialized membrane microdomains enriched with sphingomyelin-saturated phospholipids and cholesterol typical of lipid rafts and binds components of the endosomal sorting complexes required for transport (ESCRT) pathway (see Fig. 362-4). The ESCRT pathway is normally involved in intracellular membrane remodeling and scission processes necessary for events such as organelle biogenesis, lysosome formation, and cytokinesis. By recruiting ESCRT to sites of HIV assembly on the plasma membrane, HIV engages a highly specialized pathway to execute budding. Elegant studies of HIV transmission have suggested these events may also participate in cell-cell transmission of HIV at "virologic synapses," specialized areas of cell-cell contact.

During the budding process, HIV undergoes several maturation events, including proteolytic processing of the Gag and GagPol precursor proteins by HIV protease (see Fig. 362-4). Protease is embedded as part of the GagPol

precursor, cleaves itself from the precursor, and then proceeds to process Gag and GagPol into component proteins. Processing is essential for virion infectivity, and protease inhibitors are highly effective agents in HIV therapy. During processing, the core lattice begins to bend by introducing pentamers of CA at critical points of the hexagonal lattice, effectively folding the structure into a fullerene-like cone that encapsidates dimeric HIV RNA-tRNA[lys] and HIV enzymes. Maturation inhibitors that block processing by binding Gag instead of inhibiting protease represent a new antiviral target.

HIV Env precursor glycoprotein is processed by a cellular furin-like protease into mature products, gp120 (SU) and gp41, which traffic to plasma membranes through Golgi and post-Golgi membranes. Because the cellular receptor CD4 is also processed through similar mechanisms, intracellular Env-CD4 binding can effectively block Env from reaching the cell surface. The HIV Vpu protein, which directly binds and redirects CD4 to proteolytic degradation, thereby increases the proportion of Env reaching the cell surface and sites of HIV budding.

Bone marrow stromal cell antigen-2 (BST-2/tetherin) transmembrane protein prevents HIV-1 particles release by virion retention at membranes of infected cells. Single nucleotide polymorphisms in *BST-2*/tetherin are associated with a reduced risk for mother-to-child transmission of HIV-1 and AIDS progression in adults.[12]

New restriction factors, serine incorporator proteins (SERINC) 3 and 5, have been identified that reduce virion infectivity. SERINC3 and SERINC5 are integral plasma membrane proteins that reduce infectivity when incorporated into virions during the budding process. The HIV protein Nef effectively redirects SERINC3/5 from the surface, thereby enhancing infectivity. These studies reveal new potential targets for further antiviral development.

⬤ SUMMARY

By the completion of the infectious cycle, HIV has produced progeny for the next round of infection, obstructed adaptive and innate immune responses, and established a proviral state in the infected cell. Despite multiple mechanisms of immune evasion, the majority of infected cells (>99.9%) die within 1 to 2 days of infection. Thus, the virus has a strikingly short period to engage critical cell pathways to complete replication, while the cells are undergoing destruction. A minority of cells survive infection and persist for prolonged periods. As a consequence, current antiretroviral therapy that targets active steps in HIV replication does not eradicate HIV infection. Mechanisms of persistence remain poorly understood but likely include transcriptional and immunologic mechanisms. Additional research will be essential to determine mechanisms of persistence[13] and to identify new strategies to cure HIV infection.

GENERAL REFERENCES

For the General References and other additional features, please visit Expert Consult at https://expertconsult.inkling.com.

363

PREVENTION OF HUMAN IMMUNODEFICIENCY VIRUS INFECTION

CARLOS DEL RIO AND MYRON S. COHEN

More than 35 years have passed since the first report of a case of human immunodeficiency virus (HIV) infection, and, at the end of 2017 there were approximately 36.9 million people worldwide living with HIV/AIDS and over 35 million have died as a consequence of acquired immunodeficiency (AIDS). HIV prevention efforts have been "front and center" since the virus was discovered as the cause of AIDS, as summarized in Figure 363-1. Behavioral interventions focused on HIV-negative persons have played a role in the falling population-level incidence in some countries, but it is the scale-up of antiretroviral therapy, with more than 18 million people now on treatment, that has made a significant impact on the number of new infections. Nevertheless, there were still 1.8 million new infections in 2017, and we have made little

Four Prevention Opportunities

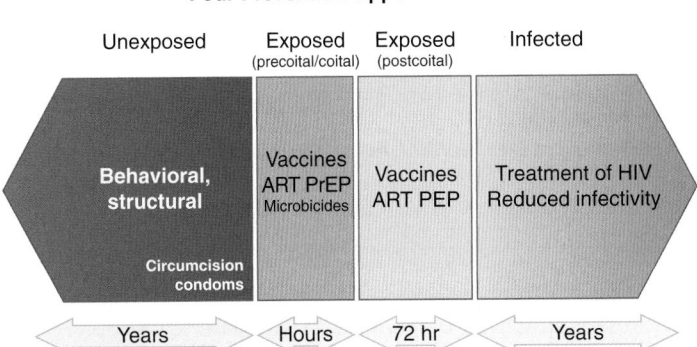

FIGURE 363-1. Opportunities for human immunodeficiency virus (HIV) prevention. ART = antiretroviral therapy; PEP = postexposure prophylaxis; PrEP = pre-exposure prophylaxis. (Modified from Cohen MS. Recent developments in HIV prevention. *AIDS.* 2008, Abstract TUPL0102.)

Risk for HIV Transmission per Coital Act

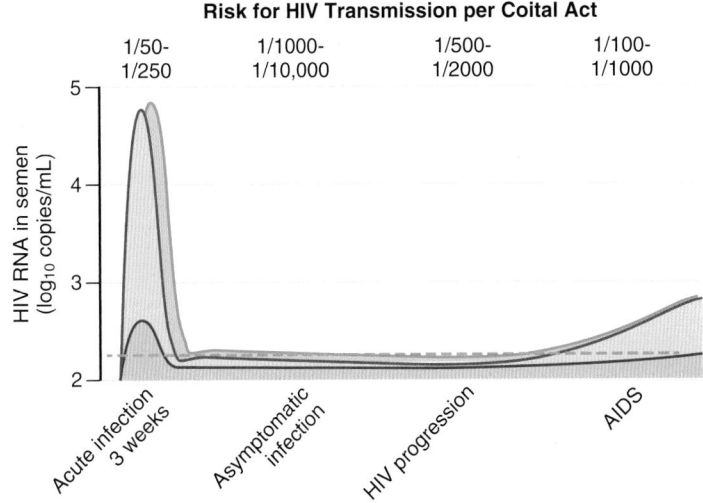

FIGURE 363-2. Prediction of the efficiency of human immunodeficiency virus (HIV) transmission according to HIV burden in the genital tract. Probability of male-to-female HIV transmission per coital act, as a function of HIV disease stage in the index case. Dashed line = a potential threshold for HIV transmission; orange = theoretical effect of a biologic intervention designed to reduce viral excretion; blue = expected distribution of viral burden in semen among men over time. (Modified from Cohen MS, Pilcher CD. Amplified HIV transmission and new approaches to HIV prevention. *J Infect Dis.* 2005;191:1391-1393.)

progress in reducing HIV incidence in the groups at highest risk. In the past few years, several promising new prevention strategies have demonstrated efficacy in clinical trials and are now being implemented. This chapter will provide a detailed view of HIV prevention approaches that are useful to the practicing clinician.

MODES OF TRANSMISSION AND PREVENTION

Sexual Transmission

The primary mode of HIV transmission throughout the world is sexual contact. However, the geographic distribution of cases attributable to homosexual or heterosexual transmission varies markedly. In the United States, most sexually transmitted cases of HIV are observed in men who have sex with men (MSM), and heterosexual transmission accounts for a smaller number of new infections except among women. However, heterosexual transmission is the leading mode of transmission worldwide and remains the primary mode of disease acquisition in Africa. Sexual transmission of HIV is relatively inefficient, but behavioral and biologic factors influence the likelihood of HIV transmission in a given sexual encounter. In particular, coinfection with classical sexually transmitted infections (STIs) (especially genital ulcerative diseases such as herpes simplex) greatly increases the infectiousness and the susceptibility of an individual. STIs increase the concentration of HIV in genital secretions, which increases the likelihood for transmission.

The risk for acquisition of HIV per coital act has been estimated to be 5 per 10,000 for insertive unprotected penile-vaginal intercourse to 50 per 10,000 for receptive unprotected anal intercourse. However, the risk is not stable and varies depending on the stage of infection and other amplifying cofactors. HIV transmission risk is highest in early HIV infection and in advanced infection (Fig. 363-2), demonstrating that the viral concentration in the genital secretions is the strongest predictor of the risk for transmission.

Prevention Strategies

Traditional strategies for the prevention of sexual transmission of HIV have focused on encouraging abstinence, reducing unsafe sexual behaviors (especially unprotected anal intercourse and concurrent relationships), encouraging proper condom use, and treating STIs. These interventions primarily focus on HIV-negative persons.

In situations in which a decision to engage in sexual activity has been made and the HIV status of the partner is positive, unknown, or in doubt, safe sexual practices ("safe sex") should be implemented. Consistent use of latex condoms has been shown to be effective in preventing HIV transmission at both individual and population levels. The condom should be made of latex and must be used properly. Natural skin condoms should not be used because they do not prevent transmission of HIV. Petroleum-based lubricants enhance the likelihood of rupture of latex condoms and should be avoided. If needed, water-based lubricants such as K-Y jelly should be used.

The effectiveness of condoms in preventing heterosexual transmission of HIV has been estimated to be 87%, but it may be as low as 60% or as high as 96%. The effectiveness of condoms during anal intercourse is probably lower because the frequency of condom breakage and slippage may be considerably higher than during vaginal intercourse. Circumcision represents an alternative strategy to protect men from HIV. Randomized clinical trials have demonstrated a protective benefit of male circumcision, with the risk for acquisition

of HIV infection through heterosexual intercourse decreasing by approximately 60%, with increasing reduction in HIV acquisition over time. However, this benefit has not been confirmed for MSM.

Antiretroviral Prevention

Antiretroviral therapy is a powerful tool in decreasing HIV replication and thus infectivity and the subsequent risk for transmission through sexual contact. In the HPTN 052 study, early antiretroviral therapy of HIV-infected patients beginning at a CD4 count of 350 to 550 cells/μL reduced sexual transmission of HIV-1 by 96%.[A1] Observational studies also suggest that broader antiretroviral use at a population level can reduce HIV incidence. Antiretrovirals also are effective for the prevention of HIV when administered prophylactically to HIV-uninfected at-risk individuals as pre-exposure prophylaxis (PrEP). In a randomized trial, daily administration of co-formulated tenofovir plus emtricitabine as PrEP among MSM decreased the risk for HIV infection by 44%.[A2] Other studies using tenofovir with emtricitabine show a decrease of as much as 85% in infections,[1] although findings have varied across studies depending on adherence.[A3-A6] Based on these studies, in 2013 the U.S. Food and Drug Administration approved the use of co-formulated tenofovir plus emtricitabine for PrEP to prevent sexual transmission of HIV. A tenofovir-containing vaginal gel led to a 39% reduction in the risk for HIV infection among women in one study,[A7] but not in an intention-to-treat analysis in a large randomized trial.[A8] Use of a monthly vaginal ring containing dapivirine has been shown to reduce HIV infection by about 30%; however, such a product is not yet commercially available.[A9]

The U.S. Centers for Disease Control and Prevention (CDC) and the International Antiviral Society-USA Panel (Table 363-1) have issued guidelines for clinicians for PrEP with antiretroviral drugs for the prevention of HIV-infection in the United States. PrEP with frequent screening and prompt treatment for those who become infected can reduce HIV burden among persons who inject drugs (PWID) and can provide health benefits for the entire population, but it remains a very expensive intervention at current drug prices.[2]

Four placebo-controlled randomized clinical trials have demonstrated that PrEP with daily dosing of tenofovir disoproxil fumarate (TDF)/emtricitabine (300/200 mg) significantly decreases HIV acquisition in MSM, high-risk heterosexuals, and injection drug users who share injection equipment. The efficacy of daily TDF/emtricitabine is greater than 90% but is highly correlated with degree of compliance.[3] TDF/emtricitabine is safe and well tolerated.[4] In trials in which women were adherent to oral PrEP, PrEP was equally efficacious in men and women. However, in studies of oral PrEP exclusively in women, adherence was low, and it was not efficacious.[5] Compliance similarly has been found to be a problem in women using other forms of PrEP, such

TABLE 363-1 PRE-EXPOSURE PROPHYLAXIS REGIMENS

PrEP should be considered in HIV-negative persons:
- in whom the population incidence of HIV is ≥2% per year or who are HIV-seronegative partners of HIV-infected persons whose HIV is not fully suppressed
- who do not have osteopenia, osteoporosis, or a creatinine clearance <60 mL/min; PrEP should be used cautiously in patients with chronic hepatitis B virus infection

The preferred regimen is tenofovir disoproxil fumarate/emtricitabine.

HIV = human immunodeficiency virus; PrEP = pre-exposure prophylaxis.
Data from Günthard HF, Saag MS, Benson CA, et al. Antiretroviral drugs for treatment and prevention of HIV infection in adults: 2016 recommendations of the International Antiviral Society-USA panel. *JAMA.* 2016;316:191-210.

TABLE 363-2 POSTEXPOSURE PROPHYLAXIS REGIMENS

NUMBER OF ANTIRETROVIRAL DRUGS

A two-drug regimen is effective, but three drugs are preferred; 28 days of treatment are recommended

PREFERRED ANTIRETROVIRAL REGIMEN

TDF + 3TC (or FTC) as the first two drugs
LPV/r or ATV/r is the preferred third drug, but RAL, DRV/r, or EFV are alternatives

3TC = lamivudine; ATV = atazanavir; DRV = darunavir; EFV = efavirenz; FTC = emtricitabine; HIV = human immunodeficiency virus; LPV = lopinavir; /r = boosted with ritonavir; RAL = raltegravir; TDF = tenofovir.
Adapted from Ford N, Mayer KH. World Health Organization guidelines on postexposure prophylaxis for HIV: recommendations for a public health approach. *Clin Infect Dis.* 2015;60(Suppl 3):S161-S164.

as topical PrEP, including vaginal tenofovir gel and the monthly dapivirine ring,[A10] thus leading to the conclusion that focused research is needed to identify the most acceptable and effective agents and modes of delivery of PrEP to women.

Postexposure Prophylaxis

In addition, antiretrovirals can be given after exposure to prevent HIV acquisition (postexposure prophylaxis [PEP]). The CDC, the Canadian Institutes of Health Research (CIHR) Canadian HIV Trials Network, the World Health Organization, and professional organizations have published guidelines for antiretroviral PEP after sexual assault, injection drug use, and other nonoccupational exposures to HIV.[6-8] In these guidelines it is recommended that persons seek care 72 hours or sooner after nonoccupational exposure to the blood, genital secretions, or other potentially infected body fluids of a person known or suspected to have HIV infection and be offered a 28-day course of antiretroviral therapy (Table 363-2).[9]

Transmission in Injection Drug Users

The primary mode of HIV transmission in PWID is sharing of contaminated needles and syringes. Sharing of injection paraphernalia ("works") is commonplace among injection drug users and is reinforced by the cultural, economic, and legal environment in that community. The risk for transmission of HIV is highest in injection drug users who share needles and use drugs that are injected more frequently, such as cocaine or methamphetamines.

Prevention Strategies

The primary mode of preventing HIV transmission in PWID is to stop the use of intravenous drugs. Education programs that are culturally sensitive and geared to young audiences have the best chance of preventing drug use.[10] Access to treatment centers for injection drug users is the best approach. However, approximately 80% of active drug users in the United States are not in substance abuse treatment because of either choice or the unavailability of treatment centers. For injection drug users who do not wish to seek treatment or who are unable to gain access to treatment, the most effective way to prevent HIV infection is to avoid sharing needles and paraphernalia. Some communities have adopted programs that provide free needles and syringes for injection drug users, and there is strong evidence that these programs, when implemented properly, are effective in reducing HIV transmission and do not result in increased drug use among participants. Where supplies cannot be obtained, needles and syringes should be cleaned after each use, preferably with readily accessible virucidal cleansers such as chlorine bleach (diluted 1 : 10). As with sexual transmission, data from Vancouver, Canada, suggest that antiretroviral treatment of injection drug users decreases the incidence of HIV infection among drug users. A randomized controlled trial conducted in PWID in Thailand demonstrated a 49% reduction in HIV acquisition when tenofovir was given as PrEP. As a result the CDC issued guidance for the use of PrEP among injection drug users but has recommended the use of co-formulated tenofovir plus emtricitabine rather than tenofovir alone as the preferred PrEP regimen among injection drug users. However, this is an off-label indication. A recent outbreak of HIV among PWID and persons who were addicted to prescription opioids in rural Indiana is a reminder that the current opioid epidemic can lead to rapidly spreading outbreaks of HIV.

Transmission Through Blood Products and Other Tissues

HIV has been transmitted through the transfusion of single-donor blood and blood products, including whole blood, fresh-frozen plasma, packed red blood cells, cryoprecipitate, clotting factors, and platelets (Chapter 167). Confidential donor exclusion, as well as the institution of HIV antibody screening in 1985, followed by additional testing for antibodies to HIV-2 and p24 antigen in 1996 and nucleic acid testing in 2002, has reduced the risk for HIV infection through the transfusion of blood or blood products to approximately 1 in 2,135,000. Transmission of HIV by liver, heart, kidney, pancreas, bone, and possibly skin transplantation has been reported. In contrast, relatively avascular tissues such as corneas and processed tissues have not been associated with transmission.

Prevention Strategies

The institution of HIV antibody testing of donated blood and blood products in 1985 has had the most dramatic effect on lowering the incidence of transfusion-related transmission (Chapter 167). When combined with voluntary self-deferral and nucleic acid testing, the blood supply in most countries has become virtually free of HIV. Heat inactivation processes for cryoprecipitate and clotting factor concentrates have eliminated transmission of HIV through use of these products. Other products, such as immunoglobulin preparations and hepatitis B vaccines, are produced by fractionation methods that remove HIV and have never been associated with transmission of HIV. Organ and tissue donors should be evaluated and serologically screened in a manner similar to blood donors. In addition, donations of semen and bone from a living donor may be quarantined until subsequent testing has definitively ruled out the possibility of delayed seroconversion in the donor.

Transmission to Health Care Workers

Detailed studies examining the risk associated with specific exposures to health care workers, such as needlestick injuries and mucous membrane exposure, have demonstrated low risk for acquisition of disease in the workplace. More than 3628 health care workers have been prospectively examined in carefully designed surveillance studies at 10 high-incidence medical centers. The overall risk for seroconversion after a percutaneous needlestick from a known HIV-infected source is 0.3% per exposure. A retrospective study conducted by the CDC found that the risk for transmission of HIV to health care workers is increased when the device causing the injury is visibly contaminated with blood, when the device has been used for insertion into a vein or artery, when the device causes a deep injury, or when the source patient dies within 2 months after the exposure. Exposure of mucous membranes to HIV-infected blood has resulted in seroconversion only rarely, and the risk for transmission is estimated to be 0.09% per exposure.

Prevention Strategies

In August 1987, the CDC published guidelines recommending that the principles of "universal precautions" be incorporated into health care settings to minimize exposure of health care workers to blood and body fluids that may be infected with blood-borne pathogens such as HIV. Universal precautions are based on the premise that any patient may be infected with blood-borne infectious agents and it may be difficult, if not impossible, to differentiate those with infection from their uninfected counterparts. All specimens containing blood or blood-tinged fluids obtained from *any* patient should be considered hazardous and handled as such. The use of universal precautions helps minimize the transmission of many transmissible diseases in addition to HIV.

Gowns, protective eyewear, and masks are not usually needed except in circumstances in which splattering or splashing of blood-containing fluids is likely to occur. Health care workers with denuded skin, open lesions, or active dermatitis should avoid direct patient contact and should not process contaminated equipment or materials. Handling of sharp instruments ("sharps") represents the greatest risk for transmission of HIV to health care workers. Although injuries from sharps cannot be eliminated entirely, the number of exposures can be reduced substantially by adhering to guidelines put forth in universal precautions. Before a sharp instrument is used, thought should be given to where the instrument will be disposed of after use. Impervious containers should be readily available in all patient care areas and identified by the health care worker *before* the use of sharps. These containers should be checked frequently and should not be allowed to overfill. Used needles should never be manipulated, bent, broken, or recapped. Recapping of needles is the single most common activity that results in needlestick injuries. Technologic developments that do not rely on health care worker compliance, such as self-sheathing needles, also have been important in decreasing the risk for needlestick injury.

Antiretroviral agents are also used for PEP in health care workers. A case-control study suggested that risk for HIV seroconversion after occupational exposure was decreased by approximately 81% with the use of zidovudine alone. Subsequent recommendations have incorporated the newer antiretroviral drugs, as well as risk stratification for the type of exposure, in the management of occupational exposure to HIV. In 2013, the CDC issued revised recommendations for the use of PEP after exposure to HIV among health care workers. The essential elements of management of a health care worker after a needlestick or mucous membrane exposure include appropriately evaluating the donor (patient) and recipient (health care worker) at the time of exposure, counseling of the health care worker, and providing follow-up HIV testing. There is no longer the need to determine the severity of exposure to direct the number of antiretroviral drugs to be used; a regimen containing three or more drugs is now recommended with co-formulated tenofovir/emtricitabine plus raltegravir as the preferred regimen. Antiretroviral drugs for PEP should be initiated within 72 hours of exposure and continued for 4 weeks. The U.S. Public Health Service has established a National Clinicians' Post-Exposure Prophylaxis Hotline (PEPline) to provide expert consultation about the management of health care workers with potential HIV exposure. The PEPline can be accessed at 1-888-448-4911 or through the Internet at http://nccc.ucsf.edu/clinician-consultation/pep-post-exposure-prophylaxis/.

PREVENTION INTERVENTIONS FOR INFECTED INDIVIDUALS

Antiretroviral therapy administered to HIV-infected individuals decreases the risk for HIV transmission by over 96%, and thus suppression of HIV replication to undetectable levels is the most effective intervention to decrease HIV transmission from an HIV-infected person (undetectable = untransmittable or U = U). As a result, the U.S. Department of Health and Human Services antiretroviral treatment guidelines now recommend initiation of antiretroviral treatment regardless of the CD4 cell count and monitoring for viral suppression.

In addition, the CDC, Health Resources and Services Administration, National Institutes of Health, and Infectious Diseases Society of America have published joint recommendations for incorporating HIV prevention into the HIV medical care setting. These guidelines reflect four basic priorities: (1) screening for risky behavior and STIs; (2) providing general and tailored risk reduction messages to patients; (3) when indicated, referring patients for additional risk reduction services and other services that may affect risk reduction (e.g., substance abuse treatment); and (4) ensuring that patients are provided with partner counseling and referral services. HIV-infected persons should be screened and treated for STIs. The CDC's 2010 sexually transmitted disease treatment guidelines recommend that all patients with newly diagnosed HIV infection undergo screening for gonorrhea, chlamydial infection, hepatitis B and C virus infection, and syphilis. Screening for curable STIs (gonorrhea, chlamydial infection, and syphilis) should be performed at least annually in sexually active patients. More frequent screening for STIs might be appropriate depending on individual risk behaviors, the local epidemiology of STIs, and whether incident STIs are detected by screening or by the presence of symptoms.

PREVENTION IN DEVELOPMENT

As shown in Figure 363-1, many prevention strategies are available, and some are in development. Vaccine strategies are increasingly focused on the generation of different types of antibodies. Broad neutralizing antibodies offer almost complete protection in macaques from infection for several months, suggesting the feasibility of a protective vaccine.[11] Injectable antiretroviral agents in different classes may serve as an advance for PEP and PrEP, and such agents are in phase 2 testing. Delivering of slow-release topical tenofovir from a cervical ring is being examined in two clinical trials.

Grade A References

A1. Cohen MS, Chen YQ, McCauley M, et al. Prevention of HIV-1 infection with early antiretroviral therapy. *N Engl J Med.* 2011;365:493-505.
A2. Grant RM, Lama JR, Anderson PL, et al. Preexposure chemoprophylaxis for HIV prevention in men who have sex with men. *N Engl J Med.* 2010;363:2587-2599.
A3. Baeten JM, Donnell D, Ndase P, et al. Antiretroviral prophylaxis for HIV prevention in heterosexual men and women. *N Engl J Med.* 2012;367:399-410.
A4. Thigpen MC, Kebaabetswe PM, Paxton LA, et al. Antiretroviral preexposure prophylaxis for heterosexual HIV transmission in Botswana. *N Engl J Med.* 2012;367:423-434.
A5. Choopanya K, Martin M, Suntharasamai P, et al. Antiretroviral prophylaxis for HIV infection among people who inject drugs in Bangkok, Thailand: a randomized, double-blind, placebo-controlled trial. *Lancet.* 2013;381:2083-2090.
A6. Molina JM, Capitant C, Spire B, et al. On-demand preexposure prophylaxis in men at high risk for HIV-1 infection. *N Engl J Med.* 2015;373:2237-2246.
A7. Abdool Karim Q, Abdool Karim SS, Frohlich JA, et al. Effectiveness and safety of tenofovir gel, an antiretroviral microbicide, for the prevention of HIV infection in women. *Science.* 2010;329:1168-1174.
A8. Marrazzo JM, Ramjee G, Richardson BA, et al. Tenofovir-based preexposure prophylaxis for HIV infection among African women. *N Engl J Med.* 2015;372:509-518.
A9. Baeten JM, Palanee-Phillips T, Brown ER, et al. Use of a vaginal ring containing dapivirine for HIV-1 prevention in women. *N Engl J Med.* 2016;375:2121-2132.
A10. Nel A, van Niekerk N, Kapiga S, et al. Safety and efficacy of a dapivirine vaginal ring for HIV prevention in women. *N Engl J Med.* 2016;375:2133-2143.

GENERAL REFERENCES

For the General References and other additional features, please visit Expert Consult at https://expertconsult.inkling.com.

364

ANTIRETROVIRAL THERAPY FOR HUMAN IMMUNODEFICIENCY VIRUS AND ACQUIRED IMMUNODEFICIENCY SYNDROME

ROY M. GULICK

The development of effective antiretroviral therapy (ART) for human immunodeficiency virus (HIV) infection is one of the most notable achievements in modern medicine. Triple-drug therapy was first introduced in the mid-1990s and resulted in a two-thirds decrease in HIV-related deaths within 2 years in developed countries and a continued decrease subsequently. Today, a total of 32 antiretroviral drugs are approved by the U.S. Food and Drug Administration (FDA), and three-drug combination regimens are the standard of care. The benefits of ART have been extended to developing countries, and more than 21 million people currently are taking ART worldwide. The life expectancy of an HIV-infected individual appropriately treated with ART is now estimated to be nearly that of the general population, both in developed[1] and developing countries.[2]

WHEN TO START ART?

ART for the treatment of HIV infection should be started as soon as possible. Large, randomized clinical trials conducted in both developed and developing countries demonstrated consistently decreased clinical progression in individuals who started ART immediately compared with delaying treatment, regardless of their CD4 cell count.[A1-A3] In addition, it is now well established that ART in an HIV-infected individual with suppressed viremia reduces the risk for transmission to others by more than 90%.[A4]

Current guidelines from around the world now recommend starting ART in *all* HIV-infected patients, because of both clinical benefits to the HIV-infected person and reduction in HIV transmission to others. Current ART regimens are potent, convenient, and generally well tolerated.

TABLE 364-1 ANTIRETROVIRAL DRUGS

MECHANISTIC DRUG CLASS	GENERIC NAME	ABBREVIATION(S)	TRADE NAME	YEAR OF U.S. FDA APPROVAL
HIV NUCLEOSIDE ANALOGUE REVERSE TRANSCRIPTASE INHIBITORS (NRTIs)				
	zidovudine	ZDV, AZT	Retrovir	1987
	didanosine	ddI	Videx	1991*
	zalcitabine	ddC	Hivid	1992†
	stavudine	d4T	Zerit	1994*
	lamivudine	3TC	Epivir	1995
	abacavir	ABC	Ziagen	1998
	tenofovir disoproxil fumarate	TDF	Viread	2001
	emtricitabine	FTC	Emtriva	2003
	tenofovir alafenamide	TAF	Descovy‡	2015
HIV NON-NUCLEOSIDE ANALOGUE REVERSE TRANSCRIPTASE INHIBITORS (NNRTIs)				
	nevirapine	NVP	Viramune	1996
	delavirdine	DLV	Rescriptor	1997*
	efavirenz	EFV	Sustiva	1998
	etravirine	ETR	Intelence	2008
	rilpivirine	RPV	Edurant	2010
	doravirine	DOR	Pifeltro	2018
HIV PROTEASE INHIBOTIRS (PIs)				
	saquinavir	SQV	Invirase	1995
	ritonavir	RTV	Norvir	1996
	indinavir	IDV	Crixivan	1996
	nelfinavir	NFV	Viracept	1997
	amprenavir	APV	Agenerase	1999†
	lopinavir/ritonavir	LPV/r	Kaletra	2000
	atazanavir	ATV	Reyataz	2003
	fosamprenavir	FPV	Lexiva	2003
	tipranavir	TPV	Aptivus	2005
	darunavir	DRV	Prezista	2006
HIV ENTRY INHIBITORS (EIs)				
	enfuvirtide	ENF, T-20	Fuzeon	2003
	maraviroc	MVC	Selzentry	2007
	ibalizumab	IBA	Trogarzo	2018
HIV INTEGRASE INHIBITORS (INSTIs)				
	raltegravir	RAL	Isentress	2007
	elvitegravir	EVG	Vitekta	2011
	dolutegravir	DTG	Tivicay	2013
	bictegravir	BIC	Biktarvy	2018‡

*Withdrawal from the market planned.
†Withdrawn from the market.
‡Currently available only as part of a fixed-dose combination (e.g., with TAF/emtricitabine).
U.S. FDA = U.S. Food and Drug Administration; HIV = human immunodeficiency virus.

WHAT TO START?

Since 1987, the FDA has approved 32 antiretroviral drugs from seven mechanistic classes (Table 364-1). The goals of ART are to suppress viral replication, prevent the emergence of drug-resistant viral strains, enhance immunologic responses, decrease clinical events, and prolong healthy life.[3-7] Antiretroviral drugs interfere with individual steps in the HIV replication cycle (Fig. 364-1). The first step of the life cycle is HIV entry, a three-step process starting with binding of the HIV external membrane glycoprotein (gp120) to the CD4 receptor on the surface of the CD4$^+$ T lymphocyte. This binding induces a conformational change in gp120, permitting the second step of HIV entry, which is binding to a second cellular receptor, the chemokine receptor, either CCR5 (bound by R5 viruses) or CXCR4 (bound by X4 viruses). Some HIV strains are dual-tropic and can bind to either the CCR5 or CXCR4 receptor, and some individuals are infected with a mixed population of R5 and X4 viral strains. HIV binding to the chemokine receptor induces an additional conformational change, allowing the viral protein gp41 to pierce the target cell membrane and then fold in on itself in a coil-on-coil interaction, leading to fusion of the viral and cellular membranes and extrusion of the viral particle contents (viral RNA, viral proteins) into the cytoplasm of the cell.

Inside the cell, viral RNA is transcribed to viral DNA by a viral-specific enzyme called *HIV reverse transcriptase*. Following transcription, two strands of viral DNA form a double-stranded complex catalyzed by a second viral-specific enzyme called *HIV integrase*, which also promotes transport of the viral DNA complex into the nucleus of the cell and DNA strand transfer—the random integration of the viral DNA into the cellular genome. At the point

of viral DNA integration, the cell is infected for life. The cell may enter a latent period, with a cellular lifespan as long as 60 years, or may be activated to transcribe both cellular and viral DNA into RNA and then translate RNA into proteins, including viral proteins, which assemble at the surface of the cell and then bud off into new viral particles. After budding, a third viral-specific enzyme, *HIV protease*, cleaves viral precursor proteins, a step that is necessary for viral maturation and infectivity. One infected cell can produce hundreds to thousands of viral particles, and many will be capable of starting the process again on encountering another CD4$^+$ T lymphocyte.

Antiretroviral drugs inhibit steps of the HIV replication cycle (see Fig. 364-1). Three kinds of HIV entry inhibitors target the first step in the HIV life cycle, viral entry, by inhibiting either conformation changes after CD4 receptor attachment (CD4 post-attachment inhibitors), CCR5 chemokine receptor binding (CCR5 antagonists), or membrane fusion (fusion inhibitors). The nucleoside analogue reverse transcriptase inhibitors (NRTIs) target the viral-specific enzyme *HIV reverse transcriptase*. A second class of HIV reverse transcriptase inhibitors are the non-nucleoside analogue reverse transcriptase inhibitors (NNRTIs), which bind to a different part of the same enzyme. The integrase strand transfer inhibitors (INSTIs) inhibit the viral-specific enzyme *HIV integrase* by specifically targeting the transfer of viral DNA to the host cell genome. The HIV protease inhibitors (PIs) bind to the active site of the *HIV protease* enzyme and prevent precursor protein cleavage, viral maturation, and infectivity.

Currently, there are nine FDA-approved, one-pill, once-daily regimens; these are popular with providers and patients and lead to excellent adherence, with virologic suppression rates of more than 85% in some groups

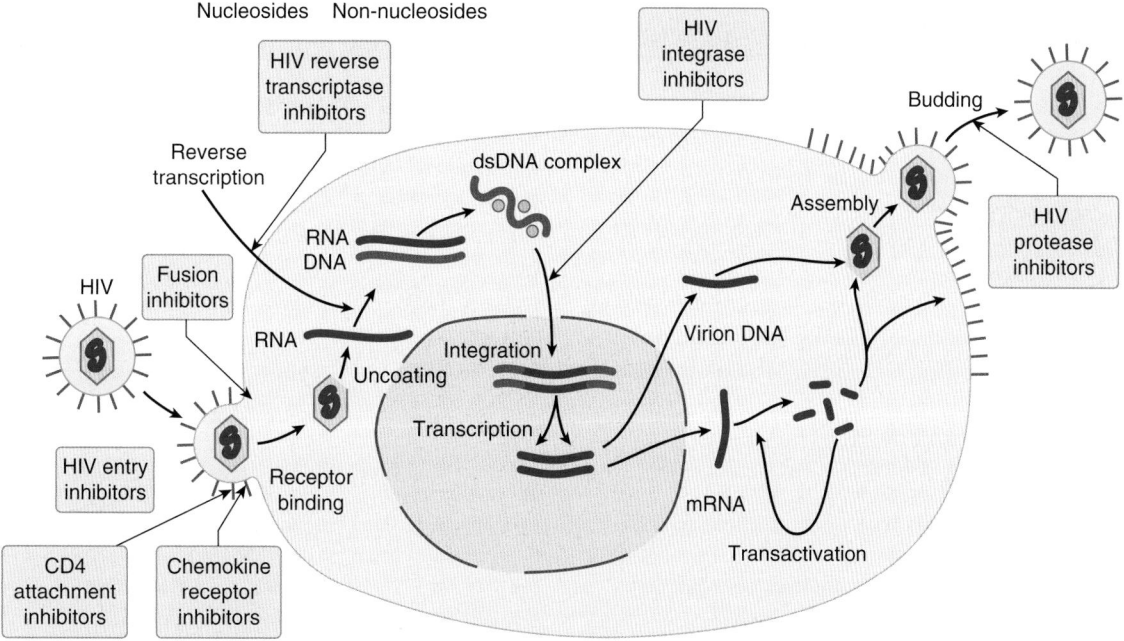

FIGURE 364-1. Life cycle of human immunodeficiency virus (*HIV*) and mechanisms of action of the seven antiretroviral drug classes. See text (What to Start? section) for details.

(Table 364-2).[A5-A9] However, some 2-drug antiretroviral regimens, given either as initial or maintenance therapy, achieved non-inferior efficacy to standard 3-drug regimens in phase 3 randomized studies, including the combination of dolutegravir with lamivudine or rilpivirine.[A10][A11] Potency, convenience, and tolerability are essential qualities of current antiretroviral drug regimens and account for the durable clinical benefits. Current recommended initial regimens in the U.S. ART guidelines (Table 364-3) are combinations of two nucleoside analogues together with a third drug (integrase inhibitor). Globally, the most widely used antiretroviral regimen is two nucleoside analogues combined with a non-nucleoside analogue (NNRTI), efavirenz.

WHEN TO CHANGE ANTIRETROVIRAL THERAPY?

In a stable patient on ART, HIV RNA should be monitored every 3 to 6 months. Even with virologic suppression rates of more than 85%, some patients will experience virologic failure, with a once-suppressed viral load level now being repeatedly detectable above the limit of the HIV RNA assay (20, 40, or 50 copies/mL). The reasons for regimen failure can include suboptimal adherence, baseline drug resistance or cross-resistance, prior use of ART, use of less potent antiretroviral drug regimens, drug levels and drug-drug interactions, penetration into tissue reservoirs (e.g., genital tract, central nervous system [CNS]), suboptimal provider experience, and other, unknown reasons. Also, more than one factor may play a role in an individual patient. One of the challenges with treatment failure is to try to determine the cause of failure and then select the next regimen that can address and overcome the reason for failure.

U.S. ART guidelines recommend addressing virologic failure by changing antiretroviral regimens promptly when failure is confirmed. Virologic failure can be defined as repeated detection of HIV RNA levels in a drug-adherent patient. HIV RNA levels suppressed below the level of detection of the assay are unlikely to result in the emergence of drug-resistant viral strains. Levels confirmed greater than 200 copies/mL (and certainly greater than 500 copies/mL) will lead to the selection of drug-resistant viral strains and result in treatment failure. More controversial are repeated HIV RNA levels between the level of detection and 200 copies/mL (low-level viremia) that may represent a higher virologic set point rather than ongoing viral replication and may not necessitate treatment change.

HIV is prone to errors in gene replication, and thus an individual is infected with not just one virus but a "swarm" of related viral strains with distinct genetic mutational patterns. Drug resistance is conferred by viral strains with specific amino acid substitutions in viral proteins (HIV reverse transcriptase, HIV integrase, HIV protease) that are selected for in the presence of an antiretroviral drug. For example, with ongoing viral replication in the presence of the HIV nucleoside analogue emtricitabine or lamivudine, a viral strain

with the substitution of valine for methionine at amino acid position 184 (denoted M184V) of HIV reverse transcriptase will be selected and confer complete resistance to these drugs. Drugs with which single substitutions confer resistance are considered to have a low barrier to resistance and include the nucleoside analogues emtricitabine and lamivudine, the NNRTIs efavirenz and nevirapine, and the integrase inhibitors elvitegravir and raltegravir. Drugs that require multiple substitutions are considered to have a higher barrier to resistance, including the nucleoside analogue zidovudine, most of the HIV protease inhibitors, and the integrase inhibitors bictegravir and dolutegravir. Drugs with overlapping resistance patterns lead to cross resistance. For example, a patient who develops resistance to emtricitabine with the M184V substitution will have complete cross resistance to lamivudine, even though the patient never took lamivudine. Drug resistance can be assessed by an HIV genotype that identifies amino acid substitutions that must be correlated with drug resistance or an HIV phenotype that assesses viral growth in the presence of each of the antiretroviral drugs.[8]

Another common clinical conundrum is immunologic failure—a patient taking ART who achieves virologic suppression but fails to increase the CD4 cell count. The cause of immunologic failure is not clear, but associations with various factors, including CD4 count less than 200 cells/μL at the time of ART initiation, older age, coinfections, older medications (e.g., zidovudine; the combination of didanosine and tenofovir), persistent immune activation, and loss of regenerative potential have been reported. There is no accepted treatment for immunologic failure. Neither changing nor adding antiretroviral drugs results in an improved CD4 cell response. Immune-based therapies have been studied but are not effective. For example, in two large randomized clinical trials, interleukin-2 was associated with increased CD4 cell counts but failed to demonstrate associated clinical benefits. Current management is to continue antiretroviral therapy, optimize opportunistic infection prophylaxes, and follow the patient closely.

WHAT ANTIRETROVIRAL THERAPY TO CHANGE TO?

The current goal for all HIV-infected patients taking ART, regardless of treatment experience, is to maximally suppress the viral load level below the level of assay detection. In a treatment-experienced patient, this is done by reviewing the ART history with a focus on adherence, tolerability, and possible drug-drug interactions; conduct drug-resistance testing (HIV genotype for first or second failure; HIV genotype and phenotype for more advanced failure); identify susceptible drugs and drug classes; and, ultimately, design a subsequent regimen with at least two (and preferably three) fully active antiretroviral agents.

In recent years, a number of newer antiretroviral drugs have made this goal possible, including drugs in existing mechanistic classes with activity against

TABLE 364-2   ANTIRETROVIRAL FIXED-DOSE COMBINATIONS

DRUG CLASS(ES)	GENERIC NAMES	ABBREVIATION(S)	TRADE NAMES	DOSING	YEAR OF U.S. FDA APPROVAL
2 NRTI	zidovudine + lamivudine	ZDV/3TC	Combivir	Twice daily	1997
3 NRTI	abacavir + zidovudine + lamivudine	ABC/ZDV/3TC	Trizivir	Twice daily	2000
Boosted PI	lopinavir + ritonavir	LPV/RTV	Kaletra	Once or twice daily	2000
2 NRTI	tenofovir disoproxil fumarate + emtricitabine	TDF/FTC	Truvada	Once daily	2004
2 NRTI	abacavir + lamivudine	ABC/3TC	Epzicom	Once daily	2004
2 NRTI + NNRTI	tenofovir disoproxil fumarate + emtricitabine + efavirenz*	TDF/FTC/EFV*	Atripla	Once daily	2006
2 NRTI + NNRTI	tenofovir disoproxil fumarate + emtricitabine + rilpivirine*	TDF/FTC/RPV*	Complera	Once daily	2011
2 NRTI + boosted INSTI	tenofovir disoproxil fumarate + emtricitabine + elvitegravir + cobicistat*	TDF/FTC/EVG/c*	Stribild	Once daily	2012
2 NRTI + INSTI	abacavir + lamivudine + dolutegravir*	ABC/3TC/DTG*	Triumeq	Once daily	2014
Boosted PI	atazanavir + cobicistat	ATV/c	Evotaz	Once daily	2015
Boosted PI	darunavir + cobicistat	DRV/c	Prezcobix	Once daily	2015
2 NRTI + boosted INSTI	tenofovir alafenamide + emtricitabine + elvitegravir + cobicistat*	TAF/FTC/EVG/c*	Genvoya	Once daily	2015
2 NRTI + NNRTI	tenofovir alafenamide + emtricitabine + rilpivirine*	TAF/FTC/RPV*	Odefsey	Once daily	2016
2 NRTI	tenofovir alafenamide + emtricitabine	TAF/FTC	Descovy	Once daily	2016
2 NRTI + INSTI	tenofovir alafenamide + emtricitabine + bictegravir*	TAF/FTC/BIC*	Biktarvy	Once daily	2018
2 NRTI + boosted PI	tenofovir alafenamide + emtricitabine + darunavir + cobicistat*	TAF/FTC/DRV/c*	Symtuza	Once daily	2018
2 NRTI + NNRTI	tenofovir disoproxil fumarate + lamivudine + doravirine*	TDF/3TC/DOR*	Delstrigo	Once daily	2018

*One pill, once-daily antiretroviral therapy (ART) regimen.
INSTI = integrase inhibitor; NNRTI = non-nucleoside reverse transcriptase inhibitor; NRTI = nucleoside analogue reverse transcriptase inhibitor; PI = protease inhibitor.

TABLE 364-3   RECOMMENDED INITIAL ANTIRETROVIRAL DRUG REGIMENS

REGIMEN*	DRUGS
Integrase strand transfer inhibitor (INSTI)-based	bictegravir/tenofovir alafenamide/emtricitabine (co-formulated)
	dolutegravir/abacavir†/lamivudine (co-formulated)
	dolutegravir + either tenofovir disoproxil fumarate/emtricitabine (co-formulated) or tenofovir alafenamide/emtricitabine (co-formulated)
	raltegravir + either tenofovir disoproxil fumarate/emtricitabine (co-formulated) or tenofovir alafenamide/emtricitabine (co-formulated)

*From Panel on Antiretroviral Guidelines for Adults and Adolescents. Guidelines for the use of antiretroviral agents in HIV-1-infected adults and adolescents. Department of Health and Human Services. http://aidsinfo.nih.gov/contentfiles/lvguidelines/AdultandAdolescentGL.pdf. October 25, 2018. Also see the International Antiviral Society—USA (IAS-USA) Guidelines,[4] European AIDS Clinical Society (EACS) Guidelines[5] and the World Health Organization Consolidated Guidelines.
†For patients who are HLA-B*5701 negative.

class-resistant virus (the HIV protease inhibitor darunavir and the HIV NNRTI etravirine) and drugs with new mechanisms of action (the HIV fusion inhibitor enfuvirtide; the CCR5 antagonist maraviroc; the CD4 post-attachment inhibitor ibalizumab; and the HIV integrase inhibitors). Some studies show that new active antiretroviral regimens result in virologic suppression in a majority of treatment-experienced patients for extended periods.[A12] One study also found that including nucleoside analogues in subsequent regimens is not necessary if the regimen contains more than two active antiretroviral drugs.[A13]

⬤ SIDE EFFECTS AND TOXICITY

Antiretroviral drugs (like all drugs) are associated with side effects and toxicity. Probably the most common side effect of ART as a group is gastrointestinal (nausea, vomiting, diarrhea), although some drugs are more associated than others (e.g., zidovudine, ritonavir). Toxicities may be divided according to seriousness and drug classes. Life-threatening toxicities occur and include drug-related hepatitis associated with NNRTIs and protease inhibitors. Of these, the NNRTI nevirapine is unique in causing drug-related hepatitis more frequently in patients with higher CD4 counts (>250 cells/μL in women and >400 cells/μL in men), likely owing to an immunologic mechanism. A hypersensitivity reaction characterized by rash and constitutional symptoms that can be life-threatening is associated with the nucleoside analogue abacavir and, less commonly, with the NNRTIs etravirine and nevirapine. An elegant study linked the abacavir-associated hypersensitivity reaction to a genetic locus that can be screened for in patients (HLA-B*5701, at a cost of approximately $50); if the drug is avoided in patients with the genetic marker, the risk for a

hypersensitivity reaction is minimized. Lactic acidosis is associated with the older nucleoside analogues (particularly stavudine and zalcitabine). The NNRTIs, although structurally unrelated, all are associated with rash; Stevens-Johnson syndrome is rarely described with etravirine or nevirapine. Although teratogenicity is described with efavirenz (FDA pregnancy category D), newer recommendations allow using or continuing[9] the drug in a pregnant woman. A preliminary report linked neural tube defects in babies born to mothers who took dolutegravir at the time of conception. Efavirenz also is linked to a small but increased risk for suicidality.

Acute side effects can be troubling to the patient and can lead to suboptimal adherence. Providers should be in close contact with a patient starting a new antiretroviral regimen and have a low threshold to substitute offending drugs for side effects or toxicities. As noted, probably the most common side effect of antiretroviral drugs is gastrointestinal toxicity, though this often can be managed by taking ART with food. Zidovudine causes anemia, neutropenia, and fatigue. Efavirenz causes CNS side effects (e.g., vivid dreams, somnolence) in up to 50% of people and should be dosed fasting at bedtime. Atazanavir causes increased indirect bilirubin by inhibiting uridine 5′-diphospho-glucuronosyltransferase, which can be associated with frank jaundice but is not associated with other liver test abnormalities.

With the current expectation that ART is lifelong, chronic and cumulative toxicities also are important. Increased cardiovascular events are associated with some, but not all, protease inhibitors[10] and, controversially, with abacavir. Indinavir and atazanavir cause renal stones. Metabolic changes, including hyperglycemia and frank diabetes, hyperlactatemia, and/or hyperlipidemia, are associated with stavudine and some protease inhibitors. Morphologic changes occur and can be very distressing for patients, including lipoatrophy (loss of fat in the face and extremities) associated with stavudine and zidovudine, and lipoaccumulation (gain of fat in the breasts, abdomen, and/or dorsocervical fat pad [buffalo hump]) associated with some protease inhibitors. Some NRTIs, including didanosine and stavudine, cause a progressive toxic peripheral neuropathy. Tenofovir disoproxil fumarate is associated with proximal renal tubular dysfunction (Fanconi syndrome) characterized by hypophosphatemia, proteinuria, glycosuria, and, eventually, elevated creatinine. Tenofovir disoproxil fumarate and protease inhibitors have also been associated with loss of bone mineral density over the first year of treatment that appears to stabilize thereafter.[11] A newer formulation of tenofovir, tenofovir alafenamide, is associated with less renal and bone toxicity. Newer antiretroviral drugs and investigational antiretroviral agents often are developed and selected for better tolerability and less toxicity.

SPECIAL POPULATIONS

Acute Infection and Prophylaxis

Current guidelines recommend that an individual identified with acute HIV infection start three-drug ART. ART reduces signs and symptoms of acute HIV and also prevents ongoing HIV transmission. Because of the risk for acquiring drug-resistant HIV, estimated at about 17% in the United States, ART should be started while awaiting the results of the HIV genotype. Guidelines recommend starting a protease inhibitor- or dolutegravir-containing regimen and then adjusting when the genotypic results are available.

Acute Opportunistic Infection

An untreated HIV-infected patient presenting with an acute opportunistic infection should be started on ART. One study of patients with a treatable opportunistic infection diagnosed in the previous 2 weeks (the majority with *Pneumocystis* pneumonia) randomized them to start ART within 48 hours or to wait at least 4 weeks. There were significantly fewer clinical events (disease progression and death) in the group that started ART earlier. Additional studies of patients with tuberculosis also demonstrated clinical benefits to starting ART earlier, particularly in patients with CD4 counts less than 50 cells/μL.[12] Starting ART within 2 weeks of an opportunistic infection is now considered the standard of care. However, caution should be taken with CNS opportunistic infections (e.g., cryptococcal or tuberculous meningitis) because some studies in developing countries have demonstrated increased mortality in patients who started ART earlier.

Coinfection with Hepatitis B

If treatment is started for either viral infection, both need to be treated optimally: two active drugs for hepatitis B and three active drugs for HIV. The antiretroviral drugs emtricitabine, lamivudine, and tenofovir have activity against both viruses; thus, a suitable regimen to treat both infections would be tenofovir (either formulation), emtricitabine (or lamivudine), and a third antiretroviral drug. Stopping drugs with activity against hepatitis B may result in a serious hepatitis flare.

Coinfection with Hepatitis C

The optimal time to treat hepatitis C infection in a patient with HIV infection is not known. The newer hepatitis C protease inhibitors are unrelated to the HIV protease inhibitors and have no activity against HIV. Significant drug interactions can occur between antiretrovirals and hepatitis C drugs, and consultation with an expert is required.

Pregnancy

The U.S. Perinatal Treatment Guidelines recommend ART for prevention of mother-to-child transmission of HIV for all pregnant women, regardless of CD4 cell count or HIV RNA level.[13] Based on efficacy, tolerability, convenience, and safety, preferred drugs in pregnancy include the NRTI pairs of abacavir/lamivudine, or tenofovir disoproxil fumarate/emtricitabine (or lamivudine) combined with a third drug: the ritonavir-boosted PI atazanavir or darunavir; or the integrase inhibitors, dolutegravir (after the first trimester) or raltegravir. Other drugs are considered alternatives, and insufficient data are available on newer drugs (the integrase inhibitors bictegravir). U.S. guidelines also recommend continuing efavirenz in a woman found to be pregnant if she is maximally virologically suppressed.

ANTIRETROVIRAL THERAPY FOR PREVENTION

One of the most successful HIV prevention strategies is the use of ART, both in HIV-infected and HIV-uninfected people (also see Chapter 363). The first

example of this was the prevention of HIV-infected mother-to-child transmission by giving the mother ART. In a classic study from the mid-1990s, the use of a single drug, zidovudine, by an HIV-infected mother reduced the risk for transmission to her infant from 25 to 8%. Current standard of care is to treat the mother with three-drug ART, with a resultant reduction in the risk for transmission to less than 0.5%.

A large multinational study randomized HIV-infected individuals with CD4 counts of 350 to 550/μL who were members of a committed couple with an HIV-uninfected partner to start ART immediately or to wait until the CD4 count decreased to less than 250 cells/μL and followed the seronegative partners for HIV infection. Of 46 linked HIV infections, 43 occurred in the group not on ART versus only 3 in individuals randomized to ART (none of whom had detectable drug concentrations); thus, treating the HIV-infected partner with ART was associated with at least a 93% reduction in transmission to the HIV-uninfected partner.

Giving ART to at-risk HIV-uninfected individuals to avoid infection is a strategy that has been explored. Postexposure prophylaxis (PEP) is recommended on the basis of an older case-control study of health care workers exposed to HIV in which taking zidovudine was associated with an 81% decrease in the risk for seroconversion compared with no prophylaxis. The U.S. Centers for Disease Control and Prevention (CDC) recommend administering three-drug ART within 72 hours for 4 weeks following significant exposure (occupational or nonoccupational) to HIV.[14]

Preexposure prophylaxis (PrEP)[15] is a strategy in which two-drug ART is given to at-risk HIV-uninfected individuals to reduce their risk for acquiring HIV infection. Recent studies in men who have sex with men showed more than an 85% reduction in new HIV infections. Other studies demonstrate PrEP efficacy in African heterosexuals[A16][A17] and Thai injection drug users.[A18] Notably, other PrEP studies in African women failed to show a benefit, mainly owing to suboptimal adherence.[A19][A20] Current CDC guidance recommends PrEP for high-risk individuals with two-drug ART with tenofovir disoproxil fumarate/emtricitabine (co-formulated) following exclusion of acute or chronic HIV infection together with ongoing monitoring of HIV status and renal function, screening for sexually transmitted infections, and risk-reduction counseling and condom distribution.

CURE

Although current ART is highly effective, it is not curative. Soon after infection, HIV establishes a latent-CD4+ T-lymphocyte cell reservoir that can persist for decades. Even with years of ART-induced prolonged virologic suppression, the latent-cell reservoir does not decrease significantly. Strategies of intensification of ART by changing or adding additional antiretroviral drugs have not been successful in decreasing the viral reservoir. HIV cure is aspirational and could be sterilizing (complete elimination of HIV) or functional (suppression of HIV without ART).[16] The best documented sterilizing cure is the case of a man with well-controlled HIV infection on ART who developed acute myelogenous leukemia and underwent radiation and cytotoxic chemotherapy, and ultimately received a bone marrow transplant from a donor with a deletion in the gene that codes for the CCR5 receptor that is required for HIV entry. After more than 10 years off of ART with no detectable HIV, he is considered to be cured. An example of functional cure is the VISCONTI cohort, 14 HIV-infected individuals treated during acute infection who discontinued ART and whose viremia remained suppressed. HIV cure currently is an active area of research.

 Grade A References

A1. Severe P, Juste MA, Ambroise A, et al. Early versus standard antiretroviral therapy for HIV-infected adults in Haiti. *N Engl J Med.* 2010;363:257-265.

A2. Lundgren JD, Babiker AG, Gordin F, et al. Initiation of antiretroviral therapy in early asymptomatic HIV infection. *N Engl J Med.* 2015;373:795-807.

A3. TEMPRANO ANRS 12136 Study Group; Danel C, Moh R, et al. A trial of early antiretrovirals and isoniazid preventive therapy in Africa. *N Engl J Med.* 2015;373:808-822.

A4. Cohen MS, Chen YQ, McCauley M, et al. Antiretroviral therapy for the prevention of HIV-1 transmission. *N Engl J Med.* 2016;375:830-839.

A5. Lennox JL, Landovitz RJ, Ribaudo HJ, et al. Efficacy and tolerability of 3 nonnucleoside reverse transcriptase inhibitor-sparing antiretroviral regimens for treatment-naive volunteers infected with HIV-1: a randomized, controlled equivalence trial. *Ann Intern Med.* 2014;161:461-471.

A6. Molina JM, Clotet B, van Lunzen J, et al. Once-daily dolutegravir versus darunavir plus ritonavir for treatment-naive adults with HIV-1 infection (FLAMINGO): 96 week results from a randomised, open-label, phase 3b study. *Lancet HIV.* 2015;2:e127-e136.

A7. Sax PE, Wohl D, Yin MT, et al. Tenofovir alafenamide versus tenofovir disoproxil fumarate, coformulated with elvitegravir, cobicistat, and emtricitabine, for initial treatment of HIV-1 infection: two randomised, double-blind, phase 3, non-inferiority trials. *Lancet.* 2015;385:2606-2615.

A8. Gallant J, Lazzarin A, Mills A, et al. Bictegravir, emtricitabine, and tenofovir alafenamide versus dolutegravir, abacavir, and lamivudine for initial treatment of HIV-1 infection (GS-US-380-1489): a double-blind, multicentre, phase 3, randomised controlled non-inferiority trial. *Lancet.* 2017;390:2063-2072.

A9. Sax PE, Pozniak A, Montes ML, et al. Coformulated bictegravir, emtricitabine, and tenofovir alafenamide versus dolutegravir with emtricitabine and tenofovir alafenamide, for initial treatment of HIV-1 infection (GS-US-380-1490): a randomised, double-blind, multicentre, phase 3, non-inferiority trial. *Lancet.* 2017;390:2073-2082.

A10. Llibre JM, Hung CC, Brinson C, et al. Efficacy, safety, and tolerability of dolutegravir-rilpivirine for the maintenance of virological suppression in adults with HIV-1: phase 3, randomised, non-inferiority SWORD-1 and SWORD-2 studies. *Lancet.* 2018;391:839-849.

A11. Cahn P, Madero JS, Arribas JR, et al. Dolutegravir plus lamivudine versus dolutegravir plus tenofovir disoproxil fumarate and emtricitabine in antiretroviral-naive adults with HIV-1 infection (GEMINI-1 and GEMINI-2): week 48 results from two multicentre, double-blind, randomised, non-inferiority, phase 3 trials. *Lancet.* 2019;393:143-155.

A12. Eron JJ, Cooper DA, Steigbigel RT, et al. Efficacy and safety of raltegravir for treatment of HIV for 5 years in the BENCHMRK studies: final results of two randomised, placebo-controlled trials. *Lancet Infect Dis.* 2013;13:587-596.

A13. Tashima KT, Smeaton LM, Fichtenbaum CJ, et al. HIV salvage therapy does not require nucleoside reverse transcriptase inhibitors: a randomized, controlled trial. *Ann Intern Med.* 2015;163:908-917.

A14. Molina JM, Capitant C, Spire B, et al. On-demand preexposure prophylaxis in men at high risk for HIV-1 infection. *N Engl J Med.* 2015;373:2237-2246.

A15. McCormack S, Dunn DT, Desai M, et al. Pre-exposure prophylaxis to prevent the acquisition of HIV-1 infection (PROUD): effectiveness results from the pilot phase of a pragmatic open-label randomised trial. *Lancet.* 2016;387:53-60.

A16. Baeten JM, Donnell D, Ndase P, et al. Antiretroviral prophylaxis for HIV prevention in heterosexual men and women. *N Engl J Med.* 2012;367:399-410.

A17. Thigpen MC, Kebaabetswe PM, Paxton LA, et al. Antiretroviral preexposure prophylaxis for heterosexual HIV transmission in Botswana. *N Engl J Med.* 2012;367:423-434.

A18. Choopanya K, Martin M, Suntharasamai P, et al. Antiretroviral prophylaxis for HIV infection in injecting drug users in Bangkok, Thailand (the Bangkok Tenofovir Study): a randomised, double-blind, placebo-controlled phase 3 trial. *Lancet.* 2013;381:2083-2090.

A19. Van Damme L, Corneli A, Ahmed K, et al. Preexposure prophylaxis for HIV infection among African women. *N Engl J Med.* 2012;367:411-422.

A20. Marrazzo JM, Ramjee G, Richardson BA, et al. Tenofovir-based preexposure prophylaxis for HIV infection among African women. *N Engl J Med.* 2015;372:509-518.

GENERAL REFERENCES

For the General References and other additional features, please visit Expert Consultn at https://expertconsult.inkling.com.

365

MICROBIAL COMPLICATIONS IN PATIENTS INFECTED WITH HUMAN IMMUNODEFICIENCY VIRUS

HENRY MASUR AND COLLEEN HADIGAN

MICROBIAL COMPLICATIONS

Despite the widespread availability of effective antiretroviral regimens in the United States since the late 1990s, AIDS-related opportunistic infections are still seen frequently at many health care facilities, especially those serving populations with poor access to health care.

Approximately 10% of HIV-infected patients in the United States are unaware of their retroviral infection. This group often presents to health care facilities with opportunistic infections as their initial clue that they have HIV infection.

In addition, a substantial number of patients are aware of their HIV infection but are not in care as a result of economic, behavioral, or social factors. These patients also present with initial or serial opportunistic infections because they are not benefitting from stable and effective antiretroviral therapy (ART).

Even for patients who initiate ART and adhere carefully to their regimens, opportunistic infections can occur. Within the first few weeks or months after ART is started, opportunistic infections may develop due to immune reconstitution or unmasking (immune reconstitution inflammatory syndrome), that is, infectious syndromes can occur due to enhanced immunologic response to latent organisms or to residual antigen (see Chapter 367). In addition, even for the many patients who have sustained viral suppression and CD4 rise due to ART, such patients continue to be at enhanced risk lifelong for certain infections such as pneumococcal disease and tuberculosis, although the magnitude of the enhanced risk declines as the CD4 count rises. Finally, some opportunistic infections occur rarely at unexpectedly high CD4 counts.

As patients live longer they are developing increasing chronic morbidity and mortality due to certain latent viruses such as human papillomavirus (HPV) (Chapter 349),[1] hepatitis C virus (HCV),[2] and hepatitis B virus (HBV) (Chapter 140),[3] as well as JC virus, and human herpes-virus 8 (HHV-8) (Chapter 367).[4] HCV and HBV progression is accelerated in HIV-infected patients compared to HIV-uninfected patients, leading to earlier development of cirrhosis, liver failure, and hepatoma. HPV is associated with cervical carcinoma and anal carcinoma, as well as oral cancers. JC virus is associated with progressive neurologic disease, and HHV-8 is associated with Kaposi sarcoma and other neoplastic processes including multicentric Castleman disease. These chronic processes related to latent viruses are causing increasing morbidity and mortality.

In addition to opportunistic infections and malignant neoplasms, an unexpected complication of chronic HIV disease even in patients who have suppressed HIV viral loads has been a persistent inflammatory state that appears to be related to HIV viremia. This viremia is often below the level of detection of standard clinical assays for blood and may be related to viral replication in poorly understood reservoirs. The persistent inflammatory state appears to accelerate atherosclerotic cardiovascular and cerebrovascular disease, renal disease, and hepatic disease. This persistent inflammatory state interacts with the AIDS-related metabolic dysfunctions, including dysglycemias and dyslipidemias, which exacerbate and complicate the inflammation-induced accelerated atherosclerosis (see Chapter 366).[5]

PATHOBIOLOGY

HIV infection causes cellular immune dysfunction by multifaceted mechanisms that include reducing the number and function of CD4 lymphocytes. The immune defect in patients with HIV infection is unique: in no other population does the constellation of PCP, toxoplasma encephalitis, CMV retinitis, disseminated *Mycobacterium avium* complex (MAC), cryptococcal meningitis, cryptosporidiosis, microsporidiosis, and Kaposi sarcoma occur so frequently. It is also remarkable that some infections that might be expected to occur in patients with HIV infection and low CD4 counts are in fact unusual. It is rare to diagnose pneumonia due to CMV or MAC, bacteremia or meningitis due to *Listeria monocytogenes*, or disseminated HSV or VZV.

The opportunistic infections that occur in patients with HIV infection differ substantially not only in their incidence, but also in their natural history compared with opportunistic infections that occur in patients with other immunodeficiencies such as those due to corticosteroids or calcineurin inhibitors. For instance, PCP is a much more indolent disease characteristically in patients with HIV infection than in stem cell transplant recipients or patients receiving cancer chemotherapy. Toxoplasmosis is much more likely to be a central nervous system process in patients with HIV infections, but is more often disseminated in transplant recipients. Effective therapy may require longer courses of treatment of patients with HIV/AIDS than other immunosuppressive diseases. Moreover, subsequent to clinical response to therapy, relapses are unusually common for HIV-infected patients with PCP, CMV retinitis, MAC bacteremia, or cryptococcal meningitis if the patients are not reconstituted immunologically with ART.

The number of circulating CD4 cells is an excellent indicator of patient prognosis and of susceptibility to opportunistic infection for patients with HIV/AIDS (Fig. 365-1). Monitoring CD4 counts prospectively has thus become a cornerstone of patient management. The blood HIV viral load is also an independent predictor of host susceptibility to opportunistic infection, but is not nearly as sensitive and specific for estimating survival or for assessing susceptibility to opportunistic infection as are CD4 counts. Although CD4 cells are enormously important to host defenses in all patients, the circulating CD4 count is much more useful in predicting susceptibility to infection for patients with HIV infection than in any other patient population.

The specific opportunistic infections that an HIV-infected person develops are influenced not only by the person's specific immunologic defects but also by environmental factors. For instance, in areas of the world where exposure to *M. tuberculosis* is common, tuberculosis is the major cause of morbidity and mortality in patients with HIV infection regardless of CD4 count, although the incidence of disease increases as the CD4 count declines. In contrast, however, in areas of the world such as the United States where tuberculosis exposure is relatively uncommon, tuberculosis is rarely seen except in

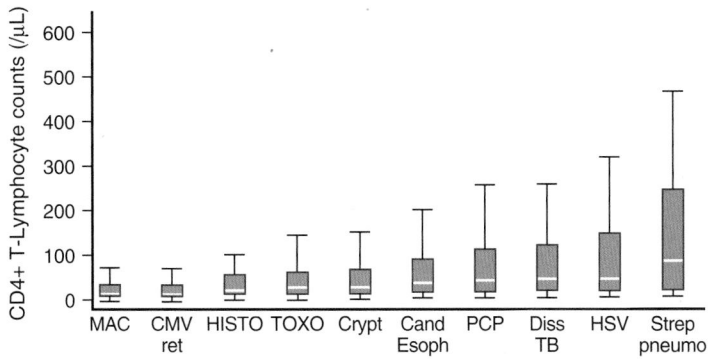

FIGURE 365-1. Distribution of CD4+ lymphocyte counts at diagnosis of opportunistic infection.

immigrants and patients exposed to special populations, such as those in prisons or homeless shelters. MAC is more common than tuberculosis in the United States (although the incidence of *M. avium* disease in patients with HIV infection appears to have declined in the United States in recent years partially due to more widespread viral suppression with ART). Similarly, in many areas of the developing world, patients are exposed to salmonella, toxoplasma, and *Cryptococcus* more frequently than in the United States, and as a result, disease in HIV-infected patients is much more common in those areas than in the United States.

Studies of the human microbiome provide an interesting perspective on factors that could influence the range of pathogens causing diseases among patients with HIV infection.[6] For instance, HIV-infected patients with lower CD4 counts have demonstrable changes in their respiratory microbiome compared to other patient populations—changes that tend to reverse with effective HIV treatment.

Behavioral factors are also important determinants of which opportunistic infections occur. Individuals who inject drugs are more likely to be infected with HCV and HBV than matched patients without injection drug use histories. They are also more likely to develop certain nonopportunistic processes such as *Staphylococcus aureus* because of their parenteral exposures. Men who have sex with men who develop proctitis or colitis are more likely to have rectal disease due to *Neisseria gonorrhoeae*, *Chlamydia trachomatis* (especially lymphogranuloma venereum strains), or *Shigella* than individuals who are not men who have sex with men.

The pathogens that cause active disease in patients with HIV infection may be organisms that were acquired recently or may represent reactivation of latent organisms acquired months or years previously. *Mycobacterium tuberculosis*, *Pneumocystis jiroveci*, *Trypanosoma cruzi*, *Leishmania donovani*, *Histoplasma capsulatum*, *Coccidioides immitis*, Herpes simplex, Herpes zoster, and CMV are examples of pathogens that can cause acute disease either soon after exposure or after many months or years of latency as determined by molecular typing or clinical epidemiology. Thus, many pathogens need to be considered as possible etiologic agents despite exposure that may have occurred in the distant past.

CLINICAL MANIFESTATIONS

One of the early observations about clinical disease in patients with AIDS was that the clinical manifestations of opportunistic infections were not identical to the presentations in other immunosuppressed patients. In patients with AIDS, for instance, PCP is much more likely to manifest with subacute symptoms over weeks or months than in HIV-uninfected patients with cancer or transplant recipients who most often present acutely over a few days. When patients are diagnosed with PCP, those with AIDS are usually less hypoxemic and have less impressive radiographic infiltrates despite the longer duration of symptoms before diagnosis. The number of organisms found in sputum or bronchoalveolar lavage specimens is also greater in patients with AIDS than in other immunosuppressed individuals, such as patients with cancer or transplant recipients, despite the less severe symptoms. Patients with AIDS also are more likely to develop treatment-limiting toxicity associated with trimethoprim-sulfamethoxazole than patients with cancer or transplant recipients. They are also more likely than other immunosuppressed populations to have multiple recurrences if they are not placed on chemoprophylaxis.

For infections due to *Toxoplasma gondii*, patients with HIV/AIDS characteristically develop toxoplasma encephalitis. Other immunosuppressed populations more often develop disseminated visceral disease involving the liver, spleen, or kidneys. Similarly, CMV in patients with HIV/AIDS causes retinitis and colitis. In patients with stem cell transplants, however, CMV retinitis is relatively uncommon and pneumonia is frequent.

Some pathogens that have been recognized to cause frequent disease among patients with HIV/AIDS, such as *M. avium*, *Cryptosporidium*, *Microsporidium*, *Bartonella*, and HHV-8, were rarely recognized as causes of life-threatening human disease before the HIV/AIDS epidemic. Even as diagnostic studies have improved for these pathogens, these organisms are far more often recognized among patients with HIV/AIDS than among other highly immunosuppressed patient populations. Conversely, as noted above, some pathogens that were deemed likely to be AIDS associated based on the mechanisms for host immune response, such as *Listeria monocytogenes*, disseminated herpes simplex or herpes zoster, and disseminated *Strongyloides stercoralis*, are rarely seen in patients with HIV/AIDS. The reasons why some pathogens are unexpectedly frequent, or unexpectedly unusual despite similar environmental exposures, have not been fully elucidated.

DIAGNOSIS

For any infection in any patient population, management is likely to be more effective and to be associated with fewer complications if the specific cause is conclusively identified, the appropriate therapy is started quickly, and unnecessary drugs are avoided. For patients with HIV infection, such an approach is especially appropriate for opportunistic complication given the broad range of opportunistic and nonopportunistic infections that could cause a particular syndrome, as well as the noninfectious causes, including drug toxicities, that can masquerade as infections.

Although the diagnostic approach always should be individualized to the specific patient considering the current CD4 count, past and current exposures, prior infections, the history, physical findings, and routine laboratory tests of the current illness, certain tests are consistently useful. Blood cultures for routine bacteria and fungi, a serum cryptococcal antigen test, or a syphilis serologic test often provide useful information. If the patient has pulmonary dysfunction, Gram stain and routine culture of expectorated or induced sputum is usually useful. If a history of appropriate geographic exposure is present, serum and urine histoplasma antigen and *Coccidioides* antibodies also can be useful, as can a *Toxoplasma* IgG test.

The utility of specific tests needs to be validated in each patient population to determine their positive and negative predictive value. Certain tests that are useful in other patient populations or for research purposes are not necessarily useful to clinically diagnose opportunistic infections. For instance, blood polymerase chain reaction (PCR) for CMV is very useful for managing patients who have received stem cell transplants, because their positive and negative predictive values are high. However, blood CMV PCR in patients with HIV infections correlates mainly with the degree of immunosuppression and does not have sufficient positive and negative predictive value to be useful for assessing the cause of end organ disease. Blood PCR for Epstein-Barr virus (EBV), varicella zoster virus (VZV), or herpes simplex virus (HSV) also would not be useful in most circumstances for similar reasons. An increasing number of laboratories are offering other molecular tests for opportunistic pathogens, but care must be taken to be certain that the predictive value of these tests is proved. For instance, PCR for *Pneumocystis* in bronchoalveolar lavage may have excellent negative predictive value, but its positive predictive value is very low because many immunosuppressed patients appear to be colonized with *Pneumocystis* and thus a positive result does not prove with any confidence that *Pneumocystis* is the cause of the pulmonary dysfunction.

Imaging is an important aspect of patient evaluation. Patients with HIV infection may have pathologic processes despite a paucity of symptoms or normal readings on routine chest radiographs, for example. Computerized tomography (CT) of the lungs may reveal unexpected pathologic findings such as diffuse interstitial infiltrates suggestive of PCP despite the absence of cough, shortness of breath, or oxygen desaturation. Such a finding could lead to an induced sputum or bronchoalveolar lavage diagnosis of the process at a time when disease is mild and the likelihood of successful treatment is high. CT of the abdomen also should be considered in patients with prolonged fever or wasting and low CD4 counts even in the absence of abdominal symptoms, because such a study may reveal unexpected adenopathy or organ infiltration that could be readily biopsied more feasibly than other more obvious clinical manifestations. Positron emission tomography and nuclear scans may have roles for identifying the infectious cause of clinical syndromes.

TREATMENT   Rx

Empirical Management

For the initial management of a presumed infectious syndrome in a patient with HIV infection or AIDS, clinicians need to determine the urgency of starting therapy before the specific causative process is definitively identified. Given the range of processes that can cause disease in patients with HIV infection or AIDS, the optimal approach is to establish the specific cause before starting therapy. However, some patients will be too sick or deteriorating too quickly to permit withholding therapy until a diagnosis can be established. Thus, for some patients, empirical therapy may be the best management strategy, with careful monitoring of the patient to determine if the therapy is effective.

When assessing an HIV-infected patient with any clinical syndrome, especially a syndrome associated with fever, opportunistic infections are immediate considerations. However, the likelihood of an opportunistic infection depends on the current CD4 count: if the patient's current CD4 count is greater than 200 to 300 cells/μL, the likelihood of most opportunistic infections (other than tuberculosis and pneumococcal disease) is low (but not zero). For any patient, regardless of CD4 count, common community-acquired, nonopportunistic infections also must be considered because HIV-infected patients are equally susceptible to these as their HIV-uninfected counterparts. In addition, noninfectious syndromes must be considered, especially as the patient population ages and congestive heart failure, cerebrovascular disease, or chronic renal disease occur, potentially accelerated by the HIV-related inflammatory state. Patients also may have more than one process occurring concurrently. A familiar scenario, for instance, for a patient with documented PCP, would be the failure to recognize that the reason for pulmonary deterioration is not progressive PCP, but superimposed heart failure, pulmonary hypertension, pulmonary emboli, or secondary lung infection due to methicillin-resistant *Staphylococcus aureus* (MRSA, Chapter 272), *Streptococcus pneumoniae* (Chapter 273), or *Cryptococcus neoformans* (Chapter 317).

For some syndromes, empirical therapy is appropriate, with response to therapy providing a presumptive diagnosis. For instance, an empiric 2-week course of pyrimethamine plus sulfadiazine would be appropriate for a patient with AIDS with a CNS mass lesion, CD4 count less than 100 cells/μL, and positive antitoxoplasma serum immunoglobulin G (IgG), before considering a diagnostic brain biopsy. Given the potential morbidity of a brain biopsy, and the high probability that a patient with AIDS with cerebral toxoplasmosis would demonstrate clinical and radiologic improvement within 14 days, such an approach has been considered preferred compared to immediate brain biopsy or even, if the patient has increased intracranial pressure or a potential to herniate, lumbar puncture. Similarly, for a patient with a CD4 count less than 200 cells/μL who presents with fever, cough, shortness of breath, severe hypoxemia, and diffuse bilateral interstitial pulmonary infiltrates, empirical therapy with ceftriaxone or vancomycin, plus azithromycin, plus trimethoprim-sulfamethoxazole to adequately provide coverage against common causes of community-acquired pneumonia as well as PCP would often be appropriate if the patient were too unstable to tolerate bronchoscopy without a high risk for intubation.

Definitive Therapy

The NIH-CDC-HIVMA Guidelines for the Prevention and Treatment of Opportunistic Infections in HIV-Infected Adults and Adolescents and other chapters in this text provide details on the diagnostic, therapeutic, and preventive approaches to specific syndromes. The drugs of choice are also listed in Table 365-1, adapted from the CDC-NIH-IDSA Guideline on Management of Opportunistic Infections in Adults and Adolescents, which is updated regularly online throughout the year (http://www.aidsinfo.nih.gov).

The treatments for opportunistic infections change as new drugs and new data become available. Thus major AIDS guidelines are now updated promptly online (www.aidsinfo.nih.gov). For hepatitis-C (Chapter 140), recommendations are changing so rapidly that the online site should be consulted before therapy is initiated unless the provider is very familiar with current data (www.hcvguidelines.org).

HIV-infected patients are also at risk for a variety of sexually transmitted diseases (Chapters 269, 299, and 303). In general, treatment for such infections usually is similar to what is recommended in HIV-uninfected patients.

The institution of therapeutic or preventive drugs requires careful considerations of pharmacokinetics and drug-drug interactions. Patients with HIV infection often have organ dysfunction that may alter absorption or excretion of drugs. These patients are also often on multiple drugs (both AIDS related and AIDS unrelated) that can interact with clinically important consequences for drug effectiveness or toxicity. Such therapy thus requires considerable experience and consultation with up-to-date references for guidance.

When a patient with HIV/AIDS who has not been receiving ART develops an opportunistic infection, prospective studies demonstrate that the patient will have longer survival and fewer AIDS-defining complications if the patient is put promptly on ART.[A1] The definition of "prompt," that is, the decision as to how soon to start ART, is a complex analysis that must factor in the patient's willingness and ability to take ART, the evolution of the opportunistic infection if ART is not initiated, access to medical care and drugs after hospitalization, ability to absorb the drugs, potential interactions of ART with other drugs, including those used to treat the opportunistic infection, the patient's ability to tolerate potential drug toxicities, and the possible consequences if immune reconstitution inflammatory syndrome occurs. The general principle is to start ART as soon as possible, but each patient will require individual assessment to determine the optimal interval between recognition of an opportunistic infection and initiation of ART. HIV-infected patients who present with tuberculosis or cryptococcal meningitis who are not on ART require special considerations in terms of determining when to start ART, and which antiretroviral agents to use. For example, ART can be delayed safely until after 6 months of tuberculosis treatment if the CD4 count is 200 cells/μL or higher, and it may be safer to delay ART until 5 to 6 weeks after starting antifungal therapy in patients with cryptococcal meningitis.[A2][A3]

When patients who are already receiving ART develop an opportunistic infection or any other complication not directly related to the drug itself, ART should be continued. The regimen should be reassessed to ensure that it is optimal in terms of antiviral activity, tolerability, potential toxicity and drug interactions, and the patient's ability to attain adequate serum levels given their ability to absorb oral drugs.

PREVENTION

Soon after the initial recognition of AIDS, before the era of ART or pathogen specific chemoprophylaxis, clinicians recognized that PCP ultimately occurred in 60 to 80% of HIV-infected patients in North America. Moreover, many of the patients who survived their first episode of PCP had one or more subsequent episodes. One of the first interventions demonstrated to prolong life was the institution of anti-*Pneumocystis* prophylaxis for patients who had oral thrush, oral hairy leukoplakia, a prior episode of PCP, or a CD4 count less than 200 cells/μL. Subsequently, the concept of primary chemoprophylaxis and chronic suppressive therapy was extended to other pathogens such as *M. avium* complex (MAC) and toxoplasma.

These observations about *Pneumocystis*, MAC, and toxoplasma led to the development of a comprehensive preventive strategy to minimize the impact of opportunistic infections on those HIV-infected individuals who are immunologically vulnerable as measured by their CD4 count and viral load or by prior experience with an opportunistic infection (CDC-NIH-IDSA Guideline on Management of Opportunistic Infections in Adults and Adolescents, http://www.aidsinfo.nih.gov).[A4] Specific chemotherapy for primary prevention is indicated for the duration of immunosuppression, with the CD4 count thresholds depending on the pathogen. Chronic suppressive therapy should be continued for durations that depend on the pathogen and the patient's CD4 count. Recommendations for primary prophylaxis are summarized in Table 365-2; more complete information on primary and secondary prophylaxis is available in the CDC-NIH-IDSA Guideline on Management of Opportunistic Infections in Adults and Adolescents (http://www.aidsinfo.nih.gov). As the management of HIV infection evolves, criteria for starting and stopping prophylaxis are being modified. For instance, there is growing recognition that MAC disease is less and less common in the United States, and thus MAC prophylaxis is no longer recommended.

Although immune reconstitution with ART (Chapter 367) is the most effective method to prevent opportunistic infections, many patients with low CD4 counts and uncontrolled viremia will continue to benefit from chemoprophylaxis. Such prophylaxis can be discontinued when patients meet the criteria for ART-induced reduction in viral load and increase in CD4 counts, as outlined for each individual pathogen in the guideline (https://aidsinfo.nih.gov/guidelines/html/4/adult-and-adolescent-oi-prevention-and-treatment-guidelines/0).

Preventive strategies focus not only on chemoprophylaxis but also on immunization and reducing exposure to opportunistic pathogens. Examples of exposure reduction interventions likely to be effective would include immunizing household members of HIV-infected patients for pneumococcus and hemophilus to prevent spread of these respiratory pathogens in the home setting, reducing the likelihood of cryptosporidiosis by decreasing exposure for HIV-infected patients to kittens and puppies, reducing the likelihood of toxoplasmosis by avoiding exposure to cat feces for HIV-infected patients whose cats spend time outdoors, and limiting exposure to patients who might present unexpectedly with tuberculosis for HIV-infected health care workers.

TABLE 365-1 PROPHYLAXIS TO PREVENT FIRST EPISODE OF OPPORTUNISTIC DISEASE

OPPORTUNISTIC INFECTIONS	INDICATION	PREFERRED	ALTERNATIVE
Pneumocystis pneumonia (PCP)	• CD4 count <200 cells/µL, *or* • CD4 <14%, *or* • CD4 count >200 but <250 cells/µL if monitoring CD4 cell count every 3 months is not possible **Note:** Patients who are receiving pyrimethamine/sulfadiazine for treatment or suppression of toxoplasmosis do not require additional PCP prophylaxis.	• TMP-SMX 1 double-strength (DS) PO daily *Or* • TMP-SMX 1 single-strength (SS) daily	• TMP-SMX 1 DS PO three times weekly *Or* • Dapsone 100 mg PO daily or 50 mg PO BID *Or* • Dapsone 50 mg PO daily + (pyrimethamine 50 mg + leucovorin 25 mg) PO weekly *Or* • Dapsone 200 mg + pyrimethamine 75 mg + leucovorin 25 mg PO weekly *Or* • Aerosolized pentamidine 300 mg via Respirgard II™ nebulizer every month *Or* • Atovaquone 1500 mg PO daily *Or* • Atovaquone 1500 mg + pyrimethamine 25 mg + leucovorin 10 mg PO daily
Toxoplasma gondii encephalitis	• Toxoplasma IgG-positive patients with CD4 count <100 cells/µL **Note:** All regimens recommended for primary prophylaxis against toxoplasmosis are also effective as PCP prophylaxis.	TMP-SMX 1 DS PO daily	• TMP-SMX 1 DS PO three times weekly *Or* • TMP-SMX 1 SS PO daily *Or* • Dapsone 50 mg PO daily + (pyrimethamine 50 mg + leucovorin 25 mg) PO weekly *Or* • Dapsone 200 mg + pyrimethamine 75 mg + leucovorin 25 mg PO weekly *Or* • Atovaquone 1500 mg PO daily *Or* • Atovaquone 1500 mg + pyrimethamine 25 mg + leucovorin 10 mg PO daily
Mycobacterium tuberculosis infection (TB) (i.e., treatment of latent TB infection [LTBI])	• (+) screening test for LTBI, with no evidence of active TB, and no prior treatment for active TB or LTBI *Or* • Close contact with a person with infectious TB, with no evidence of active TB, regardless of screening test results.	• INH 300 mg + pyridoxine 25-50 mg PO daily × 9 months *Or* • INH 900 mg PO BIW (by DOT) + pyridoxine 25-50 mg PO daily × 9 months	• Rifampin 600 mg PO daily × 4 months *Or* • [Rifapentine (see dose below) PO + INH 900 mg PO + pyridoxine 50 mg PO] once weekly × 12 weeks *rifapentine dose—* • 32.1 to 49.9 kg: 750 mg • 50 mg: 900 mg Rifapentine only recommended for patients receiving raltegravir or efavirenz-based ART regimen For patients exposed to drug-resistant TB, select anti-TB drugs after consultation with experts or public health authorities.
Streptococcus pneumoniae infection	For individuals who have not received any pneumococcal vaccine, regardless of CD4 count, followed by: • if CD4 count ≥200 cells/µL • if CD4 count <200 cells/µL For individuals who have previously received PPV23 Re-vaccination • If age 19-64 years and ≥5 years since the first PPV23 dose • If age ≥65 years, and if ≥5 years since the previous PPV23 dose	PCV13 0.5 mL IM × 1 PPV23 0.5 mL IM at least 8 weeks after the PCV13 vaccine PPV23 can be offered at least 8 weeks after receiving PCV13 or can wait until CD4 count increased to ≥200 cells/µL. One dose of PCV13 should be given at least 1 year after the last receipt of PPV23. • PPV23 0.5 mL IM or SC × 1 • PPV23 0.5 mL IM or SC × 1	PPV23 0.5 mL IM × 1
Influenza A and B virus	All HIV-infected patients	Inactivated influenza vaccine annually (per recommendation for the season) Live-attenuated influenza vaccine is ***contraindicated*** in HIV-infected patients	
Histoplasma capsulatum infection	CD4 count ≤150 cells/µL and at high risk because of occupational exposure or lives in a community with a hyperendemic rate of histoplasmosis (>10 cases/100 patient-years)	Itraconazole 200 mg PO daily	
Coccidioidomycosis	A new positive IgM or IgG serologic test in patients who live in a disease-endemic area and with CD4 count <250 cells/µL	Fluconazole 400 mg PO daily	

TABLE 365-1 PROPHYLAXIS TO PREVENT FIRST EPISODE OF OPPORTUNISTIC DISEASE—cont'd

OPPORTUNISTIC INFECTIONS	INDICATION	PREFERRED	ALTERNATIVE
Varicella-zoster virus (VZV) infection	Preexposure prevention: Patients with CD4 counts ≥200 cells/µL who have not been vaccinated, have no history of varicella or herpes zoster, or who are seronegative for VZV **Note:** Routine VZV serologic testing in HIV-infected adults and adolescents is not recommended. Post-exposure prevention: Close contact with a person with chickenpox or herpes zoster; and is susceptible (i.e., no history of vaccination or of either condition, or known to be VZV seronegative)	Preexposure prevention: Primary varicella vaccination (Varivax™), 2 doses (0.5 mL SC each) administered 3 months apart. If vaccination results in disease because of vaccine virus, treatment with acyclovir is recommended. Post-exposure prevention: Varicella-zoster immune globulin (VariZIG™) 125 international units per 10 kg (maximum 625 international units) IM, administered as soon as possible and within 10 days after exposure **Note:** VariZIG is exclusively distributed by FFF Enterprises at 800-843-7477. Individuals receiving monthly high-dose IVIG (>400 mg/kg) are likely to be protected if the last dose of IVIG was administered <3 weeks before exposure.	Preexposure prevention: VZV-susceptible household contacts of susceptible HIV-infected patients should be vaccinated to prevent potential transmission of VZV to their HIV-infected contacts. Alternative post-exposure prevention: • Acyclovir 800 mg PO 5 ×/day for 5-7 days *Or* • Valacyclovir 1 g PO TID for 5-7 days These alternatives have not been studied in the HIV population. If antiviral therapy is used, varicella vaccines should not be given until at least 72 hours after the last dose of the antiviral drug.
Human Papillomavirus (HPV) infection	Aged 9-26 years	For patients who have completed a vaccination series with the recombinant bivalent or quadrivalent vaccine, providers may consider additional vaccination with recombinant 9 valent vaccine • HPV 9-valent vaccine 0.5 mL IM at months 0, 1-2, and 6	
Hepatitis A virus (HAV) infection	HAV-susceptible patients with chronic liver disease, or who are injection-drug users, or MSM	Hepatitis A vaccine 1 mL IM × 2 doses at 0 and 6-12 months IgG antibody response should be assessed 1 month after vaccination; non-responders should be revaccinated when CD4 count >200 cells/µL.	For patients susceptible to both HAV and hepatitis B virus (HBV) infection (see below): Combined HAV and HBV vaccine (Twinrix®), 1 mL IM as a 3-dose (0, 1, and 6 months) or 4-dose series (days 0, 7, 21 to 30, and 12 months)
Hepatitis B virus (HBV) infection	• Patients without chronic HBV or without immunity to HBV (i.e., anti-HBs <10 international units/mL) • Patients with isolated anti-HBc and negative HBV DNA • Early vaccination is recommended before CD4 count falls below 350 cells/µL). However, in patients with low CD4 cell counts, vaccination should not be deferred until CD4 count reaches >350 cells/µL, because some patients with CD4 counts <200 cells/µL do respond to vaccination.	• HBV vaccine IM (Engerix-B 20 µg/mL or Recombivax HB 10 µg/mL), 0, 1, and 6 months *Or* • HBV vaccine IM (Engerix-B 40 µg/mL or Recombivax HB 20 µg/mL), 0, 1, 2, and 6 months *Or* • Vaccine conjugated to CpG (Heplisav-B)9H at 0 and 1 month *Or* • Combined HAV and HBV vaccine (Twinrix®), 1 mL IM as a 3-dose (0, 1, and 6 months) or 4-dose series (days 0, 7, 21 to 30, and 12 months) Anti-HBs should be obtained 1 month after completion of the vaccine series. Patients with anti-HBs <10 international units/mL at 1 month are considered non-responders.	Some experts recommend vaccinating with 40-µg doses of either HBV vaccine.

Guidelines for the Prevention and Treatment of Opportunistic Infections in HIV-Infected Adults and Adolescents. http://aidsinfo.nih.gov/guidelines.

DOT = directly observed therapy; HIV = human immunodeficiency virus; IM = intramuscularly; IV = intravenously; MSM = men who have sex with men; PO = orally.

TABLE 365-2 TREATMENT OF ACQUIRED IMMUNODEFICIENCY VIRUS–ASSOCIATED OPPORTUNISTIC INFECTIONS (INCLUDES RECOMMENDATIONS FOR ACUTE TREATMENT AND SECONDARY PROPHYLAXIS/CHRONIC SUPPRESSIVE/MAINTENANCE THERAPY)

OPPORTUNISTIC INFECTION	PREFERRED THERAPY	ALTERNATIVE THERAPY	OTHER COMMENTS
Pneumocystis pneumonia (PCP)	Patients who develop PCP despite TMP-SMX prophylaxis can usually be treated with standard doses of TMP-SMX. Duration of PCP treatment: 21 days *For moderate-to-severe PCP:* • TMP-SMX: [TMP 15-20 mg and SMX 75-100 mg]/kg/day IV given q6h or q8h, may switch to PO after clinical improvement *For mild-to-moderate PCP:* • TMP-SMX: [TMP 15-20 mg and SMX 75-100 mg]/kg/day, given PO in 3 divided doses *Or* • TMP-SMX: (160 mg/800 mg or DS) 2 tablets PO TID *Secondary prophylaxis, after completion of PCP treatment:* • TMP-SMX DS: 1 tablet PO daily *Or* • TMP-SMX (80 mg/400 mg or SS): 1 tablet PO daily	*For moderate-to-severe PCP:* • Pentamidine 4 mg/kg IV daily infused over ≥60 minutes; can reduce dose to 3 mg/kg IV daily because of toxicities • Primaquine 30 mg (base) PO daily + (clindamycin 600 mg q6h IV or 900 mg IV q8h) or (clindamycin 450 mg PO q6h or 600 mg PO q8h) *For mild-to-moderate PCP:* • Dapsone 100 mg PO daily + TMP 5 mg/kg PO TID *Or* • Primaquine 30 mg (base) PO daily + (clindamycin 450 mg PO q6h or 600 mg PO q8h) *Or* • Atovaquone 750 mg PO BID with food *Secondary prophylaxis, after completion of PCP treatment:* • TMP-SMX DS: 1 tablet PO three times weekly *Or* • Dapsone 100 mg PO daily *Or* • Dapsone 50 mg PO daily + (pyrimethamine 50 mg + leucovorin 25 mg) PO weekly *Or* • Dapsone 200 mg + pyrimethamine 75 mg + leucovorin 25 mg PO weekly *Or* • Aerosolized pentamidine 300 mg monthly via Respirgard II™ nebulizer *Or* • Atovaquone 1500 mg PO daily *Or* • Atovaquone 1500 mg + pyrimethamine 25 mg + leucovorin 10 mg PO daily	*Indications for adjunctive corticosteroids:* • PaO₂ <70 mm Hg at room air, or • Alveolar-arterial O₂ gradient >35 mm Hg *Prednisone doses (beginning as early as possible and within 72 hours of PCP therapy):* • Days 1-5: 40 mg PO BID • Days 6-10: 40 mg PO daily • Days 11-21: 20 mg PO daily IV methylprednisolone can be administered as 75% of prednisone dose. Benefit of corticosteroid if started after 72 hours of treatment is unknown, but some clinicians will use it for moderate-to-severe PCP. Whenever possible, patients should be tested for G6PD before use of dapsone or primaquine. Alternative therapy should be used in patients found to have G6PD deficiency. Patients who are receiving pyrimethamine/sulfadiazine for treatment or suppression of toxoplasmosis do not require additional PCP prophylaxis. If TMP-SMX is discontinued because of a mild adverse reaction, reinstitution should be considered after the reaction resolves. The dose can be increased gradually (desensitization), reduced, or the frequency modified. TMP-SMX should be permanently discontinued in patients with possible or definite Stevens-Johnson Syndrome or toxic epidermal necrosis.

Toxoplasma gondii encephalitis	*Treatment of acute infection:*
	• Pyrimethamine 200 mg PO 1 time, followed by weight-based therapy:
	  • If <60 kg, pyrimethamine 50 mg PO once daily + sulfadiazine 1000 mg PO q6h + leucovorin 10-25 mg PO once daily
	  • If ≥60 kg, pyrimethamine 75 mg PO once daily + sulfadiazine 1500 mg PO q6h + leucovorin 10-25 mg PO once daily
	  • Leucovorin dose can be increased to 50 mg daily or BID.
	Duration for acute therapy:
	• At least 6 weeks; longer duration if clinical or radiologic disease is extensive or response is incomplete at 6 weeks
	• After completion of acute therapy, all patients should be initiated on chronic maintenance therapy
	Chronic maintenance therapy:
	• Pyrimethamine 25-50 mg PO daily + sulfadiazine 2000-4000 mg PO daily (in 2-4 divided doses) + leucovorin 10-25 mg PO daily
		Treatment of acute infection:
		• Pyrimethamine (leucovorin) + clindamycin 600 mg IV or PO q6h
		Or
		• TMP-SMX (TMP 5 mg/kg and SMX 25 mg/kg) IV or PO BID
		Or
		• Atovaquone 1500 mg PO BID with food + pyrimethamine (leucovorin)
		Or
		• Atovaquone 1500 mg PO BID with food + sulfadiazine 1000-1500 mg PO q6h (weight-based dosing, as in preferred therapy)
		Or
		• Atovaquone 1500 mg PO BID with food
		Chronic maintenance therapy:
		• Clindamycin 600 mg PO q8h + (pyrimethamine 25-50 mg + leucovorin 10-25 mg) PO daily
		Or
		• TMP-SMX DS 1 tablet BID
		Or
		• TMP-SMX DS 1 tablet once daily
		Or
		• Atovaquone 750-1500 mg PO BID + (pyrimethamine 25 mg + leucovorin 10 mg) PO daily
		Or
		• Atovaquone 750-1500 mg PO BID + sulfadiazine 2000-4000 mg PO daily (in 2-4 divided doses)
		Or
		• Atovaquone 750-1500 mg PO BID with food
			Refer to http://www.daraprimdirect.com for information regarding how to access pyrimethamine.
			If pyrimethamine is unavailable or there is a delay in obtaining it, TMP-SMX should be utilized in place of pyrimethamine-sulfadiazine.
			For patients with a history of sulfa allergy, sulfa desensitization should be attempted using one of several published strategies.
			Atovaquone should be administered until therapeutic doses of TMP-SMX are achieved.
			Adjunctive corticosteroids (e.g., dexamethasone) should only be administered when clinically indicated to treat mass effect associated with focal lesions or associated edema; discontinue as soon as clinically feasible.
			Anticonvulsants should be administered to patients with a history of seizures and continued through acute treatment, but should not be used as seizure prophylaxis.
			If clindamycin is used in place of sulfadiazine, additional therapy must be added to prevent PCP.
			Pyrimethamine and leucovorin doses are the same as for preferred therapy.

TABLE 365-2 TREATMENT OF ACQUIRED IMMUNODEFICIENCY VIRUS–ASSOCIATED OPPORTUNISTIC INFECTIONS (INCLUDES RECOMMENDATIONS FOR ACUTE TREATMENT AND SECONDARY PROPHYLAXIS/CHRONIC SUPPRESSIVE/MAINTENANCE THERAPY)—cont'd

OPPORTUNISTIC INFECTION	PREFERRED THERAPY	ALTERNATIVE THERAPY	OTHER COMMENTS
Mycobacterium tuberculosis (TB) disease	After collecting specimen for culture and molecular diagnostic tests, empiric TB treatment should be started in individuals with clinical and radiographic presentation suggestive of TB. *Initial phase (2 months, given daily, 5-7 times/week by DOT):* • INH + [RIF or RFB] + PZA + EMB Continuation phase: • INH + (RIF or RFB) daily (5-7 times/week) Total duration of therapy (for drug-susceptible TB): • Pulmonary, drug-susceptible TB: 6 months • Pulmonary TB and culture-positive after 2 months of TB treatment: 9 months • Extrapulmonary TB w/CNS infection: 9-12 months; • Extrapulmonary TB w/bone or joint involvement: 6 to 9 months; • Extrapulmonary TB in other sites: 6 months • Total duration of therapy should be based on number of doses received, not on calendar time	*Treatment for drug-resistant TB* Resistant to INH: • (RIF or RFB) + EMB + PZA + (moxifloxacin or levofloxacin) for 2 months; followed by (RIF or RFB) + EMB + (moxifloxacin or levofloxacin) for 7 months Resistant to rifamycins +/− other drugs: • Regimen and duration of treatment should be individualized based on resistance pattern, clinical and microbiological responses, and in close consultation with experienced specialists.	Adjunctive corticosteroid improves survival for TB meningitis and pericarditis. See text for drug, dose, and duration recommendations. All rifamycins may have significant pharmacokinetic interactions with antiretroviral drugs. Therapeutic drug monitoring should be considered in patients receiving rifamycin and interacting ART. Paradoxical IRIS that is not severe can be treated with NSAIDs without a change in TB or HIV therapy. For severe IRIS reaction, consider prednisone and taper over 4 weeks based on clinical symptoms. For example: • If receiving RIF: prednisone 1.5 mg/kg/day for 2 weeks, then 0.75 mg/kg/day for 2 weeks • If receiving RFB: prednisone 1.0 mg/kg/day for 2 weeks, then 0.5 mg/kg/day for 2 weeks A more gradual tapering schedule over a few months may be necessary for some patients.
Disseminated *Mycobacterium avium complex* (MAC) disease	*At least 2 drugs as initial therapy with:* • Clarithromycin 500 mg PO BID + ethambutol 15 mg/kg PO daily Or • (Azithromycin 500-600 mg + ethambutol 15 mg/kg) PO daily if drug interaction or intolerance precludes the use of clarithromycin *Duration:* • At least 12 months of therapy, can discontinue if no signs and symptoms of MAC disease and sustained (>6 months), CD4 count >100 cells/µL in response to ART	Addition of a third or fourth drug should be considered for patients with advanced immunosuppression (CD4 counts <50 cells/µL), high mycobacterial loads (>2 log CFU/mL of blood), or in the absence of effective ART. *Third or fourth drug options may include:* • RFB 300 mg PO daily (dosage adjustment may be necessary based on drug interactions), • Amikacin 10-15 mg/kg IV daily or Streptomycin 1 g IV or IM daily Or • Moxifloxacin 400 mg PO daily Or • Levofloxacin 500 mg PO daily	Testing of susceptibility to clarithromycin and azithromycin is recommended. NSAIDs can be used for patients who experience moderate to severe symptoms attributed to IRIS. If IRIS symptoms persist, short-term (4-8 weeks) systemic corticosteroids (equivalent to 20-40 mg prednisone) can be used.
Salmonellosis	• Ciprofloxacin 500-750 mg PO (or 400 mg IV) q12h, if susceptible *Duration of therapy:* For gastroenteritis without bacteremia: • If CD4 count ≥200 cells/µL: 7-14 days • If CD4 count <200 cells/µL: 2-6 weeks For gastroenteritis with bacteremia: • If CD4 count ≥200/µL: 14 days; longer duration if bacteremia persists or if the infection is complicated (e.g., if metastatic foci of infection are present) • If CD4 count <200 cells/µL: 2-6 weeks *Secondary prophylaxis should be considered for:* • Patients with recurrent *Salmonella* gastroenteritis +/− bacteremia Or • Patients with CD4 <200 cells/µL with severe diarrhea	• Levofloxacin 750 mg (PO or IV) q24h Or • Moxifloxacin 400 mg (PO or IV) q24h Or • TMP, 160 mg-SMX 800 mg (PO or IV) q12h Or • Ceftriaxone 1 g IV q24h Or • Cefotaxime 1 g IV q8h	All HIV-infected patients with salmonellosis should receive antimicrobial treatment due to an increased risk of bacteremia (by 20- to 100-fold) and mortality (by up to 7-fold) compared with HIV negative individuals. Oral or IV rehydration if indicated. Antimotility agents should be avoided. The role of long-term secondary prophylaxis in patients with recurrent *Salmonella* bacteremia is not well established. Must weigh benefit against risks of long-term antibiotic exposure. Effective ART may reduce the frequency, severity, and recurrence of *Salmonella* infections.

Infection	Preferred Therapy	Alternative Therapy	Comments
Mucocutaneous candidiasis	*For oropharyngeal candidiasis; initial episodes (for 7-14 days):* Oral therapy • Fluconazole 100 mg PO daily Topical therapy • Clotrimazole troches, 10 mg PO 5 times daily Or • Miconazole mucoadhesive buccal 50-mg tablet—apply to mucosal surface over the canine fossa once daily (do not swallow, chew, or crush) *For esophageal candidiasis (for 14-21 days):* • Fluconazole 100 mg (up to 400 mg) PO or IV daily Or • Itraconazole oral solution 200 mg PO daily *For uncomplicated vulvovaginal candidiasis:* • Oral fluconazole 150 mg for 1 dose Or • Topical azoles (clotrimazole, butoconazole, miconazole, tioconazole, or terconazole) for 3-7 days *For severe or recurrent vulvovaginal candidiasis:* • Fluconazole 100-200 mg PO daily for ≥7 days Or • Topical antifungal for ≥7 days	*For oropharyngeal candidiasis; initial episodes (for 7-14 days):* Oral therapy • Itraconazole oral solution 200 mg PO daily Or • Posaconazole oral suspension 400 mg PO BID for 1 day, then 400 mg daily Topical therapy • Nystatin suspension 4-6 mL QID or 1-2 flavored pastilles 4-5 times daily *For esophageal candidiasis (for 14-21 days):* • Voriconazole 200 mg PO or IV BID Or • Anidulafungin 100 mg IV 1 time, then 50 mg IV daily Or • Caspofungin 50 mg IV daily Or • Micafungin 150 mg IV daily Or • Amphotericin B deoxycholate 0.6 mg/kg IV daily Or • Lipid formulation of amphotericin B 3-4 mg/kg IV daily *For uncomplicated vulvovaginal candidiasis:* • Itraconazole oral solution 200 mg PO daily for 3-7 days	Chronic or prolonged use of azoles may promote development of resistance. Higher relapse rate for esophageal candidiasis seen with echinocandins than with fluconazole use. Suppressive therapy usually will not recommended unless patients have frequent or severe recurrences. *If decision is to use suppressive therapy:* Oropharyngeal candidiasis: • Fluconazole 100 mg PO daily or three times weekly Or • Itraconazole oral solution 200 mg PO daily Esophageal candidiasis: • Fluconazole 100-200 mg PO daily Or • Posaconazole 400 mg PO BID Vulvovaginal candidiasis: • Fluconazole 150 mg PO once weekly
Cryptococcosis	*Cryptococcal meningitis* Induction therapy (for at least 2 weeks, followed by consolidation therapy): • Liposomal amphotericin B 3-4 mg/kg IV daily + flucytosine 25 mg/kg PO QID (**Note:** Flucytosine dose should be adjusted in patients with renal dysfunction.) Consolidation therapy (for at least 8 weeks, followed by maintenance therapy): • Fluconazole 400 mg PO (or IV) daily Maintenance therapy: • Fluconazole 200 mg PO daily for at least 12 months *For non-CNS, extrapulmonary cryptococcosis, and diffuse pulmonary disease:* • Treatment same as for cryptococcal meningitis *Non-CNS cryptococcosis with mild-to-moderate symptoms and focal pulmonary infiltrates:* • Fluconazole, 400 mg PO daily for 12 months	*Cryptococcal meningitis* Induction therapy (for at least 2 weeks, followed by consolidation therapy): • Amphotericin B deoxycholate 0.7 mg/kg IV daily + flucytosine 25 mg/kg PO QID Or • Amphotericin B lipid complex 5 mg/kg IV daily + flucytosine 25 mg/kg PO QID Or • Liposomal amphotericin B 3-4 mg/kg IV daily + fluconazole 800 mg PO or IV daily Or • Amphotericin B deoxycholate 0.7 mg/kg IV daily + fluconazole 800 mg PO or IV daily Or • Fluconazole 400-800 mg PO or IV daily + flucytosine 25 mg/kg PO QID Or • Fluconazole 1200 mg PO or IV daily Consolidation therapy (for at least 8 weeks, followed by maintenance therapy): • Itraconazole 200 mg PO BID for 8 weeks—less effective than fluconazole Maintenance therapy: • No alternative therapy recommendation	Addition of flucytosine to amphotericin B has been associated with more rapid sterilization of CSF and decreased risk for subsequent relapse. Patients receiving flucytosine should have either blood levels monitored (peak level 2 hours after dose should be 30-80 µg/mL) or close monitoring of blood counts for development of cytopenia. Dosage should be adjusted in patients with renal insufficiency. Opening pressure should always be measured when an LP is performed. Repeated LPs or CSF shunting are essential to effectively manage increased intracranial pressure. Corticosteroids and mannitol are ineffective in reducing ICP and are NOT recommended. Corticosteroid should not be routinely used during induction therapy unless it is for the management of IRIS.

TABLE 365-2 TREATMENT OF ACQUIRED IMMUNODEFICIENCY VIRUS–ASSOCIATED OPPORTUNISTIC INFECTIONS (INCLUDES RECOMMENDATIONS FOR ACUTE TREATMENT AND SECONDARY PROPHYLAXIS/CHRONIC SUPPRESSIVE/MAINTENANCE THERAPY)—cont'd

OPPORTUNISTIC INFECTION	PREFERRED THERAPY	ALTERNATIVE THERAPY	OTHER COMMENTS
Histoplasmosis	*Moderately severe to severe disseminated disease* Induction therapy (for at least 2 weeks or until clinically improved): • Liposomal amphotericin B 3 mg/kg IV daily Maintenance therapy *Less severe disseminated disease* Induction and maintenance therapy: • Itraconazole 200 mg PO TID for 3 days, then 200 mg PO BID Induction and maintenance therapy: • Itraconazole 200 mg PO TID for 3 days, then 200 mg PO BID Duration of therapy: • At least 12 months *Meningitis* Induction therapy (4–6 weeks): • Liposomal amphotericin B 5 mg/kg/day Maintenance therapy: • Itraconazole 200 mg PO BID to TID for ≥1 year and until resolution of abnormal CSF findings Long-term suppression therapy: For patients with severe disseminated or CNS infection after completion of at least 12 months of therapy; and those who relapse despite appropriate therapy: • Itraconazole 200 mg PO daily	*Moderately severe to severe disseminated disease* Induction therapy (for at least 2 weeks or until clinically improved): • Amphotericin B lipid complex 3 mg/kg IV daily Or • Amphotericin B cholesteryl sulfate complete 3 mg/kg IV daily Alternatives to itraconazole for maintenance therapy or treatment of less severe disease: • Voriconazole 400 mg PO BID for 1 day, then 200 mg BID Or • Posaconazole 400 mg PO BID Or • Fluconazole 800 mg PO daily *Meningitis:* • No alternative therapy recommendation Long-term suppression therapy: • Fluconazole 400 mg PO daily	Itraconazole, posaconazole, and voriconazole may have significant interactions with certain ARV agents. These interactions are complex and can be bidirectional. Therapeutic drug monitoring and dosage adjustment may be necessary to ensure triazole antifungal and ARV efficacy and reduce concentration-related toxicities. Random serum concentration of itraconazole + hydroxyitraconazole should be >1 µg/mL. Clinical experience with voriconazole or posaconazole in the treatment of histoplasmosis is limited. Acute pulmonary histoplasmosis in HIV-infected patients with CD4 counts >300 cells/µL should be managed as non-immunocompromised host.
Cytomegalovirus (CMV) disease	*CMV retinitis* Induction therapy (followed by chronic maintenance therapy) For immediate sight-threatening lesions (within 1500 microns of the fovea): • Intravitreal injections of ganciclovir (2 mg) or foscarnet (2.4 mg) for 1–4 doses over a period of 7–10 days to achieve high intraocular concentration faster; plus • Valganciclovir 900 mg PO BID for 14–21 days, then 900 mg once daily For peripheral lesions • Valganciclovir 900 mg PO BID for 14–21 days, then 900 mg once daily Chronic maintenance • Valganciclovir 900 mg PO daily for 3–6 months until ART induced immune recovery *CMV esophagitis or colitis:* • Ganciclovir 5 mg/kg IV q12h; may switch to valganciclovir 900 mg PO q12h once the patient can tolerate oral therapy • Duration: 21–42 days or until symptoms have resolved • Maintenance therapy is usually not necessary, but should be considered after relapses. *Well-documented, histologically confirmed CMV pneumonia:* • Experience for treating CMV pneumonitis in HIV patients is limited. Use of IV ganciclovir or IV foscarnet is reasonable (doses same as for CMV retinitis). • The optimal duration of therapy and the role of oral valganciclovir have not been established. *CMV neurologic disease* **Note: Treatment should be initiated promptly.** • Ganciclovir 5 mg/kg IV q12h + (foscarnet 90 mg/kg IV q12h or 60 mg/kg IV q8h) to stabilize disease and maximize response, continue until symptomatic improvement and resolution of neurologic symptoms • The optimal duration of therapy and the role of oral valganciclovir have not been established. • Optimize ART to achieve viral suppression and immune reconstitution	*CMV retinitis* For immediate sight-threatening lesions (within 1500 microns of the fovea): Intravitreal therapy as listed in the Preferred section, plus one of the following: Alternative systemic induction therapy (followed by chronic maintenance therapy) • Ganciclovir 5 mg/kg IV q12h for 14–21 days Or • Foscarnet 90 mg/kg IV q12h or 60 mg/kg q8h for 14–21 days Or • Cidofovir 5 mg/kg/week IV for 2 weeks; saline hydration before and after therapy and probenecid, 2 g PO 3 hours before dose, followed by 1 g PO 2 hours and 8 hours after the dose (total of 4 g). **(Note:** This regimen should be avoided in patients with sulfa allergy because of cross hypersensitivity with probenecid.) Chronic maintenance (for 3–6 months until ART induced immune recovery): • Ganciclovir 5 mg/kg IV 5–7 times weekly Or • Foscarnet 90–120 mg/kg IV once daily Or • Cidofovir 5 mg/kg IV every other week with saline hydration and probenecid as above *CMV esophagitis or colitis:* • Foscarnet 90 mg/kg IV q12h or 60 mg/kg q8h for patients with treatment-limiting toxicities to ganciclovir or with ganciclovir resistance Or • Valganciclovir 900 mg PO q12h in milder disease and if able to tolerate PO therapy Or • Duration: 21–42 days or until symptoms have resolved • For mild disease, if ART can be initiated without delay, consider withholding CMV therapy	*CMV retinitis* The choice of therapy for CMV retinitis should be individualized, based on location and severity of the lesions, level of immunosuppression, and other factors (e.g., concomitant medications and ability to adhere to treatment). Given the evident benefits of systemic therapy in preventing contralateral eye involvement, reduce CMV visceral disease, and improve survival, whenever feasible, treatment should include systemic therapy The ganciclovir ocular implant, which is effective for treatment of CMV retinitis, is no longer available. For sight-threatening retinitis, intravitreal injections of ganciclovir or foscarnet can be given to achieve higher ocular concentrations faster. Routine (i.e, every 3 months) ophthalmologic follow-up is recommended after stopping chronic maintenance therapy for early detection of relapse or IRU, and then periodically after sustained immune reconstitution IRU may develop in the setting of immune reconstitution. *Treatment of IRU* • Periocular corticosteroid or short courses of systemic steroid. Initial therapy in patients with CMV retinitis, esophagitis, colitis, and pneumonitis should include initiation or optimization of ART.

Herpes simplex virus (HSV) disease

Orolabial lesions (for 5-10 days):
- Valacyclovir 1 g PO BID

Or
- Famciclovir 500 mg PO BID

Or
- Acyclovir 400 mg PO TID

Initial or recurrent genital HSV (For 5-14 days):
- Valacyclovir 1 g PO BID

Or
- Famciclovir 500 mg PO BID

Or
- Acyclovir 400 mg PO BID

Severe mucocutaneous HSV:
- Initial therapy acyclovir 5 mg/kg IV q8h
- After lesions begin to regress, change to PO therapy as above.
- Continue until lesions are completely healed.

Chronic suppressive therapy:
For patients with severe recurrences of genital herpes or patients who want to minimize frequency of recurrences:
- Valacyclovir 500 mg PO BID
- Famciclovir 500 mg PO BID
- Acyclovir 400 mg PO BID
- Continue indefinitely regardless of CD4 cell count.

For acyclovir-resistant HSV
Preferred therapy:
- Foscarnet 80-120 mg/kg/day IV in 2-3 divided doses until clinical response

Alternative therapy:
- IV cidofovir (dosage as in CMV retinitis), *or*
- Topical trifluridine, *or*
- Topical cidofovir, *or*
- Topical imiquimod
- Duration of therapy: 21-28 days or longer

Patients with HSV infections can be treated with episodic therapy when symptomatic lesions occur, or with daily suppressive therapy to prevent recurrences.

Topical formulations of trifluridine and cidofovir are not commercially available.

Extemporaneous compounding of topical products can be prepared using trifluridine ophthalmic solution and the IV formulation of cidofovir.

Varicella zoster virus (VZV) disease

Primary varicella infection (Chickenpox)
Uncomplicated cases (for 5-7 days):
- Valacyclovir 1 g PO TID

Or
- Famciclovir 500 mg PO TID

Severe or complicated cases:
- Acyclovir 10-15 mg/kg IV q8h for 7-10 days
- May switch to oral valacyclovir, famciclovir, or acyclovir after defervescence if no evidence of visceral involvement

Herpes zoster (shingles)
Acute localized dermatomal:
- For 7-10 days; consider longer duration if lesions are slow to resolve
- Valacyclovir 1 g PO TID

Or
- Famciclovir 500 mg TID

Extensive cutaneous lesion or visceral involvement:
- Acyclovir 10-15 mg/kg IV q8h until clinical improvement is evident
- May switch to PO therapy (valacyclovir, famciclovir, or acyclovir) after clinical improvement or improvement of signs and symptoms of visceral VZV), to complete a 10-14 day course

Progressive outer retinal necrosis (PORN):
- (Ganciclovir 5 mg/kg +/- foscarnet 90 mg/kg) IV q12h + (ganciclovir 2 mg/0.05 mL +/- foscarnet 1.2 mg/0.05 mL) intravitreal injection BIW,
- Initiate or optimize ART

Acute retinal necrosis (ARN):
- (Acyclovir 10-15 mg/kg IV q8h) + (ganciclovir 2 mg/0.05 mL intravitreal injection BIW × 1-2 doses) for 10-14 days, followed by valacyclovir 1 g PO TID for 6 weeks

Primary varicella infection (chickenpox)
Uncomplicated cases (for 5-7 days):
- Acyclovir 800 mg PO 5 times/day

Herpes zoster (shingles)
Acute localized dermatomal:
- For 7-10 days; consider longer duration if lesions are slow to resolve
- Acyclovir 800 mg PO 5 times/day

In managing VZV retinitis, consultation with an ophthalmologist experienced in management of VZV retinitis is strongly recommended.

Duration of therapy for VZV retinitis is not well defined, and should be determined based on clinical, virologic, and immunologic responses and ophthalmologic responses.

Optimization of ART is recommended for serious and difficult-to-treat VZV infections (e.g., retinitis, encephalitis).

ART = antiretroviral therapy; ARV = antiretroviral; CNS = central nervous system; DOT = directly observed therapy; EMB = ethambutol; ICP = intracranial pressure; IRIS = immune reconstitution inflammatory syndrome; IRU = immune recovery uveitis; NSAIDs = nonsteroidal antiinflammatory drugs; PI = protease inhibitor; PZA = pyrazinamide; RFB = rifabutin; RIF = rifampicin; TMP-SMX = trimethoprim/sulfamethoxazole.

Immunizations such as HPV vaccine and hepatitis B vaccine also can be important, for preventing the development of neoplastic processes. Live virus vaccines must be avoided in patients with low CD4 counts.

Grade A References

A1. Uthman OA, Okwundu C, Gbenga K, et al. Optimal timing of antiretroviral therapy initiation for HIV-infected adults with newly diagnosed pulmonary tuberculosis: a systematic review and meta-analysis. *Ann Intern Med.* 2015;163:32-39.

A2. Mfinanga SG, Kirenga BJ, Chanda DM, et al. Early versus delayed initiation of highly active antiretroviral therapy for HIV-positive adults with newly diagnosed pulmonary tuberculosis (TB-HAART): a prospective, international, randomized, placebo-controlled trial. *Lancet Infect Dis.* 2014;14:563-571.

A3. Eshun-Wilson I, Okwen MP, Richardson M, et al. Early versus delayed antiretroviral treatment in HIV-positive people with cryptococcal meningitis. *Cochrane Database Syst Rev.* 2018;7:CD009012.

A4. Aberg J, Powderly W. HIV: primary and secondary prophylaxis for opportunistic infections. *BMJ Clin Evid.* 2010;2010:1-34.

GENERAL REFERENCES

For the General References and other additional features, please visit Expert Consult at https://expertconsult.inkling.com.

366

SYSTEMIC MANIFESTATIONS OF HIV/AIDS

SAMUEL T. MERRICK, SIAN JONES, AND MARSHALL J. GLESBY

Morbidity and mortality from opportunistic infections (OIs) dominated the early years of the HIV epidemic until the mid-1990s when the first protease inhibitors were introduced and combination antiretroviral therapy (cART) began to achieve durable viral suppression and immune reconstitution. Because of the side effects, pill burden, and toxicities of the early combination regimens, or patient preference, clinicians often continued to wait to start antiretroviral therapy (ART) until immune suppression had progressed to the 200 to 350 CD4 cells/μL range. This strategy occasionally led to the development of OIs, although with much less frequency. With the advent of better tolerated, less toxic regimens, including fixed-dose combinations and single-tablet regimens, followed by the definitive answer to the long-debated question of when to start ART with the results of the Strategic Timing of Antiretroviral Therapy (START) trial (the earlier the better),[A1] OIs are now typically only seen in patients unaware of their HIV status or in those who are poorly adherent or have no access to appropriate treatment.

However, many complications may arise that are either unique to HIV infection or happen at a younger age or with greater frequency than in HIV-negative individuals. To some degree, this may be from the high prevalence in the HIV-infected population of traditional risk factors for systemic disease, for example, substance use, poor dietary habits, or smoking. Additionally, it is becoming clearer that the chronic inflammatory state and immune activation caused by HIV infection, even when fully suppressed, may play a large role in the noninfectious systemic complications seen in people living with HIV (PLWH). This chapter addresses both the infectious and noninfectious complications that can arise in the course of HIV infection, with less emphasis on the OIs that are addressed in detail in a separate chapter.

AGING-RELATED SYNDROMES

In most resource-rich countries, including the United States, more than half of PLWH are now 50 years or older. Many comorbidities are more common in the HIV population at any given age, and aging-related syndromes, such as frailty and falls, may also occur at earlier ages than in the general population.[1] There is controversy about whether HIV or its associated inflammation and immune activation accelerates the aging process or is merely an additional risk factor for comorbidities and aging-related disorders. Nonetheless, multimorbidity—having two or more chronic conditions—is common in older HIV-infected adults. The higher prevalence of potentially confounding factors such as smoking, alcohol and substance use, depression, hepatitis C virus (HCV) infection, poverty,

and unstable housing further complicates the attribution of multimorbidity and aging-related syndromes to HIV infection per se.

In older adults with HIV infection, clinicians should pay attention to polypharmacy, functional decline, fall risk, cognitive dysfunction, depression, social isolation, and frailty. Geriatric consultation, or adopting the principles of geriatric assessment and care, may be of value.

NEUROPSYCHIATRIC MANIFESTATIONS OF HIV

HIV enters the central nervous system (CNS) early during infection, and indeed aseptic meningitis may be a presenting sign in primary infection.[2] There is also likely ongoing seeding of the CNS in the presence of ongoing systemic viremia. Discordance between the plasma and cerebrospinal fluid (CSF) viral concentrations has been demonstrated, and up to 10% of individuals with suppressed plasma HIV viral loads may have detectable CSF virus.[3] The presence of HIV in the CSF causes a pro-inflammatory state as evidenced by increased levels of neopterin and pro-inflammatory cytokines in the CSF. This state of chronic inflammation is ameliorated, but does not fully resolve with ART.

PLWH may develop complications in any part of the neurologic axis. Unlike opportunistic infections of the nervous system, some of these manifestations may actually be increasing in incidence since the introduction of effective cART as a function of the increased survival and aging of the HIV-infected population.

Neurocognitive Disorders

Diffuse white matter changes occur more commonly in PLWH than in HIV-uninfected individuals. These changes become more extensive the longer the duration of HIV infection and have been associated with neurocognitive deficits. In the pre-cART era, up to 20 to 30% of patients developed AIDS dementia, which is characterized by memory deficits, psychomotor slowing, and personality changes. In the cART era, this condition, now renamed *HIV-associated dementia* (HAD), is much less common and has an incidence of less than 5%. However, a milder form of cognitive dysfunction, *HIV-associated neurocognitive disorder* (HAND), may affect as many as 50% of PLWH.

HAND is subdivided into asymptomatic neurocognitive impairment (ANI) and mild neurocognitive disorder (MND) based on the Frascati criteria.[4] The criteria for both ANI and MND are a score on standardized neuropsychiatric testing of 1 or more standard deviations (SD) below the mean in at least two cognitive domains. Whereas patients with ANI are asymptomatic and have no functional impairment, individuals with MND will be at least mildly symptomatic. Patients who have HAD, however, have a score that is 2 or more SD below the mean on neuropsychiatric testing and significant impairment in activities of daily living. It is important to note that HAD is a diagnosis of exclusion.

Active HIV replication, as measured by plasma viral load, is an independent risk factor for HAND. However, while virologic suppression is the most important treatment for HAD, it is not sufficient to prevent the development of HAND. Chronic inflammation related to activated monocytes and macrophages is thought to be an important mechanism behind the development of HAND. Increased levels of neopterin and neurofilament light chain can be found in the CSF of patients with HAND, consistent with macrophage activation, supporting this hypothesis. Magnetic resonance imaging (MRI) findings early on show white matter changes that progress to atrophy and reduced brain volume.[5] These findings on imaging have been shown to correlate with the degree of neurocognitive impairment.

Antiretroviral (ARV) agents differ in their ability to penetrate into the CSF, and a CNS penetration effectiveness (CPE) score has been developed. Each drug is assigned a score between 1-4 based upon available pharmacokinetic data and achievable CSF concentrations (Table 366-1). It still remains controversial whether using drugs with higher CPE scores is beneficial. Some studies show neurocognitive improvement when ARV agents with higher CPE score are used, but others fail to show benefit.

"AIDS mania" is a unique condition that has been described in individuals with advanced AIDS and is rarely seen now. Unlike classical mania, this condition is characterized more by irritability than euphoria and does not remit if left untreated.

Efavirenz, a non-nucleoside reverse transcriptase inhibitor (NNRTI), has been commonly associated with neuropsychiatric side effects such as sleep disorder, depression, and seizure. Typically these side effects are worst in the first 4 to 6 weeks after starting treatment, and many patients adjust to efavirenz with time. Some patients, however, are never able to tolerate efavirenz. There are data that this may, at least in part, be due to a genetic polymorphism in cytochrome CYP2B6, which is the main pathway for the metabolism of

TABLE 366-1 CNS PENETRATION EFFECTIVENESS (CPE) SCORES OF ANTIRETROVIRAL MEDICATIONS

ANTIRETROVIRAL CLASS	CPE SCORE*			
	1	2	3	4
Nucleoside reverse transcriptase inhibitors (NRTIs)	Tenofovir Zalcitabine (ddC)	Didanosine (ddI) Lamivudine (3TC) Stavudine (d4T)	Abacavir Emtricitabine (FTC)	Zidovudine (AZT)
Non-nucleoside reverse transcriptase inhibitors (NNRTIs)			Efavirenz Etravirine	Nevirapine
Protease inhibitors	Nelfinavir Ritonavir Saquinavir/ritonavir Saquinavir Tipranavir/ritonavir	Atazanavir Fosamprenavir	Darunavir/ritonavir Fosamprenavir/ritonavir Lopinavir/ritonavir Indinavir	Indinavir/ritonavir
Integrase strand transfer inhibitors		Elvitegravir	Raltegravir	Dolutegravir
Entry inhibitor			Maraviroc	
Fusion inhibitor	Enfuvirtide (T20)			

*CPE scores: 1 = below average; 2 = average; 3 = above average; 4 = much above average.

efavirenz. A base-pair change from G to T at position 516 results in significantly higher efavirenz plasma concentrations and more side effects. This polymorphism is overrepresented in individuals of African ancestry. Rilpivirine is a second-generation NNRTI, which is better tolerated and has fewer CNS side effects than efavirenz, although depression has been reported with the use of this medication as well.

Unsurprisingly, because intravenous drug use is a risk factor for HIV, PLWH have a higher prevalence of substance abuse relative to the general population. There is also a higher prevalence of comorbid psychiatric conditions in PLWH; individuals who have underlying mental health issues may be more prone to high-risk behavior. Conversely, PLWH with no premorbid mental health diagnoses may develop depression and/or anxiety as a result of the stress of coping with their illness. Distinguishing the effects of illicit substances (Chapter 31) from underlying organic psychiatric conditions can be challenging. Active drug use with methamphetamine or cocaine, for example, may cause someone to be erroneously diagnosed with bipolar disorder. Appropriate management of mental health and substance abuse (Chapter 31) issues is very important, not just for the health and general well-being of the patient, but also because these conditions will have a significant negative impact on adherence if not adequately treated.

Immune reconstitution inflammatory syndrome (IRIS) (Chapter 367) has been described with a variety of opportunistic infections shortly after the start of ART. In general, patients who have low nadir CD4 cell counts, particularly if less than 50 cells/μL, or a rapid virologic response to ARV drugs, are at higher risk for IRIS. IRIS has also been described as an encephalitic process complicating HAND in patients who have started ART. HAND IRIS may present as worsening of preexisting HAND or may be the cause of new-onset cognitive dysfunction. White matter lesions may be seen on MRI and are typically in a perivascular distribution. A rare, but fulminant, presentation with CD8 cell infiltration in the brain and demyelination has been described. This condition has been fatal in 4 of the 10 reported cases.

As with other presentations of IRIS, corticosteroids may be used to dampen the inflammatory response in HAND IRIS; however, there have been no controlled trials that demonstrate a clear benefit to the use of corticosteroids.

Peripheral Neuropathy

Peripheral neuropathy (Chapter 392) is the most common neurologic condition affecting PLWH. Distal symmetrical peripheral polyneuropathy (HIV-DSP) is by far the most common of the peripheral neuropathies seen, and 30 to 67% of PLWH may have this condition. Patients typically present with numbness, burning pain, and paresthesias in a glove-and-stocking distribution. HIV-DSP may result either from indirect effects of infection with HIV or from ARV therapy. In the pre-cART era, HIV-DSP was associated with a lower CD4 count and higher HIV viral load. The pathologic findings are distal degeneration in the peripheral nerves of predominantly small myelinated and unmyelinated fibers. Because HIV does not infect Schwann cells or axons directly, the damage has been thought to be due to indirect mechanisms related to pro-inflammatory cytokines. The presence of infiltrating macrophages on biopsy supports this hypothesis, although biopsies are rarely performed for clinical purposes.

HIV-DSP related to ART is referred to as antiretroviral toxic neuropathy (ATN) and is thought to result from the differential inhibition of the mitochondrial DNA polymerase by certain nucleoside reverse transcriptase inhibitors (NRTIs) such as didanosine (ddI), zalcitabine (ddC), and stavudine (d4T). These agents, known as the "d-drugs," are infrequently used now, and the newer NRTI agents are much less likely to cause these symptoms. The diagnosis is typically made clinically, based on symptoms and a neurologic exam that reveals absent ankle reflexes and abnormal vibratory and pinprick sensation in the feet. Nerve conduction studies (NCS) and electromyography (EMG) are reserved for cases with atypical presentations. Findings on NCS typically show reduced sensory nerve action potentials and conduction velocities, whereas EMG reveals features of acute or chronic denervation. It is difficult, if not impossible, to differentiate HIV-DSP based on the underlying etiology for PLWH who have taken d-drugs.

In the case of ATN, removal of the offending agent may result in improvement, although not necessarily complete resolution of symptoms. Success with agents typically used to treat neuropathic pain such as antidepressants and anticonvulsants have been poor. The agents that have shown the most promise, topical capsaicin, lamotrigine, smoked cannabis, and recombinant human nerve growth factor, all have significant barriers to their use. Lamotrigine must be carefully dose-titrated to avoid developing a severe rash or even Stevens-Johnson syndrome, and some guidelines do not recommend its use because of the poor risk-to-benefit ratio. Capsaicin may cause pain on administration that is severe enough to require opiates for analgesia. It is important to exclude potentially treatable causes of distal neuropathy such as diabetes, hypothyroidism, or B_{12} deficiency.

A less commonly seen type of peripheral neuropathy is mononeuritis multiplex (Chapter 392). In the early stages of HIV infection, mononeuritis multiplex is typically due to HIV-related inflammation, whereas with more advanced immunosuppression, it is important to exclude opportunistic infections, notably cytomegalovirus (CMV). Patients typically present with a painful, asymmetrical polyneuropathy involving multiple nerves in a progressive fashion. Diagnosis is confirmed by electrophysiologic testing. For patients with the early-onset form, treatment is typically supportive because the condition is self-limited. However, if vasculitis is seen on nerve biopsy, then treatment with corticosteroids, intravenous immunoglobulin (IVIG), or plasma exchange is indicated.

PLWH may also rarely develop mononeuropathies of either cranial or peripheral nerves. Patients with acute HIV infection may present with unilateral or bilateral facial nerve palsy (Bell palsy). Other manifestations include sensorineural hearing loss and foot or wrist drop. Diagnosis is confirmed by electrophysiologic testing. Treatment with corticosteroids may be helpful, but ART has not been shown to be of benefit.

PLWH may rarely develop an inflammatory demyelinating polyneuropathy (IDP). IDP may present acutely as a rapidly progressive ascending, symmetrical flaccid paralysis similar to Guillain-Barré syndrome. Patients have areflexia and weakness but do not have sensory loss. They may also have autonomic dysfunction and even develop respiratory failure. Symptoms peak at about 4, weeks with recovery shortly thereafter.

AIDP typically develops early during HIV infection and may occur at the time of seroconversion. The CSF in HIV-associated AIDP may have a mild lymphocytic pleocytosis (10 to 50 cells/μL) and a slightly elevated protein. This is in distinction to Guillain-Barré syndrome, in which CSF analysis will typically show an elevated protein but no pleocytosis.

A chronic form, *chronic inflammatory demyelinating polyneuropathy* (CIDP), has a relapsing and remitting course over more than 8 weeks. Treatment for these conditions is similar to HIV-uninfected individuals with IVIG, corticosteroids, and potentially plasma exchange.

Autonomic Neuropathy

Autonomic neuropathy is typically seen with advanced AIDS and may be asymptomatic or may be a cause of orthostatic hypotension, impotence, and abnormalities in sweating. Resting tachycardia may be seen in asymptomatic individuals. Pathologic examination of the sympathetic ganglia reveals neuronal degeneration and perivascular infiltration by T cells and macrophages. It is important to consider other treatable conditions in patients who present with these findings, such as cardiomyopathy and adrenal insufficiency, which have also been associated with HIV infection.

Treatments that have been tried for orthostatic hypotension include sodium chloride tablets, midodrine, mineralocorticoids, and compression stockings.

Myelopathy

Infection with HIV has been associated with the development of a vacuolar myelopathy. This entity may occur at any stage of HIV infection but is more common with advanced disease. In the pre-cART era, most patients died within 6 months of developing symptoms. The typical presentation is that of a slowly progressive (over weeks to months) spastic paraparesis with loss of vibration and position sense. Some patients may have spasticity in their legs but still have preserved strength. Patients will also typically have a wide-based gait. Symptoms usually do not involve the upper extremities. Urinary symptoms such as frequency, urgency, and incontinence are often seen. Since HIV dementia was previously a common finding in advanced AIDS, it is thought that its coexistence might have obscured the symptoms of concomitant myelopathy. MRI of the spine is usually normal but may show spinal cord atrophy or patchy abnormalities on T2-weighted images. The upper thoracic spine is typically involved. CSF findings are nonspecific, such as slight elevation of protein levels or mild pleocytosis, both of which may be seen in the setting of HIV infection even in the absence of known neurologic disease. Measurement of somatosensory evoked potentials (SEPs) is often prolonged and may be abnormal even before the development of clinical disease.

The pathogenesis of HIV-associated myelopathy is unknown. On pathologic examination, demyelination of the dorsal and dorsolateral columns is seen with prominent vacuoles in the myelin sheaths. Virus is not thought to directly invade the spinal cord, so the changes are considered to be related to inflammatory cytokines produced by macrophages.

HIV-associated myelopathy is a diagnosis of exclusion, and it is important to look for other, potentially treatable causes. In particular, the clinical and pathologic presentation of HIV-associated myelopathy is very similar to that seen with B_{12} deficiency (Chapter 155).

Human T-lymphotropic virus 1 (HTLV1) (Chapter 354) is endemic in areas of South America, southern Japan, the Caribbean, parts of the Middle East, and Papua, New Guinea. Individuals who use injection drugs may also be infected, and PLWH may be coinfected with HTLV1. HTLV1 may cause a myelopathy known as HTLV1-associated myelopathy (HAM) or, alternatively, tropical spastic paraparesis. On pathologic examination, the lateral corticospinal, spinocerebellar, and spinothalamic tracts are typically involved, with relative sparing of the posterior columns. Examination of CSF for intrathecal production of antibodies to HTLV1 can help to make the diagnosis.

A defined sensory level is not typically seen with HIV-associated myelopathy, and an alternative diagnosis should be sought if this is found (Chapter 372). In addition, patients who present with other atypical features, such as rapid progression of disease, back pain, or constitutional symptoms, should have a detailed evaluation for the broad range of infectious conditions and malignancies that may involve the spinal cord.

The benefit of cART is unclear in HIV-associated myelopathy, and the mainstay of treatment is to manage symptoms related to spasticity. The most common treatments include baclofen, tizanidine, and botulinum toxin.

Myopathy

The NRTI zidovudine (AZT) has been associated with a toxic myopathy in 0.4% of patients receiving the drug. Patients typically develop proximal shoulder and hip girdle weakness after more than 6 months of therapy. The mechanism

of toxicity is due to inhibition of the mitochondrial DNA polymerase in muscles, and muscle biopsy is notable for ragged red fibers and abnormal mitochondria. Discontinuation of AZT usually results in improvement of myalgia or weakness, although symptoms may initially progress before improving.

Of note, unlike the d-drugs NRTIs, AZT has not been associated with peripheral neuropathy. This is thought to be due to different affinities of the NRTI for binding to mitochondrial DNA polymerase in different tissues.

It is important to be mindful of potential toxicity related to statin use, particularly in patients on HIV protease inhibitors or the pharmacokinetic enhancer cobicistat, because drug-drug interactions can result in increased blood levels of all statins except pitavastatin.

HIV-associated polymyositis (HIV-PM) is a rare condition, with an incidence of less than 1%, but presents similarly to autoimmune polymyositis (Chapter 253). Indeed, the two entities are essentially indistinguishable both clinically and pathologically. HIV-PM can be seen at any stage of HIV infection, and patients present with a slowly progressive symmetrical proximal muscle weakness. Twenty-five to 50% of patients complain of myalgias, and 90% will have an elevated creatine phosphokinase (CPK). CPK levels do not correlate with the degree of muscle weakness. Because these findings are nonspecific, additional testing with EMG or muscle biopsy is required to confirm the diagnosis. EMG may be normal despite biopsy-proven HIV-PM, however. Muscle biopsy typically reveals inflammation with an infiltration of CD8 lymphocytes and rare scattered necrosis. As with autoimmune polymyositis, treatment is typically with corticosteroids. Second-line therapies include IVIG, methotrexate, and azathioprine.

Cerebrovascular

Several observational cohort studies have shown higher rates of both ischemic and hemorrhagic stroke in PLWH in the cART era.[6] The prevalence of traditional risk factors such as diabetes, hyperlipidemia, smoking, and hypertension is increased in PLWH compared with the general population. However, after adjusting for these classical risk factors, the increased risk has still been estimated to be 20 to 80%. Increased immune activation and chronic inflammation have been impugned as likely causes.

● RENAL MANIFESTATIONS OF HIV

The prevalence of kidney disease in PLWH has been reported as between 2.4 to 12% and that of proteinuria as 10 to 30%. Both acute kidney injury (AKI) and chronic kidney disease (CKD) occur more commonly in PLWH and are associated with increased morbidity and mortality.[7] AKI is most commonly a result of systemic infection, sepsis, or medication-related adverse effects. CKD is defined as decreased renal function with a glomerular filtration rate (GFR) of less than 60 mL/minute lasting more than 3 months. CKD may be related to HIV infection itself, medications used to treat HIV, or comorbid conditions, such as diabetes mellitus and hypertension, which are becoming more prevalent as the population of PLWH ages.[8]

HIV infection also disproportionately affects African Americans, a group that is similarly predisposed to renal disease. Coinfection with HCV and HIV may predispose to renal complications because HCV infection itself is associated with immune complex formation and membranoproliferative glomerulonephritis.

In addition to the HIV-specific causes of CKD, membranous nephropathy may be seen in PLWH who also have syphilis (Chapter 303) or chronic hepatitis B virus (HBV) infection (Chapter 140).

Guidelines for the screening and management of renal disease in patients infected with HIV have been developed by the HIV Medicine Association (HIVMA) of the Infectious Disease Society of America. In summary, it is recommended that GFR be monitored at baseline, when cART is started or changed, and at least twice a year in PLWH who are otherwise stable. In individuals who are at higher risk for developing CKD, more frequent measurement should be considered. Urinalysis and spot microalbumin/creatinine should be checked at baseline, when cART is initiated or changed, and at least annually in patients who are stable.

Patients should be referred to a nephrologist for evaluation if there is a persistent decrease in GFR of more than 25%, which results in a clearance of less than 60 mL/minute, and when proteinuria exceeds 300 mg/day or is associated with hematuria. Patients with advanced CKD and GFR less than 30 mL/minute should also be referred (Fig. 366-1).

Adequate control of comorbid conditions such as diabetes mellitus and hypertension is also important to mitigate against progression of renal disease. The goal for blood pressure control should be 130/80 mm Hg. Angiotensin-converting enzyme (ACE) inhibitors or angiotensinogen receptor blockers

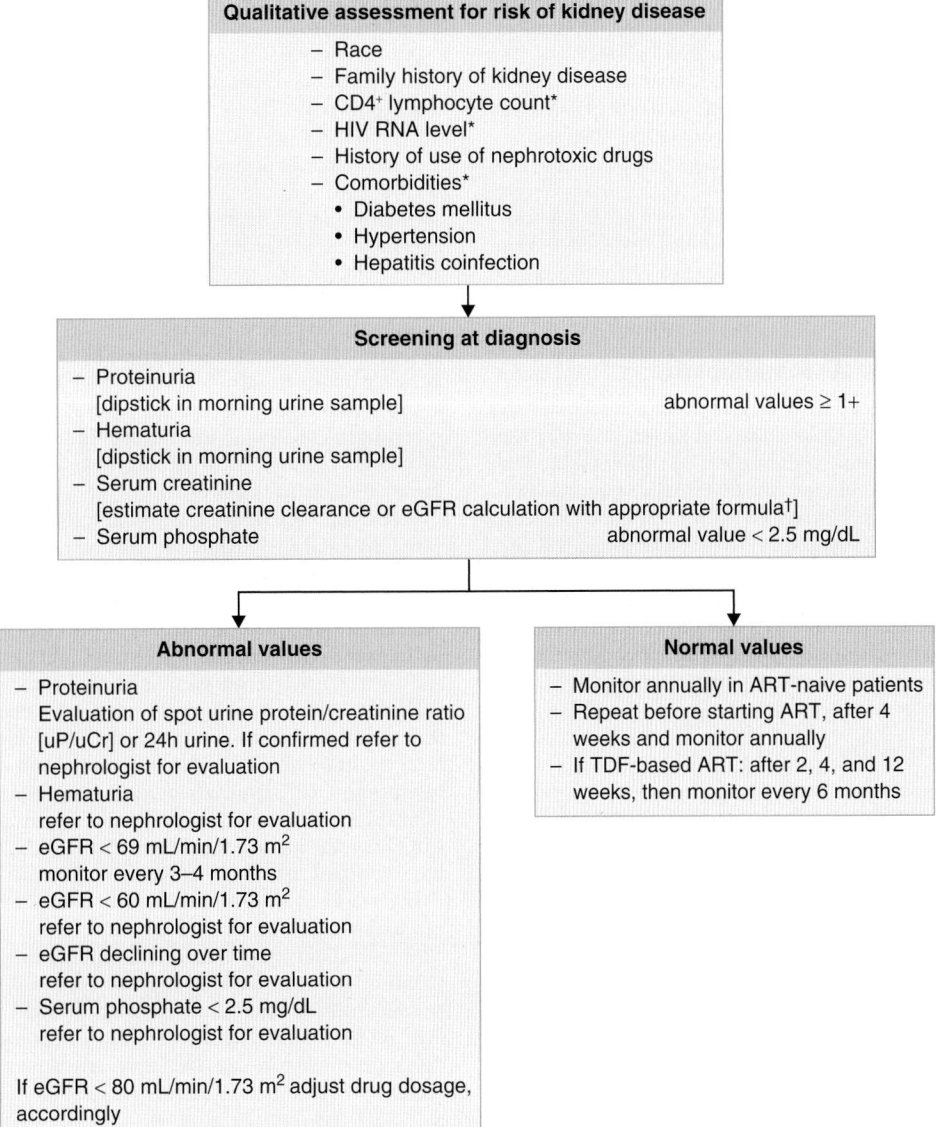

FIGURE 366-1. Guidelines for screening and management of renal disease in patients infected with HIV. *Periodical reevaluation. †Use Cockcroft-Gault or MDRD; use CKD-EPI only if creatininemia is estimated with Roche enzymatic IDMS. ART = antiretroviral therapy; CKD-EPL = chronic kidney disease epidemiology collaboration; eGFR = estimated glomerular filtration rate; MDRD = modification of diet in renal disease; TDF = tenofovir. (Adapted from the HIV Medicine Association of the Infectious Diseases Society of America. From Maggi P, Bartolozzi D, Bonfanti P, et al. Renal complications in HIV disease: between present and future. *AIDS Rev.* 2012;14:37-53.)

(ARBs) are typically used as first-line agents because of their beneficial effects on proteinuria.

HIV-Associated Nephropathy

HIV-associated nephropathy (HIVAN) was first described in 1984 and can present either as AKI or CKD. Typically, patients present with nephrotic-range proteinuria. Before cART, it almost always progressed rapidly to end-stage renal disease (ESRD). In contrast to patients with nephrotic-range proteinuria from other etiologies, patients with HIVAN typically do not have peripheral edema. This is thought to be due to a concomitant salt-wasting component to the nephropathy in HIVAN. HIVAN occurs almost exclusively in individuals of African origin and is more commonly seen with advanced AIDS. Up to 90% of individuals with HIVAN are of African origin. The next most common demographic group is Hispanic. It is exceedingly rare to see HIVAN in a white individual. The genetic basis for this observation has been attributed to polymorphisms on chromosome 22q12. A gene on this chromosome encodes for apolipoprotein L1 (*APOL1*). APOL1 has been found in podocytes and in proximal renal tubular and arterial cells, among others. It has been shown that overexpression of *APOL1* can result in autophagy and cell death. The *APOL1* risk alleles are due to missense mutations of the G1 and G2 variants. The frequency of these polymorphisms varies geographically, with the highest frequency seen in West Africa.[9] APOL1 has been associated with decreased susceptibility to infection by *Trypanosoma brucei*, and the variants seen in individuals of West African background likely afforded a survival advantage at one time.

The pathogenesis of HIVAN is attributed to the direct infection of renal podocytes by HIV, leading to dedifferentiation and apoptosis with effacement of the podocyte foot processes. Both tubular and glomerular epithelial cells may be infected. Inflammation related to chronic viral infection and immune dysregulation are also thought to contribute to the pathogenesis. The pathology on renal biopsy is very characteristic in HIVAN and reveals focal segmental glomerulosclerosis (FSGS) with collapsing glomeruli and microcystic tubular dilation. The accumulation of proteinaceous material results in atypically larger kidneys in ESRD. Other conditions that may result in larger, rather than shrunken, kidneys in ESRD are diabetes mellitus, polycystic kidney disease, and amyloidosis.

The risk for HIVAN has decreased by 60% after cART, and cART is the mainstay of treatment for HIVAN. ACE inhibitors are frequently used as adjunctive therapy. Corticosteroids have been used in patients who have progressive kidney failure despite these therapies. Decreases in proteinuria and improved GFR have been noted with steroid use but at the expense of an increased risk for infection.

HIV-Associated Immune Complex Renal Disease

HIV-associated immune complex renal disease (HIVICK) refers to a heterogeneous group of conditions characterized by immunoglobulin G (IgG) or immune complex deposition and is the second most common diagnosis made on renal biopsy.[10] Immune complex glomerulonephropathies, IgA nephropathy, and lupus-like glomerulonephritis all fall under the umbrella of HIVICK. The renal manifestations of this disorder depend on the location and extent of the glomerular deposits. Proteinuria may be nephrotic in range. Hematuria, decreased GFR, and low serum levels of complement are also often seen.

Unlike HIVAN, there does not appear to be an association with APOL1, and thus HIVICK may be seen in multiple different ethnic groups. Biopsy typically reveals immune complex deposition in the mesangial and perimesangial regions. Patients with HIVICK usually have milder renal disease and less advanced immunosuppression at the time renal disease is recognized than those with HIVAN. HIVICK is also far less likely to progress to end-stage renal disease than HIVAN. The role of ARV therapy is unclear.

HIV-Associated Thrombotic Microangiopathy

The thrombotic microangiopathies (TMAs) include thrombotic thrombocytopenic purpura (TTP), which may be hereditary, acquired, or medication related, and atypical hemolytic-uremic syndrome (aHUS). TMAs occur with increased frequency in PLWH but present similarly to HIV-uninfected individuals. The classical pentad for TTP is described as fever, thrombocytopenia, hemolytic anemia, neurologic abnormalities, and renal abnormalities (Chapter 163). However, renal findings are much less common in TTP than they are in aHUS, where renal abnormalities predominate. Mechanistically, these two syndromes are quite different, and although TTP typically responds to plasma exchange, aHUS is treated with eculizumab, a monoclonal antibody to complement C5. (Also see "Thrombotic Microangiopathy" under the heading "Hematology and Oncology" below.)

Drug-Induced Nephrotoxicity

The ARV agent currently most associated with nephrotoxicity is tenofovir disoproxil fumarate (TDF). TDF is a widely used NRTI that is used both for treatment of HIV and for pre-exposure prophylaxis (PrEP), where it is administered as a co-formulated medication with emtricitabine (FTC) as Truvada.

Tenofovir (TFV) excretion requires a combination of glomerular filtration and active tubular secretion. Tenofovir influx is mediated by the human organic anion transporters (hOAT) 1 and 3 on the basolateral side of the proximal renal tubular cell. Efflux is through the multidrug resistance proteins (MRPs) 2 and 4. TDF characteristically causes proximal renal tubular damage, particularly after prolonged use. Individuals who are older, have a lower body mass, or have comorbidities predisposing to renal complications, such as hypertension and diabetes, are at increased risk for TDF renal toxicity. Patients may present with a typical Fanconi syndrome with euglycemic glycosuria, proteinuria, hypokalemia, hypouricemia, hypophosphatemia, and metabolic acidosis, or with only one of these findings, most commonly isolated glycosuria or hypokalemia.

Given the high prevalence of diabetes and prediabetes in the developed world, it can be challenging to determine whether isolated glycosuria is due to prediabetes or nephrotoxicity from TDF. If there is concern for TDF nephrotoxicity, additional testing for tubular damage, such as measurement of the fractional excretion of phosphorus, can be helpful. Glomerular dysfunction with a decrease in GFR may be seen as an isolated finding or may coincide with the tubular abnormalities described previously.

TDF toxicity may be increased because of drug-drug interactions that lead to increased plasma levels of TFV. Ritonavir and cobicistat are intentionally used as pharmacokinetic enhancers with certain ARV drugs but can also adversely increase the plasma concentration of TFV. Similarly, ledipasvir/sofosbuvir (Harvoni), which is used for the treatment of HCV, can cause elevated TFV levels in coinfected patients.

Polymorphisms in the gene ABCC2, which encodes the cellular transporter MRP2, have been implicated in a heightened risk for TDF toxicity in individuals who have the alleles CC rather than CT or TT at position 24. More recent studies have also found that polymorphisms in ABCC4, which codes for the other transporter involved in tenofovir efflux, may similarly have an impact on toxicity.[11]

The diagnosis of TDF nephrotoxicity is based on clinical presentation and only requires renal biopsy if the presentation is atypical. Prompt discontinuation of TDF is critical if nephrotoxicity is suspected to prevent potentially irreversible damage. A new formulation of TDF, tenofovir alafenamide (TAF), is less nephrotoxic because of lower circulating levels of the metabolite tenofovir and increased uptake into immune cells at low plasma concentration. TAF therefore does not lead to accumulation of TFV in proximal

tubular cells. TAF has been approved for use in patients down to a GFR of 30 mL/minute.

All HIV protease inhibitors exhibit low solubility in the urine. However, only indinavir and atazanavir have been associated with crystalluria and frank nephrolithiasis (Chapter 117) with any frequency. The likelihood of developing crystalluria appears to increase with increased duration of therapy.

A reported 20% of patients on indinavir may develop crystalluria, but a much smaller percentage (3%) will actually have nephrolithiasis. Patients may be asymptomatic or complain of flank pain or discomfort/irritation when urinating. The stones are in large part made up of indinavir or atazanavir crystals and are radiolucent, so a routine flat-plate radiogram will not be revealing. Patients can be instructed to strain their urine to collect crystals/stones for analysis, or other radiographic imaging (e.g., computed tomography [CT] scans or sonograms) can be obtained. Interstitial nephritis (Chapter 114) presenting as sterile pyuria has also been described with indinavir and to a much lesser extent with atazanavir. If not recognized and the medication discontinued, this may progress to chronic scarring and CKD. Trimethoprim-sulfamethoxazole (TMP-SMX) is another medication frequently used in PLWH that is a known cause of interstitial nephritis.

Foscarnet and cidofovir are medications that are used to treat infection with CMV and are infrequently used now; however, they are associated with a significant potential for nephrotoxicity.

Unlike protease inhibitors (PIs) and NNRTIs, NRTIs (with the exception of abacavir) are primarily excreted by the kidneys and must be dose-adjusted for impaired renal function. Conversely, other ARV agents, such as rilpivirine and dolutegravir, an integrase strand transfer inhibitor, and the pharmacokinetic enhancer, cobicistat, may artifactually raise creatinine levels by interfering with the tubular secretion of creatinine. The change in creatinine measurement is on the order of 0.14 mg/dL. Rilpivirine and dolutegravir inhibit the renal transporter OCT2, which is located at the basolateral membrane of proximal tubular cells, whereas cobicistat predominantly inhibits the renal transporter MATE1 in the luminal membrane. Actual GFR, however, is not diminished. It is important to be aware of this finding so that medications are not erroneously underdosed. Measurement of cystatin C may help clarify whether there is actual nephrotoxicity in this situation.

Some patients may use protein supplements and, in particular, creatine. Creatine is another cause of an artifactually raised creatinine. It is important to query patients about all supplements that they use because this information may not be volunteered. There is also a frequent misconception by patients that supplements are safe, but supplements may have interactions with ARV agents and other medications, as well as potentially causing toxicity.

End-Stage Renal Disease

PLWH and ESRD are candidates for either peritoneal or hemodialysis, and the mortality associated with starting dialysis has decreased dramatically in the cART era. As with ESRD in the general population, it is important to anticipate when renal replacement therapy might need to be started. An arteriovenous graft or fistula should be placed in advance to avoid or minimize the time that a vascular catheter will be required for hemodialysis given the attendant risk for infection. Similarly, allowing sufficient time for a Tenckhoff catheter to mature can obviate the need for temporary hemodialysis in those patients planning to start peritoneal dialysis.

In addition to the need for dose adjustment based on GFR, it is important to note that NRTIs, other than abacavir, are not tightly protein bound and may be removed by dialysis, so they should be administered after dialysis. Integrase inhibitors, NNRTIs, and protease inhibitors, however, are not typically removed by dialysis.

PLWH should also be considered for transplantation evaluation because both graft survival and mortality compare favorably to HIV-uninfected individuals. An ongoing trial, the HOPE study, is designed to evaluate the safety of transplanting HIV-infected donor kidneys into HIV-infected recipients.

Given the shortage of kidneys available for transplantation, if this study is successful, it could significantly decrease the wait time for PLWH in need of renal transplantation.

The additional complexity of drug-drug interactions between ARV agents and frequently used immunosuppressants, which are also metabolized by the cytochrome P-450 pathway, such as tacrolimus, necessitates close follow-up and monitoring of drug levels where possible. Close communication between the transplant team and HIV treating physician is critical before ARV drugs are adjusted to avoid potentially catastrophic consequences. Depending on the ARV drug changes, immunosuppressant medications may also need to be adjusted to avoid transplant rejection due to a sudden decrease in immunosuppressant levels, or conversely drug toxicity from supratherapeutic immunosuppressant levels.

HEMATOLOGY AND ONCOLOGY

Cytopenia

Any hematopoietic cell line may be decreased in the setting of infection with HIV, and this may present with either a single or with multiple cell lines being affected. The pathogenesis of HIV-related cytopenias is multifactorial.[12] HIV can directly infect hematopoietic progenitor cells. Furthermore, the bone marrow milieu, which affects the development of cell lines, is affected by the inflammatory cytokines engendered by the immune dysregulation that results from infection with HIV. As such, cytopenias tend to increase in incidence with more advanced immunosuppression and improve after cART.

Cytopenias may also result from bone marrow infiltration from malignancy or opportunistic infection in the setting of advanced AIDS. Disseminated mycobacterial, especially *Mycobacterium avium* complex, or fungal infections, notably histoplasmosis, should be common pathogens to consider. In parts of the globe where visceral leishmaniasis is endemic, this is another important potential etiology. Most PLWH with either Hodgkin lymphoma or non-Hodgkin lymphoma (NHL) (Chapters 176 and 177) have bone marrow involvement at the time of presentation. Multicentric Castleman disease is associated with cytokine dysregulation and high levels of the pro-inflammatory cytokine interleukin-6 (IL-6). Individuals with this illness typically have high fevers, lymphadenopathy, and profound cytopenias.

Medications used both in the treatment of HIV and its complications are also important etiologies to consider. Zidovudine (AZT) was the first ARV agent to be used in the treatment of HIV and frequently caused a macrocytic anemia as well as neutropenia. This agent is rarely used currently because newer agents have more favorable toxicity profiles. Interestingly, AZT is not associated with thrombocytopenia and instead has been shown to be beneficial in the treatment of HIV-associated thrombocytopenia, as further discussed later. Other medications still widely used, such as TMP-SMX and ganciclovir, commonly cause cytopenias, particularly when used in treatment rather than prophylactic doses for opportunistic infections.

Nutritional deficiencies, in particular B_{12}, folate, and iron, are more common in resource-poor settings but are still important etiologies to consider in resource-rich settings and are eminently treatable.

Anemia

The highest incidence of anemia is seen in PLWH who are not yet on ARV therapy, and anemia is more common in those individuals who have symptomatic AIDS. The prevalence of anemia has decreased from 23% in the pre-cART era to 4% in individuals on cART. In addition to the factors discussed earlier, isolated anemia may result from antibody-mediated or drug-related hemolysis and certain infections (Table 366-2).

Autoantibodies to red blood cell antigens are seen relatively commonly in PLWH. One study noted that 18% of PLWH had a positive direct Coombs test compared with only 0.6% of the HIV-uninfected group. Clinically significant autoimmune hemolytic anemia (Chapter 151) is rare, however. Individuals who are glucose-6-phosphate dehydrogenase (G6PD) deficient (Chapter 152) are at risk for hemolysis with certain medications used in PLWH, most notably dapsone and primaquine. It is therefore very important to screen for G6PD deficiency before use of medications that might cause an oxidative stress. Hemolytic anemia from ribavirin is thought to be due to oxidative damage to erythrocyte membranes leading to increased extravascular hemolysis by the reticuloendothelial system.

Malaria (Chapter 324) is an important cause of anemia in coinfected patients in sub-Saharan Africa. Infection with parvovirus B19 (Chapter 347) can cause severe anemia, including aplastic crisis or pure red cell aplasia, but is readily treatable with IVIG.

Erythropoiesis-stimulating agents (ESAs) have been approved by the U.S. Food and Drug Administration (FDA) for the treatment of refractory anemia. ESAs have been shown to be effective for refractory anemia in PLWH who have serum erythropoietin (EPO) levels of less than 500 IU/L. However, the postmarketing recognition of an association between ESA use and increased cardiovascular complications in patients with CKD or malignancy has led to a significant decrease in their use in PLWH as well.

Leukopenia

HIV infection has been associated with a decrease in endogenous granulocytic colony-stimulating factor (G-CSF), with a resultant decrease in granulocytic

TABLE 366-2	EVALUATION AND MANAGEMENT OF ANEMIA IN HIV-INFECTED INDIVIDUALS	
ETIOLOGY	**EVALUATION**	**TREATMENT**
Uncontrolled HIV infection	HIV viral load	Antiretroviral therapy
Chronic inflammation	Exclude other etiologies as below	Erythropoiesis-stimulating agents for refractory anemia
Nutritional	B_{12}, folate, iron studies Endoscopy as indicated if iron low	Supplementation Treatment of underlying condition
Medication related	**Review medication list** Bone marrow suppression: AZT, TMP-SMX, chemotherapy Hemolysis (see below): Dapsone, primaquine, ribavirin	Change medication where possible, support with erythropoiesis-stimulating agents
Thrombotic microangiopathy	Peripheral smear for schistocytes, ADAMTS13 level	Plasmapheresis for TTP Eculizumab for atypical HUS
Hemolytic anemia	LDH, reticulocyte count, haptoglobin, indirect bilirubin	
1. Autoimmune	Coombs test	Corticosteroids
2. Medication-related	Dapsone, primaquine (G6PD deficiency)	Discontinue dapsone, primaquine Reduce ribavirin dose
Parvovirus B19	Parvovirus B19 PCR Bone marrow biopsy (pronormoblasts)	Intravenous immune globulin
Bone marrow infiltration	Histoplasma urine/blood antigen Blood culture for MAI LDH for lymphoma Bone marrow biopsy if noninvasive tests are unrevealing	Treatment of underlying etiology

and macrophage progenitor cells. Treatment with ARV drugs has been associated with an improvement in leukopenia in this setting.

Medications such as AZT, TMP-SMX, and ganciclovir have also been frequently implicated as causative agents for leukopenia. Although the risk for bacterial infection has been shown to be increased with an absolute neutrophil count (ANC) of less than 1000 cells/μL, and in particular if less than 500 cells/μL, the absolute risk for bacterial infection in PLWH still appears to be relative low at three to five infections per person-month in one study. Nevertheless, it seems reasonable to consider the use of G-CSF (Chapter 147) in patients who have profound neutropenia despite removal of the offending agent. In support of this, a randomized controlled study of 258 subjects with an ANC of less than 0.200 cells/μL showed a decrease in mortality in the G-CSF arm compared with the control group.

Thrombocytopenia

Thrombocytopenia was commonly seen in the pre-cART era, with up to 40% of PLWH developing thrombocytopenia at some point during their life. cART has also led to a significant decrease in the incidence of thrombocytopenia.

Patients may present with thrombocytopenia at any stage of HIV infection; however, it is more commonly seen with advanced disease. When seen during early stages of HIV infection, autoimmunity with the development of cross-reactive antibodies between the HIV envelope glycoprotein gp160/120 and the platelet glycoprotein IIb/IIIa is thought to be an important contributor to the pathogenesis.

For those individuals who present with thrombocytopenia during the later stages of AIDS, direct infection of megakaryocytes is thought to be a more important mechanism.

The state of immune activation seen with chronic HIV infection is also associated with elevated C-reactive protein (CRP) levels. CRP is known to be an important factor in IgG-mediated platelet destruction by virtue of enhancing phagocytosis of opsonized platelets.

In the absence of a superimposed coagulation disorder or the use of medications that affect platelet activity such as nonsteroidal inflammatory agents (NSAIDs), it is unusual to see significant bleeding in patients with platelet counts above $10 \times 10^3/\mu L$.

The treatment for HIV-associated thrombocytopenia (Chapter 163) is virologic suppression with ARV therapy. For those individuals who do not respond to this, corticosteroids, IVIG, or anti-D immune globulin (if the patient is not splenectomized and is Rh positive) have all shown to be of benefit. Corticosteroids increase platelet counts in 40 to 80% of individuals; however, only 10 to 20% have long-term remission. IVIG is expensive and of short-term benefit, so it is typically reserved for use before invasive procedures or in the setting of acute bleeding. Surgical splenectomy and splenic irradiation have both been used in particularly refractory cases. It is important to make sure patients are appropriately vaccinated against encapsulated organisms such as *Neisseria meningitidis*, *Haemophilus influenzae*, and *Streptococcus pneumoniae* before removal or irradiation of the spleen.

More recently, thrombopoietin receptor analogues such as eltrombopag and romiplostim have been used with some success in cases of refractory HIV-related thrombocytopenia. Because of concerns about the potential increased risk for thrombosis, it is important to use the lowest dose of these medications needed to obtain an acceptable platelet count.

Thrombotic Microangiopathy

TTP is characterized by fever, thrombocytopenia, hemolytic anemia, neurologic abnormalities, and renal abnormalities (Chapter 163). aHUS is not typically associated with neurologic symptoms, but renal injury is a major finding. It can be difficult to differentiate between these two entities, and together these two syndromes make up the TMAs. One potential differentiating feature is that TTP, but not aHUS, is associated with a decreased level of von Willebrand factor cleaving enzyme ADAMTS13. In HIV-uninfected individuals, the decrease in ADAMTS13 is mediated by autoantibodies and responds to therapy with plasma exchange. Severely low levels of ADAMTS13 have also been described in HIV-associated TTP. Treatment with ART is thus important in the management of this condition. Indeed, the incidence of TMA has decreased in PLWH from 1.4 to 7% in the pre-cART era to 0.3% after widespread use of cART. It is important to distinguish aHUS from TTP because the former is not associated with antibodies to ADAMTS13 and does not respond to plasma exchange but may respond to eculizumab, a monoclonal antibody to complement C5.

Hypercoagulable State

Several factors have been implicated in the prothrombotic tendency in PLWH. One of the major contributing factors is likely to be the pro-inflammatory state and immune activation seen with chronic HIV infection. Other factors include antiphospholipid antibodies, such as lupus anticoagulant, and acquired protein S and C deficiency (Chapter 73). Up to 64% of PLWH have been found to have anticardiolipin antibodies.

Of note, the classical risk factors for thrombosis, such as obesity, hyperlipidemia, and hypertension, also occur disproportionately in the HIV-infected population.

Megestrol acetate was used frequently in the pre-cART era for appetite stimulation and as a treatment for HIV wasting. The prothrombotic effect of this medication has been well described.

AIDS-Defining Malignancies

Systemic non-Hodgkin lymphoma (NHL), Kaposi sarcoma (KS), and invasive cervical cancer are seen at substantially higher rates in PLWH than the general population and make up what historically have been called the *AIDS-defining malignancies*.[13] Before cART, the risk for KS was 2800-fold higher in PLWH than in the general population, and for NHL and cervical cancer, it was 10-fold and three- to four-fold higher, respectively. These malignancies are all associated with specific oncogenic viral infections. KS is associated with human herpesvirus 8 (HHV8), also known as Kaposi sarcoma–associated herpesvirus (KSHV), NHL with Epstein-Barr virus (EBV), and cervical cancer with human papillomavirus (HPV). As such, the degree of immunosuppression is a major factor leading to the increased incidence of these malignancies that results from the lack of immunologic control of the respective oncogenic viruses. Apart from cervical cancer, the incidence of the other AIDS-defining malignancies has decreased significantly since the introduction of cART.

Most PLWH will be able to tolerate standard chemotherapy regimens. However, it is important to be mindful of the potential for drug-drug interactions in patients who are on HIV protease inhibitor regimens or a regimen that contains the pharmacokinetic booster cobicistat. If there are concerns for significant toxicity, it may be necessary to hold ARV therapy during chemotherapy. In general, however, it is preferable to continue ARV therapy whenever possible.

Non-Hodgkin Lymphoma

The AIDS-defining NHLs are all mature B-cell lymphomas (Chapter 176) and include diffuse large B-cell lymphoma (DLBCL), primary CNS lymphoma (PCNSL), Burkitt lymphoma, primary effusion lymphoma, and plasmablastic lymphoma (PBL). Diffuse large B-cell lymphoma (DLBCL) and primary central nervous system lymphoma (PCNSL) are closely associated with EBV infection and occur with more advanced immunosuppression. PCNSL, in particular, is typically seen when CD4 counts are less than 50 cells/μL. Burkitt lymphoma is associated with EBV in 25 to 40% of cases and may occur earlier in the course of HIV infection. The incidence of NHL has decreased substantially in the setting of cART, most notably for PCNSL; however, NHL still remains the most common AIDS-defining malignancy seen.

Of the HIV-associated NHLs, DLBCL is the one most commonly seen and is typically treated with either R-CHOP (rituximab, cyclophosphamide, doxorubicin, vincristine, prednisone) or R-EPOCH (rituximab, etoposide, prednisone, vincristine, cyclophosphamide, doxorubicin).

Although there are no randomized controlled trials evaluating these two regimens in PLWH, many experts prefer R-EPOCH. Two to 11% of newly diagnosed DLBCL patients will have rearrangements in both *BCL2* and *MYC*. These so-called double-hit lymphomas are highly aggressive and associated with a poor prognosis. HIV infection is not a contraindication to autologous stem cell transplantation (Chapter 168) for relapsed or refractory lymphoma because outcomes are comparable to the general population. Burkitt lymphoma is an obligate *MYC* gene–expressing lymphoma. It makes up 1 to 2% of NHLs in the HIV-negative population but 10% of those in PLWH. Treatment is with a high-dose cyclophosphamide regimen and prophylactic intrathecal chemotherapy due to the high propensity for CNS involvement. Burkitt lymphoma in PLWH is considered highly curable because patients are able to tolerate intensive chemotherapy such as CODOX-M/IVAC (cyclophosphamide, vincristine, doxorubicin, high-dose methotrexate/ifosfamide, etoposide, and high-dose cytarabine) well. Outcomes with CODOX-M/IVAC in PLWH and Burkitt lymphoma were similar to those in the HIV-uninfected group in one small study.

Primary CNS lymphoma is a rare variant of DLBCL that is limited to the brain and has no systemic symptoms. Typically, PCNSL occurs when CD4 cell counts are less than 50 cells/μL, and the prognosis has historically been very poor. Previously, the main treatment modality used, in addition to cART, was whole brain radiation (WBR). However, progression of disease was common with WBR, and there was a significant risk for late-onset encephalopathy. Currently, there has been a move to avoid use of WBR and use intravenous high-dose methotrexate instead.

Plasmablastic lymphoma is an EBV-associated CD20-negative lymphoma that typically involves the oropharynx. In pre-cART times, PBL was associated with a poor prognosis, but survival rates have improved. There is no standard of care for chemotherapy, but although EPOCH, HyperCVAD (cyclophosphamide, vincristine, doxorubicin, dexamethasone), and CODOX-M/IVAC have all been used, CHOP is felt to be inadequate. Some experts favor treatment with EPOCH followed by autologous stem cell transplantation as first-line treatment.

Primary Effusion Lymphoma

HHV8 infection has also been associated with the much less common primary effusion lymphoma (PEL) and multicentric Castleman disease (MCD). Primary effusion lymphoma is a rare B-cell NHL that makes up 2 to 4% of HIV-associated lymphomas and may also be associated with EBV infection. PEL presents as a malignant effusion involving the peritoneal, pleural, or pericardial spaces without evidence of a primary tumor mass. PEL typically occurs with advanced AIDS and has been associated with prior KS in 27 to 71% of patients. CHOP is often used to treat PEL, but there is no standard of care, and the overall prognosis remains poor, with a mean survival of 6 months.

Multicentric Castleman Disease

MCD is also associated with HHV8 infection, and up to 70% of patients with MCD may have concomitant KS. MCD is a lymphoproliferative disorder with a high risk for progression to lymphoma. Patients typically present with fever, weight loss, diffuse lymphadenopathy, and hepatosplenomegaly. Anemia and hypergammaglobulinemia are common laboratory findings. Although infection with HHV8 is universal in HIV-associated MCD, only 40 to 50% of HIV-negative individuals have HHV8 infection. The underlying basis for these symptoms is related to the high production of the inflammatory cytokine IL-6, which is upregulated by viral products. HHV8 has been shown to infect B cells, which then proliferate as plasmablasts and secrete a virally encoded from of IL-6 (vIL-6) that can activate the human IL-6 receptor.

POEMS syndrome (polyneuropathy, organomegaly, endocrinopathy, M component, and skin changes) and TAFRO syndrome (thrombocytopenia, anasarca, fever, reticulin fibrosis, and organomegaly) have also been reported in conjunction with MCD.

KS in PLWH is associated with latent HHV8 infection; however, MCD in PLWH is thought to be associated with lytic HHV8 replication and is associated with high serum viral loads of HHV8 that correlate with the severity of clinical disease. Because HHV8 replication is sensitive to the antiviral agents foscarnet, ganciclovir, and cidofovir in vitro, recommended treatment in PLWH and MCD is with ganciclovir and rituximab. Etoposide is sometimes included for patients with more aggressive disease.

Biologic agents that directly target IL-6 production have only been studied in HIV-negative patients so far and have not been recommended for use in HIV-infected patients with MCD. Currently, siltuximab, a monoclonal antibody to IL-6, is considered first-line therapy for MCD in HIV-uninfected individuals who are also HHV8 seronegative. Tocilizumab, which targets the IL-6 receptor, has been approved for this use in Japan and the United States.[14]

Kaposi Sarcoma

KS, in the setting of HIV infection, is seen primarily in men who have sex with men (MSM) and rarely in women or individuals who have intravenous drug use as a risk factor for HIV infection.[15] PLWH who develop KS typically have CD4 cell counts of less than 200 cells/μL, although it can occur, less commonly, with higher CD4 cell counts. The most common manifestation is characteristic purplish lesions on the skin, which may appear as nodules or plaques. KS may affect mucosal surfaces as well, and in the oropharynx lesions are most often seen on the gingiva and hard palate. The color of the lesions reflects the underlying pathology because KS is an angioproliferative tumor. Proliferation of vessels and spindle-shaped tumor cells of endothelial origin are evident on biopsy. With more developed KS lesions, there may be a background chronic inflammatory infiltrate composed of lymphocytes, plasma cells, and dendritic cells. It should be noted that in dark-skinned individuals, these lesions may be harder to identify and may be confused with dermatofibromas. Bacillary angiomatosis may also be similar in appearance to KS lesions and require biopsy to be distinguished. It is therefore necessary to have a low threshold for biopsy of skin lesions in PLWH.

Most patients who have visceral involvement will have evidence of cutaneous disease, but it is possible to have isolated visceral disease. The most common sites for visceral KS are the lungs and the gastrointestinal (GI) tract. In the lungs, KS may present with parenchymal disease with or without associated effusions. Pleural effusions are characteristically bloody, carry a poor prognosis, and may require pleurodesis to control respiratory symptoms. Lesions similar to those seen on the skin may be seen on bronchoscopy. Biopsy is not recommended, however, owing to the highly vascular nature of these lesions. Similarly, endoscopy of the upper or lower GI tract may also reveal the classical lesions of KS. Although routine endoscopy is not recommended in the absence of symptoms, it is important to evaluate patients with KS for evidence of GI blood loss such as iron deficiency or guaiac-positive stools because endoscopy to rule out visceral KS would be indicated in this setting. Similarly, a chest x-ray should be obtained to rule out asymptomatic pulmonary KS in any individual diagnosed with KS elsewhere.

cART is the mainstay of treatment for KS, and decreased serum HHV8 viral loads have been documented after the start of cART. Although KS may resolve with cART alone, patients who have diffuse or disseminated disease and those who do not respond to cART will require additional therapy. Radiation therapy has been used for treatment in the past, but chemotherapy is the preferred method of treatment now. The agents most commonly used are pegylated doxorubicin, liposomal daunorubicin, and paclitaxel.

Patients may have "unmasking" of previously unrecognized KS or worsening of previously diagnosed disease because of IRIS, which may be seen soon after starting cART (Chapter 367). Although corticosteroids have been used for other manifestations of severe IRIS reactions, it is not recommended to use corticosteroids with KS because corticosteroids will increase replication of HHV8. Instead, it is recommended that cART be continued, and chemotherapy should be started if the patient is not already on treatment.

Cervical Cancer

Women with HIV infection are less able to clear infection with HPV (Chapter 349) and are at a three- to four-fold increased risk for cervical cancer compared with HIV-uninfected women. This risk has not decreased despite the introduction of cART. Cervical cancer (Chapter 189) remains a particular problem in resource-limited settings where women do not have ready access to screening and early treatment and is a leading cause of cancer-related mortality in these countries.

The screening recommendations for women with HIV infection are slightly different from HIV-negative women[16]; in particular, it is recommended that HIV-infected women be screened throughout their lifetime and not to stop screening at age 65 years, as with HIV-negative women. A cervical Papanicolaou (Pap) test should be done within 1 year of sexual activity and no later than age 21 years. If the baseline test is normal, it should be repeated 6 to 12 months later. If the results of three consecutive tests are normal, then the patient may be screened every 3 years thereafter. If any cervical Pap test is abnormal, the patient should be referred for immediate colposcopy. For ASCUS (atypical cells of undetermined significance) cytologic results, however, it is acceptable to repeat cytology in 6 to 12 months and defer colposcopy. Co-testing (i.e., cervical cytology and concomitant HPV testing) is not recommended for women younger than 30 years, and there are no specific guidelines for its use. However, if a woman has an ASUCS cervical cytology result and tests positive for high-risk HPV, she should proceed to colposcopy immediately.

Treatment for cervical dysplasia is the same as for HIV-uninfected women. Because women with HIV are more likely to have persistent or recurrent dysplasia after treatment, it is important that they have ongoing close follow-up. Women with cervical dysplasia should also have anal Pap tests performed to screen for anal cancer (see later).

Non-AIDS-Defining Cancers

Several malignancies, which do not qualify as AIDS-defining malignancies, nevertheless occur at an increased prevalence in PLWH.[17] The risk for developing solid tumors and non-AIDS-defining lymphomas is two- to three-fold higher than in the general population. As the average age of PLWH is increasing, the prevalence of these non-AIDS-defining cancers is also increasing. Some are associated with underlying viral infections; others may be attributed to increased behavioral risk factors, such as smoking and alcohol consumption. The potential role of immunosuppression or chronic inflammation related to chronic immune activation has not been well defined but is thought to be a factor. It is important to be aware of this increased risk so that appropriate screening can be performed.

Hodgkin lymphoma (Chapter 177) is not considered an AIDS-defining malignancy, yet a five- to 20-fold higher rate occurs in PLWH compared with the general population, and the incidence has not decreased despite the introduction of cART. PLWH more commonly present with advanced disease and B symptoms, such as fever, sweats, and weight loss. Moreover, there is a higher incidence of more aggressive subtypes, such as mixed cellularity and lymphocyte depletion, in PLWH compared with the general population and a higher association with EBV infection. ABVD (doxorubicin, bleomycin, vinblastine, and dacarbazine) is the first-line chemotherapy regimen for HIV-uninfected individuals and is also used for PLWH with relapsed or refractory Hodgkin lymphoma.

Anal cancer (Chapter 184) is associated with HPV infection and in the general population is seen more commonly in women in their 50s and 60s. In the setting of HIV infection, however, anal cancer is seen most commonly in MSM. Decreased clearance of HPV has been associated with lower CD4 cell counts. Although uncommon in the general population, the rate of anal cancer in PLWH was 30-fold higher than in HIV-uninfected individuals in the Swiss Cohort study.

Screening programs have been developed that parallel those for cervical cancer in an attempt to prevent anal dysplasia from progressing to invasive cancer. Guidelines vary, but screening with anal Pap tests is recommended for HIV-infected MSM, women with a history of abnormal cervical histology, or anyone with a history of anogenital warts. Other guidelines include women with abnormal Pap test or a history of receptive anal intercourse. Some experts would recommend screening for anyone with HIV regardless of sexual orientation or history of sexual practice given that current guidelines are felt to underestimate the risk. Primary care providers perform anal cytology (anal Pap tests) and refer any patient with ASCUS or higher grade cytologic abnormalities for high-resolution anoscopy with biopsy of abnormal tissue identified by ascetic acid staining. High-grade anal dysplasia can be treated by infrared coagulation or, less commonly, surgery. More widespread lesions, which are not amenable to infrared coagulation, may be treated with topical 5-fluorouracil or imiquimod. The benefit of this approach, however, has not been validated. The ANCHOR (Anal Cancer/HSIL Outcomes Research) study is a randomized trial currently enrolling PLWH with high-grade squamous intraepithelial lesions on anoscopy to immediate treatment (as determined by provider preference) or close monitoring with treatment only if there is progression of disease. Results from this study will better define the standard of care for this condition in the future.

Lung cancer (Chapter 182) is the most common cause of non-AIDS-defining cancer in PLWH and the leading cause of malignancy-related deaths in a large population-based registry in the United States. Cigarette smoking is the leading risk factor for lung cancer, and the prevalence of tobacco use in PLWH is two to three times higher than in the general population. Studies have shown, however, that the risk for lung cancer in PLWH is also increased independent of smoking status.

Colorectal cancer (Chapter 184) has been found to develop earlier and present with more advanced disease in PLWH.

Hepatocellular carcinoma (Chapter 186) has a three- to six-fold increased risk in PLWH compared with the general population, which is likely related to the high rates of HBV and HCV coinfection seen with HIV. Furthermore, PLWH who have chronic hepatitis may develop liver fibrosis more rapidly.

Skin cancers are known to occur at a much higher frequency in immunocompromised individuals. For example, solid organ transplant recipients have between 65 and 250 times higher risk than the general population. In the Swiss Cohort study of PLWH, basal cell carcinoma was seen more commonly than squamous cell carcinoma, and the overall rate was three-fold higher in PLWH than in the general population. There was no specific association with CD4 cell count, however.

Merkel cell carcinoma is a rare primary neuroendocrine tumor of the skin that is associated with polyoma virus infection. It is a very aggressive tumor and prone to local recurrence. A 13-fold higher rate of occurrence has been reported in the setting of HIV infection.

Cancer of the head and neck (Chapter 181) occurs at a four-fold increased incidence and is also associated with HPV infection as well as smoking and alcohol consumption. Management does not differ substantially from the HIV-uninfected patient.

Notably, breast and prostate cancer are not increased in PLWH.

SCREENING AND PREVENTION

In addition to cervical Pap tests for women with HIV infection, all PLWH who are MSM, have a history of anogenital warts, or have abnormal cervical histology should have anal Pap tests performed to screen for anal cancer. Mammograms, colonoscopy, and chest CT scans, to screen for breast, colon, and lung cancer, respectively, should be performed based on age and risk factors, as per guidelines for the general population. PLWH who have chronic HBV infection should be screened for hepatocellular carcinoma with hepatic imaging every 6 months. Individuals who have chronic HCV infection should be similarly screened if they have evidence of cirrhosis, even if they have achieved a sustained virologic response after HCV treatment.

The importance of counseling for smoking cessation cannot be overstated because tobacco has an impact on several malignancies other than lung cancer in addition to its adverse cardiovascular and pulmonary effects. Patients should also be counselled on the use of sunblock with high SPF and have annual skin cancer screenings if they are at high risk.

The HPV vaccine is safe and effective in PLWH and should be administered to individuals between the ages of 9 and 26 years for prevention of cervical and anal cancer. Similarly, HBV vaccine should be given to all PLWH who do not show serologic evidence of prior HBV infection. Because it has been shown that PLWH with CD4 cell counts of less than 200 cells/μL respond less robustly to vaccinations, it is reasonable to defer immunizing patients who have low CD4 cell counts until they improve.

● CARDIOVASCULAR MANIFESTATIONS OF HIV
Coronary Heart Disease

PLWH have higher rates of myocardial infarction than the general population, even after adjustment for traditional cardiovascular risk factors.[18] This increased risk is also present in the subset of people without major cardiovascular risk factors and in those with asymptomatic, controlled HIV infection. Although

data are limited, the risk for sudden cardiac death may also be increased in the HIV-infected population.

Among traditional cardiovascular risk factors, smoking accounts for a considerable proportion of the risk among PLWH. The prevalence of smoking is higher than the general population, and its adverse effects may be potentiated by HIV.

Dyslipidemia (Chapter 195) is another important modifiable cardiovascular risk factor in PLWH. Advanced HIV disease is associated with low total cholesterol, low-density lipoprotein (LDL) cholesterol, and high-density lipoprotein (HDL) cholesterol levels as well as elevated triglycerides and a higher relative proportion of proatherogenic small, dense LDL cholesterol. Initiation of cART in advanced HIV disease often increases total and LDL cholesterol to levels that might be expected absent HIV infection, sometimes termed a "return to health" phenomenon. Increases in HDL cholesterol are variable, however, and may remain persistently low in some individuals despite virologic control. Hypertriglyceridemia is the most common lipid abnormality in HIV-infected patients, especially those on certain protease inhibitor-containing ARV drug regimens.

Certain nontraditional cardiovascular risk factors may play important roles in HIV infection because of their higher prevalence in some populations. These include HCV coinfection—more common in patients with histories of injection drug use and MSM—which may be associated with increased subclinical atherosclerosis. Cocaine use may also contribute to the incidence of myocardial infarction.

As with certain autoimmune diseases, such as systemic lupus erythematosus, inflammation and immune activation are thought to contribute to atherosclerosis and the occurrence of cardiovascular events in HIV infection, even in the setting of virologic suppression with ART. PLWH are more likely to have noncalcified, vulnerable atherosclerotic plaque on coronary computed tomography angiography, as well as increased aortic inflammation on positron emission tomography scanning. Both radiographic features have been associated with markers of macrophage activation, as have other measures of subclinical atherosclerosis, such as increased carotid artery intima media thickness on ultrasonography.

Observational data suggest that current or recent use of certain ARV drugs is associated with increased risk for myocardial infarction after statistical adjustment for cardiovascular risk factors and potential confounding variables. Of ARV drugs that are commonly in use now, the signal has been strongest with the NRTI abacavir and with the protease inhibitors darunavir and lopinavir/ritonavir. Although definitive evidence from randomized, controlled trials is lacking, and the potential mechanisms by which these medications may increase cardiovascular risk are not understood, clinicians almost always have the option of selecting other ARV drugs from the same or different classes without sacrificing virologic efficacy.

Although not unique to HIV, insulin resistance, diabetes mellitus, metabolic syndrome, and nonalcoholic steatohepatitis (NASH) may be more prevalent than in the general population and contribute to cardiovascular risk. As discussed later (see Endocrine Manifestations of HIV), some PLWH have excess visceral adipose tissue, which is linked to subclinical atherosclerosis.

Although there may be unique pathogenetic mechanisms in PLWH, the approach to prevention of cardiovascular disease mirrors that of the general population with a few caveats. Traditional risk stratification tools, such as the American Heart Association/American College of Cardiology Pooled Cohort Equations, may underestimate cardiovascular event rates in the HIV population but are commonly used in the absence of validated HIV-specific risk equations. The National Lipid Association Guidelines permit counting HIV as a major cardiovascular risk factor when risk-stratifying. Statins are the mainstay of lipid-lowering therapy, although clinicians must be mindful of drug-drug interactions with certain ARV agents. Protease inhibitors and cobicistat inhibit the metabolism of most statins; lovastatin and simvastatin should not be coadministered with these drugs (Table 366-3), whereas atorvastatin and rosuvastatin may be used cautiously starting at low doses. Pitavastatin does not interact significantly with ARV drugs. Pravastatin is generally safe to use, although only at low doses when coadministered with the protease inhibitor darunavir. Fluvastatin appears to be safe to use with protease inhibitors, although data are limited.

Although it does not specifically dampen HIV-related inflammation and immune activation, clinicians may extrapolate from guidelines from the general population to consider low-dose aspirin for primary prevention of cardiovascular disease in moderate- to high-risk HIV-infected patients who do not have contraindications. There are clinically significant interactions between certain antiplatelet agents and both protease inhibitors and

TABLE 366-3 DRUGS THAT SHOULD NOT BE COADMINISTERED WITH SPECIFIC ANTIRETROVIRALS DUE TO PROVEN OR SUSPECTED DRUG-DRUG INTERACTIONS

ANTIRETROVIRAL	CARDIAC DRUGS	LIPID-LOWERING DRUGS	PULMONARY ARTERIAL HYPERTENSION DRUGS	COPD/ASTHMA DRUGS	ANTIPLATELET/ ANTICOAGULANT DRUGS
ALL PROTEASE INHIBITORS	Dronedarone Eplerenone Ivabradine Ranolazine	Lovastatin Simvastatin	Sildenafil	Inhaled budesonide*, fluticasone*, mometasone* Prednisone* Salmeterol	Apixaban Dabigatran if CrCl <50 mL/min Edoxaban Rivaroxaban Ticagrelor Vorapaxar
Fosamprenavir ± ritonavir	Above plus: Flecainide Propafenone				
Saquinavir/ritonavir	Above plus: Amiodarone Disopyramide Dofetilide Flecainide Lidocaine Propafenone Quinidine				
Tipranavir/ritonavir	Above plus: Amiodarone Flecainide Propafenone Quinidine				
NNRTI					
Etravirine					Clopidogrel
InSTI					
Dolutegravir	Dofetilide				
Elvitegravir/cobicistat	Eplerenone Ivabradine Ranolazine	Lovastatin Simvastatin	Sildenafil	Salmeterol	Apixaban Dabigatran if CrCl <50 mL/min Edoxaban Rivaroxaban Ticagrelor Vorapaxar

Note: This table focuses on contraindications. Other medications may need to be used with caution or at lower doses based on drug-drug interactions.
*Do not co-administer unless potential benefits outweigh the risks of systemic corticosteroid adverse effects.
CrCl = creatinine clearance; InSTI = integrase strand transfer inhibitor; NNRTI = non-nucleoside reverse transcriptase inhibitor.
Adapted from tables from the Panel on Antiretroviral Guidelines for Adults and Adolescents. Guidelines for the use of antiretroviral agents in HIV-1-infected adults and adolescents. Department of Health and Human Services. Available at http://www.aidsinfo.nih.gov/ContentFiles/AdultandAdolescentGL.pdf. Accessed September 3, 2017.

NNRTIs that could result in increased risk for bleeding or reduced antiplatelet efficacy.

Cardiomyopathy and Congestive Heart Failure

Before the availability of effective combination ARV therapy, dilated cardiomyopathy (Chapter 52) was a common complication of advanced HIV disease and attributed to direct cardiac involvement by HIV, opportunistic infections, micronutrient deficiencies, or autoimmunity. Anecdotal data and animal models also implicated mitochondrial toxicity from early NRTI drugs, such as zidovudine, that are seldom if ever used today in resource-rich settings.

Echocardiography studies have shown that diastolic dysfunction is now far more common than systolic dysfunction in PLWH, presumably because of better control of HIV disease.[19] Diastolic dysfunction in this population has largely been attributed to traditional risk factors, such as age, increased body mass index, hypertension, hypercholesterolemia, and diabetes mellitus. Congestive heart failure with preserved ejection fraction is consequently more common than that attributable to reduced ejection fraction. Cardiac steatosis and fibrosis may also be more prevalent in PLWH. Management of impaired ventricular function and heart failure does not differ from the general population (Chapter 53).

Hypertension

In some studies, initiation of ART is associated with elevations in systolic and diastolic blood pressure, although data are conflicting. The prevalence of hypertension (Chapter 70) may also be increased in PLWH relative to demographically similar controls. In addition to traditional risk factors, there is some evidence that lower nadir CD4 cell count, weight gain, and elevated waist circumference are associated with incident hypertension. There are no definitive data linking specific ARV drugs or classes of drugs to hypertension.

Although management of hypertension is not fundamentally different in the setting of HIV infection, protease inhibitors may increase the concentrations of coadministered calcium-channel blockers. Furthermore, certain protease inhibitors (atazanavir, lopinavir/ritonavir, saquinavir) may prolong the PR interval, necessitating caution with coadministration of calcium-channel blockers and β-blockers.

Pericardial Disease

Before the availability of combination ARV therapy, pericardial disease, including symptomatic pericarditis and cardiac tamponade (Chapter 68), was an important cardiovascular issue in PLWH, especially those with advanced immunodeficiency. The prevalence of pericardial effusion among PLWH in this era was approximately 20%. Presently, asymptomatic pericardial effusion is uncommon in studies using echocardiography, although the prevalence may be higher by MRI.

The causes of acute pericarditis in HIV-infected patients who are not severely immunocompromised are similar to the general population, with approximately 80% considered idiopathic (presumed to be mostly of viral etiology). In settings with reduced access to ARV therapy and in patients with advanced HIV disease, infectious causes (primarily mycobacterial) and AIDS-related malignancy predominate. Evaluation and management of pericardial disease is as per the general population.

Pulmonary Arterial Hypertension

The prevalence of pulmonary arterial hypertension in PLWH is approximately 10-fold higher than that of idiopathic pulmonary arterial hypertension in the general population (Chapter 75). The prognosis of the HIV-associated condition in the setting of effective ART appears to be similar to that of the general population.

The pathogenesis of HIV-associated pulmonary arterial hypertension is poorly understood. Investigators have not found evidence of direct viral invasion of endothelial cells. Direct adverse effects of the HIV-1 viral proteins *nef*, *vpr*, and *tat* on the pulmonary vasculature and indirect effects of HIV through generation of proinflammatory cytokines may play important roles. Other cofactors such as injection drug use and coinfection with HCV or HBV may contribute.

Clinicians should consider pulmonary arterial hypertension in the differential diagnosis of dyspnea on exertion in the HIV-infected patient. Secondary causes of pulmonary arterial hypertension in this population include chronic venous thromboembolic disease, obstructive sleep apnea, and portopulmonary hypertension due to chronic viral hepatitis or other etiologies.

As with many comorbidities, the unique aspects of management of pulmonary arterial hypertension in PLWH relate to potential drug-drug interactions. Sildenafil, tadalafil, and bosentan should not be coadministered with protease inhibitors or cobicistat.

Cardiac Conduction Abnormalities

Although PLWH may be at higher risk for sudden death, the contribution, if any, of abnormal cardiac conduction is unclear. QTc prolongation may be more prevalent among PLWH, largely attributable to traditional risk factors, including concurrent use of methadone and other medications. Ritonavir-boosted saquinavir prolongs the QTc interval in healthy volunteers, but this is not a class effect of protease inhibitors. Interactions between medications known to prolong the QTc interval and protease inhibitors or cobicistat could theoretically predispose to torsades de pointes. Furthermore, psychotropic medications, some of which prolong QTc, are commonly used in HIV-infected patients because of a high prevalence of psychiatric comorbidity.

Valvular Disease

There are no HIV-specific concerns related to valvular heart disease. In particular, the incidence of infective endocarditis in people who inject drugs does not differ by HIV serostatus. Mortality rates, however, are higher among HIV-infected patients with bacterial endocarditis and advanced immunosuppression. Clinical management does not differ by HIV serostatus, and HIV infection is not a contraindication for valve replacement surgery that is otherwise indicated.

● ENDOCRINE MANIFESTATIONS OF HIV
Adrenal Function

Primary adrenal insufficiency (Chapter 214) was a common complication of AIDS before the availability of effective ART. CMV adrenalitis was the most common identifiable cause at autopsy, although other opportunistic infections and malignancies capable of infiltrating the adrenal glands, or in some cases the hypothalamus or pituitary, were also described, including mycobacteria (*Mycobacterium tuberculosis*, *M. avium* complex), fungi (*Cryptococcus*, *Histoplasma*), KS, and lymphoma. Iatrogenic adrenal insufficiency can also be caused by medications used in advanced HIV disease. For example, itraconazole and ketoconazole impair adrenal steroid production; megestrol acetate, used as an appetite stimulant in wasting, can suppress the hypothalamic-pituitary-adrenal axis; and rifampin can increase the catabolism of cortisol.

Drug-drug interactions between exogenously administered corticosteroids and ARV drugs are now the primary causes of cortisol-related problems in PLWH. Protease inhibitors and the pharmacokinetic-boosting drug cobicistat inhibit the metabolism of commonly used corticosteroids, including fluticasone, budesonide, and triamcinolone, which can lead to systemic exposure to corticosteroids that are administered topically or by injection into joint spaces, for example. Concurrent use of protease inhibitors also increases conversion of prednisone to prednisolone. These interactions can cause transient symptoms of corticosteroid excess followed by symptoms of adrenal insufficiency due to inhibition of endogenous cortisol production. Based on a drug interaction study in healthy volunteers, beclomethasone is the inhaled corticosteroid of choice for patients taking protease inhibitors and, by extension, cobicistat.

Thyroid Disorders

Clinically apparent thyroid gland dysfunction does not appear to be more prevalent in PLWH, although subclinical dysfunction may be more common, especially in advanced HIV disease. The latter includes euthyroid sick syndrome, subclinical hypothyroidism, and isolated low T4 levels. In advanced HIV disease, various pathogens and malignancies may infiltrate the thyroid gland, including *Pneumocystis jiroveci*, tuberculosis, *Cryptococcus*, *Coccidioides*, KS, and lymphoma.

Graves disease (Chapter 213) may occur in the setting of initiation of ART as a manifestation of IRIS. Unlike most infectious manifestations, which occur within the initial months, Graves disease may develop up to 3 years after initiation of ART.

Altered Fat Distribution

Shortly after the availability of protease inhibitors, clinicians began reporting cases of altered fat distribution associated with dyslipidemia and insulin resistance, commonly termed *HIV-associated lipodystrophy syndrome*. While initial reports included cases that had both subcutaneous lipoatrophy and abdominal fat accumulation (sometimes termed *lipohypertrophy* or *visceral adiposity*) with or without dorsocervical fat pad enlargement, subsequent studies have clarified that some HIV-infected patients have lipoatrophy, some have fat accumulation, and some have a combination of both.

Lipoatrophy tends to be diffuse but is most visible in the face, limbs, and buttocks. It is generally attributed to mitochondrial toxicity from exposure to thymidine analogue NRTIs (stavudine or zidovudine). Although these drugs were thought to specifically inhibit the reverse transcriptase enzyme of HIV, they were later found to have the off-target effect of inhibiting host mitochondrial DNA polymerase. Some HIV-infected patients previously treated with thymidine analogues have residual lipoatrophy. Incident cases are thought to be uncommon with contemporary ARV drug regimens, although efavirenz has been associated with loss of limb fat in some studies.

Patients with facial lipoatrophy may have low self-esteem and reduced adherence to ART, and they may feel that their HIV serostatus is readily apparent to others. There is no specific pharmacologic treatment for lipoatrophy, although the rare patient who is still taking stavudine and zidovudine should switch to an alternative drug. Investigators have demonstrated modest gains in limb fat in randomized comparisons of switches from stavudine or zidovudine to other NRTIs, such as abacavir or tenofovir disoproxil fumarate, which have less inhibitory effects on mitochondrial DNA polymerase in vitro. Two temporary injectable facial fillers are approved by the FDA—poly-L-lactic acid and calcium hydroxylapatite. Trained clinicians inject these substances into the deep dermis at regular intervals to induce collagen growth.

PLWH may have abnormal fat accumulation, typically visceral abdominal fat but sometimes dorsocervical fat pad enlargement, fat accumulation in the trunk and upper chest wall, and breast enlargement. The prevalence of abnormal fat accumulation varies greatly among studies, and one large epidemiologic study found that men and women with HIV infection did not have greater amounts of visceral fat compared with uninfected controls. The same study also did not find a reciprocal relationship between quantities of subcutaneous and visceral fat, suggesting that the causes of lipoatrophy and fat accumulation differ. Other studies have demonstrated increases in visceral fat with initiation of ART regardless of the type of regimen.

The pathogenesis of fat accumulation is unknown. No specific ARV class or drug is clearly associated with fat accumulation, and switching from various types of regimens, such as protease inhibitor–based to alternative regimens, has not been efficacious, suggesting that the process may be indirectly related to control of HIV infection rather than specific drugs.

On physical examination, increased visceral abdominal fat may be difficult to distinguish from generalized obesity, although disproportionate gain of fat in the visceral compartment may result in a firmer abdomen with relatively less "pinchable" subcutaneous fat. Measuring serial waist and hip circumferences, along with weight and body mass index, may be useful to monitor changes in body composition in patients who complain of altered appearance. Clinicians should also monitor fasting glucose, lipid panels, and liver enzymes in patients with fat accumulation because metabolic derangements, including dyslipidemia, prediabetes/diabetes, and nonalcoholic fatty liver disease (NAFLD), are common.

Management options for fat accumulation are limited.[20] Clinicians should counsel patients on diet and exercise in an analogous fashion to how they advise obese patients without HIV infection. Liposuction of dorsocervical fat pads can be efficacious, although fat may reaccumulate. The visceral nature of the fat accumulation precludes abdominal liposuction. Some women may benefit from reduction mammoplasty if breast enlargement causes symptoms such as low back pain.

Tesamorelin is a growth hormone–releasing hormone analogue that is approved by the FDA for treatment of HIV-associated abdominal fat accumulation. Tesamorelin stimulates the pituitary to release growth hormone, which increases circulating insulin-like growth factor-I (IGF-I) levels, resulting in increased lipolysis. In randomized, placebo-controlled trials, daily subcutaneous injection of tesamorelin reduced abdominal fat by approximately 15% over 26 weeks, although fat reaccumulated rapidly after cessation.[A2] Lipid profiles tend to improve, and liver fat is reduced on tesamorelin. There are no long-term safety data on this drug. Elevations of IGF-I are associated with increased malignancy risk in epidemiologic studies, which may be of concern in HIV-infected patients who are already at higher risk for certain cancers. Because the overall risk-to-benefit ratio of tesamorelin is uncertain, clinicians should not continue it if there is no objective reduction in waist circumference after 6 months. Some advocate monitoring IGF-I levels every 6 months and stopping tesamorelin if the levels exceed the upper limit of normal for age. Although tesamorelin has only minor adverse effects on glucose homeostasis, clinicians should monitor glycosylated hemoglobin levels at baseline and every 3 to 4 months.

Diabetes Mellitus

The incidence of diabetes mellitus may be higher in PLWH, although epidemiologic data are conflicting. Both traditional and HIV-specific factors may contribute to risk. Increasing age, higher body mass index, male sex, nonwhite race, HCV coinfection, and opioid use are associated with incident diabetes in the HIV population. Older studies implicated both early NRTIs, such as stavudine and zidovudine, and first-generation protease inhibitors, such as indinavir, in the development of insulin resistance and diabetes.

Limited data suggest that HIV itself may directly cause insulin resistance and diabetes, possibly through the effects of HIV proteins such as *vpr* on glucocorticoid sensitivity. More compelling data support an indirect role of the virus through generation of pro-inflammatory cytokines that may directly affect insulin signaling. Indinavir directly inhibits the GLUT-4 glucose transporter, and a single dose of the drug can induce demonstrable reductions in insulin sensitivity in healthy volunteers. Protease inhibitors that are in common use now do not appear to induce insulin resistance. Older NRTIs, such as stavudine, likely induced insulin resistance through mitochondrial toxicity, which is not a significant concern with drugs in this class that are in current use. Subcutaneous lipoatrophy induced by older NRTIs, specifically those in the thymidine analogue category (stavudine, zidovudine), may cause insulin resistance by virtue of an inability of this fat depot to store triglycerides, leading to ectopic fat deposition in the liver and skeletal muscle. Increased visceral adiposity (lipohypertrophy) in some PLWH may also contribute to insulin resistance and diabetes risk. The more common concomitant use of certain diabetogenic medications in HIV-infected patients is an additional contributor to the incidence of diabetes. Before effective ART, patients with wasting frequently took megestrol acetate as an appetite stimulant; the glucocorticoid effects of this drug can precipitate diabetes. In the same era, intravenous pentamidine for *Pneumocystis* pneumonia sometimes caused β-cell injury and ultimately diabetes. Presently, certain statins and atypical antipsychotic drugs are more common culprits.

Treatment guidelines recommend screening HIV-infected patients for diabetes annually using fasting glucose or glycosylated hemoglobin levels. An important caveat to both screening for and monitoring of diabetes in HIV infection is a concern that glycosylated hemoglobin may underestimate ambient glycemia in this population. Several studies have identified use of NRTIs (specifically abacavir), higher red cell mean corpuscular volume, and lower CD4 cell counts as factors associated with greater discordance between glycosylated hemoglobin levels and glucose values. Some experts advocate measuring fasting glucose and possibly performing oral glucose tolerance tests instead of measuring glycosylated hemoglobin to screen for diabetes in this population.

The management of diabetes (Chapter 216) does not differ in PLWH, with a few exceptions. Metformin is typically the first-line drug for treating both diabetes and prediabetes, if indicated. Dolutegravir, an integrase strand transfer inhibitor, increases exposure to metformin, necessitating dose reduction of the latter drug. Similarly, exposure to the dipeptidyl peptidase-4 inhibitor saxagliptin is increased when this drug is used concurrently with protease inhibitors or the pharmacokinetic enhancer cobicistat.

Vitamin D Deficiency

Data are conflicting as to whether vitamin D deficiency is more common in HIV-infected patients relative to the general population. Nonetheless, vitamin D insufficiency or deficiency are common in HIV infection. In addition to traditional risk factors, immune activation and inflammation may play a role. Efavirenz, an NNRTI, can reduce circulating levels of the active form of vitamin D by inducing cytochrome P-450 enzymes that increase the catabolism of vitamin D to an inactive form. Protease inhibitors may inhibit the conversion of vitamin D to active metabolites. There are insufficient data to recommend universal screening or supplementation of vitamin D in HIV-infected patients. Clinicians should check 25-hydroxyvitamin D levels in patients with low bone mineral density or history of fracture.

Bone Disorders

HIV infection is associated with greater risk for low bone mineral density and fragility fracture. One meta-analysis demonstrated a three-fold higher prevalence of osteoporosis among HIV-infected individuals compared with uninfected controls, with higher rates among those on ARV drugs and specifically protease inhibitors. Initiation of ART results in an average lost bone mineral density of 2 to 6%, akin to that seen in women going through menopause. HIV-specific risk factors for decreased bone mineral density in some studies include low nadir CD4 cell count, HIV viremia, and use of protease inhibitors and tenofovir disoproxil fumarate. A newer pro-drug of tenofovir, tenofovir alafenamide, has less adverse effects on bone mineral density. Inflammation and immune activation in untreated and treated HIV infection may also contribute to osteopenia and osteoporosis.

U.S. guidelines recommend screening for osteoporosis by dual X-ray absorptiometry (DXA) scanning in men 50 years and older and postmenopausal women living with HIV. Some experts additionally advocate calculating 10-year fracture risk using the Fracture Risk Assessment Tool (FRAX) in men 40 to 49 years old and women older than 40 years, followed by DXA scanning if the risk for major osteoporotic fracture exceeds 10%.[21] Data support counting HIV as a secondary cause of osteoporosis when using this risk calculator. Patients who have had fragility fractures, are at high risk for falls, or have used glucocorticoids chronically (the equivalent of 5 mg or more per day of prednisone for more than 3 months) should also be screened by DXA. Clinicians should evaluate patients with osteoporosis for secondary causes as in the general population. As part of routine care, patients 50 years and older should have heights measured every 1 to 2 years to screen for height loss from vertebral fractures.

Criteria for initiating osteoporosis therapy (Chapter 230) in HIV-infected patients do not differ from the general population. Investigators have demonstrated the expected increases in bone mineral density with alendronate and zolendronic acid. Patients taking tenofovir disoproxil fumarate should be switched to tenofovir alafenamide or an alternative drug based on treatment history. Protease inhibitors should also be switched to alternative drugs when possible.

In one randomized, placebo-controlled trial, calcium and vitamin D supplementation abrogated loss of bone mineral density associated with initiation of ART with the combination of tenofovir disoproxil fumarate, emtricitabine, and efavirenz in treatment-naïve patients.[A3] This strategy has not been studied with other ARV drug regimens but may be considered for patients with known baseline abnormal bone mineral density or multiple risk factors for osteoporosis who are initiating HIV therapy.

Tenofovir disoproxil fumarate uncommonly causes Fanconi syndrome, and the associated urinary phosphate wasting and hypophosphatemia can lead to defective bone mineralization (osteomalacia) (Chapter 231), manifesting as bone pain, weakness, myopathy, low bone mineral density, and fragility fracture. Osteomalacia is also caused by severe vitamin D deficiency and has been reported rarely in HIV-infected patients taking inducers of cytochrome P-450 that reduce levels of active vitamin D, such as efavirenz and rifabutin.

Male Hypogonadism

Hypogonadism is less prevalent in the era of cART, although some estimate that 15 to 20% of HIV-infected men are hypogonadal in the current era. Risk factors include low CD4 cell count and use of certain medications such as megestrol acetate, glucocorticoids, and ketoconazole. Patients may present with classic symptoms and signs, including fatigue, low energy, depressed mood, decreased libido, erectile dysfunction, weight loss, testicular atrophy, and gynecomastia. Bone mineral density may also be reduced.

Although most cases of hypogonadism in HIV-infected men are secondary to pituitary or hypothalamic dysfunction (Chapter 211), primary hypogonadism may also be seen. In patients with CD4 cell counts less than 100 cells/µL, various opportunistic pathogens and malignancies can infiltrate the pituitary, hypothalamus, or testes. These include *M. avium* complex, *Toxoplasma*, CMV, KS, and lymphoma. Elevations in pro-inflammatory cytokines such as tumor necrosis factor-α (TNF-α) may also contribute to hypogonadism at all stages of HIV disease.

Sex hormone–binding globulin levels are often elevated in HIV infection, which may result in normal total testosterone levels when free testosterone levels are actually below normal (Chapter 221). Consequently, clinicians should screen symptomatic men with morning free testosterone levels. Repletion of testosterone by intramuscular injections or topical preparations may result in symptomatic improvement and improved quality of life. It is important to exclude occult prostate cancer with a digital rectal examination and screening prostate-specific antigen test before starting therapy with testosterone.

Ovarian Function

Some studies have noted an earlier onset of menopause in HIV-infected women relative to controls, although whether ovarian failure per se is associated with HIV infection is controversial. Menstrual irregularities are common in HIV-infected women, which may complicate the diagnosis of menopause based on history. Low CD4 cell count has been associated with early menopause in some studies. Women living with HIV also appear to report a greater number of menopausal symptoms.

The prevalence of infertility is increased in HIV-infected women, and response rates to in vitro fertilization are also reduced. Investigators have reported reduced ovarian reserve in women with HIV infection as assessed by antimüllerian hormone levels. This state has been associated with increased monocyte activation and subclinical atherosclerosis.

● PULMONARY MANIFESTATIONS OF HIV

The epidemiology of HIV-associated pulmonary manifestations has shifted from predominantly infectious to noninfectious complications with the advent of potent ART. The incidence of bacterial pneumonia, most commonly caused by *S. pneumoniae*, and pneumonia caused by the fungus *P. jiroveci* have declined dramatically, although the latter remains a concern in those with low CD4 cell counts. Pulmonary tuberculosis remains prevalent in many resource-limited settings, although its incidence, too, is reduced with effective ART and the use of isoniazid preventive therapy. Chronic obstructive pulmonary disease (COPD), pulmonary arterial hypertension, and lung cancer (discussed earlier under Non-AIDS-Defining Cancers) have emerged as key noninfectious complications.

Chronic Obstructive Pulmonary Disease

Multiple epidemiologic studies have shown dramatically higher prevalence rates of smoking in HIV-infected populations compared with the general population. Even after adjustment for cigarette exposure, several studies have demonstrated higher rates of COPD (Chapter 82) in PLWH relative to uninfected controls. HIV is a risk factor for emphysema, with data supporting onset at an earlier age and lower smoking threshold in pack-years. HIV infection is associated with greater severity and diffuseness of emphysema, a higher rate of ongoing lung destruction, and accelerated decline in pulmonary function.

The pathogenesis of COPD in PLWH is multifactorial. Aside from cigarette-induced lung injury, HIV viremia, low nadir CD4 cell count, and colonization with *P. jiroveci* may play roles. Monocyte activation, increased expression of matrix metalloproteinase enzymes involved in lung tissue destruction, alterations in the microbiome, and oxidant-antioxidant imbalance likely contribute. Prior lung injury from inhaled or injected illicit drugs may also predispose some patients to COPD. The role of coinfections that may induce immune activation, such as CMV, is uncertain.

In a substudy of the START trial, rates of decline in pulmonary function over a median of 2 years of follow-up did not differ in patients with CD4 cell counts higher than 500 cells/μL randomized to immediate initiation of ART versus deferred initiation until the CD4 count fell to below 350 cells/μL.[A4] These data suggest that ART itself does not cause a decline in pulmonary function.

The management of COPD in PLWH does not differ fundamentally from the general population, with a few exceptions. Acute exacerbations of COPD may be more common even in the setting of well-controlled HIV infection. As noted earlier (see Endocrine Manifestations of HIV), certain inhaled corticosteroids interact with protease inhibitors and cobicistat; beclomethasone is the preferred agent to coadminister. Because of the potential increased risk for adverse cardiovascular events, salmeterol should not be coadministered with protease inhibitors and cobicistat.

Venous Thromboembolic Disease

The incidence of venous thromboembolism (Chapter 74) is higher in PLWH relative to the general population. Risk factors include low CD4 cell count, the presence of opportunistic infections, and the use of older protease inhibitors (indinavir, nelfinavir, ritonavir, or saquinavir). Furthermore, HIV infection predisposes to hypercoagulability that may in part be related to chronic inflammation.

The management of venous thromboembolic disease in HIV infection is complicated by drug-drug interactions. Warfarin exposure may increase with coadministration of protease inhibitors or cobicistat, necessitating careful monitoring of the international normalized ratio. Among the novel anticoagulant drugs, edoxaban and rivaroxaban should not be coadministered with protease inhibitors or cobicistat, whereas dabigatran is likely safe if the creatinine clearance rate is at least 50 mL/minute. Some clinicians avoid apixaban with protease inhibitors or cobicistat, although others use it at 50% reduced dose.

Obstructive Sleep Apnea

Data on obstructive sleep apnea in PLWH are limited, with some data in men suggesting a similar prevalence relative to uninfected controls, although body mass indices tended to be lower in the HIV-infected group. Sleep apnea is likely underdiagnosed in PLWH, and clinicians should consider this in the differential diagnosis of fatigue and daytime somnolence. Some patients with abnormal fat deposition in the neck and abdomen may be predisposed to sleep apnea for anatomic reasons.

Pneumonitis

Several forms of noninfectious interstitial lung disease, both symptomatic and asymptomatic, were prevalent before the availability of effective ART; these are largely of historical interest in the current treatment era.

Lymphocytic interstitial pneumonitis classically affects HIV-infected infants, although it may also affect adults, even at CD4 cell counts greater than 350 cells/μL. While usually asymptomatic, patients may present with cough, dyspnea, and constitutional symptoms such as fever and weight loss. The radiographic appearance includes reticulonodular infiltrates, alveolar infiltrates, or a miliary pattern. The pathogenesis is unknown, and diagnosis depends on lung biopsy. Initiation of ART in an untreated patient may lead to resolution. Otherwise, corticosteroid treatment with concurrent *Pneumocystis* prophylaxis may be indicated.

Nonspecific interstitial pneumonitis (Chapter 86) is commonly an asymptomatic finding but may present with fever, dyspnea, and cough typically in people with CD4 cell counts less than 200 cells/μL, thus mimicking *Pneumocystis* pneumonia. Although approximately half of patients will have normal chest radiographs, the spectrum of abnormalities on chest x-ray includes interstitial or alveolar infiltrates, ground-glass opacities, and consolidation. An interstitial infiltration of mononuclear cells is seen on pathology, although it is typically less dense than that seen with lymphocytic interstitial pneumonitis. The differential diagnosis includes community-acquired bacterial pneumonia, *Pneumocystis* pneumonia, tuberculosis, mycobacteria other than tuberculosis, toxoplasmosis, fungal pneumonia, KS, and lymphoma. Nonspecific interstitial pneumonitis is typically self-limited and responds to ART.

Diffuse infiltrative (CD8) lymphocytosis syndrome is a chronic systemic disorder with pulmonary involvement in half of patients. It shares clinical features with lymphocytic interstitial pneumonitis with the addition of Sjögren-like features, including sicca, lymphadenopathy, parotid gland enlargement (sometimes dramatic), and hepatosplenomegaly. There may be associated neurologic manifestations, including facial nerve palsy, aseptic meningitis, and polyneuropathy. The pathologic appearance is characterized by CD8 cell infiltration. ART, sometimes with adjunctive corticosteroids, often leads to improvement or resolution of symptoms.

Other Pulmonary Conditions

PLWH are not at higher risk for asthma, although the issue of drug-drug interactions between protease inhibitors or cobicistat and both salmeterol and many inhaled corticosteroids applies to this group of patients. Bronchiectasis may complicate recurrent pneumonia in PLWH and is typically diagnosed by high-resolution CT. Sarcoidosis may manifest as an immune reconstitution inflammatory syndrome in the setting of recently initiated ART.

● GASTROINTESTINAL MANIFESTATIONS OF HIV

Wasting was so prevalent in Africa in the early 1980s at the dawn of what was to be the HIV pandemic that this new and mysterious illness with no known cause was called "slim disease." The incidence and type of GI manifestations associated with HIV infection have traced the arc of treatment advances, shifting from the opportunistic infections of the early epidemic, to the sometimes profound drug toxicities of early cART in the late 1990s, to the present where, in patients on suppressive therapy, coinfections such as HBV and HCV, and metabolic complications such as NAFLD and NASH are the predominant GI-related complications. Gastrointestinal symptoms and illnesses remain important contributors to morbidity in PLWH, particularly in patients who are unable to maintain viral suppression through nonadherence or lack of access to ART, or who present with advanced disease at initial diagnosis.

Although newer first-line ARV medications have very minimal GI side effects, some patients may remain on older therapies or be on second- or third-line drugs because of acquired treatment resistance. Older ARV drugs are also still commonly used in resource-constrained settings.

The GI tract itself is now an active area of research because of the role it may play in the chronic inflammatory state that seems to contribute to many of the non-AIDS-related complications of HIV such as cardiovascular disease, malignancies, and metabolic disorders. With its abundant gut-associated lymphoid tissue, one of the largest reservoirs of T lymphocytes in the body, it is an important target for HIV, particularly in acute infection. At the time of infection, there is a rapid and massive CD4 cell depletion in the gut due to both direct and indirect viral cytopathicity, in contrast to the slower depletion of circulating CD4 lymphocytes. Although the chronically immune-activated state and resultant altered T-cell homeostasis found in HIV-infected patients are clearly multifactorial, it is now felt that microbial translocation due to the damaged host intestinal epithelial barrier may be a central contributor. Translocation occurs when luminal bacteria or other microbes traverse the epithelial barrier and lamina propria and are unable to be contained in the mesenteric lymph nodes, thus disseminating to a variety of extranodal sites. This activity is most pronounced in acute infection and may be the cause of gastrointestinal symptoms during acute and early infection. Early treatment may diminish but not interrupt this pathogenic process; it will continue, albeit at a slower rate during chronic infection, even in those on effective therapy.[22,23]

Although patients with well-controlled HIV are at risk for all the usual diseases that can happen to immune-competent individuals, they continue to have complications specifically related to their HIV infection. Most of the infectious complications are seen with increasing incidence as immune suppression progresses, particularly at CD4 counts below 100 cells/µL, whereas the noninfectious complications can occur at any CD4 cell count.

This section addresses both noninfectious and infectious causes of gastrointestinal disease, although infectious causes are discussed in more detail elsewhere.

Gastrointestinal Side Effects of Antiretroviral Drugs
NUCLEOSIDE AND NUCLEOTIDE REVERSE TRANSCRIPTASE INHIBITORS
All of the medications used to treat HIV can cause nausea or mild GI distress, although earlier drugs such as the NRTIs zidovudine (AZT), stavudine (d4T), and didanosine (ddI) were more difficult to tolerate than the newer and more commonly used NRTIs such as tenofovir disoproxil fumarate (TDF), tenofovir alafenamide (TAF), and abacavir. Lamivudine (3TC) and emtricitabine (FTC) are well-tolerated and remain mainstays of combination therapies, particularly in fixed-dose combination regimens. Pancreatitis, sometimes fatal, can occur with the ARV drugs d4T and ddI. Because of this and other side effects such as neuropathy and catastrophic lactic acidosis with organ failure, these so-called d-drugs are no longer used in resource-rich settings. Lactic acidosis (Chapter 110) often presents initially with vague symptoms such as fatigue, myalgias, and few signs on routine blood tests but can present with dramatic tachypnea and markedly elevated serum lactate levels. Although uncommonly seen now given the shift away from older drugs such as d4T and ddI, diagnosis requires a very high index of suspicion because of the high morbidity and mortality associated with late diagnosis. The etiology is attributed to mitochondrial toxicity due to cross-inhibition of mitochondrial DNA polymerase. While all nucleoside or nucleotide analogues can cause mitochondrial toxicity, lactic acidosis is rarely seen with drugs other than d4T and ddI. Abacavir can cause a subtle hypersensitivity syndrome with low-grade fever, abdominal discomfort, nausea and vomiting, and sometimes mild rash, early after initiation of therapy; interruption with subsequent rechallenge in patients who have manifested signs and symptoms of hypersensitivity can lead to rapid, severe non-IgE-mediated anaphylactoid reactions and death. Testing for HLA-B-5701 allele positivity before initiation of therapy has largely eliminated this risk. Patients previously labeled with abacavir hypersensitivity based on non-specific symptoms can be safely rechallenged with abacavir if they are HLA-B-5701 negative.

NON-NUCLEOSIDE REVERSE TRANSCRIPTASE INHIBITORS
Most NNRTIs are well tolerated from a GI standpoint, but nevirapine, still in use in resource-poor settings, in addition to having a higher rate of severe systemic reactions such as Stevens-Johnson syndrome, has been reported to cause transaminitis and rarely hepatic failure, particularly in men with a CD4 count higher than 400 cells/µL and women with a CD4 count higher than 250 cells/µL at the time of initiation of ART.

PROTEASE INHIBITORS
The first-generation protease inhibitors saquinavir (SQV), indinavir (IDV), nelfinavir (NFV), and ritonavir (RTV) often cause significant GI problems, including nausea, vomiting, and, particularly in the case, of RTV and NFV, diarrhea. RTV was so poorly tolerated at treatment doses that it was fairly quickly relegated to low-dose therapy in combination with other protease inhibitors as a pharmacokinetic booster given its strong inhibition of the cytochrome P-450 pathways. Atazanavir (ATV) has been associated with cholelithiasis and almost always causes a benign mild indirect hyperbilirubinemia, similar to Gilbert disease, owing to inhibition of UDP-glucuronyltransferase. Because it can occasionally rise to levels resulting in scleral icterus, it is important to warn patients in advance of this potential phenomenon, which is reversible on cessation of the drug. Protease inhibitors, particularly RTV and RTV-lopinavir, are more likely to cause hypertriglyceridemia, which may be quite significant and possibly contribute to the risk for pancreatitis and fatty liver disease.

INTEGRASE STRAND TRANSFER INHIBITORS
Drugs in this class are generally well tolerated, but there are reports of dermatologic reaction with eosinophilia and systemic symptoms (DRESS) with concomitant transaminitis and liver failure in patients taking raltegravir.

OTHER
The entry inhibitor maraviroc and the fusion inhibitor enfuvirtide have few GI side effects but are often used in treatment-experienced patients with advanced HIV and multiclass ARV resistance when patients may either have, or develop, other GI manifestations common to patients with profound immunosuppression. Pentamidine, even in the aerosol form used to prevent *Pneumocystis* pneumonia, can also cause pancreatitis but has not been associated with lactic acidosis. High-dose TMP-SMX used in the treatment of *Pneumocystis* pneumonia or for the treatment of methicillin-resistant staphylococcal infections can cause a significant hepatitis.

Oral
Patients with HIV can have a variety of noninfectious complications in the oral cavity and salivary glands; this easily examined area can often serve as an early indication of undiagnosed HIV infection or progression of existing disease. The prevalence of oral complications related to immune suppression such as candidiasis, oral hairy leukoplakia (associated with Epstein-Barr virus as an etiologic agent), necrotizing ulcerative gingivitis or periodontitis, and malignancies such as KS has decreased with more widespread ART, but other conditions related to dry mouth (xerostomia), smoking, and poor access to dental care have increased. The prevalence of HPV-related and ulcerative disease such as herpes simplex virus (HSV) or idiopathic aphthous ulcers has remained stable relative to the early years of the epidemic.

The lesions of oral hairy leukoplakia (Fig. 366-2) cannot be scraped off, in contrast to the whitish coating seen with oral candidiasis, or thrush (Fig. 366-3). The latter can be treated with oral nystatin suspension or clotrimazole troches in the absence of concomitant esophageal symptoms (see later); oral azoles are rarely required and should be discontinued after thrush has resolved to avoid development of azole resistance. Oral hairy leukoplakia is limited to the lateral tongue and does not appear on the oral mucosal surfaces; it requires no specific treatment other than effective ART, and it is rarely necessary to perform a biopsy for diagnosis. Linear gingival erythema can present as a brightly inflamed, well-demarcated line of gingiva. Gram-negative and enteric organisms, as well as candida, can be involved. The treatment is débridement and antibiotics such as penicillin or metronidazole. Necrotizing ulcerative gingivitis or periodontitis can present as a rapid, painful destruction of bone and soft tissue with the same microbiologic flora that is present in linear gingival erythema. Urgent débridement, pain control, and antibiotics, as in linear gingival erythema, are required to preserve alveolar bone. Oral antifungal agents may also be added. KS typically involves the hard palate or gingiva (Fig. 366-4) and may cause ulcerative disease. Biopsy may be required if the diagnosis has not yet been made based on biopsy of cutaneous or other visceral lesions.

Idiopathic oral aphthous ulceration (Fig. 366-5) can be a severe and refractory problem in advanced HIV, placing patients at nutritional risk and sometimes requiring topical steroids or, in more extensive disease, systemic corticosteroids or thalidomide for treatment. Appearing as deep, well-circumscribed ulcerations, often solitary as opposed to the multiple ulcerations more characteristic of herpes simplex, they happen with the same frequency as seen

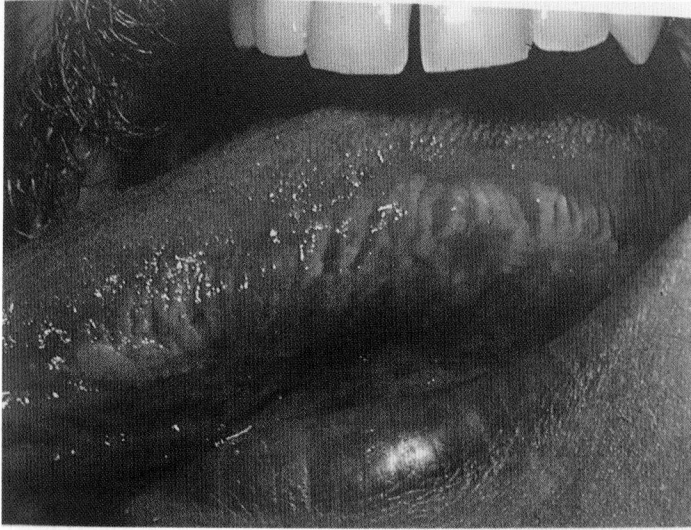

FIGURE 366-2. Lesions of oral hairy leukoplakia.

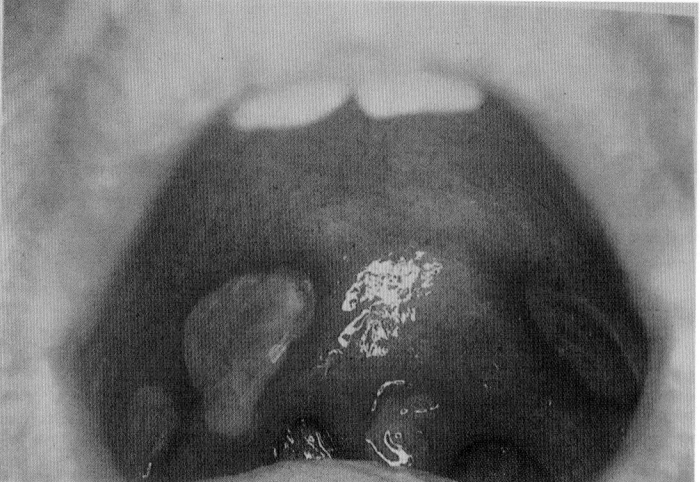

FIGURE 366-5. Oral aphthous ulcer.

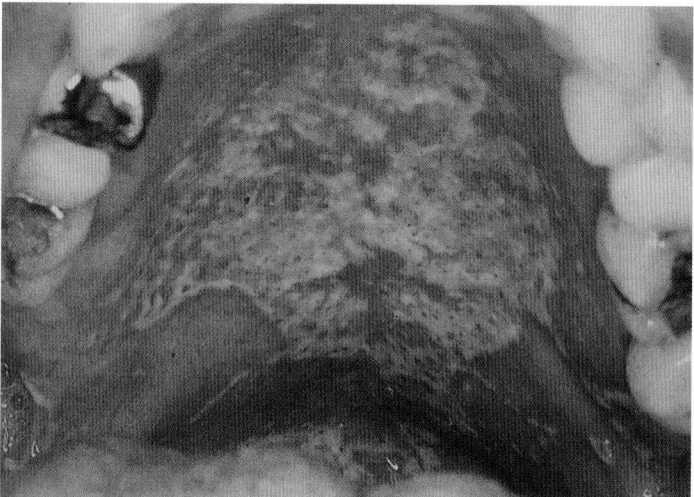

FIGURE 366-3. Oral candidiasis or thrush.

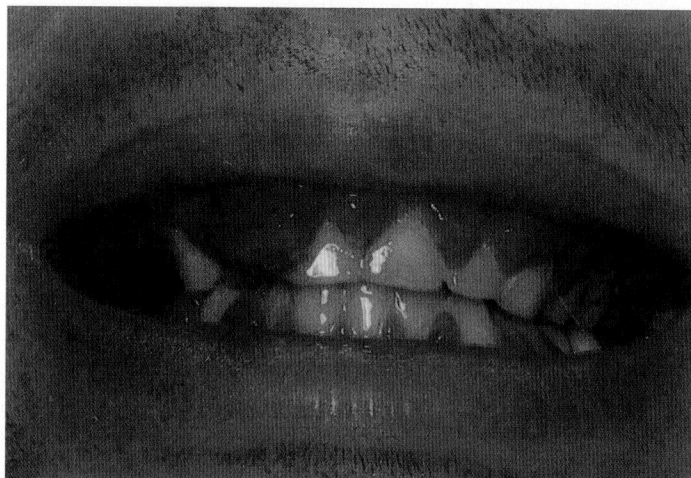

FIGURE 366-4. Gingival Kaposi sarcoma.

in immune-competent patients but can be more severe and take longer to resolve. They should be differentiated from HSV-related, premalignant, or malignant lesions using culture or biopsy as indicated. Aphthous ulcerations may also be seen as part of acute HIV infection. Premalignant or malignant ulcers are often painless in contrast to other ulcerative lesions. Xerostomia can

be the result of drug side effects or lymphocytic infiltration of the salivary glands manifested by painless parotid enlargement and subsequent salivary hypofunction, sometimes as part of diffuse infiltrative lymphocytosis syndrome (DILS). DILS is more commonly seen in the pediatric population or in advanced disease, but it can occur at any stage in the course of HIV infection. Bilateral parotid enlargement due to lymphocytic or fatty infiltration has a characteristic radiologic appearance, and biopsies are rarely necessary to establish the diagnosis. Xerostomia has a large impact on quality of life as well as tooth and gum health and can be quite difficult to treat. Typically, over-the-counter lubricating agents in the form of gels, lozenges or mouthwash can provide some relief. Artificial salivary fluid by prescription can also be tried.

Esophageal

Dysphagia and odynophagia can be common complaints in patients with HIV and are most typically related to either the common infectious complications of HIV in more advanced disease such as candidiasis and HSV (CD4 <200 cells/μL) or CMV (CD4 <50 cells/μL) and, rarely, histoplasmosis (typically CD4 <150 cells/μL with median CD4 <50 cells/μL). However, they can also be caused by idiopathic aphthous ulcerations such as those seen in the oral cavity, which may happen at any CD4 cell count but are more severe in advanced disease. Eosinophilic esophagitis is an increasingly recognized entity that can cause dysphagia and retrosternal discomfort on swallowing. Gastroesophageal reflux disease (GERD) is a common complaint in those with HIV and can complicate ART therapy because medications used to treat GERD (proton-pump inhibitors [PPIs] and histamine-2 receptor antagonists) are contraindicated or must be used with caution with commonly used ARV drugs such as atazanavir and rilpivirine. Concomitant use of calcium- or magnesium-containing acids can reduce the serum concentrations of the integrase inhibitors raltegravir, dolutegravir, and elvitegravir. They are contraindicated with raltegravir. Empirical therapy with fluconazole for typical symptoms of candidal esophagitis, which may present without oral thrush, or a trial of a PPI for GERD or symptoms consistent with eosinophilic esophagitis such as dysphagia may be indicated. Persistent symptoms referable to the esophagus will require motility studies and/or endoscopic evaluation with biopsies as appropriate and treatment directed at the underlying cause.

Gastric

Many of the more serious gastric complications of HIV are infectious and seen only in advanced disease with CD4 counts of less than 50 cells/μL: CMV gastritis, *M. avium* complex gastritis or enteritis, and gastric candidiasis. Gastritis and peptic ulcer disease can be seen with the same frequency and for the same reasons as in those without HIV infection. Similar considerations with regard to PPI and antacid use for GERD symptoms apply to the treatment of gastritis and ulcer disease, sometimes necessitating temporary or permanent ARV medication changes if the patient is taking atazanavir or rilpivirine. Gastroparesis is a late complication of diabetes, which is increasingly prevalent in the HIV-infected population. It can complicate effective ART because of nausea and vomiting. Radiologic imaging, video esophagrams, endoscopic evaluation, and transit studies may help elucidate the cause of gastric symptoms with treatment directed at the specific underlying cause.

Small Bowel

In areas of the world where ART is widely available and prescribed, some of the most devastating infectious diarrheal illnesses such as cryptosporidiosis, a lethal complication of advanced HIV, have diminished to the point that they are seen occasionally only as the typical self-limited traveler's diarrhea that cryptosporidium can still cause. Similarly, chronic refractory microsporidiosis was difficult to cure in the absence of immune reconstitution with ART. *Cyclospora* and *Cystoisospora belli* (formerly known as *Isospora belli*) can also cause prolonged diarrhea and weight loss in advanced HIV, making proper diagnosis paramount because they can be treated effectively with TMP-SMX. Most other infectious causes of diarrhea tend to be similar in their presentation and course to those seen in immune-competent patients, such as viral gastroenteritides, or *Giardia*, which has a higher incidence in MSM. HIV enteropathy is an entity that can cause the typical symptoms of small bowel disease such as bloating, gas, abdominal pain, and watery diarrhea but is established as a diagnosis of exclusion after more typical bacterial or parasitic causes have been ruled out. The conditions for HIV enteropathy may be established early in disease, with HIV disrupting the mucosa and ultimately causing villous atrophy and reducing the effective area of small bowel. Although this is more typical in patients with low CD4 cell counts, patients may experience symptoms due to HIV enteropathy at any CD4 cell count, particularly if symptoms developed before immune reconstitution, even if the patient is receiving ART and is fully suppressed. Medication toxicity can usually be ruled out by taking a careful history to establish the timing of onset, in which case switching therapy may lead to resolution of symptoms. Work-up of diarrheal illnesses should always include stool studies with appropriate stains, or, if available, multiplex polymerase chain reaction (PCR) assays, which have greater sensitivity particularly for protozoal causes of disease. Treatment should be directed at the underlying pathogen or, in the case of HIV enteropathy, treatment of the underlying HIV infection along with antimotility agents and nutritional support.

Large Bowel

There are no major noninfectious causes of large bowel pathology specific to HIV infection. Patients can have diverticulosis, inflammatory bowel diseases, chronic constipation (particularly if on methadone maintenance therapy or chronic opiates for pain control), and colon cancer or other malignancies such as lymphoma, although lymphoma is more commonly seen in the small bowel. More common infectious causes of HIV-related colitis such as CMV occur only at CD4 counts in the less than 50 cells/μL range and must be diagnosed by biopsy during direct examination of the colon. On histopathologic examination, infected cells are up to four-fold larger than normal cells and show thickened membranes with classic basophilic intracytoplasmic inclusion bodies. Similarly, with advanced disease, KS can involve any part of the gastrointestinal lumen from the oral cavity to large bowel. *Clostridium difficile* infection has been reported as the most commonly isolated bacterial infection in patients with HIV; however, this has also decreased with time as patients are being hospitalized less frequently and requiring less antimicrobial treatment.[24] It is also possible that impaired gut integrity and both humoral and cell-mediated immune response may play a role in the high incidence of *C. difficile* infection.

Other bacterial infections such as *Campylobacter*, *Salmonella*, and *Shigella* present with typical symptoms of frequent, small volume, bloody, or nonbloody stool. Resistance to *Campylobacter* species is variable. In patients with CD4 cell counts of more than 200 cells/μL with mild diarrhea, no treatment may be needed unless symptoms persist. More severe disease, or disease in patients with lower CD4 cell counts, should be treated with a macrolide such as azithromycin as empirical therapy, pending antibiotic susceptibilities. The risk for *Salmonella* bacteremia is higher in PLWH, so all patients should receive treatment with a fluoroquinolone; recurrence is common in patients with lower CD4 cell counts and may require suppressive antibiotic therapy. *Shigella* occurs with greater frequency and severity in HIV-infected MSM, and in addition to supportive care, antibiotics are indicated both to shorten duration of symptoms and potentially prevent spread to others. Multidrug antimicrobial resistance is a problem outside of the United States and is being seen with more frequency here as well. Treatment of *Shigella* should be based on antimicrobial sensitivity testing. When empirical therapy is warranted, a fluoroquinolone is appropriate in areas with low or no reports of resistance, or a third-generation cephalosporin is used if resistance is suspected. *Entamoeba dispar* and

Blastocystis hominis are generally nonpathogenic parasites and do not require treatment. Patients with asymptomatic *Entamoeba histolytica* found on stool microscopy or by PCR should receive a luminal agent such as paromomycin to clear the cysts. Patients with symptomatic disease should receive metronidazole followed by a luminal agent to prevent recurrence of infection. Diagnosis of infectious diarrhea other than CMV depends on stool studies (bacterial culture and stains for parasites, antigen tests, or if available, multiplex PCR including for viruses) and assays for *C. difficile* as per local laboratory protocol. If no etiology is found and symptoms persist, particularly if the CD4 count is less than 50 cells/μL, colonoscopy should be performed for direct visualization and biopsy of any lesions seen. CMV is typically treated with a 2- to 3-week induction course of ganciclovir followed by oral valganciclovir until immune reconstitution is achieved and therapy is no longer needed.

Hepatic

Liver disease remains a major cause of morbidity and mortality in patients with HIV in part due to the high prevalence of chronic HBV and HCV coinfection resulting from shared transmission routes. With the advent of well-tolerated and highly efficacious direct-acting ARV drugs for the treatment of HCV, it is hoped that widespread treatment will create the same "treatment as prevention" effect that is seen with fully suppressive HIV therapy, leading to lower rates of new HCV infections. Although many of the drugs used to treat HIV can have direct liver toxicity, especially in the setting of chronic hepatitis, it is unusual and avoidable with proper monitoring and prompt discontinuation of the offending agent. As mentioned earlier, nevirapine and, rarely, the integrase inhibitors, notably raltegravir, have been associated with fulminant hepatic failure, the latter as part of DRESS. There have been reports of noncirrhotic portal hypertension associated with ddI, another reason beyond risk for lactic acidosis, pancreatitis, and peripheral neuropathy to avoid its use. Acute fulminant liver failure has occurred in patients with chronic active HBV in the setting of IRIS, even while on ART that is also active against HBV. Close follow-up of liver enzymes is required during initiation of therapy in these patients. HIV-infected patients with HBV should have ARV medication regimens that include drugs active against HBV (i.e., TDF, TAF, 3TC, or FTC), and providers should be aware that if ART interruption is necessary, liver disease may flare. Autoimmune hepatitis is uncommon in HIV infection but has been reported.

NAFLD and NASH are important and growing causes of morbidity in patients with effectively treated HIV who now in most cases have normal life expectancies. The prevalence of NAFLD in the general population is now estimated to be as much as 25%, rising to 35% in those with HIV monoinfection (no coinfection with HCV). NAFLD is the accumulation of triglycerides in hepatocytes, similar to alcoholic steatosis, but with low or no alcohol consumption. Progression to NASH with frank inflammation and fibrosis or cirrhosis appears to occur at a higher rate than in the HIV-uninfected population. Traditional risk factors such as the metabolic syndrome (insulin resistance, central obesity, and dyslipidemia) and obesity are at play, but other unknown factors may increase the incidence and rate of progression in HIV, including disruption of the gut microbiome or drug toxicity, especially with NRTIs. Radiologic appearance can be pathognomonic, but assessment of fibrosis has traditionally relied on liver biopsy. Noninvasive markers are being explored for staging of disease. Treatment has relied on modification of risk factors, but studies are underway to identify drug candidates for more effective therapy, including in those with HIV. Over the next decade, cirrhosis from fatty liver disease may supplant HCV as the most common reason for liver transplantation.[25,26]

Pancreatic

As mentioned earlier, d4T and ddI were common causes of toxic pancreatitis and are no longer recommended for use in ARV medication regimens for this and other reasons. The decreased incidence of *Pneumocystis* pneumonia and the reduced need for prophylaxis have sharply curtailed the need for pentamidine, also a known cause of pancreatitis. Other opportunistic infections such as CMV have been felt to be possible causes of pancreatitis. Hypertriglyceridemia has a known association with pancreatitis and is more prevalent in the HIV-infected population, particularly in those taking early NRTIs such as AZT, d4T, and ddI as well as the first-generation protease inhibitors. Patients with hypertriglyceridemia should be treated in the same fashion as those without HIV, and ARV medication changes should be made as appropriate.

Presentation and treatment of pancreatitis are similar to the HIV-uninfected population and require withdrawal of the offending agent, treatment of the underlying infectious catalyst, or treatment of HIV itself after the patient has recovered from the acute illness.

Biliary

As mentioned previously, atazanavir has been associated with cholelithiasis and benign indirect bilirubinemia. In cases in which scleral icterus develops, patients may prefer to switch to a different therapy for cosmetic reasons. HIV cholangiopathy, a result of biliary strictures from opportunistic pathogens such as microsporidium or CMV, is rarely seen in the current era of effective ART. Endoscopic retrograde cholangiopancreatography can be used to investigate biliary disease.

Anorectal

Proctitis or proctocolitis as a result of the common sexually transmitted pathogens *Neisseria gonorrhoeae*, *Chlamydia trachomatis* (both *Lymphogranuloma venereum* [LGV] and non-LGV serovars), HSV, and *Treponema pallidum* (syphilis) may present in the same fashion as in the general population. However, LGV, formerly seen primarily in temperate regions of the world as an ulcerative proctitis with subsequent painful inguinal lymphadenopathy and occasional rupture and drainage, may present as a painful, hemorrhagic proctocolitis without ulceration or adenopathy. It has been increasingly seen in the MSM population throughout the world, although predominantly in HIV-infected MSM. Caused by the L1, L2, and L3 serovars of chlamydia, definitive diagnosis is challenging given the inability to distinguish LGV serovars from non-LGV chlamydia infections on routine testing. Treatment may be based on presentation and clinical suspicion alone. Culture is neither sensitive nor widely available. IgG or IgA antibodies or titers by complement fixation or microimmunofluorescence can be used to rule out infection if negative, but positive titers are only supportive, not diagnostic, because they do not differentiate past from recent infection. Rising titers over time, if done, can be confirmatory in hindsight. If available, nucleic acid amplification testing for chlamydia, although not FDA-approved, can be used to support the diagnosis in the setting of a compatible proctocolitis. Treatment for LGV is the same as for HIV-uninfected patients (doxycycline for 21 days) but may require more prolonged therapy for complete resolution of symptoms in some cases. Non-LGV chlamydia infections can be treated with azithromycin orally as a one-time dose, or with doxycycline for 7 days. Ulcerative disease from HSV is common; CMV and recurrent multiple aphthous ulcerations are seen less outside of advanced HIV disease but are important causes of morbidity in patients with CD4 counts of less than 50 cells/μL. HPV-related condyloma and anal dysplasia can occur at all stages of disease. They are more common in MSM, with the prevalence of oncogenic HPV infection exceeding 50% in this population (see Non-AIDS-Defining Cancers). Anal fissures, fistulas, and perirectal abscesses are also more common in MSM (Table 366-4).

DERMATOLOGIC MANIFESTATIONS OF HIV

Cutaneous issues are extraordinarily common in those with HIV infection, with up to 90% of patients developing some complication in the course of

---

TABLE 366-4 GASTROINTESTINAL MANIFESTATIONS OF HIV

ORAL	PRESENTATION/DIAGNOSIS	TREATMENT
Candidiasis	Clinical appearance (see Fig. 366-3) Culture and sensitivities rarely for suspected resistance	Nystatin suspension or clotrimazole troches Oral fluconazole for extensive disease; discontinue when resolved to avoid resistance
Oral hairy leukoplakia	Clinical appearance (see Fig. 366-2)	No specific treatment other than ART; various topical treatments have been studied
Kaposi sarcoma	Clinical appearance (see Fig. 366-4) Biopsy indicated if diagnosis not established previously May have disease elsewhere	ART, intralesional injection Chemotherapy or radiation sometimes indicated for extensive cutaneous or concomitant visceral disease
Aphthous ulcerations	Clinical appearance (see Fig. 366-5) Biopsy	Topical steroids Oral steroids or thalidomide for extensive or refractory ulcers
HSV	Clinical appearance Culture	Oral antivirals
Parotid enlargement	Clinical appearance Imaging may be helpful	ART
ESOPHAGEAL	**PRESENTATION/DIAGNOSIS**	**TREATMENT**
Candidiasis	Dysphagia, odynophagia Clinical appearance and brushings at EGD	Oral azoles
HSV	Odynophagia Biopsy at EGD	Oral antivirals
CMV	Odynophagia Biopsy at EGD	Ganciclovir, valganciclovir
Aphthous Ulcerations	Odynophagia Biopsy at EGD	Oral steroids and/or thalidomide
GASTRIC	**PRESENTATION/DIAGNOSIS**	**TREATMENT**
Infectious (CMV, MAC, *Candida*)	Advanced disease; nausea, dyspepsia Endoscopy	ART Treat underlying organism
GERD, gastritis, peptic ulcer disease	Dyspepsia, abdominal pain, bleeding Endoscopy	PPI, H2RA (attention to drug-drug interactions with ART)
SMALL BOWEL	**PRESENTATION/DIAGNOSIS**	**TREATMENT**
Infectious (*Cryptosporidium*, *Microsporidium*, *Cyclospora*, *Giardia*)	Advanced disease Watery large volume diarrhea, bloating Stool studies	Primarily immune reconstitution with ART Metronidazole for giardia
Enteropathy	Weight loss, bloating, diarrhea Exclude other causes	Primarily immune reconstitution with ART Antimotility agents, nutritional support
LARGE BOWEL	**PRESENTATION/DIAGNOSIS**	**TREATMENT**
CMV	Crampy abdominal pain, small volume diarrhea Advanced disease Colonoscopy with biopsy	Ganciclovir, valganciclovir ART
Clostridium difficile	Crampy abdominal pain, diarrhea, fever Stool studies	Oral metronidazole, vancomycin

TABLE 366-4 GASTROINTESTINAL MANIFESTATIONS OF HIV—cont'd

LIVER	PRESENTATION/DIAGNOSIS	TREATMENT
Chronic hepatitis B and C	Transaminitis Serologies and PCR for viremia	HBV: antivirals (e.g., TAF, lamivudine) HCV: direct-acting antiviral combination therapy
NAFLD, NASH	Transaminitis Imaging, liver biopsy	Weight loss, referral to specialist
Drug toxicity	Transaminitis	Withdrawal or change of offending agent
PANCREAS	**PRESENTATION/DIAGNOSIS**	**TREATMENT**
Pancreatitis	Mid-epigastric pain, nausea, vomiting, metabolic derangements	NPO, withdrawal of offending agent if present
BILIARY	**PRESENTATION/DIAGNOSIS**	**TREATMENT**
Drug (atazanavir)	Indirect hyperbilirubinemia	Benign, can change ART based on patient concerns
Cholangiopathy (infectious)	Advanced disease Elevated alkaline phosphatase, RUQ discomfort ERCP	ART
ANORECTAL	**PRESENTATION/DIAGNOSIS**	**TREATMENT**
Proctitis (chlamydia, syphilis, gonorrhea)	Pain, discharge, can be asymptomatic Serologies, nucleic acid testing	Treatment of underlying organism
Ulcerative disease	HSV; culture In advanced disease CMV, aphthous; biopsy	Antivirals Antivirals, steroids, thalidomide
Anal dysplasia	Asymptomatic; Pap, HRA with acetic acid stain and biopsy	Topical, IRC
Condyloma	Clinical appearance Biopsy	Topical, surgical
Fissure, fistula, abscess	Pain, drainage	Fissure: topical compounded diltiazem Fistula, abscess: surgical

ART = antiretroviral therapy; CMV = cytomegalovirus; EGD = esophagogastroduodenoscopy; ERCP = endoscopic retrograde cholangiopancreatography; GERD = gastroesophageal reflux disease; HBV = hepatitis B virus; HCV = hepatitis C virus; HRA = high-resolution anoscopy; H2RA = H₂ receptor antagonists; HSV = herpes simplex virus; IRC = infrared cautery; MAC = *Mycobacterium avium* complex; NAFLD = nonalcoholic fatty liver disease; NASH = nonalcoholic steatohepatitis; NPO = nothing by mouth; PCR = polymerase chain reaction; PPI = proton pump inhibitor; RUQ = right upper quadrant; TAF = tenofovir alafenamide.

their disease. Skin conditions may be the first presenting sign of HIV infection. Given that missed opportunities to diagnose HIV are common, primary care providers and dermatologists should be alert to atypical, more fulminant, or persistent presentations of common skin conditions as well conditions seen less often in HIV-negative patients. They can be broadly divided into infectious, noninfectious, and inflammatory conditions, with presentations typically similar to what is seen in immune-competent individuals but at times more severe and prolonged and possibly requiring more intensive therapy (see Chapters 407-413). As with many other areas of HIV medicine, the incidence and prevalence of certain conditions has decreased as more patients are diagnosed early and started on ART. This section focuses on the noninfectious and inflammatory conditions, although mention is made of the infectious problems that are discussed in more detail elsewhere.

Approach to the Patient

Proper characterization of skin lesions, along with an assessment of current immune status, can help narrow the diagnosis in patients with HIV infection. Papules (<1 cm diameter) and plaques (>1 cm diameter) are raised, well-circumscribed lesions involving the dermis and epidermis, whereas nodules involve deeper tissues and are typically greater than 2 cm. These lesions can be associated with any of the broad categories of cutaneous disease in HIV. Vesicles and bullae are raised, fluid-filled lesions that are again distinguished by size less than or greater than 1 cm, respectively. Macules and patches are flat with defined borders either alone or in groups.[27] Approach to skin diseases in general is provided in Chapter 407.

Pruritus with and without Physical Findings

Pruritus is the most common dermatologic complaint in the modern cART era and often has a significant impact on quality of life. Common conditions such as xerosis, seborrheic dermatitis, fungal infections, and eczema may present in a more persistent refractory fashion in patients with HIV, even at higher CD4 cell counts, and may also represent the presenting manifestation in undiagnosed HIV. Pruritus may be present with no other findings on physical examination, so a diligent search for underlying disease should be undertaken; for instance, it may be seen in a subset of patients with chronic HCV (Table 366-5).[28]

Malignancies

KS (Fig. 366-6) was the first AIDS-defining cancer to be reported 1981 when cases were seen in MSM. The incidence and prevalence in the United States have declined in the modern treatment era. KS is a vascular tumor that can affect any organ system but often presents with cutaneous lesions, including the oral cavity. It may, however, present with visceral disease, such as pulmonary or gastrointestinal disease, in the absence of cutaneous lesions. It is etiologically associated with HHV8 (KSHV) and in the United States is found predominantly in gay, transgender, and bisexual MSM, but it can also affect women. It presents as violaceous papular or nodular lesions, and although it has a typical appearance, biopsy, typically showing fascicles of spindle-shaped tumor cells, should be performed to establish the diagnosis and differentiate it from bacillary angiomatosis, which can present with similar lesions either alone or in conjunction with KS. KS that presents in untreated patients, including visceral KS, may regress with initiation of ART and immune reconstitution but sometimes will require local therapy such as cryotherapy or intralesional injections of chemotherapeutic agents or, in more advanced cases of symptomatic disease, systemic chemotherapy. KS may be induced or exacerbated by concomitant corticosteroids such as the doses used to treat *Pneumocystis* pneumonia or idiopathic immune thrombocytopenia. Regression or stabilization occurs with withdrawal of steroids.

HIV-infected individuals share the typical risk factors for squamous cell and basal cell carcinomas as HIV-uninfected individuals but get these cancers at a two- to three-fold higher rate, at a younger age, in multiple locations, and sometimes in areas of the skin that are not exposed to the sun.[29] Bowen disease and bowenoid papulosis can occur in the genital area of young sexually active males and females, typically presenting as raised, erythematous plaques and associated with HPV infection. Bowenoid papulosis often has a benign course and responds to locally destructive treatment or topical agents but can progress to Bowen disease, which has a 5% risk for developing into invasive squamous cell carcinoma. Malignant melanoma occurs at an increased frequency and is usually more advanced and aggressive in patients living with HIV. Merkel cell tumors can present at a younger age than is typically seen in immunocompetent, older, light-skinned individuals. Associated with Merkel polyomavirus, it presents as a rapidly enlarging,

TABLE 366-5 APPROACH TO CUTANEOUS LESIONS ASSOCIATED WITH HIV

LOCALIZED VS. GENERALIZED	LESION DESCRIPTION	DIFFERENTIAL DIAGNOSIS	CLINICAL FINDINGS
Localized skin findings *Can be generalized in immunosuppressed patients	Papules and nodules	Molluscum ecthyma	2- to 3-mm skin-colored umbilicated papules Eroded, ulcerated papules with overlying crust
		Furuncle/carbuncle	Inflammatory papules and nodules, tender
		Bacillary angiomatosis	Friable, red, purple, or flesh-colored papules and nodules
		Verruca vulgaris	Verruciform hyperkeratotic papules
		Condylomas	Skin-colored, often pedunculated verruciform papules
		Prurigo nodularis	Excoriated, often hyperkeratotic papules and nodules
		Nonmelanoma skin cancer: SCC	Erythematous papules with variable hyperkeratosis, crusting, and ulceration
		BCC	Pearly papules with overlying telangiectasias
		Kaposi sarcoma	Red-to-brown macules, papules, and plaques
	Plaques	Cellulitis	Erythematous plaques; increased warmth, tenderness
		Intertrigo	Erythematous thin papules and plaques with superficial erosions and fine scale; skin folds
		Thrush	White plaque of the oral mucosa, can be removed by scraping
		Oral hairy leukoplakia	Nonpainful white plaque along the lateral tongue
		Other fungal or bacterial infections	Variable cutaneous presentation
		Erythematous plaques with scale: seborrheic dermatitis	Erythematous plaques with greasy scale in a seborrheic distribution
		Psoriasis	Well-demarcated erythematous plaques with silvery scale, often on extensor surfaces
	Vesicles and bullae	Bullous impetigo	Superficial vesicles, erosions, honey-colored crust
		Folliculitis	Follicular pustules and papules
		Herpes simplex	Grouped vesicles on erythematous base
		Herpes zoster	Grouped vesicles in dermatomal distribution
		Bullous tinea or candida	Predominantly erosions and few superficial vesicles on erythematous background
	Exanthem ± enanthem	Viral diseases, acute HIV exanthem	Morbilliform macular eruptions, often associated with systemic symptoms
Generalized skin findings	Exanthem ± enanthem	Drug reaction	Often generalized morbilliform macular eruptions
	Erythema with desquamation	SJS, TEN	Erythematous to dusky macules and patches; check for mucosal involvement
	Papules, plaques	Pruritic papular eruption	Widespread skin-colored to erythematous papule with signs of excoriation
		Scabies	Widespread hyperkeratotic, scaly papules; severe pruritus
	Erythema with scaling	Eczema/dermatitis, xerosis	Erythematous scaly papules and plaques, often worse in the winter

BCC = basal cell carcinoma; SCC = squamous cell carcinoma; SJS = Stevens-Johnson syndrome; TEN = toxic epidermal necrolysis.
From Altman K, Vanness E, Westergaard RP. Cutaneous manifestations of human immunodeficiency virus: a clinical update. *Curr Infect Dis Rep.* 2015;17:464.

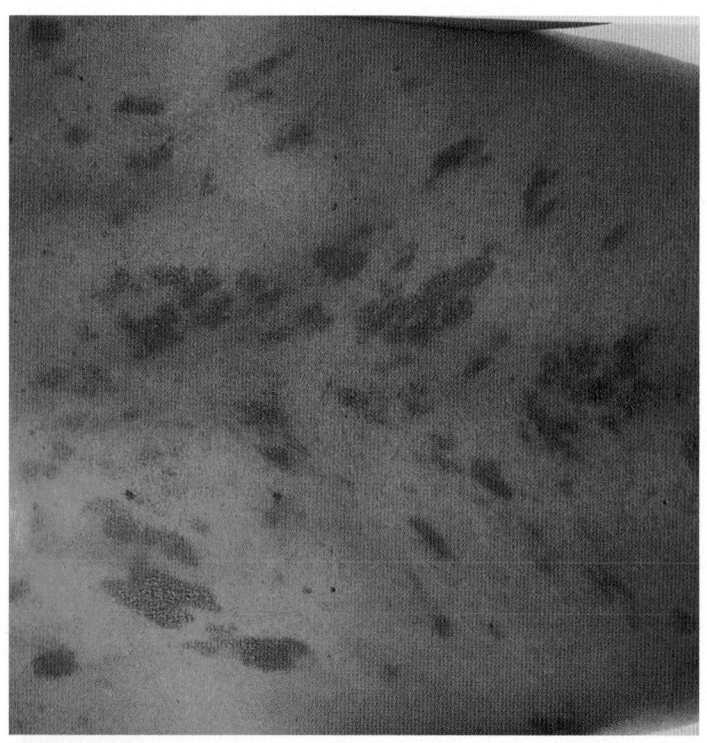

FIGURE 366-6. Cutaneous Kaposi sarcoma.

painless, nodular flesh-toned or bluish lesion and requires a high index of suspicion and biopsy for diagnosis. Treatment of melanoma and nonmelanoma skin cancers in HIV-infected individuals is similar to that in HIV-uninfected individuals.

Inflammatory Conditions

Many of the more severe inflammatory skin conditions are no longer seen as frequently, given the more widespread availability of ART and recommendations to start all HIV-infected patients at any CD4 cell count. Eosinophilic pustular folliculitis (Fig. 366-7) can be intensely pruritic, presenting as multiple papular or pustular lesions arising from hair follicles, usually on the face, neck, trunk, and upper extremities, although it may be found anywhere on the body. It is typically a complication of more advanced disease and can be particularly extensive in the setting of immune reconstitution when starting ART in patients with low CD4 cell counts and high viral loads. It is so common in this setting that the provider should alert the patient to the possibility in advance to make clear that it is not related to the drugs themselves unless this result in misdiagnosis of a drug allergy. It may last as long as several months but will generally subside. Topical antibiotics such as erythromycin, along with topical corticosteroids, may help; itraconazole has been used with some success. Ultraviolet B therapy has also been tried. Antihistamines can help with the pruritus, especially at night. Papular pruritic eruption of HIV is most common in sub-Saharan Africa and is thought to be caused by an exaggerated response to arthropod bites. Other conditions that may be included in the differential diagnosis are bacterial folliculitis and acne.

Psoriasiform dermatitis and frank psoriasis (Fig. 366-8) with or without arthritis can occur in HIV and may be quite severe, particularly in those with more advanced immunosuppression. It is felt to have a much higher incidence

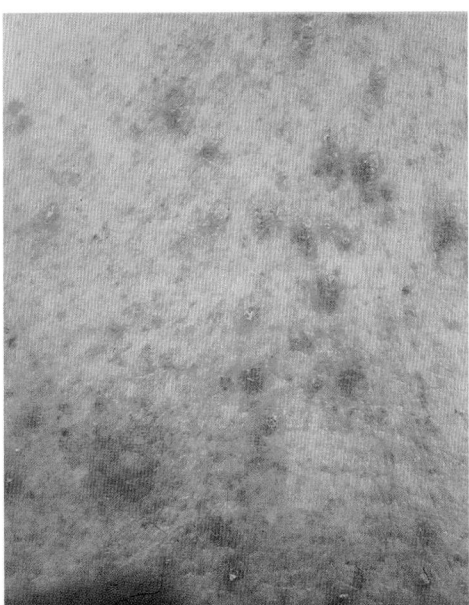
FIGURE 366-7. Eosinophilic pustular folliculitis.

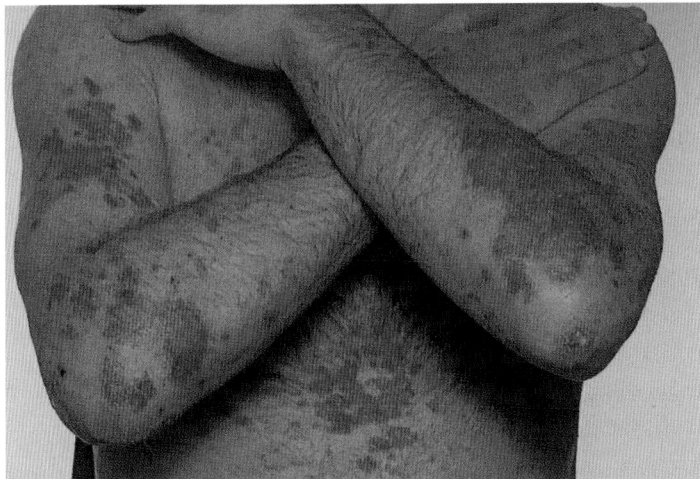
FIGURE 366-8. Psoriasis.

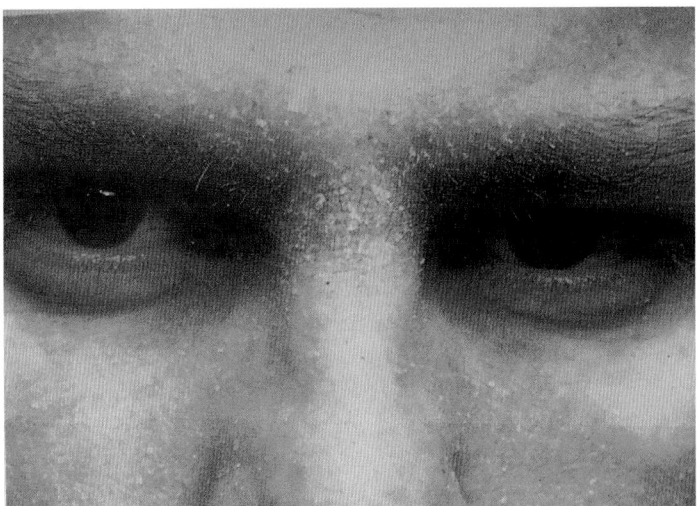
FIGURE 366-9. Seborrheic dermatitis.

in HIV and also involves the joints in a larger percentage of patients compared with those without HIV. It is sometimes the presenting condition of undiagnosed HIV. The ideal therapy is ART because the disease will often improve or go into remission with reconstitution of the immune system. Therapy is similar to treatment in immune-competent patients, including topical steroids, topical and oral retinoids, light therapy, and drugs such as cyclosporine and methotrexate in more severe disease, although patients taking these agents should be followed very closely for potential toxicity. TNF-α inhibitors such as etanercept and infliximab have not been studied in randomized clinical trials but have been used safely in patients who have failed or are intolerant of other therapies.[30] All patients treated with these drugs should be screened for tuberculosis before initiation of therapy.

Seborrheic dermatitis (Fig. 366-9), presenting as reddish orange plaques with scale, typically affecting the scalp, forehead, eyebrows, nose, and cheeks, has a much higher incidence in patients with HIV than in the general population. Although it may be more severe and refractory with advanced HIV, it can occur at any CD4 cell count and may be a sign of undiagnosed HIV. Combination therapy with topical corticosteroids and topical antifungal agents is usually effective. Atopic dermatitis also has a higher incidence in patients with HIV and is treated with topical steroids and antihistamines. Photodermatitis is also more common in patients with HIV, presenting as pruritic plaques in sun-exposed areas, especially in those taking photosensitizing drugs such as TMP-SMX or dapsone for *Pneumocystis* prophylaxis. Other lesions that can start on sun-exposed areas are prurigo nodularis, distinguished by

the nodular hyperpigmented character and intense pruritis, or porphyria cutanea tarda, presenting with bullous lesions on the backs of the hands, forearms, or face. Prurigo nodularis is almost exclusively seen in very advanced HIV disease, whereas porphyria cutanea tarda has a strong association with chronic HCV infection.

Infectious
BACTERIAL
Even with adequate virologic control, infectious complications of HIV occur commonly. Community-acquired methicillin-resistant *Staphylococcus aureus* (CA-MRSA) can be a serious and life-threatening infection sometimes requiring urgent surgical intervention if occurring in a closed space or in deep tissue. Colonization rates are higher in HIV-infected patients compared with the general population, particularly in MSM, thus explaining the higher incidence of serious infections. Superficial furuncles can be incised and drained or may spontaneously drain, but deep infections require urgent intervention given the rapidity of progression. The mainstay of therapy is intravenous vancomycin, and in less severe infections, community strains are often sensitive to doxycycline or TMP-SMX. Linezolid should be reserved for use in those patients who have contraindications to first-line antibiotics. Bacillary angiomatosis or peliosis hepatis, caused by *Bartonella* species (Chapter 299), is an uncommon but serious illness that can present with lesions very similar to KS—vascular, nodular, or plaque-like lesions—accompanied by fever and constitutional symptoms. This is typically only seen in advanced disease and responds well to erythromycin or doxycycline. Diagnosis can be made at biopsy. Anyone presenting with a diffuse new nonpruritic cutaneous eruption should be tested for syphilis. The typical chancre of primary syphilis may be absent or missed by the patient, so presentation with a rash during secondary syphilis is very common. All sexually active patients with HIV should be screened at least annually, even in the absence of signs or symptoms, and more frequently for those with multiple partners in high-risk groups such as MSM.[31] Patients should be educated that oral sex alone can transmit syphilis. Serology is reliable in HIV-infected patients, and syphilis will respond well to intramuscular benzathine penicillin 2.4 million units, with doxycycline the second-line agent in patients with penicillin allergy. Patients who report vague penicillin allergies should be skin-tested proactively because penicillin is the preferred treatment.

VIRAL
The rash of acute HIV occurs in up to 70% of patients, typically a few days after the onset of fever, with a maculopapular appearance affecting the face, trunk, and sometimes the extremities including the palms and soles. Any sexually active patient who presents with a maculopapular erythematous rash in the setting of a flu- or mono-like illness should be tested for HIV.

Herpes zoster (varicella-zoster virus [VZV]) (Fig. 366-10) is far more common in HIV-infected patients at all CD4 cell counts than in the general population and in younger patients should prompt consideration of HIV testing (Table 366-6). It will most commonly present in the typical dermatomal fashion seen in those without HIV but can be seen in multiple dermatomes or become disseminated. Oral antiviral therapy should be initiated at the time

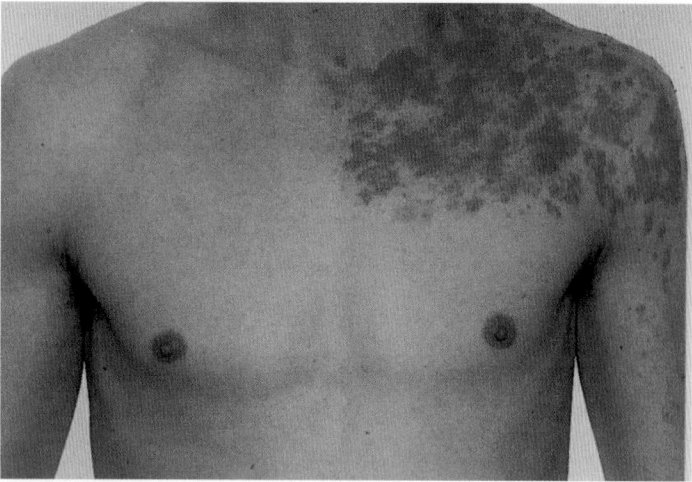

FIGURE 366-10. Herpes zoster (varicella-zoster virus).

FIGURE 366-11. Molluscum contagiosum.

TABLE 366-6	CUTANEOUS MANIFESTATIONS THAT SHOULD PROMPT CONSIDERATION OF HIV TESTING

Oral candidiasis
Secondary syphilis
Psoriasis
Seborrheic dermatitis
Viral exanthem with or without enanthem
Herpes zoster (disseminated)

of diagnosis, which is typically made by visual inspection of classical clustered vesicular lesions in a dermatomal distribution; for multidermatomal or disseminated VZV, intravenous therapy is the treatment of choice. For atypical presentations, direct fluorescent antibody staining of scrapings from the lesions is a rapid and specific method of diagnosis, although less sensitive than PCR. In patients with CD4 counts of more than 200 cells/μL and suppressed viral load, VZV vaccination has been found in one small study to be safe, although no efficacy studies have been done. It is reasonable to consider vaccination in patients older than 50 years with HIV after demonstrating previous VZV infection through serology. Given the severity of the disease in adults with immune compromise, patients without demonstrated VZV immunity should be vaccinated when the CD4 cell count is higher than 200 cells/μL, ideally with an undetectable HIV viral load as well. Patients should discontinue chronic ARV drugs such as acyclovir, famciclovir, and valacyclovir before vaccination and for 14 days after vaccination to allow an adequate immune response.

HSV, particularly anogenital infection, is common in HIV-infected patients and typically responds well to standard antiviral therapy. Prophylaxis with daily ARV agents is safe and effective, has few drug interactions, and has not been shown to lead to the development of resistant virus. HSV in advanced disease can be difficult to treat, requiring longer courses, higher doses, or intravenous therapy. When refractory to treatment, drug resistance to first-line therapy should be considered and tested for. Foscarnet or cidofovir can be tried in cases of suspected resistance. Although foscarnet is not widely used in the modern cART era, there have been reports of foscarnet-induced penile and vulvar ulceration due to local irritation from the drug itself during urination, more commonly in women. It may be confused with worsening of disease but does not require treatment cessation and can be mitigated by careful hygiene. Compounded topical cidofovir, although expensive and not widely available, can be effective in limited disease. Initiation of ART can lead to worsening of cutaneous infections, including VZV and HSV, and to a higher incidence of shingles as well as an increased frequency of HSV type 2 outbreaks in the first few months of ARV therapy.[32]

HPV is ubiquitous in sexually active men and women (Chapter 349). The nononcogenic types 6 and 11 are responsible for genital warts, which can sometimes be quite extensive and can involve the anal canal. Cryotherapy, infrared coagulation, topical treatments such as salicylic acid, imiquimod or podophyllin, and intralesional chemotherapeutic agents have been used to treat warts, although surgical excision may be required. The oncogenic types,

of which there are 14, are associated with both cervical and anal dysplasia and cancers. Testing for HPV is rarely indicated other than in triage of ASCUS cervical Pap tests. Diagnosis and treatment are usually based on cytology and histology. Vaccination is strongly recommended using the nine-valent HPV vaccine on a three-shot schedule in men and women aged 9 to 26 years.[33] Utility of vaccination at older ages remains unproved.

Molluscum contagiosum can cause umbilicated lesions (Fig. 366-11) that may be widespread but typically responds to ART and immune reconstitution. Curettage or cryotherapy has been used for more immediate treatment. Epstein-Barr virus is felt to be the cause of oral hairy leukoplakia, a painless plaque found on the lateral tongue in more advanced HIV. No specific treatment is indicated other than ART.

FUNGAL

The presence of oral candidiasis should always prompt consideration of HIV testing (see Table 366-6). Caused by *Candida albicans*, it is one of the most common manifestations of decreasing immune function in patients with HIV and is easily treatable with nystatin suspension or clotrimazole troches used on an as-needed basis for short courses until cleared. Fluconazole may be used in more refractory cases, but continuous use can lead to resistant infection necessitating alternative intravenous antifungal agents, such as echinocandins or in some cases amphotericin. Oral itraconazole or voriconazole is sometimes used with varying results to treat refractory candidiasis. The full range of tinea infections may be seen in patients with HIV, and these are sometimes difficult to eradicate in the absence of immune reconstitution. Topical antifungal agents are the treatment of choice, although oral drugs are sometimes necessary for more refractory infections. In the modern era, cutaneous cryptococcal lesions are quite rare. They present as umbilicated papules similar in appearance to molluscum but are usually part of a clinical picture consistent with severe disseminated cryptococcal disease. Disseminated cutaneous histoplasmosis may present as widespread papulopustular lesions associated with systemic disease.[34] The skin lesions associated with infection by *Talaromyces marneffei* (formerly *Penicillium marneffei*) have a similar appearance. Talaromycosis is typically seen in those with severe immune compromise and is endemic to Southeast Asia, South Asia, China, and Northern Australia.

OTHER

Scabies presents in similar fashion to patients without HIV, marked by the classical burrows in the webs between the fingers and toes as well as more widespread excoriations and papules in the axillae and on the nipples and genitalia. Topical treatment such as permethrin is usually adequate after demonstration of the mite on direct examination. "Norwegian" scabies is characterized by thick crusts of skin teeming with mites and may require oral ivermectin in addition to topical therapies; it is typically seen in very advanced HIV disease only and is highly infectious. Diffuse alopecia and alopecia areata may occur in PLWH and have been seen in association with some protease inhibitors; they may be either transient or persistent. Discoloration of the nailbeds may be present with zidovudine use. Hyperpigmented areas, usually on the palms and soles and almost exclusively in patients of African origin, may rarely develop as a result of emtricitabine therapy. Atypical mycobacterial infections such as *Mycobacterium marinum*, *M. haemophilum*, *M. fortuitum*, and *M. chelonae* can cause skin disease ranging from pustular erythematous nodules to ulcerating nonhealing wounds, although much less frequently in the era of widespread ART. The vasculitis associated with cryoglobulinemia, often associated with chronic HCV and found more often in HIV coinfection, can cause purpuric skin lesions and Raynaud phenomenon. Treatment of underlying HCV will lead to clinical improvement and resolution in most cases, although cryoglobulinemia not associated with HCV can be more difficult to treat.

Drug Reactions

Toxic epidermal necrolysis and Stevens-Johnson syndrome are devastating complications that occur much more commonly in HIV-infected than in HIV-uninfected individuals. The two major culprits are TMP-SMX and nevirapine, the latter of which is no longer used in resource-rich settings. Other drugs such as fluconazole and clindamycin have been implicated less commonly. Stevens-Johnson syndrome presents with diffuse and severe erythroderma and may progress to exfoliation of skin and mucous membrane involvement. It is a systemic disease requiring treatment similar to that for burn victims and carries a high mortality rate in large part because of a risk for bacterial superinfection and sepsis. Typical morbilliform drug reactions are more common in PLWH and happen with higher frequency at lower CD4 cell counts, with TMP-SMX again being a very common cause. In the era before effective ART, desensitization to TMP-SMX was sometimes undertaken given its effectiveness at *Pneumocystis* prophylaxis, although not if there was a prior history of Stevens-Johnson syndrome.

● MUSCULOSKELETAL MANIFESTATIONS OF HIV

Much as in the general population, musculoskeletal complaints are common throughout the course of HIV disease, with a high incidence of pain in general and muscle or joint pain specifically. Whether HIV itself is an etiologic agent in these disorders is still debated. Pain in general, and musculoskeletal pain in particular, was a frequent complaint in patients with advanced HIV in the early epidemic; it is not clear if the prevalence is currently higher in treated patients versus the general population. However, there are several distinct entities either unique to HIV or occurring at a higher incidence in HIV-infected individuals, including those on suppressive therapy, such as HIV-associated arthropathy and painful articular syndrome.

There have been descriptions of HIV arthritis as a self-limited, large-joint, seronegative sterile arthritis. Particularly in Africa, the incidence of asymmetrical seronegative arthritis, sometimes termed *painful articular syndrome*, seems to have increased, primarily in patients naïve to ART. There is some indirect evidence to suggest that HIV may cause direct joint inflammation, such as detection of p24 antigen in joint fluid at levels up to 10-fold higher than in serum; however, there is no conclusive evidence at this time of a direct causal link.[35] Patients with acute HIV infection often have myalgias and arthralgias as part of their presenting complaints, but these are typically nonspecific and self-limited. Much of the literature on rheumatic complications of HIV was reported in the era before effective ART, describing conditions more commonly seen in advanced HIV disease. Early in the epidemic, a myopathy was described characterized by muscular pain, typically in the proximal muscles of the extremities, accompanied by elevated muscle enzymes. This was often associated with zidovudine use, later presumed to be from dose-dependent mitochondrial toxicity, and would usually resolve with withdrawal of the drug. Similarly, lactic acidosis, primarily due to the use of stavudine or didanosine, could cause marked muscle inflammation as part of the syndrome of mitochondrial toxicity and organ damage or failure. With the avoidance of these particular agents, the incidence of isolated myopathies and myositis is no longer a common problem.

Another clinical entity, seen more commonly in advanced disease, is pyomyositis. It is usually caused by *S. aureus* but occasionally by other organisms. Pyomyositis typically starts as localized muscle pain, progressing to swelling, fever, and induration, then subsequently the development of one or more abscesses in large striated muscle. The bacteria are believed to seed traumatized muscle; diagnosis is made by imaging and aspiration. Antibiotics and surgical drainage are the mainstays of treatment.

Diffuse infiltrative lymphocytosis syndrome (DILS) appears to be unique to HIV-infected individuals. A Sjögren-like syndrome, it is thought to be caused by an oligoclonal expansion of circulating CD8⁺ lymphocytes, causing an infiltrative disease that more commonly involves the parotids and lung, but in many cases there is visceral infiltration as well. Symptoms are similar to Sjögren syndrome with unilateral or bilateral parotid enlargement, xerostomia,

and xerophthalmia. Pulmonary infiltrates may resemble those found in *Pneumocystis* pneumonia. Additional findings could include a lymphocytic infiltrative myositis and hepatitis as well as a painful peripheral neuropathy and nephropathy. Demonstration of CD8⁺ cell infiltrates on biopsy, typically of the salivary gland, differentiates this entity from Sjögren syndrome, which is caused by CD4⁺ lymphocytic infiltration. The disease was reported predominantly in African Americans and West Africans and has decreased significantly with the introduction of effective ART.

Osteoporosis, osteopenia, and vitamin D deficiency are common in PLWH (see Endocrine Manifestations of HIV).

Osteonecrosis, or avascular necrosis (AVN), most commonly affects the hip. It is characterized by interruption of the blood supply to the joint, ultimately leading to bone death and destruction of the joint. Trauma is a recognized cause of AVN, but there are also a variety of atraumatic etiologies associated with osteonecrosis, the most common being prior glucocorticoid use and excessive alcohol consumption. There is debate about whether HIV itself is an independent risk factor for the development of AVN; however, most studies have shown an incidence higher than that of the general population, even in the absence of other traditional risk factors. It affects both men and women, is often bilateral, and may be present radiographically before the onset of symptoms.[36] Patients may present with hip pain that radiates to the groin and symptoms are typically progressive. Bisphosphonates have been used with mixed results to attempt to slow the progression of disease, and there are a variety of joint-sparing procedures such as core decompression or wedge osteotomy. Definitive treatment involves total hip arthroplasty.

Psoriatic arthritis (Chapter 249) has had an increase in severity in white HIV-infected individuals but not an increase in prevalence, in contrast to Africa where, once rare, the overall prevalence has increased in those with HIV. Rheumatoid arthritis (Chapter 248) has been reported to become symptomatically improved with lower CD4 cell counts, with concomitant exacerbation or new presentation in patients who start ART.

Rhabdomyolysis (Chapter 105) in HIV-infected patients has been seen with raltegravir and certain protease inhibitors with a higher risk when used in conjunction with statin therapy due to inhibition of the cytochrome pathway by the ARV drugs and resultant higher levels of circulating drug. Careful attention should be paid to drug-drug interactions with statins and ART, including drugs that contain cobicistat, another pharmacokinetic booster used primarily in single-tablet regimens or in combination with the protease inhibitors atazanavir and darunavir as single-tablet boosted protease inhibitors.

Reactive arthritis (Chapter 249) occurs with similar frequency and is due to the same causes as in the HIV-negative population. Typically caused by a genitourinary or enteric infection, such as *Shigella*, *Salmonella*, *Yersinia*, or *Campylobacter*, the manifestations are similar, including most typically an oligoarthritis affecting the lower extremities, although sometimes affecting joints in the upper extremities and occasionally the small joints of the hands or feet, occasionally accompanied by enthesitis. Extra-articular manifestations can include conjunctivitis, urethritis, uveitis, and skin changes such as keratoderma blennorrhagica (hyperkeratotic skin lesions on soles and palms) and erythema nodosum. Diagnosis is made by establishment of a preceding infection in the presence of the typical clinical findings as described previously. Disease is often self-limited and may respond to NSAIDs. More refractory disease may necessitate intra-articular or oral corticosteroid use, keeping in mind the potential for drug-drug interactions with protease inhibitors. In chronic cases not responding to NSAIDs or steroids, disease-modifying agents such as sulfasalazine or TNF-α inhibitors may be used. Data are limited, but both nonbiologics and biologics can be safely used with close monitoring in selected patients. Cryoglobulinemia, often associated with concurrent chronic HCV, can cause arthralgias in the absence of cutaneous manifestations.

Grade A References

A1. The INSIGHT START Study Group. Initiation of antiretroviral therapy in early asymptomatic HIV infection. *N Engl J Med.* 2015;373:795-807.

A2. Mangili A, Falutz J, Mamputu JC, et al. Predictors of treatment response to tesamorelin, a growth hormone-releasing factor analog, in HIV-Infected patients with excess abdominal fat. *PLoS ONE.* 2015;10:1-14.

A3. Overton ET, Chan ES, Brown TT, et al. Vitamin D and calcium attenuate bone loss with antiretroviral therapy initiation: a randomized trial. *Ann Intern Med.* 2015;162:815-824.

A4. Kunisaki KM, Niewoehner DE, Collins G, et al; INSIGHT START Pulmonary Substudy Group. Pulmonary effects of immediate versus deferred antiretroviral therapy in HIV-positive individuals: a nested substudy within the multicentre, international, randomised, controlled Strategic Timing of Antiretroviral Treatment (START) trial. *Lancet Respir Med.* 2016;4:980-989.

GENERAL REFERENCES

For the General References and other additional features, please visit Expert Consult at https://expertconsult.inkling.com.

367

IMMUNE RECONSTITUTION INFLAMMATORY SYNDROME IN HIV/AIDS

MARTYN A. FRENCH AND GRAEME MEINTJES

DEFINITION

Treatment of human immunodeficiency virus (HIV) infection with combination antiretroviral therapy (ART) results in the restoration of protective pathogen-specific immune responses and the regression or prevention of opportunistic infections (OIs) and cancers in most individuals (Chapter 365). However, restoration of an immune response against a pathogen may also result in immunopathology at body sites infected by the pathogen. This has been referred to as immune restoration disease (IRD) to differentiate it from immunodeficiency disease, but it is now commonly known as immune reconstitution inflammatory syndrome (IRIS) because an inflammatory illness is the most common clinical feature.[1,2]

Essentially any pathogen that causes an infection as a result of HIV-induced cellular immunodeficiency may be associated with IRIS after ART is commenced.[3] However, the clinical characteristics and severity of IRIS associated with each type of pathogen vary greatly (Table 367-1). For example, IRIS associated with Mycobacterium tuberculosis, cryptococcal, or JC polyomavirus (JCV) infection is manifested differently from an OI caused by these pathogens, and the resulting illness is often severe and may result in death. In contrast, herpes zoster after ART is usually indistinguishable from that occurring before ART, and it is only the timing of onset and its increased frequency during early ART that suggest that it results from IRIS.

IRIS develops mainly during the first 3 months of ART but occasionally later. Two patterns are recognized. Paradoxical IRIS refers to the worsening or atypical manifestation (or both) of an established OI after ART is commenced. In most cases the infection had been treated before ART was initiated, and the immune response appears to be against residual antigens of the pathogen or the dying organism. Unmasking IRIS refers to disease that occurs for the first time after ART is commenced and appears to result from an immune response against a subclinical infection by an opportunistic pathogen or a missed diagnosis of an OI. Typically, unmasking IRIS manifests with accelerated or exaggerated inflammatory presentations of the infection.

EPIDEMIOLOGY

The reported incidence of IRIS has varied from 8% to over 40% in different studies. To some extent, the large variation reflects the lack of universally accepted diagnostic criteria. It also probably reflects differences in risk factors in the populations of patients studied. The most important risk factors for IRIS are a low CD4$^+$ T-cell count when ART is initiated and, in patients in whom paradoxical IRIS develops, disseminated infection and a short time interval between treatment of the infection and commencement of ART.

PATHOGENESIS

Information about the pathogenesis of IRIS has been obtained mostly by studying patients who experience disease associated with a mycobacterial infection.[4] Both clinicopathologic and immunologic studies have shown an association with a T_H1 cellular immune response against mycobacterial antigens, which has been demonstrated by measuring delayed-type hypersensitivity skin test responses or the frequency of circulating antigen-specific T cells that produce interferon (IFN)-γ. However, there is increasing evidence that innate immune responses by myeloid cells (monocytes, macrophages, and neutrophils) and their mediators also contribute to the immunopathology, particularly in paradoxical tuberculosis (TB)-IRIS. The immunopathogenesis of IRIS

TABLE 367-1 EXAMPLES OF IMMUNE RECONSTITUTION INFLAMMATORY SYNDROME

PATHOGEN	NOMENCLATURE	TYPICAL CHARACTERISTICS OF THE DISEASE
Mycobacterium tuberculosis	TB-IRIS	Paradoxical exacerbation of TB
Nontuberculous mycobacteria (NTM)	NTM-IRIS	Mainly lymphadenitis, also pulmonary and abdominal disease
Bacille Calmette-Guérin (BCG)	BCG-IRIS	Necrotizing regional lymphadenitis
Mycobacterium leprae	Leprosy-associated IRIS	Borderline and type 1 reactional state
Cryptococcus neoformans	C-IRIS	Mainly meningitis, also lymphadenitis
Pneumocystis jiroveci	Pneumocystosis-associated IRIS	Paradoxical exacerbation of pneumonitis
Cytomegalovirus (CMV)	CMV retinitis after ART or immune recovery uveitis	Acute retinitis after commencing ART or uveitis
JC polyomavirus	PML-IRIS	Multifocal leukoencephalopathy with inflammatory features
Human herpesvirus 8	KS-IRIS	Rapid progression of existing and/or new KS lesions
Hepatitis B or C virus	Hepatitis B or C virus-associated IRIS (that may mimic DILI)	Hepatitis flare and/or liver enzyme elevation
Varicella-zoster virus		Dermatomal or multidermatomal zoster and rarely myelitis after ART
Herpes simplex virus		Herpes lesions with exaggerated inflammation and rarely myelitis or encephalitis after ART
Molluscum contagiosum virus	Inflammatory molluscum contagiosum	Inflamed molluscum lesions
Malassezia spp.	Inflammatory seborrheic dermatitis	Abnormally inflamed seborrheic dermatitis

ART = antiretroviral therapy; DILI = drug-induced liver injury; C= cryptococcosis; IRIS = immune reconstitution inflammatory syndrome; KS = Kaposi sarcoma; PML = progressive multifocal leukoencephalopathy; TB = tuberculosis.

associated with other pathogens is less well understood and appears to vary depending on the provoking pathogen.[5] For example, IRIS associated with JCV infection (progressive multifocal leukoencephalopathy IRIS [PML-IRIS]) is characterized by an inflammatory cell infiltrate dominated by CD8$^+$ T cells in affected areas of the brain. Other forms of IRIS associated with virus infections also appear to be CD8$^+$ T-cell mediated.

CLINICAL MANIFESTATIONS

The clinical manifestations of IRIS are different for each associated pathogen and will therefore be described for individual pathogens. Only disease that presents a significant patient management problem will be discussed.

TB-IRIS

M. tuberculosis is the most common pathogen involved in IRIS, with estimates of paradoxical TB-IRIS incidence ranging from 4 to 54% of patients with HIV infection and treated TB. Most TB-IRIS develops within the first 3 months after the initiation of ART. Patients in whom paradoxical TB-IRIS develops typically give a history of having improved with treatment of TB before initiation of ART. After starting ART, recurrent, worsening, or new clinical or radiologic manifestations of TB develop. Common manifestations include fever, enlargement of lymph nodes, and worsening radiographic pulmonary infiltrates. Tracheal compression by intrathoracic lymph nodes or massive pleural effusions can cause life-threatening dyspnea. Respiratory failure as a result of worsening pulmonary infiltrates and acute respiratory distress syndrome have occasionally been reported. In a prospective case series from South Africa, neurologic TB-IRIS accounted for 12% of cases of paradoxical TB-IRIS. Meningitis, tuberculoma, or both were the most common manifestations. TB-IRIS may cause granulomatous hepatitis, typically with tender hepatomegaly and cholestatic liver function derangement. Peritonitis due to IRIS-mediated peritoneal inflammation and peritonitis secondary to bowel perforation or splenic rupture are other unusual presentations. Although usually negative, mycobacterial cultures may be positive, particularly if IRIS occurs early during anti-TB therapy and in patients with multidrug-resistant TB. Histologic examination often reveals necrotizing granulomas.

High rates of TB have been reported during ART, especially in the initial months of treatment in ART programs in resource-limited settings. This type of TB has been referred to as ART-associated TB because the mechanisms underlying the manifestations of TB after initiating ART are likely to be heterogeneous. Diagnoses of active TB before initiation of ART may be missed because of the inherent insensitivity of TB diagnostics in this patient group and only later be diagnosed during ART. Because ART-induced immune recovery is a time-dependent process and some patients fail to respond immunologically, a proportion of cases may develop as a result of persisting immunodeficiency. Other patients may have active subclinical disease at the time of ART initiation or a missed TB diagnosis, and progression to symptomatic disease may be accelerated with exaggerated inflammatory features by ART-induced restoration of a cellular immune response against *M. tuberculosis* antigens. Of patients in this latter group, some have exuberant inflammatory clinical features that are consistent with a diagnosis of unmasking TB-IRIS.

NTM-IRIS

Atypical manifestations of *Mycobacterium avium* complex (MAC) disease in patients who had commenced zidovudine monotherapy were the first indication that IRIS may be a complication of ART. MAC and other nontuberculous mycobacteria have been associated with IRIS in up to 4% of patients who commence combination ART with a $CD4^+$ T-cell count lower than $100/\mu L$. Disease is usually localized, as opposed to the disseminated nontuberculous mycobacterial disease of patients with acquired immunodeficiency syndrome (AIDS) not on ART, and is most commonly manifested as fever, night sweats, and lymphadenitis. Unmasking disease is most common. Peripheral lymphadenitis may suppurate and sometimes cause chronically discharging fistulas to the skin. Abdominal disease frequently causes pain, which is usually associated with lymphadenitis and occasionally with omental masses, hepatitis, and inflammation of the spleen (Fig. 367-1). Pulmonary and thoracic disease

usually causes cough that is sometimes associated with chest pain. Microscopic examination of biopsy material or aspirates from affected tissues often reveals mycobacteria, but these may not be cultured.

In HIV-seropositive children vaccinated with bacille Calmette-Guérin (BCG), a BCG-associated lymphadenitis with or without abscess formation may develop after starting ART (Fig. 367-2).

Leprosy-associated IRIS is usually manifested as unmasking of previous subclinical *Mycobacterium leprae* infection, with a borderline and type I reactional state (Chapter 310).

Cryptococcosis-IRIS

The proportion of patients with HIV infection and treated cryptococcosis in whom cryptococcosis-IRIS (C-IRIS) develops ranges from 8 to 49%. The majority represent a recurrence of previously treated cryptococcal meningitis. Unmasking inflammatory reactions to unrecognized meningeal infection during the first few weeks of ART have also been reported.[6] The time of onset of C-IRIS varies from 4 days to around 3 years after initiation of ART. In addition to recurrent meningitis, the central nervous system (CNS) features of C-IRIS include intracranial cryptococcoma or abscesses, spinal cord abscesses, recalcitrant raised intracranial pressure, optic disc swelling, cranial nerve lesions, dysarthria, hemiparesis, and paraparesis. Extracranial manifestations of C-IRIS include lymphadenitis, eye disease, suppurating soft tissue lesions, and pulmonary disease that may include cavitating or nodular lesions.

At the diagnosis of cryptococcal meningitis, cerebrospinal fluid (CSF) white blood cell counts of 25 cells/μL or less and protein levels of 50 mg/dL or less are associated with the development of C-IRIS. On the other hand, CSF profiles at the moment of paradoxical C-IRIS may show an increased white blood cell count and an increased opening pressure of greater than 25 cm H_2O, but these features overlap significantly with those observed in patients with non–IRIS-related relapses of cryptococcal meningitis. A positive CSF cryptococcal culture prior to commencing ART is a predictor for paradoxical C-IRIS. Cultures of CSF or tissue samples obtained at the time of paradoxical C-IRIS are usually negative even when cryptococci can be seen on microscopy.

The importance of C-IRIS is emphasized by the finding that earlier (1 to 2 weeks) ART initiation in cryptococcal meningitis results in higher mortality compared with deferred (5 weeks) ART initiation likely due to enhanced immune cell recruitment and activation when ART is started very early in the context of a partially treated CNS infection.[7,8]

Pneumocystosis-IRIS

Patients who have been treated for *P. jiroveci* pneumonitis (PJP) may experience pulmonary inflammation after ART is commenced. It is usually characterized by fever, cough, dyspnea, chest discomfort, and patchy alveolar infiltrates on the chest radiograph (Fig. 367-3). In some patients, organizing pneumonia develops. This condition is relatively rare, occurring in less than 5% of patients treated for PJP prior to ART.

PML-IRIS

PML of the brain occurs when cellular immune responses fail to control JCV infection of oligodendrocytes and astrocytes. It is characterized by a paucity of inflammatory cells in brain lesions. ART is effective in some patients,

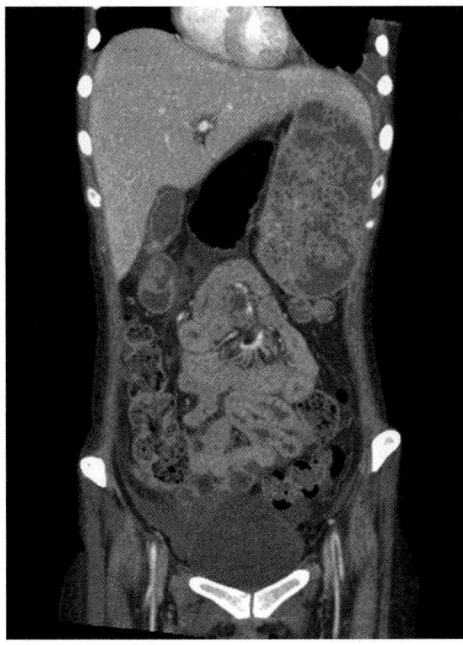

FIGURE 367-1. *Mycobacterium avium* complex–associated immune reconstitution inflammatory syndrome manifested as necrotizing inflammation in the spleen and abdominal lymph nodes.

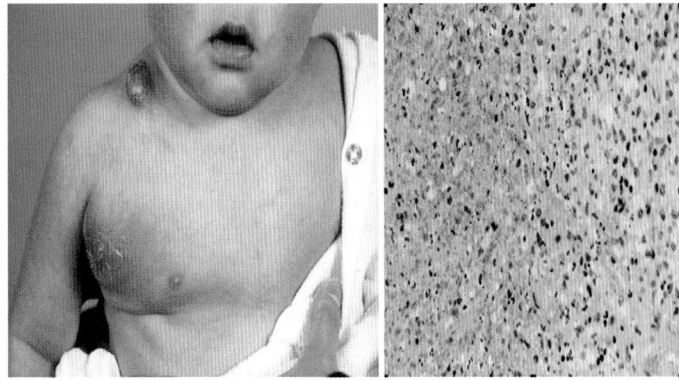

FIGURE 367-2. Bacille Calmette-Guérin (BCG)–associated immune reconstitution inflammatory syndrome after starting antiretroviral therapy for human immunodeficiency virus infection in a child who received BCG vaccination shortly after birth. A biopsy specimen from the larger lesion demonstrated necrotizing granulomatous inflammation.

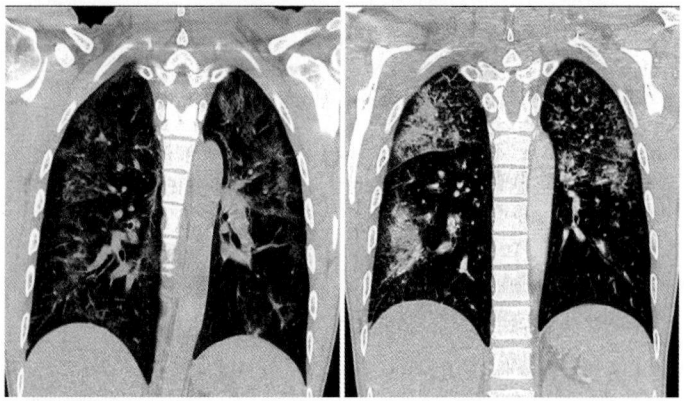

FIGURE 367-3. Pneumocystosis-associated immune reconstitution inflammatory syndrome. *Left,* Before treatment of the *P. jiroveci* infection. *Right,* After treatment of the *P. jiroveci* infection and commencing antiretroviral therapy.

presumably because it enhances cellular immune responses against JCV antigens. However, ART may also result in a paradoxical worsening of established PML or in unmasking of subclinical JCV infection and appearance of PML for the first time. These manifestations of PML on ART are often atypical in that imaging studies of the brain demonstrate changes associated with inflammation, and brain biopsy specimens demonstrate inflammatory cell infiltrates with a prominence of CD8+ T cells. Between 19 and 23% of cases of PML in HIV-infected patients are due to paradoxical or unmasking PML-IRIS. The median time at onset is 7 weeks on ART, and most cases occur within the first 3 months but very occasionally as late as 26 months after commencing ART. Predictors of PML-IRIS have not been identified.

Other CNS manifestations of IRIS, which vary greatly in incidence following ART, may include cryptococcal meningitis and meningoencephalitis, cerebral toxoplasmosis, primary CNS lymphoma, and HIV encephalitis,[9] as well as stroke.[10]

KS-IRIS

A prospective study of Kaposi sarcoma (KS) in patients from Mozambique commencing ART found that paradoxical KS-IRIS developed in 31% of patients with pre-ART KS, and that unmasking KS-IRIS developed in 7% of patients without pre-ART KS. Clinical manifestations included an increased number of preexisting skin lesions that sometimes exhibited increased nodularity and ulceration, new skin or mucosal lesions, and lymphedema. Independent risk factors for the development of KS-IRIS were KS before ART, human herpesvirus 8 DNA detectable in plasma, a hematocrit of less than 30%, and a plasma HIV RNA level greater than 5 $\log_{10}$ copies/mL. This form of IRIS may be life-threatening when there is worsening of pulmonary KS or airway obstruction due to enlarging KS lesions.

Some cases of KS-IRIS will resolve without treatment, but chemotherapy is usually necessary.

Cytomegalovirus-associated IRIS

Eye disease is the most common manifestation of IRIS associated with cytomegalovirus (CMV) infection. Retinitis usually develops during the first few weeks of ART as a "paradoxical" worsening of treated retinitis or as a new manifestation of CMV retinitis. Previously treated CMV infection is the most common cause of immune recovery uveitis (IRU), which presumably results from the restoration of an immune response against residual CMV antigens in the eye. The risk for development of CMV-associated IRU is greatest in patients who had a large proportion of the retina affected by CMV infection. It may develop up to 21 months after ART is commenced, and the clinical manifestations vary in severity from a transient vitreitis to persistent uveitis, papillitis, cystoid macular edema, and detachment of epiretinal membranes.

Liver Disease after ART Associated with Hepatitis B and C Virus Infection

Elevations of serum liver enzyme levels occur in up to 18% of patients after ART is initiated. Several causes have been defined, but the most important risk factor is concomitant infection with hepatitis B virus (HBV) or hepatitis C virus (HCV). Prospective studies of patients with HIV infection who are coinfected with HBV, HCV, or both, who commenced ART demonstrated that 22 to 24% of patients with HBV coinfection, 13.5% of patients with HCV

coinfection, and 50% of patients with both HBV and HCV coinfection experienced a "flare" of hepatitis. Flares of HBV hepatitis were associated with increased plasma levels of several immune mediators, suggesting that at least some of these cases were due to IRIS related to hepatitis B in the liver. Patients who experienced flares of HBV hepatitis had higher plasma HBV DNA levels and serum alanine transaminase levels before ART was commenced. Severe hepatitis after ART in patients with HIV infection and coinfection with HBV or HCV is uncommon but can occasionally result in liver decompensation and death. It is difficult to determine with certainty in an individual case whether this phenomenon is due to direct drug hepatoxicity or IRIS associated with hepatitis viruses.

Herpes Simplex Virus and Varicella Zoster Virus Disease after ART

Recurrence or exacerbation of mucocutaneous herpes simplex virus (HSV) disease may occur after ART is initiated. Sometimes lesions become hemorrhagic and exhibit significant tissue necrosis. Rarely HSV infection of the brain or spinal cord may be unmasked by commencing ART and be manifested as encephalitis or myelitis. Dermatomal or multidermatomal zoster lesions may also develop after commencing ART and are usually indistinguishable from zoster that occurs in patients not receiving ART. Rarely, myelitis may be associated with varicella-zoster virus infection.

DIAGNOSIS

Immunologic tests for diagnosing IRIS are currently not available for routine use. In the absence of diagnostic tests, IRIS may be established with diagnostic criteria that take into consideration the timing, clinical characteristics, and pathology of the disease, as well as the virologic response to the ART as measured by HIV viral load.

TREATMENT   Rx

The general approach to the treatment of IRIS is to continue ART and provide appropriate antimicrobial therapy for the provoking infection. Cessation of ART should be considered only in patients with life-threatening disease when all other measures have failed. Anti-inflammatory therapy should not be given routinely but be reserved for patients with severe inflammation, particularly when it is life-threatening, or significant symptoms. Corticosteroid therapy is used most often, but its effectiveness may vary from one type of IRIS to another. Thus, a randomized controlled trial in South Africa demonstrated that corticosteroids (prednisone 1.5 mg/kg/day for 2 weeks, then 0.75 mg/kg/day for 2 weeks) are a safe and effective treatment option for paradoxical TB-IRIS.[A1] In contrast, in an analysis of data from previously reported cases of PML-IRIS, it was suggested that corticosteroid therapy is not effective, although it was indicated that it may be effective if used early in the course. There is anecdotal evidence suggesting that corticosteroid therapy can be effective in other types of IRIS, but there are potential risks to using corticosteroid therapy in HIV patients who are already very immunodeficient, and it should be started only after weighing all considerations. Corticosteroid therapy for IRIS affecting the eye should be supervised by an ophthalmologist. Corticosteroid therapy may cause worsening of KS.

PREVENTION

Given that a low CD4+ T-cell count is a major risk factor for the development of IRIS, commencing ART at a CD4+ T-cell count higher than 350/μL, as recommended by treatment guidelines, will prevent most cases. However, this is not possible in patients who are seen for the first time with an OI or low CD4+ T cell count. Other strategies to prevent paradoxical IRIS are therefore under investigation. A randomized controlled trial demonstrated that the risk of paradoxical TB-IRIS could be reduced by 30% in high-risk patients (CD4+ T-cell count ≤100 cells/μL) with HIV-associated TB starting ART by prescribing prednisone for the first 4 weeks of ART (40 mg daily for 2 weeks then 20 mg daily for 2 weeks).[A2]

Several observations indicate that a high pathogen load is an important risk factor for IRIS, including the association with disseminated TB, a shorter duration of treatment of TB or cryptococcal meningitis, and positive CSF cultures for cryptococcal or *Mycobacterium tuberculosis* infections prior to commencing ART. Therefore, delaying the introduction of ART so that the OI can be fully treated might be beneficial. However, doing so may increase the risk for development of other OIs or cancers and of mortality. The results of an AIDS Clinical Trial Group study provided evidence supporting the introduction of ART within 1 to 2 weeks of starting antimicrobial therapy, particularly in patients with PJP. In addition, randomized controlled trials demonstrated that for patients with HIV-associated TB and CD4$^+$ T-cell count less than 50 cells/μL, the survival benefit of starting ART within the first 2 weeks of TB therapy outweighs the risk for IRIS and other adverse events.[A3-A6] Nevertheless, a more recent clinical trial of the effect of timing of ART initiation on TB treatment outcomes for HIV-positive patients with CD4$^+$ T-cell counts of 220 cells/μL or more showed that ART can be delayed until after completion of 6 months of TB treatment in this population.[A7] In contrast, commencing ART at the same time as treatment of cryptococcal meningitis has been shown to increase mortality when compared with delaying ART until 5 to 6 weeks after starting antifungal treatment.[A8] It seems probable that IRIS affecting the CNS is more likely than other types of IRIS to result in morbidity and mortality. Therefore, a single approach to this issue may not be possible, and a strategy for commencing antimicrobial therapy and ART may have to be determined for each pathogen or for infections of the CNS.

PROGNOSIS

The prognosis for patients in whom IRIS develops is highly variable because of differences in the extent of the infection by the provoking pathogen, the characteristics of the immunopathology caused by the restored immune response, and the body site affected. Most cases of IRIS are self-limited, and outcomes are usually good. However, mortality rates of up to 66% have been reported for C-IRIS. The mortality rate for TB-IRIS is much lower, but hospital admissions are common. Mortality and hospitalization rates are particularly high when TB-IRIS or C-IRIS affects the CNS. Indeed, involvement of the CNS by any type of IRIS may result in death or permanent neurologic disability. For example, mortality rates of 53% have been reported for paradoxical PML-IRIS and 31% for unmasking PML-IRIS. Furthermore, patients who survive PML-IRIS may have neurologic sequelae such as hemiparesis or seizures. Patients with lymphadenitis resulting from TB-IRIS[11] or NTM-IRIS and those with meningitis or cerebral lesions resulting from C-IRIS may experience recurrent relapses.

Autoimmune Disease and Sarcoidosis

Patients with HIV infection who are receiving ART have an increased susceptibility to some autoimmune diseases, mainly Graves disease, and sarcoidosis. Although sometimes referred to as types of IRIS, they appear to have a different immunopathogenesis.

Grade A References

A1. Meintjes G, Wilkinson RJ, Morroni C, et al. Randomized placebo-controlled trial of prednisone for paradoxical tuberculosis-associated immune reconstitution inflammatory syndrome. *AIDS.* 2010;24:2381-2390.

A2. Meintjes G, Stek C, Blumenthal L, et al. PredART Trial Team. Prednisone for the prevention of paradoxical tuberculosis-associated IRIS. *N Engl J Med.* 2018;379:1915-1925.

A3. Abdool Karim SS, Naidoo K, Grobler A, et al. Timing of initiation of antiretroviral drugs during tuberculosis therapy. *N Engl J Med.* 2010;362:697-706.

A4. Blanc FX, Sok T, Laureillard D, et al. CAMELIA (ANRS 1295–CIPRA KH001) Study Team. Earlier versus later start of antiretroviral therapy in HIV-infected adults with tuberculosis. *N Engl J Med.* 2011;365:1471-1481.

A5. Havlir DV, Kendall MA, Ive P, et al. AIDS Clinical Trials Group Study A5221. Timing of antiretroviral therapy for HIV-1 infection and tuberculosis. *N Engl J Med.* 2011;365:1482-1491.

A6. Uthman OA, Okwundu C, Gbenga K, et al. Optimal timing of antiretroviral therapy initiation for HIV-infected adults with newly diagnosed pulmonary tuberculosis: a systematic review and meta-analysis. *Ann Intern Med.* 2015;163:32-39.

A7. Mfinanga SG, Kirenga BJ, Chanda DM, et al. Early versus delayed initiation of highly active antiretroviral therapy for HIV-positive adults with newly diagnosed pulmonary tuberculosis (TB-HAART): a prospective, international, randomized, placebo-controlled trial. *Lancet Infect Dis.* 2014;14:563-571.

A8. Eshun-Wilson I, Okwen MP, Richardson M, et al. Early versus delayed antiretroviral treatment in HIV-positive people with cryptococcal meningitis. *Cochrane Database Syst Rev.* 2018;7:CD009012.

GENERAL REFERENCES

For the General References and other additional features, please visit Expert Consult at https://expertconsult.inkling.com.

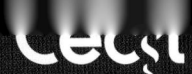

XXVI

NEUROLOGY

368

APPROACH TO THE PATIENT WITH NEUROLOGIC DISEASE

GABRIELE C. DELUCA AND ROBERT C. GRIGGS

INTRODUCTION

Neurologic diseases are encountered in all spheres of clinical practice. Many symptoms of nervous system diseases are a part of everyday experience for most healthy people, whether it be slips of the tongue, headache, numbness, muscle twitches, tremors, or mood swings with feelings of elation and depression. The challenge is to decipher whether symptoms fall within the spectrum of health or warrant further investigation. Neurology demands a pragmatic and skillful approach embedded in core principles of the clinical medicine.

CLINICAL MANIFESTATIONS

Knowledge of the structure and function of the nervous system is essential to the diagnostic method in neurology. Through a careful history and neurologic examination, the clinician can elicit the key symptoms and signs to formulate problems within an anatomic and pathophysiologic framework, thereby targeting appropriate evaluation.[1] The seasoned clinician can often swiftly arrive at the neurologic diagnosis by extracting the most relevant historical details and generating a hypothesis that can be tested and refined through a reliable neurologic examination. In evaluating a patient's symptoms and signs, it is valuable to arrive at a clinical diagnosis without reference to neurodiagnostic laboratory findings, which can often be normal when symptoms first appear. Furthermore, the widespread availability of neurodiagnostic imaging and electrophysiologic, biochemical, and genetic testing can lead to the detection of incidental "abnormalities" that often cause unnecessary concern, further evaluation, and potentially harmful treatment. In general, the adage that it is difficult to improve an asymptomatic patient should be kept in mind.

A practical approach to understand the basis of a patient's neurologic symptoms involves addressing three key questions:

1. *Are the symptoms neurologic?*

A patient may present with a constellation of symptoms that masquerade as neurologic (such as "dizziness" in a patient with cardiovascular disease, or perioral tingling in a patient with panic attacks) or as non-neurologic (such as intractable hiccups in a patient with a lesion in the area postrema of the medulla, or abdominal discomfort caused by a thoracic myelopathy). It is important to allow patients to describe symptoms in their own words. Direct questions are often necessary to characterize the problem fully. Terms such as weakness, numbness, heaviness, cramps, and tiredness may each mean pain, weakness, or alteration of sensation to some patients. Clarification of described symptoms provides critical clues to ascertain whether there is an underling neurologic basis for their presentation.

Context is also relevant, because a history of general medical and psychiatric problems may lead one to consider a non-neurologic cause. A history of physical abuse (Chapter 228) or alcohol (Chapter 30) and drug abuse (Chapter 31) can add a challenging layer of complexity to the interpretation of symptoms.

2. *Where is the lesion?*

The organization of the nervous system is such that diseases affecting a neuroanatomic structure usually give rise to specific constellations of neurologic symptoms and signs in keeping with the disrupted function of that structure. For this reason, the clinician should formulate a diagnostic opinion in anatomic terms. The neurologic history and clinical examination are best viewed as a search to detect a pattern of dysfunction where symptoms suggest a lesion of particular neuroanatomic units. The clinician should aim to discern which level of the nervous system is involved—the central nervous system (supratentorial [Videos 368-1 through 381-4], posterior fossa [Videos 368-5 and 386-6], spinal cord/column [Video 368-7]) or the peripheral nervous system (anterior horn cell [Video 368-8], nerve root, plexus [Video 368-9 and E-Fig. 368-1], peripheral nerve [Video 368-10 and E-Fig. 368-2], neuromuscular junction [Video 368-11], muscle [Videos 368-12 and 368-13 and E-Figs. 368-3 through 368-6])—and whether the process is focal (midline or lateralized) or diffuse. Relevant questions include

the following: Can one disease account for all of the symptoms and signs? A second issue is whether the history is suggestive of a single focus (e.g., stroke or tumor) or multiple sites of nervous system involvement (e.g., multiple sclerosis), or part of a systemic disease (e.g., vitamin B_{12} deficiency, myopathy, or polyneuropathy).

3. *What is the lesion?*

In neurologic diagnosis, the history usually indicates the nature of the disease or the diagnosis, whereas the neurologic examination localizes it and quantitates its severity. In arriving at a diagnosis, the following points are useful: consider the patient's entire medical history; consider the tempo and duration of the symptoms; determine whether the symptoms have been progressive without remission, or whether there have been plateaus or periods of return to normal. Symptoms with an acute onset suggest a vascular cause (Chapter 378) or seizure (Chapter 375); symptoms that are subacute in onset suggest a mass lesion, such as tumor (Chapter 180) or abscess (Chapter 385); symptoms that have a waxing and waning course with exacerbations and remissions suggest a central demyelinating cause (Chapter 383); and symptoms that are chronic and progressive suggest a degenerative disorder. Toxic and metabolic syndromes (Chapter 388) are typically diffuse and can manifest acutely or chronically.

DIAGNOSIS

History

The neurologic history is the most important component of neurologic diagnosis. For many diseases, the history is almost the only avenue to explore. Examples of such disorders include headaches (Chapter 370), seizures (Chapter 375), developmental disorders (Chapter 389), memory disorders (Chapter 374), and behavioral diseases (Chapter 369). A careful history frequently determines the cause. When a neurologic problem is suspected, the physician should begin to try to localize the lesion, a process that aids in establishing whether the disease is diffuse or focal.

The history is often the only way of diagnosing neurologic illnesses that typically have normal or nonfocal findings on neurologic examination. Such illnesses include paroxysmal disorders (such as many seizure disorders [Chapter 375], narcolepsy [Chapter 377], migraine, and most other headache syndromes [Chapter 370], as well as the various causes of dizziness), and most types of dementia. The neurologic history may often provide the first clues that a symptom is psychological (Chapter 369) in origin.

To guide the clinician in obtaining a meaningful neurologic history, the following are points to consider:

- *Carefully identify the chief complaint or problem.* Not only is the chief complaint important in providing the first clue to the physician about the differential diagnosis, but it is also the reason the patient is seeking medical advice and treatment. If the chief complaint is not properly identified and addressed, the correct diagnosis may be missed and an inappropriate diagnostic evaluation may be undertaken. Establishing a diagnosis that does not incorporate the chief complaint frequently focuses attention on a coincidental process irrelevant to the patient's concerns.

- *Begin with open-ended questions and listen carefully to the patient as long as necessary.* The patient often volunteers the most important information at the start of the history. A good rule of thumb is to listen initially for at least 5 minutes without interrupting the patient. During this time, insight into the patient's mental status (including level of alertness, cognitive function, and behavior), cranial nerve function (e.g., ocular movements [Video 368-5], facial asymmetry [Video 368-13], speech disturbances [Video 368-11]), and motor function (e.g., increase or paucity of spontaneous movements as seen with movement disorders [Video 368-4]) can be gleaned. This period of intent listening and observation allows the physician to follow up with focused and relevant questions and clinical examination maneuvers to formulate an accurate diagnostic opinion.

- *Obtain a collateral history from surrogate historians.* Surrogate historians often provide key or missing information about the onset and evolution of neurologic disorders that alter mental status, whether episodic (e.g., loss of consciousness in syncope [Chapter 56] or epilepsy [Chapter 375, Videos 368-1 and 368-2]) or progressive (e.g., degenerative dementia [Chapter 374] or cerebral tumor [Chapter 180]) or influence a patient's awareness of disease (e.g., anosognosia in nondominant hemispheric lesions). Importantly, surrogate historians can provide real-life context that casts light onto the severity and impact of the patient's symptoms on his or her functional status.

- *Take a complete past medical, medication, psychiatric, family, and social and occupational history.* Many neurologic illnesses are complications of underlying medical disorders or are due to adverse effects of drugs. For example, posterior reversible vasoconstriction syndrome can be a complication of renal disease (Chapter 121) and encephalopathy after bariatric surgery can be secondary to thiamine deficiency (Chapter 388). Parkinsonism (Chapter 381) is a frequent complication of the use of antinausea medicines (e.g., metoclopramide or prochlorperazine) and many neuroleptic agents (Chapter 406). A large number of neurologic disorders have a hereditary component, so a positive family history often can help establish the diagnosis. Occupational exposures play a role in various neurologic disorders, such as carpal tunnel syndrome (e.g., repetitive injury in machine operators or people who use keyboards), peripheral neuropathy (e.g., lead or other toxin exposure), and parkinsonism (e.g., heavy metal exposure).

- *Summarize the history for the patient.* A summary of the history is an effective way to ensure that all details were covered sufficiently for a tentative diagnosis to be made. This summary provides an opportunity for the physician to fill in historical gaps not apparent when the history was initially taken, as well as for the patient or surrogate to correct any historical misinformation.
- *End by asking if the patient had considered or was concerned about a particular diagnosis and what the patient's expectations are for the visit.* These questions allow the physician to evaluate the patient's concerns about and insight into his or her symptoms and/or condition. Some patients have a specific diagnosis in mind that spurs them to seek medical attention. Multiple sclerosis (Chapter 383, Videos 368-5 and 368-6), amyotrophic lateral sclerosis (Chapter 391, Video 368-8), Alzheimer disease (Chapter 374), and brain tumors (Chapter 180) are diseases that patients often suspect may be the cause of their neurologic symptoms. The discussion will also help guide how to discuss prognosis, especially in patients with advanced neurologic disease.
- *Avoid referral bias and keep an open mind.* Often patients come to a consultation with a neurologic diagnosis already in mind, whether it be self-generated or from the referring physician. In these situations, it is important to steer the patient away from discussions of previous diagnostic test results and the opinions of previous health care professionals. Abnormal results on laboratory and imaging studies may be incidental to the patient's primary problem or, in some instances, may simply represent a normal variant. In addition, patients often browse websites and fit their symptoms to a diagnostic entity. Clinicians can sometimes be influenced by the opinion of their colleagues and, as a result, potentially overlook key historical elements that may prove central to the diagnosis.

Important Considerations: Physical Abuse and Substance Abuse

Traumatic injury (Chapter 371) and substance abuse (Chapters 30 and 31) are usually difficult to detect by the medical history and examination. Physically, sexually, and/or emotionally abused individuals are often unable or unwilling to report abuse even though such harm may cause or contribute to symptoms. People who abuse alcohol (Chapter 30) or toxins (Chapters 31 and 102) do not typically give an accurate account of their use of these agents, which themselves may cause a host of neurologic disorders. Therefore a systematic and sensitive consideration of the possibility of these frequent causes of neurologic symptoms is important in every patient. Awareness of and attention to the often-subtle signs that suggest physical trauma (Chapter 228) is of paramount importance.

ACUTE NEUROLOGIC DISORDERS REQUIRING IMMEDIATE DIAGNOSIS AND TREATMENT

Most neurologic diagnoses are made by a careful, thorough history and an appropriately complete examination. However, the tempo of illness and the availability of life-saving treatment that is effective only if administered within minutes of evaluating a patient dictate rapid action in several specific circumstances. Coma (Chapter 376), repetitive seizures (Chapter 375), acute stroke (Chapters 379 and 380), suspected meningitis and encephalitis (Chapters 384 and 386), head and spine trauma (Chapter 371), and acute spinal cord compression are diagnosed by clinical and laboratory assessment, and urgent treatment must be instituted as soon as ventilation and cardiac status are stabilized.

For acute spinal cord compression, the differential diagnosis includes transverse myelopathy (Chapter 383), spinal shock (Chapter 371), central cord syndrome (Chapter 371), hemicord (Brown-Séquard) syndrome (Chapter 371), conus medullaris syndrome (Chapter 372), and cauda equina syndrome (Chapters 346 and 372). The cause may be acute spinal trauma (Chapter 371), a spinal epidural abscess (Chapter 385), or a spinal epidural hematoma

(Chapter 372). Emergent imaging followed, if possible, by targeted surgical therapy is indicated.[2]

NEUROLOGIC EXAMINATION

The neurologic examination is an extension of the history that can affirm the presence of disease; detect unsuspected or subclinical findings; localize the process, when there is a fixed lesion; and provide a clue to etiology. For these reasons, many tests of neurologic function are routinely indicated in all patients. For practical purposes, however, there is no "complete" neurologic examination; the skilled clinician implements a core examination and adds/subtracts layers, as clinically indicated.

The neurologic examination should be tailored to the clinical setting of the patient. The approach to an ambulatory office patient is considerably different than the approach to a critically ill patient. The examination of a patient with specific complaints focuses on findings pertinent to that patient. Thus more detailed testing of cognition is indicated in patients with behavioral or memory disturbance, and more detailed testing of sensation should be performed in patients with complaints of pain, numbness, or weakness. It is important to perform all routine tests in patients with abnormalities in one sphere of neurologic dysfunction; otherwise, erroneous localization of a lesion or disease process can occur. For deviations from normal to be recognized and quantitated, a physician must have extensive experience in the routine assessment of healthy individuals.

The General Examination

Specific neurologic symptoms or signs should prompt a general physical examination focused on conditions that may have neurologic significance. Examination of the scalp and skull should focus on any abnormalities of the contour or symmetry. Localized thickening of the skull or a cluster of abnormal blood vessels could suggest an underlying meningioma (Chapter 180) or arteriovenous malformation (Chapter 380); depressions in the skull may represent the consequence of fracture (Chapter 371). An enlarged head circumference in an adult (greater than 55 to 60 cm) is occasionally a normal, often hereditary variant, but could point toward a long-standing anomaly of the brain or spinal cord in a patient with underlying central nervous system disease. Neck range of motion, straight leg raising, and spinal curvature (scoliosis; Chapter 92) should be assessed. Deformities of the spinal column or extremities may suggest the cause of presenting neurologic signs or provide an adequate non-neurologic explanation for the chief complaint.

The skin should be inspected for neurofibromas and café au lait maculae (e.g., neurofibromatosis type I; Chapter 389), adenoma sebaceum (e.g., tuberous sclerosis; Chapter 389), lipomas (e.g., lipomatosis), vascular nevi (e.g., Sturge-Weber syndrome [Chapter 389] if in trigeminal nerve distribution), and brown hair nevi/pad of fat or skin dimple (e.g., spina bifida or myelodysplasia when found over the sacral region). Peripheral nerve lesions may be associated with vasomotor or trophic changes to the overlying skin and/or irregular hair or nail growth.

Assessment of blood pressure and heart rate (with orthostatic measurements, where indicated) should be routinely performed. Carotid auscultation for bruits is indicated in older adults, especially in the presence of focal neurologic symptoms or signs. Evaluation of peripheral pulses may provide important clues relevant to sensory or motor complaints.

In patients with bladder, bowel, or leg symptoms, evaluation of rectal sphincter tone is usually indicated. Limitation of joint range of motion or painless swelling of joints may be a sign of an unsuspected neurologic lesion. The presence of enlarged lymph nodes should raise suspicion of underlying infection or malignancy affecting not only those nodes but also parts of the nervous system.

Components of the Neurologic Examination

The neurologic examination begins with the first sight of the patient and continues throughout the consultation. The handshake, manner of walking and seating, nature of clothing, and general comportment can provide useful clues that help guide the history and examination. Facial features such as prominent supraorbital ridges and jaw (acromegaly; Chapter 211), protruding ocular globes and eyelid retraction with staring expression (exophthalmic goiter; Chapter 213), frontal balding, ptosis, and drooping mouth (myotonic dystrophy; Chapter 393, Video 368-12, E-Fig. 368-3), fatigable ptosis and snarling expression (myasthenia gravis; Chapter 394, Video 368-11), and masked facies with reduced blink frequency (Parkinson disease; Chapter 381, Video 368-4) should alert the clinician along specific lines of inquiry and examination.

The various aspects of the detailed neurologic examination are considered in specific symptom and disease sections noted later. The major divisions of the examination include mental status, cranial nerves, motor (including reflexes), sensory, cerebellar/coordination, and gait and should form part of the clinician's "core" examination and be assessed in all patients.

A careful medical history usually provides an adequate assessment of mental status: level of consciousness, orientation, memory, language function, affect, and judgment[3]; abnormalities in any of these functions demand more detailed testing. Detailed mental status testing is also indicated when the chief complaint suggests a cognitive problem.

Cranial nerve function that should be tested in all patients includes visual acuity (with and without correction); optic fundi; visual fields; pupils (size and reactivity to direct and consensual light); ocular motility (Video 368-5); jaw, facial, palatal, neck, and tongue movement (e.g., tongue fasciculations, Video 368-8); and hearing.

Examination of motor function (Chapter 393) is essential in all patients. The patient should be observed for tremor (Chapter 382, Videos 368-4 and 368-10) and other abnormal movements, and the muscles inspected for fasciculations (Video 368-8). Muscle bulk (atrophy or hypertrophy) and tone (flaccid, spastic, or rigid) and muscle strength can be assessed rapidly. The distribution of weakness often sheds light on localization based on the pattern (e.g., upper motor neuron, myotomal, peripheral [Videos 368-9 through 368-11 and 368-13]). Strength testing should include assessment of specific functional activities, including the ability to sit up from a supine position, to rise from a deep knee bend or deep chair, to walk on heel and toe, to lift the arms over the head, and to make a tight fist.

Muscle stretch reflexes are the most objective component of the motor examination and are useful in confirming the localization (i.e., central versus peripheral) of motor dysfunction. Reflexes and plantar responses should take into account right-left symmetry and disparity between proximal and distal reflexes in a limb or between arm and leg reflexes. Biceps, triceps, brachioradialis, quadriceps, and ankle reflexes should be quantitated from 0 to 4 (0 = absent; 1 = hypoactive; 2 = normal; 3 = brisk; 4 = clonus).

Sensory testing (Chapter 392) need not be detailed unless there are sensory symptoms. However, the evaluation of at least one large fiber (e.g., vibration or joint position sense with use of tuning fork or by moving a distal joint, respectively) and one small fiber (e.g., pain or temperature with respective use of a single-use pin or warmed tuning fork) should be performed. If sensory changes do not follow a peripheral pattern, cortical sensory function should be tested (i.e., two point discrimination, graphesthesia, stereognosis).

Appendicular (finger-nose-finger, heel-to-shin) and truncal (station) function (Video 368-6) should be assessed. Rapid alternating movements of the tongue, hands, fingers, and feet can point to a pyramidal, extrapyramidal, or cerebellar lesion if the rate, amplitude (Video 368-4), or rhythm is affected. Asymmetry of movement should be noted.

The assessment of a patient's ability to stand and walk provides important clues about motor, sensory, and cerebellar function. The patient should be instructed to walk across the room normally, then on his or her heels, then toes, and then in tandem (heel to toe) (Videos 368-4, 368-6, and 368-10). If an ambulatory patient is able to rise from a deep knee bend and walk on heels and toes, lower limb strength is likely normal and may preclude the need for individual muscle testing. Postural instability should be evaluated (Videos 368-4 and 368-6).

The Comatose Patient

In the patients with reduced level of consciousness, lesions in the ascending reticular activating system, thalamus, or diffuse injury to the cerebral hemispheres should be considered. To evaluate these possibilities, a rapid examination that differs considerably from an alert, aware individual is required (Chapter 376). In such patients, many aspects of the neurologic examination cannot be tested, but considerable information can still be gleaned. On inspection, attention should focus on the examination of the level of consciousness, respiratory pattern, position of eyelids and eyes in primary gaze, size of pupils, and spontaneous eye and limb movements. Signs of injury related to seizures, including tongue biting, should be sought. Assessment of the optic fundi should look for hemorrhage (Fig. 395-22) or papilledema (Fig. 395-25), and examination of cranial nerve reflexes, including pupillary, corneal, vestibulocular, and gag reflexes, can provide valuable insight into possible contributory intracranial processes and brainstem function. The nature and distribution of motor responses to (painful) stimuli provide localization value. Muscle stretch reflexes when obviously asymmetrical suggest dysfunction of the motor unit. However, minor asymmetries are much less important than in an awake patient, especially given that reflexes are likely to fluctuate from one moment to the next. Particular elements of the general examination must also be assessed quickly: evidence of cranial and spinal trauma, tenderness of the skull to percussion, nuchal rigidity (but not in patients with head or neck trauma), and evidence of physical abuse.

⬤ COMMON COMPLAINTS OF POSSIBLE NEUROLOGIC ORIGIN

Spontaneous Movements

Muscle tremors, jerks, twitches, cramps, and spasms (Chapter 382) are frequent symptoms. The cause of spontaneous movements can reside at any level of the nervous system. In general, movements that occur in an entire limb or in more than one muscle group concurrently are caused by central nervous system disease. Movements confined to a single muscle are likely to be a reflection of disease of the motor unit (including the motor neurons of the brainstem and spinal cord; Video 368-8). When spontaneous movements of a muscle are associated with severe pain, patients often use the term "cramp." Cramp is a medically defined disorder that reflects the intense contraction of a large group of motor units. Leg cramps are occasionally a sign of an underlying disease of the anterior horn cell, nerve roots, or peripheral nerve; however, cramps are frequent in normal persons and particularly common in older patients, and they are usually benign. When cramps are severe, they can produce such intense muscle contraction that muscle injury is caused and muscle enzyme (e.g., creatine kinase) levels are elevated in blood.

The rare muscle diseases in which an enzyme deficiency interferes with substrate use as fuel for exercise (e.g., McArdle disease; Chapter 393) are often associated with severe exercise-provoked muscle contractures. These contractures are electrically silent on electromyography, in contrast to the intense motor unit activity seen with cramps. Such contractures should not be confused with the limitation of joint range of motion resulting from long-standing joint disease or long-standing weakness, also termed *contractures*.

The intense muscle contractions of tetany are frequently painful. Although tetany is usually a reflection of hypocalcemia (Chapter 232), it can occasionally be seen without demonstrable electrolyte disturbance. Tetany results from hyperexcitability of peripheral nerves. Similarly, in the syndrome of tetanus produced by a clostridial toxin (Chapter 280), intensely painful life-threatening muscle contractions arise from hyperexcitable peripheral nerves. A number of toxic disorders, such as strychnine poisoning and black widow spider envenomation, produce similar neurogenic spasms.

Muscle Pain

Acute muscle pain in the absence of abnormal muscle contractions is an extremely common symptom. When such pain occurs after strenuous exercise or in the context of an acute viral illness (e.g., influenza), it probably reflects muscle injury. In such patients, the serum creatine kinase level is often raised. It is uncommon for this frequent and essentially normal sign of muscle injury to be associated with weakness or demonstrable ongoing muscle disease. Chronic muscle pain is a common symptom but is seldom related to a definable disease of muscle. Muscle pain in the presence of progressive proximal muscle weakness should suggest an underlying inflammatory or immune-mediated myopathy (Chapters 253 and 393).

Weakness

It is axiomatic that patients typically have motor signs before motor symptoms and, conversely, sensory symptoms before sensory signs. Thus patients with even severe weakness may not report symptoms of weakness. Somewhat paradoxically, patients who complain of "weakness" often do not have confirmatory findings on examination that document the presence of weakness.

When weakness is confirmed to be a symptom of underlying neurologic disease, a lesion of the peripheral nervous system (i.e., motor unit) is the frequent culprit (Chapters 391, 393, and 394). The pattern of weakness (i.e., upper motor neuron versus lower motor neuron) and associated neurologic signs and symptoms help localize the responsible lesion (Videos 368-3 and 368-6 through 368-13; E-Figs. 368-1 through 368-6). The symptom of weakness in the absence of objective weakness on neurologic examination is more likely to be a symptom of disease outside of the nervous system altogether (Table 368-1) than to be attributable to neuromuscular disease.

Episodic and Intermittent Weakness

The complaint of attacks of severe weakness or paralysis in a patient with normal baseline strength is uncommon and suggests an underlying ion channelopathy (e.g., periodic paralysis; Chapter 393) or neuromuscular junction disorder (e.g., myasthenia gravis [Video 368-11] or the myasthenic syndrome; Chapter 394). Patients with narcolepsy also occasionally complain of intermittent paralysis as a reflection of sleep paralysis (Chapter 377). Exposure to heat in a patient with a demyelinating disease such as multiple sclerosis (Chapter

TABLE 368-1 DISORDERS COMMONLY ACCOMPANIED BY WEAKNESS

NEUROLOGIC CAUSES
Central Nervous System
- Upper motor neuron lesions—spasticity (e.g., amyotrophic lateral sclerosis, multiple sclerosis, stroke)
- Basal ganglia disorders—rigidity (e.g., Parkinson disease)

Peripheral Nervous System
- Disorders of the motor unit (e.g., peripheral neuropathy, myopathy)

NON-NEUROLOGIC CAUSES
- Heart failure
- Respiratory insufficiency
- Renal, hepatic, and other metabolic disease
- Alcoholism and other toxin-related disease
- Functional disorders
- Psychiatric disorders (e.g., depression, factitious disorders, malingering)

TABLE 368-2 CHARACTERISTIC GAIT DISORDERS

SPECIFIC DISORDER	LOCATION OF LESION	CHARACTERISTICS
Spastic gait	Bilateral corticospinal pathways within the thoracic or cervical cord or in the brain	Legs stiff, feet turning inward, "scissoring"
Hemiparetic gait	Unilateral central nervous system, cervical cord, or brain	Affected leg circumducted, foot extended, arm flexed
Sensory ataxia	Posterior columns of the spinal cord or peripheral nerve	Wide-based, high steps; Romberg sign present
Cerebellar ataxia	Brainstem or cerebellum	Wide-based steps; Romberg sign absent
Parkinsonian gait	Basal ganglia	Shuffling, small steps
Dystonic gait	Basal ganglia; also corticospinal pathways	Abnormal posture of the arms, head, neck
Gait disorder of the elderly	Multifactorial: bihemispheric disease, spinal cord disease, impaired proprioception, muscle weakness	Stooped posture, wide-based steps; often retropulsion
Steppage gait	Distal muscle weakness	High steps ("steppage")
Waddling gait	Proximal muscle weakness	Both legs circumducted to allow locking of the knees
Antalgic gait	Non-neurologic; reflects disease of joints, bones, or soft tissue	Minimizes pain in the hip, spine, leg
Hysterical gait	Psychiatric or behavioral disorder	Reeling side to side, associated astasia-abasia, bizarre arm and trunk movements

383) also may cause intermittent weakness, but other features of an underlying upper motor neuron lesion are typically seen (Videos 368-6 and 368-7).

Dizziness
Dizziness is a vague term that can mean one of many things to a patient, including vertigo (illusion of world spinning; Chapter 400), unsteadiness (imbalance without abnormal head sensation), lightheadedness (sense of impending faint; Chapter 56), or a sensation of wooziness (a difficult to describe floating sensation; Chapter 56).[4,5] Vertigo (Fig. 400-3) suggests disease of the labyrinth, vestibular nerve, brainstem, or cerebellum as a probable cause. When unsteadiness and loss of balance are not associated with vertigo, particularly if the unsteadiness appears to be out of proportion to other symptoms of the patient, a widespread disorder of sensory or motor function is likely (e.g., multiple sclerosis [Video 368-6] or Charcot-Marie-Tooth disease [Video 368-10]). In the unsteady patient, one should also consider extrapyramidal (Video 368-4) (e.g., Parkinson disease), cerebellar, and endocrine (e.g., hypothyroidism) disorders. Lightheadedness is typically not from a focal neurologic disorder and should prompt the clinician to consider cardiac dysrhythmias, neurally mediated syncope (e.g., vasovagal), endocrine, or autonomic causes (Chapter 56).

Abnormal Gait and Posture
The ability to stand and walk in a well-coordinated, effortless fashion requires integrity of the entire nervous system.[6] Relatively subtle deficits localized to one part of the nervous system produce characteristic abnormalities (Table 368-2 and Videos 368-4, 368-6, and 368-10).

Sensory Symptoms and Pain
Sensory symptoms, which can be negative or positive, and pain are among the most common neurologic complaints. Negative symptoms refer to a loss of sensation, such as numbness, whereas positive symptoms, which can occur either spontaneously or when evoked by stimulation of sensory receptors, include paresthesias and dysesthesias. Paresthesias refer to a feeling of tingling, crawling, itching, compression, tightness, cold, or heat. Dysesthesias refer to abnormal, unpleasant sensations, often tingling, discomfort, or pain. Dysesthesias include hyperalgesia (increased pain from a stimulus that normally provokes pain) and allodynia (pain evoked by innocuous stimuli). In contrast, hypoesthesia denotes decreased sensitivity to stimulation (e.g., loss or impairment of touch), with hypoalgesia specifically referring to a diminished pain response to a normally painful stimulus.

For pain (Chapter 27), the initial goal is to ascertain whether the pain is secondary to a lesion in the nervous system (neuropathic pain), disease of visceral or somatic structures (nociceptive pain), or without identifiable organic cause (idiopathic pain). Neuropathic pain most commonly originates from lesions of the peripheral nerves and spinal roots, but interruption of sensory fibers in the central nervous system are also an important cause.

Peripheral neuropathies lead to sensory disturbances that depend on the population of affected nerves (Chapter 392). In large-fiber predominant neuropathies, paresthesias are common; on examination, vibration and joint position sense are impaired. In contrast, pain and temperature appreciation are relatively preserved. Movement can become clumsy and ataxic, and tendon reflexes are lost early. With severe loss of proprioception, patients may develop pseudoathetoid movements of the outstretched hands, sensory ataxia, or postural and action tremors (Video 368-10). In contrast, small-fiber predominant neuropathies commonly present with spontaneous pain that may be burning, lancinating, or aching in quality. Pain and temperature are disproportionately affected in these neuropathies, and autonomic dysfunction may be a feature. Examples of small-fiber neuropathies include diabetes (Chapter 216) and alcoholism (Chapter 30). Most sensory neuropathies have sensory loss that begins distally and is dependent on the distance of the nerve ending from the spinal cord. By comparison, lesions affecting the dorsal root ganglia, which give rise to sensory neuronopathies, may also involve the trunk and face. Sensory changes in a radiculopathy owing to a nerve root lesion (Chapter 372) conform to a dermatome. Root pain is typically aggravated or intensified by maneuvers that stretch the involved nerve root, such as the straight-leg raising test or by bending forward via traction on the sciatic nerve. With distal nerve root involvement, as in the cauda equine syndrome, sensory deficits involve multiple roots and may lead to saddle anesthesia and reduced sensation associated with the passage of urine or feces.

Spinal cord lesions can lead to sensory symptoms, the nature of which depends on the part of the cord affected. With involvement of the dorsal columns, such as occurs in multiple sclerosis (Chapter 383), vitamin B_{12} deficiency (Chapter 388), and cervical spondylosis (Chapter 372), patients commonly report a feeling of compression or bandlike tightness in the affected region. They may also experience Lhermitte sign (paresthesia radiating down the back and/or limbs on neck flexion). Examination reveals ipsilateral impairment of vibration and joint position senses, with relative sparing of pain and temperature sensation. Conversely, with involvement of the spinothalamic tracts in the anterolateral columns (as in cordotomy) or central cord where spinothalamic fibers decussate (as in syringomyelia; Chapter 389), patients will have impaired pain and temperature sensation with relative preservation of vibration, joint position sense, and light touch. Thalamic lesions cause dense hemibody (i.e., face, arm, trunk, and leg) sensory loss and can be associated with a thalamic pain syndrome. Somatosensory cortical lesions cause contralateral sensory loss of varying distribution; lateral cortical involvement leads to sensory alteration in the face and arm compared with medial cortical involvement, which causes predominant leg symptoms. Dysfunction of cortical sensory modalities, including trouble with two-point discrimination, graphesthesia, and stereognosis, is a typical feature. For both central and peripheral lesions, motor deficits may also be present and help localize the lesion.

Fatigue

Complaints of fatigue, tiredness, and lack of energy are usually symptoms of disease outside the nervous system. Medical conditions associated with a complaint of "weakness" (e.g., anemia, endocrine dysfunction, or inflammatory disease) and psychiatric and behavioral disorders (Chapter 369) are all frequent causes of fatigue. Chronic fatigue syndrome and many cases of fibromyalgia (Chapter 258) have fatigue as a predominant and disabling symptom. These disorders are defined in part by the absence of consistent neurologic findings and lack of demonstrable disease in the nervous system.

Neurologic disorders associated with fatigue through mechanisms that are not known include multiple sclerosis (Chapter 383; Videos 368-6 and 368-7), Parkinson disease (Chapter 381; Video 368-4), and motor neuron disease (Chapter 391; Video 368-8). Sleep disorders (Chapter 377) may also include fatigue as a prominent symptom.

NEUROLOGIC DIAGNOSTIC PROCEDURES

Lumbar Puncture

Lumbar puncture accesses cerebrospinal fluid (CSF) in the lumbar cistern of the subarachnoid space for both diagnostic and therapeutic purposes. On average, a patient's discomfort should be only slightly greater than for a blood draw.[7] Ultrasonography can help identify the optimal site for the procedure,[A1] and atraumatic needles can reduce pain and the incidence of post–lumbar puncture headache.[A2]

Laboratory evaluation of CSF is crucial for the accurate diagnosis of meningeal infections and carcinomatosis and is useful in the assessment of inflammatory and demyelinating diseases. CSF analysis is also helpful to evaluate for hemorrhage, particularly when imaging studies are inconclusive (Fig. 368-1). For example, the combination of less than 2000 red blood cells/μL and the absence of xanthochromia excludes the diagnosis of aneurysmal subarachnoid hemorrhage with a sensitivity of 100% and a specificity of 91%.[8] The measurement of β-amyloid-42/total tau and β-amyloid-42/hyperphosphorylated tau can identify early Alzheimer disease with high accuracy.[9] In terms of therapeutic uses, lumbar puncture allows removal of CSF to lower intracranial pressure (as seen in idiopathic intracranial hypertension; Chapter 370) and access to the CSF for drug delivery.

Lumbar puncture is otherwise contraindicated in patients with evidence of raised intracranial pressure (e.g., secondary to obstructive noncommunicating hydrocephalus, focal mass lesion, or hemorrhage), a bleeding diathesis (e.g., thrombocytopenia or a prolonged international normalized ratio [INR]), local skin infection, or developmental anomaly (e.g., myelomeningocele). In patients with suspected meningitis or encephalitis, emergent lumbar puncture is critical. However, the administration of empiric antibiotic or antiviral therapy should not be delayed if the lumbar puncture is delayed to obtain brain imaging in patients who have focal findings or papilledema or if there are technical difficulties in performing the lumbar puncture itself (Chapter 384).[10] Neuroimaging should be performed before lumbar puncture in patients who are over age 60 years; are immunocompromised; or have papilledema, a reduced level of consciousness, or focal findings on the neurologic examination.

The CSF formula often provides an important clue to the pathologic process involved (Table 368-3). An elevated white blood cell count is seen with infections and other inflammatory diseases, as well as with carcinomatosis. The differential white blood cell count may point to a specific class of pathogen;

polymorphonuclear leukocytes suggest a bacterial process, whereas mononuclear cells suggest a viral, fungal, or immunologic cause. The CSF glucose concentration is typically reduced to less than 50% of a simultaneous serum concentration in bacterial and fungal infections, as well as with certain viral infections (e.g., mumps virus) and sarcoidosis. The CSF protein concentration is elevated in a variety of disorders, including most infections and demyelinating neuropathies. If malignancy is being considered, CSF cytology is useful in the detection of primary brain tumors, metastatic lesions, and lymphomas.

CSF polymerase chain reaction (PCR) is a rapid, sensitive, and specific test that is useful for suspected viral infections, including herpes simplex types 1 and 2, varicella zoster, Epstein-Barr virus, cytomegalovirus, and enterovirus.[11] PCR for tuberculosis is more specific than a smear for acid-fast bacilli, but its lack of sensitivity makes cultures the diagnostic gold standard. The CSF Venereal Disease Research Laboratory (VDRL) assay is a relatively specific although insensitive test for neurosyphilis (Chapter 303).

Specialized CSF tests for oligoclonal bands that are more abundant in the CSF than a paired serum sample are found in most patients with multiple sclerosis (Videos 368-6 and 368-7) but are not specific to this disease and can be seen in other inflammatory and noninflammatory conditions, including systemic lupus erythematosus, neurosarcoidosis, cerebral angiitis, paraneoplastic disorders, human immunodeficiency virus infection, and stroke. The detection of antibodies in the CSF is helpful to diagnose an expanding number of autoimmune neurologic diseases and encephalitides (Chapter 383).

Electroencephalography

Electroencephalography, which is the recording and measurement of scalp electrical potential, provides useful information about baseline brain function and paroxysmal brain electrical activity suggestive of a seizure disorder.[12] A

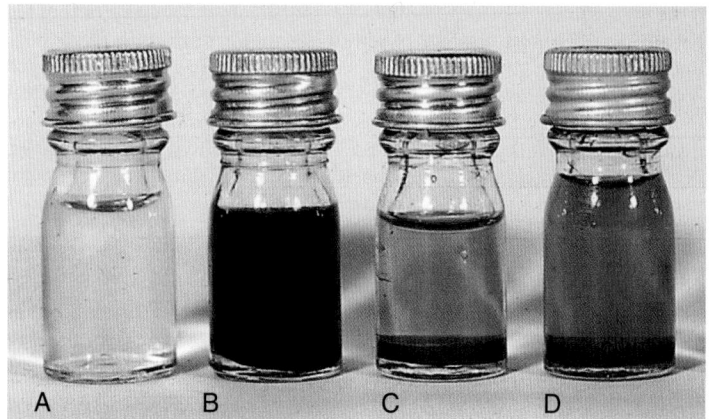

FIGURE 368-1. Cerebrospinal fluid (CSF) examination. **A,** Normal crystal-clear CSF. **B,** Blood in the CSF, which could result from a traumatic (bloody) tap or from subarachnoid hemorrhage. In a traumatic tap, subsequent tubes of CSF are usually less bloody. **C,** Centrifuged CSF in a traumatic tap. The supernatant is nearly clear. **D,** CSF from a patient with subarachnoid hemorrhage. There is blood at the bottom of the tube and the supernatant is yellow (xanthochromic) as a result of breakdown of blood cells in the CSF before the lumbar puncture. (From Forbes CD, Jackson WD. *Color Atlas and Text of Clinical Medicine.* 3rd ed. London: Mosby; 2003, with permission.)

TABLE 368-3 CHARACTERISTIC CEREBROSPINAL FLUID FORMULAS

	TURBIDITY AND COLOR	OPENING PRESSURE	WBC COUNT	DIFFERENTIAL CELLS	RBC COUNT	PROTEIN	GLUCOSE
Normal	Clear, colorless	70-180 mm H$_2$O	0-5 cells/μL	Mononuclear	0	<60 mg/dL	>½ serum
Bacterial meningitis	Cloudy, straw colored	↑	↑↑	PMNs	0	↑↑	↓
Viral meningitis	Clear or cloudy, colorless	↑	↑	Lymphocytes	0	↑	Normal
Fungal and tuberculous meningitis	Cloudy, straw colored	↑	↑	Lymphocytes	0	↑↑	↓↓
Viral encephalitis	Clear or cloudy, straw colored	Normal to ↑	↑	Lymphocytes	0 (herpes ↑)	Normal to ↑	Normal
Subarachnoid hemorrhage	Cloudy, pink	↑	↑	PMNs and lymphocytes	↑↑	↑	Normal (early); ↓ (late)
Guillain-Barré syndrome	Clear, yellow	Normal to ↑	0-5 cells/μL	Mononuclear	0	↑	Normal

PMN = polymorphonuclear leukocyte; RBC = red blood cell; WBC = white blood cell.

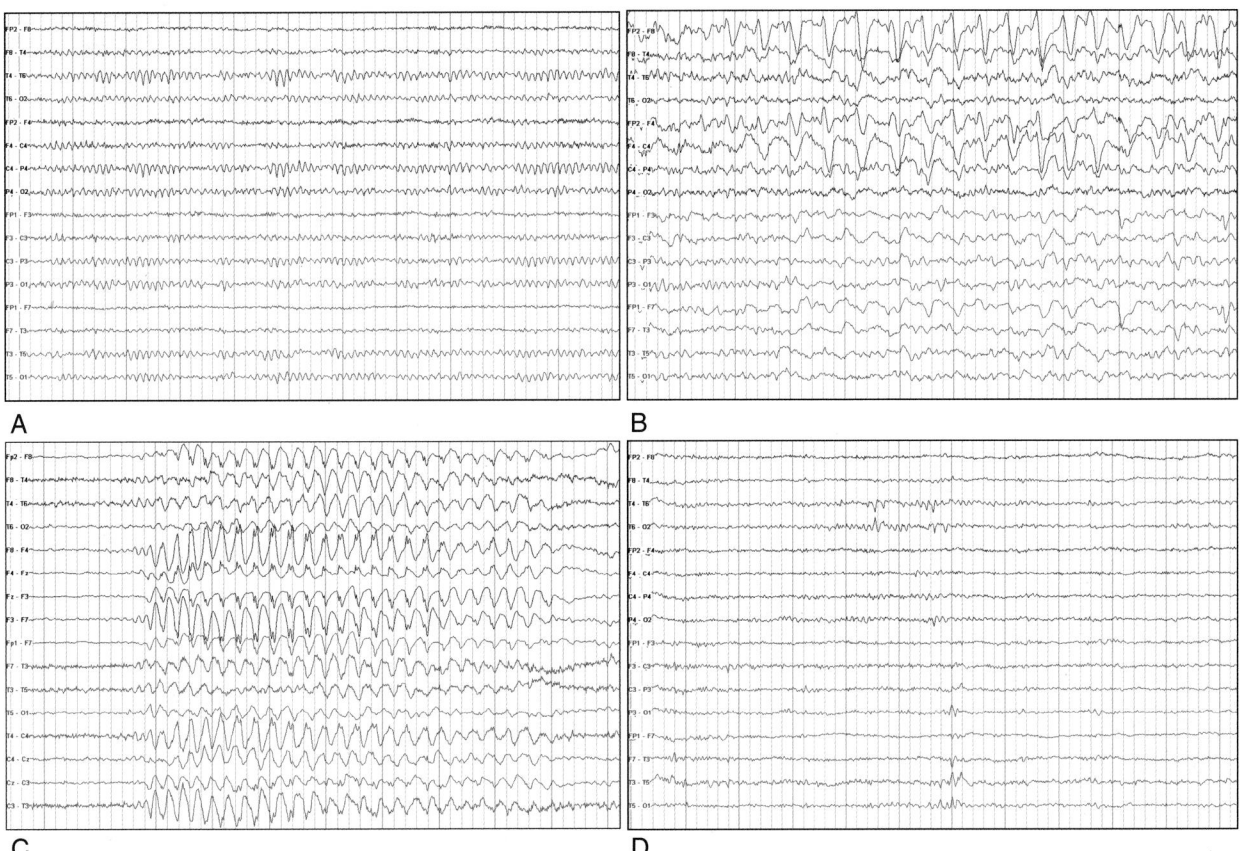

FIGURE 368-2. Normal and abnormal electroencephalograms. **A,** The EEG of a normal awake adult with evidence of a posterior 9 Hz alpha rhythm with eye closure. **B,** Focal slowing over the right frontal region due to underlying gliosis from a resected metastatic melanoma (Focal intermittent rhythmic delta activity [FIRDA]). **C,** Generalized 3 to 4 Hz spike and wave paroxysmal discharges (maximal in frontal regions) in a patient with a primary generalized (absence) epilepsy syndrome. **D,** Bilateral temporal lobe sharp waves (left midtemporal and right posterior temporal) in a patient with temporal lobe epilepsy.

standard electroencephalograph (EEG) typically records around 30 minutes of brain activity, both in the awake state and in the first two stages of sleep. Activation procedures, including hyperventilation and photic stimulation, are routinely performed to increase the frequency of epileptogenic discharges. Electroencephalographic frequencies are divided into four categories: delta (<4 Hz), theta (4 to 7 Hz), alpha (8 to 13 Hz), and beta (>13 Hz). The presence of spikes (20 to 70 ms) and sharp waves (70 to 200 ms) may indicate a seizure focus.

In the occipital leads, the normal awake EEG contains an alpha rhythm that attenuates with eye opening. In normal sleep, EEG activity shows typical features of different stages of light, deep, and rapid eye movement (REM) sleep. Abnormalities seen on EEG can be broadly classified into changes in background activity or paroxysmal discharges (Fig. 368-2 and Table 368-4).

Electroencephalography plays a major role in the diagnosis and categorization of a seizure disorder and can aid in determining the probability of recurrent seizures. EEG studies are neither highly sensitive nor completely specific for a seizure diagnosis. Only about 50% of patients with seizures show epileptiform activity on a single EEG recording. Repeating the EEG with provocative maneuvers such as sleep deprivation, hyperventilation, and photic stimulation may increase this percentage to 90%. Conversely, about 1% of adults and 3.5% of children who are neurologically normal and who have never had a seizure have pseudoepileptiform activity on EEG.

An EEG also can provide important clues about the diagnosis and prognosis in patients with disorders of consciousness, such as coma (Chapter 376) and encephalopathy, and can be a useful adjunct in the determination of brainstem death (Chapter 376) and diagnosing sleep disorders (Chapter 377). In addition, specific EEG patterns lend support to specific neurologic diagnoses (see Table 368-4; Videos 368-1 and 368-2). More recently, a wearable EEG device has shown promise for objectively recording seizures in ambulatory patients.[13]

TABLE 368-4	ELECTROENCEPHALOGRAPHIC ABNORMALITIES
ELECTROENCEPHALOGRAPHIC ABNORMALITY	**CLINICAL CORRELATE**
BACKGROUND RHYTHM ABNORMALITIES	
Generalized slowing	Most metabolic encephalopathies
Triphasic waves	Hepatic, renal, and other metabolic encephalopathies
Focal slowing	Large mass lesions (tumor, large stroke)
Electrocerebral inactivity with lack of response to all stimuli	Neocortical death, hypothermia, drug overdose
PAROXYSMAL ABNORMALITIES	
3-Hz spike and wave, augmented by hyperventilation	Primary generalized epilepsy (e.g., childhood absence epilepsy)
3- to 4-Hz spike and wave in light sleep or with photic stimulation	Primary generalized epilepsy (e.g., juvenile myoclonic epilepsy)
Central to midtemporal spikes	Benign epilepsy with centrotemporal spikes
Anterior temporal spikes or sharp waves	Focal epilepsy (e.g., mesial temporal lobe seizures)
Periodic lateralizing epileptiform discharges	Stroke, herpes simplex encephalitis
Generalized periodic sharp waves	Creutzfeld-Jakob disease
Burst suppression	Severe anoxic brain injury, barbiturate coma

TABLE 368-5 NERVE CONDUCTION STUDY ABNORMALITIES

ABNORMALITY	CLINICAL CORRELATE
Reduced CMAP amplitude	Axonal neuropathy
Prolonged terminal latency	Demyelinating neuropathy Distal compressive neuropathy
Conduction block	Severe focal compressive neuropathy Severe demyelinating neuropathy
Slowed conduction velocity	Demyelinating neuropathy

CMAP = compound muscle action potential.

TABLE 368-6 ELECTROMYOGRAPHIC ABNORMALITIES

ABNORMALITY	CLINICAL CORRELATE
INSERTIONAL ACTIVITY	
Prolonged	Acute denervation Active (usually inflammatory) myopathy
SPONTANEOUS ACTIVITY	
Fibrillations and positive waves	Acute denervation Active (usually inflammatory) myopathy
Fasciculations	Chronic neuropathies Motor neuron disease (rare fasciculations may be normal)
Myotonic discharges	Myotonic disorders Acid maltase deficiency
VOLUNTARY ACTIVITY	
Neuropathic potentials: large-amplitude, long-duration, polyphasic potentials	Chronic neuropathies and anterior horn cell diseases
Myopathic potentials: small-amplitude, short-duration, polyphasic potentials	Chronic myopathies Neuromuscular junction disorders
RECRUITMENT	
Reduced	Chronic neuropathic disorders
Rapid	Chronic myopathies

Nerve Conduction Study

Nerve conduction can be measured in motor and sensory nerves.[14] A nerve conduction study, which is the recording and measurement of the compound nerve and muscle action potentials elicited in response to an electrical stimulus, can glean information only from medium- to large-diameter myelinated fibers, which include motor fibers and sensory fibers that convey sensation to vibration and joint position sense. Small unmyelinated fibers responsible for pain and temperature are not assessed.

Abnormalities on a nerve conduction study can document a neuropathy and demarcate its distribution (i.e., whether it is distal, proximal, or diffuse). In addition, it can decipher the modality involved (i.e., motor versus sensory or both) and whether the underlying process is predominantly axonal or demyelinating (E-Fig. 368-7 and Table 368-5).

Repetitive Stimulation Study

To diagnose disorders that affect the neuromuscular junction, repetitive stimulation repeatedly delivers a supramaximal electrical stimulus to a nerve and serially records the amplitude of the compound muscle action potential. In myasthenia gravis (Chapter 394), these amplitudes become progressively smaller with repetitive stimulation in affected muscles (Video 368-11). In contrast, fast repetitive stimulation evokes an increment in these amplitudes in presynaptic myasthenic syndromes.

Electromyography

Electromyography (EMG) assesses the properties of the motor unit by recording variations of electrical potential detected by a needle electrode inserted into skeletal muscle. During EMG, the electrical activity of muscle is studied in four settings: insertional activity (occurs within the first second of needle insertion), spontaneous activity (electrical activity at rest), voluntary activity (electrical activity with muscle contraction), and recruitment pattern (change in electrical activity with maximal contraction; Table 368-6). EMG can help support or exclude a diagnosis, but no EMG findings are pathognomonic for a specific disease. If a patient has weakness, EMG is helpful in localizing the abnormalities to determine whether the weakness is due to disease of the anterior horn cell (e.g., motor neuron disease; Video 368-8), nerve root (radiculopathy), plexus (plexopathy; Video 368-9), an individual peripheral nerve (mononeuropathy), or multiple peripheral nerves (polyneuropathy; Video 368-10). EMG can also detect muscle disease by distinguishing active (inflammatory) myopathies (e.g., dermatomyositis, polymyositis, inclusion body myositis; E-Fig. 368-5) from chronic myopathies (e.g., congenital myopathies and some metabolic myopathies). Myotonic discharges on EMG may point to certain muscle diseases, including myotonic dystrophy (Video 368-12 and E-Fig. 368-3), myotonia congenita, or paramyotonia. It is important to note that it may take several weeks for a muscle to develop EMG signs of acute degeneration after nerve transection. For this reason, EMG performed in the acute setting after nerve injury should be interpreted with caution, and it may need to be repeated at a later date.

Evoked Potentials

Evoked potentials measure conduction velocities of sensory pathways from the periphery through the central nervous system.[15] Three types of evoked potentials are routinely performed in clinical practice: visual, brainstem auditory, and somatosensory.

Pattern Reversal Visual Evoked Potentials

The function of the anterior visual pathway, particularly the optic nerve, is assessed by the pattern reversal visual evoked potential. A prolonged latency in the absence of ocular disease implies slowed conduction velocity in the optic nerve and suggests underlying demyelination (E-Fig. 368-8). When multiple sclerosis is suspected, evoked potential testing is helpful to document the presence of a demyelinating lesion that may not be clinically evident.

Brainstem Auditory Evoked Potentials

The electrophysiologic response to auditory stimuli is measured by brainstem auditory evoked potentials. Brainstem auditory evoked potential testing is helpful in the diagnosis of acoustic neuroma (Chapter 180) and other cerebellopontine angle tumors.

Somatosensory Evoked Potentials

The somatosensory evoked potential assesses conduction after stimulation of a mixed or cutaneous peripheral nerve. The recorded responses reflect activity of large-diameter, myelinated cutaneous and muscle afferents in the peripheral nervous system and the dorsal columns of the spinal cord, medial lemniscus of the brainstem, ventroposterior lateral nucleus of the thalamus, and somatosensory cortex of the contralateral cerebral hemisphere. Somatosensory evoked potential testing is helpful when multiple sclerosis (Chapter 383) is suspected clinically, and it is necessary to document the presence of a demyelinating lesion in the central nervous system that may not be clinically or radiographically evident. Somatosensory evoked potential testing is also useful for prognostication in comatose patients and for intraoperative monitoring of spinal cord function in patients undergoing spinal surgery.

Imaging

On the basis of the relative advantages and disadvantages of computed tomography (CT), magnetic resonance imaging (MRI), and other neuroimaging modalities, different clinical entities can and should be assessed differently (Table 368-7). In acute ischemic stroke (Chapter 379) without bleeding, CT abnormalities typically appear within 4 to 12 hours and are seen even earlier with larger infarctions and embolic infarctions (E-Fig. 368-9).[16] The addition of CT angiography in acute ischemic stroke helps guide the need for thrombectomy. CT detects hemorrhagic stroke (Chapter 380) acutely and can estimate its age. CT is also the preferred initial imaging modality for detection of intraparenchymal hemorrhage and subarachnoid hemorrhage, and it often suggests whether an aneurysm is the likely cause. Either CT angiography or magnetic resonance angiography can display the three-dimensional anatomy of aneurysms with sufficient detail for therapy to be planned, but surgical/endovascular treatment generally requires catheter arteriography. CT is the first-line method for evaluation of brain trauma and diagnosis of subdural or epidural hematoma (Chapter 371), usually without requiring intravenous contrast material. Many brain tumors are initially recognized on CT scans, but MRI is the preferred modality for detection and characterization of all

TABLE 368-7	STRENGTHS AND WEAKNESSES OF SELECTED IMAGING MODALITIES	
MODALITY	**STRENGTHS**	**WEAKNESSES**
Computed tomography (CT)	Fast; good at bony pathology; preferred for trauma, acute neurologic symptoms, and decreased level of consciousness	Poorer soft tissue contrast resolution than MRI; ionizing radiation exposure
Conventional angiography	Best spatial resolution for vessels, useful in aneurysms, vascular malformations, and vasculitis; provides information about flow and arteriovenous shunting	Invasive and often lengthy; risk of stroke and other complications
CT myelography and cisternography	Useful in CSF leaks with intracranial hypotension to identify point of leak	Invasive, with risk of complications from lumbar puncture and instillation of contrast material
Magnetic resonance imaging (MRI)	Noninvasive; no radiation; multiplanar; high soft tissue contrast resolution	Less sensitive for bony pathology; contraindicated in patients with ferromagnetic devices or foreign bodies; patient must be able to cooperate and tolerate confined space; time-consuming relative to CT
Magnetic resonance angiography (MRA)	Noninvasive; good for screening extracranial and intracranial vascular disease; may be performed with or without contrast agent	Technically demanding; may overestimate the degree of vascular stenosis (noncontrast MRA); cannot image distal vessels optimally without contrast agent
Magnetic resonance spectroscopy (MRS)	May help differentiate tumor grade or tumor from nontumor (e.g., tumefactive demyelination); may help diagnose and classify dementias such as Alzheimer disease	Low spatial resolution; low specificity; time-consuming
Positron emission tomography (PET)	Provides information as to metabolic activity dependent on the tracer used; Fludeoxyglucose (FDG) most commonly used—can help in diagnosis of Alzheimer disease, epilepsy, and radiation necrosis	Requires a cyclotron to generate radioisotopes with a short half-life; lower resolution and less available than MRI and CT; high radiation exposure
Single-photon emission computed tomography (SPECT)	Occasionally useful in epilepsy; sensitive for diffuse pathologic processes	Lower resolution than PET, MRI, or CT
Ultrasonography	Fast; easy to use; can be performed at the bedside to assess vessel patency	Limited field of view due to bone; cannot visualize vessels in the upper neck and cranial base; operator dependent
Transcranial Doppler (TCD)	Fast; easy to use; assesses vascular velocities quantitatively; can assess cerebral vasospasm and occluded vessels	Does not provide images of vessels

brain tumors (Chapter 180),[17] including those that might be the cause of new-onset seizures in adults.

Imaging often detects asymptomatic findings,[18] including subclinical cerebrovascular lesions of unclear immediate significance. However, even very small (<3 mm) subclinical cerebrovascular lesions portend about a 3-fold increased risk of a subsequent stroke.

Grade A References

A1. Dussourd L, Martinon B, Candille C, et al. Ultrasonography helps emergency physician identify the best lumbar puncture site under the conus medullaris. *Scand J Trauma Resusc Emerg Med.* 2017;25:1-3.
A2. Nath S, Koziarz A, Badhiwala JH, et al. Atraumatic versus conventional lumbar puncture needles: a systematic review and meta-analysis. *Lancet.* 2018;391:1197-1204.

GENERAL REFERENCES

For the General References and other additional features, please visit Expert Consult at https://expertconsult.inkling.com.

369

PSYCHIATRIC DISORDERS IN MEDICAL PRACTICE

JEFFREY M. LYNESS

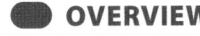

OVERVIEW

Disorders in Psychiatry

Psychiatric disorders, also known as mental illnesses, are extraordinarily common and have a profound impact on well-being and functional status. Collectively, psychiatric disorders account for more aggregate disability than do those involving any other organ system, with depression alone being second only to cardiovascular disorders.

Psychiatric disorders are defined as disorders of the psyche—that is, conditions that affect thoughts, feelings, or behaviors. By definition, such mental disturbances must be sufficient to produce significant distress in the patient or impairment in role or other functioning. Because the pathogeneses of most psychiatric disorders are incompletely understood, classification is based on clinical syndromes that are defined by diagnostic criteria with high interrater reliability because they emphasize discrete reportable or observable symptoms and signs. Interestingly, however, many underlying pathophysiologic mechanisms probably cut across these descriptive diagnostic categories, although current knowledge of such mechanisms rarely directly informs predictions of course or therapeutic decision making.[1]

Specific Syndromes

Because many psychiatric disorders result from the direct influence of neurologic conditions, systemic diseases, or drugs on brain functioning, assessment of any new or worsened psychiatric condition must include evaluation for their potential contributions (Table 369-1). Delirium (Chapter 25) and dementia (Chapter 374), which are neurocognitive disorders defined by impairment in intellectual functions such as attention, memory, or language, are always the result of neurologic abnormalities, systemic illnesses, or drugs. Although intellectual impairment is the hallmark of neurocognitive disorders, these conditions also may manifest as alterations in other aspects of mental status, including mood, thought content, thought process, and behavior. If a noncognitive psychiatric syndrome is caused by an identifiable underlying condition, it is known as a secondary psychiatric disorder (e.g., "major depression due to hypothyroidism").

The major nonsecondary, noncognitive psychiatric syndromes (Table 369-2) can coexist with multiple syndromes. For example, a patient suffering major depression with psychotic features may have depressive, anxiety, and psychotic syndromes simultaneously. Addictive disorders are considered in Chapters 30 and 31.

Comorbid Conditions in Psychiatry

It is common for persons who suffer from mental disorders to meet the diagnostic criteria for more than one condition. Although such comorbidity may reflect the limitations of current approaches to diagnosis, psychiatric comorbidity influences the choices or sequence of indicated treatments and may worsen the overall prognosis. Comorbidity with other medical conditions also is common, probably reflecting complex bidirectional causal relationships between physical and mental illnesses, and such comorbidity also often worsens the prognosis for both conditions.

Treatments in Psychiatry

Treatments in psychiatry are intended to reduce or eliminate symptoms, thereby improving the patient's distress and dysfunction and averting suicidal behavior. Maintenance therapies reduce the frequency or severity of recurrent episodes. Pharmacotherapy remains an evidence-based mainstay of the treatment of many psychiatric conditions. The evidence for a number of forms of psychotherapy administered in individual, group, or family modalities also strongly support their use as primary treatment or co-treatment of many conditions. Other psychosocial interventions, ranging from self-help groups to the use of structured treatment or residential programs, are often important components

of treatment. Nonpharmacologic evidence-based somatic therapies include electroconvulsive therapy, light therapy, and vagal nerve stimulation for particular forms of major depression. Studies are ongoing regarding other methods for selected cases of severe depressive or obsessive-compulsive disorders, including deep brain stimulation, transcranial direct-current stimulation, and repetitive transcranial magnetic stimulation.

Mood Disorders

Mood disorders are categorized as either depressive (also termed *unipolar*), characterized by depressive episodes only, or bipolar, characterized by manic or hypomanic episodes, typically with depressive episodes as well.

⬤ MAJOR DEPRESSIVE DISORDER

DEFINITION

Major depressive disorder is characterized by one or more episodes of idiopathic major depressive syndrome (Table 369-3).

EPIDEMIOLOGY

In the United States major depression has a 12-month prevalence of approximately 7%, and it is at least 1.5 times more common in females than males, only in part because of the 6 to 13% prevalence of postpartum depression.[2] Lifetime prevalence is up to 10% in males and 20 to 25% in females. New depressive episodes have an annual incidence of approximately 3%. Depression accounts for more than twice as much disability in midlife as any other medical condition, and its overall cumulative burden is greater than that from all but cardiovascular disorders. The economic impact is also enormous, with U.S. estimates of annual costs for depression exceeding $12 billion for treatment, $8 billion for associated morbidity, and $33 billion for lost earnings and work productivity.

PATHOBIOLOGY

Major depression is not a single disease entity but rather a heterogeneous group of conditions with multiple pathogenic mechanisms. It is both multifactorial and polygenic: genetic factors account for approximately 40% of the risk for depression, but multiple gene loci, most of which are currently unknown, are probably involved in a complex interplay with developmental and environmental influences. Alterations in the brain's noradrenergic and serotonergic systems are likely related to the efficacy of current antidepressant medications. The hypothalamic-pituitary-adrenal axis is hyperactive in depression, as

TABLE 369-1	IMPORTANT CAUSES OF PSYCHIATRIC SYNDROMES
CENTRAL NERVOUS SYSTEM DISEASES	
Trauma	
Tumor	
Toxins	
Seizures	
Vascular	
Infections	
Genetic/congenital malformations	
Demyelinating diseases	
Neurodegenerative diseases	
Hydrocephalus	
SYSTEMIC DISEASES	
Cardiovascular	
Pulmonary	
Endocrine	
Metabolic	
Nutritional	
Infections	
Cancer	
DRUGS (e.g., recreational, prescription, or over-the-counter drugs)	
Drug intoxication	
Drug withdrawal	

TABLE 369-2	IMPORTANT PSYCHIATRIC SYNDROMES AND DISORDERS	
SYNDROME	**MAIN SYMPTOMS AND SIGNS**	**MAY OCCUR AS PART OF THESE DISORDERS**
Neurocognitive	Deficits in intellectual functions (e.g., level of consciousness, orientation, attention, memory, language, praxis, visuospatial, executive functions)	Neurocognitive disorders Intellectual disability (if onset in childhood)
Mood: depressive	Lowered mood, anhedonia, negativistic thoughts, neurovegetative symptoms	Neurocognitive disorders Mood disorders (bipolar or depressive) (primary or secondary) Psychotic disorders (schizoaffective disorder)
Mood: manic	Elevated or irritable mood, grandiosity, goal-directed hyperactivity with increased energy, pressured speech, decreased sleep need	Neurocognitive disorders Bipolar disorder (primary or secondary) Psychotic disorders (schizoaffective disorder)
Anxiety	All include anxious mood and associated physiologic symptoms (e.g., palpitations, tremors, diaphoresis); may include various types of dysfunctional thoughts (e.g., catastrophic fears, obsessions, flashbacks) and behavior (e.g., compulsions, avoidance behavior)	Neurocognitive disorders Mood disorders (bipolar or depressive) (primary or secondary) Psychotic disorders (primary or secondary) Trauma- and stressor-related disorders Anxiety disorders (primary or secondary) Obsessive-compulsive and related disorders
Psychotic	Impairments in reality testing: delusions, hallucinations, thought process derailments	Neurocognitive disorders Mood disorders (bipolar or depressive) (primary or secondary) Psychotic disorders
Somatic symptom syndromes	Somatic symptoms with associated distressing thoughts, feelings, or behaviors	Mood disorders (bipolar or depressive) (primary or secondary) Anxiety disorders (primary or secondary) Obsessive-compulsive and related disorders Trauma- and stressor-related disorders Somatic symptom disorders
Personality pathology	Enduring patterns of dysfunctional emotional regulation, thought patterns, interpersonal behavior, impulse regulation	Neurocognitive disorders (dementia) Personality change due to another medical condition Personality disorders

Author summary based on categories and criteria from American Psychiatric Association. *Diagnostic and Statistical Manual of Mental Disorders.* 5th ed. (DSM-5) Washington, DC: American Psychiatric Association; 2013.

TABLE 369-3	SYMPTOMS/SIGNS OF AN EPISODE OF MAJOR DEPRESSIVE SYNDROME

DIAGNOSTIC CRITERIA (*a minimum of five symptoms must be present for a minimum of 2 consecutive weeks*)

Depressed mood (may be irritable mood in children and adolescents) most of the day, nearly every day, *OR*
Markedly diminished interest or pleasure most of the day, nearly every day *AND*
Weight loss or gain, or change in appetite (decrease or increase) nearly every day
Change in sleep (insomnia or hypersomnia) nearly every day
Psychomotor agitation or retardation nearly every day
Fatigue or loss of energy nearly every day
Feeling of worthlessness or guilt nearly every day
Diminished concentration or indecisiveness nearly every day
Recurrent thoughts of death or suicidal ideation, or a suicide attempt, or a specific suicide plan

MNEMONIC TO AID RECALL OF DIAGNOSTIC CRITERIA: "*SIG: E CAPS*" (*i.e., prescribe energy capsules*) for depressed mood

Sleep change
Interests decreased
Guilt
Energy decreased
Concentration decreased
Appetite/weight disturbance
Psychomotor changes
Suicide thoughts

DEPRESSIVE SYMPTOMS/SIGNS GROUPED CONCEPTUALLY, WITH ADDITIONAL COMMON PHENOMENA

Emotional

Depressed mood, sadness, tearfulness
Irritability (seen in all ages, perhaps most commonly in children/adolescents and the elderly)
Anxiety
Loss of interests or pleasure (anhedonia)

Ideational

Worthlessness/lowered self-esteem
Guilt
Hopelessness/nihilism
Helplessness
Thoughts of death, dying, suicide

Somatic/Neurovegetative

Change in appetite/weight
Change in sleep
Anergia
Decreased libido
Trouble concentrating
Diurnal variation in symptoms (*mornings—worst pattern is most characteristic*)

Other

Ruminative thinking (tendency to dwell on one [negativistic] theme)
Somatic symptoms or somatic worry
Psychotic symptoms (negativistic delusions most characteristic)—defines the subtype "Major Depression with Psychotic Features"

Based on criteria from American Psychiatric Association. *Diagnostic and Statistical Manual of Mental Disorders.* 5th ed. (DSM-5) Washington, DC: American Psychiatric Association; 2013.

TABLE 369-4	TREATMENTS FOR DEPRESSION
NAME OF PSYCHOTHERAPY	**APPROACH**
Cognitive psychotherapy	Identify and correct negativistic patterns of thinking
Interpersonal psychotherapy	Identify and work through role transitions or interpersonal losses, conflicts, or deficits
Problem-solving therapy	Identify and prioritize situational problems; plan and implement strategies to deal with top-priority problems
Psychodynamic psychotherapy	Use therapeutic relationship to maximize use of the healthiest defense mechanisms and coping strategies

be seen without a depressed mood, albeit by definition they then must have loss of interest or pleasure in their usually desired activities. They may also exhibit prominent anxiety, irritability, or somatization. Although the mildest forms of major depression in the community may remit spontaneously within a few months without medical care, patients may have persistent symptoms for months or years, too often without seeking treatment.

DIAGNOSIS

The diagnosis is made clinically by elicitation of findings from the history and mental status examination to determine the presence of major depressive syndrome. The differential diagnosis includes other idiopathic disorders with episodes of major depression, such as bipolar disorder (distinguished by a history of manic episodes) and schizoaffective disorder (distinguished by a history of psychotic episodes in the absence of depression). Major depression may accompany delirium or dementia, and secondary depression also commonly accompanies serious medical illnesses; these comorbid conditions require careful, well-coordinated care. Screening instruments (see Table 24-3 in Chapter 24) can help identify cases of depression. For example, using the two-item version of the Patient Health Questionnaire, the screener asks the patient the following questions: Over the past 2 weeks, how often have you (1) had little interest or pleasure in doing things, or (2) been feeling down, depressed, or hopeless? Responses for each question are scored as follows: 0 = not at all, 1 = several days, 2 = more than half the days, 3 = nearly every day. A score of 3 points or higher on the two-item screen is associated with 75% probability of having a depressive disorder.

TREATMENT Rx

The three phases of treatment are (1) acute, in which treatment is provided to resolve the major depressive episode; (2) continuation, in which the acute treatment is continued for 6 to 12 months to prevent relapse; and (3) maintenance, for those with two to three or more episodes of recurrent depression, for whom treatment is maintained indefinitely to reduce the frequency and severity of future recurrences.[3,4]

Acute treatment of depression includes focused psychotherapies (Table 369-4), which are more efficacious than usual care and equivalent to medications when used for patients in primary care settings.[A1-A3] Based on the patient's preference, psychotherapy rather than medication may be the initial treatment of mild to moderate major depression, perhaps especially for individuals with prominent psychosocial stressors. Involvement of family members for education, support, and sometimes formal family therapy may be an important adjunctive or primary therapeutic approach. These therapies may be administered with decreased frequency during the continuation or maintenance phases of treatment. However, psychotherapies alone are insufficient for more severe forms of depression, including major depression with psychotic features. Meta-analyses suggest that the combination of medication with psychotherapy is more effective than medication alone in the initial treatment of mild to moderate major depression.[A4]

Medications should be used as initial treatment for most patients with more severe forms of major depression. Antidepressant medications (Table 369-5) are also effective for acute, continuation, and maintenance therapy. Overall data suggest that no second-generation agent is predictably better than others,[A5] although agents targeting noradrenergic as well as serotonergic systems may be more efficacious in more severe depression. Because antidepressant medications typically do not begin to improve symptoms for at least 1 to 2 weeks, with maximal benefit accruing up to at least 6 to 8 weeks, it is crucial

evidenced by a nonsuppressed response to the dexamethasone suppression test, although this test is too insensitive and nonspecific for clinical use as a diagnostic tool. Neuroimaging studies in subjects with depression show an array of findings, including smaller hippocampal volumes that may be the result of exposure to chronically elevated cortisol levels, and altered cerebral metabolic activity in regions including frontal-striatal circuitry and the anterior cingulate cortex. Cognitive psychology studies have demonstrated dysfunctional patterns of negative thinking, with distorted thoughts about self, the future, and the environment. Poor quality or absence of social relationships, and stressful life events, particularly events such as deaths, separations, or functional impairment, are powerfully associated with depression as well.

CLINICAL MANIFESTATIONS

The symptoms of depression (see Table 369-3) may be conceptually grouped as alterations in mood, ideation (i.e., thought content), and somatic/neurovegetative functioning. Importantly, patients with depressive illness may

TABLE 369-5 COMMONLY USED ANTIDEPRESSANT MEDICATIONS*

NAME OF CLASS/ SPECIFIC MEDICATION	IMMEDIATE MECHANISM OF ACTION	INITIAL ADULT DOSE	TARGET ADULT DOSE RANGE[†]	SIDE EFFECTS	COMMENTS
Selective serotonin reuptake inhibitors (SSRIs)	Inhibit presynaptic reuptake of serotonin			Nausea, diarrhea, sexual dysfunction, serotonin syndrome	
Citalopram		20 mg daily	20-40 mg daily (maximum 20 mg daily in patients age >60 yr)	Risk of QTc prolongation/ torsade de pointes in at-risk patients	Few drug-drug interactions
Escitalopram		10 mg daily	10-20 mg daily		Enantiomer of citalopram
Fluoxetine		20 mg daily	20-40 mg daily (depression), up to 80 mg daily (OCD)		Long half-life; tends to be activating
Paroxetine		20 mg daily	20-50 mg daily	Anticholinergic effects	Tends to be sedating
Sertraline		25-50 mg daily	50-200 mg daily		Few drug-drug interactions
Serotonin and norepinephrine reuptake inhibitors (SNRIs)	Inhibit presynaptic reuptake of serotonin and norepinephrine			Nausea, diarrhea, serotonin syndrome, sinus tachycardia, mild elevation in blood pressure, tremor	
Duloxetine		30-60 mg daily	30-60 mg daily on a twice-daily schedule, maximum of 120 mg/ day		
Venlafaxine		37.5 mg bid	150-375 mg/day on bid schedule		XR form allows once-daily dosing
Desvenlafaxine		50 mg daily	50 mg daily, maximum of 100 mg ER daily		Metabolite of venlafaxine
Tricyclic antidepressants (TCAs)	Inhibit presynaptic reuptake of serotonin and norepinephrine (in varying proportions depending on the specific TCA)			Anticholinergic effects, sedation, orthostatic hypotension, tremor, cardiac conduction delays, ventricular arrhythmias	
Amitriptyline		25-75 mg qhs	150-300 mg qhs		Strongly anticholinergic and sedating; aim for combined amitriptyline/nortriptyline blood level of 120-250 ng/mL
Desipramine		25-75 mg daily	150-300 mg daily		Aim for blood level of 115-250 ng/mL
Doxepin		25-75 mg qhs	150-300 mg qhs		Strongly sedating
Imipramine		25-75 mg daily	150-300 mg daily		Strongly anticholinergic; aim for combined imipramine/ desipramine blood level of 180-350 ng/mL
Nortriptyline		25-50 mg qhs	50-150 mg qhs		Aim for blood level of 50-150 ng/mL; least anticholinergic of the TCAs
Monoamine oxidase inhibitors (MAOIs)	Inhibit monoamine oxidase, the enzyme that catalyzes oxidative metabolism of monoamine neurotransmitters			Need for tyramine-free diet to avoid sympathomimetic (hypertensive) crisis; sedation, anticholinergic effects, tremor, orthostatic hypotension	
Isocarboxazid		10 mg bid	20-60 mg/day in bid-qid dosing		
Phenelzine		15 mg tid	45-90 mg/day in tid or qid dosing		
Selegiline	(selective MAO-B inhibitor)	5 mg bid	5 mg bid	Tyramine-free diet not required	Take with meals
Tranylcypromine		10 mg tid	30-60 mg/day in tid dosing		
Other					
Bupropion	Unknown, although it is a weak inhibitor of presynaptic reuptake of norepinephrine and dopamine	75-150 mg/day	300-450 mg/day	Activating; risk for seizures reduced by divided dosing and careful dosage titration	Divided dosing required unless using SR or XL forms
Mirtazapine	Antagonist at α_2 and 5-HT$_2$ receptors	15 mg qhs	30-45 mg qhs; maximum of 45 mg qhs	Sedation, hyperphagia	Becomes more stimulating at higher doses
Trazodone	Inhibits presynaptic reuptake of serotonin; antagonist at 5-HT$_2$ and 5-HT$_3$ receptors	25-50 mg qhs	300-600 mg qhs for depression, 25-100 mg qhs for insomnia	Sedation, priapism	Few sexual side effects
Vilazodone	Inhibits presynaptic reuptake of serotonin; agonist at 5-HT$_{1A}$ receptors	10 mg daily	40 mg daily	Nausea, diarrhea, sexual side effects	Dosage must be increased slowly
Vortioxetine	Inhibits presynaptic reuptake of serotonin; agonist at 5-HT$_{1A}$ receptors, antagonist at 5-HT$_3$ receptors	10 mg daily	20 mg daily	Nausea, diarrhea, sexual side effects	

*Patients on any of these medications must be monitored for suicidal thoughts.
[†]Target doses in the elderly may be lower.
ER = extended release; 5-HT$_2$ = 5-hydroxytryptamine; OCD = obsessive-compulsive disorder; qhs = at bedtime; SR = sustained release; XR = extended release.

to see patients regularly (every 1 to 2 weeks initially) to monitor their clinical status, provide support and education, and foster adherence. Antidepressant medications appear to increase the relative risk for suicidal behavior in adolescents and young adults, so such patients require careful benefit/risk assessments and close monitoring. By comparison, the relative risk for suicidal behavior is not increased by drug treatment in individuals older than age 25 and is substantially lowered in older adults. For patients with a psychotic depression, the addition of an antipsychotic medication (see Table 369-12) to an antidepressant may be more efficacious than either alone. Growing evidence suggests that a single intravenous dose of ketamine may rapidly reduce severe depressive symptoms within 24 hours,[A6] and esketamine nasal spray is FDA-approved for treatment-resistant depression. Electroconvulsive therapy is preferred for the most severe forms of major depression, including major depression with psychotic features, and is also used for depression refractory to other forms of treatment. Deep brain stimulation is an investigational therapy for otherwise refractory depression. Overall evidence to date does not support the efficacy of repetitive transcranial magnetic stimulation for depression.

Mindfulness-based cognitive therapy, behavioral activation, and maintenance antidepressant treatment can reduce the rate of relapsing or recurrent depressive symptoms, with approximately equal efficacy.[A7] In highly recurrent depression, however, maintenance pharmacotherapy may have the best outcomes. Optimal care for depression in primary care and other treatment settings may be enhanced by the use of collaborative care models,[A8] although the lack of reimbursement mechanisms often limits their implementation.

PROGNOSIS

Optimal guideline-based treatment of major depression results in full remission in up to 80% of patients, and the expectation is that patients with major depression will return to baseline functioning after resolution of the depressive episodes. However, at least 50 to 70% of patients will suffer recurrent episodes, up to 20% may experience chronic major depression, and many more will achieve only partial remission with persistent lower-level symptoms because of a variety of factors, including limited access to care, nonadherence, or insufficiently assertive treatments.

BIPOLAR DISORDER

DEFINITION AND EPIDEMIOLOGY

Bipolar disorder is characterized by recurrent episodes of idiopathic mania. Most persons with bipolar disorder also have recurrent episodes of major depression.

The 12-month prevalence of bipolar disorder is approximately 0.6%. Males are affected slightly more often than females. The average age at first onset is late adolescence or early adulthood. Childhood onset is possible, but diagnosis may be difficult because of symptomatic overlap with other conditions of childhood, such as the attention-deficit/hyperactivity disorder. Onset in midlife to late life is also possible, although most late-onset mania is secondary to other medical conditions or drugs rather than idiopathic bipolar disorder.

PATHOBIOLOGY

Even though the pathogenesis of bipolar disorder remains unclear, genetic factors play a greater role than in unipolar depressive conditions. Heritability has been traced to several specific loci in rare families, but genetic screening is not yet clinically useful, and the gene associations have to date revealed no unifying pathophysiologic themes. Most cases of bipolar disorder are polygenic and multifactorial, with genetic factors accounting for approximately 50% of the risk for the disorder. Dysregulation of the frontostriatal systems is probably involved in the manifestations of the illness. Though not specific enough to be diagnostic, structural neuroimaging studies show increased ventricular-brain ratios suggestive of parenchymal atrophy. Phase advance of central circadian rhythms can precipitate episodes of mania, so the decreased sleep need of persons with incipient mania may produce a vicious cycle in which phase-advanced circadian cycles lead to a further decreased need for sleep, thereby resulting in further phase advancement. Psychosocial stressors also often play a role in precipitating episodes of both mania and depression.

CLINICAL MANIFESTATIONS AND DIAGNOSIS

The symptoms of mania include a distinct period of abnormally and persistently elevated (euphoric) or irritable mood; goal-directed hyperactivity, often for pleasurable activities, with poor judgment that leads to long-lasting adverse financial, psychosocial, or medical consequences (e.g., sprees of spending, sexual activity, or gambling); increased energy; decreased need for sleep; pressured speech; and distractibility.[5]

TABLE 369-6 SYMPTOMS/SIGNS OF AN EPISODE OF MANIA

DIAGNOSTIC CRITERIA

A distinct period of abnormally, persistently elevated, expansive, or irritable mood; and abnormally and persistently increased goal-directed activity or energy lasting ≥1 week and present most of the day, nearly every day, _AND_

3 or more of the following symptoms/signs (4 or more if the mood abnormality is only irritability):

Inflated self-esteem/grandiosity
Decreased need for sleep
More talkative or pressure to keep talking
Subjective experience of racing thoughts or flight of ideas observed on examination
Distractibility
Increase in goal-directed activity or psychomotor agitation
Excessive involvement in activities with a high potential for painful consequences

MANIC SYMPTOMS/SIGNS GROUPED CONCEPTUALLY, WITH ADDITIONAL COMMON PHENOMENA

Emotional

Euphoria
Irritability
Labile affect

Ideational

Grandiosity

Somatic/Neurovegetative

Increased energy
Psychomotor agitation
Decreased need for sleep
Distractibility

Other

Goal-directed hyperactivity
Pressured speech
Impaired judgment
Flight of ideas
Psychotic symptoms (may include delusions, hallucinations, or derailment of thought processes such as loose associations)—defines the subtype "mania with psychotic features"

From *Diagnostic and Statistical Manual of Mental Disorders.* 5th ed. (DSM-5) Washington, DC: American Psychiatric Association, 2013, with permission.

As with major depression, the diagnosis is based on findings from the history and examination revealing a pattern of recurrent manic episodes (Table 369-6) that are usually interspersed with major depressive episodes and cannot be explained by other medical conditions, medications, or other substances. Although persons with bipolar disorder may become psychotic while in manic or depressed states, a history of psychotic symptoms in the absence of mania or depression indicates a diagnosis other than bipolar disorder. Manic and depressive episodes may also be seen in the course of delirium (Chapter 25) and dementia (Chapter 374), in which case the psychiatric symptoms are accompanied by the neurocognitive impairment that is the hallmark of the latter conditions.

TREATMENT   Rx

The mainstay of treatment for bipolar disorder is mood stabilizer medications to reduce the frequency and severity of recurrent manic and depressive episodes.[6] Mood stabilizers with substantial evidence base to support their use include lithium (typical dose of 600 to 1500 mg/day or higher given in two or three divided doses as needed to achieve plasma levels of 0.6 to 1.2 mEq/L [up to 1.4 mEq/L in acute mania]), valproic acid (typical dose of 500 to 1500 mg/day or higher as tolerated to achieve plasma levels of 50 to 100 μg/mL), and carbamazepine (typical dose of 400 to 1200 mg/day as tolerated to achieve plasma levels of 4 to 12 μg/mL). The combination of lithium plus valproate is superior to valproate alone for prevention of relapses. Lithium treatment is, however, associated with a decline in renal function, hypothyroidism, and hypercalcemia, especially in patients with higher lithium concentrations.[7] A number of other anticonvulsants have been tried but generally with less empirical support for their use, although lamotrigine (starting at 25 mg/day, maximum dose of 200 mg/day, titrated slowly to minimize the risk for Stevens-Johnson syndrome) can be used for prophylaxis against depressive episodes. Several second-generation antipsychotic medications have received approval by the

U.S. Food and Drug Administration (FDA) for their mood-stabilizing properties, but their potential to precipitate metabolic syndrome (and to a lesser extent tardive dyskinesia) should limit their use as maintenance medications to patients for whom other mood stabilizers are inefficacious or poorly tolerated.[A9] For acute episodes of mania, second- or first-generation antipsychotics are more rapidly efficacious than mood stabilizers, with doses similar to their use for acute psychosis (see Table 369-12). For acute treatment of depressive episodes, antidepressants may be required, but they may precipitate mania. Therefore patients should receive therapeutic doses of a mood stabilizer first, and exposure to antidepressant medication should be for the minimum dose and duration required. Electroconvulsive therapy is useful for refractory mania or depression and for patients with relative contraindications to medications, such as pregnancy.

Supportive psychotherapy fosters compliance with maintenance treatments and helps patients manage psychosocial stressors, thereby minimizing their impact on precipitating mania or depression.[A10] For acute treatment of bipolar depression, evidence-based psychotherapies for unipolar depression also may be used.

PROGNOSIS

Most patients with bipolar disorder return to baseline functioning between episodes. Some patients may experience frequent debilitating episodes (known as "rapid cycling," defined as four or more episodes per year), and others may experience deterioration in overall functioning over time.

OTHER MOOD DISORDERS

Although the diagnosis of chronic major depression should be made in patients with long-lasting major depressive episodes, others may have chronic (≥2 years) lower-level depressive symptoms known as persistent depressive disorder (dysthymia), which may be treated with a combination of antidepressant medication and psychotherapy. Other patients may have "less than major depression" episodes of shorter duration, often referred to as subsyndromal or subthreshold depression. Broad psychotherapeutic interventions may prevent progression to full-fledged major depression in such patients. Premenstrual dysphoric disorder manifests as cyclical depressive and anxiety symptoms that resolve in the week after menses and recur in the week before the onset of menses; this is the only mood disorder that may respond to brief cyclical administration of antidepressant medication.

Less severe bipolar-related disorders include bipolar II disorder, which is characterized by episodes of hypomania (i.e., low-level manic symptoms without substantial functional impairment and without psychosis) and episodes of major depression. Such patients typically seek care during depressive episodes rather than during hypomania, but antidepressant medication may worsen the manic symptoms. It is therefore imperative to ask about a history of manic or hypomanic symptoms in the evaluation of all patients with depression. Cyclothymic disorder, which includes episodes of hypomania and low-level depressive episodes, may be difficult to distinguish from the mood instability seen in cluster B personality disorders (see later).

ANXIETY DISORDERS

DEFINITION

The anxiety disorders (Table 369-7) are a group of conditions whose hallmark is idiopathic anxiety, typically accompanied by psychological (i.e., thought content) and somatic symptoms.[8] Anxiety is a common accompanying symptom in many other psychiatric disorders, but the primary anxiety disorders lack the neurocognitive deficits, depressive or manic symptoms, or psychosis seen in the other disorders. Trauma- and stressor-related and obsessive-compulsive disorders are classified separately from the anxiety disorders.

EPIDEMIOLOGY

Anxiety disorders are a worldwide problem. Panic disorder has a 12-month prevalence of 2 to 3%. Generalized anxiety disorder has a 12-month prevalence of approximately 3%, and the phobias collectively have a prevalence of 10 to 15% in the adult population. Cumulatively, anxiety disorders may have the highest prevalence of all primary psychiatric disorders in primary care settings. Clear data on incidence rates are not available. Primary anxiety disorders typically begin in adolescence through the mid-30s. Most anxiety symptoms with new onset in later life are due to mood or neurocognitive disorders or are secondary to medical illnesses or drugs; true late-onset primary anxiety disorders are often triggered by traumatic or other stressful life events.

TABLE 369-7　TYPES OF ANXIETY DISORDERS

ANXIETY DISORDER	MAJOR CLINICAL CHARACTERISTICS
Panic disorder	Recurrent unexpected panic attacks, typically with anticipatory anxiety and avoidance behavior
Generalized anxiety disorder	Excessive anxiety and worry, not meeting the criteria for other anxiety disorders, lasting ≥6 months
Phobias:	
Agoraphobia	Anxiety about or avoidance of places or situations from which escape might be difficult or embarrassing or in which help might not be available in the event of panic symptoms
Social phobia (social anxiety disorder)	Anxiety provoked by exposure to social situations, typically with ensuing avoidance behavior; may be generalized (i.e., in response to many interpersonal situations) or specific in response to a particular social situation (e.g., using a public restroom, public speaking)
Specific phobia	Anxiety provoked by exposure to a specific feared object or (nonsocial) situation, typically with ensuing avoidance behavior

Author summary based on categories and criteria from American Psychiatric Association. *Diagnostic and Statistical Manual of Mental Disorders.* 5th ed. (DSM-5) Washington, DC: American Psychiatric Association; 2013.

PATHOBIOLOGY

Anxiety may be understood in part as inappropriate triggering of the stress response system, commonly referred to as the "fight-or-flight" response. However, it is important to recognize that the responses involve a wide range of cognitive, motor, neuroendocrine, and autonomic systems and thus are not limited to manifestations of sympathetic nervous system activity. The "salience network" is believed to play a crucial role in the neurobiologic coordination of anxiety. The amygdala receives excitatory glutamatergic input from several cortical areas and from the thalamus, thereby allowing it to respond to a wide variety of stimuli, including sensory input from the external world, as well as stressors that are processed and recognized by cortical association areas. The amygdala in turn projects to the many brain regions that subserve the clinical manifestations of the anxiety response, in part through its direct projections to the important centers of monoaminergic systems: dopaminergic neurons of the ventral tegmental area in the midbrain, noradrenergic neurons in the locus coeruleus, and serotonergic neurons in the raphe nuclei.

From a cognitive psychology perspective, the pathogenesis of many anxiety disorders, particularly panic, may be understood as catastrophic misinterpretations of normal somatic sensations. A vulnerable individual may become aware of a normal or minimally abnormal body sensation, which is interpreted as something concerning, thereby leading to sympathetic and other autonomic arousal, which in turn leads to further somatic sensations (e.g., tachycardia, sweating) in what becomes a vicious cycle of thoughts and somatic symptoms.

CLINICAL MANIFESTATIONS

Most individuals experience one or more somatic symptoms (Table 369-8) that accompany psychic anxiety, regardless of whether the anxiety is normal or part of a pathologic condition. Such somatic symptoms may be referable to virtually every body organ system.

Many anxiety disorders include acute, discrete periods of symptoms known as panic attacks. In a panic attack, the patient experiences an abrupt surge in anxiety, fear-related thoughts, and somatic symptoms in the space of a few minutes ("crescendo onset"). The acute symptoms resolve quickly, typically within an hour or less.

Panic Disorder

Panic disorder consists of recurrent panic attacks. Although some panic attacks may be precipitated by situations known to be stressful, at least some attacks must be unexpected ("out of the blue"). Patients also exhibit anticipatory anxiety in which they experience ongoing psychic distress by worrying about their next panic attack or the attack's effects (e.g., humiliation if the attack were to happen in public view). In addition, patients manifest avoidance behavior by staying away from known triggers or from situations in which having a panic attack might be dangerous (e.g., driving) or particularly distressing (e.g., in public spaces). For many patients, the anticipatory anxiety and avoidance behavior may be more disabling than the panic attacks themselves. Avoidance behavior may overlap with agoraphobia, which is defined as a distressing and disabling fear of places or situations from which escape might be difficult or embarrassing or from which help might not be available in the event of panic-like symptoms. Common agoraphobic foci include being outside one's home alone, being on bridges or in tunnels, traveling by vehicle, or being in crowds or lines. A third or more of patients with panic disorder have comorbid agoraphobia, whereas others have agoraphobia alone or comorbid with other conditions.

Generalized Anxiety Disorder

This more heterogeneous condition is defined by the presence of clinically significant anxiety and associated somatic symptoms for 6 or more months. Generalized anxiety disorder[9] is often overridden in the diagnostic hierarchy by other conditions that produce anxiety.

Social Anxiety and Phobias

The phobias are a group of conditions defined by the consistent ability of a specific environmental stimulus to elicit a pathologic anxiety response. Exposure to such a stimulus nearly always produces this response, so the patient avoids the stimulus whenever possible or endures the stimulus with considerable distress. In addition to agoraphobia, the other main types of phobias are social phobia (social anxiety disorder)[10] and specific phobias (see Table 369-7).

DIAGNOSIS

Diagnosis of anxiety disorders must rest on consideration of both syndromic and etiologic perspectives. From a syndromic perspective, a careful history and mental status examination are required to determine the pattern of anxiety and associated symptoms and to determine whether the phenomenology fits the pattern for any of the anxiety disorders as described earlier. The history and mental status examination must also assess for the presence of any other psychiatric disorder that might truly be comorbid with the anxiety disorder but might also supersede the anxiety disorder in the diagnostic hierarchy. For example, generalized anxiety may be seen as part of neurocognitive disorders (delirium or dementia), depressive or bipolar disorders, and psychotic disorders.

From an etiologic perspective, it is important to determine whether the anxiety disorder is primary (idiopathic) or secondary to a systemic or neurologic condition (see Table 369-1), drug intoxication, or withdrawal state. The evaluation should include laboratory tests (e.g., toxic drug screen) as guided by the differential diagnosis generated from the clinical evaluation.

TABLE 369-8	COMMON SOMATIC MANIFESTATIONS OF ANXIETY
CARDIORESPIRATORY	
Palpitations	
Chest pain	
Dyspnea or sensation of being smothered	
GASTROINTESTINAL	
Sensation of choking	
Dyspepsia	
Nausea	
Diarrhea	
Abdominal bloating or pain	
GENITOURINARY	
Urinary frequency or urgency	
NEUROLOGIC/AUTONOMIC	
Diaphoresis	
Warm flushes or chills	
Dizziness or presyncope	
Paresthesias	
Tremor	
Headache	

TREATMENT   Rx

Empirical evidence from controlled trials demonstrates the efficacy of cognitive-behavioral psychotherapies for most of the anxiety disorders.[A11] Such therapies, which use the principles of learning theory to extinguish unhelpful behavior and positively reinforce more functional behavior, help the patient learn to identify and correct the dysfunctional patterns of thinking ("automatic thoughts") that underlie or trigger the cognitive-physiologic cascade of pathologic anxiety responses. Cognitive behavioral therapy may be used as sole therapy, particularly for specific phobias, or in combination with pharmacotherapy. Frequently, cognitive behavioral therapy may be administered as part of family therapy (e.g., to help family members avoid behavior that inadvertently reinforces the patient's symptoms) or in group therapy settings.

Although anxiolytic drugs such as the benzodiazepines (Table 369-9) will usually relieve acute anxiety symptoms, concerns about their long-term efficacy and side effects (e.g., risk for abuse, risk for neurocognitive impairment or falls) make antidepressant medications the more attractive pharmacologic agents for most anxiety disorders (see Table 369-5).[A12] Most antidepressants, with the probable exception of bupropion, are helpful for panic disorder, generalized anxiety disorder, and social phobia.

TABLE 369-9	SELECTED ANTIANXIETY AND HYPNOTIC DRUGS*				
DRUG	**TRADE NAME**	**INITIAL DOSE**	**TARGET DOSE RANGE†**	**SIDE EFFECTS**	**COMMENTS**
Benzodiazepines				Sedation, ataxia, risk for falls	Potential for abuse/dependence
Lorazepam	Ativan	0.5 mg bid-qid	2-6 mg/day, tid-qid dosing		Reliable IM absorption
Diazepam	Valium	2-5 mg bid-tid	10-40 mg/day, bid-tid dosing		Long half-life of drug and active metabolites
Triazolam	Halcion	0.125 mg qhs	0.125-0.25 mg qhs	Rebound insomnia	Used as hypnotic
Chlordiazepoxide	Librium	5 mg bid-tid	10-40 mg/day, bid-tid dosing		Long half-life of drug and active metabolites
Temazepam	Restoril	7.5 mg qhs	7.5-30 mg qhs		Used as hypnotic
Alprazolam	Xanax	0.25 mg tid-qid	2-8 mg/day, tid-qid dosing	Possibly greater addictive potential	
Clorazepate	Tranxene	7.5-15 mg bid-tid	15-60 mg/day, bid-tid dosing		
Flurazepam	Dalmane	15-30 mg qhs	15-30 mg qhs	Daytime somnolence	Used as hypnotic
Oxazepam	Serax	10-15 mg tid-qid	10-30 mg tid-qid		
Clonazepam	Klonopin	0.5 mg bid-tid	0.5-5 mg bid-tid		Long duration of action
Zaleplon	Sonata	5-10 mg qhs	5-20 mg qhs		"Nonbenzodiazepine" hypnotic
Zolpidem	Ambien	5-10 mg qhs	5-10 mg qhs		"Nonbenzodiazepine" hypnotic
Eszopiclone	Lunesta	1-2 mg qhs	1-3 mg qhs		"Nonbenzodiazepine" hypnotic
β-Blockers					
Propranolol	Inderal	20 mg bid	Individualize, 40-120 mg/day	Bradycardia, hypotension, potential for mental slowing	Only helps with sympathetically mediated somatic symptoms of anxiety

*Antidepressants (see Table 369-5) are often first-line agents of choice for primary anxiety disorders.
†Target doses in the elderly may be lower.
qhs = at bedtime.

TABLE 369-10 COMMON TYPES OF OBSESSIONS AND COMPULSIONS IN OBSESSIVE-COMPULSIVE DISORDER

OBSESSIONS

Aggressive (fears of harming self or others, of blurting out obscenities, or of other unwanted aggressive acts; unwanted violent or horrific images)

Contamination (concerns about dirt, germs, body waste or secretions, environmental contaminants, or animals/insects)

Sexual (concerns about unwanted sexual images or impulses)

Hoarding/saving

Religious (scrupulosity) (excessive concerns about sacrilege, blasphemy, right/wrong, morality)

Need for symmetry/exactness

Somatic (excessive concern about illness, body part, or appearance)

COMPULSIONS

Cleaning/washing (excessive or ritualized handwashing, showering, or other grooming)

Checking (checking locks, stove, appliances; checking body in relation to somatic obsessions; checking that did not or will not harm self or others)

Repeating rituals (rereading or rewriting; routine activities such as going through a door or arising from a chair)

Counting

Ordering/arranging

Hoarding/saving

Adapted from Goodman WK, Price LH, Rasmussen SA, et al. The Yale-Brown Obsessive Compulsive Scale. I. Development, use, and reliability. *Arch Gen Psychiatry.* 1989;46:1006-1011.

PROGNOSIS

In general, most persons with ongoing anxiety disorders tend to have a chronic course of waxing and waning symptoms. Maintenance therapies should often be used for patients with more chronic anxiety disorders, although evidence to support long-term therapies is not as robust as for mood and psychotic disorders.

Obsessive-Compulsive Disorder

Although anxiety is often prominent in obsessive-compulsive disorder (OCD), OCD has a distinct pathogenesis that is likely more closely related to other conditions such as body dysmorphic disorder, hoarding disorder, trichotillomania (hair-pulling), and excoriation (skin-picking) disorder.

Patients with OCD have recurrent obsessions or compulsions (Table 369-10), and most patients have both. OCD should not be confused with obsessive-compulsive personality traits or disorder, described later under "Personality Disorders." Obsessions, not to be confused with obsessing (ruminating) on a topic, are recurrent, persistent, and typically distressing thoughts that at some point during the course of the disorder are experienced as intrusive and unwanted. The latter quality may be described in language such as "I don't know where this thought comes from" or "I don't know why I have this thought, I would never actually do such a thing!" Compulsions are repetitive behaviors or mental acts the individual feels driven to perform in response to an obsession or according to rigid rules. For example, compulsive handwashing may relate to obsessional thoughts about germs or contamination. Patients with OCD typically attempt to ignore, suppress, or neutralize their obsessions, but doing so causes great psychic distress. OCD patients may spend many hours per day related to their obsessions and compulsions.

The 12-month prevalence of OCD is approximately 1%, with onset typically in childhood, adolescence, or young adulthood. Remission rates are low in adults, with most persons experiencing a chronic waxing and waning course. Pathogenesis probably involves altered functioning of the striatofrontal systems, as well as a prominent role for central serotonergic systems. Obsessions and compulsions may represent inappropriate triggering of neural "scripts" involving thoughts and behaviors that have been analogized to the scripts involved in animal grooming and other complex but stereotypical behaviors.

The only efficacious antidepressants in OCD are those with strong activity on serotonergic systems, such as the selective serotonin reuptake inhibitors and the tricyclic compound clomipramine. Cognitive-behavioral therapies also have well-demonstrated efficacy, often in combination with pharmacotherapy.[11] Deep brain stimulation[12] targeting the ventral capsule/ventral striatum is FDA approved (as a humanitarian device exemption) for severe treatment-refractory OCD, although its precise role remains to be determined. Focused ultrasound is another experimental possibility in refractory cases.[13]

Acute Stress Disorder and Post-Traumatic Stress Disorder

Acute stress disorder and post-traumatic stress disorder (PTSD) are specific manifestations of symptoms referable to an extremely traumatic event. The event by definition must involve exposure to actual or threatened death, serious injury, or sexual violence, as reported directly by the patient or by family members or friends. Patients suffer from repeated or extreme exposure to aversive details of the event. It is important to recognize that acute stress disorder or PTSD does not develop in all individuals exposed to a single traumatic event (e.g., a natural or man-made disaster). Some individuals may instead develop other anxiety disorders, major depression, mania, or psychosis, and many may never develop diagnosable psychopathology.

PTSD symptoms by definition persist for more than 1 month after the traumatic event and include the following types of clinical phenomena: (1) intrusion, such as intrusive memories, dreams, flashbacks, or intensely distressing psychological or physiologic responses to reminders of the trauma; (2) avoidance of distressing memories or external reminders of the trauma; (3) negative cognitions and mood, such as amnesia for aspects of the event, negativistic thoughts about oneself in general or blame related to the event, persistent negative emotions, diminished interests or activities, or feelings of detachment; and (4) alterations in arousal and reactivity.[14] Acute stress disorder by definition resolves in less than 1 month, with symptoms of intrusion, avoidance, or arousal as well as negative mood or dissociative symptoms (e.g., "in a daze").

The 12-month prevalence of PTSD in the United States is about 3%, with projected lifetime risk approaching 9%. About half of adults with PTSD have complete recovery within 3 months, but PTSD may persist for many months or years. Both cognitive-behavioral and psychodynamic psychology perspectives are useful in informing psychotherapeutic treatments.[A13] Antidepressants also have demonstrated efficacy in PTSD. Ketamine (0.5 mg/kg intravenously) can provide rapid relief in patients with chronic PTSD.[A14] Other agents have been used as well, including prazosin (primarily for nightmares and insomnia) and second-generation antipsychotics, such as risperidone and quetiapine.

PSYCHOTIC DISORDERS

Psychotic symptoms, defined as a loss of reality testing, include delusions (fixed false beliefs), hallucinations (false sensory perceptions), and major derailments in thought processes (e.g., loose associations). Psychotic symptoms may be seen in the course of neurocognitive, secondary, and mood disorders. The psychotic disorders are defined by the presence of psychotic symptoms in the absence of prominent mood disturbance or of neurocognitive deficits consistent with delirium or dementia. In general, the diagnosis and treatment of patients with psychotic disorders should be conducted in mental health specialty settings, but primary care settings are common points of entry to care.

Schizophrenia

DEFINITION AND EPIDEMIOLOGY

Schizophrenia, the prototypical psychotic disorder, necessarily includes symptoms of psychosis ("positive" symptoms) and also often includes "negative symptoms" such as affective flattening, abulia, apathy, and social withdrawal. The level of functioning is impaired in one or more realms (e.g., occupational, interpersonal, or self-care). The lifetime prevalence of schizophrenia is slightly less than 1%, and its chronic debilitating course takes a considerable toll on patients, families, and society. Peak onset is in late adolescence to young adulthood, slightly younger for males than females. The annual incidence is approximately 15 per 100,000, but with marked variability across study samples and populations. When narrowly defined as above, the condition is slightly more common in males than in females.

PATHOBIOLOGY

The pathogenesis of schizophrenia remains unknown. Twin studies show that the disease is multifactorial. Genetic factors account for up to 50% of the risk, and multiple gene loci appear to be involved. Studies of postmortem brains indicate a nongliotic neuropathologic process with subtle disruptions of cortical cytoarchitecture. It is likely that psychosocial factors and neurodevelopment interact with a nonlocalizable brain "lesion" that is either present at birth or acquired early in life. Dopaminergic mesocortical and mesolimbic pathways as well as glutamatergic systems are important in the production of psychotic symptoms.

DIAGNOSIS

The diagnosis of schizophrenia is based on the presence of delusions, hallucinations, and disorganized speech and behavior, often accompanied by apathy and social withdrawal and resulting in major impairment in functioning for at least 6 months (Table 369-11).[15] In patients with single schizophrenia-like psychotic episodes of briefer duration, with subsequent return to asymptomatic baseline functioning, brief psychotic disorder (<1 month) or schizophreniform disorder (1 to 6 months) is diagnosed.

TABLE 369-11 SYMPTOMS AND SIGNS OF MAJOR PSYCHOTIC DISORDERS

SCHIZOPHRENIA

Delusions
Hallucinations
Disorganized speech (i.e., thought process derailments)
Grossly disorganized or catatonic behavior
Negative symptoms: affective flattening, alogia, avolition
Major impairment in social or occupational functioning
Duration of at least 6 months

SCHIZOAFFECTIVE DISORDER

During the course of illness, at least one episode of schizophrenia-like psychotic symptoms *with* a mood syndrome (either major depression or mania), AND
During the course of illness, at least 2 weeks of schizophrenia-like psychotic symptoms *in the absence of* a mood syndrome

DELUSIONAL DISORDER

One or more delusions for at least 1 month, most often nonbizarre (i.e., potentially plausible, such as delusions of being followed, poisoned, infected, loved at a distance, deceived by a spouse or lover, or having a disease)
Not meeting full criteria for an acute episode of schizophrenia
Functioning *not* markedly impaired other than as related to the impact of the delusion(s) and its ramifications

Based on criteria from American Psychiatric Association. *Diagnostic and Statistical Manual of Mental Disorders.* 5th ed. (DSM-5) Washington, DC: American Psychiatric Association; 2013.

TREATMENT Rx

Antipsychotic medications (Table 369-12), often with adjunctive benzodiazepines, are used to treat acute psychotic episodes, commonly in acute inpatient settings so that the patient can be managed safely until the acute symptoms improve.[16] Although maintenance antipsychotic medications help reduce the severity and frequency of acute psychotic episodes, comprehensive psychosocial rehabilitation programs are required to improve functional outcomes; assertive use of such programs after first-onset psychosis may improve the longer-term course of the illness. Second-generation ("atypical") antipsychotic medications have replaced first-generation antipsychotics in common U.S. practice because of their lower rates of extrapyramidal side effects, including tardive dyskinesia, although their efficacy is generally not better than that of first-generation drugs.[A15] However, second-generation drugs contribute to the increase in obesity and metabolic syndrome in patients with chronic schizophrenia (Chapter 406).[17] A large trial found that clozapine and long-acting injectable antipsychotics are associated with the greatest reduction in relapse rates.[A16] Data suggest that cariprazine, a new-generation antipsychotic, is preferable to risperidone for patients with predominantly negative symptoms (withdrawal, apathy, etc.).[A17]

PROGNOSIS

The prognosis of individuals with schizophrenia is often poor, with recurrent episodes of psychotic exacerbations superimposed on progressively deteriorating baseline functioning. However, antipsychotic drugs significantly reduce relapse rates. Some patients have a more favorable course, and a small proportion of individuals may recover completely. Male sex, prominent negative symptoms, younger age at first onset, and enduring psychosocial stressors and family discord all predict poorer outcomes. Average life expectancy is shortened by 10 to 15 years because of poor health behaviors, higher rates of other medical disorders (including metabolic syndrome), and a lifetime suicide risk of approximately 5 to 6%.

TABLE 369-12 COMMONLY USED ANTIPSYCHOTIC MEDICATIONS

DRUG NAME	INITIAL DOSE FOR PSYCHOSIS IN SCHIZOPHRENIA*	TARGET DOSE FOR PSYCHOSIS IN SCHIZOPHRENIA†	SIDE EFFECTS	CHLORPROMAZINE DOSAGE EQUIVALENCE (FIRST-GENERATION DRUGS ONLY)/OTHER COMMENTS
First-generation drugs			Low-potency drugs: anticholinergic effects, orthostatic hypotension, prolongation of QT interval, cholestatic jaundice High-potency drugs: extrapyramidal side effects (dystonias, akathisia, parkinsonism, neuroleptic malignant syndrome), hyperprolactinemia with galactorrhea	
Chlorpromazine	100 mg qd	300-1000 mg/day, qd-bid dosing		100 mg
Thioridazine	50-100 mg qd	300-800 mg/day, qd-bid dosing	Pigmentary retinopathy at higher doses	100 mg
Thiothixene	2-5 mg qd	5-60 mg/day, qd-bid dosing		5 mg
Trifluoperazine	2-5 mg qd	5-40 mg/day, qd-bid dosing		5 mg
Perphenazine	4-8 mg qd	8-64 mg/day, qd-tid dosing		8 mg
Haloperidol	0.5-2 mg qd	2-10 mg/day (up to 40 mg/day or higher in refractory cases), qd-bid dosing		2 mg; available in depot IM form
Fluphenazine	1-2.5 mg qd	2.5-10 mg/day (up to 40 mg/day in refractory cases), qd-bid dosing		2 mg; available in depot IM form
Second-generation drugs			Metabolic syndrome, risk for stroke and mortality in older patients with dementia, QT prolongation	
Risperidone	0.5-1 mg qd-bid	2-4 mg/day, qd-bid dosing	Extrapyramidal side effects at higher doses	Available in depot IM form
Olanzapine	5 mg qd	5-10 mg qd (up to 20 mg/day in refractory cases)		
Ziprasidone	20 mg bid	20-80 mg bid		
Quetiapine	25-50 mg bid-tid	300-800 mg/day, bid-tid dosing		Extended-release form for qd dosing
Asenapine	5 mg bid	5-10 mg bid		Sublingual form only
Paliperidone	3-6 mg qd	6-12 mg qd		
Iloperidone	1 mg bid	2-12 mg bid		
Lurasidone	40 mg qd	40-160 mg qd		
Aripiprazole	10-15 mg qd	10-30 mg qd		Partial agonist/antagonist at D_2 receptors
Clozapine	12.5 mg qd-bid	300-900 mg/day, qd-bid (titrate dose slowly by 25-50 mg/day every 3-7 days)	Risk for agranulocytosis, requires ongoing monitoring of complete blood count	Efficacy superior to that of other antipsychotics, but hematologic risks and need for monitoring limit its use

*Doses for other indications, such as agitation in delirium or dementia, may be much lower.
†Target doses in the elderly may be lower.

Schizoaffective Disorder

Schizoaffective disorder is a chronic recurrent disorder with a lifetime prevalence of approximately 0.3%. It is characterized by episodes of psychosis in the absence of mania or depression, and also by mood episodes (manic or depressed) with psychotic features. As a result, the diagnosis of schizoaffective disorder requires knowledge of the patient's course over time and cannot be based on the patient's clinical findings at any one point in time. Treatment is symptomatic and involves the use of antipsychotic medications (see Table 369-12), mood stabilizers (see the Treatment box for bipolar disorders), and antidepressant medications (see Table 369-5) to target specific psychotic and mood symptoms. The outcomes of schizoaffective disorder are heterogeneous but on average intermediate between those of schizophrenia and mood disorders.

Delusional Disorder

Delusional disorders are characterized by one or more delusions in the absence of a thought process disorder, prominent hallucinations, or the negative symptoms seen in schizophrenia. The most characteristic types of delusions are potentially plausible ("nonbizarre"), such as unfounded beliefs of a partner's infidelity. Delusional disorder has a lifetime prevalence of approximately 0.2%. The pathogenesis of delusional disorder remains largely unknown. It is often only partially responsive to antipsychotic medications (see Table 369-12), but patients' functioning may be largely unimpaired if they are able, with the aid of antipsychotics and psychotherapy, to avoid acting on their delusions.

● SOMATIC SYMPTOM AND RELATED DISORDERS

Formerly termed *somatoform disorders,* the somatic symptom disorders include both somatic symptoms and associated thoughts, feelings, or behaviors that are distressing and disabling (Table 369-13). Although identifiable physical disease is insufficient to explain the patient's presentation fully, in all these conditions (other than factitious disorder) the patient's distress and dysfunction are *not* consciously produced and thus are just as distressing and baffling to patients as would be similar symptoms produced by physical disease. Malingering is the conscious feigning of illness for conscious gain and is therefore not considered to be a mental disorder at all.

TREATMENT ℞

Management of patients with somatic symptom disorders is often difficult because physicians must simultaneously maintain an appropriate level of vigilance for undiagnosed physical illness while avoiding unnecessary interventions. Keys to ongoing care include maintaining an ongoing therapeutic alliance, setting regular office visits, conveying empathy for the patient's very real distress without colluding with the patient's belief in an identifiable physical disorder, and assertively treating depression, anxiety, or other comorbid psychopathology. Antidepressant medications may benefit selected patients (e.g., some chronic pain syndromes), even in the absence of other comorbid psychiatric disorders.

● PERSONALITY DISORDERS

Personality is defined as the repertoire of enduring patterns of inner mental experience and behavior, including affect and impulse regulation, defense and coping mechanisms, and interpersonal relatedness. Dimensional models of personality (i.e., using multiple continuous measures of constructs such as neuroticism, extraversion, and openness to experience) likely are a more accurate representation of the spectrum of human personality, but categorical diagnostic categories (i.e., personality disorders) are more useful for clinicians to determine prognosis and treatments.[18] Personality and personality disorders are the result of complex interactions among genetic, environmental, and developmental factors. The cumulative point prevalence of all personality disorders in the general adult population is approximately 10 to 15%, with rates as high as 50% in patients receiving care in psychiatric treatment settings.

CLINICAL MANIFESTATIONS AND DIAGNOSIS

A personality disorder is diagnosed when enduring personality traits lead to pervasive (if variable) distress or dysfunction in a range of situations (Table 369-14). In diagnosing personality disorders, care must be taken to distinguish personality *traits,* which by definition are enduring, from time-limited *states.* Most persons can regress to less adaptive personality styles not characteristic of their baseline personality traits in the context of substantial psychosocial stressors.

TREATMENT

In many affected individuals, trying to alter the fundamental personality structure is not a realistic goal. Instead, a more realistic goal is to help patients maximize use of their personality strengths while minimizing the harmful effects of emotional dysregulation, dysfunctional defenses, and destructive behavior. Dialectic behavior therapy is an evidence-based, focused psychotherapy based on specific cognitive-behavioral techniques that reduce self-injurious behavior and suicidality in patients with borderline personality disorder.

Although pharmacotherapy is not the mainstay of treatment of most personality disorders, drugs can be useful in selected patients. Antipsychotic drugs may be used to target escalating paranoia in paranoid personality disorder or for short-term reduction in emotional and impulse regulation with a wide range of (often cluster B, see Table 369-14) personality disorders in times of crisis. For longer-term treatment of emotional dysregulation in borderline and other cluster B personality disorders, mood stabilizers or antidepressants may be used.

TABLE 369-13	SOMATIC SYMPTOM AND RELATED DISORDERS
TYPE	**MAIN CLINICAL MANIFESTATIONS**
Somatic symptom disorder	One or more distressing somatic symptoms, together with excessive thoughts, feelings, or behaviors related to these symptoms; subsumes most of the former terms somatization disorder, pain disorder, undifferentiated somatoform disorder, and many with the former diagnosis of hypochondriasis
Illness anxiety disorder	Illness preoccupation and excessive health-related behaviors in the absence of or disproportionate to somatic symptoms; subsumes some patients with the former diagnosis of hypochondriasis
Conversion disorder (functional neurologic symptom disorder)	Neurologic somatoform symptoms (other than pain) with clinical evidence incompatible with recognized neurologic or general medical conditions (e.g., paralysis, blindness, dyscoordination, convulsion-like phenomena, memory or other neurocognitive complaints)
Psychological factors affecting other medical conditions	Psychological factors adversely affecting a (non–mental disorder) medical symptom or condition by worsening the course, interfering with treatment, adding to known health risks, or influencing underlying pathophysiology
Factitious disorder (commonly called Munchausen syndrome)	Falsification of physical or psychological signs or symptoms, with health- or help-seeking behaviors, in the absence of clear external rewards

Author summary based on criteria from American Psychiatric Association. *Diagnostic and Statistical Manual of Mental Disorders.* 5th ed. (DSM-5) Washington, DC: American Psychiatric Association; 2013.

● SUICIDE AND EVALUATION OF SUICIDALITY

Suicide is a leading cause of death worldwide.[19] Suicide rates in the United States average approximately 11 per 100,000 per year, with considerable variability geographically and demographically. Of all age-, gender-, and race-based demographic groups, the highest U.S. suicide rates occur in older white men, while suicide is the third leading cause of death in adolescents and young adults and the tenth leading cause of death in the population overall. Suicide attempts, more than 10 times more common than death by suicide, lead to considerable morbidity and utilization of health care resources.

Suicide is a potentially preventable cause of death, but despite considerable research on risks for suicidal behavior, specific predictions about an individual's

TABLE 369-14 PERSONALITY DISORDERS

TYPE OF PERSONALITY DISORDER	MAIN IDENTIFYING CHARACTERISTICS
CLUSTER A: ODD/ECCENTRIC	
Schizoid personality disorder	Detachment from social relationships, restricted emotional expression
Schizotypal personality disorder	Discomfort with close relationships, cognitive or perceptual distortions, eccentric behavior
Paranoid personality disorder	Pervasive distrust and suspiciousness of others' motives as malevolent
CLUSTER B: DRAMATIC/EMOTIONAL/ERRATIC	
Borderline personality disorder	Instability of interpersonal relationships, self-image, and affects, and marked impulsivity
Narcissistic personality disorder	Grandiosity, need for admiration, and lack of empathy
Antisocial personality disorder	Pervasive disregard for and violation of the rights of others, lack of true remorse ("conscience")
Histrionic personality disorder	Pervasive excessive emotionality (theatricality) and attention seeking
CLUSTER C: ANXIOUS/FEARFUL	
Avoidant personality disorder	Social inhibition, feelings of inadequacy, and sensitivity to negative views from others
Dependent personality disorder	Pervasive and excessive need to be taken care of, resulting in submissive and clinging behavior and fears of separation
Obsessive-compulsive personality disorder	Pervasive preoccupation with orderliness, perfectionism, and mental and interpersonal control

Author summary based on criteria from American Psychiatric Association. *Diagnostic and Statistical Manual of Mental Disorders.* 5th ed. (DSM-5) Washington, DC: American Psychiatric Association; 2013.

TABLE 369-15 SOME IMPORTANT RISKS FOR SUICIDE AND SUICIDE ATTEMPTS

Mental disorder, particularly depressive, bipolar, substance use, psychotic, and personality disorders

Other symptoms of acute psychic distress, particularly hopelessness and panic attacks

Previous history of suicide attempt

Family history of suicide or suicide attempt (and, to a lesser degree, of any mental disorder)

Family violence, including physical or sexual abuse

Access to firearms or other lethal methods

Incarceration

Exposure to suicidal behavior of others (family, peers, public figures)

Social isolation

Interpersonal discord or other psychosocial stressors

Demographic factors, including male, non-Hispanic white or American Indian/ Alaska Native race, older age

behavior cannot be made with certainty. The linchpin of the clinical evaluation is a methodical assessment of risks for suicide (Table 369-15), together with direct questioning of the patient regarding thoughts of death, dying, and suicide; specific plans (in ideation or action) for suicide; and the details of any attempts. Although most persons who attempt suicide do not die, a previous history of a suicide attempt is a powerful risk for subsequent death by suicide. Suicide attempts and verbal threats should always be evaluated carefully and never dismissed as "gestures" or "attention-seeking" behavior. Patients at increased risk for suicide should be referred for psychiatric evaluation, with emergency referral if the risk is deemed to be imminent or increasing.

WHEN TO REFER A PATIENT FOR PSYCHIATRIC EVALUATION

Clinical decisions to refer a patient for specialty psychiatric evaluation must be made on an individual basis by taking into account the patient's clinical

TABLE 369-16 GENERAL CONSIDERATIONS IN DECIDING TO REFER A PATIENT FOR PSYCHIATRIC SPECIALTY CARE

Diagnosis or ongoing care of severe/chronic mental disorders, including bipolar disorder, psychotic disorders such as schizophrenia, and psychotic symptoms in other disorders

Management of more severe forms of other mental disorders and those refractory to treatment, including depression, anxiety disorders, and substance use disorders

Need for safety evaluation or management, including suicidality, homicidality or other aggressivity, or inability to care for self

Evaluation of decision-making capacity

Diagnostic uncertainty

Psychiatric comorbid conditions complicating diagnosis or treatment, including personality and substance use disorders coexisting with other psychiatric disorders

Psychiatric-medical comorbid conditions complicating diagnosis or treatment, including management of psychiatric disorders during pregnancy

Need for expertise in psychopharmacologic treatment

Need for expertise in other somatic therapies (e.g., electroconvulsive therapy, light therapy)

Need for expertise in psychotherapy or other psychosocial interventions

findings, including any previous history and immediate needs, and the clinician's own experience and expertise in assessing and managing the disorder (Table 369-16).

Grade A References

A1. Qaseem A, Barry MJ, Kansagara D. Nonpharmacologic versus pharmacologic treatment of adult patients with major depressive disorder: a clinical practice guideline from the American College of Physicians. *Ann Intern Med.* 2016;164:350-359.

A2. Gartlehner G, Gaynes BN, Amick HR, et al. Comparative benefits and harms of antidepressant, psychological, complementary, and exercise treatments for major depression: an evidence report for a clinical practice guideline from the American College of Physicians. *Ann Intern Med.* 2016; 164:331-341.

A3. Cipriani A, Furukawa TA, Salanti G, et al. Comparative efficacy and acceptability of 21 antidepressant drugs for the acute treatment of adults with major depressive disorder: a systematic review and network meta-analysis. *Lancet.* 2018;391:1357-1366.

A4. Cuijpers P, Sijbrandij M, Koole SL, et al. Adding psychotherapy to antidepressant medication in depression and anxiety disorders: a meta-analysis. *World Psychiatry.* 2014;13:56-67.

A5. Amick HR, Gartlehner G, Gaynes BN, et al. Comparative benefits and harms of second generation antidepressants and cognitive behavioral therapies in initial treatment of major depressive disorder: systematic review and meta-analysis. *BMJ.* 2015;351:1-10.

A6. Wilkinson ST, Ballard ED, Bloch MH, et al. The effect of a single dose of intravenous ketamine on suicidal ideation: a systematic review and individual participant data meta-analysis. *Am J Psychiatry.* 2018;175:150-158.

A7. Richards DA, Ekers D, McMillan D, et al. Cost and outcome of behavioural activation versus cognitive behavioural therapy for depression (COBRA): a randomised, controlled, non-inferiority trial. *Lancet.* 2016;388:871-880.

A8. Grochtdreis T, Brettschneider C, Wegener A, et al. Cost-effectiveness of collaborative care for the treatment of depressive disorders in primary care: a systematic review. *PLoS ONE.* 2015;10:1-19.

A9. McGirr A, Vöhringer PA, Ghaemi SN, et al. Safety and efficacy of adjunctive second-generation antidepressant therapy with a mood stabiliser or an atypical antipsychotic in acute bipolar depression: a systematic review and meta-analysis of randomised placebo-controlled trials. *Lancet Psychiatry.* 2016;3:1138-1146.

A10. Chiang KJ, Tsai JC, Liu D, et al. Efficacy of cognitive-behavioral therapy in patients with bipolar disorder: a meta-analysis of randomized controlled trials. *PLoS ONE.* 2017;12:1-19.

A11. Cuijpers P, Sijbrandij M, Koole S, et al. Psychological treatment of generalized anxiety disorder: a meta-analysis. *Clin Psychol Rev.* 2014;34:130-140.

A12. Slee A, Nazareth I, Bondaronek P, et al. Pharmacological treatments for generalised anxiety disorder: a systematic review and network meta-analysis. *Lancet.* 2019;393:768-777.

A13. Reiter K, Andersen SB, Carlsson J. Neurofeedback treatment and posttraumatic stress disorder: effectiveness of neurofeedback on posttraumatic stress disorder and the optimal choice of protocol. *J Nerv Ment Dis.* 2016;204:69-77.

A14. Feder A, Parides MK, Murrough JW, et al. Efficacy of intravenous ketamine for treatment of chronic posttraumatic stress disorder: a randomized clinical trial. *JAMA Psychiatry.* 2014;71:681-688.

A15. Leucht S, Cipriani A, Spineli L, et al. Comparative efficacy and tolerability of 15 antipsychotic drugs in schizophrenia: a multiple-treatments meta-analysis. *Lancet.* 2013;382:951-962.

A16. Tiihonen J, Mittendorfer-Rutz E, Majak M, et al. Real-world effectiveness of antipsychotic treatments in a nationwide cohort of 29823 patients with schizophrenia. *JAMA Psychiatry.* 2017;74:686-693.

A17. Németh G, Laszlovszky I, Czobor P, et al. Cariprazine versus risperidone monotherapy for treatment of predominant negative symptoms in patients with schizophrenia: a randomised, double-blind, controlled trial. *Lancet.* 2017;389:1103-1113.

GENERAL REFERENCES

For the General References and other additional features, please visit Expert Consult at https://expertconsult.inkling.com.

370

HEADACHES AND OTHER HEAD PAIN

KATHLEEN B. DIGRE

DEFINITION

Headache, which is a very common symptom, can be secondary to an underlying abnormality but is usually a primary headache disorder such as migraine headache, tension-type headache, cluster headache, and paroxysmal hemicrania.

EPIDEMIOLOGY

About 90% of all adults experience headache at some time in their lives, and over 75% of children have complained of headaches by the age of 15 years. In the United States, the direct and indirect costs associated with migraine are over $20 billion annually. The World Health Organization lists migraine in the top 10 most disabling conditions. Patients at most risk for lost days of employment are those with chronic migraine and daily headache.

In large population-based studies, the relative risk of having migraine, tension-type headaches, or cluster headaches increases up to four times if a first-degree relative has the same kind of headaches. Studies of twins, especially identical twins, also show a similar susceptibility.

PATHOBIOLOGY

Headache pain is initiated by primary trigeminal afferents that innervate the blood vessels, mucosa, muscles, and tissues. Fibers from these sources coalesce in the trigeminal ganglion, especially the first division. The trigeminal afferents terminate in the primary sensory nucleus of cranial nerve V and its spinal nucleus, which has several small subnuclei, the most important of which is the subnucleus caudalis. This subnucleus receives afferents from meningeal vessels, dura-sensitive neurons, and even the upper cervical cord and then projects them to the lateral and medial thalamus by way of the spinothalamic tract and to diencephalic and brain stem regions that are involved in the regulation of autonomic functions. Thalamic nociceptive information ascends to the sensory cortex, as well as to other areas of the brain.

Although secondary headaches may stimulate the pathway by way of processes such as inflammation and compression, primary headache disorders occur spontaneously by means of chemical mediators such as calcitonin gene–related peptide. The sequence of events commences with peripheral activation caused by neurogenic plasma extravasation activated spontaneously or by cortical spreading depression. The trigeminocervical complex, especially the nucleus caudalis, is then activated, and patients can experience allodynia, a condition in which a non-noxious stimulus is sensed as painful.

Aura is defined as a focal visual, sensory, or motor neurologic disturbance that may occur with or without headache. Aura is thought to occur when cortical spreading depression causes depolarization of membranes. Both neurons and glia can mediate both constriction and dilation of blood vessels. Migraine headache clearly has a genetic component. Familial hemiplegic migraine can be caused by mutations in the *CACNA1A* gene, which is located on chromosome 19p13.2-p13.1 and encodes for voltage-gated neuronal calcium channels. Mutations in the *CACNA1A* gene also cause episodic ataxia and epilepsy. Another mutation is in *ATP1A2*, also called the familial hemiplegia migraine 2 (*FHM2*) gene, which is located on chromosome 1q21-q23 and encodes for the sodium-potassium adenosine triphosphatase (Na^+,K^+-ATPase) transport protein. A third genetic locus is the *SCN1A* gene on chromosome 2q24.3, which is a voltage-gated sodium channel. In addition, many single nucleotide polymorphisms have been associated with migraine.[1] Although there are linkages to many genetic loci for more common forms of migraine, migraine and other headaches also probably have multiple epigenetic interactions[2] with environmental factors, and it is clear that the genetic contributions are complex.

CLINICAL MANIFESTATIONS

Patients with headache may describe the pain as throbbing, bandlike, or aching. The pain is frequently unilateral but can be bilateral. Migraine headache is often associated with nausea, vomiting, photophobia, and phonophobia. It is invariably moderate to severe and interferes with activities. Other autonomic manifestations that can accompany migraine, cluster, and other headache variants include ptosis, conjunctival injection, tearing, rhinorrhea, Horner

TABLE 370-1	REASONS FOR FURTHER EVALUATION TO LOOK FOR SECONDARY HEADACHES

Beginning of headaches at an older age, without a previous history or a positive family history

Unexplainable and abnormal worsening of previously existing migraines

Dramatic or unusual change in character of the prodrome or the headache previously present

Headaches awakening the patient in the middle of the night (except for a cluster headache)

Headaches much worse when recumbent, only when upright, or with coughing, sneezing, or the Valsalva maneuver

Unusually severe headache of sudden onset ("worst headache of my life")

Focal deficits that do not disappear after the headache is over

Any abnormal neurologic or new psychiatric finding on examination

A new headache in a patient with human immunodeficiency virus infection, malignancy, or pregnancy

syndrome, and facial edema. Secondary headaches sometimes may appear to be similar to tension-type or migraine headaches, but "red flags" may suggest a secondary rather than a primary headache disorder (Table 370-1). Particular attention should be paid to the sudden onset of severe headaches, which frequently have an underlying secondary cause.[3]

DIAGNOSIS

Five elements of the history are key for evaluating headaches. The family history helps determine whether a person has a genetic predisposition to headache. The life history of headache determines whether the headache is new or has evolved over the course of a lifetime. The attack history provides the clinical features of the headache or headaches. The medical and psychiatric history determines whether there are comorbid conditions that can cause or worsen the headache. The medication and drug history determines whether the headache could be caused by or worsened by medications or drugs the person has ingested.

Diagnosis of the type of headache is based on the type of pain, the duration of headache, and accompanying features (Table 370-2). Secondary headaches are usually due to an underlying condition such as a brain tumor (Chapter 180), increased or low intracranial pressure, sinus disease (Chapter 398), or a vascular malformation (Chapter 380); on removing the cause, the headache generally improves. Headaches that occur at a frequency of less than 15 days a month are called episodic, whereas headaches that occur more than 15 days a month are considered chronic.

The diagnostic evaluation for headache depends on the clinical findings. If the history is typical and if the neurologic examination is completely normal, no further evaluation is needed. The features of the history that are most likely to predict migraine headache without a secondary disorder include photophobia, nausea, and disabling nature. However, if there are atypical features of the history or any abnormality on neurologic examination, further evaluation is indicated. Patients with cluster headache types and headaches of undetermined cause need imaging to exclude secondary causes.

In patients with acute onset headache, computed tomography (CT) is best for assessing acute hemorrhage as the cause of the headache, whereas magnetic resonance imaging (MRI) is best for assessing most persistent headaches to look for mass lesions, evidence of intracranial hypertension or hypotension, hemosiderin (old hemorrhage), and congenital abnormalities (e.g., Chiari malformation). In individuals older than 60 years with an unexplained new or unusual headache, the erythrocyte sedimentation rate (ESR) and/or C-reactive protein (CRP) level should be measured to evaluate for giant cell arteritis (Chapter 69). Cerebrospinal fluid (CSF) analysis, including opening pressure, protein, glucose, cells, culture, and cytology, is indicated in patients with suspected intracranial hypertension or meningitis.

TREATMENT   Rx

Treatment of acute headache depends on the type and severity of the headache. For mild headaches, simple analgesics such as acetaminophen[A1] (500 to 1000 mg), acetaminophen with caffeine, aspirin (250 to 1000 mg),[A2] and nonsteroidal anti-inflammatory drugs[A3] ([NSAIDs]; e.g., ibuprofen, 400 to 800 mg; naproxen sodium, 220 to 500 mg, diclofenac 50-100 mg) will suffice.

TABLE 370-2 DIFFERENTIAL DIAGNOSIS OF HEADACHE

HEADACHE TYPE	GENETICS	EPIDEMIOLOGY	CHARACTERISTIC FEATURES	LENGTH	ACCOMPANYING SYMPTOMS
Migraine headache	Complex genetics but usually a family history	More frequent in women	Unilateral, bilateral; throbbing; moderate to severe; worsens with activity	Hours to days	Photophobia, phonophobia, nausea and/or vomiting
Tension-type headache	Usually a family history	Equal frequency in men and women	Tight band–like pain; bilateral; pain may be mild to moderate; improves with activity	Hours to days	No nausea or vomiting; small amount of light or sound sensitivity, but not both
Cluster headache	May have a family history	More frequent in men	Unilateral severe pain in the face	Minutes to hours	Ipsilateral ptosis, miosis, rhinorrhea, eyelid edema, tearing
Paroxysmal hemicrania	Usually no family history	More frequent in women	Unilateral pain in the face	Minutes	Ipsilateral ptosis, miosis, rhinorrhea, eyelid edema, tearing; responds to indomethacin
Short unilateral headache with conjunctival injection, tearing	No family history	More frequent in men	Unilateral eye pain; orbit pain	Seconds to 240 seconds	Conjunctival injection, tearing
Hemicrania continua	No family history	More frequent in women	Unilateral continuous headache with episodic stabbing pains	Continuous	Ipsilateral autonomic features: ptosis, miosis, rhinorrhea, eyelid edema, tearing; responds to indomethacin

TABLE 370-3 PREVENTIVE MEDICATIONS FOR HEADACHE

DRUG	RATIONAL USE	DOSAGE	SIDE EFFECTS	CONTRAINDICATIONS/ CAUTION
β-Blockers (e.g., propranolol, nadolol, timolol)	Migraine, anyone with elevated blood pressure	Propranolol, 20-80 mg; may increase	Lethargy, depression	Asthma, low blood pressure
Calcium-channel antagonists: verapamil, amlodipine	Cluster headache, elevated blood pressure	Verapamil, 120-480 mg/day	Low blood pressure	
Nonsteroidal anti-inflammatory drugs:				
Naproxen, ibuprofen	Migraine, tension-type, and menstrual migraine	Naproxen, 200-600 mg/day; Ibuprofen, 600-800 mg bid-tid;	Gastrointestinal	Ulcers, sensitivity, allergy
Indomethacin	Paroxysmal hemicrania, hemicrania continua	Indomethacin, 25-50 mg tid	Gastrointestinal	Ulcers; renal insufficiency
Tricyclic antidepressants: amitriptyline, nortriptyline, imipramine	Migraine, tension-type headache, anyone with poor sleep	10-25 mg qhs; may increase	Dry mouth, orthostatic hypotension, weight gain	Sensitivity
Anticonvulsants: topiramate valproate	Migraine, cluster headache	Topiramate, 25-50 mg bid; valproate, 250-500 mg bid	Topiramate: weight loss, kidney stones, intraocular hypertension Valproate: weight gain	Pregnancy—both U.S. FDA classification D
Calcitonin gene–related peptide antibodies: erenumab, fremanezumab, galcanezumab	Migraine, chronic migraine	Erenumab 70-140 mg SC monthly; fremanezumab 225 mg SC monthly; galcanezumab 120 or 240 mg SC monthly	Injection site redness; nasal symptoms	Unknown pregnancy effect

bid = twice daily; FDA = Food and Drug Administration; qhs = at bedtime; SC = subcutaneously; tid = three times daily.

PREVENTION

Preventive medications are recommended when headaches are frequent or severe enough to interfere with quality of life. The choice of medications should be based on the type of headache (migraine, tension-type), their side effect profiles, and the patient's comorbid conditions (Table 370-3).

PROGNOSIS

The natural history of headache depends on many factors, including the type of headache, comorbid conditions that accompany the headache, and success of treatment.[4] Risk factors for chronic headache include female sex, migraine-type headaches, frequent headaches, obesity, low education and socioeconomic level, overuse of medication, depression, anxiety, stressful life events, and sleep apnea.

MIGRAINE HEADACHE

DEFINITION

Migraine is an inherited headache disorder that is typically unilateral but sometimes bilateral, moderate to severe, worsens by routine physical activity, associated with nausea and/or vomiting, and accompanied by photophobia and phonophobia. The headache occurs anytime and persists from 4 to 72 hours. It may occur with or without an aura (a focal neurologic symptom that may be visual, sensory, or motor). Visual auras may have positive (photopsias) and negative (scotomas) features.

EPIDEMIOLOGY

The prevalence of migraine is 15 to 20% in women and 4 to 7% in men. In children the prevalence may be as high as 17% and is equal in boys and girls. At puberty, the prevalence rises in girls and remains higher throughout their lifespan. The highest prevalence occurs between the ages of 25 and 55. Migraine with aura affects 5% of the adult population, and 90% of auras are visual. Migraine is more prevalent in white persons and in those with a lower socioeconomic status or income.

Comorbid conditions that may be associated with migraine headache include epilepsy, stroke, depression, anxiety, myocardial infarction, patent foramen ovale, Raynaud phenomenon, irritable bowel syndrome, and pain disorders such as fibromyalgia. Menstruation and ovulation may increase the frequency of headache.

PATHOBIOLOGY

The aura of a migraine headache is thought to be due in part to cortical spreading depression, which is associated with a brief reduction in blood flow followed by hyperemia.[5] These changes do not seem to correlate with the phase of the headache. Pain occurs when trigeminal afferents of the dura are stimulated.

CLINICAL MANIFESTATIONS

Migraine headache often begins with a prodrome that may persist for hours to days, when patients note difficulty concentrating or fatigue without headache. An aura may or may not occur but is generally present before the headache begins. The headache may be unilateral or bilateral, throbbing, moderate to severe, and worsened with activity. Accompanying clinical features include nausea, vomiting, and sensitivity to light and sound. Other clinical features include neck pain, occasionally dizziness, osmophobia (sensitivity to odors), and difficulty thinking clearly.

The migraine aura is generally visual but can be sensory or include aphasia or vertigo. Migraine aura without headache begins with a neurologic disturbance (e.g., a visual phenomenon), but without a subsequent headache. Although an aura is traditionally thought to precede the headache, it can be present during the headache phase.

DIAGNOSIS

The diagnosis of migraine is based on the history. The differential diagnosis includes tension-type headache, but most moderate to severe headaches are migraine.[6] In patients with a history suggestive of a secondary headache, further evaluation with MRI should be considered (see Table 370-2). However, if the headache is typical of migraine and the findings on neurologic examination are normal, no further studies are needed.

TREATMENT   Rx

Treatment of migraine is divided into treatment of the acute headache and prevention of subsequent migraine attacks. Acute treatment is most effectively accomplished with migraine-specific care: a nonspecific analgesic agent or combination analgesic therapy for milder migraine, and most frequently aggressive migraine-specific therapy for migraine (Table 370-4). For example, mild attacks can generally be treated successfully with over-the-counter analgesics such as acetaminophen (suggested dose, 650 to 1000 mg) or NSAIDs (aspirin, 250 mg to 1000 mg; ibuprofen, 1000 mg to 1200 mg; naproxen, 500 mg to 825 mg; diclofenac 50 mg, or ketoprofen, 75 mg). If the migraine headaches are moderate to severe, patients benefit from migraine-specific therapies (see Table 370-4) such as triptans (sumatriptan, zolmitriptan, rizatriptan, almotriptan, naratriptan, frovatriptan, and eletriptan), ergotamine (dihydroergotamine, ergotamine tartrate), or isometheptene,[7] and the combination of naproxen plus sumatriptan may be better than either alone[A4] (see Table 370-4).

During pregnancy, mild to moderate attacks can be treated with acetaminophen. Moderate headaches may respond to the combination of acetaminophen, isometheptene mucate (a mild vasoconstrictor, 65 mg), and dichloralphenazone (a mild sedative, 100 mg). Antinausea agents include prochlorperazine (10 to 25 mg) and metoclopramide (2.5 to 10 mg).

Stratification of care, including tailoring the treatment according to the type of headache, results in fewer days of disability and use of medications. Which migraine-specific drug will work for any individual patient depends on the patient. It is important to avoid overuse of analgesic and other medications (especially opiates) because overuse can cause chronic daily headache in susceptible individuals. Prompt treatment improves the outcome of headache when compared with late treatment. Contraindications to use of triptans (see Table 370-4) include uncontrolled hypertension, clinical evidence of ischemic heart disease, and Prinzmetal angina.

Opioids such as N-acetyl-p-aminophenol (APAP) with codeine, or butorphanol, benefit some patients, but meperidine is not effective. Oral opiates should not be used for chronic recurrent, primary headaches, although sometimes opiates (e.g., acetaminophen, 325 mg, with codeine, 30 mg) are often the only option during pregnancy or in patients with severe vascular disease. When opiates are used, caution is required, and the associated risks of rebound headache and dependency must be recognized by both the patient and physician. Barbiturates (with caffeine and aspirin or acetaminophen) have not been efficacious in controlled trials but may be helpful in individual patients in whom other migraine-specific drugs cannot be used or are contraindicated.

For moderate to severe attacks, options include dihydroergotamine (1 to 2 mg intranasally); oral, intranasal, or subcutaneous administration of sumatriptan (25 to 100 mg orally, 20 mg intranasally, or 4 to 6 mg subcutaneously); or other triptans (e.g., naratriptan, 2.5 mg; zolmitriptan, 5 mg; rizatriptan, 10 mg; eletriptan, 40 mg; frovatriptan, 2.5 mg; or almotriptan, 12.5 mg).[A5] Ergotamine (2 mg sublingually or 1 to 2 mg orally), when given early in the migraine attack, can be effective if the associated nausea and peripheral vasoconstriction are tolerable.

TABLE 370-4 SPECIFIC TRIPTAN MEDICATIONS FOR THE TREATMENT OF ACUTE MIGRAINE

	SUMATRIPTAN	ZOLMITRIPTAN	NARATRIPTAN	RIZATRIPTAN	ALMOTRIPTAN	FROVATRIPTAN	ELETRIPTAN
Trade name	Imitrex, Zecuity	Zomig	Amerge	Maxalt	Axert	Frova	Relpax
Forms	SC, nasal (NS), oral	Oral: tablet/ZMT, NS	Oral	Oral: tablet/MLT	Oral	Oral	Oral
Dose	Oral: 50-100 mg (200 mg/24 hr max.) SC: 4-6 mg (12 mg/24 hr max.) NS: 5-20 mg (40 mg/24 hr max.) Nasal delivery device (22 mg)	2.5-5 mg (10 mg/24 hr max.) 5 mg (10 mg/24 hr max.)	1-2.5 mg (5 mg/24 hr max.)	5-10 mg (30 mg/24 hr max.)	6.25-12.5 mg (25 mg/24 hr max.)	2.5 mg (7.5 mg/24 hr max.)	20-40 mg (80 mg/24 hr max.)
Half-life	2-3 hr	3-4 hr	6-8 hr	2-3 hr	3-4 hr	26 hr	4-6 hr
Crosses blood-brain barrier	–	+	+	+	+	+	+
Use with monoamine oxidase inhibitor (MAOI)	–	–	+	–	+	+	–
Good for recurrences	–	–	+	–	–	+	+
Rapid response	SC, 10-15 min NS, 15-20 min Oral, 30 min	30 min	1-4 hr	30 min	60 min	1-4 hr	20-30 min
Menstrual migraine	+	+	+	+	+	+	+
Other	In combination with naproxen (Treximet)			Decrease dose by half with propranolol			Do not use with CYP3A4 drugs (ketoconazole and some macrolide antibiotics)

max. = maximum; MT = Maxalt Melting tablet; NS = nasal spray; SC = subcutaneous; ZMT = Zolmitriptan melting tablet.

For very severe attacks, dihydroergotamine (1 mg subcutaneously or 0.5 to 1 mg intravenously [IV]) is usually effective but generally requires an antiemetic (e.g., promethazine, 25 mg) before intravenous use. Ketorolac (60 mg intramuscularly [IM] or 30 mg IV), prochlorperazine (10 to 25 mg IM or 10 mg IV[A6] delivered over a 5-minute period), or metoclopramide (10 mg IV)[A7] is useful for patients who are nonresponsive or have contraindications to vasoactive abortive agents. An experimental approach is electrical skin stimulation of the upper arms, especially if applied within the first 20 minutes of the onset of pain.[A8]

PREVENTION

Preventive treatment (see Table 370-3) is often recommended when the headaches interfere with activities on 3 or more days per month, the headaches are severe or prolonged, or migraine is complicated by events such as cerebral infarction. Prophylactic options include β-adrenergic blockers, calcium-channel antagonists, NSAIDs, tricyclic antidepressants, valproate, and topiramate. Topiramate, divalproex, timolol, propranolol, metoprolol, atenolol, nadolol, acebutolol, captopril, lisinopril, and candesartan reduce migraine frequency by 50% or more compared with placebo, with no statistically significant differences among them.[A9] Other alternatives include the serotonergic drug cyproheptadine (4 to 20 mg) or the monoamine oxidase inhibitor phenelzine (30 to 60 mg). Acupuncture and biofeedback have been used successfully. OnabotulinumtoxinA injection is also effective for prophylaxis of chronic migraine.[A10] Supraorbital nerve stimulation[A11] also is approved by the Food and Drug Administration (FDA) to prevent migraines. A new and very promising approach is calcitonin gene–related peptide antibodies.[8] Erenumab is currently approved (70 to 140 mg subcutaneously monthly),[A12][A13] and similarly beneficial results have been seen with fremanezumab (225 mg subcutaneously monthly or 675 mg quarterly)[A14][A15] and galcanezumab (240 mg loading and 120 mg monthly).[A16]

PROGNOSIS

The prognosis for patients with migraine is variable. In many patients, headaches decrease in severity with age, but migraine aura without headache becomes more frequent with older age. Modification of inciting factors such as avoiding dietary triggers (tyramine, phenylethylamine, ethanol), ameliorating or preventing insomnia, and averting environmental triggers (light, sound, odor) may improve outcome. Migraines may become chronic, defined as more than 15 days per month, especially when associated with obesity, snoring, depression, and low socioeconomic status. Since there appears to be shared genetic susceptibility to migraine with aura and ischemic stroke, careful attention to cardiovascular risk factors is important.

TENSION-TYPE HEADACHE

DEFINITION

Tension-type headache is defined as a mild or moderate holocranial headache without nausea or vomiting. Patients may have either photophobia or phonophobia but not both, and the headache does not worsen with activity.

EPIDEMIOLOGY

The 1-year prevalence is 14 to 93 per 100,000 individuals for episodic tension-type headache and 8.1 per 100,000 for chronic tension-type headache. Tension-type headaches are more common in women than in men, regardless of age, race, and educational level. Tension-type headaches are more common in Western countries and less frequent in Asian countries, and they are more common in white persons than in African Americans.

PATHOBIOLOGY

The pathophysiology of tension-type headache is less well understood than that of the other types of headache. Myofascial tenderness is increased, especially in chronic tension-type headache. Genetic factors are uncertain. Migraine and tension-type headache often coexist. Although tension-type headaches are not due to emotion or muscle contraction, triggers of a tension-type headache are similar to those associated with migraine: stress, fatigue, and lack of sleep. Comorbid conditions in patients with tension-type headache include depression and anxiety in more than 50% of individuals.

CLINICAL MANIFESTATIONS

Tension-type headaches are usually mild to moderate in severity, and most individuals do not seek care. Tension-type headache can be episodic (occurring

<15 days per month) or chronic (occurring >15 days per month). In many patients headaches remain episodic, but about 25% progress to chronic headache. Of the patients with chronic tension-type headache, about a quarter to a third continue as chronic, half can improve to episodic, and in about a quarter medication overuse headache can develop. Episodic tension-type headaches can last minutes, hours, or days.

DIAGNOSIS

Headaches that can be misdiagnosed as tension-type headache include migraine, hemicrania continua, new daily persistent headache, and headaches caused by brain tumors, elevated or low intracranial pressure, or giant cell arteritis. A careful history is the best way to distinguish other types of headaches.

TREATMENT

Episodic tension-type headaches are generally treated successfully[9] with acetaminophen (650 to 1000 mg) or NSAIDs (aspirin, 250 to 1000 mg; naproxen, 250 to 500 mg; ibuprofen, 200 to 800 mg; or ketoprofen, 12.5 to 75 mg). However, analgesic use for more than 3 days per week can worsen headaches and lead to medication-induced headache.

PREVENTION

Chronic tension-type headaches may benefit from prophylactic treatment with amitriptyline (starting with 10 mg at bedtime and increased slowly up to 100 mg until the patient improves or intolerable side effects develop), nortriptyline (25 to 100 mg each evening), doxepin (25 to 75 mg/day), maprotiline (10 to 25/mg/day), or fluoxetine (10 to 20 mg/day). Tricyclics are generally more efficacious than serotonin reuptake inhibitors.[A17] Muscle relaxants, physical therapy, localized botulinum toxin injection, and acupuncture can be useful.[A18]

PROGNOSIS

Tension-type headache has a variable prognosis. Adolescents with tension-type headache and two or more psychiatric factors (e.g., depression and anxiety) have a worse prognosis.

CLUSTER HEADACHE AND OTHER TRIGEMINAL AUTONOMIC CEPHALALGIAS

DEFINITION

Trigeminal autonomic cephalalgias, including cluster headaches, are unilateral headaches associated with ipsilateral autonomic features. Other trigeminal autonomic cephalalgias include paroxysmal hemicrania, which is characterized by bouts of headache that persist for 5 to 30 minutes, is generally unilateral, and usually occurs in women; they typically respond to indomethacin. Hemicrania continua, another indomethacin-responsive headache seen in both men and women, is characterized by continuous unilateral pain and mild associated autonomic features; it frequently coexists with a form of chronic daily headache. Short unilateral neuralgiform headache with conjunctival injection and tearing is a rare trigeminal autonomic cephalalgia that occurs in men; individual headaches persist for only a short time (seconds to 2 minutes).

EPIDEMIOLOGY

Cluster headache occurs in 56 to 401 per 100,000 persons and is more frequent in men (3:1 to 7:1). Attacks usually begin between 20 and 30 years of age. Paroxysmal hemicrania occurs in 56 to 381 per 100,000 persons; it affects women more often (2:1) and can begin at any age but usually commences at 34 to 41 years. Short unilateral neuralgiform headache with conjunctival injection and tearing is rare, with a slight male preponderance (2:1).

PATHOBIOLOGY

Cluster headache may have a genetic predisposition. Imaging studies such as positron emission tomography and functional MRI show inferior posterior hypothalamic activation at the onset of cluster headache and other trigeminal autonomic cephalalgias. In addition, the trigeminovascular complex and the cranial autonomic system are activated. The pathophysiology of hemicrania continua is unknown, and there is debate whether it is associated with hypothalamic involvement or whether it resembles migraine.

CLINICAL MANIFESTATIONS

Cluster headache is almost always unilateral, rarely bilateral, and has characteristic ipsilateral autonomic features, commonly including lacrimation and

TABLE 370-5 DISTINGUISHING CHARACTERISTICS OF THE TRIGEMINAL AUTONOMIC CEPHALALGIAS

CHARACTERISTIC	CLUSTER	PAROXYSMAL HEMICRANIA	HEMICRANIA CONTINUA	SHORT UNILATERAL NEURALGIFORM HEADACHE WITH CONJUNCTIVAL INJECTION AND TEARING
Sex—F:M	1:3-7	2:1	2:1	1:2
Unilateral	+	+	+	+
Attack frequency	1-8/day	1-40/day	3-200/day	3-200/day
Attack duration	15-80 min	2-30 min	Continuous with episodic exacerbations	5-240 sec
Autonomic features	+	+	+ with exacerbations	+
Indomethacin effect	–	+++	+++	–
Acute treatment at onset	Oxygen, sumatriptan SC, DHE nasal spray; sumatriptan or zolmitriptan nasal spray (A-level evidence)	None	None	None
Preventive medications	Verapamil, lithium, corticosteroids, anticonvulsants (A level)	Indomethacin (A level)	Indomethacin (A level)	Lamotrigine, topiramate, gabapentin (B level)

DHE = dihydroergotamine; SC = subcutaneous.

conjunctival injection and occasionally nasal congestion, rhinorrhea, ptosis, miosis, flushing, and eyelid edema (Table 370-5). The location of the pain is usually behind or above the eye or in the temple but can include the forehead, cheek, teeth, or jaw. The pain reaches its maximum intensity in about 9 minutes and tends to end abruptly. Attacks occur one to eight times a day and are usually described as "boring" or "stabbing" excruciating pain that persists for 15 minutes to 2 hours. Migraine symptoms may coexist, including unilateral photophobia, phonophobia, and rarely, an aura. Unlike migraine patients, who usually try to rest, patients with cluster headaches pace and are unable to sit or lie down. Cluster headaches, often precipitated by alcohol, histamine, or nitroglycerin, have a daily periodicity and may also have a seasonal periodicity. For example, episodic cluster headache may occur annually or every 2 years, often in the same season each time. Chronic cluster headache occurs without a remission.

Paroxysmal hemicrania is pain of short duration, usually 2 to 30 minutes, and occurs unilaterally around the eye, temple, or maxillary region, sometimes precipitated by head movements. Autonomic features similar to cluster headache can occur. The usual attack rate is up to 40 episodes each day. Bouts of pain may be episodic, separated by a remission, but most patients have daily chronic paroxysmal hemicrania without a remission.

Short unilateral neuralgiform headache with conjunctival injection and tearing attacks are unilateral and consistently on the same side. Although the pain is excruciating, the attack is brief, usually seconds; most patients are free of pain between attacks, although a dull ache can be present. Associated autonomic features include ipsilateral conjunctival injection and tearing.

DIAGNOSIS

The diagnostic criteria for cluster headache include severe unilateral orbital, supraorbital, or temporal pain persisting for 15 to 180 minutes with at least one of the following: ipsilateral conjunctival injection or lacrimation, nasal congestion or rhinorrhea, eyelid edema, forehead and facial sweating, miosis with or without ptosis, and restlessness or agitation.[10] Attacks occur between once and as often as eight times each day. There is no other cause of the disorder.

Paroxysmal hemicrania is defined by unilateral pain persisting for 2 to 30 minutes, about five times each day, with one or more autonomic features such as conjunctival injection, nasal congestion, eyelid edema, forehead and facial sweating, and miosis or ptosis (or both). Complete prevention may be achieved with indomethacin.

Hemicrania continua is a unilateral headache that occurs daily and continuously without pain-free periods; its intensity is moderate, with exacerbations of severe pain. During the exacerbations, at least one ipsilateral autonomic feature is present: conjunctival redness, lacrimation, nasal congestion, ptosis, or miosis. It responds to indomethacin.

Short unilateral neuralgiform headache with conjunctival injection and tearing is diagnosed by unilateral orbital, supraorbital, temporal stabbing pain persisting for 5 to 240 seconds at a frequency of three to 200 per day. It is associated with conjunctival injection and tearing.

An imaging procedure such as MRI is indicated for all patients at the onset of cluster headaches or other trigeminal autonomic cephalalgias because they can be the result of infection (Chapters 384 to 386), vascular malformation (Chapter 380), carotid dissection, or neoplasm, especially a pituitary tumor (Chapter 180). Other possibilities in the differential diagnosis include migraine, hypnic headache (rare short-lasting headaches exclusively during sleep in the elderly), and trigeminal neuralgia.

TREATMENT Rx

Because the course of the headache is brief, oral medications take too long to work to be effective. The use of 100% oxygen at 7 to 10 L/minute for 15 to 30 minutes benefits some patients.[A19] Sumatriptan or zolmitriptan nasal spray or sumatriptan subcutaneously (4 to 6 mg) can be helpful.[11] Dihydroergotamine can be helpful when given nasally, IM, or even IV. Vagal nerve stimulation was recently approved for acute cluster headache.[A20] Refractory cases may respond to sphenopalatine ganglion and occipital nerve stimulation. Chronic paroxysmal hemicranias and hemicrania continua are characterized by a response to indomethacin, 25 to 50 mg three times daily. Short unilateral neuralgiform headache with conjunctival injection and tearing attacks is so brief that there are no medications to treat it acutely.

PREVENTION

Preventive medications should be started at the beginning of a cluster bout. Verapamil, 240 to 480 mg, is the drug of choice. Lithium (300 mg twice daily) is an alternative. Corticosteroids (e.g., prednisone, 40 mg/day, or dexamethasone, 4 mg twice daily for 2 weeks) act rapidly as a bridge to prevent cluster headache while other preventive medications are started. Valproic acid (500 to 1500 mg/day in divided doses), topiramate (50 to 100 mg/day), melatonin (4 mg at bedtime), and gabapentin (300 mg three times daily) are sometimes beneficial. Surgical approaches, including suboccipital steroid injections, occipital nerve stimulators, sphenopalatine ganglion stimulation, hypothalamic stimulation, and destructive procedures, are sometimes necessary for this disabling headache.

Paroxysmal hemicrania and hemicrania continua respond to daily indomethacin (25 to 50 mg three times daily). If the patient cannot tolerate indomethacin, calcium-channel blockers (e.g., verapamil, 240 to 480 mg/day) or melatonin may be helpful. Preventive treatment of short unilateral neuralgiform headache with conjunctival injection and tearing includes lamotrigine (100 to 400 mg/day), topiramate (50 to 100 mg), gabapentin (300 to 900 mg), or intravenous lidocaine (starting at 1-2 mg/minute with cardiac monitoring).

Short unilateral neuralgiform headache with conjunctival injection and tearing is regarded as a more difficult headache to prevent. Lamotrigine and topiramate may be helpful.

PROGNOSIS

Cluster headache is often a lifelong problem, but remissions may persist for longer periods as the patient ages. The other trigeminal autonomic cephalalgias are probably lifelong; nevertheless, symptomatic treatment combined with preventive medications is helpful.

CHRONIC DAILY HEADACHE

DEFINITION

Though not a specific disorder, chronic daily headache, defined as a headache that is present on more than 15 days per month, is challenging for both patients and physicians. These headaches may be chronic migraine, chronic tension-type headache, new daily persistent headache, or chronic cluster headache, with or without overuse of medications.

EPIDEMIOLOGY

Up to 5% of the population suffers from chronic daily headache, most commonly chronic tension-type or chronic migraine. Trigger factors such as a previous infection, mild head injury, or stressful life event are present in 40 to 60% of patients with new daily persistent headache. Risk factors for chronic daily headache include medication overuse, history of migraine headache, frequent headache, depression, female sex, obesity, snoring, stressful life events, and low educational level.

PATHOBIOLOGY

Chronic daily headache is probably related to migraine, with both central and peripheral abnormalities. Once migraine has been prolonged and headache occurs on a daily basis, allodynia, a sense that a usually nonpainful stimulus is becoming painful, often develops. Use of an opiate for more than 8 days per month, especially in men, use of barbiturates for more than 5 days per month, especially in women, or use of triptans for more than 10 to 14 days per month can often lead to chronic migraine headache or at least worsening of headaches.

CLINICAL MANIFESTATIONS

New daily persistent headache is characterized by daily occurrence, onset at specific time, and an unrelenting course. It is generally bilateral, nonpulsating, mild to moderate, and associated with features of migraine, photophobia, phonophobia, or nausea. Severe nausea or vomiting is rare. New daily persistent headache can be disabling and is difficult to treat. Chronic daily headache is often associated with profound psychiatric comorbidity, especially depression and anxiety; such psychiatric comorbidity predicts intractability.

DIAGNOSIS

Diagnosis of chronic daily headache is based on the history. It is important to identify the underlying type of primary chronic daily headache: chronic migraine, chronic tension-type headache, new daily persistent headache, or hemicrania continua. Headaches of less than 4 hours' duration can also be chronic and daily: cluster headache, paroxysmal hemicrania, hypnic headaches occurring every night (usually in the elderly), and episodic stabbing headache.[12] It is most important to exclude secondary headaches (including post-traumatic headache), headaches associated with vascular disorders (e.g., giant cell arteritis, arteriovenous malformations, carotid and vertebral artery dissections), and headaches associated with nonvascular disorders (e.g., intracranial hypertension or hypotension, infections). MRI and laboratory studies (e.g., ESR in an elderly individual) are commonly recommended. Lumbar puncture (LP) to assess intracranial pressure may also be indicated in selected patients.

TREATMENT   Rx

The most common cause of chronic daily headache is overuse of medications, so patients must be weaned off the overused symptomatic medication.[13] Treatment of underlying depression, anxiety, and pain may also be helpful. Occasionally, hospital admission is necessary to break the headache cycle. Acute migraine-specific treatments (see earlier), especially intravenous dihydroergotamine (0.5 to 2 mg), are helpful in terminating migrainous attacks.

PREVENTION

Medications that are helpful in preventing chronic daily headache include tricyclic antidepressants, selective serotonin reuptake inhibitors if patients are depressed, anticonvulsants, β-blockers, and calcium-channel blockers (see Tables 370-3 and 370-4). For hemicrania continua, indomethacin (25 to 50 mg three times daily) is the preferred treatment.

PROGNOSIS

The prognosis depends on the underlying headache diagnosis. Depression, anxiety, poor sleep, stress, medication overuse, and poor self-efficacy are associated with a worse prognosis among patients with chronic headaches. If medication overuse is the cause and the patient is successfully detoxified, about 75% of patients improve when treated with preventive medications. Treatment may fail if the diagnosis is incorrect or because of continued overuse of medications, overuse of caffeine, lack of sleep, dietary or other life triggers, hormonal factors, or psychiatric factors. Explaining medication overuse headache to the patient, inpatient and outpatient detoxification, and multidisciplinary care treatments have been found helpful. New daily persistent headache often does not respond to medical therapy.

SECONDARY CAUSES OF HEADACHES

Sinus Headache

Rhinosinusitis (Chapter 398) is characterized by inflammation or infection of the nasal mucosa and sinuses. The sinuses themselves are relatively insensate, but ducts, turbinates, blood vessels, and ostia are the painful structures.

Headaches attributed to rhinosinusitis are frontal headaches with pain in the face, ears, or teeth. The onset of pain is simultaneous with the rhinosinusitis, and the headache and face pain resolve within 7 days after successful treatment. The diagnosis requires imaging and clinical evidence that support the diagnosis of acute rhinosinusitis. Many acute and most chronic headaches that are initially thought to result from sinus disease are found to be migraine or tension-type headache.

The headache should resolve with treatment of acute sinusitis (Chapter 398). If it does not, an underlying primary headache disorder is likely.

Temporal (Giant Cell) Arteritis

Temporal arteritis (Chapter 255) is an inflammatory process seen almost exclusively in elderly individuals. Headache, especially pain in the jaw when chewing, is one of the most common features. Its incidence is approximately 12 per 100,000 and increases with age to 51 per 100,000 in individuals older than 80. It affects women more often than men (3 : 1) and is more common in white individuals, especially those of Scandinavian and British descent. It is associated with polymyalgia rheumatica.

The headache has no specific feature, but the pain is usually continuous, generalized, and occasionally throbbing. The temples are generally painful, and patients complain of pain when performing certain activities of daily living, such as chewing food or combing their hair. Transient monocular blindness, permanent blindness, and diplopia can occur.

Elevation of the ESR and CRP occurs almost invariably. The diagnosis is made by finding giant cells in a temporal artery biopsy specimen. Immediate treatment with corticosteroids, sometimes before the biopsy result is available, is necessary in doses between 40 and 80 mg daily, with the dose then titrated downward while monitoring the ESR or CRP. Used early enough, corticosteroids (Chapter 255) generally prevent the complications of temporal arteritis, including blindness. Tocilizumab (162 mg subcutaneously weekly or every other week) is FDA approved to provide sustained corticosteroid-free remission in patients with temporal arteritis.[A21] The disorder can be long lasting.

Intracranial Hypertension and Pseudotumor Cerebri

Intracranial hypertension can be primary and idiopathic or secondary to cerebral venous thrombosis (Chapter 379), a mass in the brain (Chapter 180), hydrocephalus, or other intracranial processes. *Pseudotumor cerebri* is an all-encompassing term referring to increased intracranial pressure without obvious mass lesions. Primary idiopathic intracranial hypertension occurs in obese women of childbearing age. Secondary pseudotumor cerebri causes a similar syndrome but is due to an offending agent such as medications (e.g., tetracycline, minocycline, lithium, fluoroquinolones, vitamin A–related medications, growth hormone), endocrine disorders (e.g., parathyroid dysfunction), and sleep apnea.

Idiopathic increased intracranial pressure occurs in one to two per 100,000 individuals but in 19 to 20 per 100,000 individuals (15 to 55 years of age) who are obese. Women are affected more frequently than men (6 to 8 : 1). Onset is usually in young adulthood.

The cause of the increased pressure is poor CSF absorption, as is thought to be the problem in idiopathic intracranial hypertension; venous hypertension, as is seen in venous thrombosis; or a mass that causes an increase in pressure. A genetic component is also likely because there are reports of the condition occurring in families.

CLINICAL MANIFESTATIONS

Idiopathic intracranial hypertension is characterized by headache in more than 90% of individuals, about 90% of whom are obese. The headache may be pulsatile and is frequently felt behind the eyes. Patients often report neck pain, upper back pain, or even radicular pain. The intensity of headache does not correlate with the height of the intracranial pressure. Pulse-synchronous tinnitus is a frequent accompaniment, as are transient visual obscurations and diplopia. Vision-specific quality of life is often reduced.

On examination, papilledema (Chapter 395, Fig. 395-25) may be found. The remainder of the general and neurologic examination is usually normal in patients with idiopathic intracranial hypertension, but abnormalities on examination may point to a secondary cause, such as underlying venous sinus thrombosis (Chapter 379), ischemic stroke, central nervous system infection (Chapters 384 and 385), or brain tumor (Chapter 180). Although idiopathic intracranial hypertension often persists for years, the condition can be self-limited. In about a third of patients, there are permanent visual sequelae related to the effect of papilledema.

DIAGNOSIS

The diagnosis of intracranial pressure is made by the symptoms and signs such as papilledema (Chapter 395, Fig. 395-25), but up to 40% of cases of presumptive intracranial hypertension are not confirmed by specialist evaluation, usually because of an initially inaccurate diagnosis of papilledema.[14] MRI is necessary to exclude secondary causes of increased intracranial pressure. MR or CT venography is often needed to exclude venous sinus thrombosis (Chapter 379). LP must be performed unless patients have a contraindication such as an intracranial mass lesion, and CSF pressure should be measured. The diagnosis can be made if the pressure is elevated (CSF >250 mm H_2O) and the fluid itself is normal in terms of its protein level, glucose level, and cell count. Visual fields must be examined formally because visual acuity is not affected until late in the course of the disorder.

TREATMENT   Rx

Acetazolamide (doses ranging from 500 to 4000 mg daily) combined with a weight loss program is more efficacious for individuals with idiopathic intracranial hypertension and mild to moderate visual loss than is placebo.[A22][A23] Any underlying secondary cause should also be treated (e.g., stopping an offending medication, treatment of sleep apnea [Chapter 377]). Weight loss is beneficial in obese subjects. If visual loss progresses, surgical procedures should be considered. Optic nerve sheath fenestration allows CSF to escape through slits or windows in the orbit; sometimes the treatment of one side decreases the optic disc swelling on the other side as well. Complications include visual loss or diplopia, so visual fields must be followed carefully to anticipate and prevent visual loss. Lumbar or ventricular peritoneal diversion procedures also reduce intracranial pressure, but their complications include infection and shunt obstruction. Venous sinus stenting has occasionally been used for fixed stenoses.[15]

PROGNOSIS

The prognosis of patients with idiopathic intracranial hypertension is good with treatment, but up to a third of inadequately treated patients can experience permanent defects of visual fields or loss of visual acuity. Individuals are susceptible to recurrence if they suddenly gain weight.

Intracranial Hypotension

Intracranial hypotension (or CSF hypovolemia) causes a headache that is characteristically better when the patient is supine and worse when the patient is upright. It can be primary (spontaneous) or secondary to another underlying cause, most commonly a previous LP.

Intracranial hypotension was once considered rare, but modern imaging techniques suggest an incidence of about five per 100,000 per year; it is slightly more common in women than men. The onset is usually at about 40 years of age, but it can occur in children and the elderly. Post-LP headaches occur more commonly but only infrequently persist.

PATHOBIOLOGY

The cause of primary intracranial hypotension is thought to be a small leak or tear in the dura, usually in the lumbar region around cystic structures called Tarlov cysts. The cause of intracranial hypotension may not be the tear itself but rather the low CSF volume and low epidural venous pressure that assists in development of the lower pressure and hence the leak. The leaks frequently occur in the thoracic and cervicothoracic junction spine. Previous trauma history is reported in only one third of cases. Genetic and connective tissue disorders (e.g., Ehlers-Danlos syndrome, Marfan syndrome [Chapter 244]) may predispose individuals to have these leaks.

CLINICAL MANIFESTATIONS

Intracranial hypotension is characterized clinically by a positional headache. The location of the pain is variable, and the most constant characteristic is the orthostatic change in the pain. If the leak is untreated for a long time, the headache may lose the orthostatic characteristic. Posterior neck pain can also occur. Changes in hearing, taste, and balance, as well as blurred vision and diplopia, can develop if hindbrain herniation occurs. If very severe hindbrain herniation occurs, changes in consciousness, subdural hygromas, ataxia, a pseudo-frontotemporal dementia can occur.

DIAGNOSIS

The diagnosis of intracranial hypotension is made by MRI showing pachymeningeal enhancement, venous engorgement, dural thickening, pituitary fossa enlargement, and herniation of the hindbrain (Fig. 370-1). Hindbrain herniation appears as a downward descent of the posterior fossa along with loss of the prechiasmatic cistern, flattening of the pons against the clivus, and descent of the cerebellar tonsils, which is often misconstrued as a Chiari I malformation. LP may also show low (<50 mm H_2O) CSF pressure, but it also may be normal. The diagnosis is most commonly made by clinical characteristics and imaging, so the decision as to whether or not to do an LP should be made on a case-by-case basis because there is at least a theoretical risk of more hindbrain herniation. The differential diagnosis includes new daily persistent headache, chronic migraine, or another secondary headache. The diagnosis is confirmed if a CSF leak is demonstrated by isotope studies, CT myelography, or MR myelography.

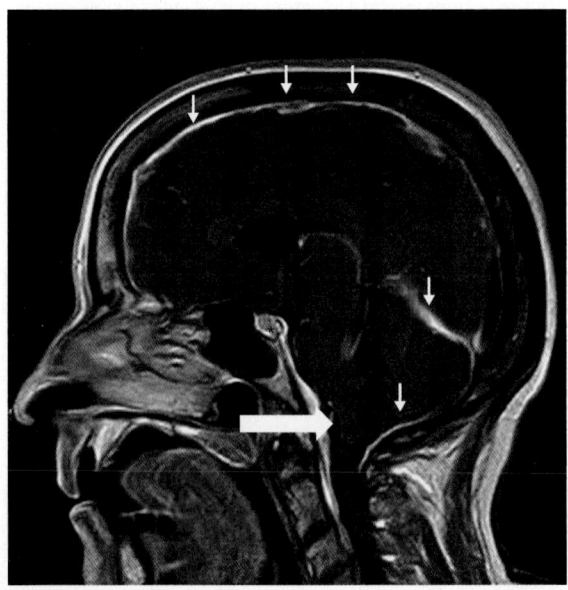

FIGURE 370-1. **Intracranial hypotension.** This 56-year-old woman had headaches that initially were positional. Gadolinium-enhanced magnetic resonance imaging shows characteristic findings of engorgement of the pituitary (*), slumping of the posterior fossa with tonsillar herniation (*large arrow*), and meningeal enhancement (*smaller arrows*).

TREATMENT AND PROGNOSIS

For spontaneous intracranial hypotension, the recommended treatment is bed rest and an epidural blood patch (blind or directed).[16] Treatment of CSF leaks includes bed rest, caffeine (200 to 300 mg two to three times daily), an abdominal binder wrapped around the abdomen to increase central pressure, and generous intake of oral fluids. For post–dural puncture headache and most spontaneous episodes, an epidural blood patch usually improves the symptoms within days.[17] Surgical repair is rarely required. With treatment, the symptoms and MRI findings should resolve completely. Recurrence is infrequent.

Trigeminal Neuralgia

Trigeminal neuralgia is a distinct, excruciatingly painful condition provoked by sensory stimuli in the distribution of the trigeminal nerve.[18] Trigeminal neuralgia occurs in four per 100,000 individuals, most commonly in persons between 50 and 70 years of age and in women slightly more than in men (1.5 : 1).

In younger individuals, multiple sclerosis (Chapter 383) can be associated with the condition. In older individuals, an ectatic artery in the vertebrobasilar system often causes the syndrome. The trigeminal nerve root entry zone is thought to be the site of pathology. Either demyelination or compression of this region increases the firing of trigeminal afferents. When a specific cause can be defined, the term *symptomatic trigeminal neuralgia* is often used.

CLINICAL MANIFESTATIONS

Trigeminal neuralgia pain is characteristically sharp, lancinating (shooting), and electric shock–like in the distribution of the trigeminal nerve: cheek (V2), chin or lower teeth (V3), and around the eye (V1). A combination of V2 and V3 is the most common. The paroxysms are brief—usually seconds but up to 2 minutes. Some patients have a dull and continuous interictal pain, whereas most have only staccato-like volleys of pain. Pain is usually triggered by stimuli such as touching the face, brushing the teeth, air moving across the face, or masticating food. Once a volley of pain is triggered, there is usually a refractory period in which pain will not occur.

DIAGNOSIS

Diagnostic criteria include paroxysmal attacks of pain persisting for a second to 2 minutes and affecting one or more divisions of the trigeminal nerve. To make the diagnosis, the pain must be intensely sharp, stabbing, or precipitated by a trigger. Each attack is stereotypical, and there are usually no other neurologic defects. Idiopathic trigeminal neuralgia by definition has no causative lesion, whereas symptomatic trigeminal neuralgia has a cause such as vascular compression of the trigeminal nerve root exit zone. The differential diagnosis includes trigeminal autonomic cephalgia, which has autonomic accompaniments that are not associated with trigeminal neuralgia. Atypical facial pain, idiopathic stabbing headache, and Tolosa-Hunt syndrome, an inflammatory syndrome of the anterior cavernous sinus, are also included in the differential. MRI is recommended to evaluate possible secondary causes of trigeminal neuralgia, such as demyelination, tumors, and vascular loops on the trigeminal nerve exit zone.

TREATMENT

Trigeminal neuralgia is treated with medications or surgery.[19] Carbamazepine (400 to 1200 mg) is considered the first-line agent for the neuralgia. Phenytoin (200 to 300 mg), baclofen (40 to 80 mg), clonazepam (2 to 6 mg), valproic acid (500 to 1500 mg), lamotrigine (100 to 400 mg), gabapentin (900 to 1800 mg), oxcarbazepine (300 to 1800 mg), levetiracetam 2 to 4 g), and topiramate (50 to 200 mg) are also used. Botulinum toxin may be effective for this disorder. Surgical treatments include microvascular decompression, which may alleviate the symptoms and preserve sensory function. Other treatments include partial destruction of the trigeminal nerve with heat (radio frequency lesions) or with glycerol (chemical destruction).

PROGNOSIS

Patients with trigeminal neuralgia can have spontaneous or medication-induced remissions. Microvascular decompression is often curative. In patients whose pain is triggered by mastication, weight loss and inanition may develop; prompt treatment is essential.

Glossopharyngeal Neuralgia

Less common than trigeminal neuralgia, glossopharyngeal neuralgia is unilateral pain in the distribution of the glossopharyngeal and vagal nerves in the ear, jaw, throat, and base of the tongue. This neuralgia is rare, with a prevalence of less than one per 100,000. The cause is thought to be compression of the glossopharyngeal nerve by blood vessels, tumor, or aneurysm and demyelination or infection.

The pains are paroxysmal and persist for less than seconds to 2 minutes, but patients can experience 30 to 40 attacks in a day. As in trigeminal neuralgia, the pain is triggered by chewing, swallowing, or talking.

The diagnosis is made clinically. MRI should be done to evaluate the glossopharyngeal nerve to exclude a tumor or vascular abnormality. The differential diagnosis includes trigeminal neuralgia, geniculate neuralgia, and atypical pain syndrome.

Pharmacologic therapy is similar to that for trigeminal neuralgia, and carbamazepine (200 to 800 mg) is usually the drug of choice. Surgical therapy and microvascular decompression or radio frequency ablation should be considered in patients whose weight loss does not respond promptly to medication.

Grade A References

A1. Stephens G, Derry S, Moore RA. Paracetamol (acetaminophen) for acute treatment of episodic tension-type headache in adults. *Cochrane Database Syst Rev.* 2016;6:CD011889.
A2. Derry S, Wiffen PJ, Moore RA. Aspirin for acute treatment of episodic tension-type headache in adults. *Cochrane Database Syst Rev.* 2017;1:CD011888.
A3. Derry S, Wiffen PJ, Moore RA, Bendtsen L. Ibuprofen for acute treatment of episodic tension-type headache in adults. *Cochrane Database Syst Rev.* 2015;7:CD011474.
A4. Law S, Derry S, Moore RA. Sumatriptan plus naproxen for the treatment of acute migraine attacks in adults. *Cochrane Database Syst Rev.* 2016;4:CD008541.
A5. Cameron C, Kelly S, Hsieh SC, et al. Triptans in the acute treatment of migraine: a systematic review and network meta-analysis. *Headache.* 2015;55(suppl 4):221-235.
A6. Friedman BW, Irizarry E, Solorzano C, et al. Randomized study of IV prochlorperazine plus diphenhydramine vs IV hydromorphone for migraine. *Neurology.* 2017;89:2075-2082.
A7. Friedman BW, Garber L, Yoon A, et al. Randomized trial of IV valproate vs metoclopramide vs ketorolac for acute migraine. *Neurology.* 2014;82:976-983.
A8. Yarnitsky D, Volokh L, Ironi A, et al. Nonpainful remote electrical stimulation alleviates episodic migraine pain. *Neurology.* 2017;88:1250-1255.
A9. Silberstein SD. Preventive migraine treatment. *Continuum (Minneap Minn).* 2015;21:973-989.
A10. Bruloy E, Sinna R, Grolleau JL, et al. Botulinum toxin versus placebo: a meta-analysis of prophylactic treatment for migraine. *Plast Reconstr Surg.* 2019;143:239-250.
A11. Schoenen JE. Migraine prevention with a supraorbital transcutaneous stimulator: a randomized controlled trial. *Neurology.* 2016;86:201-202.
A12. Tepper S, Ashina M, Reuter U, et al. Safety and efficacy of erenumab for preventive treatment of chronic migraine: a randomised, double-blind, placebo-controlled phase 2 trial. *Lancet Neurol.* 2017;16:425-434.
A13. Goadsby PJ, Reuter U, Hallstrom Y, et al. A controlled trial of erenumab for episodic migraine. *N Engl J Med.* 2017;377:2123-2132.
A14. Silberstein SD, Dodick DW, Bigal ME, et al. Fremanezumab for the preventive treatment of chronic migraine. *N Engl J Med.* 2017;377:2113-2122.
A15. Dodick DW, Silberstein SD, Bigal ME, et al. Effect of fremanezumab compared with placebo for prevention of episodic migraine: a randomized clinical trial. *JAMA.* 2018;319:1999-2008.
A16. Stauffer VL, Dodick DW, Zhang Q, et al. Evaluation of galcanezumab for the prevention of episodic migraine: the EVOLVE-1 randomized clinical trial. *JAMA Neurol.* 2018;75:1080-1088.
A17. Jackson JL, Mancuso JM, Nickoloff S, et al. Tricyclic and tetracyclic antidepressants for the prevention of frequent episodic or chronic tension-type headache in adults: a systematic review and meta-analysis. *J Gen Intern Med.* 2017;32:1351-1358.
A18. Zhao L, Chen J, Li Y, et al. The long-term effect of acupuncture for migraine prophylaxis: a randomized clinical trial. *JAMA Intern Med.* 2017;177:508-515.
A19. Petersen AS, Barloese MC, Lund NL, et al. Oxygen therapy for cluster headache. A mask comparison trial. A single-blinded, placebo-controlled, crossover study. *Cephalalgia.* 2017;37:214-224.
A20. Silberstein SD, Mechtler LL, Kudrow DB, et al. Non-invasive vagus nerve stimulation for the acute treatment of cluster headache: findings from the randomized, double-blind, sham-controlled ACT1 study. *Headache.* 2016;56:1317-1332.
A21. Stone JH, Tuckwell K, Dimonaco S, et al. Trial of tocilizumab in giant-cell arteritis. *N Engl J Med.* 2017;377:317-328.
A22. Wall M, McDermott MP, Kieburtz KD, et al. Effect of acetazolamide on visual function in patients with idiopathic intracranial hypertension and mild visual loss: the idiopathic intracranial hypertension treatment trial. *JAMA.* 2014;311:1641-1651.
A23. Bruce BB, Digre KB, McDermott MP, et al. Quality of life at 6 months in the idiopathic intracranial hypertension treatment trial. *Neurology.* 2016;87:1871-1877.

GENERAL REFERENCES

For the General References and other additional features, please visit Expert Consult at https://expertconsult.inkling.com.

371

TRAUMATIC BRAIN INJURY AND SPINAL CORD INJURY

JEFFREY J. BAZARIAN AND GEOFFREY S.F. LIN

EPIDEMIOLOGY

Traumatic brain injury and traumatic spinal cord injury are common preventable diseases. An estimated 54 to 60 million people sustain a traumatic brain injury worldwide each year, and it is projected to become the third largest cause of disease burden worldwide by 2020. In the United States, traumatic brain injury results in over 2.5 million emergency department visits and 52,000 deaths each year, thereby making it the single leading cause of traumatic death and disability (Chapter 103). Between 2000 and 2015, over 300,000 soldiers were diagnosed with traumatic brain injury, and estimates of sports-related traumatic brain injury range from 1.6 to 3.8 million annually. The prevalence of traumatic brain injury in the U.S. population is estimated at 5 million, but the magnitude is likely greater because this injury is often underreported by patients and overlooked by acute care providers. Over 85% of all traumatic brain injuries are mild injuries, commonly known as concussions. The majority of traumatic brain injuries are due to falls (Chapter 22), motor vehicle accidents, and assaults. An additional approximately 11,000 cases of severe spinal cord injury occur each year in the United States, resulting from motor vehicle accidents, falls, sports-related injuries, and work-related accidents (Chapter 103). The majority of patients with traumatic brain and spinal cord injuries are young adult males.

Over the past 20 years, overall mortality associated with traumatic brain injury and spinal cord injury has decreased because of prompt neurosurgical intervention, improved care in intensive care units (ICUs), and prevention of complications such as deep vein thrombosis and decubitus ulcers. The almost 5.5 million survivors of traumatic brain injury and spinal cord injury in the United States often require extended rehabilitation. Because the majority of these patients are young and otherwise in good physical health at the time of injury, many need chronic care for decades. Even relatively minor injury can lead to major disability. If untreated, many patients with traumatic brain injury continue to have residual symptoms months later, and many are unable to return to gainful employment.

PATHOBIOLOGY

Traumatic injury to the central nervous system has two phases. The first is neuronal injury and occurs as a direct result of the initiating traumatic event. The second or late phase, caused by multiple neuropathologic processes, can continue for days to weeks after the initial injury.

Primary Injury Phase

The primary injury phase is immediate, and its damage, which can cause death almost instantaneously, is often complete by the time medical care can be instituted. In closed compartment injury to the head or spine, the direct impact of neuronal tissue against the bony vault and shearing of neurovascular structures result in neuronal damage. Because brain neuronal structures reside in a fluid-filled compartment, these structures can lag behind the bony structure as it moves during sudden stopping of the body in motion. Thus the structures will strike both anteriorly and posteriorly against the inner bony table, and a coup-contrecoup lesion will result. If a rotational component is present—which is nearly universal in the case of traumatic brain injury—intracranial structures will torque and twist, thereby resulting in excessive shear strain (i.e., stretch). Neuronal axons and blood vessels are most susceptible to sheer strain owing to their elongated microstructure. Thus the primary injury phase results in damage to axons (axonal injury) and blood vessels (hemorrhage). Motor vehicle accidents are particularly injurious because of the sudden deceleration.

Secondary Injury Phase

The secondary injury phase begins immediately after the primary phase and can continue for a prolonged period. This phase involves progression of axonal injury, with shifts in ionic flux leading to axonal swelling, loss of axonal transport, and altered neurotransmission (E-Fig. 371-1). Mitochondrial failure results in energy crisis for the neuron, thereby leading to loss of neuronal function and/or apoptosis (programmed cell death). This secondary phase continues over days to weeks and also involves necrosis and neuronal demyelination. A neuroinflammatory response involving microgliosis starts within hours after traumatic brain injury and may continue for months or even years. Injury-induced dysfunction of the blood-brain barrier allows elements of the peripheral immune system to participate in this process. Diffuse microvascular damage, dysfunction of the blood-brain barrier, and loss of autonomic regulation result in both hyperperfusion and hypoperfusion, thereby contributing to ischemia and cerebral edema. The destruction of intra-axonal structures can result in abnormal accumulations of neurotoxic proteins, such as beta-amyloid and phosphorylated tau, which in combination with persistent abnormal neuroinflammation may contribute to early-onset neurodegeneration or dementia.

CLINICAL MANIFESTATIONS

Traumatic Brain Injury

The clinical hallmark of acute traumatic brain injury is an alteration in the level of consciousness, often associated with amnesia, confusion, or disorientation at the time of injury. Additional clinical manifestations vary with the severity of the injury, typically assessed by the Glasgow Coma Scale (Table 371-1), which measures a person's ability to open his or her eyes and respond to spoken questions or physical prompts for movement.

Patients with moderate to severe traumatic brain injury have readily recognizable alterations in consciousness ranging from confusion to agitation to somnolence. The physical examination may reveal signs of elevated intracranial pressure or brainstem herniation with vomiting, unequal pupils, decorticate or decerebrate posturing, hypopnea, hypertension, and bradycardia. Signs of open/depressed skull fracture or basilar skull fracture (hemotympanum, cerebrospinal fluid rhino/otorrhea, periorbital ecchymosis, postauricular ecchymosis) are often associated with intracranial hemorrhage. Focal cerebral injury may manifest as seizures or focal limb weakness/numbness. Patients with mild traumatic brain injury may be briefly confused or amnestic (repeating questions to providers) but will have a normal sensorium within several hours of injury. In mild traumatic brain injury, vomiting and seizures do not occur, blood pressure and heart rate are normal, and the skull is not fractured.

After resolution of the acute alteration in consciousness, most patients with traumatic brain injury experience one or more symptoms such as headache, dizziness, difficulty with memory and concentration, difficulties with balance, and fatigue. These symptoms are thought to reflect axonal injury involving several functional domains, including regulation of head and neck pain (producing headache), regulation of sleep, regulation of mood, cognitive function, vestibular function, and near-vision function. On physical examination, patients with traumatic brain injury may display abnormal postural stability, unsteady tandem gait, abnormal smooth pursuit or saccadic eye movements, abnormal vestibulo-ocular reflex, convergence insufficiency, or accommodative insufficiency. Neurocognitive testing may reveal deficits in immediate and delayed recall, concentration, information processing, executive functioning, and reaction time. In addition, patients who survive moderate-severe traumatic brain injury can have deficits of motor function, sensation, and language.

Postinjury symptoms that persist beyond 3 months are referred to as the postconcussion syndrome. The symptoms are similar to the subacute symptoms of concussion, but complaints of altered mood and sleep are more common. The cause of postconcussion syndrome is not known, but both the physiologic effects of brain injury and emotional reactions to these effects appear to play a role.

TABLE 371-1   GLASGOW COMA SCALE SCORE

BEST MOTOR RESPONSE	BEST VERBAL RESPONSE	BEST EYE OPENING
1 = No motor response	1 = No verbal response	1 = No eye opening
2 = Extension to pain	2 = Incomprehensible sounds	2 = Eye opening to pain
3 = Flexion to pain	3 = Inappropriate words	3 = Eye opening to verbal command
4 = Withdrawal from pain	4 = Confused	4 = Eyes open spontaneously
5 = Localizes pain	5 = Oriented	
6 = Obeys commands		

To calculate the score, sum the numbers from each of the three columns. A score of 3-8 indicates a severe head injury; 9-12 indicates moderate injury; and 13-15 is classified as mild injury.

Traumatic Spinal Cord Injury

There are three main spinal cord syndromes: Brown-Séquard, central cord, and anterior cord syndromes. In Brown-Séquard syndrome, the deficits are referable to a lesion of a lateral half of the cord; findings consist of loss of ipsilateral motor, touch, proprioception, and vibration sensation, as well as contralateral loss of pain and temperature sensation. Central cord syndrome is manifested as bilateral loss of motor function involving the upper extremities but sparing the lower extremities and is sometimes referred to as "man in a barrel syndrome." Proximal weakness is greater than distal weakness. Pain and temperature sensation is reduced, whereas proprioception and vibration are usually spared. Anterior cord syndrome is manifested by deficits referable to bilateral anterior and lateral spinal cord columns or funiculi. There is loss of touch, pain, and temperature sensation and motor function below the level of the lesion, but the posterior column functions of proprioception and vibratory sensation remain intact.

After acute traumatic spinal cord injury, patients may suffer from spinal shock or temporary loss of spinal reflexes below the level of injury, including loss of muscle stretch reflexes, the bulbocavernosus reflex, and the anal wink. In high cervical injuries, the lower reflexes (bulbocavernosus and anal wink) may be preserved. Some patients demonstrate the Schiff-Sherrington phenomenon, in which reflexes are affected above the level of injury. Patients with spinal shock also may lose autonomic reflexes, thereby leading to neurogenic hypotension, peripheral vasodilation, ileus, and urinary retention. If the lesion is at T3 or above, sympathetic tone to the heart is compromised. In this setting, hypotension is accompanied by bradycardia, thus producing dysautonomia and the neurogenic shock triad of bradycardia, hypotension, and peripheral vasodilation.

DIAGNOSIS

Traumatic Brain Injury

The diagnosis of traumatic brain injury is primarily clinical. Two necessary elements are the injury and a change of mental state at time of injury. Examples of mental status change include loss of consciousness, amnesia, confusion, and disorientation. Physical examination findings, neurocognitive testing, and neuroimaging can substantiate the initial clinical impression and determine the severity of the injury, but none of them is sensitive enough to exclude traumatic brain injury. Mental status changes are readily recognized in severe traumatic brain injury but are more difficult to detect in milder forms.[1] A standardized protocol (Table 371-2) can help first responders identify more subtle mental status changes. Any decline compared with a baseline, preinjury score suggests concussion, because normal subjects tend to do better on retesting.

The Glasgow Coma Scale score (see Table 371-1) should be calculated to estimate the severity of the traumatic brain injury. The physical examination should also assess evidence of unequal pupils, open or depressed skull fracture, basilar skull fracture, seizure, focal limb weakness, or numbness. Findings consistent with milder forms of traumatic brain injury include abnormal postural stability, unsteady tandem gait, abnormal smooth pursuit and saccadic

eye movements, abnormal vestibulo-ocular reflex, convergence insufficiency, and accommodative insufficiency.[2] Neurocognitive tests, which are not designed to diagnose traumatic brain injury but can be used to substantiate the diagnosis and to track recovery, assess memory, concentration, information processing, executive functioning, reaction time, and problem solving.

Biomarkers and Imaging

Biomarkers such as ubiquitin carboxyl-terminal hydrolase isozyme L1 precursor and glial fibrillary acid protein are approved by the U.S. Food and Drug Administration to aid in the rapid diagnosis of brain injury,[3] with a sensitivity of about 98% and specificity of 99.6% for finding intracranial lesions on a computed tomography (CT) head scan. All patients with a Glasgow Coma Scale score below 15 should have a noncontrast CT scan of their head to detect clinically important intracranial injuries such as trauma-related fractures, hemorrhage, and brain tissue swelling. Early detection of expanding hemorrhage is key for rapid neurosurgical decompression, which can be lifesaving. For patients with a Glasgow Coma Scale score of 15, in whom the prevalence of intracranial injury is less than 10%,[4] clinical decision rules can be used to identify high-risk patients in need of head CT scanning (Table 371-3).[5] Typical postinjury CT findings include subdural hematoma (Fig. 371-1), epidural hematoma, intraparenchymal hemorrhage, contusion, and traumatic subarachnoid hemorrhage

TABLE 371-2 STANDARDIZED ASSESSMENT OF CONCUSSION

TASK	POSSIBLE SCORE
ORIENTATION	
Month, date, day of week, year, time (1 point for each correct answer)	0-5
IMMEDIATE MEMORY	
Patient repeats a 5-word list spoken by examiner; 3 trials (1 point for each word correctly remembered)	0-15
CONCENTRATION	
Digits backward; 3-, 4-, 5-, and 6-digit strings (1 point for each digit string correctly repeated backward)	0-4
Months of the year in reverse order (1 point for repeating backward in correct sequence)	0-1
DELAYED MEMORY RECALL	
Patient repeats the 5 words from Immediate Memory test (1 point for each word correctly recalled)	0-5
TOTAL SCORE	0-30

TABLE 371-3 DECISION RULES FOR DETERMINING THE NEED FOR A COMPUTED TOMOGRAPHY (CT) SCAN IN HEAD-INJURED ADULTS

INDICATION FOR CT SCANNING	CANADIAN	NEW ORLEANS	ACEP
GCS	<15 at 2 h	<15	<15
Amnesia	Retrograde >30 min	Anterograde	Any
Suspected skull fracture	Yes	Yes	Yes
Vomiting	Recurrent	Any	Any
Age	≥65	>60	>60*
Coagulopathy	—	—	Yes
Focal deficit	—	—	Yes
Seizure	—	Any	Yes
Loss of consciousness	If GCS = 14	—	Yes?
Visible trauma above the clavicles	—	Any	Any
Headache	—	Yes	Yes
Dangerous injury mechanism†	Yes	—	Only if no LOC
Suspected intoxication	—	Drug, alcohol	Drug, alcohol
Sensitivity/specificity‡	0.99/0.51	0.99/0.33	unknown

*Age >65 if no loss of consciousness, otherwise positive only if loss of consciousness or amnesia.
†Pedestrian vs. motor vehicle, ejection from motor vehicle, fall from height >1 m or 5 stairs.
‡For detection of traumatic intracranial injury on head CT scan.
ACEP = American College of Emergency Physicians; GCS = Glasgow Coma Scale; LOC = loss of consciousness.

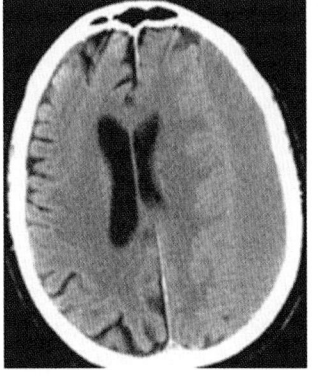
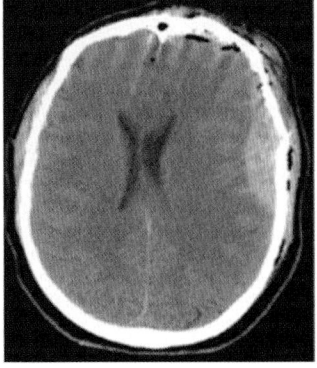

FIGURE 371-1. Computed tomography image of subdural hematoma (*left*) and epidural hematoma (*right*).

(Chapter 380).[6] An associated skull fracture, especially at the temporoparietal junction, increases the likelihood of epidural hematoma, usually by disruption of the middle meningeal artery. Magnetic resonance imaging (MRI) is a more sensitive test that can detect subtle changes not visible on CT. Most patients with mild traumatic brain injury will have normal neuroimaging, because axonal injury is largely invisible on CT and standard MRI. However, susceptibility weighted MRI can detect microhemorrhages, and diffusion tensor imaging can visualize disrupted white matter tracts.

Traumatic Spinal Cord Injury

A detailed neurologic examination is needed to identify the level of the injury and the severity of any deficits, as well as to document the degree of neurologic dysfunction at the earliest time possible. The level of the injury is the lowest spinal cord segment with intact motor and sensory function. Normal neurologic findings in patients with a clear sensorium obviate the need for imaging studies. However, any complaints of pain over the spine, numbness, tingling, or weakness should raise suspicion of spinal cord injury. In particular, a complaint of "burning hands" suggests traumatic spinal cord injury.

The time of injury should be recorded as accurately as possible. The prognosis for neurologic improvement is better if the lesion is incomplete as opposed to complete. During the acute period, serial examinations must be performed frequently.

If spinal cord injury is suspected, the patient should be appropriately immobilized, such as with a rigid collar and back board. In patients who are able to cooperate with a neurologic examination, are not intoxicated, and do not have painful distracting injuries (e.g., femoral fracture, which would interfere with the leg motor and sensory examination), normal neurologic findings effectively exclude cervical spinal cord disease.

Imaging

In patients who are alert and stable, the Canadian C-Spine Rule (Fig. 371-2) can be used to reduce unnecessary spinal imaging without any adverse effect on patients' outcomes. In other patients, the radiologic evaluation should begin with plain radiographs of the bony spine, with further neuroimaging of any abnormalities that are found. Bony vertebrae should be examined with CT, whereas the spinal cord and intervertebral and paravertebral soft tissue are best studied with MRI. After blunt trauma, negative results from a well-interpreted, high-quality CT scan is probably a safe and efficient way to exclude cervical spine injury in obtunded patients.[7] A chest radiograph is usually indicated to provide images of the lower cervical and thoracic vertebrae; the presence of a pleural effusion in the setting of a possible thoracic spine injury suggests a hemothorax.

Ligamentous Injury versus Spinal Cord Injury

If plain radiographs and CT of the cervical spine are normal but the patient still complains of neck pain, a ligamentous injury should be considered. Patients should be kept in a rigid cervical collar until one of the following conditions is met: (1) pain and muscle spasm resolve, (2) dynamic flexion/extension radiographs are normal, or (3) MRI obtained within 48 hours of injury is normal. Abnormal imaging or persistent pain warrant surgical evaluation to determine whether further immobilization or surgical correction is necessary.

TREATMENT　　　　　　　　　　　　　　　　　　　**Rx**

Traumatic Brain Injury

The approach to treatment varies based on the severity of the injury. For moderate to severe traumatic brain injury, the immediate goals of therapy are to limit secondary injury phase insults such as hypoxia and ischemia, preserve and if possible restore neurologic function, and avoid secondary medical complications.[8,9] Treatment requires airway support, mechanical ventilation, and rapid identification of neurosurgically manageable injuries with a head CT scan (Table 371-4). Early neurosurgical evacuation of hemorrhage can be lifesaving. Close monitoring of blood pressure and cerebral perfusion pressure in an ICU

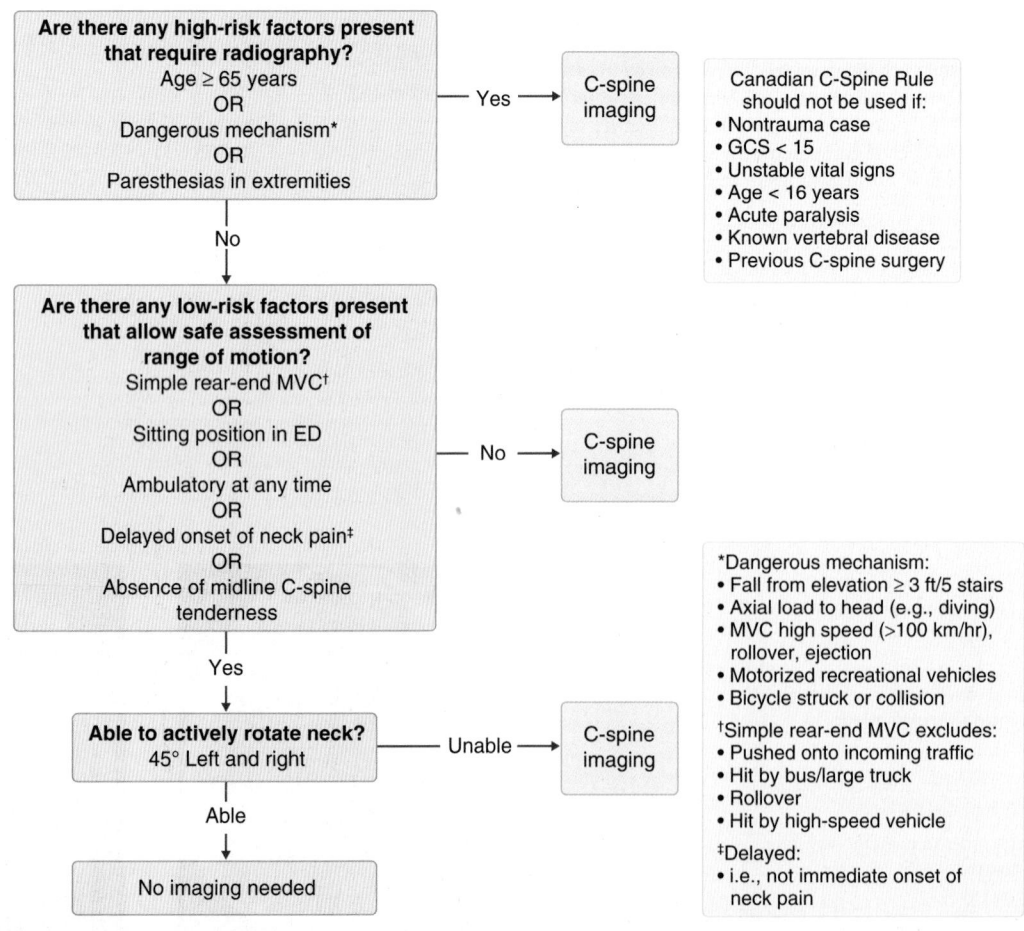

FIGURE 371-2. Canadian C-Spine Rule. For alert (Glasgow Coma Scale ≥15) and stable trauma patients in whom cervical spine injury is a concern. ED = emergency department; GCS = Glasgow Coma Scale (see Table 371-1); MVC = motor vehicle collision. (Modified from Stiell IG, Clement CM, McKnight RD, et al. Comparative validation of the Canadian C-Spine Rule and the NEXUS low-risk criteria in alert and stable patients. *N Engl J Med.* 2003;349:2510-2518; and Stiell IG, Wells GA, Vandemheen KL, et al. The Canadian C-Spine Rule for radiography in alert and stable trauma patients. *JAMA.* 2001;286:1841-1848.)

TABLE 371-4 MONITORING AND TREATMENT RECOMMENDATIONS FOR SEVERE TRAUMATIC BRAIN INJURY*

MONITORING	INDICATION AND/OR RECOMMENDATION
Intracranial pressure (ICP)	GCS ≤8 *AND* abnormal head CT[†] *OR* any 2 of the following: age >40, motor posturing, SBP <90 mm Hg. Treatments should aim to keep ICP ≤22 mg Hg.
Cerebral perfusion pressure (CPP)	Treatments should aim for a CPP of 60-70 mm Hg.
Advanced cerebral monitoring	Jugular bulb monitoring of AV oxygen difference. Treatments should aim to keep venous saturation ≥50%.
SBP	Treatments should aim to keep SBP ≥110 mm Hg in those 18-49 and >70 years old, ≥100 mm Hg in those 50-69 years old.
TREATMENT	
Decompressive craniectomy	Not recommended to improve outcome, but may shorten ICU stay and result in less ICP-targeting interventions.
Prophylactic hypothermia	Does not improve outcome.[A2]
Hyperosmolar therapy	Mannitol for signs of herniation or progressive neurologic deterioration.
CSF drainage	Within first 12 hours in those with GCS <6. Continuous drainage is better than intermittent.
Ventilation	Short-term hyperventilation can be used to reduce elevated ICP, but avoid in the first 24 hours after injury. Prolonged hyperventilation with PaCO$_2$ ≤25 mm Hg is not recommended; if used, monitor jugular venous saturation.
Sedation	Propofol to control ICP. High-dose barbiturate administration is restricted to ICP refractory to standard surgical and medical treatments.
Corticosteroids	Not recommended (high-dose methylprednisolone is associated with increased mortality risk).
Nutrition	Achieving basic caloric replacement by postinjury day 5-7 to reduce mortality risk. Transgastric jejunal feeding tube reduces ventilator-associated pneumonia.
Prophylactic antibiotics	Povidone-iodine oral care does not reduce ventilator-associated pneumonia. Antimicrobial-impregnated catheters may prevent catheter-related infections during external ventricular drainage.
DVT prophylaxis	LMWH or low-dose unfractionated heparin may be used (in combination with compression stockings) if the traumatic brain injury is stable and the benefit outweighs the increased risk of intracranial hemorrhage expansion.
Seizure prophylaxis	Phenytoin to prevent early post-traumatic seizures (within 1 week of injury), although early seizures are not associated with worse outcome; antiepileptic drugs are not recommended to prevent late seizures.

*Brain Trauma Foundation Guidelines.
[†]Hematoma, contusion, swelling, herniation, or compressed basal cisterns.
AV = arteriovenous; CSF = cerebrospinal fluid; CT = computed tomography; DVT = deep venous thrombosis; GCS = Glasgow Coma Scale; ICU = intensive care unit; LMWH = low-molecular-weight heparin; SBP = systolic blood pressure.

setting is recommended, regardless of need for neurosurgery. Despite major research efforts, current clinical treatment is largely confined to supportive measures: maintaining cerebral perfusion pressure, minimizing intracranial pressure, and indirectly treating edema. Recalcitrant elevated intracranial pressure despite these interventions is an ominous sign. In such cases, bifronto-temporoparietal craniectomy can reduce intracranial pressure and the length of ICU stay but has not been shown to improve outcomes, in part because any reduction in mortality is offset by an increase in very severe disability and persistent vegetative state, with no significant differences in the rate of good recovery or good recovery plus moderate disability.[A1]

For mild traumatic brain injury, the acute treatment priority is identification of those at risk for traumatic intracranial injuries such as skull fracture, hemorrhage, and edema. Patients who have intracranial injury should be evaluated by a neurosurgeon and observed in a hospital setting for neurologic deterioration or expansion of the hematoma. Patients without intracranial injury or at low risk for it can be managed as an outpatient but should be removed from play or work[10] and, by law, should not return until a detailed evaluation with written authorization can be made by an appropriately experienced physician. Most patients with mild traumatic brain injury will experience one or more postconcussive symptoms such as headache, dizziness, difficulty with memory and concentration, difficulties with balance, and fatigue. Despite a common belief that mild traumatic brain injury is not a treatable injury, targeted, symptom-based treatments (Table 371-5) can improve head and neck pain, cognition, vestibular function, near-vision, and overall recovery.

Traumatic Spinal Cord Injury

Initial Management

Emergency management of traumatic injury to the spinal cord begins with the basics of airway, breathing, and circulation. Cervical lesions above C5 and sometimes below C5 are associated with impaired ventilatory capability, and emergency intubation is required if there is any concern that the airway or ventilatory effort is compromised. If the cervical spine has not yet been imaged, the preferred method is nasotracheal intubation under fiberoptic guidance.

Hypotension can be either neurogenic shock or hypovolemia. For neurogenic shock, vasopressive pharmacologic agents such as phenylephrine (beginning as a continuous IV infusion at 100 µg/min with titration to clinical effect) may be needed. If tachycardia is present, hypovolemia is more likely, so fluid resuscitation would be more appropriate (Chapter 98).

Targeted Therapy

Methylprednisolone is no longer advocated for the treatment of acute spinal cord injury.[12] Systemic administration of a blood-brain barrier–permeable

TABLE 371-5 ASSESSMENT AND TREATMENT RECOMMENDATIONS FOR MILD TRAUMATIC BRAIN INJURY

FUNCTION	ASSESSMENT	TREATMENT
Overall recovery	Standardized symptom checklist	Physical rest 1-2 days[A3] followed by subsymptomatic aerobic exercise[11]
Headache	Determine the type (Chapter 370)	HA persisting more than 3-4 days may require abortive treatment tailored to phenotype (migraine, tension-type, occipital neuralgia, etc.) (Chapter 370)
Vertigo	Romberg test, dynamic standing, tandem gait (see Chapter 400)	If Hallpike Dix is normal, or if Epley maneuver (Chapter 400) does not relieve symptoms, consider physical therapy for vestibular rehabilitation
Eye movements	Examine cranial nerves 3, 4, 6 for tracking, saccades, diplopia, nystagmus (Chapter 396)	Physical therapy evaluation for vestibular rehabilitation
Near-vision	Near-point accommodation and binocular convergence	Ophthalmologic evaluation for vision therapy
Cognitive function	Symptoms, cognitive testing, neuropsychologist evaluation (Chapters 25 and 374)	Sleep hygiene, neuropsychology evaluation for cognitive rehabilitation[A4]

HA = headache.

microtubule-stabilizing drug, epothilone B, has been beneficial in animal models, but its utility in humans is unknown.

Surgical intervention within 8 hours should be based on the stability of the anterior (anterior half of the vertebral body and the vertebral disc), middle (posterior half of the body and disc), and posterior (the arch, facets, and ligaments) vertebral columns.[A5] In general, if two of the three columns are damaged, surgical stabilization is needed. If immediate surgery is not indicated, the patient should be admitted to the ICU for further management.[13]

Acute and Subacute Management

Patients with severe spinal cord injury require close cardiovascular and ventilatory care, supportive care for bladder and bowel function, approaches to avoid pressure ulcers,[14] and general measures similar to those used for patients with traumatic brain injury.

Neurogenic Shock and Dysautonomia

Initial therapy for dysautonomia should be fluid administration to restore an adequate circulating volume with a target central venous pressure of 4 to 6 mm Hg. A hematocrit of 30 is optimal for perfusion of the central nervous system, so blood can be used if the patient is anemic. If blood is not required, either colloid (e.g., albumin solutions) or crystalloid (e.g., normal saline) may be used. If there is a suspicion of cardiac or pulmonary disease, a pulmonary artery catheter may be needed briefly to assess fluid status and the relationship between pulmonary pressure and central venous pressure.

Once adequate circulating volume has been achieved, hypotension should be managed with vasopressors such as phenylephrine, norepinephrine, or dopamine (beginning at 1 µg/kg/min by continuous IV infusion) (Chapter 98), with the goal of a mean arterial pressure of 85 mm Hg or greater to maintain a spinal cord perfusion pressure of 50 mm Hg or greater.[15] Symptomatic bradycardia can be treated with atropine (1 mg IV).

Ventilatory Compromise

An injury at C5 or higher can result in diaphragmatic denervation and requires complete ventilatory assistance. Proper management requires endotracheal or nasotracheal intubation and mechanical ventilation, with an appropriate tidal volume (6 to 10 mL/kg), an FiO_2 to achieve a Po_2 between 80 and 100 mm Hg, and a rate to give a Pco_2 of 40 mm Hg (Chapter 97). Positive end-expiratory pressure should also be given to minimize atelectasis. If the patient does not show signs of ventilatory recovery within 2 weeks of intubation, a tracheostomy should be considered.

Lesions below C5 may also be associated with inadequate spontaneous ventilation. Midcervical lesions may be associated with intact but compromised diaphragm function. If suspected, a "sniff" test under fluoroscopy can be performed to determine whether both hemidiaphragms are functioning properly. If not, intubation/tracheostomy with volume-controlled ventilation may be needed. If intact, pressure support ventilation may be sufficient (Chapter 97) to achieve an appropriate tidal volume.

Cervical lesions at C6 and below spare the phrenic nerves but may disrupt innervation of the intercostal muscles. The primary finding is decreased cough and an inability to increase ventilation when needed, thereby leading to atelectasis and pneumonia; assisted elimination of tracheal secretions is essential.

Thromboembolic Disease

Thromboembolic disease (Chapter 74) is a leading cause of morbidity and mortality after traumatic spinal cord injury. Prolonged immobility of the lower extremities leads to deep venous thrombosis in up to 70% of spinal cord–injured patients. Patients should receive prophylaxis with low-molecular-weight heparin (e.g., enoxaparin 30 mg twice daily subcutaneously) within 72 hours of injury (Chapter 76). Anticoagulation can be held on the day of surgery but should be resumed 24 hours after surgery. A less effective alternative is intermittent compression devices (e.g., pneumatic stockings) with low-dose unfractionated heparin. An inferior vena cava filter may be placed if anticoagulation therapy is contraindicated.

Visceral Function and Nutrition

The abdominal wall musculature is innervated by T7 to T12. The stomach, small bowel, liver, pancreas, and proximal two thirds of the colon receive innervation from T5 to L2. Spinal cord injury at these levels or above may impair visceral function. For ileus, a nasogastric tube should be placed to decompress the stomach. Parenteral nutrition should be started as soon as possible. Enteral feeding should be delayed until gastrointestinal motility returns, usually within 2 to 3 weeks. Until enteral feeding can begin, total or peripheral parenteral nutrition should be used (Chapter 204). In comparison with conservative bowel management, transanal irrigation improves constipation, fecal incontinence, and symptom-related quality of life in patients with spinal cord injuries.

Stress-induced peptic ulcer disease occurs in nearly a third of patients without prophylaxis. H_2-receptor antagonists (e.g., ranitidine 50 mg IV three times daily) or a proton pump inhibitor (e.g., omeprazole 20 mg/day PO) reduce the incidence of ulcers.

Bladder tone may be lost because of spinal shock. A Foley catheter should be placed for a minimum of 5 to 7 days to drain the bladder and evaluate urine output. After spinal shock has resolved, autonomic dysreflexia may occur as a result of bladder distention. Clinical signs such as sweating, skin flushing, and hypertension may be present. Clinical examination with palpation and percussion will reveal a distended bladder, which can be treated by bladder training or intermittent catheterization.

Other Therapy

In a randomized trial, pregabalin, 150 to 600 mg/day, was effective in reducing central neuropathic pain after spinal cord injury.[A6] Patients with traumatic spinal cord injury often develop decubitus ulcers and pressure sores (Chapter 22). Mechanical kinetic beds, regular log rolling (every 2 hours), and padded orthotics are all useful for minimizing this complication. Orthotics, physical therapy, and occupational therapy (for cervical cord injury) are also important to minimize contractures and begin the rehabilitation process.

PROGNOSIS

Traumatic Brain Injury

The most useful prognostic indicators after traumatic brain injury are the Glasgow Coma Scale and the neurologic examination at the initial evaluation. For patients with moderate to severe traumatic brain injury, the lower the initial Glasgow Coma Scale score, the less likely a patient will have meaningful neurologic or functional recovery; 40% of patients with a score of 8 have a good recovery versus only 7% when the score is 3. Furthermore, only 27% of patients with a score of 3 survive versus 88% of patients with a score of 8. Patients in whom the Glasgow Coma Scale score remains the same or worsens over a period of 6 hours do worse clinically than those whose score improves. Further prognostic stratification at 24 hours can be based on pupillary responses, motor responses, and age (Chapter 376). Of patients who survive for 3 to 5 years after traumatic brain injury, approximately 6% will have severe disability, 18% will have moderate disability, and 75% will have a good recovery. Most clinical recovery occurs during the first 6 months, although significant recovery can take place up to 2 years after injury.[16]

Most patients with mild traumatic brain injury make a full recovery within 2 to 3 months. However, symptoms persist for longer than 3 months in 15 to 20% of such patients, with some experiencing symptoms for several years. A subsequent head injury before full recovery from even a mild traumatic brain injury may occasionally result in "second impact syndrome," which can worsen the clinical outcome. When seen (mostly in children and adolescents), coma develops rapidly after the second injury, often within minutes. There is decreased autoregulation, diffuse cerebral edema, and intracranial hypertension. Second impact syndrome is associated with a high mortality rate.

Even a single, mild traumatic brain injury is associated with increased risk of later development of symptoms resembling Alzheimer disease,[17] and individuals who have sustained moderate to severe traumatic brain injury are four times more likely to develop dementia than are people without traumatic brain injury.[18,19] Mounting evidence indicates a clear association between repetitive head hits sustained in contact sports and a form of early-onset dementia called chronic traumatic encephalopathy. Symptoms of chronic traumatic encephalopathy include memory loss, confusion, impaired judgment, impulse control problems, aggression, depression, anxiety, suicidality, parkinsonism, and, eventually, progressive dementia. As with Alzheimer disease–like dementia, the symptoms of chronic traumatic encephalopathy often begin years after the last head impact. Individuals with one or more E4 alleles of the apolipoprotein E genes may be at particular risk for postinjury neurodegenerative disease.

Traumatic Spinal Cord Injury

After traumatic spinal cord injury, the completeness of the injury is the most useful prognostic predictor (Table 371-6), and complete motor and sensory

TABLE 371-6	AMERICAN SPINAL INJURY ASSOCIATION IMPAIRMENT SCALE		
GRADE	**INJURY TYPE**	**DEFINITION**	**LIKELIHOOD OF RECOVERY***
A	Complete	No motor or sensory function below the lesion	15.5% (cervical) and 7% (thoracic)
B	Incomplete	Sensory but no motor function	47%
C	Incomplete	Some motor strength (<3)	84%
D	Incomplete	Motor strength >3	84%
E	None	Sensory and motor function normal	100%

*Data from Coleman WP, Geisler FH. Injury severity as primary predictor of outcome in acute spinal cord injury: retrospective results from a large multicenter clinical trial. *Spine J.* 2004;4:373-378.

deficit below the lesion has a poor prognosis. If a complete lesion persists for 24 hours, there is little likelihood of meaningful recovery. Conversely, even severe partial injuries have a higher probability of recovery. Most patients initially show some improvement but usually do not continue to improve after 2 years.[20]

Grade A References

A1. Zhang D, Xue Q, Chen J, et al. Decompressive craniectomy in the management of intracranial hypertension after traumatic brain injury: a systematic review and meta-analysis. *Sci Rep.* 2017;7:1-10.

A2. Lewis SR, Evans DJ, Butler AR, et al. Hypothermia for traumatic brain injury. *Cochrane Database Syst Rev.* 2017;9:CD001048.

A3. Thomas DG, Apps JN, Hoffmann RG, et al. Benefits of strict rest after acute concussion: a randomized controlled trial. *Pediatrics.* 2015;135:213-223.

A4. Cooper DB, Bowles AO, Kennedy JE, et al. Cognitive rehabilitation for military service members with mild traumatic brain injury: a randomized clinical trial. *J Head Trauma Rehabil.* 2017;32:E1-E15.

A5. Lee DY, Park YJ, Kim HJ, et al. Early surgical decompression within 8 hours for traumatic spinal cord injury: is it beneficial? A meta-analysis. *Acta Orthop Traumatol Turc.* 2018;52:101-108.

A6. Cardenas DD, Nieshoff EC, Suda K, et al. A randomized trial of pregabalin in patients with neuropathic pain due to spinal cord injury. *Neurology.* 2013;80:533-539.

GENERAL REFERENCES

For the General References and other additional features, please visit Expert Consult at https://expertconsult.inkling.com.

372

MECHANICAL AND OTHER LESIONS OF THE SPINE, NERVE ROOTS, AND SPINAL CORD

J.D. BARTLESON AND RICHARD L. BARBANO

Disorders of the spine, nerve roots, and spinal cord are frequent reasons for seeking health care. Low back pain is the most common cause of disability for persons under the age of 45 years in the United States. At any one time, 1% of the U.S. population is chronically disabled by lower back pain and another 1% temporarily disabled. Lower back pain is the number one cause of years lived with disability in the United States, and neck pain is the number four cause.

PATHOBIOLOGY

The 7 cervical vertebrae, 12 thoracic vertebrae, 5 lumbar vertebrae, the sacrum, and the coccyx comprise the spine (Fig. 372-1). Each vertebra has an anterior cylinder-shaped body, which is flattened posteriorly and held together by intervertebral discs, as well as by anterior and posterior longitudinal ligaments (Fig. 372-2A). Each disc consists of an outer annulus fibrosus, which receives some blood supply, and an inner, softer nucleus pulposus, which is avascular. The vertebral arch is composed of two short, round, rod-like bones called pedicles, which project backward from the dorsolateral surface of a vertebral body. Each pedicle meets a broad lamina. At one level, two laminae are angled posteriorly and medially to meet in the midline behind the vertebral (or spinal) foramen, where they fuse and form the posteriorly projecting spinous process. The ligamenta flava connect vertically adjacent laminae. At the junctions of the pedicles and laminae, paired superior and inferior articular processes articulate with similar processes from above and below. These so-called zygapophyseal joints are true synovium-covered joints that help to protect the spine while permitting a limited amount of movement. The overlapping facet joints and multiple sets of longitudinal ligaments give the spine stability during its ranges of motion and prevent excess motion. The posterolaterally placed intervertebral or neural foramina allow the exit of spinal nerves.

The spinal cord has 31 spinal segments, with one more cervical cord segment (8) than vertebra. Each segment gives rise to a bilateral pair of spinal nerves. Spinal nerves C1 to C7 exit the canal above their corresponding vertebral body, whereas the C8 nerve exits below the C7 vertebra. Subsequent inferior spinal nerves in the thoracic and lumbar spine exit below the vertebra with the same number. Spinal cord segments lie progressively superior to the vertebrae, so that the end of the spinal cord and conus medullaris is at about the L1 vertebral level in adults. Below this level, the spinal nerves travel as the cauda equina within the subarachnoid space before exiting through their respective foramina. The spinal cord is wider in the cervical and lumbar cord segments because of the increased number of motor and sensory neurons supplying the upper and lower extremities.

Spinal nerves are formed by joining of the anterior (or ventral) and posterior (or dorsal) spinal nerve roots, which directly enter and exit the spinal cord (Fig. 372-2B). The anterior or ventral root is derived from axons of the anterior horn cells and lateral columns. The posterior or dorsal root mostly derives axons from the dorsal root ganglion. The sensory root is twice as thick as the motor root. The spinal nerves exit and enter the spinal canal through the intervertebral or neural foramina formed by the upper and lower pedicles, the vertebral body, and the laminae (Fig. 372-2A).

CLINICAL MANIFESTATIONS

The majority of spine disorders are related to spondylosis, which results from wear and tear that takes place in the vertebrae, intervertebral discs, facets, and other true joints of the spine, associated ligaments, and secondarily the paraspinal and other muscles. Pain-sensitive structures in the spine include the periosteum of the bony spine (vertebrae), the dura, facet and other true joints, the annulus fibrosus (but not the nucleus pulposus), blood vessels, ligaments, and paraspinal muscles.

The most frequent complaint related to spondylosis is axial spine pain affecting the low back more than the neck and more than the midback. With compression or irritation of the spinal nerves, patients can develop tingling, prickling, or burning sensations (termed paresthesias if they occur spontaneously or dysesthesias if they are provoked by stimulation); loss of sensation; weakness; and sometimes autonomic dysfunction (most commonly difficulty with bowel or bladder control).

When it affects a myotome (the group of muscles served by motor neurons of a single spinal cord segment), the motor deficit associated with a spinal root disorder is of the lower motor neuron type. Typical findings are weakness, hypotonia, depressed or absent reflexes, fasciculations, and, if the syndrome has persisted for at least several weeks, muscle atrophy (Table 372-1 and Table 372-2). Sensation at the spinal nerve level is diminished or absent for all modalities in a characteristic dermatomal pattern (Fig. 372-3). Sensation below and above the affected root is intact.

Conversely, disorders of the spinal cord produce a "level" below which sensation is abnormal and motor deficits are of the upper motor neuron type, with weakness without atrophy (unless caused by disuse), hypertonia, and increased reflexes. At the level of a spinal cord lesion, the motor deficits can be of the lower motor neuron type owing to injury to anterior horn cells or nerve roots; but below this level, an upper motor neuron syndrome will predominate. As with strokes (Chapter 378) and other central nervous system (CNS) insults, the full upper motor neuron syndrome of spasticity and hyperreflexia may be absent in the acute phase of spinal cord injury.

DIAGNOSIS

Knowledge of the usual patterns of the sensory, motor, and reflex innervation of the spinal nerves greatly aids in diagnosis of the patient with possible radiculopathy. The history of sensory loss or motor weakness may be more important than findings on the physical examination. The patient should be asked about, and the neurologic examination focus on, sensory, motor, and reflex functions. Careful side-to-side comparisons can help detect subtle deficits. All muscles receive innervation from more than one spinal nerve and all nerve roots innervate multiple muscles, so individual muscles are rarely profoundly weak when a single root is affected. Give-way weakness, whereby a patient does not give a full effort, can be due to pain, lack of understanding, the patient trying to help the provider, conversion disorder, and malingering; in this setting it may be best to interpret strength as being at least equivalent to when it gave way, but the presence or absence of some weakness cannot be known. Overlap of sensory dermatomes explains why sharp demarcations and complete sensory loss rarely occur. All sensory loss is subjective, thereby making the sensory examination less reliable. Typical symptoms and signs are associated with cervical and lumbosacral radiculopathies Tables 372-1 and 372-2.

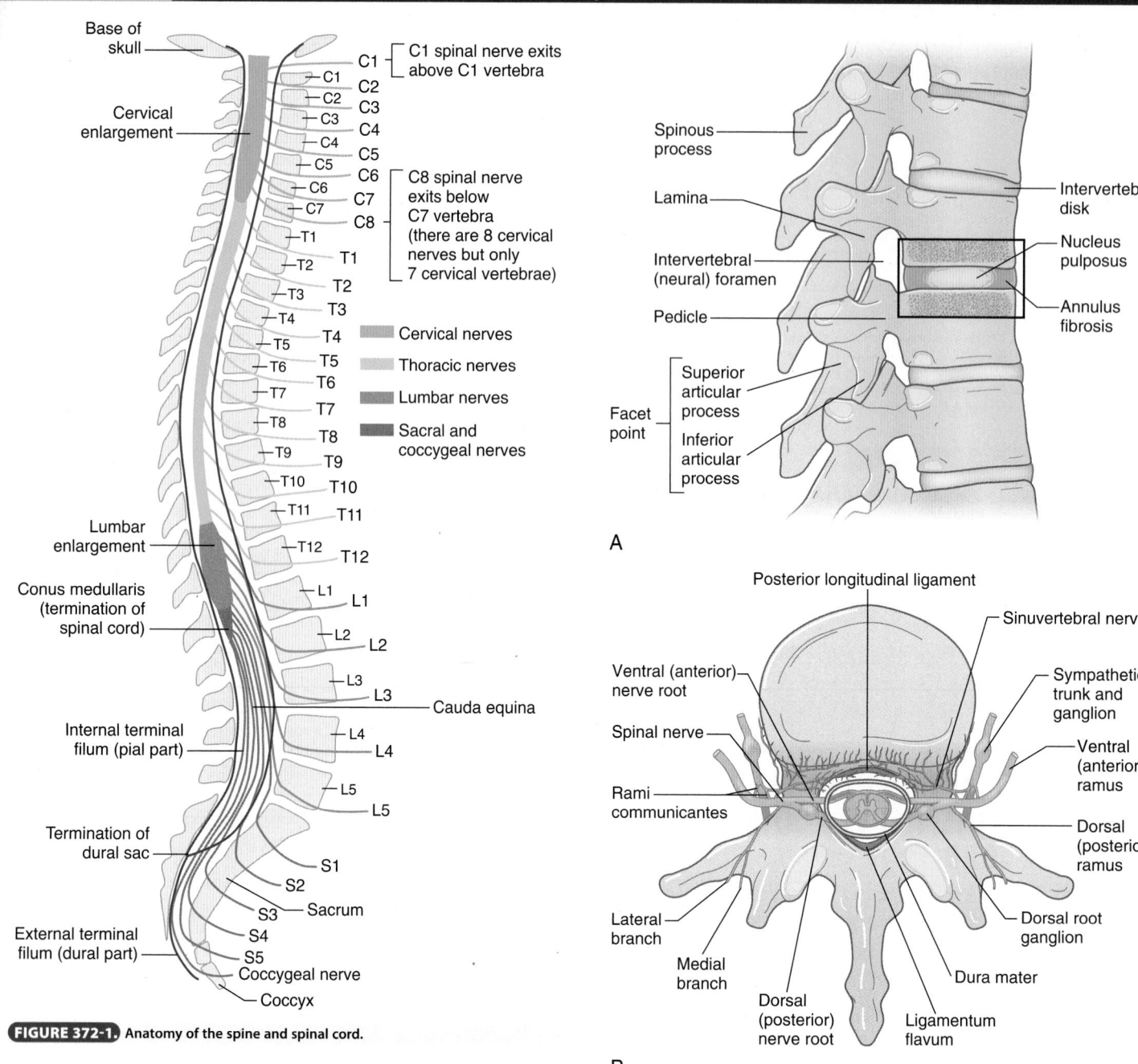

FIGURE 372-1. Anatomy of the spine and spinal cord.

FIGURE 372-2. A, Anatomy of the thoracic spine. B, Cross-section of the spine, spinal cord, spinal nerves and nerve roots.

TABLE 372-1	SYMPTOMS AND SIGNS ASSOCIATED WITH CERVICAL AND HIGH THORACIC RADICULOPATHY			
	USUAL LOCATION OF:			
DISC LEVEL/ROOT	**PAIN**	**SENSORY ABNORMALITIES**	**WEAKNESS**	**AFFECTED REFLEX**
C3-4/C4	Neck	Suprascapular, supraclavicular, and top of shoulder	Usually none	None
C4-5/C5	Neck, scapula, shoulder, anterior arm	Lateral arm and forearm	Shoulder abduction, elbow flexion, forearm pronation	Biceps, brachioradialis
C5-6/C6	Neck, scapula, shoulder, lateral arm, and forearm	Anterolateral arm, forearm, hand, thumb, and forefinger	Shoulder abduction, elbow flexion, and forearm pronation	Biceps, brachioradialis
C6-7/C7	Neck, shoulder, lateral arm, medial scapula, extensor surface of forearm	Dorsolateral forearm and hand, forefinger, and long finger	Extension of elbow, wrist, and fingers	Triceps
C7-T1/C8	Neck; medial scapula, arm, and forearm	Medial forearm and hand, ring, and little fingers	Finger abduction, adduction, and flexion	None or finger flexor
T1-2/T1	Anterior chest, medial arm, and forearm	Medial arm and forearm	Finger abduction, adduction, and flexion	None or finger flexor

Adapted from *Spine Disorders: Medical and Surgical Management* by JD Bartleson and HG Deen; Cambridge University Press, 2009. Copyrighted and used with permission of Mayo Foundation for Medical Education and Research.

TABLE 372-2 SYMPTOMS AND SIGNS ASSOCIATED WITH LUMBOSACRAL RADICULOPATHIES

| | USUAL LOCATION OF: | | | |
DISC LEVEL/ROOT	PAIN	WEAKNESS	AFFECTED REFLEXES	SENSORY ABNORMALITIES
L1-2/L1	Inguinal	None	Cremasteric	Inguinal
L2-3/L2	Inguinal and anterior thigh	Hip flexion, hip adduction, some knee extension	Cremasteric, thigh adductor	Proximal anterior thigh
L2-3/L3	Anterior thigh and knee	Knee extension, hip flexion, hip adduction	Knee, thigh adductor	Anterior and anteromedial thigh including knee
L3-4/L4	Anterior thigh, anteromedial leg	Knee extension, hip flexion, hip adduction	Knee	Anterior knee and medial leg
L4-5/L5	Posterolateral thigh, lateral leg, medial foot	Foot dorsiflexion, inversion and eversion, knee flexion, hip abduction, toe extension and flexion	Internal hamstring	Lateral leg, dorsal foot, and great toe
L5-S1/S1	Posterior thigh and leg, heel, and lateral foot	Foot plantar flexion, toe flexion, knee flexion, hip extension	Ankle, external hamstring	Posterolateral leg and lateral foot, heel
L5-S1/S2	Buttock	Foot plantar flexion, hip extension	Anal reflex, ankle	Posterior leg and thigh, medial buttock

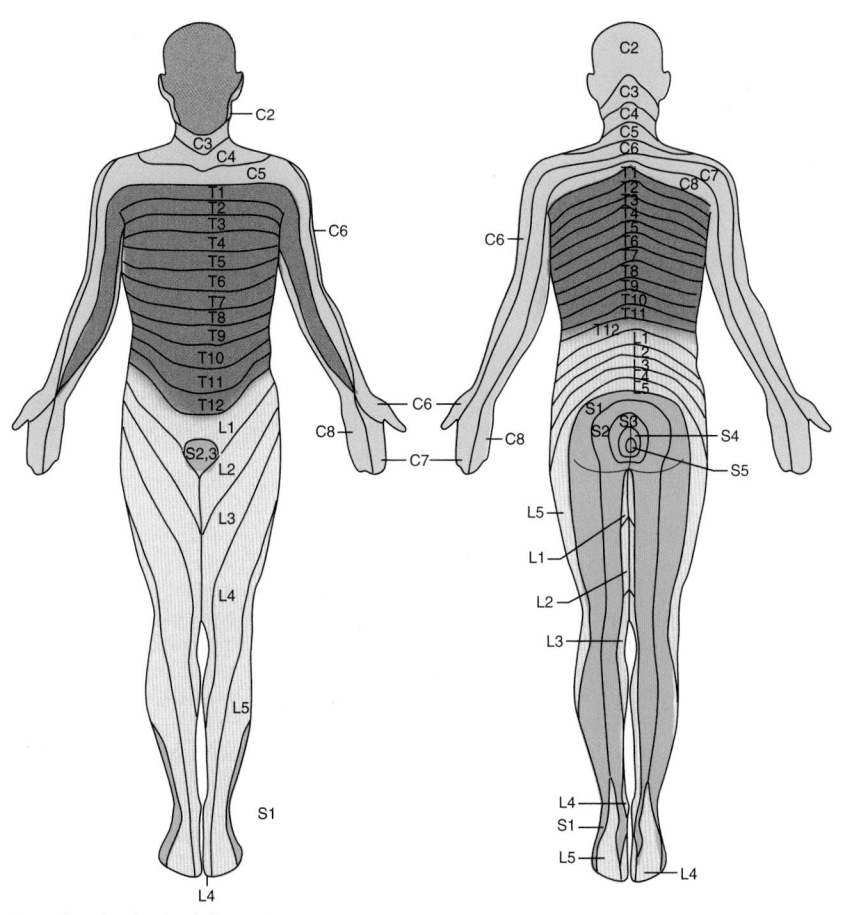

Levels of principal dermatomes

C5	Clavicles
C5,6,7	Lateral parts of upper limbs
C8, T1	Medial sides of upper limbs
C6	Thumb
C6,7,8	Hand
C8	Ring and little fingers
T4	Level of nipples
T10	Level of umbilicus
T12	Inguinal or groin regions
L1,2,3,4	Anterior and inner surfaces of lower limbs
L4,5 S1	Foot
L4	Medial side of great toe
S1,2, L5	Posterior and outer surfaces of lower limbs
S1	Lateral margin of foot and little toe
S2,3,4	Perineum

FIGURE 372-3. Schematic demarcation of levels of principal dermatomes shown as distinct segments. There is actually considerable overlap between any two adjacent dermatomes.

DISORDERS OF THE SPINE
Neck and Low Back Pain

DEFINITION

Most neck and low back pain is mechanical and attributable to the structural elements of the spine, which are the vertebrae, discs, ligaments, true joints, tendons, and muscles. Pain referred to the spine may arise from internal structures in the neck, upper chest, abdomen, or pelvis. Pain of spinal origin may be referred to the upper or lower extremity. In the lower limbs, conditions affecting the upper lumbar spine tend to refer pain to the groin and/or anterior thigh (from the hip to the knee). Conditions affecting the lower lumbar spine tend to cause referred pain in the buttock, posterior thigh, leg (from the knee to the ankle), or foot. Referred pain can be unilateral or bilateral. Pain that follows a dermatomal distribution is likely to be due to nerve root pathology.

EPIDEMIOLOGY

Lower back pain is more common than neck pain.[1] The thoracic spine, possibly because of rib attachments and limited range of motion, is a less common location for spine pain. An exception to this rule is the condition of diffuse idiopathic skeletal hyperostosis (Chapter 257), which is a noninflammatory, age-related condition of unknown etiology, characterized by ossification of paravertebral ligaments and peripheral entheses. It is more common in men and increases with age. Pain in the thoracic spine region occurs in up to 80% of patients with diffuse idiopathic skeletal hyperostosis.

In the general population, the incidence of self-reported neck pain is 213 per 1000; the 12-month prevalence of any neck pain is typically between 15 and 50%, and pain severe enough to limit activity is between 1.7 and 11.5%. The prevalence is higher in women. Risk factors for neck pain include heredity, poor psychological health, occupations such as dentistry, and tobacco use. The presence of disc degeneration does not correlate with the incidence of neck pain.

More than 70% of people will experience lower back pain significant enough to inhibit their participation in daily activities at some time in their life. The highest prevalence is in the 45- to 64-year age group, without a gender difference. Tobacco use is an associated risk factor. Physical work–related factors (e.g., heavy lifting, prolonged sitting, repetitive twisting) increase risk. Prospective studies show that psychosocial issues such as work monotony, job dissatisfaction, and depression also are major predisposing factors for chronic lower back pain.

PATHOBIOLOGY

Neck and lower back pain can occur with or without radicular pain. In the low back, radicular lower limb pain usually affects the L5 or S1 nerve root. In the cervical spine, the C7 nerve root is most commonly affected. Radicular upper or lower limb pain is usually caused by compression and irritation of the spinal nerve, typically by a protruding disc or osteoarthritic change. The cause of axial neck and lower back pain is more difficult to determine. The degenerative process of spondylosis is thought to be responsible for both acute and chronic axial spine pain, whereas the intervertebral disc is thought to account for a minority of symptoms. Intervertebral disc degeneration has a genetic predisposition, with heritability estimates in the range of about 35 to 75%.

Spondylosis is accompanied by disc degeneration, the formation of osteophytes, ligamentous hypertrophy, facet joint arthropathy, and vertebral subluxation (spondylolisthesis) of one vertebral body forward (anterolisthesis) or backward (retrolisthesis) on its mate below. The vast majority of people develop spondylosis, which includes disc desiccation and loss of elasticity of the annulus fibrosus. Congenital or acquired fractures of the pars interarticularis on both sides of one lumbar spinal level, termed spondylolysis, promote the development of spondylolisthesis. Spondylolisthesis is graded by the amount of maximal shift in quartiles from 0 being normal to 5 being total dissociation of the vertebral body with an adjacent vertebra. Stability of the spondylolisthesis is estimated by plain radiographs of the spine with the patient in flexion and extension.

Whiplash, an acute flexion or extension injury (or both) of the cervical spine, is common, especially after motor vehicle accidents. The acute whiplash syndrome is thought to be a result of mechanical irritation of pain-sensitive mostly musculoskeletal structures in the cervical spine, typically without spinal cord or spinal nerve injury. More severe trauma can cause fracture and vertebral instability, which often requires urgent surgical intervention.

CLINICAL MANIFESTATIONS

Acute neck pain and lower back pain are commonly limited to the axial region, although radicular signs and symptoms can occur in the presence of nerve root irritation. The most common radicular pain occurs in the distribution of a dermatome. Other radicular signs and symptoms can include dysesthesias or sensory loss in the affected dermatome, decreased strength in muscles of the affected myotome, and one or more decreased reflexes. Cranial nerve findings, diffuse weakness throughout a limb or in more than one limb, hemisensory symptoms, autonomic symptoms, and diffuse increase in reflexes are not typical manifestations of spine disease in the absence of spinal cord compression; these characteristics should prompt more extensive evaluation for other conditions that affect the brain, brain stem, or spinal cord. Bowel and bladder symptoms should prompt urgent evaluation for cauda equina compression or a myelopathy.

Acute spine problems can also cause referred pain at sites other than their anatomic source. More often, the term *referred pain* denotes the situation in which other structures, usually internal organs, refer pain to the spine or limbs. Areas of referred pain usually share the same embryologic origin and the same sensory pathways. Differentiation of referred pain from localized spine pain is aided by the history and examination. Mechanical pain is often exacerbated by spinal movement, whereas referred pain tends to be independent of such activities. Sciatica, which is defined as pain in the distribution of the sciatic nerve, often includes pain in the back as well as the buttock, posterior thigh, leg, and foot.[2] Although sciatica can be caused by a lesion anywhere along the course of the sciatic nerve, it is most commonly caused by injury of one of the exiting spinal nerves that contribute to the sciatic nerve (L4-S2).

DIAGNOSIS
History and Clinical Examination

The history and physical examination are essential for the initial evaluation and triage of patients with neck and lower back pain, with or without possible radicular upper or lower limb pain. "Red flags"[3] help identify patients who may have a serious underlying cause for their spinal pain and generally warrant very prompt diagnostic evaluation and possibly earlier medical or surgical intervention (Table 372-3). Red flags for neck or upper limb pain are similar to those for lower back pain with the addition of conditions unique to the cervical spine (rheumatoid arthritis, Down syndrome, and spondyloarthropathy); neck pain associated with chest pain, diaphoresis, or dyspnea, which can occur with myocardial ischemia (Chapter 63); and signs or symptoms of myelopathy. In the absence of red flags, guidelines usually recommend a wait-and-see approach for at least 4 to 6 weeks after the onset of neck or lower back pain.

On clinical examination, inspection should assess for evidence of trauma, muscle wasting, fasciculations, erythema, rashes, and scars. Palpation should look for areas of point tenderness, muscle spasm, and masses. If light percussion of the spinous process evokes significant pain, a focal lesion, such as fracture, tumor (Chapter 180), or infection (Chapter 385), should be considered. Active and passive range of motion for flexion, extension, rotation, and side-to-side bending should be tested.

Many provocative tests have been described for the evaluation of spine and limb pain, but few have undergone formal evaluation of their diagnostic accuracy. For neck and upper limb pain, an increase in symptoms with contralateral rotation of the neck and extension of the arm and fingers (Video 372-1) suggests cervical root involvement, as does the Spurling maneuver, in which the patient's head is bent backward and flexed (bent) laterally to the symptomatic side. Provocation of radicular pain or paresthesias with or

---

TABLE 372-3   "RED FLAGS" IN THE EVALUATION OF SPINE PAIN

Recent significant trauma or minor trauma at age >50 years
Unexplained weight loss
Unexplained fever
Immunosuppression
History of cancer
History of prior local surgery
Systemic disorder, bone or arthritic disorder
Intravenous drug use
Prolonged use of corticosteroids or osteoporosis
Age >70 years
Focal neurologic deficit with progressive symptoms
Duration >6 weeks
Thoracic spine pain

Modified from Davis PC, Wippold FJ, Brunberg JA, et al. ACR Appropriateness Criteria on low back pain. *J Am Coll Radiol.* 2009;6:401-407.

without downward pressure onto the top of the patient's head suggests cervical nerve root impingement or irritation (Video 372-2). Diagnostic tests also can reduce symptoms. In the cervical distraction test, the examiner's hands are placed under the jaw and occiput. Gentle upward pulling of the head can temporarily reduce or alleviate the symptoms of cervical spinal nerve impingement (Video 372-3).

Provocative tests that can be helpful in the patient with low back and lower limb pain include straight leg raising performed with the patient supine. The examiner flexes the thigh at the hip while the leg is held in extension at the knee. The test is positive if pain along the course of the sciatic nerve is provoked. Further increase in pain with foot dorsiflexion provides additional evidence of lumbosacral nerve root impingement.

For lower back pain, the straight leg raise (Video 372-4) has sensitivity of 0.85 to 0.91 but a specificity of only 0.26 to 0.52 for the diagnosis of sciatica due to a herniated disc. The crossed straight leg raise test (Video 372-5), which has a lower sensitivity of 0.23 to 0.34 but a much higher specificity of 0.86 to 0.90, is often positive in the presence of a disc extrusion. Positive seated straight leg raising when the knee is fully extended is about as useful as a positive test when the patient is supine at 65 degrees elevation (Video 372-6). In reverse straight leg raising, the examiner maximally flexes the knee while the patient is prone; provocation of same-sided pain, usually in the anterior thigh, is highly suggestive of impingement of the L2, L3, or L4 nerve roots, which contribute to the femoral nerve and are stretched by this maneuver.

Ancillary Testing

For acute and subacute neck and lower back pain, observation and conservative treatment are recommended if no red flags are present.[4] If the patient's symptoms are unchanged after 4 to 6 weeks, then further investigation can be considered. Magnetic resonance imaging (MRI) is the diagnostic test of choice for patients with neck and lower back pain, especially if they have radicular pain. MRI is recommended only in patients who have major or progressive neurologic deficits, in whom a serious underlying condition is expected, or in whom surgery or epidural corticosteroid injections are being considered. Even in patients age 65 years and older, the value of early diagnostic imaging in patients without radiculopathy is uncertain. However, MRI abnormalities are common in asymptomatic patients, so MRI has a very high false-positive rate when imaging the cervical or lumbar spine. Findings include loss of disc signal intensity, disc protrusion, narrowing of the disc space, and central or foraminal stenosis.

Care must be taken to ensure correlation with the clinical syndrome, because more than half of asymptomatic patients will have more than one potentially symptomatic cervical or lumbar finding on MRI. This number approaches 100% with age older than 50 to 60 years. Modic changes in the vertebrae, anterolisthesis, and lumbar disc extrusion are more strongly associated with low back pain than is disc degeneration without end plate changes. Discography is an invasive procedure which can be of some help in diagnosing lumbar internal disc disruption, a condition which has no known effective treatment. Discography is not recommended in the cervical spine.

Computed tomography (CT) is not as accurate as MRI but is the test of choice for patients intolerant of or unable to undergo MRI. CT myelography can be complementary to MRI, and one imaging study may be positive when the other is not. Otherwise, with few exceptions, MRI is the test of choice given its superiority in evaluating soft tissue structures and its lack of radiation exposure.

For stress fracture (Chapter 230), plain CT and single-photon emission computed tomography (SPECT) are more sensitive than MRI. CT can also be used to evaluate scoliosis, bone graft integrity, implanted instrumentation, and union of surgical fusion.

Plain radiography is of some use for judging the presence of spondylosis, normal cervical and lumbar lordosis and alignment, and absence of gross fracture and spinal instability. For patients in whom only a benign lumbar compression fracture is suspected, plain radiography may suffice if the results are normal and no other abnormalities are present.

Electrodiagnostic testing is not usually helpful in axial spine pain without neurologic symptoms. It can, however, be useful in documenting the presence and activity of radiculopathy and in diagnosing other conditions (e.g., brachial plexus neuritis, carpal tunnel syndrome, and sciatic neuropathy.) Furthermore, it is a lagging indicator and may not become abnormal until four weeks have elapsed from the onset of nerve injury.

Differential Diagnosis

The differential diagnosis of neck pain (Table 372-4) and lower back pain (Fig. 372-4) is very broad. Acute mechanical neck pain is most often caused

---

TABLE 372-4 CAUSES OF ACUTE AND CHRONIC NECK PAIN

Spondylotic/degenerative disease of intervertebral discs, facet joints, ligaments, bones, muscles

Rheumatologic conditions (e.g., rheumatoid arthritis [Chapter 248], spondyloarthropathies [Chapter 249], diffuse idiopathic skeletal hyperostosis, polymyalgia [Chapter 255], crystal deposition diseases [Chapter 257], fibromyalgia [Chapter 258])

Trauma (Chapter 371)

Neurogenic (Chapter 368) owing to spinal cord, nerve roots, meninges

Tumors of the spinal cord (Chapter 180), bone (Chapter 192), head and neck (Chapter 181), lung (Chapter 182) (primary or metastatic)

Infection (Chapter 385) (e.g., osteomyelitis, epidural, meninges, spinal cord)

Other (e.g., thyroid disease [Chapter 213], carotid or vertebral artery dissection [Chapter 379], upper esophageal abnormalities [Chapter 129], throat and laryngeal [Chapter 401])

Psychogenic [Chapter 369], usually with an additional source of pain

Malingering

---

by neck muscle strain, a herniated nucleus pulposus, or whiplash. Up to 97% of cases of low back pain are due to mechanical causes (see Table 372-5) or are idiopathic. For neck pain of gradual onset, osteoarthritis and cervical spinal stenosis are leading causes. For low back pain, muscle strain and a herniated nucleus pulposus are possible acute causes, whereas insidious causes include osteoarthritis, lumbar spinal stenosis, spondylolisthesis, and scoliosis. Queries regarding the aforementioned red flags will help identify serious and nonmechanical causes of neck and low back pain.

Abdominal and pelvic structures can refer pain to the low back. Abdominal aortic aneurysms (Chapter 69) can present with mid- or low back pain that may radiate to the hips or anterior thighs. Dissection of the thoracic aorta (Chapter 69) can cause sudden severe pain in the front and back of the chest including the spine. Cholecystitis (Chapter 146) can cause pain in the mid-thoracic area. Pancreatic disease (Chapter 135) can cause pain in the L1 region. Diverticulitis (Chapter 133) can cause lower abdominal and diffuse low back pain. Genitourinary disorders (Chapter 117) can cause colicky pain referred to the flank and costovertebral angle. Bladder disorders can occasionally refer pain to the sacral area, as can prostate problems (Chapter 120). Pelvic disorders in women that can cause referred low back pain include endometriosis (Chapter 223), ectopic pregnancy, and pelvic inflammatory disease (Chapters 283 and 302). Most of these disorders have additional signs and symptoms to aid in the diagnosis.

Myocardial ischemia (Chapters 62 to 64) can be associated with anterior neck pain, although less commonly than with left arm or jaw pain. Arterial dissections (Chapter 69) are more commonly associated with neck pain. For example, about 25% of patients with carotid dissections (Chapter 379) complain of anterolateral neck pain, and about 50% of patients with vertebral dissections have posterior neck pain. Patients with arterial dissections can have signs and symptoms of stroke (Chapter 379). Disorders of the esophagus (Chapter 129) and mass lesions of the neck and throat (Chapters 181 and 401) can present with neck pain.

Acute radicular pain can precede the rash in herpes zoster (Chapter 351). Sickle cell anemia can cause severe pain in almost any location, including the spine (Chapter 154). Infections of the disc (Chapter 385) cause severe back pain worsened by movement. Arachnoiditis (Chapter 384), an inflammatory process of the arachnoid membrane, can cause chronic back and radicular pain, often after spine surgery or the introduction of a foreign substance into the intrathecal space. Twenty to 50% of patients with depression (Chapter 369) will complain of back pain that is often diffuse and described in emotionally laden terms. Complaints of low back pain are also common in malingering patients.

TREATMENT   Rx

Patients with neck or lower back pain, with or without limb pain, should try to continue routine activities insofar as possible.[5]

Medications

Medication options include nonsteroidal anti-inflammatory drugs (NSAIDs) (e.g., ibuprofen 600 mg three times daily for up to a few weeks),[A1] exercise, and physical therapy. Acetaminophen is of no help for lower back pain, and its benefit for neck pain is uncertain.[A2] Skeletal muscle relaxants (e.g., cyclobenzaprine 5

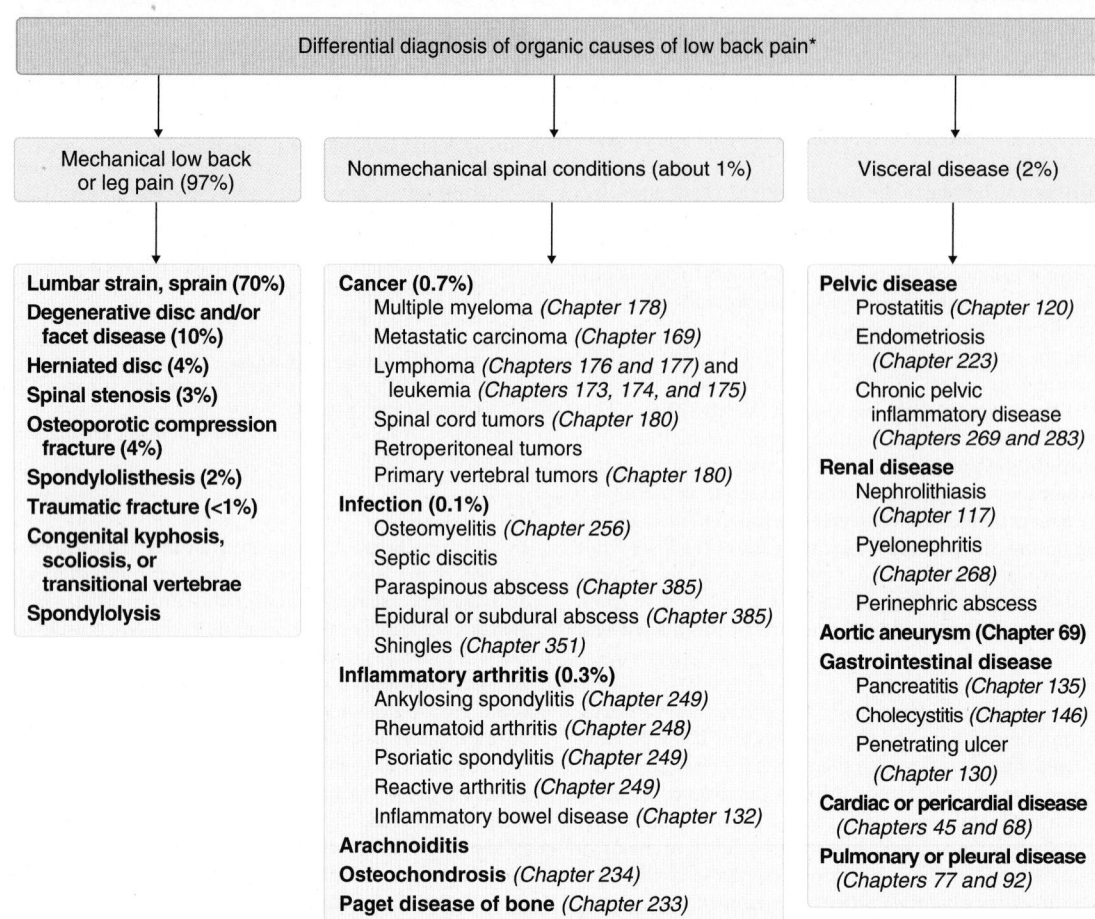

FIGURE 372-4. Differential diagnosis of organic causes of low back pain. *Percentages are approximations and may vary substantially in different practices. (Data from Deyo RA, Weinstein JN. Low back pain. *N Engl J Med.* 2001;344:363-370.)

TABLE 372-5　MECHANICAL LOW BACK PAIN

	MUSCLE STRAIN	HERNIATED NUCLEUS PULPOSUS	OSTEOARTHRITIS	SPINAL STENOSIS	SPONDYLOLISTHESIS	SCOLIOSIS
Age (yr)	20-40	30-50	>50	>60	20	30
Pain pattern location	Back (unilateral)	Back (unilateral)	Back (unilateral)	Leg (bilateral)	Back	Back
Onset	Acute	Acute (prior episodes)	Insidious	Insidious	Insidious	Insidious
Standing	↑	↓	↑	↑	↑	↑
Sitting	↓	↑	↓	↓	↓	↓
Bending	↑	↑	↓	↓	↑	↑
Straight leg	−	+	−	+ (stress)	−	−
Plain radiography	−	−	+	+	+	+

From Borenstein DG, Wiesel SW, Boden SD. *Low Back Pain: Medical Diagnosis and Comprehensive Management.* 2nd ed. Philadelphia: WB Saunders; 1995.

to 10 mg three times daily, tizanidine 2 to 6 mg three times daily, or carisoprodol 250 to 350 mg three times daily for up to a few weeks) are of short-term help but can cause sedation. Duloxetine (60 mg once daily) can be helpful for chronic lower back pain. Systemic corticosteroids do not seem to be effective, and the use of opioid analgesics is controversial and of uncertain benefit for chronic lower back pain.[A3]

Nonsurgical Interventions

No data support corticosteroid injections into facet joints for axial neck or lower back pain, although transforaminal and interlaminar epidural corticosteroid injections are indicated for radicular pain. Temporary pain relief with medial branch nerve blocks can help determine which facet joints are responsible for axial neck and lower back pain. If medial branch blocks are helpful, radiofrequency ablation of the identified nerves can provide months of pain relief, especially for chronic neck pain.

Heat, massage, physical therapy, acupuncture, and spinal manipulation are helpful for acute and subacute lower back and possibly for axial neck pain, but bed rest is not recommended for acute neck or lower back pain. For chronic neck pain, yoga therapy provides modest to significant pain relief. Cervical collars and traction are not of established benefit. Chiropractic manipulation is more helpful for lower back pain than for neck pain and better for acute than chronic pain.

Helpful therapies for chronic lower back pain include Tai Chi, mindfulness-based stressed reduction, and yoga.[A4] Psychological therapies, multidisciplinary rehabilitation, massage, cognitive behavioral therapy, and acupuncture also are helpful for chronic lower back pain.[A5]

Surgery

Even in the absence of radicular pain or myelopathy, surgical intervention for neck pain is indicated in cases of vertebral instability, such as caused by fracture, tumor, or infection. For neck pain that is accompanied by signs or symptoms of radiculopathy, surgery should be considered but is not usually the initial treatment. If a cervical spine lesion is causing spinal cord compression, evaluation for possible surgery is indicated.

When persistent nonradicular lower back pain is accompanied by degenerative spine changes, surgical fusion is often performed. However, randomized controlled studies have shown that lumbar spinal fusion is only modestly helpful compared with no treatment, and lumbar fusion is not beneficial compared with an active physical therapy program.[A6][A7] Total disc arthroplasty (artificial disc) can be useful for cervical radiculopathy or myelopathy but not for neck pain alone. Total lumbar disc arthroplasty is available but little used for chronic lower back pain.

PROGNOSIS

Between 50 and 85% of patients who have neck pain that persists for more than 1 day report recurrence of symptoms in 1- and 5-year follow-up. About 50% of patients recover within 3 months. Patients who remain symptomatic generally have relatively mild pain and disability. Factors that increase the likelihood of developing persistent or recurrent neck pain include prior neck injury, psychopathology, low work satisfaction, poor workplace environment, female gender, concomitant low back and other pain disorders, poor coping skills, catastrophization, neck trauma, sedentary lifestyle, and weight gain. Patients with neck pain following a whiplash injury are especially likely to experience protracted symptoms.

Mechanical low back pain, even with radicular symptoms, resolves without specific intervention within 30 days in the majority of patients and within 3 months in 90% of patients. Exercise alone or in combination with education is effective for preventing low back pain.[A8] Recurrence is frequent, however, and about 50% of patients will experience another episode within one year. Many patients will have lingering fluctuating or intermittent low back pain, but only a minority develop significant chronic low back pain.

Long-term disability is more common with obesity, low education level, tobacco use, high levels of pain at the onset, tendency to somatization, job dissatisfaction, lack of availability of light-duty employment, and need to perform heavy lifting at work. Genetic variability, such as in polymorphisms of catechol *O*-methyltransferase, also may play a role in the development of chronic pain.

Lumbar Spinal Stenosis

DEFINITION

Lumbar spinal stenosis occurs when narrowing of the lumbar spinal canal, its lateral recesses, or neural foramina causes symptomatic or asymptomatic compression of the lumbosacral nerve roots. L4-5 is the most common level of stenosis, followed by L3-4, L2-3, L5-S1, and L1-2; however, most patients have stenosis at more than one vertebral level.

EPIDEMIOLOGY

Congenital spinal stenosis occurs in about 7% of the general population, and midsagittal degenerative stenosis occurs in about 30%. More severe stenosis is associated with older age and more low back pain. About 10% of patients have spinal stenosis in both the cervical and lumbar levels. Patients with diffuse idiopathic skeletal hyperostosis are especially likely to develop spinal stenosis.

PATHOBIOLOGY

Primary lumbar spinal stenosis is caused by congenital narrowing of the spinal canal, whereas causes of secondary stenosis include degenerative spondylotic changes, which increase with age. Patients with congenital lumbar spine stenosis typically do not have symptoms until they develop additional degenerative changes in the spine. Structures that can hypertrophy and lead to canal narrowing include disc bulging and vertebral osteophytic spurring, enlargement of the facet joints, thickening of the ligamenta flava, thickening of the posterior longitudinal ligament, and spondylolisthesis.

In addition to static narrowing of the lumbar spinal canal, dynamic narrowing accounts for the postural provocation of symptoms. With extension, the inferior articular processes, which form the upper half of facet joints, slide backward and downward on the superior articular processes, which form the lower half of the facet joints. Movement of the facet joints narrows the lumbar spinal canal and intervertebral foramina. The lumbar discs and posterior longitudinal ligaments may bulge posteriorly into the spinal canal, and the ligamenta flava can buckle forward into the canal. These mechanical changes

further narrow the lumbar spinal canal and compress the spinal nerves. Intervertebral foramina also narrow when the lumbar spine is extended, thereby causing compression of individual lumbosacral spinal nerves.

CLINICAL MANIFESTATIONS

Lumbar spinal stenosis causes a syndrome of pseudoclaudication, which can mimic the symptoms of lower limb vascular claudication (Chapter 71). Pseudoclaudication typically affects the entire lower limb, usually the posterior aspect, but can affect the thigh alone or leg alone. Patients report lower limb numbness, weakness, or pain, with or without back pain, when standing or walking. The absence of pain when seated and the improvement of symptoms when bending forward at the waist are typical. Patients also can develop fixed neurologic deficits, usually in the distribution of the L5 and S1 nerve roots, especially if they have a concomitant peripheral neuropathy. Bowel and bladder function are usually unaffected.

DIAGNOSIS

Plain CT can be used as a screening test, but MRI is the diagnostic test of choice. CT myelography has the advantage of allowing imaging with the patient in an upright position (Fig. 372-5). Plain lumbar spine radiographs with the patient in flexion and extension can detect any spondylolisthesis. Electromyography (EMG) typically shows evidence of radiculopathy rather than peripheral neuropathy (unless the patient has both). Vascular laboratory testing of the lower extremity arteries can help exclude peripheral arterial disease. The differential diagnosis includes any mass in the thecal sac (e.g., large lumbar disc, tumor), vascular claudication (usually due to atherosclerosis), osteoarthritis (Chapter 246) of the hips and/or knees, arteriovenous malformation of the spinal cord, multiple sclerosis (Chapter 383), and peripheral neuropathy (Chapter 392).

TREATMENT AND PROGNOSIS   Rx

Treatment includes physical, pharmacologic, and surgical approaches.[A9] Exercises to strengthen the abdominal muscles and reduce lumbar lordosis may be helpful. Use of a short cane or walker can allow the patient to stand longer and walk farther. Lumbar corsets and braces may help to reduce lumbar lordosis when standing and delay the onset of symptoms. Very substantial weight loss in the obese patient can reduce the degree of lumbar lordosis that occurs with standing and reduce the axial load on the lumbar spine. Analgesics are not very helpful because pain is intermittent and can be relieved by changing posture. Epidural corticosteroid injections, though often tried, are of no benefit.[A10]

Without surgery, most patients gradually worsen, although some stabilize, and a small percentage improves. For patients who have appropriate symptoms for more than three months, have symptoms that interfere with their work or leisure activities, have progressive neurologic deficits, and have stenosis at one or more levels, the mainstay of treatment is elective surgical decompression, typically consisting of laminectomy with or without medial facetectomies at one or more levels. Lumbar fusion is of no incremental benefit, except perhaps in patients with spondylolisthesis.[A11][A12] About 80% of patients improve after surgery, but postural low back pain may persist. Despite adequate decompression, about 30% of patients develop recurrent lumbar stenosis at another level after a number of years, and this risk is higher in patients with diffuse idiopathic skeletal hyperostosis.[6]

● CERVICAL SPINAL STENOSIS AND SPONDYLOTIC MYELOPATHY

DEFINITION

Cervical spinal stenosis is narrowing of the cervical spinal canal owing to congenital factors, acquired conditions (mostly spondylosis), or a combination of the two. Cervical spondylotic myelopathy occurs when cervical spondylosis causes spinal cord injury.

EPIDEMIOLOGY

The prevalence of cervical spondylosis is 95% in men and 89% in women over age 60 years. In one autopsy study of presumably asymptomatic patients, 7.5% were found to have spondylotic compression of their spinal cord. Risk factors include repeated trauma, male gender, older age, stenosis at another spinal level, and a positive family history.

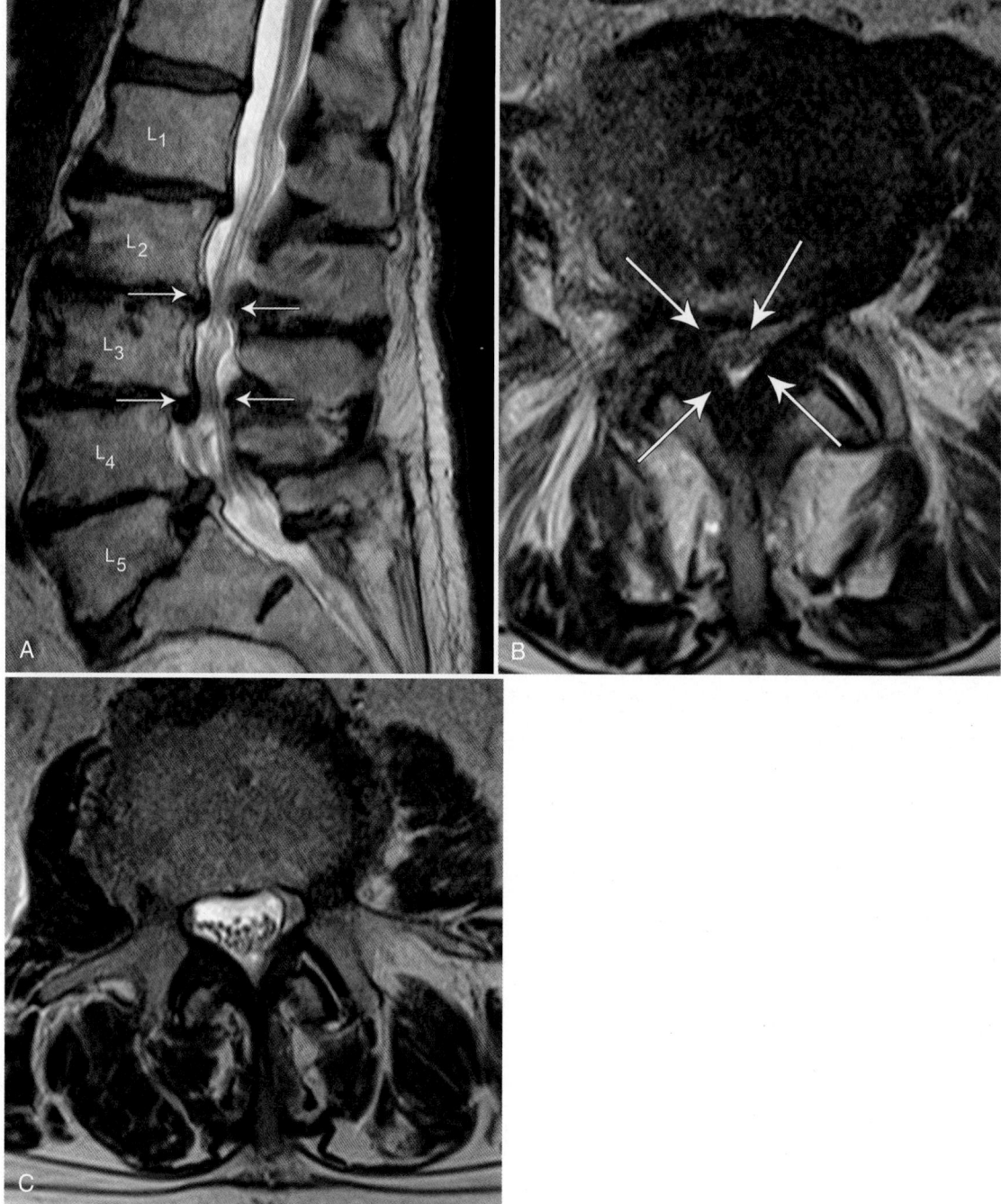

FIGURE 372-5. **A,** Sagittal T-2 weighted MRI of lumbar spine shows severe stenosis at L2-3 and L3-4 (*arrows*). **B,** Axial T-2 weighted MRI of lumbar spine shows severe stenosis at L3-4 level (*arrows*). **C,** Axial T-2 weighted MRI of lumbar spine shows no significant stenosis at L1-2 level.

PATHOBIOLOGY

Narrowing of the cervical spinal canal is due to bulging discs, which generate osteophytic spurring in the vertebral bodies, thickening of the posterior longitudinal ligament anterior to the spinal canal, thickening of the ligamenta flava posterior to the canal, enlargement of the uncovertebral processes, and enlargement of the facet joints. When the disc or hypertrophic spur projects posteriorly, the spondylotic bar compresses the spinal cord. The C5-6 level is most commonly affected, followed by C6-7 and then by C4-5; however, more than one level is characteristically involved. Compression of one or more spinal nerves causes radiculopathy. In addition to static narrowing of the spinal canal, neck flexion (when the spinal cord is pulled over the spondylotic osteophytes and bulging discs) and neck extension (when the spinous process may get close to the most posterior aspect of the vertebral disc osteophyte complex and pinch the spinal cord) can cause dynamic symptoms. The mechanism of cord and nerve root injury is a combination of direct mechanical compression and impaired circulation.

CLINICAL MANIFESTATIONS

Symptoms include neck pain; unilateral or bilateral upper limb pain; upper limb weakness, numbness, and loss of dexterity; lower limb stiffness, weakness, or sensory loss; urgency of bladder more likely than bowel; and the Lhermitte sign (electric-like pain or tingling down the spine or limbs with neck flexion or extension). The condition may be painless, and severe pain is uncommon. Neurologic symptoms are typically steady and persistent rather than transient or fluctuating.

On physical examination, the patient can have increased or reduced upper or lower limb reflexes, upper or lower limb weakness or sensory loss, abnormal reflexes, gait disturbance, and lower more often than upper limb spasticity.

DIAGNOSIS

MRI of the cervical spine is the diagnostic test of choice followed by CT myelography (Fig. 372-6). The physician must recognize that cervical spondylosis and cervical spinal stenosis are common, often asymptomatic, and

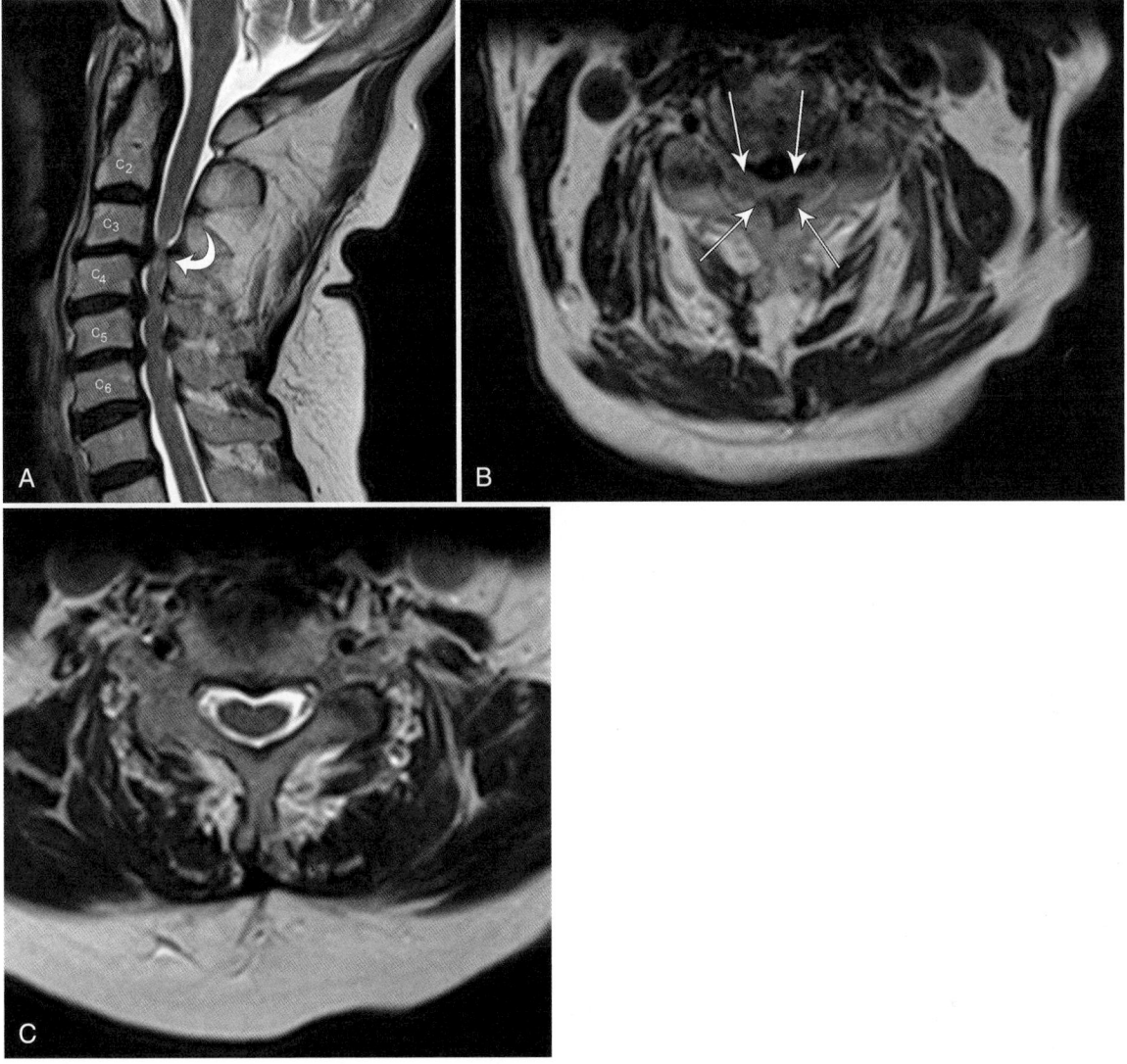

FIGURE 372-6. **A,** Sagittal T-2 weighted MRI of cervical spine shows multi-level spinal stenosis worse at C3-4 than at C4-5 than at C5-6. There is increased T-2 signal within the spinal cord just below the C3-4 level indicating myelomalacia (*arrow*). **B,** Axial T-2 weighted MRI of cervical spine at C3-4 level shows severe cord compression and deformity (*arrows*). **C,** Axial T-2 weighted MRI of cervical spine at C6-7 level, away from severe stenosis shows a nearly normal appearance.

not necessarily the cause of a patient's symptoms. Signal abnormality within the spinal cord on MRI indicates that some cord injury has occurred. EMG can be helpful in excluding carpal tunnel syndrome, brachial plexus neuritis, and motor neuron disease and in documenting the presence of one or more cervical radiculopathies. Blood and cerebrospinal fluid (CSF) testing may be helpful to exclude, for example, tabes dorsalis (Chapter 303) and neuromyelitis optica (Chapter 383).

approach and always includes fusion when performed anteriorly. An artificial cervical disc is an option for 1- or 2-level stenosis. Patients who have undergone iatrogenic fusion or have congenital fusion develop new or additional spondylotic degeneration at a level above or below their fusion, with potential root or cord impingement, at a rate of about 3% per year and may require additional surgery.

TREATMENT AND PROGNOSIS   Rx

Conservative treatment is aimed at controlling any pain, maintaining function (e.g., physical therapy, a gait aid), protecting the spinal cord from additional injury by avoiding head and neck trauma, and monitoring for neurologic worsening. Nonoperative therapy with little or no evidence includes a cervical collar during the day and a cervical pillow at night. Physical therapy should be directed at neurologic signs and symptoms (e.g., imbalance, weakness). Vigorous neck range-of-motion exercises should be avoided.

Medical treatments include acetaminophen and NSAIDs if any pain control is needed (Chapter 27). Cervical epidural corticosteroid injections can be tried for radicular pain.

Decompressive surgery, which is indicated for moderate to severe neurologic deficits or progressively worsening myelopathy,[7] results in neurologic improvement in 50 to 70% of patients. Recovery is typically incomplete and plateaus at about six months. Some patients have late deterioration with or without recurrent spinal stenosis. Surgery can be performed from an anterior or posterior

PROGNOSIS

Without surgery, a small number of patients with cervical spondylotic myelopathy improve, 20 to 60% worsen either gradually or in a stepwise fashion, and many are stable for long periods.[8]

DISORDERS OF THE NERVE ROOTS

DEFINITION

Disorders of the spinal nerve or nerve root, which is the short segment of nerve after the ventral and dorsal nerve roots have joined and before the spinal nerve divides into its ventral and dorsal rami are termed *radiculopathies.* Symptoms depend on the specific spinal level and the side(s) involved.

EPIDEMIOLOGY

The average annual age-adjusted incidence rate for cervical radiculopathy is about 83/100,000. Men are affected nearly twice as often as women, and the peak age is 50 to 54 years. The annual incidence of new-onset lumbosacral radicular pain ranges from about 1.5% to 18.5%. The estimated prevalence of cauda equina syndrome among all patients with lower back pain is about 1 in 2500. Strenuous physical activity, cigarette smoking, and genetic factors are thought to increase the risk of disc herniation.

PATHOBIOLOGY

Irritation of the spinal sensory nerve root or dorsal root ganglion causes symptoms referable to that dermatome. Mechanical compression of the nerve contributes to the syndrome. In addition, inflammatory cytokines can leak from the nucleus pulposus into the epidural space, where they result in endoneurial edema and pain. The pro-inflammatory cytokine TNF-α is a likely key contributor. Herniation of the nucleus pulposus releases phospholipase A_2, which also plays an important role in the inflammatory process. The inflammatory process itself can cause pain in the absence of frank root compression.

Sciatica is pain in the distribution of the sciatic nerve, which receives contributions from the L4, L5, S1, and S2 nerve roots and innervates the ipsilateral buttock, posterior thigh, leg, and foot. Disc herniations, which are a frequent cause of sciatica, are most common at L4-5 and L5-S1. A herniated disc characteristically protrudes posterolaterally and impinges on the nerve that is migrating laterally to exit beneath the pedicle of the next lower vertebral segment. For this reason, a disc rupture usually compresses the nerve root that is one higher in number (and one lower in the spine). Hence, an L4 disc typically impinges on the L5 nerve, and an L5 disc compresses the S1 nerve. A far lateral disc protrusion can compress the spinal nerve at the same level as the protruded disc, and a large disc can compress more than one nerve root. In addition to disc herniation, sciatica can be caused by direct sciatic nerve injury anywhere along its course. The *cauda equina syndrome* results from disease involving multiple roots of the lower lumbar and sacral spinal levels as they travel downward within the spinal canal on their way to exit through their respective intervertebral (or neural) foramina.

CLINICAL MANIFESTATIONS

The symptoms of radiculopathy depend on the affected root (see Tables 372-1 and 372-2). Root involvement is likely if pain radiates beyond the shoulder or the knee. In the thoracic region, root involvement often produces symptoms that "wrap around" the trunk. Radicular pain is often worsened by activities that increase intraspinal pressure, such as coughing, sneezing, straining, and other Valsalva maneuvers. The character of the pain varies, but it is often described as sharp, shooting, electrical, or tingling. When reporting symptoms, patients may point to or rub the dermatome where they are experiencing the discomfort (perceived pain). Patients also may report specific positions that increase or decrease pain; for example, sitting will often worsen the pain of acute lumbar disc herniation, and neck extension can produce radiating pain in cervical disc herniation or other processes that narrow the intervertebral foramen. Radicular pain often worsens when the patient is supine and frequently wakes the patient from sleep. Referred cervical root pain may affect only the scapula.

Patients often note hypesthesia (diminished sensation), which often follows a dermatome but also can be described as affecting a limb diffusely. Complaints of weakness may be difficult to localize to a particular muscle, except when the patient complains of a weak grip (C8 or T1) or a foot drop (L5).

Weakness can be asymptomatic (especially the triceps, C7, and the gastrocnemius, S1, muscles). Side-to-side strength testing aids in the detection of weakness. Mild weakness is more readily appreciated if the muscle is placed in a position of mechanical disadvantage (e.g., testing the triceps with the elbow flexed at ≥90 degrees). Slight weakness can also be identified by asking patients to walk on their toes, walk on their heels, and go up and down stairs or a step-stool. Sensory examination should test all potential root distributions. Testing pinprick is often sufficient. Hyperreflexia is not expected in a spinal nerve disorder and should raise questions about pathology in the spinal cord or brain (Chapter 371). Patients who are older than 65 years or who have a peripheral neuropathy (Chapter 392) can have reduced or even absent ankle and knee reflexes.

Cauda equina syndrome manifests as unilateral or bilateral leg weakness, saddle anesthesia, sexual dysfunction, urinary dysfunction with hesitancy or retention, and, less commonly, bowel dysfunction. Depending on the cause, it is frequently accompanied by low back pain. The syndrome can be accompanied by severe sciatica, which can be unilateral or bilateral and also involve perineal pain. Lower limb weakness, which may be asymmetrical, is of the lower motor neuron type.

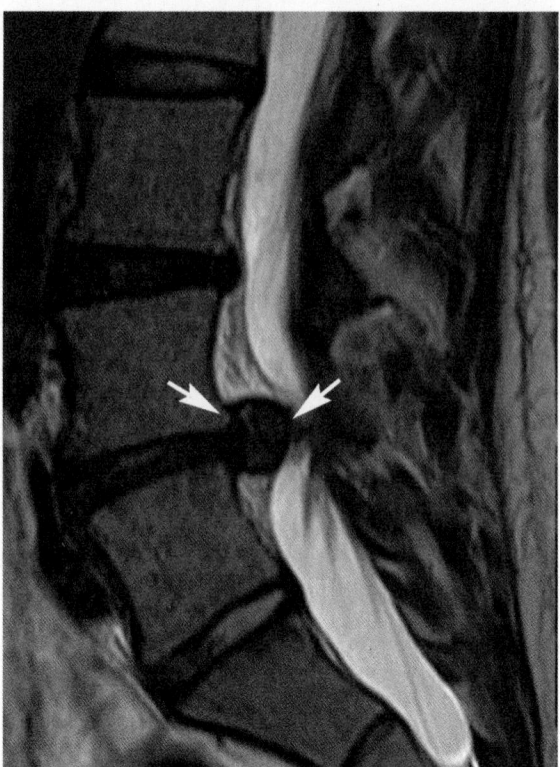

FIGURE 372-7. Magnetic resonance imaging of a large lumbar disc herniation. (From *Spine Disorders: Medical and Surgical Management* by JD Bartleson and HG Deen; Cambridge University Press, 2009. Copyrighted and used with permission of Mayo Foundation for Medical Education and Research.)

DIAGNOSIS

The history and physical examination for suspected radiculopathy is similar to the evaluation of neck and lower back pain (see earlier), with special emphasis on finding evidence of nerve root deficits.

The patient should be asked about bowel and bladder dysfunction. Frank incontinence (Chapter 23) suggests either the cauda equina syndrome or a myelopathy. If the patient reports any loss of perineal sensation, such as might be noted during or after voiding or passing stool, the examination should test perianal sensation, anal sphincter strength and tone, and the anal reflex. Because the cauda equina syndrome involves nerve roots, reflexes should be normal or decreased; hyperactive reflexes or a Babinski sign suggest myelopathy.

Imaging to evaluate a potential radiculopathy is similar to the evaluation for neck and back pain (see above), and MRI (Fig. 372-7) is the best test in almost all instances. However, many imaging findings are asymptomatic and should be ignored. For example, MRI performed 1 year after disc herniation with sciatica cannot determine which patients continue to be symptomatic and which are symptom-free. EMG, which can be very helpful in determining whether a finding on MRI is truly associated with neurologic signs and symptoms, can localize radicular abnormalities, judge their severity, and determine comorbid or alternative neurologic diseases, such as diffuse peripheral or focal entrapment neuropathies. EMG may not show abnormalities for 3 to 4 weeks following nerve root injury but has a high sensitivity and specificity for identifying chronic denervation when the motor component of the root is involved. However, EMG is less sensitive (about 30 to 70%) if only the sensory component of the root is involved by the lesion. An EMG is unnecessary if the diagnosis is clear from the history, physical examination, and MRI. In other situations, its high specificity complements the high sensitivity of MRI.

Many of the conditions that cause neck and lower back pain can also cause radiculopathy, including sciatica (Table 372-6). Spondylosis is the most common cause of radiculopathy, sciatica, and cauda equina syndrome, but the same symptoms and signs can be caused by infections (e.g., herpes zoster; Chapter 351), tumor (e.g., mass effect or leptomeningeal spread; Chapter 180), and scarring (e.g., post-surgical arachnoiditis). Disorders of the brachial plexus (e.g., brachial plexus neuritis) and lumbosacral plexus (e.g., diabetic radiculoplexus neuropathy; Chapter 392) also can simulate spondylotic radiculopathy.

Non-neurologic disorders, such as fibromyalgia (Chapter 258) and polymyalgia rheumatica (Chapter 255), can cause pain that mimics radiculopathy.

TABLE 372-6	DIFFERENTIAL DIAGNOSIS OF LOWER LIMB PAIN SUGGESTIVE OF SCIATICA

Neurogenic within the spine
- Spondylotic
  - Herniated nucleus pulposus
  - Stenosis of central canal, lateral recess, or intervertebral foramen
  - Synovial cyst
- Arachnoid or perineural cyst
- Sterile inflammatory arachnoiditis
- Tumor: primary (e.g., neurofibroma, ependymoma) or metastatic (bone or epidural space, meningeal)
- Infection: disc, epidural, herpes zoster, Lyme disease
- Inflammatory radiculopathy (e.g., sarcoidosis, paraneoplastic)

Neurogenic outside of the spine (e.g., lumbosacral plexus, sciatic neuropathy, peripheral neuropathy)

Non-neurogenic
- Musculoskeletal
- Peripheral vascular disease

Cervical radiculopathy also can be mimicked by acromioclavicular joint arthropathy, shoulder bursitis, rotator cuff disease, thoracic outlet syndrome, and the shoulder impingement syndrome. Lumbar radiculopathy can be mimicked by hip arthritis, trochanteric bursitis, sacroiliac joint disease, piriformis syndrome, iliotibial band syndrome, and hamstring tendinitis (Chapter 247).

The most common cause of cauda equina syndrome is a very large L4-5 or L5-S1 disc herniation. Other causes include tumor, abscess, epidural hematoma, and scarring. Depending on the rate of progression, cauda equina syndrome should be considered an emergency. Unless the onset is gradual, emergent or possibly urgent lumbar spine MRI and neurosurgical consultation should be obtained.

TREATMENT   Rx

Acute radicular symptoms are usually self-limited and resolve. Treatment with medications[A13] and physical therapies are as for neck and lower back pain. Pregabalin is not helpful for acute or chronic sciatica.[A14]

If radiculopathy is associated with the cauda equina syndrome or with an underlying lesion other than spondylosis, such as infection (Chapter 385) or tumor (Chapter 180), treatment should be directed toward that underlying process. If symptoms or neurologic dysfunction progress or persist for more than 4 to 6 weeks, intervention should be considered. Early surgery is indicated for spinal instability, severe or progressive neurologic deficits, myelopathy, neurologic deficits critical to the patient's vocation or avocation, or uncontrollable severe radicular pain in the presence of root compression.

In cervical radiculopathy, transforaminal epidural corticosteroid injections can provide short-term pain relief with an acceptable risk. In cervical spondylosis with radiculopathy, surgery provides more rapid pain relief than does physical therapy, but little or no long-term benefit. Anterior cervical discectomy with fusion or placement of an artificial disc (arthroplasty) provides symptomatic benefit, and cervical laminectomy and discectomy from a posterior approach is also effective.

For lumbar radiculopathy, epidural corticosteroid injections may provide relatively minor short-term pain relief for 2 to 6 weeks, but they do not improve function or relieve pain beyond 3 months.[A15] In some cases, temporary relief of symptoms may help confirm the causal link with an injected anatomic site. There is no evidence that epidural injections prevent eventual surgical intervention.[A16] For symptomatic lumbar radiculopathy due to a herniated disc, either open surgical discectomy or microdiscectomy (Video 372-7) is superior to nonsurgical therapy for at least 3 months[9] but not necessarily in the medium- or long-term. If the condition is isolated to a single disc and no significant degenerative changes are present, longer duration of benefit is more likely. Patients who derive a greater benefit from surgery include those in whom MRI shows a herniated disc with compression of the thecal sac of one third or more, or those with nerve root compression. Minimally invasive procedures are not clearly better than standard approaches.[A17]

DISORDERS OF THE SPINAL CORD

DEFINITION AND OVERVIEW

A disorder of the spinal cord is termed a *myelopathy*. A myelopathy can be intramedullary, as the result of a disorder intrinsic to the cord, or extramedullary,

TABLE 372-7	CAUSES OF MYELOPATHY

Extramedullary but Compressing the Spinal Cord
- Cervical stenosis (spondylosis, congenital)
- Cervical disc herniation
- Diffuse idiopathic skeletal hyperostosis
- Tumor
- Synovial or arachnoid cyst
- Infection (e.g., epidural abscess [Chapter 385], osteomyelitis [Chapter 256])
- Trauma
- Rheumatoid arthritis (Chapter 248), ankylosing spondylitis (Chapter 249)
- Other: Paget disease (Chapter 233), epidural lipomatosis, ossification of posterior longitudinal ligament

Intramedullary and Intrinsic to Spinal Cord
- Tumor
- Infection (e.g., syphilis [Chapter 303]; HIV-associated [Chapter 366], HTLV-1 [Chapter 354])
- Demyelinating (e.g., multiple sclerosis [Chapter 383], neuromyelitis optica [Chapter 396], acute disseminated encephalomyelitis [Chapter 383], acute transverse myelitis [Chapter 383])
- Inflammatory (e.g., systemic lupus erythematosus [Chapter 250], Sjögren syndrome [Chapter 252], Behçet disease [Chapter 254], sarcoidosis [Chapter 89], paraneoplastic [Chapter 169])
- Metabolic
- Deficiency of vitamin B_{12}, folic acid, vitamin E, copper
- Post-radiation myelopathy
- Hereditary spastic paraparesis
- Vascular (e.g., spinal cord infarction, vascular malformation)
- Syringomyelia
- Nitrous oxide
- Sarcoidosis
- Motor neuron disease

HIV = human immunodeficiency virus; HTLV = human T-lymphotropic virus.

as the result of an abnormality that is extrinsic to the cord but compressing it. Extramedullary lesions can be further divided into intradural (within) and extradural (outside) the dura.

EPIDEMIOLOGY AND PATHOBIOLOGY

Spinal cord disorders can be caused by a wide range of conditions (Table 372-7), but cervical spondylotic myelopathy is the most common cause.

The functional elements of the spinal cord (Fig. 372-8) include tracts descending to motor and autonomic neurons, as well as ascending sensory tracts. The anterior horn cell motor neuron is the cell body for the axon that will become the anterior nerve root and continue directly to innervate skeletal muscle. The cell bodies for the primary sensory neurons reside in the dorsal root ganglia outside the spinal cord itself.

CLINICAL MANIFESTATIONS

The clinical manifestations of myelopathy correlate with the spinal level of the lesion. The majority of signs will be bilateral, but asymmetry, or even unilaterality, does not exclude a spinal cord lesion.

In general, the three major functions affected are motor, sensory, and autonomic, especially bowel, bladder, and erectile function. If anterior horn cells are involved at the lesion level, the corresponding myotome will exhibit lower motor neuron findings (hypotonic weakness), and reflexes may be decreased at that level. Below the lesion, patients will have hypertonic weakness that can progress to spastic paralysis, hyperreflexia, and the Babinski sign. Sensation will be decreased at and below the level of the lesion. Increased tone and spasticity often develop over time, so they may not be prominent at the initial clinical presentation. If the posterior columns are compromised, patients may lose joint position sense and develop ataxia, especially of gait. If the posterior columns of the cervical cord are impaired, patients may have pseudoathetosis of the fingers, manifested as unconscious, slow, writhing (athetotic) movements of the fingers of the outstretched arm when the eyes are closed.

The anterior cord syndrome is manifested as lower motor neuron weakness at the level of the lesion (anterior horn); upper motor neuron weakness and spasticity below the lesion (corticospinal tracts); autonomic dysfunction below the level of the lesion (lateral horn), most often difficulty with bowel and bladder control; and loss of pain and temperature sensation below the level of the lesion (spinothalamic tract). Vibration and joint position sense remain intact (posterior columns). The major causes of this syndrome are vascular,

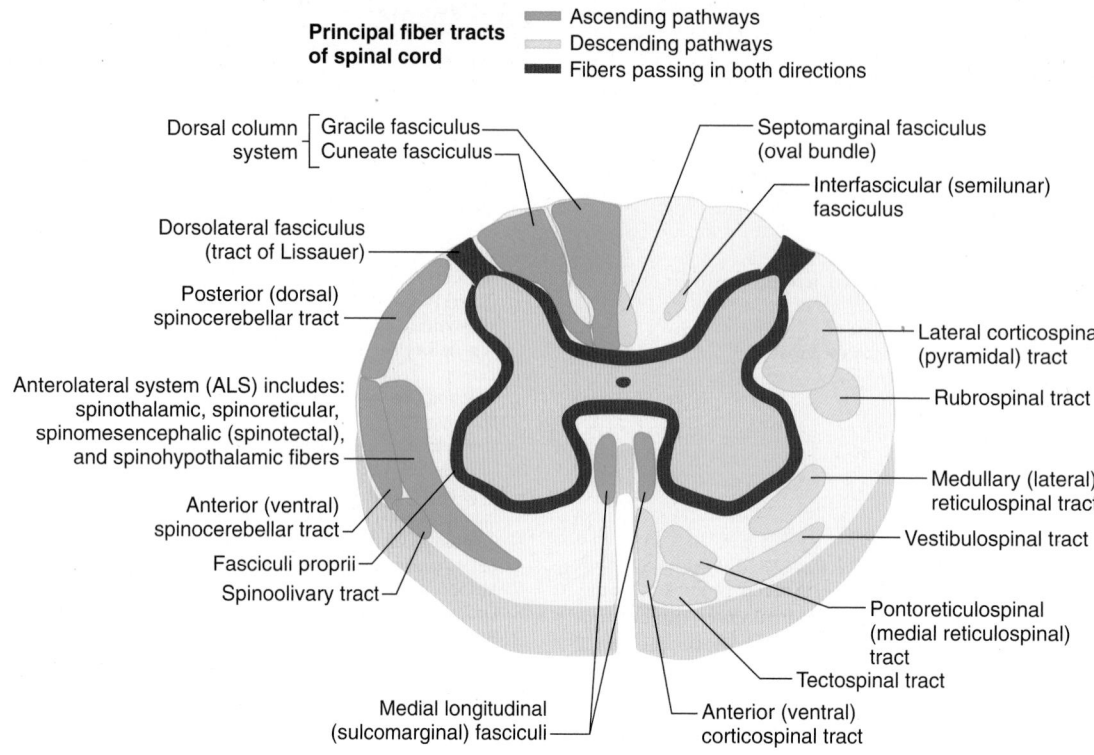

FIGURE 372-8. Principal fiber tracts of the spinal cord.

such as an anterior spinal artery occlusion, or an anteriorly impinging mass lesion, such as a disc or vertebral body mass.

The central cord syndrome is characterized by lower motor neuron signs and symptoms at the level of the lesion (anterior horn cells) and upper motor neuron signs and symptoms below the lesion (corticospinal tracts), urinary retention, and a band of loss of temperature and pain sensation at the level of the lesion (anterior white commissure decussation of these fibers). In the midcervical level, this syndrome is typical of syringomyelia (Chapter 389). Other major causes include cervical trauma (Chapter 371), especially when patients with preexisting cervical spondylosis sustain a hyperextension injury, and intramedullary tumors (Chapter 180).

The posterior cord syndrome is manifested by imbalance, especially in the dark or with eyes closed, and an examination notable for sensory ataxia, presence of the Romberg sign, and loss of vibration and position sense below the level of the lesion (posterior columns), with preservation of pain and temperature sensation. Patients are seldom weak. Posterior cord dysfunction may be caused by spondylotic disease, but other causes include deficiency of vitamin B_{12}, copper deficiency (which can be caused by excess zinc intake), vitamin E deficiency (Chapters 205 and 388), syphilis (Chapter 303), AIDS-associated vacuolar myelopathy (Chapter 366), and nitrous oxide inhalation (Chapter 404).

The Brown-Séquard (cord hemisection) syndrome combines features of these syndromes. At the level of the lesion, patients exhibit ipsilateral lower motor weakness (anterior horn) and loss of all sensation (posterior root entry zone). Below the level of the lesion, patients have ipsilateral upper motor neuron weakness and spasticity (corticospinal tract) and ipsilateral loss of vibration sense and proprioception (posterior columns), with contralateral loss of pain and temperature (spinothalamic tract, the fibers of which have crossed from the opposite side through the anterior white commissure). The Brown-Séquard syndrome is often caused by trauma (Chapter 371) or eccentric compression.

The conus medullaris syndrome refers to dysfunction of the distal-most tapered portion of the spinal cord, which anatomically lies at approximately the T12-L1 vertebral spine level. The arms are normal; weakness in the legs is variable but often symmetrical when it is present. The main signs and symptoms are sexual dysfunction, loss of bowel and bladder control, and perianal anesthesia with loss of the anal reflex. The major causes are disc herniation, lumbar stenosis, trauma, and neoplasm.

With high cervical spine lesions, paresis or paralysis of the diaphragm and respiratory failure can occur. In lesions of the thoracic level or above, interruption of the lateral column autonomic pathways can lead to autonomic instability, including labile blood pressure. At any level, but especially at the conus and cauda equina levels, acute urinary retention can occur.

DIAGNOSIS

Symptoms of bilateral involvement of the arms or legs suggest a myelopathy, although bilateral lower limb involvement can be seen in lumbar spinal stenosis and the cauda equina syndrome. Complaints of leg stiffness or incoordination suggest spasticity from myelopathy. Other symptoms include a recent change in bowel or bladder function, erectile dysfunction, imbalance (especially in the dark or with eyes closed), and catching of the feet when walking. These central symptoms can also reflect lesions of the brain stem and higher, so the patient should be asked about cortical and brain stem symptoms (e.g., cognitive function, vision, facial strength, sensation, and swallowing). Focal cervical or thoracic spine pain supports a myelopathy.

Examination for a potential myelopathy must include an evaluation of anal tone and perineal sensation. The patient should be examined in a gown to allow inspection of the spine and overlying skin. A sensory level, which represents a point where distal sensation is altered, should also be sought but is not always found. Joint position sense can be reduced if the posterior columns are involved. Tandem gait testing identifies possible ataxia. Finally, the patient should be examined for spasticity by testing limb muscle tone and deep tendon reflexes. In acute spinal cord lesions, however, a state of "spinal shock" can cause hyporeflexia or even flaccid paralysis.

Ancillary Testing

MRI is the test of choice because it provides anatomic detail of the spine and subarachnoid space as well as the spinal cord. MRI can also show evidence of demyelination or metastatic disease. If MRI is normal, lumbar puncture and blood tests can be useful for diagnosing conditions that resemble or cause myelopathy (e.g., Guillain-Barré syndrome) (Chapter 392), infectious or carcinomatous meningitis (Chapter 384), syphilis, herpes simplex, varicella zoster virus, deficiency states, and paraneoplastic conditions.

Differential Diagnosis

Many causes of myelopathy can occur at any spinal level, but certain conditions predominate at specific spinal levels. Any lesion that has an upper cervical localization must be evaluated for disorders of the craniocervical junction, especially disorders that can produce atlantoaxial instability, such as rheumatoid arthritis and ankylosing spondylitis (Chapter 248). After trauma, cervical or odontoid fracture must be excluded. Disorders at the base of the skull, such as Chiari I and other congenital malformations (Chapter 389), can sometimes affect the upper cervical cord. Syringomyelia (Chapter 389), which may or may not be associated with Chiari malformation, also has a predilection for the cervical cord.

The thoracic cord is relatively protected from all but direct trauma but is the most common site for metastatic cord compression. Transverse myelitis most commonly affects the thoracic level, and the thoracic cord also is particularly vulnerable to a watershed ischemic myelopathy due to severe hypotension. Epidural lipomatosis often is most symptomatic at the thoracic level. Ossification of the posterior longitudinal ligament has a predilection for the cervical spine.

The rapidity of onset helps in diagnosis. Acute or relatively acute myelopathy suggests vascular causes, disc herniation, trauma, demyelinating lesions, or a pathologic fracture. In a young person with no other comorbid illnesses, a demyelinating illness, such as multiple sclerosis, neuromyelitis optica (Chapter 383), or acute disseminated encephalomyelitis (Chapter 386), is suggested. In older persons or patients with known vascular risk factors, hypotension, or onset in the immediate postoperative period, spinal cord infarction is possible. Sudden sharp back pain suggests mechanical disorders (e.g., pathologic fracture, sudden worsening of spondylolisthesis) or spinal cord infarction, whereas demyelinating lesions are often painless.

Myelopathy developing subacutely, especially accompanied by back pain, can be caused by metastatic disease (Chapter 180) and epidural abscess (Chapter 385). Both of these conditions must be evaluated and treated as emergencies to prevent permanent paralysis. Subacute or chronic myelopathies include vitamin B_{12} deficiency (Chapter 388), although nitrous oxide inhalation may cause an acute expression of the disorder; syringomyelia (Chapter 389); and slowly growing tumors, such as meningiomas (Chapter 180), ependymomas, and neurofibromas (Chapter 389).

In the setting of known malignant disease or unexplained weight loss, metastatic cord compression (Chapter 180) must be considered.[10] Weight loss, back pain, and fever can be seen in infection (Chapters 384 and 385) and occasionally spondyloarthropathies (Chapter 249). Infectious causes also include tropical spastic paraparesis (human T-lymphotropic virus type 1 [HTLV-1; Chapter 354]). Syphilis (Chapter 303) is the cause of tabes dorsalis; patients may have lancinating pains, ataxia, depressed lower limb reflexes, and Argyll Robertson pupils. Myelopathies that follow an infectious illness include acute disseminated encephalomyelitis and transverse myelitis (Chapter 383). Myelopathy accompanied by evidence of multifocal central nervous system dysfunction suggests multiple sclerosis or acute disseminated encephalomyelitis (Chapter 383). An accompanying peripheral neuropathy is seen in vitamin B_{12} deficiency myelopathy (Chapter 388), which tends to cause gait ataxia. Rheumatoid arthritis (Chapter 248) and ankylosing spondylitis can cause atlantoaxial instability and C1-C2 subluxation. Other systemic illnesses, such as systemic lupus erythematosus (Chapter 250), Behçet syndrome (Chapter 254), and sarcoidosis (Chapter 89), can also cause myelopathies. In patients with exogenous or endogenous hypercortisolemia (Chapter 214), epidural deposition of fat can cause dorsal epidural lipomatosis that can compress the spinal cord. A remote history of cord trauma raises the possibility of post-traumatic syringomyelia.

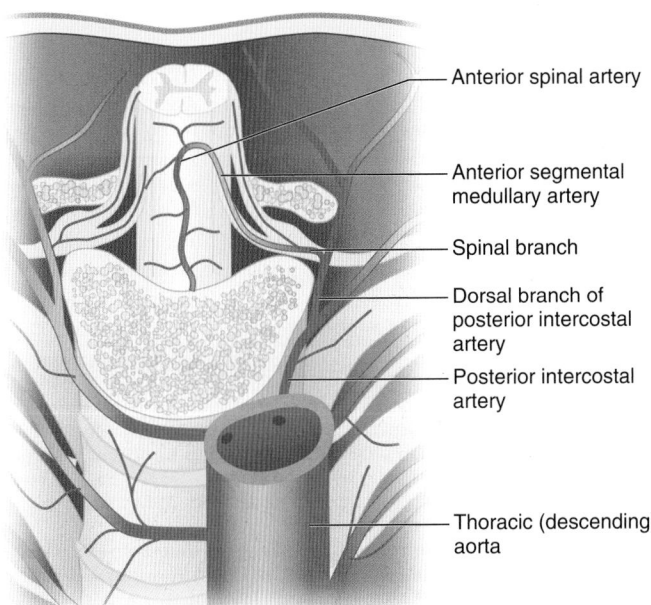

FIGURE 372-9. Blood supply of the spinal cord: section through thoracic level, antero-superior view.

TREATMENT AND PROGNOSIS ℞

Depending on the rate of worsening, patients with spinal cord lesions may need urgent or emergent assessment and treatment to prevent further deterioration and hopefully to restore lost function. Surgery may be needed for cord compression (e.g., disc, tumor, abscess).[11] Other specific causes require targeted treatment. Prognosis depends on the diagnosis, severity of the condition, and the patient's response to appropriate treatment. Long-term complications of spinal cord injury include osteoporosis (Chapter 230), orthostatic hypotension (Chapter 56), deep vein thrombosis (Chapter 74), decubitus ulcers, autonomic dysreflexia (Chapter 390), and chronic neuropathic pain (Chapter 27).

Specific Causes of Myelopathies
VASCULAR MYELOPATHIES
The spinal cord is as intolerant of ischemia as the brain is. Vascular myelopathy occurs when there is loss of blood flow to the spinal cord, whether it is acute or chronic and whether the cause is ischemic or hemorrhagic.[12]

The blood supply to the spinal cord comes from one anterior and two posterior spinal arteries that run longitudinally along the length of the spinal cord (Fig. 372-9). The paired posterior spinal arteries arise rostrally as branches of the vertebral arteries at the level of the medulla and run inferiorly along the posterolateral surface of the spinal cord. The anterior spinal artery is formed superiorly when branches of the vertebral artery join to form a single anterior spinal artery, which then runs down the midline of the anterior surface of the spinal cord. The main caudal anterior spinal blood supply is from a large artery of Adamkiewicz that enters the spinal canal through an intervertebral foramen somewhere between T5 and L1, usually on the left, and supplies most of the lower spinal cord and conus medullaris.

Spinal cord compression and compromise of the microvascular supply to the cord underlie the gliotic changes in many slowly progressive myelopathies such as spondylotic myelopathy. Ischemic causes include hypotension, atherosclerotic disease, embolic events, vasculitis (Chapter 254), decompression sickness (Chapter 88), and vascular steal.

Spinal dural arteriovenous fistulas are the most common type of spinal cord vascular malformation. Vascular malformations can cause myelopathy by acting as mass lesions that compress local structures, by interfering with normal venous drainage, by diverting blood as part of a vascular steal with exercise of muscles that compete for blood flow, or by bleeding. Spinal cord hemorrhage, which is rare, can be caused by trauma, bleeding into a tumor, an intramedullary vascular malformation, or a complication of anticoagulant therapy. Epidural hematomas cause cord compression and can occur as a complication of surgery or a lumbar puncture, especially in patients with a bleeding diathesis.

CLINICAL MANIFESTATIONS
Occlusion of the artery of Adamkiewicz usually presents with signs of thoracic watershed ischemia—paraplegia with relative sparing of the sacral roots and dorsal columns. Infarction in the anterior spinal artery distribution results in dysfunction of the anterior two thirds of the cord, including the anterior horns, spinothalamic tracts, and corticospinal tracts. Patients usually present with acute paraparesis and impaired bowel and bladder function. Below the level of the lesion, temperature and pain sensation are lost, but vibration and joint position sense are preserved.

Infarction of the posterior arteries is less common because of their better collateral circulation. Clinical manifestations include loss of vibration and joint position sense, ataxia, gait disturbance, and positive Romberg sign. Reflexes may be depressed at the level of the infarction.

Vascular malformations most often have a chronic or stepwise progressive clinical course. Pain is common. Arteriovenous fistulas commonly occur in the thoracic cord, and present as progressive paraplegia.

DIAGNOSIS

Vascular malformations are initially evaluated by MRI. If embolization or surgery is being considered, spinal angiography is needed to identify feeding and draining vessels. Intramedullary arteriovenous malformations are more commonly found in the cervical and thoracic levels and may require angiography to be visualized. When imaging is equivocal, lumbar puncture can be considered; an elevated leukocyte count (>10 cells/µL of CSF) suggests an inflammatory myelopathy rather than a vascular lesion.

TREATMENT AND PROGNOSIS   Rx

Treatment options for spinal cord ischemia are limited and include reversal of the cause of ischemia, such as by correcting hypotension (Chapter 98). Prognosis for most cases of spinal cord infarct is poor unless blood flow is restored rapidly. In one study, for example, 3-year mortality was 23%, 42% of survivors needed wheelchairs, but 40% of those in wheelchairs at hospital discharge were able to walk at a 3-year follow-up.

Arteriovenous fistulas are treated by occluding the shunt with embolization or surgery. Successful treatment may arrest and improve symptoms. Patients with suspected epidural hematomas (Chapter 371) require emergency surgery if they have severe or progressive neurologic dysfunction.

INFLAMMATORY, METABOLIC, AND INFECTIOUS MYELOPATHIES

Transverse myelitis,[13] multiple sclerosis, neuromyelitis optica, and other demyelinating diseases are considered in Chapter 383. Metabolic myelopathies can be caused by vitamin B_{12}, vitamin E, and copper deficiencies (Chapter 205).

Acute disseminated encephalomyelitis is mostly a monophasic disorder of demyelination of the spinal cord and brain. If it is isolated to the spinal cord, it is termed *transverse myelitis*. Extensive evaluation of presumed idiopathic transverse myelitis frequently leads to a more precise diagnosis, such as multiple sclerosis (Chapter 383) or sarcoidosis (Chapter 89) affecting the spinal cord.

Connective tissue diseases can infrequently cause myelopathy. Systemic lupus erythematosus (Chapter 250) with or without antiphospholipid antibody can cause myelitis in 1 to 3% of patients. Sjögren syndrome (Chapter 252), Behçet syndrome (Chapter 254), sarcoidosis (Chapter 89), mixed connective tissue disease (Chapter 254), and systemic sclerosis (Chapter 251) can be associated with inflammatory myelitis.

HIV can cause a vacuolar myelopathy which is not always symptomatic. Human T-lymphotropic virus type 1 (HTLV-1)–associated myelopathy, also known as tropical spastic paraparesis (Chapter 354), is a chronic progressive myelopathy that can cause leg weakness, spasticity, loss of vibratory sense, and bladder dysfunction. More than 90% of infected persons remain asymptomatic, with transformation to a symptomatic condition thought to be largely related to the host's immune response. Tertiary syphilis (Chapter 303) affecting the spinal cord is called tabes dorsalis and is rarely seen today.

DIAGNOSIS

In general, diagnosis of these myelopathies is based on the history, clinical examination, MRI, analysis of the CSF, and blood tests. With inflammatory myelopathies, MRI often shows increased T2 signal and focal enlargement of the spinal cord.

TREATMENT   Rx

Intravenous corticosteroid infusions (e.g., methylprednisolone, 1 g intravenously daily for 5 days) are used to treat acute attacks of inflammatory myelopathy. In patients who do not respond to corticosteroids, plasma exchange can be effective. About 60% of patients show improvement at 6 months. Factors predicting improvement are initiation of treatment within 15 days of the onset of symptoms and evidence of early improvement.

Metabolic deficiencies can be replaced. Aggressive antiretroviral therapy can lead to improvement in HIV myelopathy. No effective treatment is available for HTLV-1 associated myelopathy (Chapter 354).

METASTATIC SPINAL CORD COMPRESSION

When metastatic cancer invades the spine or epidural space, the resultant destruction and tumor growth compress the spinal cord and lead to a myelopathy. The prevalence of metastatic spinal cord compression may be as high as 5% in patients with cancer, depending on the type of malignant neoplasm and its tendency to metastasize to bone. Prostate (Chapter 191), breast (Chapter 188), and lung (Chapter 182) cancers each account for approximately 15 to 20% of cases, and non-Hodgkin lymphoma (Chapter 176), renal cell cancer (Chapter 187), and multiple myeloma (Chapter 178) account for about 5 to 10% each.

Metastatic spinal disease usually causes compression as a result of an extradural lesion, although a smaller number of metastatic lesions can be intradural-extramedullary. Intramedullary metastases are rare. Symptoms can be caused by direct compression of the cord and roots in the epidural space as a result of direct extension from a hematogenous metastasis to the vertebral body. However, some tumors (e.g., lymphomas) may grow through the intervertebral foramen without causing significant bone destruction. Vertebral destruction can make the spine unstable and cause pathologic fractures that lead to damage of the cord and root.

CLINICAL MANIFESTATIONS

About 90% of patients present with pain that is classically worse on lying down and increases with the Valsalva maneuver. If the nerve root is involved, the pain will have a radicular component; if there is bone collapse, pain can be made worse by movement. At the time of diagnosis, muscle weakness is present in 35 to 75% of patients, sensory deficits in 50 to 70% of patients, and autonomic dysfunction in 50 to 60% of patients. Signs and symptoms depend on the level of compression.

DIAGNOSIS

Spinal cord compression, which must be suspected when any patient with cancer complains of spine pain even in the absence of neurologic signs or symptoms, is a neurologic emergency. MRI is the test of choice because of its ability to detect soft tissue masses, spinal cord and nerve root damage, and bone pathology. CT myelography should be used if MRI cannot be performed. Because up to 35% of patients have more than one site of metastasis, the entire spine should be imaged.

Differential Diagnosis

For extradural lesions, the differential diagnosis includes lipomas, neurofibromas (Chapter 389), meningiomas (Chapter 180), and chordomas as well as vascular malformations and abscesses. Intradural-extramedullary lesions include neurofibromas (Chapter 389), neurinomas, meningiomas, vascular malformations, and (less often) metastases. Arachnoid cysts, usually benign, can cause cord compression. Finally, intramedullary lesions that can present as a myelopathy and must be considered in the differential of metastatic cord compression include vascular malformations, ependymomas, astrocytomas, syringomyelia, and intramedullary metastases.

TREATMENT   Rx

Prompt initiation of corticosteroids (e.g., dexamethasone, loading dose of 10 to 16 mg followed by tapering over 10 to 14 days) and radiation therapy are the mainstays of initial therapy. Patients with an unstable spine, limited disease burden, and a relatively favorable prognosis may benefit from decompressive resection and spinal stabilization.[14] Vertebroplasty and kyphoplasty may provide symptomatic help for patients who are not candidates for radical spine surgery.

PROGNOSIS

Metastatic spinal cord compression usually occurs in the setting of metastases to multiple locations, and the expected prognosis for survival is generally less than 6 months. Prognosis is improved in patients with neoplasms that are sensitive to corticosteroid therapy (especially lymphoma and leukemia) or are radiosensitive (e.g., multiple myeloma, small cell lung cancer). Patients who are ambulatory at the time of diagnosis, have a single site of compression, and have a slower onset of symptoms also have a better prognosis.

Grade A References

A1. Chou R, Deyo R, Friedly J, et al. Systemic pharmacologic therapies for low back pain: a systematic review for an American College of Physicians clinical practice guideline. *Ann Intern Med.* 2017;166:480-492.

A2. Machado GC, Maher CG, Ferreira PH, et al. Efficacy and safety of paracetamol for spinal pain and osteoarthritis: systematic review and meta-analysis of randomised placebo controlled trials. *BMJ.* 2015;350:1-13.

A3. Krebs EE, Gravely A, Nugent S, et al. Effect of opioid vs nonopioid medications on pain-related function in patients with chronic back pain or hip or knee osteoarthritis pain: the SPACE randomized clinical trial. *JAMA.* 2018;319:872-882.

A4. Chou R, Deyo R, Friedly J, et al. Nonpharmacologic therapies for low back pain: a systematic review for an American College of Physicians clinical practice guideline. *Ann Intern Med.* 2017;166:493-505.

A5. Qaseem A, Wilt TJ, McLean RM, et al. Noninvasive treatments for acute, subacute, and chronic low back pain: a clinical practice guideline from the American College of Physicians. *Ann Intern Med.* 2017;166:514-530.

A6. Hedlund R, Johansson C, Hagg O, et al. The long-term outcome of lumbar fusion in the Swedish lumbar spine study. *Spine J.* 2016;16:579-587.

A7. Mannion AF, Brox JI, Fairbank JC. Comparison of spinal fusion and nonoperative treatment in patients with chronic low back pain: long-term follow-up of three randomized controlled trials. *Spine J.* 2013;13:1438-1448.

A8. Steffens D, Maher CG, Pereira LS, et al. Prevention of low back pain: a systematic review and meta-analysis. *JAMA Intern Med.* 2016;176:199-208.

A9. Delitto A, Piva SR, Moore CG, et al. Surgery versus nonsurgical treatment of lumbar spinal stenosis: a randomized trial. *Ann Intern Med.* 2015;162:465-473.

A10. Friedly JL, Comstock BA, Turner JA, et al. A randomized trial of epidural glucocorticoid injections for spinal stenosis. *N Engl J Med.* 2014;371:11-21.

A11. Försth P, Ólafsson G, Carlsson T, et al. A randomized, controlled trial of fusion surgery for lumbar spinal stenosis. *N Engl J Med.* 2016;374:1413-1423.

A12. Ghogawala Z, Dziura J, Butler WE, et al. Laminectomy plus fusion versus laminectomy alone for lumbar spondylolisthesis. *N Engl J Med.* 2016;374:1424-1434.

A13. Machado GC, Maher CG, Ferreira PH, et al. Non-steroidal anti-inflammatory drugs for spinal pain: a systematic review and meta-analysis. *Ann Rheum Dis.* 2017;76:1269-1278.

A14. Mathieson S, Maher CG, McLachlan AJ, et al. Trial of pregabalin for acute and chronic sciatica. *N Engl J Med.* 2017;376:1111-1120.

A15. Chou R, Hashimoto R, Friedly J, et al. Epidural corticosteroid injections for radiculopathy and spinal stenosis: a systematic review and meta-analysis. *Ann Intern Med.* 2015;163:373-381.

A16. Bicket MC, Horowitz JM, Benzon HT, et al. Epidural injections in prevention of surgery for spinal pain: systematic review and meta-analysis of randomized controlled trials. *Spine J.* 2015;15:348-362.

A17. Phan K, Xu J, Schultz K, et al. Full-endoscopic versus micro-endoscopic and open discectomy: a systematic review and meta-analysis of outcomes and complications. *Clin Neurol Neurosurg.* 2017;154:1-12.

GENERAL REFERENCES

For the General References and other additional features, please visit Expert Consult at https://expertconsult.inkling.com.

373

REGIONAL CEREBRAL DYSFUNCTION: HIGHER MENTAL FUNCTIONS

DAVID S. KNOPMAN

DEFINITION

Higher mental function is at the core of what defines competent, independent individuals. Impairment of higher mental function can be broadly classified into four categories. Intellectual developmental disorder is a form of cognitive impairment that is present from infancy. Acquired forms of cognitive impairment are delirium, dementia, and focal cognitive disorders. Delirium (Chapter 25) is defined by its acute or subacute onset and coexistent alterations in alertness. Dementia (Chapter 374) represents an acquired cognitive impairment that is usually gradual in onset and not associated with alterations in alertness. Focal cognitive disorders involve only one aspect of cognition: memory, language, visuospatial cognition, psychomotor speed, or executive cognitive functioning, each of which is supported by a different cerebral region.

For the majority of patients outside of a neurology or psychiatry practice, a global description such as "normal mental function" or "cognitively impaired" will suffice. Cognitive impairment then becomes a diagnosis that subsumes all forms of altered higher mental function regardless of which domains are affected or how severely they are affected.

CLINICAL MANIFESTATIONS AND DIAGNOSIS

An informal conversation with a patient lacks sensitivity for detecting cognitive impairment. If cognitive impairment is suspected from the patient's history, formal assessments should be performed. Bedside evaluations of orientation, memory, language, reasoning, and visuospatial function can be used to derive an overall view of cognitive function but do not automatically translate into diagnoses, because alertness, cooperation, education, native language, sensorimotor function, and mood must be taken into account. Although scores on bedside mental status examinations correlate strongly with severity and prognosis, they provide only rough guides to cognitive ability and cannot localize a cognitive deficit anatomically in the brain. The Mini-Cog Test (Chapter 24, Table 24-5) is among the most brief of available bedside examinations. If cognitive dysfunction is discovered in the course of the bedside examination, further exploration of individual cognitive domains must be undertaken.

MEMORY FUNCTION AND AMNESIC DISORDERS

DEFINITION

Declarative memory describes the type of learning and retrieval of facts and information that occur with conscious attention and intent; examples include remembering conversations, events, and intentions. Declarative memory has semantic and episodic components. Semantic memory refers to the brain's storehouse of knowledge, words, and facts. Episodic memory refers to learning and recall of specific events. Retention of information for more than a few seconds in the face of exposure to additional facts, details, or events requires declarative episodic memory to store and organize the information suitable for later recall. It is this declarative episodic memory system that is assessed as "memory" in the clinical setting. Anterograde amnesia is the clinical manifestation of disturbances in declarative episodic memory. Anterograde refers to failure to learn, and hence recall, new information on an ongoing basis. Most disorders of memory also exhibit retrograde amnesia, a disturbance of the ability to retrieve information from the past.

Immediate recall of information with zero delay and zero intervening information is a very short-term declarative memory function. Immediate memory is capable of storing an image of an auditory message in exact form, but only a small amount and for a short period. The fidelity of immediate memory recall accuracy drops off dramatically over seconds, particularly if intervening sensory stimuli attract attention. A comparable system exists in the visual modality in that the memory acts like a photograph that fades rapidly. From a clinical perspective, immediate memory is separate from declarative episodic memory. Immediate recall is generally used as a marker of attention and alertness and not memory per se.

PATHOBIOLOGY

The hippocampal formations are the anatomic structures of importance for the declarative episodic memory system. The hippocampal formations are imaged well with magnetic resonance imaging (MRI) (E-Fig. 373-1). The principal input to the hippocampus comes through the entorhinal cortex from multimodal association areas in the frontal, parietal, and temporal neocortices. A second important input is a cholinergic pathway that originates in the septum of the medial-orbital frontal lobe. There are two principal output circuits of the hippocampal formations. One is via the subiculum back to multimodal association areas. The other hippocampal efferent pathway projects via the fornix to the mammillary bodies. The projection from the mammillary bodies passes through the medial thalamus to the ventral anterior nucleus of the thalamus, then to the posterior cingulate, and then back to the entorhinal cortex. The hippocampal circuit is believed to facilitate the formation of memory in association neocortices. The hippocampus does not store a particular learned fact, but rather it enables the appropriate region in a multimodal association cortical region to do so.

Lesions in one hippocampal formation will not generally have as devastating an impact on episodic memory as bilateral lesions will. However, in older persons who may have subclinical bilateral hippocampal pathology, a unilateral lesion, particularly in the dominant hemisphere, may produce dense anterograde amnesia. Lesions in the columns of the fornix, mammillary bodies, and medial thalamus have also been linked to anterograde amnesia.

CLINICAL MANIFESTATIONS AND DIAGNOSIS

The diagnosis of anterograde amnesia begins with a complaint of memory impairment from the patient or someone close to the patient. Patients with anterograde amnesia have poor or no recollection of events, conversations, or observations in a manner that exceeds normal forgetting. Family members report that patients repeat themselves in conversation or re-ask the same questions over the course of a few minutes to hours. Patients will generally forget important events and conversations, even when they were fully engaged in them. They will lose track of the date and time of day. They will forget appointments, even with reminders. Generally, patients with anterograde amnesia will fail to encode most events and happenings around them. The consequences of such memory failure are usually more evident to the family and acquaintances of patients with the disorder than they are to the patients themselves. Anosognosia (lack of awareness) for the deficit of anterograde amnesia is very common, though not universal. Patients who most vehemently complain of memory loss are often suffering from depression rather than focal cognitive dysfunction. Testing of memory can be performed at the bedside in alert patients. The patient is asked to learn three or four words and recall them after 1 or 2 minutes. A patient with severe anterograde amnesia will recall none or at most one of the words, whereas individuals with normal memory can recall all of the words or all but one.

In patients with questionable memory difficulties, assessment by an experienced neuropsychologist is often a necessary part of the evaluation. Standardized tests of memory have greater precision and reliability than "bedside" tests and involve the use of lengthier material to be remembered and a longer delay between learning and recall.

Determining the Cause

Alzheimer disease is the most common disorder in which anterograde amnesia occurs (Chapter 374). In Alzheimer disease, anterograde amnesia is usually the dominant cognitive symptom, not only as the earliest symptom but also as a very prominent symptom across the duration of the disease. Hippocampal atrophy is common (Chapter 374, Fig. 374-3). Anterograde amnesia also occurs in other dementing illnesses, such as vascular dementia and dementia with Lewy bodies.

Strokes can damage regions involved in episodic memory. Occlusion of the medial temporal branch of the posterior cerebral artery causes infarction of the hippocampus. Infarction in the territory of penetrating branches of the tip of the basilar artery causes bilateral medial thalamic infarcts.

Anterograde amnesia may be a major residual deficit after herpes simplex encephalitis (Chapter 350). Herpes simplex encephalitis has a predilection for damaging structures at the base of the cerebral hemispheres; frequently, the temporal lobes are severely damaged. Korsakoff syndrome, the residual of the encephalopathy of thiamine deficiency (Chapter 388), is characterized by profound anterograde amnesia. Hemorrhagic necrosis of the mammillary bodies occurs in Korsakoff syndrome. Survivors of closed head injuries (Chapter 371) may have anterograde amnesia because the medial temporal lobes are vulnerable to trauma as a result of their close proximity to the temporal bone. Survivors of an episode of anoxic-ischemic encephalopathy may also have dense anterograde amnesia. The pyramidal neurons of the CA1 region of the hippocampus are particularly vulnerable to hypoxic injury.

The syndrome of transient global amnesia involves anterograde amnesia, but the duration of the amnesia is a matter of 6 to 12 hours rather than the weeks or months seen in post-traumatic amnesia or the permanent deficits in patients with Alzheimer disease or Korsakoff syndrome. Patients with transient global amnesia remain alert though inattentive; the key element of the syndrome is that they lay down no new memories during the event. As a consequence, they are amnestic for the several hours of the episode. Transient global amnesia generally affects middle-aged or elderly individuals. Its cause is not known, although it is not usually due to typical cerebrovascular disease or epilepsy. Electroencephalography is typically not specifically abnormal, but diffusion-weighed MRI often shows distinctive abnormalities of the hippocampus a day or more after the onset of transient global amnesia. Data suggest that the relapse rate is low, the risk of stroke and seizures is not considerably increased, and cognitive outcome is generally good.[1]

THE APHASIAS

DEFINITION

Aphasia is a disorder of language at the conceptual level. Aphasics may have difficulty producing language, comprehending language, or both.

PATHOBIOLOGY

In more than 99% of right-handed individuals, language is localized to the left hemisphere. In left-handed individuals, language is also predominantly localized to the left hemisphere, although varying degrees of bilateral or rarely right hemispheric dominance may be seen. The hemisphere involved in language is referred to as the dominant hemisphere. Anatomic differences in the temporal and parietal lobes of the dominant hemisphere versus the other hemisphere also reflect its specialization for language.

Different aspects of language processing can be localized to specific regions within the dominant hemisphere. Lesions in the dominant hemisphere's auditory association areas cause receptive language dysfunction. The critical regions are located in the superior temporal lobes adjacent to the primary auditory cortex and in the adjacent supramarginal and angular gyri of the inferior parietal lobule, an area known as the Wernicke area.[2] Lesions in the dominant hemisphere's lateral inferior posterior frontal lobes, often referred to as the Broca area, result in expressive language deficits. Loss of access to one's vocabulary for either understanding spoken language or expressing oneself results from lesions in any portion of the region around the sylvian fissure of the dominant hemisphere, including the lateral posterior inferior frontal lobe, the inferior parietal lobule, and the superior and middle temporal gyri.

CLINICAL MANIFESTATIONS AND DIAGNOSIS

The language comprehension difficulties in persons with aphasia must be distinguished from hearing disorders (Chapter 400), and the motor speech dysfunction in aphasia must be distinguished from dysarthria. Errors of articulation in persons with aphasia reflect altered conceptual selection of what is to be said. In aphasia, mispronunciation of a sound within one word may be followed by perfect pronunciation of the same sound in a different word. In dysarthria, by comparison, the errors in articulation or phonation are consistent.

Aphasia has three principal components: impaired verbal comprehension, disordered verbal expression, and impaired naming. Disorders of reading, writing, and sentence repetition are additional elements of the aphasia syndrome. The disordered verbal comprehension may range from profound to mild. When profound, patients are unable to grasp the meaning of single words. In milder forms of disordered comprehension, patients may be able to follow one-step but not two- or three-step commands. Usually, the comprehension difficulty involves both spoken and written language, but each can be affected separately. Anomia, which is an inability to produce names of people or objects, is common in almost all aphasic syndromes. Naming can be tested by asking the patient to name a series of common objects, such as the parts of the hand and arm (e.g., thumb, palm, knuckles, wrist, elbow). In general, the more commonly a word is used in the language, the easier it will be to name, whereas infrequent words are harder for aphasics.

In expressive aphasic syndromes, written material and spoken speech are most often but not always affected in parallel. Speech is labored in the expressive aphasias, and it lacks the normal melody and variation in intonation that characterize normal speaking. Melody and intonation are referred to as the prosody of speech. Speech is often grammatically impoverished. The number of words per utterance is greatly reduced, thus giving the speech a choppy, staccato character. These features are referred to as speech apraxia. *Nonfluency* is a related term that describes the reduced number of words and the terseness of verbal output. In some aphasic syndromes, speech is often degraded by anomia and paraphasic errors (word or syllable substitutions), even when fluency, melody, and intonation are preserved.

Specific Aphasic Syndromes

Specific common aphasic syndromes exhibit various combinations of receptive and expressive difficulty (Table 373-1).

Aphasia occurs in two principal settings: acute stroke and its aftermath and as a chronic and insidious process owing to neurodegenerative disease referred to as primary progressive aphasia.[3]

WERNICKE APHASIA

In Wernicke aphasia, verbal comprehension of both written and verbal language is severely impaired. Patients with Wernicke aphasia have difficulty understanding the meaning of individual words and may not be able to follow any command consisting of greater than one step. Their speech is fluent but marred by paraphasia and anomia. Wernicke aphasics tend to lack awareness of the extent of their communicative difficulties and are often unaware that the words they are uttering are fundamentally incorrect. Embolic strokes are the most common cause of Wernicke aphasia. The location that typically causes Wernicke aphasia is the dominant posterior superior temporal lobe or inferior supramarginal gyrus (see E-Fig. 373-1).

TABLE 373-1 MAJOR APHASIC SYNDROMES

APHASIA SYNDROME	REGIONAL LOCALIZATION	SPONTANEOUS SPEECH ABNORMALITIES	AUDITORY COMPREHENSION	CONFRONTATION NAMING	SENTENCE REPETITION
Broca aphasia	Lateral inferior frontal lobe	Nonfluent, labored, agrammatic	Preserved	Poor	Poor
Wernicke aphasia	Posterior superior temporal-parietal supramarginal gyrus	Fluent, many paraphasic errors, very little information content	Very impaired	Poor	Poor
Global aphasia	Major portions of the frontoparietal operculum and superior temporal lobe	Nonfluent or virtually absent	Very impaired	Poor	Poor
Anomic aphasia	Small lesion somewhere in the perisylvian region	Fluent, may contain some paraphasias	Normal or mildly impaired	Poor to moderately impaired	Preserved or impaired

SEMANTIC VARIANT OF PRIMARY PROGRESSIVE APHASIA

The aphasic disturbance of semantic variant of primary progressive aphasia is characterized by a loss of access to the meaning of words. Spontaneous speech melody, intonation, and grammatical integrity are preserved, but patients have marked difficulties with production of nouns and verbs. This condition is usually caused by left anterior temporal lobe degeneration owing to one of the frontotemporal lobar degenerations or Alzheimer disease (Chapter 374).[4]

BROCA APHASIA

Broca aphasia is a syndrome in which expressive language is prominently affected. Patients with Broca aphasia have nonfluent labored speech. The location of the lesion that typically causes Broca aphasia is the dominant posterior inferior frontal lobe (see E-Fig 373-1). The typical syndrome is usually due to embolic strokes. Patients with Broca aphasia have largely preserved comprehension and as a result are acutely aware of their difficulties and become frustrated with them. Depression is common in Broca aphasics.

NONFLUENT/AGRAMMATIC VARIANT OF PRIMARY PROGRESSIVE APHASIA

The nonfluent/agrammatic variant of primary progressive aphasia is characterized by the gradual onset of labored, hesitant, sparse speech that is often grammatically impoverished. Comprehension of spoken speech is typically preserved. This syndrome is usually caused by one of the frontotemporal lobar degenerations (Chapter 374).

GLOBAL APHASIA

Global aphasia occurs when both expressive and receptive problems are present. Global aphasia often appears acutely after a major infarction, hemorrhage, or traumatic brain injury involving the dominant hemisphere. Global aphasia may also be present in the context of severe dementia.

ANOMIA

Anomia is at the milder end of the spectrum of language disorders. Some anomic aphasics also have difficulty with sentence repetition, even in the presence of relatively preserved comprehension and verbal expressive abilities. There is some controversy whether this latter syndrome, called conduction aphasia, represents a disconnection between the perisylvian centers for comprehension and expression or whether it represents a lesion in the cortical auditory areas involved in immediate auditory memory.

IDEOMOTOR APRAXIA

Ideomotor apraxia is a disorder at the interface between comprehension and execution of facial or limb motor actions. Patients with ideomotor apraxia have no paresis of the face or limb musculature and are able to carry out simple tasks, but they are unable to execute more complex tasks or commands. For example, in a woman who is able to name a comb and use her right hand to point to parts of her body, ideomotor apraxia can be demonstrated if she is unable to indicate through her actions how she would use the comb.

STUTTERING

The left pars opercularis is a locus where the intrinsic functional architecture of speech-language processes is altered in patients with persistent developmental stuttering.

DIAGNOSIS

The diagnosis of aphasia is made by listening to the patient speak and by examining comprehension, naming ability, reading, and writing in a standardized fashion. Frequently the diagnosis of aphasia is made during attempts to obtain a history from the patient. It is helpful to prompt patients to speak about a neutral topic such as what they had for their last meal or what they did the previous day. Listening to their spontaneous speech allows the examiner to characterize its fluency, grammatical form, articulation, melody, and intonation, as well as difficulty finding words, the presence of paraphasias, and the overall information content.

Comprehension should be examined formally by asking the patient to perform tasks that range from one to at least three steps.

Determining the Cause

Portions of the dominant perisylvian cerebral cortex may be damaged by infarction (Chapters 379 and 380), hemorrhage, and other space-occupying brain lesions such as neoplasms (Chapter 180) and abscesses (Chapter 385). Aphasia secondary to stroke has an abrupt onset, usually with some subsequent improvement. Aphasia due to stroke is often but not always accompanied by other neurologic signs, such as hemiparesis or hemianopia.[5] Recovery from aphasia after a stroke may occur as ischemic zones around an infarction eventually regain function. Regions remote from the infarction may also be synaptically depressed acutely after a stroke (diaschisis) but eventually regain function. Finally, regions in the nondominant hemisphere may become more active over the course of recovery. Aphasia that has a gradual and slowly progressive onset occurs in the neurodegenerative syndromes of primary progressive aphasia (Chapter 374).

TREATMENT Rx

Speech therapy may be helpful for patients in the first few months after a brain injury that causes aphasia. In fact, 3 weeks of intensive speech and language therapy can significantly improve verbal communication in stroke survivors under age 70 years with chronic aphasia.[A1]

CORTICAL DISORDERS OF VISUAL FUNCTION AND HEMISPATIAL NEGLECT

DEFINITIONS

Cortical disorders of vision and spatial cognition are caused by lesions in the occipitoinferotemporal or occipitoposteroparietal lobes. The principal disorders of cortical visual functioning are alexia (impaired reading), object agnosia (impaired recognition of visual forms), and prosopagnosia (impaired face recognition). The principal disorders of spatial cognition are simultanagnosia (impaired integration of complex visual scenes), dressing apraxia, and visual hemispatial neglect (lack of awareness of the personal or extrapersonal hemispace). In order to consider a cortical visual disorder diagnostically, a clinician should verify the integrity of primary visual function from the cornea to the lateral geniculate nuclei.

PATHOBIOLOGY

Higher visual function is localized to a network centered in the occipital lobe and includes the inferior temporal and posterior parietal lobes (see E-Fig. 373-1). From area 17, processing of visual information passes to visual association areas 18 and 19. From there it proceeds in several directions. Disorders of higher visual function can be related to a ventral or dorsal pathway. The

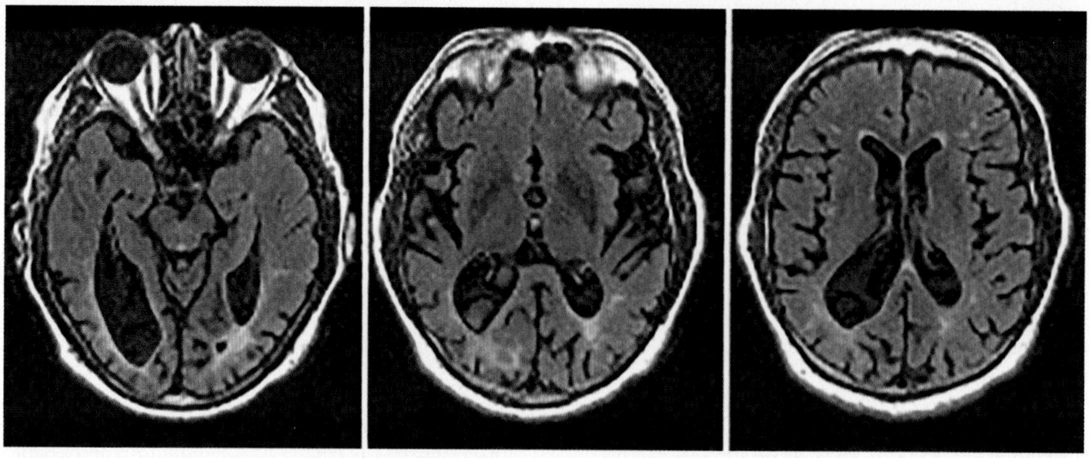

FIGURE 373-1. Magnetic resonance imaging (MRI) scans of a patient with the syndrome of posterior cortical atrophy caused by Alzheimer disease. The MRI scans show marked atrophy of the primary visual areas and parieto-occipital association areas. The right hemisphere (*left side of each image*) is more affected than the left (*right side of each image*).

ventral pathway from the visual centers to the medial temporal lobe links visual information to meaning ("What is the object?"). The dorsal visual processing pathway has several target regions. One links the visual centers to the parietal lobes and is concerned with locating objects in space and determining spatial relationships among objects in order to grasp a complete visual scene ("Where is the object?"). Another integral part of the dorsal visual processing stream is the cortical control of the extraocular muscles in the parietal and prefrontal regions, whereby the eyes are directed to various elements of a visual scene so that the individual elements are synthesized into a coherent ensemble. Yet a third part of the dorsal visual pathway leads to premotor areas that, in conjunction with eye movement control, facilitate visually guided limb motor actions.

Alexia occurs as a result of lesions in the ventral pathway of the dominant hemisphere. Object agnosia may also occur with lesions, usually bilateral, in the ventral pathway. Alexia and object agnosia occur with neurodegenerative diseases that affect the parieto-occipital cortex. Simultanagnosia, dressing apraxia, and hemispatial neglect are syndromes caused by lesions in the dorsal pathway. Limb apraxia and impaired visuomotor activities may result from disruption of the premotor pathways that interact with the dorsal visual system. Simultanagnosia usually requires bilateral posterior parietal lesions. Dressing apraxia and hemispatial neglect arise from unilateral lesions, most often in the nondominant hemisphere. Cortical blindness is a consequence of bilateral occipitoparietal pathology.

CLINICAL MANIFESTATIONS AND DIAGNOSIS

Alexia may occur as an isolated deficit, or it may occur in the context of other evidence of aphasia. Patients may be able to recognize individual letters but are unable to recognize a string of letters as a word. Patients with cortical disorders usually have difficulty with visuoconstructional tasks such as copying figures or drawing simple objects such as a flower, house, or clock. Dressing apraxia represents a deficit of practical significance in which patients are unable to comprehend the orientation of articles such as a shirt or a blouse and to manipulate them. The most severe form of a cortical disorder of visuospatial processing is cortical blindness. In this condition, in which the anterior visual pathways can be reasonably believed to be intact, patients appear functionally blind.

Hemispatial neglect occurs in the setting of acute strokes involving the nondominant perisylvian region. Even when there is no hemianopia as measured by single visual stimuli, presentation of double simultaneous stimuli to the patient reveals unawareness in the nondominant field. Hemispatial neglect can be demonstrated at the bedside with a task such as drawing a clock. A patient with hemispatial neglect will fail to place the numbers on the nondominant side (i.e., the left side in a right-handed person). Patients with hemispatial neglect may sometimes deny that their paretic limb belongs to them.

Bedside tests that screen for visuospatial deficits include either copying a simple geometric design or drawing an object. Intersecting pentagons and a cube are objects used clinically. Clock drawing is a brief but informative exercise. Reading of words or commands and naming of objects can be done at the bedside as well. Formal testing of visuospatial function in the neuropsychology laboratory involves the use of specially designed instruments to characterize visual processing.

Determining the Cause

The etiology of lesions that cause deficits in cortical vision and spatial cognition ranges from focal cerebrovascular disease, neoplasms, infectious processes, and brain trauma to neurodegenerative disorders. Patients with posterior cortical atrophy, which is usually due to Alzheimer disease, show marked atrophy and dysfunction of the occipital and parieto-occipital lobes (Fig. 373-1).

● PSYCHOMOTOR SPEED, EXECUTIVE COGNITIVE DYSFUNCTION, AND CONTROL OF PERSONAL BEHAVIOR

DEFINITIONS

Speed of mental processing is a necessary function that supports all cognitive functions. Integrative abilities that are broadly referred to as executive cognitive function include mental agility, abstract reasoning, and problem solving. Executive cognitive function represents processes that support mental flexibility, adaptability, focus, and tenacity. Control of personal actions and regulation of interpersonal relationships are also major functions that are part of integrative abilities. The term *comportment* denotes how a person behaves, particularly toward other people.

PATHOBIOLOGY

The anatomic basis of psychomotor speed and executive cognitive function is a network of brain regions anchored by the prefrontal neocortex. The control of personal actions and behavior also is centered in the prefrontal regions as well as the anterior temporal lobes (see E-Fig. 373-1). These regions receive input from multiple cortical and subcortical regions. Although psychomotor speed, executive function, and maintenance of comportment and interpersonal relationship are often referred to as frontal lobe functions, the anatomic basis of these alterations is often more broadly distributed throughout the temporal and parietal gray and white matter, as well as subcortical nuclei such as the caudate.[6]

CLINICAL MANIFESTATIONS AND DIAGNOSIS

Psychomotor slowing, executive cognitive dysfunction, and alteration in the control and regulation of behavior often occur concurrently. Patients with executive dysfunction are deficient in goal-oriented behavior; they lose the ability to predict the consequences of their actions or words. Patients with executive dysfunction also exhibit poor mental agility and inflexibility in their thinking and control of their actions. They are easily distracted and exhibit a tendency to perseverate, in which the answer to a prior question is repeated in response to subsequent questions. They are disinhibited; as a consequence, when asked to recall a specific event, they may glibly answer with a fabrication, a phenomenon referred to as confabulation.

Patients with lateral prefrontal pathology exhibit poor performance on tests of abstract reasoning and mental agility. In a test such as verbal similarities, they tend to be very concrete and narrowly focused. They become easily distracted and are slow in performing tasks that require sustained attention.

Because of their mental rigidity and difficulty in set shifting, they do poorly on tests that require the ability to vary their response strategies, such as verbal fluency tests.

Patients with medial frontal lesions are often profoundly apathetic and lack initiative and motivation. They may be laconic and completely unable to express emotion, whether it be anger, sadness, or elation. They tend to be indifferent to their surroundings, a state referred to as abulia. The majority of patients with substantial prefrontal or anterior temporal lobe pathology lack insight into the extent of their inappropriate behavior.

Patients with diseases of the frontal lobes or of the anterior portions of the temporal lobes often exhibit changes in personality and dysregulation of personal actions and interpersonal behavior. These alterations may include difficulty controlling impulsivity, poor social graces (manifested as rude behavior or caustic comments), a disregard for the feelings of others (loss of empathy), and a general failure to understand what constitutes acceptable behavior in a particular social context. If the underlying disease is progressive, gross alterations in table manners and loss of interest in maintaining personal hygiene may appear. Inappropriate sexual behavior may occur. Patients with prominent disease of the frontal lobes may also exhibit hyperorality, which is a compulsion to put nonfood objects into their mouths. Hyperorality can be life-threatening, depending on the substance ingested.

Bedside testing of executive cognitive dysfunction provides only a superficial view of the cognitive domain. Assessment in the neuropsychology laboratory gives a more refined estimate of the degree of psychomotor slowing and executive dysfunction.

Determining the Cause

Space-occupying lesions of the frontal lobes (e.g., neoplasms, brain abscesses) can lead to the cognitive and behavioral syndromes of frontal lobe dysfunction. With these diseases, executive cognitive dysfunction and alteration of control of personal behavior develop over a period of weeks.

In patients with acute brain trauma (Chapter 371), brain imaging at the time of initial medical and surgical evaluation will reveal whether the brain suffered acute traumatic lesions. Chronically, traumatic brain injury may later lead to encephalomalacia of the frontal lobes.

Neurodegenerative diseases such as frontotemporal lobar degeneration (Chapter 374) are associated with dysfunction and brain loss in the prefrontal and anterior temporal lobes (Chapter 374, Fig. 374-8). These disorders may produce the entire spectrum of executive cognitive dysfunction and altered control of personal behavior over a period of a year or longer.

Some diseases that do not directly damage the frontal or anterior temporal neocortex may cause executive cognitive dysfunction and alteration of control of personal behavior because of the interconnectedness of the frontal and anterior temporal lobes with other cortical and subcortical regions. Multiple sclerosis (Chapter 383), a disorder of white matter pathways, may cause abnormalities in cognition and behavior of the frontal type. Similarly, Huntington disease (Chapter 382) and progressive supranuclear palsy, which affect the caudate nuclei, may also resemble a frontal cognitive and behavioral syndrome and result in executive cognitive dysfunction and alterations in comportment.

TREATMENT Rx

Cognitive-behavioral therapies offer modest but definite benefit for patients with aphasia and for patients with mild attention deficits and mild memory deficits caused by brain injury.

FUTURE DIRECTIONS

The assessment of cognition is being supplemented by new imaging techniques. Functional magnetic resonance imaging can provide an unprecedented view into cortical connectivity patterns, which are influenced by aging and disease.

 Grade A Reference

A1. Breitenstein C, Grewe T, Floel A, et al. Intensive speech and language therapy in patients with chronic aphasia after stroke: a randomised, open-label, blinded-endpoint, controlled trial in a health-care setting. *Lancet.* 2017;389:1528-1538.

GENERAL REFERENCES

For the General References and other additional features, please visit Expert Consult at https://expertconsult.inkling.com.

374

COGNITIVE IMPAIRMENT AND DEMENTIA

DAVID S. KNOPMAN

THE SPECTRUM OF MILD COGNITIVE IMPAIRMENT TO DEMENTIA

DEFINITION

Dementia is a cognitive disorder that leads to interference with daily functioning and results in loss of independence (Table 374-1). Dementia can range in severity from mild, when a patient may still be independent in a few activities, to severe, when total dependence occurs. Mild cognitive impairment is the term that describes the earlier phase of symptomatic cognitive impairment that precedes mild dementia (Table 374-2). The definitional boundary between mild cognitive impairment and dementia is based on the preservation or loss of independence in daily life. Given the diversity of life experiences and circumstances, the concept of the distinction between mild cognitive impairment and dementia has more conceptual clarity than operational precision. Indeed, the spectrum of symptomatic cognitive impairment is a continuum.

The majority of conditions that result in symptomatic cognitive impairment are of gradual onset, are progressive in course, and occur in persons with previously normal cognition. Some diseases that lead to dementia, such as those caused by an acute neurologic illness secondary to stroke (Chapter 378), encephalitis (Chapter 386), or head trauma (Chapter 371), may begin abruptly and then remain static for long periods. Conversely, a small subset of dementias, such as Creutzfeldt-Jakob disease (Chapter 387), has a rapid onset and a course that can run for less than a year. Dementia may also occur in persons with developmental disabilities and long-standing cognitive deficits.

EPIDEMIOLOGY

The prevalence and incidence of mild cognitive impairment and dementia increase with advancing age. Both are uncommon before 50 years of age. In individuals older than 65 years, the prevalence of dementia of all types is about 7%. In the age range of 65 to 69, the prevalence of dementia is only 1 to 2%, but it increases to 20 to 25% in the 85- to 89-year age range and

TABLE 374-1 DEFINITION OF DEMENTIA

Dementia is cognitive impairment that interferes with the ability to function at work or at usual activities; *and*
  It represents a decline from prior levels of functioning and performing; *and*
  The cognitive impairment and impaired functioning are not explained by delirium or major psychiatric disorder

The cognitive impairment of dementia is detected and diagnosed through a combination of:
  a. History-taking from the patient and a knowledgeable informant; *and*
  b. Objective cognitive assessment, either a "bedside" mental status examination or neuropsychological testing

The cognitive or behavioral impairment of dementia involves *at least two* of the following domains:
  Impaired ability to acquire and remember new information
  Impaired reasoning and handling of complex tasks; poor judgment
  Impaired visuospatial abilities
  Impaired language functions (speaking, reading, writing)
  Changes in personality, behavior, or comportment

Adapted from McKhann GM, Knopman DS, Chertkow H, et al. The diagnosis of dementia due to Alzheimer's disease: recommendations from the National Institute on Aging-Alzheimer's Association workgroups on diagnostic guidelines for Alzheimer's disease. *Alzheimers Dement.* 2011;7:263-269.

TABLE 374-2 DIAGNOSTIC CRITERIA FOR AMNESIC MILD COGNITIVE IMPAIRMENT

The presence of a new memory complaint, preferably corroborated by an informant

Objective evidence of an impairment in episodic declarative memory (for age)

Normal general cognitive functions

No substantial interference with work, usual social activities, or other activities of daily living

No dementia

Adapted from Albert MS, DeKosky ST, Dickson D, et al. The diagnosis of mild cognitive impairment due to Alzheimer's disease: recommendations from the National Institute on Aging-Alzheimer's Association workgroups on diagnostic guidelines for Alzheimer's disease. *Alzheimers Dement.* 2011;7:270-279.

continues to rise steadily thereafter. The incidence of new cases of dementia is about 1 per 100 per year at the age of 70 and rises to about 2 to 3 new cases per 100 per year by about the age of 80. Incidence rates continue to rise into the ninth and tenth decades of life. The incidence and prevalence of mild cognitive impairment are roughly the same as those of dementia. This means, for example, that the prevalence of symptomatic cognitive impairment after age 65 years is about 14%. With the dramatic increase in longevity, the societal burden of dementia has risen substantially. Interestingly, however, in some studies, the incidence rate of dementia has declined over the past three decades, perhaps in part to better and earlier treatment of cardiovascular risk factors.[1]

In absolute numbers, far more women than men have dementia because women live longer. However, men and women have an equal age-adjusted risk for the development of dementia. There are no racial or ethnic differences in the risk for dementia. Risk factors include the *APOE* ε4 allele, current depressive symptoms, midlife onset of diabetes, hypertension or hyperlipidemia, and vascular diseases such as atrial fibrillation or stroke. A parental history of dementia before age 80 years increases the risk for dementia by about two- to six-fold independent of all currently known genetic risk factors.[2]

PATHOBIOLOGY

Symptomatic cognitive impairment is the culmination of dysfunction in the cerebral hemispheres, especially the association cortices, hippocampal formations, their supporting subcortical nuclear structures (e.g., caudate nuclei, thalamus), and their white matter interconnections (see Fig. 373-1 in Chapter 373). Specific diseases that cause mild cognitive impairment and dementia do so by affecting particular parts of the cerebral cortex, subcortical nuclei, or the underlying white matter pathways linking different cortical regions.

CLINICAL MANIFESTATIONS

Any of the major domains of cognition—declarative episodic memory, executive cognitive functioning, visuospatial function, or language—may be affected in dementia (Chapter 373). Because Alzheimer disease is the most common cause of mild cognitive impairment and dementia, anterograde amnesia is typically present first and most intensely in the majority of dementia patients. In other dementing illnesses, deficits in the other cognitive domains may be dominant. Although persons with mild cognitive impairment often retain some sense of their loss of cognitive capacities, a pervasive and nearly invariant aspect of dementia is a loss of insight (anosognosia) into the extent of one's cognitive and functional losses.

Neuropsychiatric symptoms are also common in dementia. Apathy and loss of initiative are almost always present. Depression and anxiety are frequent, as are irritability, paranoia, delusional thinking, and hallucinations. Daily functioning of patients with dementia is compromised. In early dementia, difficulty is likely to be present in management of finances and medications, independent travel, preparation of meals, and keeping of appointments. In more advanced disease, difficulty becomes evident in basic activities of daily living such as bathing, dressing, toileting, and feeding oneself. Dementias secondary to cerebrovascular or Lewy body disease are often associated with specific abnormalities in strength, coordination, gait, or balance. Alzheimer disease typically has no associated motor abnormalities.

DIAGNOSIS

Clinical Examination

Mild cognitive impairment and dementia are strictly clinical diagnoses based on evidence of cognitive dysfunction in both the history and the mental status examination.[3] The key elements of the history flow from their definitions: What is the evidence for impairment in one or more domains of cognition?

What is the evidence that daily functioning is affected? The mental status examination is necessary to establish that alertness is preserved (i.e., the patient does not have delirium [Chapter 25]) and to determine what specific areas of cognition exhibit directly observable impairment. For diagnosis of the syndrome of dementia, no laboratory test supersedes the clinical history and mental status examination. Laboratory testing is critical, however, to determine the cause of the cognitive disorder.

Bedside testing of mental status is based on the principles of cognitive neurology (Chapter 373). For moderate or severe dementia to be distinguished from normal cognitive states, a bedside mental status examination such as the Mini-Cog test (see Table 24-5 in Chapter 24) is accurate. However, for mild cognitive impairment and mild dementia, bedside mental status examinations lack sensitivity (i.e., they fail to diagnose some cases at the milder end of the spectrum).[4] For patients with suspected mild cognitive impairment or dementia, neuropsychometric testing is a useful adjunct to the bedside examination. The neurologic examination is also important for evaluation of signs of specific diseases, including signs of cerebrovascular disease (e.g., hemiparesis [Chapter 378]) and signs of extrapyramidal disease (e.g., rigidity, bradykinesia, resting tremor [Chapter 381]).

Differential Diagnosis

Mild cognitive impairment and dementia must be distinguished from other disorders of cognition (Fig. 374-1).[5] Delirium (Chapter 25) also affects cognition directly; key features distinguishing it from dementia include impaired arousal and attention. Delirium is almost always of sudden onset, whereas the majority of cases of dementia are of gradual onset.

Primary psychiatric diseases (Chapter 369) such as major depression, bipolar disorder, and schizophrenia may also impair cognition. In mild cognitive impairment and dementia, however, the impairment in cognition is typically equivalent to or more pervasive than the changes in mood and behavior.

The principal diseases that cause mild cognitive impairment and dementia are three neurodegenerative diseases—Alzheimer disease, Lewy body disease, and frontotemporal lobar degeneration—and cerebrovascular disease (Fig. 374-2). The neurodegenerative diseases are typically slow and insidious in onset and inexorably progressive. Mild cognitive impairment and dementia secondary to cerebrovascular disease may be of either sudden or gradual onset.

Many much less common secondary causes account for less than 2% of all dementias. Drug intoxication (Chapters 31 and 388), metabolic disorders (Chapter 194), central nervous system infections (Chapters 384 to 386), and brain structural lesions (Chapter 373) are typically subacute in onset; if they are diagnosed and treated early, the cognitive deficits improve or resolve completely. A number of medications such as sedatives, pain medications, corticosteroids, digoxin, and others cause mental confusion, particularly but not always at toxic levels (Chapter 102). Metabolic disorders that may also cause subacute confusion and produce a cognitive disorder include hypothyroidism or hyperthyroidism (Chapter 213), vitamin B_{12} deficiency (Chapter 388), chronic liver disease (Chapter 144), chronic renal failure (Chapter 121), and hypocalcemia or hypercalcemia (Chapter 232). Chronic viral infections of the brain, especially human immunodeficiency virus infection, frequently cause dementia (Chapter 366). Chronic meningitides in the differential diagnosis of dementia include cryptococcal meningitis (Chapter 317), tuberculous meningitis (Chapter 308), and tertiary syphilis (Chapter 303). Finally, structural lesions of the brain, including primary and metastatic tumors (Chapter 180), chronic subdural hematomas (Chapter 371), and normal-pressure hydrocephalus, can cause a syndrome resembling dementia that consists of a subacute or slowly progressive decline in cognition with few or no other neurologic symptoms or signs.

PROGNOSIS

Except for the secondary causes of mild cognitive impairment and dementia and the rare dementing illnesses caused by single episodes of brain injury (e.g., severe head trauma, anoxic encephalopathy), dementia is a condition that invariably leads to worsening of cognition and function. Almost all patients who have more than mild cognitive impairment worsen over the course of several years if they do not die from other causes. The rate of cognitive decline is variable among individuals and, of course, also varies with the specific disease. In general, dementia can be said to decrease life expectancy by half compared with the life expectancy of nondemented individuals.

End-of-Life Care

The terminal stage and end-of-life care issues (Chapter 3) associated with the common dementias are usually similar. Dementia itself does not directly cause

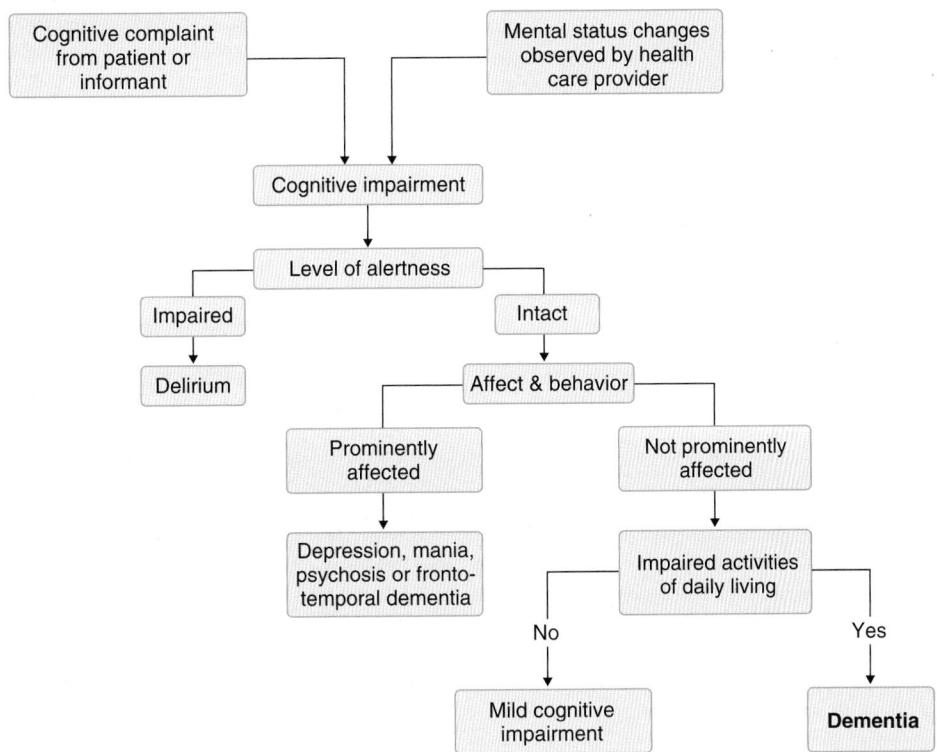

FIGURE 374-1. Flow diagram to establish the diagnosis of dementia.

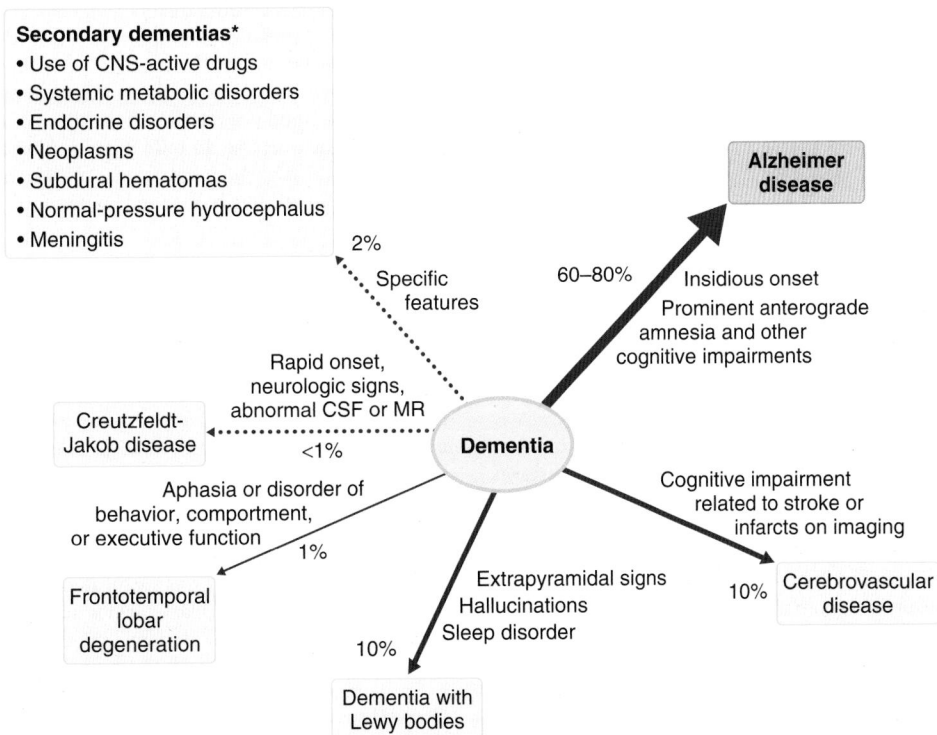

FIGURE 374-2. Flow diagram for the differential diagnosis of mild cognitive impairment and dementia. The percentage contributions of various diagnoses are approximate. *The list of secondary causes of dementia is not exhaustive. CNS = central nervous system; CSF = cerebrospinal fluid; MR = magnetic resonance imaging.

death, but it is strongly linked to reduced survival. Patients with dementia typically die of the same illnesses that affect debilitated individuals, such as sepsis, pneumonia, pulmonary embolism, or heart disease.

Most patients with dementia experience their terminal illnesses in hospitals or extended care facilities. Given the inexorably progressive nature of most dementing illnesses and their likelihood of producing severe and completely disabling cognitive and functional impairment, it is widely accepted that patients with end-stage dementia should receive conservative care. Feeding tubes and ventilatory support should not generally be considered.

MANAGEMENT OF PERSONS WITH MILD COGNITIVE IMPAIRMENT OR DEMENTIA

Pharmacologic treatment of persons with mild cognitive impairment or dementia should be focused on the specific disease causing the cognitive disorder. Unfortunately, symptomatic treatments are currently available only for Alzheimer disease dementia. Management of persons with symptomatic cognitive impairment, on the other hand, involves issues that are common to all etiologies. Principles of care include disclosure of the diagnosis; education

TABLE 374-3 DIAGNOSTIC CRITERIA FOR PROBABLE ALZHEIMER DISEASE DEMENTIA

The clinical diagnosis of probable Alzheimer disease dementia is made when:

Criteria for dementia met (see Table 374-1), and the illness has the following characteristics:
  Insidious onset: symptoms have a gradual onset over months to years; *and*
  Clear-cut history of worsening of cognition by report or observation; *and*
  The initial and most prominent cognitive deficits are evident on history and examination consistent with an amnestic disorder (most common) or a nonamnestic cognitive disorder (less common) (aphasia, visuospatial disorder, or behavioral/dysexecutive disorder)

The diagnosis of probable Alzheimer disease dementia *should not* be applied when there is substantial evidence for another neurodegenerative disease, extensive cerebrovascular disease, or a non-neurologic medical comorbidity or medication use that could have a substantial impact on cognition

Research criteria for probable Alzheimer disease dementia with higher certainty when imaging or cerebrospinal fluid biomarkers are available:

Alzheimer disease is considered the cause of cognitive impairment when β-amyloid markers (in cerebrospinal fluid or by PET imaging) are abnormal and tau markers (cerebrospinal fluid phospho-tau or tau PET) are abnormal

Alzheimer disease pathophysiology is considered present but of uncertain etiologic significance when β-amyloid markers (in cerebrospinal fluid or by PET imaging) are abnormal but tau markers are normal

PET = positron emission tomography; MR = magnetic resonance.
Adapted from McKhann GM, Knopman DS, Chertkow H, et al. The diagnosis of dementia due to Alzheimer's disease: recommendations from the National Institute on Aging-Alzheimer's Association workgroups on diagnostic guidelines for Alzheimer's disease. *Alzheimers Dement.* 2011;7:263-269; and Jack CR, Jr., Bennett DA, Blennow K, et al. NIA-AA research framework: toward a biological definition of Alzheimer's disease. *Alzheimers Dement.* 2018;14:535-562.

and support of caregivers; assessment of functional status; screening and management of behavioral and psychiatric symptoms; addressing safety concerns; assessing driving status; advance care planning; pain assessment; and pharmacologic treatment of dementia.[6]

ALZHEIMER DISEASE

DEFINITION

Alzheimer disease, which is a pathophysiologic process involving β-amyloidosis and limbic and isocortical neurodegeneration with tauopathy, produces a cognitive disorder that usually progresses to severe dementia in which anterograde amnesia is the initial dominant symptom (Table 374-3).[7,8] The clinical diagnosis implies that the causative pathologic process is of the Alzheimer type, whereas the pathologic diagnosis rests on the findings of characteristic histopathologic features.

EPIDEMIOLOGY

Between 60 and 80% of all dementing illness is due to Alzheimer disease. Among all individuals older than 65 years, the prevalence of Alzheimer disease is estimated to be about 5%. As with dementia in general, the prevalence doubles in every 5-year interval after age 65, and the incidence continues to rise into the 10th and 11th decades of life. Men and women may be equally affected, although on an absolute basis, far more women have prevalent Alzheimer disease because women live longer than men. There are no ethnic or racial differences in the predilection for Alzheimer disease.

Risk Factors

Established risk factors for Alzheimer disease include advancing age and a family history. Putative risk factors include diabetes mellitus, hypertension, cardiovascular disease, and head trauma. Evidence for and against each of these four conditions is inconclusive, but the consensus is that at least diabetes and hypertension may play a role in the pathogenesis of Alzheimer disease. Midlife vascular risk factors and elevated low-density lipoprotein (LDL) levels specifically may be associated with elevated brain β-amyloid later in life. Low educational achievement is also a consistent risk factor, but most experts believe educational level is a proxy for some other factor, such as socioeconomic status or the early childhood medical and psychosocial environment. Protective factors have also been proposed, but their status is much debated.

PATHOBIOLOGY

The histopathologic diagnosis of Alzheimer disease is based on the joint presence of a substantial cerebral burden of neuritic plaques and neurofibrillary tangles. Neuritic plaques consist of a core of aggregated β-amyloid peptide surrounded by degenerating neurites, which are fragments of axons and dendrites. β-Amyloid contains 39 to 42 amino acids and is proteolytically derived from a larger protein, the amyloid precursor protein. Neurofibrillary tangles are intracellular aggregations of an excessively phosphorylated form of the microtubule-associated protein tau. The altered tau protein self-aggregates and forms neurofibrillary tangles. In a low-powered microscopic section of frontal, temporal, or parietal cortex, at least six neuritic plaques and neurofibrillary tangles should be visible for the diagnosis of Alzheimer disease to be made.

Pathophysiology

The progression of changes of β-amyloidosis follows a roughly predictable pattern in Alzheimer disease. Positron emission tomography (PET) imaging with ligands that bind to β-amyloid shows that β-amyloid begins to accumulate in the neocortex as long as 20 years before dementia occurs. Soluble aggregates of β-amyloid in oligomeric (consisting of a small number of monomers) forms may be the key pathogenic molecules that eventually induce or accelerate neuronal injury. By the time clinical dementia due to Alzheimer disease is present, large numbers of β-amyloid peptide–containing deposits invariably are found in neuritic plaques in the neocortex. Neuritic plaques represent the end stage of the Alzheimer process. Because β-amyloidosis begins well before clinical symptoms appear and probably reaches a plateau in terms of abundance, the amount of β-amyloidosis does not closely mirror the severity of dementia in Alzheimer disease.

The regional extent of neurofibrillary tangles in Alzheimer disease anticipates and parallels the clinical progression of the disease from an amnestic disorder to a multidomain cognitive disorder. Neurofibrillary tangles appear in the medial temporal lobe and brain stem in cognitively normal persons by the fourth decade of life. In persons destined to develop Alzheimer disease, a critical part of the pathophysiology involves transsynaptic spread of neurofibrillary tangle pathology to cortical association areas. At the time clinical symptoms develop, neurofibrillary tangles are found in association neocortices of the frontal, parietal, and temporal lobes. It is only in the most severe and final stages that neurofibrillary tangles are found in the occipital lobes and primary motor and sensory cortices. The location of neurofibrillary tangles corresponds faithfully to the clinical evolution of specific symptoms and severity of Alzheimer disease. In mild cognitive impairment, the earliest clinical manifestation of Alzheimer disease, the most intense burden of neurofibrillary tangles is in the entorhinal cortex and hippocampi, precisely the regions involved in declarative episodic memory. Hippocampal atrophy is characteristic, and reductions in hippocampal volumes may be observed on magnetic resonance imaging (MRI; Fig. 374-3). Involvement of the association neocortices with neurofibrillary tangles represents the histopathologic correlate of the progression to dementia. Quantitative MRI in patients with mild cognitive impairment who later progress to dementia shows increasing atrophy of key cortical association areas, such as the lateral temporal lobes, inferior parietal lobes, posterior cingulate cortex, and lateral frontal lobes. Reflecting the spread to association neocortex, language functions, visuospatial functions, and executive cognitive functions typically become impaired some time after declarative episodic memory dysfunction occurs.

The most consistent neurotransmitter deficit in Alzheimer disease is in cholinergic neurotransmission. The cells of origin of hippocampal and neocortical cholinergic projections are located in the septum, diagonal band, and nucleus basalis. Neurofibrillary tangles accumulate in the neurons in these regions as Alzheimer disease develops, but there is also neurochemical evidence that these neurons are stressed much earlier in the disease.

Genetics

The overwhelming majority of Alzheimer disease is due to sporadic (not genetic) disease. However, in a very small number of instances, Alzheimer disease occurs as an autosomal dominant disease. The three known genes involved in autosomal dominant Alzheimer disease all are directly involved in the production of β-amyloid peptide. The first is the amyloid precursor protein (*APP*) gene, located on chromosome 21q21.3. Eighteen known mutations in this gene lead to excess production of β-amyloid and are reliably associated with a very early onset (20 to 50 years of age) of Alzheimer disease. Another line of evidence implicating the *APP* gene in Alzheimer disease is the invariable appearance of the pathologic process of Alzheimer disease in individuals with Down syndrome (trisomy 21 [Chapter 36]) who have an extra copy of the *APP* gene as a result of the trisomy.

The other two genes associated with autosomal dominant Alzheimer disease are the presenilin 1 and 2 genes, located on chromosomes 14q24.3 and 1q31.42. A large number of presenilin 1 mutations account for the majority of autosomal

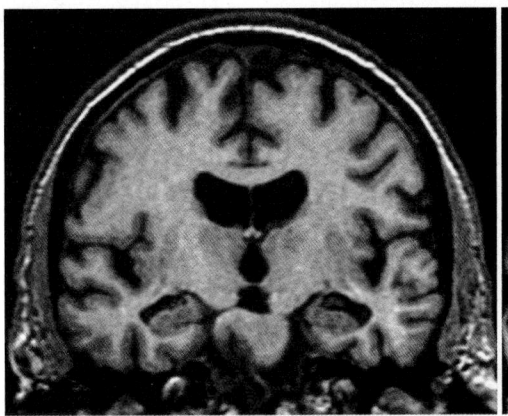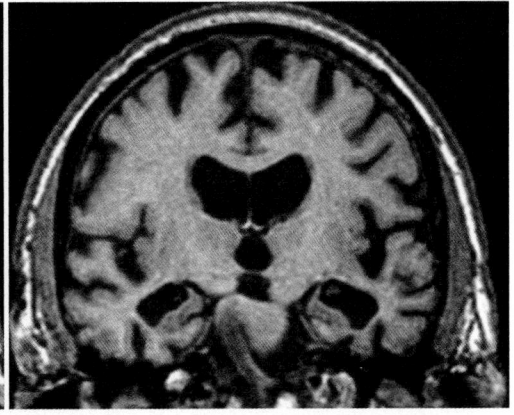

FIGURE 374-3. Serial coronal images from magnetic resonance imaging of a patient with Alzheimer disease. The scan on the *left* was performed when the patient was clinically normal. The scan on the *right* was performed 11 years later when the patient was demented. Hippocampal atrophy has increased dramatically from the first to the subsequent scan. (Courtesy Maria Shiung and Clifford Jack.)

dominant Alzheimer disease. Both genes code for a similar protein known as presenilin. Presenilin is involved in the proteolysis of the APP molecule at the gamma cleavage site. Presenilin mutations alter the balance of APP cleavage products, including β-amyloid and other peptides that may influence synaptic functioning. The presenilin mutations are also associated with early-onset (age 40 to 60 years) Alzheimer disease.

Studies of the familial aggregation of Alzheimer disease have shown that later onset disease also displays genetic risks, but only a few genes have been definitively linked to later onset Alzheimer disease. The most prominent gene related to later onset Alzheimer disease, located on chromosome 19q13.2, encodes apolipoprotein E (apo E), a protein involved in lipid transport. In humans, three allelic variants of apolipoprotein gene (*APOE*) are determined by differences in the amino acids cysteine and arginine at positions 112 and 158 of the 299–amino acid protein. One of the allelic variants, with arginine at both positions, designated the ε4 variant, is strongly associated with a 14-fold increased risk for Alzheimer disease in homozygotes and a three-fold increase in heterozygotes. In many series, almost 50% of Alzheimer disease dementia patients, but only about 25% of nondemented controls, have at least one copy of the *APOE* ε4 allele. The presence of an *APOE* ε4 allele does not always cause Alzheimer disease in that the disease never develops in some carriers of the genotype. The mechanism by which the *APOE* ε4 allele predisposes to Alzheimer disease is not established, but the tertiary structure of the APOE protein with arginine at positions 112 and 158 may lead to impaired binding to β-amyloid, which in turn reduces the clearance of β-amyloid from cells.

A rare missense mutation in the *TREM2* gene also increases the risk for Alzheimer disease. The pathophysiology appears to be impaired containment of inflammatory processes rather than a direct effect on neurologic function. Rare loss-of-function mutations in *ABCA7* uniformly lead to classical Alzheimer disease, but with a widely variable age of onset.

CLINICAL MANIFESTATIONS

The early course of symptomatic cognitive impairment due to Alzheimer disease is dominated by difficulties with anterograde amnesia. Some of the usual complaints include forgetting recent events and conversations, misplacing items, problems with keeping track of the date, getting lost in familiar surroundings, and problems with remembering to complete tasks. The frequency and severity of the memory lapses progress from occasional difficulty to more pervasive and consistent failure.

In mild cognitive impairment and mild dementia due to Alzheimer disease, declarative episodic memory function may be lost.[9] Familiarity and access to previous knowledge may allow patients to function in their usual daily routines as long as nothing out of the ordinary is required of them. They may still retain the ability to prepare simple meals and take walks in their neighborhood without getting lost. However, even in mild Alzheimer disease, medication-taking errors and difficulty managing money or balancing a checkbook are likely to occur. Traveling to unfamiliar places often accentuates confusion. Changes in personality commonly accompany the cognitive losses. Apathy, loss of initiative, and loss of interest in previous hobbies and pastimes are ubiquitous in early symptomatic Alzheimer disease.

As the disease progresses, the ability to perform necessary daily tasks becomes more and more difficult to the point that the patient will need assistance preparing meals, paying bills, taking transportation, and keeping house. As the disease moves into the severe stages, assistance and supervision in basic activities such as bathing, dressing, toileting, and eating become necessary.

In the terminal stages of the disease, all communicative abilities may be lost. Mobility may still be preserved until late in the disease. Alzheimer disease dementia patients commonly die of illnesses that strike other debilitated elderly individuals, such as sepsis, pneumonia, and heart failure.

The duration of the course of dementia due to Alzheimer disease is long but variable. The time from mild dementia to death may be as short as 2 to 3 years or may be well over a decade. For patients in whom mild dementia is diagnosed, about 10% per year reach the stage of severe dementia.

Rarely, Alzheimer disease is associated with prominent symptoms in cognitive domains other than memory. The most common of the atypical syndromes is one in which profound visuospatial deficits occur without the typical severe anterograde amnesia. This syndrome is referred to as posterior cortical atrophy.

DIAGNOSIS

The diagnosis of mild cognitive impairment or dementia due to Alzheimer disease is largely a clinical one based on the history and examination. The key elements in the history are a gradual onset and insidious progression of cognitive impairment, especially anterograde amnesia. The mental status examination should demonstrate impairment in short-term memory and other cognitive deficits. The clinical diagnosis of Alzheimer disease should be thought of as a diagnosis of inclusion: if the history and examination are compatible with Alzheimer disease and if certain exclusions can be verified, the diagnosis can be made with moderate confidence. Recent PET imaging studies have shown that non-Alzheimer disease etiologies can sometimes mimic the amnestic syndrome of Alzheimer disease.

Cerebrospinal fluid (CSF) protein markers (β-amyloid and tau) (see Table 374-3)[10] and brain imaging (structural MRI, [18]fluorodeoxyglucose PET [Fig. 374-4], amyloid positron emission tomography [Fig 374-5], and tau positron emission tomography [Fig 374-6][11]) are being used in research settings to enhance the precision of a diagnosis of Alzheimer disease as a cause of symptomatic cognitive impairment. For example, amyloid PET scanning and CSF Aβ42/t-tau and Aβ42/p-tau can identify early-stage Alzheimer disease with sensitivities of about 97% and specificities of about 83%. For experimental therapeutics, efforts are now underway to use CSF or imaging biomarkers to diagnose Alzheimer disease before individuals develop symptoms.

Differential Diagnosis

A number of other conditions that bear similarity to Alzheimer disease must be excluded on clinical or laboratory grounds (see Fig. 374-2). One is dementia with Lewy bodies, which is suggested by the presence of parkinsonism, prominent visual hallucinations, and a specific sleep disorder. At autopsy, the pathologic processes of Lewy body disease and Alzheimer disease often coexist, thus suggesting that the diagnoses overlap. Frontotemporal lobar degeneration is suggested by prominent behavioral and personality changes or by prominent language difficulties early in the course. Hippocampal sclerosis has unique neuropathologic findings but is virtually impossible to distinguish from Alzheimer disease by clinical features. Other neurodegenerative conditions in the differential diagnosis of Alzheimer disease include Huntington disease (Chapter 382), progressive supranuclear palsy (Chapter 382), corticobasal degeneration (Chapter 382), amyotrophic lateral sclerosis (Chapter 391), and Wilson disease (Chapter 200); however, these diseases invariably

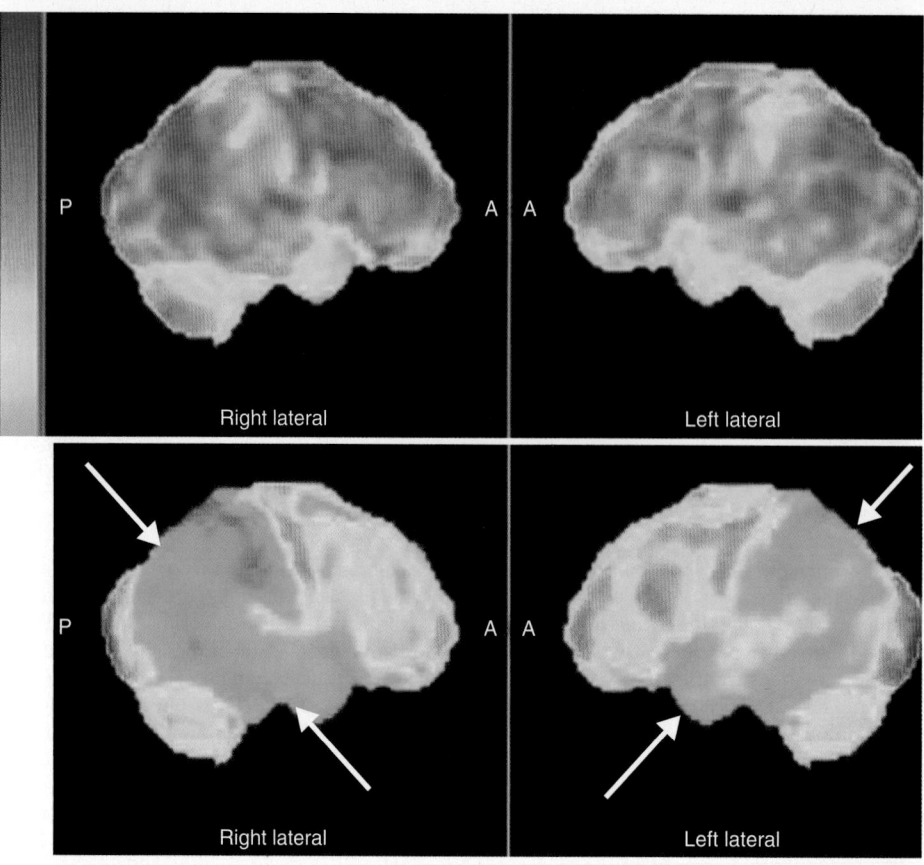

FIGURE 374-4. ¹⁸Fluorodeoxyglucose positron emission tomographic scan of a patient with Alzheimer disease dementia. Computerized reconstructions of the regional glucose uptake ratio (using pons as reference) of the cortical surface show hotter colors (*yellow* and *orange*) in areas of normal glucose uptake, whereas cooler colors (*green* and *blue*) indicate hypometabolism. The scan on the top is from a normal individual of the same age. The scan on the bottom is from a patient with typical Alzheimer disease dementia, and it shows hypometabolism in the temporal and parietal cortical regions (*arrows*).

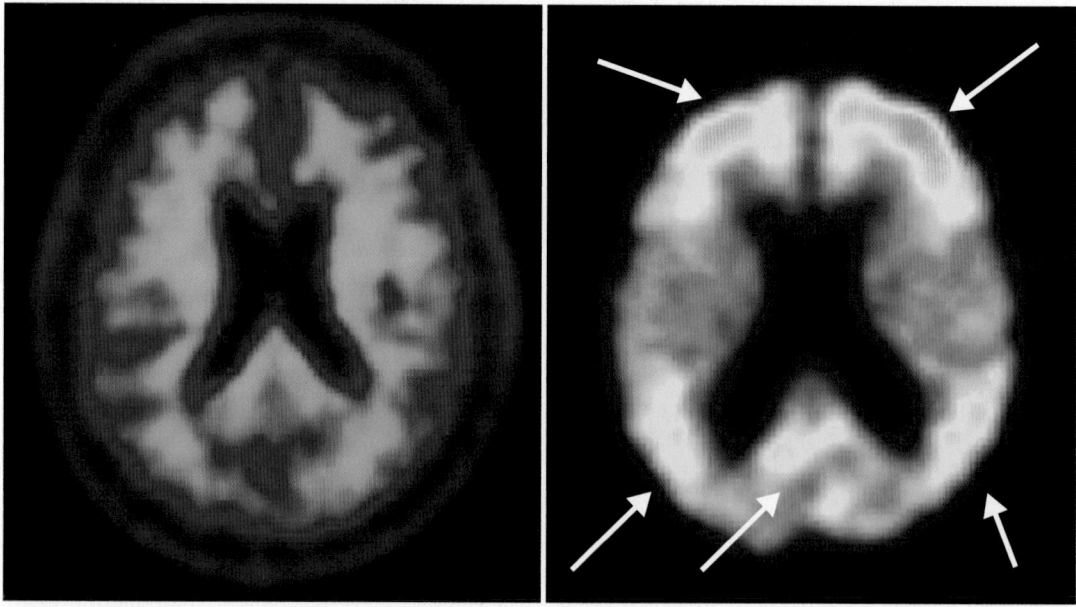

FIGURE 374-5. Amyloid positron emission tomographic (PET) scan of a patient with Alzheimer disease dementia. On this axial image of a ¹¹C Pittsburgh compound B PET scan, the *left* scan is from an individual with no cortical amyloid retention. The *green* signal represents low levels of nonspecific white matter binding. On the *right*, a scan of a patient with Alzheimer disease dementia shows the prominent retention of the amyloid imaging agent in the frontal, parietal, and posterior cingulate cortices (*arrows*).

have prominent motor manifestations early in their course. Normal-pressure hydrocephalus (see later) is a rare cause of dementia associated with a gait disorder.

It is particularly challenging to distinguish dementia caused by cerebrovascular disease from Alzheimer disease (see later). The fact that Alzheimer disease and cerebrovascular disease often coexist requires clinicians to consider both simultaneously.

PREVENTION AND TREATMENT   Rx

There are no established preventive therapies for mild cognitive impairment or dementia due to Alzheimer disease.[A1] Although a healthy diet, physical exercise, and stimulating cognitive leisure activities are sensible, evidence supporting their value in the prevention of dementia is limited. There also currently

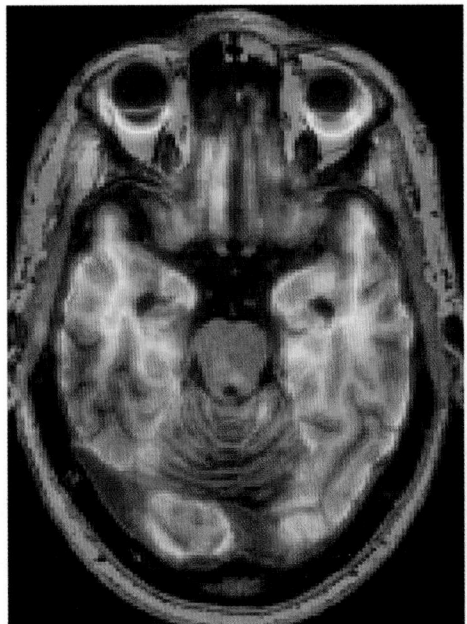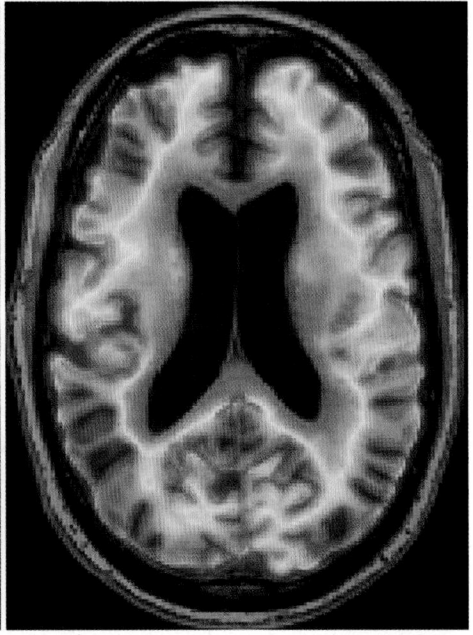

FIGURE 374-6. AV1451 (tau) positron emission tomographic (PET) scan of a patient with Alzheimer disease dementia. On axial images, the tau PET signal can be seen in the temporal and parietal lobes. The *left* scan at the level of the temporal lobes shows the increased signal (*red* and *yellow*) representing tau deposition. The *right* scan at the level of the lateral ventricles shows the tau deposition to be widespread in the parietal lobes, including the precuneus in the medial parietal lobes and lateral frontal lobes.

is insufficient evidence to recommend any diet, physical activity program, or cognitive activities program for the treatment of symptomatic cognitive impairment. A multidomain intervention has been shown to delay cognitive decline in an elderly Finnish population who had existing cardiovascular risk factors.[12] However, another intervention trial in France (including cognitive training, physical activity, and nutrition) failed to show any benefits.[13]

Evidence-Based Treatments

Two classes of drugs are approved for the treatment of Alzheimer disease: cholinesterase inhibitors and memantine, a glutamate receptor antagonist. The rationale for use of cholinomimetic drugs (donepezil, 5 or 10 mg/day; immediate release galantamine, 16 or 24 mg/day) or rivastigmine (6 to 12 mg/day orally or 4.5 to 9 mg/day by skin patch) is the reduced levels of cholinergic markers in the neocortex of patients dying of Alzheimer disease. All three agents delay the progression of symptoms to a statistically significant but clinically marginal extent at 6 to 12 months in patients with mild to moderate dementia due to Alzheimer disease.[A2] For example, donepezil shows some benefits in reducing the development of dementia among patients with mild cognitive impairment at 1 year but not at 3 years. Furthermore, community-dwelling patients whose moderate or severe Alzheimer disease had been treated with donepezil for at least 3 months and who continue donepezil at 10 mg daily may have functional benefits over the next 12 months compared with patients who discontinue it.[A3] Memantine, which is a low- to moderate-affinity uncompetitive *N*-methyl-D-aspartate receptor antagonist that acts on glutamate neurotransmission, appears to delay the progression of functional decline in patients with moderate to severe Alzheimer disease at a dose of 10 mg twice daily. Individual patients, however, often do not show any clear benefits of treatment.

Except in patients who have folate or vitamin B$_{12}$ deficiency, vitamin B supplementation is not effective in slowing cognitive decline. Treatment of diabetes (Chapter 216) and hypertension (Chapter 70) is beneficial for other reasons, but it is not clear that such treatment alters the course of Alzheimer disease.

One study of patients with moderately severe Alzheimer disease showed that vitamin E was effective in delaying progression, and it may also benefit patients with mild to moderate Alzheimer disease.[A4][A5] Multivitamins are not efficacious,[A6] and trials of drugs to bind β-amyloid peptides or block the 5-hydroxytryptamine 6 receptor have been unsuccessful.[A7-A10] Antidepressants generally are ineffective and increase adverse events when used to treat patients with Alzheimer disease. Humanized monoclonal antibodies that bind soluble forms of amyloid, inhibit the formation of amyloid plaques, or inhibit β-amyloid production have not shown any clinical benefit.

After Alzheimer disease becomes symptomatic, exercise is not helpful for preventing progression.[A11] Support for family caregivers is a critical intervention that cannot be overemphasized. Support groups through the Alzheimer Association (available at www.alz.org) can benefit families coping with the disease.

Important safety issues include supervision of medications, supervision of finances, and close scrutiny of motor vehicle operation. Operation of other potentially dangerous tools, firearms, appliances, and equipment should also

TABLE 374-4	DIAGNOSTIC CRITERIA FOR THE SYNDROME OF DEMENTIA CAUSED BY CEREBROVASCULAR DISEASE (VASCULAR COGNITIVE IMPAIRMENT)

Mild cognitive impairment as defined in Table 374-1 or dementia as defined in Table 374-1

Clinically important cerebrovascular disease is demonstrable by *either* of the following:
Onset of the cognitive disturbance or dramatic worsening of an existing disturbance that occurred within 3 months of a stroke, where stroke is defined as a focal neurologic deficit of acute onset in which the symptoms and signs persist for more than 24 hours
Neuroimaging evidence of bilateral brain infarctions rostral to but including the thalamus

be carefully monitored or avoided. Patients with Alzheimer disease often wander and can become lost long distances from home. Identification of patients can prevent tragic occurrences.

PROGNOSIS

Alzheimer disease is inevitably progressive, and severe cognitive impairment and complete dependence on others develop in virtually all patients unless they die prematurely. Alzheimer disease also contributes to premature death; the mortality rate in patients with Alzheimer disease is about 10% per year. In patients with advanced dementia, the 6-month mortality rate is about 55%; pneumonia, fever, and eating problems are associated with poor prognosis.

COGNITIVE IMPAIRMENT DUE TO CEREBROVASCULAR DISEASE

DEFINITION

Cerebrovascular disease makes an important contribution to late life cognitive impairment. For a cognitive disorder to be attributed to cerebrovascular disease from a neuropathologic perspective, there must be sufficient cerebral infarction in locations known to be responsible for the cognitive deficits in the absence of other neurodegenerative neuropathologic changes (Table 374-4).

When cerebrovascular disease produces cognitive impairment that is not severe enough to meet the criteria for dementia, it is referred to as vascular cognitive impairment.

EPIDEMIOLOGY

In clinical studies, as many as 20% of dementia patients have cerebrovascular disease. Like Alzheimer disease, it is less common in patients younger than 65 years and increases steadily thereafter. In neuropathologic studies, about 25% of all cases of dementia have some vascular component. Roughly half that number are relatively pure vascular dementia; the remainder consists of vascular disease mixed with Alzheimer disease. Men and women are equally affected.

Risk Factors

Risk factors for vascular cognitive impairment include cardiovascular disease, atrial fibrillation, higher glucose levels, diabetes, and hypertension. There are no known protective factors other than treatment of these risk factors. Populations with high rates of generalized vascular disease should have higher rates of vascular dementia, but competing mortality from cardiovascular disease may obscure part of the relationship. Microinfarcts contribute to brain atrophy and cognitive impairment, particularly before dementia is clinically evident. In the first year after a stroke, the risk for development of dementia is about nine-fold higher than the rate in persons without a stroke; the risk remains about two-fold higher in subsequent years.

PATHOBIOLOGY

The majority of vascular disease causing cognitive impairment is due to atherosclerosis. One mechanism is through large infarctions, such as those secondary to occlusive disease in major cerebral vessels, including the carotid arteries and the anterior, middle, and posterior cerebral arteries (Chapter 379). A second mechanism of infarction is at the arteriolar level, with lacunar infarctions in the thalamus, basal ganglia, and subcortical white matter. Both these processes can be detected by brain MRI. Infarcts in the hippocampal formations, medial thalamus, caudate nuclei, and parietal association areas are highly likely to produce cognitive impairment but not necessarily dementia. Microinfarcts, which are small zones of infarction that are not visible to the naked eye but can be observed with light microscopy, may also contribute to the dementia. Lacunar infarction and microinfarcts are far more commonly represented in series of patients with vascular dementia than are large infarctions. The simultaneous presence of Alzheimer disease is common in vascular dementia.

There are other uncommon causes of vascular cognitive impairment. Cerebral autosomal dominant arteriopathy with subcortical infarcts and leukoencephalopathy (CADASIL) is a very rare inherited disease that usually becomes clinically evident between the ages of 30 and 50 years and causes severe white matter disease, headaches, and dementia. The cause of CADASIL is mutations in the *notch3* gene on chromosome 19q12. Cerebral amyloid angiopathy, a β-amyloidosis in which the β-amyloid peptide accumulates in the media of small to medium-sized arteries in the leptomeninges and superficial cortex, causes cerebral hemorrhages that may lead to dementia if it occurs in sufficient number and in critical locations. Cerebral amyloid angiopathy is also seen in Alzheimer disease, but its hemorrhagic manifestations may occur in individuals with little evidence of Alzheimer disease clinically and modest evidence pathologically. Cerebral vasculitis (Chapter 254) is a very rare cause of dementia.

CLINICAL MANIFESTATIONS

The spectrum of cognitive changes in patients with cerebrovascular disease is broad. The more common cognitive syndromes in cerebrovascular disease include mild cognitive impairment, a dementia with prominent anterograde amnesia, and a dementia with prominent changes in personality and executive function. Some patients with vascular cognitive impairment without dementia may have deficits in only one domain (Chapter 373). A number of aphasia syndromes are a result of cerebral infarction or hemorrhage in the perisylvian regions of the dominant hemisphere. Infarction or hemorrhage in the occipitotemporal or occipitoparietal regions may produce one of the disorders of visual cognition, such as alexia or visual agnosia. Infarcts in the caudate nuclei, particularly if they are bilateral, may produce a cognitive syndrome that includes both amnesia and disordered executive function, thus mimicking dementia. Large infarcts in the right parietal lobe can also produce dementia. Infarcts in the medial thalami or in the hippocampal formations can produce isolated amnesia.

The evolution of symptoms in vascular cognitive impairment does not follow a stereotypical pattern. In some, the cognitive syndrome may remain static. In others, new strokes may lead to substantial declines in cognition and function. Some patients with vascular cognitive impairment may experience a gradually declining illness. Patients with vascular cognitive impairment without dementia or vascular dementia may also have other neurologic signs typical of patients with cerebrovascular disease, such as hemiparesis, hemianopia, hemisensory changes, or cranial nerve abnormalities.

DIAGNOSIS

The diagnosis of vascular cognitive impairment is based on the neurologic history and examination. Brain imaging, preferably with MRI, is essential to establish the presence of infarcts.[14] The cardinal diagnostic features of vascular cognitive impairment are that (1) the cognitive disorder should have begun within 3 months of a clinical stroke event and (2) there should be multiple bilateral infarcts in the cerebral hemispheres visible on brain imaging studies (Fig. 374-7). A temporal link between the onset or worsening of cognitive impairment and a stroke is important in demonstrating that cerebrovascular disease is etiologically relevant to the cognitive impairment. Brain imaging of infarcts in the cerebral cortex, basal ganglia, thalamus, and cerebral white matter has obvious value for establishment of cerebrovascular disease. In contrast to actual infarcts on imaging, the presence of white matter hyperintensities without infarcts on brain MRI is much less specific.

The accuracy of the clinical diagnosis of cerebrovascular disease as a cause of cognitive impairment is generally lower than that of Alzheimer disease. The combination of (1) a temporal relationship between dementia and a stroke and (2) imaging evidence of bilateral infarcts is diagnostically specific for vascular dementia but is insensitive. Broader diagnostic criteria (see Table 374-4) are more sensitive but less specific. The usual alternative diagnosis is Alzheimer disease, and there is typically no way to be certain whether and how much Alzheimer disease is simultaneously present.

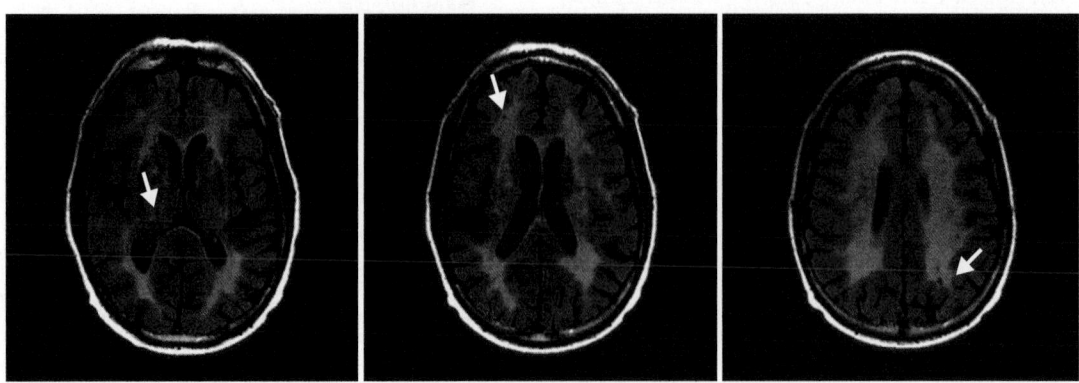

FIGURE 374-7. Axial magnetic resonance images of a patient with extensive cerebrovascular disease. The images show extensive white matter hyperintensities bilaterally. There are also lacunar infarcts (*arrows*).

PREVENTION AND TREATMENT

The burden of cerebrovascular disease in later life can be mitigated by treatment of vascular risk factors in midlife. With early lifelong aggressive treatment of diabetes (Chapter 216), hypertension (Chapter 70), and hyperlipidemia (Chapter 195), as well as the use of prophylactic anticoagulation in patients with atrial fibrillation (Chapter 58), the number of cerebral infarcts should be reduced, with a corresponding reduction in the number of cases of vascular dementia. Evidence for this link comes from large-scale studies in which the treatment of hypertension reduced the frequency of strokes and incident dementia. After vascular dementia develops, cholinesterase inhibitors have shown some benefit, but the major goal is to prevent future strokes.

PROGNOSIS

Patients with vascular dementia can often be expected to have severe cardiovascular disease and a greater likelihood of future strokes and cardiac ischemic events. Survival of patients with vascular dementia is poorer than that of patients with Alzheimer disease dementia.

DEMENTIA WITH LEWY BODIES

DEFINITION

Dementia with Lewy bodies is a multifaceted dementing disorder in which the underlying pathologic process includes Lewy bodies in limbic and cortical structures (Table 374-5). Some clinicians make a distinction between patients in whom parkinsonism preceded the cognitive disorder and those in whom the cognitive disorder occurred either simultaneously with or before the movement disorder. This distinction may be somewhat useful in clinical practice, but there are few clinical or neuropathologic differences based on different sequences of signs and symptoms. The diagnosis of dementia with Lewy bodies is similar in principle to diagnosis of both dementia and Parkinson disease (Chapter 381) in the same individual, but *dementia with Lewy bodies* is a term with broader connotations because of other features

---

TABLE 374-5	DIAGNOSTIC CRITERIA FOR THE DEMENTIA SYNDROME ASSOCIATED WITH LEWY BODY PATHOLOGY

Mild cognitive impairment as defined in Table 374-1 or dementia as defined in Table 374-1

Core clinical features (The first three typically occur early and may persist throughout the course.)
1. Fluctuating cognition with pronounced variations in attention and alertness
2. Recurrent visual hallucinations that are typically well formed and detailed
3. REM sleep behavior disorder, which may precede cognitive decline
4. One or more spontaneous cardinal features of parkinsonism: bradykinesia (defined as slowness of movement and decrement in amplitude or speed), rest tremor, or rigidity

Supportive clinical features
Severe sensitivity to antipsychotic agents; postural instability; repeated falls; syncope or other transient episodes of unresponsiveness; severe autonomic dysfunction, e.g., constipation, orthostatic hypotension, urinary incontinence; hypersomnia; hyposmia; hallucinations in other modalities; systematized delusions; apathy, anxiety, and depression

Indicative biomarkers
Reduced dopamine transporter uptake in basal ganglia demonstrated by SPECT or PET
Abnormal (low uptake) ^{123}iodine-MIBG myocardial scintigraphy
Polysomnographic confirmation of REM sleep without atonia

Probable dementia with Lewy bodies can be diagnosed if:
a. Two or more core clinical features of dementia with Lewy bodies are present, with or without the presence of indicative biomarkers, or
b. Only one core clinical feature is present, but with one or more indicative biomarkers

Probable dementia with Lewy bodies should not be diagnosed on the basis of biomarkers alone.

MIBG = meta-iodobenzylguanidine; PET = positron emission tomography; REM = rapid eye movement; SPECT = single-photon emission computed tomography.
From McKeith IG, Boeve BF, Dickson DW, et al. Diagnosis and management of dementia with Lewy bodies: fourth consensus report of the DLB Consortium. *Neurology.* 2017;89:88-100.

(hallucinations, fluctuations, and sleep disorder) that may be more apparent than the movement disorder.

EPIDEMIOLOGY

Mild cognitive impairment or dementia with Lewy bodies is about one fourth as common as Alzheimer disease dementia. Lewy body disease becomes more common with advancing age, and the prevalence of dementia with Lewy bodies increases with advancing age as well. As with the other dementias, there are no known ethnic or racial differences, but dementia with Lewy bodies may be more common in men. There are no known risk factors for dementia with Lewy bodies. Dementia develops in up to 30% of patients with Parkinson disease, and advancing age is the major risk factor.

PATHOBIOLOGY

The pathology of dementia with Lewy bodies is a mixture of Lewy body disease and Alzheimer disease. In general, the more intense the Lewy body disease, the less abundant the Alzheimer disease. Lewy bodies, which are intraneuronal inclusions that contain α-synuclein, are found in the nucleus basalis, pars compacta of the substantia nigra, locus caeruleus, other brain stem structures, amygdala, cingulate gyrus, and neocortex. The earliest locations of Lewy bodies are the brain stem, where they affect nuclei involved in sleep and arousal, and the substantia nigra, the locus caeruleus, and cranial nerve nuclei IX and X. Typically, the nucleus basalis, transentorhinal cortex, cingulate gyrus, and neocortex become involved later.

In Lewy body disease, the α-synuclein protein becomes misfolded and aggregates intraneuronally. Mutations in the α-synuclein gene have been seen in a few families with autosomal dominant Parkinson disease, but most cases of dementia with Lewy bodies are sporadic.

CLINICAL MANIFESTATIONS

The clinical manifestations of mild cognitive impairment and dementia with Lewy bodies include four major abnormalities: the cognitive disorder, the neuropsychiatric disorder, the motor disorder, and the disorder of sleep and wakefulness. The cognitive disorder may differ from Alzheimer disease dementia, although there is considerable overlap.[15] In a typical patient with dementia with Lewy bodies, visuospatial deficits, impaired concentration, and impaired attention dominate the picture. In some patients, the deficits in executive functions may be similar to what is seen in frontotemporal lobar degeneration. Anterograde amnesia is usually present but milder than in Alzheimer disease dementia. Language deficits are not prominent. The neuropsychiatric manifestations of dementia with Lewy bodies, including prominent apathy, loss of initiative, and depression, may be more disabling than the cognitive symptoms. The motor manifestations include bradykinesia, gait disturbances, postural disturbances, and rigidity. Rest tremor is less common in dementia with Lewy bodies in patients in whom the cognitive disorder appears before the parkinsonism. Visual hallucinations, fluctuations in alertness, and rapid eye movement (REM) sleep disorders are part of a broader disorder of the regulation of sleep and wakefulness. Visual hallucinations are often graphic, detailed, and bizarre, perhaps because the sleep phenomenon of dreaming intrudes into wakefulness. Patients with dementia with Lewy bodies have large fluctuations in their alertness and arousal from day to day.

REM sleep behavior disorder (Chapter 377) is a parasomnia in which patients exhibit dream enactment behavior, often with violent, threatening overtones. Patients typically relate that they feel as though they are being chased by something or someone. Their behavior while they are asleep consists of excessive talking, calling out or shouting, and thrashing about, often to the point of striking a bed partner or falling out of bed. The REM sleep behavior disorder may precede the development of Parkinson disease and dementia with Lewy bodies by years.

DIAGNOSIS

The diagnosis of dementia with Lewy bodies is based on clinical information that corroborates the presence of abnormalities in cognition, motor function, neuropsychiatric behavior, and regulation of sleep and wakefulness.[16] Formal neuropsychological testing is often helpful in evaluating memory, executive function, and visuospatial function in a detailed manner. Neuroimaging has only a limited role in the diagnosis of dementia with Lewy bodies.

Differential Diagnosis

Other disorders that must be considered in patients with dementia and a movement disorder include progressive supranuclear palsy (Chapter 382), which can resemble dementia with Lewy bodies in terms of both the dementia and the motor disorder. In progressive supranuclear palsy,[17] patients are much less likely to have disorders of arousal and typically have other distinctive signs and symptoms, including the characteristic supranuclear gaze palsy and other brain stem findings. The corticobasal degenerations, which are members of the family of frontotemporal lobar dementias (see later), may also produce a movement disorder and dementia. Huntington disease (Chapter 382) is associated with dementia and a movement disorder, but the movement disorder of Huntington disease includes prominent chorea and athetosis, neither of which is present in dementia with Lewy bodies.

Normal-pressure hydrocephalus, which is very rare relative to dementia with Lewy bodies and Alzheimer disease, is typically characterized by the triad of a gait disorder, dementia, and urinary incontinence. Altered dynamics of CSF flow in the ventricular system appear to reduce periventricular metabolism and also induce damage in periventricular axons. Normal-pressure hydrocephalus can be suspected when computed tomography or MRI shows ventricular enlargement that is out of proportion to the amount of sulcal widening. Predicting a favorable response to ventriculoperitoneal shunting in suspected normal-pressure hydrocephalus has proved to be difficult. Imaging studies that measure CSF flow through the aqueduct of Sylvius or that measure flow of radiolabeled CSF with radionuclide cisternography have not been useful. Clinical response to the removal of a high volume (e.g., 30 mL) of CSF through lumbar puncture is sometimes used to select patients for surgery, although its positive and negative predictive values are unclear. Only about one third of patients who initially respond to shunting have persistent benefits at 3 years.[18]

TREATMENT Rx

Management of patients with cognitive impairment with Lewy bodies is challenging because of the simultaneous appearance of a cognitive disorder, a neuropsychiatric disorder, a motor disorder, and a sleep and wakefulness disorder. Treatment of the motor disorder is accomplished with antiparkinsonian drugs such as levodopa and dopaminergic agonists (Chapter 381). Treatment with these agents should be instituted for dementia with Lewy bodies if there are prominent gait or balance problems that threaten safety and interfere with independence. These medications may worsen hallucinations and exacerbate confusional states, but this concern should not preclude a treatment trial if the motor symptoms pose safety risks or interfere with independence.

Cholinesterase inhibitors, which do not exacerbate parkinsonian symptoms, have a beneficial effect on neuropsychiatric symptoms and perhaps on the cognitive disorder. [A12] Autonomic disturbances such as urinary incontinence can be challenging to treat in persons with cognitive impairment due to Lewy body disease because the usually prescribed medications have anticholinergic pharmacologic profiles. Anticholinergic drugs have a definite risk for increasing confusion.

Hallucinations and agitation impair quality of life for the patient and family and often require treatment. Some antipsychotic agents that might otherwise control these symptoms dramatically exacerbate the parkinsonism in dementia with Lewy bodies. Atypical antipsychotics are usually recommended, but there is insufficient experience from controlled clinical trials. Many movement disorder specialists prefer to use quetiapine in doses of 25 to 200 mg/day or clozapine at 6.25 to 50 mg/day because these agents appear to have the lowest rate of extrapyramidal side effects. However, it is not possible to make any strong statements about the relative efficacy of atypical antipsychotics in treating the hallucinations in dementia with Lewy bodies, especially in view of the possibility that atypical antipsychotic agents may be associated with higher than expected mortality.

REM sleep behavior disorder (Chapter 377) can be disabling, but there are no controlled clinical trials to inform treatment. Some sleep disorder specialists typically use either melatonin, 3 to 12 mg, or clonazepam, 0.5 to 2 mg, at bedtime.

Treatment of depressive symptoms may substantially improve a patient's functioning. Use of one of the newer generation antidepressants, such as sertraline (25 to 100 mg/day) or citalopram (10 to 20 mg/day), may be beneficial and does not necessarily interfere with management of the other symptoms (Chapter 369).

PROGNOSIS

As opposed to patients with Alzheimer disease dementia, some studies show that patients with dementia with Lewy bodies have a more rapidly progressive course and poorer survival. As a result of the combination of manifestations, patients with dementia with Lewy bodies may become disabled sooner in their course.

FRONTOTEMPORAL LOBAR DEGENERATION

DEFINITION

The frontotemporal lobar degenerations are a group of neurodegenerative disorders with distinctive clinical manifestations and a predilection for the prefrontal and anterior temporal neocortices. The most common clinical syndrome is a disorder of behavior and personal relationships (comportment) with a loss of executive functions (Table 374-6). This syndrome is referred to as behavior-variant frontotemporal dementia. Other syndromes in the clinical spectrum of frontotemporal lobar degeneration involve different aspects of language or motor dysfunction of the limbs.

EPIDEMIOLOGY

Unlike Alzheimer disease, the frontotemporal lobar degenerations have a peak age at onset in the 50- to 70-year range, and the incidence declines after the age of 70. In patients with dementia who are younger than 70 years, frontotemporal lobar degeneration makes up 10 to 20% of cases. However, across the entire age spectrum, the frontotemporal lobar degenerations are much less common than Alzheimer disease dementia, dementia with Lewy bodies, or vascular dementia. Both men and women are affected equally. There are no known risk factors for the frontotemporal lobar degenerations except a family history.

PATHOBIOLOGY

The clinical syndrome in frontotemporal lobar degeneration is determined by the lobar location of the pathologic process. Right prefrontal or anterior temporal disease and brain atrophy produce behavioral syndromes like frontotemporal dementia. Left frontal involvement tends to produce progressive nonfluent aphasia. Predominant left anterior temporal lobe involvement may produce semantic dementia.

On histopathologic grounds, patients with frontotemporal lobar degeneration can be divided into three groups: those whose inclusions contain the microtubule-associated protein tau, those whose inclusions contain the TAR DNA-binding protein 43 (TDP-43), and those whose inclusions contain the fused in sarcoma (FUS) protein, another ribonucleic acid–binding protein. The latter is much less common than the first two. Each type includes both genetically determined and sporadic forms.

TABLE 374-6 DIAGNOSTIC CRITERIA FOR BEHAVIOR-VARIANT FRONTOTEMPORAL DEMENTIA

The following symptom must be present to meet criteria for behavior-variant frontotemporal dementia:

  Shows progressive deterioration of behavior and/or cognition by observation or history (as provided by a knowledgeable informant)

Three of the following behavioral/cognitive symptoms that are persistent or recurrent must be present **within 3 years of onset** to meet criteria for **possible** behavior-variant frontotemporal dementia:

  Early behavioral disinhibition such as socially inappropriate behavior, loss of manners or decorum, or impulsive, rash, or careless actions
  Early apathy or inertia
  Early loss of sympathy or empathy
  Early perseverative, stereotyped, or compulsive/ritualistic behavior
  Hyperorality and dietary changes such as altered food preferences, binge eating, increased consumption of alcohol or cigarettes, or oral exploration or consumption of inedible objects
  Neuropsychological profile exhibits executive/generation deficits with relative sparing of memory and visuospatial functions

Probable behavior-variant frontotemporal dementia is diagnosed when **all of the following** are present:

  Criteria met for possible behavior-variant frontotemporal dementia
  Significant functional decline present by caregiver report
  Imaging results that demonstrate frontal and/or anterior temporal atrophy on MRI or CT, or frontal hypoperfusion or hypometabolism on PET or SPECT

The diagnosis of behavior-variant frontotemporal dementia **should not** be applied when the pattern of deficits is better explained by a psychiatric diagnosis, other nondegenerative nervous system disorders, or medical disorders.

CT = computed tomography; MRI = magnetic resonance imaging; PET = positron emission tomography; SPECT = single-photon emission computed tomography.
Adapted from Rascovsky K, Hodges JR, Knopman D, et al. Sensitivity of revised diagnostic criteria for the behavioural variant of frontotemporal dementia. *Brain*. 2011;134:2456-2477.

Among the tau-positive varieties are Pick disease, in which intracellular tau-positive inclusions known as Pick bodies are seen. Several other pathologic tau-positive subtypes occur, including progressive supranuclear palsy, corticobasal degeneration, and the disorder associated with mutations in the tau gene. Nearly 50 mutations in the *MAPT* gene on chromosome 17q21 are associated with autosomal dominant frontotemporal lobar degeneration syndromes, each with a slightly different clinical and neuropathologic phenotype. The most common is a proline-to-leucine mutation at codon 301, located in exon 10. The tau gene undergoes alternative splicing, resulting in six isoforms of the tau protein. Pathologic mutations appear to disrupt splicing of alternative isoforms of tau protein, which in turn adversely affects the binding of tau to microtubules in neurons. Reduced binding of tau to microtubules is deleterious to microtubule function and neuronal integrity.

The TDP-43-positive frontotemporal lobar degenerations are almost equally common. Immunostaining shows that there are distinctive TDP-43-containing inclusions. Mutations in the granulin (*GRN*) gene, also located on chromosome 17q21, cause familial autosomal dominant forms of frontotemporal lobar degeneration with TDP-43-positive inclusions. Nearly 70 different mutations in the granulin gene are linked to frontotemporal lobar degenerations. All of the mutations lead to premature degradation of the messenger RNA, a process termed *haploinsufficiency*. Granulin mutation carriers have an abnormally low amount of the protein progranulin. The normal function of granulin in the brain is unclear, and the pathophysiologic basis for dementia in persons with granulin gene mutations is unknown. The link between alterations in TDP-43 and *GRN* mutations is also unknown at this time.

A third important gene mutation involved in frontotemporal lobar degenerations associated with TDP-43 inclusions is the hexanucleotide repeat expansion in *C9ORF7* gene located on chromosome 9p21. This latter mutation is the most common of the mutations causing frontotemporal lobar degeneration and amyotrophic lateral sclerosis (Chapter 391).

Frontotemporal lobar degenerations that are FUS positive are much less common. At this time, all FUS-positive cases have had the behavioral variant of frontotemporal dementia.

CLINICAL MANIFESTATIONS

The clinical manifestations of the syndrome of frontotemporal dementia begin insidiously. Apathy, loss of initiative, and flattening of affect are common early symptoms. As the disease progresses, the entire spectrum of behavioral changes associated with dysfunction of the frontal and anterior temporal lobes appears.[19] On cognitive assessments, patients may have preserved memory functions, but they typically have difficulty with tests of executive cognitive function. When frontotemporal dementia progresses to moderate or severe stages, the behavioral changes remain prominent, but the disease becomes more difficult to distinguish from other dementias such as Alzheimer disease. The neuropathology of behavior-variant frontotemporal dementia may be either tau positive or TDP-43 positive.

In some patients with frontotemporal lobar degeneration, signs and symptoms of motor neuron disease (Chapter 391) develop, such as weakness, atrophy, and fasciculation in the limbs or the bulbar musculature.[20] In other patients with frontotemporal lobar degeneration, asymmetrical limb apraxia develops that is part of the corticobasal syndrome. Features of progressive supranuclear palsy may also appear in patients with behavior-variant frontotemporal dementia.

Aphasic disturbances are often the presenting manifestation of patients with frontotemporal lobar degeneration. The two most characteristic syndromes are a nonfluent/agrammatic variant of primary progressive aphasia or the semantic variant of primary progressive aphasia. The nonfluent/agrammatic primary progressive aphasia variant is seen in patients who exhibit hesitancy in selecting words in their speech, a problem that may be difficult for others to appreciate at first. Anomia is an early sign. Gradually, the patient's speech becomes laconic and labored. Eventually, a nonfluent, apractic, agrammatic speech develops. In other cognitive domains, patients often have no deficits. Other nonfluent/agrammatic primary progressive aphasic patients may eventually become virtually mute even though they may appear to have preserved memory and visuospatial functions. Patients with nonfluent/agrammatic primary progressive aphasia often have tau-positive neuropathologic findings.

The semantic variant of primary progressive aphasia, previously known as semantic dementia, is a disorder that involves dissolution of the meaning of words or objects. A patient with semantic variant primary progressive aphasia may also become unable to access knowledge about objects (object agnosia) and people's faces (prosopagnosia). The most striking demonstration of the deficit in semantic variant primary progressive aphasia is when a patient can produce the name of an object—a watch, for example—but then cannot say what a watch is for when asked. Often, patients with semantic variant primary progressive aphasia have preservation of the ability to learn a list of words, even if their knowledge of the meaning of the words is diminished. Patients with semantic variant primary progressive aphasia usually have TDP-43-positive neuropathologic findings.

Not all patients with primary progressive aphasia fit neatly into a well-delineated syndrome. Although the semantic and nonfluent/agrammatic variants of primary progressive aphasia are almost always due to frontotemporal lobar degenerations, other variants, especially one in which word-finding problems predominate (the logopenic variant of primary progressive aphasia), may be due to Alzheimer disease.

DIAGNOSIS

Frontotemporal lobar degeneration as a cause for a cognitive or behavioral disorder must first be suspected on clinical grounds, based on the appearance of one of the distinctive clinical syndromes such as frontotemporal dementia (see Table 374-6) or one of the aphasic subtypes.[21] Neuropsychological testing can also aid in the diagnosis by detecting abnormalities in executive function and verifying that memory function is preserved, as it often is. For all frontotemporal lobar degeneration syndromes, MRI showing focal atrophy of the frontal (Fig. 374-8) or temporal lobes (Fig. 374-9) is highly likely to be diagnostic. Imaging with fluorodeoxyglucose PET can also be useful when the clinical diagnosis is uncertain and MRI is nondiagnostic.

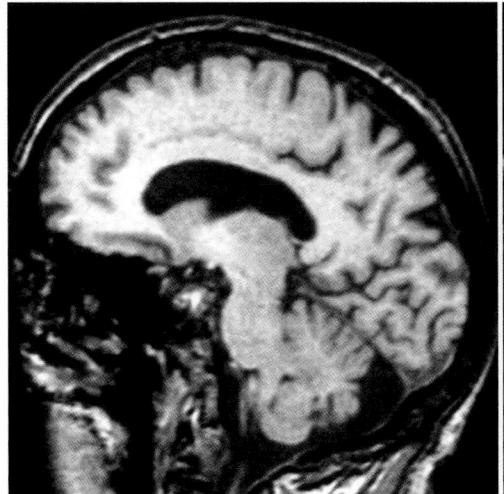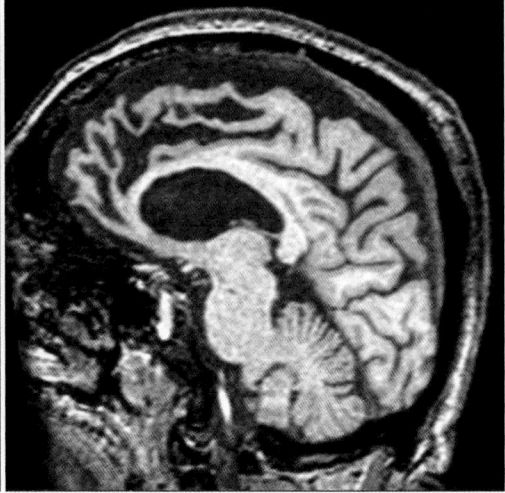

FIGURE 374-8. Parasagittal image from magnetic resonance imaging of a patient with frontotemporal dementia (*right*). Atrophy of the frontal lobes is dramatic compared with the brain of a normal individual (*left*). (Courtesy Maria Shiung and Clifford Jack.)

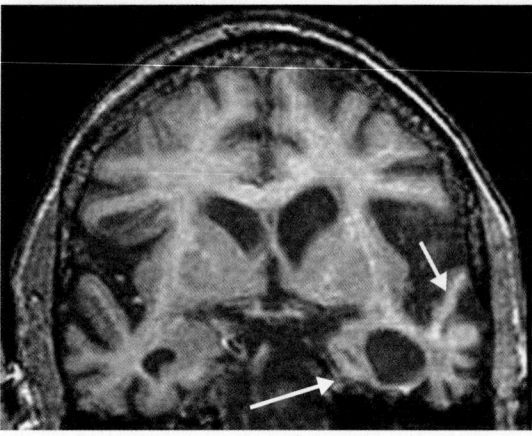
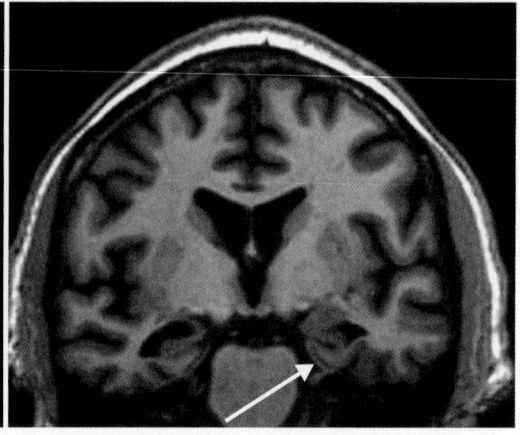

FIGURE 374-9. Coronal images from magnetic resonance imaging of a patient with semantic variant of primary progressive aphasia (*left*). There is prominent asymmetrical atrophy of the left anterior temporal lobe involving the amygdala, head of the hippocampus, and the lateral temporal lobe neocortex. By comparison, on the scan of a patient with Alzheimer disease dementia (*right*), the neocortex is preserved even though there is atrophy involving the amygdala and head of the hippocampus (*arrows*).

TREATMENT　　　　　　　　　　　　　　　　Rx

There is no symptomatic therapy specifically for frontotemporal lobar degeneration.[22] In patients with agitation, paranoia, delusions, or obsessive behavior, atypical antipsychotics (e.g., quetiapine, 25 to 200 mg/day) are used, but no controlled clinical trials are available. There are no preventive or disease-modifying treatments of frontotemporal lobar degeneration.

PROGNOSIS

Specific frontotemporal lobar degeneration syndromes have dramatic differences in their clinical course and outcome. In patients with motor neuron signs and symptoms, the prognosis is usually poor, with survival of only about 2 years from the time of diagnosis. Patients with semantic variant and nonfluent variant primary progressive aphasia have much more protracted and gradual trajectories; survival for more than 10 years is not uncommon. Behavior variant frontotemporal dementia itself can also exhibit a more protracted course.

Grade A References

A1. Kane RL, Butler M, Fink HA, et al. AHRQ Comparative Effectiveness Reviews. Interventions to prevent age-related cognitive decline, mild cognitive impairment, and clinical Alzheimer's-type dementia. Rockville (MD): Agency for Healthcare Research and Quality (US); 2017.
A2. Tricco AC, Ashoor HM, Soobiah C, et al. Comparative effectiveness and safety of cognitive enhancers for treating Alzheimer's disease: systematic review and network metaanalysis. *J Am Geriatr Soc.* 2018;66:170-178.
A3. Renn BN, Asghar-Ali AA, Thielke S, et al. A systematic review of practice guidelines and recommendations for discontinuation of cholinesterase inhibitors in dementia. *Am J Geriatr Psychiatry.* 2018;26:134-147.
A4. Farina N, Llewellyn D, Isaac M, et al. Vitamin E for Alzheimer's dementia and mild cognitive impairment. *Cochrane Database Syst Rev.* 2017;4:CD002854.
A5. Dysken MW, Sano M, Asthana S, et al. Effect of vitamin E and memantine on functional decline in Alzheimer disease: the TEAM-AD VA cooperative randomized trial. *JAMA.* 2014;311:33-44.
A6. Grodstein F, O'Brien J, Kang JH, et al. Long-term multivitamin supplementation and cognitive function in men: a randomized trial. *Ann Intern Med.* 2013;159:806-814.
A7. Honig LS, Vellas B, Woodward M, et al. Trial of solanezumab for mild dementia due to Alzheimer's disease. *N Engl J Med.* 2018;378:321-330.
A8. Egan MF, Kost J, Tariot PN, et al. Randomized trial of verubecestat for mild-to-moderate Alzheimer's disease. *N Engl J Med.* 2018;378:1691-1703.
A9. Atri A, Frolich L, Ballard C, et al. Effect of idalopirdine as adjunct to cholinesterase inhibitors on change in cognition in patients with Alzheimer disease: three randomized clinical trials. *JAMA.* 2018;319:130-142.
A10. Egan MF, Kost J, Voss T, et al. Randomized trial of verubecestat for prodromal Alzheimer's disease. *N Engl J Med.* 2019;380:1408-1420.
A11. Lamb SE, Sheehan B, Atherton N, et al. Dementia and physical activity (DAPA) trial of moderate to high intensity exercise training for people with dementia: randomised controlled trial. *BMJ.* 2018;361:1-11.
A12. Wang HF, Yu JT, Tang SW, et al. Efficacy and safety of cholinesterase inhibitors and memantine in cognitive impairment in Parkinson's disease, Parkinson's disease dementia, and dementia with Lewy bodies: systematic review with meta-analysis and trial sequential analysis. *J Neurol Neurosurg Psychiatry.* 2015;86:135-143.

GENERAL REFERENCES

For the General References and other additional features, please visit Expert Consult at https://expertconsult.inkling.com.

375

THE EPILEPSIES

SAMUEL WIEBE

DEFINITION

A seizure is defined by transient focal or generalized signs or symptoms due to abnormal excessive or synchronous neuronal activity in the brain. Focal seizures, which originate within neuronal networks limited to one cerebral hemisphere, produce signs and symptoms corresponding to the specific region of the brain affected by the seizure. Generalized seizures rapidly affect extensive neuronal networks on both cerebral hemispheres, and their signs and symptoms are consistent with substantial involvement of both sides of the brain.

Seizures are not synonymous with epilepsy. The epilepsies should be distinguished from situations in which acute brain insults (e.g., infections, trauma, intoxication, metabolic disturbances) cause one or more seizures without a resulting chronic seizure tendency. Acute symptomatic seizures, or provoked seizures, constitute about 40% of all incident cases of nonfebrile seizures, typically respond to treatment of the provoking factor, and do not require long-term treatment with antiepileptic drugs.

The epilepsies are a group of conditions in which an underlying neurologic disorder results in a chronic tendency to have recurrent unprovoked seizures.

The diagnosis of epilepsy is established if one of the following three criteria is met: two or more unprovoked or reflex seizures occurring more than 24 hours apart; a single unprovoked or reflex seizure in a person whose risk of recurrence is at least 60% over the next 10 years (e.g., brain tumor, hemorrhage, or infection); or a known epilepsy syndrome (e.g., benign epilepsy with centrotemporal spikes, reflex epilepsy).[1]

The causes, types, and clinical expression of the epilepsies are numerous and varied. However, some of the epilepsies conform into identifiable epileptic syndromes, which consist of clusters of clinical and electroencephalographic (EEG) features that have specific causes, respond to particular treatments, and may have specific prognostic implications.

EPIDEMIOLOGY

Incidence and Prevalence

Seizures are common in the general population, and about 1 in 10 people will experience a seizure in their lifetime. Most of these seizures are provoked by acute events and are not related to epilepsy. The overall annual incidence of acute symptomatic seizures, excluding febrile seizures, in developed countries is about 39 per 100,000 people. The incidence is higher in men and follows a bimodal age distribution, with its highest peak in the first year of life (up to 300 per 100,000), a nadir of 15 per 100,000 in the third and fourth decades of life, and a second peak rising to 123 per 100,000 after 75 years of age. These differences are attributable to the high incidence of acute symptomatic seizures associated with metabolic, infectious, and encephalopathic causes during the neonatal period, and of cerebrovascular, neoplastic, and degenerative diseases in elderly persons.

After headache, the epilepsies are the most frequent chronic neurologic condition seen in general practice worldwide. In developed countries, the prevalence of active epilepsy ranges from 5 to 7 per 1000 persons, and the median annual incidence is 45 per 100,000 (range, 30 to 67), varying by age and socioeconomic status.[2] One in 26 people will develop epilepsy during their lifetime (1 in 21 males and 1 in 28 females). The incidence of epilepsy peaks in children younger than 5 years at 60 to 70 per 100,000, decreases throughout adolescence to 30 per 100,000 in early adulthood, and rises again after the sixth decade, reaching a peak of 150 to 200 per 100,000 persons older than 75 years. The overall incidence of epilepsy appears to be increasing in recent decades because of a larger proportion of elderly persons in the population and an increasing incidence rate of epilepsy within the elderly population. Overall, the incidence and prevalence of the epilepsies are higher in developing countries, largely owing to a higher frequency of perinatal insults, trauma, and infectious disorders of the brain and to suboptimal treatment. In these countries, the median prevalence of active epilepsy is 12.5 per 1000 (range, 5 to 57 per 1000), and the annual incidence ranges from 78 to 190 per 100,000. Furthermore, the patterns of age-specific incidence are quite different in developing countries, where incidence peaks in young adults, not in elderly persons.

Risk Factors

Among all age groups, the top five risk factors for developing acute symptomatic seizures are head trauma (16%), stroke (16%), infectious disorders (15%), toxic-metabolic disorders (15%), and drug and alcohol withdrawal (14%) (Table 375-1).

The risk factors for developing epilepsy differ in adults and children. In childhood, excluding inherited epilepsies, the risk is increased by febrile seizures, head trauma, infections of the brain, mental retardation, cerebral palsy, and attention-deficit/hyperactivity disorder. Perinatal insults do not carry an increased risk for epilepsy unless they are accompanied by mental retardation or cerebral palsy.

In adults, risk factors for developing epilepsy can be identified in only one third of patients, in whom head trauma, brain infections, stroke, and dementia are the most common. The risk of developing epilepsy is increased more than 500-fold by a history of a military head injury, 30-fold by a severe civilian head injury (Chapter 371), 20-fold each by stroke (Chapter 379) and brain infections (Chapters 384 to 386), and 10-fold each for Alzheimer disease (Chapter 374), migraine (Chapter 370), and hypertension. In Latin America, the most frequently identified risk factor is brain infection. In endemic areas, neurocysticercosis (Chapter 333) accounts for about 10% of all newly diagnosed cases of epilepsy.

Pathobiology
Pathogenesis

The pathologic substrates and mechanisms underpinning initiation and propagation differ for focal and generalized seizures. In focal seizures, an aggregate of cortical or subcortical neurons develop high-frequency bursts of sodium-dependent action potentials caused by a shift in calcium conductance, thereby resulting in the typical EEG spike discharge (Fig. 375-1). Spread of bursting activity to other neurons is normally prevented by surrounding inhibitory mechanisms, such as hyperpolarization and inhibitory interneurons. When

TABLE 375-1	COMMON CAUSES OF ACUTE SYMPTOMATIC (PROVOKED) SEIZURES

METABOLIC

Hypernatremia, hyponatremia, hypocalcemia, hypoxia, hypoglycemia, nonketotic hyperosmolar hyperglycemia, renal failure

DRUG INDUCED

Theophylline, meperidine, tricyclic antidepressants, ephedra, ginkgo, phenothiazines, quinolones, β-lactams, isoniazid, antihistamines, cyclosporine, interferons, tacrolimus, cocaine, lithium, amphetamines

DRUG WITHDRAWAL

Alcohol, benzodiazepines, barbiturates

ENDOCRINE

Hyperthyroidism, hypothyroidism, peripartum

OTHER SYSTEMIC CONDITIONS

Sickle cell crisis, hypertensive encephalopathy, systemic lupus erythematosus, polyarteritis, eclampsia, high fever

CENTRAL NERVOUS SYSTEM DISORDERS

Trauma, stroke, intracerebral hemorrhage, encephalitis, abscess, bacterial meningitis

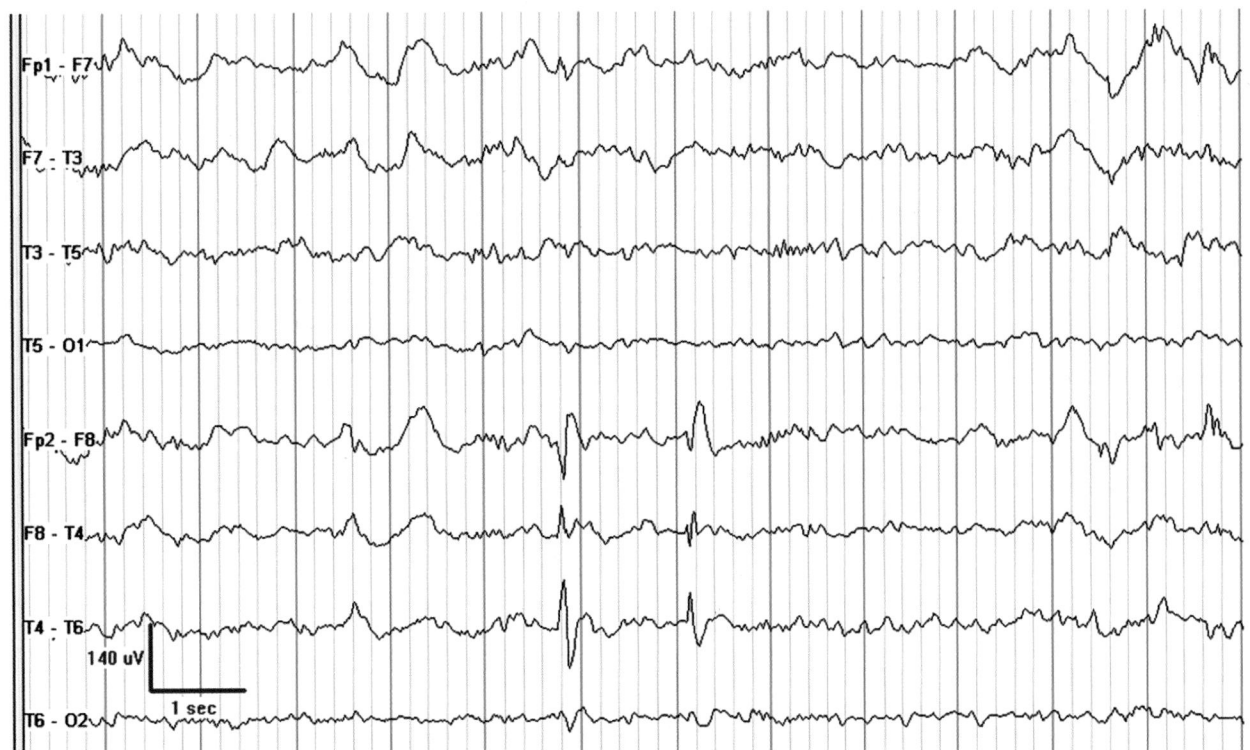

FIGURE 375-1. Selected electroencephalogram channels showing a typical right anterior temporal spike, the archetypal interictal footprint of temporal lobe epilepsy. The patient had right hippocampal sclerosis.

a sufficient number of neurons are engaged in sustained bursting, further excitatory phenomena ensue, including the increased release of excitatory neurotransmitters owing to presynaptic accumulation of Ca^{2+}, depolarization of surrounding neurons owing to increased extracellular K^+, and further neuronal activation caused by depolarization-induced activation of N-methyl-D-aspartate (NMDA) receptors. As excitation increases and inhibition decreases, additional neurons are recruited regionally and distantly, thereby resulting in seizure propagation. The mechanisms by which neurons develop a tendency toward anomalous bursting activity include alterations in neurotransmitters, membrane receptors, ion channels, second-messenger systems, and gene expression of various proteins.

Considerably less is known about the basic mechanisms underlying generalized seizures, which depend prominently on thalamocortical circuits. In absence seizures, the classic generalized spike-and-wave discharges seen on EEG (Video 375-1) are related to alterations in oscillatory rhythms generated by circuits that connect the thalamus and cortex and that involve T-type Ca^{2+} channels, which are located in the reticular nucleus of the thalamus. In generalized convulsive seizures, cortical neurons exhibit prolonged depolarization during the tonic phase, followed by rhythmic depolarization and repolarization during the clonic phase. Activation of NMDA receptors increases calcium Ca^{2+} influx, thereby leading to further neuronal excitation. The initiation and modulation of generalized convulsive seizures involve cholinergic, noradrenergic, serotonergic, and histaminergic afferents from the brain stem and basal forebrain structures, which modulate excitability of hemispheric motor mechanisms.

Genetics

One or more genetic factors play a role in 70% of people with epilepsy, and the risk of epilepsy is higher in first-degree relatives of patients with epilepsy than in the general population. For example, about 15% of patients have one or more first-degree relatives who also suffer from epilepsy, and 75% of those have just one affected relative. In a large population-based study, the cumulative incidence of epilepsy to age 20 years was 2.5-fold higher in siblings and 3.4-fold higher in offspring of patients with epilepsy. Transcranial magnetic stimulation shows increased cortical excitability in siblings of patients with epilepsy, even when these epilepsies are acquired.

Genetic causes of epilepsy may arise at a chromosomal or molecular level. Important chromosomal disorders producing epilepsy include the following syndromes: Angelman (15q11-q13), Down (trisomy 21), Klinefelter (XXY), Miller Dieker (17p), Pallister Killian (12p), Wolf-Hirschhorn (4p), and Ring 14 and 20.

All modes of inheritance are involved in epilepsy: mendelian epilepsy genes, which are rare but carry a high risk of epilepsy; rare variants associated with an intermediate risk and frequency of epilepsy; and common variants, which occur frequently but have a low independent risk of epilepsy.[3]

1. Conditions in which epilepsy forms part of a mendelian disorder (e.g., autosomal dominant, autosomal recessive, X-linked) comprise over 200 rare conditions with a high risk. These conditions include neurocutaneous disorders (Chapter 389), neurodegenerative disorders, inherited malformations of cortical development (Chapter 389), and inherited metabolic disorders. For example, genes have been identified in progressive myoclonic epilepsies (e.g., Unverricht-Lundborg disease, Lafora disease, and the neuronal ceroid lipofuscinosis), X-linked myoclonic epilepsy with mental retardation, and cortical malformation syndromes (e.g., polymicrogyria, pachygyria, periventricular nodular heterotopia).

2. Epilepsies that can be directly explained by single gene mutations are rare and account for only about 1% of all epilepsy cases. Over 30 genes have been identified in at least 15 epilepsy syndromes, including genetic epilepsy with febrile seizures plus, severe myoclonic epilepsy of infancy and related syndromes, benign familial neonatal convulsions, benign familial neonatal-infantile seizures, benign familial infantile seizures, juvenile myoclonic epilepsy, childhood absence epilepsy, West syndrome, early infantile epileptic encephalopathy with suppression burst, malignant migrating partial seizures of infancy, autosomal dominant nocturnal frontal lobe epilepsy, familial infantile myoclonic epilepsy, epilepsy + paroxysmal exercise-induced dyskinesia, familial lateral temporal lobe epilepsy, and familial focal epilepsy with variable foci. Genetic mutations may affect neuronal excitability, neuronal metabolism, synaptic function, or network development. Although most of these gene mutations affect ion channels (*SCN1A, SCN1B, SCN2A, KCNQ2, KCNQ 3, KCNT1, KCTD7*), other cellular functions affected include neurotransmitter release (*STXBP1*), neurotransmitter receptors (*CHRNA, CHRNB, GABRD, GABRG2, GRIN2A,*

GRIN2B), synaptic function (*SYN1*), glutamate transport (*SLC25A22*), gene regulation and transcription (*ARX*), cell adhesion (*PCDH19*), cell membrane function (*PRRT2, TBC1D24, DEPDC5*), protein kinase and cell energy function (*CDKL5, BCKDK, ATP1A2*), glucose transporter GLUT1 deficiency (*SLC2A1*), the mTOR pathway for cell growth and differentiation (*TSC1, TSC2*),[4] and neuronal signaling (*EFHC1, LGI1, PLCB1*). An increased genetic predisposition for epilepsy is associated with specific genotypes (*MTHFR, C677T*) in patients who develop post-traumatic epilepsy.

3. In some patients, the epilepsy is associated with "complex" disease genes. In this large group, which constitutes about 50% of all patients with epilepsy, multiple genes (common variants) with individually small but additive effects act in combination with environmental factors to produce an increased risk for epilepsy. Genes associated with generalized epilepsy in this category include *CHRM3, VRK2, ZEB2, SCN1A,* and *PNPO*.

CLINICAL MANIFESTATIONS

The clinical expression of seizures varies widely depending on the type of seizure and the areas of the brain involved by the epileptic activity. Accurate identification of the specific type of seizures is crucial because it dictates the type of medication the patient should receive. The signs and symptoms at the onset of individual seizures describe three categories: focal, generalized, and unknown onset (Fig. 375-2 and www.epilepsydiagnosis.org).[5]

Focal seizures are further subclassified according to their clinical expression. If awareness is impaired at any point, they are referred to as *focal impaired awareness seizures*. For example, patients who formerly were classified as having simple partial seizures are now classified as having *focal aware seizures*. Focal seizures are also subclassified by the presence or absence of motor phenomena at the onset into *focal motor or nonmotor seizures*. More granular categorizations of motor and nonmotor seizures are then provided according to the clinical expression.

Generalized seizures are classified primarily into *motor* (e.g., tonic, tonic-clonic, myoclonic seizures) and *nonmotor* (absence seizures). Finally, when it is not possible to determine whether the onset of seizures is focal or generalized, because of lack of information or ambiguous features, seizures are termed *unknown onset seizures*.

Focal Seizures

The seizure warning often consists of sensory, autonomic, or emotional symptoms that are experienced at the start of an observable seizure. The warning symptom is a focal seizure itself, and it is often missed because patients and clinicians focus on the more dramatic aspects of awareness or convulsion that follow. Careful inquiry about the occurrence of a warning is of crucial importance for three reasons. First, it points to a focal as opposed to a generalized onset, thereby implying an underlying focal structural or functional brain abnormality (e.g., a tumor) that requires further investigation. Second, focal seizures have important implications for therapy and for prognosis (see below). Third, the nature of the symptoms points to the area of the brain that gives rise to the seizure and that could be a target for surgical treatment (Table 375-2).

The neuronal discharge causing the focal seizure may remain confined to the region where it began (as a warning symptom or more objective focal event), or it may spread to involve additional brain areas. Thus a focal seizure originating in the cortical area that represents sensation of the hand (rolandic area) may begin with contralateral hand tingling and then progress to involve additional cortical regions ipsilaterally, producing more extensive sensory symptoms as well as clonic motor signs. Seizures of rolandic origin in particular exhibit a peculiar type of propagation, in which the seizure activity "marches" from hand to arm to leg area ipsilaterally, a process referred to as a jacksonian march. After the clonic motor activity ends, patients are often weak; a postictal or Todd paralysis may last hours or even a day or two, with gradual resolution (Video 375-2). The seizure may also propagate to distant ipsilateral or contralateral regions along known anatomic pathways.

In focal impaired awareness seizures, the person is not aware of self or environment during the seizure because of sufficient propagation of seizure activity to limbic and bilateral structures to cause alteration of awareness (Videos 375-3 and 375-4). Focal seizures originating from any region can impair awareness, and unilateral focal seizures can progress to involve bilateral brain areas and cause a bilateral convulsive seizure (Video 375-5). Such convulsive seizures usually take the form of bilateral tonic-clonic events rather than another type of generalized seizure (Table 375-3).

The evolution of the focal clinical seizure reflects the evolution of the EEG changes, which in turn reflects the pathophysiology of the process. A

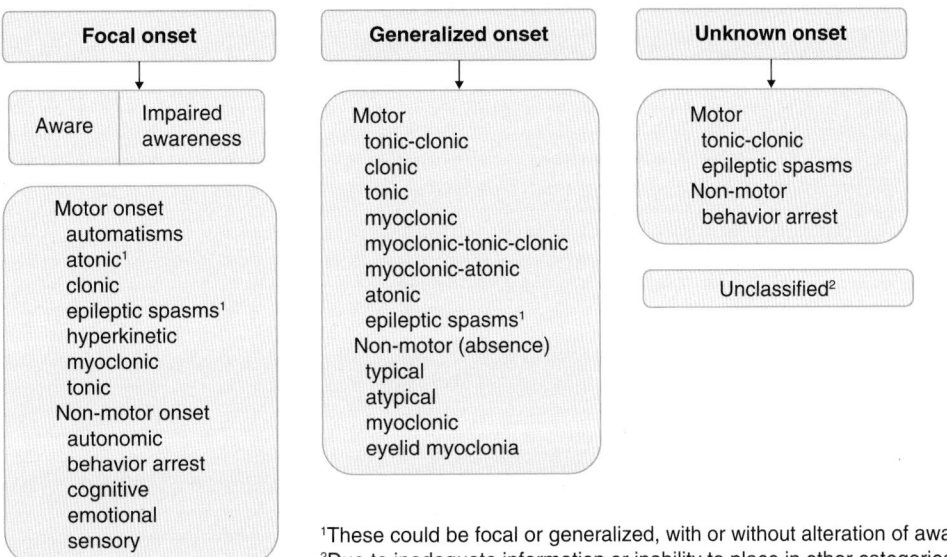

[1]These could be focal or generalized, with or without alteration of awareness
[2]Due to inadequate information or inability to place in other categories

FIGURE 375-2. International League Against Epilepsy Classification of Seizures. Seizures are classified by the earliest clinical signs and symptoms. The first question is whether the onset is focal, generalized, or unknown. *Focal* seizures can be described based on whether the most prominent feature at the onset consists of motor or nonmotor phenomena, or whether awareness is impaired at any point during the seizure. *Generalized* seizures are divided into motor and nonmotor.[6]

TABLE 375-2	CLINICAL MANIFESTATIONS OF DIFFERENT TYPES OF FOCAL SEIZURES AND AREAS OF THE BRAIN INVOLVED	
SEIZURE TYPE	**AREAS OF BRAIN INVOLVED**	**CLINICAL EXPRESSION**
MOTOR		
Clonic	Precentral rolandic	Contralateral regional clonic jerking, usually rhythmic and sustained, may spread to other body segments in jacksonian motor march; often accompanied by sensory symptoms in the same area
Tonic and Dystonic	Supplementary sensory-motor	Unilateral or bilateral tonic contraction of limbs causing postural changes; may exhibit classic fencing posture; may have speech arrest or vocalization
	Frontal	Contralateral head and eye version, salivation, speech arrest or vocalization; may be combined with other motor signs (as above) depending on seizure spread
NONMOTOR		
Somatosensory	Postcentral rolandic; parietal	Contralateral intermittent or prolonged tingling, numbness, sense of movement, desire to move, heat, cold, electric shock. Sensation may spread to other body segments.
	Parietal	Contralateral agnosia of a limb, phantom limb, distortion of size or position of body part
	Second sensory; supplementary sensory-motor	Ipsilateral or bilateral facial, truncal or limb tingling, numbness, or pain. Often involve lips, tongue, fingertips, feet
Gustatory	Parietal; rolandic operculum; insula; temporal lobe	Often unpleasant taste, acidic, metallic, salty, sweet, smoky
Olfactory	Mesial temporal; orbitofrontal	Often unpleasant, often with gustatory symptoms
Vestibular	Occipitotemporal-parietal junction; frontal lobe	Sensation of body displacement in various directions
Visual	Occipital	Contralateral static, moving, or flashing colored or uncolored lights, shapes, or spots. Contralateral or bilateral, partial or complete loss of vision
	Temporal; occipitotemporal-parietal junction	Formed visual scenes, faces, people, objects, animals
Autonomic, Cognitive and Emotional	Limbic structures: amygdala, hippocampus, cingulum, olfactory cortex, hypothalamus	Autonomic: abdominal rising sensation, nausea, borborygmi, flushing, pallor, piloerection, perspiration, heart rate changes including asystole, chest pain, shortness of breath, cephalic sensation, lightheadedness, orgasm Cognitive: déjà vu, jamais vu, depersonalization, derealization, dreamlike state, forced memory or forced thinking, apraxia, aphasia Emotional: fear, elation, sadness, anxiety, pleasure, crying, laughing, anger
Impaired Awareness	Usually extensive or bilateral involvement of limbic structures (see above)	Previously known as "complex partial seizures," characterized by lack of perception, knowledge or memory of events occurring during the seizure

Note: Focal seizures may evolve into bilateral tonic-clonic seizures.

simultaneous rhythmic, localized discharge (often in the 4- to 7-Hz range) becomes higher in amplitude and lower in frequency as the seizure continues (see Video 375-5). Some seizures that begin in the association cortex (e.g., frontal or parietal lobes) have bizarre or extremely brief clinical manifestations without postictal deficits and create diagnostic challenges (Videos 375-6, 375-7, and 375-8). The stereotyped nature of the clinical events, with identification of EEG changes if present, may be the only way to make an appropriate diagnosis. The diagnosis can be even more challenging if the seizure spreads to different cortical regions during different seizure episodes, thereby producing variable constellations of clinical findings at different times.

Focal seizures with or without impaired awareness can also occur as a series of single events without intervening normal behavior, thereby resulting in focal status epilepticus. Focal status epilepticus with impaired awareness seizures is characterized by prolonged confused behavior. EEG findings may be normal in a focal seizure without altered awareness, even in patients with status epilepticus, but the diagnosis is usually evident from the clinical features.

TABLE 375-3 GENERALIZED SEIZURES: CLASSIFICATION AND CLINICAL EXPRESSION

TYPE OF SEIZURE	SUBTYPE	CLINICAL EXPRESSION
MOTOR		
Tonic		Sustained increase in muscle contraction persisting for a few seconds to minutes
Clonic		Sustained regularly repetitive contractions involving the same muscle groups at a rate of 2-3 cycles per second
Tonic-clonic		A sequence consisting of a tonic followed by a clonic phase
Myoclonic	Myoclonic	Sudden, brief (<100 msec), shock-like, involuntary, single or multiple contractions of muscle groups of various locations
	Myoclonic atonic	A sequence consisting of a myoclonic followed by an atonic phase
	Myoclonic-tonic-clonic	A sequence consisting of a few myoclonic jerks followed by a tonic-clonic seizure, commonly seen in juvenile myoclonic epilepsy
Atonic		Sudden loss or diminution of muscle tone persisting 1-2 seconds, involving head, trunk, jaw, or limb muscles
NONMOTOR		
Absence	Typical	Abrupt cessation of activities, motionless, blank stare, and loss of awareness persisting about 10 seconds; attack ends suddenly, and patient resumes normal activities immediately.
	Atypical	Longer duration than typical absence, gradual onset and offset, often accompanied by myoclonic, tonic, atonic, and autonomic features as well as automatisms
Myoclonic	Myoclonic	Sudden, brief (<100 msec), shock-like, involuntary, single or multiple contractions of muscle groups of various locations
	Myoclonic atonic	A sequence consisting of a myoclonic followed by an atonic phase

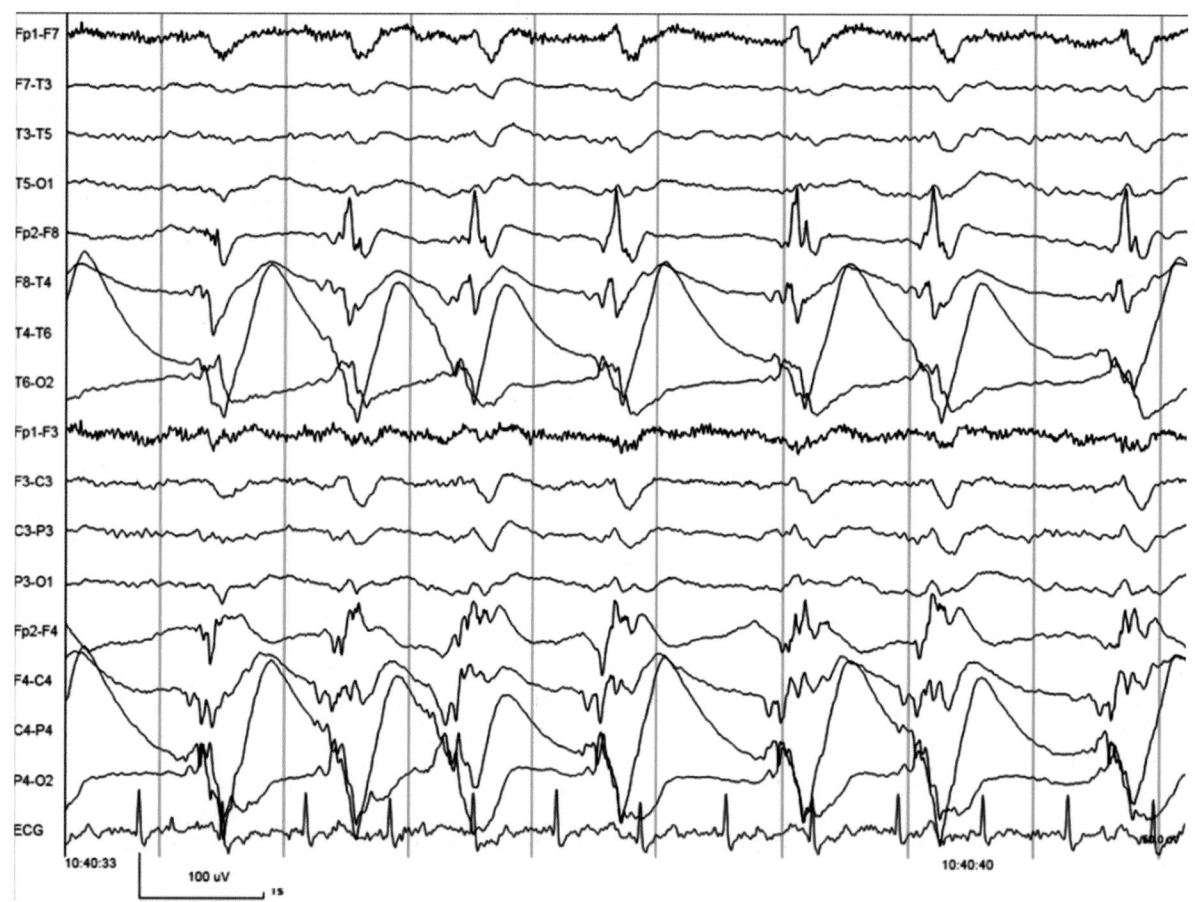

FIGURE 375-3. Focal right hemisphere nonconvulsive status epilepticus in a comatose patient with a large right hemisphere infarct.

In status epilepticus of focal impaired awareness seizures, EEG recordings show continuous abnormalities that are different than those seen in single seizures in that individual. The most common are a slow background with superimposed rhythmic high-amplitude sharp waves or repetitive rhythmic seizure discharges (Fig. 375-3). This type of status epilepticus is most frequent with frontal lobe seizures but can occur in temporal lobe or other seizures as well. The factors that precipitate status epilepticus are not well defined, nor are the implications for treatment or prognosis.

Nonconvulsive status epilepticus consists of a state of confusion or impaired mental status in patients with various neurologic diagnoses (e.g., trauma, stroke) in the acute intensive care unit setting (Video 375-9). It also denotes a

condition that can occur de novo in older adults without a precipitating cause and that is characterized by prolonged confusional episodes, which are caused by generalized slow spike-and-wave status epilepticus. Clinical suspicion should prompt an EEG study, which is essential for diagnosis.

Generalized Seizures
Generalized seizures rapidly affect both cerebral hemispheres, and their clinical expression is consistent with substantial involvement of both sides of the brain (see Table 375-3). Convulsive seizures, which are also referred to as grand mal seizures, consist of excessive abnormal muscle contractions that may be sustained or interrupted and usually are a combination of tonic and

clonic phases (generalized tonic-clonic seizures). This type of seizure may involve both hemispheres at the onset or may result from propagation of a focal seizure. These dramatic seizures often frighten witnesses and cause severe disruption of social interaction and development. They may begin with a "cry" as a result of abrupt air movement across the glottis from sudden tonic muscle contraction. The patient becomes diffusely stiff, usually with limb and body extension (Video 375-10). Breathing is suspended, cyanosis occurs, and urinary incontinence is common. After 15 to 45 seconds, the tonic activity gives way to clonic, rhythmic, sometimes asymmetrical jerking of all four extremities (Video 375-11). The rhythmic contractions gradually become slower in frequency until the event stops; the patient is apneic, comatose, and diaphoretic, but breathing with stridor and gasping begins within 60 seconds. Patients who have generalized tonic-clonic seizures in public often prompt bystanders to initiate resuscitation efforts, although such patients begin spontaneous respiration within 1 minute or so. Postictal stupor persists for a variable length of time. The patient generally sleeps for 2 to 8 hours and then complains of severe headache, sore muscles, a bitten tongue, and the inability to concentrate for a day or more. After generalized tonic-clonic seizures, some individuals have severe memory loss that gradually improves, sometimes over a period of weeks. Generalized tonic-clonic seizures also are a common expression of many metabolic, toxic, traumatic, or ischemic insults (see Table 375-1), but these provoked seizures do not qualify for the diagnosis of epilepsy.

Absence seizures, which are the second most common type of generalized seizure, are classified as typical or atypical (see Table 375-3). In typical absence seizures, patients experience an abrupt onset and termination of a momentary lapse of awareness. Patients have no perception of any aspect of the event and may or may not realize that some time was lost, although individuals often lose their train of thought. Because consciousness is abruptly lost and immediately regained, there is neither an initial symptom nor residual postictal symptoms. These seizures begin in childhood, and school teachers are often the first to notice them. In absence seizures, patients stop abruptly, stare vacantly, may have brief eye blinking or myoclonic movements, particularly if the event extends beyond 10 seconds (as judged by EEG), and regain function instantly (see Video 375-1). These seizures can occur many times a day but are not associated with progressive neurologic disease. Absences can also occur in a more continuous form as nonconvulsive status epilepticus with resultant confusion.

Atypical absence seizures occur in patients with extensive bilateral brain disease. The events are similar to typical absence seizures in terms of loss of contact, but the onset and termination are gradual instead of abrupt; the duration is longer; and there is more motor, autonomic, or automatic activity.

Myoclonic seizures consist of brief, irregular, unsustained episodes of sudden motor contraction (see Table 375-3) that can be focal (Video 375-12), with one limb involved, or bilateral and massive, with involvement of the face, both upper extremities, and the trunk. Consciousness may be preserved but can be difficult to evaluate because of the brevity of these seizures. Myoclonic seizures form part of three main clinical entities: juvenile myoclonic epilepsy, which starts in childhood or adolescence and often persists into adulthood; epilepsy with various combinations of absence and myoclonic seizures; and progressive myoclonic epilepsy, which occurs in the setting of degenerative or inherited syndromes with bilateral cerebral involvement and abnormal cerebral function. Myoclonic seizures most commonly occur in the morning after awakening and often increase in frequency to culminate in a generalized tonic-clonic seizure.

Atonic and tonic seizures are brief but extremely disabling motor events that are characterized by a sudden increase or decrease in muscle tone. They can result in falls and injuries with variable impairment of awareness. Such seizures frequently begin in children with diffuse central nervous system (CNS) disease and multiple types of seizures, but they persist during adulthood (Videos 375-13 and 375-14).

DIAGNOSIS

The basic diagnosis of seizures is established by the clinical history.[6] Although EEG, imaging, and laboratory studies are commonly required to determine the type of epilepsy, epilepsy syndrome, site of origin of focal seizures, and occurrence of nonepileptic seizures, the answer to the basic question of whether the patient's episodes are seizures or not rests almost entirely on a careful clinical history. The diagnosis of epilepsy can also be established by history, because epilepsy is defined as the occurrence of two unprovoked seizures or one unprovoked seizure in the context of a high underlying risk of recurrence or an epileptic syndrome.[7]

Differential Diagnosis

The first question facing clinicians is whether the episodes under consideration are indeed seizures. The diverse clinical expression of seizures encompasses a large differential diagnosis among conditions that produce episodic neurologic dysfunction (Table 375-4). Common conditions resembling seizures include syncope (Chapters 45 and 56), transient ischemic attacks (Chapter 379), migraine (Chapter 370), movement disorders (Chapter 382), and psychogenic nonepileptic seizures (see Table 375-4).[8]

A number of historical elements dramatically change the likelihood of this diagnosis. Three essential elements help determine whether an episode is a seizure (Table 375-5) and distinguish seizures from other causes of temporary loss of consciousness, especially syncope (Chapters 45 and 56).

TABLE 375-4 DISORDERS RESEMBLING SEIZURES

VASCULAR AND PERFUSION DISORDERS

Migraine, syncope, transient ischemic attack, transient global amnesia, arrhythmia/hypoperfusion

PSYCHIATRIC DISORDERS

Psychogenic nonepileptic seizures, panic disorder, dissociative disorder

MOVEMENT DISORDERS

Tics, paroxysmal dystonia, paroxysmal choreoathetosis, paroxysmal ataxia

SLEEP DISORDERS

Night terrors, sleep walking, sleep myoclonus, narcolepsy/cataplexy, rapid eye movement sleep intrusions

METABOLIC DISTURBANCES

Alcoholic blackouts, delirium tremens, hypoglycemia, hallucinogenic drugs, renal or hepatic encephalopathy

OTHER

Breath-holding spells in children, paroxysmal vertigo, migraine with recurrent abdominal pain and cyclic vomiting

TABLE 375-5 CLINICAL FEATURES THAT HELP DISTINGUISH A GENERALIZED TONIC CLONIC SEIZURE FROM SYNCOPE

	SEIZURE	SYNCOPE
Clinical context and circumstances	Neurologic or systemic conditions that predispose to seizures, family history of seizures. Mental fatigue, sleep deprivation, alcohol use or withdrawal, systemic illness	Cardiovascular disorders, dehydration, anemia. Family history of syncope
Triggers	Usually none (unless reflex epilepsy)	Orthostatic hypotension, venipuncture, painful and noxious stimuli, emotional stress, micturition, Valsalva maneuver
Clinical features		
• Onset	No warning unless there is a warning symptom. Abrupt loss of consciousness, generalized stiffening, and fall. Occurs in any position	Tiredness, nausea, diaphoresis, tunneling of vision. Loss of consciousness over few seconds and fall. Occurs usually standing
• Course	Prominent tonic phase then clonic movements lasting about 1 minute, cyanosis, labored breathing, may bite tongue or cheeks, sometimes urinary incontinence	Usually loss of tone, pallor, multifocal myoclonic jerks lasting <15 seconds, sometimes urinary incontinence, usually no tongue or cheek biting
• Offset	Postictal sleepiness and confusion lasting up to hours, headache, myalgia	Rapid recovery over seconds to less than few minutes, no confusion, headache, or myalgia. May have fatigue

1. The clinical context, including medical and family history and circumstances under which the episode occurred. For example, a strong family history of seizures and an event after sleep deprivation support a diagnosis of epileptic seizures. Conversely, a family history of syncope and an event occurring upon standing or with painful stimuli support a diagnosis of syncope.
2. Specific triggers or provoking factors. For example, events occurring with exposure to bright or flashing lights support a diagnosis of epileptic seizures.
3. A detailed clinical description of the event, including four key components:
   - What is the first symptom or sign (presence and type of warning symptom, evidence of focal seizure at onset)?
   - How does it evolve after onset (what happens during the seizure proper, what are the signs or symptoms, how long does it last)?
   - How does it end (gradually or abruptly)?
   - Are there any neurologic deficits after the seizure ends?

Because patients have limited or no recall, the history from others is crucial. Observers can contribute important information about the patient's activity, responses, and appearance, including changes in color, diaphoresis, respirations, vocalization, and muscle tone. Cell-phone videos obtained by witnesses can be very helpful in this regard. This information is required to characterize the type of seizure and to distinguish seizures from conditions that resemble seizures.

Migraine (Chapter 370) and focal seizures not only resemble each other but also coexist as comorbid conditions and share genetic susceptibility loci. Features that favor a diagnosis of seizures over classic migraine include an inconsistent occurrence of headache during the event, a brief duration, and the occurrence of more severe seizures. Myoclonus (Chapter 382) occurs in a variety of settings (e.g., metabolic encephalopathies) without any association with epilepsy or the EEG changes seen in myoclonic epilepsy.

Frontal lobe seizures arise predominantly during sleep and can have dramatic motor expression. They can be confused with nonepileptic psychogenic seizures, sleep disorders (Chapter 377), or movement disorders (Chapters 381 and 382). Video EEG monitoring may be necessary for diagnosis (see Videos 375-7 and 375-8).

Patients with panic attacks (Chapter 369) can experience events that mimic focal seizures with autonomic and emotional features. However, panic attacks usually have a longer duration, do not progress to more severe seizures, and can be linked to specific circumstances. Nevertheless, focal seizures with emotional symptoms are often misdiagnosed as panic attacks.

Psychogenic nonepileptic seizures are behaviors that resemble seizures and are often part of a conversion reaction (Chapter 369) precipitated by underlying psychological distress. Psychogenic seizures can be difficult to diagnose because they can mimic almost any type of epileptic seizure, and they often coexist with epilepsy in the same patient. An erroneous diagnosis of nonepileptic seizures poses a risk for inappropriate discontinuation of medication, resulting in status epilepticus. Conversely, an erroneous diagnosis of epileptic seizures in a patient with psychogenic seizures can result in complications of unnecessary therapy, excessive sedation, and consequent cardiorespiratory depression, often requiring intubation and respiratory support. Features suggesting nonepileptic psychogenic seizures include variable clinical manifestations across episodes, frequent and prolonged episodes, lack of response to antiseizure medication, out-of-phase upper and lower body movements, prominent pelvic thrusting, eye closure during convulsive movements, and lack of rigidity. Secondary gain is often evident, and there may be a history of sexual abuse. Nevertheless, the peculiarities of these attacks may require continuous video EEG monitoring for diagnosis.

Diagnostic Investigations

A detailed history, EEG recordings, and magnetic resonance imaging (MRI) can lead to a definitive diagnosis of epilepsy and can identify a cause in up to 50% of patients. In other patients, the information is insufficient or inconsistent, but the physiologic and CNS abnormalities surrounding the actual event allow it to be placed provisionally into a specific diagnostic category in about another 30% of patients. Continuous video EEG monitoring in an inpatient epilepsy unit can increase diagnostic accuracy.

Single Seizures

Single seizures can be classified as *unprovoked* (with no apparent immediate cause), or *acute symptomatic* (see Table 375-1), which are the known consequence of an acute condition, and investigations should be directed at the possible cause of these seizures. Evaluation of patients who present with a first unprovoked seizure, which may be an indicator of the onset of epilepsy,[9] includes either brain computed tomography (CT) or preferably MRI, which

reveals a possible cause in about 10% of patients. An EEG obtained after the seizure will demonstrate abnormalities with prognostic significance in 20 to 25% of these patients. Blood tests (including levels of serum electrolytes, glucose, calcium, and magnesium; tests of liver and kidney function; a complete blood cell count; and screening for suspected toxins) will reveal abnormalities in up to 15% of these patients but are often nonspecific. Lumbar puncture is indicated if CNS infections are suspected and in all patients infected with human immunodeficiency virus (HIV), even in the absence of clinical findings suggestive of infection.

Epilepsy
Electroencephalogram

The EEG is the keystone investigation in all patients with seizures and epilepsy. Between seizures, the EEG can assess overall brain function and the type, location, and amount of epileptiform (spike) discharges (see Fig. 375-1). The EEG is crucial in determining the epilepsy syndrome and choosing appropriate antiepileptic drugs. In focal epilepsies, the EEG often demonstrates focal slowing and spike discharges in the area of abnormality.

The EEG can establish the definitive diagnosis of epilepsy if electrical changes consistent with a seizure are recorded during a clinical seizure. However, the EEG may fail to demonstrate electrical changes during a typical clinical seizure if the seizure focus is too small (at least $10\ cm^2$ of cortical involvement is needed to create an EEG epileptiform change), if the seizure focus is deep or in the mesial or inferior surfaces of the brain, or if the event in question is not an epileptic seizure. The EEG is always abnormal during generalized convulsive and absence seizures.

The interictal initial EEG is normal in up to 60% of people with known epilepsy. However, epileptiform abnormalities occur in more than 80% of individuals with focal epilepsy if three or more EEG studies are performed. Interictal epileptiform discharges are more common and are easier to capture on the EEG when they are a manifestation of generalized rather than focal epilepsies (see Video 375-1).

The type of abnormality points to the epileptic syndrome. For example, the EEG can show hypsarrhythmia in West syndrome (see later) or the classic 3-Hz generalized spike wave in generalized epilepsies with absence seizures (see Table 375-3 and Video 375-1). In atypical absence seizures, the EEG demonstrates discharges that are slower than the 3-Hz spike and wave of typical absence seizures.

In some circumstances, it is imperative to record seizures with video EEG, such as in the evaluation of patients for epilepsy surgery and when the diagnosis of seizures is in question (Video 375-15; also see Video 375-7). Continuous video EEG monitoring for prolonged periods has made it possible to capture these events. Continuous EEG is also used in comatose patients in the intensive care unit setting when nonconvulsive seizures or status epilepticus are suspected and to monitor the effect of treatment.

Magnetoencephalography

Magnetoencephalography measures the small magnetic fields that are generated by electrical activity in the brain and approximates their location using mathematical models. Its use is largely restricted to the evaluation of patients for epilepsy surgery, in whom it is used for mapping interictal discharges and the localization of brain function when superimposed on brain MRI.

Imaging Studies

Brain MRI, which can demonstrate lesions in most patients whose epilepsy is associated with a structural cause, should be performed in essentially all patients with new-onset seizures. The most common lesions in adults with new-onset focal seizures are post-stroke or post-traumatic gliosis or encephalomalacia (50%), tumors (15%), vascular abnormalities (15%), developmental abnormalities (15%), and mesial temporal sclerosis (9%). The use of fluid-attenuated inversion recovery (FLAIR) (Fig. 375-4A) sequences increases the sensitivity to detect abnormalities of cortical development as well as hippocampal sclerosis, which point to the need for chronic anticonvulsant therapy or possible surgical treatment. Functional imaging procedures such as positron emission tomography (PET) for analysis of metabolism and single-photon emission computed tomography (SPECT) (see Fig. 375-4B) for determination of blood flow are also used to help localize areas of the brain to be targeted with epilepsy surgery.

Genetic Testing

Based on genetic test accuracy, implications for diagnosis and management, and ability to offer genetic counseling, an international consensus panel has

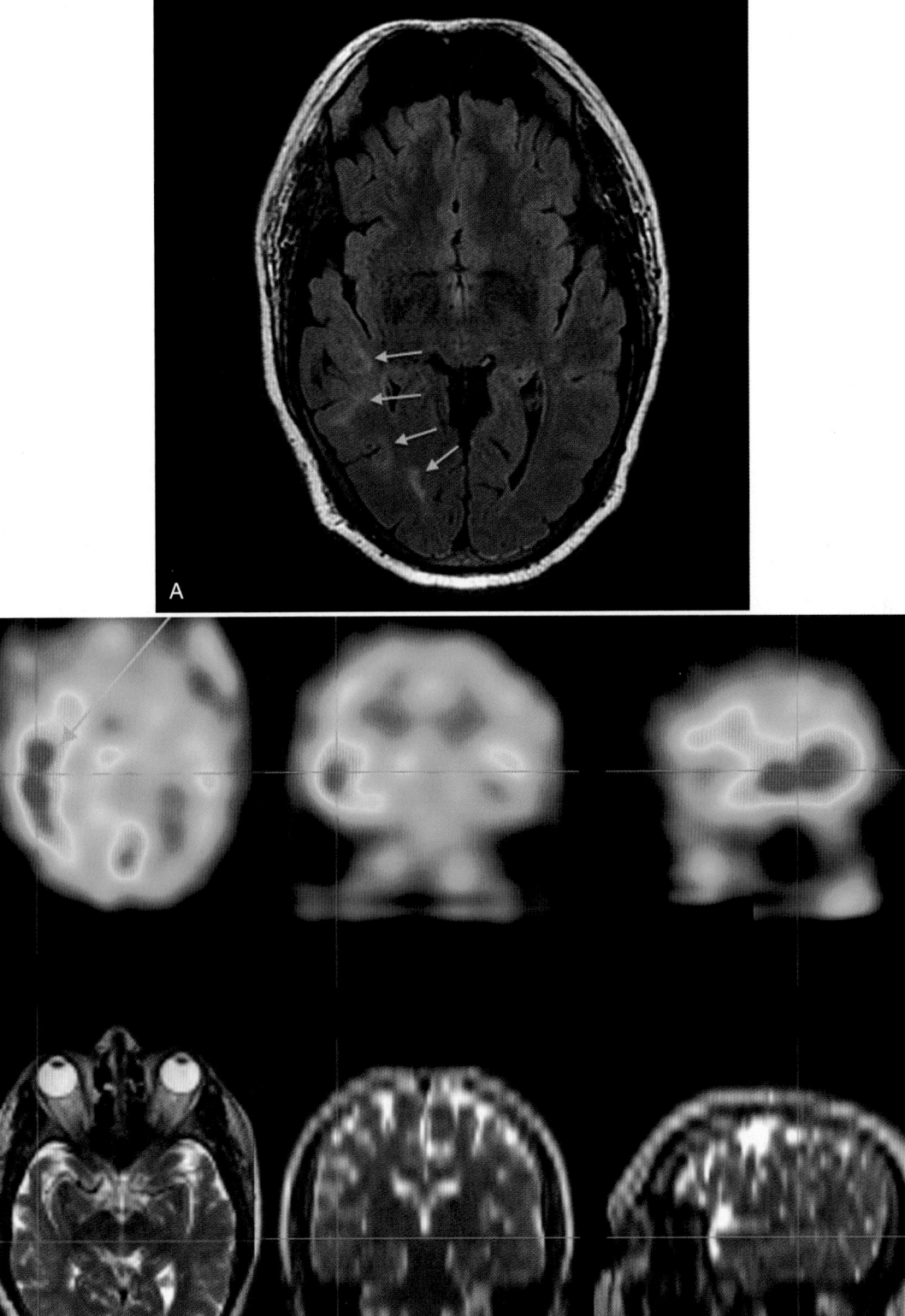

FIGURE 375-4. Imaging studies from a patient with dramatic motor seizures that were initially attributed incorrectly to psychogenic nonepileptic events (see Video 375-7). **A,** Fluid-attenuated inversion recovery (FLAIR) axial magnetic resonance image (MRI) demonstrating a large developmental cortical abnormality involving the midposterior right temporal lobe. **B,** Ictal SPECT during a seizure demonstrating an area of hyperperfusion that corresponds to the abnormality seen on the MRI and confirms the area where the seizure originated.

identified eight epilepsy syndromes of genetic origin for which genetic testing of patients is most useful: Ohtahara syndrome, early-onset infantile spasms, X-linked infantile spasms, Dravet syndrome, epilepsy and mental retardation limited to females, early-onset absence epilepsy, autosomal dominant nocturnal frontal lobe epilepsy, and epilepsy with paroxysmal exercise-induced dyskinesia. As with other conditions, the ethical aspects, the potential harms and benefits

of genetic testing, and the need for pre- and post-testing counseling must be carefully considered.

Specific Epileptic Syndromes and Clinical Entities
There are a large number of age-related epileptic syndromes, of which all but six begin or occur in infancy and childhood (Table 375-6). In addition, specific

TABLE 375-6 EPILEPTIC SYNDROMES AND DISTINCTIVE CLINICAL ENTITIES

BY AGE AT ONSET

Neonatal Period
Benign familial neonatal epilepsy
Early myoclonic encephalopathy
Ohtahara syndrome

Infancy
Epilepsy of infancy with migrating partial seizures
West syndrome
Myoclonic epilepsy in infancy
Benign infantile epilepsy
Benign familial infantile epilepsy
Dravet syndrome
Myoclonic encephalopathy in nonprogressive disorders

Childhood
Genetic epilepsy with febrile seizures plus (GEFS+, these can also start in infancy)
Panayiotopoulos syndrome
Epilepsy with myoclonic atonic (previously astatic) seizures
Benign epilepsy with centrotemporal spikes
Autosomal dominant nocturnal frontal lobe epilepsy
Late-onset childhood occipital epilepsy
Epilepsy with myoclonic absences
Lennox-Gastaut syndrome
Epileptic encephalopathy with continuous spike and wave during sleep
Landau-Kleffner syndrome
Childhood absence epilepsy

Adolescence-Adult
Juvenile absence epilepsy
Juvenile myoclonic epilepsy
Epilepsy with generalized tonic-clonic seizures alone
Progressive myoclonus epilepsies
Autosomal dominant partial epilepsy with auditory features
Other familial temporal lobe epilepsies

LESS SPECIFIC AGE RELATIONSHIP

Familial focal epilepsy with variable foci (childhood to adult)
Reflex epilepsies

DISTINCTIVE CLINICAL ENTITIES

Mesial temporal lobe epilepsy with hippocampal sclerosis
Rasmussen syndrome
Gelastic seizures with hypothalamic hamartoma
Hemiconvulsion-hemiplegia-epilepsy

GEFS+ = generalized epilepsy with febrile seizures plus.

clinical entities represent diagnostically meaningful forms of epilepsy, with specific implications for treatment, especially surgery, and also categorize for structural-metabolic causes, epilepsies of unknown cause, and conditions characterized by seizures that are not a form of epilepsy (e.g., febrile seizures). The diagnosis of epileptic syndromes and clinical entities is based on the types of seizures, the setting in which seizures occur, the patient's neurologic and cognitive status, age at onset, family history, and results of diagnostic studies, including EEG and MRI. The selection of specific drugs and surgical treatment depends on the types of seizures present (Table 375-7). The need for lifelong treatment, the risk for genetic transmission, the likelihood of concurrent neurologic diseases, the risk for comorbid conditions, and the long-term prognosis are critical factors that can be addressed only with knowledge of the specific epileptic syndrome or entity.

Neonatal and Infantile Epilepsy Syndromes

Self-limited neonatal convulsions occur in previously healthy newborns on about day 5 as focal or generalized tonic seizures. Mutations in two potassium channel genes (*KCNQ2, KCNQ3*) have been associated with this syndrome. Potassium channel regulation may be age dependent and therefore account for the age-related appearance of the seizures. The EEG shows rhythmic slow-wave activity or spiking with seizures. The seizures are refractory to treatment, are recurrent over a brief interval, and disappear within a month. About 90% of such infants subsequently have normal development, whereas 10 to 20% have subsequent seizures.

Genetic epilepsy with febrile seizures plus, which can start in infancy or childhood, is a syndrome that consists of febrile seizures in combination with other nonfebrile types of seizures, including myoclonic, absence, atonic, tonic-clonic,

and focal seizures, expressed with variable severity in different families. Mutations have been identified in at least four genes for voltage-gated ion sodium channels (*SCN1A, SCN9A, SCN1B, SCN2A*), two for GABA receptors (*GABRD, GABRG2*), one for synaptic vesicle function (*STX1B*), and one for cell adhesion function (*PCDH19*).

Dravet syndrome (severe myoclonic epilepsy of infancy) starts in the first year of life with myoclonic seizures plus other seizure types, including absence, atonic, and focal. In this devastating syndrome, the seizures are resistant to treatment and are accompanied by developmental and cognitive decline. Mutations in the *SCN1A* sodium channel have been identified and occur de novo in 95% of patients.

West syndrome comprises a triad of epileptic spasms, developmental arrest, and an EEG pattern called hypsarrhythmia (a markedly abnormal EEG pattern with high-amplitude slowing and superimposed multifocal spikes, polyspikes, and spike and slow-wave complexes). It appears before the age of 12 months and ceases by 5 years of age, often to be replaced by other epilepsy syndromes such as Lennox-Gastaut syndrome. Tuberous sclerosis (Chapter 389) and hypoxia are among the common causes, but a cause may not be found. Associated abnormalities often include developmental delay, porencephaly, atrophic lesions, calcifications, and agenesis of the corpus callosum. West syndrome and early infantile epileptic encephalopathy have been associated with mutations in genes involved in a number of neurotransmitter and cellular functions (*ARX, CDKL5, STXBP1*).

Childhood Epilepsy Syndromes

Childhood absence epilepsy begins before age 12 years, and its onset peaks at age 5 to 7 years, with a strong genetic tendency. It is more common in girls than boys and is characterized by very frequent daily absence seizures (up to hundreds per day), rarely with other types of generalized seizures. It occurs in the setting of otherwise normal brain structure and function, and it is self-limited in about 40% of cases. The seizures are accompanied by a characteristic 3-Hz spike-and-wave EEG discharge, which appears in short bursts between seizures and in continuous runs during seizures. Remission usually occurs before the age of 12 years, but generalized tonic-clonic seizures occasionally may develop in adolescence. In early-onset absence epilepsy, mutations have been found in genes related to GABA receptors (*GABRA1, GABRG2*) and GLUT1 glucose transporter (*SLC2A1*).

Lennox-Gastaut syndrome is one of the most severe childhood epilepsies. It starts before age 8 years (peak from 3 to 5 years) and is characterized by a triad of mental retardation, multiple types of generalized seizures (atypical absence, generalized tonic-clonic, tonic, atonic), focal seizures that are highly resistant to treatment, and a typical EEG pattern of slow spike and wave (slower than the typical 3 Hz associated with absence seizures) and bursts of fast rhythms at 10 to 12 Hz during sleep. Structural brain abnormalities account for about 70% of cases, and it evolves from earlier syndromes such as West or Ohtahara in up to 30% of patients.

Childhood epilepsy with centrotemporal spikes (benign rolandic epilepsy) starts between 3 and 13 years of age and is characterized by almost exclusively nocturnal focal motor or sensory seizures that have a facial or oral onset and often evolve to convulsive seizures. Nearly 50% of cases have a family history of epilepsy, but most patients have no known brain abnormality. The EEG shows spiking in the centrotemporal region. Behavioral and cognitive deficits, which occur during the period of active epilepsy, resolve when epilepsy remits. The disorder does not always require treatment, and it usually remits spontaneously.

Adolescence and Adult Epilepsy Syndromes and Entities

Juvenile myoclonic epilepsy is one of the most common generalized genetic epilepsies. It usually starts in the second decade with myoclonic and generalized tonic-clonic seizures in cognitively intact males and females. Mutations in γ-aminobutyric acid (GABA) receptors (*GABRG1*) and in genes related to neuronal signaling (*EFHC1*) can be found. Seizures typically occur in the morning immediately after awakening. The seizures are especially linked to sleep deprivation and tend to appear in college students. A proportion of these patients have absence seizures as well. The EEG typically shows fast (4 to 6 Hz) generalized spike and wave. Lifetime treatment is generally needed.

Mesial temporal lobe epilepsy with hippocampal sclerosis is the most common epilepsy to produce focal impaired awareness seizures in adults. It is characterized by recurrent focal limbic seizures (see Table 375-2), with and without impaired awareness, that originate in mesial temporal and limbic structures. Up to 70% of patients have a risk factor such as lengthy and complicated seizures before the age of 4 years, frequently associated with fever or encephalitis, meningitis, or trauma. However, the characteristic seizures generally begin

TABLE 375-7 ANTIEPILEPTIC DRUG SELECTION BY SEIZURE TYPE

SEIZURE TYPE	COMMONLY USED (ALPHABETICAL ORDER)	LESS COMMONLY USED (ALPHABETICAL ORDER)	EFFECTIVENESS (GRADE A RECOMMENDATION)	
			NEW-ONSET SEIZURES	REFRACTORY SEIZURES
Focal seizures with or without impaired awareness or evolution to bilateral tonic clonic seizures	Carbamazepine Gabapentin Lacosamide Lamotrigine Levetiracetam Oxcarbazepine Phenytoin Tiagabine Topiramate Valproate Zonisamide Clobazam	Acetazolamide Brivaracetam Clonazepam Clorazepate Eslicarbazepine Felbamate Perampanel Phenobarbital Primidone Rufinamide	Carbamazepine*† Gabapentin*† Lamotrigine*† Levetiracetam† Oxcarbazepine*† Phenobarbital* Phenytoin*† Topiramate* Valproate* Zonisamide†	Carbamazepine† Gabapentin* Lamotrigine* Levetiracetam* Oxcarbazepine* Phenobarbital† Phenytoin† Tiagabine* Topiramate* Valproate† Zonisamide*
Generalized convulsive seizures (clonic, tonic or tonic-clonic seizures)	Carbamazepine Lamotrigine Levetiracetam Oxcarbazepine Phenytoin Topiramate Valproate Zonisamide	Acetazolamide Clonazepam Clorazepate Felbamate Phenobarbital Primidone	Carbamazepine† Lamotrigine* Levetiracetam* Phenytoin† Valproate*	Carbamazepine† Lamotrigine* Levetiracetam* Phenytoin† Topiramate* Valproate*
Absence seizures	Ethosuximide Lamotrigine Valproate Topiramate	Acetazolamide Clonazepam Phenobarbital Primidone	Ethosuximide*† Lamotrigine* Valproate*†	
Myoclonic seizures	Clonazepam Levetiracetam Valproate Zonisamide	Phenobarbital	Valproate†	

*Supported by class I evidence, American Academy of Neurology.
†Supported by class I evidence for initial monotherapy, International League Against Epilepsy.
‡Often the "standard" of comparison, without evidence of effectiveness by randomized controlled trials.

some years later. Although most cases are sporadic, familial forms of mesial temporal lobe epilepsy have been associated with a susceptibility locus on chromosome 18(P11.31).

Various components of the mesial temporal limbic network (including the hippocampus, entorhinal cortex, amygdala, neocortical areas of the frontal and temporal lobes, and dorsal medial thalamus) are probably involved in the pathogenesis of these seizures. Mesial temporal sclerosis, also called hippocampal sclerosis, is characterized by neuronal loss and gliosis, mostly in the CA1 and CA3 regions of the hippocampus, with mossy fiber reorganization that is seen as sprouting of neuropeptide Y and dynorphin interneurons into the inner third of the dentate molecular layer. Whether hippocampal sclerosis is the cause or the result of seizures (or both) is not known. However, up to 12% of children with febrile status epilepticus have MR evidence of hippocampal injury, thereby suggesting a causal association. The seizures of mesial temporal lobe epilepsy often begin at 5 to 15 years of age. Typical seizures with impaired awareness and emotional symptoms predominate, often starting with a warning of a rising epigastric sensation or a feeling of déjà vu, followed by oral and alimentary automatisms and later by contralateral arm dystonia and ipsilateral arm automatisms. The seizures persist for several minutes, rarely generalize, and typically occur several times a month. Warning symptoms without subsequent seizures are common. Hippocampal atrophy and increased hippocampal signal are best seen on T2-weighted and FLAIR coronal MRI sequences, and interictal hypometabolism is seen in the temporal lobe on PET. Verbal or visual memory impairment corresponds to primary involvement of the dominant or nondominant hippocampus, respectively. EEG recordings show temporal lobe spikes interictally as well as rhythmic 4- to 7-Hz rhythmic discharges over the appropriate temporal lobe during seizures.

Seizures with Less Specific Age Relationship

Reflex seizures are triggered reliably by specific simple (e.g., flashing lights, sound) (see Video 375-15) or elaborate (e.g., reading) stimuli. The mechanisms are diverse and may involve cortical and brain stem pathways, cortical dysregulation of extracellular calcium concentrations, and an imbalance between excitatory and inhibitory neurotransmitters. Most patients have no structural abnormalities. Visual-sensitive seizures (triggered by light or visual patterns) are the most common type of reflex seizures. They occur most commonly in females, and their incidence peaks around puberty, when they represent 4%

to 7% of all new cases of epilepsy. Other triggers of reflex seizures include specific thoughts, actions, reading, tactile stimuli, adopting certain positions, eating, listening to music, startle, and contact with hot water. The triggered seizures can be myoclonic, convulsive, atonic, or focal, depending on the triggering stimulus. Avoiding the offending stimulus is crucial to avoid seizures, emphasizing the importance of careful questioning about seizure triggers in patients with epilepsy.

TREATMENT

The treatment of seizures and epilepsy is guided by accurate knowledge of the type of seizure and epileptic syndrome, the probability of recurrent seizures, the likelihood and severity of psychosocial or physical consequences with further seizures, and whether the benefit from treatment substantially outweighs the risks for side effects.[10] It is important to identify and correct any environmental, physiologic, or lifestyle factors, such as sleep deprivation and irregular sleep habits, and alcohol abuse, which can lower the seizure threshold and trigger seizures in patients with epilepsy.

Single Unprovoked Seizures

The decision to treat single unprovoked seizures depends on the likelihood of recurrence according to prognostic variables (see Prognosis) and on the individual patient's profile and preference.[11] The risk of recurrence (20 to 45%) is highest in the first 2 years and is higher in patients with prior brain insults or abnormalities on EEG or MRI. Antiepileptic drug treatment after a first seizure reduces the absolute risk of having a second seizure in the short term by 33%, corresponding to a number needed to treat (NNT) of 3. However, at least two randomized trials have shown that deferring antiepileptic drug treatment until additional seizures occur achieves a similar long-term seizure outcome as does treating the first seizure.[A1] Therefore the decision to treat the first seizure should be individualized based on the patient's preference, the risk for and impact of recurrent seizures (e.g., driving and employment), and the risk for medication side effects, which occur in 7 to 30% of patients (Table 375-8).

Acute Provoked Seizures

Seizures that are provoked by specific exposures are usually self-limited and not associated with an enduring seizure tendency, so the primary therapeutic consideration should be identification and treatment of the underlying disorder (see Table 375-1). However, the risk of developing epilepsy after febrile seizures is about 10 times that of the general population. If antiepileptic drugs are

TABLE 375-8 CHARACTERISTICS OF MAJOR ANTIEPILEPTIC DRUGS

NAME	TOTAL MILLIGRAMS PER DAY (USUAL SCHEDULE)	THERAPEUTIC RANGE (µg/mL)	PROMINENT SIDE EFFECTS	OTHER EFFECTS	OTHER ISSUES
Brivaracetam	50-200 (bid)	Not well established	Mood change, irritability, lethargy	Serum concentration is decreased by phenytoin and carbamazepine	Can be up-titrated rapidly
Carbamazepine	400-1600 (bid)	4-12	Diplopia, fatigue, hyponatremia	Mood stabilizer	Enzyme inducer
Clobazam	10-40 (od, bid)	0.25-0.75	Sedation, depression	Metabolite desmethylclobazam has significant clinical effect	
Ethosuximide	750-1250 (daily, bid)	40-100	Ataxia, lethargy	Rash, bone marrow suppression	
Gabapentin	600-6000 (tid, qid)	2-12	Fatigue	Treatment of pain	No drug interactions
Lacosamide	200-400 (bid)	Not well established	Dizziness, diplopia, tremor	Minor prolongation of PR interval	Low risk of drug interaction
Lamotrigine	100-600 (bid)	4-18	Insomnia, headache, tremor, anxiety	Mood stabilizer	Risk for Stevens-Johnson syndrome; slow start-up
Levetiracetam	500-3000 (bid)	3-63	Mood change, irritability, lethargy		No drug interactions
Oxcarbazepine	300-2400 (tid)	6-40	Diplopia, hyponatremia, sedation	Mood stabilizer	
Perampanel	2-12 (od)	Not well established	Psychiatric and behavioral adverse reactions	Serum concentration is decreased by phenytoin and carbamazepine	Hormonal contraceptives may be less effective
Phenobarbital	60-240 (at bedtime)	15-40	Fatigue, depression, sedation	Joint pain	Enzyme inducer
Phenytoin	200-600 (bid)	10-20	Fatigue, hirsutism, gingival hypertrophy	Treatment of some pain	Enzyme inducer
Rufinamide	400-3200 (bid)	5-48	Mood change, irritability, lethargy	Contraindicated in familial short QT syndrome	Hormonal contraceptives may be less effective
Topiramate	50-600 (bid)	2-12	Anorexia, weight loss, kidney stones, speech disturbance, distal paresthesias	Headache prophylaxis, mood stabilizer	Enzyme inducer
Valproate	4000 (bid or tid)	50-100	Weight gain, hair loss, tremor	Headache prophylaxis, mood stabilizer	Enzyme inhibitor, parkinsonian effects in elderly patients
Zonisamide	100-600 (at bedtime)	10-40	Anorexia, kidney stones, dizziness, distal paresthesias	Mood stabilizer	

needed to treat seizures acutely, they usually can be discontinued after the patient has recovered from the primary illness. Some acute conditions like stroke (Chapter 379), brain infections (Chapters 384 to 386), and trauma (Chapter 371) can produce both acute provoked seizures and a higher than 60% risk of recurrent seizures (which establish the diagnosis of epilepsy), thereby warranting the consideration of long-term antiepileptic drug treatment to prevent or reduce future seizures. To date, however, randomized controlled trials have not been able to demonstrate that antiepileptic drugs prevent the development of epilepsy in these conditions.

Epilepsy Syndromes with a Favorable Course

In syndromes such as childhood epilepsy with centrotemporal spikes and some types of childhood occipital epilepsy, seizures are mild, infrequent, or exclusively nocturnal, and they remit spontaneously, thereby making treatment generally unnecessary. In selected cases, treatment may be desirable to prevent recurrences and to help alleviate parental concerns. In such cases, drug treatment is usually limited to 1 to 2 years regardless of interictal EEG abnormalities, which can persist long after seizures have remitted. The recommended antiepileptic drugs are those used in focal epilepsy in children, including oxcarbazepine, carbamazepine, valproate, gabapentin, lamotrigine, and topiramate. Some patients with reflex seizures may require antiseizure medication, which should be chosen according to seizure type (see Table 375-7).

Choice of Antiepileptic Drugs

The ultimate goal of treatment is to obtain complete freedom from seizures without side effects. Some of the newer antiepileptic drugs (see Table 375-8) are better tolerated and have better pharmacokinetics than older drugs, but there is no evidence to support superior efficacy of one drug over another. The choice of medication depends on the type of seizure and epilepsy syndrome (thereby making a correct diagnosis crucial) and the medication's side effects, cost, and ease of use.[A2] Specific drugs are effective for specific types of seizures, and some drugs can worsen other types of seizures. Knowledge of individual drugs as they relate to age, sex, comorbid conditions, drug interactions, sedation, tolerance, mood, and withdrawal is critical in the drug selection process (see Table 375-7). For example, levetiracetam is effective and generally well-tolerated for partial-onset epilepsy.[A3]

Drugs that cause enzyme induction (e.g., carbamazepine, phenytoin, phenobarbital, oxcarbazepine, topiramate) or inhibition (e.g., valproic acid) can be difficult to manage when additional medications, such as oral contraceptives and oral anticoagulants, are used for independent conditions. For these clinical settings and in elderly patients, drugs such as gabapentin, levetiracetam, and brivaracetam are particularly useful because they have fewer drug interactions.

In patients with newly diagnosed focal epilepsy, the underlying cause influences the response to antiepileptic drugs. The likelihood of achieving seizure freedom is higher for patients with vascular malformations, stroke, and tumors (63 to 78%), and lower for patients with hippocampal sclerosis and malformations of cortical development (40 to 50%). Among patients presenting with a new diagnosis of epilepsy, about 65% achieve seizure remission on antiepileptic drug treatment. Of these patients, about 45 to 50% achieve seizure remission with the first antiepileptic drug, 10 to 15% with the second, 1% with the third, and 3% with a combination of two or more antiepileptic drugs.

Effective treatments are emerging using novel antiseizure targets and mechanisms. In a randomized trial comparing the mTOR inhibitor everolimus versus placebo in patients with tuberous sclerosis (Chapter 389), for example, everolimus reduced seizures by 25%.[A4] Cannabidiol can significantly reduce seizures in patients with Dravet syndrome and Lennox Gastaut syndrome.[A5,A6] Stiripentol, a lactate dehydrogenase inhibitor in astrocytes and neurons, also may be useful in epilepsy.

Because the likelihood of achieving subsequent seizure remission is small if two drug trials fail, the 35% or so of patients who fail adequate trials of two antiepileptic drugs are considered to be drug resistant. In these patients, other forms of treatment, including surgery, should be considered. The first consideration in managing apparently drug-resistant patients is to ensure that the diagnosis is correct and the antiepileptic drug is appropriate. Other common causes of a poor response to drugs include poor adherence to antiepileptic drugs, sleep deprivation, alcohol use, fatigue, emotional stress, systemic illnesses, use of concurrent medications, and nonepileptic seizures. After addressing these factors, patients who remain drug resistant should be considered potential candidates for surgical therapy.[12]

Surgical Treatment

Surgical treatment entails resection or disconnection of the cerebral region that contains the seizure focus.[13] Removal of an epileptogenic region requires accurate identification of the region as well as documentation of a lack of functional consequences after its removal. Video EEG monitoring with seizure recording from scalp electrodes, MRI protocols with special attention to areas commonly associated with refractory seizures (e.g., the medial temporal and frontal lobes), and functional neuroimaging, including PET and SPECT, are used to make the assessment. In temporal lobe epilepsy, neuropsychological evaluation is essential to localize dysfunction and establish the level of function in the region considered for resection. EEG localization of the region of seizure onset and mapping of brain function may require the surgical implantation of intracranial electrodes for recording and for stimulating cortical tissue. These procedures are performed by multidisciplinary teams in specialized epilepsy centers.

Epilepsy surgery interventions that have been subjected to rigorous randomized trials include temporal lobe resection compared with medical therapy for mesial temporal lobe epilepsy,[A7] radiosurgery ablation, and neurostimulation (of the vagal nerve, trigeminal nerve, thalamus, hippocampus, or cerebral cortex). The most dramatic surgical effect is seen for temporal lobe resection compared with medical therapy. In one randomized trial, 64% of surgical patients and only 8% of medical patients became seizure free at 1 year. Among these patients, clinically meaningful improvement in quality of life was achieved in 56% of patients treated surgically compared with only 11% of patients treated medically.[A8] In another randomized trial of patients with drug-resistant temporal lobe epilepsy, surgery plus continued antiepileptic medications was successful in eliminating seizures in 11 of 15 patients at 2 years, whereas all medically treated patients continued to have seizures at 2 years. As a result, patients with drug-resistant temporal lobe epilepsy should be evaluated for epilepsy surgery. In a randomized trial of children undergoing various types of surgical procedures, freedom from seizures was achieved in 37% of patients after surgery compared with none of the patients treated with medication.[A9] Nonrandomized studies demonstrate enduring freedom from seizures at 10 years or more after hemispheric disconnection (61%), temporal lobe resection (64%), parieto-occipital resection (46%), and frontal lobe resection (27%). In the long term, about 65% of patients undergoing surgery achieve sustained seizure freedom (40 to 50% immediately after surgery, and 15% after a period of initial seizures), 16% have a fluctuating course of relapsing-remitting seizures, and 18% never become seizure free. Palliative surgical procedures such as callosotomy and multiple subpial transections have lower success rates and are used when surgical resection of the seizure focus is not possible. Promising less invasive surgical therapies for epilepsy include various types of electrical brain stimulation,[A10] laser interstitial therapy, and focused ultrasound. However, standard surgical resection may be preferable to radiosurgery in patients with temporal lobe epilepsy.[A11]

Status Epilepticus

Status epilepticus is a medical emergency in which seizures occur continuously or repeatedly without intervening resumption of consciousness. The diagnosis is established after 5 minutes in generalized tonic-clonic seizures and 10 minutes in focal impaired awareness seizures, although long-term neurologic consequences are not likely to occur unless status epilepticus persists for 30 minutes for generalized tonic-clonic seizures or 60 minutes for focal impaired awareness seizures. Most episodes of status epilepticus are caused by an acute brain insult in persons without underlying epilepsy, so a cause should be sought promptly. In one study, the most common cause was autoimmune encephalitis, but 50% remained cryptogenic even after detailed evaluation. After securing the airway and stabilizing cardiovascular function, immediate intervention with parenteral agents is needed to stop the seizures. In adults in status epilepticus treated before arriving at the hospital, 10 mg of intramuscular midazolam is more effective and at least as safe as 4 mg of intravenous (IV) lorazepam for stopping seizures. Early status epilepticus (first 5 to 10 minutes) can be controlled in about 70% of patients with IV lorazepam (0.1 mg/kg given at 2 mg/min), diazepam (5 to 10 mg IV bolus given at 5 mg/min), clonazepam (1 mg IV bolus, given at 0.5 mg/min), or phenobarbital (10 mg/kg, given at 100 mg/min). Established status epilepticus (10 to 30 minutes) that does not respond to such treatment can be successfully treated in 15% of patients with IV phenytoin (15 mg/kg at a rate of 50 mg/min), fosphenytoin (15 to 20 mg/kg at a rate of 150 mg/min), valproate (30 mg/kg at 5 mg/kg/min), levetiracetam (30 mg/kg over 10 minutes), or lacosamide (200 to 400 mg over 3 to 5 minutes). Patients who do not respond to these measures have refractory status epilepticus and require treatment in an intensive care unit with respiratory support and IV sedation sufficient to suppress the epileptic EEG discharges, as well as continuous IV infusion of midazolam (0.1 to 0.4 mg/kg/hour), propofol (1 to 3 mg/kg/hour), pentobarbital (0.5 to 3 mg/kg/hour), or thiopental (3 to 5 mg/kg/hour). In refractory cases, general anesthesia for 24 hours is used. In children, convulsive status epilepticus can be controlled within 10 minutes in 70 to 75% of patients treated with either IV diazepam (0.2 mg/kg) or IV lorazepam (0.1 mg/kg). Therapeutic hypothermia is not beneficial.[A12]

Activity Restrictions in Epilepsy

Complete prevention of seizures is the goal of treatment. Patients with even infrequent seizures are at risk for harm to themselves or others while driving, operating machinery, working near depths or heights, swimming, or doing activities that entail risk of injuries. Patients with inadequately controlled seizures should be advised to avoid such activities. Some jurisdictions require patients or physicians to notify authorities if they have a condition that alters consciousness. The duration of restriction of activities after seizures are controlled varies among jurisdictions, and physicians must be aware of these requirements. Once seizures are controlled, these restrictions are unnecessary, and it is important to encourage normal activities to avoid stigmatization.

Considerations in Women

Changes in hormone levels during the menstrual cycle may aggravate seizures perimenstrually in some women (i.e., catamenial epilepsy). The administration of oral contraceptives (Chapter 225), Depo-Provera, acetazolamide (250 to 500 mg/day), or clobazam (10 to 20 mg/day) may reduce perimenstrual seizures. Enzyme-inducing antiepileptic drugs (see Table 375-8) that reduce estrogen levels by enhancing its metabolism require patients to be treated with higher doses of estrogen or alternative methods of contraception.

Pregnancy poses challenges with regard to seizure control, teratogenesis, and outcomes of pregnancy.[14] Nevertheless, pregnancy itself has no consistent effect on the frequency of seizures, and more than 90% of pregnancies in women with epilepsy are safe and successful. Freedom from seizures for at least 9 months preceding pregnancy is associated with a high probability of freedom from seizures during the pregnancy. Serum levels of lamotrigine, phenytoin, carbamazepine, levetiracetam, and oxcarbazepine may change during pregnancy and should be monitored. Valproate carries a higher risk for major congenital malformations and an enduring reduction in cognitive abilities in children exposed to this medication in utero; therefore its use should be avoided during pregnancy if seizure control permits it. Similarly, polytherapy and high doses of antiepileptic drugs should be avoided if possible, but antiepileptic drugs should not be discontinued. There is no increased risk for cesarean section or premature contractions, and epilepsy itself does not increase the risk for cognitive impairment in the child. Supplementation with at least 0.4 mg of folic acid daily should be given before conception and during pregnancy to reduce the risk for neural tube defects.

Considerations in the Elderly

The incidence and prevalence of epilepsy in the elderly is rising, and its management poses special considerations because of increased frailty, multiple coexisting conditions, and polypharmacy with potential for adverse drug interactions, for example, between antihypertensives, lipid-lowering drugs, anticoagulant drugs, and enzyme-inducing antiepileptic drugs. There is evidence that newer antiepileptic drugs with fewer interactions are better tolerated in the elderly. An unblinded randomized trial found that more elderly patients remained on levetiracetam than on valproate or carbamazepine, supporting the efficacy and tolerability of the newer drug.[A13]

Discontinuing Antiepileptic Drugs

About 60% of patients have seizures that are easy to control with antiepileptic drugs. Medications may be slowly tapered over 4 to 6 months in patients who have remained free of seizures for 2 years or longer, have had few seizures before treatment started, and who have a normal neurologic examination and EEG. However, the increased absolute risk for recurrent seizures after withdrawal of medication is about 20% (number needed to harm of 5). The consequences of a recurrent seizure, the costs and side effects of drugs, and aspects such as personal preferences influence the decision to withdraw antiepileptic drugs in patients who have been free of seizures. Evidence-based algorithms can assist in estimating the risk of recurrence after the withdrawal of medications.[15]

PROGNOSIS

The prognosis is favorable in the majority of patients who experience either unprovoked seizures or one of the epilepsies.

Prognosis after Febrile Seizures

Febrile seizures are common and usually consist of generalized tonic-clonic seizures. They are provoked by fever and therefore are not considered epilepsy. The seizures begin after 6 months of age and stop before 6 years of age. Usually, febrile seizures are left untreated because the prognosis is benign. When febrile seizures occur in the setting of a neurologic abnormality or are prolonged or complicated, the risk for later epilepsy is increased.

Prognosis after a Single Unprovoked Seizure

The risk of experiencing recurrent seizures after a first unprovoked seizure ranges from 21 to 69% at 2 years and from 34 to 70% at 5 years. The risk is lower in the general population than in hospital-based studies (36% at 1 year and 45% at 2 years). The probability of a relapse decreases with time; about 50% of recurrences occur within 6 months of the initial seizure, and 76 to 96% occur within 2 years. The two most consistent predictors of recurrence are the presence of a neurologic cause for the seizure, which is often uncovered on brain MRI or by the neurologic examination and history, and an epileptiform or slow EEG. The 2-year risk for recurrence is lowest for patients without an identified neurologic cause and with a normal EEG (about 25%), intermediate for patients with an identified neurologic cause or without a cause but with an abnormal EEG (48%), and highest for those with a neurologic cause and an abnormal EEG (about 65%). The risk rises dramatically if more than one seizure has occurred; after a second unprovoked seizure, the risk for a third seizure is 73%, and after a third seizure, the risk for a fourth seizure is 76%.

Prognosis of Epilepsy

The natural history of untreated epilepsy, mostly in developing countries, shows that 30 to 40% of patients obtain 5- to 10-year remissions without treatment. In developed countries, where treatment is generally started after two unprovoked seizures have occurred, the likelihood of 5-year remission is about 60% when patients are followed for 10 years, and about 70% when patients are followed for 20 years. The rate of 5-year remission in children is about 75%. In the long term, sustained freedom from seizures is achieved in about 60% of patients (early remission in about 35 to 40% of patients and late remission in about 20 to 25%), about 16% of patients fluctuate between relapses and remissions, and about 25% never achieve seizure remission. Epilepsy is considered to be resolved in patients who had an age-dependent epilepsy syndrome and are now past the applicable age, or in patients who have been seizure free for at least 10 years, with no seizure medications for the last 5 years.

Conversely, the duration of active epilepsy before achieving control is one of the most powerful predictors of remission. If seizures remain uncontrolled during the first year after diagnosis, the chance of ever achieving control is only 60%. If the period of uncontrolled seizures extends to 4 years, the chance of ever achieving control is only 10%. The presence of multiple seizure types and frequent generalized tonic-clonic seizures is associated with a lower likelihood of remission. Less than 40% of patients with newly diagnosed mesial temporal lobe epilepsy will be controlled with medications, although familial cases are more easily managed medically.

Children whose seizures remain uncontrolled are at risk of developing cognitive impairment, especially at a younger age, thereby emphasizing the importance of prompt seizure control. In children with absence epilepsy, the 12-month probability of seizure control and remaining on medication is about 35 to 40% overall, but it is higher for ethosuximide (45%) and valproic acid (44%) than for lamotrigine (21%). In longitudinal population studies of children with newly diagnosed epilepsy, quality of life improves over time in about 50%, remains stable in 30%, and deteriorates in 20%.

Patients with epilepsy are at risk for poor psychosocial outcomes, depression, and increased mortality.[16] The risk for death is two to three times higher in epilepsy than in the general population, and it can be up to five times higher in patients with frequent generalized convulsions and drug-resistant epilepsy. The major causes of death are underlying conditions such as stroke and pneumonia, although unnatural deaths from unintentional injury and poisoning are also more common.[17] Sudden unexpected death in epilepsy occurs in about 1 per 1000 patient-years in adults and is particularly devastating because it affects young individuals with frequent uncontrolled seizures. Complete control of seizures is a major way to decrease mortality in epilepsy. Patients who undergo successful epilepsy surgery, the most effective treatment for drug-resistant focal epilepsy, have a 66% decrease in mortality compared with medically treated patients.[18]

Grade A References

A1. Krumholz A, Wiebe S, Gronseth GS, et al. Evidence-based guideline: management of an unprovoked first seizure in adults: report of the Guideline Development Subcommittee of the American Academy of Neurology and the American Epilepsy Society. *Neurology.* 2015;84:1705-1713.

A2. Nevitt SJ, Sudell M, Weston J, et al. Antiepileptic drug monotherapy for epilepsy: a network meta-analysis of individual participant data. *Cochrane Database Syst Rev.* 2017;12:CD011412.

A3. Hu Q, Zhang F, Teng W, et al. Efficacy and safety of antiepileptic drugs for refractory partial-onset epilepsy: a network meta-analysis. *J Neurol.* 2018;265:1-11.

A4. French JA, Lawson JA, Yapici Z, et al. Adjunctive everolimus therapy for treatment-resistant focal-onset seizures associated with tuberous sclerosis (EXIST-3): a phase 3, randomised, double-blind, placebo-controlled study. *Lancet.* 2016;388:2153-2163.

A5. Devinsky O, Cross JH, Laux L, et al. Trial of cannabidiol for drug-resistant seizures in the Dravet syndrome. *N Engl J Med.* 2017;376:2011-2020.

A6. Thiele EA, Marsh ED, French JA, et al; GWPCARE Study Group. Cannabidiol in patients with seizures associated with Lennox-Gastaut syndrome (GWPCARE4): a randomised, double-blind, placebo-controlled phase 3 trial. *Lancet.* 2018;391:1085-1096.

A7. Jobst BC, Cascino GD. Resective epilepsy surgery for drug-resistant focal epilepsy: a review. *JAMA.* 2015;313:285-293.

A8. Fiest KM, Sajobi TT, Wiebe S. Epilepsy surgery and meaningful improvements in quality of life: results from a randomized controlled trial. *Epilepsia.* 2014;55:886-892.

A9. Dwivedi R, Ramanujam B, Chandra PS, et al. Surgery for drug-resistant epilepsy in children. *N Engl J Med.* 2017;377:1639-1647.

A10. Sprengers M, Vonck K, Carrette E, et al. Deep brain and cortical stimulation for epilepsy. *Cochrane Database Syst Rev.* 2017;7:CD008497.

A11. Barbaro NM, Quigg M, Ward MM, et al. Radiosurgery versus open surgery for mesial temporal lobe epilepsy: the randomized, controlled ROSE trial. *Epilepsia.* 2018;59:1198-1207.

A12. Legriel S, Lemiale V, Schenck M, et al. Hypothermia for neuroprotection in convulsive status epilepticus. *N Engl J Med.* 2016;375:2457-2467.

A13. Pohlmann-Eden B, Marson AG, Noack-Rink M, et al. Comparative effectiveness of levetiracetam, valproate and carbamazepine among elderly patients with newly diagnosed epilepsy: subgroup analysis of the randomized, unblinded KOMET study. *BMC Neurol.* 2016;16:1-12.

GENERAL REFERENCES

For the General References and other additional features, please visit Expert Consult at https://expertconsult.inkling.com.

376
COMA, VEGETATIVE STATE, AND BRAIN DEATH

DAVID M. GREER AND JAMES L. BERNAT

Disorders of consciousness (Table 376-1) encompass a range of conditions, from mild encephalopathy or confusion to coma and brain death. Although not all causes of encephalopathy lead to poor outcomes, the rapid and comprehensive evaluation of a patient with altered consciousness remains one of the most important goals in all of medicine. Depending on the cause, a patient with altered mental status or coma may suffer irreversible brain injury or even death; conversely, with prompt diagnosis and treatment, many if not most patients will recovery, often fully.

Consciousness arises from the ascending reticular activating system, an ill-defined group of neurons that originates in the rostral portion of the brain stem tegmentum and projects to the thalami and then to both cerebral cortices. For consciousness to be disrupted, the underlying pathologic process must affect the brain stem or thalami primarily (e.g., a structural injury such as an intracerebral hemorrhage or ischemic stroke), affect both cerebral cortices simultaneously (e.g., global anoxic brain injury or encephalitis), or both (e.g., drug intoxication or toxic-metabolic insult).

Consciousness comprises two elements: wakefulness and awareness. Wakefulness represents the ability to establish an alertness response to internal need or external stimulation. Awareness of the self and environment is established by a diffuse network of thalamocortical and corticocortical circuits. Patients in coma have neither wakefulness nor awareness. Patients in persistent vegetative state (or unresponsive wakefulness syndrome as it is also called) have wakefulness, including sleep-wake cycles, but no awareness.

COMA

Coma is a state of pathologic unresponsiveness from which the patient cannot be aroused by any form of stimulation.

EPIDEMIOLOGY

The most common causes of coma include trauma, toxic-metabolic, global anoxia, and lesions that result in herniation and compression of the brain stem (Table 376-2).

PATHOBIOLOGY

Wakefulness arises from the ascending reticular activating system, which is a neural network that originates in the central tegmentum of the pons and midbrain in the rostral brain stem, receiving input at each level as it ascends into the central basal forebrain, thalami, and cerebral cortices. Awareness requires not only wakefulness but also a normal functioning parallel network of reverberating neuronal circuits between the thalamus and multiple cortical regions to create an integrated and unified experience. Arousal can be affected by damage or dysfunction anywhere along these pathways, but thalamic and cortical neurons are more susceptible to damage because of their higher metabolic demands. The classic scenario is a global anoxic insult from a cardiac arrest, which selectively injures specific cortical laminae, the thalami, basal ganglia, and the hippocampus owing to their high oxygen demands and relatively high metabolic activity. By comparison, phylogenetically older and less metabolically demanding neurons of the ascending reticular activating system are relatively spared. This selective injury helps explain the unresponsive wakefulness syndrome (also called the vegetative state), which is characterized by wakefulness without awareness.

Coma is caused by (1) structural damage resulting from trauma, edema, inflammation, ischemia, hemorrhage, or mass lesions or (2) diffuse toxic and/or metabolic effects on neurons. Structural lesions can affect the ascending reticular activating system directly by neuronal damage or indirectly by extrinsic pressure or displacement, thereby causing ischemia and/or edema. Metabolic and toxic encephalopathies diffusely affect all brain neurons but preferentially the metabolically sensitive neurons in the cortex and thalamus. However, several acute metabolic derangements or toxicities can also cause structural brain injury by altering blood pressure or oxygenation (e.g., opioid toxicity [Chapter 31]), brain edema (e.g., acute hepatic failure [Chapter 145] with

TABLE 376-1 COMPARISON OF DISORDERS OF CONSCIOUSNESS*

	AWARENESS	WAKEFULNESS	BRAIN STEM/ RESPIRATORY	MOTOR	EEG	EVOKED POTENTIALS	PET/fMRI	PROGNOSIS
Brain death	Absent	Absent	Absent	Absent	ECS	Absent	Absent cortical metabolism	The person has died
Coma	Absent	Absent	Depressed, variable	Reflex or posturing	Polymorphic delta, burst suppression	BAER variable; cortical ERPs often absent	Resting <50%	Variable
Vegetative state	Absent	Present, intact sleep-wake cycles	Intact	Reflex, nonpurposeful	Delta, theta, or ECS	BAER preserved; cortical ERPs variable	Resting <50%; primary areas stimulatable	Poor, when chronic
Minimally conscious state	Intact but poorly responsive	Intact	Intact	Variable with purposeful movements	Nonspecific slowing	BAER preserved; cortical ERPs often preserved	Reduced; secondary areas also stimulatable	Variable
Locked-in syndrome	Intact but communication difficult	Intact	Intact breathing; often brain stem signs	Quadriplegia, pseudobulbar palsy	Usually normal	BAER variable; cortical ERPs normal	Normal or nearly normal	Poor

BAER = brain stem auditory evoked response; ECS = electrocerebral silence; EEG = encephalography; ERP = event-related potential; fMRI = functional magnetic resonance imaging; PET = positron emission tomography.
*The table lists typical findings, which are not necessarily present in all patients. Locked-in syndrome may be mistaken for a disorder of consciousness.
From Bernat JL. *Ethical Issues in Neurology.* 3rd ed. Philadelphia: Lippincott Williams & Wilkins; 2008:292.

TABLE 376-2 CAUSES OF STUPOR AND COMA

Traumatic brain injury*
  Contusion
  Intracerebral, epidural, subdural, or subarachnoid hemorrhage
  Diffuse axonal injury
  Raised intracranial pressure
Neoplasms and other mass lesions
Infections
  Meningitis
  Encephalitis
  Brain abscess or empyema
  Sepsis or other infection, especially in the elderly or a demented patient*
Cerebrovascular disease
  Intracerebral hemorrhage
  Infarction in the brain stem or cerebellum or large hemispheric infarction
  Hemorrhage in the brain stem or cerebellum or large hemispheric hemorrhage
  Vasculitis, disseminated intravascular coagulation, thrombotic thrombocytopenic purpura
Seizures
  Status epilepticus
  Spike-wave stupor
  Postictal state
Metabolic encephalopathies*
  Hypoglycemia, hyperglycemia
  Hypercalcemia
  Hyponatremia, hypernatremia
  Hypoxemia, including anoxia after cardiac arrest
  Acidosis
  Organ system failure: hepatic, renal, pulmonary, cardiac
  Endocrinopathy (e.g., myxedema coma)
Toxic encephalopathies
  Drug intoxications*: alcohol, barbiturates, benzodiazepines, opioids, stimulants, salicylates, anticonvulsants, anticholinergics, psychotropic drugs, or others
  Poisoning: carbon monoxide, industrial toxins
Other encephalopathies
  Hypertensive encephalopathy
  Acute hydrocephalus
  Pituitary apoplexy
Other
  Conversion, malingering, catatonia

*Most common causes.

hyperammonemia), or acute demyelination (e.g., central pontine myelinolysis owing to rapid osmolar shifting, such as seen in rapid correction of chronic hyponatremia [Chapter 108]).

Structural lesions causing coma typically present with clinically recognizable herniation syndromes, in which shifts in intracranial pressure produce caudal and lateral displacement and ischemia of the midbrain and medial temporal lobe through the tentorial incisura. Herniation results in dysfunction of cranial nerves (first pupillary dilation, followed by more complete third nerve palsy), breathing, and motor systems. Most commonly, central herniation occurs with global events such as meningoencephalitis (Chapter 386), global anoxic brain injury, massive brain swelling from toxic-metabolic insults, or hydrocephalus. Uncal herniation results from rapidly expanding and laterally placed lesions that trap the ipsilateral oculomotor nerve against the uncus of the temporal lobe. Lateral displacement of brain structures can match or exceed downward displacement. Brain stem compression can also result from structural lesions in the posterior fossa. The ascending reticular activating system can also be damaged directly by primary brain stem injuries, such as from hemorrhage or infarction, or indirectly by downward-directed pressure produced by hemispheric mass lesions, such as from brain trauma (Chapter 371), neoplasms (Chapter 180), abscesses (Chapter 385), hemorrhages (Chapter 380), or large infarctions (Chapter 379).

Encephalopathy in the setting of metabolic disturbances results from perturbation of the neuronal microenvironment by altering the precise metabolic conditions necessary for normal neuronal conduction and excitability. These disturbances can occur due to changes in blood flow, oxygen delivery, glucose concentration, temperature (hyperthermia or hypothermia), electrolyte concentrations, and intracranial pressure. Other causes include meningitis, seizures, and organ failure. The severity of the insult matches the impact: more profound metabolic insults cause greater encephalopathy. The rapidity of onset also is an important factor. Sudden metabolic changes, such as in serum sodium concentration, may result in seizures and coma, whereas a slow decline, even to a low level, may cause little clinical impact (Chapter 108). Toxic encephalopathies, with indistinguishable clinical manifestations, can result from exogenous poisoning with illicit (e.g., opiates, hallucinogenics) or therapeutic (e.g., antidepressants, anticholinergics) substances, or endogenous toxins that result from renal or hepatic failure. Acute meningoencephalitis, with inflammation of both the meninges and cerebrum, causes coma by direct inflammation, vascular insults, cerebral edema, and hydrocephalus.

CLINICAL MANIFESTATIONS

A patient in coma displays neither wakefulness nor awareness. There is no purposeful response to noxious stimulation. Reflexive posturing may be present. The eyes are typically closed, except in the rare situation of "eyes open coma," which occasionally follows cardiac arrest (Chapter 57) with global anoxic brain injury. The eyes do not open in response to noxious stimulation. The patient does not express any interpretable sounds reflective of responsiveness, only sounds associated with attempts at breathing.

Coma should be differentiated from stupor, in which the patient is able to be aroused temporarily during vigorous stimulation but then immediately resumes unresponsiveness once stimulation is stopped.

Coma may have multiple levels of depth graded by the presence and degree of brain stem and motor reflexes. However, this differentiation serves only to distinguish levels of brain stem dysfunction and does not imply reversibility, which depends on the underlying etiology. The pattern of brain stem dysfunction usefully localizes the anatomic extent of a structural injury or impingement.

DIAGNOSIS

Rapid diagnosis of the etiology of coma is crucial for expeditious and targeted treatment (Table 376-3).[1] A detailed history, physical examination, laboratory testing, and neuroimaging should be performed in a parallel manner. Immediate attention should be focused on whether the patient has any signs of trauma (cranial or cervical), meningitis (fever, nuchal rigidity), drug intoxication (which may be rapidly reversed), seizures (including nonconvulsive status epilepticus, which may manifest only with eye deviation), or focal findings suggestive of a mass or vascular event.

The history should focus on any witnessed events or recent history according to others, such as feeling unwell or suffering any trauma or medication changes. Information should be obtained regarding any preceding headache, vomiting, confusional state, prescription and illicit drug use, alcohol use, fever, metabolic disturbances (including a history of diabetes), seizure history, abnormal recent behavior, and preexisting medical conditions, particularly atrial fibrillation or prior neurologic events (e.g., stroke, hemorrhage).

The general physical examination should include assessment of vital signs, otoscopy, funduscopic examination, and a search for physical signs of head trauma, nuchal rigidity, or needle track marks. The respiratory rate and pattern should be carefully noted (Table 376-4). Cheyne-Stokes respiration is a periodic breathing pattern whose amplitude forms a sine wave, with 5- to 45-second periods of apnea alternating with periods of hyperpnea. It can be seen in patients with primary cardiac/respiratory disorders or in patients with metabolic encephalopathy, and it is typically reversible by treating the underlying cause. Central neurogenic hyperventilation consists of continuous hyperpnea and tachypnea that leads to a pure respiratory alkalosis; it occurs with lesions of the rostral brain stem tegmentum at the level of the midbrain, or damage to the central pons. Kussmaul respiration, which consists of rapid deep breathing, is seen as a compensatory mechanism in the setting of severe metabolic acidosis, often with hyperglycemia (Chapter 216). Ataxic or irregular breathing patterns, with or without apneic periods, are associated with lower brain stem dysfunction and can represent an agonal pattern.

A detailed neurologic examination is important to discern if there are localizing signs that may point to a structural etiology to assess the level of brain function and to look for evidence of trauma or drug use.

The patient's limbs should be uncovered to view any movements, either spontaneously or in response to stimulation. Responsiveness should be checked by increasingly noxious stimulation, starting with loud auditory stimulation. Noxious physical stimulation should include not only stimulation of the extremities (typically starting with pressure on the nail bed), but also on the cranium, including the supraorbital ridge and temporomandibular joint. Only when adequate stimulation has been provided can one say that the patient is truly unresponsive and comatose.

Cranial Nerve Examination

In a detailed cranial nerve examination, the eyes should be held open, and any spontaneous eye movements, deviation, nystagmus, or dysconjugance should be noted. The patient should be asked to look up and down, so that pseudocoma from a locked-in state can be detected. A blink to visual threat should be tested with the hand flat (so as to avoid creating a wind wave that would stimulate a corneal reflex) approaching the eye, first laterally (to test the visual field), and then centrally if there is no response laterally. The pupillary light reflex should be tested with a bright light, and a magnifying glass or pupillometer may be helpful to evaluate questionable responsiveness or briskness and degree of response. A corneal reflex may be tested initially with a squirt of water or saline and then a light cotton wisp; however, if these minor stimuli are not successful, a more potent stimulus, such as pressing on the eye with a cotton-tipped applicator, may be necessary.

TABLE 376-3	SOME INITIAL CLINICAL CLUES TO THE DIAGNOSIS OF STUPOR AND COMA

STRUCTURAL CAUSES

History
  Abrupt onset of unconsciousness
  Sudden headache
  Vomiting
Examination
  Focal neurologic signs (hemiparesis, posturing, asymmetrical reflexes)
  Abnormal pupillary light reflexes

METABOLIC OR TOXIC CAUSES

History
  Gradual onset of unconsciousness
  Preceding confusional state
  Seizures
  Known cognitive impairment
  Taking insulin or street drugs
Examination
  Absence of focal neurologic signs
  Presence of frontal release signs
  Intact pupillary light reflexes
  Tremor, asterixis, or multifocal myoclonus
  Evidence of systemic infection
  Needle tracks

MENINGITIS

History
  Worsening headache
  Neck stiffness and pain
  Fever, chills
  Progressive stupor and coma
Examination
  Fever, rigors
  Nuchal rigidity and signs of meningeal inflammation

TABLE 376-4	BRAIN FUNCTIONAL LEVELS DETERMINED BY FINDINGS IN CLINICAL SYSTEMS

FUNCTIONAL LEVEL	CONSCIOUSNESS	RESPIRATION	PUPILS	VESTIBULO-OCULAR REFLEXES	MOTOR RESPONSES
CENTRAL TRANSTENTORIAL HERNIATION					
High diencephalic	Light stupor	Eupnea, yawning, post-hyperventilation apnea	Small, reactive	Loss of checking component	Paratonia, grasp
Low diencephalic	Deep stupor	Cheyne-Stokes	Small, reactive	Loss of checking component	Decorticate posturing
Midbrain	Coma	Central neurogenic hyperventilation	Midposition, fixed	Loss of medial rectus function	Decerebrate posturing
Upper pons	Coma	Central neurogenic hyperventilation	Midposition, fixed	Loss of medial rectus function	Decerebrate posturing
Lower pons	Coma	Ataxic	Midposition, fixed	Absent	Flaccid
Medulla	Coma	Apnea	Midposition, fixed	Absent	Flaccid
UNCAL TRANSTENTORIAL HERNIATION					
Early third nerve	Unreliable	Normal	Ipsilateral dilated, fixed	Normal	Contralateral hemiparesis
Late third nerve	Coma	Cheyne-Stokes or central neurogenic hyperventilation	Ipsilateral dilated, fixed; contralateral dilated, fixed	Medial rectus dysfunction	Ipsilateral hemiparesis and contralateral decerebrate posturing
Midbrain-pons	Coma	Central neurogenic hyperventilation or ataxic	Midposition, fixed	Absent	Bilateral decerebrate posturing

Pupillary responses to bright light assess the pathways of the optic nerve, oculomotor nerves, midbrain, and sympathetic nerves. Pupillary reactivity helps distinguish structural from toxic-metabolic causes of coma. Pupils remain reactive to light and usually symmetrical through varying depths and causes of toxic-metabolic coma, whereas pupillary reflexes are abnormal, and often asymmetrical, with structural causes of coma such as transtentorial herniation with compression of the third nerve. With asymmetrical pupils, it is important to distinguish which eye is the abnormal one; the larger pupil may not necessarily be the abnormal side, such as in the setting of Horner syndrome, in which there is loss of sympathetic input. However, in the setting of a compressive lesion or other cause of third nerve dysfunction, pupillary enlargement occurs before ophthalmoplegia because the parasympathetic pupilloconstrictor fibers course on the outside of the nerve and are compressed first. With progressive herniation, the brain stem sympathetic tracks are also damaged, so the pupil may return to be midposition and remain unreactive. Primary structural injuries to the pons (e.g., hemorrhage or infarction) cause "pinpoint" pupils owing to loss of sympathetic tracts; however, they are typically still reactive with a magnifying glass or pupillometer. The examiner should consider the potential for preexisting pupillary abnormalities (e.g., diabetes, postsurgical), as well as locally applied medications that can impair pupillary reflexes.

A dilated funduscopic examination is helpful to look for ocular pathology as well as evidence of increased intracranial pressure. However, if pharmacologic dilation is performed, it is important that all caregivers know that it has been performed so erroneous conclusions do not result.

Spontaneous eye movements may have localizing value. Horizontally and conjugately deviated eyes owing to a hemispheric lesion follow the rules of "look toward a stroke, look away from a seizure" because of ablation or stimulation of the frontal lobe gaze center. With lesions in the brain stem, however, the eyes often will deviate in the opposite direction because of damage to the parapontine reticular formation. Tonic downward eye deviation is sometimes seen in patients with global anoxic brain injury. Ocular bobbing, with rapid downward movement followed by a slow return upward, can occur with pontine lesions. "Reverse" ocular bobbing with slow downward but rapid upward movement ("ocular dipping") may be seen after primary brain stem insults or with global anoxia or toxic-metabolic states. "Ping-pong" gaze with alternative conjugate horizontal movements is nonspecific, but a slower and similar disorder of periodic alternating gaze can be seen with hyperammonemia owing to portosystemic encephalopathy.

Horizontally dysconjugate gaze should be placed in the clinical context because it may be secondary to a brain stem injury or it may simply be an uncovering of a preexisting esotropia or exotropia. However, vertical dysconjugation ("skew") is almost always abnormal and should signal a structural problem at the level of the rostral brain stem.

The vestibulo-ocular reflex can be tested using ice-water caloric stimulation of the external auditory canals. Before doing the ice-water test, otoscopic evaluation should reveal an intact tympanic membrane and a clear auditory canal, and the head of bed should be elevated to 30 degrees. Ice water is instilled in one ear at a time for 60 seconds continuously, and the eyes are observed for any movement. With an intact brain stem, the eyes will tonically deviate toward the cold-irrigated ear, sometimes with nystagmus in the opposite direction. Both ears should be tested, but there should be an interval of at least 5 minutes before testing the second ear. If a cervical spine computed tomography (CT) scan shows cervical spine stability, it can also be tested using sudden head movements. For this test, the head is briskly rotated, laterally as well as vertically to elicit the oculocephalic reflex. In an intact brain stem, the eyes move in the opposite direction from which the head is turned.

Facial movement is tested as above with noxious stimulation, which can also include stimulation of the nasal hair and septum with a cotton-tipped swab, which may elicit a grimace response. Lower cranial nerve function is tested with posterior pharyngeal stimulation to test for a gag reflex, and deep bronchial suctioning to test for a cough reflex.

Motor Examination

The motor response can give a clue to localization. The motor examination includes observing the patient for spontaneous movements and then responses elicited by noxious stimulation of the extremities, typically starting with deep nail bed pressure, and then with noxious stimulation more proximally on the limb. The movement in response to stimulation in both locations should be noted, including whether they are symmetrical. Stereotyped responses are most consistent with a posturing reflex. Responses can be graded as localization, purposeful withdrawal, reflex flexor (decorticate) posturing, reflex extensor (decerebrate) posturing, and none.

TABLE 376-5 FOUR SCORE COMA ASSESSMENT SCALE*

EYE RESPONSE

E4 = Eyelids open or closed, tracking or blinking to command
E3 = Eyelids open but not tracking
E2 = Eyelids closed but open to pain
E1 = Eyelids remain closed with pain stimuli

MOTOR RESPONSE

M4 = Thumbs up, fist, or peace sign
M3 = Localizing to pain
M2 = Flexion response to pain
M1 = Extension response to pain
M0 = No response to pain or generalized myoclonic status epilepticus

BRAIN STEM REFLEXES

B4 = Pupillary and corneal reflexes present
B3 = One pupil dilated and unreactive to light
B2 = Pupillary or corneal reflexes absent
B1 = Pupillary and corneal reflexes absent
B0 = Absent pupillary, corneal, or cough reflexes

RESPIRATION

R4 = Regular breathing pattern
R3 = Cheyne-Stokes breathing pattern
R2 = Irregular breathing pattern
R1 = Triggers or breathes above the ventilator rate
R0 = Apnea or breathes at the ventilator rate

*For nontraumatic coma and other disorders of consciousness.
From Wijdicks EFM. *The Comatose Patient.* 2nd ed. New York: Oxford University Press; 2014.

Decorticate or flexor posturing suggests a lesion above the level of the red nucleus in the brain stem, whereas decerebrate or extensor posturing suggests a brain stem lesion. Symmetrical findings are more consistent with a toxic-metabolic or global insult, whereas asymmetrical findings suggest a focal structural injury. However, exceptions include hypoglycemia and hyponatremia, which notoriously can cause focal neurologic findings in the absence of a structural injury and which are often reversible. Other motor findings include tonic or clonic movements consistent with seizure, or myoclonic (nonrhythmic) jerking, which is a nonspecific finding associated with many disease states. Unrelenting myoclonic jerking (myoclonic status epilepticus) in the setting of a global anoxic brain injury tends to carry a poorer prognosis.

Grading Coma

Multiple scales are helpful for grading and evaluating coma, estimating prognosis, and assessing changes over time. The Glasgow Coma Scale (Table 371-1) is widely used, especially to evaluate patients with traumatic brain injury; its components include verbal, motor, and eye responses. The more recent FOUR score (Table 376-5) is more comprehensive for brain stem function (including respiratory patterns) and responsiveness, and it is useful in evaluating all causes of coma.

Laboratory Testing

Emergency laboratory testing should include a complete blood count, electrolytes, serum glucose, liver and kidney function tests, a coagulation profile, thyroid function tests, an ammonia level, arterial blood gas analysis, a blood alcohol concentration, and blood and urine drug screens. If intoxication is likely, particularly in the absence of ketones, uremia, or an elevated lactate level, anion and osmolar gaps should be measured. Urine or blood serum for opioids, benzodiazepines, and other toxins (e.g., pesticides, heavy metals, and atypical alcohols) should be obtained. Blood, urine, and sputum cultures should be obtained, as should an electrocardiogram and chest radiograph.

Expeditious neuroimaging often starts with a noncontrast head CT, but a CT angiogram should be performed if a vascular lesion is suspected. If the patient was found unconscious or if there is any question of trauma, a cervical spine CT can be obtained concomitantly. Magnetic resonance imaging (MRI) typically is not helpful in the acute setting and may be contraindicated in an unstable patient in whom close monitoring is required. The one exception would be a possible acute brain stem or posterior fossa infarction, which may not be seen on noncontrast head CT but should be detected by MRI with diffusion-weighted imaging.

If the head CT shows no evidence of mass lesion or edema, a lumbar puncture should be performed to exclude meningitis (Chapter 384) or other causes of central nervous system inflammation. An urgent electroencephalogram (EEG) should be considered to exclude nonconvulsive seizures or status epilepticus.

TREATMENT   Rx

Management of coma requires simultaneous diagnostic, supportive, and treatment measures (Table 376-6).[2] Specific treatments relate to the underlying cause, and some conditions require urgent attention, such as head trauma (Chapter 371), cerebrovascular events (Chapter 378), severe hypoglycemia or hypoglycemia (Chapter 216), meningitis (Chapter 384), and encephalitis (Chapter 386). Emergency stabilization of respiratory and circulatory functions is paramount for all patients. Early treatment of seizures (Chapter 375) can prevent progression to status epilepticus.

In patients without focal findings or obvious meningitis, 50% dextrose (25 g IV for potential hypoglycemia), empiric thiamine (100 mg IV to prevent glucose-induced Wernicke-Korsakoff syndrome), naloxone (0.4 to 2 mg IV for potential opioid overdose), and flumazenil (0.2 mg IV to reverse the action of benzodiazepines) can be administered during the diagnostic evaluation. If fever, nuchal rigidity, or leukocytosis are present, the patient should empirically be treated for bacterial meningitis (Chapter 384) and viral encephalitis (Chapter 386) while awaiting the results of polymerase chain reaction testing and/or cultures of the cerebrospinal fluid.

Raised intracranial pressure must be treated urgently. Hyperventilation by bag or ventilator to a goal PCO_2 of 30 mm Hg will rapidly lower the intracranial pressure, but the effect is transient. If this maneuver is undertaken, care must be given to reestablish normocapnia slowly and at the appropriate time. Hyperosmolar therapy with mannitol (0.5 to 1.5 g/kg every 6 hours) or hypertonic saline (1.5 to 7% as a continuous drip or 23.4% as a bolus) has a more durable effect. Glucocorticoids may be used in patients with brain tumors (Chapter 180) or bacterial meningitis (Chapter 384), but they are not effective in traumatic brain injury, vascular insults, or metabolic causes of coma. For refractory elevations in intracranial pressure, barbiturates (typically pentobarbital, with the dose titrated based on EEG findings) may be helpful; but at that stage (or earlier), a surgical craniectomy should be considered for decompression[A1] or evacuation of any mass lesion. For global anoxic brain injury after cardiac arrest (Chapter 57), therapeutic hypothermia for 24 hours is considered beneficial, with a target temperature of 32° to 36° C.[3]

PROGNOSIS

The prognosis of coma, which is highly variable, depends on the cause, stage, degree of structural brain damage, and potential reversibility. Prediction rules apply only to specific causes, and common sense must prevail. For example, patients with isolated respiratory arrest who never lose perfusion may be comatose for extended periods of time but usually achieve a good neurologic recovery.

For global anoxic brain injury owing to cardiac arrest, however, reliable predictors of poor outcome include absent pupillary or corneal reflexes 72 hours after arrest (or 72 hours after rewarming, if the patient undergoes therapeutic hypothermia), as well as bilateral absence of cortical responses on somatosensory evoked potential testing 48 hours after arrest (or 48 hours after rewarming, if the patient undergoes therapeutic hypothermia). Other potential prognostic factors include malignant patterns (burst-suppression, severe attenuation) on the EEG,[4] elevated serum neuron-specific enolase levels, and evidence of severe anoxic injury on CT or MRI.

Some patients may recover within the first few days after a hypoxic event but then regress days to weeks later with a syndrome of delayed posthypoxic leukoencephalopathy, which is thought to be a demyelinating process. This outcome is more common in patients with prolonged hypoxia/anoxia followed by cardiac arrest with ischemia. Neuroimaging shows diffuse bilateral hemispheric demyelination that spares the cerebellum and brain stem. Some patients can recover slowly over 3 to 12 months, but often with substantial neurologic sequelae. Others may be left in a vegetative or minimally conscious state.

VEGETATIVE STATE/UNRESPONSIVE WAKEFULNESS SYNDROME

Vegetative state, recently renamed the unresponsive wakefulness syndrome, is a disorder of consciousness in which wakefulness is achieved but awareness of the self or environment is absent on clinical testing (Table 376-7).[5] The unresponsive wakefulness syndrome can be transient or permanent, depending on the underlying cause and degree of injury. It is a state into which comatose patients may emerge, but it may also be the final state. Adjectives such as "persistent" or "permanent" should be avoided, because they are arbitrary and lead to confusion by confounding the diagnosis and prognosis.

EPIDEMIOLOGY

The unresponsive wakefulness syndrome is caused by diffuse or multifocal brain lesions that disrupt the thalamocortical pathways but spare the brain stem and hypothalamus. The prevalence of the transient unresponsive wakefulness syndrome is unknown, but the prevalence of a chronic, stable unresponsive wakefulness syndrome is about 19 per million population.

PATHOBIOLOGY

Causative lesions can be located in the bilateral thalami, diffusely in the cerebral cortices, or diffusely in the white matter that connects the thalami to the cortex. The two most common underlying causes are hypoxic-ischemic injury to the thalami and cortex in the setting of cardiac arrest (Chapter 57) and diffuse axonal injury caused by traumatic brain injury (Chapter 371) with torque force. These causes have different pathologies. Hypoxic-ischemic injury affects cortical, thalamic, basal ganglia, and cerebellar neurons, whereas diffuse axonal injury shears and disconnects the axons at the gray matter–white matter junctions diffusely and multifocally, often with profound white matter injury that includes the brain stem.

CLINICAL MANIFESTATIONS AND DIAGNOSIS

Patients have wakefulness but no evidence of responsiveness.[6] A careful clinical examination is mandatory to search for any evidence of awareness, because up to 40% of patients diagnosed with the unresponsive wakefulness syndrome are actually in a minimally conscious state (see below).

TABLE 376-6	EMERGENCY MANAGEMENT OF COMATOSE PATIENTS

1. Ensure oxygenation
2. Maintain the circulation
3. Administer 50% dextrose, 25 g IV, and control glucose
4. Lower raised intracranial pressure
5. Stop seizures with lorazepam, 1-2 mg IV
6. Search for and treat infections
7. Restore acid-base and electrolyte balance
8. Normalize body temperature
9. Administer thiamine, 50 mg IV, and multivitamins
10. Consider administration of opioid antagonists (naloxone, 0.4-2 mg IV)
11. Consider administration of benzodiazepine antagonists (flumazenil, 0.2 mg IV)
12. Control agitation
13. Protect the eyes
14. Consider inducing therapeutic hypothermia for neuroprotection following cardiac arrest

Modified from Posner JB, Saper CB, Schiff ND, et al. *Plum and Posner's Diagnosis of Stupor and Coma.* 4th ed. New York: Oxford University Press; 2007:311.

TABLE 376-7	DIAGNOSIS OF THE VEGETATIVE STATE

I. Absence of:
  Awareness of self or environment
  Purposeful or voluntary behavioral response to all stimuli
  Language comprehension or expression

II. Presence of:
  Intermittent wakefulness manifested by the presence of sleep-wake cycles
  Autonomic functions
  Cranial nerve and spinal reflexes

III. Potential behavioral repertoire:
  Breathe spontaneously
  Spontaneous roving eye movements
  Utter sounds but no words
  Grimace to pain, make facial expressions
  Yawn, make chewing jaw movements, swallow saliva
  Move limbs nonpurposefully, arch back, decorticate limb posturing
  Flexion withdrawal from noxious stimuli
  Move head or eyes briefly toward sound or movement
  Auditory startle

As a clinical syndrome, unresponsive wakefulness presents as a spectrum of severity. Most patients have slow wave activity on EEG, but the most severely affected patients may have nearly flat EEGs. However, some patients in the unresponsive wakeful state can generate appropriate EEG responses to distinct commands, thereby suggesting residual cognitive function and conscious awareness. A subset of patients who are thought to have the unresponsive wakefulness syndrome possess awareness based on their ability to perform ideational tasks on command with corresponding changes on functional MRI. Such findings identify patients who are more appropriately categorized as minimally conscious.

TREATMENT AND PROGNOSIS   Rx

There are no proven treatments to reverse or improve the chronic, stable unresponsive wakefulness syndrome. Aggressiveness of treatment should ideally be guided by a patient's previously stated wishes (Chapters 2 and 3),[7] which unfortunately are often unknown. Patients in the unresponsive wakefulness state often require nearly the same nursing, physical therapy, and nutritional care as patients in coma. Referral to specialized neurorehabilitation centers may be appropriate.

Patients who have some recovery from unresponsive wakefulness usually have initially preserved pupillary light reflexes and nociceptive responses, paroxysmal sympathetic hyperactivity, and preserved cortical somatosensory evoked potential responses. If patients with unresponsive wakefulness from nontraumatic causes do not regain awareness within 3 months of the insult, they have only a small chance of experiencing neurologic improvement. The prognosis with unresponsive wakefulness owing to head trauma (Chapter 371) is less clear, and patients typically require at least a year or two to provide a similar level of certainty. Functional neuroimaging is a promising but as yet unproven way to help to identify patients who may be destined to recover awareness, particularly after traumatic brain injury.

The minimally conscious state, which is a profound disorder of consciousness, is distinguished from the unresponsive wakefulness syndrome by clear partial or intermittent evidence of awareness of self and environment (E-Table 376-1).[8-10] Patients with the minimally conscious state have necessarily suffered a less severe injury than patients with unresponsive wakefulness, and the minimally conscious state is much more common.

Disruptions in an underlying functionally connected network that is involved in consciousness, the "default mode network," can be explored by neuroimaging as well as by EEG. Some patients have behaviors that imply preservation of language function, which may be evidenced by the reproducible ability to follow commands after object recognition or intelligible verbalization.

Patients in the minimally conscious state may respond to environmental and sensory stimuli in a nonreflexive manner. They also respond to stimulants, such as levodopa/carbidopa (25/100 mg, which stimulates thalamic dopaminergic neurons, thereby likely leading to improvement in consciousness and responsiveness) and amantadine.[11] Amantadine (100 mg twice daily initially, later increased to 200 mg twice daily) can accelerate the pace of early recovery, but may not ultimately affect overall prognosis.[A2]

Patients in the minimally conscious state require extensive rehabilitation services, and their prospects of recovery are better than for patients with unresponsive wakefulness syndrome, likely because of their ability to participate, at least at a minimal level.

Prognostic data are limited for the minimally conscious state, other than for recovery in the subset of patients with traumatic brain injury (Chapter 371). Both FDG-positron emission tomography and functional MRI are useful tools for evaluating patients, and the EEG may also provide information about the extent of brain injury and likelihood of recovery.

THE LOCKED-IN SYNDROME

The locked-in syndrome, a state of profound paralysis, is not a disorder of consciousness but may be mistaken for one. In its classic form, it is produced when a large infarction or hemorrhage in the pontine tegmentum and base produces quadriplegia, pseudobulbar palsy, and paralysis of horizontal eye movements. Once the acute encephalopathy resolves, locked-in patients usually remain awake and alert, breathe spontaneously, and have normal consciousness and cognition, to the extent that they can be tested accurately. Inexperienced examiners may incorrectly diagnose locked-in patients as being comatose because of their profound paralysis, pinpoint pupils, and seeming unresponsiveness. A similar state of profound global paralysis with intact cognition can be produced by advanced amyotrophic lateral sclerosis (Chapter 391), Guillain-Barré syndrome (Chapter 392), or critical illness polyneuropathy (Chapter 392).

Patients can be taught to communicate with voluntary vertical eye movements and eyelid movements, because they are controlled rostral to the pons. Most affected patients, particularly older patients with comorbid illnesses, die within a few months, but some otherwise healthy young patients who have become locked in as a result of basilar artery occlusion have survived for many years. Occasional patients may recover function to become independent. Computerized systems targeting remaining voluntary eye movements and other intact voluntary movements can help patients communicate.

BRAIN DEATH

Brain death is not only a state of unconsciousness, it is a state of complete and irreversible loss of all brain function that constitutes legal death in the United States and most of the developed world.[12,13] Diagnosis of brain death is a medical imperative, with medical, legal, and ethical implications, as well as a potential for organ donation (Chapter 2). It is a diagnosis that must be made with 100% accuracy.

EPIDEMIOLOGY AND PATHOBIOLOGY

The most common causes of brain death include traumatic brain injury (Chapter 371), global anoxic brain injury (e.g., cardiac arrest, Chapter 57), intracranial hemorrhage (including subarachnoid hemorrhage [Chapter 380] and primary intracerebral hemorrhage), meningitis (Chapter 384), or ischemic stroke (Chapter 379). Cerebral edema and/or hydrocephalus leads to severely elevated intracranial pressure. When the mean arterial pressure equals the intracranial pressure, the cerebral perfusion pressure is thus zero, meaning that there is no effective forward intracranial flow, which is incompatible with life. Widespread ischemic neuronal death ensues.

CLINICAL MANIFESTATIONS AND DIAGNOSIS

Before clinical testing for brain death, strict criteria must be met (Table 376-8). The cause of the neurologic catastrophe must be known, and the state must be known to be completely irreversible. If there is any question as to the potential for reversibility, the patient should not be tested for brain death. There must be an absence of confounding, including from drug/alcohol intoxication; metabolic, acid-base, or endocrine disturbances; or pharmacologic

TABLE 376-8	TESTS FOR BRAIN DEATH IN ADULTS

I. Preconditions showing irreversibility: all necessary
- Presence of a structural brain lesion sufficient to produce all the clinical signs
- No neuromuscular blockade (use electroneurography if uncertain)
- Absence of reversible significant toxic or metabolic encephalopathy:
  No depressant drug intoxication
  No severe acid-based, electrolyte or endocrine disorders, or severe hyperammonemia
  Temperature at least 36° C
  Systolic blood pressure at least 100 mm Hg

II. Signs showing complete cessation of all clinical brain functions: all necessary
- Coma: no spontaneous movements, no response to any stimuli, and no brain-mediated movements
- Brain stem areflexia: all necessary
  Absent pupillary light and dark reflexes
  Absent corneal reflexes
  Absent facial movement to noxious stimuli, both on corpus and cranium
  Absent oculocephalic reflexes (only tested in patients with integrity of the cervical spine)
  Absent vestibulo-ocular reflexes tested by caloric irrigation of the external auditory canal with ice water for 60 seconds continuously
  Absent pharyngeal and tracheal reflexes to pharyngeal stimulation and deep bronchial suctioning
- Apnea: no breathing or respiratory effort when the $PaCO_2 \geq 60$ mm Hg while preserving the PaO_2

III. Ancillary tests: performed only when the clinical examination cannot be adequately or confidently completed
- Neuroimaging showing complete absence of intracranial blood flow (preferred over electrophysiology testing):
  Conventional angiography
  Transcranial Doppler ultrasound
  Single-photon emission computed tomography (SPECT)
- Electrophysiologic testing showing absence of brain potentials (both required)
  Electroencephalography
  Brain stem evoked responses

paralysis. The patient must be normotensive (adult systolic blood pressure at least 100 mm Hg) and normothermic (at least 36° C).

Brain dead patients have no clinical evidence of brain function whatsoever. There are three cardinal clinical features: coma, brain stem areflexia, and apnea. The patient must have complete unresponsiveness, with the testing methods as described above, including both cranial and corporeal noxious stimulation, which should produce only spinally mediated responses, if any. The pupils are typically midposition (3 to 7 mm) and fixed, even when checked with an arduous method, such as a magnifying glass or pupillometer; small pupils should alert the clinician to the possibility of intoxication or a pontine lesion. The corneal reflex, likewise, should be tested with a potent stimulus, such as pressing the cornea at the iris-sclera junction with a cotton-tipped applicator and with enough pressure to see the eye move. Oculocephalic and maximal oculovestibular testing should show no eye movement in brain death, and no gag or cough reflexes should be present.

A number of motor signs of spinal origin can be seen in brain death, such as intact deep tendon reflexes, triple flexion (stereotyped flexion at the ankle, knee, and hip to noxious stimulation at multiple locations), and Babinski sign, as well as other movements that fall under the term "Lazarus signs" (including head turning, arching of the back, and crisscrossing of the arms across the body). However, decorticate posturing and decerebrate posturing are brain-mediated responses and are not consistent with brain death.

To test for apnea, the ventilator should be adjusted to achieve normocarbia and preoxygenation to a PaO_2 of greater than 200 mm Hg. The patient is observed for at least 8 to 10 minutes off the ventilator for any respiratory effort, and the test should be aborted if a breath is observed or if the patient develops hypotension (systolic blood pressure <90 mm Hg) or hypoxia (O_2 saturation <85% for at least 30 seconds). The PCO_2 must rise to greater than or equal to 60 mm Hg (or at least 20 mm Hg above baseline for a patient who chemically retains CO_2 owing to lung disease). The time of death is when an arterial blood gas consistent with apnea is reported by the laboratory.

If clinical testing, including the apnea test, cannot be performed or is precluded by hemodynamic instability, currently accepted alternative tests include intracranial blood flow studies (conventional angiography, transcranial Doppler, or single-photon emission computed tomography [SPECT]). When alternative testing is required, the time of death is the time the study is formally interpreted and signed by the attending physician.

TREATMENT Rx

Once brain death is diagnosed, the patient is legally dead. Further management is pursued only in the setting of possible organ donation. Otherwise, the ventilator is removed and all lines and monitors are discontinued. Physicians should be aware of local laws or policies that may restrict diagnosing death by brain criteria in patients who belong to certain religious groups that do not adhere to the concept of brain death.

Grade A References

A1. Hutchinson PJ, Kolias AG, Timofeev IS, et al. Trial of decompressive craniectomy for traumatic intracranial hypertension. *N Engl J Med.* 2016;375:1119-1130.
A2. Giacino JT, Whyte J, Bagiella E, et al. Placebo-controlled trial of amantadine for severe traumatic brain injury. *N Engl J Med.* 2012;366:819-826.

GENERAL REFERENCES

For the General References and other additional features, please visit Expert Consult at https://expertconsult.inkling.com.

377

SLEEP DISORDERS

BRADLEY V. VAUGHN AND ROBERT C. BASNER

DEFINITION

Sleep is essential to good health and a sense of well-being.[1] This normal state of decreased responsiveness restores bodily processes, and it also promotes alertness, memory, and learning. Conversely, the disruption of sleep is associated with a variety of health issues, as well as impaired performance and psychosocial interactions. Second in frequency only to pain, sleep-wake complaints lead one in three individuals to seek medical attention. Untreated sleep disorders and disruption may also exacerbate symptoms of other diseases by worsening a preexisting disorder or impairing the ability to cope with or counter the symptoms of the original disease. Thus clinicians should recognize that such signs and symptoms may be related to dysfunctional sleep.

PATHOBIOLOGY

Complex humoral, neurochemical, and neuronal networks determine the sleep-wake state. Dynamic in organization, sleep is composed of non–rapid eye movement (NREM) sleep and rapid eye movement (REM) sleep (denoted as Stage R). NREM is divided into three stages (N1, N2, and N3). Each stage has a distinct physiologic regulation, and each contributes to health and improved brain function.

Wakefulness involves activation of the monoaminergic neuronal groups, basal forebrain cholinergic neurons, and the brainstem reticular activating system (E-Fig. 377-1). The reticular activating system promotes the relay of sensory information to the cerebral hemispheres, and the forebrain cholinergic and monoaminergic neurons promote attention of the hemispheric networks to sensory information.

With the onset of sleep, information from two major drives (homeostatic, the chemicals that build during wakefulness; and circadian, the internal body clock) influence the ventral lateral preoptic nucleus to actively suppress the networks of wakefulness and allow the initiation of NREM sleep (E-Fig. 377-2). NREM sleep typically starts as stage N1, with slowing of the electroencephalogram (EEG), and slow eye movements (Table 377-1). Stage N1, which is associated with the feeling of drowsiness, accounts for about 5% of nocturnal sleep time. Although minimal sensory processing can occur, memory is not stored. Blood pressure may decrease slightly, and breathing becomes more periodic.

The hallmark of stage N2 sleep is an EEG with sleep spindles and K complexes. N2 typically represents about 50% of a night's sleep. Although stage N2 is considered light sleep, it is associated with less responsiveness to stimuli and to changes in CO_2 and O_2 than stage N1. Stage N3 is characterized by slow waves (0.5 to 2.0 Hz, >75 μV) in the EEG. These slow waves are more prominent in brain areas that are more heavily used during the preceding awake period. In stage N3, which constitutes 20% of nocturnal sleep, the individual is difficult to arouse and has rhythmic breathing that is less responsive to elevated CO_2 and low O_2 than during stage N2. This stage is also associated with metabolic rebalancing of the neurons, synapses, and glia.

REM sleep (stage R) is generated by cholinergic neurons in the subcoeruleus nucleus in the brainstem, which then activate other neuronal groups to produce the associated rapid eye movements, active theta and alpha frequency EEG waveforms, skeletal muscle paralysis, and reduced temperature regulation. Most vivid dreaming occurs in stage R, but dreams can occur in other stages. Because most skeletal muscles are paralyzed in Stage R, ventilation is solely dependent on the diaphragm. This stage is associated with the least amount of responsiveness to low O_2 and elevated CO_2. Stage R typically encompasses about 20% of the night's sleep and is ended by activation of norepinephrine and serotonergic neurons (E-Fig. 377-3). Age influences the distribution of sleep stages: REM sleep occupies 50% of sleep at birth and then gradually declines to 20 to 25% by age 3 years. Similarly, slow wave sleep is prominent in children and declines in men in their 30s and in women by age 40 to 50 years.

Sleep stages graphed through the night demonstrate the dynamic interplay of the various stages. As seen in a hypnogram (Fig. 377-1), sleep has repeating cycles of approximately 90 minutes. These cycles show a predominance of stage N3 in the first two cycles, and a gradual lengthening of the periods of stage R through the night.

TABLE 377-1 SLEEP STAGE PARAMETERS*

STAGE	EEG FINDINGS	EYE MOVEMENTS (EOG)	SUBMENTAL EMG	ASSOCIATED PHYSIOLOGY
Wakefulness (W)	**More than 50% of an epoch has the posterior dominant rhythm present**	**Rapid eye movements** to slow movements. **Blinking** may be present	**Normal to high muscle tone**	Memory registration, voluntary control over breathing
Stage N1	**Attenuation of the posterior dominant rhythm with mixed theta frequency low-amplitude background activity**	*Slow rolling eye movements*	*Variable but less than wake*	Automatic behavior can occur; diminished cognitive processing, periodic breathing
Stage N2	**K-complexes and/or sleep spindles.** *Low-amplitude mixed-frequency EEG*	*No eye movements, but slow eye movements may persist*	*Variable amplitude, typically lower than W and higher than R*	No memory, decreased arousal to stimuli, less response to elevated CO_2 and low oxygen
Stage N3	**Slow wave activity (0.5-2 Hz, >75 μV) for >20% of an epoch.** Sleep spindles and K complexes may persist	*No eye movements seen*	*Variable amplitude, typically lower than N2 and can be as low as R*	No memory, monotonous breathing pattern with less responsiveness to elevated CO_2 or low O_2
Stage R (REM sleep)	**Low-amplitude mixed-frequency EEG.** *Sawtooth waves*	**Rapid eye movements**	**Low muscle tone**	Similar response to stimuli as light sleep, irregular breathing pattern, least response to elevated CO_2 or low O_2

*Sleep staging requirements. **Boldfaced** items are requirements for staging. *Italicized* items are nonrequired associated findings that may be present in that stage.
CO_2 = carbon dioxide; EEG = electroencephalogram; EMG = electromyogram; EOG = electro-oculogram; O_2 = oxygen.
Adapted from the American Academy of Sleep Medicine. *The AASM Manual for the Scoring of Sleep and Associated Events.* 2nd ed. version 2.4. Westchester, IL: American Academy of Sleep Medicine; 2017.

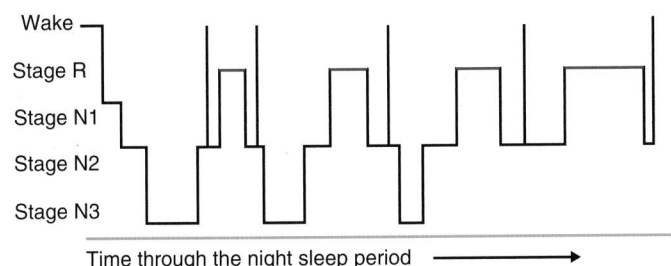

FIGURE 377-1. Hypnogram showing sleep stages across a sleep period.

Many models that consider the array of neurochemical pathways that influence sleep can theoretically explain its physiologic regulation. The most accepted two-driver model uses the homeostatic and circadian drivers to explain sleep-wake state. Other issues such as psychological status also play a role. The homeostatic drive is the accumulation of substances that promote sleepiness while the person is awake and are metabolized during sleep. Mental and physical activities increase this drive by producing neuronal byproducts (e.g., adenosine), whereas caffeine blunts this drive by blocking adenosine. In contrast, the circadian rhythm drive promotes wakefulness and, through its predictable cycle, prepares the body for anticipated activities. The circadian rhythm is a naturally occurring rhythm that is slightly longer than 24 hours but is readjusted each day to maintain alignment with the natural day-night cycle. This cycle is driven by a genetic transcription feedback loop that occurs in every cell of the body. These cells are synchronized by a master clock in the suprachiasmatic nucleus by complex signaling and the hormone melatonin, which is released in response to darkness. The circadian rhythm is primarily adjusted by bright light and to a lesser extent by exercise, food, and social interactions. When the circadian rhythm is stronger than the homeostatic drive, the person is awake, and when the homeostatic drive is stronger than the circadian rhythm, the person is sleepy (E-Fig. 377-4). This theoretical model helps explain aspects of sleep-wake regulation, such as the periods of postlunch sleepiness or evening wakefulness.

CLINICAL MANIFESTATIONS

Most patients who seek medical help for sleep issues present with one of three complaints: (1) excessive sleepiness, (2) difficulty attaining or sustaining sleep, (3) or unusual events associated with sleep. Excessive sleepiness may be confused with fatigue or lack of energy. Difficulty with sleep at night may be a clue to daytime issues, and nocturnal events may be a clue to possible neurologic issues. Other common presenting symptoms include morning headaches, lapses of attention, or diffuse muscle aches.

DIAGNOSIS

Both subjective information and objective tests are used to investigate sleep complaints. Questionnaires such as the Pittsburgh Sleep Quality Index provide a broad overview of sleep symptoms, including bedtime, wake time, activities, medications, and other substances that could influence sleep. Sleep diaries can also give a subjective report of the daily schedule (Fig. 377-2).

Objective testing of sleep includes polysomnography, actigraphy, multiple sleep latency testing, and maintenance of wakefulness testing. Polysomnography (Fig. 377-3) assesses both sleep stage and associated physiology. Sleep stage is determined by EEG, electro-oculogram, and submental electromyogram activity. Measures assessing physiology include respiratory function (airflow, effort, and gas exchange), limb muscle activity, and electrocardiogram. Polysomnography is most useful for sleep disruption, including sleep apnea, excessive movements, parasomnias, and unexplained excessive sleepiness (Table 377-2). More limited overnight recordings may focus on strictly respiratory measurements. Actigraphy monitors movement, typically of a nondominant extremity, over 7 to 28 days (Fig. 377-4). When combined with a sleep diary, actigraphy estimates total sleep time and assesses the sleep-wake schedule.

Two daytime tests can help estimate the degree of physiological sleepiness. The multiple sleep latency test quantifies objective sleepiness based on the time to onset of sleep across five daytime naps; it is most useful for diagnosing narcolepsy. The maintenance of wakefulness test quantifies the propensity to stay awake across four 40-minute epochs, and it can provide objective evidence of daytime efficacy of stimulant therapy.

HYPERSOMNIA

Sleepiness is normal just before a typical sleep period or after prolonged wakefulness. In 5 to 20% of adults, sleepiness occurs in inappropriate settings and affects quality of life, because of lapses of attention, decreased mood, and diminished cognitive abilities. After chronic sleep deprivation, the perception of sleepiness is reduced such that these individuals become accustomed to their impairment and fail to recognize their degree of sleepiness.

DIAGNOSIS

Clinicians should question hypersomnic patients for clues about sleep restriction, sleep disruption, neurologic issues, medication effect, or medical or psychiatric causes (Fig. 377-5). Information regarding sleep habits, including week and weekend schedules, as well as environment, may disclose important contributing factors. Patients with sleep apnea, narcolepsy, excessive periodic limb movements, circadian rhythm disorders, and parasomnias may have excessive daytime sleepiness as their main complaint. A history of snoring, observed apnea, morning headaches, cataplexy, sleep paralysis, hypnogogic hallucinations, or altered sleep schedule suggests other specific sleep disorders. Excessive sleepiness can also result from many medical disorders and medications. Patients with heart (Chapter 52), kidney (Chapter 122), or liver failure (Chapter 144), rheumatologic disease, or endocrinologic disorders such as

TWO WEEK SLEEP DIARY

INSTRUCTIONS:
1. Write the date, day of the week, and type of day: Work, School, Day Off, or Vacation.
2. Put the letter "C" in the box when you have coffee, cola or tea. Put "M" when you take any medicine. Put "A" when you drink alcohol. Put "E" when you exercise.
3. Put a line (I) to show when you go to bed. Shade in the box that shows when you think you fell asleep.
4. Shade in all the boxes that show when you are asleep at night or when you take a nap during the day.
5. Leave boxes unshaded to show when you wake up at night and when you are awake during the day.

SAMPLE ENTRY BELOW: On a Monday when I worked, I jogged on my lunch break at 1 PM, had a glass of wine with dinner at 6 PM, fell asleep watching TV from 7 to 8 PM, went to bed at 10:30 PM, fell asleep around Midnight, woke up and couldn't get back to sleep at about 4 AM, went back to sleep from 5 to 7 AM, and had coffee and medicine at 7:00 in the morning.

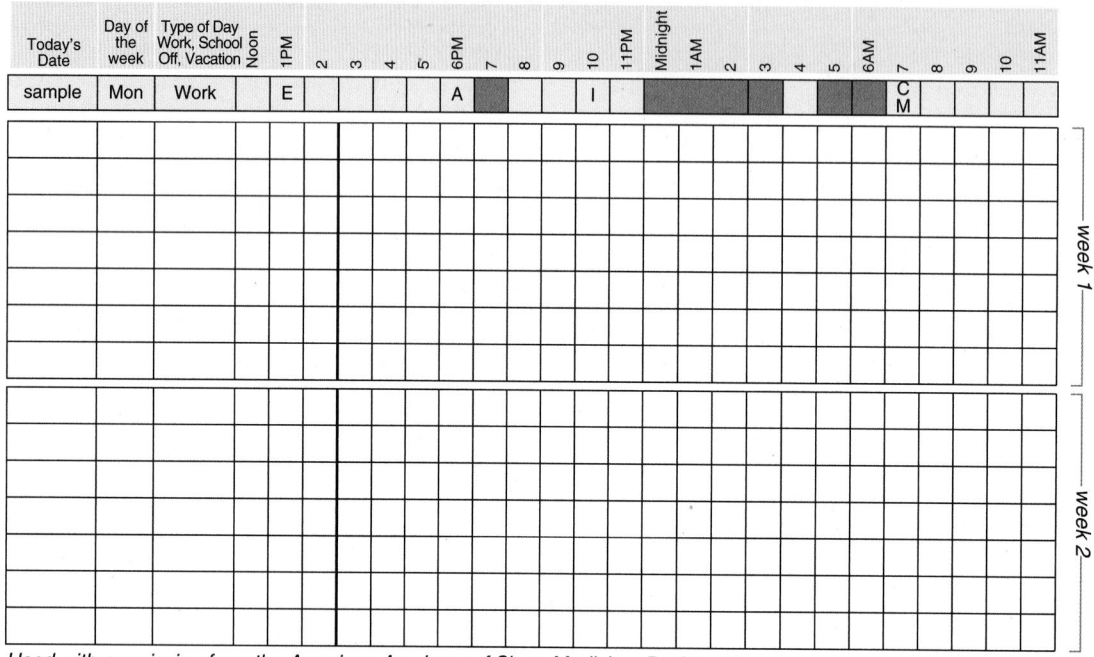

Used with permission from the American Academy of Sleep Medicine, Darien, Illinois.

FIGURE 377-2. Example of a sleep diary. Patients record their daily schedule, work, and medications.

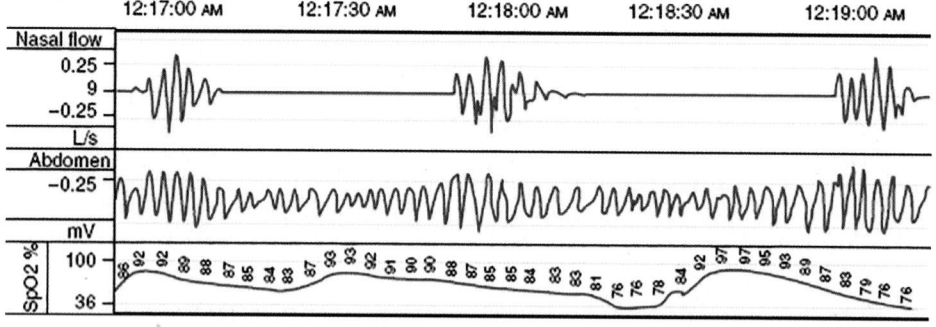

FIGURE 377-3. Polysomnographic tracing of a patient with obstructive sleep apnea during 2 minutes of non–rapid eye movement sleep. Displayed are airflow in the upper airway ("nasal flow"), recorded with a nasal pressure transducer; respiratory effort ("abdomen"), recorded by inductance plethysmography; and oxygen saturation of hemoglobin (Sp_{O_2}), recorded with pulse oximetry.

hypothyroidism (Chapter 213) and diabetes (Chapter 216) may note sleepiness and fatigue. Neurologic disorders such as stroke (Chapters 379), degenerative diseases (Chapters 374 and 381), tumor (Chapter 180), demyelinating disease (Chapter 383), and head trauma (Chapter 371) can cause excessive sleepiness.[2]

Sleepiness can be quantified subjectively by questionnaires or by physiologic measures such as a multiple sleep latency test. The Epworth Sleepiness Scale quantifies sleepiness by asking the subject to rate on a scale of 0 to 3 (0, no chance; 3, high likelihood) the chance of dozing in eight situations (Table 377-3). A score of 7 is considered average, whereas a score of 10 or more is consistent with subjective sleepiness. This score has a modest correlation with objective measures of sleepiness and better correlation with the severity of obstructive sleep apnea. The multiple sleep latency test is a valid test for narcolepsy, and the maintenance of wakefulness test gives a snapshot of the patient's ability to stay awake.

Narcolepsy

DEFINITION

Narcolepsy includes a tetrad of excessive sleepiness, cataplexy, sleep paralysis, and hypnogogic hallucinations. Narcolepsy has been divided into patients with low neurotransmitter hypocretin-1 (also known as orexin) or cataplexy (type 1), and patients without cataplexy or low hypocretin-1 (type 2).

EPIDEMIOLOGY

Narcolepsy type 1 affects 1 in 2000 to 6000 individuals; 40 to 80% have the complete tetrad, and approximately 50% complain of sleep disruption. Over 90% of individuals in the United States with cataplexy have the HLA-DQB1*0602 gene. Narcolepsy type 2 occurs in about 2 per 1000 individuals; approximately 40% have the HLA-DQB1*0602 gene, and some exhibit intermediate cerebrospinal fluid (CSF) hypocretin-1 levels. Despite the connection to a gene,

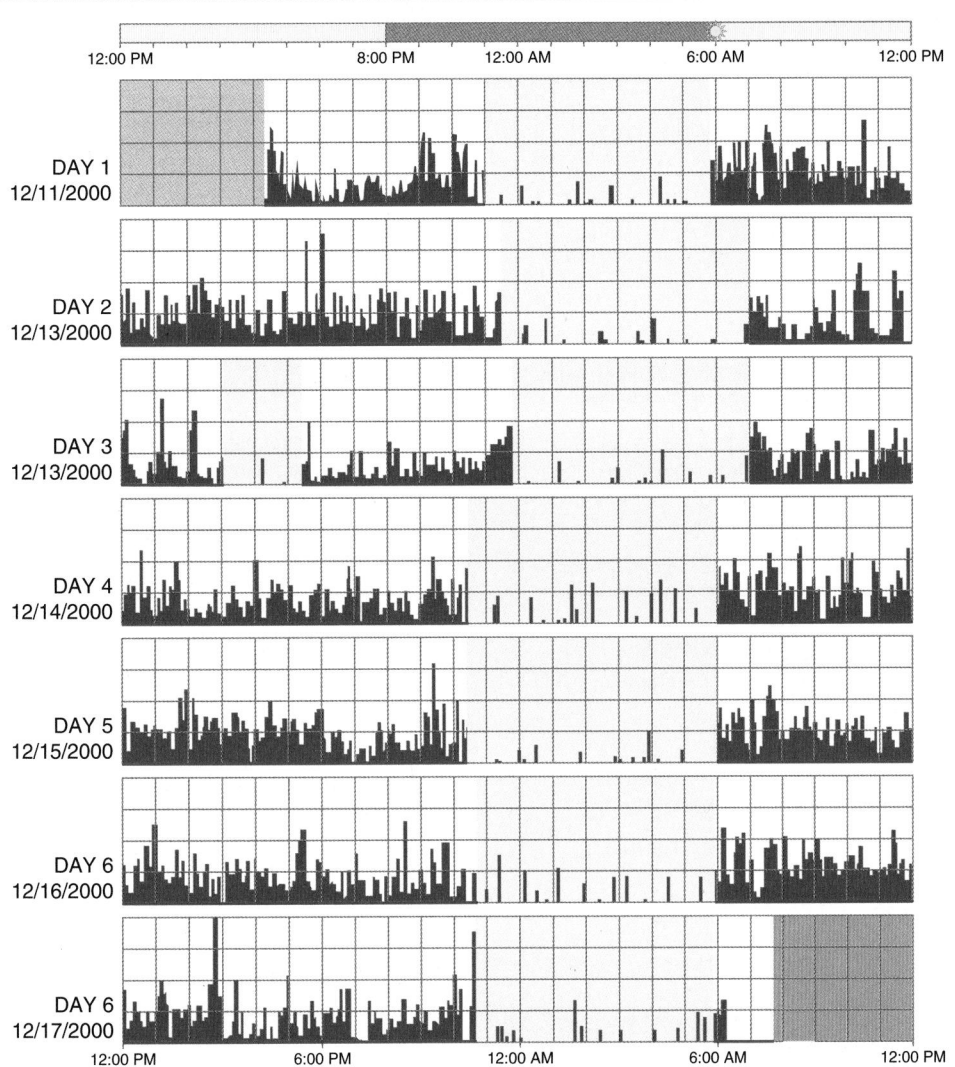

FIGURE 377-4. Actigraphy report. The shaded areas are scored as rest time; in this instance, the bedtime is 11 PM to 12 midnight, and wake time about 6 AM. One nap is observed on day 3 in the middle of the afternoon.

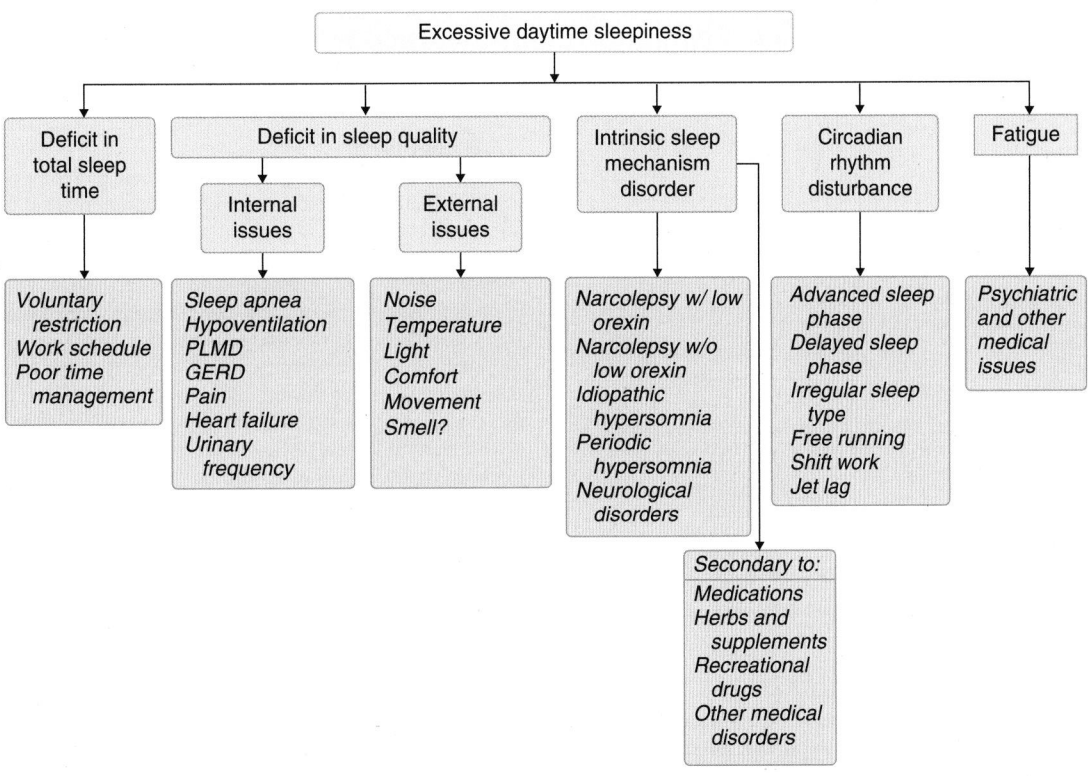

FIGURE 377-5. Differential diagnosis of excessive daytime sleepiness. GERD = gastroesophageal reflux disease; PLMD = periodic limb movement disorder.

TABLE 377-2   INDICATIONS FOR POLYSOMNOGRAPHY

POLYSOMNOGRAPHY IS ROUTINELY INDICATED FOR:

Diagnosis of sleep-related breathing disorders (SRBDs), including suspected obstructive sleep apnea (OSA) in patients with heart, brain, neuromuscular, or lung disease

Patients with sleep-related symptoms and heart, brain (stroke), neuromuscular, lung, or other major organ disease

Positive airway pressure (PAP) titration in patients with sleep-related breathing disorders

A preoperative clinical evaluation to evaluate for the presence of OSA before upper airway surgery or oral appliance therapy for OSA

Patients suspected of nocturnal movement disorders

Patients suspected of narcolepsy or unexplained excessive daytime sleepiness may require polysomnography and multiple sleep latency test on the ensuing day

Follow-up Polysomnography:

After titration of oral appliance treatment or final fitting in patients with OSA

Following surgical treatment of patients with moderate to severe OSA

After surgical or dental treatment of patients with SRBDs whose symptoms return

Substantial weight gain or loss in patients on PAP for SRBD

Insufficient clinical response to PAP therapy

Evaluation of patients with sleep behaviors that are potentially injurious or suggestive of unusual or atypical parasomnias or in which specific motor patterns are in question

POLYSOMNOGRAPHY IS *NOT* ROUTINELY INDICATED FOR:

Patients whose symptoms resolve with continuous positive airway pressure (CPAP) treatment

Diagnosis of chronic lung disease

Diagnosis of typical, uncomplicated, and noninjurious parasomnias when the diagnosis is clearly delineated

Patients with a seizure disorder who have no specific complaints consistent with a sleep disorder

Diagnosis or treatment of restless legs syndrome, except where diagnostic uncertainty exists

Establishing the diagnosis of depression

Diagnosis of circadian rhythm sleep disorders

TABLE 377-3   EPWORTH SLEEPINESS SCALE

How likely are you to doze off or fall asleep in the following situations, in contrast to just feeling tired? This refers to your usual way of life in recent time. Even if you have not done some of these things recently, try to work out how they would have affected you. Use the following scale to choose the most appropriate number for each situation.

0 = would never doze
1 = slight chance of dozing
2 = moderate chance of dozing
3 = high chance of dozing

SITUATION	CHANCE OF DOZING
Sitting and reading	_____
Watching TV	_____
Sitting and inactive in a public place (theater or meeting)	_____
As a passenger in a car for an hour without a break	_____
Lying down to rest in the afternoon when circumstances permit	_____
Sitting and talking to someone	_____
Sitting quietly after lunch (without alcohol)	_____
In a car, while stopped for a few minutes in traffic	_____
Total	_____

Adapted from Johns MW. A new method for measuring daytime sleepiness: the Epworth Sleepiness Scale. *Sleep.* 1991;14:540-545.

the risk to first-degree relatives is only 1 to 2%, or about a 10- to 50-fold increased risk compared with the general population. Some data suggest a link to infectious antigens such as the 2009 H1N1 influenza vaccine used in Europe and China.[3]

PATHOBIOLOGY

Narcolepsy type 1 reflects the loss of hypocretin-producing neurons in the lateral hypothalamus. This neurotransmitter is important for stabilizing the sleep-wake state and for motor control. Thus the manifestations of the disease are related to frequent stage shifts and intrusion of fragments of REM sleep into wakefulness. Why these neurons are lost is not known, but immune mechanisms are postulated.

CLINICAL MANIFESTATIONS

The tetrad of excessive sleepiness, cataplexy, hypnogogic hallucinations, and sleep paralysis is the major clinical manifestation. Cataplexy is abrupt loss of muscle tone triggered by strong emotional stimuli such as laughter, surprise, or anger. Patients are aware of their surroundings but lose muscle control, first in the face and neck, followed by the arms and then the trunk and legs. Hypnogogic (sleep-onset) and hypnopompic (sleep-offset) hallucinations are vivid and often frightening visual or auditory events. Sleep paralysis is an inability to move or speak, typically during the transition out of sleep when individuals have complete or partial awareness of their surroundings. Patients may describe a strong feeling of impending doom or having to escape imminent danger. Patients with narcolepsy often feel brief naps are refreshing. Frequently, their sleep is fragmented, with sleep intruding into daily activities and wakefulness interrupting nighttime sleep. Sleep paralysis and hypnogogic hallucinations can occur in normal individuals, especially after sleep deprivation, but cataplexy is virtually pathognomonic for narcolepsy.

DIAGNOSIS

The diagnosis of narcolepsy type 1 and type 2 is based on a mean sleep latency of less than 8 minutes and the presence of REM sleep on at least two of the five naps of a multiple sleep latency test. The multiple sleep latency test is predicated on the documentation of at least 6 hours of sleep before the study. The previous night's polysomnography must also not show other sleep pathologies. Low CSF hypocretin level in the setting of excessive sleepiness can also confirm of the diagnosis of narcolepsy type 1.

TREATMENT   Rx

Treatment of narcolepsy focuses on improving symptoms of excessive sleepiness, cataplexy, and REM sleep intrusion into wakefulness (Table 377-4).[4] Sleepiness requires a three-pronged approach of improving the quality of sleep, prescribing stimulants, and controlling cataplexy. Nighttime sleep may be improved with sodium oxybate (4.5 to 9.0 grams in divided nighttime doses), which improves daytime alertness and reduces cataplexy.[A1] Planned naps may help some patients, and stimulants such as modafinil (100 to 600 mg/day), armodafinil (50 to 250 mg/day), methylphenidate (5 to 60 mg/day), and dextroamphetamine (5 to 60 mg/day) can improve but do not eliminate daytime sleepiness. To avoid further sleep disruption, patients should not use stimulants in the evening and night hours. Solriamfetol (a selective dopamine and norepinephrine inhibitor at 75 to 300 mg daily) can reduce daytime sleepiness.[A2] Selective serotonin reuptake inhibitors (SSRIs) (Chapter 369, Table 369-5) and combined serotonin-norepinephrine reuptake inhibitors (SNRIs) (Chapter 369, Table 369-5) also reduce cataplexy, as well as sleep paralysis and hallucinations.

PROGNOSIS

Narcolepsy is a lifelong disorder. Patients who present in adolescence or young adulthood may progress to more severe symptoms, but the disorder does not affect longevity.

Other Hypersomnias

Idiopathic hypersomnia is a disorder in which hypersomnia cannot be explained by another disorder, is characterized by unrelenting hypersomnia, and is only minimally improved with therapy. Patients find that their symptoms persist despite long sleeping periods. These patients have average sleep latencies of less than 8 minutes, typically do not display REM sleep, but may have stage N3 on their multiple sleep latency test studies. Periodic hypersomnia can also occur in in Kleine-Levin syndrome (a syndrome of periodic hypersomnia, hyperphagia, and hypersexuality) and in perimenstrual hypersomnia.

TREATMENT   Rx

Treatment of sleepiness should focus on correcting the underlying cause. One early step is to extend the total sleep time to see if sleep deprivation plays a role. Stimulants such as modafinil (100 to 600 mg)[A3] should be used only in individuals who are impaired by the symptoms and in whom other therapies have failed to correct the hypersomnia. Some patients with Kleine-Levin syndrome respond to lithium.

TABLE 377-4 THERAPIES FOR NARCOLEPSY			
MODALITY	**STARTING DOSE**	**HIGHEST DAILY DOSE**	**DOSE AT**
Scheduled naps	10-15 minutes	1-3 naps	Just before time needing to be awake
OVER-THE-COUNTER STIMULANT			
Caffeine	25 mg	300 mg	AM
STIMULANTS			
Modafinil	100-200 mg	600 mg	AM and noon
Armodafinil	50-150 mg	250 mg	AM
Methylphenidate	5-10 mg	120 mg	AM and noon
Methylphenidate ER	10-20 mg	120 mg	AM
Dextroamphetamine	5-10 mg	60 mg	AM and noon
Combination dextroamphetamine/amphetamine	5-10 mg	60 mg	AM and noon
IMPROVE NIGHTTIME SLEEP, DAYTIME ALERTNESS, AND CATAPLEXY			
Sodium oxybate	2.25 grams	9.0 grams	Bedtime and 4 hr into sleep
THERAPIES FOR CATAPLEXY (NOT FDA APPROVED)			
Fluoxetine	10-20 mg	40 mg	AM
Venlafaxine	75 mg	225 mg	AM at lower dose or divided
Protriptyline	5 mg	30 mg	AM at lower dose or divided

SLEEP-RELATED BREATHING DISORDERS

Sleep-related breathing disorders in adults include obstructive sleep apnea, the central sleep apneas (including Cheyne-Stokes breathing), and the sleep-related hypoventilation disorders (including obesity-hypoventilation, congenital and idiopathic central alveolar hypoventilation, and hypoventilation due to medical disorders and respiratory suppressants). These categories and clinical disorders can overlap, but each has distinctive features. Obstructive sleep apnea and Cheyne-Stokes breathing are common in patients with heart failure (Chapters 52 and 53). Patients with brainstem dysfunction may have central apneas, whereas patients with obesity (Chapter 207), chest wall (Chapter 92), neuromuscular (Chapter 394), and central nervous system disorders with hypoventilation will often manifest sleep-related hypoventilation and hypoxemia in association with central or obstructive apneas.

Sleep Apnea

Obstructive sleep apnea is characterized by episodes of absent (apnea) or attenuated (hypopnea) upper airway airflow for at least 10 seconds with continued, and typically increasingly forceful, ventilatory effort followed by arousal and resumption of ventilation. Repetitive, often cyclic, asphyxia and sleep fragmentation is the hallmark of this disorder. *Central sleep apnea* is defined by repetitive episodes, either periodic, intermittent, or erratic, of at least 10 seconds of absent respiratory effort.

SLEEP-RELATED HYPOVENTILATION

Sleep-related alveolar hypoventilation is defined by intermittent or sustained elevation of arterial PCO_2 levels—either ≥55 mm Hg, or ≥10 mm Hg above awake—with or without outright apnea. Alveolar hypoventilation may occur only during sleep, or it may be exacerbated during sleep in patients who have hypoventilation disorders while awake. Both central and obstructive sleep apneas may be present; in the absence of such apneas, sleep-related hypercapnia and hypoxemia are typically more prolonged than are seen with the sleep apneas.

PATHOBIOLOGY

In patients with obstructive sleep apnea, particularly those with obesity, chest wall movement is restricted, with resultant mechanical and reflex upper airway narrowing, increased upper airway compliance, ventilatory instability, and an impaired ability to compensate for increased upper airway resistance. All these abnormalities may contribute to the obstruction of the upper airway during sleep, as well as NREM sleep-wake cycling and respiratory periodicity. During REM sleep, erratic neural drive and descending neural inhibition of accessory ventilatory and upper airway muscles may lead to severe alveolar hypoventilation and/or obstructive apnea.

With each obstructive event, the combination of progressive asphyxia, increasingly negative intrathoracic pressure, and autonomic and behavioral arousal leads to acute cardiac and cerebrovascular perturbations, including increased afterload of both the left and right ventricles, decreased left ventricular compliance, increased pulmonary artery pressure, decreased coronary artery blood flow, and increased myocardial oxygen demand (see Fig. 377-3). The abrupt arousal at the termination of obstructive events is associated with peripheral vasoconstriction and an increase in the heart rate and in systemic blood pressure, even as cardiac output continues to fall.

Central sleep apnea in patients who have heart failure is characteristically of the Cheyne-Stokes breathing type, mediated by interacting physiologic variables, including lung volume changes, circulatory timing, and a higher than normal gradient between inspired and arterial carbon dioxide tensions (PCO_2). The ventilatory response to a change in blood gases is augmented. The net effect is oscillation of ventilation between central apnea and hyperpnea, as sleep and awake states oscillate. Central apneas in other circumstances may be linked to dysfunctional neural chemosensitivity responses resulting in subsequent apnea, as is seen in the idiopathic, medication-related, and central alveolar hypoventilation syndromes. Sleep-related hypoventilation without central or obstructive apnea is pathogenetically linked to neural inhibition of postural respiratory muscles and perturbed respiratory mechanics.

CLINICAL MANIFESTATIONS
Obstructive Sleep Apnea

The cardinal manifestations of obstructive sleep apnea include loud, chronic snoring; excessive daytime somnolence; and witnessed sleep-related choking or gasping (E-Fig. 377-5). Excessive daytime somnolence is present in approximately 50% of patients with obstructive sleep apnea and may be quantified by laboratory tests that monitor the propensity to fall asleep during the day or by questionnaires or subjective scales that assess sleepiness or decrements in quality of life. Resolution of obstructive sleep apnea does not necessarily resolve excessive daytime somnolence, thereby suggesting the possibility of sustained neurologic perturbation from chronic intermittent hypoxemia and highlighting the association of obstructive sleep apnea with metabolic, neurocognitive, respiratory, and cardiovascular abnormalities. Mood disorders, including depression and irritability, as well as perturbations in visual memory and working memory appear to be related to the severity of sleep fragmentation and hypoxemia. Morning dry mouth is a common symptom, as is morning headache. Insomnia may be associated with the repetitive interruption of sleep characteristic of sleep apnea. Transient arousals during N3 sleep may result in confusional parasomnias, such as sleepwalking and sleep talking. Arousals and increased work of breathing may result in restless sleep and night sweats. Nocturia, possibly mediated via atrial natriuretic receptors, may resolve with treatment.

Upper airway abnormalities associated with obstructive sleep apnea include nasal congestion, rhinitis, chronic sinusitis, nasopharyngeal anatomic abnormalities, and craniofacial abnormalities such as micrognathia and retrognathia. Large tonsils, redundant soft palate tissue, and a large tongue may all be associated with a "crowded" oropharynx, but the precise role of these upper airway abnormalities in the pathogenesis of the disorder is unclear.[5]

Obstructive sleep apnea is commonly associated with major medical disorders, including cardiovascular (e.g., heart failure [Chapters 52 and 53], systemic [Chapter 70][6] and pulmonary hypertension [Chapter 75], dysrhythmias including atrial fibrillation [Chapter 58][7] and coronary artery disease), cerebrovascular (e.g., stroke and transient ischemic attack [Chapter 379]), pulmonary (e.g., chronic obstructive pulmonary disease [COPD; Chapter 82], asthma [Chapter 81], and interstitial lung disease [Chapter 86]), and metabolic (e.g., metabolic syndrome) disorders. These conditions tend to have a worse prognosis when concomitant obstructive sleep apnea is not treated.

Central Sleep Apnea

Central sleep apnea is prevalent in patients who use opiates (Chapter 31), during which cluster breathing with central apneas is characteristic, and in patients with congenital and acquired central nervous system and/or cervical spine disorders, in which Biot-type breathing is characteristic (E-Fig. 377-6). Cheyne-Stokes breathing, the most common form of central sleep apnea, is manifested as a crescendo-decrescendo breathing pattern with central apnea or hypopnea as the nadir of the breathing effort cycle (E-Fig. 377-7); central sleep apnea with Cheyne-Stokes breathing is prevalent in patients with heart failure (Chapter 52), in which it is an independent predictor of increased mortality. Patients with heart failure and Cheyne-Stokes breathing tend to have lower awake arterial carbon dioxide tensions ($Paco_2$) than other patients who have heart failure. The increased mortality in this setting has been correlated with the severity of the associated nocturnal hypoxemic burden.

Sleep-Related Hypoventilation

Patients with sleep-related hypoventilation may note daytime sleepiness, fatigue, morning headache, or unrefreshing sleep. Sleep-related hypoventilation is common in individuals with central obesity (often in association with obesity-hypoventilation syndrome), neuromuscular and chest wall disease, central hypoventilation disorders (with disordered respiratory control), COPD, and narcotic use.

DIAGNOSIS

Screening is not indicated in asymptomatic patients,[8] but a high degree of clinical suspicion in symptomatic patients[9] should prompt the physician to obtain polysomnography, which generally involves all-night monitoring at home or in a sleep laboratory (or at the bedside in hospitalized patients). In a sleep laboratory or hospital setting, data are gathered via electroencephalography, electro-oculography (primarily to determine rapid eye movements characteristic of REM sleep), electrocardiography, leg and chin electromyography, and measures of respiratory effort (airflow, hemoglobin oxygen saturation, and alveolar or arterial carbon dioxide levels). Audiovisual recordings can identify crescendo snoring and thoracoabdominal paradoxical breathing efforts to help differentiate obstructive from nonobstructive hypopnea. Home sleep studies, which monitor only basic respiratory parameters, are as good for making the diagnosis at a lower cost in patients who are suspected of having obstructive sleep apnea without major hypoventilation, cardiovascular, or cerebrovascular comorbidities.[A4] In-laboratory polysomnography has the advantages of recording more parameters, such as carbon dioxide in a controlled setting, and of allowing for objective titration of positive airway pressure and/or oxygen during the same night as the diagnostic portion of study.

TREATMENT   Rx

For obstructive sleep apnea, weight loss and avoidance of supine sleep are important components of treatment.[10] The mainstay of immediate and effective reversal of the disorder is positive airway pressure (PAP), usually in a continuous mode (continuous positive airway pressure [CPAP]). This therapy requires a significant commitment for compliance, and the physician must closely monitor and work with the patient to ensure its usage. Both continuous and bilevel PAP are also effective in improving sleep-related and awake hypoventilation and quality of life in the obesity hypoventilation syndrome.[A5][A6] Although positive airway pressure can improve symptoms, it does not reduce future cardiovascular events or death.[A7]

Neither supplemental oxygen alone nor medication provides optimal benefit. A mandibular advancement device may also be effective therapy[A8]; conversely, surgical uvulopalatopharyngoplasty, radiofrequency volumetric tissue reduction of the palate or tongue (or both), and laser-assisted uvuloplasty are not

recommended as first-line therapy to treat symptomatic patients. Promising evolving therapeutic modalities include proprietary implantable neurostimulation of the hypoglossal nerve,[A9] nasal expiratory positive airway pressure, and oral pressure therapy.

In patients with heart failure (Chapter 53), the increased mortality associated with Cheyne-Stokes breathing can be reduced by an effective response to CPAP. Adaptive servo-ventilation can improve the Cheyne-Stokes breathing, quality of life, and functional status in patients with heart failure but does not reduce mortality, and in one study was shown to increase mortality.[A10] Transvenous phrenic nerve stimulation also can normalize Cheyne-Stokes breathing but again without a demonstrated reduction in mortality.[A11]

Some patients with sleep-related hypoventilation may be treated with noninvasive ventilation, with supplemental oxygen as needed and titrated to address primarily obstructive apneas (common in patients with both the obesity hypoventilation syndrome and COPD) as well as nonapneic hypoventilation and hypoxemia. Noninvasive ventilation alone should *not* be considered safe therapy in patients with central alveolar hypoventilation, in whom tracheostomy and 24-hour assured ventilation should be considered standard of care.

Insomnia

DEFINITION

Insomnia is the complaint of difficulty initiating or maintaining sleep, or of unrefreshing sleep that results in daytime symptoms of excessive fatigue or impairment of performance. Some individuals may need less sleep and have no daytime sequelae, thereby differentiating them from individuals with insomnia. Chronic insomnia is defined by symptoms that persist more than 3 months regardless of the underlying cause or associations.

EPIDEMIOLOGY

Most individuals have occasional nights with difficulty falling asleep or maintaining sleep, often provoked by psychological challenges or sudden changes in their environment. Approximately 35% of individuals complain of intermittent difficulty with sleep, and approximately 10% have chronic insomnia. Women, older individuals, and patients with psychiatric or chronic medical illness are predisposed to develop insomnia. Insomnia is also more common in individuals with lower socioeconomic status and poor education. Patients with behavioral traits such as obsessive-compulsive tendency, frequent rumination, or poor coping strategies are also at greater risk for insomnia.

PATHOBIOLOGY

Patients with insomnia frequently give historical clues directed toward the mechanisms behind their insomnia. Studies of patients with insomnia show that these individuals are in a state of hyperarousal with increased brain metabolic rates during NREM sleep. Most patients have multiple factors that contribute to the insomnia, including features that predispose them to insomnia, events that precipitated the insomnia, and maladaptive behaviors that perpetuate the insomnia. Many patients have a coincident psychiatric disorder (Chapter 369) or psychological or medical issues. Patients with depression or anxiety may have insomnia for years before other characteristics of affective disorders. Patients with organ failure, such as heart failure, commonly complain of insomnia and may note difficulty remaining in bed owing to breathing issues. Restless legs syndrome, pain of any origin, and diseases that limit mobility (e.g., muscular dystrophy [Chapter 393] or Parkinson disease [Chapter 381]) can interrupt sleep. Sleep schedules also may be influenced by diseases (e.g., dementia [Chapter 374] in which circadian rhythm abnormalities promote nighttime awakenings).

CLINICAL MANIFESTATIONS

The patient or bed partners may give clues to a poor sleep environment, maladaptive behaviors, psychological stress, psychiatric or neurologic disease, primary sleep disorders, or other medical issues that cause insomnia. Insomnia may be initiated by events that shift schedules or by a change in medications. Initiating events may play little role in long-term insomnia, but these also give important clues to preventing further recurrence of the insomnia. When insomnia persists, many patients adopt behaviors that help perpetuate it. Maladaptive behaviors that may occur during the day or night include heavy daytime caffeine or alcohol use, watching television or playing video games while in bed, or eating or exercising near the sleep period. A subgroup of patients may develop mental rumination or even sleep phobias. This expectation of poor sleep promotes apprehension about sleep and may perpetuate counterproductive

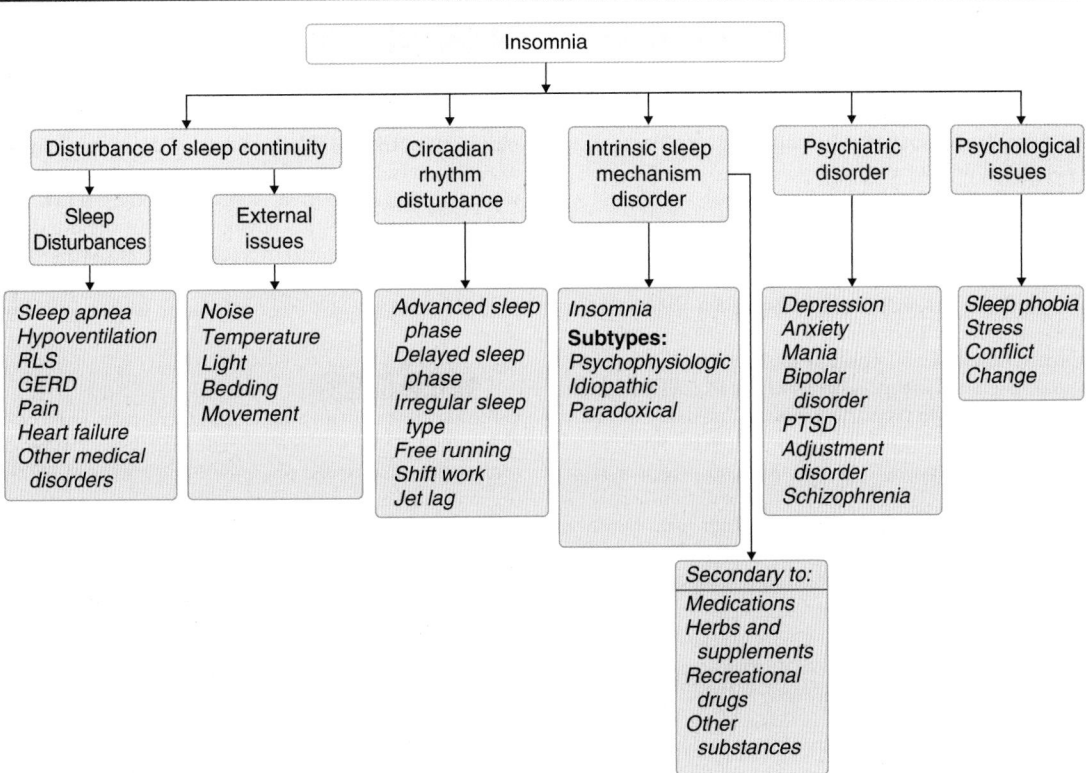

FIGURE 377-6. Differential diagnosis of insomnia. GERD = gastroesophageal reflux disease; PTSD = post-traumatic stress disorder; RLS = restless legs syndrome.

TABLE 377-5	CLASSIFICATION OF ADULT INSOMNIA

INSOMNIA

Subtypes:

Psychophysiologic insomnia—maladaptive behaviors conditioned in response to associating the bed environment or thoughts of bedtime with heightened arousal; patients typically sleep better in a different environment, such as away on vacation.

Idiopathic insomnia—insomnia beginning in infancy or childhood, with a persistent unremitting course and no improvement with change in environment

Paradoxical insomnia (sleep state misperception)—insomnia characterized by a marked mismatch between the patient's description of sleep duration and objective polysomnographic findings

INSOMNIA ASSOCIATED WITH

Adjustment insomnia—associated with an acute or active psychosocial stressor

Inadequate sleep hygiene—associated with lifestyle habits that impair the ability to sleep

Insomnia comorbid with a psychiatric disorder—associated with an active psychiatric disorder such as anxiety or depression

Insomnia comorbid with a medical condition—associated with a condition such as renal failure, hepatic failure, chronic pain, nocturnal cough or dyspnea, or hot flashes

Insomnia caused by a drug or substance—secondary to consumption or discontinuation of medications, drugs of abuse, alcohol, or caffeine

sleep rituals. These maladaptive behaviors become the predominant feature of the subtype of psychophysiologic insomnia (Table 377-5).

Some patients may not perceive that they are asleep. Individuals with the subtype of paradoxical insomnia have normal physiologic sleep but do not recognize that they have been asleep. Other patients may have the unrealistic expectation that sleep should not be interrupted by any arousals or that they must sleep a set number of hours.

The less common subtype of idiopathic insomnia starts in childhood and continues as a lifelong difficulty of sleep. These patients may have defective sleep mechanisms. Noting the timing of the insomnia during the sleep period may also be helpful. Difficulty with the onset of sleep suggests an underlying delayed sleep phase, and insomnia with early morning arousal suggests underlying depression or advanced sleep phase. Documentation of schedule changes (e.g., from jet lag or shift work) can be useful in determining links to circadian rhythm issues.

DIAGNOSIS

The diagnosis of insomnia is based on the patient's history that difficulty with sleep results in daytime sequelae (Fig. 377-6).[11] Although a patient may have more than one insomnia subtype, evidence is lacking that subtypes should direct therapy.

The history should include a review of the patient's 24-hour schedule, meals, and caffeine, tobacco, and medicine intake; sleep environment; attitudes about sleep; and the sleep experience. In addition, a thorough history from the bed partner may disclose features the patient is unaware of, such as snoring, limb movements, and sleep habits. Patients should be asked to keep a 2-week diary of their daily events, which often will show specific patterns or provide clues that can guide interventions. Polysomnography should be considered only if the patient has symptoms of sleep apnea or has failed therapeutic trials.

TREATMENT   Rx

Insomnia is generally treated as a single disorder even though it has been divided into subtypes (Table 377-6), but effective treatment requires identifying factors that contribute to insomnia. Treatment is multipronged and includes improving behaviors that promote sleep, addressing the perpetuating factors, and deciding if hypnotic medication is appropriate. Every patient with insomnia should practice routines that appropriately promote good sleep and wake habits. Cognitive-behavioral therapy provides long-term success for insomnia (see Table 377-6).[A12] The cognitive portion focuses on restructuring beliefs about sleep, whereas behavioral therapies focus on actions that may mitigate maladaptive behaviors and promote better sleep behaviors: progressive relaxation techniques, stimulus control, or sleep or time-in-bed restriction (Table 377-7).

Hypnotics are best used for short-term treatment in conjunction with cognitive-behavioral therapy (see Table 377-7).[12] Agents with rapid onset and a short half-life are typically used to address difficulties initiating sleep, whereas agents with a longer half-life or continuous-release are used to improve sleep maintenance. Benzodiazepines are preferred first-line agents, but a melatonin receptor agonist (ramelteon, 8 mg) and antidepressant medications (Chapter 369, Table 369-5) may also be used for insomnia. A newer agent, suvorexant (10 to 20 mg), improves sleep by blocking hypocretin to promote sleep maintenance.[A13] In patients with insomnia and coexisting depression or anxiety, the combination of the short-term use of a hypnotic, such as a benzodiazepine, and long-term antidepressant or anxiolytic is better for both the insomnia and the affective disorder than either therapy alone.[A14]

PROGNOSIS

Most patients will improve, although some will relapse. Intractable insomnia often heralds an affective disorder (Chapter 369). Except for very rare patients with the prion-induced fatal familial insomnia (Chapter 387), patients with insomnia have only a slightly lower life expectancy.

Circadian Rhythm Disorders

DEFINITION

Circadian rhythm disorders cause misalignment of the person's sleep-wake cycle and the naturally occurring day-night cycle. Pathologic symptoms must be persistent or recurrent, and the patient must incur some social, occupational, or additional impairment. Individuals may note insomnia, excessive daytime sleepiness, or both. Circadian rhythm sleep-wake disorder is typically classified by comparing the patient's rhythm to the naturally occurring day. Circadian rhythm sleep-wake disorders are subtyped into advanced phase type (early to bed and rise), delayed phase type (late to bed and rise), irregular type (no clear pattern), and free-running type (a rhythm that is not entrained to the environment). Induced disorders include jet lag and shift work. Another disorder related to circadian rhythm involves the gastrointestinal cycle: night eating syndrome, in which individuals consume over half of their caloric intake after 9 PM.

TABLE 377-6 NONPHARMACOLOGIC THERAPIES FOR INSOMNIA

COGNITIVE-BEHAVIORAL THERAPY with or without relaxation therapy (Standard)
The combination of multiple modalities noted below
STIMULUS-CONTROL THERAPY (Standard)
Go to bed only when sleepy.
Use the bedroom only for sleeping and sex.
Go to another room when unable to sleep in 15-20 minutes, read or engage in other quiet activities, and return to bed only when sleepy; repeat if necessary.
Have a regular wake time regardless of the duration of sleep.
Avoid daytime napping.
SLEEP-RESTRICTION THERAPY (Guideline)
Reduce time in bed to the estimated total sleep time (minimum, 5 hr).
Increase time in bed by 15 minutes every week when the patient estimates the sleep efficiency is at least 85% (ratio of time asleep to time in bed).
RELAXATION THERAPY (Standard)
Physical component: progressive muscle relaxation, autogenic training
Mental component: reducing intrusive thoughts through imagery training, meditation, or hypnosis
PARADOXICAL INTENTION (Guideline for sleep-onset difficulties)
Instruct the patient to remain passively awake in bed and avoid any effort to fall asleep.
COGNITIVE THERAPY (Insufficient evidence as a single therapy)
Education to alter maladaptive or unrealistic beliefs and attitudes about sleep, such as that a minimum of 8 hours of sleep per night is required for health
SLEEP HYGIENE EDUCATION (Insufficient evidence as a single therapy)
Correction of extrinsic factors and behaviors that affect sleep, such as environmental disruption (pets, music, or television); bedroom temperature; fixation on the bedside clock; use of alcohol, nicotine, or caffeine; lack of exercise or exercise too close to bedtime

---

EPIDEMIOLOGY

The prevalence of circadian rhythm disorders is not known. Some patterns of sleep are inherent in specific age groups. Advanced sleep phase issues are more common in the elderly, and delayed sleep phase issues are more common in adolescents. Purposeful shifting of the circadian rhythm, such as with shift work or jet lag, is common. Although about 30% of the U.S. workforce works nights or rotating shifts, only one third of these individuals have a clinical circadian rhythm disorder. A free-running circadian rhythm is more common among blind persons, of whom about 25% have the disorder. Irregular sleep-wake disorder appears more commonly in patients with neurodegenerative diseases, in which it may be an early symptom.

PATHOBIOLOGY

Circadian rhythm sleep-wake disorders may be more prevalent in today's "24-hour society," which offers constant stimuli to remain awake. Teens are more vulnerable to the phase-delaying effects of light in the evening. The human "master clock," which resides in the suprachiasmatic nucleus of the hypothalamus, synchronizes the body's peripheral tissue clocks, possibly mediated by melatonin. About 10% of genes are expressed with circadian rhythmicity. Abnormalities in genetic clock genes may contribute to circadian rhythm disorders. Variations in the *Clock*, *Per2*, and *Per3* genes appear to influence the morning/evening preference. Advance sleep phase type has been associated with the *Per2* S662G mutation and the *Ck1d* T44A mutation, whereas delayed sleep phase type is associated with the *Per3* V647G and *Ck1e* S408N mutations. The latter mutation is also associated with free-running type. Free-running type in individuals who are blind appears to be related to the loss of the photoreceptive ganglion cell input to the hypothalamus and not into the retina itself.

CLINICAL MANIFESTATIONS

Patients with circadian rhythm disorders typically complain of insomnia and/or excessive sleepiness, and they may incur sleep deprivation by trying to maintain schedules that are not consistent with their inherent clocks.[13] Some individuals "catch up" on the weekends by sleeping during their preferred times. Once asleep, the patient sleeps well. Circadian rhythm sleep-wake disorders are associated with an increased risk of accidents and impaired quality of life.

Delayed sleep phase–type patients typically have trouble falling asleep and may not fall sleep for over 2 hours later than the conventional bedtime (E-Fig. 377-8A). They then have trouble arousing in the morning, preferring late wake times. Advanced sleep phase–type patients fall asleep early in the evening and awaken several hours earlier than the conventional morning awakening (E-Fig. 377-8B). Patients complain of early morning awakening and the inability to maintain wakefulness during evening activities. Free-running type individuals have a circadian rhythm that continues to run on the 24.3- to 25-hour cycle. In this disorder, also known as non–24-hour sleep-wake rhythm disorder, patients have alternating episodes of insomnia and excessive sleepiness, depending on the phase of the endogenous sleep-wake cycle. This disorder can be confused with a periodic hypersomnia. Irregular-type patients have both excessive sleepiness and insomnia, with deceased functioning and a decreased sense of well-being[14] during the waking period.

TABLE 377-7 MEDICATIONS FOR INSOMNIA

NAME	DOSE	TIME OF DOSE	FDA INDICATION	COMMON SIDE EFFECTS	HALF-LIFE	MECHANISM
Zolpidem SL	1.75-10 mg	Bedtime	Yes	Sleepiness, amnesia, falls, parasomnias	1-2 hr	Benzodiazepine receptor agonist (BZRA)
Zolpidem reg	5-10 mg	Bedtime	Yes	Sleepiness amnesia, falls, parasomnias	1-2 hr	BZRA
Zolpidem CR	6.25-12.5 mg	Bedtime	Yes	Sleepiness, amnesia, falls	1-2 hr but continued release	BZRA
Temazepam	7.5-30 mg	Bedtime	Yes	Sleepiness, dizziness	8-10 hr	Benzodiazepine
Zaleplon	5-20 mg	Bedtime	Yes	Sleepiness, dizziness, parasomnias	1 hr	BZRA
Eszopiclone	1-3 mg	Bedtime	Yes	Sleepiness, dizziness	4-8 hr	BZRA
Doxepin	3-6 mg	Bedtime	Yes	Drowsiness, dizziness, nausea	17 hr	Histamine receptor antagonist
Mirtazapine	7.5-15 mg	Bedtime	No	Drowsiness, dizziness, weight gain	20 hr	Histamine receptor antagonist
Ramelteon	4-8 mg	Bedtime	Yes	Sleepiness, headache	1-2 hr	Melatonin receptor agonist
Subvorexant	10-20 mg	Bedtime	Yes	Sleepiness	12 hr	Blocks orexin

FDA = U.S. Food and Drug Administration.

DIAGNOSIS

The diagnosis of a circadian rhythm disorder is made by history and a 2-week sleep diary or actigraphy recording. Normal individuals have a tendency toward "morningness" or "eveningness," so the diagnosis requires documentation of a negative impact of circadian rhythm on quality of life.

TREATMENT

Most therapy is directed toward aligning the disordered circadian rhythm with the desired sleep-wake schedule. Shifting the schedule, known as chronotherapy, can be accomplished by allowing a gradual delay or advancing of the inherent schedule to the desired time, and then using clues to maintain the schedule.

The circadian rhythm is susceptible to time clues only if such clues are given at an appropriate time of the endogenous circadian rhythm. Using the temperature cycle nadir (which typically occurs approximately 2 hours before the natural wake up time) as a reference, bright light, exercise, food, and social interactions delivered before the temperature nadir will delay the cycle, whereas these stimuli delivered after the temperature nadir will advance the cycle. Melatonin has an opposite effect and typically advances the cycle if given 4 to 6 hours before the onset of sleep. Melatonin therapy may delay the cycle if used after the temperature nadir.

Once the circadian rhythm is realigned, patients benefit from strictly maintaining their schedule and time clues to reinforce the new circadian timing. Although short-term hypnotics and stimulants are commonly used to help adjustment, these medications do not realign the circadian rhythm.

Parasomnia

DEFINITION

Parasomnias are undesirable behavioral events or experiential phenomena occurring during entry into, within, or as part of arousal from sleep. These events include abnormal movements, behaviors, emotions, perceptions, dreaming, and activities of the autonomic nervous system. Parasomnias are typically subdivided into those arising from NREM sleep, REM sleep–related parasomnias, and other parasomnias. NREM events include sleep-related eating disorder and disorders of arousal (sleepwalking, sleep terrors, and confusional arousals). REM-related parasomnias include nightmare disorder, REM sleep behavior disorder, and recurrent sleep paralysis.

EPIDEMIOLOGY

Approximately 3% of adults and 15% of children have a sleep-related abnormal behavior. Although some parasomnias, such as disorders of arousal from NREM sleep (sleepwalking, sleep terrors, and confusional arousals), are more common in children, REM-related parasomnias, such as nightmare disorder, are common among all ages and are especially common in individuals with post-traumatic stress disorder (Chapter 369). REM sleep behavior disorder, which is another REM sleep–related parasomnia, is more common in the elderly and may predate other features of synucleinopathy neurodegenerative disorders such as Parkinson disease (Chapter 381), dementia with Lewy bodies (Chapter 374), and multiple-system atrophy (Chapter 381).

CLINICAL MANIFESTATIONS AND DIAGNOSIS

The history is the mainstay of the diagnosis of most parasomnias. Key features include age of onset, time of night of the events, memory for the events, and family history (Table 377-8). Because NREM parasomnias are a mixture of deep NREM sleep with the awake state, these events are more common in the first third of the night, are associated with no or little memory for the event, and are not stereotypical. Events are more likely to occur with sleep deprivation, alcohol ingestion, sleeping in strange environments, and coincidental conditions that predispose to arousals, such as sleep apnea. Patients are neurologically and psychiatrically normal during wakefulness.

REM sleep behavior disorder usually begins in late adulthood, but it can occur in children. In this disorder, patients lose the muscle atonia of REM sleep and thus act out during their dreams, sometimes injuring themselves or bed partners.[15] This nonstereotypical motor activity is often associated with vivid recall of a dream that correlates with the witnessed behavior. Patients can have multiple events typically in the latter half of the night. This behavior disorder can be provoked by medications such as tricyclic antidepressants, monoamine oxidase inhibitors, and serotonin reuptake inhibitors.

The diagnosis is based on the documented excessive electromyographic activity during REM sleep and the history of dream enactment. If the patient demonstrates stereotypic sleep motor behavior, rather than the characteristic nonstereotypical behavior of REM sleep behavior disorder, the possibility of epilepsy (Chapter 375) should be considered. Because chronic REM sleep behavior disorder has been linked to the subsequent development of Parkinson disease (Chapter 381), multiple system atrophy (Chapter 381), and Lewy

TABLE 377-8 KEY FEATURES OF NOCTURNAL EVENTS

DISORDER	SYMPTOMS	TIME OF NIGHT	DURATION	FREQUENCY	STEREOTYPICAL	MEMORY	POLYSOMNOGRAPHIC FINDINGS
Sleepwalking	Slow, deliberate, complex behaviors	First half of sleep period	Seconds to minutes	Less than one per night to fewer	No	No or partial vague memory	Arousal from slow wave sleep
Sleep terrors	Piercing scream, followed by fight or flight response	First half	Seconds to minutes	Less than one per night or fewer	No	No or partial vague memory	Arousal from slow wave sleep
Confusional arousals	Variety of unusual behaviors upon sudden awakening	Anytime	Seconds to minutes	Less than one per night or fewer	No	No or partial vague memory	Arousal from slow wave sleep
Sleep-related eating	Eating of high-calorie or strange foods in a messy manner	First half	Minutes	May occur nightly	No	No or partial vague memory	Arousal typically from NREM sleep
Nightmares	Frightening dreams associated with anxiety	Latter half	Seconds to minutes	Variable	No, but may have a common theme	Yes	Events occur in REM sleep
REM sleep behavior disorder	Dream enactment, may be violent	Latter half	Seconds	Multiple times per night	No	Yes	Excessive EMG activity in REM sleep
Rhythmic movement disorder	Rocking, head banging	Near sleep onset but may be throughout the night	Minutes to hours	Multiple times per night	Yes	Yes	Rhythmic movement in transition from waking to sleeping
Catathrenia	Nocturnal prolonged moaning	Intermittent throughout the night	Minutes to hours	Multiple	Yes	No	Prolonged expiratory moans and groans, with slowed respiratory rate
Exploding head syndrome	Loud painless sound of explosion inside the head	Near the onset of sleep	Seconds	Rare, typically infrequent	Yes	Yes	Typically events are close to sleep onset

EMG = electromyogram; NREM = non–rapid eye movement; REM = rapid eye movement.

body dementia (Chapter 374), patients should have a detailed neurologic examination to look for subclinical features.

Other nocturnal events can present as sensory phenomena or sleep-related movements. Nightmares are emotionally disturbing dreams associated with fear, anxiety, anger, or sadness. Nightmares most commonly occur after a psychologically disturbing event, but may also occur as a result of antihypertensive medications, antidepressants, or dopamine agonists. Exploding head syndrome is the painless perception of a loud sound or sense of an explosion, typically in light sleep. Bruxism is a disorder of jaw clenching or grinding that can cause tooth damage and headaches. Rhythmic movement disorder is associated with body rocking or head banging in the transition from wake to sleep.

Patients who have nocturnal events with atypical features, a risk of harm, signs or symptoms of other sleep disorders, or excessive daytime sleepiness should undergo in-laboratory video polysomnography, with extended EEG recording if seizures are being considered.

TREATMENT   Rx

Therapy first should focus on ensuring safety for individuals who may injure themselves or others (e.g., placing the bed on the floor, blocking windows, or moving the patient's bedroom to the ground floor), decreasing factors that may provoke events such as NREM parasomnia by causing arousals, and avoiding inciting factors such as sleep deprivation, alcohol, and short-acting hypnotic agents. Pharmacologic treatment with clonazepam (0.5 to 2) mg and tricyclic antidepressants (Chapter 369, Table 369-5) has been tried for NREM parasomnias with varying success. Treatment of sleep apnea reduces both NREM and REM events. For REM sleep behavior disorder, most patients respond well to clonazepam (0.25 to 3 mg) or melatonin (3 to 20 mg). Rhythmic movement disorder is typically refractory to medication therapy. Nightmares may respond to removal of the provocative substance or may require prazosin (5 to 15 mg) or imagery rehearsal therapy.

RESTLESS LEGS SYNDROME

Restless legs syndrome (Chapter 392) is characterized by four essential features: discomfort or urge to move the legs, worsening with rest, improvement with movement, and worsening in the evening. Patients with restless legs syndrome may report that the discomfort can be torturously debilitating and cause them to walk or continuously move their legs until the early morning hours. Some patients note that their legs will move on their own, thereby indicating periodic limb movements in wakefulness. About 85 to 90% of restless legs syndrome patients will have periodic limb movements in sleep, but only a minority of patients with periodic limb movements in sleep will meet the clinical criteria of restless legs syndrome.

U.S. Food and Drug Administration–approved therapies for restless legs syndrome are dopamine agonists (pramipexole 0.125 to 1.5 mg or ropinirole 0.25 to 3 mg), transdermal rotigotine (1 to 3 patch/24 hours), and gabapentinoid medications (e.g., gabapentin-encarbil 600 to 1800 mg).[A15,16] Dopamine agonists can augment the intensity and duration of daily symptoms; in such patients the agent should be carefully withdrawn, and another agent, such as pregabalin (25 to 300 mg daily), can be tried.[A16] In some patients, restless legs syndrome has been linked to low iron levels in the central nervous system and may improve with iron replacement.[A17] More intractable symptoms may require chronic narcotics (Chapter 27, Table 27-4).

Grade A References

A1. Dauvilliers Y, Roth T, Guinta D, et al. Effect of sodium oxybate, modafinil, and their combination on disrupted nighttime sleep in narcolepsy. *Sleep Med.* 2017;40:53-57.
A2. Thorpy MJ, Shapiro C, Mayer G, et al. A randomized study of solriamfetol for excessive sleepiness in narcolepsy. *Ann Neurol.* 2019;85:359-370.
A3. Philip P, Chaufton C, Taillard J, et al. Modafinil improves real driving performance in patients with hypersomnia: a randomized double-blind placebo-controlled crossover clinical trial. *Sleep.* 2014; 37:483-487.
A4. Corral J, Sánchez-Quiroga MÁ, Carmona-Bernal C, et al. Conventional polysomnography is not necessary for the management of most patients with suspected obstructive sleep apnea. Noninferiority, randomized controlled trial. *Am J Respir Crit Care Med.* 2017;196:1181-1190.
A5. Howard ME, Piper AJ, Stevens B, et al. A randomised controlled trial of CPAP versus non-invasive ventilation for initial treatment of obesity hypoventilation syndrome. *Thorax.* 2017;72:437-444.
A6. Masa JF, Mokhlesi B, Benitez I, et al. Long-term clinical effectiveness of continuous positive airway pressure therapy versus non-invasive ventilation therapy in patients with obesity hypoventilation syndrome: a multicentre, open-label, randomised controlled trial. *Lancet.* 2019;393:1721-1732.
A7. Yu J, Zhou Z, McEvoy RD, et al. Association of positive airway pressure with cardiovascular events and death in adults with sleep apnea: a systematic review and meta-analysis. *JAMA.* 2017;318:156-166.
A8. Schwartz M, Acosta L, Hung YL, et al. Effects of CPAP and mandibular advancement device treatment in obstructive sleep apnea patients: a systematic review and meta-analysis. *Sleep Breath.* 2018;22:555-568.
A9. Woodson BT, Soose RJ, Gillespie MB, et al. Three-year outcomes of cranial nerve stimulation for obstructive sleep apnea: the STAR trial. *Otolaryngol Head Neck Surg.* 2016;154:181-188.
A10. Cowie MR, Woehrle H, Wegscheider K, et al. Adaptive servo-ventilation for central sleep apnea in systolic heart failure. *N Engl J Med.* 2015;373:1095-1105.
A11. Costanzo MR, Ponikowski P, Javaheri S, et al. Transvenous neurostimulation for central sleep apnoea: a randomised controlled trial. *Lancet.* 2016;388:974-982.
A12. Ritterband LM, Thorndike FP, Ingersoll KS, et al. Effect of a web-based cognitive behavior therapy for insomnia intervention with 1-year follow-up: a randomized clinical trial. *JAMA Psychiatry.* 2017;74:68-75.
A13. Herring WJ, Connor KM, Snyder E, et al. Suvorexant in patients with insomnia: pooled analyses of three-month data from phase-3 randomized controlled clinical trials. *J Clin Sleep Med.* 2016;12:1215-1225.
A14. Manber R, Buysse DJ, Edinger J, et al. Efficacy of cognitive-behavioral therapy for insomnia combined with antidepressant pharmacotherapy in patients with comorbid depression and insomnia: a randomized controlled trial. *J Clin Psychiatry.* 2016;77:e1316-e1323.
A15. Garcia-Borreguero D, Allen R, Hudson J, et al. Effects of rotigotine on daytime symptoms in patients with primary restless legs syndrome: a randomized, placebo-controlled study. *Curr Med Res Opin.* 2016;32:77-85.
A16. Allen RP, Chen C, Garcia-Borreguero D, et al. Comparison of pregabalin with pramipexole for restless legs syndrome. *N Engl J Med.* 2014;370:621-631.
A17. Deng Y, Wu J, Jia Q. Efficacy of intravenous iron sucrose in hemodialysis patients with restless legs syndrome (RLS): a randomized, placebo-controlled study. *Med Sci Monit.* 2017;23:1254-1260.

GENERAL REFERENCES

For the General References and other additional features, please visit Expert Consult at https://expertconsult.inkling.com.

378

APPROACH TO CEREBROVASCULAR DISEASES

LARRY B. GOLDSTEIN

DEFINITION

The term *cerebrovascular disease* refers to a group of conditions in which injury to the brain or spinal cord occurs from a vascular cause. The onset is generally abrupt, but it also can be insidious. Clinical manifestations depend on the location and extent of damage to neural structures.[1] Although risk factors and treatments may overlap, cerebrovascular diseases are pathophysiologically divided into those in which an insufficiency in the blood supply causes ischemic injury and those in which bleeding, either into the parenchyma (intracerebral or much more rarely intraspinal hemorrhage) or into the space between the pial and arachnoid coverings over the brain or spinal cord (subarachnoid hemorrhage), causes direct neural injury, leads to secondary ischemic injury, or acts as a space-occupying lesion. Cerebrovascular disease is often both preventable and treatable.

EPIDEMIOLOGY

Nearly 800,000 Americans have a stroke each year, and about 75% are first strokes.[2] Stroke is the underlying cause of death of about 130,000 Americans each year, corresponding to approximately 1 in 20 deaths in the country.

Measured in terms of disease-attributed healthy years of life lost, cerebrovascular disease ranks seventh in the United States and third worldwide.[3] Stroke, which is a generic term for cerebrovascular disease, has fallen from the third to the fifth leading cause of death in the United States (behind diseases of the heart, cancer, chronic lower respiratory diseases, and unintentional injuries/accidents), because of a dramatic reduction in stroke-related mortality combined with a reclassification of pulmonary diseases. From 2004 to 2014, the age-adjusted stroke death rate decreased nearly 30% and the actual number of stroke deaths declined 11%. However, the annual decrease slowed from 0.9% per year between 2001 and 2007 to 0.5% per year, and U.S. stroke-related mortality has recently been rising.[4]

The overall prevalence of stroke is estimated at 2.7%, with 7.2 million Americans over age 20 years having had a stroke. Even though the incidence of stroke has declined substantially, largely because of better prevention, the declining case-fatality rate, until recently, has kept the population prevalence reasonably stable.

The risk for stroke generally increases with age, and it doubles for every decade after the age of 55 years. Symptoms consistent with transient focal cerebral ischemia (a transient ischemic attack, TIA) in which there is no evidence of permanent tissue injury, have a 9 to 17% risk of stroke by 90 days. A retinal vein occlusion increases the risk of stroke in the next 30 days by about 2.6-fold.

About 60% of stroke deaths occur in women, but the rates are actually highest in African American men. It is estimated that someone in the United States has a stroke about once every 40 seconds. In addition, blacks, people with lower levels of education, individuals who reside in the southeastern portion of the country (the "Stroke Belt"), and individuals with a first-degree relative who had a stroke before the age of 65 years have a higher risk for stroke and stroke-related mortality. Poor diet, lack of exercise (Chapter 13), cigarette smoking (Chapter 29), exposure to environmental tobacco smoke, obesity (Chapter 207), and excess alcohol consumption (Chapter 30) are lifestyle factors that greatly increase the risk for stroke. Of the medical conditions that increase the risk for stroke, hypertension (Chapter 70) has the highest population-attributable risk.[5] Other stroke risk factors include atrial fibrillation (Chapter 58), diabetes (Chapter 216), dyslipidemia (Chapter 195), inflammatory states, elevated homocysteine levels, high lipoprotein (a), carotid artery stenosis, patent foramen ovale (Chapter 61), other congenital heart defects, sleep apnea (Chapter 377), and chronic kidney disease. Coagulation

disorders (Chapter 73), oral contraceptive agents (Chapter 225), and migraine headache with aura (Chapter 370) also may contribute to the risk. Mendelian diseases associated with stroke include sickle cell disease (Chapter 154); mitochondrial encephalopathy, lactic acidosis, and stroke (MELAS); cerebral autosomal dominant arteriopathy with subcortical infarcts and leukoencephalopathy (CADASIL; Chapter 374); Fabry disease (Chapters 197 and 259); and Marfan syndrome (Chapter 244). In addition, autosomal dominant polycystic kidney disease (Chapter 118) is associated with intracranial aneurysms and fibromuscular dysplasia. Ehlers-Danlos type IV (Chapter 244) is also associated with intracranial aneurysms as well as cervical arterial dissection. Several genetic polymorphisms also have been associated with stroke (e.g., variants on chromosomes 9p21 and 4q25), although these genetic markers are not yet clinically relevant.

▶ PATHOBIOLOGY

Anatomy

An understanding of vascular anatomy and its normal variants as well as their relationships to functional neuroanatomy can provide important clues for identifying the cause of cerebrovascular symptoms and signs in individual patients and can also help guide treatment.

Aortic Arch

Paired carotid and vertebral arteries normally supply the brain (Fig. 378-1). The right common carotid artery arises from the brachiocephalic trunk

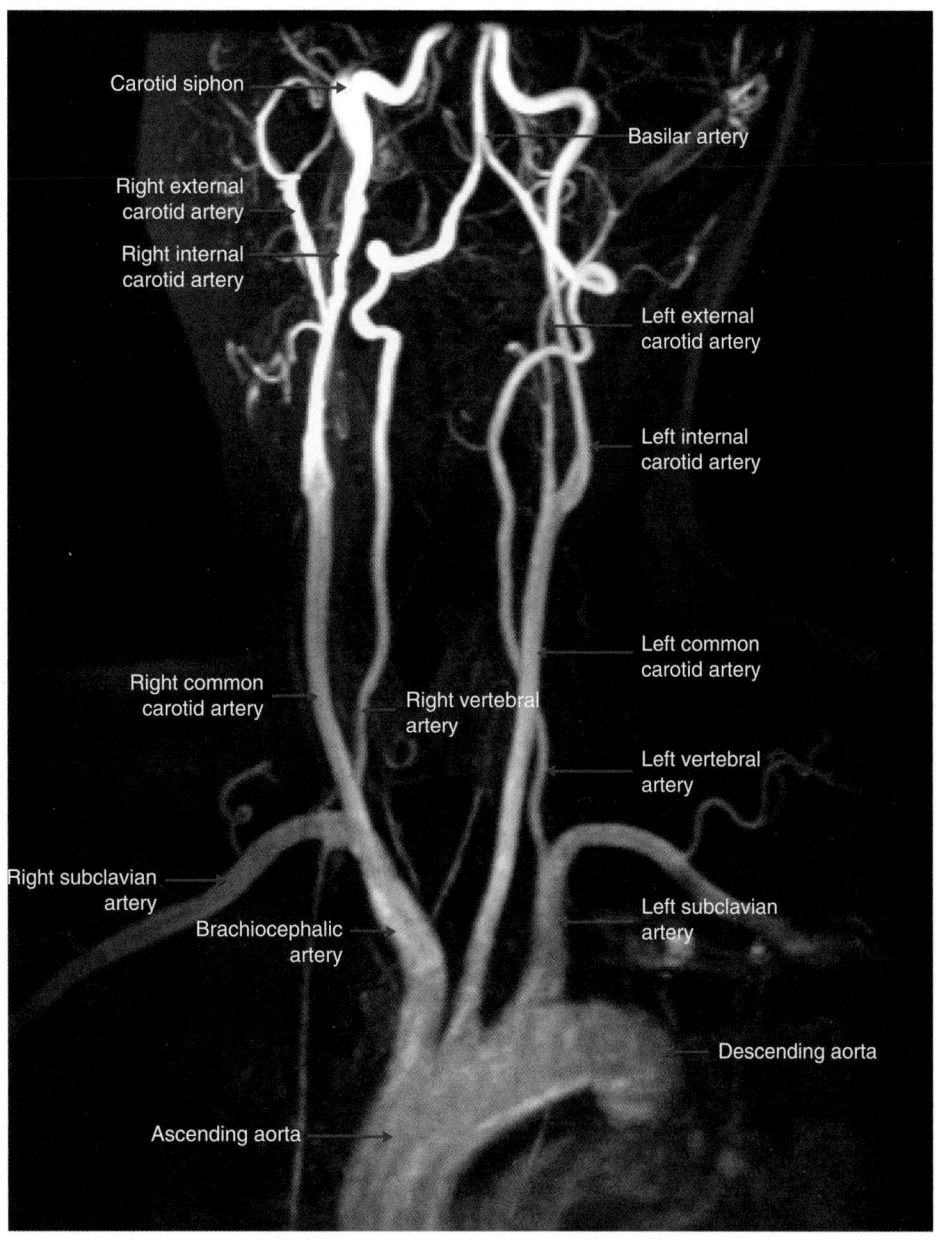

FIGURE 378-1. Magnetic resonance angiogram of normally configured aortic arch.

(innominate artery), which then gives rise to the right subclavian artery. The right vertebral artery generally arises from the proximal portion of the right subclavian artery. The left common carotid artery usually arises directly from the aortic arch; but in some individuals, it may arise from the proximal portion of the brachiocephalic trunk ("bovine" anatomy). The left subclavian artery originates from the aortic arch distal to the left common carotid artery and also supplies the left vertebral artery.

Internal Carotid Arteries

The common carotid arteries bifurcate into the internal carotid artery and external carotid artery in the neck, generally at the level of the thyroid cartilage. The bifurcation may less commonly occur above the lower level of the mandible or lower in the neck. The internal carotid artery enters the skull through the foramen lacerum and travels through the petrous bone adjacent to the inner ear. It then enters the cavernous sinus, ascends in an S shape (carotid siphon), penetrates the dura, and finally divides into the anterior cerebral artery and middle cerebral artery (Fig. 378-2). The ophthalmic artery can originate from the internal carotid artery in the carotid siphon, but it more commonly arises from the supraclinoid internal carotid artery, followed by the posterior communicating and anterior choroidal arteries.

External Carotid Arteries

In contrast to the internal carotid arteries, the external carotid arteries have extracranial branches. The superficial temporal arteries (palpable anterior to the ears) and facial arteries can anastomose with the intracranial circulation through branches of the ophthalmic artery and can be clinically important in the setting of a proximal internal carotid artery occlusion.

Vertebral Arteries

Although the vertebral arteries generally arise from the subclavian arteries, they can also originate from the aortic arch or thyrocervical trunk. They most commonly enter the C6 transverse process but may also enter at the C4, C5, or C7 levels. They exit the transverse processes at C1, turn posteriorly behind the atlantoaxial joint, and then pass through the dura at the foramen magnum. Intracranially, they typically join at the pontomedullary junction to form the single basilar artery, although the vertebral artery can end in the posterior inferior cerebellar artery in some individuals (Fig. 378-3). The portion of the vertebral artery between its origin and its entry into the transverse process is referred to as the V1 segment. The V2 segment refers to the portion of the artery traveling through the transverse foramina; the V3 segment, the portion between where the artery exits the transverse foramina and penetrates the dura; and the V4 segment, the intracranial portion of the artery. One vertebral artery may be hypoplastic (E-Fig. 378-1). Clues are that the ipsilateral transverse foramina are generally smaller on the side of the hypoplastic artery and that the proximal portion of the basilar artery can be displaced ipsilateral to the hypoplastic artery. The V3 segment is particularly vulnerable to mechanical injury that can lead to dissection. The vertebral arteries have medial branches that unite to form the anterior spinal artery and lateral branches that supply the dorsolateral medulla and inferior portion of the cerebellum, which also supplies the vestibular nuclei (Fig. 378-4). Other medial branches of the vertebral artery supply the medullary pyramid, inferior olivary nucleus, medial lemniscus, and hypoglossal nerve fibers. Longer circumferential branches from the vertebral arteries and posterior cerebral arteries supply the spinothalamic tracts and sympathetic fibers as they traverse the medulla, the sensory nuclei,

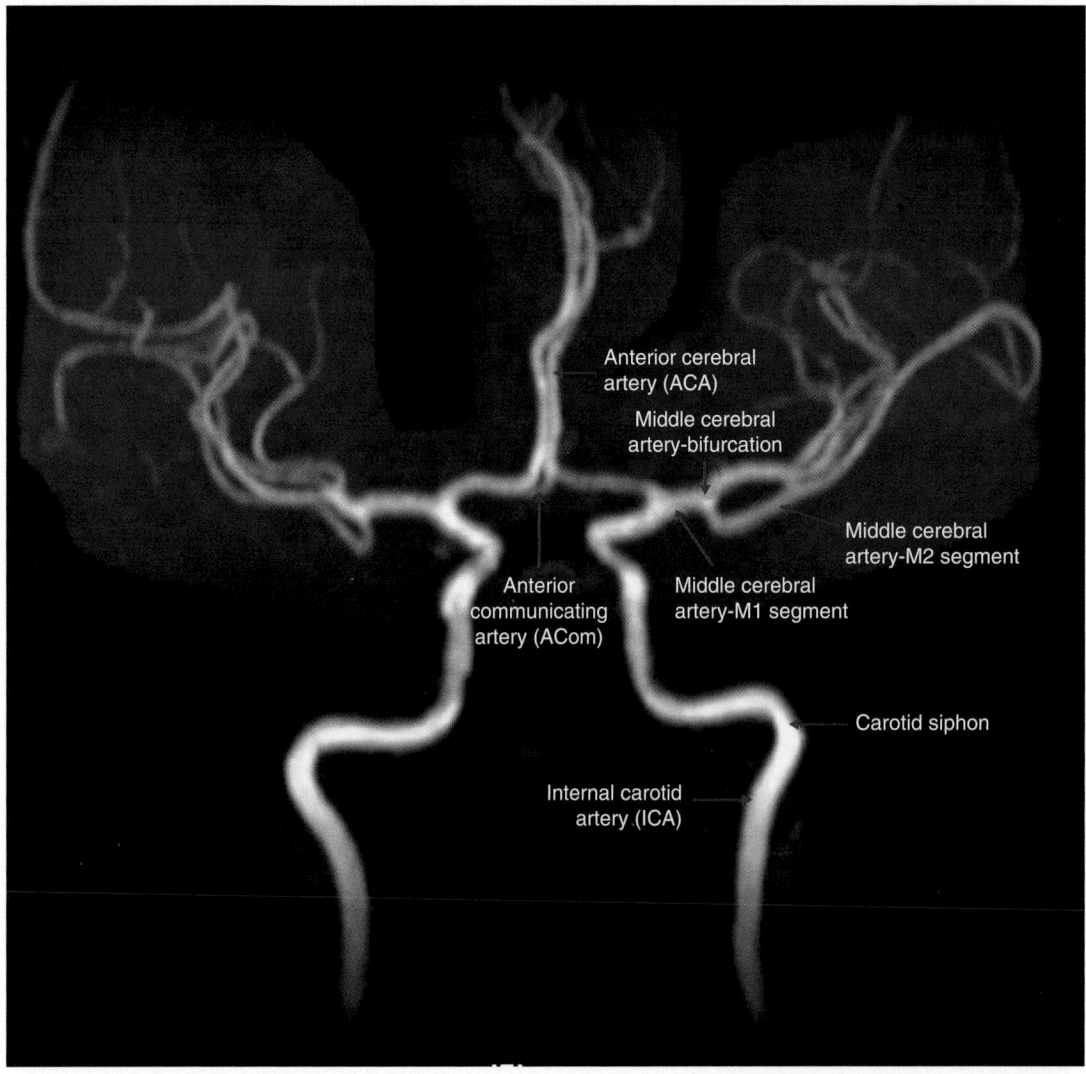

FIGURE 378-2. Magnetic resonance angiogram of the intracranial portion of the internal carotid artery and its main branches.

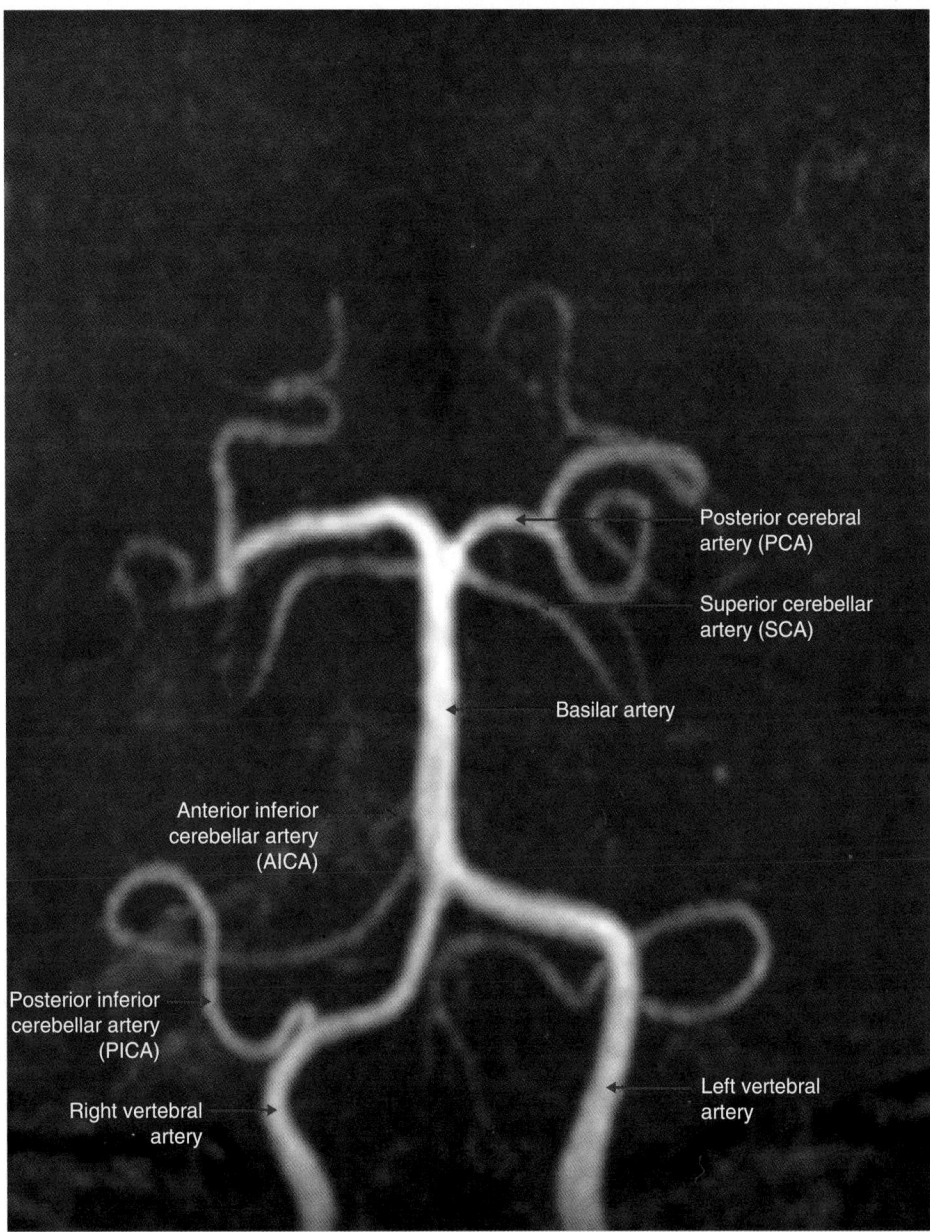

FIGURE 378-3. Magnetic resonance angiogram of the intracranial portion of the vertebrobasilar system.

and the descending tracts from cranial nerve V as well as emerging fibers from the vagus and glossopharyngeal nerves.

Basilar Artery

The basilar artery has small penetrating branches supplying the dorsal portions of the pons and midbrain (see Figs. 378-3 and 378-4). The anterior inferior cerebellar arteries originate from the mid-basilar artery. They supply portions of the cerebellar hemispheres in addition to the lateral pons; cranial nerves V, VII, and VIII; and pontine portions of the spinothalamic tracts and sympathetic fibers. The two superior cerebellar arteries arise from the distal basilar artery at the level of the midbrain proximal to the common origin of the two posterior cerebral arteries. The oculomotor nerve exits the midbrain between the superior cerebellar artery and posterior cerebral artery. The superior cerebellar arteries give branches supplying the dorsal midbrain, including the colliculi and the superior portions of the cerebellar hemispheres and vermis. The long circumferential vessels also supply the dorsolateral brain stem.

In addition to the anterior inferior cerebellar artery and superior cerebellar artery, the basilar artery has paramedian vessels supplying the middle portion of the basis pontis and midline pontine structures, including the corticospinal tracts, medial longitudinal fasciculus, and pontine reticular nuclei. At the midbrain level, paramedian branches of the basilar artery supply the cerebral

peduncles, cranial nerve III nuclei and fibers, and medial portions of the red nucleus and medial lemniscus. Short circumferential branches supply the ventrolateral pons and midbrain.

Circle of Willis

The arterial anastomosis at the base of the brain is termed the circle of Willis (see E-Fig. 378-1). The two anterior cerebral arteries are connected by the anterior communicating artery. The posterior communicating arteries connect the supraclinoid internal carotid arteries with the proximal posterior cerebral arteries. In persons with an intact circle of Willis, the entire intracranial circulation can be supplied by a single patent internal carotid artery or vertebral artery. The majority of individuals, however, have an incomplete circle of Willis (see Fig. 378-2). One common variant is for the portion of the anterior cerebral artery between the internal carotid artery and the anterior communicating artery (A1 segment) to be hypoplastic or absent. In this case, both anterior cerebral arteries can be supplied from a single internal carotid artery. Another common variant is for the portion of the posterior cerebral artery between its normal origin from the basilar artery and the posterior communicating artery (P1 segment) to be absent or hypoplastic (termed a "fetal" posterior cerebral artery). In these individuals, the distal posterior cerebral artery territory is supplied by the carotid rather than by the vertebrobasilar arteries.

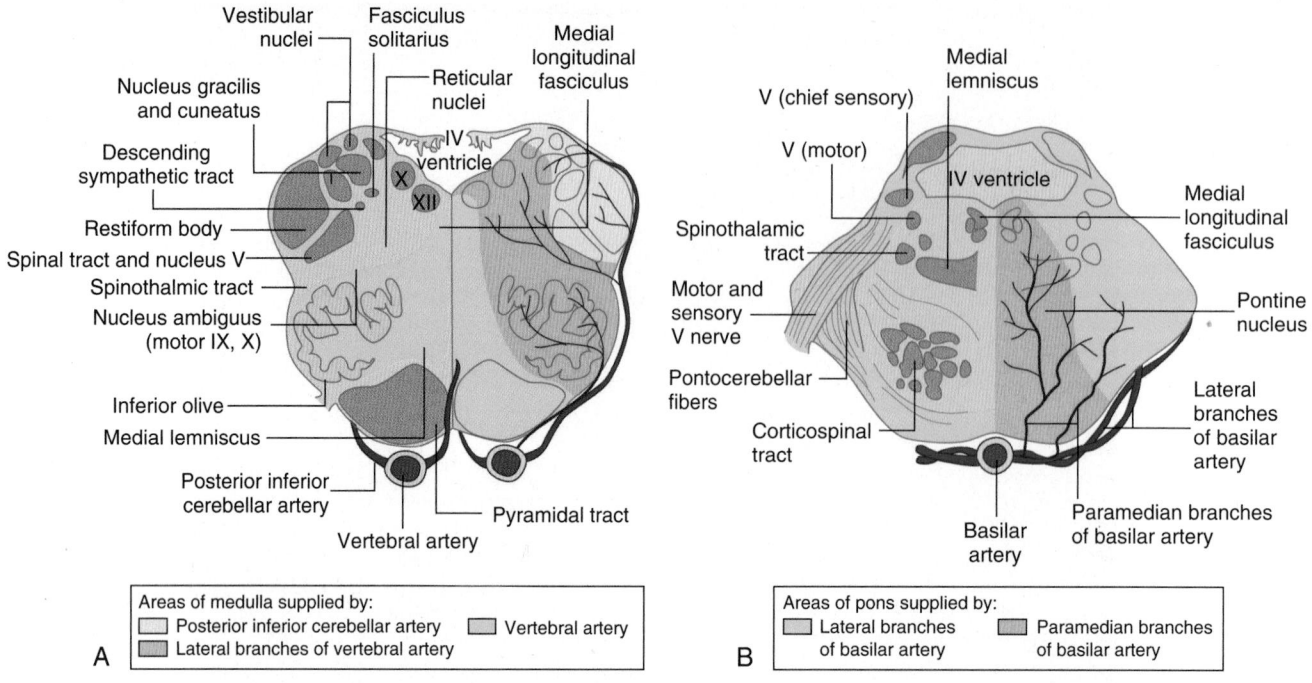

FIGURE 378-4. Brain stem blood supply. **A,** Cross section of the medulla oblongata at the level of the hypoglossal nuclei (cranial nerve XII). Short branches of the vertebral and anterior spinal arteries supply the medulla. Longer circumferential branches, including the posterior inferior cerebellar artery, supply the lateral portions of the medulla. **B,** Cross section of the midpons region. The medial portion receives blood supply from short, perforating basilar artery branches. More laterally, the blood supply comes from lateral basilar artery branches. (From Zivin JA. Approach to cerebrovascular diseases. In: Goldman L, Schafer AI. *Goldman's Cecil Medicine.* 24th ed. Philadelphia: Elsevier Saunders; 2012.)

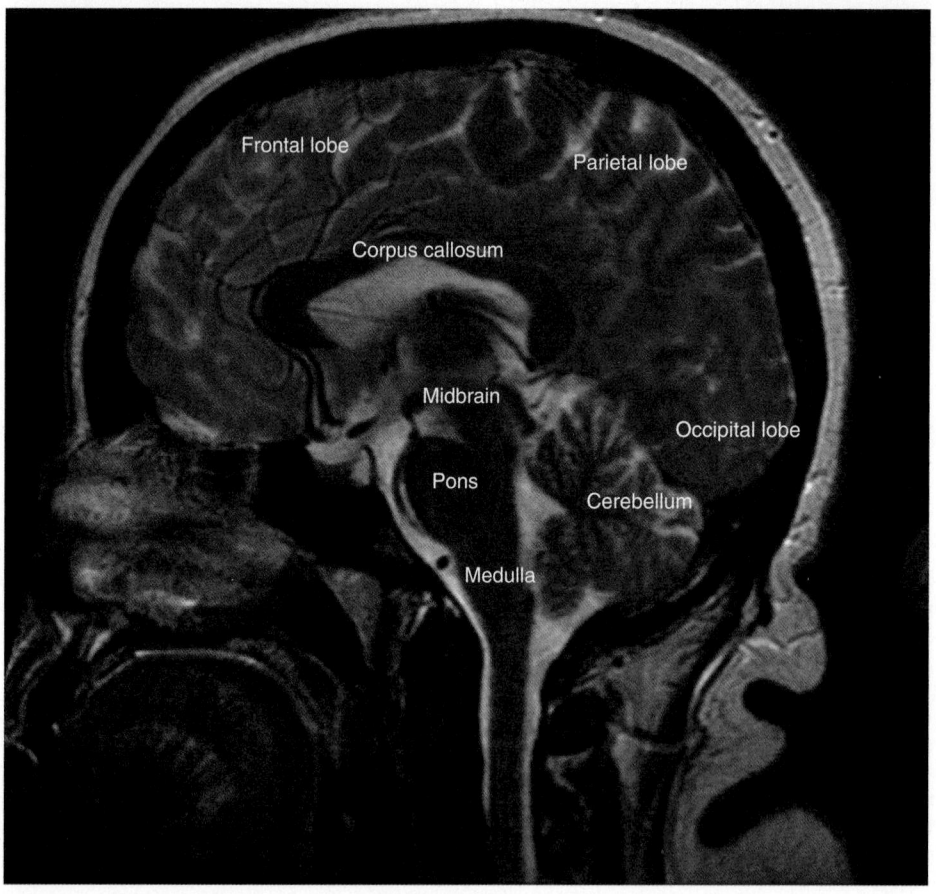

FIGURE 378-5. Parasagittal T2-weighted magnetic resonance image showing midline structures.

Anterior Cerebral Arteries

The anterior cerebral arteries travel anteriorly and then turn posteriorly with leptomeningeal branches supplying the medial portions of the frontal and parietal lobes (Figs. 378-5 to 378-7; see also Fig. 378-2). In about half of people, the anterior cerebral artery divides into pericallosal and callosal marginal branches. Terminal portions of the latter artery supply the medial cortex between the parietal and occipital lobes. Damage to this area can be confused with "watershed" hypoperfusion injury. A series of small lenticulostriate arteries originate from the A1 and A2 (between the anterior communicating artery and corpus callosum) segments of the anterior cerebral artery. The recurrent artery of Heubner is a large, important medial striate artery that provides blood supply to the anterior and inferior portions of the anterior limb of the

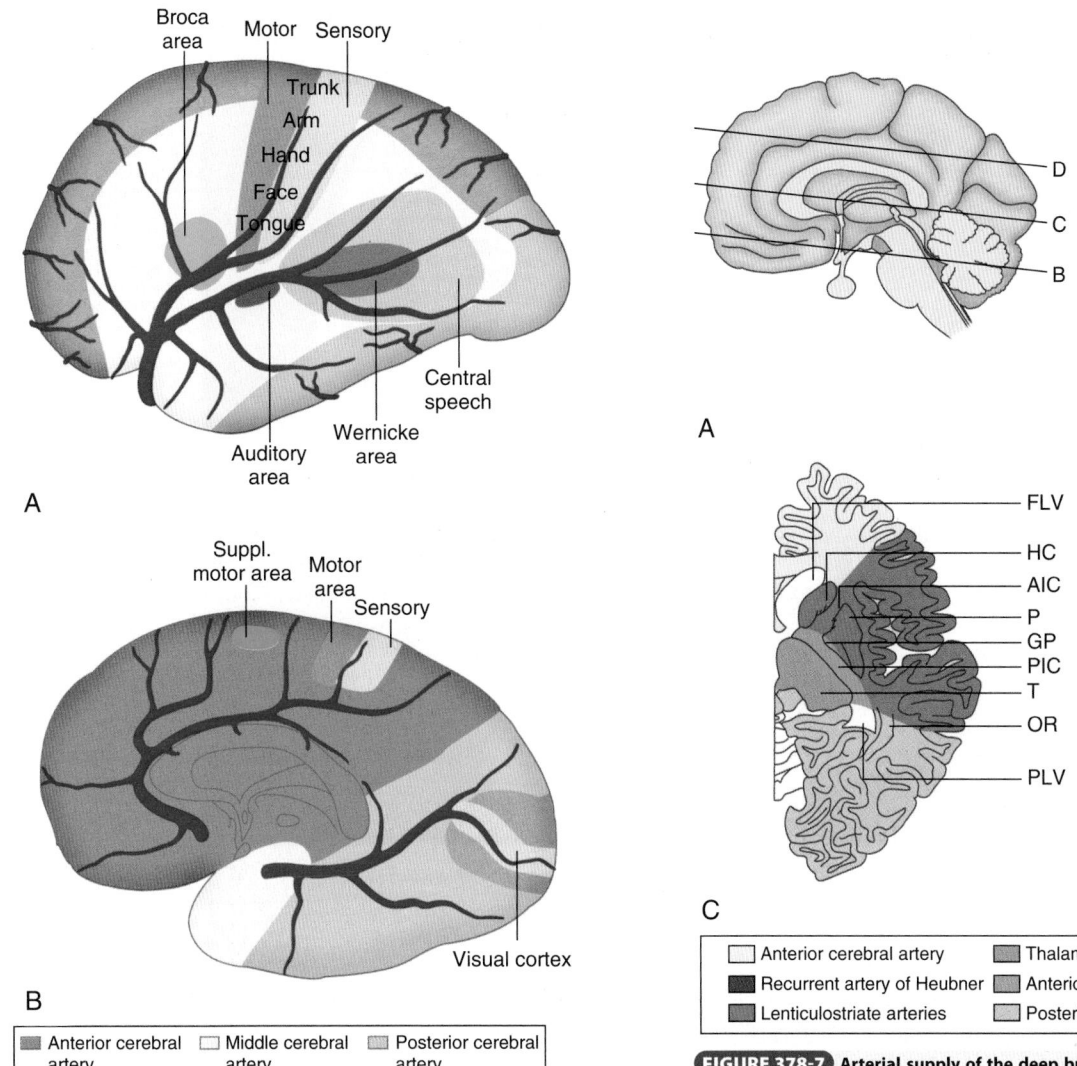

FIGURE 378-6. Surface cerebral arterial anatomy. Lateral (A) and medial (B) views of the cerebral hemisphere show the surface distributions of the anterior, middle, and posterior cerebral arteries. (From Zivin JA. Approach to cerebrovascular diseases. In: Goldman L, Schafer AI. *Goldman's Cecil Medicine.* 24th ed. Philadelphia: Elsevier Saunders; 2012.)

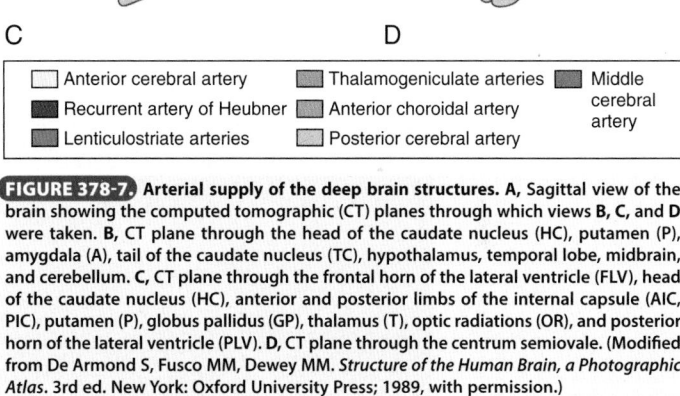

FIGURE 378-7. Arterial supply of the deep brain structures. **A,** Sagittal view of the brain showing the computed tomographic (CT) planes through which views **B, C,** and **D** were taken. **B,** CT plane through the head of the caudate nucleus (HC), putamen (P), amygdala (A), tail of the caudate nucleus (TC), hypothalamus, temporal lobe, midbrain, and cerebellum. **C,** CT plane through the frontal horn of the lateral ventricle (FLV), head of the caudate nucleus (HC), anterior and posterior limbs of the internal capsule (AIC, PIC), putamen (P), globus pallidus (GP), optic radiations (OR), and posterior horn of the lateral ventricle (PLV). **D,** CT plane through the centrum semiovale. (Modified from De Armond S, Fusco MM, Dewey MM. *Structure of the Human Brain, a Photographic Atlas.* 3rd ed. New York: Oxford University Press; 1989, with permission.)

internal capsule, anterior and inferior portions of the caudate nucleus, anterior globus pallidus, putamen, hypothalamus, olfactory bulbs and tracts, and uncinate fasciculus. It can be inadvertently damaged during surgical clipping of an anterior communicating artery aneurysm.

Anterior Choroidal Artery

The anterior choroidal artery (medial striate artery) commonly arises from the supraclinoid internal carotid artery distal to the posterior communicating artery. It travels posteriorly over the medial optic tract and enters the brain at the choroidal fissure. It gives branches to the optic tract, anterior hippocampus, amygdala, tail of the caudate nucleus, geniculate body, and inferior portion of the posterior limb of the internal capsule (see Fig. 378-7). Ischemic lesions in this area can be confused with lesions arising from the middle cerebral artery.

Middle Cerebral Artery

The middle cerebral artery supplies the bulk of the frontal, parietal, and lateral portions of the temporal lobes (Figs. 378-8 and 378-9; see also Figs. 378-6 and 378-7). The M1 segment refers to the portion of the middle cerebral artery between its origin from the supraclinoid internal carotid artery and its distal branches (see Fig. 378-2). The middle cerebral artery bifurcates in the Sylvian fissure in 20 to 30% of individuals and trifurcates in about 70% of individuals. The superior division supplies the frontal and parietal lobes, and the inferior division supplies the lateral portion of the temporal lobe. The M1 segment gives rise to some medial and all of the lateral lenticulostriate arteries.

These arteries supply the head and body of the caudate nucleus, the putamen, and the globus pallidus as well as the anterior limb, genu, and superior portions of the posterior limb of the internal capsule (see Fig. 378-7).

Posterior Cerebral Artery

The distal portion of the posterior cerebral artery divides into an anterior and a posterior division (see Fig. 378-3). The anterior division supplies the inferior and medial portions of the temporal lobe in the middle cranial fossa, with distal branches anastomosing with those of the middle cerebral artery (see E-Fig. 378-1). The posterior division supplies the occipital lobe, including the calcarine cortex, with terminal branches anastomosing with those of the middle cerebral artery and anterior cerebral artery. The proximal portions of both the posterior cerebral artery and the posterior communicating artery give off small penetrating arteries to the thalamus (thalamoperforators). In some individuals, a single common artery arising from the P1 segment (artery of Percheron) can supply both thalami. Unless the posterior cerebral artery has a fetal-type origin from the internal carotid artery, thalamic strokes are generally related to the vertebrobasilar circulation. Two posterior choroidal arteries arise separately from the posterior cerebral artery and supply the choroid plexus, posterior thalamus, fornix, and midbrain tectum. Posterior cerebral artery perforators also supply the medial portions of the cerebral peduncles, substantia nigra, red nuclei, hippocampus, and posterior hypothalamus.

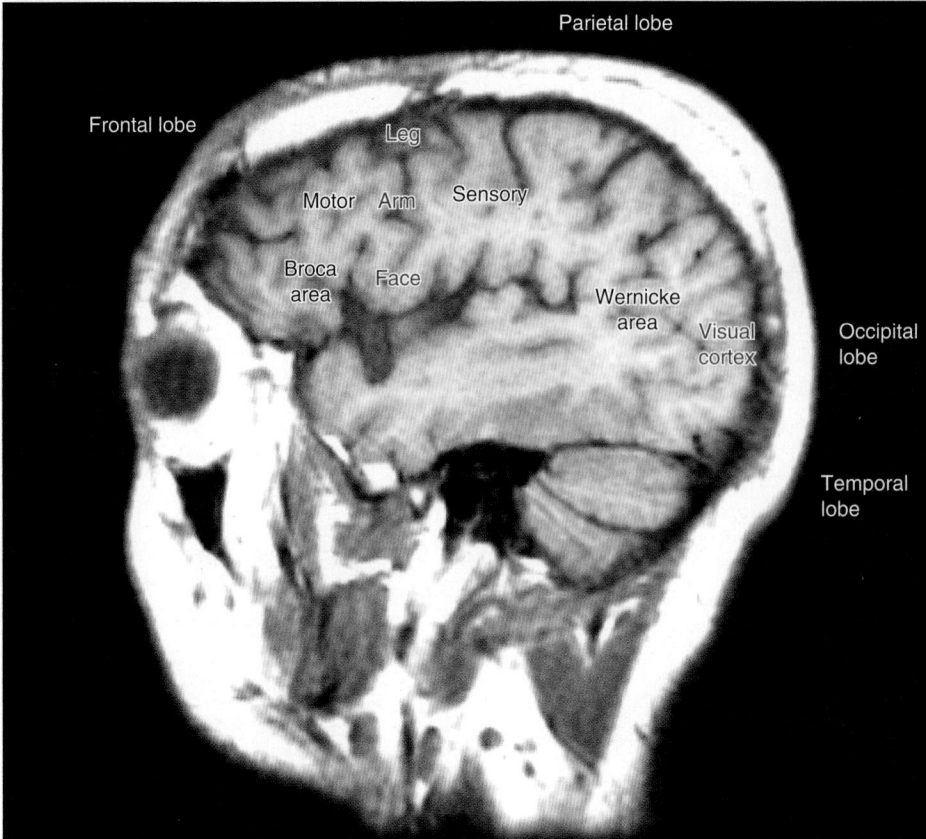

FIGURE 378-8. Sagittal, lateral T1-weighted magnetic resonance image showing cortical motor, sensory, visual, and language areas.

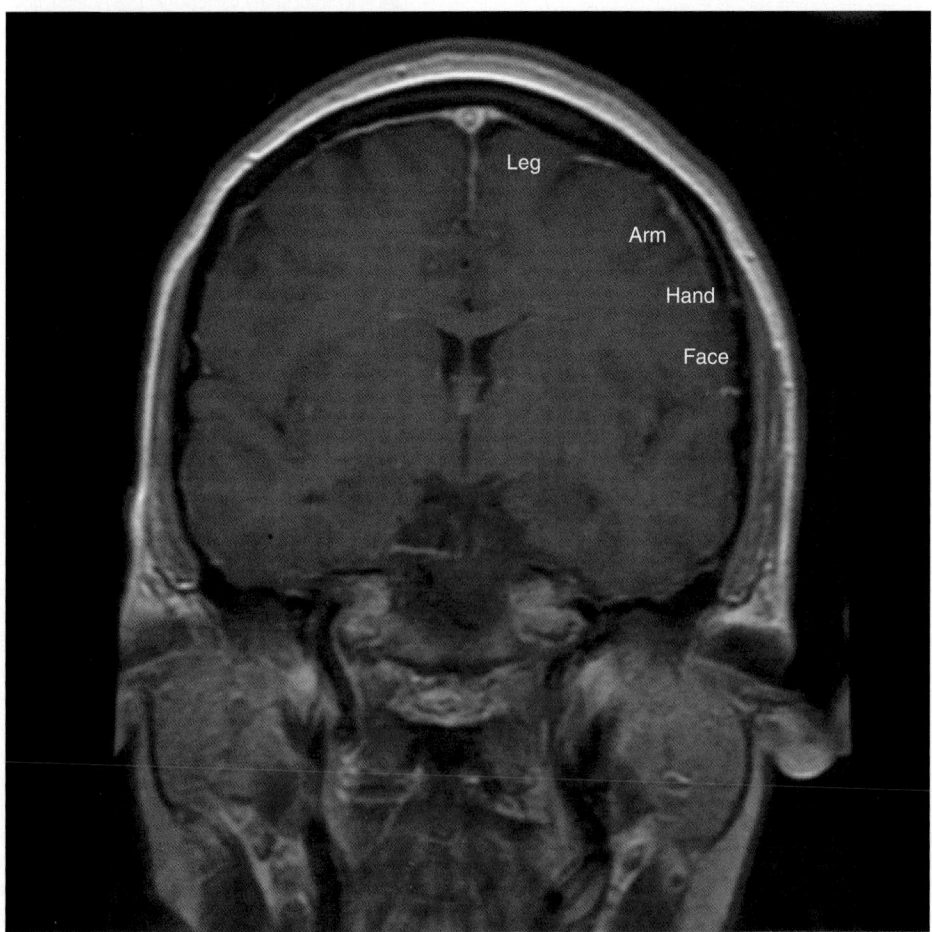

FIGURE 378-9. Coronal T1-weighted magnetic resonance image showing cortical areas for the leg, arm, hand, and face.

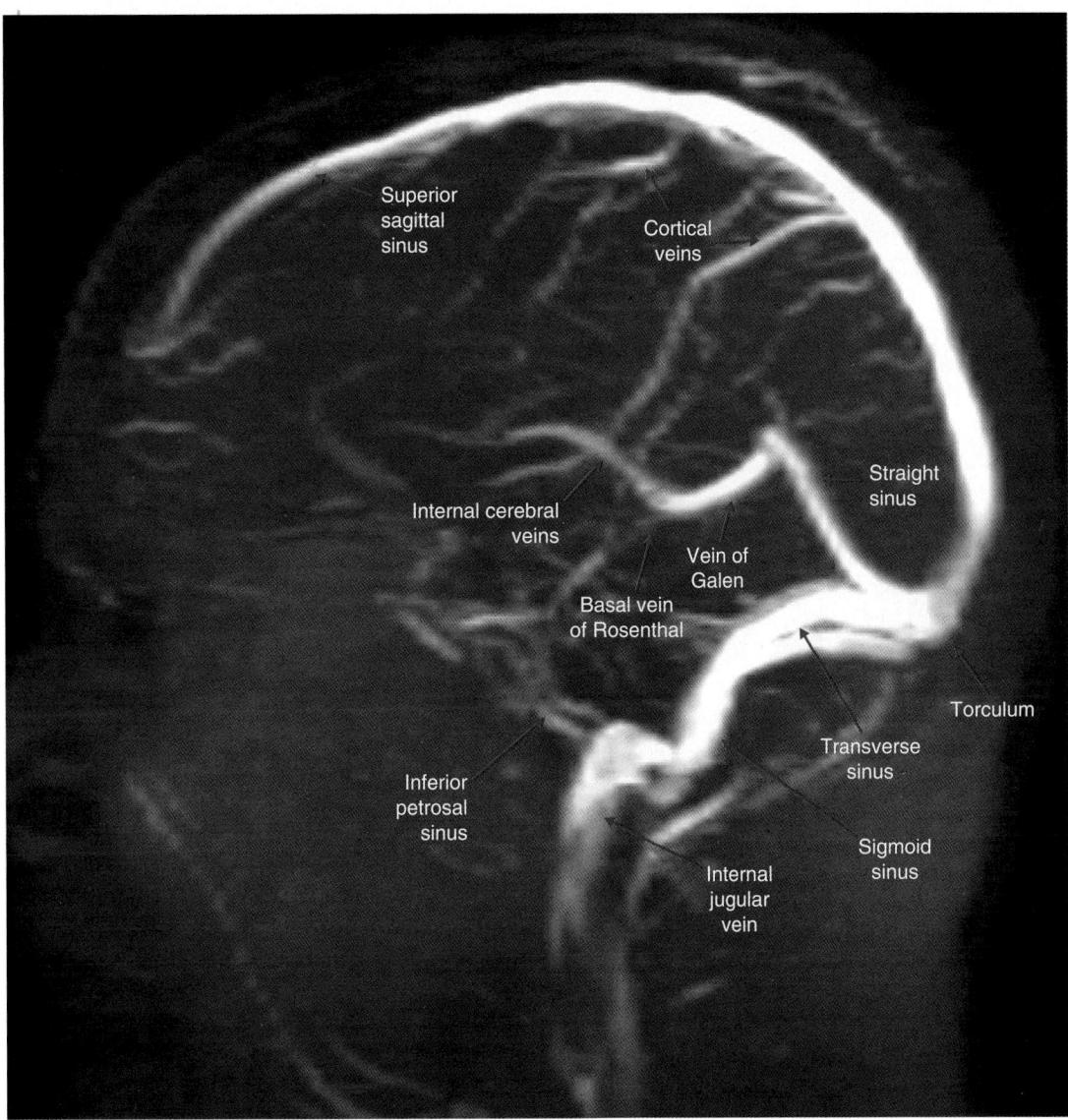

FIGURE 378-10. Parasagittal magnetic resonance venogram showing venous structures.

Venous System

The venous drainage of the brain is divided into superficial and deep systems (Figs. 378-10 and 378-11). Deep structures drain into the inferior sagittal sinus and vein of Galen that join to form the straight sinus, which runs along the tentorium to join the superior sagittal sinus at the torcula. The cerebral veins drain into the sagittal sinus. The two transverse sinuses extend laterally from the torcula into the sigmoid sinus, which then forms the jugular vein. Often, one hypoplastic transverse sinus can cause confusion if a sinus thrombosis is suspected. In these cases, the jugular notch in the occipital bone and jugular foramen may be smaller on the side of the hypoplastic transverse sinus. Each cavernous sinus surrounds the ipsilateral internal carotid artery. Fibers from cranial nerve VI run within the cavernous sinus inferior to the carotid artery, with fibers from cranial nerves III, IV, V1, and V2 running in its lateral wall. The two cavernous sinuses connect to each other and drain into the petrosal sinus and then the sagittal sinus.

Physiology
Cerebral Blood Flow

The brain, which is among the body's most metabolically active tissues, receives about 14% of resting cardiac output. Normal resting metabolism of brain tissue requires 140 μmol of oxygen and 24 μmol of glucose per 100 g of tissue per minute. Although total blood flow to the brain remains constant in normal conditions, regional flow changes with mental activity, often manifested by changes in synaptic activity, and provides the basis for functional magnetic resonance imaging or positron emission tomography imaging studies. Approximately 80% of glucose is used to generate energy, with the remainder metabolized to lactate or used for synthetic activities. Little glucose is stored in the

brain, and the brain's high metabolic demand makes it particularly vulnerable to reductions in oxygen and blood supply. Cerebral blood flow at rest averages 50 to 100 mL per 100 g of brain tissue per minute. If blood flow falls below this level, normal neuronal function is suppressed (i.e., neurons become electrically quiescent). If the deficit persists, irrevocable neural injury can result.

Cerebral blood flow is regulated though a variety of mechanisms in addition to mental activity. Constant, overall cerebral blood flow is maintained through autoregulation. This autoregulatory relationship is reflected in the equation cerebral blood flow = cerebrovascular resistance/mean arterial pressure. If the mean arterial pressure is decreased, there is a compensatory decrease in cerebrovascular resistance (through dilation of cerebral arterioles) to maintain cerebral blood flow constant. If the mean arterial pressure is increased, there is a compensatory increase in cerebrovascular resistance (through constriction of cerebral arterioles). There are, however, limits to cerebral autoregulation. At mean arterial pressures greater than about 150 mm Hg, cerebral arterioles are maximally constricted, and cerebral blood flow rises. At mean arterial pressures below about 50 mm Hg, cerebral arterioles are maximally dilated, and cerebral blood flow falls. In the setting of chronic hypertension, the autoregulatory relationship between cerebrovascular resistance and mean arterial pressure is shifted to higher critical mean arterial pressures (i.e., cerebral blood flow falls at a higher mean arterial pressure).

Metabolic factors can also affect cerebral blood flow. Hypercapnia causes cerebral vasodilation, and hypocapnia causes cerebral vasoconstriction that is mediated by changes in the pH of the brain's extracellular fluid. Cerebral blood flow declines by approximately 2% for every 1 mm Hg decline in P_{CO_2}. In patients who have increased intracranial pressure and threatened herniation, a short period of hyperventilation (target arterial P_{CO_2} of 30 to 35 mm Hg)

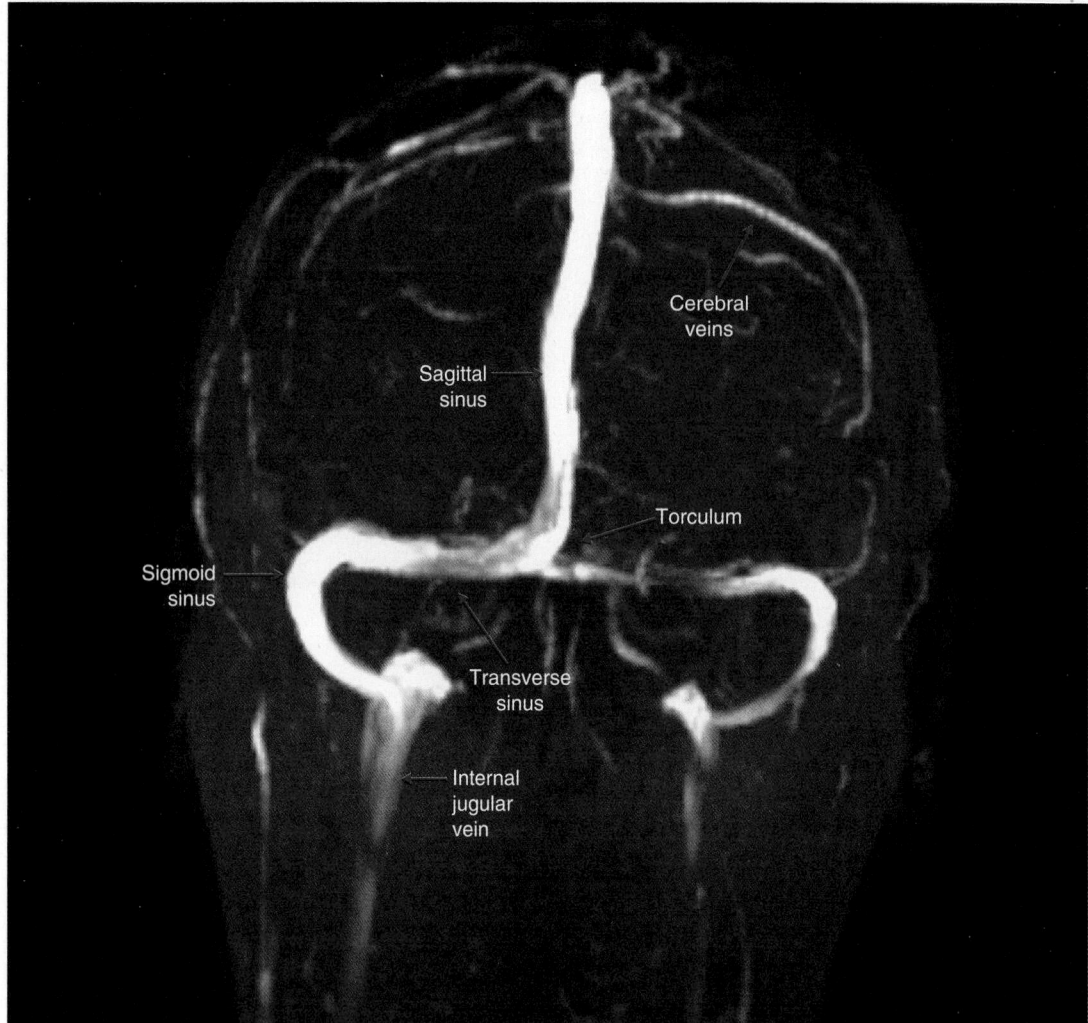

FIGURE 378-11. Anteroposterior magnetic resonance venogram showing venous structures.

can be used as a temporary measure until more definitive treatment can be instituted. The response is only transient because of compensation by the choroid plexus, and a rebound increase in $Paco_2$ can lead to a rise in intracranial pressure when hyperventilation is discontinued.

Blood-Brain Barrier

The triggering of a neuronal action potential depends on the relative concentrations of Na^+, K^+, and Ca^{2+}, and it is also modulated by Mg^{2+} and a variety of neurotransmitters. The blood-brain barrier is critical for maintaining the environment necessary for normal neuronal function.[6] The blood-brain barrier consists anatomically of the capillary endothelial cells, a basement membrane with pericytes, and astrocytic perivascular footplates. The brain's vascular endothelial cells, which are the principal component of the blood-brain barrier, are joined by tight junctions and generally lack the transport channels found elsewhere in the body. As a result, the blood-brain barrier prevents hydrophilic polar and large molecules in the blood from entering the brain. By comparison, oxygen and carbon dioxide rapidly cross the blood-brain barrier. Nutrients, toxins, and drugs can cross the blood-brain barrier by simple diffusion, by transport through carrier molecules based on concentration gradients (facilitated transport), or by energy-dependent mechanisms (active transport). Glucose is the brain's sole source of energy. Glucose transport into the brain is through non–energy-dependent facilitated transport (glucose transporter isotype 1, Glut1). In the setting of ischemia, endothelial cell function can be compromised, and the blood-brain barrier can fail.

The Neurovascular Unit

The concept of the neurovascular unit has become important for understanding the complex relationships between anatomic structures and the integrity of brain function. The term reflects the physiologic interrelatedness of the brain's various components, including endothelial cells, vascular smooth muscle, adventitial cells, glia, and neurons. The concept reflects the observation that local pH as well as neural activity can affect local cerebral blood flow. In addition to linking neural activity with blood flow and maintaining the blood-brain barrier, the neurovascular unit can secrete a variety of immunologic and neurotrophic factors that further affect both normal function and the brain's response to injury.

CEREBRAL ISCHEMIA

Because of its high metabolic demands, brain function is completely dependent on its supply of blood and oxygen. Clinical symptoms ensue when global or regional blood supply falls below the critical 50 mL per 100 g per minute. Permanent neural injury does not occur if the supply of blood and oxygen is quickly restored, such as with a faint (Chapter 56) in the setting of a global reduction in the supply of blood or oxygen or a transient ischemic attack (Chapter 379) with brief, local reductions in cerebral blood flow. Certain groups of neurons may be particularly vulnerable to hypoxic-ischemic injury (i.e., regions of the hippocampus, cerebellar Purkinje cells, and neocortical layers III, V, and possibly VI). Hypoxic-ischemic injury can be global, diffuse, or focal. In stable patients who are not hypoxemic, supplemental oxygen administration is not helpful.[A1]

Global Ischemic Injury

Global ischemic injury occurs in the setting of complete cardiovascular collapse, such as with ventricular fibrillation, electromechanical dissociation, and asystole (Chapter 57). Some neurons are particularly vulnerable to ischemic injury and will be selectively damaged, whereas neurons only millimeters away may be spared. In the setting of hypotension, areas of brain between the territories of major arteries (i.e., between the anterior cerebral artery and middle cerebral artery in the frontal cortex and adjacent subcortical white matter), between the middle cerebral artery and posterior cerebral artery (in the parieto-occipital cortex and adjacent subcortical white matter), and between penetrating arteries from distal branches of the middle cerebral artery and lenticulostriate arteries (deep hemispheric white matter, centrum semiovale) are especially vulnerable and are termed watershed areas.

The duration of anoxia, the duration of cardiopulmonary resuscitation (CPR), and the cause of cardiac arrest are related to outcome after CPR (Chapters 57 and 376), but none of these factors accurately discriminate between patients who will have a poor or a favorable outcome. Prognosis also cannot be based on the circumstances of CPR or on elevated body temperature alone. Myoclonic status epilepticus within the first day after cardiac arrest implies a poor prognosis, as does the absence of pupillary or corneal reflexes or extensor motor responses 3 days after cardiac arrest in patients who remain comatose. Bilateral absence of cortical somatosensory evoked responses within 1 to 3 days also portends a poor prognosis.

Out-of-hospital cardiac arrest carries a poor prognosis if effective CPR is not rapidly instituted. A period of therapeutic hypothermia to 36° C may improve neurologic outcome after resuscitated cardiac arrest if it can be instituted rapidly after hospital admission (Chapter 57), but data are conflicting and the absolute benefit is uncertain.[A2] Therapeutic hypothermia to 36° C is as good as cooling to 33° C or 34° C.[A3][A4] Current recommendations are for cooling to 32° C to 36° C, maintained for 24 hours, then followed by gradual rewarming but not to above 37° C.[7] If the cerebral cortex is irreversibly damaged but the relatively resistant brain stem control of respiration and cardiovascular regulation is preserved, the patient can enter a persistent vegetative state (Chapter 376).

Diffuse Hypoxic Injury

Diffuse hypoxia can alter cognition, cause confusion, impair consciousness, and lead to coma, which can be irreversible. Causes include travel to high altitudes, severe anemia, and pulmonary disease. Symptoms are generally present when the PaO_2 abruptly falls to less than 40 mm Hg. Increases in cerebral blood flow can partially compensate for slow declines in PaO_2, which may still cause symptoms with further or rapid reductions.

Focal Ischemic Injury

Focal ischemic injury is caused by occlusion of a cervical or intracranial artery that supplies the brain. Although this injury can occur from many causes (including infection, inflammation, metabolic disorders, trauma, and hematologic disorders), the majority of strokes are related to thrombotic or embolic occlusion (Fig. 378-12). If flow is not restored within minutes, a core area of irreversible brain injury is commonly produced. A surrounding area of variable size, depending on the artery involved and the integrity of collaterals in which blood flow is reduced, will suffer injury that is not irreversible. The brain in this area, termed the penumbra, is electrically quiescent and contributes to the resulting neurologic deficit. Because the pH of the extracellular fluid in the penumbral zone is low, vessels are maximally dilated and the cerebral autoregulatory response is inoperative. Because cerebrovascular resistance in

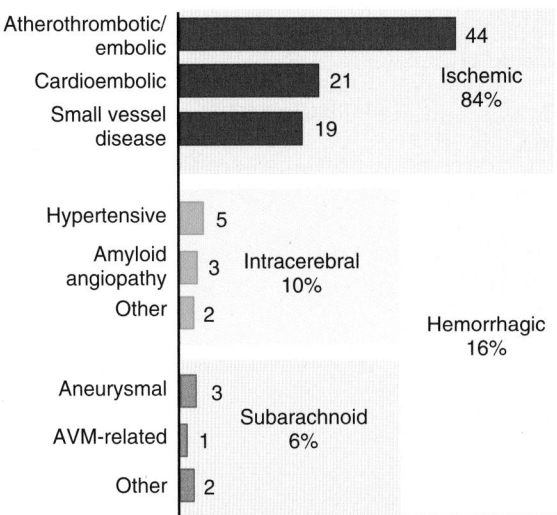

FIGURE 378-12. Classification of cerebrovascular disease by cause. AVM = arteriovenous malformation. (From Zivin JA. Approach to cerebrovascular diseases. In: Goldman L, Schafer AI. *Goldman's Cecil Medicine.* 24th ed. Philadelphia: Elsevier Saunders; 2012.)

the penumbral zone is fixed, any decline in mean arterial pressure can further reduce its cerebral blood flow, thereby extending the volume of infarcted brain tissue. A variety of neuroimaging techniques can help distinguish penumbral from infarcted brain tissue (i.e., magnetic resonance diffusion-perfusion mismatch, computed tomographic perfusion imaging) but have not been standardized and have not been proved essential for clinical decisions regarding the use of intravenous thrombolytic therapy. Identification of viable tissue in areas of reduced perfusion can guide the use of endovascular thrombectomy in the setting of large vessel occlusions.[8] Many putative neuroprotective strategies aimed at preserving ischemic brain tissue until it can be reperfused through collateral flow have failed in clinical trials.

PATHOLOGY

Permanent occlusion of a cerebral artery results in necrosis of its supplied neurons, glia, and endothelial cells (pan-necrosis). In gross appearance, the area of infarcted brain may be pale or hemorrhagic if secondary bleeding occurred. Over time, the lesion becomes cavitary (encephalomalacia). On microscopic examination, ischemic neurons initially appear small and angular. The cytoplasm becomes homogeneously eosinophilic, and the nucleus becomes dark and pyknotic. As endothelial cells die, associated areas of petechial hemorrhage may appear. An initial inflammatory reaction may lead to microvascular occlusions, such that flow to ischemic tissue may not be restored even if a proximal thrombus is removed (no-reflow phenomenon). Leukocytes that infiltrate ischemic tissue can also release interleukins and cytokines, which can contribute to cytotoxic injury. Blood macrophages begin to reach the infarcted tissue, and neovascularization peaks after about 2 weeks. Macrophage-mediated removal of cellular debris peaks at about 3 to 4 weeks after the infarct. Astrocytes then form a glial scar around the area of infarction.

PATHOPHYSIOLOGY

Because the brain has no reserve energy supply, energy-dependent neuronal and glial processes stop soon after acute deprivation of blood and oxygen. Calcium ions enter depolarized neurons and glia, where they activate second messengers, including lipases and proteases, thereby releasing free fatty acids and generating free radicals that degrade cellular organelles and membranes. Depolarized neurons also release high levels of excitatory neurotransmitters, such as glutamate into synapses, which leads to further neuronal depolarization and calcium entry. Once this cascade has been initiated, neurons may still degenerate over time by apoptosis (programmed cell death) even if blood flow is restored. Although promising in the laboratory, all attempts to block the ischemic cascade pharmacologically have failed in clinical trials to date.

● CEREBRAL HEMORRHAGE

Subarachnoid hemorrhage, which is bleeding between the pial and arachnoid coverings over the brain, is most commonly related to a ruptured aneurysm (Chapter 380). Cerebral aneurysms may occur spontaneously or be acquired as a result of infection or trauma. They are more common in first-degree relatives of patients who have a cerebral aneurysm and with certain conditions, such as autosomal dominant polycystic kidney disease (Chapter 118) and type IV Ehlers-Danlos syndrome (Chapter 244). Noninfectious aneurysms are typically situated at branch points of major cerebral arteries: anterior cerebral artery–anterior communicating artery, internal carotid artery–posterior communicating artery, middle cerebral artery bifurcation, basilar artery tip. Initial brain injury can be caused by an acute increase in intracranial pressure, with delayed ischemic injury related to the development of vasospasm after 7 to 10 days. Interference with the absorption of cerebrospinal fluid though the arachnoid granulations can lead to communicating hydrocephalus. Clot within the third or fourth ventricle or cerebral aqueducts can cause obstructive hydrocephalus.

The most common causes of intracerebral parenchymal brain hemorrhages are hypertension (Chapter 70) and cerebral amyloid angiopathy. Myriad other potential vascular and nonvascular causes, including vascular malformations, vasculitis (Chapter 254), venous sinus thrombosis, and coagulopathies (Chapters 163, 164, and 165), are less common. Some tumors (e.g., melanoma [Chapter 193] and renal cell carcinoma [Chapter 187]) can initially present as an intracerebral hemorrhage. Hypertension-related intracerebral hemorrhage occurs in typical areas of the brain (i.e., basal ganglia, thalamus, basis pontis, and cerebellum). In contrast, intracerebral hemorrhage related to cerebral amyloid angiopathy is typically lobar and located closer to the cortical surface. Without sequential neuroimaging studies showing an initial area of ischemic injury, lobar hemorrhages may be difficult to distinguish from a hemorrhagic infarction. Susceptibility-weighted brain magnetic resonance imaging sequences may reveal prior microhemorrhages at the gray-white junction in patients with cerebral amyloid angiopathy.

CEREBRAL EDEMA

When neurons and glia are injured by ischemia, energy metabolism fails and the cells can no longer maintain normal ion gradients between the intracellular and extracellular compartments. The result is cytotoxic edema, in which cells swell soon after the injury. Neurons, glia, and endothelial cells can be affected. Vasogenic edema, which may occur as a result of disruption of the blood-brain barrier due to injury to the endothelium, allows large molecules to pass through the blood-brain barrier and gain access to the brain. Edema generally peaks between 48 and 72 hours after the onset of ischemic injury. In patients with ischemic stroke, the development of cytotoxic edema can lead to an increase in intracranial pressure and, when severe, herniation. In selected patients, craniotomy can be considered to relieve the pressure until the edema subsides.

Neurons, glia, and endothelial cells are also damaged in the setting of intracerebral hemorrhage. The hemorrhage itself is a space-occupying lesion that can also be associated with both cytotoxic and vasogenic edema. Mass effect from cerebellar hemorrhages can compress the fourth ventricle (thereby leading to obstructive hydrocephalus), compress the brain stem (thereby compromising the reticular activating system and impairing consciousness), or cause herniation. Emergent evacuation of cerebellar hemorrhages can be life-saving and leave surviving patients with little or no long-term functional impairment. By comparison, surgical evacuation of intracerebral hemorrhage is not of proven value (Chapter 380), although minimally invasive surgery shows promise.

Grade A Reference

A1. Roffe C, Nevatte T, Sim J, et al. Effect of routine low-dose oxygen supplementation on death and disability in adults with acute stroke: the stroke oxygen study randomized clinical trial. *JAMA.* 2017;318:1125-1135.

A2. Hakim SM, Ammar MA, Reyad MS. Effect of therapeutic hypothermia on survival and neurological outcome in adults suffering cardiac arrest: a systematic review and meta-analysis. *Minerva Anestesiol.* 2018;84:720-730.

A3. Kim F, Nichol G, Maynard C, et al. Effect of prehospital induction of mild hypothermia on survival and neurological status among adults with cardiac arrest: a randomized clinical trial. *JAMA.* 2014;311:45-52.

A4. Lilja G, Nielsen N, Friberg H, et al. Cognitive function in survivors of out-of-hospital cardiac arrest after target temperature management at 33 degrees C versus 36 degrees C. *Circulation.* 2015;131:1340-1349.

GENERAL REFERENCES

For the General References and other additional features, please visit Expert Consult at https://expertconsult.inkling.com.

379

ISCHEMIC CEREBROVASCULAR DISEASE

LARRY B. GOLDSTEIN

DEFINITION

Ischemic cerebrovascular disease is caused by a reduction of blood supply to the brain. The injury may be focal (related to occlusion of a single artery), multifocal (related to occlusion of several arteries), or diffuse. Although certain clinical features (e.g., severe hypertension, headache, impaired consciousness) may suggest brain hemorrhage (Chapter 380) rather than ischemia, it is not possible to differentiate the two sets of conditions without a brain imaging study. In the absence of an inflammatory disease such as vasculitis or other rare conditions, simultaneous involvement of more than one vascular distribution suggests a proximal source of embolism (i.e., a cardiogenic or a proximal arterial source). Involvement of a single vascular territory may be due to either local steno-occlusive disease (e.g., atherosclerosis) or a proximal source of embolism. Involvement in the distribution of a single penetrating artery suggests small-vessel type intracranial disease, but ischemic strokes in this

distribution may also be caused by proximal arterial steno-occlusive disease or embolism.

The definition of ischemic stroke is brain, spinal cord, or retinal cell death attributable to ischemia with neuropathologic, neuroimaging, or clinical evidence of permanent injury. Overall, approximately 85% of strokes are related to ischemic disease, with 44% attributable to atherosclerosis, 21% to cardiogenic embolism, and 20% to small-vessel disease.

Transient ischemic attack (TIA) is defined as a brief episode of neurologic dysfunction resulting from focal cerebral ischemia with no evidence of corresponding tissue injury. Symptoms are similar to those of ischemic stroke. Previously characterized as a transient deficit with symptoms persisting for less than 24 hours, evidence of corresponding tissue injury can be seen on brain magnetic resonance imaging (MRI) in 30 to 40% of patients who otherwise fulfill the clinical definition of TIA.

EPIDEMIOLOGY

Stroke (ischemic and hemorrhagic) is the second leading cause of death worldwide and the fifth leading cause of death in the United States.[1] It is also a leading cause of adult disability. In addition to age, race or ethnicity, and family history, certain lifestyle factors and medical conditions increase the risk of stroke (Chapter 378; Table 379-1). Of these, hypertension is the single most important (Chapter 70; Table 379-1), and the risk of stroke increases with increasing blood pressure with no threshold effect. Diabetes (Chapter 216) is associated with a doubling of the risk of stroke (Table 379-1). Atrial fibrillation (Chapter 58; Table 379-1) is associated with up to 25% of ischemic strokes, with the absolute risk varying by concomitant risk factors.

Extracranial carotid artery stenosis is found in 5 to 10% of individuals older than 65 years and is associated with about 10% of all ischemic strokes. Untreated asymptomatic carotid stenosis carries only a 1 to 2% annual risk of stroke, and the risk is decreased to as low as 0.5% annually with standard medical therapy. Stroke is also a complication of sickle cell disease (Chapter 154), with risk dramatically reduced with transfusion therapy in high-risk children. Unlike with coronary heart disease, the overall association between high cholesterol concentration and the risk of stroke is less certain. Ischemic stroke risk is associated with higher levels of total cholesterol, whereas the risk of hemorrhagic stroke is increased with lower cholesterol levels.

Other factors associated with the risk of stroke include migraine headaches with aura (Chapter 370), particularly in women who smoke and are receiving oral contraceptives; elevated homocysteine level; high lipoprotein (a) level; postmenopausal hormone replacement therapy (Chapter 227); coagulation disorders (Chapter 73); systemic infection (Chapter 67); renal impairment (Chapter 121); low vitamin D levels (Chapters 205 and 231); and environmental factors, including high levels of air pollution.

PATHOBIOLOGY

For patients who have a TIA and who are by definition at increased risk of having an ischemic stroke during the next few days or weeks or who have an

TABLE 379-1	COMMON STROKE RISK FACTORS	
FACTOR	**POPULATION-ATTRIBUTABLE RISK**	**RISK REDUCTION WITH TREATMENT**
LIFESTYLE		
Cigarette smoking	12-14%	50% within 1 year of quitting
Physical inactivity	30%	?
Excess alcohol consumption	7%	?
MEDICAL		
Hypertension	>90%	32%
Diabetes	5-27%	—
Atrial fibrillation	2-24%	64%
Carotid stenosis	2-7%	50%
Sickle cell disease	—	91% with transfusion therapy in children

Data from Goldstein LB, Bushnell CD, Adams RJ, et al. Guidelines for the primary prevention of stroke: a guideline for healthcare professionals from the American Heart Association/American Stroke Association. *Stroke.* 2011;42:517-584.

ischemic stroke, distinguishing among the major pathophysiologic causes (i.e., atherothrombotic, cardioembolic, small vessel) is critical to guide secondary prevention. Atherothrombosis due to atherosclerosis is the most common cause of a TIA or stroke that is related to steno-occlusive disease in a single artery. The ischemia may be caused when progressive stenosis at the site of an atherosclerotic plaque leads to hemodynamic compromise affecting distal brain tissue. Sometimes bleeding into the plaque can lead to abrupt arterial occlusion, and sometimes a thrombus that has formed on an ulcerated plaque may embolize and occlude a distal artery. Occlusion of a cerebral artery, however, does not necessarily lead to ischemic brain injury. Blood may still reach the supplied territory through collaterals, either through the circle of Willis or from extracranial-intracranial anastomoses (see E-Fig. 378-1).

Arterial dissection is now recognized frequently on the basis of noninvasive vascular imaging such as MR angiography or computed tomography (CT) angiography. Other arteriopathies, such as fibromuscular dysplasia (Chapters 70, 72, and 116), may also lead to single, large-vessel distribution, ischemic stroke. Atherosclerosis of the ascending aorta or aortic arch can lead to the formation of thrombus, which can then embolize to a cerebral artery.

Atrial fibrillation is the single most common cause of cardioembolic stroke, with annual risks of 3 to 5% if it is not treated with anticoagulation but declining to about one fourth of that risk with anticoagulation (Chapter 58). The use of extended cardiac rhythm monitoring (i.e., 30-day event-triggered loop monitoring or an implanted monitor; Chapter 56) reveals occult atrial fibrillation in up to 25% of patients with an otherwise cryptogenic stroke. Other cardiac causes of cerebral embolism include clots or vegetations in patients with valvular heart disease (Chapter 66), such as mechanical prosthetic heart valves (Chapter 66), infectious endocarditis (Chapter 67), and nonbacterial endocarditis (Chapter 67); and mural thrombi in patients with a cardiomyopathy (Chapter 54) or myocardial infarction (MI), particularly anteroseptal MI (Chapter 64). Paradoxical embolism of a venous clot across a congenital heart defect, such as a patent foramen ovale or an atrial septal defect (Chapter 61), is another cause of embolic stroke.

Small-vessel intracranial disease may result in ischemic stroke in the distribution of a single penetrating vessel. These strokes commonly affect deep structures (e.g., centrum semiovale, basal ganglia, thalamus, internal capsule, pons) and occur more frequently in patients with hypertension and diabetes. Classically, small-vessel strokes are caused by lipohyalinosis, which is a thickening of the vessel wall resulting in a diminished luminal area, but they also can be caused by atherothrombosis or embolism.

Symptoms of ischemic stroke may worsen during the first hours or days through various mechanisms. For example, decreases in systemic blood pressure may decrease cerebral blood flow to marginally perfused, ischemic brain. In the setting of atherothrombotic disease, a partially occluded artery may progress to complete occlusion. Recurrent embolism may occur from a proximal arterial or cardiac source. Cerebral edema may develop during the first few days after an ischemic stroke, and the resulting mass effect can lead to clinical deterioration (Chapter 378). Secondary bleeding can occur in an area that was primarily the site of an ischemic injury when reperfusion, either through collateral vessels or as the result of a therapeutic intervention, restores blood flow into vessels in which the endothelium was damaged by the original ischemic insult.

CLINICAL MANIFESTATIONS

Neurologic deficits that occur in the setting of ischemic stroke depend on the involved vascular territory (Table 379-2) and underlying cause. Embolic stroke is generally characterized by the presence of a maximal deficit at onset, whereas the onset may be more gradual or stuttering in the setting of an atherothrombotic stroke. The distinction, however, is not of great use for diagnosis in individual patients. Transient symptoms in the same distribution can be caused by TIA if there is no permanent tissue injury.

Internal Carotid Artery

The bifurcation of the common carotid artery into the internal and external carotid arteries in the neck is a common site of atherosclerotic disease (see Fig. 378-1). With occlusion of the internal carotid artery, patients who have an incomplete circle of Willis can suffer profound contralateral loss of motor and sensory function affecting the face, arm, and leg. In patients with an intact anterior communicating artery that can supply the ipsilateral anterior cerebral artery (see Fig. 378-2), the leg may be relatively spared, and an internal carotid artery occlusion may be clinically indistinguishable from a middle cerebral artery occlusion. If the A1 segment of the anterior cerebral artery is absent on the side opposite an internal carotid artery occlusion in a patient with an

TABLE 379-2 CLINICAL MANIFESTATIONS OF ISCHEMIC CEREBROVASCULAR DISEASE

OCCLUDED ARTERY	TYPICAL MAJOR CLINICAL MANIFESTATIONS*
Internal carotid artery	Ipsilateral visual loss Ipsilateral middle cerebral artery syndrome
Anterior choroidal artery	Contralateral hemiparesis Contralateral sensory impairment Contralateral visual field defect
Anterior cerebral artery	Contralateral leg > arm paresis Contralateral leg > arm sensory deficit
Middle cerebral artery	Contralateral hemiparesis affecting face and arm > leg Contralateral sensory deficit affecting face and arm > leg Contralateral visual field defect Aphasia (dominant hemisphere) Contralateral hemispatial neglect (nondominant or dominant hemisphere)
Posterior cerebral artery	Contralateral homonymous hemianopia (or homonymous superior or inferior quadrantanopia) Contralateral sensory deficits (thalamic involvement)
Basilar artery tip	Bilateral central visual loss Confusion
Basilar artery	Ipsilateral cranial nerve deficit Contralateral hemiparesis Contralateral sensory impairment affecting arm and/or leg Coordination deficit
Vertebral artery, posterior inferior cerebellar artery	Ipsilateral sensory impairment over the face Dysphagia Ipsilateral Horner syndrome Ataxia
Superior cerebellar artery	Gait ataxia Ipsilateral limb ataxia Variable contralateral limb weakness

*Note: not all may be present.

intact anterior communicating artery, the ipsilateral leg may also be affected, and the presentation may be confused with a cardioembolic cause because both hemispheres are involved. Occlusion of the ipsilateral ophthalmic artery can lead to blindness in that eye. Transient symptoms of retinal ischemia, classically described by patients as a "shade coming down over my vision," indicate amaurosis fugax. Other common symptoms include a darkening or blurring of vision in the affected eye. Transient hypoperfusion ipsilateral to a high-grade internal carotid artery stenosis can cause limb-shaking TIAs that can be confused with seizures. Systemic hypotension in the setting of a high-grade carotid stenosis can lead to ischemic injury in watershed zones between the major intracranial arteries and in the border zone between the distal territories of cortical and lenticulostriate penetrating vessels (Chapter 378).

Anterior Choroidal Artery

The anterior choroidal artery generally arises from the supraclinoid portion of the internal carotid artery. Causes of occlusion of the anterior choroidal artery are similar to those of occlusion of the small intracranial arteries. Symptoms can include contralateral motor and sensory deficits and contralateral visual field deficits, the latter of which can occur in isolation.

Cerebral Arteries

About 2% of strokes are related to isolated occlusion of the anterior cerebral artery (see Figs. 378-6 and 378-7). Occlusion of the A1 segment in patients in whom the contralateral A1 segment is hypoplastic or absent can lead to bilateral leg involvement, abulia, and urinary incontinence because of infarction of both frontal lobes.

The middle cerebral artery is the most common artery involved in occlusions related to cardiogenic embolism. It supplies the lateral portions of the frontal, parietal, and temporal lobes as well as the basal ganglia and the anterior limb and genu of the internal capsule. Middle cerebral artery occlusions are characterized by involvement of the contralateral face and arm to a greater extent than of the leg (see Figs. 378-6, 378-7, and 378-8), often accompanied by a contralateral hemispatial neglect. When the dominant hemisphere is involved, the patient may have an aphasia. With frontal lobe involvement, patients often have an ipsilateral conjugate deviation of the eyes, which can be forced past the midline with vigorous encouragement, oculocephalic maneuvers, or caloric stimulation.

Branch middle cerebral artery occlusions can result in partial syndromes. For example, a branch middle cerebral artery occlusion with intact collaterals can cause a global aphasia without an accompanying motor deficit (i.e., "global aphasia without hemiparesis"). Anterior branch dominant hemisphere middle cerebral artery occlusions can cause an expressive cortical-type motor (Broca) aphasia with sparing of comprehension. Occlusion of the angular branch of the middle cerebral artery can cause receptive cortical-type (Wernicke) aphasia. Borderzone infarcts can result in transcortical aphasias, characterized by relatively preserved repetitions.

Both posterior cerebral arteries arise from the basilar artery in about 75% of people (see E-Fig. 378-1). In the other 25%, one or both P1 segments are hypoplastic or absent, with the posterior cerebral arteries arising from the ipsilateral internal carotid artery (so-called fetal circulation). Without vascular imaging, it is not possible to determine if a posterior cerebral artery distribution infarct (see Figs. 378-6 to 378-8) is related to carotid or vertebrobasilar circulation disease. The posterior cerebral artery and posterior communicating arteries supply the thalamus. Thalamic infarctions can result in contralateral hemianesthesia and ataxia. Contralateral hemiballismus can result if the subthalamic nucleus is damaged. Infarction of the ipsilateral occipital lobe causes a contralateral homonymous hemianopia that can be partial, depending on the extent of injury. The visual field deficit tends to become more congruous in the two eyes as the area of injury becomes more posterior (i.e., the closer to the occipital pole).

Vertebral and Basilar Arteries

Occlusion of the basilar artery (see Figs. 378-3 and 378-4B) can lead to "locked-in syndrome" (Chapter 376) in which the patient is awake and alert, because the periaqueductal gray can receive a separate blood supply, but unable to move or to communicate except for vertical eye movements, because of sparing of the collicular nuclei in the midbrain. The top of the basilar artery is a common location for embolic occlusion. Symptoms can include visual field defects due to unilateral or bilateral occipital injury and confusional states due to thalamic involvement.

Occlusions of penetrating and circumferential branches of the basilar artery and vertebral artery can produce a variety of symptoms (see Table 379-2) depending on the portion of the artery involved, several of which constitute eponymic midbrain (E-Fig. 379-1), pontine (E-Fig. 379-2), or medullary (E-Fig. 379-3) syndromes. Occlusion of the superior cerebellar artery can cause truncal ataxia because of infarction of the cerebellar vermis, with or without ataxia of the ipsilateral limbs, which can be caused by infarction of the ipsilateral cerebellar hemisphere.

Small Vessels

Occlusion of a small penetrating intracranial vessel can result in one of the classic lacunar syndromes (Table 379-3). These syndromes are not otherwise localizing and can occur with occlusions of small penetrating vessels in either the anterior or vertebrobasilar circulations. Lacunar syndromes are not pathognomonic of small-vessel intracranial disease and can be caused by a variety of other conditions, including emboli from a more proximal arterial or cardioembolic source or brain hemorrhage (Chapter 380).

DIAGNOSIS

The diagnosis of ischemic stroke depends on acquiring an accurate history, eliciting key findings on general and neurologic examinations, and obtaining supporting data from selected laboratory studies (Fig. 379-1). An initial anatomic and pathophysiologic differential diagnosis is usually established on the basis of the patient's history. Findings on physical and neurologic examinations can support or refute initial conclusions based on the history and can further refine the differential diagnosis.[2]

History

The abrupt onset of a focal neurologic deficit in the distribution of a specific vascular territory is the hallmark of acute ischemic stroke. The differential and most likely diagnosis can often be determined on the basis of history alone. For example, a patient with a history of atrial fibrillation who abruptly develops word-finding difficulties associated with a right hemiparesis and sensory impairment most likely had a cardiogenic embolus to the left middle cerebral artery. A patient with the acute onset of diplopia, vertigo, and a hemiparesis most likely has a lesion in the brain stem.

Goals of the immediate history include determining the exact time when symptoms began or the last time the patient was known to be well, concomitant medical illnesses, risk factors, medications, allergies, and other potential causes for symptoms that might mimic acute ischemic stroke. Because a stroke may affect a patient's ability to communicate, the history may require input from a witness. Additional details of the patient's past medical, family, and social history may need to be deferred in the emergent setting, but these issues can be explored if the information is important for acute treatment decisions.

TABLE 379-3	LACUNAR SYNDROMES

Pure motor stroke
Pure sensory stroke
Ataxic hemiparesis
Clumsy hand–dysarthria

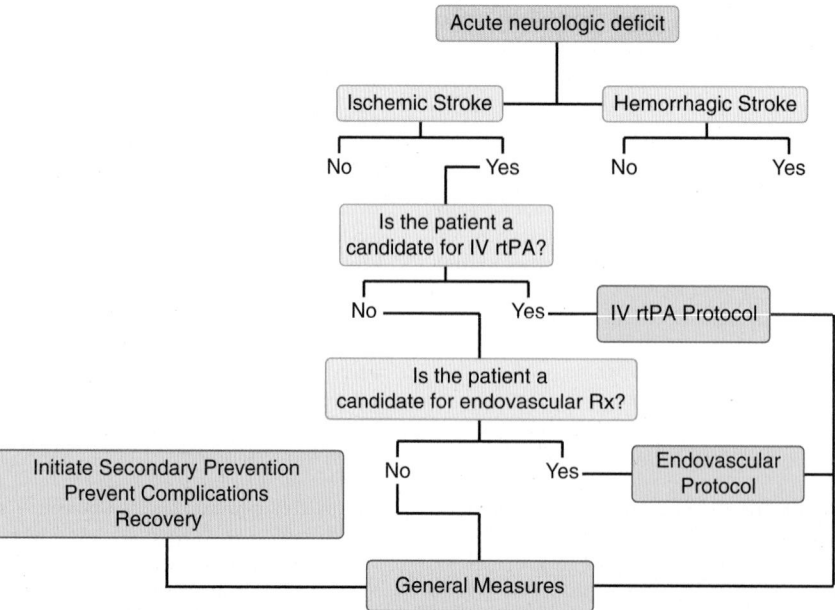

FIGURE 379-1. Approach to ischemic stroke. IV rtPA = intravenous tissue plasminogen activator; Rx = therapy. (Modified from Goldstein LB. Modern medical management of acute ischemic stroke. *Methodist DeBakey Cardiovasc J.* 2014;10:99-104.)

Physical Examination

Severely elevated blood pressures in the setting of neurologic deficits referable to the basal ganglia, thalamus, pons, or cerebellum increase the likelihood of a brain hemorrhage (Chapter 380). In a patient with transient vertigo associated with left arm movement, a reduced blood pressure in that arm suggests subclavian steal syndrome. Detection of an anterior cervical bruit contralateral to symptoms and signs indicative of a middle cerebral artery distribution infarct increase the likelihood of symptomatic carotid stenosis. An irregularly irregular heart rhythm with or without a cardiac murmur may indicate atrial fibrillation and a cardioembolic etiology. Finding a cholesterol embolus on funduscopic examination can be consistent with a proximal source of atheroembolism. Funduscopy can also show evidence of a small-vessel disease related to diabetes or hypertension (see Figs. 395-23 and 395-24).

A general neurologic examination (Chapter 368) including evaluations of cognition, language, spatial neglect, cranial nerves, motor function, sensation, coordination, gait, and reflexes is important both for documenting stroke-related deficits and for providing information critical for determining the area of the brain affected by the stroke and the severity of the injury. The use of a standardized graded neurologic impairment assessment provides a tool for measuring the severity of the stroke, determining the risks and benefits of treatment interventions, assessing prognosis, and observing patients objectively over time. The National Institutes of Health Stroke Scale (Table 379-4), which is the most commonly used approach, is both reliable and well validated. The individual items are summed to provide a total score.

Initial Laboratory Tests

Laboratory testing can help exclude conditions that may mimic, complicate, or lead to an acute ischemic stroke (Table 379-5). Tests that should be obtained in all patients with suspected ischemic stroke include a complete blood count and platelet count, prothrombin time/international normalized ratio (INR), activated partial thromboplastin time, blood glucose level, serum electrolytes, tests of renal function, troponin level, and oxygen saturation. An electrocardiogram should be obtained urgently.

The patient should be sent for a CT brain scan or MRI as soon as possible. CT or MR angiography should be obtained in patients suspected of

---

TABLE 379-4 NATIONAL INSTITUTES OF HEALTH STROKE SCALE

Administer stroke scale items in the order listed. Record performance in each category after each subscale exam. Do not go back and change scores. Follow directions provided for each exam technique. Scores should reflect what the patient does, not what the clinician thinks the patient can do. The clinician should record answers while administering the exam and work quickly. Except where indicated, the patient should not be coached (i.e., repeated requests to patient to make a special effort).

INSTRUCTIONS	SCALE DEFINITION	SCORE
1a. **Level of Consciousness:** The investigator must choose a response if a full evaluation is prevented by such obstacles as an endotracheal tube, language barrier, orotracheal trauma/bandages. A 3 is scored only if the patient makes no movement (other than reflexive posturing) in response to noxious stimulation.	0 = **Alert**; keenly responsive. 1 = **Not alert**; but arousable by minor stimulation to obey, answer, or respond. 2 = **Not alert**; requires repeated stimulation to attend, or is obtunded and requires strong or painful stimulation to make movements (not stereotyped). 3 = Responds only with reflex motor or autonomic effects or totally unresponsive, flaccid, and areflexic.	_____
1b. **LOC Questions:** The patient is asked the month and his/her age. The answer must be correct—there is no partial credit for being close. Aphasic and stuporous patients who do not comprehend the questions will score 2. Patients unable to speak because of endotracheal intubation, orotracheal trauma, severe dysarthria from any cause, language barrier, or any other problem not secondary to aphasia are given a 1. It is important that only the initial answer be graded and that the examiner not "help" the patient with verbal or nonverbal cues.	0 = **Answers** both questions correctly. 1 = **Answers** one question correctly. 2 = **Answers** neither question correctly.	_____
1c. **LOC Commands:** The patient is asked to open and close the eyes and then to grip and release the nonparetic hand. Substitute another one-step command if the hands cannot be used. Credit is given if an unequivocal attempt is made but not completed due to weakness. If the patient does not respond to command, the task should be demonstrated to him or her (pantomime), and the result scored (i.e., follows none, one, or two commands). Patients with trauma, amputation, or other physical impediments should be given suitable one-step commands. Only the first attempt is scored.	0 = **Performs** both tasks correctly. 1 = **Performs** one task correctly. 2 = **Performs** neither task correctly.	_____
2. **Best Gaze:** Only horizontal eye movements will be tested. Voluntary or reflexive (oculocephalic) eye movements will be scored, but caloric testing is not done. If the patient has a conjugate deviation of the eyes that can be overcome by voluntary or reflexive activity, the score will be 1. If a patient has an isolated peripheral nerve paresis (CN III, IV, or VI), score a 1. Gaze is testable in all aphasic patients. Patients with ocular trauma, bandages, preexisting blindness, or other disorder of visual acuity or fields should be tested with reflexive movements, and a choice made by the investigator. Establishing eye contact and then moving about the patient from side to side will occasionally clarify the presence of a partial gaze palsy.	0 = **Normal.** 1 = **Partial gaze palsy**; gaze is abnormal in one or both eyes, but forced deviation or total gaze paresis is not present. 2 = **Forced deviation**, or total gaze paresis not overcome by the oculocephalic maneuver.	_____
3. **Visual:** Visual fields (upper and lower quadrants) are tested by confrontation, using finger counting or visual threat, as appropriate. Patients may be encouraged, but if they look at the side of the moving fingers appropriately, this can be scored as normal. If there is unilateral blindness or enucleation, visual fields in the remaining eye are scored. Score 1 only if a clear-cut asymmetry, including quadrantanopia, is found. If patient is blind from any cause, score 3. Double simultaneous stimulation is performed at this point. If there is extinction, patient receives a 1, and the results are used to respond to item 11.	0 = **No visual loss.** 1 = **Partial hemianopia.** 2 = **Complete hemianopia.** 3 = **Bilateral hemianopia** (blind including cortical blindness).	_____
4. **Facial Palsy:** Ask—or use pantomime to encourage—the patient to show teeth or raise eyebrows and close eyes. Score symmetry of grimace in response to noxious stimuli in the poorly responsive or noncomprehending patient. If facial trauma/bandages, orotracheal tube, tape, or other physical barriers obscure the face, these should be removed to the extent possible.	0 = **Normal** symmetrical movements. 1 = **Minor paralysis** (flattened nasolabial fold, asymmetry on smiling). 2 = **Partial paralysis** (total or near-total paralysis of lower face). 3 = **Complete paralysis** of one or both sides (absence of facial movement in the upper and lower face).	_____

TABLE 379-4 NATIONAL INSTITUTES OF HEALTH STROKE SCALE—cont'd

INSTRUCTIONS	SCALE DEFINITION	SCORE
5. **Motor Arm**: The limb is placed in the appropriate position: extend the arms (palms down) 90 degrees (if sitting) or 45 degrees (if supine). Drift is scored if the arm falls before 10 seconds. The aphasic patient is encouraged using urgency in the voice and pantomime, but not noxious stimulation. Each limb is tested in turn, beginning with the nonparetic arm. Only in the case of amputation or joint fusion at the shoulder, the examiner should record the score as untestable (UN) and clearly write the explanation for this choice.	0 = **No drift**; limb holds 90 (or 45) degrees for full 10 seconds. 1 = **Drift**; limb holds 90 (or 45) degrees, but drifts down before full 10 seconds; does not hit bed or other support. 2 = **Some effort against gravity**; limb cannot get to or maintain (if cued) 90 (or 45) degrees, drifts down to bed, but has some effort against gravity. 3 = **No effort against gravity**; limb falls. 4 = **No movement**. UN = **Amputation** or joint fusion, explain: _____ 5a. **Left Arm** 5b. **Right Arm**	_____
6. **Motor Leg**: The limb is placed in the appropriate position: hold the leg at 30 degrees (always tested supine). Drift is scored if the leg falls before 5 seconds. The aphasic patient is encouraged using urgency in the voice and pantomime, but not noxious stimulation. Each limb is tested in turn, beginning with the nonparetic leg. Only in the case of amputation or joint fusion at the hip, the examiner should record the score as untestable (UN) and clearly write the explanation for this choice.	0 = **No drift**; leg holds 30-degree position for full 5 seconds. 1 = **Drift**; leg falls by the end of the 5-second period but does not hit bed. 2 = **Some effort against gravity**; leg falls to bed by 5 seconds, but has some effort against gravity. 3 = **No effort against gravity**; leg falls to bed immediately. 4 = **No movement**. UN = **Amputation** or joint fusion, explain: _____ 6a. **Left Leg** 6b. **Right Leg**	_____
7. **Limb Ataxia**: This item is aimed at finding evidence of a unilateral cerebellar lesion. Test with eyes open. In case of visual defect, ensure testing is done in intact visual field. The finger-nose-finger and heel-shin tests are performed on both sides, and ataxia is scored only if present out of proportion to weakness. Ataxia is absent in the patient who cannot understand or is paralyzed. Only in the case of amputation or joint fusion, the examiner should record the score as untestable (UN) and clearly write the explanation for this choice. In case of blindness, test by having the patient touch nose from extended arm position.	0 = **Absent**. 1 = **Present in one limb**. 2 = **Present in two limbs**. UN = **Amputation** or joint fusion, explain: _____	_____
8. **Sensory**: Sensation or grimace to pinprick when tested, or withdrawal from noxious stimulus in the obtunded or aphasic patient. Only sensory loss attributed to stroke is scored as abnormal, and the examiner should test as many body areas (arms [not hands], legs, trunk, face) as needed to accurately check for hemisensory loss. A score of 2, "severe or total sensory loss," should only be given when a severe or total loss of sensation can be clearly demonstrated. Stuporous and aphasic patients will, therefore, probably score 1 or 0. The patient with brain stem stroke who has bilateral loss of sensation is scored 2. If the patient does not respond and is quadriplegic, score 2. Patients in a coma (item 1a = 3) are automatically given a 2 on this item.	0 = **Normal**; no sensory loss. 1 = **Mild-to-moderate sensory loss**; patient feels pinprick is less sharp or is dull on the affected side; or there is a loss of superficial pain with pinprick, but patient is aware of being touched. 2 = **Severe to total sensory loss**; patient is not aware of being touched in the face, arm, and leg.	_____
9. **Best Language**: A great deal of information about comprehension will be obtained during the preceding sections of the examination. For this scale item, the patient is asked to describe what is happening in the attached picture, to name the items on the attached naming sheet, and to read from the attached list of sentences. Comprehension is judged from responses here, as well as to all of the commands in the preceding general neurological exam. If visual loss interferes with the tests, ask the patient to identify objects placed in the hand, repeat, and produce speech. The intubated patient should be asked to write. The patient in a coma (item 1a = 3) will automatically score 3 on this item. The examiner must choose a score for the patient with stupor or limited cooperation, but a score of 3 should be used only if the patient is mute and follows no one-step commands.	0 = **No aphasia**; normal. 1 = **Mild-to-moderate aphasia**; some obvious loss of fluency or facility of comprehension, without significant limitation on ideas expressed or form of expression. Reduction of speech and/or comprehension, however, makes conversation about provided materials difficult or impossible. For example, in conversation about provided materials, examiner can identify picture or naming card content from patient's response. 2 = **Severe aphasia**; all communication is through fragmentary expression; great need for inference, questioning, and guessing by the listener. Range of information that can be exchanged is limited; listener carries burden of communication. Examiner cannot identify materials provided from patient response. 3 = **Mute, global aphasia**; no usable speech or auditory comprehension.	_____
10. **Dysarthria**: If patient is thought to be normal, an adequate sample of speech must be obtained by asking patient to read or repeat words from the attached list. If the patient has severe aphasia, the clarity of articulation of spontaneous speech can be rated. Only if the patient is intubated or has other physical barriers to producing speech, the examiner should record the score as untestable (UN) and clearly write an explanation for this choice. Do not tell the patient why he or she is being tested.	0 = **Normal**. 1 = **Mild-to-moderate dysarthria**; patient slurs at least some words and, at worst, can be understood with some difficulty. 2 = **Severe dysarthria**; patient's speech is so slurred as to be unintelligible in the absence of or out of proportion to any dysphasia, or is mute/anarthric. UN = **Intubated** or other physical barrier, explain: _____	_____
11. **Extinction and Inattention (formerly Neglect)**: Sufficient information to identify neglect may be obtained during the prior testing. If the patient has a severe visual loss preventing visual double simultaneous stimulation, and the cutaneous stimuli are normal, the score is normal. If the patient has aphasia but does appear to attend to both sides, the score is normal. The presence of visual spatial neglect or anosognosia may also be taken as evidence of abnormality. Since the abnormality is scored only if present, the item is never untestable.	0 = **No abnormality**. 1 = **Visual, tactile, auditory, spatial, or personal inattention** or extinction to bilateral simultaneous stimulation in one of the sensory modalities. 2 = **Profound hemi-inattention or extinction to more than one modality**; does not recognize own hand or orients to only one side of space.	_____

From http://www.ninds.nih.gov/doctors/nih_stroke_scale.pdf. Accessed February 26, 2015.

TABLE 379-5	IMMEDIATE DIAGNOSTIC STUDIES: EVALUATION OF A PATIENT WITH SUSPECTED ACUTE ISCHEMIC STROKE

ALL PATIENTS

Noncontrast brain CT or brain MRI
Blood glucose
Oxygen saturation
Serum electrolytes/renal function tests*
Complete blood count, including platelet count*
Markers of cardiac ischemia*
Prothrombin time/INR*
Partial thromboplastin time*
ECG*

SELECTED PATIENTS

Thrombin time and/or ecarin clotting time if it is suspected the patient is taking
    direct thrombin inhibitors or direct factor Xa inhibitors
Hepatic function tests
Toxicology screen
Blood alcohol level
Pregnancy test
Arterial blood gas tests (if hypoxia is suspected)
Chest radiography (if lung disease is suspected)
Lumbar puncture (if meningitis is suspected or subarachnoid hemorrhage is
    suspected but the CT scan is negative for blood)
Electroencephalogram (if seizures are suspected)

*Although it is desirable to know the results of these tests before giving intravenous recombinant tissue-type plasminogen activator, fibrinolytic therapy should not be delayed while awaiting the results unless (1) there is clinical suspicion of a bleeding abnormality or thrombocytopenia, (2) the patient has received heparin or warfarin, or (3) the patient has received other anticoagulants (direct thrombin inhibitors or direct factor Xa inhibitors).
CT = computed tomography; ECG = electrocardiogram; INR = international normalized ratio; MRI = magnetic resonance imaging.
From Jauch EC, Saver JL, Adams HP Jr, et al. Guidelines for the early management of patients with acute ischemic stroke: a guideline for healthcare professionals from the American Heart Association/American Stroke Association. *Stroke.* 2013;44:870-947.

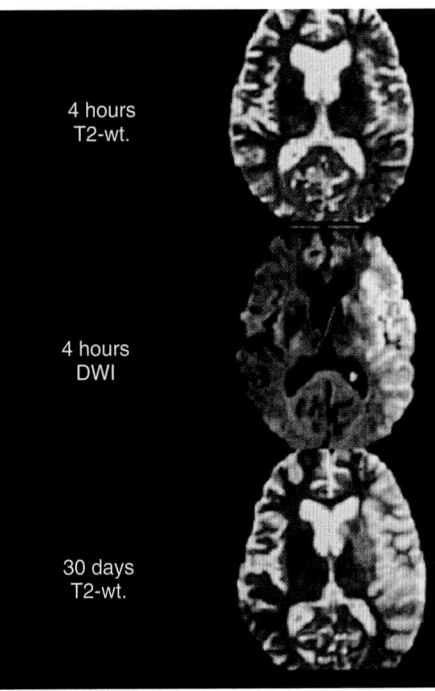

FIGURE 379-2. Magnetic resonance imaging (MRI) showing possible advantages of diffusion-weighted imaging (DWI) relative to conventional MRI at early times after vascular occlusion. *Top,* Conventional T2-weighted MRI 4 hours after symptom onset that appears normal. *Middle,* At the same time, a DWI scan shows abnormalities in the left hemisphere. *Bottom,* Repeated T2-weighted MRI 1 month later showed an infarction in the same location as the initial DWI scan. (Courtesy Gregory W. Albers, Stanford University, Stanford, Calif.)

having a large-vessel occlusion.[3] In many stroke centers, patients are taken for neuroimaging directly from the ambulance after a very brief assessment. Mobile stroke units with CT brain scans also are being used in some communities.[A1]

Additional tests are indicated in selected patients. For example, women of childbearing age should have a pregnancy test. A toxicology screen and blood alcohol levels should be obtained if drug or alcohol abuse is suspected. In patients who may be receiving a direct thrombin inhibitor or a factor Xa inhibitor, a thrombin time or ecarin clot time may be helpful in determining whether the patient is anticoagulated. An elevated erythrocyte sedimentation rate may point to an inflammatory cause or systemic infection.

The complete blood count can provide information about both the potential cause of the stroke and possible therapeutic interventions. An elevated white blood cell count may indicate an infectious cause of stroke, such as infective endocarditis (Chapter 67). Systemic infection may also cause a recrudescence of prior stroke symptoms in a patient who had previously recovered or in whom a stroke had not been previously recognized. Polycythemia (Chapter 157) can cause hyperviscosity that leads to occlusion of small intracranial vessels. Thrombocytopenia, either primary or secondary, can lead to platelet thrombi. The prothrombin time/INR and activated thromboplastin time provide indices that may reveal an underlying coagulation disorder, and thrombocytopenia and coagulation disorders may preclude treatment with intravenous recombinant tissue plasminogen activator (rtPA).

Both hypoglycemia (Chapter 217) and hyperglycemia (Chapter 216) may cause stroke-like symptoms. Impaired renal function (Chapter 121) is a risk factor for ischemic stroke and may increase the risks of using thrombolytic and anticoagulant medications. Abnormalities of other serum electrolytes (e.g., hyponatremia; Chapter 108) can also cause neurologic symptoms.

The electrocardiogram may reveal changes suggestive of acute myocardial ischemia as well as atrial fibrillation, the most common cause of embolic stroke. Stroke may also cause a variety of cardiac arrhythmias. Acute MI, especially anteroseptal MI, is associated with a higher risk of cardiogenic embolism, and an acute stroke may also precipitate an MI. A troponin level is usually adequate for this purpose, especially because it remains elevated for several days after the MI when embolism from a mural thrombus is most likely to occur. Patients with acute stroke should be placed on telemetry monitoring. Urgent echocardiography is used selectively.

Brain Imaging

CT or MRI brain imaging is an essential part of the evaluation of all patients with suspected ischemic stroke. Imaging can locate the area of damage, distinguish a brain hemorrhage from an ischemic stroke, and identify mass lesions such as tumor (Chapter 180), abscess (Chapter 385), or subdural hematoma that can present acutely and mimic a stroke. Brain CT is widely and rapidly available and provides the information necessary for the treatment of most patients with acute stroke. Brain MRI can detect areas of acute ischemic injury not apparent on CT brain imaging (Fig. 379-2), but it cannot be performed in patients with metal implants and devices such as cardiac pacemakers and is a challenge to perform in unstable patients.

The changes on brain CT, such as loss of gray-white distinction, loss of the insular ribbon, and blurring of the borders of the basal ganglia, can be subtle. The area of ischemic injury on brain CT scan appears as a relative hypodensity (Fig. 379-3), in contrast to brain hemorrhage, which appears hyperdense compared with the surrounding brain parenchyma (see Fig. 380-3). CT can also show acute hemorrhage in the subarachnoid space, which can be indicative of aneurysmal rupture (see Fig. 380-1). The dense middle cerebral artery sign or the dot sign, in which an artery in the Sylvian fissure may appear dense, can indicate thrombus in these vessels.

The findings on CT are often normal in the acute phase of ischemic stroke, and MRI is more sensitive for detecting acute ischemic injury (Fig. 379-4). Because brain CT imaging of posterior fossa structures is often obscured by beam hardening artifact from the petrous bones, MRI is also more sensitive for visualizing the brain stem and cerebellum. MRI signal patterns also can distinguish acute from subacute and remote ischemic injury, distinguish acute and remote brain hemorrhage, and identify other nonvascular conditions. However, MRI is not required before treatment with intravenous rtPA because CT can reliably exclude parenchymal brain hemorrhage and can detect other common conditions that may mimic a stroke, such as a mass lesion. Depending on time since the onset of symptoms, CT or MR perfusion can identify patients who might benefit from endovascular clot removal.

Lumbar Puncture

Lumbar puncture is rarely necessary in the evaluation of patients with acute stroke. In occasional patients, meningitis, especially septic meningitis from cardiogenic embolism in a patient with infective endocarditis, may cause stroke or stroke-like symptoms and be an indication for an urgent lumbar puncture.

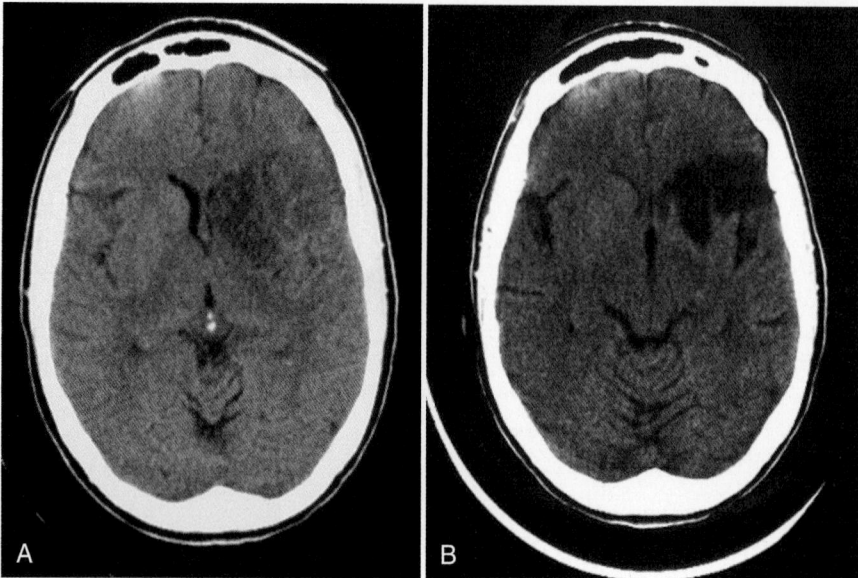

FIGURE 379-3. Computed tomographic imaging. **A,** A computed tomography (CT) scan of a patient with a left hemisphere infarction 6 to 24 hours after the onset of symptoms shows a hypodense area in the basal ganglia region and compression of the frontal horn of the lateral ventricle. **B,** A CT scan shows the chronic infarction 1 year later; atrophy and loss of tissue volume are visible. (Courtesy Gregory W. Albers, Stanford University, Stanford, Calif.)

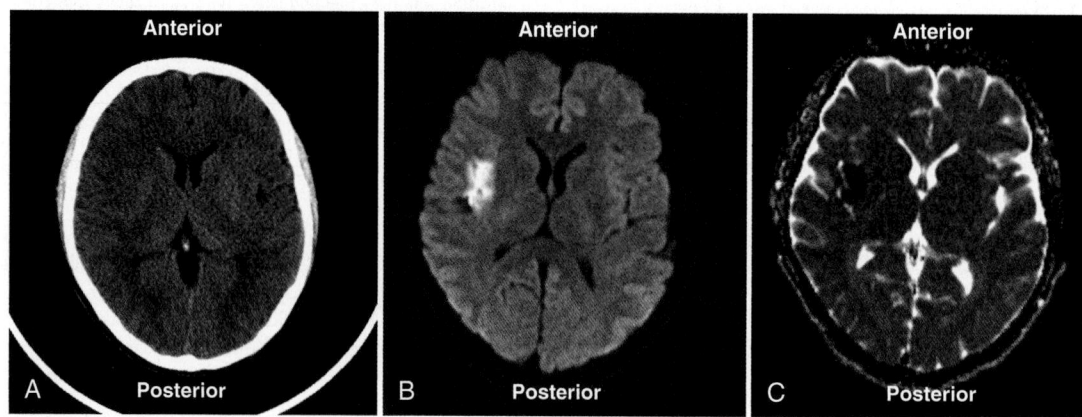

FIGURE 379-4. **A,** Computed tomographic imaging. **B,** Magnetic resonance imaging, diffusion sequence. **C,** Magnetic resonance imaging, apparent diffusion coefficient (ADC) map. Computed tomography shows no evidence of ischemic injury. There is an obvious area of restricted diffusion in the right frontotemporal cortex that is dark on the ADC map, consistent with an area of acute ischemic injury.

Brain CT usually demonstrates blood in the subarachnoid space in patients presenting with symptoms and signs of subarachnoid hemorrhage (Chapter 380), such as headache and meningismus. If, however, brain CT fails to visualize a subarachnoid hemorrhage in a patient in whom the clinical suspicion of subarachnoid hemorrhage is high, lumbar puncture should still be obtained.

Other Imaging

Carotid duplex ultrasonography, which combines B-mode vascular imaging with measures of blood flow velocity, is commonly used to screen for extracranial carotid artery stenosis but is rarely indicated in the acute setting. Both CT and MR angiography provide noninvasive vascular imaging of the extracranial and intracranial cerebral circulation, and one of these studies should be obtained emergently in patients who have suspected large-vessel occlusion and who might be candidates for endovascular thrombectomy. CT or MR angiography may be helpful in identifying cervical artery dissections in a patient with headache, neck pain, and symptoms and signs consistent with ipsilateral ischemic injury. Venous sinuses should be imaged if a sinus thrombosis is being considered. Transcranial Doppler ultrasonography is an alternative for evaluating the proximal cerebral vessels, but it cannot be obtained in some patients because of inadequate sonographic windows.

Diagnostic catheter angiography carries about a 0.5 to 1.5% risk of causing a stroke. For screening for large-vessel occlusion in the acute setting, it has largely been supplanted by noninvasive vascular imaging. Catheter angiography is, however, superior to CT or MR angiography for visualizing smaller

intracranial vessels and for detecting intracranial vasculopathies such as vasculitis (Chapter 254).

Differential Diagnosis

The hallmark of acute ischemic stroke is the abrupt onset of a focal neurologic deficit, frequently attributable to an area of brain supplied by a specific artery or arteries. In some patients, however, the onset of ischemic stroke may be stuttering, and the stroke symptoms may have been heralded by a prior TIA. The detection of an ipsilateral cervical artery bruit may also support the diagnosis. Embolic stroke typically has its maximal severity at onset, but it can involve multiple vascular territories. The diagnosis of an embolic stroke may be further suggested by finding a cardiac murmur, an irregularly irregular heart rhythm, or signs of emboli in other vascular territories.

A variety of other neurologic conditions may also be manifested acutely. Migraine with aura (Chapter 370) can be associated with focal neurologic deficits, including speech impairment, visual changes, vertigo, weakness, numbness, and imbalance. Partial seizures (Chapter 375) may have negative symptoms, including aphasia and paresis, and a patient with a postictal Todd paralysis may appear to have had a stroke. As a further challenge in diagnosis, seizures may occur in patients who are having an acute stroke. In a patient without a previous diagnosis, the first episode of multiple sclerosis (Chapter 383) can mimic a stroke. Mass lesions such as neoplasms (Chapter 180) and abscesses (Chapter 385) are generally associated with a slowly progressive worsening of neurologic symptoms but may occasionally be manifested acutely. Metabolic disorders such as hypoglycemia (Chapter 217) or hyperglycemia (Chapter 216), toxin exposures (Chapters 19 and 102), and drug intoxications (Chapter 31) can cause focal symptoms similar to stroke. Stroke-like symptoms may also be a manifestation of malingering, a conversion disorder, or other psychiatric illness.

TREATMENT Rx

After initial respiratory and hemodynamic stabilization (Chapter 98), the management of patients with acute ischemic stroke is directed at determining expeditiously (Table 379-6) whether treatment with intravenous rtPA (total dose 0.9 mg/kg, maximum 90 mg, 10% bolus with the remainder given over 1-hour) or endovascular thrombectomy is appropriate (Table 379-7; see also Fig. 379-1).[4] Current guidelines recommend treatment with intravenous rtPA even if intra-arterial treatments are available, but endovascular therapy is recommended and considered usual therapy in selected patients who have an emergent large-vessel occlusion and who can be treated at centers with such capabilities.[5]

Intravenous rtPA

Intravenous rtPA, administered within 4.5 hours of the onset of symptoms, does not reduce mortality but results in higher odds of a better neurologic outcome at 3 months compared with placebo.[A2] The benefit of rtPA declines over time within this 4.5-hour treatment window (E-Fig. 379-4), with the odds ratio for a favorable 3-month outcome declining from 2.55 for treatment within 0 to 90 minutes, to 1.64 for 91 to 180 minutes, to 1.26 for 181 to 270 minutes, and to no statistical benefit for treatment beyond 4.5 hours except that patients with ischemic but not yet infarcted brain tissue on imaging can still benefit between 4.5 and 9 hours.[A3] Registry studies support a benefit in routine clinical practice similar to that in randomized trials. As a result, current guidelines recommend that treatment with intravenous rtPA (Food and Drug Administration approved up to 3 hours after symptom onset) not be given if more than 4.5 hours have elapsed since the onset of symptoms. Treatment with rtPA is efficacious and safe among patients who are chronically treated with warfarin, provided their INR is 1.7 or lower, and is contraindicated with an INR higher than 1.7. The prothrombin time may be normal in patients who have received a direct oral anticoagulant (direct thrombin inhibitor or direct factor Xa inhibitor), and rtPA should not be administered unless appropriate assays are normal.

Treatment increases the risk of intracranial hemorrhage, but the overall benefit includes these adverse events, which do not significantly increase in frequency during the 4.5-hour treatment window. Treatment with intravenous rtPA is absolutely contraindicated in some patients (Table 379-8), with additional relative contraindications for treatment between 3 and 4.5 hours (Table 379-9).[6] In patients without contraindications, treatment should begin as soon as possible in either treatment window. Prehospital magnesium sulfate is of no benefit.

Endovascular Therapy

Strokes caused by large proximal occlusions tend to benefit less from treatment with intravenous rtPA compared with more distal or small-vessel obstructions. One randomized trial showed additional benefit of infusing rtPA directly into a proximal intracranial occlusion in the anterior circulation.[A4] In randomized trials, patients had improved neurologic outcomes and potentially lower mortality when treated acutely with devices to remove clots from brain blood vessels, especially if they had proximal intracranial occlusions,[A5,A6] with potentially salvageable tissue on CT perfusion angiography,[A7] even if they had already received rtPA.[A8] Overall data for mechanical thrombectomy indicate improved functional outcomes but no significant difference in symptomatic intracranial hemorrhage or all-cause mortality at 90 days and two years compared with standard care (including intravenous rtPA).[A9,A10] Improvement is more likely if endovascular therapy is provided earlier,[7] but functional benefit is seen even when patients with middle cerebral artery or internal carotid artery occlusion are treated between 6 and 16 hours after the onset of symptoms if the affected brain is ischemic but not infarcted.[A11] When thrombectomy is being considered, thrombolysis with tenecteplase may be preferable to alteplase.[A12]

Other Treatments

Regardless of whether the patient received intravenous rtPA or endovascular therapy, care in a comprehensive specialized stroke unit that incorporates rehabilitation is associated with better patient outcomes. Urgent anticoagulation to prevent recurrent stroke, to prevent worsening, or to improve functional outcome of patients with acute ischemic stroke is not recommended. Aspirin generally should not be started within 24 hours of treatment with intravenous rtPA unless its benefit for the treatment of concomitant conditions outweighs the risk of bleeding. For patients with high-risk TIA or a minor, nondisabling ischemic stroke, a short course of dual antiplatelet therapy with aspirin and clopidogrel is reasonable.[A13] Aspirin should otherwise be started at 325 mg daily within 24 to 48 hours after the onset of stroke.[A13] Long-term dual or triple antiplatelet therapy increases bleeding without reducing the risk of recurrent stroke.[A14] Hemicraniectomy can increase survival in patients with extensive middle cerebral artery strokes, but most survivors will require assistance with their body needs.

Antihypertensive medications to reduce blood pressure acutely by 10 to 25% in the first 24 hours with a goal of blood pressure to below 140/90 mm Hg by 1 week does not improve outcomes compared with discontinuation of all antihypertensive medications.[A15,A16] Current guidelines recommend that antihypertensive medications not be given unless the blood pressure rises to more than 220/120 mm Hg or higher in the absence of other indications. An exception is that blood pressure can be lowered in patients who are otherwise candidates for intravenous rtPA with a goal of maintaining blood pressures below 180/105 mm Hg after treatment (Fig. 379-5). Disability after acute stroke is similar for patients who lie flat for the first 24 hours compared with those who sit up with the head elevated to at least 30 degrees for 24 hours.

Several potential complications of acute stroke can often be avoided. Patients with stroke in any vascular distribution are at risk of aspiration pneumonia (Chapter 91). Stroke patients should not receive oral medications or nutrition until their ability to swallow safely has been assessed. Urinary tract infections

---

TABLE 379-6	**TIME GOALS FOR EVALUATION AND TREATMENT OF PATIENTS WITH ACUTE ISCHEMIC STROKE**
TIME AFTER EMERGENCY DEPARTMENT ARRIVAL	**GOALS**
10 minutes	Assess ABCs, vital signs Provide oxygen if hypoxemic Obtain intravenous access Obtain laboratory studies 　CBC, coagulation, electrolytes 　Check glucose level, treat if indicated Perform screening neurologic assessment Activate stroke team Order "stroke code" brain CT or MRI Obtain 12-lead ECG
25 minutes	Review history Establish time at onset or last known normal Perform neurologic examination NIH Stroke Scale
45 minutes	Review laboratory studies Review brain CT or MRI results Evaluate inclusion and exclusion criteria (see Tables 379-8 and 379-9)
60 minutes	Review risks and benefits Obtain consent Begin infusion

ABCs = airway, breathing, circulation; CBC = complete blood count; CT = computed tomography; ECG = electrocardiogram; MRI = magnetic resonance imaging; NIH = National Institutes of Health.

TABLE 379-7	**ADMINISTRATION OF rtPA FOR ACUTE ISCHEMIC STROKE**

Infuse 0.9 mg/kg (maximum dose 90 mg) over 60 minutes, with 10% of the dose given as a bolus over 1 minute.

Admit the patient to an intensive care or stroke unit for monitoring.

If the patient develops severe headache, acute hypertension, nausea, or vomiting or has a worsening neurological examination, discontinue the infusion (if IV rtPA is being administered) and obtain emergent CT scan.

Measure blood pressure and perform neurological assessments every 15 minutes during and after IV rtPA infusion for 2 hours, then every 30 minutes for 6 hours, then hourly until 24 hours after IV rtPA treatment.

Increase the frequency of blood pressure measurements if systolic blood pressure is >180 mm Hg or if diastolic blood pressure is >105 mm Hg; administer antihypertensive medications to maintain blood pressure at or below these levels.

Delay placement of nasogastric tubes, indwelling bladder catheters, or intra-arterial pressure catheters if the patient can be safely managed without them.

Obtain a follow-up CT or MRI scan at 24 hours after IV rtPA before starting anticoagulants or antiplatelet agents.

CT = computed tomography; IV = intravenous; MRI = magnetic resonance imaging; rtPA = recombinant tissue plasminogen activator.
From Jauch EC, Saver JL, Adams HP Jr, et al. Guidelines for the early management of patients with acute ischemic stroke: a guideline for healthcare professionals from the American Heart Association/American Stroke Association. *Stroke.* 2013;44:870-947.

TABLE 379-8	INCLUSION AND EXCLUSION CHARACTERISTICS OF PATIENTS WITH ISCHEMIC STROKE WHO COULD BE TREATED WITH IV rtPA WITHIN 3 HOURS FROM SYMPTOM ONSET

INCLUSION CRITERIA

Diagnosis of ischemic stroke causing measurable neurological deficit
Onset of symptoms <3 hours before beginning treatment
Aged ≥18 years

EXCLUSION CRITERIA

Significant head trauma or prior stroke in previous 3 months
Symptoms suggest subarachnoid hemorrhage
Arterial puncture at noncompressible site in previous 7 days
History of previous intracranial hemorrhage
Intracranial neoplasm, arteriovenous malformation, or aneurysm
Recent intracranial or intraspinal surgery
Elevated blood pressure (systolic >185 mm Hg or diastolic >110 mm Hg)
Active internal bleeding
Acute bleeding diathesis, including but not limited to
   Platelet count <100,000/μL
   Heparin received within 48 hours, resulting in aPTT greater than the upper limit
     of normal
   Current use of anticoagulant with INR >1.7 or PT >15 seconds
   Current use of direct thrombin inhibitors or direct factor Xa inhibitors with
     elevated sensitive laboratory tests (such as aPTT, INR, platelet count, and
     ECT; TT; or appropriate factor Xa activity assays)
Blood glucose concentration <50 mg/dL (2.7 mmol/L)
CT demonstrates multilobar infarction (hypodensity > ⅓ cerebral hemisphere)

RELATIVE EXCLUSION CRITERIA

Recent experience suggests that under some circumstances—with careful
  consideration and weighting of risk to benefit—patients may receive fibrinolytic
  therapy despite 1 or more relative contraindications. Consider risk to benefit of IV
  rtPA administration carefully if any of these relative contraindications are present:
    Only minor or rapidly improving stroke symptoms (clearing spontaneously)
    Pregnancy
    Seizure at onset with postictal residual neurological impairments
    Major surgery or serious trauma within previous 14 days
    Recent gastrointestinal or urinary tract hemorrhage (within previous 21 days)
    Recent acute myocardial infarction (within previous 3 months)

NOTES:

- The checklist includes some FDA-approved indications and contraindications for administration of IV rtPA for acute ischemic stroke. Recent guideline revisions have modified the original FDA-approved indications. A physician with expertise in acute stroke care may modify this list.
- Onset time is defined as either the witnessed onset of symptoms or the time last known normal if symptom onset was not witnessed.
- In patients without recent use of oral anticoagulants or heparin, treatment with IV rtPA can be initiated before availability of coagulation test results but should be discontinued if INR is >1.7 or PT is abnormally elevated by local laboratory standards.
- In patients without history of thrombocytopenia, treatment with IV rtPA can be initiated before availability of platelet count but should be discontinued if platelet count is <100,000/μL.

aPTT = activated partial thromboplastin time; CT = computed tomography; ECT = ecarin clotting time; FDA = Food and Drug Administration; INR = international normalized ratio; IV = intravenous; PT = partial thromboplastin time; rtPA = recombinant tissue plasminogen activator; TT = thrombin time.
From Jauch EC, Saver JL, Adams HP Jr, et al. Guidelines for the early management of patients with acute ischemic stroke: a guideline for healthcare professionals from the American Heart Association/American Stroke Association. *Stroke.* 2013;44:870-947.

TABLE 379-9	RELATIVE CONTRAINDICATIONS TO IV rtPA IN PATIENTS WITHIN 3 TO 4.5 HOURS AFTER ONSET OF SYMPTOMS OF ACUTE ISCHEMIC STROKE

National Institutes of Health Stroke Scale >25 (see Table 379-4)
Age >80 years old
Taking an oral anticoagulant regardless of INR
History of diabetes *and* a prior ischemic stroke

INR = international normalized ratio; IV = intravenous; rtPA = recombinant tissue plasminogen activator.
Adapted from Jauch EC, Saver JL, Adams HP, Jr., et al. Guidelines for the early management of patients with acute ischemic stroke: a guideline for healthcare professionals from the American Heart Association/American Stroke Association. *Stroke.* 2013;44:870-947.

(Chapter 268) are a potential complication; the routine placement of indwelling bladder catheters should be avoided. Patients who require an indwelling bladder catheter should have it removed as soon as feasible. Any infectious complications should be treated aggressively, and antipyretics should be used to maintain euthermia because fever is associated with more ischemic injury and poorer outcomes.[8] Immobilized patients should receive deep venous thrombosis prophylaxis with subcutaneous unfractionated heparin or low-molecular-weight heparin (see Table 76-2) if it is not contraindicated, with mechanical intermittent pneumatic compression if anticoagulation is contraindicated, or with both.

UNUSUAL CAUSES OF STROKE

Ischemic strokes may be caused by a variety of rarer conditions. Specific treatments, many of which are not supported by extensive clinical trial data, vary accordingly (E-Table 379-1).

Cerebral Venous Thrombosis

Thrombosis of a cerebral venous sinus can cause headache, focal stroke-like manifestations, seizures, altered mental status, and papilledema owing to raised intracranial pressure.[9] With superior sagittal sinus obstruction (see Fig. 378-10), patients can develop bilateral leg weakness and sensory changes. Obstruction of a transverse sinus or one of the major veins over the cerebral convexity (see Fig. 378-11) can also produce symptoms, depending on the area of the brain that is injured. Cerebral venous sinus thrombosis is an uncommon condition that is usually seen in patients with coagulopathies, disseminated cancer, or a prior inner ear infection. It can also occur in the peripartum period. Venous obstruction can mimic an ischemic arterial stroke, but symptoms and signs are often more diffuse and resemble encephalitis (Chapter 386) or meningitis (Chapter 384). The diagnosis can be suspected on routine CT or MRI and confirmed by CT or MR venography (Fig. 379-6). Initial acute treatment options include either body weight–adjusted subcutaneous low-molecular-weight heparin (see Table 76-2) or dose-adjusted intravenous heparin (see Table 74-6), even if patients have some degree of hemorrhage. One small randomized trial found that treatment with low-molecular-weight heparin was associated with lower mortality compared with unfractionated heparin.[A17] Oral warfarin anticoagulation should be started and continued for at least 3 months, with an INR target of 2.0 to 3.0. Data on the efficacy of newer oral anticoagulants (Chapter 76) are limited, but they appear to be equivalent to warfarin. Longer periods of anticoagulation may be considered, depending on the cause of the sinus thrombosis.

Cervical Artery Dissection

A cervical artery dissection or cerebral artery dissection, each of which can be associated with the formation and subsequent longitudinal extension of an intramural hematoma, can narrow or obstruct the arterial lumen. These dissections can be spontaneous, or they can be associated with major neck injury, relatively minor trauma (such as a chiropractic neck manipulation or neck hyperextension), or otherwise innocuous activities, such as coughing, sneezing, or lifting. Patients may have underlying fibromuscular dysplasia (Chapters 70 and 72); inherited conditions, such as Marfan syndrome (Chapter 244), Ehlers-Danlos syndrome, or tuberous sclerosis (Chapter 389); an elevated blood homocysteine level; or no identified underlying cause. The diagnosis can be challenging but should be considered especially in an otherwise healthy young patient who has neck or facial pain in conjunction with a stroke. MR angiography may show a hyperintense mass adjacent to a flow void, and MR angiography or catheter angiography can show a tapered lumen leading to an obstruction or even a double lumen. Antiplatelet and anticoagulation therapy provide equivalent outcomes.[A18] Treatment also may include thrombolysis, or endovascular or surgical repair, depending on individual circumstances.

Vasculitis

Vasculitis (Chapters 250, 254, and 255) can cause focal or multifocal cerebral ischemia due to local inflammation, stenosis, and even necrosis of extracranial or intracranial blood vessels.[10] Patients can have preexisting or concurrent headaches, cognitive changes, and seizures. Because vasculitis often involves multiple arteries, multiple foci of ischemic injury on neuroimaging studies may mimic multiple emboli. Cerebral angiography classically shows multiple areas of beadlike segmental narrowing, but findings may be normal. Similar findings may occur with other causes of intracranial vasculopathy, and the angiographic appearance is not specific. The diagnosis may require leptomeningeal/cortical biopsy, which may be negative because the inflammatory process can

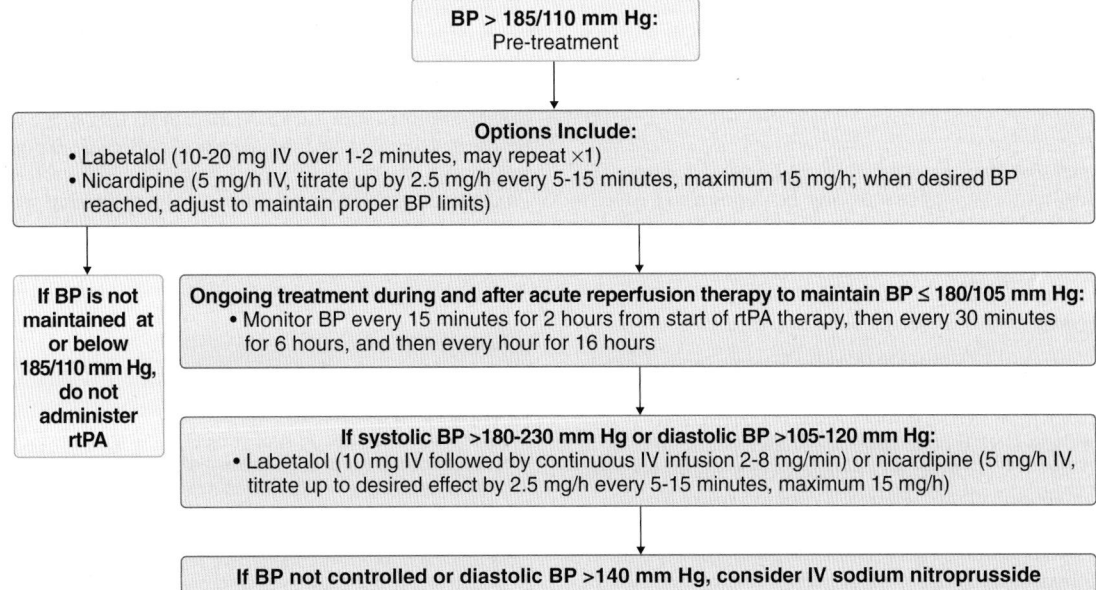

BP > 185/110 mm Hg:
Pre-treatment

Options Include:
- Labetalol (10-20 mg IV over 1-2 minutes, may repeat ×1)
- Nicardipine (5 mg/h IV, titrate up by 2.5 mg/h every 5-15 minutes, maximum 15 mg/h; when desired BP reached, adjust to maintain proper BP limits)

If BP is not maintained at or below 185/110 mm Hg, do not administer rtPA

Ongoing treatment during and after acute reperfusion therapy to maintain BP ≤ 180/105 mm Hg:
- Monitor BP every 15 minutes for 2 hours from start of rtPA therapy, then every 30 minutes for 6 hours, and then every hour for 16 hours

If systolic BP >180-230 mm Hg or diastolic BP >105-120 mm Hg:
- Labetalol (10 mg IV followed by continuous IV infusion 2-8 mg/min) or nicardipine (5 mg/h IV, titrate up to desired effect by 2.5 mg/h every 5-15 minutes, maximum 15 mg/h)

If BP not controlled or diastolic BP >140 mm Hg, consider IV sodium nitroprusside

Abbreviations: BP, blood pressure; IV, intravenously; and rtPA, recombinant tissue plasminogen activator.
Adapted from Jauch EC, Saver JL, Adams HP, Jr., et al. Guidelines for the early management of patients with acute ischemic stroke: a guideline for healthcare professionals from the American Heart Association/ American Stroke Association. *Stroke.* 2013;44:870–947.

FIGURE 379-5. Potential approaches to arterial hypertension in acute ischemic stroke patients who are candidates for acute reperfusion therapy.

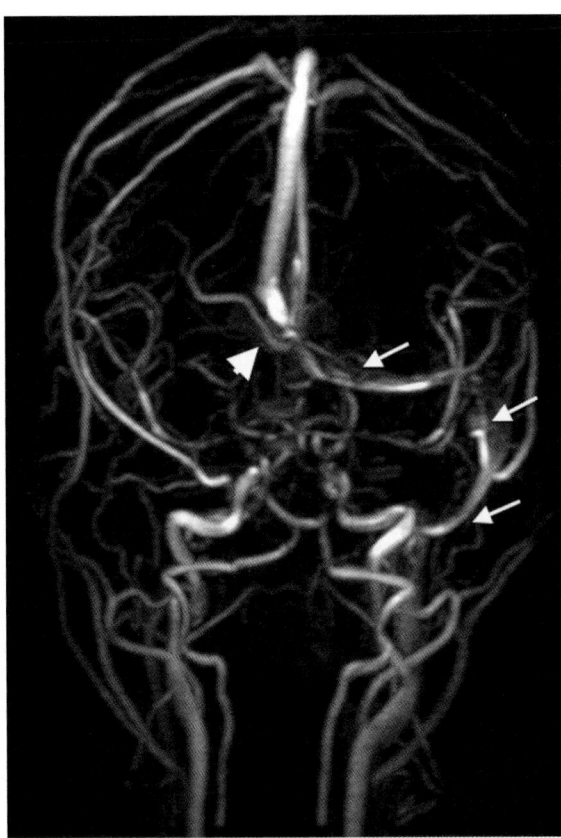

FIGURE 379-6. Magnetic resonance venogram showing absent flow in the right transverse sinus (*arrowhead*) and sigmoid sinus and intact flow in the left transverse sinus and sigmoid sinus (*arrows*).

be multifocal rather than diffuse. Examples of vasculitides that can cause stroke-like symptoms include primary central nervous system vasculitis, systemic lupus erythematosus (Chapter 250), rheumatoid vasculitis (Chapter 248), Behçet disease (Chapter 254), Takayasu arteritis (Chapters 69 and 254), temporal arteritis (Chapter 255), fibromuscular dysplasia (Chapters 67 and 72),

granulomatosis with angiitis (Chapter 254), sarcoidosis (Chapter 89), meningovascular syphilis (Chapter 303), and lymphomatoid angioendotheliomatosis.

Sickle Cell Disease

Strokes occur in about 8 to 17% of patients with sickle cell disease and in about 2% of individuals with sickle cell trait (Chapter 154). Ischemic strokes are more common in children, whereas hemorrhagic strokes are more common in adults. Transfusion therapy can markedly reduce the risk of a first or recurrent stroke. When adults with sickle cell disease have an acute ischemic stroke, treatment with IV rtPA can be beneficial.

Drug-Related Causes of Stroke

A variety of legal and illicit drugs (Chapter 31) can precipitate an ischemic stroke. Intravenous drug users are more likely to develop bacterial endocarditis (Chapter 67), which can cause embolic stroke and lead to mycotic aneurysms that can cause subarachnoid hemorrhage. Solid adulterants in injected material can reach the brain through an existing shunt, such as a patent foramen ovale, or they can cause local pulmonary arteriolitis that damages the endothelium and results in arteriovenous shunts through which microemboli can reach the brain. Potent vasoconstricting drugs (e.g., cocaine, ephedrine, phenylpropanolamine, and fenoxazoline) and dietary supplements (e.g., ephedra) may precipitate cerebral vasospasm and ischemic stroke, although hemorrhagic strokes are more common (Chapter 380). These drugs have been used in high doses as appetite suppressants, and case reports suggest that stroke may occur even after the first use of these products.

Rare Genetic Causes

Several relatively rare genetic diseases can cause ischemic stroke. *Cerebral autosomal dominant arteriopathy with small subcortical infarcts and leukoencephalopathy* (CADASIL) can cause multiple deep infarcts and dementia in patients without other risk factors for stroke. A mutation in the Notch3 receptor gene on the short arm of chromosome 19 leads to an accumulation of Notch3 protein in vascular smooth muscle cells. The mean age at onset is about 40 years, although migraine with aura often antedates strokes by several years. Dementia usually develops within 10 to 15 years. Antenatal diagnosis is recommended in affected families. Treatment is symptomatic, with CADASIL-associated headaches potentially responding to acetazolamide (125 to 500 mg daily).

X-linked *Fabry disease* (angiokeratoma corporis diffusum) (Chapter 197) frequently includes cerebrovascular occlusion due to the accumulation of glycolipids in small and medium-sized arteries. Enzyme replacement therapy is recommended, although it is not proven to reduce the risk of stroke.

Neurofibromatosis (Chapter 389) can occlude the internal carotid arteries or the proximal part of the anterior cerebral circulation. Marfan syndrome (Chapter 244) can cause ischemic stroke due to dissection of the carotid arteries or related valvular heart disease.

Fat Embolism

Fat embolism (Chapter 74) after trauma to the long bones (Chapter 103), orthopedic procedures, and severe trauma to large fat deposits can cause a stroke, usually several days later. Diffuse embolization can produce encephalopathy or seizures, but more focal emboli can be manifested as an ischemic stroke.

Cryptogenic Stroke

An echocardiogram may reveal an undiagnosed patent foramen ovale (Chapter 61) as a potential cause of a cryptogenic stroke. For example, transesophageal echocardiography in adult patients with embolic stroke of undetermined source may positively affect the selection of an appropriate therapeutic strategy in approximately 1 in 7 patients by detecting a patent foramen ovale, bacterial endocarditis, or other abnormalities.[11] Despite a comprehensive evaluation (Fig. 379-7), however, no definitive cause of stroke is found in 15 to 40% of patients with strokes.[12] Randomized trials confirm that prolonged ECG monitoring with an event-triggered recorder or an insertable monitor increases the detection of atrial fibrillation to 9 to 16% compared with 1 to 3% with just 24-hour monitoring.[A19] Other initially cryptogenic strokes may be due to embolism from either a cardiac or other proximal arterial source. In these patients, neither dabigatran nor rivaroxaban is preferable to aspirin prophylaxis.[A20][A21]

RECOVERY/REHABILITATION

The process of recovery begins even before the sequelae of acute brain injury have resolved.[13] Multidisciplinary physiotherapy should include assessments by speech pathologists, physical therapists, and occupational therapists.

Organized inpatient multidisciplinary rehabilitation is associated with a 34% lower odds of death, a 30% lower odds of death or institutionalization, and a 35% lower odds of death or dependency for patients with deficits warranting these services, but aggressive mobilization within 24 to 48 hours is of no benefit compared with usual care. All patients with stroke-related deficits should be assessed for rehabilitative interventions. Because depression can complicate stroke and affect recovery, all patients should be screened for depression. Prophylactic antibiotics are not effective for preventing post-stroke pneumonia, even in patients with dysphagia.

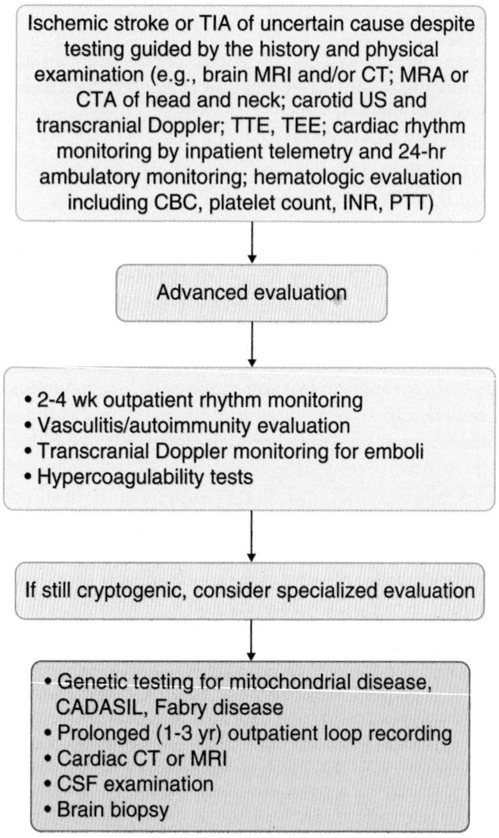

PREVENTION   Rx

Primary Prevention

Because more than 75% of strokes are first events, primary prevention of stroke is of paramount importance. Following a healthy lifestyle (not smoking, following a diet low in sodium and rich in fruits and vegetables, getting at least 30 minutes of moderate or vigorous physical activity daily, having a body mass index below 25 kg/m^2, and consumption of no more than one alcoholic drink per day for women and one or two for men) is associated with an 80% lower risk of a first stroke compared with people who do not follow these lifestyles. The effect is graded, with increasing benefit depending on the number of healthy lifestyles an individual follows. There is no evidence that prophylactic treatment with aspirin or other antiplatelet drugs reduces the risk of stroke in low-risk individuals.

Risk factors that are amenable to treatment (see Table 379-1) include hypertension, diabetes, atrial fibrillation, and carotid stenosis. Treatment of hypertension dramatically reduces the risk of stroke.[14] Regular blood pressure screening and treatment of hypertension (see Tables 70-5 and 70-7) is recommended, and aggressive treatment (goal systolic blood pressure less than 120 mm Hg) may prevent an additional 100,00 deaths in the United States each year compared with a goal of 140/90 mm Hg (Chapter 70).[15] Blood pressure treatment and the use of a statin in patients with diabetes (Chapter 216) are recommended to lower the risk of a first stroke. Statins (Chapter 195) are also recommended to prevent a first ischemic stroke in patients with coronary heart disease. Although microvascular complications of diabetes are reduced with adequate glycemic control (target glycated hemoglobin level <7%), there is no evidence that tight control reduces the risk of stroke or coronary heart events. Patients who have atrial fibrillation are at increased risk of embolism and benefit from treatment with a direct oral anticoagulant or warfarin (Chapter 58). In patients with a mechanical prosthetic heart valve (Chapter 66), direct oral anticoagulants are contraindicated, and anticoagulation with warfarin is recommended to prevent stroke. The U.S. Preventive Services Task Force recommends against screening for asymptomatic carotid artery stenosis. Folic acid does not prevent stroke in Western countries, but does reduce the risk of stroke in Chinese adults with hypertension, among whom absolute or relative folate deficiency is more common.[A22]

Prevention of Stroke in the Patient with Asymptomatic Carotid Stenosis

The benefit of carotid endarterectomy for patients with asymptomatic carotid stenosis is currently uncertain because of advances in medical therapy. The risk of ipsilateral stroke associated with an asymptomatic carotid stenosis may be considerably less than 1% per year on the basis of observational studies and clinical trials, and the reported benefit of carotid endarterectomy depends on surgical success and complication rates that may not be widely achievable outside of randomized trials. Clinical trials are in progress comparing carotid revascularization in asymptomatic patients with current best medical therapy. Population screening for asymptomatic carotid stenosis is not recommended.

Secondary Prevention after a Transient Ischemic Attack or Stroke

Although clinical trials demonstrating the efficacy of lifestyle interventions for secondary stroke prevention are generally lacking, the same lifestyle behaviors associated with a reduced risk of a first stroke are an essential part of secondary stroke prevention.[16] Patients should routinely be prescribed an antiplatelet agent unless there are contraindications. The exception is the patient who has a specific indication for treatment with an anticoagulant, such as atrial fibrillation or a prosthetic heart valve, or in whom antithrombotic therapy is contraindicated. The choice of agent needs to be individualized, but aspirin (50 to 325 mg daily), clopidogrel (75 mg daily), ticagrelor (180 mg loading dose on day 1 followed by 90 mg twice daily), or aspirin plus sustained-release dipyridamole (25/200 mg twice daily) are options. Ticagrelor alone is no better than aspirin in reducing the rate of stroke, myocardial infarction, or death at 90 days. Short-term dual antiplatelet therapy with aspirin and clopidogrel may be more efficacious than single-agent therapy, but long-term therapy increases the risk of serious bleeding.

FIGURE 379-7. Diagnostic evaluation of patients with cryptogenic ischemic stroke or transient ischemic attack. CADASIL = cerebral autosomal dominant arteriopathy with subcortical infarcts and leukoencephalopathy; CBC = complete blood count; CSF = cerebrospinal fluid; CT = computed tomography; CTA = computer tomographic angiography; INR = international normalized ratio; MRA = magnetic resonance angiography; MRI = magnetic resonance imaging; PTT = partial thromboplastin time; TEE = transesophageal echocardiography; TIA = transient ischemic attack; TTE = transthoracic echocardiography; US = ultrasound. (Data from Saver JL. Clinical practice. Cryptogenic stroke. *N Engl J Med.* 2016;374:2065-2074.)

Blood pressure reduction is recommended to lower the risk of recurrent stroke and other vascular events. The precise timing of initiation of antihypertensive therapy after ischemic stroke is not established, but it can begin once the patient is stabilized after the acute period, generally after at least 24 hours. An average reduction of 10/5 mm Hg is associated with about a 25% reduction in the risk of recurrent stroke. In a randomized trial of patients with MRI-defined symptomatic lacunar infarctions, reducing systolic blood pressure to a target of less than 130 mm Hg starting 2 weeks later significantly reduced the rate of intracerebral hemorrhage and insignificantly reduced all subsequent stroke compared with a target of 130 to 149 mm Hg.[A23] The choice of a specific antihypertensive regimen for secondary prevention should be individualized (see Tables 70-5 and 70-7). Treatment recommendations are for a diuretic, calcium channel antagonist, angiotensin-converting enzyme inhibitor, or angiotensin receptor blocker.

Patients with a prior stroke or TIA and known atherosclerotic disease, diabetes, or hyperlipidemia meeting criteria for statin therapy should be treated with a high-potency statin (e.g., 40 to 80 mg of atorvastatin or 20 to 40 mg of rosuvastatin daily; see also Table 195-3), unless contraindicated,[A24] to reduce the risk of recurrent stroke and of other cardiovascular events.[A24] Stopping a statin in the setting of an acute ischemic stroke is associated with increased morbidity and mortality.

In one randomized trial of patients who had a recent history of ischemic stroke or TIA and who also had insulin resistance but not diabetes, the subsequent risk of stroke or myocardial infarction was lower among patients who received pioglitazone (target dose, 45 mg daily) than among patients who received placebo. Additional data are necessary before such treatment is recommended for routine use. In addition to these general measures, additional specific treatment for secondary stroke prevention depends on the cause of the stroke. Atrial fibrillation–related stroke is associated with a high risk of recurrence (i.e., 6 to 10% annually). Patients with atrial fibrillation–related stroke should be treated with a direct oral anticoagulant or warfarin. Anticoagulation with warfarin is indicated in patients with stroke related to acute MI and in those with valvular heart disease.

Procedures and Devices

The rate of recurrent stroke after stroke or TIA related to a high-grade (70 to 99%) extracranial carotid artery stenosis may be as high as 25% during the ensuing 2 years, with the highest risk in the first weeks after the index event. Because this risk of recurrence is decreased by 50% with successful carotid revascularization, selected patients with stroke associated with 70 to 99% extracranial carotid artery stenosis within the prior 6 months benefit from carotid revascularization, provided the procedure can be performed with less than 6% morbidity. Patients with a 50 to 69% symptomatic stenosis also appear to benefit, but with about a 16% relative reduction in subsequent events.[A25] Patients with less than 50% carotid stenosis do not benefit from carotid revascularization.

For a combined endpoint of stroke, MI, and death, carotid stenting appears to be as efficacious as endarterectomy in patients with a symptomatic or asymptomatic extracranial carotid artery stenosis,[A26][A27] but stenting tends to be associated with a higher risk of stroke. Younger patients seem to do somewhat better with stenting, whereas patients over age 70 years seem to do better with endarterectomy.[A28] For patients with cryptogenic stroke and a patent foramen ovale, transcatheter closure of the patent foramen ovale with or without antiplatelet therapy may be considered for reducing the risk of subsequent transient ischemic attacks and strokes compared with antiplatelet therapy alone.[A29] Extracranial-intracranial bypass does not reduce the risk of recurrent strokes in patients with complete occlusion of an extracranial carotid artery and may be associated with a higher risk of stroke than medical therapy.[A30][A31] Similarly, vertebral artery angioplasty or stenting is not beneficial even in symptomatic patients.[A32]

PROGNOSIS

TIA is a major risk factor for stroke and requires urgent evaluation to detect specific causes that may require immediate treatment. Overall, approximately 10% of patients who have a TIA will have a stroke within 90 days, with almost half occurring within 2 days. The strokes that occur are frequently fatal or associated with disabling deficits (E-Table 379-2). Factors associated with higher risk include age older than 60 years, diabetes, impaired speech or weakness, symptoms lasting more than 10 minutes, and evidence of ischemic injury on brain MRI. After the acute period, about 20% of patients who had a TIA will have a stroke during the next 10 years.

Stroke-related mortality varies by age. The 30-day stroke mortality rate is estimated to be 9% for patients aged 65 to 74 years, 13% for patients aged 74 to 84 years, and 23% for patients older than 85 years. About 30% of patients who have had a stroke will have a recurrent stroke within 5 years. Stroke is also a leading cause of disability. Among stroke survivors, approximately 45% have cognitive deficits, 30% are unable to walk without assistance, 25% are institutionalized, and 25% are dependent in activities of daily living after 6 months.

Grade A References

A1. Ebinger M, Winter B, Wendt M, et al. Effect of the use of ambulance-based thrombolysis on time to thrombolysis in acute ischemic stroke: a randomized clinical trial. JAMA. 2014;311:1622-1631.

A2. Emberson J, Lees KR, Lyden P, et al. Effect of treatment delay, age, and stroke severity on the effects of intravenous thrombolysis with alteplase for acute ischaemic stroke: a meta-analysis of individual patient data from randomised trials. Lancet. 2014;384:1929-1935.

A3. Ma H, Campbell BCV, Parsons MW, et al. Thrombolysis guided by perfusion imaging up to 9 hours after onset of stroke. N Engl J Med. 2019;380:1795-1803.

A4. Berkhemer OA, Fransen PS, Beumer D, et al. A randomized trial of intraarterial treatment for acute ischemic stroke. N Engl J Med. 2015;372:11-20.

A5. Goyal M, Demchuk AM, Menon BK, et al. Randomized assessment of rapid endovascular treatment of ischemic stroke. N Engl J Med. 2015;372:1019-1030.

A6. Jovin TG, Chamorro A, Cobo E, et al. Thrombectomy within 8 hours after symptom onset in ischemic stroke. N Engl J Med. 2015;372:2296-2306.

A7. Campbell BC, Mitchell PJ, Kleinig TJ, et al. Endovascular therapy for ischemic stroke with perfusion-imaging selection. N Engl J Med. 2015;372:1009-1018.

A8. Saver JL, Goyal M, Bonafe A, et al. Stent-retriever thrombectomy after intravenous t-PA vs. t-PA alone in stroke. N Engl J Med. 2015;372:2285-2295.

A9. Goyal M, Menon BK, van Zwam WH, et al. Endovascular thrombectomy after large-vessel ischaemic stroke: a meta-analysis of individual patient data from five randomised trials. Lancet. 2016;387:1723-1731.

A10. van den Berg LA, Dijkgraaf MG, Berkhemer OA, et al. Two-year outcome after endovascular treatment for acute ischemic stroke. N Engl J Med. 2017;376:1341-1349.

A11. Albers GW, Marks MP, Kemp S, et al. Thrombectomy for stroke at 6 to 16 hours with selection by perfusion imaging. N Engl J Med. 2018;378:708-718.

A12. Campbell BCV, Mitchell PJ, Churilov L, et al. Tenecteplase versus alteplase before thrombectomy for ischemic stroke. N Engl J Med. 2018;378:1573-1582.

A13. Rothwell PM, Algra A, Chen Z, et al. Effects of aspirin on risk and severity of early recurrent stroke after transient ischaemic attack and ischaemic stroke: time-course analysis of randomised trials. Lancet. 2016;388:365-375.

A14. Bath PM, Woodhouse LJ, Appleton JP, et al. Antiplatelet therapy with aspirin, clopidogrel, and dipyridamole versus clopidogrel alone or aspirin and dipyridamole in patients with acute cerebral ischaemia (TARDIS): a randomised, open-label, phase 3 superiority trial. Lancet. 2018;391:850-859.

A15. He J, Zhang Y, Xu T, et al. Effects of immediate blood pressure reduction on death and major disability in patients with acute ischemic stroke: the CATIS randomized clinical trial. JAMA. 2014;311:479-489.

A16. Anderson CS, Huang Y, Lindley RI, et al. Intensive blood pressure reduction with intravenous thrombolysis therapy for acute ischaemic stroke (ENCHANTED): an international, randomised, open-label, blinded-endpoint, phase 3 trial. Lancet. 2019;393:877-888.

A17. Misra UK, Kalita J, Chandra S, et al. Low molecular weight heparin versus unfractionated heparin in cerebral venous sinus thrombosis: a randomized controlled trial. Eur J Neurol. 2012;19:1030-1036.

A18. Markus HS, Levi C, King A, et al. Antiplatelet therapy vs anticoagulation therapy in cervical artery dissection: the cervical artery dissection in stroke study (CADISS) randomized clinical trial final results. JAMA Neurol. 2019;76:657-664.

A19. Gladstone DJ, Spring M, Dorian P, et al. Atrial fibrillation in patients with cryptogenic stroke. N Engl J Med. 2014;370:2467-2477.

A20. Diener HC, Sacco RL, Easton JD, et al. Dabigatran for prevention of stroke after embolic stroke of undetermined source. N Engl J Med. 2019;380:1906-1917.

A21. Hart RG, Sharma M, Mundl H, et al. Rivaroxaban for stroke prevention after embolic stroke of undetermined source. N Engl J Med. 2018;378:2191-2201.

A22. Huo Y, Li J, Qin X, et al. Efficacy of folic acid therapy in primary prevention of stroke among adults with hypertension in China: the CSPPT randomized clinical trial. JAMA. 2015;313:1325-1335.

A23. Benavente OR, Coffey CS, Conwit R, et al. Blood-pressure targets in patients with recent lacunar stroke: the SPS3 randomised trial. Lancet. 2013;382:507-515.

A24. Koskinas KC, Siontis GCM, Piccolo R, et al. Effect of statins and non-statin LDL-lowering medications on cardiovascular outcomes in secondary prevention: a meta-analysis of randomized trials. Eur Heart J. 2018;39:1172-1180.

A25. Orrapin S, Rerkasem K. Carotid endarterectomy for symptomatic carotid stenosis. Cochrane Database Syst Rev. 2017;6:CD001081.

A26. Brott TG, Howard G, Roubin GS, et al. Long-term results of stenting versus endarterectomy for carotid-artery stenosis. N Engl J Med. 2016;374:1021-1031.

A27. Rosenfield K, Matsumura JS, Chaturvedi S, et al. Randomized trial of stent versus surgery for asymptomatic carotid stenosis. N Engl J Med. 2016;374:1011-1020.

A28. Howard G, Roubin GS, Jansen O, et al. Association between age and risk of stroke or death from carotid endarterectomy and carotid stenting: a meta-analysis of pooled patient data from four randomised trials. Lancet. 2016;387:1305-1311.

A29. De Rosa S, Sievert H, Sabatino J, et al. Percutaneous closure versus medical treatment in stroke patients with patent foramen ovale: a systematic review and meta-analysis. Ann Intern Med. 2018;168:343-350.

A30. Derdeyn CP, Chimowitz MI, Lynn MJ, et al. Aggressive medical treatment with or without stenting in high-risk patients with intracranial artery stenosis (SAMMPRIS): the final results of a randomised trial. Lancet. 2014;383:333-341.

A31. Zaidat OO, Fitzsimmons BF, Woodward BK, et al. Effect of a balloon-expandable intracranial stent vs medical therapy on risk of stroke in patients with symptomatic intracranial stenosis: the VISSIT randomized clinical trial. JAMA. 2015;313:1240-1248.

A32. Markus HS, Larsson SC, Kuker W, et al. Stenting for symptomatic vertebral artery stenosis: the vertebral artery ischaemia stenting trial. Neurology. 2017;89:1229-1236.

GENERAL REFERENCES

For the General References and other additional features, please visit Expert Consult at https://expertconsult.inkling.com.

380

HEMORRHAGIC CEREBROVASCULAR DISEASE

STEPHAN A. MAYER

Approximately 20% of all strokes are due to spontaneous intracranial hemorrhage. About three quarters of intracranial hemorrhages are intracerebral, and one quarter are subarachnoid. Intracerebral hemorrhage is most frequently caused by the rupture of small penetrating arteries that are within the brain parenchyma, thereby resulting in a focal collection of clot within the parenchyma. Subarachnoid hemorrhage is caused by rupture of vessels on the surface of the brain, most often by a congenital berry aneurysm (Fig. 380-1), with blood extending diffusely throughout the cerebrospinal fluid (CSF) spaces. In 40% of both forms of hemorrhagic stroke, blood extends into the brain's ventricles—a devastating complication known as intraventricular hemorrhage. Hemorrhagic stroke has high mortality rates, depending on subtype and location, but recovery and survival have improved with advances in neurocritical care.

SUBARACHNOID HEMORRHAGE

EPIDEMIOLOGY

In the United States the incidence of spontaneous subarachnoid hemorrhage is approximately 1 in 10,000 individuals per year. The 30,000 annual cases of subarachnoid hemorrhage predominantly involve young adults.[1] Women are affected more than men, and the rate is twice as high in African Americans as in whites. In 10% of patients, a first-degree relative has also had subarachnoid hemorrhage, often despite the absence of an identifiable genetic predisposition such as polycystic kidney disease (Chapter 118), Marfan disease (Chapter 244), or Ehlers-Danlos syndrome (Chapter 244). Modifiable risk factors include cigarette smoking, heavy alcohol use, arterial hypertension, and use of sympathomimetic agents such as cocaine and phenylpropanolamine.

PATHOBIOLOGY

In 80% of cases, the cause of subarachnoid hemorrhage is rupture of an intracranial saccular or berry aneurysm. Saccular aneurysms most often occur at the circle of Willis or its major branches, especially at bifurcations, where the arterial elastic lamina and tunica media are defective, tend to enlarge with age, and can become paper-thin. Saccular aneurysms, which are rarely detected in children, increase with age, likely because congenital wall defects develop into aneurysms over time. The point of rupture is usually through the dome of the aneurysm. Approximately 15% of patients who present with a subarachnoid hemorrhage from an identifiable aneurysm also harbor another unruptured intracranial aneurysm. Individuals with autosomal dominant polycystic kidney disease (Chapter 118) represent about 1% of all patients with intracranial aneurysms. These individuals present about 10 years younger than other patients with intracerebral aneurysm and have about a 6-fold higher annual risk of rupture (about 1.3% per year versus about 0.2% per year).[2]

About 2% of adults have saccular aneurysms, thereby suggesting that approximately 2 to 3 million Americans have such an aneurysm. However, more than 90% of these aneurysms are small (less than 10 mm) and remain asymptomatic throughout life. The annual risk of rupture of an asymptomatic intracranial aneurysm is approximately 0.7%. Important risk factors for the initial rupture of an intracranial aneurysm include increasing size, prior hemorrhage from another aneurysm, active cigarette smoking, and aneurysms in the basilar apex and posterior communicating artery.

CLINICAL MANIFESTATIONS

The classic symptom of subarachnoid hemorrhage is a very rapidly developing, severe "thunderclap" headache, which the patient typically calls the "worst headache of my life." The headache is usually generalized, but focal pain may refer to the site of aneurysmal rupture (e.g., periorbital pain related to an ophthalmic artery aneurysm). Commonly associated symptoms include stiff neck, loss of consciousness, nausea, vomiting, back or leg pain, and photophobia.[3] In patients who lose consciousness, tonic posturing may occur and may be difficult to differentiate from a seizure. Although aneurysmal rupture often occurs during periods of exercise or physical stress, subarachnoid hemorrhage can occur at any time, including sleep. More than one third of patients give a history of a "sentinel headache" in the prior days to weeks. These prodromal symptoms are usually due to minor "warning leaks" of blood from the aneurysm or to acute thrombosis or expansion of an aneurysm.

The most important determinant of outcome after subarachnoid hemorrhage is the patient's neurologic condition on arrival at the hospital. A patient's score on a standardized risk stratification scale on their initial neurologic examination (Table 380-1) generally correlates with the overall extent of bleeding and the likelihood of developing obstructive hydrocephalus. Severe primary brain injury related to the acute effects of hemorrhage is the leading cause of death and disability after subarachnoid hemorrhage. Focal neurologic signs occur in a minority of patients but may point to the site of bleeding and clot formation. Hemiparesis or aphasia suggests a middle cerebral artery aneurysm, and paraparesis or abulia suggests an aneurysm of the proximal anterior cerebral artery. An isolated third cranial nerve palsy is typically the result of oculomotor nerve compression from a large posterior communicating artery aneurysm.

Aneurysmal rebleeding is a catastrophic complication of subarachnoid hemorrhage: approximately 50% of affected patients die immediately, and another 30% suffer incremental brain injury. The risk of rebleeding is highest

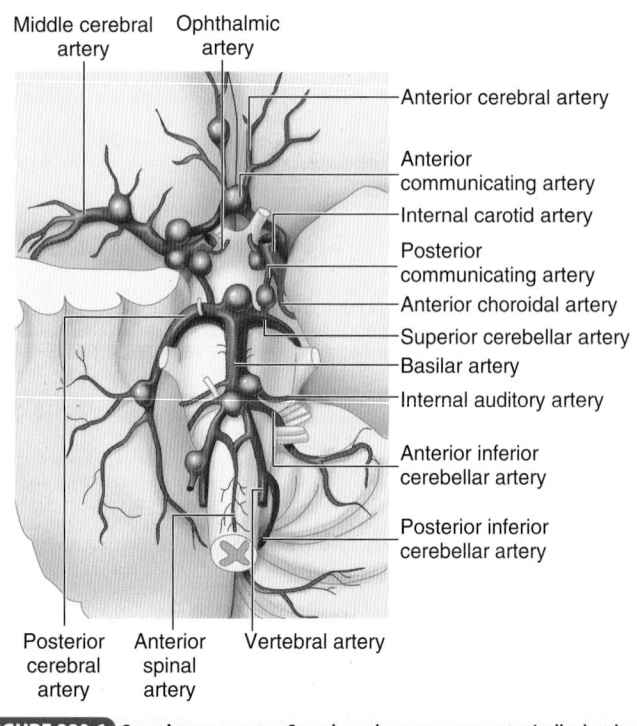

Middle cerebral artery — Ophthalmic artery

— Anterior cerebral artery

— Anterior communicating artery
— Internal carotid artery
— Posterior communicating artery
— Anterior choroidal artery
— Superior cerebellar artery
— Basilar artery
— Internal auditory artery

— Anterior inferior cerebellar artery

— Posterior inferior cerebellar artery

Posterior cerebral artery — Anterior spinal artery — Vertebral artery

FIGURE 380-1. Saccular aneurysms. Saccular or berry aneurysms typically develop at the bifurcations of arteries on the undersurface of the brain. (Courtesy Dr. Justin Zivin)

TABLE 380-1	MORTALITY ACCORDING TO THE HUNT-HESS GRADING SCALE FOR ANEURYSMAL SUBARACHNOID HEMORRHAGE	
GRADE	CLINICAL FINDINGS	HOSPITAL MORTALITY (%)
I	Asymptomatic or mild headache	3
II	Moderate to severe headache, or oculomotor palsy	3
III	Confused, drowsy, or mild focal signs	9
IV	Stupor (localized to pain)	24
V	Coma (posturing or no motor response to pain)	70
TOTAL		18

Data are from 580 patients treated at Columbia University Medical Center.

TABLE 380-2 MODIFIED FISHER CT RATING SCALE FOR THE PREDICTION OF SYMPTOMATIC VASOSPASM

GRADE	CRITERIA	PERCENTAGE OF AFFECTED PATIENTS		
		FREQUENCY	DELAYED CEREBRAL ISCHEMIA*	INFARCTION
0	No subarachnoid hemorrhage or intraventricular hemorrhage	5%	0%	0%
1	Minimal/thin subarachnoid hemorrhage, no biventricular intraventricular hemorrhage	30%	12%	6%
2	Minimal/thin subarachnoid hemorrhage, *with* biventricular intraventricular hemorrhage	5%	21%	14%
3	Thick subarachnoid hemorrhage,† no biventricular intraventricular hemorrhage	43%	19%	12%
4	Thick subarachnoid hemorrhage,† *with* biventricular intraventricular hemorrhage	17%	40%	28%
	All patients	100%	20%	12%

*Defined as symptomatic deterioration, cerebral infarction, or both resulting from vasospasm.
†Thick subarachnoid hemorrhage is defined as completely filling at least one cistern or fissure.
Adapted from Claassen J, Bernardini GL, Kreiter K, et al. Effect of cisternal and ventricular blood on risk of delayed cerebral ischemia after subarachnoid hemorrhage: the Fisher scale revisited. *Stroke*. 2001;32:2012-2020.

within the first 24 hours after the initial aneurysmal rupture (4%) and remains elevated (approximately 1% to 2% per day) for the next 4 weeks. The cumulative risk of rebleeding in untreated patients is 20% at 2 weeks and 30% at 1 month. Poor clinical grade and larger size aneurysms are the strongest risk factors for in-hospital rebleeding.

Delayed cerebral ischemia from vasospasm accounts for a large proportion of morbidity and mortality after subarachnoid hemorrhage. Progressive arterial narrowing develops in approximately 70% of patients, but delayed ischemic deficits develop in only 20 to 30%. The process begins 3 to 5 days after the hemorrhage, becomes maximal at 5 to 14 days, and gradually resolves over 2 to 4 weeks (E-Fig. 380-1). The most important risk factor for symptomatic vasospasm is thick cisternal or intraventricular clot, which can be graded using the Modified Fisher scale (Table 380-2).

DIAGNOSIS

If a patient who presents with acute headache peaking within one hour of onset has none of the features on the Ottawa Subarachnoid Hemorrhage Rule (Fig. 380-2), subarachnoid hemorrhage is effectively excluded and imaging is not needed.[4] Otherwise, a high degree of vigilance is required to establish the diagnosis, either by computed tomography (CT) or by lumbar puncture if the initial CT is negative. Initial misdiagnosis of subarachnoid hemorrhage occurs in approximately 15% of patients, especially patients with the mildest symptoms. Approximately 40% of misdiagnosed patients experience subsequent neurologic deterioration, which is associated with increased morbidity and mortality, owing to rebleeding, hydrocephalus, or vasospasm before reaching medical attention.

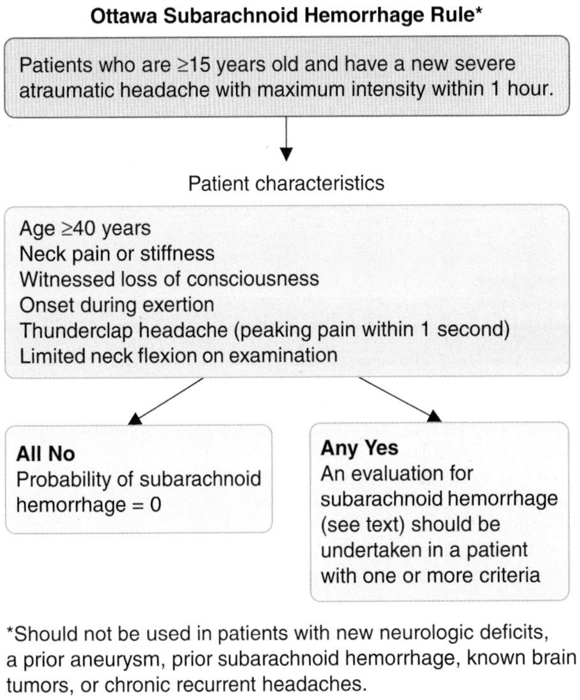

Computed Tomography

Any patient with suspected subarachnoid hemorrhage should be sent immediately for emergency CT. A scan performed within 24 hours of onset will almost always reveal blood within the basal cisterns (Fig. 380-3). Sensitivity of CT declines, however, as time passes from the clinical onset of bleeding to the time of imaging. By 48 hours after onset of symptoms, the sensitivity of CT declines to about 75%. For this reason lumbar puncture is mandatory if a CT is negative but the index of suspicion remains high.

Lumbar Puncture

The CSF is usually grossly bloody. Subarachnoid hemorrhage can be differentiated from a traumatic tap by a xanthochromic (yellow-tinged) appearance of the supernatant fluid after centrifugation. The combined finding of less than 2000 red blood cells/μL and the absence of xanthochromia excludes the diagnosis of aneurysmal subarachnoid hemorrhage with a sensitivity of close to 100% and a specificity of 91%.[5] However, xanthochromia may take up to 12 hours to appear. The CSF pressure is nearly always high, and the protein level is elevated. Initially, the proportion of CSF leukocytes to erythrocytes is that of peripheral blood, with a usual ratio of 1:700; after several days, however, a reactive pleocytosis and low glucose levels may arise owing to a sterile chemical meningitis caused by the blood. Red blood cells and xanthochromia disappear in about 2 weeks, unless hemorrhage recurs.

Ottawa Subarachnoid Hemorrhage Rule*

Patients who are ≥15 years old and have a new severe atraumatic headache with maximum intensity within 1 hour.

↓

Patient characteristics

Age ≥40 years
Neck pain or stiffness
Witnessed loss of consciousness
Onset during exertion
Thunderclap headache (peaking pain within 1 second)
Limited neck flexion on examination

All No
Probability of subarachnoid hemorrhage = 0

Any Yes
An evaluation for subarachnoid hemorrhage (see text) should be undertaken in a patient with one or more criteria

*Should not be used in patients with new neurologic deficits, a prior aneurysm, prior subarachnoid hemorrhage, known brain tumors, or chronic recurrent headaches.

FIGURE 380-2. The Ottawa Subarachnoid Hemorrhage Rule.

Angiography

Cerebral angiography is the definitive diagnostic procedure for detecting intracranial aneurysms and defining their anatomy (see Fig. 380-1). Although the increasing availability and image quality of CT and magnetic resonance (MR) angiography has allowed some centers to use these tests to make the initial diagnosis, a four-vessel (bilateral internal carotid and vertebral artery injections) angiogram is mandatory when those tests are negative.

In approximately 20% of cases of subarachnoid hemorrhage, the initial angiogram is negative. In half of subarachnoid hemorrhages in which an aneurysm is not identified, the blood has a focal "perimesencephalic" distribution around the midbrain or anterior to the pons. In these cases, the source of bleeding is felt be venous. Patients are neurologically intact, there is no risk of rebleeding or symptomatic vasospasm, and full recovery is the rule. In the remainder of cases of nonaneurysmal subarachnoid hemorrhage (Table 380-3), the bleeding source is usually a thin-walled arterial "blister" that is not amenable to surgical clipping or endovascular coiling. Other nonaneurysmal causes of spontaneous subarachnoid hemorrhage include arteriovenous malformations; mycotic aneurysms (Chapter 67); vasculitis (Chapter 254); tumors (Chapter 180); and severe coagulation disorders, such as hemophilia (Chapter

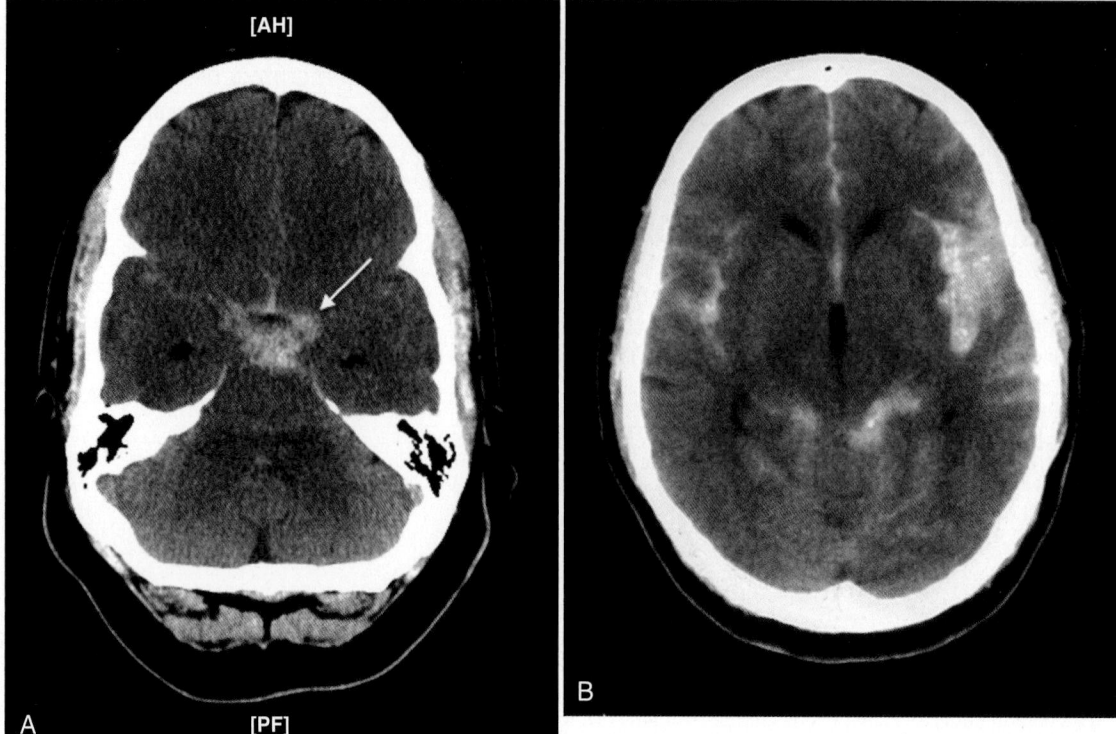

FIGURE 380-3. Two CT images of subarachnoid hemorrhage. **A,** Diffuse thick subarachnoid hemorrhage is seen in the anterior interhemispheric and bilateral sylvian fissures and the quadrigeminal cistern. A left middle cerebral artery aneurysm was identified. **B,** Perimesencephalic subarachnoid hemorrhage; only a small focus of blood in the interpeduncular cistern is identified. No aneurysm was identified. (Part A Courtesy Dr. Larry B. Goldstein)

TABLE 380-3	NON-ANEURYSMAL CAUSES OF SUBARACHNOID HEMORRHAGE

Trauma
Idiopathic perimesencephalic subarachnoid hemorrhage
Arteriovenous malformation
Intracranial arterial dissection (Chapter 379)
Cocaine and amphetamine use (Chapter 31)
Mycotic aneurysm (Chapter 67)
Pituitary apoplexy (Chapter 211)
Moyamoya disease (Chapter 379)
Central nervous system vasculitis (Chapter 254)
Sickle cell disease (Chapter 154)
Coagulation disorders (Chapters 163, 165, and 166)
Primary or metastatic neoplasm (Chapter 180)

Causes are listed in approximate order of frequency.

165), marked thrombocytopenia (Chapter 163), and disseminated intravascular coagulation (Chapter 166).

Vasospasm, local thrombosis, or poor technique can lead to a false-negative angiogram. For this reason, patients with a high clinical suspicion but an initially negative angiogram should have a follow-up study 1 to 2 weeks later; an aneurysm will be demonstrated in about 5% of these cases.

Magnetic Resonance Imaging

Conventional magnetic resonance imaging (MRI) sequences (T1- or T2-weighted scans) are generally less sensitive than CT scans for detecting blood. Susceptibility-weighted imaging may be useful for documenting a completely thrombosed aneurysm in selected patients who have subarachnoid hemorrhage but a negative angiogram.

Laboratory Testing

In addition to routine admission laboratory tests, patients should have: an international normalized ratio (INR), partial thromboplastin time, and platelet count to diagnose a potential coagulopathy; an electrocardiogram (ECG) and serum troponin level to diagnose sympathetically mediated cardiac injury; and a chest radiograph to look for neurogenic pulmonary edema or aspiration pneumonitis. In patients with ECG abnormalities (typically peaked T-waves

with QTc segment prolongation) or an elevated troponin level, an echocardiogram should be performed.

Vasospasm

Symptomatic vasospasm usually involves a decrease in level of consciousness, hemiparesis, or both. Transcranial Doppler ultrasonography is widely used to diagnose vasospasm of the larger cerebral arteries after subarachnoid hemorrhage, but CT angiography is rapidly gaining acceptance to diagnose large-vessel spasm and reductions in tissue blood flow.

TREATMENT   Rx

The initial goals of treatment are to: minimize early brain injury in high-risk patients with a depressed level of consciousness (e.g., Hunt and Hess grades 3 to 5 [see Table 380-1]); prevent rebleeding; perform definitive surgery expeditiously; and rapidly but safely transfer the patient to an intensive care unit, preferably at a high-volume regional center with access to skilled interventionalists and specialized neurocritical care for postoperative management of secondary complications, the most important of which is delayed cerebral ischemia owing to vasospasm.[6]

Minimizing Early Brain Injury

In the emergency department, the immediate concern in high-risk patients is reducing intracranial pressure and preventing secondary cerebral hypoxic-ischemic injury. Patients with impaired ability to protect the airway should be intubated, given supplemental oxygen as needed, and treated aggressively with fluids and vasopressors to maintain a mean arterial pressure of 90 mm Hg (Table 380-3). Stuporous or comatose patients with extensive subarachnoid blood, intraventricular hemorrhage, acute obstructive hydrocephalus, or global cerebral edema should be empirically treated for intracranial hypertension with 1.0 g/kg of 20% mannitol prior to emergent placement of an external ventricular drain. Further doses of bolus osmotherapy should be directed at reducing intracranial pressure to less than 20 mm Hg.

Prevention of Rebleeding

Medical interventions that may reduce the risk of acute aneurysmal rebleeding prior to a definitive repair of the aneurysm include intravenous loading with an antifibrinolytic agent (e.g., epsilon aminocaproic acid 4 g followed by 1 g/hr until 4 hours prior to angiography for a maximum of 72 hours after the onset of subarachnoid hemorrhage)[A1] and control of arterial hypertension (e.g., a nicardipine infusion to maintain systolic blood pressure <160 mm Hg; see Table 70-9). Desmopressin (0.3 μg/kg intravenous push) is useful to boost platelet function in patients on antiplatelet agents.[7] Administration of an anticonvulsant to minimize the risk of an acute seizure (phenytoin 20 mg/kg IV or levetiracetam 2 g IV are most commonly used as a loading dose) is also recommended.[8]

Definitive Surgery

Complete obliteration of a ruptured berry aneurysm by either surgical clipping or endovascular coiling is the definitive treatment for prevention of rebleeding and should be performed as an emergency procedure. The only exception to this rule is in patients who are Hunt and Hess grade 5 and who have an extremely poor neurologic prognosis. Early aneurysm repair not only prevents rebleeding, it also permits treatment of symptomatic vasospasm with hypertensive hypervolemic therapy (see Vasospasm), a treatment that would not be safe in the context of an unprotected aneurysm.

For small-to-medium sized anterior circulation aneurysms in good-grade patients, endovascular coil embolization results in better 6-month outcomes than does surgical clipping. Endovascular coil embolization involves packing of the ruptured aneurysm with soft, thrombogenic detachable platinum coils. This procedure leads to complete obliteration of small-to-medium sized aneurysms (<10 mm in diameter) in 80 to 90% of cases, with an acceptable complication rate of approximately 10%. Approximately 5% of patients will develop recurrent dilation at the neck of the original aneurysm and will require either repeat coil embolization or delayed surgical clipping. Surgical clipping, which involves an open craniotomy to expose the aneurysm and fully exclude it from the parent artery, carries a 5 to 15% risk of major morbidity or mortality, especially the inadvertent occlusion of an adjacent vessel, thereby resulting in stroke or intraoperative rebleeding.

Vasospasm

To *prevent* vasospasm, blood pressure control can be liberalized after the aneurysm has been repaired and brain perfusion becomes the dominant consideration. Patients should receive isotonic fluid resuscitation (i.e., 1 mL/kg/hr of 0.9% saline) to maintain a euvolemic state guided by total fluid balance, central venous pressure, and other measures of volume status. In poor-grade patients (Hunt-Hess 4 and 5), early goal-directed fluid therapy using transpulmonary thermodilution monitoring to maintain the cardiac index above 3 L/min^{-1}/m^{-2} can reduce the risk of delayed cerebral ischemia and improve outcome compared with standard management.[A2] Nimodipine (60 mp PO every 4 hours) reduces the frequency of delayed ischemic deterioration and infarction by about 30%.[9]

Treatment of acute symptomatic vasospasm relies on increasing blood volume, blood pressure, and cardiac output in an attempt to improve cerebral blood flow through arteries that have lost the capacity to autoregulate. Hypertensive hypervolemic therapy involves administration of isotonic crystalloid solutions to maintain central venous pressure above 10 mm Hg and pressors such as norepinephrine or phenylephrine to elevate systolic blood pressure to levels as high as 180 to 220 mm Hg (Chapter 98). Short-term clinical improvement occurs in about 70% of patients; cerebral angioplasty can lead to dramatic improvement in patients who have severe deficits that are refractory to hemodynamic augmentation.

Cerebral Edema

After subarachnoid hemorrhage, brain edema may be focal (usually related to a space-occupying hematoma) or global (an ominous pattern that implies severe primary brain injury and a poor prognosis). Treatment should be guided by continuous monitoring of intracranial pressure.[10] Neither dexamethasone nor other steroids are beneficial for the treatment of brain swelling after subarachnoid hemorrhage.

Hydrocephalus

Patients with subarachnoid hemorrhage can present acutely with acute obstructive hydrocephalus, which can lead to dangerous elevations in intracranial pressure and precipitate transtentorial herniation. Later in the course, most patients with acute hydrocephalus transition to a chronic form of normal pressure hydrocephalus—characterized by psychomotor slowing, confusion, and gait instability—that responds to permanent ventriculoperitoneal shunting.

Seizures

Generalized tonic-clonic seizures occur in about 10% of cases: about 5% at the onset and about 5% later during hospitalization. Prehospital seizures and focal pathology on CT (i.e., subdural hematoma or cerebral infarction) are risk factors for in-hospital seizures. Antiepileptic therapy (phenytoin 20 mg/kg IV or levetiracetam 2 g IV are most commonly used as a loading dose) is typically started at the time of diagnosis to minimize the risk of rebleeding but can be safely discontinued in good-grade patients on postoperative day 1. Continued prophylactic antiepileptic therapy (e.g., phenytoin 300 mg daily or levetiracetam 1,000 mg twice daily) until ICU discharge is a treatment option for comatose patients who remain at risk for nonconvulsive seizures, which occur in 15% of comatose patients monitored with continuous EEG.

Medical Complications

Subarachnoid hemorrhage places patients at risk for a variety of common medical complications that occur as a consequence of homeostatic derangements. The most common are fever, anemia, hyperglycemia, and hyponatremia. The extent and severity of these derangements are independently correlated with poor outcome and should be actively managed according to an established protocol (see Table 380-4). Many poor-grade patients develop acute cardiopulmonary dysfunction owing to massive sympathetic outflow at the time of bleeding. Electrocardiographic QT segment prolongation with T-wave inversion and minor troponin elevations signal the possibility of cardiac injury. The most common important clinical manifestations are pulmonary edema (Chapter 53) and left ventricular neurogenic stunning (Chapter 54) that resolve over the first week. Treatment is supportive.

TABLE 380-4 MANAGEMENT PROTOCOL FOR ACUTE SUBARACHNOID HEMORRHAGE

Blood pressure	• Control elevated blood pressure during the preoperative phase (systolic BP <160 mm Hg) with IV labetalol or nicardipine to prevent rebleeding
Rebleeding prophylaxis	• ε-aminocaproic acid 4 g IV upon diagnosis followed by 1 g/hr until aneurysm repair, for a maximum of up to 72 hours after ictus
Intravenous hydration	• Normal (0.9%) saline at 1.0-1.5 mL/kg/hr
Laboratory testing	• Periodically check complete blood count and electrolytes • Obtain serial ECGs and check admission cardiac troponin level to evaluate for cardiac injury; perform echocardiography in poor-grade patients (i.e., Hunt-Hess IV-V), ECG findings, or elevated cardiac troponin level.
Seizure prophylaxis	• Fosphenytoin or phenytoin IV load (15-20 mg/kg); discontinue on post-op day 1 unless patient has seized, is poor grade, or has focal cortical pathology or is otherwise unstable.
Vasospasm prophylaxis	• Nimodipine 60 mg PO every 4 hours until day subarachnoid hemorrhage 21 or discharge
Physiologic homeostasis	• Cooling blankets to maintain temperature ≤37.5° C • Insulin drip if needed to maintain glucose 100-120 mg/dL • Transfuse to maintain hemoglobin >7.0 g/dL (in the absence of active cerebral or cardiac ischemia)
Ventricular drainage	• Emergent external ventricular drain placement in all stuporous/comatose patients (Hunt-Hess IV/V), as well as lethargic patients with hydrocephalus • Begin trials of clamping external ventricular drain and monitoring intracranial pressure on day 3 after placement. • Perform ventriculoperitoneal shunting during subacute phase of illness in patients with persistent cognitive dysfunction and ventriculomegaly
Vasospasm diagnosis	• Transcranial Doppler sonography every one to two days until the tenth day after subarachnoid hemorrhage • Computed tomographic angiography and perfusion on day 4-8 after subarachnoid hemorrhage or for neuroworsening
Therapy for symptomatic vasospasm	• Place patient in Trendelenberg (head down) position. • Infuse 1 liter normal saline over 30 minutes. • If the deficit persists, raise the systolic blood pressure with phenylephrine or norepinephrine until the deficit resolves (target 180-220 mm Hg). • If refractory, monitor cardiac output and add dobutamine or milrinone to maintain cardiac index ≥4.0 L/min/m². • Transfuse to maintain hemoglobin >10.0 g/dL • Emergency angiogram for intra-arterial verapamil or cerebral angioplasty unless the patient responds well to the above measures.

PREVENTION

Secondary prevention of subarachnoid hemorrhage requires surgical or endovascular repair of any coexisting unruptured aneurysms. Risk factor control, especially control of blood pressure (Chapter 70) but also cessation of cigarette smoking (Chapter 29) and heavy alcohol use (Chapter 30), are critical.

PROGNOSIS

Approximately 20% of patients treated at high-volume centers do not survive to discharge. Important risk factors for mortality include poor clinical grade, advanced age, large aneurysmal size, aneurysm rebleeding, cerebral infarction from vasospasm, and global cerebral edema. Half of survivors remain disabled by a neurocognitive syndrome that includes prominent memory loss, fatigue, inability to concentrate, depression, and anxiety. Cognitive and physical rehabilitation are essential for maximizing recovery in severely affected patients.

The risk of subsequent rupture of an existing unruptured aneurysm depends on its size. The annualized risk of rupture is close to zero for aneurysms 3 mm and smaller, less than 0.5% for aneurysms 5 mm or smaller, and less than 1% for aneurysms 7 mm and smaller.[11]

OTHER CAUSES OF SUBARACHNOID HEMORRHAGES

Fusiform Aneurysms

Fusiform aneurysms are elongated, atherosclerotic ectasias of large arteries. They are usually in the basilar artery but can be seen in the internal, middle, and anterior cerebral arteries. As fusiform aneurysms progressively dilate, they compress surrounding structures and cause focal neurologic dysfunction, such as facial pain (cranial nerve V), hemifacial spasm (cranial nerve VII), and hearing loss with vertigo (cranial nerve VIII). Fusiform aneurysms can even mimic pituitary (Chapter 211) and suprasellar mass lesions or cerebellopontine angle tumors (Chapter 180). Fortunately, fusiform aneurysms rarely rupture; but if they do, total occlusion is usually required because their stiff walls and shape make surgical clipping difficult.

Mycotic Aneurysms

An infected embolism, usually from infectious endocarditis (Chapter 67), may lodge in a distal branch of a cerebral artery, where it causes microinfarction or microabscesses. The artery may rupture acutely, or focal arteritis and mycotic aneurysms may develop. Up to 10% of these aneurysms, which are often multiple and in distal cerebral arteries, may eventually rupture, but treatment other than as for the endocarditis itself is uncertain. As a result, diagnostic imaging usually is undertaken only after symptoms appear, and the potential value of serial imaging is controversial. Anticoagulation is contraindicated in the setting of acute septic emboli to the brain because of the high risk of hemorrhagic complications.

Other Causes of Subarachnoid Hemorrhage

In patients who suffer subarachnoid hemorrhage from other causes, treatment is aimed at the underlying condition. In patients with an idiopathic perimesencephalic venous subarachnoid hemorrhage, rebleeding is rare, symptomatic vasospasm does not occur, and no specific treatment is indicated. Coagulation and platelet disorders require prompt treatment (Chapters 163-165) to prevent further bleeding. Arteriovenous malformations, which more commonly cause intracerebral rather than subarachnoid hemorrhage, are discussed later.

INTRACEREBRAL HEMORRHAGE

Intracerebral hemorrhage is defined as acute spontaneous bleeding into the brain parenchyma.[12] Primary intracerebral hemorrhage results from microscopic small-artery degeneration in the brain caused by either chronic poorly controlled hypertension (80% of cases) or amyloid angiopathy (20% of cases). Secondary intracerebral hemorrhage refers to intraparenchymal bleeding from a diagnosable anatomic vascular lesion or coagulopathy (Table 380-5).

EPIDEMIOLOGY

Intracerebral hemorrhage is responsible for 10 to 15% of all strokes in Western countries but up to 20 to 30% of strokes among Asian populations. The incidence of intracerebral hemorrhage in the United States is approximately 60,000 per year. By far the most important risk factor is hypertension, particularly when it is poorly controlled. The risk of intracerebral hemorrhage is about

TABLE 380-5	CAUSES OF SECONDARY INTRACEREBRAL HEMORRHAGE

Trauma
Arteriovenous malformation
Intracranial aneurysm
Coagulopathy
Hemorrhagic conversion of cerebral infarct
Dural sinus thrombosis
Intracranial neoplasm
Cavernous angioma
Dural arteriovenous fistula
Venous angioma
Cocaine or sympathomimetic drug exposure
Central nervous system vasculitis

40% higher in blacks than in whites. Worldwide, the incidence of intracerebral hemorrhage ranges from 10 to 40 per 1 million people, with the rate in Japan being at the top end of this range. Age-adjusted rates for men are about 50% higher than those for women. Other than hypertension, age, race/ethnicity, and male gender, additional risk factors for intracerebral hemorrhage include heavy alcohol use, coagulopathy, and low serum cholesterol levels.

PATHOBIOLOGY

Primary intracerebral hemorrhage typically consists of a large, space-occupying confluent area of blood that has clotted within the brain parenchyma (E-Fig. 380-2). Abrupt arterial rupture leads to rapid accumulation of blood within the brain parenchyma, thereby causing increased local tissue pressure, physical distortion, and displacement of the brain. After the bleeding has ceased, the blood clots; plasma rich in thrombin and other clotting factors then seeps into the surrounding brain tissue, where it triggers a cascade of secondary brain injury that evolves over days to weeks. This unique form of neurohemoinflammation causes local brain edema, neuronal and glial cell apoptosis, and breakdown of the brain-blood barrier.

The arterial pathology that results in primary intracerebral hemorrhage is microscopic. Poorly controlled chronic hypertension (Chapter 70) causes a small-vessel vasculopathy characterized by fragmentation, degeneration, and the eventual rupture of penetrating arteries within the brain. The most commonly affected structures are the basal ganglia and thalamus (50%), followed by the lobar regions (33%), brainstem, and cerebellum (17%) (Fig. 380-4). In 40% of cases, blood also ruptures into the ventricular system, where it results in intraventricular hemorrhage.

Cerebral *amyloid angiopathy* is a distinctive cause of nonhypertensive lobar intracerebral hemorrhage in the elderly. The deposition of beta-amyloid protein in small- to medium-sized blood vessels of the brain and leptomeninges can be demonstrated by birefringence after application of Congo red stain on microscopic examination of brain tissue. It usually occurs as a sporadic disorder, and it is unrelated to systemic amyloidosis.

CLINICAL MANIFESTATIONS

Primary intracerebral hemorrhage usually presents as an acute focal neurologic deficit that is clinically indistinguishable from ischemic stroke (Chapter 379), except that the onset and evolution of the deficit tend to be more violent. Unlike aneurysmal subarachnoid hemorrhage, which often causes a dramatic surge in intracranial pressure with sudden loss of consciousness at its onset, intracerebral hemorrhage tends to produce progressive headache, vomiting, and depressed consciousness over several hours. In fulminant cases, however, catastrophic bleeding can lead to a massive hematoma and brain death within 6 hours of onset.

The putamen is the site most frequently affected. When the expanding hematoma involves the adjacent internal capsule, a dense contralateral hemiparesis develops, usually hemianesthesia and hemianopia. Larger hemorrhages progressively affect the overlying cortex, thereby resulting in aphasia, hemispatial neglect, and contralateral gaze paresis. When the hemorrhage arises in the thalamus, hemianesthesia can initially precede the hemiparesis. The completed syndrome is usually characterized by a dense contralateral sensorimotor deficit that may be accompanied by a contralateral visual field deficit, impaired upward gaze, or both.

Lobar hemorrhages usually originate at the junctions between gray and white matter in the cerebral hemispheres. The clinical manifestations depend on the location of the hemorrhage. Lobar hemorrhages may result from either

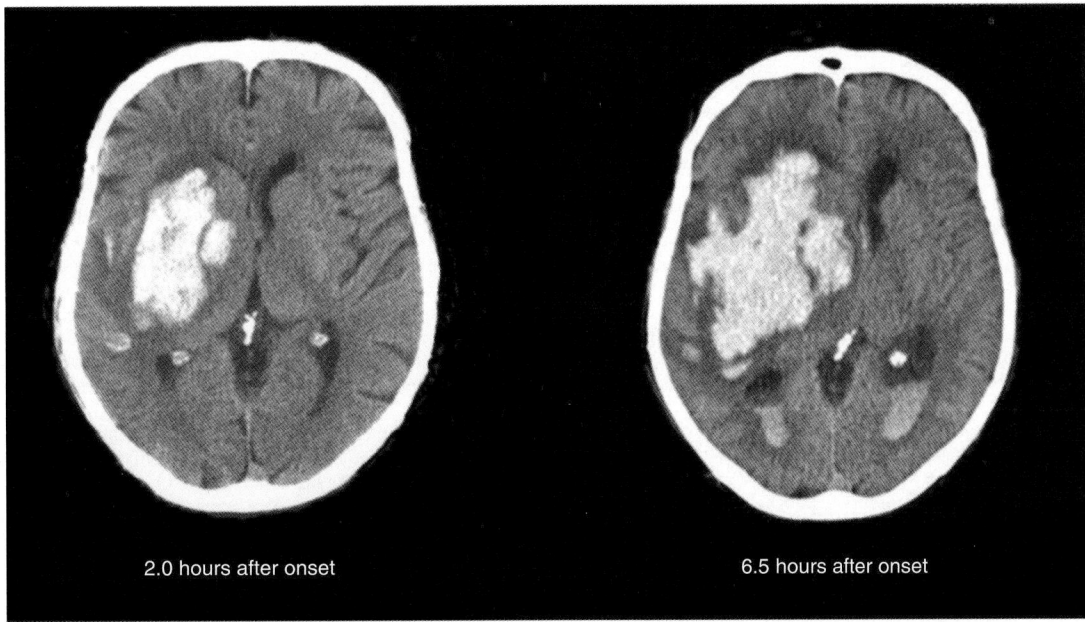

2.0 hours after onset 6.5 hours after onset

FIGURE 380-4. **Early hematoma growth in a 48-year-old chronically hypertensive woman.** *Left,* The baseline computed tomography scan shows a moderate-sized intracerebral hemorrhage in the right putamen. At this point, she is stuporous with a left hemiparesis. *Right,* A follow-up computed tomography scan performed after she deteriorated to coma with bilateral decerebrate posturing shows massive expansion of the hematoma as well as new intraventricular hemorrhage and obstructive hydrocephalus. Within 24 hours, she was declared brain dead. (From Mayer SA, Rincon F. Treatment of intracerebral haemorrhage. *Lancet Neurol.* 2005;4:662-672).

hypertension or amyloid angiopathy. In addition to lobar intracerebral hemorrhage, patients with amyloid angiopathy may present with dementia, gait disturbances, complex partial seizures due to multiple microbleeds, or small multifocal inflammatory lesions that are thought to represent an autoimmune response to beta-amyloid.

In 40% of cases, deep parenchymal bleeding ruptures into the ventricular system, thereby causing intraventricular hemorrhage. Blood occluding the third or fourth ventricles blocks the normal anterograde flow of CSF through the ventricular system, thereby resulting in acute hydrocephalus and intracranial hypertension. Left untreated, massive intraventricular hemorrhage results in rapid descent into coma (Chapter 376), with motor posturing and rostrocaudal loss of brain stem reflexes.

Pontine hemorrhage typically causes coma with quadriparesis and grossly disconjugate ocular motility disorders, although small hemorrhages may mimic syndromes of infarction. Cerebellar hemorrhage usually begins abruptly with vomiting and severe ataxia, which usually prevents standing and walking. Cerebellar hemorrhage is occasionally accompanied by dysarthria, adjacent cranial nerve (mostly sixth and seventh) dysfunction, and paralysis of conjugate ipsilateral gaze.

Expansion of a hematoma because of active bleeding is an important cause of early neurologic deterioration, especially within 3 to 6 hours after intracerebral hemorrhage. Enlargement of the mass does not change the clinical picture until there is enough brainstem compression to precipitate coma, which can happen abruptly.

Convulsive seizures complicate the course of intracerebral hemorrhage in 12% of patients. Although the risk is higher when the cortex is the primary site of bleeding, seizures can complicate deep intracerebral hemorrhage as well.

DIAGNOSIS

Intracerebral hemorrhage cannot be distinguished from ischemic stroke (Chapter 379) based on clinical findings alone, although fulminant onset, early changes in level of consciousness, vomiting, and extreme hypertension are suggestive. Nonenhancing CT imaging of the brain is the method of choice for making the emergency diagnosis of intracerebral hemorrhage. CT readily demonstrates the size and location of the hematoma, any extension into the ventricular system, the degree of surrounding edema, and midline shift owing to a mass effect. The volume of the hematoma, which is a powerful predictor of 30-day mortality, can be easily calculated by CT. CT angiography may reveal secondary intracerebral hemorrhage owing to an aneurysm or arteriovenous malformation, or active contrast extravasation into the clot ("spot sign"), which implies an increased risk of early growth of the hematoma when identified soon after the onset of symptoms.

MRI also is highly sensitive for the diagnosis of intracerebral hemorrhage. The diagnosis of probable amyloid angiopathy is made clinically in patients with the appropriate clinical picture when an MRI reveals multiple cortical microbleeds. Patchy white-matter lesions are also commonly seen. Conventional contrast cerebral angiography should be reserved for patients in whom secondary causes of intracerebral hemorrhage are suspected (e.g., aneurysms, arteriovenous malformations, cortical vein or dural sinus thrombosis, or vasculitis).

TREATMENT ℞

Treatment in an intensive care unit or stroke unit is strongly recommended for at least the first 24 hours when the risk of neurologic deterioration is highest.[13] The most urgent treatment consideration for intracerebral hemorrhage is whether to proceed emergently with surgical evacuation or the placement of a ventricular drain. Owing to the irreversible nature of secondary brain injury related to herniation and intracranial pressure, outcomes are always better when definitive measures to reverse these processes are performed as soon as possible. Delayed surgical intervention triggered by clinical deterioration must always be tempered by realization that an earlier procedure would have been the better plan.

Surgical Management

Although intracerebral hemorrhage has traditionally been considered a neurosurgical problem, craniotomy and surgical evacuation of the hematoma does not improve the outcome of supratentorial intracerebral hemorrhage compared with initial medical management, even in patients with larger bleeds within 1 cm of the cortical surface.[A3] However, randomized trials have not enrolled patients in whom emergency surgery was felt to be a life-saving intervention, so urgent craniotomy may improve the outcome of younger patients with large lobar hemorrhages and a deteriorating course owing to a mass effect.

In contrast to supratentorial intracerebral hemorrhage, patients with cerebellar hemorrhages exceeding 3 cm in diameter appear to benefit from emergent surgical evacuation, especially because abrupt and dramatic deterioration can occur within the first 24 hours. For this reason, it is generally unwise to defer surgery until further clinical deterioration in these patients.

Ventricular Drainage

External ventricular drainage is indicated in all stuporous or comatose patients who have intraventricular hemorrhage and ventricular enlargement and in whom aggressive support is indicated. This life-saving procedure, which can be performed at the bedside, decompresses the intracranial vault and arrests the process of downward brain stem herniation by allowing drainage of bloody CSF into a drainage receptacle. Connecting the drainage system to a pressure transducer also allows measurement of intracranial pressure. The use of tissue

TABLE 380-6 MEDICAL MANAGEMENT PROTOCOL FOR ACUTE INTRACEREBRAL HEMORRHAGE

Blood pressure	• Maintain mean arterial pressure <140 mm Hg with continuous infusion labetolol (2-10 mg/min), nicardipine (5-15 mg/hr), or clevidipine (2-6 mg/hr) • If stuporous or comatose, measure ICP and maintain CPP >70 mm Hg.
Reversal of anticoagulation	• For elevated INR: Vitamin K 10 mg IV push and 4F-PCC 　INR 2 to <4: 25 units/kg; not to exceed 2500 units 　INR 4-6: 35 units/kg; not to exceed 3500 units 　INR >6: 50 units/kg; not to exceed 5000 units • For heparin: protamine sulfate 10 to 50 mg slow IV push (1 mg reverses approximately 100 units of heparin) • For dabigatran: Idarucizumab 5g IV (Praxibind®) • For the factor Xa inhibitors (rivaroxaban, apixaban and edoxaban): Andexanet-alpha IV. Low dose (≤10 mg rivaroxaban or ≤5 mg apixaban per dose): 400 mg IV bolus, followed by 4 mg/kg for 2 hrs. High dose (higher doses given within 8 hours): 800 mg bolus, followed by 8 mg/kg for 2 hrs. • For thrombocytopenia or platelet dysfunction: Desmopressin 0.3 µg/kg intravenous push. Platelet transfusion is reasonable in the setting of thrombocytopenia but is not effective and may be harmful when given to patients on NSAIDs or other antiplatelet agents. • Expedited INR reversal for life-saving neurosurgical intervention: recombinant activated factor VII 40-80 µg/kg (approximately 3.0-6.0 mg) intravenous push
Intracranial hypertension	• Elevate head of bed to 30° • Mannitol 1.0-1.5 g IV • Hyperventilate to pCO$_2$ of 30 mm Hg
Fluids and nutrition	• Normal (0.9%) saline at 1.0 mL/kg/hr • Begin enteral feeding via nasoduodenal tube within 24 hours
Seizure prophylaxis	• For coma with intracranial hypertension or acute seizures: fosphenytoin or phenytoin IV load (15-20 mg/kg); 300 mg IV daily for 7 days
Physiologic homeostasis	• Cooling blankets to maintain temperature ≤37.5° C • Insulin drip as needed to maintain glucose 120-180 mg/dL

CPP = cerebral perfusion pressure; FEIBA = factor VIII inhibitor bypass activity; 4F-PCC = four factor prothrombin complex concentrate, containing factors II, VII, IX, and X; NSAIDs = non-steroidal anti-inflammatory drugs.

plasminogen activator to hasten clearance of intraventricular hemorrhage is not beneficial.[A4]

Emergency Reversal of Anticoagulation

Fifteen percent of intracerebral hemorrhages are associated with the use of oral anticoagulants, and these patients face a high risk of progressive bleeding.[14] For warfarin-associated intracerebral hemorrhage, immediate treatment with a 4-factor prothrombin-complex concentrate and intravenous vitamin K (Table 380-6) to normalize the INR to below 1.4 reduces the risk of progressive bleeding more rapidly and safely than does fresh frozen plasma.[A5] A single 3- to 6-mg intravenous dose of recombinant activated factor VII normalizes the INR within minutes, promotes hemostasis, and is an attractive option for expediting life-saving neurosurgical intervention, but at the cost of a 5% risk of a thromboembolic complication such as myocardial infarction or stroke. In intracerebral hemorrhage with normal coagulation, factor VII does not improve outcome. Patients who had been anticoagulated with unfractionated or low-molecular-weight heparin should be reversed with protamine sulfate (Chapter 76). Patients with thrombocytopenia or platelet dysfunction can be treated with a single dose of desmopressin (0.3 µg/kg IV). Platelet transfusion (Chapter 167) is reasonable in the setting of thrombocytopenia but is not effective and appears to be harmful when given to patients on anti-platelet therapy.[A6]

For intracerebral hemorrhage associated with the direct oral thrombin inhibitor dabigatran, idarucizumab 5g IV rapidly reverses the anticoagulant effect and has shown benefit in uncontrolled studies. For reversal of factor Xa inhibitors (rivaroxaban, apixaban, and edoxaban). Andexanet-alpha is a promising agent that has been shown to reverse the anticoagulant effect of Xa inhibition in laboratory assays in either a low-dose or high-dose regimen (see Table 380-6).

Blood Pressure Control

Acute intracerebral hemorrhage often leads to extreme arterial hypertension. Excessive reduction of blood pressure can exacerbate ischemic injury in the setting of impaired autoregulation, whereas poor blood pressure control can exacerbate the early growth of the hematoma and contribute to vasogenic edema. Current guidelines recommend a systolic blood pressure target of lower than 180 mm Hg and mean blood pressure target of lower than 130 mm Hg. Lowering of systolic blood pressure to lower than 140 mm Hg compared with lower than 180 mm Hg within 6 hours of onset results in no difference in mortality, a slight reduction in the growth of a hematoma, and possible borderline improvement in disability among survivors,[A7][A8] perhaps at the cost of an increase in acute kidney injury. Given the need to control blood pressure levels precisely in the setting of impaired autoregulation, continuous infusion of fast-acting agents with intra-arterial monitoring is recommended. Agents of choice are labetolol plus nicardipine or clevidipine (see Table 70-9). Sodium nitroprusside should be avoided owing to the lack of a reliable dose-response effect and its tendency to increase intracranial pressure directly.

Antifibrinolysis

Despite the theoretical appeal, antithrombolytic therapy with tranexamic acid has not been shown to reduce deaths or improve functional status in patients with intracerebral bleeds.[A9]

Cerebral Edema

Brain swelling can progress for many days after the onset of intracerebral hemorrhage, but it is especially concerning within the first 72 hours in patients whose hemorrhages exceed 30 mL in volume. Management of cerebral edema should be guided by maintaining intracranial pressure below 20 mm Hg and cerebral perfusion pressure higher than 70 mm Hg. Dexamethasone and other corticosteroids do not effectively treat intracerebral hemorrhage-related brain edema and are contraindicated. Hypotonic intravenous fluids should be strictly avoided because the free water in these solutions can aggravate brain edema.

Medical and Neurologic Complications

To combat malnutrition and muscle wasting in patients who lack the capacity to swallow, early enteral feeding (Chapter 204) should be initiated via a naso-duodenal feeding tube. Body temperature should be maintained at less than 37.5° C with surface cooling, and a continuous insulin infusion should be used as needed to keep the blood glucose level between 120 and 180 mg/dL. Prophylactic anticonvulsant therapy (phenytoin 20 mg/kg IV or levetiracetam 2 g IV loading dose; then phenytoin 300 mg daily or levetiracetam 1 gram twice daily) is reasonable for patients with lobar bleeding, stupor, or coma. If seizures have not occurred, anticonvulsants should be discontinued at discharge because they can hamper neurologic recovery during rehabilitation. Even with anticonvulsant therapy, continuous EEG monitoring reveals electrographic seizure activity in about 20% of comatose patients. It is unclear whether a midazolam infusion (Chapter 375) or other aggressive measures to eliminate these seizures can improve outcome.

PREVENTION

Blood pressure reduction (Chapter 70), which significantly decreases the risk of intracerebral hemorrhage and other forms of stroke, is by far the most effective method for preventing recurrent intracerebral hemorrhage.[15] Angiotensin-converting enzyme inhibitors (Table 70-5) are particularly effective. Antiplatelet agents and anticoagulants of all types should be meticulously avoided in patients with multiple lobar microbleeds caused by amyloid angiopathy.

PROGNOSIS

Factors that consistently predict death or functional disability at 30 days include a large-volume intracerebral hemorrhage, a depressed level of consciousness, intraventricular hemorrhage, an infratentorial location, and older age. A simple clinical grading scale (Table 380-7) incorporating these variables can give a reliable prediction of 30-day mortality.

Except in the most severe cases, however, caution is warranted when communicating a hopeless prognosis before aggressive efforts have been made to resuscitate victims of intracerebral hemorrhage. It has become increasingly evident that physicians tend to underestimate the chances of a good outcome and that many poor outcomes result from self-fulfilling prophesies of doom. Mortality after intracerebral hemorrhage is lower in patients who receive care in a neurologic intensive care unit, presumably because a team of experts adheres to best medical practices, including early transition to rehabilitation.

TABLE 380-7	THE INTRACEREBRAL HEMORRHAGE SCORE
COMPONENT	**SCORE POINTS**
GCS Score (See Table 371-1)	
3-4	2
5-12	1
13-15	0
Intracerebral hemorrhage (Volume, cm³)	
≥30	1
<30	0
Intraventricular hemorrhage	
Yes	1
No	0
Infratentorial intracerebral hemorrhage	
Yes	1
No	0
Age, years	
≥80	1
<80	0

Estimated 30-day Mortality is 0% for a score of 0, 13% for a score of 1, 26% for a score of 2, 72% for a score of 3, 97% for a score of 4, and 100% for a score of 5+.
GCS = Glasgow Coma Scale.
From: Hemphill JC, 3rd, Bonovich DC, Besmertis L, et al. The ICH score: a simple, reliable grading scale for intracerebral hemorrhage. *Stroke.* 2001;32:891-897.

BRAIN VASCULAR MALFORMATIONS

Brain vascular malformations are space-occupying congenital anomalies that can often exist for a lifetime without symptoms. The most feared and dangerous complication is rupture, which can be manifested as intracerebral hemorrhage, as intraventricular hemorrhage, or less often as subarachnoid hemorrhage.

EPIDEMIOLOGY

About 10% of intracerebral hemorrhages but only about 1% of strokes are caused by vascular malformations. The prevalence of an arteriovenous malformation is about 0.5%, and the annual incidence of hemorrhage is between 1 and 3 cases per 100,000 people. Hemorrhage from an arteriovenous malformation is most common during the second through fourth decades. The risk of rebleeding is about 7% acutely. For the next 5 years, the risk of bleeding is about 2% per year, and it then falls to about 1 to 2% annually thereafter. Over a lifetime, a young person therefore has a 50 to 60% probability of another hemorrhage, each of which carries a 10 to 15% risk of acute death. Unlike with some causes of cerebral hemorrhage, preexisting hypertension does not seem to be a risk factor.

PATHOBIOLOGY

Cerebrovascular malformations are characterized on the basis of their histologic appearance and the intervening neural parenchyma. The most frequent type of vascular malformation is an arteriovenous malformation, in which a core or nidus of dysplastic vessels is fed by arteries and drained by veins without intervening capillaries. The result is a low-resistance, high-flow shunt that leads to progressive arterial dilation and venous wall thickening. The nidus usually does not contain any intervening neural tissue. Bleeding from a feeding artery aneurysm usually results in subarachnoid hemorrhage, bleeding from the nidus itself usually results in intracerebral hemorrhage, and bleeding from a draining vein usually is manifested as intraventricular hemorrhage.

The next most common vascular malformations are cavernous angiomas or hemangiomas.[16] These malformations, which also do not contain neural tissue, are composed of small-caliber sinusoidal vascular channels that are commonly thrombosed.

Dural arteriovenous fistulas are typically acquired lesions that result from the formation of small arteriovenous shunts in the wall of a cavernous sinus as a consequence of dural sinus thrombosis. Over time, flow through the fistula increases, leading to pulsatile expansion of regional veins and subsequent rupture. Rare familial cases have been described. In over 60% of patients with arteriovenous malformation, an activating *KRAS* mutation appears to be pathogenic.[17]

CLINICAL MANIFESTATIONS

About 50% of arteriovenous malformations are manifested with intracranial hemorrhage, about 30% initially are manifested as seizures, and about 20% may be manifested with progressive neurologic disability. An increasing proportion, however, are now detected by brain imaging as part of the evaluation of headaches (Chapter 370), to which arteriovenous malformations may or may not be causally related.

Because an arteriovenous malformation can bleed into the subarachnoid space, the brain parenchyma, or the ventricular system, symptoms and signs depend on the location and severity of bleed. Post-bleeding cerebral vasospasm, which is less common than aneurysmal bleeding, occurs in less than 5% of cases and is typically linked to thick cisternal clot or extensive intraventricular hemorrhage.

Patients who develop seizures as a result of these arteriovenous malformations often have focal seizures (Chapter 375). Even without seizures, patients can develop focal neurologic deficits due to vascular thrombosis or the shunting of blood through the malformation rather than allowing it to perfuse normal brain tissue.

DIAGNOSIS

A noncontrast CT scan may show bleeding, sometimes in a location that is unusual for a primary intracerebral hemorrhage or a ruptured aneurysm. Contrast-enhanced CT may show marked enhancement of the feeding arteries and draining veins. Another option is MRI with signal void on T1- or T2-weighted images. However, angiography is the definitive test to identify an arteriovenous malformation and to delineate its size, gross morphology, feeding arteries, and draining veins. Even if an arteriovenous malformation is found by unilateral carotid injection, four-vessel angiography is indicated because malformations can be multiple and can be associated with saccular aneurysms.

When cavernous angiomas or hemangiomas hemorrhage, they tend to produce minor focal syndromes that appear on MRI as a classic target lesion that results from multiple previous minor bleeding events. The low flow rate through these lesions makes them difficult to detect by angiography.

TREATMENT Rx

In a patient who survives the initial hemorrhage, the two therapeutic goals are to avoid neurologic deterioration and to remove the arteriovenous malformation completely.[18] General medical treatment measures for intracranial hemorrhage related to arteriovenous malformation are the same as for intracerebral hemorrhage (see Table 380-6). Removal of the arteriovenous malformation can be curative, but surgery is challenging for malformations in critical neurologic areas. Options include selective embolization of the feeding arteries, surgical resection, and radiation-induced thrombosis, alone or sometimes in combination. Selective embolization can reduce the size of the malformation and blood flow through it but rarely can obliterate it completely. Stereotactic radiosurgery is used only for small lesions, and its therapeutic effect depends on the gradual shrinkage of abnormal vessels after the procedure.

Microsurgical removal of an arteriovenous malformation is often performed in stages until a postoperative angiogram shows no residual malformation. However, recanalization and recurrent hemorrhage can occur, and long-term success rates are unknown.

PREVENTION AND PROGNOSIS

The prognosis of an unruptured arteriovenous malformation varies according to its location, size, and morphology. In a randomized trial, medical management emphasizing control of hypertension, avoidance of anticoagulants, and use of anticonvulsants to control seizures was superior to multimodality intervention with surgery, embolization, or radiotherapy, with a 10% rate of death or stroke at 33 months compared with a 30% risk in the intervention group.[A10] Until further data are available, routine interventional treatment of unruptured arteriovenous malformations is not justified.

Grade A References

A1. Gaberel T, Magheru C, Emery E, et al. Antifibrinolytic therapy in the management of aneurismal subarachnoid hemorrhage revisited. A meta-analysis. *Acta Neurochir (Wien).* 2012;154:1-9.
A2. Mutoh T, Kazumata K, Terasaka S, et al. Early intensive versus minimally invasive approach to postoperative hemodynamic management after subarachnoid hemorrhage. *Stroke.* 2014;45:1280-1284.
A3. Mendelow AD, Gregson BA, Rowan EN, et al. Early surgery versus initial conservative treatment in patients with spontaneous supratentorial lobar intracerebral haematomas (STICH II): a randomised trial. *Lancet.* 2013;382:397-408.

A4. Hanley DF, Lane K, McBee N, et al. Thrombolytic removal of intraventricular haemorrhage in treatment of severe stroke: results of the randomised, multicentre, multiregion, placebo-controlled CLEAR III trial. *Lancet.* 2017;389:603-611.

A5. Sarode R, Milling TJ Jr, Refaai MA, et al. Efficacy and safety of a 4-factor prothrombin complex concentrate in patients on vitamin K antagonists presenting with major bleeding: a randomized, plasma-controlled, phase IIIb study. *Circulation.* 2013;128:1234-1243.

A6. Baharoglu MI, Cordonnier C, Salman RA, et al. Platelet transfusion versus standard care after acute stroke due to spontaneous cerebral haemorrhage associated with antiplatelet therapy (PATCH): a randomised, open-label, phase 3 trial. *Lancet.* 2016;387:2605-2613.

A7. Anderson CS, Heeley E, Huang Y, et al. Rapid blood-pressure lowering in patients with acute intracerebral hemorrhage. *N Engl J Med.* 2013;368:2355-2365.

A8. Qureshi AI, Palesch YY, Barsan WG, et al. Intensive blood-pressure lowering in patients with acute cerebral hemorrhage. *N Engl J Med.* 2016;375:1033-1043.

A9. Sprigg N, Flaherty K, Appleton JP, et al. Tranexamic acid for hyperacute primary intracerebral haemorrhage (TICH-2): an international randomised, placebo-controlled, phase 3 superiority trial. *Lancet.* 2018;391:2107-2115.

A10. Mohr JP, Parides MK, Stapf C, et al. Medical management with or without interventional therapy for unruptured brain arteriovenous malformations (ARUBA): a multicentre, non-blinded, randomised trial. *Lancet.* 2014;383:614-621.

GENERAL REFERENCES

For the General References and other additional features, please visit Expert Consult at https://expertconsult.inkling.com.

381

PARKINSONISM

MICHAEL S. OKUN AND ANTHONY E. LANG

Parkinsonism is a clinical syndrome that consists of four cardinal signs: tremor, rigidity, akinesia, and postural disturbances (TRAP). Parkinson disease is a common cause of the TRAP syndrome, but there are numerous other causes (Table 381-1).

PARKINSON DISEASE

EPIDEMIOLOGY

Parkinson disease, which is the second most common neurodegenerative disorder after Alzheimer disease, occurs in approximately 1 in 1000 in the general population and in 1% of persons older than 65 years. Men are affected slightly more often than women (3 : 2). Traumatic brain injury severe enough to cause an emergency department visit or hospitalization in later life is associated with about a 55% increased risk of developing Parkinson disease.[1]

PATHOBIOLOGY

The cause of Parkinson disease is believed to be a variable combination of poorly understood genetic and environmental factors, including dose-dependent manganese exposure primarily in welders (Chapter 19).[2] Both autosomal dominant and recessive genes can cause classic Parkinson disease. The protein α-synuclein, which is the chief constituent of the hallmark cytoplasmic inclusion, the Lewy body (Chapter 374), is critical in the pathogenesis of Parkinson disease. Abnormal aggregation of the protein, either from mutations in the α-synuclein gene or as a result of excessive production of the normal protein because of gene duplications or triplications, is associated with varying disease phenotypes. Other defined genetic abnormalities may be associated with classic later-onset Parkinson disease, including *LRRK2*,[3] which is currently the most common cause of autosomal dominantly inherited Parkinson disease, or with early-onset parkinsonism, typically found in the autosomal recessive forms associated with *parkin*, *DJ1*, and *PINK1*. The *PARK10* haplotype on chromosome 1 also is strongly associated with Parkinson disease. Other genes in which mutations may increase the risk for development of Parkinson disease include the glucocerebrosidase gene (*GBA*), which appears to be associated with faster cognitive decline.[4]

Strong support for the "environmental hypothesis" of sporadic Parkinson disease relates to the observation that the selective neurotoxin 1-methyl-4-phenyl-1,2,3,6-tetrahydropyridine (MPTP) causes acute parkinsonism due to loss of dopamine neurons in the substantia nigra pars compacta (SNc). MPTP is oxidized to the active toxin MPP$^+$, which is a selective inhibitor of

complex I of the mitochondrial electron transport chain. This knowledge, combined with recognition of the importance of dopamine (see later), has implicated oxidative stress in the pathogenesis of Parkinson disease. Other proposed pathogenetic factors include mitochondrial dysfunction, protein misfolding or aggregation, excitotoxicity, inflammation, apoptotic cell death, and loss of trophic support.

Pathology

Many of the features of Parkinson disease are due to loss of dopamine in the neostriatum (especially the putamen) secondary to loss of pigmented dopaminergic neurons in the SNc of the midbrain. Approximately 60% of these dopaminergic neurons will have degenerated before clinical features of the disease develop.

In addition to the prominent degenerative changes in the SNc (cell loss, gliosis, abnormal deposition of aggregated α-synuclein as Lewy bodies and Lewy neurites), pathologic changes are also evident in other brainstem nuclei, in cortical regions, and in peripheral autonomic neurons. Indeed, it has been suggested that Parkinson disease may begin in the lower brainstem and the olfactory system, where it causes early loss of the sense of smell and only later

---

TABLE 381-1	DIFFERENTIAL DIAGNOSIS OF PARKINSONISM

PARKINSON DISEASE

Sporadic
Genetic
    Autosomal dominant (e.g., α-synuclein gene mutations, duplications, triplications; *LRRK2* mutations)
    Autosomal recessive (e.g., *parkin*, *DJ1*, *PINK1*)
    Associated with genetic mutations (e.g., glucocerebrosidase deficiency [GBA])

SECONDARY PARKINSONISM

Neurodegenerative diseases (sporadic or genetic)
    Progressive supranuclear palsy* (Videos 381-3 through 381-6)
    Multiple system atrophy* (Videos 381-7 through 381-9)
    Corticobasal degeneration* (Videos 381-10 and 381-11)
    Dementia with Lewy bodies*
    Alzheimer disease*
    ALS-parkinsonism-dementia complex of Guam
    Huntington disease
    Rapid-onset dystonia-parkinsonism
    Pallidopyramidal degeneration (including PARK9 and PARK15)
    Neuroacanthocytosis
    Spinocerebellar ataxias (e.g., SCA-3, SCA-2)
    Wilson disease
    Pantothenate kinase–associated neurodegeneration (Hallervorden-Spatz syndrome)
    Neuroferritinopathy
    Calcification of the basal ganglia (Fahr disease)
    Dopa-responsive dystonia (not a degenerative disorder)
Drugs*
    Neuroleptics, metoclopramide, prochlorperazine, tetrabenazine, reserpine, cinnarizine, flunarizine, α-methyldopa, lithium
Toxic
    MPTP, manganese (including illicit use of ephedrone), carbon monoxide, mercury
    Copper (Wilson disease)
Infectious
    Encephalitis lethargica
    Other encephalitis, including HIV associated
    Subacute sclerosing panencephalitis
    Creutzfeldt-Jakob disease
Vascular*
    Atherosclerosis
    Amyloid angiopathy
Neoplastic
    Brain tumor
    Other mass lesions
Normal-pressure hydrocephalus*
Head trauma
Multiple sclerosis

*See Table 381-4 for additional details.
ALS = amyotrophic lateral sclerosis; HIV = human immunodeficiency virus; MPTP = 1-methyl-4-phenyl-1,2,3,6-tetrahydropyridine.
Modified from Cloutier M, Lang AE. Movement disorders: an overview. In: Factor SA, Lang AE, Weiner WJ, eds. *Drug Induced Movement Disorders.* Malden, Mass: Blackwell; 2005:3-19.

involves the substantia nigra. Independent of the order of involvement, it is likely that the widespread extranigral neurodegenerative changes account for the many symptoms that do not respond to dopamine replacement and that become increasingly problematic as the disease progresses. How the disease progresses and spreads in the nervous system is unknown. Genetic causes account for approximately 10% of cases, and environmental interactions have been shown to be closely associated with the disease. Mechanisms such as oxidative stress, mitochondrial dysfunction, and neuroinflammation have all been shown to play a role in neurodegeneration. Cell-to-cell transmission of a form of α-synuclein may induce abnormal folding and aggregation of the normal protein in a "permissive templating" fashion similar to prion diseases (Chapter 387).[5] Both epidemiologic and experimental data suggest that the beta-2 adrenoreceptor regulates the α-synuclein gene and that agonists of the receptor may protect against the development of Parkinson disease.[6]

CLINICAL MANIFESTATIONS

Typically, the symptoms begin in one limb. This asymmetry often persists into later stages of the disease.

Motor Symptoms
Tremor
The classic "resting tremor" of Parkinson disease has characteristic clinical features but occurs in only one in five patients. The tremor has a slow frequency of 4 to 6 cycles per second, typically with a "pill-rolling" character when it involves the hand; but its characteristics, including frequency, can be widely variable.[7] It is generally present with the limb in complete repose and typically subsides when the limb moves and takes up a new position, although the tremor may reemerge ("reemergent tremor") within a short time after maintaining the new position (Video 381-1). Because resting tremor diminishes or subsides with action, it may not be disabling but can be embarrassing and may be associated with aching or fatigue of the affected limb. Resting tremor is usually accentuated by stress (e.g., by asking the patient to perform mental calculations). It is also characteristically present in the upper limbs while walking. A higher-frequency (e.g., 7 to 10 Hz) postural and kinetic tremor is also common in patients with various causes of parkinsonism, and younger patients tend to have a higher frequency tremor.

Rigidity
Rigidity is a form of increased muscle tone appreciated best on slow passive movements. It may be characterized as "cogwheel" when a tremor is superimposed or as "lead pipe" when it is not. Rigidity is "activated" or accentuated on examination by asking the patient to move the limb opposite the one being tested. Patients may complain of stiffness, but the rigidity is not usually disabling.

Akinesia
Akinesia or bradykinesia comprises a variety of disturbances in movement, including slowness, reduced amplitude, fatiguing, and interruptions in ongoing movement. This aspect of parkinsonism interferes with all voluntary activities and accounts for many of the well-known features of parkinsonism: lack of facial expression with reduced blinking (hypomimia or masked facies—the "reptilian stare"), soft monotonous speech (hypophonia), impaired swallowing resulting in drooling (sialorrhea), small handwriting (micrographia), reduced arm swing while walking, shortened stride and shuffling gait, difficulty arising from a low chair, and problems turning over in bed. Arrest in ongoing movement ("motor block") can interfere with a variety of activities, but it is best appreciated as freezing of gait (Video 381-2). Bradykinesia is evident on inspection and elicited by testing rapid repetitive and alternating movements: finger tapping, opening and closing the fist, pronating and supinating the wrist, and toe and heel tapping.

Postural Disturbances
Postural disturbances include a flexed posture in the limbs and trunk (stooped posture) as well as postural instability resulting in imbalance and falls.[8] Patients may complain of being unable to stop themselves from going forward (propulsion, festination) or backward (retropulsion). Assessment of postural instability includes the "pull test," in which the examiner stands behind and abruptly pulls the patient by the shoulders while protecting the patient from a fall.

Other Symptoms
In addition to the motor features of parkinsonism, a variety of non–motor-related features are common.[9] These include pain and other sensory disturbances; dysautonomic complaints, such as urinary urgency and frequency; orthostatic faintness; constipation; male erectile dysfunction; sleep abnormalities, including rapid eye movement behavioral disorder (Chapter 377); anxiety; fatigue; depression; and cognitive disturbances, including dementia.[10] As the disease progresses, more resistant features develop, including "axial" motor disturbances (speech and swallowing abnormalities, freezing, and postural instability) as well as neurobehavioral and cognitive dysfunction.

Complications
In addition to the manifestations of the disease itself, complications of drug therapy include motor- and non–motor-related fluctuations and psychiatric or behavioral disturbances. Thus in the later stages of the disease, the clinical picture often fluctuates from hour to hour and even from minute to minute. Accordingly, patients exhibit a mixture of the classic features of parkinsonism, which may improve considerably in response to medication; symptoms that persist despite the peak benefit of medication; and symptoms that occur as a complication of dopaminergic medication (Table 381-2).

DIAGNOSIS

Testing for the approximately 10% of genetic forms of Parkinson disease are becoming available, but genetic diagnosis has not dramatically changed therapeutic approaches. Given the classic clinical manifestations, the diagnostic evaluation focuses largely on ways to exclude other causes of parkinsonism (Table 381-3).[11] Young-onset patients should have Wilson disease excluded by determination of 24-hour urine copper excretion, a serum ceruloplasmin, and slit lamp examination (Chapter 200). Findings on magnetic resonance imaging (MRI) are generally normal in Parkinson disease, but MRI can be useful to exclude other diagnoses (Table 381-4), including multiple-system atrophy that is characterized by progressive autonomic failure with parkinsonian,

TABLE 381-2 PROBLEMS IN LATE-STAGE PARKINSON DISEASE

PROBLEM	SYMPTOMS
LATER TREATMENT-RESISTANT SYMPTOMS	
Motor	Dysarthria Dysphagia Freezing of gait (on-period freezing) Postural instability with falls
Non–motor	Dysautonomia, weight loss Sensory symptoms, including pain (some may be responsive to levodopa) Changes in mood or behavior (depression, anxiety), apathy, sleep disturbances (excessive daytime sleepiness often caused by or aggravated by dopaminergic medication) Rapid eye movement sleep behavior disorder (may develop before parkinsonism) Fatigue Cognitive dysfunction and dementia
RELATED TO TREATMENT AND DISEASE	
Motor fluctuations	Wearing off of drug effect (predictable end-of-dose deterioration, morning akinesia), increased latency to benefit ("delayed-on"), dose failures ("no-on") On-off phenomenon, more rapid and unpredictable fluctuations Concomitant fluctuations of non–motor-related symptoms ("nonmotor fluctuations") that may be as disabling as motor symptoms (or more so)
Dyskinesias (abnormal involuntary movements)	Peak-dose dyskinesias: chorea, athetosis, and, less often, more prolonged dystonia, typically worse on the initially affected side (Video 381-12) Diphasic dyskinesia ("beginning-of-dose" and "end-of-dose" dyskinesias): mixtures of choreoathetosis, ballism, dystonia, alternating movements (especially in the legs) Off-period dystonia: most often involving the legs and feet (including morning foot dystonia)
Psychiatric disturbances	Vivid dreams and nightmares Visual hallucinations with a clear sensorium Hallucinations with confusion Mania, impulse control disorders (e.g., hypersexuality, problem gambling), dopaminergic drug addiction Paranoid psychosis

Modified from Lang AE, Lozano AM. Parkinson's disease—second of two parts. *N Engl J Med.* 1998;339:1130-1143.

TABLE 381-3	CLINICAL CLUES TO AN ALTERNATIVE (NON–PARKINSON DISEASE) CAUSE OF PARKINSONIAN SIGNS AND SYMPTOMS

Extraocular movements—e.g., nystagmus, limitation of vertical gaze, especially with slowing of downward saccadic eye movements (see Video 381-4)

Early and prominent dysarthria or dysphagia

Prominent or early abnormal neck postures: flexion or extension (see Video 381-8)

Ataxia—limb, gait (impaired tandem gait)

Lower body distribution with relative sparing of upper limb function

Early postural instability, falls, or freezing (see Video 381-3)

Dysautonomia (early and prominent), prominent hypotensive response to dopaminergic medication

Pyramidal tract signs—very brisk reflexes, clonus, extensor plantar responses

Peripheral nerve dysfunction—loss of reflexes, distal sensory loss, weakness

Apraxia and cortical sensory changes

Early severe dementia

Poor response to levodopa

cerebellar, and pyramidal features in various combinations. Positron emission tomography, which can assess the presynaptic and postsynaptic sides of the nigrostriatal dopamine system, is useful for research, but the most common ligand, [^{18}F]fluorodopa, does not reliably distinguish Parkinson disease from many other neurodegenerative diseases that mimic it. The same limitations apply to evaluation of the dopamine transporter by single-photon emission computed tomography, which is available for clinical use.

TREATMENT Rx

Early treatment in a patient with little or no disability may entail only education, psychological support, encouragement to remain active and to become involved in an exercise program, and ongoing follow-up. For example, tai chi training improves balance and lowers the incidence of falls in patients with mild to moderate Parkinson disease. Treadmill and resistance exercises also appear to be beneficial.[A1][A2]

There is some evidence that early treatment, even when patients are only mildly symptomatic, may preserve quality of life, and therapy is typically initiated when quality of life is impaired or when there is a risk of physical injury. Such treatment is directed at slowing progression ("neuroprotective" or "disease-modifying" treatments); improving symptoms, typically by restoring dopaminergic tone medically or by correcting basal ganglia neurophysiology surgically

TABLE 381-4	DISEASES THAT MUST BE DISTINGUISHED FROM PARKINSON DISEASE	
DIAGNOSIS	**IMPORTANT DISTINGUISHING CLINICAL FEATURES**	**RESPONSE TO LEVODOPA/COMMENTS (INCLUDING IMAGING)**
Multiple-system atrophy (MSA) (includes older terms: striatonigral degeneration, sporadic olivopontocerebellar atrophy, and Shy-Drager syndrome) (a "synucleinopathy") MSA-P, a predominant parkinsonian manifestation MSA-C, a predominant cerebellar manifestation (mixed features are common)	Early dysautonomia (including orthostatic hypotension and sexual impotence) and bladder dysfunction (with autonomic and nonautonomic components) Cerebellar dysfunction Pyramidal tract signs Stimulus-sensitive myoclonus of the hands and face Extreme forward neck flexion (anterocollis) Mottled, cold hands Inspiratory stridor (see Video 381-9) Prominent dysarthria	Good response initially evident in 20% and sustained partial response in ≈15% Dyskinesias or motor fluctuations possible; cranial dystonia may be prominent (see Video 381-7) Patient is wheelchair bound despite response to levodopa (early loss of postural reflexes, with or without ataxia) MRI (including diffusion-weighted imaging and gradient-echo sequences) often shows diagnostic changes in the striatum in MSA-P and "hot cross bun sign" in the pons and hyperintensity in middle cerebellar peduncles in MSA-C
Progressive supranuclear palsy (a "tauopathy")	Supranuclear vertical ophthalmoplegia (see Video 381-4) Other oculomotor and eyelid disturbances (see Video 381-6) Axial rigidity greater than limb rigidity Early falls, speech and swallowing disturbances Nuchal extension Cognitive or behavioral changes Progressive nonfluent aphasia Possibly a higher incidence of hypertension than in Parkinson disease and other neurodegenerative causes of parkinsonism	Good response rarely evident; benefit only for classic parkinsonian features, such as limb rigidity, classic bradykinesia with fatiguing of amplitude of repetitive movements, and rare examples of tremor at rest MRI often demonstrates profound midbrain atrophy ("hummingbird sign" on a midline sagittal view, "morning glory sign" on axial view)
Corticobasal (cortical-basal ganglionic) degeneration (a "tauopathy")	Apraxia, cortical sensory loss, alien limb phenomenon (see Video 381-10) Pronounced asymmetrical rigidity Limb dystonia Stimulus-sensitive myoclonus (see Video 381-11) Aphasia (progressive nonfluent aphasia) Cognitive dysfunction (frontotemporal dementia)	Usually negligible MRI may show pronounced asymmetrical cortical atrophy
Vascular parkinsonism	"Lower-half" parkinsonism with gait disturbances predominating, often with minimal or much milder upper body involvement Additional neurologic deficits (e.g., pyramidal tract signs, pseudobulbar palsy)	Usually poor, but some respond well Imaging demonstrates multiple infarcts involving the basal ganglia and subcortical white matter
Dementia with Lewy bodies (a "synucleinopathy")	Early dementia (cognitive profile somewhat different from that of Alzheimer disease) Spontaneous hallucinations, fluctuating cognitive status, falls, orthostatic hypotension, RBD Pronounced sensitivity to the extrapyramidal side effects of neuroleptic drugs Parkinsonism may be similar to typical Parkinson disease, although rigidity may be more prominent than bradykinesia or tremor	Motor features may respond well; psychiatric side effects of dopaminergic drugs are typically dose limiting

TABLE 381-4 DISEASES THAT MUST BE DISTINGUISHED FROM PARKINSON DISEASE—cont'd

DIAGNOSIS	IMPORTANT DISTINGUISHING CLINICAL FEATURES	RESPONSE TO LEVODOPA/COMMENTS (INCLUDING IMAGING)
Alzheimer disease	Early dementia (memory loss, apraxia, aphasia) Tremor uncommon Spontaneous hallucinations less common than in dementia with Lewy bodies	Poor
Normal-pressure hydrocephalus	"Lower-half" parkinsonism ("gait apraxia") Urinary complaints (frequency, urgency, incontinence) Cognitive disturbances	Generally poor Imaging demonstrates ventriculomegaly out of proportion to cortical atrophy
Drug-induced parkinsonism	All the classic features of parkinsonism (tremor may be less common than in Parkinson disease) Usually symmetrical signs and symptoms Other drug-induced movement disorders (e.g., tardive dyskinesia with neuroleptics)	Usually poor because of ongoing dopamine receptor blockade; may aggravate movements of tardive dyskinesia

MRI = magnetic resonance imaging; RBD = rapid eye movement sleep behavior disorder.

("symptomatic"); or attempting to restore or to regenerate the damaged neurons ("neurorestorative" or "neuroregenerative" therapy).[12-14]

Medical Treatment
Disease-Modifying Treatment
The selective monoamine oxidase B inhibitors selegiline and rasagiline[A3] have shown some potential as disease-modifying agents, but medical treatment (Table 381-5) has not been proven to modify the progressive course of Parkinson disease. In one trial, exenatide (a glucagon-like peptide-1 receptor agonist at 2 mg subcutaneously weekly) improved motor scores during and after treatment,[A4] but it is not clear whether it modifies the long-term course of disease. Whether the early initiation of symptomatic therapy bolsters the brain's compensatory mechanisms is uncertain.

Alleviating Symptoms
Levodopa is the most effective symptomatic treatment of Parkinson disease,[A5] but it does not alter the course of the disease[A6] and is associated with a variety of side effects (see Table 381-2). For the first year or more, the benefit of levodopa lasts throughout the day with little symptomatic variability. However, in time, the duration of benefit declines, with worsening of symptoms the first thing in the morning (morning akinesia) and for a variable time before scheduled daytime doses (wearing-off/end-of-dose akinesia). Within 2 to 5 years of initiation of treatment, up to 50% of patients may also experience involuntary movements (chorea, athetosis, dystonia), most often at the peak action of the medication. These complications, which are generally more prominent and occur earlier in patients with an onset of disease at a younger age, reflect the short half-life of levodopa combined with the underlying progressive loss of presynaptic dopamine neurons and result in nonphysiologic "pulsatile" stimulation of striatal dopamine receptors, which then induces "neuroplastic" changes in postsynaptic striatal neurons. Initially, these complications rarely cause major disability.

Although initiation of therapy with a dopamine agonist rather than with levodopa may be associated with a delay in the onset of these motor problems, the clinical benefit is generally less than with levodopa,[A7] and all patients eventually require the addition of levodopa to control symptoms. No data support delaying treatment with levodopa, and some data suggest that levodopa could have a neuroprotective effect. Even as Parkinson disease progresses, most of the classic features continue to respond after 20 years or more of treatment. It is not clear that delaying motor complications in the first 5 years of treatment by the initial use of a dopamine agonist improves long-term outcome or quality of life; indeed, clinical status, including the incidence of motor complications, may be no different after 10 years of treatment in those initiating therapy with a dopamine agonist and those starting with levodopa.

There is no clear advantage to starting initial treatment with a controlled-release rather than with an immediate-release preparation of levodopa or combining levodopa with a catechol O-methyltransferase inhibitor. When motor fluctuations develop during levodopa therapy, however, they can be managed by a number of approaches (see Table 381-5), including increasing the frequency of the dose, using a controlled-release preparation, prolonging the action by blocking metabolism (monoamine oxidase B or catechol O-methyltransferase inhibition), or adding a dopamine agonist. For example, adding rasagiline or entacapone to levodopa provides significant incremental benefits.

Newer levodopa formulations that provide more reliable, sustained plasma levels are in active development.[A8] A formulation that provides continuous infusion into the duodenum (Duodopa) can significantly improve symptoms during "off" time without increasing dyskinesias compared with immediate-release levodopa[A9]; this formulation is available in most European countries and was recently approved in Canada and the United States for patients with problematic motor fluctuations. Dyskinesias improve when doses of dopaminergic medications are reduced, but the parkinsonism often increases to an intolerable level. Amantadine may improve the dyskinesias without worsening the parkinsonism. Agents under study include the α_2-adrenergic receptor antagonist fipamezole as well as the combination of dextromethorphan plus quinidine. Antagonists of the adenosine A_{2A} receptor are being actively studied but with variable results. One of these, istradefylline, is marketed in Japan for the treatment of wearing-off phenomenon.

Mildly effective drugs such as a monoamine oxidase B inhibitor and amantadine may provide adequate benefit in mildly symptomatic patients (see Table 381-5). Although anticholinergics may be used for tremor, their cognitive side effects make them a less desirable choice. When symptoms are more pronounced or inadequately controlled with these approaches, dopaminergic therapy should be introduced. In patients younger than 65 years who are cognitively intact and lack other major medical problems, initial therapy with a dopamine agonist may be reasonable. However, these drugs result in more excessive sleepiness, leg edema, "impulse control disorders" (such as pathologic gambling, hypersexuality, binge eating, and shopping), and hallucinations than levodopa. Impulse control disorders occur in one of six patients, so monitoring by a family member is highly encouraged. If a full dose of a dopamine agonist does not provide adequate clinical benefit or has intolerable side effects, levodopa should be initiated. In older patients, in those with cognitive dysfunction (more prone to hallucinations with dopamine agonists), and in circumstances that require more rapid improvement of pronounced disability, levodopa should be the initial drug.

Medical management of Parkinson disease often includes a variety of other agents, including medications directed at the treatment of orthostatic hypotension (Chapter 56), depression (Chapter 369), anxiety (Chapter 369), urinary frequency and urgency (Chapters 23 and 120), and male erectile dysfunction (Chapter 221). Pimavanserin (40 mg daily) is an option for treating psychosis related to Parkinson disease.[A10] Management of late-stage Parkinson disease requires skill in polypharmacy and an understanding of the complicated benefit-risk ratios of the many drugs needed.

Surgical Treatment
Bilateral deep brain stimulation of the subthalamic nucleus or globus pallidus improves the symptoms of Parkinson disease, often permits lower doses of antiparkinson medications to be used, and improves self-reported quality of life.[A11] Earlier use of subthalamic nucleus deep brain stimulation, at a time when patients are just beginning to develop motor complications (mean duration of disease, 7.5 years), provides significantly greater benefit than best medical therapy, but there is no consensus as to the most appropriate time to intervene surgically. Thalamic deep brain stimulation is of limited utility because it is effective only for tremor. The best predictor of a good response to deep brain stimulation of the subthalamic nucleus or globus pallidus internus is the patient's ongoing clinical response to levodopa. Apart from tremor, which may be resistant to the highest tolerable dose of levodopa but generally responds well to surgery, symptoms that are resistant to the peak effect of levodopa (e.g., dysarthria, postural instability with falls) also fail to respond to deep brain stimulation. The typical good candidate for deep brain stimulation of the subthalamic nucleus or globus pallidus is an otherwise healthy, relatively young, cognitively intact, and psychiatrically stable patient who still responds well to levodopa (apart from tremor) but is suffering from disabling tremor, off time, motor fluctuations, and dyskinesias. Double-blind randomized trials of transplantation of fetal substantia nigra into the striatum have failed to show significant efficacy and also have been associated with the side effect of transplant-induced off-medication "runaway" dyskinesias.

TABLE 381-5   DRUGS FOR PARKINSON DISEASE

CLASS	DRUG	USUAL STARTING DOSE	USUAL FINAL DOSAGE	IMPORTANT ADVERSE EFFECTS	COMMENTS	INDICATIONS
Anticholinergic	Many (e.g., benztropine, trihexyphenidyl)	Benztropine or trihexyphenidyl, 1-2 mg 2-3 times per day	Varied	Peripheral effects, e.g., dry mouth, blurred vision, constipation, difficulty with urination Central effects, e.g., confusion, memory problems, hallucinations	Relatively contraindicated in the elderly and contraindicated in patients with cognitive disturbances	Early treatment of tremor
Miscellaneous	Amantadine	100 mg once per day	100 mg 2 or 3 times per day	Confusion, visual hallucinations; livedo reticularis, swelling of the ankles; dose reduction or drug withdrawal necessary in patients with renal failure	Previously considered a dopaminergic drug, now thought to act primarily through NMDA antagonist effects	Early treatment; later for dyskinesias
	Memantine	5 mg once daily	10 mg twice daily	Confusion, fatigue, dizziness, headache	NMDA antagonist	Possibly effective for cognitive dysfunction in PDD
Dopamine precursor	Levodopa given with peripheral dopa decarboxylase inhibitor (DDCI) (carbidopa [in 4:1 and 10:1 ratios] or benserazide [4:1]*)	50 (levodopa) / 12.5 (DDCI) mg (4:1 preparation) 3 times per day (with meals to reduce nausea and vomiting)	Varied; begin with 3-times-daily schedule (controlled-release levodopa-carbidopa may be given twice daily at first); late in the disease, patients may require multiple doses per day (sometimes >2 g/day) Initially give with meals to reduce GI upset; later avoid meals to improve absorption and reliability of response	Peripheral and central dopaminergic side effects Peripheral: nausea, vomiting, and orthostatic hypotension Central: motor fluctuations, dyskinesias, psychiatric disturbances	Peripheral side effects often controlled by additional carbidopa or the peripheral dopamine receptor blocker domperidone* Controlled-release formulations often less bioavailable with less reliable absorption (more "dose failures" later on)	Formulations: immediate-release—for early and later treatment Controlled-release (with carbidopa [4:1] or benserazide [4:1]*)—for predictable motor fluctuations (wearing off) and nighttime akinesia Stalevo (with carbidopa and entacapone)—for wearing off Parcopa (orally disintegrating tablets for faster absorption)—for patients with problematic long latency to benefit with individual doses Melevodopa* (methyl ester of levodopa; effervescent prodrug with much higher water solubility than tablets of levodopa; available in Italy) Duodopa* (used with a pump for duodenal infusions)—for problematic motor fluctuations

	Drug	Starting dose	Dose/day	Side effects	Comments	Indication
Dopamine agonists **Ergot derived**	Bromocriptine	1.25 mg 3 times per day with meals	30-40 mg/day	Peripheral and central dopaminergic side effects; pedal edema, excessive daytime sleepiness Pleuropulmonary reaction, retroperitoneal fibrosis, erythromelalgia Impulse control disorders probably equally common with all dopamine agonists	Peripheral side effects often well controlled with domperidone* Rare pulmonary, retroperitoneal, and skin effects possibly caused by ergot derivation (drug withdrawal usually required)	Early and adjunctive therapy
	Pergolide	0.05 mg once per day × 2 days, increasing slowly thereafter	3-5 mg/day	As for bromocriptine; cardiac valvulopathy	As for bromocriptine; cardiac valvulopathy	Not the first agonist because it causes restrictive cardiac valve disease
	Cabergoline*	0.5-1 mg once per day	2-6 mg/day	As for pergolide	As for pergolide Long half-life allows once-daily dosage	As for pergolide, although advantage of a long half-life may outweigh this concern
	Lisuride*	0.1-0.2 mg 1-3 times per day	2-5 mg/day	As for bromocriptine	As for bromocriptine	Uncertain whether cardiac valve abnormalities occur Parenteral formulations allow chronic infusion (pump) therapy
Non-ergot derived	Ropinirole	0.25 mg 3 times per day	Up to 24 mg/day in 3 divided doses Once-daily extended/ prolonged-release formulation available	Peripheral and central dopaminergic side effects similar to those of ergot-derived dopamine agonists, with the probable exceptions of pleuropulmonary reaction, retroperitoneal fibrosis, erythromelalgia, and cardiac valvulopathy	Effective as first-line and adjunctive therapy; dopamine D_3 agonist effects may contribute to efficacy Some patients withdrawing from the drug (especially those with impulse control disorders) experience symptoms similar to an addictive drug withdrawal ("dopamine agonist withdrawal syndrome")	De novo therapy shown to be associated with fewer motor complications than with levodopa Implications of less progressive loss of dopamine terminal function on imaging uncertain
	Pramipexole	0.125 mg 3 times per day	Up to 4.5 mg/day in 3 divided doses Once-daily extended/ prolonged-release formulation available	As for ropinirole	As for ropinirole, possibly greater "D_3-preferring" effects—may account for antidepressant effect	As for ropinirole
	Rotigotine	Nominal dose: 2.0 mg/day (10 cm² containing 4.5 mg)	Transdermal patch nominal dose 4.0-16 mg/day (patch content 9-36 mg; 20-80 cm²)	As for ropinirole Additional adverse effects related to skin patch application (dermatitis)	May be effective for both first-line and adjunctive therapy	As for ropinirole
	Piribedil*	50 mg once/day	150-250 mg/day (in 3-5 doses per day)	As for ropinirole	As for ropinirole	As for ropinirole
	Apomorphine	3-5 mg SC injection	Parenteral agent given as needed or as continuous infusion	Peripheral and central dopaminergic side effects Local skin reactions, including nodule formation	Concomitant antiemetic (eg, domperidone,* trimethobenzamide) needed	Late-stage problematic motor fluctuations Long-term use of infusions may reduce dyskinesias as well as motor fluctuations

TABLE 381-5 DRUGS FOR PARKINSON DISEASE—cont'd

CLASS	DRUG	USUAL STARTING DOSE	USUAL FINAL DOSAGE	IMPORTANT ADVERSE EFFECTS	COMMENTS	INDICATIONS
Monoamine oxidase B inhibitors	Selegiline	5 mg once per day	5 mg 2 times per day	Dopaminergic effects of other drugs possibly accentuated, insomnia, confusion	Last dose given at midday to avoid insomnia	Early mild disease Some controversial evidence suggesting disease-modifying effects Predictable motor fluctuations (wearing off)
	Zydis selegiline	1.25 mg once per day	1.25 or 2.5 mg/day (wafer formulation)	As for selegiline	As for selegiline Absorbed from the buccal mucosa, thereby avoiding first-pass hepatic metabolism and methamphetamine metabolite of selegiline	As for selegiline
	Rasagiline	1 mg once per day	1-2 mg once per day	As for selegiline		Possible disease-modifying effects As for selegiline
Catechol O-methyltransferase (COMT) inhibitors	Tolcapone	100 mg 3 times per day	100 or 200 mg 3 times per day (at 6-hour intervals)	Effects of levodopa accentuated Diarrhea in approximately 5% of patients Hepatotoxicity Urine discoloration	Dose of levodopa may have to be reduced by as much as 25%; diarrhea (sometimes explosive) typically forces discontinuation Ongoing monitoring of liver function tests required (second-line COMT inhibitor)	Motor fluctuations, especially wearing off (probably more effective than entacapone)
	Entacapone	200 mg with each dose of levodopa	200 mg 4-10 times per day (given with doses of levodopa)	Effects of levodopa accentuated 10% note brown/orange urine discoloration	As for tolcapone; diarrhea possibly less frequent Liver function monitoring unnecessary	As for tolcapone Available in a combination tablet with levodopa/carbidopa (Stalevo)
A₂ₐ antagonist	Istradefylline* (Japan only)	20 mg once per day	20 mg once per day	Increased dyskinesias		
Atypical neuroleptics	Clozapine	12.5 mg hs	Wide range (6.25-150 mg/day), usually <75 mg/day	Agranulocytosis, sedation, hypotension, sialorrhea	Very low risk of worsening parkinsonism; agranulocytosis rare (<1%) and reversible if discovered early (requires regular monitoring of complete blood count)	Drug-induced psychosis Other "off-label" indications include drug-resistant tremor and possibly levodopa-induced dyskinesias
	Quetiapine	12.5-25 mg hs	25-150 mg/day	Sedation May worsen parkinsonism	Probably less effective than clozapine	Drug-induced psychosis
Acetylcholinesterase inhibitors	Donepezil	5 mg once per day	5-10 mg/day	Peripheral cholinergic side effects: nausea, vomiting, diarrhea, syncope, bradycardia Increased tremor, worsening of other Parkinson features		Dementia Possibly effective for psychotic symptoms, especially hallucinations
	Rivastigmine	1.5 mg twice per day	3-12 mg/day	As for donepezil	Patch formulation available for transdermal administration—tolerability may be improved over oral formulation	As for donepezil

*Unavailable in the United States.

GI = gastrointestinal; NMDA = N-methyl-ᴅ-aspartate; PDD = Parkinson disease dementia.

382

PROGNOSIS

Parkinson disease progresses inexorably during a period of many years; the speed and course of progression vary considerably from patient to patient. So far, genotypic information has not helped predict outcomes or change treatment. Some patients maintain an excellent response to treatment and seem to change very little during prolonged follow-up, but most note increasing disability, with the development of many symptoms that are poorly responsive to medications. Factors such as poor postural stability, falls, dysarthria, dysphagia, dysautonomia, excessive daytime sleepiness, apathy, and dementia contribute to the disability and increased mortality. Approximately half of patients who have normal cognition at baseline develop cognitive impairment within 6 years, and patients who develop mild cognitive impairment commonly progress to dementia within 5 years. Whether deep brain stimulation improves survival is uncertain, and most Parkinson patients die of causes directly related to Parkinson disease.[15]

FUTURE DIRECTIONS

Gene therapies directed at either modifying neurotransmitter function or inducing neuroregeneration and other cell-based therapies are under development. Vaccine based approaches and improvements to deep brain stimulation devices are being studied. Future treatments must also address the widespread, multisystemic nature of the disease, especially symptoms that are unrelated to nigrostriatal dopamine deficiency and that fail to respond to current therapies.

● OTHER CAUSES OF PARKINSONISM

The numerous causes of parkinsonism (see Table 381-1) are sometimes termed *akinetic-rigid syndrome, Parkinson syndrome, atypical parkinsonism,* or *Parkinson-plus syndrome* to emphasize that these patients commonly demonstrate additional clinical features indicative of the more widespread and particularly more severe pathologic involvement of areas beyond the dopaminergic SNc. These other parkinsonism conditions are generally associated with "postsynaptic" changes that result in a poor or unsustained response to levodopa, and this unresponsiveness serves as one of the most important of several clues that the parkinsonism features are caused by conditions other than Parkinson disease (see Table 381-4) (e.g., "parkinsonism minus," a levodopa response; see Table 381-3).

Grade A References

A1. Rafferty MR, Prodoehl J, Robichaud JA, et al. Effects of 2 years of exercise on gait impairment in people with Parkinson disease: the PRET-PD randomized trial. *J Neurol Phys Ther.* 2017;41:21-30.

A2. Mak MK, Wong-Yu IS, Shen X, et al. Long-term effects of exercise and physical therapy in people with Parkinson disease. *Nat Rev Neurol.* 2017;13:689-703.

A3. Chen F, Jin L, Nie Z. Safety and efficacy of rotigotine for treating Parkinson's disease: a meta-analysis of randomised controlled trials. *J Pharm Sci.* 2017;20:285-294.

A4. Athauda D, Maclagan K, Skene SS, et al. Exenatide once weekly versus placebo in Parkinson's disease: a randomised, double-blind, placebo-controlled trial. *Lancet.* 2017;390:1664-1675.

A5. Xie CL, Zhang YY, Wang XD, et al. Levodopa alone compared with levodopa-sparing therapy as initial treatment for Parkinson's disease: a meta-analysis. *Neurol Sci.* 2015;36:1319-1329.

A6. Verschuur CVM, Suwijn SR, Boel JA, et al. Randomized delayed-start trial of levodopa in Parkinson's disease. *N Engl J Med.* 2019;380:315-324.

A7. Gray R, Ives N, Rick C, et al. Long-term effectiveness of dopamine agonists and monoamine oxidase B inhibitors compared with levodopa as initial treatment for Parkinson's disease (PD MED): a large, open-label, pragmatic randomised trial. *Lancet.* 2014;384:1196-1205.

A8. Hauser RA, Hsu A, Kell S, et al. Extended-release carbidopa-levodopa (IPX066) compared with immediate-release carbidopa-levodopa in patients with Parkinson's disease and motor fluctuations: a phase 3 randomised, double-blind trial. *Lancet Neurol.* 2013;12:346-356.

A9. Olanow CW, Kieburtz K, Odin P, et al. Continuous intrajejunal infusion of levodopa-carbidopa intestinal gel for patients with advanced Parkinson's disease: a randomised, controlled, double-blind, double-dummy study. *Lancet Neurol.* 2014;13:141-149.

A10. Wilby KJ, Johnson EG, Johnson HE, et al. Evidence-based review of pharmacotherapy used for Parkinson's disease psychosis. *Ann Pharmacother.* 2017;51:682-695.

A11. Tan ZG, Zhou Q, Huang T, et al. Efficacies of globus pallidus stimulation and subthalamic nucleus stimulation for advanced Parkinson's disease: a meta-analysis of randomized controlled trials. *Clin Interv Aging.* 2016;11:777-786.

GENERAL REFERENCES

For the General References and other additional features, please visit Expert Consult at https://expertconsult.inkling.com.

OTHER MOVEMENT DISORDERS

MICHAEL S. OKUN AND ANTHONY E. LANG

DEFINITION

Movement disorders are first divided into hypokinetic and hyperkinetic categories. *Hypokinetic disorders,* which are characterized by akinesia, bradykinesia, and rigidity, are parkinsonian syndromes and are discussed in Chapter 381. The common *hyperkinetic movement* disorders (Table 382-1) are defined by specific clinical phenomena.

CLINICAL MANIFESTATIONS AND DIAGNOSTIC APPROACH

The traditional approach to a neurologic symptom is first to address localization within the nervous system (i.e., "Where is the lesion?"), followed by an evaluation of the origin ("What is the lesion?"). The neurologic examination is critical in determining the localization of the lesion, and generally the history, including the nature of onset and the progression of the symptoms, will determine the most likely diagnosis. However, when a movement disorder is the predominant problem, the approach is somewhat different. The pathophysiology of most movement disorders is complex. Many of these disorders are the result of dysfunction of different circuits in the brain, and it is often impossible to ascertain a specific anatomic localization. Instead, an accurate appreciation of the clinical phenomena is the first important step in evaluation. The clinician must observe and examine the patient to define the type of movement disorder that best describes the clinical picture. This accurate characterization then allows the generation of a differential diagnosis for the specific movement disorder. The age and nature of onset, the distribution, the progression of symptoms, a family history of similar or related symptoms, and the presence of other neurologic and systemic signs aid in determining the most likely explanation.

● TREMOR

Tremor, which is a rhythmic, sinusoidal movement of a body part, is caused by regular, either synchronous or alternating, contractions of reciprocally innervated muscles. Tremors are classified based on whether they occur at rest (weight fully supported against gravity) or in action. Resting tremors are typically seen in Parkinson disease and other parkinsonism syndromes, but this is not an absolute rule[1] (see Table 381-1). Action tremors are further divided into postural, kinetic, or intention tremors. A postural tremor is seen with the maintenance of a posture against gravity (e.g., when the arms are outstretched in front of the body). A *kinetic tremor* is seen with a voluntary movement of the limb (e.g., a tremor in an upper limb when performing the finger-to-nose test). An intention tremor increases in amplitude on approaching a target.

CLINICAL MANIFESTATIONS

Most action tremors (Table 382-2) combine postural and kinetic components. Most tremors worsen with stress, including performing an affected activity in public. Initially, a tremor may be evident only when one attempts fine,

TABLE 382-1	HYPERKINETIC MOVEMENT DISORDERS
Tremor	
Chorea	
Ballism	
Dystonia	
Athetosis	
Tics	
Myoclonus	
Startle	
Stereotypies	
Miscellaneous	

TABLE 382-2 DIFFERENTIAL DIAGNOSIS OF TREMOR AND RHYTHMIC MOVEMENT DISORDERS

ENHANCED PHYSIOLOGIC TREMOR

Metabolic disorders
   Hyperthyroidism
   Hyperparathyroidism
   Hypoglycemia
   Pheochromocytoma
Drugs
   Caffeine
   Theophylline
   Amphetamines
   Lithium
   Valproic acid
   Antidepressants
   Amiodarone
   β-Agonists
   Others
Withdrawal of drugs
   Benzodiazepines
   Alcohol
   Others
Fever, sepsis
Anxiety, stress, fatigue

PRIMARY OR IDIOPATHIC TREMOR

Essential tremor
Task-specific tremor
Orthostatic tremor
Idiopathic palatal tremor

TREMOR ASSOCIATED WITH CENTRAL NERVOUS SYSTEM DISEASES

Tremor with parkinsonian syndromes
   Idiopathic Parkinson disease
   Multiple system atrophy
   Progressive supranuclear palsy
   Corticobasal degeneration
   Neuroleptic-induced parkinsonism
Wilson disease
Multiple sclerosis
Fragile X premutation-tremor/ataxia syndrome
Stroke
Arteriovenous malformation
Tumor
Head trauma
Midbrain tremor (Holmes tremor)

TREMOR ASSOCIATED WITH PERIPHERAL NEUROPATHIES

PSYCHOGENIC TREMOR

OTHER RHYTHMIC MOVEMENT DISORDERS

Rhythmic movements in dystonia (dystonic tremor)
Rhythmic myoclonus (including myoclonic tremor)
Asterixis
Clonus
Epilepsia partialis continua
Hereditary chin quivering
Spasmus nutans
Head bobbing with hydrocephalus
Nystagmus

Modified from Cloutier M, Lang AE. Movement disorders: an overview. In: Factor SA, Lang AE, Weiner WJ, eds. *Drug Induced Movement Disorders.* Malden, Mass: Blackwell; 2005:3-19.

---

the foot up to a target (e.g., the examiner's hand) and then perform a heel-knee-shin test.

Most upper limb action tremors affect many activities to a similar extent. Less commonly, tremors can affect a single task in isolation (task-specific tremors), the most common being a primary writing tremor. Orthostatic tremor is apparent in the legs and in antigravity muscles only when the patient is standing in one spot and subsides during walking or leaning against a wall; these patients commonly complain of a tremendous sense of insecurity while standing and a fear of falling. Electrophysiologic assessment demonstrates a very characteristic high-frequency tremor (14 to 18 Hz).

Enhanced Physiologic Tremor

A 7- to 12-Hz tremor is detectable by electrophysiologic recordings in all humans. This physiologic tremor is enhanced and may become symptomatic in a variety of circumstances, including fatigue, anxiety, and excitement. This same tremor may be accentuated by drugs and systemic processes.

Essential Tremor

Essential tremor affects up to 5% of the general population after the age of 60 years.[2,3] Essential tremor is often inherited in an autosomal dominant fashion, with the phenotype showing genetic heterogeneity from at least six different genes, as well as environmental influences. Recent pathology studies have variably demonstrated microscopic abnormalities of cerebellar decreased Purkinje cells, changes in axon thickness, and decreased axonal branching. The age of onset may be as early as the first or second decade of life, but senile tremor may be delayed until the mid-60s. Patients first become aware of a mild postural and action tremor in the hands, which is indistinguishable from an enhanced physiologic tremor and may result in little functional impairment for many years until it gradually interferes with activities. Older patients with large-amplitude, lower frequency tremors can have a resting component that is often misdiagnosed as Parkinson disease (see Table 381-1) (Video 382-1).

TREATMENT

Treatment of essential tremor does not influence the course of the illness and therefore is justified only when the tremor interferes with function. At least 50% of patients note improvement or complete amelioration of tremor following the ingestion of a small amount of ethanol.

First-line drug treatment includes trials of a noncardioselective β-adrenergic blocker (e.g., propranolol, ≤320 mg/day), primidone (starting in a low dose of 25 to 62.5 mg at night and increasing to 500 to 750 mg/day), or topiramate (≤400 mg/day).🄰🄸 Other drugs that have been shown probably to be effective in double-blind crossover trials include gabapentin (1200 to 1800 mg/day), atenolol (50 to 150 mg/day), alprazolam (0.125 to 3 mg/day), and sotalol (75 to 200 mg/day). However, sotalol is associated with ventricular arrhythmias and dose-related QT interval prolongation, so it is not routinely considered as treatment of essential tremor. The medications that have been shown to be of possible benefit include nadolol (120 to 240 mg/day), nimodipine (120 mg/day), and clonazepam (0.5 to 6 mg/day), but many patients remain resistant to all drugs. Botulinum toxin may be effective, but it also may result in dose-dependent weakness and pain at the injection site. If disability is substantial, thalamic deep brain stimulation or thalamotomy can be of major benefit, with significant reductions following unilateral or bilateral treatment.[4] Recently unilateral ultrasound thalamotomy has been used successfully.🄰🄲

However, a few patients suffer permanent neurologic sequelae such as speech and gait dysfunction even with unilateral procedures, and even more suffer such problems after bilateral procedures.

---

dexterous tasks such as threading a needle, soldering, or using a screwdriver. More severe tremors interfere with activities such as handwriting, fastening buttons, shaving, eating soup with a spoon, or drinking from a cup. Patients often adapt or use compensatory measures, such as switching an activity to a less affected hand (e.g., shaving with the nondominant hand), using two hands to drink, drinking only from an incompletely filled glass or cup, or completely avoiding more challenging feeding activities in public. Severe action and intention tremors can cause handwriting to become completely illegible and can result in dependence on others for care.

Head tremors, which may be side to side, up and down, or mixed, are rarely disabling but are often a source of embarrassment. Tremor of the larynx, which causes the voice to quaver, is best appreciated by asking the patient to sustain a note. Action tremor of the lower limbs is assessed by having the patient hold

⬤ CHOREA

Chorea (Table 382-3) consists of irregular, random, brief, flowing movements that often flit from one body part to another in an unpredictable and purposeless sequence. Patients may incorporate choreiform movements into a voluntary movement to mask them. The severity varies from the appearance of being slightly fidgety or restless, to striking, continuous movements involving the whole body. Many patients with chorea seem unaware of their movements, whereas others can be very troubled and disabled.

Huntington Disease

DEFINITION AND EPIDEMIOLOGY

Huntington disease is a fully penetrant autosomal dominant neurodegenerative disorder caused by an expanded trinucleotide (CAG) repeat in the gene

TABLE 382-3 DIFFERENTIAL DIAGNOSIS OF CHOREA

GENETIC DISORDERS

Benign hereditary chorea
Huntington disease
Huntington-like conditions
Neuroferritinopathy
Neuroacanthocytosis, including McLeod syndrome
Dentatorubropallidoluysian atrophy
Wilson disease
Neurodegeneration with brain iron accumulation 1 (NBIA 1) (previously
    Hallervorden Spatz disease)
Spinocerebellar ataxias
Ataxia-telangiectasia
Ataxia-oculomotor apraxia type 1
Tuberous sclerosis

INFECTIONS/PARAINFECTIOUS CAUSES

Sydenham chorea
Acquired immunodeficiency syndrome (including complications)
Encephalitis and postencephalitic disorders
Creutzfeldt-Jakob disease

DRUGS

Levodopa
Dopaminergic agonists used for Parkinson disease
Amphetamines
Anticholinergics
Anticonvulsants (especially phenytoin)
Neuroleptics
Tricyclic antidepressants
Selective serotonin reuptake inhibitors (occasionally)
Oral contraceptives (typically in patients with a prior history of Sydenham chorea)
Antihistaminics

ENDOCRINOLOGIC/METABOLIC CONDITIONS

Hyperthyroidism
Hypoparathyroidism
Chorea gravidarum
Acquired hepatolenticular degeneration

IMMUNOLOGIC DISORDERS

Systemic lupus erythematosus
Antiphospholipid syndrome
Henoch-Schönlein purpura

VASCULAR DISORDERS

Stroke
Hemorrhage
Arteriovenous malformation
Polycythemia rubra vera

OTHER CONDITIONS

Cerebral palsy
Kernicterus
Head trauma
Cardiopulmonary bypass with hypothermia
Neoplastic and paraneoplastic syndromes
Paroxysmal dyskinesias

Modified from Cloutier M, Lang AE. Movement disorders: an overview. In: Factor SA, Lang AE, Weiner WJ, eds. *Drug Induced Movement Disorders.* Malden, Mass: Blackwell; 2005:3-19.

combination of a movement disorder, psychiatric disturbances, and cognitive dysfunction. Early on, the movement disorder is predominantly chorea, but parkinsonism and dystonia develop later (Video 382-2). Some patients, especially those with juvenile onset, have a more rapidly progressive akinetic-rigid and dystonic form (the Westphal variant). Psychiatric manifestations, which are universal but widely variable, include personality changes, impulsiveness, aggressive behavior, depression, and paranoid psychosis. These psychiatric symptoms may precede the motor manifestations, and psychotropic drug therapy may be incorrectly blamed for the subsequent development of the movement disorder. Cognitive changes result in progressive subcortical dementia with disturbed attention, concentration, judgment, and problem solving that differs from the typical cortical dementia of Alzheimer disease. Oculomotor dysfunction, most often manifested by difficulties with refixating the gaze and a resulting tendency to use blinks and head thrusts, is another common feature.

DIAGNOSIS

The diagnosis is confirmed by genetic testing. Normal alleles of the *IT15* gene have fewer than 30 CAG repeats, whereas 40 or more repeats invariably result in clinical illness. An earlier age of onset correlates with larger numbers of CAG repeats. Patients with intermediate alleles (27 to 35) have more behavioral abnormalities, such as apathy and suicidal ideation, than unaffected individuals. Mutant huntingtin protein levels, detected by ultrasensitive single-molecule counting, are associated with the onset of symptoms and diminished cognitive and motor function.[5]

TREATMENT AND PROGNOSIS Rx

Current care for patients with Huntington disease involves a multidisciplinary team of clinical geneticists, neurologists, psychiatrists, psychologists, social workers, occupational and physical therapists, speech therapists, nutritionists, and nurses.[6] Genetic counseling for patients and family members is critical. Chorea may be extremely responsive to drugs that reduce central dopamine activity, especially tetrabenazine, starting at 12.5 mg two or three times daily and gradually increasing to up to 100 to 200 mg/day, or deutetrabenazine (starting at 6 mg/day and increasing weekly by 6 mg/day until chorea is adequately controlled or up to maximum 48-mg daily dose).[A3] Patients should be monitored for depression, parkinsonism, and weight gain. Other agents should be reserved for patients with disabling chorea because they may be associated with increased parkinsonism, postural instability, depression, sedation, and other adverse effects[7]; these options include amantadine (300 to 400 mg/day) and possibly riluzole (200 mg/day). Other potential agents that work by blocking dopamine receptors include haloperidol (3 to 30 mg/day), pimozide (0.5 to 10 mg/day), fluphenazine (0.5 to 20 mg/day), and reserpine (0.75 to 5 mg/day). Data suggest that RAN proteins could be future therapeutic targets.

Unfortunately, physical function may not improve significantly even when the chorea is controlled. Psychiatric symptoms (e.g., anxiety, psychosis, depression) can be managed effectively with the same strategies as in other psychiatric diseases (Chapter 369).

Disease-modifying strategies are under active development. For example, an experimental approach is the intrathecal administration of an antisense oligonucleotide to reduce the concentration of the mutant huntingtin protein.

Progression can be monitored by clinical changes and by following changes in gray matter volumes on brain magnetic resonance imaging (MRI) in both premanifest and early-stage patients. Patients inexorably decline at a relatively constant rate, and the disease progresses to institutionalization and death over the course of approximately 15 years. However, this prognosis is variable depending largely on the burden of disease.

for the protein huntingtin located on chromosome 4. The worldwide 2.71 per 100,000 prevalence ranges from 5.7 per 100,000 for individuals of European descent to 0.4 per 100,000 for Asians. The age at diagnosis is driven by the longest expanded allele and as yet unidentified genetic or environmental factors.

PATHOBIOLOGY

Huntington disease is characterized neuropathologically by neuronal loss accompanied by intraneuronal inclusions and gliosis, especially in the caudate nucleus and putamen (the striatum) and the cerebral cortex. Understanding how these changes result from the expanded polyglutamine tract in the mutated huntingtin protein is the goal of current research.

CLINICAL MANIFESTATIONS

Symptoms typically begin between the ages of 30 and 55 years, but 5 to 10% of patients have an onset before the age of 20 years (juvenile Huntington disease) and a few patients begin to have symptoms late in life. Symptoms include a

Other Choreas

Most of the non-neurodegenerative causes of chorea (see Table 382-3) can be established or excluded by a careful history (including a detailed drug history) and a focused set of investigations, including, in appropriate circumstances, wet preparation of peripheral blood for acanthocytes (which are associated with neurodegeneration), immunologic studies (including anticardiolipin antibodies), endocrine assessment (hyperthyroidism, pregnancy), neuroimaging, and genetic testing. Mutations in the *NKX2-1* gene and the *ADCY5* gene can cause benign hereditary chorea.[9] Heterozygous hexanucleotide expansions in the *C9orf72* gene or in the *RNF216* gene can cause a Huntington-like disorder, and *C9orf72* may co-occur with the Huntington gene.[10] Among 36 adult cases of autoimmune chorea seen at one institution in 5 years, 50% had a coexisting autoimmune disorder, especially systemic lupus erythematosus (Chapter 250), and most of the remainder had a paraneoplastic cause, especially small cell carcinoma of the lung and adenocarcinoma.

TABLE 382-4	DIFFERENTIAL DIAGNOSIS OF BALLISM

Focal lesions in basal ganglia
  Vascular: Stroke (including infarction and hemorrhage), cavernous angioma, postsurgical complications
  Neoplastic: Metastases, primary central nervous system tumors
  Infections: Cryptococcosis, toxoplasmosis, tuberculoma
  Inflammatory: Multiple sclerosis
  Iatrogenic: Subthalamotomy, thalamotomy

Immunologic: Systemic lupus erythematosus, scleroderma; Behçet disease

Nonketotic hyperglycemia (high-intensity lesions in striatum on T1 MRI)

Hypoglycemia

Sydenham chorea

Head injury

Drugs
  Anticonvulsants
  Oral contraceptives
  Levodopa

Modified from Cloutier M, Lang AE. Movement disorders: an overview. In: Factor SA, Lang AE, Weiner WJ, eds. *Drug Induced Movement Disorders.* Malden, Mass: Blackwell; 2005:3-19.
MRI = magnetic resonance imaging.

Sydenham chorea, which is a late component of rheumatic fever (Chapter 274), is presumably the result of immunologic cross-reactivity between the causative group A β-hemolytic streptococcus and the basal ganglia. However, not all patients with Sydenham chorea have a history of rheumatic fever. This disorder is infrequently seen in North America but is more common in developing countries. Sydenham chorea usually affects children and young adults, and it is more common in girls before puberty. Adults with a history of Sydenham chorea in childhood may develop chorea during pregnancy or in response to taking oral contraceptive agents or estrogen preparations. They also may have a higher rate of subsequent psychiatric disturbances and impaired executive neurologic function even when in remission.

Drugs that can cause chorea should be withdrawn if possible. Tetrabenazine and deutetrabenazine, as prescribed for Huntington disease, may be useful for these other choreas.[11]

Ballism

Ballism, which is considered an extreme form of chorea, involves large-amplitude, random, often violent flinging movements of the proximal limbs (Table 382-4). It is most often a consequence of an acute cerebral insult, such as a stroke, and it usually involves one side of the body, particularly the arm, hence the term *hemiballism* (Video 382-3). When a causative lesion can be demonstrated, it typically involves the region of the subthalamic nucleus, the thalamus, or the striatum. When the condition is caused by a stroke, movements usually subside spontaneously over days to weeks, although they may persist indefinitely in some patients. Ballism also may be a side effect after deep brain stimulation or ablative procedures that target the subthalamic region. Treatment often requires the use of medication that antagonizes the effects of dopamine in the brain, including dopamine receptor blockers (neuroleptics such as haloperidol, 3 to 30 mg/day) or dopamine depleters (e.g., tetrabenazine, 50 to 200 mg/day). Functional neurosurgery (e.g., pallidotomy, deep brain stimulation) can be considered in patients with refractory, persistent symptoms.

⬤ DYSTONIA

DEFINITION AND PATHOBIOLOGY

In dystonia, sustained muscle contractions, often initiated or worsened by voluntary action, result in repetitive twisting and sometimes tremulous movements and abnormal postures. Dystonia can be classified as primary dystonia, dystonia-plus, secondary dystonia, and heredogenerative dystonia (Table 382-5). One classification uses five descriptors to specify the clinical characteristics: age at onset, body distribution, temporal pattern, and whether dystonia occurs in isolation (or only accompanied by tremor; "pure dystonia") or coexists with other movement disorders (typically parkinsonism and myoclonus). *Etiology* is defined as the presence or absence of degenerative or structural nervous system pathologic process and by whether the mode of inheritance is autosomal dominant, autosomal recessive, X-linked recessive, mitochondrial,

or acquired.[12] A commonly used classification scheme for the genetic dystonias involves applying the "DYT" prefix followed by a number (e.g., 1 to 25); however, several shortcomings have encouraged an active reevaluation of this approach. Acquired causes include drugs, toxins, infections, vascular disease, neoplasia, trauma, and psychogenic.

CLINICAL MANIFESTATIONS

Common forms of dystonia include eyelid closure (blepharospasm), jaw opening or closing (oromandibular dystonia), pulling or turning of the neck in any one or combination of directions (cervical dystonia: rotatory torticollis, laterocollis, retrocollis, anterocollis), hyperadduction and less often excessive abduction of the vocal cords (laryngeal dystonia or spasmodic dysphonia), abnormal posturing and tightness of the hand while writing or using the hand for other tasks (writer's cramp, manual dystonia), abnormal posturing of the trunk or pelvis (axial dystonia), or abnormal posturing of the lower limb, including plantar flexion and inversion of the foot (Videos 382-4, 382-5, 382-6, and 382-7). The movements are often slow and sustained, although they also may be rapid (dystonic spasms). Slower, sinuous writhing dystonic movements, particularly present in the distal limbs, are referred to as *athetosis*. Dystonia is often made worse by activity (action dystonia), and a unique aspect of dystonia is that only selected acts may be affected, with complete sparing of all other activities in the same limb (task-specific dystonia, including writer's cramp and musician's cramp) (Video 382-8). Task specific dystonia (e.g., golfing, running) may occur only during specific activities. In some patients, dystonia remains isolated and action specific over many years; in others, it progresses to involve adjacent muscles (overflow dystonia) and may eventually be present at rest, in which case joint contractures may result. Another common feature of dystonia is its transient improvement with the use of a sensory trick (geste antagoniste), such as lightly touching the chin to relieve severe cervical dystonia or the lid to relieve disabling blepharospasm (Video 382-9). Patients with dystonia, independent of cause, often have additional postural and action tremors, phenotypically similar to those in essential tremor. Some patients also demonstrate more irregular, coarse, lower frequency rhythmic movements called *dystonic tremor*.

Dystonia is often classified according to the site of involvement: focal, only one body part (e.g., blepharospasm, cervical dystonia, writer's cramp); segmental, two or more contiguous body parts; multifocal, two or more noncontiguous body parts; generalized, trunk and at least two other sites (with or without leg involvement); and hemidystonia, unilateral (generally a causative focal brain lesion is found most often involving the putamen).

DIAGNOSIS AND PROGNOSIS

For diagnostic and prognostic purposes, dystonia also may be distinguished by age of onset as childhood-onset, adolescent-onset, or adult-onset dystonia. The younger the age of onset, the more likely a cause can be defined. Conversely, isolated dystonia beginning in adult life is most often an idiopathic disorder; further investigations are typically unrewarding and are usually not indicated. Likewise, independent of the cause, dystonia beginning in childhood commonly progresses to segmental or generalized involvement whereas adult-onset dystonia usually remains focal or segmental.

Specific Dystonias
PRIMARY (IDIOPATHIC) OR ISOLATED DYSTONIAS

Primary dystonia accounts for up to 90% of patients with a pure dystonic syndrome, in which dystonia either is the only motor feature or is accompanied only by tremor. To date, no consistent neuropathologic changes have been found in the small numbers of brains affected by primary dystonia that have been studied.

When symptoms begin in childhood, a definable genetic cause is often identified, one of the most common being DYT1, usually resulting from the autosomal dominant inheritance of a GAG deletion in the *torsin A* gene (Oppenheim dystonia). This disorder is more common in persons of Ashkenazi Jewish descent. The dystonia often begins in the first decade of life and can progress to severe disability, although the spectrum of disease, even within the same family, can be quite varied and penetrance is relatively low (about 40%) (Video 382-10). Other genetic forms of dystonia include *THAP1* mutations for DYT6 and *TUBB4A* mutations for DYT4 or "whispering dystonia." Genetic testing is available but in the case of DYT1 is recommended only when the age of onset in the patient or another affected family member is less than 26 years. Among the many other potential genes and gene variants are the rare *KMT2B* missense mutation in generalized dystonia.[13]

TABLE 382-5 CLASSIFICATION AND CAUSES OF DYSTONIA

PRIMARY DYSTONIAS (PRIMARY TORSION DYSTONIA)	HEREDODEGENERATIVE DYSTONIAS

Familial (several genetic causes and types)
 Sporadic, usually adult onset, focal, or segmental
	X-linked
	    Lubag disease
	    Deafness-dystonia-optic atrophy (Mohr-Tranebjaerg) syndrome
	    Pelizaeus-Merzbacher disease
	    Lesch-Nyhan syndrome
	 Autosomal dominant
	    Rapid-onset dystonia-parkinsonism
	    Juvenile parkinsonism (e.g., from mutations in the *parkin* gene)
	    Huntington disease
	    Machado-Joseph disease (SCA3) and other SCAs
	    Dentatorubropallidoluysian atrophy
	 Autosomal recessive
	    Wilson disease
	    Niemann-Pick disease type C
	    GM₁ gangliosidosis
	    GM₂ gangliosidosis
	    Metachromatic leukodystrophy
	    Homocystinuria
	    Glutaric acidemia
	    Triose-phosphate isomerase deficiency
	    Hartnup disease
	    Ataxia-telangiectasia
	    Neurodegeneration with brain iron accumulation (NBIA 1) (previously
	       Hallervorden-Spatz disease)
	    Juvenile neuronal ceroid lipofuscinosis
	    Neuroacanthocytosis
	    Intranuclear hyaline inclusion disease
	    Hereditary spastic paraplegia with dystonia
	 Probably autosomal recessive
	    Familial basal ganglia calcifications (also dominantly inherited)
	    Progressive pallidal degeneration
	    Rett syndrome
	 Mitochondrial
	    Leigh disease
	    Leber disease
	    Other mitochondrial cytopathies
	 Sporadic, with parkinsonism
	    Parkinson disease
	    Progressive supranuclear palsy
	    Multiple system atrophy
	    Corticobasal degeneration

DYSTONIA-PLUS	

Dystonia with parkinsonism
    Dopa-responsive dystonia
    Dopamine agonist–responsive dystonia (e.g., aromatic acid decarboxylase deficiency)
 Myoclonus dystonia	

SECONDARY DYSTONIAS	

Perinatal cerebral injury
    Athetoid cerebral palsy
    Delayed-onset dystonia
    Pachygyria
    Kernicterus
 Encephalitis
    Reye syndrome
    Subacute sclerosing leukoencephalopathy
    Wasp sting
    Creutzfeldt-Jakob disease
    Human immunodeficiency virus infection
 Head trauma
 Thalamotomy
 Brainstem lesion
 Primary antiphospholipid syndrome
 Stroke
 Arteriovenous malformation
 Hypoxia
 Brain tumor
 Multiple sclerosis
 Central pontine myelinolysis
 Cervical cord injury
 Peripheral injury
 Drugs
 Toxins
 Hypoparathyroidism
 Psychogenic conditions	

Modified from Cloutier M, Lang AE. Movement disorders: an overview. In: Factor SA, Lang AE, Weiner WJ, eds. *Drug Induced Movement Disorders*. Malden, Mass: Blackwell; 2005:3-19.

ADULT-ONSET IDIOPATHIC DYSTONIA

Adult-onset idiopathic dystonia is the most common type of dystonia seen in general neurologic practice. The dystonia typically begins in the face, neck, or arm and may remain focal and nonprogressive or spread only to contiguous muscles after many years. The cause of this disorder is not known, although a positive family history may be noted if multiple family members can be examined. Genetic forms of adult-onset focal or segmental dystonia include *ANO3* and *GNAL* mutations for craniocervical dystonia and possibly *CIZ1* mutations for cervical dystonia.

DYSTONIA-PLUS

The term *dystonia-plus* refers to a small number of disorders characterized by dystonia with other neurologic signs that result from a known or presumed genetic defect without an underlying progressive neurodegenerative process. In the newer classification, these conditions are included in the group of disorders with dystonia combined with other neurologic features.

Dopa-responsive dystonia, which usually results in dystonia beginning in the first decade of life, most often in the lower limbs, sometimes can be mistaken for hereditary spastic paraplegia or cerebral palsy. Most patients with dopa-responsive dystonia have a mutation in the *GCH1* gene, which results in reduced production of dopamine. Approximately 75% of patients have notable worsening of dystonia as the day progresses (diurnal variation). Exercise often aggravates the dystonia. Patients commonly demonstrate some degree of bradykinesia (especially in the legs) and postural instability. Rare adult-onset disease may result in a pure parkinsonian phenotype. Dopa-responsive dystonia should be considered in all children with dystonia. Symptoms are

exquisitely sensitive to low doses of levodopa (typically as little as 50 mg/day of levodopa), and this treatment allows patients to live a normal life without the usual complications seen in Parkinson disease (Chapter 381).

Myoclonus dystonia, which usually begins within the first decade of life, combines dystonia with separate multifocal myoclonic jerks. Myoclonus dystonia is genetically heterogeneous; the most common definable cause is a mutation in the *epsilon-sarcoglycan* gene. The dystonia in these patients most often involves the neck or upper limbs, is mild, and is often overlooked. The disorder also can include psychopathology, such as obsessive-compulsive behavior. A characteristic feature of this disorder is the marked ameliorative effect of ethanol on both the myoclonus and the dystonia, a feature that sometimes results in alcohol abuse.

OTHER DYSTONIAS

Dystonia may be a symptom of many diseases. The nature and extent of the investigations undertaken depend on such factors as age at onset, clues provided on the history, and additional neurologic or systemic features on examination. Wilson disease (Chapter 200) is an important consideration in the diagnosis of dystonia beginning in children and young adults. Another potentially treatable form of dystonia caused by a mutation in the *SLC30A10* gene, which codes for a manganese transporter. The phenotype is similar to that of Wilson disease, with generalized dystonia, cirrhosis, and hyperintensities in the basal ganglia on T1 MRI scans.

Some patients with dystonia, chorea, or a mixture of the two (choreoathetosis) have intermittent symptoms (paroxysmal dyskinesias) and may be normal between episodes. The duration of symptoms can be as brief as a few seconds to a few minutes or persist for several hours. Symptoms triggered by sudden movement, which are termed *kinesigenic*, are typically brief; prolonged episodes are commonly triggered by exercise, stress, fatigue, caffeine, or alcohol. Paroxysmal dyskinesias may be genetically determined, idiopathic, the manifestation of another disorder (e.g., head injury, brain tumor, or stroke), or even psychologically based. A mutation of the *PRRT2* gene has been described in a large proportion of genetically determined paroxysmal kinesigenic dystonia.

TREATMENT   Rx

Ideally, treatment is directed at the underlying cause, such as dopa-responsive dystonia, which is treated with levodopa (usually up to 300 mg/day) or Wilson disease by copper chelation (Chapter 200). Patients with mutations in the manganese transporter gene may benefit from chelation with ethylenediaminetetraacetic acid (EDTA) (see Table 19-2). Unfortunately, cause-specific treatment usually is not possible, so a variety of symptomatic treatments may be tried, often unsuccessfully, in an attempt to reduce disability.

Focal injections of botulinum toxin are now usually the first choice for treatment of focal and segmental dystonias.[A4] This approach can improve symptoms of patients with cranial (blepharospasm, oromandibular dystonia) and cervical dystonia. Patients with task-specific limb dystonias (e.g., writer's cramp) often benefit less because weakness of the treated muscles, which is the most common side effect of this therapy, can impair other important upper limb functions.

Young patients in particular can tolerate and benefit from high doses of anticholinergic drugs such as trihexyphenidyl (6 to 40 mg/day, but sometimes as much as 100 mg/day). However, high doses may affect school performance. Muscle relaxants, including benzodiazepines (diazepam, 5 to as much as 100 mg/day) and baclofen (40 to 120 mg/day), may provide some benefit. Dopamine-depleting (e.g., tetrabenazine, 50 to 200 mg/day) and dopamine-blocking (e.g., haloperidol, 3 to 30 mg/day) agents are occasionally helpful (more often effective in tardive dystonia than in other types). Paroxysmal kinesigenic dyskinesia usually responds well to anticonvulsant drugs. Paroxysmal exercise-induced dyskinesias are associated with mutations in the *SLC2A1* gene, which encodes the glucose transporter GLUT1, and may respond to a ketogenic diet. Deep brain stimulation of the internal segment of the globus pallidus, thalamus, and the subthalamic nucleus,[14] can be considered in medically refractory, disabling dystonia, especially in patients with idiopathic dystonia (e.g., DYT1, adult-onset cervical dystonia). However, the target should be chosen based on symptoms and clinical findings.

TICS

EPIDEMIOLOGY AND PATHOBIOLOGY

Tics are repetitive, stereotyped movements (motor tics) or vocalizations (vocal tics). Transient tics are extremely common in childhood, and simple tics may begin in childhood and persist throughout adult life. Most tics (Table 382-6) are primary or idiopathic and have no identifiable cause. Secondary tics are caused by a defined underlying brain disease or environmental factor. The tics of Tourette syndrome are now classified as a neurodevelopmental disorder.

CLINICAL MANIFESTATIONS

Tics vary in terms of complexity, from abrupt, brief, meaningless movements or sounds (simple motor tics such as eye blinking, nose wrinkling, or head jerking; simple vocal-phonic tics such as sniffing, throat clearing, or grunting) to more sustained, more deliberate, almost meaningful gestures or utterances (complex motor tics such as touching, hand shaking, and jumping; complex vocal tics such as echolalia [repeating others], palilalia [repeating oneself], and coprolalia [uttering profanities]). The frequency of the tics in an individual patient varies markedly over minutes, hours, days, weeks, and years.

DIAGNOSIS

Various characteristics help to differentiate tics from other abnormal movements. Tics are often described by patients as being "semivoluntary" in response to an inner, irresistible urge. Premonitory sensory symptoms occasionally precede the tic, usually in the same general anatomic area as the tic itself. Relief is often associated with the production of the tic. Tics can be partially or completely voluntarily suppressed for variable periods, but often at the expense of mounting inner tension and psychological discomfort. Performing the tic or sometimes even substituting another more acceptable behavior for the socially inappropriate tic alleviates the tension. Many patients report that

TABLE 382-6   ETIOLOGIC CLASSIFICATION OF TICS
PRIMARY OR IDIOPATHIC TICS
Transient motor or phonic tics
Chronic motor or phonic tics
Adult-onset tics
Tourette syndrome
SECONDARY TICS
Genetic disorders
Neuroacanthocytosis
Huntington disease
Neurodegeneration with brain iron accumulation 1 (NBIA 1) (previously Hallervorden-Spatz disease)
Idiopathic dystonia*
Tuberous sclerosis*
Chromosomal disorders
Infections
Sydenham chorea
PANDAS†
Encephalitis and postencephalitic disorders
Creutzfeldt-Jakob disease
Neurosyphilis
Drugs
Methylphenidate
Amphetamines
Cocaine
Levodopa
Carbamazepine
Phenytoin
Phenobarbital
Lamotrigine
Neuroleptics
Developmental disorders
Mental retardation
Pervasive developmental disorders/autism
Other causes
Head trauma
Stroke
Carbon monoxide poisoning
Cardiopulmonary bypass with hypothermia
RELATED DISORDERS
Mannerisms, stereotypies
Compulsions
Self-injurious behavior

Modified from Cloutier M, Lang AE. Movement disorders: an overview. In: Factor SA, Lang AE, Weiner WJ, eds. *Drug Induced Movement Disorders*. Malden, Mass: Blackwell; 2005:3-19.
*Tics have been described with these conditions but may simply be coincidental.
†Pediatric autoimmune neuropsychiatric disorders associated with streptococcal infections. The existence of this disorder remains somewhat controversial.

some tics occur in response to a typical urge, whereas the same or different tics may be unexpected and totally involuntary.

Tourette Syndrome
EPIDEMIOLOGY AND PATHOBIOLOGY

The exact relationship between childhood tics and Gilles de la Tourette syndrome remains uncertain. Tourette syndrome is a common disorder, with an overall prevalence of 7.7 per 1000 children. There is a male preponderance of 3:1 for the classic syndrome, but female patients manifest obsessive-compulsive features more often than tics. A functional mutation in the *HDC* gene encoding L-histidine decarboxylase can be a rare cause of Tourette syndrome, thereby suggesting a role for histaminic neurotransmission in its pathogenesis (Video 382-11). Two new copy number variants, NRXN1 and CNTN6, increase the risk of Tourette syndrome.[15]

CLINICAL MANIFESTATIONS AND DIAGNOSIS

The criteria for this disorder include the presence of multiple motor and at least one vocal tic beginning before the age of 21 years (typically between ages 2 and 10 years) and lasting for more than 1 year, waxing and waning symptoms over time (new tics replacing old ones; previous tics sometimes recurring years after they had originally resolved), and the absence of other explanatory medical conditions. Involuntary swearing (coprolalia), a highly publicized feature of the syndrome, is present in fewer than 10% of patients.

Patients commonly exhibit a variety of comorbid disorders, including obsessive-compulsive disorder, attention-deficit disorder (with or without hyperactivity), impulse control problems, and other behavioral disturbances.

TREATMENT   Rx

Most patients who fulfill diagnostic criteria for Tourette syndrome have mild symptoms that do not require drug treatment; education, reassurance, behavioral therapy,[16] and follow-up are often sufficient. When tics (isolated or as part of Tourette syndrome) interfere with social and physical function, low-dose clonazepam (0.5 to 4 mg/day) may be effective. Clonidine (0.05 to 0.5 mg/day) is variably effective in controlling tics and may be useful for impulse control and symptoms of attention-deficit/hyperactivity disorder (ADHD); alternatively, guanfacine (0.5 to 4 mg/day) can be used. The most effective treatments for disabling tics are the dopamine receptor blockers such as risperidone (0.5 to 16 mg/day), haloperidol (0.5 to 20 mg/day), pimozide (0.5 to 10 mg/day), fluphenazine (0.5 to 20 mg/day), and aripiprazole (5 to 15 mg/day),[17] but caution is required in view of the potential for important side effects, rarely including tardive dyskinesia, with long-term use. An alternative without this complication is the dopamine depleter tetrabenazine (50 to 200 mg/day). Injected botulinum toxin may be effective for simple motor tics of the face and neck and may also reduce the urge to perform the tic. More aggressive use of botulinum toxin in neck muscles should be considered in patients with very forceful neck tics, which have rarely been associated with complications such as noncompressive myelopathy and vertebral artery dissection. Comorbid ADHD can be treated safely with stimulant therapy (e.g., methylphenidate, 2.5 to 60 mg/day) without increasing the severity of tics. Obsessive-compulsive symptoms may respond well to selective serotonin reuptake inhibitors (e.g., clomipramine, 25-250 mg/day; paroxetine, 10 to 60 mg/day; or citalopram, 10 to 40 mg/day). Behavioral disorders, which remain a major therapeutic challenge, may require a variety of psychotherapeutic or behavioral modification approaches. Even in the absence of behavioral disturbances, comprehensive behavioral intervention therapy, which incorporates habit reversal training, can be very effective as first-line therapy for tic disorders. Promising preliminary reports of deep brain stimulation require confirmation in controlled clinical trials.

PROGNOSIS

The natural history of Tourette syndrome is to stabilize and in the majority of cases to improve in adolescence. Approximately half of patients have a complete or partial remission at this time.

● MYOCLONUS

DEFINITION

Myoclonus (or myoclonic jerks) consists of sudden, brief, shocklike, involuntary movements that result from both active muscle contraction (positive myoclonic jerks) and brief inhibition of ongoing muscle activity (negative myoclonic jerks). The most common form of a negative myoclonic jerk is asterixis.

PATHOBIOLOGY

Myoclonus generally arises in the central nervous system, although rare peripheral causes are described, and it is distinct from abnormal muscle activity associated with peripheral nervous system diseases, such as fasciculations or myokymia. Myoclonus can be classified according to origin (E-Table 382-1), including physiologic, essential, epileptic, and symptomatic forms. Physiologic myoclonus, such as hypnic (sleep) jerks and hiccups, occurs in normal healthy subjects. Patients with essential myoclonus, which may be sporadic or inherited, often have additional postural tremor or dystonia, and this disorder is probably the same as what is now referred to as myoclonus dystonia (see Dystonias, earlier). Epileptic myoclonus arises in the context of seizures (Chapter 375), including many inherited generalized epileptic syndromes and the progressive myoclonic epilepsies. Symptomatic myoclonus occurs in association with a large number of encephalopathic states.

CLINICAL MANIFESTATIONS

Myoclonic jerks are very short, typically persisting for less than 100 msec, although occasional patients have longer muscle bursts. Myoclonus can be spontaneous, action induced, reflex (induced by various sensory stimuli), or a combination. Spontaneous myoclonus occurs at rest, without any provocation. Action myoclonus occurs during purposeful movement and is often very disabling owing to its interference with volitional activity. Reflex myoclonus

can be triggered by visual, auditory, or somesthetic stimuli. The distribution of myoclonus may be focal, segmental, multifocal, or generalized. When myoclonus involves more than one body area, the movements may be synchronous or asynchronous. Myoclonus can be intermittent or repetitive, and it sometimes is rhythmic (e.g., usually originating in the brainstem or spinal cord). Palatal myoclonus, now referred to as palatal tremor, is a rhythmic movement disorder originating in the brainstem and involving the soft palate as well as the eyes, facial muscles, neck, and limbs; it is commonly the result of a focal lesion (e.g., stroke, demyelination) in the connections between the dentate nucleus of the cerebellum and the inferior olives of the medulla (symptomatic palatal tremor), and it may persist during sleep.

DIAGNOSIS

Myoclonus can be classified according to the anatomic site of origin, usually with the assistance of detailed electrophysiologic assessments.[18] These sites may be cortical, subcortical (e.g., thalamic, lower brainstem [reticular myoclonus]), or spinal (two types: spinal segmental and propriospinal).

TREATMENT   Rx

Management of myoclonus, when possible, should be directed specifically at the underlying cause. Drug treatment includes a variety of anticonvulsant medications, most notably clonazepam (1.5 to 15 mg/day), valproic acid (10 to 15 mg/kg/day), carbamazepine (600 to 1200 mg/day), and levetiracetam (1000 to 4000 mg/day). Lacosamide (200 to 400 mg/day) is also effective in select patients. Postanoxic action myoclonus (the Lance-Adams syndrome) in some patients who survive severe cerebral anoxia also may respond to 5-hydroxy-tryptophan (400 to 2800 mg/day) given with carbidopa (75 to 300 mg/day). Acetazolamide (250 to 1000 mg/day) may be useful for patients with action myoclonus. Zonisamide (300 mg/day) improves myoclonus and related disability in patients with myoclonus-dystonia.^{A5}

● HYPEREXPLEXIA

Hyperexplexia, which is a disorder related to myoclonus, manifests as an excessive startle response to tactile, visual, and/or auditory stimulations. Genetic causes are mainly abnormalities in synaptic transmission of the inhibitory neurotransmitter glycine, including glycine receptor α_1 gene (*GLRA1*), glycine receptor subunit gene (*GLRB*), and the presynaptic glycine transporter 2 gene *SLC6A5*. Some patients demonstrate only generalized body jerking or an exaggerated startle response that habituates poorly after repeated stimuli. By comparison, other patients experience disabling stiffness in response to sudden unexpected stimuli, such as a loud sound. The disorder typically responds well to clonazepam (1.5 to 15 mg/day) therapy. Additional medications that have been tried with mixed results include clobazam, levetiracetam, valproic acid, and phenobarbital.

● OTHER MOVEMENT DISORDERS
Drug-Induced Movement Disorders

All the movements listed in Table 382-1 can be induced by medications. Neuroleptic drugs, which block postsynaptic dopamine receptors, particularly the D2 subtype, can result in a variety of movement disorder syndromes, including acute dystonic reactions, akathisia, drug-induced parkinsonism (including the "rabbit syndrome" with perinasal and perioral rest tremor), the neuroleptic malignant syndrome, and a variety of later-onset, often persistent, movements referred to as tardive dyskinesia. Metronidazole also rarely can cause an encephalopathy that typically manifests as dysarthria and gait instability.

ACUTE DYSTONIC REACTIONS

Acute dystonic reactions (Chapter 406) are most often seen in young patients who are receiving potent antipsychotic agents (e.g., young male patients receiving high doses of haloperidol for acute psychosis), but they also occur in patients receiving dopamine receptor blockers, including metoclopramide as antiemetic therapy. Symptoms range from overt dystonic postures of the face and neck, to involuntary prolonged deviation of the eyes (oculogyric crises), to simple slurring of speech and difficulty coordinating the tongue. Symptoms often vary from moment to moment and can increase with anxiety and improve with relaxation or reassurance. Acute dystonic reactions are self-limited and respond rapidly to a parenteral injection of an anticholinergic drug such as benztropine (2 mg intravenously [IV] followed by 2 mg three orally [PO] times daily for a variable duration depending on neuroleptic use) or an antihistaminic such as diphenhydramine (50 mg IV followed by oral benztropine).

AKATHISIA

Akathisia refers to a sense of restlessness and a need to move. Typically, the patient performs a variety of purposeful or semipurposeful, often complex, movements in response to an uncomfortable subjective restlessness, including pacing when standing, marching in place, rocking, shifting weight, moving legs when sitting, picking at clothing or hair, rubbing body parts with hands, and other similar movements. Akathisia is most often a side effect of medications, especially neuroleptic drugs and selective serotonin reuptake inhibitors (Chapter 369). Symptoms occur in a dose-related fashion and usually resolve on drug withdrawal. Akathisia is a common reason for psychiatric patients to comply poorly with their medications; management includes adjustment of the dose or type of antipsychotic agent and trials of β-blockers (e.g., propranolol, 80 mg/day) or antiparkinson agents, such as anticholinergics (e.g., benztropine (6 mg/day) or amantadine (200 to 300 mg/day). Rare patients experience a very disabling and persistent form referred to as tardive akathisia. Akathisia is also sometimes seen in patients with Parkinson disease.

NEUROLEPTIC MALIGNANT SYNDROME

The neuroleptic malignant syndrome (Chapters 404 and 406) is an uncommon but severe, sometimes fatal, complication of neuroleptic therapy. Patients usually manifest a combination of features including fever, marked rigidity, changes in level of arousal, and autonomic instability. Laboratory abnormalities include a marked increase in the serum creatine kinase level and the blood leukocyte count. Management involves early recognition, withdrawal of the causative agent, systemic supportive therapy, a dopamine agonist (most experience has been with the older agent bromocriptine, ≤60 mg/day), and, when necessary, dantrolene sodium (50 to 600 mg/day PO or ≤10 mg/kg/day IV) to reduce muscle contraction.

TARDIVE DYSKINESIA

EPIDEMIOLOGY AND PATHOBIOLOGY

The term *tardive dyskinesia* encompasses a wide variety of abnormal movements caused by chronic neuroleptic therapy (Chapter 406). The cumulative 5-year incidence rate in patients taking classic neuroleptics is approximately 25%, and the incidence may continue to increase almost linearly beyond that point. The annualized risk is estimated to be 5% in haloperidol-treated patients compared with 2% in patients treated with atypical neuroleptics (Video 382-12). The pathophysiology commonly has been attributed to hypersensitivity or upregulation of dopamine D2 receptors induced by chronic blockade. However, this explanation is generally felt to be inadequate, especially for more persistent symptoms, and other proposed mechanisms include oxidative stress from increased dopamine turnover and a maladaptive synaptic plasticity.

CLINICAL MANIFESTATIONS

Tardive dyskinesia generally begins after a minimum of 6 weeks of treatment. One of the most common forms involves the lower facial muscles and has been given a variety of names, including orobuccolinguomasticatory dyskinesia.[19] The movements generally include repetitive chewing and smacking movements with the tongue either protruding between the lips (fly-catching movements) or pushing into the cheek (bonbon sign). Although the movements are somewhat choreic, they are not as random as true chorea. The more stereotypical, repetitive nature of the movements, involving not only face but also the limbs (e.g., piano playing movements of the fingers, rocking or thrusting of the pelvis), has encouraged the more recent term *tardive stereotypies*. This term, however, fails to fulfill the definition of stereotypy owing to the lack of distractibility and the unpredictability of the sequence of movements. Many patients with classic orofacial tardive dyskinesia seem unaware of the presence of the movements and are not disabled by them, but others are embarrassed or otherwise impaired.

Tardive akathisia and tardive dystonia are less common but particularly disabling subtypes of tardive dyskinesia. Rarer forms include tardive tics (tourettism), tardive tremor, tardive myoclonus, and even tardive oral or genital pain.

TREATMENT AND PROGNOSIS

Rx

Treatment is often unsatisfactory, but the dopamine depleters deutetrabenazine (starting at 6 mg daily and increasing up to 48 mg daily), [AG] valbenazine (40 mg daily for the week, then 40 mg or 80 mg daily),[20] and tetrabenazine (50 to 200 mg/day) can be very effective. Other drugs that possibly provide benefit include amantadine, propranolol, zolpidem, ginkgo biloba, and clonazepam. Consideration should be given to discontinuing concurrent anticholinergic medications. Prevention is the most important consideration. The physician must regularly reassess the need for ongoing neuroleptic therapy, consider switching to an atypical agent when possible (particularly quetiapine and clozapine; Chapter 369), and routinely evaluate the patient for the presence of early subtle clinical features, such as mild pursing of the lips or rolling movements of the tongue in the mouth. Unfortunately, tardive dyskinesia may persist for many years despite withdrawal of neuroleptic treatment in up to 50% of patients. Several atypical neuroleptics, such as risperidone and olanzapine, nevertheless block dopamine D2 receptors sufficiently to cause drug-induced parkinsonism and tardive dyskinesias.

Restless Legs Syndrome

EPIDEMIOLOGY

Restless legs syndrome (Chapter 377) is now recognized as an extremely common disorder affecting between 3 and 29% of the general population. Women are affected more frequently than men. Although the incidence increases with age, it also can affect children, in whom it may be confused with "growing pains" or ADHD.

PATHOBIOLOGY

Restless legs syndrome is most often primary or idiopathic, in which case it is frequently inherited in an autosomal dominant fashion. Eight genetic loci associated with restless legs syndrome include variants in *MEIS1, BTBD9, MAP2K5/LBXCOR1, PTPRD,* and *PCDHA3,* as well as loci on 2p14 and 16q12.1. Restless legs syndrome also may be secondary to other causes, including peripheral neuropathy, uremia, pregnancy, and iron deficiency, and it may occur more commonly than by chance in some neurodegenerative disorders such as Parkinson disease. The pathophysiology of restless legs syndrome is uncertain, but central iron dysregulation may somehow alter central dopamine. Serum ferritin levels are often low, even in the presence of normal values of hemoglobin, hematocrit, iron, and iron-binding capacity.

CLINICAL MANIFESTATIONS AND DIAGNOSIS

In restless legs syndrome, as in akathisia, movements occur because of the subjective need to move. However, unlike in akathisia, the patient typically complains of a variety of sensory disturbances in the legs, including pins and needles, creeping or crawling sensations, aching, itching, stabbing, heaviness, tension, burning, or coldness.[21] Occasionally, similar symptoms are appreciated in the upper limbs or other areas of the body. These symptoms are usually experienced during periods of prolonged inactivity, especially with recumbency in the evening, and are often associated with insomnia (Chapter 377). The discomfort appears particularly during the transition from wake to sleep in the evening and often follows a circadian pattern, peaking between midnight and 4 AM. Symptoms are typically relieved only by movement or stimulation of the legs; although these maneuvers are effective while they are being performed, the discomfort usually returns as soon as the individual becomes inactive or returns to bed to try to sleep. Patients often have significant problems with immobility during long automobile drives or plane flights.

In approximately 80% of patients, this condition is associated with another movement disorder, periodic leg movements in sleep, sometimes inappropriately called nocturnal myoclonus. These periodic, slow, sustained (1 to 2 seconds) movements range from synchronous or asynchronous dorsiflexion of the toes and feet to triple flexion of one or both legs. In 15% of patients, more rapid myoclonic movements or slower, prolonged dystonic-like movements of the feet and legs are present while patients are awake. In the absence of evidence of a secondary cause of restless legs syndrome, the only useful routine test is a serum ferritin level.

TREATMENT   Rx

Dopamine agonists (e.g., pramipexole, 0.125 to 1.5 mg at bedtime), ropinirole (0.25 to 3 mg at bedtime), and transdermal rotigotine (1 to 3 mg/24 hours) are the treatments of choice in moderate-to-severe restless legs syndrome and can be very effective.[22] Impulse control disorders are an occasional side effect. Levodopa preparations (100 to 300 mg of levodopa at bedtime; consider controlled-release preparation) are also effective but are more often associated with disabling rebound symptoms early in the morning or during the day (augmentation). Gabapentin enacarbil (a gabapentin prodrug at 600 to 1200 mg/day) is also effective and approved in the United States at the 600-mg dose.[A7] Patients with milder symptoms may respond to gabapentin (300 to 2400 mg/day). Opiate agonists (e.g., oxycodone, 5 mg at bedtime; codeine, 30 mg at bedtime; propoxyphene, 65 mg or N-100 mg at bedtime) and less often benzodiazepines (e.g., clonazepam, 0.5 to 2 mg at bedtime) also may be effective. Tolerance or loss of original benefit may occur with all these treatments. Iron replacement is indicated in patients with reduced serum ferritin levels (325 mg ferrous sulfate two or three times per day for 3 to 4 months until ferritin levels exceed 50 mg/L and iron saturations exceed 20%). Deep brain stimulation may be effective but is rarely required.[23]

Painful Legs and Moving Toes

Another uncommon but well-defined movement disorder of the lower limbs has been termed *painful legs and moving toes*. Patients typically complain of a deep pulling or searing pain in the lower limbs, associated with continuous involuntary wriggling or writhing of the toes. Occasionally, the ankle and less commonly more proximal muscles of the legs are involved. Rarely, a similar problem is seen in the upper limbs as well. Although a peripheral nerve trigger, such as a radiculopathy, may be evident, the pain and movements probably are generated centrally in the spinal cord or brainstem. Various treatments have been tried without much benefit to the pain, which is typically the major concern of the patient.

Other Abnormal Movements

Numerous abnormal movements are caused by dysfunction of the peripheral nerves (e.g., fasciculations, myokymia); these movements are usually easily separated from the movement disorders described earlier. *Hemifacial spasm* is a common disorder in which irregular clonic and tonic movements involve the muscles innervated by the facial nerve, usually owing to compression of the seventh nerve as it exits the brainstem, most often by a normal small artery or vein and less often by a mass lesion or inflammatory process. Eyelid twitching is usually the first symptom, followed at variable intervals by lower facial muscle involvement. MRI with careful assessment of the posterior fossa is necessary to exclude secondary causes. Treatment usually involves injections of botulinum toxin into selected facial muscles, although surgical decompression can be curative (Video 382-13).

Cerebellar Ataxias and Spastic Paraplegias

There are an extremely large number of causes of cerebellar ataxia (Table 382-7). Many are hereditary, with the full spectrum of possible inheritance patterns. Sporadic or noninherited ataxias are common; in many cases, a cause can be defined and treatment may be effective in halting or even reversing the process. However, a large proportion of ataxias in adults are progressive, presumably owing to a degenerative cause, many of which remain to be determined.

HEREDITARY CEREBELLAR ATAXIAS

The hereditary cerebellar ataxias, which may begin in childhood or adulthood, can progress at widely varying rates. During the preclinical stage, subtle abnormalities may be detected on a careful clinical examination.[24] These ataxias are divided into early-onset ataxias, which are usually inherited as autosomal recessive disorders, and adult-onset ataxias, which are usually autosomal dominant. A small number are X-linked.[25] Because most of these ataxias are untreatable, it is important to recognize the rare causes of treatable or preventable progressive ataxias.

Friedreich Ataxia
EPIDEMIOLOGY AND PATHOBIOLOGY

The most common progressive inherited ataxia in children is Friedreich ataxia. Friedreich ataxia is a trinucleotide-repeat disorder that affects the central and

TABLE 382-7	DIFFERENTIAL DIAGNOSIS OF ADULT-ONSET ATAXIA

Inherited
  Autosomal dominant, including the spinocerebellar ataxias (SCAs)
  Autosomal recessive, including Friedreich ataxia
  X-linked, including fragile X tremor ataxia syndrome (FXTAS)
  Mitochondrial
  Episodic ataxias
  Ataxia telangiectasia
Autoimmune (e.g., paraneoplastic, anti-GAD antibodies, postinfectious)
Degenerative (e.g., multiple system atrophy [MSA-C])
Demyelinating (e.g., multiple sclerosis)
Infectious
Metabolic (e.g., hypothyroidism, vitamin E deficiency)
Stroke
Trauma (e.g., closed head injury)
Toxic (e.g., alcoholic cerebellar degeneration, lithium)
Tumor: Primary and secondary brain tumors

GAD = glutamate decarboxylase.

peripheral nervous systems, the heart, and many other organs. Friedreich ataxia is an autosomal recessive disorder with no anticipation. It has an estimated carrier frequency in the population of approximately 1 in 100 and a resulting disease prevalence of approximately 1 per 50,000.

The normal length of the GAA repeat on the long arm of chromosome 9 (9q13-q21) is 10 to 21 copies, but expansion in individuals with Friedreich ataxia results in 200 to 900 copies and disrupts the expression of the protein frataxin. GAA unstable expansion, which occurs on an intron, leads to gene silencing rather than to the production of an abnormal protein. Higher numbers of copies correlate with more severe neurologic deficits. Frataxin appears to be critical for iron export and mitochondrial function. Because accumulation of mitochondrial iron affects the production of oxygen radicals, loss of frataxin may lead to oxidative mitochondrial damage. The pathology of Friedreich ataxia includes spinal cord atrophy, which often is evident on MRI, with loss of neurons in Clarke columns and the dorsal root ganglia. Degeneration occurs in spinocerebellar tracts, pyramidal tracts, dorsal column tracts, and peripheral nerves, with minor cell loss in the brainstem and cerebellum. Cardiomyopathy is associated with ventricular hypertrophy and chronic interstitial myocardial fibrosis.

CLINICAL MANIFESTATIONS AND DIAGNOSIS

Typical Friedreich ataxia first manifests clinically during puberty with progressive ataxia, loss of lower extremity deep tendon reflexes, and extensor plantar responses (i.e., Babinski signs).[26] Other common clinical features include nystagmus, dysarthria, stocking-glove sensory loss, and weakness in the lower extremities. Patients frequently have kyphosis, scoliosis, and pes cavus. Interstitial myocardial disease may cause a typical hypertrophic cardiomyopathy (Chapter 54). A small number of patients have a later onset and a less severe and progressive course, sometimes with retained or even brisk reflexes.

The diagnosis is made by genetic testing for the trinucleotide repeat expansion, which usually is present on at least one allele. Point mutations are sometimes present in the other allele and are more difficult to detect. Potentially treatable conditions with similar clinical manifestations include vitamin B_{12} deficiency (Chapter 205), abetalipoproteinemia (Chapter 131), and a selective defect in vitamin E absorption (Chapter 205).

TREATMENT AND PROGNOSIS   Rx

No effective disease-modifying treatments are available, so treatment consists of supportive measures. Intensive inpatient rehabilitation can improve overall function. Nicotinamide can increase frataxin concentrations, but whether it alters the clinical course of the disease is unproven. Future treatments may include histone deacetylase inhibitors that may increase frataxin gene expression. The disorder is progressive, and patients usually are wheelchair bound by their mid-20s. The average age at death is 37 years, and the major cause of death is hypertrophic cardiomyopathy (Chapter 54).

Other Spinocerebellar Ataxias

The hereditary spinocerebellar ataxias are routinely classified by their specific molecular diagnosis. At least 20 autosomal recessive and more than 35 autosomal dominant cerebellar ataxias have been identified. Clinical features, ethnic origin, and family history may suggest an autosomal recessive, autosomal dominant, or X-linked inheritance and often narrow the search for the genetic mutation. As the molecular pathogenesis of many of the hereditary ataxias is unraveled, the current numerical classification, which largely reflects the chronology of the identification of causative mutations, is likely to be replaced by a gene-specific or pathophysiologic approach. Spinocerebellar ataxias 1, 2, 3, 6, 7, and 17 are caused by trinucleotide expansions in or adjacent to a protein-coding region of a gene. These expansions result in polyglutamine expansions in the protein product, which likely results in a toxic gain of function in a manner analogous to the pathogenesis of Huntington disease. Approximately 40 spinocerebellar ataxias have been described, but clear genotype-phenotype associations have not been confirmed for every type.[27,28]

CLINICAL MANIFESTATIONS AND DIAGNOSIS

The predominant clinical features of the spinocerebellar ataxias are ataxia and dysarthria. Other cerebellar signs include titubation, dysdiadochokinesia, and dysmetria. With increasing ataxia, patients can become wheelchair bound. Additional clinical signs include ophthalmoplegia, dementia, optic atrophy, retinal pigmentary degeneration, deafness, dysphagia, and peripheral neuropathy. Extrapyramidal features include masked facies, cogwheel rigidity, dystonia, athetosis, and chorea. Levodopa-responsive parkinsonism (Chapter 381) may be seen in some patients, particularly in spinocerebellar ataxias 2 and 3. Pyramidal dysfunction includes spastic limbs, especially legs; hyperreflexia; and Babinski response. Diagnosis is based on genetic testing.

TREATMENT AND PROGNOSIS Rx

In a small randomized trial, varenicline (a partial agonist of 24β2 neuronal nicotinic acetylcholine receptors, at 1 mg/day for 2 weeks, then 2 mg/day) improved gait, stance, and timed 25-foot walk but did not improve appendicular function, except for rapid alternating movements, in adults with genetically confirmed SCA3. However, these results have not been reproduced, and the drug is often poorly tolerated. Docosahexaenoic acid (600 mg daily) is effective for spinocerebellar ataxia 38, in which polyunsaturated fat metabolism is altered.[29] No treatment is currently available for the other spinocerebellar ataxias, although preliminary data indicate that physiotherapy may improve gait and balance. Cerebello-spinal direct current stimulation is a potential new option for the neurodegenerative ataxias.[A8] The spinocerebellar ataxias are progressive, with worsening gait, hand coordination, speech, and eye movements, but with preserved mental function in most forms. Pneumonia is a common cause of death.

HEREDITARY SPASTIC PARAPLEGIAS

Hereditary spastic paraplegias, also known as Strümpell disease, are a group of clinically and genetically heterogeneous monogenic neurodegenerative disorders. The prevalence is approximately 1 per 10,000 in the population. Over 70 different genetic loci have been identified; approximately 20 autosomal dominant, over 45 autosomal recessive, 5 X-linked, and 1 a maternal trait of inheritance. The most common forms of hereditary spastic paraplegia are autosomal dominant mutations in one of four proteins: spastin (SPG4), atlastin-1 (SPG3A), *REEP1* (SPG31), and reticulon-2 (SPG12). These proteins are involved in the endoplasmic reticulum network, whose morphology and distribution in neurons has a special importance for their normal function. Defects of ganglioside biosyntheses and defects in glucocerebrosidase functions are present in some forms. At autopsy, patients with hereditary spastic paraplegia have axonal degeneration of the pyramidal tracts and dorsal column tracts with lesser involvement of the spinocerebellar tracts. The neurons of origin are intact. The peripheral nervous system is unaffected.

CLINICAL MANIFESTATIONS

Patients with hereditary spastic paraplegia have a progressive gait disturbance with spasticity of lower extremities, hyperreflexia, clonus, and extensor plantar responses. Cranial nerves, speech, swallowing, and upper extremities remain normal. Although patients can experience weakness of their lower extremities, spasticity is usually the disabling component. The progressively increased leg spasticity results in tripping and an inability to run. Pain is infrequent, and sensation is normal. Other clinical features include pes cavus (30 to 50%),

TABLE 382-8	DIFFERENTIAL DIAGNOSIS OF SPASTIC PARAPLEGIAS

Hereditary
    Dopa-responsive dystonia
    Spinocerebellar ataxias
    Adult-onset adrenoleukodystrophy (Chapters 214 and 383)
Structural lesions of the spinal cord (Chapter 372)
Cervical spondylosis (Chapter 372)
Tumor (Chapter 169)
Arteriovenous malformation (Chapter 380)
Syringomyelia (Chapter 389)
Multiple sclerosis (Chapter 383)
Primary lateral sclerosis (Chapter 391)
Vitamin B$_{12}$ deficiency (Chapter 388)
Copper deficiency (Chapter 388)
Infections
    Human immunodeficiency virus (Chapter 366)
    Human T-lymphotropic virus type 1 (Chapter 354)
    Tertiary syphilis (Chapter 303)

decreased vibratory sensation, and urinary frequency, urgency, and hesitancy. Pure hereditary spastic paraplegia is limited to symptoms and signs of spasticity, whereas complex or complicated hereditary spastic paraplegia can include cognitive impairment, dementia, epilepsy, extrapyramidal disturbances, cerebellar involvement, retinopathy, optic atrophy, deafness, polyneuropathy, or skin lesions.

DIAGNOSIS

Hereditary spastic paraplegia is diagnosed when patients meet clinical criteria and when other causes of spasticity are excluded. MRI may show spinal cord atrophy, but cerebrospinal fluid analysis and nerve conduction studies are normal. The differential diagnosis of spastic paraplegia includes other genetic conditions, spinal cord disease from structural lesions, multiple sclerosis, and vitamin deficiencies or retroviral infections (Table 382-8). Even a positive family history does not obviate the need to exclude potentially treatable alternative diagnoses.

TREATMENT AND PROGNOSIS Rx

No specific treatment is available. Symptomatic therapy is aimed at decreasing disability and preventing complications, such as contractures. Antispastic agents, such as oral baclofen (usually 10 to 20 mg three times daily), improve spasticity but should be used with caution because they may worsen weakness. Some reports suggested an improved therapeutic response to intrathecal baclofen, but no controlled trials have addressed this issue. Preliminary data also raise the possible utility of injected botulinum neurotoxin type A injections for improving spasticity. Most patients become nonambulatory between 60 and 70 years of age. Patients with complicated hereditary spastic paraplegia often have other disabling features. Some patients with parkinsonism may benefit from dopaminergic therapies such as levodopa.

Grade A References

A1. Bruno E, Nicoletti A, Quattrocchi G, et al. Topiramate for essential tremor. *Cochrane Database Syst Rev.* 2017;4:CD009683.
A2. Elias WJ, Lipsman N, Ondo WG, et al. A randomized trial of focused ultrasound thalamotomy for essential tremor. *N Engl J Med.* 2016;375:730-739.
A3. Frank S, Testa CM, Stamler D, et al. Effect of deutetrabenazine on chorea among patients with Huntington disease: a randomized clinical trial. *JAMA.* 2016;316:40-50.
A4. Hallett M, Albanese A, Dressler D, et al. Evidence-based review and assessment of botulinum neurotoxin for the treatment of movement disorders. *Toxicon.* 2013;67:94-114.
A5. Hainque E, Vidailhet M, Cozic N, et al. A randomized, controlled, double-blind, crossover trial of zonisamide in myoclonus-dystonia. *Neurology.* 2016;86:1729-1735.
A6. Fernandez HH, Factor SA, Hauser RA, et al. Randomized controlled trial of deutetrabenazine for tardive dyskinesia: the ARM-TD study. *Neurology.* 2017;88:2003-2010.
A7. Kume A. Gabapentin enacarbil for the treatment of moderate to severe primary restless legs syndrome (Willis-Ekbom disease): 600 or 1,200 mg dose? *Neuropsychiatr Dis Treat.* 2014;10:249-262.
A8. Benussi A, Dell'Era V, Cantoni V, et al. Cerebello-spinal tDCS in ataxia: a randomized, double-blind, sham-controlled, crossover trial. *Neurology.* 2018;91:e1090-e1101.

GENERAL REFERENCES

For the General References and other additional features, please visit Expert Consult at https://expertconsult.inkling.com.

383

MULTIPLE SCLEROSIS AND DEMYELINATING CONDITIONS OF THE CENTRAL NERVOUS SYSTEM

PETER A. CALABRESI

The disorders of myelin encompass a wide range of diseases in which myelin is not produced (hypomyelination), myelin is not formed in a normal fashion (dysmyelinating disease), or normally formed myelin is destroyed or not maintained appropriately (demyelinating disease and myelinolysis) (Table 383-1).[1] Hypomyelinating and dysmyelinating diseases are uncommon and include an array of leukodystrophies that have a genetic basis and may affect the formation of myelin as a primary or secondary result. Demyelinating diseases are much more common and include multiple sclerosis (MS), which represents more than 95% of all types of disorders of central nervous system (CNS) myelin.

Some disorders of myelin have a distinct pathogenesis in which the disruption of myelin is secondary. Further, in many of the diseases of myelin, the axon degenerates as a result of decreased trophic support from loss of myelin, impaired health of the oligodendrocyte, or increased susceptibility to injury in the absence of myelin. This observation led to the recent hypothesis that axonal loss is the underlying substrate for permanent disability in MS, adrenoleukodystrophy, and perhaps other diseases of myelin.

MULTIPLE SCLEROSIS

DEFINITION

MS is a disease characterized by multifocal areas of demyelination in the brain and spinal cord, with associated inflammatory cell infiltrates, reactive gliosis, and axonal degeneration. It typically manifests in young adults with episodic neurologic dysfunction. Although the exact origin of MS remains enigmatic, evidence suggests that it is an immune-mediated attack on myelin, with secondary disruption of axons leading to progressive disability over time in most afflicted patients.

TABLE 383-1 DISEASES OF MYELIN

IDIOPATHIC

Recurrent or chronic progressive demyelination (multiple sclerosis and its variants)
Monophasic demyelination (may be the first clinical episode of multiple sclerosis)
Optic neuritis
Acute transverse myelitis
Acute disseminated encephalomyelitis; acute hemorrhagic leukoencephalopathy

VIRAL INFECTIONS

Progressive multifocal leukoencephalopathy
Subacute sclerosing panencephalitis (Chapter 346)

NUTRITIONAL AND METABOLIC DISORDERS (Chapter 388)

Combined systems disease (vitamin B_{12} deficiency)
Copper deficiency (dorsal columns and subacute optic neuropathy)
Demyelination of the corpus callosum (Marchiafava-Bignami disease)
Central pontine myelinolysis

ANOXIC-ISCHEMIC SEQUELAE (Chapter 376)

Delayed postanoxic cerebral demyelination
Progressive subcortical ischemic encephalopathy

LEUKODYSTROPHIES PRIMARILY AFFECTING CENTRAL NERVOUS SYSTEM MYELIN

Adrenoleukodystrophy (Schilder disease)
Pelizaeus-Merzbacher disease (sudanophilic leukodystrophies)
Spongy degeneration
Vanishing white matter disease
Others (Alexander disease, Canavan disease)
Leukodystrophies of the central and peripheral nervous system
Metachromatic leukodystrophy
Globoid cell leukodystrophy (Krabbe disease)

EPIDEMIOLOGY

The annual incidence of MS varies by location and ranges between 1.5 and 11 per 100,000 people. MS is second only to trauma as the most common cause of neurologic disability in young adults. Recent studies suggest that the incidence rate has increased, in part because of recognition of more cases at an earlier stage, but probably also because of a truly rising incidence, especially in women. The prevalence is estimated at 150 per 100,000 in the adult U.S. population, which translates to about 400,000 cases in the United States and more than 2 million worldwide, but these numbers may be underestimates owing to incomplete recognition of the disease, even in developed countries, and the increased incidence since these estimates were made.

MS occurs two- to 2.5-fold more frequently in women than in men, a sex predilection that is common in autoimmune diseases. The disease most often manifests in the third to fourth decades of life, but with an incidence age range from postpubertal teenagers to persons in their 50s. Rare cases occur in infants or in patients in their 60s, but extreme caution is warranted in these situations to exclude alternative processes. In many of the late-onset MS cases, symptoms were present in younger years and were attributed to other causes.

MS is most common in people of Northern European descent. In many areas of the world, MS is more prevalent in temperate latitudes (approaching one in 500 in some locations) and becomes less common toward the Equator (one in 20,000 or rare case reports only in some locations), perhaps explained in part by migration patterns of people with the same gene pools. However, the absence of complete genetic penetrance in monozygotic twin studies and recent increases in incidence in genetically stable populations strongly suggest an environmental component to the disease. Indeed, an outbreak of MS was documented on the Faroe Islands following World War II, and numerous other clusters have been reported, although a single environmental trigger has not been identified.

Several studies have linked cigarette smoking with risk for MS. High levels of vitamin D and early exposure to excessive sunlight (sunburns) have been linked with lower risk for MS, possibly related to the beneficial effects of cholecalciferol (vitamin D) on regulating immune cell responses.

PATHOBIOLOGY AND GENETICS

Monozygotic twins with MS show a concordance rate of between 15 and 50%, compared with only 3 to 5% concordance in dizygotic twins, consistent with a strong but incomplete role for genes in causing MS. The lifetime risk for MS is increased to 2 to 4% in individuals with a first-degree relative with MS, compared with the general population risk of 0.1%. In addition, between 10 and 20% of patients with MS have a first-degree relative with another autoimmune disease, commonly rheumatoid arthritis, systemic lupus erythematosus, or autoimmune thyroid disease. Psoriasis (Chapter 409) and inflammatory bowel disease (Chapter 132) also may be more common in patients with MS. Genetic modeling of the disease strongly argues against a single MS gene and suggests that many different genes predispose to MS and account for its many phenotypes and its overlap with other autoimmune diseases. Linkage and association studies have identified the human leukocyte antigen (HLA) or major histocompatibility complex (MHC) region on chromosome 6p21 as one genetic determinant for MS. The MHC class II region, involved in presentation of antigen to CD4$^+$ T cells, is the most strongly associated locus. The HLA-DR2 allele and, more specifically, the molecular haplotype HLA-DRB1*1501 allele have repeatedly been implicated. Multiple single-nucleotide polymorphisms (SNPs) in the interleukin-2 (IL-2) receptor-α gene and the IL-7 receptor-α gene also appear to be associated with a higher risk for MS. Over 200 other gene SNPs have been identified, most of which are related to immune function. Although patterns are emerging to suggest dysregulation of differing immune cell subsets, the associations to date are not strong enough to have clinical predictive value.

PATHOLOGY

Most cases are characterized by multifocal areas of demyelination and gross gliotic scar in the brain and spinal cord. Classic locations of these lesions, called *plaques*, are the optic nerves, periventricular white matter, deep white matter, juxtacortical white matter, corpus callosum, cerebellar peduncles, and dorsolateral spinal cord. However, there is a bias toward recognition of lesions in white matter because of the relative ease of detecting demyelination and inflammation in white compared with gray matter. Indeed, more recent pathologic studies have confirmed demyelination, neuritic damage, and atrophy in the cerebral cortex (pial surface and intracortical or juxtacortical) and deep gray matter structures, especially the thalamus. At the microscopic level, one usually sees multiple areas of perivenular inflammatory cell infiltrates with extravasation into the surrounding tissue parenchyma. In the acute active plaque, CD4 helper T (T$_H$) cells are prominent in the perivenular areas. Proinflammatory cytokines released from T$_H$1 (interferon-γ [IFN-γ]) and T$_H$17 (IL-17, tumor necrosis factor [TNF], and granulocyte-macrophage colony-stimulating factor [GM-CSF]) cells are thought to mediate damage. Increasingly, large numbers of CD8 cytotoxic T cells have been documented in brain tissue, especially in the parenchyma, and these cells may mediate direct damage to axons and oligodendrocytes through release of proteases such as granzyme B. Most parenchymal inflammatory cells, especially in chronic plaques, are CD68$^+$ macrophages and microglia. In addition to the influx of circulating immune cells, prominent astroglial activation and in some cases oligodendrocyte precursor cell differentiation occur in response to injury. Over time, the inflammation becomes less prominent in the center of the plaque, but a chronic active rim of inflammation with microglial activation exists at a well-demarcated border between abnormal and normal unharmed myelin. This characteristic of MS is seldom seen in other disorders of myelin. Although oligodendrocytes may survive, proliferate, and result in partial remyelination (shadow plaques) in some early cases, this process is hardly ever complete in MS. Over time, remyelination is less successful, and oligodendrocyte precursor cells appear unable to differentiate into mature myelinating oligodendrocytes.

The number of damaged axons correlates with the extent of inflammation. Further, axonal damage and even neuronal apoptosis and loss are seen in the cortex and retina. Atrophy of both the brain and spinal cord, which occurs more rapidly in MS than in normal aging, reflects loss of both myelin and axons.

No consistent microbial cause has been discerned from careful examination of MS tissues for known infectious pathogens. Differential expression of human herpesvirus type 6, which is acquired by most people in childhood, has been noted in oligodendrocytes of patients with MS, but whether this virus is a cofactor in demyelination or just a bystander remains unclear. Evidence suggests the possibility that the earliest event in MS may be an insult to the oligodendrocytes, with subsequent activation of resident immune cells and secondary recruitment of other immune cells only at later stages.

Some pathologists believe that four distinct subtypes of MS can be discerned, in which the pathologic characteristics are consistent in every lesion, thereby allowing classification of patients with differing pathologic categories rather than just describing evolution of lesions over time. Type I lesions are characterized by typical perivenular inflammatory infiltrates consisting mainly of T cells, with early preservation of oligodendrocytes. Type II lesions are similar to type I but have an additional humoral component with immunoglobulin G (IgG) deposition and complement activation. Type III lesions are distinguished by not being based around venules and by prominent loss of myelin-associated glycoprotein, with evidence for oligodendrocyte apoptosis. Type IV lesions have inflammatory infiltrates more similar to those in types I and II but also have oligodendrocyte loss as in type III. These varying pathologic features may begin to explain clinical subtypes of the disease.

PATHOGENESIS

It remains possible that the autoimmune hypothesis is wrong and that the inflammation observed in MS is secondary to an as yet uncharacterized primary degenerative process. Proponents of this theory cite evidence from pathologic features of hyperacute cases, in which the oligodendrocytes appear to die before any systemic immune response occurs, as well as recent data revealing neuronal and axonal death or demyelination in the absence of inflammation.

Macrophages and microglia, which make up the majority of cells within the parenchymal infiltrate in chronic MS plaques, are potent antigen-presenting cells and express HLA and costimulatory molecules. Activated macrophages and microglia also have effector functions, including release of cytokines that are partly (IL-6, TNF-α) or completely distinct from the T cells (IL-1β, IL-12, and IL-23). In high concentrations, these cytokines may damage oligodendrocytes and neurons and activate T cells.

CLINICAL MANIFESTATIONS
Presenting Symptoms

MS, which can manifest in many ways across a broad age range, may initially masquerade as a variety of different illnesses (Table 383-2; see Table 383-1).[2] In a classic presentation, a young white person, more often a woman, will have the acute to subacute onset of impaired vision or sensation. Fatigue, depression, bladder urgency, weakness, impaired balance, and impaired

TABLE 383-2	CONDITIONS THAT CAN BE MISTAKEN FOR MULTIPLE SCLEROSIS AND OTHER DISEASES OF MYELIN

VASCULAR DISEASE

Small-vessel cerebrovascular disease
Vasculitides
Arteriovenous malformation
CADASIL, CARASIL, COL4A1
Antiphospholipid antibody syndrome

STRUCTURAL LESIONS

Craniocervical junction, posterior fossa, or spinal tumors
Cervical spondylosis or disc herniation
Chiari malformation or syrinx

DEGENERATIVE DISEASES

Hereditary myelopathy
Hereditary neuropathy
Spinocerebellar degeneration

INFECTIONS

HTLV-1 infection
HIV myelopathy or HIV-related cerebritis
Neuroborreliosis (e.g., Lyme disease)
JC virus/progressive multifocal leukoencephalopathy
Neurosyphilis

OTHER INFLAMMATORY CONDITIONS

Systemic lupus erythematosus
Sjögren syndrome
Sarcoidosis
Autoimmune encephalitis

MONOFOCAL OR MONOPHASIC DEMYELINATING SYNDROMES

Transverse myelitis
Optic neuritis
Neuromyelitis optica/Devic disease
Acute disseminated encephalomyelitis

OTHER CONDITIONS

Hashimoto thyroiditis with or without encephalopathy
Nonspecific MRI abnormalities related to migraine, aging, or trauma
Leukodystrophy

CADASIL = cerebral autosomal dominant arteriopathy with subcortical infarcts and leukoencephalopathy; CARASIL = cerebral autosomal recessive arteriopathy with subcortical infarcts and leukoencephalopathy; COL4A1 = collagen type IV alpha 1 chain gene mutation; HIV = human immunodeficiency virus; HTLV = human T-cell lymphotropic virus; MRI = magnetic resonance imaging.

coordination also are common symptoms. The often remarkably mild nature of the first symptoms often dissuades the patient from seeking medical attention or is insufficiently impressive to stimulate the physician to order diagnostic tests. Furthermore, patients may initially have few objective neurologic findings, especially between attacks.

Paresthesias of a limb that are circumferential and do not follow a dermatome suggest a spinal cord lesion; these symptoms often manifest distally and then ascend to involve more proximal parts of the limb, spread to the contralateral limb, or progress from a leg to an arm. Similarly, bandlike painful sensations around a limb or the torso also suggest a myelopathic process.

Incomplete transverse myelitis is a focal (partial) spinal cord syndrome that is usually inflammatory and does not follow vascular territories. It is a common presentation of MS.

Lhermitte sign, an electrical sensation moving down the spine into the limbs on flexion of the neck, is characteristic of cervical myelitis from any cause, including MS. Frank loss of sensation is less common as an early symptom or sign but is seen in more advanced cases. Burning, electrical, or deep aching sensations are also common in MS.

Sensory Abnormalities

On examination, the most common sensory findings are loss of vibration perception, most prominent in the feet, and incomplete spinal cord levels to pinprick or vibration, which are often more notable in a graded fashion rather than at a distinct level. Such sensory levels may be asymmetrical and differ by sensory modality because of isolated demyelination in the dorsal columns compared with the spinothalamic tracts. Patchy or seemingly nonanatomic focal areas of impaired sensation can occur, and some patients describe bizarre sensations such as water dripping or bugs crawling on an area of the body.

Visual Effects

Optic neuritis (Chapter 396) is a classic manifesting syndrome, typically with visual symptoms in one eye. In optic neuritis, patients often complain of pain over the temporal eyebrow and worsening on lateral eye movement. The visual impairment may be described as looking through frosted glass or a veil. The scotoma or area of greatest loss often can be mapped in a centrocecal distribution (central focal point to the blind spot laterally), which in mild cases may be evident only as desaturation to red color using the head of a pin. More severe cases may result in total loss of light perception. In most acute cases of optic neuritis, the inflammation is retrobulbar (behind the disc), so no immediate changes are visible on the optic disc, thereby leading to the aphorism "the patient sees nothing, and the doctor sees nothing." However, there should be a relative afferent papillary defect (Marcus-Gunn pupil; Chapter 396) with paradoxical dilation of the affected eye to direct light on swinging a flashlight from the unaffected eye in which consensual constriction was induced. In cases of bilateral optic neuritis (new or old), this abnormality may not be seen. Patients usually spontaneously recover substantial vision after weeks to months. Later, the optic disc may become pale, especially in the temporal region, a finding reflecting damage to the axons following inflammation and demyelination, even with recovery of normal visual acuity. Patients often have more subtle chronic visual impairment for colors, low-contrast visual acuity, and contrast sensitivity. Visual testing using low-contrast letter acuity charts commonly reveals substantial visual loss after clinical optic neuritis, which manifests clinically as nyctalopia (night blindness).

Visual impairment from impaired tracking of eye movements owing to brain stem or cerebellar disease most commonly occurs in the setting of an acute lesion affecting the medial longitudinal fasciculus, which is the neurologic pathway that yokes the eyes together on lateral saccades. Patients may experience frank diplopia or just blurred vision, especially when they look off to one side rapidly, such as when looking over one's shoulder while driving. The neurologic sign of this problem is called *internuclear ophthalmoplegia* (Chapter 396) and manifests as slowed or absent adduction of one eye with abducting nystagmus of the other eye. It may occur bilaterally or may exist in milder forms, such that the adduction lag is imperceptible to the human observer. Blurred vision from cerebellar damage with nystagmus is very common in MS and is often worse on extreme lateral or vertical gaze. *Oscillopsia*, the sensation that the environment is moving when it actually is not, is another symptom of impaired cerebellar coordination of the eyes. Saccadic eye movement or loss of smooth pursuit is common in MS and also can be seen in numerous neurologic conditions or with aging.

Motor Symptoms

The most common motor symptoms of MS are weakness and impaired coordination in a leg, with ascending involvement from distal to proximal and commonly spreading to the contralateral leg or ipsilateral arm. The lesion causing these symptoms is more commonly in the cervical spinal cord rather than the thoracic spinal cord, even when the first sign is partial footdrop. It is likely that axons that must conduct impulses over the longest distance (entire length of the spinal cord) from a site of inflammatory demyelination will become symptomatic before axons delivering signals to closer synapses (adjacent anterior horn cells in the cervical cord). Clinically, the weakness may be severe and may result in an obvious paralysis or be so subtle as to be undetectable. Heat-induced fatigue and weakness, as manifested by focal symptoms (slapping of a foot or dragging a leg) occurring after 15 to 20 minutes of exercise and resolving with rest, are characteristic of early demyelinating disease. The early absence of associated hyperreflexia and plantar extensor responses (Babinski sign) may make it difficult to document corticospinal tract involvement. Later, in more established MS, classic corticospinal tract signs are often evident and manifest clinically as spastic gait (either hemiparetic or paraparetic), muscle cramps, and clonus (sustained reflex loop), sometimes occurring with positional changes and mistaken for signs of a cerebellar tremor.

Ataxia may occur as a result of impaired delivery of sensory information up the spinal cord or from demyelination of cerebellar pathways in the brain stem or cerebellum. Often, the two are mixed and may be confounded further by visual loss and impaired ability to compensate by fixing on the environment; this combination commonly causes dizziness in crowds, in which fixation may be further obscured. Appendicular dysmetria resulting in tremor on reaching for an object is a common cause of impaired coordination and dexterity. Lower extremity and truncal ataxia may result in a wide-based (drunk) gait.

Other movement disorders, such as postural tremor and titubation (head tremor), are much less common in MS. *Myokymia* (wormlike muscle movements) under the skin, especially around the face, however, is fairly common. Pseudoathetosis and parkinsonism can be seen in severe cases.

Cognitive and Behavioral Symptoms

Over 50% of patients with MS experience bouts of moderate-to-severe depression (Chapter 369). There is also increased incidence of bipolar disease, which may manifest after treatment of depression or treatment with corticosteroids. Pseudobulbar affect, either pathologic laughing or crying, is seen in patients with more advanced disease. Numerous cognitive symptoms, including short-term memory loss, word-finding difficulty, trouble with multitasking, and cognitive fatigue, may be mistaken for depression but are well-recognized primary symptoms of MS pathology. Most patients do not progress to dementia (Chapter 374), but cognitive and behavioral impairments are major causes of losing employment and marital discord.

Organ Dysfunction

Bladder symptoms are extremely common, but often are not volunteered, so specific questions must be asked concerning urinary frequency, urgency, incontinence, or retention. Careful discrimination of a spastic bladder (detrusor muscle spasm) causing incontinence from an atonic bladder or spasm of the external sphincter (the latter two causing retention) leading to overflow incontinence is critical to designing treatment (Chapter 23). Urinary tract infections (Chapter 268) owing to bladder dysfunction may aggravate symptoms of MS.

Bowel dysfunction commonly manifests as constipation (Chapter 127), which may be primary (related to spinal cord involvement) or secondary (related to self-induced dehydration to manage urinary frequency or to side effects of anticholinergic drugs). Bowel incontinence secondary to an incompetent anal sphincter is less common and most often occurs as an isolated episode of fecal urgency, sometimes related to dietary change or diarrheal illness, or as a sequela of prolonged compaction.

Sexual dysfunction is common and underdiscussed in MS. In men, erectile dysfunction is frequent. In women and men, loss of libido and inability to achieve orgasm can occur as a result of medication, loss of sensation, heat-induced worsening of symptoms, physical barriers to intercourse (impaired mucosal moisture, spasticity, and pain), depression, or disorders of body image.

Systemic Symptoms

Fatigue is common in MS. It may be linked to depression but often occurs independently and can be the most disabling symptom of the disease. A sleep history is important to exclude daytime fatigue resulting from disrupted sleep secondary to pain, cramps, bladder frequency, sleep apnea, periodic limb movements, depression, or disrupted sleep-wake cycles. Daytime fatigue even after a good night of sleep may occur in mid-afternoon and may be described as being "unplugged" or completely drained. Many patients obtain benefit from a short daytime nap.

Sensitivity to heat, which is a classic symptom of MS, occurs only in some patients. Even minor elevations of the body temperature can dramatically worsen symptoms (Uhthoff phenomenon). Some patients complain of worsened symptoms in cold weather, likely related to increased dysfunction of already stiff muscles or signal blockade consistent with the known physiology of nerve conduction, which has an inverted U-shaped temperature versus conduction curve.

Pregnancy

Women with MS may have children, and the activity of MS lessens during the course of pregnancy, especially by the third trimester, when the frequency of exacerbations is reduced by approximately two thirds. Relapses are more frequent in the first 6 postpartum months, but no evidence indicates that pregnancy changes the natural history of the disease. Whether breast-feeding alters the course of MS is unclear, but it is contraindicated for patients who resume disease-modifying drugs following delivery.

Types of Multiple Sclerosis

The three major clinical types of MS are relapsing remitting, secondary progressive, and primary progressive. Approximately 85 to 90% of patients present with relapsing-remitting MS, characterized by acute or subacute episodes of new or worsening old neurologic symptoms that increase in severity, plateau, and then partly or completely remit. Patients may have no detectable residual deficit, or they may accumulate significant permanent disability from an attack.

TABLE 383-3	2017 REVISIONS TO THE MCDONALD DIAGNOSTIC CRITERIA FOR MULTIPLE SCLEROSIS	

CLINICAL PRESENTATION	ADDITIONAL DATA NEEDED FOR DIAGNOSIS OF MULTIPLE SCLEROSIS
Two or more attacks; objective clinical evidence of two or more lesions; or one lesion with a prior attack	None*
Two or more attacks; objective clinical evidence of one lesion	Dissemination in space, demonstrated by: 1. MRI (see Table 383-4), or 2. Two or more MRI-detected lesions consistent with MS plus positive CSF specific oligoclonal bands, or 3. Await further clinical attack implicating a different site
One attack; objective clinical evidence of two or more lesions	Dissemination in time, demonstrated by: 1. MRI (see Table 383-4), or 2. Second clinical attack
One attack; objective clinical evidence of one lesion (monosymptomatic presentation; clinically isolated syndrome)	1. Dissemination in space, demonstrated by: a. MRI (see Table 383-4), or b. Two or more MRI-detected lesions consistent with MS plus positive CSF-specific oligoclonal bands, and 2. Dissemination in time, demonstrated by: a. MRI (see Table 383-4), or b. Second clinical attack or c. Demonstration of CSF-specific oligoclonal bands

*Must rule out other causes (e.g., see Table 383-2).
CSF = cerebrospinal fluid; MRI = magnetic resonance imaging; MS = multiple sclerosis.
Modified from Thompson AJ, Banwell BL, Barkhof F, et al. Diagnosis of multiple sclerosis: 2017 revisions of the McDonald criteria. *Lancet Neurol.* 2018;17:162-173.

TABLE 383-4	MAGNETIC RESONANCE IMAGING CRITERIA IN MULTIPLE SCLEROSIS (INTERNATIONAL PANEL RECOMMENDATIONS: 2017)

DISSEMINATION

Dissemination in space can be demonstrated by one or more T2-hyperintense lesions that are characteristic of multiple sclerosis in two or more of four areas of the CNS: periventricular, cortical or juxtacortical, and infratentorial brain regions, and the spinal cord.

Dissemination in time can be demonstrated by the simultaneous presence of gadolinium-enhancing and non-enhancing lesions at any time or by a new T2-hyperintense or gadolinium-enhancing lesion on follow-up MRI, with reference to a baseline scan, irrespective of the timing of the baseline MRI.

DIAGNOSIS OF PRIMARY PROGRESSIVE MULTIPLE SCLEROSIS

Primary progressive multiple sclerosis can be diagnosed in patients with:
- 1 year of disability progression (retrospectively or prospectively determined) independent of clinical relapse

Plus two of the following criteria:
- One or more T2-hyperintense lesions characteristic of multiple sclerosis in one or more of the following brain regions: periventricular, cortical or juxtacortical, or infratentorial
- Two or more T2-hyperintense lesions in the spinal cord
- Presence of CSF-specific oligoclonal bands

CNS = central nervous system; CSF = cerebrospinal fluid; MRI = magnetic resonance imaging.
From Thompson AJ, Banwell BL, Barkhof F, et al. Diagnosis of multiple sclerosis: 2017 revisions of the McDonald criteria. *Lancet Neurol.* 2018;17:162-173.

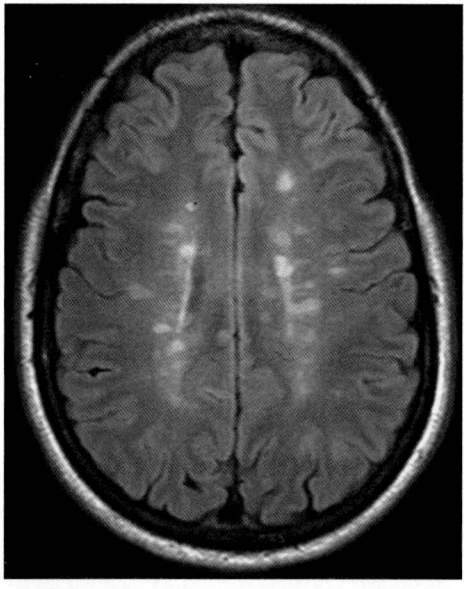

FIGURE 383-1. Axial fluid attenuation inversion recovery image of the brain from a patient with multiple sclerosis revealing classic multiple periventricular and deep white matter high-signal lesions.

Most patients with relapsing-remitting MS convert to secondary progressive MS after 20 to 40 years. This stage of the disease, which is characterized by at least 6 months of progressive worsening without evidence of a relapse, can be diagnosed with confidence only retrospectively. Some patients with secondary progressive MS also have interposed relapses distinct from their periods of progressive worsening, although these episodes become less frequent with time. Primary progressive MS, which is characterized by progressive deterioration from the onset for at least 1 year without a history of distinct relapses, occurs in approximately 10 to 15% of patients. It is more common in middle-aged men and typically has more involvement of the spinal cord and fewer inflammatory brain lesions.

Acute progressive MS (Marburg disease) causes acute or subacute progressive neurologic deterioration leading to severe disability within days to a month in a patient with no prior history of MS. This rare form of the disease may progress to a quadriplegic, obtunded state with death as a result of intercurrent infection, aspiration, or respiratory failure from brain stem involvement.

DIAGNOSIS

The diagnosis of MS rests on demonstrating evidence of at least two inflammatory demyelinating lesions referable to different locations within the CNS, occurring at different times (usually ≥1 month apart), and for which no better explanation exists. Diagnostic criteria allow for the diagnosis to be made on clinical grounds alone as long as appropriate exclusionary testing is performed (Table 383-3).[3] Clinical evidence of a lesion requires objective findings on examination, not just a symptom. Further, repeated episodes of neurologic dysfunction that could be explained based on one lesion (e.g., a cervicomedullary junction lesion causing brain stem, cerebellar, and corticospinal tract dysfunction) is not enough evidence to diagnose MS.

Magnetic Resonance Imaging

No definitive diagnostic laboratory test exists for MS, but magnetic resonance imaging (MRI) of the brain is extremely useful and should be performed in all patients in whom MS is a diagnostic consideration.[4] More than 95% of patients with clinically definite MS have an abnormal brain MRI, and the presence of high-signal, bright lesions is so characteristic of MS that a normal brain MRI should suggest an alternative diagnosis. Brain MRI is also useful in predicting future MS at the time of a clinically isolated demyelinating syndrome. Specific MRI findings allow for confirmation of disease disseminated in time and space (different parts of the brain or spinal cord) and fulfilling evidence for dissemination in time (Table 383-4). MS plaques typically appear as high-signal (white) areas on fluid attenuation inversion recovery (FLAIR) T2-weighted images, which allow for the best discrimination of the supratentorial lesions by suppressing high signal from cerebrospinal fluid (CSF) in the ventricles (Fig. 383-1). Lesions generally range in size from 2 mm to 2 cm; larger plaques occasionally resemble a tumor. Features of an MRI lesion suggesting MS include an elliptical shape, discrete borders, lack of mass effect, and gadolinium enhancement. Typical locations include the periventricular area (perpendicular to or abutting the walls of the ventricles) (Fig. 383-2), the corpus callosum, the cerebellar peduncles, the brain stem, the juxtacortical area, and the dorsolateral spinal cord (Fig. 383-3). Cortical and deep gray matter lesions also occur but are less clearly seen on conventional MRI. Gadolinium enhancement, which suggests permeability

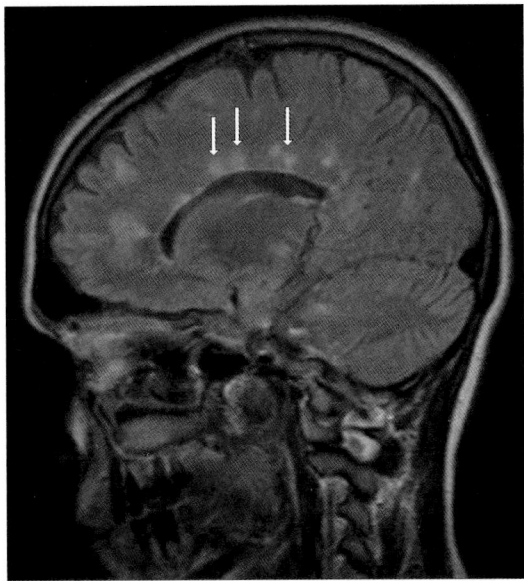

FIGURE 383-2. Sagittal fluid attenuation inversion recovery image of the brain from a patient with multiple sclerosis revealing classic periventricular lesions radiating outward from the ventricles (*arrows*).

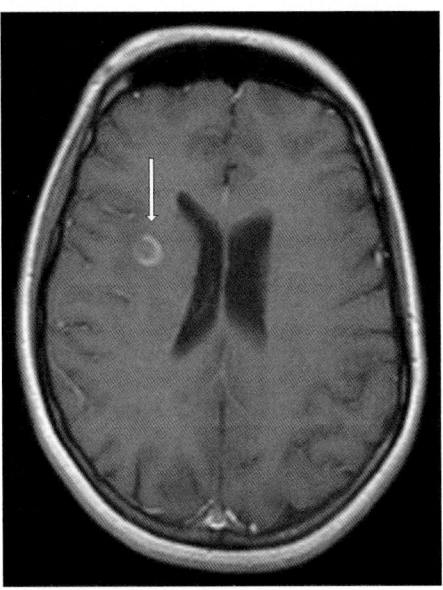

FIGURE 383-4. Axial T1-weighted image after gadolinium contrast showing an actively inflamed ring-enhancing lesion (*arrow*) in a patient with multiple sclerosis.

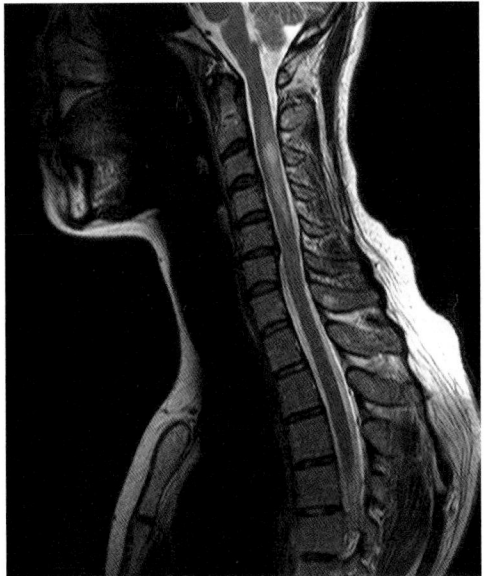

FIGURE 383-3. Sagittal T2-weighted image of the brain and cervical spine from a patient with multiple sclerosis. The image shows a high-signal plaque from C3-C5 in the spinal cord.

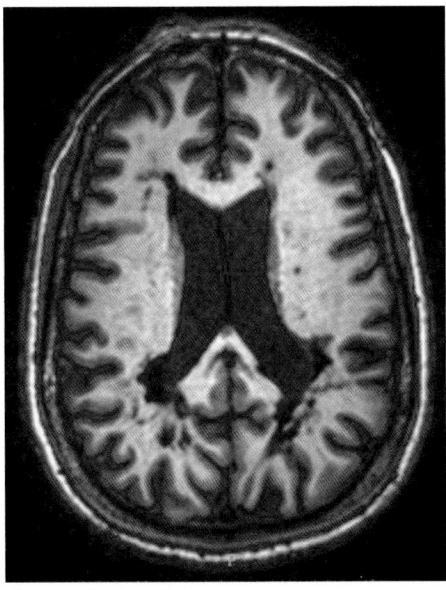

FIGURE 383-5. Axial T1-weighted image showing numerous areas of T1 low signal ("black holes"), ventricular enlargement, and diffuse atrophy.

of the blood-brain barrier, is correlated with new or active inflammation in lesions (Fig. 383-4). Lesions that enhance on a T1-weighted sequence usually have a concomitant lesion in the same location on a T2-weighted image. However, T2-weighted lesions may form without evident enhancement. Gadolinium enhancement may be homogenous, central, or in a ring pattern; it typically persists for 2 to 8 weeks and thus may be missed on intermittent scans. Persistent areas of low signal on T1-weighted images before contrast ("black holes") correlate with pathologic evidence of axonal loss and atrophy (Fig. 383-5).

Cerebrospinal Fluid

Examination of the CSF is useful in many cases but is not mandatory in patients with a typical clinical presentation and MRI evidence of disseminated disease. CSF evaluation includes cell counts, total protein, glucose, IgG index, and electrophoresis to assess for an oligoclonal banding pattern with a paired serum sample. The presence of myelin basic protein is not specific for MS because it can be elevated secondary to any disruption of CNS tissue. Oligoclonal IgG bands in the CSF or an elevated IgG index provides evidence for intrathecal

production of immunoglobulins. However, although oligoclonal bands are common in MS, they also can occur with infection or other immune-mediated processes. As a result, the test lacks specificity for MS and has a sensitivity of only approximately 85 to 90% of patients with clinically definite MS. In clinically isolated demyelinating syndromes (see later), the sensitivity is even lower (~50%). Further, the sensitivity depends on local laboratory techniques. Oligoclonal mirror bands, in the serum and CSF, may signal a systemic immune process with CNS involvement.

CSF evaluation is generally recommended if an alternative diagnosis is considered, especially if one suspects an infectious or neoplastic process (e.g., fever, sweats, unusual travel history, tick bite, or rash). CSF analysis also may be useful if clinical or MRI criteria are incomplete to provide confirmation of the diagnosis.

Evoked Potential Tests

Evoked potentials (Chapter 368) may be useful in some situations to document objective evidence of slowed conduction owing to demyelination in locations different from those recognized clinically. However, visual evoked potentials (VEPs), brain stem auditory evoked potentials, and somatosensory evoked potentials are less sensitive and less specific for MS than is high-resolution MRI. Multifocal VEPs may be more sensitive than global VEPs in revealing focal areas of abnormal conduction along the optic nerve.

Optical Coherence Tomography

Optical coherence tomography is performed with an office-based device that uses the reflection of infrared light (from an exogenous source directed through the pupil) off the back of the eye to quantify the thickness of retinal tissues, including the peripapillary retinal nerve fiber layer and macular layers. This test, which has been widely used in glaucoma, can monitor axonal and retinal ganglion cell damage, both in the setting of acute optic neuritis and in detecting subclinical neuroaxonal damage (E-Fig. 383-1). Retinal nerve fiber layer thinning correlates with brain atrophy and may be useful as a surrogate marker of more global neurodegeneration in MS.

Differential Diagnosis

The diagnosis of MS may be so clear that it is recognized by the patient and is readily confirmed by the primary physician or so obscure that even experienced specialists disagree.[5] Many processes (see Table 383-2) can mimic the clinical, radiologic, and CSF findings associated with MS, and there is no "gold standard" diagnostic test that is 100% sensitive and specific for the disease. The most common conditions misdiagnosed as MS in one study were migraine (Chapter 370), fibromyalgia (Chapter 258), and conversion or psychogenic disorders (Chapter 369).[6]

Processes that mimic MS include structural lesions, especially of the base of the brain and of the spinal cord, in which one lesion can cause symptoms referable to many different tracts and at different perceived locations in the body. Chiari malformations with or without syrinx (Chapter 389), disc herniation (Chapter 372), cervical spondylosis, and low-grade tumors (Chapter 180) can produce symptoms of MS both in newly presenting patients and in patients who truly have MS but who also have a second process.

Various infectious diseases can mimic MS. Examples include human T-cell lymphotropic virus types I and II (virally associated myelopathy or tropical spastic paraparesis; Chapter 354), human immunodeficiency virus (neuropathy, myelopathy, cognitive impairment, CNS white matter changes; Chapter 366), neuroborreliosis (Lyme disease; Chapter 305), neurosyphilis (Chapter 303), Epstein-Barr virus (Chapter 353), cytomegalovirus (Chapter 352), herpes simplex virus (Chapter 350), varicella-zoster virus myelitis (Chapter 351), and JC virus (progressive multifocal leukoencephalopathy; Chapter 346).[7]

Inflammatory diseases that usually involve other parts of the body can concomitantly affect or, rarely, manifest in the CNS. Examples include sarcoidosis (Chapter 89), systemic lupus erythematosus (Chapter 250), Sjögren syndrome (Chapter 252), and vasculitides (Chapter 254). Autoimmune encephalitis, although usually more fulminant and with distinguishing features such as seizures and behavioral disturbance, may be mistaken for MS. Ischemic vascular disease secondary to any cause also can resemble MS. Metabolic and nutritional disorders that can mimic MS include vitamin B_{12} deficiency and methylmalonic acidemia (in some cases distinct from cyanocobalamin deficiency). Rarely, central pontine myelinolysis (Chapters 108 and 388) is mistaken for MS. Thyroid disease (Chapter 213) may mimic the fatigue of MS and may cause dysesthesias and disorders of the optic nerve and muscles. Nutritional deficiency (Chapter 203) and malabsorption have been associated with demyelination and may mimic MS. Copper deficiency can cause dorsal column pathology, neuropathy, anemia, and optic neuropathy. Vitamin D deficiency (Chapter 231), which is becoming increasingly common, can cause proximal weakness, fatigue, asthenia, bone loss, and impaired immune function. Vitamin A deficiency, although not common in industrialized countries, can cause night blindness and immune dysfunction.

Monophasic demyelinating syndromes with or without multiple other lesions often, but not always, progress to become MS (see later). Spinocerebellar atrophy and hereditary myelopathy cause slowly progressive disease but do not cause sensory and visual abnormalities.

Hereditary diseases are increasingly recognized as mimicking MS. Spinocerebellar atrophy may manifest as progressive myelopathy and ataxia. A variety of genetic neuropathies (type 2 CMT mitofusinopathies, adult-onset polyglucosan body disorder; Chapter 392), ataxias (Friedreich, ataxia telangiectasia; Chapter 382), mitochondrial diseases (progressive optic atrophy, Leber, mitochondrial encephalopathy, lactic acidosis, and strokelike episodes [MELAS], myoclonic epilepsy with ragged red fibers [MERRF]; Chapter 393),

and metabolic diseases (urea cycle disorders; Chapter 194) can have CNS manifestations that could lead to misdiagnosis.

TREATMENT　　Rx

The treatment of MS can be divided into drugs designed to relieve symptoms, drugs designed to modify the course of the disease, and nondrug measures.[8] Numerous drugs target specific aspects of MS: depression, fatigue, muscle spasticity, pain, insomnia, and bladder, bowel, and sexual dysfunction. Before considering a symptomatic therapy, the patient should be educated about the purpose of the drug and its side effect profile. On learning that these drugs have no long-term impact on disease activity, patients may elect not to use them for relief of symptoms alone. Symptomatic therapies are best started at low doses and frequently require titration to obtain the optimal balance between efficacy and side effects.

Treatment of Specific Symptoms

Depression and emotional lability are common symptoms of MS. In addition to appropriate supportive care and counseling, antidepressant therapy with one of the "activating" serotonergic or noradrenergic drugs (fluoxetine, sertraline, citalopram, escitalopram, venlafaxine, or bupropion) can be of benefit for depression as well as for anxiety and panic symptoms (see Table 369-5) Most patients do not seem to tolerate paroxetine well long term; fluoxetine and sertraline work for panic and anxiety. Patients with pain or insomnia may benefit more from a sedating antidepressant (amitriptyline, nortriptyline, or trazodone) given at bedtime, which may have the added anticholinergic benefits on urinary bladder urgency.

Spasticity can be managed by physical therapy, stretching, and institution of either baclofen (5 to 160 mg in divided doses) or tizanidine (2 to 32 mg in divided doses). Either drug should be started as a single agent at a low dose at bedtime, gradually increasing to three to four times daily, with a larger dose at bedtime to target nocturnal symptoms. Decreasing muscle tone can result in weakness. Baclofen should never be discontinued abruptly because of the potential for a severe withdrawal reaction.

Bladder urgency resulting from detrusor muscle spasm can be managed effectively with anticholinergics (antimuscarinic) such as oxybutynin (5 to 20 mg in divided doses) or tolterodine (1 to 4 mg) or focal intravesicular injections of botulinum toxin, but these agents can cause temporary urinary hesitancy or retention. Bladder ultrasonography permits accurate bedside assessment of postvoid residual volume to determine whether a patient is retaining excessive amounts of urine (>50 mL is abnormal but >300 mL requires intervention). Urinary retention may be improved by removing drugs known to induce it (e.g., anticholinergics and opioids). Primary urinary retention is difficult to treat with drugs, but external sphincter spasm can be treated with α_{1a}-adrenergic receptor blockers such as tamsulosin (0.4 to 0.8 mg) and doxazosin (1 to 8 mg). Bethanechol (10 to 150 mg in divided doses) may be tried for an atonic bladder, but intermittent catheterization is often required. Alternative causes of bladder symptoms such as urinary tract infections, prostatic enlargement, or anatomic changes following pregnancy should be considered and managed separately. Prolonged urinary retention predisposes to infections, structural damage to the bladder and kidneys, and malignancy. Persistent postvoiding residual volumes greater than 300 mL should be treated medically, with intermittent straight catheterization recommended for patients with large volume retention refractory to medical therapy.

Painful dysesthesias and paroxysmal dystonic spasms may be managed effectively with antiepileptic drugs (gabapentin, 300 to 5400 mg/day in divided doses; pregabalin, 75 to 600 mg/day in divided doses; or oxcarbazepine, 300 to 2400 mg/day in divided doses) or tricyclic antidepressants (amitriptyline, 10 to 150 mg; or nortriptyline, 10 to 50 mg). Patients with trigeminal neuralgia (Chapter 370) may respond to these drugs or to baclofen, misoprostol, botulinum toxin, or decompression surgery; consideration of intravenous loading with an antiepileptic drug (Chapter 375) is worthwhile for severe acute pain attacks.

Sexual dysfunction in MS is often multifactorial. Patients with erectile dysfunction usually respond well to the phosphodiesterase type 5 inhibitors, which enhance penile vasodilation (Chapter 221). Education regarding the use of lubrication, alternative sensory stimulation, and the adverse effect of heat can improve sexual function.

Symptoms related to heat sensitivity may improve on cooling. Cooling devices can prevent this phenomenon, but there is no persistent benefit of inducing hypothermia.

Systemic Treatments

Corticosteroids (e.g., methylprednisolone, 1 g/day orally or intravenously [IV] for 3 to 5 days) are equivalent[A1] to each other for shortening the duration and severity of symptoms from an acute exacerbation, but they have no proved effect on long-term disability. Intravenous immunoglobulin (IVIG) and plasma exchange may occasionally benefit steroid-refractory patients, but large randomized placebo-controlled trials in relapsing MS have failed to show consistent benefits, perhaps because only patients with type II disease (humoral component) are likely to respond.

Approved Disease-Modifying Treatments

Multiple disease-modifying agents have been approved by the U.S. Food and Drug Administration (FDA): IFN-β1b (Betaseron and Extavia), IFN-β1a (Avonex), IFN-β1a (Rebif), pegylated IFN-β1a (Plegridy), glatiramer acetate (Copaxone and Glatopa), natalizumab (Tysabri), alemtuzumab (Lemtrada), mitoxantrone (Novantrone), fingolimod (Gilenya), teriflunomide (Aubagio), dimethyl fumarate (Tecfidera), and ocrelizumab (Ocrevus). All of these agents are approved for relapsing-remitting MS, and mitoxantrone is indicated for worsening forms of MS and for secondary progressive MS. Ocrelizumab is the only drug approved for primary progressive MS.[9,10]

The five IFN-β drugs reduce the relapse rate by approximately one third.[A2] IFN-β1b (8 million international units [IU], subcutaneously [SC] every other day [Betaseron and Extavia]) and IFN-β1a (30 μg intramuscularly [IM] weekly [Avonex] or 22 to 44 μg SC three times weekly [Rebif]) and pegylated IFN-β1a (125 μg every 14 days, SC [Plegridy]) appear to have a more rapid onset of action, perhaps based on their dosing regimen, compared with weekly IFN-β1a (30 μg IM weekly). However, weekly IFN-β1a (Avonex) and pegylated IFN-β1a (Plegridy) are less immunogenic and result in only a 3 and 1% incidence of neutralizing antibodies, respectively, which reduce efficacy, compared with 20 to 30% for the other IFN-β preparations. The major side effects of IFN-β are a flulike reaction (low-grade fever, chills, and myalgias 6 to 24 hours after the injection), local reactions at the injection site (pain, erythema, and rarely necrosis), and elevated aminotransferase levels (rarely severe hepatitis). These side effects can be managed by initiating the drug slowly and by prophylaxis with acetaminophen and nonsteroidal anti-inflammatory agents, and they improve in most patients after 3 to 6 months. Side effects remained typical of the IFN-β drugs but seem to be more severe than other IFN-β1a preparations in some patients.

Glatiramer acetate is a copolymer of four amino acids designed to mimic myelin basic protein; given as 20 mg/day SC or as 40 mg SC three times a week, it also reduces relapses by about one third and is well tolerated by most patients.[A3] Major side effects are local reactions at the injection site, (swelling, hives, and delayed lipoatrophy) and a rare, self-limited (15 to 20 minutes) systemic reaction consisting of chest pain, palpitations, and anxiety. No monitoring of blood tests is required for this medication. The effect of glatiramer acetate on MRI T2-weighted and gadolinium-enhancing lesions is less dramatic than for the IFNs (30% reduction), perhaps because its primary effect is not at the blood-brain barrier.

Natalizumab is a monoclonal antibody directed against the α4-integrin chain of the leukocyte adhesion molecule VLA-4. At a dose of 300 mg IV every 4 weeks, it reduces relapses by 68% compared with placebo and reduces gadolinium-enhancing lesions by 92%.[A4] It also may slightly reduce progression in secondary progressive MS.[A5] However, approximately one in 500 patients develop JC virus brain infection (Chapter 346) after 24 months of exposure, which causes progressive multifocal leukoencephalopathy (PML). The risk for PML appears to be significantly higher in patients with JC virus serum antibody titers greater than 0.9 (one in 100 to 200) compared with low-titer or seronegative patients, in whom the risk is less than one in 1000. Such data can help guide the safety of long-term usage; however, the results may change over time, so patients require repeated testing.

Alemtuzumab, a monoclonal antibody that targets CD52 on lymphocytes and monocytes, reduces annualized relapse rates by approximately 50% and also can reduce the progression of disability compared with IFN-β1a.[A6] The drug is given as yearly courses at 12 or 24 mg daily for 5 consecutive days in year 1 and for 3 days in years 2 and 3. Serious side effects associated with alemtuzumab include a 20 to 25% risk for developing autoimmune thyroid disease and rare cases of immune thrombocytopenic purpura (Chapter 163), autoimmune hemolytic anemia (Chapter 151), autoimmune neutropenia (Chapter 158), and Goodpasture syndrome (Chapter 113).

Mitoxantrone, which is an anthracenedione antineoplastic agent with potent immunosuppressive activity, is approved to slow the progression of neurologic disability and reduce the relapse rate in patients with relapsing-remitting MS and secondary progressive MS.[A7] The recommended dose is 5 to 10 mg/m² intravenous infusion every 3 months, and the lifetime use of this drug is limited to 2 to 3 years (or a cumulative dose of 120 to 140 mg/m²) because of its cardiotoxicity.

Fingolimod is a sphingosine-1 phosphate receptor modulator that is given orally once daily at 0.5 mg. Fingolimod reduces relapse rates and the progression of disease compared with placebo and compared with IFN therapy.[A8] It generally is not considered first-line therapy because its risks, including type 2 heart block and herpes encephalitis, are concerning, especially in young, otherwise healthy people with MS. Fingolimod side effects include first-dose bradycardia, macular edema, and respiratory infections.

Teriflunomide is approved as an oral agent for MS based on two phase 3 trials in which the annualized relapse rate was reduced by 31% compared

with placebo, and disability also was reduced.[A9] It is dosed at 7 or 14 mg/day orally and requires monitoring of blood tests for rare liver and kidney toxicities.

Oral dimethyl fumarate (240 mg twice daily)[A10] reduces the annualized relapse rate and disease progression in addition to suppressing active MRI lesions. Rare cases of PML have been reported in patients with prolonged severe lymphopenia (<500/μL), and close monitoring is recommended.

The only approved therapy for primary progressive MS is ocrelizumab (Ocrevus 600 mg IV every 6 months), which is a humanized anti-CD20 monoclonal antibody that rapidly depletes B cells and significantly reduces the annualized relapse rate by about 45% compared with IFN-β1a.[A11][A12] In addition, ocrelizumab reduces gadolinium-enhancing lesions by about 95%. Infusion-related side effects are common but can be managed with corticosteroids (e.g., prednisone 100 mg before the infusion) and antihistamines (e.g., diphenhydramine 50 mg before infusion). Ocrelizumab also reduces the rate of progression of disability by about 25% in patients with primary progressive MS.

Several other B-cell–depleting strategies are being tested in MS. Ataxicept, a targeted B-cell therapy, has no effect on MS or actually worsens it, thereby raising questions regarding the subset of memory B cells that might be pathogenic. Furthermore, the long-term side effects of sustained B-cell depletion remain unclear.

Other Therapies

Rituximab (1000 mg IV 2 weeks apart repeated every 6 months) is a monoclonal antibody that depletes B-cell lymphocytes and can significantly reduce inflammatory brain lesions and relapse by approximately 50% for up to 48 weeks in patients with relapsing-remitting MS.[A13] However, it has not been effective in primary progressive MS. Cladribine (2-chlorodeoxyadenosine, 3.5 or 5.25 mg/kg/day) given as a short course once per year reduces the annualized relapse rate by 55% and disease progression by one third compared with placebo.[A14] Both these drugs may have a role in treating MS, but they also have global immunosuppressive effects that increase the risk for serious infections and possibly other systemic complications.

Sustained-release dalfampridine, a potassium-channel Kv1.4 blocker at 10 mg twice daily, improves walking in 35% of patients compared with only 8% of patients receiving placebo. It is approved by the FDA as a symptomatic therapy for MS.[A15] Only a subset of patients appears to benefit, and dalfampridine is contraindicated in patients with a history of seizures and may cause dizziness, insomnia, and an increase in painful paresthesias. Siponimod, which is a selective sphingosine 1-phosphate receptor modulator, can reduce the risk of progressive disability in patients with the label specified "active" secondary progressive MS.[A16]

Other forms of immunosuppression, including laquinimod, methotrexate, azathioprine, mycophenolate mofetil, and cyclophosphamide, may have some efficacy in MS, although either no definitive clinical trials have been done with these agents or safety profiles have outweighed risks, and none is as yet approved for MS by the FDA.

Choosing the Best Treatment Options

No specific treatment algorithm can be recommended because the disease is heterogeneous, there are few head-to-head studies between medications, and reported effect sizes of the approved drugs versus placebo depend on the varying characteristics of patients in different trials.[11] As a result, the treatment decision is best made in conjunction with the patient based on the patient's disease, the side effect and safety profiles of the various drugs, and the physician's assessment of severity and prognosis. Older drugs such as IFN-β or glatiramer acetate have provided variable responses, with some patients doing well for many years. For the typical newly diagnosed patient with relapsing MS but no early signs of poor prognosis (e.g., high relapse rate with early accrual of disability, African American ancestry, high lesion load, T1 black holes on MRI, multiple spinal cord lesions), one reasonable strategy is to start with one of the older, relatively safe drugs such as IFN-β1b or glatiramer acetate and then switch to the other if the patient experiences a severe relapse, multiple small relapses, or new MRI lesions, before escalating to one of the newer, more potent drugs associated with more potential risk. Increasingly, the oral agents and even monoclonal antibodies are being considered as first-line therapies in some patients.[12]

Prevention

Patients who present with a first demyelinating event such as optic neuritis, transverse myelitis, or another brain stem, cerebral, or cerebellar myelopathy are at risk for developing full-blown MS. In one randomized trial, minocycline (100 mg twice daily) substantially reduced the short-term progression to MS but was no longer effective at 2 years.[A17]

Other Approaches to Well-Being

Patients with MS are at high risk for developing osteopenia or osteoporosis (Chapter 230), so prophylaxis with vitamin D and calcium and treatment with bisphosphonates or other proved approaches should be considered.

Patients with suboptimal 25-OH vitamin D levels (<30 ng/mL) on standard 1000-IU cholecalciferol replacement therapy should consider increasing to 4000 to 5000 IU/day or 50,000 IU every other week or, in some cases, weekly, with appropriate monitoring of vitamin D and serum plus urine calcium levels. If osteoporosis has already been diagnosed, bisphosphonate therapy, such as alendronate (10 mg/day or 70 mg/week) or a similar drug, is generally indicated.

Nonmedical treatment of MS is a critical part of managing the disease. Patients derive benefit from a health care team approach consisting of an experienced MS physician, nurse, social worker, therapist, and counselor, with appropriate referral to other subspecialties as needed. Alternative and complementary therapies (Chapter 34) are commonly used by patients with MS, and the risks and benefits of these approaches must be discussed with the patient. No diet has yet proved effective in MS.

PROGNOSIS

The annual risk of death for patients with MS is about twice as high as in the overall population,[13] and the average lifespan of patients with MS is approximately 8 years less than normal, a finding reflecting a bimodal distribution in which many patients live a normal lifespan and a few die earlier owing to aggressive disease, severe disability, infection, or suicide. About 85% of patients commence with a relapsing and remitting pattern of disease, whereas 15% progress from what is initially felt to be primary progressive MS. Most patients presenting with relapsing-remitting MS convert to secondary progressive MS after 20 to 40 years. Only one third of patients will require use of a wheelchair, but 50% may need assistive devices and nearly two thirds will have disability that prevents them from working. African Americans and men of all races tend to have a more aggressive course and are more likely to become disabled. Immunomodulating therapy early in the course of the disease appears to slow progression of disability, but long-term follow-up data are open-label and uncontrolled, so it is difficult to quantify the extent of this benefit.

OTHER DISEASES OF MYELIN
Monofocal and Monophasic Demyelinating Processes

OPTIC NEURITIS AND TRANSVERSE MYELITIS
Optic neuritis (Chapter 396) and transverse myelitis are inflammatory processes that can occur as entities distinct from MS or as part of MS (see earlier).[14] In addition, optic neuritis and transverse myelitis can occur together in the syndrome called *neuromyelitis optica* (Devic disease).

Optic Neuritis
Optic neuritis (Chapter 396) is an inflammatory disease that usually involves the retrobulbar portion of the optic nerve and sometimes parts of the optic chiasm. Although optic neuritis is most often associated with MS (50 to 75%), it also can be seen as an isolated idiopathic disorder (25 to 50%), as part of neuromyelitis optica, or associated with other inflammatory and infectious diseases such as chronic relapsing inflammatory optic neuropathy, systemic lupus erythematosus, Sjögren syndrome, sarcoidosis, Lyme disease, syphilis, and human immunodeficiency virus infection. The pathobiologic features are thought to be similar to those of MS and are characterized by idiopathic inflammatory demyelination followed by secondary axonal injury. Hereditary optic neuropathies may be unmasked during periods of stress and manifest as an acute monocular visual loss.

CLINICAL MANIFESTATIONS AND DIAGNOSIS
The clinical presentation, which typically is monocular visual loss with pain over the brow that worsens with lateral eye movement, is similar regardless of whether it manifests as part of MS (see the earlier discussion of the visual effects of MS) or not. Retinal axonal and neuronal damage develops quickly after the onset of acute optic neuritis. When it involves the optic nerve head, it is called *papillitis* and, in bilateral cases, can be impossible to differentiate from papilledema. Optic neuritis also can be mimicked by anterior segment, choroidal, or retinal diseases. Optic neuritis is distinguished from optic neuropathy, which is a chronic, generally noninflammatory condition of the optic nerve caused by tobacco or nutritional amblyopia, ischemia, Leber disease, Charcot Marie Tooth type 2a (mitofusinopathy; Chapter 392), or a number of other rare hereditary diseases (Chapter 396). Subclinical optic neuropathy in the absence of painful monocular visual loss may result in retinal nerve fiber layer thinning over time.

Among patients with optic neuritis, the 15-year risk for developing MS is 25% in patients without lesions on their baseline brain MRI but 72% in patients with one or more baseline MRI lesions. Treatment with intravenous methylprednisolone as in MS or with bioequivalent doses of oral corticosteroids[A18] may shorten the duration and severity of the attack, but no definitive evidence indicates that it changes the long-term outcome. Data support the use of IFN-β drugs and glatiramer acetate in patients whose optic neuritis is at high risk for conversion to MS (one or more typical brain MRI lesions).

Transverse Myelitis
Transverse myelitis is a rare (approximately one in 100,000 people) monophasic inflammatory process of the spinal cord that is usually distinct from MS in that it either involves the entire cross section or is longitudinally extensive along three vertebral body segments rostrocaudally.[15] Transverse myelitis or myelopathy may be idiopathic or associated with inflammatory diseases (neuromyelitis optica, systemic lupus erythematosus, Sjögren syndrome, vasculitis, or MS), infectious diseases, or vascular diseases (antiphospholipid antibody syndrome or dural venous fistula).

CLINICAL MANIFESTATIONS AND DIAGNOSIS
In its fulminant form, transverse myelitis causes complete loss of motor and sensory function below the affected level of the spinal cord and causes concomitant bowel, bladder, and sexual dysfunction. Autonomic involvement can be seen in cervical and high thoracic spine cases. Transverse myelitis also may manifest in an incomplete or partial form, which is more commonly associated with MS. In older patients, patients with vascular risk factors, or patients with central cord edema pattern on MRI, spinal angiography should be considered to exclude spinal cord ischemia or infarction (Chapter 372).

Treatment of the inflammatory process is usually with methylprednisolone (1000 mg IV for 3 to 5 days), followed by specific treatment of any identifiable underlying disease process. The prognosis is worse than in MS in that significant recovery is seen in fewer than 50% of patients and many patients remain completely paralyzed after the initial attack. Plasma exchange or cyclophosphamide may be considered in steroid-refractory cases.

NEUROMYELITIS OPTICA
Neuromyelitis optica is now recognized as an entity distinct from MS and is characterized by an optic neuritis, often bilateral and temporally associated with a fulminant multilevel transverse myelitis.[16] A specific serum IgG (NMO-IgG) directed against aquaporin 4 strongly predicts this process. Brain lesions may be seen on MRI and have a predilection for the brain stem. Neuromyelitis optica may be similar to what is called *opticospinal MS* in Japan, although the latter overlaps with MS. There is no proved effective treatment, but patients are usually given anti-inflammatory and immunosuppressive medications (e.g., azathioprine 2 to 3 mg/kg or prednisone 1 mg/kg). Therapies directed against B cells (e.g., rituximab 1000 mg IV 2 weeks apart every 6 months),[17] humoral factors (complement), or nonpathogenic antibody blockers of aquaporin 4–IgG binding also have shown efficacy, but no placebo-controlled trials have been completed as of yet because of considerations. The prognosis is generally poor; if not treated, most patients develop sustained disabling visual loss and weakness.

ACUTE DISSEMINATED ENCEPHALOMYELITIS
Acute disseminated encephalomyelitis and its hyperacute form, acute necrotizing hemorrhagic encephalopathy, are thought to be forms of monophasic immune-mediated inflammatory demyelination. They differ from MS in that they are typically monophasic, whereas MS is by definition multiphasic or chronically progressive. However, no reliable clinical or pathologic criteria are available to differentiate the two processes, which may represent a continuum. Patients may present with fever, headache, meningeal signs, and altered consciousness, which are exceedingly rare in MS. There is no known effective treatment. Large numbers of patients, especially children, make remarkable

recoveries, but the necrotizing form can be severely disabling or fatal. Relapsing forms of the disease in children are more likely to become MS.

Leukodystrophies

The leukodystrophies represent a variety of diseases characterized by progressive hereditary CNS white matter degeneration thought to be related to abnormal production or maintenance of myelin. Many of these diseases now have a defined biochemical and genetic basis, are caused by primary pathology in other CNS components (including astrocytes, microglia, axons, and blood vessels), and are no longer considered exclusively to be primary myelin disorders.[18]

ADRENOLEUKODYSTROPHY AND ADRENOMYELONEUROPATHY

Adrenoleukodystrophy and adrenomyeloneuropathy, which are caused by impaired ability of the peroxisomes to metabolize very-long-chain fatty acids, represent different phenotypes resulting from the same X-linked, incompletely recessive genetic defect. Impaired oxidation of very-long-chain fatty acids results from deficient function of the enzyme lignoceroyl–coenzyme A ligase. The defective gene maps to Xq28 and codes for a peroxisomal membrane protein (ALDP), which is a member of a large family of proteins referred to as the adenosine triphosphate–binding cassette (ABC) transporters, specifically *ABCD1*.

Childhood cerebral adrenoleukodystrophy, which is the most common form of the disorder, represents 45% of all cases; it is seen only in male patients, with an onset at ages 4 to 11 years. Adolescent (5%) and adult (3%) cerebral forms progress at a similar or slower rate than the childhood form.

CLINICAL MANIFESTATIONS

Adrenomyeloneuropathy begins in young men as slowly progressive paraparesis with hypogonadism, impotence, sphincter disturbances, variable adrenal insufficiency, and axonal neuropathy affecting mainly the lower extremities. A rare acute inflammatory form with rapid progression and dementia may occur. A similar, but usually milder, disorder can be seen in up to 20% of women who are hemizygous for the disease.

DIAGNOSIS

Diagnosis is established in male patients by finding elevated very-long-chain fatty acids in the plasma. DNA-based diagnosis in carriers is reliable and is recommended in women because of false-negative results using the plasma assay.

TREATMENT   Rx

Treatment is unsatisfactory. A 4:1 mixture of glyceryl trioleate and glyceryl trierucate (i.e., "Lorenzo oil") normalizes plasma very-long-chain fatty acids within 4 weeks and has few side effects. Although clinical trials suggested that treatment in presymptomatic patients delayed or prevented the onset of disease, this treatment is ineffective after symptoms have begun and the disease progresses relentlessly. Hematopoietic stem-cell gene therapy may be an effective alternative to allogeneic stem cell transplantation in boys with early-stage diseases.[19]

Pelizaeus-Merzbacher Disease

Pelizaeus-Merzbacher disease is a rare, chronic, familial leukodystrophy usually caused by a genetic defect in the X-linked myelin proteolipid protein (PLP) gene. In classic Pelizaeus-Merzbacher disease, age at onset varies between 3 months and 9 years, and the age at death varies between 6 years and 25 years. However, milder forms of spastic paraplegia 2 are now well recognized in adults. The disease manifests as a slowly progressive myelopathy, often with cerebellar and cognitive involvement, and the diagnosis is established by genetic testing for mutations in the *PLP* gene. A variety of different types of PLP mutations account for the variability in clinical phenotypes. An autosomal recessive disease called Pelizaeus-Merzbacher–like disease 1 and the less severe spastic paraplegia 44, caused by mutations of the gap junction protein gamma-2 gene (*GJC2*), are recognized variants. No specific treatment exists beyond supportive therapy.

Metachromatic Leukodystrophy

Metachromatic leukodystrophy usually results from a recessively inherited defect in the lysosomal enzyme arylsulfatase A. Absence of arylsulfatase A results in the accumulation of sulfatide in both central and peripheral myelin and myelin-forming cells; instability of the myelin membranes results in the breakdown of myelin. Metachromatic leukodystrophy is generally divided into four subtypes: congenital, late infantile (most common), juvenile, and adult. It appears in all ethnic groups and has an overall frequency of one in 40,000.

The clinical manifestations are variable and may include progressive spastic paraparesis, extrapyramidal signs, seizures, and peripheral neuropathy. Brain MRI usually shows large confluent symmetrical high-signal areas in the cerebral white matter, brain stem, and cerebellum, but a more patchy appearance resembling MS is occasionally seen in adult cases. At present, no satisfactory treatment exists. A case series suggests that hematopoietic stem cell gene therapy can potentially prevent the onset of symptoms in presymptomatic patients and may slow or even halt progression of the disease.[20]

Globoid Cell Leukodystrophy

Globoid cell leukodystrophy (Krabbe disease; Chapter 197) is characterized biochemically by accumulation of galactocerebroside in cerebral white matter as a result of deficient galactocerebroside β-galactosidase activity. The disease is transmitted as an autosomal recessive trait and affects infants in the first 2 to 3 months of life, initially manifesting with behavioral changes and failure to achieve developmental milestones. Rare late-onset cases manifest with progressive motor impairment and, less frequently, visual failure. Neuropathologic examination reveals marked loss of myelin throughout the brain, with the presence of round or oval macrophages and large, irregular, multinucleated cells, termed *globoid cells*, that are filled with galactocerebroside. Accumulation of galactosylsphingosine (psychosine) is thought to cause destruction of oligodendrocytes and marked reduction of myelin formation.

Canavan Disease

Canavan disease is a fatal, progressive leukodystrophy with an autosomal recessive inheritance, caused by mutations in the gene for aspartoacylase, an enzyme that hydrolyzes *N*-acetylaspartate into L-aspartate and acetate. Aspartoacylase deficiency results in elevated levels of its substrate molecule, *N*-acetylaspartate, brain edema, and dysmyelination. Clinically, the disease manifests with retardation, seizures, and diffuse, symmetrical white matter degeneration in the subcortical areas, with involvement of the globus pallidum on MRI. No treatment is available.

Vanishing White Matter Disease

Vanishing white matter disease is an increasingly recognized autosomal recessive disorder with a broad range of clinical manifestations from rapidly progressive presentations in infants to slowly progressive disease in adults. The disease is caused by mutations in the eukaryotic translation initiation factor 2B (*eIF2B*) genes 1 to 5, which code for proteins involved in the integrated stress response of cells. Pathologic characteristics include vacuolated myelin with cystic appearance on MRI. No specific therapy, other than avoidance of stress, is known.

⬤ AUTOIMMUNE ENCEPHALITIS

Autoimmune encephalitis is increasingly recognized as a treatable cause of brain dysfunction distinct from infectious encephalitis.[21] It can be caused by number of autoantibodies and is also an infrequent complication of treatment with PD-1 checkpoint inhibitors.

CLINICAL MANIFESTATIONS AND DIAGNOSIS

The clinical presentation is typically acute or subacute alteration of mental status characterized by change in behavior, memory, and awareness. Seizures also are common. An expanding number of IgG autoantibodies is useful both for the definitive diagnosis of the type of autoimmune encephalitis and also for guiding subsequent evaluation, including the search for an occult malignancy and the potential escalation of immunotherapy.

There are three characteristic clinical syndromes: limbic encephalitis, *N*-methyl-D-aspartate (NMDA)-receptor encephalitis, and brain stem encephalitis.[22] A diagnosis of autoimmune limbic encephalitis is suggested by the subacute onset of a loss of working memory, seizures, or psychiatric symptoms in a person with no other clear explanation. Typical supportive findings include CSF with low level of lymphocytes (5 to 100/μL) but no identifiable infection, electroencephalography with epileptiform activity, and MRI with bilateral medial temporal signal changes. Autoantibody testing from both serum and CSF can identify the immunologic subtype. An underlying cancer is found in more than 95% of patients who have antibodies directed against the intracellular antigens anti-Hu (small cell lung carcinoma) or Ma2 (testicular seminoma), whereas only 25% of patients who have high-titer anti–glutamic acid decarboxylase (GAD) antibodies will be found to have a cancer (thymomas or small cell lung carcinoma). GAD antibodies also occur in the setting of diabetes mellitus and other endocrine disorders.[23]

NMDA-receptor encephalitis is characterized by the presence of cognitive and psychiatric manifestations (often prominent), frequently with seizures, but also with speech dysfunction (mutism or rapid speech), movement disorders (dyskinesias and rigidity), and autonomic nervous system dysfunction. CSF analysis detects antibodies directed against the GluN1 subunit of the NMDA receptor, but false-negative results can occur on serum analysis. This diagnosis is frequently associated with ovarian teratomas, and resection of the teratoma in conjunction with immunotherapy is associated with favorable outcomes. Special consideration of NMDA receptor encephalitis should be pursued in cases of recurrent herpes simplex virus encephalitis (Chapters 350 and 386), which can follow herpes simplex virus brain infection. Other autoimmune encephalitides with antibodies directed against synaptic receptors carry a moderately high risk of malignancy, including γ-aminobutyric acid (GABA) B (small cell lung cancer), mGlu-R5 (Hodgkin lymphoma), and α-amino-3-hydroxy-5-methyl-4-isoxazolepropionic acid (AMPA) receptor (thymomas and small cell lung cancer). The differential diagnosis of autoimmune encephalitis includes consideration of acute disseminated encephalomyelitis, anti-MOG childhood demyelinating syndromes, anti–thyroid (thyroglobulin or tissue peroxidase) antibody Hashimoto encephalopathy, and Susac syndrome (encephalopathy with branched retinal artery occlusion and hearing loss).

Brain stem encephalitis should be considered in patients with an acute or subacute decline in sensorium with prominent symmetrical cerebellar signs and ophthalmoparesis in the absence of another explanation. Pyramidal tract dysfunction, bulbar signs, and pupillary abnormalities are common. This syndrome, which often follows infections, is monophasic with a good prognosis. Anti-GQ1b antibodies are present in the majority of cases. Granulomatous diseases (sarcoidosis), malignancy (lymphoma), and viral encephalitis need to be excluded.

Several other characteristic syndromes are associated with specific autoantibodies. Patients with IgG antibodies directed against surface proteins such as the voltage-gated potassium channels (VGKC) include patients with antibodies against anti–leucine-rich glioma-inactivated (LGI)-1 (cognitive impairment and seizures—especially faciobrachial dystonic seizures) or contactin-associated protein-like (CASPR)-2 (peripheral nerve hyperexcitability and less commonly encephalitis). Two clinical syndromes, Morvan (fibrillary chorea, encephalopathy, autonomic instability, and neuromuscular hyperexcitability) and Isaac (progressive neuromyotonia), are strongly linked with VGKC antibodies. The presence of VGKC antibodies in the absence of LGI-1 or CASPR-2 is nonspecific and can be benign.

CHRONIC AUTOIMMUNE SYNDROMES

Chronic autoimmune neurologic syndromes with either cerebral or extracerebral symptoms and signs include stiff person syndrome, which is characterized by chronic progressive axial rigidity and spasticity and is associated with high titer anti-GAD65, antiamphiphysin (women), and anti–glycine receptor antibodies. Stiff person syndrome, which may be mistaken for progressive supranuclear palsy (Chapter 381), is associated with diabetes and other

endocrine disorders. Progressive encephalomyelitis with rigidity and myoclonus is a distinct process that may be confused with stiff person syndrome but is often more acute in onset and rapidly progressive; patients also may have brain stem features such as ataxia, dysphagia, dysarthria, and ophthalmoparesis. Rasmussen encephalitis is a refractory epilepsy syndrome with hemispheric dysfunction associated with CD8 T-lymphocyte infiltration.

Grade A References

A1. Liu S, Liu X, Chen S, et al. Oral versus intravenous methylprednisolone for the treatment of multiple sclerosis relapses: a meta-analysis of randomized controlled trials. *PLoS ONE.* 2017;12:1-13.
A2. Melendez-Torres GJ, Auguste P, Armoiry X, et al. Clinical effectiveness and cost-effectiveness of beta-interferon and glatiramer acetate for treating multiple sclerosis: systematic review and economic evaluation. *Health Technol Assess.* 2017;21:1-352.
A3. La Mantia L, Di Pietrantonj C, Rovaris M, et al. Interferons-beta versus glatiramer acetate for relapsing-remitting multiple sclerosis. *Cochrane Database Syst Rev.* 2016;11:CD009333.
A4. Saida T, Kira JI, Kishida S, et al. Efficacy, safety, and pharmacokinetics of natalizumab in Japanese multiple sclerosis patients: a double-blind, randomized controlled trial and open-label pharmacokinetic study. *Mult Scler Relat Disord.* 2017;11:25-31.
A5. Kapoor R, Ho PR, Campbell N, et al. Effect of natalizumab on disease progression in secondary progressive multiple sclerosis (ASCEND): a phase 3, randomised, double-blind, placebo-controlled trial with an open-label extension. *Lancet Neurol.* 2018;17:405-415.
A6. Zhang J, Shi S, Zhang Y, et al. Alemtuzumab versus interferon beta 1a for relapsing-remitting multiple sclerosis. *Cochrane Database Syst Rev.* 2017;11:CD010968.
A7. Martinelli Boneschi F, Vacchi L, Rovaris M, et al. Mitoxantrone for multiple sclerosis. *Cochrane Database Syst Rev.* 2013;5:CD002127.
A8. La Mantia L, Tramacere I, Firwana B, et al. Fingolimod for relapsing-remitting multiple sclerosis. *Cochrane Database Syst Rev.* 2016;4:CD009371.
A9. He D, Zhang C, Zhao X, et al. Teriflunomide for multiple sclerosis. *Cochrane Database Syst Rev.* 2016;3:CD009882.
A10. Xu Z, Zhang F, Sun F, et al. Dimethyl fumarate for multiple sclerosis. *Cochrane Database Syst Rev.* 2015;4:CD011076.
A11. Montalban X, Hauser SL, Kappos L, et al. Ocrelizumab versus placebo in primary progressive multiple sclerosis. *N Engl J Med.* 2017;376:209-220.
A12. Hauser SL, Bar-Or A, Comi G, et al. Ocrelizumab versus interferon Beta-1a in relapsing multiple sclerosis. *N Engl J Med.* 2017;376:221-234.
A13. Castillo-Trivino T, Braithwaite D, Bacchetti P, et al. Rituximab in relapsing and progressive forms of multiple sclerosis: a systematic review. *PLoS ONE.* 2013;8:1-8.
A14. Comi G, Cook S, Rammohan K, et al. Long-term effects of cladribine tablets on MRI activity outcomes in patients with relapsing-remitting multiple sclerosis: the CLARITY Extension study. *Ther Adv Neurol Disord.* 2018;11:1-11.
A15. Jensen HB, Nielsen JL, Ravnborg M, et al. Effect of slow release-fampridine on muscle strength, rate of force development, functional capacity and cognitive function in an enriched population of MS patients. A randomized, double blind, placebo controlled study. *Mult Scler Relat Disord.* 2016;10:137-144.
A16. Kappos L, Bar-Or A, Cree BAC, et al. Siponimod versus placebo in secondary progressive multiple sclerosis (EXPAND): a double-blind, randomised, phase 3 study. *Lancet.* 2018;391:1263-1273.
A17. Metz LM, Li DKB, Traboulsee AL, et al. Trial of minocycline in a clinically isolated syndrome of multiple sclerosis. *N Engl J Med.* 2017;376:2122-2133.
A18. Morrow SA, Fraser JA, Day C, et al. Effect of treating acute optic neuritis with bioequivalent oral vs intravenous corticosteroids: a randomized clinical trial. *JAMA Neurol.* 2018;75:690-696.

GENERAL REFERENCES

For the General References and other additional features, please visit Expert Consult at https://expertconsult.inkling.com.

384

MENINGITIS: BACTERIAL, VIRAL, AND OTHER

AVINDRA NATH

BACTERIAL MENINGITIS

DEFINITION

Meningitis is an inflammation of the arachnoid membrane, the pia mater, and the intervening cerebrospinal fluid (CSF). The inflammatory process extends throughout the subarachnoid space around the brain and spinal cord and involves the ventricles. Pyogenic meningitis is usually an acute bacterial infection that evokes a polymorphonuclear response in CSF. By comparison, tuberculous meningitis (Chapter 308) is often subacute and characterized initially by a modest polymorphonuclear pleocytosis that rapidly evolves to lymphocytic predominance.

EPIDEMIOLOGY

The incidence of bacterial meningitis has dropped dramatically to about one to two cases per 100,000 adults in developed countries since the introduction of vaccines against bacterial pathogens such as *Haemophilus influenzae* type b (Chapter 282), *Streptococcus pneumoniae* (Chapter 273), and *Neisseria meningitidis* (Chapter 314). Since the advent of the *Haemophilus* vaccine, *S. pneumoniae* has become the most common pathogen, accounting for about 70% of cases, and the disease is now more common in older adults than children; mortality rates (~15%) have not changed.[1] Worldwide, however, bacterial meningitis remains a major cause of mortality and morbidity. Although all human microbes have the potential to cause meningitis, only a few organisms account for most cases of bacterial meningitis.

The clinical setting in which meningitis develops may provide a clue to the specific bacterial cause. *H. influenzae* (Chapter 284) affects primarily children, whereas *S. pneumoniae* (Chapter 273) affects predominantly adults older than age 50 years with comorbid conditions. Meningococcal meningitis (Chapter 282) often occurs in outbreaks. In developed countries, *Listeria monocytogenes* (Chapter 277) is emerging as the most common cause of bacterial meningitis, with peak frequencies in the neonatal period and in persons older than 60 years of age. Simultaneous mixed bacterial meningitis is rare but may occur after neurosurgical procedures, penetrating head injury, head trauma with fracture of the cribriform plate, erosion of the skull or vertebrae by adjacent neoplasm, extension of osteomyelitis, or intraventricular rupture of a cerebral abscess. Isolation of anaerobes should strongly suggest the latter two of these situations. In approximately 10% of patients with pyogenic meningitis, the bacterial cause cannot be defined.

Over the past several decades, gram-negative bacillary meningitis has doubled in frequency in adults, a change reflecting more frequent and extensive neurosurgical procedures, as well as other nosocomial factors. *L. monocytogenes* has increased eight- to 10-fold as a cause of bacterial meningitis. *Listeria* infections are most often food-borne via dairy products, processed meats, uncooked vegetables, and precut salads. Although *Listeria* meningitis may occur in immunocompetent individuals, it occurs most frequently in individuals who are immunocompromised owing to organ transplantation, hemodialysis, corticosteroid therapy, cytotoxic drugs for treatment of cancer or autoimmune diseases, liver disease, alcoholism, uncontrolled diabetes, and pregnancy. Meningitis caused by coagulase-negative staphylococci, which represents approximately 3% of cases in large urban hospitals, occurs as a complication of neurosurgical procedures and is often caused by methicillin-resistant strains.

In large tertiary care hospitals, approximately 40% of cases of bacterial meningitis in adults are of nosocomial origin.[2] The leading causes are gram-negative bacilli (primarily *Escherichia coli* and *Klebsiella*), which account for approximately 40% of nosocomial episodes, as well as various streptococci, *Staphylococcus aureus*, and coagulase-negative staphylococci, each responsible for approximately 10% of nosocomial cases.

Meningococcal disease, including meningitis, may occur sporadically and in cyclic outbreaks. High-risk groups include individuals who live in close quarters such as crowded classrooms, college dormitories, military barracks, or jails. In children the greatest risk is in the first year of life. With the introduction of the meningococcal vaccine, the incidence meningococcal meningitis has decreased drastically, although vaccinated populations remain vulnerable to the serotypes that are not covered by the vaccine. Antibiotic-resistant strains of meningococcus also have emerged. The incidence of meningococcal meningitis was probably underestimated historically when the diagnosis was based on isolation of the organism. Polymerase chain reaction (PCR) testing suggests twice the number of cases.

Predisposing factors for the development of pneumococcal meningitis include acute otitis media (Chapters 273 and 398), with or without mastoiditis, in approximately 20% of adult patients. Pneumonia is present in approximately 15% of patients with pneumococcal meningitis, a much higher frequency than in meningitis caused by *H. influenzae* or *N. meningitidis*. Acute pneumococcal sinusitis (Chapter 398) is occasionally the initial focus from which infection spreads to the meninges. A recent or remote major head injury (Chapter 371) precedes approximately 10% of episodes of pneumococcal meningitis, and CSF rhinorrhea (usually caused by a defect or fracture in the cribriform plate) is present in approximately 5% of patients. Cochlear implants, particularly those that include a positioner, have been implicated in childhood bacterial meningitis caused by *S. pneumoniae*. Occasionally, meningitis caused by *S. pneumoniae* develops in patients with central nervous system (CNS) shunts.

Splenectomy or splenic dysfunction, as in sickle cell anemia (Chapter 154), cirrhosis (Chapter 144) with portal hypertension, or defects in humoral immunity also predispose patients to pneumococcal meningitis. Alcoholism (Chapter 30) is an underlying risk factor in 10 to 25% of adults with pneumococcal meningitis in urban hospitals. The estimated annual incidence of bacterial meningitis (primarily pneumococcal) in patients infected with human immunodeficiency virus (HIV) is 150-fold higher than in the general population. However, cryptococcal meningitis and tuberculous meningitis are much more common in HIV-infected patients.

S. aureus meningitis may occur as a complication of a neurosurgical procedure, after penetrating skull trauma, or occasionally secondary to staphylococcal bacteremia and endocarditis. Meningitis caused by gram-negative bacilli takes one of three forms: neonatal meningitis, meningitis after trauma or neurosurgery, or spontaneous meningitis in adults (e.g., bacteremic *Klebsiella* meningitis in a patient with diabetes mellitus). The most common causes of gram-negative bacillary meningitis in adults are *E. coli* (≈30%) and *Klebsiella-Enterobacter* (≈40%). Meningitis caused by group A streptococci is uncommon but occasionally occurs after acute otitis media, more often in children than in adults. *H. influenzae* type b meningitis in an adult suggests an underlying anatomic or immunologic defect.

PATHOBIOLOGY

Pathology

On gross examination, purulent exudate in the subarachnoid space is most abundant in the cisterns at the base of the brain and over the convexities of the rolandic and sylvian sulci, which are expansions of the subarachnoid space. Although neither the infecting organism nor the inflammatory exudate directly invades cerebral tissue, the subjacent brain becomes congested and edematous. The pial barrier generally prevents bacterial meningitis from causing a cerebral abscess; when these two processes coexist, the sequence is usually that an initial abscess leaks its contents into the ventricular system and produces secondary ventriculitis and meningitis.

The inflammatory exudate can extend around the perivascular spaces to adjacent structures, especially the arteries and veins that carry a layer of pia mater and arachnoid membrane as they enter the brain from the cortical surface. *Cortical thrombophlebitis* results from venous stasis and adjacent meningeal inflammation. Infarction of cerebral tissue may follow. *Involvement of cortical and pial arteries* by peripheral aneurysm formation and vascular occlusion or narrowing (related to spasm, arteritis, or both) of the supraclinoid portion of the internal carotid artery at the base of the brain occurs in approximately 15% of patients with meningitis. The anterior and middle cerebral arteries may have markedly increased intracerebral blood flow velocity (an index of stenosis or arterial spasm) on transcranial Doppler ultrasonography, a finding corresponding to focal cerebral signs. In fulminating cases, particularly meningococcal meningitis, *cerebral edema* may be marked even though the pleocytosis is only moderate. Rarely, temporal lobe herniation through the tentorium develops in such patients and compresses the midbrain, thereby leading to ipsilateral third nerve palsy and contralateral hemiparesis; or cerebellar herniation through the foramen magnum with compression of the medulla, which results in apnea, hemodynamic instability, and coma. *Damage to cranial nerves* occurs in areas where dense exudate accumulates around the nerves; the third and sixth cranial nerves are also vulnerable to damage by increased intracranial pressure. *Ventriculitis* accompanies most cases of bacterial meningitis and may rarely progress to *ventricular empyema*. As the exudates continue to accumulate, obstruction of the flow of CSF may result in *hydrocephalus*. Obstruction of the foramina of Magendie and Luschka at the base of the fourth ventricle results in noncommunicating or obstructive hydrocephalus, whereas obstruction at the level of the arachnoid granulations in the venous sinuses results in communicating hydrocephalus. *Subdural effusions* are sterile transudates that develop over the cerebral cortex and can be demonstrated readily by computed tomography (CT) as low-density areas about the cerebrum. On magnetic resonance imaging (MRI), they appear as high signal intensity lesions of T2 or fluid-attenuated inversion recovery (FLAIR) sequences. Rarely, such effusions become infected and produce subdural empyema.

Pathogenesis

Bacteria may gain access to the meninges by several routes: (1) hematogenous spread from a distant site; (2) direct ingress from the upper respiratory tract or skin through an anatomic defect (e.g., skull fracture, meningocele, sequela of surgery); (3) passage intracranially through venules in the nasopharynx; or (4) spread from a contiguous focus of infection (infection of the paranasal sinuses, leakage of a brain abscess). Bacteremic spread of *H. influenzae, N. meningitidis,* and *S. pneumoniae* is probably the most frequent path of infection. Bacteremia is usually initiated by pharyngeal adhesion and colonization by an infecting strain. Adhesion of such strains, as well as of *S. pneumoniae,* to mucosal surfaces is abetted by their capacity to produce proteases that cleave immunoglobulin A, thus inactivating this local antibody defense. Adhesion of *N. meningitidis* to nasopharyngeal cells is affected by fimbriae or pili and promoted by previous damage to ciliated cells such as from smoking or viral infections. Meningococci invade the nasopharyngeal mucosal cells by means of endocytosis and are transported to the abluminal side in membrane-bound vacuoles. *H. influenzae,* in contrast, invades intercellularly by causing separation of the apical tight junctions between columnar epithelial cells. When these meningeal pathogens gain access to the blood stream, their intravascular survival is aided by the presence of polysaccharide capsules that inhibit phagocytosis and confer resistance to complement-mediated bactericidal activity.

Bacteria also may travel along nerve tracts to invade the brain. For example, *L. monocytogenes* invades the intestine, and animal models suggest that these bacteria can travel along the vagus nerve to the brain stem, from where they also may invade the meninges in the posterior fossa.

Bacteria can gain access to the subarachnoid spaces from blood cells, either by disruption of the blood brain barrier or via the choroid plexus, also termed the blood-CSF barrier. Once established in any part of the meninges, infection quickly extends throughout the subarachnoid space. Bacterial replication proceeds relatively unhindered because the low CSF levels of immunoglobulin and complement early in meningeal inflammation result in minimal or no opsonic or bactericidal activity and because surface phagocytosis of unopsonized organisms is meager in such a fluid environment. During meningitis, the concentrations of immunoglobulins in CSF increase but still remain relatively low. Secondary bacteremia may follow meningeal infection and may itself contribute to continuing further inoculation of CSF.

Bacterial meningitis following head trauma occurs because of a dural fistula from the nasal cavity, paranasal sinuses, or middle ear to the subarachnoid space. The most frequent site is at the cribriform plate, where the bone is thin and the dura is tightly adherent to the bone. Leakage of CSF results in CSF rhinorrhea and loss of smell.

Bacterial components (e.g., pneumococcal cell walls or lipoteichoic acid, *H. influenzae* lipo-oligosaccharide) are major elicitors of meningeal inflammation by causing release into the subarachnoid space of various pro-inflammatory cytokines such as interleukin-1 and tumor necrosis factor (TNF) from endothelial and meningeal cells, macrophages, and microglia. Cytokines appear to enhance the passage of leukocytes by inducing several families of adhesion molecules that interact with the corresponding receptors on leukocytes. Cytokines also can increase the binding affinity of a leukocyte selectin, leukocyte adhesion molecule, for its endothelial cell receptor and may thereby further contribute to trafficking of neutrophils into the subarachnoid space.

In bacterial meningitis, neutrophils move into the subarachnoid space but are not able to control the bacterial infection because their phagocytic properties are inefficient as a result of a lack of opsonic and bactericidal activity. Within the subarachnoid space, neutrophils release prostaglandins, matrix metalloproteinases, and free radicals that disrupt the endothelial intercellular tight junctions and the subendothelial basal lamina. The increased local vascular permeability of the blood-brain barrier may cause cerebral edema, which also can be caused by increased CSF pressure as a result of obstruction of CSF outflow because of interstitial inflammation at the level of the arachnoidal villi.

Cerebral blood flow, which depends on mean arterial pressure, is increased in the early stages of meningitis, but it subsequently decreases, substantially in some patients, which may cause ischemic neurologic injury. Localized regions of marked hypoperfusion, attributable to focal vascular inflammation or thrombosis, can occur in patients with normal blood flow. Impairment of cerebral blood flow autoregulation, as measured by transcranial Doppler ultrasonography of the middle cerebral artery, occurs early in acute bacterial meningitis and causes cerebral blood flow to correspond directly to mean arterial blood pressure, with attendant hyperperfusion or hypoperfusion of the brain. On recovery, the ability of the cerebral vasculature to maintain a constant level of perfusion despite variations in mean arterial pressure is restored.

Genetics

Patients with defects in cell-mediated immunity are susceptible to the development of CNS infections with intracellular organisms such as *L. monocytogenes.* Patients with defective humoral immunity and an inadequate antibody response are particularly vulnerable to meningitis with *S. pneumoniae* and *H. influenzae.* For example, deficiencies in the complement system predispose patients to

meningitis, and 50 to 60% of adults with pneumococcal meningitis may have C2 deficiency. Meningococcal meningitis is associated with polymorphisms in CD32, CD16, mannose-binding lectin, toll-like receptor 4 (TLR4), and the B-2 adrenoceptor gene. Patients with neutropenia are at higher risk for meningitis with *Pseudomonas aeruginosa* and members of the Enterobacteriaceae family.

CLINICAL MANIFESTATIONS

History

Acute-onset fever, generalized headache, vomiting, and stiff neck are common to many types of meningitis (Table 384-1). Most patients with community-acquired pyogenic meningitis have had an antecedent or accompanying upper respiratory tract infection or nonspecific febrile illness, acute otitis (or mastoiditis), or pneumonia. Myalgia, particularly in patients with meningococcal disease, backache, and generalized weakness are common symptoms. The illness usually progresses rapidly, with the development of confusion, obtundation, and loss of consciousness. Occasionally, the onset may be less acute, with meningeal signs being present for several days to a week.

General Physical Findings

Evidence of meningeal irritation is usually present, as evidenced by a stiff neck, Kernig sign (inability to straighten the leg when the hip is flexed to 90 degrees), and Brudzinski sign (involuntary flexion of the hip and knee when the neck is passively flexed). Neck stiffness, Kernig sign, and Brudzinski sign each have sensitivities of approximately 30% or lower for diagnosing acute

TABLE 384-1	SYMPTOMS AND SIGNS OF BACTERIAL MENINGITIS*	
CHARACTERISTIC	**EPISODES OF MENINGITIS**
Duration of symptoms <24 hr	48%
Predisposing conditions	
Otitis or sinusitis	25%
Pneumonia	12%
Immunocompromise[†]	16%
Symptoms at initial evaluation	
Headache	87%
Nausea	74%
Neck stiffness	83%
Triad of fever, neck stiffness, and change in mental status	44%
Focal neurologic deficits	33%
Aphasia	23%
Hemiparesis	7%
Indices of CSF inflammation	
Opening pressure (mm H_2O)[†]	370 ± 130
White cell count[§]	
Mean (cells/μL)	$7753 \pm 14,736$
<100/μL	7%
100-999/μL	14%
>999/μL	78%
Protein (g/L)	4.9 ± 4.5
CSF/blood glucose ratio	0.2 ± 0.2
Positive blood culture[‖]	66%
Blood tests	
ESR (mm/hr)[¶]	46 ± 37
C-reactive protein (g/L)**	225 ± 132
Platelet count (platelets/μL)[††]	$198,000 \pm 100,000$

*Data from 696 cases reported in van de Beek D, de Gans J, Spanjaard L, et al. Clinical features and prognostic factors in adults with bacterial meningitis. *N Engl J Med.* 2004;351:1849-1859. The study included 671 patients who had a total of 696 episodes of community-acquired meningitis. Plus-minus values are means ± standard deviation.

[†]Immunocompromise was defined by the use of immunosuppressive drugs, a history of splenectomy, or the presence of diabetes mellitus or alcoholism, as well as patients infected with human immunodeficiency virus.

[†]CSF pressure was measured in 216 patients.

[§]The CSF leukocyte count was determined in 659 patients; CSF specimens from 14 patients had too many leukocytes for an exact count to be performed.

[‖]Blood culture was performed in 611 patients.

[¶]The ESR was determined in 549 patients.

**C-reactive protein levels were determined in 394 patients.

[††]The thrombocyte count was determined in 653 patients.

CSF = cerebrospinal fluid; ESR = erythrocyte sedimentation rate.

bacterial meningitis in adults. Although the classic triad of fever, stiff neck, and change in mental status is initially present in only 44% of episodes, a combination of two of four symptoms (headache, fever, stiff neck, and altered mental status) is found in 95% of patients. The findings of meningitis may be easily overlooked in infants, obtunded patients, elderly patients with heart failure or pneumonia, or immunosuppressed individuals, who may have meningitis without prominent meningeal signs; in such patients, lethargy should be investigated carefully, meningeal signs should be sought, and examination of CSF is indicated if any doubt exists. In elderly patients, neck stiffness may be difficult to evaluate because of osteoarthritis in the neck or stiffness of neck muscles secondary to basal ganglia disorders. When neck stiffness is caused by meningitis, the neck resists flexion but can be rotated passively from side to side; with cervical spine disease, however, resistance is present in all directions of neck movement. Neck stiffness disappears during coma.

The presence of a petechial or ecchymotic rash (see Fig. 282-3) in a patient with meningeal findings almost always indicates meningococcal infection and requires prompt treatment because of the rapidity with which this infection can progress (Chapter 282). Rarely, extensive petechial and ecchymotic lesions occur in meningitis caused by *S. pneumoniae, H. influenzae,* or echovirus type 9. Very rarely, skin lesions almost indistinguishable from those of meningococcal bacteremia occur in patients who have acute *S. aureus* endocarditis (see Fig. 67-1) and who also have meningeal signs and pleocytosis (secondary to either staphylococcal meningitis or embolic cerebral infarction). Usually, one or two of the lesions in such a patient represent purulent purpura; aspiration of material reveals staphylococci on Gram staining. In the summer, viral aseptic meningitis may produce meningeal signs, macular and petechial skin lesions, and a pleocytosis of several hundred cells, sometimes with neutrophils predominating initially.

Fulminant meningococcal septicemia may cause hemorrhages within the adrenal glands and result in Waterhouse-Friderichsen syndrome (Chapter 214), a condition characterized by the sudden onset of a febrile illness, large petechial hemorrhages in the mucous membranes and skin, cardiovascular collapse, and disseminated intravascular coagulation. In contrast, hyponatremia and the syndrome of inappropriate secretion of antidiuretic hormone may develop in patients with meningitis attributable to *H. influenzae.* A concurrent respiratory tract infection or acute otitis media may be present with either *H. influenzae* or *S. pneumoniae.*

In patients with a basilar skull fracture, the potential for development of a dural fistula and bacterial meningitis is indicated by the presence of CSF rhinorrhea, periorbital ecchymoses, bruising behind the ear (Battle sign), hemotympanum, or blood in the external auditory canal. Meningitis complicating neurosurgical procedures may be insidious in onset and difficult to distinguish from the altered consciousness and signs of meningeal irritation that are expected in the postoperative period. However, fever or prolonged obtundation is an indication for evaluation of CSF.

Neurologic Findings and Complications

Neurologic complications in patients with inadequately treated bacterial meningitis can be severe and disabling.[3] Cranial nerve abnormalities, involving principally the third, fourth, sixth, or seventh nerve, occur in 5 to 10% of adults with community-acquired meningitis and usually disappear shortly after recovery. Persistent sensorineural hearing loss occurs in 10% of children with bacterial meningitis, and another 16% have transient conductive hearing loss. The most likely sites of involvement in patients with persistent sensorineural deafness appear to be the inner ear (infection or toxic products possibly spreading from the subarachnoid space along the cochlear aqueduct) and the acoustic nerve. In children, permanent hearing impairment is more common after meningitis caused by *S. pneumoniae* than by *H. influenzae* or *N. meningitidis.*

Seizures (focal or generalized; Chapter 375) occur in 20 to 30% of patients and may result from reversible causes (high fever or hypoglycemia in infants, penicillin neurotoxicity when large doses are administered intravenously (IV) to patients with renal failure) or, more commonly, from focal cerebral injury related to arterial hypoperfusion and infarction, cortical venous thrombosis, or focal edema and cerebritis. Seizures can occur during the first few days or can appear with associated focal neurologic deficits caused by vascular inflammation some days after onset of the meningitis. In adults with seizures accompanying meningitis, *S. pneumoniae* is more commonly the cause, but alcohol withdrawal is a confounding factor.

Increased CSF pressure, which can be caused by brain swelling or hydrocephalus, is associated with seizures, vomiting, sixth and third nerve dysfunction, abnormal reflexes, reduced consciousness or coma, dilated and poorly reactive pupils, and the Cushing response of decerebrate posturing, hypertension,

bradycardia, and irregular respirations. In approximately a fourth of fatal cases of community-acquired meningitis in adults, cerebral edema accompanied by temporal lobe herniation is observed at autopsy.

Papilledema (see Fig. 395-25) occurs in less than 1% of patients with bacterial meningitis, even with high CSF pressure, probably because the patient is seen early in the process before changes in the nerve head have occurred. The presence of this sign should indicate the possibility of another associated or independent suppurative intracranial process, such as subdural empyema or brain abscess or a more chronic process such as fungal or tuberculous meningitis. Marked central hyperpnea sometimes occurs in patients with severe bacterial meningitis; CSF acidosis, which is principally due to increased lactic acid levels, provides much of the respiratory stimulus.

Focal cerebral signs (principally hemiparesis, dysphasia, visual field defects, and gaze preference) occur in approximately a third of adults with community-acquired bacterial meningitis. These signs may develop because of arterial or venous occlusion. In addition, cerebral blood flow velocity may be decreased in patients with increased intracranial pressure and may lead to temporary or lasting neurologic dysfunction. It is important to distinguish these vascular effects from postictal changes (Todd paralysis), which usually persist for less than a day. Meningitis may cause the syndrome of inappropriate secretion of antidiuretic hormone.

DIAGNOSIS

Bacterial meningitis is a medical emergency that requires immediate diagnosis and rapid institution of antimicrobial therapy.[4] Delay in treatment is the most critical factor in determining the morbidity and mortality of patients with bacterial meningitis. The diagnosis of bacterial meningitis is not difficult in a febrile patient with meningeal symptoms and signs developing in the setting of a predisposing illness. The diagnosis may be less obvious in an elderly, obtunded patient with pneumonia or a confused alcoholic patient in impending delirium tremens.

When the diagnosis of bacterial meningitis is entertained, blood cultures should be performed, CSF examined and cultured, and antimicrobial therapy instituted promptly. Observational data suggest that the prompt performance of a lumbar puncture before CT scanning is associated with significantly earlier treatment and favorable outcomes.[5] If a mass lesion (cerebral abscess, subdural empyema) is suspected from the history, clinical setting, or physical findings (papilledema, focal cerebral signs), CT with or without contrast enhancement or MRI should be performed because of the danger of brain herniation with lumbar puncture. Antibiotics can and commonly should be started immediately, with the goal of a door to antibiotics time of less than 1 hour, even before performing lumbar puncture, because it takes approximately 2 hours for antibiotics to affect CSF cultures. Empiric corticosteroids (see Treatment) also should be given at this same time. Diagnostic lumbar puncture should not be delayed to perform CT or MRI except in patients who have focal neurologic findings suggestive of a parameningeal collection or other intracranial mass lesions; in such patients, it is critical to initiate antimicrobial therapy for meningitis of unknown origin or brain abscess before CT or MRI is performed. Patients with community-acquired meningitis rarely have important abnormalities detected on CT in the absence of focal neurologic findings.

Laboratory Findings
Cerebrospinal Fluid Examination

Initial CSF pressure is usually moderately elevated (200 to 300 mm H_2O in adults). Striking elevations ($\geq$450 mm H_2O) occur in occasional patients with acute brain swelling complicating meningitis in the absence of an associated mass lesion. Findings on CSF analysis are strikingly abnormal in patients with meningitis, and such findings help suggest the cause even before the results of culture are available (Table 384-2). In patients with skull fractures, CSF rhinorrhea can be distinguished from nasal secretions by the presence of glucose.

Gram-Stained Smear

By the time of hospitalization, most patients with pyogenic meningitis have large numbers ($\geq$10^5/mL) of bacteria in their CSF. Careful examination of the Gram-stained smear of the spun sediment of CSF reveals the etiologic agent in 60 to 80% of cases. In most instances in which gram-positive diplococci (or short-chain cocci) are observed on a stained CSF smear, they are pneumococci. *Enterococcus,* an occasional cause of nosocomial meningitis, is detected by latex particle agglutination. Rarely, three species may morphologically mimic *Neisseria* in CSF or may suggest a mixed infection with short

TABLE 384-2 COMMON CEREBROSPINAL FLUID FINDINGS IN PATIENTS WITH MENINGITIS

MICROORGANISM	CSF OPENING PRESSURE (cm H$_2$O)	CELL COUNT (CELLS/µL)	PROTEIN (mg/dL)	GLUCOSE (mg/dL)
Normal	10-20	<5	20-40	40-60
Bacteria*	>20	>1000	>100	<10
Mycobacterium tuberculosis	>20	100-500	>100	10-45
Borrelia burgdorferi	<20	100-500	50-150	10-45
Treponema pallidum	<20	5-500	50-150	10-45
Fungi	<20	5-500	>100	10-45
Viruses	<20	5-500	50-150	Normal

Ranges of biochemical tests may vary in different laboratories.
*Group B streptococci, *Escherichia coli*, *Listeria monocytogenes*, *Streptococcus pneumoniae*, *Neisseria meningitidis*, and *Haemophilus influenzae* type b.
CSF = cerebrospinal fluid.
Modified from Kim KS. Acute bacterial meningitis in infants and children. *Lancet Infect Dis.* 2010;10:32-42.

gram-negative rods and meningococci: *Acinetobacter baumannii*, *Moraxella* sp, and *Pasteurella multocida*.

Rapid Bacteriologic Diagnosis
Broad-range PCR testing, which can be performed on CSF within 1.5 hours, can diagnose bacterial meningitis in patients in whom cultures will be negative. Overall reported sensitivities in various studies range from 87 to 100%, with specificities of 98 to 100%.[6] PCR also can rapidly diagnose viral meningitis, which overall is far more common than bacterial meningitis,[7] thereby establishing an alternative diagnosis so that antibiotics can be discontinued because a combined viral and bacterial meningitis is highly unlikely. However, because a totally negative PCR result does not exclude bacterial meningitis, other tests (cell count; glucose, protein, and lactic acid levels), which served as proxies while awaiting culture results in an earlier era, still remain very useful in such patients.

In resource-poor countries, a urine reagent strip that detects cells, proteins, and glucose in CSF has a sensitivity of 92% and a specificity of 98% for diagnosing bacterial meningitis.[8] In many parts of the world, it may be especially useful for distinguishing bacterial meningitis from CNS malaria (Chapter 324). Culture of CSF reveals the etiologic agent in 80 to 90% of patients with bacterial meningitis if CSF is obtained before or within 1 to 2 hours of the initiation of antibiotics, but its sensitivities declined to less than 50% with longer delays. For therapeutic decisions, a positive PCR or a positive culture mandates a full course of antibiotic treatment.

Cell Count
Cell counts should be determined promptly because the cells will begin to lyse after 90 minutes. The normal CSF white blood cell count is less than 5/µL (all mononuclear). The cell count in untreated meningitis usually ranges between 100 and 10,000/µL, with polymorphonuclear leukocytes predominating initially (>80%) and lymphocytes appearing subsequently.

Extremely high cell counts (>50,000/µL) should raise the possibility of intraventricular rupture of a cerebral abscess. Cell counts as low as 10 to 20/µL may be observed early in bacterial meningitis, particularly that caused by *N. meningitidis* and *H. influenzae*. Occasionally, in granulocytopenic patients or in elderly persons with overwhelming pneumococcal meningitis, CSF may contain very few leukocytes and yet may appear grossly turbid because of the presence of a myriad of organisms and an elevated protein level. Meningitis caused by several bacterial species (*Mycobacterium tuberculosis*, *Borrelia burgdorferi*, *Treponema pallidum*, *Leptospira* sp, *Francisella tularensis*, *Brucella* sp) is characteristically associated with a lymphocytic pleocytosis. With *L. monocytogenes* meningitis in an adult, there is usually a polymorphonuclear response but lymphocytes may predominate in rare instances.

Glucose
CSF glucose is reduced to values of 40 mg/dL or less (or <50% of the simultaneous blood level) in 50% of patients with bacterial meningitis; this finding helps distinguish bacterial meningitis from most viral meningitides or parameningeal infections. However, a normal CSF glucose value does not exclude the diagnosis of bacterial meningitis. The blood glucose level should be determined simultaneously because patients with diabetes mellitus (or those who are receiving intravenous glucose infusions) have an elevated CSF glucose level that can be appreciated only by comparison with the simultaneous blood

level; however, it may take 90 to 120 minutes for equilibration to occur after major shifts in the level of glucose in the circulation.

Protein
The level of protein in lumbar CSF is usually elevated to greater than 100 mg/dL, and higher values are more commonly observed in pneumococcal meningitis. Extreme elevations, 1000 mg/dL or greater, may indicate subarachnoid block with obstruction of CSF flow. Values higher than 15 mg/dL in ventricular CSF are considered abnormal. If the lumbar puncture is traumatic, the CSF protein level is corrected by subtracting 1 mg/dL for every 1000 red blood cells.

Lactic Acid
Elevated levels of lactic acid occur in pyogenic meningitis. The diagnostic accuracy of a CSF lactate level is at least as good as a cell count for differentiating bacterial from aseptic meningitis, a value above 3.0 mmol/L has a sensitivity and specificity of 94 to 95% for bacterial meningitis. However, the CSF lactate level is less useful in patients who have received antibiotics, and it also may be increased in other conditions such as cerebral ischemia, stroke, and head trauma.

Blood and Respiratory Tract Cultures
Bacteremia is demonstrable in approximately 80% of patients with *H. influenzae* meningitis, 50% of patients with pneumococcal meningitis, and 30 to 40% of patients with meningococcal meningitis. Hence, blood cultures should be performed routinely in patients suspected of having bacterial meningitis. Cultures of the upper respiratory tract are not helpful in establishing an etiologic diagnosis.

Determination of serum creatinine and electrolyte levels is important in view of the gravity of the illness, the occurrence of specific abnormalities secondary to the meningitis (syndrome of inappropriate secretion of antidiuretic hormone), and problems with therapy in patients with renal dysfunction (seizures and hyperkalemia with high-dose penicillin therapy). In patients with extensive petechial and purpuric skin lesions, evaluation for coagulopathy is indicated.

Radiologic Studies
Because of the frequency with which pyogenic meningitis is associated with primary foci of infection in the chest, nasal sinuses, or mastoid, radiographs of these areas should be taken when clinically indicated at the appropriate time after antimicrobial therapy is begun. Initial head CT or MRI is not indicated in most patients with bacterial meningitis. For example, in patients who undergo head CT or MRI before lumbar puncture for suspected meningitis, only approximately 5% have a mass effect identified on CT. Baseline clinical features associated with abnormal findings on CT include age older than 60 years, history of CNS disease, seizure within the previous week, abnormal level of consciousness, abnormal visual fields, limb drift, and aphasia. In patients without any of these clinical findings, only approximately 1% have a mass effect identified on CT or MRI that would raise concern regarding lumbar puncture.

Specific changes that may be observed on CT or MRI during meningitis include cerebral edema and enlargement of the subarachnoid spaces, contrast enhancement of the leptomeninges and the ependyma, or patchy areas of diminished density as a result of associated cerebritis and necrosis. In patients with meningitis whose clinical status deteriorates or fails to improve, CT or MRI may help demonstrate suspected complications—that is, sterile subdural collections or empyema; ventricular enlargement secondary to communicating or obstructive hydrocephalus; prominent persisting basilar meningitis; extensive areas of cerebral infarction resulting from occlusion of major cerebral arteries, veins, or venous sinuses; or marked ventricular wall enhancement suggesting ventriculitis or ventricular empyema. MRI is superior to CT for visualizing these abnormalities. Rarely, cerebral hemorrhage identifiable on CT may complicate acute bacterial meningitis in adults. In approximately 10% of adults with bacterial meningitis, findings on cranial CT (mastoid or sinus wall defect, eroding retrobulbar mass, pneumocephalus) are indicative of disruption of the dural barrier.

Rarely, paraparesis or tetraparesis resulting from myelitis may complicate bacterial meningitis. In this situation, T2-weighted or short tau inversion recovery (STIR) sequences on MRI can be helpful to exclude spinal cord compression by an extramedullary mass.

Differential Diagnosis

Headache, fever, stiff neck, confusion, vomiting, and pleocytosis are features of meningeal inflammation and are common to many types of meningitis (e.g., bacterial, fungal, viral, chemical) and also some parameningeal processes. The CSF findings are most helpful in distinguishing among these processes (Chapters 385 and 386), and PCR can usually provide a rapid diagnosis. In most modern studies of adults, viral meningitis or encephalitis is about four times more common than bacterial meningitis (Table 384-3).[9] Although a lymphocyte-predominant pleocytosis without hypoglycorrhachia is characteristic of viral (usually enteroviral or herpes simplex virus type 2 [HSV-2]) meningitis or meningoencephalitis, the initial CSF finding may be a polymorphonuclear response (of ≤60%) that quickly becomes mononuclear. HSV-1 encephalitis is suggested by neurologic findings (dysphasia, hemiparesis, olfactory hallucinations, other temporal lobe signs, seizures), abnormalities in the orbitofrontal and medial temporal lobes on MRI, and distinctive electroencephalographic changes in the temporal lobe or lobes. The rash, fever, and headache of Rocky Mountain spotted fever (Chapter 311) may suggest meningococcal infection, but the geographic and seasonal predilections of the former can provide clues. Approximately 10% of patients hospitalized with Rocky Mountain spotted fever have CSF cell counts higher than 100/μL (>70% polymorphonuclear), and thus the condition initially may be confused with bacterial meningitis. The rash associated with enteroviral infections typically consists of erythematous macules and papules on the face, neck, and trunk.

Acute subarachnoid hemorrhage (Chapter 380) may be confused with bacterial meningitis because of headache, stiff neck, and vomiting. However, subarachnoid hemorrhage usually has a more abrupt onset without a prodromal fever but with evidence of subarachnoid blood on CT or CSF examination. In patients with neuroleptic malignant syndrome (Chapters 382 and 390), fever, generalized rigidity, and a fluctuating level of consciousness with autonomic instability and leukocytosis may develop. The most specific laboratory abnormality in these patients is a markedly elevated creatine kinase level.

In patients who have meningitis but whose CSF does not reveal the etiologic agent on a Gram-stained smear or PCR test, particularly when the CSF glucose level is normal and the polymorphonuclear pleocytosis is atypical, certain treatable processes that can mimic bacterial meningitis should be considered in the differential diagnosis:

1. *Parameningeal infections.* The presence of infections (chronic ear or nasal accessory sinus infections, lung abscess) predisposing to brain abscess, epidural (cerebral or spinal) abscess, subdural empyema, or pyogenic venous sinus phlebitis should be considered (Chapter 385). Neurologic symptoms may appear in the course of primary bacterial meningitis, but their presence may indicate the presence of a space-occupying infectious process in the CNS. Neurologic symptoms or findings antedating the onset of meningeal symptoms may suggest a parameningeal infection. Isolation of an anaerobic organism should suggest the possibility of intraventricular leakage of a cerebral abscess.

2. *Bacterial endocarditis.* Bacterial meningitis may occur during bacterial endocarditis (Chapter 67) caused by pyogenic organisms such as *S. aureus* and enterococci. In subacute bacterial endocarditis, sterile embolic infarctions of the brain may produce meningeal signs and a pleocytosis consisting of several hundred cells, including polymorphonuclear leukocytes. A history of dental manipulation, fever, and anorexia antedating the meningitis should be sought; careful examination for heart murmurs and peripheral stigmata of endocarditis is indicated.

3. *"Chemical" meningitis.* The clinical and CSF findings (polymorphonuclear pleocytosis and even reduced glucose level) of bacterial meningitis may be produced by chemically induced inflammation. Acute meningitis after diagnostic lumbar puncture or spinal anesthesia may result from bacterial or chemical contamination of equipment or anesthetic agent. Chemical meningitis, characterized by polymorphonuclear pleocytosis, hypoglycorrhachia, and a latent period of 3 to 24 hours, occurs after 1% of metrizamide myelograms. Endogenous chemical meningitis resulting from material from an epidermoid tumor or a craniopharyngioma leaking into the subarachnoid space, a glioblastoma invading the ventricles (Chapter 180), or carcinomatous meningitis (see later) can produce polymorphonuclear pleocytosis and hypoglycorrhachia.

Complications
Non-neurologic Complications
Shock
When shock occurs in patients with pyogenic meningitis, it is usually a manifestation of the accompanying intense bacteremia, as in fulminant meningococcemia, rather than a manifestation of the meningitis itself. Management is guided by the principles of septic shock therapy (Chapter 100), with appropriate modifications in patients with heart failure (Chapter 53).

Coagulation Disorders
Coagulopathies (Chapter 165) are frequently associated with the intense bacteremia (usually meningococcal, occasionally pneumococcal) and hypotension that can accompany meningitis. The changes may be mild, such as thrombocytopenia (with or without prolongation of the prothrombin and partial thromboplastin times), or more marked, with clinical evidence of disseminated intravascular coagulation (Chapter 166).

Septic Complications
Endocarditis
In patients with pneumococcal meningitis, particularly those with concomitant bacteremia and pneumonia, acute endocarditis (Chapter 67) can develop, most commonly on the aortic valve. In such patients, febrile relapse and a new cardiac murmur may appear shortly after the completion of antimicrobial therapy for meningitis.

Pyogenic Arthritis
Septic arthritis may result from the bacteremia associated with meningitis caused by *S. pneumoniae*, *N. meningitidis*, or *H. influenzae*.

Prolonged Fever
With appropriate antimicrobial treatment of community-acquired bacterial meningitis, patients become afebrile within 2 to 5 days. Sometimes, however, the fever persists or recurs after an afebrile period. In a patient with persisting headache, obtundation, and cerebral findings, inadequate drug therapy or neurologic sequelae (cortical venous thrombophlebitis, ventriculitis, subdural collections) are important considerations. Re-evaluation of CSF, particularly Gram-stained smear and culture, is essential in these circumstances. Drug-induced fever (Chapters 239 and 264) should be suspected in patients who continue to show clinical improvement in all other respects. Metastatic infection (septic arthritis, purulent pericarditis, thoracic empyema, endocarditis) may be the cause of continuing or recurrent fever. A syndrome, probably immunologic, consisting of fever, arthritis, and pericarditis 3 to 6 days after the initiation of effective antimicrobial therapy for meningococcal meningitis occurs in approximately 10% of patients (Chapter 282).

TABLE 384-3	CAUSES OF NON-NOSOCOMIAL MENINGITIS AND ENCEPHALITIS IN U.S. ADULTS	
Enterovirus		51%
Unknown cause		19%
Bacterial		14%
Herpes simplex		8%
Noninfectious		3%
Fungal		3%
Other viruses		2%

Hasbun R, Rosenthal N, Balada-Llasat JM, et al. Epidemiology of meningitis and encephalitis in the United States, 2011-2014. *Clin Infect Dis.* 2017;65:359-363.

Recurrent Meningitis

Repeated episodes of bacterial meningitis generally indicate a host defect, either in local anatomy or in antibacterial and immunologic defenses (e.g., recurrent *N. meningitidis* infections in patients with congenital or acquired deficiencies of complement, particularly the late-acting components). Approximately 10% of episodes of pneumococcal meningitis in adults are recurrent meningitis, but only 0.5% of patients with community-acquired meningitis caused by other microorganisms have recurrent attacks. *S. pneumoniae* is the cause of a third of episodes of community-acquired recurrent meningitis; various streptococci, *H. influenzae*, and *N. meningitidis* are the cause of another third of episodes. In contrast, in nosocomial recurrent meningitis, gram-negative bacilli and *S. aureus* are the cause of approximately 60% of episodes. A history of head trauma is frequent in patients with recurrent meningitis. Organisms may enter the subarachnoid space directly, through a defect in the cribriform plate (the most common site), in association with the empty sella syndrome, by means of a basilar skull fracture, through an erosive sequestrum of the mastoid, through congenital dermal defects along the craniospinal axis (usually evident before adult life), or as a consequence of penetrating cranial trauma or neurosurgical procedures. The anatomic defect may produce a frank CSF leak (rhinorrhea or, less commonly, otorrhea) or may entrap a vascular cuff of meninges that may subsequently serve as a direct route for organisms to reach the meninges. CSF rhinorrhea may be intermittent, and meningitis may occur months or years after head injury.

Any patient with bacterial meningitis, particularly if the meningitis is recurrent, should be evaluated for congenital or post-traumatic defects. The presence of CSF rhinorrhea should be sought at admission and subsequently (rhinorrhea may clear during active meningitis only to recur when the inflammation has resolved). Clinical clues suggesting the presence of a CSF fistula through the cribriform plate, pericranial air sinuses, or temporal bone include (1) a salty taste in the throat; (2) positionally dependent rhinorrhea (rhinorrhea only in the lateral recumbent or prone position suggests an otic or sphenoid origin); (3) anosmia (cribriform plate leak); and (4) hearing loss or full feeling in the ear, often with a finding of fluid or bubbles behind the tympanic membrane (leakage into the middle ear). Quantitative determination of the glucose and chloride content of nasal secretions and detection of a transferrin band unique to CSF by protein electrophoresis can definitively establish the presence of CSF rhinorrhea.

Recurrent pneumococcal meningitis may develop without apparent predisposing circumstances, and cryptic CSF leaks should be sought actively in such patients by CT of the frontal and mastoid regions and by radioisotope techniques. Radioiodine-labeled albumin is introduced intrathecally, and pledgets of cotton placed in the nares are subsequently examined for the radionuclide. Intrathecal introduction of fluorescein as a visual tracer (under ultraviolet light) can similarly be used to detect active leaks. Surgical closure of CSF fistulas should be performed to prevent further episodes of meningitis. Extracranial approaches through the ethmoidal sinuses can be used to repair cribriform plate or sphenoidal sinus dural defects and avoid the higher morbidity associated with craniotomy.

In most patients with CSF otorrhea and rhinorrhea after an acute head injury, the leak ceases in 1 or 2 weeks. *Persistent rhinorrhea for more than 4 to 6 weeks is an indication for surgical repair.* Prolonged administration of penicillin does not prevent pneumococcal meningitis and may encourage infection with more drug-resistant species.

TREATMENT   Rx

Antimicrobial Agents

Antimicrobial therapy should be initiated promptly in this life-threatening emergency, even before performing an emergent lumbar puncture and within 1 hour of hospital arrival.[10] Subsequent management should be undertaken with close monitoring, often in an intensive care unit. Treatment should be aimed at the most likely causes based on clinical clues, such as the age of the patient, the presence of a petechial or purpuric rash, a recent neurosurgical procedure, and CSF rhinorrhea. However, it is difficult to distinguish among the various causes of bacterial meningitis on clinical grounds alone, although patients with pneumococcal meningitis frequently have altered mental status and progress rapidly to coma, often with recurrent seizures and the rapid development of focal neurologic deficits. If the infecting organism is observed on examination of a Gram-stained smear of the CSF sediment, specific therapy is initiated. If the etiologic agent is not seen on a smear from a patient with suspected bacterial meningitis or if lumbar puncture is delayed because head CT is needed, empirical antimicrobial therapy should be initiated (Table 384-4).

Adequate CSF bactericidal activity, which is critical to cure the meningitis, depends on the ability of the antibiotic to penetrate CSF and maintain its activity in the purulent exudate, as well as on its metabolism and rate of clearance from CSF. The ability of the antibiotic to penetrate CSF depends on its lipid solubility, protein binding in serum, molecular size, and the status of the blood-CSF barrier. For example, chloramphenicol has very high lipid solubility, whereas β-lactam antibiotics have poor solubility. With the exception of rifampin and chloramphenicol, the commonly used antimicrobial agents do not readily penetrate the normal blood-brain barrier, but the passage of penicillin and other antimicrobial agents is enhanced in the presence of meningeal inflammation (Table 384-5). Antimicrobial drugs should be administered IV throughout the treatment period; the dose should not be reduced as the patient improves because normalization of the blood-brain barrier during recovery reduces the achievable CSF drug levels. Bactericidal drugs (penicillin, ampicillin, third-generation cephalosporins) are preferred whenever possible, and CSF levels of antibiotics at least 10 to 20 times the minimal bactericidal concentration are needed for optimal therapy. Some antibiotics are removed from CSF by active transport into blood via the epithelium of the choroid plexus; by comparison, third-generation cephalosporin antibiotics persist in CSF for longer

---

TABLE 384-4	INITIAL EMPIRICAL THERAPY FOR COMMUNITY-ACQUIRED AND NOSOCOMIAL PURULENT MENINGITIS BASED ON AGE AND CLINICAL SETTING (SEE TABLE 384-8 FOR DOSING SCHEDULES)		
PREDISPOSITIONS	**LIKELY PATHOGENS**	**PREFERRED ANTIMICROBIALS**	**ALTERNATIVE ANTIMICROBIALS**
Age			
<1 mo	Group B streptococcus, *Escherichia coli*, *Listeria monocytogenes*	Amoxicillin/ampicillin plus cefotaxime	Amoxicillin/ampicillin plus aminoglycoside
1-23 mo	*Streptococcus pneumoniae*, *Neisseria meningitidis*, group B streptococci, *Haemophilus influenzae*, *E. coli*	Vancomycin* plus ceftriaxone or cefotaxime	Meropenem (? plus vancomycin*)
2-50 yr	*N. meningitidis*, *S. pneumoniae*	Vancomycin* plus ceftriaxone or cefotaxime	Meropenem (? plus vancomycin*)
>50 yr	*S. pneumoniae*, *N. meningitidis*, *L. monocytogenes*, aerobic gram-negative bacilli	Vancomycin* plus ceftriaxone or cefotaxime plus ampicillin	Vancomycin* plus ceftriaxone or cefotaxime plus trimethoprim-sulfamethoxazole
Impaired immunity	*L. monocytogenes*, gram-negative bacilli, *S. pneumoniae*, *Staphylococcus*, *Salmonella*	Ampicillin plus cefapime or meropenem plus vancomycin*	Trimethoprim-sulfamethoxazole plus meropenem
Cerebrospinal fluid leak or basilar skull fracture	*S. pneumoniae*, various streptococci, *H. influenzae*	Vancomycin* plus cefotaxime or ceftriaxone	Vancomycin* plus meropenem
After neurosurgery or penetrating trauma	*S. aureus*, coagulase-negative staphylococci, aerobic gram-negative bacilli (including *P. aeruginosa*)	Vancomycin* plus cefepime	Vancomycin* plus ceftazidime or vancomycin* plus meropenem
Cerebrospinal fluid shunts (external or internal)	Coagulase-negative staphylococci, *S. aureus*, aerobic gram-negative bacilli (including *P. aeruginosa*), *Propionibacterium acnes*	Vancomycin* plus cefepime	Vancomycin* plus ceftazidime or vancomycin* plus meropenem

*If dexamethasone is also administered, consideration should be given to the addition of rifampin.
Modified from van de Beek D, Brouder MC, Thwaites GE, et al. Advances in treatment of bacterial meningitis. *Lancet.* 2012;380:1693-1702.

TABLE 384-5 PERMEABILITY OF ANTIBIOTICS INTO CEREBROSPINAL FLUID

GOOD CONCENTRATIONS IN CSF WITH AND WITHOUT MENINGITIS	ADEQUATE CONCENTRATIONS IN CSF IN MENINGITIS	FAIR TO POOR CONCENTRATIONS IN CSF IN MENINGITIS
Chloramphenicol	Penicillin	Early cephalosporins
Sulfonamides	Ampicillin	Cephalothin
Cephalosporins	Methicillin	Cefoxitin
Cefotaxime	Oxacillin	Aminoglycosides
Ceftriaxone	Nafcillin	Gentamicin
Ceftazidime	Carbenicillin	Tobramycin
Moxalactam	Ticarcillin	Amikacin
Cefepime	Tetracycline	Clindamycin
Metronidazole	Erythromycin	Benzathine penicillin
Trimethoprim-sulfamethoxazole	Ethambutol	
Isoniazid	Rifampin	
Linezolid	Vancomycin	
Fluconazole	Meropenem	
Fluoroquinolones		

CSF = cerebrospinal fluid.
Courtesy Allen Aksamit, Mayo Clinic, Rochester, MN.

TABLE 384-6 ANTIMICROBIAL THERAPY FOR COMMUNITY-ACQUIRED BACTERIAL MENINGITIS OF KNOWN CAUSE IN ADULTS OR CHILDREN (SEE TABLE 384-8 FOR DOSING SCHEDULES)

ORGANISM	PREFERRED ANTIMICROBIAL THERAPY	ALTERNATIVE ANTIMICROBIAL THERAPY
Streptococcus pneumoniae		
Penicillin MIC <0.1 µg/mL	Penicillin G or ampicillin	Cefotaxime, or ceftriaxone, or vancomycin, or chloramphenicol
Penicillin MIC 0.1-1 µg/mL	Ceftriaxone or cefotaxime	Vancomycin,* or meropenem, or cefepime
Penicillin MIC ≥2.0 µg/mL	Vancomycin* (plus cefotaxime or ceftriaxone)	Moxifloxacin or gatifloxacin
Cefotaxime or ceftriaxone MIC ≥1.0 µg/mL	Vancomycin* (plus cefotaxime or ceftriaxone)	Moxifloxacin or gatifloxacin
Neisseria meningitidis		
Penicillin MIC <0.1 µg/mL	Penicillin G or ampicillin	Ceftriaxone, or cefotaxime, or chloramphenicol
Penicillin MIC 0.1-1.0 µg/mL	Ceftriaxone or cefotaxime	Chloramphenicol, or meropenem, or gatifloxacin, or moxifloxacin
Haemophilus influenzae		
β-Lactamase negative	Ampicillin	Ceftriaxone, or cefotaxime, or cefepime, or chloramphenicol
β-Lactamase positive	Ceftriaxone or cefotaxime	Cefepime, or chloramphenicol, or gatifloxacin, or moxifloxacin
Listeria monocytogenes	Ampicillin† or penicillin G†	Trimethoprim-sulfamethoxazole or meropenem
Streptococcus agalactiae (group B streptococci)	Ampicillin† or penicillin G†	Cefotaxime or ceftriaxone

*Addition of rifampin should be considered. Consider intrathecal (or intraventricular vancomycin, 5 to 20 mg/day) if not responding to intravenous therapy.
†Addition of intravenous gentamicin should be considered.
MIC = minimal inhibitory concentration.

periods. First- or second-generation cephalosporins and clindamycin do not provide effective levels in CSF and should not be used.

Empirical Treatment

Initial treatment of presumed bacterial meningitis when the etiologic agent cannot be identified on a Gram-stained smear of CSF is based on the available clinical clues.[11] In older children and adults, therapy with vancomycin and a third-generation cephalosporin (cefotaxime or ceftriaxone) is recommended (see Table 384-4). In adults older than 50 years and in high-risk groups, ampicillin is also added because of the possibility of the presence of *L. monocytogenes*, which is susceptible to ampicillin or amoxicillin but not to third-generation cephalosporins. In a penicillin-allergic individual, trimethoprim-sulfamethoxazole is a suitable alternative for *Listeria* meningitis. In special settings, such as nosocomial meningitis associated with neurosurgical procedures or penetrating head trauma, more resistant species such as methicillin-resistant *S. aureus* (MRSA), coagulase-negative staphylococci, and *P. aeruginosa* may be responsible; in these situations, vancomycin and a β-lactam such as cefepime, ceftazidime, or meropenem is indicated as initial therapy. If β-lactams are contraindicated, aztreonam or ciprofloxacin is recommended for gram-negative coverage.

Meningitis of Specific Bacterial Cause
Pneumococcal Meningitis

The treatment of choice for pneumococcal meningitis in adults has historically been penicillin, with vancomycin (or chloramphenicol) being a reasonable alternative in patients allergic to penicillin (see later). However, penicillin-resistant pneumococcal strains are found worldwide, including 25% of clinical isolates in the United States. Thus, antimicrobial susceptibilities should be determined for all pneumococcal isolates from CSF, blood, or sterile body fluids (see Table 384-5). Approximately 9% of pneumococcal isolates from patients with meningitis in the United States are resistant to third-generation cephalosporins, with a minimal inhibitory concentration of 2 µg/mL or greater. If the minimal inhibitory concentration for cefotaxime or ceftriaxone (≤1.0 µg/mL) indicates

a susceptible isolate, cefotaxime or ceftriaxone would be the drug of choice. If the isolate is highly penicillin resistant or is resistant to 1 µg/mL ceftriaxone or cefotaxime, alternative therapy (vancomycin with or without rifampin IV) is indicated. Because of the increasingly wide distribution of highly resistant strains, initial therapy (pending susceptibility testing) with cefotaxime (or ceftriaxone) in addition to vancomycin IV is recommended as per guidelines by the Infectious Disease Society of America. When initial adjunctive therapy with dexamethasone is used (see later) along with vancomycin, it should be borne in mind that vancomycin levels in CSF may be reduced by concomitant corticosteroid use.

Although resistance to chloramphenicol is unusual in pneumococcal isolates from the United States, chloramphenicol has poor bactericidal activity against penicillin-resistant isolates from children with meningitis in South Africa. The relative chloramphenicol resistance of such strains may not be discerned on usual laboratory testing, but it is revealed when the minimum bactericidal concentration is determined. For this reason, vancomycin is preferred over chloramphenicol for the initial treatment of pneumococcal meningitis in a highly penicillin-allergic patient.

The β-lactam antibiotic meropenem is as effective as cefotaxime for meningitis caused by *S. pneumoniae*, *N. meningitidis*, and *H. influenzae* in adults and in children. Cefepime is also similar to ceftriaxone and cefotaxime for infection with *S. pneumoniae, N. meningitidis,* and *H. influenzae,* and it has greater activity than these antibiotics against *Enterobacter* sp and *P. aeruginosa* (Table 384-6).

Meningococcal Meningitis

Intravenous administration of penicillin G and ampicillin, in doses used to treat meningitis caused by penicillin-susceptible pneumococci, successfully treats *N. meningitidis* meningitis resulting from susceptible strains. Meningococci resistant to penicillin have occasionally been isolated in Spain (≤50% of strains), South Africa, and Canada but rarely in the United States. Most of these isolates have been only intermediately resistant to penicillin (minimal inhibitory concentration of 0.1 to 1.0 µg/mL), although rare strains have had high-level resistance related to β-lactamase production and require third-generation cephalosporins such as ceftriaxone, which is as effective as the potentially more toxic chloramphenicol. Nevertheless, "meningitis doses" of penicillin or ampicillin may provide CSF levels that are sufficient for infections with some strains of intermediately penicillin-resistant N. meningitidis. Usually, a 7-day course of antibiotics is sufficient.

Haemophilus influenzae Meningitis

At present, 25 to 35% of isolates of H. influenzae type b in the United States are β-lactamase producers and are ampicillin resistant; cefotaxime or ceftriaxone is the initial therapy of choice (see Table 384-6). Alternatives include cefepime or the combination of chloramphenicol and ampicillin; if the isolate proves susceptible to ampicillin, chloramphenicol may be discontinued. Although more than 50% of isolates are chloramphenicol resistant in some areas of Spain, less than 1% of isolates have been found to be resistant in the United States. A 10-day course of antibiotics is usually sufficient.

Staphylococcal Meningitis

For the treatment of adult meningitis caused by methicillin-susceptible S. aureus, nafcillin or oxacillin is recommended. For MRSA or in a penicillin-allergic patient, vancomycin is the alternative of choice (Tables 384-7 and 384-8). Because penetration of vancomycin into CSF is limited, adjunctive intrathecal (or

---

TABLE 384-7 THERAPY FOR NOSOCOMIAL MENINGITIS OF KNOWN BACTERIAL CAUSE IN ADULTS

ORGANISM	THERAPY OF CHOICE	ALTERNATIVE THERAPY
Staphylococcus aureus		
Methicillin susceptible	Nafcillin or oxacillin; in difficult cases may add rifampin	Vancomycin or meropenem
Methicillin resistant	Vancomycin; in difficult cases may add rifampin	Daptomycin, linezolid, or trimethoprim-sulfamethoxazole
Coagulase negative	Vancomycin; may consider addition of rifampin	Daptomycin
Enterococcus sp		
Ampicillin susceptible	Ampicillin plus gentamicin	Vancomycin plus gentamicin
Ampicillin resistant	Vancomycin plus gentamicin	Daptomycin
Ampicillin and vancomycin resistant	Daptomycin	
Escherichia coli and other	Cefotaxime, ceftriaxone, or cefepime	Meropenem, aztreonam, ampicillin, or trimethoprim-sulfamethoxazole
Enterobacteriaceae*		
*Pseudomonas aeruginosa**	Cefepime or ceftazidime	Meropenem, aztreonam, or ciprofloxacin
Acinetobacter sp		
Meropenem susceptible	Meropenem	
Meropenem resistant	Colistimethate or polymyxin B	

*Selection of specific antimicrobial drug should be based on in vitro susceptibility results, with consideration given to the addition of an aminoglycoside (e.g., tobramycin, gentamicin, or amikacin).
Modified from van de Beek D, Drake JM, Tunkel AR. Nosocomial bacterial meningitis. *N Engl J Med.* 2010;362:146-154.

TABLE 384-8 DOSES OF ANTIMICROBIAL DRUGS FOR TREATMENT OF BACTERIAL MENINGITIS*

ANTIMICROBIAL DRUG	ADULTS (24-HR DOSE)	INFANTS AND CHILDREN (24-HR DOSE)
β-LACTAMS		
Penicillin G	24 million U, q4h aliquots	300,000 U/kg, q4h aliquots
Ampicillin	12 g, q4h aliquots	300 mg/kg, q4h aliquots
Nafcillin	10-12 g, q4h aliquots	200 mg/kg, q4h aliquots
Oxacillin	10-12 g, q4h aliquots	200 mg/kg, q4h aliquots
Aztreonam (a monobactam)	6-8 g, q6-8h aliquots	
Meropenem (a carbapenem†)	6 g, q8h aliquots	120 mg/kg, q8h aliquots
CEPHALOSPORINS		
Cefotaxime	12 g, q4h aliquots	200-300 mg/kg, q6h aliquots
Ceftriaxone‡	4 g, q12h aliquots	80-100 mg/kg, q12h aliquots
Ceftazidime	6 g, q8h aliquots	150 mg/kg, q8h aliquots
Cefepime	6 g, q6-8h aliquots	150 mg/kg, q8h aliquots
Ceftaroline	600 mg, q12h aliquots	Safety not established in children
AMINOGLYCOSIDES		
Gentamicin§	5 mg/kg, q8h aliquots	7.5 mg/kg, q8h aliquots
Tobramycin§	5 mg/kg, q8h aliquots	7.5 mg/kg, q8h aliquots
Amikacin§	15 mg/kg, q8h aliquots	20-25 mg/kg, q8h aliquots
FLUOROQUINOLONES		
Ciprofloxacin	800-1200 mg, q8-12h aliquots	—
Gatifloxacin‖	400 mg, q24h dosing	—
Moxifloxacin‖	400 mg, q24h dosing	—
OTHERS		
Chloramphenicol	4-6 g, q6h aliquots	75-100 mg/kg, q6h aliquots
Vancomycin¶	2-3 g, q6-8h aliquots	50-60 mg/kg, q6h aliquots
Rifampin	600 mg, q24h dosing	10-20 mg/kg, q12-24h aliquots
Trimethoprim-sulfamethoxazole**	20 mg/kg, q6h aliquots	20 mg/kg, q6h aliquots
Daptomycin	8-10 mg/kg, q24h dosing	6 mg/kg, q24h dosing
Polymyxin B*	7,500-12,500 U/kg, q12h dosing	7,500-12,500 U/kg, q12h dosing
Colistimethate*	1.25 mg/kg, q6-12h dosing	—

*Dosages are intravenous and for patients with normal renal and hepatic function.
†Use may be associated with seizures, but much less so than with imipenem.
‡Four-gram maximum daily dose.
§Peak and trough serum levels should be monitored.
‖No data are available on the optimal dosage required for bacterial meningitis.
¶Monitoring of trough serum levels is advisable; they should be maintained at concentrations of 15 to 20 μg/mL. If the patient is not responding well, one may need to monitor cerebrospinal fluid levels and, if low, temporarily increase the daily dose accordingly or add adjuvant intrathecal vancomycin (5 to 20 mg), as for the treatment of methicillin-resistant *Staphylococcus aureus* meningitis.
**Dosage based on the trimethoprim component of the combination.

intraventricular) therapy with vancomycin (without preservative) is occasionally used when CSF cultures have remained positive after 48 hours of intravenous therapy alone and CSF levels can be monitored. For adult meningitis caused by MRSA, intravenous vancomycin (with adjunctive intrathecal vancomycin as needed) is the treatment of choice. If β-lactam agents or vancomycin cannot be used, linezolid, daptomycin, or trimethoprim-sulfamethoxazole is recommended. In severe or refractory cases, the addition of rifampin is warranted. Rifampin is also recommended as part of combination therapy for patients with intracranial or spinal hardware such as a CSF shunt or drain.

Listeria Meningitis

Ampicillin is the drug of choice for *Listeria* meningitis. When combined with gentamicin, it can have a synergistic bactericidal effect. Third-generation cephalosporins and vancomycin are not effective. In patients allergic to ampicillin, intravenous trimethoprim-sulfamethoxazole may be used, followed by oral trimethoprim alone.

Gram-Negative Bacillary Meningitis

Cefotaxime or ceftriaxone (see Tables 384-7 and 384-8) is used to treat meningitis known to be caused by susceptible gram-negative bacilli (e.g., *E. coli, Klebsiella, Proteus*), but they should not be used to treat meningitis caused by less susceptible species such as *P. aeruginosa* and *Acinetobacter*. After identifying the specific pathogen and determining its drug susceptibilities, alterations in antimicrobial therapy may be indicated. If the organism is *P. aeruginosa,* ceftazidime or cefepime is recommended and may be combined with vancomycin (see Tables 384-7 and 384-8). An alternative is aztreonam or a fluoroquinolone with in vitro activity. For *Acinetobacter* species, meropenem is recommended; for strains that demonstrate carbapenem resistance, colistimethate sodium or polymyxin B (see Table 384-8) administered by the intravenous or intraventricular routes is recommended. Intraventricular administration of polymyxin B is recommended at a dose of 50,000 U once daily for 3-4 days, then every other day for 2 weeks after the CSF cultures are negative. Concomitant use of muscle relaxants should be avoided.

Zoonotic Meningitis

Brucella meningitis (Chapter 294) is a subacute or chronic process that is often accompanied by other manifestations of neurobrucellosis (encephalitis, polyradiculitis, myelitis). Infection is transmitted to humans in endemic areas (Central and South America, Mediterranean littoral, Arabian peninsula) from the ingestion of unpasteurized milk or cheese or direct contact with domestic animals. Neurobrucellosis occurs in 2 to 5% of patients with brucellosis. CSF findings consist of a lymphocytic pleocytosis (<500 cells/μL), hypoglycorrhachia, and an elevated protein level, findings that could mistakenly suggest tuberculous meningitis. The diagnosis is based on demonstration of antibody in serum and CSF or by isolation of *Brucella* from blood; the microorganism is isolated from CSF in only a minority of cases. Treatment of adults involves the three-drug combination of doxycycline (200 mg/day), rifampin (600 mg/day), and trimethoprim-sulfamethoxazole (20 mg/kg/day IV, based on trimethoprim component, in 6-hour aliquots) for several months, depending on the clinical and CSF responses.

Streptococcus suis is an uncommon cause of meningitis seen in pig breeders, butchers, and abattoir workers in Europe, Canada, and China. *S. suis* meningitis, which is an acute illness with a brisk neutrophilic pleocytosis, is often initially mistaken for pneumococcal meningitis on the basis of Gram stain of CSF. Treatment of adults consists of penicillin (12 to 24 million units [U]/day in 4-hour aliquots) or ampicillin (12 g/day in 4-hour aliquots) IV for 10 to 14 days.

Bacillus anthracis (Chapter 278) is a rare cause of meningitis that most often develops as a complication of inhalation anthrax following exposure to aerosols of anthrax spores in the setting of large-scale processing of wool and hides or a bioterrorism attack (Chapter 18). Anthrax meningitis is an acute process characterized by hemorrhagic or serohemorrhagic CSF with a neutrophilic predominance (several thousand cells per cubic millimeter), hypoglycorrhachia, an elevated protein level, and prominent large gram-positive bacilli on stained smear. Treatment of adults initially includes ciprofloxacin (400 mg at 12-hour intervals) in addition to penicillin (24 million U/day in 4-hour aliquots) and chloramphenicol (4 g/day in 6-hour aliquots) IV. Alternatively, treatment could substitute levo- or moxifloxacin for ciprofloxacin, meropenem for penicillin, and linezolid or chloramphenicol (Chapter 262). Whether all drugs are continued (or treatment is narrowed to one or two antimicrobials) and the duration of treatment depend on whether the meningitis is of suspected bioterrorist origin (Chapter 18) or caused by cutaneous anthrax resulting from animal (or animal product) exposure (Chapter 278). Consultation with infectious disease and public health authorities should be sought.

Duration of Therapy

The frequency of CSF examination depends on the clinical course, but examination should be repeated in 24 to 48 hours if there has not been satisfactory improvement or if the causative microorganism is a more resistant gram-negative bacillus or a highly penicillin-resistant (or cephalosporin-resistant) *S. pneumoniae* strain, especially in patients who are receiving adjunctive dexamethasone therapy. Routine "end-of-treatment" CSF examination is unnecessary in most

patients with the common types of community-acquired bacterial meningitis. Although 5 days of ceftriaxone treatment is as good as 10 days in children who are stable at 5 days, longer courses are still recommended in adults. Meningococci are rapidly eliminated from the circulation and CSF with appropriate antimicrobial therapy, which should be continued for 4 to 7 days after the patient becomes afebrile. *H. influenzae* meningitis should be treated for 7 to 10 days. In pneumococcal meningitis, antimicrobial treatment should be continued for 10 to 14 days and follow-up examination of CSF should be performed, particularly when the patient has coexistent mastoiditis. More prolonged therapy is indicated with concomitant parameningeal infection. Meningitis caused by *L. monocytogenes* should be treated for 21 days. Treatment of gram-negative bacillary meningitis with parenteral antimicrobials is prolonged, usually for a minimum of 3 weeks (particularly in patients after a recent neurosurgical procedure) to prevent relapse. Repeated examinations of CSF are necessary both during and at the conclusion of treatment to determine whether bacteriologic cure has been achieved.

Other Aspects of Treatment

Adjunctive Corticosteroids

In children, the routine use of dexamethasone administered IV (either 0.15 mg/kg every 6 hours for 4 days or 0.4 mg/kg every 12 hours for 2 days), either at the time of or 10 to 20 minutes before initiating antimicrobial therapy (third-generation cephalosporin), has no effect on mortality but reduces the incidence of neurologic sequelae (primarily bilateral sensorineural hearing loss).[A1] In adults with community-acquired bacterial meningitis, adjunctive dexamethasone therapy (10 mg every 6 hours IV for 4 days) significantly reduces the proportion of patients with an unfavorable neurologic outcome from 25 to 15% or a fatal outcome from 15 to 7%, with the beneficial effect most evident in patients with pneumococcal meningitis.[A2] In a study of adolescents and adults with bacterial meningitis in Vietnam, dexamethasone significantly reduced death and disability by approximately 54% at 6 months in patients with confirmed disease. By comparison, adjunctive corticosteroids were not effective in treating bacterial meningitis in a large trial of predominantly HIV-positive patients in sub-Saharan Africa. Based on these data, adjunctive dexamethasone (0.15 mg/kg every 6 hours for 2 to 4 days, with the initial dose given 10 to 20 minutes before or simultaneously with the initial dose of antimicrobial therapy) is recommended in adults with suspected or demonstrated pneumococcal meningitis and perhaps routinely in all cases of bacterial meningitis, at least in non–HIV-infected patients in high-income countries,[A3] and its benefits extend for at least 13 years after the event[A4] (see Table 384-5).

Elevated Cerebrospinal Fluid Pressure (Brain Swelling)

Occasional patients with acute bacterial meningitis experience marked brain swelling (CSF pressure >450 mm H_2O), which may lead to temporal lobe or cerebellar herniation after lumbar puncture. To decrease the possibility of this complication when the pressure is found to be this high, only a small amount of CSF should be removed for analysis (the amount present in the manometer), and a 20% solution of mannitol (0.25 to 0.5 g/kg IV) should be infused over a period of 20 to 30 minutes while monitoring (if possible) for a decline in CSF pressure to a lower level before the spinal needle is removed. Continued control of increased intracranial pressure, if needed thereafter, may be effected with additional mannitol; dexamethasone (10 mg IV, followed by 0.15 mg/kg every 6 hours) should be used in patients with brain swelling regardless of the suspected bacteriologic cause of meningitis.

In a stuporous patient or one with respiratory insufficiency and markedly increased intracranial pressure, use of a ventilator to reduce the arterial carbon dioxide pressure to between 25 and 32 mm Hg is reasonable, and the patient's head should be elevated 30 to 45 degrees. Intubation should be performed with minimal stimulation to avoid an appreciable further rise in pressure; pharmacologic aids to intubation are recommended, such as succinylcholine and opioids, with the possible use of adjunctive intravenous lidocaine. Subsequently, transient increases in intracranial pressure associated with hyperactive airway reflexes can be mitigated by intratracheal instillation of lidocaine before vigorous suctioning. With continued marked and fluctuating elevations in intracranial pressure, use of a continuous intracranial monitoring device may be warranted. Induced hypothermia is not beneficial and may be harmful.

Hypotension

Initial hypovolemia or hypotension, if present, should be treated with fluid to prevent significantly decreased cerebral blood flow. Over the next 24 to 48 hours, inappropriate secretion of antidiuretic hormone may contribute to further brain swelling; in such cases, fluid should be restricted to 1200 to 1500 mL daily in adults if possible, although a study in children suggests that routine fluid restriction does not improve outcome and that the resulting decrease in extracellular water may increase the likelihood of hypovolemia and an adverse outcome.

Supportive Care

Patients with acute bacterial meningitis should receive constant nursing attention in an intensive care unit to ensure prompt recognition of seizures and to prevent aspiration. If seizures occur, they should be treated acutely in adults with diazepam (administered slowly IV at a dose of 5 to 10 mg) or lorazepam (4 to 8 mg). Maintenance anticonvulsant therapy can be continued thereafter with intravenous phenytoin (Chapter 375) until the medication can be administered orally (PO). Sedation should be avoided because of the danger of respiratory depression and aspiration.

Surgery

Surgical treatment of an accompanying pyogenic focus such as mastoiditis should be undertaken when recovery from the meningitis is as complete as possible but under continuing antibiotic administration. Rarely, the mastoid infection (e.g., Bezold abscess) is so hyperacute that early drainage may be required after 48 hours or so of antibiotic therapy when the acute meningeal process has subsided somewhat.

PROGNOSIS

Prompt treatment of bacterial meningitis usually results in rapid recovery of neurologic function. Persistent or late-onset obtundation and coma without focal findings suggest brain swelling, subdural effusion, hydrocephalus, loculated ventriculitis, cortical thrombophlebitis, or sagittal sinus thrombosis. The last three conditions are commonly associated with fever and continuing pleocytosis.

The mortality rate for community-acquired bacterial meningitis in adults varies with the etiologic agent and clinical circumstances. With current antimicrobial therapy, the mortality rate for *H. influenzae* meningitis is less than 5% and that for meningococcal meningitis is approximately 10%. The highest mortality is seen with pneumococcal (20%) and *L. monocytogenes* (20 to 30%) meningitis.

The mortality rate for gram-negative bacillary meningitis, commonly nosocomial in origin, has been 20 to 30% in adults, but may be decreasing. The mortality rate for recurrent community-acquired meningitis in adults ($\approx$5%) is lower than the 20% rate for nonrecurrent episodes. Poor prognostic factors include advanced age, the presence of other foci of infection, underlying diseases (leukemia, alcoholism), obtundation, seizures within the first 24 hours, and delay in instituting appropriate therapy.

Residual neurologic damage is seen in 10 to 20% of patients who recover from bacterial meningitis. Approximately 25% of adults considered clinically well recovered (expected to function independently and resume activities of daily life, including work) from pneumococcal meningitis show neuropsychological abnormalities, mainly loss of cognitive speed, when they are examined 6 to 24 months after hospital discharge. Developmental delay and speech defects are each observed in approximately 5% of children, and bacterial meningitis is associated with lower subsequent educational achievement and economic self-sufficiency in adulthood.

PREVENTION

Vaccination

Adherence to recommended vaccination (Chapter 15) substantially reduces the risk of bacterial meningitis. For example, effective vaccines for *H. influenzae* (Chapter 340) have nearly eliminated this formerly common cause of meningitis. The meningococcal vaccine is approximately 85% protective against four of the strains that cause illness: A, C, Y, and W-135 (Chapters 15 and 282), and recombinant serogroup B vaccination is now available for high-risk individuals. All 11- to 12-year-olds should be vaccinated with the MenACWY conjugate vaccine, and a booster dose should be given at age 16 to 18 years (Chapter 15). It should also be given to any previously unvaccinated college freshmen who will live in dormitories, military recruits, or people traveling to sub-Saharan Africa. The MenB vaccine is currently recommended only for immunocompromised individuals or those exposed during an outbreak (Chapter 15). For adolescents who receive the first dose at age 13 through 15 years, a one-time booster dose should be administered, preferably at age 16 through 18 years, before the peak in increased risk. Adolescents who receive their first dose of quadrivalent meningococcal conjugate vaccine at or after age 16 years do not need a booster dose. At age 65 years, all adults should receive pneumococcal PCV13 vaccination, followed about 1 year later by PPSV23 vaccination. For people who smoke, have underlying lung disease, or are immunosuppressed, vaccination is recommended after age 19 years (Chapter 15). Some immunocompromised patients, such as those taking eculizumab, remain at high risk for infection despite vaccination.

Chemoprophylaxis

Prompt prophylaxis of close contacts (individuals who frequently slept and ate in the same household with the patient, girlfriend, or boyfriend) is warranted because up to a third of secondary cases of meningococcal disease develop within 2 to 5 days of illness in the initial case. Only hospital personnel who were in close contact with a patient (mouth-to-mouth resuscitation, initial examination before institution of respiratory precautions) are at special risk. Commonly, oral rifampin is used for prophylaxis: for adults (other than pregnant women), 600 mg twice daily for 2 days; for children, 10 mg/kg twice daily for 2 days. Alternatively, for adults, ciprofloxacin (500 mg), ofloxacin (400 mg), or azithromycin (500 mg), each given PO as a single dose, may be used. Another choice is ceftriaxone intramuscularly as a single dose in adults (250 mg) or children (125 mg).

Widespread use of *H. influenzae* type b polysaccharide protein-conjugate vaccine in developed countries has largely eliminated the need for chemoprophylaxis of close childhood contacts of patients with *H. influenzae* meningitis or invasive infection. However, prophylaxis would be indicated for unimmunized close household contacts of an index patient (e.g., recent immigrant) younger than 6 years. If two or more cases of invasive *H. influenzae* type b disease occur in children at a daycare center, prophylaxis of other unimmunized attendees is warranted with rifampin (20 mg/kg/day PO) for 4 days.

VIRAL MENINGITIS

DEFINITION

The nonspecific term *aseptic meningitis* describes an inflammatory process involving the meninges, usually accompanied by a mononuclear pleocytosis, without evidence of pyogenic bacterial infection on Gram stain or culture. The definition encompasses various processes that produce similar clinical pictures and inflammatory responses: viral meningitis, atypical and nonpyogenic bacterial and fungal meningitis, chemically induced meningitis, drug-induced meningitis, neoplastic meningitis, meningeal inflammation caused by adjacent pyogenic infections, and meningitis associated with autoimmune hypersensitivity diseases. Aseptic meningitis, which is usually an acute or subacute process, can be further divided into types by the duration of illness (chronic versus chronic-intermittent) and distinctive cellular responses in CSF (e.g., eosinophilic meningitis).

Many of the viruses causing meningitis also may cause infection of the brain parenchyma (encephalitis; Chapter 386) or spinal cord. Sometimes, parenchymatous involvement and meningeal involvement occur simultaneously in the same patient and are referred to as meningoencephalitis and meningomyelitis.

EPIDEMIOLOGY

Most cases of community-acquired aseptic meningitis are the result of viruses, principally enteroviruses, which account for more than 60% of viral meningitides and for 90% of those for which an etiologic agent is identified (Table 384-9). Enteroviruses are members of the Picornaviridae (small RNA) family, which consists of more than 60 serotypes: 28 echoviruses, 23 group A and 6 group B coxsackieviruses, four numbered enteroviruses (68 to 71), and three polioviruses. The most common serotypes implicated in viral meningitis from year to year have been echoviruses 4, 6, 9, 11, 16, and 30 (most recently 13 and 33) and coxsackie B serotypes 2 to 5. Currently, poliovirus infections (Chapter 355) are limited to parts of Asia and Africa, although rare cases occur secondary to attenuated vaccine strains.

Many viruses that produce the clinical picture of aseptic meningitis, such as arthropod-borne viruses, HSV-1, enterovirus 71, lymphocytic choriomeningitis virus, mumps virus, HIV-1, cytomegalovirus, and Epstein-Barr virus, also can produce the clinical picture of meningoencephalitis and encephalitis (Chapter 386). In addition, some viruses involve the spinal cord, including the anterior horn cells (poliovirus, West Nile virus) or the dorsal root ganglia (HSV-2).

Enterovirus

An estimated 10 to 15 million clinical enteroviral infections (Chapter 355) occur annually in the United States, and these include an estimated 50,000 to 75,000 cases of enteroviral meningitis. In temperate climates, enteroviral meningitis peaks during the summer and fall, especially in children. Serotypes tend to cycle with varying periodicity, and outbreaks are related to lack of previous exposure to a particular serotype. Serotype-specific protective antibodies

TABLE 384-9	AGENTS OF VIRAL MENINGITIS

COMMON

Nonarthropod Viruses

Picornavirus (RNA)
   Enterovirus
      Enterovirus 70, 71, 68, D68
      Coxsackie A, B
      Echovirus
Herpes simplex virus type 2 (HSV-2) (DNA)

LESS COMMON

Arthropod-Borne Viruses (Arboviruses)

Togavirus (alphavirus, RNA)
   Eastern equine encephalitis
   Western equine encephalitis
   Venezuelan equine encephalitis
Flavivirus (RNA)
   West Nile virus (WNV)
   Dengue
   St. Louis encephalitis
   Japanese B encephalitis
   Zika virus
Bunyavirus (RNA)
   California encephalitis

UNCOMMON

Arenavirus (RNA)
   Lymphocytic choriomeningitis
Paramyxovirus (RNA)
   Mumps
Retrovirus (RNA)
   Human immunodeficiency virus (HIV-1)

RARE

Enterovirus—poliovirus
Herpesvirus (DNA)
   Herpes simplex virus type 1 (HSV-1)
   Epstein-Barr virus
   Cytomegalovirus
   Varicella-zoster virus
   Human herpesvirus type 6 (HHV-6)
Adenovirus (DNA)
Coltivirus (RNA)
   Colorado tick fever
Bunyavirus (RNA)
   Toscana virus (a Phlebovirus)
Filoviruses
   Ebola virus

develop following infection, so subsequent episodes of enteroviral meningitis are uncommon and are caused by a different serotype.

Humans are the only known reservoir of enteroviruses. Enteroviral infection is spread predominantly by the fecal-oral route and occasionally by the respiratory route.

Herpes Simplex Virus

HSV (Chapter 350) accounts for 1 to 3% of all episodes of aseptic meningitis and occurs most commonly in sexually active adults or adolescents. In individuals with primary genital herpes (HSV-2) infection, up to 36% of women and 13% of men have symptoms of aseptic meningitis. Recurrences of genital herpes are common and are sometimes accompanied by aseptic meningitis. More than 80% of cases of benign recurrent aseptic meningitis are caused by HSV-2. In contrast, HSV-1 CNS infection almost always manifests as encephalitis rather than aseptic meningitis. Herpesviruses also may be reactivated in patients taking immunomodulatory drugs, which are often used to treat autoimmune diseases.

Arboviruses

Although the most common form of CNS infection caused by arboviruses (Chapters 359 and 386) is encephalitis, aseptic meningitis also may occur. These vector-borne viruses are introduced subcutaneously by a mosquito (e.g., West Nile virus, Japanese B encephalitis), tick (e.g., Colorado tick fever), or sandfly (e.g., Toscana virus). Birds, which are vectors of mosquito-borne arboviruses,

may not be obviously sick, although West Nile virus may cause prominent die-offs of corvine species, especially crows and blue jays, which can provide clues to an outbreak affecting humans.

The geographic spread of alphavirus infections (Eastern equine encephalitis, Western equine encephalitis, Venezuela equine encephalitis) in the United States is determined by the range of their individual mosquito vectors. Eastern equine encephalitis occurs sporadically or as focal outbreaks in the summer in the eastern and Gulf coasts, most frequently in children and elderly persons. Western equine encephalitis occurs predominantly in the western states, and Venezuela equine encephalitis is found in Florida. St. Louis encephalitis infections were originally recognized in the Midwest, but sporadic cases and outbreaks have occurred more recently in most parts of the United States; it is the most common arbovirus causing aseptic meningitis in the United States. West Nile virus infections first appeared in the United States in 1999 and now account for approximately 3000 cases of meningitis and another 3000 cases of encephalitis annually. Meningitis is a rare manifestation of Zika virus infection.

Mumps

Mumps virus (Chapter 345) was the leading identifiable cause of viral meningitis before widespread immunization in the 1960s. Episodes occurred most frequently in the winter and spring. It is now an uncommon cause of viral meningitis in the United States.

Lymphocytic Choriomeningitis

Lymphocytic choriomeningitis virus is transmitted to humans by rodents through direct contact, through ingestion of animal-contaminated food, or via aerosol or an animal bite. Cases tend to occur in early winter when mice seek shelter in homes. Outbreaks have occurred following exposure to pet or laboratory hamsters. Currently, lymphocytic choriomeningitis virus is infrequently a cause of aseptic meningitis.

PATHOBIOLOGY

The two basic routes for virus to gain access to the CNS are hematogenous (enteroviral infection) or neuronal (HSV infection). Enteroviruses pass through the stomach, where they resist the acid pH, and proceed to the lower gastrointestinal tract. Some virus also undergoes replication in the nasopharynx and spreads to regional lymphatics. After presumably binding to specific enterocyte receptors, the virus breaches the epithelial lining and undergoes primary replication in a permissive cell. From there, the virus progresses to Peyer patches, where further replication occurs. A minor enterovirus viremia then seeds the CNS, heart, liver, and reticuloendothelial system. Following extensive replication at the latter sites, a major viremia ensues, often accompanying the onset of clinical illness. The mechanism by which enterovirus enters the CNS is presumed to involve crossing the blood-CSF barrier's tight endothelial junctions and then entering CSF, probably at the choroid plexus.

In contrast, HSV infections may reach the CNS via the neuronal route: in HSV-1 encephalitis, from oral sites via the trigeminal and olfactory nerve; in HSV-2 (and the rare HSV-1) aseptic meningitis, by spread from a primary genital lesion and ascent along the sacral nerve roots to the meninges. After subsidence of the primary infection, HSV-1 may remain dormant in the trigeminal or olfactory root ganglia only to reactivate at a later date, enter the temporal lobe, and produce encephalitis. Similarly, HSV-2 may remain latent in the sacral root ganglia until subsequent reactivation causes later episodes of aseptic meningitis.

CLINICAL MANIFESTATIONS
Enteroviral Meningitis

The clinical features of enteroviral meningitis (Chapter 355) in older children and adults often begin abruptly with headache (85 to 100%), fever (80 to 100%), and stiff neck (50 to 80%). In some patients the course is biphasic, with the initial prodromal phase being characterized by low-grade fever and nonspecific symptoms (malaise, sore throat, diarrhea), followed by a second phase at which time the meninges are seeded, with the development of higher fever, nausea, vomiting, myalgia, photophobia, and stiff neck. Other enteroviral syndromes may coexist, particularly pleurodynia or pericarditis resulting from coxsackieviruses. Rash may be a manifestation of infections caused by echoviruses, particularly echovirus type 9, coxsackieviruses A9 and A16, and enterovirus 71; the latter three cause hand-foot-and-mouth disease, which may occur alone or accompany aseptic meningitis. Echovirus 9 epidemics often produce syndromes of exanthem, enanthem (small, grayish white lesions resembling Koplik spots on the buccal mucosa), and aseptic meningitis, either alone or in combination; a macular and petechial rash in the presence of a meningitic syndrome must be differentiated from meningococcal meningitis.

The clinical course of enteroviral meningitis is usually benign, even in the minority of patients in whom the onset is acute and even fulminant. Symptoms typically subside within a week in children but may continue for several weeks in adults.

However, some patients have encephalitis or meningoencephalitis, rather than enteroviral meningitis, with neurologic abnormalities affecting the cerebrum. In agammaglobulinemic individuals in whom enteroviral CNS infection develops, meningitis may progress to a chronic meningoencephalitis with multiple neurologic features, including headache, seizures, ataxia, weakness, hearing loss, obtundation, and coma. Enterovirus D68 is associated with an acute flaccid myelitis.

Herpes Simplex Virus Type 2 Meningitis

Aseptic meningitis is a common complication of primary genital HSV-2 infection (Chapter 350); up to 36% of women and 13% of men have headache (developing over 2 to 3 days), stiff neck, and photophobia. Clinical features of meningitis occur 3 to 12 days after the appearance of genital lesions and usually last for 4 to 7 days. Neurologic complications occur in up to 37% of patients and include dysesthesia or paresthesia in the perineum or sacral area, urinary retention, and constipation; evidence of transverse myelitis with motor weakness in the lower extremities, hyporeflexia, and paraparesis occasionally ensues. Recurrent episodes of HSV-2 meningitis may occur at intervals of months or years in 20% of patients. In recurrent HSV-2 meningitis, fever may develop but is not as prominent as in bacterial or acute enteroviral meningitis. Recurrent vesicular lesions, paresthesia, or dysesthesia in areas of previous genital herpes may or may not precede individual recurrences of meningitis. Between recurrences, CSF findings and clinical manifestations return to normal. In patients who have had neurologic complications with a first episode of HSV-2 meningitis, the findings subside within 6 months.

Mumps Meningitis

Symptomatic CNS disease, principally meningitis or meningoencephalitis, occurs in 1 to 10% of patients with mumps parotitis (Chapter 345), but pleocytosis occurs in more than 50% of patients with mumps, most of whom lack CNS symptoms. When meningitis occurs in patients with mumps, it usually follows parotitis by 4 to 10 days, but it may precede parotitis by up to 1 week. The typical features of viral meningitis (headache, fever, vomiting) are each present in 50 to 100% of patients. Stiff neck (40 to 90%) is common, and abdominal pain (perhaps complicating pancreatitis or oophoritis) or orchitis (in ≤20% of men with mumps) may be present. Other complications of mumps may involve the nervous system (eighth nerve damage, transient facial nerve paralysis, and rarely, fifth nerve palsy) but are usually independent of mumps meningitis or meningoencephalitis. The incubation period for mumps is 18 to 21 days. When mumps meningitis occurs in the absence of clinical parotitis, it is difficult to distinguish it from other forms of viral meningitis.

When meningitis complicates mumps, fever, which had been low grade, rises to 103° F or higher and persists at this level for 3 or 4 days. Most cases are uncomplicated, with approximately a 10-day duration of illness and then complete recovery. However, symptomatic mumps meningitis may persist for more than 14 days in some patients.

Meningitis Caused by Lymphocytic Choriomeningitis Virus

Lymphocytic choriomeningitis virus infections are uncommon, and clinical illness occurs after an incubation period of 1 to 3 weeks. Illness begins with a grippe-like syndrome of fever, rigors, malaise, myalgia, anorexia, and photophobia. Sore throat and arthralgia or arthritis of the digits are noted by some patients. Orchitis or parotitis occurs rarely. This grippe-like illness lasts 1 to 3 weeks in humans, but 15% of patients have a biphasic illness consisting of transient improvement and then recrudescence, 1 to 2 days later, of fever, photophobia, and more prominent headache. Meningeal signs are observed during the second phase. The duration of meningitis caused by lymphocytic choriomeningitis virus, like that of mumps meningitis, tends to be longer than the 7 to 10 days for enteroviral meningitis.

Meningitis Caused by Human Immunodeficiency Virus

Initial infection with HIV-1 (Chapter 360) is symptomatic in 40 to 90% of patients but is frequently overlooked. The interval between exposure and onset of symptoms is 2 to 4 weeks. This acute illness resembles mononucleosis, with fever, malaise, lymphadenopathy, arthralgia, myalgia, anorexia, nausea, headache, and morbilliform rash. A few patients with this initial syndrome have manifestations of aseptic meningitis (headache, photophobia, nausea, vomiting, and stiff neck). Occasionally, encephalopathy or cranial nerve palsies (seventh, eighth, and fifth) develop. Symptoms of the initial HIV-1 aseptic meningitis syndrome last several weeks and then subside. Occasionally, manifestations similar to those of the initial infection may appear later in the course of untreated infection.

DIAGNOSIS

Cerebrospinal Fluid Examination

Neuroimaging with an MRI or CT scan can be helpful if there is accompanying encephalitis as manifested by focal neurological signs or to look for obstructive hydrocephalus prior to performing a lumbar puncture. CSF findings in all types of viral meningitis are similar and consist of a predominantly lymphocytic pleocytosis, usually 50 to 1000/μL but occasionally up to several thousand per cubic millimeter, a normal glucose concentration, and a mildly elevated protein level, usually less than 150 mg/dL. During the first 24 to 48 hours of enteroviral meningitis, a predominance of neutrophils (55 to ≤90%) is observed in approximately 50% of patients; subsequently, the principal cells in CSF change to lymphocytes. Occasionally, no pleocytosis is noted in patients proved by culture or PCR to have early enteroviral meningitis. Rarely, hypoglycorrhachia occurs in meningitis resulting from mumps or lymphocytic choriomeningitis virus or in infants with enterovirus.

Polymerase Chain Reaction versus Culture or Antibody Detection

Rapid PCR testing of the CSF has a sensitivity for detecting viruses of 85 to 100%, with a specificity of 95 to 100%, depending on the laboratory, and has been standardized for a select number of clinically relevant pathogens in the same sample.[12] For example, reverse-transcription PCR for enteroviruses can reduce detection time to 5 hours or less, thereby shortening hospital stay and minimizing the unnecessary use of antimicrobial agents. By comparison, viral culture of enterovirus from CSF has a sensitivity of only 65 to 75% and takes 4 to 8 days.

PCR for HSV-2 DNA is usually positive in the CSF of patients with initial episodes of meningitis and is positive in approximately 80% of patients with benign recurrent meningitis caused by lymphocytic choriomeningitis virus.

Recent advancements include the use of next-generation sequencing which maybe particularly useful for identification of rare and unusual organisms when routine testing fails to identify a cause.

The diagnosis can be made retrospectively by demonstrating seroconversion in antibody to gG-2 antigen in HSV-2 meningitis. A four-fold rise in titer to mumps or lymphocytic choriomeningitis virus between acute and convalescent sera is also diagnostic. Serodiagnosis is not practical for sporadic enteroviral meningitis because of the lack of specificity of antibodies to individual serotypes.

Differential Diagnosis

The most important process to distinguish from viral meningitis is bacterial meningitis. A predominance of CSF neutrophils, hypoglycorrhachia, and bacteria on Gram-stained smear or culture indicate bacterial meningitis. An early neutrophilic predominance in CSF combined with a macular and petechial rash in enteroviral meningitis may mimic meningococcemia with meningitis. Occasional bacteria and fungi cause meningitis with a predominantly lymphocytic pleocytosis similar to that of most viral meningitides (Table 384-10). Epidemiologic considerations and clinical findings aid in distinguishing leptospiral, Lyme *Borrelia*, and syphilitic meningitis, whereas hypoglycorrhachia suggests tuberculous and cryptococcal meningitis.

PREVENTION AND TREATMENT   Rx

The introduction of live attenuated mumps vaccine in the United States reduced mumps from the leading cause of aseptic meningitis and meningoencephalitis to the point at which it occurs only rarely. Chronic enteroviral meningitis and meningoencephalitis in agammaglobulinemic patients have been controlled by parenteral (even intrathecal) administration of immune globulin.

No approved antiviral chemotherapy is available for enteroviral meningitis.[13] Pleconaril, a drug that prevents attachment of virus to host cells, can produce clinical improvement in agammaglobulinemic patients with chronic enteroviral meningoencephalitis.

Intravenous acyclovir (5 to 10 mg/kg three times daily) is used to treat hospitalized, symptomatic patients with HSV-2 meningitis, particularly when the

TABLE 384-10	NONVIRAL INFECTIOUS CAUSES OF ASEPTIC MENINGITIS

UNCOMMON	RARE
BACTERIAL	
Leptospira interrogans serovars	*Mycoplasma pneumoniae*
Borrelia burgdorferi	*Ehrlichia chaffeensis*
Treponema pallidum	*Listeria monocytogenes*
Mycobacterium tuberculosis	*Borrelia recurrentis* and *Borrelia hermsii*
Brucella sp	*Chlamydia psittaci*
Parameningeal infections	Staphylococcal enterotoxin or TSST-1
Subacute bacterial endocarditis	*Rickettsia rickettsii* and *Rickettsia prowazekii*
Partially treated bacterial (pyogenic) meningitis	
FUNGAL	
Cryptococcus neoformans	*Blastomyces dermatitidis*
Coccidioides immitis	*Sporothrix schenckii*
Histoplasma capsulatum	*Candida* sp
PROTOZOAN	
	Trypanosoma brucei sp
	Toxoplasma gondii
	Acanthamoeba sp

TSST-1 = toxic shock syndrome toxin 1.

TABLE 384-11	NONINFECTIOUS CAUSES OF ASEPTIC MENINGITIS

Drug hypersensitivity

Systemic disease
  Systemic lupus erythematosus
  Familial Mediterranean fever
  Behçet syndrome
  Granulomatosis with polyangiitis (formerly Wegener)
  Cogan syndrome
  Sarcoidosis
  Still disease
  Kawasaki disease
  Lead poisoning

Neoplastic disease
  Metastatic carcinomatous meningitis
  Central nervous system tumors (meningeal gliomatosis, dysgerminomas, ependymomas)
  Tumors that leak inflammatory material into cerebrospinal fluid (squamous cells in epidermoid tumors of the posterior fossa, cholesteatomas)

Inflammatory processes involving central nervous system structures primarily
  Chemical meningitis following myelography (water-soluble nonionic contrast material)
  Continuous spinal and epidural anesthesia, inflammation after neurosurgery
  Granulomatous cerebral vasculitis
  Vogt-Koyanagi-Harada syndrome

disease is associated with primary genital herpes, although it has not been shown in clinical trials to alter the course of illness. In patients with frequent recurrences of HSV meningitis, it is reasonable to attempt prophylaxis with oral antivirals: valacyclovir (500 mg/day),[AS] famciclovir (250 mg twice daily), or acyclovir (400 mg twice daily).

PROGNOSIS

The course and outcome in patients with enteroviral meningitis are almost always benign, although approximately 1% of patients have subsequent abnormalities, probably reflecting a meningoencephalitic process. Most viral meningitides are self-limited, but some cause chronic or recurrent illness. Persistent meningitis or meningoencephalitis, sometimes fatal, can occur in individuals with hereditary (usually X-linked agammaglobulinemia or common variable immunodeficiency) deficiencies in B-lymphocyte function. HIV-1 may produce a prolonged meningeal inflammation. HSV-2 infection is the most common viral cause of recurrent episodes of aseptic meningitis.

OTHER MENINGITIDES
Nonviral Infectious Causes of Aseptic Meningitis

Categories of aseptic meningitis other than the viral meningitides include nonviral infectious processes (see Table 384-10), noninfectious processes (Table 384-11), chronic meningitides (Table 384-12), recurrent meningitis (Table 384-13), and eosinophilic meningitis (Table 384-14). Nonviral infectious causes are uncommon or rare in comparison to viral or acute suppurative meningitis. Some of the bacterial causes (e.g., *Leptospira* serovars, *B. burgdorferi*, *Brucella* sp, *T. pallidum*) produce a lymphocytic pleocytosis; others (partially treated bacterial meningitis, subacute bacterial endocarditis with embolic cerebral infarcts) produce a mixed neutrophilic-mononuclear pleocytosis; and *M. tuberculosis*, though producing a lymphocytic response with developing hypoglycorrhachia, may show a predominantly neutrophilic response in a minority of patients early in the disease. Although patients with *L. monocytogenes* infection usually have neutrophilic pleocytosis, this infection may suggest aseptic meningitis because of its sometimes indolent onset and, occasionally, an early predominantly lymphocytic response in young children. Fungal (e.g., *Cryptococcus neoformans*, *Coccidioides immitis*, *Histoplasma capsulatum*) meningitides are associated with a predominantly mononuclear response, sometimes with a small percentage of eosinophils, particularly in coccidioidal meningitis (Chapter 316). Patients with Rocky Mountain spotted fever (Chapter 311), an acute disease with a macular and petechial rash, may exhibit confusion. When examined, the CSF in approximately 20% of such patients shows a pleocytosis of 10 to 100 or more cells/μL, with either a neutrophilic or lymphocytic predominance. The clinical picture may suggest either enteroviral or meningococcal disease.

Epidemiologic factors are important in raising suspicion for nonviral aseptic meningitis. Leptospirosis (Chapter 307) may be suggested by a history of recent direct or indirect exposure to animals (e.g., dogs, rodents, dairy cattle) and their urine. Neurobrucellosis (Chapter 294) is suggested by the recent ingestion of unpasteurized cheese from the Mediterranean littoral, Middle East, or Mexico or by work as a veterinarian or in an abattoir. Specific endemic mycoses may be a consideration with residence in the southwestern United States (coccidioidomycosis; Chapter 316) and the Mississippi River valley (histoplasmosis; Chapter 316). The setting of immunosuppression by drugs or illness such as acquired immunodeficiency syndrome would raise the possibility of *C. neoformans* (Chapter 317) or *L. monocytogenes* (Chapter 277). Sexual promiscuity and the macular rash of secondary syphilis could suggest *T. pallidum* (Chapter 303) as the cause in a patient with lymphocytic meningitis.

Noninfectious Causes of Aseptic Meningitis

Noninfectious causes fall into four principal categories (see Table 384-11): drug hypersensitivity; systemic processes such as systemic lupus erythematosus and other collagen-vascular diseases; neoplastic disease, primary or metastatic, infiltrating the leptomeninges; and inflammatory processes primarily involving the CNS. Although a mononuclear cell predominance is found in the CSF in most noninfectious aseptic meningitides, there are several important exceptions. Drug hypersensitivity meningitis usually causes a neutrophilic response, although occasionally mononuclear cells or eosinophils predominate. In systemic lupus erythematosus (Chapter 250), the pleocytosis may be predominantly lymphocytic or neutrophilic (sometimes several thousand per cubic millimeter) with a normal CSF glucose level. Hypoglycorrhachia is a feature of few noninfectious aseptic meningitides and suggests malignant disease or sarcoidosis. Various drugs, most commonly the nonsteroidal anti-inflammatory drugs, have also been implicated in aseptic meningitis.

Chronic (Persistent) Meningitis

Chronic meningitis is defined by the clinical syndrome of headache, stiff neck, altered mental status, nausea and vomiting, evidence of myelopathy or radiculopathy with or without cranial nerve palsies (e.g., III, IV, VI, VII, VIII), and an inflammatory response in the CSF for 4 weeks or longer. Obstruction of CSF flow may produce hydrocephalus and papilledema.

Infectious Causes

Among the more common bacterial causes of chronic meningitis, *M. tuberculosis* (Chapter 308) is the most important to identify because if untreated, it is almost always fatal within 4 to 8 weeks (see Table 384-12). Similarly,

TABLE 384-12 INFECTIOUS CAUSES OF CHRONIC (PERSISTENT) LYMPHOCYTIC MENINGITIS

CAUSATIVE CONDITIONS	OTHER CSF FINDINGS
BACTERIAL	
Mycobacterium tuberculosis	Usually <500 white blood cells/μL, low glucose, high protein
Borrelia burgdorferi (Lyme disease)	Normal glucose, elevated protein
Treponema pallidum (secondary syphilitic meningitis, tertiary meningovascular syphilis)	Elevated protein; Venereal Disease Research Laboratory positive in CSF and serum
Brucella sp (uncommon)	Often low glucose; elevated protein
Tropheryma whippelii (rare)	Cells positive for periodic acid–Schiff on meningeal biopsy
Partially treated bacterial meningitis	Mixture of PMNs and lymphocytes, bacteria on Gram stain and culture
Parameningeal infections	Lymphocytes or mixed lymphocytic-PMN response, normal glucose
FUNGAL	
Cryptococcus neoformans	Low glucose, elevated protein, budding yeast on fungal wet mount, antigen detectable
Coccidioides immitis	Often low glucose, may have 10-20% eosinophils, elevated protein, presence of complement-fixing antibody
Histoplasma capsulatum	Low glucose; complement-fixing antibodies in CSF; antigen detectable in urine, CSF, serum
Blastomyces dermatitidis	Low glucose
Candida sp	Low glucose, may have PMN or lymphocyte predominance, fungal stain may be positive
Aspergillus sp	Lymphocytes or PMNs predominate
Sporothrix schenckii (sporotrichosis)	Low glucose; protein, 200-800 mg/dL
PROTOZOAL	
Toxoplasma gondii	Usually, picture is that of an encephalitis; often in patients with AIDS; pleocytosis is mild (<60 cells/μL) and protein is mildly elevated
Trypanosoma gambiense or Trypanosoma rhodesiense	Meningoencephalitis is stage II of disease, elevated protein and immunoglobulin M, trypanosomes on Giemsa-stained smear
VIRAL	
Mumps	Rarely, low glucose
Lymphocytic choriomeningitis	Rarely, low glucose
Echovirus (in patients with congenital agammaglobulinemia)	Occasionally, low glucose
HIV-1	Cell counts lower (10-20/μL) than in acute self-limited meningitis at clinical onset of HIV infection or may develop during course of AIDS

AIDS = acquired immunodeficiency syndrome; CSF = cerebrospinal fluid; HIV = human immunodeficiency virus; PMN = polymorphonuclear leukocyte.

TABLE 384-13 CAUSES OF CHRONIC (RECURRENT) MENINGITIS

Infections
  Herpes simplex virus type 2

Leakage of contents from central nervous system tumors (chemical meningitis)
  Epidermoid tumors
  Craniopharyngiomas
  Cholesteatomas

Drug hypersensitivity with repeated use of agent

Inflammatory processes
  Behçet syndrome
  Systemic lupus erythematosus
  Mollaret meningitis
  Vogt-Koyanagi-Harada syndrome

TABLE 384-14 CAUSES OF EOSINOPHILIC MENINGITIS*

CAUSATIVE CONDITIONS	SOURCE
PARASITIC DISEASE	
Angiostrongylus cantonensis	Ingestion of raw shellfish; Pacific
Taenia solium (cysticercosis)	Fecal-oral transmission of T. solium eggs
Gnathostoma spinigerum	Ingestion of raw fish; Japan, Southeast Asia
Baylisascaris procyonis	Accidental ingestion of B. procyonis eggs from raccoon feces
Trichinella spiralis (trichinosis)	Ingestion of poorly cooked pork
Schistosoma sp	Exposure of skin to fresh water; Africa, Middle East
Echinococcus granulosus	Contact with infected dogs passing eggs in feces
Toxoplasma gondii	Ingestion of meat containing cysts or food contaminated with oocysts from cat feces
Toxocara canis (visceral larva migrans)	Ingestion of infective eggs from dog feces
FUNGAL INFECTIONS	
Coccidioides immitis	Southwestern United States
NEOPLASTIC DISEASE	
Lymphoma, leukemia, metastatic carcinoma	
Hypereosinophilic syndrome (myeloproliferative disorder)	
INFLAMMATORY PROCESSES	
Sarcoidosis	
Drug hypersensitivity	
Presence of foreign body in the central nervous system	

*The percentage of eosinophils varies from as little as 6% to the majority of cells.

parameningeal infections (Chapter 385) must be recognized and treated promptly because surgery often is necessary to provide a specific bacteriologic diagnosis and prevent neurologic residua. Tuberculosis should be suspected in patients with a previous history of a tuberculous illness, a history of recent exposure, HIV infection or another immunosuppressed state, particularly the use of drugs and biologics that block TNF-α and that are often used to treat autoimmune diseases. Clinical manifestations include fever and night sweats, sixth cranial nerve palsies, stroke related to arteritis, or lesions on the chest radiograph.[14] The purified protein derivative skin test may be negative in patients who are severely immunosuppressed or who have recently acquired or overwhelming disease. Acid-fast smear and culture of concentrated CSF can provide the diagnosis, and modern PCR testing has a sensitivity above 90% and a specificity close to 100%.[15] Measurement of CSF levels of adenosine deaminase has both a sensitivity and specificity of about 90%.[16] When clinical and CSF testing findings suggest the diagnosis, treatment (Chapter 308) should be initiated while awaiting the culture results. There is no benefit from adding levofloxacin (10 mg/kg, maximum 500 mg) or using high-dose rifampicin (15 mg/kg as compared with 10 mg/kg) routinely,[A6] but such therapy can improve survival in drug-resistant cases.[A7] Drug resistance and coinfection with HIV infection can be major impediments to adequate treatment. Rifampicin resistance can be easily detected by PCR, because almost all the mutations that confer rifampicin resistance are contained within a well-defined segment of the *rpoB* gene. Resistance to other drugs is less easily detected by these methods. Adjunctive corticosteroids (e.g., dexamethasone 0.3 to 0.4 mg/kg IV daily for 1 week, then 0.2 to 0.3 mg/kg IV for another week, then a taper from 4 mg daily to 1 mg daily PO over 4 weeks) reduce mortality by about 25%, but do not significantly alter the risk of neurologic sequelae among survivors.[A8]

Parameningeal infections (Chapter 385) should be suspected when chronic meningitis with focal neurologic signs develops in the setting of chronic otitis media or sinusitis, pleuropulmonary infection, or right-to-left cardiopulmonary shunting. Contrast-enhanced CT or MRI of the head is important to delineate brain abscess, sinus infection, and epidural or subdural infections.

Meningitis may accompany the skin, mucous membrane, and lymph node features of secondary syphilis (Chapter 303), or it may occur alone. Individual cranial nerves (II to VII) may be involved; visual abnormalities, hearing loss, and facial palsy are most frequent. The fluorescent treponema antibody absorption test or microhemagglutination T. pallidum serologic studies are helpful in distinguishing the process from biologic false-positive Venereal Disease Research Laboratory (or rapid plasma reagent) results in serum.

Lyme disease meningitis (Chapter 306) should be suspected on the basis of epidemiologic grounds (geographic location, season, tick exposure) and associated clinical features (erythema migrans rash, Bell palsy, radiculopathy). The diagnosis is made by enzyme-linked immunosorbent assay with Western blot confirmation.

A variety of fungal infections can cause a chronic meningitis. Cryptococcal meningitis (Chapter 317) is common in immunosuppressed individuals and can be diagnosed by detection of cryptococcal antigen in the CSF. Histoplasmosis (Chapter 316) should be suspected in endemic regions. Aspergillosis (Chapter 319) is angiocentric and can cause associated cerebral infarcts. Mucormycocis (Chapter 320) is common in patients with poorly controlled diabetes mellitus. Flucytosine is superior to fluconazole when used with amphotericin B for treatment of cryptococcal meningitis (Chapter 317).[A9] Unlike bacterial and tuberculous meningitis, adjunctive corticosteroids are not beneficial and even seem to be detrimental,[A10] except in patients with immune reconstitution inflammatory syndromes (Chapter 367), in which corticosteroids may be beneficial if given concomitantly with antimicrobial agents.

Noninfectious Causes

Noninfectious causes of meningitis include malignant disease, chemical meningitis, and primary inflammatory conditions (Table 384-15). Malignant disease may be diagnosed by cytologic examination of large volumes of CSF. Contrast-enhanced MRI may disclose thickening of the meninges and nerve roots, but meningeal biopsy may be required for diagnosis. Chemical meningitis from previous subarachnoid injection may persist, with xanthochromia noted in CSF; meningeal inflammation may be identified on contrast-enhanced CT or MRI.

Meningeal or CNS sarcoid (Chapter 89) may be isolated or occur with other organ involvement, such as pulmonary granulomas, lymphadenopathy, or myopathy. Neurologic findings can include diabetes insipidus and cranial nerve palsies. Granulomatosis with polyangiitis (Chapter 254) may produce meningeal inflammation and cranial nerve palsies, often in association with air sinus disease. The diagnosis is suggested by lesions on the chest radiograph, microscopic hematuria, skin lesions, peripheral neuropathy, and serum antineutrophil cytoplasmic antibodies. Aseptic meningitis associated with systemic lupus erythematosus (Chapter 250) may be accompanied by other neurologic manifestations (seizures, encephalopathy, stroke, transverse myelopathy),

systemic manifestations (rash, arthritis), and antinuclear and anti-DNA antibodies.

Chronic (Intermittent) Meningitis

In chronic intermittent meningitis, all clinical and CSF abnormalities resolve completely between episodes without antimicrobial therapy (see Table 384-12). Uncommonly, a patient may have several episodes resulting from different viral agents. The major causes of recurrent aseptic meningitis are infections (almost always viral and resulting from HSV-2), endogenous chemical meningitis, drug hypersensitivity (including the use of intravenous immunoglobulins) with meningitis following each use, and inflammatory and autoimmune diseases.

In HSV-2 recurrent meningitis, lymphocytes predominate, with the cell numbers being approximately 40% higher in the initial episode than in recurrences. Leakage of material from intracranial epidermoid cysts produces 1000 to 5000 cells/μL (≈80% polymorphonuclear leukocytes) initially, with a subsequent mononuclear cell predominance. Occasionally, polarizing microscopy may demonstrate keratin and cholesterol crystals in the CSF of patients with endogenous chemical meningitis. In Behçet syndrome (Chapter 254), the CSF may have predominantly mononuclear cells or polymorphonuclear leukocytes. Mollaret meningitis, a syndrome of benign recurrent meningitis usually caused by HSV-2, is initially associated with neutrophils and monocytes in the CSF without hypoglycorrhachia but subsequently transitions to a predominantly lymphocytic pleocytosis. However, prolonged treatment with valacyclovir 1 g/day does not prevent recurrences of HSV-2–associated meningitis. Vogt-Koyanagi-Harada syndrome, a rare uveomeningoencephalitis, consists of recurrent meningitis/meningoencephalitis and anterior or posterior uveitis, followed by vitiligo, poliosis, alopecia, and dysacousia; the CSF cellular response is mononuclear, and an autoimmune origin, directed against a melanocyte antigen, has been suggested.

Chronic Meningitis with Predominantly Neutrophilic Pleocytosis

Chronic persistent neutrophilic meningitis (E-Table 384-1) is defined by the following combination: (1) clinical features consistent with meningitis; (2) initial CSF examination showing greater than 50% neutrophils, hypoglycorrhachia, and elevated protein concentration; (3) antimicrobial therapy that would be appropriate for the usual causes of bacterial meningitis; (4) negative smears and cultures for bacteria on the initial CSF specimen; and (5) repeated CSF examination 7 days or more after initial analysis showing 50% or greater neutrophils, hypoglycorrhachia, and elevated protein concentration.

Among the bacterial causes (see E-Table 384-1) are organisms (*Actinomyces israelii* and *Arachnia propionica* [Chapter 313]) that can be isolated by culture only under anaerobic conditions. Coexisting pulmonary lesions may suggest *Nocardia* (Chapter 314) or *M. tuberculosis* (Chapter 308) as the cause, although the initial polymorphonuclear pleocytosis present in some cases uncommonly persists much beyond a week before changing to a lymphocytic predominance. *Brucella* (Chapter 294) and endemic invasive mycotic infections would be suggested by epidemiologic considerations. Other fungal causes may be diagnosed, particularly in immunocompromised patients, by antigen testing with enzyme-linked immunosorbent assay (*Aspergillus* sp galactomannan; Chapter 319), or meningeal biopsy may be required.

Occasionally, exogenous chemical meningitis secondary to intrathecal injection of antimicrobials, chemotherapeutic agents, or contrast media may produce persisting pleocytosis and hypoglycorrhachia resulting from sclerosing arachnoiditis well after the inciting medication has been withdrawn. Systemic lupus erythematosus (Chapter 250) can produce a variety of meningitides, including acute lymphocytic or neutrophilic aseptic meningitis, as well as chronic persistent lymphocytic or neutrophilic CSF responses.

Eosinophilic Meningitis

The presence of 5% or greater eosinophils in CSF is uncommon and suggests parasitic disease, certain fungal infections such as coccidioidal or candidal meningitis, neoplastic diseases, or a few inflammatory processes (see Table 384-14).[17] In most cases, eosinophils are mixed with lymphocytes, which predominate; the highest percentage of eosinophils is seen with meningitis caused by migrating larvae of the raccoon ascarid *Baylisascaris procyonis* (Chapter 335) and the rat lung worm *Angiostrongylus cantonensis* (Chapter 335). In fungal meningitides, particularly those resulting from *C. immitis* (Chapter 316), the CSF response is primarily mononuclear with 6 to 20% eosinophils; hypoglycorrhachia may be a feature of *C. immitis* and *Candida* meningitis (Chapter 318) and of neoplastic processes and sarcoid.

TABLE 384-15	NONINFECTIOUS CAUSES OF CHRONIC (PERSISTENT) LYMPHOCYTIC MENINGITIS
CAUSATIVE CONDITIONS	**OTHER CSF FINDINGS**
NEOPLASMS	
Metastatic: Lung, breast, stomach, pancreas, lymphoma, melanoma, leukemia	Low glucose; elevated protein, cytologic examination; polarizing microscopy; clonal lymphocyte markers
Central nervous system: Meningeal gliomatosis, meningeal sarcoma, cerebral dysgerminoma; epidermoid tumors/cysts	
CHEMICAL INFLAMMATION	
Endogenous: Epidermoid tumor, craniopharyngioma	Low glucose, elevated protein
Exogenous: Recent injection into the subarachnoid space	Low glucose, elevated protein
PRIMARY INFLAMMATORY PROCESSES	
Central nervous system sarcoid	Often low glucose, elevated protein, elevated angiotensin-converting enzyme levels in CSF (and serum)
Granulomatosis with polyangiitis (formerly Wegener)	Elevated protein
Behçet syndrome	Elevated protein
Isolated granulomatous angiitis of the central nervous system	Elevated protein
Systemic lupus erythematosus	Elevated protein
?Chronic idiopathic benign meningitis	Elevated protein

CSF = cerebrospinal fluid.

Most patients with eosinophilic meningitis, except those with cases resulting from trichinosis (Chapter 335) or drug hypersensitivity, have prolonged symptoms suggesting chronic meningitis. Most patients with meningitis of parasitic or neoplastic origin have evidence of cerebral involvement as well.

Grade A References

A1. Wang Y, Liu X, Wang Y, et al. Meta-analysis of adjunctive dexamethasone to improve clinical outcome of bacterial meningitis in children. *Childs Nerv Syst.* 2018;34:217-223.

A2. van de Beek D, Farrar JJ, de Gans J, et al. Adjunctive dexamethasone in bacterial meningitis: a meta-analysis of individual patient data. *Lancet Neurol.* 2010;9:254-263.

A3. Brouwer MC, McIntyre P, Prasad K, et al. Corticosteroids for acute bacterial meningitis. *Cochrane Database Syst Rev.* 2015;9:CD004405.

A4. Fritz D, Brouwer MC, van de Beek D. Dexamethasone and long-term survival in bacterial meningitis. *Neurology.* 2012;79:2177-2179.

A5. Aurelius E, Franzen-Röhl E, Glimåker M, et al. Long-term valacyclovir suppressive treatment after herpes simplex virus type 2 meningitis: a double-blind, randomized controlled trial. *Clin Infect Dis.* 2012;54:1304-1313.

A6. Heemskerk AD, Bang ND, Mai NT, et al. Intensified antituberculosis therapy in adults with tuberculous meningitis. *N Engl J Med.* 2016;374:124-134.

A7. Heemskerk AD, Nguyen MTH, Dang HTM, et al. Clinical outcomes of patients with drug-resistant tuberculous meningitis treated with an intensified antituberculosis regimen. *Clin Infect Dis.* 2017;65:20-28.

A8. Prasad K, Singh MB, Ryan H. Corticosteroids for managing tuberculous meningitis. *Cochrane Database Syst Rev.* 2016;4:CD002244.

A9. Day JN, Chau TTH, Wolbers M, et al. Combination antifungal therapy for cryptococcal meningitis. *N Engl J Med.* 2013;368:1291-1302.

A10. Beardsley J, Wolbers M, Kibengo FM, et al. Adjunctive dexamethasone in HIV-associated cryptococcal meningitis. *N Engl J Med.* 2016;374:542-554.

GENERAL REFERENCES

For the General References and other additional features, please visit Expert Consult at https://expertconsult.inkling.com.

385

BRAIN ABSCESS AND PARAMENINGEAL INFECTIONS

AVINDRA NATH AND JOSEPH R. BERGER

Brain abscess affects the brain's parenchyma directly, whereas parameningeal infections produce suppuration in potential spaces covering the brain and spinal cord (epidural abscess and subdural empyema) or produce occlusion of the contiguous venous sinuses and cerebral veins (cerebral venous sinus thrombosis).

BRAIN ABSCESS

EPIDEMIOLOGY

The frequency of various causes of brain abscess (Table 385-1) in the population is difficult to ascertain because of wide variations among case series, in part owing to referral patterns. The incidence is about two in 100,000 person years.[1] Brain abscesses account for less than 1% of intracranial mass lesions in developed countries but are significantly more common in developing countries. Males predominate in virtually all series of brain abscess.

Children with brain abscesses often have cyanotic congenital heart disease (Chapter 61) or otogenic infection.[2] Brain abscess also occurs in patients with pulmonary arteriovenous malformation, as is seen in hereditary hemorrhagic telangiectasia (Chapter 164).[3] Cryptogenic abscesses account for a greater percentage of cases perhaps related to the presence of a patent foramen ovale. On average, 90% of brain abscesses are a consequence of a focus of suppuration elsewhere in the body, with the remainder due to introduction of the infection from head wounds or neurosurgical procedures.

PATHOBIOLOGY

Brain abscesses are collections of purulent material (neutrophils and necrotic tissue) caused by infection with bacterial, fungal, or parasitic organisms. When contiguous to the brain, infection enters by direct extension or by traveling along veins with associated thrombophlebitis of pial veins and sinuses. More commonly, the brain is seeded hematogenously by the offending microorganism from a distant site. Within the brain, the infection begins as a cerebritis with perivascular infiltrates and infiltration of neutrophils into the brain parenchyma. With time, the developing abscess is characterized by a purulent exudate that includes necrotic brain tissue as well as viable and necrotic neutrophils. Granulation tissue develops at the interface between necrotic and viable tissue, and eventually, the abscess is walled off by a fibrous capsule. Formation of the capsule depends on the virulence of the organism and the immune status of the individual. More virulent organisms cause larger lesions, more necrosis, earlier ependymitis, and a greater degree of inflammation outside the collagen capsule. Hematogenous dissemination typically results in lesions located at the junction of white and gray matter.

CLINICAL MANIFESTATIONS

The clinical picture reflects a triad of the infectious nature of the lesion, focal brain involvement, and an increasing intracranial mass effect (Table 385-2). One or two elements may be absent, particularly early in the course. Among infectious symptoms, fever is present at onset or early in the course in only about 60% of cases. Neck stiffness is an infrequent complaint, and meningeal signs are elicited in about 30% of cases. The absence of classical signs may delay diagnosis.[4]

Focal neurologic deficits depend on the site and size of the lesion, which in turn will be determined by the causative agent and any underlying condition that may predispose to the development of brain abscess. In some patients, seizures precede the diagnosis. Temporal lobe lesions, which are often caused by spread of an otogenic abscess, may manifest as contralateral homonymous

TABLE 385-1	CONDITIONS THAT PREDISPOSE TO THE DEVELOPMENT OF BRAIN ABSCESS
Otogenic	
Otitis media	
Mastoiditis	
Dental	
Cardiac	
Cyanotic heart disease	
Tetralogy of Fallot	
Patent foramen ovale	
Infective endocarditis	
Pulmonary	
Pulmonary arteriovenous fistula	
Lung infection	
Esophageal strictures	
Cerebral infarcts and tumors	
Penetrating and nonpenetrating head injury	
Postoperative neurosurgical procedure	
Dermal sinus tracts	
Sepsis	
Immunosuppression	
Unknown mechanism	

TABLE 385-2	BRAIN ABSCESS: INITIAL FEATURES IN 123 CASES
Fever	58%
Headache	55%
Disturbed consciousness	48%
Hemiparesis	48%
Nausea, vomiting	32%
Nuchal rigidity	29%
Dysarthria	20%
Seizures	19%
Sepsis	17%
Visual disturbance	15%

superior quadrantic visual field defects and, if in the dominant hemisphere, with aphasia. Motor deficits eventually occur in 40 to 50% of supratentorial abscesses. Cerebellar abscesses, which are often caused by aural-mastoid infections, are characterized by ipsilateral limb ataxia; there may also be abnormal head positioning (forward and away from the side of the lesion) and nystagmus that is slow and coarse on gaze to the side of the abscess and rapid in the opposite direction. Patients with multiple brain abscesses may have multifocal signs or encephalopathy. Patients with *Toxoplasma* species (Chapter 328) brain abscesses often have movement disorders because these abscesses frequently localize to the basal ganglia. In fact, nearly all patients with human immunodeficiency virus (HIV) infection in whom hemiballism or hemichorea is present have *Toxoplasma* species brain abscesses.

Headache is an important initial symptom in 80 to 90% of patients with bacterial abscess but is less frequent (≈20%) in patients with fungal abscesses. Symptoms of increased intracranial pressure, such as nausea, depressed level of consciousness, and papilledema, occur less often. The development of headache in a patient with a known chronic anaerobic infection, such as aural-mastoid, paranasal sinus, or pulmonary suppuration, suggests the possibility of brain abscess. Similarly, the development of headache in a child with cyanotic congenital heart disease is often related to a brain abscess. Tetralogy of Fallot (Chapter 61) is the most common congenital heart anomaly associated with brain abscess.

DIAGNOSIS

Examination of the cranium, ears, paranasal sinuses, oral cavity, heart, and lungs may provide important clues to the etiology, as may overt signs of infection at other sites. Cultures of blood and sputum may identify the organism and its antimicrobial sensitivity. In patients with signs of raised intracranial pressure, lumbar puncture may be contraindicated because of the risk of herniation.

Magnetic resonance imaging (MRI) can detect early changes such as brain edema and is preferable to computed tomography (CT).[5] In the early cerebritis stage, T2-weighted MRI shows abnormally high signal intensity corresponding to low signal intensity on the T1-weighted images. The fluid-attenuated inversion recovery (FLAIR) sequence provides superior visualization of brain edema. On T1-weighted images, the area of cerebritis that is seen initially as a low-signal-intensity, ill-defined area later progresses to a central cavity with slightly higher signal intensity than cerebrospinal fluid (CSF), surrounded by edema that is slightly hypointense in comparison to brain parenchyma. Later stages of infection show central necrosis and formation of a rim of slightly high signal intensity on T1-weighted images (Fig. 385-1). With gadolinium administration, there is a ring-enhancing lesion owing to leakage of the contrast material at the rim of the lesion where there is breakdown of the blood-brain barrier. Diffusion-weighted imaging helps differentiate abscesses from brain tumors (Chapter 180); pus in the abscess cavity demonstrates high signal with decreased apparent diffusion coefficient values, whereas necrotic tumor cavities demonstrate the opposite.

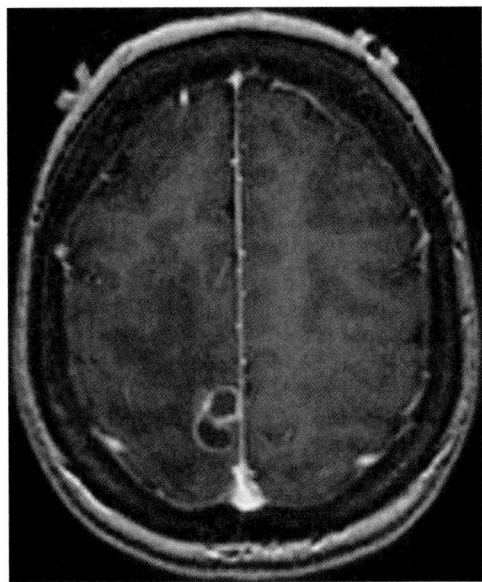

FIGURE 385-1. Brain abscess. Magnetic resonance imaging with gadolinium shows a multiloculated ring-enhancing lesion caused by *Nocardia* species infection.

Surgical aspiration or excision of the lesion may be necessary to establish a microbial diagnosis. Gram stain and culture from abscess fluid, with proper handling, have high yield, with or without previous antibiotic therapy. If immediate surgery is planned, antibiotics can be deferred until culture material has been acquired. Multiplex polymerase chain reaction testing is being developed for rapid identification of bacterial organisms and detection of antibiotic resistance genes.

TREATMENT Rx

Brain abscess requires urgent intervention. Surgical intervention has the advantage of establishing a definitive diagnosis, identifying the causative organism, and determining antibiotic susceptibility.

Because of the risk for cerebral herniation with large lesions, treatment of cerebral edema (intravenous [IV] dexamethasone, 16 to 24 mg/day in four divided doses) may be needed even while initiating surgical intervention.[6] Corticosteroids often decrease edema within 8 hours but may retard the formation of a capsule around the brain abscess, suppress the immune response to the infection, and decrease penetration of antibiotics. Hence, they should be used for short periods, usually only until surgical decompression by needle drainage or surgical removal is possible.

Brain abscesses caused by *Toxoplasma* species (Chapter 328) usually occur in immunocompromised patients (e.g., patients with HIV infection), are not accompanied by capsule formation, and hence respond well to antibiotic therapy alone. As a result, patients with acquired immunodeficiency syndrome and suspected cerebral toxoplasmosis (Chapter 328) should receive antimicrobial therapy initially.

For other abscesses, empirical antibiotic therapy (Table 385-3) is recommended prior to surgery, based on the likely source of infection, knowledge of proved or suspected pathogens, as well as familiarity with a drug's spectrum of activity and penetration into the central nervous system.[7] Because abscesses may include multiple organisms, antibiotic coverage should include both aerobic and anaerobic bacteria.

However, antibiotics may not penetrate the cavity of more advanced brain abscesses owing to the absence of blood supply in the necrotic lesion. Therefore, surgical drainage is usually the treatment of choice.[8]

When surgery cannot be performed (e.g., in a remote location where neurosurgical expertise may not be available), empirical antibiotic therapy is the

TABLE 385-3 COMMON PATHOGENS AND EMPIRICAL THERAPY FOR BRAIN ABSCESS

PREDISPOSING CONDITION	COMMON PATHOGENS	ANTIMICROBIAL AGENTS*
Dental abscess	Streptococci, *Bacteroides fragilis*	Penicillin + metronidazole
Chronic otitis	*Bacteroides fragilis; Pseudomonas, Proteus, Klebsiella* species	Cefotaxime or ceftriaxone + metronidazole; ceftazidime or cefepime for *Pseudomonas* species
Sinusitis	Streptococci; *Haemophilus, Staphylococcus* species	Cefotaxime, ceftriaxone, or nafcillin + metronidazole
Penetrating trauma or postsurgical	*Staphylococcus, Pseudomonas, Enterobacter* species; streptococci	Nafcillin or vancomycin + ceftriaxone or cefotaxime + metronidazole
Bacterial endocarditis or drug use	Mixed flora, streptococci, *Staphylococcus* species	Nafcillin or vancomycin + ceftriaxone or cefotaxime + metronidazole
Congenital heart disease	Streptococci	Cefotaxime or ceftriaxone
Pulmonary infection	*Nocardia* species, *Bacteroides fragilis*, streptococci, mixed flora	Penicillin + metronidazole + trimethoprim-sulfamethoxazole
HIV infection	*Toxoplasma gondii*	Pyrimethamine + sulfadiazine + folinic acid

*See Table 271-4 in Chapter 271 for dosing schedules.
HIV = human immunodeficiency virus.

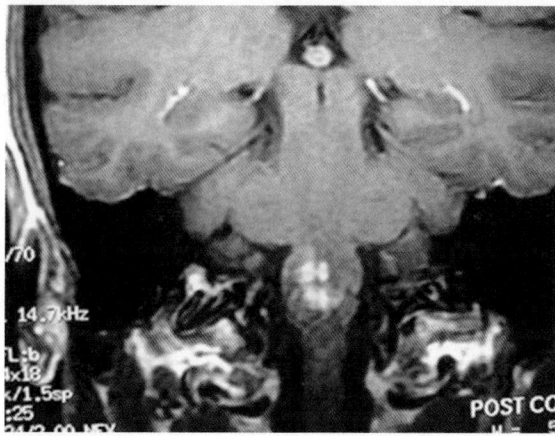

FIGURE 385-2. Brain stem abscess. Magnetic resonance imaging with gadolinium shows an enhancing lesion in the brain stem caused by *Listeria* species infection.

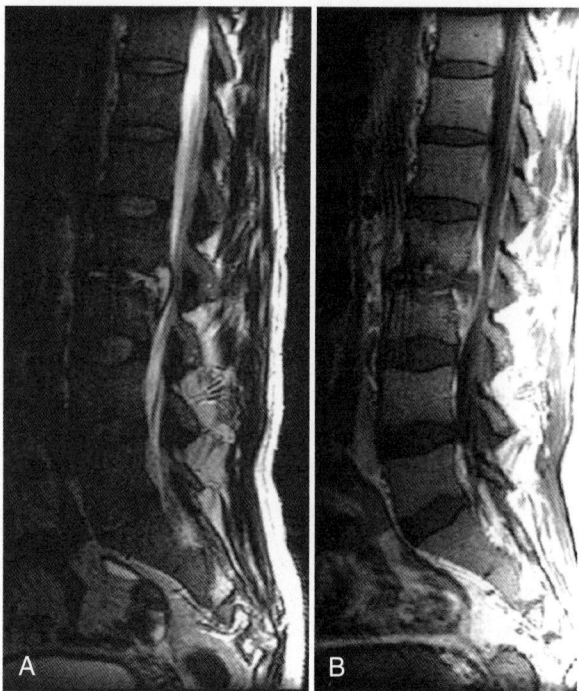

FIGURE 385-3. Spinal epidural abscess. A and B, Magnetic resonance images of the lumbosacral spine show a lesion in the epidural space compressing the thecal sac.

only alternative. A trial of nonsurgical treatment may also be considered in patients with (1) small lesion size; (2) an already identified pathogen; (3) no symptoms or signs of increased intracranial pressure requiring neurosurgical intervention; (4) a deep or inaccessible lesion; (5) multiple abscesses; (6) a contraindication to surgery (e.g., a bleeding diathesis); (7) a short duration of symptoms, which suggests that the lesion is in the cerebritis stage; and (8) availability of monitoring with MRI.

In patients who are suspected of having a brain stem abscess, the possibility of listerial infection (Chapter 277) should be considered (Fig. 385-2), even in the absence of a clear immunodeficiency. Empirical parenteral antibiotics to cover *Listeria* species should be started (Chapter 277).

PROGNOSIS

Before the CT scan era, the mortality of brain abscesses ranged from 40 to 60%, and even in the era of modern neuroimaging, the mortality rate remains about 10%. About 70% of patients recover fully. In post-transplantation patients and those with deep hemispheric or brain stem abscesses, mortality rates may exceed 80%. Other factors associated with a poor prognosis include extremes of age, multiple abscesses, and diagnostic delay in the absence of systemic signs of infection. An impaired level of consciousness is a poor prognostic sign even with early hospitalization and rapid diagnosis. Anaerobic and gram-negative organisms and culture-negative cases also have a poor prognosis. Seizures (Chapter 375) develop in up to 50% of patients, sometimes after latencies as long as 5 years.

SPINAL EPIDURAL ABSCESS

DEFINITION

Infection within the epidural space around the spinal cord is an uncommon, but often readily treatable potential cause of paralysis and death. The epidural space surrounds the dural sac and is limited by the posterior longitudinal ligament anteriorly, the ligamenta flava and the periosteum of the laminae posteriorly, and the pedicles of the spinal column and the intervertebral foramina containing their neural elements laterally. The space communicates with the paravertebral space through the intervertebral foramina. Superiorly, the space is closed at the foramen magnum. Caudally, the space is closed by the sacrococcygeal ligament. The epidural space contains loose areolar connective tissue, semiliquid fat, lymphatics, arteries, an extensive plexus of veins, and the spinal nerve roots.

EPIDEMIOLOGY

Spinal epidural abscesses can result from hematogenous spread of infection; risk factors include IV drug use, organ transplantation, chronic steroid use, malignancy, and diabetes. Local infection after acupuncture for back pain or epidural analgesia can also cause epidural abscesses. Cutaneous sites of infection are the most common remote sources, especially in IV drug users. Abdominal, respiratory tract, and urinary sources are also common. Osteomyelitis may be a cause of either direct extension or hematogenous spread, particularly when associated with sepsis. Contiguous spread may occur from epidurally placed catheters, psoas abscesses, decubitus ulceration, perinephric and

retropharyngeal abscesses, or surgical sites. Minor back trauma has been implicated in causing a paraspinal hematoma, which may be seeded hematogenously. *Staphylococcus aureus* is the most common organism isolated from spinal epidural abscesses.[9]

PATHOBIOLOGY

Because the dura mater around the cord is adherent to the vertebral column anteriorly, more epidural abscesses lie posteriorly, and because no anatomic barriers separate the spinal segments in the posterior epidural space, such abscesses usually extend over several vertebral segments. Spinal cord dysfunction probably reflects toxic processes secondary to inflammation, as well as venous thrombosis, thrombophlebitis, ischemia secondary to compression of the spinal arteries, and edema.

CLINICAL MANIFESTATIONS

The presence of a risk factor (>80% of patients) in the setting of neurologic deficits or back or radicular pain should suggest a spinal epidural abscess.[10] The clinical manifestations can be divided into four stages (E-Table 385-1). Back pain (71%), fever (66%), tenderness of the spine with focal percussion (17%), spinal irritation (20%), and headache (3%) are common. Radicular pain can be mistaken for sciatica, a visceral abdominal process, chest wall pain, or cervical disc disease. Clinical signs are often substantially greater than would be predicted from the anatomic extent of pus or granulation tissue.

Unfortunately, as many as 75% of patients with spinal epidural abscess are misdiagnosed at the time of initial presentation. If the condition goes unrecognized, symptoms can evolve over a period of hours to days to paralysis below the spinal level of infection.

DIAGNOSIS

The differential diagnosis includes compressive and inflammatory processes involving the spinal cord: transverse myelitis (Chapter 383), herniation of an intervertebral disc (Chapter 372), epidural hemorrhage (Chapter 372), or metastatic tumor (Chapter 180), none of which are associated with evidence of systemic infection.[11] Blood leukocytosis may not be present, but the sedimentation rate is often elevated. Other infectious processes that may produce back or neck pain or tenderness must be excluded: bacterial meningitis (Chapter 384), perinephric abscess, disc space infection, and bacterial endocarditis (Chapter 67).

Lumbar puncture should be avoided in patients suspected of having a spinal epidural abscess, for fear of spreading the infection to the subarachnoid space and causing meningitis. Gadolinium-enhanced MRI (Fig. 385-3) is the method of choice for diagnosis, and paraspinal edema on MRI is the most sensitive feature for a spinal epidural abscess, but MRI findings in patients undergoing epidural analgesia can resemble those of epidural spinal abscess even when no infection is present.

PROGNOSIS

The mortality rate of spinal epidural abscess is about 15%. Approximately 50% of survivors have residual neurologic deficits. More severe preoperative neurologic deficits and deficits of longer duration are associated with a worse prognosis. In general, patients who develop paralysis that persists for longer than 36 hours do not recover function.

SUBDURAL EMPYEMA

Subdural empyema is an infection in the space between the dura and the arachnoid. It usually results from infected paranasal sinuses and rarely from infected mastoid sinuses by extension of thrombophlebitis from the sinuses into the subdural space. The infection is often unilateral because bilateral spread is prevented by the falx. The empyema may result in cortical vein thrombosis, cerebral abscesses, or purulent meningitis.

CLINICAL FEATURES AND DIAGNOSIS

The most common symptoms are headache, fever, a neurologic deficit, and a stiff neck. However, subdural empyema may progress and cause signs of raised intracranial pressure, such as vomiting, altered level of consciousness, seizures, and papilledema. A high degree of suspicion is needed to establish the diagnosis early in the course of the illness. In patients with sinusitis (Chapter 398), the symptoms of subdural empyema may be incorrectly attributed to the sinusitis.

MRI with gadolinium enhancement and diffusion-weighted images is useful in visualizing the subdural infection as a crescent-shaped mass with an enhancing rim over the cerebral convexities and below the inner table of the skull (Fig. 385-4). CSF evaluation is useful only if there is accompanying meningitis. In a patient with signs of raised intracranial pressure, lumbar puncture should be avoided because of the risk for herniation.

PROGNOSIS

The mortality rate is about 25%, with severe residual neurologic sequelae in about 20% of survivors. Accompanying venous sinus thrombosis or brain abscess carries a poor prognosis.

VENOUS SINUS THROMBOSIS SECONDARY TO INFECTION

The venous sinus system (Fig. 385-5) lacks valves, thereby permitting retrograde propagation of clots or infections that emanate from structures located in the central portion of the face or the middle ear.[14]

Septic Cavernous Sinus Thrombosis

DEFINITION

The cavernous sinuses, which are the most caudal dural venous chambers at the base of the skull, lie on either side of the pituitary fossa immediately above the midline sphenoid sinus. The cavernous sinus encloses the "cavernous portion" of the internal carotid artery as well as the third, fourth, and sixth cranial nerves.

EPIDEMIOLOGY AND PATHOBIOLOGY

The infection usually spreads from the paranasal sinuses, dental abscesses, or other infections affecting the orbit or middle third of the face. *S. aureus* is the most common organism. Streptococci, pneumococci, and gram-negative bacilli are less common; anaerobic infection has also been reported.

CLINICAL MANIFESTATIONS

Cavernous sinus thrombosis may be manifested as an acute fulminant disease or have an indolent subacute manifestation. Fever and other systemic symptoms from sepsis may be present. Clinical symptoms and signs are related to anatomic structures within the cavernous sinuses or drained by them: unilateral periorbital edema, headache, photophobia, proptosis, ophthalmoplegia, pupillary dilation, decreased corneal reflex, and periorbital sensory loss. Obstruction of venous drainage from the retina can result in papilledema, retinal hemorrhages, and visual loss. The infection can spread rapidly (24 to 48 hours) through the intercavernous sinuses to the contralateral cavernous sinus. Thrombus can extend to other dural venous sinuses, adjacent vascular structures, or the brain parenchyma.

DIAGNOSIS

The diagnosis is made on clinical findings and confirmed by radiographic studies. Radiologic evaluation includes sinus imaging, particularly the sphenoid

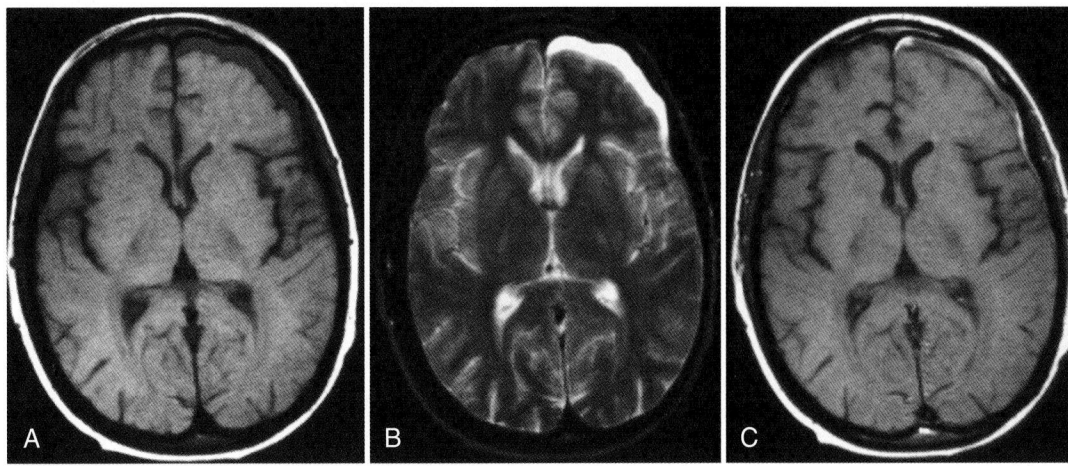

FIGURE 385-4. Subdural abscess. **A,** T1-weighted magnetic resonance imaging shows a hypodense area in the left frontal region. **B,** T2-weighted image shows increased signal intensity in the same region. **C,** A contrast scan shows enhancement in the same region.

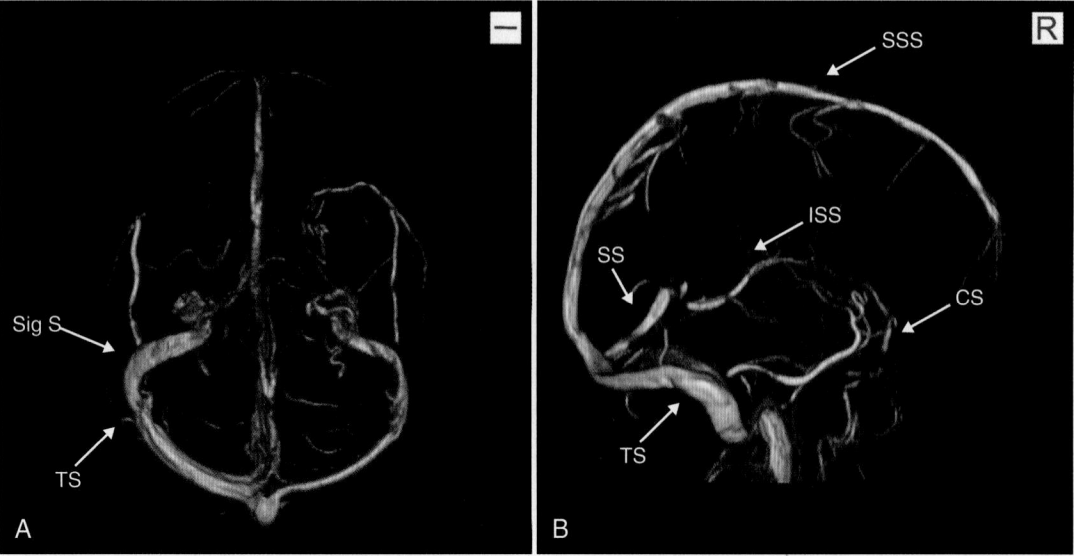

FIGURE 385-5. Anatomy of major venous sinuses. Magnetic resonance venography of the brain shows the normal venous sinuses. **A** shows sigmoid sinus (Sig S) and transverse sinus (TS). **B** shows superior sagittal sinus (SSS), inferior sagittal sinus (ISS), straight sinus (SS), transverse sinus (TS), and cavernous sinus (CS).

and ethmoid sinuses. MRI using flow parameters and MR venogram is sensitive and may reveal deformity of the cavernous portion of the internal carotid artery, a heterogeneous signal from the abnormal cavernous sinus, and an obvious hyperintense signal of thrombosed vascular sinuses. MRI with IV gadolinium can demonstrate venous thrombosis by illustrating a lack of the normal "flow void" within vascular structures. Cranial CT scans are less helpful but may show a subtle increase in the size and enhancement of the thrombosed sinus. MR angiography may demonstrate extrinsic narrowing of the intracavernous portion of the internal carotid artery.

TREATMENT AND PROGNOSIS   Rx

Blood cultures are often negative, so delays in diagnosis are common. Even when the diagnosis is established, empirical antimicrobial treatment may not provide full coverage.

Treatment consists of prompt drainage of infected paranasal sinuses or other identifiable source of infection, as well as specific antistaphylococcal agents (Chapter 272). Heparin anticoagulation without a loading dose is sometimes initiated to reduce morbidity from associated brain ischemia, but experience in septic venous thrombosis is limited compared with the more frequent use of anticoagulation in nonseptic venous thromboses. Hemorrhage caused by anticoagulation is rare in this setting. Despite modern therapy, mortality rates may approach 50%.

Lateral Sinus Thrombosis

Septic thrombosis of the lateral sinus results from acute or chronic infections of the middle ear.

CLINICAL MANIFESTATIONS AND DIAGNOSIS

Symptoms consist of ear pain and fever followed by headache, nausea, vomiting, loss of hearing, and vertigo, usually evolving over a period of several weeks. Symptoms or signs suggestive of otitis media (Chapter 398), including mastoid swelling, may be seen. Sixth cranial nerve palsies can occur, but other focal neurologic signs are rare. In some patients with nonseptic lateral sinus thrombosis, headache may be the only symptom. Papilledema occurs in 50% of cases, and elevated CSF pressure is present in most, especially with occlusion of the right lateral sinus, which is the major venous conduit from the superior sagittal sinus (Fig. 385-6).

CSF is usually normal, although a parameningeal inflammatory profile (mild pleocytosis, slight elevation in protein level, and a normal glucose level) may be seen. The diagnosis is confirmed by MR venography.

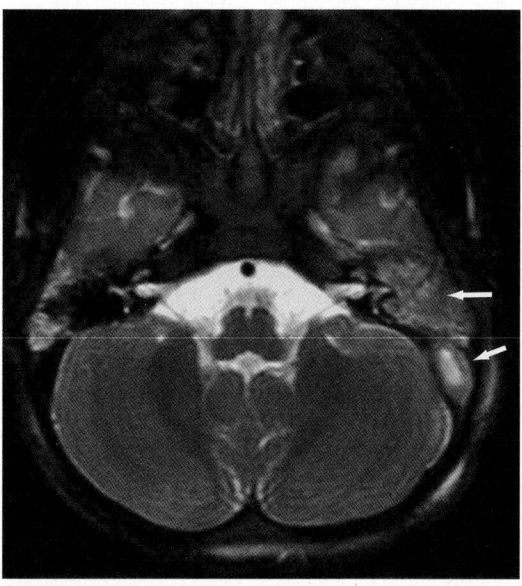

FIGURE 385-6. Lateral sinus thrombosis. Magnetic resonance imaging shows a thrombus in the lateral sinus (*short arrow*) with accompanying mastoiditis (*long arrow*).

TREATMENT   Rx

Treatment includes IV antibiotics to cover staphylococci, anaerobes, and gram-negative bacilli such as *Proteus* species and *Escherichia coli* (nafcillin, 2 g every 6 hours, or vancomycin, 1 g every 12 hours; plus cefotaxime, 2 g every 6 hours, or ceftriaxone, 2 g every 12 hours; plus metronidazole, 7.5 mg/kg every 6 hours, or clindamycin, 300 mg every 6 hours; plus ciprofloxacin, 400 mg every 12 hours). Surgical drainage (mastoidectomy or tympanoplasty) may be required to eradicate the nidus of infection and determine the antibiotic susceptibility of the organism. If the sinus contains pus, it must be opened so the septic thrombus can be removed. Unless vision is compromised, increased intracranial pressure seldom requires drainage or placement of a shunt.

PROGNOSIS

Broad IV antibiotic coverage and eradication of the perisinus infection, which may require surgical drainage, early in the course of the illness lead to a good prognosis. Neurologic sequelae may include a sixth nerve palsy, ataxia, and hearing loss.

Septic Sagittal Sinus Thrombosis

Although superior sagittal sinus thrombosis is the most common form of venous sinus thrombosis and is frequently associated with the use of oral contraceptives, septic sagittal sinus thrombosis is an uncommon condition that occurs as a consequence of purulent meningitis, infections of the ethmoid or maxillary sinuses spreading through venous channels, compound infected skull fractures, or (rarely) neurosurgical wound infections.

CLINICAL MANIFESTATIONS AND DIAGNOSIS

Symptoms are primarily related to the elevated intracranial pressure and can evolve rapidly to stupor and coma. Seizures and hemiparesis may result from cortical infarction. Early recognition and treatment are necessary because septic sagittal sinus thrombosis carries a high mortality rate. The rate of progression, severity of symptoms, and prognosis are all related to the location of thrombosis. Obstruction of the anterior third of the sinus produces less intense symptoms and evolves more slowly.

CSF abnormalities are frequent, including enough red blood cells that the CSF can sometimes be mistaken for a subarachnoid hemorrhage; the opening pressure is increased in proportion to the extent of sagittal sinus involvement. A septic sagittal sinus is best visualized during the venous phase of cerebral angiography or MR venography. The diagnosis can also be made by MRI, which demonstrates an abnormal increase in signal intensity (absent flow void) within the affected venous sinus. Contrast-enhanced CT scanning may reveal a contrast void lying at the junction of the transverse and sagittal sinuses (the region of the torcular); this so-called delta sign is an intraluminal clot surrounded by contrast material.

TREATMENT — Rx

IV antibiotics should be directed at organisms recovered from the meningeal process or the meningeal site. *S. aureus* (Chapter 272), β-hemolytic streptococci (Chapter 274), pneumococci (Chapter 273), and gram-negative aerobes such as *Klebsiella* species (Chapter 290) are the most common organisms. Associated paranasal sinusitis should be drained surgically.

PROGNOSIS

If the thrombosis progresses to involve the middle and posterior thirds of the sinus, deterioration progresses rapidly. The prognosis is poor, with a mortality rate of nearly 30%.

NEUROLOGIC COMPLICATIONS OF INFECTIOUS ENDOCARDITIS

Neurologic complications develop in nearly one third of patients with infective endocarditis (Chapter 67), and neurologic manifestations are the initial symptom in 20% of patients with infective endocarditis. In nearly 30% of patients, the neurologic complications occur within 2 weeks after the initiation of treatment. Ischemic stroke owing to cerebral embolization is the most common[15] manifestation of infectious endocarditis. Stroke may occur in 20 to 40% of cases, and it is the presenting manifestation in about 20% of patients. Hemorrhagic stroke is much less common in patients with infectious endocarditis. Infective endocarditis should always be considered in a patient with a fever and stroke.

PATHOBIOLOGY

Cerebral embolization occurs as a result of dislodgement or disruption of the cardiac vegetations and frequently causes occlusion of cerebral blood vessels. Emboli occurring before the initiation or completion of treatment with antibiotics may contain microorganisms capable of causing metastatic infections such as abscesses, arteritis, meningitis, or mycotic aneurysms. Most cerebral emboli involve small or moderate-sized blood vessels, and multiple cerebral emboli are common. Intracranial hemorrhage is usually due to rupture of a mycotic aneurysm (Chapter 380), septic erosion of the arterial wall without the formation of an aneurysm, or hemorrhagic transformation of a large cerebral infarct. Mycotic aneurysms occur in approximately 2 to 3% of patients with infective endocarditis. About 20% of patients have multiple aneurysms; involvement of the middle cerebral artery and its branches occurs in more than 75% of patients, unlike congenital aneurysms, which occur predominantly in the circle of Willis. Mycotic aneurysms develop as a result of either septic embolization into the vasa vasorum or direct penetration of the microorganism into the wall of the artery. Streptococci and staphylococci account for nearly 90% of all mycotic aneurysms.

CLINICAL MANIFESTATIONS

Embolic stroke typically causes an acute onset of a focal neurologic deficit. Seizures may also occur. Multiple microemboli result in an altered or fluctuating level of consciousness not adequately explained by other abnormalities.

Most patients with mycotic aneurysms have a sudden, often fatal, subarachnoid or intracerebral hemorrhage without warning signs. Warning signs, if present, include severe localized headache, ischemic events, seizures, and cranial nerve abnormalities. In some patients, mycotic aneurysms may be asymptomatic and resolve with antibiotic therapy. Some patients develop micro- or macroabscesses, septic or aseptic meningitis (Chapter 384), or a generalized toxic metabolic encephalopathy.

DIAGNOSIS

MRI is the modality of choice for the diagnosis of cerebral infarcts and brain abscesses related to endocarditis. Gradient echo sequences on the MRI may be more sensitive than a CT scan for detecting intracranial hemorrhage and can also detect microbleeds. MRI should include diffusion-weighted sequences for detection of infarcts. An MR angiogram is preferred for diagnosing an aneurysm. CSF evaluation is useful if accompanying meningitis or a slow leak from an aneurysm is suspected but not visualized with these imaging tests.

TREATMENT — Rx

Treatment of patients with infective endocarditis and cerebral emboli requires prevention of embolization with appropriate antibiotic therapy and sometimes cardiac surgery (Chapter 67). Anticoagulation is contraindicated in patients with cerebral infarcts and septic emboli because of the high risk for complications from intracerebral bleeding.

Patients with unruptured aneurysms smaller than 7 mm in diameter, proximal aneurysms, multiple aneurysms, ruptured aneurysms without an intracerebral hematoma, and aneurysms for which excision is likely to cause a neurologic deficit can be monitored conservatively with serial MRI and MR angiography. All other aneurysms require surgical excision of the aneurysm and the adjacent septic vessel wall. Patients who cannot undergo surgery may be candidates for endovascular embolization of the aneurysmal vessel.

PROGNOSIS

Mortality rates in patients with infective endocarditis and cerebral emboli range from 30 to 80%. Mortality is high if there is hemorrhagic transformation of the infarct. Mortality in patients with ruptured mycotic aneurysms is 80%, and even patients with unruptured aneurysms have a mortality rate of 30%.

GENERAL REFERENCES

For the General References and other additional features, please visit Expert Consult at https://expertconsult.inkling.com.

386

ACUTE VIRAL ENCEPHALITIS

ALLEN J. AKSAMIT, JR.

DEFINITION

Encephalitis is a diffuse or focal inflammation of the parenchyma of the brain. The term *encephalitis* indicates that the predominant clinical syndrome arises from infection and inflammation in the parenchyma of the brain rather than in the leptomeninges. When both the leptomeninges and brain parenchyma are involved, the term *meningoencephalitis* is used.

In the United States, about 50% of cases of encephalitis are viral in origin and about 25% are autoimmune (Chapter 383).[1] The remaining 25% or so

TABLE 386-1	COMMON CAUSES OF VIRAL ENCEPHALITIS

I. Causes of viral encephalitis
  A. Nonseasonal
    Herpes simplex virus type 1 (herpes simplex encephalitis)
    Herpes simplex virus type 2 (neonatal encephalitis or adult
      meningoencephalitis)
  B. Seasonal—summer and fall—arboviruses (arthropod borne)
    West Nile virus
    St. Louis encephalitis virus
    Eastern equine encephalitis virus
    Western equine encephalitis virus
    La Crosse/California encephalitis virus
    Powassan encephalitis virus
    Chikungunya virus
  C. Seasonal—non–arthropod borne
    Summer and fall: enteroviruses (including coxsackieviruses, echoviruses,
      polioviruses, and enterovirus 71)
    Winter: influenza virus
  D. Immunosuppressed patients
    Human immunodeficiency virus (chronic HIV encephalitis)
    Varicella-zoster virus (subacute encephalitis)
    JC virus (progressive multifocal leukoencephalopathy)
    Cytomegalovirus (ventriculitis or encephalitis)
    Human herpesvirus 6 (subacute encephalitis)
    Epstein-Barr virus (subacute encephalitis)

II. Uncommon causes in the United States
    Powassan encephalitis virus
    Zika virus
    Chikungunya virus
    Variegated squirrel bornavirus
    Lymphotropic choriomeningitis virus
    Rabies
    Measles (subacute sclerosing panencephalitis)
    Mumps
    Adenovirus
    Herpes B virus (of monkeys)
    Rubella (progressive rubella panencephalitis)

III. Causes outside the United States
    Zika virus (Africa, Asia, Caribbean, Central America, Pacific Islands, South
      America)
    Chikungunya virus (Africa, Asia, Central America, Pacific Islands, South
      America, Western Europe)
    Tick-borne encephalitis virus (Russia, Asia)
    Japanese encephalitis virus (Japan, Southeast Asia, Malaysia)
    Venezuelan equine encephalitis virus (Central and South America)
    Dengue virus (Southern Asia, Africa, South America)
    Rift Valley fever virus (east central Africa)
    Murray Valley encephalitis virus (Australia)
    Powassan encephalitis virus (Canada)
    Nipah virus (Malaysia and Bangladesh)

are currently of unknown cause, although advances in diagnostic technology may reduce this percentage in the future.

EPIDEMIOLOGY

Viral encephalitis has an estimated incidence of seven per 100,000 per year. Many viruses (Table 386-1) are implicated, and testing by serologic or nucleic acid identification (by polymerase chain reaction [PCR]) is required to identify the specific virus. The epidemiology of each virus responsible for central nervous system infection (see Table 386-1) is distinct in terms of the patients who are at highest risk, geographic distribution, and seasonal occurrence, especially the arboviruses (Chapter 359) and enteroviruses (Chapter 355), which are covered in separate chapters.[2]

In the United States, the most common cause of nonepidemic encephalitis is herpes simplex encephalitis, which is caused by herpes simplex virus type 1 (Chapter 350). The most common epidemic virus in the United States is now West Nile virus (Chapter 359), which is a mosquito-transmitted Flavivirus related to St. Louis encephalitis virus and its Asian counterpart Japanese encephalitis virus. There is serologic cross-reactivity among St. Louis encephalitis, Japanese encephalitis, and West Nile viruses. Recent emerging infections that are capable of causing encephalitis in the United States are Chikungunya and Zika.[3,4] A novel cause recently reported is variegated squirrel

bornavirus, which has been associated with fatal human encephalitis in three squirrel breeders.

PATHOBIOLOGY

In general, gross pathologic inspection of an encephalitic brain does not reveal purulence visible to the naked eye. If focal purulence is present, *cerebritis* is the more correct term. If frank necrosis and purulence are present, the correct pathologic term is *brain abscess* (Chapter 385). Encephalitis, however, can be associated with substantial necrosis, and patients with severe acute viral encephalitis frequently have microscopic evidence of necrosis. Certain viral encephalitides, such as herpes simplex encephalitis, can be both focal and hemorrhagic. Viruses that cause acute encephalitis may often also cause meningitis (Chapter 384). Indeed, patients with encephalitis virtually always have some microscopic inflammatory changes in the leptomeninges. Conversely, patients with viral meningitis will inevitably have some component of microscopic encephalitis. The degree of inflammatory change present in the brain is determined by the individual viral pathogen and by host immune factors, which are responsible for the reaction to the invading virus.

CLINICAL MANIFESTATIONS

The clinical findings in patients with acute viral encephalitis start with a prodrome of fever, headache, malaise, myalgia, and nonspecific symptoms. Nausea, vomiting, diarrhea, cough, sore throat, and rash can precede the neurologic symptoms as part of the systemic initial manifestations of the infection. Invasion of the nervous system is typically accompanied by headache, photophobia, and altered consciousness, with symptoms progressing over a period of a few days. Seizures are a common heralding symptom. Signs of meningeal irritation may be present but are an unreliable finding in encephalitis.

Focal brain dysfunction is seen with some viruses. For example, West Nile virus (Chapter 359) can cause a brain stem encephalitis with an early onset of coma. Herpes simplex virus (Chapter 350) tends to cause focal cortical neurologic deficits, including hemiparesis, aphasia, and seizures. Limbic parts of the brain commonly involved by herpes simplex encephalitis or rabies can lead to prominent behavioral changes at the beginning of the illness before the patient's level of consciousness is depressed. Focal or generalized seizures are particularly common when encephalitis affects the cerebral cortex, especially the hippocampus and limbic system. Rabies is typically associated with brain stem–mediated laryngospasm, hydrophobia, and depressed consciousness. Because of spinal cord anterior horn cell involvement, West Nile virus, St. Louis encephalitis virus, Japanese encephalitis virus, poliovirus, and rabies virus infections can cause focal or asymmetrical weakness with areflexia.

DIAGNOSIS

In patients with coma or focal deficits, computed tomography (CT) of the head should usually be performed before spinal fluid analysis to exclude substantial mass effect and to avoid the risk of herniation during lumbar puncture. In patients without focal findings, however, lumbar puncture should be performed immediately to: establish the diagnosis; distinguish viral from bacterial, fungal, and parasitic causes; and allow early empirical treatment. Opening pressures should be measured because increased intracranial pressure can occur with all forms of viral encephalitis and may need additional treatment.

Spinal fluid analysis typically reveals an elevated protein level, which usually is less than 2 g/dL. The cerebrospinal fluid (CSF) glucose level is typically normal and greater than 40% of the coincident serum value, but rare patients may have a low CSF glucose level similar to what is seen in patients with bacterial infection (Chapter 384). The CSF white blood cell count is typically elevated, usually in the range of 10 to 500 cells/μL. The cell type is usually a lymphocytic predominance. However, a polymorphonuclear predominance is seen in some cases, especially in some patients with West Nile encephalitis or cytomegalovirus ventriculitis.

Serologic, PCR testing, or next-generation sequencing on spinal fluid is helpful (Table 386-2). PCR testing has the advantage of proving direct viral infection within the central nervous system,[5] but serologic testing is more appropriate for some infections like West Nile virus encephalitis, which is best confirmed by an immunoglobulin M (IgM) antibody response in spinal fluid. Next-generation sequencing can detect viral pathogens for which PCR assays are insensitive, not established, or not readily available.[6]

Magnetic resonance imaging (MRI) of the brain is the most sensitive technique for defining structural abnormalities in patients with viral encephalitis.[7] However, frank viral encephalitis can occur with normal findings on MRI. MRI findings also can suggest the responsible virus. For example, herpes simplex encephalitis has a characteristic pattern involving the mesiotemporal,

TABLE 386-2	SELECTED TESTS FOR VIRAL ENCEPHALITIS	
ORGANISM/ SYNDROME	**TEST**	**COMMENT**
WEST NILE VIRUS		
West Nile encephalitis	IgM in CSF	Diagnostic of CNS invasive disease including encephalitis or acute flaccid paralysis
HERPES SIMPLEX VIRUS TYPE 1		
Herpes simplex encephalitis	PCR in CSF	Sensitive and specific in the acute phase
HERPES SIMPLEX VIRUS TYPE 2		
Neonatal encephalitis	PCR in CSF	Confirmatory, high sensitivity
Relapsing meningitis	PCR in CSF	Sensitive and specific in first 3 days of illness
HUMAN HERPESVIRUS 6		
Limbic encephalitis	PCR in CSF	Confirmatory, sensitivity unknown
VARICELLA-ZOSTER VIRUS		
Meningoencephalitis	PCR in CSF	Confirmatory when used with clinical and spinal fluid findings; sensitivity unclear
JC VIRUS		
Progressive multifocal leukoencephalopathy	PCR in CSF	Diagnostic but incompletely (70%) sensitive
CYTOMEGALOVIRUS		
CMV ventriculitis	PCR in CSF	Sensitive and specific

CNS = central nervous system; CSF = cerebrospinal fluid; IgM = immunoglobulin M; PCR = polymerase chain reaction.

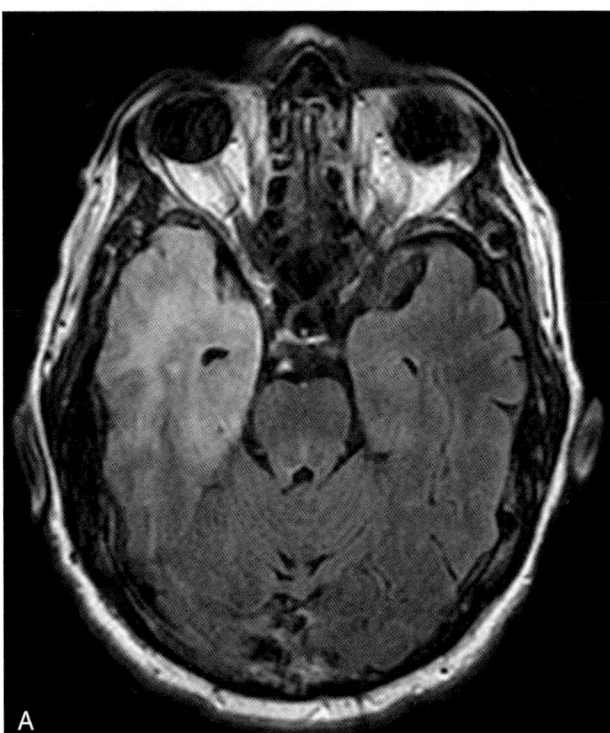

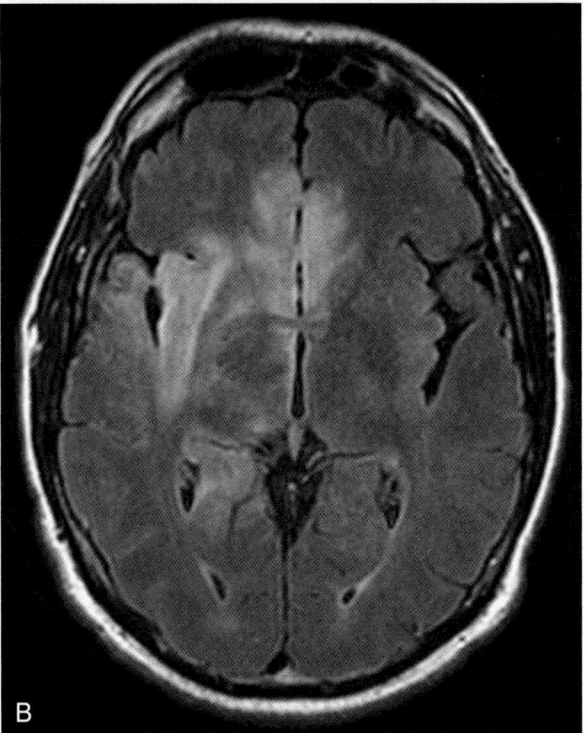

FIGURE 386-1. Magnetic resonance imaging (MRI) in herpes simplex encephalitis. Fluid-attenuated inversion recovery (FLAIR) MRI scan of the brain, showing increased signal in the right mesiotemporal lobe (including the amygdala, hippocampus, and uncus) **(A)** and in the bilateral inferofrontal lobes (cingulate gyrus and orbital frontal cortex) and the right insular cortex **(B)**.

inferofrontal, and insular cortices, usually unilateral or asymmetrically bilateral (Fig. 386-1).

Differential Diagnosis
A number of nonviral pathogens can cause encephalitis that is clinically and pathologically indistinguishable from viral encephalitis. Examples include *Rickettsia* (Chapter 311), *Borrelia* (Chapter 306), Whipple disease (Chapters 131 and 259), *Toxoplasma* (Chapter 328), *Mycoplasma* (Chapter 301), and *Acanthamoeba* (Chapter 331). Other forms of infectious nonviral causes mimicking viral encephalitis include bacterial cerebritis, meningovascular syphilis, and cerebral cysticercosis.

Additionally, autoimmune encephalitides can mimic viral encephalitis,[8] including limbic paraneoplastic encephalitis, especially associated with antibodies against the voltage-gated potassium channel complex, Hashimoto encephalopathy associated with autoimmune thyroiditis (Chapter 213), and encephalitis associated with anti–N-methyl-D-aspartate (NMDA) receptor antibodies.

In parainfectious encephalitis, a systemic viral infection is associated with a febrile encephalopathy, sometimes with inflammatory spinal fluid but without direct evidence of brain invasion by the virus. Examples of parainfectious encephalitis include infection and encephalopathy associated with influenza virus (Chapter 340), varicella virus (Chapter 351), and Epstein-Barr virus (Chapter 353). Furthermore, primary demyelinating disease (Chapter 383), particularly in the form of acute disseminated encephalomyelitis, overlaps clinically with viral encephalitis.

SELECTED SPECIFIC VIRUSES
Herpes Simplex Encephalitis
EPIDEMIOLOGY
Herpes simplex (Chapter 350) encephalitis, which is second only to West Nile encephalitis (Chapter 359) as the most common form of encephalitis in the United States, has an annual incidence of two to four cases per million people per year. There is no seasonal or gender predisposition. The encephalitis can strike children but is most commonly a disease of adults.

PATHOBIOLOGY
Herpes simplex encephalitis usually occurs in immunocompetent patients, but immunosuppressed patients may also be affected. Patients who are deficient in toll-like receptor 3 in the immune system may be selectively vulnerable to herpes simplex encephalitis.

Herpes simplex virus type 1 infects and establishes latency in the trigeminal ganglion in a majority of the population. Whether herpes simplex encephalitis arises from reactivation of a latent viral infection or is a primary nasopharyngeal infection that ascends into the olfactory nervous system is uncertain.

The pathology of herpes simplex encephalitis is a necrotizing hemorrhagic inflammatory encephalitis in a characteristic pattern affecting the mesiotemporal, inferofrontal, and insular cortices, with gray matter predominance. Even if the brain is affected bilaterally, the pathologic features are usually asymmetrical, a pattern that helps distinguish herpes simplex from other forms of limbic encephalitis.

CLINICAL MANIFESTATIONS

The clinical manifestations of herpes simplex encephalitis usually begin with a nonspecific febrile prodrome that is followed within hours to days by the symptoms of headache, malaise, nausea, and vomiting. A reduced level of consciousness may occur early. Seizures may be the first manifestation of this encephalitis. Focal neurologic deficits, such as hemiparesis or aphasia, appear early and can be mistaken for stroke. More specific manifestations of herpes simplex encephalitis are symptoms of limbic system–associated behavioral changes, such as behavioral or emotional lability and inappropriateness. Memory is affected early if consciousness is preserved. As the encephalitis progresses, symptoms of increased intracranial pressure, lethargy, and coma are usual. Focal findings alone in the context of clinical encephalitis are not sufficient to confirm a diagnosis of herpes simplex encephalitis.

DIAGNOSIS

Spinal fluid analysis is necessary in the diagnosis of herpes simplex encephalitis. In a patient with focal encephalitis or coma, however, CT of the brain should be performed before spinal fluid analysis to avoid the risk of herniation. Elevation of the CSF protein level and the white blood cell count, with a predominance of lymphocytes, is the most frequent pattern; red blood cells are also commonly seen. The CSF glucose level is usually normal but is less than 50% of the blood glucose level in about 5% of patients.

The best and most accurate test for proof of herpes simplex encephalitis is the presence of herpes simplex virus type 1 DNA amplified by PCR of the spinal fluid. Herpes simplex virus type 1 can be distinguished from herpes simplex virus type 2 by specific primer amplification, applied as part of the PCR analysis. Because herpes simplex type 2 can cause encephalitis in neonates and meningoencephalitis in adults, this distinction may guide therapy.

MRI typically shows characteristic focal involvement with increased T2 and fluid-attenuated inversion recovery (FLAIR) signal in the mesiotemporal lobes (including the amygdala, hippocampus, and uncus), the inferofrontal lobes (cingulate gyrus and orbital frontal cortex), and the insular cortex (see Fig. 386-1).[9] MRI abnormalities are often unilateral but can be bilateral and asymmetrical. Focal MRI abnormalities must be distinguished from brain abscess (Chapter 385), cerebral infarction (Chapter 379), cerebral hemorrhage (Chapter 380), brain tumors (Chapter 180), and paraneoplastic limbic encephalitis. Radiographically detected involvement of the mesiotemporal rather than the lateral temporal areas and involvement of the gray matter rather than the white matter suggest herpes simplex encephalitis as the diagnosis. Early gadolinium contrast enhancement may occur but is not universal.

CT of the head is less sensitive than MRI for detecting mild cases of herpes encephalitis. However, because herpes simplex encephalitis can be hemorrhagic, CT may sometimes identify the hemorrhage more accurately than MRI can.

Electroencephalography is an adjunctive test that can show periodic lateralized epileptiform discharges ipsilateral to the involved temporal lobe. However, the findings are not specific for herpes simplex encephalitis and commonly occur in patients with cerebral infarction (Chapter 379) and occasionally other forms of viral encephalitis.

TREATMENT   Rx

Multicenter prospective trials emphasize that early treatment affects outcome. When suspicion for herpes simplex encephalitis is raised in the acute setting by the presence of focal signs or symptoms, early empirical treatment is recommended even while the diagnostic evaluation is proceeding.

Intravenous acyclovir (10 mg/kg every 8 hours for 14 to 21 days) is the therapy of choice. No prospective data support a longer duration of therapy or higher doses of acyclovir to improve neurologic outcomes. Autoimmune post–herpes simplex encephalitis may respond to corticosteroids, intravenous immunoglobulin, or plasma exchange, but no randomized trials are available.

Rabies

Human rabies is an encephalitic illness caused by the rabies virus, usually transmitted by an animal bite. It produces a fatal encephalitis, although the latency between animal bite exposure and occurrence of neurologic symptoms may sometimes obscure the diagnosis.[10]

EPIDEMIOLOGY AND PATHOBIOLOGY

Rabies is a rare illness in the United States and developed world. However, initially unsuspected cases have been transmitted via trivial bites by infected bats, which are widely distributed in every state in the United States except Hawaii. Rabies virus variants in bats are now responsible for the majority of recent human cases in the United States and Canada.

Canine rabies is still endemic in much of the developing world, including Africa, Latin America, Eastern Europe, and Asia, and the vast majority of human rabies cases occur as a result of untreated dog bites from endemic areas. Rare cases of transmission of rabies to transplant organ recipients have occurred in the United States.

The presence of Negri bodies (intracytoplasmic viral inclusions) in neurons of the brain stem, cerebellum (especially the Purkinje cells), or hippocampus defines rabies pathologically. These inclusions are often not present, and more sensitive detection of antigen by immunohistochemistry aids in the pathologic diagnosis.

CLINICAL MANIFESTATIONS

Human rabies usually develops 20 to 90 days after a bite, although rarely disease develops after only a few days or after a year or more following bite exposure. Multiple bites and facial bites are associated with shorter incubation times.

Nonspecific prodromal symptoms include fever, chills, malaise, fatigue, insomnia, anorexia, headache, and irritability. In the majority of patients, migratory pain or paresthesias will develop in the limb that was affected by the bite. Following the prodromal illness, an encephalitic form develops in about 80% of patients and causes behaviors ranging from episodes of agitated arousal to quiet lethargy. Fever is a common accompaniment but not universal at this phase. Disinhibition of brain stem reflexes leads to hydrophobia with laryngospasm and an inability to deal with salivation, swallowing of water, or other oral intake. When the brain stem encephalitis affects the bulbar, cardiovascular, and respiratory centers, autonomic dysfunction, cardiopulmonary complications, and respiratory failure occur.

Another form of rabies that affects up to a third of patients is known as paralytic rabies. This form of rabies is manifested as acute flaccid paralysis, which may be multifocal and affect the limbs and the bulbar musculature, thereby resembling poliomyelitis (Chapter 355) because of its multifocality. It can be confused with Guillain-Barré syndrome (Chapter 392). Paralytic rabies typically occurs in conjunction with febrile encephalitis.

DIAGNOSIS

Findings on spinal fluid analysis may be abnormal in human rabies. A lymphocytic pleocytosis, usually less than 100 white cells/µL, is found in more than 50% of patients in the first week of illness. The CSF protein concentration usually is mildly elevated, and the glucose level is usually normal.

Imaging of patients with rabies is sometimes useful. MRI may show gray matter involvement, particularly involvement of the brain stem, with increased T2 signal, commonly without enhancement. Spinal cord MRI in patients with paralytic rabies may show multifocal increased T2 signal mimicking acute disseminated encephalomyelitis. Involvement of brain gray matter, including the hippocampus and basal ganglia structures, indicates the gray matter predilection and often bilateral involvement of supratentorial structures. However, MRI cannot be relied on to exclude rabies.

Serum antibodies against rabies virus are not usually present in unimmunized patients until the second week of illness, and patients can die before having a detectable serum antibody level. Antibodies may also be detected in spinal fluid, but their absence is unreliable in excluding the diagnosis. Classically, staining a skin biopsy sample taken from an area near the nape of the neck for rabies antigen in the sensory nerves can confirm the diagnosis of rabies. Alternatively, rabies RNA can be detected by PCR testing. Typical specimens to detect virus include saliva, brain tissue, or spinal fluid. A positive result confirms the diagnosis, but the exclusionary value of negative results is unknown.

TREATMENT   Rx

After an animal bite, local treatment with antirabies immunoglobulin and systemic treatment with vaccination are typically offered.[11] Rabies postexposure prophylaxis includes local wound cleansing, passive immunization with immunoglobulin, and active immunization with rabies vaccine. Inactivated cell culture rabies vaccines are used for active immunization, and the risk for vaccination-induced acute disseminated encephalomyelitis has been markedly reduced by the use of these vaccines. However, once rabies encephalitis is manifested, it is unclear whether vaccination, although regularly used, has any role in improving outcome. Antiviral therapy and a variety of immunotherapies, including ribavirin and interferon alfa, have been tried in the treatment of rabies, usually without success. Although one patient has survived with the use of therapeutic coma without vaccination, subsequent reports of patients treated in similar fashion have been associated with a fatal outcome. Treatment is otherwise supportive, and outcome is essentially always fatal.

Health care workers can occasionally have high-risk exposures related to broken skin contact or mucosal splash with the patient's secretions. Given the lack of documented human-to-human rabies transmission, a conservative approach seems appropriate. An mRNA vaccine is currently being tested for primary prophylaxis in high-risk individuals.[12]

Rare Causes of Encephalitis

Lymphocytic choriomeningitis (Chapter 384) virus is a human infection acquired from mice. Typically, humans acquire the infection by contact with food or dust that is contaminated by excreta of the common house mouse. Most commonly, human disease occurs in winter, when the natural host tends to move indoors. It can also be acquired as a consequence of laboratory exposure by human caretakers.

Mumps virus (Chapter 345) is typically acquired by the respiratory route. Infection can occur throughout the year, but the incidence is higher during the spring. Although mumps virus infects both sexes equally, meningoencephalitis develops in males three times more frequently than in females. Vaccination programs in the United States have made mumps encephalitis rare.

Autoimmune encephalitis is described in Chapter 383.

TREATMENT Rx

Effective antiviral therapy does not exist for most forms of viral encephalitis, except for herpes simplex encephalitis. However, because of the usual delay in establishing or excluding the diagnosis of herpes simplex encephalitis, patients suspected of having encephalitis should start acyclovir therapy (10 mg/kg intravenously every 8 hours for 2 weeks) while specific serologic and spinal fluid analyses are being performed to make a diagnosis.

Supportive measures for patients with encephalitis typically include intensive care unit treatment in the initial phases of the illness. Seizures are common and frequently refractory to antiepileptic drugs; however, the seizures themselves can increase morbidity and mortality, so vigorous treatment attempts are required (Chapter 375).

In patients who are immunosuppressed (see Table 386-1), the spectrum of possible infections is broader and potentially more treatable. Examples include varicella-zoster virus (Chapter 351), with acyclovir administered at doses similar to those used for herpes simplex virus, and cytomegalovirus (Chapters 346 and 352), with ganciclovir administered at 5 mg/kg intravenously every 12 hours for 2 weeks or cidofovir administered at 5 mg/kg intravenously weekly for 2 weeks, although some patients require long-term oral valganciclovir (900 mg every 24 hours) or intravenous cidofovir (5 mg/kg every 2 weeks). HIV encephalitis (Chapter 366) responds in variable degree to triple antiretroviral therapy. By comparison, no specific treatments are currently effective for Epstein-Barr virus (Chapters 346 and 353) and JC virus (progressive multifocal leukoencephalopathy [Chapter 346]). Variable success has been reported for treatment of human herpesvirus 6 encephalitis in hematopoietic stem cell transplant recipients using ganciclovir, foscarnet, or valganciclovir alone or in combination (Chapter 336, Table 336-4).

PROGNOSIS

The prognosis of encephalitis is dependent on the cause, with an overall mortality rate of about 6 to 10% in the United States. Herpes simplex encephalitis, even with adequate treatment, has a 20% mortality, and the likelihood of major persistent morbidity with seizures or defects in memory and behavior is 35 to 40%. Each of the arboviruses has a different mortality rate, with eastern equine encephalitis virus associated with the highest mortality. La Crosse encephalitis virus has the lowest mortality.

Some forms of encephalitis have specific sequelae, such as sensorineural deafness or hydrocephalus associated with mumps encephalitis. About 50% of survivors will have significant clinical sequelae. In one large observational study of acute encephalitis, factors that portended a worse prognosis included advanced age, immunocompromised state, coma, mechanical ventilation, and acute thrombocytopenia. Conversely, the cause of encephalitis, the development of seizures or a focal neurologic deficit, and MRI findings were not associated with clinical outcomes.

GENERAL REFERENCES

For the General References and other additional features, please visit Expert Consult at https://expertconsult.inkling.com.

387

PRION DISEASES

PATRICK J. BOSQUE

DEFINITION

Prion diseases are a group of closely related neurodegenerative conditions of humans and other mammals. In prion diseases, a normal brain protein known as the prion protein (PrP) aggregates in an abnormal conformation.[1] This abnormal form of the protein can act as an infectious agent called a prion and transmit disease to another host. The prion is thus an infectious protein conformation that contains no specific nucleic acid. The name Creutzfeldt-Jakob disease (CJD) is applied to most human forms of prion disease, although other names are used for some forms.

EPIDEMIOLOGY

Prion diseases occur worldwide, with an incidence of 1 to 2 cases per million annually. These conditions can be acquired sporadically, genetically, or infectiously, but sporadic disease accounts for about 90% of cases, and genetic forms represent almost all the remainder. Both dietary and iatrogenic exposure have transmitted prion disease to humans, but these infectiously acquired forms are extremely rare, representing less than 1% of cases in most human populations.

Sporadic prion disease is typically a disease of late-middle or late life, with a peak incidence in the eighth decade. However, apparently sporadic cases have been reported in individuals as young as 16 years of age and as old as 98 years of age. Genetic forms tend to have a younger onset, with a peak in the sixth decade.

Two human outbreaks of prion disease, kuru and variant CJD, were caused by dietary exposure. Kuru was epidemic in tribes of the Fore language group in the highlands of New Guinea. It probably arose as a case of sporadic prion disease, and then was spread by the practice of ritual cannibalism. The last exposures are thought to have occurred in the late 1950s, but new clinical cases have occurred as recently as 2009, thereby indicating a maximum incubation period of at least 50 years.

Variant CJD is caused by eating meat from cattle infected with the prion disease known as bovine spongiform encephalopathy. Variant CJD first arose in Great Britain in 1994, about 10 years after an outbreak of a massive bovine spongiform encephalopathy epidemic there. Despite the exposure of millions of people to meat contaminated with bovine spongiform encephalopathy prions, only 228 people worldwide are known to have contracted variant CJD.[2] The incidence of variant CJD has decreased in recent years as the bovine spongiform encephalopathy outbreak in cattle has been contained and the entry of contaminated meat into the food supply has been restricted.

Scrapie in sheep and chronic wasting disease in deer and elk are endemic prion diseases in some populations of these animals. In contrast to bovine spongiform encephalopathy, neither disease is known to have been transmitted to humans.

Prion-contaminated cadaveric dura mater allografts and pituitary-derived growth hormone injections have each caused more than 200 iatrogenic cases of CJD. Most dura mater–associated cases have been from a single product, Lyodura, manufactured before May 1987.[3] All growth hormone cases involve product derived from cadaveric pituitaries before recombinant growth hormone became available in the 1980s. Blood and blood products derived from donors with variant CJD have transmitted the illness, but, perhaps surprisingly, sporadic CJD has not been transmitted through blood products.[4] Other modes of iatrogenic spread of CJD are quite rare. Contaminated surgical instruments are persuasively documented to have transmitted CJD on six occasions, and corneal transplants have been documented to transmit CJD only twice.

PATHOBIOLOGY

PrP is a cell surface glycoprotein normally produced in the brain and several other tissues. Its function is unknown, but it may play a role in copper metabolism. An abnormally aggregated form of PrP, termed PrP^{Sc}, accumulates in the brain in prion disease. Remarkably, PrP^{Sc} is able to recruit the normal form of PrP into the pathologic aggregate. The precise structure of PrP^{Sc} aggregates and the mechanism of prion propagation are incompletely understood, but a basic conceptual model proposes that the normally α-helical regions of PrP directly interact with the β sheets of PrP^{Sc}, lose their normal α-helical structure, and then join the aggregate. At some point, the growing aggregate fractures, thereby creating additional aggregate particles. In this way, an aggregate of PrP^{Sc} can propagate as an infectious agent. A curious feature of prion diseases is that more than one aggregated structure of PrP^{Sc} can be stably propagated, and these various "strains" of prions can give rise to distinct clinical manifestations.

Predominantly β-sheet aggregates of other proteins are implicated as the causes of more common neurodegenerative diseases (e.g., the β-amyloid protein in Alzheimer disease [Chapter 374] and synuclein in Parkinson disease [Chapter 381]). Although these other diseases are not known to be infectiously transmitted, recent studies suggest that a mechanism of self-propagation like that described above for prion diseases may play a role in their pathogenesis.[5]

What precisely initiates sporadic or genetic prion diseases is not known. In infectious forms of prion disease that are transmitted by the alimentary route, prions first replicate in the enteric lymphatic system, including Peyer patches. From the lymphatic system, prions spread to the central nervous system (CNS) via sympathetic nerves in lymphatic tissue. Once in the CNS, prions appear to spread trans-synaptically. As with other neurodegenerative diseases associated with accumulations of aggregated proteins, the mechanism by which the PrP aggregates cause neuronal dysfunction and death is unknown.

Pathology

Traditionally, prion diseases are recognized by a combination of vacuolization (status spongiosus) of the gray matter, astrocytic gliosis, and loss of neurons. In modern practice, histologic diagnosis rests on demonstrating the presence of PrP^{Sc}, using techniques that exploit the enhanced resistance to degradation displayed by these PrP aggregates. Certain forms of prion disease have a distinct and characteristic histochemical appearance. For example, variant CJD produces a peculiar type of amyloid plaque surrounded by vacuoles, the so-called florid plaque.

Genetics

All inherited forms of prion disease are caused by mutations in the PrP coding sequence of the gene *PRNP*. Mutations associated with familial forms of prion disease include more than 20 missense mutations, two premature stop mutations, and a series of insertions in a region of a repeated eight–amino acid sequence. Genetic forms of prion disease are transmitted in an autosomal dominant pattern, usually with high but incomplete penetrance. Three distinctive forms of prion disease are associated with certain *PRNP* mutations. First, the Gerstmann-Sträussler-Scheinker syndrome is caused by any of several mutations in *PRNP*, the most common of which codes for a substitution of leucine for proline at codon 102 (P102L). Pathologically, there are accumulations of plaques of PrP amyloid in the brain, especially in the cerebellum. Second, fatal familial insomnia is caused by a D178N mutation on the same allele as a methionine at the polymorphic codon 129 of *PRNP*. Pathologically, there is neuronal loss and accumulation of PrP^{Sc} in the thalamus. In contrast, the D178N mutation on an allele with valine at codon 129 causes a disease that is indistinguishable from sporadic CJD. Third, some *PRNP* mutations cause slowly progressive dementia. The most common of these mutations are large expansions of the octapeptide repeat region.

Certain common genotypes affect susceptibility to prion disease. Codon 129 of *PRNP* is polymorphic, with alleles coding for either valine or methionine. Persons who are homozygous (129VV or 129MM) at this allele are

overrepresented among victims of sporadic CJD, and all victims of variant CJD carry 129M on both *PRNP* alleles.

CLINICAL MANIFESTATIONS

Sporadic CJD is the most common prion disease in humans.[6] In about 25% of cases, patients or their families report a prodrome of a psychiatric disturbance such as anxiety, depression, or altered sleep. Cognitive dysfunction is usually the most prominent neurologic sign; but unlike Alzheimer disease, prion disease typically causes motor signs (e.g., ataxia, bradykinesia, spasticity) and vague somatic sensory disturbances. Myoclonus is a characteristic but not pathognomonic sign. Perhaps the most distinctive feature of prion disease is the pace of its progression. Typically, clear decrements in neurologic function can be observed over a period of weeks.

Variations on this typical presentation can occur and are common in genetic and infectiously transmitted disease. In Gerstmann-Sträussler-Scheinker syndrome, ataxia is the most prominent initial sign, and dementia occurs only late in the course of the disease. The disease worsens slowly compared with sporadic CJD (typically 5 to 6 years from onset to death). Fatal familial insomnia begins with anxiety, depression, and sleep disturbance followed by ataxia and other motor signs; dementia occurs relatively late. Some familial forms of prion disease are so slowly progressive as to have clinical manifestations similar to those of familial Alzheimer disease (Chapter 374) or Huntington disease (Chapter 382).

Variant CJD, acquired by exposure to bovine spongiform encephalopathy prions, is distinguished clinically from sporadic CJD by a much younger mean age at onset (mean, 26 years; range, 12 to 74 years), more prominent psychiatric and sensory signs early in the disease, and later emergence of dementia and motor signs. Iatrogenic CJD usually resembles sporadic CJD, but a subset of patients may have an ataxic form that clinically and pathologically shares some features with Gerstmann-Sträussler-Scheinker syndrome. Kuru begins with limb pain followed by cerebellar ataxia and tremor ("kuru" means "shiver" in the Fore language). Overt dementia occurs late in the disease.

On occasion, sporadic CJD will present with atypical clinical features, such as cases that clinically and biochemically are indistinguishable from fatal familial insomnia, without any mutation in *PRNP*. Another such example is "variable protease encephalopathy," which presents similarly to a frontal lobe dementia. At least some of these clinical variations in sporadic prion disease are caused by the propagation of prion strains that are different than the strain usually associated with sporadic CJD.

DIAGNOSIS

The diagnosis of prion disease should be considered for any patient with rapidly worsening cognitive impairment, but it is important to know that certain treatable structural, inflammatory, metabolic, endocrine, and nutritional disorders can mimic prion disease (Table 387-1). In particular, any signs of inflammation in the cerebrospinal fluid (CSF) should prompt consideration of a diagnosis other than prion disease. The clinician may also need to consider special tests to search for some rare but treatable conditions (Table 387-2).

Methods for amplifying prions in vitro, such as RT-QuIC, now have specificities that approach 99%,[7] thereby greatly diminishing the chances of a

TABLE 387-1	DIFFERENTIAL DIAGNOSIS OF RAPIDLY PROGRESSIVE DEMENTIA
Neurodegenerative diseases that may mimic CJD	Alzheimer disease (Chapter 374), diffuse Lewy body disease (Chapter 374), frontotemporal dementia (Chapter 374), corticobasal ganglion degeneration (Chapter 374), progressive supranuclear palsy (Chapter 381)
Treatable diseases that mimic CJD	**Autoimmune:** CNS vasculitis (Chapter 254), limbic encephalitis (Chapter 386), Hashimoto encephalopathy (Chapter 386), anti–voltage-gated potassium channel encephalopathy, sarcoidosis (Chapter 89), steroid-responsive autoimmune encephalopathy (Chapter 386) **Infections:** viral encephalitis (Chapter 386), chronic meningitis (Chapter 384), Whipple disease (Chapter 259) **Neoplasms:** primary CNS lymphoma (Chapter 176), intravascular lymphoma (Chapter 176) **Vascular:** dural arteriovenous fistula **Nutritional:** Wernicke encephalopathy (Chapter 388) **Toxicities:** lithium, bismuth, methotrexate

CJD = Creutzfeldt-Jakob disease; CNS = central nervous system.

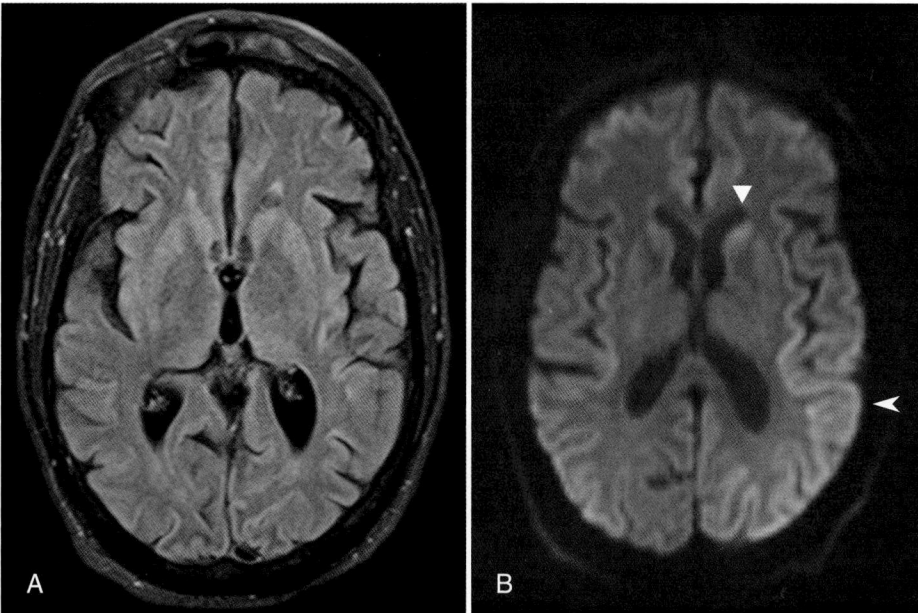

FIGURE 387-1. MRI appearance of sporadic Creutzfeldt-Jakob disease. The figure depicts FLAIR (A) and diffusion-weighted images (B) of the brain of a patient with sporadic Creutzfeldt-Jakob disease. An excess of brightness is barely detectable in the FLAIR image but is readily apparent in the diffusion-weighted image in several regions of cortical gray matter, particularly in the left parietal region (*notched arrowhead*). Also, the left caudate (*triangular arrowhead*) is abnormally bright.

TABLE 387-2	EVALUATION OF RAPIDLY PROGRESSIVE DEMENTIA
Initial screening	**History:** review for exposure to tricyclic antidepressants, lithium, bismuth, methotrexate, etc.; consider blood levels if toxicity suspected **Blood tests:** levels of glucose, sodium, calcium, blood urea nitrogen, creatinine, hepatic aminotransferases, albumin, vitamin B$_{12}$, thyroid stimulation hormone; international normalized ratio, antinuclear antigen, HIV testing, and syphilis serology **Imaging:** brain MRI, including DWI sequences **CSF:** glucose, protein, cell counts, VDRL
Further tests to consider	**Serum:** antibodies against thyroglobulin, thyroid peroxidase, voltage-gated potassium channel, Hu (ANNA-1) **CSF:** cytology, flow cytometry **EEG** **Brain biopsy**
Test findings supporting a diagnosis of prion disease	**CSF:** prion amplification assay (e.g. RT-QuIC)* Levels of 14-3-3 and tau proteins* **MRI:** T2 hyperintensity in the basal ganglia, sometimes in the cortex **EEG:** periodic sharp wave complexes

CJD = Creutzfeldt-Jakob disease; CSF = cerebrospinal fluid; DWI = diffusion-weighted imaging; EEG = electroencephalography; HIV = human immunodeficiency virus; MRI = magnetic resonance imaging; TSH = thyroid-stimulating hormone; VDRL = Venereal Disease Research Laboratory test.
*In the United States, available through National Prion Disorders Pathology Service Center.

false-positive diagnosis. In the United States, testing of CSF using one such method is available through the National Prion Disorders Pathology Service Center (available at http://www.cjdsurveillance.com).

The diagnosis of prion disease also can be suggested by certain tests. An unusual hyperintensity of the basal ganglia and thalamus and sometimes the cortical gray matter on certain magnetic resonance imaging (MRI) sequences (T2-weighted, fluid-attenuated inversion recovery, and diffusion-weighted weighting) occurs in about two thirds of CJD cases (Fig. 387-1). The electroencephalogram (EEG) in patients with CJD may show a pattern of periodic large-amplitude triphasic complexes. The specificity of these tests is about 80%, and these same abnormalities sometimes occur in treatable conditions that mimic prion disease. Elevated CSF levels of the neuronal proteins 14-3-3 and

tau can complement the amplification assays, but, like MRI and EEG, must be interpreted with careful consideration of alternative diagnoses.

The definite diagnosis of prion disease can be made by biochemical and histologic examination of brain tissue, obtained by biopsy or at autopsy. National or regional specialized prion disease centers, such as the National Prion Disorders Pathology Service Center in the United States, can assist pathologists in tissue analysis. In patients with a family history of neurodegenerative disease consistent with prion disease, determining the sequence of the protein-coding region of the prion protein gene can be diagnostic if a mutation is found.

TREATMENT AND PROGNOSIS   Rx

Prion diseases are incurable, and no treatment significantly improves the course of disease. Most patients with sporadic CJD die within a year of the onset of symptoms after progressing to a state of akinetic mutism. Patients with Gerstmann-Sträussler-Scheinker syndrome and certain other genetic or variant forms of prion disease may live longer. Excellent animal models of prion disease exist, and a number of novel therapeutic approaches are under active investigation. It is worthwhile to consider enrolling patients in experimental clinical trials if they are available (http://clinicaltrials.gov).

PREVENTION

Most cases of prion disease occur sporadically and cannot be prevented. Genetic cases can potentially be prevented through genetic counseling and prenatal testing, although whether such measures are warranted to prevent a disease that may not manifest until midlife or later is an ethically complex question. Infectiously transmitted cases are currently amenable to preventive measures, including avoidance of surgical transmission as a result of contaminated instruments or tissue grafts and protection of the human food supply from meat products contaminated with bovine spongiform encephalopathy or other ruminant prions. Chronic wasting disease is epidemic among deer and elk in certain regions of the United States, and scrapie, which affects sheep and goats, is endemic at low levels in the United States and many other countries. Neither of these prion diseases has been convincingly linked to human illness, but prudence dictates that humans should avoid eating any prion-infected animal.

GENERAL REFERENCES

For the General References and other additional features, please visit Expert Consult at https://expertconsult.inkling.com.

388

NUTRITIONAL AND ALCOHOL-RELATED NEUROLOGIC DISORDERS

BARBARA S. KOPPEL

Vitamins and minerals, which are essential elements to cellular function, must be obtained from the environment because the body cannot produce them. They are necessary for embryonic and early development as well as the subsequent maintenance of metabolic function of both the central and peripheral nervous systems. Deficiencies can cause a variety of neurologic syndromes (Table 388-1), each with a well-described constellation of symptoms that are dependent on the location(s) of the resulting pathology, the duration of the deficiency, and the potential presence of multiple deficiencies.

Acquired vitamin deficiency (Chapter 205) can be caused by either malnutrition (Chapter 203) or malabsorption (Chapter 131). Functional deficiency can result from increased demand owing to sepsis (Chapter 100), chronic inflammatory conditions, renal dialysis (Chapter 121), or other stress onset.

Inherited (genetic) conditions present early in life, even infancy, owing to the failure to absorb vitamins from the intestine or to bind and transport them to their site of action, such as mitochondria, neurons, and glia. Exposure to alcohol, chemotherapy, cassava, or other neurotoxins in the setting of certain vitamin deficiencies (usually B$_1$) synergistically contributes to neuropathology.[1] Genetic predisposition also may explain why not all patients who consume the same food or ingest the same amount of alcohol develop deficiencies.

Malnutrition is the most common cause of vitamin deficiency in economically disadvantaged geographic locations, especially in seasons of drought. Overreliance on a single food source, particularly one that has lost its nutritional value—such as polished rice, untreated corn, or spoiled grain—can precipitate disease. In contrast, attempts to deal with obesity,[2] such as following a fad diet or undergoing restrictive bariatric surgery without supplemental vitamins, can cause disease. Even when adequate food supplies are readily available, malnutrition may be caused by inadequate consumption owing to mechanical obstruction from cancer of the mouth or gastrointestinal tract, unbalanced diets, fasting, anorexia, chronic nausea, or recurrent or persistent vomiting.

Iatrogenic causes include failure to feed patients who are comatose, are not self-sufficient (from dementia [Chapter 374], brain injury [Chapter 371], psychiatric illness [Chapter 369]), or have dysphagia, as can occur following a stroke or spinal cord injury. Vitamin deficiency can also result from failure to include adequate amounts of vitamin and mineral supplements in parenteral or liquid enteral diets.

Malabsorption (Chapter 131) over long periods can cause deficiency of fat-soluble vitamins such as vitamin E and even substances with higher body stores, such as vitamin B$_{12}$ and copper.[3] As bariatric surgery becomes more common in the treatment of morbid obesity (Chapter 207), patients who do not maintain their vitamin supplementation after bypass-type procedures, or those who extremely limit intake after undergoing restrictive procedures ("lap band," sleeve gastrectomy), are at high risk of vitamin deficiency syndromes, primarily acute thiamine deficiency but also delayed cases of copper and B$_{12}$ deficiency.

DEFICIENCY OF WATER-SOLUBLE VITAMINS
Thiamine (Vitamin B$_1$) Deficiency

Thiamine is converted to thiamine pyrophosphate, which is a coenzyme required in glucose and lipid metabolism for energy production and in the synthesis of neurotransmitters from branched-chain amino acids (Chapter 205). Storage is exhausted after 2 to 3 weeks, and even sooner in conditions of high demand, such as pregnancy, lactation, or infection. Daily requirements of about 1 mg (0.33 mg per 1000 calories) can be obtained from food sources such as whole grains, legumes, meat, and fortified bread or cereals.

BERI-BERI

In developing countries, the most common manifestation of thiamine deficiency is beri-beri, which is characterized by a peripheral sensorimotor axonal neuropathy with numbness, paresthesias, or burning pain, occasionally accompanied by peripheral edema from heart failure ("wet beri-beri").[4] Other causes

of thiamine deficiency include reliance on foods in which the vitamin has been inactivated by processing (e.g., polished rice), overcooking, or eating foods that contain thiaminase-producing bacteria (e.g., raw fish). Deficiency also contributes to the neuropathy of chemotherapy.[5] Thiamine deficiency has been reported to cause the postural orthostatic tachycardia syndrome.

WERNICKE ENCEPHALOPATHY

Even short-term thiamine deficiency can result in Wernicke encephalopathy, a syndrome characterized by the insidious development and progression (over days to weeks) of confusion or delirium, abnormal eye movements, and ataxia as early as 2 weeks after thiamine stores have been depleted, especially in seriously ill patients. Wernicke encephalopathy occurs most often in the setting of poor nutrition and prolonged vomiting in patients with chronic alcohol abuse. Based on pathologic changes discovered at autopsy, only about 25% of cases are detected before death. Other at-risk patients include those with excessive vomiting from any cause, including bariatric surgery[6]; AIDS or cancer patients with cachexia and poor nutrition; or people who are chronically malnourished.[7] The symptoms and signs of Wernicke encephalopathy reflect the preferential dysfunction of brain regions that have a high demand for thiamine, a cofactor in energy-producing cycles, including the blood-brain barrier, anterior and centromedian thalamus, mammillary bodies, periaqueductal gray matter, superior and inferior colliculi, and floor of the fourth ventricle. The most common pathologic changes in these regions include neuronal swelling and microscopic hemorrhages, followed by gliosis. Rarely, the cerebral cortex and hypothalamus may be involved as well. Deficiency of α-ketoglutamate dehydrogenase activity in astrocytes leads to microglial activation and glutamatergic toxicity.

CLINICAL MANIFESTATIONS AND DIAGNOSIS

The full triad of mental status change, abnormal eye movements, and ataxia occurs in only about one third of cases. Acute symptoms may be provoked if intravenous (IV) glucose or food is given before thiamine has been replaced. Because a medical history may be unobtainable until the patient's confusion clears, physical signs of chronic alcoholism (e.g., gynecomastia, skin angiomata, pulmonary erythema, ascites, jaundice) (Chapters 137 and 143) must be sought.

Mental status changes range from mild memory impairment or inattention to delirium, often with apathy or abulia. Eye movement abnormalities include nystagmus, dysconjugate gaze, and gaze palsies (Video 388-1). Especially in alcoholic patients, ataxia can affect the limbs (legs more than arms), trunk, and gait. Nonalcoholic patients are more likely to have ocular dysfunction (Video 388-2).[8] Patients with Wernicke encephalopathy can also have autonomic and hypothalamic dysfunction, with bradycardia and hypothermia, as well as papilledema, optic neuropathy, seizures, and myoclonus.

In symptomatic patients, T2-weighted magnetic resonance imaging (MRI) can be normal but often demonstrates symmetrical increased signal due to edema or hemorrhage in affected areas, most often periventricular thalamus, periaqueductal regions in the floor of the fourth ventricle or cerebellum, and in the mammillary bodies.[9] If a patient is too sick to undergo MRI, computed tomography (CT) is a less sensitive alternative (Fig. 388-1). Low thiamine levels (<50 mg/mL) are common, although levels may be normal in about 10% of cases. Because thiamine deficiency disrupts carbohydrate metabolism, serum levels of lactate and pyruvate can be elevated.

KORSAKOFF SYNDROME

Korsakoff syndrome becomes apparent in up to 80% of patients who survive Wernicke encephalopathy. It is more likely to follow in the setting of alcoholism than in pure nutritional deficiency, thereby implying a synergistic mechanism that may be due to repeated episodes of alcohol withdrawal with associated glutamate neurotoxicity, compounded by lack of thiamine. The primary pathologic findings occur in the limbic system, especially the mamillary bodies, amygdala, and dorsomedial and anterior thalamus. Cortical involvement may be related to alcohol neurotoxicity rather than thiamine deficiency.

As confusion and delirium of Wernicke syndrome improve, an amnestic state in which patients are often unaware of their memory impairment becomes apparent. Korsakoff syndrome can be reliably identified only when patients can cooperate with neuropsychologic testing following resolution of acute delirium and global confusional states. It is characterized by disproportionate retrograde and anterograde episodic amnesia, transient confabulation, and hallucinations. Occasionally, Korsakoff psychosis is present clinically or pathologically without documented episodes of Wernicke encephalopathy, perhaps because Wernicke encephalopathy was subclinical or went unrecognized.

TABLE 388-1 SUMMARY OF VITAMIN AND MINERAL DEFICIENCIES

VITAMIN AND MINERAL DEFICIENCIES	NEUROLOGIC SYNDROME(S)	SUPPORTING TESTS	TREATMENT	CAUSES (OTHER THAN MALNUTRITION)
A (retinol)	Blindness from retinal or corneal damage	Visual fields, visual acuity Serum level <30-65 µg/dL	30,000 IU vitamin A daily × 1 wk or 60,000 µg × 2 days, repeated in 2 weeks	Hypothyroidism, diabetes, renal or liver failure
B₁ (thiamine)	Wernicke encephalopathy: ataxia, nystagmus, ophthalmoparesis, confusion, delirium Korsakoff syndrome: amnesia, confabulation Beri-beri: axonal neuropathy	MRI: symmetrical lesions of midbrain (periaqueductal area), pons, hypothalamus, thalamus, cerebellum MRI: necrosis of mamillary bodies, dorsomedial and anterior thalamus Nerve conduction tests: decreased amplitude Serum thiamine level <20 ng/dL Decreased erythrocyte transketolase	Prevent by 100 mg PO daily before and 1 year after bariatric surgery, 100 mg IV before glucose administration or refeeding after starvation Treat Wernicke encephalopathy with 5 days of thiamine, 100-500 mg IV or IM daily, until improvement stabilizes, then PO 100 mg daily Antioxidants (N-acetylcysteine)	Alcoholism, bariatric or other major GI surgery, prolonged vomiting, hemodialysis, diuretic treatment of heart failure, cachexia, 5-fluorouracil, other blockers of thiamine phosphate production
B₃ (niacin)	Pellagra: confusion, dementia, weakness, ataxia, spasticity, myoclonus, glossitis, dermatitis, photosensitivity	Erythrocyte NAD, plasma niacin, urinary N1-methylnicotinamide	Nicotinic acid, 50 mg PO tid or 25 mg IV tid; nicotinamide, 50-100 mg IM or PO tid	Alcoholism, corn- or cereal-based diet, Hartnup syndrome, carcinoid syndrome
B₅ (pantothenic acid)	Dysesthesias, foot paresthesias	Deficient coenzyme A	5 mg PO daily	Severe malnutrition
B₆ (pyridoxine)	Neuropathy, sensory ataxia, depression Infantile and adult pyridoxine-deficient epilepsy	Plasma PLP <27 nmol/L; urinary 4-pyridoxic acid, <3 nmol ↑ Homocysteine after methionine loading challenge ↑ α-AASA in urine, plasma, CSF	50-100 mg PO daily for neuropathy (preventive use if taking B₆ antagonist) 100-200 mg daily for adult epilepsy	Diverticulosis, isoniazid, cycloserine, other antagonists Genetic defects in antiquitin (aldehyde dehydrogenase), pyridoxal synthesis
B₁₂ (cobalamin)	Myelopathy with spastic paraparesis and sensory ataxia, peripheral neuropathy, optic neuropathy, memory loss, dementia; indirect contributor to stroke	Blood level <200 pg/mL ↑ Methylmalonic acid >145 nmol/L Intrinsic factor antibodies Megaloblastic anemia (bone marrow) Delayed somatosensory evoked potentials ↑ Homocysteine, total >12.5 µmol/L	IM B₁₂, 1000 µg daily for 1 week, then weekly for 1 month, then monthly; or oral B₁₂, 1000 µg daily; or nasal B₁₂, 500 µg weekly for lifetime if abnormal absorption, 50-100 µg daily if normal absorption	Achlorhydria, pernicious anemia, gastric or ileal resection, blind loop syndrome, sprue, HIV infection, nitrous oxide anesthesia (especially abuse), fish tapeworm, vegan diet
D (calciferol)	Proximal myopathy, often painful; cognitive impairment Secondary compression of spinal cord, plexus, or peripheral nerves from rickets or osteomalacia	25-(OH) vitamin D₃ level <10 ng/ mL in urine Serum calcium ↑ PTH >54 pg/mL Osteopenia/osteoporosis on bone densitometry	Daily supplementation with 400 IU cholecalciferol (D₃) or 50,000 IU ergocalciferol (D₂) 3 times per wk if malabsorption; use blood level or urine calcium excretion to guide (should be >100 mg/day)	Lack of exposure to sunlight, including sunblock protection; chronic antiepileptic drug use
E (tocopherol)	Spinal and cerebellar ataxia, Babinski sign, ophthalmoplegia, peripheral neuropathy, retinitis pigmentosa	Vitamin E level <2.5 mg/L (normal, 6-15 with normal lipid level) ↑ A-β-lipoprotein levels, antigliadin antibodies Genetic analysis to rule out other spinocerebellar ataxias such as Friedreich ataxia	Supplement with 6-800 IU or 5-10 mg/kg twice daily, for ataxia of genetic causes, water-soluble 200 mg/kg/day or IM α-tocopherol for malabsorption to normal serum level	Biliary atresia, celiac sprue, Genetic: ↓ α-tocopherol transport protein (8q13), microsomal triglyceride transfer protein
Folate	Dementia, B₁₂ deficiency, stroke	↑ Homocysteine, plasma level <2.5 µg/L	1 mg 3 times daily until normal level, then maintenance of 1 mg/day Pregnancy: 1-4 mg/day during first trimester if taking a folate antagonist or at risk of neural tube defects	Malabsorption or use of antagonist (methotrexate) or antiepileptic medication
K (phytonadione)	Intracranial hemorrhage	INR or PT elevation	IM phytonadione at birth, maternal vitamin K for last month of pregnancy	Medication use that increases metabolism (e.g., phenytoin)
Copper	Myelopathy, neuropathy	Serum Cu <75 µg/dL, ↓ urinary Cu, ceruloplasmin <23 mg/dL MRI: ↑ T2 signal in cervical cord, dorsal column Mutation in ATP7A gene (Menkes disease)	Elemental Cu, 8 mg/day PO or 2 mg/day IV week 1, 6 mg/day week 2, 4 mg/day week 3, 2 mg/ day ongoing malabsorption Menkes disease: 250 mg copper histidine SC bid, 1-2 mg in a multivitamin postbariatric surgery	Wilson disease, Menkes disease, alcoholism, malabsorption, gastric bypass, zinc toxicity
Magnesium	Seizures, encephalopathy	Serum magnesium <1.5 mg/dL, correct for low albumin	Magnesium sulfate IV or PO to normal level Avoid magnesium-wasting drugs	Alcoholism, especially beer
Potassium	Muscle weakness, chronic, acute	Serum potassium <3.5 mEq/L, ECG	IV or PO KCl until normalized	Diuretic use, bulimia

AASA = aminoadipic semialdehyde; CSF = cerebrospinal fluid; ECG = electrocardiography; GI = gastrointestinal; IM = intramuscular; INR = international normalized ratio; IV = intravenous; MRI = magnetic resonance imaging; NAD = nicotinamide adenine dinucleotide; PLP = pyridoxal-5-phosphate (active coenzyme of pyridoxine); PO = by mouth; PT = prothrombin time; PTH = parathyroid hormone; SC = subcutaneous.

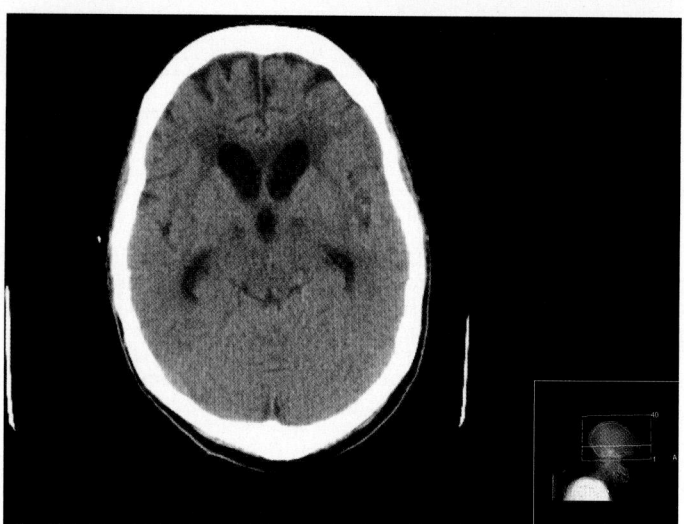

FIGURE 388-1. Computed tomography scan of the brain showing bilateral thalamic hypodensities, which are typical of Wernicke encephalopathy.

The memory deficit, which precludes learning new information or acquisition of new memories, is disproportionately severe in relation to other aspects of cognitive function. For example, alertness, attention, social interactions, and motor learning (procedural memory) are generally well preserved. There may be mild disorientation with respect to time and place, and sometimes apathy and other emotional changes are present. Confabulation, in which the intrusion of errors in response to questions leads to fabrication of answers without the intention to deceive, is sometimes present spontaneously in the first weeks after Wernicke encephalopathy. Since it is most likely a compensatory mechanism, it usually lessens over time. Neuropsychological testing frequently demonstrates emotional changes and mild problems in executive function, which are indicative of frontal lobe involvement.

TREATMENT AND PROGNOSIS Rx

Prophylactic treatment (i.e., more than 100 mg daily) of anyone at risk and timely thiamine replacement (see Table 388-1) can prevent or treat Wernicke encephalopathy as well as beri-beri.[10] In the acute setting, high-dose IV or intramuscular (IM) thiamine, which is recommended to circumvent any problems with swallowing or absorption, will lead rapidly—often within hours—to complete resolution of nystagmus and oculomotor paresis, followed by resolution of the ataxia and eventually of the mental status changes attributable to thiamine deficiency. Magnesium (Chapter 111) and sodium must also be replaced if deficient.

However, many alcoholic patients may have residual ataxia and cognitive impairment, including memory dysfunction, owing to the toxic effects of alcohol itself. As a result, about 50% of treated patients die within 8 years.[11] Because Korsakoff syndrome does not respond to thiamine replacement, prevention by timely recognition of Wernicke encephalopathy is essential. Untreated, Wernicke encephalopathy is fatal in 90% of cases, and the mortality rate is 25% among known cases.

Cobalamin (Vitamin B₁₂) Deficiency

Cobalamin is involved in methionine pathways that regulate myelination during development and maintain myelin throughout life (Chapter 205). Deficiency results in combined system disease (peripheral neuropathy and spinal cord degeneration) or subacute combined degeneration of the dorsal (sensory) and lateral (motor) tracts (i.e., myelopathy). The spinal cord tracts that are dysfunctional result in impaired position and vibratory sensation and spastic paraparesis.

Cobalamin deficiency is rarely due to inadequate dietary intake (e.g., a vegan diet for several years), because it is stored in fat and found in many foods, especially animal protein. Cobalamin deficiency (Chapter 155) is most common in individuals over age 60 years because the prevalence of atrophic gastritis (Chapter 130) and achlorhydria rises in older individuals.[12] Long-term use of proton pump inhibitors can also cause the same lack of gastric acid and the need for B₁₂ supplementation. A more common cause in recent years is bypass (Roux-en-Y, not restrictive) surgery for weight loss. Nitrous oxide ("laughing gas") toxicity, usually from illicit use rather than administration as

an anesthetic, can cause cobalamin deficiency by inactivating the cobalamin-dependent enzyme methionine synthase. Long-term treatment of diabetes with metformin also can lower B₁₂ levels. Low vitamin B₁₂ levels have been associated with increased homocysteine levels, but a relationship to vascular disease or vascular dementia has not been established.

CLINICAL MANIFESTATIONS

Demyelination of the dorsal columns causes proprioceptive loss that can result in sensory ataxia owing to loss of position sense in the feet. Romberg sign (failure to maintain balance with the eyes closed) distinguishes sensory from cerebellar ataxia. An axonal peripheral neuropathy causing numbness and tingling in the hands and feet is almost always present. Motor nerve function eventually becomes impaired as well. The optic nerve is the most commonly involved cranial nerve, but vagal neuropathy has also been reported. Signs of cerebral involvement include memory loss, personality changes, and occasionally hallucinations and psychosis. Encephalopathy and dementia may be present, but B₁₂ deficiency may be a secondary phenomenon in a patient with another cause of memory impairment, or both conditions may coexist without a causative relationship. Neurologic abnormalities may be present without anemia, although the anemia is severe in 20% of patients with vitamin B₁₂ deficiency. Symptoms generally progress slowly, but they can appear rapidly after exposure to nitrous oxide anesthesia in individuals with preexisting subclinical cobalamin deficiency.

DIAGNOSIS

Serum vitamin B₁₂ levels are usually low (<300 pg/mL) but can rarely be normal in symptomatic patients. In such cases, serum levels of methylmalonic acid and homocysteine are useful ancillary tests because these levels are increased as a result of impaired cobalamin-dependent reactions. Pernicious anemia (Chapter 155) is severe in about 20% of patients. However, both the hematocrit and mean corpuscular volume are sometimes normal because the hematologic effects of cobalamin deficiency can be partially masked by folate supplementation.

Low levels of cobalamin are sometimes present in normal people, especially the elderly, in which dementia, peripheral polyneuropathy, and myelopathy may be due to a myriad of causes. Therefore a low cobalamin level may reflect poor nutrition or absorption rather than being the cause of these conditions. Causality is definitively confirmed by clinical improvement after cobalamin replacement, which usually begins after several weeks and may continue for up to a year.

TREATMENT Rx

Treatment usually begins with subcutaneous or IM injections of 500 to 1000 µg of cobalamin daily for 1 week and then weekly for 1 month. After that time, oral supplementation with 50 to 100 µg daily of cyanocobalamin usually suffices in patients with achlorhydria or other causes of malabsorption; 1000 µg daily should be used in patients with intrinsic factor antibodies. Sublingual, transdermal patch, and nasal gel forms (500 µg weekly) have not been adequately studied. The anemia can be corrected by high-dose folate replacement, but the neurologic damage will progress unless vitamin B₁₂ is administered.

PROGNOSIS

Neurologic symptoms, especially paresthesias, typically improve to some extent within 3 months of achieving adequate B₁₂ serum levels. Numbness and areflexia often persist, especially if treatment was delayed. If there is no improvement whatsoever, causes other than vitamin B₁₂ deficiency are likely, such as copper deficiency or human immunodeficiency virus (HIV)–associated myelopathy. Similarly, vitamin B₁₂ supplementation does not affect cognitive performance in hyperhomocysteinemic elderly people without evidence of B₁₂ deficiency.[13]

Folate Deficiency

Folate is an important coenzyme in the metabolism of nucleic and amino acids (Chapter 205). Maternal deficiency accounts for 50% of babies born with neural tube defects and may cause more subtle neurologic problems. Inborn errors of folate metabolism cause seizures and intellectual disability, especially when there has been no history of birth injury. Other signs include psychomotor retardation, autism, dyskinesias, and irritability. In adults, folate deficiency can cause retrobulbar optic neuropathy in conjunction with other B vitamin deficiencies. Folate deficiency also results in elevated levels of homocysteine, which is associated with an increased risk for ischemic heart disease and stroke. Patients with genetic folate deficiency due to lack of methylenetetrahydrofolate reductase, which converts ingested folate to the active metabolic cofactor, have an increased risk of intracerebral hemorrhage.

The supplementation of flour with folate has greatly reduced the risk of folate deficiency, and all pregnant women are now prescribed supplemental folate. Women of childbearing age should be treated even before pregnancy if they have any conditions that predispose to folate deficiency, such as the use of antiepileptic medication.

Folate deficiency also leads to megaloblastic anemia (Chapter 155). Before correction of megaloblastic anemia with folate alone, vitamin B_{12} levels should be checked to avoid ongoing neurologic injury resulting from unrecognized cobalamin deficiency. Folate deficiency is treated with 1 mg three times daily for 1 month, followed by 1 mg daily. However, return of folate and homocysteine serum levels to normal has not shown benefit for preventing progressive cognitive impairment, for preventing stroke, or for reducing adverse vascular events except in patients with classic homocysteinemia (Chapter 198).

Pyridoxine (Vitamin B_6) Deficiency

Pyridoxine is a coenzyme in multiple reactions that involve gluconeogenesis, biosynthesis of neurotransmitters, and the metabolism of amino acids, nucleic acids, and lipids. Pyridoxine deficiency can be caused by genetic defects, such as defective antiquitin, that lead to increased utilization of pyridoxine. In adults, low serum levels of pyridoxine are well tolerated, so symptomatic deficiency is rare. However, symptomatic deficiency can occur in the setting of renal failure (Chapter 121), dialysis (Chapter 122), or cirrhosis (Chapter 144), or with medications such as isoniazid for antitubercular therapy (Chapter 308) or hydralazine for heart failure (Chapter 53) if patients do not receive concurrent supplementation. Deficiency is also seen with extreme malnutrition, especially diets consisting predominantly of white rice.

CLINICAL MANIFESTATIONS AND DIAGNOSIS
Prolonged pyridoxine deficiency causes a painful peripheral axonal neuropathy that leads to weakness and sensory ataxia. Some patients have skin thickening, seborrheic dermatitis, or glossitis, which can resemble pellagra. Serum levels of the active form of pyridoxine, pyridoxal 5'-phosphate, and urine levels of the metabolite 4-pyridoxic acid are low. Ancillary tests include nerve conduction studies, which show significantly reduced amplitudes in sensory and motor action potentials with normal conduction velocity times, typical of an axonal neuropathy.

In epilepsy caused by pyridoxine deficiency, seizures begin in the neonatal period and may persist, along with intellectual disability. Electroencephalography shows a highly disorganized pattern with excessive slow frequency activity and abundant multifocal and generalized spikes, similar to hypsarrhythmia. Pyridoxine deficiency in pregnancy can be caused by hyperemesis gravidarum and may rarely produce neurologic disease in offspring, but routine supplementation is not recommended for all pregnancies.

Toxicity due to excess pyridoxine intake (>200 mg daily), which results from competition between the inactive pyridoxine form and the active form of pyridoxal-5'-phosphate, leads to a ganglioneuropathy manifested by pure sensory symptoms, including sensory loss, ataxia, areflexia, and the presence of a Romberg sign. However, this syndrome, which can result from an overdosing of vitamin supplements, is generally less common than deficiency-related neurologic disease.

TREATMENT [Rx]

Patients in whom symptoms of pyridoxine deficiency develop or who take pyridoxine antagonists should receive supplemental pyridoxine (50 to 100 mg daily). Children with pyridoxine-dependent epilepsy require immediate and lifelong supplementation with at least 100 mg of pyridoxine daily. Antisense therapy against the mutant gene is being tested.

For pyridoxine toxicity, simply stopping excess oral vitamin intake will eventually reverse the damage. The only exception is if a very large IV dose was administered, in which case neuropathy is not reversible.

Other B Vitamins
B_2 (Riboflavin)
Oxidation-reduction reactions require flavins, which are present in dairy products, meat, fish, vegetables, and fortified cereal and bread. Deficiencies are therefore rare, but some inherited mitochondrial myopathies respond to supplementation with this vitamin.

B_3 (Niacin)
Pellagra is a symptom complex of photosensitive dermatitis, delirium or dementia, neuropathy, and diarrhea. It occurs in patients with malabsorption or in patients undergoing dialysis. The syndrome can be confused with alcohol withdrawal (delirium tremens) or psychosis.[14] Pellagra is also seen in Hartnup syndrome, a recessively inherited failure to transport tryptophan, which is converted to niacin. In utero genetic deficiencies cause malformations of many organ systems,[15] but it is often difficult to isolate the effects of niacin from other B vitamins.

B_5 (Pantothenic Acid)
Deficiency of vitamin B_5 is rare and hard to prove, because this vitamin is found in many different foods and is produced by bacteria in the colon. The neurologic syndrome is a small-fiber neuropathy with dysesthesias and paresthesias that result in "burning feet."

DEFICIENCY OF FAT-SOLUBLE VITAMINS
Vitamin E (Tocopherol) Deficiency

Although vitamin E is composed of several tocopherols, it is the α form that is biologically active in humans and contained in most foods (vegetable oils, leafy vegetables). Because it is so widely available, deficiency is almost never due to inadequate dietary consumption (malnutrition). Rather, vitamin E deficiency is the result of prolonged malabsorption in the setting of biliary and pancreatic disease (Chapters 146 and 135), cystic fibrosis (Chapter 83), celiac disease (Chapter 131), Crohn disease (Chapter 132), extensive small bowel resection, and blind loop syndrome (Chapter 131). In inherited forms, vitamin E deficiency is associated with defects in the α-tocopherol transfer protein gene on chromosome 8q12.3 whose product binds the vitamin to protein, or of absorption of lipids (hypolipoproteinemia and abetalipoproteinemia).

CLINICAL MANIFESTATIONS AND DIAGNOSIS
Neurologic manifestations of vitamin E deficiency include a spinocerebellar syndrome with ataxia of gait or limbs (dysmetria); abnormal eye movements (nystagmus or dysconjugate gaze); loss of vibration and position senses (sensory ataxia or pseudoathetosis); distal sensory neuropathy with hyporeflexia; and, rarely, cognitive dysfunction, myopathy, or blindness owing to retinopathy.[16]

Serum levels of vitamin E can vary with the serum lipid levels. Especially in patients with extreme hyperlipidemia, such as cholestasis, the ratio of vitamin E to cholesterol will be more reliable than the absolute vitamin E level.

Although generally not toxic, excessive intake of vitamin E causes bleeding, including hemorrhagic infarcts, in adults, probably owing to its effects on platelet function. During pregnancy, high doses of vitamin E can interfere with oxidation in the fetus and cause growth retardation.

TREATMENT [Rx]

The amount of vitamin E replacement required depends on the cause of the deficiency. Malabsorption syndromes require 1000 to 2000 mg daily for infants and 100 mg/kg/day (10 to 20 g) for adults, with 300 mg daily considered adequate supplementation after bariatric surgery. Genetic causes can be treated with 5 to 10 g/day. For vitamin E, 1 mg is equivalent to 1.49 IU. Supplementation probably does not benefit neurodegenerative diseases, including Alzheimer disease.

Vitamin D (Calciferol) Deficiency

Vitamin D deficiency is being widely diagnosed because screening is encouraged in primary care settings (Chapter 205). It results from inadequate exposure to sunlight, dietary insufficiency, or malabsorption caused by celiac disease, inflammatory bowel disease, or extensive small bowel resection. The average multivitamin contains 400 IU of combined D_2 (ergocalciferol) and D_3 (cholecalciferol), whereas 20 minutes of full-body summer sun exposure provides 10,000 IU of D_3, the form used in the body. Vitamin D deficiency causes rickets in children and osteomalacia (Chapter 231) in adults. Bone remodeling may lead to compression of the spinal cord or roots (Chapter 372) owing to changes in vertebral bodies and foramina. Abrupt lack of vitamin D causes hypocalcemia with secondary hyperparathyroidism (Chapter 232). Hypocalcemia, in turn, can cause tetany, encephalopathy, and generalized seizures. Deficiency also causes a proximal myopathy (owing to impaired calcium influx or actin and troponin production), which is worse in the legs and pelvic girdle than the arms and which can lead to peculiar patterns of gait as a result of weakness and fear of falling. This myopathy is associated with sleep disorders and fibromyalgia without weakness. Vitamin D deficiency is also associated with an increased incidence of Alzheimer and all-cause dementia. Prenatal deficiency may be associated with autism and schizophrenia in children. Vitamin D receptors are found in the substantia nigra, and deficiency allows more rapid progression of Parkinson disease.

Vitamin D plays a role in immune modulation of regulatory T cells, which may explain the relationship of vitamin D deficiency to an earlier onset, higher prevalence, higher relapse rate, and more severe manifestations of multiple sclerosis (Chapter 383). Other autoimmune diseases, such as narcolepsy (Chapter 377), are more common in patients with low levels of vitamin D.

Individuals whose dietary absorption is normal require 400 to 600 IU (10 to 15 μg) of vitamin D_3 daily, but persons with malabsorption may need more than twice that amount. Reliance on sunlight is not recommended owing to risks of skin cancer (Chapter 193) as well as variability in personal environmental exposure. Supplementation doses depend on the degree of deficiency, with high doses (50,000 units, 1.25 mg) of ergocalciferol (D_2) given weekly to patients whose 25-OH-calciferol level is very low (<20 ng/mL) for 8 weeks, followed by daily 400 to 800 IU of cholecalciferol (D_3). In patients with malabsorption, 1000 IU should be given daily indefinitely. Serum levels should be monitored after reaching at least 20 ng/mL. Clinical trials are ongoing to determine whether vitamin D supplementation can protect patients who are receiving neurotoxic chemotherapy from developing neuropathy.

Toxicity from excess absorption of vitamin D, as is seen in sarcoidosis (Chapter 89) or other granulomatous conditions or from excessive intake, is rare. Like deficiency states, vitamin D toxicity causes muscle and bone pain (Chapter 232). Very high doses have been associated with an increased risk of falls.

Vitamin A Deficiency

Deficiency in vitamin A, which is required to bind opsin to produce the retinal transmitter rhodopsin, leads to abnormal fetal development. In adults, the absence of retinol or retinoids and carotenoids impairs vision in conditions of low light. In abetalipoproteinemia, in which vitamin E is also lacking, complete blindness may occur (Chapter 195). The ability to taste is also impaired, and skin and cornea damage can occur. Deficiency has occasionally been associated with raised intracranial pressure in children. Malabsorption must be very prolonged to produce vitamin A deficiency because this fat-soluble vitamin has large body stores.

Vitamin A toxicity is rare but can occur in patients who use isotretinoin for acne or have excessive dietary intake owing to the consumption of liver (especially from fish-eating mammals such as polar bear, seal, and walrus). Toxicity can cause idiopathic intracranial hypertension (Chapters 180 and 370) with headache and papilledema that leads to diminished vision or even blindness in severe cases.

Vitamin K Deficiency

Vitamin K deficiency, a rare consequence of malabsorption, is most often seen in patients who have compromised liver synthesis or who are taking the antagonist warfarin (Chapter 205). Vitamin K deficiency causes excessive bleeding and increases the risk of intracerebral hemorrhage. Hemorrhagic disease of the newborn is better prevented by routinely giving all newborns an injection of vitamin K rather than by maternal supplementation using 5 mg daily for the last month of pregnancy. Because vitamin K levels are difficult to obtain, functional testing of the international normalized ratio is typically used to guide dose adjustments.

⬤ DEFICIENCY OF MISCELLANEOUS ELEMENTS AND NUTRIENTS

Copper Deficiency

Acquired copper deficiency (Chapter 205) is rare and can be difficult to recognize. It occurs most often in premature or malnourished infants and in patients with very prolonged malabsorption owing to celiac disease, cystic fibrosis (Chapter 83), Crohn disease (Chapter 132), or intestinal blind loops after surgery (e.g., a Whipple procedure for pancreatic cancer or other malignancy, or bypass surgery for weight loss). It can also occur in patients with nephrotic syndrome (Chapter 113) and intestinal bacterial overgrowth (Chapter 131). Copper deficiency is also a well-recognized consequence of excessive intake of zinc (from denture paste, wound cream, or herbal therapy for colds) or as a consequence of parenteral overload during hemodialysis (Chapter 122), which competitively upregulates copper loss in the intestine.

The most common neurologic complication of copper deficiency is a myelopathy that is clinically very similar to that seen with cobalamin deficiency. The most prominent features are spastic paraparesis and sensory ataxia. An insidious peripheral polyneuropathy, initially sensory and eventually motor, of the axonal type is usually present as well. Optic neuropathy with hallucinations or visual loss, wrist drop, and foot drop have also been reported. Copper levels, including excreted urinary copper, should be measured in patients who have symptoms suspicious for vitamin B_{12} deficiency but have normal vitamin B_{12} levels or who fail to respond to cyanocobalamin replacement. Treatment consists of oral copper supplementation, 8 mg/day tapering by 2 mg weekly over 3 weeks, followed by maintenance of 2 mg/day for life. Zinc overexposure should be sought and stopped.

Menkes disease, an X-linked recessive copper deficiency caused by mutations in the *ATP7A* gene needed for absorption, is characterized by severe intellectual disability and kinky hair. The diagnosis is made by finding low serum copper levels or changes in the ratio of dopamine to norepinephrine. Large doses of copper histidine (250 mg twice daily until age 1, then daily until age 3) must be delivered subcutaneously, but improvement is variable. Patients survive to adulthood only if copper injections are begun in the neonatal period.

Toxicity from copper is indirectly caused by Wilson disease. Wilson disease is an autosomal recessive disorder caused by mutation in the *ATP7B* gene that encodes ceruloplasmin, a copper-transporting protein. Symptoms result from excessive copper accumulation, primarily in the liver and brain, as a result of failed transport and impaired copper excretion. Psychiatric features such as personality change, disinhibition, depression, and psychosis sometimes overshadow neurologic manifestations such as dementia, dysarthria, chorea, tremor, and dystonia. Deposition of copper in the eye's Descemet membrane causes the characteristic Kayser-Fleischer ring, which is seen in the iris in over 95% of patients (Chapter 200, Fig. 200-2). Serum ceruloplasmin levels are low. Accumulation of copper in the liver leads to chronic liver failure. Wilson disease is treated by copper chelation with penicillamine or zinc (Chapter 200) and by minimizing dietary intake.

Other Nutritional Disorders

Biotin deficiency is caused by lack of protein in the diet, accidentally failing to add it to total parenteral nutrition, and an autosomal recessive disorder affecting biotinidase, which prevents biotin from being accessible for use. Genetic causes result in developmental delay, seizures or myoclonus, ataxia, and deafness if supplementation is not begun in the newborn period. Dietary deficiencies lead to lethargy, myalgias, and paresthesias, along with rash.

Iodine deficiency leads to hypothyroidism (Chapter 213), which causes varying degrees of cretinism.

Overreliance on one hardy food source (grass peas, chick peas) may lead to spastic paraparesis from lathyrism owing to oxalyldiaminoproprionic acid, which is a neurotoxic glutamate agonist. In older Nigerian men, cassava tuberis (konzo), which can potentiate neurotoxicity from cyanate and glucoside (Chapter 102), causes sensory neuropathy, ataxia, optic atrophy, and sensorineural deafness. In contrast, women and children develop spasticity, presumably from the same toxin. Amyotrophic lateral sclerosis and Parkinson-dementia complex in Guam are probably caused by cycad toxins in flour. Occasional epidemics that combine toxins such as alcohol or smoking with malnutrition and then respond clinically to vitamin B supplementation are presumed to reflect deficiencies of various nutrients. Examples are Strachan Jamaican neuropathy and Cuban tobacco-alcohol amblyopia with optic neuropathy.

⬤ ALCOHOL-RELATED DISORDERS

Alcohol (Chapter 30) is responsible for a wide spectrum of neurologic disorders. At one extreme, it can cause irreversible dementia, cerebellar degeneration, optic neuropathy, and peripheral polyneuropathy. Syndromes are "dose dependent" in the sense that greater durations and amounts of alcohol use produce more serious complications.[17] Binge drinking, combined with B-vitamin deficiencies and electrolyte derangements, also contribute to neurologic disease. Intoxication and withdrawal states may obscure other serious conditions such as osmotic demyelination syndromes and Wernicke encephalopathy, thereby delaying treatment.

Acute intoxication can range from mild euphoria to vestibular and cerebellar dysfunction to coma and death. Intoxication may also affect judgment and coordination, thereby contributing to subsequent vehicular accidents, falls, traumatic brain injury, violence, and other unsafe behaviors. After chronic excessive alcohol intake, cessation or lowering of intake leads to withdrawal, which presents with overexcitation syndromes such as seizures, tremors, hallucinosis, and autonomic overload, and sometimes fatal delirium tremens.

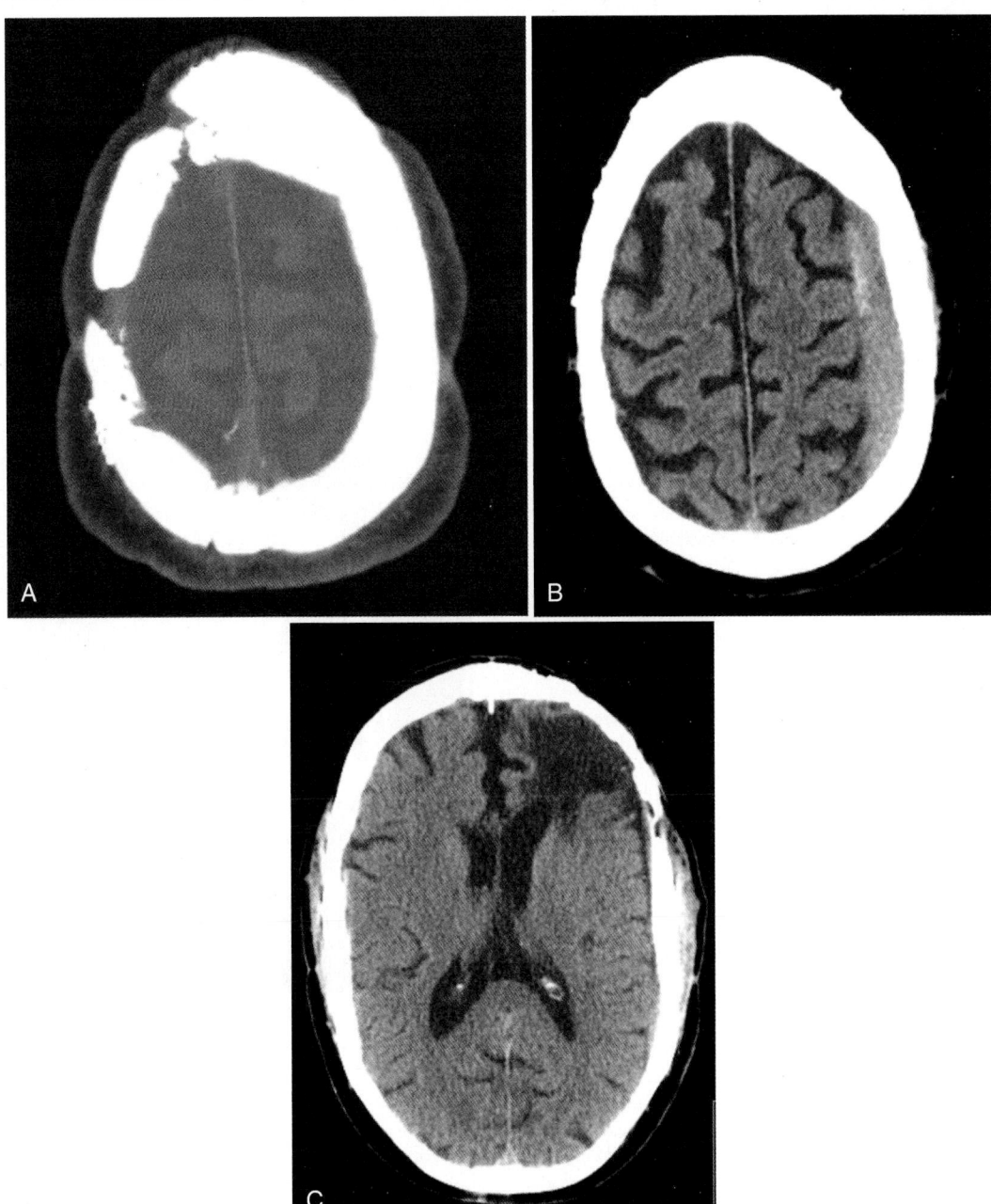

FIGURE 388-2. **Complications of remote and acute head trauma in an alcoholic patient.** Alcoholic man admitted after a seizure, with no clinical signs of head trauma, lateralized weakness, or aphasia, but drowsy several hours after receiving lorazepam 2 mg intravenously. Computed tomography axial brain scan shows (**A**) craniotomy defect on right, (**B**) mixed chronic and acute subdural hematoma on left, and (**C**) left frontal encephalomalacia from prior trauma.

Alcohol-induced liver toxicity results in hepatic encephalopathy and hepatolenticular degeneration. Coagulopathy caused by liver disease or suppressed platelet production raises the risk for subdural or intracranial hematoma (Fig. 388-2). Fetal alcohol syndrome reflects the vulnerability of the developing nervous system to the toxic effects of alcohol.

Signs of intoxication correlate with blood alcohol levels: 50 mg/dL for personality changes; 150 mg/dL for ataxia, vestibular dysfunction, and nystagmus; 300 mg/dL for stupor; 400 mg/dL for coma; and up to 500 mg/dL for respiratory depression or apnea. However, the effects vary greatly depending on the chronicity of intake and the rate at which high levels develop. Intoxication alone should never be assumed to be the sole cause of a depressed mental state, because alcoholics are at increased risk for other causes of coma such as intracranial hemorrhage (Fig. 388-2).

Specific Clinical Syndromes

Seizures and status epilepticus (Chapter 375) can be a direct consequence of intoxication, withdrawal, hyponatremia (Chapter 108), and hypomagnesemia (Chapter 111), or they can result from epileptogenic foci owing to previous head trauma (Fig. 388-2) (Chapter 371) or stroke (Chapter 379). Withdrawal seizures, which precede the autonomic excitation of delirium tremens by several hours, warrant observation and benzodiazepine therapy at the time of the seizure (e.g., lorazepam 2 mg intravenously) followed by a tapering dose to suppress withdrawal symptoms (e.g., oxazepam, usually starting at 30 mg every 4 hours and then reducing the dose as the patient's response dictates) for about 3 days. Even in patients with obvious withdrawal seizures, other causes of seizures should be investigated and treated appropriately with antiepileptic medications.

Hepatic encephalopathy is most often seen in patients with alcoholic cirrhosis (Chapter 144), especially patients who have bleeding esophageal varices. It is characterized by irritability alternating with depressed mental status, seizures, tremor, and asterixis. Encephalopathy can be iatrogenic in patients placed on detoxification protocols with standing doses of benzodiazepines instead of dosing in response to symptoms of withdrawal. Although temporary reversal of encephalopathy with flumazenil (2 mg IV) can confirm the diagnosis, treatment focuses on trying to reduce the serum ammonia level, usually with lactulose (15 to 30 mL orally twice daily) and nonabsorbable antibiotics such as rifaximin (550 mg twice daily), neomycin (500 mg to 1 g three times daily), or metronidazole (250 mg two to four times daily). Closure of spontaneous portosystemic shunts by embolization may be effective for reducing intractable encephalopathy in some patients.

Dementia, not the memory disorder of Korsakoff syndrome, develops even when nutrition is well maintained because of alcohol's direct and irreversible neurotoxic effects, although the absolute amounts of alcohol necessary to produce dementia are unclear. In younger patients with dementia, 10 to 25% of cases are attributed to alcohol. In the elderly, excessive alcohol consumption is associated with faster cognitive decline compared with light to moderate alcohol consumption. Frontal lobe dysfunction results in executive dysfunction (planning, abstract reasoning) rather than the amnesia that is prominent in Korsakoff syndrome. Additional damage from head injury, status epilepticus, and cerebrovascular disease contribute to cognitive dysfunction. The appearance of cerebral atrophy is further evidence of alcohol's deleterious effect on cortical and white matter fibers. Abstinence is advised to limit degeneration; standard dementia therapies such as memantine and acetylcholinesterase inhibitors are not very effective.

Marchiafava-Bignami syndrome, which was first described in postmortem studies of Italian chianti wine drinkers, can occur in persons who consume any type of alcohol. Acute signs include nonspecific encephalopathy or coma, abnormal gait, pyramidal signs (such as weakness and spasticity), and death. After recovery, neuropsychologic evaluation may detect hemispheric disconnection ("split brain") syndrome. The most severe pathology involves demyelination and necrosis of sections of the corpus callosum. Findings on MRI include increased T2- and diffusion-weighted signals in the corpus callosum, especially the splenium.

Wernicke encephalopathy and Korsakoff syndrome (see above) are seen in alcoholic patients, especially binge drinkers, owing to thiamine deficiency.

Osmotic demyelination syndromes (central and extrapontine myelinolysis) may also be related to thiamine deficiency, as well as to rapid correction of extreme hyponatremia (Chapter 108). Beer drinkers are at increased risk owing to their tendency to hyponatremia. If confusion and delirium persist despite treatment of alcohol withdrawal, or if ocular and cerebellar signs emerge after recovery from withdrawal, central pontine myelinolysis should be suspected. On CT scanning, the base of the pons is affected in a nonvascular pattern, but hypodensities can extend rostrally into the thalamus and midbrain or basal ganglia (Fig. 388-3 and Video 388-3).

Cerebellar degeneration and ataxia result from alcohol-induced loss of Purkinje cells, mainly in the anterior superior part of the cerebellar vermis; the cerebellar hemispheres are less affected. As a result, the clinical picture is one of mainly truncal and gait ataxia, with a wide-based unsteady gait and inability to walk tandem. The arms are usually spared, with no intention tremor; nystagmus and dysarthria are rare when the patient is not intoxicated. Findings are exacerbated by concurrent thiamine deficiency, potentially causing Wernicke encephalopathy. Alcohol may activate antibodies against Purkinje cells in individuals with gluten intolerance.

Optic neuropathy, which occurs with severe chronic alcohol abuse, is manifested as progressive painless visual loss and sometimes visual hallucinations as a result of damage to the optic nerve fibers. The macular region is most affected.

Peripheral neuropathy (Chapter 392) ("alcoholic neuropathy") is the most common neurologic complication of chronic alcoholism. It is an axonal sensorimotor neuropathy that causes dysfunction of small nerve fibers, thereby presenting with painful sensory symptoms such as burning and paresthesias of the soles of the feet. Numbness develops in a stocking-glove distribution, with loss of ankle reflexes. Mild distal weakness eventually occurs in some patients. Involvement of the autonomic nervous system frequently causes impotence as well as urinary or bowel complaints. Neurophysiologic testing reveals both axonal and demyelination patterns. Although supplements of thiamine and pyridoxine may lead to some improvement, especially in the painful paresthesias, complete resolution is rare. If abstinence from alcohol is not also achieved, the symptoms persist, thereby implying that a direct toxic effect of alcohol is likely.

Compressive neuropathies, especially of the radial nerve ("Saturday night palsy") or peroneal nerve, can result after prolonged pressure on a nerve while the patient is obtunded from heavy alcohol consumption. Recovery takes many weeks but is generally complete.

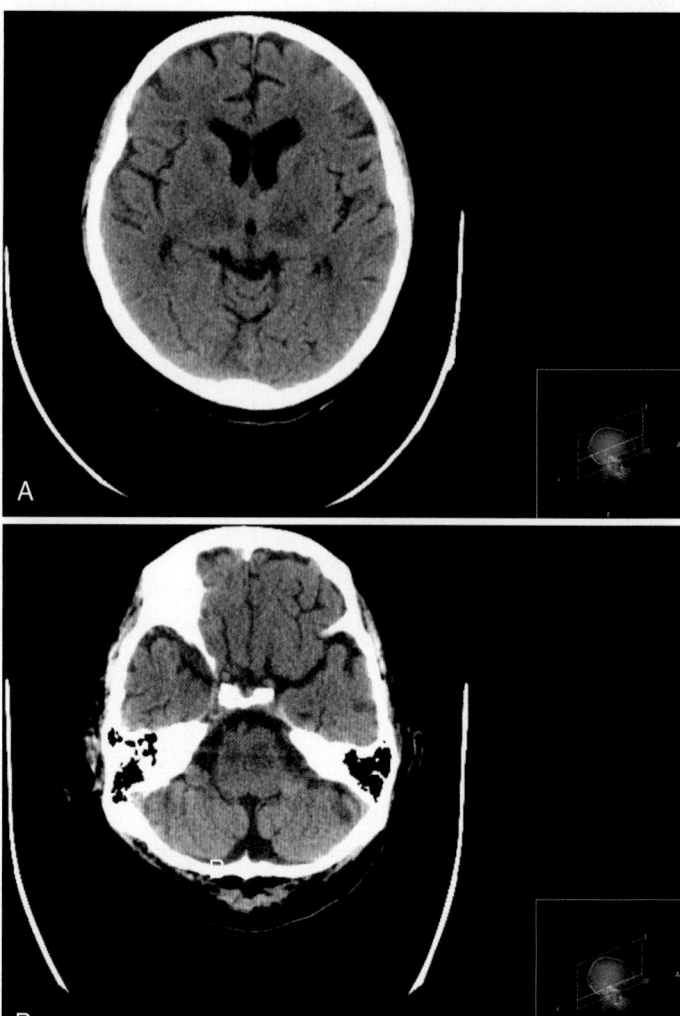

FIGURE 388-3. Osmotic demyelination syndrome. (A) Computed tomography shows scattered hypodensities in the basal ganglia and thalamus and temporal lobes. (B) Central pontine hypodensity.

Myopathy occurs in binge drinkers, in whom severe muscle injury with rhabdomyolysis (Chapter 105) can develop, especially in the setting of fasting and prolonged absence of movement. Myoglobinuria can result in kidney damage. Heavy alcohol consumption is also associated with cardiomyopathy (Chapter 54), which can lead to arrhythmias even in the absence of hypokalemia. Chronic steady (not binge) alcohol abuse causes a symmetrical proximal weakness (Chapter 393) that is not usually severe enough to prevent walking or standing. It can be detected in up to 50% of heavy users.

Fetal alcohol syndrome is recognized at birth in infants whose mothers consumed significant amounts of alcohol in the early stages of pregnancy, but the quantity required to place a fetus at risk has not been definitively determined.[18] Rates as high as 55 per 1000 births have been described. The characteristic findings are growth retardation, microcephaly, hypotonia, skeletal and cardiac anomalies, and characteristic facial features (micrognathia, small palpebral fissures). Exposure of the developing brain to alcohol can also lead to subtle or severe neurocognitive defects and attention-deficit disorder, which may not be detected until later in childhood. Although malnutrition and excess alcohol have synergistic deleterious effects, the teratogenic effects of alcohol are not prevented by adequate amounts of thiamine, folate, and other vitamins.

GENERAL REFERENCES

For the General References and other additional features, please visit Expert Consult at https://expertconsult.inkling.com.

389

CONGENITAL, DEVELOPMENTAL, AND NEUROCUTANEOUS DISORDERS

JONATHAN W. MINK

CONGENITAL DISORDERS

Malformations of Cerebral Cortex

Developmental malformations of the cerebral cortex arise from a wide variety of etiologies, including genetic mutations, intrauterine infections, intrauterine ischemia, toxic exposures, or their interactions.[1] These malformations are heterogeneous and can result from disrupted neuronal proliferation, migration, or cortical organization. In general, disorders that arise early in development are more severe than those that arise after the basic architecture of the brain has developed. When small areas of the brain are involved, the patient may have minor impairment of neurologic function. When larger areas of the brain are involved, patients often have cognitive deficits and more severe neurologic dysfunction. Epilepsy (Chapter 375), which is the most common manifestation of abnormal cortical development, may occur with or without other neurologic signs or symptoms.

Abnormal cortical development may also manifest as cerebral palsy. This nonprogressive abnormality of the developing brain causes permanent disorders of movement and posture. In most affected children, it follows easily diagnosed perinatal insults, including asphyxia, intrauterine infection, hemorrhage, prematurity, and brain infarction, or it is associated with obvious anatomic abnormalities in brain development, such as congenital absence of the corpus callosum. About 20% of cases, are idiopathic, and about one third of such cases have clinically significant, usually de novo, copy number variants.[2] Intrathecal baclofen, deep brain stimulation, and ventral and dorsal rhizotomy are potential therapies for managing hypertonia in cerebral palsy.[3]

Disorders of Neuronal Proliferation

Neuronal proliferation can be abnormally increased or decreased owing to a variety of mechanisms. These disorders can manifest with megalencephaly or microcephaly, or head size can be normal. Abnormal proliferation can involve specific cell types, thereby resulting in focal or multifocal areas of dysplasia or in the formation of hamartomas (see Tuberous Sclerosis, later).

FOCAL CORTICAL DYSPLASIA WITH BALLOON CELLS

Focal cortical dysplasia is caused by abnormal proliferation of both neurons and glia. Its neuropathology is characterized by the presence of giant dysmorphic neurons and "balloon cells" associated with altered cortical lamination, but some lesions have abnormal cortical layering with ectopic neurons in white matter. Affected patients typically present with partial seizures that may be intractable to medical therapy. These seizures can begin at any age but most commonly present during childhood or adolescence. The type of seizure depends on the anatomic location of the dysplasia. Other neurologic manifestations such as sensory, motor, or cognitive impairments depend on the extent of the dysplasia and whether multiple brain regions are affected. The diagnosis of focal cortical dysplasia is usually made with brain magnetic resonance imaging (MRI), which demonstrates focal thickening of a gyrus or alteration of the gray-white matter junction. Management includes medical treatment of seizures, but surgical resection of the epileptic focus may be required for complete remission (Chapter 375).

Disorders of Neuronal Migration

Disorders of neuronal migration typically result in disruption of the normal laminar organization of the cerebral cortex. Defects include impaired initiation of neuronal migration, impaired orderly migration, and impaired termination of migration. All result in abnormal cortical organization and function.

LISSENCEPHALY AND BAND HETEROTOPIA

The lissencephalies (smooth brain) are a group of disorders that are caused by arrested migration of neurons to the cerebral cortex. Lissencephaly, which is typically diagnosed in infancy or early childhood, is usually accompanied by microcephaly, severe global developmental delay, cerebral palsy, and intractable epilepsy. At least 19 lissencephaly genes have been identified, most of which are involved in the regulation of microtubule organization and function. The most important of these are *PAFAH1B1* (also known as *LIS1*), *DCX*, and *TUBA1A*.[4] Individuals with mutations of *LIS1* typically have severe malformations that are most prominent in the posterior cerebrum. More extensive mutations in the region of *LIS1* result in Miller-Dieker syndrome, a condition characterized by lissencephaly and distinctive facial features that include a prominent forehead, midface hypoplasia, low-set and abnormally shaped ears, and a small jaw. Males with *DCX* mutations typically have a severe lissencephaly that is most prominent in the anterior cerebrum. Individuals with *TUBA1A* mutations may have isolated lissencephaly or may have lissencephaly with cerebellar hypoplasia. Diagnosis of lissencephaly is made by brain MRI showing a smooth cortex with minimal sulcation. Genetic testing is necessary to determine etiology. Management consists of seizure control, genetic counseling, and supportive care.

Band heterotopia (double cortex) is a less severe form of lissencephaly that is seen in females with *DCX* mutation. Clinical manifestations of band heterotopia range from mild to severe and include seizures, intellectual disability, and developmental delay. Women with a *DCX* mutation are at risk of having male children with severe lissencephaly. Brain MRI demonstrates a band of gray matter underlying a nearly normal-appearing cerebral cortex. Management consists of seizure control and genetic counseling.

NODULAR HETEROTOPIA

Nodular heterotopias are characterized by collections of neurons and glia in the subependyma or in the subcortical white matter. The most important form is subependymal nodular heterotopia, a condition characterized by multiple gray matter nodules in the walls of the lateral ventricles bilaterally. This X-linked condition is due to a mutation in *FLNA*, which codes for filamin A, an actin-cross-linking phosphoprotein. As a result of this mutation, many neurons do not migrate out of the subventricular zone. Most affected individuals are heterozygous females. Males are severely affected and often die in infancy. Most affected females present with seizures during childhood or adolescence. They may be intellectually normal or have mild disability. Individuals with subependymal nodular heterotopia are at increased risk for aortic or carotid dissection and for cardiac valvular abnormalities.

The diagnosis is based on brain MRI, which shows gray matter nodules along the walls of the lateral ventricles, followed by genetic testing for *FLNA*. Management consists of seizure control and genetic counseling.

Disorders of Cortical Organization

Disorders of cortical organization include conditions such as polymicrogyria and schizencephaly. These disorders are not due to abnormal numbers of neurons or impaired migration but instead include abnormalities of gyration, sulcation, connectivity, or synaptogenesis. The best-understood of these disorders are polymicrogyria and schizencephaly.

POLYMICROGYRIA

Polymicrogyria is characterized by regions of complex cortical convolutions with miniature gyri that are fused and superimposed together. Polymicrogyria is caused by failure of cortical organization as a result of in utero injury or genetic mutation; it has been associated with prenatal infections (e.g., cytomegalovirus) and possible vascular abnormalities, but often it is idiopathic. A single gene, *GPR56* (chromosome 16q13), has been associated with bilateral frontoparietal polymicrogyria. *GPR56* codes for a G protein–coupled receptor that appears to be important for human cerebral cortical development. Clinical manifestations include epilepsy, developmental delay, cerebral palsy, and intellectual disability, depending on the location and extent of the abnormality. The diagnosis of polymicrogyria is made by brain MRI. Clinical management consists of seizure management and supportive therapies.

SCHIZENCEPHALY

Schizencephaly is characterized by infolding of cortical gray matter along a hemispheric cleft near the primary cerebral fissures. In most cases, the cause cannot be determined, but it has been associated with in utero insult. A rare familial form has been described, but no gene has been identified. Clinical features include developmental delay, cerebral palsy, dysarthria, and epilepsy. The clinical abnormalities are more severe with large open-lip schizencephaly and with bilateral lesions than with small unilateral closed-lip schizencephaly. Diagnosis is made by brain MRI. Management consists of seizure control and supportive therapies when indicated.

Malformations of Cerebellum and Brain Stem

Developmental abnormalities of the hindbrain are less well understood than are abnormalities of cerebral cortical development.[5] Two of the better known and important syndromes are Joubert syndrome and Dandy-Walker malformation.

JOUBERT SYNDROME

Joubert syndrome is characterized by a distinctive pattern of cerebellar and brain stem developmental malformation. Four causative genes (*NPHP1*, *CEP290*, *AHI1*, and *TMEM67* [*MKS3*]) together account for approximately 30% of cases. Clinical features include hypotonia, truncal ataxia, developmental delay, abnormal eye movements, and disordered breathing. The combination of signs and severity can be variable. Some individuals with Joubert syndrome also have retinal dystrophy, renal disease, ocular colobomas, occipital encephalocele, or hepatic fibrosis. No formal diagnostic criteria exist. The diagnosis is usually based on the combination of hypotonia in infancy with later development of ataxia, intellectual impairment, and abnormal breathing pattern, or abnormal eye movements in combination with a characteristic MRI finding known as the molar tooth sign. The molar tooth sign results from hypoplasia of the cerebellar vermis and accompanying brain stem abnormalities on axial imaging through the junction of the midbrain and pons. Genetic testing is available for the four identified genes. Management is supportive. Caffeine can be helpful for periodic hypoventilation, but some patients require tracheostomy.

DANDY-WALKER MALFORMATION

Dandy-Walker malformation is characterized by cerebellar vermis hypoplasia, cystic dilation of the fourth ventricle, and enlargement of the posterior fossa. Rare familial cases have been reported, but a genetic basis has not been identified. This heterogeneous disorder is usually accompanied by hypotonia, delayed motor development, and ataxia. Intellectual disability is present in about 50% of affected individuals. In some cases, hydrocephalus requires shunting. Diagnosis is based on characteristic findings on brain MRI. Treatment is supportive, with cerebrospinal fluid (CSF) shunting when indicated.

CHIARI MALFORMATIONS

Four types of Chiari malformation have been described. The most common of these are Chiari types I and II. Chiari I malformations are most often diagnosed in adulthood, whereas Chiari II malformations are associated with spina bifida and are usually diagnosed in childhood.

Chiari I malformations are characterized by downward displacement of the cerebellar tonsils through the foramen magnum, often first accompanied by compression of the tonsils. Chiari I is a developmental abnormality that is thought to be congenital in most cases, even though symptoms may not present until adulthood, typically in the third or fourth decade of life. The abnormality is often asymptomatic and discovered only as an incidental finding. However, clinical manifestations can result from compression of neural structures at the cranial-cervical junction or obstruction of CSF flow. Signs and symptoms include headaches that worsen with straining or coughing, lower cranial nerve findings, downbeat nystagmus, ataxia, or long-tract signs. Chiari I malformations are accompanied by syringomyelia (see later) in up to 80% of cases. Diagnosis is made with brain MRI, which shows the cerebellar tonsils extending through the foramen magnum 5 mm or more (Fig. 389-1). Unfortunately, no MRI findings can clearly differentiate symptomatic from asymptomatic individuals.[6] Surgical treatment with craniocervical decompression is recommended for symptomatic patients but usually not for asymptomatic or mildly symptomatic individuals[7] or patients whose only symptom is headache.

Chiari II malformations, commonly called Arnold-Chiari malformations, are characterized by descent of the cerebellar tonsils, the inferior vermis, and portions of the cerebellar hemispheres into the spinal canal, along with elongation and displacement of the brain stem and fourth ventricle. Chiari II malformations are almost always associated with meningomyelocele and spina bifida. Hydrocephalus requiring shunting occurs in most cases. Brain stem dysfunction may result from intrinsic malformation or from compression of neural structures at the craniocervical junction. Treatment is surgical repair of the myelomeningocele, relief of hydrocephalus, and occasionally cervical bone decompression. The prognosis depends on the level and extent of the myelomeningocele and on the severity of brain anomalies.

Malformations of Spinal Cord

TETHERED SPINAL CORD

Tethered spinal cord syndrome is a disorder caused by an anomalous filum terminale that restricts the normal ascent of the conus medullaris and limits

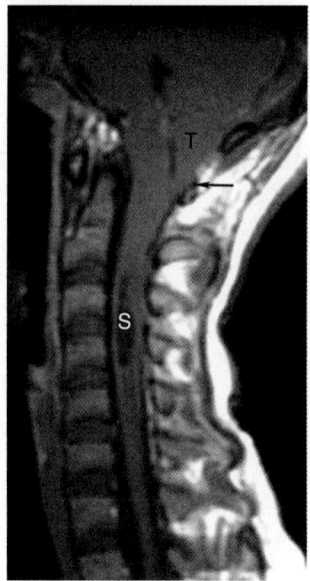

FIGURE 389-1. Chiari I malformation. A sagittal magnetic resonance image shows low, pointed cerebellar tonsils (i.e., Chiari I malformation, T) that extend to the level of C1 (*arrow*) and a dilated central canal of the spinal cord (i.e., syringohydromyelia [S]). (From Barkovich AJ, Kuzniecky RI. Congenital, developmental, and neurocutaneous disorders. In Goldman L, Ausiello D, eds. *Cecil Textbook of Medicine.* 23rd ed. Philadelphia: Saunders Elsevier; 2008:2790.)

the movement of the spinal cord within the spinal column. The result is an abnormal stretching of the spinal cord, with neurologic symptoms referable to the lower spinal cord. Tethering may also develop after spinal cord injury. Associated spinal anomalies are common and may include diastematomyelia, spinal lipomas, dermal sinuses, and fibrolipomas of the filum terminale. Symptoms can occur at any age but usually develop during periods of rapid growth in childhood or adolescence. However, tethered spinal cord syndrome may go undiagnosed until adulthood, when sensory and motor problems and loss of bowel and bladder control emerge. Erectile dysfunction may occur in males. Symptoms are typically progressive. Diagnosis is made with MRI, which shows a low conus medullaris (i.e., below the bottom of the L2 vertebral body) or a thickened or fat-containing filum terminale. Diminished pulsations of the spinal cord may also be seen. Treatment consists of surgical release of the tethered cord. With successful surgery, symptoms typically do not progress and may improve.

SYRINGOHYDROMYELIA

Syringohydromyelia is a condition in which the central canal of the spinal cord (hydromyelia) or the substance of the spinal cord (syringomyelia) is expanded by the accumulation of CSF. In many cases, both hydromyelia and syringomyelia are present (syringohydromyelia). The proximate cause of syringes probably is altered flow of CSF, with pressure variations in different parts of the subarachnoid space. This altered flow creates forces that drive CSF into the spinal cord. Possible causes include narrowing of the foramen magnum, Chiari I and II malformations, intramedullary and extramedullary spinal cord tumors, and subarachnoid scarring. Subsequent extension of the cyst may result from rapid changes in intraspinal pressure owing to such events as coughing or sneezing. Symptoms of syringohydromyelia most commonly begin in late adolescence or early adulthood and progress irregularly, with long periods of stability. The classic presentation is asymmetrical weakness and atrophy in the upper extremities, loss of upper limb deep tendon reflexes, and loss of pain and temperature sensation (with preservation of vibration and proprioception) in the neck, arms, and upper part of the trunk. With progression, spasticity and hyperreflexia develop in the lower extremities. Progressive ascending and descending levels of weakness and sensory impairment typically occur over time. The diagnosis is made by spinal MRI (see Fig. 389-1). If syringohydromyelia is identified, it is important to perform a brain MRI to look for associated abnormalities of the craniocervical junction. Occasionally, mild central canal dilation is discovered incidentally in patients without spinal cord symptoms or signs. If no associated cause is found, the prognosis of such incidentally discovered anomalies is generally good. Treatment is directed at the cause if one can be identified. Syringopleural or syringoperitoneal shunting is sometimes performed, with variable benefit.

DEVELOPMENTAL DISORDERS

Disorders associated with impaired postnatal neurodevelopmental function range from specific disorders such as fragile X syndrome and Rett syndrome, to complex syndromes such as autism, to nonspecific developmental delay and learning disabilities.

Fragile X Syndrome

Fragile X syndrome is an X-linked trinucleotide repeat disorder that is characterized by intellectual disability in most affected males. It is the most common genetic cause of intellectual disability, affecting 1 per 4000 males and 1 per 8000 females. The classic disorder is seen in males with full mutations (>200 repeats) in the *FMR1* gene.[8] Fragile X syndrome may present as isolated intellectual disability, but it is often associated with a prominent forehead, large ears, prominent jaw, and macro-orchidism. Postpubertal males often have poor impulse control, perseveration, and poor eye contact. Up to 25% of affected males have autism. Heterozygous females may be asymptomatic or may have a syndrome similar to what is seen in males, depending on repeat size and random X-inactivation.

Other disorders associated with *FMR1* include the fragile X ataxia syndrome, which is characterized by the late onset, usually after age 50 years, of progressive cerebellar ataxia and intention tremor in individuals who have an *FMR1* premutation (60 to 200 repeats). It occurs equally in males and females. Diagnosis of *FMR1* disorders is by molecular genetic testing. Cytogenetic testing for fragile sites is no longer recommended because it is less sensitive and more expensive than molecular testing. Treatment is symptomatic and supportive. Genetic counseling is recommended for affected individuals and their families.

Rett Syndrome

Rett syndrome is a neurodevelopmental disorder that occurs classically in females with mutations in the *MECP2* gene. *MECP2* mutations are generally lethal in male embryos, but Rett syndrome has been reported in males with XXY karyotype or with somatic mosaicism. *MECP2* is thought to mediate transcriptional silencing of methylated DNA. Most mutations are probably de novo or may reflect germline mosaicism; 99% of cases represent a single occurrence within a family. Affected girls are usually normal at birth and have apparently normal development for the first 6 to 18 months of life. Brain growth decelerates, and development stagnates, followed by rapid regression of language and motor skills. A classic feature of Rett syndrome is the loss of purposeful hand use and the development of repetitive stereotyped hand movements that usually have the appearance of wringing or clapping. Other features present to variable degree are bruxism, episodic apnea and hyperpnea, seizures, gait disorders, and tremor. Non-neurologic features include growth failure and wasting, bowel dysmotility, scoliosis, osteopenia, and vasomotor changes in the limbs. Diagnosis is by clinical criteria followed by molecular genetic testing. Treatment is symptomatic.

Autism

Autism or autism spectrum disorder is characterized by impaired social communication and interactions as well as restricted and repetitive behaviors. Autism is associated with many different causes and is often idiopathic. No evidence links autism to vaccinations.[9] Fragile X syndrome and tuberous sclerosis are two important entities in which an autistic phenotype can occur and in which autism may be the most prominent feature.

Symptoms typically present before 3 years of age and persist into adulthood.[10] Autism is a spectrum ranging from severe, with impairment in all domains, to mild with normal intellect and language but with impaired social interactions and repetitive behaviors or restricted interests. Autism has many causes but in most cases is idiopathic. Epilepsy is common in autism but may not emerge until adolescence. Diagnosis is based on careful diagnostic interview and examination (Table 389-1).[11] When epilepsy is present, treatment with antiepileptic medications is indicated. Behavioral therapy can help individuals learn rules for social interaction and can improve communication. It can also help with problematic behavior. Educational support is important. Medications such as atypical antipsychotics, selective serotonin reuptake inhibitors, and anxiolytics (Chapter 369) can help with aggressive behavior, repetitive behaviors, and anxiety.

NEUROCUTANEOUS DISORDERS

Neurocutaneous disorders are congenital syndromes characterized by dysplastic and neoplastic lesions primarily involving the nervous system and skin. The

TABLE 389-1	DIAGNOSTIC CRITERIA FOR AUTISM SPECTRUM DISORDER

1. Deficits in Social Communication/Interaction (must have all three criteria):
   a. Problems reciprocating social or emotional interaction, including difficulty establishing or maintaining back-and-forth conversations and interactions, inability to initiate an interaction, and problems with shared attention or sharing of emotions and interests with others
   b. Severe problems maintaining relationships—ranges from lack of interest in other people to difficulties in pretend play and engaging in age-appropriate social activities, and problems adjusting to different social expectations
   c. Nonverbal communication problems such as abnormal eye contact, posture, facial expressions, tone of voice and gestures, as well as an inability to understand these

2. Restricted and Repetitive Behavior (at least two criteria must be met):
   a. Stereotyped or repetitive speech, motor movements, or use of objects
   b. Excessive adherence to routines, ritualized patterns of verbal or nonverbal behavior, or excessive resistance to change
   c. Highly restricted interests that are abnormal in intensity or focus
   d. Hyper- or hyporeactivity to sensory input or unusual interest in sensory aspects of the environment

Symptoms must be present in early childhood but may not become fully manifest until social demands exceed capacities. Symptoms need to be *functionally impairing* and not better described by another DSM-5 diagnosis.

DSM-5: *Diagnostic and Statistical Manual of Mental Disorders.* 5th ed.
From American Psychiatric Association. *Diagnostic and Statistical Manual of Mental Disorders.* 5th ed. Arlington, VA: American Psychiatric Publishing; 2013.

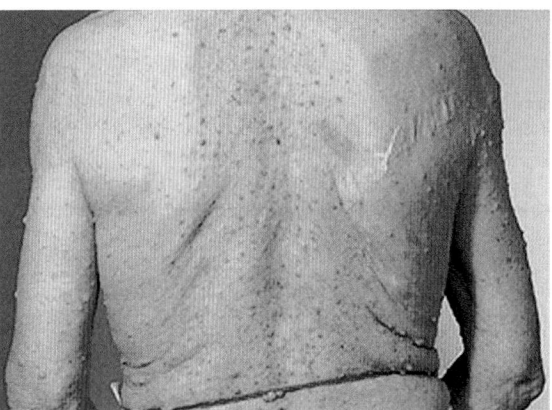

FIGURE 389-2. Multiple neurofibromas covering the back of a patient with neurofibromatosis type 1.

more than 40 described syndromes include neurofibromatosis, tuberous sclerosis, Sturge-Weber syndrome, and von Hippel-Lindau disease.

Neurofibromatosis

Neurofibromatosis encompasses a spectrum of syndromes with distinctive neural and cutaneous lesions. The two major forms of neurofibromatosis are genetically and clinically distinct.

NEUROFIBROMATOSIS TYPE 1

Neurofibromatosis type 1, the classic disorder described by von Recklinghausen, is an autosomal dominant condition with an incidence of 1 per 2500 to 3000 births.[12] It is an autosomal dominant disorder, but approximately 50% of cases are due to new mutations. Most mutations in *NF1* occur in the parental germline. The *NF1* gene, which is located on chromosome 17q11.2, codes a protein called neurofibromin, which is thought to function as a tumor suppressor by acting as a negative regulator of the Ras signaling pathway. Neurofibromatosis type 1 is characterized by multiple café au lait spots, axillary and inguinal freckling, multiple discrete cutaneous neurofibromas (Fig. 389-2), and Lisch nodules (Table 389-2). Subcutaneous neurofibromas may be painful or disfiguring. Learning disabilities are present in at least 50% of individuals. Other manifestations include plexiform neurofibromas, tibial dysplasia, and vasculopathy. The risk of optic nerve and other central nervous system (CNS) gliomas and malignant peripheral nerve sheath tumors is markedly increased, but the risk of other tumors is also elevated, with a 60% lifetime risk of cancer.[13]

TABLE 389-2 DIAGNOSTIC CRITERIA FOR NEUROFIBROMATOSIS TYPE 1

Two or more of the following clinical features signify the presence of neurofibromatosis type 1:

Six or more café au lait macules (>0.5 cm at largest diameter in prepubertal individuals or >1.5 cm in individuals past puberty)

Axillary freckling or freckling in inguinal regions

Two or more neurofibromas of any type or ≥1 plexiform neurofibroma

Two or more Lisch nodules (iris hamartomas)

A distinctive osseous lesion

A first-degree relative with neurofibromatosis type 1 diagnosed by using the above-listed criteria

TABLE 389-3 RECOMMENDED SURVEILLANCE IN PATIENTS WITH NEUROFIBROMATOSIS TYPE 1

Annual physical examination by a physician who is familiar with the individual and with the disease

Annual ophthalmologic examination in early childhood, less frequent examination in older children and adults

Regular developmental assessment by screening questionnaire (in childhood)

Regular blood pressure monitoring

Other studies only as indicated on the basis of clinically apparent signs or symptoms

Monitoring of those who have abnormalities of the central nervous system, skeletal system, or cardiovascular system by an appropriate specialist

TABLE 389-4 DIAGNOSTIC CRITERIA FOR NEUROFIBROMATOSIS TYPE 2

Presence of one or more of the following makes the diagnosis of neurofibromatosis type 2:

- Bilateral vestibular schwannomas
- A first-degree relative with neurofibromatosis type 2, *and* Unilateral vestibular schwannoma, *or* Any two of: meningioma, schwannoma, glioma, neurofibroma, posterior subcapsular lenticular opacities*
- Unilateral vestibular schwannoma, *and* Any two of: meningioma, schwannoma, glioma, neurofibroma, posterior subcapsular lenticular opacities*
- Multiple meningiomas, *and* Unilateral vestibular schwannoma, *or* Any two of: schwannoma, glioma, neurofibroma, cataract*

*"Any two of" refers to two individual tumors or cataracts.

TABLE 389-5 DIAGNOSTIC CRITERIA FOR TUBEROUS SCLEROSIS COMPLEX

Definite—Two major features or one major feature plus two minor features
Probable—One major feature plus one minor feature
Possible—One major feature or two or more minor features

MAJOR FEATURES

Facial angiofibromas or forehead plaque
Nontraumatic ungual or periungual fibromas
More than three hypomelanotic macules (ash leaf spots)
Shagreen patch (connective tissue nevus)
Multiple retinal nodular hamartomas
Cortical tuber
Subependymal nodule
Subependymal giant cell astrocytoma
Cardiac rhabdomyoma, single or multiple
Lymphangiomyomatosis
Renal angiomyolipoma

MINOR FEATURES

Multiple dental enamel pits
Hamartomatous rectal polyps
Bone cysts
Cerebral white matter radial migration lines
Gingival fibromas
Nonrenal hamartoma
Retinal achromic patch
"Confetti" skin lesions
Multiple renal cysts

Management of patients depends on the specific manifestations and often requires multidisciplinary collaboration. Most patients with neurofibromatosis type 1 do not require treatment, but all require surveillance (Table 389-3). Subcutaneous, intraspinal, and intracranial tumors can be treated surgically. Selumetinib (an oral selective inhibitor of mitogen-activated protein kinase [MAPK] 1 and 2 at 20 to 30 mg/m^2 twice daily in 28-day cycles) may reduce the size of inoperable plexiform neurofibromas in patients with neurofibromatosis type 1.[14] Optic nerve gliomas may be treated with chemotherapy; both cisplatin and temozolomide have shown some benefit. Radiation is not recommended. Genetic counseling should be provided to all patients and their families.

NEUROFIBROMATOSIS TYPE 2

Neurofibromatosis type 2 is an autosomal dominant condition with an incidence of approximately 1 in 25,000 individuals. The *NF2* gene is located on chromosome 22q12.2. Its gene product merlin is a cytoskeletal protein thought to act as a membrane-stabilizing protein. The specific function of merlin is unknown. Neurofibromatosis type 2 is characterized by bilateral vestibular schwannomas, which usually present with symptoms of tinnitus, hearing loss, and imbalance. The age at onset is usually in young adulthood, but some individuals may develop posterior subcapsular lens opacities or mononeuropathy in childhood. Almost all affected individuals develop bilateral vestibular schwannomas by age 30 (Table 389-4). Affected individuals may also develop schwannomas of other cranial and peripheral nerves, meningiomas, and (rarely) ependymomas or astrocytomas. Posterior subcapsular lens opacities are the most common ocular abnormality.

Management depends on the specific manifestations and complications. In individuals who either have tested positive for known *NF2* mutations or have a family history of neurofibromatosis type 2 and whose genetic status cannot be determined with genetic testing, annual brain MRI is recommended starting between ages 10 and 12 years and continuing until at least age 40 years. Hearing evaluations may be useful in detecting changes in auditory nerve function before changes can be visualized by MRI. Routine complete eye examinations should be part of the care of all individuals.

Bevacizumab, a vascular endothelial growth factor inhibitor (5 mg/kg intravenously every 2 weeks), can improve hearing in some patients with neurofibromatosis type 2 and vestibular schwannomas.[15] Surgical treatment of schwannomas and meningiomas may be indicated to preserve function or to relieve compression of adjacent structures, especially in patients with intramedullary spinal tumors. Genetic counseling should be provided to affected individuals and their families.

Tuberous Sclerosis

Tuberous sclerosis complex is characterized by abnormalities of the brain, kidney, and heart.[16] Tuberous sclerosis may occur as an autosomal dominant syndrome or result from spontaneous mutation. Two tuberous sclerosis genes have been identified. *TSC1* (chromosome 9q34) codes for a protein called hamartin, a protein that interacts with the product of the *TSC2* gene to inhibit the mammalian target of rapamycin (mTOR). *TSC2* (chromosome 16p13) codes for tuberin, which interacts with hamartin. *TSC2* mutations account for about 60% of individuals with clinical tuberous sclerosis.

Specific findings vary across individuals, and severity ranges from minimal to severe. Skin lesions are seen in almost 100% of affected individuals, but CNS lesions are the leading cause of morbidity and mortality. Epilepsy is seen in as many as 80% of patients with CNS lesions. Intellectual impairment and developmental delay are common, and up to 40% of patients have an autism spectrum disorder. Giant cell astrocytoma is the leading cause of death. Up to 80% of children with tuberous sclerosis have an identifiable renal lesion (Chapter 187) by 10.5 years of age, and renal disease is the second leading cause of early death in individuals with tuberous sclerosis. Cardiac rhabdomyomas, which can occur in up to 50% of patients, are usually present at birth and typically regress over time. Diagnosis of tuberous sclerosis (Table 389-5) is usually clinical and confirmed by identification of calcified or uncalcified hamartomas on imaging studies (Fig. 389-3).

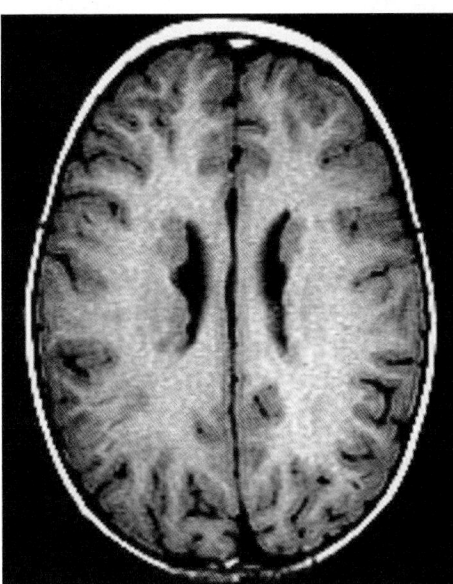

FIGURE 389-3. Subependymal nodules and multiple cortical tubers in a patient with tuberous sclerosis.

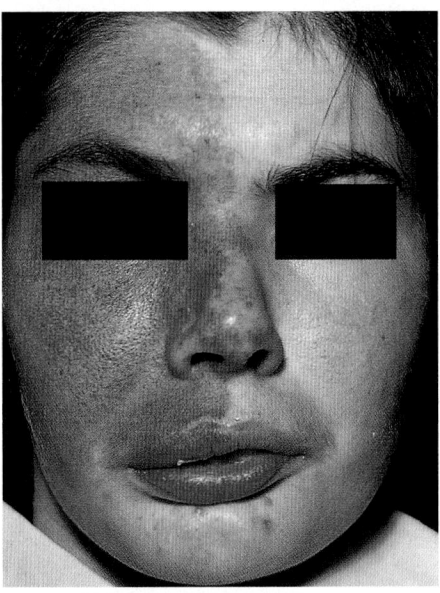

FIGURE 389-4. Sturge-Weber syndrome. This patient has a classic diffuse capillary hemangioma in the distribution of the ophthalmic, nasociliary, and maxillary branches of the trigeminal nerve. The lesion extends backward over the anterior two thirds of the crown of the head. (From Forbes CD, Jackson WD. *Color Atlas and Text of Clinical Medicine.* 2nd ed. London: Mosby; 1996.)

Treatment is directed at complications of the disease, particularly epilepsy (Chapter 375). Neurosurgical intervention may sometimes be indicated for epilepsy and for symptomatic treatment of complications such as hydrocephalus, which results from midline giant cell tumors. In a randomized controlled trial, treatment with everolimus (10 mg/day) reduced the size of the angiomyolipomas in 42% of participants receiving active drug as compared with 0% of participants receiving placebo.[A1] Everolimus titrated to 9 to 15 ng/mL as an adjunct therapy can also reduce the frequency of focal-onset seizures that are otherwise resistant to treatment.[A2] Everolimus titrated to a concentration of 5 to 15 ng/mL was also effective in reducing the size subependymal giant cell astrocytomas by at least 50% in 35% of participants receiving active drug as compared with 0% of participants receiving placebo.[A3] At similar doses, everolimus also can change fractional anisotropy and radial diffusivity, suggesting that the genetic defect of tuberous sclerosis complex in the brain may be modified pharmacologically. Topical 1% rapamycin is a safe and effective treatment for the facial angiofibromas that are seen in about 75% of patients.[A4] Serial brain MRI and renal ultrasound screening may be indicated in some patients because benign tumors of these organs may enlarge rapidly. Genetic counseling is an important part of management.

Sturge-Weber Syndrome

Sturge-Weber syndrome is a sporadic disorder characterized by facial vascular nevi, epilepsy, cognitive impairment, and sometimes hemiparesis, hemianopia, or glaucoma. It is most commonly due to somatic mutation in *GNAQ* (chromosome 9q21).[17] The characteristic CNS feature of this disorder is capillary angiomatosis of the pia mater. Cerebral cortical calcifications are generally seen in a pericapillary distribution and are progressive. Most patients with Sturge-Weber syndrome have epilepsy. The diagnosis is usually based on the presence of a facial nevus (Fig. 389-4), which is manifested as a typical port-wine stain, and confirmatory imaging on a contrast brain MRI showing leptomeningeal enhancement.

Regular ophthalmologic examination is warranted because of the risk for glaucoma. Treatment is usually aimed at the epilepsy, which can be medically intractable. In patients with intractable epilepsy and infantile-onset hemiplegia, hemispherectomy can improve the seizures and the neurodevelopmental outcome.

Von Hippel-Lindau Disease

Von Hippel-Lindau disease (i.e., CNS angiomatosis) is an autosomal dominant disorder caused by a defective tumor suppressor gene (*VHL*) at chromosome 3p25-p26.[18] It is characterized by retinal angiomas, brain (usually cerebellar) and spinal cord hemangioblastomas, renal cell carcinomas, endolymphatic sac tumors, pheochromocytomas, papillary cystadenomas of the epididymis, angiomas of the liver and kidney, and cysts of the pancreas, kidney, liver, and epididymis. Both sexes are affected equally.

Symptoms typically begin during the third or fourth decade. Retinal inflammation with exudate, hemorrhage, and retinal detachment from the retinal angiomas typically precedes the cerebellar complaints, but the order is not constant. The ocular findings are nonspecific, and the retinal detachment may mask the underlying lesion. Headache, vertigo, and vomiting result from cerebellar tumors. Cerebellar signs such as ataxia, dysdiadochokinesis, and dysmetria are common. Rare patients present with symptoms of spinal cord or visceral lesions or may have hearing loss from tumors of the endolymphatic sac.

Clinical diagnosis is established if the patient has more than one CNS hemangioblastoma, one hemangioblastoma with a visceral manifestation of the disease, or one manifestation of the disease and a known family history. Molecular genetic testing detects mutations in the *VHL* gene in nearly 100% of affected individuals.

For patients with von Hippel-Lindau disease and for those with a disease-causing *VHL* mutation, surveillance is recommended with annual ophthalmologic examination, annual blood pressure monitoring, measurement of urinary catecholamine metabolites beginning at age 5 years in families with pheochromocytoma, and annual abdominal ultrasound examination beginning at age 16 years, with evaluation of suspicious lesions by computed tomography or MRI. Treatment is symptomatic. Retinal detachments and tumors are treated by laser therapy. Large brain tumors (Chapter 180), renal cell carcinomas (Chapter 187), pheochromocytomas (Chapter 215), epididymal tumors (Chapter 190), and endolymphatic sac tumors are treated surgically; smaller CNS tumors may be treated by gamma knife. Pazopanib, which is a tyrosine kinase inhibitor that inhibits angiogenesis, may be useful for patients with progressive lesions.[19]

Grade A References

A1. Bissler JJ, Kingswood JC, Radzikowska E, et al. Everolimus for angiomyolipoma associated with tuberous sclerosis complex or sporadic lymphangioleiomyomatosis (EXIST-2): a multicentre, randomised, double-blind, placebo-controlled trial. *Lancet.* 2013;381:817-824.

A2. French JA, Lawson JA, Yapici Z, et al. Adjunctive everolimus therapy for treatment-resistant focal-onset seizures associated with tuberous sclerosis (EXIST-3): a phase 3, randomised, double-blind, placebo-controlled study. *Lancet.* 2016;388:2153-2163.

A3. Franz DN, Belousova E, Sparagana S, et al. Efficacy and safety of everolimus for subependymal giant cell astrocytomas associated with tuberous sclerosis complex (EXIST-1): a multicentre, randomised, placebo-controlled phase 3 trial. *Lancet.* 2013;381:125-132.

A4. Koenig MK, Bell CS, Hebert AA, et al. Efficacy and safety of topical rapamycin in patients with facial angiofibromas secondary to tuberous sclerosis complex: the TREATMENT randomized clinical trial. *JAMA Dermatol.* 2018;154:773-780.

GENERAL REFERENCES

For the General References and other additional features, please visit Expert Consult at https://expertconsult.inkling.com.

390

AUTONOMIC DISORDERS AND THEIR MANAGEMENT

WILLIAM P. CHESHIRE, JR.

TABLE 390-1	BRAIN DYSAUTONOMIAS
Autonomic failure	Multiple system atrophy
	Lewy body dementia
	Parkinson disease
Autonomic dysregulation	Autonomic storms
	Takotsubo cardiomyopathy
	Tachycardia or bradycardia
	Neurogenic hypertension
	Overactive bladder

Below the level of conscious awareness, the autonomic nervous system continuously regulates bodily functions to maintain homeostasis and respond to stress. Many diseases can impair autonomic responses and, in turn, affect cardiovascular, thermal, metabolic, gastrointestinal (GI), urinary, reproductive, or other organ functions. Examples include brain lesions that involve the central autonomic network, disorders that damage peripheral nerves, and systemic illnesses or drugs that affect autonomic neurons.

EPIDEMIOLOGY

The most frequently disabling manifestation of autonomic failure is orthostatic hypotension, which increases in prevalence with aging and is associated with decreased functional capacity and a two-fold increased risk for falls (Chapters 21 and 22). Its prevalence is about 5% among ambulatory elderly persons, 30% among all persons older than 75 years, and greater than 50% in frail individuals who live in nursing homes.

Neurally mediated syncope, also termed *vasodepressor* or *vasovagal syncope* (Chapter 56), is an episodic phenomenon, with a lifetime prevalence of about 20%.[1] Various types of situational syncope, which can occur in response to emotional distress, micturition, defecation, coughing, carotid sinus stimulation, and other factors, are episodic phenomena.

Diabetes mellitus (Chapter 216) is the most common cause of autonomic neuropathy in the developed world. Within 10 to 15 years of the onset of diabetes, laboratory evidence of autonomic neuropathy can be detected in 25 to 30% of patients.[2] Symptomatic orthostatic hypotension occurs in about 5% of diabetic patients (Chapter 216).

PATHOBIOLOGY

The peripheral autonomic nervous system comprises three main divisions: (1) the sympathetic outflow from the thoracolumbar segments of the spinal cord; (2) the parasympathetic outflow from cranial nerves III, VII, IX, and X and the sacral spinal segments; and (3) the enteric ganglionated plexuses intrinsic to the wall of the gut. Sympathetic and parasympathetic responses, though generally antagonistic, can be localized and are not always equally counterbalanced.

Sympathetic noradrenergic denervation causes orthostatic hypotension, which is a hallmark of autonomic disorders and which renders a standing patient unable to constrict the splanchnic and other peripheral vascular beds in response to the pooling of blood volume (300 to 800 mL) owing to gravity. Sympathetic noradrenergic failure may also impair pupillary dilation, the ability to mount a tachycardia in response to exercise or hypotension, the mobilization of energy substrates, and male erectile function.

Sympathetic cholinergic denervation impairs sweating. Whereas patients may complain if sweating is excessive, they usually do not notice anhidrosis, which is more concerning because it can predispose to heat stress or heat stroke (Chapter 101).[3] Parasympathetic denervation may, depending on the site of the lesion, impair pupillary constriction, lacrimal or salivary secretion, reflex bradycardia, or bladder detrusor contraction.

BRAIN DISORDERS

Many diseases can disrupt central autonomic function at the level of the hypothalamus, ventrolateral medulla, nucleus of the solitary tract, parabrachial nucleus, periaqueductal gray matter, amygdala, and insular or prefrontal cortices. The result may be autonomic hypofunction or hyperfunction (Table 390-1).[4]

General autonomic failure occurs in neurodegenerative disorders characterized by abnormal neuronal (Lewy body disorders [Chapter 374], including Parkinson disease [Chapter 381]) or glial (multiple system atrophy) accumulation of α-synuclein. The most severe is multiple system atrophy, in which autonomic failure accompanies parkinsonism (Shy-Drager syndrome; Chapter 381) or cerebellar ataxia (Chapter 382).[5,6]

Other brain disorders may disturb individual autonomic responses or, by releasing inhibition of downstream functions, give rise to autonomic hyperactivity. Cerebral small vessel white matter disease may be associated with an overactive bladder (Chapter 23). Bilateral damage to the carotid baroreceptors, which signal blood pressure changes to the nucleus of the solitary tract in the brain stem, causes a central deafferentation syndrome characterized by volatile hypertension and orthostatic hypotension. Some insular strokes may destabilize sympathoregulatory balance and occasionally contribute to adverse cardiac events. Seizures (Chapter 375) arising from the mesial temporal lobe may induce ictal tachycardia or, more rarely, bradycardia or asystole. Damage to the medulla oblongata may cause hypertension, orthostatic hypotension, or syncope. Medullary ischemia or compression can cause acute neurogenic hypertension (Cushing response). Lateral medullary infarction (Wallenberg syndrome) typically produces ipsilateral Horner syndrome and occasionally bradycardia, acute hypertension, supine hypotension, or central hypoventilation.

Catastrophic conditions such as subarachnoid hemorrhage (Chapter 380), head trauma (Chapter 371), status epilepticus (Chapter 375), or acute hydrocephalus with increased intracranial pressure can profoundly stimulate sympathetic responses with cardiovascular consequence. These paroxysmal sympathetic storms are characterized by episodic sympathetic hyperactivity with hypertension, tachycardia, hyperventilation, pupillary dilation, flushing, and diaphoresis.

Autonomic responses are closely linked to emotional states via the amygdala, insular, and anterior cingulate cortices. Extreme stress generating a catecholamine surge can cause takotsubo cardiomyopathy, a typically reversible syndrome of left ventricular dysfunction (Chapter 54).

SPINAL CORD DISORDERS

Lesions of the spinal cord (Chapter 372), whether compressive, demyelinating, vascular, or neoplastic, commonly result in an overactive bladder (Chapter 23) with symptoms of frequency, urgency, and sometimes incontinence. Lesions that involve the sacral cord segments or cauda equina result in an underactive bladder with incomplete emptying, overflow incontinence, sphincter atonia, and sexual dysfunction.

After spinal cord injuries above the level of splanchnic sympathetic outflow at T5, sprouting of afferent fibers in the thoracolumbar dorsal horns and necrosis of the descending white matter connections to sympathetic preganglionic neurons result in autonomic dysreflexia. In these patients, strong peripheral sensory stimuli such as bladder or bowel distention can induce a reversible state of sympathetic hyperresponsiveness that may present with hypertension, diaphoresis, flushing, or headache.

PERIPHERAL NEUROPATHIES

Autonomic dysfunction can arise at the level of the autonomic ganglia or peripheral nerves (Table 390-2). Peripheral autonomic nerves are generally small in caliber and unmyelinated or thinly myelinated. Peripheral neuropathies that selectively involve small nerve fibers can cause various combinations of sensory, sympathetic, or parasympathetic signs and symptoms.

Diabetic neuropathy (Chapter 216) involves autonomic nerves early in its course, and about 20% of patients advance to a clinically consequential cardiovascular autonomic neuropathy. The glycemic burden appears to represent a continuum of risk, because some patients with impaired glucose regulation or newly diagnosed diabetes may already have evidence of small fiber neuropathy. Another peripheral dysautonomia is pure autonomic failure, an α-synucleinopathy that presents insidiously with severe, generalized autonomic failure as the sole clinical feature.

Disorders of neurologic autoimmunity include Guillain-Barré syndrome, in which antiganglioside antibodies mediate an acute inflammatory demyelinating polyradiculoneuropathy that may be associated with tachycardia, blood pressure lability, and pupillomotor, sudomotor, and vasomotor disturbances (Chapter 392). Acute pandysautonomia develops dramatically over a period of days to weeks as combined sympathetic and parasympathetic failure with

TABLE 390-2 SOME CAUSES OF PERIPHERAL AUTONOMIC NEUROPATHY

Metabolic	Diabetes mellitus Alcohol Acute intermittent porphyria Uremia
Autoimmune	Autoimmune autonomic ganglionopathy Guillain-Barré syndrome Paraneoplastic Morvan syndrome Lambert-Eaton myasthenic syndrome Chronic inflammatory demyelinating polyradiculoneuropathy Sjögren syndrome Systemic lupus erythematosus Mixed connective tissue diseases
Paraproteinemic	Amyloidosis
Nutritional	Cyanocobalamin deficiency Thiamine deficiency Gluten-sensitive neuropathy
Toxic	Heavy metals Organic solvents Organophosphates Vacor Acrylamide
Drug induced	Cisplatin Vincristine Amiodarone Metronidazole Perhexiline Paclitaxel
Infectious	Human immunodeficiency virus Leprosy Chagas disease Botulism Diphtheria Lyme disease
Genetic	Hereditary sensory and autonomic neuropathies types I, II, III, IV, V Fabry disease
Idiopathic	Adie syndrome Ross syndrome Acute cholinergic neuropathy Chronic idiopathic anhidrosis Amyotrophic lateral sclerosis

GI dysmotility and, in contrast to Guillain-Barré syndrome, spares the somatic nerves. An antecedent (presumably viral) infection is reported in about 50% of cases. The finding of antibodies against the nicotinic acetylcholine receptor in the autonomic ganglia in many of these patients has established autoimmune autonomic ganglionopathy as a definable disease entity.

Autoimmune neuromyotonia is characterized by peripheral nerve hyperexcitability, insomnia, fluctuating delirium, and prominent dysautonomia with hyperhidrosis and orthostatic intolerance. Most patients have antibodies to voltage-gated potassium channels (Chapter 394).

Paraneoplastic autonomic neuropathies, which can predate the diagnosis of malignancy, are a rare epiphenomenon of malignancy, most frequently small cell lung carcinoma (Chapter 182),[7] and can occur also in association with other cancers. The most commonly encountered paraneoplastic antibody is antineuronal nuclear antibody type 1 (ANNA-1 or anti-Hu), which binds to a 35- to 40-kD family of neuronal nuclear RNA-binding proteins, including those in autonomic and enteric ganglia. Antibodies against collapsing response mediator proteins (CRMP-5 or anti-CV2) have also been associated with paraneoplastic autonomic neuropathy. Dysautonomia occurs in approximately 10 to 30% of patients with ANNA-1 and in 30% of patients with CRMP-5 seropositivity. Small cell lung cancer (Chapter 182) has been found in more than 80% of patients seropositive for ANNA-1 or CRMP-5.

Amyloidosis (Chapter 179) results from the focal deposition of insoluble fibrillary proteins arranged in β-pleated sheet configurations within the extracellular space of various tissues, which may include the vasculature of peripheral autonomic nerves and sympathetic ganglia. Amyloid neuropathy is typically manifested as a painful distal small fiber sensory and severe autonomic neuropathy. Autonomic dysfunction frequently occurs in primary AL (amyloid

light-chain), immunoglobulin light chain–associated disease, and hereditary amyloidosis,[8] but only rarely in reactive or AA (amyloid A) amyloidosis.

Among the infectious neuropathies, tetanus infection (Chapter 280) causes sympathetic overactivity in a third of patients because of the exotoxin tetanospasmin, which is taken up by peripheral nerve terminals and transported across synaptic junctions to reach the central nervous system. There it binds to gangliosides at presynaptic junctions to disinhibit preganglionic neurons and damages autonomic brain stem nuclei. Sympathetic hyperactivity results in labile or persistent hypertension or hypotension, tachyarrhythmias, peripheral vasoconstriction, fever, and profuse sweating. Diphtheritic neuropathy (Chapter 276) causes bulbar weakness and may be associated with cardiovagal impairment but not usually with orthostatic hypotension.

The acute cholinergic neuropathy of botulism (Chapter 280) occurs along with bulbar and generalized neuromuscular paralysis 12 to 36 hours after the ingestion of food contaminated with the gram-positive anaerobic bacterium *Clostridium botulinum*. Botulinum toxin binds with high affinity to presynaptic receptors of cholinergic nerve terminals and inhibits the release of acetylcholine, thereby blocking neuromuscular and cholinergic autonomic transmission. Autonomic manifestations include anhidrosis, dry eyes, dry mouth, paralytic ileus, gastric dilation, urinary retention, and sometimes orthostatic hypotension with fluctuating blood pressure and vasomotor tone.

Human immunodeficiency virus infection commonly causes autonomic disturbances, particularly in its advanced stages. Manifestations can include orthostatic hypotension, tachycardia, urinary dysfunction, impotency, diarrhea, and cardiac conduction defects. Perivascular mononuclear inflammatory infiltrates and neuronal degeneration in biopsy specimens of sympathetic ganglia suggest an autoimmune pathogenesis.

Chagas disease (Chapter 326) causes a predominantly parasympathetic neuropathy characterized by megaesophagus, megaduodenum, and megacolon, as well as sympathetic cardiovascular failure with cardiomegaly and conduction defects. The autonomic neuropathy develops years to decades after primary infection with *Trypanosoma cruzi*.

Leprosy (Chapter 310), one of the most common causes of neuropathy worldwide, frequently causes peripheral autonomic neuropathy as a result of an immune reaction against *Mycobacterium leprae*. Focal anhidrosis occurs in areas of hypopigmented and hypoesthetic skin. Cardiac denervation and orthostatic hypotension have been described.

Nutritional deficiencies that lead to autonomic neuropathy include alcoholic neuropathy, which is a dying-back neuropathy identical to that of beriberi that is caused by thiamine deficiency (Chapter 388). Distal parts of the vagus nerve are affected early, and orthostatic hypotension may occur in more advanced stages. Subacute combined degeneration from vitamin B_{12} deficiency (Chapter 205) results in axonal degeneration and is occasionally manifested as orthostatic hypotension. Autonomic neuropathy has been described in some cases of celiac disease (Chapter 131).

Notable among the hereditary sensory and autonomic neuropathies is familial dysautonomia, which is an autosomal recessive disorder linked to mutations in the I-κB kinase–associated protein gene (*IKBKAP*). It occurs in about 1 in 3600 live births to parents of Ashkenazi Jewish descent. Affected children cry without tears, feed poorly, lack lingual fungiform papillae, have depressed patellar reflexes, and are subject to orthostatic hypotension and autonomic storms owing to impaired baroreflex afferent neurons. Holmes-Adie syndrome, which consists of tonic pupils with asymmetrical or absent tendon reflexes, has been described in patients with Ross syndrome, a partial dysautonomia consisting of the clinical triad of unilateral or bilateral tonic pupils, tendon hyporeflexia, and segmental body anhidrosis.

CLINICAL MANIFESTATIONS

Some patients present with generalized autonomic failure, whereas others present with regional or system-selective autonomic dysfunction. Orthostatic hypotension without a compensatory tachycardia (Chapter 56) is the hallmark of generalized autonomic failure. It is typically worse in the morning and aggravated by dehydration, deconditioning, prolonged standing, physical exertion, heat, carbohydrate ingestion, or menstruation. Early symptoms typically include lightheadedness on arising in the morning or following a warm shower, physical exercise, or a large meal. Neurogenic orthostatic hypotension is often accompanied by supine hypertension, and the normal diurnal decrease in blood pressure during sleep is reversed. Other common symptoms include male erectile dysfunction, decreased sweating, dry mouth, constipation, and bladder dysfunction. Gastroparesis (Chapter 127) may manifest as early satiety, nausea, anorexia, bloating, and sometimes pain and weight loss. Intestinal dysmotility may cause severe constipation (Chapter 127).

Autonomic symptoms may or may not reflect a disorder of the autonomic nervous system. Panic disorder (Chapter 369), for example, manifests its symptoms through a normally functioning autonomic nervous system. Some patients have a functional dysautonomia, in which a medical or psychosomatic condition impairs normal autonomic function in the absence of a known structural neurologic deficit. Examples include neurally mediated syncope (Chapter 56), irritable bowel syndrome (Chapter 128), and some forms of orthostatic intolerance and pain.

DIAGNOSIS

Clinical evaluation of autonomic dysfunction begins with a detailed history. Autonomic disorders are quite diverse, so it is helpful to recognize which organ systems are affected; distinguish whether symptoms and signs are the result of hypofunction or hyperfunction; probe for factors that make symptoms better or worse; and then to gauge the evolution, severity, and impact of symptoms on the patient's daily function. Progressive or episodic phenomena must be distinguished from chronic and stable conditions.

Bedside Evaluation

Blood pressure and heart rate should be measured with the patient resting supine and again after standing for 1 to 3 minutes and correlated with symptoms. Orthostatic hypotension is defined as a reduction in systolic blood pressure of at least 20 mm Hg or a reduction in diastolic blood pressure of at least 10 mm Hg, with or without symptoms, within 1 to 3 minutes of assuming an erect posture. Measurements taken immediately on standing can be misleading, because healthy young persons without orthostatic hypotension will sometimes exhibit transient hypotension that resolves within 30 seconds of standing. Neurogenic orthostatic hypotension is typically sustained with continued standing. Except in patients treated with β-blockers, orthostatic hypotension without reflex tachycardia is evidence of generalized adrenergic failure. If reflex tachycardia occurs, dehydration or excessive venous pooling should be considered.

Some patients with orthostatic intolerance on standing experience an abnormal rise in heart rate rather than a drop in blood pressure. Postural tachycardia syndrome[9] is defined as a sustained increase in heart rate by more than 30 beats per minute in adults (40 beats per minute in adolescents) and often greater than 120 beats per minute when standing.

Laboratory Evaluation

Appropriate laboratory testing depends on the type and distribution of autonomic dysfunction. Investigations may include a complete blood cell count, fasting glucose, electrolytes, morning cortisol, thyroid function testing, vitamin B_{12} level, serum protein electrophoresis, and, when indicated, autoimmune markers.

In a patient with an autonomic neuropathy, seropositivity for antibodies to the alpha-3 ganglionic neuronal acetylcholine receptor is diagnostic of autoimmune autonomic ganglionopathy. The most sensitive screening test for pheochromocytoma is the plasma free metanephrine level (Chapter 215). Manometry and scintigraphic studies are useful in the diagnosis of GI dysmotility. Postvoiding residual volumes or urodynamic studies can clarify patterns of urinary bladder dysfunction (Chapter 23). Suspected amyloidosis may require biopsy (Chapter 179).

Ambulatory blood pressure testing (Chapter 70), usually over a period of 24 hours, is useful to detect patterns of nocturnal hypertension, postprandial hypotension, and the labile hypertension of baroreflex failure. Adrenergic function is assessed by tilt table testing (Chapter 56) or beat-to-beat blood pressure responses to the Valsalva maneuver. Cardiovagal function is assessed by analyzing heart rate variability. Sudomotor dysfunction, which is often a sign of autonomic involvement in small fiber neuropathies,[10] can be assessed functionally by quantitative sudomotor axon reflex testing or structurally by epidermal biopsy examining nerve fiber density.

TREATMENT ℞

Treatment begins with educating patients about the underlying physiology, helping them avoid exacerbations, and managing their symptoms. Elderly patients may be able to use regular physical exercise to compensate for some of the age-associated decline in autonomic function. Efforts at treating the underlying cause of an autonomic neuropathy should be pursued. Good control of glucose in patients with diabetes mellitus (Chapter 216) reduces the rate of complications, including neuropathy.

Medications are not always indicated. In some cases, prescribed medications or over-the-counter supplements are the cause of autonomic symptoms and should be scrutinized carefully. Hyperhidrosis may improve with reduction or elimination of opioids or serotonin reuptake inhibitors. Anhidrosis may improve with the discontinuation of any medications with anticholinergic effects.

In treating orthostatic hypotension, the first step is to reduce, or eliminate, if appropriate, antihypertensive, diuretic, or α-receptor antagonist medications. The goals of treatment are to increase the time the patient is able to stand without developing orthostatic symptoms, while simultaneously avoiding excessive recumbent hypertension. Mild orthostatic hypotension often responds to conservative measures such as increasing oral hydration (2 to 2.5 L/day), drinking sports beverages, and adding dietary salt or sodium tablets to increase daily salt intake to 10 to 20 g. Prolonged bedrest and medications that could potentially exacerbate orthostatic hypotension should be avoided if possible. Elevating the head of the bed by inserting 4-inch blocks under the head posts can improve orthostatic tolerance in some patients by reducing nocturnal natriuresis and stimulating the release of renin. Water bolus treatment (drinking 16 oz. of water) can increase systolic blood pressure in patients with orthostatic hypotension by 20 mm Hg for 1 to 2 hours by a sympathetic reflex.[11] Education about physical countermaneuvers (leg crossing, squatting, bending forward, or placing one foot on a chair) can help patients increase venous return to the heart and improve orthostatic tolerance by activating leg muscles. Compressive stockings (which may be poorly tolerated in warm climates) are effective if they are tightly fitting, and abdominal compression is also helpful. Postprandial hypotension may be managed by dividing meals to avoid large carbohydrate loads.

For the treatment of severe neurogenic orthostatic hypotension, two drugs currently are approved: midodrine (5 to 10 mg three times daily), which constricts capacitance vessels,[A1] and droxidopa (100 to 600 mg three times daily), which is an orally active synthetic precursor of norepinephrine.[A2] Frequently used, but not currently approved by the U.S. Food and Drug Administration, are fludrocortisone (0.1 to 0.4 mg/day) to expand plasma volume and sensitize peripheral vascular α-adrenergic receptors,[A3] and pyridostigmine (30 to 60 mg two to three times daily) to enhance sympathetic ganglionic outflow.[A4] Pyridostigmine has a more modest pressor effect but is less problematic in terms of supine hypertension. These pharmacologic measures are of variable benefit, and some patients stop taking them because of lack of symptomatic improvement or the development of adverse reactions.[12] Aldose reductase inhibitors (e.g., epalrestat [50 mg three times daily]) may provide some benefit for patients with diabetic cardiovascular autonomic neuropathy. Tafamidis, a transthyretin stabilizer at 20 mg daily, has demonstrated safety and efficacy in slowing the progression of the hereditary transthyretin amyloid neuropathy,[A5] and patisiran (an RNA interference agent at 0.3 mg/kg every 3 weeks) is also effective for such patients.[A6]

Nocturnal hypertension may be minimized by avoiding pressor agents within several hours of bedtime and by elevating the head of the bed. In severe cases, bedtime clonidine (0.1 mg), hydralazine (25 mg), nifedipine (10 mg), amlodipine (2.5 to 5 mg), or a nitroglycerin patch (0.1 mg/hour) may be needed. Paroxysmal hypertension in patients with arterial baroreflex denervation may improve on clonidine (0.1 mg three times daily orally or by transdermal patch).

PROGNOSIS

The prognosis depends on the nature of the autonomic disorder. Among patients with pure autonomic failure, about one third will develop dementia with Lewy bodies, Parkinson disease, or multiple system atrophy within the next 5 or so years.[13] Hospital admission for orthostatic hypotension increases the subsequent likelihood of death by about 15%, even after adjusting for other known risk factors.[14]

The most grave diagnoses are amyloid autonomic neuropathy, which portends a median survival of less than 1 year, and multiple system atrophy, which carries an estimated life expectancy of 7 to 9 years. Diabetic cardiovascular autonomic neuropathy is associated with an approximately two-fold increased risk for silent myocardial ischemia and overall mortality.

Regional Sympathetic Dysfunction

Regional sympathetic dysfunction may accompany the pain that sometimes follows peripheral nerve injuries. For example, sympathetic activation can occur as a normal physiologic response to any painful state.

Complex regional pain syndrome is characterized by severe ongoing neuropathic pain that is disproportionate in intensity, duration, and distribution to the expected sequela of limb trauma.[15] About 80% of affected patients are female, and about 70% of cases affect the upper limbs.[16] In this syndrome, allodynia (pain in response to normally nonpainful stimuli, such as light touch or cold) or hyperalgesia (increased sensitivity to painful stimuli) accompany cutaneous vasomotor or sudomotor abnormalities. The vasomotor changes are manifested as vasodilation with a warm, red, or swollen limb, or alternatively as vasoconstriction with a cold pale limb. The sudomotor findings range from regional hyperhidrosis to anhidrosis. Regional dystrophic changes, such as dry atrophic skin, sparse or coarse hair, brittle nails, and osteopenia, may also develop. Although sympathetic dysfunction may be pronounced, it does not appear to cause the pain. The mechanisms of pain and sympathetic dysfunction in this condition are incompletely understood and may result from crosstalk among aberrantly regenerated peripheral nerve fibers, expression of a new α-adrenergic receptors on sensory nerve fibers and sweat glands, release of substance P and pro-inflammatory peptides at the site of injury, and sensitization of pain-mediating structures at multiple levels within the central nervous system.

Mobilization of the affected limb is of paramount importance in the early treatment of complex regional pain syndrome. A primary goal of analgesic medication or regional anesthesia in early treatment is to facilitate participation in physical therapy, which can be helpful.[A7] Small studies have reported improvement with the use of bisphosphonates (e.g., alendronate, 40 mg orally or 7.5 mg intravenously daily), steroids (e.g., prednisone, 40 mg daily, or methylprednisolone, 8 mg four times daily initially and then tapered), dimethyl sulfoxide (50% cream one to four times daily), epidural clonidine (300 to 700 μg daily), intrathecal baclofen (25 to 75 μg daily), and epidural spinal cord stimulation. Intravenous immunoglobulin (0.5 g/kg) is not effective.[A8]

Grade A References

A1. Izcovich A, Gonzalez Malla C, Manzotti M, et al. Midodrine for orthostatic hypotension and recurrent reflex syncope: a systematic review. *Neurology.* 2014;83:1170-1177.

A2. Strassheim V, Newton JL, Tan MP, et al. Droxidopa for orthostatic hypotension: a systematic review and meta-analysis. *J Hypertens.* 2016;34:1933-1941.

A3. Schreglmann SR, Buchele F, Sommerauer M, et al. Pyridostigmine bromide versus fludrocortisone in the treatment of orthostatic hypotension in Parkinson's disease—a randomized controlled trial. *Eur J Neurol.* 2017;24:545-551.

A4. Byun JI, Moon J, Kim DY, et al. Efficacy of single or combined midodrine and pyridostigmine in orthostatic hypotension. *Neurology.* 2017;89:1078-1086.

A5. Waddington Cruz M, Amass L, Keohane D, et al. Early intervention with tafamidis provides long-term (5.5-year) delay of neurologic progression in transthyretin hereditary amyloid polyneuropathy. *Amyloid.* 2016;23:178-183.

A6. Adams D, Gonzalez-Duarte A, O'Riordan WD, et al. Patisiran, an RNAi therapeutic, for hereditary transthyretin amyloidosis. *N Engl J Med.* 2018;379:11-21.

A7. Smart KM, Wand BM, O'Connell NE. Physiotherapy for pain and disability in adults with complex regional pain syndrome (CRPS) types I and II. *Cochrane Database Syst Rev.* 2016;2:CD010853.

A8. Goebel A, Bisla J, Carganillo R, et al. Low-dose intravenous immunoglobulin treatment for long-standing complex regional pain syndrome: a randomized trial. *Ann Intern Med.* 2017;167:476-483.

GENERAL REFERENCES

For the General References and other additional features, please visit Expert Consult at https://expertconsult.inkling.com.

391

AMYOTROPHIC LATERAL SCLEROSIS AND OTHER MOTOR NEURON DISEASES

PAMELA J. SHAW AND MERIT E. CUDKOWICZ

DEFINITION

The motor neuron diseases (Table 391-1) are a heterogeneous group of disorders in which selective loss of function of upper motor neurons, lower motor neurons, or both results in impairment of the nervous system's control of voluntary movement.[1] The most common acquired motor neuron disease, amyotrophic lateral sclerosis (ALS), is a combined upper and lower motor neuron disorder. The features of lower motor neuron involvement are muscle wasting, fasciculations, and flaccid weakness, with normal or depressed tendon reflexes. Upper motor neuron dysfunction may cause increased muscle tone, clonus, weakness in a pyramidal distribution, and extensor plantar responses. Recent advances in the molecular genetics of hereditary motor neuron diseases have improved their classification and enhanced the careful diagnosis that is essential for genetic counseling, guidance, treatment, and advising patients about prognosis.

TABLE 391-1 CLASSIFICATION OF MOTOR NEURON DISORDERS

COMBINED UPPER AND LOWER MOTOR NEURON DISORDERS

Amyotrophic lateral sclerosis
  Familial adult onset
  Familial juvenile onset
  Sporadic
  ALS-plus syndromes
    ALS with frontotemporal dementia
    Western Pacific ALS–parkinsonism-dementia complex

UPPER MOTOR NEURON DISORDERS

Primary lateral sclerosis
Hereditary spastic paraplegias
Neurolathyrism
Konzo

LOWER MOTOR NEURON DISORDERS

Hereditary
  Spinal muscular atrophies (SMAs)
    Proximal autosomal recessive SMA (associated with *SMN* mutations) types I to IV
    Other forms of SMA not associated with *SMN* mutations
    Distal spinal muscular atrophies/hereditary motor neuronopathies
      Kennedy disease (X-linked spinobulbar neuronopathy)
      Hexosaminidase deficiency (GM2 gangliosidosis)
Acquired
  Monomelic focal and segmental spinal muscular atrophies
  Multifocal motor neuropathies
  Acute motor axonal neuropathy (AMAN)
  Postpolio syndrome
  Postirradiation syndrome
Infective disorders
  Acute poliomyelitis
  West Nile fever
  Other viral infections (e.g., enterovirus 71 and rabies virus)
  Human immunodeficiency virus–associated motor neuron disorder
  Lyme disease
  Creutzfeldt-Jakob disease (amyotrophic forms)

DISORDERS OF THE BULBAR MOTOR SYSTEM

Kennedy disease (X-linked bulbospinal neuronopathy)
Brown-Vialetto-Van Laere syndrome
Fazio-Londe disease

TOXIC DISORDERS OF THE MOTOR NEURON

Neurolathyrism
Konzo
Heavy metal toxicity (lead, mercury)
Western Pacific ALS–parkinsonism-dementia complex
Postirradiation motor neuron injury

DISORDERS OF MOTOR NEURON OVERACTIVITY

Neuromyotonia
Stiff person syndrome

MISCELLANEOUS MOTOR NEURON DISORDERS

Endocrinopathies (e.g., hyperthyroidism, hyperparathyroidism, hypoglycemia)
Copper deficiency syndrome
Benign cramp-fasciculation syndrome

AMYOTROPHIC LATERAL SCLEROSIS

EPIDEMIOLOGY

ALS is a neurodegenerative disorder that causes progressive injury and cell death of lower motor neurons in the brain stem and spinal cord, as well as upper motor neurons in the motor cortex.[2] ALS has an incidence of about 2 per 100,000 and a prevalence of 6 to 8 per 100,000. The global incidence is fairly uniform, with the exception of a few high-incidence foci such as the Western Pacific island of Guam. The disease affects predominantly middle-aged and elderly individuals, with a mean age at onset of 55 to 60 years, although younger individuals can also be affected. Increasing age, male sex (male/female ratio ≈ 1.6 : 1), and genetic susceptibility are the only proven risk factors, although ongoing research is assessing the effects of athleticism/physical exercise and other potential environmental risk factors. Approximately 90%

of cases of ALS occur sporadically, but 5 to 10% are familial, usually with an autosomal dominant mode of inheritance.

The process of neuronal degeneration in ALS is complex, and more than 40 ALS susceptibility genes have been identified. GGGGCC hexanucleotide intronic expansions in the chromosome 9 *C9ORF72* gene are the most common genetic cause of ALS identified to date, accounting for up to 40 to 50% of familial ALS cases and 7 to 10% of sporadic ALS. Accumulating evidence suggests that defective RNA processing likely plays a key role in the pathogenesis of *C9ORF72* ALS as well as other genetic subtypes. The pathobiology of C9-ALS is not yet completely understood, but the sequestration of RNA binding proteins by RNA foci and altered nucleocytoplasmic transport that allows the expansion RNA to translate into dipeptide repeat proteins in the cytoplasm are clearly of key importance.[3]

The subtype of disease caused by *SOD1* mutations accounts for 20% of familial ALS cases and 2% of ALS overall. Mutant *SOD1* appears to transmit templated propagation in a prion-like (Chapter 387)[4] fashion, with these aggregates then triggering a complex interplay of multiple pathogenic processes, including oxidative stress, protein aggregation, mitochondrial dysfunction, excitotoxicity, and impaired axonal transport. Non-neuronal cells in the vicinity of motor neurons may contribute importantly to neuronal injury. Genetically engineered mouse models of *SOD1*-related ALS have shown that normal astrocytes can protect motor neurons expressing mutant *SOD1* and that removing the expression of mutant *SOD1* from microglia or astrocytes slows the progression of disease in these murine models. Astrocytes expressing mutant *SOD1* exert toxic effects on neighboring motor neurons through as yet undefined mechanisms.

Familial motor neuron disease has been linked to mutations involving alsin, senataxin, angiogenin, *VAPB*, dynactin, *TARDBP, TBK1, FUS/TLS*, and multiple other genes.[5] Intermediate length polyQ expansions (27-33Q) in ataxin 2 are found as a risk factor for ALS in approximately 5% of patients. Associations have been reported with alterations in at least eight other genes in cases that appear sporadic. Large combined genome-wide association studies suggest that rare genetic variants underpin 15 to 20% of cases of sporadic ALS.[6]

Pathology

At autopsy, the gross pathologic features of ALS consist of atrophy of the cerebral precentral gyrus, as well as sclerosis and pallor of the corticospinal tracts of the spinal cord. Thinning of the hypoglossal nerves and ventral spinal roots may be observed, and muscle atrophy is obvious. Microscopically, ALS patients will typically have lost at least 50% of their spinal motor neurons and have diffuse astrocytic gliosis in the spinal gray matter. By comparison, motor neurons in Onuf nucleus in the sacral spinal cord (which innervate the pelvic floor muscles) and the motor nuclei of cranial nerves III, IV, and VI (which control eye movements) are relatively preserved. A cardinal feature in residual motor neurons is the presence of ubiquitinated proteinaceous inclusions, which may be compact or skeinlike. TDP-43 has been recognized as a major protein constituent of these aggregates. In the motor cortex, there is variable loss of upper motor neurons and astrocytic gliosis. In the descending corticospinal tracts, axonal loss, myelin pallor, and gliosis are seen. The atrophied skeletal muscle shows clusters of angular atrophic fibers and fiber-type grouping that results from serial denervation and reinnervation. The selectivity of the disease process for the motor system is now recognized to be relative, and involvement of extramotor parts of the central nervous system can be found, especially in the sensory and spinocerebellar pathways, substantia nigra neurons, and dentate granule cells in the hippocampus. In the ALS variant caused by C9ORF72 expansions, the characteristic extramotor system pathology demonstrates cerebellar and hippocampal inclusions that are P62+ and TDP-43-negative by immunostaining. Some of these inclusions comprise dipeptide proteins generated by aberrant translation of the G4C2 repeats.

ALS is characterized by a combination of upper and lower motor neuron degeneration. Lower motor neuron degeneration causes weakness, atrophy, and fasciculation of the limb and bulbar musculature. Features of upper motor neuron dysfunction include the incongruous presence of active or brisk tendon reflexes in a wasted limb, increased muscle tone, and sometimes the presence of Babinski sign. Upper motor neuron bulbar disease causes pseudobulbar palsy, with emotional lability, a brisk jaw jerk, slowing of repetitive tongue movements, and strained effortful speech. Fatigue and weight loss are also common symptoms. With end-stage disease, most patients will have features

of upper and lower motor neuron dysfunction affecting all four limbs and the bulbar musculature.

In approximately 75% of patients, the disease starts distally, focally, and asymmetrically in an upper or lower limb (Video 391-1), followed by progressive spread of injury in an anatomically logical progression to contiguous groups of motor neurons. Affected individuals may notice weakness, wasting or clumsiness of one hand, or unilateral footdrop. Muscle cramps may precede other clinical features, and fasciculations are most noticeable in the large proximal limb muscles. In the upper limbs, the thenar and intrinsic hand muscles tend to be severely affected, whereas the triceps and finger flexors are relatively spared until late in the disease. In the lower limbs, the pattern of weakness is often in a pyramidal distribution (flexors weaker than extensors), with early weakness of hip flexion and ankle dorsiflexion and severe involvement of the distal muscles.

Bulbar symptoms, which are the initial feature in approximately 25% of patients, are especially common in elderly women with ALS (Video 391-2). The first problem is usually slurring of speech, initially apparent only when the individual is tired. Patients often have a mixed spastic/flaccid dysarthria in which speech develops a tight strangled quality because of the upper motor neuron component, with a superimposed nasal quality as a result of the flaccid lower motor neuron weakness of the palate and nasopharynx. In patients with bulbar disease, examination often reveals weakness of the facial muscles; a spastic, weak, wasted, and fasciculating tongue; and a brisk jaw jerk. Dysphagia, initially more pronounced for liquids than for solids, usually follows the dysarthria within a few weeks or months (Video 391-3). Complications include weight loss and prolonged and arduous meal times with frequent episodes of coughing, drooling of saliva, and aspiration pneumonia.

Respiratory muscle weakness is rarely the initial feature of ALS. More commonly, respiratory muscle weakness develops insidiously and causes dyspnea and orthopnea. Diaphragmatic weakness may be apparent from the paradoxical movement of the abdominal wall during inspiration and a marked decline in forced vital capacity in the supine position. Symptoms of nocturnal carbon dioxide retention may develop, including interrupted sleep, morning headaches, anorexia, and daytime somnolence.

Neck muscle weakness, which is common later in the course of disease, causes difficulty holding the head upright (dropped head syndrome). Eye movements tend to be spared even in advanced disease, thereby permitting limited communication by movements of the eyes. Similarly, the strength of the pelvic floor muscles is relatively preserved, so patients with ALS usually remain continent throughout the course of the disease.

Overt features of frontotemporal dementia (Chapter 374), with progressive deterioration in personality and behavior, will develop in approximately 5% of patients with ALS.[7] Cognitive dysfunction may precede, follow, or coincide with the features of motor dysfunction. Up to 50% of ALS patients without overt dementia may show more subtle features of frontal lobe dysfunction. The C9ORF72-ALS variant causes both ALS and/or frontotemporal dementia (Chapter 374), and patients with this subtype of ALS are more likely to have cognitive disturbances as well as a family history of dementia or psychosis.

About 5 to 10% of ALS patients have the progressive muscular atrophy variant with clinical features reflecting only degeneration of lower motor neuron groups in the spinal cord. In primary lateral sclerosis, patients have pure upper motor neuron degeneration. Although severe spastic spinobulbar paresis ultimately develops in these patients, the duration of survival is commonly 10 to 15 years after the onset of symptoms. The progressive bulbar palsy variant usually progresses to involve the limbs, although limb signs may not be present initially.

Several ALS variants follow a more segmental pattern than is typical in ALS. Up to 10% of patients with ALS have flail arm syndrome, which is more common in men and is associated with a longer median survival than seen in those with typical ALS. A similar focal manifestation in the lower limbs, flail leg syndrome, is another recognized segmental variant.

The diagnosis of ALS is essentially clinical, and there currently is no specific diagnostic test. Nevertheless, biomarkers of motor neuron injury, including elevated levels of neurofilament light and phosphorylated neurofilament heavy in cerebrospinal fluid (CSF), have promise for the future.[8]

Diagnosis requires evidence of lower motor neuron degeneration by clinical, electrophysiologic (Chapter 368), or neuropathologic examination; upper motor neuron degeneration by clinical examination; and progressive spread of symptoms or signs within a region or to other regions, as determined by the history or examination. The diagnosis also requires the absence of other disease processes as determined by electrophysiologic testing, neuroimaging, and (if performed) biopsy. Generally accepted criteria (Table 391-2) classify patients as having definite, probable, or possible ALS. However, a number of other conditions may mimic ALS (Table 391-3), and about 8% of patients in whom ALS is initially diagnosed have other lower motor neuron syndromes, such as multifocal motor neuropathy with conduction block, Kennedy disease, or mixed spinal cord and root compression (Chapter 372). Conversely, 10 to 15% of patients in whom ALS is ultimately diagnosed may first undergo inappropriate surgery for presumed spinal cord or root compression abnormalities.

Blood tests that may be helpful in distinguishing ALS from mimic syndromes (see Table 391-3) include a complete blood count and serum calcium level, thyroid function tests, parathyroid hormone, serum protein electrophoresis, Venereal Disease Research Laboratory test, creatine kinase level, inflammatory markers (erythrocyte sedimentation rate and C-reactive protein), and levels of anti-GM1 ganglioside and anti–myelin-associated glycoprotein (MAG) antibodies. Further testing, which is guided by the patient's clinical findings, might include acetylcholine receptor antibody; mutation screening in patients with familial disease, suspected Kennedy disease, or spinal muscular atrophy (SMA); heavy metal screening; urinary porphyrins; serum hexosaminidase A and B levels; Borrelia titers; and testing for human immunodeficiency virus.

Typical features of ALS on electromyography (EMG) include evidence of active denervation (i.e., positive sharp waves, fibrillation, and fasciculation potentials) and chronic denervation, as evidenced by large motor unit potentials that cannot be explained by a single nerve, root, or plexus lesion. Neuroimaging of the brain and spinal cord is usually needed to exclude structural pathology.

Baseline respiratory function tests should be performed on all patients. Muscle biopsy is indicated only in atypical cases when diagnostic uncertainty persists.

TABLE 391-2 AWAJI-SHIMA CONSENSUS CRITERIA FOR DIAGNOSING AMYOTROPHIC LATERAL SCLEROSIS

The diagnosis of ALS requires:
1. Evidence of LMN loss (reduced interference pattern on full contraction and increased firing rate)
2. Evidence of reinnervation (motor units of large amplitude and longer duration)
3. Fibrillation and sharp waves or fasciculation potentials (fibrillation and sharp waves are required in weak limb muscles)

Number of muscles affected by region:
Cervical and lumbar-sacral region: a minimum of 2 muscles innervated by different roots and nerves
Bulbar and thoracic region: a minimum of 1 muscle

Diagnostic classification: Awaji-Shima Consensus Recommendations and the Revised El Escorial Criteria
Clinically definite ALS:
clinical or electrophysiologic evidence of the presence of LMN as well as UMN signs in the bulbar region and at least 2 spinal regions or the presence of LMN and UMN signs in 3 spinal regions
Clinically probable ALS:
clinical or electrophysiologic evidence of LMN and UMN signs in at least 2 regions, with some UMN signs necessarily rostral to (above) the LMN signs
Clinically possible ALS:
clinical or electrophysiologic signs of UMN and LMN dysfunction are found in only 1 region, or UMN signs are found alone in ≥2 regions, or LMN signs are found rostral to UMN signs.

ALS = amyotrophic lateral sclerosis; LMN = lower motor neuron; UMN = upper motor neuron.
UMN signs: clonus, Babinski sign, absent abdominal reflexes, hypertonia, loss of dexterity.
LMN signs: atrophy, weakness. If only fasciculation, search with EMG for active denervation.
Regions reflect segmental motor neuron pools: bulbar, cervical, thoracic, and lumbosacral.
Adapted from Costa J, Swash M, de Carvalho M. Awaji criteria for the diagnosis of amyotrophic lateral sclerosis: a systematic review. *Arch Neurol.* 2012;69:1410-1416.

TABLE 391-3 DISORDERS THAT CAN MIMIC AMYOTROPHIC LATERAL SCLEROSIS/MOTOR NEURON DISEASE

FORM OF MOTOR NEURON DISEASE	MIMIC SYNDROMES	CLINICAL CLUES
Progressive muscular atrophy (PMA)/LMN-predominant phenotype	Multifocal motor neuropathy	Weakness out of proportion to wasting. Neurophysiology identifies conduction block. Anti-GM1 antibodies may be raised.
	Kennedy disease	Gynecomastia, distal sensory features, perioral fasciculation, indolent progression.
	Spinal muscular atrophy	SMA can be adult onset. Pure LMN syndrome. Slower progression than PMA. Probably no family history.
	Chronic idiopathic demyelinating polyneuropathy	Electrophysiology identifies peripheral nerve demyelination.
	Benign cramp-fasciculation syndrome	Predominantly middle-aged men. Largely calf involvement. Failure to progress. No active denervation on EMG.
	Postpolio syndrome	Pure LMN syndrome. Past history of an illness compatible with poliomyelitis. Indolent progression.
	Lead poisoning	Extramotor clinical features, e.g., constipation, nail and buccal signs.
	Acute motor axonal neuropathy (AMAN—a Guillain-Barré syndrome variant)	Acute onset, with progression ceasing after a few weeks. Nerve conduction studies show features of motor axonopathy.
	Hereditary motor neuropathies	Pure LMN syndrome. Family history, clinical signs indicating chronicity, slower rate of progression.
	Porphyria	Extramotor clinical features, family history, episodic exacerbations.
	Compressive focal motor neuropathies	Pure motor disorders can result from compression of the deep palmar branch of the ulnar nerve and posterior interosseous branch of the radial nerve. Failure to extend beyond territory of one nerve. Electrophysiology with or without imaging helpful.
Amyotrophic lateral sclerosis	Multilevel spinal cord and root compression by discs, osteophytes, or tumor	Sensory symptoms and pain are common. UMN signs often caudal to LMN signs.
	Thyrotoxicosis	Systemic symptoms and signs.
	Combined peripheral neuropathy and cervical myelopathy	MRI of the spine and electrophysiology will differentiate.
	Inclusion body myositis	Rarer than ALS. Characteristic pattern of weakness with early involvement of the long finger flexors and quadriceps.
	Paraneoplastic syndromes, especially lymphoma	History of malignancy or systemic features.
	Sjögren syndrome	Non–motor-related symptoms.
	Radiation myelopathy	History of radiotherapy.
	Structural lesions of the bulbar region (e.g., tumor of the tongue base)	Pain, failure of features to extend outside the bulbar territory.
Primary lateral sclerosis	Hereditary spastic paraplegia	Family history. Symptoms rarely extend beyond the lower limb territory. Prominent bladder dysfunction.
	Multiple sclerosis	Non–motor-related symptoms and signs (e.g., eye, bladder, cerebellar, and sensory involvement).
	Spinal cord compression by disc or tumor	Pain and sensory involvement usually present.

ALS = amyotrophic lateral sclerosis; EMG = electromyography; LMN = lower motor neuron; MRI = magnetic resonance imaging; SMA = spinal muscular atrophy; UMN = upper motor neuron.

TREATMENT   Rx

ALS is best managed in specialized centers that offer multidisciplinary care. Teams typically include a neurologist, nurse specialist, occupational therapist, physical therapist, speech and language therapist, and dietitian. During the course of the disease, patients frequently require referral for placement of a gastrostomy tube[9] and to provide respiratory support.[10]

There currently is no therapy that stops the progression of ALS.[11] Riluzole, a sodium channel blocker whose primary mechanism of action is to reduce excitotoxicity through inhibition of presynaptic glutamate release, prolongs survival by approximately 3 months when given at 50 mg twice daily.[A1] It may cause fatigue, nausea, and dizziness, but these effects are frequently transient. Liver function tests should be performed at baseline and monthly for the first 3 months of therapy. Edaravone (an intravenous injection, initially daily for 14 days, then 14 days off, and then given as cycles thereafter) is an antioxidant that is approved in Japan, South Korea, and the United States; it can slow the progression of disease by approximately one third in patients with early ALS and a preserved vital capacity.[A2] Other phase III trials of potential neuroprotective therapies have so far proved negative. New experimental approaches include gene therapy and antisense oligonucleotide technology to reduce the expression of disease-causing genes, small molecules to improve muscle contraction, and cell-based therapy aimed primarily at providing a supportive environment to prolong the survival of endogenous motor neurons.

Good clinical care must focus on symptoms and preservation of independence and quality of life. In one randomized trial, mexiletine (300 mg/day) resulted in large dose-dependent reductions in the frequency and severity of muscle cramps.[A3] In patients with progressive bulbar problems, optimal positioning, attention to food and fluid consistency, and protective swallowing techniques are helpful. Nuedexta (a combination of 20 mg dextromethorphan and 10 mg quinidine once daily) has been shown to improve symptoms of pseudobulbar affect (inappropriate tearfulness and laughter) and is also currently under study for symptoms of swallowing and speech dysfunction.[A4] If weight loss continues, high-calorie nutritional supplements are added between meals. In ALS patients with dysphagia due to upper motor neuron impairment of the upper esophageal sphincter, local injection of botulinum toxin type A can significantly improve the dysphagia and may represent an alternative to percutaneous endoscopic gastrostomy.[A5] Placement of a gastrostomy tube via endoscopy or under radiologic guidance is recommended in patients in whom dehydration, weight loss of 10 to 15%, frequent distressing choking episodes, prolonged and tiring mealtimes, or aspiration pneumonia develop. Tube placement is higher risk in patients with respiratory insufficiency. Tubes should ideally be placed before the patient's forced vital capacity falls below 50% of expected. Some evidence suggests that radiologically guided gastrostomy insertion may be safer in frail patients in the late stages of ALS.

Respiratory muscle weakness, which can develop insidiously during the course of ALS, causes breathlessness, orthopnea, daytime somnolence, morning headaches, and interrupted sleep. Management must emphasize detection and prevention of aspiration pneumonia, assistance in clearing of secretions by agents to reduce saliva production (e.g., anticholinergic drugs such as glycopyrrolate, 1 to 2 mg 3 to 4 times daily, or intrasalivary botulinum toxin injections), providing a suction machine, use of a mucolytic agent such as carbocisteine (in a dose of up to 750 mg three times daily), adoption of a semi-upright position for sleep, and aggressive antibiotic therapy for chest infection (Chapters 90 and 91). A small dose of sublingual lorazepam (0.5 to 1 mg) may be useful if the dyspnea is accompanied by extreme anxiety; opiate therapy (e.g., morphine, diamorphine, fentanyl [Chapter 27, Table 27-4]) may be given orally, transdermally, or by subcutaneous infusion to relieve respiratory distress during the later stages of the disease.

As respiratory function worsens, noninvasive ventilation can alleviate symptoms of chronic hypoventilation, significantly improve quality of life, and prolong survival,[A6] especially in patients with orthopnea, daytime hypercapnia, and nocturnal oxygen desaturation. Full 24-hour ventilation via a tracheostomy is an option that is chosen uncommonly by fully informed patients. Diaphragm muscle pacing appears to worsen the course of the disease in ALS.[A7] Ongoing clinical research is evaluating the value of cough assist devices as well as the optimal way to manage respiratory symptoms at the end of life. An experimental fully implanted brain-computer interface has allowed communication at the equivalent of two letters per minute in a locked-in patient with ALS. Palliative care teams and hospices can contribute substantially to the care of ALS patients in the later stages of the disease. In the absence of ventilatory support, ALS patients will almost always die in their sleep from hypercapnic coma. In the terminal phases (Chapter 3), the aim of treatment is to ensure comfort by prescribing opiates and anxiolytic medications as required to alleviate discomfort or distress.

PROGNOSIS

Clinical features associated with a worse prognosis include older age at onset of symptoms, compromise of respiratory function,[12] bulbar symptoms, and more rapid presentation to medical attention. The mean duration from the onset of symptoms to death in patients with sporadic ALS ranges from 27 to 43 months. The average 5-year survival rate is 25%, and approximately 5% of patients will survive for more than 10 years. The usual cause of death is respiratory failure, which may be accompanied by bronchopneumonia.

● SPINAL MUSCULAR ATROPHIES

DEFINITION

The term *spinal muscular atrophy* encompasses a group of pure lower motor neuron disorders that cause progressive symmetrical muscle weakness and wasting. Because the bulbar musculature may be affected, an alternative term, *hereditary motor neuronopathy*, has been proposed. The time of onset is variable and ranges from in utero to adult life.

EPIDEMIOLOGY AND PATHOBIOLOGY

The most common type of SMA is caused by mutations in the survival motor neuron (*SMN*) gene and is inherited as an autosomal recessive disorder. The estimated carrier frequency of an *SMN* mutation is 1 in 50. Type 1 SMA (Werdnig-Hoffmann disease) has an incidence of 1 in 8000 births. SMA is divided into subtypes I to IV according to age at onset and severity of the phenotype.

The human *SMN* gene on chromosome 5q13 exists in two forms, with 5–base pair differences between *SMN1* and its centromeric homologue *SMN2*. A change in exon 7 of *SMN2* leads to skipping of exon 7, and as a result, 80% of the protein encoded by *SMN2* is truncated and nonfunctional rather than full length. The majority of patients with SMA have homozygous absence of *SMN1* exon 7, but *SMN1* may be replaced by a copy of *SMN2* during DNA replication by a process known as gene conversion. An individual may have one to four copies of *SMN2*, with a proportional increase in the amount of full-length SMN protein. A molecular basis for the wide variation in the phenotypic severity of SMA, which can range from in utero onset (SMA type I) to adult onset (SMA type IV), is the number of copies of *SMN2* and the SMN protein levels, although other disease-modifying factors have also been implicated.

The SMN protein oligomerizes and associates with other proteins to form the SMN complex, which in turn has an important role in the assembly of spliceosomal small nuclear ribonucleoproteins that have a function in pre-mRNA splicing in the nucleus. These cellular processes are ubiquitous, so either the clinical features of SMA may be caused by a particular susceptibility of lower motor neurons to defects in RNA processing or SMN may have functions that are specific to the motor neuron, including axonal transport of mRNA molecules essential for the health of the distal axon. Recent work has highlighted the role of dysregulation of ubiquitin homeostasis and β-catenin signaling, as well as genes involved in motor neuron synaptogenesis in the pathophysiology of SMA.

At autopsy, patients with SMA have atrophic spinal cords with loss of α-motor neurons and evidence of motor neuron degeneration and gliosis. The ventral roots are atrophic, and muscle atrophy is apparent with microscopic evidence of denervation and reinnervation.

CLINICAL MANIFESTATIONS

Type I SMA (Werdnig-Hoffman disease) is characterized by severe generalized muscle weakness and hypotonia at birth or by the age of 6 months; affected children never sit or walk. Type II is an intermediate form with an onset of muscle weakness before the age of 18 months; patients can sit but are never able to walk unaided. Type III SMA (Wohlfart-Kugelberg-Welander disease) appears after 18 months of age; patients acquire the ability to stand and walk but often become wheelchair dependent in adolescence or adult life, although life expectancy is normal. Patients with type IV SMA have an onset of muscle weakness in adult life.

DIAGNOSIS

The diagnosis of SMA caused by changes in *SMN* can be made by genetic testing in a patient with appropriate clinical signs and symptoms; 95% of affected individuals have *SMN* deletions. Prenatal diagnosis is available. Electrophysiology and muscle biopsy reveal evidence of denervation.

Other disorders can present in infancy or childhood as hypotonia, and a pattern of weakness similar to *SMN*-related SMA can be distinguished by associated clinical features such as early respiratory distress or vocal cord paralysis, or an atypical distribution of motor features such as upper limb– or lower limb–predominant or scapuloperoneal involvement. The etiologic relationship of these disorders to classic SMA can be clarified by testing for *SMN* mutations.

It is important to distinguish SMA type I from infantile botulism, which can have a similar initial clinical picture. EMG with high-frequency repetitive nerve stimulation shows a decrement in botulism, and testing for the presence of botulinum toxin can confirm the diagnosis (Chapter 280). SMA II and SMA III can be distinguished from chronic inflammatory demyelinating polyneuropathy (Chapter 392) by the presence of normal CSF protein and normal nerve conduction studies in SMA. Patients with SMA type III can have clinical features that are similar to those of the hereditary motor and sensory neuropathies, but it can be distinguished by neurophysiologic assessment and genetic testing.

TREATMENT AND PROGNOSIS Rx

Approaches to upregulate expression of the SMN protein include the intravenous infusion of an adenoviral vector that contains the DNA that codes for SMN.[13] Nusinersen (an antisense oligonucleotide drug that modifies the pre–messenger RNA splicing of the *SMN2* gene) promotes increased production of full-length SMN protein and improves motor function in infants and children with spinal muscular atrophy.[A8][A9]

Children with SMA may benefit from passive and active physical therapy, lightweight braces, surgical correction of scoliosis, and respiratory support measures. Untreated patients with type I SMA usually die by the age of 18 months, untreated patients with type II typically survive into adolescence, and patients with type III and type IV have a normal life expectancy. New treatments hold great promise for changing this prognosis.[14]

SPINOBULBAR MUSCULAR ATROPHY/KENNEDY DISEASE

EPIDEMIOLOGY

Kennedy disease, or spinobulbar muscular atrophy (SBMA), is an X-linked degenerative disorder of the lower motor neurons. Though rare, it is important not to miss the diagnosis because of the genetic implications for the family and a more benign course than occurs with ALS. The diagnosis should be considered in any male patient with a pure lower motor neuron disorder, particularly when the disease course is relatively indolent, gynecomastia is present, or there is evidence of a mild accompanying sensory neuropathy.

PATHOBIOLOGY

SBMA is a trinucleotide repeat disorder in which a CAG expansion encodes for a polyglutamine tract in the first exon of the androgen receptor gene on chromosome Xq11-12. The androgen receptor, which contains three functional domains, is transported to the nucleus, where it binds to DNA and acts as a transcription factor. Expansion of the polyglutamine tract results in reduced target gene transactivation, and neurodegeneration occurs when the polyglutamine tract reaches a critical length of approximately 40 repeats. The neurodegeneration in patients with SBMA is considered to result from a ligand-dependent toxic gain of function of the mutant androgen receptor protein. Complete loss of its function, as seen in testicular feminization syndrome (Chapter 220), does not lead to motor neuron degeneration. The toxicity has not been fully characterized, but protein aggregation, impairment of protein degradation pathways, disruption of gene transcription, impairment of axonal transport, and altered neurotrophic factor signaling may all contribute.

Pathologic examination reveals mild spinal cord atrophy with ventral horn gliosis and loss of α-motor neurons. Misfolding of the polyglutamine (Q)–expanded protein leads to the formation of nuclear inclusions that contain the amino-terminal epitopes of the mutant androgen receptor within motor neurons and certain non-neuronal tissues.

CLINICAL MANIFESTATIONS AND DIAGNOSIS

The mean age at onset of SBMA is 30 years, with a range of 15 to 60 years, and the severity of the disease and its age at onset correlate with the size of the repeat expansion. Initial symptoms consist of hand tremors, fasciculations, and muscle cramps, followed by progressive weakness and atrophy of the limb and bulbar muscles. Limb muscle weakness tends to be proximal and predominantly involves the lower limbs. There are no clinical signs of upper motor neuron dysfunction. Weakness of the lower facial and tongue muscles causes dysarthria, and jaw weakness may cause the mouth to hang open. The presence of perioral fasciculations with quivering of the chin is a characteristic feature. Pharyngeal involvement can cause dysphagia, and respiratory muscle weakness causes breathlessness. Mild distal sensory loss is frequently present in the lower limbs. Features of mild androgen insensitivity are frequent: gynecomastia, testicular atrophy, and erectile dysfunction. Heterozygous female carriers of SBMA may show mild clinical manifestations of the disease.

EMG and muscle biopsy, which are often performed because the creatine kinase level tends to be elevated, reveal evidence of chronic denervation. Genetic screening for the CAG repeat expansion in exon 1 of the androgen receptor gene is diagnostic.

TREATMENT AND PROGNOSIS Rx

Because there are no established disease-modifying therapies for SBMA, current therapy consists of supportive care to prevent complications. The course of the disease is slowly progressive in comparison to ALS and is compatible with normal life expectancy, although some patients may die of respiratory failure. Patients may become wheelchair dependent over a period of 2 to 3 decades, but some remain ambulatory until late in life.

Grade A References

A1. Miller RG, Mitchell JD, Moore DH. Riluzole for amyotrophic lateral sclerosis (ALS)/motor neuron disease (MND). *Cochrane Database Syst Rev.* 2012;2:CD001447.
A2. Writing Group; Edaravone (MCI-186) ALS 19 Study Group. Safety and efficacy of edaravone in well defined patients with amyotrophic lateral sclerosis: a randomised, double-blind, placebo-controlled trial. *Lancet Neurol.* 2017;16:505-512.
A3. Weiss MD, Macklin EA, Simmons Z, et al. A randomized trial of mexiletine in ALS: safety and effects on muscle cramps and progression. *Neurology.* 2016;86:1474-1481.
A4. Smith R, Pioro E, Myers K, et al. Enhanced bulbar function in amyotrophic lateral sclerosis: the nuedexta treatment trial. *Neurother.* 2017;14:762-772.
A5. Restivo DA, Casabona A, Nicotra A, et al. ALS dysphagia pathophysiology: differential botulinum toxin response. *Neurology.* 2013;80:616-620.
A6. Radunovic A, Annane D, Rafiq MK, et al. Mechanical ventilation for amyotrophic lateral sclerosis/motor neuron disease. *Cochrane Database Syst Rev.* 2017;10:CD004427.
A7. Gonzalez-Bermejo J, Morélot-Panzini C, Tanguy ML, et al. Early diaphragm pacing in patients with amyotrophic lateral sclerosis (RespiStimALS): a randomised controlled triple-blind trial. *Lancet Neurol.* 2016;15:1217-1227.
A8. Finkel RS, Mercuri E, Darras BT, et al. Nusinersen versus sham control in infantile-onset spinal muscular atrophy. *N Engl J Med.* 2017;377:1723-1732.
A9. Mercuri E, Darras BT, Chiriboga CA, et al. Nusinersen versus sham control in later-onset spinal muscular atrophy. *N Engl J Med.* 2018;378:625-635.

GENERAL REFERENCES

For the General References and other additional features, please visit Expert Consult at https://expertconsult.inkling.com.

392

PERIPHERAL NEUROPATHIES

GORDON SMITH AND MICHAEL E. SHY

APPROACH TO PERIPHERAL NEUROPATHY

The term *peripheral neuropathy* is used to describe a group of disorders that share in common injury to the peripheral nervous system, which encompasses the final pathways of motor, sensory, and autonomic function.[1]

EPIDEMIOLOGY

As a group, peripheral neuropathies are among the most common neurologic problems encountered in medical practice. The prevalence of peripheral neuropathy increases with age from 2 to 3% in individuals who are 50 to 60 years of age to 13% among individuals who are 70 to 80 years of age and greater than 30% among individuals over age 80 years. The age-adjusted population prevalence of peripheral polyneuropathy in the United States is 9%.[2] The most common cause of polyneuropathy is diabetes, which accounts for approximately 50% of cases. Most of the remainder have cryptogenic sensory peripheral neuropathy, although over 50% of this population has prediabetes. Other common causes of neuropathy include genetic, inflammatory, metabolic, and toxic etiologies.[3]

PATHOBIOLOGY

Motor neurons extend from their cell body in the ventral horn of the spinal cord through the ventral nerve roots and peripheral nerves to the neuromuscular junctions at the muscle that they innervate. The cell bodies of primary sensory neurons lie outside the spinal cord in the dorsal root ganglia, where they extend peripherally to specialized sensory end organs, including nociceptors (pain receptors), thermoreceptors, and mechanoreceptors. Central projections from dorsal root ganglia enter the spinal cord through the dorsal roots to carry sensory information to the central nervous system (CNS). At each spinal segment, the ventral roots, which carry motor axons, and the dorsal roots, which carry sensory axons, join to form mixed sensorimotor nerves. In the proximal upper and lower extremities, the mixed spinal nerves form the brachial and lumbar plexuses from which arise the major anatomically defined limb nerves. Each mixed nerve is composed of a spectrum of nerve fibers, damage to which causes specific but overlapping symptoms and signs. Large-diameter myelinated fibers are responsible for motor function, proprioception, and touch sensation, whereas small-diameter lightly myelinated and unmyelinated axons are responsible for pain and autonomic function. Preganglionic sympathetic autonomic fibers begin in the intermediolateral column of the spinal cord and synapse in ganglia of the sympathetic trunk. Preganglionic parasympathetic fibers travel long distances from their cell bodies in the brain stem or sacral spinal cord to reach terminal ganglia near the organs that the parasympathetic fibers innervate.

Although positive sensory symptoms occur with injury to both large- and small-diameter fibers, severe painful sensations, particularly burning, usually suggests preferential injury to small-diameter axons. Because motor axons are capable of reinnervating denervated muscle fibers via collateral sprouting, weakness does not develop in axonal neuropathies until about 50% of axons have been injured.

CLINICAL MANIFESTATIONS

The clinical features of a peripheral neuropathy are dependent on the involved regions. Most patients with peripheral neuropathy have a chronic axonal sensory greater than motor peripheral polyneuropathy and present with slowly progressive sensory symptoms.

Sensory and motor symptoms may be divided into negative (loss of function) and positive (abnormal function). Common negative sensory symptoms include a general sense of numbness or loss of sensation, such as feeling as if feet are "walking on pebbles" or "ice cold," difficulty determining whether bath water is hot or cold with the foot, and loss of balance, particularly in the dark when visual compensation is difficult. Positive symptoms include painful dysesthesias, such as feeling as though the feet are "on fire," "on hot coals," or "stuck with pins." If severe, the symptoms may reach the level of

the knee, at which point the fingers may become involved. Motor symptoms and signs are typically mild and limited to subtle weakness of toe extension and flexion, with atrophy of foot muscles. There may be mild gait instability that does not require the use of assistive devices. Foot ulceration is absent. Gait imbalance owing to a sensory ataxia (instability worse with eyes closed) indicates large fiber involvement or dysfunction of the dorsal columns of the spinal cord. Sensory ataxia involving the upper extremities is manifest by impaired coordination and finger-nose-finger testing that is worse with eyes closed, when there are often writhing, "pseudoathetoid" movements of the fingers with arms outstretched.

Involvement of motor nerves results in muscle weakness and, over time, atrophy. In peripheral polyneuropathies weakness involves distal muscles in the legs more than the arms. Deep and superficial muscles that are innervated by the peroneal nerve, such as the tibialis anterior and peroneus brevis and longus muscles, are usually affected first. As a result, tripping on a carpet or curb and ankle sprains are frequent symptoms. In the hands, symptoms typically involve fine movements, such as using buttons or zippers and inserting and turning keys in locks.

Peripheral neuropathies that involve nerve roots (polyradiculopathies, such as acute inflammatory demyelinating polyradiculoneuropathy, the most common cause of the Guillain-Barré syndrome) usually cause proximal muscle weakness that results in difficulty arising from a chair, climbing stairs, or working with the arms over the head (e.g., washing or combing hair). Positive motor symptoms, which are less common, include cramps and fasciculations, which are characteristic of disorders involving the motor neuron (e.g., amyotrophic lateral sclerosis) but may also be seen in peripheral neuropathies.

Careful examination of deep tendon reflexes is an important part of the clinical examination. Absence of reflexes often reflects a demyelinating neuropathy. In patients with acute numbness or weakness, this finding suggests Guillain-Barré syndrome. Length-dependent reduction or loss of reflexes (e.g., in Achilles tendons) is common in peripheral polyneuropathies. Because both the afferent and efferent limbs of the deep tendon reflexes involve large myelinated fibers, reflexes are often normal in neuropathies that preferentially involve small-diameter lightly myelinated and unmyelinated axons.

Autonomic symptoms (Chapter 390) are frequent in neuropathies associated with diabetes (Chapter 216) or amyloidosis (Chapter 179) and include urinary retention or incontinence, abnormalities of sweating, constipation alternating with diarrhea, and lightheadedness when standing. Erectile dysfunction is frequent in men.

DIAGNOSIS

A Systematic Approach to Patients with Neuropathy

Diagnosis of peripheral neuropathies is founded on neuroanatomical localization (Table 392-1). The pattern of involvement is often appreciable with a careful history. The most common form of neuropathy is peripheral polyneuropathy. Polyneuropathies cause length-dependent, "stocking glove" symptoms and signs. Most polyneuropathies are sensory predominant, although some forms, particularly inherited polyneuropathies, cause more weakness than sensory loss. Multifocal and asymmetrical distal predominant motor and sensory signs and symptoms usually suggest a disorder involving multiple

TABLE 392-1	TYPES OF NEUROPATHIES		
PERIPHERAL NERVOUS SYSTEM LOCALIZATION	**SYSTEMS INVOLVED**	**ANATOMIC DISTRIBUTION**	**EXAMPLES**
Acquired peripheral polyneuropathy	Positive sensory symptoms and sensory signs; usually less motor involvement	Symmetrical and length dependent ("stocking glove") sensory loss and weakness	Diabetes, cryptogenic sensory peripheral neuropathy, chemotherapy-induced peripheral neuropathy
Genetic peripheral polyneuropathy	Motor greater than sensory, with primarily negative sensory symptoms (numbness), high arched feet, and hammer toes	Symmetrical and length dependent ("stocking glove") weakness and sensory loss	Charcot-Marie-Tooth disease
Mononeuritis multiplex	Motor and sensory, often painful	Asymmetrical, usually distal predominant	Vasculitis (systemic and primary peripheral nervous system)
Polyradiculopathy	Motor greater than sensory involvement	Proximal and distal; usually symmetrical but may be asymmetrical	Acute or chronic inflammatory demyelinating polyradiculoneuropathy (symmetrical); diabetic radiculoplexus neuropathy (asymmetrical)
Sensory neuronopathy (dorsal root ganglionopathy)	Sensory only, usually with ataxia and often painful	Proximal and distal, and asymmetrical	Sjögren syndrome, paraneoplastic (anti-Hu), idiopathic

Most peripheral neuropathies are polyneuropathies, which cause injury to the longest nerve fibers, thereby resulting in length-dependent numbness and weakness. Other patterns suggest different diagnoses with distinct treatments.

individual peripheral nerves ("mononeuritis multiplex"). Polyradiculopathies, which involve multiple nerve roots, cause non–length-dependent motor and sensory signs and symptoms that involve both proximal and distal locations. Recognition of a specific pattern can suggest a diagnosis. For example, a patient with stepwise development of asymmetrical distal weakness, pain, and numbness likely has a mononeuritis multiplex, which is usually caused by a vasculitis (Chapter 134).

Approximately 50% of patients with an acquired peripheral polyneuropathy have diabetes (Chapter 216), and most of the remainder have cryptogenic sensory peripheral neuropathy. Over half of patients with cryptogenic sensory peripheral neuropathy have prediabetes or previously unrecognized mild diabetes, and up to 80% have the metabolic syndrome. Every patient with this pattern of polyneuropathy should be evaluated for diabetes and prediabetes, paraproteinemia (Chapter 178), and vitamin B_{12} deficiency (Chapter 205). In the absence of clinical evidence of a systemic disorder or history of toxic exposure associated with peripheral polyneuropathy (see Table 392-6), additional diagnostic evaluation is usually unhelpful.

Disorders of the peripheral nervous system usually conform to one of ten patterns, which reflect the underlying neuroanatomic pattern of impairment of sensory, motor, and/or autonomic function caused by the specific disorder. Recognition of a specific pattern narrows the differential diagnosis and focuses the diagnostic evaluation (Table 392-2).

Any pattern other than typical neuropathy, or the presence of any atypical "red flag" (e.g., an acute onset suggestive of inflammatory, infectious, or toxic causes; proximal involvement; motor predominance; significant ataxia; or asymmetry) should prompt additional diagnostic evaluation to assess the neuroanatomic localization, underlying physiology (demyelinating versus axonal), and structural changes.

Nerve Conduction Studies and Electromyography

Nerve conduction studies and electromyography (Chapter 368) should be performed in all patients with diagnostic red flags or patterns other than distal, symmetrical, sensory-predominant polyneuropathy. On nerve conduction studies, axonal polyneuropathies reduce the action potential amplitudes of sensory nerves and, if there is motor axonal involvement, muscle action potential amplitudes as well; however, conduction velocities and latencies remain normal. Demyelinating neuropathies slow conduction velocities and prolong distal latencies. Genetic demyelinating polyneuropathies cause uniform conduction slowing, but acquired demyelinating neuropathies cause nonuniform slowing.

On electromyography, abnormal insertional and spontaneous activity, such as fibrillations or positive sharp waves, suggests acute or active axon injury. The presence of large, polyphasic motor units suggests partial reinnervation of muscle by regenerating axons (i.e., a more chronic process). Recruitment of motor units (firing too few motor units at a higher than normal frequency) is reduced in patients with demyelinating and axonal neuropathies.

Nerve and Skin Biopsy

The most common indications for biopsy of a distal sensory nerve, usually the sural or superficial peroneal sensory nerve, is peripheral nerve vasculitis (E-Fig. 392-1). A simultaneous muscle biopsy increases diagnostic yield by 15%. The second most common indication for nerve biopsy is evaluation for suspected light chain amyloidosis (Chapter 179). Nerve masses usually require a biopsy to diagnose a potential tumor. Rarely, nerve biopsy may be useful in the diagnosis of other infiltrative or inflammatory disorders.

Skin biopsies are routinely performed to confirm the presence of a small fiber neuropathy in patients with distal symmetrical sensory loss with neuropathic pain (E-Fig. 392-2), in which nerve conduction studies are usually normal, with an antibody that binds to all axons (PGP 9.5). The diagnosis of small fiber neuropathy is based on demonstrating a reduced density of intraepidermal nerve fibers.

Laboratory Testing

A hemoglobin A_{1c} level is usually the best first test in all patients with distal symmetrical polyneuropathy, but 2-hour glucose tolerance may be performed when the suspicion for prediabetes is high (Chapter 216). Paraproteinemia is most easily evaluated by measuring serum globulin levels and performing a serum protein electrophoresis (Chapter 178). The vitamin B_{12} level should also be measured; if it is borderline, a methylmalonic acid level may be required to confirm deficiency. Other common disorders associated with polyneuropathy include hepatitis C (Chapter 140) and HIV (Chapter 366). Heavy alcohol users (Chapters 30 and 388) are also at risk for polyneuropathy owing to a combination of direct ethanol toxicity and associated vitamin deficiency, particularly vitamin B_1 (thiamine).

In selected patients, electrodiagnostic studies will suggest the need to test for specific antibodies, such as antibodies reacting to ganglioside GM1 (multifocal motor neuropathy) or myelin-associated glycoprotein (MAG— distal demyelinating neuropathy with weakness and tremor). Genetic testing

TABLE 392-2 TEN TYPICAL PATTERNS OF NERVOUS SYSTEM DISORDERS

ANATOMIC PATTERN	NEUROANATOMIC LOCALIZATION	DIFFERENTIAL DIAGNOSIS
1. Symmetrical proximal and distal weakness with sensory loss	Polyradiculoneuropathy	Acute inflammatory demyelinating polyradiculoneuropathy if acute and maximal involvement within the first 4 weeks, chronic inflammatory demyelinating polyneuropathy if progressive over >8 weeks
2. Symmetrical distal sensory loss with or without distal weakness	Peripheral polyneuropathy	Cryptogenic sensory peripheral neuropathy, diabetes or other metabolic disorders, toxic, hereditary such as Charcot-Marie-Tooth
3. Asymmetrical distal weakness with sensory loss	Mononeuritis multiplex	Vasculitis, hereditary neuropathy with predisposition to pressure palsies, multifocal acquired demyelinating sensory and motor neuropathy, infections (e.g., leprosy)
	Mononeuropathy or radiculopathy	Compression, trauma, or tumor
4. Asymmetrical proximal and distal weakness with sensory loss	Polyradiculopathy	Polyradiculopathy or plexopathy due to diabetes (diabetic lumbosacral radiculoplexus neuropathy) or a meningeal disorder (carcinoma, lymphoma, sarcoidosis, chronic infection)
5. Asymmetrical distal weakness without sensory loss	Motor neuronopathy with upper motor neuron signs (brisk reflexes, spasticity, Babinski responses)	Amyotrophic lateral sclerosis
	Motor neuronopathy (lower motor neurons) or motor neuropathy	Progressive muscular atrophy, multifocal motor neuropathy, monomelic amyotrophy ("Hirayama Disease").
6. Symmetrical sensory loss with distal areflexia with upper motor neuron findings	Mixed myelopathy and polyneuropathy	Severe combined degeneration due to vitamin B_{12} or copper deficiency or to inherited disorders (adrenomyeloneuropathy, metachromatic leukodystrophy, Freidreich ataxia)
7. Symmetrical weakness without sensory loss	Motor neuronopathy	Proximal and distal: spinal muscular atrophy or progressive muscular atrophy
	Motor neuropathy	Distal predominant: hereditary motor neuropathy
8. Focal midline proximal weakness	Motor neuronopathy, neuromuscular junction disorder, myopathy	Neck extensor weakness (head drop): amyotrophic lateral sclerosis, myasthenia gravis, myopathy
		Bulbar weakness: amyotrophic lateral sclerosis, myasthenia gravis
9. Asymmetrical sensory loss with sensory ataxia without weakness	Sensory neuronopathy	Sjögren, paraneoplastic (anti-Hu antibody), idiopathic
	Sensory polyradiculoneuropathy	Chronic immune sensory polyradiculoneuropathy
10. Autonomic symptoms and signs	Autonomic neuropathy	Diabetes, amyloid, autoimmune autonomic neuropathies

is most cost-effective when the selection of candidate genes is based on the patient's nerve conduction studies, inheritance pattern, and clinical findings.

INHERITED NEUROPATHIES

Inherited neuropathies can be divided into those that affect the peripheral nervous system in isolation, such as Charcot-Marie-Tooth (CMT) disease, and those that involve multiple organ systems.[4]

Charcot-Marie-Tooth Disease

EPIDEMIOLOGY AND PATHOBIOLOGY

CMT has a prevalence of 1 : 2500 and is caused by mutations that affect myelin formation. Autosomal dominant CMT is subdivided into demyelinating (CMT1) and axonal (CMT2) forms based on electrophysiologic criteria. Many patients have de novo mutations. X-linked (CMTX) and autosomal recessive (CMT4) forms are also seen. Each type is further subdivided by the specific genetic cause. The most common form, CMT1A, is caused by a duplication of a fragment of chromosome 17 containing the peripheral myelin protein 22-kD (*PMP22*) gene. The most common form of CMT2 is a mutation in the mitofusin gene (CMT2A). Overall, CMT1A accounts for 60 to 70% of CMT1, CMT1X accounts for 10 to 20%, CMT1B for less than 5%, and CMT2 for 20%. However, mutations have been identified in more than 90 genes, and this number is likely to increase substantially in the future. In severe cases of congenital hypomyelination, myelination is disrupted during embryologic development.

CLINICAL MANIFESTATION

CMT1 and CMT2 cause distal weakness and sensory loss in the first 2 decades. Children are often slow runners and have impaired balance (e.g., skating, walking across a log). Ankle-foot orthoses are frequently required by the third decade. Fine hand movements (e.g., turning a key or using buttons and zippers) may be impaired. Most patients have distal leg atrophy ("inverted champagne bottle") with high arched feet (pes cavus) and hammer toes (E-Fig. 392-3). Nevertheless, most patients remain ambulatory throughout life and have a normal lifespan. A minority of patients have a more severe phenotype with delayed motor milestones and onset in infancy (Dejerine-Sottas neuropathy).

Patients with hereditary motor neuropathies sometimes have mild sensory abnormalities, and patients with hereditary sensory and autonomic neuropathies usually have some weakness. The same mutations in the same gene (*GARS*) cause both CMT2D and hereditary motor neuropathy type V (Video 392-1).

DIAGNOSIS

Clinically directed molecular testing suggests probable candidate genes (www.geneclinics.org), but not all identified genetic variants are pathogenic. In nerve conduction studies, CMT1 causes uniformly slow conduction velocity of about 20 m/sec, but virtually all forms of CMT1 have axonal loss as well as demyelination. CMT2 is characterized by axonal loss and reduced compound muscle action potential or sensory nerve action potential amplitudes. On nerve biopsy, onion bulbs of concentric Schwann cell lamellae are usually present, with loss of both small- and large-diameter myelinated axons.

Differential Diagnosis

Inherited neuropathies must be distinguished from acquired neuropathies. Other genetic disorders of the CNS, such as hereditary spastic paraplegia or leukodystrophies, may mimic inherited neuropathies by causing distal weakness, sensory loss, and foot deformities such as pes cavus; these patients often have upper motor neuron signs, and do not have neurophysiologic evidence of neuropathy.

TREATMENT   Rx

Clinical and genetic counseling and symptomatic and rehabilitative treatment are important. A detailed family history and examination of family members may be required for prognosis and genetic counseling. Ankle-foot orthoses may return gait and balance to normal for years. Foot surgery is occasionally offered to correct inverted feet, pes cavus, and hammer toes to improve walking, alleviate pain over pressure points, and prevent plantar ulcers. Ascorbic acid, progesterone antagonists, and subcutaneous injections of neurotrophin 3 have improved animal models of CMT1A but have not proven successful in human studies.

Familial Amyloid Polyneuropathy

Familial amyloid polyneuropathy (Chapter 179) is caused by dominantly inherited mutations in at least three genes: transthyretin, apolipoprotein A1, and gelsolin. Pathogenic mutations in transthyretin cause a conformational change that destabilizes its normal tetramers, thereby resulting in intracellular aggregates that form amyloid deposits in peripheral nerve, heart, and other tissues.

Familial amyloid polyneuropathy typically presents as a painful sensory neuropathy in mid to late adulthood, with prominent autonomic features including sexual dysfunction, gastrointestinal disturbances, and cardiac arrhythmias, followed by weakness, weight loss, and inanition.[5] Certain mutations commonly cause neuropathy (Val30Met), whereas others (Val122Ile) usually present with heart disease.

Diagnosis is based on genetic testing supported by tissue evidence of amyloid because mutations are not always penetrant.

TREATMENT   Rx

Tafamidis (20 mg daily) acts to stabilize the variant transthyretin polymer to prevent its dissociation and can delay progression of the polyneuropathy.[A1] Other effective options for polyneuropathy include patisiran (30 mg intravenously every 3 weeks)[A2] and inotersen (284 mg subcutaneously weekly).[A3] Diflunisal (a Food and Drug Administration–approved generic nonsteroidal anti-inflammatory drug that complexes to the thyroxine binding sites on the tetrameric form of transthyretin, stabilizes it, and thus inhibits the release of the transthyretic monomer required for amyloidogenesis; at 250 mg twice daily, it can slow the rate of progression of familial amyloidosis-associated polyneuropathy.[A4]

PROGNOSIS

Death typically occurs within a decade of diagnosis owing to cardiac or autonomic failure unless patients undergo liver transplantation. Other experimental therapies designed to reduce transthyretin expression (antisense oligonucleotides, RNA interference) may further improve prognosis.

INFLAMMATORY AND IMMUNOLOGIC NEUROPATHIES

Autoimmune disorders of the peripheral nervous system include primary inflammatory neuropathies (Guillain-Barré syndrome and chronic inflammatory demyelinating polyneuropathy) and those related to vasculitis and other systemic autoimmune disorders.

Guillain-Barré Syndrome

DEFINITION

Guillain-Barré syndrome refers to acquired, inflammatory polyradiculoneuropathies that share an acute onset, elevated cerebrospinal fluid (CSF) protein levels with low cell counts (cytoalbuminologic dissociation), and a monophasic course.[6,7] Guillain-Barré syndrome is subdivided into demyelinating (acute inflammatory demyelinating polyradiculoneuropathy), and axonal (acute motor and sensory axonal neuropathy and acute motor axonal neuropathy) variants, and the Miller-Fisher syndrome.

EPIDEMIOLOGY

The annual incidence of Guillain-Barré syndrome is 1 to 2 per 100,000, although in some areas the incidence may be higher. Acute inflammatory demyelinating polyradiculoneuropathy accounts for 97% of cases in North America and Europe with an incidence of 0.6 to 1.9 cases per 100,000. Men are more often affected than women (1.4 : 1). In 60% of patients, a respiratory tract infection or gastroenteritis precedes Guillain-Barré syndrome. Patients with axonal variants are particularly likely to have had a prior *Campylobacter jejuni* diarrheal illness. In Belgium and the Netherlands, 5 to 10% of patients have a preceding hepatitis E infection (Chapter 139), thereby emphasizing the regional variability in infectious triggers.[8] Zika virus (Chapter 359) has been associated with a significant increased risk of all forms of Guillain-Barré syndrome,[9] as well as a transient polyneuritis pattern of mild distal sensory symptoms (acute peripheral polyneuropathy).

PATHOBIOLOGY

All forms of Guillain-Barré syndrome probably result from postinfectious molecular mimicry, in which the immune system attacks peripheral nerve antigens because they resemble antigens presented by microbes, in particular, *C. jejuni*. For example, the HS/0:19 serotype of *C. jejuni* is common in patients with the acute motor axonal neuropathy form of Guillain-Barré syndrome in northern China and other countries. However, it is not clear that molecular mimicry causes acute inflammatory demyelinating polyradiculoneuropathy, which is the most common form in the United States and Europe.

CLINICAL MANIFESTATIONS

Weakness is the most common initial symptom. It can be mild, such as difficulty walking, or severe, with total quadriplegia and respiratory failure. The most common manifestation is leg weakness that progresses into the arms. Bilateral facial weakness occurs in 50% of patients and may lag behind limb weakness. Although Guillain-Barré syndrome has been described as an "ascending paralysis," proximal weakness is common, and 5% of patients have isolated cranial nerve involvement that subsequently descends into the limbs. Slight sensory loss occurs in most patients. The autonomic nervous system is involved in about 65% of cases.

Acute motor sensory axonal neuropathy is clinically similar to acute inflammatory demyelinating polyradiculoneuropathy except it is typically more severe because of primary injury to axons rather than to myelin. Autonomic dysfunction is more common. Weakness without sensory loss develops in acute motor axonal neuropathy, including cranial nerve involvement in about 25% of patients.

The Miller-Fisher syndrome consists of the triad of ophthalmoplegia, ataxia, and areflexia. Facial weakness, ptosis, and pupillary abnormalities may be present. Nerve conduction velocities in Miller-Fisher syndrome are normal, unlike acute inflammatory demyelinating polyradiculoneuropathy.

DIAGNOSIS

The diagnosis of acute inflammatory demyelinating polyradiculoneuropathy and acute motor sensory axonal neuropathy is based on the history, physical examination, CSF evaluation, and nerve conduction studies. Weakness is symmetrical, and deep tendon reflexes are decreased or absent. The presence of other CNS abnormalities should cast doubt on the diagnosis.

CSF analysis typically reveals high protein with a paucity of white blood cells (WBCs). The CSF should have less than 5 WBCs/mL; a CSF cell count greater than 50 WBCs/mL suggests HIV seroconversion (Chapter 366) or infections such as Lyme disease (Chapter 305). Acute inflammatory demyelinating polyradiculoneuropathy is distinguished from acute motor sensory axonal neuropathy by nerve conduction studies. Because elevated CSF protein and abnormal nerve conduction studies may not be apparent in the first 7 to 10 days of the illness and because CSF protein remains normal in up to 10% of cases, the initial treatment decision often must be made based on clinical judgment. Most Miller-Fisher syndrome patients (>85%) have polyclonal antibodies that react to the ganglioside GQ_{1b}.

Differential Diagnosis

Guillain-Barré syndrome usually causes symmetrical proximal and distal weakness with milder sensory loss that reaches maximum severity in less than 4 weeks. A number of warning signs suggest further evaluation for an alternative diagnosis (Table 392-3). Other causes for symmetrical acute weakness include acute toxic neuropathies; fulminant myopathies, particularly immune-mediated necrotizing myopathy (the serum creatine kinase level is usually markedly elevated); and myasthenia gravis (ptosis, diplopia and dysphagia/dysarthria; Chapter 394). Botulism (Chapter 280) causes ophthalmoplegia, unreactive pupils, bulbar weakness, dry mouth, constipation, and orthostatic hypotension, without sensory symptoms. Asymmetrical weakness can be seen with viral encephalomyelitis (Chapter 386). In North America, polio has been eradicated, but other viral illnesses may induce polio-like syndromes including ECHO 70, coxsackievirus (Chapter 355), and West Nile virus (Chapter 358). Though very rare, rabies (Chapter 386) also may present with rapidly progressive paralysis. Tick paralysis (Chapter 359), caused by a toxin within the tick, can mimic Guillain-Barré syndrome, particularly in children. Usually, removal of the tick is associated with improvement within hours, although progression can occur, particularly in Australia where the toxin differs from that found in North America.

Acute myelopathies such as transverse myelitis (Chapter 383), neuromyelitis optica, and vascular myelopathies (Chapter 253) may also cause rapidly

TABLE 392-3	WARNING SIGNS SUGGESTING AN ALTERNATIVE DIAGNOSIS IN PATIENTS WITH SUSPECTED GUILLAIN-BARRÉ SYNDROME
WARNING SIGN	**DIFFERENTIAL DIAGNOSIS**
Sensory predominant	Sensory neuronopathy
Prominent bowel and bladder symptoms	Myelopathy
Spinal sensory level	Myelopathy
Persistently asymmetrical weakness	Viral encephalomyelitis (enteroviral), mononeuritis multiplex (vasculitis), radiculoplexus neuropathy (diabetic amyotrophy)
Distal predominant weakness and sensory loss (peripheral polyneuropathy pattern)	Toxic neuropathies (e.g., arsenic)
Slow progression	Chronic inflammatory demyelinating polyradiculoneuropathy
CSF: >50 WBCs/μL	HIV seroconversion

CSF = cerebrospinal fluid; HIV = human immunodeficiency virus; WBCs = white blood cells.

progressive symmetrical weakness and sensory loss. Brisk reflexes and a sensory level are often observed, and bowel and bladder dysfunction are apparent. Carcinomatous or lymphomatous meningitis can also cause a rapidly developing quadriparesis owing to an acute polyradiculopathy.

Nerve conduction studies and electromyography are helpful in excluding myopathies and disorders of the neuromuscular junction. Other acute neuropathies cause axonal injury, so neurophysiologic findings share features with axonal variants of Guillain-Barré syndrome. CSF analysis can be helpful in excluding infectious causes.

PREVENTION

Although there was an increased risk of Guillain-Barré syndrome following the H1N1 influenza vaccination program in 1977, subsequent studies have demonstrated a significantly reduced risk among vaccinated individuals compared with unvaccinated individuals. More limited data suggest the risk of recurrent Guillain-Barré syndrome following influenza or pneumococcal vaccination is extremely low.

TREATMENT   Rx

Patients with Guillain-Barré syndrome require hospitalization because of the risk of respiratory compromise, and the decision to admit a patient to an intensive care unit should be based on the trajectory of change in respiratory function and clinical assessment. A vital capacity of less than 1 L or a negative inspiratory force of less than −70 suggests the need for ventilator support (Chapter 97) in an intensive care unit. Autonomic and swallowing function should also be monitored.

Guillain-Barré syndrome can be treated within 2 weeks of onset with either intravenous immunoglobulin (IVIG, 2 g/kg divided over 2 days or longer if necessary because of the patient's cardiac function or fluid status)[A5] or therapeutic plasma exchange of 5 plasma volumes over 10 days.[A6] Patients are significantly more likely to complete a full course of IVIG, so this treatment is generally preferred. Methylprednisolone (500 mg/day for 5 days) plus IVIG has a slight initial advantage but no long-term benefit compared with IVIG alone[A7]; given its risks, it generally is not recommended. The prognosis of Miller-Fisher syndrome is generally excellent, and there is controversy regarding the necessity of treatment with IVIG or plasma exchange.

PROGNOSIS

Fifty percent of patients progress to maximum disability within 2 weeks of the onset of symptoms, 75% within 3 weeks, and greater than 90% within 4 weeks. With supportive care, mortality is 3% at 6 months, primarily in the elderly and severely affected patients, and especially during the recovery phase. After a brief period of stabilization, slow recovery occurs over weeks to months. Most patients recover completely or are left with minor sequelae; 20% have a persistent disability. The prognosis is poorer in patients with axonal variants or with acute inflammatory demyelinating polyradiculoneuropathy with significant axonal loss as reflected by reduced compound muscle action potential amplitudes in the upper extremities. Other predictors of a poor prognosis include older age, preceding diarrheal illness, and severity of weakness.

Chronic Inflammatory Demyelinating Polyradiculoneuropathy

DEFINITION

Chronic inflammatory demyelinating polyradiculoneuropathy is usually slowly progressive but may be monophasic or relapsing. By definition, it develops over at least 2 months and more slowly than acute inflammatory demyelinating polyradiculoneuropathy, which it otherwise resembles.

EPIDEMIOLOGY

Chronic inflammatory demyelinating polyradiculoneuropathy[10] occurs in all age groups, with a mean age of 30 to 50 years. Women are more likely to be affected. Antecedent events in about 30% of patients include upper respiratory infections, gastrointestinal infections, vaccinations, surgery, and trauma. In some patients it is a paraneoplastic phenomenon, especially with non-Hodgkin lymphoma (Chapter 176).[11]

PATHOBIOLOGY

Chronic inflammatory demyelinating polyradiculoneuropathy is considered an autoimmune disorder based on its pathology and experimental models, in which a similar disorder follows immunization with peripheral nervous system myelin components and Freund adjuvant. Nerve biopsy shows macrophage-mediated segmental demyelination, occasional endoneurial lymphocytic T-cell infiltrates, and endoneurial edema. Major histocompatibility complex class I and II antigens are upregulated, and there are often deposits of immunoglobulins and complement on the outer Schwann cell membranes or myelin sheaths. Chronic inflammatory demyelinating polyradiculoneuropathy can be passively transferred to animals by patient sera, but no clear autoantigen has been identified.

CLINICAL MANIFESTATIONS

Weakness and sensory loss begin insidiously and progress over a period of months to years. Weakness, which involves both proximal and distal muscles, is usually symmetrical. The absence of proximal weakness suggests a polyneuropathy. Patients often require assistance with ambulation. Loss of proprioception from damage to large-diameter sensory nerves may affect balance. Deep tendon reflexes are usually absent or markedly decreased. Facial weakness (15%), ptosis, or ophthalmoparesis (5%) may occur. Variants include pure motor, pure sensory, and multifocal forms (multifocal acquired demyelinating sensory and motor neuropathy).

DIAGNOSIS

Diagnosis is based on clinical symptoms and signs, CSF examination, and electrodiagnostic studies. CSF results resemble those of acute inflammatory demyelinating polyradiculoneuropathy: WBC counts are usually less than 10 cells/μL, and protein greater than 60 mg/dL. CSF WBC count greater than 50/μL suggest another diagnosis, such as HIV infection or hematologic malignancy.

Nonuniform, asymmetrical slowing of motor nerve conduction velocity with prolonged F wave latencies is typical. Compound muscle action potential amplitudes are generally reduced because of secondary axonal degeneration. Sensory nerve action potential amplitudes are usually reduced or absent.

Many patients, however, do not meet formal electrophysiologic criteria for chronic inflammatory demyelinating polyradiculoneuropathy. The combination of symmetrical onset of weakness involving all four limbs with proximal weakness in at least one limb has a comparable diagnostic accuracy (sensitivity 83%, specificity 97%). Different clinical patterns should suggest a broader differential diagnosis.

A subset of patients with severe disability and ataxia have antibodies reactive against contactin or neurofascin.[12] These antibodies, which are usually of the IgG4 isotype, bind to the nodal and paranodal region.

Differential Diagnosis

Chronic inflammatory demyelinating polyradiculoneuropathy, which is distinguished from acute demyelinating polyneuropathy by its time course, may be associated with monoclonal gammopathies (Chapter 178). However, it does not appear to be related to diabetes.

TREATMENT Rx

A standard approach is oral prednisone (1 mg/kg/day) for 6 to 8 weeks, followed by slow tapering over a 3- to 12-month period to a maintenance level of about 0.1 mg/kg/day.[A8] A response to prednisone may take months to occur, and occasional patients may worsen before they respond. Other alternatives are pulsed dexamethasone (6 cycles of 40 mg/day orally for 4 days) or short-term prednisolone (60 mg/day for 5 weeks, then tapering to zero).

IVIG at a dose of 1 g/kg every 3 weeks is also effective. Most patients respond within the first three treatments, and a failure to do so suggests a low likelihood of future response. IVIG is more frequently effective than corticosteroids initially, but it may have a less durable benefit.[A9] Although plasma exchange also is effective, it is difficult to use as a chronic therapy.

Because of the side effects of long-term corticosteroids, azathioprine 2 mg/kg and mycophenolate mofetil 1000 to 1500 mg in divided doses twice daily are often used as steroid-sparing agents. Cyclosporine, cyclophosphamide, methotrexate, rituximab, and interferon-α or -β have been used with variable success in uncontrolled reports.

Patients with contactin or neurofascin antibodies may respond to corticosteroids or IVIG. However, some patients have been reported to respond better to rituximab, most often administered at a dose of 325 mg/m² weekly for four doses.

Multifocal Motor Neuropathy

DEFINITION

Multifocal motor neuropathy is characterized by progressive, distal more than proximal, asymmetrical limb weakness, mostly affecting the upper limbs with minimal or no sensory impairment.

EPIDEMIOLOGY

The prevalence of multifocal motor neuropathy is estimated at 2 per 100,000. Men are more frequently affected than women (2.6 : 1). Initial symptoms develop in 80% between 20 and 50 years, with a mean age at onset of 40 years.

PATHOBIOLOGY

Multifocal motor neuropathy is considered to be an autoimmune neuropathy based on clinical improvement with immunotherapies and because patients often have serum antibodies that react with ganglioside GM_1 and because this antibody titer decreases during effective treatment. GM_1 is highly represented in neural membranes at the nodes of Ranvier, compact myelin, and the motor end plate at the neuromuscular junction.

CLINICAL MANIFESTATIONS

The usual pattern is progressive, distal, asymmetrical arm weakness, often in the distribution of a single nerve. In a minority of patients, weakness may start proximally or in the legs. Multifocal motor neuropathy frequently affects multiple nerve distributions, occasionally with a crossed distribution (i.e., one arm and the contralateral leg). Asymmetry and predominance of arm weakness may become less evident over time. Localized muscle atrophy, which may be mild or absent initially, becomes prominent later as a result of axonal degeneration.

DIAGNOSIS

The diagnosis is established by the presence of multifocal, persistent, partial conduction block on motor but not sensory nerve conduction studies. Conduction block can be hard to find, however, and multifocal motor neuropathy should be considered in patients with a typical clinical pattern in the absence of upper motor neuron signs. Anti-GM_1 ganglioside antibodies are detectable in 50% of patients with multifocal motor neuropathy.

Differential Diagnosis

Multifocal motor neuropathy shares many diagnostic features with amyotrophic lateral sclerosis (Chapter 391), including distal asymmetrical upper extremity weakness and atrophy. Key differentiating features include the time course (multifocal motor neuropathy is slowly progressive whereas amyotrophic lateral sclerosis progresses rapidly) and the absence of respiratory or bulbar weakness and of upper motor neuron features. In patients with suspected multifocal motor neuropathy but without apparent conduction block or GM_1 antibodies, magnetic resonance imaging or ultrasound of peripheral nerves may help distinguish multifocal motor neuropathy from amyotrophic lateral sclerosis (Chapter 391).[13] Multifocal motor neuropathy may also be confused with multifocal chronic inflammatory demyelinating polyradiculoneuropathy, which causes sensory loss as well as motor weakness and which is associated with more severe sensory abnormalities on nerve conduction studies.

TREATMENT   Rx

IVIG (2 g/kg) is the initial treatment for multifocal motor neuropathy, and almost 80% of patients respond within a week. However, improvement is typically brief (3 to 6 weeks), so repeated treatments are required indefinitely.[14] Clinical improvement is often accompanied by a reduction or resolution of motor conduction block in some nerves, but it does not consistently correlate with a reduction in GM_1 titers. In patients who may eventually become refractory to IVIG, either pulse cyclophosphamide (1 g/m² monthly for 6 months) or rituximab (e.g., 375 mg/m² weekly for 4 weeks) have been effective in case reports. Mycophenolate and corticosteroids are ineffective.

VASCULITIC NEUROPATHIES

Vasculitic neuropathies typically present as a subacute painful mononeuritis multiplex with acute motor and sensory loss in multiple nerve territories.

EPIDEMIOLOGY

Systemic vasculitic neuropathy is more common than nonsystemic vasculitic neuropathy, but about 10% of patients who initially have nonsystemic peripheral nerve vasculitis ultimately develop a systemic vasculitis. Peak age at onset of both are between the ages of 40 and 70 years, but vasculitis can occur at any age. Rheumatoid arthritis (Chapter 248) evolves into systemic rheumatoid vasculitis in 5 to 15% of patients, and vasculitic neuropathy develops in about 50% of these cases. More than 50% of patients with Churg-Strauss syndrome, 40 to 50% with granulomatosis with polyangiitis (Chapter 254), 35 to 75% with polyarteritis nodosa (Chapter 254), and a majority with mixed cryoglobulinemia have neuropathy. Patients with Sjögren syndrome (Chapter 252) are often initially found to have sensory neuropathies. By comparison neuropathies are uncommon in systemic lupus erythematosus (Chapter 250).

PATHOBIOLOGY

In patients with mononeuritis multiplex, axonal degeneration develops as a result of nerve ischemia. Inflammation and necrosis of blood vessel walls occlude the lumen, thereby resulting in ischemic damage. Peripheral nerve vasculitides can be divided into those that affect large-diameter arterioles (75 to 300 μm), small-diameter arterioles (<40 μm), and capillaries. Systemic vasculitis typically involves the former, and nonsystemic peripheral nerve vasculitis the latter.[15]

The immune-mediated inflammation is associated with antibody-antigen complexes that are deposited in the vessel wall. Antibodies also bind directly to endothelial cell antigens. In both circumstances, complement is activated. Chemotactic factors then recruit neutrophils, which release proteolytic enzymes and generate toxic oxygen free radicals.

The sensory neuropathy of Sjögren syndrome (Chapter 252) probably results from the infiltration of dorsal root ganglia by cytotoxic T cells. Some patients with systemic vasculitis have symmetrical neuropathies rather than mononeuritis. The pathogenesis of such cases is not defined.

CLINICAL MANIFESTATIONS

Patients typically have a relatively sudden onset of painful focal or multifocal weakness or of sensory loss. These symptoms reflect ischemia anywhere along the length of the nerves, most often in the lower extremities. Up to 30% of patients have a progressive symmetrical pattern of involvement. Patients with large arteriole, systemic vasculitis often have systemic symptoms including fatigue, myalgias, fevers, and arthralgias in addition to the organ involvement that is typical for the specific disorder (Table 392-4). For example, certain forms of vasculitis may affect cranial nerves (polyangiitis with granulomatosis and Sjögren syndrome) or cause autonomic neuropathy (Sjögren syndrome). Mononeuritis multiplex can occur in systemic vasculitis that involves other organ systems, in association with underlying viral infection, or as an organ-specific (nonsystemic) peripheral nerve vasculitis.

DIAGNOSIS

Diagnostic clues are the subacute and progressive time course, as well as the presence of distal weakness and pain. The number of nerves involved may be extensive enough to make the distinction between a multifocal and diffuse neuropathy difficult, and many patients have a mildly asymmetrical or symmetrical confluent mononeuritis multiplex.

Nerve biopsy of clinically affected sensory nerves (sural, superficial peroneal, or superficial radial) is the gold standard for diagnosis, especially because aggressive, long-term therapy may be required. The addition of muscle biopsy may increase diagnostic yield by 15%. Diagnostic pathologic features of vasculitis are seen in about 60% of patients, including destruction of the vessel and inflammation within the vessel wall. Fibrinoid necrosis, vessel wall scarring, recanalization, neovascularization, and hemosiderin are common but not essential histopathologic features.

Electrophysiologic findings can also suggest the diagnosis. For example, electromyography and nerve conduction studies can distinguish between mononeuritis multiplex and a symmetrical neuropathy.

Differentiation of systemic versus isolated peripheral nervous system vasculitis depends on clinical and serologic evaluation. The erythrocyte sedimentation rate is usually elevated in systemic vasculitis but is often normal in nonsystemic vasculitis. Perinuclear and cytoplasmic antineutrophil cytoplasmic antibodies (p-ANCA and c-ANCA) suggest granulomatosis with polyangiitis or Churg-Strauss syndrome (Chapter 254). Hepatitis C (Chapter 140) is usually associated with cryoglobulinemia. Serum complement levels,

TABLE 392-4   CLINICAL AND SEROLOGIC FINDINGS OF SYSTEMIC AND NONSYSTEMIC VASCULITIS INVOLVING THE PERIPHERAL NERVOUS SYSTEM

DIAGNOSIS	SEROLOGIC FEATURES	ASSOCIATED CLINICAL FEATURES	USUAL TYPE OF NEUROPATHY	PREVALENCE OF NEUROPATHY
Rheumatoid arthritis (Chapter 248)	RF (80-90%)	Arthritis frequent; multiple organs often affected	Mononeuritis multiplex and sensorimotor neuropathy	50%
Eosinophilic granulomatosis with polyangiitis (formerly Churg-Strauss syndrome) (Chapter 254)	c-ANCA (<30%), p-ANCA (<50%), eosinophilia (100%), elevated ESR (85%)	Eosinophilia, asthma, sinusitis (60-80%), skin lesions (50-70%)	Mononeuritis multiplex	20%
Granulomatosis with polyangiitis (Chapter 254)	c-ANCA (75-90%) p-ANCA (<20%)	Pulmonary and renal involvement	Mononeuritis multiplex	15%
Polyarteritis nodosa	Elevated ESR (85%), positive serology, hepatitis B (30%), ANCA (<10%)	Multiple organs (skin, joints, renal, gastrointestinal)	Mononeuritis multiplex	60%
Mixed cryoglobulinemia (Chapter 178)	Hepatitis C (80-90%), reduced complement (70-90%), RF (70-90%), elevated ESR (70%).	Skin (purpura, livedo), joints, Raynaud phenomenon	Mononeuritis multiplex	20-90%
Sjögren syndrome (Chapter 252)	α-Ro/SS-A (60%), α-La/SS-B (50%)	Dry eyes, dry mouth; 90% are women	Multiple patterns	25%
Nonsystemic peripheral nerve vasculitis	Elevated ESR (50%), positive ANA (25%), reduced complement (5%)	Muscle disease (25%)	Mononeuritis multiplex	100%

α-Ro/SS-A and α-La/SS-B = antibodies to the Ro/SS-A and La/SS-B antigens; ANA = antinuclear antibodies; ESR = erythrocyte sedimentation rate; p- and c-ANCA = perinuclear and cytoplasmic antineutrophil cytoplasmic antibodies; RF = rheumatoid factor.

extractable nuclear antigen, angiotensin-converting enzyme levels, serum protein electrophoresis, and HIV serology are generally indicated. CSF analysis may be needed to exclude infectious (e.g., Lyme disease; Chapter 305) or other inflammatory causes.

Differential Diagnosis

Acute or subacute mononeuritis multiplex may also result from diabetic and nondiabetic lumbosacral radiculoplexus neuropathy, which usually causes proximal greater than distal weakness in the legs, sarcoidosis (Chapter 89), Lyme disease (Chapter 305), and malignant infiltration of nerves. Multifocal motor neuropathy and multifocal acquired demyelinating sensory and motor neuropathy cause asymmetrical weakness, but neither causes pain; furthermore, multifocal motor neuropathy does not cause sensory loss. Asymmetrical isolated sensory loss occurs in some forms of sensory neuronopathy that are caused by dorsal root ganglionopathy (Chapter 372).

TREATMENT   Rx

Treatment for vasculitic neuropathy should be based on the specific form and clinical situation. Patients with large arteriole systemic vasculitis are at risk for rapid progression and disability, so treatment should be more aggressive, for example, oral prednisone (1 mg/kg) or intravenous methylprednisolone (1000 mg/day for 3 to 5 days) as induction therapy. Oral prednisone is continued at this dose for 1 to 2 months before instituting a slow taper. Maintenance cyclophosphamide (1 g/m² IV monthly for 6 months, or 2 mg/kg orally daily) is usually required for 3 to 6 months. If ongoing therapy is needed, cyclophosphamide may be replaced with oral methotrexate (e.g., starting at 7.5 to 15 mg/week) or azathioprine (e.g., starting at 2 to 3 mg/kg/day), with the dose ultimately decreased if the treatments prove effective. Patients with refractory vasculitis may benefit from rituximab (usually at a dose of 325 mg/m² weekly for four doses), IVIG (typically 1 g/kg every 3 to 4 weeks), or plasma exchange.

Because patients with nonsystemic vasculitic neuropathy usually have a more benign course than do patients with systemic vasculitis, alternate-day oral prednisone (e.g., 60 to 80 mg every other day) is often adequate therapy. Azathioprine or weekly methotrexate can be used as a glucocorticoid-sparing agent.

Patients with viral-induced peripheral nerve vasculitis, such as hepatitis C–associated cryoglobulinemia, require treatment of the underlying viral illness. Clinically significant vasculitic neuropathy can be treated as previously outlined.

PROGNOSIS

Most systemic and nonsystemic vasculitis cases respond at least partially to treatment. For systemic vasculitic neuropathy, the prognosis is linked to that of the causative disease, whereas isolated peripheral nervous system vasculitis has a better prognosis.

● NEUROPATHIES ASSOCIATED WITH MONOCLONAL GAMMOPATHIES AND MULTIPLE MYELOMA

Monoclonal gammopathy and multiple myeloma (Chapter 178) are associated with multiple patterns of neuropathy, including a distal symmetrical polyneuropathy; polyneuropathy, organomegaly, endocrinopathy, myeloma protein, and skin changes (POEMS) syndrome; light chain amyloidosis; and distal acquired demyelinating syndrome, which is a variant of chronic inflammatory demyelinating polyradiculoneuropathy characterized by antibodies to myelin-associated glycoprotein in 50% of patients. Multifocal motor neuropathy may occur with IgM gammopathies with specificity for GM₁ ganglioside (reviewed earlier). Patients with typical chronic inflammatory demyelinating polyradiculoneuropathy have a monoclonal gammopathy in the absence of the specific syndromes reviewed later; however, treatment and the response to it are similar to patients without gammopathy.

Monoclonal Gammopathy of Uncertain Significance

Monoclonal gammopathy refers to the presence in the β-γ region of serum protein electrophoresis of an abnormal spike (variably termed a paraprotein, monoclonal protein, or M protein) consisting of immunoglobulins of the same isotype, all produced by a single clone of abnormally proliferating lymphocyte/plasma cells. In some cases, the M protein is part of a malignant lymphoproliferative disease such as multiple myeloma, solitary plasmacytoma (IgG and IgA), Waldenström IgM macroglobulinemia (Chapter 178), chronic lymphocytic leukemia (Chapter 174), primary amyloidosis (Chapter 179), or cryoglobulinemia (Chapter 178). In most instances, however, monoclonal gammopathy is not initially associated with any of these disorders and is classified as a monoclonal gammopathy of uncertain significance (MGUS; Chapter 178), although patients with MGUS have a 1% per year risk of progressing to myeloma or another hematologic disease.

▮ EPIDEMIOLOGY

Monoclonal gammopathy occurs in 5 to 8% of patients with peripheral neuropathy of unknown etiology. However, MGUS is frequent, being found in 1% of the population older than 50 years and in 3% older than 70 years, and most subjects with MGUS do not have neuropathy. In some cases, the co-occurrence of neuropathy and M protein may be a coincidence.

The prevalence of neuropathy is higher in patients with IgM versus IgG or IgA M proteins. The prevalence of symptomatic neuropathy associated with IgM monoclonal gammopathy in patients older than 50 years is approximately 20 per 100,000. In half of such patients, the M protein reacts with either the HNK1 carbohydrate moiety of MAG or with other glycoproteins (MPZ, PMP22) and glycolipids (sulfoglucuronylparagloboside [SGPG] and lactos-aminylparagloboside [SGLPG]). IgM M proteins associated with neuropathy may also bind to other neural antigens.

In patients with IgG monoclonal gammopathy and neuropathy, the relationship is less clear than with IgM. Although about 10% of patients with multiple myeloma have neuropathy, in most cases, the M protein does not react with a neural antigen, and patients do not improve with immunotherapy (see later).

▮ PATHOBIOLOGY

The underlying pathobiology of neuropathy associated with MGUS and multiple myeloma is unknown.

▮ CLINICAL MANIFESTATIONS

Patients with MGUS typically present with a slowly progressive distal symmetrical peripheral polyneuropathy that is clinically indistinguishable from cryptogenic sensory peripheral neuropathy. Patients with multiple myeloma also typically have a slowly progressive sensory greater than motor peripheral polyneuropathy, although motor-predominant forms have been described.

▮ DIAGNOSIS

Diagnosis is based on demonstration of a monoclonal gammopathy on serum protein or immunoelectrophoresis. Immunoelectrophoresis has a higher sensitivity than serum protein electrophoresis, but serum protein electrophoresis is required to define the heavy and light chain of MGUS. Patients with a non-IgG gammopathy, anemia, constitutional symptoms, or a high weight gammopathy (>15 g/L) require a full hematologic evaluation (Chapter 178). Patients with a distal symmetrical sensory polyneuropathy, a low level of monoclonal IgG or IgM, and normal hematologic values can be followed with yearly paraprotein measurements. The presence of distal weakness, tremor, severe pain, autonomic dysfunction, or rapid progression should prompt a more extensive evaluation for another cause for neuropathy, either related to the monoclonal gammopathy (e.g., POEMS, see later) or as a distinct disorder.

TREATMENT   Rx

Treatment of MGUS neuropathy is largely symptomatic. Treatment of the underlying monoclonal gammopathy does not improve the neuropathy. In contrast, treatment of multiple myeloma may improve the neuropathy.

PROGNOSIS

In patients whose myeloma responds to treatment, more than 50% have improvement in neuropathy. Prognosis is as for the myelitis itself. Patients with MGUS usually have a disease course similar to cryptogenic sensory peripheral neuropathy, with slow progression and minimal disability.

POEMS Syndrome

The component features of POEMS syndrome are *P*olyneuropathy, *O*rganomegaly, *E*ndocrinopathy, *M*yeloma protein, and *S*kin changes. POEMS syndrome is a rare paraneoplastic neuropathy associated with osteosclerotic myeloma or Castleman disease (Chapters 176 and 366).[16]

EPIDEMIOLOGY

Approximately 50% of patients with the osteosclerotic form of myeloma have neuropathy.

PATHOBIOLOGY

The underlying mechanism of neuropathy in POEMS syndrome is unknown, although the very frequent elevation of vasoactive growth factors such as vascular endothelial growth factor (VEGF), the levels of which correlate with disease severity, suggest vascular permeability as a contributing mechanism.

CLINICAL MANIFESTATIONS

Neuropathy typically presents with distal numbness and pain progressing to weakness that is often in the pattern of a length-dependent polyneuropathy. The progressive nature and severity of weakness often suggest chronic inflammatory demyelinating polyradiculoneuropathy, although proximal weakness is less common in POEMS. The general physical examination should evaluate possible organomegaly (hepatomegaly, splenomegaly, or lymphademopathy), features of volume overload (edema, ascites, or pleural effusions), endocrinopathy (diabetes, hypothyroidism, gynecomastia, amenorrhea, and hypogonadism), and skin changes.

DIAGNOSIS

The monoclonal protein usually has a lambda light chain, and any patient with a progressive neuropathy or suspected chronic inflammatory demyelinating polyradiculoneuropathy with a lambda monoclonal gammopathy should be carefully examined and evaluated for POEMS syndrome, as should patients who are thought to have chronic inflammatory demyelinating polyradiculoneuropathy but fail to respond to immunotherapy. Important diagnostic clues include common skin changes such as hyperpigmentation or hypertrichosis, edema, gynecomastia, and papilledema. However, most patients do not manifest the full syndromic spectrum of POEMS (Table 392-5).[17]

Nerve conduction studies often demonstrate some features of demyelination, although axon loss is common. Blood levels of VEGF are elevated to greater than 200 pg/mL in many patients (sensitivity of 68% and specificity of 95%), and the concentration increases as the disease progresses.

TREATMENT 〈Rx〉

Treatment of POEMS syndrome is based on directing therapy at the clonal plasma cell expansion. Modalities include radiation of osteosclerotic lesions, systemic chemotherapy (Chapter 178), and autologous stem cell transplantation. Treatments typically recommended for chronic inflammatory demyelinating polyradiculoneuropathy are usually ineffective.

Light Chain Amyloidosis

Light chain amyloidosis (Chapter 179), which shares many features with hereditary forms of amyloidosis, affects peripheral nerve in about 20% of patients. The heart and kidney are commonly affected.

TABLE 392-5	DIAGNOSTIC CRITERIA FOR POEMS SYNDROME
Mandatory major criteria (both must be present)	Polyneuropathy Monoclonal plasma cell-proliferative disorder (almost always lambda)
Other major criteria (1 required)	Castleman disease Sclerotic bone lesions Elevated vascular endothelial growth factor
Minor criteria (1 required)	Organomegaly (splenomegaly, hepatomegaly, or lymphadenopathy) Extravascular volume overload (edema, pleural effusion, ascites) Endocrinopathy (diabetes, hypothyroidism, gynecomastia, amenorrhea, and hypogonadism) Skin changes (hyperpigmentation, hypertrichosis) Papilledema Thrombocytosis or polycythemia

POEMS = Polyneuropathy, Organomegaly, Endocrinopathy, Myeloma protein, Skin changes.

EPIDEMIOLOGY

Light chain amyloidosis is more common in men (2 : 1 ratio) and has a median age at onset in the seventh decade.

PATHOBIOLOGY

Monoclonal light chains, either lambda or kappa, misfold and aggregate into beta-pleated sheets, which deposit in susceptible tissues. The most commonly involved tissues are kidneys, liver, heart, the carpal tunnel, and the peripheral nervous system.

CLINICAL MANIFESTATIONS

Patients typically present with a relentlessly progressive, distal, symmetrical polyneuropathy that is usually painful and associated with autonomic dysfunction, often with fatigue and unexplained weight loss. Orthostatic hypotension is common, and men often note erectile dysfunction. A minority of patients have a painless neuropathy or do not have prominent autonomic symptoms (Chapter 390). Other organ systems are usually involved, most often leading to renal failure and heart failure.

DIAGNOSIS

Most patients with light chain amyloidosis have free light chains in the urine. Confirmation requires tissue diagnosis, usually with bone marrow biopsy and fat pad biopsy or aspiration (Chapter 179). Biopsy of other affected tissues may be necessary.

TREATMENT 〈Rx〉

Treatment (Chapter 179) consists of systemic chemotherapy and, for patients who are candidates, stem cell transplantation. When successful, treatment may result in stabilization of the neuropathy.

Distal Acquired Demyelinating Syndrome

Distal acquired demyelinating syndrome, which is a variant of chronic inflammatory demyelinating polyradiculoneuropathy, preferentially affects the distal nerve segments, where it results in distal weakness and numbness, often with tremor.

PATHOBIOLOGY

In patients with IgM M proteins that immunoreact with MAG, nerve biopsy demonstrates segmental demyelination with deposits of M protein and complement. The myelin lamellae are often widened on sural nerve biopsies, but a biopsy is not necessary for diagnosis. High titers (>1 : 10,000) of anti-MAG IgM antibodies are associated with neuropathy, and intraneural or systemic injection of anti-MAG IgM M proteins causes complement-mediated demyelination of nerves in animals.

CLINICAL MANIFESTATIONS

Most patients with anti-MAG neuropathies are initially seen in their sixth to seventh decade of life with dysesthesias and paresthesias in their legs and unsteadiness while walking because of loss of proprioception. Distal weakness subsequently develops, and many patients develop a coarse postural and action tremor. Disability and reduced quality of life are determined by weakness, tremor, ataxia, and fatigue.[18] Physical examination shows a length-dependent large fiber sensory neuropathy.

DIAGNOSIS

Nerve conduction studies demonstrate evidence of distal demyelination with markedly prolonged motor distal latencies. The presence of an IgM monoclonal gammopathy with high titer anti-MAG antibodies is observed in 50% of patients.

TREATMENT 〈Rx〉

Patients with anti-MAG neuropathy and distal acquired demyelinating syndrome do not respond as well to immunotherapy as do patients with typical chronic inflammatory demyelinating polyradiculoneuropathy. One small trial of rituximab failed to show substantial improvement. Multiple other agents have been tried without success.[A10]

PARANEOPLASTIC NEUROPATHIES

DEFINITION

Paraneoplastic neuropathies are a "remote effect of cancer" not caused by metastatic invasion of neural tissue; radiation therapy or chemotherapy; metabolic, vascular, or hormonal disturbances; or opportunistic infections. It is hypothesized that they are the result of host immune responses to a tumor antigen or antigens that are also present in neural tissues.

EPIDEMIOLOGY

Paraneoplastic syndromes occur in less than 1% of patients with cancer; peripheral neuropathy is only one of the paraneoplastic syndromes. Although more than 25% of patients with cancer have evident neuropathy on neurologic examination, the relationship to malignancy is unclear in most. Paraneoplastic neuropathy may develop before, during, or after the tumor is diagnosed. In certain tumors, neuropathies are distinctive and should prompt a thorough investigation for cancer. Small cell carcinoma of the lung is by far the most common underlying neoplasm, followed by carcinoma of the stomach, breast, colon, rectum, ovary, and prostate.

PATHOBIOLOGY

Subacute sensory neuropathy, the most characteristic paraneoplastic neuropathy, results from an immune-mediated ganglionitis that destroys sensory neurons in the dorsal root ganglia. Mononuclear inflammatory infiltrates composed of $CD4^+$ and prominent $CD8^+$ T cells, along with plasma cells, are found in the stroma surrounding the dorsal root ganglion neurons. Other findings include atrophy of the dorsal roots; loss of sensory neurons, which appear to be replaced by a proliferation of satellite cells (Nageotte nodule); axonal degeneration; and secondary degeneration of the dorsal column of the spinal cord. Inflammatory infiltrates can also be found in peripheral nerves or muscle. Sural nerve biopsies typically reveal only loss of myelinated nerve fibers and are not useful for diagnosis.

CLINICAL MANIFESTATIONS

Subacute sensory neuropathy is characterized by subacute, progressive impairment of all sensory modalities and is associated with severe sensory ataxia and areflexia. Subacute sensory neuropathy may precede the diagnosis of tumor by months or even years. At onset, patients may have shooting pain and burning sensations. Other symptoms include numbness, tingling, and a progressive sensory loss that may be asymmetrical. Symptoms usually progress rapidly to involve all four limbs, the trunk, and face. Findings may then stabilize, although by this time the patient is often totally disabled. Occasional patients have an indolent course.

Neurologic examination reveals loss of deep tendon reflexes and involvement of all modalities of sensation; large fiber modalities such as vibration and joint position sense are most severely affected. The loss of position sense may lead to severe sensory ataxia with pseudoathetoid movements of the hands and an inability to walk despite normal strength. Cranial nerve involvement includes sensorineural deafness, loss of taste, and facial numbness. The asymmetrical pattern of symptoms sometimes suggests a radiculopathy or plexopathy.

A paraneoplastic encephalomyelitis characterized by patchy, multifocal neuronal loss in regions of the cerebral hemispheres, the limbic system, the cerebellum, the brain stem, the spinal cord, and autonomic ganglia often develops in patients with subacute sensory neuropathy. Autonomic symptoms include impotence, dry mouth, and constipation.

DIAGNOSIS

The diagnosis is based on recognizing the typical neuropathy in the setting of malignancy. The results of routine laboratory studies are generally normal. The diagnosis is supported by finding serum polyclonal IgG anti-Hu antibodies, also called antineuronal antibodies type 1, or by indirect immunofluorescence or immunohistochemistry and confirmed by Western blot analysis.

Subacute painful, asymmetrical neuropathy or neuronopathy in an elderly patient should prompt a search for carcinoma of the lung because small cell lung cancer accounts for more than 80% of the associated tumors.[19] Subacute sensory neuropathy has also been reported in patients with adenocarcinoma of the lung, breast, ovary, stomach, colon, rectum, and prostate, as well as Hodgkin and non-Hodgkin lymphoma. In patients with no evidence of cancer, detection of anti-Hu antibodies should prompt a computed tomography study of the chest with special attention to the mediastinal lymph nodes. The use of whole body positron emission tomography with fluorodeoxyglucose has been advocated for early diagnosis in patients with anti-Hu antibodies or clinical suspicion of subacute sensory neuropathy because it may reveal neoplastic adenopathy months before computed tomography or magnetic resonance imaging.

TREATMENT   Rx

Subacute sensory neuropathy responds poorly to plasma exchange, IVIG, or immunosuppressant medications, even when such treatment is started early in the course of the disease. Successful treatment of the tumor rarely induces remission of subacute sensory neuropathy, but it may stabilize symptoms.

THE DIABETIC NEUROPATHIES

Diabetes causes a broad spectrum of neuropathies that can be divided into chronic (distal symmetrical polyneuropathy and autonomic neuropathy) and acute forms (diabetic amyotrophy, acute cranial mononeuropathies and truncal radiculopathy, and treatment-induced neuropathy of diabetes). Patients with prediabetes, obesity, and the metabolic syndrome are at risk for cryptogenic sensory peripheral neuropathy.

EPIDEMIOLOGY

Diabetes (Chapter 216) is the most common cause of neuropathy in the world. Distal symmetrical polyneuropathy, which occurs in about 50% of patients, is one of the most costly and disabling diabetic complications. Autonomic neuropathy is also common (erectile dysfunction develops in 20 to 60% of diabetic men), but widespread autonomic dysfunction (Chapter 390) develops in less than 5% of patients.

Distal Symmetrical and Autonomic Polyneuropathy
PATHOBIOLOGY

The pathogenesis of distal symmetrical and autonomic polyneuropathy involves both microvascular and metabolic abnormalities. In type 1 diabetes, increased blood glucose levels are clearly linked to the risk of neuropathy. In type 2 diabetes, other metabolic features including hyperlipidemia and obesity are important contributors to the risk of neuropathy. Specific pathogenic mechanisms, ultimately leading to mitochondrial injury and axon loss in both types of diabetes, include activation of the polyol pathway, formation of advanced glycation end products, altered diacylglycerol/protein kinase activity, and oxidative stress.

CLINICAL MANIFESTATIONS

Distal symmetrical polyneuropathy can be symptomatic or asymptomatic.[20] Patients with symptoms develop numbness, tingling, and, in 20% of cases, neuropathic pain in the feet that over time progresses proximally toward the knees. In type 2 diabetes, small-diameter axons responsible for pain sensation are injured first. With time, injury to large-diameter fibers results in loss of proprioception and touch sensation, leading to gait instability and risk of ulceration and amputation. Patients with asymptomatic neuropathy often present later in the disease with large-fiber neuropathy and severely reduced sensation in the feet. Weakness is minimal, even in the distal foot muscles. Once numbness reaches the knees, the fingers and hands may become involved. Ankle reflexes are generally absent, although patellar reflexes may be present.

Autonomic neuropathy (Chapter 390) typically presents after years of diabetes with gastroparesis (Chapter 127), constipation that may alternate with diarrhea, orthostatic hypotension, anhidrosis, cardiac arrhythmias, and erectile dysfunction. Autonomic abnormalities, which can be the most disabling component of diabetic neuropathy, pose a significant risk of cardiac mortality.

DIAGNOSIS

Diagnosis is based on a combination of symptoms and signs of polyneuropathy. Distal symmetrical polyneuropathy may be the first symptom of diabetes, with the diagnosis apparent only after careful evaluation. Nerve conduction studies or skin biopsy can confirm the diagnosis if there is diagnostic uncertainty but are not routinely recommended.

TREATMENT   Rx

Aggressive glycemic control reduces the risk of neuropathy in type 1 diabetes[A11] but not in type 2 diabetes, in which control of other metabolic risk factors may be equally important. Several studies suggest diet and exercise may reduce neuropathic symptoms, including pain, and slow their progression.[21] Gabapentin (up to 3600 mg/day in divided doses 3 to 4 times per day), pregabalin (150 to 300 mg/day in 2 or 3 divided doses), duloxetine (60 to 120 mg/day), and tricyclic antidepressants (e.g., amitriptyline, desipramine or nortriptyline at doses of 25 to 100 mg daily) may be partially effective for treatment of neuropathic pain.[A12][A13] Patients with loss of touch and protective sensation are at risk for foot ulceration and amputation.

Diabetic Lumbosacral Radiculoplexus Neuropathy

Diabetic lumbosacral radiculoplexus neuropathy, commonly referred to as "diabetic amyotrophy," develops acutely or subacutely, most commonly in type 2 diabetes, with asymmetrical proximal leg pain that is typically severe. Atrophy and weakness of proximal thigh muscles ensues, and symptoms often spread to the contralateral side. Distal leg weakness is common, and some patients develop hand weakness. Diagnosis is based on clinical features. Nerve conduction studies and EMG demonstrate an axonal polyradiculoneuropathy with frequent denervation in paraspinal muscles. CSF examination reveals an elevated protein with normal cell counts. Although not necessary for diagnosis, cutaneous sensory nerve biopsy demonstrates a small vessel vasculitis, thereby suggesting an autoimmune etiology. Half of patients require opiate analgesia and a wheelchair to assist with ambulation. Spontaneous recovery is typical, although up to 50% of patients do not regain baseline function. It is unclear if immunosuppressant therapy can alter the natural history, although a brief course of corticosteroids (e.g., 1 g solumedrol 3 times weekly with a tapering dose over 12 weeks) may improve pain.

Treatment-Induced Neuropathy of Diabetes

Treatment-induced neuropathy of diabetes develops after rapid correction of severe hyperglycemia. Patients present with a subacute painful neuropathy with autonomic features. The distribution and severity of symptoms are proportional to the magnitude of rapid decline in the hemoglobin A_{1c} level. Patients whose hemoglobin A_{1c} drops by 2 to 3% over 3 months have a 20% risk of a distal predominant painful neuropathy, and patients with a drop of 4% or more have an 80% risk, often with more proximal involvement and severe pain. Treatment-induced neuropathy of diabetes is often associated with worsening diabetic retinopathy, suggesting a common microvascular mechanism, although the time course is also consistent with an inflammatory etiology. Neuropathy improves gradually, although most patients require symptomatic pain management.

Acute Focal Neuropathies

Truncal radiculopathy is characterized by the subacute onset of focal pain and sensory loss over a region of the trunk, with some patients developing segmental abdominal weakness appreciable as a bulge. Symptoms are similar to post-herpetic neuralgia. As with diabetic lumbosacral radiculoplexus neuropathy, many patients require aggressive pain management, and at least partial improvement occurs after a period of months.

Cranial neuropathies classically manifest as an acute oculomotor nerve palsy in which retro-orbital pain is followed by diplopia and ptosis. Pupillary fibers are often spared, thereby distinguishing the disorder from lesions that compress the oculomotor nerve and cause a dilated pupil. Similar findings may occur with the trochlear or abducens nerves. Bell palsy is more frequent in diabetic patients and is less likely to involve taste than in patients without diabetes.

⬤ INFECTIOUS NEUROPATHIES
Neuropathies Associated with HIV Infection

The peripheral nervous system may be involved in all phases of HIV infection (Chapter 366). The most common peripheral neuropathy is a distal, painful, sensory axonal polyneuropathy that is similar to the toxic neuropathy caused by nucleoside reverse transcriptase inhibitors (NRTIs), including zidovudine, zalcitabine, didanosine, stavudine, and lamivudine. When an iatrogenic neuropathy is suspected, discontinuation of NRTIs may improve symptoms. Conversely, a neuropathy caused by HIV is likely to stabilize or improve with antiretroviral treatment.

Inflammatory neuropathies such as chronic or acute inflammatory demyelinating polyradiculoneuropathy can also occur in the early stages of HIV infection at the time of seroconversion; the CSF cytoalbumin dissociation usually seen with these conditions may not be evident in these patients because of a mild CSF mononuclear pleocytosis. The response of these neuropathies

to plasma exchange or IVIG is generally good. In later stages of HIV infection, cytomegalovirus (Chapter 352) may cause either an acute lumbosacral polyradiculopathy as a result of direct invasion of nerve roots or a mononeuritis multiplex through a vasculitic mechanism.

Neuropathies Associated with Herpes Zoster

Varicella-zoster virus (Chapter 351) usually remains latent in cranial or spinal ganglia after resolution of a systemic infection. Reactivation, which is more frequent in elderly and immunocompromised patients, causes a vesicular skin eruption accompanied by pruritus and dysesthesias. Herpes zoster resolves spontaneously but is frequently followed by post-herpetic neuralgia, which is characterized by severe pain persisting for more than 6 weeks after the rash appears. Early treatment with oral acyclovir (800 mg, five times daily for 7 days) may reduce both the duration of the acute phase and the risk for post-herpetic neuralgia. The use of concomitant corticosteroids in addition to acyclovir improves acute pain without exacerbating viral spread but does not reduce the incidence or severity of post-herpetic neuralgia. Vaccination with the herpes zoster subunit vaccine reduces the risk of post-herpetic neuralgia (Chapter 351).[A14]

Neuropathy Associated with Lyme Disease

Borrelia burgdorferi (Chapter 305) causes a disease with three stages. In the first stage, shortly after and in the same area of a tick bite, a nonpruritic rash (erythema migrans) appears and spontaneously disappears after a few weeks. The second stage is frequently associated with neurologic complications such as lymphocytic meningitis and focal and multifocal peripheral and cranial neuropathies; characteristic manifestations are unilateral or bilateral facial palsy and radiculitis. The third stage is associated with severe neurologic complications, including encephalopathy, encephalomyelitis, and a predominantly sensory axonal polyneuropathy. A lymphocytic pleocytosis in CSF and demonstration of *B. burgdorferi* infection in serum or CSF are the main laboratory findings. Treatment is discussed in Chapter 305.

Neuropathy Associated with Leprosy

Leprosy (Chapter 310) is infrequent in the United States but is a common cause of peripheral neuropathy in some developing countries. Leprosy presents in different forms, depending on the host's immune system. Patients with normal cell-mediated immunity are more likely to have a tuberculoid form characterized by hypopigmented skin lesions associated with decreased sensation. In patients with abnormal cell-mediated immunity, the more severe lepromatous form with large disfiguring lesions may develop. A mononeuritis multiplex pattern with prominent superficial sensory loss is the most typical clinical manifestation of leprosy. If treated early, neuropathies in leprosy improve. World Health Organization recommendations call for combination therapy that includes dapsone (50 to 100 mg/day or 200 to 250 mg/week), rifampicin (600 mg monthly), and clofazimine (100 mg/day).

Neuropathy Associated with Diphtheria

Vaccination has made diphtheria (Chapter 276) rare in developed countries, but it is an important cause of subacute neuropathy in developing countries. Some strains of *Corynebacterium diphtheriae* produce a potent neurotoxin that causes palatal weakness, lens accommodation deficits, and extraocular palsies. These acute manifestations are followed by limb paralysis that resembles acute inflammatory demyelinating polyradiculoneuropathy (see earlier). The neuropathy caused by the neurotoxin usually resolves with resolution of the infection. The diphtheria organism can be eradicated by therapy with antibiotics such as erythromycin (2 g/day intravenously divided twice daily for adults) or penicillin (procaine penicillin G, 1.2 million U/day intramuscularly divided twice daily for 14 days). However, the neuropathy, as with other manifestations of the disease, generally requires treatment with diphtheria antitoxin, a hyperimmune antiserum produced in horses. Depending on the severity of the disease, antitoxin is administered intramuscularly or intravenously (80,000 to 120,000 units for extensive disease for 3 or more; Chapter 276) days.

⬤ TOXIC AND DEFICIENCY SYNDROMES

In Western countries, toxic neuropathies are frequently the side effects of medications[22] rather than a result of environmental exposure (Table 392-6). In most cases, iatrogenic neuropathy is manifested as a length-dependent or "dying-back" axonal neuropathy. Treatment requires a correct diagnosis (see Table 392-5) and discontinuation of the drug. The most common category of drugs associated with neuropathy are antineoplastic agents (especially paclitaxel and oxaliplatin). In some cases, the neuropathy progresses for weeks

TABLE 392-6	SELECTED CAUSES FOR TOXIC NEUROPATHIES
TOXIN CATEGORY	**SPECIFIC AGENTS**
Antineoplastic agents	Paclitaxel, cisplatin, oxaliplatin, bortezomib, thalidomide
Antimicrobials	Chloroquine, dapsone, isoniazid, metronidazole, nitrofurantoin
Cardiac medications	Amiodarone, perhexiline, hydralazine
Other medications	Colchicine, gold salts, phenytoin, disulfiram, pyridoxine
Heavy metals	Lead (wrist drop), arsenic, thallium (alopecia), mercury
Organic solvents	Hexane, acrylamide, vacor

following discontinuation of exposure (hexane and cisplatin), a phenomenon referred to as "coasting," and improvement often requires many months.

Treatment is symptomatic. Duloxetine (30 mg orally once daily for 1 week, then 60 mg daily for 4 weeks) improves pain in chemotherapy-induced peripheral neuropathy.[A15]

Peripheral polyneuropathy may also develop with deficiency of a number of vitamins and nutrients (Chapter 388). Deficiency of vitamin B_{12} results in severe combined degeneration of the spinal cord and peripheral nerves, accompanied by tingling feet and a sensory ataxia. Copper deficiency (Chapter 205), often due to zinc overload, causes a similar syndrome. Vitamin E deficiency causes ataxia and a phenotype similar to Friedreich ataxia (Chapter 382). Vitamin B_1 (thiamine) deficiency may cause a severe sensorimotor axonal neuropathy in addition to the classic triad of Wernicke encephalopathy (ataxia, ophthalmoparesis, and encephalopathy; Chapter 388). Vitamin B_6 (pyridoxine) is unique in that neuropathy may develop with either deficiency or overload. Excessive doses of B_6 result in a sensory neuronopathy that ranges in severity from mild distal numbness and tingling with modest exposure to severe sensory ataxia with higher doses.

An acute axonal sensorimotor peripheral polyneuropathy with ataxia and areflexia in the setting of nutritional deficiency has been described in alcoholic patients and in patients who fail to follow the recommended nutritional supplementation plan following bariatric surgery (Chapter 388). Some patients develop significant weakness. Serum thiamine and vitamin B_6 levels are often reduced,[23] and most patients respond to nutritional repletion.

● CRITICAL ILLNESS NEUROPATHY

Critical illness polyneuropathy is an acute or subacute axonal length–dependent axonal neuropathy that occurs in critically ill patients with sepsis. It is often associated with critical illness myopathy (Chapter 393), which has resulted in some confusion regarding the extent to which clinical symptoms are attributable to the neuropathy or the myopathy. Up to 70% of critically ill patients with sepsis (Chapter 100) develop some degree of critical illness neuropathy, and patients with the systemic inflammatory response syndrome are at particular risk. Treatment is directed at the underlying systemic disorder that led to critical illness and sepsis. Most patients experience at least some degree of recovery, with the ultimate disability determined by the degree of persistent weakness.

● NEURALGIC AMYOTROPHY (IDIOPATHIC BRACHIAL PLEXITIS)

Neuralgic amyotrophy, also known as idiopathic brachial plexitis, typically presents with acute severe shoulder and proximal arm pain followed by rapidly progressive arm weakness and atrophy within several days. Hereditary neuralgic amyotrophy is due to autosomal dominant mutations in the SEPT9 gene, which encodes the Septin 9 protein. Idiopathic neuralgic amyotrophy is thought to be inflammatory because 50% of patients describe a preceding infection.

Initially thought to be very uncommon, recent data suggest the incidence may be as high as 1 : 1000.[24] Although 70% of patients have a typical presentation, the remainder present with other focal variants, including involvement of individual upper extremity peripheral nerves, including the phrenic and laryngeal nerves. Recurrent episodes occur in 25% of idiopathic cases. Treatment is focused on management of neuropathic pain (Chapter 27).

● COMPRESSIVE MONONEUROPATHIES

Peripheral nerves are vulnerable to compression at specific anatomic sites. The most common are median nerve compression at the wrist within the carpal tunnel (carpal tunnel syndrome), ulnar nerve compression at the elbow (cubital tunnel syndrome), and peroneal nerve compression over the lateral fibular head.

Carpal Tunnel Syndrome

Carpal tunnel syndrome, which is caused by compression of the median nerve at the wrist, is the most common compressive mononeuropathy. The carpal tunnel is bounded by the carpal bones and carpal ligament, and it is traversed by the median nerve and flexor tendons. Risk factors include repetitive motion of the wrist and fingers, as well as structural abnormalities within the tunnel such as osteoarthritis, synovial cysts, myxedema, and (rarely) amyloid deposition. Carpal tunnel syndrome is also common during pregnancy, but it usually resolves following delivery.

Symptoms typically include paresthesias of the first three fingers, often at night, and are relieved by shaking or elevating the hand. Patients also commonly experience subjective numbness in a broader distribution including the medial hand (ulnar distribution) and as proximal as the shoulder. In severe cases, patients have objective sensory loss in the median nerve distribution as well as atrophy and weakness of median-innervated thenar muscles (abduction and opposition). Provocative maneuvers such as the *Tinel* (tapping the carpal tunnel) and *Phalen* (sustained flexion of the wrist) signs have poor diagnostic utility compared with nerve conduction studies. Neutral splinting of the wrist during sleep is effective for most patients. Subacute painful, asymmetrical neuropathy or neuronopathy in an elderly patient should prompt a search for carcinoma of the lung because small cell lung cancer (Chapter 182) accounts for more than 80% of the associated tumors. Methylprednisolone injections can provide temporary relief,[A16] as can injection of 5% dextrose,[A17] but patients who fail to respond or whose symptoms recur usually obtain relief from endoscopic or open decompressive surgery.[25]

● BELL PALSY

Unilateral facial paralysis of acute onset frequently occurs on an idiopathic basis (Bell palsy). The diagnosis is one of exclusion. Facial nerve palsies also occur in the setting of *herpes zoster oticus* and are associated with otalgia and varicelliform lesions affecting the external ear, ear canal, or tympanic membrane. Facial paralysis of a lower motor neuron type can be caused by carcinomatous meningitis (Chapter 384), sarcoidosis (Chapter 89), Lyme disease (Chapter 305), and HIV infection (Chapter 366).

Primary tumors of the facial nerve can cause rapidly developing facial paralysis. Facial paralysis can also occur in *CNS disease* affecting the pontomedullary junction, such as stroke or multiple sclerosis (Chapter 383).

CLINICAL MANIFESTATIONS AND DIAGNOSIS

Most cases of facial paralysis are idiopathic. Patients typically notice facial paralysis on inspection in the mirror in the morning. Facial paralysis may be heralded or accompanied by pain behind the ear. The severity of paralysis varies widely.

TREATMENT   Rx

Ten days of oral corticosteroids (prednisolone 25 mg twice daily for 10 days) administered early in the course increases the return of facial function from 63 to 83% at 3 months in patients with idiopathic Bell palsy.[A18] Acyclovir is of no independent benefit, but adding it (at a dose of 400 mg five times daily for 7 days, or twice this dose for varicella zoster) to corticosteroid therapy appears to improve outcomes in severe cases.[A19] In severe cases, protection of the cornea from drying and injury is essential.

PROGNOSIS

Most patients improve, but about 10% of patients have little recovery. Aberrant regeneration of the facial nerve can cause synkinesias, such as "jaw winking" (when the eye is closed) or tearing accompanying salivation ("syndrome of crocodile tears").

● TRIGEMINAL NEURALGIA (TIC DOULOUREUX)

Trigeminal neuralgia and other painful cranial neuralgias are discussed in Chapter 370.

Grade A References

A1. Barroso FA, Judge DP, Ebede B, et al. Long-term safety and efficacy of tafamidis for the treatment of hereditary transthyretin amyloid polyneuropathy: results up to 6 years. *Amyloid.* 2017;24:194-204.

A2. Adams D, Gonzalez-Duarte A, O'Riordan WD, et al. Patisiran, an RNAi therapeutic, for hereditary transthyretin amyloidosis. *N Engl J Med*. 2018;379:11-21.

A3. Benson MD, Waddington-Cruz M, Berk JL, et al. Inotersen treatment for patients with hereditary transthyretin amyloidosis. *N Engl J Med*. 2018;379:22-31.

A4. Berk JL, Suhr OB, Obici L, et al. Repurposing diflunisal for familial amyloid polyneuropathy: a randomized clinical trial. *JAMA*. 2013;310:2658-2667.

A5. Hughes RA, Swan AV, van Doorn PA. Intravenous immunoglobulin for Guillain-Barré syndrome. *Cochrane Database Syst Rev*. 2014;9:CD002063.

A6. Chevret S, Hughes RA, Annane D. Plasma exchange for Guillain-Barré syndrome. *Cochrane Database Syst Rev*. 2017;2:CD001798.

A7. Hughes RA, Brassington R, Gunn AA, et al. Corticosteroids for Guillain-Barré syndrome. *Cochrane Database Syst Rev*. 2016;10:CD001446.

A8. Hughes RA, Mehndiratta MM, Rajabally YA. Corticosteroids for chronic inflammatory demyelinating polyradiculoneuropathy. *Cochrane Database Syst Rev*. 2017;11:CD002062.

A9. Oaklander AL, Lunn MP, Hughes RA, et al. Treatments for chronic inflammatory demyelinating polyradiculoneuropathy (CIDP): an overview of systematic reviews. *Cochrane Database Syst Rev*. 2017;1:CD010369.

A10. Lunn MP, Nobile-Orazio E. Immunotherapy for IgM anti-myelin-associated glycoprotein paraprotein-associated peripheral neuropathies. *Cochrane Database Syst Rev*. 2016;10:CD002827.

A11. Dy SM, Bennett WL, Sharma R, et al. AHRQ Comparative Effectiveness Reviews. Preventing complications and treating symptoms of diabetic peripheral neuropathy. Rockville (MD): Agency for Healthcare Research and Quality (US); 2017. https://www.ncbi.nlm.nih.gov/books/NBK442335/pdf/Bookshelf_NBK442335.pdf. Accessed May 29, 2019.

A12. Waldfogel JM, Nesbit SA, Dy SM, et al. Pharmacotherapy for diabetic peripheral neuropathy pain and quality of life: a systematic review. *Neurology*. 2017;88:1958-1967.

A13. Wiffen PJ, Derry S, Bell RF, et al. Gabapentin for chronic neuropathic pain in adults. *Cochrane Database Syst Rev*. 2017;6:CD007938.

A14. Cunningham AL, Lal H, Kovac M, et al. Efficacy of the herpes zoster subunit vaccine in adults 70 years of age or older. *N Engl J Med*. 2016;375:1019-1032.

A15. Smith EM, Pang H, Ye C, et al. Predictors of duloxetine response in patients with oxaliplatin-induced painful chemotherapy-induced peripheral neuropathy (CIPN): a secondary analysis of randomised controlled trial—CALGB/alliance 170601. *Eur J Cancer Care (Engl)*. 2017;26:1-19.

A16. Chesterton LS, Blagojevic-Bucknall M, Burton C, et al. The clinical and cost-effectiveness of corticosteroid injection versus night splints for carpal tunnel syndrome (INSTINCTS trial): an open-label, parallel group, randomised controlled trial. *Lancet*. 2018;392:1423-1433.

A17. Wu YT, Ke MJ, Ho TY, et al. Randomized double-blinded clinical trial of 5% dextrose versus triamcinolone injection for carpal tunnel syndrome patients. *Ann Neurol*. 2018;84:601-610.

A18. Madhok VB, Gagyor I, Daly F, et al. Corticosteroids for Bell's palsy (idiopathic facial paralysis). *Cochrane Database Syst Rev*. 2016;7:CD001942.

A19. Gagyor I, Madhok VB, Daly F, et al. Antiviral treatment for Bell's palsy (idiopathic facial paralysis). *Cochrane Database Syst Rev*. 2015;11:CD001869.

GENERAL REFERENCES

For the General References and other additional features, please visit Expert Consult at https://expertconsult.inkling.com.

393

MUSCLE DISEASES

DUYGU SELCEN

DEFINITION

Muscle diseases, which are also called myopathies, are disorders of skeletal muscle structure or function. Myopathies can be primary and occur in isolation, or they can be part of a multisystem disorder.

EPIDEMIOLOGY

Many muscle diseases (Table 393-1) are inherited as autosomal dominant, autosomal recessive, X-linked, or maternal (mitochondrial) conditions.[1] Environmental factors that may precipitate myopathies include recent infection, foreign travel, exposure to medications such as statins, and alcohol abuse (Chapter 30). Exercise commonly precipitates symptoms in patients with metabolic myopathies, whereas exposure to cold and high-carbohydrate or potassium-rich food can precipitate weakness in muscle channelopathies.

The prevalence of muscle disease is estimated to be about 1 per 1000 people, including acute and transient disorders (e.g., myositis owing to infectious or toxic causes) and chronic inflammatory or genetic disorders that cause substantial morbidity over decades or a lifetime. Myopathies can cause premature death owing to neuromuscular weakness and secondary respiratory infections or to involvement of other organs in multisystem diseases. Myocardial involvement, which is particularly common in some muscle diseases, can cause heart failure or life-threatening arrhythmias.

TABLE 393-1 CLASSIFICATION OF MYOPATHIES

HEREDITARY

Muscular dystrophies
Congenital myopathies
Myotonia and channelopathies
Metabolic myopathies
Mitochondrial myopathies

ACQUIRED

Inflammatory myopathies
Endocrine myopathies
Myopathies associated with systemic illness
Drug-induced/toxic myopathies

Adapted from Goldman L, Schafer AI, eds. *Cecil Medicine*. 24th ed. Philadelphia: Elsevier; 2012.

PATHOBIOLOGY

Muscle disease can result from a perturbation in the anatomy or any of the physiologic processes required for muscle contraction or the genes that control them. Skeletal muscle is part of a motor unit, which is defined as the anterior horn cell body, its axon, the neuromuscular junction, and the skeletal muscle fibers innervated by the one axon. The motor unit is coordinated in a manner that allows efficient muscle contraction and function. The number of muscle fibers innervated by each motor unit varies from a few (e.g., in muscles controlling very precise movements, such as extraocular muscles) to more than 1000 (e.g., large and powerful but less precise muscles, such as the quadriceps).

Skeletal muscle is composed of myriad muscle fibers. Muscle fibers, which are multinucleated cells formed by fusion of myoblasts during development, are surrounded by a plasma membrane, the sarcolemma, which is surrounded by a basal lamina and endomysial connective tissue. Groups of muscle fibers compose the fascicles, which are surrounded by perimysium, and the groups of fascicles in turn are surrounded by epimysium. Nerve branches, blood vessels, muscle spindles, and fat cells lie within the connective tissue of the muscle.

Each muscle fiber is composed of myofibrils, which themselves are composed of repeat units a few microns long called sarcomeres. The sarcomere consists of a highly organized protein network that gives the muscle fiber its characteristic striated appearance. Each sarcomere is flanked by two Z discs. Z discs are composed of multiple proteins, including α-actinin. Emanating from the Z disc are thin filaments, composed of actin, troponin, and tropomyosin. Thick filaments consist of myosin. Other structures comprise subcellular organelles, including the mitochondria, which are the principal energy source, the endoplasmic reticulum, and the transverse tubules that communicate with the extracellular space.

Muscle function (E-Fig. 393-1) is dependent on chemical energy from adenosine triphosphate (ATP). In the first 30 minutes of sustained activity, ATP is produced by the breakdown of glycogen (glycolysis), and after 30 minutes ATP is produced by fatty acid β-oxidation and oxidative phosphorylation within the mitochondria. The process that leads to muscle contraction begins with the generation of the muscle fiber action potential (Chapter 47), which initiates muscle contraction after it is propagated into the interior of muscle fiber through the transverse tubular system. The release of calcium from the endoplasmic reticulum triggers a coordinated series of events that lead to the coupling of excitation to contraction. Calcium binds to troponin, which interacts with tropomyosin and results in actin-myosin binding. The repeated formation and cleavage of actin-tropomyosin cross-bridges, in an ATP-dependent process, results in sliding of thick and thin filaments and shortening of the sarcomere.

The structural integrity of the muscle fiber surface membrane is maintained by a network of proteins within the muscle. Dystrophin is a key component of the subsarcolemmal cytoskeleton. In combination with several glycoproteins called sarcoglycans (α, β, δ, γ), dystroglycans (α,β), and syntrophins (α,β1, β2), which form the dystrophin-sarcoglycan complex, it anchors the contractile elements of the muscle fiber to the sarcolemma and to the extracellular basal lamina. The basal lamina contains several important proteins, such as collagen, fibronectin, and laminin, which includes merosin and related proteins. The intermediate filament proteins, including desmin, connect the Z disc and other organelles to the subsarcolemmal cytoskeleton.

CLINICAL MANIFESTATIONS

Muscle diseases often present with localized or diffuse muscle weakness, reduced exercise tolerance, resting or exercise-induced muscle pain, muscle enlargement or atrophy, cramps, delayed relaxation, or, rarely, myoglobinuria. These symptoms and signs can be masked by other neurologic or systemic features in patients with multisystem diseases.

History

The assessment of patients with neuromuscular diseases begins with a careful history, general physical examination, and detailed neurologic examination. The age of onset, the rate of progression, and whether the process is episodic, static, or progressive can provide important clues. Congenital and childhood-onset myopathies can be associated with reduced fetal movements, breech delivery, weak cry or suck, and the delayed acquisition of motor milestones. Weakness is the most common presenting symptom, but other symptoms of muscle disease include muscle pain, reduced exercise intolerance, change in the muscle bulk (hypertrophy or atrophy), abnormal spontaneous muscle activity, delayed relaxation, fatigue, or myoglobinuria. Weakness may be relatively static as in some congenital myopathies, progressive as in muscular dystrophies, intermittent as in periodic paralysis, fluctuating as in neuromuscular junction disorders (Chapter 394), or exercise related as in metabolic myopathies. The most common distribution of weakness is proximal or limb-girdle weakness, which results in difficulties in getting out of low chairs, a bathtub, or a car seat; climbing up and down stairs; arising from squat; or getting off the floor. Proximal arm weakness manifests as difficulty reaching to shelves, washing or brushing hair, or raising arms to put on a shirt. Distal leg weakness can lead to difficulty walking on uneven surfaces, tripping over curbs, difficulty standing on the toes, or slapping feet owing to footdrop. Distal upper limb weakness results in difficulty opening jars, typing at a keyboard, writing, or buttoning clothes. Bilateral facial weakness can result in difficulty whistling, blowing up balloons, or drinking through a straw. Predominant involvement of ocular muscles can produce ptosis and diplopia. Weakness of the bulbar muscles manifests as difficulties with speech and swallowing, neck weakness that can lead to a dropped head, and respiratory muscle weakness that can lead to symptoms suggestive of nocturnal hypoventilation or respiratory failure. The early recognition of progressive respiratory failure is essential because it is treatable with noninvasive positive-pressure ventilation.

Fatigue and exercise intolerance can be presenting symptoms of muscle diseases, but they can also be multifactorial and nonspecific. In isolation, these symptoms usually do not indicate a primary muscle disease.

Muscle pain is another nonspecific symptom that can arise from many systemic and psychiatric conditions. Sometimes patients describe aching, stiffness, numbness, or burning as pain. Muscle diseases rarely cause diffuse, generalized, or persistent muscle pain. Muscle pain without muscle weakness is often a feature of fibromyalgia (Chapter 258) or chronic fatigue syndrome. Diffuse myalgia can occur in inflammatory muscle disease such as polymyositis or dermatomyositis, vasculitis, or viral or parasitic myositis. Muscle pain precipitated by exercise usually suggests a metabolic myopathy.

Muscle cramps are involuntary painful contractions that may occur in healthy individuals. Dehydration, renal failure (Chapter 121), and electrolyte imbalances (Chapters 108, 109, 111, and 232) can also produce muscle cramps. Muscle stiffness can occur in inflammatory, metabolic, and ion-channel diseases as well as in conditions such as multiple sclerosis (Chapter 383), polymyalgia rheumatica (Chapter 255), and connective tissue diseases (Chapter 241).

Fasciculations are caused by spontaneous firing of muscle fibers that are innervated by a single motor unit. Fasciculations may occur in normal persons, in whom they are usually exacerbated by stress and increased caffeine intake.

Fasciculations in association with muscle weakness suggest anterior horn cell disease. Myotonia, often described as muscle stiffness, is characterized by prolonged contraction and delayed relaxation of muscle.

Myotonia can affect limb, facial, or bulbar muscles, and it can lead to persistent limb muscle contraction, eyelid closure, or dysphagia. Myotonic dystrophy is the most common muscle disease associated with myotonia, but patients usually complain more of weakness than the myotonia. Conversely, the myotonia associated with sodium and chloride channelopathies can be disabling. Patients who describe locking of their hands but do not have objective myotonia rarely have a physical explanation for their symptoms.

Tetany is the most severe form of sustained muscle contraction. Tetany occurs in patients with hypocalcemia and hypomagnesemia (Chapter 111), and it is aggravated by metabolic or respiratory alkalosis (Chapter 110).

Severe acute muscle damage, termed *rhabdomyolysis* (Chapters 105), results in myoglobinuria that presents as dark brown or red urine. Such discoloration must be distinguished from other causes of pigmenturia (Chapter 106) such as hemolysis or porphyria.

The detailed family history should include questions about muscle disease, including specific questions about the use of canes, braces, or wheelchairs. It also should assess whether family members have had a cardiomyopathy, unexpected sudden death, diabetes, or cataracts.

Physical Examination

A full physical examination must look for signs that may suggest any of the systemic diseases that are associated with myopathies. The skin examination can give clues to systemic illness, such as the heliotrope rash of dermatomyositis (Chapter 253).

A comprehensive neurologic examination should be performed in each patient to exclude possible central or peripheral nervous system disorders (Table 393-2). The examination begins as soon as the patient enters the examination room. Proximal leg muscle weakness may be evident if patients push themselves up on their thighs or have a waddling gait. Patients should be examined for possible facial muscle weakness or wasting, ptosis, or characteristic dysmorphic features, such as with myotonic dystrophy (Fig. 393-1), that can lead to an immediate clinical diagnosis.

Patients should be asked to rise from a squatting position and walk on their toes to assess possible calf weakness and on their heels to assess ankle dorsiflexion weakness. Patients should be asked to stand to assess posture and any evidence of rigidity or scoliosis. Joints should be moved passively to assess for contractures.

All muscle groups should be inspected for evidence of involuntary movements, atrophy, or hypertrophy. Muscles should be palpated for tenderness or unusual texture. Myotonia can be assessed by the inability to relax the muscle belly after percussion with a reflex hammer or the inability to relax the fingers from a firm grip.

Strength should be graded (Table 393-3) in each muscle group. Observing children and infants when they play with toys and how they stand up and walk usually reveals more than formal manual muscle strength testing. The pattern of muscle involvement can provide clues for the diagnosis of a specific myopathy.

DIAGNOSIS

Neurophysiologic testing, measurement of serum creatine kinase (CK), muscle biopsy, and genetic testing help guide the diagnosis of muscle diseases (Table 393-4).

TABLE 393-2   CLINICAL FINDINGS DIFFERENTIATING MUSCLE FROM NERVE DISEASE

FINDING	MYOPATHY	ANTERIOR HORN CELL DISEASE	PERIPHERAL NEUROPATHY	NEUROMUSCULAR JUNCTION DISEASE
Distribution	Usually proximal and symmetrical but can be distal or asymmetrical at onset	Proximal, asymmetrical, and bulbar	Distal, symmetrical	Extraocular, bulbar, proximal limb, but sometimes distal
Atrophy	Slight early, marked late	Marked early	Moderate	Absent
Fasciculations	Absent	Frequent	Sometimes present	Absent
Reflexes	Lost late	Variable, can be hyperreflexic	Lost early	Normal or hyporeflexic
Pain	Variable	Absent	Variable, distal when present	Absent
Cramps	Rare	Frequent	Occasional	Absent
Sensory loss	Absent	Absent	Usually present	Absent
Serum creatine kinase	Usually elevated	Occasionally mildly elevated	Normal	Normal

Adapted with revision from Goldman L, Schafer AI, eds. *Cecil Medicine*. 24th ed. Philadelphia: Elsevier; 2012.

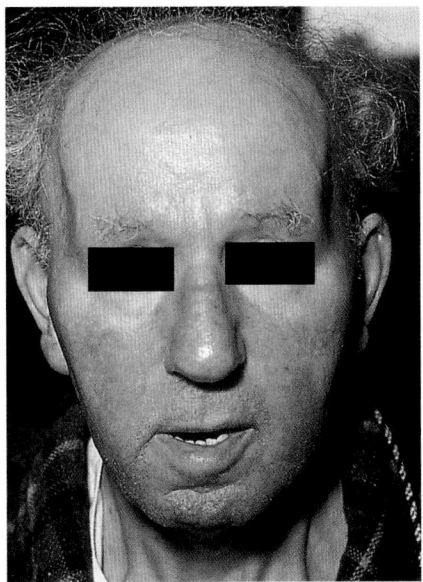

FIGURE 393-1. Myotonic dystrophy in a 50-year-old man. His appearance is typical with facial weakness, atrophy of the temporal muscles and sternocleidomastoids, and frontal baldness, which gives a monklike appearance. (From Goldman L, Schafer AI, eds. *Cecil Medicine.* 24th ed. Philadelphia: Elsevier; 2012.)

TABLE 393-3	MEDICAL RESEARCH COUNCIL SCALE OF MUSCLE STRENGTH

GRADE	DEGREE OF STRENGTH
5	Normal power
4	Active movement against gravity and resistance (often subdivided into 4−, 4, and 4+)
3	Active movement against gravity, but not against resistance
2	Active movement, with gravity eliminated
1	Observable muscle contraction, but not capable of initiating movement
0	No contraction

Adapted from Goldman L, Schafer AI, eds. *Cecil Medicine.* 24th ed. Philadelphia: Elsevier; 2012.

A complete blood count and serum levels of alanine aminotransferase, aspartate aminotransferase, and creatinine can assess possible systemic involvement. An elevated erythrocyte sedimentation rate or C-reactive protein level is found in some inflammatory myopathies and is typical of connective tissue disorders (Chapters 241 and 242). Additional tests to evaluate patients suspected of having inflammatory myopathy or connective tissue disease can include antinuclear antibodies, extractable nuclear antigens, rheumatoid factor, antineutrophilic cytoplasmic antibodies, anti-Jo-1, anti-Mi2, anti-MDA5, anti-3-hydroxy-3-methylglutaryl-coenzyme A reductase, or anti–signal recognition particle antibodies (Chapter 242).

The muscle isoform (MM) of CK is frequently elevated in patients with muscle disease, although a normal level is seen in metabolic myopathies and in some chronic myopathies. A mild to moderate increase in the serum CK level can occur in patients with peripheral neuropathy, radiculopathy, and anterior horn cell diseases. The serum CK level is markedly increased in dystrophinopathies, dysferlinopathy, some of the sarcoglycanopathies, α-dystroglycanopathies, and during rhabdomyolysis (Chapter 105). However, it can decline later in muscular dystrophies as the disease progresses. When the serum CK level exceeds the upper limit of normal by about 10-fold, levels of alanine aminotransferase, aspartate aminotransferase, and lactate dehydrogenase also can be elevated, and some patients can be initially misdiagnosed as having hepatitis (Chapters 138 and 139) before the serum CK level is measured. The blood lactate level can be increased in patients with a mitochondrial myopathy, but a normal value does not exclude this diagnosis. In patients with acute muscle pain and/or weakness, electrolytes and thyroid function tests should be checked.

In patients who are diagnosed with dermatomyositis (Chapter 253), the evaluation should include a search for an underlying malignancy. In patients with suspected mitochondrial cytopathy, a serum and/or spinal fluid lactate level should be obtained. In patients with suspected fatty acid β-oxidation defects, blood acylcarnitine profile may be useful for the diagnosis.

TABLE 393-4	GUIDING PRINCIPLES FOR ASSESSING MUSCLE DISEASES

1. History
　Age of onset (most inherited and acquired disorders have a characteristic age of onset)
　Rate of progression (acute suggests an acquired, often inflammatory cause)
　Fluctuating weakness (may indicate a neuromuscular junction disorder, metabolic myopathy, or a channelopathy)
　Relationship to exercise (may indicate metabolic myopathy or channelopathy)
　Muscle pain (may indicate inflammatory or metabolic myopathy)
　Relevant multisystem involvement (may indicate a mitochondrial cytopathy or myotonic dystrophy)
　Family history (may indicate a genetically determined chronic muscle disease)

2. Pattern of weakness
　Limb-girdle weakness is relatively nonspecific.
　Inherited disorders often have specific patterns of muscle involvement.
　Fluctuating weakness may indicate a neuromuscular junction disorder, metabolic myopathy, or a channelopathy.

3. Testing
　The serum creatine kinase can be normal.
　Electromyography is often normal in metabolic myopathies.
　All patients with muscular dystrophy should have an electrocardiogram and echocardiogram to look for cardiomyopathy and/or conduction defect.
　Muscle magnetic resonance imaging is increasingly being used to guide muscle biopsy and may sometimes reveal diagnostic patterns of muscle involvement.
　Some inherited muscle diseases can be diagnosed clinically and confirmed by genetic testing without requiring other investigations (e.g., myotonic dystrophy; Duchenne, Becker, and facioscapulohumeral dystrophy).
　Muscle biopsy will reveal the cause in most cases; it identifies specific inflammatory myopathies and muscular dystrophies and often provides diagnostic clues for other muscle and neurogenetic disorders.

Adapted with revision from Goldman L, Schafer AI, eds. *Cecil Medicine.* 24th ed. Philadelphia: Elsevier; 2012.

Electromyography

Electromyography (EMG) consists of nerve conduction studies, repetitive nerve stimulation, and needle examination of muscles (Chapter 368). Nerve conduction studies (Chapter 392) are normal in patients with myopathies. In myopathies, the needle examination typically shows complex, polyphasic, low-amplitude motor unit potentials. Myotonia is caused by recurrent depolarization of the muscle fiber surface membrane and has characteristic waxing and waning rhythmical discharges or fibrillation potentials during the needle examination on an EMG. Contractures are electrically silent on EMGs, but muscle cramps are associated with high-amplitude, high-frequency bursts of motor unit activity. The EMG can be normal in some focal myopathies (such as inflammatory myositis), in metabolic myopathies, and in some congenital myopathies.

Genetic Testing

The widespread availability of molecular genetic testing with commercial panels and whole exome sequencing has revolutionized the approach to patients who are suspected of having hereditary muscle disease. Dystrophin genetic testing can identify the defects in dystrophin in 90 to 95% of the patients with Duchenne and Becker muscular dystrophy. The sensitivity of the whole exome sequencing is higher if multiple affected and some unaffected family members and more than one family are analyzed at the same time. Novel genes causing muscular dystrophies are still being discovered.

Muscle Biopsy

Despite advances in genetics and molecular biology, muscle biopsy remains a key component in the diagnosis of most muscle diseases. The biopsy site should be carefully chosen from a clinically affected but not too severely involved muscle. Fresh-frozen sections of the specimens should be used for histochemical studies because even marked morphologic alterations may be undetected in paraffin-embedded tissue. Immunocytochemical localization of specific proteins is useful and diagnostic in some forms of muscular dystrophies. Specific enzyme histochemistry and biochemistry can be used for metabolic myopathies. Genetic analysis of the muscle specimen can be more informative than blood specimens for mitochondrial myopathies.

Imaging

Muscle computed tomography (CT) and magnetic resonance imaging (MRI) are of limited utility for evaluating muscle diseases but can be very useful in excluding spinal cord abnormalities that may cause weakness. Some inherited myopathies are associated with patterns of atrophy and the replacement of muscle with fat. In patchy or focal inflammatory myopathy, MRI can guide muscle biopsy. Functional MRI is sometimes useful in patients with suspected mitochondrial disorders.

SPECIFIC MUSCLE DISEASES

Inherited Muscle Diseases

The four main categories of inherited muscle diseases are muscular dystrophies (E-Table 393-1), congenital myopathies (E-Table 393-2), muscle ion-channel disorders (E-Table 393-3), and metabolic myopathies (E-Table 393-4). Some gene defects cause specific phenotypes that are instantly recognizable at the bedside by an experienced clinician, but less specific phenotypes can be caused by defects in more than one gene. A systematic approach is critical for an efficient and successful investigation of these disorders.

Muscular Dystrophies

The term *muscular dystrophy* refers to the primary degeneration of the muscle fiber, usually associated with an increase in fatty and fibrous connective tissue. The common clinical presentation is progressive muscle weakness.[2]

DYSTROPHINOPATHIES

Duchenne and Becker muscular dystrophies are caused by mutations in the dystrophin gene, which is located on the X chromosome. Female carriers can develop variable phenotypes, including a severe Duchenne-like presentation, mild adult-onset limb-girdle weakness, asymptomatic CK elevation, and cardiomyopathy.

Duchenne Muscular Dystrophy

Duchenne muscular dystrophy is the most common inherited muscle disease, with an incidence of about 1 in 5000 male births. About one third of patients carry a de novo mutation without a family history. In most patients, a frameshift mutation in the dystrophin gene results in a complete absence of the dystrophin protein. This absence of dystrophin disrupts the mechanical link between the sarcomere and the sarcolemma, thereby causing a calcium leak that leads to necrosis of muscle fibers.

CLINICAL MANIFESTATIONS

Duchenne dystrophy typically presents in young boys who are between 2 and 5 years of age with delayed motor milestones, difficulty running, increasing falls, and enlarged calves. The disorder is relentlessly progressive and can cause a cardiomyopathy (Chapter 54) that leads to heart failure and fatal arrhythmias.[3] Intellectual disability, learning disorders, autism, and attention-deficit/hyperactivity disorder can be associated features. By 12 years of age, most affected individuals can no longer ambulate. By the age of 20 years, most patients develop joint contractures and kyphoscoliosis that lead to further respiratory compromise.

DIAGNOSIS

Affected individuals have a 20- to 100-fold elevation of their serum CK level. Confirmation of diagnosis requires DNA analysis of the dystrophin gene. Genetic test is positive in about 90 to 95% of patients. If genetic testing is negative, a muscle biopsy is indicated. The pathologic features are typical of a chronic myopathy. Immunostaining shows an absence of dystrophin except in revertant fibers that express dystrophin (E-Fig. 393-2).

TREATMENT ℞

Management requires a multidisciplinary team approach, including physical therapy to prevent contractures and the timely provision of appropriate devices and wheelchairs.

Eteplirsen, a phosphorodiamidate morpholino oligomer designed to skip DMD exon 51, slows the rate of decline in ambulation on a 6-minute walk test compared with placebo over 3 years of treatment compared with nonrandomized controls and has been approved by the Food and Drug Administration at 30 to 50 mg/kg/day.[4] Prednisone (0.75 mg/kg/day or weekend 10 mg/kg/day) prolongs the ability to ambulate despite its significant side effects (Chapter 32). Both prednisone (0.75 mg/kg/day) and deflazacort (0.9 mg/kg/day) improve muscle strength, with less weight gain from deflazacort.[A1] Prednisone may also help respiratory function and slow the progression of scoliosis. Ataluren does not significantly change the 6-minute walk distance compared with placebo.[A2]

The cardiomyopathy is typically managed by using β-blockers and angiotensin-converting enzyme inhibitors (Chapter 53), the latter of which can slow the progression of myocardial fibrosis,[A3] which in turn is associated with a poorer prognosis. An orthopedic surgeon should help with monitoring of scoliosis and spinal fusion if indicated. A pulmonologist should assess and follow respiratory function, including the initiation and monitoring of noninvasive ventilation.[5]

Additional gene-therapy approaches are being developed.[6] For example, removal of the mutation in the gene encoding the dystrophin protein in mice using CRISPR-Cas9 technology delivered to muscle by an adeno-associated virus can initially correct about 2% of the protein but then apparently spreads enough over time to improve strength.[7]

PROGNOSIS

With ventilatory support, patients often live well into the third or even fourth decades. Chronic respiratory failure is the primary cause of death in the late 20s or early 30s, with most patients succumbing to pneumonia, heart failure, or arrhythmias.[8]

Becker Muscular Dystrophy

Becker dystrophy is a milder form of Duchenne dystrophy caused by an in-frame mutation in the dystrophin gene.

CLINICAL MANIFESTATIONS AND DIAGNOSIS

Becker dystrophy can present in boys older than age 5 years, teenagers, or even in adults. Typical findings are symmetrical proximal weakness and prominent calf hypertrophy. Heart failure is common and may be the initial manifestation in some patients. The CK is elevated, although not to the same degree as seen in Duchenne dystrophy. Muscle biopsy findings are similar to those of Duchenne dystrophy but less severe: immunohistochemistry shows decreased dystrophin expression, and immunoblotting reveals decreased expression and/or a lower molecular weight dystrophin protein.

TREATMENT AND PROGNOSIS ℞

Management is largely supportive. Corticosteroids are rarely used. Similar to Duchenne dystrophy, screening for respiratory function and cardiac monitoring is indicated. Heart transplantation (Chapter 53) has been performed in patients with severe restrictive cardiomyopathy (Chapter 54).

Many patients have a normal lifespan, although some develop respiratory failure and have a shortened lifespan owing to respiratory complications. Heart failure and arrhythmias occur late in the course of disease.

Female Carriers of Duchenne or Becker Dystrophy

Female carriers of a dystrophin gene mutation are usually totally asymptomatic. However, about 2.5 to 10% of carriers can develop symptoms, including myalgias, proximal muscle weakness, and cardiomyopathy. Rarely, they present with a Duchenne phenotype owing to an XO karyotype (Turner syndrome) or skewed X-chromosome inactivation. If a specific mutation is identified in the family, targeted DNA analysis can confirm the diagnosis. Immunostaining of the muscle specimens shows a mosaic pattern, in which some fibers express dystrophin normally and others show decreased or even absent expression. Management of symptomatic carriers is similar to the management of Duchenne and Becker dystrophy patients with similar disease severities.

Facioscapulohumeral Muscular Dystrophy

Facioscapulohumeral muscular dystrophy is an autosomal dominant disorder with variable penetrance.[9] It is the third most common dystrophy after the dystrophinopathies and myotonic muscular dystrophy, with a prevalence of about 1 in 15,000. About 95% of patients have a truncated D4Z4 tandem repeat region in chromosome 4q35. The other 5% have hypomethylation of the D4Z4 region along with a mutation in the *SMCHD1* gene, which is critical for the structural maintenance of chromosome-flexible hinge-domain-containing protein 1.

CLINICAL MANIFESTATIONS

Facioscapulohumeral muscular dystrophy has a highly variable penetrance within the same family. Some gene carriers never present with clinical symptoms or signs. The muscle weakness initially affects the face, where it causes difficulty smiling or whistling. Patients then develop scapular, humeral, truncal, and lower limb weakness leading to footdrop. Scapular winging is a typical feature. Muscle involvement is often asymmetrical.

Associated symptoms can include high-frequency hearing loss and retinal telangiectasia. Rare patients with retinal vascular abnormalities can develop retinal exudation leading to retinal detachment (Chapter 395). Infants with profound facial diplegia can also have intellectual disability and intractable epilepsy.

DIAGNOSIS

The CK level ranges from normal to mildly elevated. EMG shows typical myopathic features. Muscle biopsy shows chronic myopathic changes sometimes with an inflammatory exudate. Definite diagnosis is based on genetic testing.

TREATMENT AND PROGNOSIS [Rx]

Management is supportive, and corticosteroids are of no benefit. Patients do benefit, however, from physical therapy for motion exercises for the shoulder girdle, molded ankle-foot orthoses for the footdrop, hearing aids for patients with hearing loss, and scapular fixation surgery to improve shoulder range of motion. Cardiac features are not prominent, and respiratory muscle weakness is a late feature. The prognosis is highly variable, depending on the severity and age of onset. Many patients have a normal lifespan.

Myotonic Dystrophies

Myotonic dystrophies, which are the second most common inherited muscle disease, affect about 1 in 8000 of the population. The two types, DM1 and DM2, are inherited in an autosomal dominant manner. Both cause multisystem disease and can be difficult to distinguish from each other. DM1 is caused by an abnormal expansion of CTG nucleotide repeats in an untranslated region of the dystrophia myotonica protein kinase (*DMPK*) gene on chromosome 19q. DM2 is caused by an abnormal expansion of CCTG nucleotide repeats in intron 1 of the zinc finger protein 9 (*ZNF9*) gene on chromosome 3q.

CLINICAL MANIFESTATIONS

Patients typically have frontal balding, ptosis, and temporal and masseter muscle wasting.[10] Speech is nasal in quality, and patients display a high-steppage gait owing to their distal myopathy. On neurologic examination, myotonia is seen with percussion (inability to relax the muscle after percussion with a reflex hammer), after a grip (inability to relax the fingers after a firm grip), and in the eyelids (inability to open forcibly closed eyelids). Weakness in DM1 predominantly affects facial, oropharyngeal, forearm flexor, and foot dorsiflexor muscles. In DM2, weakness is predominantly proximal, although deep finger flexors are frequently affected. Muscle pain and stiffness are common in DM2 but can be seen in DM1 as well. Systemic features include premature subcapsular lens cataracts, testicular atrophy, intellectual disability, impotence, and hypersomnolence mediated by both central and neuromuscular mechanisms. Endocrine dysfunction is common, including diabetes mellitus and thyroid abnormalities. Dysphagia and constipation are common. Progressive cardiac conduction defects can lead to sudden death. Patients may require ventilation support after general anesthesia. Women who transmit DM1 are at high risk for having a child with a severe congenital form, including hypotonia at birth, respiratory failure, failure to thrive, and globally delayed developmental milestones with mild to severe intellectual disability.

DIAGNOSIS

Classical myotonic dystrophy usually can be diagnosed clinically by a patient's essentially pathognomonic facial features (see Fig. 393-1). The CK may be normal or mildly elevated. EMG, which is useful when the diagnosis is unsuspected or unclear, reveals myopathic features and myotonic discharges. Molecular genetic analysis of the nucleotide repeats confirms the diagnosis.

TREATMENT [Rx]

All patients should have an annual electrocardiogram and a Holter monitor to detect conduction system abnormalities (Chapter 56). An echocardiogram should be performed at diagnosis and repeated about every 2 to 4 years. Respiratory function testing also is usually recommended about every 2 to 4 years, and a sleep study is useful to detect nocturnal hypoventilation for symptomatic patients.

Mexiletine (150 to 200 mL three times daily) is well tolerated and can improve muscle relaxation.[11] Hypersomnolence (Chapter 377) can be treated with overnight positive-pressure ventilation. Methylphenidate (20 mg daily) may be preferable to modafinil (200 mg daily) for excessive daytime sleepiness, but neither provides dramatic results. Cardiac pacing, which is frequently required, can reduce the incidence of paroxysmal atrial fibrillation. Physical therapy can help to prevent contractures.

OTHER MUSCULAR DYSTROPHIES

Limb-girdle muscular dystrophies are a diverse group of myopathies caused by gene defects or deficiencies of muscle proteins that are critical for the normal function of the muscle cell membrane and especially the dystrophin-sarcoglycan complex. Inheritance can be autosomal dominant or recessive. Although most patients have classical limb-girdle muscle weakness at the onset, some can present with distal leg muscle involvement that may initially be misdiagnosed as sensorimotor neuropathy. Some causes can be identified clinically by an experienced clinician. However, EMG can help to differentiate these conditions from neuropathies, and muscle biopsy, immunohistochemistry studies, and genetic analysis are often required to make a precise diagnosis.

Myofibrillar myopathies present with progressive distal or proximal muscle weakness and characteristic morphologic features on muscle biopsy (E-Fig. 393-3). Cardiomyopathy and neuropathy can be associated features.

Emery-Dreifuss muscular dystrophy was originally X-linked and was initially shown to be caused by mutations in the emerin gene, a nuclear membrane protein. However, mutations in other genes can cause a similar phenotype. Patients have a distinctive phenotype, including progressive joint contractures, scapuloperoneal distribution weakness, and cardiomyopathy with a progressive cardiac conduction disorder. The CK is often elevated but can be normal. Cardiac function needs to be monitored periodically. As with the dystrophinopathies, female carriers of the X-linked forms may develop weakness and cardiac disease.

Oculopharyngeal muscular dystrophy is an autosomal dominant myopathy caused by a trinucleotide repeat expansion of the poly(A)-binding protein, nuclear 1 (*PABPN1*) gene. Onset typically occurs in the fifth or sixth decade of life with dysphagia and marked ptosis. Marked distal and proximal weakness occurs later in the disease course. Surgical correction of ptosis often yields excellent results, but the dysphagia can be more difficult to manage. Patients often have a normal lifespan.

CONGENITAL MUSCULAR DYSTROPHIES

Congenital muscular dystrophies (see E-Table 393-2) are a rare group of autosomal recessive muscle diseases that present in infancy or childhood with hypotonia and muscle weakness. The main differential diagnosis is spinal muscular atrophy (Chapter 391) and congenital myasthenia (Chapter 394). Affected infants can have joint contractures, which can be severe at birth. Some have a pure muscle phenotype and survive into adulthood. Others have severe central nervous system and eye involvement, which are associated with hypoglycosylation of α-dystroglycan that may be fatal in early childhood.

Congenital Myopathies

Congenital myopathies (see E-Table 393-2) are rare inherited muscle diseases that are generally less severe than congenital muscular dystrophies. Most patients present at birth with hypotonia, myopathic facies, and delayed motor milestones. The weakness is usually slowly progressive. Respiratory muscle weakness can occur, and patients can present with ventilator failure at birth or insidiously in adult life. The most severely affected patients present in utero with reduced fetal movements and polyhydramnios. Muscle biopsy is diagnostic (E-Figs. 393-4 to 393-6). Patients with central core myopathy can develop malignant hyperthermia (Chapter 404).

No specific treatments are available. Management requires a multidisciplinary team approach similar to muscular dystrophies.

Ion Channelopathies

Ion channelopathies (see E-Table 393-3) are genetically determined disorders in which the muscle membrane functions abnormally. The combined prevalence of the various skeletal muscle channelopathies is about 1.1 per 100,000.[12] Each has a specific molecular cause, but the phenotypes overlap.

CHLORIDE CHANNELOPATHIES

Mutations in the muscle chloride-channel gene *CLCN1* cause autosomal dominant (Thomson) and autosomal recessive (Becker) myotonia congenita. Patients present with painless myotonia, muscle stiffness that may be slightly worse in the cold and improves with exercise (the warm-up phenomenon), muscle hypertrophy, and grip and percussion myotonia. EMG shows myotonic discharges. The myotonia responds to mexiletine (150 to 200 mg up to three times a day).[A4] Patients have a normal lifespan.

SODIUM CHANNELOPATHIES

Mutations in *SCN4A*, which is the voltage-gated sodium-channel gene, cause a range of autosomal dominant phenotypes, including hyperkalemic periodic paralysis, paramyotonia congenita, and potassium aggravated myotonia. Periodic paralysis is typically precipitated by sustained exercise that leads to weakness during the rest period, by potassium-rich food, or sometimes by emotional stress or cold. The attacks can persist for hours, during which the patient can be quadriplegic with depressed tendon reflexes but normal sensation, eye movements, and respiration. The serum potassium level may be high or normal during the attack. The physical examination is usually normal between attacks, but some patients develop fixed proximal weakness later in the disease. In patients with paramyotonia, the muscle stiffness paradoxically increases with exercise and is often painful. Cold sensitivity is typically more extreme than that seen in myotonia congenita, and cold can precipitate the muscle weakness. The diagnosis is made clinically, although patients with fixed proximal muscle weakness, which can be confused with other myopathies, have vacuolar changes and sometimes tubular aggregates on muscle biopsy. For both phenotypes, management involves avoidance of precipitating factors such as cold or strenuous exercise. If the myotonia is disabling, medications that act on sodium channels such as dichlorphenamide (50 to 200 mg daily), acetazolamide (250 mg twice daily), mexiletine (150 mg three times a day), phenytoin (300 to 600 mg daily), and carbamazepine (400 to 800 mg daily) can be considered. Life expectancy is normal.

CALCIUM CHANNELOPATHIES

Hypokalemic periodic paralysis is usually caused by autosomal dominant mutations in the voltage-dependent calcium channel gene *CACNA1S* but in about 10% of cases is caused by dominant mutations in *SCN4A*. The attacks of weakness, which are usually more severe and prolonged than in hyperkalemic period paralysis, generally persist for hours to days before gradually resolving. Attacks occur spontaneously or during prolonged rest after vigorous exercise and also can be precipitated by a high-carbohydrate meal. The serum potassium level is reduced or low-normal during the attack. Avoidance of high carbohydrate loads and treatment with acetazolamide (125 to 1000 mg/day) or dichlorphenamide (50 to 200 mg/day)[A5] are effective in hypokalemic periodic paralysis. Patients may develop permanent muscle weakness if they have frequent attacks.

OTHER FORMS OF PERIODIC PARALYSIS AND MUSCLE STIFFNESS

Periodic paralysis can occur in a wide range of metabolic and electrolyte disorders (Table 393-5).[13] Mutations in the *KCNJ2* gene, which encodes the inward rectifier potassium channel Kir2.1, cause *Andersen-Tawil syndrome*, an autosomal dominant, usually hypokalemic, periodic paralysis that is associated with distinctive facial features, including hypertelorism and low-set ears, as well as a propensity for cardiac arrhythmias. Treatment includes acetazolamide (250 mg twice daily) and dichlorphenamide. For patients with sulfa allergy, potassium-sparing diuretics such as spironolactone (25 to 100 mg/day) or triamterene (25 to 100 mg/day) can be used. The patients should be treated as indicated for the cardiac arrhythmia and prolonged QT interval (Chapter 59). *Brody disease*, an autosomal recessive disorder caused by mutations in the SR calcium ATPase gene (*ATP2A1*), is characterized by exercise-induced muscle stiffness that is electrically silent on EMG. There are case reports of treatment with dantrolene, verapamil, or nifedipine with varying success.

Neuromyotonia (Isaac syndrome) is an autoimmune disorder associated with peripheral nerve hyperexcitability. It is caused by voltage-gated potassium-channel antibodies and is part of a spectrum of disorders, including limbic

TABLE 393-5	SECONDARY CAUSES OF PERIODIC PARALYSIS

HYPOKALEMIC

Thyrotoxicosis
Primary hyperaldosteronism (Conn syndrome)
Renal tubular acidosis (e.g., Fanconi syndrome)
Juxtaglomerular apparatus hyperplasia (Bartter syndrome)
Gastrointestinal potassium wastage
Villous adenoma
Pancreatic non–insulin-secreting tumors with diarrhea
Nontropical sprue
Barium intoxication
Potassium-depleting diuretics
Amphotericin B
Licorice
Corticosteroids
Toluene toxicity
p-Aminosalicylic acid
Carbenoxolone

HYPERKALEMIC

Addison disease
Hypoaldosteronism
Excessive potassium supplementation
Potassium-sparing diuretics
Chronic renal failure

From Goldman L, Ausiello DA, eds. *Cecil Textbook of Medicine*. 23rd ed. Philadelphia: Elsevier; 2008.

encephalitis. Oral immunomodulatory therapy, intravenous immunoglobulin, plasmapheresis, and symptomatic therapy with carbamazepine or phenytoin have been used with varying response. *Rippling muscle syndrome,* which can be caused by mutations in the *CAV3* gene, is characterized by rippling muscles triggered by exercise or percussion. Rippling muscle syndrome and neuromyotonia can be paraneoplastic phenomena, and a search for malignancy should be considered in these patients.

Metabolic Myopathies

Metabolic myopathies (see E-Table 393-4) are caused by enzyme defects that affect the three principal stages of muscle metabolism: (1) carbohydrate disorders due to a defect of glucose-glycogen metabolism; (2) disorders of fatty acid oxidation; and (3) disorders of mitochondrial oxidative phosphorylation. Muscle dysfunction can be acute, recurrent, and reversible, but the exercise intolerance can cause progressive weakness or even rhabdomyolysis (Chapter 105).

DISORDERS OF CARBOHYDRATE METABOLISM

Because glucose and glycogen are the primary energy sources for muscle contraction, any defects of glucose-glycogen metabolism cause muscle pain, cramps, contracture, and weakness within the first 30 minutes of exercise. The most common form is myophosphorylase deficiency (Chapter 196), and other forms are extremely rare. Most of these disorders are inherited autosomal recessively, although phosphoglycerate kinase deficiency is X-linked. Patients also note exercise intolerance and become deconditioned. Severe episodes are associated with very high CK levels, rhabdomyolysis, and myoglobinuria.

Phosphorylase Deficiency

Phosphorylase deficiency (McArdle disease, type IV glycogenosis) typically presents with muscle pain or cramps after short bursts of exercise. Some patients present with recurrent rhabdomyolysis. Persistent exercise beyond 30 minutes leads to the "second-wind" phenomenon, when fatty acids become the primary source of muscle energy. Clinical examination and the CK can be normal between the attacks, although some patients develop fixed proximal muscle weakness with myopathic features on EMG. Histochemical and enzyme analysis of muscle confirms the diagnosis. A high-protein diet and 37 g or 75 g of oral sucrose shortly before exercise and graded exercise may improve symptoms, but patients are at risk for developing contractures. The life expectancy is normal.

Acid Maltase Deficiency

Acid maltase deficiency (type II glycogenosis, α-1,4-glucosidase), also called Pompe disease, may present in infancy as a very severe generalized muscle disease that is fatal before age 2 years, as a juvenile variant that causes muscle weakness and death by the second or third decade owing to respiratory failure, or as an adult-onset form that presents with limb-girdle muscle weakness or sometimes with respiratory failure (Chapter 197). In each type, EMG reveals myotonic discharges. Abnormal glycogen storage and acid phosphatase–positive vacuoles are seen on muscle biopsy. The disorder can be diagnosed by measuring the enzyme activity in leukocytes or in muscle, but the use of dried blood samples to measure enzyme activity is increasingly becoming the standard practice. Mutation analysis is also clinically available. Enzyme replacement therapy appears promising in children and in the late-onset form.[A6]

DISORDERS OF FATTY ACID METABOLISM

After about 30 minutes of exercise, when the muscle glycogen reserves become exhausted, fatty acids become the principal source of muscle energy. Fatty acid metabolism involves the transport of fatty acids from the serum into the muscle and mitochondria, where both carnitine and carnitine palmitoyltransferase are key components of the β-oxidation pathway.

Fatty acid oxidation disorders can present with a proximal myopathy, exercise intolerance, muscle pain, rhabdomyolysis, and cardiomyopathy. Other features can include neuropathy, pigmentary retinopathy, recurrent hypoketotic hypoglycemia, seizures, and intellectual disability. There may be a family history of sudden unexpected death syndrome. The most common fatty acid oxidation defect is *medium-chain acyl-CoA dehydrogenase (MCAD) deficiency*. *Carnitine palmitoyltransferase I deficiency* presents in childhood with an encephalopathy and liver failure associated with hypoglycemia and a high blood ammonia during metabolic crises. *Carnitine palmitoyltransferase II deficiency* can present as a fatal infantile onset form or more commonly between first to sixth decade of life with muscle pain, exercise intolerance, and myoglobinuria, typically after a long period of fasting or sustained exercise.

Carnitine deficiency can be primary or secondary. *Primary carnitine deficiency* causes myopathy, cardiomyopathy, and encephalopathy in association with hypoketotic hypoglycemia, although pure muscle presentations have been described. The diagnosis can be made by finding a low blood level, although prominent fat deposition in muscle is another clue. Other metabolic myopathies that can cause a secondary carnitine deficiency include disorders of β-oxidation and mitochondrial oxidative phosphorylation and may cause similar symptoms as the primary carnitine deficiency. Analysis of serum acylcarnitines, urine organic acids, and urine acylglycines and specific enzyme assays in fibroblasts can help to pinpoint the enzyme defect.

TREATMENT   Rx

General treatment approach is avoidance of precipitating factors, such as prolonged fasting or prolonged exercise. Carbohydrate intake is advised before exercise, and patients should be prescribed a high-carbohydrate, low-fat diet with frequent feedings. Both primary and secondary carnitine deficiencies respond well to oral carnitine replacement (200 to 400 mg/kg/day in divided doses). Some patients have a multiple acyl-coenzyme A dehydrogenase deficiency (also called trifunctional enzyme deficiency, or glutaric aciduria type II), which responds well to riboflavin (100 mg daily).

DISORDERS OF MITOCHONDRIAL OXIDATIVE PHOSPHORYLATION

Disorders of mitochondrial oxidative phosphorylation (see E-Table 393-4), which are among the most common causes of inherited metabolic diseases, can present with isolated myopathy but often are multisystemic with cardiac involvement, diabetes mellitus, and both central and peripheral neurologic features. Abnormal fatigability or exercise intolerance is a frequent complaint. Common CNS manifestations include epilepsy, migraine, strokelike episodes, myoclonus, ataxia, neuropathy, pigmentary retinopathy, dementia, and psychomotor regression.

Mitochondrial oxidative phosphorylation requires five respiratory chain complexes that are located on the inner mitochondrial membrane. Mitochondrial dysfunction results in energy deficits, which can lead to organ failure. Mitochondrial proteins can be coded by mitochondrial DNA (mtDNA), which is maternally inherited, and nuclear DNA, which can be inherited in an autosomal dominant, recessive, or X-linked manner. Phenotypic presentation of mtDNA defects depends on heteroplasmy, which is the amount and tissue distribution of the mutant mtDNA. If the amount of heteroplasmy exceeds a certain threshold, symptoms become apparent. Mitochondrial DNA disorders affect the structure or amount of the respiratory chain proteins, whereas nuclear

DNA disorders can affect the proteins, the assembly of the respiratory chain, or the maintenance of mtDNA.

CLINICAL MANIFESTATIONS

Mitochondrial diseases should be considered in all patients who have a complex multisystemic myopathy, especially patients with neuromuscular, ocular, and endocrine involvement.[14]

Mitochondrial encephalomyopathy with lactic acidosis and strokelike episodes (MELAS) is most frequently caused by a point mutation of mtDNA (m.3243A>G). Patients can have myopathy, cardiomyopathy, strokelike attacks, and encephalopathy. Some patients have one or only a few of these characteristics, some only have diabetes and deafness, and some only have cardiomyopathy.

Myoclonic epilepsy with ragged-red fibers (MERRF) is usually caused by a point mutation of mtDNA (m.8344A>G). It presents with a proximal myopathy associated with slowly progressive ataxia, epilepsy, peripheral neuropathy, and myoclonus.

Leber hereditary optic neuropathy (Chapter 396) predominantly affects young adult men, more than 95% of whom have mtDNA point mutations in m.3460G>A, m.11778G>A, or m.14484T>C. Patients develop subacute bilateral visual failure in both eyes within 2 to 3 months.

Chronic progressive external ophthalmoplegia with ptosis and gradual limitation of eye movements is seen in up to 20% of mitochondrial disorders.[15] About 95% of patients have sporadic mtDNA point mutations or deletions, but the disease can be inherited as either an autosomal dominant or recessive trait. Mutations in *POLG* gene, which encodes the mitochondrial polymerase γ, are the most common causes of autosomal dominant or recessive progressive external ophthalmoplegia. *Kearns-Sayre syndrome* (Chapter 396) is characterized by the triad of external ophthalmoplegia, retinitis pigmentosa, and onset before the age of 20 years plus at least one of the following: heart block, cerebellar ataxia, or cerebrospinal fluid protein greater than 100 mg/dL. Kearns-Sayre syndrome is usually sporadic and caused by a single deletion of mtDNA.

Mitochondrial DNA depletion syndromes can present in neonatal period or infancy with subacute necrotizing encephalomyopathy (*Leigh syndrome*), hepatorenal failure, cardiomyopathy, and severe lactic acidosis. Children with *Pearson syndrome*, which is caused by accumulation of mtDNA deletions, typically present with pancytopenia, sideroblastic anemia, and exocrine pancreatic failure. *Primary coenzyme Q10 (ubiquinone) deficiency* is a rare autosomal recessive disorder that can present with encephalopathy, lipid storage myopathy, myoglobinuria, seizures, and cerebellar ataxia, or as an isolated nephrotic syndrome or an isolated myopathy.

DIAGNOSIS, TREATMENT, AND PROGNOSIS

The investigation of suspected mitochondrial disorders involves a systematic screen for multisystem complications, especially diabetes and cardiomyopathy; muscle biopsy to look for ragged red fibers, cytochrome c oxidase deficiency, or biochemical evidence of respiratory chain dysfunction; search for mitochondrial deletion or depletion in muscle; and molecular genetic tests. Some primary mtDNA defects are not detectable in blood, so skeletal muscle is often required for the biochemical and genetic tests. For example, diagnosis of primary coenzyme Q10 (CoQ10) deficiency is made by measuring CoQ10 in muscle but not in blood.

Patients with primary CoQ10 deficiency can respond dramatically to CoQ10 supplementation (30 mg/kg/day in children and up to 2400 mg/day in adults in three divided doses). Vitamins and cofactors, including thiamine, riboflavin, and CoQ10, have shown varying degrees of benefit in different mitochondrial diseases. Management is largely supportive with monitoring and treatment of complications. Prognosis varies depending on the phenotype, ranging from the relatively normal life expectancy with chronic external ophthalmoplegia to a relatively rapid demise with Leigh syndrome.

OTHER METABOLIC AND TOXIC MYOPATHIES

Myopathy can complicate many metabolic disorders, including hypothyroidism (Chapter 213), Addison disease (Chapter 214), hyperaldosteronism (Chapter 214), hyperparathyroidism (Chapter 232), vitamin D deficiency (Chapter 231), and liver and renal failure (Chapters 121 and 144). The myopathy is often subtle, the CK level and EMG are often normal, and the muscle biopsy may be nonspecifically abnormal.

Alcohol (Chapters 30 and 388)[16] and many drugs cause myopathy (Table 393-6) with proximal muscle weakness, muscle pain, and exercise intolerance. The CK and EMG can be normal, and muscle biopsy findings may be nonspecific. The diagnosis may depend on the resolution of symptoms after the

TABLE 393-6 TOXIC MYOPATHIES

INFLAMMATORY	**MALIGNANT HYPERTHERMIA**
Cimetidine	Halothane
d-Penicillamine	Ethylene
Procainamide	Diethyl ether
L-Tryptophan	Methoxyflurane
L-Dopa	Ethyl chloride
NONINFLAMMATORY NECROTIZING OR VACUOLAR	Trichloroethylene
	Gallamine
Statins	Succinylcholine
Chloroquine	**MITOCHONDRIAL**
Colchicine	
Emetine	Zidovudine
ε-Aminocaproic acid	**MYOTONIA**
Labetalol	
Cyclosporine	2,4-d-Chlorophenoxylacetic acid
Tacrolimus	Anthracene-9-carboxylic acid
Isoretinoic acid (vitamin A analog)	Cholesterol-lowering agents
Vincristine	Chloroquine
Alcohol	Cyclosporine
Programmed death-1 (PD-1) inhibitors	**MYOSIN LOSS**
RHABDOMYOLYSIS AND MYOGLOBINURIA	Nondepolarizing neuromuscular blocking agents*
	Intravenous glucocorticosteroids*
Statins	**CORTICOSTEROID INDUCED**
Alcohol	
Heroin	
Amphetamine	
Toluene	
Cocaine	
ε-Aminocaproic acid	
Pentazocine	
Phencyclidine	

*In the setting of critical illness.
Adapted with revisions from Goldman L, Ausiello DA, eds. *Cecil Textbook of Medicine.* 23rd ed. Philadelphia: Elsevier; 2008.

TABLE 393-7 CRITERIA SUPPORTING THE DIAGNOSIS OF INFLAMMATORY MYOPATHIES

CRITERION	DERMATOMYOSITIS	POLYMYOSITIS	NECROTIZING AUTOIMMUNE MYOPATHY	INCLUSION-BODY MYOSITIS
Pattern of muscle weakness	Subacute symmetrical proximal weakness with characteristic skin rash	Subacute symmetrical proximal weakness	Acute or subacute severe proximal weakness	Slow onset of proximal and distal weakness after age 50; atrophy of quadriceps, forearms, and facial muscles; frequent falls
Creatine kinase level	Usually elevated, up to 50-fold	Elevated up to 50-fold	Elevated more than 50-fold	Usually elevated up to 10-fold
Autoantibodies	Anti-MDA-5, anti-Mi-2; anti-TIF-1 and anti-NXP-2 in cancer-associated dermatomyositis	Antisynthetase antibodies associated with interstitial lung disease, arthritis, and fever	Anti-SRP and anti-HMGCR	Anti-cN1A
Electromyography	Active and chronic myopathic units	Active and chronic myopathic units	Active myopathic units	Active and chronic myopathic units
Magnetic resonance imaging	May show active inflammation	May show active inflammation	May show active inflammation	Shows selective muscle involvement
Muscle biopsy	Perivascular, perimysial, and perifascicular inflammation; necrotic fibers in "wedge-like" infarcts; perifascicular atrophy; reduced capillaries	CD8+ cells invading healthy fibers; widespread expression of MHC class I antigen; no vacuoles	Scattered necrotic fibers with macrophages; no CD8+ cells or vacuoles; deposits of complement on capillaries	CD8+ cells invading healthy fibers; widespread expression of MHC class I antigen; autophagic vacuoles

Anti-cN1A = anti–cytosolic 5′-nucleotidase 1A; anti-HMGCR = anti–3-hydroxy-3-methylglutaryl–coenzyme A reductase; anti-MDA-5 = anti–melanoma differentiation–associated protein-5; anti-NXP-2 = anti–nuclear matrix protein 2; anti-SRP = anti–signal recognition particle; anti-TIF-1 = anti–transcriptional intermediary factor 1; MHC = major histocompatibility complex.
Adapted from Dalakas MC. Inflammatory muscle diseases. *N Engl J Med.* 2015;372:1734-1747.

toxic agent is removed. Perhaps the most commonly incriminated medications are statins (Chapter 195), which can cause mild muscle symptoms or a severe autoimmune myopathy with a symmetrical proximal weakness, muscle pain, a markedly increased CK level, and, rarely, myoglobinuria. The presence of anti-HMG-CoA reductase antibodies is diagnostic.[17] Steroid-induced myopathy (Chapter 32) is characterized by symmetrical weakness predominantly of proximal muscles.[18]

● INFLAMMATORY MUSCLE DISEASES

Inflammatory or immune myopathies are a heterogeneous group of acquired muscle diseases (E-Table 393-5) that usually present with muscle weakness

and exercise intolerance, with or without pain (Chapter 253).[19,20] Careful evaluation can help distinguish among the most common possible causes (Table 393-7). Most patients have an elevated CK level and an abnormal EMG. Muscle biopsy shows an inflammatory infiltrate. However, the inflammatory process can be patchy and missed on the EMG or muscle biopsy, especially if the specimen is small or if a clinically unaffected muscle is biopsied. Similarly, a short period of corticosteroid therapy can mask the findings. MRI guidance can help to identify high-yield locations for muscle biopsy.

Systemic diseases associated with an inflammatory myopathy include polymyositis,[21] dermatomyositis, inclusion body myositis[22] (Chapter 253), systemic lupus erythematosus (Chapter 250), mixed connective tissue disease

TABLE 393-8	CLASSIFICATION OF INFLAMMATORY MYOPATHIES

IDIOPATHIC

Polymyositis
Dermatomyositis
Inclusion body myositis
Overlap syndromes with other connective tissue disease (scleroderma, systemic
    lupus erythematosus, mixed connective tissue disease, Sjögren syndrome,
    rheumatoid arthritis, polyarteritis nodosa)
Sarcoidosis and other granulomatous myositis
Behçet disease
Inflammatory myopathies and eosinophilia
    Eosinophilic polymyositis
    Diffuse fasciitis with eosinophilia
Focal myositis
Myositis ossificans

INFECTIOUS

Bacterial: *Staphylococcus aureus*, streptococci, *Escherichia coli, Yersinia* spp., *Legionella*
    spp., gas gangrene (*Clostridium welchii*), leprous myositis, Lyme disease (*Borrelia
    burgdorferi*)
Viral: acute myositis after influenza or other viral infections (adenovirus,
    coxsackievirus, echovirus, parainfluenza virus, Epstein-Barr virus, arbovirus,
    cytomegalovirus), retrovirus-related myopathies (HIV, HTLV-1), hepatitis B and
    C
Parasitic: trichinosis (*Trichinella spiralis*), toxoplasmosis (*Toxoplasma gondii*),
    cysticercosis, sarcosporidiosis, trypanosomiasis (*Taenia solium*)
Fungal: *Candida* spp., *Cryptococcus* spp., sporotrichosis, actinomycosis,
    histoplasmosis

HIV = human immunodeficiency virus; HTML-1 = human T-lymphotrophic virus 1.
From Goldman L, Ausiello DA, eds. *Cecil Textbook of Medicine.* 23rd ed. Philadelphia: Elsevier;
2008.

(Chapter 68), Sjögren syndrome (Chapter 252), rheumatoid arthritis (Chapter 248), and sarcoidosis (Chapter 89). Systemic viral illnesses and other infectious microorganisms (Table 393-8) frequently cause muscle pain and an elevated CK, which rarely are major clinical problems.

Sarcopenia and Muscle Wasting

Muscle wasting is a common problem in elderly people (Chapter 22), partly related to hormonal changes and largely related to underuse. Critically ill patients rapidly lose muscle owing to inactivity and reduced protein synthesis,[23] with some potential to slow this process with protein-calorie nutrition (Chapter 103). Sarcopenia is also a prominent feature of many cancers, end-stage heart failure (Chapter 52) and renal failure (Chapter 122), and eating disorders (Chapter 206).

 Grade A References

A1. Griggs RC, Miller JP, Greenberg CR, et al. Efficacy and safety of deflazacort vs prednisone and placebo for Duchenne muscular dystrophy. *Neurology.* 2016;87:2123-2131.
A2. McDonald CM, Campbell C, Torricelli RE, et al. Ataluren in patients with nonsense mutation Duchenne muscular dystrophy (ACT DMD): a multicentre, randomised, double-blind, placebo-controlled, phase 3 trial. *Lancet.* 2017;390:1489-1498.
A3. Silva MC, Magalhaes TA, Meira ZM, et al. Myocardial fibrosis progression in Duchenne and Becker muscular dystrophy: a randomized clinical trial. *JAMA Cardiol.* 2017;2:190-199.
A4. Statland JM, Bundy BN, Wang Y, et al. Mexiletine for symptoms and signs of myotonia in nondystrophic myotonia: a randomized controlled trial. *JAMA.* 2012;308:1357-1365.
A5. Sansone VA, Burge J, McDermott MP, et al. Randomized, placebo-controlled trials of dichlorphenamide in periodic paralysis. *Neurology.* 2016;86:1408-1416.
A6. Case LE, Bjartmar C, Morgan C, et al. Safety and efficacy of alternative alglucosidase alfa regimens in Pompe disease. *Neuromuscul Disord.* 2015;25:321-332.

GENERAL REFERENCES

For the General References and other additional features, please visit Expert Consult at https://expertconsult.inkling.com.

394

DISORDERS OF NEUROMUSCULAR TRANSMISSION

AMELIA EVOLI AND ANGELA VINCENT

DEFINITION

Neuromuscular transmission depends on the release of acetylcholine from synaptic vesicles that are stored in the terminal boutons of the motor nerve axon (Fig. 394-1). Invasion of the motor nerve terminal by the action potential opens voltage-gated calcium channels, resulting in the Ca^{2+}-dependent release of acetylcholine into the synaptic space. Acetylcholine binds to the acetylcholine-gated ion channels (acetylcholine receptors [AChRs]) on the postsynaptic membrane, thereby leading to the opening of these channels and a local depolarization, the end-plate potential. If the end-plate potential exceeds the critical firing threshold, voltage-gated sodium channels (sited at the bottom of the postsynaptic folds) open to generate the muscle action potential that propagates along the muscle fiber and activates muscle contraction. The action of acetylcholine is terminated by its dissociation from the AChRs, which close spontaneously after 1 to 4 milliseconds, hydrolysis of acetylcholine by acetylcholinesterase, and acetylcholine diffusion from the synaptic cleft. Meanwhile, in the motor nerve terminal, the voltage-gated calcium channels close spontaneously, and the resting membrane potential is restored through the transient opening of voltage-gated potassium channels.

The extent to which the amplitude of the end-plate potential exceeds the threshold for activation of the voltage-gated sodium channels is called the safety factor. In healthy individuals, the amplitude decreases during repeated activity but does not fall below this threshold; thus, neuromuscular transmission is not compromised. However, if there is an abnormally low end-plate potential amplitude, failure of neuromuscular transmission may occur. Causes include defects in the release of acetylcholine, the postsynaptic response to acetylcholine, or the number or sensitivity of the voltage-gated sodium channels. Morphologic changes to the presynaptic or postsynaptic components, or to the basal lamina between them, may also influence the efficacy of transmission. Although myasthenia gravis and some neurotoxic envenomations (Chapter 104) are the most common disorders of neuromuscular transmission, a number of genetic myasthenic syndromes also should be considered (Table 394-1).

AUTOIMMUNE DISEASES
Myasthenia Gravis
EPIDEMIOLOGY

Myasthenia is the most common disorder of neuromuscular transmission, with a prevalence of about 15 per 100,000 in Western countries.[1] All races can be affected, and it can occur at any age from year 1 onward. There is a small peak of incidence rate in women in the third decade and a larger peak, the majority males, at later ages. The annual incidence rises to about 5 per 100,000 above age 70 years. It is important, therefore, to differentiate myasthenia gravis from other causes of limb or bulbar muscle weakness in elderly people. Myasthenia gravis is also a complication of therapy with immune checkpoint inhibitors.[2]

Myasthenia gravis itself is heterogeneous and can be divided into different subtypes; the relative frequency of these different forms is not known, but relatively mild childhood forms are frequent in Asian countries. Neonatal myasthenia gravis, due to the placental transfer of maternal antibodies to the AChR or to muscle-specific kinase (MuSK), can affect up to one in eight babies born to mothers with myasthenia gravis. Autoimmune myasthenia gravis must be distinguished from congenital myasthenic syndromes, which are caused by gene mutations.

PATHOBIOLOGY
Pathophysiology

Myasthenia gravis is the result of a defect in neuromuscular transmission. The postsynaptic response to acetylcholine, the end-plate potential, is reduced so that the threshold for activation of the muscle action potential is not reached. At a severely affected end plate, this deficiency can occur at the initiation of

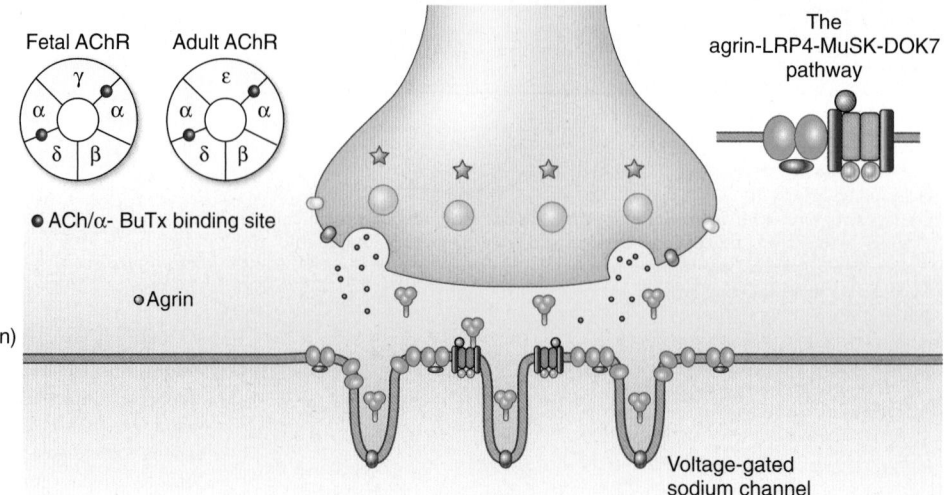

Known targets for autoantibodies

- Acetylcholine receptor (AChR)
- Muscle-specific kinase (MuSK)
- Lipoprotein-related receptor protein 4 (LRP4)
- Voltage-gated calcium channel (VGCC)
- Voltage-gated potassium channel (VGKC)

Main targets for genetic defects

- Acetylcholine receptor (AChR)
- Receptor aggregating protein at the synapse (Rapsyn)
- Choline acetyltransferase (CHAT)
- Acetylcholinesterase (AChE)
- DOK7

FIGURE 394-1. Diagrammatic representation of the neuromuscular junction, indicating the ion channels, receptors, enzymes, and associated proteins that are the most frequent targets for autoimmune diseases (*left*) or mutations in genetic diseases (*right*). The acetylcholine (ACh) receptor (AChR) exists in fetal and adult isoforms as illustrated at *top left*. The replacement of the fetal form by the adult form takes place toward the end of gestation in humans. The agrin–lipoprotein-related receptor protein 4–muscle-specific kinase–downstream of kinase 7 (DOK7) pathway associated with AChRs on the postsynaptic membrane is illustrated at *top right*. α-BuTx = α-bungarotoxin, the snake toxin that binds with high specificity to the two ACh binding sites on the AChRs.

TABLE 394-1 DISORDERS OF NEUROMUSCULAR TRANSMISSION

DISEASE	TARGET	PATHOBIOLOGY
AUTOIMMUME		
Myasthenia gravis	AChRs	Antibodies to AChR in 85% reduce AChR numbers and EPP amplitude
	MuSK	Antibodies to MuSK in 5-8% reduce MuSK-LRP4 binding
	LRP4	Antibodies to LRP4 in a small proportion of patients reduce LRP4-agrin binding
Transient neonatal myasthenia	AChRs, MuSK	Maternal antibodies cause transient disease in neonate
Arthrogryposis	Fetal AChR	Maternal antibodies that inhibit fetal AChR function resulting in paralysis in the fetus in utero, leading to multiple joint contractures.
Lambert-Eaton myasthenic syndrome	VGCCs	Antibodies to VGCC in 90% reduce VGCC numbers, ACh release and EPP amplitude
Acquired neuromyotonia	VGKC-complex	Antibodies to VGKC-complex (mainly CASPR2) in 40% lead to increased and spontaneous ACh release
GENETIC		
Presynaptic	ChAT, ChT, SYT2, SNAP25	Different mutations (mostly recessive) reduce acetylcholine release. ChAT mutations are the most common
Synaptic	ColQ, laminin β2	Mutations in the collagen tail (*COLQ*) that anchors AChE at the neuromuscular junction cause absence of AChE
		Rare mutations of LAMB2 reduce ACh release and EPP amplitude
	AChR	Recessive mutations in AChR-subunits (mostly in the ε-subunit) cause reduced AChR expression
Postsynaptic	AChR	Dominant or recessive mutations in AChR-subunits cause kinetic defects—"slow" and "fast" channel syndromes
	Na,1.4	Mutations in SCN4A sodium channel reduce muscle fiber excitability
Defects in end-plate development and maintenance	Rapsyn, DOK7, agrin, MuSK, LRP4	Recessive mutations cause structural alterations of the end plate. DOK7 and rapsyn defects are the most common.
Glycosylation defects	GFPT1, DPAGT1, ALG2, ALG14	Recessive mutations cause glycosylation defects of end-plate proteins. GFPT1 defect is the most common
Arthrogryposis, multiple pterygium, Escobar syndrome	Rapsyn, AChR δ- and γ-subunits, DOK7, MuSK, GFPT1	Recessive mutations cause a prenatal defect of neuromuscular transmission with fetal akinesia
NEUROTOXIC		
Botulism	SNARE (SNAP receptor) proteins	Botulinum toxin gains entry into the presynaptic motor nerve and cleaves proteins involved in ACh release mechanism
Envenomation following bites from snakes, spiders, scorpions, etc.	Varied sites of action	Neurotoxins specific for VGCCs, VGKCs, AChE, AChRs, voltage-gated sodium channels, and other targets are frequent in many animal venoms and generally inhibit function
Drugs and insecticides	Varied sites of action	Muscle relaxants and other drugs
		Many antibiotics and quinine-related drugs can alter neuromuscular transmission at high dose
		Organophosphates block AChE and have complicated acute and chronic actions

AChE = acetylcholinesterase; AChR = acetylcholine receptor; ALG2 = alpha-1,3-mannosyl transferase; ALG14 = uridine diphosphate-*N*-acetylglucosaminyl-transferase subunit; CASPR2 = contactin-associated protein 2; ChAT = choline acetyltransferase; ChT = high-affinity choline transporter 1; ColQ = collagen like tail of acetylcholinesterase; DOK7 = downstream of kinase 7; DPAGT1 = dolichyl-phosphate *N*-acetylglucosaminephosphotransferase 1; EPP = end-plate potential; GMPPB = guanosine diphosphate mannose pyrophosphorylase B; GFPT1 = glutamine fructose-6-phosphate transaminase; LRP4 = low-density lipoprotein-related receptor protein 4; MuSK = muscle-specific kinase; Na,1.4 = muscle sodium channel; SCN4A = sodium voltage-gated channel alpha subunit 4; SNAP25 = synaptosomal nerve-associated protein 25; SYT2 = synaptotagmin 2; VGCC = voltage-gated calcium channel; VGKC-complex = voltage-gated potassium channel and associated proteins.

contraction, but it is most common during repetitive activity when the release of acetylcholine naturally declines. This phenomenon, occurring across many end plates within a muscle, is responsible for the decrement in the amplitude of the compound muscle action potential on repetitive nerve stimulation, a finding that is diagnostic of a disorder of neuromuscular transmission.

In myasthenia gravis, the reduced end-plate potentials result from loss of AChRs on the postsynaptic membrane and from simplification of the postsynaptic folds, which contain the voltage-gated sodium channels. In most patients, these changes are caused by antibodies against the AChRs. The pathophysiology in patients with antibodies to other postsynaptic proteins,

Direct block of function preventing ACh binding and ion channel opening

Cross-linking of AChRs by divalent antibodies leading to increased internalization and degradation

Complement-mediated lysis of the postsynaptic membrane leading to morphologic damage and loss of AChRs

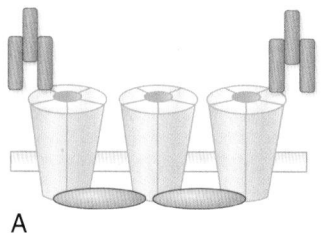
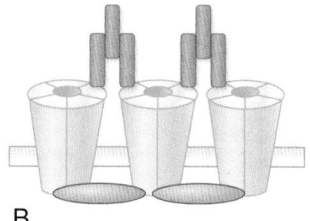
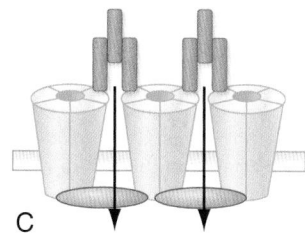

A   B   C

FIGURE 394-2. **Effects of antibodies on the acetylcholine (Ach) receptor (AChR).** In myasthenia gravis, complement-dependent lysis is likely to be the most important mechanism overall. Interestingly, there is no evidence of complement-dependent mechanisms in either the Lambert-Eaton myasthenic syndrome or acquired neuromyotonia, in which cross-linking of the respective ion channels with increased internalization seems to be the main mechanism.

such as MuSK and the low-density lipoprotein–related receptor protein 4 (LRP4), involves intracellular pathways that are crucial for neuromuscular junction maintenance and AChR clustering. Like most synapses, the neuromuscular junction is highly regulated. If the nerve is cut, leading to loss of neuromuscular transmission, the muscle responds by upregulating the expression of AChR that revert to a fetal phenotype (see Fig. 394-1). Alternatively, if the activity of the postsynaptic muscle decreases, both muscle and motor nerve attempt to compensate. Consequently, the synthesis of AChRs in the muscle fiber and the release of acetylcholine from the motor nerve are generally increased in myasthenia gravis.

Pathogenesis

Myasthenia gravis is associated with other autoimmune disorders, most often thyroid disease (Chapter 213). Younger AChR antibody–positive patients have an increased prevalence of the human leukocyte antigen (HLA)-B8 and -DR3 haplotype that is often associated with autoimmunity. AChR antibodies are immunoglobulin G (IgG), have high affinity, are highly specific for the native human AChR, and act by three main mechanisms (Fig. 394-2). First, a few antibodies directly inhibit the binding of acetylcholine to the AChR, thereby causing a pharmacologic-like blockade of function. Second, because of their divalence, antibodies can bind simultaneously to two adjacent AChRs, through the α-subunits that are present in duplicate in each receptor, to form AChR-antibody complexes that are internalized and degraded, thereby leading to loss of AChRs. Third, most of the antibodies are IgG1 subclass that bind and activate complement. The result is activation of the membrane attack complex with destruction of the postsynaptic membrane and morphologic damage. These effects are strictly limited to the neuromuscular junction; the remainder of the muscle fiber is essentially normal.

Specific antibody production requires helper T cells that recognize AChR epitopes. The thymus gland, which is often abnormal in myasthenia, is thought to have a relevant role in the immune response. In patients with early-onset disease, the thymus is often the site of follicular hyperplasia, with T- and B-cell lymphocytic infiltrates in an expanded medulla. These infiltrates, which are very similar to the germinal centers found in lymph nodes, contain B cells that express surface immunoglobulin specific for AChRs and plasma cells that synthesize AChR antibodies. In the thymic medulla, muscle-like "myoid" cells have AChRs on their surface in both normal and myasthenic individuals; these cells may be an early target of complement and antibodies, thereby providing the antigenic stimulus responsible for chronic germinal center formation and a proportion of antibody production.

In late-onset myasthenia gravis and in patients with MuSK antibodies the thymus is mostly normal for age. However, some patients without AChR or MuSK antibodies on standard assays have thymic hyperplasia and antibodies that bind to tightly clustered AChRs on transfected cells.

Thymomas, which are epithelial cell tumors, occur in 10 to 15% of myasthenic patients and nearly always are associated with AChR antibodies. Thymomas associated with myasthenia gravis correspond mainly to the World Health Organization types B1 and B2 and are characterized by active thymopoiesis (i.e., the capacity to promote T-cell maturation and export). Thymoma epithelial cells express muscle antigens and AChR subunits, and they are thought to be responsible for defective negative selection, thereby resulting in export to the periphery of autoreactive T lymphocytes. Rarely, myasthenia gravis arises after removal of a thymoma.

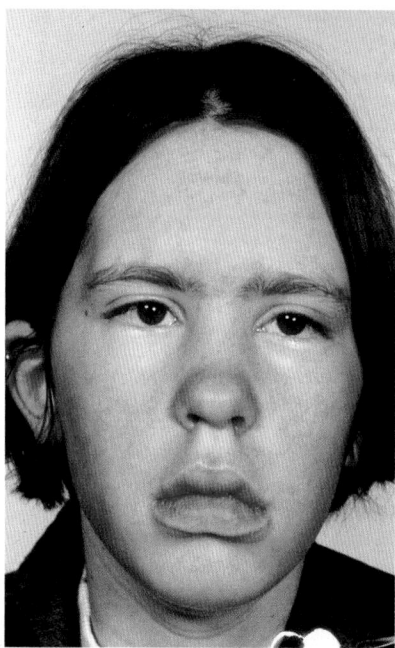

FIGURE 394-3. Marked ocular and facial muscle weakness in a young female with myasthenia gravis.

About 40% of AChR antibody–negative patients have antibodies to MuSK. MuSK is activated by nerve-secreted agrin through its coreceptor LRP4; MuSK phosphorylation and dimerization induce an intracellular signaling cascade that leads to AChR clustering. In animal models, MuSK antibodies cause AChR loss and reduced postsynaptic folds, as well as a lack of presynaptic compensatory increase in the release of acetylcholine. MuSK antibodies, which are predominantly IgG4, act mainly through direct interference with MuSK-LRP4 binding, but IgG1, 2, and 3 MuSK antibodies coexist and may play an additional role.

Lastly, a small number of AChR and MuSK antibody–negative patients have serum antibodies to LRP4. LRP4 antibodies may interfere with LRP4-agrin binding and reduce AChR clustering in vitro.

CLINICAL MANIFESTATIONS

Myasthenia gravis presents clinically with painless muscle weakness that increases with muscle use and improves after rest. In many patients, the weakness starts in the eye muscles, where it results in double vision and ptosis (drooping eyelids). In others, it may first affect bulbar muscles or limb muscles (Fig. 394-3). Virtually any skeletal muscle may be involved as the illness progresses. Typically, the weakness varies in distribution and severity from day to day or from week to week, and it is often worse in the evening. It may first appear following an infection. Established weakness can increase with anxiety, with infection, or with the menstrual period.

Ptosis, which is often asymmetrical, and diplopia can initially be transient and first noticed while driving, for example. Severity can range from mild unilateral ptosis or minimal diplopia to profound bilateral ptosis combined with almost complete ophthalmoplegia. Bulbar symptoms include weakness of facial muscles with difficulties in closing eyes and a "snarling" smile, difficulty in chewing, nasal or slurred speech that can noticeably deteriorate as speech continues, impaired swallowing sometimes associated with nasal regurgitation of fluids, reduced tongue movements, and head droop related to neck weakness.

Limb muscle involvement is common, and proximal muscles are usually more involved than distal. Weakness of the legs can lead to collapse when walking and can be misinterpreted as a functional (psychogenic) disorder. Weakness of elbow extension and of finger abduction may be prominent. By contrast, ankle dorsiflexion is rarely affected except in severe disease. Respiratory dysfunction is less common but can be life-threatening, especially if associated with dysphagia. Selective involvement of the diaphragm can cause severe breathlessness in the supine posture. Wasting is uncommon but can affect the facial muscles and tongue, for example, in long-standing disease. Tendon reflexes are typically brisk. Bladder disturbances are rare, and sensory symptoms do not occur.

Subtypes of Myasthenia Gravis

Several subgroups can be distinguished on the basis of clinical and pathologic criteria and can help to inform treatment.

Ocular Myasthenia Gravis

Ocular myasthenia gravis is confined to extraocular muscles; if it remains localized for at least 2 years, subsequent generalization is unlikely. AChR antibody levels are generally low and are undetectable in about 50% of patients. This subgroup rarely is associated with a thymoma. The neuromuscular junction of ocular muscles shows structural and physiologic differences from limb muscles. Ocular weakness is often the presenting symptom not only in myasthenia gravis but also in neurotoxin poisoning, for example, botulism (Chapter 280). Thus, physiologic factors or accessibility of the neuromuscular junctions of ocular muscles to circulating factors may make them particularly vulnerable to antibodies in myasthenia gravis.

Generalized Myasthenia Gravis with Acetylcholine Receptor Antibodies

Among patients with generalized disease and AChR antibodies, there are three clinical subgroups.[3] Early-onset myasthenia gravis is more frequent in females and associates strongly with HLA-A1, -B8, -DR3 and with thymic hyperplasia.

AChR antibody titers are usually high and decline to varying degrees after successful treatments, including thymectomy.

Late-onset myasthenia gravis is becoming increasingly common with the aging of the population and, when associated with bulbar weakness, may be mistaken for amyotrophic lateral sclerosis (Chapter 391) or brain stem cerebrovascular disease. Among older patients, males are more frequently affected.

Thymoma-associated myasthenia gravis is an important distinction because thymectomy or other specific tumor therapy is required. Most patients with thymomas and myasthenia gravis present between the ages of 40 and 60 years.

Myasthenia Gravis with Muscle-Specific Kinase Antibodies

About 15% of myasthenic patients with generalized symptoms do not have detectable AChR antibodies. Up to 40% of these patients have antibodies to MuSK. MuSK antibodies are absent or very infrequent in patients with AChR antibodies and in patients with persistent ocular symptoms. In comparison with typical myasthenia gravis, MuSK antibody–positive disease is characterized by high prevalence in younger females, predominant bulbar, neck, and respiratory muscle weakness, and more frequent facial and tongue muscle atrophy. There is no evidence of a pathogenic role of the thymus in patients with MuSK antibodies.

Myasthenia Gravis with Neither Acetylcholine Receptor nor Muscle-Specific Kinase Antibodies

Some patients with thymic hyperplasia and a good response to treatment, including thymectomy, may have antibodies that bind only to clustered AChRs on AChR-expressing cells. Some individuals, generally affected with mild disease, have LRP4 antibodies with unclear thymic pathology.

DIAGNOSIS

Diagnosis is based on the clinical features, serologic testing for specific antibodies, electromyography (EMG), and, if doubt still remains or specialized facilities are not available, the clinical response to anticholinesterase medication (Table 394-2).[4] Mediastinal imaging is needed to exclude a thymoma, especially in patients with AChR antibodies.

If AChR antibodies are absent, especially in patients with generalized symptoms, testing for MuSK antibodies is recommended. Both AChR and MuSK antibodies are very specific, and their detection in symptomatic patients confirms the diagnosis.[5] Whether testing for LRP4 or "clustered AChR" antibodies, which can be measured only in specialized centers, will improve the diagnosis of myasthenia is unclear at present.

The electrophysiologic abnormality is an abnormally large decrement (>10%) in the amplitude of the compound muscle action potential on low-rate (3-Hz)

TABLE 394-2 DIAGNOSTIC EVALUATION (EXCLUDES NEUROMYOTONIA)

	AChR MG	MuSK MG	LRP4-MG SN-MG	NEONATAL MG	LEMS	CMS	BoTx	MM
Onset at birth, recovery of muscle strength within 2 mo	−	−		+	−	AChR γ-subunit mutations, variable severity	−	−
Onset at birth plus arthrogryposis	−	−		+	−	Rapsyn, AChR δ-subunit, DOK7, MuSK mutations	−	−
Onset at <1 yr and persistent	−	−		−	−	Any CMS DOK7, rapsyn deficiency, and SCS may present later	+	+/−
Infantile apneas	−	−		+/−	−	Fast channel syndrome, rapsyn, ChAT, CHT mutations		
AChR Ab positive	+	−	−	+/−	−	−	−	−
MuSK Ab positive	−	+	−	+/−	−	−	−	−
VGCC Ab positive	−	−	−	−	+	−	−	−
EMG decrement >10%	+	+/−	+/−	+	+	+	+/−	−
Jitter increased at single-fiber EMG	+	+ Especially face muscles	+	+	+	+	+	+/−
Post-tetanic potentiation	−	−		−	+		+	−
AChE inhibitor response	+	−	+	+	Often weak	Except SCS, COLQ, or DOK7 mutations	+/−	−
Thymoma	+/−	−		−	−	−	−	−

Ab = antibody; AChE = acetylcholinesterase; AChR = acetylcholine receptor; BoTx = botulism; ChAT = choline acetyltransferase; ChT = high-affinity choline transporter 1; CMS = congenital myasthenic syndromes; DOK7 = downstream of kinase 7; EMG = electromyography; LEMS = Lambert-Eaton myasthenic syndrome; LRP4 = low-density lipoprotein-related receptor protein 4; MG = myasthenia gravis; MM = mitochondrial myopathy; MuSK = muscle-specific kinase; SCS = slow-channel syndrome; SN = seronegative for AChR and MuSK antibodies; VGCC = voltage-gated calcium channel.

repetitive nerve stimulation or increased jitter on single-fiber EMG. In patients with MuSK antibodies, EMG abnormalities may be detectable only in facial muscles. These EMG changes are not specific for myasthenia gravis but can occur in any disorder that interferes with neuromuscular transmission.

Intravenous administration of up to 10 mg of edrophonium (Tensilon), a short-acting cholinesterase inhibitor, transiently improves myasthenic weakness but requires an appropriate medical setting, including resuscitative facilities and the availability of atropine, because of the risk of a severe cholinergic reaction, including syncope. An alternative pharmacologic test in adults is a single dose of subcutaneous or intramuscular neostigmine (1 to 2.5 mg) or of oral pyridostigmine (60 mg). The administration of cholinesterase inhibitors should be preceded by the administration of a placebo, and only clear and objective responses should be regarded as positive.

Differential Diagnosis

Congenital myasthenic syndromes (see later) should be considered in patients who have clinical and EMG evidence of myasthenia but are negative on antibody assays. Lambert-Eaton myasthenic syndrome almost always begins with difficulty in walking; ocular symptoms are rare, and specific laboratory tests are available (see later). The ocular muscle involvement that characterizes Miller-Fisher syndrome is more rapid in onset than is usual in myasthenia gravis and is associated with GQ1b antibodies (Chapter 392). Mitochondrial myopathy may show signs that are similar to those of myasthenia gravis (e.g., asymmetrical ptosis and limitation of eye movements), and there may be increased jitter on single-fiber EMG, but this condition and oculopharyngeal dystrophy can be distinguished from myasthenia gravis by the nonfluctuating weakness and by muscle biopsy (Chapter 393). In neurasthenia and chronic fatigue syndrome (Chapter 258), the laboratory tests for myasthenia gravis are negative.

TREATMENT Rx

Most patients with AChR antibodies respond to oral pyridostigmine, 30 to 60 mg four or five times daily; in patients with mild disease, this dose may adequately control symptoms. Doses in excess of 90 mg are likely to cause gastrointestinal side effects, abdominal cramps and diarrhea, which can be controlled with oral propantheline bromide, 15 mg, or loperamide, 2 mg. Patients with MuSK antibodies generally have an unsatisfactory response. In some of these patients, pyridostigmine, even at low doses, can increase weakness and cause nicotinic side effects (muscle cramps and diffuse fasciculations).

Neonatal Myasthenia Gravis

Pyridostigmine, 3 to 5 mg, can be given every 4 hours to about an hour before a feeding. Close monitoring and respiratory support in a special unit may be required.

Ocular Myasthenia

Diplopia can sometimes be helped by the use of prisms. Ocular symptoms that respond incompletely to pyridostigmine are generally improved by low-dose prednisone therapy (e.g., 5 mg every other day) increasing by 5 mg at weekly intervals either until symptoms are completely controlled or until a ceiling dose (e.g., 1 mg/kg) is reached. When remission is established, the dose can be slowly reduced (e.g., by 5 mg every 2 weeks) until symptoms recur and then adjusted upward to define the effective minimal dose. Full withdrawal of prednisone is usually followed by a symptomatic relapse. Thymectomy is not considered beneficial for nonthymomatous ocular myasthenia gravis. In patients who fail to respond adequately to prednisone or who are intolerant of the medication, the addition of azathioprine (2 to 2.5 mg/kg body weight) or ocular muscle surgery is an option. However, the diagnosis should be questioned in patients who show no improvement with high-dose prednisone treatment.

Thymoma

Thymoma is usually an indication for surgery, but removal of the tumor seldom improves muscle weakness. If the tumor is locally invasive, postoperative radiotherapy is indicated. If tumor spread is more extensive, chemotherapy with cisplatin-containing regimens can be considered. Thymoma-associated myasthenia gravis is generally severe, and most patients need long-term immunosuppressive treatment.

Generalized Nonthymomatous Myasthenia Gravis

Immunoglobulin infusion and plasmapheresis are equally efficacious for providing short-term improvement, typically persisting 4 to 6 weeks, and can be used in preparation for thymectomy to cover the initiation of prednisone therapy or to control disease exacerbations. An immunoglobulin infusion of 1 g/kg given on day 1 only is as effective as 1 g/kg given on day 1 and again

on day 2.[A1] Because of the short-lived benefits of these therapies, they must be accompanied by additional immunosuppressive therapy.

When generalized symptoms are inadequately controlled by pyridostigmine, thymectomy can improve symptoms and reduce the need for corticosteroids and for immunosuppressive drugs in patients aged 18 to 65 years with generalized nonthymomatous myasthenia gravis of less than 5 years' duration.[A2][A3] By comparison, thymectomy is not beneficial in patients who have MuSK antibodies and in whom the thymus is generally normal for age. As a general rule, thymectomy, even in the presence of a thymoma, should never be an emergency treatment but rather should be postponed until a stable control of myasthenic symptoms is achieved.

Immunosuppressive therapy with prednisone is usually administered in the initial phases of treatment owing to its short-latency effect. Most patients respond to alternate-day prednisone, started at a low dose (e.g., 10 mg every other day) and increasing by 5 to 10 mg per dose to 1.0 to 1.5 mg/kg. Because starting prednisone can temporarily exacerbate the disease, patients are usually best managed in the hospital, especially if they have bulbar or respiratory muscle involvement. When remission is established, the dose can be reduced by 5 to 10 mg every 2 weeks (or more slowly) to the effective minimal dose. Prophylactic treatment for osteoporosis (Chapter 230) and careful follow-up for other side effects are mandatory in all patients.

For long-term treatment, immunosuppressive medication is required in patients who do not respond satisfactorily to prednisone or who need high maintenance doses.[6] Because these agents have a long latency of effect, they are generally combined with prednisone (see earlier) during initial treatment and then used as monotherapy if steroids can be withdrawn or are contraindicated. Azathioprine (2.5 mg/kg/day) is the preferred treatment; compared with prednisone alone, combination treatment is better tolerated and associated with fewer relapses. Cyclosporine (3 to 5 mg/kg daily) is effective as monotherapy or combined with corticosteroids and is used as a second- or third-choice immunosuppressant. Although the efficacy of mycophenolate mofetil in association with prednisone is questioned, this agent at the standard dose of 2000 mg/day is used in patients who are unresponsive to or intolerant of azathioprine. Tacrolimus is considered a third-line immunosuppressant.[A4] Methotrexate (5 to 15 mg weekly) has shown variable efficacy as a steroid-sparing agent.[A5] When remission has been achieved, doses of these agents can be reduced slowly and cautiously; full withdrawal is likely to be followed by relapse.

High-dose intravenous cyclophosphamide (500 mg/m^2/monthly) and rituximab, a chimeric monoclonal antibody that depletes circulating B cells (usually administered at 375 mg/m^2/once a week for 4 consecutive weeks),[7] have been used successfully in patients with refractory disease.[8] In a randomized trial, eculizumab (a humanized monoclonal antibody that binds C5 to prevent complement activation, given as 1200 mg intravenously every 2 weeks) also was effective in AChR antibody–positive patients with refractory disease.[A6]

PROGNOSIS

The increasing use of immunosuppressive therapies, coupled with advances in critical care, has greatly improved the prognosis of myasthenia gravis. Patients with myasthenic crisis are at high risk for recurrences,[9] but many patients achieve optimal control of symptoms with a normal life expectancy. The prognosis is less good, however, in patients with invasive thymoma, who have a 5-year survival rate of about 80%, or with invasive thymic carcinomas, who have a 5-year survival rate of only about 40%.

Lambert-Eaton Myasthenic Syndrome

DEFINITION AND EPIDEMIOLOGY

The Lambert-Eaton myasthenic syndrome, which is a rare disorder[10] that affects all races, can occur in paraneoplastic and nonparaneoplastic forms. The incidence of the paraneoplastic form is higher, but its shorter survival results in a similar prevalence of the two types. The associated tumor is usually a small cell lung cancer (about 2% of patients with small cell lung cancer develop Lambert-Eaton myasthenic syndrome) and more rarely lymphoma. The nonparaneoplastic form associates with HLA-A1, -B8, and -DR3, as in early-onset myasthenia gravis.

PATHOBIOLOGY

Lambert-Eaton myasthenic syndrome is an antibody-mediated presynaptic disorder characterized by a reduced number of acetylcholine quanta (vesicles) released by each nerve impulse. End-plate potentials recorded from intercostal muscle biopsies are consequently much reduced in amplitude. During high-frequency repetitive nerve stimulation, the end-plate potential amplitude increases, probably because build-up of calcium in the motor nerve terminal leads to increased release of acetylcholine. Freeze-fracture electron microscopic studies of motor nerve terminals show that the "active zone" particles, which correspond to voltage-gated calcium channels, are reduced in number and disorganized. The antibodies in Lambert-Eaton myasthenic syndrome bind to the presynaptic nerve terminal at the sites of acetylcholine release and appear to act principally by cross-linking the voltage-gated calcium channels, thereby leading to their clustering and internalization. The antibodies also interfere with transmitter release from postganglionic parasympathetic and sympathetic neurons in injected mice, providing an explanation for the autonomic dysfunction observed in many patients.

CLINICAL MANIFESTATIONS

Almost all patients present with difficulty in walking,[11] which exhibits a rolling characteristic. Weakness in ocular, bulbar, and respiratory muscles is less common than in myasthenia gravis. Weakness predominantly affects proximal muscles, which may show augmentation of strength during the first few seconds of a maximal contraction. Reflexes are absent or depressed but can increase after 10 seconds of maximal contraction of the muscle (post-tetanic potentiation). Autonomic symptoms such as dry mouth, constipation, and erectile dysfunction are present in most patients. Cerebellar ataxia may be present, usually in association with small cell lung cancer (Chapter 182). Patients with nonparaneoplastic Lambert-Eaton myasthenic syndrome may have other autoimmune diseases, notably vitiligo.

DIAGNOSIS

Diagnosis is based on the clinical features, on a positive serum voltage-gated calcium-channel antibody test, and on the characteristic EMG findings (see Table 394-2). Antibodies specific for the α1A (P/Q) subtype of voltage-gated calcium channels are found in 90% of patients, both with and without small cell lung cancer. Patients may not respond convincingly to intravenous edrophonium. On EMG, the amplitude of the resting compound muscle action potential is reduced; it decreases further during low-rate repetitive nerve stimulation but increases by more than 100% immediately after 10 seconds of voluntary contraction of the muscle or during high-frequency (40-Hz) nerve stimulation.[12] Single-fiber EMG is less specific, because an increased jitter does not distinguish between myasthenia gravis and Lambert-Eaton myasthenic syndrome. Upon diagnosis, an extensive search for malignancy is necessary. All patients should undergo thoracic computed tomography and fluorodeoxyglucose positron emission tomography (FDG-PET). If tumor screening is negative, it should be repeated periodically for at least 2 years after the onset of neurologic symptoms.

Differential Diagnosis

Botulinum poisoning (Chapter 280) causes blockade of presynaptic transmitter release at the neuromuscular junction, as well as EMG changes similar to those in the Lambert-Eaton myasthenic syndrome. Botulism is detected by finding the toxin in serum or the *Clostridium botulinum* bacteria in the wound or feces. Muscle diseases (Chapter 393) can mimic Lambert-Eaton myasthenic syndrome clinically, but autonomic changes do not occur and EMG findings are different.

TREATMENT   Rx

Plasmapheresis and intravenous immunoglobulin (1 g/kg for 2 days) can induce a rapid response in acutely ill patients. Symptomatic treatment is based on 3,4-diaminopyridine (10 to 20 mg four times daily). Both the base form and a phosphate version of the drug, which has been licensed in Europe, are effective. [A7][A8] Immunosuppressive treatment with prednisone and azathioprine may be required in patients with severe weakness, using doses similar to those prescribed for myasthenia gravis. Rituximab has been used in few patients with severe weakness. In the paraneoplastic form, specific tumor treatment often leads to improvement of the neurologic disorder.

PROGNOSIS

Prognosis mainly depends on that of the associated malignancy. Patients with paraneoplastic Lambert-Eaton myasthenic syndrome tend to have a progressive disease and a less satisfactory response to treatment.

ACQUIRED NEUROMYOTONIA

DEFINITION AND EPIDEMIOLOGY

Neuromyotonia, or Isaacs syndrome, is a rare disorder primarily characterized by myokymia (spontaneous undulating muscle contractions) that can be intermittent or continuous and may be present during sleep or general anesthesia. It results from the hyperexcitability of motor nerves. A milder variant, the cramp-fasciculation syndrome, is more common.

PATHOBIOLOGY

Neuromyotonia may be associated with other autoimmune diseases or other autoantibodies, and cerebrospinal fluid analysis may show oligoclonal bands. In about 15% of patients, it is paraneoplastic, usually associated with thymoma and, more rarely, with lung cancer. Occasionally, neuromyotonia follows infection or allergic reactions, and it may improve spontaneously within weeks to months in these cases.

In neuromyotonia, peripheral nerve hyperexcitability is caused by dysfunction of voltage-gated potassium channel (Kv1) whose activation, within milliseconds of nerve depolarization, limits the depolarizing afterpotential and prevents the generation of repetitive discharges.

CLINICAL MANIFESTATIONS

The clinical presentation is variable: muscle stiffness, cramps, myokymia, fasciculations, pseudomyotonia (e.g., failure to relax after fist clenching), and weakness. Increased sweating is common. In the cramp-fasciculation syndrome, symptoms are milder and mostly induced by exertion. Some patients have sensory symptoms, including neuropathic-type pain, or less severe paresthesias, dysesthesia, and numbness, and a few have autonomic and central nervous system features of an encephalopathy, with insomnia, hallucinations, delusions, and mood change (Morvan syndrome).

DIAGNOSIS

EMG shows spontaneous motor unit discharges: distinctive doublet, triplet, or multiplet bursts with high intraburst frequency (40 to 300 per second), longer continuous bursts, and postactivation contraction. The abnormal muscle activity may be generated at different sites throughout the length of the nerve but is usually distal. Many patients have serum antibodies to voltage-gated potassium channel complex (Kv1 channel and associated proteins), predominantly to contactin-associated protein-2, which is required for clustering Kv1 channels at the iuxtaparanodal areas. The differential diagnosis includes neuromyotonia caused by acquired and inherited neuropathies and by voltage-gated potassium-channel gene mutations (Kv1.1) causing neuromyotonia and episodic ataxia.

TREATMENT AND PROGNOSIS   Rx

Neuromyotonia can be improved by anticonvulsant drugs, such as carbamazepine (up to 800 to 1000 mg daily), phenytoin (up to 300 mg daily), or lamotrigine (up to 100 mg daily), that depress sodium channel function and reduce the hyperexcitability of nerves. Plasmapheresis and intravenous immunoglobulins, using the same regimen as for myasthenia gravis, may be followed by short-term improvement. Immunosuppressive medications (as for myasthenia gravis) are effective in some patients. Neuromyotonia is often a monophasic disease that can be successfully managed with symptomatic treatment. When it is associated with myasthenia gravis, the administration of pyridostigmine can increase symptoms of motor nerve hyperexcitability. Prognosis is less favorable in cases with central nervous system involvement, but the neurologic symptoms often improve with immunomodulating medications.

GENETIC MYASTHENIC SYNDROMES

Congenital myasthenic syndromes are inherited disorders that result from mutations in genes encoding key proteins at the neuromuscular junction.[13] In the United Kingdom, their prevalence is at least 6 per 1 million population.

PATHOBIOLOGY

Congenital myasthenic syndromes are classified by the site of the mutated protein (see Table 394-1).[14] Postsynaptic disorders are more frequent and most commonly involve the AChR ε-subunit gene, in which single nucleotide missense substitutions or frameshift mutations result in complete loss of function of the AChR ε-subunit. Because this subunit replaces the AChR γ-subunit around the time of birth, infants are normal in development but show weakness during late pregnancy and in the neonatal period. Survival depends on the continued expression of the γ-subunit, whereas homozygous mutations in the other subunits are probably lethal. AChR deficiency can also result from defects of rapsyn, a cytoplasmic protein required for the clustering of the AChRs, as well as from synaptopathies (see later) and glycosylation defects. Single nucleotide changes in genes for AChR subunits can affect affinity for acetylcholine and gating efficiency, thereby leading to kinetic defects. In the fast-channel syndrome (recessive), AChR openings are abnormally brief, whereas the opposite occurs in the slow-channel syndrome (dominant), where the channel opens for prolonged periods, thereby resulting in subsynaptic accumulation of cations and degenerative changes with loss of AChR.

Mutations in the *COLQ* gene, which encodes the collagen tail that anchors acetylcholinesterase in the synaptic cleft, are less common. The absence of acetylcholinesterase is responsible for reduced quantal release and for continuous exposure of the postsynaptic membrane to acetylcholine leading to cation overload and junctional fold degeneration. Mutations in choline acetyltransferase, the enzyme responsible for the synthesis of acetylcholine, do not always lead to dysfunction at rest; during repetitive activity, however, the amount of acetylcholine in each packet decreases, with consequent failure of neuromuscular transmission. Mutations in *DOK7* cause a "synaptopathy" with small, simplified neuromuscular junctions. DOK7 binds MuSK, and the mutations are thought to impair the signaling that maintains the synaptic structure. Other mutations are much less common.

CLINICAL MANIFESTATIONS

Clinical manifestations may vary from death in utero in severe cases to mild symptoms that present in adulthood.[15] Although most cases present in infancy with ptosis, hypotonia, and difficulties with feeding and breathing, the slightly different patterns of muscle weakness provide clues that point to which gene is involved. Arthrogryposis multiplex congenita, indicative of fetal akinesia, occurs more commonly with rapsyn mutations. Life-threatening episodic apnea can occur with mutations in choline acetyltransferase or rapsyn or in fast-channel syndromes. Severe ophthalmoplegia occurs in end-plate acetylcholinesterase deficiency, AChR deficiency due to AChR subunit mutations, and fast-channel syndromes but is rarely seen in the other genetic syndromes. Motor symptoms with *DOK7* mutations usually appear at about 2 years of age after the child first learns to walk and are characterized by a limb-girdle weakness associated with ptosis and facial and bulbar muscle involvement. Defects in glycosylation enzymes (particularly GFPT1; Table 394-1) are typically associated with limb-girdle weakness and tubular aggregates on muscle biopsy.

DIAGNOSIS

A congenital myasthenic syndrome should be considered when symptoms are evident at birth or during early infancy and other relatives are affected. However, a negative family history does not exclude the diagnosis, and the onset can be later in the slow-channel syndrome, rapsyn, and *DOK7* mutations. Impaired neuromuscular transmission can be detected by a decremental response on repetitive nerve stimulation and increased jitter on single-fiber EMG. In the slow-channel and acetylcholinesterase deficiency syndromes, the prolonged end-plate potential outlasts the refractory period of the muscle fiber, and a single nerve stimulus is usually followed by a repetitive compound muscle action potential (double response) (see Table 394-2).

Genetic analysis is essential to confirm the diagnosis and help in treatment, prognosis, and counseling, although the faulty gene has not been identified in all families.

The principal differential diagnoses are spinal muscular atrophy, infant botulism, hereditary neuropathies, and congenital myopathies or muscular dystrophies. Onset in early childhood, adolescence, or adulthood may lead to the incorrect diagnosis of seronegative myasthenia gravis.

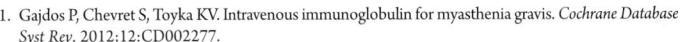

TREATMENT AND PROGNOSIS

Many of the congenital myasthenic syndromes respond to acetylcholinesterase inhibitors, as used for myasthenia gravis, and to 3,4-diaminopyridine (1 mg/kg/day in four divided doses). Patients with the slow-channel syndrome respond to quinidine (at doses corresponding to serum levels of 1 to 2.5 mg/L) or to fluoxetine (60 to 100 mg/day in adults, though some patients may respond to doses as low as 20 mg), but the use of fluoxetine in children or adolescents requires psychiatric supervision. For syndromes in which the neuromuscular junction is destabilized or there are degenerative changes, such as for DOK7 or end-plate acetylcholinesterase deficiency, treatment with ephedrine (75 to 100 mg/day in adults, 3 mg/kg/day in children) or salbutamol (0.5 to 2 mg, three times a day) can be remarkably effective. The beneficial effects of this treatment are not seen immediately but build up over a period of 6 months or more.

Although congenital disorders can be fatal during infancy, usually because of apneic episodes during infections, most tend to be nonprogressive or even may improve during adolescence or adult life. The exceptions are the slow-channel syndrome and acetylcholinesterase deficiency, which, owing to the excess AChR activations, can be associated with end-plate progressive degenerative changes, although this risk is mitigated with treatment.

Grade A References

A1. Gajdos P, Chevret S, Toyka KV. Intravenous immunoglobulin for myasthenia gravis. *Cochrane Database Syst Rev.* 2012;12:CD002277.

A2. Wolfe GI, Kaminski HJ, Cutter GR. Randomized trial of thymectomy in myasthenia gravis. *N Engl J Med.* 2016;375:2006-2007.

A3. Wolfe GI, Kaminski HJ, Aban IB, et al. Long-term effect of thymectomy plus prednisone versus prednisone alone in patients with non-thymomatous myasthenia gravis: 2-year extension of the MGTX randomised trial. *Lancet Neurol.* 2019;18:259-268.

A4. Wang L, Zhang S, Xi J, et al. Efficacy and safety of tacrolimus for myasthenia gravis: a systematic review and meta-analysis. *J Neurol.* 2017;264:2191-2200.

A5. Pasnoor M, He J, Herbelin L, et al. A randomized controlled trial of methotrexate for patients with generalized myasthenia gravis. *Neurology.* 2016;87:57-64.

A6. Howard JF Jr, Utsugisawa K, Benatar M, et al. Safety and efficacy of eculizumab in anti-acetylcholine receptor antibody-positive refractory generalised myasthenia gravis (REGAIN): a phase 3, randomised, double-blind, placebo-controlled, multicentre study. *Lancet Neurol.* 2017;16:976-986.

A7. Oh SJ, Shcherbakova N, Kostera-Pruszczyk A, et al. Amifampridine phosphate (Firdapse®) is effective and safe in a phase 3 clinical trial in LEMS. *Muscle Nerve.* 2016;53:717-725.

A8. Sanders DB, Juel VC, Harati Y, et al. 3,4-Diaminopyridine base effectively treats the weakness of Lambert-Eaton myasthenia. *Muscle Nerve.* 2018;57:561-568.

GENERAL REFERENCES

For the General References and other additional features, please visit Expert Consult at https://expertconsult.inkling.com.

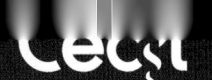

XXVII

EYE, EAR, NOSE, AND THROAT DISEASES

395

DISEASES OF THE VISUAL SYSTEM

GEORGE A. CIOFFI AND JEFFREY M. LIEBMANN

The eye is a compact, complicated structure (Fig. 395-1) that is remarkably stable throughout life. Once the growth of the eye is complete, at approximately age 7 to 8 years, the structure of the eye changes very little for the next 60 to 80 years.

The eyelids physically protect the eye. The pathway of light through the eye, termed the *visual axis*, ideally contains no opaque structures such as blood vessels. Light passes through the tear film, cornea, aqueous humor, crystalline lens, vitreous, and inner retina, all of which, except for the crystalline lens, remain essentially transparent throughout life. Delicate intraocular structures are protected by a tough collagenous "eye wall" composed of the cornea and sclera. The optic nerve, which is composed of axons from the retinal ganglion cells, is enveloped by dura, arachnoid, and pia mater, which are contiguous with the brain. The optic nerve is long enough to allow free excursions of the eye through a 100-degree arc under the influence of six coordinated and critically placed rectus muscles. All these functional components are housed in a bony cavity, the orbit, which protects the eye from external injury.

The eyelid skin, only loosely connected to underlying structures, is among the thinnest of the body. The eyelid is unique because it contains the highest density of sebaceous glands in the body. These meibomian glands produce a sebaceous (lipid) material that is the principal evaporation retardant for the tear film. Malorientation of the eyelid margin or malorientation of the lashes (trichiasis) may cause scarring of the anterior surface of the eye, even to the point of blindness, owing to diminished transparency of the cornea. The upper eyelid is opened by contraction of the levator muscle. The tendon of the levator tends to degenerate over time to produce mechanical ptosis ("drooping eyelids"). The soft tissue of the eyelid is separated from the soft tissue of the orbit by the orbital septum, a major collagenous barrier that protects intraorbital soft tissue from extension of preseptal eyelid inflammation. Extension of inflammation from preseptal cellulitis or ethmoiditis may cause orbital cellulitis, thereby resulting in potential consequences such as cavernous sinus thrombosis. The elastic tissue supporting the skin of the anterior eyelid is reduced over time, thereby causing dermatochalasis ("baggy eyelids"). Redundant tissue may be sufficient in quantity to restrict the visual field, particularly superiorly.

The conjunctiva is a mucous membrane with an outer layer of stratified, nonkeratinizing squamous epithelium containing goblet cells. The epithelium is supported by delicate fibrovascular tissue that contains lymphatic channels. The conjunctival epithelium also contains melanocytes. Squamous carcinoma or malignant melanoma originating in the conjunctiva may extend through these channels to regional lymph nodes or beyond. Immune processing cells are present in the epithelium (Langerhans cells) and in the stroma as collections of non-nodal B and T lymphocytes. Non-nodal primary lymphomas, which tend to have an indolent course in this location, may arise from this tissue. The aqueous portion of tears is formed constantly by accessory lacrimal glands in the conjunctiva as well as by reflex action from the lacrimal gland. Symptoms of itching and burning, as well as periodic disturbance of vision, may result from inadequacies of the tear film layer.

Tears drain through two puncta located at the nasal eyelid margin (one in the upper lid and one in the lower lid) into the nasolacrimal duct, which exits into the nasal cavity inferior under the inferior turbinate. The epithelium of the nasolacrimal duct also contains melanocytes and is supported by a resting lymphocyte population. Neoplasms including lymphoma, concretions (dacryoliths), and tissue injury from trauma may occlude the puncta and nasolacrimal system in adults.

The cornea is avascular and lined anteriorly by epithelial cells and posteriorly by endothelial cells. Lack of an adequate tear film (dry eye syndrome) may seriously alter the ability of the cornea to transmit light, thereby affecting visual acuity. The posterior cellular lining of the cornea is a single layer of highly modified corneal endothelial cells that maintain tissue dehydration. Lack of effective pumping by the endothelial cells will allow excess hydration of the corneal stroma, that is, corneal edema, which diminishes its clarity. The corneal stroma is particularly sensitive to proteolysis from collagenases found with certain inflammatory conditions, such as herpes simplex and zoster keratitis. The cumulative effect of multiple episodes of corneal inflammation may be corneal thinning and even perforation of the cornea.

Intraocular pressure is measured by tonometry. The amount of pressure necessary to flatten the central cornea is proportional to the intraocular pressure.

The anterior chamber is bounded by the posterior surface of the cornea, the anterior surface of the iris, and the anterior surface of the crystalline lens within the pupillary space. The posterior chamber is bounded by the posterior surface of the iris, the ciliary body circumferentially, and the anterior surface of the vitreous. Aqueous humor normally flows from the posterior chamber into the anterior chamber through the pupil and exits into the general circulation through the trabecular meshwork and a series of collector veins. Most causes of pathologically increased intraocular pressure and optic nerve damage (e.g., glaucoma) are due to abnormalities of filtration through the trabecular meshwork. The crystalline lens is located entirely in the posterior chamber.

The anterior segment is composed of the cornea and the anterior and posterior chambers. Most of the anterior segment is derived from the skin and neural crest tissue. The posterior segment is the remainder of the eye. Most of the posterior segment structures are derived from the central nervous system and neural crest tissue.

When first formed, the crystalline lens is a totally cellular structure bounded by a true basement membrane. Throughout life, the new cells that are continuously added from the outer layer epithelial cells that compress the central cells, thereby resulting in cell degeneration in the central core (nucleus). The lens doubles in volume from birth to age 70 years at the cost of both pliability (presbyopia) and clarity (cataract). The lens is suspended in the posterior chamber by fibers (zonules) attached to the ciliary body.

The ciliary body is comprised of the middle layer of the eye wall, the uveal tract. The uveal tract extends under the retina as a vascular plexus, the choroid, and the iris. The surface cells of the ciliary body produce aqueous humor, and its muscles function in accommodation.

The vitreous is composed primarily of water and type II collagen. The vitreous makes up the majority of the volume and weight of the eye. It functions as a biochemical sink as well as to maintain neural retinal attachment. With time, the vitreous shrinks and separates from the retina (posterior vitreous detachment). Condensed vitreous opacities, which cast shadows on the retina, are perceived by the patient as "floaters."

The retina is the site of photochemical conversion of light to electrical energy. Ganglion cells and their axons in the internal retina aggregate at the optic disc to form the optic nerve. Only the inner half of the retina is supplied by intraretinal vessels that are seen by ophthalmoscopy. The outer half of the retina is supplied by large-caliber capillary vessels in the choroid (the choriocapillaris). Only a 500-μm area of the posterior retina, the central macula (about 3 to 5% of the total retina), has the ability to resolve images to 20/20. The remainder of the retina has much less sensitive image resolution. Extensive biochemical support and control of stray light are performed by the retinal pigment epithelium located between the choriocapillaris and the photoreceptor outer segments. The blood-retinal barrier, which protects the biochemical integrity of the retina, is composed of anatomic attachments between neighboring retinal pigment epithelial cells, as well as attachments between vascular endothelial cells of the retinal circulation. The retina is held in place by physiologic forces that may be compromised by holes in the retina (rhegmatogenous retinal detachment) or by fluid accumulating in the subretinal space without a retinal hole (nonrhegmatogenous retinal detachment).

The optic nerve is composed of approximately 1 million axons from retinal ganglion cells. Axons are separated into bundles by pial septa, which are in turn enclosed in an arachnoid layer. The dura is contiguous with the posterior sclera and the periosteum of the optic canal. Delicate vessels extending from the dura across the arachnoid to the pial septa supply the optic nerve. The central retinal artery is present in the axial layer of the optic nerve near the eye but does not supply blood to the optic nerve itself. The optic nerve axons travel through a collagenous sieve in the plane of the posterior sclera, the lamina cribrosa. The choroid is that portion of the uveal tract external to the retina. This layer is composed of various calibers of blood vessels that ultimately supply blood for the choriocapillaris.

The sclera is composed of dense, relatively disorganized collagen. It is opaque because of the nonhomogeneous structure of the collagen and the degree of hydration relative to the cornea. There are multiple scleral ostia for the passage of arteries, veins, and nerves, both posteriorly and anteriorly.

The orbit is composed of bones of the facial skeleton. Sutures between major bones exist in the superior nasal and superior temporal quadrants. Multiple vessels and nerves extend through the thin ethmoid bone from nasal

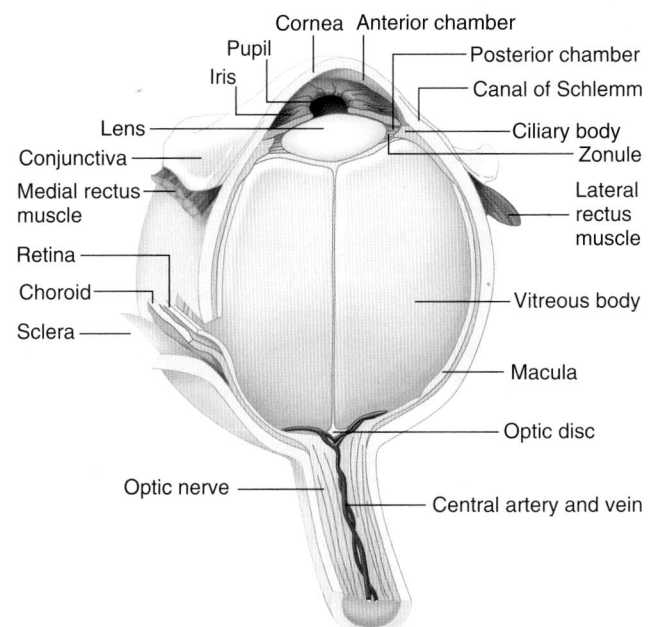

FIGURE 395-1. Anatomy of the eye.

Cornea · Anterior chamber
Pupil
Iris
Posterior chamber
Canal of Schlemm
Lens
Conjunctiva
Ciliary body
Zonule
Medial rectus muscle
Lateral rectus muscle
Retina
Choroid
Sclera
Vitreous body
Macula
Optic disc
Optic nerve
Central artery and vein

TABLE 395-1	VISUAL ACUITIES REQUIRED FOR COMMON DAILY TASKS
20/20	Physiologic vision
20/30-20/100	Driver's license, varies by state
20/50	Newspaper print
20/70	Large-print *Reader's Digest*
20/100	Check writing
20/200	Legal blindness
20/400	Paper currency

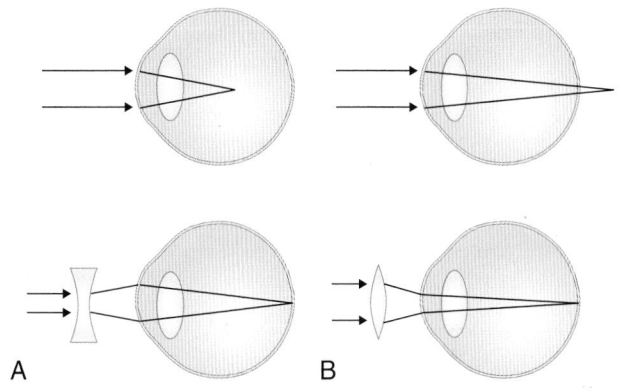

A   **B**

FIGURE 395-2. **Myopia/hyperopia. A,** In the myopic eye, parallel rays of light are focused anterior to the retina. A divergent lens can be used to compensate for the mismatch between refracting power and axial length. **B,** The hyperopic eye requires the additional power of a convergent lens to bring images into focus on the retina.

sinus tissue medially. The orbital floor, which is a relatively thin layer of bony support over the maxillary sinus, may rupture with increased intraorbital pressure. The nasolacrimal duct travels through a portion of the lacrimal bone. Portions of the sphenoid bone protect the optic nerve. Major cranial nerves travel through the adjacent superior orbital fissure, also a portion of the sphenoid bone. There is no normal lymphoid tissue in the orbit outside of the lacrimal gland. The rectus muscle may be enlarged by inflammation in thyroid eye disease, but the tendinous insertion into the sclera is usually not inflamed early in the course of the disease.

CLINICAL MANIFESTATIONS AND DIAGNOSIS

Patients may present with complaints of diminished vision, eye pain, redness, or pain around the eye. The causes may be primarily ophthalmic (e.g., cataract) or systemic (e.g., diabetic retinopathy). A comprehensive ophthalmologic examination also should evaluate for possible asymptomatic local (e.g., choroidal melanoma) or systemic (e.g., hypertensive retinopathy) abnormalities in patients with normal acuity and no subjective complaints.

Functional Evaluation

The most objective and common measure of ocular function is line letter acuity, with normal vision (Table 395-1) defined as the ability to see at 20 feet what a normal person sees at 20 feet, known as 20/20 vision (E-Fig. 395-1). Less than 20/20 vision can be caused by an abnormality anywhere from the tear film to the visual cortex of the occipital lobe (see Fig. 395-1). However, normal vision also includes other functions, such as the perception of color, motion, contrast, brightness, field, and depth, for which there is greater variation among individuals. Normal visual acuity is potentially achievable in essentially all individuals, either naturally or with the correction of the refractive error. Although effective treatments are available for refractive errors, cataracts, glaucoma, and other eye conditions, there is no evidence that routine screening for impaired visual acuity is associated with improved visual or clinical outcomes.[A1]

Correction of vision is based on the refraction of light (Fig. 395-2). The diopter (D) is the unit of measurement of the ability of an optical system to refract (bend) light. The normal human eye has a refractive capacity of approximately 60 D, which is accomplished by the cornea and the crystalline lens. This refractive capacity is needed to focus light onto the central retina, the macula. If the eye is too short, light will be focused behind the eye (hyperopia). If the eye is too long, light will be focused in the vitreous in front the retina (myopia). Normally, a person can involuntarily control the crystalline lens, alternating between near and distant tasks. At approximately age 45 years, the lens becomes less pliable, and the eye loses it ability to alter its shape (presbyopia). Refraction is the method of determining the amount of optical correction (strength of glasses) needed to establish 20/20 (6/6) vision.

Examination of pupillary response assesses whether neural function is intact (see Figs. 396-2 and 396-4). Confrontational visual field testing (see Fig. 396-1 in Chapter 396) should be performed in each eye to detect gross quadrantic defects. Extraocular motility should be assessed to exclude nerve or muscle abnormalities (see Table 396-6). Color vision testing plates are a sensitive indicator of optic nerve function and for detecting genetic variations that result in deficiencies of color perception.

Diagnostic testing during a routine eye examination also includes external examination of the lids and adnexa, applanation tonometry to determine intraocular pressure, biomicroscopy (slit lamp examination) of the anterior segment, and ophthalmoscopic examination of the ocular fundus (the retina and associated structures). Other tests include exophthalmometry (measurement of proptosis), visual field and electrophysiologic testing, and imaging (fluorescein angiography, mainly in diabetic patients; optical coherence tomography [OCT] to investigate retinal disease and glaucomatous damage); and corneal topography.

The conjunctiva, cornea, lens, and anterior chamber are evaluated using a slit lamp biomicroscope. The slit lamp is composed of a binocular microscope with variable magnification (40× and 80×) in conjunction with adjustable light sources. An increased concentration of protein can be detected in the anterior chamber because of the Tyndall (flare) effect, indicating vascular incompetence associated with either inflammation or ischemia. Even individual inflammatory cells can be resolved with the slit lamp. A cobalt blue filter can be used to detect fluorescein dye that accumulates in regions of abnormal epithelium (dendrite of herpes simplex keratitis or a corneal abrasion). The slit beam is used to examine the crystalline lens to determine the depth of the anterior chamber and the degree of opacification from a cataract. By using a green filter with the 90-D lens, the retinal vessels and retinal vascular abnormalities such as microaneurysm can be seen at relatively high magnification.

COMMON CLINICAL CONDITIONS
Chronic Abnormal Vision

MYOPIA

Nearsightedness (myopia; Fig. 395-2) is usually discovered during childhood when children cannot perform distant tasks during school (reading the blackboard) or during school screening. Myopia usually progresses until age 20 to 25 years. Rapidly progressing myopia during childhood or at any time after age 25 years requires evaluation for juvenile glaucoma, diabetes mellitus (reversible metabolic changes in the crystalline lens), trauma (development of a cataract), or use of corticosteroids (development of a cataract). Nonpathologic forms of myopia are usually fully correctable with eye glasses or contact lenses, or can be permanently corrected to a visual acuity of 20/40 or better in 95% or more of patients by various forms of laser in situ keratomileusis (LASIK).[A2] Complications of LASIK include glare symptoms, dry eye, and undercorrection or overcorrection.[1] Rare but serious complications include epithelial ingrowth, diffuse keratitis, and flap dislocation. In patients who undergo subsequent cataract surgery, special attention is needed to calculate the parameters for the intraocular lens.

Pathologic myopia is a partly heritable condition causing progressive weakening of the posterior sclera and resulting increases in the axial length of the eye. Localized areas of deformation arise where there is an abrupt increase in the posterior radius of curvature of the eye (posterior staphyloma). The axial length of a normal eye is typically between 20 and 24 mm, whereas it can increase to above 25 mm in pathologic myopia and may be as high as 40 mm in severe cases. Abnormal physical forces in pathologic myopia may lead to retinal hole formation, retinal detachment, choroidal neovascularization, or intraocular hemorrhage. Associated systemic conditions include trisomy 21, Cornelia de Lange syndrome, Stickler syndrome, and Marfan syndrome. Clinical surveillance is important to identify treatable complications such as retinal holes and detachment. Pathologic myopia is treated palliatively with eye glasses or contact lenses. Refractive procedures are less successful in pathologic myopia because of the severity of the refractive errors and the presence of posterior segment abnormalities. Surgical and laser procedures may be required to treat retinal and choroidal lesions.

HYPEROPIA

In hyperopia (farsightedness; see Fig. 395-2), in contrast to myopia, the eye tends to have a shorter than the average axial length. Compensatory mechanisms of the crystalline lens may functionally correct small degrees of hyperopia until age 40 years, when the crystalline lens loses its pliability. The initial pair of glasses may have to correct for both distance and near tasks (bifocals). Refractive surgical procedures can correct up to 5 D of hyperopia.

PRESBYOPIA

Presbyopia typically presents in the fourth to sixth decades of life and manifests as a progressive decrease in the ability to focus clearly on near objects. Presbyopia results when the crystalline lens loses its pliability, thereby preventing light rays from close objects from focusing onto the retina. The lens is suspended by fibers (zonules) attached to the ciliary body. In youth, the musculature of the ciliary body, acting via the zonules, alters the shape of the lens to provide increased near focusing power. As the lens hardens and presbyopia ensues, symptoms include difficulty reading small print, eyestrain, headaches, and the inability to read material unless it is farther away. Treatment is typically with eye glasses, such as bifocals, to provide adequate magnification to replace the lost ability of the eye.

ASTIGMATISM

Astigmatism derives from changes in the radius of curvature of the cornea and from the lens. Symptoms are predominantly blurry vision with "shadowing" and difficulty seeing fine detail. Regular astigmatism is not a pathologic state, but rather a variation in anatomy; most people have some degree of regular astigmatism that can be corrected with eye glasses or contact lenses. Irregular astigmatism is usually from changes on the cornea (e.g., from scarring owing to infections or trauma) or from adjacent tissue on the cornea (e.g., pterygia or limbal masses that induce changes in the corneal curvature). Some forms of regular astigmatism can be corrected with corneal laser ablation, but irregular astigmatism often requires correction with rigid contact lenses.

KERATOCONUS

Keratoconus is an acquired thinning of the cornea that induces irregularities of the corneal surface and irregular astigmatism; its cause is controversial but probably is partly genetic. Chronic eye rubbing has been associated with progressive disease. Onset generally is during adolescence, and the process often evolves over 5 to 10 years. The prevalence in the United States is approximately 55 cases per 100,000, but this figure may underestimate subclinical cases. Corneal surface mapping (computerized videokeratography and Scheimpflug tomography) allows earlier and more precise diagnosis.

Patients with keratoconus typically report a progressive worsening of vision, sometimes severe. The condition is usually bilateral but not symmetrical. Mild

degrees of early keratoconus can be corrected with glasses or contact lenses. The condition is typically progressive, but corneal collagen cross-linking can halt the progression in early to moderate cases and provide a sustained improvement in vision. For severe cases with significant corneal scarring and intolerance to contact lenses, corneal transplantation (graft) is the primary therapy.

STRABISMUS

The control of simultaneous orientation of the two eyes to ensure that the visual axes of both eyes are aligned is not complete until 6 to 12 months following birth. Misalignments of the two eyes (strabismus) may be the result of abnormalities in the central oculomotor nuclei of the brain, malfunction of one or several oculomotor nerves, or intrinsic abnormalities of the rectus or oblique muscles (see Fig. 396-6). If the eyes are not simultaneously stimulated with the images of the same degree of clarity or complexity, there is a risk that only one eye will develop normal vision (amblyopia). In most cases, only the central vision is affected. The peripheral vision in both eyes is likely to be equal and normal. Binocular vision can be disrupted with amblyopia, with a loss in depth perception that may become permanent if the normal eye alignment is not restored.

Amblyopia also may be caused by a marked difference in refractive error between the two eyes (anisometropic amblyopia), congenital cataracts, or eyelid ptosis (deprivational amblyopia). Ptosis may be neurogenic or mechanical (e.g., congenital eyelid hemangioma). To avoid amblyopia, it is extremely important to refer a child with strabismus to an ophthalmologist as soon as the strabismus is noted.

Treatment options include patching or atropine eye-drops (1%, typically daily but effective if used as infrequently as twice per week) to blur the better seeing eye, thereby strengthening the amblyopic eye. These therapies have been shown to be equally effective in providing good vision if patients are treated before age 7 years. The outcome of treatment is more favorable if amblyopia is detected before age 2 to 3 years but may be occasionally successful into the teenage years depending on the severity. Success is directly related to compliance and the timeliness of diagnosis.

Esotropia is a deviation of one eye inward ("crossed eyes"). Although intermittent esotropia may be a normal finding in infancy, it should not be present beyond 6 months of age. Delay in facial maturation (underdeveloped nasal bridge) may give the appearance of esotropia, even though the visual axes are correctly aligned. In true strabismus, the corneal light reflex will be in the center of one cornea and decentered in the other.

Exotropia is deviation of one eye outward. Exotropia is often intermittent and less likely to result in amblyopia compared to esotropia. Like esotropia, intermittent exotropia may also be a normal developmental finding in infancy.

In some cases, esotropia or exotropia may be treated by using appropriate corrections of refractive error with glasses (occasionally bifocals). It is critically important to recognize that strabismus may be the presenting sign of vision loss due to other causes (e.g., retinoblastoma). Extraocular muscle surgery may be necessary to correct alignment.

DIPLOPIA (DOUBLE VISION)

Acute onset of diplopia is an ominous sign suggestive of a cranial nerve palsy (i.e., III, IV, or VI) or pathology in the orbit (Chapter 396). Diplopia of any kind is usually an intolerable symptom, which is often worse with vertical deviations than horizontal deviations.

COLOR VISION CHANGE

Most cases of congenital color blindness are genetically determined and go undetected for many years. Acquired color deficiency at any age may be caused by a cataract or optic nerve disease.

CHANGE IN VISION

If only one eye has a change in vision, the problem, such as a cataract or retinal detachment, is most likely in that eye. If both eyes have a change in vision, the problem generally is outside of the eye, such as homonymous hemianopia (Chapter 396). Improvement of near vision in middle age may be a sign of cataract ("second sight") or hyperglycemia. Transient complete or partial unilateral or bilateral loss of vision may be caused by vascular abnormalities inside or outside of the eye (Table 395-2).

Acute Eye Abnormalities
PAIN

The most severe eye pain (Table 395-3), typically associated with a red eye, is caused by acute angle-closure glaucoma. Sharp, intermittent pain is usually caused by ocular surface abnormalities (e.g., corneal foreign body). Burning pain that clears with blinking generally relates to tear film abnormalities (dry eyes). Deep boring pain most often is associated with an ocular abnormality (e.g., uveitis).

RED EYE

A red or inflamed eye can be caused by conjunctivitis, iritis (anterior uveitis), acute glaucoma, corneal trauma, or infection (Table 395-4).[2] Of these causes, all are typically painful, with the occasional exception of conjunctivitis.

DISTORTED VISION

Distorted vision (metamorphopsia), which is the perception that straight lines are distorted or bowed, results from macular dysfunction. Causes include fluid under the retina; exudative macular degeneration, which tends to elevate the retina; and an epiretinal membrane, which tends to contract the retina.

NIGHT BLINDNESS

Retinitis pigmentosa, vitamin A deficiency, and systemic medications such as phenothiazines can cause true night blindness, in which patients have difficulty seeing any stars in the sky on a clear night and may be unable to ambulate without assistance in a dark environment. Patients with cataracts may have difficulty driving at night because of excessive glare and visual distortion.

Gene therapy using adeno-associated virus vectors carrying the *RPE65* gene has been shown to increase retinal sensitivity and to improve night vision in patients with retinitis pigmentosa.

SENSATION OF FLASHING LIGHTS

The sudden onset of flashes (photopsia) in the peripheral visual field suggests traction of the vitreous on the peripheral retina, sometimes with a resulting retinal tear. The flashes, which may be more pronounced in the dark and with rapid eye movement, may be associated with the sudden onset of floaters, which can indicate debris or blood in the vitreous cavity. Because a tear in the retina can lead to a retinal detachment, urgent consultation with an ophthalmologist is required.

Flashing light with a migraine (Chapter 370) is described as scintillations or zigzagging lights that march across the visual field for a few minutes or as long as 30 minutes, sometimes associated with transient visual field loss. Headache is not universal.

FLOATERS

Floaters, which are caused by small aggregates or opacities in the vitreous cavity, result from the normal aging of the vitreous. The acute onset of vitreous floaters may be associated with uveitis or with the sudden onset of bleeding in the vitreous cavity owing to diabetes or sickle cell anemia. Acute floaters, however, particularly if associated with flashing lights, may indicate a posterior vitreous detachment and/or a retinal tear with an impending retinal detachment. Urgent ophthalmic referral is essential.

PHOTOPHOBIA

Photophobia, particularly if associated with eye pain, redness, and decreased vision, is a symptom of intraocular inflammation (uveitis) from trauma or other causes. Photophobia is also typical of acute migraine and meningeal irritation. Prompt ophthalmologic referral is prudent.

HALOS AROUND LIGHTS

Patients with cataracts commonly see halos around lights, particularly when driving at night. Episodic decreased vision, redness, and halos around lights may be symptoms of impending angle-closure glaucoma owing to increased intraocular pressure with resulting corneal edema and loss of corneal clarity. Halos also can occur as a complication of refractive eye surgery.

FOREIGN BODY SENSATION

A foreign body sensation is commonly caused by ocular surface diseases such as dry eye syndrome (see later). Entropion (see Fig. 395-3) or misdirected lashes (trichiasis) also can cause a foreign body sensation. Most corneal abrasions cause severe pain, but minor corneal abrasions may be associated with a foreign body sensation rather than the severe pain. An arc welder burn causes a punctate corneal keratopathy, and foreign body sensation may be a prominent symptom. A true conjunctival or corneal foreign body also may be present.

EXCESSIVE TEARING (EPIPHORA)

Tearing can occur because of the overproduction of tears or impairment of tear drainage. Any abnormalities in upper or lower lid laxity, position, or closure can impair the lacrimal pump system. Obstruction of the nasolacrimal tear

TABLE 395-2	DIFFERENTIAL DIAGNOSIS OF SUDDEN VISUAL LOSS
UNILATERAL	**BILATERAL**
Amaurosis fugax (carotid artery stenosis or vascular occlusion)	Eclampsia
Central retinal artery occlusion	Vertebrobasilar infarct
Occipital lobe infarct	Trauma
Temporal arteritis	
Nonarteritic anterior ischemic optic neuropathy	
Hemorrhage	
Preretinal (high altitude, Valsalva)	
Vitreous	
Aqueous (hyphema)	
Trauma	

TABLE 395-3	CAUSES OF EYE PAIN
Blepharitis	Glaucoma
Blocked tear duct	Hordeolum (stye)
Chalazion	Iritis
Conjunctivitis	Keratoconus
Corneal abrasion	Optic neuritis
Dry eyes	Scleritis
Ectropion	Trauma
Entropion	Uveitis
Foreign object	

TABLE 395-4	DIFFERENTIAL DIAGNOSIS OF COMMON CAUSES OF INFLAMED EYE*			
FEATURE	**ACUTE CONJUNCTIVITIS**	**ACUTE IRITIS†**	**ACUTE GLAUCOMA‡**	**CORNEAL TRAUMA OR INFECTION**
Incidence	Extremely common	Common	Uncommon	Common
Discharge	Moderate to copious	None	None	Watery or purulent
Vision	No effect on vision	Slightly blurred	Markedly blurred	Usually blurred
Pain	None	Moderate	Severe	Moderate to severe
Conjunctival injection	Diffuse: more toward fornices	Mainly circumcorneal	Mainly circumcorneal	Mainly circumcorneal
Cornea	Clear	Usually clear	Steamy	Change in clarity related to cause
Pupil size	Normal	Normal or small	Moderately dilated and fixed	Normal or small
Pupillary light response	Normal	Normal or reduced	None	Normal
Intraocular pressure	Normal	Variable	Elevated	Normal
Smear	Causative organisms	No organisms	No organisms	Organisms found only in corneal ulcers related to infection

*Less common causes of red eyes include endophthalmitis, foreign body, episcleritis, and scleritis.
†Acute anterior uveitis.
‡Angle-closure glaucoma.

drainage system owing to age, inflammation, infection, or neoplasm can prevent appropriate tear drainage. Finally, ocular surface irritants such as trichiatic eyelashes touching the cornea can stimulate excessive tear production. Treatment depends on the underlying condition.

EYELID TWITCHING

Any irritation of the conjunctiva or cornea can cause the eyelids to twitch. Occasional twitching of the lids usually is associated with stress or adrenergic stimulation. Benign essential blepharospasm is severe spasm of the lids leading to functional impairment. Multiple sclerosis (Chapter 383) also can cause lid spasm.

CONJUNCTIVITIS

Any ocular inflammation, including corneal ulcers, angle-closure glaucoma, endophthalmitis, and uveitis, can be associated with secondary conjunctival hyperemia. Conjunctivitis usually involves the entire conjunctiva, is associated with a discharge, and usually is not associated with pain (see Table 395-4).

PTOSIS (DROOPY EYELID)

Ptosis (Fig. 395-4) is typically due to age-related disinsertion of the levator palpebrae superioris muscle. However, it also can be caused by a third nerve palsy, Horner syndrome, myasthenia gravis (Chapter 394), or other neurologic conditions. Third nerve palsy is usually associated with diplopia and a large pupil. Horner syndrome (see Fig. 396-5) is associated with a small pupil and ipsilateral anhydrosis. With myasthenia gravis (Chapter 394), other typical features of muscle weakness and fatigability are usually present or can be elicited. Non-neurologic causes of ptosis include age-related dehiscence of the levator muscle.

PROPTOSIS (EXOPHTHALMOS)

Proptosis, or a prominent globe, can be a manifestation of thyroid eye disease, which in turn is associated with thyroid abnormalities, especially Graves disease (Chapter 213). In this setting, proptosis can be subacute and asymmetrical. Any orbital inflammation, infection, or neoplasm can cause unilateral proptosis;

in the case of inflammation or infection, proptosis is typically acute in onset. All orbital processes can affect orbital cranial nerves, with associated diplopia or optic neuropathy. Orbital infection, or cellulitis, typically presents with concurrent severe eye redness, pain, sinusitis and an elevated white blood cell count (Fig. 395-5). Idiopathic orbital inflammation can cause acute, usually unilateral proptosis, with severe pain, particularly with eye movement, and often with decreased vision. An optic nerve tumor causes chronic, unilateral proptosis associated with a slow onset of visual field loss. Acute cellulitis can be associated with unilateral proptosis, severe redness, and moderate to severe pain, commonly with sinusitis and an elevated white blood cell count.

SMALL PUPIL

A unilateral small pupil is best detected in dark conditions. Causes include Horner syndrome, associated with ptosis on the same side; the bilaterally small, poorly reacting pupils of tertiary syphilis (Argyll Robertson pupils), which accommodate with normal constriction to a near object; miotic drops (e.g., pilocarpine); traumatic iritis; uveitis; and recent eye surgery.

LARGE PUPIL

Any α-adrenergic or anticholinergic agent placed into the eye can cause a large pupil. With eye trauma, the iris sphincter muscle can be damaged, and an abnormally large pupil can result. Tears in the iris sphincter can sometimes be appreciated on slit lamp examination. Third nerve palsy may cause a dilated pupil associated with ptosis and decreased elevation, depression, and medial eye movement. Adie pupil (see Fig. 396-3) is an idiopathic, unilateral large pupil that is hypersensitive to weak cholinergic stimulation. Recent eye surgery, uveitis, an acute angle-closure glaucoma attack, and traumatic iritis can cause a large pupil.

LEUKOCORIA

Leukocoria (white pupil) in a young child is a critically important because it may be a sign of retinoblastoma. Some of the more common nonretinoblastoma conditions presenting with leukocoria (Table 395-5) include cataracts, retinal detachment, persistent fetal vasculature (a developmental anomaly of

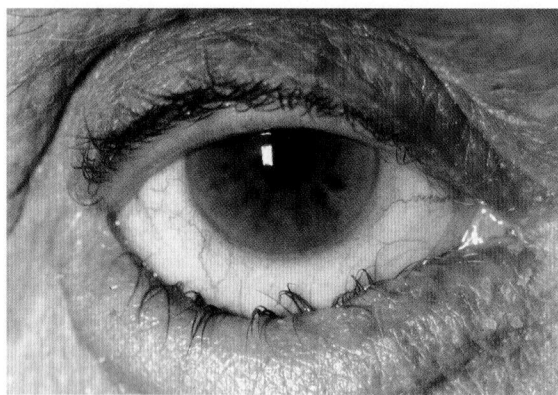

FIGURE 395-3. Involutional entropion. (From Palay DA, Krachmer JH. *Primary Care Ophthalmology*, 2nd ed. Philadelphia: Elsevier Mosby; 2005.)

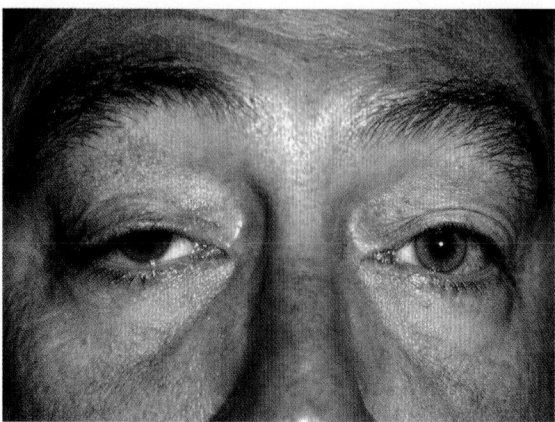

FIGURE 395-4. Ptosis of the right upper lid. (From Palay DA, Krachmer JH. *Primary Care Ophthalmology*, 2nd ed. Philadelphia: Elsevier Mosby; 2005.)

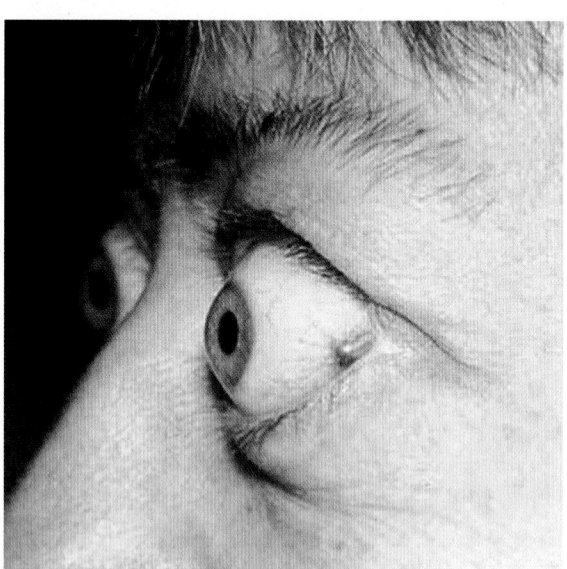

FIGURE 395-5. Thyroid eye disease (Graves) with characteristic exophthalmos and eyelid retraction.

TABLE 395-5 DIFFERENTIAL DIAGNOSIS OF LEUKOCORIA
Retinoblastoma
Cataract
Persistent hyperplastic primary vitreous
Retinopathy of prematurity (retrolental fibroplasia)
Coats disease (retinal telangiectasia)
Retinal detachment
Toxocariasis
Familial exudative vitreoretinopathy (FEVR)

the vitreous resulting in intraocular fibrosis and retinal detachment), Coats disease (a developmental vascular malformation of the retina leading to exudative retinal detachment), and ocular toxocariasis (a parasitic intraocular nematode infection, which leads to intraocular scarring and retinal detachment).

Eyelid Abnormalities

ECTROPION AND ENTROPION

An ectropion is an out-turning of the eyelid, typically the lower lid (Fig. 395-6), with exposure of the undersurface of the lid. Causes include aging, scarring, a mass on the eyelid, and seventh nerve palsy. Common symptoms, which derive from corneal exposure and drying, include burning, itching, tearing, and the sense of a foreign body. Treatment is surgical, although mild symptoms may be managed conservatively with lubrication.

An entropion, which is an in-turning of the eyelid (see Fig. 395-3), is usually age related and associated with irritation, burning, and a foreign body sensation because the eyelashes touch the cornea. If it leads to trichiasis, in which the eyelashes rub or abrade the cornea, the lashes can be removed with forceps or surgery to correct the eyelid malposition. Botulinum toxin can be injected into the orbicularis muscle to temporarily correct the entropion.

CHALAZION

A chalazion (Fig. 395-7) is a localized lipogranulomatous inflammation owing to an occluded sebaceous (meibomian) gland. The retained, lipid-rich sebaceous material acts as a foreign material that stimulates a lipogranulomatous foreign body inflammatory reaction. A painless or slightly tender, nonmobile nodule forms under the eyelid skin. Most lesions resolve over days to weeks with warm compresses or without specific treatment. If the chalazion persists, it may be surgically débrided. Some individuals may have recurrent chalazia. A recurrent chalazion in the same spot may point to an underlying carcinoma.

HORDEOLUM (STYE)

A hordeolum (stye) (Fig. 395-8) is an extremely painful abscess in a hair or eyelash follicle or in a sebaceous gland. Styes are usually self-limited infections that respond to warm compresses and topical antibiotics (e.g., bacitracin or erythromycin ointment or moxifloxacin or gatifloxacin drops). An ophthalmologist may perform incision and drainage if symptoms do not improve within 48 hours.

BLEPHARITIS

Blepharitis (Fig. 395-9) is a common, nonspecific inflammation of the eyelid margin or skin. The condition is usually bilateral and symmetrical. Rosacea (Chapter 410) is the most common associated cutaneous condition, and *Staphylococcus aureus* is the most common infectious agent. If untreated, blepharitis becomes chronic and may lead to corneal and conjunctival inflammation (blepharoconjunctivitis). Effective supportive care for blepharitis includes warm compresses and maintenance of good lid hygiene. Ophthalmic antibiotic ointment (e.g., bacitracin or erythromycin) is more efficacious than eye-drops, but systemic antibiotics (e.g., minocycline, 50 to 100 mg, or doxycycline, 100 mg, once daily; tetracycline, 250 mg twice daily; or erythromycin, 250 mg three times daily) may infrequently be recommended, particularly if there is any evidence of inflammation of the cornea or conjunctiva.

In seborrheic blepharitis, exfoliated keratinous debris accumulates along the eyelid margin, particularly at the follicles of the eyelashes, and irritates the conjunctiva. Treatment of this chronic condition is directed at mechanically removing the keratinous debris by scrubbing the eyelid and eyelashes daily with a mild detergent ("baby shampoo") in warm water applied with a soft cloth.

BENIGN EYELID NEOPLASMS

Skin tags, also known as squamous papillomas, are the most common benign skin lesions. Other skin lesions include seborrheic keratitis, actinic keratitis, inverted follicular keratitis, and benign lesions of the eccrine and apocrine systems. Most of these benign lesions are cured by simple excision.

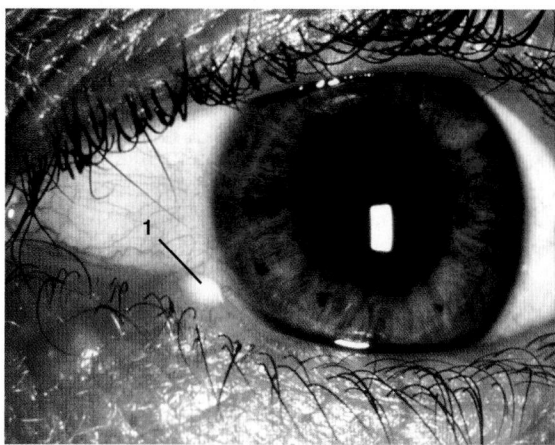

FIGURE 395-8. A lower lid stye *(1)*. (From Palay DA, Krachmer JH. *Primary Care Ophthalmology,* 2nd ed. Philadelphia: Elsevier Mosby; 2005.)

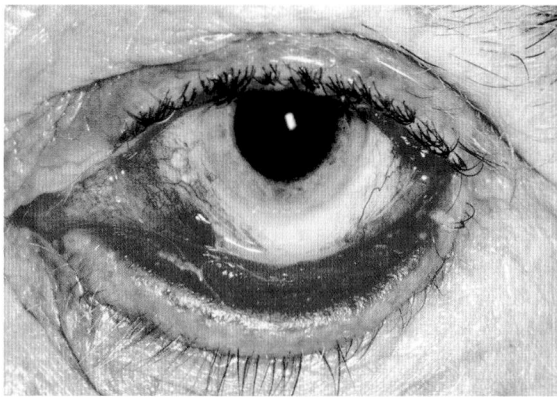

FIGURE 395-6. Involutional ectropion. (From Palay DA, Krachmer JH. *Primary Care Ophthalmology,* 2nd ed. Elsevier Mosby, Philadelphia, 2005.)

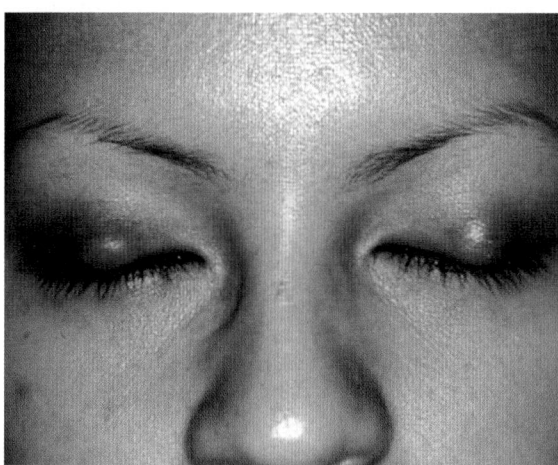

FIGURE 395-7. Bilateral chalazion in the upper eyelids.

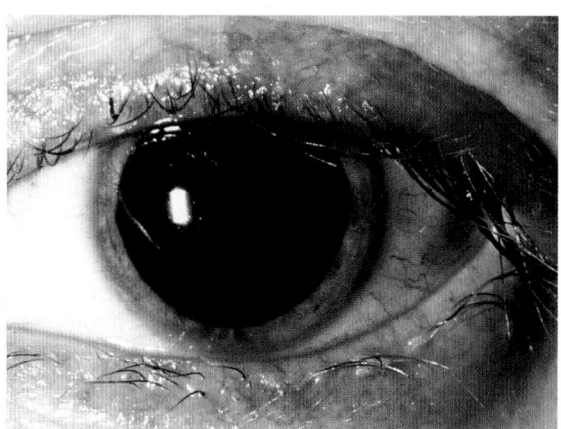

FIGURE 395-9. Staphylococcal blepharitis. The lid margins are very red and under high magnification demonstrate tiny ulcerations. (From Palay DA, Krachmer JH. *Primary Care Ophthalmology,* 2nd ed. Philadelphia: Elsevier Mosby; 2005.)

SEBACEOUS CARCINOMA

Sebaceous carcinoma originates from sebaceous glands either in the tarsal plate (meibomian gland) or associated with eyelashes (glands of Zeis) and is capable of producing widespread metastasis resulting in death. Muir-Torre syndrome is a syndrome of sebaceous tumors associated with visceral malignancy. Except for chronic, unilateral blepharitis, owing to the peculiar manner of spread of this tumor in the plane of the skin epithelium (pagetoid spread) without causing the formation of nodules, few symptoms occur early in the course of the disease. The tumor may progress to involve the tarsal conjunctiva, the bulbar conjunctiva, and even the corneal epithelium. A characteristic sign is regional loss of eyelashes. When the mass thickens, it may have the appearance of a chalazion, and a history of multiple chalazia in the same region of the eyelid is suggestive of sebaceous carcinoma. Diagnostic delay is common because the lesion often has only modest clinical features.

Treatment is complete surgical excision. Map biopsies to determine the extent of tumor spread can be useful for definitive surgical planning. Topical mitomycin C has been suggested as treatment for pagetoid invasion of the conjunctiva. Cryotherapy can also be a useful adjuvant to surgery for eyelid and conjunctival lesions. In advanced cases, removal of the eyelids, eye, and orbital contents (exenteration) may be necessary. Imaging for local and distant metastases is critical.

BASAL CELL CARCINOMA

Basal cell carcinoma (E-Fig. 395-2), which originates from the basal cell layer of the epithelium, is the most common cutaneous malignancy (Chapter 193). The lesion, which usually is asymptomatic, is often a well-demarcated, elevated nodule that may have a central region of ulceration and fine cutaneous vascular channels (telangiectasias). Occasionally, lesions may be more subtle and present only with eyelid margin thickening, a focal loss or disruption of the eyelashes, or a mild out-turning (ectropion) of the eyelid. A common benign cutaneous lesion, sometimes confused clinically with basal cell carcinoma, is seborrheic keratosis (Chapter 411), which tends to be soft and appear hyperpigmented; the most common site is the lower eyelid, especially in the nasal quadrant. Basal cell carcinoma, particularly near the medial canthus, may extend posteriorly into the soft tissues of the orbit. Imaging before surgical excision for medial canthal lesions may be necessary to determine the true extent of the tumor. Basal cell carcinoma is treated by surgical excision, using Mohs' technique with intraoperative histologic evaluation to determine adequate margins of excision, if possible.

Metastasis is extremely rare. With early detection and adequate excision of the local lesion, the prognosis is excellent.

EYELID SQUAMOUS CELL CARCINOMA

Eyelid squamous cell carcinoma, which is much less common than basal cell carcinoma, arises from the surface squamous epithelium. Ultraviolet light exposure is the major risk factor. In contrast to basal cell carcinoma, squamous cell carcinoma can metastasize, most often to regional lymph nodes. It also can invade the orbit and cavernous sinus via perineural spread from untreated lesions on the eyelids. Treatment is surgical excision, often with the Mohs micrographic surgical technique. Except in rare circumstances, such as in immunosuppressed patients or patients with xeroderma pigmentosa, the prognosis is excellent.

Ocular Surface Abnormalities
DRY EYES

Even minor disturbances in the tear film can cause itching, burning, a foreign-body sensation, and transient changes in vision.[3] Dry eyes that cause conjunctival hyperemia without purulent discharge particularly disturb some patients. Paradoxically, decreased tearing can result in irritation and secondary increased (reflux) tearing.

Most daily tear production is not by the lacrimal gland but by small collections of lacrimal glands, mucus-producing glands, and sebaceous glands located throughout the conjunctiva, eyelid, and anterior orbital soft tissue. Over time, particularly in women, production of tear film diminishes. Because tear film production is lower during sleep, patients often note symptoms on awakening followed by slow resolution over minutes or hours. Wind and low-humidity environments, such as in commercial airliners, can exacerbate symptoms. The reduction in aqueous components of tears is often associated with a compensatory increase in mucus production, which tends to blur vision until the patient blinks or uses supplemental tears. These symptoms are particularly prominent in persons who have autoimmune diseases, including

rheumatoid arthritis (Chapter 248), Sjögren syndrome (Chapter 252), Stevens-Johnson syndrome (Chapter 411), and ocular cicatricial pemphigoid.

Dry eye disease can be divided by etiology into aqueous tear deficiency and evaporative tear dysfunction. Evaporative tear dysfunction is most commonly secondary to tear film instability and is the result of meibomian gland dysfunction (Fig. 395-10).

Treatment is not definitive and is rarely satisfactory. No medication increases the production of tears. Low-viscosity artificial tears (e.g., polyethylene glycol 400 0.4%), which do not tend to blur vision but have a short duration of action, are best used during visually important tasks. High-viscosity tears (e.g., carboxymethylcellulose sodium) have a longer duration of action but tend to blur vision; they are best used at bedtime to maintain lubrication of the ocular surface during sleep. When artificial tears do not control symptoms, occlusion of the nasolacrimal duct with synthetic plugs or permanent surgical occlusion tends to retain the tears that are produced. Anti-inflammatory drugs (e.g., cyclosporine 0.05% drops, every 12 hours indefinitely) can preserve glandular tissue that may be affected by local inflammation. Topical lifitegrast, given topically twice daily indefinitely, is also thought to work through anti-inflammatory mechanisms by inhibiting T-cell activation. For patients with systemic disease associated with dry eyes, effective treatment of the systemic disease sometimes improves the eye abnormalities.

PINGUECULA AND PTERYGIUM

A pinguecula (Fig. 395-11) consists of a limbal (at junction of cornea and sclera) and bulbar conjunctival degenerative process caused by ultraviolet light damage to the subepithelial tissue. It is very common and rarely causes symptoms. If the supportive tissue degeneration extends into the cornea, it becomes a pterygium (Fig. 395-12), which may cause corneal astigmatism and require surgical excision. About 2 to 10% with a pterygium have a coexisting squamous carcinoma, which often is clinically unsuspected and diagnosed only by histopathologic examination.

RECURRENT EROSION

Recurrent corneal erosion most often manifests as a delayed reaction to a minor traumatic corneal abrasion. The abrasion heals abnormally, resulting in a weakness of the epithelial attachment to its underlying tissue. Weeks to months to years later, the patient awakens with ocular pain on opening the eye, sometimes with recurrent episodes of pain every morning. The epithelium has become "stuck" to the overlying upper lid and is mechanically abraded. The condition is treated with hyperosmotic drops and ointment. If the erosions continue to occur despite drops and ointment, surgical options include superficial keratectomy (where the epithelium is mechanically débrided), phototherapeutic keratopathy, or stromal micropuncture. All three techniques work by trying to scar or adhere the weak epithelium to the underlying cornea.

ACCIDENTAL TRAUMA

With ocular trauma, many tissues of the eye can be easily disrupted, and the effects of trauma may not be manifest for months or even years after the episode of trauma. If the traumatic episode disrupts the eye wall (cornea and sclera), surgical repair is necessary, usually urgently. If the eye wall is intact, surgical treatment is often not necessary, at least initially.

CORNEAL ABRASION

The corneal epithelium is very delicate, and contact by any object can result in shearing or irregularity of the epithelium. Corneal abrasion is one of the most common forms of ocular injury. Symptoms are often intense and intolerable. Healing (i.e., re-epithelialization) of the cornea occurs within 24 to 48 hours. Rust from metallic fragments is toxic to the epithelium and should be removed. Bacterial or fungal keratitis may complicate injuries from fingernails or vegetable matter, such as tree branches. Treatment usually consists of a topical antibiotic (e.g., fluoroquinolone antibiotics or antibiotic ointment, four times daily for 10 to 14 days) to prevent bacterial keratitis. Subsequent scarring usually does not occur unless deeper structures, such as the Bowman membrane, are affected. Topical anesthetics never should be prescribed to control pain because they increase the risk for microbial keratitis and scarring and may delay healing.

MAJOR OCULAR TRAUMA

Hyphema (Fig. 395-13) is hemorrhage into the anterior chamber usually caused by blunt trauma. If the patient is supine, such as in an intensive care unit, the blood will distribute uniformly over the iris to cause the appearance of increased pigmentation of the iris (heterochromia iridis). If the patient

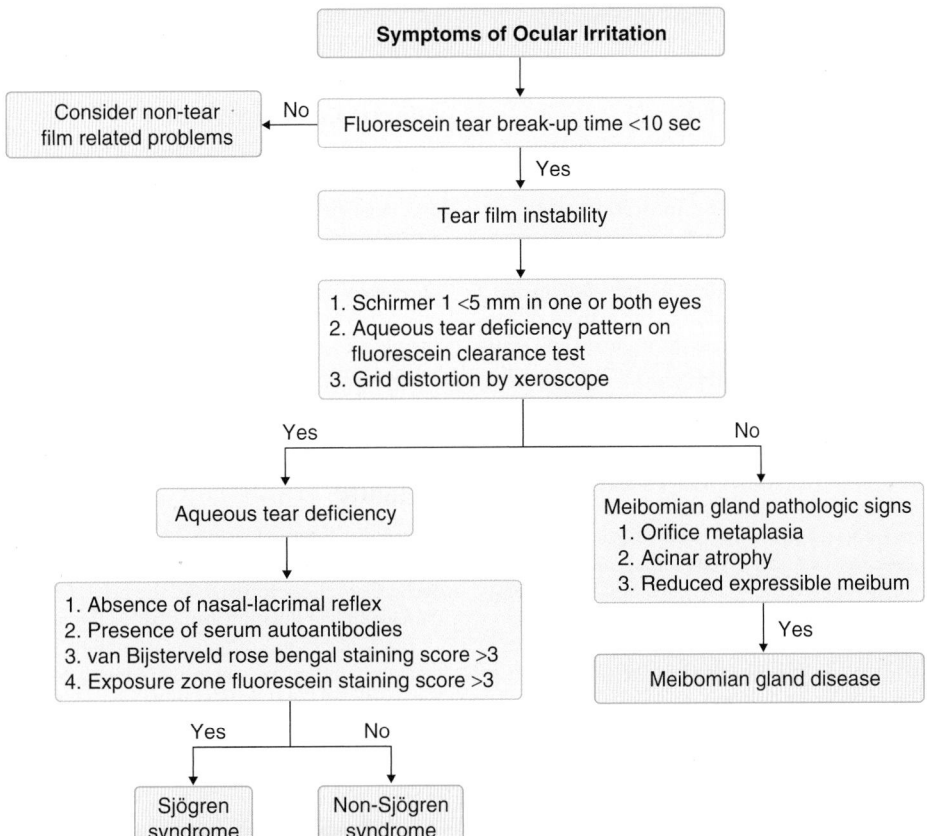

Symptoms of Ocular Irritation

Fluorescein tear break-up time <10 sec

No → Consider non-tear film related problems

Yes ↓

Tear film instability

1. Schirmer 1 <5 mm in one or both eyes
2. Aqueous tear deficiency pattern on fluorescein clearance test
3. Grid distortion by xeroscope

Yes ↓

Aqueous tear deficiency

1. Absence of nasal-lacrimal reflex
2. Presence of serum autoantibodies
3. van Bijsterveld rose bengal staining score >3
4. Exposure zone fluorescein staining score >3

Yes → Sjögren syndrome
No → Non-Sjögren syndrome

No ↓

Meibomian gland pathologic signs
1. Orifice metaplasia
2. Acinar atrophy
3. Reduced expressible meibum

Yes ↓

Meibomian gland disease

FIGURE 395-10. Diagnostic algorithm for ocular irritation. (Modified from Pflugfelder SC, Tseng SC, Sanabria O, et al. Evaluation of subjective assessments and objective diagnostic tests for diagnosing tear-film disorders known to cause ocular irritation. *Cornea.* 1998;17:38-56.)

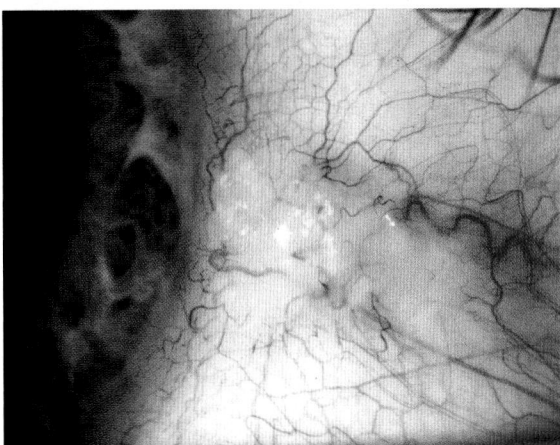

FIGURE 395-11. **Pinguecula.** These lesions are found at the 3-o'clock and 9-o'clock positions and are extremely common, especially in older patients. (From Palay DA, Krachmer JH. *Primary Care Ophthalmology,* 2nd ed. Philadelphia: Elsevier Mosby; 2005.)

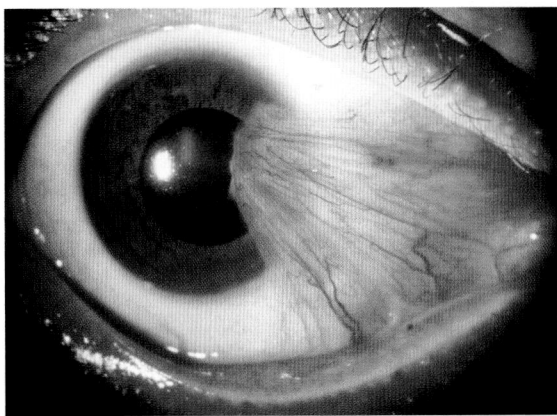

FIGURE 395-12. **Pterygium.** These lesions are found in the horizontal meridian, most common nasally. (From Palay DA, Krachmer JH. *Primary Care Ophthalmology,* 2nd ed. Philadelphia: Elsevier Mosby; 2005.)

has been sitting, the blood may settle by gravity to form an aqueous-blood interface with the blood in the dependent portion of the anterior chamber. Hyphema, which is a sign of serious ocular damage, may lead to secondary glaucoma and blood staining of the cornea. It requires prompt evaluation by an ophthalmologist.

The most common site of rupture of a globe is at the limbus (junction of cornea and sclera), where a pigmented mass may be noted. The mass may be either a blood clot or an anteriorly displaced uveal tract (usually iris). Any manipulation of the globe may force the remaining intraocular tissue through the wound and may make the injury irreparable. Emergent surgical repair is usually indicated.

Cataract and retinal detachment are not common except in severe accidental trauma. A unilateral cataract or unilateral glaucoma may occur decades after the injury, even when an injury is too minor to be recalled. Traumatic cataract

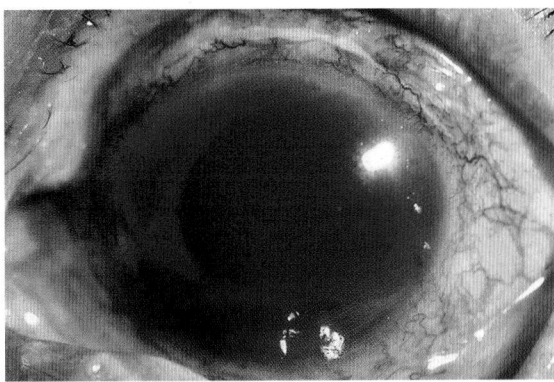

FIGURE 395-13. Hyphema following cataract surgery. (Courtesy of Dr. Myron Yanoff.)

and traumatic glaucoma are treated in the same manner as other forms of these conditions.

INFLAMMATORY EYE DISORDERS
Uveitis

Inflammation of any part or parts of the uveal tract (iris, ciliary body, and choroid) may be called anterior or posterior uveitis, iritis, iridocyclitis, or choroiditis. Symptoms include a red eye (see Table 395-4), decreased vision, and photophobia. The inflammation may be acute or chronic, and an underlying systemic cause is found in approximately 50% of cases. Uveitis accompanies many autoimmune diseases, often without correlation to the activity of the systemic inflammation. Anterior uveitis or conjunctivitis is nearly universal in patients with reactive arthritis (Chapter 249). About 25% of patients with ankylosing spondylitis (Chapter 249) develop acute, recurrent anterior uveitis. Two to 12% of patients with inflammatory bowel disease (Chapter 132) develop anterior uveitis, which is also common with psoriatic arthritis but not with psoriasis alone (Chapters 249 and 409). Treatment with topical corticosteroids (e.g., prednisolone acetate 1%, one drop in the affected eye or eyes every 1 to 6 hours while awake) is often sufficient to control ocular disease, but some patients will require more aggressive local therapy, including intravitreal or periocular steroid injections. Systemic immunosuppression[4] with oral corticosteroids (e.g., 10 to 35 mg prednisone daily)[A3] or steroid-sparing immunosuppressive agents (e.g., adalimumab 80 mg loading dose then 40 mg every 2 weeks)[A4][A5] is an effective alternative that can may also be necessary to reduce flares and visual loss in patients with chronic disease.

Endophthalmitis

Endophthalmitis is extensive inflammation within the eye from any cause. Most cases of endophthalmitis involve a breach in the eye wall (cornea and sclera), associated with either accidental trauma (incidence of approximately 5%) or surgical procedures (incidence of approximately <0.03%). The initial symptom is usually decreased vision followed by dull ocular pain. The initial sign is often evidence of inflammatory cells either within the aqueous (anterior uveitis) or within the vitreous (vitritis). The cells can be seen only by slit lamp biomicroscopy. Common microbial organisms include toxin-producing gram-positive species and gram-negative species that are often associated with rapidly destructive course. Other organism of relatively low virulence, *Propionibacterium acnes* and *Staphylococcus epidermidis*, follow a more indolent course with less potential destruction. Metastatic endophthalmitis infection from a primary source outside of the eye is an unusual cause.

Diagnosis is established by sampling anterior chamber fluid or preferably vitreous fluid (vitreous tap) and evaluation of that fluid by Gram stain and culture. Prophylaxis against endophthalmitis includes preoperative topical instillation of povidone-iodine and intracameral antibiotic injection at the end of cataract surgery.

Systemic antibiotics are not generally effective. Initial management is with intravitreal antibiotics[5] (e.g., commonly used, but not limited to, vancomycin 1 mg/0.1 mL and ceftazidime 2.25 mg/0.1 mL) and in certain instances, corticosteroids. If there are external signs of infection (e.g., corneal ulcer), topical antibiotics are also used simultaneously. Severe cases may require surgical debulking of the infection (vitrectomy) to reduce the microbial and inflammatory debris burden and to treat associated vitreoretinal pathology.

Allergic Conjunctivitis

Allergic conjunctivitis (Table 395-6) is commonly associated with atopy, hay fever, and allergic rhinitis.[6] Itching, a foreign body sensation, and a watery discharge are common. Treatment includes cool compresses and topical or antihistamines (e.g., olopatadine, once to twice per day until symptoms resolve). Long-term treatment with mast cell stabilizers (e.g., pemirolast drops, four times daily during the allergic season) or the combination of an antihistamine plus a mast cell stabilizer (e.g., olopatadine drops, two times daily during the allergic season) can be extremely effective in treating chronic symptoms. Oral antihistamines (e.g., cetirizine 5 to 10 mg per day until symptoms resolve) can also be useful.

INFECTIOUS EYE DISORDERS
Cellulitis

Preseptal cellulitis (Fig. 395-14) is soft tissue inflammation of the eyelid anterior to the orbital septum. The orbital septum divides the soft tissues of the eyelid from the soft tissues of the orbit. Orbital tissue is more susceptible to damage by the inflammation than is the preseptal tissue.

The clinical signs of preseptal cellulitis include soft tissue swelling, hyperemia, and conjunctival chemosis (edema). Movement of the eye is not restricted. Extension of inflammation posterior to the orbital septum is indicated by proptosis of the globe and ophthalmoplegia (restricted motion). Treatment of preseptal cellulitis includes oral antibiotics (e.g., commonly used, but not

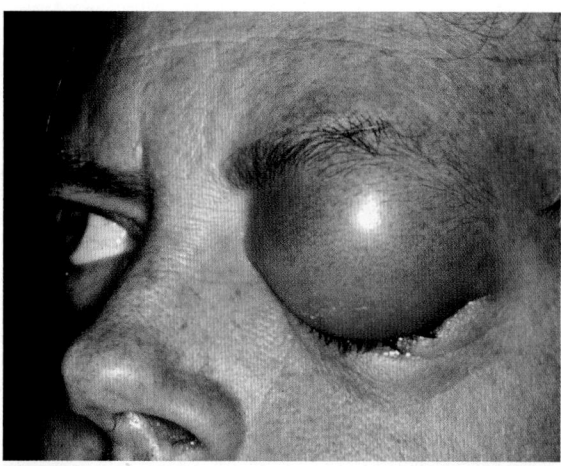

FIGURE 395-14. Eyelid abscess. Preseptal cellulitis, commonly resulting from minor penetrating trauma, may evolve into an abscess. Treatment requires incision and drainage followed by systemic antibiotics.

TABLE 395-6 OPHTHALMIC DISORDERS ASSOCIATED WITH CONJUNCTIVITIS

DISORDER	ACUTE OR CHRONIC	UNILATERAL OR BILATERAL	KEY SYMPTOMS	DEGREE OF INJECTION	DISCHARGE TYPE	OTHER FEATURES
Viral conjunctivitis	Acute	Bilateral, possibly asymmetrical	Itching, burning, soreness	4+	Watery	Preauricular lymphadenopathy
Bacterial conjunctivitis	Acute	Unilateral or bilateral	Burning	3+	Heavy, mucopurulent	Lids possibly adherent
Chlamydial conjunctivitis	Subacute, chronic	Usually unilateral	Burning, irritation	2+	Scant, mucopurulent	Usual occurrence in young, sexually active adults
Herpes simplex conjunctivitis	Acute	Unilateral	Photophobia, irritation	1-2+	None	Dendritic ulcer on the cornea or vesicles on the lid possible
Allergic conjunctivitis	Chronic	Bilateral	Itching	2+	Stringy, mucoid	Usual occurrence in atopic persons, possible seasonal symptoms
Blepharitis	Chronic	Bilateral	Itching, burning, foreign body sensation	1-2+	Usually none	Inflammation and crusting of lid margins
Dry eye	Chronic	Bilateral	Foreign body sensation	1+	Mucoid in severe cases	Punctate fluorescein staining of the cornea

Adapted from Palay DA, Krachmer JH. *Primary Care Ophthalmology*, 2nd ed. Philadelphia: Elsevier Mosby; 2005.

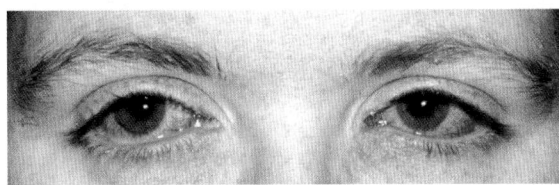

FIGURE 395-15. Diffuse injection of the conjunctiva with a watery discharge is evident in this case of viral conjunctivitis. (From Palay DA, Krachmer JH. *Primary Care Ophthalmology,* 2nd ed. Philadelphia: Elsevier Mosby; 2005.)

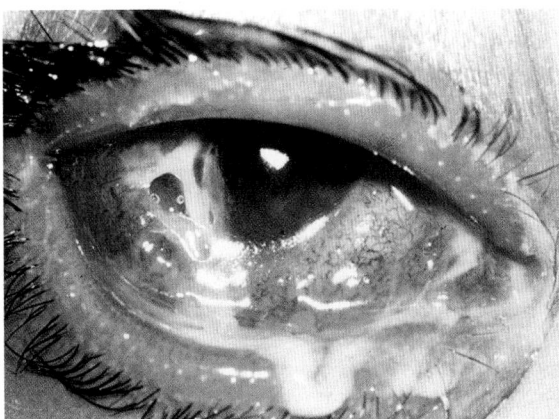

FIGURE 395-16. Bacterial conjunctivitis. Purulent discharge and conjunctival hyperemia suggest bacterial conjunctivitis. Viral conjunctivitis produces watery discharge, foreign body sensation, preauricular lymphadenopathy, and conjunctival follicles seen on slit lamp examination. (Reproduced with permission from the American Academy of Ophthalmology.)

TABLE 395-7	TOPICAL ANTIBIOTICS FOR EYE INFECTIONS		
DRUG	**TYPE**	**CONCENTRATION**	**DOSE**
Moxifloxacin	Drops	0.5%	1 drop bid × 7 days
Gatifloxacin	Drops	0.5%	1 drop q2h × 24 hours; then qid × 6 days
Ciprofloxacin	Drops	0.3%	1 drop q2h × 48 hours; then q4h × 5 days
Gentamicin	Drops	0.3%	1 drop 4 times daily
Ofloxacin	Drops	0.3%	1 drop 2h × 48h; then qid × 5 days
Bacitracin	Ointment	500 U/g	Put in eye, for several days
Tobramycin	Ointment	0.3%	Put in eye, for several days
Erythromycin	Ointment	0.5%	Put in eye, for several days

bid = twice a day; qid = four times a day.

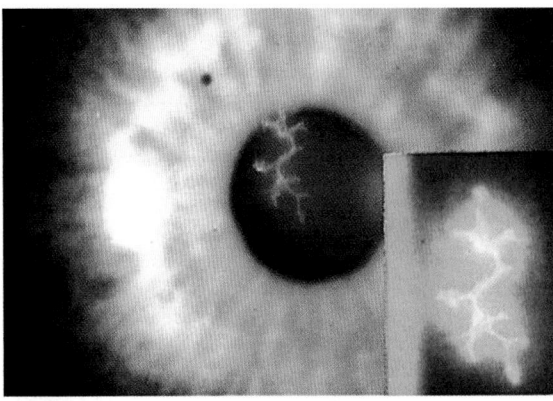

FIGURE 395-17. Herpes simplex corneal epithelial keratitis in diffuse light and in light passed through a cobalt blue filter after fluorescein staining (*inset*). Note the dendritic staining pattern characteristic of herpes simplex.

limited to, amoxicillin-clavulanate, 500 mg orally every 8 hours for 10 days, or Bactrim 500 mg orally twice a day for cases of suspected methicillin-resistant *S. aureus* [MRSA]). Treatment of orbital cellulitis, which can lead to septic optic neuritis, intracranial spread, and cavernous sinus thrombosis, may require intravenous antibiotics and surgical drainage of a paraorbital abscess.

Adenoviral Conjunctivitis

Viral conjunctivitis (Fig. 395-15) is commonly (Table 395-6) caused by adenoviruses (especially subtypes 7, 11, and 18). The condition is highly contagious through direct contact or inhalation of respiratory particles. After an incubation period of 3 to 7 days, the patient presents with red eyes (Table 395-4), itching, burning, foreign body sensation, and often a discharge, which persist for 5 to 15 days. Preauricular lymphadenopathy may be present, and a history of upper respiratory tract infection is common. The disease is self-limited, and treatment is aimed at patients' comfort. Cool compresses are often soothing. Patients are advised to wash their hands frequently. Topical antibiotics are not required.

Bacterial Conjunctivitis

Fewer than 5% of cases of conjunctivitis are caused by bacteria, mostly *Staphylococcus, Haemophilus,* or *Streptococcus* species. Patients have a mucoid or purulent discharge (Fig. 395-16), often with crusting and edema of the conjunctiva (chemosis) and lids. Bacterial conjunctivitis responds to broad-spectrum antibiotic solutions or ointments (e.g., topical erythromycin ointment three times daily for 2 weeks) (Table 395-7).

Chlamydial Conjunctivitis

Adult inclusion conjunctivitis is a chronic conjunctivitis caused by sexual transmission of *Chlamydia trachomatis* (Chapter 302). Patients often have preauricular lymphadenopathy. Oral erythromycin (500 mg orally, four times daily for 7 days) or azithromycin (1 g orally twice daily for 7 days) is required. Trachoma, which is a chronic cicatricial conjunctivitis after repeated chlamydial infection (Chapter 302), is the world's leading cause of corneal blindness. It causes an entropion, inversion of the eyelashes (trichiasis), corneal vascularization, and opacification. Topical erythromycin or tetracycline, twice daily for 3 to 4 weeks, can be effective, but surgical epilation or eyelid reconstruction may be required.

Herpes Simplex Keratitis

Herpes simplex keratitis is the most common cause of central corneal ulcer (Fig. 395-17). Herpes simplex virus also can cause vesicular eyelid dermatitis. Initially, the main signs of primary herpes simplex keratitis are a red eye and a corneal epithelial dendritic ulcer. With appropriate antiviral therapy (e.g., ganciclovir 0.15% ophthalmic gel five times daily for at least 1 week or oral acyclovir 800 mg five times per day for 7 to 10 days), the keratitis usually heals without scarring. Herpes simplex keratitis can recur and may extend into the corneal stroma and cause a red eye, ocular discomfort, blurred vision, and corneal scarring. Patients with recurrent disease may benefit from chronic low-dose antivirals (e.g., oral acyclovir 800 mg per day indefinitely) for suppression. Stromal involvement is multifactorial and can be recalcitrant. Corneal transplantation is occasionally needed for scarring.

Herpes Zoster Ophthalmicus

Herpes zoster ophthalmicus (shingles, Chapter 351) has a propensity to involve one or more branches of the trigeminal nerve. The virus also can affect the uveal tract and, in immunosuppressed patients, the retina (i.e., acute retinal necrosis). When the trigeminal nerve is involved, spread to the inside of the eye (uveitis) is most likely if vesicles are present in the inner corner of the eyelids or on the nose, especially the tip of the nose (Hutchinson sign). If the uvea is not involved, the skin lesions heal with some scarring but no long-term effects. In patients with moderate to severe skin involvement, treatment can be started with oral acyclovir (800 mg orally five times per day for 7 to 10 days) or valacyclovir (1 g three times a day for 10 to 14 days). If uveitis develops, the treatment (e.g., prednisolone acetate drops 1% four times daily and atropine 1.0% once or twice daily) can be extended and difficult. Like herpes simplex virus, herpes zoster can affect the cornea and patients should be monitored for recurrent disease.

Pseudomonal and Gonococcal Keratitis

Keratitis, which is inflammation of the corneal stroma, can be caused by spread of pathogens internally from a corneal ulcer. *Pseudomonas aeruginosa* (Chapter

290), which causes a particularly virulent keratitis, is the most common gram-negative pathogen and is especially common in people who wear contact lenses. To avoid intraocular spread, urgent and aggressive antibiotic treatment is necessary (e.g., fortified tobramycin [9 mg/mL] or a fourth-generation fluoroquinolone (e.g., moxifloxacin), every hour for 3 to 7 days. The dosage and duration of the treatment depend on the response.

Another gram-negative cause of a virulent keratitis is *Neisseria gonorrhoeae* (Chapter 282), especially in neonates. Corneal infection is accompanied by copious tearing and a characteristic hyperpurulent discharge. Prompt treatment with topical irrigation (normal saline to remove mucopurulent material) and penicillin G (100,000 units/kg/day given intravenously in four divided doses for 7 days) is essential to prevent corneal perforation.[7]

Cytomegalovirus Retinitis

Cytomegalovirus retinitis (Chapter 352) is unusual except in immunosuppressed patients and human immunodeficiency virus (HIV) infection but is increasing among patients who have undergone solid organ or hematopoietic stem cell transplantation. Clinically, a central retinochoroiditis is seen. The presumptive diagnosis is made on the characteristic intense, retinal, wedge-shaped reaction, with considerable exudates and hemorrhages, giving the terms "pizza pie retinitis" and "hemorrhagic cottage cheese retinitis" to the entity. Treatment is with antiviral drugs: ganciclovir (5 mg/kg intravenously twice daily, two to three times per week), foscarnet (90 mg/kg intravenously twice daily, twice per week), or cidofovir (5 mg/kg intravenously, weekly for 3 weeks) with follow-up maintenance. Intravitreal injections with an appropriately reduced dose are also used in selected cases.

Acanthamoeba Keratitis

Acanthamoeba species (Chapter 331) can cause a severe, blinding keratitis. Contact lens wearing is a major risk factor. A characteristic stromal ring infiltrate develops, and uveitis may occur. When patients are examined early in their disease course, they may only have a slight epitheliopathy and have pain out of proportion to findings on examination. Swimming or using fresh water with contact lens wear can often be elicited in the history. Using a confocal microscope, the acanthamebic parasite can be observed clinically as a pear-shaped cyst (11 to 15 µm). Numerous treatment protocols exist (e.g., poly-hexamethyl biguanide 0.02% drops every hour). The duration and dose depend on the response. Corneal transplantation may be necessary in cases of severe corneal scarring.

Toxoplasmic Retinitis

Toxoplasma gondii (Chapter 328) causes both a congenital and an acquired retinochoroiditis, which is more common in immunosuppressed patients. The lesions begin as an acute retinitis that atrophies centrally and pigments peripherally as it heals. The protozoa are found both in free and encysted forms within the retina. The condition may be self-limited and diagnosed as a healed incidental finding that does not need treatment. Standard treatment of vision-threatening toxoplasmosis remains controversial. When active lesions are in the macula or a severe vitreitis causes at least a two-line decrease in vision, 4 to 6 weeks of quadruple therapy (pyrimethamine, 200 mg oral loading dose, then 25 mg orally daily; folinic acid, 10 mg orally every other day; sulfadiazine, 2 g oral loading dose, then 1 g four times daily; and oral corticosteroids, e.g., prednisone, 20 to 60 mg orally daily beginning at least 24 hours after antibiotic therapy is started and tapered 10 days before stopping antibiotics) usually produces good results. Alternative regimens may include trimethroprim-sufamethoxazole (800/160 mg orally twice daily), clindamycin (150 to 450 mg orally three to four times daily), or atovaquone (1 g oral loading dose, then 500 mg daily).

Fungal Endophthalmitis

Fungal endophthalmitis is infrequent (7% of microbial endophthalmitis) but is a potentially disastrous infection of the inside of the eye, often leading to blindness. The primary organisms are *Candida*, *Coccidioides*, and *Aspergillus* species, which can gain access inside the eye either by traumatic introduction or through hematogenous spread. The patient presents with floaters and/or decreased vision. In advanced cases, the patient develops red eye and ocular pain. Multiple abscesses tend to be caused by fungi, whereas a solitary abscess is more likely caused by bacteria. Systemic antifungal agents (e.g., fluconazole 100 to 200 mg daily for 2 months) are often effective in treating localized fungal abscesses, but if the infection has progressed into the vitreous body, vitrectomy and intravitreal antifungal therapies are indicated.

Tuberculosis

About 1% of patients with pulmonary tuberculosis (Chapter 308) have uveal involvement, usually as iridocyclitis or diffuse choroiditis. Painless progressive visual loss is the most common symptom. Small yellow choroidal lesions may be seen, and retinal periphlebitis may occur secondarily. Treatment is as for the primary disease.

Syphilis

About 5% of patients with secondary syphilis (Chapter 303) develop anterior uveitis or neuroretinitis. In tertiary syphilis, the miotic Argyll Robertson pupil reacts poorly to light but briskly to accommodation. Treatment is as for the systemic disease.

● STRUCTURAL AND AGE-RELATED DISORDERS
Cataract

A cataract is an opacification of the crystalline lens. The lens doubles in volume between birth and age 70 years as new lens "fiber cells" are laid down on the external aspect of the lens cortex, beneath the lens capsule. The older fibers in the center of the lens cannot be desquamated into the surrounding aqueous and thus are compressed into the center of the lens. At birth, the lens is pliable and totally transparent. By age 45 years, the lens loses its pliability, which compromises near vision. As the process progresses, the lens loses its transparency, beginning at the center of the lens (nuclear sclerosis). The concurrent change in density of the lens nucleus may alter the optical characteristics of the eye to cause acquired nearsightedness ("second sight"). Ultimately, the cataract may become so dense that cataract surgery is necessary to restore vision.

Symptoms are typically loss of vision, especially at night, and glare.[8] Cataract surgery, performed as an outpatient, is elective and depends on how much the decreased vision interferes with the normal lifestyle of the patient. A synthetic intraocular lens implant is inserted into the eye during surgery. Prognosis for restoration of vision is excellent, depending on the function of the retina. In general, cataracts develop asymmetrically. The worst eye (vision-wise) should have surgery first. As the second eye's cataract worsens, decreasing vision and monocularity are indications for cataract surgery in the second eye.

Glaucoma

Glaucoma is an optic neuropathy in which progressive damage to retinal ganglion cells and their axons results in the characteristic loss of optic nerve tissue and damage to the peripheral and central visual field.[9] The primary site of damage is at the lamina cribrosa, where the axons of the optic nerve leave the eye.

Aqueous humor is produced by the nonpigmented ciliary epithelium of the pars plicata of the ciliary body. Aqueous fluid leaves the eye through the trabecular meshwork and uveoscleral pathways into the venous circulation. If the drainage function does not match production, the intraocular pressure increases. If the elevated intraocular pressure is high enough or is present long enough, ganglion cells in the retina are damaged, causing loss of their axons. Loss of axons can best be appreciated clinically at their normal exit from the eye, the optic disc. Bulk loss of axons will lead to enlargement of the optic cup, which is recorded as increase in the cup-to-disc ratio.

Intraocular pressure is the principal risk factor for the onset and progression of glaucoma. In general, the higher the pressure, the greater the risk. An intraocular pressure greater than 2 standard deviations above the population mean (21 mm Hg) is termed *ocular hypertension*, but there is no fully protective intraocular pressure, and many individuals develop glaucoma despite a statistically normal intraocular pressure. Additional risk factors for glaucoma include African ancestry, older age, low blood pressure, genetic predisposition, disc hemorrhage, myopia, and anterior segment abnormalities and systemic associations.

In open-angle glaucoma, there is apparent free anatomic access to the trabecular meshwork. In closed-angle glaucoma, there is a relative or absolute anatomic barrier to the flow of aqueous. For most individuals, glaucoma is asymptomatic until late in the disease, and the only way to detect it is by an ophthalmologic examination.

PRIMARY OPEN-ANGLE GLAUCOMA

The most common type of glaucoma in elderly people is primary open-angle glaucoma. For many patients, the first symptom may be difficulty reading, loss of contrast sensitivity, or glare. Peripheral visual fields may be reduced considerably before the patient notes loss of function. Most cases of primary open-angle glaucoma are identified during routine eye examinations, either

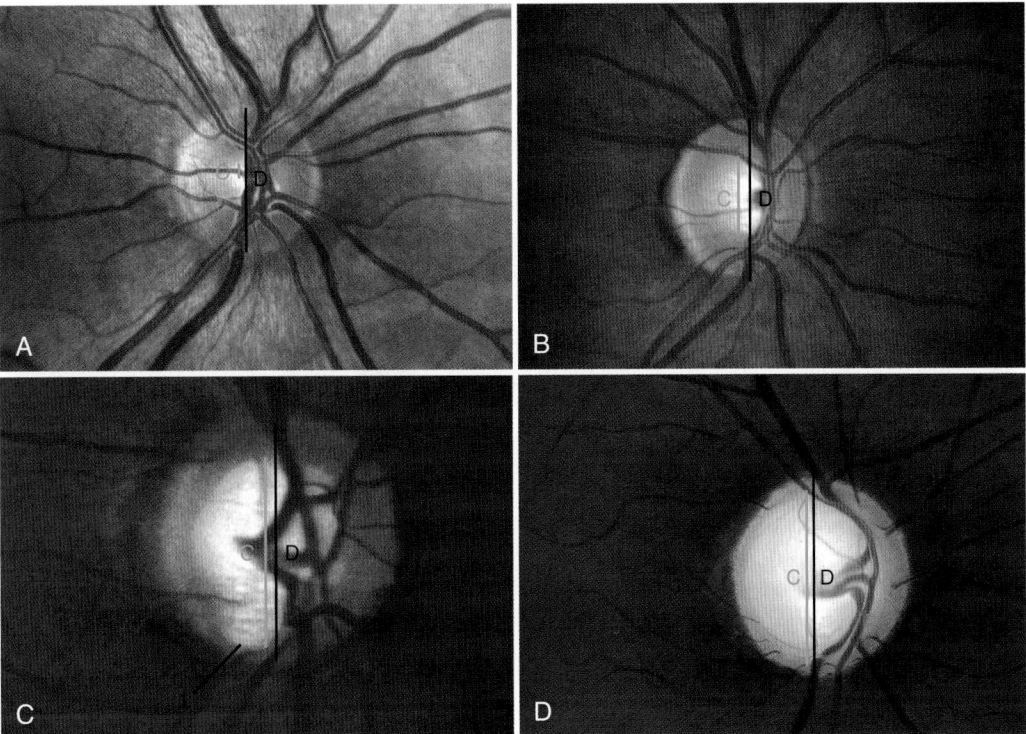

FIGURE 395-18. Cup-to-disc ratios. **A,** Normal cup-to-disc (C/D) ratio of 0.1. **B,** Likely normal C/D ratio of 0.5. **C,** C/D ratio of 0.8 vertically with inferior notching (1) of the nerve (glaucomatous change). **D,** C/D ratio of 0.90 vertically (glaucomatous change). C = cup; D = disc. (From Palay DA, Krachmer JH. *Primary Care Ophthalmology,* 2nd ed. Philadelphia: Elsevier Mosby; 2005.)

by discovery of abnormally high intraocular pressure or by the presence of a high cup-to-disc ratio (Fig. 395-18). Average intraocular pressure is generally at or below 21 mm Hg, but exceptions exist depending on corneal thickness (causing artifacts of measurement in patients with excessively thin or thick corneas) and genetic disposition. The diagnosis of glaucoma is confirmed by characteristic visual field loss as determined by automated perimetry.

The treatment goal is to reduce intraocular pressure, initially with pharmacologic agents: β-blockers (e.g., betaxolol drops 0.5% twice daily), carbonic anhydrase inhibitors (e.g., dorzolamide drops two or three times daily), α-agonists (e.g., brimonidine drops twice or twice daily), and prostaglandin analogues (e.g., travoprost[A6] 0.004% or latanoprost 0.005% drops once daily). Generally, the drops are taken for a lifetime. Applying energy to the structures of the trabecular meshwork with a laser (laser trabeculoplasty) often results in years of control of intraocular pressure, and this procedure may become first-line therapy because it can maintain normal pressure without medications.[A7] In resistant cases, mechanical filtration is accomplished surgically by bypassing the trabecular meshwork either by creating a fistula (trabeculectomy) between the anterior chamber and the episcleral tissue or by implanting a synthetic filtration device (a tube-shunt)[A8] from the anterior chamber through the sclera into a collection reservoir located at the equator of the eye in the soft tissues of the orbit.

SECONDARY OPEN-ANGLE GLAUOMA

Secondary causes of elevated intraocular pressure also can lead to glaucomatous nerve damage. The most common is pseudoexfoliation syndrome, a genetically determined biochemical abnormality of the basement membrane protein, fibrillin. The syndrome occurs among people throughout the world but is especially prominent in Scandinavians and Saudi Arabians. Affected individuals are identified by accumulation of abnormal fibrillogranular material (exfoliative material) on the surface of the crystalline lens, most easily seen in the pupillary space or pupillary border. Pseudoexfoliative glaucoma greatly increases the risk for developing open-angle glaucoma. Treatment is as for open-angle glaucoma.

ANGLE-CLOSURE GLAUCOMA

An acute attack of angle-closure glaucoma (Fig. 395-19) may occur over a short period of time and cause extreme, debilitating symptoms. Alternatively, symptoms may develop over a long period of time with few specific symptoms.

The risk factors for angle-closure glaucoma are based on the anatomic configuration of the components of anterior chamber. Persons who are farsighted

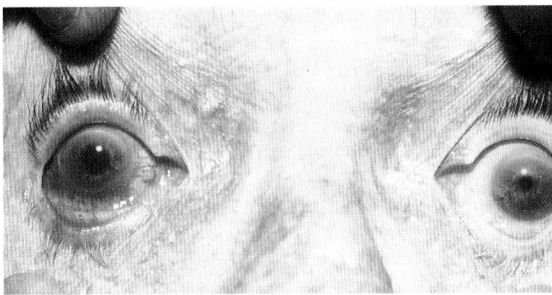

FIGURE 395-19. Acute angle-closure glaucoma. The left eye is normal. The red right eye has a nonreactive pupil. (Courtesy of Dr. Myron Yanoff.)

(hyperopia) have a shortened anterior-to-posterior axis of the eye, indicated clinically by a shallow anterior chamber that may be noted with penlight illumination but often requires slit lamp examination. As the crystalline lens increases in volume with time, the iris is displaced anteriorly. At some point, the posterior surface of the iris may come in relatively tight contact with the anterior surface of the lens. Aqueous flow is restricted, and fluid accumulates in the posterior chamber, where it displaces the diaphanous peripheral iris anteriorly. When the peripheral iris comes in contact with the posterior cornea, the anterior chamber angle is suddenly occluded. Acute angle closure may be precipitated by pharmacologic dilation of the pupil. Patients who are farsighted (hyperopia) or have cataracts should be dilated with caution. The intraocular pressure may increase from 21 mm Hg to 50 to 70 mm Hg (nearly equaling diastolic arterial pressure). The symptoms of acute angle closure may include extreme pain, which may be poorly localized to the eye, nausea, and vomiting. Persistent vomiting may cause abdominal pain, simulating an acute abdomen.

Initial treatment is with topical (e.g., timolol 0.5% in one dose) and systemic pressure-lowering agents (e.g., carbonic acetazolamide, 250 to 500 mg intravenously or two 250-mg tablets orally in one dose if intravenous access or drug is not available), followed by creation of a fistula in the peripheral iris with a laser (laser iridectomy) between the posterior chamber and the anterior chamber to bypass the obstruction. Most patients require a laser iridectomy prophylactically in the second eye to prevent angle-closure glaucoma. Another potential option is lens extraction[A9] because age-related growth in the lens contributes to angle closure.

Secondary glaucoma may also occur after intraocular hemorrhage, intraocular trauma, and intraocular inflammation. Some developmentally related secondary glaucomas, such as the iridocorneal endothelial syndrome, may not become evident until adulthood.

Retinal Detachment

A retinal detachment is a separation of the neural (sensory) retina from the underlying retinal pigment epithelium. The main types are rhegmatogenous, caused by a retinal tear or hole, as typically occurs with a posterior vitreous detachment; tractional, caused by fibrosis, such as in advanced proliferative diabetic retinopathy; or serous, when fluid accumulates under neural retina because of breakdown of the blood-retinal barrier in conditions such as malignant hypertension or eclampsia of pregnancy.

The classic symptoms are a sensation of flashes of light, floaters in the involved eye owing to the causative vitreous detachment, and a shadow in the field of vision. Urgent treatment usually is needed to prevent macular involvement or deterioration. Most cases require a scleral buckle and/or vitreous surgery, although select cases may be successfully treated by in-office procedures such as laser photocoagulation and pneumatic tamponade. The latter involves the intravitreal injection of a gas bubble that, with proper head positioning on the part of the patient, effectively closes a retinal break; permanent sealing of the break is accomplished laser photocoagulation. In contrast, serous retinal detachments generally resolve without direct intervention when the underlying cause is successfully treated.

Age-Related Macular Degeneration

Age-related macular degeneration is a neurodegenerative disease that initially affects the retinal pigment epithelium of the macula, mainly in the sixth to ninth decades of life.[10] About 8.5% of the world's blindness is caused by age-related macular degeneration, mainly in industrialized countries. In the United States, age-related macular degeneration affects more than 1.75 million persons, and its prevalence increases with each decade after the age of 55 years. The exact genetic influence has not yet been determined, but abnormalities of complement factor H appear to play a role. Environmental factors such as smoking are known to accelerate this degenerative process.

Two forms of age-related macular degeneration predominate: the "dry" or non-exudative type, and the "wet" or neovascular type. The dry form usually precedes the wet form, which usually causes the most profound vision loss, especially if untreated.

The first clinical sign of age-related macular degeneration is an attenuated or mottled appearance of the retinal pigment epithelium in the macula, usually accompanied by *drusen*, which are abnormal lipoprotein deposits within the retinal pigment epithelial basement membrane complex (Bruch membrane). Lipofuscin, a complex mixture composed mainly of the oxidation products of polyunsaturated fatty acids and vitamin A dimers, accumulates in stressed retinal pigment epithelial cells. Significant macular degeneration is typically characterized by soft drusen that are greater than 60 μm and appear on examination as deep, hypopigmented spots. This non-exudative age-related macular degeneration may antedate subjective alteration in vision by years to several decades.

Symptoms of age-related macular degeneration are confined to deterioration of central visual function, because the peripheral retina is not involved. As the process progresses, individuals with advanced disease will be able to walk down a street without apparent difficulty (a peripheral retinal function) but will not be able to recognize facial features of people whom they meet (a macular retinal function). Visual aids and other devices, such as special glasses and television aids, often allow patients to continue with daily functions and to continue to live independently.

Dry age-related macular degeneration advances at a variable rate (months to decades), during which patients develop retinal features of well-defined pigment loss (geographic retinal atrophy; Fig. 395-20). No current treatment exists for the dry phase of the disease, except for a possible positive influence of dietary supplements (antioxidants). Vitamin supplementation with vitamins C and E, lutein, zeaxanthin, zinc, and copper may retard the progression of moderate age-related macular degeneration to severe age-related macular degeneration.[A10] β-Carotene (a vitamin A precursor) of this quantity is not recommended for cigarette smokers because of an increased risk for lung cancer. Cessation of smoking, control of blood sugar, control of blood lipid levels, and control of systemic blood pressure are particularly important behavioral modifications. Patients with dry age-related macular degeneration who are at higher risk for developing choroidal neovascularization should be advised to monitor themselves by means of Amsler grid or

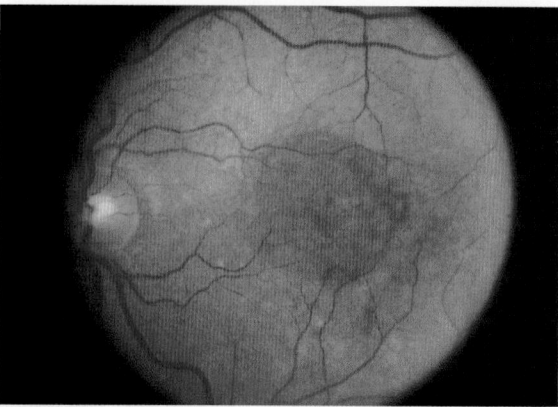

FIGURE 395-20. Dry age-related macular degeneration. Drusen are present in the posterior pole around a large area of geographic atrophy of the retinal pigment epithelium.

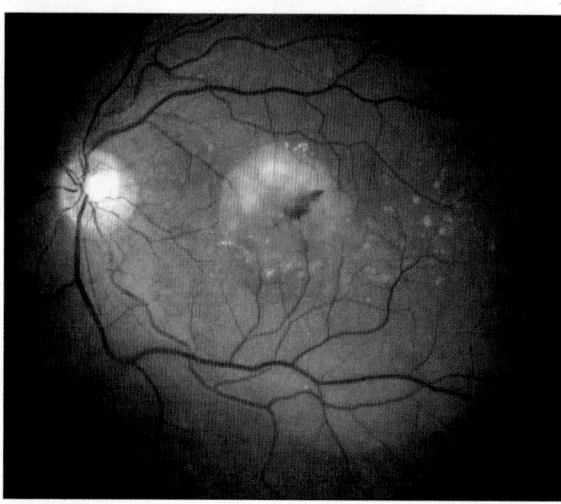

FIGURE 395-21. Wet age-related macular degeneration. A "dirty gray" neovascular membrane is present under the central macular area.

similar testing strategies and urgently seek treatment if new visual symptoms develop.

In the "wet phase" of age-related macular degeneration (Fig. 395-21), frail, neovascular channels originating from the established vascular system of the choroid may extend through a breach in Bruch membrane into the subretinal space (subretinal or choroidal neovascularization). Spontaneous hemorrhage of the vessels adds to the loss of photoreceptors. Hemorrhage is accompanied by acute, and often permanent, loss of central visual acuity (i.e., the wet phase of age-related macular degeneration). Both eyes are typically affected to a similar degree. Neovascularization can be identified by fluorescein angiography and ocular coherence tomography. Intraocular injections of antivascular endothelial growth factors (e.g., ranibizumab, bevacizumab, or aflibercept)[A11] reduce the risk for visual loss in patients with neovascular age-related macular degeneration and can result in gains in vision, especially when administered on a timely basis. Other treatments include photodynamic therapy or, in advanced cases, vitrectomy to remove massive subretinal hemorrhage.

● SYSTEMIC DISEASES WITH OCULAR SYMPTOMS DURING ADULTHOOD

Diabetes Mellitus

Diabetic retinopathy is one of the leading causes of blindness in the United States. More than 75% of the blind are women. Background diabetic retinopathy, with microaneurysms, hemorrhages, exudates (Fig. 395-22), and macular edema, accounts for most cases of decreased vision but rarely causes profound vision loss. With acute hyperglycemia, accumulation of sorbitol may lead to swelling of the lens; secondary refractive errors may persist for 6 to 8 weeks. Most diabetic patients never develop the more severe proliferative diabetic retinopathy (Fig. 395-23), which generally occurs only after 15 years or more of diabetes and causes a profound loss of vision.

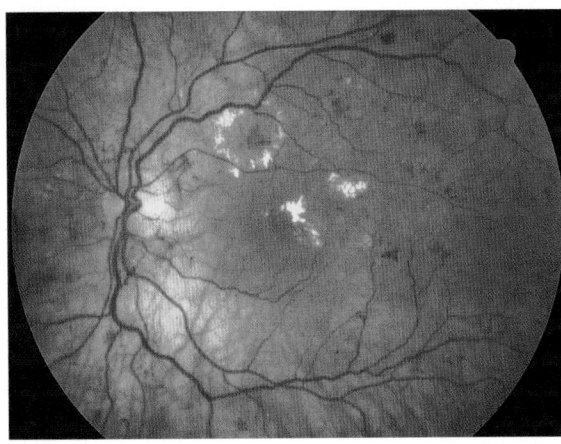

FIGURE 395-22. Background diabetic retinopathy. Exudates, microaneurysms, and small hemorrhages are seen in the posterior pole (left eye).

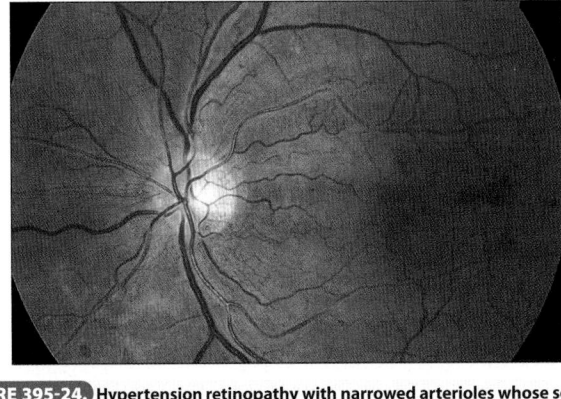

FIGURE 395-24. Hypertension retinopathy with narrowed arterioles whose sclerosed walls create the appearance of "nicking" when the arterioles cross venules. (From Yanoff M, Duker JS, eds. *Ophthalmology.* Philadelphia: Mosby Elsevier; 2009.)

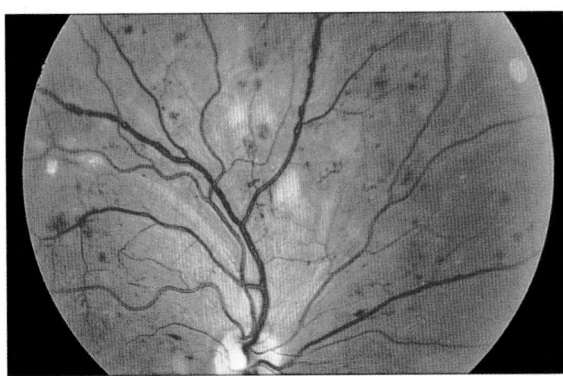

FIGURE 395-23. Severe nonproliferative diabetic retinopathy with cotton-wool spots, intraretinal microvascular abnormalities, and venous beading. (From Yanoff M, Duker JS, eds. *Ophthalmology.* Philadelphia: Mosby Elsevier; 2009.)

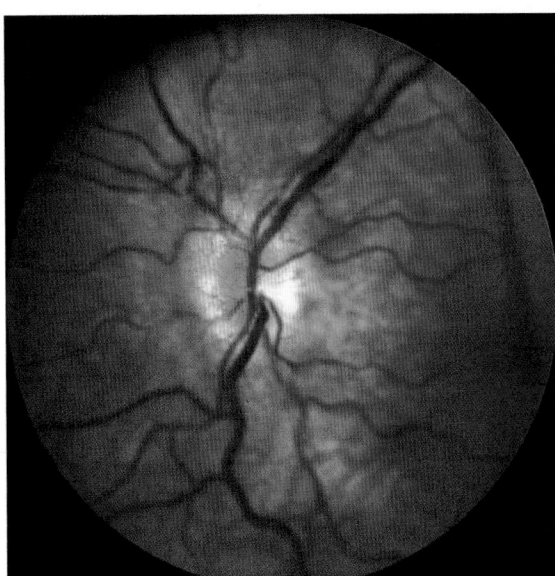

FIGURE 395-25. Papilledema. (Courtesy of Dr. Kathleen Digre.)

Diabetic retinopathy is closely correlated with the duration of diabetes mellitus (Chapter 216). The prevalence of diabetic retinopathy is approximately 27% among patients who have had type 1 diabetes for 5 to 10 years, 70 to 90% among patients who have had diabetes for more than 10 years, and 95% among patients who have had diabetes for 20 to 30 years. In patients with type 2 diabetes (Chapter 216), the prevalence of diabetic retinopathy is about 23% after 12 years and 60% after 16 years. Tight control of blood glucose greatly reduces the risk for the development of diabetic retinopathy.

The treatment of diabetic retinopathy includes control of the diabetes and any hyperlipidemia (Chapter 195). Intensive diabetes therapy reduces the risk of future ocular surgery in type 1 diabetes.[A12] Antiangiogenic therapy (e.g., ranibizumab, bevacizumab, or aflibercept[A13][A14]) is generally superior to laser therapy for diabetic macular edema and has often replaced it as first-line therapy.[11] However, laser photocoagulation remains particularly useful for proliferative diabetic retinopathy, for clinically significant macular edema that does not involve the foveal center, or when antiangiogenic therapy does not provide a complete response. Intravitreal steroid injection may also be beneficial.

Hypertension

In chronic systemic hypertension (Chapter 70), the characteristic retinal vascular findings can assess the severity of hypertension. As the severity increases, patients develop arterial narrowing, arteriovenous nicking (Fig. 395-24), nerve fiber layer infarcts, and intraretinal hemorrhages. Moderately sclerosed arterioles have a "copper wiring" appearance, whereas severely sclerosed vessels demonstrate "silver wiring." Acute hypertension may cause optic nerve edema ("papilledema"; Fig. 395-25) and serous retinal detachments that usually resolve without significant sequelae if blood pressure is controlled.

Other Systemic Diseases

In bacterial endocarditis (Chapter 67), emboli may cause retinal hemorrhages or the characteristic Roth spot (Fig. 395-26). Accumulation of copper in the

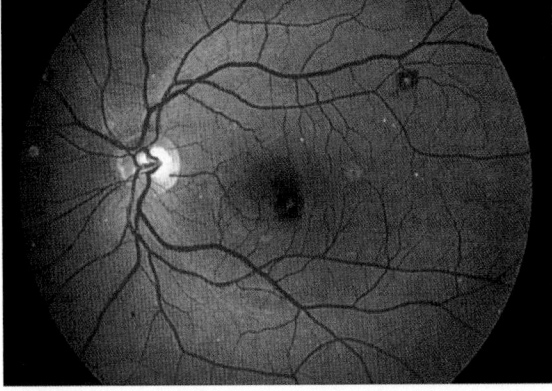

FIGURE 395-26. Roth spots. Multiple white-centered hemorrhages in a man with recurrent subacute bacterial endocarditis. White-centered hemorrhages are also seen with leukemia and diabetes. The small white scars are probably the residua of previous episodes.

posterior cornea may aid in the diagnosis of Wilson disease (Chapter 200), although its clinical diagnosis usually precedes the characteristic Kayser-Fleischer ring (see Fig. 200-2), which fades after treatment. Tay-Sachs and Niemann-Pick diseases (Chapter 197) are associated with a foveal cherry-red spot owing to the accumulation of gangliosides within perifoveal ganglion cells. Pseudoxanthoma elasticum (Chapter 244) is often associated with characteristic angioid streaks of the retina.

VASCULAR ABNORMALITIES OF THE EYE

The major vessels of the retina enter the eye at a point of relative constriction in the tissues of the lamina cribrosa of the optic disc. In persons who have generalized vascular disease, particularly systemic hypertension, occlusion of either the artery or vein may lead to a sudden loss of vision. Partial occlusion of either the artery or vein is associated with less visual loss but still increases the risk for developing neovascular glaucoma.

Occlusion of the central retinal artery (Fig. 395-27) presents as painless acute loss of vision. The ischemic retina generally has a pale gray appearance except at the fovea, where the normal color is preserved (cherry-red spot). The clinical appearance of edema resolves over time, but vision generally does not recover.

Venous occlusion of the central retinal vein (Fig. 395-28) presents as painless loss of vision. The appearance of the fundus is characterized by extensive intraretinal hemorrhages and a variable degree of retinal ischemia. Macular edema is common, but intravitreal anti–vascular endothelial growth factor injections can provide significant and sustained visual improvement.[A15] Ischemic central vein occlusion is a major risk factor for developing secondary neovascular glaucoma.

Giant cell arteritis (temporal arteritis [Chapter 255]) can occlude the blood supply of the optic disc by inflammation of the short posterior ciliary arteries. This occlusion causes acute, painless loss of vision. Presenting symptoms before visual loss often include scalp tenderness or jaw claudication, which may be accompanied by weight loss and a vague sensation of fatigue. Diagnostic suspicion is further raised by an elevated erythrocyte sedimentation rate or C-reactive protein level. Temporal artery biopsy showing granulomatous inflammation in the region of the internal elastic lamina confirms the diagnosis.

Because of the significant risk of visual loss in the initial and contralateral eye, even before laboratory or pathologic studies are known, systemic corticosteroid therapy (e.g., oral prednisone 40 to 60 mg per day) should be administered for a protracted period until the sedimentation rate normalizes and symptoms are relieved (Chapter 255). Unfortunately, treatment usually does not restore lost vision in the presenting eye.

Nonarteritic ischemic optic neuropathy is caused by occlusion of the posterior ciliary arteries and infarction of the optic disc, resulting in acute, usually unilateral, painless loss of vision. There often are no antecedent symptoms except those systemic signs and symptoms associated with systemic nonarteritic vascular disease such as systemic hypertension. Occlusion is thought to be due to atherosclerosis or some other lumen-compromising mechanism. No treatment restores vision. There is a risk for the same process affecting the second eye.

IDIOPATHIC INFLAMMATORY AND AUTOIMMUNE DISORDERS

Ocular or periocular tissues may be the primary focus of isolated idiopathic or autoimmune inflammation. Pain is common, and changes in vision may occur.

Keratoconjunctivitis Sicca

Keratoconjunctivitis sicca, or the dry eye syndrome, results from deficiency of any of the tear film layers. Symptoms include gritty, foreign body sensations, burning, photophobia, and decreased visual acuity. Idiopathic inflammation in keratoconjunctivitis sicca and xerostomia represents Sjögren syndrome (Chapter 252). Recurrent corneal erosion, keratitis, and corneal opacification can occur. Many medications can also cause dry eyes (Table 395-8).

Artificial tears, up to four times daily, and lubricating ointments are helpful. Corticosteroids (e.g., loteprednol 0.5% eye-drops four times a day) are also effective as an initial treatment. Cyclosporine eye-drops (0.05%, one drop in each eye every 12 hours) are useful when other measures fail.

Scleritis

Episcleritis, which is an inflammation immediately underlying the conjunctiva, is distinguished from conjunctivitis because its radially oriented vessels do not move with the conjunctiva. Mild pain may be present. Episcleritis is self-limited. Instillation of 10% phenylephrine is helpful in making the diagnosis because it causes blanching in episcleritis but not in scleritis. Oral or topical nonsteroidal anti-inflammatory medications such as flurbiprofen or diclofenac may hasten resolution.

Scleritis, which presents as severe pain and redness, is associated with infectious or autoimmune connective tissue disease in about 50% of cases. Vision may be reduced if the posterior sclera is involved. Diffuse or sectoral hyperemia is nonmobile and does not blanch with instillation of phenylephrine. Secondary uveitis and keratitis may occur. Diagnostic evaluation includes ultrasonography or magnetic resonance imaging and laboratory tests to identify

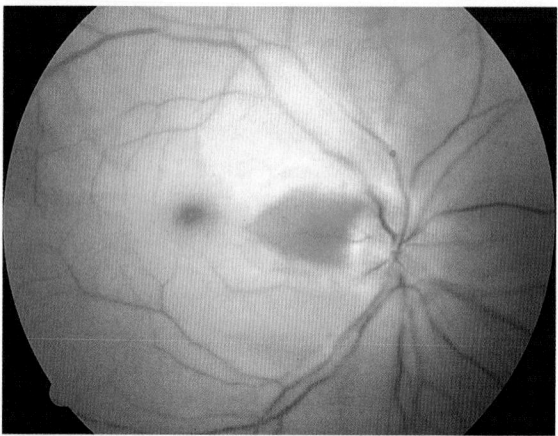

FIGURE 395-27. Central retinal artery occlusion. Fundus photograph shows the fovea, which lacks inner retinal layers, as a cherry-red spot, in contrast to extrafoveal retina, which appears white because of inner retinal infarction. In this case, a small area of retina adjacent to the optic disc is spared, owing to the presence of a cilioretinal artery.

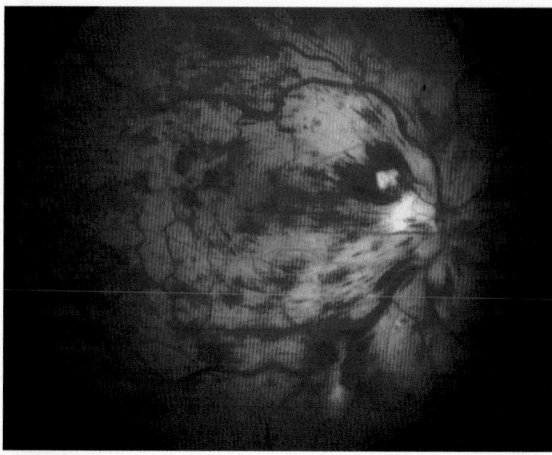

FIGURE 395-28. Central retinal vein occlusion with diffuse intraretinal hemorrhages in all four quadrants.

TABLE 395-8	PARTIAL LIST OF SYSTEMIC MEDICATIONS CAUSING DRY EYE
MEDICATION	**CLASS**
Ibuprofen	Nonsteroidal anti-inflammatory
Diphenhydramine	Antihistamine
Triprolidine	Antihistamine
Chlorpheniramine	Antihistamine
Atenolol	β-Blocker
Metoprolol	β-Blocker
Propranolol	β-Blocker
Clonidine	α-Agonist
Scopolamine	Anticholinergic
Amiodarone	Antiarrhythmic
Thiabendazole	Antinematode
Isotretinoin*	Retinoid

*Severe, long-term dry eye with onset up to several years after treatment. All others tend to abate with cessation.
From Goldman L, Ausiello DA, eds. *Cecil Textbook of Medicine*, 23rd ed. Philadelphia: Saunders Elsevier; 2008:2852.

potential underlying conditions. Treatment may require topical or oral nonsteroidal anti-inflammatory medications or corticosteroids.

Mooren Ulcer

Mooren ulcer is idiopathic, progressive, peripheral corneal thinning, likely autoimmune. It can be unilateral or bilateral, and pain is common. Topical corticosteroids, mucolytics, and cytotoxic agents have been used. Bandage contact lenses and conjunctival recession or advancement have also been used with variable success.

Orbital Pseudotumor

Nonspecific, idiopathic orbital inflammation involving the lacrimal gland (dacryoadenitis), extraocular muscles (myositis), orbital fat, sclera, or optic nerve sheath (optic perineuritis) can be caused by orbital pseudotumor. Some of the cases of idiopathic orbital inflammation have been recently associated with immunoglobulin G4 autoimmune disease. Pain is frequent. Patients may present with proptosis, limited ocular movements, or decreased acuity. Orbital ultrasonography or magnetic resonance imaging excludes a mass lesion. Patients respond dramatically to systemic corticosteroids within 24 hours, but the steroids must be tapered slowly over months to prevent recurrence.

Iritis

Iritis presents with pain, photophobia, and blurred vision, with about 50% of cases related to systemic disease. Slit lamp examination shows inflammatory cells and protein exudate in the anterior chamber. Symptomatic treatment is with prednisolone acetate 1% suspension four times a day and cycloplegic drugs (cyclopentolate 1 or 2% twice daily) is usually effective, but repeated episodes require evaluation for autoimmune and infectious causes.

Rheumatoid Arthritis

Juvenile rheumatoid arthritis (Chapter 248) is the most common specific childhood entity associated with uveitis. In adults, the ocular manifestations of rheumatoid arthritis mainly affect the anterior part of the eye, cornea, and sclera. Nearly 50% of patients who have peripheral ulcerative keratitis of the cornea have an associated systemic disease, mainly collagen vascular disease, and especially rheumatoid arthritis. Similarly, almost half of patients who have scleritis have an associated systemic disease, and about 15% of these are connective tissue diseases. Scleromalacia perforans, which is aseptic necrosis of the sclera, is associated with rheumatoid arthritis about 46% of the time.

Systemic Lupus Erythematosus

Systemic lupus erythematosus (Chapter 250) causes eye manifestations from both the primary disease and its treatment with derivatives of chloroquine. Patients may have retinal vasculitis and can develop an ischemic or nonischemic optic neuritis, both of which can result in severe and permanent loss of vision. Hydroxychloroquine therapy can cause a toxic retinal degeneration, but this complication is rare during the first 10 years of use and lower at a dose of 5 mg/kg per day. Screening with visual fields or retinal imaging can detect toxicity before the patient complains of visual loss or any signs are seen on examination of the fundus.

Sarcoidosis

About 25% of patients with sarcoidosis (Chapter 89) develop chronic uveitis. Sarcoid also can involve the lids, conjunctiva, optic nerve, cranial nerves, and lacrimal glands. Anterior uveitis is treated topically with prednisolone acetate in decreasing doses, depending on degree of inflammation, and with daily cycloplegics (cyclopentolate 2%, atropine 1%). Posterior uveitis, dacryoadenitis, and neurologic manifestations require systemic corticosteroids, but the doses have not been standardized.

Sympathetic Ophthalmia

Sympathetic ophthalmia is an autoimmune disease characterized by bilateral, granulomatous uveitis following trauma to one eye. The condition is very rare, occurring in less than 1 per 10,000 cases of ocular surgical procedures and 1 per 1000 cases of accidental trauma.

The identified antigen within the eye is thought to be located in the outer retina. The disease is recognized clinically by signs of inflammation in the uninjured eye, generally 2 weeks or longer after the injury. Generally, removal of the injured eye within these 2 weeks will protect against the development of sympathetic ophthalmia in the uninjured eye, but once the uninjured eye is involved, removal of the originally injured eye is not likely to influence the process. Left untreated, inflammation may destroy the function of both eyes.

When sympathetic ophthalmia is established, the patient will require anti-inflammation treatment (e.g., prednisolone, 1.0 to 1.5 mg/kg orally per day), most likely for an extended period. Most patients retain useful vision if treated at an early stage.

● GENETICALLY DETERMINED DISEASES THAT MAY BECOME SYMPTOMATIC DURING ADULTHOOD
Corneal Stromal Dystrophy

Most corneal dystrophies are autosomal dominant and bilateral, progress slowly, and primarily affect one layer of an otherwise normal cornea. Common types of dystrophies are anterior basement membrane, macular, granular, lattice, and Fuchs endothelial. Some result from mutations within the same gene. For example, the *BIGH3* on 5q31 is associated with granular and lattice dystrophy and corneal dystrophy of Bowman. The main symptom, caused by opaque corneal deposits, is blurred vision. If the decreased vision interferes with activities of normal living, a corneal transplantation can be performed.

Choroidal Dystrophy

Choroidal dystrophies are progressive, inherited disorders characterized by atrophy of the retinal pigment epithelium and choroid. The main entities are central areolar choroidal sclerosis (autosomal dominant or recessive), gyrate atrophy (deficiency of the mitochondrial matrix enzyme ornithine-δ-aminotransferase), and choroideremia (deficiency of component A of Rab geranylgeranyl transferase). No treatment exists for central areolar choroidal sclerosis or choroideremia. An arginine-restricted diet may be helpful in treating gyrate atrophy, and gene therapy trial has shown promising results for choroideremia.[12] An arginine-restricted diet may also be helpful in treating gyrate atrophy.

Retinitis Pigmentosa

Retinitis pigmentosa (Fig. 395-29) is bilateral and symmetrical, starts in early adult life, and is progressive. Retinitis pigmentosa can be an autosomal dominant or recessive disease, X-linked, digenic, mitochondrial, or sporadic. The primary defect, apoptotic in nature, appears to be in the neural retinal receptors. The main findings consist of the tetrad of bone-corpuscular retinal pigmentation; a pale, waxy optic nerve; attenuation of retinal arterioles; and a posterior subcapsular cataract. Night blindness is the primary symptom. The electroretinogram usually shows no electrical evidence of retinal function. Vitamin A palmitate supplementation (15,000 IU daily) may slow the rate of progression. Gene therapy is under investigation.

● COMMON PEDIATRIC OR ADOLESCENT DISEASES THAT MAY PERSIST INTO ADULTHOOD
Retinopathy of Prematurity

Retinal vascular development is not complete until 40 weeks of gestational age, so a premature infant is at risk of developing retinopathy of prematurity,

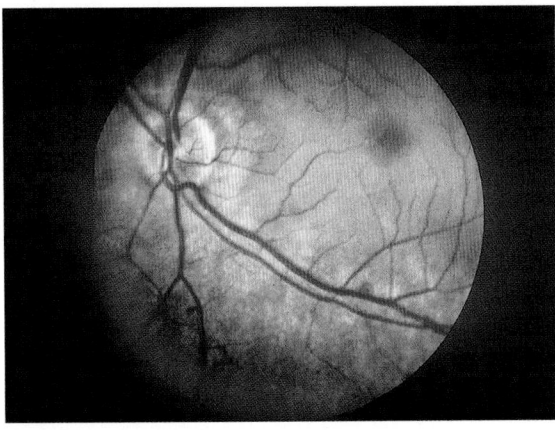

FIGURE 395-29. Retinitis pigmentosa. Fundus photograph shows "bone spicule" pigmentation of the midperipheral fundus, waxy pallor of the optic disc, and attenuated retinal vessels, the most consistent finding in retinitis pigmentosa. (Courtesy of Dr. John I. Loewenstein.)

in which blood vessels of the immature retina may leave the plane of the retina and grow into the adjacent vitreous body. The resulting tractional forces can cause total, irreversible retinal detachment and, ultimately, blindness. Myopia, strabismus, and amblyopia also are sequelae of retinopathy of prematurity. The primary risk factors for retinopathy of prematurity are early gestational age, low birth weight, and the use of supplemental oxygen. Early recognition and treatment (typically with laser photocoagulation) of retinal neovascularization are essential to halt progressive disease and prevent blindness.

Hemangioma of the Eyelid

Hemangioma of the eyelid is a hamartomatous (tissue normally found in the area) malformation of vessels in the soft tissues of the eyelid. The abnormal vascular lesion is usually insignificant at birth but grows in size over the first several months of life. The expanding hemangioma may cause astigmatism or mechanical ptosis, placing the infant at risk of amblyopia. The lesions rarely grow beyond 1 year of age, and typically involute over time. If hemangiomas are small and not visually significant, observation is appropriate. Oral propranolol (1.5 to 3 mg/kg per day in two divided doses for up to 1 year), which is the treatment of choice for larger lesions or those at risk of causing amblyopia, can result in complete regression of the hemangioma.

Congenital Cataract

Congenital cataracts, which can be inherited as an autosomal dominant trait, are opacifications of the crystalline lens at birth. In congenital rubella (Chapter 344), the opacity is relatively limited to the fetal nucleus and has a pearl-like appearance. The cataract of galactosemia (Chapter 194) is potentially reversible with dietary restriction of galactose. Small cataracts can be observed, whereas dense cataracts that obstruct vision should be excised at an early age to prevent amblyopia.

● TUMORS OF THE EYE
Retinoblastoma

Retinoblastoma, the most common intraocular malignant tumor of childhood, results from uncontrolled proliferation of retinoblasts, which are pluripotential neuroectodermal cells that will differentiate into the various components of mature retina. A genetic deletion of the *Rb* (retinoblastoma) gene occurs in the chromosomal region 13q14. The tumor initially proliferates in the plane of the retina but is capable of involving all structures within the eye. Retinoblastoma may spread to the central nervous system through the optic nerve and vasculature to tissues at distant sites.

Approximately 40% of cases of retinoblastoma are heritable germline tumors generally diagnosed before the age of 12 months. In 80% of heritable retinoblastomas, tumors are bilateral and multiple in each eye. These patients also have a significant risk for developing a secondary primary malignant tumor (e.g., osteogenic sarcoma).

The nonheritable sporadic retinoblastomas arise spontaneously and represent about 60% of cases. The average age at presentation is 24 months and patients generally have only a single tumor in one eye. Except in patients with mosaicism, the absence of germline mutations means that the risk for retinoblastoma in succeeding generations is low and the risk for a second primary tumor is the same as in the general population.

Retinoblastoma is often discovered by parents or relatives who notice a light reflex in one eye relative to the other either (white pupil or "cat's eye" reflex; leukokoria). Children with retinoblastoma also may present with strabismus, pseudocellulitis, iris neovascularization, dilated fixed pupil, secondary glaucoma, or tumor accumulation in the anterior chamber (neoplastic hypopyon). More advanced cases may present with signs of intraocular inflammation or ruptured globe with orbital extension. In some cases of spontaneously regressed retinoblastoma, the sole clinical sign may be a small, calcified tumor in the plane of the retina with surrounding retinal pigment epithelial scarring. Magnetic resonance imaging is the diagnostic test of choice.

Most children are treated with chemotherapy, sometimes with intraocular laser or cryotherapy. Enucleation is used for advanced cases in eyes with no visual potential.

Malignant Melanoma

Malignant melanoma (Chapter 193) of the conjunctiva is rare. Individuals at risk are middle aged and lightly pigmented. Melanoma of the conjunctiva arises most commonly from primary acquired melanosis but can occur as a de novo lesion, and, rarely, from a preexisting conjunctival nevus. The regions of greatest risk are in the conjunctiva at the limbus (junction of cornea and

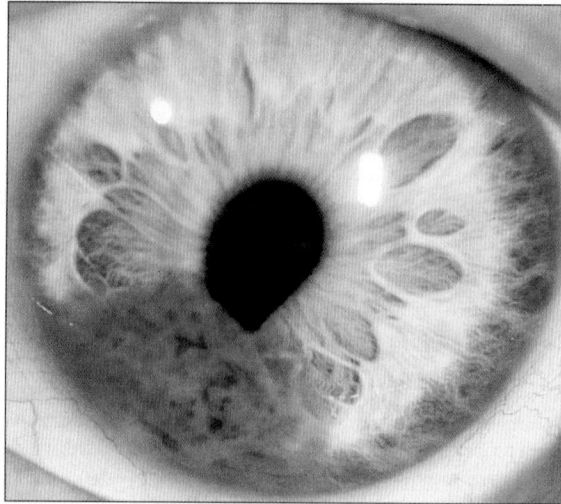

FIGURE 395-30. Iris melanoma that has prominent intrinsic blood vessels. Note peaking of the pupil toward the tumor. (From Yanoff M, Duker JS, eds. *Ophthalmology.* Philadelphia: Mosby Elsevier; 2009.)

sclera), in the conjunctival fornix (deep peripheral recesses of the conjunctiva), and in the caruncle (elevated nodule between the nasal lid margins). Extensions onto the corneal surface or formation of a nodule or loss of pigmentation are indications for excisional biopsy. Proliferation and hyperpigmentation of melanocytes without nuclear or cellular atypia is not associated with progression to melanoma, whereas associated nuclear or cellular atypia, particularly coupled with mitotic activity, is highly linked with progression to melanoma. Frank melanoma with a thickness of more than 0.8 mm is a risk factor for metastatic melanoma. Treatment is surgical excision, often supplemented with cryoablation. The long-term outcome is less favorable than for cutaneous melanoma because the tumor may metastasize early when the primary tumor is very small (e.g., 2 mm).

Malignant melanoma of the uveal tract is the most common primary intraocular malignancy of adults, but its incidence is only 2 to 6 per 1 million per year in high-risk populations (blue-eyed, light-skinned persons). The tumor, which arises from preexisting nevi or dendritic melanocytes anywhere in the uveal tract, is almost always unilateral, unicentric, and nodular and is usually diagnosed at an asymptomatic phase during routine screening examination of the dilated fundus. Symptomatic tumors arise near sensitive portions of the retina (e.g., the macula) or cause retinal detachment or cystoid macular edema. Iris tumors (Fig. 395-30) are generally pigmented and elevated above the surrounding contour, where they are recognized early in their course. Posterior tumors may be completely amelanotic and occasionally may have a bilobed appearance. Accuracy in diagnosing melanoma of the uveal tract by clinical means alone is greater than 98%. Treatment is controversial; options include enucleation of the eye, proton beam and plaque (iodine-125) radiation, thermal laser ablation, photodynamic therapy, and en bloc resection. The survival rate can be as low as 50% at 15 years for large lesions. Risk factors for metastasis, most commonly to the liver, include tumor size, cell type, angiogenic mimicry, the presence of monosomy 3, and other genetic markers.

Orbital Tumors

Primary tumors in the orbit of adults include cavernous hemangioma, schwannomas, and various proliferations of fibrous tissue (solitary fibrous tumor). Rhabdomyosarcoma may arise from ectopic rests of mesenchyme rather than from mature rectus muscle. Orbital tumors usually are diagnosed by imaging techniques. The treatment is orbital exploration and surgical removal.

Lymphoma

Orbital and conjunctival lymphomas are usually small (marginal zone B-cell lymphomas; Chapter 176). Approximately 50% of cases ultimately include systemic disease that may not be clinically diagnosed. External beam radiation is used to treat isolated periocular disease, whereas systemic chemotherapy (Chapter 176) is required for symptomatic, systemic involvement.

Large-cell B-cell lymphoma may present in the eye as a form of vitreitis (cells suspended in the vitreous) or a subretinal or intraretinal infiltrate before it is discovered in the central nervous system. The diagnosis may be verified by cytologic examination of vitrectomy specimens. Treatment is generally systemic (Chapter 176), but the outcome is usually poor.

The eye may infrequently be involved in multiple myeloma (Chapter 178). Retinal hemorrhages and vitreous opacification may occur. Periorbital osteolytic lesions of bone may be present.

Lacrimal Gland Tumors

The lacrimal gland contains a resting population of non-nodal lymphocytes and is a common site for lymphomas. Epithelial neoplasms may arise from components of the acini and ducts of the lacrimal gland. Malignant epithelial tumors (adenoid cystic carcinoma) may metastasize at an early stage through perineural spaces of large peripheral nerves to adjacent bone. Most epithelial tumors are treated with total surgical removal of the lacrimal gland because of the risk for recurrence and malignant transformation of residual tumor. The prognosis for malignant lacrimal gland tumors is generally poor.

Ocular Metastasis

Metastasis to the orbit in adults is very uncommon because of its relatively small vascular volume. Metastasis to the rectus muscles present with adult-onset strabismus. Metastasis to the orbit is more common in childhood leukemia than adult leukemia.

Metastasis to the uveal tract is common, especially from primary breast and lung tumors. Metastatic lesions often grow rapidly and disturb visual function; serous retinal detachment is common. Treatment of the underlying malignancy can be effective on the choroidal lesions, but supplemental radiation or photodynamic therapy can be used to try to restore or preserve vision.

OCULAR EFFECTS OF SYSTEMIC MEDICATIONS

Innumerable medications may cause ocular side effects (Table 395-9). Therefore patients taking systemic medications often require periodic surveillance to identify ocular toxicity.

The most common cause of drug-induced glaucoma is topical corticosteroid therapy of more than 4 to 6 weeks' duration in the 5 to 6% of the population that is genetically predisposed. Nonsteroidal drugs usually cause narrow-angle glaucoma. Sulfa-containing drugs may induce glaucoma as an idiosyncratic reaction in persons with either narrow or open anterior chamber configuration. Treatment is the same as for non–drug-induced glaucoma.

Chloroquine and *hydroxychloroquine* may cause decreased color vision and visual field defects at high doses. Chloroquine toxicity is thought to occur after a cumulative dose of 300 g, whereas hydroxychloroquine may cause symptoms after long-term maintenance of 750 mg/day. The macular portion of the fundus develops a typical bull's-eye pattern of pigment disturbance. Corneal whorls composed of epithelial intracellular pigment may be seen. Vision loss from retinal toxicity is not reversible and tends to progress even after cessation of hydroxychloroquine treatment. Annual fundus examination with color testing, macular function tests, and automated visual field test may be indicated.

Ethambutol is often used for chronic pulmonary infection. The dose of drug is dependent on body weight. Toxic optic neuropathy is rare but unpredictable in incidence and outcome. Careful follow-up with close ophthalmic clinical surveillance is required.

Any of the commonly used antituberculous medications may cause optic neuropathy, although *ethambutol* carries the greatest risk. Pupillary response, color vision, acuity, and visual fields are the clinical parameters used to assess optic nerve function.

Cornea verticillata may be seen in patients taking *amiodarone* because of lysosomal accumulations within the epithelial basement membrane. *Fabry disease* produces similar changes, as can other medications. Corneal whorls are usually reversible when caused by drug toxicity, and they rarely interfere with vision.

Grade A References

A1. Chou R, Dana T, Bougatsos C, et al. Screening for impaired visual acuity in older adults: updated evidence report and systematic review for the US Preventive Services Task Force. *JAMA.* 2016; 315:915-933.

A2. Wen D, McAlinden C, Flitcroft I, et al. Postoperative efficacy, predictability, safety, and visual quality of laser corneal refractive surgery: a network meta-analysis. *Am J Ophthalmol.* 2017;178:65-78.

A3. Kempen JH, Altaweel MM, Holbrook JT, et al. Association between long-lasting intravitreous fluocinolone acetonide implant vs systemic anti-inflammatory therapy and visual acuity at 7 years among patients with intermediate, posterior, or panuveitis. *JAMA.* 2017;317:1993-2005.

A4. Nguyen QD, Merrill PT, Jaffe GJ, et al. Adalimumab for prevention of uveitic flare in patients with inactive non-infectious uveitis controlled by corticosteroids (VISUAL II): a multicentre, double-masked, randomised, placebo-controlled phase 3 trial. *Lancet.* 2016;388:1183-1192.

A5. Jaffe JA, Dick AD, Brezin AP, et al. Adalimumab in patients with active noninfectious uveitis. *N Engl J Med.* 2016;375:932-943.

A6. Lerner SF, Park KH, Hubatsch DA, et al. Efficacy and tolerability of travoprost 0.004%/timolol 0.5% fixed-dose combination for the treatment of primary open-angle glaucoma or ocular hypertension inadequately controlled with beta-blocker monotherapy. *J Ophthalmol.* 2017;2017:1-8.

A7. Gazzard G, Konstantakopoulou E, Garway-Heath D, et al. Selective laser trabeculoplasty versus eye drops for first-line treatment of ocular hypertension and glaucoma (LiGHT): a multicentre randomised controlled trial. *Lancet.* 2019;393:1505-1516.

A8. Tseng VL, Coleman AL, Chang MY, et al. Aqueous shunts for glaucoma. *Cochrane Database Syst Rev.* 2017;7:CD004918.

A9. Azuara-Blanco A, Burr J, Ramsay C, et al. Effectiveness of early lens extraction for the treatment of primary angle-closure glaucoma (EAGLE): a randomised controlled trial. *Lancet.* 2016;388: 1389-1397.

A10. Chew EY, Clemons TE, Sangiovanni JP, et al. Secondary analyses of the effects of lutein/zeaxanthin on age-related macular degeneration progression: AREDS2 report No. 3. *JAMA Ophthalmol.* 2014;132:142-149.

A11. Gillies MC, Hunyor AP, Arnold JJ, et al. Effect of ranibizumab and aflibercept on best-corrected visual acuity in treat-and-extend for neovascular age-related macular degeneration: a randomized clinical trial. *JAMA Ophthalmol.* 2019;137:372-379.

A12. Aiello LP, Sun W, Das A, et al. Intensive diabetes therapy and ocular surgery in type 1 diabetes. *N Engl J Med.* 2015;372:1722-1733.

A13. Wells JA, Glassman AR, Ayala AR, et al. Aflibercept, bevacizumab, or ranibizumab for diabetic macular edema. *N Engl J Med.* 2015;372:1193-1203.

A14. Sivaprasad S, Prevost AT, Vasconcelos JC, et al. Clinical efficacy of intravitreal aflibercept versus panretinal photocoagulation for best corrected visual acuity in patients with proliferative diabetic retinopathy at 52 weeks (CLARITY): a multicentre, single-blinded, randomised, controlled, phase 2b, non-inferiority trial. *Lancet.* 2017;389:2193-2203.

A15. Scott IU, VanVeldhuisen PC, Ip MS, et al. Effect of bevacizumab vs aflibercept on visual acuity among patients with macular edema due to central retinal vein occlusion: the SCORE2 randomized clinical trial. *JAMA.* 2017;317:2072-2087.

GENERAL REFERENCES

For the General References and other additional features, please visit Expert Consult at https://expertconsult.inkling.com.

396

NEURO-OPHTHALMOLOGY

ROBERT W. BALOH AND JOANNA C. JEN

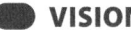

A mechanistic understanding of vision impairment along with disturbances in pupillary and oculomotor control lies close to the heart of diagnosing neurologic disorders.

VISION

One of the most difficult diagnostic problems is vision loss that cannot be explained by obvious abnormalities of the eye. To evaluate such a patient properly, the examining physician must be familiar with the anatomy and physiology of the afferent visual system. The afferent visual pathways cross

TABLE 395-9	SYSTEMIC MEDICATIONS WITH OCULAR EFFECTS
AGENT	**EFFECT**
Chloroquine	Dyschromatopsia, visual field defects
Hydroxychloroquine	Dyschromatopsia, visual field defects; bull's-eye maculopathy
Thioridazine	Blurred vision
Chlorpromazine	Blurred vision
Digoxin	Yellow vision
Ethambutol	Optic neuritis
Amiodarone	Corneal whorls, pigmentary retinopathy
Corticosteroids	Glaucoma, cataract
Tamoxifen	Maculopathy
Neuroleptics	Nystagmus
Compazine	Oculogyric crisis
Vitamin A	Pseudotumor cerebri
5-Fluorouracil	Canalicular stenosis (tearing)
Isotretinoin	Severe dry eye (long-term effect)

the major ascending sensory and descending motor systems of the cerebral hemispheres and in their anterior portion are intimately related to the vascular and bony structures at the base of the brain. Not surprisingly, localization of lesions within the afferent visual pathways has great value in neurologic diagnosis.

Anatomy of the Visual Pathways

Light entering the eye falls on the retinal rods and cones, which transduce the stimulus into neural impulses to be transmitted to the brain. The distribution of visual function across the retina takes a pattern of concentric zones increasing in sensitivity toward the center, the fovea. The fovea consists of a "rod-free" central grouping of approximately 100,000 slender cones. The ganglion cells subserving these cones send their axons directly to the temporal aspect of the optic disc, where they form the papillomacular bundle. Axons originating from ganglion cells in the temporal retina curve above and below the papillomacular bundle and form dense arcuate bands.

The arteries supplying the optic nerve and retina derive from branches of the ophthalmic artery. The central retinal artery approaches the eye along each optic nerve and pierces the inferior aspect of the dural sheath about 1 cm behind the globe to enter the center of the nerve. The artery emerges in the fundus at the center of the nerve head, from which it nourishes the inner two thirds of the retina by superior and inferior branches. Anastomotic branches derived from the choroidal and posterior ciliary arteries, the ciliary system, supply the choroid, optic nerve head, and outer retinal layers, including the photoreceptors. In about 10% of the population, the macula is supplied by a retinociliary artery, a branch of the ciliary system. Venous drainage from the retina and nerve head flows primarily through the central retinal vein, whose course of exit from the eye parallels that of entry of the artery.

What each eye "sees" is termed its *visual field* (Fig. 396-1). The nasal side of the left retina and the temporal side of the right see the left side of the world, and the upper half of each retina sees the lower half of the world. Behind the eyes, the optic nerves pass through the optic canal to form the optic chiasm. In the chiasm, nerves from the nasal half of each retina decussate and join the fibers from the temporal half of the contralateral retina. From the chiasm, the optic tracts pass around the cerebral peduncles to reach the lateral geniculate ganglia. The orientation of the visual field is rotated 90 degrees in the lateral geniculate such that images from the inferior visual field project to the medial half, whereas images from the superior visual field project to the lateral half. The geniculocalcarine radiation initially fans out into superolateral and inferolateral projections, the latter passing around the lateral ventricle and for a short distance into the temporal lobe (Meyer loop) before turning posteriorly to reach the striate cortex of the occipital lobe. In the occipital lobe, the striate cortex (area 17) lies along the superior and inferior bands of the calcarine fissure, with macular fibers projecting most posteriorly to the occipital pole and more peripheral retinal projections lying more anteriorly.

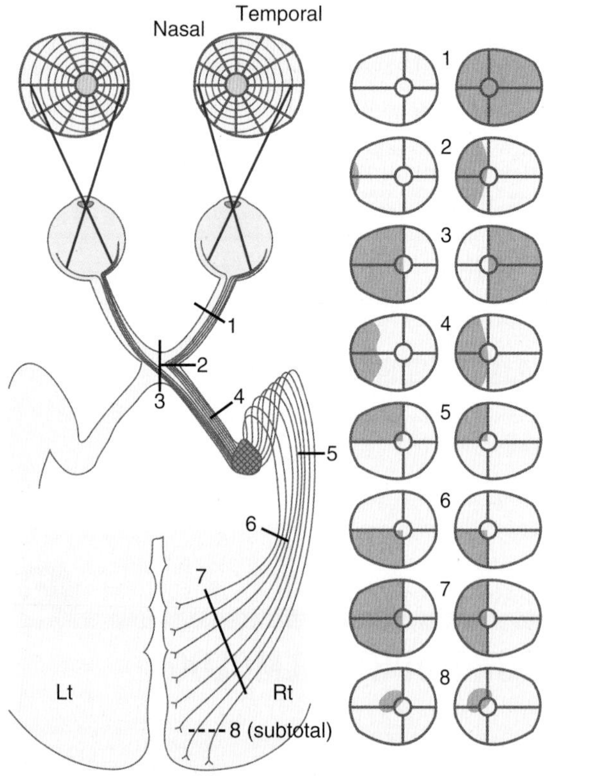

Localization of Lesions within Visual Pathways

Monocular vision loss is due to a lesion in one eye or optic nerve. Binocular visual loss, on the other hand, can result from disease located anywhere in the visual pathways from the corneas to the occipital poles. Lesions involving the optic chiasm produce nonhomonymous visual abnormalities (e.g., the bitemporal hemianopia illustrated by lesion 3 in Fig. 396-1). Optic tract abnormalities are comparatively rare but produce characteristic visual changes. The fibers serving identical points in the homonymous half fields do not fully commingle in the optic tract, so lesions damaging this structure produce incongruous homonymous hemianopia. Lesions of the geniculate nuclei, optic radiations, or visual cortex produce congruent hemianopic field defects that may go unrecognized unless the hemianopia intrudes on macular vision. Postgeniculate visual loss can be differentiated from pregeniculate visual loss by (1) a normal funduscopic appearance, (2) intact pupillary light reactions, and (3) appropriate lesions on brain imaging.

Examination of the Afferent Visual System

Visual function is most commonly assessed by "best-corrected visual acuity" (Chapter 395). If visual acuity is not normal, it must be determined whether acuity can be improved with lenses or at least with the use of a pinhole. The normal reference is recognition of letters at an idealized 20 feet, and acuity charts are designed with even larger letters that are normally recognized at proportionally greater distances. Thus, if one reads letters at 20 feet no better than those normally perceived at 40 feet, vision is recorded as 20/40. Small visual charts that are easily carried in the physician's case permit quick and fairly accurate bedside appraisal of acuity.

Visual fields can be tested at the bedside by confrontation, and rough estimates of their integrity can be made even in patients with reduced alertness. The fields should be tested individually for each eye because the pattern of visual field defects can provide important localizing information. A quick screen of the visual fields can be made by having the patient fixate on the examiner's nose and identify the number of fingers flashed in each of the four visual field quadrants.

Common Causes of Visual Loss

Eye

The cause of monocular vision loss secondary to ocular and retinal lesions can often be detected by ophthalmoscopic examination or by measurement of intraocular pressure (Chapter 395). *Glaucoma* caused by impaired absorption of aqueous humor results in a high intraocular pressure that usually produces gradual loss of peripheral vision, "halos" seen around lights, and occasionally, pain and redness in the affected eye. *Retinal tears* and *detachments* give rise to unilateral distortions of the visual image seen as sudden angulations or curves of objects containing straight lines (metamorphopsia). *Hemorrhages* into the vitreous humor or infections or inflammatory lesions of the retina can produce scotomas that resemble those resulting from primary disease of the central visual pathway.

Binocular vision loss secondary to retinal disease in younger subjects is often due to *heredodegenerative conditions.* Vascular diseases, diabetes (Chapter 216), and age-related macular degeneration are causes in older patients. In most cases of *pigmentary retinal degeneration*, visual loss begins peripherally and slowly proceeds centrally. By contrast, *macular degeneration* (see Figs. 395-20 and 395-21) impairs central vision early in its course. A common variant in the complement factor H (*CFH*) gene is associated with a markedly increased risk for the development of age-related macular degeneration.

FIGURE 396-1. Visual fields that accompany damage to the visual pathways. *1,* Optic nerve: unilateral amaurosis. *2,* Lateral optic chiasm: grossly incongruous, incomplete (contralateral) homonymous hemianopia. *3,* Central optic chiasm: bitemporal hemianopia. *4,* Optic tract: incongruous, incomplete homonymous hemianopia. *5,* Temporal (Meyer) loop of the optic radiation: congruous partial or complete (contralateral) homonymous superior quadrantanopia. *6,* Parietal (superior) projection of the optic radiation: congruous partial or complete homonymous inferior quadrantanopia. *7,* Complete parieto-occipital interruption of the optic radiation: complete congruous homonymous hemianopia with psychophysical shift of the foveal point, often sparing central vision and resulting in "macular sparing." *8,* Incomplete damage to the visual cortex: congruous homonymous scotomas, usually encroaching at least acutely on central vision. Lt = left; Rt = right.

TABLE 396-1	COMMON CAUSES OF TRANSIENT MONOCULAR VISION LOSS	
CATEGORY (TYPICAL DURATION)	CAUSES	DIFFERENTIAL FEATURES
Thromboembolism (1-5 min)	Atherosclerosis	Other atherosclerotic vascular disease, associated contralateral hemiparesis, angiography (carotid atheroma)
	Cardiac	Valvular disease, mural thrombi, atrial fibrillation, recent myocardial infarction
	Blood dyscrasia	Blood tests positive for sickle cell anemia, macroglobulinemia, multiple myeloma, polycythemia, other
Vasospasm (5-30 min)	Migraine	Ipsilateral headache, other classic aura, family history
Vascular compression (few seconds)	Increased intracranial pressure	Precipitated by position change, Valsalva maneuver, or pressure waves
	Tumor	Associated slowly progressive monocular visual loss
Vasculitis (1-5 min)	Temporal arteritis	Associated headache, polymyalgia rheumatica, palpable temporal artery, elevated sedimentation rate

TABLE 396-2	DIFFERENTIATION OF OPTIC NEURITIS FROM PAPILLEDEMA	
	OPTIC NEURITIS	PAPILLEDEMA
Central-cecocentral vision loss	Present	Absent
Distribution	Usually unilateral	Usually bilateral
Ocular pain on movement	Present	Absent
Direct light reflex	±Reduced	Intact
CT and MRI of head	White matter plaques	Tumor, venous occlusion, etc.
Visual evoked responses	Abnormal	Normal
Lumbar puncture pressure	Normal	Elevated

CT = computed tomography; MRI = magnetic resonance imaging.

Optic Nerve

Acute or subacute monocular vision loss (Table 396-1) as a result of optic nerve disease is most commonly produced by demyelinating disorders, vascular obstruction, neoplasm, or hereditary optic neuropathy.[1,2] Demyelinating disease of the nerve head (optic neuritis or papillitis) produces disc edema along with loss of central vision in the affected eye only; subjectively unrecognized scotomas may sometimes be found in the other eye. Demyelination of the optic nerve behind the point where the retinal vein emerges (retrobulbar neuritis) initially leaves a normal-looking disc but a central or paracentral scotoma. With chronic demyelinating disorders, the optic disc becomes pale and atrophic.

Optic neuritis can be an isolated syndrome or a manifestation of systemic diseases.[3] The clinical course and therapeutic response of optic neuritis depend on the underlying inflammatory mechanism. In more than 50% of patients initially seen with optic neuritis, typical symptoms and signs of multiple sclerosis eventually develop (Chapter 383). Optic neuritis caused by multiple sclerosis is not responsive to steroids,[A1] but the underlying multiple sclerosis should be treated promptly.[4] Some data suggest that phenytoin may be neuroprotective in patients with acute optic neuritis when used in doses of 4 to 6 mg/kg/day.[A2] Optic neuritis related to systemic lupus erythematosus (Chapter 250),[5] vasculitis (Chapter 254), or sarcoidosis (Chapter 89) may be steroid responsive.

Optic neuritis with an associated transverse myelitis is the clinical hallmark of neuromyelitis optica,[6] which is a severe demyelinating disease often mistaken for multiple sclerosis but now recognized to be caused by anti–aquaporin 4 autoantibodies. The recommended treatment options include rituximab (1 g infusions at an interval of 2 weeks) or azathioprine (3 mg/kg/day orally). Doses should be adjusted based on response and immune suppression.

Intraocular arterial occlusion may produce either central visual loss or an altitudinal field defect (ischemic optic neuropathy). Nonarteritic anterior ischemic optic neuropathy results from disease of the small vessels supplying the anterior portion of the optic nerve. The most common systemic disorders associated with it are hypertension (present in 50% of patients) and diabetes mellitus (present in 25%). Arteritic ischemic optic neuropathy is most commonly caused by giant cell arteritis (Chapters 69 and 255) and should be considered in all patients who are older than 50 years of age. Oral glucocorticoids are the cornerstone of treatment for giant cell arteritis but are not helpful in patients with nonarteritic anterior ischemic optic neuropathy.[A3]

Tumors (Chapter 180) invading the optic nerve or space-occupying lesions compressing it anywhere between the orbit and chiasm cause gradually decreasing central vision or a sector defect of the peripheral visual field. With such chronic lesions, the affected optic nerve becomes visibly atrophic.

Acute binocular vision loss resulting from bilateral optic nerve disease is most often caused by demyelinating disease or by toxic (methanol, tobacco, isoniazid) or nutritional factors (B vitamin deficiency, particularly of thiamine; Chapter 388). In younger persons and those lacking a clear history of toxic exposure, demyelinating lesions overwhelmingly predominate. Symptoms are of abrupt or subacute onset with visual blurring, which may progress rapidly to blindness within hours or days. There may be pain about the eyes, particularly with movement. Leber optic neuropathy, caused by a mutation in mitochondrial DNA, typically begins painlessly and centrally in one eye, with the second eye affected weeks to months later. Gene therapy can improve retinal sensitivity, albeit modestly, but only for 3 years or so.[7]

Papilledema is disc edema secondary to increased intracranial pressure (Table 396-2). Vision is normal except under one of two circumstances: (1) acute transient episodes of amaurosis lasting a few seconds and attributable to acute increases in intracranial pressure (plateau waves); and (2) progressive loss of peripheral vision with long-standing, severe papilledema caused by compression of the optic nerve head. Idiopathic intracranial hypertension (Chapter 180) is commonly seen in overweight women of childbearing age. Optical coherence tomography can help establish the diagnosis and differentiate papilledema from other optic disc abnormalities.[8] Subacute or chronic binocular vision loss secondary to optic nerve disease can result from toxic and nutritional causes or from inherited optic atrophy. Visual loss is painless and primarily affects central vision; ophthalmoscopy shows optic atrophy.

Chiasm and Optic Tract

Patients with lesions of the optic chiasm or optic tract are often unaware of visual impairment until the deficit encroaches on central vision in one or both eyes. Intrinsic or extrinsic neoplasms and parachiasmal arterial aneurysms are the most common lesions in this location. Gliomas that arise within the chiasm or optic tract are rare in adulthood. Extrinsic lesions compressing the chiasm or tract include pituitary adenomas (Chapter 211), dysgerminomas, craniopharyngiomas, meningiomas (Chapter 180), and large aneurysms of the carotid or basilar artery (Chapter 380). The diagnosis rests on finding the characteristic visual field abnormalities (bitemporal hemianopia for chiasm and incongruous homonymous hemianopia for optic tract lesions) and identifying the lesion with computed tomography or magnetic resonance imaging. Pituitary apoplexy secondary to acute hemorrhage into the gland (Chapter 211) can result in sudden vision loss; prompt neurosurgical intervention under steroid coverage is required for most patients.

Visual Radiations and Occipital Cortex

Lesions involving the postgeniculate visual pathways most often result from vascular damage, traumatic injuries, neoplasms, or rarely, inflammatory or degenerative disorders involving the cerebral white matter. Their localization can be deduced by the resulting visual field defects. Vascular disease of the occipital lobes is the most common cause of homonymous visual field defects in middle-aged and elderly people. Anton syndrome refers to cerebral visual loss with denial of a visual defect. Affected patients not only deny that they are blind but also confabulate details of their visual environment from memory. Anton syndrome results from bilateral lesions involving the parieto-occipital lobes or in the setting of metabolic encephalopathy. The reversible posterior leukoencephalopathy syndrome, which is characterized by headache, seizures, confusion, and cortical visual loss, is associated with an abrupt increase in blood pressure, such as may be seen with eclampsia and with immunosuppressive therapy after transplantation.

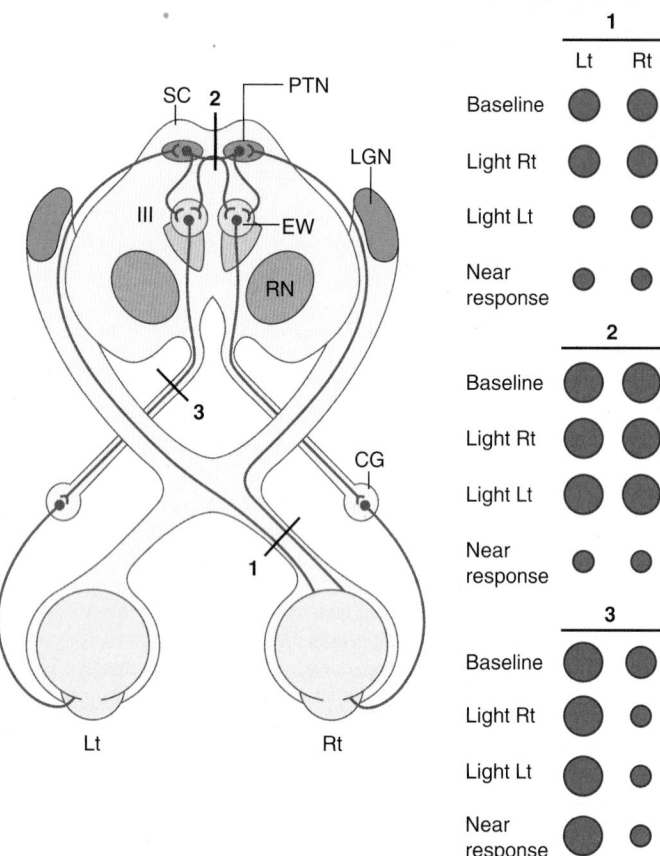

FIGURE 396-2. Pupillary responses associated with lesions of the *(1)* optic nerve, *(2)* pretectum, and *(3)* oculomotor nerve. Baseline is obtained with fixation on a distant target and the near response with a target in front of the nose. CG = ciliary ganglion; EW = Edinger-Westphal nucleus; LGN = lateral geniculate nucleus; Lt = left; PTN = pretectal nucleus; RN = red nucleus; Rt = right; SC = superior colliculus.

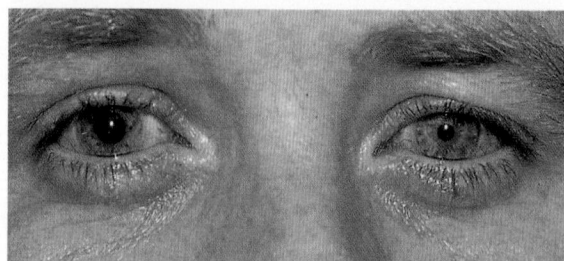

FIGURE 396-3. Adie tonic pupil in the right eye of a young woman. The affected pupil is "tonic"; that is, it responds slowly to light and accommodation but on rapid testing appears unresponsive. The site of the lesion is usually obscure, but the condition is benign. There may be associated areflexia. (From Forbes CD, Jackson WF. *Color Atlas and Text of Clinical Medicine,* 3rd ed. London: Mosby; 2003.)

PUPILLARY CONTROL

The neuromechanisms that control pupil size and reactivity are complex, yet they can be evaluated by simple clinical procedures. The diameter of the pupil is determined by the antagonistic actions of the iris sphincter and dilator muscles, with the latter playing a minor role. If the sphincter muscle is severed or ruptured, it does not retract toward one quadrant but rather continues to function, except in the altered segment. Therefore, pupillary response can be evaluated even in the presence of significant damage to the iris.

Anatomy and Localization of Lesions within Pupillary Pathways

The size of the pupil is governed by tonic balance between sympathetic and parasympathetic innervation of the muscles of the iris. Sympathetic stimulation dilates the pupil, whereas parasympathetic stimulation constricts it. In the normal resting state, light entering the eye provides the major stimulus governing the size of the pupil (Fig. 396-2). Light activates the retinal rods and cones, with maximal sensitivity in the macular area. The optic nerve fibers follow the crossed and uncrossed visual pathways to the pregeniculate portion of the optic tracts, where the receptor fibers for light diverge to the pretectal nucleus located at the midbrain-diencephalic junction. Interneurons project from this nucleus to the Edinger-Westphal nuclei atop the midbrain third nerve nuclear complex of either side. From that point, paired parasympathetic efferents leave the midbrain in the third nerves, travel in the interpeduncular space across the petroclinoid ligament and edge of the tentorium, traverse the cavernous sinus, and then enter the orbit through the superior orbital fissure. In the orbit, the parasympathetic efferents synapse in the ciliary ganglion, from which ciliary nerves enter the eye to reach the pupillary muscles.

The principal sympathetic control of the pupil originates in the ventral lateral hypothalamus (first-order neuron), from which fibers descend ipsilaterally through the brain stem tegmentum and thence to the cervical cord, where they synapse with preganglionic neurons in the intermedial lateral column of the upper three thoracic segments. Preganglionic fibers (second-order neurons) emerge with the ventral roots of C8, T1, and T2 and ascend in the neck to synapse in the superior cervical ganglion adjacent to the base of the skull. Postganglionic (third-order neurons) pupillary fibers accompany the internal carotid artery through the skull and then leave it to follow the ophthalmic branch of the trigeminal nerve to reach the pupillodilator muscle of the eye.

Examination of the Pupil

The pupillary response to light should be examined in a dimly lighted room, where the pupils are naturally dilated. First, the size and symmetry of the pupils are assessed by shining a dim light onto the face from below so that both pupils are seen simultaneously in the indirect illumination. To test light reactivity, gaze is directed at a distant object (so that constriction secondary to convergence is minimal), and first one and then the other pupil is illuminated with a bright light source. If a pupil reacts poorly to direct light, it is observed as the opposite eye is illuminated (consensual response). Pupils that react poorly to light should be tested for reactivity to the near reflex by first having the patient gaze at a distant object and then quickly fixate on an object just in front of his or her nose. *Light-near dissociation* refers to a pupil that does *not* react to light but does accommodate by constricting to a near target.

Common Causes of Pupillary Abnormalities

With so-called benign pupillary dilation or *physiologic anisocoria,* there is a long-standing difference in the size of the two pupils with normal reflex reactions; the disparity remains constant during constriction and dilation. Lesions compressing or damaging the pretectal region interrupt the afferent light reflex bilaterally to produce dilated and light-fixed pupils (e.g., lesion 2; see Fig. 396-2). Pupillary constriction to the near response is preserved until late stages. Tumors of the pineal gland (e.g., dysgerminomas) and *localized infarctions* are the most common lesions in this location. *Adie tonic pupil* (Fig. 396-3) is a medium to large (3 to 6 mm) pupil that constricts little or not at all to light and very slowly to accommodation but constricts with the instillation of dilute (0.125%) pilocarpine (Fig. 396-4). The condition usually affects one eye (occasionally both), is more common in women 25 to 45 years of age, and carries no serious implications. It most likely results from postviral denervation of the pupillary muscles. Unexplained unilateral or bilateral dilated pupils as an isolated finding can result from *accidental or intentional instillation of mydriatic drugs.* Transdermal scopolamine is a common cause. Failure of the pupil to constrict promptly with pilocarpine (1%) gives the diagnosis if the history is unclear. Interruption of the emerging third nerve in the ventral midbrain or along the proximal part of its course produces a dilated pupil 6 to 7 mm in diameter. Important causes of compression of the third nerve in this region are *aneurysms* (Chapter 380), *neoplasia* (Chapter 180), and *brain herniation* (Chapter 180) as a result of increased intracranial pressure. In nearly all cases, the pupillary involvement is associated with other signs of third nerve involvement (see later text).[9]

Sympathetic paralysis of the eye with ptosis, anhidrosis, and miosis (Horner syndrome; Fig. 396-5) can result from lesions anywhere along the pathway of the sympathetic innervation to the eye (Table 396-3). The diagnosis can sometimes be made by identifying associated signs in the brain stem or neck or along the carotid artery. *Argyll Robertson pupils* are small (1 to 2 mm), unequal, irregular, and fixed to light; they constrict minimally to accommodation. Their principal cause is tertiary neurosyphilis (Chapter 303).

OCULOMOTOR CONTROL

Abnormal eye movements can result from disturbances at several levels. Disconjugate eye movements result from lesions in the individual ocular muscles, the myoneural junctions, the oculomotor nerves and their three paired nuclei

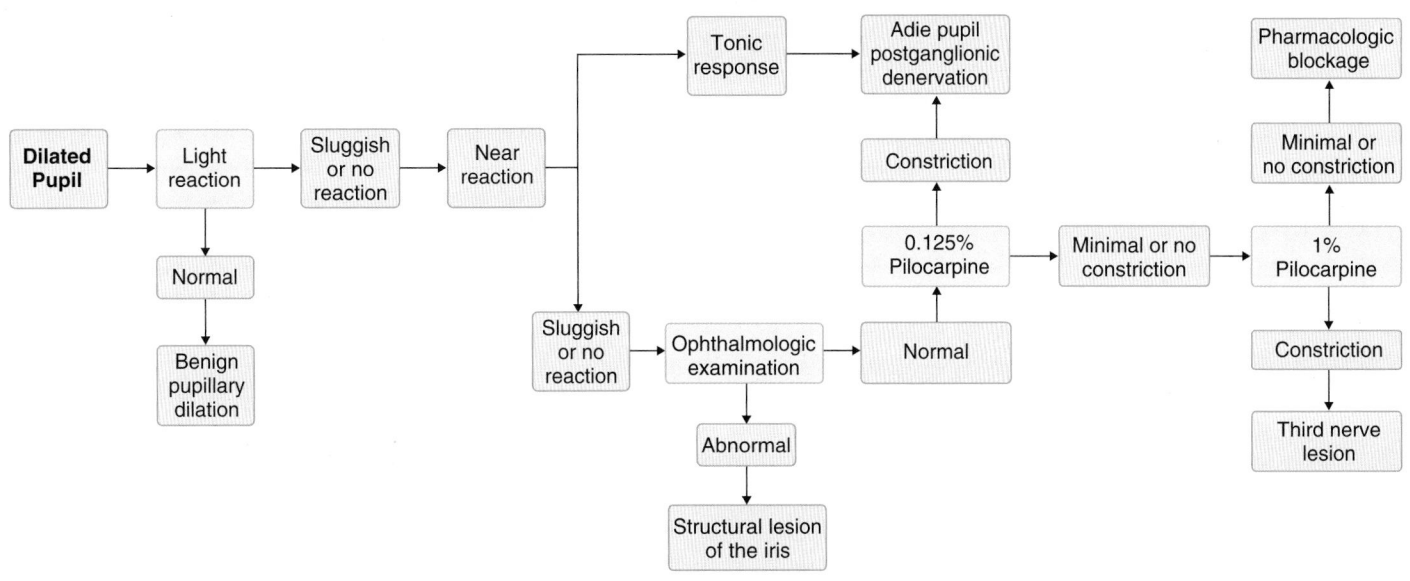

FIGURE 396-4. Use of pilocarpine to help differentiate between different causes of a dilated pupil.

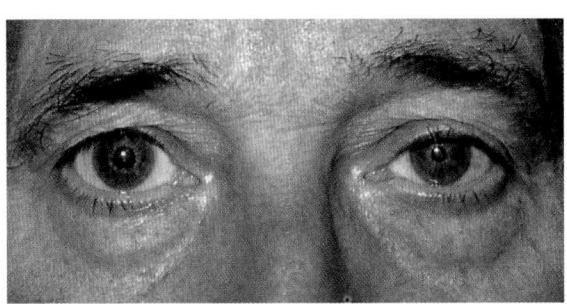

FIGURE 396-5. Horner syndrome. Note the characteristic ptosis of the left eye associated with constriction of the pupil (miosis). This patient had syringomyelia, but Horner syndrome has many possible causes. (From Forbes CD, Jackson WF. *Color Atlas and Text of Clinical Medicine,* 3rd ed. London: Mosby; 2003.)

TABLE 396-3 HORNER SYNDROME RESULTS FROM LESIONS IN MULTIPLE LOCATIONS

LOCATION OF LESION	NEURON INVOLVED	TYPE OF LESION	ASSOCIATED SYMPTOMS AND SIGNS
Lateral brain stem	1st order	Infarction, glioma	Vertigo, nystagmus, imbalance, numbness, weakness
Apex of lung	2nd order	Lung cancer, trauma	Often none
Neck	3rd order	Carotid dissection or inflammation	Pain, monocular visual loss, hemiparesis

in the brain stem, and the internuclear medial longitudinal fasciculus (MLF), which yokes the eyes in horizontal movements. Supranuclear lesions typically produce disorders of conjugate gaze (gaze palsies).

Anatomy and Localization of Lesions within the Oculomotor Pathways
Nuclear and Internuclear Pathways
The abducens (sixth) nerve supplies the lateral rectus muscle. Selective involvement of the abducens nerve anywhere along its pathway leads to isolated weakness of abduction of the affected eye. Destruction of the abducens nucleus in the brain stem results in a conjugate gaze paralysis (ipsilateral) because, in addition to oculomotor neurons, the nucleus contains interneurons destined for the contralateral medial rectus nucleus. The trochlear (fourth) nerve supplies the contralateral superior oblique muscle, which turns in and depresses the eye. Patients with superior oblique weakness note an increase in diplopia

with head tilt toward the side of weakness and often tilt their head in the opposite direction. At rest, there is slight upward deviation of the involved eye, and downward movement is impaired when the affected eye is turned in. Patients typically complain of diplopia when reading or going down stairs. The third (oculomotor) cranial nerve supplies the remaining ocular muscles. Involvement of the third nerve nucleus in the midbrain always produces at least some bilateral oculomotor weakness; the superior rectus division of the nucleus supplies the contralateral superior rectus muscle (all other divisions supply ipsilateral muscles). Peripheral third nerve paralysis can result from lesions damaging the structure anywhere from its course within the ventral midbrain to where it enters the orbit through the superior orbital fissure. When complete, third nerve palsy produces a widely dilated pupil, severe ptosis, and an externally deviated eye held in position by unopposed contraction of the lateral rectus muscle. In such conditions, the continued trochlear action reveals itself by intorsion of the eye when the subject attempts to look down.

The MLF interconnects the abducens nucleus in the pons with the contralateral oculomotor nuclear complex in the midbrain. It terminates cephalad in the interstitial nucleus in the rostral midbrain and can be traced as far caudad as the thoracocervical region of the spinal cord (coordinating nuchal-ocular control). Lesions involving the MLF characteristically produce internuclear ophthalmoplegia, in which the eyes are conjugate in the primary position but disconjugate on lateral gaze. With fully developed internuclear ophthalmoplegia on lateral gaze away from the side of the lesion, the contralateral eye abducts and shows nystagmus, whereas the ipsilateral adducting eye does not move nasally because of failure of ascending impulses to reach the medial rectus division of the third nerve nucleus. Adduction for convergence is usually relatively maintained.

Supranuclear Pathways
Pathways descending from the frontal eye fields in the frontal lobe through the superior colliculi to the contralateral brain stem regulate rapid voluntary eye movements (saccades; E-Table 396-1).[10] Pathways descending from the parieto-occipital and frontal regions to the ipsilateral brain stem subserve slow visual tracking (smooth pursuit—foveal target; optokinetic—full-field target). For the vestibulo-ocular reflex, primary afferent neurons in the inner ear synapse with neurons in the vestibular nuclei, which in turn synapse with appropriate oculomotor neurons to produce compensatory eye movements. The *convergence* center is located in the rostral-dorsal midbrain near the vertical gaze center.

Examination of Eye Movements
Fixation and gaze holding are tested by having the patient look center, right, left, up, and down. Each position should be held steady and unwavering with the observer carefully documenting abnormal movements or ocular disconjugacies. Each supranuclear oculomotor control system is examined separately. *Saccades* are tested by having the patient alternately fixate on two targets such as the examiner's finger and nose; the speed and accuracy are noted. *Smooth*

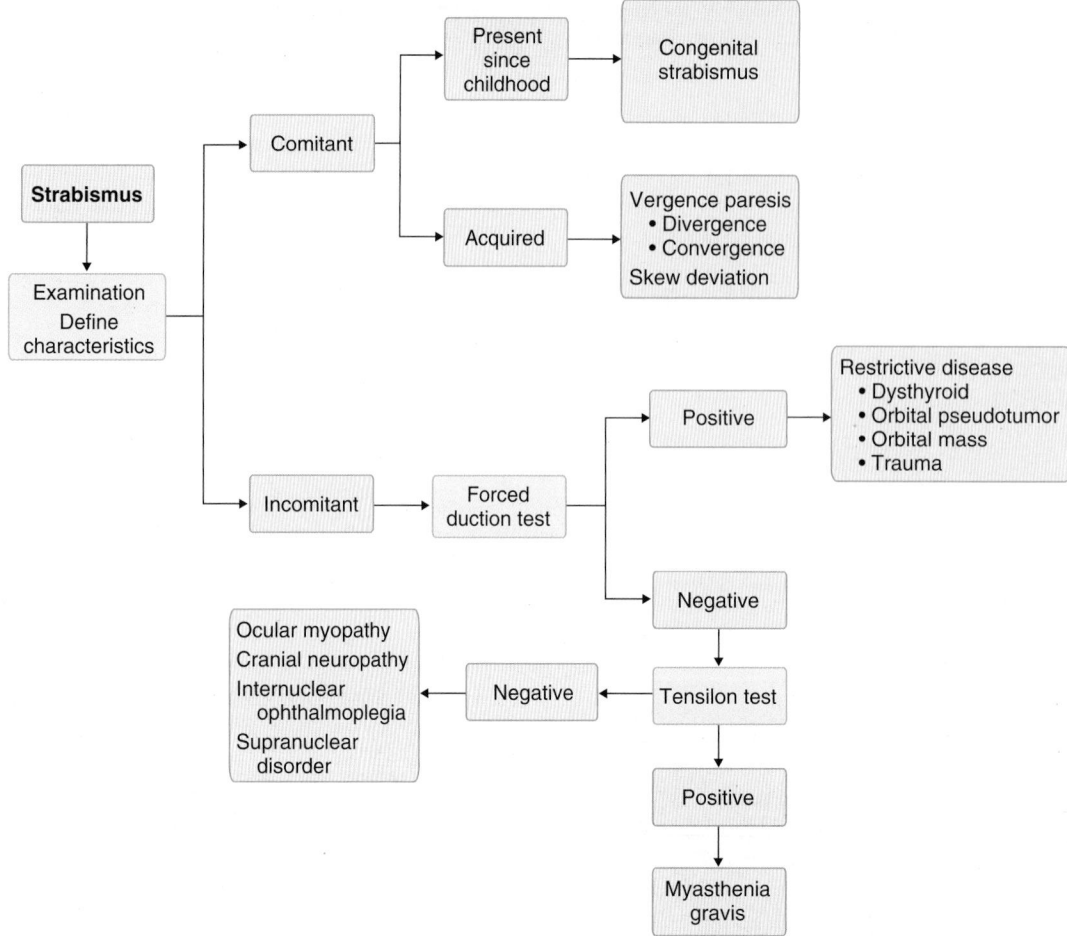

FIGURE 396-6. Diagnostic tests that help differentiate among common causes of strabismus.

pursuit is tested by slowly moving a target back and forth and up and down and observing the patient's ability to produce smooth tracking movements. If the target velocity is low, normal subjects should be able to pursue without requiring catch-up saccades. The *vestibulo-ocular reflex* is evaluated with the head-thrust test (Chapter 400). *Convergence* is tested by having the patient follow a target moving from far to near. The degree of convergence depends to some extent on the cooperation of the patient. A clear sign that the patient is attempting to converge is simultaneous pupillary constriction.

Common Causes of Abnormal Oculomotor Control
Strabismus (Ocular Misalignment)

A comitant (same in all directions of gaze) strabismus present since childhood is usually a benign *congenital disorder.* Latent congenital strabismus can become manifested in adulthood in association with a systemic illness. An acquired skew deviation (vertical displacement of the ocular axes) indicates a lesion within the otolith-ocular pathways (generally the brain stem). Incomitant strabismus can result from restrictive disease of the orbit or from abnormal muscle or oculomotor nerve function. The presence of mechanical restriction is confirmed by the use of forced duction testing (Fig. 396-6; After a topical anesthetic is applied to the eye, the ophthalmologist grasps the muscle insertion with large blunt-toothed forceps. Failure of the eye to deviate fully in the pulled direction implies restriction.) Common causes of *orbital restrictive disease* include dysthyroid ophthalmopathy (Chapter 213), orbital pseudotumor, trauma, and orbital mass lesions (Chapter 395). Variable strabismus that increases with fatigue suggests *myasthenia gravis* (Chapter 394). A Tensilon test can usually confirm the diagnosis (see Fig. 396-6). If both restrictive disease and myasthenia gravis (Chapter 394) have been excluded, most patients with incomitant strabismus have processes affecting the oculomotor nuclei, their fascicles, or the cranial nerves themselves. Common causes of an *isolated third nerve palsy* in an adult include aneurysm (Chapter 380), small-vessel occlusive disease (including diabetes mellitus [Chapter 216]), trauma (Chapter 371), and neoplasm. Typically, third nerve lesions secondary to vascular disease spare the pupil. Vascular disease and trauma are by far the

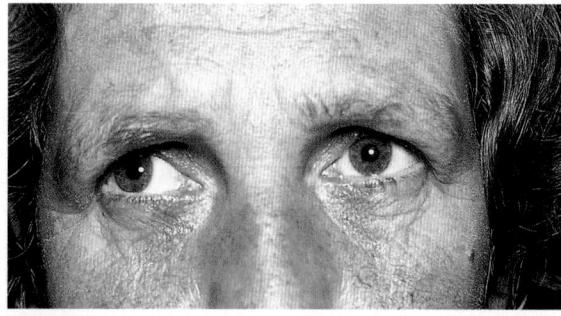

FIGURE 396-7. Internuclear ophthalmoplegia may be an initial feature of brain stem involvement in multiple sclerosis. On lateral gaze to the right, adduction of the left eye is incomplete. On convergence, eye movement was normal. The lesion is in the left medial longitudinal bundle, between the nucleus in the pons and the third nerve nucleus on the opposite side. (From Forbes CD, Jackson WF. *Color Atlas and Text of Clinical Medicine,* 3rd ed. London: Mosby; 2003.)

most common causes of *isolated trochlear nerve palsy.* The abducens nerve is particularly vulnerable to isolated traumatic involvement because of its long pathway outside the brain stem. Lesions that produce increased intracranial pressure (Chapter 180) can lead to abducens nerve dysfunction regardless of the location and produce a "false localizing sign." Other common causes of *isolated sixth nerve palsy* are vascular disease (Chapter 379), trauma (Chapter 371), and neoplasm. Progressive external ophthalmoplegia, with worsening bilateral ptosis and diffuse reduction in ocular motility, is a manifestation of a mitochondrial myopathy.[11,12]

Internuclear Ophthalmoplegia

Internuclear ophthalmoplegia (Fig. 396-7) may be unilateral or bilateral, partial or complete, depending on the location of the lesion and the degree of damage to the MLF. *Demyelinating* and small *vascular lesions* are the most common causes of unilateral internuclear ophthalmoplegia unaccompanied by other ocular palsies or brain stem signs. Myasthenia gravis (Chapter 394) can produce an ophthalmoparesis resembling internuclear ophthalmoplegia as a result of greater involvement of the medial rectus than the lateral rectus. Demyelinating diseases (Chapter 383) are the most common causes of bilateral internuclear ophthalmoplegia involvement.

Disorders of Conjugate Gaze

Acute lesions involving a frontal eye field (e.g., hemorrhage or infarction [Chapters 379 and 380]) result in a transient inability to direct the eyes contralaterally. Vertical eye movements are not affected by unilateral lesions. Bilateral damage to the frontal eye fields or their descending pathways may produce an inability to move the eyes voluntarily (horizontally or vertically) despite preserved reflex eye movements, a condition called *oculomotor apraxia.* Lesions involving the horizontal gaze center in the pons produce an ipsilateral paralysis of conjugate gaze and tonic deviation of the eyes to the contralateral side (Chapter 395). Lesions of the pretectum selectively impair vertical gaze, with the vertical upgaze center being slightly rostral and dorsal to the vertical downgaze center. Patients with the *dorsal midbrain syndrome* (Parinaud syndrome) have a conjugate upgaze paresis. When they attempt to make upward saccades, convergence retraction nystagmus develops. As noted earlier, impaired convergence and light-near dissociation of the pupillary reflexes are also part of the syndrome. The most common causes of the dorsal midbrain syndrome include tumors of the pineal gland (Chapter 210; dysgerminomas), hydrocephalus (Chapter 180), and localized infarction.

Nystagmus

Spontaneous nystagmus can be congenital or acquired. *Congenital nystagmus* typically has a high frequency and variable waveform (usually pendular) and is highly fixation dependent. It generally remains horizontal in all positions of gaze. The lifelong history and lack of symptoms confirm the diagnosis. Spontaneous nystagmus resulting from a *peripheral vestibular* lesion (i.e., in the labyrinth or vestibular nerve) usually has combined horizontal and torsional components (Table 396-4). The nystagmus resolves within a few days of the acute lesion. Acquired persistent spontaneous nystagmus indicates a lesion in the brain stem or cerebellum, or both. The latter is often purely vertical, horizontal, or torsional. Spontaneous *downbeat nystagmus* is commonly seen with lesions of the cerebellum or cervicomedullary junction (e.g., Arnold-Chiari malformation [Chapter 389]).

Gaze-evoked nystagmus is always in the direction of gaze and is usually present with and without fixation. It is most commonly produced by the ingestion of *drugs* such as phenobarbital, phenytoin, alcohol, and diazepam (Chapter 102). It can also occur in patients with such varied conditions as myasthenia gravis (Chapter 394), multiple sclerosis (Chapter 383), and cerebellar atrophy. Asymmetrical horizontal gaze-evoked nystagmus is caused by a structural brain stem or cerebellar lesion (particularly at the cerebellopontine angle), with the lesion generally being on the side of the larger amplitude nystagmus (Bruns nystagmus). *Rebound nystagmus* is a type of gaze-evoked nystagmus that either disappears or reverses direction as the eccentric gaze position is held. When the eyes are returned to the primary position, nystagmus occurs in the direction of the return saccade. Rebound nystagmus occurs in patients with cerebellar atrophy and focal structural lesions of the cerebellum; it is the only variety of nystagmus thought to be specific for cerebellar involvement.

Disconjugate gaze–evoked nystagmus most commonly results from lesions of the MLF (see earlier discussion), but it can also occur with other lesions of the brain stem involving the oculomotor nuclei. Positional nystagmus is discussed in Chapter 400.

Other Ocular Oscillations

Ocular bobbing consists of a fast conjugate downward eye movement followed by a slow return to the primary position. The phenomenon accompanies severe displacement or destruction of the pons or, less often, metabolic central nervous system depression. *Ocular myoclonus* consists of continuous rhythmic pendular oscillations, most often vertical, at a rate of one to three beats per second; it often accompanies palatal myoclonus and has a similar pathogenesis. *Square-wave jerks* and *ocular flutter* consist of brief, intermittent, horizontal oscillations (back-to-back saccades) arising from the primary gaze position. These types of ocular oscillation are most commonly seen with cerebellar disease but can also accompany more diffuse central nervous system disorders. *Opsoclonus* consists of rapid, chaotic, conjugate, repetitive saccadic eye movements (dancing eyes). Opsoclonus accompanies the cerebellar dysfunction, with the most chaotic varieties associated with brain stem encephalitis or the remote effects of systemic neoplasm, especially neuroblastoma in children. *Ocular dysmetria* refers to overshooting and undershooting of saccadic eye movements, often followed by multiple attempts at refixation. It reflects cerebellar dysfunction.

Grade A References

A1. Gal RL, Vedula SS, Beck R. Corticosteroids for treating optic neuritis. *Cochrane Database Syst Rev.* 2015;8:CD001430.
A2. Raftopoulos R, Hickman SJ, Toosy A, et al. Phenytoin for neuroprotection in patients with acute optic neuritis: a randomised, placebo-controlled, phase 2 trial. *Lancet Neurol.* 2016;15:259-269.
A3. Saxena R, Singh D, Sharma M, et al. Steroids versus no steroids in nonarteritic anterior ischemic optic neuropathy: a randomized controlled trial. *Ophthalmology.* 2018;125:1623-1627.

GENERAL REFERENCES

For the General References and other additional features, please visit Expert Consult at https://expertconsult.inkling.com.

397

DISEASES OF THE MOUTH AND SALIVARY GLANDS

TROY E. DANIELS AND RICHARD C. JORDAN

More than 200 primary lesions or diseases occur in the oral mucosa, gingiva, teeth, jaws, and minor or major salivary glands. In addition, secondary abnormalities of the oral mucosa or salivary glands can be caused by systemic diseases or drugs. The most common or important of these diseases may be observed during physical examination.[1]

ORAL MUCOSAL DISEASES
Acute Ulcerations

Painful, short-lasting ulcerations can be caused by mechanical trauma, immunologic mechanisms, or bacterial or viral infections (Table 397-1). Soon after formation, oral mucosal ulcers become covered by a white to gray pseudomembrane, analogous to scabs on dry epidermis. Pseudomembrane-covered ulcers are distinguished from white hyperkeratotic lesions by their clinical features: pain, a flat surface, and an erythematous periphery. Traumatic ulcers are characteristically located on the tongue or inside the cheeks or lips, usually close to the chewing surfaces of the teeth.

APHTHOUS STOMATITIS ("CANKER SORES")

These idiopathic recurrent ulcers, which afflict up to 20% of the population, are found on all nonkeratinized mucosa: the buccal mucosa, ventral tongue, lips, and alveolar mucosa (Fig. 397-1). They form well-defined circular lesions that may be single or multiple. There are three clinical forms: (1) minor, which

TABLE 396-4 KEY DISTINGUISHING FEATURES OF PERIPHERAL AND CENTRAL TYPES OF SPONTANEOUS AND POSITIONAL NYSTAGMUS

TYPE OF NYSTAGMUS	PERIPHERAL (END ORGAN AND NERVE)	CENTRAL (BRAIN STEM AND CEREBELLUM)
Spontaneous	Unidirectional, fast phase away from the lesion, combined horizontal torsional, inhibited with fixation	Bidirectional or unidirectional; often pure horizontal, vertical, or torsional; *not* inhibited with fixation
Static positional	Fixed or changing direction, inhibited with fixation	Fixed or changing direction, *not* inhibited with fixation
Paroxysmal positional	Vertical-torsional, occasionally horizontal-torsional, vertigo prominent, fatigability, latency	Often pure vertical, vertigo less prominent, no latency, nonfatigable

TABLE 397-1 ORAL MUCOSAL ULCERS

TYPE/DISEASE	CLINICAL FEATURES
INSIDIOUS ONSET, CHRONIC	
Multiple or Bilateral	*Shallow ulcers on mucosa, skin, or both*
Pemphigus vulgaris	Begin as short-duration blisters
Mucous membrane pemphigoid	Begin as short-duration blisters
Lichen planus	Bilaterally symmetrical lesions (white with or without erythema)
Lupus erythematosus	Asymmetrical lesions, with or without systemic lupus (white with or without erythema)
Lichenoid drug reaction	Variable lesions; history of medication use
Epidermolysis bullosa	Begin as blisters; lifelong history
Solitary	*Indurated or cratered ulcers*
Squamous cell carcinoma	Most common on tongue, oropharynx, lip, mouth floor
Adenocarcinomas, various	Salivary tumors most common; on palate, cheeks, mouth floor
Tuberculosis	Usually painful
Actinomycosis	Often associated with draining sinus tract
Deep mycoses (particularly histoplasmosis, coccidioidomycosis)	Associated with systemic infection
Midline (lethal) granuloma	Associated with necrosis, may perforate palate; usually an NK/T-cell lymphoma or granulomatosis with polyangiitis
Bony osteonecrosis	Associated with prior cancer, radiation therapy or bisphosphonate/antiresorptive agent use
ACUTE ONSET, OFTEN SELF-LIMITING	
Clusters	*Usually small and shallow ulcers; history of blisters*
Primary herpes simplex	Any oral mucosal site, associated with fever, malaise
Recurrent herpes simplex	Unilateral, only on keratinized mucosa (gingiva, hard palate, or lip)
Varicella-zoster	Unilateral lesions along neural distribution
Herpangina	Usually on soft palate
Measles (rubeola)	Precede skin rash; associated with fever, malaise
Solitary or Multiple (without Clustering)	*Variable, usually without history of blisters*
Traumatic ulcers	Usually solitary; history of trauma
Aphthous stomatitis (canker sores)	Circular, often multiple, only on nonkeratinized mucosa
Behçet syndrome	Oral lesions similar to recurrent aphthae
Erythema multiforme	Multiple lesions, often involve lower labial mucosa; can be recurrent or chronic
Drug reaction	Appropriate history of drug use
Necrotizing sialometaplasia	Deep ulcers, usually on palate
Primary syphilis	Solitary, indurated, painless, any site
Gonorrhea	Painful, surrounded by erythema, usually in oropharynx

TABLE 397-2 ORAL LESIONS ASSOCIATED WITH HUMAN IMMUNODEFICIENCY VIRUS INFECTION

Kaposi sarcoma (human herpesvirus type 8)

Candidiasis (pseudomembranous, hyperplastic and/or erythematous lesions)

Other opportunistic fungal infections (e.g., histoplasmosis or coccidioidomycosis)

Aphthous ulcers (increased frequency, duration, or size)

Virus-associated epithelial hyperplasias
 Hairy leukoplakia (Epstein-Barr virus)
 Oral wart (human papillomavirus type 11 and other types)
 Focal epithelial hyperplasia (Heck disease) (human papillomavirus types 13 and 32)
 Condyloma acuminatum (human papillomavirus types 6 and 11)

Herpes zoster (varicella-zoster virus)

Exaggerated forms of gingivitis and inflammatory periodontal disease

Decreased salivary gland function

Parotid gland enlargement (lymphoepithelial lesion)

Non-Hodgkin lymphoma (e.g., plasmablastic lymphoma)

are flat and less than 1 cm in diameter and last 5 to 10 days; (2) major, which have raised borders, are greater than 1 cm, and often last for weeks or months; and (3) herpetiform, which are usually clusters of very small ulcers that resemble recurrent herpetic lesions but are not preceded by vesicles and do not occur on keratinized mucosa. A viral or bacterial pathogenesis has not been established for any of these forms. Lesions clinically identical to minor aphthae occur in Behçet syndrome (Chapter 254). Aphthae are occasionally associated with anemias or gluten-sensitive enteropathy and may become more frequent and severe in association with human immunodeficiency virus (HIV) infection (Table 397-2).

Minor or herpetiform aphthous ulcers are generally self-limiting within a week or two and may not require treatment unless they occur frequently. Topical steroids, such as fluocinonide gel or ointment, can reduce the severity and duration of the lesions only if applied with prodromal symptoms or earliest signs. A suspension of tetracycline or doxycycline in water used as a mouth rinse at the onset of symptoms also reduces the severity and duration of disease.[A1] Unfortunately, none of these treatments prevent recurrent ulcers.[2] Major aphthae usually require treatment with prednisone (e.g., 40 mg daily for 3 days); failure to respond significantly should prompt incisional biopsy to exclude neoplasia. Unfortunately, no treatment will cure a patient of recurrent aphthous stomatitis.[A2]

VIRAL ULCERS
Several types of virus (most commonly herpes simplex type 1; Chapter 350) cause multiple oral mucosal vesicles that last only a few hours or days and then become irregular shallow ulcers. In the initial infection by herpes simplex virus, usually in children, numerous vesicles may appear on any oral mucosal site (primary herpetic gingivostomatitis), accompanied by malaise, headache, fever, and cervical lymphadenopathy. Patients previously exposed to this virus may develop recurrent (secondary) lesions as clusters of small vesicles, most commonly on the lips (herpes labialis) and less commonly on the keratinized mucosa of the gingiva or hard palate (Fig. 397-2). Such lesions contain live virus and tend to recur at the same site but less frequently with increasing age.

Although widespread vaccination has reduced the incidence, similar mucosal vesicles may also accompany the initial infection by the varicella-zoster virus in children with chickenpox (Chapter 351), and unilateral lesions may occur if herpes zoster (Chapter 351) affects branches of the trigeminal nerve. Uncommonly, oral mucosal ulcers may be caused by different types of coxsackievirus (Chapter 355), appearing on any oral site in hand-foot-and-mouth disease or on the soft palate or pharynx in herpangina. After infection by the measles (rubeola) virus, small ulcers (Koplik spots; see Fig. 343-2) may form on the inside of the cheeks 1 to 2 days before development of the skin rash (Chapter 343).

ERYTHEMA MULTIFORME
In this potentially recurrent disease, painful oral mucosal ulcerations develop rapidly, with or without target-like skin lesions. It may be associated with a previous viral infection or hypersensitivity to a food or drug. The affected patients, usually young adults with minimal or no systemic symptoms, have irregularly shaped ulcers that can be small and few or involve large areas of the mucosa; the most common sites are the lower labial mucosa and vermilion. On

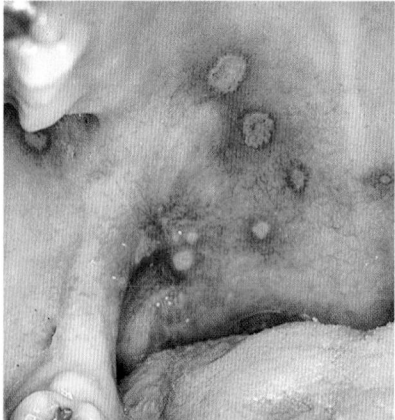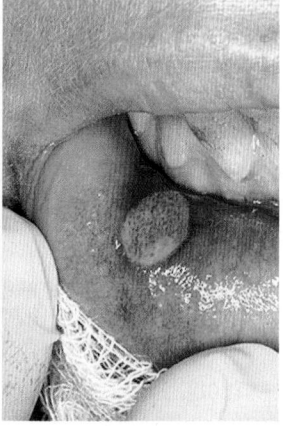

FIGURE 397-1. Aphthous ulcers. *Left,* A cluster of minor aphthae on the soft palate and buccal mucosa, present about 1 week. *Right,* A major aphthous ulcer on the labial mucosa, present about 3 weeks.

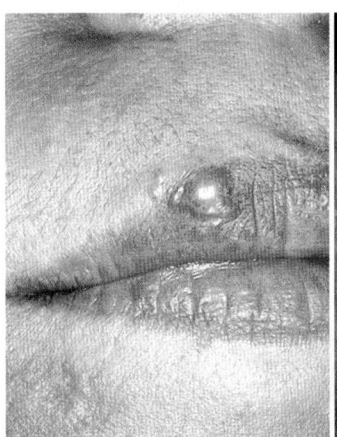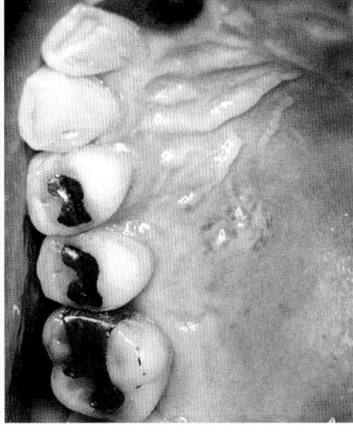

FIGURE 397-2. Clusters of recurrent herpes simplex vesicles. *Left,* on the lip; *right,* on the hard palate, both present 2 to 3 days, in different patients.

the vermilion, bilateral hemorrhagic crusting is a characteristic finding. These lesions can be distinguished from those of primary herpes by the absence of oral vesicles and systemic symptoms or by the presence of characteristic skin lesions (Chapter 410). A major variant of this disease is Stevens-Johnson syndrome, in which ocular, genital, and other lesions may accompany the oral lesions.

VENEREAL INFECTIONS

Primary syphilis may arise as a solitary, indurated, painless ulcer on the oral mucosa that resolves spontaneously in 4 to 6 weeks (Chapter 303). Uncommonly, *Neisseria gonorrhoeae* (Chapter 283) may cause oral ulcers, usually in the pharynx, which may be confused with oral ulcers of other causes.

Oral Squamous Cell Carcinoma

About 4% of all cancers occur in the mouth, commonly as squamous cell carcinomas of the mucosal epithelium (Chapter 181). Oral carcinoma occurs usually in the fifth decade or beyond, in men twice as frequently as in women, and is associated with long-term use of tobacco in more than 80% of cases.

Oral carcinoma usually arises as a chronic, indurated, cratered ulcer, but white (leukoplakia) and especially red (erythroplakia) macular lesions (Table 397-3; Fig. 397-3) frequently exhibit premalignant dysplasia or early carcinoma. Oral carcinomas spread to cervical lymph nodes. The overall 5-year survival rate is about 40%, but early treatment of small, localized lesions can lead to survival rates as high as 90%. Nevertheless, current guidelines find insufficient evidence to recommend for or against screening in asymptomatic adults.

Over the past two decades, there has been a rapid increase in a type of head and neck cancer associated with the human papillomavirus (HPV) type 16 (Chapter 349).[3] Occurring primarily at the base of tongue and tonsillar region of the oropharynx, this form of nonkeratinizing squamous cell carcinoma is seen in younger patients who typically lack the history of smoking and alcohol that is usually associated with more traditional forms of oral cancer. Other features of the disease include advanced stage at presentation and its good response to radiation and chemotherapy (Chapter 181). In the absence of concurrent tobacco use, the 5-year survival rate is over 80%.

Other Chronic Ulcerations

Prescription drugs that can be responsible for chronic oral mucosal ulcerations include barbiturates, β-blockers, nonsteroidal anti-inflammatory drugs, allopurinol, isoniazid, and many others.[4] Several mucocutaneous diseases can cause chronic multifocal oral mucosal lesions composed of ill-defined areas of erythema and ulceration. They are among the most difficult oral lesions to diagnose and are discussed later with the red lesions (see Table 397-3). Several microbial infections or underlying osteonecrosis (e.g., with the use of bisphosphonates and other antiresorptive medications) can lead to indurated, chronic oral mucosal ulcerations with moderate symptoms (see Table 397-1).

White Lesions

White plaques are commonly found in the mouth but, like ulcerations, have a wide variety of causes and outcomes (see Table 397-3). The clinical descriptor term *leukoplakia* applies to a white plaque that does not rub off and whose appearance does not indicate another disease. Leukoplakia can occur in any area of the mouth and usually exhibits benign hyperkeratosis on biopsy. On

TABLE 397-3	WHITE AND RED/BLUE ORAL MUCOSAL LESIONS

WHITE LESIONS (PLAQUES)

Squamous cell carcinoma (early)
Frictional keratosis (buccal mucosa at dental occlusal line)
Leukoplakia (with or without dysplasia)
Smokeless tobacco–associated lesions
Nicotine stomatitis (palate)
Lichen planus (reticular and plaque types)
Pseudomembranous candidiasis (thrush)
Hyperplastic candidiasis (candidal leukoplakia)
Hairy leukoplakia (often HIV associated; usually on lateral tongue)
Geographic tongue
Mucous patch or condyloma latum of secondary syphilis
Pseudomembrane-covered ulcers (see Table 397-1)

RED OR BLUE LESIONS (MACULAR, MACULOPAPULAR)

Squamous cell carcinoma (early)
Erythroplakia (epithelial dysplasia)
Erythematous (atrophic) candidiasis
Median rhomboid glossitis
Mucocutaneous diseases (see Table 397-1)
Angular cheilitis
Telangiectasias and purpuras (red to blue)
Kaposi sarcoma (blue to purple)

HIV = human immunodeficiency virus.

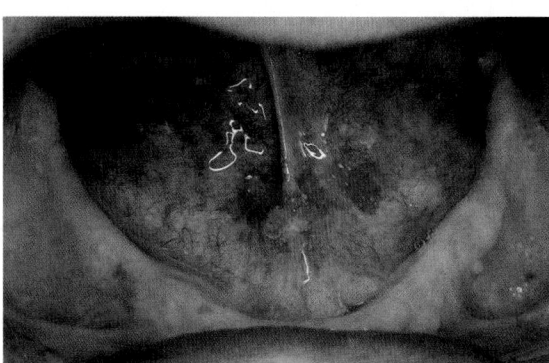

FIGURE 397-3. Squamous cell carcinoma. Biopsy of this area of erythroplakia with slight induration in the anterior mouth floor exhibited squamous cell carcinoma.

long-term follow-up, 2 to 6% of these lesions undergo malignant transformation into squamous cell carcinoma. Leukoplakias that are shown on biopsy to contain epithelial dysplasia have a higher rate of transformation to cancer than those that do not, thereby emphasizing the important role of biopsy for these lesions. Areas of leukoplakia with a corrugated surface or mixed with areas of erythema are often found in the lower labial or buccal vestibule of patients who use smokeless tobacco.

Frictional keratoses are often found posterior to the lower molar teeth as irregular white plaques and on the buccal mucosa as white lines adjacent to the dental occlusion. Unlike leukoplakia, these lesions rarely become malignant.

LICHEN PLANUS

Oral lesions of lichen planus (Chapter 409) occur in about 1% of the population, usually as multiple, bilaterally symmetrical reticular white plaques, with or without adjacent areas of erythema (atrophy or erosion) or irregular ulcers (Fig. 397-4). The presence of mucosal atrophy, erosion, or ulceration usually causes pain and sensitivity to certain foods. Most lesions can be adequately controlled by topical application of fluocinonide or clobetasol gel or ointment (0.05%, three times a day) for periods of several weeks,[A3] although recurrence is common.

ORAL CANDIDIASIS

This common fungal disease (Chapter 318) has three clinical forms: pseudomembranous (thrush), erythematous (atrophic), and hyperplastic (candidal leukoplakia).[5] Pseudomembranous candidiasis, usually of relatively short duration, occurs on any site and consists of white fungal plaques that can be rubbed off, leaving a red or bleeding base. Lesions of hyperplastic candidiasis

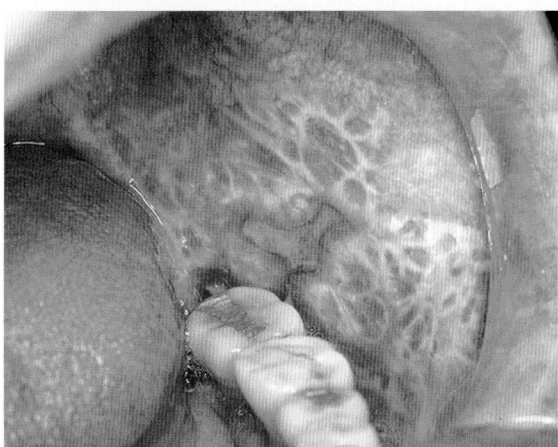

FIGURE 397-4. Lichen planus. A similar-appearing lesion is also present on the right buccal mucosa. Note central pseudomembrane-covered ulceration.

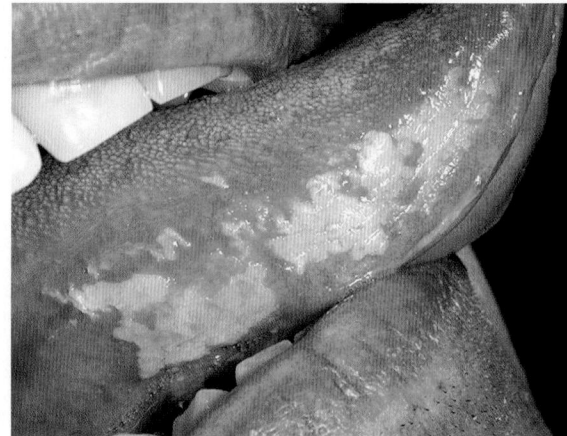

FIGURE 397-5. Hairy leukoplakia. These white plaques were the first visible sign of human immunodeficiency virus infection.

are white, have fungal hyphae within the surface layers of hyperkeratotic epithelium, do not rub off, and are most often found on the anterior buccal mucosa or on the tongue. Erythematous candidiasis is discussed under Red Lesions. All forms of oral candidiasis represent overgrowth or superficial infection by *Candida* species from the oral flora, induced by a variety of causes, including suppression of bacterial flora by systemic antibiotics, chronic salivary dysfunction, uncontrolled diabetes mellitus or anemia, and immunosuppression (especially in HIV-infected patients). The condition can be managed with topical or systemic antifungal agents, although acquired resistance to fluconazole (discussed later) therapy can occur.

HAIRY LEUKOPLAKIA

The lesion of hairy leukoplakia, which is caused by Epstein-Barr virus, is a white plaque occurring most frequently on the lateral surfaces of the tongue bilaterally in immunosuppressed persons, usually but not always HIV infected (Fig. 397-5). *Candida* may be present in the surface layers, but the lesion is not eliminated by effective antifungal therapy. The diagnosis of hairy leukoplakia by biopsy should raise suspicion of HIV infection or other forms of systemic or local immunosuppression.

GEOGRAPHIC TONGUE

Also called *benign migratory glossitis*, this benign idiopathic condition affects the dorsal tongue of about 2% of the population. It is characterized by well-defined areas of atrophied filiform papillae bordered by arcs of normal or hyperplastic filiform papillae and by gradual changes in the location of these lesions over time (Fig. 397-6). There is no association with psoriasis. Treatment is usually not necessary.

SECONDARY SYPHILIS

Secondary syphilis may manifest as a well-defined white plaque on the labial or palatal mucosa, called *condyloma latum* (or "split papule," because of its lobulated periphery), or as a mucous patch.

Red Lesions

Solitary red macules or plaques (*erythroplakia*) are less common in the mouth than white lesions but should be viewed with concern because they may exhibit premalignant dysplasia, carcinoma in situ, or squamous cell carcinoma (see Table 397-3 and Fig. 397-3). One exception is a red macule occurring in the midline of the posterior dorsal tongue, classified as *median rhomboid glossitis*, which is an idiopathic but uniformly benign condition that is often associated with localized overgrowth of *Candida* species.

ERYTHEMATOUS (ATROPHIC) ORAL CANDIDIASIS

Erythematous (atrophic) oral candidiasis is a chronic condition characterized by erythema and atrophy of the filiform papillae on the dorsal tongue or by patchy, ill-defined erythema on the palate, tongue, or buccal mucosa (Fig. 397-7). It is usually accompanied by symptoms of oral mucosal burning and sensitivity to spicy foods. It occurs most commonly in patients with chronic salivary hypofunction (e.g., Sjögren syndrome or anticholinergic drug effects), but it also occurs in patients who wear removable dentures infected with *Candida*, in whom mucosal erythema is confined to the denture-bearing area.

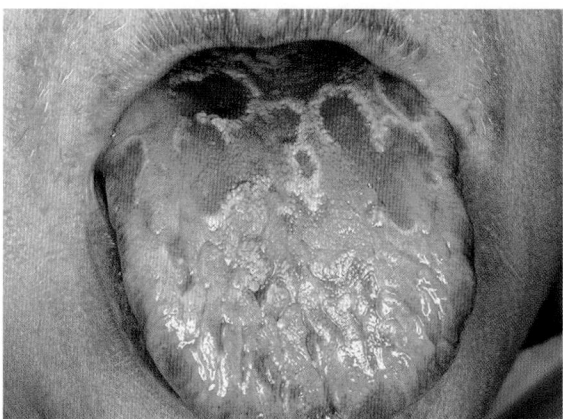

FIGURE 397-6. Geographic tongue. The distribution of these changes on the dorsal tongue may change over time, but they are asymptomatic and diagnosed by their characteristic appearance.

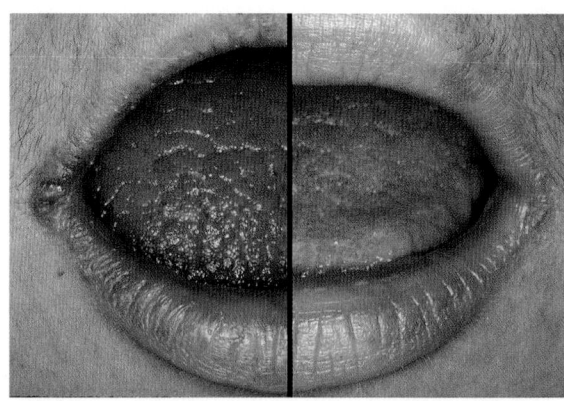

FIGURE 397-7. Erythematous oral candidiasis. *Left,* Erythematous candidiasis in a 26-year-old woman with primary Sjögren syndrome, exhibiting symptomatic angular cheilitis, atrophic mucositis, and lingual papillary atrophy. *Right,* Asymptomatic and normal-appearing mucosa after treatment with appropriate topical antifungal drugs (see text).

For acute or chronic oral candidal infections, systemic or topical antifungal drugs are necessary to resolve the associated lesions.[6] In patients who have clinically apparent salivary production, fluconazole (200 mg on the first day, then 100 mg every day for 2 to 4 weeks) is the drug of choice. However, systemic antifungal drugs may not be effective in patients who have severe salivary hypofunction and insufficient saliva to convey the drug from the blood stream to oral mucosa. In such patients, with remaining natural teeth, *oral antifungal preparations* (troches or pastilles), all of which contain cariogenic amounts of sucrose or glucose, *must not be used* to avoid enhancing dental caries. Instead, slow oral dissolution (15 to 20 minutes for 2 weeks) of vaginal nystatin tablets (twice daily) or miconazole tablets (50 mg daily), which contain little or no caries-supporting carbohydrates, is safe and effective; patients usually need frequent sips of water to aid in dissolving the tablets. Effective topical or systemic treatment significantly improves oral symptoms. Treatment of denture-associated candidiasis requires concurrent treatment of the denture.

The treatment end point is reached when mucosal burning symptoms cease, the patient can again tolerate acidic or spicy foods, and filiform papillae on the dorsal tongue have returned to normal; this recovery takes 2 to 12 weeks, depending on patients' salivary production and treatment compliance. Recurrence is common in patients with chronic salivary hypofunction or immunosuppression, which necessitates recurring or long-term treatment using a noncariogenic topical antifungal drug that provides a sufficient duration of oral mucosal contact (e.g., nystatin or miconazole tablets).

ANGULAR CHEILITIS
Erythema or crusting of the labial angles is usually caused by *Candida* species (see Fig. 397-7) and is usually associated with intraoral candidiasis. In such cases, topical treatment of the angular cheilitis with clotrimazole (1% cream) should be accompanied by intraoral or systemic antifungal treatment, as described previously.

MUCOCUTANEOUS DISEASES
The mucocutaneous diseases of pemphigus vulgaris, mucous membrane pemphigoid, atrophic or erosive lichen planus, and lupus erythematosus can cause similar-appearing oral lesions. Their diagnosis requires examination of a biopsy specimen by routine histopathology and direct immunofluorescence to identify characteristic deposits of various inflammatory proteins.

The first lesions of pemphigus vulgaris are usually oral mucosal vesicles that rapidly rupture, leaving painful erosions or ulcerations. These are followed by development of skin lesions. Rarely, the lesions remain confined to the mouth (Chapter 410).

Lesions of mucous membrane (cicatricial) pemphigoid are usually confined to the oral mucosa or conjunctivae and occur in patients older than 50 years. They begin as vesicles that quickly rupture, leaving ulcers that are chronic but only moderately symptomatic. Use of topical fluocinonide or clobetasol (0.05% gel or ointment, three times a day, 4 to 12 weeks) for several months, as described for lichen planus, is sometimes sufficient to treat the oral lesions, but many patients also need systemic treatment (Chapter 410).

Oral mucosal lesions of lupus may occur in patients who have systemic lupus erythematosus (SLE), in patients who do not have SLE but later develop that disease, or in patients who do not develop SLE (Chapter 250). In this last group, the lesions of mucosal lupus may be analogous to the skin lesions of chronic discoid lupus. They take the form of reticular hyperkeratotic figures associated with erythema, often resembling lichen planus, but unlike lichen planus are usually solitary or bilaterally asymmetrical. They can be controlled by topical fluocinonide (0.05%, three times a day, 2 to 4 weeks) or intralesional triamcinolone suspension (5 mg/mL), or respond to systemic treatment of SLE.

Pigmentations

Brown or gray-black macules on the oral mucosa are relatively common and range from benign to highly malignant. They may be caused by localized increase in melanin production, proliferation of melanin-producing cells, or deposition of local or systemically distributed pigmented substances (Table 397-4). Mucosal pigmentation may occur after long-term administration of hydroxychloroquine, minocycline, ketoconazole, methyldopa, or cyclophosphamide. Malignant melanomas can occur at any oral mucosal site, but about 85% develop on the hard palatal mucosa or gingiva, or both. Diagnosis of any of these conditions is established by biopsy and knowledge of relevant underlying conditions.

Lesions of Kaposi sarcoma associated with HIV infection often appear first on the oral mucosa, especially the palate. They begin as macules with a blue or purple color, at which time they must be distinguished from purpura. Later, they spread radially and expand vertically (Chapter 366).

⬤ ORAL SOFT TISSUE TUMORS
A range of oral benign soft tissue tumors should be treated by excisional biopsy.

Connective Tissue Hyperplasias

The most common oral soft tissue tumors are small, pedunculated masses of hyperplastic fibrous connective tissue covered by normal-appearing mucosa (Table 397-5). Solitary lesions are usually found on the inside of the cheeks or lips. Similar lesions may be present at the border of an ill-fitting denture

TABLE 397-4	PIGMENTATIONS OF THE ORAL MUCOSA (BROWN OR GRAY-BLACK IN COLOR)

INCREASED MELANIN PRODUCTION (FLAT LESIONS)

Oral melanotic macule
Ephelis (vermilion border)
Systemic diseases: Addison disease, von Recklinghausen disease of skin, Albright syndrome, Peutz-Jeghers syndrome

PROLIFERATION OF MELANIN-PRODUCING CELLS (FLAT OR RAISED LESIONS)

Melanocytic nevi
Melanoma in situ
Malignant melanoma

NONMELANIN PIGMENTATION

Amalgam tattoo
Focal deposition of systemically distributed metal (lead, bismuth, mercury, others) usually at sites of chronic inflammation
Systemically administered drugs (chloroquine, minocycline, ketoconazole, cyclophosphamide)

TABLE 397-5	ORAL SOFT TISSUE TUMORS

CONNECTIVE TISSUE HYPERPLASIA (NORMAL-APPEARING OVERLYING MUCOSA)

Irritation fibroma
Denture-associated hyperplasia
Palatal papillomatosis (papillary hyperplasia)
Generalized gingival hyperplasias
Drug-induced (phenytoin, nifedipine, cyclosporine)
Hereditary

REACTIVE HYPERPLASIA (ERYTHEMATOUS OVERLYING MUCOSA)

Pyogenic granuloma/pregnancy tumor
Peripheral giant cell granuloma
Inflammatory gingival hyperplasia
Hyperplastic lingual tonsil

EPITHELIAL MASSES (USUALLY IRREGULAR WHITE SURFACE)

Papilloma/oral wart
Squamous cell carcinoma
Verrucous carcinoma
Focal epithelial hyperplasia (Heck disease)
Condyloma acuminatum (venereal wart)
Keratoacanthoma (on lips)

SALIVARY DUCT OBSTRUCTION (MINOR SALIVARY GLANDS)

Mucocele/ranula (usually fluctuant)
Salivary stone (sialolith)

SUBEPITHELIAL NEOPLASMS

Primary connective tissue or salivary gland tumors
Metastatic lesions (especially in the mandible)
Lymphoma (especially in the palate or posterior mandible)
Focal or generalized leukemic infiltrates in the gingiva (especially with acute monocytic leukemia)

or may occur in clusters on the hard palate under an ill-fitting denture (palatal papillomatosis).

Generalized or multifocal enlargement of the gingiva (gingival hyperplasia) may be caused by chronic administration of phenytoin, cyclosporine, and many of the calcium-channel blocking drugs (e.g., diltiazem, verapamil, or nifedipine; Fig. 397-8). It can also be associated with a hereditary defect or be caused by an infiltration of atypical white blood cells in some types of leukemia (particularly acute monocytic leukemia; Chapter 173) or by uncontrolled diabetes mellitus (Chapter 216).

Reactive Hyperplasias

Small masses with surfaces that are ulcerated or only partially covered by normal-appearing mucosa usually represent reactive lesions in the form of pyogenic granulomas (whose frequency increases during pregnancy), peripheral giant cell granulomas, or lymphoid hyperplasia of the lingual or other tonsillar tissue. The granulomas are most often located on the gingiva. Rarely, such lesions may represent a metastatic neoplasm.

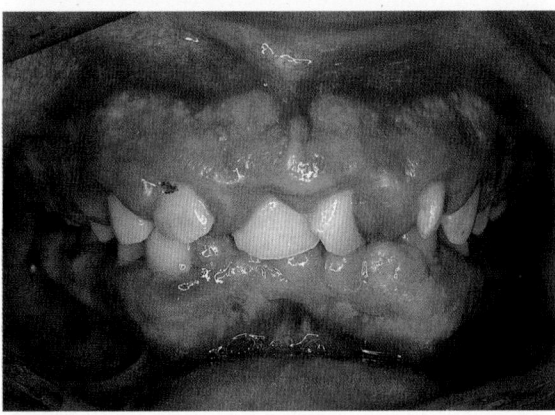

FIGURE 397-8. Drug-induced gingival hyperplasia. Similar clinical lesions may occur with prolonged use of various drugs or as a hereditary condition (see text).

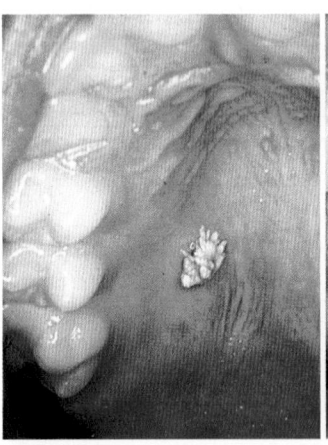 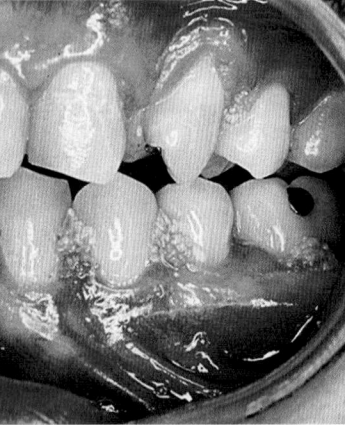

FIGURE 397-9. Papillary epithelial tumors. *Left,* A solitary squamous papilloma. *Right,* multiple gingival papillomas, occurring in all quadrants, from condyloma acuminatum, associated with papillomavirus subtype 6 or 11.

Epithelial Proliferations

Small, white, wartlike epithelial masses are common and can occur in any area of the oral mucosa (Fig. 397-9). They are occasionally classified as epithelial neoplasms, but most do not continue to grow. Human papillomavirus types 2, 6, 11, 13, 32, and 57 have been identified in these wartlike lesions, which are usually classified generically as squamous papillomas. A large wartlike lesion on the oral mucosa should raise suspicion of verrucous carcinoma.

Mucous Retention Lesions (Mucoceles)

Mucoceles are small, chronic, or recurring vesicles or bullae that occur commonly on the inside of the cheeks and lips, the posterior palate, and the mouth floor. They are caused by injury to one of the many submucosal minor salivary glands, resulting in extravasation of mucus, which causes granulomatous inflammation or blockage of the excretory duct, leading to cyst formation. Both types of lesions require conservative surgical excision because simple incision and drainage are usually followed by recurrence.

● SALIVARY GLAND DISEASES
Primary Diseases of Salivary Glands

Unilateral major salivary gland enlargement that is markedly painful or tender to palpation and has a purulent exudate or nothing expressible from the duct suggests bacterial sialadenitis. Any exudate should be cultured, and initial treatment should be with an oral penicillinase-resistant antibiotic, such as cloxacillin or dicloxacillin, 500 mg, every 6 hours.

Painful sialolithiasis usually occurs in submandibular gland ducts, less commonly in the parotid gland and much less commonly in sublingual and minor salivary glands.[7] Peak incidence is in the third to sixth decades, almost always with pain but occasionally with painless swelling. Diagnosis is clinical, supplemented by ultrasound or computed tomography. Small stones may be

TABLE 397-6 CAUSES OF SALIVARY GLAND ENLARGEMENT
USUALLY UNILATERAL
Benign or malignant salivary gland neoplasms (more than 30 different histopathologic types)
Bacterial infection
Chronic sialadenitis (single gland)
USUALLY BILATERAL AND ASSOCIATED WITH SALIVARY HYPOFUNCTION
Viral infection (mumps, cytomegalovirus, influenza, Coxsackie A)
Sjögren syndrome
Chronic granulomatous diseases (sarcoidosis, tuberculosis, leprosy)
Recurrent parotitis of childhood
Human immunodeficiency virus infection/acquired immunodeficiency syndrome
BILATERALLY SYMMETRICAL, SOFT, NONTENDER, PAROTID ONLY
Sialadenosis (asymptomatic parotid enlargement), idiopathic or associated with:
Diabetes mellitus
Hyperlipoproteinemia
Hepatic cirrhosis
Anorexia/bulimia
Chronic pancreatitis
Acromegaly
Gonadal hypofunction
Phenylbutazone use

expressible or treated by extracorporeal shock wave lithotripsy or endoscopic removal. Larger stones require incisional surgery.

More than 20 types of benign or malignant neoplasms appear as firm and nontender unilateral or bilateral enlargement of a major gland or as a firm submucosal nodule on the palate or the labial or buccal mucosa (Table 397-6). Their causes are unknown, except for Warthin tumor (papillary cystadenoma lymphomatosum), which has a strong association with cigarette smoking. Uncommonly, unilateral major gland enlargement may be reactive—for example, chronic sialadenitis from duct obstruction or inadequately treated bacterial sialadenitis.

Salivary gland tumors are relatively uncommon and usually present as a swelling in one of the major paired salivary glands or in one of the minor glands of the mouth.[8] Most occur in the major glands, with approximately 90% developing in the parotid. The most common benign salivary gland tumor is the pleomorphic adenoma. Most salivary gland tumors in the parotid gland are benign, in contrast to the sublingual gland, where more than 90% are malignant. Approximately half of tumors in the submandibular and minor glands are malignant. Benign tumors are generally slowly growing, not fixed to the skin, and do not show ulceration. Malignancies generally grow more quickly, are often fixed to the skin or adjacent normal structures, and tend to show ulceration. Adenoid cystic carcinoma has a characteristic local infiltration by perineural spread. Detection of any salivary gland mass lesions should be followed by appropriate imaging, cytology, and biopsy. Both benign and malignant tumors are generally treated by surgery.

Secondary Diseases of Salivary Glands
BILATERAL SALIVARY GLAND ENLARGEMENT AND DECREASED SALIVARY SECRETION ASSOCIATED WITH SYSTEMIC DISEASES

The best-known cause of bilateral salivary gland enlargement is infection by the mumps virus (Chapter 345) in children. However, the prevalence of mumps decreased in the United States by more than 98% after the introduction of an effective vaccine in 1967, and now there are only a few hundred to a few thousand cases per year. Uncommonly, a less acute, mumps-like illness may occur in adults in association with cytomegalovirus (Chapter 352), influenza (Chapter 340), or Coxsackie A (Chapter 355) virus infection.

About 15% of patients who meet the criteria for Sjögren syndrome (Chapter 252) may gradually develop chronic bilateral enlargement of major salivary glands, which feel firm and nontender or only slightly tender to palpation. Histologically, the tumors begin as a benign lymphoepithelial lesion but after years of chronicity, some transform into an extranodal marginal zone lymphoma (Chapter 176).

In most patients with Sjögren syndrome, gradually progressive salivary hypofunction can impair speech and swallowing and cause a characteristic pattern of progressive dental caries that leads to excessive tooth loss if not actively prevented. In severe cases, the oral mucosa becomes dry and sticky, saliva is not expressible from the major ducts, and about one third of patients

TABLE 397-7	CAUSES OF DECREASED SALIVARY SECRETION

TEMPORARY

Effects of short-term drug use (e.g., antihistamines)
Virus infections (e.g., mumps)
Dehydration
Psychogenic conditions (e.g., anxiety)

CHRONIC

Effects of chronically administered drugs (particularly antidepressants, monoamine oxidase inhibitors, neuroleptics, parasympatholytics, some combinations of drugs for treating hypertension)
Chronic diseases
   Sjögren syndrome
   Sarcoidosis
   Human immunodeficiency virus or hepatitis C infection
   Depression
   Diabetes mellitus (uncontrolled)
   Amyloidosis (primary or secondary)
   Central nervous system diseases
Other effects of treatment
   Therapeutic radiation to the head and neck
   Graft-versus-host disease
Absent or malformed glands (rare)

have signs and symptoms of chronic erythematous candidiasis (see earlier discussion and Fig. 397-7).

The salivary component of Sjögren syndrome is diagnosed from a labial salivary gland biopsy specimen that contains three to five minor glands and exhibits focal lymphocytic sialadenitis in the absence of nonspecific chronic sialadenitis or another disease, such as noncaseating granuloma. A patient's symptoms of oral dryness (xerostomia) can be caused by a wide variety of conditions (Table 397-7).

Several chronic granulomatous diseases, such as sarcoidosis (Chapter 89), tuberculosis (Chapter 308), and leprosy (Chapter 310), can cause bilateral enlargement and decreased function of salivary glands. The clinical and serologic features of sarcoidosis may occasionally closely mimic those of Sjögren syndrome, and the distinction is best made by minor salivary gland biopsy.

A few adult patients with HIV infection and most children who are infected in utero develop major salivary gland enlargement and reduced salivary secretion that are caused by lymphocytic infiltration. Parotid gland enlargement usually represents a solid or cystic lymphoepithelial lesion (see Table 397-2).

Recurrent parotitis of childhood includes episodes of unilateral or bilateral parotid enlargement. During flares of this illness, salivary secretion may be reduced, but usually without prominent secondary symptoms or signs. This condition, of unknown cause, usually subsides after puberty.

ASYMPTOMATIC PAROTID ENLARGEMENT (SIALADENOSIS, SIALOSIS)

Parotid glands can develop bilateral, symmetrical enlargement that is soft and nontender to palpation and associated with normal salivary function (see Table 397-6). Diagnosis is established by this clinical presentation and the presence of one of the systemic diseases known to be associated with it: diabetes mellitus (Chapter 216), hyperlipoproteinemia (Chapter 195), hepatic cirrhosis (Chapter 144), anorexia or bulimia (Chapter 206), chronic pancreatitis (Chapter 135), acromegaly (Chapter 211), and gonadal hypofunction. It can also result from use of phenylbutazone or be a reaction to iodine-containing contrast media. Biopsy of the affected glands is not indicated for diagnosis.

Impaired Salivary Secretion without Gland Enlargement

The common symptom of dry mouth (xerostomia) is most often a side effect of chronically administered drugs.[9] Many classes of drugs reduce unstimulated salivary secretion through anticholinergic or other mechanisms (see Table 397-7). Patients experience these symptoms soon after beginning to use the drug but produce enough saliva during a meal for normal chewing and swallowing. However, the symptoms and associated dental caries are dose dependent and gradually increase with prolonged use of the drug. The classes of drugs producing the most profound effects are most tricyclic antidepressants, most neuroleptics, monoamine oxidase inhibitors, and all anticholinergics. A combination of drugs for treatment of hypertension may also cause symptoms of dry mouth.

Several systemic diseases affect salivary secretion. As noted earlier, most patients with Sjögren syndrome, some with sarcoidosis, and a few patients with HIV infection experience symptoms of dry mouth to various degrees, with or without salivary gland enlargement. In addition, patients who have primary or secondary *amyloidosis* with salivary gland amyloid deposits may develop impaired secretion. The symptom of xerostomia is more prevalent in individuals who exhibit symptoms of depression, even in those not taking drugs for its treatment. Studies done before the availability of antidepressant drugs showed that symptoms of depression were associated with decreased salivary secretion.

Irradiation of the head and neck region to treat a malignant tumor usually produces profound dry mouth during therapy. Secretory capacity recovers only slightly in the months after treatment for patients with solid tumors but recovers significantly for those with multifocal tumors (e.g., Hodgkin disease).

TREATMENT

Significant chronic salivary hypofunction from any cause produces a risk for dental caries (decay) in approximate proportion to the secretory impairment, but caries can largely be prevented if appropriate measures are taken as soon as the hypofunction begins. Remaining teeth should be protected by a comprehensive dental caries prevention program, monitored by a dentist and including frequent application of appropriate topical fluorides, removal of dental plaque, counseling on control of cariogenic dietary carbohydrates, and placement of appropriate dental restorations as necessary.

Symptomatic treatment of mild to moderately severe salivary hypofunction can include sialagogues such as sugar-free hard candies or chewing gum, regular sips of water, and use of saliva substitutes at night, but no topical therapy is reliably helpful. If not contraindicated, symptoms of severe hypofunction can be improved by prescribing pilocarpine (5 mg four times a day). Such treatment alone, however, will not prevent dental caries.

Chronic erythematous oral candidiasis is a frequent sequela of chronic salivary hypofunction, and its treatment and retreatment, as noted earlier, substantially improve the patient's oral symptoms.

PERIODONTAL DISEASE

Periodontal diseases are a group of oral infections that affect the periodontium, which are the hard and soft tissues that support and maintain teeth in the jaws. A worldwide problem, it is the most common cause of tooth loss. Periodontal disease in its most prevalent form is associated with excessive build-up of plaque on teeth and roots. Most cases of periodontal disease begin with inflammation of the gingiva—termed *gingivitis*—that may progress to loss of the supporting bone around the roots of the teeth. Other subtypes of periodontal disease are recognized with differing risk factors and natural histories. The mainstay of treatment is the removal of subgingival calculus and biofilm deposits using mechanical methods (tooth brushing, flossing, scaling, and root planing). Referral for appropriate dental care is indicated. Despite ongoing concerns, there is no current evidence that periodontal disease is an independent risk factor for coronary artery disease.

ACUTE DENTAL INFECTIONS

Localized dental infections respond well to local surgical treatment. Analgesia and nonsteroidal anti-inflammatory drugs are helpful. Antibiotics should be prescribed only in patients with signs of local or systemic spread or in patients who are moderately or severely immunocompromised. Amoxicillin (250 mg three times daily for 3 days) is the first-choice medication, and clindamycin (150 mg four times daily for 3 days) is an alternative in patients who are allergic to it.[10] Spreading dental infections require evacuation of pus without delay, including exploration of all affected fascial spaces and removal of necrotic debris. Parenteral broad-spectrum antibiotics are indicated (e.g., a broad spectrum β-lactam, metronidazole, or gentamicin; see Chapter 263).

Grade A References

A1. Staines K, Greenwood M. Aphthous ulcers (recurrent). *BMJ Clin Evid.* 2015;2015:1-30.
A2. Nasry SA, El Shenawy HM, Mostafa D, et al. Different modalities for treatment of recurrent aphthous stomatitis. A randomized clinical trial. *J Clin Exp Dent.* 2016;8:e517-e522.
A3. Davari P, Hsiao HH, Fazel N. Mucosal lichen planus: an evidence-based treatment update. *Am J Clin Dermatol.* 2014;15:181-195.

GENERAL REFERENCES

For the General References and other additional features, please visit Expert Consult at https://expertconsult.inkling.com.

398

APPROACH TO THE PATIENT WITH NOSE, SINUS, AND EAR DISORDERS

ANDREW H. MURR

Patients with nose, sinus, and ear disorders may have a variety of chief complaints. Nasal symptoms most commonly relate to rhinorrhea or congestion, both of which may be due to allergic, infectious, inflammatory, neoplastic, or structural causes. Sinus disorders, which commonly arise as a feeling of stuffiness or congestion but are sometimes also manifested as pain or even headache (Chapter 370), have a similar set of causes. Common ear complaints include pain, tinnitus, loss of hearing (Chapter 400), and vestibular symptoms (Chapter 400). Epistaxis, which is bleeding from the nose, is usually easy to distinguish from hemoptysis from the bronchial tree (Chapter 77) or hematemesis from the gastrointestinal tract (Chapter 126).

NASAL AND SINUS COMPLAINTS
Rhinitis and Sinusitis

DEFINITION

Rhinitis is generally defined as any inflammatory process in the nose, with the common result being a sensation of excess mucous or nasal congestion. Anterior nasal drainage may be perceived by the patient as being accompanied by an activity such as eating (gustatory rhinitis) and may be visible to an observer. Posterior nasal drainage is more nebulous and subjective, but it is very common and is referred to as postnasal drip.

In general, acute rhinitis and sinusitis describe inflammatory conditions of the nose and sinuses that last less than 4 weeks. Chronic rhinitis and sinusitis persist for more than 12 weeks despite treatment. Recurrent acute rhinitis and sinusitis are defined by episodes that occur four or more times per year and persist for 7 to 10 days per episode, but symptoms clear completely between episodes. Subacute rhinitis and sinusitis define symptoms that persist between 4 and 12 weeks and resolve completely with treatment.[1]

EPIDEMIOLOGY

The most common reason for a patient to seek the advice of a physician in the United States concerns problems relating to rhinitis and sinusitis. More than 30 million patient visits per year are devoted to this complaint, and billions of dollars are spent on medications that are expected to improve the condition.

Allergic rhinitis affects between 10 and 30% of adults and up to 40% of children. Each year, nearly 80 million people in the United States experience 7 days or more of nasal or ocular symptoms as a result of allergic rhinitis. The impact of allergic rhinitis also reflects its association with a variety of comorbid conditions, including asthma (Chapter 81), acute and chronic sinusitis, nasal polyposis, secretory otitis media, and sleep disorders (Chapter 377).

PATHOBIOLOGY

Humans normally produce about 2 L of mucus per day from their nasal lining. The nose functions primarily as a humidification and filtration system, with a clean and refreshed nasal mucous blanket serving to trap particulate matter and organisms. The nasal and sinus lining consists of ciliated respiratory epithelium; the cilia function in a highly organized and orderly fashion under normal circumstances to transport particulate matter trapped in the mucous blanket in a consistent fashion so that the mucus can be swallowed, thereby avoiding deposition in the bronchi. The nose also serves as the organ of olfaction (Chapter 399) to allow patients to discern tastes and avoid spoiled foods that could cause illness.

The parasympathetic nervous system controls both vascular tone and mucus production in the nose. Inflammatory conditions, such as the common cold, can cause the nasal and sinus lining to swell, thus highlighting the nasal cycle governed by parasympathetic neural control. In a normal state, one side of the nose is relatively decongested and one side is relatively congested because of vascular engorgement. This vascular dilation allows humidification and warming of inspired air and can also affect the ability to discern odors in the process of olfaction. During rhinitis, the inflammation exaggerates the normal

TABLE 398-1	ALLERGENS CAUSING ALLERGIC RHINITIS
COMMON NAME	**SEASON**
SEASONAL ALLERGENS	
Trees	
Birch	March–May
Cottonwood	April–May
Elm	February–May
Cedar	March–May
Oak	May–June
Maple	March–May
Grasses	
Kentucky blue	Mid-May–June
Timothy	Mid-May–June
Orchard	Mid-May–June
Sweet vernal	Mid-May–June
Fescue	Mid-May–June
Bermuda	Mid-May–June
Weeds	
Ragweed	August–September
Kochia	July–September
Russian thistle	July–September
Sage	July–September
Marsh elder	July–September
English plantain	July–September
Outdoor Molds	
Alternaria	Spring–fall
Cladosporium	Spring–fall
PERENNIAL ALLERGENS	
Household Allergens	
Cockroaches (German and American)	
Dust mites: *Dermatophagoides farinae, D. pteronyssinus, Blomia tropicalis*	More active in summer and humid months
Other insects (spiders, ladybugs)	
Animals	
Cats	
Dogs	
Other pets (guinea pigs, ferrets, hamsters, horses)	
Rodents	
Indoor Molds	
Aspergillus	
Cladosporium	
Penicillium	

relative comparison between the decongested and congested sides of the nose and can be perceived as an uncomfortable nasal stuffiness that shifts from side to side over a period of several hours.

Sinusitis differs from rhinitis in that the term implies an infectious cause rather than physiologic dysfunction. Nevertheless, many different mechanisms of inflammation besides infection may give rise to what is currently generally termed sinusitis.

Airborne Allergens

Allergic respiratory diseases result from a hypersensitivity immune reaction to airborne allergens (Table 398-1). Perennial allergic rhinitis may occur year-round. The most common causes include indoor fungi, which are related to periods of high indoor humidity; animal danders, particularly cats, but rodents (mice, rats, guinea pigs, ferrets, hamsters), rabbits, dogs, and birds may also be significant; dust mites of the genus *Dermatophagoides,* which grow in bedding and pillows and are semiseasonal, with maximal levels from August to December; and other insects (the best studied is the cockroach, but gypsy moths, crickets, ladybugs, spiders, and beetles may be locally important). Dust mites and cats produce the most important indoor allergens. Dust mites grow well only with a relative humidity higher than 50%. Dust mite allergy is probably relevant in all areas with more than 6 humid months in the year.

Within minutes of allergen exposure, immunoglobulin E (IgE)–sensitized mast cells degranulate and release preformed and newly synthesized mediators, including histamine, proteases (tryptase and chymase), cysteinyl leukotrienes, prostaglandins, platelet-activating factor, and cytokines. Some of these mediators produce the characteristic early-phase symptoms of allergic rhinitis, namely, sneezing, pruritus, rhinorrhea, and, to some extent, congestion. Other mediators stimulate infiltration of the nasal mucosa with inflammatory cells, including basophils, eosinophils, neutrophils, additional mast cells, and mononuclear cells. This infiltration of inflammatory cells and their subsequent release of a secondary wave of mediators sustain the inflammatory reaction and produce the late-phase response of allergic rhinitis.

Eosinophils represent an important component of the inflammation that develops in allergic rhinitis. Eosinophils release a wide variety of proinflammatory mediators that are major components of the chronic allergic response.

CLINICAL MANIFESTATIONS

When normal nasal mucosal function is lost, patients often complain of nasal crusting or obstruction, hypersecretion or postnasal drip, coughing, facial pressure, and fatigue. Nasal obstruction that shifts from side to side during the day is common in many types of rhinitis and may be considered an exaggeration of normal physiology.

Rhinitis is characterized by sneezing, which is often paroxysmal; rhinorrhea with clear, watery secretions; nasal congestion; and itching in the nares and palate. In allergic rhinitis, these symptoms are generally associated with allergic conjunctivitis manifested by ocular itching, lacrimation, and conjunctival injection. Severe conjunctivitis is less common in perennial allergic rhinitis than in seasonal allergic rhinitis. Lethargy, fatigue, arthralgias, myalgias, and cognitive impairment frequently accompany allergic rhinitis. Fever is not a feature of allergic rhinitis, even though the lay term for this condition is *hay fever,* which reflects the influenza-like nature of this disease. The natural history of allergic rhinitis is for symptoms to worsen inexorably during several weeks in the presence of ongoing allergen exposure. Symptoms often do not peak until well after the peak in pollen counts, and then they persist after pollen counts have declined.

Cardinal symptoms of *acute sinusitis* (Table 398-2) include purulent nasal drainage; nasal obstruction; and facial pain, pressure, or fullness.[2] Additional signs and symptoms include fever, cough, fatigue, reduced or absent sense of smell, dental pain, and ear symptoms such as pressure and fullness. The sign with the highest diagnostic value is purulent nasal discharge or posterior pharyngeal discharge. The presence of purulent nasal drainage generally supports the diagnosis of acute bacterial sinusitis, but culture of the drainage does not necessarily correlate well with actual pathogenic bacteria found on direct sinus culture.

Pain is a frequent complaint with acute bacterial sinusitis but infrequent with chronic sinusitis in the absence of other nasal signs and symptoms. Patients with chronic sinusitis often note a dull facial pressure that seems to worsen with dependency. Other factors favoring a diagnosis of bacterial sinusitis over viral sinusitis include length of illness beyond 10 days or when a patient's symptoms worsen within 10 days after an initial improvement in symptoms.

DIAGNOSIS

History

A thorough history should probe whether patients have tried over-the-counter or prescription medications, including antihistamines, decongestants, mucolytics, analgesics, mast cell stabilizers, and even steroids, and whether they have helped improve the condition. In addition, other prescription medications have side effects that affect nasal physiology, including antihypertensive medications that cause systemic vasodilation, aspirin, steroids, and antibiotics. Specific questions regarding allergies are important, including seasonality or environmental triggers, the presence or absence of pets, food sensitivities, recent changes in environment, and living conditions, with a focus on old or new carpets, mattresses, furnace filters, or freshly painted interior walls. A patient should be questioned about past allergy skin testing or other testing.

A recent history of other family members or coworkers being ill with an upper respiratory viral infection suggests an infectious over an environmental process. A careful past medical history should allow one to determine whether relevant conditions such as previous nasal surgery or trauma, granulomatous diseases, cystic fibrosis (Chapter 83), rheumatologic conditions, immune deficiencies (Chapter 236), or other problems may be contributing factors. Unilateral nasal congestion raises concern for either an anatomic abnormality, such as septal deviation, perhaps related to previous trauma, a polyp or other neoplastic mass, or perhaps even a foreign body.

Physical Examination

The nose should be inspected with a nasal speculum to assess nasal septal anatomy (Fig. 398-1), the most caudal aspect of the inferior turbinates (Fig. 398-2), and the possibility of large nasal polyps (Fig. 398-3) or other masses.

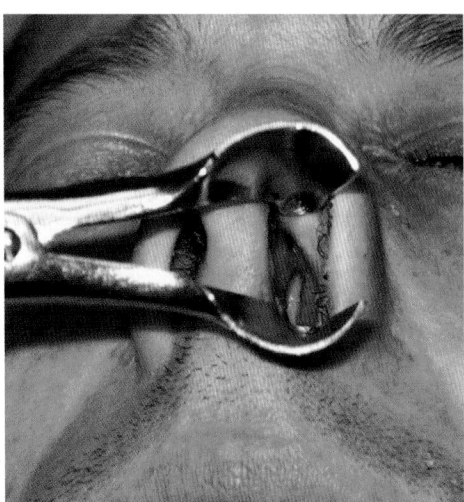

FIGURE 398-1. Purulent drainage from the middle meatus seen on anterior rhinoscopy.

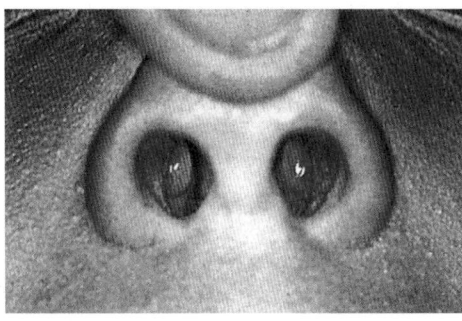

FIGURE 398-2. Edematous inferior turbinates narrowing the nasal airway in a patient with hay fever. Physical examination. (From Dhillon RS, East CA, eds. *Ear, Nose and Throat and Head and Neck Surgery,* 2nd ed. Edinburgh: Churchill Livingstone; 1994:34.)

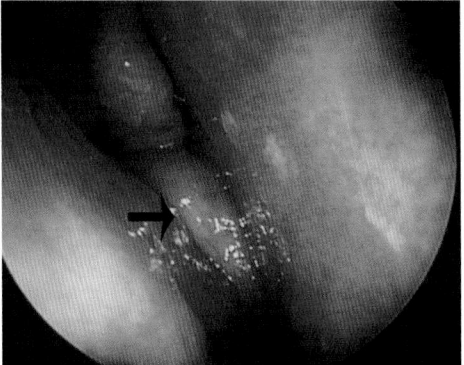

FIGURE 398-3. Nasal polyp in the right nasal cavity. A polyp is seen on the right side just inferior to the middle turbinate, next to the nasal septum. It is paler than the surrounding tissue.

TABLE 398-2 CARDINAL SYMPTOMS OF ACUTE SINUSITIS	
CARDINAL SYMPTOMS	**OTHER SIGNS/SYMPTOMS**
Facial pain, pressure, or fullness	Hyposmia/anosmia
Nasal obstruction	Fatigue
Nasal purulent discharge	Dental pain
	Fever
	Cough
	Ear pressure or fullness

In patients with allergic rhinitis, the physical examination may reveal pale and swollen inferior turbinates, whereas copious nasal secretions are more apparent with viral infections. By spraying the nose with a topical decongestant such as phenylephrine (Neo-Synephrine) or oxymetazoline, the middle meatus, which is the air space between the middle turbinate and lateral nasal wall, can often be visualized to assess for nasal polyps or purulent discharge. Examination of the mouth and oropharynx, including the posterior pharyngeal wall, with a tongue blade if necessary, can sometimes identify a stream of postnasal discharge or pus. Sinus palpation and transillumination, although part of the art of medicine, are not sufficiently reliable for diagnosis. The patient's ability to open the mouth without limitation helps exclude trismus, which can sometimes be caused by a dental infection or a deep neck infection.

A complete examination of the head and neck should be performed to look for signs of recent or old trauma such as ecchymosis under the eyelids, swelling of the soft tissue of the face, or deviation of the nasal dorsum. The neck should be palpated for adenopathy (Chapter 159) or other masses.

A basic eye examination should be performed to assess pupillary function, extraocular movements, and possible nystagmus (Chapter 396). An ear examination should be conducted to assess the tympanic membranes bilaterally. In patients with an abnormality of the tympanic membrane or concomitant complaints of hearing loss or disequilibrium (Chapter 400), pneumatoscopy using an air bulb attached to the otoscope can be used to insufflate the ear canal and assess for mobility of the tympanic membrane; decreased mobility suggests a middle ear effusion. Weber and Rinne testing using a 512-Hz tuning fork screens for conductive hearing loss, especially unilateral loss.

Endoscopic examination of the nose, almost always performed by a specialist, is the "gold standard" for evaluating rhinitis and sinusitis. A flexible or rigid fiberoptic scope can allow fine inspection of the septum, turbinates, middle meatus, and sphenoethmoid recess, as well as direct inspection of the nasopharynx, orifice of the eustachian tube, and fossa of Rosenmüller, which is just rostral to the eustachian tube in the nasopharynx and is often the site of origin of nasopharyngeal carcinoma (Chapter 181). Flexible endoscopy can be used to further inspect the oropharynx, larynx, and most of the hypopharynx (Chapter 401).

Laboratory Findings
Cultures
Cultures of the nostril or lower nasal cavity are not typically useful and are not recommended. An endoscopically guided culture of the middle meatus by a specialist may help guide treatment for acutely ill immunocompromised patients, for patients suspected of having acute bacterial rhinosinusitis, for patients with refractory chronic rhinosinusitis, or for those whose sinusitis is suspected of causing secondary meningitis, epidural or subdural abscess, brain abscess, orbital involvement, or cavernous sinus thrombosis.

Other Tests
A nasal smear can reveal eosinophils, which is consistent with allergic rhinitis. Likewise, skin testing or radioallergosorbent testing can help pinpoint allergic triggers (Chapter 235). In patients with acute sinusitis, a white blood cell count with differential may be useful. In patients with chronic sinusitis, serum immunoglobulin levels can be helpful: highly elevated IgE levels can raise suspicion for allergic fungal sinusitis, whereas low levels of IgG and other subclasses suggest immunodeficiency (Chapter 236). If the patient has chronic nasal crusting as a primary complaint, screening serologic tests for sarcoid (Chapter 89), granulomatosis with polyangiitis (Chapter 254), T-cell lymphomas (Chapter 176), syphilis (Chapter 303), tuberculosis (Chapter 308), Sjögren syndrome (Chapter 252), and other chronic inflammatory diseases can be considered. Relatively rare infections such as rhinoscleroma may also be present, so biopsy and cultures may be indicated to help reveal a diagnosis. Use of illicit substances should be considered because cocaine and other illicit drugs may cause chronic nasal crusting. Toxicology screening can be useful if substance abuse (Chapter 31) is suspected. In a patient with a lifelong history of sinusitis since childhood, cystic fibrosis should also be considered (Chapter 83).

Imaging
Non–contrast-enhanced computed tomography (CT) is indicated for patients with known or suspected rhinitis and sinusitis. CT is generally performed to document the presence of disease or the effects of treatment to improve the disease. A CT with contrast is used to evaluate complications of sinusitis. Finally, CT is critical before any surgical treatment of the sinuses because of the anatomic information that it provides the surgeon. Opacification or other

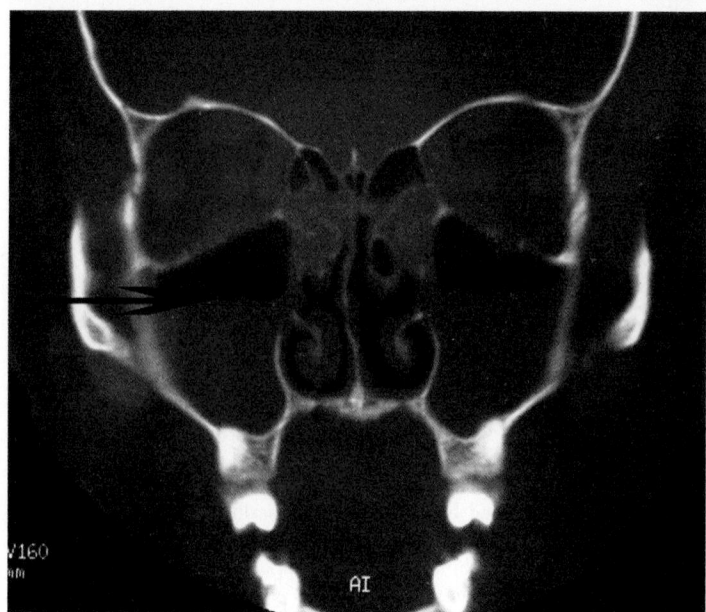

FIGURE 398-4. Coronal computed tomography showing bilateral acute pansinusitis. There are bilateral fluid levels in the maxillary sinuses that, if aspirated, can be sent for microbiology.

findings on CT (Fig. 398-4) can sometimes differentiate among the various causes of sinusitis. Plain films have little utility and are not generally recommended. Magnetic resonance imaging (MRI) is occasionally helpful, especially when evaluating tumors or processes that erode bone and are proximate to the brain or eye.

Differential Diagnosis
Rhinitis is primarily a clinical diagnosis with multiple specific causes (Fig. 398-5 and Table 398-3) based on symptoms and exposure history. Physical examination reveals the nasal mucosa to be cyanotic and swollen, with clear secretions.

The diagnosis of *allergic rhinitis* is confirmed by the demonstration of specific IgE antibodies reactive to the relevant allergen through either positive allergy skin test responses or IgE immunoassays (Video 398-1). Prick skin testing is safe, specific, and rapid, and it is the diagnostic test of choice for identifying relevant allergens. IgE immunoassays are an appropriate alternative that can be used by primary care physicians who manage patients with allergic rhinitis. However, a negative IgE immunoassay with a strong clinical suspicion suggests the need for a specialty referral.

Viral rhinitis may be difficult to distinguish from seasonal allergic rhinitis. In contrast to the pervasive eosinophilia in allergic rhinitis, viral rhinitis produces thicker, purulent secretions, with neutrophils present on the nasal smear. Conjunctival symptoms are less pronounced, and on physical examination, the nasal mucosa is erythematous and swollen.

Abuse of topical nasal decongestants (e.g., oxymetazoline), with chronic reflex vasodilation, has historically been the most common cause of rhinitis medicamentosa; however, cocaine and nasal narcotic abuse is another frequent cause of this condition. Chronic unilateral nasal blockage suggests an anatomic defect, typically a deviated or fractured septum, but such blockage can also result from polyps, foreign bodies, and tumors, which can be malignant. This history necessitates referral for rhinoscopy (Video 398-2) and possibly CT of the nose and sinuses.

An abnormal neurogenic response to irritants (e.g., cold air, pollutants, cigarette smoke, strong odors, alcohol, foods) is the predominant feature of vasomotor rhinitis. Patients with vasomotor rhinitis typically have chronic nasal congestion and posterior pharyngeal drainage, but they lack the paroxysmal sneezing, rhinorrhea, pruritus, conjunctivitis, and systemic complaints typical of patients with allergic rhinitis. In addition, eosinophils are absent in their nasal mucus.

An increasingly recognized cause of perennial nasal congestion and posterior pharyngeal drainage that often occurs in association with cough and hoarseness can be ascribed to laryngopharyngeal reflux. These patients are often otherwise asymptomatic from ("silent") gastroesophageal reflux (Chapter 129), making recognition challenging. Because symptoms may not resolve

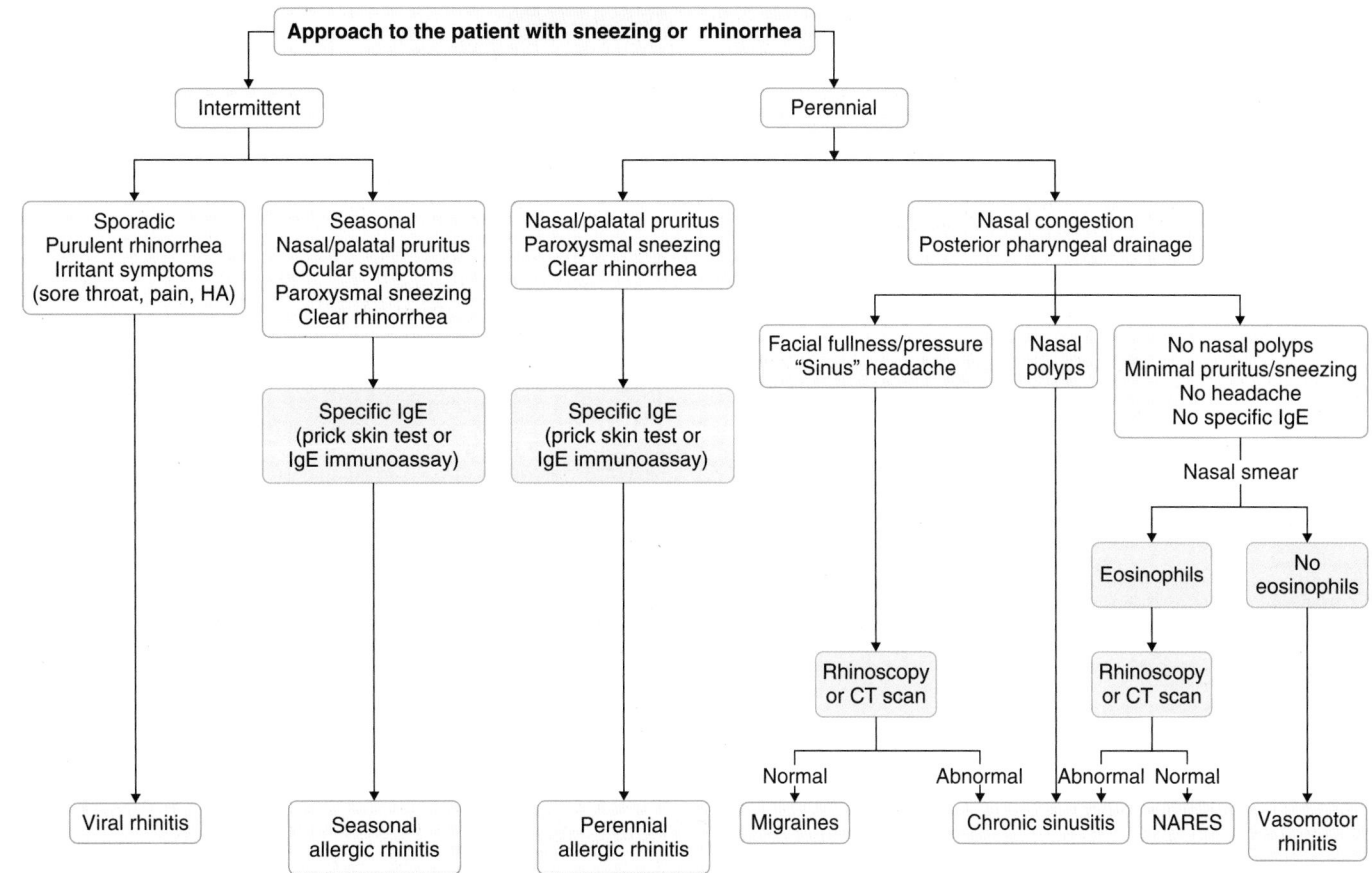

FIGURE 398-5. Approach to the patient with rhinitis symptoms. CT = computed tomography; HA = headache; IgE = immunoglobulin E; NARES = nonallergic rhinitis with eosinophilia syndrome.

TABLE 398-3	DIFFERENTIAL DIAGNOSIS OF RHINITIS

ALLERGIC

Seasonal allergic rhinitis
Perennial allergic rhinitis

INFLAMMATORY

Infectious rhinitis (viral)
Nonallergic rhinitis with eosinophilia syndrome
Chronic sinusitis with or without nasal polyposis
Laryngopharyngeal reflux

HORMONAL

Pregnancy, oral contraceptives, perimenopause
Hypothyroidism
Hyperthyroidism

RHINITIS MEDICAMENTOSA

Topical or, less commonly, oral decongestants
Antihypertensives
Antidepressants
Cocaine

VASOMOTOR

Irritant induced (pollution, cigarette smoke)
Cold air induced
Gustatory (food induced)

ANATOMIC

Nasal septal deviation
Tumor, neoplasm
Foreign body
Cerebrospinal fluid leak
Atrophic (postsurgical or trauma)

until after several months of aggressive reflux treatment and because proton pump inhibitors by themselves may not prevent reflux of digestive enzymes (e.g., pepsin) or other stomach-derived irritants, proper diagnosis can be daunting.

Atrophic rhinitis is characterized by atrophy of the nasal epithelium and is associated with complaints of nasal congestion and a perceived bad odor. It is observed in elderly patients, but the most common cause is devascularization secondary to nasal surgery or trauma.

A disease termed *nonallergic rhinitis with eosinophilia syndrome* presents with symptoms similar to those of vasomotor rhinitis. The syndrome is diagnosed by performing a nasal smear for eosinophils; however, a CT scan or rhinoscopy is required to exclude chronic sinusitis or nasal polyposis because these conditions may be minimally symptomatic. In contrast to vasomotor rhinitis, nonallergic rhinitis with eosinophilia syndrome is more responsive to intranasal cromolyn and intranasal corticosteroids.

Differential Diagnosis, Sinusitis

Sinusitis must be differentiated from rhinitis. Sinusitis may be caused by viral infection, bacterial infection, fungal infection, and allergy (Table 398-4).

A rapid onset of sinus-related symptoms suggests a viral upper respiratory infection, especially if the patient also has typical systemic symptoms, such as arthralgia, myalgia, fever, chills, gastrointestinal symptoms, and cough in addition to nasal congestion, postnasal drip, and headache. By comparison, acute bacterial rhinosinusitis causes facial pressure and purulent postnasal discharge. Viral disease can progress to a secondary bacterial infection, which can become chronic. An acute onset of inhalant allergy is often seasonal or can be traced to a particular precipitant.

Chronic sinusitis is a term that encompasses multiple pathophysiologic mechanisms and implies a prolonged course of sinus symptoms that have been refractory to symptomatic treatment over a period of at least 3 months. Chronic sinusitis presents with nasal congestion, nasal drainage, facial pressure,

TABLE 398-4 HETEROGENEITY OF CHRONIC SINUSITIS

PHENOTYPE	CHARACTERISTIC
Infectious	Very unusual as a cause of chronic sinusitis
Inflammatory	Develops secondary to anatomic obstruction of the sinus ostia; often resolves after surgical correction Bacterial biofilms contribute to presence and severity Infrequently associated with nasal polyps
Hyperplastic eosinophilic	Prominent eosinophilic infiltrate with systemic eosinophilia Frequent association with allergies and asthma Usually associated with nasal polyps
Allergic fungal	Often unilateral; presents as expansive, dense infiltrate on CT scan Associated with elevated total IgE and specific IgE to colonizing fungi
Aspirin-exacerbated respiratory disease	Intense eosinophilic infiltrate Usually associated with nasal polyps and asthma Exacerbations of upper and lower respiratory disease (asthma) after ingestion of aspirin and nonselective COX1 inhibitors

COX1 = cyclooxygenase 1; CT = computed tomography; IgE = immunoglobulin E.

TABLE 398-5 DIAGNOSTIC CRITERIA FOR CHRONIC SINUSITIS

Symptoms for more than 3 months:

- Mucopurelent nasal drainage
- Nasal obstruction
- Reduced sense of smell
- Facial pressure, or fulness

Supported by an objective finding:

- Nasal or middle meatus polyps
- Edema or purulence in middle meatus
- Paranasal *sinusitis* on endoscopy or CT scan

CT = computed tomography.
Data from Fokkens WJ, Lund VJ, Mullol J, et al. EPOS 2012: European position paper on rhinosinusitis and nasal polyps 2012. A summary for otorhinolaryngologists. *Rhinology.* 2012;50:1-12; Desrosiers M, Evans GA, Keith PK, et al. Canadian clinical practice guidelines for acute and chronic rhinosinusitis. *Allergy Asthma Clin Immunol.* 2011;7:1-38; Rosenfeld RM, Piccirillo JF, Chandrasekhar SS, et al. Clinical practice guideline (update): adult sinusitis. *Otolaryngol Head Neck Surg.* 2015;152:S1-S39.

TABLE 398-6 INTRANASAL CORTICOSTEROIDS*

GENERIC NAME	DOSE (PER ACTUATION)	MINIMUM APPROVED AGE	USUAL DOSING
Beclomethasone AQ	42 µg	6 yr	Twice daily
Beclomethasone HFA	80 µg	12 yr	Once daily
Flunisolide	25 µg	6 yr	Twice daily
Triamcinolone	55 µg	2 yr	Once daily
Budesonide	32 µg	6 yr	Twice daily
Fluticasone furoate	27.5 µg	2 yr	Once daily
Fluticasone propionate	50 µg	4 yr	Once daily
Mometasone	50 µg	2 yr	Once daily
Ciclesonide	50 µg	6 yr	Once daily
Ciclesonide HFA	37 µg	12 yr	Once daily

*Intranasal corticosteroids are generally administered at 2 sprays per nostril.

and sometimes anosmia (see Table 398-2). In contrast to acute (infectious) sinusitis, headaches are an unusual manifestation of either perennial rhinitis (allergic or nonallergic) or chronic sinusitis, and virtually all patients who complain of "sinus headaches" suffer from atypical migraines (Chapter 370), headaches that occur in a bilateral distribution involving the maxillary or ophthalmic branches of the trigeminal nerve. This distribution, especially when it is combined with vasomotor symptoms such as nasal congestion, rhinorrhea, and conjunctival injection, often leads to misdiagnosis as chronic sinusitis or rhinitis. Because of this overlap in symptoms among chronic sinusitis, perennial rhinitis, and atypical migraines and their synergistic influences on each other, objective evaluation with either CT or rhinoscopy is usually required to establish the diagnosis of chronic sinusitis (Table 398-5).

Endoscopically guided culture techniques combined with CT are the best way to diagnose or exclude *infectious* sinusitis. CT can reveal mucoceles, which are blocked individual sinuses that continue to secrete mucus and can slowly erode bone, expand to involve the eye and brain, or become acutely infected. A mycetoma, which is an isolated "fungus ball" in a sinus, has a characteristic hyperdensity within a sinus opacification. Mycetomas (Chapter 322) are noninvasive but may erode bone through pressure necrosis over a long period.

Mucus retention cysts, often present in the maxillary sinus, are manifested as a spherical opacification; an estimated 10% of the population has a mucus retention cyst, which is usually asymptomatic.

TREATMENT   Rx

Medical Therapy
Rhinitis

Antihistamines are considered first-line therapy for allergic rhinitis because they reduce rhinorrhea even though they do not generally improve nasal congestion. Episodic symptoms are treated with oral or nasal H₁-antihistamines, with an oral or nasal decongestant if needed. Mild seasonal or perennial symptoms should be treated with an intranasal glucocorticoid, an oral or nasal H₁-antihistamine, or a leukotriene-receptor antagonist. Moderate-to-severe symptoms are treated with an intranasal glucocorticoid, an intranasal glucocorticoid plus a nasal H₁-antihistamine, or allergen immunotherapy.

The benefit of antihistamines diminishes in patients with continuous allergen exposures, such as perennial allergic rhinitis caused by indoor allergens or after several days of continuous exposure to seasonal allergens; in such settings, these drugs often prove to be little better than placebo.[3]

Second-generation antihistamines have a long duration of action and are nonsedating. These once-daily agents include cetirizine (10 mg), levocetirizine (5 mg), fexofenadine (180 mg), desloratadine (5 mg), and loratadine (10 mg). The intranasal antihistamines azelastine and olopatadine have a more rapid onset of action than oral antihistamines and also are effective for nonallergic forms of rhinitis.

Decongestants such as pseudoephedrine treat nasal stuffiness but are mild stimulants and even in oral formulations may produce rebound congestion and headaches. These drugs are usually used in combination with antihistamines to control the full spectrum of allergic rhinitis symptoms. Antihistamines and decongestants alone generally do not provide satisfactory relief in patients with moderate to severe allergic rhinitis.

Intranasal corticosteroids, including triamcinolone acetonide (two sprays [55 µg] to each side of the nose every day), mometasone furoate (two sprays [50 µg] to each naris every day), fluticasone propionate (two sprays [50 µg] to each naris every day), and budesonide (two sprays [32 µg] to each naris every day) (Table 398-6), are the treatments of choice for patients with moderate to severe seasonal allergic rhinitis or perennial allergic rhinitis.[A1] Intranasal corticosteroids provide a 50 to 90% reduction in symptoms compared with 20 to 30% for oral antihistamines.

Leukotriene modifiers (zileuton [1200 mg twice daily], zafirlukast [20 mg twice daily], montelukast [10 mg once daily]) have a confirmed efficacy in allergic rhinitis that is comparable to that of antihistamines but do significantly improve sneezing, rhinorrhea, nasal congestion, ocular symptoms, and quality of life in patients with seasonal allergic rhinitis and perennial allergic rhinitis.

Nasal *cromolyn* stabilizes mast cells and mediates additional anti-inflammatory activities. Although it is not as effective as intranasal corticosteroids, cromolyn provides relief in patients with mild to moderate symptoms. The value of cromolyn is mitigated by the need for frequent doses (four times/day), a lack of efficacy in approximately 30 to 40% of recipients, and the superior efficacy of intranasal corticosteroids in controlled studies. Cromolyn may be especially useful preventively (e.g., immediately before cat exposure). Ocular cromolyn has been especially useful in the treatment of allergic conjunctivitis. No significant side effects are associated with its use.

Infectious Rhinitis and Sinusitis

Viral rhinitis is treated with supportive care, including fluid replacement and treatment of the febrile component of the syndrome with acetaminophen or nonsteroidal anti-inflammatory medications. Steam has a mild decongestant effect, and vitamin C and good nutrition may help hasten the resolution of symptoms. Oral decongestants (e.g., pseudoephedrine, 120 mg every 12 hours for several days), mucolytics (e.g., guaifenesin, 200 to 400 mg every 4 to 6 hours for several days), and ipratropium bromide (0.03 or 0.06%, two sprays on each side of the nose every 12 hours for several days) are of potential benefit.

Acute bacterial maxillary sinusitis confirmed by a CT scan usually requires surgical decompression, as do some cases of refractory sinusitis in immuno-compromised patients or patients in the intensive care unit, where direct culture can guide antibiotic therapy. For clinically diagnosed acute purulent rhinitis or acute rhinosinusitis of less than 10 days' duration, antibiotics are of little benefit because a diagnosis of bacterial rhinosinusitis based on the history and physical examination is quite inaccurate.[A2] For example, a 10-day course of amoxicillin does not reduce symptoms at day 3 or 10 compared with placebo among patients with acute rhinosinusitis, and it only slightly improves symptoms at day 7.[A3]

Because the potential side effects of antibiotics are not trivial, they should be reserved for patients with a high probability of bacterial infection.[4] The best clinical predictors of the presence of *acute* bacterial rhinosinusitis rather than viral rhinosinusitis include persistent symptoms for 7 or more days without evidence of clinical improvement; high fever (>39° C or 102° F) with puru-lent nasal discharge or facial pain for at least 3 to 4 consecutive days; or the onset of worsening symptoms more than 5 days after the onset of an apparent viral upper respiratory tract infection. In patients who meet one or more of those three criteria, empirical antibiotic therapy is recommended,[5] preferably with amoxicillin-clavulanate (875 mg/125 mg orally twice daily, increasing to 2000 mg/125 mg orally twice daily in patients with fever greater than 39° C or 102° F, immunocompromise, or recent antibiotic use). In patients who are allergic to penicillin, the best alternative is doxycycline (100 mg orally twice daily), with a fluoroquinolone (e.g., levofloxacin 500 mg orally daily or moxi-floxacin 400 mg orally daily) reserved for patients who cannot tolerate it or do not respond because of their poorer side-effect profiles. By comparison, macrolides, trimethoprim-sulfamethoxazole, and second- and third-generation oral cephalosporins are not recommended because of high levels of resistance. The usual course of therapy is 5 to 7 days, regardless of the medication chosen. Intranasal saline irrigations, using either physiologic or hypertonic saline, may be a useful adjunct in patients with acute bacterial, rhinosinusitis, but neither topical decongestants nor antihistamines are useful. If patients worsen despite 72 hours of treatment or do not improve after 5 to 7 days, further evaluation should include CT to localize the infection and detect complications, and cul-tures—either by direct sinus aspiration or endoscopically guided cultures of the middle meatus; other cultures are unreliable.

Chronic Rhinosinusitis

The mainstay of treating the symptoms of chronic rhinosinusitis are corticoster-oids, either as a *topical spray* (e.g., triamcinolone acetonide, two 55-μg sprays to each side of the nose every day; mometasone furoate, two 50-μg sprays to each naris every day; fluticasone propionate, two 50-μg sprays to each naris every day; or budesonide, two 32-μg sprays to each naris every day) for 6 weeks or an *oral tapering dose* (prednisone 40 mg per day for 5 days, followed by 30 mg per day for 5 days, followed by 20 mg per day for 5 days, followed by 10 mg per day for 5 days; or methylprednisolone 4 mg tablets begin-ning with 24 mg the first day and tapering by 4 mg each subsequent day for 6 days).[A4] Hypertonic saline irrigation may be of some help,[A5] but courses of oral antibiotics are of little value.[A6] Endoscopically obtained cultures of the middle meatus can help define which patients may improve with culture-guided antibiotic treatment. Antifungal agents, including itraconazole in an oral or aerosolized form and amphotericin B in an aerosolized form, do not appear beneficial in the treatment of typical chronic sinusitis.

Surgical Therapy

Patients who have severe symptoms, who fail to respond to therapy, or who have unusual, or resistant, or recurrent infections should be sent to a specialist for further evaluation and treatment (Table 398-7). Surgery is recommended in patients with benign neoplasms, mucoceles, juvenile nasopharyngeal angio-fibroma, and some types of malignancies. Surgery can correct septal deviations and anatomically related nasal obstruction. Surgery on the inferior turbinates may be beneficial for refractory rhinitis. Functional endoscopic surgery, which is designed to preserve mucociliary function and is performed with endoscopes through the nostril without skin incisions, can be useful for recurrent acute sinusitis and chronic rhinosinusitis.

Avoidance and Environmental Control

When it is feasible, avoidance or elimination of the source of the allergen is the treatment of choice for patients with allergic rhinitis. Dust mite avoidance involves removing reservoirs for mite growth (i.e., use allergen-impermeable

TABLE 398-7	WHEN TO REFER A PATIENT WITH PRESUMED BACTERIAL RHINOSINUSITIS TO AN EAR, NOSE, AND THROAT SPECIALIST

- Temperature >39° C (>102° F); orbital edema; severe headache, visual disturbance, altered mental status, meningeal signs
- Failure to respond to more than two courses of antimicrobial therapy
- Nosocomial infection, anatomic abnormalities
- Immunocompromise or multiple comorbidities
- Unusual or resistant pathogens
- Fungal sinusitis or granulomatous disease
- Recurrent episodes suggesting chronic sinusitis

Adapted from Chow AW, Benninger MS, Brook I, et al. IDSA clinical practice guideline for acute bacterial rhinosinusitis in children and adults. *Clin Infect Dis.* 2012;54:e72-e112.

mattress and pillow covers), keeping the relative humidity lower than 50%, washing bedding in hot water (130° F) to kill mites, and wearing a simple mask when dust is being disturbed. Many of the measures suggested for mites are also helpful for fungi, especially dehumidification. Windows, shower cur-tains, and indoor plants are important sites for fungal growth and can be treated with mild fungicides (dilute household bleach).

In some houses, and particularly urban apartment blocks, large numbers of cockroaches are present, and IgE sensitivity is common. Although it may be difficult to kill cockroaches in an apartment, it is usually possible to keep a house clear of cockroaches by using chemical sprays and traps. Air-conditioning with closed windows is useful for reducing seasonal allergens, and the dehu-midification provided by air-conditioning also mitigates the mite and indoor mold load.

Pets, especially cats and dogs, are the most preventable source of allergic diseases. The dominant rodent allergen is a urinary protein, and rodents, like cats, can deposit large quantities of allergen in a house.

Immunotherapy

Subcutaneous immunotherapy decreases the severity of allergic rhinitis, reduces the need for pharmacotherapy, and significantly improves quality of life. Patients should normally go through at least one full pollen season before considering immunotherapy. Efficacy depends on delivery of the correct antigen, regular injections for 3 to 5 years, and administration of an adequate dose of the allergen (10 to 15 μg, a dose much higher than that used historically). Immu-notherapy is associated with a small risk of fatal anaphylaxis (about 3 fatalities/year in the United States, of 2 million people receiving this form of treatment) and must be administered in a facility where resuscitation equipment and trained personnel are available.

Immunotherapy is indicated primarily in patients with refractory rhinitis or in those experiencing unacceptable side effects from standard medications. The effects of immunotherapy persist for many years after a 3- to 5-year course of treatment has been discontinued, and they could be lifelong.

Sublingual immunotherapy provides significant clinical benefit along with reduced need for pharmacologic therapy for numerous allergens including grass, ragweed, and dust mites.[A7] For example, administration of a house dust mite sublingual allergen immunotherapy tablet (6 or 12 development units) is an experimental option for reducing asthma exacerbations in patients who are allergic to house dust mites.[A8] In comparison to subcutaneous administra-tion, sublingual immunotherapy is sufficiently safe to permit home administra-tion. As with subcutaneous immunotherapy, long-term clinical benefits are observed after it is discontinued, although recurrences are common after 5 to 10 years and some sublingual preventive treatments may lose efficacy within 3 years.[A9]

Nasal Polyps

During the evaluation of symptoms of rhinitis or sinusitis, the physical exami-nation may reveal nasal polyps. Nasal polyps often present with symptoms of nasal blockage and anosmia along with typical symptoms of rhinitis. When polyps are present, the nasal congestion is often unrelenting. Sometimes, patients with prolonged symptoms will present with a visible mass in their nostril. Rarely, facial asymmetry or orbital involvement will be the presenting sign of long-ignored nasal polyps. Patient with nasal polyps may be more likely to complain of facial or ear pain than patients with rhinitis without polyps.

Nasal polyps typically begin near the ethmoid sinuses in the middle meatus and extend into the nose, where they block the nasal airway and/or the sinuses. Nasal polyps may be caused by chronic inflammation and also often occur as part of a rare metabolic disorder of arachidonic acid metabolism triggered by exogenous aspirin intake—known as aspirin-exacerbated respiratory disease. Also historically known as Samter's triad, patients with this syndrome have asthma that is exacerbated by aspirin ingestion, a skin rash precipitated by aspirin, and often have difficult-to-control chronic nasal polyposis. This constellation of symptoms is thought to be caused by inflammation elicited by leukotrienes, which are upregulated by the prostaglandin blockade caused by aspirin and sometimes by other nonsteroidal anti-inflammatory drugs. Human papillomavirus (Chapter 349) may cause an inverted papilloma, which presents as a polyp causing unilateral nasal obstruction. This initially benign neoplasm responds to surgical excision but can transform to frank malignancy. Polyps are also seen in patients with cystic fibrosis, especially patients with the delta F508 mutation (Chapter 83). They are also seen in allergic fungal sinusitis, which is manifested by an elevated IgE level, positive fungal cultures (usually for aspergillosis), Charcot-Leyden crystals on histopathology, characteristic densities on CT, and nasal polyposis that is often, but not always, unilateral. Antral choanal polyps may extend into the nasal cavity or nasopharynx and cause obstruction.

Nasal polyps will be visible in a careful examination (see Fig. 398-3 and E-Fig. 398-1), and their extent can be shown on a CT scan (Fig. 398-6). Unilateral nasal polyposis is suggestive of antral choanal polyps, malignancy, inverted papilloma, or allergic fungal sinusitis; early biopsy is recommended.

Benign inflammatory nasal polyps frequently respond to oral steroids, either in a tapered burst dose or, in rare cases, in small amounts of titrated daily oral steroids such as prednisone (40 mg per day for 5 days, followed by 30 mg per day for 5 days, followed by 20 mg per day for 5 days, followed by 10 mg per day for 5 days) or methylprednisolone (beginning with 24 mg the first day and tapering by 4 mg each subsequent day for 6 days). The combination of systemic steroids with doxycycline (e.g., 100 mg twice daily) may be even more effective, and the leukotriene antagonist montelukast (10 mg once daily) can be helpful as well.[A10] Topical steroids are also efficacious for treating nasal polyps.[A11] In adults with symptomatic chronic sinusitis and nasal polyps that are refractory to intranasal corticosteroids, the addition of subcutaneous dupilumab (600 mg loading dose followed by 300 mg weekly) to a corticosteroid nasal spray can reduce endoscopic polyp burden after 16 weeks compared with a corticosteroid spray alone[A12] and may become a useful therapy.

Surgery for benign nasal polyposis can improve symptomatic control and reduce the need for oral steroids. Surgery is always recommended for inverted papillomas, antral choanal polyps, and mucoceles, and surgery is likely to be helpful if acute sinusitis has caused central nervous system complications such as brain abscess (Chapter 385), meningitis (Chapter 384), epidural abscess, subdural abscess, or orbital abscess. Occasionally, surgery will be required when an untreated and aggressively growing polyp causes orbital or skull base erosion. Allergic fungal sinusitis is often treated with a combination of surgery, corticosteroids, and sometimes immunotherapy.

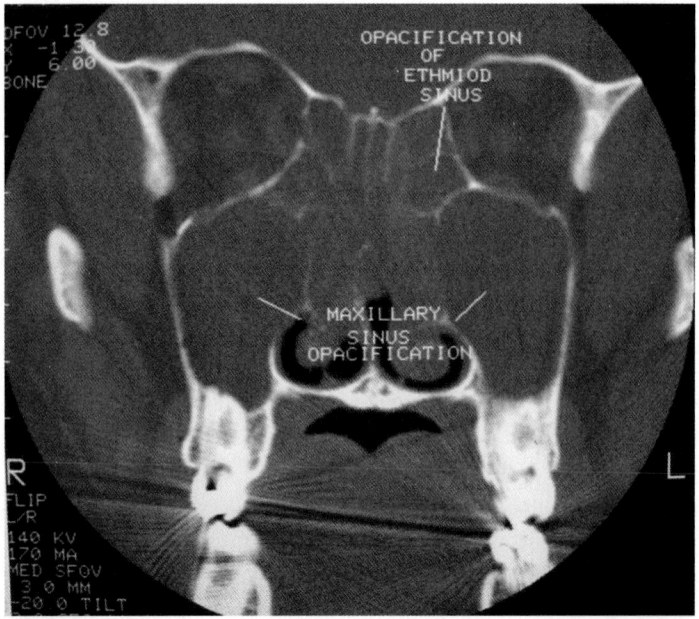

FIGURE 398-6. Computed tomography showing bilateral nasal polyposis of a chronic nature.

Epistaxis

For a patient with epistaxis, it is first critical to determine the severity of the blood loss. Persistent bleeding may result from warfarin, antiplatelet agents, or any underlying platelet (Chapters 163 and 164) or clotting deficiency (Chapter 165). Physical examination should focus on inspection of the anterior septum, which is the most frequent point of origin for epistaxis. Frequently, dilated blood vessels on the caudal septum can be seen with anterior rhinoscopy (Fig. 398-7 and E-Fig. 398-2). The combination of unilateral otitis media, epistaxis, nasal congestion, and a neck mass would be concerning for nasopharyngeal carcinoma. Rare tumors that can arise with bleeding include juvenile nasopharyngeal angiofibromas in male patients.

Epistaxis can be treated by local pressure, packing (using nasal sponges, balloons, or by ½-inch by 72-inch gauze impregnated with petroleum jelly), humidification, and hydration.[6] Hospitalization and transfusion are rarely required. Offending medications should be reduced in dose or discontinued temporarily if possible.[7] Topical vasoconstrictive medication such as oxymetazoline spray, two sprays on each side of the nose every 12 hours for 3 days, can help prevent persistent epistaxis. Hemostatic agents such as gelfoam-thrombin combination products can also be useful in treating refractory epistaxis or epistaxis in the presence of coagulopathy. However, topical bevacizumab, estriol, and tranexamic acid are not effective for reducing the frequency of epistaxis in patients with hereditary hemorrhagic telangiectasia. Occasionally, lasers or other types of cautery are used to improve the problem. At times, surgical arterial clipping or interventional neuroradiologic arterial occlusion can address a specific bleeding area.

⬤ EAR PAIN

❰ DEFINITION ❱

Ear pain (Table 398-8) is discomfort perceived by a patient in the area of the temporal bone. Although the discomfort can often be localized by the patient, at times the cause of the discomfort may in fact be distant from the site where the pain is felt. This referred pain can be due to problems in the oral cavity, oropharynx, hypopharynx, or larynx.

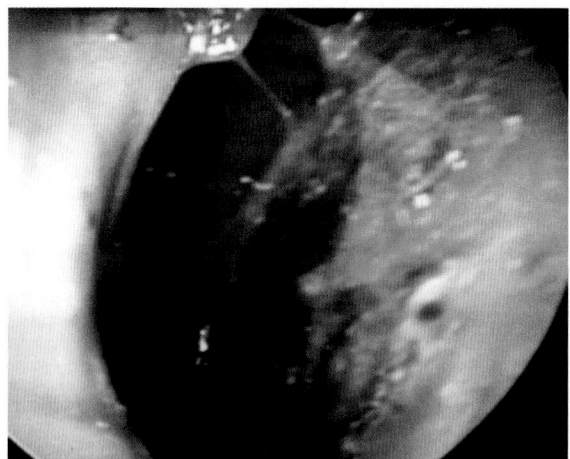

FIGURE 398-7. Dilated nasal vessels and crusting typical of a patient with epistaxis.

TABLE 398-8	CAUSES OF OTALGIA		
CAUSES OF OTALGIA	**EXTERNAL EAR**	**MIDDLE EAR**	**UPPER AERODIGESTIVE TRACT**
Likely	Otitis externa	Acute otitis media	Tonsillitis
	Herpes zoster oticus	Acute eardrum perforation	Tonsil abscess
	Chondritis	Barotrauma	Deep neck abscess
	Foreign body	Chronic otitis media with impending complication	Tumor (especially base of the tongue, tonsil, hypopharynx, larynx, nasopharynx)
Unlikely	Malignant otitis externa	Tumor	
	Tumor		

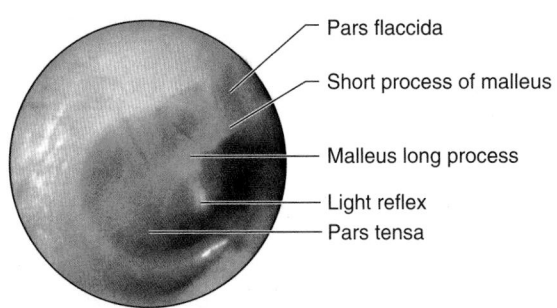

FIGURE 398-8. A normal tympanic membrane. (From Dhillon RS, East CA, eds. *Ear, Nose and Throat and Head and Neck Surgery,* 2nd ed. Edinburgh: Churchill Livingstone; 1994:2.)

PATHOBIOLOGY

The ear is well supplied with sensory nerves and is positioned on the side of the skull. The ear is divided into the outer ear, or pinna, and the ear canal; the middle ear, which encompasses the tympanic membrane and ossicles (Fig. 398-8); and the inner ear, which consists of the cochlea and the vestibular canals, including the utricle and saccule. In general, otalgia is due to problems in the outer or middle ear. The trigeminal nerve innervates the anterior-superior quadrant of the pinna, whereas the C2 and C3 cervical cutaneous nerves innervate the rest of the majority of the outer ear. However, there are contributions by the 9th and 10th nerves in the ear canal and even a small patch of sensory innervation by the 7th nerve in the posterior superior ear canal. It is the overlap in distribution of the 9th and 10th cranial nerves that establishes the anatomic basis for referred otalgia in diseases of the oral cavity, oropharynx, and larynx. Additionally, otalgia may be caused by disorders of the temporal mandibular joint, which is located just anterior to the external auditory canal. Therefore ear pain may be due to inflammatory conditions of the skin of the outer ear, the ear canal, or the middle ear, or it may be due to disease processes unrelated to the ear itself.

CLINICAL MANIFESTATIONS

Patients with ear pain often have complaints referable directly to the ear itself. In cases of otitis externa, frankly obvious erythema and swelling of the skin of the ear canal may be present. Even minute physical manipulation of the ear may be excruciating. In chondritis of the pinna, which may be related to rheumatologic disorders, infection, or trauma, the entire pinna may be swollen and painful (E-Fig. 398-3). Hearing loss accompanying otalgia may indicate middle ear disease, especially otitis media. Patients sometimes complain of pain in the ear after air travel or driving from a mountainous region. Quick changes in pressure, such as encountered in scuba diving, may indicate barotrauma (Chapter 88), in which the eustachian tube is unable to compensate rapidly enough for the changes in pressure that are encountered. Pain may also be a posttraumatic symptom from relatively minor percussion injury, more severe head trauma, or percussion injury related to a blast. Pain related to noise exposure may also indicate damage to the middle ear or even the inner ear. Deep-seated boring pain over the temporal area accompanied by retro-orbital pain can be due to petrous apex disease, including petrous apicitis.

DIAGNOSIS

History

A patient with ear pain should be asked to reveal the location of the discomfort, the duration of the symptoms, and any activities related to onset of the condition. As an example, recent swimming would make otitis externa ("swimmer's ear") more likely, whereas a recent upper respiratory infection with hearing loss would suggest otitis media. Questions should address possible hearing loss, vertigo, otorrhea, hoarseness, voice change, dysphagia, odynophagia, dyspnea, hemoptysis, hematemesis, and weight loss. A social history with specific concentration on tobacco and alcohol use should be obtained. A possible family history of upper aerodigestive tract and nasopharyngeal carcinoma should be sought. A past surgical history can reveal distant ear or throat surgery.

Physical Examination

A complete head and neck examination, including general assessment for trauma and a basic eye examination, is required. The outer ear and pinna should be examined first. The ear canal should first be palpated and then inspected. An otoscope with a pneumatic bulb attachment is critical to establish the presence or absence of a middle ear effusion. Inspection of the tympanic

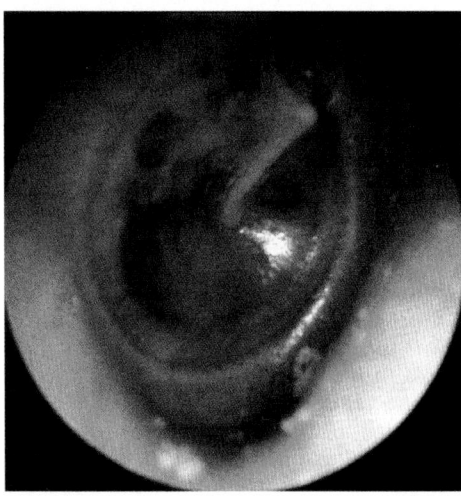

FIGURE 398-9. Otoscopic appearance in otitis media with effusion. The handle and short process of the malleus are brought into relief by retraction of the eardrum. There is a slightly yellow appearance of the eardrum related to the middle ear effusion. (From Dhillon RS, East CA, eds. *Ear, Nose and Throat and Head and Neck Surgery,* 2nd ed. Edinburgh: Churchill Livingstone; 1994:7.)

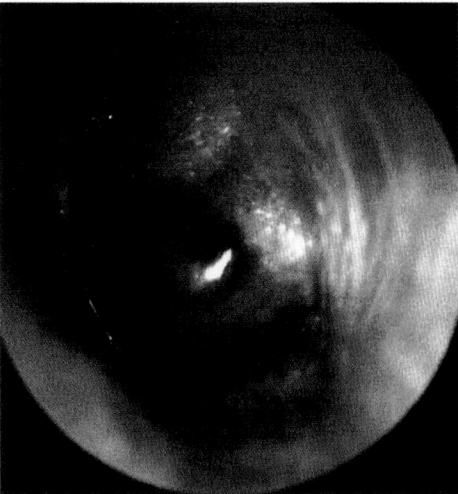

FIGURE 398-10. Blood in the middle ear (hemotympanum). Causes include otitic barotrauma, secretory otitis media, and a high jugular bulb. (From Dhillon RS, East CA, eds. *Ear, Nose and Throat and Head and Neck Surgery,* 2nd ed. Edinburgh: Churchill Livingstone; 1994:26.)

membrane should be accomplished with notations made about patency and perforation, translucency of the eardrum, position and definition of the malleus, and the eardrum's mobility with the ear canal sealed and a puff of air delivered by the pneumatic bulb (pneumotoscopy). Abnormalities may be caused by infection (Fig. 398-9) or barotrauma (Fig. 398-10). Examination with a 512-Hz tuning fork should be performed to determine lateralization of the sound (Weber test) and whether air conduction is superior to bone conduction (Rinne test). Facial nerve function should be assessed (Chapter 368) by determining whether the patient can raise the eyebrows, close the eyes, wrinkle the nose, and purse the lips. The presence or absence of nystagmus should be recorded. Inspection of the nose, oral cavity, oropharynx, and neck should be accompanied by cranial nerve examination (Chapter 368). Palpation of the tongue and tonsils is especially important if the ear pain is intense and persistent. A careful neck examination should be performed to look for masses. Oral cavity infections (Chapter 397), such as a peritonsillar abscess or severe tonsillitis, may arise as ear pain, and the physical examination should reveal trismus, erythema, mass effect, and other common signs of pharyngitis.

Laboratory

An audiogram can assess hearing loss (Chapter 400). A tympanogram measures compliance of the middle ear system and is an accurate method for diagnosis of otitis media. Cultures are rarely performed because they require tympanocentesis, and cultures of the external ear can reveal a vast variety of organisms that are often treated empirically with antibiotics. If a fever and middle ear effusion are present and neck stiffness is found on physical examination, lumbar puncture may rarely be recommended because of the small chance that otitis media can cause central nervous system complications such as meningitis.

Imaging

In general, imaging is indicated if complications of acute or chronic otitis media are suspected or to look for occult causes of otalgia in the upper aerodigestive tract. If a patient is suspected of having meningitis, epidural or subdural abscess, brain abscess, or sagittal sinus thrombosis, contrast imaging is mandatory. Imaging is also useful for operative planning in patients with chronic otitis media or (rarely) to evaluate for the presence of tumors in the middle or external ear.

Differential Diagnosis

Otitis externa, which is an infection of the skin of the ear canal, is often due to manipulating the ear after swimming or trying to scratch an ear canal that itches because of skin irritation. Patients exhibit erythema of the canal skin and extreme pain on manipulation of the ear canal. In the presence of concomitant cranial neuropathies, especially in diabetic or otherwise immunocompromised patients, malignant otitis externa with osteomyelitis should be suspected. Inspection of the tympanic membrane may reveal fluid consistent with otitis media; the tuning fork examination should support the presence of conductive hearing loss. Vesicles on the conchal portion of the pinna, especially when accompanied by facial nerve paralysis, strongly suggest herpes zoster oticus with Ramsay Hunt syndrome (Chapter 351). Perforation of the eardrum suggests either acute or chronic otitis media, traumatic perforation, or possibly cholesteatoma (Chapter 400) if the perforation is in the posterior-superior quadrant. Chronic draining otorrhea of long standing with a deep boring pain and perforation of the tympanic membrane suggests a complication of otitis media.

If findings on ear and cranial nerve examination are negative but the patient's complaints of otalgia are persistent, special effort needs to be made to visualize the upper aerodigestive tract, including the nasopharynx, oral cavity, oropharynx, larynx, and hypopharynx, to be sure that infection or tumor is not present in these hard-to-examine areas. Flexible fiberoptic nasopharyngoscopy is a standard examination in these circumstances, and imaging such as MRI with contrast also can be very useful.

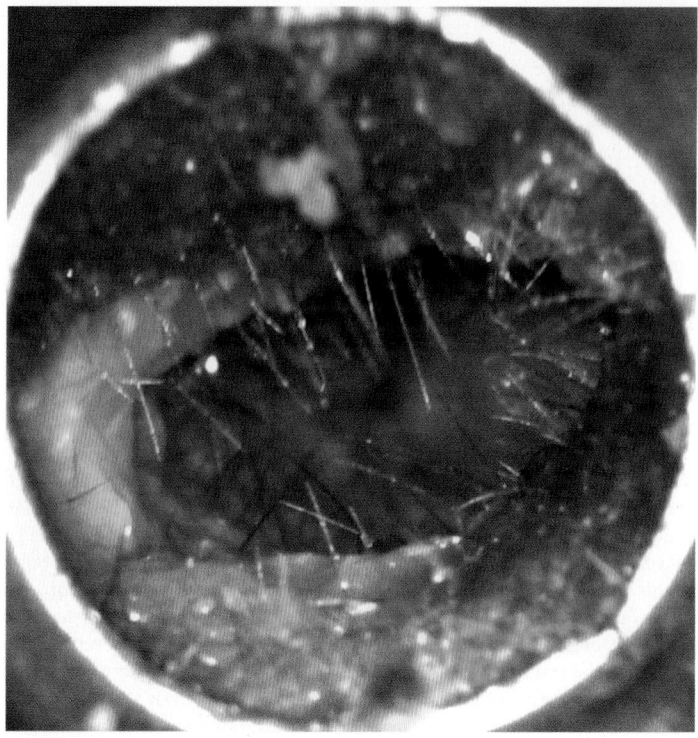

FIGURE 398-11. Otitis externa. Otitis externa in a patient's left ear with the tympanic membrane in the distance. Exudate and erythema are present. The ear canal is quite painful, and a wick may be necessary to maintain patency of the external auditory canal.

TREATMENT　Rx

Otitis externa is often treated with office suctioning of debris under a microscope and the application of antibiotic drops (ciprofloxacin, tobramycin, neomycin, polymyxin B), with or without hydrocortisone in various combinations.[8] Frequently, a small wick or sponge is placed in the ear canal to help maintain patency of the canal and allow facile application of the medications (Fig. 398-11).[9]

For otitis media, oral antibiotic treatment is directed at eradicating *Haemophilus influenzae*, *Moraxella catarrhalis*, *Streptococcus pneumoniae*, and *Staphylococcus aureus* with amoxicillin or erythromycin as for sinusitis.[10] The benefit is notable for children 2 years or younger with bilateral otitis media and for older children with otitis plus otorrhea, whereas other patients can be observed without antibiotics. In general, antibiotics provide somewhat better short-term outcomes but at the expense of significantly more diarrhea and rashes. In patients with middle ear effusions, antimicrobial treatment may effectively reduce the duration of effusion, but whether it improves hearing is unknown.[A13] Interestingly, the natural history of acute otitis media is acute perforation of the eardrum, which often results in otorrhea and relief of pain. Most middle ear effusions clear spontaneously within 3 months regardless of whether they are treated. Most perforations of an eardrum caused by trauma heal without surgical intervention, but if an eardrum perforation persists for more than about 3 months, surgical closure and the use of tympanoplasty with or without mastoidectomy can be contemplated. Chronic draining perforations, especially if located in the posterior-superior quadrant of the tympanic membrane, may portend the presence of cholesteatoma and may require tympanomastoid surgery. Earwax, which may cause reduced hearing (Chapter 400) or ear pain, may be treated with removal of the wax and over-the-counter ceruminolytic agents.[11]

In patients in whom herpes zoster is suspected, acyclovir can be started at 800 mg by mouth five times per day for 7 days, with or without prednisone (Chapter 351). Intracranial complications of otitis media often need to be addressed surgically.

Grade A References

A1. Juel-Berg N, Darling P, Bolvig J, et al. Intranasal corticosteroids compared with oral antihistamines in allergic rhinitis: a systematic review and meta-analysis. *Am J Rhinol Allergy.* 2017;31: 19-28.

A2. Kenealy T, Arroll B. Antibiotics for the common cold and acute purulent rhinitis. *Cochrane Database Syst Rev.* 2013;6:CD000247.

A3. Garbutt JM, Banister C, Spitznagel E, et al. Amoxicillin for acute rhinosinusitis: a randomized controlled trial. *JAMA.* 2012;307:685-692.

A4. Chong LY, Head K, Hopkins C, et al. Intranasal steroids versus placebo or no intervention for chronic rhinosinusitis. *Cochrane Database Syst Rev.* 2016;4:CD011996.

A5. Chong LY, Head K, Hopkins C, et al. Saline irrigation for chronic rhinosinusitis. *Cochrane Database Syst Rev.* 2016;4:CD011995.

A6. Head K, Chong LY, Piromchai P, et al. Systemic and topical antibiotics for chronic rhinosinusitis. *Cochrane Database Syst Rev.* 2016;4:CD011994.

A7. Di Bona D, Plaia A, Leto-Barone MS, et al. Efficacy of grass pollen allergen sublingual immunotherapy tablets for seasonal allergic rhinoconjunctivitis: a systematic review and meta-analysis. *JAMA Intern Med.* 2015;175:1301-1309.

A8. Virchow JC, Backer V, Kuna P, et al. Efficacy of a house dust mite sublingual allergen immunotherapy tablet in adults with allergic asthma: a randomized clinical trial. *JAMA.* 2016;315: 1715-1725.

A9. Scadding GW, Calderon MA, Shamji MH, et al. Effect of 2 years of treatment with sublingual grass pollen immunotherapy on nasal response to allergen challenge at 3 years among patients with moderate to severe seasonal allergic rhinitis: the GRASS randomized clinical trial. *JAMA.* 2017;317: 615-625.

A10. Rudmik L, Soler ZM. Medical therapies for adult chronic sinusitis: a systematic review. *JAMA.* 2015;314:926-939.

A11. Head K, Chong LY, Hopkins C, et al. Short-course oral steroids as an adjunct therapy for chronic rhinosinusitis. *Cochrane Database Syst Rev.* 2016;4:CD011992.

A12. Bachert C, Mannent L, Naclerio RM, et al. Effect of subcutaneous dupilumab on nasal polyp burden in patients with chronic sinusitis and nasal polyposis: a randomized clinical trial. *JAMA.* 2016;315: 469-479.

A13. Tapiainen T, Kujala T, Renko M, et al. Effect of antimicrobial treatment of acute otitis media on the daily disappearance of middle ear effusion: a placebo-controlled trial. *JAMA Pediatr.* 2014;168: 635-641.

GENERAL REFERENCES

For the General References and other additional features, please visit Expert Consult at https://expertconsult.inkling.com.

399

SMELL AND TASTE

ROBERT W. BALOH AND JOANNA C. JEN

Millions of people suffer from disorders of taste and smell,[1] but these disorders are often neglected because they are not fatal and, unlike abnormalities of vision and hearing, are not considered serious handicaps.

DEFINITION

The sensory receptor for taste, the taste bud, is made up of 50 to 150 cells arranged to form a pear-shaped organ. The lifespan of these cells is 10 to 14 days, and they are constantly being renewed from dividing epithelial cells surrounding the bud. Taste buds are located on the tongue, soft palate, pharynx, larynx, epiglottis, uvula, and upper third of the esophagus. The taste buds located on the anterior two thirds of the tongue and on the palate are innervated by the chorda tympani branch of the seventh cranial nerve. The ninth cranial nerve innervates the posterior third of the tongue. The ninth and tenth nerves innervate taste buds in the pharynx and larynx. Afferent signals from the taste buds project to the nucleus of the solitary tract in the medulla and then through a series of relays to the thalamus and postcentral somatosensory cerebral cortex (primary ipsilateral). Free nerve endings of the fifth cranial nerve are found on the tongue and in the oral cavity, and lesions involving these pathways can also alter taste perception.

Olfactory receptors lie in a roughly dime-sized area of specialized pigmented epithelium that arches along the superior aspect of each side of the nasal mucosa. Specialized bipolar sensory cells in this region thrust short receptor hairs into the overlying mucosa to detect aromatic molecules as they dissolve. Like taste buds, the specialized receptor portion of the bipolar neuron undergoes continuous renewal, with turnover occurring approximately every 30 days. Thin axons of the bipolar neurons course through small holes in the cribriform plate of the ethmoid bone to form connections in the overlying olfactory bulb on the ventral surface of the frontal lobe. From there,

second- and third-order neurons project directly and indirectly to the prepiriform cortex and parts of the amygdaloid complex of both sides of the brain, which represents the primary olfactory cortex.

PATHOBIOLOGY

Disorders of taste interfere with digestion because taste stimulants alter salivary and pancreatic flow, gastric contractions, and intestinal motility. Smell also contributes to the anticipation and ingestion of food because much of what is tasted is derived from olfactory stimulation during ingestion and chewing. An inability to detect noxious tastes and odors can result in food or gas poisoning, particularly in elderly subjects. In the extreme, chemosensory disorders can lead to overwhelming stress, anorexia, and depression. Genes that encode chemoreceptor proteins belong to the G protein–coupled receptor superfamily, which accounts for up to 1% of mammalian genomes. Sequence diversity in these genes encodes unique structural motifs that bind to different ligands signaling different odors and tastes. Distinct and dedicated taste receptor cells express unique receptors to detect each of the five basic tastes: sweet (sensed by the heterodimers T1R1 and T1R3), umami (detected by the heterodimers T1R2 and T1R3), bitter (sensed by an estimated 30 T2Rs), sour (sensed by PKD2L1, with membrane-tethered carbonic anhydrase IV sensing carbonation), and salty (epithelial sodium channel). The taste receptor cells transform and transmit information to primary afferents through multiple cranial nerves (VII, IX, and X) that project to the solitary tract nucleus in the brain stem, with relay in the thalamus, and then onward to the primary cortex (Fig. 399-1).

Disorders of taste and smell can be divided into local, systemic, and neurologic categories (Table 399-1). The taste buds and the specialized receptor portion of the bipolar olfactory cells are constantly being renewed, and the process of renewal can be affected by nutritional, metabolic, and hormonal states as well as by therapeutic radiation, drugs, and age. For example, with interruption of mitosis by antiproliferative agents, return of normal taste function takes a minimum of 10 days, whereas return to normal olfactory function takes more than 30 days. Diuretics can block apical ion channels on a taste bud, and antifungal drugs inhibit cytochrome P-450–dependent enzymes at the level of the receptors.[2] Numerous local conditions, such as colds and allergies, chronic sinusitis, and nasal polyposis, can influence the sense of smell by restricting airway patency. Accidental blows to the head can shear the fine

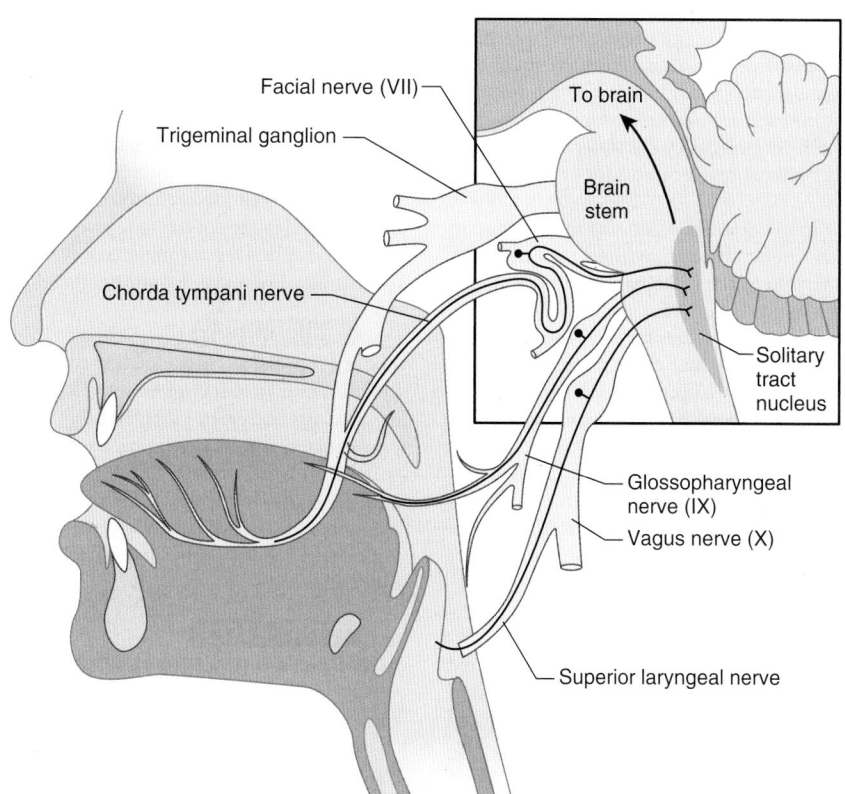

FIGURE 399-1. Anatomy of peripheral taste pathways. Taste information is transmitted from the mouth and the pharynx through multiple cranial nerves that project to the solitary tract nucleus in the brain stem, with relay in the thalamus before reaching the cortex. (Copyright 1999-2000 David Klemm. Reproduced from Bromley SM. Smell and taste disorders: a primary care approach. *Am Fam Physician.* 2000;61:427-436, 438.)

TABLE 399-1	COMMON CAUSES OF LOSS OF TASTE AND SMELL	
	TASTE	**SMELL**
Local	Radiation therapy, oral infections, dentures, dental procedures	Allergic rhinitis, sinusitis, nasal polyposis, upper respiratory infection
Systemic	Cancer, renal failure, hepatic failure, nutritional deficiency (vitamin B_3, zinc), Cushing syndrome, hypothyroidism, diabetes mellitus, infection (viral), drugs (antirheumatic and antiproliferative, e.g., corticosteroids, cisplatin, carboplatin, cyclophosphamide, doxorubicin, and methotrexate)	Renal failure, hepatic failure, nutritional deficiency (vitamin B_{12}), Cushing syndrome, hypothyroidism, diabetes mellitus, infection (viral hepatitis, influenza), drugs (nasal sprays, antihistamines, decongestants, antibiotics, and antirheumatic and antiproliferative drugs that affect taste)
Neurologic	Bell palsy, familial dysautonomia, multiple sclerosis	Head trauma, multiple sclerosis, Parkinson disease, Alzheimer disease, frontal tumor

axons of the bipolar olfactory neurons and result in loss of smell. Lesions of the fifth, seventh (chorda tympani), and ninth nerves can lead to disordered taste sensation. Olfactory and gustatory disturbances can serve as important diagnostic signs for focal neurologic lesions (e.g., frontal lobe tumors). Hallucinations of smell and taste occur in persons with epileptogenic lesions affecting the mesial temporal lobe and insular region, respectively. Finally, olfactory disturbances and hallucinations occur with a number of psychiatric illnesses (particularly depressive illness and schizophrenia).

CLINICAL MANIFESTATIONS

An inability to smell or a diminished sense of smell is present in 3 to 20% of the population.[3] The most frequently encountered causes of loss of smell are local obstructive disease, viral infections, head injuries (Chapter 371), and normal aging (Chapter 22). Patients can lose their sense of smell not only from chronic allergies and sinusitis[4] (Chapter 398) but also from the nasal sprays and drops that they use to treat these conditions.

The most common causes of loss of the sense of taste are viral infections and drug ingestion, particularly antirheumatic and antiproliferative drugs (see Table 399-1). Many of the systemic disorders listed in Table 399-1 probably produce their effect by decreasing the rate of turnover of sensory receptors on the tongue and olfactory epithelia. In pregnancy (Chapter 226), taste is often altered, perhaps because taste buds express receptors for hormones that are altered during pregnancy.[5]

Disturbances of smell and taste in malnourished patients may be due to specific deficiencies in vitamins and minerals, such as zinc. Viral illnesses, such as influenza (Chapter 340), viral hepatitis (Chapter 139), and allergic rhinitis, are the most common causes of loss of both taste and smell. Multifocal neurologic disorders such as multiple sclerosis (Chapter 383) and traumatic head injuries (Chapter 371) can affect the central olfactory and gustatory pathways at multiple levels; as a result, abnormalities in taste and smell are common in such patients. Loss of smell is increasingly being recognized by the fifth decade of life[6] and especially in patients with depression[7] and in the early stages of many neurodegenerative disorders, including Parkinson disease, motor neuron disease, Huntington disease, Alzheimer dementia,[8] and even mild cognitive impairment.[9] An irritative lesion from a neoplastic,[10] inflammatory, or demyelinating process may lead to a persistent disturbance rather than to a loss of taste.

DIAGNOSIS

Olfaction can be tested grossly at the bedside with a few easily recognized odors, such as coffee, chocolate, and the roselike aroma of the compound phenylethyl alcohol. Nasal irritants should be avoided. Each nostril is tested separately to determine whether the problem is unilateral or bilateral. Gustatory sensation is typically tested with weak solutions of sugar, salt, and acetic acid or vinegar. The patient must keep the tongue protruded and respond to questions by nodding the head or by pointing to names of the tastes written on cards. The anterior two thirds and posterior third of the tongue should be tested separately.

Treatment of olfactory dysfunction secondary to nasal disease is aimed at opening the air passageways while preserving the olfactory epithelium (Chapter 398). Intranasal steroids for rhinosinusitis (Chapter 398), antibiotics as needed for sinusitis, and therapies for seasonal allergies are useful in selected cases. Drugs known to affect taste or smell (see Table 399-1) should be discontinued for a trial. Vitamin and mineral therapies are of unproven benefit.[A1] Impaired odor identification, particularly in the anosmic range, is associated with increased mortality in older adults even after controlling for dementia and medical comorbidity.

Grade A Reference

A1. Kumbargere Nagraj S, George RP, Shetty N, et al. Interventions for managing taste disturbances. *Cochrane Database Syst Rev.* 2017;12:CD010470.

GENERAL REFERENCES

For the General References and other additional features, please visit Expert Consult at https://expertconsult.inkling.com.

400

HEARING AND EQUILIBRIUM

ROBERT W. BALOH AND JOANNA C. JEN

DISORDERS OF THE AUDITORY SYSTEM

DEFINITION

The normal ear can detect sound frequencies ranging between 20 and 20,000 Hz; the upper range drops off fairly rapidly with advancing age. The ear is most sensitive between 500 and 4000 Hz, which roughly corresponds to the frequency range most important for understanding speech. The hearing level in this range has several practical implications in terms of the degree of handicap and the potential for useful correction with amplification. A 30- to 40-dB hearing level in the speech range would impair normal conversation, whereas an 80-dB hearing level would make everyday auditory communication almost impossible (the social definition of deafness).

EPIDEMIOLOGY

About 5% of the world population suffers from disabling hearing loss (defined by the World Health Organization as greater than 40 dB in the better hearing ear in adults and greater than 30 dB in the better hearing ear in children). The prevalence of disabling hearing loss is twice as high in poorer countries compared with richer countries. The prevalence increases with every age decade, and it is higher in men than in women across all age decades. Hearing loss is independently associated with accelerated cognitive decline, incident cognitive impairment, and a higher risk of accidental injury[1] in community-dwelling older adults.

PATHOBIOLOGY

Localization of Lesions within the Auditory Pathways

Conductive hearing loss results from lesions involving the external or middle ear. It is typically characterized by an approximately equal loss of hearing at all frequencies and by well-preserved speech discrimination once the threshold for hearing is exceeded. Patients with conductive hearing loss can hear speech in a noisy background better than in a quiet background because they can understand loud speech as well as anyone.

Sensorineural hearing loss results from lesions of the cochlea or auditory division of the eighth cranial nerve, or both. With sensorineural hearing loss,

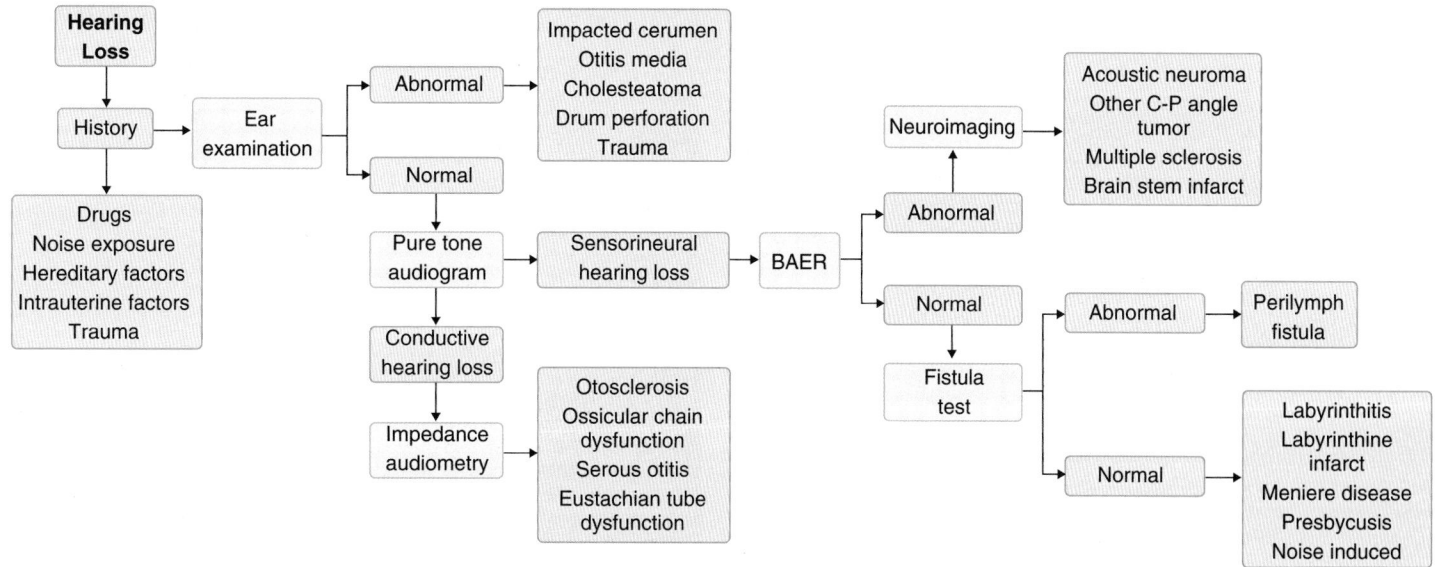

FIGURE 400-1. Evaluation of hearing loss. BAER = brain stem auditory evoked response; C-P = cerebellopontine.

the hearing levels for different frequencies are usually unequal, typically resulting in better hearing for low- than for high-frequency tones. Patients with sensorineural hearing loss often have difficulty in hearing speech that is mixed with background noise and may be annoyed by loud speech. Three important manifestations of sensorineural lesions are diplacusis, recruitment, and tone decay. Diplacusis and recruitment are common with cochlear lesions; tone decay usually accompanies eighth nerve involvement.

Central hearing disorders result from lesions of the central auditory pathways. As a rule, patients with central lesions do not have impaired hearing for pure tones, and they can understand speech as long as it is clearly spoken in a quiet environment. If the listener's task is made more difficult with the introduction of background noise or competing messages, performance deteriorates more markedly in patients with central lesions than in normal subjects.

DIAGNOSIS
Evaluation
Bedside Test
A quick test for hearing loss in the speech range is to observe the response to spoken commands at different intensities (whisper, conversation, shouting). Tuning fork tests permit a rough assessment of the hearing level for pure tones of known frequency. The clinician can use his or her own hearing level as a reference standard. In the Rinne test, nerve conduction is compared with bone conduction by holding a tuning fork (preferably 512 Hz) against the mastoid process until the sound can no longer be heard. It is then placed 1 inch from the ear and, in normal subjects, can be heard about twice as long by air as by bone. If bone conduction is better than air conduction, the hearing loss is conductive, but care must be taken to ensure that the bone conduction is not heard in the normal ear. In the Weber test, the tuning fork is placed on the patient's forehead or upper teeth. Normally, this sound is referred to the center of the head. If it is referred to the side of unilateral hearing loss, the hearing loss is conductive; if it is referred away from the side of unilateral hearing loss, the loss is sensorineural.

Audiometry
Pure tone testing is the cornerstone of most auditory examinations. Pure tones at selected frequencies are presented through either earphones (air conduction) or a vibrator pressed against the mastoid portion of the temporal bone (bone conduction), and the minimal level that the subject can hear (threshold) is determined for each frequency. Two speech tests are routinely used. The *speech reception threshold* is the intensity at which the patient can correctly repeat 50% of the words presented. The speech reception threshold is a test of hearing sensitivity for speech and should reflect the hearing level for pure tones in the speech range. The *speech discrimination test* is a measure of the patient's ability to understand speech when it is presented at a level that is easily heard. In patients with eighth nerve lesions, speech discrimination scores can be severely reduced, even when pure tone thresholds are normal or nearly

normal; by comparison, in patients with cochlear lesions, discrimination tends to be proportional to the magnitude of hearing loss.

Brain stem auditory evoked responses can be recorded from scalp electrodes at 0 to 10 msec (early), 10 to 50 msec (middle), and 50 to 500 msec (late) following a click (a high-frequency stimulus). The early potentials reflect electrical activity at the cochlea, eighth cranial nerve, and brain stem; the later potentials reflect cortical activity. Computer averaging of the responses to 1000 to 2000 clicks separates the evoked potential from background noise. Early evoked responses may be used to estimate the magnitude of hearing loss and to differentiate among cochlea, eighth nerve, and brain stem lesions.

Differential Diagnosis
Conductive Hearing Loss
The history, examination, and audiometry usually provide the key differential features for identifying common causes of hearing loss (Fig. 400-1). Asymmetric hearing loss in adults in usually idiopathic.[2]

Otosclerosis commonly produces progressive conductive hearing loss by immobilizing the stapes with new bone growth in front of and below the oval window. The hearing loss is typically conductive, although in some persons the cochlea may be invaded by foci of otosclerotic bone, producing an additional sensorineural hearing loss. Otosclerosis usually stabilizes when the hearing level reaches 50 to 60 dB and rarely progresses to deafness.

The most common cause of reversible conductive hearing loss is *impacted cerumen* in the external canal. This benign condition is usually first noticed after bathing or swimming when a droplet of water closes the remaining tiny passageway. The most common serious cause of conductive hearing loss is inflammation of the middle ear, *otitis media*, either infective (suppurative; see Fig. 398-9) or noninfective (serous). Chronic otitis media with perforation of the tympanic membrane can result in an invasion of the middle ear and other pneumatized areas of the temporal bone by keratinizing squamous epithelium (*cholesteatoma*). Cholesteatomas can produce erosion of the ossicles and bony labyrinth, thereby resulting in a mixed conductive and sensorineural hearing loss. Barotrauma to the middle ear arises with otalgia and hearing loss and can be associated with serous effusion or hematotympanum (see Fig. 398-10). Other causes of conductive hearing loss include trauma, congenital malformations of the external and middle ear, and glomus body tumors.

Sensorineural Hearing Loss
Hereditary Deafness
Genetically determined deafness, usually from hair cell aplasia or deterioration, may be present at birth or may develop in adulthood. The diagnosis of *hereditary deafness* rests on the finding of a positive family history. Mutations in connexin 26, a key component of gap junctions in the inner ear, account for most cases of recessively inherited deafness. *Intrauterine factors* resulting in congenital hearing loss include infection (especially rubella); toxic, metabolic,

and endocrine disorders; and anoxia associated with Rh incompatibility and difficult deliveries.

Cochlear Damage

Acute unilateral deafness usually has a cochlear basis. *Bacterial or viral infections* of the labyrinth, *head trauma* with fracture or hemorrhage into the cochlea, or *vascular occlusion* of a terminal branch of the anterior inferior cerebellar artery can extensively damage the cochlea and the vestibular labyrinth. An isolated sudden unilateral sensorineural hearing loss is presumed to reflect a viral infection of the cochlea and auditory nerve terminals. High-dose steroids followed by a rapid taper are recommended (see Treatment).

Sudden unilateral hearing loss often associated with vertigo and tinnitus can result from a *perilymphatic fistula*. Such fistulas may be congenital or may follow stapes surgery or head trauma.

Drugs

Drugs cause acute and subacute bilateral hearing impairment. Salicylates, furosemide, and ethacrynic acid have the potential to produce transient deafness when they are taken in high doses. More toxic to the cochlea are aminoglycoside antibiotics (gentamicin, tobramycin, amikacin, kanamycin, streptomycin, and neomycin). These agents can destroy cochlear hair cells in direct relation to their serum concentrations. Some antineoplastic chemotherapeutic agents, particularly cisplatin, cause severe ototoxicity.

Meniere Disease

Subacute relapsing cochlear deafness occurs with *Meniere disease*, a condition associated with fluctuating hearing loss and tinnitus, recurrent episodes of abrupt and often severe vertigo, and a sensation of fullness or pressure in the ear. Recurrent endolymphatic hypertension (hydrops) is believed to cause the episodes. On pathologic examination, the endolymphatic sac is dilated, and the hair cells become atrophic. The resulting deafness is subtle and reversible in the early stages but subsequently becomes permanent and is characterized by diplacusis and loudness recruitment. The disorder is usually unilateral, but in about 20 to 40% of patients, bilateral involvement eventually occurs.

Presbycusis

The gradual, progressive, bilateral hearing loss commonly associated with advancing age is called presbycusis. Presbycusis is not a distinct disease entity but rather represents multiple effects of aging on the auditory system. It may include conductive and central dysfunction, although the most consistent effect of aging is on the sensory cells and neurons of the cochlea. The typical audiogram of presbycusis is a symmetrical high-frequency hearing loss gradually sloping downward with increasing frequency. The most consistent pathologic finding associated with presbycusis is degeneration of sensory cells and nerve fibers at the base of the cochlea.

Noise

The recurrent trauma of *noise-induced hearing loss* affects approximately the same region at the base of the cochlea and is also common, particularly among those with exposure to loud explosive or industrial noises. Loud, blaring, modern music has become a recent offender. The loss almost always begins at 4000 Hz and does not affect speech discrimination until late in the disease process. With only brief exposure to loud noise (hours to days), there may be only a temporary threshold shift, but with continued exposure, permanent injury begins. The duration and intensity of exposure determine the degree of permanent injury, but estimates suggest that nearly 25% of American adults have some degree of noise-induced hearing damage or loss.[3]

Acoustic Neuroma

Progressive unilateral hearing loss, which arises insidiously, initially in the high frequencies, and worsens by almost imperceptible degrees, is characteristic of benign neoplasms of the cerebellopontine angle, most commonly *acoustic neuromas*. In about 10% of cases, the hearing loss can be acute, apparently due to either hemorrhage into the tumor or compression of the labyrinthine vasculature. Magnetic resonance imaging (MRI) with contrast enhancement reliably identifies small acoustic neuromas.

Central Hearing Loss

Central hearing loss is unilateral only if it results from damage to the pontine cochlear nuclei on one side of the brain stem from conditions such as *ischemic infarction* of the lateral brain stem (e.g., occlusion of the anterior inferior cerebellar artery [Chapter 379]), a plaque of *multiple sclerosis* (Chapter 383), or,

rarely, invasion or compression of the lateral pons by a *neoplasm* or *hematoma* (Chapters 180 and 371). Bilateral *degeneration* of the cochlear nuclei accompanies some of the rare recessive inherited disorders of childhood. As noted, clinically important unilateral hearing loss never results from neurologic disease arising rostral to the cochlear nucleus. Although bilateral hearing loss could, in theory, result from bilateral destruction of central hearing pathways, in practice this is rare because involvement of neighboring structures in the brain stem or hemisphere would usually produce overwhelming neurologic disability.

TREATMENT   Rx

If an underlying disorder has not yet destroyed the auditory system and can be ameliorated medically or surgically, hearing may be improved or preserved.[4] Most patients with otosclerosis respond to stapedectomy. Closure of a perilymph fistula may improve hearing. Antibiotic and decongestive treatment of otitis media (Chapter 398) should prevent permanent hearing loss.

A brief course of high-dose steroids is commonly used for patients with idiopathic sudden unilateral sensorineural deafness, but the evidence to support this approach is limited. Intratympanic corticosteroid treatment (four doses of 40 mg/mL of methylprednisolone during 2 weeks) is not inferior to oral treatment (60 mg/day of oral prednisone followed by a 5-day taper) for idiopathic sudden sensorineural hearing loss,[A1] and combination oral and intratympanic therapy may be better than either alone.[A2] A low-salt diet and diuretics are effective in selected cases of Meniere disease. Folic acid supplementation appears to reduce the rate of hearing loss in the elderly. Hearing aids amplify sound, usually with the goal of making speech intelligible. Patients with conductive hearing loss require simple amplification, but those with sensorineural hearing loss often need frequency-selective amplification to make hearing aids useful. Cochlear implants can markedly help patients of all ages with profound hearing loss if they have some intact auditory nerve fibers.[5] Intense postoperative speech recognition training is required.

PREVENTION

Noise-induced hearing loss can be prevented with the use of ear plugs and other noise-reducing interventions.[A3] Recent evidence also suggests that ebselen (a glutathione peroxidase 1 mimic at 400 mg twice daily 2 days before and 2 days after a noise challenge) can prevent noise-induced damage.[A4]

Tinnitus

DIAGNOSIS

As many as 10% of U.S. adults may complain of tinnitus. The evaluation of common causes of tinnitus (Fig. 400-2) begins with a careful history to identify common offending drugs.[6]

Objective Tinnitus

With objective tinnitus, the patient hears a sound arising external to the auditory system, a sound that can usually be heard by the examiner with a stethoscope. Objective tinnitus usually has benign causes, such as noise from temporomandibular joints, opening of eustachian tubes, or repetitive muscle contractions. Sometimes, in a quiet room, the patient can hear the pulsatile flow in the carotid artery or a continuous hum of normal venous outflow through the jugular vein. The latter can be obliterated by compression of the jugular vein or extreme lateral rotation of the neck. Pathologic objective tinnitus occurs when patients hear turbulent flow in vascular anomalies or tumors (e.g., glomus jugulare tumor). Objective tinnitus may also be an early sign of increased intracranial pressure. Such tinnitus, which probably arises from turbulent flow through compressed venous structures at the base of the brain, is usually overshadowed by other neurologic abnormalities.

Subjective Tinnitus

Subjective tinnitus can arise from sites anywhere in the auditory system. The sounds most frequently reported are metallic ringing; buzzing; blowing; roaring; or, less often, bizarre clanging, popping, or nonrhythmic beating. Tinnitus heard as a faint, moderately high pitched, metallic ring can be observed by almost anyone who concentrates attention on auditory events in a quiet room. Sustained louder tinnitus accompanied by audiometric evidence of deafness occurs in association with both conductive and sensorineural hearing loss. Tinnitus observed with otosclerosis tends to have a roaring or hissing quality, and that associated with Meniere disease often produces sounds that vary widely in intensity with time and quality, sometimes including roaring or clanging. Tinnitus with auditory nerve lesions tends to be higher pitched and

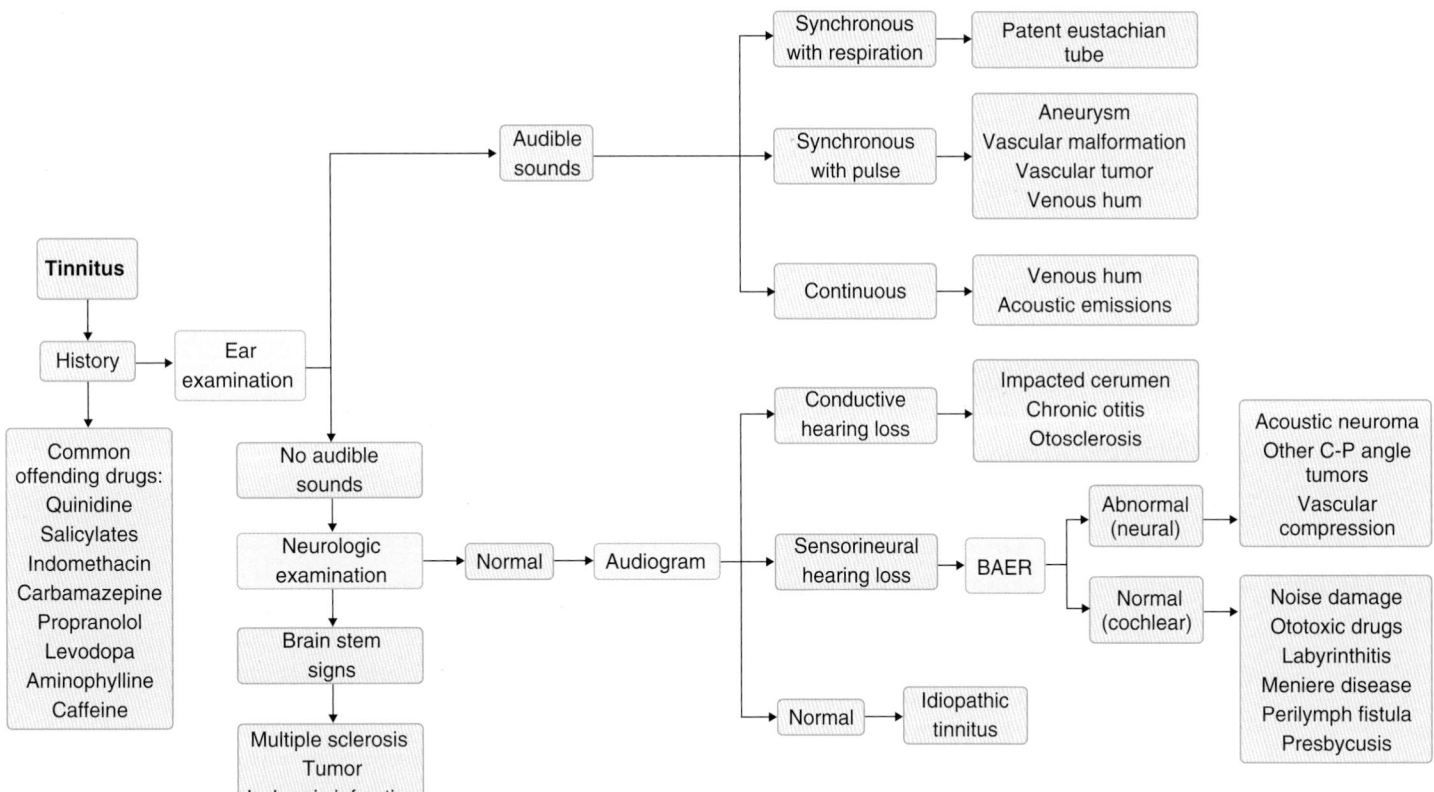

FIGURE 400-2. Evaluation of tinnitus. BAER = brain stem auditory evoked response; C-P = cerebellopontine.

ringing in quality. Audiometric and brain stem evoked response testing can help distinguish between lesions involving the conducting apparatus, the cochlea, and the auditory nerve. Tinnitus without observable deafness appears sporadically and for variable lengths of time in many persons without other evidence of an ongoing pathologic process.

TREATMENT

Most patients with tinnitus can be helped by a careful evaluation to exclude serious underlying conditions and by subsequent reassurance when appropriate.[7] Often, exacerbating factors such as chronic anxiety and depression can be treated. In patients with hearing loss and tinnitus, a hearing aid may improve tinnitus because the amplification of ambient sound may effectively mask the tinnitus. This mechanism probably explains the frequent observation that removal of cerumen from the external auditory canal to improve ambient hearing also improves tinnitus. Also, when cerumen is attached to the tympanic membrane, tinnitus may result from local mechanical effects on the conductive system. For patients who find their tinnitus most obtrusive when trying to sleep, recorded masking sounds (e.g., white noise, rainfall, mountain stream) can be helpful. A careful drug history should be taken (see Fig. 400-2), and a drug-free trial period should be considered when possible.

No medications are approved for the treatment of tinnitus in the United States or Europe. Benzodiazepines (e.g., diazepam, 2 to 5 mg every 8 hours) or tricyclic amines (e.g., amitriptyline, 25 to 75 mg at bedtime) may provide temporary symptomatic relief of tinnitus, but cognitive-behavioral therapy, which can be administered face-to-face or via the Internet, is a more effective long-term approach that can significantly decrease tinnitus and improve health-related quality of life.[A5][A6] Furthermore, some patients have varying degrees of spontaneous improvement.[8] In patients with concomitant profound bilateral sensorineural hearing loss, cochlear implants can improve hearing and often decrease tinnitus.

EQUILIBRIUM–VESTIBULAR SYSTEM

PATHOBIOLOGY
Anatomy and Physiology of the Vestibular System
The paired vestibular end organs lie within the temporal bones next to the cochlea. Each organ consists of three semicircular canals that detect angular acceleration and two otolith structures, the utricle and saccule, that detect linear acceleration (including gravitational). Like the cochlea, these organs possess hair cells that act as force transducers, converting the forces associated with head acceleration into afferent nerve impulses. The hair cells of the three semicircular canals, each of which is oriented at right angles to the others, are located in the crista, where their cilia are embedded in a gelatinous mass called the *cupula*. Movement of the head causes the endolymph to flow either toward or away from the cupula, bending the cilia and, depending on the direction of endolymphatic movements, either exciting or inhibiting the afferent nerves at the base of the hair cells. The hair cells of the utricle and saccule are located in an area called the *macule*. The macule of the utricle lies approximately in the plane of the horizontal canal, and the macule of the saccule is approximately in the plane of the anterior canal. The hair cell cilia are embedded in a membrane that contains calcium carbonate crystals or otoliths; the density of otoliths is considerably greater than that of the endolymph. Linear accelerations of the head combine with the linear acceleration of gravity to distort the otolith membrane, thereby bending the cilia of the hair cells and modulating the activity of the afferent nerve terminals at the base of the hair cells.

The afferent vestibular nerves have their cell bodies in the Scarpa ganglion. The nerve fibers travel in the vestibular portion of the eighth cranial nerve contiguous to the acoustic portion. Fibers from different receptor organs terminate in different vestibular nuclei at the pontomedullary junction. There are also direct connections with many portions of the cerebellum, the greatest representation being in the flocculonodular lobe, the so-called vestibular cerebellum.

DIAGNOSIS
Evaluation
History
Most vestibular problems presented to the physician are episodic, and often there are neither symptoms nor signs when the physician examines the patient. The history therefore can become paramount for identifying vestibular dysfunction. The history should attempt to distinguish vertigo (the illusion of movement in space) from other types of dizziness (see later).

About 12% of patients with vertigo have a central cause, and about 88% have a problem with the peripheral vestibular apparatus. In general, peripheral vertigo is more severe, is more likely to be associated with hearing loss and tinnitus, and often leads to nausea and vomiting. Nystagmus associated with peripheral vertigo is usually inhibited by visual fixation. Central vertigo is

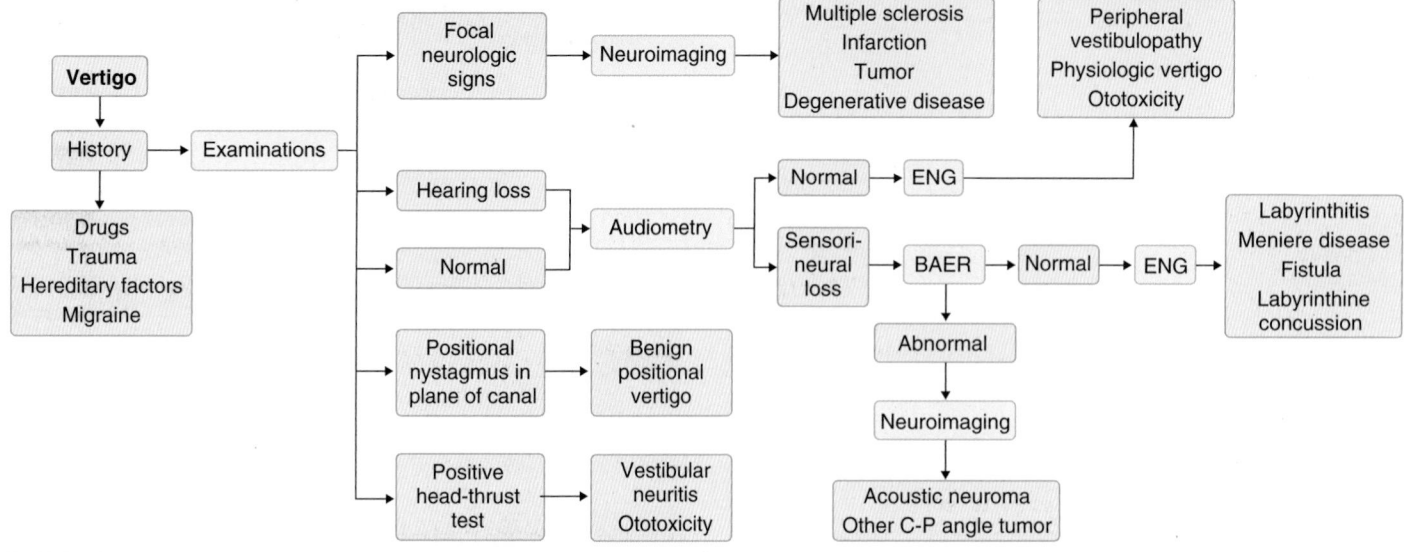

FIGURE 400-3. Evaluation of vertigo. BAER = brain stem auditory evoked response; C-P = cerebellopontine; ENG = electronystagmography.

generally less severe than peripheral vertigo and is often associated with other signs of central nervous system disease.[9] The nystagmus of central vertigo is not inhibited by visual fixation and frequently is prominent when vertigo is mild or absent.

Common Causes of Vertigo
Physiologic Vertigo
Physiologic vertigo includes common disorders that occur in healthy people, such as *motion sickness, space sickness,* and *height vertigo* (Fig. 400-3). In these conditions, vertigo (defined as an illusion of movement) is minimal while autonomic symptoms predominate. With height vertigo, patients may experience acute anxiety and panic reaction. Individuals with motion sickness and space sickness typically develop perspiration, nausea, vomiting, increased salivation, yawning, and generalized malaise. Gastric motility is reduced and digestion impaired. Even the sight or smell of food is distressing. Hyperventilation is a common sign, and the resulting hypocapnia leads to changes in blood volume, with pooling in the lower parts of the body predisposing to postural hypotension and syncope. An unusual variant of motion-induced dizziness occurs when the subject returns to stationary conditions after prolonged exposure to motion (*mal de débarquement syndrome*). Typically, affected patients report that they feel the persistent rocking sensation of a boat long after returning to solid ground. Rarely, the syndrome can last for months to years after exposure to motion and can even be incapacitating. The cause is unknown.

Physiologic vertigo can often be suppressed by supplying sensory cues that help to match the signals originating from different sensory systems. Thus motion sickness, which is caused by a mismatch of visual and vestibular signals, is exacerbated by sitting in a closed space or reading (giving the visual system the miscue that the environment is stationary). It may be improved by looking out at the horizon. Height vertigo, caused by a mismatch between sensation of normal body sway and lack of its visual detection, can often be relieved either by sitting or by visually fixating a nearby stationary object.

Benign Paroxysmal Positional Vertigo (Canalithiasis)
Benign paroxysmal positional vertigo is by far the most common cause of vertigo.[10] Patients with this condition develop brief episodes of vertigo (less than 1 minute) with position change, typically when turning over in bed, getting in and out of bed, bending over and straightening up, or extending the neck to look up (so-called top-shelf vertigo). Benign paroxysmal positional vertigo results when otolith debris inadvertently enters one of the semicircular canals. It can occur after head trauma or inner ear infection but most commonly occurs spontaneously in older people and particularly in older women with osteoporosis. The diagnosis rests on finding characteristic positional nystagmus in the plane of the affected canal (see later). It is important to recognize this syndrome because, in most patients, it can be cured by simple bedside maneuvers (Fig. 400-4). If the history or findings are atypical, the condition must be distinguished from other causes of positional vertigo that may occur with tumors or infarcts of the posterior fossa.

Acute Peripheral Vestibulopathy (Vestibular Neuritis)
One of the most common clinical neurologic syndromes at any age is the acute onset of vertigo, nausea, and vomiting lasting for several days and not associated with auditory or neurologic symptoms. A viral origin is suspected, but attempts to isolate an agent have been unsuccessful, except for occasional findings of a herpes zoster infection. Pathologic studies showing atrophy of one or more vestibular nerve trunks, with or without atrophy of their associated sense organs, are evidence of a vestibular nerve site and, probably, viral cause for most patients with this syndrome. Patients gradually improve during 1 to 2 weeks, but residual dizziness and imbalance can persist for months.

Meniere Disease
Meniere disease (see earlier) accounts for about 10% of all patients with vertigo.[11] The diagnosis is based on documenting episodic severe attacks accompanied by fluctuating hearing levels on audiometric testing beginning in the low frequencies.

Migraine
Vertigo is a common symptom with migraine (Chapter 370). It can occur with headaches or in separate isolated episodes, and it can predate the onset of headache. So-called benign paroxysmal vertigo of childhood is often the first symptom of migraine. The mechanism of vertigo with migraine is not clear, but both peripheral and central types of nystagmus can occur with attacks. A few develop typical features of Meniere disease.

Post-traumatic Vertigo
Vertigo, hearing loss, and tinnitus often follow a blow to the head (Chapter 371) that does not result in temporal bone fracture, termed *labyrinthine concussion*. Blows to the occipital or mastoid region are particularly likely to produce labyrinthine damage. *Transverse fractures* of the temporal bone typically pass through the vestibule of the inner ear, tearing the membranous labyrinth and lacerating the vestibular and cochlear nerves. Complete loss of vestibular and cochlear function is the usual sequela, and the facial nerve is interrupted in approximately 50% of cases. Examination of the ear often reveals hemotympanum (see Fig. 398-10), but bleeding from the ear seldom occurs because the tympanic membrane usually remains intact. As noted earlier, *benign paroxysmal positional vertigo* is also a common sequela of head trauma. *Fistulas* of the oval and round windows can result from impact noise, deep-water diving, severe physical exertion, or blunt head injury without skull fracture. Clinically, the rupture leads to the sudden onset of vertigo or hearing loss, or both. Surgical exploration of the middle ear is warranted when there is a clear relationship between the onset of vertigo or hearing loss, or both, and the onset of severe exertion, barometric change, head injury, or impact noise.

Postconcussion Syndrome
The so-called postconcussion syndrome refers to a vague dizziness (not vertigo) associated with anxiety, difficulty in concentrating, headache, and photophobia induced by a head injury resulting in concussion (Chapter 371). On occasion,

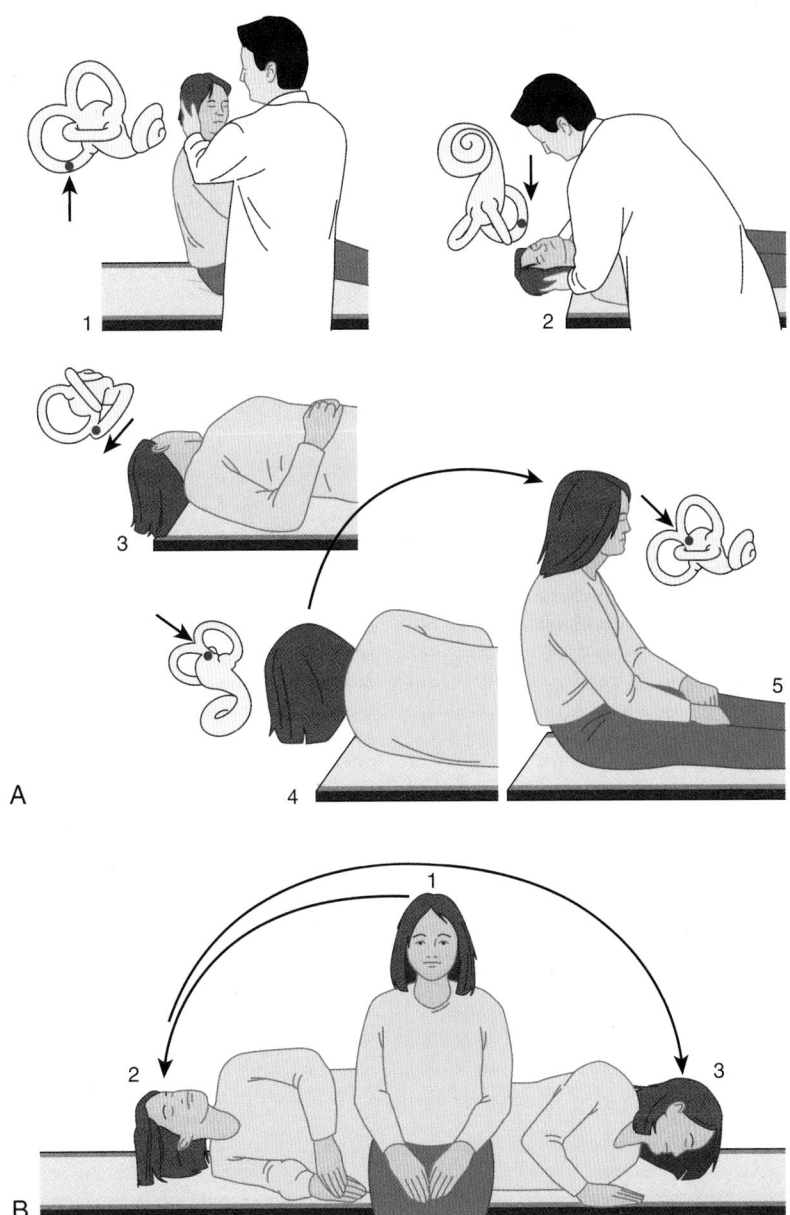

FIGURE 400-4. Modified Epley (A) and Semont (B) maneuvers for benign positional vertigo affecting the right posterior semicircular canal. The procedure is reversed to treat the left posterior semicircular canal. The entire sequence should be repeated until no nystagmus is elicited. (From Fife TD, Iverson DJ, Lempert T, et al. Practice parameter: therapies for benign paroxysmal positional vertigo [an evidence-based review]: report of the Quality Standards Subcommittee of the American Academy of Neurology. *Neurology.* 2008;70:2067-2074.)

similar but less pronounced symptoms are associated with mild head injury judged to be trivial at the time. The cause is unknown, but animal studies indicate that small multifocal brain lesions (petechiae) commonly occur after concussive brain injury.

Other Peripheral Causes of Vertigo

Vertigo can be associated with *chronic bacterial otomastoiditis,* either from direct invasion of the inner ear by the bacteria or by erosion of the labyrinth by a cholesteatoma. Radiographic studies of the temporal bone readily identify these disorders. *Autoimmune inner ear disease* typically arises with episodic vertigo and fluctuating hearing levels similar to Meniere disease, but it is more fulminant with early bilateral involvement. It can occur in isolation or with other systemic features of autoimmune disease. About two thirds of patients have antibodies directed against heat shock protein 70. The aminoglycosides streptomycin and gentamicin are remarkably selective for vestibular ototoxicity. The patient may suffer acute vertigo if the toxic effect is asymmetrical. More often, there is a progressive symmetrical loss of vestibular function leading to imbalance but not vertigo. Unfortunately, many patients being treated with ototoxic drugs are initially bedridden and unaware of the vestibular impairment until they recover from their acute illness and try to walk. They then discover that they are unsteady on their feet and that the environment tends to jiggle in front of their eyes (*oscillopsia*). The diagnosis can be made

at the bedside with a head-thrust test (bilateral corrective saccades; see later). Caloric and rotational testing can confirm the vestibular loss. The best treatment is prevention. If the drug is discontinued early during the course of symptoms, the disorder may stabilize or improve.

Vascular Insufficiency

Vertebrobasilar insufficiency is a common cause of vertigo in older people. Whether the vertigo originates from ischemia of the labyrinth, brain stem, or both structures is not always clear because the blood supplies to the labyrinth, eighth cranial nerve, and vestibular nuclei originate from the same source, the basilar vertebral circulation (Chapter 378). Vertigo with *vertebrobasilar insufficiency* is abrupt in onset, usually lasting several minutes, and is frequently associated with nausea and vomiting. Associated symptoms resulting from ischemia in the remaining territory supplied by the posterior circulation include visual illusions and hallucinations, drop attacks and weakness, visceral sensations, visual field defects, diplopia, and headache. These symptoms occur in episodes either in combination with the vertigo or alone. Vertigo may be an isolated initial symptom of vertebrobasilar ischemia, but repeated episodes of vertigo without other symptoms should suggest another diagnosis. Vertebrobasilar insufficiency is usually caused by atherosclerosis of the subclavian, vertebral, and basilar arteries. MRI of the brain is usually normal because the vascular insufficiency is transient and function returns to normal between episodes. Magnetic resonance angiography can identify occlusive vascular disease most commonly involving the vertebral-basilar junction.

Vertigo is a common symptom with *infarction of the lateral brain stem* or *cerebellum* (Chapter 379), or both. The diagnosis is usually clear, based on the characteristic acute history and pattern of associated symptoms and neurologic findings. On occasion, cerebellar infarction or hemorrhage arises with severe vertigo, vomiting, and ataxia without associated brain stem symptoms and signs that might suggest the erroneous diagnosis of an acute peripheral vestibular disorder. The key differential is the finding of clear cerebellar signs (extremity and gait ataxia); direction-changing, gaze-evoked nystagmus; and a normal head-thrust test. Such patients must be watched carefully for several days because they may develop progressive brain stem dysfunction due to compression by a swollen cerebellum.

Cerebellopontine Angle Tumors

Most tumors growing in the cerebellopontine angle (e.g., *acoustic neuroma, meningioma, epidermal cyst*) grow slowly, allowing the vestibular system to accommodate so that they produce only a vague sensation of disequilibrium rather than acute vertigo (Chapter 180). On occasion, however, episodic vertigo or positional vertigo heralds the presence of a cerebellopontine angle tumor. In virtually all patients, retrocochlear hearing loss is present, best identified by audiometric testing. MRI with contrast enhancement is the most sensitive diagnostic study for identifying a cerebellopontine angle tumor.

Other Central Causes of Vertigo

Acute vertigo may be the first symptom of *multiple sclerosis* (Chapter 383), although only a small percentage of young patients with acute vertigo eventually develop multiple sclerosis. Vertigo in multiple sclerosis is usually transient and often associated with other neurologic signs of brain stem disease, in particular, internuclear ophthalmoplegia or cerebellar dysfunction. Vertigo may also be a symptom of *parainfectious encephalomyelitis* or, rarely, *parainfectious cranial polyneuritis*. In this instance the accompanying neurologic signs establish the diagnosis. The *Ramsay Hunt syndrome* (geniculate ganglion herpes) is characterized by vertigo and hearing loss associated with facial paralysis and, sometimes, pain in the ear. The typical lesions of herpes zoster (Chapter 351), which may follow the appearance of neurologic signs, are found in the external auditory canal and over the palate in some patients. Rarely is herpes zoster responsible for vertigo in the absence of the full-blown syndrome. *Granulomatous meningitis* (Chapter 384) or *leptomeningeal metastasis* and cerebral or systemic *vasculitis* (Chapter 254) may involve the eighth nerve, producing vertigo as an early symptom. In these disorders, cerebrospinal fluid analysis usually suggests the diagnosis (Chapter 368). Patients suffering from *temporal lobe epilepsy* (Chapter 375) occasionally experience vertigo as the aura. Vertigo in the absence of other neurologic signs or symptoms is never caused by epilepsy or other diseases of the cerebral hemispheres.

Bedside Tests
Hyperventilation

If the history is not clear, bedside provocative tests to mimic the symptom may assist in making a pathophysiologic diagnosis. Hyperventilation, which lowers the arterial partial pressure of carbon dioxide ($Paco_2$) and decreases cerebral blood flow, causes a lightheaded sensation associated with syncope. Patients with compressive lesions of the vestibular nerve, such as with an acoustic neuroma or cholesteatoma, or with demyelination of the vestibular nerve root entry zone may develop vertigo and nystagmus after hyperventilation. Presumably, metabolic changes associated with hyperventilation trigger the partially damaged nerve to fire inappropriately.

Vestibulospinal Function

Bedside tests of vestibulospinal function are often insensitive because most patients can use vision and proprioceptive signals to compensate for any vestibular loss. Patients with acute unilateral peripheral vestibular lesions may past-point or fall toward the side of the lesion, but within a few days, balance returns to normal. Patients with bilateral peripheral vestibular loss have more difficulty compensating and usually show some imbalance on the Romberg and tandem walking tests (Chapter 368), particularly with eyes closed.

Doll's-Eye and Head-Thrust Tests

The vestibulo-ocular reflex can be tested at the bedside with the doll's-eye and head-thrust tests. In an alert human, rotating the head back and forth in the horizontal plane induces compensatory horizontal eye movements that are dependent on both the visual and vestibular systems. The doll's-eye test

is a test of vestibular function in a comatose patient (Chapter 376) because such patients cannot generate pursuit or corrective fast components. In this setting, conjugate compensatory eye movements indicate normally functioning vestibulo-ocular pathways. Because the vestibulo-ocular reflex has a much higher frequency range than the smooth pursuit system, a qualitative bedside test of vestibular function can be made with the *head-thrust test*. It is performed by grasping the patient's head and applying brief, small-amplitude, high-acceleration head thrusts first to one side and then the other. The patient fixates on the examiner's nose and the examiner watches for corrective saccades, which are a sign of an inappropriate compensatory slow phase.

Caloric Test

The caloric test induces endolymphatic flow in the horizontal semicircular canal and horizontal nystagmus by creating a temperature gradient from one side of the canal to the other. With a cold caloric stimulus, the column of endolymph nearest the middle ear falls because of its increased density. This causes the cupula to deviate away from the utricle (ampullofugal flow) and produces horizontal nystagmus with the fast phase directed away from the stimulated ear. A warm stimulus produces the opposite effect, causing ampullopetal endolymph flow and nystagmus directed toward the stimulated ear (a mnemonic is COWS, meaning cold opposite, warm same). Because of its ready availability, ice water (approximately 0° C) can be used for bedside caloric testing. To bring the horizontal canal into the vertical plane, the patient lies in the supine position with head tilted 30 degrees forward. Infusion of 1 to 3 mL of ice water induces a burst of nystagmus usually lasting about a minute. Greater than a 20% asymmetry in nystagmus duration suggests a lesion on the side of the decreased response. The ice water caloric test is a useful way to test the integrity of the oculomotor pathways in a comatose patient. In this case ice water induces only a slow tonic deviation toward the side of stimulation.

Positional Tests

Examination for pathologic vestibular nystagmus should include a search for spontaneous and positional nystagmus (see Table 396-4). Because vestibular nystagmus secondary to peripheral vestibular lesions is inhibited with fixation, the yield is increased by impairing fixation with +30 lenses (Frenzel glasses) or infrared video recordings. Two types of positional testing are typically performed: moving the patient from the sitting to head-hanging-right and head-hanging-left positions (Dix-Hallpike test) and turning the head to the right and left while the patient lies supine.[12] Induced positional nystagmus may be paroxysmal or persistent, and it may be in the same direction in all positions or change directions in different positions. The most common cause of positional nystagmus is otolith debris in the semicircular canals, either free floating (paroxysmal) or attached to the cupula (persistent). This type of nystagmus always occurs in the plane of the affected canal—vertical torsional for the vertical canals and horizontal torsional for the horizontal canal. By contrast, central positional nystagmus is often pure vertical or horizontal and cannot be explained by stimulating a single semicircular canal.

Nystagmography

Nystagmography tests oculomotor control by inducing and recording eye movements. A standard test battery includes (1) tests of visual ocular control (saccades, smooth pursuit, and optokinetic nystagmus), (2) a careful search for pathologic nystagmus with fixation and with eyes open in darkness, and (3) the measurement of induced vestibular nystagmus (caloric and rotational). Nystagmography can be helpful in identifying a vestibular lesion and localizing it within the peripheral and central pathways.

Evaluating the "Dizzy" Patient

The history is key because it determines the type of dizziness (Table 400-1), associated symptoms (neurologic, audiologic, cardiac, psychiatric), precipitating factors (position change, trauma, stress, drug ingestion), and predisposing illness (systemic viral infection, cardiac disease, cerebrovascular disease).[13] The history provides direction for both the examination and the diagnostic evaluation. When focal neurologic signs are found, neuroimaging usually leads to a specific diagnosis. When vertigo is present without focal neurologic symptoms or signs, head-thrust and positional testing are key to localizing the lesion to the labyrinth or eighth nerve.[14] Audiometry and nystagmography are useful if the cause of vertigo is not clear after the history and examination. Patients with psychogenic dizziness (also called chronic subjective dizziness or persistent perceptual-postural dizziness) should be identified early so that needless tests are not obtained. A detailed cardiac evaluation (including loop monitoring) often identifies the cause of episodic near-fainting (Chapters 45 and 56).

TABLE 400-1	DESCRIPTION, MECHANISM, AND FOCUS OF DIAGNOSTIC WORK-UP FOR COMMON TYPES OF DIZZINESS		
TYPE OF DIZZINESS	**DESCRIPTION**	**MECHANISM**	**FOCUS OF DIAGNOSTIC EVALUATION**
Vertigo	Spinning (environment moves), tilt, drunkenness	Imbalance in tonic vestibular activity	Auditory and vestibular systems
Near-faint	Lightheaded, swimming	Decreased blood flow to entire brain	Cardiovascular system
Psychogenic	Dissociated from body, spinning inside (environment still)	Impaired central integration of sensory signals	Psychiatric assessment
Disequilibrium	Off balance, unsteady on feet	Loss of vestibulospinal, proprioceptive, cerebellar, or motor function	Neurologic assessment

TABLE 400-2	TREATMENT OF COMMON VERTIGO SYNDROMES	
SYNDROME	**TREATMENT**	
Benign positional vertigo		
Posterior canal variant	Epley maneuver (see Fig. 400-4)	
Horizontal canal variant	Barbecue roll toward normal side (side with less nystagmus), sleep with normal ear down	
Vestibular neuritis	Methylprednisolone, 100 mg × 3 days, gradual taper during 22 days (must start within 3 days of onset)	
Meniere disease		
Medical	Low salt (1-2 g salt/day) *and* either hydrochlorothiazide 25-50 mg/day *or* hydrochlorothiazide 25 mg/day plus triamterene 50 mg/day	
Surgical	Intratympanic gentamicin, vestibular nerve section	

TREATMENT Rx

Treatment of vertigo can be divided into three general categories: specific, symptomatic, and rehabilitative. When possible, treatment should be directed at the underlying disorder (Table 400-2). Specific therapies include particle repositioning maneuvers (the Epley and Semont maneuvers; see Fig. 400-4) for benign paroxysmal positional vertigo.[A7] For vestibular neuritis, steroids (e.g., methylprednisolone, 1 mg/kg/day for 5 days, then tapered during the next 15 days) are effective, at least for the short term, but antiviral agents are not. For Meniere disease, a low-salt diet and diuretics (e.g., 25 mg hydrochlorothiazide and 50 mg triamterene daily) are effective in some cases. Intratympanic methylprednisolone can significantly reduce vertiginous attacks in patients with refractory unilateral Meniere disease.[A8] Another option is intratympanic gentamicin, which also can significantly reduce vertigo in patients with refractory unilateral Meniere disease, but its ototoxicity will cause a permanent vestibular defect. Endolymphatic duct blockage is a potential option for medically refractory Meniere disease.[A9]

In many cases, however, symptomatic treatment either is combined with specific therapy or is the only treatment available. Many different classes of drugs have been found to have antivertiginous properties, and in most instances, the exact mechanism of action is uncertain. All these agents produce potentially unpleasant side effects, and the decision concerning which drug or combination to use is based on their known complications and on the severity and duration of the vertigo. An episode of prolonged, severe vertigo is one of the most distressing symptoms that a patient can experience. Affected patients prefer to lie still with eyes closed in a quiet, dark room. Antivertiginous drugs, such as dimenhydrinate (25 mg) or diazepam (5 mg), may be helpful. Promethazine suppositories (25 mg) are useful in patients with vomiting.

In more chronic vertiginous disorders, when the patient is trying to carry on normal activity, less sedating antivertiginous medications, such as meclizine (25 mg) or transdermal scopolamine (0.5 mg every 3 days), may provide relief. Chronic use of these drugs should be avoided.

Vestibular rehabilitation exercises are designed to help the patient compensate for permanent loss of vestibular function.[A10] As the acute stage of nausea and vomiting subsides, the patient should attempt to focus the eyes and to move and hold them in the direction that provokes the most dizziness. A useful exercise involves staring at a visual target while oscillating the head from side to side or up and down, slow at first and then fast. The patient should try to stand and walk, at first in contact with a wall or with an assistant, and make slow supported turns. As improvement occurs, head movements should be added while standing and walking.

PROGNOSIS

Vertigo commonly resolves, either because patients become truly asymptomatic or adjust to occasional symptoms. Among patients diagnosed with a peripheral cause of vertigo, the 30-day risk of accidental injury is less than 0.2%, as is the 30-day risk of stroke.[15]

Grade A References

A1. Qiang Q, Wu X, Yang T, et al. A comparison between systemic and intratympanic steroid therapies as initial therapy for idiopathic sudden sensorineural hearing loss: a meta-analysis. *Acta Otolaryngol.* 2017;137:598-605.

A2. Han X, Yin X, Du X, et al. Combined intratympanic and systemic use of steroids as a first-line treatment for sudden sensorineural hearing loss: a meta-analysis of randomized, controlled trials. *Otol Neurotol.* 2017;38:487-495.

A3. Tikka C, Verbeek JH, Kateman E, et al. Interventions to prevent occupational noise-induced hearing loss. *Cochrane Database Syst Rev.* 2017;7:CD006396.

A4. Kil J, Lobarinas E, Spankovich C, et al. Safety and efficacy of ebselen for the prevention of noise-induced hearing loss: a randomised, double-blind, placebo-controlled, phase 2 trial. *Lancet.* 2017; 390:969-979.

A5. Zenner HP, Delb W, Kroner-Herwig B, et al. A multidisciplinary systematic review of the treatment for chronic idiopathic tinnitus. *Eur Arch Otorhinolaryngol.* 2017;274:2079-2091.

A6. Beukes EW, Andersson G, Allen PM, et al. Effectiveness of guided internet-based cognitive behavioral therapy vs face-to-face clinical care for treatment of tinnitus: a randomized clinical trial. *JAMA Otolaryngol Head Neck Surg.* 2018;144:1126-1133.

A7. Zhang X, Qian X, Lu L, et al. Effects of Semont maneuver on benign paroxysmal positional vertigo: a meta-analysis. *Acta Otolaryngol.* 2017;137:63-70.

A8. Patel M, Agarwal K, Arshad Q, et al. Intratympanic methylprednisolone versus gentamicin in patients with unilateral Ménière's disease: a randomised, double-blind, comparative effectiveness trial. *Lancet.* 2016;388:2753-2762.

A9. Saliba I, Gabra N, Alzahrani M, et al. Endolymphatic duct blockage: a randomized controlled trial of a novel surgical technique for Ménière's disease treatment. *Otolaryngol Head Neck Surg.* 2015; 152:122-129.

A10. McDonnell MN, Hillier SL. Vestibular rehabilitation for unilateral peripheral vestibular dysfunction. *Cochrane Database Syst Rev.* 2015;1:CD005397.

GENERAL REFERENCES

For the General References and other additional features, please visit Expert Consult at https://expertconsult.inkling.com.

401

THROAT DISORDERS

PAUL W. FLINT

Nearly every systemic and infectious disease results in head and neck manifestations, with the majority affecting the upper aerodigestive tract. Diseases of the upper aerodigestive system include infection (acute and chronic; viral, bacterial, and fungal), systemic disease, and neoplasm (Chapter 181), some of which require urgent care or referral to an otolaryngologist.

Abnormalities of swallowing, respiratory function, voice, and speech are influenced by the anatomic site involved, the host's immune status and inflammatory response, the severity of the disease process, and the presence or absence of neurologic involvement.

In a patient with hoarseness, current clinical practice guidelines recommend visualization of the larynx for symptoms that persist for 3 months or longer; however, warning signs of a potentially serious or emergent throat condition warrant referral regardless of duration. These conditions include persistent throat pain with or without trismus, difficulty in swallowing, difficulty in breathing, hemoptysis, and ear pain with normal ear examination findings.

Diagnostic testing options, which include fiberoptic examination, imaging, pulmonary function studies, and laboratory testing, are directed by history, symptoms, and physical findings.

● ANATOMY OF THE UPPER AERODIGESTIVE TRACT

The pharynx is divided into three anatomic regions (Fig. 401-1). The *nasopharynx* is the region above the soft palate and uvula. Its anatomic components include the adenoids, the openings of the eustachian tubes, Rosenmüller fossa at the junction of the posterior and lateral walls, and the posterior aspect of the inferior turbinates of the nasal cavity. Diseases of the nasopharynx typically produce few symptoms until the process is well advanced and causes nasal obstruction (Chapter 398), epistaxis (Chapter 398), ear pain (Chapter 398), headache (Chapter 370), or cranial nerve abnormalities due to extension to the skull base. The *oropharynx* begins at the level of the soft palate and extends inferiorly to the tip of the epiglottis. This region includes the faucial tonsils, the base of the tongue, the lingual tonsils, the soft palate, the uvula, and part of the posterior pharyngeal wall. The *hypopharynx*, which extends from the tip of the epiglottis to the upper esophagus (the cricopharyngeus muscle) below, includes the larynx (epiglottis, arytenoids, glottis or true vocal cords), the piriform sinuses (pharyngeal folds lateral to the larynx), and the posterior pharyngeal wall. The tip of the epiglottis can be visualized by an experienced examiner with use of a laryngeal mirror or sometimes even on a routine oral examination with just a flashlight and tongue blade. The nasopharynx and hypopharynx are best visualized with a flexible fiberoptic nasopharyngoscope.

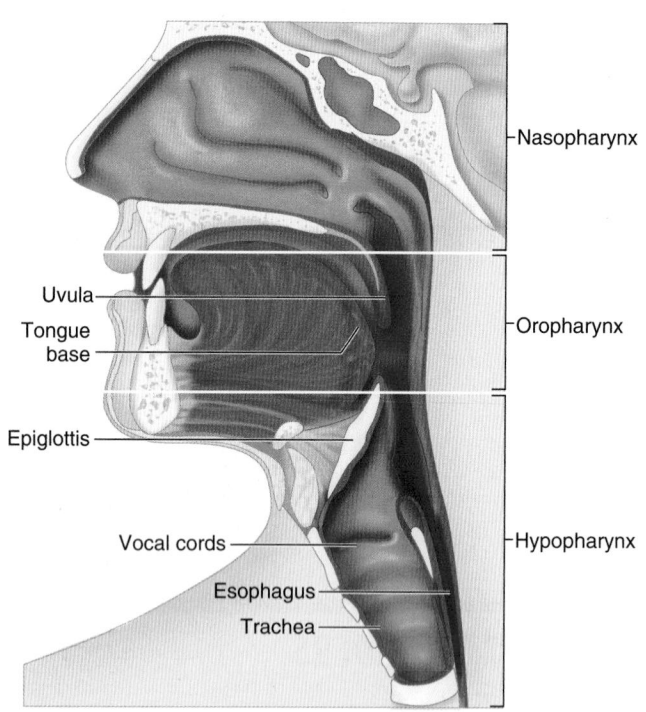

FIGURE 401-1. The pharynx (throat) is typically divided into three distinct anatomic regions (nasopharynx, oropharynx, and hypopharynx). (Courtesy Thomas A. Tami, MD.)

● INFECTIOUS DISEASES OF THE UPPER AERODIGESTIVE SYSTEM

Infectious disorders of the upper aerodigestive tract typically are manifested as sore throat (pharyngitis), changes in voice (laryngitis), or both.[1] The clinical evaluation must differentiate among bacterial (usually streptococcus [Chapter 274]), viral, and other infections and systemic causes (Table 401-1). Clinical differentiation of sore throat is critical to primary care and emergency management of the airway.

Pharyngitis

Bacterial infection accounts for approximately 5 to 10% of pharyngitis in adults compared with 30 to 40% in children. Unfortunately, as many as two thirds of adults with a sore throat are prescribed antibiotics.

STREPTOCOCCAL INFECTIONS

Group A β-hemolytic *Streptococcus pyogenes* (Chapter 274) is the most common cause of bacterial pharyngitis in adults, although it accounts for only 10% of all pharyngitis in adults. Infection is manifested with the rapid onset of sore throat, often accompanied by pain with swallowing, fever, chills, malaise, headache, mild neck stiffness, and anorexia. Hypertrophic tonsils with exudates, foul breath, and tender cervical adenopathy are hallmark findings. Some patients have palatal petechiae or a scarlatiniform rash. Rhinorrhea, hoarseness, cough, conjunctivitis, diarrhea, and ulcerative oral lesions are less common.

Untreated group A β-hemolytic *S. pyogenes* pharyngitis usually resolves within 3 to 7 days. The administration of antibiotics within 24 to 48 hours reduces pain by approximately 1 day,[A1] whereas both immediate and delayed antibiotics reduce the risk for suppurative complications.[A2] Antibiotics also reduce the contagious period from 2 weeks to 24 hours after administration. For prevention of rheumatic fever (Chapter 274), antibiotic therapy must be started within 10 days after the onset of symptoms. The risk for acute poststreptococcal glomerulonephritis (Chapter 113), however, is not affected by antibiotics.

To minimize the potential side effects and costs of unnecessary antibiotics, antibiotic therapy should be based on the presence of fever, tender anterior cervical adenopathy, tonsillar swelling or exudates, age, and the absence of cough. A rapid antigen test should be obtained in patients with three or more (or perhaps two or more) criteria (Table 401-2),[2] and a negative result is sufficiently accurate to avoid the use of unnecessary antibiotics.[3] If the rapid antigen test result is negative but the clinical suspicion remains high, a throat culture specimen should be obtained for confirmation before starting antibiotics.

Antibiotic options (Chapter 274) include penicillin (penicillin VK, 250 mg three times a day or 500 mg twice a day for 5 to 10 days), which is usually chosen to treat acute bacterial pharyngitis,[A3] although cefuroxime axetil (250 mg twice a day for 5 to 10 days) is even more effective for primary treatment and can be effective for persistent infection. In patients with proven recurrent infections, clindamycin (300 mg orally three times a day for 10 days) or amoxicillin–clavulanic acid (875 mg orally twice a day, or 500 mg three times a day for 10 days) is recommended. For patients who are allergic to penicillin, azithromycin (500 mg/day for 3 days) is another alternative. Evidence also suggests that a single dose of oral or intramuscular corticosteroids given at the start of treatment will reduce the pain of severe pharyngitis, especially in children.[A4] In patients with recurrent symptomatic episodes despite appropriate antimicrobial therapy, tonsillectomy can decrease future throat infections, at least in the short-term compared with continued observation.[A5]

TABLE 401-1 CLINICAL DIFFERENTIATION OF COMMON CONDITIONS ARISING AS SORE THROAT				
FEATURE	**VIRAL PHARYNGITIS**	**BACTERIAL TONSILLITIS**	**PERITONSILLAR ABSCESS**	**EPIGLOTTITIS**
Tonsillar enlargement	Usual	Often	None	None
Tonsillar exudates	Occasional (infectious mononucleosis)	Usual	Often	None
Tonsillar asymmetry	None	None	Usual	None
Trismus (inability to open jaw)	None	None	Usual	None
Cervical adenopathy	Occasional	Usual (tender)	Usual (tender)	None
Tender larynx	Rare	None	None	Usual

From Tami TA. Throat disorders. In: Goldman L, Schafer AI, eds. *Goldman's Cecil Medicine.* 24th ed. Philadelphia: Elsevier Saunders; 2012.

TABLE 401-2	GUIDELINES FOR THE MANAGEMENT OF PHARYNGITIS	
CENTOR SCORE*	**PERCENTAGE POSITIVE FOR *STREPTOCOCCUS* INFECTION**	**ACP/CDC GUIDELINES†**
0	7%	Do not test, do not treat
1	12%	Do not test, do not treat
2	21%	} Treat if rapid test result positive
3	38%	
4	57%	

*Calculated as follows: 1 point each for temperature >38° C, absence of cough, presence of swollen and tender anterior cervical nodes, tonsillar swelling or exudate, or age 3 to 14 years; and −1 point for age ≥45 years.
†See Harris AM, Hicks LA, Qaseem A. Appropriate antibiotic use for acute respiratory tract infection in adults: advice for high-value care from the American College of Physicians and the Centers for Disease Control and Prevention. *Ann Intern Med.* 2016;164:425-434.
ACP = American College of Physicians; CDC = Centers for Disease Control.

Non–group A β-hemolytic streptococcal infections (Chapter 274), including groups B, C, and G, can cause acute pharyngitis with a clinical picture that mirrors that of group A β-hemolytic streptococcal pharyngitis. Glomerulonephritis is a known sequela, whereas rheumatic fever is not. Penicillin or clindamycin, as prescribed for group A β-hemolytic streptococcus, provides adequate coverage.

NONSTREPTOCOCCAL BACTERIAL PHARYNGITIS
A variety of bacteria other than streptococci can infect the throat. For example, *Fusobacterium necrophorum*-positive pharyngitis, which clinically resembles streptococcal pharyngitis, occurs more frequently than group A β-hemolytic streptococcus–positive pharyngitis in a student population.[4] *Staphylococcus aureus* (Chapter 272) infections, whether caused by methicillin-resistant (MRSA) or methicillin-sensitive (MSSA) strains, usually are manifested with chronic hoarseness. About 30% of patients with bacterial laryngitis will have MRSA infection.[5] Laryngoscopy typically reveals thickened erythematous vocal folds with edema, whitish debris, and crusting, which may resemble leukoplakia (Fig. 401-2). Trimethoprim-sulfamethoxazole (160 mg/800 mg twice daily for 2 to 4 weeks) is generally effective, but treatment should be guided by antibiotic sensitivities.

Bordetella pertussis (Chapter 297) infections have become more common in adults because of their gradual loss of immune protection after vaccination. Adults typically present with cough, often but not always accompanied by nonspecific upper respiratory symptoms, fever, and leukocytosis. A *B. pertussis* serum immunoglobulin G titer higher than 27 IU/mL is highly predictive of recent infection. Erythromycin (500 mg four times a day for 14 days) or azithromycin (500 mg single dose orally on day 1, then 250 mg daily on days 2 through 5) is effective treatment.

Neisseria gonorrhoeae (Chapter 283) can cause sexually transmitted gingivitis, stomatitis, glossitis, and pharyngitis, especially in men who have sex with men. Treatment is the same as for urogenital disease and should include treatment for chlamydia. Options include ceftriaxone, 250 mg intramuscularly in a single dose; azithromycin, 1 g orally in a single dose; and doxycycline, 100 mg orally twice daily for 7 days. *Treponema pallidum* (Chapter 303) can cause oral and oropharyngeal ulcerations that involve the lips, tongue, and tonsil. Treatment is the same as that recommended for systemic disease. *Chlamydia* (Chapter 302), which is commonly associated with pneumonia and bronchitis, also can cause pharyngitis and hoarseness, sometimes as its presenting symptoms. *Mycoplasma pneumoniae* (Chapter 301), which frequently accounts for 15 to 20% of cases of community-acquired pneumonias, also can cause sore throat, nasal congestion, and coryza. Treatment of chlamydia and mycoplasma infections with tetracyclines, macrolides, and quinolones is the same as for the pneumonias they cause (Chapters 301 and 302).

Francisella tularensis (Chapter 295) is a gram-negative bacillus that causes tularemia. Oropharyngeal involvement is associated with fever, pharyngeal erythema, exudative tonsillitis, and tender lymphadenopathy. A false-positive monospot test result and atypical lymphocytosis can mimic infectious mononucleosis. The organism is sensitive to macrolides, fluoroquinolones, and tetracyclines.

Corynebacterium diphtheriae infection (Chapter 276) involves the mucosal surfaces of the upper respiratory tract, where it causes a patchy gray-black pseudomembrane in the nasopharynx, oropharynx, larynx, and trachea. About 75% of patients complain of throat pain. Airway obstruction and severe

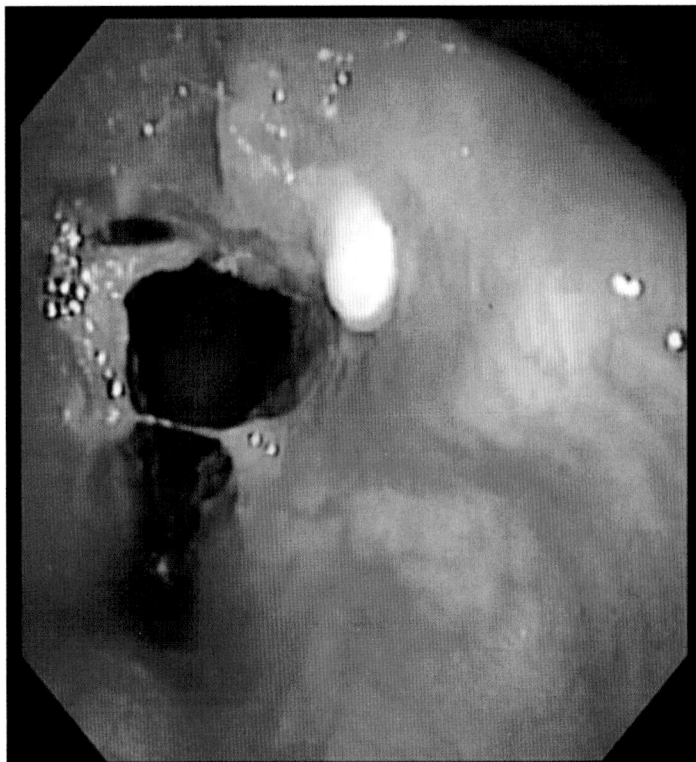

FIGURE 401-2. Fiberoptic laryngoscopy demonstrating chronic laryngitis secondary to methicillin-sensitive *Staphylococcus aureus* infection. Diagnosis is based on culture and biopsy.

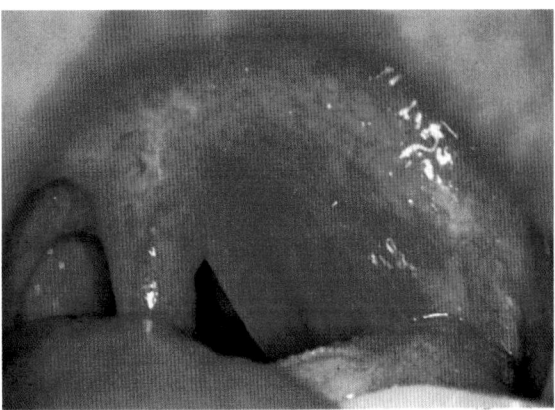

FIGURE 401-3. Left peritonsillar abscess identified by bulging anterior pillar and soft palate with midline shift. (Courtesy Thomas A. Tami, MD.)

dysphagia are life-threatening sequelae. Antitoxin is given in combination with penicillin, erythromycin, tetracycline, clindamycin, or rifampin.

Arcanobacterium haemolyticum (Chapter 276) is a gram-positive bacillus that can cause pneumonia, meningitis, osteomyelitis, brain abscess, and peritonsillar abscess in both normal and immunocompromised patients. Uncomplicated pharyngitis may be treated with erythromycin (250 mg four times a day). Complicated infections require intravenous dosing with vancomycin, clindamycin, or cephalexin, with or without gentamicin (see Table 271-4 in Chapter 271).

PERITONSILLAR ABSCESS AND DEEP SPACE INFECTIONS
Only about 1% of patients with acute bacterial pharyngitis develop serious suppurative complications.[6] The best predictors are severe tonsillar inflammation and severe earache, but most complications occur in patients with neither of these findings. Peritonsillar abscesses usually can be diagnosed on physical examination (Fig. 401-3) and managed by an otolaryngologist in an outpatient setting by surgical drainage, needle drainage, or medical therapy.

In uncomplicated patients without trismus, medical therapy appears to be equally safe and efficacious. Patients treated with medical therapy also experience less pain, use fewer opioids, and miss fewer days of work.[7] Oral antibiotics, such as penicillin (1 million IU three times daily for 7 days), amoxicillin (500 mg orally twice a day for 10 days), clindamycin (300 to 600 mg three times a day for 14 days), or amoxicillin-clavulanate (875 mg orally twice a day for 10 days), are recommended. The addition of metronidazole does not add benefit in otherwise healthy adults who are treated with incision and drainage, and it can increase adverse events.[A6]

By comparison, patients with deep neck abscesses often have swelling of the external neck, trismus, torticollis, and even a compromised airway due to infection that has spread to the fascial planes of the neck and chest. These infections require urgent evaluation, usually with a computed tomography scan with contrast enhancement. Aggressive management includes incision and drainage as well as broad-spectrum intravenous antibiotics that cover aerobic and anaerobic bacteria (e.g., clindamycin, 600 mg intravenously every 8 hours; ampicillin-sulbactam, 3 g every 6 hours; or penicillin G, 2 million units every 4 hours plus metronidazole 500 mg every 6 hours).

Severe infections of the pharynx can cause septic thrombophlebitis of the internal jugular vein (Lemierre syndrome), an uncommon but serious complication. Patients typically present with persistent fever, difficulty in swallowing, neck pain, and a neck mass due to an underlying peritonsillar, retropharyngeal, or parapharyngeal abscess. Diagnosis is best established with a contrast-enhanced computed tomography scan of the neck. This potentially life-threatening condition is almost always associated with anaerobic infection, especially with *F. necrophorum* or *A. haemolyticum* (Chapter 281). Infection can extend into the intrathoracic vasculature, and patients can develop bacteremia and septic pulmonary emboli. Treatment should be directed toward anaerobic coverage (e.g., clindamycin, 600 mg every 8 hours, or metronidazole, 500 mg every 6 hours). Anticoagulation with heparin is controversial and generally reserved for persistent septic emboli. Surgical intervention includes drainage of the abscess. Ligation or excision of the jugular vein may be indicated for persistent septic emboli unresponsive to medical management. Mortality rates can be as high as 5%.

VIRAL INFECTIONS

In adults, the common cold (Chapter 337) causes 30 to 60% of cases of pharyngitis, with rhinovirus (Chapter 337) accounting for the majority of cases, followed by coronavirus (Chapter 342) and parainfluenza (Chapter 339) (see Table 401-2). U.S. adults experience an average of 2.5 episodes per year of noninfluenza upper respiratory infections, each with a 7.4-day average duration of symptoms. For the entire U.S. population, these 500 million episodes cost an estimated $40 billion annually, in part because of associated systemic symptoms such as fever, cough, and sinusitis and in part because of associated exacerbations of allergies, asthma, and chronic obstructive pulmonary disease.

The viral infection that is most likely to be confused with a bacterial infection is mononucleosis. Mononucleosis is caused by Epstein-Barr virus (Chapter 353), which has a seroprevalence of 67% in U.S. children and adolescents aged 6 to 19 years. After an incubation period of 3 to 7 weeks, patients present with initial malaise, fever, and chills followed by sore throat, fever, and anorexia.[8] Some patients have associated abdominal discomfort due to splenomegaly or hepatomegaly, headache, stiff neck, and rash. On physical examination, patients have erythematous pharyngitis with exudative tonsillar hypertrophy (Fig. 401-4), prominent lingual tonsils, and adenoid hypertrophy (Waldeyer ring). Aphthous-type ulcerations and petechiae may be seen, especially at the junction of the hard and soft palate. Impressive cervical adenopathy is typical, and 50% of patients have splenomegaly. Lymphoid hyperplasia can cause some degree of upper airway obstruction in about 5% of patients.

A blood count will show lymphocytosis, usually with more 10% atypical lymphocytes. The heterophil antibody test result is often positive, and Epstein-Barr virus–specific antibody tests are diagnostic. β-Lactam antibiotics, which may mistakenly be prescribed, will cause a maculopapular rash in 95% of patients. Laryngeal obstruction may require hospitalization and intravenous corticosteroids (e.g., dexamethasone, 8 to 10 mg intravenously three times a day).

Influenza virus infection can include nonexudative pharyngitis, but the predominant symptoms are tracheobronchial, usually accompanied by fever, headache, rhinorrhea, cough, and myalgia, without lymphadenopathy. Adenovirus (Chapter 341) can cause pharyngitis associated with fever, nonproductive cough, nasal congestion, myalgia, headache, nausea, vomiting, and diarrhea, especially in outbreaks, such as among military recruits, or in immunocompromised patients.

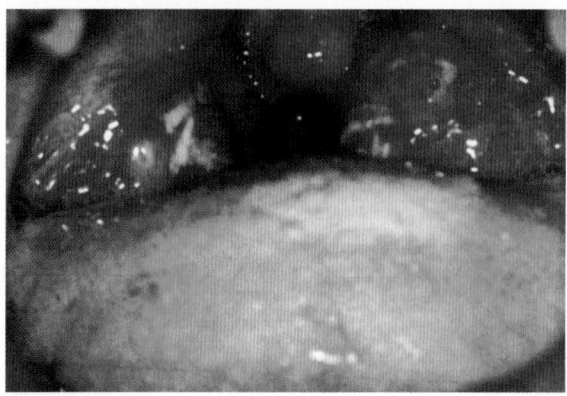

FIGURE 401-4. Mononucleosis with symmetrical exudative tonsillitis. (Courtesy Thomas A. Tami, MD.)

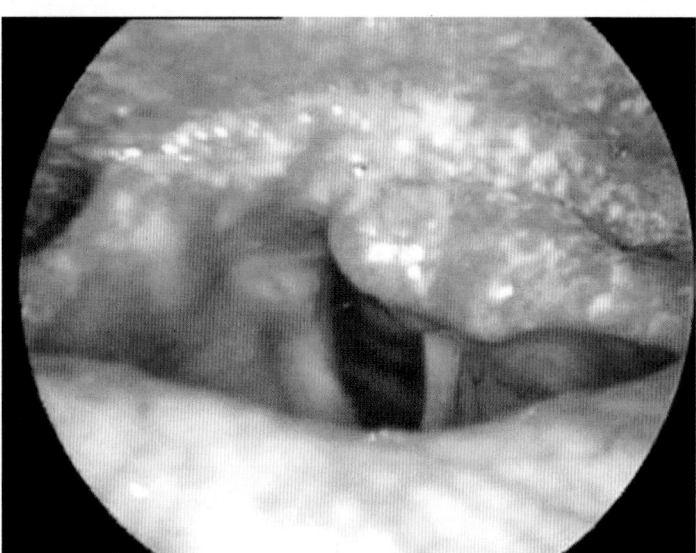

FIGURE 401-5. Fiberoptic laryngoscopy demonstrating characteristic erythema and white pseudomembrane secondary to *Candida* infection.

Primary herpes simplex virus (Chapter 350) infection is characterized by pharyngitis with or without gingival stomatitis. Symptoms include sore throat, fever, and malaise; physical findings include erythema and hypertrophy of the tonsils with exudates, often with enlarged, tender cervical nodes. It may be difficult to distinguish clinically from group A β-hemolytic streptococcal pharyngitis unless patients have herpes-like lesions of the oral cavity or oropharynx.

Human immunodeficiency virus infection (Chapter 360) can be manifested as an acute retroviral syndrome that mimics infectious mononucleosis and resolves in 1 to 2 weeks. The diagnosis must be considered in febrile patients with known risk factors. Once infection is established, oral and oropharyngeal infectious ulcerations may be due to herpes simplex virus, cytomegalovirus, syphilis, cryptococcus, histoplasmosis, or mycobacteria. Large, painful, noninfectious aphthous ulcers also can involve the tonsillar fossa, floor of mouth, hypopharynx, and epiglottis (Chapter 397). In adults with a sore throat that does not warrant antibiotics, a single 10 mg oral dose of dexamethasone does not improve symptoms at 24 hours but does modestly improve symptoms at 48 hours.[A7]

FUNGAL INFECTIONS

By far, the most common fungal infection of the oropharynx and larynx is candidiasis. *Candida* (Chapter 318) is a normal commensal organism of the oral cavity and oropharynx, but it can be an opportunistic infectious agent in immunocompromised patients, patients who have received prior head and neck irradiation, patients with xerostomia or diabetes, and immunocompetent patients who have been treated with antibiotics or with systemic or inhaled steroids. *Candida* infection is manifested with sore throat, burning of the mouth and tongue, dysgeusia, dysphagia, and hoarseness. White pseudomembranes characteristic of thrush (Fig. 401-5) may involve the oral cavity, oropharynx, hypopharynx, larynx, and esophagus. Treatment includes oral hygiene, probiotics, and topical antifungals (Chapter 318). Fluconazole (200 mg orally once a day for 14 to 21 days) is indicated for laryngeal and esophageal involvement and for recurrent disease. In patients who do not respond to fluconazole, resistant *Candida albicans* and non-*albicans Candida* species are likely causes and should be treated with itraconazole (200 mg orally once a day for 14 to 21 days).[9]

Other fungal infections may affect the oropharynx and larynx in isolation or as part of a systemic infection. *Blastomycosis* (Chapter 316) involves the larynx in less than 5% of cases, in which it produces pseudoepitheliomatous hyperplasia and clinically resembles squamous cell carcinoma. *Histoplasmosis* (Chapter 316), which is endemic to the Ohio and Mississippi river valleys, can involve the oral cavity, oropharynx, and larynx in immunocompromised patients. *Cryptococcosis* (Chapter 317) can involve the larynx and occurs most often in an immunocompromised host, in whom pseudoepitheliomatous hyperplasia may occur.

Paracoccidioidomycosis (Chapter 316) is the leading cause of fungal laryngitis in South America, especially among farmers. It causes pseudoepitheliomatous hyperplasia that can be misdiagnosed initially as squamous cell carcinoma. *Coccidioidomycosis* (Chapter 316), which is endemic to southwestern United States, can involve the larynx, in which it results in hoarseness and throat pain and can progress to airway obstruction. For each of these fungal diseases, treatment is similar to what is recommended for the disseminated disease (Chapter 315) that usually accompanies pharyngeal and laryngeal disease.

MYCOBACTERIAL INFECTIONS
The risk that tuberculosis (Chapter 308) infection will involve the oropharynx and larynx is low, with only about 1 to 1.5% of infected tuberculosis patients having involvement of the tonsils or larynx. Tonsillar involvement, which most often occurs in the presence of systemic disease, is manifested as sore throat with exudative tonsillitis and cervical adenopathy. Other diseases that can have a similar clinical presentation include lymphoma (Chapter 176), squamous cell carcinoma (Chapter 181), and sarcoidosis (Chapter 89). Tuberculosis in the larynx is most likely to involve the vocal folds and supraglottis (false vocal folds). It is manifested with hoarseness and odynophagia, and its lesions mimic squamous cell carcinoma. Approximately 50% of cases occur in the presence of active disseminated disease, about one third occur with inactive disease, and the other 15% occur as primary laryngeal disease.

In contrast, *Mycobacterium leprae* infection (Chapter 310) is manifested with laryngeal disease in one third of patients with systemic disease. The clinical picture is indistinguishable from that of laryngeal tuberculosis. Atypical mycobacteria rarely involve the larynx, and infection most often is manifested as cervical adenopathy.

CHRONIC TONSILLITIS
Patients may develop deep tonsillar crypts that accumulate debris, such as food or sloughed mucosa, thereby providing an ideal environment for the growth of bacteria, especially anaerobes. Such patients commonly complain of whitish or yellow pieces of semisolid debris on or emanating from their tonsils. These tonsilliths often have a foul taste and odor, and they can cause halitosis. Some patients have chronic sore throats because of the persistent infection. Treatment includes frequent gargling of a hydrogen peroxide mouthwash and occasionally expressing this debris from the tonsil manually. Long-term amoxicillin (500 mg three times a day for 21 days) or clindamycin (300 mg orally three times a day for 21 days) may be effective; however, the presence of *Actinomyces*, a commensal organism of the oral cavity and oropharynx, is indicative of chronic infection that requires tonsillectomy because even long-term antibiotics are unlikely to be effective. Multiple episodes of acute tonsillitis, especially if accompanied by a peritonsillar abscess, can also be an indication for surgery.[10] Adenotonsillectomy decreases the number of episodes of sore throat and days with sore throat in children in the first year after surgery,[A3] but its effectiveness in adults is less clear; many adults improve spontaneously, and the potential benefit of surgery must be weighed against its risks, including hemorrhage and pain, the latter of which is more prevalent in adults.

Epiglottitis
Epiglottitis (supraglottiis) is an uncommon problem in adults and has become even less common in children because of routine *Haemophilus influenzae* vaccination in children (Chapters 15 and 284). In adults, *Streptococcus pneumoniae* (Chapter 273) is now the most common organism, and adults present with a severe sore throat, odynophagia, fever, and "hot potato" voice. Airway obstruction occurs less frequently than in children, although it should be

considered a possibility.[11] Palpation or movement of the larynx causes significant pain. On transnasal fiberoptic laryngoscopy, the larynx typically reveals swelling, erythema, and occasionally exudates of the epiglottis and other supraglottic structures. Patients with a confirmed diagnosis of epiglottitis require intravenous antibiotics (e.g., cefotaxime, 2 g every 6 hours, or ceftriaxone, 1 to 2 g/day, intravenously), and they should be observed in an intensive care unit setting until symptoms improve because of the risk for rapidly progressive airway obstruction.[12]

● NONINFECTIOUS PHARYNGITIS
Laryngopharyngeal Reflux

Patients with gastroesophageal reflux disease (Chapter 129) can develop laryngopharyngeal reflux with intermittent hoarseness, nighttime or chronic cough, postnasal drip, "globus" sensation, reactive airway disease, halitosis, and brackish or acid taste in the back of the mouth and throat. Findings on laryngoscopy, although nonspecific, may include posterior laryngitis, with swollen and erythematous arytenoid cartilages, thickening of the vocal folds, interarytenoid edema, and thickening of the mucosa. In severe cases, spasm or thickening of the cricopharyngeus muscle, also known as the upper esophageal sphincter (Chapter 129), can cause dysphagia as a result of poor pharyngeal emptying or even spillage of secretions into the larynx with aspiration.

Treatment should address dietary change, behavioral modification, elevation of the head of the bed at night, and a therapeutic trial of a proton pump inhibitor for up to 3 months (Chapter 129). Empirical treatment without laryngoscopy is reasonable in patients with classic symptoms, but patients who do not respond within 3 months or patients with warning signs (e.g., ear pain, trismus, or odynophagia) require laryngoscopy to exclude more serious causes of hoarseness. In patients with persistent symptoms and a positive pH probe or with evidence of Barrett esophagitis, an antireflux procedure (Chapter 129) should be strongly considered.

SYSTEMIC DISEASES OF THE THROAT AND LARYNGITIS
About 80% of patients with *pemphigus* (Chapter 410) will have symptoms affecting the nasal cavity, oral cavity, and oropharynx, and half of these patients will have laryngeal involvement. Shallow ulcerations with fibrinous material and surrounding erythema are characteristic. Bullous lesions are less likely to be observed because the epithelial layer sloughs during swallowing. Laryngeal involvement may result in stenosis with airway obstruction due to scarring. Upper aerodigestive tract involvement occurs in 35% of patients with *pemphigoid* (Chapter 410), and 50% of these patients will have laryngeal involvement. Treatment in both disorders consists of high-dose steroids (prednisone, 75 to 100 mg orally per day until remission) during the attack phase and then tapered to a maintenance dose. Other immunosuppressive medications, such as azathioprine, cyclophosphamide, or cyclosporine (Chapter 32), may be required in the maintenance phase. Perilesional or intralesional triamcinolone acetonide injections are recommended during the maintenance phase for new lesions.

Granulomatosis with polyangiitis (Chapter 254) includes laryngeal involvement in 20% of patients, with a predilection for the subglottis (E-Fig. 401-1). Presenting symptoms may include hoarseness, cough, dyspnea, wheezing, and stridor. Flow-volume loops are useful and demonstrate flattening of both inspiratory and expiratory loops characteristic of a fixed extrathoracic obstruction. Patients presenting with airway obstruction require surgical intervention. Active disease with granulation tissue requiring airway management is treated with endoscopic dilation and steroid injection. Systemic immunosuppression is not effective for treatment of laryngeal involvement, so open resection may be required as the disease becomes chronic with the deposition of fibrous tissue.

Relapsing polychondritis involves cartilage in the ear, nose, and upper and lower airway as well as in the articular joints and costal cartilage. About 50% of patients will develop dyspnea, cough, hoarseness, stridor, or wheezing due to the destruction of cartilage and the resulting loss of structural support of the airway (E-Fig. 401-2). Airway obstruction may necessitate stenting or tracheostomy.

About 25 to 30% of patients with rheumatoid arthritis (Chapter 248) develop hoarseness, globus symptoms, and difficulty in swallowing. Hoarseness may result from acute inflammation or chronic nodular formation. Bilateral arytenoid joint involvement may impair vocal fold motion and cause airway obstruction with stridor. Surgical intervention may be necessary to open the airway. The role of steroids (systemic or injectable) for airway stenosis in rheumatoid arthritis has not been established.

About 1 to 5% of all patients with *sarcoidosis* (Chapter 89) develop laryngeal involvement, usually manifested as hoarseness. As the disease progresses, however, it can cause a conical stenosis due to thickening of the soft tissue (E-Fig. 401-3). Laryngeal paralysis can be caused by a mass effect or by adenopathy with peripheral nerve compression along the course of the vagus or recurrent laryngeal nerve. Vocal fold involvement responds to intralesional steroid injection, but endoscopic laser excision is recommended in patients with airway symptoms.

Amyloid (Chapter 179) can deposit anywhere in the upper aerodigestive tract. In patients with localized immunoglobulin light chain amyloidosis, the most common site is the larynx (about 14% of cases).[13] Hoarseness and cough are the most common symptoms in patients with laryngeal involvement (E-Fig. 401-4), but pharyngeal involvement may be associated with pain. Airway obstruction is rare. Surgical debulking with or without external beam radiation may relieve symptoms and even resolve the lesions. Unfortunately, reports are anecdotal, and there are no large series to support treatment options.

NEUROLOGIC DISORDERS AFFECTING THE THROAT

Neurologic disorders of the oropharynx, hypopharynx, and larynx may be due to focal diseases or be a local manifestation of generalized neurologic disease. Head and neck manifestations of neurologic and neuromuscular disorders are classified as hyperfunctional and hypofunctional disorders. Hyperfunctional disorders include muscle tension dysphonia, dystonia (Chapter 382), essential tremor (Chapter 382), myoclonus, and stuttering. Hypofunctional neurologic disorders include Parkinson disease (Chapter 381), multiple sclerosis (Chapter 383), neuromuscular disorders (Chapters 391 and 394), postpolio syndrome (Chapter 355), myopathies (Chapter 393), medullary disorders, and laryngeal paralysis. Given the variety of disorders with head and neck manifestations, it is critical to identify and classify the physical findings and associated symptoms. For example, a patient who complains about the sound of the voice may in fact have a normal voice but actually have severe dysarthria and hypernasality secondary to amyotrophic lateral sclerosis. The site of the lesion associated with the neurologic disorder will result in characteristic physical findings and facilitate establishment of a correct diagnosis (Table 401-3).

Hyperfunctional Neurologic Disorders

In *dystonia* (Chapter 382), spasmodic dysphonia fluctuates moment to moment and day to day. Adductor spasms of the vocal folds produce strained, strangled vocal quality with pitch breaks. Abductor spasms produce breathy hypophonic word breaks. Nonspeech sounds (laughter) and singing voice may be normal. This condition responds well to botulinum toxin injections.

Muscle tension dysphonia, which may be difficult to distinguish from dystonia, can occur secondary to underlying weakness (paresis, aging) with compensatory hyperfunction. Speech has a rough strained quality, perhaps with pitch breaks, and does not fluctuate moment to moment. It generally responds to voice therapy.

Vocal tremor is seen in 30% of patients with *essential tremor* (Chapter 382) and may be associated with spastic dystonia. Patients have a tremulous, quavering vocal quality, with or without head or hand tremor. Because of involvement of pharyngeal and laryngeal muscles, botulinum toxin may not be effective.

Myoclonus (Chapter 382) causes rhythmic contraction of the palate, pharynx, or larynx at a rate of one or two per second. Patients may have audible clicking from the eustachian tube or larynx. Voice may or may not be affected. Palate and vocal folds may be treated with botulinum toxin.

Pseudobulbar palsy (Chapters 376 and 391) causes spasticity and hyperreflexia of the bulbar muscles (pharynx, palate, lips tongue, and larynx). Patients develop dysarthria, hypernasality, and a harsh strident strained vocal quality, which is more spastic than spasmodic.

Hypofunctional Neurologic Disorders

Parkinson disease affects speech and swallowing in more than 80% of patients. Patients have dysarthria, prosody of speech, hypophonia, tachyphemia, monotonous pitch, and absence of vocal tremor.

Laryngeal examination shows bilateral vocal fold bowing with incomplete glottic closure. In advanced disease, vocal fold motion becomes hypokinetic. Pooling of secretions occurs as swallowing dysfunction progresses. Patients benefit from early intervention by speech-language therapists to address both voice and swallowing symptoms. In *progressive supranuclear palsy*, bulbar symptoms progress more rapidly, with pronounced speech and swallowing difficulty (Chapter 381). In *multiple system atrophy* (Chapter 381), progressive airway obstruction from bilateral vocal fold motion impairment may necessitate tracheostomy. In *myasthenia gravis* (Chapter 394), hypernasal speech, palatal weakness, and hypophonia may be accompanied by difficulties with swallowing and respiration. Some patients with *amyotrophic lateral sclerosis* (Chapter 391) present with bulbar symptoms that result from buccal-labial-lingual weakness, which produces speech and swallowing dysfunction, before the definitive diagnosis is made. In *multiple sclerosis* (Chapter 383), dysphonia and dysarthria are common.

LUMP IN THE THROAT

The sensation of a lump in the throat, called *globus pharyngeus*,[14] should prompt a careful history and physical examination by an otolaryngologist to exclude a serious diagnosis. When no underlying anatomic disease is found, possible causes include gastroesophageal reflux and spasm of the cricopharyngeus. Cognitive-behavioral therapy may be helpful.

HOARSENESS

Hoarseness, also called dysphonia, is characterized by altered voice quality, pitch, loudness, or vocal effort. Relevant history includes smoking status, occupation, and recent procedures involving the neck or affecting the recurrent laryngeal nerve. Symptomatic treatment should be considered in patients who have evidence suggesting a recent bacterial infectious process or gastroesophageal reflux without any historical features, such as ear pain, dysphagia, or odynophagia, or physical findings such as adenopathy or oral lesions suggestive of tumor. Additionally, there is no evidence to support the use of antibiotics or oral corticosteroids in patients with hoarseness unless otherwise indicated for a specific cause. Hoarseness that does not resolve within 4 weeks, or a history or physical examination suggesting a serious cause, should prompt referral to an otolaryngologist for laryngoscopy.[15]

The symptom of hoarseness invariably points to the larynx as the site of disease. Benign lesions are most common, including vocal nodules (screamer's nodules), vocal cord cysts, vocal cord granulomas (usually resulting from intubation trauma or laryngeal hyperfunction), and vocal cord papillomas. Malignant neoplasms must be suspected (Chapter 181), especially in patients with a strong smoking history.[16]

Of the malignant tumors that can occur in the hypopharynx and larynx, squamous cell carcinoma is the most common and is usually associated with tobacco and ethanol use. However, the incidence of human papillomavirus–related oropharyngeal squamous cell carcinoma is increasing and should be considered in the nonsmoking population. Squamous cell carcinoma (Chapter 181) can occur on essentially any mucosal surface in the head and neck. Symptoms can range from mild sore throat to hoarseness, severe dysphagia, and

TABLE 401-3	CORRELATING SITE OF LESION WITH PHYSICAL FINDINGS IN NEUROLOGIC DISORDERS AFFECTING THE THROAT
SITE OF LESION	**SIGNS**
Cortex	Aphasia Aphonia Dysarthria Dysphonia Stridor
Extrapyramidal system	Vocal strain and pitch breaks Tremor Hypophonia/tachyphemia Spasmodic movements Focal, regional, or generalized dystonia
Cerebellum	Ataxia Dysmetria Tremor Incoordination
Brain stem	Flaccid paralysis Associated dense sensory deficit
Peripheral	Focal paresis or paralysis Other cranial nerve ± Palate involvement defines location

Modified from Blitzer A, Alexander RE, Grant NN. Neurologic disorders of the larynx. In: Flint PW, Haughey BH, Lund VJ, et al., eds. *Cummings: Otolaryngology–Head and Neck Surgery.* 6th ed. Philadelphia: Mosby Elsevier; 2015.

odynophagia. Pain is often referred to the jaw or ear. Associated cervical lymph node enlargement is also common in advanced disease. Successful management depends on early detection by a careful examination of the entire upper aerodigestive tract, biopsy with histopathologic examination, and aggressive treatment based on the clinical stage and site of the lesion.

LARYNGEAL PARALYSIS

Laryngeal paralysis most often is manifested as a unilateral paralysis as a result of a mediastinal tumor; surgical trauma during thyroid, carotid, or anterior cervical spine surgery; blunt or penetrating trauma; aortic aneurysm; progressive neurologic disease; or viral or idiopathic causes. The severity of impairment can be determined from subjective criteria based on the patient's symptoms, such as breathiness, aspiration, and exertional intolerance.

Unilateral vocal fold paralysis with a favorable prognosis occurs after blunt trauma, endotracheal intubation, idiopathic vocal fold paralysis, and paralysis associated with viral pathogens (Ramsay Hunt syndrome). In this setting, the severity of aspiration, dysphonia, and electromyographic findings can be used to determine the choice of procedure and timing of intervention. Temporary medialization with collagen injection is warranted in patients with unilateral paralysis and a good prognosis. Patients who have poor prognosis for recovery include those with injury after complete section of the nerve during a surgical resection of tumor, invasion of cranial nerves by a tumor, paralysis associated with thoracic aneurysm, or paralysis due to progressive neurologic disorders. In patients with a low likelihood of recovery, permanent medialization of the paralyzed vocal fold is warranted.

Bilateral vocal fold motion impairment, which is less common, has the same causes. Its management is most often directed toward improving the airway because the predominant symptom is airway obstruction.

Grade A References

A1. Spinks A, Glasziou PP, Del Mar CB. Antibiotics for sore throat. *Cochrane Database Syst Rev.* 2013;11:CD000023.

A2. Spurling GK, Del Mar CB, Dooley L, et al. Delayed antibiotic prescriptions for respiratory infections. *Cochrane Database Syst Rev.* 2017;9:CD004417.

A3. van Driel ML, De Sutter AI, Habraken H, et al. Different antibiotic treatments for group A streptococcal pharyngitis. *Cochrane Database Syst Rev.* 2016;9:CD004406.

A4. Sadeghirad B, Siemieniuk RAC, Brignardello-Petersen R, et al. Corticosteroids for treatment of sore throat: systematic review and meta-analysis of randomised trials. *BMJ.* 2017;358:1-10.

A5. Morad A, Sathe NA, Francis DO, et al. Tonsillectomy versus watchful waiting for recurrent throat infection: a systematic review. *Pediatrics.* 2017;139:1-11.

A6. Wiksten JE, Pitkaranta A, Blomgren K. Metronidazole in conjunction with penicillin neither prevents recurrence nor enhances recovery from peritonsillar abscess when compared with penicillin alone: a prospective, double-blind, randomized, placebo-controlled trial. *J Antimicrob Chemother.* 2016;71:1681-1687.

A7. Hayward GN, Hay AD, Moore MV, et al. Effect of oral dexamethasone without immediate antibiotics vs placebo on acute sore throat in adults: a randomized clinical trial. *JAMA.* 2017;317:1535-1543.

A8. Burton MJ, Glasziou PP, Chong LY, et al. Tonsillectomy or adenotonsillectomy versus non-surgical treatment for chronic/recurrent acute tonsillitis. *Cochrane Database Syst Rev.* 2014;11:CD001802.

GENERAL REFERENCES

For the General References and other additional features, please visit Expert Consult at https://expertconsult.inkling.com.

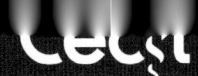

XXVIII

MEDICAL CONSULTATION

402

PRINCIPLES OF MEDICAL CONSULTATION

GERALD W. SMETANA

APPROACH TO MEDICAL CONSULTATION

A general medical or subspecialty medical physician may receive a request to perform a consultation for a variety of purposes. In some settings, a single consultative encounter will be requested, or the consultant will determine that only one visit, either in the inpatient or in the outpatient setting, is necessary. More commonly, the approach will include one or more follow-up visits to meet the goals of the consultation from the perspectives of the requesting physician, patient, and consultant. The consultant generally assumes one of four roles: cognitive consultant, procedural consultant, comanager with shared care, or comanager with principal care. The consultant as a comanager continues to care for a component of the patient's needs in an ongoing fashion while being careful to coordinate this comanagement with the continuing role of the requesting physician. Finally, in some situations, it may be most appropriate that the physician who initially requested the consultation no longer play an active role in the care of the patient but rather transfer ongoing care exclusively to the consultant.

From a practical perspective, consulting medical physicians, whether they are generalists or subspecialists, enter into the consultative mode in a relatively limited number of ways.[1] Surgeons may request a preoperative medical consultation to assess operative risk and obtain recommendations regarding perioperative care (Chapter 403) or, after surgery, to seek help in managing specific postoperative complications or assisting in the patient's long-term management. Both general medical physicians and medical subspecialists appropriately seek help from a subspecialist with particular knowledge in problems outside their own area of expertise to reduce uncertainty. Sometimes these requests are for specific medical procedures, but requests often seek cognitive guidance as well. Finally, noninternists may seek medical consultation for reasons other than perioperative care. For example, a psychiatrist may request a consultation to help determine whether the somatic symptoms of a particular patient represent important medical conditions (Chapter 406). In the peripartum setting, specific complications of pregnancy may require sophisticated medical consultation (Chapter 226).

Each of these settings raises different challenges for the medical consultant. In all settings, however, a number of general principles apply and can improve the effectiveness of consultations. Communication between physicians and other team members is critical to the process of consultation in all settings. The burgeoning patient safety movement has developed best practices for "hand-offs" that can be applied to consultations.

SETTING-SPECIFIC CONSULTATIVE ISSUES

An effective consultant must recognize the setting in which the consultation is requested and possess the required content knowledge. Distressingly, a number of studies have demonstrated that the requesting physician and the consultant often have substantially different views on the reasons that a consultation was requested, and this initial disconnection, if present, will doom any medical consultation.

Preoperative Surgical Consultation

In the preoperative setting, the medical consultant should not "clear" a patient for surgery and must avoid the temptation to do so even if asked. Clearance may incorrectly imply that the procedure has no risk or that the medical consultant will take responsibility for having misled the patient and surgeon. Instead, the medical consultant should help determine the inherent risk associated with the proposed procedure for the particular patient, whether the patient is in the best possible condition for surgery, and whether any generic or patient-specific interventions would reduce the risk (Chapter 403). Effective consultation also requires a specialized knowledge base, whether the consultation is focusing on a particular organ system or on overall perioperative risk (Chapter 403). The most important attributes of a preoperative medical consultation are a careful history and physical examination. Diagnostic testing plays only

a secondary role in this setting. The consultant can help avoid unnecessary and repetitive preoperative testing that is costly in the aggregate with essentially no benefit.[2] A poor consultant-patient interaction can have a substantial negative effect on a patient's confidence in the planned therapy.

Postoperative Surgical Consultation

Surgeons typically request a postoperative medical consultation when a complication has developed that is beyond their area of expertise (Chapter 405). These problems are commonly urgent, so the goal is expeditious consultation and prompt intervention. Management of these problems does not usually differ from management in nonoperative settings. Another reason for a postoperative consultation is to obtain assistance in post-hospitalization care or to facilitate seamless discharge planning. Consultants should aid in the transition to the outpatient or long-term care setting by taking primary or consultative roles as appropriate.

Medical-Medical Consultations

Cross-consultations between medical subspecialists or between a subspecialist and a generalist, in either direction, are quintessential examples of collaboration.[3] For subspecialty consultations, the key is to provide the requested expertise and benefit without overstepping into the domain of the expertise of the requesting physician.

Shared care, which is defined as truly joint participation of primary care physicians and specialist physicians in the delivery of care for patients with chronic conditions, can improve outcomes for hypertension, depression, and other medical conditions.[A1] For example, a randomized trial of shared care for patients with hypertension and chronic kidney disease demonstrated lower blood pressures and better use of lipid-lowering drugs in the shared care group. Infectious disease consultation also is associated with better adherence to quality measures, reduced in-hospital mortality,[4] with bacteremia and other infectious diseases.[5]

A growing example of medical-medical consultation is the situation in which a hospitalist assumes principal responsibility for an inpatient admission and then returns the patient to the primary care physician after discharge from the hospital. In this consultative interaction, close communication is critical because primary responsibility for the patient's care has shifted from the outpatient medical physician to the inpatient physician. This transfer of responsibility is not dissimilar to that occurring when a patient is submitted to the care of a subspecialist for a procedure such as cardiac catheterization or gastrointestinal endoscopy. Similar issues also arise when a critically ill patient with a condition such as a complicated myocardial infarction (Chapter 64) or shock (Chapters 98, 99, and 100) is managed principally by a critical care medical specialist and is then expected to return to the care of the primary physician after hospital discharge. However, a key difference is that the inpatient hospitalist physician, unlike the consulting subspecialist, will not typically have an ongoing comanagement role. Because of the higher risk for discontinuity, effective communication at the time of hospitalization, whenever key issues arise during hospitalization, and at the time of discharge is even more important in the inpatient hospitalist model than in the other settings in which subspecialists may take on more of a comanagement role. Effective and comprehensive hand-offs at the time of hospital discharge improve continuity and reduce the potential for errors and medicolegal liability.

Rapid Response Teams

A recent quality improvement initiative has been the development of rapid response teams. These teams aim to reduce the "failure to rescue," which often precedes an unplanned intensive care unit (ICU) transfer or non-ICU cardiac arrest. In this model, a prespecified consultative team urgently sees sick, hospitalized patients when a "trigger" abnormality indicates potential impending serious complications. The activation triggers for rapid response teams have varied somewhat among institutions, but there is substantial agreement on what constitutes an appropriate trigger (Table 402-1). Rapid response teams differ from traditional "code blue teams" in several aspects, the most important of which is their goal to rescue patients before a crisis situation occurs (Table 402-2).

Although implementation of these teams has not consistently reduced hospital mortality, most trials have shown a reduction in unplanned ICU transfers and in hospital length of stay. In a systematic review, rapid response teams reduced in-hospital mortality by 11% and unexpected mortality by about 50%.[A2]

This consultative strategy crosses specialties and may include general internal medicine, hospital medicine, and critical care physicians, as well as respiratory therapists and ICU nurses. When an emergency consultation is generated by

TABLE 402-1 TRIGGERS: CRITERIA FOR MOBILIZING AN IN-HOSPITAL RAPID RESPONSE SERVICE

VITAL SIGNS

Heart rate
- Heart rate <40 beats/min, especially if symptoms
- Heart rate >140 beats/min

Blood pressure
- Systolic blood pressure <90 mm Hg or >30-40 mm Hg below patient's usual stable blood pressure
- Systolic blood pressure >200 mm Hg for >30 min
- Diastolic blood pressure >110 mm Hg with symptoms

Respiratory rate
- Respiratory rate <8 breaths/min or >35 breaths/min
- New onset of marked dyspnea, compromised airway, cyanosis

Oxygenation
- O_2 saturation <85% for >5 min (except patients with chronic severe hypoxemia)
- Need for 100% supplemental O_2 or a nonrebreathing O_2 mask

Temperature
- Body temperature >39° C or associated with acute decompensation

NEUROLOGIC STATUS

- Acute change in mental status
- New focal findings
- Prolonged or repeated seizures
- ≥2 Point decline in Glasgow Coma Scale score

GENERAL STATUS

- Uncontrollable bleeding
- Decreased urine output to <50 mL over 4 hr

Based on criteria of The Joint Commission and on other sources.

TABLE 402-2 FEATURES OF RAPID RESPONSE TEAMS AND TRADITIONAL CODE TEAMS

FEATURE	TRADITIONAL CODE TEAM	RAPID RESPONSE TEAM
Criteria for calling team	No pulse, blood pressure, or respiratory effort; unresponsive	Low blood pressure, rapid heart rate, respiratory distress, change in mental status
Typical conditions	Cardiac arrest, respiratory arrest, airway obstruction	Sepsis, pulmonary edema, arrhythmias, respiratory failure
Typical team composition	Anesthesia fellow, ICU fellow, internal medicine house staff, ICU nurse	ICU fellow, ICU nurse, respiratory therapist, internal medicine house staff
Typical call rate (number per 1000 admissions)	0.5-5	20-40
In-hospital mortality	70-90%	0-20%

ICU = intensive care unit.
Adapted from Jones DA, DeVita MA, Bellomo R. Rapid-response teams. *N Engl J Med.* 2011;365:139-146.

TABLE 402-3 REASONS TO CONSIDER A SUBSPECIALTY CONSULTATION

To provide ongoing comanagement become a partner in inpatient care
- For an acute, unstable problem
- For a chronic condition

To perform a procedure (or advise on whether to perform it)
- Diagnostic
- Therapeutic

To provide one-time or periodic advice
- Diagnostic guidance
- Therapeutic guidance
- Reassurance
- Medicolegal issues

about the requesting physician's knowledge base regarding the specific medical issues that generate the consultation. The written report and verbal communications should be comprehensive and commonly include more basic medical content and specific recommendations than may be typical of a consultation for a medical subspecialist.

Subspecialty consultations requested by primary care physicians may be for advice, a technical procedure, or ongoing comanagement (Table 402-3). Consultations for general practitioners or family physicians generally follow the same guidelines as those for general internists. However, because both the training and ongoing practices of such physicians may or may not include the same spectrum and complexity of disease encountered by typical general internists, the subspecialty consultant must use judgment regarding both the initial consultation and the advisability of ongoing comanagement.

STRATEGIES FOR EFFECTIVE CONSULTATION

It is critical that requesting and consulting physicians agree about the reason for the consultative request. For example, the nature of a preoperative medical consultant's evaluation would differ substantially if the request were (1) routine, (2) for advice on perioperative insulin management in a patient with type 1 diabetes, or (3) to assist in determining the risks and benefits of proceeding to vascular surgery in a high-risk patient with coronary artery disease and a previous stroke. Effective communication at the time of the request will improve the value of the consultation and clarify the question. When there is doubt regarding the reason for the consultation, the consultant should speak directly to the referring physician before completing and documenting the evaluation of the patient.

Common reasons for medical consultation include assessment of perioperative risk; interpretation of a laboratory abnormality; help in performing a procedure, in obtaining advice, or in selecting therapy; and aid in providing long-term care. Prophylactic strategies (venous thromboembolism, endocarditis, and surgical site infection) infrequently generate requests for medical consultation because they are commonly standardized to conform to practice guidelines at individual institutions.

Determining the question will also help narrow the scope of the consultant's advice and minimize the number of recommendations. Adherence by the requesting physician to any of the recommendations made by the consultant is higher for consultations with fewer recommendations. Another strategy to minimize the number of recommendations is to restrict advice to pertinent issues at the time, preferably in order of their importance. For example, a consultant who is asked to aid in the care of a critically ill pregnant patient with HELLP syndrome (hemolysis, elevated liver enzymes, and low platelet count) (Chapters 151 and 226) should not also make recommendations regarding the value of cigarette cessation (Chapter 29), even though this issue will be pertinent after the mother and child have survived the acute event.

Requesting physicians are also more likely to adhere to recommendations when the patient is sicker, when the consultation is performed promptly, when advice is given to institute specific therapy rather than perform more diagnostic testing, when the consultant writes frequent follow-up notes, and when computerized order entry support systems are used to convey recommendations. When giving advice about medications, consultants should indicate specific doses and duration of treatment. If a recommendation is likely to be controversial (e.g., postpone surgery), it is always preferable to speak directly to the requesting physician before writing a consultation note in the hope that direct conversation will provide an opportunity to develop a consensus that may then be reflected in the formal consultation note. In one study of 323 physicians, the three elements of greatest perceived importance for a high-quality

a trigger event, the consultant's relationship is primarily with the patient rather than with the referring physician.

Consultations for Special Populations

When consulting for psychiatrists or in the peripartum period, the consultant requires special expertise to understand the different expressions of signs and symptoms in specific populations, as well as how and when to modify typical medical recommendations because of special circumstances (Chapters 226 and 406). Although these consultations occasionally result in long-term comanagement, more commonly they revolve around the resolution of an isolated problem. In addition, the medical consultant should not make assumptions

TABLE 402-4 GUIDELINES TO HELP MAKE CONSULTATIONS EFFECTIVE

Determine whether the goal is to obtain advice (and, if so, specifically for what) or to aid in ongoing comanagement (see Table 402-2).

Understand the urgency of the consultation so that the consultation will be performed on a timely basis that meets the needs of the requesting physician and patient.

Perform a focused but careful history and physical examination—do not rely on information gathered by others.

Do not rehash information in an overly detailed note—emphasize the key issues your evaluation reinforced or discovered.

Be sure your recommendations are clearly listed and appropriately detailed—for example, indicate specific drugs, doses, and durations.

Limit the total number of recommendations to improve adherence.

Indicate how to monitor the effectiveness of your recommendations, as well as how to contact you urgently if problems arise.

Adjust your involvement (advice vs. comanagement) as appropriate, in concert with the requesting physician.

Serve as a peer—teach as appropriate but also seek to learn.

Remember that personal contact with the requesting physician, even if very brief, may be far more helpful than the best of written notes.

Do not disappear—follow the patient as frequently as appropriate, in coordination with the requesting physician.

For a more complete discussion of this topic, see Goldman L, Lee T, Rudd P. Ten commandments for effective consultations. *Arch Intern Med.* 1983;143:1753-1755; and Salerno SM, Hurst FP, Halvorson S, et al. Principles of effective consultation: an update for the 21st-century consultant. *Arch Intern Med.* 2007;167:271-275.

consultation request were to frame the question, to indicate clearly whom to call with the response, and to establish urgency.

Consultants should be careful to restrict their advice to their particular area of expertise. For example, unless a particular antipsychotic medication is contraindicated because of a medical issue (Chapter 406), it is wisest to defer decision making regarding psychiatric management to the psychiatrist. A strongly worded consultation note that advises against a particular strategy will put another physician in a difficult medicolegal position if it differs from the physician's usual or recommended practice. The most important attributes of a consultative role are simple, concise recommendations and a clearly stated rationale for decision making. Detailed differential diagnosis is less important, and literature support is usually unnecessary.

Timely consultation reports improve physician satisfaction and patient care. For example, primary care physicians note that failure to receive timely reports from consultants limits their ability to provide high-quality care.

Salerno and colleagues have proposed modifications of Goldman's original "Ten Commandments" for effective consultations (Table 402-4). These recommendations serve as a helpful guide for consultants to improve adherence to their advice and, as a result, improve patient outcomes. Specific interactive training on the principles of consultation can increase the effectiveness of consultative communication.

SPECIAL CONSULTATIVE SITUATIONS

Curbside Consultation

Informal consultations are commonly called "curbside" consultations. In the current era, ready access to online medical references may potentially reduce curbside requests. Consultants in "cognitive" specialties such as infectious diseases, rheumatology, and endocrinology provide a disproportionate amount of informal (compared with formal) consultations. Informal consultations may occur by telephone, by e-mail, or in person. Curbside consultation is ingrained into the fabric of medical care.

Both generalists and specialists participate in an average of three to four curbside consultations per week. These consultations commonly involve questions about diagnostic tests, treatment plans, and the potential value of a formal consultation (which follows about one third of curbside consultations) in the future. To be effective, curbside consultations should be brief, involve a single question, and require no direct examination of the patient or medical records.

An important limitation of curbside consultations is that the consultant must rely on limited, secondhand information from the requesting physician rather than primary data from direct evaluation of the patient. Consultants report that such indirect information is inaccurate in as many as half of curbside consultations. This reality, along with lack of financial compensation, leads to a greater degree of dissatisfaction with the curbside process by consultants than by requesting physicians. Salaried consultants may view a request for a

curbside consultation more favorably than might those whose livelihood depends on a fee-for-service model of care.

Although requesting physicians may perceive reduced medicolegal risk when they obtain and even document a curbside consultation, consultants may fear the risk for malpractice liability themselves when offering such advice. However, courts have consistently found that curbside consultants have no liability because no direct physician-patient relationship exists. Rather, the relationship is only between the requesting and consulting physicians.

Electronic Consultations

Increasingly, physicians are using electronic communication, either as part of a shared electronic medical record or by e-mail, to supplement formal consultation requests. An obvious advantage of this approach is that the requesting and consulting physician can communicate on their own schedules. Potential benefits include saving time, reducing costs, and improving continuity and access to specialty care. However, the lack of reimbursement for such activities may be a barrier to e-consultations.

Mandatory Consultations

In some situations, mandatory consultations may help enforce a standard of care. For example, mandatory inpatient infectious disease consultations, as part of an antimicrobial stewardship program, can improve the rational use of antimicrobial agents in the hospital and after discharge. Similarly, instituting routine consultation for patients with certain sentinel conditions, such as diabetes, may improve outcomes.

Comanagement

A consultation that begins with an initial encounter or a limited number of follow-up visits may evolve into ongoing comanagement. In such an arrangement, the physician initially serving in a consultative role becomes at least coequal to the requesting physician in the provision of ongoing care. In some situations, the consultant may actually become the primary physician. This arrangement is obvious in situations in which the consultation was requested specifically for the provision of ongoing care. Other examples include situations in which an oncologist assumes principal care of a patient with a malignancy or a nephrologist assumes principal care of a patient with end-stage renal disease who is being maintained on dialysis. In some of these situations, a general internist who initially requested the consultation may now become the consultant and provide advice on preventive care and occasional help with intercurrent medical problems.

Comanagement is also increasingly common in the hospital setting. Medical consultants may become comanagers of postoperative surgical patients, with a potential for improving outcomes. In an early randomized trial of perioperative patients, formal comanagement, in which a medical physician took responsibility for managing medical problems rather than acting in a consultative role, reduced postoperative complications; in addition, both nurses and surgeons preferred this model. However, not all studies have shown that comanagement improves patient outcomes. In one study of comanagement on a neurosurgical service, for example, nursing staff perceived substantial improvement in the quality of patient care, and costs were reduced, but there were no differences in mortality, readmission rates, or length of stay. In some institutions, comanagement for orthopedic or other surgical patients has become routine and does not require a specific request for consultation. Internists currently comanage more than one third of surgical inpatients in some hospitals.

In some settings, the outpatient primary care physician may retain a comanagement role even as a cardiologist cares for a patient with acute myocardial infarction, a pulmonologist cares for a patient in the ICU, a hospitalist cares for a patient in the general medical setting, or a noninternist addresses a specific problem.

RESPONSIBILITIES OF THE CONSULTANT

The consultant is responsible to two parties: the patient and the referring physician. A paternalistic approach is not desirable. The consultant should not limit communication to the referring physician and must not withhold discussion and recommendations from the patient. However, the consultant should not usurp the role of the referring physician, who remains responsible for assembling information and advice from varied sources, as well as for developing an integrated plan with the patient. For example, in the preoperative setting, the consultant should not express a final opinion regarding the suitability of proceeding to surgery without first discussing all relevant considerations with the referring surgeon. In the trilateral deliberative model, the patient, referring physician, and consultant each have responsibilities and constraints inherent in their relationships (E-Fig. 402-1). Above all, the role of the consultant is to improve patient care and outcomes.

IMPACT OF CONSULTATIONS ON PATIENT OUTCOME

Few controlled trials have investigated the impact of medical consultations on outcomes. In one small study in the 1990s, an outpatient preoperative medical consultation reduced unnecessary admissions (those that did not result in surgery) compared with usual care (inpatient consultation at the discretion of the surgeon). In the outpatient setting, about 20% of diagnoses made by specialty consultants may be distinctly different than those made by referring physicians.[6] Other reports indicate that anywhere from 5 to 50% of preoperative medical consultations result in changes in patient management. Comprehensive preoperative geriatric consultation can also reduce postoperative complications and length of stay.[A3]

Grade A References

A1. Smith SM, Cousins G, Clyne B, et al. Shared care across the interface between primary and specialty care in management of long term conditions. *Cochrane Database Syst Rev.* 2017;2:CD004910.
A2. De Jong A, Jung B, Daurat A, et al. Effect of rapid response systems on hospital mortality: a systematic review and meta-analysis. *Intensive Care Med.* 2016;42:615-617.
A3. Partridge JS, Harari D, Martin FC, et al. Randomized clinical trial of comprehensive geriatric assessment and optimization in vascular surgery. *Br J Surg.* 2017;104:679-687.

GENERAL REFERENCES

For the General References and other additional features, please visit Expert Consult at https://expertconsult.inkling.com.

403

PREOPERATIVE EVALUATION

STEVEN L. COHN

Each year in the United States, more than 25 million inpatient surgical procedures and an additional 25 million outpatient procedures are performed. Although more than one third of these surgical patients are older than 65 years, overall morbidity and mortality are relatively low, in part because of modern anesthetic and surgical techniques. A crucial aspect of safety is careful preoperative evaluation of the patient not only by the surgeon and anesthesiologist but also, in many instances, by a general medical consultant or medical subspecialist.[1]

OPERATIVE RISK ASSESSMENT

The components of perioperative risk include those related to the patient, procedure, provider, and anesthesia. Anesthetic risk is low, with mortality less than 0.03% in a normal healthy patient—American Society of Anesthesiology (ASA) class 1—but increasing to 0.2% in ASA class 2 (mild systemic disease), 1.2% in class 3 (severe systemic disease), 8% in class 4 (severe systemic disease that is a constant threat to life), and 34% in class 5 (a moribund patient not expected to survive for 24 hours without surgery). Among adult patients undergoing major noncardiac surgery, perioperative all-cause death, acute myocardial infarction (MI), or acute ischemic stroke occurs in 3% of hospitalizations nationwide.[2] Meta-analysis suggests that when feasible, neuraxial (spinal or epidural) anesthesia may reduce postoperative complications compared with general anesthesia (Chapter 404), but decisions regarding the anesthetic technique should be the responsibility of the anesthesiologist and not be part of the preoperative medical consultation. With respect to the provider, data support a "learning curve," with better outcomes when procedures are performed by more experienced, higher-volume surgeons.

GENERAL RISK ASSESSMENT

History and Physical Examination

The medical history and physical examination are the most important components in assessing a patient's risk for surgery. The consultation should focus on pertinent medical problems, particularly cardiopulmonary symptoms and diseases that are associated with risk and are likely to influence perioperative management (Chapter 402). The importance of the past surgical history is to determine whether the patient was able to undergo major surgery in the recent past or had any perioperative medical or anesthetic-related complications that could occur again. The social history should assess and quantify the amount, duration, and last use of tobacco, alcohol, or illicit substances. It is important to document allergies to medications, foods, and latex as well as to obtain an accurate list of the patient's current prescription and over-the-counter medications, including doses and adherence. The family history is relevant primarily for any genetically associated complications such as malignant hyperthermia or a bleeding disorder. The review of systems should include the presence or absence of chest pain and dyspnea and the patient's exercise capacity. The physical examination must include the vital signs, assessment of the airway and respiratory status, cardiovascular examination, and documentation of any neurologic deficit.

Preoperative Tests

Screening preoperative test results in otherwise healthy individuals are usually normal and, even when abnormal, rarely affect management (generally <1%) (Table 403-1).[3] Most significant abnormalities can be predicted from the clinical information obtained, which then guides selective testing based on the history, the physical findings, and the planned type of surgery and anesthesia. Most patients undergoing low-risk surgery with local anesthesia require no preoperative testing. Repeat testing should be avoided if recent (within 3 months) results were normal, unless the patient's condition or medications have changed.

Perioperative Medications

Decisions regarding whether to continue a medication perioperatively should consider the drug's pharmacokinetics (Chapter 26) as well as its effects on the primary disease and perioperative risk, including potential interactions with anesthetic agents. Some medications are essential to continue (e.g., cardiac medications and corticosteroids), whereas others must be discontinued (e.g., oral hypoglycemic agents) or have their dose altered (e.g., insulin and anticoagulants). Still other medications should be started prophylactically to minimize perioperative risk (e.g., anticoagulants for prophylaxis against venous thromboembolism [Chapter 74] and antibiotic prophylaxis for surgical site infection or endocarditis [Chapter 67]). Data are often lacking or conflicting. Table 403-2 briefly summarizes "consensus" perioperative recommendations for the major classes of drugs.

CARDIAC RISK ASSESSMENT

A significant proportion of patients who undergo surgery have either known coronary artery disease or risk factors for it, and postoperative cardiac complications are second only to direct surgical complications as a cause of perioperative mortality. The goal is to risk-stratify patients clinically and to determine whether additional testing, new medications, or cardiac interventions will be beneficial.[4,5]

History and Physical Examination

Important information includes any history of previous cardiac disease (MI, angina, heart failure, arrhythmias, valvular disease), cardiac interventions (e.g., coronary artery bypass grafting; percutaneous coronary intervention, including date, indication, type, and number of stents placed), cardiac evaluation (noninvasive testing, angiography), risk factors (hypertension, diabetes mellitus, dyslipidemia, cigarette smoking), and associated diseases (peripheral arterial disease, stroke, chronic kidney disease, and chronic obstructive pulmonary disease [COPD]). Current status regarding chest pain or dyspnea, functional capacity,[6] and medications should be assessed. The physical examination serves to confirm findings in the history as well as to assess severity and control of the disease (e.g., heart failure, hypertension, valvular disease). The preoperative electrocardiogram rarely changes management unless it demonstrates evidence of a recent or silent MI, but it may be useful as a baseline against which to compare postoperative tracings.

Cardiac Risk Indices

Over the years, several risk indices have been proposed to assist in preoperative cardiac evaluation. The most widely used, the revised cardiac risk index (RCRI; Table 403-3), was derived during the evaluation of several thousand patients, was validated in thousands more, and has been incorporated into the consensus guidelines developed by the American College of Cardiology and the American Heart Association. These guidelines, which are updated

TABLE 403-1 RECOMMENDATIONS FOR PREOPERATIVE LABORATORY TESTING

TEST	% ABNORMAL	% INFLUENCING MANAGEMENT	INDICATIONS
Hemoglobin	1.8	0.1	Expected major blood loss, symptoms of anemia, chronic kidney disease
White blood count	0.7	0.0	Suspected infection, myeloproliferative disorder, myelotoxic medications
Platelet count	0.9	0.02	Bleeding diathesis, myeloproliferative neoplasm, myelotoxic medications
Prothrombin time/INR	0.3	0.0	Bleeding diathesis, liver disease, malnutrition, antibiotic use, anticoagulants
Partial thromboplastin time	6.5	0.1	Bleeding diathesis, anticoagulant use
Electrolytes	12.7	1.8	Renal disease, medications affecting electrolytes (e.g., diuretics, digoxin, ACE inhibitor, ARBs)
Glucose	9.3	0.5	Known DM, steroids, morbid obesity
Renal function	8.2	2.6	Renal disease, DM, HTN, major surgery, older age, medications affecting renal function
Liver function tests	0.4	0.1	Known liver disease, albumin level if at risk for needing postoperative parenteral nutrition
Urinalysis	19.1	1.4	No indication unless GU symptoms or instrumentation planned (although often requested before joint replacement or spine surgery)
Electrocardiogram	29.6 (19.7)	2.6	Vascular surgery; intermediate-risk surgery with at least 1 RCRI risk factor; not indicated in asymptomatic patients undergoing low-risk procedures or solely based on age
Chest radiograph	21.2 (4.9)	3.0	Acute cardiopulmonary disease suspected based on history and physical examination

ACE = angiotensin-converting enzyme; ARB = angiotensin receptor blocker; DM = diabetes mellitus; GU = genitourinary; HTN = hypertension;
INR = international normalized ratio; RCRI = Revised Cardiac Risk Index (1 point each for coronary artery disease; heart failure; prior cerebrovascular accident or transient ischemic attack; diabetes mellitus on insulin; creatinine >2.0; and abdominal, thoracic, or suprainguinal vascular surgery) (see Table 403-3).
Modified from Smetana GW, Macpherson DS. The case against routine preoperative laboratory testing. *Med Clin North Am.* 2003;87:7-40.

TABLE 403-2 PERIOPERATIVE MANAGEMENT OF MEDICATIONS

MEDICATION CLASS	RECOMMENDATION
Anticoagulants (heparins, warfarin NOACs [novel oral anticoagulants])*	Continue for minor surgery Discontinue at an appropriate interval before major surgery Consider bridging anticoagulation for patients at high risk for interim thrombosis (Chapter 76)
Antiplatelet drugs	Continue for minor surgery Discontinue clopidogrel and ticagrelor at least 5 days before surgery and prasugrel at least 7 days before surgery, except in patients with recent coronary stenting If discontinuing aspirin, do so 3-7 days before surgery
Cardiovascular medications	Continue most agents Consider starting β-blockers in select patients at high risk for perioperative cardiac morbidity Withhold diuretics on the morning of surgery, especially if signs of volume depletion are present Consider stopping ACE inhibitors or ARBs at least 12 hours before surgery unless patient has heart failure or uncontrolled hypertension Stop tamsulosin before cataract surgery (floppy iris syndrome)
Lipid-lowering agents	Continue "statins" Discontinue other agents
Pulmonary agents	Continue
Gastrointestinal agents	Continue
Diabetic agents (see text)	Withhold oral hypoglycemic agents on the morning of surgery; restart when the patient resumes eating For type 1 diabetes, continue some form of insulin (long-acting or intravenous) at all times For type 2 diabetes, decrease the dose of morning intermediate insulin; continue 80-100% of basal insulin
Thyroid agents (hypothyroidism and hyperthyroidism) (see text)	Continue thyroid replacement Continue antithyroid medication and postpone surgery until the hyperthyroidism is controlled
Oral contraceptives, hormone replacement, and SERMs	May discontinue 3 weeks before surgery only in patients at high risk for perioperative venous thromboembolism; otherwise continue
Corticosteroids (see text)	Continue chronic corticosteroids; increase the dosage to account for surgical stress
Psychotropic agents	Continue SSRIs Continue tricyclic antidepressants, benzodiazepines, lithium, and antipsychotics Usually discontinue MAOIs 10-14 days before surgery
Chronic opioids	Continue; substitute equianalgesic or higher doses for surgical pain
Rheumatologic agents	Continue methotrexate Discontinue other DMARDs and anticytokines about 2 weeks before surgery Continue hypouricemic agents
Neurologic agents	Continue antiseizure medications Continue antiparkinsonian agents Continue agents for myasthenia gravis
Herbal agents	Discontinue all agents

*See also Tables 403-5 and 403-6 for more detail.
ARB = angiotensin receptor blocker; ACE = angiotensin-converting enzyme; CNS = central nervous system; DMARD = disease-modifying antirheumatic drug; MAOI = monoamine oxidase inhibitor; SERM = selective estrogen receptor modulator; SSRI = selective serotonin reuptake inhibitor.
Adapted from Cohn SL, Macpherson DS. Perioperative medication management. In: Cohn SL, Smetana GW, Weed HG, eds. *Perioperative Medicine: Just the Facts.* New York: McGraw-Hill; 2006.

periodically, use a stepwise strategy based on clinical risk factors, surgery-specific risk, and exercise capacity, combined with a systematic approach to perioperative testing and treatment in patients with known or suspected cardiac disease (Fig. 403-1). Because the RCRI may underestimate risk in major vascular surgery and did not include many types of lower-risk surgeries (Table 403-4), newer risk indices have been developed. Although these alternatives have not been widely validated, current guidelines recommend either the RCRI or the American College of Surgeons surgical risk calculator (https://riskcalculator.facs.org/RiskCalculator/) or the MI/cardiac arrest risk calculator

derived from the National Surgical Quality Improvement (NSQIP) database (E-Table 403-1).[7] Preoperative levels of troponin and of brain natriuretic peptide (BNP) are independent predictors of postoperative cardiac complications. Although it is unclear how to use these biomarkers and whether any intervention based on these numbers will improve outcome, the Canadian Cardiovascular Society guidelines[8] recommend measuring a BNP level in patients who have an RCRI score greater than 1 or any other risk factors, and they also recommend 2 to 3 days of once-daily postoperative troponin levels if the BNP level is elevated (E-Fig. 403-1).

TABLE 403-3 CLINICAL FACTORS IMPORTANT IN ASSESSING PERIOPERATIVE CARDIAC RISK

REVISED CARDIAC RISK INDEX CRITERIA*

Ischemic heart disease defined as history of myocardial infarction, positive exercise test, current complaint of chest pain considered secondary to myocardial ischemia, use of nitrate therapy, or pathological Q waves on the electrocardiogram

Or at least two of the following:

Heart failure defined as S_3 or bilateral rales on physical examination or pulmonary edema on chest radiograph

Cerebrovascular disease defined as history of transient ischemic attack or history of cerebrovascular accident

Insulin-dependent diabetes mellitus

Chronic renal insufficiency defined as baseline creatinine of 2.0 mg/dL or greater

High-risk surgery defined as intrathoracic, intra-abdominal, or suprainguinal vascular surgery

*Lee TH, Marcantonio ER, Mangione CM, et al. Derivation and prospective validation of a simple index for prediction of cardiac risk of major noncardiac surgery. *Circulation.* 1999;100:1043-1049.

TABLE 403-4 RISKS OF VARIOUS SURGICAL PROCEDURES

HIGH (VERY ELEVATED) RISK (CARDIAC RISK >5%)

Major vascular surgery
Emergent major operations
Prolonged procedures with large fluid shifts or significant blood loss

INTERMEDIATE (BUT ELEVATED) RISK (CARDIAC RISK 1-5%)

Intraperitoneal or intrathoracic procedures
Carotid endarterectomy
Endovascular aortic aneurysm repair
Head and neck surgery
Orthopedic procedures
Prostate surgery

LOW RISK (CARDIAC RISK <1%)

Superficial operations
Cataract surgery
Breast surgery
Ambulatory surgery

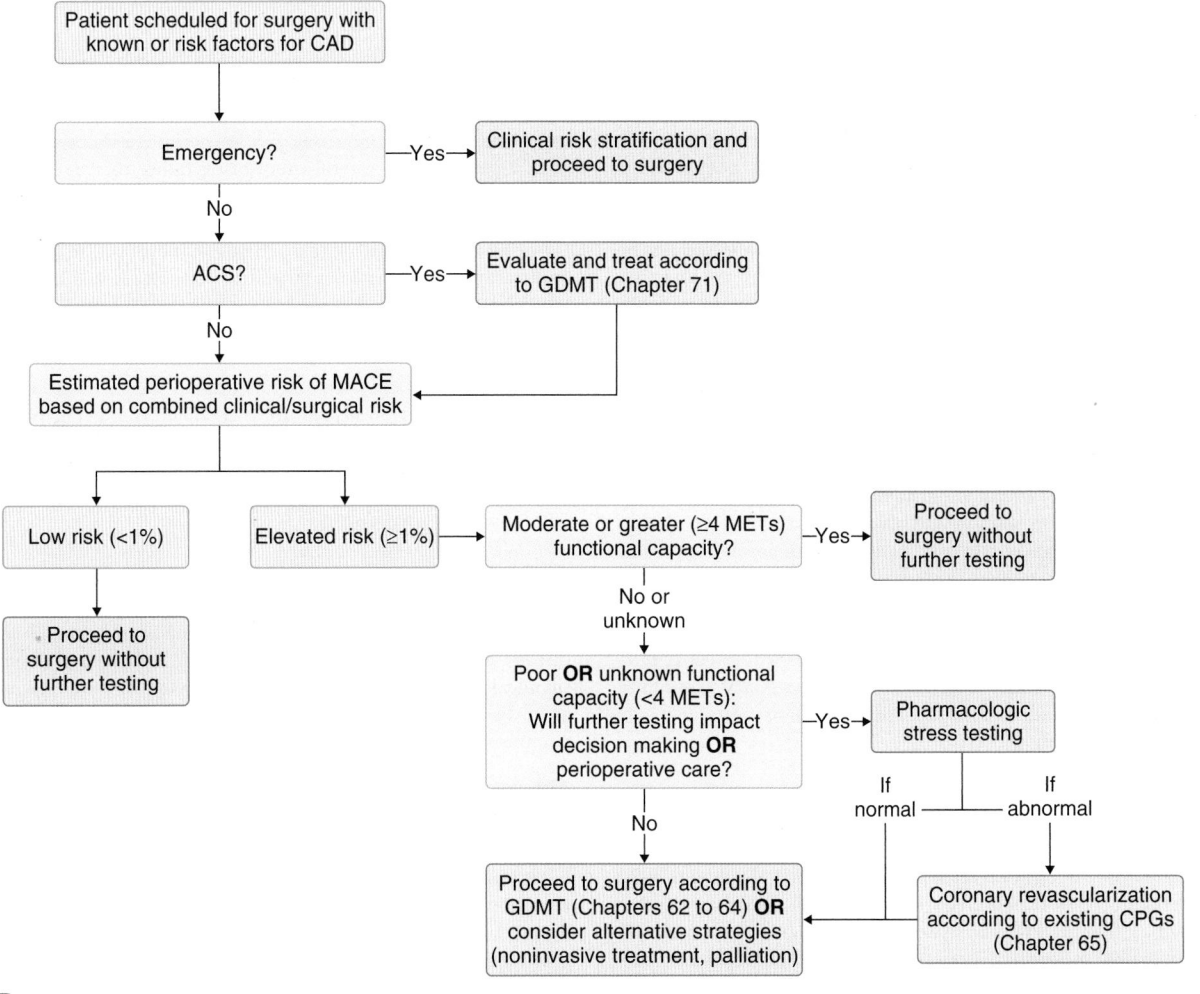

FIGURE 403-1. Stepwise approach to perioperative cardiac assessment for coronary artery disease (CAD). ACS = acute coronary syndrome (Chapter 63); CPGs = clinical practice guidelines; GDMT = guideline-directed medical therapy; MACE = major adverse cardiac event; METs = metabolic equivalents. The METS study investigators have reported that the use of scores on the Duke Activity Status Index (DASI) is more accurate for preoperative risk evaluation than subjective clinical assessment by the physician (Wijeysundera DN, Pearse RM, Shulman MA, et al.; METS study investigators. Assessment of functional capacity before major non-cardiac surgery: an international, prospective cohort study. *Lancet.* 2018;391:2631-2640.) (Adapted from Fleisher LA, Fleischmann KE, Auerbach AD, et al. 2014 ACC/AHA guideline on perioperative cardiovascular evaluation and management of patients undergoing noncardiac surgery: executive summary: a report of the American College of Cardiology/American Heart Association Task Force on Practice Guidelines. *J Am Coll Cardiol.* 2014;64:2373-2405.)

Noninvasive Tests

One emphasis of current guidelines is to minimize cardiac testing unless the results are likely to alter management. A resting echocardiogram (Chapter 49) is indicated to evaluate valvular heart disease in patients with clinically suspicious murmurs and to evaluate left ventricular function in patients with heart failure. Other than for the assessment of aortic stenosis (see later), resting echocardiography is not a reliable predictor of perioperative cardiac events.

Pharmacologic Stress Testing

Pharmacologic stress testing (either dipyridamole or adenosine with nuclear imaging [Chapters 50 and 62] or dobutamine echocardiography [Chapters 49 and 62]) is indicated when a patient who needs a stress test cannot perform adequate exercise (see Table 62-5 and Fig. 62-6 in Chapter 62). Both tests have a similar sensitivity for predicting perioperative ischemic complications, whereas stress echocardiography has fewer false-positive results. Nevertheless, local expertise commonly influences which test is selected. Dipyridamole and adenosine can cause bronchospasm and are best avoided in patients with symptomatic or severe asthma or obstructive lung disease, but they are preferred in patients with left bundle branch block, in whom exercise or stress echocardiography is more likely to give false-positive results. Quantitatively, the number and extent of reperfusion defects or wall motion abnormalities correlate with the severity of disease, likelihood of complications, and need for further evaluation by angiography.

Patients whose clinical condition would warrant stress testing independent of planned surgery should have such testing before elective operations. Otherwise, stress testing is recommended only in patients at elevated risk for noncardiac surgery and with poor functional capacity (defined as the inability to walk two to four blocks at 3 to 4 mph on level ground or to climb one flight of stairs; see Table 45-5 in Chapter 45) *if* the results will change management.

Risk Reduction Strategies for Ischemic Heart Disease

Medical Therapy

β-Blockers may reduce the risk for perioperative MI but with the side effect of increasing stroke risk and with no evidence for a reduction in overall mortality. In patients who do not have a very high risk for perioperative MI, β-blockers probably increase risk.[A1-A3] Whether it is helpful to start β-blockers before surgery in patients with intermediate- to high-risk ischemia on stress testing or with three or more RCRI risk factors is unknown, and data to support this option are insufficient. Furthermore, any benefits are more likely to be seen when β-blockers are started at least 1 week before surgery at a low dose and titrated to a heart rate of 55 to 70 beats per minute. Until more evidence is available, it seems prudent to avoid starting β-blockers immediately before surgery and to avoid them in the settings of emergency surgery, prior cerebrovascular disease, or sepsis, but to continue β-blockers in patients who are already taking them.

Neither clonidine[A4] nor aspirin[A5] is beneficial for reducing perioperative cardiac events, except continuing aspirin does appear to be beneficial in patients who have had a prior coronary stent and patients undergoing carotid endarterectomy.[9,10] Limited data on prophylactic calcium antagonists or nitrates have not shown major benefits in preventing complications after noncardiac surgery. Statins (Chapter 195) reduce endovascular inflammation and stabilize endothelial plaque. Current data suggest that they may be associated with decreased postoperative cardiac complications, should be continued perioperatively, and should be started preoperatively in patients who meet criteria for their ongoing use (Chapter 195).[A6] Aggressive fluid management to optimize cardiac output is controversial, and recent studies show no clear advantage when added to standard medical therapy.[A7]

Invasive Therapies

Prophylactic coronary revascularization in patients who have stable cardiac symptoms and no aortic stenosis and do not meet standard criteria for the procedure (Chapter 62) does not reduce perioperative MI, death within 30 days, or long-term mortality at an average of 2.7 years in patients who receive appropriate medical therapy. Preoperative coronary revascularization is indicated only if the patient meets the criteria for coronary angiography or revascularization independent of the need for surgery.

In patients with a recent coronary stent, the incremental risk for a cardiac event is increased by 3.5% and falls to 1% at 6 months and remains stable thereafter, with most of the increased risk in the first month after stent placement. For patients with bare metal stents, data suggest that elective surgery should be delayed for 4 to 6 weeks after stenting because of the risk for in-stent

thrombosis when dual antiplatelet therapy with aspirin and a P2Y12 inhibitor is discontinued early or because of the alternative risk for bleeding if surgery is performed in patients receiving such antiplatelet therapy (Chapter 65). For drug-eluting stents, elective surgery should be delayed for at least 3 months (if the risk for further delaying surgery is greater than that of stent thrombosis) and preferably 6 months if possible so that patients can complete an uninterrupted course of dual antiplatelet therapy.[11] Newer generation stents carry a lower risk for cardiac events, and shorter durations of dual antiplatelet therapy are being evaluated. However, risk is higher for stents placed in the setting of an acute MI, and dual antiplatelet therapy should be continued for 12 months in this setting. For balloon angioplasty without stenting, a delay of 2 weeks is generally recommended. If antiplatelet therapy has to be discontinued, clopidogrel is usually discontinued 5 to 7 days before the noncardiac procedure, prasugrel is stopped 7 days before, and ticagrelor is stopped 5 days before, whereas aspirin is continued, if possible. If aspirin also must be discontinued, it is usually stopped approximately 5 to 7 days before surgery, but shorter durations are being evaluated.[12]

Other Cardiovascular Diseases

Heart Failure

Heart failure, which is a major risk factor for surgery, requires treatment and optimization before surgery (Chapter 53). Patients with systolic heart failure, a reduced ejection fraction, or heart failure symptoms are at higher risk. Routine use of *pulmonary artery catheters* does not reduce morbidity or mortality in patients undergoing elective noncardiac surgery. Although an elevated BNP level is a risk factor, there is no evidence that treatment to lower the BNP level or use of β-blockers will reduce postoperative complications in patients with heart failure.

Valvular Heart Disease

Patients with *symptomatic aortic stenosis* who meet the criteria for valve replacement (Chapter 66) independent of their need for surgery should undergo the valve replacement before elective noncardiac surgery. However, patients usually survive noncardiac surgery with intensified care if they refuse valve replacement or time does not permit it.[13] An asymptomatic aortic valve area of 1.0 to 1.5 cm^2 carries an increased risk for perioperative complications but is an indication for more careful monitoring rather than requiring preoperative valve surgery. Patients with severe mitral regurgitation also have higher risks for postoperative cardiovascular complications. Endocarditis prophylaxis (Chapter 67) is appropriate for patients with mechanical heart valves, previous endocarditis, complex congenital heart disease, or valvular disease in a heart transplant recipient undergoing invasive dental or upper respiratory procedures (Chapter 67).

Hypertension

Hypertension with blood pressure lower than 110 mm Hg diastolic or 180 mm Hg systolic without significant target organ damage does not increase the risk for major perioperative cardiac complications. Even when the preoperative diastolic blood pressure is higher, limited data suggest that surgery is safe after additional antihypertensive therapy.

Arrhythmias

Although patients with arrhythmias have increased perioperative risk, the risk is increased because the arrhythmias are usually markers of more serious heart disease or cause hemodynamic problems. Patients with hemodynamically significant tachyarrhythmias and bradyarrhythmias should generally be treated as in the nonoperative setting (Chapters 58 and 59), except for the special circumstance of anticoagulation in the perioperative setting (Chapter 76).

⬤ PULMONARY RISK ASSESSMENT

Postoperative pulmonary complications are as common as cardiac complications and are associated with significant morbidity and mortality. Major complications include respiratory failure (e.g., reintubation, prolonged mechanical ventilation), pneumonia, atelectasis requiring bronchoscopy, and to a lesser degree, bronchospasm or an exacerbation of COPD requiring treatment and prolonged length of stay. Many postoperative pulmonary complications are due to exaggerations of the usual postoperative changes in pulmonary function: decreased lung volumes, diaphragmatic dysfunction, ventilation-perfusion mismatches and shunting, hypoventilation, hypoxemia, and impaired defense mechanisms. Pulmonary risk factors can be divided into patient-related and procedure-related factors, the latter of which include the type of surgery, anesthesia, and related factors.[14] Several risk indices have been developed to predict postoperative pulmonary complications, including ARISCAT (E-Table 403-2), but are not widely used.

Patient-Related Factors

COPD (Chapter 82) increases the risk for postoperative pulmonary complications approximately twofold, depending on its severity, whereas well-controlled *asthma* (Chapter 81) does not increase risk. Active cigarette smokers are at increased risk, mainly related to the number of pack years smoked; smoking cessation at least 4 to 8 weeks before surgery may reduce the risk. *Obstructive sleep apnea* (Chapter 377), typically associated with obesity, confers an increased risk for airway complications, including hypercapnia and hypoxemia. Obese patients are at increased risk for atelectasis. Patients should be screened preoperatively for obstructive sleep apnea using an approach such as STOP-BANG (E-Table 403-3). A score of 5 or higher suggests moderate to severe obstructive sleep apnea and an increased risk for hypoventilation and postoperative complications.[15,16] Advanced age, poor functional status, pulmonary hypertension, an altered mental state, and suppressed immune status from chronic steroid use, alcohol use, or diabetes may also increase the risk for postoperative pulmonary complications.

Procedure-Related Factors

The most important predictors of postoperative pulmonary complications are the type of surgery and proximity of the surgical incision to the diaphragm. Pulmonary function decreases by approximately 50% after intrathoracic and upper abdominal procedures, and it does not fully return to normal for several weeks. Lower abdominal surgery is associated with a 25% decrease in pulmonary function. Laparoscopic procedures may be associated with lower rates of postoperative pulmonary complications and shorter hospital stays than open procedures. Neuraxial anesthesia (epidural or spinal) may be associated with decreased risk when compared with general anesthesia, but the decision about which type of anesthesia to use is best left to the anesthesiologist. Emergency surgery, prolonged duration of anesthesia or surgery (>2 to 6 hours), and routine postoperative nasogastric tube use increase the risk for postoperative pulmonary complications.

Pulmonary Function Tests

In general, pulmonary function tests (Chapter 79) are no more predictive of pulmonary complications than is clinical risk assessment alone. Such testing may be more helpful in assessing risk for lung resection surgery when it can predict the function of the remaining lung mass. However, even a postoperative predicted forced expiratory volume in 1 second (FEV_1) of less than 800 mL for lung resection, which is thought to portend a very high risk for death or prolonged mechanical ventilation, is not an absolute contraindication to surgery. Preoperative arterial blood gas evaluation is also of little benefit in predicting postoperative pulmonary complications. Cardiopulmonary exercise testing for maximal oxygen consumption is useful for evaluating high-risk patients before lung resection surgery.

Risk Reduction Strategies

Unfortunately, many of the risk factors for postoperative pulmonary complications cannot be modified. Inhaled bronchodilators (β-agonists and anticholinergics) and steroids can optimize the respiratory status of patients with COPD and asthma. Broad-spectrum antibiotics should be used to treat exacerbations caused by bacterial infection. Chest physiotherapy and inspiratory muscle training may be helpful, particularly for thoracic surgery.[A8] Smoking should be stopped at least 8 weeks before surgery, if possible.

Lung expansion maneuvers (either incentive spirometry or deep-breathing exercises) can improve pulmonary function, minimize atelectasis, and reduce risk, especially for thoracic and upper abdominal surgery. Pain control (Chapter 27) improves pulmonary function by allowing deeper breathing. Epidural analgesia and patient-controlled intravenous analgesia reduce postoperative pulmonary complications and, when possible, are preferable to parenteral narcotics. Long-acting neuromuscular blockers should be avoided, and the selective rather than the routine use of a nasogastric tube may also decrease risk.

● ENDOCRINE CONDITIONS

Diabetes Mellitus

The major risks associated with surgery in diabetic patients are cardiac complications and wound infections. Complications are probably related more to associated diseases and end-organ involvement (coronary artery disease, chronic kidney disease, and autonomic neuropathy) than to the glucose level itself.

Significantly, elevated glucose levels may impair wound healing and interfere with leukocyte defense mechanisms. However, current recommendations suggest a glucose target level of 140 to 180 mg/dL rather than tight perioperative control.

Patients whose diabetes is controlled by diet require only perioperative glucose monitoring (finger sticks) with short-acting insulin coverage on an as-needed basis. Patients taking oral hypoglycemic agents (Chapter 216) should not take them on the morning of surgery and should be monitored with sliding-scale insulin coverage as needed. Patients taking insulin are most often given one half to two thirds of their usual intermediate-acting insulin on the morning of surgery and are then given short-acting insulin on a sliding scale and correction dose based on finger stick monitoring (Chapter 216). Continuous intravenous insulin, which provides tighter glucose control but is associated with more episodes of hypoglycemia and requires a monitored setting, is typically used in patients undergoing cardiac surgery and in critically ill patients. In general, long-acting basal insulin should be continued, but its dose may be reduced in patients with tight control, previous hypoglycemia, or chronic kidney disease. Regardless of the mode of treatment, frequent monitoring of the glucose level is critical.

Exogenous Corticosteroids and Adrenal Insufficiency

The stress of surgery activates the hypothalamic-pituitary-adrenal (HPA) axis, which in turn stimulates release of adrenocorticotropic hormone (ACTH) and subsequent secretion of cortisol (Chapter 214), but a patient who is taking exogenous corticosteroids may have suppression of the HPA axis and not be able to respond to this stress adequately. As a result, hypotension and shock may occur.

In general, a daily dose equivalent to 5 mg or less of prednisone (Chapter 214), alternate-day short-acting therapy, or corticosteroids given for less than 3 weeks do not cause clinically significant HPA suppression, so no supplemental therapy is indicated. Conversely, doses greater than 20 mg/day of prednisone for longer than 3 weeks usually suppress the HPA axis and warrant perioperative supplemental corticosteroids. In patients who are taking intermediate dosing regimens or who took large doses in the past year but are not taking corticosteroids or are taking lower doses now, the options are to perform an ACTH (cosyntropin) stimulation test, if time permits, and treat only patients with an inadequate response (Chapter 214) or to prescribe supplemental corticosteroids empirically.

When supplemental corticosteroids are felt to be appropriate, short-term therapy tailored to the level of expected stress can provide protection without adverse effects on wound healing and with only short-term problems with glucose intolerance and fluid retention. For minor procedures or local anesthesia, the recommended approach is to give the patient's usual dose before surgery without further supplementation. For moderate surgical stress (e.g., open cholecystectomy, lower extremity vascular surgery), a reasonable approach is 50 mg of hydrocortisone intravenously before surgery, followed by 25 mg every 8 hours for 1 to 2 days, and then the patient's usual dose. For major surgical stress, patients are typically given 75 to 100 mg of hydrocortisone intravenously before induction of anesthesia, followed by 50 mg every 8 hours for 1 to 3 days until the stressful period resolves, and then their usual dose.

Thyroid Disease

An inadequately treated or undiagnosed hyperthyroid patient is potentially at risk for thyroid storm postoperatively. Elective surgery should be postponed in patients who are symptomatic or have resting tachycardia until they are euthyroid. Treatment of a thyrotoxic patient undergoing urgent or emergency surgery includes a combination of β-blockers, antithyroid agents, and iodine to control the resting heart rate to less than 90 beats per minute, as well as prophylactic corticosteroid supplementation, as used for thyroid storm (Chapter 213). Conversely, patients with mild to moderate hypothyroidism tolerate surgery reasonably well.[17] Patients with markedly symptomatic hypothyroidism should be treated with oral levothyroxine (T_4) for several weeks before elective surgery. For emergency surgery, intravenous liothyronine (T_3) or T_4 (200 to 300 μg intravenously, then 50 to 100 μg/day) and supplemental corticosteroids (hydrocortisone, 100 mg intravenously, then 25 to 50 mg every 6 hours) should be given. Myxedema coma is a rare complication of surgery.

● LIVER DISEASE

Routine preoperative testing of liver function is not recommended, but elective surgery should be avoided in patients with acute viral, alcoholic, or drug-induced hepatitis. Patients with stable mild chronic hepatitis tolerate surgery well.

Patients with alcoholic liver disease or cirrhosis are at risk for postoperative complications, including bleeding, infection, poor wound healing, and delirium.

TABLE 403-5 SUGGESTED APPROACH TO ANTICOAGULATION IN THE PERIOPERATIVE PATIENT

Low thromboembolic risk/low bleeding risk
- Continue anticoagulant therapy with INR in therapeutic range.

High thromboembolic risk
- Discontinue VKA (warfarin) 5 days before the procedure (assuming INR 2-3).
- Start therapeutic LMWH twice daily or UFH IV 36-48 hours after warfarin interruption.
- Administer the last dose of LMWH at least 24 hr before or UFH IV at least 4-6 hr before surgery.
- Resume LMWH or UFH at the preprocedural dose 24-72 hr after the procedure depending on the risk for bleeding.
- Resume VKA anticoagulant therapy 12-24 hr after surgery according to hemostatic status.
- Continue LMWH or UFH until the INR has returned to therapeutic levels.

Intermediate thromboembolic risk
- Individualize need for bridging anticoagulation.

VKA = vitamin K antagonist; LMWH = low-molecular-weight heparin; INR = international normalized ratio; IV = intravenous; UFH = unfractionated heparin.
Adapted from Douketis JD, Spyropoulos AC, Spencer FA, et al. Perioperative management of antithrombotic therapy: antithrombotic therapy and prevention of thrombosis, 9th ed: American College of Chest Physicians Evidence-Based Clinical Practice Guidelines. *Chest.* 2012;141:e326S-350S; and Doherty JU, Gluckman TJ, Hucker WJ, et al. 2017 ACC expert consensus decision pathway for periprocedural management of anticoagulation in patients with nonvalvular atrial fibrillation: a report of the American College of Cardiology Clinical Expert Consensus Document Task Force. *J Am Coll Cardiol.* 2017;69(7):871-898.

TABLE 403-6 PREOPERATIVE MANAGEMENT OF THE NEW ORAL ANTICOAGULANTS

DRUG	CREATININE CLEARANCE (mL/min)	HALF-LIFE (hr)	WHEN TO STOP ANTICOAGULANT BEFORE SURGERY STANDARD BLEEDING RISK SURGERY	WHEN TO STOP ANTICOAGULANT BEFORE SURGERY HIGH BLEEDING RISK SURGERY*
Dabigatran	>50	13-15	1 day[†]	2 days[†]
	31-50	18	2 days	3 days
	≤30	27	3 days	4 days
Rivaroxaban	>30	7-11	1 day	2 days
	≤30	?	2 days	3 days
Apixaban	>30	8-14	1 day	2 days
	≤30	?	2 days	3 days
Edoxaban	>50	10-14	1 day	2 days
	≤50	?	2 days	3 days

*Examples include neurosurgery and spine, cardiac, major abdominal, and vascular surgery.
[†]This means 1 full day or 2 full days. For 1 full day, the last dose is given 36 hours before surgery; for 2 full days it would be given 60 hours before surgery; and so forth in this Table.

The severity of disease as assessed by Child-Turcotte-Pugh criteria and the MELD (Model for End-Stage Liver Disease) score (Chapter 145) can be used to estimate risk; the MELD score is thought to be more predictive of outcome. Child's C class and MELD score greater than 15 portend very high risk, and elective surgery is usually contraindicated. Aggressive treatment of coagulopathy, ascites, and encephalopathy is indicated before surgery.

HEMATOLOGIC PROBLEMS

Preoperative anemia, even to a mild degree, is independently associated with an increased risk for 30-day morbidity and mortality in patients undergoing major noncardiac surgery, but operative patients generally tolerate hemoglobin levels as low as 7 g/dL. Preoperative transfusion should not be triggered solely by the hemoglobin level but should also consider the expected blood loss from the surgical procedure and the patient's comorbid conditions. For patients with cardiopulmonary disease, however, a goal of 9 to 10 g/dL may be appropriate for major surgery.[A9]

Patients without a personal or family history of abnormal bleeding require no preoperative testing of coagulative function, but those with such a history should be evaluated. Ideally, the prothrombin time should be within 3 seconds of control (international normalized ratio <1.5), the partial thromboplastin time within 10 seconds of control, and the platelet count above a minimum of 50,000, depending on the type of surgery.

The approach to perioperative anticoagulation for preventing thromboembolism is described elsewhere (Chapter 76). For patients already on warfarin anticoagulation for atrial fibrillation, perioperative bridging with low-molecular-weight heparin for the prevention of arterial thromboembolism does not reduce the risk for arterial thromboembolism but does significantly increase the risk for major bleeding.[A10] Perioperative recommendations for higher risk patients (e.g., mechanical prosthetic valve or stroke, transient ischemic attack, or systemic embolism in the prior 12 weeks) depend on the short-term risks for thromboembolism and bleeding (Table 403-5),[18] but even then the need for bridging therapy has been questioned because the risk for bleeding with early postoperative anticoagulation may outweigh any potential benefit. Use of the new oral anticoagulants (dabigatran, rivaroxaban, apixaban, and edoxaban) obviates the need for bridging therapy because of their shorter half-lives and more rapid onset of action compared with warfarin (Table 403-6). They can be stopped closer to the time of surgery but should be started postoperatively only after adequate hemostasis has been ensured, usually 48 to 72 hours after major surgery. Idarucizumab (either two consecutive IV infusions with 2.5 g or two consecutive IV boluses of 2.5 g each) is an effective antidote for dabigatran, whereas andexanet (administered as a bolus plus an infusion) can safely reverse the anticoagulant activity of apixaban and rivaroxaban within minutes in patients with life-threatening bleeding (Chapter 76).

RENAL DISORDERS

Chronic kidney disease is an independent risk factor for postoperative cardiovascular events and death. Patients with chronic kidney disease typically have other comorbid diseases and may also have fluid and electrolyte abnormalities, anemia, and bleeding diatheses, which should be treated and optimized before surgery. Neither aspirin nor clonidine administered perioperatively reduces the risk for acute kidney injury.[A11] Patients maintained on dialysis should ideally undergo dialysis the day before surgery to optimize their volume status, prevent hyperkalemia, and minimize acute shifts in acid-base balance.

NEUROLOGIC AND GERIATRIC PROBLEMS

The risk for a postoperative stroke in unselected patients after general surgery is less than 0.5%, but patients with a history of stroke or atrial fibrillation, older patients, and those undergoing vascular surgery, especially cardiac and carotid surgery, have higher risk.[19] Patients with symptomatic carotid bruits require further investigation and possible intervention before elective surgery (Chapter 379). There is no evidence to support preoperative intervention in patients with asymptomatic bruits before noncardiac surgery. The general recommendation is to delay elective surgery for at least 1 to 3 months after a stroke, although some data suggest waiting up to 9 months.

The elderly are at higher risks for a variety of poor postoperative outcomes. Cognitive impairment (Chapters 24 and 25), frailty (Chapter 21), malnutrition, and prior institutionalization all are associated with a poorer prognosis.[20]

Grade A References

A1. Wijeysundera DN, Duncan D, Nkonde-Price C, et al. Perioperative beta blockade in noncardiac surgery: a systematic review for the 2014 ACC/AHA guideline on perioperative cardiovascular evaluation and management of patients undergoing noncardiac surgery: a report of the American College of Cardiology/American Heart Association Task Force on practice guidelines. *J Am Coll Cardiol.* 2014;64:2406-2425.

A2. Blessberger H, Kammler J, Domanovits H, et al. Perioperative beta-blockers for preventing surgery-related mortality and morbidity. *Cochrane Database Syst Rev.* 2018;3:CD004476.

A3. Hajibandeh S, Hajibandeh S, Antoniou SA, et al. Effect of beta-blockers on perioperative outcomes in vascular and endovascular surgery: a systematic review and meta-analysis. *Br J Anaesth.* 2017;118:11-21.

A4. Devereaux PJ, Sessler DI, Leslie K, et al. Clonidine in patients undergoing noncardiac surgery. *N Engl J Med.* 2014;370:1504-1513.

A5. Devereaux PJ, Mrkobrada M, Sessler DI, et al. Aspirin in patients undergoing noncardiac surgery. *N Engl J Med.* 2014;370:1494-1503.

A6. Antoniou GA, Fisher RK, Georgiadis GS, et al. Statin therapy in lower limb peripheral arterial disease: systematic review and meta-analysis. *Vascul Pharmacol.* 2014;63:79-87.

A7. Pearse RM, Harrison DA, MacDonald N, et al. Effect of a perioperative, cardiac output-guided hemodynamic therapy algorithm on outcomes following major gastrointestinal surgery: a randomized clinical trial and systematic review. *JAMA.* 2014;311:2181-2190.

A8. Katsura M, Kuriyama A, Takeshima T, et al. Preoperative inspiratory muscle training for postoperative pulmonary complications in adults undergoing cardiac and major abdominal surgery. *Cochrane Database Syst Rev.* 2015;10:CD010356.

A9. Docherty AB, O'Donnell R, Brunskill S, et al. Effect of restrictive versus liberal transfusion strategies on outcomes in patients with cardiovascular disease in a non-cardiac surgery setting: systematic review and meta-analysis. *BMJ.* 2016;352:1-11.

A10. Douketis JD, Spyropoulos AC, Kaatz S, et al. Perioperative bridging anticoagulation in patients with atrial fibrillation. *N Engl J Med.* 2015;373:823-833.

A11. Garg AX, Kurz A, Sessler DI, et al. Perioperative aspirin and clonidine and risk of acute kidney injury: a randomized clinical trial. *JAMA.* 2014;312:2254-2264.

GENERAL REFERENCES

For the General References and other additional features, please visit Expert Consult at https://expertconsult.inkling.com.

404

OVERVIEW OF ANESTHESIA

JEANINE P. WIENER-KRONISH AND LEE A. FLEISHER

In the United States more than 40 million procedures, including outpatient procedures that require an anesthetic, are performed annually. Additionally, many invasive procedures outside of the operating room, such as in the gastrointestinal endoscopy and electrophysiology suites, are performed using deep sedation or general anesthesia. With modern techniques, anesthesia causes or contributes to mortality in about 1 per 20,000 healthy patients. Although the worldwide perioperative mortality attributable to anesthesia has declined by more than 90% in the past several decades, the overall inpatient postoperative mortality rate remains about 4%, with large variations even among developed countries. Although mortality directly attributable to anesthesia is low, optimal perioperative management and risk reduction strategies can reduce complications related to the patient's primary disease and the stresses of surgery. Protocols to enhance recovery after surgery are one such example of risk reduction strategies.[1]

PREOPERATIVE ASSESSMENT

Important aspects of preoperative risk assessment include the type of surgery to be performed, the patient's underlying medical condition, and the particular demands for anesthesia (Chapter 403). In addition, a number of other issues are relevant to management and anesthetic evaluation.

Airway Assessment

Assessment of the airway is always necessary, even if regional anesthesia or monitored anesthesia care (local anesthesia with sedation) is planned, because unexpected complications or compromise of airway reflexes may lead to an emergent need to support ventilation. The laryngeal mask airway device allows many patients to be ventilated easily, but it is important to assess the ability to intubate the patient as well as the ability to ventilate. The prevalence of difficult intubation is about 6% for nonobese patients, and reasons for difficulty include airway pathology (e.g., tumors, previous surgery), reduced mobility of the cervical spine, obstructive sleep apnea, or the anatomic relationship between the larynx and trachea. Although the videolaryngoscope offers improved views of the larynx and is used in many patients who need difficult or emergent intubation,[A1] the device does not improve success in nonexpert hands, nor does its use prevent complications.[A2] Difficult intubations can best be accomplished by clinicians who are expert in airways and who can personalize the choice among the various methods for intubation.[A3]

Criteria for extubation in postoperative patients are similar to those in other patients who receive mechanical ventilation (Chapter 97). Older patients with more severe, comorbid diseases, especially underlying cardiac or pulmonary disease, are more likely to require postoperative reintubation, which is associated with a nine-fold increase in mortality.

MEDICATION REACTIONS

Malignant Hyperthermia

Malignant hyperthermia (Chapter 406) is characterized by acute hyperpyrexia developing during or immediately after general anesthesia. The channels that regulate the duration and amplitude of calcium efflux from the sarcoplasmic reticulum are the ryanodine receptors, which exist as three isoforms. Gain-of-function mutations affecting RyR1, the receptor expressed primarily in skeletal muscle, are present in 1 per 15,000 to 50,000 people and are associated with enhanced sensitivity to halothane and caffeine, with exertional rhabdomyolysis (Chapter 105),[2] with malignant hyperthermia and central core disease, and with bleeding abnormalities. More than 80 distinct mutations have been detected, and mutation of the adult skeletal muscle sodium channel, SCN4A, may also cause the syndrome. Patients with mutations predisposing to malignant hyperthermia function normally at resting conditions, but exposure to volatile anesthetics, including halothane, isoflurane, enflurane, desflurane, and sevoflurane, or exposure to a depolarizing muscle relaxant, succinylcholine, can precipitate life-threatening muscle contractures, increases in heart rate and body temperature, rhabdomyolysis, myoglobinuria, and metabolic acidosis. The mortality rate is 80% in untreated patients but about 5% with current treatment. Note that succinylcholine causes a release of myoglobin from muscle in small amounts even in normal patients. Patients with malignant hyperthermia do not predictably respond to triggering agents, and some patients with malignant hyperthermia have had milder symptoms of malignant hyperthermia after the administration of nontriggering agents. Malignant hyperthermia now often occurs in muted forms, probably because of the decreased use of succinylcholine by anesthesiologists, the diagnostic awareness of malignant hyperthermia by anesthesiologists, the routine use of carbon dioxide monitors so that increases in end-expiratory carbon dioxide are detected quickly, and the availability of dantrolene. If malignant hyperthermia is suspected by obtaining a family history of adverse events with the administration of anesthesia or when a patient has a reaction suspicious for malignant hyperthermia, a muscle biopsy is usually obtained for in vitro contracture testing, which evaluates the muscle contracture responses to caffeine or halothane. Genetic investigations are also recommended, but malignant hyperthermia cannot be excluded on the basis of genetic testing alone because of the diversity of mutations and genes that can be involved in this syndrome. The Malignant Hyperthermia Association of the United States, www.mhaus.org, is available for information to the public, and all medical personnel can get information 24 hours every day on the malignant hyperthermia hotline, 1-800-MHHYPER or 1-800-644-9737.

Two other rare congenital myopathies associated with mutations of the RyR1 are central core disease and multiminicore disease. Patients with central core disease present with infantile hypotonia; a muscle biopsy is needed for definitive diagnosis. Multiminicore disease is a nonprogressive congenital myopathy in which infants present with hypotonia, ophthalmoplegia, and arthrogryposis. These children develop scoliosis and eventually may require chronic ventilation. Avoidance of triggering agents is advised for these syndromes and for patients with other myopathies. Both malignant hyperthermia and central core disease are thought to be inherited as autosomal dominant diseases, but extensive genetic analysis has revealed overlapping phenotypes.

TREATMENT Rx

Dantrolene is the drug of choice to prevent and to reverse the symptoms of malignant hyperthermia.[3] Dantrolene decreases muscle sensitivity to caffeine, reduces the release of calcium from the sarcoplasmic reticulum, and produces some muscle weakness. Dantrolene comes in 20-mg bottles and must be dissolved in sterile water; the recommended dose is 2.5 mg/kg given rapidly up to 10 mg/kg, repeated every 5 to 10 minutes until symptoms subside. Other treatments for malignant hyperthermia include discontinuing the use of any volatile anesthetics; hyperventilating the patient and administering 100% oxygen; administering bicarbonate for severe acidosis; controlling fevers; and maintaining a temperature below 39° C without causing hypothermia by using iced fluids, surface cooling, and cooling of body cavities if necessary. The patient's temperature and vital signs, urinary output, muscle enzymes, glucose, coagulation studies, acid-base status, and gas exchange should be monitored for 48 hours and be observed for 72 hours to ensure there is no recrudescence.

Monoamine Oxidase Inhibitors and Serotonin Toxicity

Anesthesiologists routinely ask if patients are taking a monoamine oxidase (MAO) inhibitor because of their many drug interactions with analgesics in perioperative patients. Serotonin toxicity has features similar to malignant hyperthermia and must be distinguished from it. Serotonin toxicity is characterized as a triad of neuromuscular hyperactivity (tremor, clonus, myoclonus, hyperreflexia, and pyramidal rigidity), autonomic hyperactivity (diaphoresis, fever, tachycardia, and tachypnea), and altered mental status (agitation, excitement, and confusion). It can be precipitated by the coadministration of MAO inhibitors and selective serotonin reuptake inhibitors (SSRIs). Patients who are taking SSRIs have a higher overall perioperative mortality, a higher 30-day readmission rate, and a higher likelihood of bleeding. Rigidity, increasing arterial carbon dioxide levels, and fever above 38.5° C are associated with life-threatening toxicity. Ecstasy, or 3,4-methylenedioxymethamphetamine (MDMA), combined with MAO inhibitors, including moclobemide, can be fatal because it acts as a serotonin releaser. Tramadol, used for pain relief, and venlafaxine, an antidepressant, act as serotonin releasers and are associated with toxicity when used in patients who are taking MAO inhibitors.

Anaphylaxis in the Perioperative Period

The incidence of life-threatening hypersensitivity reactions during anesthesia is 1 : 4000 to 1 : 25,000. Anaphylaxis is caused by immunoglobulin E (IgE)–mediated reactions (Chapter 238), whereas anaphylactoid reactions produce the same clinical picture but are not mediated by IgE. Anaphylaxis during anesthesia can present as cardiovascular collapse, airway obstruction, flushing, or edema of the skin, singly or in combination, so a careful history of any previous allergic reactions to medications and the nature of the reaction must be obtained by the anesthesiologist and other members of the perioperative team. Neuromuscular blocking agents, such as succinylcholine, and opioid analgesics can cause nonimmunologic release of histamine from mast cells and produce a similar clinical syndrome. Antibiotics, protamine, and blood transfusions (Chapter 167), all given routinely during operations, also can elicit a variety of systemic reactions. About 75% of perioperative hypersensitivity reactions appear to be due to muscle relaxants, especially rocuronium and vecuronium, with a mortality rate of 3 to 6%. In patients with apparent allergic reactions, skin testing is usually performed, and IgE levels are usually obtained to determine whether the patient had an allergic reaction to a perioperative medication.

Latex Allergies

For sensitized patients (Chapter 238), exposure to even low amounts of latex-containing particles is sufficient to induce a severe anaphylactic reaction. A latex-free operating environment, in which no latex gloves or latex accessories are used, is key in patients with known allergy. Skin prick tests with latex extracts should be considered in patients at high risk for latex allergy. Early aggressive treatment with epinephrine is critical if severe anaphylaxis occurs.

⬤ INTRAOPERATIVE MANAGEMENT

There are three general classes of anesthesia: general, regional, and monitored anesthesia care. The same drugs are often used for general anesthesia and monitored anesthesia care; achievement of the two different conditions requires knowledge of the pharmacokinetics of the drugs (Table 404-1).

TABLE 404-1	COMMON ANESTHETIC APPROACHES FOR VARIOUS TYPES OF SURGERY

SURGERY ON INTRA-ABDOMINAL OR INTRATHORACIC ORGANS

Examples: cardiac surgery, lung resections, gastric bypass
   General anesthesia usually administered because mechanical ventilation is often required
   Drugs include premedication for anxiety with midazolam, general anesthesia with volatile anesthetics (desflurane, sevoflurane, nitrous oxide), neuromuscular blockade, and opioid analgesics*
   Epidural anesthesia and analgesia also used; examples include ropivacaine, lidocaine, with fentanyl

SURGERY ON LIMBS

Examples: hip replacement, knee replacement, foot or arm surgery
   Can perform with epidural or spinal anesthesia, depending on the limb. Examples of medications would include tetracaine, lidocaine, ropivacaine, and fentanyl or morphine
   Can perform axillary or scalene block; examples include lidocaine and ropivacaine
   For postoperative pain control: can perform regional blocks that leave the catheter in place, including femoral nerve block, axillary nerve blocks

CATARACT SURGERY—LOCAL ANESTHESIA ON EYE WITH OR WITHOUT SEDATION

Examples of drugs used for sedation include midazolam and fentanyl

*Includes the use of opioids given intraoperatively with effects that extend into the postanesthesia care unit (PACU) or postoperative period, opioids given in the PACU, or opioids given or intended to be given after discharge from the PACU.

General Anesthesia

General anesthesia can be achieved with a balanced drug regimen that induces a loss of consciousness, which can range from a deep sedation requiring only airway support to states requiring full ventilatory support because of weakness and loss of respiratory drive. Both intravenous[4] and inhalational drugs can be used to induce and maintain general anesthesia. In contrast, monitored anesthesia care denotes a state in which patients can still control their airway, do not require ventilatory support, but are sleepy, have less pain, and may be amnestic. The quantity of anesthesia required to achieve unconsciousness varies depending on the patient's brain function and can be titrated by using electroencephalography.

Overall, there is no evidence that major postoperative cardiac events differ depending on whether non–cardiac surgery patients receive general, spinal, or epidural anesthesia.[A4] However, careful management of the hypertensive patient[5] and individualizing the maintenance of systolic blood pressure within 10% of the patient's resting systolic blood pressure, such as by the use of intraoperative norepinephrine, can reduce the risk of postoperative organ dysfunction in high-risk patients.[A5]

Propofol

Propofol, an alkylphenol, is perhaps the most frequently used intravenous anesthetic for induction of anesthesia and is often used for maintenance of anesthesia during short procedures or to achieve deep sedation during monitored anesthesia care. It is lipid soluble and quickly cleared from the central compartment, so it is rapidly eliminated even after long periods of continuous infusion. However, the clearance of propofol is changed by gender (men have lower clearance rates than women), size (children require higher doses), age (elderly patients have decreased clearance rates and experience increased effects with the drug), and narcotics, which decrease its clearance. Because of its predilection for causing apnea, propofol should be administered only by someone with expertise in airway management. Propofol also decreases arterial blood pressure, causes pain with injection, and can precipitate myoclonus. Large quantities of propofol can cause the propofol infusion syndrome, which is associated with cardiomyopathy, metabolic acidosis, skeletal myopathy, hyperkalemia, hepatomegaly, and lipemia. Despite these issues, propofol is frequently used because the recovery from propofol is within minutes, even after it is given as a prolonged continuous infusion, in contrast to the longer duration of drug effects seen after the administration of other intravenous sedatives.

Propofol has been suggested as the preferred agent for healthy outpatients undergoing colonoscopy because it leads to earlier discharge and higher patient satisfaction compared with other agents.[A6] However, the wide variability of anesthetic practices for endoscopy has led to questions about the cost-effectiveness of this practice.[6]

Midazolam

Midazolam, a benzodiazepine that produces muscle relaxation through a central mechanism, is hypnotic, sedative, anxiolytic, amnesic, and anticonvulsant. Its amnesic and anticonvulsant effects are mediated through α_1-subunit-containing γ-aminobutyric acid A (GABA$_A$) receptors, and the anxiolytic and muscle relaxation are mediated through α_2-subunit-containing GABA$_A$ receptors. Only 20% receptor occupancy is needed to produce anxiolysis, whereas unconsciousness requires 60%. Long-term administration of benzodiazepines produces tolerance, which appears to decrease receptor binding and function. Benzodiazepines cause dose-related depression of the respiratory system, with a peak effect at 3 minutes and significant depression persisting for 60 to 120 minutes. The rate of administration of the drug affects the onset of depression: the faster the drug is given, the quicker the respiratory depression occurs. Benzodiazepines and opioids appear to produce additive respiratory depression, including apnea. Unlike propofol, benzodiazepines used alone decrease blood pressure only modestly. Other drugs, particularly drugs that affect the cytochrome P-450 3A4 enzyme (including azole antifungals, human immunodeficiency virus [HIV] protease inhibitors, and calcium-channel blockers), affect the clearance of midazolam and prolong its half-life significantly. There are several reports of prolonged amnesia in HIV patients who received midazolam for conscious sedation. Midazolam also has an active metabolite and is often associated with delirium in elderly patients (Chapter 25), perhaps because it impairs both implicit and relational memory.

Opioids

Opioids are classified as naturally occurring (morphine, codeine), semisynthetic (heroin), and synthetic (methadone, fentanyl, remifentanil). They can be administered both intravenously and in the neuraxial space (epidural or spinal). There are four opiate receptors (mu, kappa, delta, and nociceptin receptors), which are G protein–coupled receptors. Chronic exposure to agonists leads to cellular adaptation mechanisms that probably are involved in tolerance, dependence, and withdrawal. Clinically, mu agonists are used almost exclusively; mu agonists include morphine, fentanyl, and meperidine. Opioid analgesics are administered because they relieve pain, but they have other important effects, including respiratory depression, decreased gastric emptying, nausea and vomiting, sedation, constipation, pruritus, dependence, and tolerance, when given repeatedly. When opioids are given with propofol or benzodiazepines, there is a synergistic depressive effect on respiration, hence the rationale for monitoring patients who receive medications for conscious sedation. The rate of prolonged opioid use after surgery is approximately 3%, and characteristics associated with prolonged use include younger age, lower household income, diabetes, heart failure, and pulmonary disease. The recent focus on pain management as a marker of patient satisfaction and putative hospital quality may be one driver of the recent opioid crisis. For example, 70% of opioid-naïve patients who undergo low-risk surgical procedures fill a prescription for hydrocodone/acetaminophen or oxycodone/acetaminophen within 7 days after discharge or the procedure date.[7] Physicians should be careful to avoid unnecessary opiate prescriptions and to limit prescriptions to several days. Such limitations of perioperative opioid prescriptions have become a priority for both health systems and state regulators.

Ketamine

Ketamine is unique among the intravenous agents because it has analgesic properties and decreases tolerance to opiates. The metabolism of [RS]-ketamine to [2,6R]-hydroxynorketamine [HNK] is necessary and sufficient to exert antidepressant actions in mice; its antidepressant effects are N-methyl-D-aspartate (NMDA) receptor–independent but involve early and sustained activation of α-amino-3-hydroxy-5-methyl-4-isoxazole-propionic acid (AMPA) receptors. Ketamine produces dose-related analgesia, which may be profound even when patients can keep their eyes open, breathe spontaneously, and protect their own airway with conserved swallowing and cough reflex. Side effects include increased lacrimation, salivation, and muscle tone. Ketamine increases cerebral blood flow, can increase seizure activity, and can produce undesirable psychological reactions; these side effects are dose related and may be minimized by the concomitant use of benzodiazepines. Ketamine is also a bronchial smooth muscle relaxant and can prevent experimentally induced bronchospasm. Ketamine is usually associated with an increase in blood pressure, heart rate, and cardiac output. These features make ketamine a useful drug for sedating patients with hemodynamic instability and with depression.[8] Ketamine infusions (22 mg/hour for 4 days or 0.35 mg/kg/hour over 4 hours daily for 10 days) can be used as an adjuvant to reduce the need for postoperative opioids.[9]

Dexmedetomidine

Dexmedetomidine is a highly selective α_2-agonist that is associated with less respiratory depression and more cooperative behavior than is propofol. Dexmedetomidine also causes hypnosis, analgesia, sympatholysis, and inhibition of insulin secretion. Dexmedetomidine induces sedation with a respiratory pattern and electroencephalographic changes similar to natural sleep. Even high concentrations of dexmedetomidine are associated with preservation of spontaneous respiration; however, when dexmedetomidine is administered in combination with sympatholytic or cholinergic agents, there is a high risk for extreme bradycardia and sinus arrest. Dexmedetomidine is associated with less amnesia than are benzodiazepines. Although propofol and benzodiazepines commonly have been used in critically ill patients to achieve sedation for procedures or for maintenance of mechanical ventilation, dexmedetomidine appears to have significant advantages over benzodiazepines because it can provide more comfort with a similar safety profile and decrease the time that critical care patients spend on ventilators.

Volatile Anesthetics

Volatile (inhalational) anesthetics include desflurane, sevoflurane, isoflurane, and nitrous oxide, as well as halothane, which now is rarely used in the United States. Inhaled anesthetics are absorbed through the respiratory epithelium and mucous membranes of the respiratory tract, and they are excreted mainly by exhalation. Access to the circulation is almost instantaneous, owing to the large pulmonary surface area. The pharmacologic effects of inhaled anesthetics depend primarily on alveolar ventilation, the ventilation-perfusion ratio,

coadministered gases, gas flow, and the physicochemical properties of the anesthetic gas rather than on the quantity of drug administered, the extent and rate of absorption, protein binding, excretion, secretion, or metabolism. Based on the available evidence, no inhalational agent appears to be superior to any other.

All inhalational agents, with the exception of nitrous oxide, cause dose-dependent cardiovascular depression. Severe hepatotoxicity, which led to the discontinuation of the use of chloroform, carbon tetrachloride, and trichloroethylene anesthetics, is seen as fatal hepatic necrosis in 1 in 10,000 halothane anesthetics. This problem appears to occur much less frequently with isoflurane and desflurane. Mild halothane hepatotoxicity is self-limited and can occur with a single exposure, whereas fulminant halothane hepatitis occurs only after multiple exposures to the drug, has a high mortality rate (50%), and is associated with antibodies to halothane-altered antigens.

Nitrous oxide, which is the only nonhalogenated agent still used, is not metabolized in human tissues. It irreversibly oxidizes the cobalt atom of vitamin B_{12}, thereby inhibiting the activity of the cobalamin-dependent enzyme methionine synthase. Individuals with vitamin B_{12} deficiency or with mutations of methionine synthase may be at risk for neurologic injury from nitrous oxide, which should not be used in patients at risk. Exposure to high concentrations of more than 10^3 ppm may be associated with an increased incidence of abortions and decreased fertility, so exposure should be avoided in patients and personnel at risk. Nitrous oxide is safe in major noncardiac surgery. General anesthesia can be achieved only by giving combinations of drugs along with nitrous oxide to achieve the desired effects. Based on the available evidence, no one general anesthetic appears to be superior to any other.

Neuromuscular Blockers

Neuromuscular blockers are used to paralyze muscles to facilitate endotracheal intubation and mechanical ventilation, to decrease shivering during induced hypothermia, or to improve conditions for optimal surgery. Succinylcholine causes prolonged depolarization of the neuromuscular junction, thereby resulting in failure to generate an action potential. Within 9 to 13 minutes after 1 mg/kg of succinylcholine, 90% of muscle strength is restored. The very rapid onset and rapid return of muscle function make succinylcholine a useful drug for difficult intubations. Side effects of succinylcholine include hyperkalemia, myalgia, masseter spasm, sinus bradycardia and nodal rhythms, and increased intraocular pressure.

Most of the other neuromuscular drugs used by anesthesiologists are nondepolarizing in that they compete with acetylcholine for the neuromuscular junction and can be reversed by increasing the quantity of acetylcholine. These drugs are categorized by their chemical makeup: steroidal compounds, benzylisoquinolinium compounds, and other chemical compounds. Clinically, a drug is often chosen for its duration of action. Intermediate agents, which act for 20 to 50 minutes and are used most frequently, include vecuronium, rocuronium, atracurium, and cisatracurium. These drugs have different routes of metabolism, so the choice of agent depends in part on the presence of coexisting disease. Sugammadex injection is a U.S. Food and Drug Administration (FDA)–approved direct antagonist that reverses the effects of neuromuscular blockade induced by rocuronium bromide and vecuronium bromide.

The chronic administration of neuromuscular blocking agents is associated with prolonged paralysis, particularly in patients given concomitant steroids. Other notable interactions with nondepolarizing agents include that antibiotics can increase neuromuscular blockade; magnesium sulfate potentiates neuromuscular blockade; lithium can potentiate neuromuscular blockade with succinylcholine and with pipecuronium; antiepileptic drugs cause resistance to nondepolarizing muscle blockade so that larger doses must be administered to achieve paralysis; and patients receiving anticonvulsants have accelerated recovery from neuromuscular blockade.

Regional Anesthesia

Regional anesthesia involves the deposition of local anesthetics near nerves, including the deposition of local anesthetics in the epidural space and into the cerebrospinal fluid (CSF). Local anesthetics, which are aminoesters or aminoamides, affect cardiac function, as well as central nervous system function when administered systemically.

The binding of the local anesthetic to the sodium channels in the axoplasm prevents opening of the channels and conduction of nerve impulses. The rates of onset and recovery from nerve blockade are controlled by the diffusion of the local anesthetic into and out of the whole nerve.

Examples of regional anesthesia include neuraxial techniques, the deposition of local anesthetics near the brachial plexus to anesthetize the arms (axillary or intrascalene blocks), deposition near the femoral or sciatic nerves to anesthetize the legs, deposition near ulnar or radial nerves for lower arm blocks, deposition near the pudendal nerves for groin procedures, and deposition of local anesthesia in the caudal space for groin surgeries. Dentists employ this technique frequently when they inject local anesthesia near various nerves in the oral cavity. Many surgeries, including carotid surgery and the placement of fistulas for dialysis, can be performed with regional anesthesia. Regional anesthetics may also require supplementation with sedation or general anesthesia. Regional anesthesia can decrease postoperative pain and use of opioids, as well as improve pulmonary outcomes.[10]

The dangers of regional anesthesia include the injection of local anesthesia into the systemic circulation. Systemic toxicity is manifested as convulsions and respiratory depression, which can require assisted ventilation. Tinnitus, visual and auditory disturbances, and dizziness are signs of milder central nervous toxicity. Cardiac toxicity can be manifested by decreases in heart rate, prolonged conduction times, and negative inotropic effects. Bupivacaine toxicity is associated with ventricular fibrillation. Intralipid 20% at various doses (1.5 mL/kg rapid bolus [approximately 100 mL in the average adult] followed by infusion of 0.25 mL/kg/min for 10 minutes) has been reported in case reports and in animal studies to reverse these toxic effects, although the optimal dosing has yet to be determined. Furthermore, the prolonged duration of many of the local anesthetics may require the institution of cardiopulmonary bypass until the drugs are metabolized.

Neuraxial (Spinal and Epidural) Anesthesia and Analgesia

Spinal anesthesia is the instillation of local anesthetics into the CSF. Epidural anesthesia is the instillation of larger volumes of local anesthetics into the epidural space, which is the potential space that exists just before the CSF. Spinal anesthesia is associated with an increased incidence of headache in younger patients, so epidural anesthesia is often used in younger patients. Complications of epidural and spinal anesthesia and analgesia include failed blocks, postdural puncture headaches, and toxicity from the local anesthetics. Another major concern of neuraxial anesthesia is that patients on antiplatelet agents may develop epidural hematomas, although epidural hematoma remains a rare event, occurring in fewer than 1 in 150,000 operations even in the presence of potent antiplatelet agents. Other more rare complications of epidural and spinal anesthetics, in addition to the effects of local anesthesia outlined previously, include intracranial subdural hematoma, transverse myelitis, hypotension, and cardiac arrest.

Postoperative epidural analgesia, by which either local anesthesia or local anesthesia and narcotics are instilled into the epidural space for postoperative pain control, is associated with superior pain control, lower doses of opioids, improved bowel mobility, slightly decreased length of stay in the intensive care unit, and a slight decrease in the requirement for mechanical ventilation. The continuous intravenous infusion of perioperative lidocaine also may reduce pain and nausea, especially in the early postoperative period, but it is not as well studied as epidural anesthesia.[A7] Combined general-epidural anesthesia provides better control of blood sugar levels compared with general anesthesia alone.[11]

GENERAL VERSUS REGIONAL ANESTHESIA

The decision regarding what type of anesthesia should be administered often depends on the requirements of the surgery. For example, laparoscopic surgery requires general anesthesia because the insufflations of gases impair the ability to breathe adequately. General anesthesia is also required for surgeries on the airway or thorax because mechanical ventilation is usually needed to sustain adequate respiration. Low tidal volume and low positive end-expiratory pressure are preferred. Procedures that do not allow any movement (e.g., precise procedures in the brain) often require general anesthesia and paralysis. For patients in whom the intraoperative technique could include general anesthesia, regional anesthesia, or a combination of the two, regional anesthesia may minimize pulmonary complications and modestly shorten hospital length-of-stay, but there currently is no evidence that it affects mortality.

Side effects of general anesthesia depend on the drugs used to achieve anesthesia, whether neuromuscular blockade is administered, and whether mechanical ventilation is used. Complications of endotracheal intubation include local pain, trauma to the airway, swelling, vocal cord paralysis, increased bronchospasm, and death from improper placement. Volatile anesthetics are associated with postoperative atelectasis (Chapter 84), whereas regional anesthesia helps preserve respiratory dynamics. Postoperative cognitive dysfunction (Chapter 25) does not seem to depend on the type of anesthesia administered,

but it may depend on the depth of accompanying sedation and severity of comorbid conditions.

NAUSEA AND VOMITING

Postoperative nausea and vomiting are more likely with volatile anesthetics but also are common when perioperative opioids are administered. Prophylactic ondansetron, dexamethasone, and droperidol each reduce postoperative nausea and vomiting, independently, by about 25%, with the main predictor for efficacy being the patient's risk for nausea and vomiting. It should be noted that droperidol has received a "black box" warning from the FDA, so it is not used very often in the United States. Total intravenous anesthesia with propofol reduces postoperative nausea and vomiting by only about 20%, often because narcotics are still administered. The use of spinal or epidural anesthesia may decrease the incidence of nausea and vomiting. In addition to general anesthesia, risk factors for postoperative nausea and vomiting include female gender, a prior history of nausea and vomiting, a history of motion sickness, nonsmoking, and intended administration of opioids for postoperative analgesia. If three or more risk factors are present, patients generally are recommended to receive at least two prophylactic pharmacologic antiemetic agents of different classes (e.g., selected among ondansetron or another $5\text{-}HT_3$ antagonist, droperidol, dexamethasone, scopolamine, or phenothiazides) preoperatively for the prevention of nausea and vomiting.[12] Amisulpride, which is an atypical antipsychotic that reduces signaling via the dopamine D_2 receptor, is safe and efficacious for treating postoperative nausea and vomiting when given as a single 5 mg or 10 mg intravenous dose in patients who have or have not received other prophylactic therapies.[A8][A9]

Grade A References

A1. Pieters BMA, Maas EHA, Knape JTA, et al. Videolaryngoscopy vs. direct laryngoscopy use by experienced anaesthetists in patients with known difficult airways: a systematic review and meta-analysis. *Anaesthesia.* 2017;72:1532-1541.

A2. Lascarrou JB, Boisrame-Helms J, Bailly A, et al. Video laryngoscopy vs direct laryngoscopy on successful first-pass orotracheal intubation among ICU patients: a randomized clinical trial. *JAMA.* 2017;317:483-493.

A3. Lewis SR, Butler AR, Parker J, et al. Videolaryngoscopy versus direct laryngoscopy for adult patients requiring tracheal intubation: a Cochrane Systematic Review. *Br J Anaesth.* 2017;119:369-383.

A4. An R, Pang QY, Chen B, et al. Effect of anesthesia methods on postoperative major adverse cardiac events and mortality after non-cardiac surgeries: a systematic review and meta-analysis. *Minerva Anestesiol.* 2017;83:749-761.

A5. Futier E, Lefrant JY, Guinot PG, et al. Effect of individualized vs standard blood pressure management strategies on postoperative organ dysfunction among high-risk patients undergoing major surgery: a randomized clinical trial. *JAMA.* 2017;318:1346-1357.

A6. Wang D, Chen C, Chen J, et al. The use of propofol as a sedative agent in gastrointestinal endoscopy: a meta-analysis. *PLoS ONE.* 2013;8:1-12.

A7. Kranke P, Jokinen J, Pace NL, et al. Continuous intravenous perioperative lidocaine infusion for postoperative pain and recovery. *Cochrane Database Syst Rev.* 2015;7:CD009642.

A8. Candiotti KA, Kranke P, Bergese SD, et al. Randomized, double-blind, placebo-controlled study of intravenous amisulpride as treatment of established postoperative nausea and vomiting in patients who have had no prior prophylaxis. *Anesth Analg.* 2019;128:1098-1105.

A9. Habib AS, Kranke P, Bergese SD, et al. Amisulpride for the rescue treatment of postoperative nausea or vomiting in patients failing prophylaxis: a randomized, placebo-controlled phase III trial. *Anesthesiology.* 2019;130:203-212.

GENERAL REFERENCES

For the General References and other additional features, please visit Expert Consult at https://expertconsult.inkling.com.

405

POSTOPERATIVE CARE AND COMPLICATIONS

DONALD A. REDELMEIER

POSTOPERATIVE CARE

Overview

Postoperative medical complications are common, potentially fatal, and variable across different settings. Large national studies show about a two-fold difference in risk for mortality between high- and low-ranked hospitals. However, analyses disagree about how much these differences reflect a greater incidence of each complication (failure of prevention around the time of surgery), a heightened lethality of each complication (failure to rescue in the aftermath of surgery), or the differences in the severity of disease or surgical skill. Regardless of the explanation, the purpose of medical consultation is to relieve human suffering by the prevention, detection, and correction of postoperative complications. The main constraint is that the consultant often has limited ongoing direct contact with the patient before or after the perioperative interval.

Effective Teamwork

The medical consultant (Chapter 402) in the postoperative setting must have both a knowledge of medicine and an appreciation of the team psychology that can improve the outcomes of patients. In contrast to other settings, the internist is not the team leader, often does not maintain an ongoing relationship with the patient, and does not have the authority of the most responsible physician. Moreover, patients may be dispersed across diverse surgical services, each with its own orientation and culture. The challenges of coordination and communication are enormous, particularly given the many other health care professionals involved in complex surgical cases. Considerable tact is often needed to avoid antagonizing the surgeon, disrupting the team's dynamics, or inducing a cascade of cumbersome inopportune testing. The development and use of safety checklists can be an effective way for enhancing teamwork to improve outcomes.

Focusing on Recovery

Facilitating the patient's recovery from surgery differs conceptually from managing patients with acute exacerbations or chronic diseases. In the postoperative setting, many therapies must be stopped at some point because the patient has recovered, such as discontinuing a urinary catheter because the patient can now void spontaneously or discontinuing a major tranquilizer because the patient is now oriented and coherent. Discontinuation of many other interventions requires substantial judgment, such as the decision when to discontinue intravenous access, supplemental oxygen, and intermittent laxatives. Much depends on experience and reconsideration of the individual patient's situation on a regular basis.

Reading Anesthesia Records

A focused review of the anesthesia record is essential because the consultant is rarely present during the operation. Perhaps the most basic information to identify is the date of surgery because the time elapsed helps in interpreting the patient's current state of recovery. Sometimes the date is not immediately evident if more than one surgery has been performed, a planned operation was canceled, or some misquotations have arisen. Data about the duration of surgery, type of anesthesia (e.g., regional, spinal, or general [Chapter 404]), and major intraoperative events can help to establish reasonable expectations about the future course as well as the possibility of specific complications (e.g., epidural hematoma after spinal anesthesia). Sharing some of the basic data with the patient is often helpful because many individuals either benefit from repetition or are not otherwise informed.

Patterns of Mistakes

Medical errors (Chapter 10) that arise in postoperative care often seem mundane in retrospect yet can be lethal if undetected. Some patterns of mistakes have the feature of "double trouble," such as when a patient has both a potassium level of 2.0 mEq/L and an international normalized ratio of 2.0 but care focuses on only one of these two abnormalities. Other mistakes occur because a problem arises at an awkward moment, such as a patient in whom acute dyspnea develops when another patient is having a seizure. Still other mistakes relate to the fallibility of human memory and attention, such as when a normal blood glucose value in the morning leads clinicians to presume that the level is still normal at night. These errors can result in substantial harm, failures of clinicians to learn from past mistakes, and unprofessional reactions related to lingering embarrassment. None of these patterns are unique to postoperative care, yet the fast and unfamiliar terrain of surgical settings can make even simple mistakes difficult to avoid.

Checking Orders

The first method for reducing errors after surgery is to check the postoperative orders already written for the patient. Such double-checking is a tedious task, and clinicians often direct insufficient attention to this review in the faulty belief that most of the work is already done. Ironically, checking orders written by another clinician requires more than customary attention because of the challenges of following someone else's legibility, sequencing, and preferences. The set of orders may need to be read twice: once for errors of commission (e.g., a calcium-channel blocker ordered at the wrong dose) and once for errors of omission (e.g., a β-blocker inadvertently not reordered after surgery). One classic mistake on postoperative orders is failure to follow through on interventions initiated immediately before surgery (e.g., delirium tremens prophylaxis). A particularly vexing issue is the need for repeated rechecking on subsequent days (e.g., new orders for sedative drugs).

Recommended Prophylaxis

Some complications are sufficiently frequent and serious that routine prophylaxis is merited in the postoperative setting. For example, systemic anticoagulation is indicated for patients at risk for postoperative deep venous thrombosis (Chapters 74 and 76). Gastric acid suppression (Chapter 130) is justified for patients at high risk for postoperative gastric bleeding. Parenteral antibiotics are indicated for patients undergoing prosthetic joint replacement. In contrast, antibiotic prophylaxis is indicated only for selected patients who are at high risk for endocarditis (Chapter 67). The optimal method for gauging whether a patient is at high risk for each complication is contentious and thereby leads to variation in practice patterns across different settings.

Future Prevention

A postoperative consultant who maintains communication, facilitates the patient's recovery, and avoids postoperative mistakes also has the chance to initiate medical interventions for general medical care. Such opportunities for prevention might include influenza vaccination, colon cancer screening, and cholesterol reduction. The main advantage of such comprehensive care is that it conforms to the ideal of providing all services possible to the individual. The main disadvantage of such comprehensive care is the potential for creating chaos, confusion, or misquotation (Chapter 402). Such unintended consequences distract the surgical team from the primary goal and also carry some risk for side effects at a time when the patient is trying to recover from surgery. Many effective postoperative consultants will defer such opportunities for prevention to the outpatient physicians who assume long-term responsibility for the patient's care.

● COMPLICATIONS

Symptoms

Chest Pain

Chest pain is a common problem after surgery and has an extensive differential diagnosis (Chapter 45). In the postoperative setting, the immediate consideration is an acute ischemic myocardial event. The diagnosis of a perioperative myocardial infarction (MI) differs somewhat from community-acquired MI (Table 405-1). Interpretation of a patient's symptoms, examination findings, and electrocardiogram is often problematic because of changes related to surgery and anesthesia. In particular, diagnosis is heavily dependent on biomarkers, such as an elevated troponin level,[1] especially because many

---

TABLE 405-1	CRITERIA FOR DIAGNOSIS OF POSTOPERATIVE MYOCARDIAL INFARCTION

The diagnosis of perioperative MI requires any one of the following criteria.

Criterion 1: A typical rise in the troponin level or a typical fall in an elevated troponin level detected at its peak after surgery in a patient without a documented alternative explanation for an elevated troponin level (e.g., pulmonary embolism). This criterion requires that one of the following criteria be met:
Ischemic signs or symptoms (e.g., chest, arm, or jaw discomfort; shortness of breath; pulmonary edema)
Development of pathologic Q waves on an ECG
Changes on an ECG indicative of ischemia
Coronary artery intervention
New or presumed new cardiac wall motion abnormality on echocardiography or new or presumed new fixed defect on radionuclide imaging

Criterion 2: Pathologic findings of acute or healing MI

Criterion 3: Development of new pathologic Q waves on an ECG if troponin levels were not obtained or were obtained at times that could have missed the clinical event

ECG = electrocardiogram; MI = myocardial infarction.
Adapted from Devereaux PJ, Goldman L, Yusuf S, et al. Surveillance and prevention of major perioperative ischemic cardiac events in patients undergoing noncardiac surgery: a review. *CMAJ.* 2005;173:779-788.

TABLE 405-2 DISTINGUISHING AMONG COMMON CAUSES OF ACUTE POSTOPERATIVE DYSPNEA

	PULMONARY AIR SPACE	FLUID OVERLOAD/HEART FAILURE	PULMONARY THROMBOEMBOLISM
CHARACTERISTICS OF TIMING			
Days since surgery	1-7 days	0-5 days	5-28 days
Speed of onset	1-3 days	1-24 hours	1-5 minutes
PREVIOUS HISTORY			
Previous lung disease	++		
Previous heart failure		++	
Previous venous thrombosis			++
ABNORMAL VITAL SIGNS			
Temperature			
Heart rate	+	+	+
Blood pressure	+	+	++
Respiratory rate	+	++	+
Oximetry	++	+	+
PHYSICAL EXAMINATION			
Jugular venous distention		+	+
Pulmonary rales	+	++	
S$_3$ gallop		++	
RESPONSE TO TREATMENT			
Oxygen	+	+	+
Anticholinergic bronchodilators	+	+	+
Withdrawal of sedatives	+	+	+
Aggressive physiotherapy	++		
Diuretics/afterload reduction		++	

postoperative MIs are painless. Among patients undergoing noncardiac surgery, the peak postoperative troponin level during the first 3 days after surgery is significantly associated with 30-day mortality, even if patients do not have any other evidence of an acute MI.[2,3] Management priorities include supplemental oxygen, heart rate control, and correction of severe anemia. Thrombolysis is often contraindicated, but percutaneous coronary intervention may be considered, especially because of the high 30-day mortality rate for postoperative MI, although data on its benefits are lacking. Dabigatran (110 mg twice daily) can reduce the risk of major vascular complications without increasing major bleeding in patients who develop evidence of myocardial injury after noncardiac surgery.[A1] Otherwise, therapies such as aspirin, clopidogrel, nitrates, statins, and angiotensin-converting enzyme inhibitors, should be used on a case-by-case basis (Chapter 64).

Dyspnea

Shortness of breath (Chapter 77) after surgery has an extensive differential diagnosis (Table 405-2). The three key considerations are fluid overload from heart failure (Chapter 52), pulmonary embolism (Chapter 74),[4] and air space disease (a continuum encompassing atelectasis [Chapter 84], bronchitis [Chapter 90], aspiration [Chapter 88], mucous plugging, and pneumonia). Distinguishing among these considerations requires focusing on the speed of onset, timing relative to surgery, vital sign abnormalities, findings on oximetry, and physical examination (Chapter 77). Fluid overload is most commonly seen soon after the cessation of positive-pressure ventilation or vasodilating analgesia. It is also common 3 to 5 days postoperatively when fluid that had been "third spaced" is mobilized into the intravascular compartment. Interventions that are safe in most situations include administration of oxygen and withholding of sedation. The use of noninvasive ventilation can reduce the rate of reintubation in hypoxemic postoperative patients compared with the use of oxygen alone.[A2] Other interventions that will be helpful or harmful, depending on the situation, include diuretics, opioids, elaborate medical imaging, and vigorous physiotherapy. Despite its common use, incentive spirometry is of little or no benefit.[A3]

Anorexia

Loss of appetite (Chapter 123) after surgery has an extensive differential diagnosis that can be narrowed substantially if the patient was eating properly before surgery. The immediate priority is to search for and correct underlying contributors. Oral, enteral, or parenteral support is not the priority initially, although such support may eventually become necessary. Drug toxicity is a particularly common, easily detected when considered, and rapidly reversible contributor to postoperative anorexia. Anatomic abnormalities are usually evident by medical imaging studies. Common metabolic contributors include abnormalities in electrolytes, calcium, phosphorus, and magnesium. Acalculous cholecystitis (Chapter 146) is an important postoperative complication that must be considered in a patient with right upper quadrant tenderness. Constipation is another frequent contributor that sometimes justifies prophylactic laxatives.

Vomiting

Vomiting is the extreme form of nausea in the postoperative setting, and the two symptoms share the same differential diagnosis. In most patients, vomiting is unexpected and merits immediate attention. Initial management is to ensure that the patient's airway is protected, to discontinue oral medications (and find parenteral substitutes if necessary), and to consider insertion of a nasogastric tube. In patients after gastrointestinal surgery, the priority considerations include the possibility of an anastomotic leak, peritoneal abscess, or another anatomic abnormality. In patients after operations on more remote parts of the body, the priority considerations are emetogenic medications (such as postoperative chemotherapy), gastroparesis associated with autonomic neuropathy, and fecal impaction. Multiple antinausea medications are available for symptomatic relief (e.g., prochlorperazine, ondansetron, dexamethasone, droperidol) and act in an additive manner when they are used in combination (e.g., prochlorperazine 5 mg intramuscularly plus ondansetron 4 mg intramuscularly). If no reversible contributor is identified, the default diagnosis is prolonged idiopathic ileus, and a therapeutic trial of intravenous neostigmine can be considered (e.g., neostigmine 2.5 mg intravenously over 5 minutes).

Diarrhea

Diarrhea (Chapter 131) is rare after surgery and involves a limited number of possibilities if the patient's bowel movements were normal before surgery. In such cases, the situation represents an acute-onset diarrhea that is usually secretory in nature. The immediate priority is to exclude toxic megacolon, which is a potential emergency caused by overgrowth of toxigenic *Clostridium difficile*. Clinical evaluation for toxic megacolon requires assessment for tachycardia, hypotension, delirium, and other signs of sepsis rather than waiting on initial stool studies for confirmation of infection with *C. difficile.* Risk factors for antibiotic-associated diarrhea include advanced age, use of broad-spectrum antibiotics (e.g., third-generation cephalosporins), and unknown host susceptibility factors (e.g., past episodes of pseudomembranous colitis). A definitive diagnosis is frequently never established, and treatment focuses on feeding the patient a lactose-free diet while avoiding intestinal paralytics. Complete resolution is typical provided that adequate fluid and electrolyte levels are maintained.

Weakness

Generalized weakness after surgery is almost inevitable, but focal weakness may sometimes reflect nerve damage caused by intraoperative positioning (e.g., damage to the facial nerve after carotid endarterectomy) and rarely indicates a new intracranial event (e.g., intracerebral bleeding [Chapter 380] secondary to anticoagulation). Neurologic deficits are often overlooked during the initial postoperative interval and may become apparent only after the patient has regained strength elsewhere in the body. Conversely, new deficits that are evident early after surgery and resolve rapidly thereafter may reflect unmasking of an old stroke that was fully compensated during less stressful circumstances. Medical imaging of the brain is worthwhile if no explanation is apparent on initial assessment. Nonfocal weakness is usually due to deconditioning and commonly responds to physical therapy.

Delirium

Changes in mental status after surgery are common, especially in elderly patients (Chapter 25), and can be remarkably difficult to correct.[5] The immediate priorities are to determine whether the impairment is acute or chronic and to detect easily reversible contributors (such as infection, hypoglycemia, and alkalosis). A complete assessment is often unnecessary if the patient had normal mental status before surgery because many dementia syndromes are thereby excluded (such as vitamin B_{12} deficiency, tertiary syphilis, and Alzheimer disease). Multicomponent interactions that can help prevent delirium in hospitalized patients include discontinuation of medications (e.g., anticholinergics, narcotics, and tranquilizers) and the continuous presence of friends or family members who can provide frequent orientation and constant attention.[A4] In one randomized trial, intravenous dexmedetomidine (0.1 µg/kg per hour, from intensive care unit admission on the day of surgery until 8 AM on postoperative day 1) decreased the occurrence of delirium by about two thirds during the first 7 days after surgery.[A5]

A sense of patience is necessary because delirium rarely resolves instantly. The benefit of low-dose neuroleptics (e.g., risperidone, 0.5 mg by mouth twice daily) remains uncertain. Delirium after surgery is associated with a significant decline in cognitive ability during the next year, with a trajectory characterized by an initial decline and prolonged impairment.

Seizures

The development of uncontrolled seizures (Chapter 375) after surgery is rare. The immediate priorities are to exclude status epilepticus, to uncover any past history of seizures, and to identify provocative factors. Neurosurgical patients typically undergo a standardized treatment protocol, including steroids and imaging. Other conditions that can cause abnormal motor movements must be excluded, such as septic rigors, delirium tremens, Parkinson disease, major psychopathology, hypothermic shivering, and hypercapnic asterixis. Additional considerations include detection and correction of underlying metabolic abnormalities, such as hypocalcemia, hypoxemia, hyponatremia, hypophosphatemia, and drug toxicity. Treatment focuses primarily on reversing the underlying precipitating cause and providing nonspecific care with benzodiazepines, phenytoin, and ongoing monitoring.

Signs

Hypertension

Hypertension may reflect a variety of disorders and must be treated in a manner that neither overreacts nor underreacts to the situation. Hypertension is particularly common after neurosurgical procedures or carotid endarterectomy. The initial assessment focuses on whether the patient has chronic hypertension based on the past history, current electrocardiogram, or findings on funduscopy. Other potential causes include undertreated pain, agitated delirium, fluid overload, alcohol withdrawal, and inadvertent discontinuation of chronic antihypertensive medications. In uncertain cases, systemic analgesia is often helpful, along with nitrates (e.g., nitroglycerin, 0.4 mg/hour transdermally) and β-blockers (e.g., metoprolol, 5 mg intravenously). The major complication of treatment is the potential for overcorrection and inadvertent hypotension; such errors are particularly common in patients with no evidence of past hypertension.

Hypotension

Hypotension (Chapter 7) after surgery is generally an emergency, and the immediate concern is internal bleeding, especially after intra-abdominal operations or when anticoagulation is used to prevent venous thrombosis. The initial stages of hypotension are frequently unrecognized because of autonomic stress responses by patients, psychological denial by clinicians, and misattribution to the concurrent use of analgesia. Early hypotension is particularly easy to overlook if the patient has coexisting chronic hypertension and the apparently "normal" blood pressure is dismissed as unremarkable. Prompt echocardiography can almost always find the cause of undiagnosed hemodynamic instability.

Treatment usually entails volume supplementation, vasopressors as needed (Chapters 99 and 100), serial assessments, and a search for underlying causes. An extensive differential diagnosis sometimes needs to be considered if no anatomic cause related to surgery is evident (Chapter 98). Routine use of pulmonary artery catheters to guide therapy is not helpful, and goal-directed fluid therapy does not reduce mortality compared with standard care.[A6]

Hypoxemia

Postoperative hypoxemia is common after noncardiac surgery, with about 20% of patients having oxygen saturations below 90% averaged over the first 48 hours and about one third of patients having oxygen saturations below 90% for an hour or more. Many of these events are not clinically diagnosed but can be detected by continuous monitoring. The clinical implications of such undiagnosed hypoxemia are uncertain, but they may contribute to tachycardia, delirium, and cardiac sequelae.[6] Treatment generally requires supplemental oxygen, deep breathing encouragement, and a search for underlying contributing factors.

Tachycardia

Tachycardia after surgery can be caused by myriad arrhythmias (Chapters 58 and 59) and may contribute to postoperative cardiac ischemia. Distinguishing between newly detected and newly incident tachycardia can sometimes be accomplished by determining whether the patient does or does not complain of palpitations. An initial assessment also requires review of the electrocardiogram to distinguish atrial fibrillation from other disorders. The goal of treatment is to identify and correct precipitating factors, such as pain, blood loss, hypoxia, electrolyte abnormalities, fluid overload, volume depletion, pulmonary embolism, and drug withdrawal. Most arrhythmias respond to correction of the underlying abnormality. Specific antiarrhythmic treatment, when needed, is generally similar to that used in the nonoperative setting (Chapters 58 and 59). For atrial fibrillation, anticoagulation is sometimes contraindicated; in such situations, cardioversion within 48 hours merits consideration. Postoperative atrial fibrillation portends an increased long-term risk of ischemic stroke.

Fever

Fever (Chapter 264) after surgery is common, frequently perplexing, and often multifactorial. Worrisome possibilities include transfusion reactions (Chapter 167), hospital-acquired pneumonia (Chapter 91), urinary tract infection (Chapter 268), line sepsis (Chapter 266), and wound infection. In many cases, no definitive cause is found, the patient recovers spontaneously, and the default diagnosis is atelectasis. Detailed evaluation, when necessary, requires culture of blood, urine, and the surgical site to identify specific microbiologic organisms. Selection of empirical antibiotics is usually based on local practice patterns and hospital ecology, with the disadvantage of breeding resistant organisms. Hydration, nutrition, and general supportive care are important yet frequently neglected issues for patients with prolonged elevations in body temperature. Selective decontamination of the digestive tract and oropharynx appears to be beneficial, but chlorhexidine is not.[A7]

Edema

Peripheral edema (Chapter 45), which is often first noticed by nursing staff after surgery, is rarely life threatening unless it is treated with excessive diuretics. The cause is usually multifactorial and includes increased hydrostatic pressure (including heart failure and gravity from intraoperative positioning), decreased oncotic pressure (related to hypoalbuminemia from decreased liver production or increased losses), and accentuated capillary leak (potentially caused by medications or tissue reactions). Treatment focuses on correction of underlying abnormalities, maintenance of nutrition, judicious use of diuretics, monitoring of renal function, provision of systemic anticoagulation against deep venous thrombosis, and efforts toward mobilization of the patient. A low-salt diet, afterload reduction, and aldosterone antagonists (e.g., oral spironolactone, 25 mg once daily) may be helpful in patients in whom heart failure (Chapter 53) is the dominant mechanism.

Laboratory

Leukocytosis

An elevated white blood cell count (Chapter 158) can have many causes, but the immediate priority is to exclude a life-threatening septic process (Chapters 98 and 100). Direct microscopic examination of the peripheral blood smear (Chapter 148) can be helpful to check for toxic granulations (see Fig. 148-18), Döhle bodies (see Fig. 148-19), and a shift toward primitive band cells. Many cases are due to noninfectious causes, including infarcted tissue (skin, heart, intestinal tract), inflammatory conditions (renal insufficiency, diabetic keto-acidosis, lupus erythematosus), and demargination stress reactions (dehydration, systemic corticosteroids, inotropic medications). In the absence of direct evidence, some clinicians may initiate antibiotics empirically, whereas others may elect waiting. Substantial controversy remains about the proper duration of an empirical trial of antibiotics when no cause is discovered and the patient is otherwise recovering.

Anemia

Anemia (Chapter 149) is common and sometimes underappreciated because coexisting volume depletion causes the blood hemoglobin concentration to underestimate the degree of blood loss. Major perioperative hemorrhage is associated with subsequent stroke and MI in patients undergoing noncardiac, non-neurologic surgery. The initial priority is to differentiate bleeding at the surgical site from other causes. In many cases, the exact cause is unclear, and substantial uncertainty may arise over the need to initiate gastric acid suppression therapy or to interrupt systemic anticoagulation against venous thrombosis. In a large randomized trial, transfusion at a hemoglobin threshold of 10 g/dL was no better than transfusion for symptoms of anemia or at the physician's discretion for a hemoglobin level of below 8 g/dL. Guidelines for transfusion therapy depend on the patient's cardiac reserve as well as on the available blood bank supply at the particular medical center. A reasonable goal is to maintain a hemoglobin level of 7 mg/dL or higher, except in patients with cardiovascular disease, in whom a hemoglobin goal of 8 to 9 mg/dL is reasonable.[A3] The immediate postoperative interval is not usually the appropriate time to initiate erythropoietin, oral iron replacement, or detailed evaluations for other hematologic abnormalities.

Abnormalities in Platelet Count

Patients often have abnormal platelet counts after surgery yet rarely require further evaluation or treatment.[7] In most cases, the thrombocytopenia is mild, does not require transfusion therapy, resolves in a few weeks, and is not a sign of an ominous disorder (e.g., sepsis or heparin-induced thrombocytopenia). Platelet transfusions are indicated if the decrease in platelet count is extreme, accompanied by evidence of major blood loss, or related to recent surgery on the central nervous system (including the eye). Thrombocytosis is also common after surgery and is occasionally extreme. However, even postoperative thrombocytosis exceeding 1,000,000/mL rarely necessitates treatment, does not predispose patients to unwanted clotting complications, and typically resolves spontaneously after a few weeks.

Abnormal Sodium Concentration

Both hyponatremia and hypernatremia (Chapter 108) are frequent complications in the postoperative setting. The immediate priorities are to assess the patient's intravascular volume status and to correct possible volume depletion. The causes of hyponatremia are multifactorial, including excessive use of diuretics, high levels of intrinsic antidiuretic hormone (as a result of factors such as drugs, pain, and mechanical ventilation), and unmeasured osmoles (e.g., intravenous contrast agents). This risk for postoperative hyponatremia may be reduced by the administration of isotonic saline rather than by water restriction. Once hyponatremia develops, vasopressin antagonists (Chapter 108) are effective for both hypervolemic and euvolemic hyponatremia. Hypernatremia is always due to free water deficiency, which may indicate severe cognitive impairment or other factors interfering with the ability to express thirst or to ingest water. Correction is similar to that in the nonoperative setting. Abnormalities in sodium concentration require careful follow-up, can recur at any point after an operation, yet are rarely the root cause of a patient's inability to recover from surgery.

Abnormal Serum Potassium Concentration

Hyperkalemia and hypokalemia (Chapter 109) are also frequent postoperative complications. The immediate priority is to assess and to stabilize the patient's electrocardiographic findings. Hyperkalemia is usually due to cellular shifts, renal failure, and tissue destruction (including hemolysis). Hyperkalemia will generally be corrected with treatments that shift potassium into cells (e.g., intravenous glucose with or without insulin) and enhance total excretion (e.g., gastrointestinal binding agents). Hypokalemia is usually due to inadequate intake, excessive loss, or cellular shifts. Hypokalemia will generally be corrected with replacement therapy and rarely requires aldosterone antagonism. Both abnormalities can usually be treated as in the nonoperative setting (Chapter 109). The prognosis is favorable if the patient's electrocardiogram shows no major dysrhythmias and if renal function is preserved.

Alkalosis

Systemic alkalosis (Chapter 110) typically requires volume supplementation because the cause is generally intravascular volume depletion. Blood gas determinations may be necessary in some cases to exclude the possibility of concurrent carbon dioxide retention with compensatory metabolic alkalosis. Untreated, alkalosis can result in altered mentation, cardiac arrhythmias, and delayed mobilization. Most patients with postoperative alkalosis do not require carbonic anhydrase inhibitors or intravenous acid. The prognosis is usually favorable, with gradual correction during a period of several days. Rapid correction of alkalosis, unlike rapid correction of hyponatremia, is not known to cause neurologic injury.

Azotemia

The initial assessment of an elevated serum creatinine concentration (Chapter 106) focuses on reviewing previous values (to distinguish acute from chronic renal insufficiency) and identifying contributing factors (such as prerenal volume depletion, intrarenal nephrotoxins, or postrenal urethral obstruction). A trial of intravenous fluids may be useful on both a diagnostic and therapeutic basis. Treatment is the same as in the nonoperative setting. Subsequent monitoring is always necessary, with serum creatinine measurements obtained on a daily basis. Serial measurements of urinary volume and body weight as well as a urine culture are occasionally helpful in selected cases. The prognosis is dependent on the underlying factors and is less favorable after cardiac surgery.

Hyperbilirubinemia

Elevations in serum bilirubin (Chapter 138) are rare after surgery, even though abnormalities in liver enzyme levels occur frequently with general anesthesia. The most benign explanation is Gilbert syndrome, but the immediate priority is to assess for possible hepatic failure (especially in patients who have received volatile agents). As in the nonoperative setting, treatment involves withdrawing potential hepatotoxins, supporting the patient, and allowing time for liver function to recover (Chapter 144). Treatment of hepatic encephalopathy is particularly important because of the concurrent constipation and generalized catabolic state that also follow major surgery. Monitoring should include serial measurement of liver function on a daily basis because each component (e.g., bilirubin, albumen, prothrombin time) can be altered by factors unrelated to the liver. The prognosis is unfavorable if the patient's liver function fails to recover quickly.

Hypoalbuminemia

Reductions in serum albumin are common after surgery and are an ominous prognostic finding. The cause is rarely decreased production if the reduction in the albumin level occurs rapidly. Possible explanations include nephrotic syndrome, capillary leak into extravascular spaces, and occult catabolism in unrecognized sites. Treatment with albumin infusions does not usually normalize the biochemical abnormality and does not seem to improve patient survival. The main priorities are to continue nutritional support, to preserve skin integrity, to minimize the use of systemic diuretics, to correct any contributing factors, and to consider correlated serum protein deficiencies (such as reduced levels of immunoglobulins or antithrombin III). Hypoalbuminemia can also cause indirect harm by the loss of carrier proteins, which thereby predisposes patients to potential drug toxicity. The long-term prognosis is favorable for survivors because the serum albumin level will eventually fully return to normal.

Abnormalities in Blood Glucose Concentration

In patients with diabetes mellitus (Chapter 216), serum blood glucose concentrations often become unstable after surgery because of altered dietary intake, decreased physical activity, and the release of counter-regulatory hormones. The priority is to avoid hypoglycemia, severe hyperglycemia, diabetic ketoacidosis, cerebral damage, and repeated events. Intensive control of the blood glucose level increases the risk for severe hypoglycemia and death, so a target glucose level of about 140 to 200 mg/dL is recommended. Rapid reversal of sepsis or focal infection can lead to a precipitous decrease in insulin requirements; in such cases, vigilance is required because unsuspected hypoglycemia may cause permanent damage or be fatal in a patient who may otherwise seem to be sleeping. Patients need to be forewarned that temporary doses of subcutaneous insulin may be required but do not commit the patient to chronic insulin therapy. Monitoring involves serial measurement of blood glucose concentration until the patient is eating in a reliable manner.

Troponin and Natriuretic Peptide Levels

The peak postoperative troponin level during the first 3 days after noncardiac surgery is significantly associated with 30-day mortality in patients over 45 years of age, even in patients without evidence of an ischemic event.[8] However, the potential utility of routine postoperative troponin levels for patient management remains uncertain. Similarly, screening and monitoring levels of brain natriuretic peptides is favored in some guidelines and not in others.

Special Situations
Multiplicity

Some postoperative complications are difficult to classify because no single dominant problem is apparent by symptoms, signs, or laboratory test results. Instead, patients may have multiple problems that need to be addressed simultaneously. The immediate goal is to set priorities and to avoid the temptation to try to eliminate every possibility on the first day. The corollary is to continue to check progress during the subsequent days needed for a complete diagnosis and successful therapy. Because so many concerns require attention in the postoperative interval, the risk is that clinicians will lose track of a secondary issue and make an error that seems obvious in retrospect.

Redundancy

Postoperative complications sometimes generate multiple consultations with physicians who have overlapping abilities. An example might be a patient with a postoperative fever that prompts consultations from pulmonology, nephrology, dermatology, general medicine, and infectious disease specialists. In theory, gathering a critical mass of medical experts together should increase the likelihood of accurate diagnosis, timely treatment, and foolproof follow-up. In reality, however, coordination and communication are never perfect. Personal rivalries, diffusion of responsibility, and many other psychological factors may impede interactions among consultants. Opportunities for miscommunication may be further accentuated if the patient has an exotic diagnosis that is a special draw on the consultant's attention (e.g., pheochromocytoma). Arguing in front of the patient, in view of other professionals, or in the medical record can be demoralizing. The priority is to communicate effectively with the surgical team responsible for the patient and to encourage that team to make final decisions.

Ambiguity

Another vexation occurs when an urgent request is not connected to a clear rationale (Chapter 402). Diplomacy is needed to establish whether the motivation reflects a medicolegal concern rather than a biologic change in the patient. Sometimes the stimulus for the consultation can best be addressed by providing reassurance and confirmation. Sometimes the stimulus is an obscure preexisting disorder (e.g., Moyamoya disease), and the surgical team has neither the experience nor the time to investigate how this unrelated medical condition can influence recovery from surgery. Sometimes the stimulus is an unspoken political wish to transfer the care of a burdensome patient from one physician to another. A consultant should develop an understanding of how to interact with other clinicians under such ambiguous circumstances.

Setting Priorities

Requests for consultation often arrive outside conventional working hours, are usually tinged with a sense of urgency, and sometimes cluster to encompass more than one patient. Developing an effective method for prioritizing patients is a crucial clinical skill. One communication strategy is to provide an objective estimated time of arrival for the initial request from the surgical team. An often helpful treatment strategy is to make some safe suggestions at the time of the initial request so that clear-cut recommendations can be instituted during the interval before the patient is seen and used later to help evaluate the patient's status and course.

Aftermath

In many postoperative cases, the original reason for consultation may resolve and no major issues remain. The situation now provides an opportunity to review the patient, particularly for the appropriate use of unrelated medications. The consultant may often detect excessive medications that were appropriate early in the hospital course but have ceased to be necessary, thereby justifying discontinuation (e.g., diuretics, antibiotics, bronchodilators). Discontinuing medications that have become superfluous requires initiative and wisdom, and the common mistake is to propagate unnecessary medications in stable patients under the rationale of "don't mess with success." The ability to watch the patient for several hours or for a day or two often presents an ideal opportunity for the safe withdrawal of medications. Ironically, discontinuing a treatment sometimes requires more skill, time, and initiative than starting it.

Grade A References

A1. Devereaux PJ, Duceppe E, Guyatt G, et al. Dabigatran in patients with myocardial injury after noncardiac surgery (MANAGE): an international, randomised, placebo-controlled trial. *Lancet.* 2018;391:2325-2334.

A2. Jaber S, Lescot T, Futier E, et al. Effect of noninvasive ventilation on tracheal reintubation among patients with hypoxemic respiratory failure following abdominal surgery: a randomized clinical trial. *JAMA.* 2016;315:1345-1353.

A3. Pantel H, Hwang J, Brams D, et al. Effect of incentive spirometry on postoperative hypoxemia and pulmonary complications after bariatric surgery: a randomized clinical trial. *JAMA Surg.* 2017;152:422-428.

A4. Siddiqi N, Harrison JK, Clegg A, et al. Interventions for preventing delirium in hospitalised non-ICU patients. *Cochrane Database Syst Rev.* 2016;3:CD005563.

A5. Su X, Meng ZT, Wu XH, et al. Dexmedetomidine for prevention of delirium in elderly patients after non-cardiac surgery: a randomised, double-blind, placebo-controlled trial. *Lancet.* 2016;388:1893-1902.

A6. Som A, Maitra S, Bhattacharjee S, et al. Goal directed fluid therapy decreases postoperative morbidity but not mortality in major non-cardiac surgery: a meta-analysis and trial sequential analysis of randomized controlled trials. *J Anesth.* 2017;31:66-81.

A7. Price R, MacLennan G, Glen J. SuDDICU Collaboration. Selective digestive or oropharyngeal decontamination and topical oropharyngeal chlorhexidine for prevention of death in general intensive care: systematic review and network meta-analysis. *BMJ.* 2014;348:1-15.

A8. Docherty AB, O'Donnell R, Brunskill S, et al. Effect of restrictive versus liberal transfusion strategies on outcomes in patients with cardiovascular disease in a non-cardiac surgery setting: systematic review and meta-analysis. *BMJ.* 2016;352:1-11.

GENERAL REFERENCES

For the General References and other additional features, please visit Expert Consult at https://expertconsult.inkling.com.

406

MEDICAL CONSULTATION IN PSYCHIATRY

PETER MANU AND RAJESH GUPTA

HEALTH STATUS IN PSYCHIATRIC PATIENTS

The physical health of psychiatric patients is poor, with a higher risk for death at an early age than those without mental illness. Poverty, social neglect, substandard medical care, unhealthy life habits, and complications of psychiatric treatments are major contributors to the increased morbidity and mortality of patients with chronic psychiatric disorders, who have a 20-year average decline in life expectancy. Integrated care models that coordinate general medical care with psychiatric care can help meet the needs of patients with chronic psychiatric problems.[1,2]

Internists are often called on to provide consultation for patients on psychiatric inpatient units. As many as 15% of patients who are admitted for psychiatric care may be transferred to a general hospital for medical conditions that arise or deteriorate during inpatient psychiatric care. Febrile illnesses, acute neurologic changes, and falls account for nearly half of the transfers (Table 406-1). Nearly half of the patients admitted for dementia with behavioral disturbance will develop a medical complication during an inpatient psychiatric stay, a rate that is two- to three-fold higher than for other psychiatric

TABLE 406-1	COMMON REASONS FOR TRANSFERRING PSYCHIATRIC INPATIENTS WITH ACUTE MEDICAL DETERIORATION TO A GENERAL HOSPITAL
Fever	17%
Neurologic deficits, seizures, alteration of consciousness	14%
Fall, head trauma	13%
Abdominal pain, gastrointestinal bleeding	10%
Dyspnea, hypoxia	10%
Chest pain	8%
Urinary retention, azotemia, electrolyte imbalance	7%
Arrhythmia, hypotension, syncope	6%
Edema, cellulitis	5%
All others	10%

From Manu P, Asif M, Khan S, et al. Risk factors for medical deterioration of psychiatric inpatients: opportunities for early recognition and prevention. *Compr Psychiatry.* 2012;53:968-974.

patients. Renal insufficiency, anemia, poor nutritional status, and older age are also independent predictors of medical deterioration.

Medical deterioration can have major adverse consequences for psychiatric inpatients. First, it may lead to life-threatening complications if the condition is not rapidly diagnosed and treated. Second, it interrupts behavioral interventions and may require the discontinuation of psychotropic drug treatment or electroconvulsive therapy (ECT). Third, it prolongs the length of stay and can add considerable expense to the episode of psychiatric illness, especially when patients are transferred from locked psychiatric units to a general hospital, where they require constant observation by qualified personnel.

EVALUATION OF CHIEF COMPLAINTS

Medical consultation for psychiatric patients creates unique challenges in evaluation of the chief complaint. Many patients with outpatient psychiatric disorders have somatic symptoms, such as fatigue, weakness, dizziness, headache, insomnia, widespread pain, and constipation. In most of these patients, the underlying mental illnesses are mood disorders (unipolar depression and dysthymia), anxiety disorders (panic disorder and generalized anxiety disorder), somatoform disorders, substance use disorders (most often alcohol, opiates, cocaine, and benzodiazepine), and borderline personality disorder. As a group, these patients have many physical complaints and resist a psychological explanation for their symptoms even when the medical evaluation fails to identify objective abnormalities. Standardized screening approaches can help clinicians and patients alike. After careful interdisciplinary evaluations, patients whose unexplainable somatic symptoms are diagnosed as hypochondriasis may respond to treatment with fluoxetine (see Table 369-5) and cognitive-behavioral therapy.[A1]

MEDICAL COMPLICATIONS OF PSYCHIATRIC TREATMENTS

Common drug classes used in psychiatry include antidepressants (selective serotonin reuptake inhibitors [SSRIs], serotonin-norepinephrine reuptake inhibitors [SNRIs], serotonin modulators, tricyclics, monoamine oxidase inhibitors [MAOIs], and atypical antidepressants), antipsychotics (first-generation antipsychotics, also known as neuroleptics, conventional or typical antipsychotics; long-acting injectable antipsychotics and second-generation antipsychotics, also known as atypical antipsychotics [e.g., clozapine]), and anxiolytics (SSRIs, SNRIs, benzodiazepines). Patients with mania secondary to bipolar affective disorder may receive lithium, anticonvulsants (most commonly valproate), antipsychotics, and benzodiazepines. Medical consultation in psychiatry should be informed by knowledge about the serious complications of these drugs (Table 406-2).

Antipsychotic-Induced Metabolic Syndrome

Metabolic syndrome is more prevalent (range, 29 to 63%) in schizophrenic and other psychiatric patients treated with second-generation antipsychotics, especially clozapine but also olanzapine, risperidone, and quetiapine because they induce substantial weight gain. The mechanism of weight gain centers on the drug's affinity for the histamine1 (H1)–receptor and the neurobiologic

TABLE 406-2	MAJOR MEDICAL COMPLICATIONS OF PSYCHOTROPIC DRUGS
CARDIOVASCULAR	
Cardiomyopathy	Clozapine
Hypertension	MAO inhibitors, venlafaxine
Myocarditis	Clozapine
Orthostatic hypotension	Tricyclics, trazodone, antipsychotics
Venous thromboembolism	Clozapine, risperidone, phenothiazines, antipsychotics
Prolonged QTc*	Antipsychotics, tricyclics, serotonin reuptake inhibitors
RESPIRATORY	
Choking	Antipsychotics, tricyclics
Laryngospasm	Antipsychotics
Respiratory depression	Benzodiazepines, barbiturates, methadone, antidepressants, atypical antipsychotics
GASTROINTESTINAL	
Bowel obstruction	Tricyclics, antipsychotics
Dysphagia	Tricyclics, antipsychotics
Hepatic impairment	Carbamazepine, valproic acid, phenothiazines, mirtazapine, nefazodone, quetiapine, olanzapine, clozapine, MAO inhibitors, naltrexone
Pancreatitis	Carbamazepine, valproic acid, clozapine, olanzapine, risperidone
KIDNEY AND URINARY TRACT	
Renal insufficiency	Lithium, clozapine
Urinary retention	Antipsychotics, tricyclics
ENDOCRINE	
Hyperprolactinemia	First-generation antipsychotics, risperidone
Hypothyroidism	Lithium, quetiapine
Inappropriate ADH secretion	Serotonin reuptake inhibitors, methadone, tricyclics
Metabolic syndrome	Clozapine, olanzapine, risperidone, quetiapine
HEMATOLOGIC	
Leukocytosis	Lithium
Neutropenia	Clozapine, olanzapine, risperidone, carbamazepine, valproate, mirtazapine
Thrombocytopenia	Carbamazepine, valproate
MUSCULOSKELETAL	
Rhabdomyolysis†	Antipsychotics, serotonin reuptake inhibitors, MAO inhibitors
SKIN	
Stevens-Johnson syndrome	Lamotrigine, carbamazepine, barbiturates
OTHER	
Fever†	Antipsychotics, serotonin reuptake inhibitors, MAO inhibitors
Seizure	Bupropion, MAO inhibitors, tricyclics, phenothiazines, clozapine

*Also see Table 406-3.
†Includes neuroleptic malignant syndrome and serotonin syndrome (also see Tables 406-4 and 406-5).
ADH = antidiuretic hormone; MAO = monoamine oxidase.

mechanisms that regulate appetite and metabolism through the production and activity of serotonin, leptin, and tumor necrosis factor–α. As a result, up to 40% of patients receiving long-term treatment with antipsychotics have impaired glucose tolerance, and about 10% have diabetes.[3,4] Because the glucose intolerance often seen in patients treated with antipsychotic agents is due to insulin resistance (Chapter 216), it is best treated by aggressive weight reduction (Chapter 207), increasing physical activity (Chapter 13), and metformin (Chapter 216) or a combination of these. For example, in randomized trials, metformin, 850 mg twice daily, significantly reduced the weight gain and reversed the metabolic abnormalities associated with the initiation of second-generation antipsychotic drugs,[A2] and a single daily dose of 750 mg may prevent weight gain if it is initiated at the onset of olanzapine treatment. Another option is to switch from olanzapine, quetiapine, or risperidone to aripiprazole,[A3] which is less likely to cause weight gain. The administration of the glucagon-like peptide-1 receptor agonist liraglutide (starting with a dose of 0.6 mg administered subcutaneously daily and uptitrating to 1.2 mg daily after 1 week and to 1.8 mg daily in the third week) to overweight or obese patients treated with olanzapine or clozapine can lead to weight loss, decreased waist circumference and low-density lipoprotein cholesterol levels, and improved glucose tolerance.[A4]

Cardiovascular Adverse Effects of Antipsychotic Medications

Psychiatric patients have a higher rate of sudden cardiac death in part owing to the cardiovascular adverse effects of antipsychotic medications.[5,6] Antipsychotic-induced myocarditis and cardiomyopathy (Chapter 54) are most common in patients treated with clozapine (0.9%) and fluphenazine (0.4%). In contrast, the risk for these complications is only 0.1% in patients receiving haloperidol, thioridazine, and risperidone. The accepted pathophysiologic explanation for myocarditis is an immunoglobulin E–mediated acute hypersensitivity reaction, similar to the allergic myocarditis produced by penicillins, sulfonamides, and methyldopa. In a small number of patients, a competing hypothesis proposes that clozapine induces hypereosinophilic myocarditis, colitis, hepatitis, pancreatitis, alveolitis, and interstitial nephritis. A direct cardiotoxic effect of drug metabolites cannot be excluded. In patients in whom myocarditis develops, the mortality rate is as high as 50%, with almost half the deaths occurring suddenly and unexpectedly. The average duration of exposure to clozapine before diagnosis or death is 21 days, and the dosage range is 50 to 725 mg/day. Common symptoms are fever (48%), dyspnea (35%), influenza-like illness (30%), chest pain (22%), and fatigue (17%). Laboratory features include left ventricular hypokinesia or reduced ejection fraction (48%) or pericardial effusion (17%) on echocardiography, nonspecific repolarization abnormalities on electrocardiography (35%), peripheral eosinophilia (35%), elevated creatine kinase and troponin levels (22%), and radiographic evidence of heart failure (13%). The diagnosis can be confirmed by endomyocardial biopsy showing fraying of myocytes and perivascular infiltrates with degranulated eosinophils. Among survivors, symptoms resolve or substantially improve after discontinuation of clozapine and treatment with high-dose corticosteroids (e.g., prednisone, 1 mg/kg/day for 4 days, tapered to 0.33 mg/kg/day for the following 4 days).

Clozapine-induced dilated cardiomyopathy may be caused by an evolving myocarditis or by chronic injury mediated by free radicals, similar to the myocarditis produced by doxorubicin (Chapter 54). The demographic features are similar to those of myocarditis, but the mean duration of treatment before diagnosis is much longer (9 months vs. 3 weeks), and the mortality rate is lower (22% vs. 51%). Patients have clinical or echocardiographic evidence of left ventricular dysfunction without eosinophilia or enzymatic evidence of myocardial necrosis.

Significant prolongation of the QTc interval (Chapter 59) leading to ventricular tachyarrhythmias and sudden cardiac death (Chapter 57) can occur after antipsychotic treatment with the usual doses of thioridazine, haloperidol, and sertindole.[7] Abnormal myocardial repolarization has been observed during treatment with most antipsychotic medications and after intentional or accidental overdoses of tricyclic antidepressants, lithium, and methadone (Chapter 102). Antipsychotics affect the cardiac potassium channel by blocking the rapidly activating component of the rectifier potassium current (Chapter 55). This effect translates into a dose-dependent increase in the duration of phase 3 of the action potential. Compared with nonusers of antipsychotic drugs, the risk for sudden death is twice as high for current users of conventional (first-generation) antipsychotics and is 2.25 times higher for current users of atypical (second-generation) antipsychotics. Antipsychotics that do not prolong the QT interval are available (e.g., aripiprazole, paliperidone, lurasidone).

All patients about to start antipsychotic drugs should be asked about a personal history of syncope and a family history of long QT syndrome or sudden death at a young age. A baseline electrocardiogram and serum electrolyte values should be obtained before starting of antipsychotic drug therapy, tricyclic antidepressants, and methadone. Interval electrocardiograms should be obtained after each increase in medication in older patients, patients with known heart disease, and those starting other drugs known to produce QTc prolongation or hypokalemia (Table 406-3; Chapter 59). A QTc interval of 500 milliseconds or longer requires the discontinuation of all drugs that affect membrane repolarization. QTc intervals longer than 450 milliseconds in men and 470 milliseconds in women, QTc dispersion (difference between the longest and shortest QTc on a 12-lead electrocardiogram) longer than 100 milliseconds, and increase in QTc duration of more than 60 milliseconds in comparison to the baseline measurement should prompt reevaluation of the risks and benefits associated with the drugs in question.

Choking and Laryngeal Dystonia

Asphyxia deaths from choking occur at a rate of 0.8% per 1000 psychiatric patients each year, a frequency that is more than 100 times greater than in the general population.[8] In addition, videofluoroscopy demonstrates silent aspiration in 38% of psychiatric patients who survive a choking incident. Half the psychiatric patients with dysphagia have a fast-eating syndrome seen in association with restlessness, poor chewing skills, food pocketing in the cheeks, and attention deficits that characterize psychotic disorders and mental retardation. Bradykinetic dysphagia, which is seen in 25% of psychiatric patients with choking episodes, is due to the antidopaminergic and anticholinergic effects of psychotropic medications. This condition, which features reduced lingual range of motion, increased oral transit time, decreased pharyngeal peristalsis, and delayed initiation of the swallowing reflex, is seen in patients with neurologic features of drug-induced parkinsonism (Chapter 381). Dyskinetic dysphagia (7% of choking cases), which generally occurs in patients maintained with long-term antipsychotic medication, is part of the clinical spectrum of tardive dyskinesia (Chapter 382). The examination reveals involuntary contractions of the tongue and perioral musculature, clumsiness of voluntary movements of the tongue, and discontinuous bolus propulsion in the oral stage. In the remaining patients, the dysphagia is due to cerebrovascular disease (11%) or to pharyngeal or esophageal disease (7%). Laryngeal dystonia, which is a life-threatening complication of antipsychotic drug therapy, primarily with haloperidol and phenothiazines, is produced by acute spasmodic contraction of the adductor laryngeal muscles. Symptoms include respiratory distress, dysphonia, and stridor. Neuroleptic-induced bronchospasm may precede the onset of stridor. Patients typically indicate extreme subjective distress by clutching their anterior cervical area. Most patients also have other dystonias involving the head and neck, including torticollis, retrocollis, trismus, tongue protrusion, and deviation of the eyes (up, down, or sideward). In general, the symptoms and signs develop in the first week after starting or rapidly increasing the dose of neuroleptic medications. A reduction in the dose of anticholinergic or antiparkinsonian medication used to prevent or to treat extrapyramidal symptoms can also precipitate laryngeal dystonia. Nocturnal sialorrhea, a common adverse effect of clozapine and a risk factor for aspiration pneumonia, responds to anticholinergic treatment with daily doses of 2 mg oral glycopyrrolate.[A5] For drug-induced tardive dyskinesia, deutetrabenazine (12-48 mg/day) and valbenazine (12.5-100 mg/day)[A6] are effective treatments.[9]

Drug-Induced Neutropenia and Agranulocytosis

Drug-induced neutropenia with absolute neutrophil counts of less than 1500/μL has been observed during treatment with most second-generation antipsychotics (clozapine, olanzapine, risperidone, and quetiapine) and mood stabilizers (carbamazepine, valproic acid, and lamotrigine) as well as with some antidepressant drugs (tricyclic antidepressants and mirtazapine). Clozapine-induced neutropenia occurs in 4 to 5% of patients within 6 months after treatment is started and progresses to agranulocytosis in 10% or more of neutropenic patients if the drug is continued. In vitro, clozapine toxicity requires peroxide and peroxidase, and the defect in oxidation is related to abnormalities in the NQO2 (quinone oxidoreductase) gene involved in drug detoxification. Treatment with clozapine should be started only if the baseline absolute neutrophil count is higher than 1500/μL. The concomitant use of carbamazepine, angiotensin-converting enzyme inhibitors, sulfonamides, propylthiouracil, and mirtazapine should be avoided because they can produce neutropenia and increase the risk for agranulocytosis. Clozapine should be stopped and

TABLE 406-3	PSYCHIATRIC MEDICATIONS ASSOCIATED WITH QT PROLONGATION
HIGHEST RISK	
Amisulpride	
Ziprasidone	
Iloperidone	
INTERMEDIATE RISK	
Risperidone	
Olanzapine	
Quetiapine	
Haloperidol	
NO RISK	
Paliperidone	
Aripiprazole	
Lurasidone	

Adapted from Lahijani SC, Harris KA. Medical complications of psychiatric treatment: an update. *Crit Care Clin.* 2017;33:713-734.

TABLE 406-4	DIFFERENTIAL DIAGNOSIS OF NEUROLEPTIC MALIGNANT SYNDROME

Infection of the central nervous system

Infection in patients with drug-induced parkinsonism

Drug overdose (psychostimulants, antidepressants, lithium, anticholinergics)

Alcohol or drug withdrawal (benzodiazepines, barbiturates, antiparkinsonian drugs)

Side effects of nonpsychotropic dopamine-depleting drugs (reserpine, metoclopramide, prochlorperazine, promethazine)

Cholinergic rebound

Serotonin syndrome

Thyrotoxicosis

Malignant hyperthermia

TABLE 406-5	CLASSES OF MEDICATIONS THAT PRODUCE SEROTONIN SYNDROME IN PSYCHIATRIC PATIENTS

Selective serotonin reuptake inhibitors

Monoamine oxidase inhibitors

Atypical antipsychotics

Heterocyclic antidepressants

Trazodone

Dual-uptake inhibitors

Psychostimulants

Buspirone

Mood stabilizers

Analgesics

Antiemetics

Cough suppressants

Dietary supplements

the patient evaluated immediately for fever, oral ulcerations, and symptoms or signs of infection. Complete blood counts should be obtained once a week for the first 26 weeks and every other week thereafter, and clozapine should be stopped and all medications reassessed if the absolute neutrophil count drops below $1500/\mu L$. Clozapine-related agranulocytosis has been treated successfully with colony-stimulating factors (either granulocyte or granulocyte-macrophage colony-stimulating factor). Neutropenia has also been associated with olanzapine, risperidone, and quetiapine in patients who have never received clozapine. Treatment with anticonvulsant mood stabilizers, particularly carbamazepine, is associated with a dose-dependent neutropenia and thrombocytopenia in approximately 10% of patients in the first 6 months of treatment and should be monitored with complete blood counts twice each month during this period.

Neuroleptic Malignant Syndrome

Neuroleptic malignant syndrome (Chapter 105), which occurs in approximately 0.2% of patients receiving neuroleptics, must be part of the differential diagnosis of fever and rhabdomyolysis (Table 406-4). The condition is rare, and newer atypical antipsychotic agents such as aripiprazole are less likely to cause the syndrome. Newer atypical antipsychotics (e.g., aripiprazole, risperidone, and quetiapine) are associated with lower incidence of the neuroleptic malignant syndrome, milder clinical presentations, and fewer lethal outcomes compared with first-generation antipsychotic medications. The main diagnostic criteria are elevated temperature (higher than 104° F [40° C] in 40% of patients) and diffuse muscle rigidity (ranging from mild hypertonicity to severe "lead pipe" stiffness). In addition, two or more of the following are required for a definitive diagnosis: (1) autonomic instability (tachycardia, elevated or labile blood pressure, postural hypotension, diaphoresis, sialorrhea, and urinary incontinence), (2) changes in mental status (ranging from confusion to mutism or coma), (3) leukocytosis (up to 20,000/mL), and (4) elevated creatine kinase (up to 100,000 IU/L).[10] Other clinical manifestations include bradykinesia, chorea, dystonias, dysphagia, dysarthria or aphonia, seizures, and tremor. The severity of rhabdomyolysis correlates with the creatine kinase level and with the presence of myoglobinemia, myoglobinuria, metabolic acidosis, and azotemia. The electroencephalogram shows nonspecific slowing in slightly more than half of patients.

The time lag from starting of the drug to the onset of neuroleptic malignant syndrome is generally short, with 30% of cases developing within 48 hours and 96% within the first month of treatment. The exception appears to be clozapine-associated neuroleptic malignant syndrome, which has an average time lag of 50 days. Neuroleptic syndrome is sometimes confused with severe catatonia (Chapter 369), but the catatonic signs in neuroleptic malignant syndrome are usually restricted to mutism and akinesia. Furthermore, hyperthermia, rigidity, tremor, and rhabdomyolysis are not present in patients with catatonia. Nonetheless, close medical follow-up of severely catatonic patients is warranted because they are at very high risk (22%) for neuroleptic malignant syndrome.

Untreated, neuroleptic malignant syndrome has a mortality rate of 10 to 20%[11] as a result of acute renal failure, aspiration pneumonia, acute respiratory distress syndrome, disseminated intravascular coagulation, and cerebellar neuronal degeneration. Most fatalities are avoidable if the diagnosis is made early, the neuroleptic agent is discontinued rapidly, and the patient is immediately transferred to an intensive care setting for supportive and specific therapy.[12] In mild to moderate cases, benzodiazepines (e.g., lorazepam, 1 to 2 mg orally or intramuscularly every 4 to 6 hours) should be used to alleviate symptoms. Bromocriptine (starting with 2.5 mg orally or via nasogastric tube two or three times daily, and increasing the dose by 2.5 mg daily to a maximum of 45 mg/day; contraindicated in patients with uncontrolled hypertension) or amantadine (100 mg twice daily) should be used in moderately severe cases and continued until the muscle rigidity and metabolic abnormalities have significantly improved. The skeletal muscle relaxant dantrolene should be added to bromocriptine or amantadine in patients with fulminant hypermetabolic features and those with persistent muscle rigidity despite treatment with dopamine agonists.

Serotonin Syndrome

Serotonin syndrome (Chapter 404) is an adverse drug reaction primarily produced by excess serotonergic agonism of central nervous system and peripheral serotonin receptors by selected drugs (Table 406-5). In postmarketing surveillance studies of the newer antidepressants, the syndrome has an incidence of 4 cases per 10,000 patient-months in patients who start taking nefazodone, a drug that inhibits neuronal uptake of serotonin and norepinephrine and also acts as a 5-hydroxytryptamine type 2 (5-HT2) receptor antagonist. The syndrome also occurs in 15% of patients with intentional overdose of SSRIs. The serotonin syndrome is caused by overstimulation of 5-HT1A and possibly also 5-HT2 receptors through excess of serotonin precursors or agonists, increased serotonin release, reduced serotonin uptake, and decreased serotonin metabolism. Severe cases of the syndrome have been more frequently reported in patients treated with MAOIs who took over-the-counter dextromethorphan or the illegal methylenedioxymethamphetamine (Ecstasy) or who started treatment with serotonin reuptake inhibitors, meperidine, or atypical antipsychotics such as aripiprazole.

This potentially life-threatening syndrome is characterized by changes in mental status (ranging from agitation to confusion and coma), autonomic instability (tachycardia, labile or high blood pressure, diaphoresis, and diarrhea), neuromuscular abnormalities (myoclonus, mydriasis, ocular clonus, rigidity, hyperreflexia, tremors, and shivering), and hyperthermia. The symptoms occur within the first 24 hours and sometimes within minutes after the initial use of medication, a change in dose, addition of a new drug, or an overdose attempt. Death may occur as a consequence of rhabdomyolysis with renal failure, hyperkalemia, disseminated intravascular coagulation, and acute respiratory distress syndrome. The differential diagnosis includes neuroleptic malignant syndrome, viral or bacterial meningitis or encephalitis, heat stroke (Chapter 101), anticholinergic toxidrome (Chapter 102), and drug (Chapter 31) or alcohol (Chapter 30) withdrawal.

General management includes immediate discontinuation of serotonergic drugs, comprehensive supportive therapy, and benzodiazepines for control of agitation and myoclonus. Specific therapy relies on the use of cyproheptadine (an H_1-receptor antagonist with antiserotonergic and anticholinergic properties) and chlorpromazine (a 5-HT$_{1A}$ and 5-HT$_2$ receptor antagonist).

Antipsychotic-Induced Hyperprolactinemia

Drug-induced hyperprolactinemia is produced by first-generation antipsychotic medications and by risperidone, but it is rare with other atypical antipsychotics such as aripiprazole, olanzapine, and ziprasidone. In patients treated with prolactin-raising antipsychotic medications, hormone levels are above the normal limit in 60% of women and 40% of men. Symptomatic hyperprolactinemia (Chapter 209) occurs in about one third of these patients and is generally associated with a 10-fold increase above baseline levels. Excess prolactin leads to dysfunction of target tissues (galactorrhea, oligomenorrhea and amenorrhea, infertility, sexual impairment, and gynecomastia) as well as an increased risk for breast cancer, osteoporosis, and cardiovascular disease.

Psychogenic Polydipsia and Drug-Induced Hyponatremia
Hyponatremia is a common reason for referral from psychiatry inpatient units. Water intake in excess of 3 to 4 liters/day and medication-related inappropriate antidiuretic hormone (ADH) secretion are the most common causes of hyponatremia in psychiatric inpatients. Patients with psychogenic polydipsia typically have serum hypo-osmolality and a maximally dilute urine (urine osmolality less than 100 mOsm/L). The incidence of polydipsia is 20% and the incidence of water intoxication is 5% in inpatient psychiatric facilities. Urinary incontinence and nocturnal enuresis may be part of the clinical manifestation. The mechanism of increased thirst is poorly understood but may involve incomplete suppression of ADH by the hypothalamus as well as response to the mouth dryness produced by the anticholinergic effect of many psychotropic drugs. Stringent measures to restrict fluid intake are generally effective but difficult to implement in patients with severe psychosis. In schizophrenic patients with refractory water intoxication, a favorable response has been observed after switching the antipsychotic regimen to clozapine (carefully titrated up to 600 mg/day and continued for up to 6 months). The drug-induced syndrome of inappropriate antidiuretic hormone (SIADH) is predominantly related to SSRIs,[13] and animal experiments have suggested that the excess serotonin stimulates release of ADH and will lead to hyponatremia, provided water intake is sufficient. Other drugs that are commonly used by psychiatric patients and that may produce SIADH include serotonin-norepinephrine reuptake inhibitors (e.g., venlafaxine and duloxetine), second-generation antipsychotic agents with serotonergic properties (particularly aripiprazole, olanzapine, and risperidone), and mood stabilizers (e.g., carbamazepine/oxcarbazepine, valproate, and lamotrigine). Elderly patients, patients with a lower body mass index, and those with a baseline plasma sodium level of less than 138 mEq/L are at higher risk. SSRIs can be continued with careful monitoring while the patient is placed on supervised fluid restriction. For patients who cannot tolerate fluid restriction or have symptomatic hyponatremia with serum sodium levels of less than 125 mEq/L, the use of tolvaptan, a vasopressin V_2-receptor antagonist, is effective (Chapter 108).

Rechallenge after Life-Threatening Adverse Effects of Clozapine
Clozapine is widely prescribed for the treatment refractory schizophrenia, but its use is limited by many potentially life-threatening adverse effects. Rechallenge after these complications is safe and successful in about 60% of patients, but is not usually safe in patients who develop agranulocytosis, pancreatitis, or renal insufficiency after the initial exposure.[14]

Grade A References

A1. Fallon BA, Ahern DK, Pavlicova M, et al. A randomized controlled trial of medication and cognitive-behavioral therapy for hypochondriasis. *Am J Psychiatry*. 2017;174:756-764.

A2. Chen CH, Huang MC, Kao CF, et al. Effects of adjunctive metformin on metabolic traits in nondiabetic clozapine-treated patients with schizophrenia and the effect of metformin discontinuation on body weight: a 24-week, randomized, double-blind, placebo-controlled study. *J Clin Psychiatry*. 2013;74:e424-e430.

A3. Stroup TS, Byerly MJ, Nasrallah HA, et al. Effects of switching from olanzapine, quetiapine, and risperidone to aripiprazole on 10-year coronary heart disease risk and metabolic syndrome status: results from a randomized controlled trial. *Schizophr Res*. 2013;146:190-195.

A4. Larsen JR, Vedtofte L, Jakobsen MSL, et al. Effect of liraglutide treatment on prediabetes and overweight or obesity in clozapine- or olanzapine-treated patients with schizophrenia spectrum disorder: a randomized clinical trial. *JAMA Psychiatry*. 2017;74:719-728.

A5. Man WH, Colen-de Koning JC, Schulte PF, et al. The effect of glycopyrrolate on nocturnal sialorrhea in patients using clozapine: a randomized, crossover, double-blind, placebo-controlled trial. *J Clin Psychopharmacol*. 2017;37:155-161.

A6. Solmi M, Pigato G, Kane JM, et al. Treatment of tardive dyskinesia with VMAT-2 inhibitors: a systematic review and meta-analysis of randomized controlled trials. *Drug Des Devel Ther*. 2018;12:1215-1238.

GENERAL REFERENCES

For the General References and other additional features, please visit Expert Consult at https://expertconsult.inkling.com.

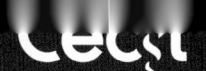

XXIX

§ SKIN DISEASES

407

APPROACH TO SKIN DISEASES

CHRISTINE J. KO

A thorough skin examination is about *sape vedere*, "knowing how to see" the skin. Although many nondermatologists feel limited to distinguishing a tumor from a neoplastic process, it is important for all clinicians to recognize common as well as morbid and life-threatening skin diseases.[1]

The American Cancer Society and the American Academy of Dermatology advocate routine skin cancer screening for adults on an annual basis, but the U.S. Preventive Services Task Force does not,[2,3] even for high risk individuals. Lesion-directed examination of patient-identified abnormalities and screening of people with atypical moles or more than 50 moles may be a reasonable middle ground.[4] Regardless of the frequency of routine total body skin examination, all clinicians should recognize concerning skin lesions, including brown/black/blue/red lesions that are asymmetric and irregular, lesions that look different than others on a given patient, and new lesions that are not healing over 3 to 4 weeks of time (Chapter 193).

STRUCTURE AND FUNCTION OF THE SKIN

A basic understanding of the structure and function of the skin provides a framework for organizing skin diseases. The functions of the skin include physical and mechanical protection, thermoregulation, immunological surveillance, and sensation. To achieve these goals, the skin is composed of the epidermis, dermis, and subcutaneous tissue. The epidermis is complex, primarily composed of keratinocytes in differentiated layers (E-Fig. 407-1). In addition to the epidermis, epithelial cells form important structures, including hair follicles, eccrine glands, apocrine glands, nails, and hair. Other cell types resident within the skin include melanocytes, Merkel cells, and immune cells. Melanocytes are critical for protecting against damage from ultraviolet light. Langerhans cells are resident immune cells that present antigens to circulating immune cells, which come in and out of the skin more transiently. Within the dermis, the fibroblast is a major cell responsible for forming collagen, which is the key structural protein. Vessels and nerves within the dermis are important for appropriate blood flow and sensation.

APPROACH TO A SKIN PROBLEM

Any new skin problem should be categorized as a tumor or a non-neoplastic process (rash).[5] Although this distinction is often simple, with tumors being solitary and rashes being more diffuse with multiple lesions, there are many exceptions. For example, tinea corporis can present as a solitary, scaling, pink plaque, as can superficial basal cell carcinoma or squamous cell carcinoma in situ (E-Fig. 407-2). Cutaneous T-cell lymphoma can present as multiple, asymptomatic pink patches and plaques, and it can easily be mistaken for a benign rash (E-Fig. 407-3). Knowledge of these pitfalls can help avoid them, with a low threshold for biopsy as clinically indicated.

THE SKIN EXAMINATION

An observational checklist (Table 407-1) can help guide the skin examination, which is aided by optimal lighting, including side lighting. Magnification can be helpful, and a simple hand lens can be used. Polarized magnifiers (dermatoscopes) can sometimes be helpful for physicians with sufficient training and experience.

The Patient

General and more specific characteristics of the patient should be observed. Age, gender, and skin type can all help direct the differential diagnosis. Skin type can be categorized (E-Table 407-1), and hair and eye color should also be noted. Red hair is associated with melanocortin-1 receptor mutations and an increased risk (about two-fold) of melanoma (Chapter 193). Occupational marks (e.g., linear burns on the arms of a baker) can sometimes be clues to job- or hobby-related diseases.

Distribution

The bodily distribution of lesions and layer of skin (epidermis, dermis, subcutaneous) they involve can be helpful in creating a differential diagnosis (E-Fig. 407-4; Table 407-2). For example, involvement of much of the face, arms, and upper chest in a photodistribution (sparing the skin under the nose, mid-chin, body folds, clothed areas) can point to sun-exacerbated diseases such as lupus erythematosus (Chapter 250) or a photo-induced drug reaction (Chapter 26). A unilateral, linear dermatomal distribution of vesicles is highly suggestive of herpes zoster (Chapter 351). Bilateral redness and swelling of the lower legs is highly unlikely to be cellulitis (Chapter 412), which is generally a unilateral disease (Fig. 407-1).

Palpation

Palpation of lesions can discern the depth of involvement, whether something is more superficial (epidermal), deeper (dermal), or even deeper (subcutaneous) (Table 407-3). Fibrosis, heat, roughness, dimpling, and firmness can also be palpated. Epidermal processes may have associated scale. Dermal disorders can have a normal-appearing surface (a clue that the process is not epidermal) or have overlying epidermal changes as well. Similarly, subcutaneous disorders may affect only the subcutaneous tissue (e.g., erythema nodosum [Chapter 411], which is the most common panniculitis, generally affecting only the adipose tissue) or may affect the epidermis and/or dermis as well (e.g., lupus profundus, in which epidermal and dermal changes are similar to discoid lupus erythematosus [Chapter 250], with necrosis and lymphocytic inflammation within the fat).

Morphology

Dermatology has its own vocabulary, and the most basic terms include those for morphology (Table 407-4; and see Table 407-1). The most important descriptions include macule, patch, papule, plaque, nodule, tumor, vesicle, bulla, and pustule. If the clinician is uncertain, descriptive language (e.g., "firm, raised bump about 0.4 cm in diameter" in place of "firm papule") is also effective for communicating among specialists.

Purpura (Fig. 407-2), which is caused by extravasation of red blood cells into the skin, results in a reddish to dark purple to black color. Small, pinpoint purpuric lesions are termed petechiae. Larger areas of purpura are termed ecchymoses. When purpura is palpable, it suggests small vessel leukocytoclastic vasculitis (Chapter 410). Larger vessel systemic vasculitis (Chapter 254) as well as occlusion of smaller vessels can produce retiform purpura, which can be a sign of a life-threatening disorder. The borders of retiform purpura form incomplete rings or nets, in a concave outline rather than the smoother, convex, scalloped, and rounded outline of palpable purpura.

Configuration

The arrangement, or configuration—linear, target, annular/serpiginous, exogenous, small net, or large net—of primary lesions is a principal diagnostic feature, as is its topography—flat-topped, smooth dome-shaped, filiform, pedunculated, verrucous, or umbilicated (Table 407-5). Each of these patterns provides clues to the diagnosis.

Color

Color can be an important guide for the differential diagnosis and sometimes is diagnostic (Table 407-6). Importantly, the background skin color can substantially influence the appearance of color within a lesion. For example, inflammation, which usually imparts a pink to red color to the skin, can be masked in darker compared with lighter skin types (E-Fig. 407-5). Lighter skin is at higher risk for skin cancer.

Secondary Changes

Normal skin does not produce visible scale. The presence of scale indicates that the stratum corneum is abnormal, and different types of scale are clues to the correct diagnosis (E-Table 407-2). Scale is an important component of conditions such as psoriasis, tinea, and pityriasis rosea (Chapter 409). Other secondary characteristics include crusting, fissures, erosion, ulceration, excoriation, atrophy, and lichenification (E-Table 407-3). Certain secondary findings are expected for a given disease—e.g., lichenification in atopic dermatitis (Chapter 409) and atrophy in lichen sclerosus (Chapter 411).

HISTORY

Because dermatologic diagnosis is, for the most part, visually based, the skin examination often precedes taking a history—or the two may be conducted simultaneously. Important factors (Table 407-7) to consider include onset/duration of the problem, systemic symptoms, and lesional symptoms including pruritus and/or pain. The past medical history, list of medications, and contactants, especially if recent or new, are important, as is a review of systems (Chapter 6).

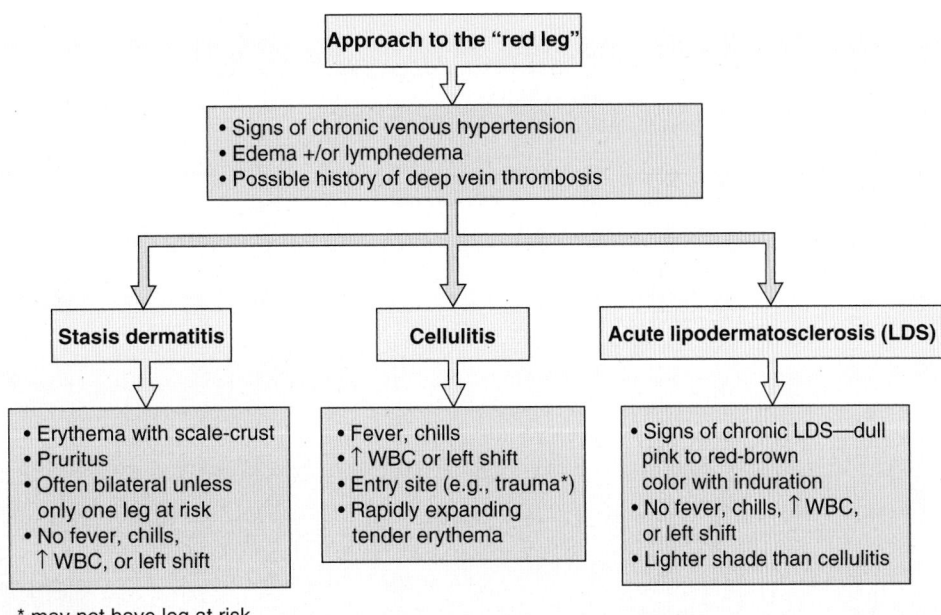

Approach to the "red leg"

- Signs of chronic venous hypertension
- Edema +/or lymphedema
- Possible history of deep vein thrombosis

Stasis dermatitis

- Erythema with scale-crust
- Pruritus
- Often bilateral unless only one leg at risk
- No fever, chills, ↑ WBC, or left shift

Cellulitis

- Fever, chills
- ↑ WBC or left shift
- Entry site (e.g., trauma*)
- Rapidly expanding tender erythema

Acute lipodermatosclerosis (LDS)

- Signs of chronic LDS—dull pink to red-brown color with induration
- No fever, chills, ↑ WBC, or left shift
- Lighter shade than cellulitis

* may not have leg at risk

FIGURE 407-1. Approach to the "red leg." WBC = white blood cells. (From Bolognia JL, Jorizzo JL, Schaffer JV. *Dermatology.* 3rd ed. Philadelphia: Saunders; 2012.)

TABLE 407-1   OBSERVATIONAL CHECKLIST

WHO?	WHERE?	WHAT?	WHEN?
The patient • General appearance • Age, degree of sun damage • Gender • Skin type, hair/eye color • Occupational marks	**Overall and local distribution** **Depth affected** (can use palpation) • Epidermal • Dermal • Subcutaneous	**Morphology of primary lesion** • Macule (Flat, <1 cm) • Patch (Flat, >1 cm) • Papule (Raised, <1 cm) • Plaque (Raised, >1 cm) • Nodule (Deeper than papule, <1 cm) • Tumor (Deeper than papule, >1 cm) • Vesicle (Fluid-filled, <1 cm) • Bulla (Fluid-filled, >1 cm) • Pustule (Pus-filled, <1 cm) **Configuration/pattern** **Color** **Secondary changes**	**Duration** • Acute • Chronic • Fixed vs. transient

An observational checklist can help guide the general skin examination (see text).

TABLE 407-2   LOCATION OF SKIN LESIONS AS A DIAGNOSTIC CLUE

LOCATION	POSSIBLE DIAGNOSES	
Unilateral	Herpes zoster Herpes simplex Deep vein thrombosis	Contact dermatitis where exposed Cellulitis Necrotizing fasciitis Solitary skin malignancies
Bilateral, widespread	Hematogenously spread process Severe drug eruption Disseminated viral, bacterial, or fungal infection Vasculitis Autoimmune disease	Psoriasis Cutaneous T-cell lymphoma Scabies Urticaria Atopic dermatitis (eczema) Other drug eruptions
Bilateral, limited sites	Stasis dermatitis Irritant contact dermatitis	Vasculitis Erythema multiforme Lipodermatosclerosis

The confidence in a diagnosis increases when the history and the skin findings point coherently to a single diagnostic entity. For example, allergic contact dermatitis (Chapter 409) seems highly likely for a new eczematous, excoriated rash that is seen on the margins of the scalp and extends slightly onto the forehead, especially if it is associated with pruritus and a recent switch to a new hairdresser and use of new hair dye. The differential diagnosis includes seborrheic dermatitis (Chapter 409), which commonly affects the scalp, though less often the forehead, and is often pruritic as well. In this specific example, patch testing (in which patches with specific allergens are placed on the patient's back for 24 to 48 hours before removal), and response to avoidance of hair dye can aid in differentiating the two disorders.

● LIFE-THREATENING EMERGENCIES

The presence of an acute fever and rash should prompt exclusion of life-threatening diseases (Table 407-8; Figs. 407-3 to 407-8). Necrotizing fasciitis (Chapter 280) can also be a life-threatening emergency that may be deceptively limited to one extremity. Widespread retiform purpura, including on sites above the waist, in an ill-appearing patient should prompt consideration of disseminated intravascular coagulation (Fig. 407-9; Chapter 166), which is seen in severe systemic infections, such as meningococcemia (Chapter 282). The widespread distribution in a sick patient is in sharp contrast to localized

Text continued on p. 2605

TABLE 407-3 REPRESENTATIVE DIAGNOSES BASED ON DEPTH OF PATHOLOGY IN THE SKIN

DEPTH	CHARACTERISTICS	DISORDERS		CLINICAL EXAMPLE
Epidermal	Distinct, even sharp margins Scaling Epidermal thickening Absence of induration May have mild erythema as well (some dermal involvement)	Seborrheic keratosis Warts In situ squamous cell carcinoma (Bowen disease) Ichthyosis Bullous impetigo Superficial basal cell carcinoma Acanthosis nigricans	Pityriasis rosea Tinea versicolor Tinea corporis Actinic keratosis	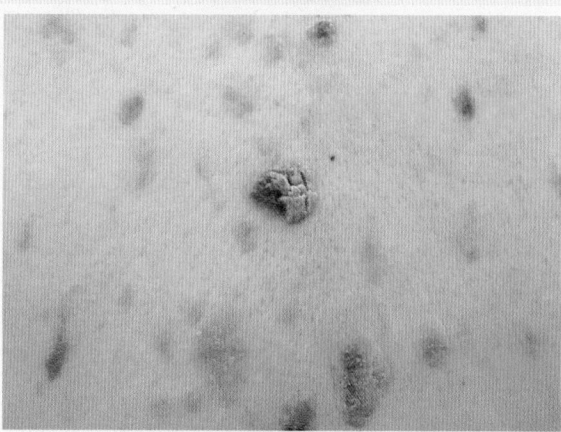 Seborrheic keratoses.
Epidermal and dermal Most skin diseases will have some degree of dermal and epidermal involvement	Margins moderately well defined Scale can be present Inflammation (erythema) Usually palpable lesions (raised)	Lichen planus Systemic lupus erythematosus Chronic cutaneous lupus Nummular (discoid) dermatitis Mycosis fungoides Pyoderma gangrenosum	Atopic dermatitis Secondary syphilis Nodular basal cell carcinoma Squamous cell carcinoma Melanoma Most vesiculobullous diseases (HSV, autoimmune)	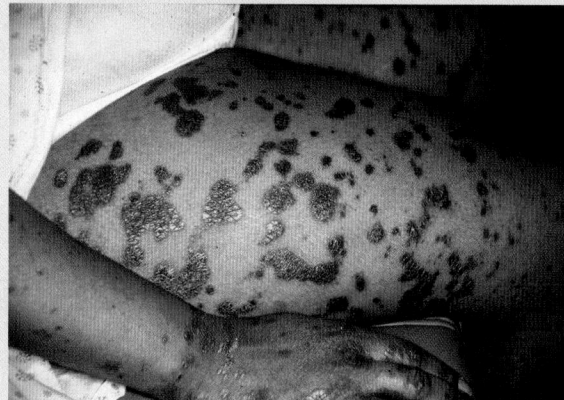 Lichen planus.
Dermal Diseases with only dermal involvement usually consist of infiltrates with inflammatory or malignant cells that do not influence epidermal function	Margins moderately defined No scale Smooth surface No ulcer Variable inflammation Usually palpable	Urticaria Sarcoidosis Granuloma annulare Leprosy Necrobiosis lipoidica Morphea Scleroderma	Cutaneous metastases Most cysts Dermal melanocytic nevi Pretibial myxedema Other cutaneous lymphomas	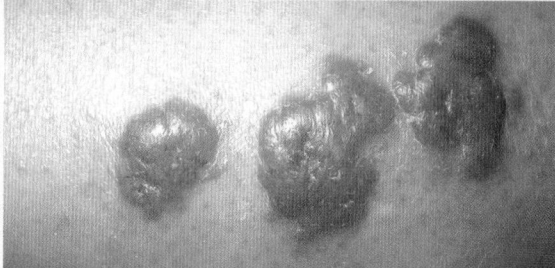 Sarcoidosis: Histiocyte collections in the upper dermis.
Subcutaneous fat	Margins rounded and/or poorly defined Variable inflammation Smooth overlying skin	Lipoma Erythema nodosum Panniculitis of any etiology Some lymphomas		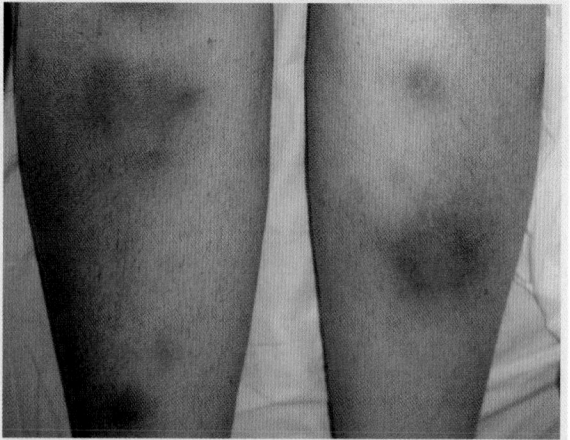 Erythema nodosum.

HSV = herpes simplex virus.
Courtesy James C. Shaw.

TABLE 407-4 MORPHOLOGIC TERMS FOR PRIMARY LESIONS

Macule: Flat, nonpalpable, <1 cm diameter

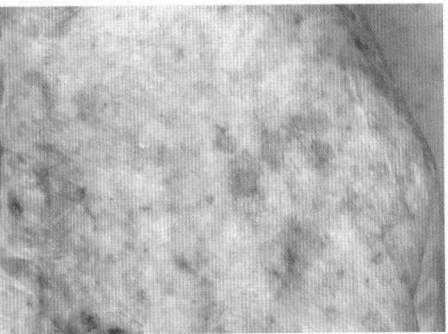

Lentigines. Light tan macules.

Papule: Superficial, raised, palpable, <1 cm diameter

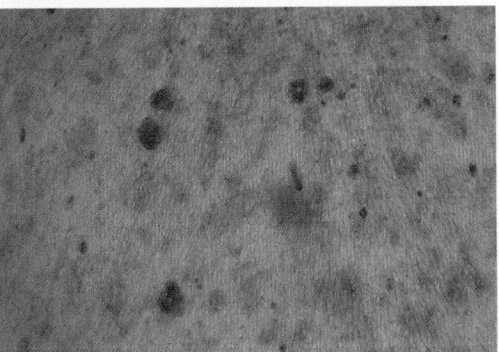

Seborrheic keratoses. Gray-brown stuck-on papules.

Patch: Large macules >1 cm diameter

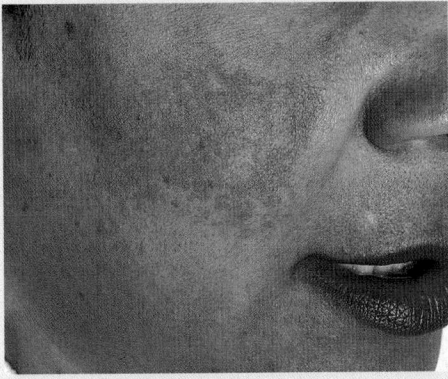

Melasma. Light tan patch on the cheek.

Plaque: Raised, palpable, >1 cm diameter

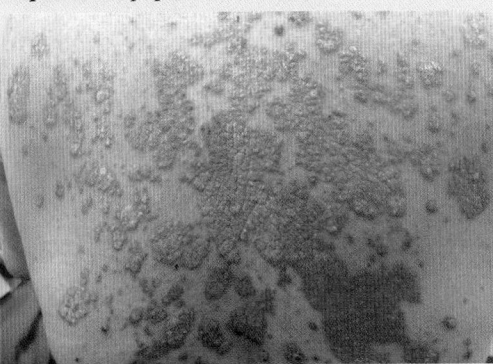

Psoriasis. Pink-red well-demarcated plaques with adherent scale.

Nodule: Deeper than a papule, usually <1 cm diameter

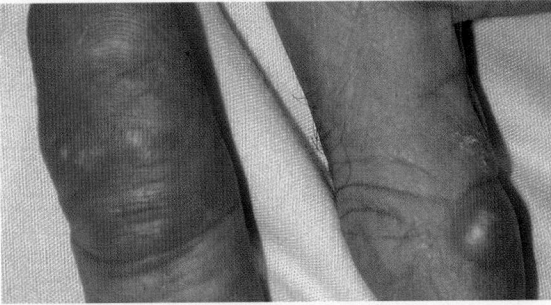

Gout. Yellow-pink nodules over and near joints.

Tumor: Large nodule, >1 cm diameter

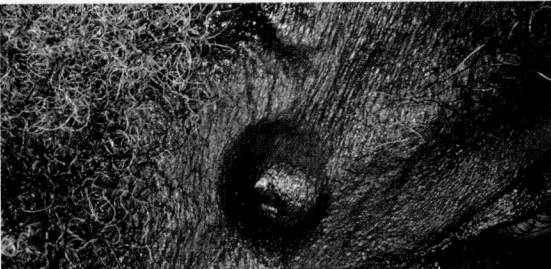

Epidermoid cyst. Tumor based in the dermis with an overlying punctum.

Vesicle: <1 cm fluid-filled, may be umbilicated or contain pus or blood

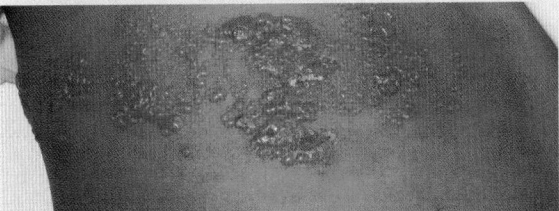

Herpes zoster. Small vesicles, some becoming confluent, with background erythema. The vesicles and erythema are unilateral in a dermatomal distribution.

Bulla: >1 cm, filled with clear fluid, pus, or blood

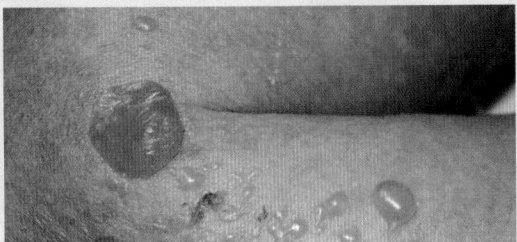

Bullous pemphigoid. Tense bullae (and some vesicles) on a pink background.

Pustule: White, pus-filled, small, raised, <1 cm diameter

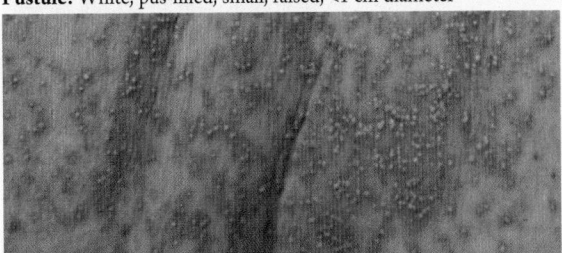

Acute generalized exanthematous pustulosis (a type of drug reaction). Small pustules over confluent erythema.

Photographs from Ko CJ. *Dermatology: Visual Recognition.* Elsevier; 2017, Bolognia JL, Jorizzo JL, Schaffer JV. *Dermatology.* 3rd ed. London: Saunders; 2012; Yale Dermatology Residents' Collection; and NYU Slide Collection.

TABLE 407-5 CONFIGURATION/PATTERN

CONFIGURATION/PATTERN/EXAMPLE

Linear
- Externally induced
- Dermatomal
- Vascular
- Blaschkoid

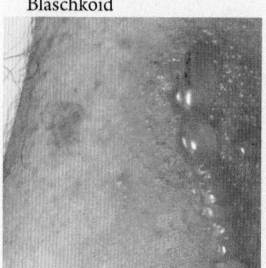

Poison ivy dermatitis.

Exogenous

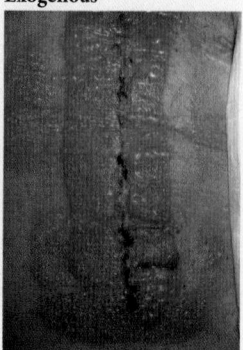

Allergic contact dermatitis.

Small net

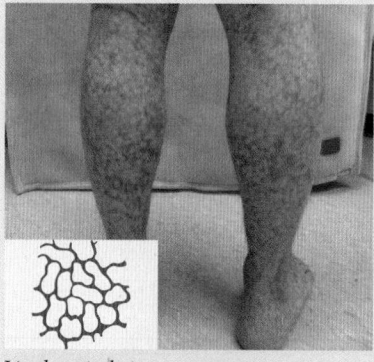

Livedo reticularis.

Large net, irregular and incomplete

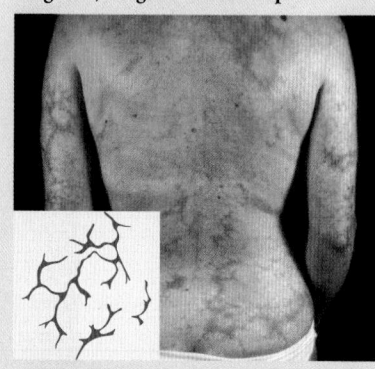

Livedo racemosa.

Target (3 zones of color)

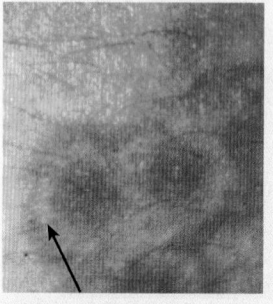

Erythema multiforme.

Annular/serpiginous

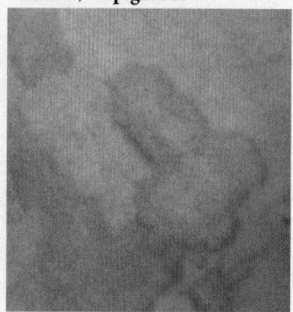

Urticaria.

Topography

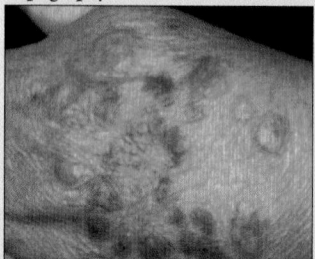

Flat-topped

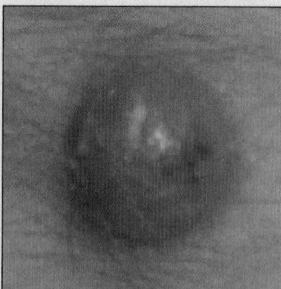

Dome-shaped, smooth

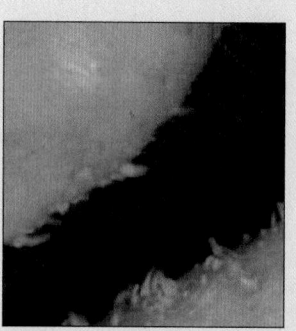

Filiform

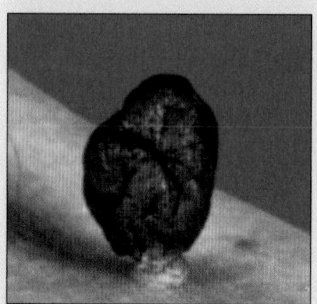

Pedunculated

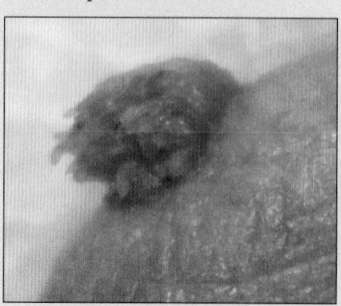

Verrucous

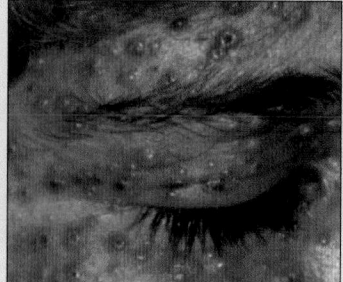

Umbilicated

Adapted from Bolognia JL, Schaffer JV, Duncan KO, Ko CJ. *Dermatology Essentials*. Elsevier; 2014. Photographs from Ko CJ. *Dermatology: Visual Recognition*. Elsevier; 2017; Bolognia JL, Jorizzo JL, Schaffer JV. *Dermatology*. 3rd ed. London: Saunders; 2012; Yale Dermatology Residents' Collection; and Kalman Watsky, MD, Peter Heald, MD, Christopher Baker, and Robert Kelly.

TABLE 407-6 COLOR CLUES IN DIAGNOSING SKIN DISEASE

COLOR		COLOR

Black

Melanin
Erythrocytes (purpura)
Necrosis (can be gray early on)
Occluded vessels
Inflammation

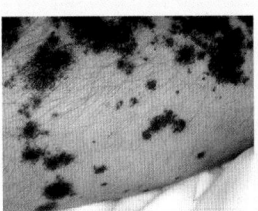

Palpable purpura. Small vessel vasculitis with papules coalescing into a larger plaque.

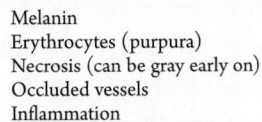
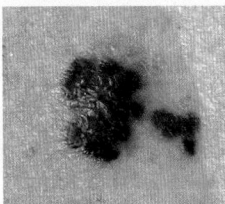

Melanoma. Irregularly shaped black papules.

Brown
Melanin
Hemosiderin

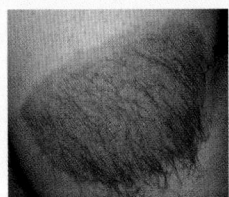

Medium-sized congenital nevus on the arm.

White

Decreased melanin
Vasospasm
Deposition (e.g., calcium)
Keratin (e.g., scale, cyst)
Sclerosis/scar

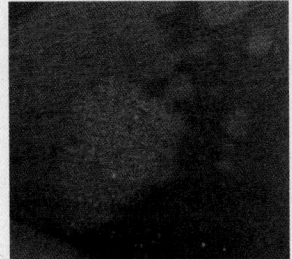

Tinea versicolor. White, powdery scale is typical with gentle scraping. The lesions are hypopigmented, thin plaques and papules.

Blue
Melanin
Vessels

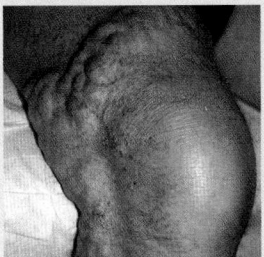

Varicose veins. Blue linear cords and papules.

Variations of pink

Pink
Vasodilation
Inflammation

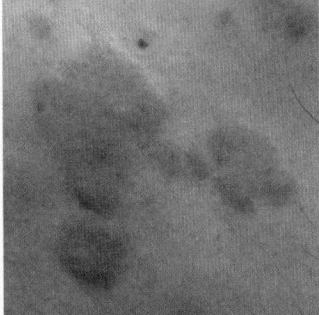

Urticaria. Light pink papules.

Pink-red (in lighter skin)
Inflammation
Vasodilation

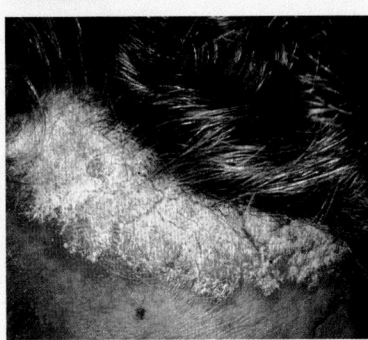

Psoriasis. Pink-red well-demarcated plaque with silvery, adherent scale.

Orange-red
Inflammation

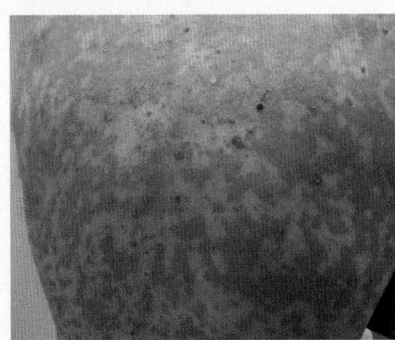

Pityriasis rubra pilaris. Orange-pink plaques with areas of uninvolved skin on the back.

Red/pink-brown
Denser inflammation, often not just lymphocytes (e.g., lymphocytes and plasma cells in secondary syphilis, granulomatous/ histiocytic disorders)

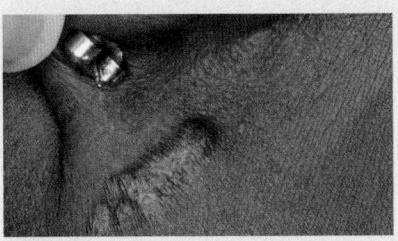

Sarcoidosis. Confluent pink-brown nodules.

Yellow to yellow-pink
Certain cell types (e.g., granulomatous/histiocytic)
Keratin (e.g., cyst)
Sebaceous lesion
Connective tissue
Lipid
Deposition (e.g., urate in gout, hemosiderin in bruise)

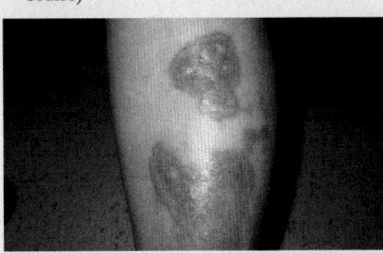

Necrobiosis lipoidica. Plaques on the shin with a characteristic slight yellow tinge).

Purple-pink
Dense lymphocytes
Vascular lesions

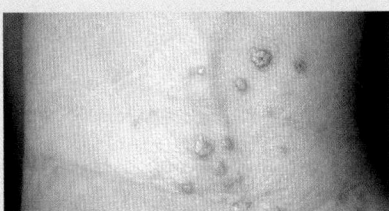

Lichen planus (pruritic purple polygonal papules; the wrist is a commonly affected site).

Photographs from Ko CJ. *Dermatology: Visual Recognition.* Elsevier; 2017, Bolognia JL, Jorizzo JL, Schaffer JV. *Dermatology.* 3rd ed. London: Saunders; 2012, and the Yale Dermatology Residents' Collection.

TABLE 407-7 IMPORTANT CLUES FROM THE HISTORY AND GENERAL HEALTH STATUS

CLUES	POSSIBLE DIAGNOSES	
Pruritus (itch)	Atopic dermatitis (eczema) Allergic contact dermatitis Urticaria Scabies	Bullous pemphigoid Lichen planus Dermatitis herpetiformis Inflammatory tinea pedis
Absence of pruritus	Acne vulgaris Rosacea Syphilis	Skin malignancies Lupus erythematosus Pemphigus vulgaris Erythema multiforme
Pain	Herpes zoster Ischemic necrosis from all causes Cellulitis Furunculosis	Carbuncles Pyoderma gangrenosum Severe systemic illnesses
Medications (especially new)	Severe drug eruptions Fixed drug eruptions Morbilliform drug eruptions Immunosuppression	Subacute cutaneous lupus Psoriasis exacerbation Urticaria Drug-induced hair loss
Cachexia/malnutrition	Paraneoplastic dermatoses Skin malignancy Alcohol exacerbated psoriasis	Nutritional deficiencies Metastatic disease Eating disorders leading to nutritional deficiencies
Obesity or weight gain	Dermatoses of diabetes Thyroid disease Cushing disease Polycystic ovarian syndrome Acne	Hirsutism Striae Acanthosis nigricans Eruptive xanthomas
Poor hygiene	Bacterial skin infections Infestations	Substance abuse
Psychiatric illness	Self-inflicted skin disease	Drug-induced dermatoses

TABLE 407-8 APPROACH TO THE ADULT WITH AN ACUTE FEVER AND RASH*

CATEGORY	DISEASES	CLUES ON SKIN EXAMINATION

Infectious	Potentially life-threatening systemic infection (viral, bacterial, fungal[†], protozoal[†])
	• Disseminated herpes zoster or herpes simplex[†] (see Fig. 407-3)
	• Meningococcemia (see Fig. 407-4)
	• Toxic shock syndrome (see Fig. 407-5)
	• Disseminated fungal diseases[†]
	   Candidiasis (see Fig. 407-6)
	   Histoplasmosis
	   Cryptococcosis
	• Protozoa1[†]
	   Strongyloidiasis
	Usually not immediately life-threatening
	• Viral exanthems due to enteroviruses, HHV-6, adenovirus; HIV, varicella; Kaposi varicelliform eruption
	• Bacterial: staphylococcal scalded skin syndrome, secondary syphilis, disseminated erythema migrans (Lyme disease)
		Multiple (>2-3 to 100s), discrete lesions, scattered over body, suggesting hematogenous spread
		Herpes viruses: primary lesion is the vesicle
		Meningococcemia: Retiform purpura affecting multiple different body sites, including above the waist
		Toxic shock syndrome: acute erythema of palms/soles
		Strongyloidiasis: periumbilical purpura

Inflammatory	Potentially life-threatening • Toxic epidermal necrolysis (see Fig. 407-7) Usually not immediately life-threatening • Drug reactions (severe drug reactions): morbilliform, serum sickness-like reaction, DRESS, AGEP, erythroderma • Erythema multiforme • Primary cutaneous disorders (e.g., pustular psoriasis) • Rheumatologic disorders (e.g., SLE, vasculitis, Still disease) • Graft-versus-host disease	Confluent erythema, scale peeling off in sheets, necrosis of skin (gray areas), widespread bullae, severe mucositis (see Fig. 407-8) **DRESS:** facial edema
Other	Potentially life-threatening • Disseminated intravascular coagulation (see Fig. 407-9) Usually not immediately life-threatening • Neoplastic (e.g., lymphoma) • Inherited (e.g., periodic fever syndromes)	Widespread retiform purpura, including above the waist

*Not a single site, as in cellulitis or necrotizing fasciitis.
[†]More likely in immunocompromised patient.
AGEP = acute generalized exanthematous pustulosis; DRESS = drug reaction with eosinophilia and systemic symptoms (also referred to as DIHS = drug-induced hypersensitivity syndrome); HHV = human herpes virus; HIV = human immunodeficiency virus; SLE = systemic lupus erythematosus.
Adapted from Bolognia JL, Schaffer JV, Duncan KO, Ko CJ. *Dermatology Essentials.* Elsevier; 2014.

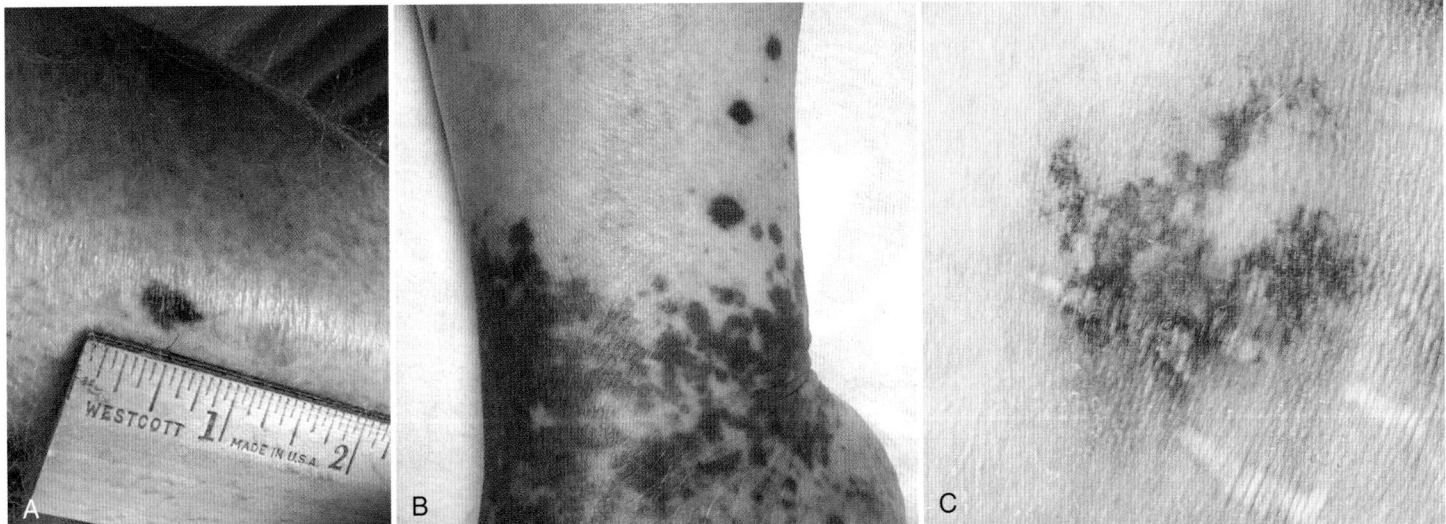

FIGURE 407-2. Purpura represents extravasated erythrocytes in the skin. **A,** Solar purpura. Bruises on the sun-exposed skin of older individuals are very common. **B,** Palpable purpura, which generally corresponds to leukocytoclastic vasculitis on biopsy. **C,** Retiform purpura in early calciphylaxis. Note the jagged, netlike outlines. This type of purpura is often associated with larger vessel systemic vasculitis or coagulopathy. (**B,** Courtesy Yale Dermatology Residents' Slide Collection. **C,** From Ko CJ. *Dermatology: Visual Recognition.* Elsevier; 2017.)

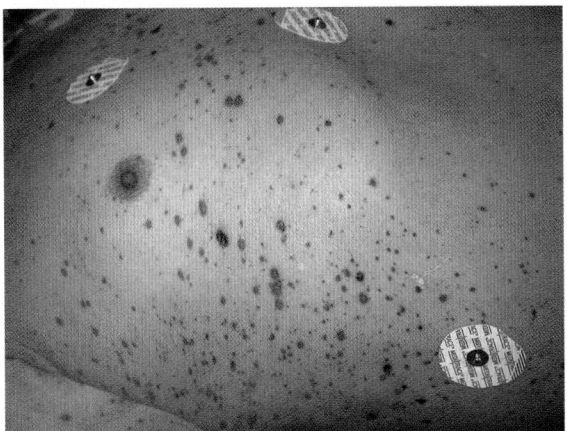

FIGURE 407-3. Disseminated varicella-zoster virus. Widespread, individual papules and vesicles, many with hemorrhage. Note the absence of coalescence into larger bullae.

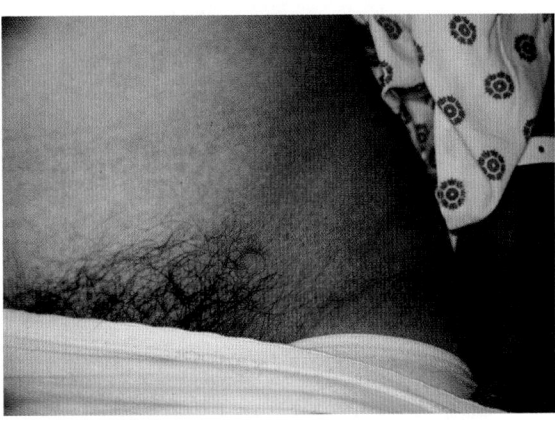

FIGURE 407-5. Toxic shock syndrome. Acute erythema in a swim-trunk distribution can be an early sign of toxic shock syndrome. Similar erythema occurs on dorsal hands and feet. Peeling of the skin in these areas occurs 1 to 2 weeks later

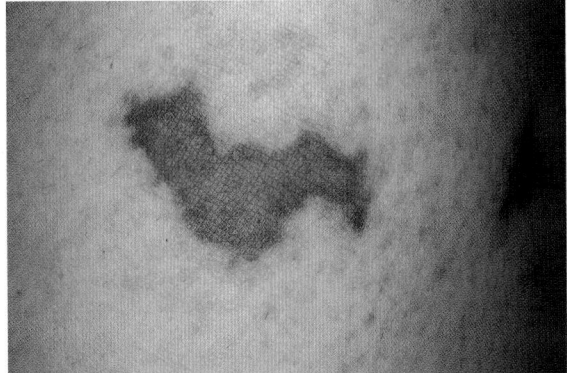

FIGURE 407-4. Acute meningococcemia. Retiform purpura with irregular outline and grayish-red color. (Courtesy Kalman Watsky, MD. From Bolognia JL, Jorizzo JL, Schaffer JV. *Dermatology.* 3rd ed. Philadelphia: Saunders; 2012.)

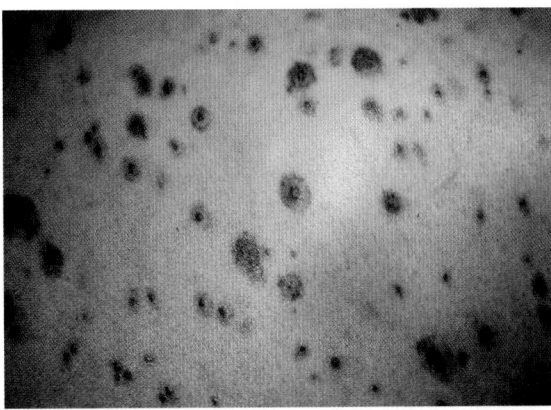

FIGURE 407-6. Disseminated candidiasis. Multiple individual small lesions, papules mostly, some with surrounding purpura, consistent with hematogenously spread disease.

purpura, which is less concerning and points to coagulation disorders, including reactions to warfarin or heparin, or the palpable purpura of small vessel leukocytoclastic vasculitis (see Fig. 407-2). Persistent skin mottling, principally in the fingers and toes, is a sign of poor circulation in a critically ill patient and is associated with increased mortality.[6] Intense pruritus accompanying an acute blistering eruption points toward bullous pemphigoid or allergic contact dermatitis (Figs. 407-10 and 407-11; Chapter 409) rather than toxic epidermal necrolysis (Chapter 411).

DIAGNOSTIC TESTS

Pressing on the skin with something transparent (termed diascopy), such as a glass slide or tube, can help confirm the status of vessels, which normally blanch and then refill. Diascopy of red-pink erythema can confirm that the color is inflammatory—the red-pink color should fade completely with pressure. This finding is in contrast to purpura (blood within the skin), which has a deep red to purple to black color that does not fade with pressure.

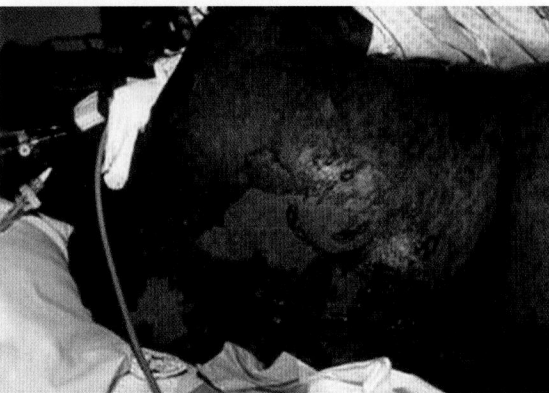

FIGURE 407-7. Bullae (toxic epidermal necrolysis). Detachment of large sheets of necrolytic epidermis (>30% body surface area), leading to extensive areas of denuded skin. A few intact bullae are still present. (From Bolognia JL, Jorizzo JL, Schaffer JV. *Dermatolog.* 3rd ed. Philadelphia: Saunders; 2012:328, Fig. 20.10A.)

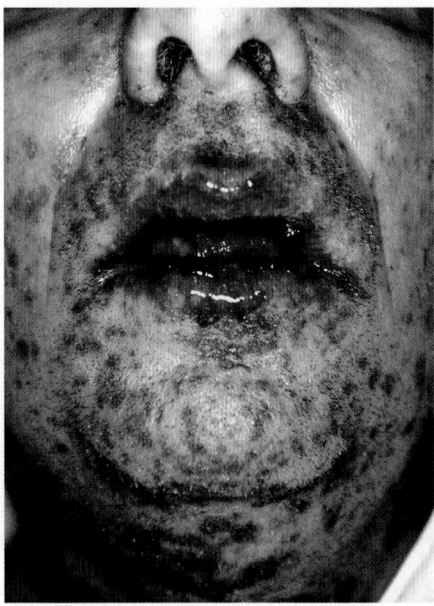

FIGURE 407-8. Mucositis (Stevens-Johnson syndrome). Extensive erosive changes on lips and oral mucosa are highly suggestive of a severe drug eruption such as Stevens-Johnson syndrome or toxic epidermal necrolysis.

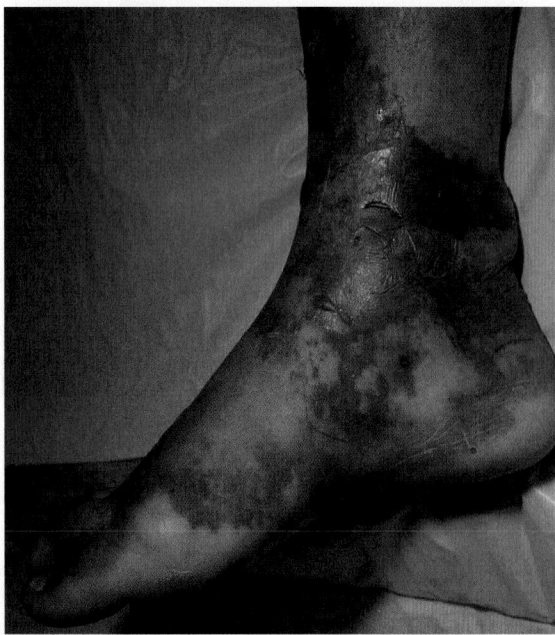

FIGURE 407-9. Disseminated intravascular coagulation. Noninflammatory (without underlying erythema) retiform purpura as well as hemorrhagic bullae in a patient with disseminated intravascular coagulation (DIC). (Courtesy Judit Stenn, MD. From Bolognia JL, Jorizzo JL, Schaffer JV. *Dermatology.* 3rd ed. Philadelphia: Saunders; 2012.)

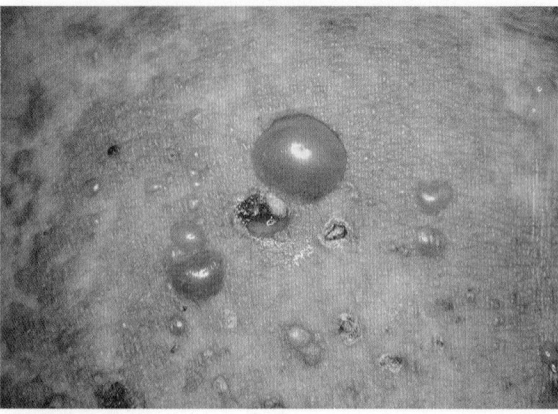

FIGURE 407-10. Vesicles and bullae (bullous pemphigoid). Large bullae as well as smaller bullae and vesicles on a background of urticaria-like erythema.

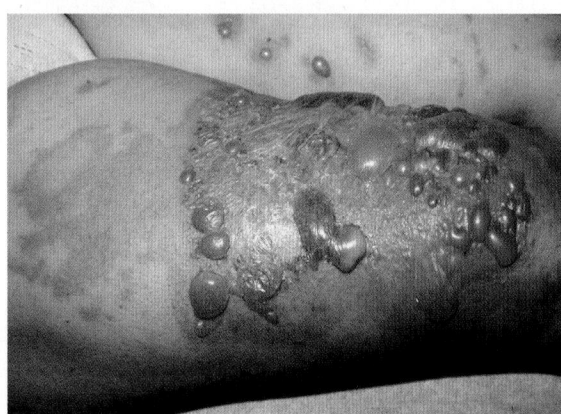

FIGURE 407-11. Severe allergic contact dermatitis. Bullae and vesicles on a background of erythema. Severe cases such as this can be mistaken for the autoimmune disease bullous pemphigoid.

Scale can always be gently scraped off onto a glass slide with a scalpel blade or even with another microscopic slide. A 10% solution of potassium hydroxide (KOH) can be applied onto the scale, then a cover slip can be placed over the scale and solution, with the bottom of the slide placed briefly over a flame (from a lighter or even a match). KOH dissolves keratin, with the heat accelerating the reaction, thereby allowing nonkeratinized structures such as fungal hyphae to be prominent on microscopic examination (E-Fig. 407-6). If scabies (Fig. 104-2) is suspected, skin lesions can be gently scraped, with scale and crust placed onto a slide covered with a small amount of mineral oil (E-Fig. 407-7).

Rapid diagnosis of herpes virus infection (without speciation) is possible with the Tzanck smear, by which vesicles are unroofed, with gentle scraping of the base of the lesion. Collected material is smeared onto a microscopic slide and briefly heated, with subsequent application of any nuclear stain (methylene blue, alanine, hematoxylin, etc.). After the slide is rinsed and blotted, microscopic examination can identify the pathognomonic multinucleated keratinocytes (E-Fig. 407-8). Other tests include direct fluorescent antibody staining, polymerase chain reaction testing, electron microscopy, and viral culture; local practice patterns often dictate which test is preferred. A Gram stain to look for bacteria is similar: pustular material is smeared and briefly heated on a slide, then four different stains are applied and rinsed (crystal violet, iodine, alcohol, safranin) in order. The slide is blotted, mounted under immersion or mineral oil, and examined under high magnification.

A skin biopsy entails taking a small piece of skin for fixation and microscopic examination. In general, the center of lesional tissue should be biopsied; the periphery should be biopsied only for ulcers, bullae, and normal skin for direct immunofluorescence studies.

● PRURITUS

Pruritus is the medical term for itch. Pruritus, especially chronic pruritus, can be likened to pain (Chapter 27), as it can be extremely disruptive and life-changing. Both pruritus and pain are mediated by the same nerve fibers, unmyelinated C fibers. Pruritus may originate in the skin (e.g., inflammatory

TABLE 407-9	APPROACH TO THE PATIENT WITH GENERALIZED PRURITUS AND NO OBVIOUS SKIN-SPECIFIC DISEASE

HISTORY

Complete history and review of systems
- Consider risk factors for scabies (e.g., nursing home resident, close contact with recent diagnosis, symptoms in household contacts)
- Ask about dermographism (exaggerated tendency to develop wheals with scratching of the skin—a type of physical urticaria), xerosis, irritants, occupational exposures
- Review all medications (prescription,* OTC, supplements, illicit)

PHYSICAL EXAMINATION

Complete skin examination
Lymph node examination

SCREENING LABORATORY TESTS

CBC with differential and platelets
ESR and LDH
TSH
BUN/creatinine
Liver function tests

ADDITIONAL EVALUATION (AS INDICATED BY AGE, HISTORY, COMORBID CONDITIONS, AND SCREENING TESTS)

Additional blood tests
- Serum fasting glucose and Hgb A_{1c}
- Serum calcium and phosphate levels
- Albumin level
- Ferritin, iron studies
- Anti–tissue transglutaminase antibodies
- Viral hepatitis screen
- HIV testing
Other tests
- Chest radiograph
- Age-appropriate cancer screening examinations
- Stool exam for ova and parasites
- Endoscopy

*Drug-induced pruritus: major culprits include calcium-channel blockers, proton pump inhibitors, narcotics, and amphetamines.

BUN = blood urea nitrogen; CBC = complete blood count; ESR = erythrocyte sedimentation rate; Hgb = hemoglobin; HIV = human immunodeficiency virus; LDH = lactate dehydrogenase; OTC = over-the-counter; TSH = thyroid-stimulating hormone.

Adapted from Bolognia JL, Schaffer JV, Duncan KO, Ko CJ. *Dermatology Essentials*. Elsevier; 2014.

TABLE 407-10	TREATMENT OF PRURITUS

TOPICAL AGENTS

Emollients
    Eucerin (e.g, Skin Calming Crème), CeraVe (e.g., Itch Relief Moisturizing Cream), Aveeno (e.g. Eczema Therapy Moisturizing Cream) as needed daily
Corticosteroid ointment (corticosteroids should be discontinued following clinical response; medium- to high-potency steroids should not be used continuously for more than 2 weeks)
    Low potency: hydrocortisone 2.5% cream, one to two times daily as needed
    Medium potency: desoximetasone cream 0.05%, 1-2 times daily as needed
    High potency: clobetasol cream 0.05%, one to two times daily as needed
Calcineurin inhibitors
    Tacrolimus 0.03 and 0.1% ointment, one to two times daily as needed
    Pimecrolimus 1% cream, one to two times daily as needed
Anesthetic agents (can be especially useful for neuropathic itch)
    Capsaicin 0.025% cream, four times daily
    Pramoxine 1%-hydrocortisone 2.5% lotion, cream, or ointment one to two times daily as needed

SYSTEMIC MEDICATIONS

Antihistamines
    Hydroxyzine 10-50 mg, four times daily
    Cetirizine 10 mg/day
    Fexofenadine 60-180 mg/day
Antidepressants
    Mirtazapine 15 mg PO at bedtime
Opioids
    Naltrexone 50 mg/day PO for cholestatic pruritus
Anticonvulsants
    Gabapentin 300 mg three times/week after dialysis for pruritus in renal dialysis patients
Ultraviolet B radiation one to three times/week for six to eight exposures

PO = orally.

Grade A References

A1. Simonsen E, Komenda P, Lerner B, et al. Treatment of uremic pruritus: a systematic review. *Am J Kidney Dis*. 2017;70:638-655.
A2. Wang W, Zhou L, Sun L. Ondansetron for neuraxial morphine-induced pruritus: a meta-analysis of randomized controlled trials. *J Clin Pharm Ther*. 2017;42:383-393.

GENERAL REFERENCES

For the General References and other additional features, please visit Expert Consult at https://expertconsult.inkling.com.

skin diseases such as atopic dermatitis and psoriasis are the most common causes of chronic itching),[7] afferent nerves (e.g., brachioradial pruritus), or the central nervous system (e.g., renal or liver failure, lymphoproliferative disorders, malignancy, delusions of parasitosis). When approaching a patient with pruritus and no signs of a specific skin disorder, a comprehensive diagnostic approach is indicated (Table 407-9) to detect causes of pruritus as diverse as occult skin disease (scabies), medications (especially calcium channel blockers, proton pump inhibitors, narcotics, and amphetamines), renal failure (Chapter 106), cholestatic liver disease (Chapter 146), hyperthyroidism (Chapter 213), myeloproliferative disorders (Chapter 157), parasitic infections, diabetes mellitus (Chapter 216), and celiac disease (Chapter 131). Anxiety and depression are often associated with chronic pruritus.[8]

Treatment of pruritus can be tailored according to its probable cause.[9] For example, gabapentin is the preferred treatment for the pruritus of renal failure,[A1] and ondansetron (4 mg intravenously) is effective for otherwise refractory morphine-induced pruritus.[A2] Itching from dry skin, such as eczema (Chapter 409), cholestatic jaundice (Chapter 146),[10] hypothyroidism (Chapter 213), or myeloproliferative diseases (Chapter 157) may respond to over-the-counter emollients (Table 407-10). A mainstay of treatment of skin inflammation causing pruritus is topical corticosteroids or topical calcineurin inhibitors. Urticaria, an inflammatory disease of the skin with histamine release from mast cells in the dermis, can be treated with oral antihistamines. Other forms of pruritus may not respond directly to antihistamines, but antihistamines nevertheless may help the patient because of their sedative effects. For pruritus that originates in afferent nerves, capsaicin can be helpful over the long term because it depletes neural stimulatory peptides. Pruritus that is more centrally caused may respond to oral medications such as naltrexone or gabapentin, and mirtazapine may be helpful for patients in whom depression or anxiety play an important role.[11] For inflammatory skin disease as well as systemic causes of pruritus, ultraviolet light therapy also can be helpful.

408

PRINCIPLES OF THERAPY OF SKIN DISEASES

VICTORIA P. WERTH

The goal of therapy is to improve a skin condition with the least toxic and most specific approach. Because many treatments or medications can be applied directly to the skin, the option for topical therapy is attractive for treating many dermatologic diseases. However, many diseases require systemic therapy, particularly when patients have widespread involvement of the skin or a disease that cannot be improved with topical therapy. Therapies work by improving barrier function, removing scale, altering inflammation in the skin, altering blood flow, providing antimicrobial effects, or affecting proliferating cells. Recent advances in the understanding of cutaneous biology have not been routinely accompanied by evidence-based documentation of the benefits of many specific therapies.

PRINCIPLES OF TOPICAL THERAPY

Soaks and Dressings

Water or saline applied by soaks and wet dressings can be beneficial for many skin conditions, including ulcers, by promoting healing of the epidermis and débridement of crusts. Soaked gauze is applied to involved areas for 15 to 30 minutes several times per day, and care should be taken not to allow the gauze to dry and adhere. If adherence occurs, the gauze should be soaked before the dressing is removed. Use of strong antiseptic solutions, including hydrogen peroxide, is not recommended because of toxicity to cells. Whirlpool action can enhance débridement. When large areas of skin are involved, baths are a convenient way to treat the skin with medications that reduce itching and inflammation. The best time to apply moisturizers that help trap water in the upper layers of skin is immediately after a bath or shower.

Wet-to-dry dressings are rarely used, except when initial vigorous wound débridement is necessary. Continued use after wounds are débrided traumatizes wounds and delays healing. Moist wound healing, which is often ideal, can be accomplished with a topical antibiotic such as a combination of polymyxin B and bacitracin (Polypore) or mupirocin (Bactrian), gauze impregnated with petrolatum (Vaseline), or an occlusive hydrocolloid dressing. Little evidence indicates that débriding enzymes are beneficial. Compression with an Unna or multilayered boot, which includes an elastic dressing such as Coban, can decrease local edema and facilitate wound healing. Polysporin/petrolatum gauze or occlusive dressings are placed underneath, an approach that is helpful for chronic venous, diabetic, and pressure ulcers, as well as for acute wounds. Closed wet dressings, in which gauze is soaked and then covered with an impervious material, can help when maceration and heat retention are needed. Biologic dressings with skin substitutes or keratinocytes can be beneficial for wounds that are resistant to healing. Skin grafts also can facilitate healing of otherwise nonhealing wounds. Platelet-derived growth factor, which is approved for use on diabetic ulcers, can modestly improve wound healing.

Topical Medications

Topical medications mix an active drug with preservatives, emulsifying agents, and an appropriate base or vehicle. Systemic absorption varies among patients, sites, and vehicles. Topically applied drugs are absorbed more readily through inflamed, thin skin. The base can be any of the following: a *powder,* which promotes dryness and is used to reduce maceration in intertriginous areas; a *lotion,* which is a suspension of oil in water; *solutions,* which include water, alcohol, and propylene glycol, but not oil; *gels,* which are solid at room temperature but melt on contact with the skin; a *cream,* which is an emulsion of oil in water that leaves a thin oil coating as the water evaporates; an *ointment,* which combines oils, such as petrolatum (Vaseline), with small amounts of water and which is more occlusive and hence increases the absorption of medication but also results in a greasier appearance; a *paste,* which is a mixture of powder and ointment; or a *spray.* Lotions, solutions, and gels provide less penetration than ointments do, but they are especially useful for the treatment of hair-bearing areas such as the scalp, where greasiness is displeasing. Creams are less greasy than ointments and are useful for the face, groin, and intertriginous areas. Ointments are often more effective for dry, scaly conditions such as eczema and psoriasis and are helpful in areas that have thick skin, such as the palms and soles, but they should be avoided in infected or intertriginous areas. The choice of base is determined by the skin condition and location. Impregnated tapes are another delivery method to provide occlusion and protect the skin from manipulation.

ANTI-INFLAMMATORY AGENTS

Glucocorticoids

Topical glucocorticoids work because of their effects on vasoconstriction, proliferation, immunosuppression, and inflammation. Assays related to the ability to vasoconstrict and clinical trials of efficacy have allowed glucocorticoids to be divided into various classes based on potency (Table 408-1). These medications are typically used twice per day. Side effects include atrophy of the skin, telangiectases, purpura, striae, local skin infections (e.g., folliculitis, tinea, and candidiasis), hypopigmentation, hypertrichosis, systemic adrenal suppression when these agents are used on as little as 20% of the skin's surface area, and glaucoma when they are used around the eye. Side effects are especially prevalent when fluorinated steroids are used on thin skin (e.g., face, groin, or scrotum), and prolonged use on the face can result in facial dermatitis, acne, and an eruption resembling acne rosacea that is often exacerbated when use of the steroid is terminated. Certain conditions are more responsive to steroids, and the potency of the steroid chosen must be based on the

condition and its location (Table 408-2). The superpotent class I agents should be restricted to patients with severe dermatoses, and their use normally should not exceed 2 weeks. Patients who receive these potent agents require frequent follow-up and must be carefully evaluated for the need to continue strong topical steroids. Use of any fluorinated steroid on the face requires an exact diagnosis and should be limited in the extent of application and duration of use. Intralesional glucocorticoids can be injected into individual lesions to improve delivery of the medication, and this method is commonly used to treat patients with acne cysts, hypertrophic scars, keloids, alopecia areata, granuloma annulare, discoid and panniculitic lupus erythematosus (Chapter 250), psoriasis, and lichen simplex chronicus. Triamcinolone acetonide is most frequently used, followed by the longer acting triamcinolone hexacetonide. It is important to use proper dilutions, such as 2.5 mg/mL on the face and 5 mg/mL elsewhere, to avoid local skin atrophy. Because these drugs vary widely in price and often require at least some out-of-pocket patient payments,[1] physicians can help their patients by being knowledgeable about their prices.

Systemic glucocorticoids are used for acute and chronic conditions in dermatology, but they should be avoided, if possible, or minimized because of their well-known side effects (Chapter 32). Acute conditions that commonly require systemic steroids include severe contact dermatitis such as poison ivy, photodermatitis, severe atopic dermatitis, and acute urticaria. Many skin conditions such as psoriasis and eczema become exacerbated when use of the steroids is tapered, so steroids should be avoided when possible in these conditions. The dose of steroid must be individualized to the condition and its severity. Steroid-sparing drugs, such as immunosuppressive agents, can be used to minimize the long-term use of steroids for selected conditions.

Nonsteroidal Anti-Inflammatory Agents

Psoriasis Therapies

Tars and anthralin are used for psoriasis (Chapter 409). Tars are most commonly used in conjunction with ultraviolet B (UVB) light. Tars also are used in shampoos and bath oils to treat seborrhea and psoriasis. Anthralin is a synthetic hydroxyanthrone that inhibits keratinocyte proliferation; it stains and can be irritating, but it can be effective therapy (Chapter 409).

Calcipotriol

Calcipotriol is a vitamin D derivative that has antiproliferative and immunomodulatory effects on skin. Hypercalcemia can occur if more than 100 g/week

TABLE 408-1	RANKING OF SOME COMMONLY USED TOPICAL STEROIDS BY POTENCY
Super potency	Clobetasol propionate (Temovate ointment and cream), betamethasone dipropionate (Diprolene cream and ointment), diflorasone diacetate (Psorcon E ointment), halobetasol propionate (Ultravate ointment)
High potency	Amcinonide, mometasone furoate ointment, diflorasone diacetate (Florone ointment), halcinonide 0.1% cream, fluocinonide, desoximetasone, triamcinolone acetonide, diflorasone diacetate ointment and cream, betamethasone dipropionate (Diprosone), betamethasone benzoate and valerate
Medium potency	Fluticasone propionate; mometasone furoate cream; halcinonide 0.25% ointment; triamcinolone acetonide 0.1% cream and lotion; fluocinolone acetonide 0.05%, and 0.1% cream, 0.1% and 0.25% ointment, and 0.5% solution; hydrocortisone valerate 0.2% ointment and cream; alclometasone dipropionate 0.5% ointment; betamethasone dipropionate 0.5% lotion; hydrocortisone butyrate 0.1% cream; betamethasone benzoate 0.25% cream; betamethasone valerate 0.1% cream and 0.5% lotion; flumethasone pivalate 0.3% cream; desonide 0.5% cream
Low potency	Hydrocortisone 1% cream

TABLE 408-2	CLINICAL APPLICATION OF TOPICAL GLUCOCORTICOIDS
Super potency and high potency	Plaque and palmoplantar psoriasis, lichen planus, dyshidrotic eczema, lichen simplex chronicus, granuloma annulare, sarcoidosis
Medium potency	Dermatitis: allergic contact, atopic, neurodermatitis
Low potency	Intertrigo, pruritus ani, seborrheic dermatitis

is used, so this agent cannot be used for widespread disease. It is applied twice daily, can be irritating on thin skin, and takes 6 to 8 weeks to be effective.

Retinoids

The retinoids are a group of compounds that include vitamin A and its derivatives. Their effects are mediated through several different classes of receptors, and the receptor-drug complex has effects on other regulatory proteins that affect growth factors, oncogenes, keratins, or transglutaminases. Retinoids affect cell growth, differentiation, and morphogenesis; inhibit tumor promotion and malignant cell growth; have immunomodulatory effects; and alter cell cohesion.

Topical retinoids include all-*trans*-retinoic acid (tretinoin), which is approved for acne (Retin-A) and photoaging (Renova 0.05% cream) and is also useful for hyperpigmentation, steroid-induced atrophy, and early stretch marks. Tretinoin is available as a cream (0.025%, 0.05%, 0.1%), a gel (0.01%, 0.025%), and a solution (0.05%). Adapalene (Differin 0.1% gel) and tazarotene (Tazorac) are used for acne (Chapter 410). Tazarotene is also used for psoriasis, often in combination with topical steroids to minimize irritation and chronic photodamage. Bexarotene (Targretin) 1% gel is used for the topical treatment of cutaneous lesions in patients who have refractory or persistent stage IA or IB cutaneous T-cell lymphoma. Topical retinoids can be irritating and frequently cause an exacerbation before improvement. However, they should be used regularly on lesion-prone skin to produce improvement. Moisturizers may be needed to minimize drying effects.

Systemic retinoids commonly used for the skin include isotretinoin, acitretin, and bexarotene (Targretin). They have many applications, but most frequently isotretinoin (Accutane) is used for cystic and conglobate acne, acitretin for severe psoriasis (especially the erythrodermic and pustular forms), and bexarotene for cutaneous T-cell lymphoma. Isotretinoin and acitretin also have been used to treat several forms of ichthyosis and lupus erythematosus and for the chemoprevention of skin cancers, particularly in immunosuppressed transplant recipients. The many side effects of systemic retinoids include teratogenicity, cheilitis, hair loss, headaches, hyperlipidemia, abnormal liver enzyme levels, vertebral hyperostosis, tendon and ligament calcification, osteoporosis, and central hypothyroidism with bexarotene. Pregnancy must be avoided, and the use of retinoids in women of childbearing age therefore requires careful monitoring. Treatment of acne is reserved for cases of cystic acne not responding to less toxic therapies; in this setting, a 4- to 5-month course of Accutane, 0.5 to 1 mg/kg/day, is curative in 85 to 90% of patients.

Other Agents
Brimonidine and Oxymetazoline Hydrochloride

Brimonidine gel is a selective α_2-adrenergic receptor agonist. Oxymetazoline hydrochloride is an α_1-adrenergic receptor agonist. Both have vasoconstrictive activity and are used topically for rosacea.[A1] Crisaborole is a boron-based phosphodiesterase 4 inhibitor that increases intracellular cAMP levels. It is applied as an ointment to treat atopic dermatitis.

Antimalarial and Antiparasitic Drugs

Aminoquinolines include hydroxychloroquine, quinacrine, and chloroquine. These agents have inhibitory effects on pro-inflammatory cytokine production, DNA replication, and chemotaxis. They are useful in patients with connective tissue diseases, polymorphous light eruption, sarcoidosis (Chapter 89), porphyria cutanea tarda (Chapters 199 and 410), sclerosing conditions, and vasculitis. Side effects include diarrhea, headache, irritability, psychosis, skin dyspigmentation, and, rarely, retinopathy. Retinopathy is rare if doses of chloroquine are 3.5 mg/kg/day or less and doses of hydroxychloroquine are 6.5 mg/kg/day or less based on ideal body weight for those not underweight or 2.3 mg/day for chloroquine and 5 mg/kg/day for hydrochloroquine based on actual body weight. Combinations of hydroxychloroquine or chloroquine with quinacrine are frequently helpful when a solitary agent is inadequate. The combination of hydroxychloroquine and chloroquine should not be used because of the additive risk for retinopathy. Ivermectin cream is a broad-spectrum antiparasitic agent used for rosacea.[A2]

Dapsone

Dapsone is a sulfone that inhibits the response of neutrophils and possibly eosinophils to chemotactic stimuli. It is useful for dermatitis herpetiformis (Chapter 410), cutaneous vasculitis (Chapter 411), pyoderma gangrenosum (Chapter 411), bullous lupus erythematosus (Chapter 250), Behçet disease (Chapter 254), and autoimmune bullous diseases (Chapter 410). Topical 5% gel is approved for use in acne. Systemic use can be associated with side effects that include hemolysis, methemoglobinemia, peripheral neuropathy,

agranulocytosis, and, rarely, a hypersensitivity syndrome with hepatitis, fevers, and rash. The glucose-6-dehydrogenase level should be checked before starting the drug, and it is common for patients with a normal glucose-6-dehydrogenase level to experience a 2-g/dL decrease in hemoglobin after achieving therapeutic doses of 100 to 200 mg/day.

Thalidomide and Lenalidomide

Thalidomide and lenalidomide have potent anti-inflammatory effects via their effects on two transcription factors that bind to cereblon. It also modifies adhesion molecules on circulating leukocytes. Thalidomide is a serious teratogen, and patients must comply with strict birth control and monitoring. It is effective at a dose of 50 to 100 mg/day, with improvement beginning in 2 weeks and a full clinical response seen in 2 to 3 months in patients with severe cutaneous lupus erythematosus (Chapter 250), erythema nodosum leprosum (Chapter 409), aphthae, Behçet disease (Chapter 254), scleromyxedema, actinic prurigo, chronic graft-versus-host disease (Chapter 168), multiple myeloma (Chapter 178), and numerous other inflammatory dermatoses. Besides teratogenesis, the main side effects include peripheral neuropathy, constipation, sedation, and, rarely, amenorrhea.

Colchicine

Colchicine, usually at a dose of 0.6 mg twice daily, is used for leukocytoclastic vasculitis (Chapter 410) and Behçet disease, as well as some patients with epidermolysis bullosa acquisita. The main side effect of this low oral dose is diarrhea.

⬤ ANTIMICROBIAL AGENTS
Antibacterials

Topical antibiotics are used to treat superficial skin diseases, such as acne and folliculitis, as well as skin wounds and ulcers. They may work by decreasing neutrophil chemotaxis and other anti-inflammatory mechanisms. Topical solutions, gels, pledgets, and ointments are available, depending on the agent, and antibiotics include erythromycin, clindamycin, tetracycline, and metronidazole.[2] Benzoyl peroxide also has antibacterial properties and is quite effective for mild-to-moderate acne, while also minimizing bacterial resistance when topical antibiotics are also used (Chapter 410). Bacitracin and Polysporin ointments are typically used for wounds, but they can cause contact hypersensitivity; neomycin should be avoided because of the high incidence of allergic reactions. Mupirocin is particularly effective against *Staphylococcus* and *Streptococcus* spp., and it can be used in the nose for carriers of staphylococci. Systemic antibiotics such as penicillins, cephalosporins, and erythromycin are used in patients with soft tissue infections such as impetigo, folliculitis, furuncles, carbuncles, cellulitis, ecthyma, erysipelas, postoperative wound infections, and necrotizing fasciitis. Tetracycline, doxycycline, and minocycline are used for acne,[3] rosacea, and perioral dermatitis. Fluoroquinolones such as ciprofloxacin are useful for the treatment of gram-negative soft tissue infections.

Antifungals

Topical antifungal agents are used in patients with limited superficial fungal infections of the skin (Chapter 409). The numerous topical antifungal drugs available include the azoles (clotrimazole, econazole, ketoconazole, oxiconazole, and miconazole), which are available as creams and lotions applied once or twice daily. The creams tend to be more effective. Topical agents used for dermatophytes, but not *Candida,* are haloprogin and tolnaftate. The newer allylamine antifungals naftifine and terbinafine have fungicidal effects. Ciclopirox 8%, efinaconazole, and tavaborole are used topically to treat and prevent relapses of onychomycosis, but they are not as efficacious as systemic therapy (Chapter 413).[A3] Nystatin creams, oral suspensions, and vaginal tablets are effective for the treatment of *Candida* infections. The combination of antifungals with potent topical steroids such as betamethasone dipropionate is not advised because of increased side effects from the steroid and decreased efficacy of the antifungal as a result of the concomitant steroid.

Systemic antifungal agents include griseofulvin, terbinafine (allylamine), ketoconazole (imidazole), itraconazole, and fluconazole. These agents are used for extensive or severe superficial skin fungal infections (Chapter 409) caused by dermatophytes, *Candida,* or *Malassezia furfur* or for local infections not responsive to topical drugs, such as those found in the nails and scalp. Itraconazole and terbinafine are the only oral antifungals approved in the United States for the treatment of onychomycosis,[A4] and griseofulvin is the only oral agent approved for tinea capitis. Griseofulvin is best taken with a fatty meal to improve absorption and is the only antifungal drug not requiring regular monitoring of liver enzymes. Griseofulvin shows weak affinity for keratin, and thus it must be used for 18 months for onychomycosis of the toenails and 6 months for the fingernails to achieve even relatively poor cure rates. Terbinafine is the only fungicidal drug; the rest are fungistatic. The number of interactions with medications is lower with terbinafine than with the triazole antifungals and ketoconazole because terbinafine does not inhibit or induce hepatic isoenzyme cytochrome P (CYP3A4) (Chapter 26). However, terbinafine affects CYP2D6, another hepatic isoenzyme, so it is relatively contraindicated in patients who are taking cyclosporine or rifampin. Itraconazole and fluconazole have been used in pulse-dosing regimens for the treatment of onychomycosis. Fluconazole and terbinafine are not dependent on gastric acidity for optimal gastrointestinal absorption. Overall, the side effects of the systemic antifungal agents are similar and include headache and gastrointestinal symptoms (griseofulvin, terbinafine), nausea and vomiting (itraconazole, fluconazole, ketoconazole), hepatitis, and lupus-like syndromes (terbinafine).

Antivirals

Verrucae are treated with various destructive modalities, including 50 to 80% dichloroacetic acid and trichloroacetic acid solutions, podophyllin resin, and podofilox. Immunosuppressed patients may benefit from treatment with intralesional cidofovir. Topical antiviral creams such as penciclovir and acyclovir do not significantly shorten the course of herpes simplex. Systemic antiviral drugs include acyclovir, valacyclovir, famciclovir, and foscarnet, which are used to treat primary and recurrent herpes simplex (Chapter 350) and herpes zoster (Chapter 351). These agents specifically block the function of herpesvirus DNA polymerase. Valacyclovir and famciclovir are available only orally in the United States, but their prolonged intracellular half-life allows less frequent dosing than with acyclovir. Patients with herpes zoster require higher doses than do patients with herpes simplex. Side effects include nausea and headaches. The varicella-zoster vaccine has significantly decreased the incidence of herpes zoster in individuals older than 50 years of age, and current recommendation is for vaccination after the age of 50 with Shingrix (Chapter 15). If possible, it should be administered before starting oral immunosuppressive agents.

Antiparasitics

Topical antiparasitic medications are used to treat pediculosis capitis, pediculosis pubis, and scabies. In addition, topical metronidazole has anti-inflammatory properties and is used to treat rosacea. For pediculosis and scabies, clothing and bedding must be washed and all family members must be treated. Effective treatment includes 1% γ-benzene hexachloride (lindane), a chlorinated hydrocarbon pesticide that should not be used on young children or on pregnant or lactating women. It is ineffective against nits and thus must be reapplied after 1 week. Permethrin 5% cream (Elimite) for scabies or 1% cream rinse is particularly effective for head lice and requires just one application; 10% crotamiton (Eurax) and 5% topical sulfur ointments are less effective. Malathion is a moderately toxic organophosphate insecticide, but it must be applied overnight to treat lice. Pyrethrins (RID, Nix) are best used twice, 1 week apart, to treat head lice and nits.

⬤ ANTIPRURITIC OR ANESTHETIC AGENTS

Topical Analgesics

Capsaicin, an active ingredient of cayenne peppers and other plants of the genus *Capsicum*, is used for postherpetic neuralgia and other painful nerve-related conditions. It causes excitation of neural afferent C fibers and reduces substance P levels. Capsaicin causes a burning sensation and is applied four or five times daily for 5 to 6 weeks. Eutectic mixture of local anesthetic (EMLA) is a mixture of lidocaine and prilocaine that is used under occlusion to induce cutaneous anesthesia before a procedure. Lidocaine can be used as a topical anesthetic, but benzocaine should be avoided because it is a sensitizer.

Antipruritic Agents

Doxepin 5% cream is used for localized pruritus. Menthol is a cyclic terpene plant alcohol used for non–histamine-related itching. Pramoxine hydrochloride is a topical anesthetic used for mild-to-moderate itching. Oral antihistamines play an important role in controlling pruritus in many skin conditions (Table 408-3), especially those mediated by histamine, such as urticaria, angioedema, and urticaria pigmentosa. The sedating and anticholinergic properties of many H1-receptor antihistamines probably account for some of their efficacy. H1-receptor antihistamines are the cornerstones of routine therapy, and if an agent from one group of H1-receptor antihistamines is ineffective, an agent from a different class should be administered or combined. Second-generation H1-receptor antihistamines are less sedating and are used if patients cannot

tolerate or do not improve after taking first-generation agents. The combination of two different H1-receptor antihistamines can be used when a solitary agent does not work; in particular, use of a sedating antihistamine at night and a second-generation antihistamine during the day can be helpful. The skin contains both H1- and H2-receptors, and occasionally combining H1- and H2-receptor antagonists can be beneficial. Usually, first-generation agents (e.g., hydroxyzine, 10 to 25 mg every 6 hours) are started at low doses and increased as tolerated, and regular continuous dosing is recommended. The tricyclic antidepressant doxepin, normally started at 10 to 25 mg at bedtime, has both anti–H1- and H2-receptor activity, but it interacts with drugs metabolized by the CYP450 pathway. Side effects of commonly used first-generation antihistamines include sedation, dry mouth, blurred vision, constipation, and urinary retention, and lower doses may be required in elderly patients. The recommended dose for second-generation antihistamines (e.g., fexofenadine, 60 mg twice daily) should not be exceeded.

⬤ AGENTS THAT IMPROVE SURFACE FUNCTIONS (LUBRICATION, SCALE)

Moisturizers

Moisturizers improve skin by diminishing scale and increasing water content. They usually contain mixtures of water and fatty substances such as petrolatum, lanolin, lanolin derivatives, and fatty alcohols. Greasy moisturizers tend to function better, but they are less acceptable cosmetically.

Keratolytics

α-Hydroxy acids (lactic acid, glycolic acid, citric acid, glucuronic acid, pyruvic acid) are extremely effective keratolytics. They are helpful in treating disorders of keratinization and photoaging, as well as acne. Propylene glycol, used in 40 to 60% aqueous solutions, can decrease scaling. Salicylic acid, which works by decreasing keratinocyte adhesion and hydrating keratins, is used in a range of concentrations with many different bases to remove scale, to soften the stratum corneum, or as destructive therapy to remove warts and calluses. Urea is used in varying concentrations to treat scaling.

TABLE 408-3 OVERVIEW OF ANTIHISTAMINES

ANTIHISTAMINE GROUP	GENERIC NAME	AVERAGE ORAL ADULT DOSES
FIRST-GENERATION H1-TYPE ANTIHISTAMINES		
Alkylamine	Brompheniramine (Dimetapp)	4 mg q4-6h
	Chlorpheniramine (Chlor-Trimeton)	4 mg q4-6h (short acting); 8-12 mg q8-12h (long acting)
Amino alkyl ether (ethanolamine)	Clemastine fumarate	1.34 mg bid or 2.68 mg qd-tid
	Diphenhydramine (Benadryl)	25-50 mg q4-6h
Ethylenediamine	Pyrilamine (Triaminic)	30 mg bid
Phenothiazine	Promethazine (Phenergan)	10-12.5 mg qid
	Trimeprazine (Temaril)	2.5 mg q6h
Piperidine	Azatadine	1-2 mg q8-12h
	Cyproheptadine	4 mg q8h
	Diphenylpyraline	2 mg tid-qid
Piperazine	Hydroxyzine (Atarax)	25-100 mg tid-qid
SECOND-GENERATION H1-TYPE ANTIHISTAMINES		
Alkylamine	Acrivastine (combined with pseudoephedrine in allergy medication)	8 mg qid
Piperidine	Astemizole (Hismanal)	10 mg qd
	Loratadine (Claritin)	10 mg qd
	Fexofenadine (Allegra)	60 mg bid or 180 mg qd
Piperazine	Cetirizine (Zyrtec)	5-10 mg/day
H2-TYPE ANTIHISTAMINES		
	Cimetidine (Tagamet)	400 mg bid
	Ranitidine (Zantac)	150 mg bid
	Famotidine	10 mg bid
	Nizatidine	300 mg hs
H1- AND H2-TYPE ANTIHISTAMINES		
	Doxepin (Sinequan)	10-25 mg hs

bid = twice daily; hs = at bedtime; qd = once daily; qid = four times daily; tid = three times daily.

IMMUNE THERAPIES

Hormonal Therapies

Systemic therapies to modulate androgen production can be beneficial in patients with acne and hidradenitis suppurativa. Such treatments for moderate acne include spironolactone and, in women, U.S. Food and Drug Administration (FDA)–approved combination oral contraceptives, such as Ortho Tri-Cyclen (norgestimate and ethinyl estradiol), Estrostep (norethindrone acetate and ethinyl estradiol), and Yaz (drospirenone and ethinyl estradiol), as they would be prescribed for contraception (Chapter 225).[4]

Immunosuppressive Agents

Topical cytotoxic drugs include 5-fluorouracil, mechlorethamine (nitrogen mustard), carmustine (BCNU), bleomycin, and the calcineurin inhibitors tacrolimus and pimecrolimus. Topical 5-fluorouracil interferes with pyrimidine metabolism and action and blocks DNA synthesis. It is used to treat actinic keratosis, superficial basal cell cancer, Bowen disease, bowenoid papulosis, actinic cheilitis, and warts. Topical use does not cause systemic toxicity, but expected side effects include local irritation, erythema, and pain. Nitrogen mustard and BCNU, which have alkylating agents that inhibit DNA, RNA, and protein synthesis, are used to treat cutaneous T-cell lymphoma (Chapter 176); they can cause cutaneous reactions and myelosuppression, and nitrogen mustard commonly causes a cutaneous hypersensitivity reaction.

Intralesional bleomycin, which disrupts DNA synthesis, has been used to treat warts. Topical tacrolimus (Prograf) and pimecrolimus, immunosuppressive macrolides that act on T lymphocytes to inhibit interleukin-2 (IL-2) transcription, are used for atopic dermatitis, allergic contact dermatitis, psoriasis, and several other inflammatory skin conditions. They frequently cause a burning sensation in the skin; although systemic absorption is minimal, ongoing studies are assessing whether the risk for cancer is increased by their topical use. Systemic immunosuppressives such as methotrexate, azathioprine, thioguanine, hydroxyurea, mycophenolate (CellCept), cyclophosphamide, chlorambucil, rapamycin, and cyclosporine are used for numerous inflammatory or immunologically mediated skin conditions, particularly for widespread psoriasis (Chapter 409) and as glucocorticoid-sparing agents for autoimmune blistering diseases.

Immunomodulatory Therapies

Imiquimod, available as a 5% cream, is an imidazoquinolinamine that has antitumor and antiviral activity. It induces local production of interferon-γ and is used to treat warts and superficial skin cancers. Topical 3% diclofenac in hyaluronic acid, which blocks the induced cyclooxygenase-2 found in precancerous lesions, is approved to treat actinic keratosis. Many systemic immunomodulatory drugs are currently used in dermatology. These include interferons and tumor necrosis factor–α (TNF-α) inhibitors such as etanercept, adalimumab, and infliximab (Remicade). Anti-IL-12/23 therapy, anti-IL-17 therapy, and anti-IL-17 receptor are effective for psoriasis (Chapter 409).[A5] PDE4 inhibitor therapy in patients with psoriasis is associated with about 2.2-fold increased risk of serious infection compared with other psoriatic treatments.[5]

Anti-CD20 antibodies have been effective in the treatment of autoimmune skin-blistering diseases, and rituximab is FDA approved for pemphigus vulgaris.[A6] Intravenous immune globulin, which is used to treat certain autoimmune skin diseases, including pemphigus vulgaris, cicatricial pemphigoid, and dermatomyositis, probably works through Fc receptor modulation and anti-idiotype interactions. Dupilumab is an IL-4 receptor antagonist[6] used in atopic dermatitis.[A7]

Interferon alfa-2b is used both intralesionally and subcutaneously to treat genital warts, high-risk melanoma, Kaposi sarcoma, hemangiomas, cutaneous T-cell lymphoma, keloids, Behçet disease, and cryoglobulinemia (Chapter 178), and perhaps basal cell and squamous cell carcinoma. Total interferon doses are generally 3 million IU or less per session, and systemic doses are usually administered 3 days per week. Side effects include flulike symptoms, leukopenia, anemia, and hepatitis. Denileukin diftitox is a fusion protein consisting of a fragment of diphtheria toxin genetically fused to IL-2. It targets IL-2 receptors on the surface of malignant cells and is approved for use in patients with resistant or recurrent cutaneous T-cell lymphoma.

Histone deacetylase inhibition increases acetylation of lysine residues that form the octomeric histone core of chromatin, thereby decreasing the ability of the histones to bind to DNA. This decreased binding allows chromatin expansion, permitting transcription of the tumor suppressor genes. However, histone deacetylase inhibitors affect acetylation globally and may have wider effects on various cellular functions. Two inhibitors (vorinostat and romidepsin) are approved by the FDA for use in patients with cutaneous T-cell lymphoma.

Extracorporeal photochemotherapy (photopheresis), which combines 8-methoxypsoralen and ultraviolet A (UVA) irradiation of lymphocytes, is used for Sézary syndrome, the leukemic form of cutaneous T-cell lymphoma (Chapter 176). Plasmapheresis, used in combination with other immunosuppressive therapies, can remove autoantibodies and immune complexes in patients in whom autoimmune disease or cryoglobulinemia is resistant to other therapies.

TREATMENT FOR SKIN CANCERS
(See Chapter 193)

Phototherapy and Laser

Ultraviolet treatments are given with different wavelengths, depending on the condition and the response to treatment. Currently, clinicians use broad-band UVB (290 to 320 nm), narrow-band 311-nm UVB, PUVA (psoralen with 320- to 400-nm UVA), and UVA1 (340 to 400 nm). Both forms of UVB and PUVA are used for psoriasis and vitiligo, but other conditions such as nummular and atopic dermatitis, pruritus resulting from uremia, and cutaneous T-cell lymphoma are treated in this way. High-dose UVA1 is used, mainly in Europe, to treat atopic dermatitis, localized scleroderma, and mastocytosis. PUVA is associated with increased risk for skin cancers, including melanoma. The risks related to long-term UVA therapy are currently unknown, but photoaging is associated with UVA, and there have been reports of an increase in melanoma associated with use of suntanning beds, in which much of the exposure is to UVA. Laser therapy is used to treat vascular lesions such as port-wine stains, tattoos, psoriasis, benign skin tumors, and photodamage, as well as to remove hair. Photodynamic therapy involves activation of a photosensitizer by illumination with visible light, which leads to photochemical tissue destruction or immunomodulation. Photodynamic therapy can be used to treat actinic keratosis,[7] Bowen disease, and superficial basal cell carcinoma by causing selective tissue necrosis and tumor destruction. Fractional lasers have been successfully used for treatment of actinic keratoses, photodamage, and scars.

Dermatologic Surgery

Although approaches such as desiccation and curettage can be used for some skin tumors, others require excisional surgery or Mohs microscopic controlled surgery to ensure complete removal of lesions. If the tumors are recurrent, of a pathologic type that increases the likelihood for recurrence, or large and requiring clearance of the tumor before repair, the Mohs approach can provide rapid documentation of full removal while sparing as much normal tissue as possible. After the margins have been cleared of tumor, flaps and grafts can be used immediately for repair of the resultant defects.

Patients with extensive actinic damage resulting in either large numbers of actinic keratoses or photodamage can be treated with various ablative approaches that use either chemical peels or laser resurfacing with the carbon dioxide laser. Chemical peels can be performed at different depths and intensities, and agents can include glycolic acid, acetic acid, or even phenol. Lasers used to remove sun-induced lentigines include Q-switched lasers such as the neodymium:yttrium-aluminum-garnet, ruby, and alexandrite lasers. Many patients seek treatment of wrinkles with soft tissue augmentation that uses human-derived collagen and hyaluronic acid or with a muscle relaxer, botulinum type A exotoxin.

Hair transplants are a surgical approach to the problem of hair loss. The process includes harvesting hair grafts from the posterior of the scalp and placing the grafts in areas of alopecia.

Sunscreen

Transparent sunscreens absorb photons of light. They are rated by the sun protection factor (SPF), which is determined by the ratio of ultraviolet exposure needed to cause erythema in protected versus unprotected skin. Most sunscreens work in the UVB range or shorter UVA wavelengths. Examples of UVB-absorptive compounds include aminobenzoates, cinnamates, salicylates, and benzophenones. Short-wavelength UVA-absorptive compounds include benzophenones and anthranilates. The best UVA blocking agent in the United States is avobenzone (Parsol 1789), which can be combined with UVB screens. Some sunscreens are water resistant or waterproof, as determined by the substantivity of the sunscreen, and these agents provide continued protection after sweating or swimming. Sunscreens can cause irritation and, rarely, contact allergic reactions. Physical sunscreens, such as zinc oxide and titanium dioxide, reflect light from the skin and include newer micronized reflecting powders that provide broad-spectrum (UVB and UVA) protection. Sunscreens decrease skin cancers and photodamage without compromising the synthesis of vitamin D.[8] UVB is partially reflected by clothing, and sun-protective clothing can provide substantial protection (Solumbra, SPF of 30).

Cosmetics: Camouflage, Bleaching, and Hair Loss

Patients with numerous skin conditions benefit from camouflage cosmetics, which can also cause contact hypersensitivity. Products such as Dermablend can be blended to match skin colors, are thicker, can cover disfiguring lesions, and can be fixed with powder. Hydroquinones, topical retinoic acid, and azelaic acid (inhibits tyrosinase) are used to treat hyperpigmented conditions such as melasma and lentigines; these agents can be irritating and cause dyspigmentation. Topical minoxidil, 2% (available over the counter) and 5% solutions, are used for androgenic alopecia and alopecia areata. Finasteride, a 5α-reductase inhibitor, is effective in men with androgenic alopecia.

Grade A References

A1. Jackson JM, Fowler J, Moore A, et al. Improvement in facial erythema within 30 minutes of initial application of brimonidine tartrate in patients with rosacea. *J Drugs Dermatol.* 2014;13:699-704.

A2. Taieb A, Ortonne JP, Ruzicka T, et al. Superiority of ivermectin 1% cream over metronidazole 0.75% cream in treating inflammatory lesions of rosacea: a randomized, investigator-blinded trial. *Br J Dermatol.* 2015;172:1103-1110.

A3. Lipner SR, Scher RK, Part II. Onychomycosis: treatment and prevention of recurrence. *J Am Acad Dermatol.* 2019;80:853-867.

A4. Kreijkamp-Kaspers S, Hawke K, Guo L, et al. Oral antifungal medication for toenail onychomycosis. *Cochrane Database Syst Rev.* 2017;7:CD010031.

A5. Jabbar-Lopez ZK, Yiu ZZN, Ward V, et al. Quantitative evaluation of biologic therapy options for psoriasis: a systematic review and network meta-analysis. *J Invest Dermatol.* 2017;137:1646-1654.

A6. Joly P, Maho-Vaillant M, Prost-Squarcioni C, et al. First-line rituximab combined with short-term prednisone versus prednisone alone for the treatment of pemphigus (Ritux 3): a prospective, multicentre, parallel-group, open-label randomised trial. *Lancet.* 2017;389:2031-2040.

A7. Blauvelt A, de Bruin-Weller M, Gooderham M, et al. Long-term management of moderate-to-severe atopic dermatitis with dupilumab and concomitant topical corticosteroids (LIBERTY AD CHRONOS): a 1-year, randomised, double-blinded, placebo-controlled, phase 3 trial. *Lancet.* 2017;389:2287-2303.

GENERAL REFERENCES

For the General References and other additional features, please visit Expert Consult at https://expertconsult.inkling.com.

409

ECZEMAS, PHOTODERMATOSES, PAPULOSQUAMOUS (INCLUDING FUNGAL) DISEASES, AND FIGURATE ERYTHEMAS

HENRY W. LIM

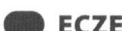

● ECZEMA

The more commonly encountered eczemas (Table 409-1) share similar histologic characteristics. They have edema within the epidermis (spongiosis) and infiltration with lymphocytes and macrophages in the superficial dermis.

Nummular Dermatitis

Nummular dermatitis occurs most frequently in patients who are in their 50s to 60s. Both sexes are affected, and it is most frequently seen in the winter. The condition tends to be more frequent and severe among East Asians. The pathogenesis is unclear, although xerosis plays a significant role.

Patients present with pruritic, coin-shaped, erythematous patches with some scales and occasionally with pinhead-sized vesicles (Figs. 409-1 and 409-2). Lesions may be excoriated and lichenified (i.e., thickened skin with accentuation of skin markings). Legs and arms are commonly affected, and the trunk is less frequently involved; facial involvement is uncommon. All patients should be educated about the use of emollients and moisturizing soaps, and avoidance of long, hot showers. Topical corticosteroid ointments (e.g., triamcinolone ointment, 0.1% twice daily for 1 to 2 weeks) are helpful for active lesions, and oral antihistamines (e.g., fexofenadine, 180 mg every morning, and hydroxyzine

---

TABLE 409-1   ECZEMAS

Nummular dermatitis
Dyshidrosis
Atopic dermatitis
Seborrheic dermatitis
Allergic contact dermatitis
Irritant contact dermatitis

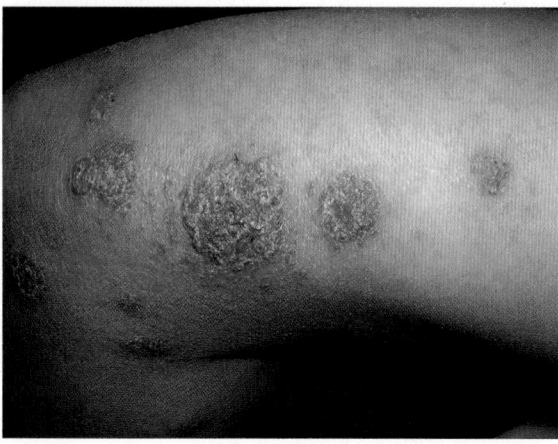

FIGURE 409-1. Nummular dermatitis. Coin-shaped erythematous patches.

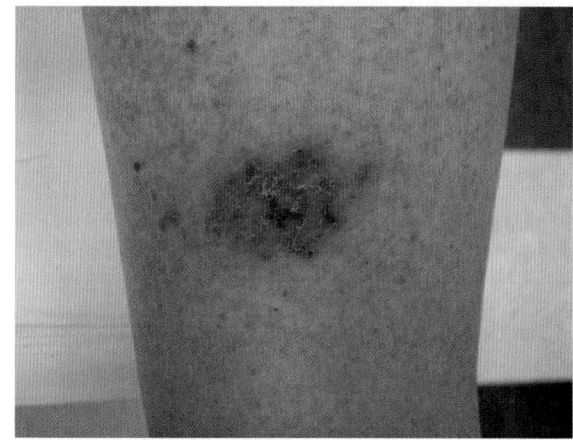

FIGURE 409-2. Nummular dermatitis. Coin-shaped erythematous patch.

25 to 50 mg at bedtime) are useful for pruritus. In severe cases, narrowband ultraviolet B (NB-UVB) phototherapy, a short course of oral corticosteroids (prednisone, 0.5 to 1 mg/kg/day, with a maximal dose of 60 mg/day, for 1 to 2 weeks, then taper in 10 to 14 days) or day hospitalization for intensive topical and NB-UVB therapy is beneficial.

Dyshidrosis

Dyshidrosis manifests as pruritic, deep-seated, pinhead-sized vesicles, most commonly along the sides of the fingers (Figs. 409-3 and 409-4). Other features include xerosis, scaliness, and fissures. In severe cases, palms and soles also may be involved. Dyshidrosis is seen in individuals who wash their hands frequently, such as food industry workers and mothers of young infants. Treatment follows a sequential order: (1) replacing soap-and-water handwashing with hand sanitizers, (2) liberal use of emollients, (3) topical corticosteroid ointments (e.g., fluocinonide ointment, 0.05% twice daily for 2 weeks), and (4) oral antihistamines (same regimen as nummular dermatitis).

Atopic Dermatitis

Atopic dermatitis is most commonly seen among young children but may persist into adulthood or even begin in adulthood.[1,2] The prevalence has been estimated at between 15 and 23%. Patients usually present with xerosis, erythematous scaly patches, small vesicles, excoriations, crusting, and, not infrequently, impetiginization (Fig. 409-5). In dark-skinned patients, a papular variant is commonly

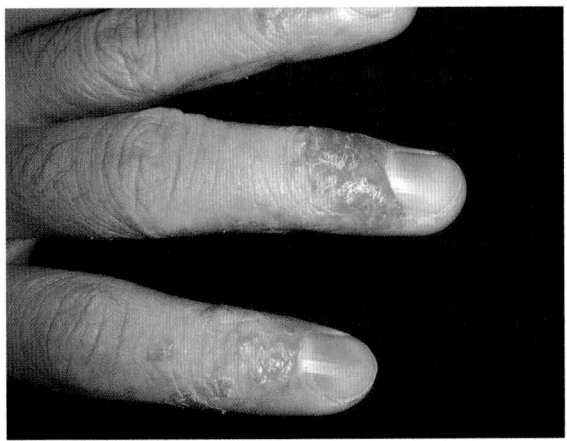

FIGURE 409-3. Dyshidrosis. Deep-seated vesicles and scaliness on fingers.

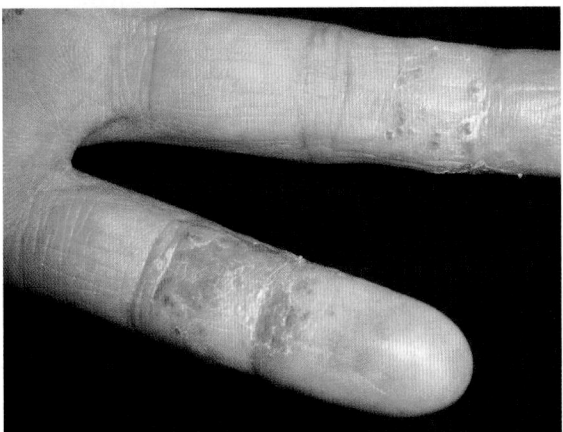

FIGURE 409-4. Dyshidrosis. Deep-seated vesicles and scaliness on fingers.

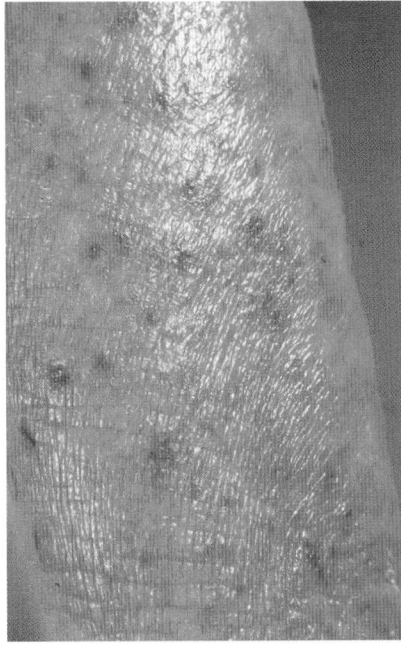

FIGURE 409-5. Atopic dermatitis. Note the erythema, excoriation, and lichenification.

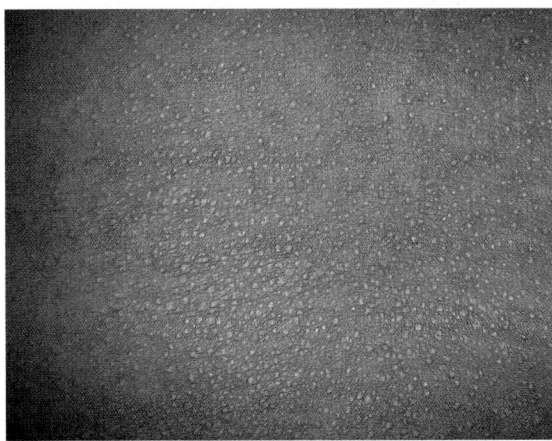

FIGURE 409-6. Atopic dermatitis in a dark-skinned patient. Note the typical papular variant commonly seen in dark-skinned individuals.

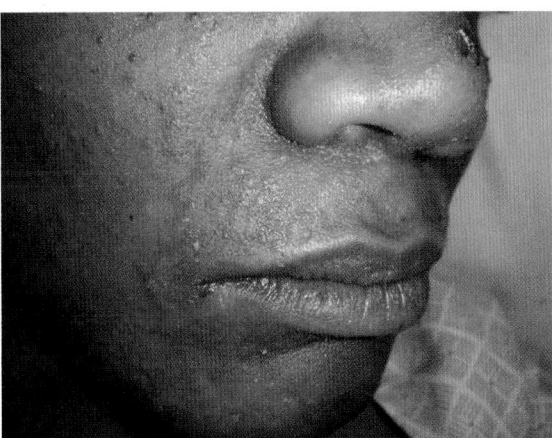

FIGURE 409-7. Seborrheic dermatitis presenting as erythematous patches and plaques with fine scales on the malar area of an HIV-positive patient.

seen (Fig. 409-6). With chronic scratching and rubbing, hyperpigmentation and lichenification occur. Commonly affected sites include the periorbital area and flexor areas such as the neck, antecubital fossa, and popliteal fossa. In severe cases, the entire skin surface may be involved. Diagnosis is made by the typical morphology, the distribution of lesions, and family and personal history of atopy. The therapeutic ladder consists of (1) emollients; (2) topical

corticosteroid ointments (e.g., triamcinolone ointment, 0.1% twice daily for 2 to 4 weeks), or topical calcineurin inhibitors (tacrolimus ointment, 0.1% for 3 to 4 weeks, or pimecrolimus cream, 1% for 3 to 4 weeks); (3) oral antihistamines (e.g., fexofenadine, 180 mg every morning, and hydroxyzine, 25 to 50 mg at bedtime, as needed); and (4) NB-UVB phototherapy.[3] Newer options for poorly responsive disease include crisaborole (a phosphodiesterase 4 inhibitor) 2% ointment applied twice daily,[A1] and dupilumab (an interleukin-4 [IL-4] receptor α-antagonist) at 300 mg subcutaneously every other week.[A2][A3] Other traditional systemic treatments include oral prednisone (0.5 to 1 mg/kg/day), cyclosporine (3 to 5 mg/kg/day), and mycophenolate mofetil (1 to 2 g/day). Nemolizumab (an IL-31 receptor A antibody) is an efficacious experimental agent.[A4]

Seborrheic Dermatitis

Seborrheic dermatitis is a common condition that presents as erythematous patches with fine, greasy-appearing scales on the malar area, midforehead, midchest, and scalp (Fig. 409-7). In dark-skinned individuals, lesions may be hypopigmented (Fig. 409-8). The pathogenesis is unknown, although *Pityrosporum ovale* is believed to play a role. Lesions are common in patients with human immunodeficiency virus (HIV) infection (Chapter 366). The diagnosis is made clinically. Topical corticosteroids (e.g., hydrocortisone cream 2.5%, twice daily for 1 to 2 weeks for facial lesions, fluocinolone acetonide 0.01% solution for the scalp, twice daily for 3 to 4 weeks) can rapidly reduce the inflammation; then topical ketoconazole cream, 2% twice daily, as needed (or shampoo 2% daily or every other day for the scalp), is safe for long-term treatment.[4]

Allergic Contact Dermatitis and Irritant Contact Dermatitis

Allergic contact dermatitis is a delayed hypersensitivity response to external allergens, whereas irritant contact dermatitis is a nonspecific toxic response to contact irritants. In both conditions, lesions occur in the exposed area. In severe cases, however, nonexposed areas may be involved, albeit less intensely. Allergic

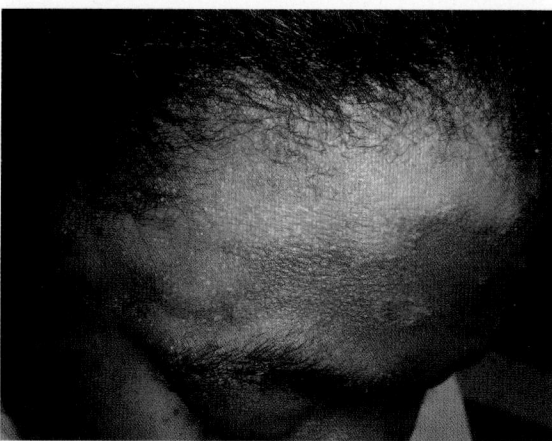

FIGURE 409-8. Seborrheic dermatitis. Hypopigmentation with fine scales on the forehead and scalp.

TABLE 409-2 SELECTED PHOTODERMATOSES

Polymorphic light eruption
Chronic actinic dermatitis
Phototoxicity and photoallergy
Porphyrias

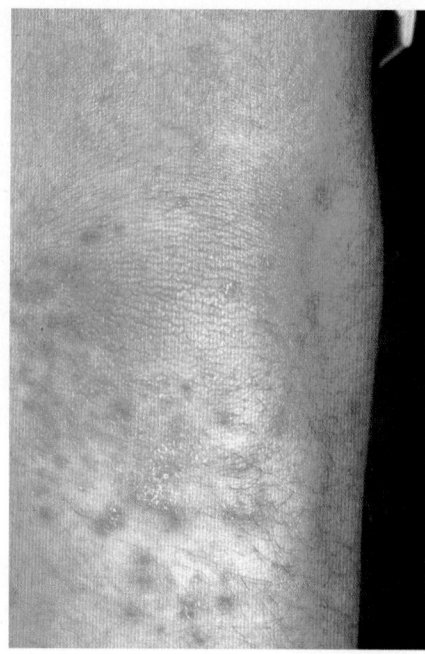

FIGURE 409-9. Polymorphic light eruption. Erythematous papules a few hours after exposure to sunlight.

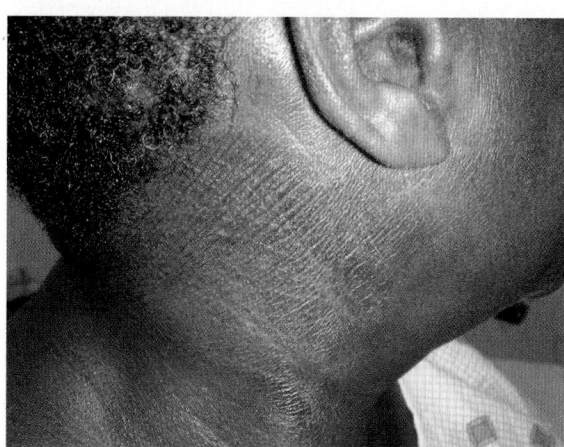

FIGURE 409-10. Chronic actinic dermatitis. Hyperpigmentation and lichenification; note sparing of the sun-protected areas of the neck and infra-auricular area.

contact dermatitis presents with erythematous pruritic papules and vesicles. Lesions resolve with fine scales. Postinflammatory hyperpigmentation may be observed. Histologically, epidermal edema and dermal histiocytic infiltrates are observed. The morphology of irritant contact dermatitis is similar to that of allergic contact dermatitis. However, irritant contact dermatitis is usually associated with a burning sensation rather than with pruritus. Postinflammatory hyperpigmentation is frequently observed. Histologic changes consist of necrotic keratinocytes, epidermal necrosis, and neutrophilic infiltrates. Management includes identification and removal of the offending agent, as well as symptomatic treatments such as topical corticosteroids and oral antihistamines.

PHOTODERMATOSES

Photodermatoses are cutaneous eruptions secondary to exposure to sunlight (Table 409-2). By convention, electromagnetic radiation in the UV region is divided into UVC (200 to 290 nm), UVB (290 to 320 nm), UVA-2 (320 to 340 nm), and UVA-1 (340 to 400 nm). Visible light extends from 400 to 760 nm. Because UVC emitted by the sun is absorbed by ozone in the stratosphere, UVC does not reach the earth's surface. UVB, UVA, and less frequently, visible light are the relevant spectra in photodermatoses.

Polymorphic Light Eruption

Polymorphic light eruption is the most common immunologically mediated photodermatosis, occurring in 10 to 20% of the general population. It usually is seen in young adults, has a slight female predominance, and has been reported worldwide. Affected individuals are less susceptible to cutaneous photoimmunosuppression and hence have an enhanced response to UV-induced neoantigens in the skin. Lesions usually occur in early spring, within a few hours of exposure to sunlight. The lesions are mildly pruritic and manifest as pinhead papules (common among dark-skinned patients), papules, papulovesicles, or, less commonly, vesicles (Fig. 409-9). They persist for several days and resolve spontaneously. The condition tends to improve as the sunny season progresses, a phenomenon known as hardening.

The course is chronic; only 11% of patients have complete resolution of the disease in 16 years and 24% in 32 years. Diagnosis is based on the typical history and morphology of the lesion. When lesions occur primarily on the face, a diagnosis of lupus must be excluded. Management consists of sun avoidance and the use of broad-spectrum sunscreens with sun protection factor (SPF) of at least 30, topical corticosteroids, and oral antihistamines. In severe cases, desensitization treatment using NB-UVB has been successful. Desensitization is usually performed in early spring by exposing patients to increasing doses of NB-UVB three times weekly for 15 treatments.

Chronic Actinic Dermatitis

Chronic actinic dermatitis is a chronic photodermatosis that occurs most commonly in men in their 60s and 70s.[5] It occurs in patients of all ethnic

groups, but in the United States it is more commonly seen in dark-skinned individuals. It is seen in 5 to 17% of patients referred for evaluation of photosensitivity. This condition has been postulated to represent a delayed hypersensitivity response to an unidentified antigen.

Patients present with lichenified plaques on sun-exposed areas (Figs. 409-10 and 409-11). Typically, sun-protected areas, such as the postauricular area, the area underneath the chin, the area above the eyes, and the trunk, are spared. Histologically, a dermal lymphohistiocytic infiltrate is seen, and atypical mononuclear cells may be observed. On phototesting, patients have increased sensitivity to UVA, UVB, and/or visible light. In a study of 178 cases, 10% resolved in 5 years and 50% in 15 years. An association with HIV infection (Chapter 366) has been reported.

The diagnosis is based on the patient's history, morphology, and distribution of the lesions. It is confirmed by phototesting.

Management is challenging. Rigorous photoprotection is a must: staying in the shade, using broad-spectrum sunscreens with SPF 50 or more, and wearing photoprotective clothing, sunglasses, and a wide-brimmed hat. Other treatment modalities, in approximate sequential order, are topical corticosteroids (fluocinonide ointment 0.05% twice daily), tacrolimus ointment (0.1% twice daily), oral mycophenolate mofetil (1 to 2 g/day), oral cyclosporine (3 to 5 mg/kg/day), and azathioprine (up to 2 to 2.5 mg/kg/day). Treatment with oral corticosteroids (e.g., prednisone, 1 mg/kg/day) may be needed for acute flare. In recalcitrant cases, low-dose PUVA or NB-UVB in conjunction with oral corticosteroids may be helpful.

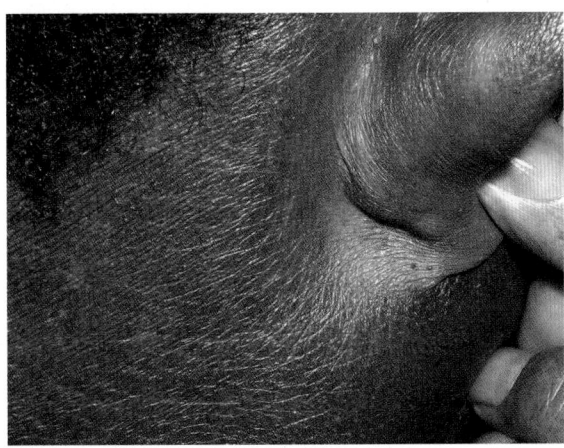

FIGURE 409-11. Hyperpigmentation and lichenification in a patient with chronic actinic dermatitis. Note sparing of the sun-protected postauricular area.

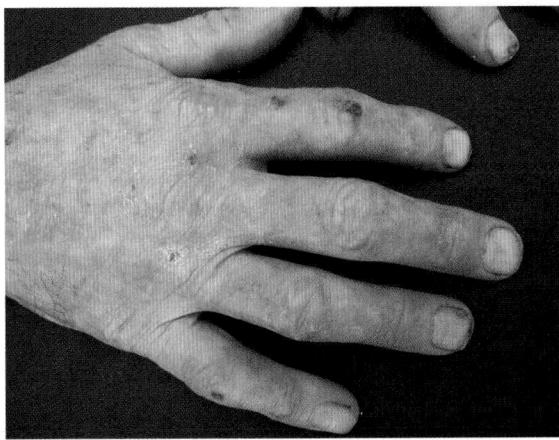

FIGURE 409-12. Erosion, crusting, and vesicles on the dorsum of the hand of a patient with porphyria cutanea tarda.

TABLE 409-3 PHOTOTOXICITY AND PHOTOALLERGY

FEATURES	PHOTOTOXICITY	PHOTOALLERGY
Lesions after first exposure	Yes	No
Onset	Minutes after sun exposure	Delayed (24-48 hr after sun exposure)
Common offending agents	Systemic medications	Sunscreen agents
Morphology	Vesicles, bulla, hyperpigmentation	Eczematous (erythema, scaliness)
Management	Symptomatic (topical corticosteroids, antihistamine)	Removal of the offending agent

Phototoxicity and Photoallergy

The terms *phototoxicity* and *photoallergy* refer to the development of skin lesions after combined exposure to an oral or topical photosensitizer and electromagnetic radiation. Phototoxicity is a nonspecific cutaneous toxic reaction, whereas photoallergy is a delayed hypersensitivity response. For all photosensitizers, the action spectrum for both lies in the UVA range (Table 409-3).

Porphyrias

The most common cutaneous porphyria is porphyria cutanea tarda, in which patients present with skin fragility and blister formation on sun-exposed areas, most commonly the dorsum of the hands and the forearms (Fig. 409-12; Chapter 199).[6] Patients have periorbital hypertrichosis and, less frequently, periorbital mottled hyperpigmentation and hypopigmentation. Sclerodermoid skin changes can occur in both sun-exposed and sun-protected areas. The defective enzyme is uroporphyrinogen decarboxylase. Porphyria cutanea tarda is associated with excessive alcohol intake, exposure to estrogens, hepatitis C infection (Chapter 140), HIV infection (Chapter 366), and hemochromatosis

TABLE 409-4 PAPULOSQUAMOUS DISEASES

Psoriasis
Pityriasis rubra pilaris
Pityriasis rosea
Lichen planus
Lichen nitidus
Secondary syphilis
Pityriasis lichenoides
Parapsoriasis
Mycosis fungoides
Acrokeratosis paraneoplastica of Bazex
Necrolytic acral erythema
Dermatophytosis
Tinea versicolor

(Chapter 201). Patients invariably have an elevated level of ferritin and frequently have elevated liver enzyme values.

The diagnosis is suggested by the typical clinical appearance and is confirmed by the characteristic porphyrin profile of elevated levels of 8-, 7-, 6-, 5-, and 4-carboxyl porphyrins in the serum and urine, and isocoproporphyrin in feces (Chapter 199). Management consists of avoidance of precipitating factors (alcohol, iron-containing vitamins, estrogen-containing birth control pills) and weekly phlebotomy. In patients who are anemic (e.g., those with HIV infection), low-dose hydroxychloroquine (200 mg/week) is beneficial (Chapter 140). In patients with concurrent chronic hepatitis C (Chapter 140), which is a susceptibility factor for clinical symptoms, effective antiviral treatment of the hepatitis C can reduce the relapse rate of skin symptoms.[7]

● PAPULOSQUAMOUS (INCLUDING FUNGAL) DISEASES

Common papulosquamous diseases are listed in Table 409-4.

Psoriasis

EPIDEMIOLOGY

Psoriasis occurs in 2 to 3% of the general population, with considerable variation in different parts of the world. It affects male and female patients equally. Approximately one third of the patients have a positive family history. Psoriasis has a bimodal peak of onset, at 22.5 years of age and again at age 55 years.

PATHOBIOLOGY

Psoriasis involves the innate and adaptive immune systems, with abnormal keratinocyte proliferation. Factors playing a role in the pathogenesis include activation of antigen-presenting cells and development of T_H1 and T_H17 cells. Mediators include IL-12, IL-17, IL-23, tumor necrosis factor-α (TNF-α), and interferon-γ.

Psoriasis has a complex, polygenetic inheritance. Cutaneous psoriasis is strongly associated with human leukocyte antigen–Cw6 (HLA-Cw6), whereas psoriatic arthritis can be associated with HLA-Cw6, HLA-B38/39, or HLA-B27. To date, genome-wide studies have identified more than 85 non–major histocompatibility complex loci that may increase the risk for psoriasis.

CLINICAL MANIFESTATIONS

Several distinct forms of psoriasis are recognized. *Psoriasis vulgaris,* the most common type, appears as a persistent erythematous papule and plaque with silvery scales most commonly on elbows, knees, and scalp (Fig. 409-13). *Guttate psoriasis* usually occurs after viral or bacterial (most commonly streptococcal) infection; it appears as small, erythematous, scaly papules scattered over a large area of the body in a raindrop distribution (*guttate* means "droplike"). *Inverse psoriasis* refers to psoriasis that occurs in skinfold areas such as the groin, axilla, and inframammary folds. It appears as an erythematous, somewhat shiny patch; because of the constant friction in the involved areas, scales are absent. *Nail psoriasis* includes nail pittings, yellowish macules underneath the nail plate ("oil drop" sign), and thickening of the nail (onychodystrophy) (Fig. 409-14). *Erythrodermic psoriasis* appears as widespread erythroderma with fine silvery scales. *Palmoplantar psoriasis* manifests as keratotic scaly patches and plaques on the palms and soles, very frequently with accompanying fissures. *Pustular psoriasis of von Zumbusch* is a rare variant of psoriasis occurring with generalized pustules that are 2 to 3 mm in diameter (Fig. 409-15) and associated with the onset of fever.

Of patients with psoriasis, 5 to 30% also may have psoriatic arthritis, which may precede the appearance of cutaneous lesions (Chapter 249). Psoriasis

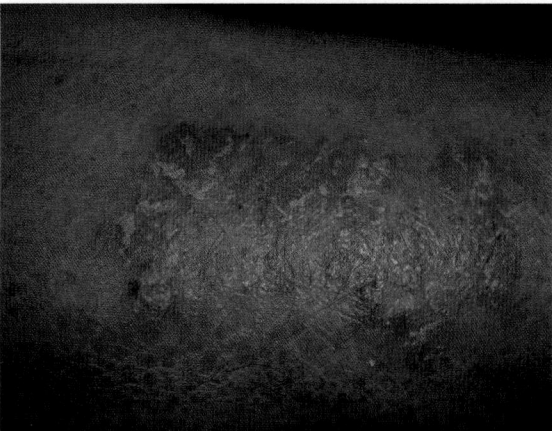

FIGURE 409-13. Psoriasis. Erythematous plaques with silvery scales.

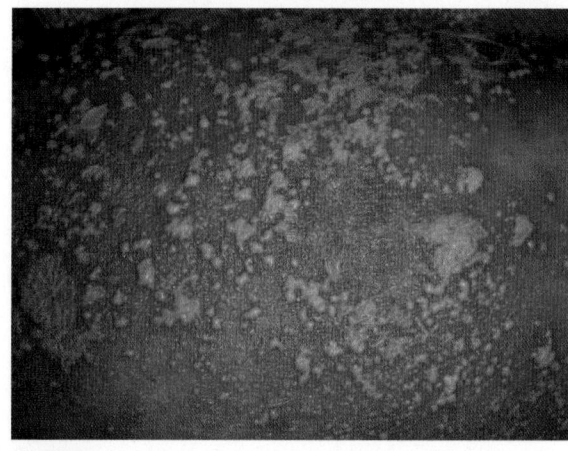

FIGURE 409-15. Pustular psoriasis. Erythematous patch with pustules in a patient with active disease.

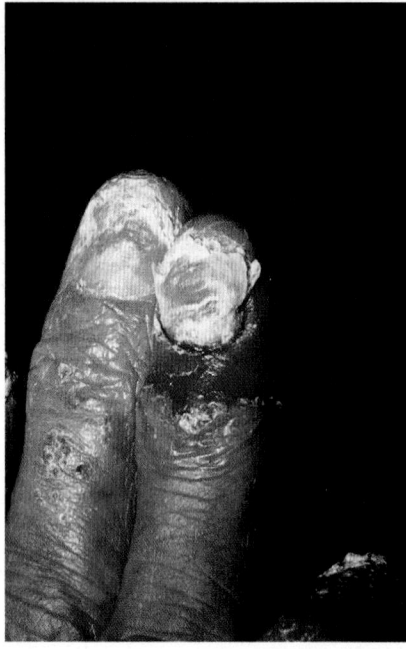

FIGURE 409-14. Psoriasis. Thickening and crumbling of the nail plate (onychodystrophy). Note the erythematous patches with silvery scales in the periungual area.

TABLE 409-5	SEQUENTIAL THERAPEUTIC APPROACH IN PSORIASIS
Topical agents	Corticosteroids (e.g., triamcinolone ointment 0.1%) Vitamin D analogues (e.g., calcipotriene cream 0.005%) Retinoids (e.g., tazarotene cream 0.1%)
Phototherapy	Narrowband ultraviolet B (three times/wk)
Traditional systemic therapy	Methotrexate (10-20 mg/wk) Cyclosporine (3-5 mg/kg/day) Acitretin (25-50 mg/day)
Oral phosphodiesterase-4 inhibitor	Apremilast (30 mg twice/day)
Biologics	TNF-α inhibitors • Etanercept (50 mg/wk SC) • Adalimumab (40 mg every 2 wk SC) • Infliximab (5-10 mg/kg every 8 wk IV) Anti–IL-12/23 • Ustekinumab (45-90 mg every 12 wk SC) Anti–IL-17 • Secukinumab (300 mg/wk for 5 weeks, followed by 300 mg every 4 wk SC) • Ixekizumab (160 mg at wk 0, followed by 80 mg every 2 wk for 12 weeks, then 80 mg every 4 wk SC) Anti–IL-17 receptor antibody • Brodalumab (210 mg at wk 0,1,2, then every 2 wk SC) Anti–IL-23 • Guselkumab (100 mg wk 0, 4, then every 8 wk SC) • Tildrakizumab (100 mg at wk 0, 4, then every 12 wk SC)
Potential future treatments*	Oral Janus kinase inhibitor • Tofacitinib

IL = interleukin; IV = intravenously; SC = subcutaneously; TNF = tumor necrosis factor.
*Doses may change if and when approved by the U.S. Food and Drug Administration.

also is associated with chronic kidney disease, inflammatory bowel disease, hepatic disease, certain malignancies, infections, and mood disorders.[8] The association of psoriasis with HIV infection (Chapter 366) has been well documented.

DIAGNOSIS

The diagnosis can usually be made based on the history and physical examination alone. However, in patients with erythrodermic psoriasis, skin biopsy is needed to exclude other causes of generalized erythroderma, such as drug eruption, cutaneous T-cell lymphoma (Chapter 176), and pityriasis rubra pilaris.

TREATMENT ℞

Treatment modalities start with topical therapy and then UV-based therapy, followed by traditional systemic therapy, an oral phosphodiesterase inhibitor, or biologic agents (Table 409-5).[9] For many patients, however, biologics are routinely more effective than placebo or traditional systemic therapies, and the most recently approved biologics—ixekizumab, tildrakizumab, guselkumab, and brodalumab—appear to be more effective than ustekinumab, etanercept, and adalimumab.[A5-A8]

Oral corticosteroids should not be used because psoriasis may worsen when they are discontinued. All of these drugs increase the risk for serious infections by about three-fold.[10] For the treatment of psoriatic arthritis, please see Chapter 249.

Pityriasis Rubra Pilaris

EPIDEMIOLOGY

Pityriasis rubra pilaris occurs equally in men and women; the incidence ranges from 1 in 5000 new dermatology patients in Great Britain to 1 in 50,000 in India. This disease most frequently occurs as the acquired form, although a familial form (autosomal dominant with variable expression) occasionally has been reported. Abnormal vitamin A metabolism and autoimmunity have been postulated as possible precipitants.

CLINICAL MANIFESTATIONS

The most common form of pityriasis rubra pilaris is type I, which is characterized by widespread salmon-colored plaques with fine scales, islands of sparing, scaliness on the scalp, waxy keratoderma of the palms and soles, and follicular hyperkeratosis (Figs. 409-16 and 409-17). In adult patients, the condition

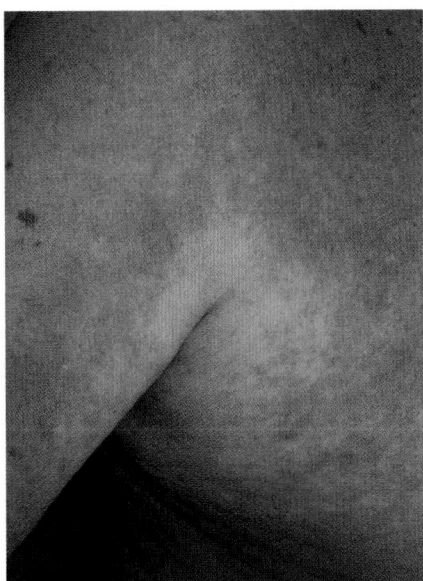

FIGURE 409-16. Pityriasis rubra pilaris. Note the erythematous orange plaques with islands of sparing.

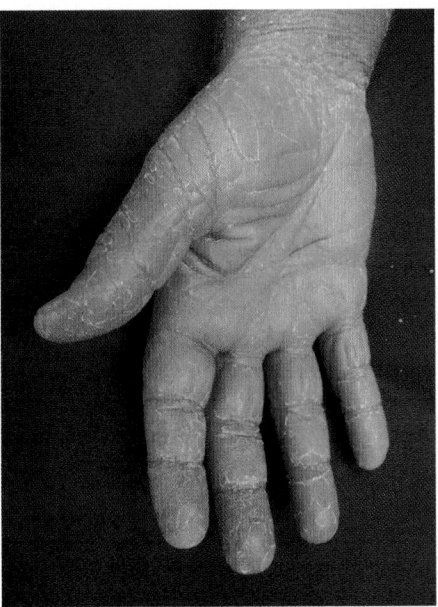

FIGURE 409-17. Pityriasis rubra pilaris. Palmar hyperkeratosis with waxy scales.

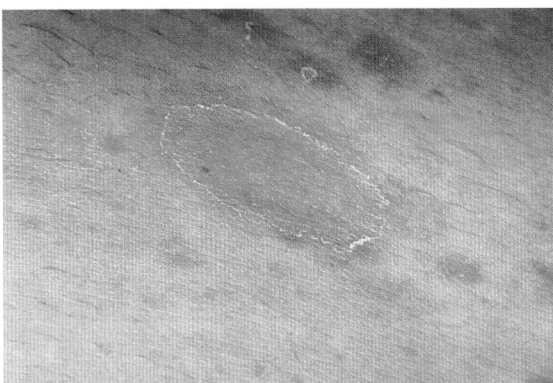

FIGURE 409-18. Pityriasis rosea. Large erythematous oval patch (herald patch) accompanied by smaller erythematous patches.

Pityriasis Rosea

EPIDEMIOLOGY AND PATHOBIOLOGY

The incidence of pityriasis rosea has been reported as 3 to 30 per 1000 patients. It occurs in all ethnic groups, most commonly in the third and fourth decades of life, with a slight female predominance. A possible association with human herpesvirus types 6 and 7 has been reported.

CLINICAL MANIFESTATIONS

In 50 to 90% of patients, pityriasis rosea starts with a primary lesion (herald patch), which is an erythematous, scaly, oval patch a few centimeters in diameter (Fig. 409-18). This lesion is usually followed within a few days by smaller, minimally pruritic, erythematous scaly patches on the trunk, less commonly on the proximal extremities. As a rule, the palms and soles are spared. The distribution of the eruption, especially on the back, tends to follow the lines of cleavage of the skin, with a resulting "Christmas tree" distribution. The eruption is self-limited and resolves within 6 to 8 weeks. In rare instances, lesions may persist.

DIAGNOSIS

The diagnosis usually can be made clinically. The most important differential diagnosis is secondary syphilis, which, in contrast to pityriasis rosea, usually involves the palms and soles. Serology testing to exclude syphilis (Chapter 303) is advisable.

TREATMENT   Rx

Treatment is primarily symptomatic, including topical corticosteroids and oral antihistamines. Acyclovir (400 mg three times daily for 7 days) has been reported to be effective.[11]

typically starts on the face and moves to the lower extremities; in the juvenile form, it usually starts in the lower half of the body. Ectropion and pruritus may occur.

DIAGNOSIS

Diagnosis is based on the clinical presentations and by the characteristic histologic findings of alternating vertical and horizontal parakeratosis in the stratum corneum.

TREATMENT   Rx

The most effective treatment is with oral retinoids (acitretin, 25 to 50 mg/day for 2 to 4 months). Some patients benefit from methotrexate (7.5 to 15 mg/week) or cyclosporine (3 to 5 mg/kg/day). TNF antagonists and apremilast, used at the same doses as for psoriasis, are helpful for patients with recalcitrant type I disease. Topical keratolytic agents, such as ammonium lactate lotion 12%, twice daily, are helpful as adjunctive therapy.

Lichen Planus

EPIDEMIOLOGY

Lichen planus occurs most commonly in patients between 30 and 60 years of age. Women are affected more frequently than men. The prevalence is approximately 1%.

PATHOBIOLOGY

Histologically, lichen planus is characterized by dense T-cell infiltrate at the dermal-epidermal junction, suggesting the pathogenic role of cell-mediated immunity. Because lichen planus or lichen planus–like eruptions can occur after exposure to drugs or chemicals (e.g., color film developer), the role of drugs and chemicals in inducing a T-cell-mediated response against the epidermis has been postulated. Lichen planus may be associated with hepatitis C infection (Chapter 140).

CLINICAL MANIFESTATIONS

Patients present with pruritic erythematous-to-violaceous flat-topped papules, often with white lacy lines (Wickham striae) on the wrists, forearms, and genitalia (Fig. 409-19). *Oral lichen planus* occurs as white reticulated lines,

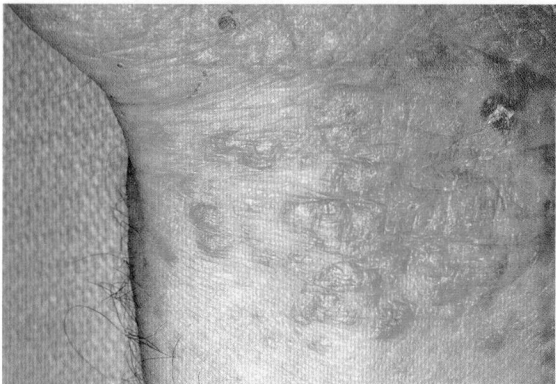

FIGURE 409-19. Lichen planus. Erythematous flat-topped papules on the wrist.

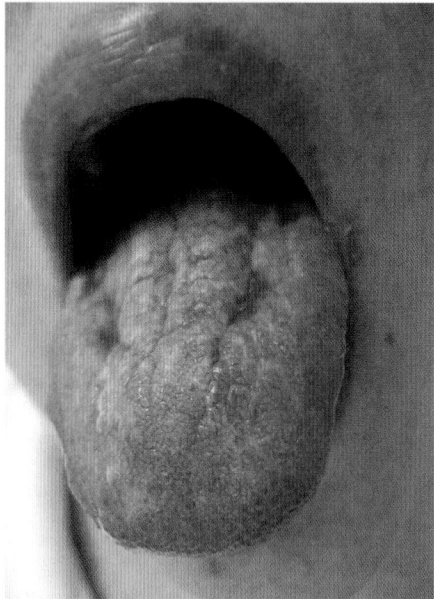

FIGURE 409-20. Lichen planus of the tongue. Note white plaques on dorsal surface of the tongue, with reticulated white line on the distal aspect of the tongue.

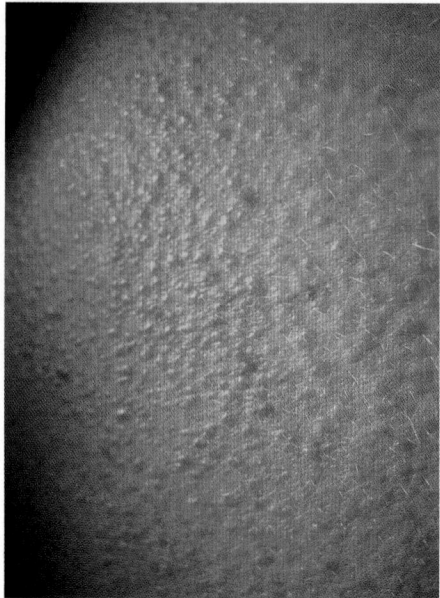

FIGURE 409-21. Lichen nitidus. Note skin-colored fine papules on the upper back.

TABLE 409-6 THERAPEUTIC OPTIONS FOR LICHEN PLANUS
CUTANEOUS LESIONS
Topical corticosteroids (triamcinolone ointment 0.1% twice/day)
HYPERTROPHIC LESIONS
Intralesional corticosteroids (triamcinolone suspension 3-5 mg/mL)
ORAL LESIONS
Corticosteroid paste (triamcinolone 0.1% paste twice/day) or cyclosporine solution (100 mg/mL, 2 mL, twice/day, swish and spit)
GENERALIZED LICHEN PLANUS, PAINFUL ORAL/GENITAL EROSIONS, RECALCITRANT DISEASE
Narrowband UVB phototherapy (two to three times/wk) Oral prednisone (0.5-1 mg/kg/day, taper in 6-8 wk) Mycophenolate mofetil (1-2 g/day) Cyclosporine (3-5 mg/kg/day) Tumor necrosis factor-α inhibitors (see Table 409-5) Apremilast (see Table 409-5)

most commonly along the bite line on the buccal mucosa. Similar lesions can be seen on the tongue (Fig. 409-20) and genital mucosa. Painful erosion may occur. *Hypertrophic lichen planus* usually occurs on the lower extremities as pruritic lichenified, violaceous plaques.

DIAGNOSIS

The diagnosis is made clinically and is confirmed by the characteristic histologic findings.

TREATMENT   Rx

Therapeutic options depend on the location of lesions (Table 409-6). Without treatment, cutaneous lesions usually resolve in approximately 1 year, whereas oral and hypertrophic lesions tend to be much more chronic, persisting for an average of 4.5 years and 8.5 years, respectively.

Lichen Nitidus

Lichen nitidus is a rather uncommon condition that usually occurs in dark-skinned children or young adults. The incidence has been estimated to be 3.4 cases per 10,000 persons. The cause is unclear.

The lesions are asymptomatic, 1- to 2-mm, shiny, skin-colored discrete papules, sometimes with fine scales on their surface, occurring most commonly on the genitalia or forearms and occasionally on the trunk (Fig. 409-21). Histologically, a dense, focal lymphocytic infiltrate is seen in the superficial dermis and at the dermal-epidermal junction.

The diagnosis can be confirmed from the typical clinical appearance and the characteristic histologic changes. The condition tends to remit spontaneously in a few years. Therapy with topical corticosteroids (e.g., triamcinolone ointment, 0.1% twice daily for 2 weeks) and oral antihistamines (e.g., fexofenadine, 180 mg every morning, and hydroxyzine, 25 to 50 mg at bedtime, as needed) should be reserved for symptomatic cases only.

Secondary Syphilis

Lesions typically occur 1 to 2 months after the development of a primary chancre lesion (Chapter 303). However, up to 25% of patients may not remember having a chancre. Once the eruption occurs, it lasts for 1 to 3 months.

Clinically, secondary syphilis may appear as erythematous macules (roseola syphilitica), erythematous-to-hyperpigmented oval or circular papules and plaques covered with scales, or a maculopapular eruption (Fig. 409-22). Nodular eruption also may occur occasionally. The lesions tend to be widespread, and the palms and soles are very frequently involved (Fig. 409-23). The diagnosis is made based on the history, physical examination, and a positive serology. Skin biopsy shows the proliferation of endothelial cells in the dermis and a dense dermal infiltrate containing many plasma cells. Intramuscular benzathine penicillin G (2.4 million U intramuscularly in a single dose) is currently the recommended treatment.

Pityriasis Lichenoides

Pityriasis lichenoides occurs as erythematous papules that may be minimally pruritic and covered with scales, scattered on all parts of the body. In the acute form (pityriasis lichenoides et varioliformis acuta [PLEVA]), the central part

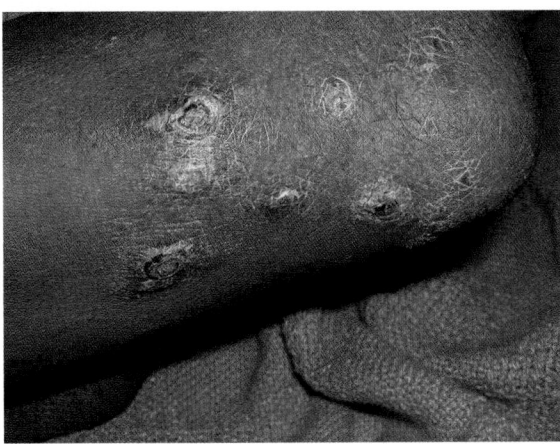

FIGURE 409-22. Secondary syphilis. Papules with crust on elbow.

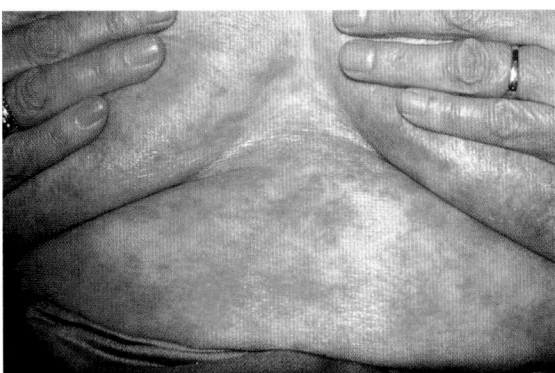

FIGURE 409-24. Large plaque parapsoriasis. Erythematous patches with fine scales.

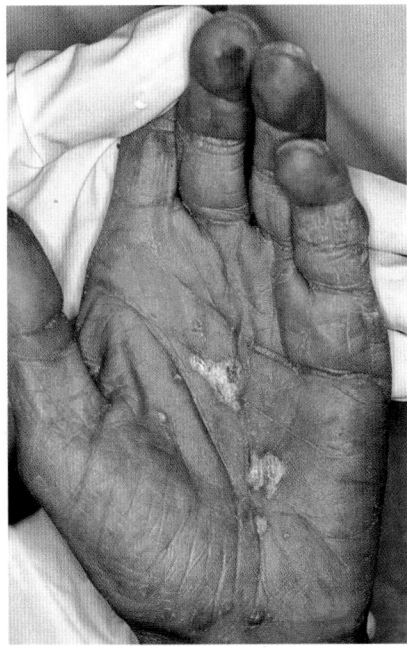

FIGURE 409-23. Secondary syphilis. Scaly papules and plaques on the palm.

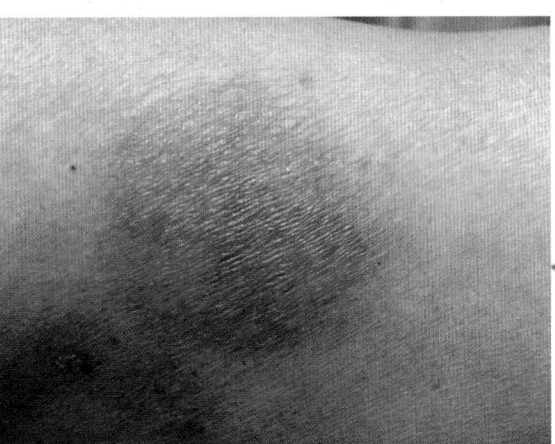

FIGURE 409-25. Mycosis fungoides. Erythematous minimally elevated plaque with "cigarette paper" wrinkling of the epidermis.

of the lesions develops vesicles, pustules, and hemorrhages, with eventual crusting of the lesions. The chronic form (pityriasis lichenoides chronica [PLC]) occurs as asymptomatic erythematous-to-hyperpigmented papules and plaques covered with fine scales; the trunk and extremities are common sites. Histologically, both PLEVA and PLC are characterized by dense lymphocytic infiltrates in the dermis, with CD8 lymphocytes predominating in PLEVA and CD4 lymphocytes in PLC.

PLEVA usually resolves in a few months, although it can persist. PLC usually lasts for a few years. Both disorders affect patients of all ages, with a slight male predominance.

Treatment generally follows a sequential order: (1) topical corticosteroids (e.g., triamcinolone ointment, 0.1% twice daily for 1 to 2 weeks) and antihistamines, (2) doxycycline (100 mg twice daily), (3) NB-UVB phototherapy (three times weekly for 8 to 10 weeks with increasing doses of NB-UVB),[12] and (4) methotrexate (7.5 to 15 mg/week).

Parapsoriasis

The two common variants of parapsoriasis are large plaque parapsoriasis and small plaque parapsoriasis. The peak incidence is in the fifth decade, although rare cases may begin in childhood. Large plaque parapsoriasis appears as minimally pruritic, oval-to-circular, erythematous-to-hyperpigmented macules and patches with fine scales and superficial atrophy (crinkling atrophy) scattered on all parts of the body (Fig. 409-24). These lesions are usually larger than 5 cm. Large plaque parapsoriasis is considered by some to be a variant of mycosis fungoides (see later). Small plaque parapsoriasis appears as circular-to-oval,

erythematous-to-hyperpigmented patches or minimally elevated plaques, with lesions smaller than 5 cm in diameter and usually covered with fine scales. A distinct variant is digitate dermatosis, in which lesions appear along the lines of cleavage, usually on the lateral aspect of the trunk in the shape of fingerprints. Histologically, large plaque parapsoriasis is characterized by a dermal lymphocytic infiltrate, which may extend into the epidermis, whereas small plaque parapsoriasis is characterized by spongiotic dermatitis, with a mild superficial lymphocytic infiltrate in the dermis. In up to one third of patients, large plaque parapsoriasis may evolve into mycosis fungoides. As a result, treatment of large plaque parapsoriasis is similar to that of early-stage mycosis fungoides: high-potency topical corticosteroids, NB-UVB phototherapy, and psoralen and UVA (PUVA). By comparison, patients with small plaque parapsoriasis have a benign course, and management should be symptomatic only, with emollients, topical corticosteroids, and if needed, NB-UVB phototherapy.

Mycosis Fungoides

This is the most common variant of cutaneous T-cell lymphoma (Chapter 176).[13] The four types of cutaneous manifestations are patch, plaque, tumor, and erythrodermic. Patch-stage disease manifests as asymptomatic skin-colored or minimally erythematous patches with fine "cigarette paper" wrinkling of the epidermis (Fig. 409-25); hyperpigmented or hypopigmented lesions are frequently seen in dark-skinned patients. The patches can vary from a few millimeters to a few centimeters in diameter; they are more common on sun-protected areas such as the buttocks. Lesions may be present for years. As the disease progresses, some of the patches may become more indurated and may evolve into plaques (Fig. 409-26). Nodular lesions may occur in patients without any patch or plaque lesions, although more commonly these lesions occur in conjunction with patches and plaques. Erythrodermic mycosis fungoides occurs as a generalized erythroderma with significant scaling and pruritus. Hyperkeratosis of the palms and soles and fissuring of hands and feet are quite common.

The diagnosis is confirmed by histologic demonstration of atypical mononuclear cells both in the epidermis and in the dermis, as well as immunophenotypic markers showing predominance of CD4 cells in the infiltrate. Treatment options are summarized in Table 409-7.[14]

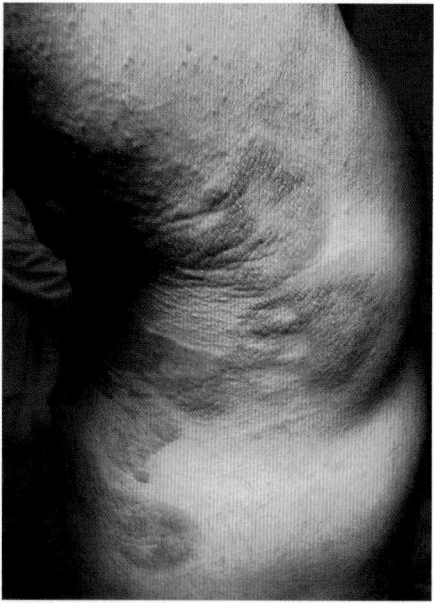

FIGURE 409-26. Mycosis fungoides. Plaque-stage disease.

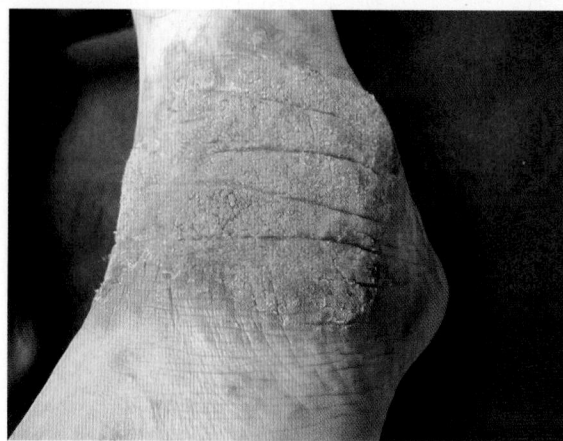

FIGURE 409-27. Necrolytic acral erythema. Lichenified plaques with fine scales on anterior lateral ankle.

TABLE 409-7	TREATMENT FOR MYCOSIS FUNGOIDES
CLINICAL TYPE	**TREATMENT**
Patch and localized plaque	Topical corticosteroids (e.g., triamcinolone ointment 0.1% q12h)
	Topical retinoids (e.g., bexarotene gel 1%, one to four times/day)
	Narrowband UVB (two to three times/wk)
Extensive plaques and Tumors	Psoralen and UVA (PUVA; two to three times/wk)
	Oral bexarotene (300 mg/m² /day)
	Methotrexate (15-25 mg/wk)
	Pegylated interferon-α2A 180 μg SC weekly
	Total skin electron beam therapy
	Histone deacetylase inhibitors: vorinostat (400 mg/day PO); romidepsin (14 mg/m² IV on days 1, 8, and 15 of a 28-day cycle)
	Low-dose pralatrexate (15 mg/m² IV, weekly for 6 wk in a 7-wk cycle)
	Brentuximab vedotin (1.2-1.8 mg/kg, maximum dose: 150 mg IV every 3 wk)
	Gemcitabine (750-1000 mg/m², IV, weekly for 3 week cycles)
	Pegylated liposomal doxorubicin (20 mg/m², IV, every 2-4 weeks)
	Radiation therapy for localized tumors
Erythrodermic	Extracorporeal photopheresis (2 consecutive days every 2-4 wk)

IV = intravenously; PO = orally; qd = daily; SC= subcutaneously; UVA = ultraviolet A; UVB = ultraviolet B.

Bazex Syndrome and Necrolytic Acral Erythema

Patients with Bazex syndrome (acrokeratosis neoplastica) present with symmetrical, scaly, erythematous-to-violaceous hyperkeratotic plaques on acral areas, such as digits, palms, soles, nose, and ears. Almost all have involvement of the ears and ridging of the nails. Bazex syndrome is associated with malignancy, especially of lips, tongue, larynx, pharynx, and esophagus, perhaps because of cross-reactivity between tumor antigens and normal keratinocytic antigens.

Necrolytic acral erythema is a marker of chronic hepatitis C infection (Chapter 140). It manifests with well-defined hyperkeratotic, lichenified plaques on the dorsum of the hands and feet (Fig. 409-27). Low serum zinc levels have been reported in some patients whose disease improved after oral zinc therapy.

Dermatophytoses

Fungal infections that occur as papulosquamous eruptions include tinea corporis, tinea manuum, tinea cruris, and tinea pedis. *Tinea corporis* manifests as

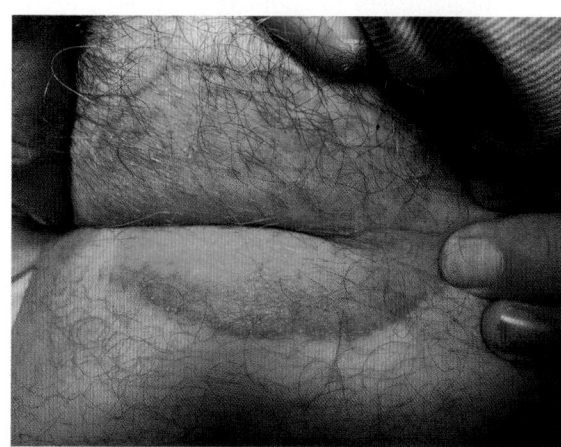

FIGURE 409-28. Tinea cruris. Erythematous patch with erythematous papules and scales at the periphery.

a polycyclic erythematous scaly patch that has elevated borders which consist of papules and pustules; the border advances centrifugally. The trunk is the most common site. *Tinea cruris* has similar morphology, except it is located in the inguinal folds (Fig. 409-28). *Tinea manuum* presents as an erythematous scaly patch with an advancing active border, usually located on the dorsum of the hands, or it may occur as diffuse scaly patches with mild hyperkeratosis involving part or the entire surface of the palm and palmar aspect of the fingers. *Tinea pedis* can occur as scaly macerated lesions with erythema in the toe webs, or as patchy or diffuse scaliness on the sole extending to the medial and lateral aspect of the foot (moccasin distribution). The latter presentation can be associated with diffuse scaliness of one but not both palms, a condition known as the "one-hand, two-feet syndrome." The diagnosis can be confirmed by examination of skin scrapings using 10% potassium hydroxide preparation or by fungal culture. Treatment consists of topical or oral antifungal medications (e.g., clotrimazole cream, 1%, twice daily for 2 to 4 weeks, or terbinafine, 250 mg for 2 to 12 weeks), depending on the site involved. Nail involvement (Chapter 413) is best treated with systemic therapy, although typical therapies can be useful as well.

TINEA VERSICOLOR

Tinea versicolor is a fungal infection of the skin caused by *Malassezia furfur*. It occurs in otherwise healthy young individuals, especially in warm and moist environments during the summer. The prevalence is estimated to be 2 to 8% in the United States and up to 50% in the tropical countries. Clinically, it appears as asymptomatic macules and patches with very fine scales; the color can be hypopigmented, skin colored, minimally erythematous, or light brown (Fig. 409-29). The patches start as perifollicular macules, with the midchest and midback the most common sites. The diagnosis is confirmed by the characteristic appearance of the fungal elements on a 10% potassium hydroxide preparation—grapelike clusters of yeast and short, septate branching hyphae ("spaghetti and meatballs" appearance). Treatment is with 2.5% selenium

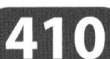

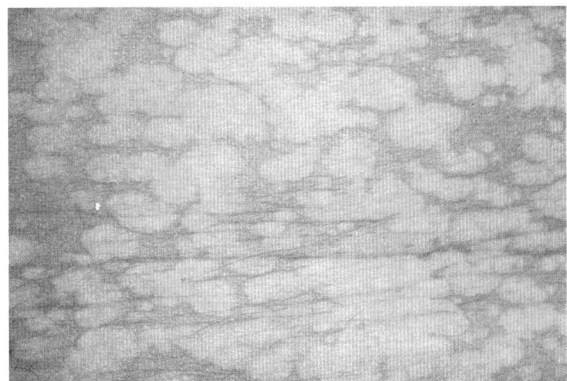

FIGURE 409-29. Tinea versicolor. Hypopigmented patches on the trunk.

sulfide shampoo (applied for 10 minutes then washed off, five times weekly for 4 to 6 weeks), topical antifungal preparations (e.g., clotrimazole cream, 1% twice daily for 4 weeks), or a 1- to 3-day course of oral ketoconazole (200 mg/day).

FIGURATE ERYTHEMIAS

The figurate erythemas (which include erythema annulare centrifugum, erythema gyratum repens, and erythema chronicum migrans) appear as erythematous circular or polycyclic plaques with central clearing and, frequently, a centrifugally migrating border. Occasionally, fine scaling also may be observed. The extremities are the most common sites. The diagnosis frequently can be made by the typical history and morphologic features.

Erythema annulare centrifugum is most commonly idiopathic; however, it also can be a manifestation of a hypersensitivity response to medications. Management includes identification of a precipitating agent (if possible) and treatment with topical or systemic corticosteroids. *Erythema gyratum repens* occurs as concentric erythematous plaques with fine scales, resembling a wood-grain pattern. This unusual form of figurate erythema has been associated with malignant hematologic diseases and with carcinomas of the breast, lung, gastrointestinal tract, prostate, and cervix. Treatment of the underlying malignant disease results in the resolution of the skin lesion in a few months. *Erythema chronicum migrans* is a cutaneous manifestation of Lyme disease and is caused by the spirochete *Borrelia burgdorferi* (Chapter 305); it appears as a concentric ring of erythema that progresses centrifugally from the site of a tick bite. Occasionally, it may appear as a circular erythematous patch. The diagnosis is made by a history of a tick bite, the characteristic cutaneous lesion, or elevated serum antibodies to *B. burgdorferi*. Management is the same as for Lyme disease.

Grade A References

A1. Paller AS, Tom WL, Lebwohl MG, et al. Efficacy and safety of crisaborole ointment, a novel, nonsteroidal phosphodiesterase 4 (PDE4) inhibitor for the topical treatment of atopic dermatitis (AD) in children and adults. *J Am Acad Dermatol*. 2016;75:494-503.

A2. Simpson EL, Bieber T, Guttman-Yassky E, et al. Two phase 3 trials of dupilumab versus placebo in atopic dermatitis. *N Engl J Med*. 2016;375:2335-2348.

A3. Blauvelt A, de Bruin-Weller M, Gooderham M, et al. Long-term management of moderate-to-severe atopic dermatitis with dupilumab and concomitant topical corticosteroids (LIBERTY AD CHRONOS): a 1-year, randomised, double-blinded, placebo-controlled, phase 3 trial. *Lancet*. 2017;389:2287-2303.

A4. Ruzicka T, Hanifin JM, Furue M, et al. Anti-interleukin-31 receptor A antibody for atopic dermatitis. *N Engl J Med*. 2017;376:826-835.

A5. Reich K, Pinter A, Lacour JP, et al. Comparison of ixekizumab with ustekinumab in moderate-to-severe psoriasis: 24-week results from IXORA-S, a phase III study. *Br J Dermatol*. 2017;177:1014-1023.

A6. Reich K, Papp KA, Blauvelt A, et al. Tildrakizumab versus placebo or etanercept for chronic plaque psoriasis (reSURFACE 1 and reSURFACE 2): results from two randomised controlled, phase 3 trials. *Lancet*. 2017;390:276-288.

A7. Reich K, Armstrong AW, Foley P, et al. Efficacy and safety of guselkumab, an anti-interleukin-23 monoclonal antibody, compared with adalimumab for the treatment of patients with moderate to severe psoriasis with randomized withdrawal and retreatment: results from the phase III, double-blind, placebo- and active comparator-controlled VOYAGE 2 trial. *J Am Acad Dermatol*. 2017;76:418-431.

A8. Lebwohl M, Strober B, Menter A, et al. Phase 3 studies comparing brodalumab with ustekinumab in psoriasis. *N Engl J Med*. 2015;373:1318-1328.

GENERAL REFERENCES

For the General References and other additional features, please visit Expert Consult at https://expertconsult.inkling.com.

410

MACULAR, PAPULAR, PURPURIC, VESICOBULLOUS, AND PUSTULAR DISEASES

DANIELA KROSHINSKY

MACULAR AND PAPULAR EXANTHEMS

An exanthem, which is an acute generalized eruption of the skin, can be scarlatiniform or morbilliform. Scarlatiniform eruptions consist of confluent blanching erythema resembling innumerable small papules. Morbilliform eruptions are erythematous macules and papules that resemble the eruption of measles. Morbilliform eruptions can be caused by viral infections or by hypersensitivity reactions to medications (Chapter 411) (Table 410-1).

Scarlatiniform Eruptions
SCARLET FEVER

Scarlet fever is usually a sequela of toxin-producing β-hemolytic streptococcal infection (Chapter 274) of the ears, nose, throat, or skin, although *Staphylococcus aureus* (Chapter 272), *Haemophilus influenzae* (Chapter 284), or *Clostridium* spp. (Chapter 280) cause occasional cases. The skin lesions often are accompanied by fever, headache, malaise, chills, sore throat, and vomiting.

On physical examination, the mucous membranes are usually erythematous with petechiae. A white membrane is often seen on the tongue, and tonsillitis may be present. The rash, which appears after the fever, is typically fine erythematous papules, beginning on the upper torso and then spreading. The face is characteristically flushed, with circumoral pallor. The rash persists for 4 to 5 days and is followed by desquamation.

Treatment is oral penicillin V 500 mg two to three times daily for 10 days or a single dose of intramuscular benzathine penicillin G (1.2 million units). Clinical recovery usually takes only 4 to 5 days, but the rash typically takes several weeks to resolve.

TOXIC SHOCK SYNDROME

Toxic shock syndrome is an acute febrile illness, usually caused by toxin-producing *S. aureus* (Chapter 272) but sometimes caused by *Streptococcus* spp. (toxic shock–like syndrome [Chapter 274]). Most cases are in previously healthy adults between 20 and 50 years of age.

CLINICAL MANIFESTATIONS

The clinical manifestations of toxic shock syndrome are a result of the massive release of tumor necrosis factor-α (TNF-α) and interleukin-1: fever, diffuse macular erythema (Fig. 407-5 in Chapter 407), severe conjunctival involvement, and erythema of the mucous membranes of the lungs, liver, gastrointestinal tract, and kidneys.[1] Blood cultures are positive in about 5 to 15% of patients who have staphylococcal toxic shock syndrome and about 50% of patients who have streptococcal toxic shock–like syndrome.

TABLE 410-1 EXANTHEMS

SCARLATINIFORM ERUPTIONS

Scarlet fever (see below)
Toxic shock syndrome (Chapter 274)
Kawasaki disease (Chapter 254)

MORBILLIFORM ERUPTIONS

Measles (Chapter 343)
Rubella (Chapter 344)
Erythema infectiosum (Chapter 347)
Roseola (Chapter 350)

For staphylococcal toxic shock syndrome caused by methicillin-sensitive organisms, treatment is oxacillin or nafcillin (2 g IV every 4 hours) or cefazolin (2 g IV every 8 hours) in the setting of a true penicillin allergy plus clindamycin (900 mg IV every 8 hours). For staphylococcal toxic shock syndrome due to methicillin-resistant *S. aureus*, treatment is vancomycin (15 to 20 mg/kg every 8 to 12 hours, not to exceed 2 g per dose) plus clindamycin (900 mg IV every 8 hours).

Streptococcal toxic shock syndrome should be empirically treated with clindamycin (900 mg IV every 8 hours) plus penicillin G (4 million units IV every 4 hours) until susceptibilities return. Alternatives to penicillin are ceftriaxone (1 to 2 g IV every 12 hours), cefazolin (1 to 2 g IV every 8 hours), vancomycin (30 mg/kg/day IV in two divided doses) or daptomycin (6 mg/kg IV every 24 hours).

PROGNOSIS

Desquamation of the skin of the palms and soles typically occurs 1 to 2 weeks after the onset of the rest. Staphylococcal toxic shock syndrome has a mortality of 5 to 15%, whereas the mortality rate for streptococcal toxic shock–like syndrome can be five times higher.

KAWASAKI DISEASE

Kawasaki disease (Chapter 254), which is a systemic vasculitis of unknown etiology, is primarily an illness of children under age 5 years, but it also can occur in adults. It is far more common in Northeast Asians than in whites.

CLINICAL MANIFESTATIONS

Patients typically present with very high fever and a scarlatiniform, morbilliform, urticarial, or targetoid rash. Other features include conjunctival infection, hemorrhagic and dry, fissured lips, a "strawberry tongue," and cervical lymphadenitis. Arthralgias, frank arthritis, urethritis, diarrhea, pneumonitis, and aseptic meningitis can occur, but the most serious complications in untreated patients are coronary artery aneurysms and myocarditis.

DIAGNOSIS

No diagnostic tests are helpful, so the diagnosis is clinical and is based on the typical rash and the development of myocarditis.

TREATMENT   **Rx**

Acute treatment is a single infusion of 2 g/kg of IV gamma globulin (IVIG) given over 8 to 12 hours within 5 to 10 days after the onset of fever.[2] Aspirin 30 to 50 mg/kg daily divided into four doses is also indicated. Patients at higher risk for resistance to IVIG should additionally receive supplemental intravenous corticosteroids for 15 days: 5 days each at the equivalent of a prednisone dose of 2 mg/kg, 1 mg/kg, and 0.5 mg/kg, with conversion to oral therapy within a day of discharge.

Morbilliform Eruptions

Acute viral infections that can cause morbilliform rashes include measles (Chapter 343), rubella (Chapter 344), erythema infectiosum (Chapter 347), and roseola (Chapter 350). With measles, the enanthem (Koplik spots; see Fig. 343-2 in Chapter 343) precedes the exanthem (Fig. 343-3 in Chapter 343) by 1 to 2 days and persists for 2 to 4 days. The exanthem begins on the fourth or fifth day, typically with papules on the face and behind the ears, with subsequent spread to the trunk and extremities. The exanthem of rubella (Fig. 344-1 in Chapter 344) starts as pink facial macules and papules that spread to the trunk and extremities and that persist for only 1 to 3 days. In erythema infectiosum (Chapter 347), a bright red erythema develops suddenly over the cheeks (Fig. 347-1 in Chapter 347), followed within 1 to 4 days by an erythematous morbilliform rash on the extremities (Fig. 410-1). In roseola (Chapter 350), 2 or so days of pink papules or blanchable macular erythema typically follow defervescence after a high fever.

These viruses are typically diagnosed on clinical grounds, but polymerase chain reaction testing is both sensitive and specific.[3,4] For each of these viruses, treatment is supportive because no antiviral therapy is efficacious.

Papular Eruptions
INFECTIOUS ERUPTIONS
Molluscum Contagiosum

In molluscum contagiosum, patients develop individual, grouped, or widely disseminated papules that are firm, smooth, frequently umbilicated, and usually 2 to 6 mm in diameter (Fig. 410-2). In patients who are infected with human immunodeficiency virus (HIV), hundreds of lesions may be seen (Chapter 366). The diagnosis is clinical.

Treatment options include cryotherapy with liquid nitrogen, curettage, cantharidin, podophyllin, and cimetidine.

Warts

Warts are benign skin and mucosal proliferations caused by over 150 types of human papillomaviruses (HPVs) (Chapter 349). Common warts, which can occur anywhere on the body, are firm, hyperkeratotic papules ranging in size from 1 mm to more than 1 cm (Fig. 410-3). Other variants include genital warts, flat warts, and deep palmoplantar warts. The diagnosis is clinical, but larger or atypical lesions should be biopsied to exclude malignant transformation. Common topical treatments include: liquid nitrogen, cantharidin, or podophyllin, as well as prescription-strength salicylic acid, imiquimod, or 5-fluorouracil. Over-the-counter liquid nitrogen is not as cold and, as a result, not as effective as in-office treatment.

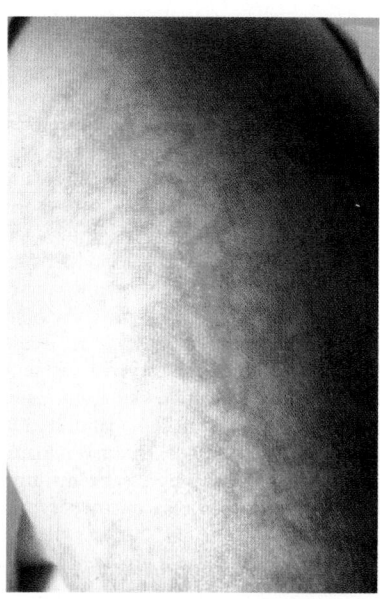

FIGURE 410-1. Reticulate macular erythema on the thigh of a patient with erythema infectiosum. (Courtesy Neil J. Korman, MD.)

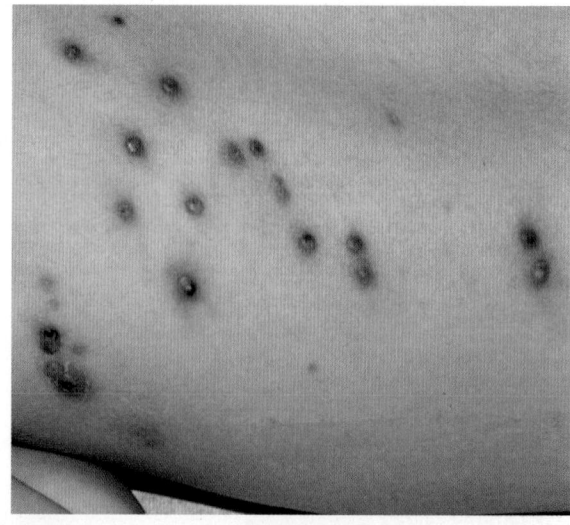

FIGURE 410-2. Pustular presentation of inflamed molluscum contagiosum. A culture revealed only normal skin flora. (From Mancini AJ, Shani-Adir A, Sidbury, R. Other viral diseases. In: Bolognia JL, Schaffer JV, Cerroni L, eds. *Dermatology.* 4th ed. Elsevier; 2018:1440.)

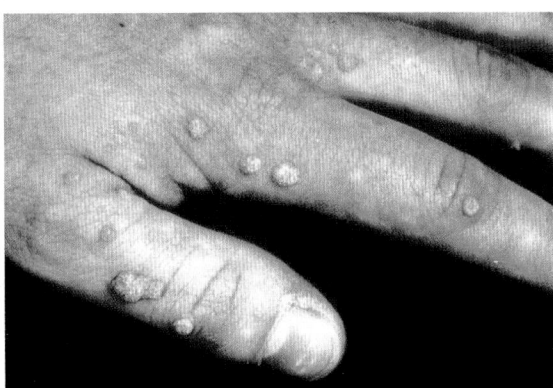

FIGURE 410-3. Hand of a patient with verruca vulgaris revealing many verrucous papules. (Courtesy Neil J. Korman, MD.)

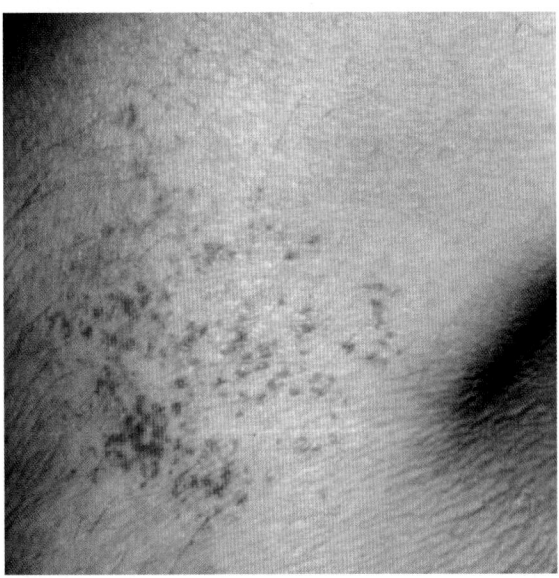

FIGURE 410-4. Round to oval petechiae, <3 mm in diameter. (From Piette WW. Purpura: mechanisms and differential diagnosis. In: Bolognia J, Schaffer J, Cerroni L, eds. *Dermatology.* 4th ed. Elsevier; 2018:377.)

TABLE 410-2 DIFFERENTIAL DIAGNOSIS OF MACULAR PETECHIAE, PURPURA, AND ECCHYMOSES

MACULAR PETECHIAE (≤4 mm IN DIAMETER)

Thrombocytopenia (platelets <50,000/μL) (Chapter 163)
Increased venous pressure
Trauma (Chapter 103)
Vitamin C deficiency (Chapter 205)
Pigmented purpuric eruptions
Waldenström macroglobulinemia (Chapter 178)

MACULAR PURPURA (5-9 mm)

Waldenström macroglobulinemia (Chapter 178)
Thrombocytopenia with infection or inflammation (Chapter 163)
Cutaneous small vessel vasculitis (Chapter 254)

MACULAR ECCHYMOSES (≥1 cm)

Anticoagulation (Chapter 76)
Hepatic insufficiency (Chapters 153 and 154)
Vitamin K deficiency (Chapter 166)
Disseminated intravascular coagulation (Chapter 166)
Actinic (solar, senile) purpura
Corticosteroid therapy, topical or systemic
Vitamin C deficiency (Chapter 205)
Systemic amyloidosis (Chapter 179)
Ehlers-Danlos syndrome (Chapter 244)
Thrombocytopenia (Chapter 163)
Platelet function defects (e.g., von Willebrand disease; Chapter 164)

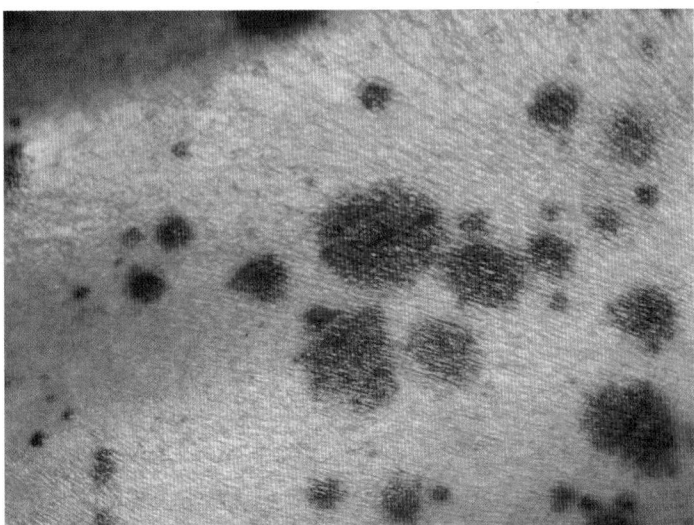

FIGURE 410-5. Palpable purpura due to cutaneous small vessel vasculitis (inflammation plus hemorrhage). (From Piette WW. Purpura: mechanisms and differential diagnosis. In: Bolognia J, Schaffer J, Cerroni L, eds. *Dermatology.* 4th ed. Elsevier; 2018:377.)

Purpuric Eruptions

Purpuric eruptions, which occur when the extravasation of blood results in visible skin or mucosal hemorrhage, are classified based on: their size as petechiae (≤4 mm; Table 410-2; Fig. 410-4), macular purpura (>4 to 10 mm; Fig. 410-5), or ecchymoses (>10 mm); and their morphology as palpable purpura (Table 410-3), and inflammatory and noninflammatory retiform purpura (Table 410-4).

NONPALPABLE PURPURA
Petechiae

A common cause of petechiae is Schamberg disease, in which petechiae result from idiopathic capillaritis. Most often seen in middle-aged to older adults, Schamberg disease presents with yellow-brown patches on the lower legs with overlying petechiae that are cayenne pepper colored. Lesions occasionally can be present on the trunk, buttocks, arms, and thighs. The lesions become hyperpigmented and then fade, with new lesions occurring over time. Topical steroids (see Table 407-10), ascorbic acid 500 mg twice daily, with or without rutoside 50 mg twice daily, can be helpful.

Systemic diseases that can result in petechiae include idiopathic thrombocytopenic purpura (Chapter 163), thrombocytopenia-caused diseases or medications that reduce platelet production (Chapter 163), abnormal platelet function as a result of renal or hepatic insufficiency (Chapters 121 and 144), and clotting factor abnormalities (Chapter 165). Treatment is for the underlying condition.

Macular Purpura

Waldenström macroglobulinemia (Chapter 178) presents with recurrent petechiae and macular purpura on the legs, typically associated with itching, stinging, or burning in the setting of a polyclonal hypergammaglobulinemia and high immunoglobulin G (IgG) or IgA rheumatoid factor titers. Some patients subsequently develop autoimmune connective tissue disease, especially Sjögren syndrome (Chapter 252) or lymphoma (Chapters 176 and 177).

Ecchymoses

Minor trauma in individuals who have lost dermal connective surrounding blood vessel tissue can result in macular ecchymoses. Solar purpura (Fig. 410-6), which is caused by aging and chronic sun exposure, is commonly seen on the forearms. Steroid purpura, which is related to prolonged treatment with topical or systemic corticosteroids, can develop anywhere on the skin (Chapter 32). Similar systemic examples include systemic amyloidosis (Chapter 179), scurvy (Chapter 205), and Ehlers-Danlos syndrome (Chapter 244).

PALPABLE PURPURA
Vasculitis

Palpable purpura is caused by inflammatory damage to small or small and medium-sized vessels, and the clinical findings depend on the size of the

TABLE 410-3 PALPABLE PURPURA: INFLAMMATORY PALPABLE PURPURA WITH PROMINENT EARLY ERYTHEMA

LEUKOCYTOCLASTIC VASCULITIS WITH IMMUNE COMPLEX DISEASE

Small Vessels Only

Idiopathic, infection-associated, or drug-associated
Waldenström macroglobulinemia (Chapter 178)
Urticarial vasculitis
Pustular vasculitis

Small- and Medium-Sized Vessels

Mixed cryoglobulinemia (Chapter 178)
Systemic lupus erythematosus (Chapter 250)
Rheumatoid arthritis (Chapter 248)
Sjögren syndrome (Chapter 252)

PAUCI-IMMUNE LEUKOCYTOCLASTIC VASCULITIS

Microscopic polyangiitis
Granulomatosis with polyangiitis (Chapter 254)
Eosinophilic granulomatosis with polyangiitis (Chapter 254)
Erythema elevatum diutinum
Sweet syndrome

OTHER

Erythema multiforme (see below)
Pityriasis lichenoides et varioliformis acuta
Pigmented purpuric eruptions (see above)
Waldenström macroglobulinemia (Chapter 178)

TABLE 410-4 DIFFERENTIAL DIAGNOSIS OF RETIFORM (ANGULATED OR BRANCHED) PURPURA

NON-INFLAMMATORY RETIFORM PURPURA

Protein C or protein S deficiency (Chapter 73)
Warfarin necrosis (Chapter 76)
Heparin necrosis
Thrombocytosis due to myeloproliferative neoplasms (Chapter 157)
Thrombotic thrombocytopenic purpura (Chapter 163)
Paroxysmal nocturnal hemoglobinuria (Chapter 151)
Cold agglutinins (Chapter 151)
Cryoglobulinemia (Chapter 178)
Cryofibrinogenemia (Chapter 72)
Vessel-invasive fungi
Ecthyma gangrenosum (Chapter 412)
Disseminated strongyloides (Chapter 335)
Postinfectious purpura fulminans (see above)
Antiphospholipid antibody (Chapter 73)
Livedoid vasculopathy
Malignant atrophic papulosis
Cholesterol emboli (Chapter 72)
Tumor emboli
Marantic endocarditis (Chapter 54)
Sickle cell disease (Chapter 154)
Malaria (Chapter 324)
Cutaneous calciphylaxis (Chapter 121)
Brown recluse spider bite (Chapter 104)
B-cell lymphoma (Chapter 176)

INFLAMMATORY RETIFORM PURPURA

Vasculitis

Systemic lupus erythematosus (Chapter 250)
Polyarteritis nodosa (Chapter 254)
Rheumatoid arthritis (Chapter 248)
Mixed cryoglobulinemia (Chapter 178)
Granulomatosis with polyangiitis (Chapter 254)
Eosinophilic granulomatosis with polyangiitis (Chapter 254)
Chilblains (Chapter 72)
Pyoderma gangrenosum (Chapter 407)

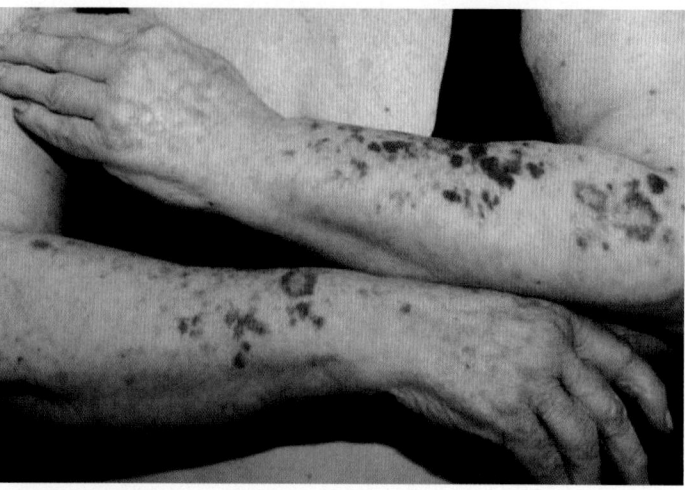

FIGURE 410-6. Solar (actinic) purpura in sites of actinic damage plus trauma. (Courtesy Kalman Watsky, MD. From Piette WW. Purpura: mechanisms and differential diagnosis. In: Bolognia J, Schaffer J, Cerroni L, eds. *Dermatology.* 4th ed. Elsevier; 2018:377.)

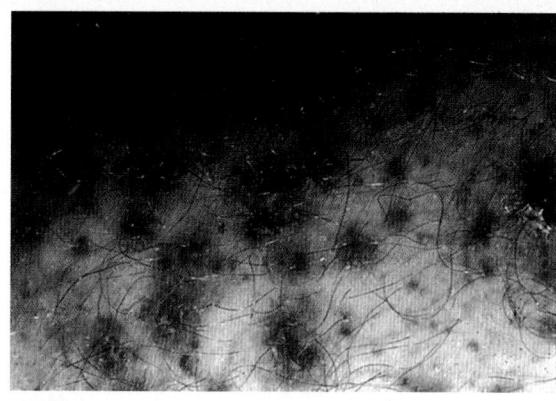

FIGURE 410-7. Palpable purpura. Leukocytoclastic vasculitis commonly causes raised purpuric and ulcerated lesions on the legs. (Courtesy Neil J. Korman, MD.)

within 48 hours of formation reveal a granular pattern of C3, IgG, IgM, and/or IgA deposits in blood vessel walls on direct immunofluorescence.

Patients with Henoch-Schönlein purpura, which usually follows a streptococcal or staphylococcal infection in adults, have perivascular deposits of IgA and C3 on skin biopsy. Patients may have fever, arthralgias, and abdominal pain, and they are at risk for renal vasculitis (Chapter 113).

Urticarial or hypocomplementemic vasculitis (Chapter 254) generally persists for more than 24 hours and is associated with arthritis, facial and laryngeal edema, and low levels of serum complement. Some patients may develop systemic lupus erythematosus (Chapter 250).

A urinalysis and renal and liver function testing should be performed. Specialized tests should be ordered based on the suspected cause (see Table 410-3).

TREATMENT   Rx

Treatment is based on the diagnosis. For idiopathic leukocytoclastic vasculitis, oral treatment options include: colchicine (0.6 mg twice daily); prednisone (1 mg/kg/day); or dapsone (up to 200 mg once daily). In severe cases, immunosuppressive options include: mycophenolate mofetil (up to 45 mg/kg); azathioprine (up to 2.5 mg/kg); or cyclophosphamide (up to 2.5 mg/kg) continued until the disease becomes inactive.

RETIFORM PURPURA

Retiform purpura is defined as large patches of purpura, each with a netlike or angulated border. Retiform purpura can be inflammatory or noninflammatory but typically is not raised.

Inflammatory Retiform Purpura

Inflammatory retiform purpura is characterized by stellate or branching purpura, but early lesions also demonstrate prominent surrounding erythema

affected vessel. Leukocytoclastic vasculitis, which is the most common form of small-vessel vasculitis (Fig. 410-7), may be idiopathic, but it also can be associated with infection, drug reactions, connective tissue disease, cryoglobulinemia, and underlying malignancy. Biopsy is often required to confirm the clinical diagnosis (E-Fig. 410-1). Skin biopsy specimens taken from lesions

(Fig. 410-8). The skin lesions can be associated with microscopic polyangiitis (Chapter 254), granulomatosis with polyangiitis (Chapter 254), and eosinophilic granulomatosis with polyangiitis (Chapter 254).

In granulomatosis with polyangiitis, palpable purpura and oral ulcerations are the most common lesions, but patients may also develop painful subcutaneous nodules and ulcers that mimic pyoderma gangrenosum. In eosinophilic granulomatosis with polyangiitis, the skin disease usually presents as palpable purpura with necrosis on the legs, but retiform purpura, urticaria, subcutaneous nodules, livedo racemosa, and papulonecrotic lesions may be seen.

Skin biopsy often is key to the diagnosis of these conditions, and treatment is for systemic disease (Chapter 254). The skin lesions generally resolve if the systemic disease responds to treatment.

Noninflammatory Retiform Purpura
Cutaneous Emboli
Cutaneous emboli, especially cholesterol emboli (Chapter 72) and infectious emboli (Chapter 67), can lead to retiform as well as palpable purpura. Cholesterol emboli, which tend to affect older patients with advanced atherosclerotic disease, can occur spontaneously upon fragmentation of an atheromatous plaque or, more commonly, acutely after catheterization, within hours to days after thrombolysis, or months after the initiation of systemic anticoagulation. Other symptoms and signs can include fever, altered mental status, myalgias, weight loss, acute kidney injury (Chapter 116), and new or worsened arterial hypertension. In addition to the acute onset of retiform purpura, patients may also develop cyanosis (Fig. 410-9), distal livedo reticularis, nodules, ulceration, and even gangrene. Up to 80% of patients have peripheral eosinophilia.

Emboli with retiform or palpable purpura can be seen in patients with infectious endocarditis (Chapter 67) and are most commonly seen in acute meningococcemia (Fig. 282-3 in Chapter 282) and disseminated gonococcal infection (Fig. 283-3 in Chapter 283). In ecthyma gangrenosum, patients infected with *Pseudomonas aeruginosa* (Chapter 290) or less commonly *Klebsiella* spp. (Chapter 289), *Escherichia coli* (Chapter 288), or *Serratia* spp. (Chapter 289) develop erythematous papules and plaques with central purpura and hemorrhagic necrosis. Fungal infections have also been implicated in immunocompromised patients.

Other emboli that may cause petechiae or purpura include fat emboli after bone trauma (Chapters 74 and 103), emboli from an atrial myxoma (Chapter 54) or ventricular thrombus, and emboli from nonbacterial thrombotic endocarditis (Chapter 54).

Thrombi
Noninflammatory retiform purpura can occur when patients with disseminated intravascular coagulation (DIC) (Chapter 166), thrombotic thrombocytopenic purpura (Chapter 163), monoclonal cryoglobulinemia (Chapter 178), and drug reactions to warfarin (Chapter 76) develop in situ thrombi. DIC also can be associated with hemorrhagic bullae and purpura fulminans (Fig. 410-10). Cryoglobulinemia (Chapter 178) may be associated with leukemia, lymphoma, multiple myeloma, and Waldenström macroglobulinemia (Chapter 178).

Another thrombotic cause of purpura is thrombotic thrombocytopenic purpura (Chapter 163).

Warfarin skin necrosis (Chapter 76), which is an uncommon complication that typically occurs between the third and tenth day of therapy in patients who are not also receiving bridging heparin anticoagulation, presents as painful erythematous to purpuric plaques (especially on the breasts, thighs, and buttocks) that can progress to hemorrhagic bullae. The course of the disease is not dependent on whether or not warfarin therapy is continued.

VESICULOBULLOUS DISEASES
Vesicles are clear, fluid-filled lesions smaller than 1 cm, whereas bullae are similar lesions larger than 1 cm. Causes of vesiculobullous lesions include genetic and immunologic conditions, infections, hypersensitivity reactions, metabolic or physical disorders, and inherited genetic defects (Table 410-5).[5]

Immunologically Mediated Blistering Diseases

Immunologically mediated blistering diseases are caused by autoantibodies that bind to components of the epidermal desmosome (pemphigoid) or hemidesmosome (pemphigus), where they activate complement and precipitate inflammation. Inflammatory cell proteases can degrade basement membrane proteins, thereby leading to the formation of subepidermal (pemphigoid) or intraepidermal (pemphigus) blisters.

Subepidermal Blistering Disorders
BULLOUS PEMPHIGOID
In bullous pemphigoid, which is an autoimmune blistering disease seen mostly in elderly individuals, patients develop pruritic, tense vesicles, bullae, and

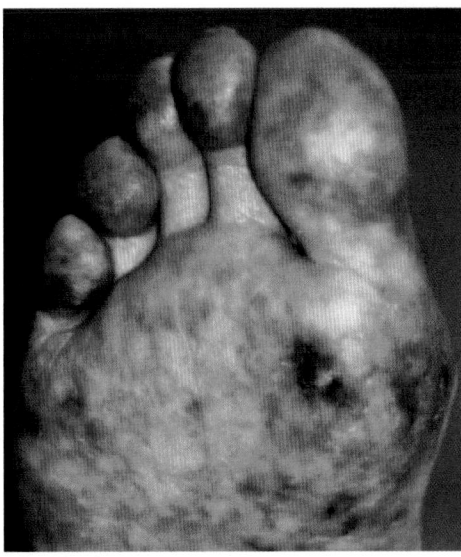

FIGURE 410-9. Cholesterol emboli. Both livedo reticularis and retiform purpura are seen distally. (Courtesy Norbert Sepp, MD. From Piette WW. Cutaneous manifestations of microvascular occlusion syndromes. In: Bolognia JL, Schaffer JV, Cerroni L, eds. *Dermatology.* 4th ed. Elsevier; 2018:399.)

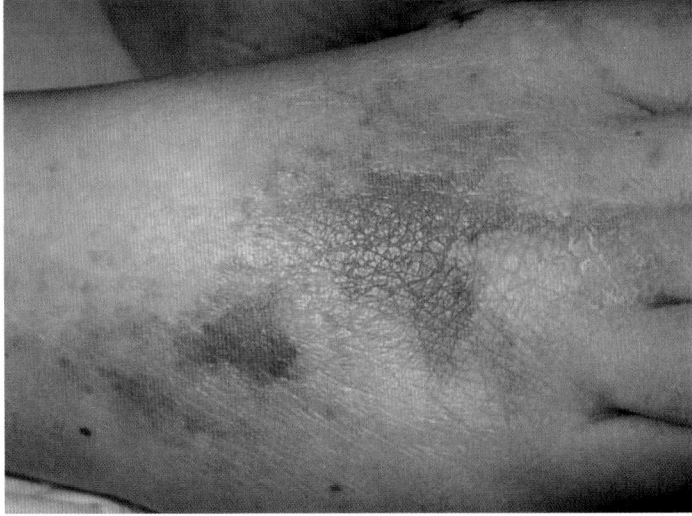

FIGURE 410-8. Polyarteritis nodosa. Retiform purpura of the dorsal foot in a patient with *systemic* polyarteritis nodosa. (From Wetter DA, Dutz JP, Shinkai K, et al. Cutaneous vasculitis. In: Bolognia JL, Schaffer JV, Cerroni L, eds. *Dermatology.* 4th ed. Elsevier; 2018:435.)

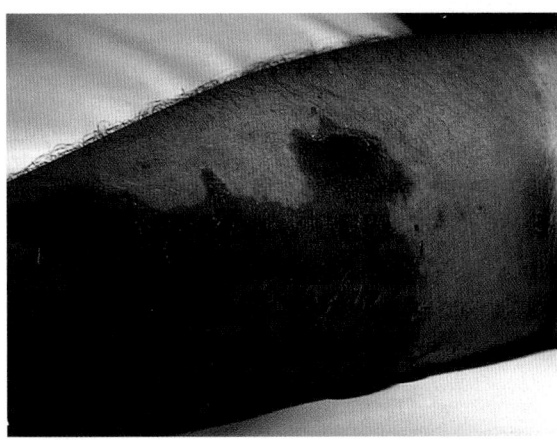

FIGURE 410-10. Purpura fulminans. Purpura and hemorrhagic blisters are seen on the arm of this patient.

TABLE 410-5 VESICULOBULLOUS DISEASES

GENETIC AND IMMUNOLOGIC

Bullous pemphigoid
Pemphigoid gestationis
Mucous membrane pemphigoid
Epidermolysis bullosa acquisita
Dermatitis herpetiformis
Linear immunoglobulin A bullous dermatosis
Pemphigus
    Vulgaris
    Foliaceus
    Paraneoplastic

INFECTIOUS DISEASES

Bullous impetigo
Herpes simplex
Varicella
Herpes zoster

HYPERSENSITIVITY

Erythema multiforme
Stevens-Johnson syndrome
Toxic epidermal necrolysis

METABOLIC/PHYSICAL

Porphyria cutanea tarda
Pseudoporphyria
Coma bulla
Bullous diabeticorum

Courtesy Neil J. Korman, MD.

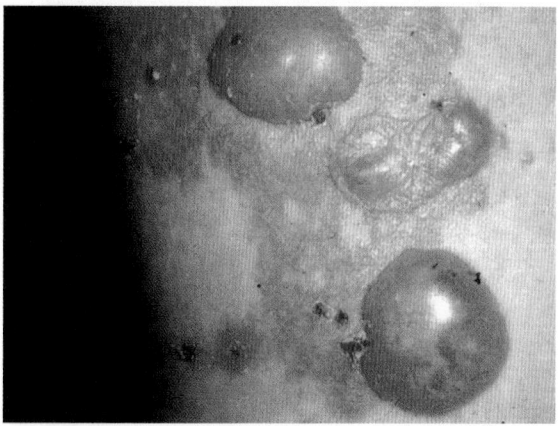

FIGURE 410-11. Bullous pemphigoid. Tense subepidermal bullae are seen on an erythematous base. (Courtesy Neil J. Korman, MD.)

urticarial or eczematous plaques on their torso and extremities, including their palms and soles. Up to 30% of patients (Fig. 410-11) also develop oral lesions.[6]

On skin biopsy, the subepidermal blisters have an eosinophilic infiltrate with linear IgG and C3 deposits at the basement membrane and IgG antibodies on the epidermal side.

TREATMENT   Rx

An ultrapotent (class 1) topical steroid can be used for patients with limited involvement, whereas oral prednisone (1 mg/kg/day) is rapidly effective in patients with moderate and severe disease. Steroid-sparing agents should be initiated to allow steroids to be tapered over several weeks after the formation of new lesions has ceased; effective options include: dapsone (up to 200 mg/day), methotrexate (up to 25 mg weekly), azathioprine (up to 2.5 mg/kg as guided by the patient's thiopurine methyltransferase level), and mycophenolate mofetil (up to 4 g divided into two daily doses). Refractory cases or patients who have side effects from these standard treatments may benefit from IVIG (2 g/kg divided over 2 to 3 days) or rituximab (375 mg/m² weekly for 4 weeks or 1000 mg given 2 weeks apart). The duration of therapy is guided by the activity of the disease and its response to medication.

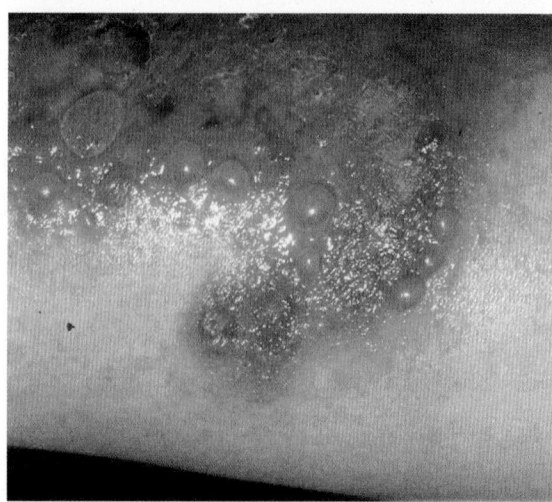

FIGURE 410-12. Pempigoid gestationis. Multiple tense blisters and erosions on an erythematous base are present. (Courtesy Neil J. Korman, MD.)

PROGNOSIS

In most patients, treatment suppresses the disease until the process fully resolves several years later. Left untreated, bullous pemphigoid generally undergoes spontaneous remissions and exacerbations with a high risk of infection.

Pemphigoid Gestationis

Pemphigoid gestationis is a rare autoimmune dermatosis predominantly arising in late pregnancy and/or immediately postpartum, although it can occur at any time during pregnancy. Intensely pruritic periumbilical urticarial plaques, which spread peripherally, progress to vesicles and blisters (Fig. 410-12). The face, palms, soles, and mucous membranes are typically spared. Skin biopsy shows bullous pemphigoid antigen II and linear C3 deposition in the basement membrane.

TREATMENT   Rx

Patients with mild disease should be treated with moderate or high-potency topical corticosteroids (see Table 407-10) twice daily to affected areas. Systemic corticosteroids (e.g., prednisone, 0.5 to 1 mg/kg once daily) should be reserved for patients who have extensive disease—usually 1 to 2 weeks of full-dose therapy, followed by a taper to the lowest effective dose. Antihistamines can be helpful in controlling itch. Women should be managed by experienced obstetricians because of the increased risk of premature labor and of the delivery of infants who are small for their gestational age.

Mucous Membrane Pemphigoid

Mucous membrane pemphigoid presents as blisters on oral, nasopharyngeal, ocular, laryngeal, anogenital, and esophageal surfaces. The scarring associated with their healing can cause major morbidity (Fig. 410-13).

Some patients with mucous membrane pemphigoid have circulating IgG autoantibodies against laminin 332 on the dermal side of skin, others have pure ocular disease with IgG antibodies against β_4 integrin, others have mucosal and skin lesions, and yet others have oral but not skin lesions. Biopsy shows subepidermal blister with basement membrane deposits of linear IgG, IgA, and C3, whereas circulating IgG and/or IgA antibodies are seen on indirect immunofluorescence.

TREATMENT   Rx

Treatment for mild disease is twice daily potent topical corticosteroids (or intralesional corticosteroids in patients with only oral disease). For ocular or significant oral disease, prednisone (1 mg/kg daily), cyclophosphamide (up to 2.5 mg/kg daily), rituximab (375 mg/m² weekly for 4 weeks or 1000 mg given 2 weeks apart), and IVIG (2 g/kg given over 2 to 3 days) may be required.

Mucous membrane pemphigoid is a chronic condition, and untreated ocular disease may lead to blindness.

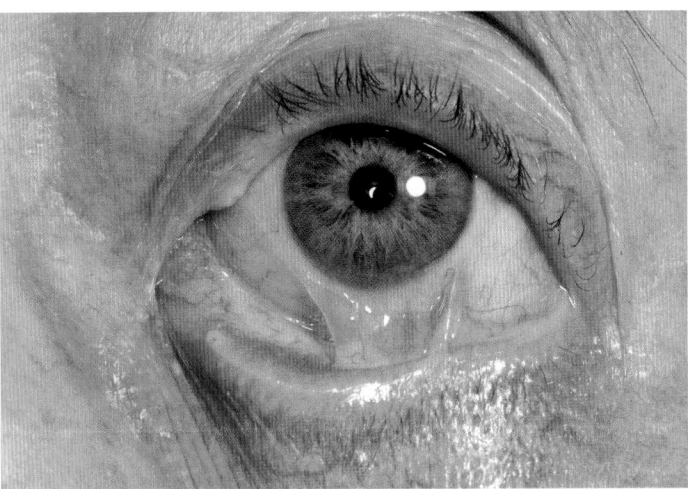

FIGURE 410-13. **Mucous membrane (cicatricial) pemphigoid.** Typical ocular involvement as manifested by fibrous tracts, representing partial or incomplete symblepharon. (From Bernard P, Borradori L. Pemphigoid group. In: Bolognia J, Schaffer J, Cerroni L, eds. *Dermatology.* 4th ed. Elsevier; 2018:521.)

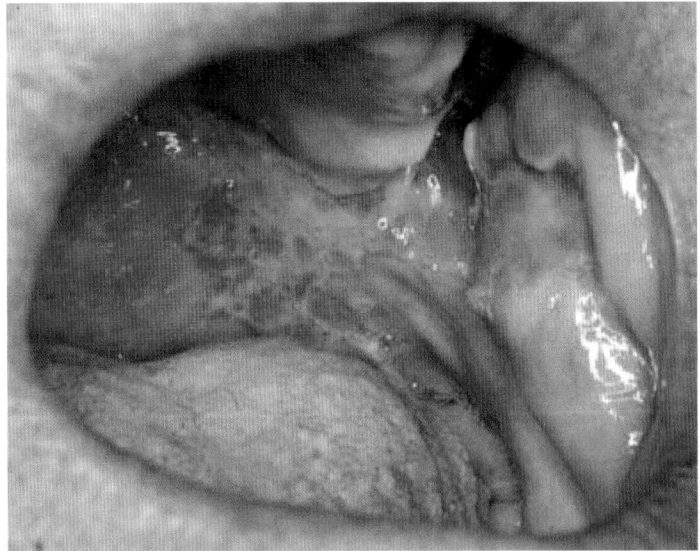

FIGURE 410-15. **Pemphigus vulgaris—oral involvement.** Essentially all patients develop painful oral mucosal erosions. The most common sites are the buccal and palatine mucosae, but lesions can also develop on the gingivae and tongue. (Courtesy Lorenzo Cerroni, MD. From Amagai M. Pemphigus. In: Bolognia JL, Schaffer JV, Cerroni L, eds. *Dermatology.* 4th ed. Elsevier; 2018:499.)

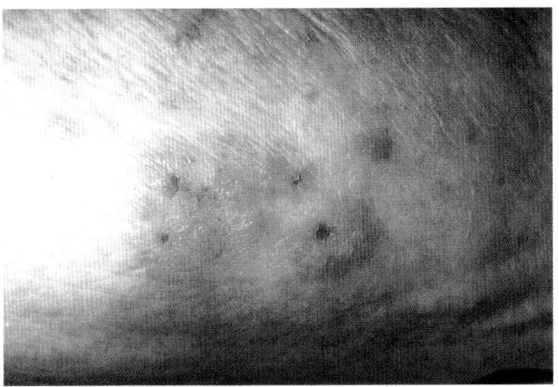

FIGURE 410-14. **Dermatitis herpetiformis.** The elbow of a patient has eroded erythematous papules and papulovesicles. (Courtesy Neil J. Korman, MD.)

EPIDERMOLYSIS BULLOSA ACQUISITA

Epidermolysis bullosa acquisita, which is an acquired autoimmune blistering disease, generally occurs in middle age. It can present as noninflammatory acral blisters, which heal with scarring, or as generalized inflammatory vesiculobullous disease. Biopsy shows subepidermal blisters with linear basement membrane IgG deposits that target collagen VII.

TREATMENT Rx

Epidermolysis bullosa acquisita is a chronic condition, and it can be refractory to treatment. Standard treatments, which are only occasionally successful, include colchicine (0.6 mg twice daily), dapsone (up to 200 mg/day), azathioprine (up to 2.5 mg/kg), or cyclophosphamide (2.5 mg/kg/day) alone or combined with prednisone (60 mg daily). For severe or refractory disease, options include cyclosporine (up to 5 mg/kg), rituximab (375 mg/m² weekly for 4 weeks or 1000 mg given 2 weeks apart), IVIG (2 g/kg given over 2 to 3 days), plasmapheresis, and extracorporeal photopheresis.

DERMATITIS HERPETIFORMIS

Dermatitis herpetiformis is an immune-mediated vesicular disease that occurs by middle age, almost always in patients who have a clinically known or subclinical gluten-sensitive enteropathy (Chapter 131). Skin lesions, which are very pruritic, can be grouped vesicles, papules, or erosions on the scalp, posterior neck, buttocks, and extensor surfaces of the elbows and knees (Fig. 410-14).[7] Many patients have other autoimmune medical conditions, such as diabetes or thyroid disease. Biopsy shows dermal papillary granular IgA deposits and neutrophilic microabscesses. In most patients, circulating IgA antibodies against tissue transglutaminase establish the diagnosis.

TREATMENT Rx

The skin disease can sometimes be controlled by diet alone, but the condition is lifelong. Treatment options also include twice-daily high-potency topical steroids (see Table 407-10) and dapsone (up to 200 mg/day) given chronically.

LINEAR IMMUNOGLOBULIN A BULLOUS DERMATOSIS

Linear IgA bullous dermatosis is an acquired autoimmune blistering disease that is usually associated with medications, especially vancomycin. Primary vesicles and bullae develop mainly on the flexural regions, but they can involve the oral mucous membranes and become generalized. Biopsy shows a subepidermal vesicle with neutrophil predominance and linear IgA specific for a portion of bullous pemphigoid antigen II at the basement membrane. Circulating IgA antibodies are detected on indirect immunofluorescence.

TREATMENT Rx

Patients usually respond to cessation of the offending medication and to dapsone (up to 200 mg/day). If the lesions do not respond, oral prednisone (1 mg/kg once daily) should be added.

Intraepidermal Blistering Disorders
PEMPHIGUS

Pemphigus refers to a group of intraepidermal autoimmune blistering diseases that affect the skin and mucous membranes.[8] Pemphigus is seen most commonly in middle age adults.

In *pemphigus vulgaris*, autoantibodies target desmoglein III. In *pemphigus foliaceus*, autoantibodies target desmoglein I. In *paraneoplastic pemphigus*, circulating antibodies react with a complex of proteins, including desmoplakin I and II, desmoglein I and III, bullous pemphigoid antigen I, envoplakin, and periplakin.

With pemphigus vulgaris, patients have flaccid blisters and erosions, which may be pruritic, in the oropharynx (Fig. 410-15), head, neck, and trunk. Patients with pemphigus foliaceus typically have erythema, scaling, and crusting on their scalp, face, and upper torso. Paraneoplastic pemphigus is characterized by ocular and oral blisters and erosions, as well as by polymorphous skin lesions that can resemble lichen planus, erythema multiforme, or pemphigoid. Associated malignancies include non-Hodgkin lymphoma (40%; Chapter

176); chronic lymphocytic leukemia (30%; Chapter 174); Castleman disease (10%; Chapters 176 and 366); thymomas (6%; Chapter 394); sarcomas (6%; Chapter 192); and Waldenström macroglobulinemia (6%; Chapter 178). Some patients can develop severe bronchiolitis obliterans.

In pemphigus vulgaris, biopsy shows suprabasilar acantholysis and deposits of IgG to desmoglein III. In pemphigus foliaceus, biopsy shows subcorneal acantholysis with IgG against desmoglein I. In patients with paraneoplastic pemphigus, biopsy shows suprabasilar acantholysis and dyskeratotic keratin-ocytes as well as antibodies to plakin proteins and IgG antibodies that are indistinguishable from those seen in pemphigus vulgaris.

TREATMENT   Rx

Treatment depends on the subtype and extent of pemphigus, as well as the rate of disease progression and the patient's age.[9] Oral prednisone (e.g., 1 mg/kg once daily) is indicated for the initial treatment of pemphigus vulgaris; topical corticosteroids (e.g., 0.05% fluocinonide ointment applied twice daily to affected areas) sometimes can control pemphigus foliaceus. Adding rituximab (375 mg/m² weekly for 4 weeks or 1000 mg IV separated by 2 weeks) to short-term (3 to 6 months) prednisone appears to be safer and more effective than longer-term prednisone alone,[A1] especially for extensive or recalcitrant disease. Steroid-sparing agents for pemphigus vulgaris include azathioprine (up to 2.5 mg/kg), mycophenolate mofetil (35 to 45 mg/kg/day divided into two daily doses), cyclophosphamide (up to 2.5 mg/kg), cyclosporine (3 to 5 mg/kg/day), and methotrexate (up to 25 mg/week). Plasmapheresis has been reported to be efficacious as well.

Systemic treatment of pemphigus foliaceus includes all of these same agents as well as dapsone (up to 200 mg/day) and hydroxychloroquine (total of <6 mg/kg of lean body mass in two divided daily doses). The duration of treatment varies with the level of disease activity.

When paraneoplastic pemphigus[10] is caused by benign tumors, such as Castleman disease,[11] it can be cured by removing the tumor (Chapter 176). Patients with associated malignant tumors should undergo treatment of their underlying condition but may have recalcitrant disease. Improvement has been reported with pulsed doses of corticosteroids (methylprednisolone, 1000 mg daily for 3 consecutive days) or cyclophosphamide (500 to 1000 mg monthly for 6 months to 1 year, often with varying doses of prednisone), rituximab (four weekly doses of 375 mg/m²), plasmapheresis, and immunoablative doses of cyclophosphamide (50 mg/kg/day for 4 days).

Morbidity and mortality are related to complications from immunosuppressive therapy. In patients with malignant tumors, the prognosis is generally poor.

Hypersensitivity Reactions Causing Blisters
ERYTHEMA MULTIFORME

Erythema multiforme is a self-limiting hypersensitivity reaction that involves the skin and sometimes mucosal surfaces in response to infection or more infrequently medication.[12] The primary findings are target lesions, which are erythematous to violaceous macules with three zones: two concentric circles and a deeply erythematous to dusky or violaceous center. Target lesions are predominantly concentrated on the distal extremities (Fig. 410-16). The lesions can become bullous or erosive, and in more severe cases erosions occur in the oral, ocular, and/or genital mucosa. The most common infectious causes of erythema multiforme are herpes simplex virus (HSV; Chapter 350) and mycoplasma pneumoniae (Chapter 301) followed by *Histoplasma capsulatum* (Chapter 316).

Biopsy demonstrates nonspecific keratinocyte necrosis, so the diagnosis is clinical.

TREATMENT   Rx

Mild cases of erythema multiforme can be treated symptomatically. Severe cases may require systemic corticosteroids (e.g., prednisone 0.5 to 1 mg/kg/day).

Lesions evolve, become fixed for up to 7 days, and then subside within 2 to 3 weeks. Recurrent episodes can occur. For recurrent erythema multiforme due to HSV, treatment is at least 6 months of antiviral treatment with acyclovir, valacyclovir, or famciclovir (Chapter 336).

Metabolic Disorders Causing Blisters
PORPHYRIA CUTANEA TARDA

Patients with porphyria cutanea tarda have fragility, erosions, and bullae in sun-exposed skin, especially of the face and the dorsal surface of the hands (Fig. 410-17) and the forearms. The cause is loss of activity of uroporphy-rinogen decarboxylase (Chapter 199).[13] Healing is associated with scars, atrophic patches, hyperpigmentation, and hypopigmentation. Hypertrichosis is commonly found over the malar and temporal areas. Diagnosis is based on elevated urinary porphyrin levels. Biopsy, though not necessary for the diag-nosis, shows a minimal dermal infiltrate, subepidermal blistering, and deposi-tion of immunoglobulin and complement at the basement membrane and in dermal capillaries.

TREATMENT   Rx

Depending on the type and cause, treatment options include phlebotomy (titrated so that the serum ferritin level declines to the lower limit of the normal range), hydroxychloroquine (100 mg—half of a 200-mg tablet), or chloroquine (125 mg—half of a 250-mg tablet) orally twice per week until porphyrin excre-tion remains normal for several months.

PSEUDOPORPHYRIA

Pseudoporphyria, which is similar to porphyria cutanea tarda histologically and clinically but is not seen with any abnormalities of porphyrin, can be associated with chronic renal insufficiency (Chapter 121) or hemodialysis (Chapter 122). It can also occur as a reaction to medications, such as nonster-oidal anti-inflammatory drugs (NSAIDs), oral contraceptives, furosemide, tetracycline, ciprofloxacin, isotretinoin, amiodarone, cyclosporine, dapsone, isotretinoin, 5-fluorouracil, oral contraceptives, and flutamide. When the offending agent is discontinued, the prognosis is good, but skin lesions may persist or recur for several months.

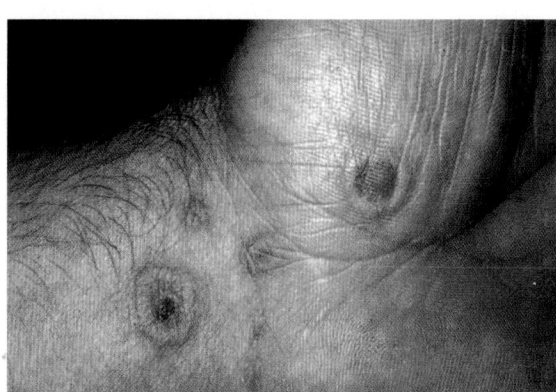

FIGURE 410-16. Erythema multiforme. Target or "bull's-eye" annular lesions with central vesicles and bullae are characteristic of erythema multiforme. (Courtesy Neil J. Korman, MD.)

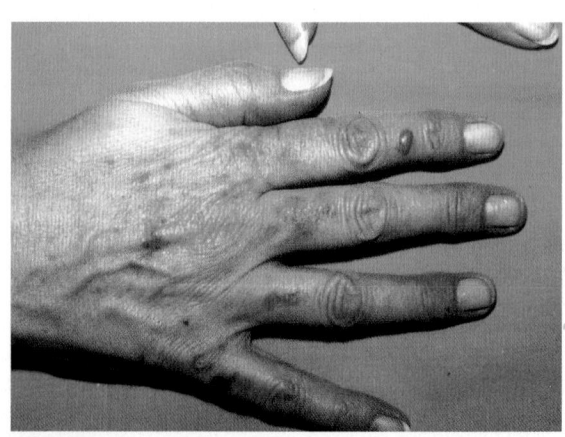

FIGURE 410-17. Porphyria cutanea tarda. A blister and erosions are present on the dorsal surface of the hand. (Courtesy Neil J. Korman, MD.)

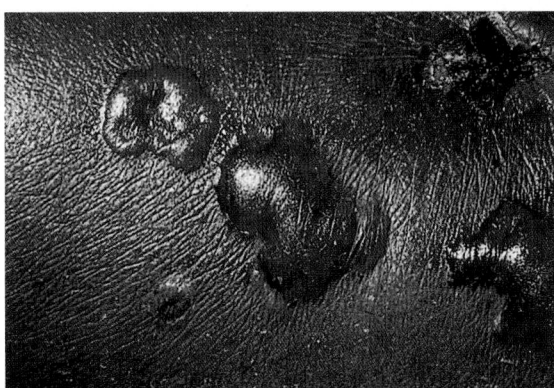

FIGURE 410-18. Bullous impetigo. Multiple blisters are present on the trunk of this patient.

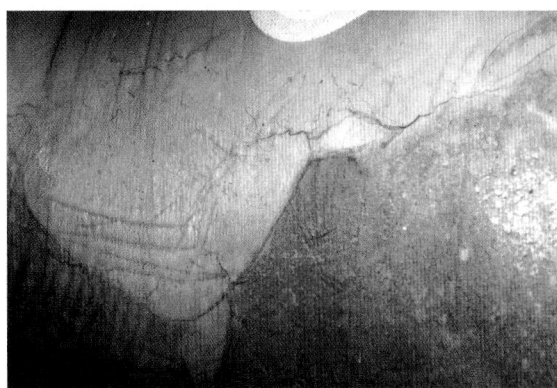

FIGURE 410-19. Staphylococcal scalded skin syndrome. Confluent erythema with exfoliation of skin is seen on the trunk. (Courtesy Neil J. Korman, MD.)

BULLOSIS DIABETICORUM

Patients with diabetes mellitus (Chapter 216) can develop blisters on their distal extremities. The pathobiology is not understood, and there is no relationship of the skin lesions with the severity, duration, or complications of diabetes. Lesions present spontaneously as large, tense, noninflammatory bulla, often with irregular shapes. Lesions may become unroofed to leave erosions. The lesions should be left in place or lanced and drained, leaving the roof in place to serve as a sterile physiologic dressing to reduce the risk of secondary infection. The condition is self-limiting.

Infectious Diseases Causing Blisters
BULLOUS IMPETIGO

Impetigo, which is an epidermal bacterial infection, can be caused by *S. aureus* (Chapter 272) and group A β-hemolytic streptococcus (Chapter 274). Exfoliative toxins A and B target epidermal protein desmoglein 1 and cause cleavage below or within the stratum granulosum. Bullous impetigo presents with superficial vesicles and bulla that easily rupture, thereby resulting in a collarette of scale (Fig. 410-18). Lesions are commonly on the face, trunk, axillae, and perineum. Diagnosis is clinical, with culture of the lesions confirming the causative bacteria.

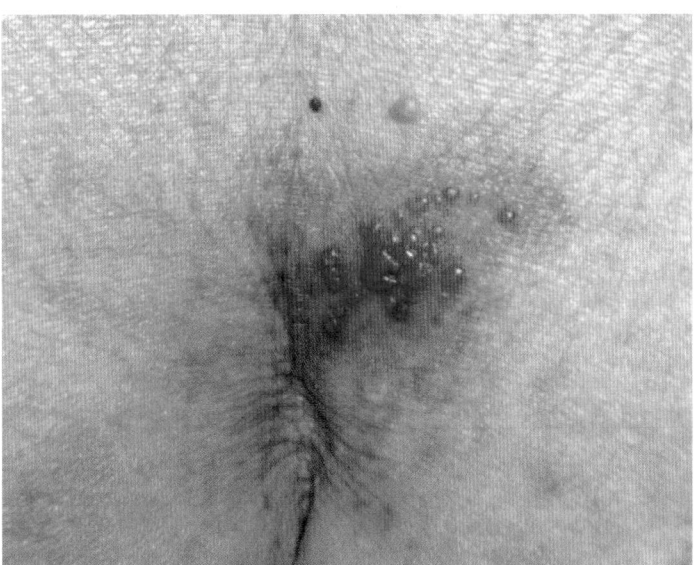

FIGURE 410-20. Recurrent genital herpes. Intact grouped vesicles and/or vesiculo-pustules with an erythematous base above the gluteal cleft. (Courtesy Kalman Watsky, MD. From Downing C, Mendoza N, Sra K, et al. Human herpesvirus. In: Bolognia JL, Schaffer JV, Cerroni L, eds. *Dermatology.* 4th ed. Elsevier; 2018:1404.)

> ## TREATMENT   Rx
>
> Gentle washing is recommended to remove any crusts. Limited cases can be treated with topical 2% mupirocin ointment. Oral antibiotics (e.g., dicloxacillin 500 mg four times daily or cephalexin 500 mg three times daily) for 7 days are indicated for extensive disease and for patients who do not respond to topical antibiotics.

STAPHYLOCOCCAL SCALDED SKIN SYNDROME

Hematogenous dissemination of exfoliative staphylococcal toxins A and B can result in staphylococcal scalded skin syndrome (Chapter 272). In adults, it is usually seen with renal insufficiency (Chapter 121) or systemic immunosuppression. Patients present with the sudden onset of fever accompanied by blanchable, tender erythema that begins over the face, the neck, and intertriginous areas and then generalizes rapidly. Unlike toxic shock syndrome, the palms, soles, and mucous membranes are not affected. Flaccid blisters, which develop within 1 to 2 days, exfoliate in large sheets and leave behind superficially denuded skin (Fig. 410-19). Skin biopsy can help to distinguish the periorificial fissuring and crusting of staphylococcal scalded skin syndrome from toxic epidermal necrolysis, which causes a subepidermal separation of the skin as well as mucosal involvement.

> ## TREATMENT   Rx
>
> Treatment for severe staphylococcal scalded skin syndrome is IV nafcillin or oxacillin 1 to 2 g every 4 hours for 7 to 14 days unless patients have methicillin-resistant staphylococci, in which case they should be treated with IV vancomycin

(starting at 1 g every 12 hours, then adjusted based on the creatinine clearance). For mild disease, oral dicloxacillin (500 mg four times daily) for 10 to 14 days is often effective, but methicillin-resistant staphylococci require antibiotics shown to be effective by sensitivity testing.

HERPES SIMPLEX VIRUS INFECTION

Herpes simplex virus (HSV) infection (Chapter 350) commonly presents as a recurrent vesicular eruption on an erythematous base (Fig. 410-20). The location is typically oral and perioral with HSV-1 but genital or sacral with HSV-2.

Traumatized areas may appear as erosions with scalloped borders. Recurrent rash can be precipitated by other infections that suppress the immune system, cold or heat, skin trauma, and menstruation. Immunocompromised patients can develop chronic erosive ulcers.

Tzanck smear from the base of an unroofed vesicle or erosion can be helpful in rapidly confirming the diagnosis by identifying multinucleated giant cells with nuclear molding and margination (see Fig. 407-8 in Chapter 407), but the diagnostic "gold standard" is viral culture or direct fluorescent antibody testing. The direct fluorescent antibody test has both high sensitivity and specificity, can yield same-day results, and can distinguish among HSV-1, HSV-2, and varicella-zoster virus (VZV).

TREATMENT

HSV infection is self-limited in healthy individuals. Antiviral treatment with acyclovir, valacyclovir, or famciclovir (see Table 336-1 in Chapter 336) can shorten the initial attack and prevent recurrences. The dose and duration of antiviral therapy depend on whether the infection is disseminated or limited and on whether the patient is immunosuppressed.

VARICELLA

Varicella (chickenpox) caused by VZV (Chapter 351) usually occurs in childhood, but it is more severe when it occurs in adulthood. Erythematous macules on the face, scalp, trunk, and proximal limbs rapidly progress to papules, vesicles, pustules, and crusting (Fig. 410-21) 10 to 21 days after exposure. The diagnosis is usually made clinically, with confirmation based on direct fluorescent antibody testing because culture results are often delayed and less sensitive. Tzanck smear can be helpful but cannot distinguish HSV from VZV.

TREATMENT

Immunocompetent adults can be treated with oral valacyclovir (1 g three times daily) or oral acyclovir (800 mg five times daily) for 5 to 7 days with extended courses in cases of delayed crusting and dose adjustments as needed for reduced kidney function. The varicella vaccine is highly effective when given once to children or twice (4 to 8 weeks apart) to previously unvaccinated persons older than 13 years of age (Chapter 15).

HERPES ZOSTER

Herpes zoster (Chapter 351), which is caused by reactivation of VZV from prior primary varicella or following varicella vaccination, most often occurs in individuals who are older or immunocompromised. Patients typically develop grouped vesicles on an erythematous base in a dermatomal distribution (Fig. 410-22). The rash is usually preceded by pain, itching, tingling, or

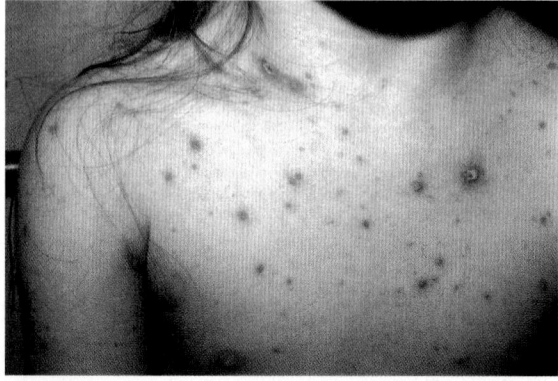

FIGURE 410-21. Erythematous macules and vesicles with crusted erosions on the chest of a patient with varicella. (Courtesy Neil J. Korman, MD.)

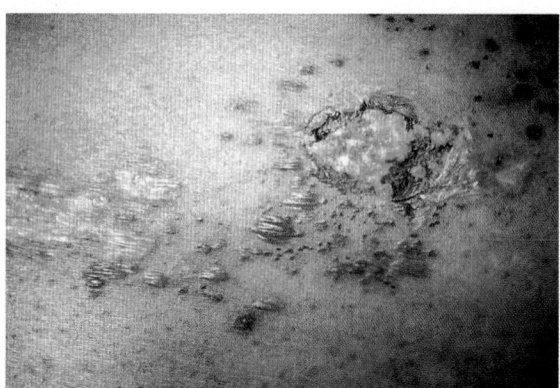

FIGURE 410-22. Herpes zoster. Necrotic blisters and erosions in a dermatomal pattern are seen on the trunk of this patient. (Courtesy Neil J. Korman, MD.)

hyperesthesia. Cutaneous dissemination, defined as more than 20 vesicles outside the primary or adjacent dermatomes and/or visceral involvement, more commonly occurs in immunocompromised patients. Dysesthesia in the affected dermatome can persist in up to 20% of patients after resolution of the skin lesions (postherpetic neuralgia).

TREATMENT

Immunocompetent adults can be treated with valacyclovir (1000 mg three times daily for 7 days), acyclovir (800 mg five times daily for 7 days), or famciclovir (500 mg three times daily for 7 days). In patients who are immunocompromised or have disseminated or visceral disease, intravenous acyclovir (10 mg/kg every 8 hours for 7 to 10 days) is indicated. The initiation of gabapentin with antiviral therapy also can decrease the incidence of postherpetic neuralgia. Varicella vaccination markedly reduces the incidences of both herpes zoster and postherpetic neuralgia (Chapter 351).

● PUSTULAR ERUPTIONS
Acne Vulgaris

Acne vulgaris affects up to 85% of teenagers, but it can persist until adulthood or even develop de novo in adults.[14] The sebum flow, which is stimulated by androgens, is physically impeded by abnormal keratinization in the pilosebaceous canal. The result is the formation of comedones, which can be open to air ("black heads"), or covered by epidermis ("white heads"). Proliferation of *Propionibacterium acnes* within the comedo can lead to rupture of the pilosebaceous unit, with resulting extravasation of its contents into the dermis, thereby creating inflammatory papules, pustules, and nodulocystic lesions.

Acne may be exacerbated or precipitated by oil-based cosmetics, hair preparations, systemic corticosteroids, and androgenic hormones. Other implicated medications include phenytoin, phenobarbital, lithium, and isoniazid. Endocrinologic conditions (e.g., polycystic ovary disease and ovarian or adrenal tumors) also may precipitate or worsen acne.

TREATMENT

Mild disease can be treated with topical benzoyl peroxide, erythromycin, or clindamycin, and/or a topical retinoid (e.g., adapalene, tretinoin, or tazarotene). Benzoyl peroxide and topical retinoids can help normalize follicular keratinization, whereas topical antibiotics help control inflammatory papules and pustules. For more serious disease, oral doxycycline or minocycline (50 to 100 mg twice daily) can be helpful.[15] In women, oral contraceptives (containing either ethinyl estradiol plus norgestimate or ethinyl estradiol plus drospirenone) and/or spironolactone can be particularly helpful in the treatment of hormonal acne that can predominantly affect the lower face, jawline, and upper neck. Isotretinoin (1.5 mg/kg given for 5 to 6 months) decreases the size of sebaceous glands as well as their production of sebum and is helpful for resistant disease, severe inflammatory cases, or extensive generalized comedonal involvement.[16]

ROSACEA

Rosacea, which is a chronic inflammatory disease, affects facial pilosebaceous units and blood vessels, generally in middle age.[17] The four main types of rosacea are erythematotelangiectatic, papulopustular, phymatous, and ocular. Erythematotelangiectatic rosacea is characterized by persistent central facial erythema and telangiectasias. Papulopustular rosacea is characterized by erythematous papules and pustules in the absence of comedones. Phymatous rosacea is characterized by thickened skin and widened pores, usually of the nose but sometimes of the forehead, chin, ears, and eyelids (Fig. 410-23). Ocular rosacea, which is characterized by dry, itchy, or gritty sensation of the eyes, conjunctivitis, blepharitis, and chalazia, should be managed by an ophthalmologist. Rosacea is more common in patients who have a tendency toward facial flushing, which can be caused by sun exposure or by other stimuli (e.g., alcohol, spicy foods, hot liquids, or emotion.)

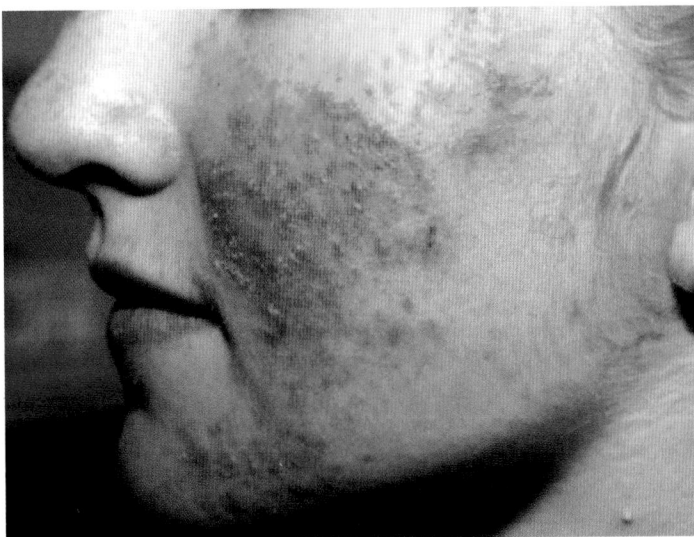

FIGURE 410-23. Rosacea dermatitis. When there is more severe disease, scaling and superficial crusting may be seen as on the cheek of this woman. (Courtesy Kalman Watsky, MD. From Powell FC, Raghallaigh SN. Rosacea and related disorders. In: Bolognia JL, Schaffer JV, Cerroni L, eds. *Dermatology.* 4th ed. Elsevier; 2018:607.)

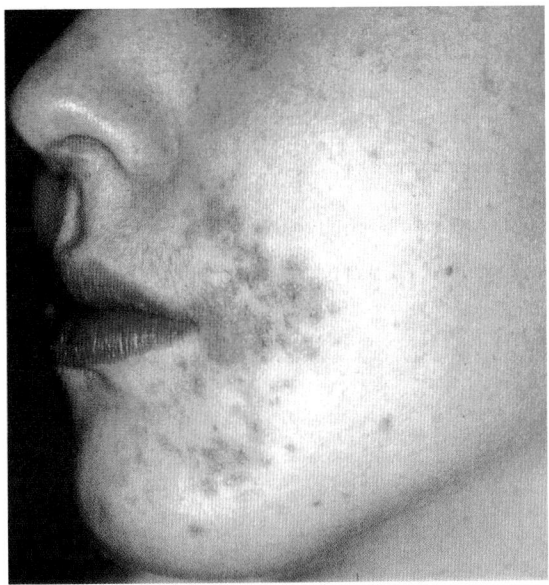

FIGURE 410-24. Perioral dermatitis. Erythematous papules and pinpoint pustules are evident around the mouth. (Courtesy Neil J. Korman, MD.)

TREATMENT   Rx

Avoidance of precipitatory causes, especially sun exposure, is recommended for all types of rosacea. Topical antibiotics (e.g., ivermectin 1% cream, azelaic acid 15% gel, or metronidazole 1% cream) are helpful in mild disease,[A2] whereas a low doxycycline dose (20 mg twice daily) is helpful for more inflamed cases.[18] For severe disease, full-dose doxycycline (100 mg twice daily) or minocycline (100 mg twice daily) are efficacious, as is low-dose isotretinoin 0.25 mg/kg.[A3]

PERIORIFICIAL DERMATITIS

In periorificial dermatitis, patients develop tiny, superficial erythematous papules and papulopustules, accompanied by occasional scaling patches around the mouth, eyes, and nose (Fig. 410-24). Patients often report an intolerance to topical agents and cosmetics, and many have inappropriately used chronic topical corticosteroids. Discontinuation of the corticosteroid often clears the rash, but a 2- to 4-week course of oral antibiotics (e.g., doxycycline 50 to 100 mg twice daily, minocycline 50 to 100 mg twice daily, erythromycin topical or 500 mg twice daily, or azithromycin 500 mg once followed by 250 mg for 4 days administered 2 weeks apart) can also clear the lesions.

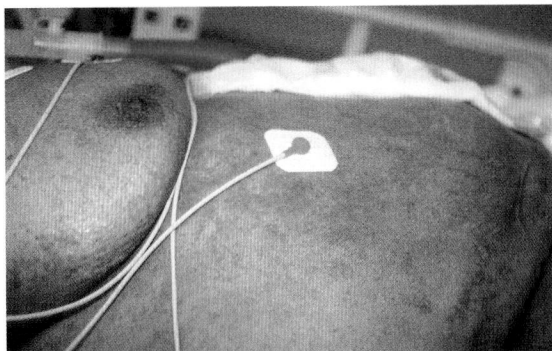

FIGURE 410-25. Acute generalized exanthematous pustulosis. Erythematous macules and numerous superficial pustules are present on the trunk of this patient. (Courtesy Neil J. Korman, MD.)

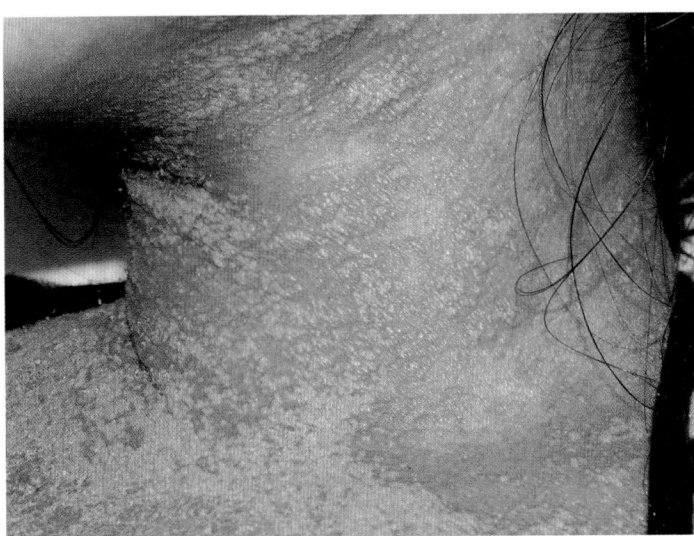

FIGURE 410-26. Generalized pustular psoriasis. Broad areas of erythema with numerous pustules and the formation of lakes of pus. (Courtesy Julie V. Schaffer, MD. From van de Kerkhof PCM, Nestlé FO. Psoriasis. In: Bolognia JL, Schaffer JV, Cerroni L, eds. *Dermatology.* 4th ed. Elsevier; 2018:145.)

ACUTE GENERALIZED EXANTHEMATOUS PUSTULOSIS

Acute generalized exanthematous pustulosis is most frequently caused by antibiotics (especially macrolides and β-lactams), calcium-channel blockers, and antimalarial agents. Edematous erythema and fever typically appear within 2 days after the drug is started, thereby suggesting a prior sensitization to the causative agent. Small sterile pustules subsequently develop on the face or in flexural areas, and they can then disseminate rapidly (Fig. 410-25). Superficial desquamation follows, and the condition usually resolves spontaneously within 2 weeks.

PUSTULAR PSORIASIS

Pustular psoriasis is a psoriatic variant (Chapter 409) that is triggered by pregnancy, infection, a rapid taper of corticosteroids, hypocalcemia, and medications such as lithium. It can be generalized (Fig. 410-26), localized to the palms and soles, annular, or acute and associated with fever and skin pain. Topical corticosteroids and/or calcipotriene may be sufficient, but systemic cyclosporine or TNF-α inhibitors are often needed for severe cases (Chapter 409).

FOLLICULITIS

Folliculitis, which is inflammation of the hair follicles caused by infection, presents as perifollicular pustules on an erythematous base. The most common cause is staphylococcal infection, but skin flora and gram-negative rods can be implicated. In addition, viral (HSV, VZV) and fungal folliculitis can occur. Folliculitis occurs more commonly in patients who are obese, are immunocompromised, or have diabetes mellitus. It most commonly affects follicles of the scalp, axilla, trunk, thighs, and inguinal area, but it also can extend deeper into the dermis where it can cause larger erythematous furuncles or carbuncles. Evaluation includes culture of the pustule's contents or base. Topical antibiotics (e.g., clindamycin solution twice daily for at least 2 weeks) and antibacterial soaps are useful for mild disease, but antibiotics (e.g., cephalexin, 500 mg twice daily for 14 days) are needed for more extensive infection.

Pseudomonas Folliculitis

Pseudomonas folliculitis manifests 1 to 2 days after using hot tubs or whirlpools contaminated with *P. aeruginosa* (Chapter 290). The typical findings are pruritic papules and pustules, mostly on the torso and accentuated in any skin areas occluded by a bathing suit (Fig. 410-27). The condition is usually self-limited in healthy individuals, but it can be treated with antibacterial soap. Ciprofloxacin (500 mg twice daily for 10 to 14 days) usually cures the infection.

Pityrosporum Folliculitis

Pityrosporum ovale folliculitis is a pruritic, acne-like eruption that develops on the face, upper chest, and arms. It is most often seen in young adults, particularly in warm weather, after sweating, and in immunosuppressed individuals. Lesions appear as itchy, follicularly based papules and sometimes pustules over the torso and shoulders. Yeast forms are identifiable on a potassium hydroxide (KOH) preparation. Treatment consists of topical antifungal cream, selenium sulfide shampoo daily for 1 month, or oral itraconazole (200 mg daily for 1 week) or fluconazole (100 to 200 mg daily for 1 to 4 weeks or 300 mg once weekly for 1 to 2 months).

Eosinophilic Pustular Folliculitis

Eosinophilic pustular folliculitis, which is seen in HIV-positive patients, is a sterile but intensely pruritic folliculitis that is usually seen on the face and torso (Chapter 366). It is accompanied by peripheral eosinophilia. Skin biopsy demonstrates eosinophils in and around the follicles. Treatment options include antihistamines, topical corticosteroids (see Table 407-10), and topical tacrolimus. Systemic options include indomethacin (50 mg/day), minocycline (100 mg twice daily), dapsone (100 to 200 mg/day), systemic corticosteroids, and colchicine (0.6 mg twice daily). Narrowband ultraviolet B phototherapy also can be helpful.

● HIDRADENITIS SUPPURITIVA

Hidradenitis suppurativa, which is a chronic and recurrent inflammatory disease, is characterized by painful, deep-seated nodules and abscesses that result from occlusion of the follicular infundibula followed by inflammation.

Hidradenitis can begin in puberty but most commonly occurs in the early 20s, with its incidence declining substantially after age 50 years. Women predominate over men 3 : 1. The pathogenesis is poorly understood, but it appears to be an inflammatory or immune disease. Cigarette smoking and obesity are risk factors. Biopsy shows atrophy of the sebaceous glands, lymphocytic inflammation of the pilosebaceous unit, destruction of the hair follicles, and granulomas.

The clinical course is chronic, with periods of flares and remissions. The typical presentation is with painful, inflamed nodules and sterile abscesses in the axilla or the groin, but lesions also often occur in the inframammary, genital, and perineal areas.[19] Sinus tracts can develop and be associated with purulent or bloody drainage; lesions may heal with scarring, sometimes cordlike. Flares are often related to menses. Lesions typically recur at the same or nearby sites despite prior incision and drainage and/or oral antibiotics (Fig. 410-28).

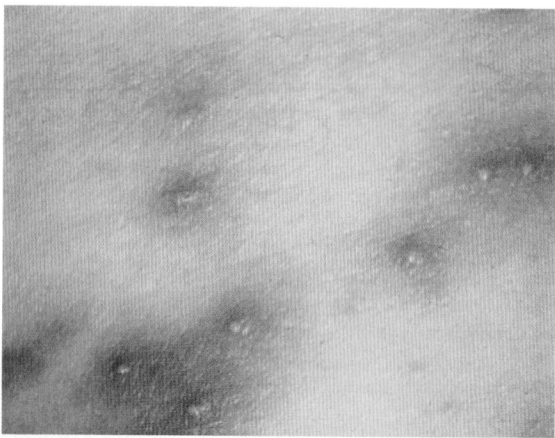

FIGURE 410-27. *Pseudomonas* **species folliculitis.** The trunk of this patient has numerous pustules on an erythematous base. (Courtesy Neil J. Korman, MD.)

TREATMENT　Rx

Treatment options have variable success. Weight loss and smoking cessation are encouraged. Moisture reduction through the use of topical aluminum chloride, powders, and loose-fitting clothing can be helpful. Antiseptic soaps and topical antibiotics (e.g., benzoyl peroxide or chlorhexidine washes or topical clindamycin/benzoyl peroxide combination products) may be beneficial for early or mild disease. Intralesional triamcinolone injections can reduce inflammation in early nodules. Systemic therapies include oral antibiotics (doxycycline, minocycline, clindamycin, rifampin, dapsone, trimethoprim-sulfamethoxazole), hormonal therapies (ethinyl estradiol plus cyproterone acetate, spironolactone, finasteride), the phosphodiesterase-4 inhibitor apremilast, and TNF-α inhibitors (e.g., adalimumab 40 mg weekly or infliximab).[A4-A6]

● SWEET SYNDROME

Sweet syndrome is an acute febrile neutrophilic dermatosis characterized by: fever; peripheral neutrophilia; and edematous, painful papules, nodules, or plaques. Sweet syndrome may be idiopathic, but it is more often seen with an underlying condition or exposure to medication.[20] In adults, Sweet syndrome is most commonly associated with hematologic malignancy, especially acute myelogenous leukemia (Chapter 173). It is also seen with inflammatory bowel disease (Chapter 132), infections, pregnancy, and exposure to medications such as all-*trans*-retinoic acid and granulocyte colony-stimulating factor. Sweet syndrome presents clinically with multiple firm, tender, deeply erythematous to violaceous papules, papulovesicles, or nodules, which may turn into edematous plaques. The most common locations are the head, neck, and upper and lower extremities (Fig. 410-29 and Chapter 411) The phenomenon of pathergy, which is the development of inflammatory lesions at sites of dermal injury, may be seen in sites such as IV insertion points and places of venipuncture. When the disease is active, patients may have fever, arthralgias, arthritis, and myalgias as well as a neutrophilic leukocytosis. Biopsy shows superficial edema and a deeper dense neutrophilic infiltrate.

TREATMENT　Rx

The skin lesions respond rapidly to oral corticosteroids (e.g., prednisone, 1 mg/kg/day). Steroid-sparing options include dapsone (100 to 200 mg/day), colchicine (0.6 mg three times daily), potassium iodide (300 mg three times daily), cyclosporine, and TNF-α inhibitors. Recurrent episodes can be a sign of recurrent cancer.

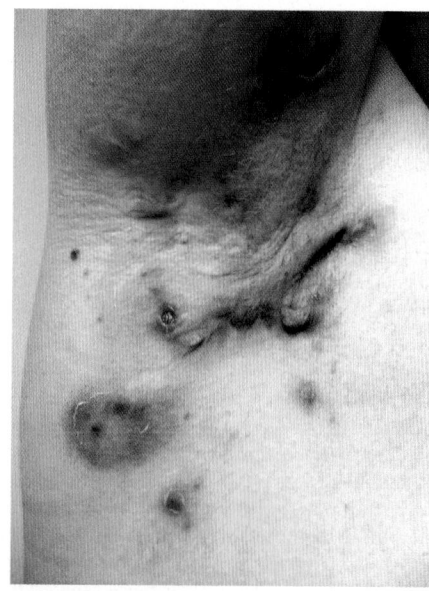

FIGURE 410-28. **Hidradenitis suppurativa.** The axilla of this patient has several erythematous nodules with draining sinus tracts. (Courtesy Neil J. Korman, MD.)

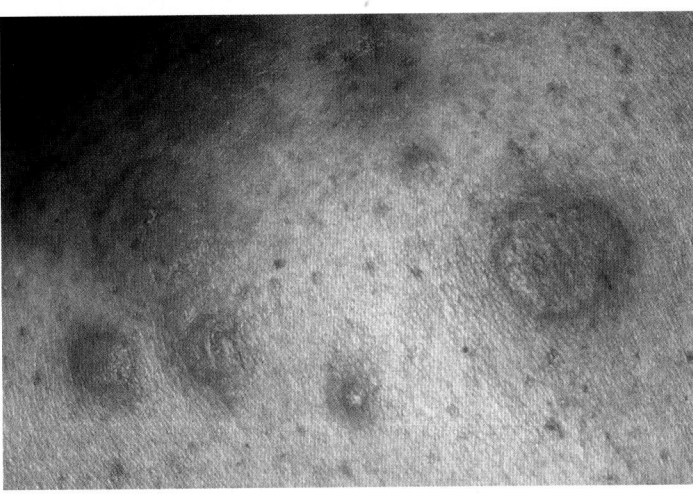

FIGURE 410-29. Sweet syndrome. The edema can be quite marked as seen in these lesions on the upper back. (Courtesy Kalman Watsky, MD. From Davis MDP, Moschella SL. Neutrophilic dermatoses. In: Bolognia JL, Schaffer JV, Cerroni L, eds. *Dermatology.* 4th ed. Elsevier; 2018:456.)

Grade A References

A1. Joly P, Maho-Vaillant M, Prost-Squarcioni C, et al. First-line rituximab combined with short-term prednisone versus prednisone alone for the treatment of pemphigus (Ritux 3): a prospective, multicentre, parallel-group, open-label randomised trial. *Lancet.* 2017;389:2031-2040.

A2. McGregor SP, Alinia H, Snyder A, et al. A review of the current modalities for the treatment of papulopustular rosacea. *Dermatol Clin.* 2018;36:135-150.

A3. Sbidian E, Vicaut E, Chidiack H, et al. A randomized-controlled trial of oral low-dose isotretinoin for difficult-to-treat papulopustular rosacea. *J Invest Dermatol.* 2016;136:1124-1129.

A4. Kimball AB, Kerdel F, Adams D, et al. Adalimumab for the treatment of moderate to severe hidradenitis suppurativa: a parallel randomized trial. *Ann Intern Med.* 2012;157:846-855.

A5. Kimball AB, Okun MM, Williams DA, et al. Two phase 3 trials of adalimumab for hidradenitis suppurativa. *N Engl J Med.* 2016;375:422-434.

A6. Vossen A, van Doorn MBA, van der Zee HH, et al. Apremilast for moderate hidradenitis suppurativa: results of a randomized controlled trial. *J Am Acad Dermatol.* 2019;80:80-88.

GENERAL REFERENCES

For the General References and other additional features, please visit Expert Consult at https://expertconsult.inkling.com.

411

URTICARIA, DRUG HYPERSENSITIVITY RASHES, NODULES AND TUMORS, AND ATROPHIC DISEASES

MADELEINE DUVIC

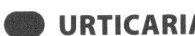

URTICARIA

DEFINITION AND EPIDEMIOLOGY

Urticaria, or hives, is one of the most common cutaneous reaction patterns (Fig. 411-1). It is triggered by a wide variety of antigens or by physical stimuli, including cold, pressure, and sunlight (Table 411-1). Urticaria is a spectrum ranging from simple wheals to angioedema. Clinical distinction between acute and chronic urticaria is important for diagnosis and treatment. Chronic urticaria is defined by recurrence over a period of 6 weeks or more and is often of unknown cause.

Urticaria is common worldwide in persons of all ages, although certain types of urticaria have a predilection for certain age groups. For example,

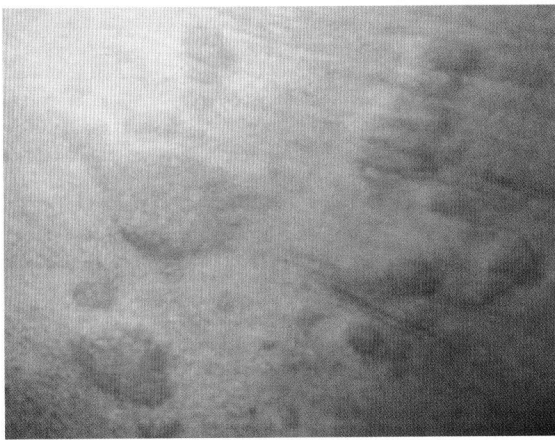

FIGURE 411-1. Urticaria. (From DermNet. Urticaria; 2014. http://www.dermnetnz.org/reactions/urticaria.html. Accessed October 23, 2014.)

TABLE 411-1	COMMON CAUSES OF URTICARIA

URTICARIA MAY BE ACCOMPANIED BY ANGIOEDEMA AND ANAPHYLAXIS

Blood products: red blood cells, platelets, gamma globulin
Drugs
    Antibiotics: penicillins, cephalosporins, sulfonamides, isoniazid
    Aspirin: salicylates, benzoates, phenylbutazone
    Anticonvulsants: hydantoin
    Chemotherapy: doxorubicin, daunorubicin, L-asparaginase, chlorambucil, cyclophosphamide, melphalan, methotrexate, nitrogen mustard, procarbazine
    Dextran
    Nonsteroidal anti-inflammatory drugs
    Opiates
    Quinidine
    Radiocontrast dyes, iodine
Environmental: animal dander or proteins, formaldehyde, pollen, mold, plants, latex, plastic tubing, exercise, heat, cold, sunlight, dermal vibration
Foods: berries, eggs, milk, nuts, tomatoes, shellfish, soy
Food additives: sodium benzoate, tartrazine (yellow dye #5)
Hormones
Infections: streptococcal, staphylococcal, sinusitis or abscesses, viral hepatitis, Epstein-Barr virus mononucleosis, *Candida* spp
Insect bites or venom: Hymenoptera, mosquitoes, mites, scabies
Mechanical stimuli (dermographism, vibratory angioedema, delayed-pressure urticaria)
Vaccines

URTICARIA-LIKE ERUPTIONS AND REACTIVE ERYTHEMAS

Erythema multiforme: herpes simplex, DNA viruses, *Mycoplasma pneumoniae*, drugs
Erythema marginatum: streptococcal rheumatic fever
Juvenile rheumatoid arthritis
Erythema chronicum migrans: *Borrelia* spp infections
Erythema annulare centrifugum: tinea, drugs
Figurate erythemas: erythema repens (often with underlying carcinoma)
Urticaria pigmentosa (mastocytosis)

whereas acute urticaria is often seen in children with atopic dermatitis, chronic urticaria peaks in the fourth decade.

PATHOBIOLOGY

Urticaria can be caused by immunologic (autoimmune, immunoglobulin E [IgE]–dependent, immune complex–mediated, complement-kinin dependent) or nonimmunologic (direct mast cell–releasing agents, vasoactive stimuli, drugs) reactions. Local degranulation of mast cells with the release of histamine and other factors, such as slow-reacting substance of anaphylaxis, precipitates urticaria. Functional IgG autoantibodies, which release histamine from mast cells and basophils, are commonly found in the blood of patients with chronic urticaria. Additionally, basophils are recruited into the wheals, where they sustain the response by releasing histamine. Eosinophils also contribute through leukotriene C_4 (LTC_4), leukotriene D_4 (LTD_4), leukotriene E_4 (LTE_4), and major basic protein. Urticaria is typically transient and self-limited, without leakage of blood cells into the skin or damage to the blood vessels. Leakage of plasma into the dermis from capillaries and small postcapillary venules correlates clinically with development of a demarcated, pink, raised lesion (hive).

CLINICAL MANIFESTATIONS

Urticarial lesions are pink to light red, blanch with pressure, and are raised above the surface of the skin. The center of the lesions may be paler than the leading edge. By definition, individual wheals come and go within 24 hours. A mosquito bite (Chapter 238) is the archetypal urticarial lesion. Individual hives can coalesce into giant plaques or annular rings called giant urticaria as is seen in serum sickness, in which they are accompanied by arthralgias and fever. Confluent urticaria may also be accompanied by swelling of the underlying soft tissue or the mucous membranes (angioedema) as well as by anaphylaxis with laryngeal edema, a life-threatening emergency. In otherwise normal individuals, pressure or writing or vibration on the skin will cause spontaneous local release of histamine, which induces a wheal-and-flare reaction known as dermatographism. Deep swelling develops at the site of sustained pressure and may remain for days in a condition known as delayed pressure urticaria. Affected individuals may develop lesions from tight-fitting clothing, shoes, socks, or sexual intercourse.

Other physical stimuli such as cold, heat, sun, or exercise may induce urticaria. Cold urticaria may be precipitated by putting an ice cube on the skin; the interval until hives develop and the duration of the hives correlate with the severity of the condition, which can be life threatening if the patient is suddenly immersed in cold water. Heat, exercise, or exertion may be accompanied by small, 2- to 3-mm urticarial lesions in a condition called cholinergic urticaria. Exercise-induced anaphylaxis may be hereditary, but the defect is unknown. Patients with vibratory angioedema develop swelling and erythema within a few minutes of exposure to a vibratory stimulus. Lesions persist for about 30 minutes. Other forms of physically induced urticaria include solar urticaria and aquagenic urticaria (urticarial lesions caused by exposure to sun and water, respectively).

Food and exercise–induced anaphylaxis is a syndrome in which a few minutes of exercise after ingestion of specific foods results in angioedema or anaphylaxis. The cause of this syndrome is still controversial, but reduced gastric acid secretion may be involved in food and exercise-induced anaphylaxis.

DIAGNOSIS

A detailed history (duration, occupation, medications, frequency of episodes, associated illness) is critical. Urticaria typically results from exposure to antigen only minutes to a few hours before the onset of the lesions. In many cases, pruritus may precede onset of the rash. The most common triggers of IgE-mediated allergic urticarial reactions are drugs (especially penicillin, sulfa drugs, antibiotics, and contrast dye), foods (shellfish, salicylates in berries, tomatoes, yeast, and penicillin in blue cheese), food additives (sodium benzoate), nuts (especially peanuts), latex, and insect bites. Nonimmunologic mediators of urticaria include aspirin and opiates as well as physical agents that work through the prostaglandin pathway or degranulate mast cells.

Acute urticaria can also be triggered by skin contact with an antigen, such as latex, and can progress to anaphylaxis. In addition, urticaria can be a sign or prodrome of a latent infection, especially streptococcal pharyngitis in children or viral hepatitis in adults. The migratory urticarial rash accompanying rheumatic fever, erythema marginatum (Fig. 411-2), is characterized by evanescent, scalloped lesions that change location over the course of hours.

When urticarial lesions are present for more than 24 hours, underlying urticarial vasculitis should be suspected. A skin biopsy is required to distinguish urticarial vasculitis from urticaria in which no damage to the blood vessels is

evident. When vascular damage is present, the lesion is termed *leukocytoclastic vasculitis,* the most severe expression of hypersensitivity reactions involving cutaneous blood vessels.

Chronic urticaria can be caused by occult infections (sinusitis, gallbladder disease, *Helicobacter pylori,* yeast infections, tooth abscesses, or silent hepatitis) as well as by collagen vascular diseases and tumors, especially Hodgkin lymphoma. Deficiency of the C1 esterase inhibitor can be manifested as chronic urticaria with angioedema. Allergy testing is recommended if the history is unrevealing. If lesions persist for more than 24 hours, skin biopsy is indicated to determine whether vasculitis or mastocytosis is present. If infection, collagen vascular disease, or a tumor is suspected, a full serologic evaluation should be undertaken. Although a thorough medical evaluation may aid in diagnosis, the cause of chronic urticaria may remain uncertain. In the absence of a known antigen, stress is often invoked as the underlying cause of chronic recurrent idiopathic urticaria

Systemic mastocytosis[1] (Chapter 240) may be accompanied by urticarial lesions and gastrointestinal symptoms. In the form of mastocytosis known as *urticaria pigmentosa,* stroking the lesions produces urticaria, known as the *Darier sign.* A skin biopsy shows an increased number of dermal mast cells. Serum tryptase and histamine levels may be elevated during an attack.

TREATMENT   Rx

Management of urticaria depends on its severity and the duration of the problem[2] (Chapter 237). For mild urticaria limited to the skin, traditional oral antihistamines (diphenhydramine) or the newer nonsedating agents (terfenadine, cetirizine, loratadine) can be administered intermittently as needed (Table 411-2). [A1][A2] Acute urticaria is often treated with diphenhydramine orally. If the urticaria is severe, short-term corticosteroids, up to 1 mg/kg, can be used. For urticaria associated with wheezing or anaphylaxis, subcutaneous epinephrine, intravenous (IV) corticosteroids, and oxygen should be administered immediately.

Finding the cause and removing the antigen of chronic recurrent urticaria is highly preferable to chronic administration of corticosteroids or antihistamines. The patient should avoid aspirin compounds and other drugs that could be the cause.

For chronic spontaneous urticaria that persists, omalizumab, an anti-IgE monoclonal antibody at 300 mg subcutaneously once per month,[A3] or cyclosporine (at doses of 3 mg/kg or higher for 8 to 16 weeks), is effective in 65 to 70% of patients who do not respond to H₁-antihistamines. H₂-antihistamines and leukotriene antagonists are no longer recommended. Prednisone is to be avoided because of long-term toxicity.

TABLE 411-2 TREATMENT OF URTICARIA

1. Avoid the inciting agent!

2. Medications based on severity

A. Mild to moderate, acute urticaria
- Oral H₁-antihistamines, e.g., diphenhydramine (Benadryl), 10-50 mg PO q12h, or hydroxyzine, 10-25 mg PO q8h; nonsedating alternatives include cetirizine (Zyrtec), 5-10 mg/day, or loratadine (Claritin), 10 mg/day
- Omalizumab (an anti-IgE antibody) at 300 mg subcutaneously monthly

B. Severe urticaria with or without angioedema
- H₁-antihistamines, e.g., diphenhydramine (Benadryl), 25-50 mg PO q6-8h or 10-50 mg IV q2-4h, not to exceed 400 mg/24 hr
- Corticosteroids, e.g., prednisone, 10-60 mg PO every morning with tapering over a 2-wk period; triamcinolone (Kenalog), 40 mg IM for one dose; or dexamethasone, 0.6-0.75 mg/m²/day IV in divided doses q6-12h, depending on severity

C. Anaphylaxis
- A—Airway (intubation)
- B—Breathing (oxygen)
- C—Circulation: parenteral aqueous epinephrine, 1 : 1000 IV, saline or volume expanders
- IV corticosteroids (e.g., methylprednisolone, 125 mg)
- Histamine H₁- and H₂-antagonists (50 mg each of diphenhydramine and ranitidine)

D. Chronic idiopathic urticaria—combination therapy
- Nonsedating H₁-antihistamine: cetirizine, 10 mg/day, or fexofenadine, 30-180 mg twice daily, alone or with montelukast, 10 mg/day, or H₁ and H₂ antagonists (50 mg each of diphenhydramine and ranitidine) and/or low-dose corticosteroids (if unavailable)
- Omalizumab (anti-IgE monoclonal antibody) at 300 mg subcutaneously once monthly and cyclosporine (doses of 3 mg/kg or higher for 8 to 16 weeks)

IM = intramuscularly; IV = intravenously; PO = orally.

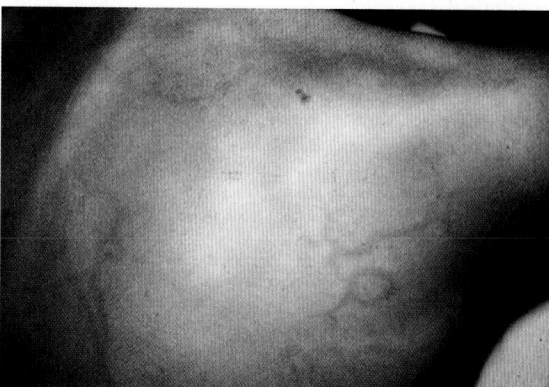

FIGURE 411-2. Erythema marginatum. (From Medscape. Urticaria; n.d. http://www.medscape.com/content/1998/00/41/73/417394/art-m5649.fig2.jpg. http://www.dermnetnz.org/reactions/urticaria.html. Accessed October 23, 2014.)

DRUG RASHES

DEFINITION

Drugs have been associated with every type of cutaneous reaction pattern ranging from mild and self-limited to severe and life threatening. Urticaria and exanthematous eruptions are common manifestations of cutaneous drug reactions. Less commonly seen are fixed drug, lichenoid, pustular, phototoxic, bullous, or vasculitic reactions, and the spectrum of erythema multiforme, Stevens-Johnson syndrome, and toxic epidermal necrolysis.

PATHOBIOLOGY

Drug rashes, which result from drug toxicity, overdose, drug-drug interactions, or products of metabolism, may be caused by immunologic or nonimmunologic mechanisms. Drugs or their metabolites can act as haptens and induce cell-mediated or humoral responses. Mechanisms include IgE-dependent anaphylaxis and urticaria, cytotoxic reactions resulting in thrombocytopenia and resultant petechiae, immune complex–mediated serum sickness, and delayed-type hypersensitivity resulting in exanthematous or fixed drug eruptions or Stevens-Johnson syndrome.

CLINICAL MANIFESTATIONS AND DIAGNOSIS

Drug rashes are either immediate (urticaria) or delayed hypersensitivity reactions (exanthems). Immediate reactions such as pruritus, hives, angioedema, and anaphylaxis occur within minutes to a few hours after the drug is taken. The most common drug-related rash (Table 411-3) is a CD8+ T-cell–mediated hypersensitivity reaction manifested as a macular, bright pink to salmon-colored exanthem that appears as early as 7 to 10 days and as late as 14 days after a drug is first administered.[3] Delayed hypersensitivity reactions can be macular or papular exanthems (or both), morbilliform eruptions, annular erythema, or confluent erythema (Fig. 411-3). After sensitization to a particular drug has occurred, readministration of the same drug may trigger an eruption within 24 to 72 hours. Drug hypersensitivity reactions are typically symmetrical. They characteristically begin on the face and upper trunk and progress to the lower extremities, where they may become purpuric. Exanthems secondary to drugs most often become confluent erythematous patches after several days.

Pruritus is the most common symptom. The differential diagnosis for drug rashes includes viral exanthems (Chapter 410), graft-versus-host disease or the leukocyte recovery rash after allogeneic bone marrow transplantation, erythematous exanthems that accompany streptococcal (scarlet fever [Chapter 274]) or staphylococcal (toxic shock syndrome [Chapter 272]) infections, and the acute manifestation of collagen vascular diseases. A similar exanthem occurs when ampicillin is administered to patients who have infectious mononucleosis. A careful drug history is critical in diagnosis and treatment.

TREATMENT AND PROGNOSIS Rx

After the offending drug is discontinued, delayed hypersensitivity reactions resolve in about 1 week. Therapy is mostly supportive. Corticosteroids, such as 0.01% triamcinolone cream, applied several times per day to the affected area and antihistamines given orally three to four times daily are helpful in reducing the itching and shortening the course.

Specific Syndromes

DRUG RASH WITH EOSINOPHILIA AND SYSTEMIC SYMPTOMS

An especially severe hypersensitivity *drug rash with eosinophilia and systemic symptoms* (DRESS) is most frequently seen with sulfonamides and anticonvulsants[4] (Fig. 411-4). This condition is thought to be caused by an alteration in drug metabolism. Activated T lymphocytes release interleukin-5 (IL-5), leading to characteristic eosinophilia. DRESS may be delayed in onset by 2 to 6 weeks, persists longer than classic drug-induced eruptions, and becomes generalized and severe even when use of the agent is discontinued. It typically begins as a morbilliform eruption, which later evolves into an edematous pustular eruption with erythroderma and purpura. The rash begins on the face, upper trunk, and extremities and later becomes generalized. Continued administration of the drug can result in exfoliative erythroderma; toxic necrolysis; and systemic hypersensitivity, including hepatitis (50%), nephritis (10%), or atypical lymphocytosis and lymphadenopathy mimicking mononucleosis

TABLE 411-3 DELAYED HYPERSENSITIVITY DRUG RASHES BY CATEGORY

MACULOPAPULAR EXANTHEMS—ANY DRUG CAN PRODUCE A RASH 7-10 DAYS AFTER THE FIRST DOSE

Allopurinol
Antibiotics: penicillin, sulfonamides
Antiepileptics: phenytoin, phenobarbital
Antihypertensives: captopril, thiazide diuretics
Contrast dye: iodine
Gold salts
Hypoglycemic drugs
Meprobamate
Phenothiazines
Quinine

DRUG RASH WITH EOSINOPHILIA AND SYSTEMIC SYMPTOMS (DRESS)

Anticonvulsants: phenytoin, phenobarbital, valproate, lamotrigine
Antibiotics: sulfonamides, minocycline, dapsone, ampicillin, ethambutol, isoniazid, linezolid, metronidazole, rifampin, streptomycin, vancomycin
Antihypertensives: amlodipine, captopril
Antidepressants: bupropion, fluoxetine
Allopurinol
Celecoxib
Ibuprofen
Phenothiazines

ERYTHEMA MULTIFORME/STEVENS-JOHNSON SYNDROME/TOXIC EPIDERMAL NECROLYSIS

Sulfonamides, phenytoin, barbiturates, carbamazepine, allopurinol, amikacin, phenothiazines
Toxic epidermal necrolysis: same as for erythema multiforme but also acetazolamide, gold, nitrofurantoin, pentazocine, tetracycline, quinidine

ACUTE GENERALIZED EXANTHEMIC PUSTULOSIS (AGEP)

Antibiotics: penicillins, macrolides, cephalosporins, clindamycin, imipenem, fluoroquinolones, isoniazid, vancomycin, minocycline, doxycycline, linezolid
Antimalarials: chloroquine, hydroxychloroquine
Antifungals: terbinafine, nystatin
Anticonvulsants: carbamazepine
Calcium-channel blockers
Furosemide
Systemic corticosteroids
Protease inhibitors

COLLAGEN VASCULAR OR LUPUS-LIKE REACTIONS

Procainamide, hydralazine, phenytoin, penicillamine, trimethadione, methyldopa, carbamazepine, griseofulvin, nalidixic acid, oral contraceptives, propranolol

ERYTHEMA NODOSUM

Oral contraceptives, penicillin, sulfonamides, diuretics, gold, clonidine, propranolol, opiates
Fixed drug reactions: phenolphthalein, barbiturates, gold, sulfonamides, meprobamate, penicillin, tetracycline, analgesics

or T-cell lymphoma. Less commonly seen are pneumonitis, myocarditis, and pericarditis. With visceral involvement, there is a 10% mortality rate, usually from hepatic failure. The initial step in management is the immediate withdrawal of the suspected drug. Systemic corticosteroids (e.g., oral prednisone at 1.0 mg/kg/day and tapered over 3 to 6 months or IV methylprednisolone at 30 mg/kg for 3 days) should be started as early as possible. For patients who develop exfoliative dermatitis, admission to a specialized unit such as a burn unit or intensive care unit is critical.

ERYTHEMA MULTIFORME, STEVENS-JOHNSON SYNDROME, AND TOXIC EPIDERMAL NECROLYSIS

Stevens-Johnson syndrome and toxic epidermal necrolysis represent a spectrum of the same disease, of which erythema multiforme (see Fig. 410-16 in Chapter 410) is the least severe. Stevens-Johnson syndrome is defined as mucosal involvement with less than 10% body surface area involvement; toxic epidermal necrolysis is defined as skin necrosis on greater than 30% of the body surface area.[5] Erythema multiforme, a hybrid of urticaria and vasculitis, consists of symmetrically distributed red macules or papules that evolve into classic target or bull's-eye lesions with deep red centers and pink urticarial rims. Erythema multiforme commonly precipitated by herpes simplex infections, other DNA viruses, or drugs. Stevens-Johnson syndrome is characterized by severe mucosal involvement with purpuric lesions. Widespread epidermal necrosis resulting from cell apoptosis is seen in toxic epidermal necrolysis. Drugs are almost always implicated when Stevens-Johnson syndrome or toxic epidermal necrolysis develops in adults (Fig. 411-5). Commonly implicated medications include nonsteroidal anti-inflammatory drugs (NSAIDs), acetaminophen, allopurinol, phenytoin, and sulfa drugs, especially trimethoprim-sulfamethoxazole. Alterations in drug metabolism (i.e., slow acetylators of sulfonamides) are often implicated. Full-thickness keratinocyte necrosis or cell apoptosis leads to separation at the dermal-epidermal junction.

Each of these conditions may start as a morbilliform drug rash and progress to skin necrosis. Symptoms include fever, severe pain, or sometimes asthenia. The condition can progress rapidly, so it is critical to determine and discontinue the causative agent immediately. Superinfection and fluid and electrolyte imbalances can lead to death in 5% of cases of Stevens-Johnson syndrome and 30% of cases of toxic epidermal necrolysis.

Management includes supportive care such as fluid and electrolyte replacement, transfer to a burn unit, and ophthalmologic evaluation. The use of corticosteroids in Stevens-Johnson syndrome and toxic epidermal necrolysis remains controversial. In Stevens-Johnson syndrome, corticosteroids (e.g., IV methylprednisolone at 60 mg every 6 hours or 1 to 2 mg/kg for a short course) are frequently used and may decrease the duration of fever and slow eruptions.

In toxic epidermal necrolysis, however, retrospective studies suggest that corticosteroids may increase mortality. IV immunoglobulin and tumor necrosis factor–α inhibitors, such as infliximab, may reduce the severity of toxic epidermal necrolysis, but no randomized control trials have been done to date. Predictors of poor outcomes include older age, malignancy, and renal failure.

LEUKOCYTOCLASTIC VASCULITIS

Severe drug reactions can also be manifested as vasculitis, neutrophilic eruptions, and ulcerations. Vasculitis is further categorized by the size of the involved vessel and the nature of the cellular reaction and immune complexes. Leukocytoclastic vasculitis, which is the most common form of vasculitis induced by drugs, is manifested as palpable purpura, usually on the lower extremities (see Figs. 410-4 and 410-5 in Chapter 410).

NEUTROPHILIC DRUG REACTIONS

Neutrophilic drug reactions include iododermas, bromodermas, acute generalized exanthematous pustulosis, and acneiform folliculitis. Sweet syndrome (acute febrile neutrophilic dermatosis; see later) also can be drug related. Epidermal growth factor receptor inhibitors and protein kinase inhibitors cause an acneiform facial or chest eruption that is associated with drugs (Fig. 411-6).

Acute generalized exanthematous pustulosis is characterized by numerous (>100), small (<5 mm), nonfollicular subcorneal pustules that arise on erythematous skin, often beginning in skin creases or on the face. High fever and peripheral neutrophilia may precede or accompany the eruption. The

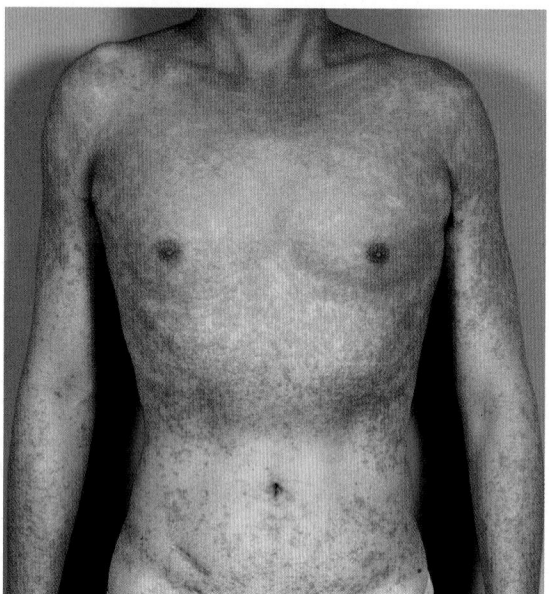

FIGURE 411-3. Morbilliform drug eruption due to trimethoprim-sulfamethoxazole (TMP-SMZ). This human immunodeficiency virus (HIV)–positive young man developed a widespread eruption of blanchable erythematous macules and papules 8 days after starting TMP-SMZ. Note the coalescence on the upper trunk. (From Bolognia. *Dermatology,* 4th ed.)

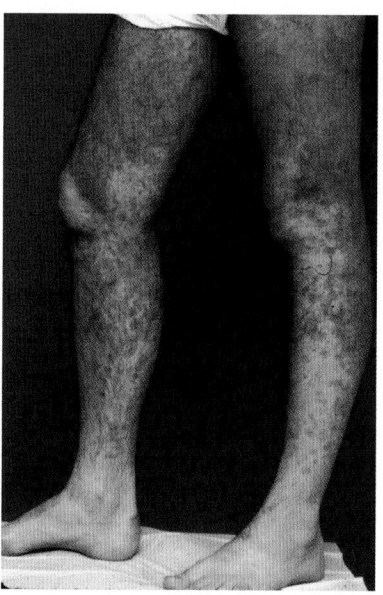

FIGURE 411-4. Hypersensitivity drug rash caused by phenytoin.

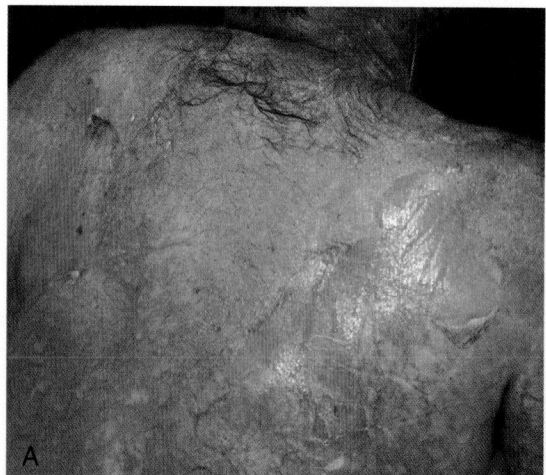
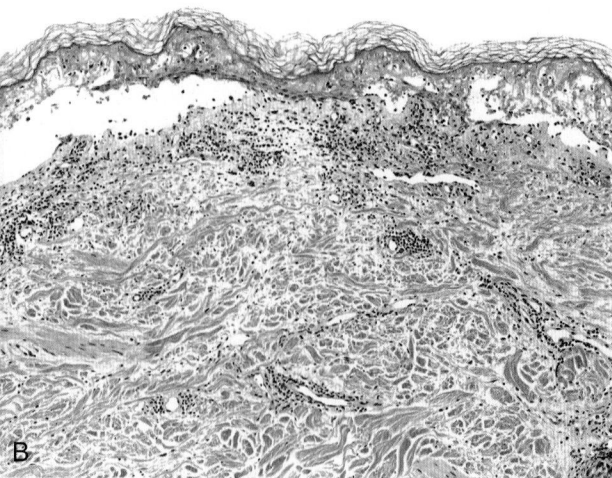

FIGURE 411-5. Toxic epidermal necrolysis. A, Detachment of necrolytic epidermis, leading to large areas of denuded skin. The glistening areas are exposed dermis. B, Full-thickness epidermal cell death results in a subepidermal separation. The normal stratum corneum points to the acute nature of the disease process. In the dermis, there is a lymphohistiocytic inflammatory infiltrate admixed with a few eosinophils. (From Bolognia. *Dermatology,* 4th ed.)

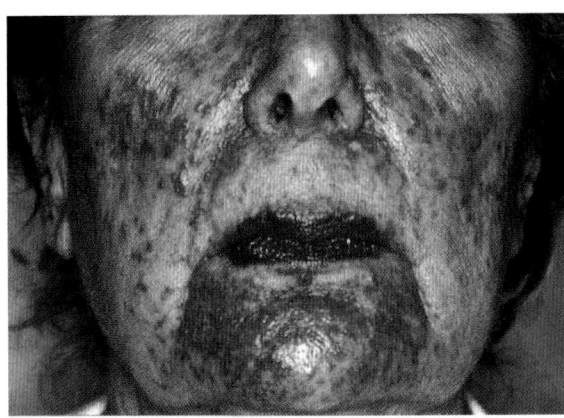

FIGURE 411-6. Epidermal growth factor receptor inhibitor–associated rash.

TABLE 411-4	DRUGS ASSOCIATED WITH SUN SENSITIVITY

PHOTOTOXIC

Chlorpromazine
Hydralazine
Levaquin
Procainamide
Psoralens
Porphyrins
Sulfonamides
Tetracyclines
Thiazide diuretics

PHOTOALLERGIC

Chlorothiazide
Griseofulvin
Hypoglycemic drugs
Promethazine

pustules are sterile, present for 5 to 10 days, and followed by desquamation. They usually appear less than 2 days after the administration of the causative drug. Ninety percent of cases are due to drugs, most commonly β-lactam antibiotics, macrolides, and calcium channel blockers. This syndrome has also been called pustular drug rash, pustular psoriasis after corticosteroid withdrawal, and toxic pustuloderma. When severe, it may be confused with toxic epidermal necrolysis, but the mortality rate is only 1 to 2%. Skin patch testing is frequently positive.

FIXED DRUG ERUPTIONS

A fixed drug reaction appears at the same location 1 to 2 weeks after first drug exposure and within 24 hours of repeat exposure. The lips, hands, face, feet, and genitalia are most commonly involved. The lesion may begin as erythema and then become gray, brown, or violaceous. Trimethoprim-sulfamethoxazole, NSAIDs, tetracyclines, and pseudoephedrine are common causes.

PHOTOSENSITIVITY AND WITHDRAWAL REACTIONS

Light combined with drugs (Table 411-4) can produce photosensitivity reactions that can be quite severe and mimic sunburn. Ultraviolet radiation interacts with a drug or its metabolite to generate reactive oxygen species, leading to cellular damage. Tetracyclines, sulfa drugs, NSAIDs, and fluoroquinolones are often implicated in photosensitivity reactions. Photosensitizing drugs may exacerbate lupus erythematosus (Chapter 250) or porphyria cutanea tarda (Chapter 199).

CONTACT DERMATITIS

Allergic contact dermatitis is a T-cell–mediated delayed hypersensitivity reaction that occurs after topical drug application or exposure to poison ivy, oak, or sumac. It is manifested by erythema and microvesiculation and may spread beyond the area of application (id reaction). Common contact sensitizers include Neosporin (polymyxin B, neomycin, and bacitracin), bacitracin, diphenhydramine, doxepin, lidocaine, lanolin, mercury, henna, ethyl cyanoacrylate (eyelash adhesive), nickel, hair dyes, latex, and p-aminobenzoic acid.

● BENIGN PAPULES, NODULES, AND TUMORS

The skin is heterogeneous, composed of epidermis, dermis, subcutaneous compartments, and blood vessels. The skin hosts a number of migrating cells (Chapter 407), all of which can give rise to benign or malignant tumors. Lesions that arise from epidermal keratinocytes are usually papules (warts, sebaceous hyperplasia) or plaques (psoriasis, Bowen disease). Nodules are deeper lesions that may be tender or asymptomatic and single or multiple, and they break down to form ulcers. Nodules are classified as inflammatory (granulomas, vasculitis, or panniculitis), infectious, vascular, or metabolic; they can be benign or malignant tumors that arise from skin cells or migrant cells (Table 411-5). Nodules that are smaller and symmetrical are more likely to be benign than lesions that grow rapidly, are larger, or invade surrounding tissue. Any rapidly changing skin nodule should be investigated with an excisional biopsy to the level of fat and sent for histology as well as for bacterial, fungal, and acid-fast cultures.

Benign Epidermal Tumors

The top layer of skin is the avascular epidermis composed of keratinocytes that undergo apoptosis from the stratum corneum. Melanocytes, Langerhans

TABLE 411-5	TUMORS AND NODULES OF THE SKIN

Benign, nonpigmented tumors and nodules
  Epidermal: warts, acrochordons, tricholemmomas, sebaceous hyperplasia
  Adnexal: epidermal cysts, syringomas, follicular cysts, pilomatricoma, apocrine or eccrine adenomas
  Dermal and subcutaneous: lipomas, angiolipomas, neurofibromas, leiomyomas

Benign, pigmented tumors and nodules
  Epidermal: seborrheic keratoses
  Melanocytic compound nevi (junctional nevi are flat)
  Spitz nevus
  Blue nevus
  Dermatofibromas

Malignant, nonpigmented tumors and nodules
  Basal cell carcinoma (nodular, superficial, morpheaform, pigmented)
  Squamous cell carcinoma (actinic keratoses, Bowen disease, keratoacanthomas)
  Cutaneous T- and B-cell lymphomas
  Amelanotic melanomas
  Merkel cell carcinomas
  Adnexal carcinomas of the sebaceous and apocrine glands

Malignant, pigmented tumors and nodules
  Pigmented basal cell carcinoma
  Malignant melanoma: in situ, superficial spreading, nodular, acral lentiginous
  Dermatofibrosarcoma protuberans

Inflammatory nodules over joints
  Gottron papules (dermatomyositis)
  Gouty tophi
  Heberden nodes (osteoarthritis)
  Multicentric reticulohistiocytosis (paraneoplastic syndrome)
  Rheumatoid nodules
  Granuloma annulare

Inflammatory nodules of the lower extremities
  Panniculitis
  Vasculitis: periarteritis nodosa

Metabolic nodules of the skin
  Amyloidosis
  Gouty tophi
  Xanthomas, necrobiotic xanthogranuloma
  Xanthelasma

Vascular lesions
  Benign: nevus flammeus, angiokeratomas, spider hemangiomas, capillary hemangiomas, cavernous hemangiomas, blue rubber bleb nevi, pyogenic granulomas
  Malignant: Kaposi sarcoma, angiosarcoma

cells, and inflammatory cells may enter the epidermis. Epidermal stem cells form adnexal organs such as hair follicles and sebaceous, eccrine, and apocrine glands that can give rise to tumors.

ACTINIC KERATOSES

Actinic keratoses are pink, scaly macules composed of sun-damaged keratinocytes and are precursors of in situ squamous cell carcinomas (Bowen disease) or invasive squamous carcinomas (Chapter 193). Actinic keratoses are 0.1 cm to 1.0 cm large and are found on sun-exposed areas such as the forearms, hands, face, and scalp (Fig. 411-7). Lesions with induration, thick crusts, ulceration, or pain are excised for biopsy to exclude invasive squamous cell carcinoma. Actinic keratoses can be treated with cryotherapy and topical fluorouracil,[A4][A5] retinoids, imiquimod, or ingenol mebutate gel.[A6] To treat and prevent actinic keratoses, sun-exposed areas may be treated topically with 5-fluorouracil cream (5%) applied daily for 2 weeks or twice weekly for 8 weeks.

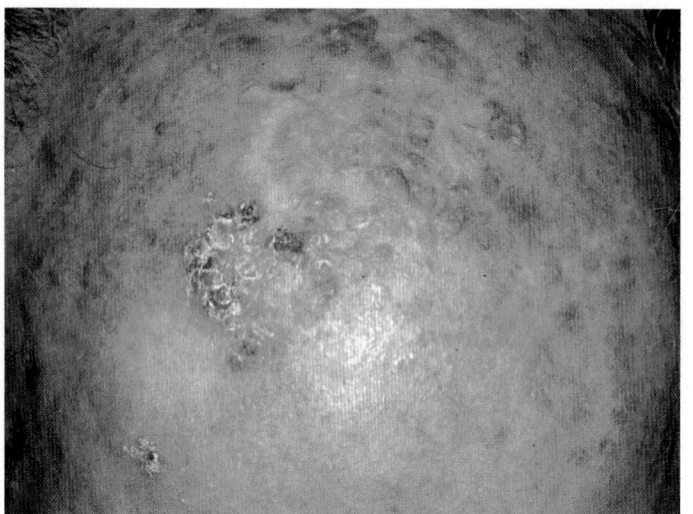

FIGURE 411-7. **Actinic keratoses.** Numerous hypertrophic actinic keratoses on the bald scalp, with hypopigmentation at sites of previous treatment. (From Bolognia. *Dermatology,* 4th ed.)

SEBORRHEIC KERATOSES

Seborrheic keratoses are common verrucous or stuck-on epidermal papules of various colors (Fig. 411-8). They are commonly seen with advancing age but may arise suddenly (sign of Leser-Trélat) in association with internal malignancy. Seborrheic keratoses consist of a single clone of keratinocytes and inherited as an autosomal dominant trait. Seborrheic keratoses have *FGFR3, PIK3CA, KRAS, EGFR, HRAS,* and *AKT* mutations but remain clinically benign. Their surface may be friable, and lesions can be scraped off. Seborrheic keratoses spare the palms, soles, and mucosal surfaces. Although benign, seborrheic keratoses must be differentiated from melanocytic nevi, melanomas, and pigmented basal cell carcinoma, usually by the presence of white to yellow horn cysts on their surface, best appreciated with dermoscopy.[6]

WARTY LESIONS

Epidermal papules include common warts (see Fig. 410-2 in Chapter 410) caused by human papillomavirus (HPV). HPV can also be detected in squamous carcinomas arising on the digits and in keratoacanthomas, which are low-grade, well-demarcated, dome-shaped papules or nodules that grow rapidly and spontaneously involute in 6 to 8 weeks. Acrodermatitis verruciformis is characterized by multiple warts with the appearance of seborrheic keratoses on the dorsal extremities and gives rise to squamous cell carcinomas. Molluscum contagiosum (Chapter 348) (Fig. 411-9), caused by a DNA virus, are small, shiny, domed-shaped, 1- to 5-mm papules with a central depression. Molluscum contagiosum lesions are common in children and immunocompromised patients. Treatment with anti-cancer BRAF inhibitors can cause warty papules, keratoacanthomas, and eruptive keratosis pilaris.

Cowden syndrome (Chapter 184), caused by mutations in *PTEN* gene, is associated with warty papules (tricholemmomas; Fig. 411-10); cobblestone papules on the gums and tongue; fibrous papules; and multiple hamartomas involving the breast, thyroid, intestines, ovary, and cerebellum.

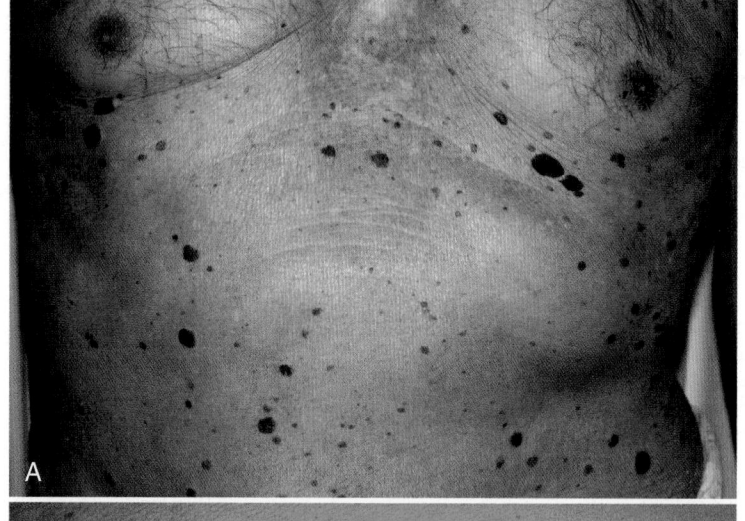

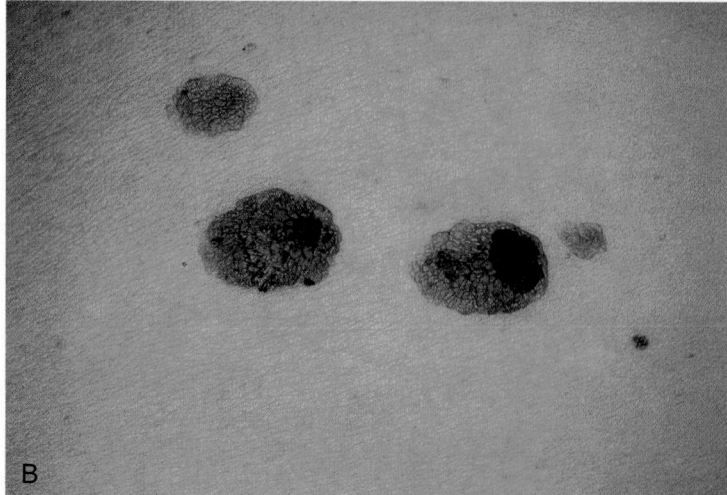

FIGURE 411-8. **Seborrheic keratoses. A,** Multiple seborrheic keratoses of the anterior trunk vary in size and color. **B,** Sharply demarcated, pigmented papules and plaques with a papillomatous surface and horn pseudocysts. Note the "stuck-on" appearance. (From Bolognia. *Dermatology,* 4th ed.)

ADNEXAL TUMORS

Adnexal tumors arise from hair follicles or glands and are commonly found on the face or scalp. Trichoepitheliomas resemble basal cell carcinomas. Sebaceous hyperplasia consists of small yellow papules with a central depression. Adnexal tumors of sebaceous origin, including sebaceous adenomas and sebaceous carcinomas, can also occur on the face, where they may be markers of the Muir-Torre syndrome of familial breast and colon cancer. Epidermal or sebaceous cysts, which are found in acne or as single firm nodules with a central pore, are filled with sebum or keratin. Epidermoid tumors of the scalp and a family history of colon cancer raise questions of a diagnosis of Gardner syndrome (Chapter 184).

DERMATOFIBROMAS AND COLLAGENOMAS

Fibroblasts, the resident cells of the dermis, produce collagen, elastin, and mucopolysaccharides. Accumulation of these products results in sclerosis,

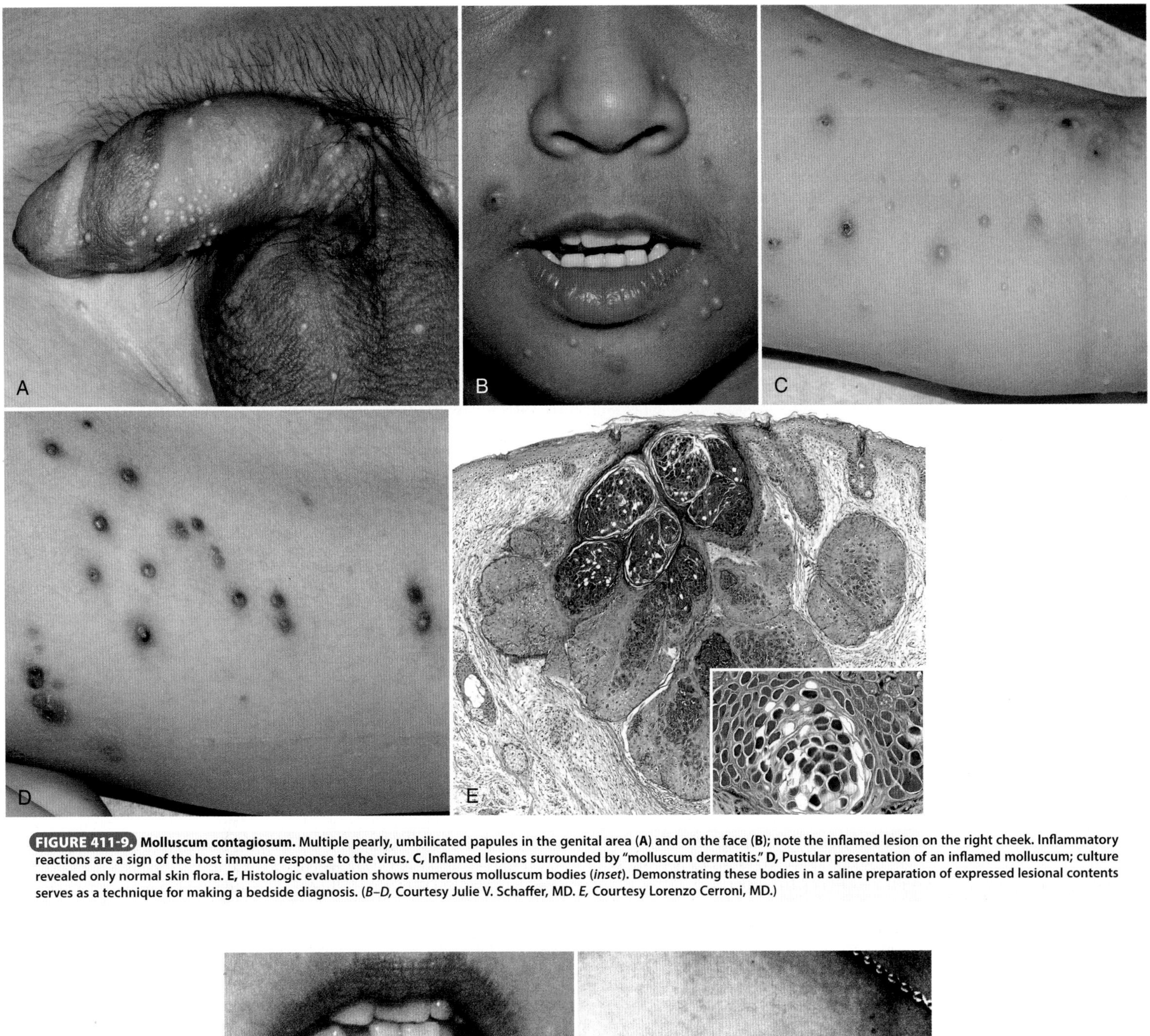

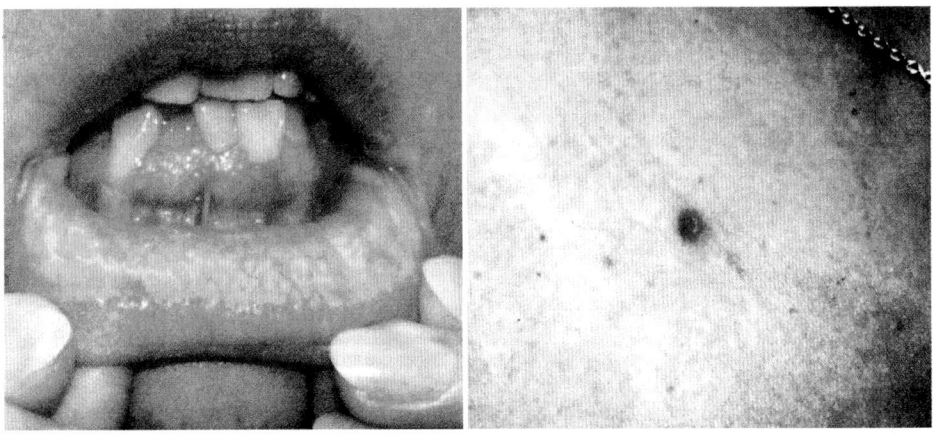

FIGURE 411-9. **Molluscum contagiosum.** Multiple pearly, umbilicated papules in the genital area (**A**) and on the face (**B**); note the inflamed lesion on the right cheek. Inflammatory reactions are a sign of the host immune response to the virus. **C,** Inflamed lesions surrounded by "molluscum dermatitis." **D,** Pustular presentation of an inflamed molluscum; culture revealed only normal skin flora. **E,** Histologic evaluation shows numerous molluscum bodies (*inset*). Demonstrating these bodies in a saline preparation of expressed lesional contents serves as a technique for making a bedside diagnosis. (*B–D, Courtesy Julie V. Schaffer, MD. E, Courtesy Lorenzo Cerroni, MD.*)

FIGURE 411-10. Cowden syndrome: cobblestone gums (*left*) and tricholemmoma (*right*).

papules, or nodules. Fibroblasts in small, dense clusters form firm brown or tan papules known as dermatofibromas. Dermatofibromas are hypertrophic scars that are commonly found on the extremities and that may form after insect bites or trauma. They are firm and well-demarcated papules, and the skin puckers when lateral pressure is applied. Dermatofibromas can be treated, but increased scarring may occur. The malignant counterpart is dermatofibroma sarcoma protuberans, which is a poorly defined, rapidly expanding, dermal, malignant tumor. Overlying erythema or hyperpigmentation is often present.

Some individuals have more pronounced and hypertrophic scar formation known as keloids, with an autosomal dominant or autosomal recessive inheritance pattern. Keloids (Chapter 412), which are shiny and firm in appearance, result from an overproduction of collagen. They are especially common on the anterior chest, neck, and earlobes and may require antineoplastic treatment, such as interferon alfa 2b, mitomycin C, bleomycin, and 5-fluorouracil (Chapter 169), and laser therapy.

Collagenomas and elastic tumors with the appearance of small white to yellow papules are found in the skin and bone of patients with Buschke-Ollendorff syndrome. *Pseudoxanthoma elasticum* (Chapter 244), an autosomal recessive disorder, is typically manifested as cutaneous yellow plaques on the neck or antecubital fossa from damaged elastin tissue. Mucin cysts are gray, shiny, well-demarcated, round nodules that generally arise on the mucosa or on the digits, where they may have an underlying connection to the joint space.

NEURAL CREST CELL TUMORS

Benign tumors in the dermis arising from neural crest cells include neurofibromas (soft, flesh-colored papules; Fig. 411-11), schwannomas (larger subcutaneous soft tumors or plaques; Fig. 411-12), and melanocytic lesions. Although solitary neurofibromas may occur, multiple lesions with café-au-lait spots (tan macules) or axillary freckling (Crowe sign) are diagnostic of neurofibromatosis type I, an autosomal dominant disorder caused by mutations in neurofibromin (Chapter 389). Schwannomas can become malignant and be manifested as dermal nodules. Merkel cell carcinoma, which is a neuroendocrine carcinoma of the skin, is a particularly aggressive small cell tumor arising from the cutaneous nerve endings or Meissner corpuscles. Merkel cell polyomavirus is associated with development of Merkel cell carcinoma.[7] Merkel cell carcinoma may present as a solitary pink to purple dome-shaped papule on the head or neck (Fig. 411-13). Sentinel lymph node biopsy is recommended in all patients with primary Merkel cell carcinoma. Treatment requires full excision, radiation therapy, and often chemotherapy because the cancer tends to recur and metastasize. For advanced Merkel-cell carcinoma, pembrolizumab (2 mg/kg every 3 weeks) provides an objective response rate of about 60% in virus-positive tumors and about 45% of virus-negative tumors.[8]

Melanocytic Lesions

Benign melanocytic moles or nevi (new) are discrete nests of melanocytes acquired during childhood and young adulthood, stimulated by sun exposure. Nevi are benign and composed of melanocytes (Chapter 193). They regress with age and change in color during pregnancy. Benign melanocytic nevi are formed by nests of melanocytes at the epidermal junction (junctional nevi), in the dermis (intradermal nevi), or in both compartments (compound nevi). Their appearance depends on type and age of the lesion. Junctional nevi (Fig. 411-14) are small, flat, and light to dark brown. Intradermal nevi are soft, flesh-colored to pink papules with smooth regular borders and surface. Compound nevi are globular papules with brown pigmentation. Blue nevi (Fig. 411-15) are flat, grayish blue, and regular. Small congenital nevi are dark brown, dysplastic nevi (Fig. 411-16), have variegated colors, and may transform into melanoma. More than 10 large, atypical moles with irregular borders and colors confer higher risk of developing melanoma, especially with a positive family history. Other recognized risk factors for melanoma include having more than 50 small nevi, red or blonde hair, or fair skin that burns and a history of blistering sunburns as a child. Patients with higher risk for melanoma should have surveillance and regular skin examinations.

Langerhans Cell Histiocytosis

Skin surveillance is mediated by antigen-presenting cells: Langerhans cells, dermal dendritic cells, and skin-homing T lymphocytes.[9] Proliferation of Langerhans cells is called histiocytosis. Childhood histiocytosis X is manifested as severe seborrheic dermatitis of the scalp and gluteal areas with underlying purpura and may result in the hemophagocytic syndrome. In adults, lesions appear in the intertriginous areas (Fig. 411-17). Patients with the non–Langerhans cell histiocytosis have lytic bone involvement (eosinophilic granulomas) or diabetes insipidus (Hand-Schüller-Christian syndrome).

Vascular Lesions
HEMANGIOMAS

Benign capillary, or cherry, hemangiomas are bright cherry-red to purple papules, generally less than 5 mm in diameter. They appear on the trunk with aging and may be numerous (Fig. 411-18). Pyogenic granulomas can resemble hemangiomas but contain polymorphonuclear leukocytes, are friable, and bleed easily. Multiple pyogenic granulomas are seen in infectious bacillary angiomatosis in immunocompromised hosts (Chapter 299). Cavernous or strawberry hemangiomas can also appear in the neonatal period as rapidly growing vascular tumors; they may obstruct the eye or the pharynx before regressing. Propranolol 2 to 3 mg/kg/day in two or three divided doses for 6 months can decrease the hemangioma's volume, color, and elevation in children younger than 5 years of age.[A7] Corticosteroids, interferon, or antiangiogenic factors also can treat these lesions if propranolol is not successful. Cavernous hemangiomas are deeper and less likely to resolve than smaller lesions. When associated with platelet consumption, Kasabach-Merritt syndrome is present (Chapter 162).

SARCOMAS

Kaposi sarcoma (Chapter 366) is a disseminated angiomatosis that arises from viral IL-8 production by herpesvirus 8.[10] Lesions are symmetrical purple, red, gray, or brown patches, papules, nodules, or ulcers (Fig. 411-19). Mucosal involvement is more common in advanced disease. Kaposi sarcoma in young African adults and Kaposi sarcoma associated with human immunodeficiency virus (HIV) infection often have a more aggressive course than Kaposi sarcoma in elderly men of Mediterranean background, whose disease is indolent and often confined to the lower extremities. Treatment of HIV disease with highly active antiretroviral therapy has been associated with a marked decreased incidence and severity of HIV-associated Kaposi sarcoma.

Angiosarcomas are malignant purple to red vascular tumor nodules that are more common in elderly individuals or on the extremities of patients with chronic lymphedema. To help distinguish cutaneous angiosarcomas from benign histologic mimics, immunohistochemistry staining for ERG, an ETS family transcription factor, is a specific and sensitive marker for endothelial differentiation.

Inflammatory and Hematopoietic Papules and Tumors

Inflammatory diseases of the skin involve the superficial or dermal vessels or subcutaneous tissue. Inflammatory infiltrates can be mixed or restricted in nature. Lymphocytes, polymorphonuclear leukocytes, histiocytes, eosinophils, and plasma cells are involved in the most common inflammatory reactions. Hematologic malignancies can present with secondary skin lesions, including patches, nodules, papules, or vasculitic lesions. Skin-homing CD4[+] T cells give rise to cutaneous T-cell lymphomas. Mycosis fungoides (Chapter 176) lesions are pleomorphic pink, white, or brown patches or plaques; alopecia; or diffuse erythroderma with blood involvement (Sézary syndrome). Early patch or plaque mycosis fungoides is indistinguishable from chronic eczematous or psoriasiform dermatitis. Tumors occur late in mycosis fungoides and can transform to a large cell lymphoma phenotype, with or without expression of CD30. Peripheral cutaneous T-cell lymphomas may also be found in subcutaneous tissue as panniculitic lesions. Lymphomatoid papulosis is characterized by crops of red to pink self-regressing papules with histologic findings similar to those of anaplastic large cell lymphoma (Chapter 176), including expression of CD30 antigen. Clinically, lymphomatoid papulosis presents as self-regressing papules, CD3[+] anaplastic T-cell lymphomas can present as tumors, and patients with transformed CD30[+] mycosis fungoides initially have patch or plaque stage disease before developing tumors. Treatment of lymphomatoid papulosis consists of topical corticosteroids, methotrexate, or bexarotene. For CD30[+] anaplastic T-cell lymphoma, therapeutic options include radiation therapy, methotrexate, bexarotene, brentuximab vedotin, and chemotherapy (Chapter 176). Natural killer T-cell lymphomas, immunoblastic lymphomas, and plasmacytoid dendritic cell tumors appear as brown to purple dermal nodules often with purpura.

Cutaneous B-cell lymphomas present as pink, infiltrated, dome-shaped shiny papules or tumors. Whereas follicular B-cell lymphoma is commonly located on the face, scalp, or upper part of the back, mucosa-associated B-cell tumors are more common on the trunk. With the exception of large B-cell lymphoma, follicular and mucosa-associated lymphoid tissue (MALT) B-cell lymphomas of the skin are indolent. Cutaneous MALT lymphomas (Fig. 411-20) have been associated with *Borrelia* spp infection (Chapter 305), *Helicobacter pylori* infection, and chronic inflammation. Plasmacytomas

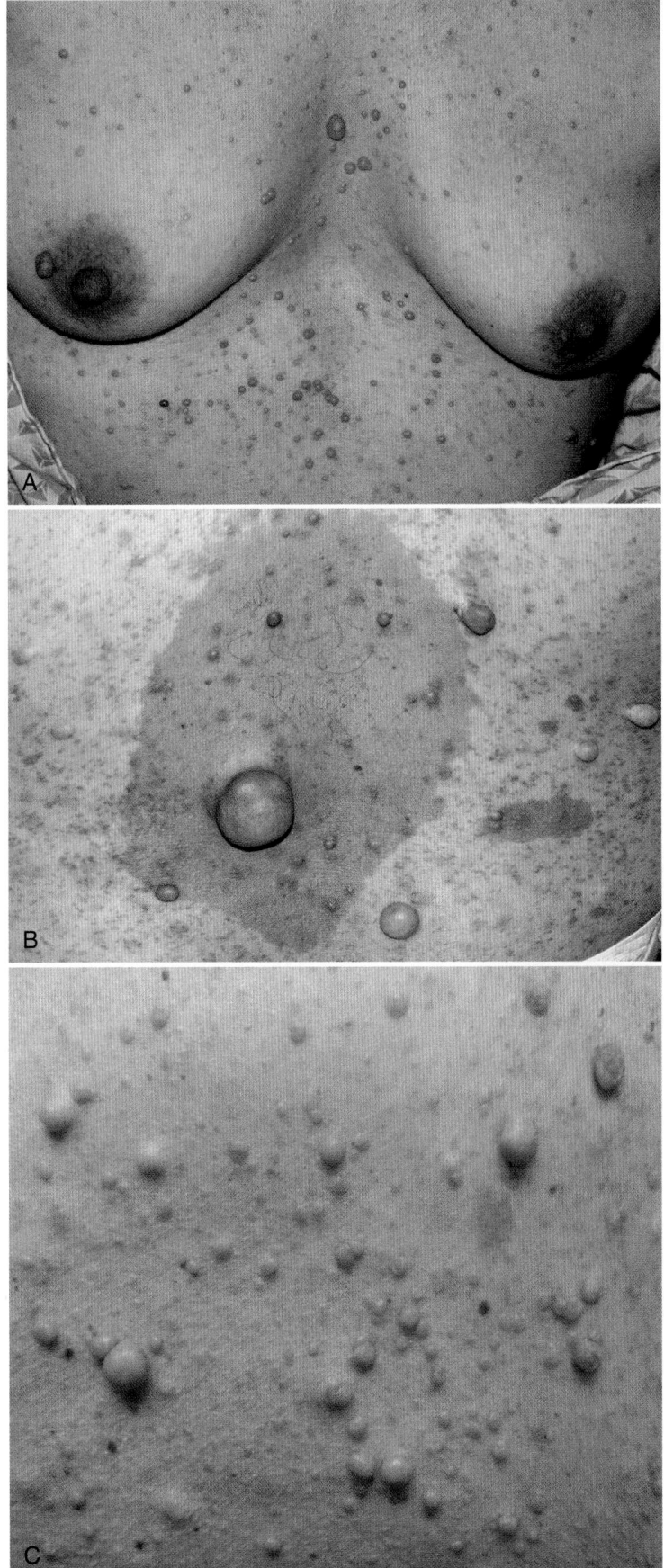

FIGURE 411-11. **Multiple cutaneous neurofibromas.** Soft, skin-colored to pinkish-tan, dome-shaped or polypoid, well-demarcated papules and nodules of various sizes (**A–C**) can occur in patients with neurofibromatosis. Neurofibromas may be superimposed on café-au-lait macules and lentigines (**B, C**). (*A, B,* Courtesy Julie V. Schaffer, MD.)

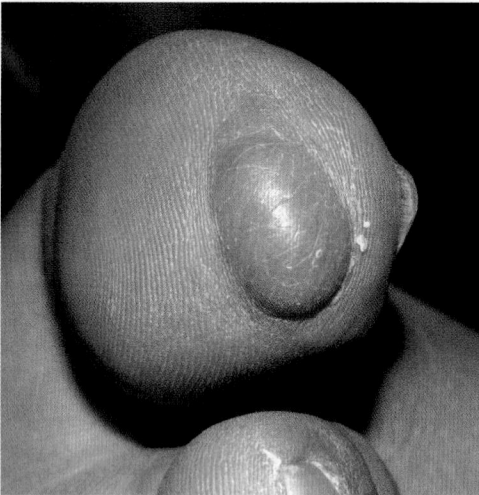

FIGURE 411-12. Solitary schwannoma. Skin-colored nodule on the plantar surface of the great toe. (Courtesy Julie V. Schaffer, MD.)

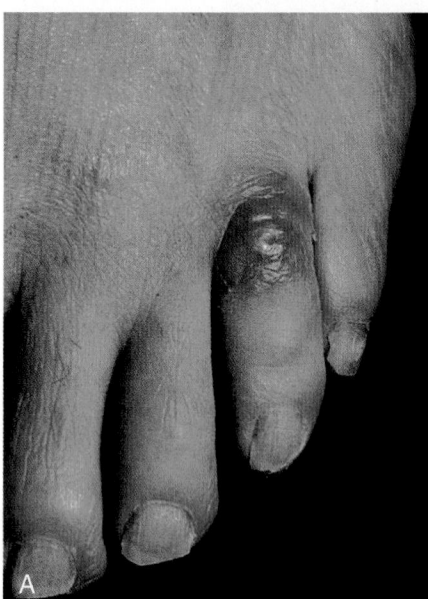

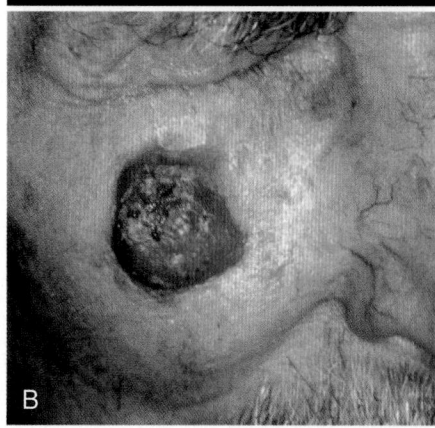

FIGURE 411-13. Merkel cell carcinoma (primary neuroendocrine carcinoma). A, A rapidly growing, violaceous nodule on the toe. B, Large, eroded, erythematous nodule arising within sun-damaged skin of the cheek. (B, Courtesy Lorenzo Cerroni, MD.)

can arise in the skin, in bone, with multiple myeloma (Chapter 178), or independently. Extramedullary hematopoiesis or endometriosis can be associated with red or brown nodules in the dermis.

Granulomatous Diseases

Sarcoidosis is an inflammatory granulomatous process manifested as ichthyosis, papules, plaques, or tumors with an apple-jelly color (Fig. 411-21). Patients with lepromatous leprosy also can have histiocytic plaques or tumors (Fig.

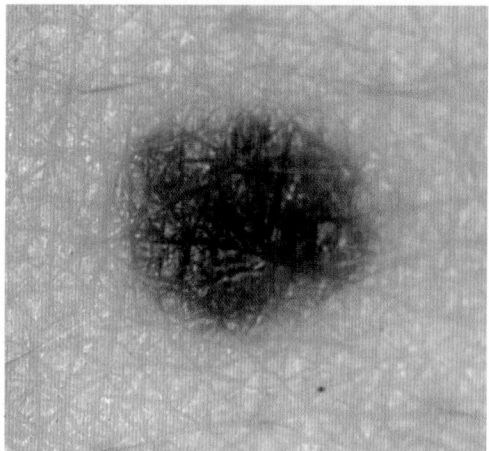

FIGURE 411-14. Junctional nevus. (From Bolognia. *Dermatology*, 4th ed.)

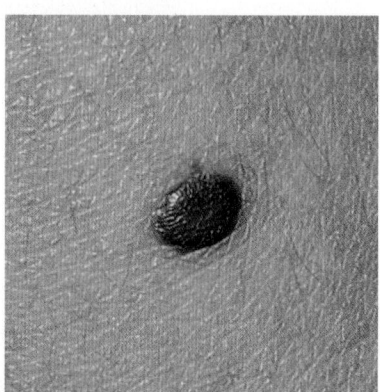

FIGURE 411-15. Benign blue nevus. Well-circumscribed, dark blue flat papule. (From Bolognia. *Dermatology*, 4th ed.)

411-22); treatment of leprosy may induce an inflammatory reaction called erythema nodosum leprosum. Granulomatous mycosis fungoides, which is a variant of cutaneous T-cell lymphoma, is difficult to diagnose and treat. Granulomatous inflammation within the dermis can result in damage to collagen, as seen in granuloma annulare (ringlike pink to red infiltrated lesions, often on the hands or elbows), rheumatoid nodules that occur on the extensor surface of the arms, and necrobiosis lipoidica on the shins of patients with diabetes. All three lesions typically include fibrin deposits within dermal blood vessels. Multicentric reticulohistiocytosis is a rare paraneoplastic syndrome in which histiocytic nodules form over joints with associated arthritis.

Inflammatory Skin Lesions and Nodules

Inflammatory skin nodules arise from inflamed blood vessels (vasculitis) or adipose tissue (panniculitis). Either can arise in response to underlying infection or antigen stimulation with influx of inflammatory cells. Vasculitis is categorized by vessel size and circulating immune complexes. Damage to blood vessels results in leakage of red blood cells with the development of purpura (nonblanching red to purple lesions; Chapter 254).

Sweet syndrome, also called febrile neutrophilic dermatosis (Fig. 411-23), is accompanied by fever, leukocytosis, and tender reddish skin plaques.[11] Some patients also have arthralgia. Biopsy shows sheets of leukocytes filling the upper dermis in the absence of infection. It can be idiopathic; drug induced; or associated with an underlying disease, typically with an underlying streptococcal infection, acute myelogenous leukemia, other malignancies, inflammatory bowel disease, or rheumatoid arthritis. Use of hematopoietic growth factors also can precipitate Sweet syndrome. Sweet syndrome, but not erythema elevatum diutinum, is highly responsive to corticosteroids (oral prednisone 1 to 2 mg/kg/day gradually tapered over 6 weeks to 3 months) or indomethacin (150 mg per day for 1 week; then 100 mg per day for 2 weeks), but oral dapsone (100 to 200 mg/day) can improve both conditions.

Erythema elevatum diutinum is manifested as multiple, infiltrated pink, yellow, red, or violaceous nodules or papules that may be painful or asymptomatic. The lesions can coalesce to form gyrate lesions on the dorsum of the hands or extensor surfaces similar to granuloma annulare. Erythema elevatum diutinum is associated with upper respiratory infections (especially *Streptococcus*

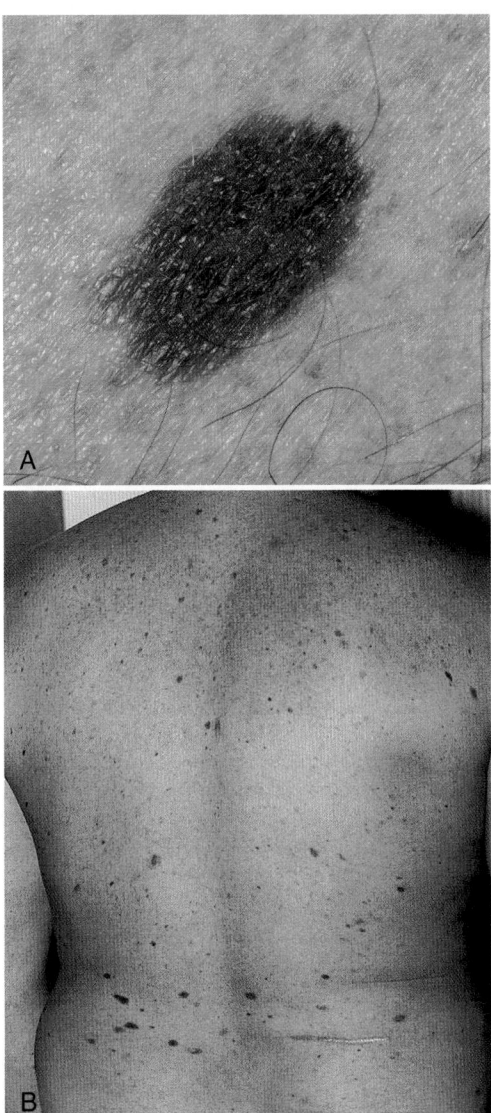

FIGURE 411-16. **Atypical melanocytic nevi. A,** There is asymmetry as well as several shades of brown, simulating the clinical features seen in cutaneous melanoma. **B,** In addition to multiple atypical nevi, patients can have numerous typical nevi. (From Bolognia. *Dermatology,* 4th ed.)

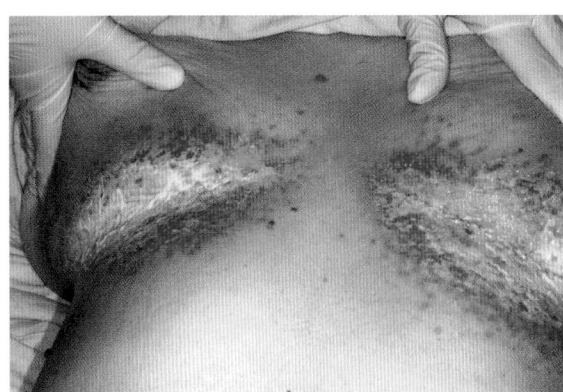

FIGURE 411-17. Histiocytosis X in intertriginous areas.

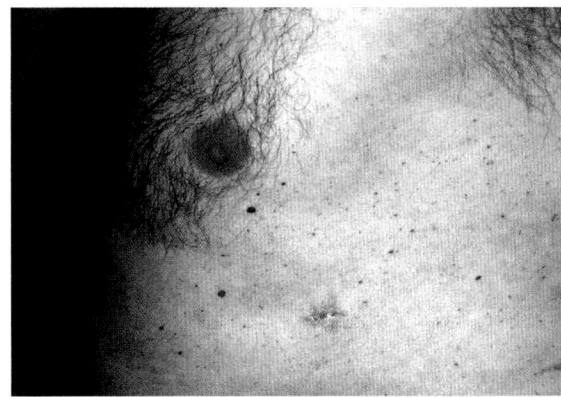

FIGURE 411-18. Benign capillary hemangioma.

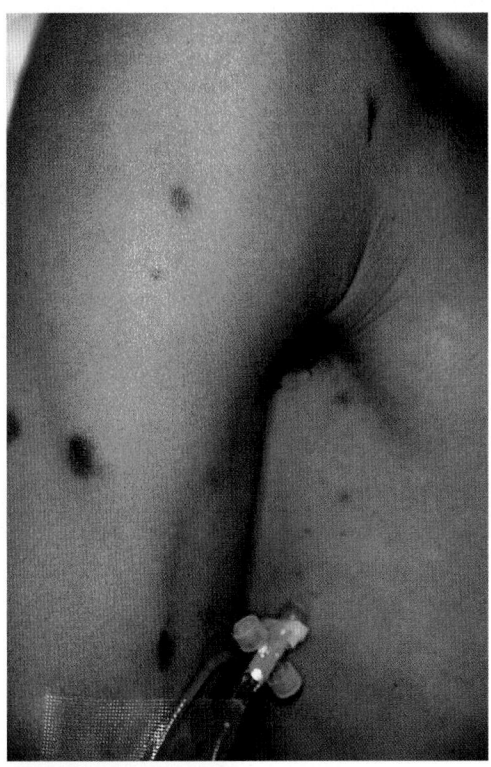

FIGURE 411-19. **Kaposi sarcoma in a patient with AIDS.** Violet-red papules or nodules are often oval to lanceolate and are usually more widely distributed than in classic Kaposi sarcoma. (From Bolognia. *Dermatology,* 4th ed.)

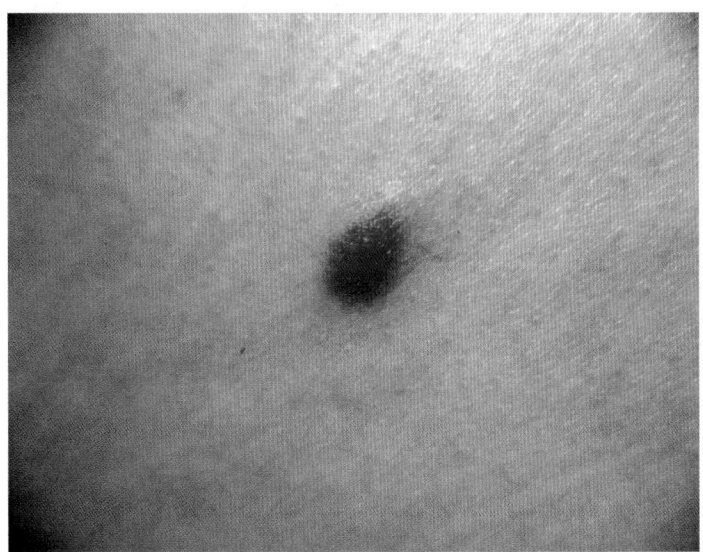

FIGURE 411-20. Cutaneous mucosa-associated lymphoid tissue (MALT) lymphoma.

spp), HIV infection, and inflammatory bowel disease. Clinically, the lesions look similar to Sweet syndrome, but their underlying histopathology (a necrotizing vasculitis with neutrophils and hyalinization of the vessels) can be distinguished from the neutrophils seen in the upper dermis in Sweet syndrome on biopsy.

Polyarteritis Nodosa and Panniculitis

Polyarteritis nodosa (Chapter 254) arises in larger arterioles and may be associated with hepatitis C infection, mesenteric aneurysms, cryoglobulinemia, cutaneous ulceration, and livedo reticularis. Polyarteritis nodosa is distinct from small vessel leukocytoclastic vasculitis, which is characterized by smaller areas (a few millimeters) of purpura.

In the clinical setting, *panniculitis* occurs more frequently than nodular vasculitis. The diagnosis of vasculitis versus septal or lobular panniculitis requires an excisional biopsy, including fat, with appropriate cultures and stains.

Erythema nodosum (Fig. 411-24) is a septal panniculitis characterized by tender nodules that are 1 to 2 cm in diameter with warm, pink, overlying epidermis. They appear in crops on the extremities. A perivascular inflammatory infiltrate is present around small intralobular vessels without vasculitis. Erythema nodosum arises frequently in response to sarcoidosis (Chapter 89), various infections, inflammatory bowel disease, or drug use and less commonly in patients with azathioprine-induced pancreatitis or primary biliary cirrhosis. Often, however, the underlying cause remains unknown (Table 411-6).

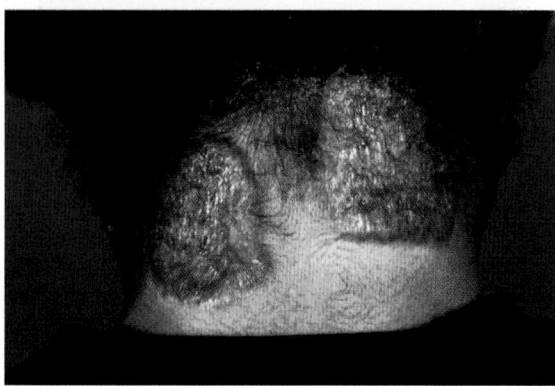

FIGURE 411-21. Cutaneous sarcoidosis.

Lobular panniculitis with necrosis and purpura is called nodular vasculitis or erythema induratum.[12] Nodular vasculitis is characterized by painful, chronic recurrent nodules on the shin or thighs that become bluish, ulcerate, and heal with scarring. Erythema induratum (Fig. 411-25) is exacerbated by cold exposure and is sometimes associated with *Mycobacterium tuberculosis* (Chapter 308). True lobular panniculitis, with or without fat necrosis, is more frequent in men with underlying pancreatitis (Chapter 135) and may precede pancreatic cancer (Chapter 185). The lesions have a predilection for the anterior aspect of the shins and may be fluctuant as a result of fat necrosis. *Lupus panniculitis,* or lupus profundus, which involves the fat, is diagnosed by overlying granular immune complex deposition of IgM along the dermal-epidermal junction and is often difficult to distinguish from subcutaneous panniculitic T-cell lymphoma. Subcutaneous panniculitic γ/δ T-cell lymphoma is more aggressive and has a poor prognosis compared with α/β panniculitic T-cell lymphoma. Lupus panniculitis of the breast, which can be mistaken for adenocarcinoma, is treated with antimalarials or corticosteroids. Lobular panniculitis with calcification of the small arterioles, which occurs in the setting of renal failure with hyperparathyroidism, is called calciphylaxis (Chapter 121). Granulomatous lobular panniculitis may also arise in the setting of schistosomiasis (Chapter 334), Sjögren syndrome (Chapter 252), Crohn disease (Chapter 132), sarcoidosis (Chapter 89), ruptured epidermal cysts, atypical mycobacterial infection (Chapter 309), or tuberculosis (Chapter 308).

Fungal Infections

In immunocompromised patients, necrotic or granulomatous lobular panniculitis can be caused by disseminated fungal infections with *Candida* spp, *Sporothrix schenckii, Cryptococcus* spp, *Histoplasma* spp, *Nocardia* spp, *Rhizopus* spp, *Aspergillus* spp, *Fusarium* spp, or chromomycosis. Fungal mycelia invade vessel walls, where they produce purpuric and painful lesions that may ulcerate. Osler nodes, which are tender nodular vasculitic lesions on the extremities, occur in the setting of bacterial endocarditis (Chapter 67). Staphylococcal or streptococcal sepsis may be manifested as pustules, papules, or panniculitic lesions.

⬤ ATROPHIC AND SCLEROTIC LESIONS
Atrophic Lesions

Atrophic lesions result from thinning or loss of the epidermal and dermal layers (Table 411-7). Examples are photoaging caused by loss of epidermal thickness

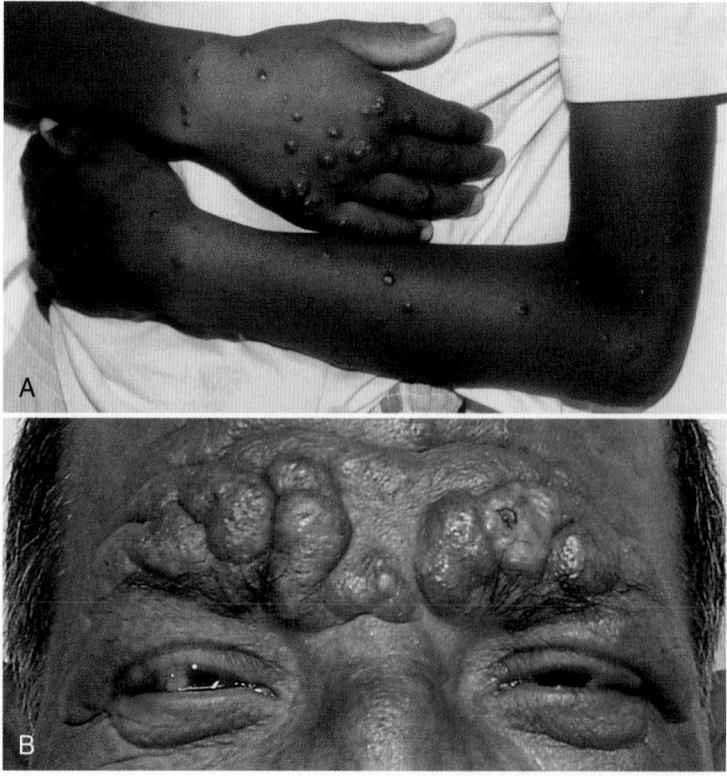

FIGURE 411-22. Lepromatous leprosy. A, Numerous erythematous papules and nodules on the forearms and hands. B, Infiltrated nodules coalescing on the forehead with leonine facies and madarosis. Note the ocular involvement.

and collagen, discoid lupus, and genetic disorders of collagen production (e.g., Ehlers-Danlos syndrome; Fig. 411-26). Epidermal wrinkling can result in a cigarette paper appearance with prominence of the underlying blood vessels. High-potency topical corticosteroids cause loss of collagen, resulting in atrophy. In Cushing syndrome (Chapter 214), striae appear as red or purple streaks because the underlying dermis can be seen through the epidermis.

Aging skin is most pronounced in sun-exposed areas, but intrinsic aging beginning as early as 30 years of age is characterized by abnormalities in the formation of elastin fibers. Aging of the skin is accompanied by decreased rete ridges and diminished circulation. Sunlight ages the skin by inducing proteolytic enzymes that digest the underlying collagen and elastin (wrinkles). In addition, sun exposure induces pigment incontinence (freckling), increased junctional nevi, and proliferation of benign keratinocyte growths (seborrheic keratoses).

Atrophy can also result from ongoing inflammatory processes that cause scarring, such as collagen vascular disease or mycosis fungoides. The cutaneous and discoid forms of lupus erythematosus (Chapter 250) are manifested

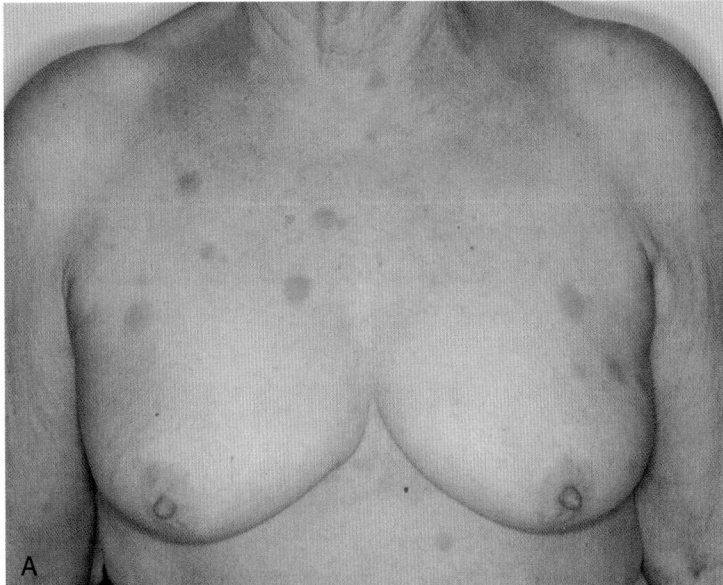

TABLE 411-6 TRIGGER FACTORS ASSOCIATED WITH ERYTHEMA NODOSUM

Infections
    Bacterial: *Streptococcus* spp, tuberculosis, leprosy, *Mycoplasma* spp, *Yersinia* spp, *Salmonella* spp, leptospirosis, tularemia
    Fungal: coccidioidomycosis, blastomycosis, histoplasmosis, dermatophytosis
    Viruses and *Chlamydia:* paravaccinia, Epstein-Barr virus, lymphogranuloma venereum, cat-scratch disease, psittacosis, hepatitis B

Drugs: sulfonamides, bromides, oral contraceptives

Malignancies: lymphoma, leukemia, carcinoma, after tumor radiation

Inflammatory: ulcerative colitis, Crohn disease, Whipple disease, Behçet syndrome, Sweet syndrome, collagen vascular diseases

Pregnancy

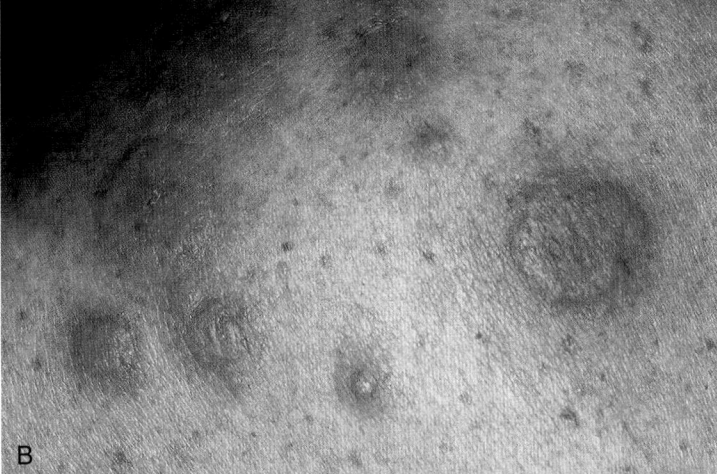

FIGURE 411-23. Sweet syndrome. **A,** Scattered tender, edematous pink papules and plaques on the chest. **B,** The edema can be quite marked as seen in these lesions on the upper back. (*B,* Courtesy Kalman Watsky, MD.)

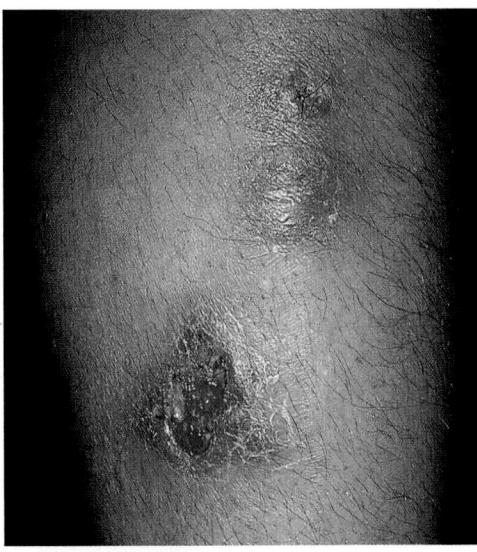

FIGURE 411-25. Erythema induratum—clinical appearance. Inflamed nodular lesions on the lower leg, with evidence of ulceration. (Courtesy Kenneth E Greer, MD.)

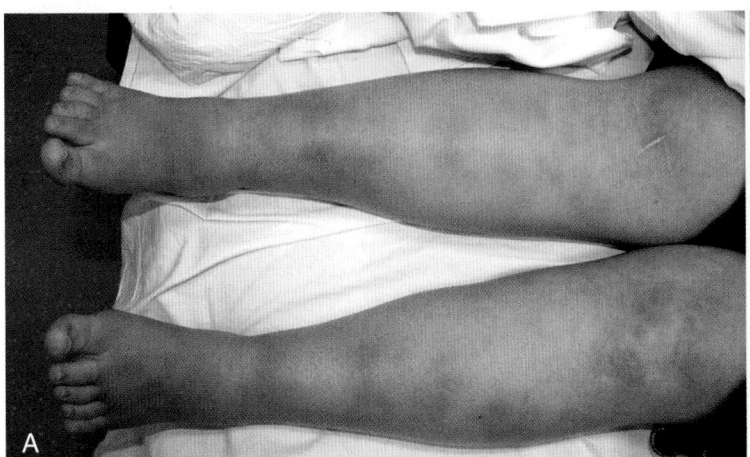
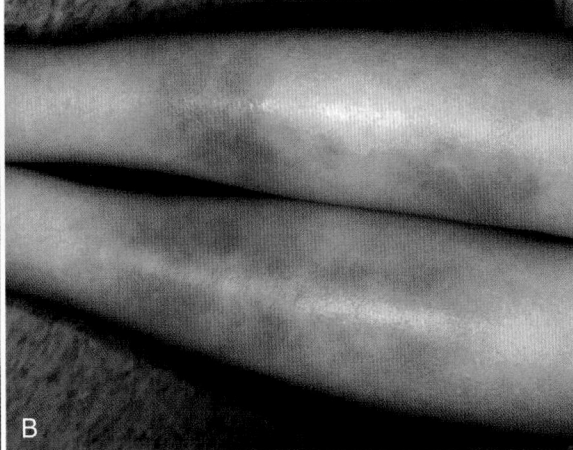

FIGURE 411-24. Erythema nodosum—clinical appearance. **A,** Erythematous, tender nodules bilaterally on the shins and dorsal feet. **B,** The nodules and plaques may develop a bruise-like appearance. (*A,* Courtesy Ian Odell, MD, PhD. *B,* Courtesy Kalman Watsky, MD.)

TABLE 411-7	ATROPHIC SKIN CONDITIONS WITH SCARRING, ULCERATIONS, OR TELANGIECTASES

ATROPHY

Epidermal: chronic corticosteroid use, photoaging, mycosis fungoides
Dermal elastin: anetoderma, cutis laxa, intrinsic aging
Dermal collagen: Ehlers-Danlos syndrome, aging
Subcutaneous: granulomatous slack skin (a mycosis fungoides variant)
Lipodystrophy (loss of fat)

SCARRING OR ATROPHY WITH TELANGIECTASIAS

Discoid and subacute cutaneous lupus erythematosus
Dermatomyositis
Keloid formation
Large plaque parapsoriasis (poikiloderma vasculare atrophicans variant of mycosis fungoides)
Photoaging
Necrobiosis lipoidica diabeticorum
Radiation dermatitis
Porphyrias
Thermal burns (erythema ab igne)

SCLEROSIS OR INFILTRATIVE PROCESSES

Amyloidosis
Systemic sclerosis, scleroderma
Localized sclerosis, morphea
Lichen sclerosis et atrophicus
Lichen myxedematosus or papular mucinosis (mucopolysaccharide deposition with paraproteinemia)
Myxedema (mucin deposits with anti–thyroid-stimulating hormone receptor antibodies)

ULCERATIONS

Secondary breakdown of any blister or nodule: infectious, inflammatory, tumor, vasculitis
Decubitus or pressure ulcers
Genital ulcers: syphilis, herpes simplex, chancroid, lymphogranuloma venereum, Behçet syndrome
Pyoderma gangrenosum, Sweet syndrome

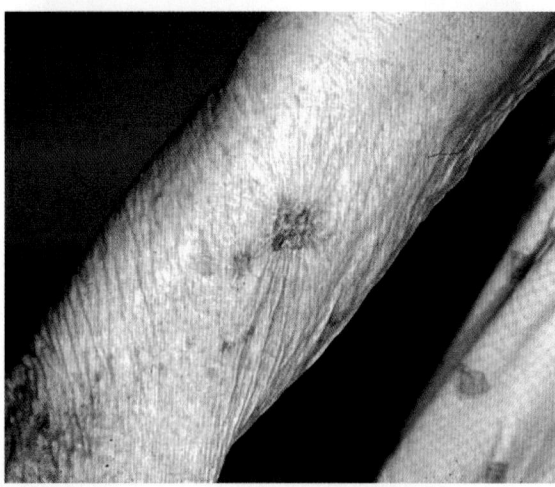

FIGURE 411-26. Atrophic skin in Ehlers-Danlos syndrome type 2.

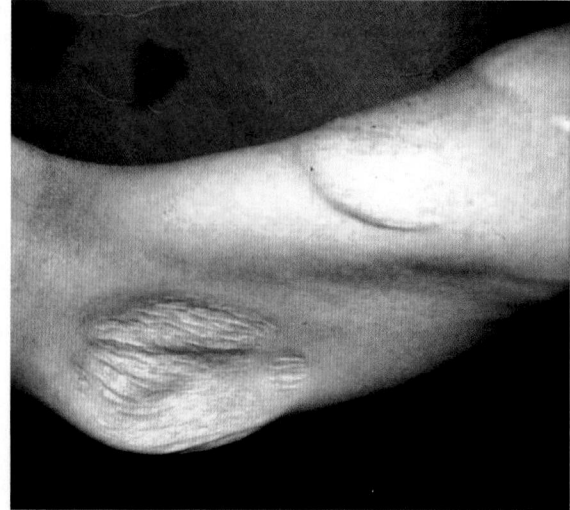

FIGURE 411-27. Anetoderma.

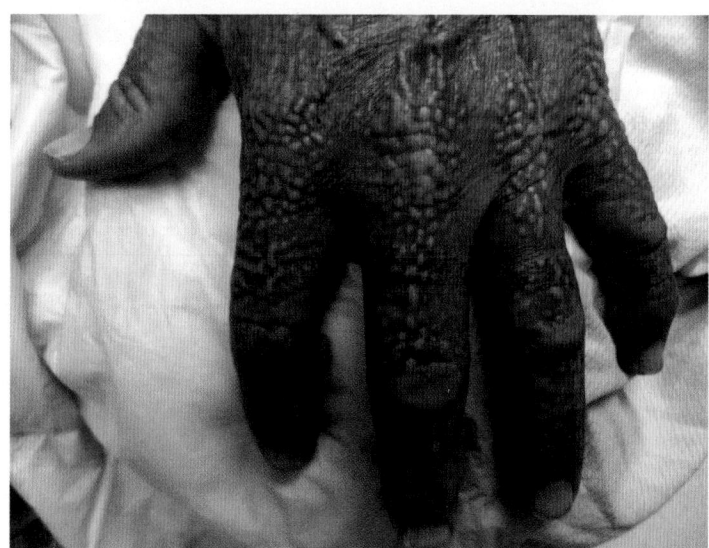

FIGURE 411-28. Lichen myxedematosus.

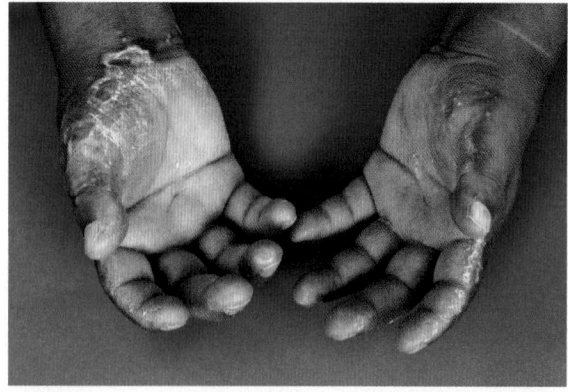

FIGURE 411-29. Nephrogenic systemic fibrosis.

as scaly plaques with atrophy or alopecia on sun-exposed areas; the systemic form is characterized by malar rash, urticaria, or vasculitic lesions. Dermatomyositis (Chapter 253) can be associated with collagen vascular disease or malignancy; periorbital suffusion, telangiectasia of the nail beds, and Gottron papules or scaly lesions over the joints are the skin manifestations. Anetodermas are localized sclerotic lesions (Fig. 411-27) with distinctive clinical features from underlying inflammation.

Eosinophilic fasciitis is accompanied by nodules or sclerosis of the lower extremities, myopathy, pulmonary disease, and eosinophilia. This syndrome, which follows the ingestion of L-tryptophan or its contaminants, resembles the panniculitis seen in systemic sclerosis, in which fat lobules are replaced by new collagen formation. Eosinophilic cellulitis, or Wells syndrome, is manifested as nodules, papules, or ulcerative lesions, as well as red plaques in which eosinophils infiltrate the area between collagen fibers.

Sclerotic Lesions

Sclerotic lesions are accompanied by more collagen production, which results in skin with a glossy appearance.[13] Sclerosis may also result from the accumulation of mucopolysaccharides in scleromyxedema (lichen myxedematosus) or from amyloid deposits. Papular mucinosis, lichen myxedematosus (Fig. 411-28), and scleromyxedema are a spectrum of diseases that are caused by deposition of hyaluronic acid. An entity associated with renal failure and gadolinium exposure, nephrogenic fibrosing dermopathy (Fig. 411-29), is also

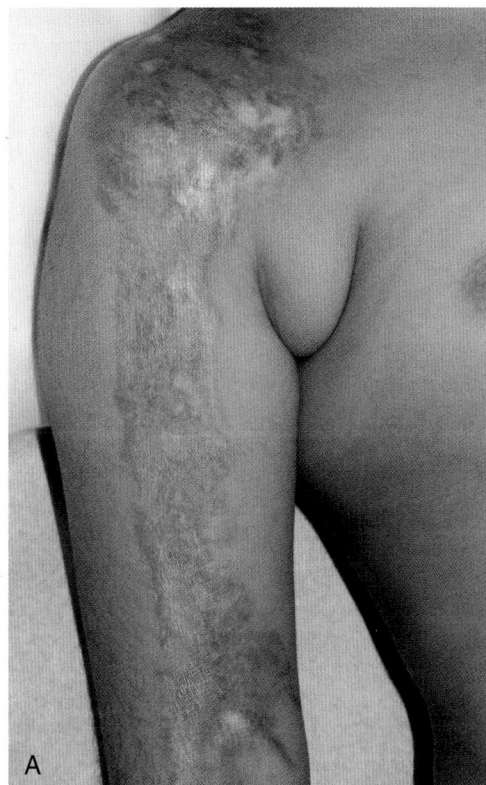

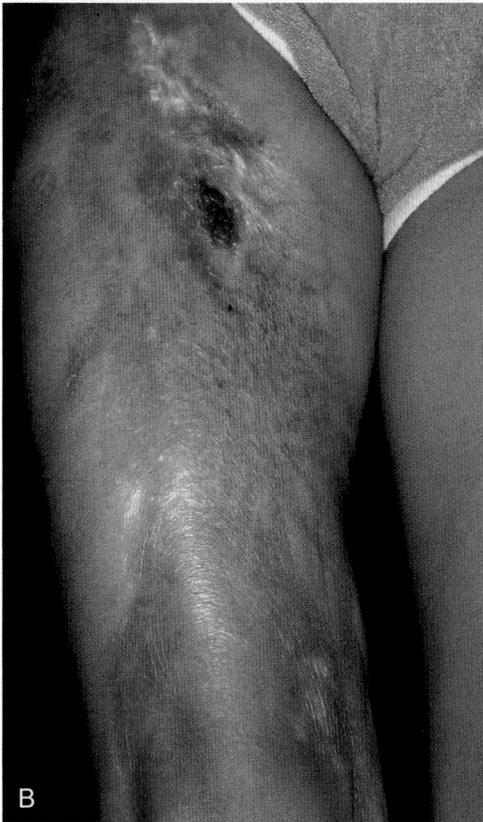

characterized by acral fibrosis and deposition of hyaluronate in the skin. In scleroderma (Chapter 251), increased collagen deposition may be associated with Raynaud syndrome, calcinosis, and telangiectasia. A localized form of scleroderma, termed *morphea,* may occur down the center of the face (coup de sabre) or as plaques on the extremities (Fig. 411-30), after radiation exposure, or with *Borrelia* spp infection. Lichen sclerosis et atrophicus is a superficial inflammatory morphea characterized by white atrophic patches, especially in the genital region. Widespread systemic sclerosis may also follow bone marrow transplantation in the setting of chronic graft-versus-host disease.

Telangiectasia

Telangiectasia is prominence of skin blood vessels that frequently accompanies atrophic as well as sclerotic processes and is common in photoaged skin and after radiation therapy. Telangiectasia of the mucous membranes is found in Osler-Weber-Rendu syndrome (Chapter 164), and vascular spiders are found both in α_1-antitrypsin deficiency and alcoholic liver disease. The presence of telangiectasia, hyperpigmentation, and hypopigmentation (poikiloderma) in sun-shielded areas of the body should alert the clinician to the diagnosis of early mycosis fungoides.

Ulcers

Ulcers are secondary skin lesions that may arise from trauma, loss of proper blood supply, aging, vasculitis, blister formation, infection, or underlying neoplasia. Ulcers may be shallow erosions (loss of the epidermis) or may be deeper and involve the dermis and underlying subcutaneous structures. Ulcers most commonly appear on the lower extremities, where they result from stasis dermatitis and venous insufficiency, arteriolar insufficiency, diabetic neuropathy, or vasculitis. *Pyoderma gangrenosum* is a trauma-induced ulcer that is part of the spectrum of Sweet syndrome, accompanies other conditions, and may require immunosuppressive therapy. Diagnosis requires skin biopsy, cultures, and serologic testing for other associated diseases. Treatment with prednisolone (0.75 mg/kg/day, maximum 75 mg/day) or cyclosporine (4 mg/kg/day, maximum 400 mg/day) is equally effective.[A8] In contrast, decubitus ulcers require débridement, elimination of local pressure, and attention to nutrition.

Grade A References

A1. Sharma M, Bennett C, Carter B, et al. H1-antihistamines for chronic spontaneous urticaria: an abridged Cochrane Systematic Review. *J Am Acad Dermatol.* 2015;73:710-716.
A2. Guillen-Aguinaga S, Jauregui Presa I, Aguinaga-Ontoso E, et al. Updosing nonsedating antihistamines in patients with chronic spontaneous urticaria: a systematic review and meta-analysis. *Br J Dermatol.* 2016;175:1153-1165.
A3. Zhao ZT, Ji CM, Yu WJ, et al. Omalizumab for the treatment of chronic spontaneous urticaria: a meta-analysis of randomized clinical trials. *J Allergy Clin Immunol.* 2016;137:1742-1750.
A4. Kulthanan K, Chaweekulrat P, Komoltri C, et al. Cyclosporine for chronic spontaneous urticaria: a meta-analysis and systematic review. *J Allergy Clin Immunol Pract.* 2018;6:586-599.
A5. Jansen MHE, Kessels J, Nelemans PJ, et al. Randomized trial of four treatment approaches for actinic keratosis. *N Engl J Med.* 2019;380:935-946.
A6. Pei S, Kaminska ECN, Tsoukas MM. Treatment of actinic keratoses: a randomized split-site approach comparison of sequential 5-fluorouracil and 5-aminolevulinic acid photodynamic therapy to 5-aminolevulinic acid photodynamic monotherapy. *Dermatol Surg.* 2017;43:1170-1175.
A7. Léauté-Labrèze C, Hoeger P, Mazereeuw-Hautier J, et al. A randomized, controlled trial of oral propranolol in infantile hemangioma. *N Engl J Med.* 2015;372:735-746.
A8. Ormerod AD, Thomas KS, Craig FE, et al. Comparison of the two most commonly used treatments for pyoderma gangrenosum: results of the STOP GAP randomised controlled trial. *BMJ.* 2015;350:1-8.

GENERAL REFERENCES

For the General References and other additional features, please visit Expert Consult at https://expertconsult.inkling.com.

FIGURE 411-30. **Linear morphea of an extremity. A,** Linear sclerotic band of the arm with both hyperpigmentation and hypopigmentation. The majority of patients with linear morphea have unilateral involvement. **B,** More inflammatory phase with ulceration in addition to induration. (*A,* Courtesy Julie V. Schaffer, MD.)

412

INFECTIONS, HYPERPIGMENTATION AND HYPOPIGMENTATION, REGIONAL DERMATOLOGY, AND DISTINCTIVE LESIONS IN BLACK SKIN

JEAN BOLOGNIA

INFECTIONS, INCLUDING CELLULITIS

Cutaneous infections can be divided into four major categories: bacterial, fungal (Chapter 409), viral, and parasitic (Table 412-1).

Bacterial Infections

Of the cutaneous bacterial infections, impetigo, folliculitis, furuncles, and cellulitis are most commonly encountered.

IMPETIGO

Impetigo, which is caused by *Staphylococcus aureus* or group A β-hemolytic streptococci, is usually seen as honey-colored crusts (Fig. 412-1); less often, subcorneal (superficial) bullae are present. This infection is most commonly found on the face in children, but it can develop at any site where the cutaneous

TABLE 412-1 SKIN INFECTIONS

BACTERIAL DISEASES

Impetigo
Ecthyma
Folliculitis
Furuncle/carbuncle
Abscess
Erysipelas
Cellulitis
Necrotizing fasciitis
Ecthyma gangrenosum
Other
   Gram-negative cocci: meningococcemia, gonococcemia
   Gram-positive bacilli: erythrasma, anaerobic cellulitis
   Spirochetes: Lyme disease, syphilis, endemic treponematoses
   Mycobacterial infections
   Rickettsial infections

VIRAL DISEASES

Herpes simplex virus: oral, genital, digital (whitlow)
Human papillomavirus: common warts, condyloma acuminata
Poxvirus: molluscum contagiosum
Varicella-zoster virus
Viral exanthems (e.g., enteroviruses, rubeola, rubella, parvovirus, Epstein-Barr virus, adenovirus, dengue virus, Zika virus, chikungunya virus, human immunodeficiency virus [seroconversion])

FUNGAL DISEASES

Candidiasis
Tinea (dermatophytoses): pedis, corporis, cruris, manuum, capitis
Pityriasis (tinea) versicolor
Emboli (e.g., *Aspergillus*, *Mucor* spp)

ECTOPARASITES/PARASITES

Scabies
Lice: scalp, pubic, body
Leishmaniasis
Schistosomiasis, human and animal
Onchocerciasis
Strongyloidiasis
Gnathostomiasis
Amebiasis
Trypanosomiasis
Hookworm infections, human and animal
Filariasis
Acanthamoebiasis

barrier has been disrupted (e.g., areas of dermatitis, sites of trauma, or arthropod bites). A deeper, but less common, bacterial infection of the skin is ecthyma, which is most frequently streptococcal in origin; it is characterized by thick hemorrhagic crusts overlying erosions or ulcerations, usually 0.5 to 1.5 cm in diameter. These lesions favor the extremities, especially in the setting of lymphedema. Ecthyma should not be confused with ecthyma gangrenosum, which represents an embolic phenomenon most often caused by bacteremia with gram-negative bacilli. Although mild cases of impetigo usually respond to topical 2% mupirocin three times daily or 1% retapamulin twice daily, more severe impetigo and ecthyma require oral antibiotics that cover *S. aureus* (e.g., dicloxacillin, 250 mg orally [PO] four times daily, or cephalexin, 250 mg PO four times daily). Compared with furuncles and abscesses, impetigo is less often due to methicillin-resistant *S. aureus* (MRSA).

FOLLICULITIS

The initial lesions of folliculitis are follicular pustules that are often surrounded by a rim of erythema (Chapter 410). Culture of pustular contents yields normal flora more often than *S. aureus* or gram-negative bacilli. *Pseudomonas* folliculitis, which favors the trunk, is usually associated with the use of hot tubs or whirlpools because their higher temperatures (vs. swimming pools) make eradication of *Pseudomonas* more difficult (see Fig. 410-27 in Chapter 410).

FURUNCLES

Furuncles, also called *boils*, represent *S. aureus* cutaneous infections that are localized primarily within the dermis. In contrast to folliculitis, the lesions are larger and manifest as tender erythematous nodules (Fig. 412-2). A central follicular structure may be noted, as may a central pustule ("pointing"). Because a furuncle is an abscess, the preferred treatment is incision and drainage followed by oral antistaphylococcal antibiotics (e.g., dicloxacillin, 250 mg PO four times daily, or cephalexin, 250 mg PO four times daily); if MRSA is likely (e.g., use of health care facilities such as dialysis units, participation in skin-to-skin contact sports, an elevated prevalence of methicillin-resistant isolates in the local community), the antibiotic should be changed to clindamycin (300 to 600 mg PO three times daily), doxycycline (100 mg PO twice daily), minocycline (100 mg PO twice daily), trimethoprim-sulfamethoxazole (160 mg/800 mg PO twice daily),**A1** or linezolid (600 mg PO twice daily), depending on local sensitivity patterns.[1] The duration of therapy is usually 10 to 14 days. Carbuncles, which are larger, more complex, and more extensive versions of furuncles, may be accompanied by systemic symptoms such as fever. In addition to incision and drainage, they may require a more prolonged course of antibiotic therapy.

CELLULITIS

Cellulitis is a fairly common cutaneous infection that occurs most often on the lower extremities. Locally, it manifests as erythema, edema, warmth, and

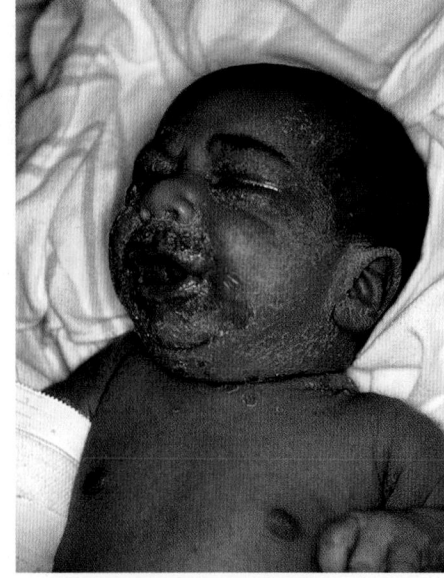

FIGURE 412-1. Impetigo in an infant and marked involvement of the face with honey-colored crusts and superficial erosions. (Courtesy Yale Dermatology Residents' Slide Collection.)

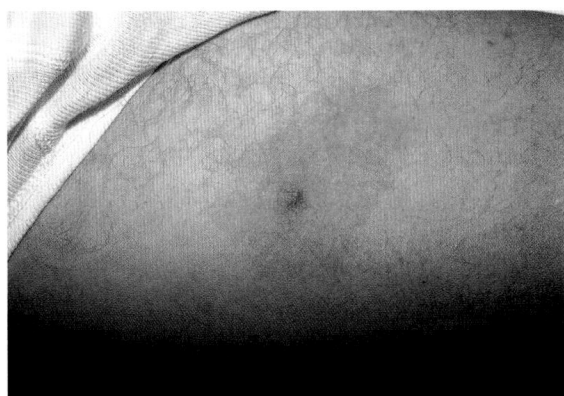

FIGURE 412-2. Furuncle with surrounding cellulitis. This common presentation of methicillin-resistant *Staphylococcus aureus* should be treated with incision and drainage as well as the administration of systemic antibiotics. (Courtesy Yale Dermatology Residents' Slide Collection.)

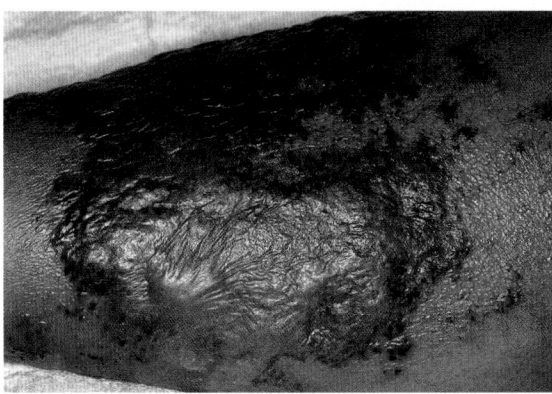

FIGURE 412-3. Bullous and hemorrhagic cellulitis of the shin. (Courtesy University of Southern California Dermatology Residents' Slide Collection.)

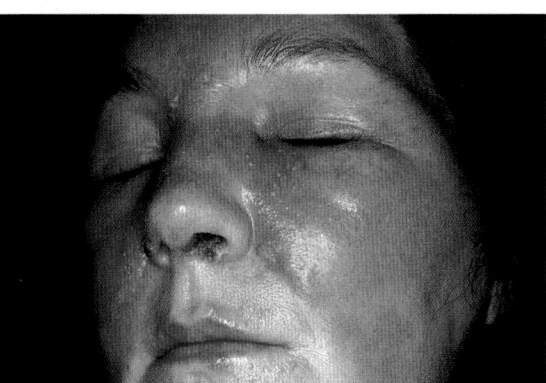

FIGURE 412-4. Erysipelas of the face with well-demarcated erythematous plaques. (Courtesy Yale Dermatology Residents' Slide Collection.)

tenderness; systemic findings can include fever, malaise, and leukocytosis. Most cases are bacterial in origin, but some are caused by fungal infections (e.g., *Cryptococcus* spp) or chemical reactions (e.g., extravasated oxacillin or calcium salts). Bacterial cellulitis is most commonly caused by group A β-hemolytic streptococci and *S. aureus*, with the former being associated with the more severe, necrotizing variant. Interestingly, the skin microbiome in the vicinity of the infection tends to be very similar to the contralateral microbiome, but both microbiomes typically differ from those of control patients. In patients who have diabetes or are immunocompromised, cellulitis can be caused by gram-negative bacilli or atypical mycobacteria. Risk factors include a preceding break in the skin barrier, edema secondary to venous hypertension, lymphedema, and previous bouts of cellulitis.

Although the diagnosis of cellulitis is usually fairly straightforward (Fig. 412-3), it can sometimes be difficult in patients with chronic lower extremity edema, especially in those who are afebrile and have persistent discoloration. One complication of chronic lower extremity edema is lipodermatosclerosis (i.e., inflammation followed by fibrosis of subcutaneous fat), which is seen acutely as erythema, warmth, and tenderness and is easily confused with cellulitis. The skin above the medial malleolus is often the initial site of involvement for lipodermatosclerosis, but the inflammation can extend onto the shin and calf. The chronic phase of lipodermatosclerosis is characterized by induration, a permanent brown-red to violet discoloration of the skin, and an "inverted wine bottle" appearance of the distal end of the lower extremity. It is important for the clinician to realize that in patients with chronic lipodermatosclerosis and superimposed cellulitis, the skin will never return to the color of uninvolved skin, even after adequate antibiotic therapy.

Unless there is an associated bacteremia, the diagnosis of cellulitis is primarily clinical. In immunocompromised hosts, a saline injection followed by aspiration and culture can be helpful. Histologically, cellulitis is characterized by an infiltrate of neutrophils within the dermis. Skin biopsy can exclude disorders that may be confused with cellulitis, such as contact dermatitis, erythema migrans, inflammatory carcinoma, toxic erythema of chemotherapy, and Wells syndrome (an idiopathic disorder in which eosinophils infiltrate the dermis).

Cellulitis resides in the middle of a spectrum of soft tissue infections that includes erysipelas (more superficial and more sharply demarcated; Fig. 412-4) at one end and necrotizing fasciitis (deeper, more necrotic, and undermining) at the other. In healthy adults, erysipelas can be treated with oral penicillin (200,000 units four times daily) or, if methicillin-sensitive *S. aureus* (MSSA) is of concern, oral dicloxacillin (500 mg four times daily) for a 10-day course.

Treatment for cellulitis should always cover *Streptococcus* and MSSA, with coverage for MRSA recommended for children, athletes, residents of long-term care facilities, military recruits, prisoners, patients with prior MRSA exposure, men who have sex with men, and intravenous drug users.[2] In general, oral antibiotic regimens are as effective as intravenous regimens.[A2] Options include oral cephalexin (250 to 500 mg four times daily for 10 to 14 days), clindamycin (300 mg three times daily for 10 days), or trimethoprim-sulfamethoxazole (160 mg/800 mg twice daily for 10 days),[A3] depending on the suspected pathogens, the host, and the severity of systemic toxicity. Penicillin (250 mg twice daily) can be effective in preventing recurrent cellulitis. Intravenous vancomycin plus intravenous ceftazidime (15 mg/kg twice daily

and 0.5 to 1 g three times daily, respectively, until clinical response allows transition to oral medications) is reserved for severe infections. Iclaprim (180 mg intravenously [IV] twice daily for 5-14 days) appears to be equally effective but is not currently approved by the U.S. Food and Drug Administration (FDA) for this indication.[A4]

Necrotizing fasciitis is usually caused by multiple organisms, including anaerobic streptococci; its diagnosis requires a high index of suspicion, and it must be considered when there are areas of painful violaceous induration or a foul-smelling discharge. Prompt surgical débridement and broad-spectrum systemic antibiotics (e.g., a β-lactam/β-lactamase inhibitor such as intravenous piperacillin-tazobactam, 4.5 g every 6 hours for a total of 18 g/day [16 g piperacillin/2 g tazobactam]) for at least 2 weeks, are mandatory; addition of ciprofloxacin (500 mg PO or 400 mg IV twice daily), metronidazole (500 mg IV three times daily), and vancomycin (15 mg/kg IV twice daily) depends on suspected pathogens. Unless only a single organism is seen on Gram stain and isolated on culture, broad-spectrum antibiotic coverage should be continued because of the polymicrobial nature of necrotizing fasciitis and the difficulty of culturing anaerobes.

Although *Clostridium perfringens* can cause anaerobic cellulitis and gas gangrene, the most common cutaneous infection by gram-positive bacilli is erythrasma, which manifests as interdigital toe web maceration with fissures as well as shiny or scaly brown-red patches in the axillae and groin. The latter is often confused with tinea cruris (Chapter 409) and seborrheic dermatitis. A diagnostic finding is the presence of coral (orange-pink) fluorescence on Wood lamp illumination (ultraviolet A). The responsible organism is *Corynebacterium minutissimum*. Treatment options include topical and oral erythromycin (e.g., 333 mg three times daily for 7 to 14 days).

TOXIC ERYTHEMAS

Eruptions caused by the release of toxins (e.g., exfoliative toxins ET-A and ET-B, erythrogenic toxin) produced by *S. aureus* and streptococci include staphylococcal scalded skin syndrome (Chapters 272 and 410), scarlet fever (Chapter 274), and toxic shock syndrome (Chapter 410). Staphylococcal scalded skin syndrome (see Fig. 410-19 in Chapter 410) is characterized by large areas of tender erythema in which superficial desquamation (peeling) develops, often with scaling and crusting in a radial array around the mouth. The areas of erythema are sterile; the conjunctivae, nasopharynx, or a distant site on the skin is the usual site of the primary staphylococcal infection. A clue to the diagnosis of scarlet fever is the presence of a strawberry tongue with prominent red papillae. Management involves treatment of the systemic infection (Chapters 272 and 410).

NEISSERIA INFECTIONS

Both gonococcemia (Chapter 283) and meningococcemia (Chapter 282) can manifest with cutaneous lesions. The former gives rise to a small number of vesicopustules on an erythematous base, generally acral in location (Fig. 412-5); these lesions represent septic emboli and are accompanied by fever, arthritis, and tenosynovitis. The earliest lesions of acute meningococcemia may be subtle (macular areas of erythema), but central hemorrhage (petechiae and purpura) and necrosis (gun-metal gray color) soon follow (Fig. 412-6). When accompanied by disseminated intravascular coagulation, large areas of retiform purpura and severe peripheral ischemia may develop. Cutaneous involvement in chronic meningococcemia is a reflection of lymphocytic or leukocytoclastic vasculitis. Management is systemic treatment (Chapters 282 and 283).

PSEUDOMONAS INFECTIONS

Pseudomonas infections of the skin vary from "hot tub" folliculitis (Chapter 410) to soft tissue infections of the external ear. Interdigital toe web infections that begin as simple tinea pedis can be complicated by superimposed *Pseudomonas* infection and result in erythema, swelling, tenderness, and drainage. Depending on its severity, treatment varies from topical antiseptics to oral or intravenous fluoroquinolones (e.g., ciprofloxacin, 500 mg PO twice daily for

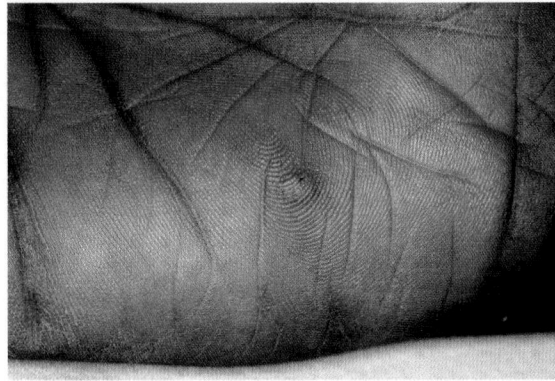

FIGURE 412-5. Disseminated gonococcal infection with an acral pustule on a red-violet base. (Courtesy Yale Dermatology Residents' Slide Collection.)

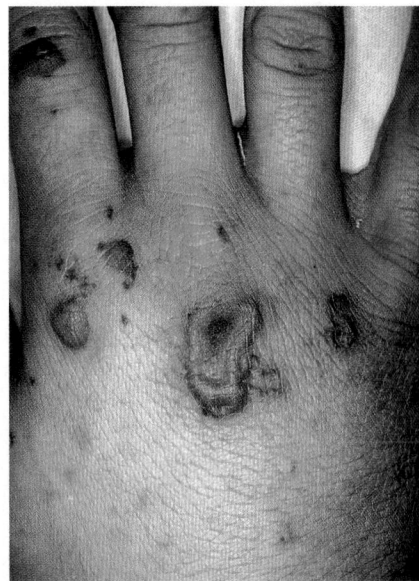

FIGURE 412-6. Purpuric and necrotic embolic lesions of meningococcemia. (Courtesy Yale Dermatology Residents' Slide Collection.)

7 to 14 days). In immunocompromised hosts, *Pseudomonas* and other gram-negative bacilli can produce cellulitis as well as secondary septic emboli in the skin. The latter begin as purpura or purpuric bullae in which central necrosis then develops. These lesions, which arise as a result of ischemic infarction of the skin, are termed *ecthyma gangrenosum*. Management is treatment of the systemic pseudomonal disease (Chapter 290).

SPIROCHETES

Spirochetal infections have a wide range of skin findings, from erythema migrans secondary to *Borrelia burgdorferi* (Chapter 305), to endemic treponematoses such as yaws and pinta (Chapter 304), to the cutaneous manifestations of the three stages of syphilis (Chapter 303). Syphilitic lesions include a firm, generally nontender ulceration (chancre) in primary syphilis; a generalized papulosquamous eruption plus alopecia, oral ulcers, and condylomata lata in secondary syphilis; and thick plaques and ulcers in tertiary disease (Chapter 409). Management involves treatment of the systemic disease.

MYCOBACTERIA INFECTIONS

Infections with *Mycobacterium tuberculosis* and mycobacteria other than *M. tuberculosis* (atypical mycobacteria) are associated with skin lesions, including verrucous or crusted papules, erythematous nodules, scarring granulomatous plaques, and draining ulcers. In immunocompetent hosts in high-income countries, *Mycobacterium marinum* (Chapter 309) is most commonly associated with skin disease, which usually manifests in a lymphocutaneous (i.e., sporotrichoid) pattern. Lower extremity furunculosis due to atypical mycobacteria can occur following pre-pedicure footbaths, and injection of tattoo ink contaminated with *Mycobacterium chelonae* can lead to erythematous papules. Treatment of cutaneous mycobacterial disease is the same as for systemic disease (Chapters 308 and 309).

Viral Infections

The most common viral infections of the skin are verrucae (warts; see Fig. 410-3 in Chapter 410), recurrent oral and genital herpes simplex (Chapters 350 and 410), molluscum contagiosum (see Fig. 411-9 in Chapter 411), and exanthems (Chapter 410). Varicella and herpes zoster are seen less frequently (Chapter 351).

Fungal Infections

A variety of fungal infections involve the skin and nails and are most commonly due to dermatophytes (tinea), *Candida* spp, and *Malassezia* spp (pityriasis versicolor, also referred to as tinea versicolor) (Chapter 409; also see Table 412-1). Although both dermatophyte infections and pityriasis versicolor are associated with scaling, cutaneous candidiasis is characterized by erythema, a more erosive appearance, and satellite pustules. Treatment is described in Chapter 409.

Septic emboli caused by *Candida* or other opportunistic fungi such as *Aspergillus* (Chapter 319) or *Fusarium* often have a clinical appearance similar to that of ecthyma gangrenosum secondary to gram-negative bacilli such as *Pseudomonas*. The responsible organisms can be detected histologically in biopsy specimens or by bedside examination of dermal scrapings; culture confirms the specific organism. While rare, cutaneous plaques secondary to *Pneumocystis jiroveci* favor the external ear canal. Treatment is for the underlying fungal infection.

Ectoparasites and Parasites
ECTOPARASITES: SCABIES AND LICE

The most common ectoparasitic cutaneous infestations are (1) scabies from the human variant of the *Sarcoptes* mite; and (2) lice, of which there are three subtypes: head, body, and pubic. Scabies is characterized by pruritus in association with papules, papulovesicles, and linear burrows as well as signs of scratching, such as excoriations and areas of dermatitis. Sites of predilection include the wrists, ankles, fingers, and toes (including the web spaces), areolae, and genitalia (especially the penis) (Fig. 412-7). The number of mites living within the stratum corneum is limited in immunocompetent hosts; when scraped and examined microscopically, linear burrows provide the highest yield of mites and eggs. In elderly and immunosuppressed patients, a form of scabies known as crusted (previously Norwegian) scabies manifests as multiple areas of scaling and crusting that are teeming with mites.

Infestations with scalp lice are seen most commonly in children, who may be symptom free or have marked pruritus. In addition to the lice, multiple egg casings ("nits") are attached to the proximal portions of scalp hairs. In high-income countries, body lice are seen primarily in homeless individuals;

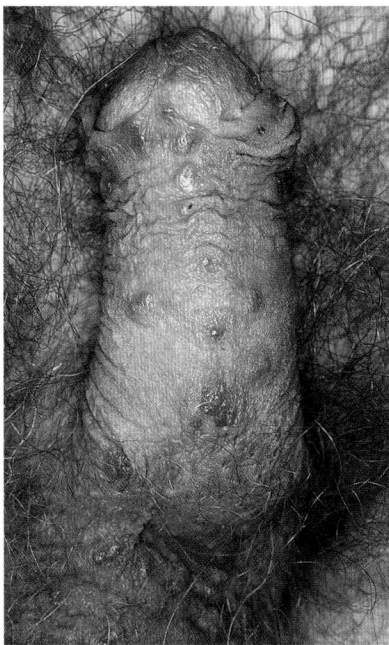

FIGURE 412-7. Scabies with involvement of the penis. (From Bolognia JL, Jorizzo JL, Schaffer JV, eds. *Dermatology,* 3rd ed. London: Elsevier; 2012.)

patients typically have multiple erythematous papules at the sites of bites as well as signs of scratching. The lice and their eggs are found in the patient's clothing. Pubic lice are sometimes called "crabs" because their bodies are shorter and broader than those of scalp or body lice and thus resemble the shape of a crab. Because of their leg span, these lice reside primarily on pubic hairs and less often on axillary hairs or eyelashes.

The first-line FDA-approved treatments for head lice, pubic lice, and routine scabies are topical 0.5% malathion lotion or gel, 5% permethrin cream, and 5% permethrin cream, respectively; each of these topical medications is applied for 8 to 12 hours on days 1 and 8. Topical ivermectin 0.5% lotion is also approved for the treatment of head lice.[3] For crusted scabies, epidemic outbreaks of scabies (e.g., in nursing homes), or difficult-to-treat head lice, oral ivermectin (250 to 400 µg/kg; off-label use) can eradicate the infestation. Treatment of body lice involves discarding egg- and lice-infested clothing; for head lice, potential sources of reinfection, such as hairbrushes, should be discarded. Sexual and household contacts of patients with pubic lice and scabies, respectively, must be treated similarly to the patient who has symptoms.

OTHER PARASITES

Cutaneous lesions are seen in leishmaniasis (Chapter 327), amebiasis (Chapter 331), schistosomiasis (Chapter 334), onchocerciasis (Chapter 335), strongyloidiasis (Chapter 335), and hookworm infections (Chapter 335). Exposure to water infested with the cercariae of animal schistosomes results in multiple erythematous papules, which occur most commonly on the feet and are termed *swimmer's itch.* Dog and cat hookworm infections lead to cutaneous larva migrans, with serpiginous erythematous tracks that correspond to the path of migration of the hookworm larvae in sites where there has been direct contact with infected sand, most commonly the feet. Both of these infections are self-limited because the parasite's life cycle cannot be completed in humans. In immunocompromised hosts, cutaneous plaques can occasionally develop from free-living amebae such as *Acanthamoeba.*

DISORDERS OF HYPOPIGMENTATION AND HYPERPIGMENTATION

Disorders of pigmentation can be divided into four major categories: diffuse, linear, circumscribed, and either reticulated (in the case of hyperpigmentation) or guttate (in the case of hypopigmentation) (Table 412-2).

Hypopigmentation
ALBINISM

For diffuse hypopigmentation, the primary disorder is oculocutaneous albinism, an autosomal recessive disorder in which there is a pigmentary dilution of melanin-containing structures (i.e., the eyes, hair, and skin). The phenotype

TABLE 412-2 DISORDERS OF PIGMENTATION

HYPOPIGMENTATION

Diffuse (Pigmentary Dilution)

Oculocutaneous albinism
Hermansky-Pudlak syndrome
Chédiak-Higashi syndrome
Generalized (total) vitiligo
Inborn errors of metabolism (e.g., phenylketonuria)

Circumscribed

Decrease in pigment
    Acquired: postinflammatory hypopigmentation (e.g., atopic dermatitis, sarcoidosis, subacute cutaneous lupus erythematosus, mycosis fungoides), pityriasis (tinea) versicolor secondary to *Malassezia* spp infection
    Congenital: nevus depigmentosus, ash-leaf spots of tuberous sclerosis
Absence of pigment
    Acquired: vitiligo, chemical or drug-induced leukoderma, leukoderma of scleroderma, leukoderma of melanoma*
    Congenital: piebaldism

Linear

Linear nevoid hypopigmentation, segmental pigmentation disorder

Guttate

Idiopathic guttate hypomelanosis
Confetti macules of tuberous sclerosis

HYPERPIGMENTATION

Diffuse

Drug reactions (e.g., cyclophosphamide, busulfan)
Addison disease
Ectopic adrenocorticotropic hormone production (e.g., small cell lung cancer)
Hemochromatosis
Scleroderma
Primary biliary cirrhosis
Hyperthyroidism
Vitamin B$_{12}$ or folate deficiency
POEMS syndrome (see Table 412-3)
Melanosis secondary to metastatic melanoma
Argyria (gray hue)

Circumscribed

Postinflammatory hyperpigmentation (e.g., acne vulgaris, arthropod bites, dermatitis, lichen planus)
Melasma
Pityriasis (tinea) versicolor
Mastocytosis
Fixed drug reactions
Deposits of drugs and their metabolites

Linear

Exposure to psoralen-containing plants (e.g., limes) plus ultraviolet A light
Drug reactions (e.g., bleomycin)
Linear nevoid hyperpigmentation
Genodermatoses (e.g., incontinentia pigmenti)

Reticulated

Erythema ab igne
Genodermatoses
Confluent and reticulated papillomatosis

*Often referred to as *vitiligo* in the oncologic literature.

varies from total absence of melanin pigment to a subtle decrease whose recognition requires comparison with first-degree relatives; the density of melanocytes in skin is normal, but their ability to produce pigment is absent or decreased. Ninety percent of patients with oculocutaneous albinism have mutations in the genes that encode either tyrosinase (type I) or P protein (type II). Complications of oculocutaneous albinism include decreased visual acuity, nystagmus, photophobia, and an increase in cutaneous carcinomas, especially squamous cell carcinoma. These signs and symptoms are most severe in those who produce the least pigment and have the greatest amount of cumulative sun exposure. The differential diagnosis includes total vitiligo (absence of melanocytes histologically) and a few inborn errors of metabolism (e.g., phenylketonuria). Treatment consists of longitudinal ophthalmologic care and minimizing sun exposure.

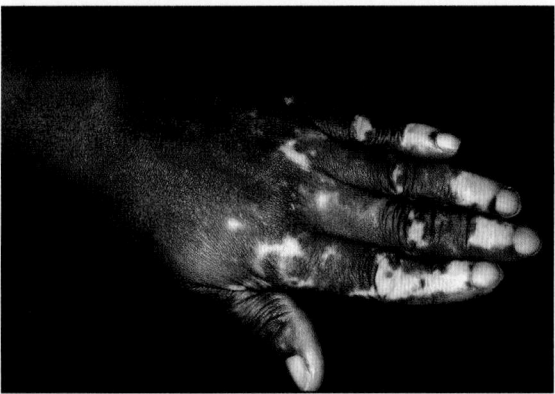

FIGURE 412-8. Striking leukoderma of the hand in a patient with vitiligo. In well-developed lesions, the skin is white, not tan, in color due to complete loss of melanin.

LINEAR HYPOPIGMENTATION

Disorders of linear hypopigmentation consist primarily of nevoid conditions caused by somatic mosaicism (e.g., linear nevoid hypopigmentation, segmental pigmentation disorder), in which streaks of hypomelanosis follow the lines of Blaschko or patients have a blocklike configuration of hypopigmented patches. A minority of patients have associated central nervous system, musculoskeletal, or ocular abnormalities.

CIRCUMSCRIBED (PATCHY) HYPOPIGMENTATION
Vitiligo

Vitiligo (Fig. 412-8) is usually slowly progressive and occurs principally in periorificial areas (around the eyes, nose, lips, genitalia) and on the hands, feet, flexor surface of the wrists, ankles, elbows, and knees and in major body folds. Vitiligo, which is caused by a loss of melanocytes within the skin, is also associated with autoimmune endocrinopathies and alopecia areata.[4]

The differential diagnosis is primarily chemical leukoderma secondary to compounds that are cytotoxic to melanocytes (e.g., catechols, phenols), drug-induced leukoderma (e.g., caused by imatinib), the leukoderma of melanoma (a good prognostic sign if seen in association with immunotherapy but an indication to exclude metastases if occurs spontaneously), and the leukoderma of scleroderma with retention of perifollicular pigmentation. T cells that recognize antigens on the surface of melanocytes (and melanoma cells) are found within the skin and in peripheral blood. Treatment includes topical corticosteroids, topical immunomodulators (e.g., tacrolimus), and phototherapy.[A5] Combinations of follicular and epidermal stem cell suspensions are an experimental approach for difficult-to-treat disease.[A6][A7]

Guttate Hypopigmentation

Idiopathic guttate hypomelanosis, in which there are well-demarcated hypopigmented macules usually measuring 2 to 4 mm in diameter, is the most common cause of guttate ("raindrop") leukoderma (Fig. 412-9). The favored sites for this common age-related disorder, which may be related to chronic sun exposure, are the shins and the extensor surface of the forearms.

Other Acquired Causes

Circumscribed hypomelanosis is seen in patients with pityriasis (tinea) versicolor (see Fig. 409-29 in Chapter 409) and postinflammatory hypopigmentation. Although postinflammatory hypopigmentation is most often associated with atopic dermatitis, it also can occur with sarcoidosis (Chapter 89), cutaneous lupus erythematosus (Chapter 250), and mycosis fungoides (Chapter 176).

Congenital Causes

Congenital circumscribed areas of hypomelanosis include *nevus depigmentosus,* a common tan "birthmark" seen in 1 in 50 infants in whom there is a partial decrease in pigment; *piebaldism,* an unusual autosomal dominant disorder with areas of complete absence of pigment caused by mutations in the *KIT* gene; *nevus anemicus,* a localized area of vasoconstriction; and the *ash-leaf spots* of tuberous sclerosis (Chapter 389), with a partial decrease in pigment.

Hyperpigmentation
DIFFUSE HYPERPIGMENTATION

Diffuse hyperpigmentation is most commonly due to drugs (e.g., cyclophosphamide, zidovudine) and endocrinopathies associated with increased circulating levels of adrenocorticotropic hormone (ACTH) (e.g., Addison

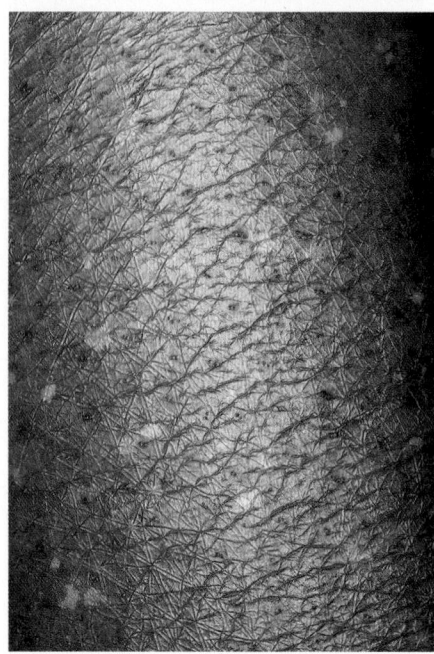

FIGURE 412-9. Idiopathic guttate hypomelanosis with small, well-demarcated hypopigmented macules on the shin.

TABLE 412-3	CUTANEOUS FINDINGS IN POEMS SYNDROME
Diffuse hyperpigmentation	
Vascular tumors, including glomeruloid hemangiomas	
Peripheral edema	
Induration (sclerodermoid)	
Hypertrichosis	
Hyperhidrosis	
Acrocyanosis	
Clubbing and/or leukonychia	
Acquired facial lipoatrophy	
Livedo reticularis	

POEMS = *polyneuropathy, organomegaly, endocrinopathy, monoclonal (M) protein, skin changes.*

disease [Chapter 214], ectopic ACTH production by tumors such as small cell lung carcinoma [Chapter 182]). ACTH, as well as melanocyte-stimulating hormone, can bind and activate the melanocortin-1 receptors on melanocytes, thereby leading to increased melanin production. Additional causes include hemochromatosis (Chapter 201), scleroderma (Chapter 251), primary biliary cirrhosis (Chapter 146), POEMS syndrome (*polyneuropathy, organomegaly, endocrinopathy, monoclonal protein, skin changes*) (Table 412-3), and hyperthyroidism (Chapter 213). Systemic exposure to silver (argyria; Chapter 19) can lead to a slate-gray color.

LINEAR AND RETICULATED HYPERPIGMENTATION

Linear streaks of hyperpigmentation can be due to nevoid conditions that reflect cutaneous mosaicism, as in linear hypopigmentation (see earlier) and several genodermatoses (e.g., incontinentia pigmenti, which is an X-linked dominant disorder caused by mutations in the gene *NEMO*), or can be due to exposure to either plant-derived psoralens (e.g., from limes) plus ultraviolet A irradiation or systemic bleomycin (flagellate pigmentation). Reticulated hypermelanosis is also seen in several genodermatoses (e.g., dyskeratosis congenita) and after chronic exposure to heat (erythema ab igne). The latter corresponds to the cutaneous venous plexus and is seen most commonly in the lumbosacral region where heating pads have been applied or on the anterior thighs from laptop computers.

CIRCUMSCRIBED (PATCHY) HYPERPIGMENTATION

The most common causes of circumscribed hypermelanosis are pityriasis (tinea) versicolor (which can present as both hypopigmentation and hyperpigmentation, hence its name), postinflammatory hyperpigmentation, and melasma. Postinflammatory hyperpigmentation (Fig. 412-10) is observed more frequently in darkly pigmented individuals and often follows acne vulgaris, arthropod bites, chronic dermatitis, and lichen planus. Additional causes of circumscribed

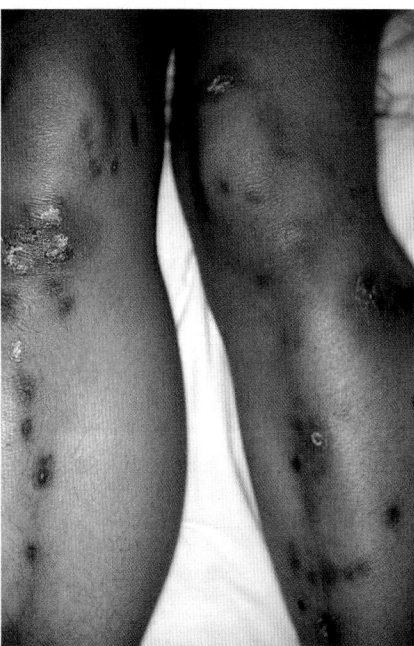

FIGURE 412-10. Postinflammatory hyperpigmentation secondary to arthropod bites. (Courtesy Yale Dermatology Residents' Slide Collection.)

TABLE 412-4	DISORDERS SEEN MORE COMMONLY IN PATIENTS OF AFRICAN ANCESTRY

HEAD AND NECK

Folliculitis decalvans/dissecting cellulitis
Tinea capitis due to *Trichophyton tonsurans*
Traction alopecia
Central centrifugal cicatricial alopecia*
Acne keloidalis nuchae
Pseudofolliculitis barbae
Pomade acne
Dermatosis papulosa nigra
Inherited patterned lentiginosis
Melasma
Discoid lupus erythematosus

PALMAR

Keratosis punctata of the palmar creases

LOWER EXTREMITIES

Ulcers secondary to sickle cell anemia

GENERALIZED

Keloids
Cutaneous sarcoidosis
Papular eczema and follicular-based inflammation

*Also *termed follicular degeneration syndrome* or *hot comb alopecia*.

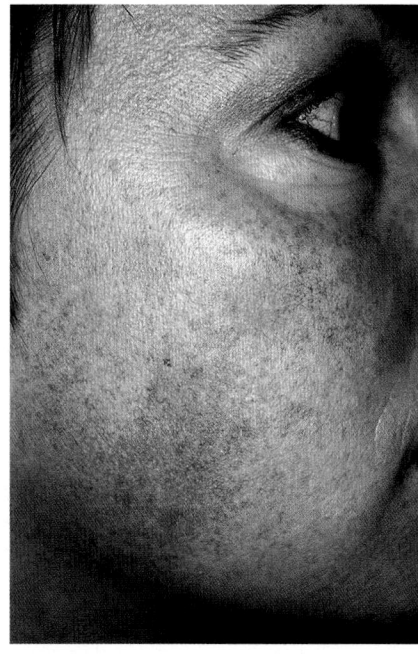

FIGURE 412-11. Hyperpigmented patches on the cheek in a patient with melasma.

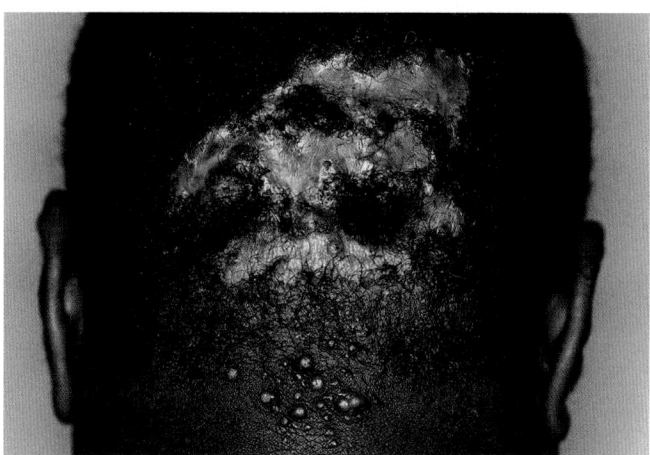

FIGURE 412-12. Acne keloidalis in an African American man. (Courtesy Kalman Watsky, MD.)

darkening of the skin are cutaneous mastocytosis (urticaria pigmentosa; Chapter 240), deposits of drugs such as antimalarials and minocycline (blue-gray discoloration), and medications that produce fixed drug reactions, most frequently trimethoprim-sulfamethoxazole and nonsteroidal anti-inflammatory drugs. In melasma (Fig. 412-11), symmetrical hyperpigmented patches are seen on the lateral aspect of the forehead, upper part of the cheek, and mandibular area. At least 90% of patients with melasma are women. The lesions are exacerbated by ultraviolet light and estrogen (oral contraceptives, pregnancy). Melasma is treated with daily broad-spectrum sunscreens plus lightening agents such as hydroquinone (4% cream) and retinoic acid (0.025 to 0.1% cream) for 3 to 4 months, often in combination with mild topical corticosteroids to reduce irritation; if irritation develops, the creams are discontinued temporarily and then restarted at a reduced frequency.

DISTINCTIVE LESIONS IN BLACK SKIN

Although some diseases are more common in patients of African ancestry (e.g., tinea capitis, pseudofolliculitis barbae, dissecting cellulitis), others are simply more noticeable (e.g., vitiligo and postinflammatory hypopigmentation) (Table 412-4). The explanation for the increased incidence is speculative in most instances, with the exception of curled hairs leading to pseudofolliculitis barbae. Tightly curled hairs, when shaved, are usually cut at an oblique angle, which results in a sharp tip at the distal end of the hair shaft that allows penetration of the skin adjacent to the hair follicle and subsequent inflammation. The patient can avoid shaving or undergo laser hair removal. Some cutaneous disorders are seen less commonly in black skin (e.g., acne rosacea and scabies).

Another entity seen more commonly in individuals of African descent is keloids (Fig. 412-12). Keloids generally appear at sites of trauma (e.g., ear piercing) but can occasionally develop spontaneously, especially on the trunk. In the former situation, they are thought to represent an exaggerated response to wound healing, with increased formation of collagen not only at the site of the trauma (as in hypertrophic scars) but also in adjacent, previously uninvolved skin. Treatment options include intralesional corticosteroids, intralesional interferon, pulsed dye laser, or excision followed by radiation therapy.[5]

REGIONAL DERMATOSES

Some common dermatoses have a predilection for particular anatomic sites (Fig. 412-13 and Table 412-5). These locations can help narrow the differential and guide further diagnostic testing and therapy in many patients.

One regional dermatosis is acanthosis nigricans (Fig. 412-14). Because of its potential systemic implications, careful medical evaluation is required (Table 412-6).

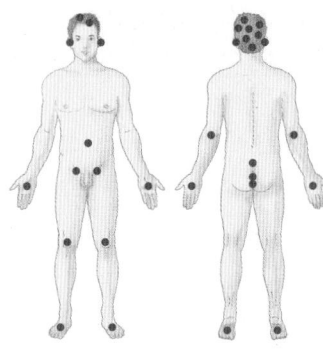

Psoriasis

Scalp, ears, scalpline
Palms, soles
Dorsal hands, feet
Elbows, knees/shins
Presacrum
Intergluteal fold
Nails

Inverse Psoriasis

Submammary
Inguinal fold
Umbilicus

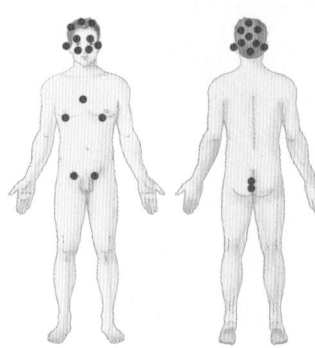

Seborrheic Dermatitis

Scalp, ears, postauricular
Eyebrows
Nasolabial folds
Central chest
Intergluteal fold
Submammary
Inguinal fold

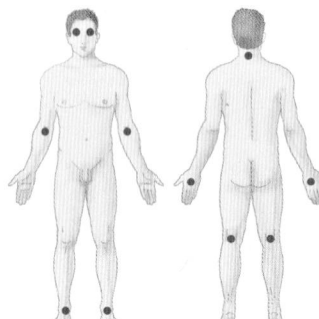

Atopic Dermatitis (adults)

Eyelids
Antecubital fossa
Popliteal fossa
Posterior neck
Ankles
Hands

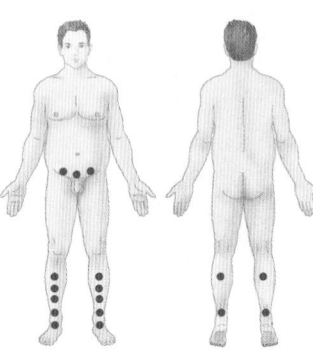

Stasis Dermatitis (adults)

Legs, below knees, but
 greater on shins than
 calves
Lower pannus

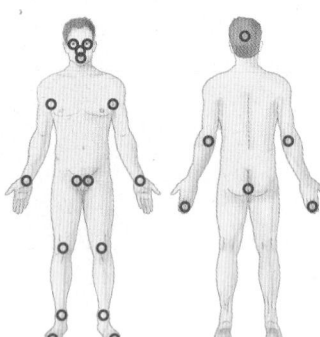

Vitiligo

Loss of color:
Around eyes
Around nose
Around mouth
Axillae, groin
Wrists (flexor)
Poliosis (streak of
 white hairs)
Elbows, knees, ankles
Backs of hands/feet
 (includes digits)
Perianal

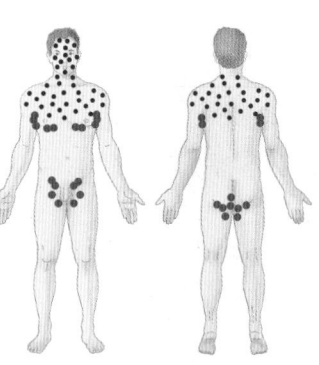

**Acne Vulgaris/
Hidradenitis Suppurativa**

∴ = papulopustules,
  blackheads or
  whiteheads
  Face/neck/upper
  trunk/shoulders

● = nodules of hidradenitis
  suppurativa

FIGURE 412-13. Regional involvement of specific skin diseases.

TABLE 412-5 REGIONAL DERMATOLOGY

REGION OF SKIN	TYPE OF SKIN LESION	DISEASE PROCESS
Scalp	Papulosquamous and eczematous	Seborrheic dermatitis, psoriasis, tinea capitis, eczema (atopic, contact [esp. hairline])
	Pustular	Folliculitis, kerion
	Papulonodular	Melanocytic nevi, seborrheic keratoses, pilar cysts, verrucae, cherry angiomas, actinic keratoses (bald scalp)
Face	Pustular	Acne, rosacea, folliculitis (beard), tinea
	Papulosquamous and eczematous	Seborrheic dermatitis, psoriasis (hairline), contact dermatitis (e.g., cosmetics), atopic dermatitis, impetigo, systemic lupus erythematosus, photodermatitis
	Vesicular	Herpes simplex, herpes zoster, bullous impetigo
	Papulonodular	Melanocytic nevi, actinic keratoses, seborrheic keratoses, sebaceous hyperplasia, basal cell carcinomas, squamous cell carcinomas, melanomas
	Atrophic and telangiectatic	Discoid lupus erythematosus
Trunk	Papulosquamous and eczematous	Psoriasis, atopic dermatitis, contact dermatitis, tinea versicolor, pityriasis rosea, scabies, secondary syphilis, subacute cutaneous lupus (upper trunk)
	Vesiculobullous	Herpes zoster, bullous pemphigoid, pemphigus, erythema multiforme, Stevens-Johnson syndrome
	Maculopapular	Morbilliform drug reactions, viral exanthems
	Papulonodular	Melanocytic nevi, seborrheic keratoses, cherry angiomas, lipomas, epidermoid inclusion cysts, basal and squamous cell carcinomas, keloids, neurofibromas, melanoma
	Pustular	Acne, folliculitis
	Urticarial	Hives, drug reactions, early herpes zoster
Arms and forearms	Eczematous and papulosquamous	Contact dermatitis (e.g., plants), atopic dermatitis, psoriasis, lichen planus, photodermatitis (drugs, contactants, dermatomyositis, subacute cutaneous lupus)
	Papulonodular	Melanocytic nevi, verrucae, seborrheic keratoses, actinic keratoses, squamous cell carcinomas, polymorphic light eruption, rheumatoid nodules (elbows), xanthomas (elbows)
	Purpuric	Actinic (solar) purpura
	Annular	Granuloma annulare, subacute cutaneous lupus

TABLE 412-5 REGIONAL DERMATOLOGY—cont'd

REGION OF SKIN	TYPE OF SKIN LESION	DISEASE PROCESS
Legs	Eczematous and papulosquamous	Stasis dermatitis, eczema craquelé (xerotic eczema), contact dermatitis, atopic dermatitis, psoriasis, lichen planus
	Papulonodular	Melanocytic nevi, dermatofibromas, erythema nodosum, melanoma, xanthomas (knees, Achilles tendon), Kaposi sarcoma
	Annular	Tinea, granuloma annulare
	Purpuric	Capillaritis, vasculitis
	Ulcerative	Stasis ulcers, arterial insufficiency, pyoderma gangrenosum, trauma, livedoid vasculopathy, squamous cell carcinoma, diffuse dermal angiomatosis
Genitalia and groin	Eczematous and papulosquamous	Seborrheic dermatitis, tinea, candidiasis, psoriasis, contact dermatitis, lichen simplex chronicus, scabies, reactive arthritis (Reiter syndrome), erythrasma, lichen planus
	Vesiculobullous	Herpes simplex
	Ulcerative	Herpes simplex, trauma, syphilis, chancroid, Behçet disease, squamous cell carcinoma
	Papulonodular	Angiokeratomas, epidermoid inclusion cysts, molluscum contagiosum, condyloma acuminata, hidradenitis suppurativa, squamous cell carcinoma
	Pustular	Folliculitis, candidiasis, hidradenitis suppurativa
Hands	Eczematous and papulosquamous	Irritant and allergic contact dermatitis, atopic dermatitis, tinea, scabies, secondary syphilis
	Vesiculobullous, pustular	Dyshidrotic eczema, psoriasis (palmar), hand-foot-and-mouth disease (palmar), herpetic whitlow, blistering dactylitis, porphyria cutanea tarda (dorsal), erythema multiforme, epidermolysis bullosa acquisita
	Papulonodular	Warts, actinic keratoses (dorsal), digital mucous cysts (dorsal fingers), squamous cell carcinomas (dorsal), granuloma annulare, pyogenic granuloma
	Depigmentation	Vitiligo, chemical leukoderma
	Cuticular telangiectases	Scleroderma, dermatomyositis, systemic lupus erythematosus, Osler-Weber-Rendu disease
Feet	Eczematous and papulosquamous	Tinea, psoriasis, contact dermatitis, atopic dermatitis, syphilis (plantar)
	Vesiculobullous	Tinea, arthropod bites, epidermolysis bullosa (inherited and acquired), erythema multiforme, hand-foot-and-mouth disease (plantar)
	Papules	Verrucae (plantar), corns, perniosis
	Ulcerative	Neuropathic ulcers (plantar)

TABLE 412-6 CLUES TO UNDERLYING SYSTEMIC CONDITIONS ASSOCIATED WITH ADULT-ONSET ACANTHOSIS NIGRICANS

Polycystic ovary syndrome	Women with acne, hirsutism, and/or menstrual irregularities
Malignancy	Sudden onset, weight loss, inflamed seborrheic keratoses, tripe palms
Endocrinopathy	Consider type 2 diabetes, Cushing syndrome (striae, hypertension, central obesity, buffalo hump), hypothyroidism
Drug-induced	Especially niacin, human growth hormone, oral contraceptive agents, corticosteroids, protease inhibitors

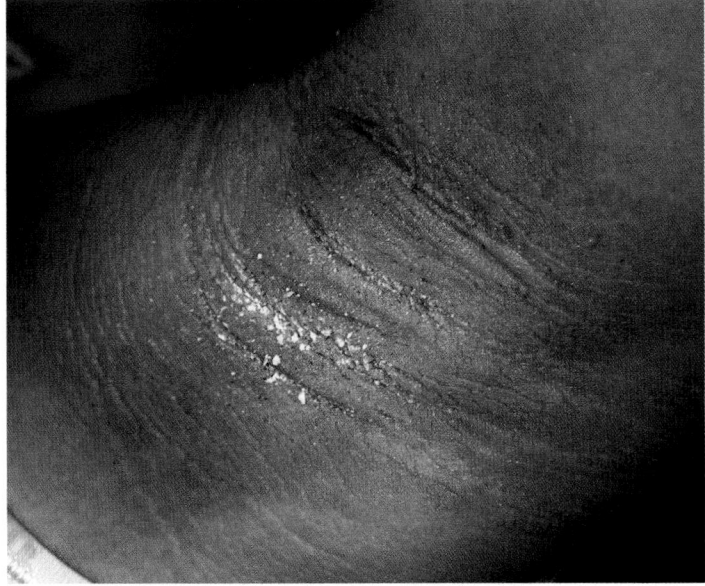

FIGURE 412-14. **Acanthosis nigricans of the axilla.** Note the velvet-like appearance of the skin. (Courtesy Yale Dermatology Residents' Slide Collection.)

 Grade A References

A1. Talan DA, Mower WR, Krishnadasan A, et al. Trimethoprim-sulfamethoxazole versus placebo for uncomplicated skin abscess. *N Engl J Med.* 2016;374:823-832.
A2. Aboltins CA, Hutchinson AF, Sinnappu RN, et al. Oral versus parenteral antimicrobials for the treatment of cellulitis: a randomized non-inferiority trial. *J Antimicrob Chemother.* 2015;70:581-586.
A3. Miller LG, Daum RS, Creech CB, et al. Clindamycin versus trimethoprim-sulfamethoxazole for uncomplicated skin infections. *N Engl J Med.* 2015;372:1093-1103.
A4. Huang DB, O'Riordan W, Overcash JS, et al. A phase 3, randomized, double-blind, multicenter study to evaluate the safety and efficacy of intravenous iclaprim vs vancomycin for the treatment of acute bacterial skin and skin structure infections suspected or confirmed to be due to gram-positive pathogens: REVIVE-1. *Clin Infect Dis.* 2018;66:1222-1229.
A5. Bae JM, Jung HM, Hong BY, et al. Phototherapy for vitiligo: a systematic review and meta-analysis. *JAMA Dermatol.* 2017;153:666-674.
A6. Razmi TM, Kumar R, Rani S, et al. Combination of follicular and epidermal cell suspension as a novel surgical approach in difficult-to-treat vitiligo: a randomized clinical trial. *JAMA Dermatol.* 2018;154:301-308.
A7. Thakur V, Kumar S, Kumaran MS, et al. Efficacy of transplantation of combination of noncultured dermal and epidermal cell suspension vs epidermal cell suspension alone in vitiligo: a randomized clinical trial. *JAMA Dermatol.* 2019;155:204-210.

GENERAL REFERENCES

For the General References and other additional features, please visit Expert Consult at https://expertconsult.inkling.com.

413

DISEASES OF HAIR AND NAILS

ANTONELLA TOSTI

HAIR DISORDERS

Normal Hair

The hair shaft is a fully keratinized structure that is produced by the hair follicle. The entire skin, with the exception of the palms and soles, contains hair follicles. Hair follicles are of two types: terminal follicles and vellus follicles. Terminal follicles, which reach the hypodermis, produce terminal hairs, which are long, thick (60 to 80 μm), and pigmented. Terminal hairs are present since

TABLE 413-1	CAUSES OF HAIR LOSS

DIFFUSE ALOPECIA

Telogen effluvium (e.g., after illness or stress)
Anagen effluvium (e.g., after chemotherapy or radiation therapy)
Medications (see Table 413-3)
Nutritional deficiency
Hair treatments
Androgenetic alopecia (in women)
Hormonal changes (e.g., menopause, discontinuation of oral contraceptives, hypothyroidism)

PATCHY ALOPECIA

Alopecia areata (probably autoimmune)
Cicatricial (scarring) alopecia (e.g., lichen planopilaris, discoid lupus erythematosus, folliculitis decalvans, central centrifugal cicatricial alopecia)
Traction alopecia (e.g., excessive hair straightening or braiding)
Trichotillomania (hair pulling)
Scalp infection (e.g., ringworm)

MARGINAL ALOPECIA

Frontal fibrosing alopecia
Traction alopecia
Alopecia areata (ophiasis variant)

TABLE 413-2	DERMATOSCOPIC SIGNS IN HAIR AND SCALP DISORDERS
Alopecia areata	Yellow dots, exclamation mark hairs, broken hairs
Androgenetic alopecia	>20% variability in the hair diameter
Lichen planopilaris/frontal fibrosing alopecia	Peripilar casts; loss of follicular openings
Trichotillomania	Broken hairs, question mark hairs
Tinea capitis	Comma hairs, corkscrew hairs
Discoid lupus erythematosus	Red dots, follicular plugs
Folliculitis decalvans	Hair tufts
Scalp psoriasis	Coiled capillaries
Seborrheic dermatitis	Arborizing vessels

birth on the scalp, eyebrows, and eyelashes and later develop after puberty on the axillae, pubis, and beard region in males. Vellus follicles are small and localized to the superficial dermis and mid-dermis, where they produce vellus hairs, which are thin (<30 μm), short (<2 cm), and not pigmented and cover all the glabrous skin.

The hair follicle is formed by an upper permanent portion and a lower dynamic transient portion that migrates during the hair cycle. The transient portion includes the hair bulb, which is surrounded by the dermal papilla and contains the hair matrix that produces the hair shaft and its sheaths. The anatomic division between the permanent and the transient portion is just below the bulge region, which corresponds to the insertion of the erector pili muscle. The bulge region contains the epithelial stem cells that regenerate the follicle in each hair growth cycle; its damage results in stem cell destruction and cicatricial alopecia.

Hair Cycle

Hair follicles have a cyclic activity, characterized by alternating periods of hair shaft production and periods of resting (anagen, catagen, telogen). During the anagen phase, the follicles produce the hair shaft. Duration of anagen, which in the scalp ranges from 2 to 7 years, determines hair shaft length. Maximal length and growth rate of terminal hair varies in the different body regions. Scalp hair grows approximately 0.4 mm/day and may reach a length of more than 1 m. Maximal hair length decreases with age. During telogen, hair production is absent, even if the shaft remains within the follicle to be shed only when, after 3 months, the follicle reenters the anagen phase.

The hair cycle of adjacent scalp follicles is not synchronized. In normal conditions, approximately 85 to 90% of follicles are in anagen and 10 to 15% in telogen.

Hair Loss and Alopecias

Hair loss distresses most patients, independently from its severity and pattern. In some cases, the decrement in quality of life attributable to hair loss is comparable with that caused by major chronic diseases. Since some causes of hair loss are readily treatable,[1] accurate diagnosis is critical.

The first diagnostic step is to assess family history, drug intake, systemic illness, and severity and duration of hair loss (Table 413-1). The second step is to establish whether the hair density is normal or decreased. The third step is to evaluate whether the rate of hair shedding is normal or increased. Acute and severe hair loss is typical of diseases that interrupt the mitotic activity of anagen follicles (drugs, alopecia areata). A normal hair density suggests telogen effluvium, which may be acute or chronic. A reduced hair density may involve the whole scalp (diffuse alopecia), may manifest with bald patches (patchy alopecia), or may be limited to specific scalp regions (patterned alopecia, marginal alopecia). In patchy alopecias, the scalp may show patches of alopecia that are completely devoid of hairs (alopecia areata, cicatricial alopecia) or have short broken hairs (trichotillomania, hair shaft disorders). Dermatoscopy is a rapid, noninvasive technique that greatly improves the clinical diagnosis of alopecias and hair shaft disorders in adults and children (Table 413-2).

TELOGEN EFFLUVIUM
Acute Telogen Effluvium

Acute telogen effluvium results from noxious events that precipitate the entry of a large number of follicles into their resting phase (telogen). Possible causes include systemic diseases, drugs (Table 413-3), fever, stress, weight loss, delivery, iron deficiency, and inflammatory scalp disorders. For drugs, the severity of hair loss depends on the drug, its dosage, and the patient's susceptibility.

Hair loss starts approximately 3 months after the causative event, a time frame that corresponds with the duration of the telogen phase. Telogen hairs are retained within the follicle during telogen, to be shed when the follicle produces a new anagen hair. Hair loss is severe when 100 to 200 hairs are shed daily. The patient usually remembers precisely when the increased shedding began. Acute telogen effluvium does not usually produce visible alopecia because approximately 50% of hairs need to be lost before reduction of hair density is evident.

TREATMENT AND PROGNOSIS   Rx

Acute telogen effluvium subsides spontaneously in a few months after removal of the cause. It may, however, unmask or aggravate androgenetic alopecia.

Chronic Telogen Effluvium

Chronic telogen effluvium mostly affects middle-aged women and frequently remains unexplained. The daily shedding is mild (<100 hairs daily), but patients are distressed and complain of progressive temporal thinning as well as decreased hair mass and volume. Scalp pain (trichodynia) is frequently reported. Patients who have a high hair density may bring in envelopes of shed hairs to prove the amount of hair loss. There is no effective treatment. Chronic telogen effluvium has a chronic course with periodic exacerbations.

DIFFUSE ALOPECIA
Anagen Effluvium

Acute hair shedding leading to diffuse alopecia is a typical side effect of cancer chemotherapy and scalp radiation. Hair loss is acute and severe and may produce loss of most of the scalp hair, eyebrows, and eyelashes; other body hairs are less commonly involved. Hair shedding usually starts 4 to 6 weeks after drug intake with up to 1000 hairs shed daily. Regrowth is usually fast after discontinuation of therapy, but hair shape and color may be different. Permanent alopecia may occur with high-dose radiation and certain drug regimens, such as busulfan and docetaxel.[2]

Scalp hypothermia prevents or reduces hair loss during chemotherapy except in patients treated with the combined docetaxel, doxorubicin, and cyclophosphamide regimen.[A1][A2] Topical minoxidil accelerates hair regrowth but does not prevent hair loss.

Patterned Alopecia (Androgenetic Alopecia)

Androgenetic alopecia, which is the most common form of hair loss, affects up to 80% of men and 50% of women in the course of their life. Androgenetic

TABLE 413-3	DRUGS REPORTED TO INDUCE HAIR LOSS
ACE inhibitors (captopril, enalapril, moexipril, ramipril)	Immunoglobulins
Allopurinol	Indanediones
Amiodarone	Indinavir*
Amphetamines*,†	Interferons*,†
Analgesics, anti-inflammatories (ibuprofen, indomethacin, naproxen)	Isonicotinic acid hydrazide‖
	Leflunomide*
Androgens*,‡	Levodopa
Anticoagulants (coumarin, dextran, heparin/heparinoids apixaban, dabigatran, rivaroxaban)*,†	Lithium*
	Maprotiline
	Mesalazine
Antiepileptics (carbamazepine, hydantoins, lamotrigine, troxidone, valproic acid, vigabatrin)*,†	Methyldopa
	Methysergide
	Metyrapone
Antipsychotics (flupenthixol decanoate, fluphenazine decanoate)	Minoxidil§
	Nicotinic acid
Antithyroid drugs (carbimazole, iodine, thiouracil)*	Nitrofurantoin
	Octreotide
Appetite suppressants	Olanzapine
Aromatase inhibitors (fadrozole, formestane [4-OHA], vorozole)*,†	Pentosan polysulfate
	Phenindione
	Piroxicam
Benzimidazoles (albendazole, mebendazole)	Placitaxel§
	Potassium thiocyanate
β-Blockers (levobunolol, metoprolol, nadolol, propranolol, timolol)*	Pyridostigmine
	Radiation (<700 Gy)*,‖
Bromocriptine	Retinol (vitamin A)*
Buspirone	Retinoids (acitretin, etretinate, isotretinoin)*,†
Busulfan§	
Butyrophenones	Risperidone
Cantharidin	Salicylates
Cholestyramine	Serotonin reuptake inhibitors (fluoxetine, fluvoxamine, paroxetine, sertraline)*
Chloramphenicol	
Cidofovir	
Cimetidine	Sonidegib*,†
Clonazepam	Sorafenib
Clotrimazole	Spironolactone
Colchicine	Strontium ranelate*,†
Contraceptives (oral)	Sulfasalazine
Danazol	Tamoxifen
Diclofenac	Terbinafine
Dixyrazine	Terfenadine
Diazoxide	Thiamphenicol
Docetaxel§	Thyroxine
Ethambutol	Tocopherol (vitamin E)
Ethionamide	Trazodone
Fibrates (clofibrate, fenofibrate)	Triazoles (fluconazole, itraconazole)
Gentamicin	Tricyclic antidepressants (amitriptyline, desipramine, doxepin, imipramine, maprotiline)
Gefitinib‖	
Glatiramer acetate	
Glibenclamide	Trimethadione
Gold salts	Triparanol
Granulocyte colony-stimulating factor	Vasopressin
Haloperidol	Vismodegib*,†

*Established by multiple reports or proved by rechallenge.
†Hair loss usually severe.
‡May produce androgenetic alopecia.
§May produce permanent alopecia.
‖May produce anagen effluvium.
¶May produce telogen effluvium 3 months after discontinuation.
ACE = angiotensin-converting enzyme inhibitor.

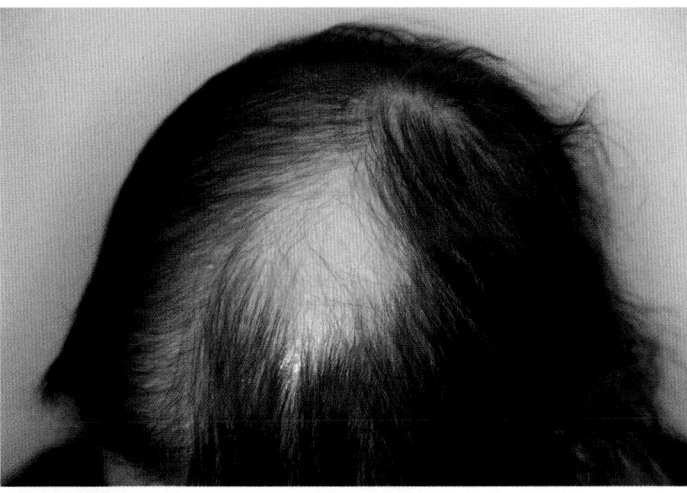

FIGURE 413-1. Alopecia areata: patchy hair loss. The alopecic area is devoid of hairs, and the scalp does not present inflammatory changes. Note diffuse thinning of the scalp surrounding the patch.

of biochemical and clinical evidence of androgen excess and may be due to excessive follicular sensitivity to androgens. Data also show that patients with androgenetic alopecia may be at increased risk for dying from diabetes and heart disease.

Androgenetic alopecia is a progressive disease that tends to worsen with time. Medical treatments include 2% topical minoxidil in women and 5% topical minoxidil and/or oral finasteride, 1 mg/day, in men.[A3] Oral dutasteride, 0.5 mg, approved in some countries, is more effective than finasteride with a similar safety profile.[A4] Clinical improvement is mostly due to thickening of the preexisting hair. Some men may report a post-finasteride syndrome characterized by persistent sexual dysfunction and depression occurring after treatment with 5α-reductase inhibitors.

Treatments for androgenetic alopecia should be continued for at least 6 months before assessing efficacy, and regular drug use is mandatory for maintaining results. Interruption of minoxidil produces an acute telogen effluvium, which becomes evident 3 to 4 months after interruption and cannot be prevented by concomitant finasteride treatment. Interruption of finasteride is followed by gradual hair loss, with return to the pretreatment status after 1 year. Hair transplantation is a good option for men with severe androgenetic alopecia, and treatment with finasteride, 1 mg/day, improves the long-term results of surgery. Hair transplantation in women is more complicated because the hair thinning is often diffuse in the parietal and occipital regions, so there is not a good hair donor area.

PATCHY ALOPECIA
Alopecia Areata

Alopecia areata is a common form of nonscarring, usually patchy hair loss affecting up to 2% of the population.[3] The etiology is unknown, but evidence is consistent with an autoimmune disease to which both a genetic predisposition and environmental factors contribute. In genetically predisposed individuals, various triggering factors cause a predominantly CD8-driven, T_H1-type T-cell autoimmune reaction against the hair follicles, thereby resulting in acute hair loss.

Alopecia areata can start at any age, but severe forms often start during childhood and are more frequent in males.[4] Clinical examination reveals one or multiple well-circumscribed smooth patches of nonscarring absence of hair that enlarge in a centrifugal way (Fig. 413-1). The margins of the patches often show 3-mm-long broken hairs with a pigmented tip (exclamation mark hairs), which indicates disease progression.

Alopecia areata may affect all hairy body areas, including the eyebrows and eyelashes (Fig. 413-2). Severe forms involve the entire scalp (alopecia totalis) or all body hair (alopecia universalis). Involvement of the scalp margins (ophiasis) is associated with a poor prognosis. Alopecia areata may be associated with other autoimmune diseases, most commonly thyroid diseases (Chapter 213). Other possible associations include celiac disease (Chapter 131), vitiligo (Chapter 412), and atopy (Chapter 409). Nail abnormalities are common, especially in children.

alopecia is caused by a progressive reduction in the diameter, length, and pigmentation of the hair. Hair thinning is not diffuse, but rather is limited to the frontal, temporal, and vertex areas, where hair follicles are sensitive to the effects of the testosterone metabolite dehydrotestosterone (DHT). This sensitivity to DHT, which requires the 5α-reductase enzymes, is genetically determined. In men, androgenetic alopecia involves the frontotemporal areas and the vertex, following a pattern that corresponds to the Hamilton-Norwood scale. In women, androgenetic alopecia produces diffuse thinning of the crown region with maintenance of the frontal hairline (Ludwig pattern), a pattern that can easily be appreciated by making a central parting and comparing hair density at the top with hair density at the occipital region. In premenopausal women, androgenetic alopecia can be a sign of hyperandrogenism, together with hirsutism and acne. In most women, however, it occurs in the absence

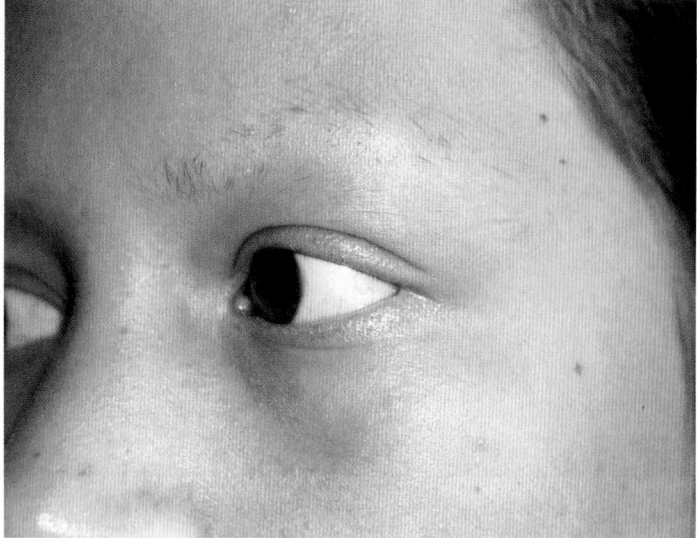

FIGURE 413-2. Alopecia areata: patchy hair loss. Hair loss involves the eyelashes and eyebrows.

The natural history of alopecia areata is unpredictable. Studies indicate that 34 to 50% of patients will recover within 1 year and 15 to 25% will progress to alopecia totalis/universalis, a condition from which full recovery is only approximately 10%. To date, available treatments may induce temporary hair regrowth but do not change the long-term prognosis.[5]

Relapses occur in a high percentage of patients, even during therapy. High-dose pulse corticosteroid therapy is effective in acute alopecia areata but is not useful in ophiasis or long-standing alopecia totalis/universalis. Intralesional steroids can be used in localized areas, including the eyebrows. High-potency topical steroids are commonly utilized and can be applied under occlusion in acute or severe disease. Topical immunotherapy with diphenylcyclopropenone (DPCP) or squaric acid dibutylester (SADBE), which is not approved by the U.S. Food and Drug Administration (FDA), is an effective option in chronic alopecia areata. Medium- and low-potency topical steroids and topical minoxidil are probably only placebo treatments. Recent data indicate that the oral Janus kinase inhibitors, ruxolitinib and tofacitinib, are highly effective in inducing hair regrowth in severe alopecia areata, but relapses can occur with drug interruption.[6]

Trichotillomania

Trichotillomania is a compulsive disorder that is more common in children. Repetitive hair pulling and plucking produces patches of irregular alopecia. The scalp is not completely bald, but rather shows broken hairs of various lengths (Fig. 413-3). The frontal, parietal, and occipital scalp are most commonly affected, but other terminal hairs can be involved, especially the upper eyelashes.

Occasionally, patients develop the habit of chewing or eating the pulled hairs. Patients with trichotillomania frequently do not admit their habit, and parents of affected children may be recalcitrant to accept the diagnosis. Psychiatric referral is indicated in adults.

Cicatricial Alopecias (Scarring Alopecia)

The hallmark of cicatricial alopecias is loss of follicular ostia. Cicatricial alopecias include diseases that primarily affect the hair follicles and diseases that affect the dermis and secondarily cause follicular destruction.

Primary cicatricial alopecias are classified as lymphocytic or neutrophilic, based on the principal inflammatory cell type seen on pathologic examination. Lymphocytic cicatricial alopecias include lichen planopilaris, frontal fibrosing alopecia, and discoid lupus erythematosus. Neutrophilic cicatricial alopecias include folliculitis decalvans and dissecting cellulitis.

Secondary cicatricial alopecias result from disorders that cause diffuse scarring of the dermis, including burns, radiation, severe skin infections, localized scleroderma, and scalp tumors. The diagnosis of primary scarring alopecia requires a scalp biopsy, which should be taken from areas with active evidence of inflammation because biopsy of atrophic scalp will typically show only follicular or dermal fibrosis. In scarring alopecias, hair loss is permanent; treatment can prevent progression but not induce hair regrowth.

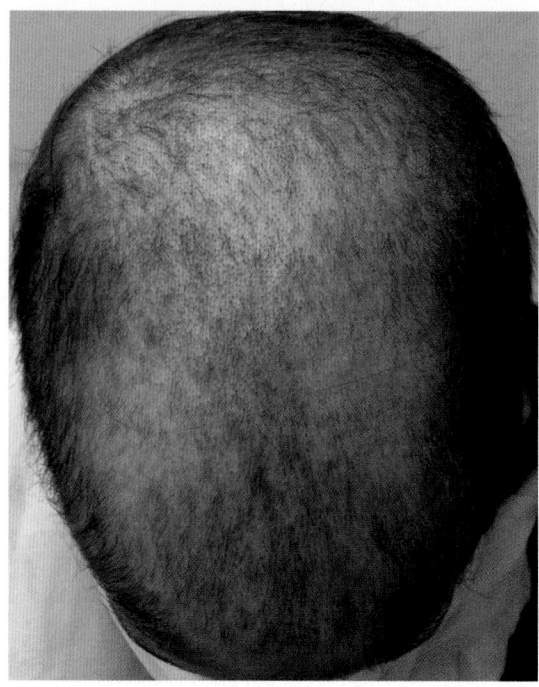

FIGURE 413-3. Trichotillomania: patchy hair loss. Irregular areas of alopecia with hairs broken at different lengths.

LICHEN PLANOPILARIS/FRONTAL FIBROSING ALOPECIA

In lichen planopilaris, which is the most common form of cicatricial alopecia, the hair follicles surrounding the alopecic patches show perifollicular erythema and scaling. The patient usually complains of severe itching. A variant of lichen planopilaris is frontal fibrosing alopecia, which typically affects postmenopausal women,[7] in which it causes recession of the frontotemporal hairline, often associated with loss of the eyebrows and hairs of the arms and legs (Fig. 413-4). Frontal fibrosing alopecia is becoming increasingly common worldwide. No therapy is consistently effective, but retrospective studies indicate that 5α-reductase inhibitors are effective in arresting disease progression in an high percentage of patients.

DISCOID LUPUS ERYTHEMATOSUS

In discoid lupus erythematosus, the alopecic area shows active inflammation with erythema, edema, scaling, and follicular plugging, as well as atrophy with variable degrees of telangiectasia and dyspigmentation (Fig. 413-5).

The disease is more common in African American women. Approximately 5 to 10% of adults with discoid lupus erythematosus will develop systemic lupus erythematosus (Chapter 250), especially those with widespread discoid lesions. In localized lesions, treatment with high-potency topical steroids (see Table 408-1) is usually effective. Antimalarials are a second-line treatment. Hair regrowth may occur when treatment is promptly started. Therapeutic strategy should include photoprotection of the involved area.

FOLLICULITIS DECALVANS

In folliculitis decalvans, the scalp shows papulopustular lesions that often coalesce to form exudative crusted areas that result in cicatricial alopecia. A typical finding is tufted folliculitis, in which tufts of 6 to 15 hairs emerge together from the scalp (Fig. 413-6). The cause is unknown, but the condition may reflect an abnormal host response to bacterial antigens. *Staphylococcus aureus* often is isolated from active lesions. Folliculitis decalvans responds to oral antibiotics (e.g., trimethoprim-sulfamethoxazole [one tablet, 160 mg/800 mg/day] or clindamycin [300 mg twice daily] with or without rifampin [300 mg twice daily] for 8 to 10 weeks) but usually relapses after interruption of therapy.

DISSECTING CELLULITIS

Dissecting cellulitis of the scalp is a follicular occlusion disorder that may progress to scarring alopecia. Patients typically complain of relapsing multifocal alopecic painful nodules, boggy plaques, and draining tracts. Possible treatments include systemic antibiotics, isotretinoin, and tumor necrosis factor–α inhibitors, but data are limited to small case series.

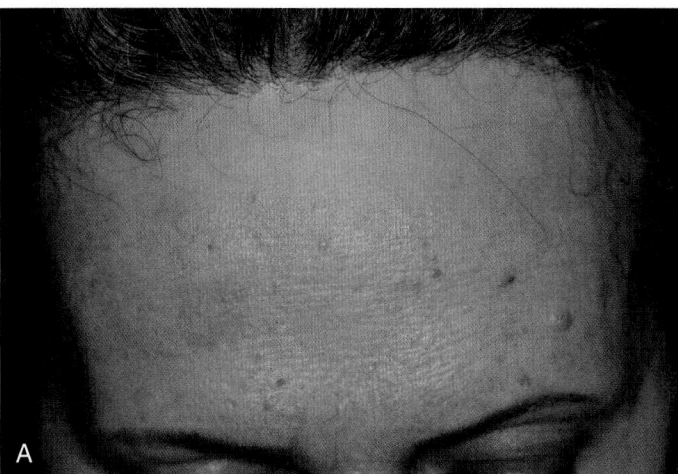

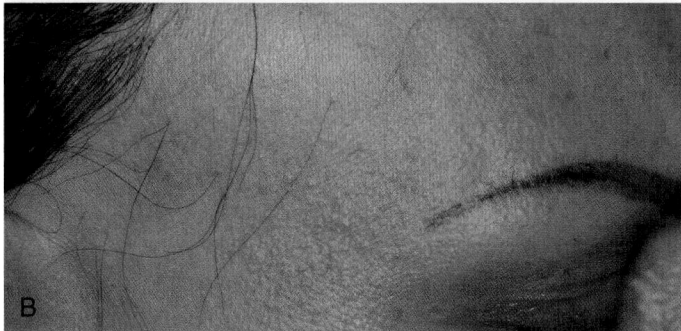

FIGURE 413-4. **A,** Frontal fibrosing alopecia. Scarring alopecia of the hair margin with recession of the frontal hairline. The alopecic area can be easily distinguished because it shows no photoaging compared with the normal forehead. **B,** Note alopecia of the eyebrows and facial papules.

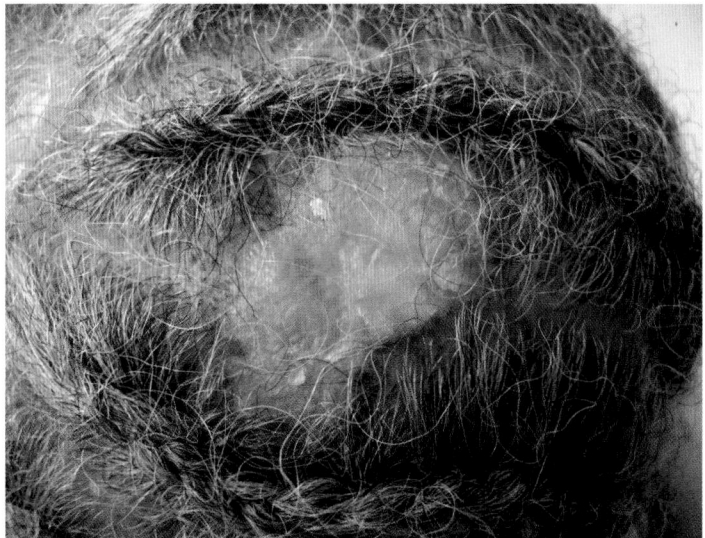

FIGURE 413-5. Discoid lupus erythematosus. The alopecic patch shows erythema, scaling, and depigmentation.

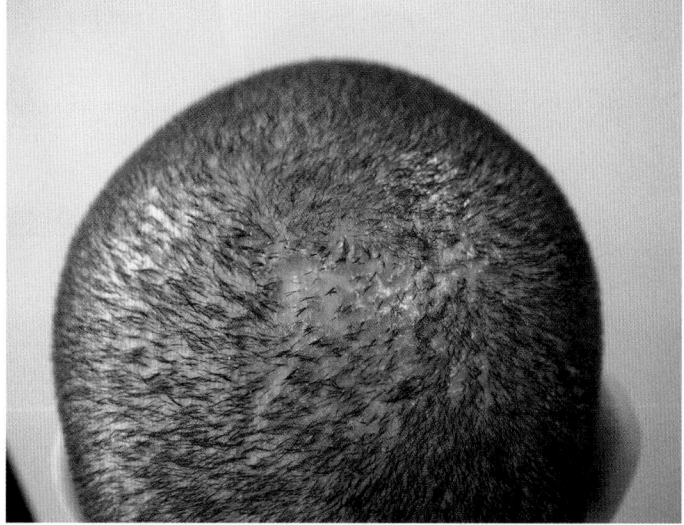

FIGURE 413-6. Folliculitis decalvans. Scarring alopecia with tufted folliculitis.

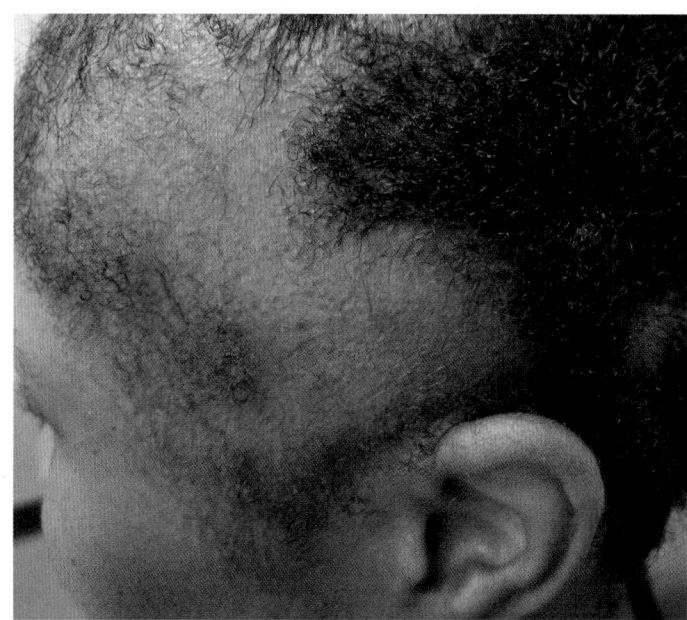

FIGURE 413-7. Traction alopecia. Hair loss involves the temporal scalp. Note presence of remaining hairs along the hairline (fringe sign).

Congenital triangular alopecia is usually noticed by the age of 6 years as an irregularly triangular patch of alopecia with vellus hairs on the frontotemporal region.

The loose anagen hair syndrome is characterized by a defective anchorage of the hair to the follicle, resulting in hairs that are easily and painlessly pulled out from the scalp. The condition is typical of children and may manifest with patchy hair loss due to hair pulling while playing.

Short anagen syndrome is a congenital disease characterized by short (<6 cm) fine hair and increased hair shedding. The condition is due to a decreased duration of the anagen phase.

HAIR DISORDERS IN CHILDREN

Hereditary and congenital alopecias are present since birth or appear in the first years of life. Aplasia cutis congenita is the most common form of focal alopecia in newborns.

Hereditary hair shaft abnormalities associated with increased hair fragility produce diffuse or patchy alopecia that appears during childhood. The most common hereditary hair shaft disorder is monilethrix, in which hair shaft fragility is associated with follicular hyperkeratosis. The hair is dull and fragile and breaks easily, especially in the nape and occipital areas. Diagnosis is confirmed by finding hair beading on dermoscopy or microscopic examination.

RACIAL DIFFERENCES

The frequency and clinical aspects of hair disorders vary in different races. Androgenetic alopecia, for instance, is more frequent in whites than in blacks and Asians, whereas black and Asian hair is more susceptible to weathering and fragility.

The black hair shaft is flat, highly twisted, and difficult to manage without strong chemical or hair styling procedures, which often cause considerable damage. Hair straightening and braiding are responsible for traction alopecia, which is common and typically produces cicatricial alopecia of the frontal and lateral margins (Fig. 413-7). Central centrifugal cicatricial alopecia is a

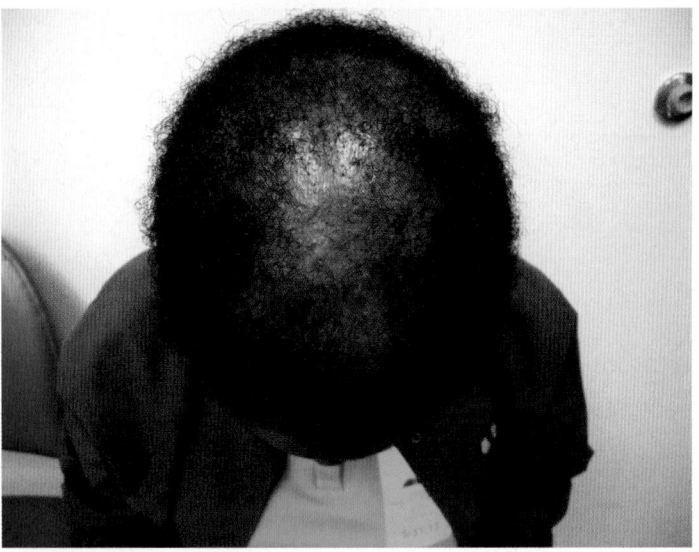

FIGURE 413-8. Central centrifugal cicatricial alopecia. The alopecic area involves the central portion of the scalp and expands centrifugally.

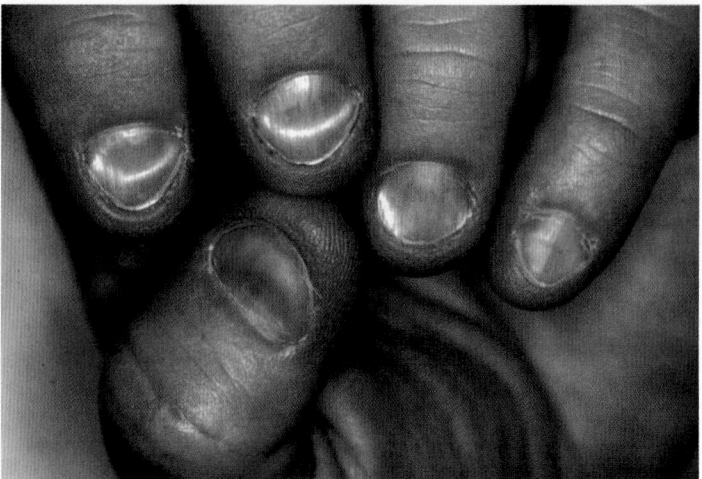

FIGURE 413-9. Spooning.

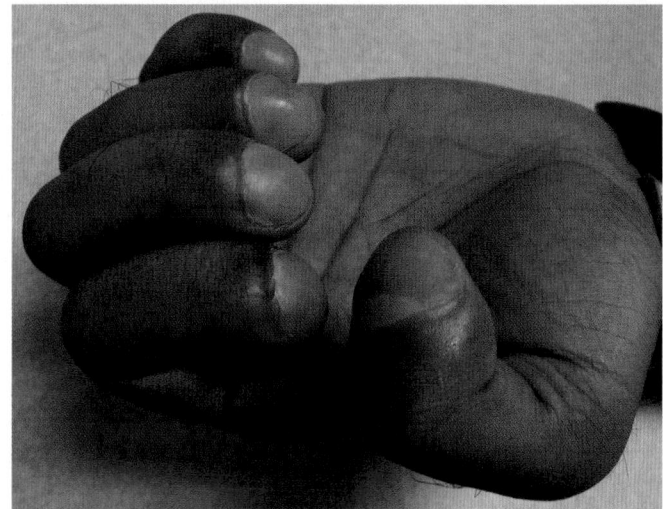

FIGURE 413-10. Clubbing.

very common cause of scarring alopecia in black women (Fig. 413-8). It manifests as slowly progressive scarring hair loss in the vertex or crown that spreads in a centrifugal pattern.

In Asians, the hair shaft is round, thick, robust, and straight. Asian hair is very difficult to style and dye, and it is often damaged by its treatment with high concentrations or long exposure to chemicals.

EXCESSIVE HAIR GROWTH

Hirsutism describes excessive terminal hair with male distribution in a female. Hirsutism should be distinguished from hypertrichosis, which is characterized by the presence of an excessive amount of hair in a non–androgen-dependent area.

Hirsutism

Hirsutism is a common condition that affects up to 10% of women and is more frequent in Hispanic and Mediterranean women. Hirsutism may be associated with hyperandrogenism and polycystic ovary syndrome (Chapters 222 and 223), but it is idiopathic in approximately 15% of cases.[8] Effective treatments include oral contraceptive agents, flutamide (250 mg twice daily), and spironolactone (100 mg daily) for severe cases. [A5]

Hypertrichosis

Hypertrichosis results from the presence of terminal hairs in anatomic areas that are normally characterized by vellus hair. Hypertrichoses can be congenital or acquired, localized or generalized. Acquired hypertrichoses are most commonly iatrogenic, metabolic (e.g., Cushing syndrome, porphyria, hyperthyroidism), nutritional (e.g., anorexia nervosa), or paraneoplastic (Chapter 169).

NAIL DISORDERS

Normal Nail

The nail plate is a keratinized hard structure produced by the nail matrix, which is a specialized epithelium located above the distal phalanx of the finger. In longitudinal sections, the matrix consists of a dorsal, an apical, and a ventral portion. The proximal matrix (dorsal portion and apex) produces the dorsal nail plate (two thirds upper plate), and the distal matrix (ventral portion) produces the ventral plate (one third lower plate). The nail plate is produced continuously throughout life. Nails grow slowly, and the nail plate can reflect illnesses that occurred several months earlier. Complete replacement takes approximately 6 months for fingernails and 12 to 18 months for toenails. Many medications (e.g., anticonvulsants, neuroleptics, antifungals), drugs (e.g., amphetamine, cocaine, doping substances), and poisons (e.g., mercury, arsenic) are retained in the nails, whose fragments (nail clippings) can be used to monitor previous exposure.

Nail abnormalities can be congenital or acquired and may be caused by developmental, traumatic, inflammatory, infective, and neoplastic disorders or by medications.[9] The diagnosis of nail dystrophies usually relies on a careful clinical examination and an accurate history, but radiographic or magnetic resonance imaging investigation of the digit and pathology may be required to guide treatment.[10]

Koilonychia (Spoon Nails)

In koilonychias (Fig. 413-9), which is also called spooning of the nails, the nail plate is thin and has a concave appearance. Koilonychia is physiologic in children. In adults, it can be occupational or, more rarely, a sign of iron deficiency (Chapter 150).

Clubbing

Clubbing (Fig. 413-10) develops when enlargement of the soft tissue of the distal digit causes a bulbous digit with an enlarged and overcurved nail plate. The angle between the proximal nail fold and the nail plate (Lovibond angle) is greater than 180 degrees. Clubbing may be congenital (i.e., in congenital heart disease; Chapter 61) or acquired. Other causes of acquired clubbing include intrathoracic (Chapter 182) and gastrointestinal neoplasms (Chapters 183 to 186), chronic intrathoracic suppurative disease (Chapter 84), inflammatory bowel disease (Chapter 132), and liver disorders.[11]

Beau Lines and Onychomadesis

Beau lines (Fig. 413-11) and onychomadesis are due to a temporary reduction or arrest of nail growth. Beau lines appear as transverse grooves of various depth; onychomadesis as a full-thickness transverse groove of the proximal nail plate. Causes include trauma, skin diseases involving the proximal nail fold and the matrix, drugs, and systemic diseases (Table 413-4). In the latter

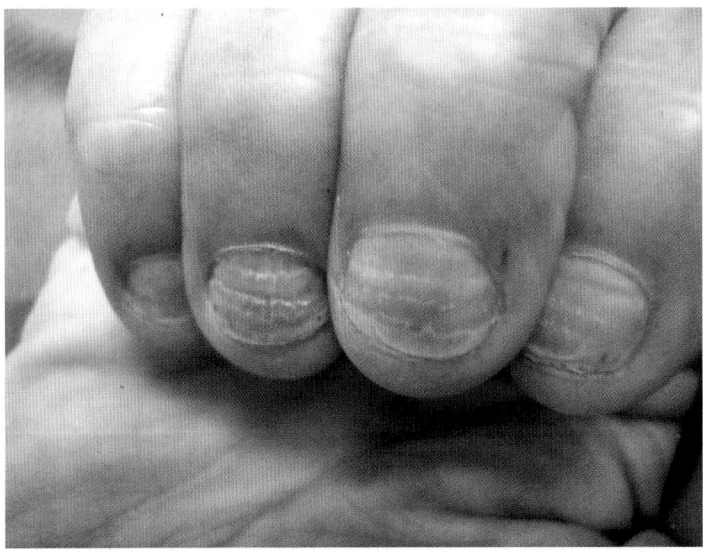

FIGURE 413-11. Beau lines due to chemotherapy. The lines affect all the nails at the same level.

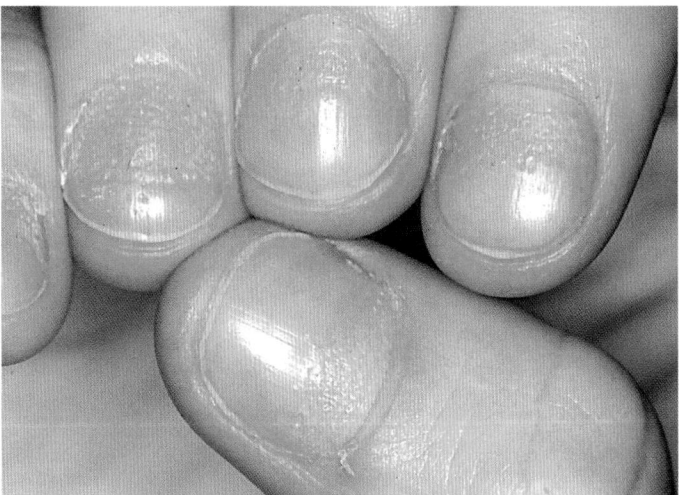

FIGURE 413-12. Pitting. Multiple punctate depressions on the nail plate surface.

TABLE 413-4	CAUSES OF BEAU LINES AND ONYCHOMADESIS

SYSTEMIC

Acrodermatitis enteropathica
Severe metabolic stress
High fever
Viral infections (Kawasaki disease, measles, hand-foot-and-mouth syndrome)
Typhus
Stevens-Johnson syndrome
Drugs
Bullous disorders (pemphigus, pemphigoids)
Deep saturation, high altitude
Hemodialysis
Myocardial infarction

LOCAL

Trauma (including manicure)
Paronychia
Congenital malalignment (big toenails)

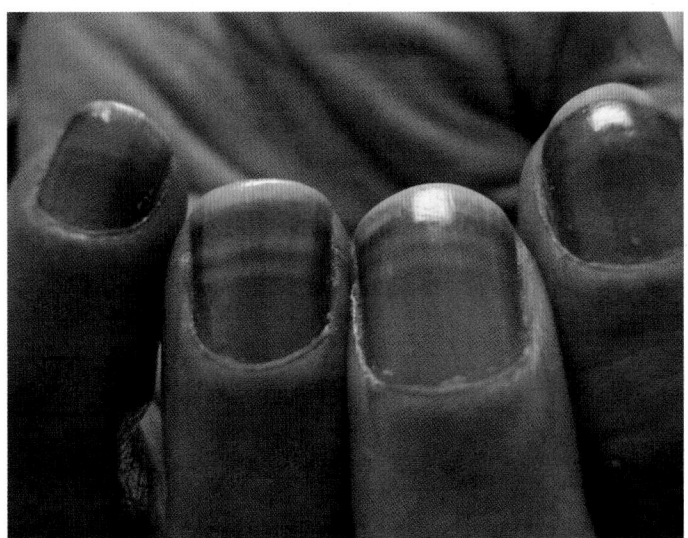

FIGURE 413-13. Muehrcke lines. Note two parallel lines of apparent leukonychia.

case, Beau lines or onychomadesis involve all the nails and are localized at the same level.

Pitting

Pitting (Fig. 413-12) appears as punctate depressions of the dorsal nail plate, with variable size and depth. Pitting is caused by inflammatory skin disorders such as psoriasis (Chapter 409), alopecia areata, and eczema (Chapter 409).

Longitudinal Grooves and Striations

Normal nails often show superficial thin longitudinal ridges that increase in number with aging. Deep longitudinal fissures, which indicate damage to the proximal matrix, can be caused by nail lichen planus, vascular insufficiency, trauma, and tumors involving or compressing the matrix.

Leukonychia

Leukonychia describes a whitish discoloration of the nail, which may be due to persistence of nuclei in the cells of the ventral nail plate (true leukonychia) or to a pallor of the nail bed (apparent leukonychia). True leukonychia, including the Mees lines of arsenic exposure (Chapter 19), does not fade with pressure and moves distally with nail growth; it is most commonly caused by trauma. Apparent leukonychia, which does not follow nail growth and fades with pressure, may be a sign of systemic diseases such as liver cirrhosis (Terry nails; Chapter 137), chronic renal diseases (half-and-half nails, characterized by apparent leukonychia of the proximal half of the nail; Chapter 121), hypoalbuminemia (Chapter 113), and systemic chemotherapy (Muehrcke lines; Fig. 413-13).

Yellow Nail Syndrome

The yellow nail syndrome is a chronic nail disorder characterized by an arrest or a reduction of nail growth, resulting in nail thickening and hardening and yellow discoloration. Fingernails and toenails are excessively curved from side to side, and cuticles are absent (Fig. 413-14). Yellow nail syndrome occasionally may be paraneoplastic (Chapter 169). The pathogenesis of yellow nail syndrome is unknown, but a congenital abnormality of the lymphatic vessels may be involved. Typical cases have associated lymphedema or respiratory disturbances. The nail abnormalities improve with treatment of the associated respiratory disorders. Oral vitamin E (1200 mg/day for several months) is useful in some cases.

Splinter Hemorrhages

Splinter hemorrhages (see Fig. 45-10) appear as longitudinal thin red-brown lines of variable length. Splinter hemorrhages are usually localized in the distal nail and are commonly seen in inflammatory diseases, including eczema (Chapter 409), psoriasis (Chapter 409), and onychomycosis (Table 413-5).[12] Multiple splinter hemorrhages localized in the proximal nail plate can be a sign of systemic diseases, including infectious or marantic endocarditis (Chapter 67), trichinosis (Chapter 335), and the antiphospholipid syndrome.

Onycholysis

Onycholysis (Fig. 413-15) describes detachment of the nail plate from the bed. The detachment usually occurs at the free lateral margins of the nail. The

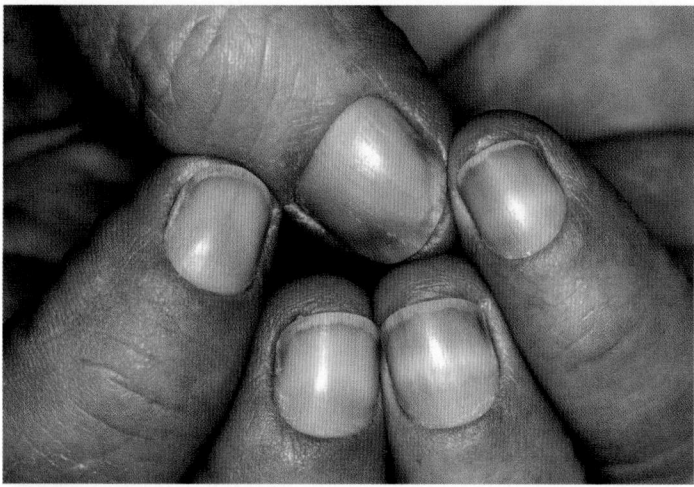

FIGURE 413-14. Yellow nail syndrome. The nails are yellow, are overcurved, and do not grow.

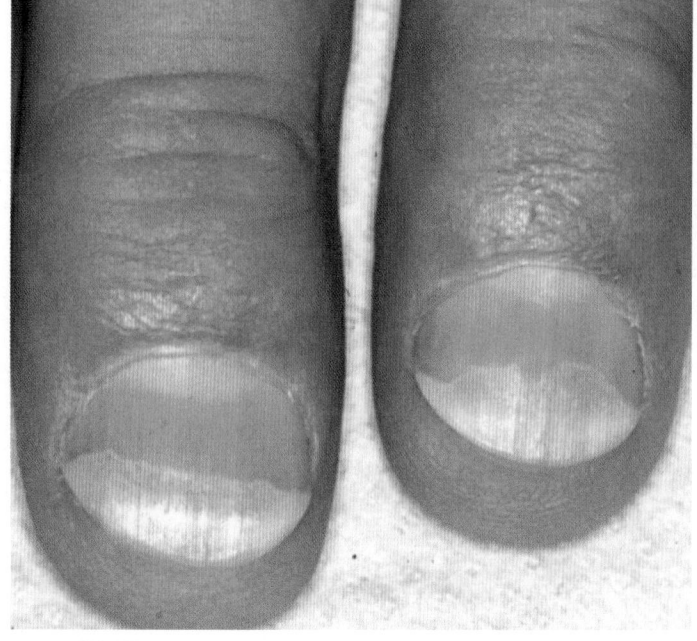

FIGURE 413-15. Onycholysis. The detached nail plate is white in color.

TABLE 413-5	CONDITIONS ASSOCIATED WITH SPLINTER HEMORRHAGE

DERMATOSIS

Psoriasis
Lichen planus
Eczema

VASCULITIS

Antiphospholipid syndrome
Thromboangitis obliterans
Granulomatosis with polyangiitis
Other small- and medium-vessel vasculitides

DRUGS

Antiangiogenic kinase inhibitors (e.g., sunitinib, sorafenib)

INFECTION

Infectious endocarditis
Psittacosis
Histoplasmosis
Meningococcemia

OTHER

Renal failure
Elderly
Amyloidosis
Marantic endocarditis
Hypereosinophilic syndrome
Langerhans cell histiocytosis
Onychomatricoma

Adapted from Haber R, Khoury R, Kechichian E, et al. Splinter hemorrhages of the nails: a systematic review of clinical features and associated conditions. *Int J Dermatol.* 2016;55:1304-1310.

onycholytic area is white owing to the presence of air, but it may acquire a green-brown color if the space if colonized by bacteria, such as *Pseudomonas aeruginosa.*

Onycholysis of the fingernails is a common sign of nail psoriasis (Chapter 409). It also may be due to prolonged and frequent contact with water, detergents, or irritants (idiopathic onycholysis). Toenail onycholysis is almost exclusively caused by trauma or onychomycosis. When onycholysis is limited to one digit, the possibility of a nail tumor always should be considered.

Paronychia

Paronychia, which describes the acute or chronic inflammation of the proximal and lateral nail folds, is common in the fingernails at any age. In acute paronychia, the affected digit is painful, with erythema, swelling, and pus discharge localized to one corner of the proximal nail fold. Acute paronychia usually follows a trauma to the nail fold, as in children who pick or bite the cuticles or in women after a manicure.

In chronic paronychia, prolonged mechanical or environmental trauma (such as contact with water and irritants) damages the cuticle, allowing penetration of dirt, bacteria, and other particles under the proximal nail fold. The result is an inflammatory reaction of the proximal nail fold and nail matrix, with edema and redness of the fold, absence of the cuticles, Beau lines, and abnormalities of the nail plate surface. Treatment includes protective measures, such as use of cotton and rubber gloves to avoid contact with irritants, as well as topical steroids and topical antimicrobials. Acute paronychia, often associated with periungual pyogenic granuloma-like lesions, is a common side effect of treatment with epidermal growth factor receptor (EGFR) inhibitors.[13]

Onychomycosis

Fungal nail infections most commonly affect the toenails of adults. Dermatophytes (particularly *Trichophyton rubrum*) are responsible for most infections.[14] The clinical presentation varies depending on the modality of the nail invasion. In distal subungual onychomycosis, the most common form, fungi spread from plantar skin and invade the nail bed. The affected nail shows subungual hyperkeratosis, onycholysis, and yellow streaks (Fig. 413-16). In white superficial onychomycosis, which only affects toenails, fungi colonize the surface of the nail plate, where they cause multiple white friable patches (Fig. 413-17). Proximal subungual onychomycosis produces a true leukonychia, owing to the presence of fungal hyphae in the deep layers of the plate. Proximal subungual onychomycosis caused by *T. rubrum* is typical in immunosuppressed patients. Diagnosis of onychomycosis must always be confirmed by mycologic examination. Treatment depends on clinical type, number of affected nails, and severity of nail involvement. A systemic treatment is preferred for proximal subungual onychomycosis and for distal subungual onychomycosis involving the proximal nail. Terbinafine (250 mg/day) for 2 months (fingernails) or 3 months (toenails) is the most effective treatment for dermatophyte infections. Topical efinaconazole and tavaborole, usually used daily for 6 months, are FDA approved for mild/moderate onychomycosis of the toenails, but these antifungal medications are not as effective as oral terbinafine.

Ingrowing Toenails

Ingrown toenails are a common condition, especially in young patients. Nail ingrowing most commonly affects one or both the big toes and is related to

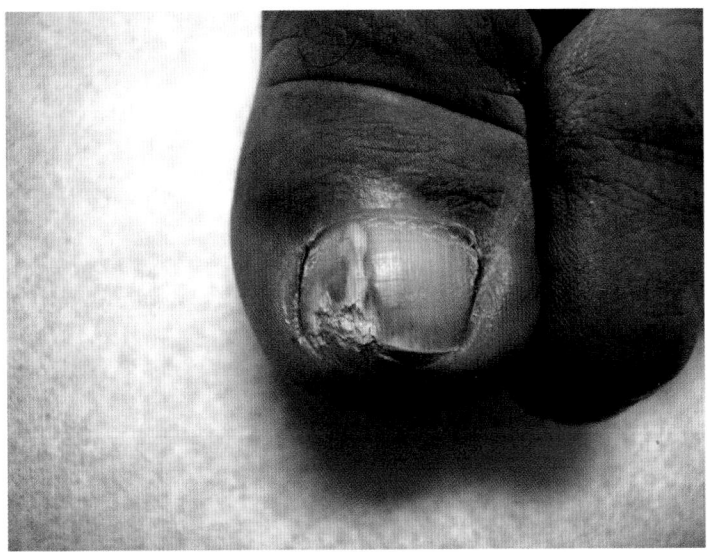

FIGURE 413-16. **Distal subungual onychomycosis.** The nail shows subungual hyperkeratosis and a yellow streak.

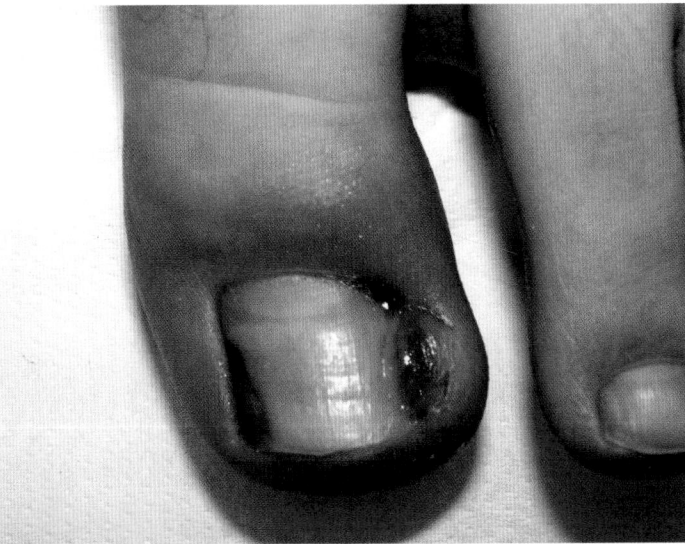

FIGURE 413-18. **Ingrowing toenail.** Penetration of the nail spicule causes inflammation and granulomatous reaction

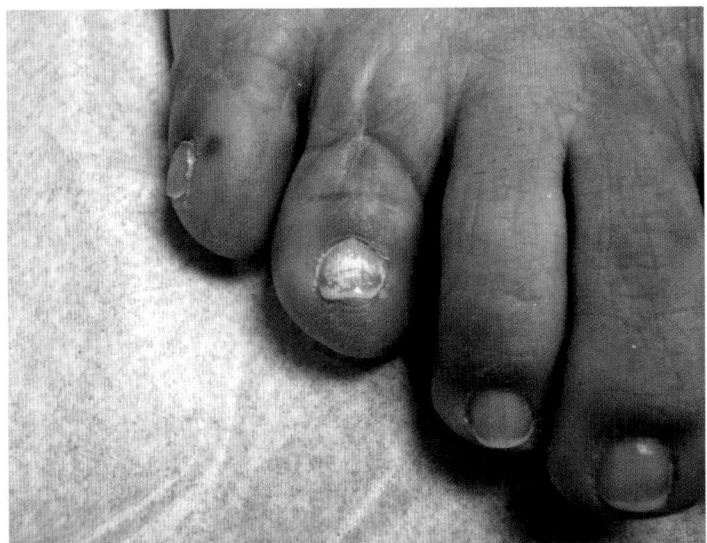

FIGURE 413-17. **White superficial onychomycosis.** The affected nail shows white superficial patches.

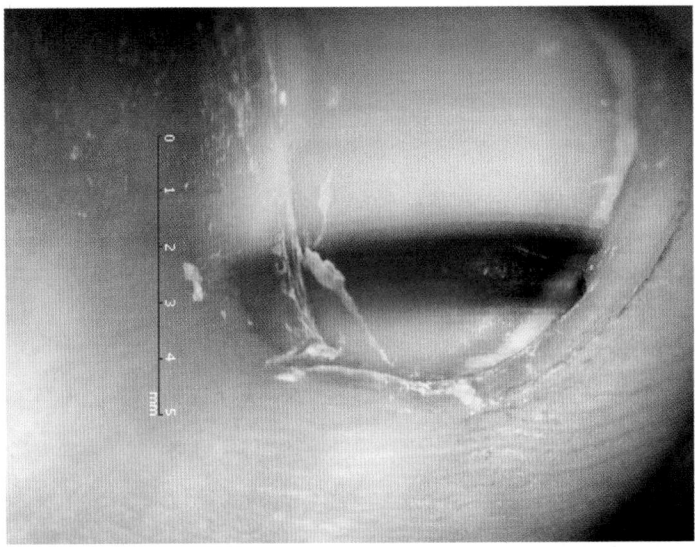

FIGURE 413-19. **Longitudinal melanonychia.** Black longitudinal pigmented band extending from the proximal nail fold to the free edge.

genetic factors, hyperhidrosis, and poorly fitting shoes. Ingrowing is usually precipitated by incorrect nail trimming, with formation of a sharp edge (spicule) of the lateral nail plate that penetrates and injures the soft tissues of the lateral nail fold (Fig. 413-18). Depending on severity, treatment varies from simple disembedding of the spicule to chemical destruction of the lateral nail matrix by phenolization.

Nail Pigmentation

Nail pigmentation is usually caused by staining from external agents, such as nicotine or hair dyes. It rarely may be due to drug deposition in the nail plate or into the nail bed (i.e., antimalarials) or systemic diseases (argyria). In these cases, the proximal margin of the pigmentation follows the shape of the lunula.

Melanonychia

Melanonychia is defined by the presence of melanin within the nail plate. It appears more often as a longitudinal brown-black band starting from the matrix and extending to the free edge of the nail plate (Fig. 413-19).

Melanonychia results from production of melanin by melanocytes of the nail matrix. Melanonychia has three main causes: simple melanocytic activation, benign melanocyte proliferations (lentigo, nevus), and malignant melanocyte proliferation (melanoma; Chapter 193).

Common causes of longitudinal melanonychia due to melanocytic activation include inflammatory and traumatic nail disorders, drugs (chemotherapy, azidothymidine, antimalarials, or psoralen and ultraviolet A [PUVA] therapy), and systemic diseases (acquired immunodeficiency syndrome [Chapter 366]; Addison disease [Chapter 214]).

Nail melanoma is rare and most frequently involves the thumb of middle-aged individuals. Diagnosis is often delayed, and the 5-year survival rate is only 15%. Hutchinson sign, extension of the pigmentation to the proximal or lateral nail folds, is an important indicator of nail melanoma (Fig. 413-20).

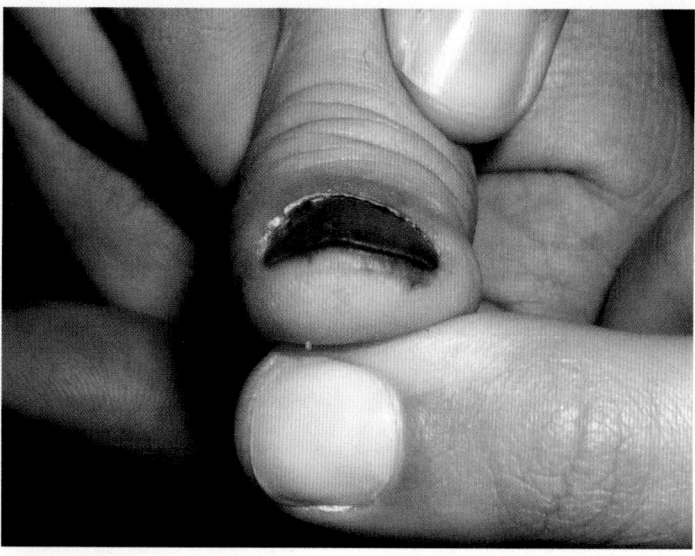

FIGURE 413-20. Nail melanoma. Melanonychia and periungual pigmentation (Hutchinson sign).

Grade A References

A1. Rugo HS, Klein P, Melin SA, et al. Association between use of a scalp cooling device and alopecia after chemotherapy for breast cancer. *JAMA.* 2017;317:606-614.

A2. Nangia J, Wang T, Osborne C, et al. Effect of a scalp cooling device on alopecia in women undergoing chemotherapy for breast cancer: the SCALP randomized clinical trial. *JAMA.* 2017;317:596-605.

A3. Adil A, Godwin M. The effectiveness of treatments for androgenetic alopecia: a systematic review and meta-analysis. *J Am Acad Dermatol.* 2017;77:136-141.

A4. Shanshanwal SJ, Dhurat RS. Superiority of dutasteride over finasteride in hair regrowth and reversal of miniaturization in men with androgenetic alopecia: a randomized controlled open-label, evaluator-blinded study. *Indian J Dermatol Venereol Leprol.* 2017;83:47-54.

A5. Barrionuevo P, Nabhan M, Altayar O, et al. Treatment options for hirsutism: a systematic review and network meta-analysis. *J Clin Endocrinol Metab.* 2018;103:1258-1264.

A6. Kreijkamp-Kaspers S, Hawke KL, van Driel ML. Oral medications to treat toenail fungal infection. *JAMA.* 2018;319:397-398.

A7. Gupta AK, Elewski BE, Rosen T, et al. Onychomycosis: strategies to minimize recurrence. *J Drugs Dermatol.* 2016;15:279-282.

A8. Elewski BE, Aly R, Baldwin SL, et al. Efficacy and safety of tavaborole topical solution, 5%, a novel boron-based antifungal agent, for the treatment of toenail onychomycosis: results from 2 randomized phase-III studies. *J Am Acad Dermatol.* 2015;73:62-69.

GENERAL REFERENCES

For the General References and other additional features, please visit Expert Consult at https://expertconsult.inkling.com.

INDEX

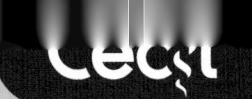

Page numbers followed by "*f*" indicate figures, "*t*" indicate tables, and "*b*" indicate boxes.

A

A blood group antigens, 218
AA amyloidosis, 763
AABB. *See* American Association of Blood Banks
Abacavir, 2256*t*
Abaloparatide, osteoporosis treated with, 1604*t*, 1606
Abatacept
  rheumatoid arthritis treated with, 1715*t*
  type 1 diabetes mellitus treated with, 1495
Abciximab, 383*t*–384*t*
Abdomen
  distention of, 944
  focal abdominal sonography in trauma study, 682*f*
  percussion of, 944, 944*f*
  physical examination of, 815
  trauma-induced injuries of, 682, 682*f*
Abdominal abscess, abdominal pain caused by, 819*t*–820*t*
Abdominal actinomycosis, 2031
Abdominal aortic aneurysm
  CT findings, 438, 439*f*
  epidemiology of, 438, 438.e2*f*
  risk factors for, 438
  screening for, 48
  treatment of, 439*b*
Abdominal compartment syndrome, 683
Abdominal examination, 27
  in cardiovascular disease, 233
  in heart failure, 279
  in liver disease, 944, 944*f*
Abdominal pain
  acute
    algorithm for, 822*f*
    causes of, 819*t*–820*t*
    clinical manifestations of, 818–821
    diagnosis of, 821–822, 822*f*
    history-taking for, 818–821
    in hospitalized patients, 821
    imaging of, 822
    jaundice associated with, 818–820
    location of, 818
    physical examination of, 821, 821*t*
    signs and symptoms of, 818
    special populations with, 821
    treatment of, 822*b*
  in acute mesenteric ischemia, 916
  in amebic liver abscess, 2109
  causes of, 819*t*–820*t*
  chronic, 818
    algorithm for, 823*f*
    causes of, 819*t*–820*t*
    description of, 822
  in chronic pancreatitis, 930
  clinical manifestations of, 818–821
  diagnostic approach to, 945*t*
  differential diagnosis of, 820*f*
  hematochezia with, 818–820
  in hospitalized patients, 821
  liver disease as cause of, 942
  pathobiology of, 818
  physical examination of, 821, 821*t*
  signs and symptoms of, 816*t*, 818
  special populations with, 821
  visceral, 818
Abdominal radiographs
  description of, 829, 830*f*
  gallbladder disease on, 1007
  in liver disease evaluations, 946
Abdominal tuberculosis, 2005
Abdominal ultrasonography
  acute pancreatitis on, 927
  in liver disease evaluations, 946
Abemaciclib, for breast cancer, 1323

Abetalipoproteinemia, 896
Abiraterone acetate, 1167*t*–1182*t*, 1186.e1*t*–1186.e26*t*
Ablation techniques, 274
Abnormal automaticity, 317
Abnormal uterine bleeding, 1553–1554, 1554*b*
Abortion, medical
  Clostridium sordellii associated with, 1892
  description of, 1568, 1574–1575
Abraxane. *See* Paclitaxel
Abscess
  amebic liver, 978*t*, 980, 980*b*, 980*f*, 2109, 2110*f*, 2110*t*
  Bartholin gland, 1908
  brain. *See* Brain abscess
  in Crohn disease, 906
  deep neck, 2568
  eyelid, 2526*f*
  perianal, 909
  peritonsillar, 2566*t*, 2567–2568, 2567*f*
  spinal epidural, 2460–2461, 2460*f*, 2460.e1*t*
Absence seizures, 2362*t*, 2363
Absolute eosinophil count, 1116
Absolute hypovolemia, 718, 718*t*
Absolute intensity, 52, 31.e4*t*
Absolute lung volumes, 521
Absolute refractoriness, 315–316
Absolute reticulocyte count, 1029*t*
Absolute risk reduction, 33*f*
Abstainers, 143
Abt-Letterer-Siwe disease, 1109
Abuse
  alcohol use disorders, 143–150
  drugs of, 150–156
Acalabrutinib, for chronic lymphocytic leukemia, 1222*t*
Acamprosate, 149*t*, 150
Acanthamoeba spp.
  description of, 2111*t*
  keratitis caused by, 2528
Acanthocytes, 1025*t*, 1027*t*
Acanthosis, 2186
Acanthosis nigricans, 943–944, 1191, 2655*f*, 2655*t*
Acarbose, for type 2 diabetes mellitus, 1499
Accelerated gastric emptying, 849
Accessory pathway tachycardia, 336–338
Accidental infection, 2183
Accidents
  radiologic, 79, 79*t*, 81
  Swiss cheese model of, 41
Accutane. *See* Isotretinoin
Acebutolol, 376*t*, 449*t*
Acetaminophen
  acute liver failure caused by, 975
  dose-response effects of, 974*t*
  metabolism of, 973.e1*f*
  toxicity, 667*t*–670*t*, 670, 674*t*–678*t*
Acetazolamide, 719, 729
  action myoclonus treated with, 2429
  altitude illness prevention using, 1850
  for altitude sickness, 579, 579*t*
  Andersen-Tawil syndrome treated with, 2506
  hypokalemia treated with, 730
  intracranial hypertension treated with, 2322*b*
  myotonia responsive to, 2504.e1*t*
  urinary alkalinization with, 737
Acetone, 738
Acetylcholine receptors
  antibodies to, 2511–2512, 2511*f*
  description of, 2509
Acetylcholinesterase inhibitors, Parkinson disease treated with, 2421*t*–2422*t*
Acetylfentanyl, 667*t*–670*t*
Achalasia, 865–866, 866*b*, 866*f*

Achilles tendinitis, 1708
Achilles tendon rupture, 1708
Achlorhydria, 1806
Achondroplasia, 1631
Acid(s)
  endogenous, overproduction of, 736
  fixed, 732
  generation of, 731–732
  nonvolatile, 732
  production of, 732
Acid-base balance
  bicarbonate in, 732
  cortical collecting duct in, 733
  kidney's role in, 732
  medullary collecting duct in, 733
  proximal tubule in, 732–733
Acid-base disorders, 731–744
  clinical manifestations of, 733–735
  compensatory changes for, 734*t*
  definition of, 731
  diagnosis of, 733–735, 734*f*, 734*t*
  epidemiology of, 731
  laboratory evaluation of, 734*t*
  pathobiology of, 731–733
Acid-fast bacillus, 2000, 2006–2007
Acid maltase deficiency, 2506–2507
Acid peptic disease. *See also* Peptic ulcer(s); Peptic ulcer disease
  anatomic diagnosis of, 875
  clinical manifestations of, 874–875
  definition of, 871
  diagnosis of, 875–877, 875*t*
  etiologic diagnosis of, 875–876
  Helicobacter pylori-associated, 878*f*
  hypersecretory syndromes as cause of, 876
  pathobiology of, 872–874
  physical examination of, 875
  prognosis for, 880
  signs and symptoms of, 874–875, 875*t*
Acidemia
  anion gap in, 735
  definition of, 731
  evaluation of, 734*f*
Acidity, 623
Acidosis
  definition of, 731
  hyperchloremic, 731*t*
  lactic. *See* Lactic acidosis
  metabolic. *See* Metabolic acidosis
  respiratory. *See* Respiratory acidosis
  uremic, 735–736
  watery diarrhea, hypokalemic, hypochlorhydric, 738
Acinetobacter spp.
  A. baumannii, 1827*t*, 1938
  bacteremia caused by, 1937
  burn infection caused by, 1937
  cellulitis caused by, 1937*f*
  clinical manifestations of, 1937
  community-acquired pneumonia caused by, 1937
  definition of, 1936
  diagnosis of, 1937
  epidemiology of, 1936–1937
  health care-associated pneumonia caused by, 1937
  laboratory tests for, 1936.e4*t*
  meningitis caused by, 1937–1938
  osteomyelitis caused by, 1937
  pneumonia caused by, 1937
  prevention of, 1938
  prognosis for, 1938
  skin and soft tissue infections caused by, 1937, 1937*f*
  structure of, 1936

Acinetobacter spp. (*Continued*)
  subspecies, 1936.e4*t*
  treatment of, 1937*b*–1938*b*
  wound infection caused by, 1937
Aclidinium bromide, 541*t*
Acne keloidalis, 2653*f*
Acne vulgaris, 2630–2632, 2654*f*
Acoustic neuromas, 1264–1265, 1265*f*, 2560
Acquired aplastic anemia, 1077–1078, 1080
Acquired cystic kidney disease, 782*t*, 787–788, 788*b*
Acquired erythrocytosis, 1090*t*
Acquired immunodeficiency syndrome. *See also* Human immunodeficiency virus; Human immunodeficiency virus infection
  acute cauda equina syndrome in, 2175
  antiretroviral therapy for, 2240.e3*f*, 2242.e2*f*, 2240.e1*f*, 2238.e3*f*, 2242.e1*f*, 2242.e3*f*, 2240.e2*f*
  brain abscesses, 2096
  candidiasis in, 2048
  cryptococcal meningitis associated with, 2047
  cryptococcosis associated with, 2046
  cytomegalovirus in, 2196–2197
  deaths caused by, 2242.e2*f*, 2242.e4*f*, 2240.e2*f*, 2238.e3*f*, 2242.e1*f*, 2242.e3*f*, 2240.e1*f*, 2240.e3*f*, 2242.e5*f*
  discovery of, 2260.e4
  fluconazole prophylaxis in, 2035
  historical perspective on, 2238.e2
  Hodgkin lymphoma in, 1245
  malignancies associated with, 2276
  non-Hodgkin lymphoma in, 1239–1240
Acquired neuromyotonia, 2514
Acquired von Willebrand disease, 1135, 1135*t*
Acral gangrene, 1956*f*
Acral lentiginous melanoma, 1345
Acrocyanosis, 469
Acrodermatitis chronica atrophicans, 1992*f*, 1994
Acrodermatitis verruciformis, 2638
Acrodynia, 89
Acrokeratosis neoplastica. *See* Bazex syndrome
Acromegaly, 1448–1449, 1448*f*, 1449*b*, 1524, 1780–1781
Acromion process, 1704*f*
Acropachy, 1468–1469
Acroparesthesia, 1371
ACT. *See* Activating clotting time
ACTHoma, 1521*t*
Actigraphy, 2377, 2379*f*
Actinic keratoses, 2637–2638, 2638*f*
Actinic keratosis, 1349
Actinomycetomas, 2031, 2071
Actinomycosis
  abdominal, 2031
  central nervous system infections caused by, 2031
  cervicofacial, 2030, 2030*f*
  clinical manifestations of, 2030–2031
  definition of, 2029–2030
  diagnosis of, 2031–2032
  epidemiology of, 2030
  pathobiology of, 2030
  pathogen that causes, 2029–2030
  pelvic, 2031
  penicillin G for, 2032
  thoracic, 2030–2031, 2031*f*
  treatment of, 2031*b*–2032*b*
Actinomycotic granulomas, 2031
Action potential
  cardiac, 241, 241*f*, 314–315, 315*f*, 345.e1*f*
  premature, 345.e1*f*
Action potential duration adaption, 315
Action tremors, 2423–2424
Activated charcoal, 667*t*–670*t*, 672, 678

Aluminum poisoning (Continued)
diagnosis of, 92
diagnostic testing for, 88t
prognosis for, 92b
treatment of, 92b
Aluminum salts, for hyperphosphatemia, 747t
Alunbrig. See Brigatinib
Alveolar-arterial oxygen gradient, 623, 623t, 2062
Alveolar damage, diffuse, 511f
Alveolar filling disorders, 552–557, 553t, 568
classification of, 557t
definition of, 552–553
general approach to, 552–553, 553f
Alveolar hemorrhage, diffuse, 553t, 555–556
Alveolar hydatid disease, 2122, 2122b
Alveolar hyperventilation, 744
Alveolar macrophages, 2163
Alveolar radiographic patterns, 513
Alveolar ventilation, 624
Alzheimer disease
anterograde amnesia in, 2344, 2348
clinical features of, 2418t–2419t
clinical manifestations of, 2351
definition of, 2350
diagnosis of, 2351–2352
epidemiology of, 2350
evidence-based treatments for, 2353
genetics of, 2350–2351
magnetic resonance imaging of, 2350, 2351f
neuritic plaques in, 2350
neurofibrillary tangles in, 2350
pathobiology of, 2350–2351
positron emission tomography of, 2352f–2353f
posterior cortical atrophy caused by, 2346f
prevention of, 2352b–2353b
prognosis for, 2353
risk factors for, 2350
treatment of, 2352b–2353b
Amanita poisoning, 974, 976
Amantadine, 2149, 2149t, 2161t, 2419
Amaurosis fugax, 2397
Ambiguous genitalia, 1536
Amblyomma africanum, 2021
Amblyomma americanum, 1991.e4, 2023.e1
Amblyomma cajennense, 2017
Amblyopia, 2520
Ambrisentan, 492–493
Ambulatory monitoring
in arrhythmias, 322–323
blood pressure monitoring, 445
24-hour tracings, 445.e1f
recommendations for, 445
Amebiasis
asymptomatic intestinal, 2107–2108
characteristics of, 2218t–2219t
clinical manifestations of, 2107–2109
definition of, 2107
diagnosis of, 2110, 2110t
epidemiology of, 2107
extraintestinal, 2110f
intestinal, 2109f
pathobiology of, 2107
pericardial, 2109
Amebic colitis, 2108–2109, 2110t
Amebic diarrhea, 2108
Amebic dysentery, 2108–2109
Amebic liver abscess, 978t, 980, 980b, 980f, 2109, 2110f, 2110t
Amenorrhea
description of, 1554–1555, 1555t, 1556f
hypergonadotropic, 1555–1557
American Association of Blood Banks, 1151, 1158.e1
American College of Cardiology, 230t
American human monocytic ehrlichiosis, 2023–2024, 2023t, 2024b
American Joint Committee on Cancer staging system, 1184
American Medical Association, 9
American Society of Anesthesiology, 2577
American Spinal Injury Association impairment scale, 2328t
American sylvatic typhus, 2018t–2019t
American Thoracic Society, 598
American trypanosomiasis. See Chagas disease
Amifostine, 81, 583, 1186.e1t–1186.e26t
Amikacin
bacterial meningitis treated with, 2450t
dosage adjustments in renal failure, 124.e1t

Amikacin (Continued)
dosage of, 1857t–1858t
nocardiosis treated with, 2033
pyelonephritis treated with, 1839t
Amiloride
dose of, 719t
Gitelman syndrome treated with, 790
hypertension treated with, 449t
Aminoglycosides, 1805
bacterial meningitis treated with, 2450t
characteristics of, 1855–1859
cystic fibrosis treated with, 1935
dosage of, 1857t–1858t
endocarditis treated with, 425
mechanism of action, 1854t
nephrotoxicity of, 1855, 1859f
resistance mechanisms, 1855t
toxicity of, 1861t
5-Aminolevulinate
acute attacks caused by, 1380
chemical structure of, 1379.e1f
synthesis of, 1380
5-Aminosalicylate, for inflammatory bowel disease, 902, 903t, 905
Aminotransferases
asymptomatic abnormalities of, 957
description of, 954–955
Amiodarone
for advanced cardiac life support, 329f
for arrhythmias, 329–330
for atrial fibrillation, 340, 342, 397
cornea verticillata caused by, 2535
dose-response effects of, 974t
doses and side effects, 339t–340t
for electrical storm, 349
for supraventricular arrhythmia, 301
thyroiditis caused by, 1472
for ventricular tachycardia, 350
Amitriptyline, 2308t
chronic pain treated with, 132
irritable bowel syndrome treated with, 855t
tinnitus treated with, 2561
AML. See Acute myeloid leukemia
Amlodipine
for acute STEMI, 399
for aortic dissection, 441
for atheromatous embolization, 465
for hypertension, 449t
for livedo reticularis, 464
for pernio, 468b
properties of, 377t
for pulmonary hypertension, 492
for Raynaud phenomenon, 467
Ammonia, 955, 992
Ammoniagenesis, 733
Ammonium, 733
Amnesic disorders, 2343–2344
Amnesic mild cognitive impairment, 2348t
Amnesic shellfish poisoning, 694
Amniotic fluid embolism, 486, 486.e1f
Amodiaquine, 2079
Amoebic encephalitis, 2073
Amoxicillin
cystitis treated with, 1839t
dosage of, 1857t–1858t
leptospirosis treated with, 2000
Lyme disease treated with, 1995t
pharmacokinetic parameters for, 122t
Amoxicillin-clavulanate
cystitis treated with, 1839t
Streptococcus pneumoniae treated with, 1870.e1t
Amoxicillin-clavulanic acid
dosage of, 1857t–1858t
for pneumonia, 599t
AmpC ß-lactamases, 1929
Amphetamines, 154
clinical manifestations of, 154
pathobiology of, 154
screening for, 671t
toxicity, 667t–670t
Amphotericin B
azotemia caused by, 2037
for bacterial endocarditis, 424t
coccidioidomycosis treated with, 2044
formulations of, 2036–2037
for hepatosplenic candidiasis, 979
histoplasmosis treated with, 2042
lipid-associated formulations of, 2037
liposomal
description of, 2074

Amphotericin B (Continued)
visceral leishmaniasis treated with, 2091–2092
mechanism of action, 2036
pulmonary histoplasmosis treated with, 2042
resistance mechanisms of, 2036
spectrum of activity, 2036
sporotrichosis treated with, 2045
visceral leishmaniasis treated with, 2092
Amphotericin B deoxycholate
acute reactions to, 2037
administration of, 2037
chronic toxicity of, 2037
cryptococcosis treated with, 2047
dosage of, 2037
formulation of, 2036
mucormycosis treated with, 2059
nephrotoxicity of, 2037
pharmacology of, 2036–2037
Ampicillin
bacterial endocarditis treated with, 424t
bacterial meningitis treated with, 2450t
dosage of, 1857t–1858t
endocarditis treated with, 425
Haemophilus influenzae treated with, 1915
leptospirosis treated with, 2000
listeriosis treated with, 1886
septic shock treated with, 657t–658t
vancomycin-resistant enterococci treated with, 1880.e1t
Ampicillin-sulbactam
for pneumonia, 599t, 601, 602t
for pyogenic liver abscess, 978
Amplatzer devices, 266.e1f
Amprenavir, 2256t
Ampullary adenomas, 1014, 1014.e1f
Ampullary tumors, 1014
Amyl nitrite, 674t–678t
Amylase, in acute pancreatitis, 927
Amyloid, 2570, 2570.e1f
Amyloid arthropathy, 1780
Amyloid neuropathy, 2483
Amyloidosis, 309, 309f–310f, 1256–1260, 2547
AA, 763
apo AI, 1257t
apo AII, 1257t
apo AIV, 1257t
arthritis and, 1780
BriPP, 1257t
cardiac involvement, 1257–1258
cardiomyopathy with, 305
clinical manifestations of, 1257–1258
cutaneous, 1260
cystatin, 1257t
definition of, 1256
diagnosis of, 309, 1258, 1259f
dialysis-associated, 806, 1257t
epidemiology of, 309
esophageal involvement in, 868
factor deficiency in, 1145
familial, 1259–1260
in familial Mediterranean fever, 1693
fibrinogen, 1257t
Finnish hereditary, 1257t
glomerular disease in, 762–763
heavy chain, 1257t
laryngeal, 1260
light chain, 1257t, 1259f, 2497, 2497b
liver involvement, 1258
localized, 1260
lysozyme, 1257t
macroglossia associated with, 1257, 1257f
pathobiology of, 309, 1256–1257
periorbital purpura in, 1257, 1258f
prognosis for, 310b, 1259
secondary, 1257t
systemic
chemotherapy for, 1258b–1259b
light chain, 1256–1259, 1259f
multiple myeloma versus, 1258
secondary, 1260
senile, 1257t, 1259
signs and symptoms of, 1257t
syndromes associated with, 1257t
treatment of, 1258b–1259b
types of, 1257t
tracheobronchial, 1260
transthyretin-related, 1260
treatment of, 310b, 1258b–1259b

Amyotrophic lateral sclerosis, 2474
bulbar symptoms in, 2486
characteristics of, 2487t
clinical manifestations of, 2486
diagnosis of, 2486–2487, 2487t
differential diagnosis of, 2487t
epidemiology of, 2485–2486
mimic syndromes of, 2487t
pathobiology of, 2486
pathology of, 2486
prognosis for, 2488
respiratory muscle weakness in, 2486, 2488
swallowing affected by, 2570
treatment of, 2488b
variants of, 2486
Anabolic-androgenic steroids, 156
Anabolic steroids, 976
Anaerobic bacteria
antimicrobial susceptibility patterns for, 1900t
bacteremia caused by, 1898
central nervous system infections caused by, 1898
clinical manifestations of, 1898–1899
culture for, 1899t
definition of, 1897
epidemiology of, 1897
head infections caused by, 1898–1899
indicators of, 1899t
intra-abdominal infections caused by, 1899
location of, 1897t, 1898f
neck infections caused by, 1898–1899
obstetric-gynecologic infections as cause of, 1899
osteomyelitis caused by, 1899
pathobiology of, 1897–1898
pleuropulmonary infections caused by, 1899
septic arthritis caused by, 1899
skin and soft tissue infections caused by, 1899
taxonomy of, 1897.e4t
treatment of, 1900b, 1900t
virulence factors in, 1898t
Anagen effluvium, 2656
Anakinra
cryopyrin-associated periodic syndromes treated with, 1696
description of, 163
Anal canal, 933
Anal cancer
clinical manifestations of, 939
diagnosis of, 939
human papillomavirus as cause of, 938, 2277
incidence of, 938
treatment of, 939b
Anal carcinoma, 834.e1f
Anal fissure, 936, 936b, 936f
Anal fistula, 935, 935b–936b, 936f
Anal warts, 938, 938b
Analgesia
critical care, 620
neuraxial, 2586
Analgesic nephropathy, 767–768, 767f
Analgesics
adjuvant, 132, 132t
antipyretic, 131–134
chronic interstitial nephritis caused by, 768
fibromyalgia treated with, 1778
opioid, 132–134, 133t–134t
renal papillary necrosis caused by, 708
topical, 2608–2609
Anamorelin, 1192
Anaphylactic shock, 1660
Anaphylactoid reactions, 2584
Anaphylatoxin receptors
anaphylatoxins, 220, 225–226
cellular responses, 225t
distribution of, 225t
Anaphylaxis, 506t–507t, 1637
systemic
algorithm for, 1656f–1657f
allergens as cause of, 1654–1655
anesthesia as cause of, 2584
aspirin as cause of, 1655
causes of, 1654t
definition of, 1654
diagnosis of, 1656–1657
differential diagnosis of, 1656–1657
epidemiology of, 1654
etiology of, 1654, 1654t
food allergy as cause of, 1654
food as cause of, 1655

Colesevelam, 896b, 1364
Colestipol, 896b
Colistimethate, 2450t
Colistin, 1929, 1934, 1938
Colitis
    amebic, 2108–2109, 2110t
    collagenous, 897
    cytomegalovirus, 2196, 2265t–2268t
    differential diagnosis of, 901t
    diverticulitis and, 912
    hemorrhagic, 1925–1926
    inflammatory, 1926
Collagen vascular disease, 608t
Collagenases, 214t
Collagenomas, 2639–2640
Collagenous colitis, 897
Collecting duct
    disorders of, 790
    natriuretics of, 719
Colloid cysts, 1267
Colon
    bleeding from. See Lower gastrointestinal
        bleeding
    diverticulitis of, 911–912, 912f, 911.e1f
    motility of, 846, 850–851
    transit in, 846
Colon cancer profile, 1194
Colon ischemia
    algorithm for, 922f
    clinical manifestations of, 921, 921.e1f
    colonoscopy evaluations, 921, 921.e1f
    computed tomography of, 922f
    conditions associated with, 921t
    diagnosis of, 921
    epidemiology of, 921
    incidence of, 921
    medications associated with, 921t
    treatment of, 921b, 922f
Colonic volvulus, 909b
Colonoscopy
    applications of, 835t, 838
    colon ischemia on, 921, 921.e1f
    colorectal cancer on, 1300f, 1301, 1301t
    gastrointestinal bleeding evaluations
        lower, 843–844
        occult, 845
    indications for, 838
    iron deficiency anemia evaluations, 845
    irritable bowel syndrome evaluations,
        853–854
    propofol as anesthesia for, 2584
    in pseudo-obstructive colonic dilation, 838
    surveillance intervals for, 1299t
Colony-forming units, 1851, 1852.e1
Color blindness, 2520
Color flow Doppler imaging, 253–254
Colorado tick fever
    clinical manifestations of, 2223
    definition of, 2222–2223
    diagnosis of, 2223
    epidemiology of, 2222–2223
    pathobiology of, 2223
    pathogen that causes, 2222–2223
    prognosis for, 2223
Colorectal cancer
    adenocarcinoma, 1299–1304, 1302b–1304b
    chemoprevention for, 1302
    colonoscopy for, 838, 1300f, 1301, 1301t
    combination therapy for, 1303
    computed tomography colography for, 1302
    diagnosis of, 1300–1302
    dietary prevention for, 1302
    epidemiology of, 1296
    familial syndromes, 1297–1298, 1297t
    fecal occult blood tests for, 1301
    flexible sigmoidoscopy for, 1301
    follow-up for, 906–907
    metastatic, 1303–1304, 1303.e1f
    microsatellite instability associated with, 1299
    molecular basis of, 1300f
    molecular biomarkers of, 1304
    nutrition and, 1395
    pathobiology of, 1299
    prevention of, 1301–1302
    prognosis for, 1304, 1304f
    radiation therapy for, 1302
    radiofrequency ablation of, 1304
    risk factors for, 1297
    screening for, 48, 1301–1302, 1301t
    sporadic, 1297

Colorectal cancer (Continued)
    staging of, 1302, 1302f
    stool DNA tests for, 1301
    surgery for, 1184, 1302
    surveillance of, 1304
    survival rates for, 1304f
    systemic therapy for, 1303
    treatment of, 1302b–1304b
    ulcerative colitis and, 906, 1301
    in women, 1565
Colovesicular fistulas, in Crohn disease, 905
Colpitis macularis, 1844
Colposcope, 1329
Colposcopy, 2188
Coma
    causes of, 2371t
    characteristics of, 2371t
    clinical manifestations of, 2371
    diagnosis of, 2372–2374
    emergency management of, 2374t
    epidemiology of, 2370
    grading of, 2373
    herniation as cause of, 2371
    laboratory testing for, 2373–2374
    motor examination in, 2373
    pathobiology of, 2370–2371
    prognosis for, 2374
    treatment of, 2374b
Comanagement, 2576
Comatose patient, neurologic examination in,
    2300
Comet sign, 575
Common cold, 2150–2152
    clinical manifestations of, 2151
    cough during, 2152
    definition of, 2150
    diagnosis of, 2151
    nasal congestion in, 2151
    pathobiology of, 2150–2151
    pathogens that cause, 2150
    pharyngitis caused by, 2568
    prevention of, 2152
    prognosis for, 2152
    treatment of, 2151b–2152b, 2151t
    viruses associated with, 2150, 2150t
Common cold illness syndrome, 2150–2151
Common couple violence, 1593
Common variable immune deficiency, 1643,
    1644t, 1780
Common ventricle, 364
Commonwealth Foundation, 37.e1t
Commotio cordis, 682
Communication
    core skills in, 14t
    nonverbal empathy, 14t
    verbal empathy, 14t
Community-acquired pneumonia, 1814
    Acinetobacter spp. as cause of, 1937
    antibiotic therapy for, 1870
    incidence of, 592.e4f
    Staphylococcus aureus as cause of, 1865
    Streptococcus pneumoniae as cause of, 1868
    treatment of
        antibiotic regimens for, 657t–658t
        empirical, 599t
Community-acquired respiratory distress
    syndrome, 1973
Community resources, 44
Compartment syndrome, 1140
Compensated cirrhosis, 992–993
Complement, 164, 212–213, 707, 1677–1678
    activation of, 221–226, 225f
        alternative pathway, 223
        classical pathway, 221–222
        lectin pathway, 222–223
        pathologic conditions associated with, 222t
        pathways of, 221–222, 222f, 224f
        regulators of, 220–221, 223, 226f
        tissue injury or degeneration and, 222t
    in glomerular disorders/diseases, 755t
    in Haemophilus influenza, 1913
Complement C5, 224f, 226
Complement C4 binding protein, 223t
Complement C3 convertase, 223
Complement C5 convertase, 223
Complement C1 inhibitor, 223t
Complement C3a, 225
Complement C5a, 225
Complement C3a receptor, 225
Complement C5a receptor, 225

Complement C5b-9, soluble, 224–225
Complement C4b/C3b receptor, 223t
Complement disorders, 1692t
Complement inhibitors, 1692t
Complement-mediated membranoproliferative
    glomerulonephritis, 757–758
Complement receptors, 199–200, 226
Complement regulating complement, 223t
Complement system
    in disease, 220–226, 221t
    features of, 220–221, 221t
    function of, 220, 221f
    in host defense, 220, 221t
Complementary and alternative treatments
    acupuncture, 167
    definition of, 166
    manual therapies, 166–167
    meditation, 166
    natural products, 167–168
    for pain, 136
    tai chi, 166
    traditional Chinese medicine, 167
    yoga, 166
Complete blood count, 1030
Complex regional pain syndrome, 2484–2485
Comportment, 2346
Comprehensive chronic disease management,
    42–45
Compression stockings, 484
Compression ultrasonography
    description of, 478, 479f
    venous thromboembolism, 478, 479f
Compressive mononeuropathies, 2500
Compulsions, 2312t
Computed tomographic pulmonary angiography,
    478, 479f, 480
Computed tomography, 81
    abdominal, 1007
    acute kidney injury findings, 706, 706f
    acute pancreatitis on, 927, 928f
    amebic liver abscess on, 980f
    analgesic nephropathy findings, 767f
    appendicitis evaluations, 911f
    cardiac, 265f, 266
    chronic obstructive pulmonary disease on,
        538, 538f
    chronic pancreatitis on, 930–931, 931f
    cirrhosis on, 994f
    colon ischemia on, 922f
    gastroenterology applications of, 830–831,
        832f, 831.e1f
    hepatic cyst on, 947f
    hepatocellular carcinoma on, 1311f
    high-resolution, 560
    Hodgkin lymphoma on, 1243f
    infectious sacroiliitis on, 1680f
    in interstitial lung disease, 560
    kidney stone findings, 777–779, 778f
    of lungs, mediastinum, and chest wall, 510
    lymphadenopathy on, 1105
    mesenteric venous thrombosis on, 917
    nephrolithiasis findings, 777–779, 778f
    neutropenic colitis on, 913.e1f
    pansinusitis on, 2550f
    peritoneal carcinomatosis on, 915
    pheochromocytoma on, 1487f
    progressive multifocal leukoencephalopathy
        on, 2176
    pyogenic liver abscess on, 977–978, 978f
    radiation dose from, 1680
    radiation exposure, 79
    renal vein thrombosis evaluations, 776
    rheumatic diseases on, 1680
    single-photon emission computed tomography
        myocardial perfusion imaging, 263–265,
        264f, 265.e1f
        for myocardial viability determination, 265
        stress-only protocol, 264
    small bowel obstruction on, 915f
    splenomegaly on, 1106f, 1107
    strengths of, 2305t
    stroke on, 2399–2401
    subarachnoid hemorrhage on, 2409, 2410f
Computed tomography angiography
    in atherosclerotic PAD, 458, 459f
    chronic mesenteric ischemia on, 920
    coronary, 265f–267f, 266, 272f, 266.e1f
    in coronary artery disease, 370
    gastrointestinal disease evaluations, 830–831
    rheumatic diseases on, 1680

Computed tomography arthrography, 1680
Computed tomography colography, 1302
Computed tomography enterography
    definition of, 831
    gastrointestinal disease evaluations, 831
Computed tomography myelography, 2305t
Computed tomography venography, 478
Computer navigation, for total joint arthroplasty,
    1787
Computerized ECG readings, automated, 252
Concussion, 2325t
Condom, 1570–1571, 2253
Conduction delays, 397–398
Conductive hearing loss, 2558–2559
Condyloma latum, 2544
Condylomata acuminatum, 2187
Condylomata lata, 1984f, 1985, 2187
Cone snails, 693
Confabulation, 2472
Confidentiality, 57
Conflicts of interest, 9–10
Confounding, 32–33
Confusion Assessment Method, 115, 115t
Confusional arousals, 2385t
Congenital abnormalities
    of aortic valve, 406
    coronary anomalies, 389t
    cystic adenomatoid malformation of the lung,
        551–552
    esophageal, 870
    of pericardium, 436
    pulmonary airway malformation, 551–552
Congenital adrenal hyperplasia
    17α-hydroxylase/17,20 lyase deficiency, 1531
    11ß-hydroxylase deficiency, 1532
    21-hydroxylase deficiency, 1531
    3ß-hydroxysteroid dehydrogenase deficiency,
        1531
    clinical presentation of, 1532f
    description of, 728t, 1432, 1477, 1481–1482
    diagnosis of, 1551
    lipoid hyperplasia, 1530
Congenital cataract, 2534
Congenital cytomegalovirus, 2196
Congenital diarrhea, 896
Congenital disorders, cystic diseases, thoracic,
    551–552
Congenital erythrocytosis, 1090t
Congenital erythropoietic porphyria, 1377, 1379,
    1381, 1384–1385
Congenital heart disease, 357–365
    assessment of, 358, 358f
    clinical manifestations of, 358
    CMR findings, 267, 270f
    echocardiographic findings, 258t–260t
    epidemiology of, 357
    exercise recommendations for, 365, 365.e2t
    exercise testing, 365
    genetic determinants, 357–358
    isolated shunt lesions, 358
    simple lesions, 358–363
    treatment of, 365b, 365.e1f
    ventricular tachycardia in, 348
Congenital Heinz body hemolytic anemia, 1061
Congenital hypogonadotropic hypogonadism, 1541
Congenital hypoventilation, central, 524
Congenital large hyperlucent lobe, 552
Congenital lobar emphysema, 552
Congenital malabsorption, 896
Congenital methemoglobinemia, 1029
Congenital muscular dystrophies, 2505–2508
Congenital myasthenic syndromes, 2514–2515,
    2515b
Congenital myopathies, 2505
Congenital neutropenia, 1098–1099, 1099t
Congenital nonspherocytic hemolytic anemia, 1052
Congenital nystagmus, 2541, 2541t
Congenital rubella syndrome
    clinical manifestations of, 2171
    diagnosis of, 2171
    epidemiology of, 2170
    pathobiology of, 2170
Congenital sideroblastic anemia, 1039, 1039t
Congenital syphilis, 1843, 1986, 1988–1989
Congenital thrombocytopenia, 1132
Congenital triangular alopecia, 2659
Congenital valvular aortic stenosis, 361
    diagnosis of, 361
    treatment of, 361b
Congestion, 649, 649t

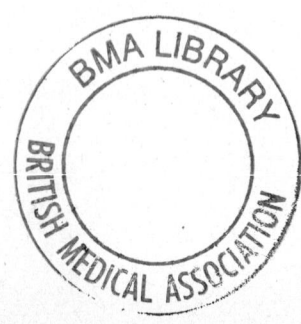

SPECIFIC TABLES OR FIGURES

SYMPTOMS

Constitutional

Fever	Tables 264-1 to 264-8 (pp. 1810-1813); Figures 265-1 (p. 1819), 265-2 (p. 1820)
Fatigue	Table 3-1 (p. 11)
Poor appetite	Table 123-1 (pp. 816-817)
Weight loss	Figure 123-4 (p. 826); Tables 123-4 (pp. 824-825), 206-1 (p. 1416), 206-2 (p. 1416)
Obesity	Figure 207-1 (p. 1425)
Snoring, sleep disturbances	Table 377-6 (p. 2384)

Head, Eyes, Ears, Nose, Throat

Headache	Tables 370-1 (p. 2316), 370-2 (p. 2317)
Visual loss, transient	Tables 395-2 (p. 2521), 396-1 (p. 2537)
Ear pain	Table 398-3 (p. 2551)
Hearing loss	Figure 400-1 (p. 2559)
Ringing in ears (tinnitus)	Figure 400-2 (p. 2561)
Vertigo	Figure 400-3 (p. 2562)
Nasal congestion, rhinitis, or sneezing	Chapter 398, pp. 2548-2556
Loss of smell or taste	Table 399-1 (p. 2558)
Dry mouth	Table 397-7 (p. 2547)
Sore throat	Figure 401-2 (p. 2567); Table 401-1 (p. 2566)
Hoarseness	Chapter 401, pp. 2570-2571

Cardiopulmonary

Chest pain	Tables 45-2 (p. 229), 128-5 (p. 858), 128-6 (p. 858)
Bronchitis	Table 84-1 (p. 550)
Shortness of breath	Figure 77-3 (p. 509)
Palpitations	Figure 56-1 (p. 319); Tables 45-4 (p. 230), 56-5 (p. 325)
Dizziness	Figure 56-1 (p. 319); Table 400-1 (p. 2565)
Syncope	Figure 56-1 (p. 319); Tables 56-1 (p. 319), 56-2 (p. 320), 56-4 (p. 324)
Cardiac arrest	Figures 57-2 (p. 329), 57-3 (p. 330)
Cough	Figure 77-1 (p. 506); Tables 77-2 (p. 505), 77-3 (p. 505)
Hemoptysis	Tables 77-6 (p. 508), 77-7 (p. 510)

Gastrointestinal

Nausea and vomiting	Figure 123-5 (p. 827); Table 123-5 (p. 827)
Dysphagia, odynophagia	Table 123-1 (pp. 816-817)
Hematemesis	Figure 126-3 (p. 843); Table 126-1 (p. 841)
Heartburn/dyspepsia	Figures 123-6 (p. 829), 129-2 (p. 861); Tables 128-3 (p. 856), 128-4 (p. 856), 130-1 (p. 873)

Abdominal pain
  Acute
  Chronic
	Figures 123-1 (p. 820), 123-2 (p. 822); Tables 123-2 (p. 820), 123-3 (p. 821), 133-1 (p. 910)
	Figure 123-3 (p. 823); Tables 123-2 (p. 820), 129-1 (p. 862)

Diarrhea	Figures 128-1 (p. 854), 131-1 (p. 884), 131-4 (p. 890)
Melena, blood in stool	Figures 126-3 (p. 843), 126-4 (p. 844), 126-6 (p. 845); Table 126-4 (p. 843)
Constipation	Figures 127-3 (p. 850), 128-1 (p. 854); Table 127-2 (p. 850)
Fecal incontinence	Figure 136-5 (p. 937)
Anal pain	Chapter 136, pp. 933-939

Genitourinary

Dysuria	Tables 268-3 (p. 1838), 268-5 (p. 1839), 269-2 (p. 1842)
Frequency	Table 268-3 (p. 1838)
Incontinence	Tables 23-1 to 23-3 (pp. 106-108)
Renal colic	Figure 117-1 (p. 778)
Vaginal discharge	Chapter 269, p. 1843
Menstrual irregularities	Figure 223-3 (p. 1556); Tables 223-3 (p. 1555), 223-4 (p. 1557)
Female infertility	Table 223-5 (p. 1560)
Hot flushes	Table 227-1 (p. 1588)
Erectile dysfunction	Figure 221-8 (p. 1546)
Male infertility	Figures 221-6 (p. 1544), 221-7 (p. 1545), 221-8 (p. 1546); Table 221-7 (p. 1543)
Scrotal mass	Figure 190-1 (p. 1336)
Genital ulcers or warts	Table 269-1 (p. 1841)

SPECIFIC TABLES OR FIGURES

Musculoskeletal

Neck or back pain	Figures 372-4 (p. 2334), 372-5 (p. 2336), 372-6 (p. 2337); Tables 372-3 to 372-5 (pp. 2332-2334)
Painful joints	Figure 241-1 (p. 1670); Tables 241-1 (p. 1668), 241-3 (p. 1671)

Extremities

Swollen feet, ankles, or legs	
Bilateral	Figure 45-8 (p. 236)
Unilateral	Figure 74-2 (p. 478); Table 74-2 (p. 477)
Claudication	Table 71-3 (p. 458)
Acute limb ischemia	Figure 71-4 (p. 460); Table 71-1 (p. 457)

Neurologic

Weakness	Tables 368-1 (p. 2301), 392-2 (p. 2491), 393-2 (p. 2502), 393-4 (p. 2503)
Sensory loss	E-Figure 392-1; Tables 392-1 (p. 2490), 392-3 (p. 2493), 392-5 (p. 2497)
Memory loss	Figures 374-1 (p. 2349), 374-2 (p. 2349); Tables 374-1 to 374-6 (pp. 2347-2356)
Abnormal gait	Table 368-2 (p. 2301)
Seizures	Tables 375-1 to 375-6 (pp. 2359-2366)

Integumentary

Abnormal bleeding	Table 162-1 (p. 1120)
Rash	Figure 407-1 (p. 2599); Tables 407-1 (p. 2599), 407-6 (p. 2603), 412-5 (pp. 2654-2655)
Hives	Figure 237-2 (p. 1651); Tables 237-1 (p. 1650), 411-1 (p. 2633), 411-2 (p. 2634)
Abnormal pigmentation	Table 412-2 (p. 2651)
Alopecia and hirsutism	Tables 413-1 (p. 2656), 413-3 (p. 2657)
Nail disorders	Table 413-4 (p. 2661)

SIGNS

Vital Signs

Fever	Figure 265-1 (p. 1819); Tables 264-1 (p. 1810), 264-8 (p. 1813), 265-2 (p. 1816)
Heat illness/hyperthermia	Tables 101-1 to 101-3 (pp. 660-661)
Hypothermia	Table 101-4 to 101-6 (pp. 662-663)
Tachycardia/bradycardia	Figures 56-2 (p. 322), 56-3 (p. 323); Tables 58-4 (p. 335), 59-2 (p. 346)
Hypertension	Tables 70-3 (p. 446), 70-7 (p. 453), 70-11 (p. 456)
Hypotension/shock	Figures 98-2 (p. 645), 100-1 (p. 655); Tables 98-1 (p. 643), 99-1 (p. 648), 99-2 (p. 649)
Altered respiration	Tables 80-1 (p. 525), 80-2 (p. 526), 96-2 (p. 627)

Head, Eyes, Ears, Nose, Throat

Eye pain	Table 395-3 (p. 2521)
Red eye	Tables 395-4 (p. 2521), 395-6 (p. 2526)
Dilated pupil	Figure 396-4 (p. 2539)
Nystagmus	Table 396-4 (p. 2541)
Papilledema	Table 396-2 (p. 2537)
Strabismus	Figure 396-6 (p. 2540)
Jaundice	Figure 138-2 (p. 958); Tables 138-1 to 138-3 (pp. 951-957)
Rhinitis	Table 398-3 (p. 2551)
Sinusitis	Tables 398-1 (p. 2548), 398-2 (p. 2549), 398-4 (p. 2552), 398-5 (p. 2552)
Oral ulcers and discolorations	Tables 397-1 to 397-4 (pp. 2542-2545)
Salivary gland enlargement	Table 397-6 (p. 2546)

Neck

Neck mass	Chapter 181, p. 1273
Lymphadenopathy	Tables 159-1 to 159-4 (pp. 1104-1105)
Thyroid nodule	Figure 213-5 (p. 1473)
Thyromegaly/goiter	Figures 213-2 (p. 1466), 213-3 (p. 1468)

Breast

Breast mass	Figure 188-1 (p. 1324)

Lungs

Wheezes	Table 77-4 (pp. 506-507)

Cardiac

Heart murmur or extra sounds	Figure 45-6 (p. 235); Tables 45-7 (p. 235), 45-8 (p. 235)
Jugular venous distention	Table 45-6 (p. 232)
Carotid pulse abnormalities	Figure 45-4 (p. 233)